Sleisenger & Fordtran's

Gastrointestinal and Liver Disease

Pathophysiology/Diagnosis/Management

7th Edition

Mark Feldman, MD
William O. Tschumy, Jr., M.D. Chair of Internal Medicine
Presbyterian Hospital of Dallas
Clinical Professor of Internal Medicine
University of Texas Southwestern Medical School
Dallas, Texas

Lawrence S. Friedman, MD
Professor of Medicine
Harvard Medical School
Physician, Gastrointestinal Unit
Chief, Walter Bauer Firm (Medical Services)
Massachusetts General Hospital
Boston, Massachusetts

Marvin H. Sleisenger, MD
Professor of Medicine, Emeritus
University of California, San Francisco, School of Medicine
Distinguished Physician
Department of Veterans Affairs Medical Center
San Francisco, California

Volume 1

SAUNDERS
An Imprint of Elsevier Science
Philadelphia London New York St. Louis Sydney Toronto

SAUNDERS
An Imprint of Elsevier Science

The Curtis Center
Independence Square West
Philadelphia, Pennsylvania 19106

SLEISENGER AND FORDTRAN'S GASTROINTESTINAL AND LIVER DISEASE **ISBN 0-7216-8973-6**

Notice

Gastroenterology is an ever-changing field. Standard safety precautions must be followed, but as new research and clinical experience broaden our knowledge, changes in treatment and drug therapy may become necessary or appropriate. Readers are advised to check the most current product information provided by the manufacturer of each drug to be administered to verify the recommended dose, the method and duration of administration, and contraindications. It is the responsibility of the treating physician, relying on experience and knowledge of the patient, to determine dosages and the best treatment for each individual patient. Neither the Publisher nor the editors assumes any liability for any injury and/or damage to persons or property arising from this publication.

THE PUBLISHER

Library of Congress Cataloging-in-Publication Data

Sleisenger & Fordtran's gastrointestinal and liver disease: pathophysiology, diagnosis, management / [edited by] Mark Feldman, Lawrence S. Friedman, Marvin H. Sleisenger.—7th ed.
p. ; cm.
Includes bibliographical references and index.
ISBN 0-7216-8973-6
1. Gastrointestinal system—Diseases. 2. Liver—Diseases. I. Title: Gastrointestinal and liver disease. II. Title: Sleisenger and Fordtran's gastrointestinal and liver disease. III. Feldman, Mark IV. Friedman, Lawrence S. (Lawrence Samuel) V. Sleisenger, Marvin H.
[DNLM: 1. Gastrointestinal Diseases. 2. Liver Diseases. WI 140 S632 2002]
RC801 .G384 2002
616.3′3—dc21 2002021046

Acquisitions Editor: Sue Hodgson
Developmental Editor: Melissa Dudlick
Project Manager: Peter Faber
Book Designer: Marie Gardocky Clifton

Printed in China.

Last digit is the print number: 9 8 7 6 5 4 3 2 1

The Editors dedicate the Seventh Edition of this textbook to the late John H. Walsh, MD, in recognition of his enormous contributions to gastroenterology in general and to Gastrointestinal and Liver Disease *in particular. Dr. Walsh contributed outstanding treatises on gastrointestinal hormones and transmitters for each of the first six editions of this book. He was also a valued advisor to and friend of the Editors, and we sorely miss him.*

We also dedicate this edition to our parents: Mildred and the late Jerome Feldman; the late Maurice and Esther Friedman; and the late Celia Levin, Louis Levin, and Abraham Sleisenger.

MARK FELDMAN, MD
LAWRENCE S. FRIEDMAN, MD
MARVIN H. SLEISENGER, MD

CONTRIBUTORS

Jane M. Andrews, MBBS, PhD, FRACP
Senior Research Fellow, Department of Medicine, Adelaide University; Consultant Gastroenterologist, Department of Gastroenterology, Hepatology, and General Medicine, Royal Adelaide Hospital, Adelaide, South Australia, Australia
Small Intestinal Motor Physiology

Paul Angulo, MD
Associate Professor of Medicine, Mayo Medical School; Senior Associate Consultant, Division of Gastroenterology and Hepatology, Mayo Clinic and Foundation, Rochester, Minnesota
Primary Biliary Cirrhosis

Thomas Anthony, MD
Associate Professor, Department of Surgery, University of Texas Southwestern Medical Center, Dallas, Texas
Gastrointestinal Carcinoid Tumors and the Carcinoid Syndrome

John E. Antoine, MD
Professor of Radiation Oncology, University of Texas Southwestern Medical Center; Chief, Radiation Oncology Service, Dallas Veterans Administration Medical Center, Dallas, Texas
Radiation Enteritis

Bruce R. Bacon, MD
James F. King, MD, Endowed Chair in Gastroenterology; Professor of Internal Medicine; Director, Division of Gastroenterology and Hepatology, St. Louis University School of Medicine, St. Louis, Missouri
Hereditary Hemochromatosis

William F. Balistreri, MD
Director, Division of Gastroenterology, Hepatology, and Nutrition, Children's Hospital Medical Center, Cincinnati, Ohio
Inherited Metabolic Disorders of the Liver

John G. Bartlett, MD
Professor of Medicine, Johns Hopkins University School of Medicine; Chief, Division of Infectious Diseases, Johns Hopkins Hospital, Baltimore, Maryland
Pseudomembranous Enterocolitis and Antibiotic-Associated Diarrhea

Nathan M. Bass, MD, PhD
Professor of Medicine, University of California, San Francisco, School of Medicine; Medical Director, Liver Transplant Program, University of California, San Francisco, Hospitals, San Francisco, California
Sclerosing Cholangitis and Recurrent Pyogenic Cholangitis; Portal Hypertension and Variceal Bleeding

Marina Berenguer, MD
Hospital Universitario La Fe, Servicio de Medicina Digestiva, Valencia, Spain
Viral Hepatitis

Patricia C. Bergen, MD
Associate Professor of Surgery, University of Texas Southwestern Medical School; Active Staff, Zale Lipshy University Hospital, Parkland Memorial Hospital, and Veterans Administration North Texas Healthcare System, Dallas, Texas
Intestinal Obstruction and Ileus

Lyman E. Bilhartz, MD, FACP
Professor of Internal Medicine, University of Texas Southwestern Medical Center; Attending Physician, Parkland Hospital and Zale Lipshy University Hospital, Dallas, Texas
Gallstone Disease and Its Complications; Acalculous Cholecystitis, Cholesterolosis, Adenomyomatosis, and Polyps of the Gallbladder

David Blumberg, MD
Assistant Professor of Surgery, University of Pittsburgh School of Medicine, Pittsburgh, Pennsylvania
Other Diseases of the Colon and Rectum

Scott J. Boley, MD
Professor of Surgery and Pediatrics, Albert Einstein College of Medicine; Emeritus Chief of Pediatric Surgery, Montefiore Medical Center, Bronx, New York
Intestinal Ischemia

Lawrence J. Brandt, MD
Professor of Medicine and Surgery, Albert Einstein College of Medicine; Chief of Gastroenterology, Montefiore Medical Center, Bronx, New York
Intestinal Ischemia; Vascular Lesions of the Gastrointestinal Tract

Robert S. Bresalier, MD
Professor of Medicine, and Chairman, Department of Gastrointestinal Medicine and Nutrition, The University of Texas MD Anderson Cancer Center, Houston, Texas
Malignant Neoplasms of the Large Intestine

Robert S. Britton, PhD
Associate Research Professor of Internal Medicine, Division of Gastroenterology and Hepatology, St. Louis University School of Medicine, St. Louis, Missouri
Hereditary Hemochromatosis

Simon J. Brookes, PhD
Senior Lecturer, Department of Human Physiology, School of Medicine, Faculty of Health Sciences, Flinders University; Senior Research Fellow, National Health and Medical Research Council of Australia, Adelaide, South Australia, Australia
Motility of the Large Intestine

William R. Brugge,, MD
Associate Professor of Medicine, Harvard Medical School; Director, Gastrointestinal Endoscopy, Massachusetts General Hospital, Boston, Massachusetts
Assistant Editor (Imaging)

J. Steven Burdick, MD
Associate Professor of Medicine, Division of Gastroenterology, University of Texas Southwestern Medical School; Director of Endoscopy and Gastroenterology, Parkland Memorial Hospital, Dallas, Texas
Anatomy, Histology, Embryology, and Developmental Anomalies of the Pancreas

Julie G. Champine, MD
Associate Professor of Radiology, University of Texas Southwestern Medical Center; Medical Director of Radiology, Parkland Memorial Hospital, Dallas, Texas
Abdominal Abscesses and Gastrointestinal Fistulas

Suresh T. Chari, MD
Assistant Professor of Medicine, Mayo Medical School; Consultant, Division of Gastroenterology and Hepatology, Mayo Clinic, Rochester, Minnesota
Acute Pancreatitis

Tsu-Yi Chuang
Professor of Dermatology Clinical Research, Indiana University School of Medicine, Indianapolis, Indiana
Oral Disease and Oral-Cutaneous Manifestations of Gastrointestinal and Liver Disease

Raymond T. Chung, MD
Assistant Professor of Medicine, Harvard Medical School; Medical Director, Liver Transplant Program, and Director, Hepatology Service, Massachusetts General Hospital, Boston, Massachusetts
Liver Abscess and Bacterial, Parasitic, Fungal, and Granulomatous Liver Disease

Ray E. Clouse, MD
Professor of Medicine and Psychiatry, Washington University School of Medicine; Physician, Barnes-Jewish Hospital, St. Louis, Missouri
Esophageal Motor and Sensory Function and Motor Disorders of the Esophagus

Robert H. Collins, Jr., MD
Associate Professor, University of Texas Southwestern Medical School; Director, Bone Marrow Transplantation, Dallas, Texas
Gastrointestinal Lymphomas, Including Immunoproliferative Small Intestinal Disease

Ian J. Cook, MD (Syd), FRACP
Associate Professor of Medicine, University of New South Wales; Head, Gastroenterology Department, St. George Hospital, Sydney, New South Wales, Australia
Motility of the Large Intestine

Diane W. Cox, PhD, FCCMG
Professor and Chair, Department of Medical Genetics, University of Alberta; Director, Medical Genetic Services, Northern Alberta; Child Health Program, Capital Health Authority, Edmonton, Alberta, Canada
Wilson Disease

Byron Cryer, MD
Associate Professor of Medicine, University of Texas Southwestern Medical School; Staff Physician, Gastroenterology Section, Dallas Veterans Administration Medical Center, Dallas, Texas
Nonsteroidal Anti-Inflammatory Drug Injury

Albert J. Czaja, MD
Professor of Medicine, Mayo Medical School; Consultant, Gastroenterology and Hepatology, Mayo Clinic, Rochester, Minnesota
Autoimmune Hepatitis

Timothy J. Davern, MD
Adjunct Assistant Professor of Medicine, University of California, San Francisco, School of Medicine, San Francisco, California
Biochemical Liver Tests

Marta L. Davila, MD
Assistant Professor of Medicine, Stanford University School of Medicine, Stanford, California
Complications of Gastrointestinal Endoscopy

Rene Davila, MD
Assistant Professor of Medicine, Gastroenterology, and Hepatology, The University of Tennessee Health Science Center, Memphis, Tennessee
Pregnancy-Related Hepatic and Gastrointestinal Disorders

Paul A. Dawson, PhD
Associate Professor of Internal Medicine, Section of Gastroenterology, Wake Forest University School of Medicine, Winston-Salem, North Carolina
Bile Secretion and the Enterohepatic Circulation of Bile Acids

Margo A. Denke, MD, FACP, FACE
Professor of Medicine, University of Texas Southwestern Medical School; Attending Physician, Veterans Affairs Medical Center, Parkland Memorial Hospital, Zale Lipshy University Hospital, and St. Paul Medical Center, Dallas, Texas
Anorexia Nervosa, Bulimia Nervosa, and Obesity

John Dent, MBBChir, PhD
Clinical Professor of Medicine, Department of Medicine, Adelaide University; Director of Gastroenterology, Hepatology, and General Medicine, Royal Adelaide Hospital, Adelaide, South Australia, Australia
Small Intestinal Motor Physiology

Nicholas E. Diamant, MDCM
Professor of Medicine and Physiology, University of Toronto; Attending Physician, Toronto Western Hospital, Division of The University Health Network, Toronto, Ontario, Canada
Esophageal Motor and Sensory Function and Motor Disorders of the Esophagus

Anna Mae Diehl, MD
Professor of Medicine, Johns Hopkins University School of Medicine; Staff, Division of Digestive Diseases, Johns Hopkins Hospital, Baltimore, Maryland
Nonalcoholic Fatty Liver Disease

Eugene P. DiMagno, MD
Professor of Medicine, Mayo School of Medicine; Consultant, Division of Gastroenterology and Hepatology, Mayo Clinic, Rochester, Minnesota
Acute Pancreatitis

Douglas A. Drossman, MD
Professor of Medicine and Psychiatry, Co-Director, Center for Functional Gastrointestinal and Motility Disorders, Division of Digestive Diseases, University of North Carolina at Chapel Hill School of Medicine, Chapel Hill, North Carolina.
Chronic Abdominal Pain (With Emphasis on Functional Abdominal Pain Syndrome); A Biopsychosocial Understanding of Gastrointestinal Illness and Disease

David E. Elliott, MD, PhD
Associate Professor of Medicine, University of Iowa School of Medicine; University of Iowa Hospitals and Clinics, Iowa City, Iowa
Intestinal Infections by Parasitic Worms

Grace H. Elta, MD
Professor of Medicine, University of Michigan School of Medicine, Ann Arbor, Michigan
Motility and Dysmotility of the Biliary Tract and Sphincter of Oddi

Geoffrey C. Farrell, MD, FRACP
Robert W. Storr Professor of Hepatic Medicine, University of Sydney; Director, Storr Liver Unit, Westmead Millennium Institute, Westmead Hospital, Westmead, New South Wales, Australia
Liver Disease Caused by Drugs, Anesthetics, and Toxins

James J. Farrell, MD
Faculty, Division of Digestive Diseases, University of California, Los Angeles, School of Medicine, Los Angeles, California
Digestion and Absorption of Nutrients and Vitamins

Richard J. Farrell, MD, MRCPI
Assistant Professor of Medicine, Harvard Medical School; Associate Physician, Division of Gastroenterology, Beth Israel Deaconess Medical Center, Boston, Massachusetts
Celiac Sprue and Refractory Sprue

Michael J. G. Farthing, DSc(Med), MD, FRCP
Executive Dean and Professor of Medicine, University of Glasgow Faculty of Medicine, Glasgow, Scotland
Tropical Malabsorption and Tropical Diarrhea

Mark Feldman, MD, FACP
Clinical Professor of Internal Medicine, University of Texas Southwestern Medical School; William O. Tschumy, Jr., M.D. Chair of Internal Medicine, Presbyterian Hospital of Dallas, Dallas, Texas
Gastric Secretion; Gastritis and Other Gastropathies

Carlos Fernández-del Castillo, MD
Associate Professor of Surgery, Harvard Medical School; Associate Visiting Surgeon, Massachusetts General Hospital, Boston, Masschusetts
Pancreatic Cancer, Cystic Pancreatic Neoplasms, and Other Nonendocrine Pancreatic Tumors

J. Gregory Fitz, MD
Waterman Professor of Medicine, University of Colorado Health Sciences Center; Head, Division of Gastroenterology and Hepatology, University of Colorado Health Sciences Center, Denver, Colorado
Hepatic Encephalopathy, Hepatopulmonary Syndromes, Hepatorenal Syndrome, Coagulopathy, and Endocrine Complications of Liver Disease

David E. Fleischer, MD
Professor of Medicine, Mayo School of Medicine; Chair, Division of Gastroenterology and Hepatology, Mayo Clinic Scottsdale, Scottsdale, Arizona
Esophageal Tumors

Chris E. Forsmark, MD
Associate Professor of Medicine, Chief of Endoscopy, Division of Gastroenterology, Hepatology, and Nutrition, University of Florida, Gainesville, Florida
Chronic Pancreatitis

Ronald Fried, MD
Staff Physician, University Hospital, Basel, Switzerland
Proctitis and Sexually Transmissible Intestinal Disease

Lawrence S. Friedman, MD
Professor of Medicine, Harvard Medical School; Physician, Gastrointestinal Unit, and Chief, Walter Bauer Firm (Medical Services), Massachusetts General Hospital, Boston, Massachusetts
A Short Treatise on Bowel Sounds; Liver Abscess and Bacterial, Parasitic, Fungal, and Granulomatous Liver Disease

Cheryl E. Gariepy, MD
Assistant Professor of Pediatrics, University of Michigan School of Medicine, Ann Arbor, Michigan
Anatomy, Histology, Embryology, and Developmental Anomalies of the Small and Large Intestine

Gregory G. Ginsberg, MD
Associate Professor of Medicine, University of Pennsylvania School of Medicine; Director of Endoscopic Services, Gastroenterology Division, Hospital of the University of Pennsylvania, Philadelphia, Pennsylvania
Foreign Bodies and Bezoars; Esophageal Tumors

Robert E. Glasgow, MD
Assistant Professor, Department of Surgery, University of Utah Health Sciences Center, Salt Lake City, Utah
Abdominal Pain, Including the Acute Abdomen; Surgical Management of Gallstone Disease and Postoperative Complications

Sherwood L. Gorbach, MD
Professor of Medicine, Family Medicine, and Community Health, Tufts University School of Medicine; Attending Physician, New England Medical Center and St. Elizabeth's Medical Center, Boston, Massachusetts
Infectious Diarrhea and Bacterial Food Poisoning

David Y. Graham, MD
Professor of Medicine and Molecular Virology and Microbiology, Baylor College of Medicine; Chief of Gastroenterology, Veterans Affairs Medical Center, Houston, Texas
Helicobacter pylori

David A. Greenwald, MD
Associate Professor of Medicine, Albert Einstein College of Medicine; Attending Physician and Fellowship Program Director, Division of Gastroenterology, Montefiore Medical Center, Bronx, New York
Vascular Lesions of the Gastrointestinal Tract

Clark R. Gregg, MD
Professor of Internal Medicine, University of Texas Southwestern Medical School; Chief, Medical Service, Veterans Affairs North Texas Health Care System, Dallas, Texas
Enteric Bacterial Flora and Small Bowel Bacterial Overgrowth Syndrome

Richard L. Guerrant, MD
Professor of Medicine and Chief, Division of Geographic and International Medicine, University of Virginia, Charlottesville, Virginia
Intestinal Protozoa

Davidson H. Hamer, MD
Assistant Professor of Medicine and Nutrition, Tufts University School of Medicine; Adjunct Assistant Professor of International Health, Boston University School of Public Health; Director, Traveler's Health Service, and Attending Physician, New England Medical Center, Boston, Massachusetts
Infectious Diarrhea and Bacterial Food Poisoning

Heinz F. Hammer, MD
Associate Professor of Internal Medicine, University of Graz, Department of Internal Medicine, Division of Gastroenterology and Hepatology, Graz, Austria
Maldigestion and Malabsorption

William Harford, MD
Professor of Internal Medicine, University of Texas Southwestern Medical School; Chief, Gastrointestinal Endoscopy, Veterans Affairs North Texas Health Care System, Dallas, Texas
Diverticula of the Hypopharynx, Esophagus, Stomach, Jejunum, and Ileum; Abdominal Hernias and Their Complications, Including Gastric Volvulus

Christoph Högenauer, MD
Fellow in Gastroenterology, Department of Internal Medicine, Division of Gastroenterology, University of Graz, Graz, Austria
Maldigestion and Malabsorption

Jay D. Horton, MD
Assistant Professor of Internal Medicine and Molecular Genetics, University of Texas Southwestern Medical Center, Dallas, Texas
Gallstone Disease and Its Complications

Tracy Hull, MD
Staff Surgeon, Colon and Rectal Surgery, and Director, Anal Physiology Section, The Cleveland Clinic Foundation, Cleveland, Ohio
Examination and Diseases of the Anorectum

Christopher D. Huston, MD
Division of Infectious Diseases, University of Virginia, Charlottesville, Virginia
Intestinal Protozoa

Steven H. Itzkowitz, MD
Dr. Burrill B. Crohn Professor of Medicine, Mount Sinai School of Medicine; Director, Dr. Henry D. Janowitz Division of Gastroenterology, Mount Sinai Hospital, New York City, New York
Colonic Polyps and Polyposis Syndromes

Robert T. Jensen, MD
Chief, Digestive Diseases Branch, National Institutes of Health, Bethesda, Maryland
Pancreatic Endocrine Tumors

Khursheed N. Jeejeebhoy, MBBS, PhD, FRCPC
Professor, University of Toronto; Director, Nutrition and Digestive Disease Program, St. Michael's Hospital, Toronto, Ontario, Canada
The Malnourished Patient: Nutritional Assessment and Management

Derek P. Jewell, DPhil, FRCP, F Med Sci
Professor of Gastroenterology, University of Oxford; Consultant Physician, John Radcliffe Hospital, Oxford, United Kingdom
Ulcerative Colitis

Rohan Jeyarajah, MD, FACS
Assistant Professor, Departments of Surgery and Internal Medicine, University of Texas Southwestern Medical Center; Attending Surgeon, Parkland Memorial Hospital, Zale Lipshy University Hospital, and Veterans Administration Medical Center, Dallas, Texas
Diverticula of the Hypopharynx, Esophagus, Stomach, Jejunum, and Ileum; Abdominal Hernias and Their Complications, Including Gastric Volvulus

Ramon E. Jimenez, MD
Fellow in Surgical Oncology, Memorial Sloan-Kettering Cancer Center, New York, New York
Pancreatic Cancer, Cystic Pancreatic Neoplasms, and Other Nonendocrine Pancreatic Tumors

Daniel B. Jones, MD, FACS
Assistant Professor, Department of Surgery, University of Texas Southwestern Medical Center; Director, Southwestern Center for Minimally Invasive Surgery, University of Texas Southwestern Medical Center, Dallas, Texas
Current Role of Surgery in Peptic Ulcer Disease

Peter J. Kahrilas, MD
Marquardt Professor of Medicine, Northwestern University Medical School; Chief, Gastroenterology and Hepatology, Northwestern Memorial Hospital, Chicago, Illinois
Gastroesophageal Reflux Disease and Its Complications, Including Barrett's Metaplasia

David J. Kearney, MD
Assistant Professor of Medicine, University of Washington School of Medicine; Staff Physician, Veterans Administration Puget Sound Health Care System, Seattle, Washington
Esophageal Disorders Caused by Infection, Systemic Illness, Medications, Radiation, and Trauma

Emmet B. Keeffe, MD
Professor of Medicine, Stanford University School of Medicine; Chief of Hepatology and Co-Director, Liver Transplant Program, Stanford University Medical Center, Stanford, California
Complications of Gastrointestinal Endoscopy

David J. Keljo, MD, PhD
Visiting Associate Professor of Pediatrics, University of Pittsburgh School of Medicine; Attending Pediatric Gastroenterologist, Children's Hospital of Pittsburgh, Pittsburgh, Pennsylvania
Anatomy, Histology, Embryology, and Developmental Anomalies of the Small and Large Intestine

Ciarán P. Kelly, MD
Associate Professor of Medicine, Harvard Medical School; Associate Physician, Division of Gastroenterology, Beth Israel Deaconess Medical Center, Boston, Massachusetts
Celiac Sprue and Refractory Sprue

Michael C. Kew, PhD, MD, DSc
Dora Dart Professor of Medicine, University of the Witwatersrand Medical School; Director, MRC/CAMSA/University Molecular Hepatology Research Unit; Consultant Hepatologist, Johannesburg Academic and Baragwanath Hospitals; Honorary Research Associate, South African Institute for Medical Research, Johannesburg, South Africa
Hepatic Tumors and Cysts

David D. Kim, MD
Senior Gastroenterology Fellow, University of California, San Francisco, San Francisco, California
Gastrointestinal Manifestations of Systemic Disease

Karen E. Kim, MD
Assistant Professor of Clinical Medicine, University of Chicago; Director, Colorectal Cancer Prevention Clinic, Chicago, Illinois
Protein-Losing Gastroenteropathy

Lawrence T. Kim, MD
Assistant Professor of Surgery and of Cell Biology and Neuroscience, University of Texas Southwestern Medical Center; Assistant Chief, Surgical Service, Veterans Administration North Texas Health Care System, Dallas, Texas
Gastrointestinal Carcinoid Tumors and the Carcinoid Syndrome

Samuel Klein, MD
William H. Danforth Professor of Medicine and Nutritional Science; Director, Center for Human Nutrition, Washington University School of Medicine, St. Louis, Missouri
The Malnourished Patient: Nutritional Assessment and Management; Enteral and Parenteral Nutrition; Assistant Editor (Nutrition)

Theodore J. Koh, MD
Assistant Professor of Medicine, University of Massachusetts Medical School, Worcester, Massachusetts
Tumors of the Stomach

Braden Kuo, MD
Instructor in Medicine, Harvard Medical School; Assistant Physician, Gastrointestinal Unit (Medical Services), Massachusetts General Hospital, Boston, Massachusetts
A Short Treatise on Bowel Sounds

Jeanne M. LaBerge, MD
Professor of Radiology, University of California, San Francisco, School of Medicine; Interventional Radiologist, Moffitt-Long and Mount Zion Hospital, San Francisco, California
Endoscopic and Radiologic Treatment of Biliary Disease

John R. Lake, MD
Professor of Medicine and Surgery, University of Minnesota School of Medicine; Department of Medicine, Fairview University Medical Center, Minneapolis, Minnesota
Gastrointestinal Complications of Solid Organ and Hematopoietic Cell Transplantation

Edward L. Lee, MD
Professor of Pathology, University of Texas Southwestern Medical Center; Chief of Pathology and Laboratory Medicine Service, Department of Veterans Affairs Medical Center, Dallas, Texas
Gastritis and Other Gastropathies; Assistant Editor (Pathology)

Makau Lee, MD, PhD
Clinical Professor of Medicine, University of Mississippi Medical Center, Jackson, Mississippi
Nausea and Vomiting

John E. Lennard-Jones, MD, DSc(Hon), FRCP, FRCS
Emeritus Professor of Gastroenterology, University of London, London; Emeritus Consultant Gastroenterologist, St. Mark's Hospital, Harrow, England
Constipation

Mike A. Leonis, MD, PhD
Fellow in Pediatric Gastroenterology, Hepatology, and Nutrition, Children's Hospital Medical Center, Cincinnati Ohio
Inherited Metabolic Disorders of the Liver

Michael D. Levitt, MD
A.C.O.S. Research, Minneapolis Veterans Affairs Medical Center; Professor of Medicine, University of Minnesota School of Medicine, Minneapolis, Minnesota
Intestinal Gas

Rodger A. Liddle, MD
Professor of Medicine, Duke University School of Medicine; Chief, Division of Gastroenterology, Duke University Medical Center, Durham, North Carolina
Gastrointestinal Hormones and Neurotransmitters

Steven D. Lidofsky, MD, PhD
Associate Professor of Medicine and Pharmacology, University of Vermont College of Medicine; Director of Hepatology, Fletcher-Allen Health Care, Burlington, Vermont
Jaundice; Acute Liver Failure

Keith D. Lillemoe, MD
Professor and Vice-Chairman, Department of Surgery, Johns Hopkins University School of Medicine; Deputy Director, Department of Surgery, Johns Hopkins Hospital, Baltimore, Maryland
Tumors of the Gallbladder, Bile Ducts, and Ampulla

Keith D. Lindor, MD
Professor of Medicine, Mayo Medical School; Chair, Division of Gastroenterology and Hepatology, and Consultant, Division of Gastroenterology and Hepatology, Mayo Clinic and Foundation, Rochester, Minnesota
Primary Biliary Cirrhosis

Peter M. Loeb, MD
Clinical Professor of Medicine, University of Texas Southwestern Medical School; Chief of Gastroenterology, Director of Gastroenterology Laboratory, Presbyterian Hospital of Dallas, Dallas, Texas
Caustic Injury to the Upper Gastrointestinal Tract

John D. Long, MD
Assistant Professor of Medicine, University of Cincinnati College of Medicine; Director, Gastrointestinal Clinic, University Hospital, Cincinnati, Ohio
Anatomy, Histology, Embryology, and Developmental Anomalies of the Esophagus

David J. Magee, MD
Assistant Professor, Division of Gastroenterology, University of Texas Southwestern Medical Center, Dallas, Texas
Anatomy, Histology, Embryology, and Developmental Anomalies of the Pancreas

Uma Mahadevan, MD
Assistant Clinical Professor of Medicine, University of California, San Francisco, School of Medicine; Director of Clinical Research, Inflammatory Bowel Disease Center, Mount Zion Hospital, San Francisco, California
Sclerosing Cholangitis and Recurrent Pyogenic Cholangitis

Jacquelyn J. Maher, MD
Associate Professor of Medicine, University of California, San Francisco, School of Medicine; Attending Physician in Medicine and Gastroenterology, San Francisco General Hospital, San Francisco, California
Alcoholic Liver Disease

Matthias Maiwald, MD
Visiting Scholar, Department of Microbiology and Immunology, Stanford University School of Medicine, Stanford, California
Whipple's Disease

Arshad Malik, MD
Fellow, University of Texas Southwestern Medical Center, Dallas, Texas
Short Bowel Syndrome

Paul Martin, MD
Professor of Medicine, University of California, Los Angeles, School of Medicine; Medical Director, Liver Transplant Program, Cedars Sinai Medical Center, Los Angeles, California
Liver Transplantation

Elizabeth J. McConnell, MD
Assistant Professor of Surgery, Mayo School of Medicine; Senior Associate Consultant, Mayo Clinic Scottsdale, Scottsdale, Arizona
Megacolon: Congenital and Acquired

George B. McDonald, MD
Professor of Medicine, University of Washington School of Medicine; Head, Gastroenterology/Hepatology Section, Fred Hutchinson Cancer Research Center, Seattle, Washington
Esophageal Disorders Caused by Infection, Systemic Illness, Medications, Radiation, and Trauma

Kenneth R. McQuaid, MD
Professor of Clinical Medicine, University of California, San Francisco, School of Medicine; Director of Endoscopy, Veterans Affairs Medical Center, San Francisco, California
Dyspepsia

Joseph P. Minei, MD
Associate Professor of Surgery, Chief, Section of Trauma and Critical Care, Division of Burn, Trauma, and Critical Care, University of Texas Southwestern Medical Center; Medical Director of Trauma Services, Surgeon-in-Chief, Parkland Health and Hospital System, Dallas, Texas
Abdominal Abscesses and Gastrointestinal Fistulas

Ginat W. Mirowski
Assistant Professor, Department of Dermatology, Oral Pathology, Medicine, and Radiology, Indiana University School of Medicine, Indianapolis, Indiana
Oral Disease and Oral-Cutaneous Manifestations of Gastrointestinal and Liver Disease

Sean J. Mulvihill, MD
Professor and Chairman, Department of Surgery, University of Utah Health Sciences Center, Salt Lake City, Utah
Abdominal Pain, Including the Acute Abdomen; Surgical Management of Gallstone Disease and Postoperative Complications

Nam P. Nguyen, MD
Clinical Assistant Professor, University of Texas Southwestern Medical Center; Radiation Oncologist, Dallas Veterans Administration Medical Center, Dallas, Texas
Radiation Enteritis

Jeffrey A. Norton, MD
Department of Surgery, University of California, San Francisco; Chief, Surgical Service, San Francisco Veterans Affairs Medical Center, San Francisco, California
Pancreatic Endocrine Tumors

Michael J. Nunez, MD
Department of Internal Medicine, Division of Gastroenterology, Presbyterian Hospital of Dallas, Dallas, Texas
Caustic Injury to the Upper Gastrointestinal Tract

Roy C. Orlando, MD
Professor of Medicine and Physiology, Tulane University Medical School; Chief, Gastroenterology and Hepatology, Tulane University Medical Center, New Orleans, Louisiana
Anatomy, Histology, Embryology, and Developmental Anomalies of the Esophagus

James W. Ostroff, MD
Clinical Professor of Medicine and Pediatrics, University of California, San Francisco, School of Medicine; Director, Endoscopy Unit and Gastrointestinal Consultation Service, Moffitt-Long and Mount Zion Hospital, San Francisco, California
Endoscopic and Radiologic Treatment of Biliary Disease

Stephen J. Pandol, MD
Professor of Medicine, University of California, Los Angeles, School of Medicine; Staff Physician, Veterans Administration Greater Los Angeles Health Care System, Los Angeles, California
Pancreatic Physiology and Secretory Testing

John E. Pandolfino, MD
Assistant Professor, Northwestern University Medical School; Attending Physician, Northwestern Memorial Hospital, Chicago, Illinois
Gastroesophageal Reflux Disease and Its Complications, Including Barrett's Metaplasia

Lisa Ann Panzini, MD
Assistant Clinical Professor of Medicine, Yale University School of Medicine; Connecticut Gastroenterology Consultants, PC, New Haven, Connecticut
Isolated and Diffuse Ulcers of the Small Intestine

Gustav Paumgartner, MD
Professor of Medicine, Department of Medicine II, Klinikum Grosshadern, University of Munich, Munich, Germany
Nonsurgical Management of Gallstone Disease

John H. Pemberton, MD
Professor of Surgery, Mayo Graduate School of Medicine; Consultant, Colon and Rectal Surgery, Mayo Clinic and Mayo Foundation, Rochester, Minnesota
Ileostomy and Its Alternatives; Megacolon: Congenital and Acquired

Walter L. Peterson, MD
Professor of Medicine, University of Texas Southwestern Medical Center; Staff Physician, Department of Veterans Affairs Medical Center, Dallas, Texas
Helicobacter pylori

Patrick R. Pfau, MD
Assistant Professor of Medicine, University of Wisconsin Medical School; Division of Gastroenterology, University of Wisconsin Hospital and Clinic, Madison, Wisconsin
Foreign Bodies and Bezoars

Sidney F. Phillips, MD
Professor of Medicine, Mayo Graduate School of Medicine; Mayo Clinic and Mayo Foundation, Rochester, Minnesota
Ileostomy and Its Alternatives

Joseph R. Pisegna, MD
Associate Professor, Department of Medicine, University of California, Los Angeles, School of Medicine; Chief, Division of Gastroenterology and Hepatology, Veterans Administration Greater Los Angeles Healthcare System, Los Angeles, California
Zollinger-Ellison Syndrome and Other Hypersecretory States

Daniel K. Podolsky, MD
Mallinckrodt Professor of Medicine, Harvard Medical School; Chief, Gastrointestinal Unit, Massachusetts General Hospital, Boston, Massachusetts
Cellular Growth and Neoplasia

Fred Poordad, MD
Assistant Professor of Medicine, University of California, Los Angeles, School of Medicine; Hepatologist, Cedars Sinai Medical Center, Los Angeles, California
Nonalcoholic Fatty Liver Disease

Deborah D. Proctor, MD
Associate Professor of Medicine, Section of Digestive Diseases, Department of Internal Medicine, Yale University School of Medicine; Attending Physician, Yale-New Haven Hospital, New Haven, Connecticut
Isolated and Diffuse Ulcers of the Small Intestine

Eamonn M. M. Quigley, MD, FRCP, FACP, FRCPI, FACG
Professor of Medicine and Human Physiology, Head of the Medical School, National University of Ireland; Consultant Physician and Gastroenterologist, Cork University Hospital, Cork, Ireland
Gastric Motor and Sensory Function, and Motor Disorders of the Stomach

Nicholas W. Read, MA, MD, FRCP
Professor of Integrated Medicine, Institute of General Practice, University of Sheffield; Consultant Gastroenterologist and Psychoanalytical Psychotherapist, Northern General Hospital, Sheffield, United Kingdom
Irritable Bowel Syndrome

Carol A. Redel, MD
Assistant Professor of Pediatrics, University of Texas Southwestern Medical School; Attending Physician, Pediatric Gastroenterology, Children's Medical Center of Dallas, Dallas, Texas
Anatomy, Histology, Embryology, and Developmental Anomalies of the Stomach and Duodenum

Robert V. Rege, MD, FACS
Professor and Chairman, Department of Surgery, University of Texas Southwestern Medical School, Dallas, Texas
Current Role of Surgery in Peptic Ulcer Disease

David A. Relman, MD
Associate Professor of Medicine, Microbiology, and Immunology, Stanford University School of Medicine, Stanford; Staff Physician, Veterans Affairs Palo Alto Health Care System, Palo Alto, California
Whipple's Disease

Joel E. Richter, MD
Chairman, Department of Gastroenterology, Cleveland Clinic Foundation; Professor of Medicine, The Cleveland Clinic Foundation Health Center of the Ohio State University, Cleveland, Ohio
Dysphagia, Odynophagia, Heartburn, and Other Esophageal Symptoms

Caroline A. Riely, MD
Professor of Medicine and Pediatrics, University of Tennessee School of Medicine, Memphis, Tennessee
Pregnancy-Related Hepatic and Gastrointestinal Disorders

Eve A. Roberts, MD, FRCPC
Professor of Pediatrics, Medicine, and Pharmacology, Division of Gastroenterology and Nutrition, The Hospital for Sick Children, Toronto, Ontario, Canada
Wilson Disease

Don C. Rockey, MD
Associate Professor of Medicine, Duke University School of Medicine; Director, Liver Center, Duke University Medical Center, Durham, North Carolina
Gastrointestinal Bleeding

Hugo R. Rosen, MD
Associate Professor of Medicine, Molecular Microbiology, and Immunology, Portland Veterans Administration Medical Center; Medical Director, Liver Transplantation Program, Portland, Oregon
Liver Transplantation

Deborah C. Rubin, MD
Associate Professor of Medicine, Washington University School of Medicine, St. Louis, Missouri
Enteral and Parenteral Nutrition

Bruce A. Runyon, MD
Professor of Medicine, University of Southern California, Los Angeles, School of Medicine, Los Angeles; Chief, Liver Unit, Rancho Los Amigos Medical Center, Downey, California
Ascites and Spontaneous Bacterial Peritonitis; Surgical Peritonitis and Other Diseases of the Peritoneum, Mesentery, Omentum, and Diaphragm

Anil K. Rustgi, MD
T. Grier Miller Associate Professor of Medicine and Genetics, University of Pennsylvania School of Medicine; Chief of Gastroenterology, University of Pennsylvania, Philadelphia, Pennsylvania
Cellular Growth and Neoplasia; Small Intestinal Neoplasms

James C. Ryan, MD
Associate Professor, University of California, San Francisco, School of Medicine, San Francisco, California
Gastrointestinal Manifestations of Systemic Disease

Hugh A. Sampson, MD
Professor of Pediatrics and Biomedical Sciences, Mount Sinai School of Medicine, New York University; Director, General Clinical Research Center, and Chief, Pediatric Allergy and Immunology, Mount Sinai Hospital, New York, New York
Food Allergies

Bruce E. Sands, MD, SM(Epidem)
Assistant Professor of Medicine, Harvard Medical School; Assistant in Medicine and Director, Clinical Research, Gastrointestinal Unit, Massachusetts General Hospital, Boston, Massachusetts
Crohn's Disease

George A. Sarosi, Jr., MD
Assistant Professor, Department of Surgery, University of Texas Southwestern Medical School; Staff Surgeon, Dallas Veterans Affairs Medical Center, Dallas, Texas
Appendicitis

R. Balfour Sartor, MD
Professor of Medicine, Microbiology, and Immunology, University of North Carolina at Chapel Hill School of Medicine; Director, Multidisciplinary Center for IBD Research and Treatment, University of North Carolina, Chapel Hill, North Carolina
Mucosal Immunology and Mechanisms of Gastrointestinal Inflammation

Daniel F. Schafer, MD
Associate Professor of Medicine, Department of Internal Medicine, University of Nebraska School of Medicine; Adult Hepatologist, University of Nebraska Medical Center, Omaha, Nebraska
Vascular Diseases of the Liver

Bruce F. Scharschmidt, MD
Adjunct Professor of Medicine, University of California, San Francisco, School of Medicine, San Francisco; Vice President, Clinical Development, Chiron Corporation, Emeryville, California
Biochemical Liver Tests; Consulting Editor

Lawrence R. Schiller, MD
Clinical Professor of Internal Medicine, University of Texas Southwestern Medical Center; Program Director, Gastroenterology Fellowship, Baylor University Medical Center, Dallas, Texas
Diarrhea; Fecal Incontinence

Michael D. Schuffler, MD
Professor, Department of Medicine, University of Washington School of Medicine; Chief of Gastroenterology, PacMed Clinics, Seattle, Washington
Chronic Intestinal Pseudo-Obstruction

Joseph H. Sellin, MD
Professor of Medicine and Integrative Biology; Director, Division of Gastroenterology, Hepatology, and Nutrition; Director, Gastroenterology Fellowship Training Program, The University of Texas Medical School–Houston; Director, Gastroenterology Service, Memorial Hermann Hospital; Director, Gastroenterology Service, Lyndon Baines Johnson General Hospital, Houston, Texas
Diarrhea; Intestinal Electrolyte Absorption and Secretion

Michael A. Shetzline, MD, PhD
Assistant Professor of Medicine, Duke University School of Medicine, Durham, North Carolina
Gastrointestinal Hormones and Neurotransmitters

G. Thomas Shires III, MD
Clinical Professor of Surgery, University of Texas Southwestern Medical Center; Chairman, Surgical Services, Presbyterian Hospital of Dallas, Dallas, Texas
Diverticular Disease of the Colon

Clifford L. Simmang, MD, MS
Associate Professor of Surgery, University of Texas Southwestern Medical Center; Attending Surgeon, Parkland Memorial Hospital and Zale Lipshy University Hospital, Dallas, Texas
Diverticular Disease of the Colon

Taylor A. Sohn, MD
Resident, General Surgery, Johns Hopkins Medical Institutions, Baltimore, Maryland
Tumors of the Gallbladder, Bile Ducts, and Ampulla

Michael F. Sorrell, MD
Robert L. Grissan Professor, University of Nebraska College of Medicine; Hepatologist, Department of Internal Medicine, University of Nebraska Medical Center, Omaha, Nebraska
Vascular Diseases of the Liver

Stuart Jon Spechler, MD
Professor of Medicine and Berta M. and Cecil O. Patterson Chair in Gastroenterology, University of Texas Southwestern Medical Center; Chief, Division of Gastroenterology, Dallas Veterans Administration Medical Center, Dallas, Texas
Peptic Ulcer Disease and Its Complications

Andrew Stolz, MD
Associate Professor of Medicine, Keck School of Medicine, University of Southern California, Los Angeles, California
Liver Physiology and Metabolic Function

Fabrizis L. Suarez, MD, PhD
Adjunct Assistant Professor, School of Allied Medical Professions, The Ohio State University; Associate Director, Medical Affairs Medical Nutrition, Ross Product Division, Abbott Laboratories, Columbus, Ohio
Intestinal Gas

José Such, MD
Consultant, Liver Unit, Hospital General Universitario, Alicante, Spain
Surgical Peritonitis and Other Diseases of the Peritoneum, Mesentery, Omentum, and Diaphragm

Frederick J. Suchy, MD
Herbert H. Lehman Professor and Chair, Department of Pediatrics, Mount Sinai School of Medicine, New York University; Pediatrician-in-Chief, Mount Sinai Hospital, New York, New York
Anatomy, Histology, Embryology, Developmental Anomalies, and Pediatric Disorders of the Biliary Tract

Christina Surawicz, MD
Professor of Medicine, University of Washington School of Medicine; Section Chief, Gastroenterology, Harborview Medical Center, Seattle, Washington
Proctitis and Sexually Transmissible Intestinal Disease

Nicholas J. Talley, MD, PhD
Professor of Medicine, University of Sydney; Head, Division of Medicine, Nepean Hospital, Penrith, New South Wales, Australia
Eosinophilic Gastroenteritis

Dwain L. Thiele, MD
Professor of Internal Medicine, Vice-Chief, Division of Digestive and Liver Diseases and Chief of Hepatology, University of Texas Southwestern Medical Center; Chief of Liver Diseases Service, Parkland Health and Hospital System; Attending Physician, Zale Lipshy University Hospital, Dallas, Texas
Hepatic Manifestations of Systemic Disease and Other Disorders of the Liver

Phillip P. Toskes, MD
Professor of Internal Medicine and Chairman, Department of Medicine, University of Florida College of Medicine, Gainesville, Florida
Enteric Bacterial Flora and Small Bowel Bacterial Overgrowth Syndrome

Richard H. Turnage, MD
Professor and Chair, Department of Surgery, Louisiana State University School of Medicine, Shreveport, Louisiana
Appendicitis; Intestinal Obstruction and Ileus

Axel von Herbay, MD
Lecturer, Institute of Pathology, University of Heidelberg, Heidelberg, Germany
Whipple's Disease

Arnold Wald, MD
Professor of Medicine, University of Pittsburgh School of Medicine; Associate Chief for Education and Training, Division of Gastroenterology, Hepatology, and Nutrition Support, University of Pittsburgh Medical Center, Pittsburgh, Pennsylvania
Other Diseases of the Colon and Rectum

Timothy C. Wang, MD
Gladys Smith Martin Professor of Medicine, Chief, Division of Digestive Diseases and Nutrition, University of Massachusetts Memorial Medical School, Worcester, Massachusetts
Tumors of the Stomach

Ian R. Wanless, MD, FRCPC
Professor of Pathology, University of Toronto; Staff Pathologist, Toronto General Hospital, Toronto, Ontario, Canada
Anatomy, Histology, Embryology, and Developmental Anomalies of the Liver

Sally Weisdorf-Schindele, MD
Associate Professor, Pediatric Gastroenterology, Hepatology, and Nutrition, University of Minnesota School of Medicine; Pediatric Gastroenterology, Hepatology, and Nutrition, University/Fairview Medical Center, Minneapolis, Minnesota
Gastrointestinal Complications of Solid Organ and Hematopoietic Cell Transplantation

Henrik Westergaard, MD
Professor of Internal Medicine, University of Texas Southwestern Medical Center, Dallas, Texas
Short Bowel Syndrome

David C. Whitcomb, MD, PhD
University of Pittsburgh Medical Center, Pittsburgh, Pennsylvania
Hereditary and Childhood Disorders of the Pancreas, Including Cystic Fibrosis

C. Mel Wilcox, MD
Professor of Medicine and Director, Division of Gastroenterology and Hepatology, University of Alabama at Birmingham, Birmingham, Alabama
Gastrointestinal Consequences of Infection with Human Immunodeficiency Virus

Teresa L. Wright, MD
Professor of Medicine, University of California, San Francisco, School of Medicine; Chief, Gastroenterology Section, Veterans Administration Medical Center, San Francisco, California
Viral Hepatitis

Francis Y. Yao, MD
Associate Clinical Professor of Medicine, University of California, San Francisco, School of Medicine; Associate Medical Director, Liver Transplant Program, University of California, San Francisco, Hospitals, San Francisco, California
Portal Hypertension and Variceal Bleeding

Hal F. Yee, Jr., MD, PhD
Assistant Professor of Medicine and Physiology, University of California, Los Angeles, School of Medicine; Attending Physician, University of California, Los Angeles, Medical Center and Greater Los Angeles Veterans Affairs Healthcare System, Los Angeles, California
Acute Liver Failure

FOREWORD

I consider it an enormous honor to be writing the foreword to this the seventh edition of Sleisenger and Fordtran's *Gastrointestinal and Liver Disease*. Those asked to write forewords to earlier editions included Franz Ingelfinger and Tom Almy. These two giants were, in Dean Acheson's words, "present at the conception" of modern, science-based gastroenterology. I was lucky enough to be "present at the conception" of the first modern, science-based textbook of gastroenterology. Marvin Sleisenger and John Fordtran, who trained with Tom Almy and Franz Ingelfinger, respectively, invited experts concerned with virtually every aspect of gastrointestinal and biliary tract disease to put together the first edition of *Gastrointestinal Disease: Pathophysiology, Diagnosis, and Management*. And what a wonderful textbook it turned out to be! It was well organized and contained authoritative, up-to-date chapters describing both scientific advances and clinical features. The scope of the book and the quality of its content assured its immediate, wholehearted, and widespread acceptance.

As they produced the next five editions, the editors refused to stand still and take the book's continuing success for granted. Instead, they kept to the task of changing with the times while sustaining excellence. More and more illustrations were added to demonstrate histologic, radiologic, and endoscopic abnormalities. Experts were recruited who came from disciplines outside traditional gastroenterology but whose interests were relevant to gastrointestinal function and disease. The scope of the book was broadened to include a section on liver disease, an entirely appropriate expansion because meaningful practice of gastroenterology is not possible without adequate knowledge of liver disease, just as the practice of hepatology requires an understanding of diseases of the gastrointestinal and biliary tracts.

And now 30 years after this remarkable textbook began, here comes the seventh edition. The tradition of excellence continues in this edition with its concise coverage of relevant basic science and pathophysiology, its meticulous, judicious chapters on disease, and—most important—the careful editing, organization, referencing, and indexing that make a textbook easy to use. Happily, I continue to see among the array of outstanding authors experts outside the mainstream of gastroenterology, such as David Relman in microbiology and John Bartlett and Sherwood Gorbach in infectious disease, to name but three. The inclusion of authorities from other disciplines adds an important dimension. The editors have further strengthened the book by increasing the number and improving the quality of diagnostic images—whether they be radiologic, endoscopic, or pathologic—that are of ever-increasing importance to gastroenterologists.

Readers will no doubt continue to use the seventh edition much as they have in the past. Practitioners will review chapters to answer questions about their patients or to prepare a talk for their colleagues. Academic gastroenterologists will bring themselves up to date in areas outside their own specific expertise and will frequently refer to the book at conferences and when supervising the work of fellows, residents, or medical students. Trainees and students of course will depend on the book, as they always have, to provide information for themselves and documentation they can use in case presentations. Of the many people who will be using the book, I envy most the students who'll be opening it for the first time to discover the astonishing world of digestive diseases. What a marvelous journey they're about to begin!

ROBERT M. DONALDSON, JR., MD
David Paige Smith Professor of Medicine Emeritus
Yale University School of Medicine

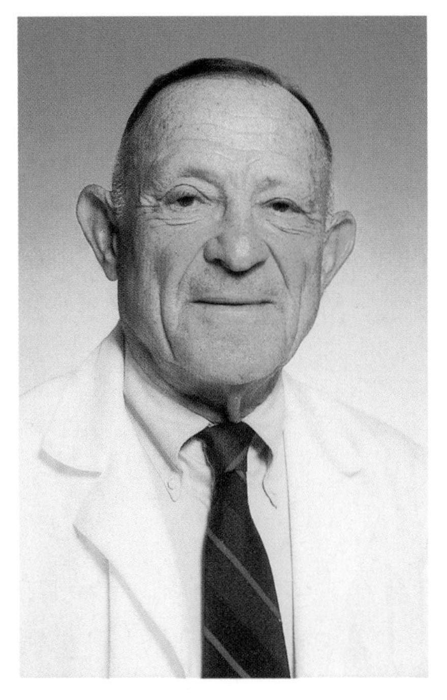

Marvin H. Sleisenger, MD
Editions 1–7

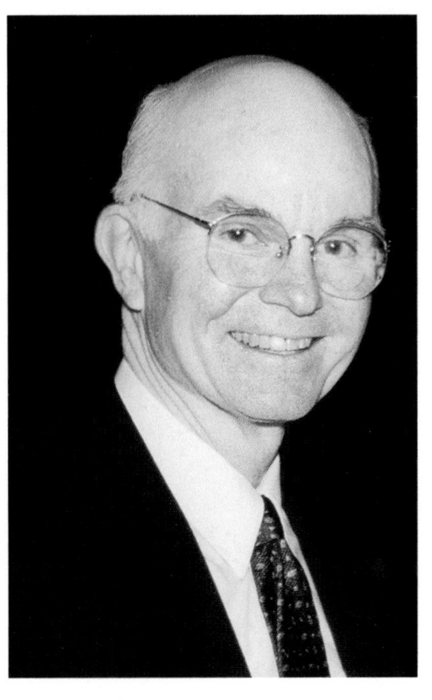

John S. Fordtran, MD
Editions 1–5

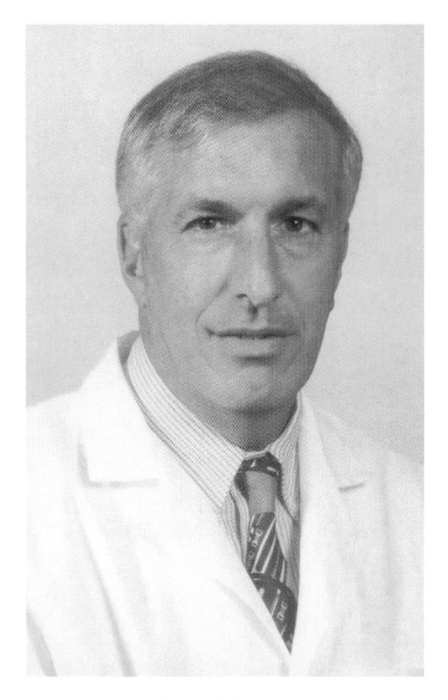

Mark Feldman, MD
Editions 5–7

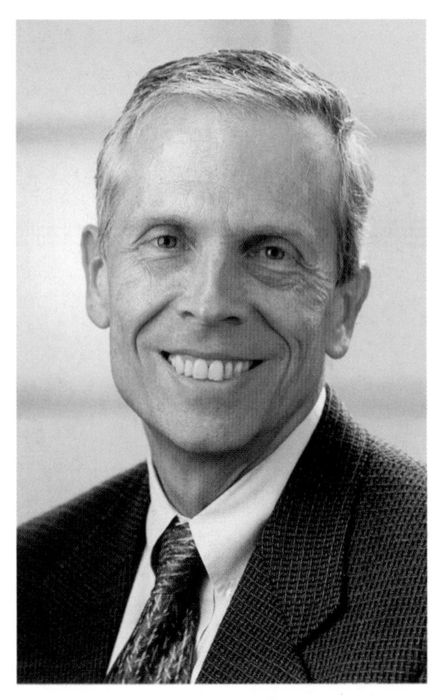

Bruce F. Scharschmidt, MD
Editions 5, 6

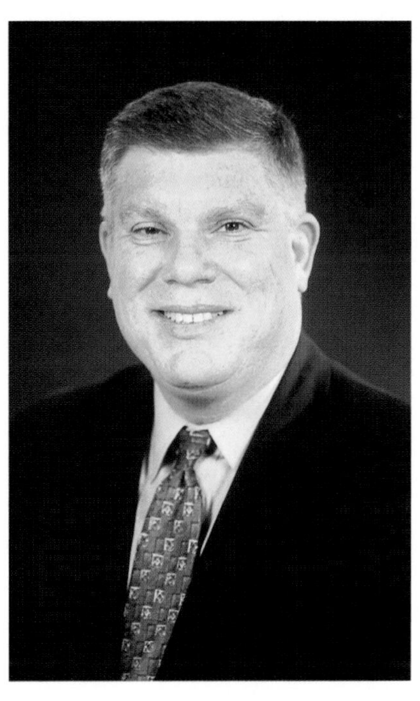

Lawrence S. Friedman, MD
Edition 7

PREFACE

The seventh edition of *Gastrointestinal and Liver Disease*, like its predecessors, is a comprehensive and authoritative textbook intended for gastroenterologists, trainees in gastroenterology, primary care physicians, residents in medicine and surgery, and medical students. The goal remains to produce a state-of-the-art, user-friendly textbook that covers disorders of the gastrointestinal tract, biliary tree, pancreas, and liver, as well as the related topics of nutrition and peritoneal disorders. Inclusion of a section on liver disease in the sixth edition was well received, and just as liver disease is integral to the practice of gastroenterology, so it has become integral to this textbook.

Considerable time and effort have been invested in improving and refining the seventh edition. A new editor, Lawrence S. Friedman, has replaced Bruce Scharschmidt, whose contributions to the fifth and sixth editions of the book and whose assistance in planning the seventh edition are gratefully acknowledged. As in the past, the editors have made a thorough and comprehensive review of the sixth edition, with the assistance of colleagues, fellows, and residents at our respective institutions, to correct deficiencies and eliminate redundancies. Because the practice of gastroenterology depends greatly on visual interpretation of endoscopic images, radiographs, and pathology specimens, a notable addition to the seventh edition is the designation of William R. Brugge as Imaging Editor and William Lee as Pathology Editor. Dr. Brugge reviewed endoscopic and radiographic figures submitted by authors to be certain that they were of the highest possible quality and, when appropriate, provided examples from his personal collection or other sources. Dr. Lee did the same for all submitted gross pathology illustrations and photomicrographs. As a result, the figures in this edition of the textbook are of exceptionally high quality and clarity. In addition, over 100 photographs that were submitted in color have been placed directly (in color) into the relevant chapters, rather than in a separate section of color plates or in a companion atlas, as was done in the sixth edition. The editors are confident that this arrangement will provide convenience and clarity for the reader.

Many aspects of the seventh edition will be familiar to the readers of previous editions. Section One deals with the Biology of the Gastrointestinal Tract and Liver with new up-to-date contributions on hormones and neurotransmitters by Dr. Liddle and on immunology and inflammation of the gastrointestinal tract by Dr. Sartor. Section Two on the Approach to Patients with Symptoms and Signs, which was reinstituted in the sixth edition, has been retained (with the addition of a short "treatise" on the history and significance of bowel sounds by Drs. Kuo and Friedman), as has Section Three on Nutrition and Gastroenterology, for which Samuel Klein again served as consulting editor. Section Four consists of Topics Involving Multiple Organs, including authoritative chapters on diverticula of the esophagus, stomach, and small bowel as well as on hernias and volvulus of the gastrointestinal tract by Drs. Harford and Jeyarajah. Sections Five through Eleven contain the chapters dealing with the broad spectrum of diseases of the esophagus, stomach and duodenum, pancreas, biliary tract, liver, small and large intestines, vascular disorders of the gut, and disorders of the peritoneum, mesentery, omentum, and diaphragm. Overall, nearly one third of the authors are new to this edition. There are now separate chapters on acute pancreatitis by Drs. DiMagno and Chari and chronic pancreatitis by Dr. Forsmark. In addition, there are separate chapters on protozoal intestinal diseases by Drs. Huston and Guerrant and on intestinal infections by worms, flukes, and other nonprotozoal parasites by Dr. Elliot. Finally, there is an eloquent concluding section on psychosocial factors in gastrointestinal disease by Dr. Drossman.

Successful features from previous editions have been retained. At the start of each chapter is a mini-outline with page citations. Each major section also contains a listing of the chapters with page citations in that section. High quality glossy paper continues to be used, and the text is amply illustrated with figures, tables, and algorithms. Chapters are appropriately cross-referenced, and the index remains extensive and useful for locating material quickly.

The seventh edition of this classic textbook remains true to the spirit of the first edition published nearly 30 years ago, namely, a critical overview of the state of gastrointestinal practice and its scientific underpinnings by eminent authorities in their respective fields. The book is truly international in scope, with authors from 11 different countries. Celebrating 30 years of excellence, this textbook remains the definitive resource for anyone involved in the care of patients with gastrointestinal and hepatic disorders.

MARK FELDMAN, MD
LAWRENCE S. FRIEDMAN, MD
MARVIN H. SLEISENGER, MD

ACKNOWLEDGMENTS

The Editors of the Seventh Edition are most grateful to more than 100 contributing authors from around the globe whose scholarship and clinical experience fill its pages. The editors also appreciate the support of our professional colleagues in Dallas, Boston, and San Francisco.

Vicky Robertson, Tracy Cooper, Hildreth Curran, and Rita Burns provided outstanding administrative support. The Editors have also greatly benefited from the contributions of the professional staff at Saunders, particularly Richard Zorab and Sue Hodgson, Melissa Dudlick, Marjory Fraser, Carol DiBerardino, and Angela Holt. We also acknowledge the valuable assistance provided by our two Assistant Editors, Edward Lee for Pathology and William Brugge for Imaging, and to Mukesh Harisinghani, who assisted Dr. Brugge. As in the sixth edition, Dr. Samuel Klein helped us immensely with the Nutrition chapters.

We are especially grateful for the constant encouragement and understanding of our wives, Barbara Feldman, Mary Jo Cappuccilli, and Lenore Sleisenger, and of our children, Matthew, Elizabeth, Daniel, and Lindsay Feldman; Matthew Friedman; and Thomas Sleisenger.

MARK FELDMAN, MD
LAWRENCE S. FRIEDMAN, MD
MARVIN H. SLEISENGER, MD

CONTENTS

Volume 1

Section One
BIOLOGY OF THE GASTROINTESTINAL TRACT AND LIVER

Section Two

APPROACH TO PATIENTS WITH SYMPTOMS AND SIGNS

Section Three
NUTRITION IN GASTROENTEROLOGY

Section Four
TOPICS INVOLVING MULTIPLE ORGANS

Section Five
ESOPHAGUS

Section Six

STOMACH AND DUODENUM

Section Seven
PANCREAS

Section Eight
BILIARY TRACT

Volume 2

Section Nine

LIVER

Section Ten

SMALL AND LARGE INTESTINE

Section Eleven
VASCULATURE AND SUPPORTING STRUCTURES

Section Twelve

PSYCHOSOCIAL FACTORS IN GASTROINTESTINAL DISEASE

Section One

BIOLOGY OF THE GASTROINTESTINAL TRACT AND LIVER

Chapter 1

GASTROINTESTINAL HORMONES AND NEUROTRANSMITTERS

Michael A. Shetzline and Rodger A. Liddle

Cells throughout the gastrointestinal tract receive information in many forms, including chemical messengers that emanate from other cells. The prototype for this type of communication came with the discovery of the first hormone, secretin. In 1902, it was observed that extracts of intestinal mucosa, when injected into the bloodstream of dogs, caused pancreatic secretion. Thus, the first hormone was a gastrointestinal peptide. It is now appreciated that gastrointestinal peptides throughout the gut play critical roles in the processes of digestion.

The initial stimulus for hormone secretion is the ingestion of food. Food provides central neural stimulation in the form of thought (anticipation) and sight, chemical stimulation in the form of odor and taste, nutrient stimulation of the epithelial cells lining the gastrointestinal tract, and mechanical stimulation. These processes all stimulate the release of peptides and other transmitters from cells of the mucosa into the bloodstream, where they circulate to distant target tissues. Therefore, chemical messengers from the gastrointestinal tract can have far-reaching effects throughout the body.

CELLULAR COMMUNICATION

Chemical transmitters of the gut are produced by discrete cells of the gastrointestinal mucosa and can be classified as endocrine, paracrine, synaptic ("neurocrine"), or autocrine (Fig. 1–1). Specialized signaling cells that secrete transmitters into the blood are known as *endocrine cells,* and the transmitters they produce are known as *hormones.* Hormones bind to specific receptors on the surface of target cells at remote sites and regulate metabolic processes.[1]

In contrast with endocrine cells that act on distant target tissues, other signaling cells of the gastrointestinal tract may produce transmitters that act on neighboring cells. This process is known as *paracrine signaling* and is typical of cells that produce somatostatin.[2] Paracrine transmitters are secreted locally and cannot diffuse far. They bind to receptors on nearby cells to exert their biologic actions. These actions are limited because they are taken up rapidly by their target cells, destroyed by extracellular enzymes, and adhere to extracellular matrix, all of which limit their ability to act at distant sites. Because paracrine signals act locally, their onset of action is generally rapid and can be terminated abruptly. In contrast, endocrine signaling takes much longer, and termination of signaling requires clearance of hormone from the circulation.

A third form of signaling in the gastrointestinal tract is neurotransmission. The enteric nervous system is a complex and sophisticated array of nerve cells and ganglia that is intimately involved in all aspects of gastrointestinal function. When neurons of the gastrointestinal tract are activated, signals in the form of neurotransmitters are released from the nerve terminals. These synapses deliver neurotransmitters to nerves, muscle cells, epithelial and secretory cells, and other specialized cells of the gastrointestinal tract. Neurotransmitters are critical for the processes of digestion and the coordination of gut motility and secretion.

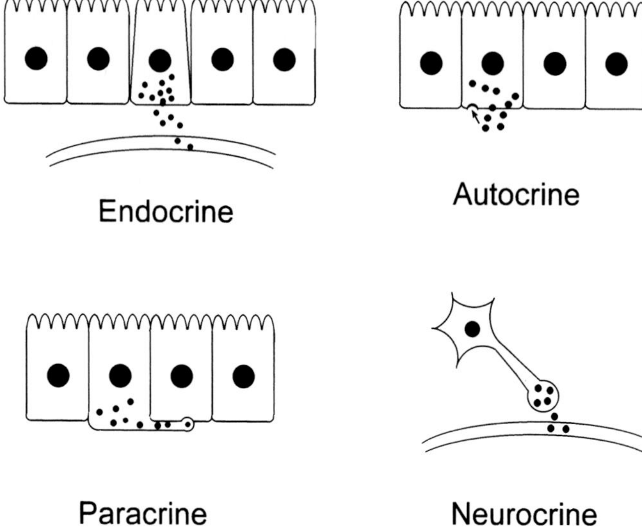

Figure 1–1. Examples of cell-to-cell communication by chemical transmitters in the gastrointestinal tract. Hormones are secreted from endocrine cells into the blood, where they are carried to distant targets. Paracrine cells secrete transmitters into the paracellular space and act locally. Neurons secrete chemical transmitters or peptides into synapses or onto other cell types. Autocrine transmitters bind to receptors on the cell from which they originate.

Many of the same transmitters are produced by endocrine, paracrine, and neural cells. For instance, cholecystokinin (CCK) is produced by typical endocrine cells of the upper small intestine and is secreted into the bloodstream on ingestion of a meal. However, CCK is also abundant in nerves of the gastrointestinal tract and brain. In neural tissue CCK functions as a neurotransmitter, although, when secreted into the blood, CCK is a classic gastrointestinal hormone. This conservation of transmitters allows the same messenger to have different physiologic actions at different locations and is made possible by the manner in which the transmitter is delivered to its target tissues. Endocrine cells secrete many different hormones into the blood, and their action depends on the specificity of the receptor on the target tissues. In contrast, in synaptic transmission the variety of neurotransmitters is more limited, and the specificity of action is dependent on the precise location where the nerves synapse with the target cells. The concentration of signaling molecules can be adjusted quickly because the transmitter can be rapidly metabolized. In the synaptic cleft, transmitters are either rapidly destroyed or taken back up by the secretory neuron. Many peptide transmitters have extremely short half-lives. Concentrations of these peptides can be regulated rapidly by changes in their rate of synthesis, secretion, or catabolism. Therefore, their duration of action may also be short-lived. This principle allows the rapid initiation and termination of signaling. In general, the circulating half-lives of gastrointestinal hormones are short, with most being on the order of several minutes.

Endocrine transmitters of the gastrointestinal tract consist predominantly of peptides such as gastrin and secretin. Paracrine transmitters can be either peptides such as somatostatin or nonpeptides such as histamine that act locally on neighboring cells. Neurotransmitters can be peptides such as vasoactive intestinal polypeptide (VIP) and tachykinins that are secreted; or small molecules such as acetylcholine and epinephrine; or nitric oxide (NO), which simply diffuses across the synaptic cleft. The major transmitters and hormones of the gastrointestinal tract are listed in Table 1–1.

Criteria for establishing whether a candidate transmitter

Table 1–1 | **Hormones and Transmitters of the Gastrointestinal Tract**

Gut Peptides That Function Mainly as Hormones
Gastrin
Glucose-dependent insulinotropic peptide (GIP)
Glucagon and related gene products (GLP-1, GLP-2, glicentin, oxyntomodulin)
Insulin
Motilin
Pancreatic polypeptide
Peptide tyrosine tyrosine (PYY)
Secretin
Gut Peptides That May Function as Hormones, Neuropeptides, or Paracrine Agents
Cholecystokinin (CCK)
Corticotropin-releasing factor (CRF)
Endothelin
Neurotensin
Somatostatin
Gut Peptides That Act Principally as Neuropeptides
Calcitonin gene-related peptide (CGRP)
Dynorphin and related gene products
Enkephalin and related gene products
Galanin
Gastrin-releasing peptide (GRP)
Neuromedin U
Neuropeptide Y
Peptide histidine isoleucine (PHI) or peptide histidine methionine (PHM)
Pituitary adenylate cyclase–activating peptide (PACAP)
Substance P and other tachykinins (neurokinin A, neurokinin B)
Thyrotropin-releasing hormone (TRH)
Vasoactive intestinal peptide (VIP)
Peptides That Act as Growth Factors
Epidermal growth factor
Fibroblast growth factor
Insulin-like factors
Nerve growth factor
Platelet-derived growth factor
Transforming growth factor-β
Vascular endothelial growth factor
Peptides That Act as Inflammatory Mediators
Interferons
Interleukins
Lymphokines
Monokines
Tumor necrosis factor-α
Gut Peptides That Act on Neurons
Cholecystokinin
Gastrin
Motilin
Nonpeptide Transmitters Produced in the Gut
Acetylcholine
Adenosine triphosphate (ATP)
Dopamine
γ-Aminobutyric acid (GABA)
Histamine
5-Hydroxytryptamine (5-HT, serotonin)
Nitric oxide
Norepinephrine
Prostaglandins and other eicosanoids
Newly Recognized Hormones or Neuropeptides
Amylin
Guanylin and uroguanylin
Leptin

functions as a true hormone requires: (1) that the peptide be released into the circulation in response to a physiologic stimulus and (2) that the target tissue response can be reproduced by infusing the transmitter into the blood, thereby producing the same blood levels that occur physiologically. If an identical target tissue response is elicited, the hormonal effect of the transmitter has been proven. These criteria have been satisfied for a limited number of gastrointestinal hormones, including gastrin, CCK, secretin, motilin, and gastric inhibitory peptide.

Somatostatin is the prototype of a paracrine transmitter. However, depending on its location, somatostatin may also exert endocrine and neural actions. For example, intestinal somatostatin is released into the local circulation on ingestion of fat and acts on the stomach as an enterogastrone to inhibit gastric acid secretion.

Some cells release messengers locally and possess cell surface receptors for the same messengers, thus enabling those cells to respond to their own secreted products. This mode of transmission, known as *autocrine signaling,* has been demonstrated for several growth factors.

NEURAL REGULATION OF THE GASTROINTESTINAL TRACT

The enteric nervous system plays an integral role in the regulation of gut mucosal and motor function. It is organized into two major plexuses[3] (Fig. 1–2). The myenteric plexus lies between the external longitudinal and internal circular muscle layers. The submucosal plexus lies between the circular muscle layer and the mucosa. Although the enteric nervous system receives input from the central and autonomic nervous systems, it can function independently. Nerves of the myenteric plexus project fibers primarily to the smooth muscle of the gut, with only a few axons extending to the submucosal plexus. Most of the fibers of the submucosal plexus project into the mucosa and the submucosal and myenteric plexuses. Various peptide and nonpeptide neurotransmitters are found in the enteric nervous system. Recent studies using immunohistochemical staining have localized neurotransmitters to specific neurons in the gastrointestinal tract. γ-Aminobutyric acid is found primarily in the myenteric plexus and is involved in regulating smooth muscle contraction. Serotonin is found within the plexus and functions as an interneuron transmitter. Adrenergic neurons originate in ganglia of the autonomic nervous system and synapse with enteric neurons. Peptides such as neuropeptide Y (NPY) are often secreted from the same adrenergic neurons and generally exert inhibitory effects such as vasoconstriction.[4] Other adrenergic neurons containing somatostatin project to the submucosal plexus, where they inhibit intestinal secretion. Coexistence of peptides and neurotransmitters in the same neurons is not unusual; in fact, the interplay among transmitters is critical for coordinated neural regulation.[5] For example, the peptides VIP and peptide histidine isoleucine (PHI) are commonly found together, as are the tachykinins substance P and substance K, where they have complementary effects.[6]

Somatostatin is found in interneurons that project caudally. The inhibitory action of somatostatin is consistent with a role in causing muscle relaxation in advance of a peristaltic wave. The abundance of VIP in the myenteric plexus also suggests that its inhibitory actions are important for smooth muscle relaxation in gut motility. VIP neurons that project from the submucosal plexus to the mucosa most likely stimulate intestinal fluid secretion. Other neurons that innervate the mucosa contain acetylcholine. Mucosal cells of the intestine contain receptors for both VIP and acetylcholine, allowing these transmitters to exert synergistic effects, because VIP increases intracellular cyclic adenosine monophosphate (cAMP) levels and acetylcholine increases intracellular calcium in the target cell.

Bipolar neurons that project to the mucosa and myenteric plexus act as sensory neurons and often contain substance P and acetylcholine as neurotransmitters. These neurons participate in pain pathways and modulate inflammation.

The ability of hormones to act on nerves locally within the submucosa of the intestine and affect more distant sites on nerves such as the vagus expands the potential organs that may be regulated by gut hormones.[7] Chemical and mechanical stimuli cause the release of hormones from endocrine cells of the intestinal mucosa. These interactions initiate a wide variety of secretomotor responses, many of which

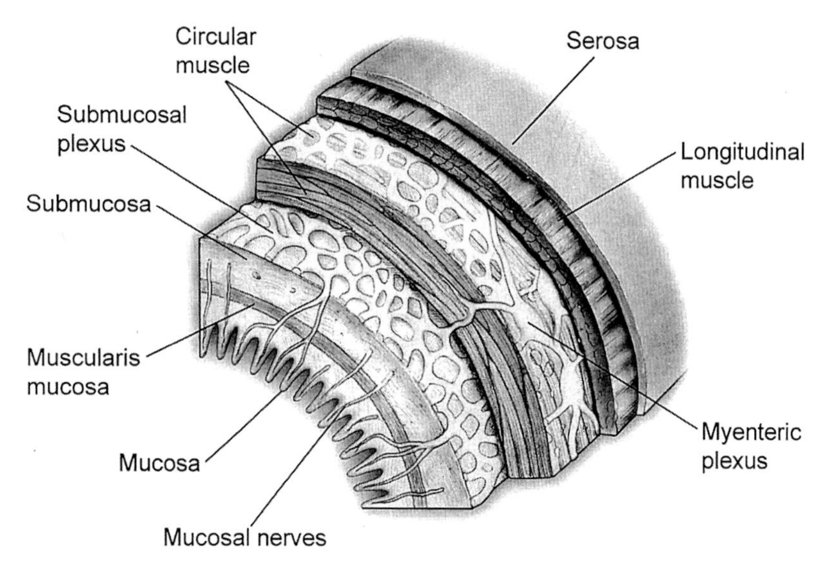

Figure 1–2. Organization of the enteric nervous system. The enteric nervous system is composed of two major plexi—one submucosal and one located between the circular and longitudinal smooth muscle layers. These neurons receive and coordinate neural transmission from the gut and central nervous system.

are mediated by enteric neurons. Secretomotor circuits consist of intrinsic primary afferent neurons with nerve endings in the mucosa and extension through the myenteric and submucosal plexuses. This circuitry allows nerves to stimulate mucosal cells to secrete fluid and electrolytes and at the same time stimulate muscle contraction. The same motor neurons also have axons that supply arterioles and can initiate vasodilator reflexes.

Extrinsic primary afferent neurons can be either of the vagus, with somal bodies in the nodose ganglia and axons that reach the gut through the vagus nerve, or of the spinal nerves of the thoracic and lumbar regions, whose cell bodies lie in the dorsal root ganglia. Information conducted by extrinsic primary afferent neurons includes pain, heat, and sensations of fullness or emptiness. These neurons are also targets for hormones. For example, the satiety effect of CCK in the bloodstream is mediated through the vagus nerve.[8] Specific CCK receptors have been identified on the vagus, and blockade of these receptors abolishes the satiation induced by peripheral CCK.

Endocrine, paracrine, and neural transmitters existing within the lamina propria modulate effects on the gut immune system.[7] Lymphocytes, macrophages, mast cells, neutrophils, and eosinophils are potential targets for endocrine and neural transmitters and participate in the inflammatory cascade. Moreover, inflammatory mediators can act directly on enteric nerves. Serotonin released from endocrine cells is involved in intestinal anaphylaxis and stimulates vagal afferent fibers that possess the 5-hydroxytryptamine 3 (5-HT_3) receptor.

PEPTIDE HORMONES OF THE GASTROINTESTINAL TRACT

Synthesis, Post-translational Modification, and Secretion

The expression of peptides is regulated at the level of the gene that resides on defined regions of specific chromosomes. The genes for most of the known gastrointestinal peptides have now been identified. Specific gene regulatory elements determine if and when a protein is produced and the particular cell in which it will be expressed. Gut hormone gene expression is generally linked to peptide production and regulated according to the physiologic needs of the organism. For example, the production of a hormone may increase when gut endocrine cells are stimulated by food, changes in intraluminal pH, exposure to releasing factors, or other transmitters or hormones. These factors may simultaneously stimulate hormone secretion and increase gene expression. Ultimately, hormones are secreted into the circulation, where they are able to bind to receptors on target tissues. Once a biologic response is elicited, signals may then be sent to the endocrine cell to "turn off" hormone secretion. This negative feedback mechanism is common to many physiologic systems and avoids excess production and secretion of hormone.

All gastrointestinal peptides are synthesized via gene transcription of DNA into messenger RNA (mRNA) and subsequent translation of mRNA into precursor proteins known as *preprohormones*. Peptides that are to be secreted contain a signal sequence that directs the transcript to the endoplasmic reticulum, where the signal sequence is cleaved and the prepro-peptide product is prepared for structural modifications.[9, 10] These precursors undergo intracellular processing and are transported to the Golgi apparatus and packaged in secretory granules. Further modifications in peptide structure may occur within the Golgi apparatus (e.g., sulfation) that is important for the bioactivity of many peptide hormones such as CCK. Secretory granules may be targeted for immediate release or stored in close proximity to the plasma membrane for release following appropriate cell stimulation. When gastrointestinal endocrine cells are stimulated, mature hormone is secreted into the paracellular space and is taken up into the bloodstream. For many hormones, such as gastrin and CCK, multiple molecular forms exist in blood and tissues. Although there is only a single gene for these peptides, the different molecular forms result from differences in pretranslational or post-translational processing (Fig. 1–3). A common mechanism of pretranslational processing includes alternative splicing of mRNA, which generates unique peptides from the same gene. Post-translational changes include cleavage of precursor molecules.

Enzymatic cleavage of the signal peptide produces a prohormone. Other post-translational features that result in mature gastrointestinal peptides include peptide cleavage to smaller forms (e.g., somatostatin), amidation of the carboxyl terminus (e.g., gastrin), and sulfation of tyrosine residues (e.g., CCK). These processing steps are usually critical for biologic activity of the hormone.[9] For example, sulfated CCK is 100-fold more potent than its unsulfated form. The vast biochemical complexity of gastroenteropancreatic hormones is evident in the different tissues that secrete these peptides. Gastrointestinal hormones are secreted from endocrine as well as nervous tissue. The distinct tissue involved often determines the processing steps for production of hormone. Many hormone genes are capable of manufacturing alternatively spliced mRNAs or proteins that undergo different post-translational processing and ultimately produce hormones of different sizes. These modifications are important

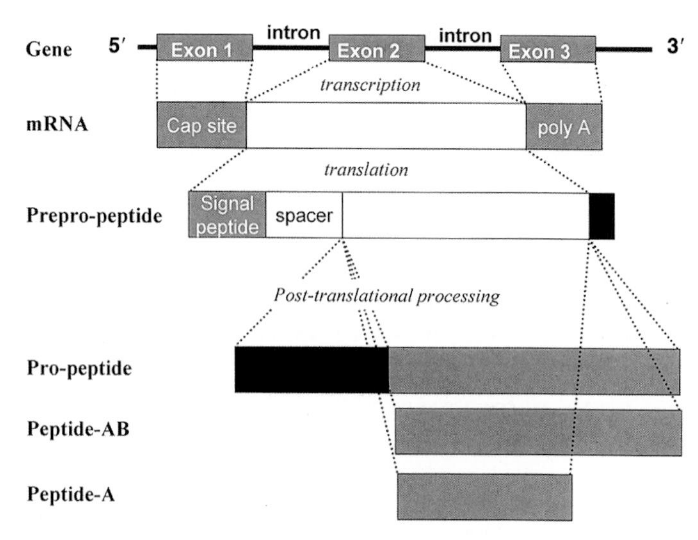

Figure 1–3. Schematic representation of the production of gastrointestinal peptides. The genetic information is transcribed into mRNA, which is translated to a prepro-peptide. Subsequent enzymatic cleavage produces peptides of various lengths.

for receptor binding, signal transduction, and consequent cellular responses.[11]

Recently, it has become possible to express human genes in other species. By introducing specific hormone-producing genes into pigs or sheep, human hormones have been produced for medicinal use.[12, 13] With the rapid sequencing of the human genome, it is likely that novel methods of gene expression will expand the therapeutic use of human proteins.[13] Moreover, drugs are being developed that inhibit the transcription of DNA into mRNA or that block the gene elements responsible for turning on specific hormone production (antisense oligonucleotides).[14–16] This technology is based on the principle that nucleotide sequences bind to critical DNA regions and prevent transcription into mRNA. Similarly, oligonucleotides can be made to interact with mRNA and alter (or inhibit) translation of a protein product. These principles may be applicable to the treatment of the growing list of diseases that result from aberrant protein processing.[17, 18]

Gastrin

As discussed in more detail in Chapter 38, gastrin is the major hormonal regulator of gastric acid secretion.[19] Its discovery at the turn of the 20th century was based on its profound effect on gastric acid secretion. The peptide was isolated and characterized in 1964 and has subsequently been found to have growth-promoting effects on gastric mucosa and possibly some cancers.[20, 21]

Human gastrin is the product of a single gene located on chromosome 17. The active hormone is generated from a precursor peptide called *preprogastrin*. Human preprogastrin contains 101 amino acids (AAs), including a signal peptide (21 AA), spacer sequence (37 AA), gastrin component (34 AA), and a 9-AA extension segment at the carboxyl terminus. The enzymatic processing of preprogastrin produces all the known physiologically active forms of gastrin.

Preprogastrin is processed into progastrin and gastrin peptide fragments of various sizes by sequential enzymatic cleavage.

The two major forms of gastrin are G_{34} and G_{17}, although smaller forms exist. The common feature of all gastrins is an amidated tetrapeptide (Try-Met-Asp-Phe-NH_2) carboxyl terminus, which imparts full biologic activity. Modification by sulfation at tyrosine residues produces alternative gastrin forms of equal biologic potency.

Most gastrin is produced in endocrine cells of the gastric antrum.[22] Much smaller amounts of gastrin are produced in other regions of the gastrointestinal tract, including the proximal stomach, duodenum, jejunum, ileum, and pancreas. Gastrin has also been found outside the gastrointestinal tract, including in the brain, adrenal gland, respiratory tract, and reproductive organs, although its biologic role in these sites is unknown.

The receptors for gastrin and CCK are related and constitute the so-called gastrin/CCK receptor family. The CCK-A (alimentary) and CCK-B (brain) receptor complementary DNAs were cloned from pancreas and brain, respectively, after which it was recognized that the CCK-B receptor was identical to the gastrin receptor of the stomach.[23]

The CCK-A receptor is present in the pancreas, in most species, and gallbladder and has a 1000-fold higher affinity for CCK than for gastrin. The CCK-A and the CCK-B/gastrin receptors have higher than 50% sequence homology and respond differentially to various receptor antagonists and to gastrin.

Gastrin is released from specialized endocrine cells (G cells) into the circulation in response to a meal. The specific components of a meal that stimulate gastrin release include protein, peptides, and AAs. Gastrin release is profoundly influenced by the pH of the stomach. Fasting and increased gastric acidity inhibit gastrin release, whereas a high gastric pH is a strong stimulus for its secretion.

Hypergastrinemia occurs in pathologic states that are associated with decreased acid production, such as atrophic gastritis. Serum gastrin levels can also become greatly elevated in patients on prolonged acid-suppressive medications, such as histamine receptor antagonists and proton pump inhibitors. Hypergastrinemia in these conditions is due to stimulation of gastrin production by the alkaline pH environment. Another important but far less common cause of hypergastrinemia is a gastrin-producing tumor, also known as Zollinger-Ellison syndrome (see Chapter 41).

The gastrin analog, pentagastrin, has been used clinically to stimulate histamine and gastric acid secretion in diagnostic tests of acid secretory capacity (see Chapter 38).

Cholecystokinin

Cholecystokinin (CCK) is a peptide transmitter produced by I cells of the small intestine and is secreted into the blood on ingestion of a meal.[24] Circulating CCK binds to specific CCK-A receptors on the gallbladder, pancreas, smooth muscle, and peripheral nerves to stimulate gallbladder contraction and pancreatic secretion, regulate gastric emptying and bowel motility, and induce satiety.[25] These effects serve to coordinate the ingestion, digestion, and absorption of dietary nutrients. Ingested fat and protein are the major food components that stimulate CCK release.

CCK was originally identified as a 33-AA peptide. However, since its discovery larger and smaller forms of CCK have been isolated from blood, intestine, and brain. All forms of CCK are produced from a single gene by post-translational processing of a preprohormone. Forms of CCK ranging in size from CCK-58 to CCK-8 have similar biologic activities.[26]

CCK is the major hormonal regulator of gallbladder contraction.[26] It also plays an important role in regulating meal-stimulated pancreatic secretion (see Chapters 46 and 53). In many species this latter effect is mediated directly through receptors on pancreatic acinar cells, but in humans, where CCK-A receptors are less abundant, CCK appears to stimulate pancreatic secretion indirectly through enteropancreatic neurons that possess CCK-A receptors. In some species CCK has trophic effects on the pancreas, although its potential role in human pancreatic neoplasia is speculative. CCK has also been shown to delay gastric emptying.[27] This action may be important in coordinating the delivery of food from the stomach to the intestine. CCK has been proposed as a major mediator of satiety and food intake, an effect that is particularly noticeable when food is in the stomach or intestine.

Clinically, CCK has been used together with secretin to stimulate pancreatic secretion for pancreatic function testing. It is also used radiographically or by nuclear medicine physicians to evaluate gallbladder contractility. There are no known diseases of CCK excess. Low CCK levels have been reported in bulimia nervosa and in individuals with celiac disease who have reduced intestinal mucosal surface area.[28, 29] Elevated levels of CCK have been reported in some patients with chronic pancreatitis, presumably owing to reduced pancreatic enzyme secretion and interruption of negative feedback regulation of CCK release.[30]

Secretin

The first hormone, secretin, was discovered when it was observed that intestinal extracts, when injected intravenously into dogs, caused pancreatic secretion.[31] This biologic action of secretin led to a search for other chemical substances that, when released from one tissue, could excite or stimulate organ function in a different location. The Greek word *hormone,* meaning "arise to activity," was used to designate these chemical messengers. It is now known that secretin is released by acid in the duodenum and stimulates pancreatic fluid and bicarbonate secretion, leading to neutralization of acidic chyme in the intestine. Secretin also inhibits gastric acid secretion and intestinal motility.

Despite knowledge of its physiologic activity, it took more than 60 years for the chemical nature of secretin to be identified.[32] Human secretin is a 27 AA peptide and, similar to many other gastrointestinal peptides, is amidated at the C-terminus. It is the founding member of the secretin/glucagon/VIP family of structurally related gastrointestinal hormones. Secretin is selectively expressed in specialized enteroendocrine cells of the small intestine called *S cells.*[33]

The secretin receptor is a member of a large family of G protein–coupled receptors (GPCRs), within which the secretin/glucagon family is structurally unique. This family consists of receptors for secretin, glucagon, calcitonin, parathyroid hormone, pituitary adenylate cyclase–activating peptide (PACAP), vasoactive intestinal polypeptide (VIP), and others. These receptors lack structural signature sequences present in the rhodopsin/β-adrenergic receptor family, which appear to be important in receptor coupling to G proteins.

One of the major physiologic actions of secretin is stimulation of pancreatic fluid and bicarbonate secretion (see Chapter 46). Pancreatic bicarbonate, on reaching the duodenum, neutralizes gastric acid and raises the duodenal pH, thereby "turning off" secretin release.[34] This series of events provides a negative feedback mechanism for regulating secretin release. It has been suggested that acid-stimulated secretin release is regulated by an endogenous intestinal secretin-releasing factor.[35] This peptide stimulates secretin release from S cells until the flow of pancreatic proteases is sufficient to degrade the releasing factor and terminate secretin release.

Although the primary action of secretin is to produce pancreatic fluid and bicarbonate secretion,[36] it is also an enterogastrone, a substance that is released when fat is present in the gastrointestinal lumen and that inhibits gastric acid secretion. In physiologic concentrations, secretin inhibits gastrin release, gastric acid secretion, and gastric motility.[37]

The most common clinical application of secretin is in the diagnosis of gastrin-secreting tumors,[38, 39] as discussed in Chapter 41.

Vasoactive Intestinal Polypeptide

Vasoactive intestinal polypeptide (VIP) is a neuromodulator that has broad significance in intestinal physiology. VIP is a potent vasodilator that increases blood flow in the gastrointestinal tract and causes smooth muscle relaxation and epithelial cell secretion.[40–42] As a chemical messenger, VIP is released from nerve terminals and acts locally on cells bearing VIP receptors. VIP belongs to a family of gastrointestinal peptides including secretin and glucagon that are structurally related. The VIP receptor is a member of class II GPCRs.

Like other gastrointestinal peptides, VIP is synthesized as a precursor molecule that is then cleaved to the active peptide of 28 AAs.[43] VIP is expressed primarily in neurons of the peripheral/enteric and central nervous systems. VIP is released along with other peptides, including primarily PHI and/or peptide histidine methionine (see Table 1–1).[44, 45]

VIP is an important neurotransmitter throughout the central and peripheral nervous systems.[46] Because of its wide distribution, VIP has effects on many organ systems.[47] Most notably, VIP stimulates gastrointestinal epithelial secretion[48, 49] and absorption[50] and promotes fluid and bicarbonate secretion from bile duct cholangiocytes.[51]

VIP, along with nitric oxide (NO), is a primary component of nonadrenergic, noncholinergic nerve transmission in the gut.[52] Gastrointestinal smooth muscle exhibits a basal tone, or sustained tension due to rhythmic depolarizations of the smooth muscle membrane potential. VIP serves as an inhibitory transmitter of this rhythmic activity, causing membrane hyperpolarization and subsequent relaxation of gastrointestinal smooth muscle. VIP is an important neuromodulator in sphincters of the gastrointestinal tract, including the lower esophageal sphincter and sphincter of Oddi. In certain pathologic conditions such as achalasia and Hirschsprung's disease, the lack of VIP innervation is believed to play a major role in defective esophageal relaxation and bowel dysmotility, respectively.[53, 54]

Unlike gastrointestinal endocrine cells that line the mucosa of the gut, VIP is produced and released from neurons, and it is likely that most measurable VIP in serum is of neuronal origin.[55] Normally, serum VIP levels are low and do not appreciably change with a meal. However, in pancreatic cholera, also known as watery diarrhea–hypokalemia–achlorhydria or Verner-Morrison syndrome,[56] VIP levels can be extraordinarily high.[48, 49] VIP-secreting tumors usually produce a voluminous diarrhea,[49, 57] as discussed in Chapter 51.

Glucagon

Glucagon is synthesized and released from pancreatic α cells and from cells of the ileum and colon (L cells). Pancreatic glucagon is a 29 AA peptide that regulates glucose homeostasis via gluconeogenesis, glycogenolysis, and lipolysis and is counter-regulatory to insulin. The gene for glucagon encodes not only preproglucagon but also glucagon-like peptides (GLPs). This precursor peptide consists of a signal peptide, a glucagon-related polypeptide, glucagon, and GLP-1 and GLP-2. Tissue-specific peptide processing occurs through prohormone convertases that produce glucagon in the pancreas and GLP-1 and GLP-2 in the intestinal L cell[58] (Fig. 1–4).

Glucagon is released from the pancreas in response to a meal and binds to receptors on skeletal muscle and the liver to exert its glucoregulatory effects. The receptors for glucagon and GLP-1 and GLP-2 are members of class II GPCRs.

Whereas glucagon and GLP-1 have long been known to participate in glucose homeostasis,[59] the physiology of this family of peptide products has expanded recently with the demonstration that GLP-2 is an intestinal growth factor.[60] GLP-2 may have therapeutic implications in the maintenance of the gastrointestinal mucosal mass and the reversal of villus atrophy.[61]

Pancreatic Polypeptide Family

Originally isolated in 1968 during the preparation of insulin, pancreatic polypeptide (PP) is the founding member of the PP family.[62, 63] The PP family of peptides includes neuropeptide Y (NPY) and peptide YY (PYY), which were discovered owing to the presence of a C-terminal tyrosine amide.[64–66] PP is stored and secreted from specialized pancreatic endocrine cells (PP cells[67]), whereas NPY is a principal neurotransmitter found in the central and peripheral nervous systems.[68–70] PYY has been localized to enteroendocrine cells throughout the gastrointestinal tract.[71]

The PP/PYY/NPY family of peptides functions as endocrine, paracrine, and neurocrine transmitters in the regulation of a number of functions that result from a multitude of receptor subtypes. There are at least five receptors identified.[72–76] PP inhibits pancreatic exocrine secretion[77] and inhibits gallbladder contraction and gut motility.[78, 79] PYY inhibits vagally stimulated gastric acid secretion and other motor and secretory functions.[80–82] NPY is one of the most abundant peptides in the central nervous system and is a potent stimulant of food intake.[83] Peripherally, NPY affects vascular and gastrointestinal smooth muscle function.[78]

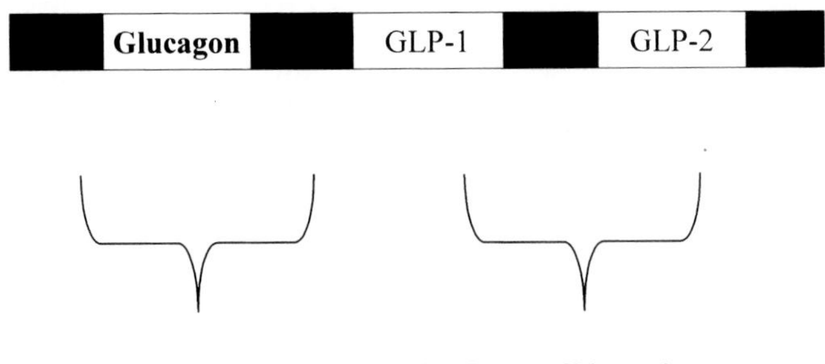

Figure 1–4. Different post-translational processing of glucagon occurs in the pancreas and small intestine. The glucagon gene transcript is transcribed and translated into a preprohormone (shown here) capable of producing glucagon, glycolipoprotein (GLP)-1, and GLP-2. However, only glucagon is produced in the pancreas owing to specific processing. In the small intestine, GLP-1 and GLP-2 are the primary products.

Substance P and the Tachykinins

Substance P belongs to the tachykinin family of peptides, which includes substance P, neurokinin A, and neurokinin B. The tachykinins are found throughout the peripheral and central nervous systems,[84] and they participate in neuropathic inflammation.[85] Tachykinins, as a group, are encoded by two genes that produce preprotachykinin A and preprotachykinin B. Common to both is a well-conserved C-terminal pentapeptide. Transcriptional and translational processing produce substance P, neurokinin A, and/or neurokinin B, which are regulated in large part by alternative splicing. These peptides function primarily as neuropeptides. Substance P is a neurotransmitter of primary sensory afferent neurons and binds to specific receptors in lamina I of the spinal cord.[86] Three receptors for this family of peptides have been identified (NK-1, NK-2, and NK-3).[87] Substance P is the primary ligand for the NK-1 receptor, neurokinin A for the NK-2, and neurokinin B for the NK-3. However, all peptides can bind and signal through all three receptor subtypes.

Substance P has been implicated as a primary mediator of neurogenic inflammation.[88] In the intestine, *Clostridium difficile*–initiated experimental colitis results from toxin-induced release of substance P and consequent activation of the NK-1 receptor.[89] These inflammatory sequelae can be blocked by substance P receptor antagonists. Substance P receptors are more abundant in the intestine of patients with ulcerative colitis and Crohn's disease.[90]

OTHER CHEMICAL MESSENGERS OF THE GASTROINTESTINAL TRACT

The enteric nervous system, through intrinsic and extrinsic neural circuits, controls gastrointestinal function. This control is mediated by a variety of chemical messengers, including motor and sensory pathways of the sympathetic and parasympathetic nervous systems. The parasympathetic preganglionic input is provided by cholinergic neurons and elicits excitatory effects on gastrointestinal motility via nicotinic and muscarinic receptors, whereas the sympathetic input occurs by postganglionic adrenergic neurons.

Acetylcholine

Acetylcholine is synthesized in cholinergic neurons and is the principal regulator of gastrointestinal motility as well as pancreatic secretion. Acetylcholine is stored in nerve terminals and released by nerve depolarization. Released acetylcholine is then able to bind to postsynaptic muscarinic and/or nicotinic receptors. Nicotinic acetylcholine receptors belong to a family of ligand-gated ion channels and are homopentamers or heteropentamers comprised of α, β, γ, δ, and ε subunits.[91] The α subunit is believed to be the mediator of postsynaptic membrane depolarization following acetylcholine receptor binding. Muscarinic receptors belong to the heptahelical GPCR family. There are five known muscarinic cholinergic receptors (M_1 to M_5). Muscarinic receptors can be further classified based on receptor signal transduction, with M_1, M_3, and M_5 stimulating adenylate cyclase and M_2 and M_4 inhibiting this enzyme.

Acetylcholine is degraded by the enzyme acetylcholinesterase, and the products may be recycled through high-affinity transporters on the nerve terminal.

Catecholamines

The primary catecholamine neurotransmitters of the enteric nervous system include norepinephrine and dopamine. Norepinephrine is synthesized from tyrosine and released from postganglionic sympathetic nerve terminals that innervate enteric ganglia and blood vessels. Tyrosine is converted to dopa by tyrosine hydroxylase. Dopa is initially converted into dopamine by dopa decarboxylase and packaged into secretory granules. Norepinephrine is formed from dopamine by the action of dopamine β-hydroxylase within the secretory granule. After an appropriate stimulus, norepinephrine-containing secretory granules are released from nerve terminals and bind to adrenergic receptors.

Adrenergic receptors are G protein coupled, have seven typical membrane-spanning domains, and are of two basic types: α and β. α-Adrenergic receptors are further classified into $\alpha 1_A$, $\alpha 1_B$, $\alpha 2_A$, $\alpha 2_B$, $\alpha 2_C$, and $\alpha 2_D$. Similarly, β receptors include β_1, β_2, and β_3. Adrenergic receptors are known to signal through a variety of G proteins, resulting in stimulation or inhibition of adenylate cyclase and other effector systems. Norepinephrine signaling is terminated by intracellular monoamine oxidase or by rapid reuptake by an amine transporter. The actions of adrenergic receptor stimulation regulate smooth muscle contraction, intestinal blood flow, and gastrointestinal secretion.

Dopamine is an important mediator of gastrointestinal secretion, absorption, and motility and is the predominant catecholamine neurotransmitter of the central and peripheral nervous systems. In the central nervous system, dopamine regulates food intake, emotions, and endocrine responses, and peripherally, it controls hormone secretion, vascular tone, and gastrointestinal motility. Characterization of dopamine in the gastrointestinal tract has been challenging for several reasons. First, dopamine can produce inhibitory and excitatory effects on gastrointestinal motility.[92] Generally, the excitatory response, which is mediated by presynaptic receptors, occurs at a lower agonist concentration than the inhibitory effect that is mediated by postsynaptic receptors. Second, localization of dopamine receptors has been hampered by identification of dopamine receptors in locations that appear to be species specific.[93, 94] Finally, studies of dopamine in gastrointestinal tract motility have often used pharmacologic amounts of this agonist. Therefore, interpretation of results has been confounded by the ability of dopamine to activate adrenergic receptors at high doses.[92]

Classically, dopamine was thought to act via two distinct receptor subtypes: type 1 and type 2. Molecular cloning has now demonstrated five dopamine receptor subtypes, each with a unique molecular structure and gene locus.[95] Dopamine receptors are integral membrane GPCRs, and each receptor subtype has a specific pharmacologic profile when exposed to agonists and antagonists. After release from the nerve terminal, dopamine is cleared from the synaptic cleft by a specific dopamine transporter.

Serotonin

Serotonin has long been known to play a role in gastrointestinal neurotransmission.[96] The gastrointestinal tract contains more than 95% of the total body serotonin, and serotonin is important in a variety of processes, including nausea, emesis, epithelial secretion, and bowel motility. Serotonin is synthesized from tryptophan, an essential AA, and is converted to its active form in nerve terminals. Serotonin is inactivated in the synaptic cleft by reuptake via a serotonin-specific transporter. Most plasma serotonin is derived from the gut, where it is found in mucosal enterochromaffin cells and the enteric nervous system. Serotonin mediates its effects by binding to a specific receptor. There are seven different serotonin receptor subtypes found on enteric neurons, enterochromaffin cells, and gastrointestinal smooth muscle (5-HT_1 to 5-HT_7). Through these receptors serotonin regulates intestinal secretion, absorption, and motility.[97]

Serotonin, and its receptor, has been implicated in the pathogenesis of irritable bowel syndrome, as well as constipation and diarrhea.[98] The myenteric plexus contains serotonic interneurons that project to the submucosal plexus as well as ganglia extrinsic to the bowel wall. Extrinsic neurons activated by serotonin participate in bowel sensation and may be responsible for abdominal pain, nausea, and symptoms associated with irritable bowel syndrome. Intrinsic neurons activated by serotonin are primary components of the peristaltic and secretory reflexes responsible for normal gastrointestinal function.[96]

Characterization of specific serotonin receptor subtypes has led to the development of selective agonists and antagonists for the treatment of gastrointestinal disorders such as irritable bowel syndrome and chronic constipation and diarrhea. For example, 5-HT_3 receptor antagonists may be useful in diarrhea-predominant irritable bowel syndrome, and the 5-HT_4 receptor agonist has prokinetic effects and may be useful in constipation or other motility disorders.[99, 100]

Histamine

In the gastrointestinal tract, histamine is best known for its central role in regulating gastric acid secretion (see Chapter 38) and intestinal motility. Histamine is produced by enterochromaffin-like cells of the stomach and intestine as well as enteric nerves. Histamine is synthesized from L-histidine by histidine decarboxylase and activates three GPCR subtypes. H_1 receptors are found on smooth muscle and vascular endothelial cells and result in activation of phospholipase C (PLC). As such, the H_1 receptor mediates many of the allergic responses induced by histamine. H_2 receptors are present on gastric parietal cells, smooth muscle, and cardiac myocytes. H_2 receptor binding stimulates Gs and activates adenylate cyclase. H_3 receptors are present in the central nervous system and gastrointestinal tract endochromaffin cells. These receptors signal through Gi and inhibit adenylate cyclase.[101] Histamine can also interact with the *N*-methyl-D-aspartate (NMDA) receptor and enhance activity of NMDA-bearing neurons independent of the three known histamine receptor subtypes.

Unlike other neurotransmitters, there is no known transporter responsible for termination of histamine's action. However, histamine is metabolized to telemethylhistamine by histamine *N*-methyltransferase, and is then degraded to telemethylimidazoleacetic acid by monoamine oxidase B and an aldehyde dehydrogenase.

Nitric Oxide

Although smooth muscle physiologists have long known of an "endothelial-derived relaxing factor" responsible for vasodilation, it took many years for the chemical nature of this substance to be identified as nitric oxide (NO). NO is a unique chemical messenger produced with citrulline from L-arginine and oxygen by the enzyme nitric oxide synthase (NOS).[102] Three types of NOS are known. Types I and III are also know as *endothelial NOS* and *neuronal NOS* and are constitutively active. Small changes in NOS activity can occur through elevations in intracellular calcium. The inducible form of NOS (type II) is apparent only when cells become activated by specific cytokines and inflammation. This form of NOS is capable of producing large amounts of NO and is calcium independent. NOS is often colocalized with VIP and PACAP in neurons of the enteric nervous system.[103]

NO, being an unstable gas, has a relatively short half-life. Unlike most neurotransmitters and hormones, NO does not act via a membrane-bound receptor. Instead, NO readily diffuses into adjacent cells to directly activate guanylate cyclase. NO activity is terminated by oxidation to nitrate and nitrite. The role of NO in gastrointestinal physiology includes stimulation of epithelial secretion, vasodilation, and mucosal defense.[104]

Adenosine

Adenosine is an endogenous nucleoside that acts through any of four GPCR subtypes.[105, 106] Adenosine causes relaxation of intestinal smooth muscle and stimulates intestinal secretion.[105] Adenosine can also cause peripheral vasodilation and activation of nociceptors that participate in pain neural pathways.

Cytokines

Cytokines are a group of polypeptides produced by a variety of immunomodulatory cells and are involved in cell proliferation, immunity, and inflammation. Cytokines are induced by specific stimuli, such as toxins produced by pathogens, and often elicit a complex variety of other cellular mediators to eradicate the foreign substance. Cytokines may be categorized as interleukins (ILs), tumor necrosis factors (TNFs), lymphotoxins, interferons, colony-stimulating factors (CSFs), and others.[107] Interleukins can be further subtyped into 17 separate substances: IL-1 to IL-17. There are two TNFs: TNF-α and TNF-β, which are also known as lymphotoxin-α. Interferons are produced during viral or bacterial infection and come in two varieties: interferon-α (also known as leukocyte-derived interferon or interferon-β) and interferon-γ. Interferon-α is produced by T lymphocytes and is used clinically in the treatment of viral hepatitis (see Chapter 68). The major CSFs are granulocyte/mononuclear phagocyte-CSF, mononuclear phagocyte-CSF, and granulocyte-CSF. These agents are used in chemotherapy-induced neutropenia and marrow support after bone marrow transplantation. Chemokines initiate and propagate inflammation and are of two groups: CXC (α chemokines) and CC (β chemokines). Other cytokines, such as transforming growth factor (TGF)-β and platelet-derived growth factor (PDGF), have proliferative effects.

SIGNAL TRANSDUCTION

Cells live in a constantly changing milieu. The structure and biochemical nature of this environment are dynamic, and for normal cellular function to proceed in a manner appropriate for the benefit of the organism, cells must be able to access this changing information. The biochemical mediators of this information are cell surface receptors and transmitters. Receptors transduce signals from the extracellular space to the intracellular compartment. Each step in the process from receptor activation to receptor desensitization, internalization, and resensitization represents a potential regulatory checkpoint and possible target for therapeutic intervention. Cell surface receptors include GPCRs, as well as ion channels and enzyme-linked receptors.

G Protein–Coupled Receptors

G protein–coupled receptors (GPCRs) are seven membrane-spanning domain proteins associated with a heterotrimeric G protein. The membrane regions consist of α-helical domains with a conserved structural motif.[108] GPCRs are classified by their structure into three distinct classes (Table 1–2). Class I, the largest, contains the receptors for rhodopsin, catecholamines, many peptide hormones, neuropeptides, and glycoproteins. These receptors share 55% to 65% sequence homology and often the presence of a "D-R-Y" (Asp-Arg-Try sequence) motif in the second intracellular loop. Class II receptors include the secretin/glucagon/VIP family. This group is distinct from class I receptors, sharing only approximately 12% sequence homology with class I and the absence of the D-R-Y motif. Class III GPCRs contain the metabotrophic receptors (calcium-sensing and glutamate receptors).

GPCRs contain an extracellular amino terminus and an

Table 1–2 | **Classification of G Protein–Coupled Receptors**

Class I
Rhodopsin, catecholamines, acetylcholine, serotonin, angiotensin, gastrin, cholecystokinin, neuropeptide Y, substance P, endothelin, opioid, chemokine, histamine, vasopressin
Class II
Secretin, calcitonin, parathyroid hormone, vasoactive intestinal polypeptide, glucagon, glucagon-like peptide 1, pituitary adenylate cyclase–activating peptide
Class III
Glutamate-metabotrophic receptors, calcium receptors

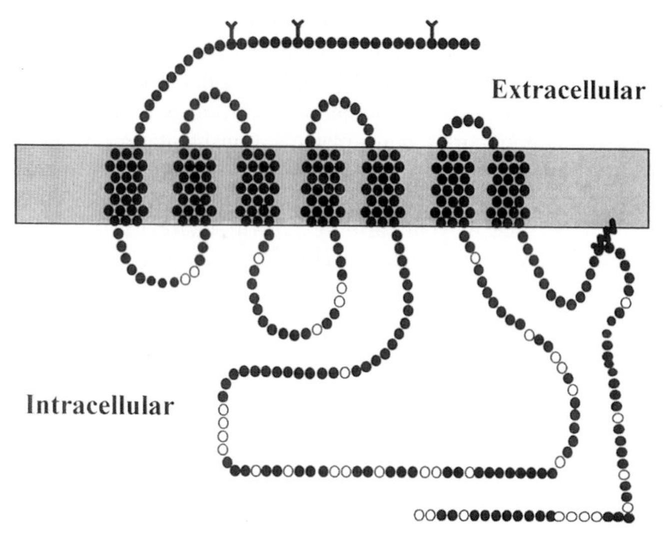

Figure 1–5. Molecular structure of a typical heptahelical G protein–coupled receptor. The amino terminus is extracellular and of variable length. It often contains *N*-linked glycosylation sites (Y) important in ligand binding. There are seven membrane-spanning domains and intracellular loops that contain sites for G protein binding and possible phosphorylation residues (*open circles*).

intracellular carboxyl terminus (Fig. 1–5). When stimulated by the appropriate chemical messenger, the GPCR undergoes a conformational change and couples to a specific G protein. Recently, the first crystal structure of a GPCR has been elucidated.[109] The three-dimensional structure of the rhodopsin receptor reveals a highly organized heptahelical transmembrane component with a portion of the C-terminus perpendicular to the seventh membrane-spanning domain.

G Proteins

G proteins are molecular intermediaries that initiate the intracellular communication process upon ligand binding to its GPCR[110, 111] (Fig. 1–6). G proteins are composed of three

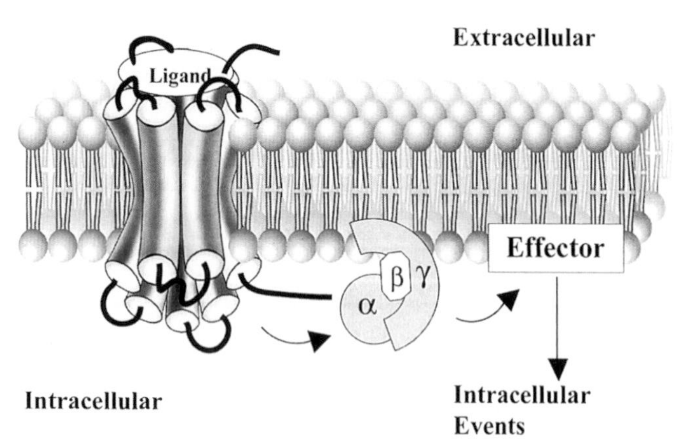

Figure 1–6. Hormones (ligands) bind to specific G protein–coupled receptors at a unique location within the receptor-binding pocket. Upon binding, the receptor conformation is altered such that a specific G protein α subunit is activated. G protein activation leads to dissociation of the α subunit from the $\beta\gamma$ subunit and activation of effector pathways. These effectors include adenylate cyclase, ion channels, and an array of other systems.

subunits: α, β, and γ.[112] When a receptor-ligand interaction occurs, the receptor changes in conformation and guanosine diphosphate (GDP) is displaced from the α subunit by guanosine triphosphate (GTP). G proteins are classified according to their α subunit and activate a variety of effector systems, including adenylate cyclase, guanylate cyclase, phospholipases, or specific ion channels.[113] G proteins that stimulate adenylate cyclase are classified as Gs; those that inhibit adenylate cyclase are called Gi.[111] Currently, 20 α subunits have been identified and are organized according to the activity of the second-messenger system.[113] Gαs couples and activates adenylate cyclase, whereas Gαi inhibits this enzyme activity.

The adenylate cyclase system represents one of the most studied effector systems of receptor activation. More than nine distinct adenylate cyclases have been cloned.[114] When an agonist binds to a Gs-coupled receptor, a conformational change occurs, allowing the receptor to associate with the Gαs subunit. Under basal (unstimulated) conditions Gαs is bound to GDP; however, with hormone binding, GDP is released and is replaced with GTP. This GTP-activated G protein then activates intracellular signaling events. Receptor activation also initiates the dissociation of the α subunit from the $\beta\gamma$ subunits. The β and γ subunits serve a vast array of signaling functions that include receptor desensitization by translocation of G protein receptor kinases to agonist-occupied receptors and stimulation of Ras-mediated mitogen-activated protein (MAP) kinase.[115] The Gs-GTP complex then activates adenylate cyclase, resulting in the generation of cAMP from adenosine triphosphate (ATP) within the cell cytoplasm. cAMP is then capable of producing effects within the cell such as phosphorylation of effector proteins that ultimately lead to responses such as secretion, cell movement, or growth.

The Gα-GTP complex is gradually inactivated by guanosine triphosphatase (GTPase) that converts GTP to GDP. This enzymatic conversion occurs spontaneously by the G protein, which is itself a GTPase. The conversion of GTP to GDP terminates G protein stimulation of adenylate cyclase and is one way by which the basal condition is restored.

Receptor activation can also stimulate a G protein to inhibit cAMP accumulation and thereby reduce cAMP levels and antagonize the effects of Gs-coupled events. The Gαi family of subunits inhibits cAMP accumulation and includes Gαi$_1$ to Gαi$_4$, transducin, and gustducin. In this manner, GPCRs can maintain fine control of the cellular cAMP concentration and subsequent intracellular signaling. Members of this GPCR family also activate phospholipases and phosphodiesterases,[116] and they participate in ion channel regulation.[115, 117] Other GPCRs couple with Gq and G12. The Gq family of G protein subunits regulates the production of inositol 1,4,5-trisphosphate (IP_3) and diacylglycerol (DAG).[118]

There are five known subtypes of the β subunit (β_1 to β_5) and two groups of γ subunits. After α-subunit dissociation, the $\beta\gamma$ subunits remain tightly associated and also act as signal transducers. It is now established that the $\beta\gamma$ subunit also participates in a vast assay of cellular signals. For example, $\beta\gamma$ subunits can activate GPCR kinases, adenylate cyclase, and/or ion channels.[119] When the α subunit is in the GDP-bound form, it reassociates with $\beta\gamma$. With re-establishment of the heterotrimer, $\alpha\beta\gamma$, along with other mechanisms of desensitization, receptor signaling via the separate subunits ceases.

Effector Systems

Following receptor occupation, G protein subunits cause activation of enzymes or other proteins, ultimately resulting in intracellular signaling events (Table 1–3). Enzymes, such as adenylate cyclase or PLC, generate specific second messengers such as cAMP and IP_3 and DAG. Some G proteins couple directly to specific ion channels, such as potassium or calcium channels, and initiate changes in ion permeability. The effector systems are not well understood for some receptors such as receptors involved with cell growth and differentiation.

Other G proteins such as Go may activate the phosphoinositide system. When bound to hormone, receptors that couple to Go activate PLC, which acts on inositol phospholipids found in the cell membrane. PLC can cause the hydrolysis of phosphatidylinositol-4,5-bisphosphate, generating 1,2-DAG and IP_3. DAG and IP_3 can regulate cell metabolism by increasing intracellular calcium levels.

Receptor Desensitization

To ensure the rapidity of hormone signaling, shortly after receptor stimulation a series of events is initiated that ultimately acts to turn off signaling. The principal events in this process involve receptor desensitization and internalization, which re-establish cell responsiveness.

Phosphorylation of the receptor is one of the initial events involved in turning off the signal after agonist binding.[120] Signal termination by phosphorylation occurs via two distinct pathways.[120, 121] *Homologous desensitization* follows ligand binding and activation of G protein receptor kinases, which phosphorylate the receptor at specific intracellular sites, generally on serine and threonine residues.[122] Heterologous desensitization does not require receptor binding and often involves protein kinases A and C.[123]

Phosphorylation of the receptor promotes binding of arrestin-like molecules, which uncouple the receptor from the G protein.[123] This uncoupling and subsequent receptor internalization (sequestration) continue the process of signal termination and eventually lead to the re-establishment of cell responsiveness.

Receptor Resensitization

Internalization or sequestration of the receptor occurs within minutes of receptor occupancy. It is best characterized as the beginning of resensitization, as opposed to the end of desensitization, because only receptors that have been internalized can be dephosphorylated and returned to the cell surface for subsequent activation.[124] Sequestration of GPCRs is facilitated by GPCR kinase–mediated phosphorylation.[125] GPCRs internalize via the clathrin-coated, vesicle-mediated endocytic pathway[126] (Fig. 1–7).

Chronic exposure of cells to high concentrations of hormones frequently leads to a decrease in cell surface–binding sites. This reduction in surface receptor expression is termed *down-regulation* and is the result of receptor internalization. The mechanisms employed by the cell that distinguish receptor internalization and recycling from down-regulation are not clear. However, long-term agonist exposure to some receptors has been shown to activate signaling molecules that may be important in receptor down-regulation. Moreover, hormone receptor complexes can be processed by either endosomes or ubiquitin-associated proteasomes. The pathway selected (or targeted) secondary to agonist stimulation may ultimately determine the fate of the receptor.

Table 1–3 | **Classification of G Protein α Subunits and Their Signaling Pathways**

CLASS	SIGNALING
Gαs	Adenylate cyclase, calcium channels
Gαi	Adenylate cyclase, cyclic guanosine monophosphate, phosphodiesterase
Gαq	Phospholipase C-β
Gα12	Sodium/hydrogen exchange

Receptors Not Coupled to G Proteins

Receptor Tyrosine Kinases

Unlike GPCRs where ligand-receptor interaction causes activation of a G protein intermediary, some ligand-receptors possess intrinsic protein tyrosine kinase activity. These membrane-spanning cell surface receptors catalyze the transfer of phosphate from ATP to target proteins. Such receptors are structurally unique in that they contain glycosylated extracellular binding domains, a single transmembrane domain, and a cytoplasmic domain. The cytoplasmic domain contains a protein tyrosine kinase region and substrate region for agonist-activated receptor phosphorylation. On activation these receptors may phosphorylate themselves or be phosphorylated by other protein kinases.[127, 128] In general, receptor tyrosine kinases exist in the cell membrane as monomers. However, with ligand binding, these receptors dimerize, autophosphorylate, and initiate other intracellular signal transduction pathways. Most receptor tyrosine kinases couple, via ligand binding, to Ras and subsequently activate MAP kinase. MAP kinase is then able to modulate the regulation of other cellular proteins, including transcription factors. Members of the receptor tyrosine kinase family include the insulin receptor, growth factor receptors (vascular endothelial growth factor, PDGF, epidermal growth factor [EGF], fibroblast growth factor [FGF], insulin-like growth factor [IGF] I, macrophage-CSF, nerve growth factor), and receptors involved in development.[127, 129]

Activated tyrosine kinase receptors participate in a number of intracellular signaling events that involve the phosphorylated cytoplasmic domain. Specific phosphorylated tyrosine residues serve as binding sites for Src homology regions 2 and 3 (SH2 and SH3 domains). The result of SH2 domain binding is activation or modulation of the signaling protein that contains this binding domain. In this manner receptor tyrosine kinases activate diverse signaling pathways.[130]

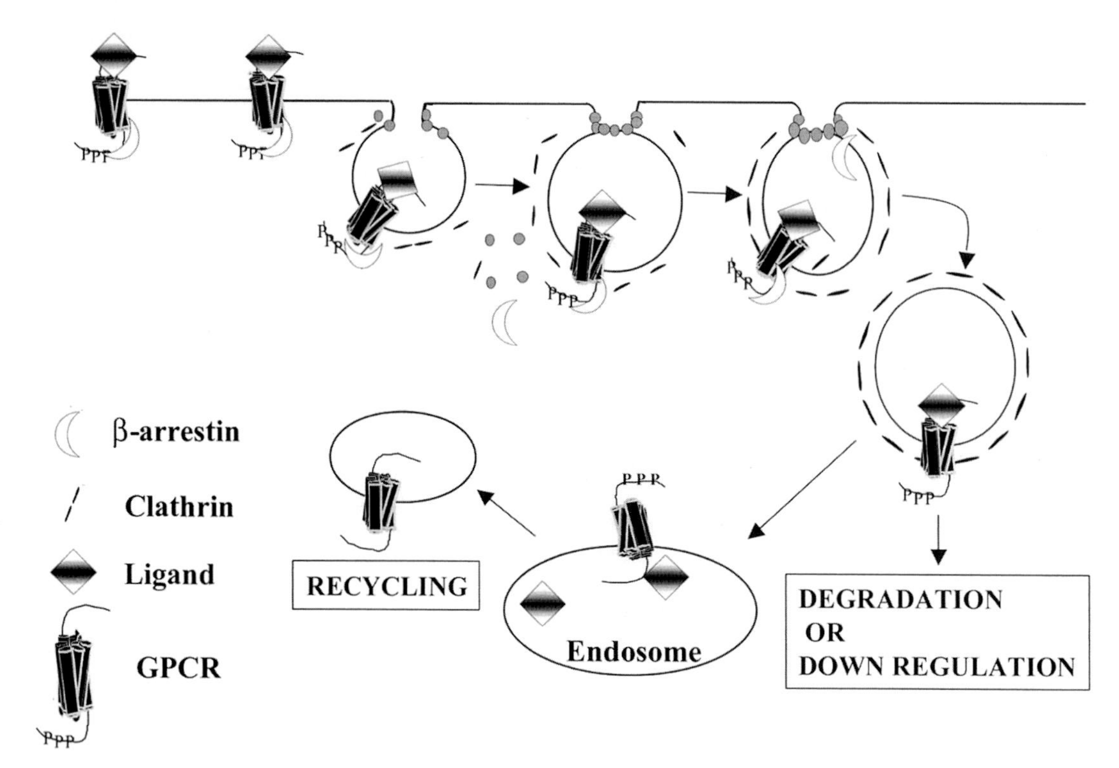

Figure 1–7. Agonist-activated receptors are phosphorylated by G protein–coupled receptor kinases at specific intracellular sites (P). The phosphorylated receptor is uncoupled from its G protein, and β-arrestin translocates from the cytosol to the receptor, thus initiating receptor endocytosis. β-Arrestin-associated G protein–coupled receptors (GPCRs) interact with other proteins (e.g., clathrin and dynamin). GPCR endocytosis leads to receptor dephosphorylation, recycling, and down-regulation.

Receptor Guanylate Cyclases

Receptor guanylate cyclases use cyclic GMP (cGMP) as a direct intracellular mediator. These cell surface receptors contain an extracellular ligand–binding region, a single transmembrane domain, and a cytoplasmic guanylate cyclase catalytic domain.[131, 132] Ligand stimulation of a receptor guanylate cyclase results in activation of cGMP-dependent protein kinase, which is a serine/threonine protein kinase. The atrial natriuretic peptide (ANP) receptor is a representative receptor guanylate kinase, whereas ANP is a potent smooth muscle–relaxing agent. Its primary function appears to be regulation of kidney sodium and water balance.[133]

Nonreceptor Tyrosine Kinases

Some cell surface receptors involved in inflammation and hematopoietic cell regulation work through tyrosine kinases but do not contain a cytoplasmic catalytic domain. The Src family of kinases is the primary component of this receptor signaling system.[134]

Receptor Tyrosine Phosphatases

Leukocyte regulation is modulated by surface receptors whose function is to remove phosphate groups from specific phosphotyrosines. CD45 is a surface protein found in white blood cells that participates in T- and B-cell activation.[135] CD45 contains a single membrane-spanning domain and a cytoplasmic region with tyrosine phosphatase activity. Depending on the substrate, dephosphorylation of signaling proteins may result in reduced or enhanced activity. Receptors in this family are important in inflammation and immune regulation and have been shown to participate in gastrointestinal development, growth, and cancer.

Receptor Serine/Threonine Kinases

TGF-β (see Growth Factor section) receptors are a unique group of surface proteins that are involved in a variety of cell functions, including chemotaxis, inflammation, and proliferation. These receptors contain a single membrane domain and a cytoplasmic serine/threonine kinase region. Receptor stimulation initiates activation of the serine/threonine kinase and subsequent modulation of cellular protein function.[136]

REGULATION OF GASTROINTESTINAL GROWTH BY HORMONES AND TRANSMITTERS

Growth of gastrointestinal tissues is a balance between cellular proliferation and senescence. Many factors participate in maintenance of the gastrointestinal mucosa. Nutrients and other luminal factors stimulate growth of the intestinal mucosa and are necessary to maintain normal digestive and absorptive functions. Hormones and transmitters serve as secondary messengers that are normally secreted in response to food ingestion and mediate many of the nutrient effects on the gastrointestinal tract. They play a key role in cellular proliferation. Alterations in intestinal proliferation are manifest by atrophy, hyperplasia, dysplasia, or malignancy.

Growth factors that have important effects on the gastrointestinal tract include peptides of the EGF family, the TGF-β family, the IGF family, the FGF family, hepatocyte growth factors, the PDGF family, trefoil factors, and many cytokines (including interleukins).[137]

Growth Factor Receptors

Growth factors regulate cellular proliferation by interacting with specific cell surface receptors. These receptors are membrane proteins that possess specific binding sites for the growth factor ligand. An unusual form of signaling occurs when the ligand interacts with its receptor within the same cell. For example, PDGF receptors present on the intracellular surface of fibroblast cell lines are activated by intracellular ligand. This process is known as intracrine signaling. Most peptide growth factors, however, interact with receptors on different cells to regulate proliferation. Growth factor receptors can be either single polypeptide chains containing one membrane-spanning region such as the receptor for EGF, or they may comprise two subunit heterodimers, with one subunit containing a transmembrane domain and the other residing intracellularly but covalently bound to the transmembrane subunit (Fig. 1–8). Heterodimers may also dimerize to form a receptor comprising four subunits. Binding of the ligand to its receptor usually causes aggregation of two or more receptors and activation of intrinsic tyrosine kinase activity. Growth factor receptors have the ability to autophosphorylate on binding of the ligand. In addition, receptor tyrosine kinase activity may phosphorylate other intracellular proteins important in signal transduction. Autophosphorylation attenuates the receptor's kinase activity and often leads to down-regulation and internalization of the receptor. Mutation of the receptor at its autophosphorylation site may lead to constitutive receptor activity and cellular transformation. Growth factor receptors may couple to a variety of intracellular signaling pathways, including adenylate cyclase, phospholipase C, calcium-calmodulin protein kinases, MAP kinase, and nuclear transcription factors. Thus, growth factors play important and varied roles in most cells of the gastrointestinal tract. It is not surprising, therefore, that mutations in growth factor receptors or downstream signaling proteins can lead to unregulated cell growth and neoplasia.

An important action of growth factors is their ability to modulate the expression of transacting transcription factors that can regulate expression of many other genes.[138] Early response genes such as *jun* and *fos*, are activated rapidly after ligand binding and control the expression of many other genes involved in cellular proliferation. Other important transcriptional factors include c-myc and nuclear factor κB (NF-κB). The latter is found in the cytoplasm in an inactive form and, on ligand binding, translocates to the nucleus where it activates other transcription factors. NF-κB is a key target for strategies to regulate cellular proliferation. Rb-1, originally identified in retinoblastoma, in its phosphorylated form is an inhibitor of cellular proliferation by complexing with the transcription factor p53. Dephosphorylation of Rb-1 releases p53, which activates other genes leading to cellular proliferation.

Virtually all growth factors of the gastrointestinal tract exert paracrine effects. However, many growth factors also possess autocrine and even intracrine actions. It has recently become apparent that growth factors and other signaling molecules secreted into the lumen of the gut can have important local biologic actions. Distant effects of growth factors found in the circulation may be important for growth of certain types of cancers, particularly lung and colon cancer.

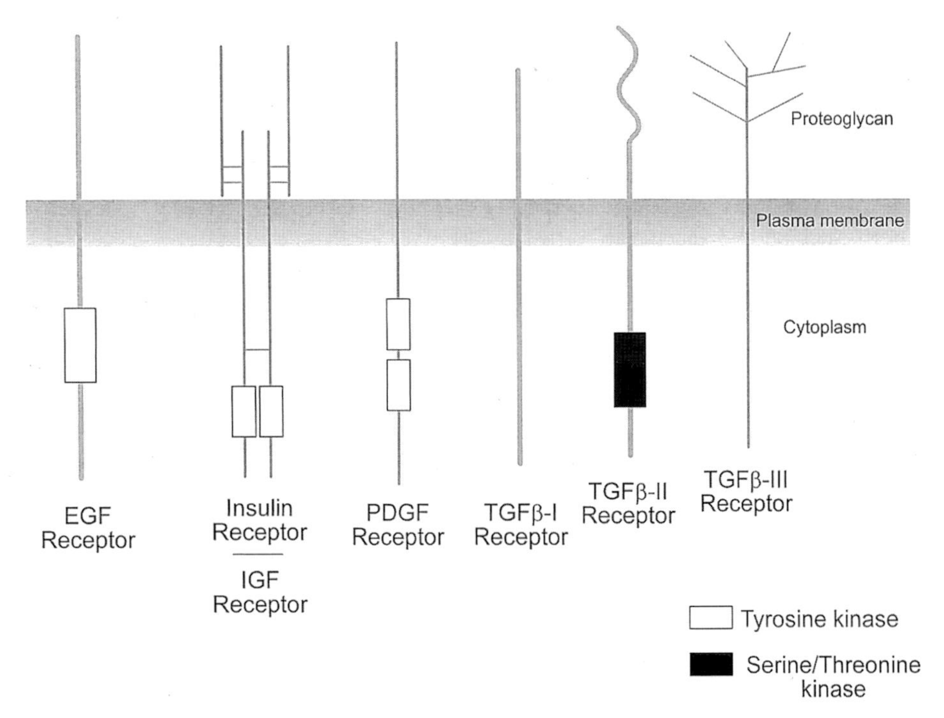

Figure 1–8. *Growth factor receptors in the gastrointestinal tract.* Schematic examples of growth factor receptor families are depicted in relation to the cell surface. Receptor regions that contain kinase activity are shown in boxes. Upon activation these receptors have the ability to autophosphorylate or phosphorylate other proteins to propagate intracellular cell signaling. (Modified from Podolsky DK: Peptide growth factors in the gastrointestinal tract. In Johnson LR: Physiology of the Gastrointestinal Tract. New York, Raven Press, 1994, pp 129–167.

Epidermal Growth Factor

Epidermal growth factor (EGF) was the first growth factor to be discovered. It is the prototype for a family of growth factors that are structurally related and have similarly related receptors. Other members of the family include TGF-α, amphiregulin, and heparin-binding EGF. EGF is identical to urogastrone (originally isolated from urine), which inhibits gastric acid secretion and promotes healing of gastric ulcers. EGF is secreted from submaxillary glands and Brunner's glands of the duodenum. It is likely that EGF interacts with luminal cells of the gastrointestinal tract and regulates proliferation. EGF has important trophic effects on gastric mucosa, and the wide distribution of EGF receptors suggests that EGF has mitogenic actions on a variety of cells throughout the gut. Recently, the EGF receptor has been reported to be responsible for gastric hyperplasia in a patient with Ménétrier's disease.[139]

Transforming Growth Factor-α

Transforming growth factor (TGF)-α is produced by most epithelial cells of the gastrointestinal tract and acts through the EGF receptor. Therefore, it shares trophic properties with EGF. It is believed to play a key role in gastric reconstitution after mucosal injury. Moreover, it appears to be important in intestinal neoplasia because most gastric and colon cancers produce TGF-α (see Chapters 44 and 115).

Transforming Growth Factor-β

A family of transforming growth factor (TGF)-β peptides exerts a variety of biologic actions, including stimulation of proliferation, differentiation, embryonic development, and formation of extracellular matrix.[140] In contrast with the TGF-α receptor, there are several distinct TGF-β receptors (TGF-βR I to TGF-βR III).[141] TGF-β modulates cell growth and proliferation in nearly all cell types and can enhance its own production from cells. It is likely that TGF-β plays a critical role in inflammation and tissue repair. Experimentally, targeted disruption of the TGF-βR I gene results in diffuse inflammation and gastric ulceration.[142] TGF-β augments collagen production by recruitment of fibroblasts through its chemoattractant properties. This action can have both beneficial and deleterious effects, depending on its site of deposition and abundance. For example, TGF-β may play a key role in the development of adhesions following surgery.[143]

Insulin-Like Growth Factor

Alternative splicing of the insulin gene produces two structurally related peptides: insulin-like growth factors (IGFs) I and II.[144] IGFs signal through at least three different IGF receptors. The IGF I receptor is a tyrosine kinase, and the IGF II receptor is identical to the mannose-6-phosphate receptor. Although the exact function of IGFs in the gastrointestinal tract is not clearly understood, they have potent mitogenic activity in intestinal epithelium. IGF II appears to be critical for embryonic development.

Fibroblast Growth Factor and Platelet-Derived Growth Factor

At least seven related fibroblast growth factors (FGFs) have been identified.[145] These peptides have mitogenic effects on a variety of cell types, including mesenchymal cells, and likely play an important role in organogenesis and neovascularization.[146] Although not unique to the gastrointestinal tract, platelet-derived growth factor (PDGF) is one of the most thoroughly studied growth factors. It is important for fibroblast growth, and its receptor is expressed in the liver and throughout the gastrointestinal tract, where it probably participates in wound healing.

Trefoil Factors

Trefoil factors (pS2, spasmolysin, and intestinal trefoil factor) are a recently identified family of proteins that is expressed throughout the gastrointestinal tract.[147] They share a common structure with six cysteine residues and three disulfide bonds, creating a cloverleaf appearance that stabilizes the peptide within the gut lumen. The pS2 peptide is produced in the gastric mucosa; spasmolysin is found both in the antrum and pancreas; and intestinal trefoil factor is produced throughout the small and large intestine.[148] These peptides are produced by goblet cells and are secreted onto the mucosal surface of the gut. It is likely that trefoil factors act on the apical surface of the epithelial cells, where they have growth-promoting properties on the gastrointestinal mucosa.

Other G Protein–Coupled Receptors and Growth

Other peptides signaling through GPCRs may also have growth-promoting effects. Three important examples include gastrin, CCK, and gastrin-releasing peptide (GRP). Gastrin stimulates the growth of enterochromaffin-like cells of the stomach and induces proliferation of the oxyntic mucosa containing parietal cells.[149] Gastrin binds to CCK-B receptors of the stomach and activates PLC and Ras pathways that ultimately result in activation of protein kinase C and MAP kinase, respectively. MAP kinase, which can also be activated by tyrosine kinase receptors typical of growth factors, causes the phosphorylation of transcription factors that are involved in cellular proliferation. In some cells, cAMP and protein kinase A exert synergistic effects on cellular growth through activation of nuclear transcription factors such as cAMP responsive element binding (protein) (CREB). However, in other cells cAMP antagonizes proliferation. Therefore, depending on the cell type, the effects of growth factors such as EGF, insulinlike growth factor (IGF), and PDGF may be enhanced by hormones that stimulate cAMP production. Certain colon cancer cells possess CCK-B receptors and respond to the proliferative effects of gastrin. Gastrin may be produced by some colon cancers, enabling it to exert an autocrine effect to promote cancer growth.[150] Whether circulating gastrin initiates colon cancer development is unknown.

CCK binds preferentially to the CCK-A type receptor, which is abundant in gallbladder, the pancreas of many spe-

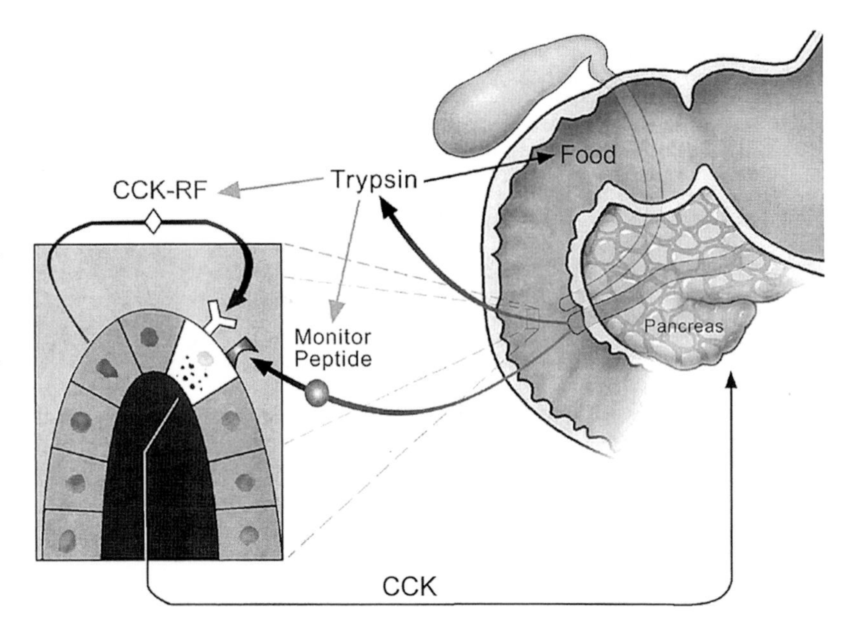

Figure 1–9. Regulation of cholecystokinin (CCK) secretion by intraluminal releasing factors. Endocrine cells containing CCK are stimulated by trypsin-sensitive releasing factors (CCK-RF) that are present in the lumen of the gut. Releasing factors secreted from the intestine are responsible for negative feedback regulation of pancreatic secretion. Under basal conditions, local trypsin inactivates CCK-RF; however, with ingestion of nutrients that compete as substrates for trypsin, CCK-RF is available to stimulate CCK secretion. The pancreatic releasing factor, monitor peptide, may contribute to sustained CCK release and pancreatic secretion after a meal.

cies, brain, and peripheral nerves of the gut. In the pancreas CCK causes both hypertrophy and hyperplasia of pancreatic acinar cells. Similar to the effects of gastrin, CCK activates PLC and small GTP-binding proteins to activate MAP kinase. In animal models CCK can promote pancreatic cancer growth.[151]

GRP (the mammalian analog of bombesin) was first recognized for its ability to stimulate gastrin secretion from the stomach. It was later appreciated that GRP stimulates proliferation of G cells. GRP has received considerable attention recently for its growth-promoting effects on small cell lung cancer, pancreatic cancer, and certain colon cancers.[152]

REGULATION OF GASTROINTESTINAL HORMONES BY INTRALUMINAL RELEASING FACTORS

Most gastrointestinal hormones are secreted into the blood on the ingestion of a meal. However, the exact mechanism by which luminal nutrients stimulate hormone secretion is unknown. Although the apical surface of most enteric endocrine cells is exposed to the intestinal lumen ("open cells"), it is unclear whether nutrients interact with specific receptors on the surface of endocrine cells or whether they are absorbed and then stimulate hormone secretion. It has recently been recognized that specific releasing factors for gastrointestinal hormones are present in the lumen of the gut (Fig. 1–9). CCK was the first hormone shown to be regulated by an intraluminal releasing factor.[153, 154] Luminal CCK-releasing factor was purified from intestinal washings and shown to stimulate CCK release when instilled into the lumen of animals. Diazepam-binding inhibitor has also been shown to stimulate CCK release, as has a pancreatic peptide known as monitor peptide.[155, 156] Secretin may also be regulated by an intraluminal releasing factor.[35] The existence of these releasing factors underscores the significance of bioactive peptides within the lumen of the gut.

REFERENCES

1. DelValle J, Yamada T: The gut as an endocrine organ. Annu Rev Med 41:447–455, 1990.
2. Larsson LI, Goltermann N, de Magistris L, et al: Somatostatin cell processes as pathways for paracrine secretion. Science 205:1393–1395, 1979.
3. Gershon MD, Erde SM: The nervous system of the gut. Gastroenterology 80:1571–1594, 1981.
4. Dockray GJ: Physiology of enteric neuropeptides. In Johnson LR (ed): Physiology of the Gastrointestinal Tract. New York, Raven Press, 1994, pp 129–167.
5. Murthy KS, Grider JR, Jin JG, et al: Interplay of VIP and nitric oxide in the regulation of neuromuscular activity in the gut. Arch Int Pharmacodyn Ther 329:27–38, 1995.
6. Makhlouf GM: Neural and hormonal regulation of function in the gut [published erratum appears in Hosp Pract (Off Ed) 25(5):15, 1990]. Hosp Pract (Off Ed) 25:79–87, 90–95, 98, 1990.
7. Furness JB, Clerc N: Responses of afferent neurons to the contents of the digestive tract, and their relation to endocrine and immune responses. Prog Brain Res 122:159–172, 2000.
8. Smith GP, Gibbs J: Satiating effect of cholecystokinin. Ann N Y Acad Sci 713:236–241, 1994.
9. Rothman JE, Orci L: Budding vesicles in living cells. Sci Am 274:70–75, 1996.
10. Corsi AK, Schekman R: Mechanism of polypeptide translocation into the endoplasmic reticulum. J Biol Chem 271:30299–30302, 1996.
11. Rehfeld JF: Processing of precursors of gastroenteropancreatic hormones: Diagnostic significance. J Mol Med 76:338–345, 1998.
12. Velander WH, Lubon H, Drohan WN: Transgenic livestock as drug factories. Sci Am 276:70–74, 1997.
13. Haseltine WA: Discovering genes for new medicines. Sci Am 276:92–97, 1997.
14. Branch AD: A good antisense molecule is hard to find. Trends Biochem Sci 23:45–50, 1998.
15. Crooke ST, Bennett CF: Progress in antisense oligonucleotide therapeutics. Annu Rev Pharmacol Toxicol 36:107–129, 1996.
16. Bennett CF: Antisense oligonucleotides: Is the glass half full or half empty? Biochem Pharmacol 55:9–19, 1998.
17. Oksche A, Rosenthal W: The molecular basis of nephrogenic diabetes insipidus. J Mol Med 76:326–337, 1998.
18. Kim PS, Arvan P: Endocrinopathies in the family of endoplasmic reticulum (ER) storage diseases: Disorders of protein trafficking and the role of ER molecular chaperones. Endocr Rev 19:173–202, 1998.
19. Edkins JS: On the chemical mechanism of gastric secretion. Proc R Soc Lond B Biol Sci 76:376, 1905.
20. Gregory RA, Tracy HJ: The constitution and properties of two gastrins extracted from hog antral mucosa. Gut 5:103–117, 1964.

21. Joshi SN, Gardner JD: Gastrin and colon cancer: A unifying hypothesis. Dig Dis 14:334–344, 1996.
22. Rehfeld JF: The new biology of gastrointestinal hormones. Physiol Rev 78:1087–1108, 1998.
23. Kopin AS, Lee YM, McBride EW, et al: Expression cloning and characterization of the canine parietal cell gastrin receptor. Proc Natl Acad Sci U S A 89:3605–3609, 1992.
24. Buchan AM, Polak JM, Solcia E, et al: Electron immunohistochemical evidence for the human intestinal I cell as the source of CCK. Gut 19: 403–407, 1978.
25. Liddle RA, Goldfine ID, Rosen MS, et al: Cholecystokinin bioactivity in human plasma: Molecular forms, responses to feeding, and relationship to gallbladder contraction. J Clin Invest 75:1144–1152, 1985.
26. Reeve JR Jr, Eysselein VE, Ho FJ, et al: Natural and synthetic CCK-58: Novel reagents for studying cholecystokinin physiology. Ann N Y Acad Sci 713:11–21, 1994.
27. Liddle RA, Morita ET, Conrad CK, et al: Regulation of gastric emptying in humans by cholecystokinin. J Clin Invest 77:992–996, 1986.
28. Calam J, Ellis A, Dockray GJ: Identification and measurement of molecular variants of cholecystokinin in duodenal mucosa and plasma: Diminished concentrations in patients with celiac disease. J Clin Invest 69:218–225, 1982.
29. Geracioti TD Jr, Liddle RA: Impaired cholecystokinin secretion in bulimia nervosa. N Engl J Med 319:683–688, 1988.
30. Slaff JI, Wolfe MM, Toskes PP: Elevated fasting cholecystokinin levels in pancreatic exocrine impairment: Evidence to support feedback regulation. J Lab Clin Med 105:282–285, 1985.
31. Bayliss WM, Starling EH: The mechanism of pancreatic secretion. J Physiol (Lond) 28:325–353, 1902.
32. Mutt V, Jorpes JE, Magnusson S: Structure of porcine secretin: The amino acid sequence. Eur J Biochem 15:513–519, 1970.
33. Leiter AB, Chey WY, Kopin AS: Secretin. In Walsh JH, Dockray GJ (series eds): Gut Peptides: Biochemistry and Physiology (Comprehensive Endocrinology, Revised Series). New York, Raven Press, 1994, pp 144–174.
34. Schaffalitzky de Muckadell OB, Fahrenkrug J: Secretion pattern of secretin in man: Regulation by gastric acid. Gut 19:812–818, 1978.
35. Li P, Lee KY, Chang TM, et al: Mechanism of acid-induced release of secretin in rats: Presence of a secretin-releasing peptide. J Clin Invest 86:1474–1479, 1990.
36. You CH, Rominger JM, Chey WY: Effects of atropine on the action and release of secretin in humans. Am J Physiol 242:G608–G611, 1982.
37. You CH, Chey WY: Secretin is an enterogastrone in humans. Dig Dis Sci 32:466–471, 1987.
38. McGuigan JE, Wolfe MM: Secretin injection test in the diagnosis of gastrinoma. Gastroenterology 79:1324–1331, 1980.
39. Brady CE III: Secretin provocation test in the diagnosis of Zollinger-Ellison syndrome. Am J Gastroenterol 86:129–134, 1991.
40. Said SI, Mutt V: Polypeptide with broad biological activity: Isolation from small intestine. Science 169:1217–1218, 1970.
41. Said SI, Mutt V: Potent peripheral and splanchnic vasodilator peptide from normal gut. Nature 225:863–864, 1970.
42. Dockray GJ: Vasoactive intestinal polypeptide and related peptides. In Walsh JH, Dockray GJ (series eds): Gut Peptides: Biochemistry and Physiology (Comprehensive Endocrinology, Revised Series). New York, Raven Press, 1994, pp 447–472.
43. Linder S, Barkhem T, Norberg A, et al: Structure and expression of the gene encoding the vasoactive intestinal peptide precursor. Proc Natl Acad Sci U S A 84:605–609, 1987.
44. Holst JJ, Fahrenkrug J, Knuhtsen S, et al: VIP and PHI in the pig pancreas: Coexistence, corelease, and cooperative effects. Am J Physiol 252:G182–G189, 1987.
45. Yasui A, Naruse S, Yanaihara C, et al: Corelease of PHI and VIP by vagal stimulation in the dog. Am J Physiol 253:G13–G19, 1987.
46. Goyal RK, Rattan S, Said SI: VIP as a possible neurotransmitter of noncholinergic, nonadrenergic inhibitory neurones. Nature 288:378–380, 1980.
47. Fahrenkrug J: Transmitter role of vasoactive intestinal peptide. Pharmacol Toxicol 72:354–363, 1993.
48. Bloom SR: Vasoactive intestinal peptide, the major mediator of the WDHA (pancreatic cholera) syndrome: Value of measurement in diagnosis and treatment. Am J Dig Dis 23:373–376, 1978.
49. Masel SL, Brennan BA, Turner JH, et al: Pancreatic vasoactive intestinal polypeptide-oma as a cause of secretory diarrhoea. J Gastroenterol Hepatol 15:457–460, 2000.
50. Barada KA, Saade NE, Atweh SF, et al: Neural mediation of vasoactive intestinal polypeptide inhibitory effect on jejunal alanine absorption. Am J Physiol 275:G822–G828, 1998.
51. Cho WK, Boyer JL: Vasoactive intestinal polypeptide is a potent regulator of bile secretion from rat cholangiocytes. Gastroenterology 117:420–428, 1999.
52. Grider JR: Interplay of VIP and nitric oxide in regulation of the descending relaxation phase of peristalsis. Am J Physiol 264:G334–G340, 1993.
53. Aggestrup S, Uddman R, Sundler F, et al: Lack of vasoactive intestinal polypeptide nerves in esophageal achalasia. Gastroenterology 84: 924–927, 1983.
54. Larsson LT, Sundler F: Is the reduction of VIP the clue to the pathophysiology of Hirschsprung's disease? Z Kinderchir 45:164–166, 1990.
55. Bitar KN, Said SI, Weir GC, et al: Neural release of vasoactive intestinal peptide from the gut. Gastroenterology 79:1288–1294, 1980.
56. Verner JV, Morrison AB: Endocrine pancreatic islet disease with diarrhea: Report of a case due to diffuse hyperplasia of non–beta islet tissue with a review of 54 additional cases. Arch Intern Med 133: 492–499, 1974.
57. Smith SL, Branton SA, Avino AJ, et al: Vasoactive intestinal polypeptide–secreting islet cell tumors: A 15-year experience and review of the literature. Surgery 124:1050–1055, 1998.
58. Mojsov S, Heinrich G, Wilson IB, et al: Preproglucagon gene expression in pancreas and intestine diversifies at the level of post-translational processing. J Biol Chem 261:11880–11889, 1986.
59. Drucker DJ: Glucagon-like peptides. Diabetes 47:159–169, 1998.
60. Drucker DJ, Erlich P, Asa SL, et al: Induction of intestinal epithelial proliferation by glucagon-like peptide 2. Proc Natl Acad Sci U S A 93:7911–7916, 1996.
61. Rubin DC: Nutrient regulation of intestinal growth and adaptation: Role of glucagon-like peptide 2 and the enteroendocrine cell [editorial; comment]. Gastroenterology 117:261–263, 1999.
62. Kimmel JR, Pollock HG, Hazelwood RL: Isolation and characterization of chicken insulin. Endocrinology 83:1323–1330, 1968.
63. Kimmel JR, Hayden LJ, Pollock HG: Isolation and characterization of a new pancreatic polypeptide hormone. J Biol Chem 250:9369–9376, 1975.
64. Tatemoto K, Mutt V: Chemical determination of polypeptide hormones. Proc Natl Acad Sci U S A 75:4115–4119, 1978.
65. Tatemoto K: Neuropeptide Y: Complete amino acid sequence of the brain peptide. Proc Natl Acad Sci U S A 79:5485–5489, 1982.
66. Tatemoto K, Carlquist M, Mutt V: Neuropeptide Y—a novel brain peptide with structural similarities to peptide YY and pancreatic polypeptide. Nature 296:659–660, 1982.
67. Larsson LI, Sundler F, Hakanson R: Pancreatic polypeptide—a postulated new hormone: Identification of its cellular storage site by light and electron microscopic immunocytochemistry. Diabetologia 12:211–226, 1976.
68. Wahlestedt C, Reis DJ: Neuropeptide Y–related peptides and their receptors—are the receptors potential therapeutic drug targets? Annu Rev Pharmacol Toxicol 33:309–352, 1993.
69. Allen YS, Adrian TE, Allen JM, et al: Neuropeptide Y distribution in the rat brain. Science 221:877–879, 1983.
70. Adrian TE, Allen JM, Bloom SR, et al: Neuropeptide Y distribution in human brain. Nature 306:584–586, 1983.
71. Lundberg JM, Tatemoto K, Terenius L, et al: Localization of peptide YY (PYY) in gastrointestinal endocrine cells and effects on intestinal blood flow and motility. Proc Natl Acad Sci U S A 79:4471–4475, 1982.
72. Eva C, Keinanen K, Monyer H, et al: Molecular cloning of a novel G protein–coupled receptor that may belong to the neuropeptide receptor family. FEBS Lett 271:81–84, 1990.
73. Rose PM, Fernandes P, Lynch JS, et al: Cloning and functional expression of a cDNA encoding a human type 2 neuropeptide Y receptor. J Biol Chem 270:29038, 1995.
74. Lee CC, Miller RJ: Is there really an NPY Y3 receptor? Regul Pept 75/76:71–78, 1998.
75. Bard JA, Walker MW, Branchek TA, et al: Cloning and functional expression of a human Y4 subtype receptor for pancreatic polypeptide, neuropeptide Y, and peptide YY. J Biol Chem 270:26762–26765, 1995.
76. Weinberg DH, Sirinathsinghji DJ, Tan CP, et al: Cloning and expression of a novel neuropeptide Y receptor. J Biol Chem 271:16435–16438, 1996.

77. Lin TM, Evans DC, Chance RE, et al: Bovine pancreatic peptide: Action on gastric and pancreatic secretion in dogs. Am J Physiol 232: E311–E315, 1977.
78. Hazelwood RL: The pancreatic polypeptide (PP-fold) family: Gastrointestinal, vascular, and feeding behavioral implications. Proc Soc Exp Biol Med 202:44–63, 1993.
79. Adrian TE, Mitchenere P, Sagor G, et al: Effect of pancreatic polypeptide on gallbladder pressure and hepatic bile secretion. Am J Physiol 243:G204–G207, 1982.
80. Lloyd KC, Grandt D, Aurang K, et al: Inhibitory effect of PYY on vagally stimulated acid secretion is mediated predominantly by Y1 receptors. Am J Physiol 270:G123–G127, 1996.
81. Sheikh SP: Neuropeptide Y and peptide YY: Major modulators of gastrointestinal blood flow and function. Am J Physiol 261:G701–G715, 1991.
82. Wen J, Phillips SF, Sarr MG, et al: PYY and GLP-1 contribute to feedback inhibition from the canine ileum and colon. Am J Physiol 269:G945–G952, 1995.
83. Hwa JJ, Witten MB, Williams P, et al: Activation of the NPY Y5 receptor regulates both feeding and energy expenditure. Am J Physiol 277:R1428–R1434, 1999.
84. Hokfelt T, Kellerth JO, Nilsson G, et al: Substance P: Localization in the central nervous system and in some primary sensory neurons. Science 190:889–890, 1975.
85. Cao T, Pinter E, Al-Rashed S, et al: Neurokinin-1 receptor agonists are involved in mediating neutrophil accumulation in the inflamed, but not normal, cutaneous microvasculature: An in vivo study using neurokinin-1 receptor knockout mice. J Immunol 164:5424–5429, 2000.
86. Mantyh PW, DeMaster E, Malhotra A, et al: Receptor endocytosis and dendrite reshaping in spinal neurons after somatosensory stimulation. Science 268:1629–1632, 1995.
87. Hershey AD, Krause JE: Molecular characterization of a functional cDNA encoding the rat substance P receptor. Science 247:958–962, 1990.
88. Otsuka M, Yoshioka K: Neurotransmitter functions of mammalian tachykinins. Physiol Rev 73:229–308, 1993.
89. Mantyh CR, Pappas TN, Lapp JA, et al: Substance P activation of enteric neurons in response to intraluminal *Clostridium difficile* toxin A in the rat ileum. Gastroenterology 111:1272–1280, 1996.
90. Mantyh CR, Gates TS, Zimmerman RP, et al: Receptor binding sites for substance P, but not substance K or neuromedin K, are expressed in high concentrations by arterioles, venules, and lymph nodules in surgical specimens obtained from patients with ulcerative colitis and Crohn disease. Proc Natl Acad Sci U S A 85:3235–3239, 1988.
91. Le Novere N, Corringer PJ, Changeux JP: Improved secondary structure predictions for a nicotinic receptor subunit: Incorporation of solvent accessibility and experimental data into a two-dimensional representation. Biophys J 76:2329–2345, 1999.
92. Willems JL, Buylaert WA, Lefebvre RA, et al: Neuronal dopamine receptors on autonomic ganglia and sympathetic nerves and dopamine receptors in the gastrointestinal system. Pharmacol Rev 37:165–216, 1985.
93. Gyorgy L, Orr Z, Doda M: Influence of dopamine and dopaminergic agonists on relaxation of isolated rabbit ileum induced by sympathetic nerve stimulation. Acta Physiol Acad Sci Hung 58:163–168, 1981.
94. Van Neuten J, Janssen P: Is dopamine an endogenous inhibitor of gastric emptying? In Duthie H (ed): Gastrointestinal Motility in Health and Disease. Lancaster, UK, MTP, 1978, pp 172–180.
95. Missale C, Nash SR, Robinson SW, et al: Dopamine receptors: From structure to function. Physiol Rev 78:189–225, 1998.
96. Gershon MD: Roles played by 5-hydroxytryptamine in the physiology of the bowel [review]. Aliment Pharmacol Ther 13 Suppl 2:15–30, 1999.
97. Kim DY, Camilleri M: Serotonin: A mediator of the brain-gut connection. Am J Gastroenterol 95:2698–2709, 2000.
98. Pandolfino JE, Howden CW, Kahrilas PJ: Motility-modifying agents and management of disorders of gastrointestinal motility. Gastroenterology 118:S32–S47, 2000.
99. Camilleri M: Management of the irritable bowel syndrome. Gastroenterology 120:652–668, 2001.
100. Bouras EP, Camilleri M, Burton DD, et al: Prucalopride accelerates gastrointestinal and colonic transit in patients with constipation without a rectal evacuation disorder. Gastroenterology 120:354–360, 2001.
101. Hill SJ, Ganellin CR, Timmerman H, et al: International Union of Pharmacology: XIII. Classification of histamine receptors. Pharmacol Rev 49:253–278, 1997.
102. Lowenstein CJ, Dinerman JL, Snyder SH: Nitric oxide: A physiologic messenger. Ann Intern Med 120:227–237, 1994.
103. Costa M, Furness JB, Pompolo S, et al: Projections and chemical coding of neurons with immunoreactivity for nitric oxide synthase in the guinea pig small intestine. Neurosci Lett 148:121–125, 1992.
104. Wallace JL, Miller MJ: Nitric oxide in mucosal defense: A little goes a long way. Gastroenterology 119:512–520, 2000.
105. Feoktistov I, Biaggioni I: Adenosine A2B receptors. Pharmacol Rev 49:381–402, 1997.
106. Fredholm BB, Abbracchio MP, Burnstock G, et al: Towards a revised nomenclature for P1 and P2 receptors. Trends Pharmacol Sci 18:79–82, 1997.
107. Curfs JH, Meis JF, Hoogkamp-Korstanje JA: A primer on cytokines: Sources, receptors, effects, and inducers. Clin Microbiol Rev 10:742–780, 1997.
108. Lefkowitz RJ: The superfamily of heptahelical receptors. Nat Cell Biol 2:E133–E136, 2000.
109. Palczewski K, Kumasaka T, Hori T, et al: Crystal structure of rhodopsin: A G protein–coupled receptor. Science 289:739–745, 2000.
110. Vaughan M: Signaling by heterotrimeric G proteins minireview series. J Biol Chem 273:667–668, 1998.
111. Neer EJ: Heterotrimeric G proteins: Organizers of transmembrane signals. Cell 80:249–257, 1995.
112. Hildebrandt JD: Role of subunit diversity in signaling by heterotrimeric G proteins. Biochem Pharmacol 54:325–339, 1997.
113. Wilkie TM, Gilbert DJ, Olsen AS, et al: Evolution of the mammalian G protein alpha subunit multigene family. Nat Genet 1:85–91, 1992.
114. Simonds WF: G protein regulation of adenylate cyclase. Trends Pharmacol Sci 20:66–73, 1999.
115. Clapham DE, Neer EJ: G protein $\beta\gamma$ subunits. Annu Rev Pharmacol Toxicol 37:167–203, 1997.
116. Hamm HE: The many faces of G protein signaling. J Biol Chem 273: 669–672, 1998.
117. Gutkind JS: Regulation of Mitogen-Activated Protein Kinase Signaling Networks by G Protein–Coupled Receptors. Science's STKE. Available at http://stke.sciencemag.org/cgi/content/full/OC_sigtrans;2000/40/re1:1–13, 2000.
118. Rhee SG, Bae YS: Regulation of phosphoinositide-specific phospholipase C isozymes. J Biol Chem 272:15045–15048, 1997.
119. Gautam N, Downes GB, Yan K, et al: The G protein $\beta\gamma$ complex. Cell Signal 10:447–455, 1998.
120. Freedman NJ, Lefkowitz RJ: Desensitization of G protein–coupled receptors. Recent Prog Horm Res 51:319–351, 1996.
121. Hausdorff WP, Caron MG, Lefkowitz RJ: Turning off the signal: Desensitization of β-adrenergic receptor function [published erratum appears in FASEB J 4(12):3049, 1990]. FASEB J 4:2881–2889, 1990.
122. Lefkowitz RJ: G protein–coupled receptor kinases. Cell 74:409–412, 1993.
123. Lohse MJ, Andexinger S, Pitcher J, et al: Receptor-specific desensitization with purified proteins: Kinase dependence and receptor specificity of β-arrestin and arrestin in the β_2-adrenergic receptor and rhodopsin systems. J Biol Chem 267:8558–8564, 1992.
124. Lefkowitz RJ, Pitcher J, Krueger K, et al: Mechanisms of β-adrenergic receptor desensitization and resensitization. Adv Pharmacol 42: 416–420, 1998.
125. Tsuga H, Kameyama K, Haga T, et al: Sequestration of muscarinic acetylcholine receptor m2 subtypes: Facilitation by G protein–coupled receptor kinase (GRK2) and attenuation by a dominant-negative mutant of GRK2. J Biol Chem 269:32522–32527, 1994.
126. Schmid SL: Clathrin-coated vesicle formation and protein sorting: An integrated process. Annu Rev Biochem 66:511–548, 1997.
127. Schlessinger J: Cell signaling by receptor tyrosine kinases. Cell 103: 211–225, 2000.
128. Hubbard SR, Mohammadi M, Schlessinger J: Autoregulatory mechanisms in protein tyrosine kinases. J Biol Chem 273:11987–11990, 1998.
129. Simon MA: Receptor tyrosine kinases: Specific outcomes from general signals. Cell 103:13–15, 2000.
130. Waksman G, Shoelson SE, Pant N, et al: Binding of a high-affinity phosphotyrosyl peptide to the Src SH2 domain: Crystal structures of the complexed and peptide-free forms. Cell 72:779–790, 1993.
131. Maack T: Receptors of atrial natriuretic factor. Annu Rev Physiol 54: 11–27, 1992.
132. Yuen PS, Garbers DL: Guanylyl cyclase–linked receptors. Annu Rev Neurosci 15:193–225, 1992.

133. Rosenzweig A, Seidman CE: Atrial natriuretic factor and related peptide hormones. Annu Rev Biochem 60:229–255, 1991.
134. Argetsinger LS, Campbell GS, Yang X, et al: Identification of JAK2 as a growth hormone receptor–associated tyrosine kinase. Cell 74: 237–244, 1993.
135. Walton KM, Dixon JE: Protein tyrosine phosphatases. Annu Rev Biochem 62:101–120, 1993.
136. Massague J: Receptors for the TGF-β family. Cell 69:1067–1070, 1992.
137. Podolsky DK: Peptide growth factors in the gastrointestinal tract. In Johnson LR (ed): Physiology of the Gastrointestinal Tract. New York, Raven Press, 1994, pp 129–167.
138. Zimmerman CM, Padgett RW: Transforming growth factor-β signaling mediators and modulators. Gene 249:17–30, 2000.
139. Burdick JS, Chung E, Tanner G, et al: Treatment of Ménétrier's disease with a monoclonal antibody against the epidermal growth factor receptor. N Engl J Med 343:1697–1701, 2000.
140. Bassing CH, Yingling JM, Howe DJ, et al: A transforming growth factor-β type I receptor that signals to activate gene expression. Science 263:87–89, 1994.
141. Massague J: The transforming growth factor-β family. Annu Rev Cell Biol 6:597–641, 1990.
142. Shull MM, Ormsby I, Kier AB, et al: Targeted disruption of the mouse transforming growth factor-β_1 gene results in multifocal inflammatory disease. Nature 359:693–699, 1992.
143. Williams RS, Rossi AM, Chegini N, et al: Effect of transforming growth factor-β on postoperative adhesion formation and intact peritoneum. J Surg Res 52:65–70, 1992.
144. Adams TE, Epa VC, Garrett TP, et al: Structure and function of the type 1 insulin-like growth factor receptor. Cell Mol Life Sci 57:1050–1093, 2000.
145. Ornitz DM: FGFs, heparan sulfate, and FGFRs: Complex interactions essential for development. Bioessays 22:108–112, 2000.
146. Kato S, Sekine K: FGF-FGFR signaling in vertebrate organogenesis. Cell Mol Biol (Noisy-le-grand) 45:631–638, 1999.
147. Podolsky DK: Mechanisms of regulatory peptide action in the gastrointestinal tract: Trefoil peptides. J Gastroenterol 35:69–74, 2000.
148. Sands BE, Podolsky DK: The trefoil peptide family. Annu Rev Physiol 58:253–273, 1996.
149. Koh TJ, Chen D: Gastrin as a growth factor in the gastrointestinal tract. Regul Pept 93:37–44, 2000.
150. Dickinson CJ: Relationship of gastrin processing to colon cancer [editorial] [see comments]. Gastroenterology 109:1384–1388, 1995.
151. Douziech N, Lajas A, Coulombe Z, et al: Growth effects of regulatory peptides and intracellular signaling routes in human pancreatic cancer cell lines. Endocrine 9:171–183, 1998.
152. Dietrich JB: Neuropeptides, antagonists, and cell proliferation: Bombesin as an example. Cell Mol Biol (Noisy-le-grand) 40:731–746, 1994.
153. Spannagel AW, Green GM, Guan D, et al: Purification and characterization of a luminal cholecystokinin-releasing factor from rat intestinal secretion. Proc Natl Acad Sci U S A 93:4415–4420, 1996.
154. Herzig KH, Schon I, Tatemoto K, et al: Diazepam-binding inhibitor is a potent cholecystokinin-releasing peptide in the intestine [published erratum appears in Proc Natl Acad Sci U S A 93(24):14214, 1996]. Proc Natl Acad Sci U S A 93:7927–7932, 1996.
155. Iwai K, Fukuoka S, Fushiki T, et al: Purification and sequencing of a trypsin-sensitive cholecystokinin-releasing peptide from rat pancreatic juice—its homology with pancreatic secretory trypsin inhibitor. J Biol Chem 262:8956–8959, 1987.
156. Li Y, Hao Y, Owyang C: Diazepam-binding inhibitor mediates feedback regulation of pancreatic secretion and postprandial release of cholecystokinin. J Clin Invest 105:351–359, 2000.

Chapter 2

MUCOSAL IMMUNOLOGY AND MECHANISMS OF GASTROINTESTINAL INFLAMMATION

R. Balfour Sartor

Increasingly complex innate and acquired defense systems that permit survival in the hostile microbial environment of the intestine have evolved. The gastrointestinal mucosal immune system has the daunting task of coexisting with an incredibly complex mix of luminal antigens, including partially digested dietary constituents, host proteins, and commensal bacteria, while maintaining the capacity to recognize and eliminate promptly pathogenic microbial organisms and transformed epithelial cells. Homeostasis is maintained by elaborate, redundant mechanisms of barrier exclusion, phagocytosis and clearance of translocating bacteria and macromolecules, immunologic tolerance to ubiquitous antigens, and coordinated, self-limited inflammatory responses leading to clearance of pathogens while limiting tissue injury. The mucosal immune system is ideally adapted to recognize and eliminate invading pathogens rapidly, while not responding to ubiquitous luminal antigens. This carefully orchestrated system depends on redundant down-regulating pathways that mediate an active state of tolerance under normal conditions. Tolerance is mediated by regulatory T cells and by early detection of invading pathogens by epithelial cells that liberate chemotactic signals to incite immigration of effector cells. These newly recruited cells are more efficient in clearing infections than the endogenous lamina propria innate cells, which have down-regulated bacterial detection systems that dampen responses to ubiquitous bacteria. Similarly, signal transduction pathways in intestinal epithelial cells are muted to prevent pathologic responses to luminal bacterial polymers. However, in susceptible individuals with genetically determined defective barrier function or altered immunoregulation, persistent infections or pathogenic immune responses can develop, resulting in chronic gastrointestinal inflammation. This chapter addresses the mechanisms of integrated, controlled immune responses to commensal antigens and invading pathogens in the normal host, as well as dysregulated immune responses that lead to chronic inflammatory sequelae in susceptible individuals. Emphasis is placed on normal immunophysiologic and immunopathogenic mechanisms as well as the clinical consequences of defective immunologic responses, diagnostic applications, and strategies for therapeutic intervention.

MUCOSAL IMMUNE RESPONSES

Luminal and Epithelial Barrier Defenses

A relatively impervious mucosal barrier provides the first line of defense against uptake of luminal dietary and bacterial antigens. Furthermore, both environmental and pathogenic ingested bacteria are largely killed in the proximal gastrointestinal (GI) tract by salivary lysozyme, gastric acid, pancreatic digestive enzymes, and the detergent effects of bile acids. As a consequence, human gastric and duodenal luminal contents contain fewer than 10^2 to 10^3 viable bacteria per milliliter, despite higher concentrations of swallowed oropharyngal flora and food organisms. Bacterial species that evade the proximal gauntlet of defenses but do not adhere to or invade epithelial cells are removed by intestinal secretion and peristalsis. The luxuriant anaerobic bacteria that populate the distal ileum and colon, consume all available nutrients, and occupy all available ecologic niches inhibit colonization by newly ingested bacterial species (colonization resistance). Colonization is further limited by antibacterial peptides secreted by Paneth and epithelial cells. A secreted mucus layer shields the epithelium from luminal bacteria and antigens, and macromolecules are excluded by epithelial tight junctions.

Recent studies[1–4] have clarified molecular characteristics of epithelial tight junctions and the mucus barrier. Tight junctions located near the apical surface of the lateral plasma membranes circumferentially fuse adjacent epithelial cells to exclude paracellular transport of macromolecules efficiently.[1] Structural proteins include two types of four-transmembrane spanning molecules—hyperphosphorylated occludin and claudin isoforms—that anchor the peripheral membrane protein zonula occludens-1 to -3, which contain PDZ domains 1 to 3.[2–4] There is evidence that hyperphosphorylated occludin and zonula occludens-1 are contained in glycolipid raftlike membrane microdomains, in contrast with the basolateral transmembrane proteins such as E-cadherin, and that occludin binds to caveolin-1, a scaffolding protein abundant in lipid rafts.[5] Fas-mediated apoptosis selectively enhances epithelial permeability to small molecules, but barrier function is maintained by rapid rearrangement of tight junctions and desmosomes.[6] Of considerable interest, mucosal dendritic cells can extend pseudopodia through intestinal tight junctions to sample luminal antigens directly without breaching barrier function; these dendritic cells accomplish this by expressing occludin, claudin-1, and zonula occludens-1, which preserve tight junction integrity.[7]

Intestinal goblet cells and gastric antral mucus cells selectively produce and secrete mucin glycoproteins and trefoil peptides that interact effectively to shield mucosal epithelial cells from harsh luminal conditions, nonmotile bacteria, and luminal antigens.[8] Predominant intestinal mucin isoforms include MUC 2, which is secreted by goblet cells,[9] and MUC 3A and B, which are membrane bound with two epidermal growth factor (EGF)-like motifs.[10] MUC 5AC, MUC 5B, and MUC 6 are found in various gastric locations.[11] Trefoil peptides interact with mucin domains synergistically to protect epithelial cells from damage by toxic lectins, bile acids, fatty acids, and *Clostridium difficile* toxins.[12] Intestinal trefoil factor, selectively produced in the intestine, and spasmolytic polypeptide, expressed in the stomach,[13] have similar protective properties.[12] Beyond their static barrier protective properties, trefoil peptides have potent capacities to stimulate protective responses in intestinal epithelial cells as demonstrated by their ability to promote migration, inhibit apoptosis, activate nuclear factor κB (NFκB) and mitogen-activated protein (MAP) kinases, and stimulate expression of the EGF receptor.[14, 15] Furthermore, intestinal trefoil factor expression is transcriptionally regulated by keratinocyte growth factor.[16] Overexpression of human growth hormone in transgenic mice leads to up-regulation of colonic intestinal trefoil factor,[17] and targeted overexpression of transforming growth factor-α (TGF-α) in the gastric mucosa stimulates local expression of spasmolytic peptide 2.[18]

Clinical Relevance

Reduction of gastric acidity and disruption of GI peristalsis can lead to bacterial overgrowth of the stomach and small intestine, resulting in clinically apparent malabsorption and potentially increased risk of aspiration pneumonia (see Chapters 38 and 90). Antibiotic treatment diminishes commensal bacterial colonization resistance, permitting growth of toxin-producing *C. difficile* (see Chapter 97) and decreasing the inoculum necessary for pathogenic species such as *Salmonella* species to colonize the intestine (see Chapter 96). *C. difficile* toxins exert their injurious activities in part by disassembling actin microfilaments through glucosylation of the rho family of proteins, leading to disruption of epithelial tight junctions.[19] Similarly, enteropathogenic *Escherichia coli* dephosphorylate and dissociate occludin from intestinal tight junctions.[20] In contrast, glucocorticoids stimulate formation of tight junctions in cultured intestinal epithelial cells.[21] The functional importance of epithelial integrity in excluding luminal molecules is elegantly demonstrated by the focal intestinal inflammation that develops when epithelial E-cadherin activity is diminished.[22] Similarly, experimental colitis is exacerbated by deletion of intestinal trefoil factor,[23] and luminal administration of recombinant trefoil peptides inhibits experimental colitis and gastric injury in multiple models.[23, 24] Finally, polymorphism of the MUC 3A gene may provide a basis for susceptibility to Crohn's disease.[10] It is highly likely that other genetic defects in barrier function and bacterial clearance are associated with GI inflammatory disorders.

Innate Defenses

When stimulated with bacterial components, epithelial, bone marrow–derived, mesenchymal, and endothelial cells actively contribute to mucosal protection by secreting antimicrobial proteins and inflammatory mediators or by engulfing and degrading invading microbial agents or toxic luminal products.

Epithelial Cells

Mucosal epithelial cells secrete antimicrobial peptides that limit luminal growth of commensal and pathogenic bacteria[25, 26] and act as sensors of microbial invasion by liberating chemotactic and inflammatory molecules that initiate protective immune responses.[27] Defensins constitute an important class of antimicrobial peptides with cytotoxic activities against bacteria, fungi, and viruses.[28] Originally described in neutrophils, defensins are peptides that contain six cysteines that form three disulfide bridges. These small cationic molecules bind electrostatically to negatively charged membranes and form pores, leading to lysis of targeted cells. Paneth cells in the small intestinal crypts secrete α-defensins (cryptins, human defensins 5 and 6), which are sequestered in secretory granules in association with lysozyme, matrilysin, and phospholipase A_2. Lysozyme splits the β-1,4 glycan backbone of peptidoglycan, the primary structural component of both Gram-positive and Gram-negative bacteria. Human defensins 5 and 6 are expressed in highest concentrations in the normal jejunum and ileum, low expression in the duodenum, and no expression in the stomach or the normal colon.[29] However, in inflammatory bowel disease[30] α-defensins are found in the inflamed colon in conjunction with Paneth cell metaplasia, and they are up-regulated in celiac disease.[29] Stored in an inactive precursor form, α-defensins are activated after cleavage by matrilysin.[31] Secretion of α-defensins is stimulated by luminal lipopolysaccharide (LPS, endotoxin),[32] and these peptides not only kill luminal bacteria, but stimulate chloride and water secretion by intestinal epithelial cells,[28] which further protect against microbial invasion. In contrast to organ-related Paneth cell localization of α-defensins, human β-defensins are produced and secreted by columnar epithelial cells throughout the GI tract.[29] Human β-defensin 1 is constitutively expressed, whereas β-

defensin 2 is induced by proinflammatory cytokines (interleukin-1β [IL-1β] and tumor necrosis factor [TNF]), invasive bacteria, or adherent pathogens through NFκB-regulated transcription.[33]

The multidrug resistance gene (mdr-1a) on chromosome 7 provides a novel mechanism of mucosal protection against bacterial products, pumping amphophilic and hydrophobic molecules across membranes, thereby eliminating toxic intracytoplasmic products.[34] The protein is expressed in epithelial cells as well as intraepithelial lymphocytes and hematopoietic and lymphoid subpopulations. Evidence that this pathway protects against bacterial stimulation is provided by development of colitis in mdr-1a deficient (knockout) mice raised in conventional conditions, with accelerated onset of colitis after *Helicobacter bilis* infection, but protection by a germ-free (sterile) environment or by antibiotic administration.[34] Bone marrow transplantation studies show that disease is conveyed by nonhematopoietic cells.

In addition to having mucosal barrier properties and secreting mucins, trefoil peptides, and antimicrobial molecules into the gut lumen, GI epithelial cells can secrete immunologically active substances that activate protective mucosal inflammatory and immune responses.[35] When stimulated by invasive bacteria (prototype *Salmonella* species), parasites (e.g., *Cryptosporidium* species), or bacterial cell wall polymers (including LPS, peptidoglycan-polysaccharide polymers), intestinal epithelial cells express a characteristic profile of chemotactic peptides, adhesion molecules, class II major histocompatibility (MHC) molecules, and proinflammatory cytokines.[36–38] Expression of these molecules is coordinately regulated in a temporal and spatial manner, leading to emigration of first neutrophils, then monocytes and T lymphocytes from the circulation. For example, IL-8, which stimulates activity and migration of neutrophils, is maximally expressed 4 to 6 hours after *Salmonella* species invasion, whereas maximal expression of epithelial neutrophil activating protein-78 (ENA-78) is delayed 18 to 24 hours after epithelial stimulation.[39] The consequence of cell migration to the injured mucosa is phagocytosis of invading pathogens and translocating luminal bacteria. Most molecules produced after epithelial activation are under the regulation of the transcription factor NFκB, which is stimulated by a variety of bacterial components, proinflammatory cytokines, and reactive oxygen metabolites (Table 2–1).[37]

Toll-like receptor (TLR) 4, which binds LPS and lipoteichoic acid to initiate signaling to NFκB, is present on native epithelial cells and most colonic epithelial cell lines,[40] although Nod-2, which transduces NFκB activation after intracellular LPS exposure, has not been detected on intestinal epithelial cells by immunohistochemical staining.[41] Stimulation of TLR4 by LPS stimulates both the NFκB and AP-1 (cJun/c-fos) pathways.[42]

Table 2–1 | **Inducing Agents and Genes Regulated by NFκB Relevant to Intestinal Injury and Inflammation**

INDUCING AGENT (RECEPTOR)	GENES REGULATED
IL-1 (IL-1RI)	Cytokines: IL-1, -2, -6, -12; TNF
TNF (TNF-RI)	Chemokines: IL-8; groα, β; RANTES; MIP-2; IP-10; MCP-1
Lymphotoxin (TNF-RII)	Membrane receptors: IL-2R; CD95/APO-1
LPS, lipoteichoic acid (TLR4)	Adhesion molecules: ICAM-1, ELAM, VCAM, P-selectin
Peptidoglycan (TLR2)	Inflammatory enzymes: COX-2, iNOS, 5-lipoxygenase, 12-lipoxygenase, SOD
Bacterial DNA (TLR9)	Immunoregulatory molecules: MHC class II
Oxygen radicals	Inhibitory molecules: COX-2, IκBα

APO, apolipoprotein; COX-2, cyclooxygenase-2; DNA, deoxyribonucleic acid; ELAM, endothelial leukocyte adhesion molecule; ICAM, intercellular adhesion molecule; IκBα, inhibitor of κBα; IL, interleukin; iNOS, inducible nitric oxide synthase; IP, inducible protein; LPS, lipopolysaccharide; MCP, macrophage chemoattractant protein; MHC, major histocompatibility complex; MIP, macrophage inflammatory protein; NFκB, nuclear factor κB; RANTES, regulated on activation, normal T cell expressed and secreted; SOD, superoxide dismutase; TLR, toll-like receptor; TNF, tumor necrosis factor; VCAM, vascular cell adhesion molecule.

Table 2–2 | **Unique Phenotypic and Functional Characteristics of Intestinal Macrophages and Blood Macrophages (A) and Mast Cells (B)**

A: MACROPHAGES/MONOCYTES	INTESTINAL MACROPHAGES	PERIPHERAL BLOOD MONOCYTES
CD14 (LPS receptor)	Low expression	High expression
CD11b (complement receptor)	Low expression	High expression
CD16 (IgG receptor)	Low expression	High expression
Phagocytosis	Reduced	Enhanced
B: MAST CELLS	**RAT MUCOSA**	**CONNECTIVE TISSUE**
Granule components	Serotonin, histamine (small amounts)	Histamine (high amounts), serotonin, heparin
Chymases	RMCP II	RMCP I, tryptase, carboxypeptidase
Cytokine profile	TNF	TNF, IL-1, IL-3, IL-4, IL-6, IL-10, IFNγ
Soluble mediators	PGD_2, NO, PAF, VIP, LTB_4	PAF, NO, PGE_2

IFN, interferon; IL, interleukin; LPS, lipopolysaccharide; LTB_4, leukotriene B_4; NO, nitric oxide; PAF, platelet-activating factor, PGD_2, prostaglandin D_2; PGE_2, prostaglandin E_2; RMCP, rat mast cell protease; TNF, tumor necrosis factor; VIP, vasoactive intestinal polypeptide.

Macrophages

Intestinal macrophages, which constitute 10% to 15% of lamina propria mononuclear cells, differ phenotypically and functionally from circulating monocytes (Table 2–2).[43, 44] Low expression of membrane receptors such as CD14 (LPS binding), CD11b (complement receptor 3), and CD16 (FcγIII receptor) leads to muted inflammatory responses to translocating bacterial cell wall polymers relative to circulating monocytes.[43] This relative nonresponsiveness to environmental stimuli helps prevent aggressive inflammatory responses and secretion of proinflammatory cytokines in response to physiologic levels of bacterial products that may reach the intestinal lamina propria under normal conditions. Similarly, intestinal macrophages have muted capacities to phagocytose and kill invading pathogens. Clearance of pathogens and generation of inflammatory responses are accelerated by entry of newly recruited monocytes and neutrophils that secrete large amounts of cytokines and reactive oxygen metabolites.[45, 46] Entry of circulating effector cells into an area of new inflammation is governed by chemotactic molecules secreted by epithelial cells and resident macrophages as well as bacterial formylated peptides.[47] Intestinal macrophages are selectively positioned under the subepithelial basement membrane, in a location ideal for responding to invading pathogens and transcellular uptake of macromolecules. Although macrophages can process and present antigens to T lymphocytes, dendritic cells are far more efficient and probably account for most antigen presenting functions in the mucosa. Macrophages and newly recruited monocytes are primary sources of proinflammatory cytokines such as IL-1, TNF, IL-6, chemokines, IL-12, and IL-18[43, 45] (see "Nonlymphoid Cells").

NFκB provides a central pathway of macrophage activation, through engagement of a variety of membrane receptors for bacterial polymers and proinflammatory mediators (Fig. 2–1).[37] The ligation of TLR4 (binding LPS and lipoteichoic acid), TLR2 (binding peptidoglycan-polysaccharide complexes), TLR9 (binding bacterial nonmethylated deoxyribonucleic acid [DNA]), IL-1RI, and $TNFR_I$ activates a series of individual signaling kinases and adaptor proteins that converge on a central pathway.[37, 42] Phosphorylation of IκBα, the primary inhibitor of NFκB, by the IKK complex leads to IκBα ubiquination and degradation. Dissociation of the NFκB homodimer from inhibitory IκBα facilitates migration of NFκB to the nucleus, where it binds to its regulatory motif in the promoter of the gene encoding many proinflammatory molecules, thereby initiating transcription of a wide range of biologically active cytokines, adhesion molecules, enzymes, and MHC class II molecules (see). Intracellular LPS stimulates a similar pathway through Nod-2.[41] An important consequence of NFκB signaling is activation of suppressive molecules such as the inhibitor of κB (IκBα), which down-regulates further NFκB activity, and inducible cyclooxygenase-2 (COX-2), which stimulates production of protective eicosanoids such as prostaglandin E_2 (PGE_2) and PGJ_2. These inhibitory molecules are important in down-regulating the inflammatory response to prevent self-perpetuating responses to invading bacteria.

Mast Cells

Around 2% to 5% of lamina propria mononuclear cells are mast cells, which are preferentially localized adjacent to nerve terminals, where they are activated by secreted neuropeptides, particularly substance P.[48] Activation of mast cells by substance P or immunoglobulin E (IgE), which binds to abundant IgE Fc receptors on the mast cell membrane, induces secretion of preformed inflammatory mediators (histamine, serotonin, and proteases) and production of proinflammatory cytokines and arachidonic acid metabolites. Mast cells are found in all layers of the intestine and stomach, with distinctive subpopulations in the mucosa versus connective tissue in rats (see Table 2–2), although such a distinction is less evident in human tissues. These subpopulations have a common hematopoietic precursor.

Mast cells are expanded during helmintic infections and are important mediators of hypersensitivity responses that promote worm clearance. Crosslinkage of IgE receptors on mast cells stimulates degranulation with release of histamine and production of PGD_2 and peptidyleukotrienes that stimulate epithelial cell chloride and water secretion, mucosal permeability, goblet cell mucus secretion, and intestinal motility. Mast cells are also important in food allergy (see Chapter 101) and perhaps in gastric acid secretion (see Chapter 38).[49] In addition to IgE, mast cells respond to activated complement fragments C3a and C5a and bear receptors for IL-3 and stem cell factor (c-kit). A spontaneous deletion in the tyrosine kinase domain of c-kit leads to deficient mucosal and connective tissue mast cells in Ws/Ws rats, although the block in mucosal mast cell production is not absolute in Ws/Ws rats infected with *Nippostrongylus brasiliensis*.[50]

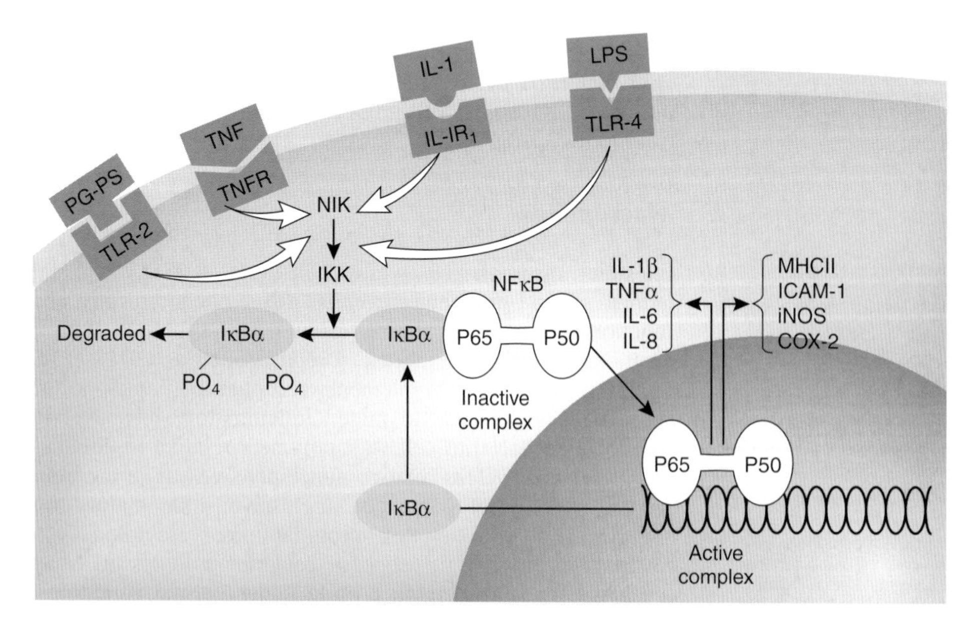

Figure 2–1. NFκB signaling. Proinflammatory cytokines such as TNF and IL-1 or bacterial polymers, including peptidoglycan-polysaccharide (PG-PS) or LPS bind to selective receptors, which converge signals on the IKK complex, which activates a central transcription factor, NFκB. NFκB is constitutively inactivated by complexing with its inhibitor, IκBα, which is phosphorylated by the IKK complex and degraded, allowing NFκB to translocate to the nucleus and initiate transcription of a number of proinflammatory and protective molecules. (See Table 2–1 also.) (Modified from the American Gastroenterological Association Teaching Project, Washington, D.C., with permission.)

Eosinophils

Mucosal eosinophils increase in helmintic infections and eosinophilic gastroenteritis (see Chapters 99 and 100). Activated eosinophils secrete prostaglandins, leukotrienes, and preformed biologically active molecules such as peroxidase, major basic protein, and eosinophilic cationic protein, which are stored in granules. Eosinophils also express membrane Fc receptors for IgE and, to a lesser extent, IgA and IgG. These migratory cells are recruited to the intestine by the C-C chemokine eotaxin, which is up-regulated in intestinal epithelial cells by IL-4, but not by interferon γ (IFNγ),[51] and facilitated by IL-5,[52] although IL-5 is not essential to eosinophilic recruitment.[53] Entry of eosinophils into the small intestine, but not into the colon, is facilitated by β_7 integrin.[54] Eosinophils contribute to clearance of helminths and help mediate GI injury, including nerve damage, after T helper 2 (T_{H2})-mediated hypersensitivity reactions to oral antigens.[55]

Natural Killer Cells

Natural killer (NK) cells are large, granular lymphocytes that function as cytotoxic cells to eliminate tumor cells and intracellular pathogens, particularly viruses.[56] Despite their morphologic similarity to lymphocytes, these cells do not express surface immunoglobulin or T cell receptors but can be modulated by T cell–derived cytokines, including IL-2. These cells may express some T cell differentiation membrane antigens such as CD2 and $\alpha\alpha$ homodimeric CD8 and can secrete IFNγ. However, they can also express monomyelocytic differentiation antigens, including CD11b and CD11c, CD14, and CD16, the receptor for the Fc component of IgG. The latter is important in one of the primary functions of NK cells, antibody-dependent cell-mediated cytotoxicity. Another important role for NK cells is cytotoxic stimulation of tumors that do not express MHC class I molecules. Human NK cells express membrane killer-inhibited receptors (KIRs) that, when bound to human leukocyte antigen (HLA)-A, -B, and -C molecules, inhibit cytotoxicity. However, in the absence of inhibitory signals for HLA class I peptides, killer-activated receptors (KARs) mediate cytotoxicity. NK cells also provide regulatory signals which inhibit T lymphocyte effector activities.[57]

Clinical Relevance

Innate defenses are critical mechanisms to maintain rapid responses to mucosal pathogens and are also key mediators of detrimental inflammatory responses to ubiquitous stimulants in chronic inflammation of the GI tract (see "Inflammatory Responses" for detailed descriptions). Descriptions of genetic polymorphisms leading to a 30-base-pair truncation of Nod-2 and subsequent defective NFκB responses to LPS in Crohn's disease[58] clearly demonstrate the importance of innate immune pathways in responding to environmental pathogens and in containing mucosal bacteria. It is entirely possible that genetic or acquired defects in defensin activity, epithelial chemotactic signaling, TLR function, and regulation of NFκB signaling pathways could similarly lead to bacterial overgrowth, microbial invasion, or inappropriately aggressive inflammatory responses. Polymorphisms in mdr-1a are associated with aggressive ulcerative colitis and Crohn's disease[59]—whether as a result of defective protective responses to luminal bacteria or of rapid excretion and inactivation of therapeutic agents remains to be determined. As discussed in detail later (see "Inflammatory Responses"), NFκB provides an attractive target for intervention by anti-inflammatory drugs.[60] Finally, defective neutrophilic killing of ingested bacteria due to absent respiratory burst generation in patients who have chronic granulomatous disease leads to ulcerative stomatitis, gastric inflammation, and a colonic inflammatory condition closely resembling Crohn's disease.[61] Indirect evidence of a defect in neutrophil function in Crohn's disease is provided by beneficial clinical responses reported in an open label pilot study of granulocyte colony stimulating factor.[62]

Acquired Immunologic Defenses

Unique Properties

Between 60% and 80% of the body's immunoglobulin-secreting cells are found within mucosal surfaces, and most are present in the GI-associated lymphoid tissues (GALT). The mucosal immune response has the unique characteristics of secretion of antibodies that complex antigen in the lumen without activating complement and of induction of tolerogenic T lymphocytes that maintain controlled local responses to commensal bacteria or dietary constituents with no systemic reactions (oral tolerance).[63, 64] These suppressive signals, which are mediated by activated T and B lymphocytes rather than clonal deletion and anergy, prevent pathologic responses to complex luminal dietary, host, and bacterial antigens, yet maintain their capacity to mount protective responses to invading microbial pathogens rapidly and to detect and eliminate neoplastic cells. Moreover, mucosal lymphoid populations are anatomically, phenotypically, and functionally compartmentalized into inductive sites (Peyer's patches and mesenteric lymph nodes) and effector sites (lamina propria and intraepithelial locations). These lymphoid tissues evolve through interaction among lymphoid, mesenchymal, and epithelial cells.[64] A carefully orchestrated trafficking system directs naive lymphoid cells from the Peyer's patch, where antigenic stimulation occurs; to draining mesenteric or caudal lymph nodes, where further antigenic exposure and clonal expansion take place; to the circulation, where mature gut-derived cells return to mucosal surfaces under the guidance of tissue-specific endothelial receptors that selectively bind mucosally derived lymphoid cells.[65] Of note, mucosal lymphocytes stimulated in one region can return to other mucosal surfaces, laying the foundation for a common mucosa-associated lymphoid tissue (MALT) in which immunization at any site (nasal, oral, rectal, inhaled) can generate protective responses at all mucosal surfaces.

Cellular Components

T LYMPHOCYTES. T lymphocytes have a crucial role in orchestrating protective immunity, leading to clearance of invading pathogens and neoplastic cells, as well as regulatory responses to endogenous bacterial and dietary antigen. T cells originate in the bone marrow and migrate to the thymus, where self-reactive (autoimmune) clones are deleted. Naive T cells expressing the $\alpha_4\beta_7$ integrin selectively home to Peyer's patches in the small intestine and homologous organized lymphoid aggregates in the colon (particularly the appendix and rectum) (discussed later). Those lymphocytes expressing the $\alpha_E\beta_7$ integrin selectively home to epithelial surfaces. Some data suggest that some intraepithelial lymphocytes (IELs) do not require thymic development but instead migrate directly from the bone marrow to the intestine (extrathymic education).[66]

T lymphocytes can be phenotypically and functionally characterized by the components of their heterodimeric glycoprotein T cell receptor (TCR$\alpha\beta$ or $\gamma\delta$) and by the presence of CD4-CD8 molecules closely associated with the TCR complex (Figs. 2–2 and 2–3). The CD3 complex of four membrane-bound subunits is intimately associated in a noncovalent fashion with the TCR complex. The CD3 complex is involved with signal transduction after the TCR binds to a peptide presented by an MHC class I or II bearing antigen presenting cell (APC) (see "Antigen Processing Cells and Antigen Presentation") or target cell. Most human T cells are TCR$\alpha\beta$; a minority of IELs contain the TCR$\gamma\delta$ phenotype. In contrast, at least 50% of murine IELs display the TCR$\gamma\delta$ marker.[67] TCR subunits (α, β, γ, δ) are composed of an extended amino-terminal extracellular domain, a transmembrane segment, and a short cytoplasmic domain. Somewhat analogous to immunoglobulins, TCRs are composed of variable (V), joining (J), constant (C), and diversity (D, present only on β and δ chains) regions. Each region is encoded by separate gene segments on chromosomes 7 (β and γ chains) and 14 (α and δ chains) that experience recombination during thymic development. These distinctive regions permit investigation of the degree of diversity or clonality (e.g., monoclonal, oligoclonal, or polyclonal) of immune responses, usually by typing the V region patterns.[68] Of interest, human gastric T lymphocytes have been shown to be oligoclonal in nature.[69] CD4 lymphocytes recognize antigens presented by MHC class II molecules,

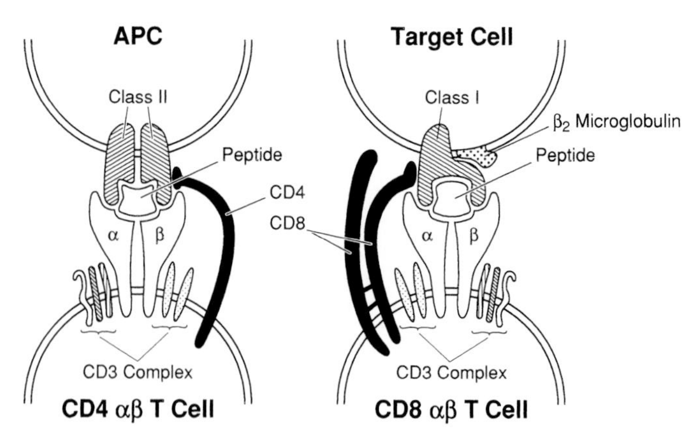

Figure 2–3. T cell interactions with MHC-bound antigen. T lymphocytes recognize antigenic peptides displayed on MHC Class I or II molecules. CD4 T cells preferentially bind to antigen presenting cells (APC) bearing MHC Class II receptors (left), whereas CD8 T lymphocytes recognize either MHC Class I bearing APC or target cells with MHC Class I-bound antigen (right). The latter interaction induces cytolytic responses. TCR/MHC ligation is stabilized by CD4 or CD8. β_2 microglobulin is part of the MHC Class I complex. MHC, major histocompatibility complex; TCR, T cell receptor.

whereas CD8 lymphocytes recognize MHC class I–presented antigens. CD8 lymphocytes frequently elicit cytotoxic responses but can also secrete cytokines with either T_{H1}, T_{H2}, or regulatory profiles (discussed later).

IELs, which migrate to epithelial surfaces, have a large, granular lymphocyte morphologic structure somewhat reminiscent of that of NK cells. Like NK cells, they bear membrane IL-2 receptor β chain, are decreased in IL-2R$\beta^{-/-}$ mice,[70] and express NK receptors.[71] IELs, as well as Peyer's patches, are virtually absent in lymphotoxin β receptor deficient mice.[72] IELs are also impaired in IL-7 receptor knockout mice, which have no $\gamma\delta$ T lymphocytes.[73] IELs almost exclusively express CD8, have a cytotoxic phenotype, and, when activated, produce cytotoxic products such as porforin, which damages membranes by creating pores, and granzyme, a serine esterase. However, resting IELs do not express these molecules or Fas ligand. Their mechanisms of action and functions remain uncertain, but they may be involved in cytotoxic clearance of transformed (neoplastic) cells or inflammatory events or may secrete IFNγ or keratinocyte growth factor.[74, 75] They are dramatically increased in frequency in lymphocytic colitis, graft-versus-host disease, protozoal infections, and celiac disease, and in celiac disease they have an activated phenotype.[76] Intestinal IELs are oligoclonal,[68, 77] suggesting that they recognize a limited antigenic repertoire. Interestingly, they are present in germ-free (sterile) hosts, indicating that their target may not be luminal bacteria.

NK T cells are described as a T cell subset bearing the surface marker NK 1.1, which may have some relation to mucosal immune responses. These cells can develop independently of the thymus and are found in the intestine and liver.[78] Many of these atypical T cells express an invariant Vα14 TCR that recognizes the glycolipid α-galactosyl ceramide presented by the nonclassic MHC CD1d.[79]

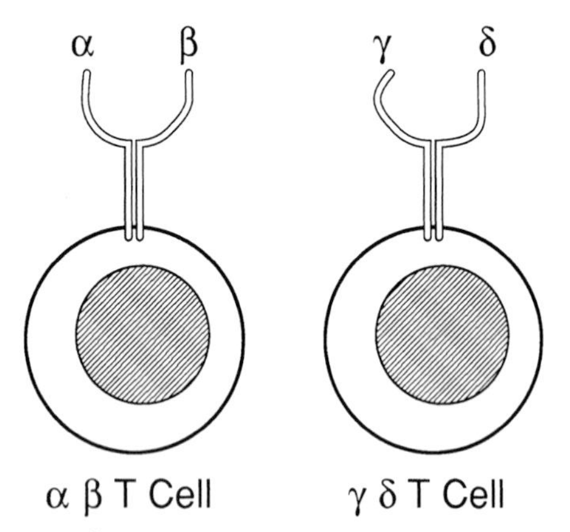

Figure 2–2. T cell receptors. Two distinct T cell populations can be defined by the types of heterodimeric T cell receptors displayed on their external membranes. Most lamina propria T cells have the $\alpha\beta$ subunits, whereas intraepithelial lymphocytes have both $\alpha\beta$ and $\gamma\delta$ receptors.

B LYMPHOCYTES. Like T cells, B cells develop from pluripotent stem cells in the bone marrow, where they begin their early stages of differentiation by undergoing a series of immunoglobulin gene locus rearrangements that yield extremely diverse antigen recognition. In early B cell differentiation, hundreds of potential V region sequences initiate random genetic rearrangement with multiple potential D and J regions by eliminating intervening DNA sequences to form a contiguous recombinant variable region. This region is fused with an IgM heavy chain. Homologous light chains are similarly formed; antigen specificity is determined by the VDJ region segment, and complement fixation and binding cellular receptors are determined by the Fc portion. Each immunoglobulin molecule is composed of two identical light chains linked to two identical heavy chains. Immature B cells express membrane-bound IgM, then mature to express membrane IgM and IgD, which is noncovalently associated with a disulfide-linked heterodimer consisting of IgA and IgB transmembrane glycoproteins that transduce activation signals when high-affinity antigen binds to the membrane IgM. This antigen-bound activation signal stimulates clonal expansion and further differentiation involving genetic rearrangement (switch differentiation) to express either IgG, IgE, or IgA under the influence of antigen specific T cells. T cells induce isotype switching by cell-cell contact through CD40-CD40 ligand (CD40L) and by the influence of secreted cytokines, including TGF-β, which selectively induces IgA. During isotype switching the epitope (antigen recognized) remains the same through insertion of the VDJ region onto a constant region of a different immunoglobulin class.

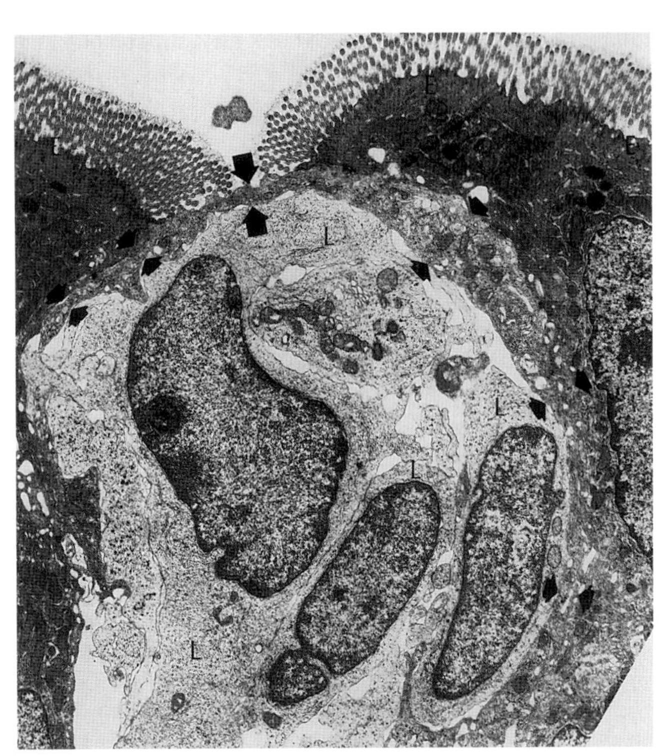

Figure 2–5. Transmission electron microscopy of an M cell. Microfold (M) cells in the dome epithelium of mucosal lymphoid aggregates lack microvilli and have closely adherent lymphocytes (L) and macrophages that receive unprocessed antigen passing by pinocytosis through the M cell. (From Owen RL, Jones AL: Epithelial cell specialization within human Peyer's patches: An ultrastructural study of intestinal lymphoid follicles. Gastroenterology 66(2):189–203, 1974.)

Peyer's Patch Organization, Development, and Antigen Uptake

Peyer's patches in the small intestine and homologous organized lymphoid follicles in the oropharynx (tonsils) and colon, especially the appendix and rectum, are sites of controlled antigen uptake and activation of naive B and T lymphocytes. Peyer's patches occur throughout the small intestine and are most frequent and well developed in the distal ileum. These lymphoid organs are anatomically organized into germinal follicles rich in B lymphocytes, thymus-dependent interfollicular areas (T cell predominant), and a specialized follicle-associated epithelium (Fig. 2–4). The epithelium covering the dome of lymphoid aggregates is unique in that villi and crypts are absent and goblet cells are rare. This epithelium contains microfold (M) cells, which are interspersed among absorptive epithelial cells. M cells are uniquely capable of sampling and transporting luminal antigens and microorganisms by a transcellular vesicular pathway to underlying B lymphocytes and dendritic cells for further processing. These specialized antigen sampling M cells have limited, short microvilli and unique microfolds on the surface membrane. M cells actively pinocytose luminal antigens but do not possess lysosomes, so antigens are not degraded or processed. Although intact commensal bacteria are rarely engulfed, numerous pathogens, including human immunodeficiency virus (HIV), reoviruses, *Vibrio cholerae*, and *Shigella* species, selectively adhere to M cells, possibly through specialized carbohydrate-binding mechanisms, and are transported without degradation.[80] The basal membrane of M cells is invaginated to form a pocket where dendritic cells and B lymphocytes are in intimate contact with extruded antigen or intact organisms (Fig. 2–5).

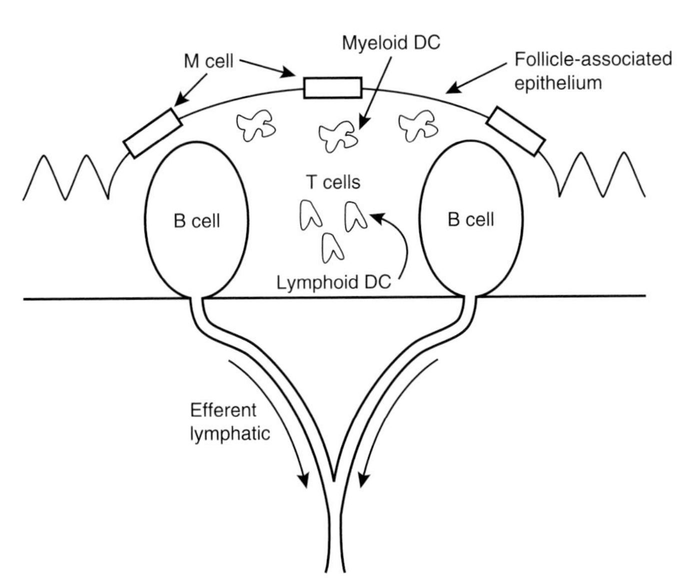

Figure 2–4. Anatomy of Peyer's patch. Peyer's patches have distinct regions composed of B cell–dominated follicles (germinal centers) and interfollicular T cell areas. Dendritic cells (DC) phenotypically distinct from T cells occupy various regions—myeloid DC, which display CD11b, are located in the subepithelial dome, whereas lymphoid DC (CD8α^+) lie in the interfollicular zone. The overlying follicle-associated epithelium is unique in structure and function.

Studies[81, 82] elucidated the development of Peyer's patches and the origin of M cells. M cells arise from pluripotential epithelial stem cells in adjacent crypts and migrate to the follicle-associated epithelium, where they differentiate into their distinctive phenotypes under the influence of lymphotoxin β receptor.[81, 82] Interaction of Peyer's patch lymphocytes, particularly B cells, facilitates M cell differentiation,[83] but M cells develop in Rag-1$^{-/-}$ mice, which lack T and B lymphocytes, indicating that lymphotoxin can arise from other sources.[81] Compartmentalization of the Peyer's patch begins at day 18.5 of gestation in mice with IL-7 receptor α^+, vascular cell adhesion molecule (VCAM)-1$^+$ and CD11c$^+$ cells that are selectively distributed in various regions of the nascent Peyer's patch.[84] Peyer's patch development requires the mutual interaction of mesenchymal cells expressing VCAM-1 and intercellular adhesion molecule (ICAM)-1 that secrete chemotactic signals that recruit IL-7 receptor$^+$ lymphoid cells that express the chemokine CXC 5 receptor and secrete lymphotoxin.[85] Mice deficient in lymphotoxin α or β, lymphotoxin β receptor, IL-7 receptor α, CXC R5, or ID2 Peyer's patches do not develop, and blockade of NFκB signaling through the lymphotoxin β receptor in IKK α deficient mice severely limits Peyer's patch formation.[86–88] Consistently with these observations, epithelial expression of IL-7 induces Peyer's patch development.[89] Of considerable functional interest, oral tolerance is absent in lymphotoxin $\alpha^{-/-}$ mice, which are devoid of both Peyer's patches and mesenteric lymph nodes.[86] Finally, GALT formation is severely impaired in mice deficient in β_7 integrin,[90] which limits lymphocyte migration to the sites, although M cell development is normal in Rag 1$^{-/-}$ (T and B cell deficient) mice, despite the small size of the lymphoid aggregates.[81] These studies demonstrate the importance of IL-7, lymphotoxin, T lymphocyte chemotactic signals, and mesenchymal cell–lymphoid cell interactions in development of Peyer's patches.

Kelsall and colleagues have demonstrated distinct anatomic locations of dendritic cell subpopulations within Peyer's patches by immunohistochemical staining.[91] Myeloid (CD11b$^+$) dendritic cells are preferentially located in the subepithelial dome region, whereas dendritic cells with lymphoid characteristics (CD8α^+) occupy the T cell rich interfollicular zone (see Fig. 2–4). The follicle-associated epithelial cells in the dome express the chemokine macrophage inflammatory protein (MIP)-3α and adjacent subepithelial dendritic cells, but not those in the interfollicular area, express the MIP-3α ligand, CCR6.[91] Supporting the concept that dome epithelial MIP-3α recruits myeloid dendritic cells to this region, CCR6 knockout mice have underdeveloped Peyer's patches, and the CD11b$^+$ dendritic cell population is not present in the subepithelial dome.[92] Furthermore, CCR6$^{-/-}$ mice have increased contact sensitivity responses, which are consistent with a relative lack of inhibitory cell induction.

Antigen Processing Cells and Antigen Presentation

Multiple cells in the GI mucosa can serve as APCs, including dendritic cells, macrophages, B lymphocytes, and epithelial cells. Although dendritic cells as "professional" APCs are more efficient than other APC populations in the GI tract,[93] they are outnumbered by B lymphocytes and epithelial cells, so the relative amount of antigen presentation performed by various APC subpopulations is unknown. In addition to their presence in Peyer's patches, dendritic cells occur in high frequency in the intestinal lamina propria, where they have been found to insert dendrites through epithelial tight junctions, presumably to sample luminal contents.[7] Antigen loaded dendritic cells from the lamina propria can migrate to draining mesenteric lymph nodes, where naive T cells entering from Peyer's patches can encounter antigen.[94] Dendritic cells in both locations express high membrane MHC class II antigens. It is probable that most physiologic uptake of antigen occurs across M cells in Peyer's patches, but when mucosal permeability is increased during inflammation, considerable presentation could occur by lamina propria dendritic cells and even macrophages.

Antigen processing occurs in two primary pathways (Fig. 2–6).[95, 96] Exogenous antigen is engulfed in coated pits, processed via the endocytic pathway into small peptides, and bound in the antigen-binding groove of complementary MHC class II molecules. Antigen binding displaces the invariant chain, which stabilizes the MHC class II molecule prior to antigen binding. This displacement of the variant chain is mediated by HLA-DM. The MHC-peptide complex is then translocated from the endosomal compartment to the

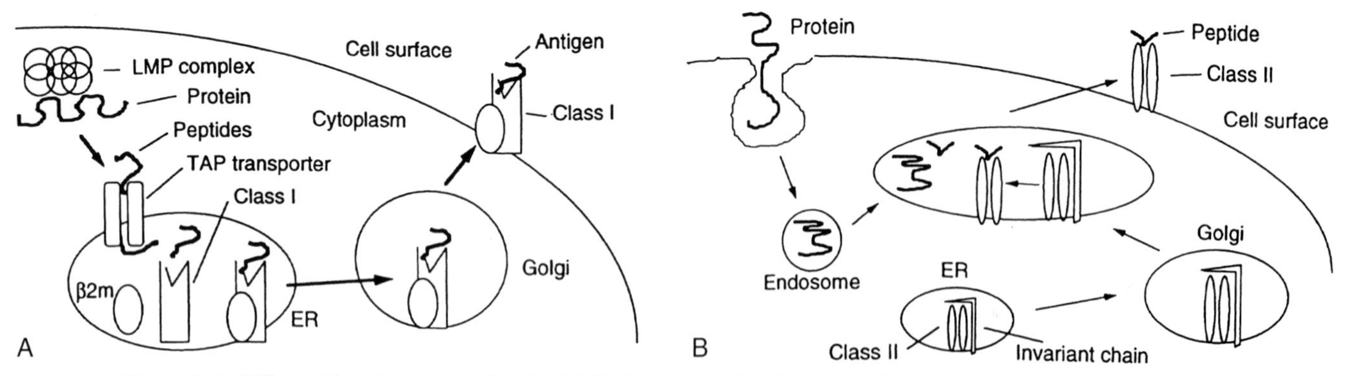

Figure 2–6. Differential antigen processing by MHC Class I– and II–bearing cells. *A*, Endogenous protein antigen is degraded in the large multifunctional proteasome (LMP) complex and transported into the endoplasmic reticulum (ER) by transport-associated proteins (TAP), where antigen binds to Class I MHC molecules. MHC Class I antigen/β_2 microglobulin complexes are then transported to the surface via Golgi. *B*, In contrast, exogenous antigen is endocytosed, degraded in the endosome, binds to MHC Class II molecules, and is transported to the surface. After being created in the ER, MHC Class II binding is blocked by invariant chain, which is removed by HLA DM. (Adapted from M. Blaser, with permission.)

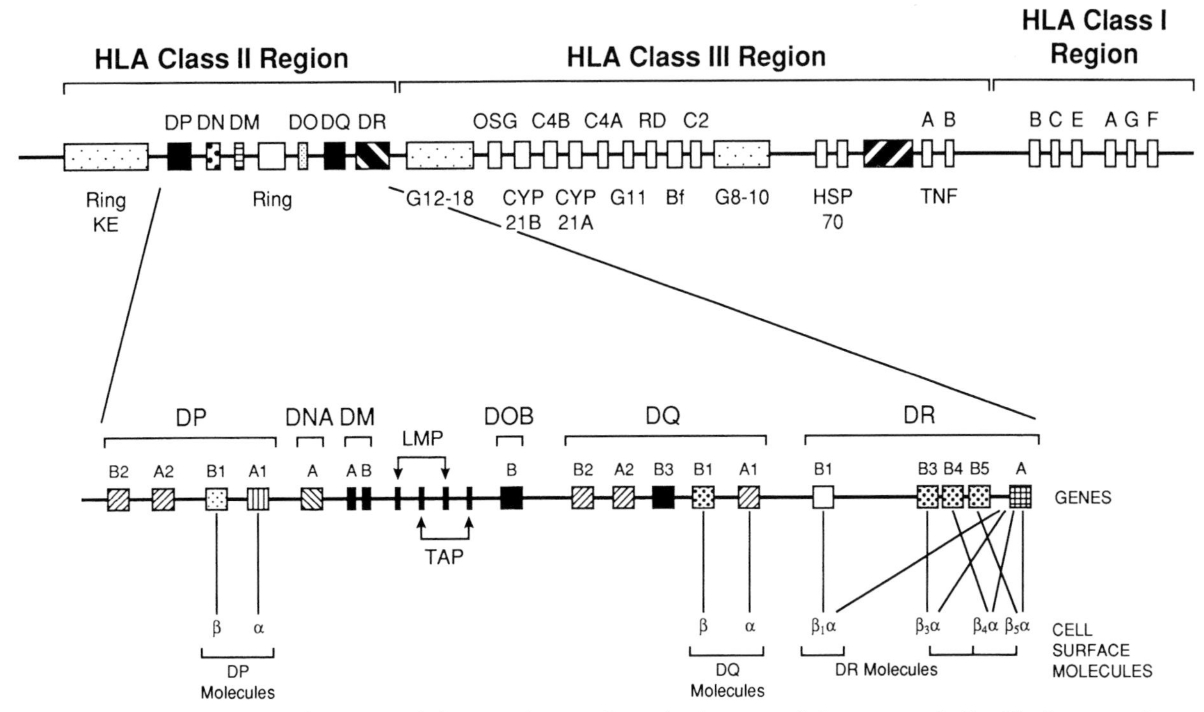

Figure 2–7. Human major histocompatibility complex (MHC) on the short arm of chromosome 6. *Top*, The human major histocompatibility complex contains several regions designated Class I, II, or III. The Class I region encodes genes for the major transplantation human leukocyte antigens (HLA-A, -B, and -C), as well as genes that encode for the less polymorphic nonclassic Class I molecules, HLA-E, -F, and -G. The Class II region (D region) encodes Class II genes (DP, DQ, DR). The HLA Class III region includes genes that code for components of complement system (C2, C4A, C4B, B1) and the enzyme steroid 21 hydroxylase (CYP 21 A and B). In addition, this region contains multiple other genes including tumor necrosis factor (TNF) and heat shock protein 70 (HSP 70). *Bottom* (expanded view), The HLA Class II D region is divided into several subregions. Each HLA-DP, -DQ, and -DR molecule contains an α chain and a β chain. DM genes code for molecules involved in peptide loading on to Class II molecules. Large multifunctional proteasome (LMP) in transport-associated protein (TAP) genes are involved in Class I antigen processing.

outer membrane, where it is recognized by CD4 T cells that bear appropriate TCR receptors that bind the presented antigen in an MHC restricted manner. In contrast, endogenous peptides produced by the host, including self-antigens or virally encoded antigens, are processed into peptides in large multifunctional proteasomes (LMPs) and transported by transport-associated proteins (TAP-1 and TAP-2) from the cytoplasm into the endoplasmic reticulum[97] (see Fig. 2–6). Here they associate with MHC class I molecules and β_2-microglobulin and then are transported to the surface membrane. CD8 T cells preferentially recognize MHC class I displayed peptides.

Because MHC class I peptides are constitutionally expressed on all cells, virtually any virally infected or transformed cell can stimulate cytolytic CD8 T cell responses. However, MHC class II expression is constitutively low on most cells, but induced by proinflammatory cytokines, particularly IFNγ. This low constitutive expression of MHC II in most cells in a noninflammatory environment limits CD4 T cell antigen presentation to dendritic cells, macrophages, B lymphocytes, and possibly intestinal epithelial cells that constitutively express MHC class II molecules. The requirement for costimulatory molecules such as CD80 ($B_{7.1}$) and CD86 ($B_{7.2}$) for T cell activation[98] further limits the repertoire of APCs. Intestinal epithelial cells express alternative nonclassic class I molecules such as CD1d, which provide an alternative mechanism for antigen presentation. A primary mechanism by which IL-10 inhibits T_{H1} responses is through down-regulation of APC activation via suppression of MHC class II and costimulatory molecules.[99]

The major histocompatibility complex encoding human HLA class I and II genes is located on chromosome 6 (Fig. 2–7).[96] This complex, which contains more than 200 genes, 40 of which comprise leukocyte antigens, also encodes proteins involved in endogenous (cytoplasmic) antigen processing and loading, such as LMP, TAP-1 and -2, and HLA-DM, and effectors of innate responses, such as TNF, inducible heat shock proteins, and complement system components, which are located in the HLA class III region. These class III molecules do not bind or present antigen and are structurally and functionally unrelated to class I and II molecules. β_2-microglobulin, involved in class I stabilization, is encoded independently on chromosome 15.

Diversity of antigens bound by MHC class I and II molecules in an individual is provided by polymorphism of class I molecules and the capacity for a wide range of combinations of class II α and β chain subunits. For example, three major class I antigens (HLA-A, -B, and -C) are present on each chromosome. The class II HLA-D region is divided into -DR, -DQ, and -DP subregions, each of which encodes an α and a β chain. The α and β chains from each region can associate with homologous subunits from the other chromosome, creating a broad array of potential binding sites. Furthermore, each HLA I or II molecule can bind multiple

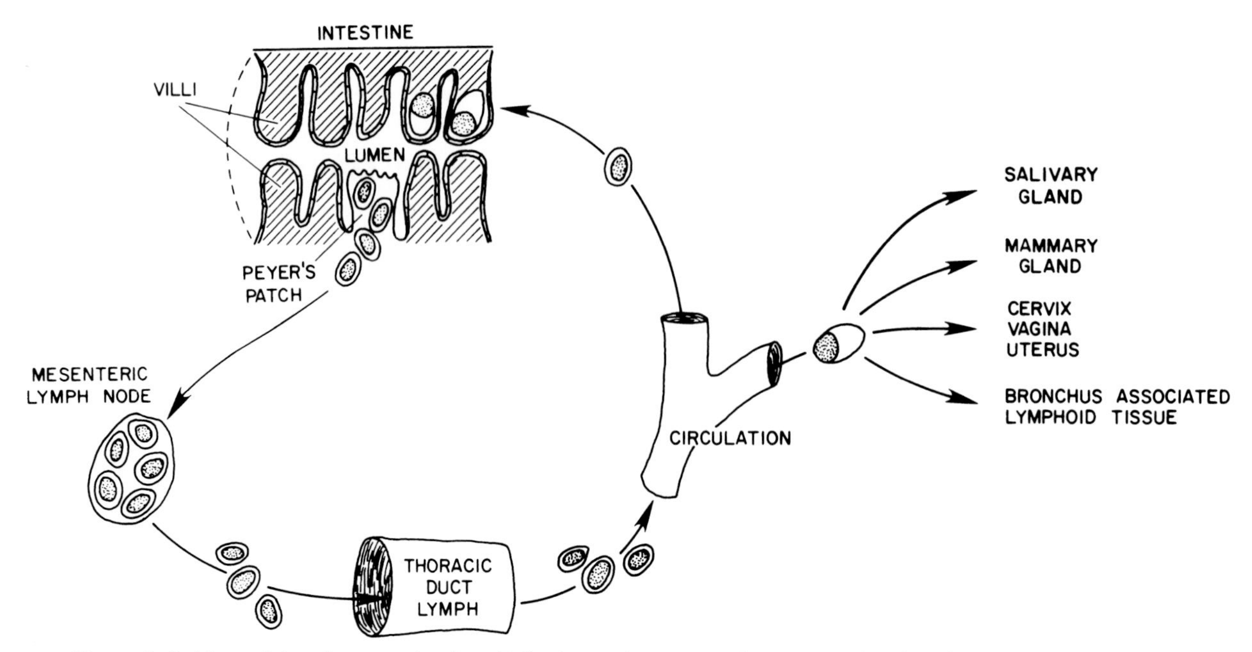

Figure 2–8. Mucosal lymphocyte migration. Following antigenic stimulation, T and B lymphocytes migrate from the intestine to the draining mesenteric lymph nodes, where they further differentiate, then reach the systemic circulation. Cells bearing the appropriate mucosal addressins then selectively home to mucosal surfaces composing the common mucosal immune system.

peptides, with affinity determined by noncovalent attraction between amino acids lining the antigen-binding groove and the degraded (processed) peptide. In this manner, an individual is genetically programmed to display a relatively predictable profile of exogenous and endogenous antigens for T cell activation. For example, HLA-DQ2, which is present in most celiac disease patients, avidly binds the glutamic acid of deamidated gluten.[100]

Migration of Lymphoid Cells

Mucosal antigen presentation to naive T lymphocytes and binding of antigen to mature but yet undifferentiated B cells that display membrane-bound IgM can occur either within Peyer's patches or homologous lymphoid aggregates in the colon and pharynx, or within draining mesenteric lymph nodes.[94] A subpopulation of bone marrow–derived native lymphocytes are predestined for mucosal targets by surface molecules that direct their distribution in a highly selective manner.[101] Most naive mucosal T and B lymphocytes display the heterodimeric membrane glycoprotein $\alpha_4\beta_7$ integrin, which avidly binds to its counterligand mucosal addressin cellular adhesion molecule (MadCAM-1). This immunoglobulin superfamily member is selectively expressed on the high endothelial postcapillary venules of Peyer's patches and mesenteric lymph nodes and on normal endothelial cells of vessels within the mucosal lamina propria. $\alpha_4\beta_7$ integrin also binds to fibronectin, which may be related to migration in the intestinal stroma after these cells translocate across blood vessels. An additional mechanism of mucosal homing is provided by L-selectin, which contains a lectin-binding domain that adheres to the sialy Lewis X blood group antigen, which can coat MadCAM-1.[102] Naive T and B lymphocytes within Peyer's patches are $\alpha_4\beta_7^{low}$, L-selectin$^+$ by flow cytometric analysis. After antigenic stimulation, these cells increase their $\alpha_4\beta_7$ expression but down-regulate L-selectin to become $\alpha_4\beta_7^{high}$, L-selectin$^-$. These activated cells migrate to the draining mesenteric lymph node, where further differentiation and clonal expansion take place. After circulating through the draining lymphatics and thoracic duct, circulating $\alpha_4\beta_7^{high}$ lymphocytes selectively home to mucosal surfaces, where endothelial cells selectively express MadCAM-1. As illustrated in Figure 2–8, mucosal sites other than the intestine attract activated lymphocytes, including salivary glands, hormonally prepared mammary and genital tissues, and the bronchus. This common mucosal homing pattern provides the foundation for targeted mucosal vaccine delivery.[103, 104] In contrast, lymphocytes that encounter antigen in peripheral sites, such as the skin or peripheral lymph nodes, display other integrins, such as $\alpha_4\beta_1$, which bind to VCAM-1, which is widely expressed and directs these activated nonmucosal lymphoid cells to return to peripheral sites. Intestinal lamina propria and intraepithelial lymphocytes selectively express a G protein–coupled receptor, GPR-9–6, which is expressed in a subset of $\alpha_4\beta_7$ memory CD4 and CD8 lymphocytes. GPR-9–6 binds to thymus expressed chemokine (TECK), which is selectively expressed in the thymus and small intestine.[105]

Most (95%) intraepithelial lymphocytes display a relatively unusual integrin, $\alpha_E\beta_7$ (human mucosal lymphocyte integrin-1 [HML-1], CD103), which binds avidly to E-cadherin, which is selectively expressed on the basolateral intestinal epithelial membrane.[106] This interaction provides a mechanism for anchoring IELs to epithelial surfaces.

Clinical Relevance

Blockade of either $\alpha_4\beta_7$, or MadCAM-1 should selectively inhibit migration of activated T and B lymphocytes into the intestine. Although this strategy may theoretically be effec-

Table 2–3 | **Distribution of Immunoglobulin Producing Cells in the Human Gastrointestinal Tract***

LOCATION	IgA+	IgM	IgG
Gastric body	74	12	14
Gastric antrum	80	8	12
Duodenum and jejunum	79	17	4
Ileum	80	11	5
Colon	90	6	4

*Percentage of total Ig-containing cells.
+These IgA producing cells secrete IgA_1 or IgA_2; percentage of IgA containing cells that secrete IgA_1 ranges from 38% (colon) to 85% (gastric antrum).
Ig, immunoglobulin.
Adapted from Mestecky J, McGhee JR, Elson CO: Intestinal IgA system. Immunol Allergy Clin North Am 8:349, 1988.

tive for reducing intestinal inflammation, the approach has the conceptual disadvantage of preventing entry of regulatory (protective) lymphocytes, thereby potentially exacerbating ongoing disease or promoting inflammation or infection in normal hosts. In practice, however, an antibody neutralizing α_4 integrin was able to decrease inflammation in a European Crohn's disease population significantly.[107] It is probable that regulatory cells expressing this integrin are limited in inflammatory bowel diseases so that use of this antibody would preferentially inhibit aggressive T cell populations.

Humoral Pathways

After antigen binds to membrane IgM, B cells are activated by signal transduction mediated by associated transmembrane Ig-α and Ig-β glycoproteins. Activated B cells can experience changes in the immunoglobulin heavy chain (switching), influenced by T cell cytokine profiles. IgA switching is mediated by TGF-β,[108] whereas IFNγ promotes human IgG_2 and murine IgG_{2a}, and IL-4 stimulates human IgG_1 and murine IgG_1. Most mucosal B cells (74% to 90%) produce IgA (Table 2–3). After final arrangement, activated B cells terminally differentiate into plasma cells, which secrete high concentrations of IgA and other immunoglobulin isoforms into the lamina propria.

Unique features of mucosal IgA include its dimeric nature and specific carrier-mediated secretion into the gut lumen. In contrast to circulating, peripherally produced monomeric IgA, IgA produced in the mucosa is predominantly dimeric bound by J chain, which is produced and secreted by plasma cells (Fig. 2–9). Dimeric IgA secreted by lamina propria plasma cells is covalently bound to the secretory component (polymeric immunoglobulin receptor, or PIgR), which is synthesized in epithelial cells and is anchored to their basal lateral membrane (Fig. 2–10). The dimeric IgA–J chain–PIgR complex is then internalized into the epithelial cell as a membrane-bound vesicle and secreted into the intestinal lumen after protease cleavage releases the extra membrane secretory component. PIgR renders dimeric IgA resistant to degradation by luminal digestive and bacterial proteases. The secreted IgA complex binds to luminal antigen to prevent mucosal contact and uptake. Secreted IgA inhibits mucosal adherence by enteropathogenic bacteria, neutralizes viruses, and enhances clearance of pathogenic organisms, although it does not bind complement or initiate cytotoxic effects. Therefore, secreted IgA functions to complex luminal antigens rather than to kill bacteria. PIgR preferentially binds polymeric Ig molecules and can facilitate secretion of pentameric IgM in a similar fashion. Analogous secretory pathways present in biliary epithelia account for very significant biliary IgA secretion by mice. Mucosal plasma cells in the distal intestine produce more IgA_2 than IgA_1, whereas circulating IgA is 85% monomeric IgA_1. Muscosal production of IgA exceeds 3 g/day.

T Lymphocyte Activation and Differentiation

T lymphocyte activation and differentiation depend on several simultaneous events, including recognition of antigen presented in the MHC antigen-binding groove of an APC; ligation of costimulatory molecules, which requires intimate contact with the APC; and secretion of cytokines from the APC (Fig. 2–11).[96] As discussed earlier, CD4 T cells preferentially recognize foreign antigens bound to MHC class II molecules, whereas CD8 lymphocytes bind to MHC class I–bound peptides (see Fig. 2–3). However, binding to MHC-antigen complexes without ligation of costimulatory molecules induces anergy rather than T cell activation. The two primary sets of costimulatory molecules include CD40/CD40 ligand and CD80 ($B_{7.1}$) or CD86 ($B_{7.2}$)/CD28 or cytotoxic T lymphocyte–associated antigen-4 (CTLA-4) (see Fig. 2–11). Both CD80 and CD86 can bind to either CD28 on cells destined to differentiate into T_{H1} cells, or to CTLA-4 on regulatory T cell precursors (T_{R1} cells). In vitro and in vivo neutralizing antibody studies demonstrate profound inhibition of T cell activation after blockade of either CD40 or CD80/86.[98] Similarly, IL-12 (or IL-18) produced by APC potently

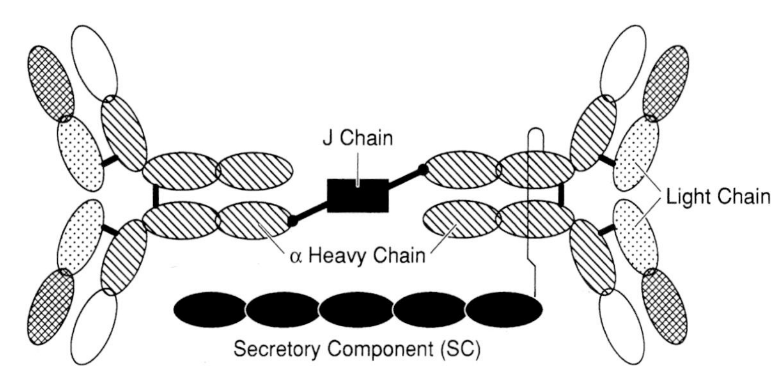

Figure 2–9. Secretory IgA complex. Two IgA molecules are linked by a J chain and stabilized by secretory component (polymeric Ig receptor) to form dimeric secretory IgA.

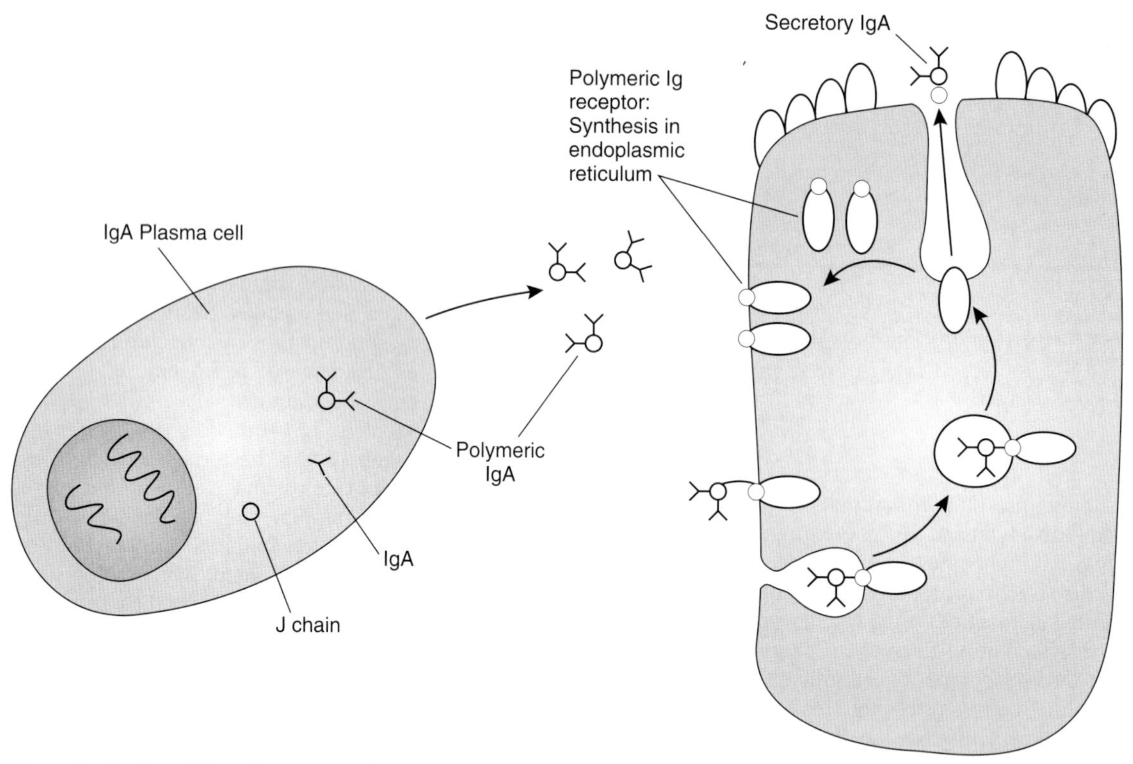

Figure 2–10. Assembly and secretion of dimeric IgA. IgA and J chain produced by IgA committed plasma cells dimerize to form polymeric IgA, which covalently binds to membrane bound polymeric Ig receptor produced by epithelial cells. This complex is transported to the apical surface of the epithelial cell and secreted into the lumen.

stimulates T_{H1} cell activation. APC cytokine production and costimulatory molecule expression are amplified by various adjuvants, including physiologically relevant bacterial cell wall polymers such as peptidoglycan-polysaccharide complexes (the active constituent of Freund's adjuvant but found in almost all bacteria) and LPS, found in Gram-negative bacteria.[109]

An alternative mechanism of luminal antigen presentation and T cell activation action is that of the intestinal epithelial cell as an APC. Several groups have demonstrated the capacity of human intestinal epithelial cells to express MHC class II molecules and to activate T lymphocytes, which preferentially have a suppressor phenotype, in an antigen specific manner.[110–112] Mayer and colleagues have demonstrated that intestinal epithelial cells preferentially induce CD8 lymphocytes through ligation with nonclassic CD1d molecules with costimulation provided by a 180-kd glycoprotein, shown to be an isoform of carcinoembryonic antigen (CEA).[113] Similarly to stimulation with other APCs, activation of epithelial stimulated T cells occurs through a cascade

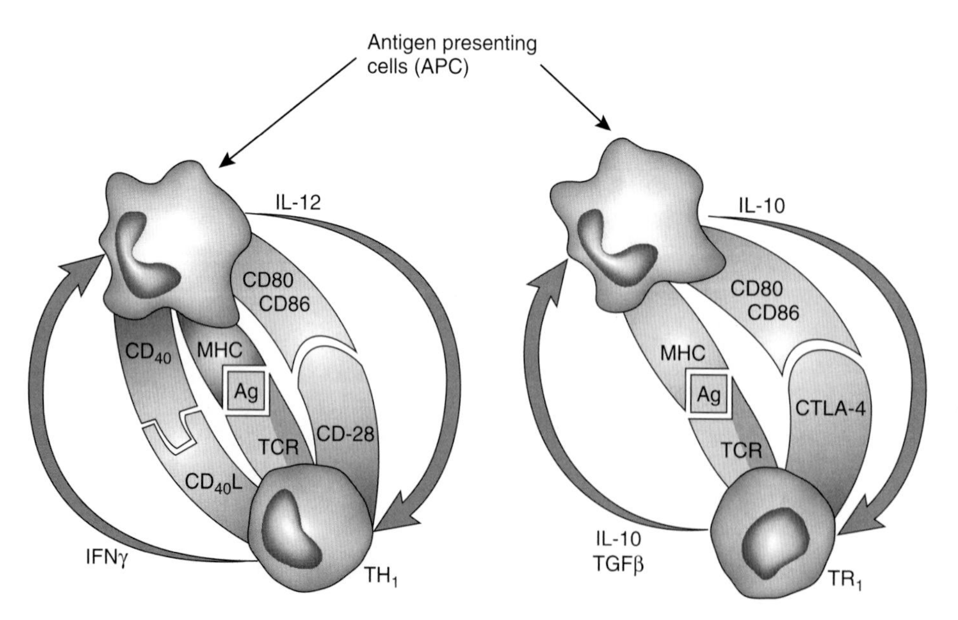

Figure 2–11. APC T cell interactions determine T cell subsets. APC-bearing MHC-bound antigen activates T cells through costimulatory molecules and secreted cytokines. A feedback loop is created by secreted products of the engaged T cell which regulate APC cell function. See text for more details.

of signaling events triggered by phosphorylation of lck by the cytoplasmic tail of engaged CD3 molecules.[114]

As T cells become activated, they display surface proteins, which can be used to phenotype their stage of activation. For example, resting murine mucosal CD4 cells express relatively high levels of L-selectin and CD45RB, but relatively low levels of $\alpha_4\beta_7$ integrin, CD25 (IL-2 receptor), and CD69. Activation decreases L-selectin and CD45RB levels but increases levels of the homing marker $\alpha_4\beta_7$, CD25, and CD69, which serve as phenotypic markers of activation. After cessation of antigen stimulation, both T and B lymphocyte clones persist as long-lived antigen specific memory cells that are capable of rapidly expanding when confronted with the same antigen or a cross-reacting antigen. This property provides the basis for immunization and is indefinitely perpetuated by periodic boosters (re-exposure to the initial antigen). As compared to peripheral blood T cells, mature lamina propria T cells proliferate poorly to antigenic, nonspecific mitogenic, or anti-CD3 antibody stimulation but actively secrete cytokines and preferentially respond to CD2 ligation.[115]

Naive CD4 and CD8 T lymphocytes can differentiate into at least three functionally different subsets that dramatically influence patterns of immune response, and hence normal mucosal homeostasis versus inflammation (Fig. 2–12). These pathways are determined in part by cytokine signals from the interacting APC and the costimulatory molecules expressed by the T cell. For example, IL-12 secreted by the APC and ligation of T cell CD28 by CD80 or CD86 ($B_{7.1}$ or $B_{7.2}$) on the APC stimulate development of T_{H1} cells that secrete IFNγ, IL-2, and TNF. These cytokines stimulate aggressive T cell–mediated immune responses and granulomatous inflammation. Alternatively, IL-10 produced by APC or ligation of T cell CTLA-4 by APC CD80 or CD86 fosters development of regulatory T lymphocyte populations that predominantly secrete TGF-β (T_{H3} cells) or IL-10 (T_{R1}) and which mediate tolerance and down-regulate pathogenic responses.[116, 117] It is controversial whether the T_{H2} pathway of cells secreting IL-4, IL-5, and IL-10 and mediating hypersensitivity responses is a default mechanism in the intestine. In mice, in which clear T_{H1} versus T_{H2} patterns of inflammation develop, these pathways are mutually exclusive, as IFNγ inhibits T_{H2} development, IL-4 down-regulates T_{H1} cells, and IL-10 and TGF-β inhibit both T_{H1} and $T_{H2}2$ responses.[118] However, the T_{H1}-T_{H2} paradigm is far less evident in humans.[119]

Table 2–4 | **Mechanisms of Immune Tolerance**

MECHANISM	DOSE OF ANTIGEN
Clonae deletion of responding cells	High
Anergy	High
Receptor down-regulation (transient)	High
Active suppression of immune response(s)	
T_{H2} lymphocytes (IL-4)	Low
T_{H3} lymphocytes (TGF-β)	Low
T_{R1} lymphocytes (IL-10)	Low
CD25+/CD4+ lymphocytes (TGF-β and IL-10)	High/low

IL, interleukin; TGF, transforming growth factor; T_{H3}, T helper 3; T_{R1}, T regulatory 1.

Modified from Weiner HL. Oral tolerance, an actine immunologic process mediated by multiple infection. Immunol Rev 127:183, 1992.

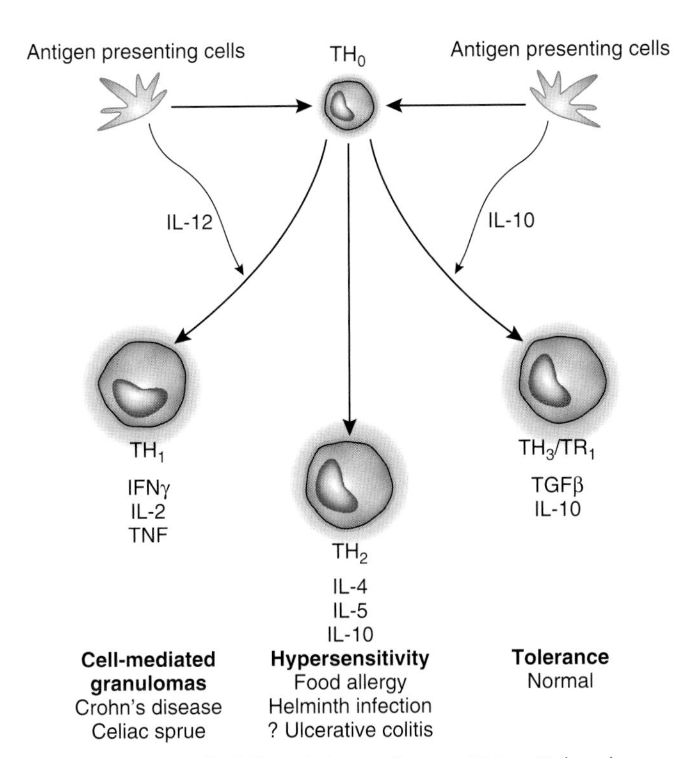

Figure 2–12. T cell differentiation pathways. Naïve T lymphocytes (THo) can differentiate into three separate subsets, with different functions being determined by secreted cytokine profiles. (Modified from the American Gastroenterological Association Teaching Project, Washington, D.C., with permission.)

Clinical Implications

As discussed later in "Inflammatory Responses," several human GI inflammatory disorders including Crohn's disease, gluten sensitive enteropathy, graft-versus-host disease, and transplant rejection have a T_{H1} profile of cytokines, whereas parasitic infections, food allergies, and eosinophilic gastroenteritis appear to be T_{H1}-mediated. Selective blockade of key cytokines (IL-12 for T_{H1} diseases, IL-4 for T_{H2} disorders), costimulatory molecules (CD40/CD40L and CD80, CD86/CD28 for T_{H1} disorders), and signal transduction pathways (STAT-3 for T_{H1}) should have a profound capacity to treat these disorders. Conversely, up-regulating intrinsic regulatory T cell populations should attenuate T_{H1}- or T_{H2}-mediated diseases with minimal toxicity.

Regulation of Tolerance

Oral tolerance is strictly defined as suppression of cellular and/or humoral immune responses to an antigen by prior oral administration of the same antigen.[120] This unresponsive state can develop from a variety of pathways and in part depends on the dose of antigen administered (Table 2–4). Feeding high doses of a foreign antigen, such as ovalbumin, leads to transient (3-day) down-regulation of TCR recognizing this antigen, followed by clonal deletion of responding cells.[121] Feeding low-dose antigen, however, activates long-lived regulatory T lymphocytes (T_{H3} or T_{R1} cells secreting

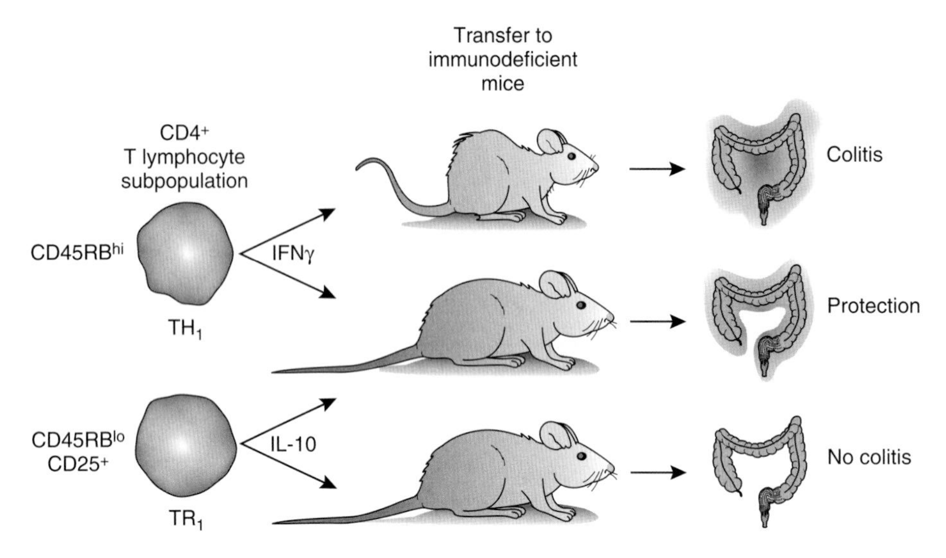

Figure 2–13. Counterbalancing effects of T cell subsets. $CD4^+$T cells isolated from the spleen of normal mice contain subsets with differentiated immunologic activities. $CD45RB^{hi}$ (naïve, undifferentiated cells) transfer colitis to immunodeficient recipients. Activated memory phenotypes ($CD45RB^{lo}$, $CD25^+$) contain IL-10 secreting regulatory cells, which prevent the onset of colitis when cotransferred with the $CD45RB^{hi}$ population. (Modified from American Gastroenterological Association Teaching Project, with permission.)

TGF-β or IL-10, respectively) that actively suppress T_{H1}, T_{H2}, and systemic antibody responses.[122, 123] Low-dose oral tolerance appears to be more analogous to intestinal conditions in which ubiquitous luminal bacterial and dietary antigens continuously bathe the GI mucosa. A study demonstrating that IL-12 induction in human Peyer's patch cells obtained after feeding suggests that human and murine tolerogenic mechanisms may be different.[124] The presence of a regulatory T cell population capable of suppressing aggressive immunologic responses to ubiquitous enteric bacteria is elegantly demonstrated by T lymphocyte subset cotransfer experiments into T cell deficient hosts in which $CD4^+$ $CD45RB^{lo}$ T cells (activated phenotype) suppress colitis induced by homologous $CD4^+$ $CD45RB^{hi}$ cells[125, 126] (Fig. 2–13). These studies clearly demonstrate that normal hosts simultaneously contain T cells capable of both inducing and preventing colitis, and that under normal conditions the suppressor phenotype is dominant.[117] This concept is relevant to other organs, because $CD4^+$ $CD25^+$ IL-2 receptor (activated phenotype) T cells are capable of suppressing autoimmune gastritis.[127] Similarly, Powrie and colleagues have demonstrated that $CD25^+$ cells convey the protective properties of $CD45RB^{lo}$ cells and that CTLA-4 is an essential determinant of suppression of these responses.[128]

The importance of the thymus in negative selection of autoreactive T lymphocytes is illustrated by the development of autoimmune gastritis in mice after neonatal thymectomy.[129] In this model inflammation is mediated by T_{H1} lymphocytes that react to H^+/K^+-adenosine triphosphatase (H^+/K^+-ATPase) on gastric parietal cells, which undergo Fas-induced apoptosis.[129, 130] Similarly, in CD3ϵ transgenic mice, which have a block in early T and B cell ontogeny and abnormal thymic development, colitis mediated by T_{H1} cells responsive to luminal bacterial antigens develops following bone marrow transplant from a normal MHC-matched donor.[131, 132] Inflammation in both of these models is presumably the result of defective thymic deletion of reactive T cells or induction of protective regulatory cells.

Clinical Relevance

The leading hypothesis of the causes of human inflammatory bowel disease (IBD), gluten sensitive enteropathy, autoimmune gastritis, and autoimmune hepatitis is loss of immunologic tolerance to commensal bacteria, a dietary protein, or self-antigens, respectively. Stimulation of effective tolerogenic responses could reverse such immunoregulatory disorders, as is currently being attempted in large clinical trials in multiple sclerosis, rheumatoid arthritis, and type I diabetes.[120] Such attempts are probably more effective when combined with antibodies to block detrimental responses (e.g., anti–IL-12) and/or with cytokines stimulating protective responses (e.g., IL-10, TGF-β). Conversely, oral tolerance must be transiently blocked in order for effective mucosal immunization to be effective. Strategies used for immunization include bacterial adjuvants (cholera toxin), microsphere encapsulation, expression in attenuated pathogens, and expression of virus-like particles in transgenic food.[103]

INFLAMMATORY RESPONSES

Mechanisms

Acute inflammation can occur in all regions of the GI tract as a result of pathogenic infections, luminal toxins, or ischemia that leads to diverse, clinically important conditions. Normal hosts promptly clear the invading pathogen and heal the injury through controlled immune responses that appropriately down-regulate potentially detrimental reactions after antigenic stimulation ceases. Chronic inflammation can arise in genetically susceptible hosts with defective mucosal host defense mechanisms or dysregulated immune responses, fostering inappropriately aggressive reactions to ubiquitous antigens.

Immune Responses That Clear Pathogens in Normal Hosts

In broad terms, bacterial and fungal infections are cleared by neutrophils, macrophages, and T_{H1} immune responses, and protection from parasitic infections is mediated by eosinophils, mast cells, and T_{H2} activation. Protection from viruses is dependent on neutralizing antibodies and cytotoxic T cells. In each situation, epithelial cells initiate the inflammatory response by secreting the appropriate profile of chemokines, that is, IL-8, macrophage chemoattractant protein-1 (MCP-1), and interferon γ inducible protein-10 (IP-10) on bacterial invasion and eotaxin after parasitic infestation, with feedback from skewed profiles of cytokines secreted by infiltrating T cell subsets.[27, 51] Plasma cell secretion of appropriate immunoglobulin classes, that is, IgM and IgG for bacterial, fungal, and viral infections, and IgE for helminths, facilitates pathogen clearance by optimizing bacterial phagocytosis by neutrophils and macrophages through IgG and IgM, activating mast cells and eosinophils through IgE, and minimizing spread of the infection by blocking the membrane-binding receptors of pathogens with IgA, IgG, and IgM. This coordinated response of the innate, cognate, and humoral effector mechanisms leads to efficient clearance of invading pathogens with minimal damage to surrounding tissues. When these clearance mechanisms are defective, the intestine can suffer chronic inflammatory consequences due to protracted infections; poorly regulated responses lead to induction of overly aggressive responses to ubiquitous luminal or self-antigens.

The study of rodents deficient in targeted chemokines, cytokines, or cell populations has clarified mechanisms of host responses to parasites. Expulsion of helminths is dependent on T lymphocytes that develop a T_{H2} profile of cytokines, including IL-4 and IL-5.[133, 134] IL-4 up-regulates the C-C chemokine eotaxin,[51] which regulates entry of eosinophils into the intestine.[55] IL-5 facilitates eosinophil entry to the intestine and contributes in a minor fashion to clearance of primary experimental *Trichinella spiralis* infection[52] but is an important determinant of protection on worm reintroduction.[135] T lymphocytes are essential for mucosal mast cell proliferation after *N. brasiliensis* infection and appear to mediate villous atrophy in this model, because epithelial damage is not altered by mast cell deficiency.[136] Intestinal mast cell accumulation after *N. brasiliensis* infection was decreased by neutralizing antibodies to $\alpha_4\beta_7$ integrin, although eosinophil entry and serum IgE levels were not affected,[137] suggesting that mast cell migration (or T cell regulation of their entry) may be dependent on this adhesion molecule. In contrast, small intestinal eosinophil accumulation and *Trichuris muris* clearance were significantly impaired in β_7 integrin$^{-/-}$ mice, with no alteration in colonic eosinophil numbers, suggesting that eosinophil entry to the small intestine is regulated by the β_7 integrin.[54] Together, these results demonstrate important interaction among eosinophils, mast cells, IgE, T_{H2} lymphocytes, and epithelial production of chemotactic cytokines (chemokines) in generating protective responses to certain helminthic infections.

Bacterial, fungal, or parasitic adherence to or invasion of intestinal epithelial cells initiates an NFκB-regulated response, culminating in production of chemokines that recruit neutrophils, macrophages, and T cells to the intestine.[27, 36] Newly recruited innate effector cells are activated by products of the invading organisms, or by LPS, formylated methionyl-leucyl-phenylalanine (FMLP), and peptidoglycan entry from the lumen secondary to enhanced mucosal permeability with the initial injury or as a consequence of disruption of epithelial tight junctions by transmigrating neutrophils.[138] Phagocytosis of the invading pathogen or translocating commensal bacteria is augmented by opsonizing IgG or IgM, which is recognized by membrane-bound IgG or IgM Fc receptors on macrophages and neutrophils. Liberation of IFNγ by microbial antigen specific T_{H1} lymphocytes further activates macrophages to facilitate clearance of the infection.

Mucosal immune responses to viral infections are less well studied, but host protection is primarily dependent on neutralizing IgG or IgM antibodies and cytotoxic T cell responses, especially CD8 lymphocytes, which recognize intracellular antigens bound to MHC class I molecules (see "Antigen Processing Cells and Antigen Presentation"). A number of enteric viruses, including reovirus, astroviruses, and HIV, selectively adhere to and enter M cells overlying Peyer's patches,[139] thereby evading the normal epithelial sensory mechanisms.

Defective host immune responses due to absent or inefficient innate or cognate immune functions, either congenital or acquired, result in a number of bacterial, fungal, parasitic, and viral infections, with predictable profiles of pathogens characteristic of each immunodeficiency state (Table 2–5).

Defective Mucosal Protection

Mucosal inflammation or infection of the GI tract can arise from dysregulated host effector immune cells or be a consequence of loss of mucosal barrier function, either acquired or genetically determined. Defective immunologic function leads to opportunistic infections; loss of barrier integrity leads to enhanced uptake of ubiquitous luminal antigens that overwhelmingly stimulate lamina propria responses.

Very different mechanisms of immunodeficiency involving decreased innate and cognate responses, either genetic or acquired, lead to similar outcomes of chronic diarrhea, malabsorption, parasitic infestation (particularly by *Giardia* species), fungal colonization (especially by *Candida* species), persistence of intracellular bacteria (by *Mycobacterium* species), and neoplasms (Kaposi's sarcoma, lymphomas) (see Table 2–5). In general, defective secreted immunoglobulin results in relatively mild parasitic infection (e.g., giardiasis), T cell defects lead to fungal and viral infections and tumors, neutrophil abnormalities result in bacterial infections, and combined deficiencies have a wider spectrum of pathologic infections. Iatrogenic immunosuppression due to chemotherapy or the increasingly widespread use of potent immunosuppressive therapeutic agents is becoming more common, generating concern about the increased frequency of opportunistic infections and neoplasms. For example, chimeric anti-TNF antibody (infliximab) for Crohn's disease has been associated with reactivation of tuberculosis, *Pneumocystis* pneumonia, mycotic aneurysms, lymphomas, and solid tumors,[140, 141] although the frequency of these complications is unknown and the incidence of neoplasms in chronic Crohn's disease patients is uncertain.

Either acquired or genetically determined defects in barrier function (Fig. 2–14) result in enhanced uptake of luminal antigens and secondary bacterial invasion.[142] Environmental toxins such as nonsteroidal anti-inflammatory drugs (NSAIDs), including to a lesser extent newer selective COX-2 inhibitors, can induce ulcers in the stomach, small intestine, and colon and block protective prostaglandins, which have cytoprotective as well as immunosuppressive activity.[143] Similarly, *C. difficile* cytotoxins A and B and enteropathogenic *E. coli* directly injure epithelial tight junctions by disassembling actin microfilaments and by dissociating occludin from intestinal tight junctions, respectively.[19, 20] The

Table 2–5 | **Gastrointestinal Manifestations of Immunodeficiency Syndromes**

SYNDROME	MECHANISM	INHERITANCE	GASTROINTESTINAL MANIFESTATIONS
IgA deficiency	80% ↓ B cell maturation, 20% ↓ T cell help	Autosomal	Variable, *Giardia* infection, NLH
Common variable immunodeficiency	↓ B cell maturation, CD40 defects, ↓ cytokines	Autosomal	*Giardia,* bacterial overgrowth, NLH, atrophic gastritis
Bruton's X-linked agammaglobulinemia	↓ Pre–B cell maturation	X-linked	*Giardia* infection, rotavirus, diarrhea
Hyper IgM syndrome	Mutations in CD40L	Autosomal	Diarrhea, oral ulcers
DiGeorge's syndrome	Thymic hypoplasia	X-linked or autosomal recessive	Diarrhea, malabsorption, *Candida* infection
Severe combined immunodeficiency	↓ Adenosine deaminase, ↓ Purine nucleoside phosphorylase, ↓ MHC class II	X-linked or autosomal recessive	Diarrhea, malabsorption, *Candida* infection, parasites
Chronic granulomatous disease	↓ NADPH oxidase	X-linked or autosomal recessive	Stomatitis, antral obstruction, Crohn's disease–like colitis, perianal abscess
Protein-losing enteropathy	↓ Ig	Nongenetic (see Chapter 25)	Variable, secondary to underlying disorder
Iatrogenic (chemotherapy, immunosuppressives)	↓ Neutrophils, T cells	Nongenetic	Fungal, parasitic, viral infections
HIV	↓ $CD4^+$ T cells, macrophages	Nongenetic (see Chapter 28)	Fungal, parasitic, viral, intracellular bacterial infections, Kaposi's sarcoma, lymphoma

HIV, human immunodeficiency virus; Ig, immunoglobulin; MHC, major histocompatibility complex; NADPH, nicotinamide-adenine dinucleotide phosphate, reduced form; NLH, nodular lymphoid hyperplasia.

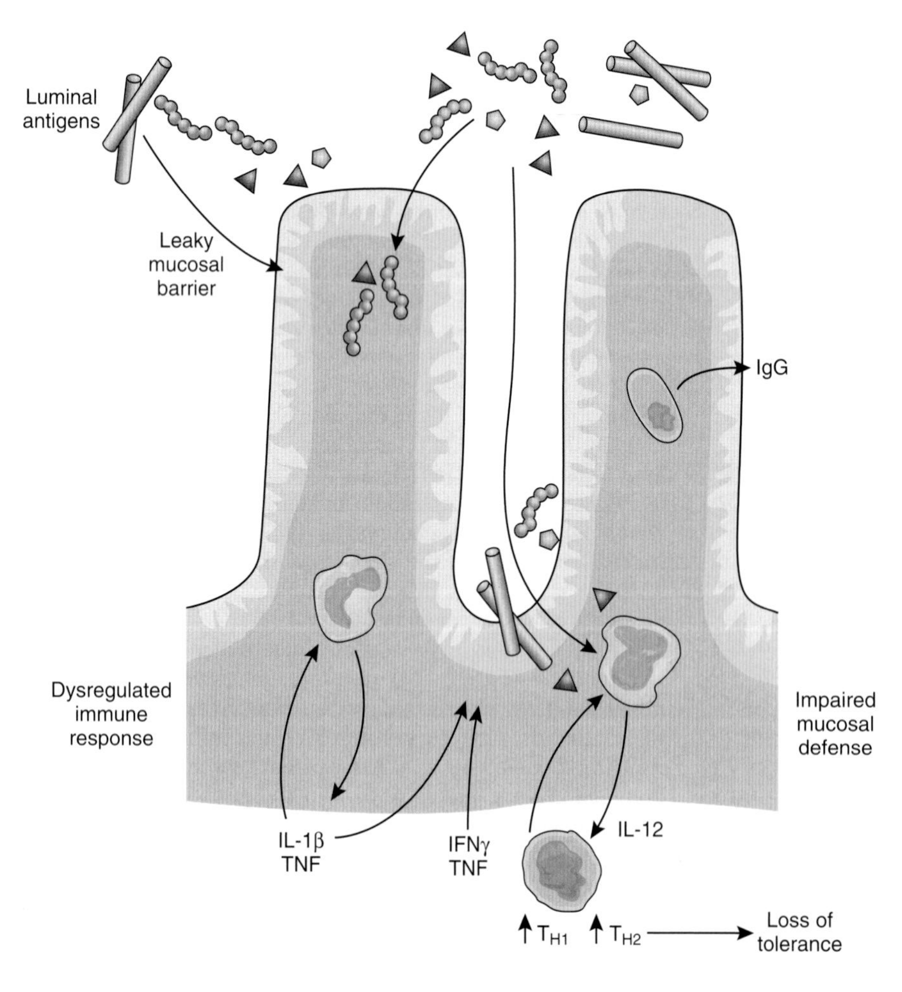

Figure 2–14. Induction of inflammation in susceptible hosts. Luminal antigens stimulate lamina propria macrophages and T cells to secrete proinflammatory cytokines with a T_{H1} profile if they cross the mucosal barrier in a host with a dysregulated immune response. Stimulation of metalloproteases and liberation of reactive O_2 metabolites in concert with secreted cytokines induce tissue destruction. (Modified from the American Gastroenterological Association Teaching Project, Washington, D.C., with permission.)

net effect of breaking the mucosal barrier is an onslaught of phlogistic luminal bacterial components, activating innate responses that recruit neutrophils, monocytes, and T cells to the area of injury, analogous to invasion of the mucosa by pathogenic microorganisms. As with transient infections, the normal host rapidly heals soon after the offending environmental toxin or microbial pathogen is cleared (as discussed later).

In contrast, genetically determined abnormalities of barrier function can lead to more protracted inflammatory events.[144] Observations in rodent models indicate that abnormalities in intercellular epithelial adhesion due to targeted deletion of N-cadherin in the small intestine lead to focal inflammation[22] and that deletion of intestinal trefoil factor had no phenotype unless colonic inflammation was initiated with dextran sodium sulfate, after which the deficient mice had exacerbated disease and enhanced mortality rates. The T cell profile of these mice is not reported, so it is unclear whether such events can induce pathologic T_{H1} or T_{H2} responses in mice with normal, protective immune function. However, it is evident that even a transient breach in the mucosal barrier can lead to long-term inflammation in genetically susceptible hosts. For example, in Lewis rats that received two subcutaneous injections of indomethacin chronic mid–small bowel ulcers that persisted for 77 days developed,[145] and NSAID treatment dramatically accelerated onset of colitis in susceptible IL-$10^{-/-}$ mice.[146]

Dysregulated Immune Responses to Ubiquitous Antigens in Susceptible Hosts

Whether mucosal homeostasis (tolerance) or chronic inflammation develops depends on the relative balance of pro- and anti-inflammatory mediators and regulatory T lymphocytes (see Figs. 2–12 and 2–15). As discussed, normal hosts exhibit active T cell–mediated suppression to commensal bacteria, tolerance, or anergy to dietary antigens, depending on the dose administered, and thymic deletion of T cells recognizing self-antigens. In contrast, genetically susceptible hosts with defective regulation of immunologic responses can mount pathogenic immune responses to ubiquitous bacterial, dietary, and self-antigens. Murine models of experimental colitis clearly illustrate this concept.[147] For example, overexpression of TNF promotes ileal inflammation, perianal fistulas, and peripheral arthritis,[148, 149] and blockade of IL-1, TNF, IL-6, IL-12, and IFNγ signaling and the chemotactic molecule leukotriene B_4 (LTB_4) inhibits intestinal inflammation.[150] In contrast, targeted deletion of IL-10 or TGF-β leads to colitis,[151, 152] and IL-1 receptor antagonist and COX-2 knockout mice have potentiated responses to injury from dextran sodium sulfate, despite having normal phenotypes in the absence of triggering agents.[153, 154] Similarly, inhibition of COX-1 inhibits recovery from radiation damage.[155] Delivery of TGF-β by nasal plasmid[156] and of IL-10 by recombinant bacteria colonizing the intestine[157] reverses experimental colitis, supporting the therapeutic potential of using novel approaches to stimulate host protective responses. Most models of chronic intestinal inflammation exhibit T_{H1} cytokine profiles with activated macrophages and B lymphocytes and are dependent on the chronic antigenic stimulation of resident enteric bacteria.[142, 147] Similarly, *Helicobacter* species–induced gastric and intestinal inflammation and *Citrobacter rodentium*–induced colitis have T_{H1} cytokine profiles.[158–160] The dominant role of commensal luminal bacteria in the pathogenesis of chronic immune-mediated intestinal inflammation is convincingly demonstrated by the lack of inflammation in the sterile (germ-free) environment in at least 13 different experimental models, induction of inflammation and immune activation after population of germ-free susceptible rodents with specific pathogen-free bacteria, attenuation of disease by broad-spectrum antibiotics, and demonstration of luminal bacterial antigen specific CD4 T cell responses in mice with colitis.[132, 142] Similarly, food antigens such as deaminated gliadin can stimulate T_{H1} mucosal responses in susceptible hosts, as demonstrated in celiac disease patients.[160, 161] Polymorphism in the CTLA-4 gene, a costimulatory molecule that determines responses after APC T cell ligation, was associated with celiac disease and a number of autoimmune disorders in studies conducted in 2000 and 2001.[162, 163] The key role of counter-regulatory T lymphocyte subsets is elegantly demonstrated by the ability of IL-10–secreting T cell clones responding to cecal bacterial antigens to prevent colitis in immunodeficient recipient mice populated with cotransferred IFNγ secreting T_{H1} clones responding to the same bacterial antigen.[164] Together, these results support the hypothesis that chronic GI inflammation is the result of overly aggressive cell-mediated immunologic responses to ubiquitous luminal bacterial or dietary antigens in genetically susceptible hosts, caused by either defective immunoregulation or abnormal host defense mechanisms.

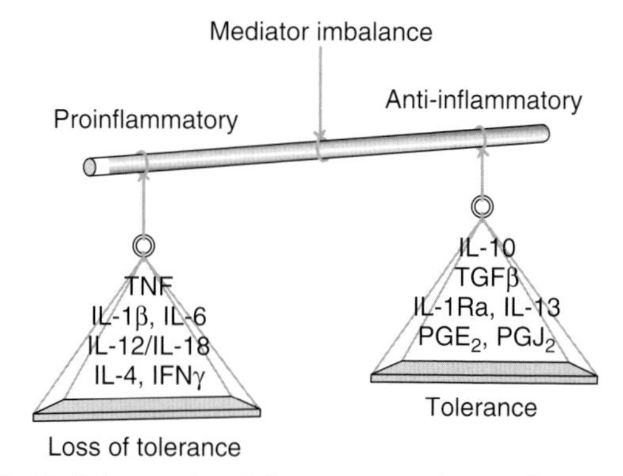

Figure 2–15. Balance of proinflammatory and anti-inflammatory cytokines. The relative balance of proinflammatory and protective cytokines and inflammatory mediators determines tissue injury (loss of tolerance) versus protection (tolerance). (Modified from the American Gastroenterological Association Teaching Project, Washington, D.C., with permission.)

Effector Pathways

Both acute and chronic phases of inflammation are mediated by a complex cascade of interacting immune and effector cells of hematopoietic, mesenchymal, endothelial, and epithelial origin; soluble inflammatory molecules; and neuroendocrine mediators. Cellular infiltration depends on the relative balance of infiltrating, newly recruited cells; egress of cells into the lumen; and apoptosis. Although superficially chaotic, each of these interactive pathways has well-described, redundant regulatory mechanisms that lead to controlled reactions in the normal, resistant host that appropriately down-regulate physiologic inflammatory responses. Less well identified are the defects in immunoregulation leading to protracted, injurious immune responses in genetically susceptible individuals caused by either overly aggressive reaction to ubiquitous antigens or, conversely, ineffective clearance of pathogenic organisms.

Soluble Mediators

Activated inflammatory cells and catalytic cascades liberate important soluble inflammatory mediators that stimulate protective mucosal responses by recruiting and activating effector cells, altering vascular and epithelial permeability, inducing peristalsis, and stimulating epithelial secretion. These mediators can be broadly characterized as lipids, nitric oxide, complement products, and kallikrein-kinin molecules.

Lipid Mediators

Lipid-derived mediators, including prostaglandins, leukotrienes, and platelet-activating factor (PAF), are immediate response elements liberated by nearly all cells in the GI tract. Although they arise from membrane phospholipid precursors, these metabolites have distinctive but overlapping functions (Fig. 2–16). The cyclooxygenase pathway received considerable attention in 2000 with development of selective COX-2 inhibitors.[165] COX-1 is constitutively expressed on almost all cells, whereas COX-2 expression is almost undetectable in noninflamed mucosal tissues but is dramatically up-regulated in inflamed tissues. COX-2 is regulated by proinflammatory mediators, most notably IL-1 and TNF, as well as bacterial polymers such as LPS and peptidoglycan-polysaccharide complexes through an NFκB-dependent activation pathway.[166] Although prostaglandins clearly contribute to enhanced vascular permeability, edema, increased motility, and chloride secretion during GI inflammation, their ability to

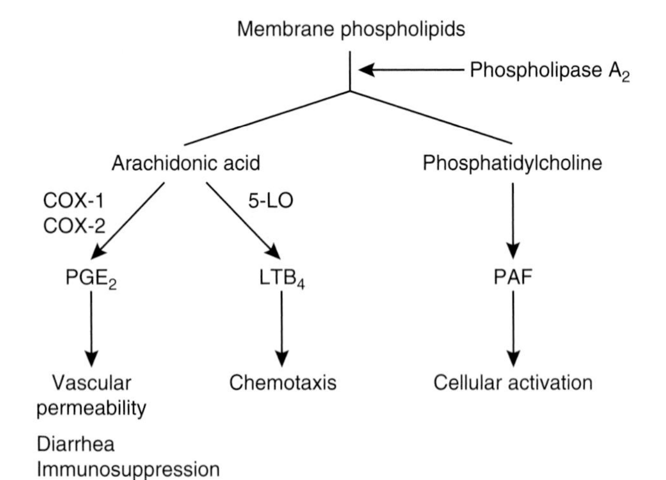

Figure 2–16. Lipid inflammatory mediators. Phospholipase A_2 cleaves phospholipids in membranes into arachidonic acid and phosphatidylcholine, which serve as substrates for enzymes, including cyclooxygenase (COX) and 5-lipoxygenase (5-LO), which in turn synthesize eicosanoids (prostaglandins and leukotrienes) and platelet activating factor (PAF), which have variable inflammatory consequences.

protect against mucosal damage is illustrated by the well documented induction of GI injury by both global and selective blockade of COX-1 and COX-2.[152, 154, 166, 167] Furthermore, stable prostaglandin agonists can prevent and treat GI injury.[168]

LTB_4, a principal product of 5-lipoxygenase, is a potent neutrophil chemotactic molecule.[169] This molecule is prominently up-regulated in mucosal inflammation and arises from activated neutrophils, macrophages, and mast cells. PAF, produced by neutrophils, macrophages, mast cells, and eosinophils, increases epithelial chloride secretion, vascular permeability, neutrophil chemotaxis, platelet aggregation, and smooth muscle contraction. PAF is degraded by acetylhydrolase, which is secreted by intestinal epithelial cells, to the inactive metabolite lyso-PAF.

The rate limiting step of synthesis of these lipid metabolites is substrate availability. Activation of phospholipase A_2 by macrophage phagocytosis, bradykinin receptor ligation, or LPS releases arachidonic acid, the substrate for prostaglandins and leukotrienes (eicosanoids), and phosphatidylcholine, the precursor of PAF (see Fig. 2–16). Enzymatic cleavage of arachidonic acid is completed within 1 to 2 minutes, leading to almost immediate responses to inciting stimuli.

Nitric Oxide

Nitric oxide synthase (NOS) oxidizes arginine to produce the volatile gas nitric oxide, which has multiple biologic properties relevant to intestinal inflammation.[170] This molecule, the principal nonadrenergic noncholinergic neurotransmitter in the intestine, is a potent vasodilator and, within phagocytic cells, kills ingested bacteria and parasites in synergy with reactive oxygen metabolites.[171] Three distinct isoforms are described, with unique signal distribution, transcriptional regulation, and function. NOS-1, found in neural tissues and circular smooth muscles, mediates peristalsis and sphincter function. High NOS-1 activity may lead to ileus and possibly toxic megacolon during intestinal inflammation.[172] NOS-3, found in vascular endothelial cells, dilates the vasculature by relaxing smooth muscles. Blockade of this enzyme in rats has regional effects, with decreased proximal blood flow in the stomach and pancreas, but no effect on the small intestine and colon.[173] NOS-1 and NOS-3 are constitutively expressed and calcium independent, whereas NOS-2 (inducible NOS [iNOS]) is dramatically induced by LPS, IL-1, TNF, IFNγ, and invasive bacteria through the NFκB signal transduction pathway[37, 174] and is dependent on calcium as a cofactor. From a quantitative standpoint, iNOS produces far more NO than NOS-1 and -2 and is consistently up-regulated during inflammation.[175] The iNOS (NOS-2) isoform is expressed in intestinal epithelial cells, macrophages, and mesenchymal cells (fibroblasts and myofibroblasts). The biologic effect of NO during inflammation is controversial, although most studies suggest a net protective effect of this molecule.[176]

Kallikrein-Kinin System

The plasma contact system, so named on the basis of the role of surface contact in activation, is a series of proteolytic cleavage steps initiated by activated factor XII.[177] A variety of environmentally relevant products can activate this path-

Table 2–6 | **Adhesion Molecules Responsible for Circulating Leukocyte (Neutrophil and Monocyte) Interactions with Endothelial Cells**

LEUKOCYTES			ENDOTHELIAL CELLS		
Adhesion Molecule(s)	**Family**	**Expression**	**Adhesion Molecule(s)**	**Family**	**Expression**
L-selectin (LAM-1)	Selectin	Constitutive	E-selectin (ELAM-1)	Selectin	Inducible
			Sialylated Lewis X	Blood group	Constitutive
			P-selectin	Selectin	Constitutive
CD11a/CD18 (LFA-1)	β_2-Integrin	Constitutive	ICAM-1, ICAM-2	IgG superfamily	Inducible
CD11b/CD18 (MAC-1)	β_2-Integrin	Constitutive	ICAM-1	IgG superfamily	Inducible

ELAM, endothelial leukocyte adhesion molecule; ICAM, intercellular adhesion molecule; IgG, immunoglobulin G; LAM, leukocyte adhesion molecule; LFA, leukocyte function–associated antigen; MAC-1, macrophage-1 antigen.

way, including the ubiquitous bacterial polymers LPS and peptidoglycan-polysaccharide. Activation of this pathway cleaves the inactive precursor prekallikrein to biologically active kallikrein, which activates neutrophils, and cleaves high-molecular-weight kininogen to bradykinin, which induces epithelial chloride secretion, stimulates pain receptors, and stimulates endothelial PGI_2 and NO (inducing vasodilatation) and HKa (inducing angiogenesis). Tissue kallikrein can also form bradykinin. Plasma kallikrein and bradykinin are activated during the acute and chronic phases of several experimental rat models of small intestinal ulceration and granulomatous enterocolitis, with a pathogenic role indicated by suppression of inflammation by a specific kallikrein inhibitor.[178, 179] Of considerable interest, genetic susceptibility to intestinal and extraintestinal inflammation in inbred rat strains correlated with activation of the contact system.[180]

Nonlymphoid Cells

In a number of nonlymphoid cells found in the intestine, including innate effector cells (neutrophils, macrophages, mast cells, and eosinophils), mesenchymal cells (fibroblasts, myofibroblasts, and myocytes), endothelial cells, and epithelial cells, inflammatory phenotypes develop and contribute to inflammatory responses.[181] These cells are activated by exposure to bacterial polymers (LPS, peptidoglycan-polysaccharide complexes) and proinflammatory cytokines, primarily IL-1 and TNF. Quantitatively, however, most inflammatory effector activities are mediated by the bone marrow–derived innate immune cell population that comprises neutrophils and newly recruited macrophages.[43, 45] Recruitment of these cells into the inflammatory focus depends on adherence of circulating cells to the vascular endothelium and migration into the injured area after a gradient of chemotactic factors.[182–184] Initial events are triggered by epithelial cell release of chemokines after bacterial invasion and direct stimulation of tissue macrophages and endothelial cells by LPS, resulting in secretion of the proinflammatory cytokines IL-1 and TNF and of chemotactic factors including IL-8 and LTB_4. The proinflammatory cytokines induce the expression of selectins (E-selectin and P-selectin) and adhesion molecules (ICAM-1 and -2) on regional vascular endothelial cells that serve as counterligands for constitutively expressed selectins and β_2 integrins on the circulating neutrophils (Table 2–6) (Fig. 2–17). After firm adhesion to the activated endothelium, diapedesis into the inflammatory focus depends on attachment of emigrating cells to extracellular matrix components (fibronectin and others) and migration that follows a chemokine gradient emanating from the inflammatory epicenter. In addition to cellular-derived chemokines of the C-C and CXC families, oligopeptides of bacterial origin, including FMLP, are potent stimulants of neutrophil chemotaxis.[47]

Resting endothelial cells constitutively express P-selectin, which binds to L-selectin (leukocyte adhesion molecule-1 [LAM-1]) and sialylated Lewis X oligosaccharides on most hematopoietic cells (see Table 2–6). Other endothelial adhesion molecules, including E-selectin (endothelial leukocyte adhesion molecule-1 [ELAM-1]), are transcriptionally regulated by NFκB after IL-1, TNF, and IFNγ release by activated cells in the inflammatory focus. These molecules bind to circulating neutrophils and monocytes that constitutively express L-selectin, sialylated Lewis X oligosaccharides, and the β_2 integrin CD11a/CD18 (leukocyte function-associated antigen [LFA]-1), which recognizes ICAM-1 and -2, and CD11b/CD18 (macrophage-1 antigen [MAC-1]), which binds to ICAM-1. Selectins are responsible for initial, loose leukocyte/endothelial interactions, resulting in rolling and adhesion, with subsequent adhesion necessary for transmigration between the endothelial cells mediated by the leukocyte integrins LFA-1 and MAC-1/endothelial cell ICAM-1 and -2 ligation. This coordinated entry of innate effector cells can be efficiently inhibited by blocking either the endothelial or leukocyte adhesion molecules.[185]

Chemotactic molecules display considerable redundancy, which fosters entry to a wide variety of cell types but also

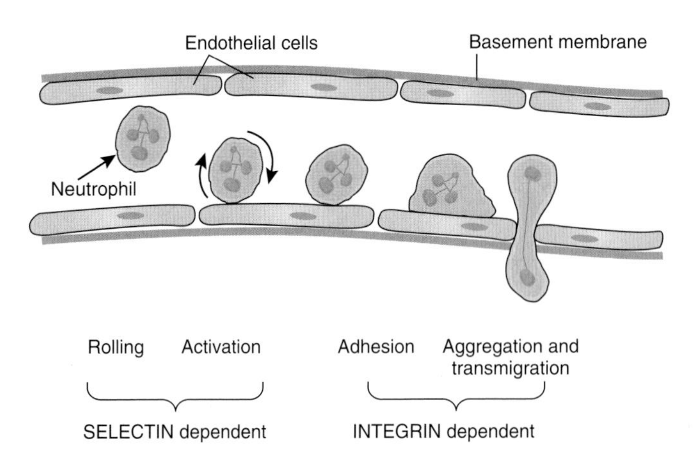

Figure 2–17. Leukocyte/endothelial interactions. Circulating leukocytes initially bind to endothelial selectins to slow their movement (rolling), then become firmly adherent to integrins, which foster transmigration into the inflammatory focus under the influence of chemotactic factors.

makes specific therapeutic targeting of this class of inhibitory molecules quite difficult. Chemotactic cytokines (chemokines) can be broadly classified by their receptor ligands, which bind multiple chemokines on defined subsets of responding cells (Table 2–7).[183] Although these receptors are also heterogeneous, they offer a somewhat more defined target for therapeutic intervention. Chemokine receptors not only provide the mechanism for cellular chemotaxis and activation, but also serve as attachment for entry of pathogens, such as HIV.[183]

Emigrating neutrophils and macrophages are activated in the inflammatory milieu by bacterial components (LPS, peptidoglycan, and FMLP), phagocytosed bacteria, and inflammatory cytokines (IL-1, TNF, and IFNγ). These stimuli transduce activation signals through NFκB and Janus kinase (JAK)/signal transducer and mediator of transcription (STAT) pathways that induce transcription of a characteristic pattern of proinflammatory cytokines, chemokines, MHC class II molecules, iNOS, COX-2, adhesion molecules, and costimulatory factors (see Table 2–1), which amplify the inflammatory responses by autocrine, paracrine, and endocrine pathways.[186] For example, IL-1 and TNF from activated macrophages stimulate ICAM-1 and ECAM-1 on vascular endothelial cells, promoting the entry of new effector cells, and in T_{H1} cells, IL-12 from macrophages dramatically up-regulates IFNγ, which in turn stimulates IL-12, TNF, and IL-1 in macrophages and other cells. Similarly, IL-1, TNF and IFNγ stimulate chemokine secretion by epithelial cells, thereby promoting entry of new effector cells. The result of such cellular interactions is induction of an inflammatory phenotype in almost all cells located in the inflamed GI area, which interact to create a massive inflammatory reaction.[181] The interplay of immune and nonimmune cells extends to cell-cell contact, in which T cell CD40L binds to intestinal fibroblast and epithelial cell CD40 to stimulate chemokine secretion by the mesenchymal cells.[187] This complex amplification involving innumerable cell lineages and countless secreted and membrane-bound receptors helps explain why it is far easier to prevent the onset of experimental intestinal inflammation than to reverse established disease,[188, 189] and also why selective blockade of a single chemokine may not have therapeutic activity.[190]

Table 2–7 | **Intestinal Chemokines and Their Receptors**

FAMILY	LIGAND	RECEPTOR	RESPONDING CELL
CXC	IL-8	CXC $R_{1,2}$	Neut, B, aEos
	ENA-78	CXC R_2	Neut
	IP-10	CXC R_3	aT, NK
	SDF-1	CXC R_4	T
C-C	MIP-1α	$CCR_{1,5}$	MΦ, B, aT, DC
	MIP-1β	CCR_1	MΦ, aT, DC
	MIP-3α	CCR_6	T, iDC
	MCP-1	CCR_2	MΦ, DC, aT, NK
	MCP-3	$CCR_{1,2,3}$	MΦ, aT, Eos
	Eotaxin	CCR_3	Eos, B, T_{H2}
	TECK	CCR_9	T
CX_3C	Fractalkine	CX_3 CR_1	CD8 T

a, activated cell; B, B lymphocyte; DC, dendritic cell; ENA-78, epithelial neutrophil activating protein-78; Eos, eosinophil; i, inactivated cell; IL-8, interleukin-8; IP-10, inducible protein-10; MΦ, macrophage; MCP-1, macrophage chemoattractant protein-1; MIP, macrophage inflammatory protein; Neut, neutrophil; NK, natural killer cell; T, T lymphocyte; T_{H2}, T helper 2.

Adapted from Papadakis KA, Targan SR: The role of chemokines and chemokine receptors in mucosal inflammation. Inflamm Bowel Dis 6:303, 2000.

Table 2–8 | **Most Common Intestinal Cytokines, Their Origin, and Their Function**

Cytokine	Primary Origin	Primary Functions
MONOKINES		
IL-1	MΦ, DC, mes, endo	Proinflammatory, ↑ adhesion molecules, activate NFκB, ↑ HPA
IL-6	MΦ, DC, mes, endo	Acute phase response, activate T_{H1}, ↑ B
TNF	MΦ, T_{H1}, DC, mes, endo	Proinflammatory, ↑ adhesion molecules, activate NFκB, ↑ apoptosis
IL-8*	MΦ, epith, mes, endo	Chemotaxic for neutrophils
IL-10	DC, MΦ	↑ Immunosuppression, ↓ DC, ↓ T_{H1}
IL-12	DC, B	Activate T_{H1}
IL-18	DC, epith, MΦ	Activate T_{H1}
TNF-β	MΦ, T	↑ NFκB, ↑ apoptosis
LYMPHOKINES		
Cytokine	**Primary Origin**	**Primary Functions**
IFN-γ	T_{H1}, NK	↑ T_{H1}, ↑ MΦ, ↓ T_{H2}
IL-2	CD4, CD8, T_{H1}	↑ T, B lymphocyte proliferation, ↑ Ig
IL-4	T_{H2}	↑ T_{H2} proliferative activity, ↑ B proliferation, Ig
IL-5	T_{H2}	↑ Eosinophils, activate eosinophils, ↑ B proliferation, ↑ IgE
IL-10	T_{R1} >T_{H3}, MΦ	↑ T_{R1}, ↓ DC, ↓ T_{H1}
TGF-β	T_{H3} > T_{R1}, MΦ	↓ T_{H1}, T_{H2}, ↑ collagen, ↑ epithelial restitution, ↑ IgA, ↓ IgG

*IL-8 is representative of a large number of chemokines.

B, B lymphocyte; DC, dendritic cell; endo, endothelial cell; epith, epithelial cell; HPA, hypothalamic-pituitary-adrenal axis; IFN-γ, interferon-γ; Ig, immunoglobulin; IL, interleukin; mes, mesenchymal cell (fibroblast, myofibroblast); MΦ, macrophage; NFκB, nuclear factor κB; NK, natural killer cell; T, T lymphocyte; TGF-β, transforming growth factor-β; T_H, T helper lymphocyte; TNF, tumor necrosis factor; T_{R1}, regulatory T lymphocyte.

Newly recruited macrophages are the primary producers of proinflammatory cytokines (Table 2–8) in an inflammatory focus,[45] because they are more responsive to LPS than native lamina propria macrophages, which have down-regulated CD14 that contributes to LPS membrane binding.[44] These proinflammatory cytokines have the ability to activate a wide spectrum of local and systemic inflammatory events, including induction of the acute phase response.[186] Activated neutrophils are short-lived cells in an inflammatory milieu, where they rapidly die or migrate through the epithelial layer to form crypt abscesses.[138] Neutrophils and macrophages secrete soluble inflammatory mediators, such as reactive oxygen metabolites and tissue metalloproteinases, which can induce tissue damage by injuring adjacent cells and degrading matrix components, respectively.

T Helper 1 and T Helper 2 Responses

In rodents, chronic experimental inflammation is characterized by well demarcated lymphokine profiles conforming to T_{H1} versus T_{H2} profiles, which are mutually exclusive. Most colitis models are T_{H1} mediated, usually with a CD4 T cell predominance,[191] regardless of whether they are induced by commensal[142] or pathogenic bacteria such as non–*H. pylori Helicobacter* species[142, 159] or *C. rodentium*.[158] Notable exceptions to this rule are the TCR deficient[192] and oxazolone-induced[193] murine models that are T_{H2} regulated. In contrast, most parasitic models are T_{H2} dependent; additional influences are provided by mucosal mast cells and eosinophils.[133] Supporting the observed cytokine T_{H1} lymphokine profiles, experimental colitis can be selectively prevented and reversed by antibody neutralization of IL-12,[150] which in some but not all models is more efficient than blockade of endogenous TNF.[194, 195] The role for luminal bacterial antigen in the induction of pathogenic T_{H1} responses is provided by in vitro cecal bacterial antigen specific stimulation of IFNγ by mesenteric lymph node CD4 T cells[132] and by transfer of colitis to T cell deficient hosts by IFNγ-secreting T_{H1} clones expanded by cecal bacterial antigen.[196] Induction of colitis in this transfer model is dependent on CD40-CD40L interactions.[98] Similarly, murine *H. pylori*–induced gastritis is associated with a T_{H1} profile of lymphokines, is potentiated in IL-4 deficient mice, and does not occur in T cell deficient hosts or resistant murine strains in which T_{H2} protective responses develop.[160]

Additional mechanisms of skewed T_{H1} or T_{H2} inflammatory responses are provided by selective entry of T_{H1} versus T_{H2} cell subsets that results from specific chemokine recruitment and selective expression of adhesion molecules. For example, P-selectin ligand is selectively expressed on T_{H1} but not T_{H2} lymphocytes,[197] and expression of this adhesion molecule is enhanced by IL-12.[198] Furthermore, T_{H1} lymphocytes selectively express certain chemokine receptors (CCR_5 and $CXCR_3$), which bind regulated on activation, normal T cell expressed and secreted (RANTES), macrophage inflammatory protein-1β (MIP-1β), IFNγ inducible protein-10 (IP-10), and monokine induced by IFNγ (Mig) produced by activated macrophages and epithelial cells.[199, 200] Of considerable interest, these chemokines are induced by IFNγ. T_{H2} cells are selectively recruited by macrophage-derived chemokine (MDC) and thymus and activation-regulated chemokine (TARC).[199, 200]

Although mucosal B lymphocytes are expanded and activated in experimental colitis, display an inflammatory phenotype with increased production of IgG subclasses relative to the usual mucosal IgA predominance,[201] and secrete autoantibodies including perinuclear-antineutrophil cytoplasmic antibody (p-ANCA),[202] B cells are not necessary for induction of inflammation. For example, B lymphocyte deficient IL-12 and IL-10 knockout mice develop colitis as aggressive as that in B cell replete controls.[203, 204] In fact, B lymphocytes were found to suppress colitis in the TCR$\alpha^{-/-}$ murine model.[205]

Observations in 2000 suggest that even in murine models, the classic T_{H1}/T_{H2} paradigms may be overly simplistic, because T_{H1} influences may be more evident in early phases of a classic T_{H1} model (the IL-10$^{-/-}$ mice) than in later stages, when IL-12 blockade is no longer effective.[206] Similarly, in mice of a stable inbred strain treated with trinitrobenzene sulfonic acid, colitis can develop with either T_{H1} or T_{H2} cytokine profiles.[207] As mentioned previously, human IBD is somewhat heterogeneous in respect to T cell cytokine profiles, although in general, Crohn's disease is characterized by elevated mucosal IL-12 and IFNγ levels and low IL-4 (T_{H1} profile), whereas ulcerative colitis is characterized by high IL-5 level in lamina propria T cells.[208, 209] However, results of biopsy of ulcers associated with early postoperative recurrence of Crohn's disease demonstrated a T_{H2} lymphokine profile,[210] and children with new onset Crohn's disease and ulcerative colitis have overlapping cytokine profiles with infectious controls.[211] Graft-versus-host disease, celiac sprue, and *H. pylori*–induced gastritis also have a predominant T_{H1} profile,[162, 212] whereas food allergy and immune responses to intestinal parasites and schistosomes appear to be T_{H2} mediated.[133, 213, 214] As discussed previously, activated T_{H2} lymphocytes are required for clearance of parasitic infections.[133]

Signaling Pathways

Binding of antigens, cytokines, growth factors, neuropeptides, and bacterial polymers activates characteristic, tightly regulated kinases that transduce signals, resulting in cellular responses. Although each receptor complex is unique, there are conserved signaling pathways leading to parallel outcomes after different initiating events. The classic example of conservation of signal transduction is the NFκB pathway, where ligation of IL-1, TNF, Fas, bacterial DNA, LPS, lipoteichoic acid, or peptidoglycan to its individual receptor activates signals that converge on a single complex (IkK) that activates NFκB (see Fig. 2–1).

Activation of the IkK complex phosphorylates the inhibitor of κB (IκBα), which in resting cells complexes cytoplasmic NFκB, thereby preventing nuclear migration.[215] When phosphorylated IκBα experiences polyubiquination and is degraded by the multifunctional proteosomal complex, heterodimeric NFκB is released to transmigrate to the nucleus. Binding of the active subunit of the heterodimer, p65 (RelA, NFκB$_1$), to specific promoter binding sites stimulates transcription of a broad array of proinflammatory molecules (see Table 2–1). Regulation of this pathway is provided by NFκB stimulated transcription of inhibitory molecules, including its own inhibitor, IκBα, and COX-2, leading to secretion of down-regulatory prostaglandins. A newly described cytoplasmic inhibitory protein, A_{20}, which is expressed in intestinal lymphoid tissues, is stimulated by TNF and effectively down-regulates TNF-induced NFκB activation and apoptosis.[216] Of considerable interest, in A_{20} knockout mice spontaneous colitis develops.[216] NFκB is activated during multiple types of experimental and clinical intestinal inflammation,[217] and inhibition of this pathway prevents and treats experimental colitis.[218, 219] Finally, polymorphism in the inhibitory IκBα-like gene is associated with more aggressive phenotypes in ulcerative colitis patients.[220] An additional inhibitory pathway is provided by peroxisomal proliferator-activated receptor γ (PPARγ), which is highly expressed in intestinal epithelial cells. Ligation of this pathway with clinically relevant agents, such as glitazone-type oral hypoglycemic agents, inhibits NFκB and treats experimental intestinal injury.[221] Finally, IL-10 can inhibit NFκB activation and its binding to DNA by several mechanisms[222] similar to the effects of 5-aminosalicylic acid (5-ASA) and glucocorticoids.[223] Intestinal epithelial cells have a uniquely adapted NFκB signaling pathway of incomplete, delayed degradation of IκBα that may allow them to maintain a

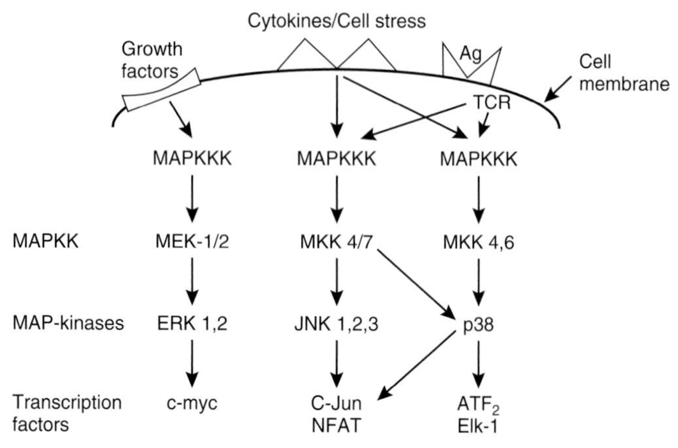

Figure 2–18. MAP-kinase signal transduction. A variety of pathophysiologically relevant stimuli, including growth factors, cytokines, cell stress, and TCR ligation by antigen, activate mitogen-activated protein-kinase kinase kinases (MAPKKK), which phosphorylate MAP kinase kinase (MAPKK) subsets. These enzymes selectively phosphorylate different MAP kinases (ERK, JNK, and p38) to activate transcription factors, which bind to promoter sequences of responsive genes. NFAT, nuclear factor of activated T cells.

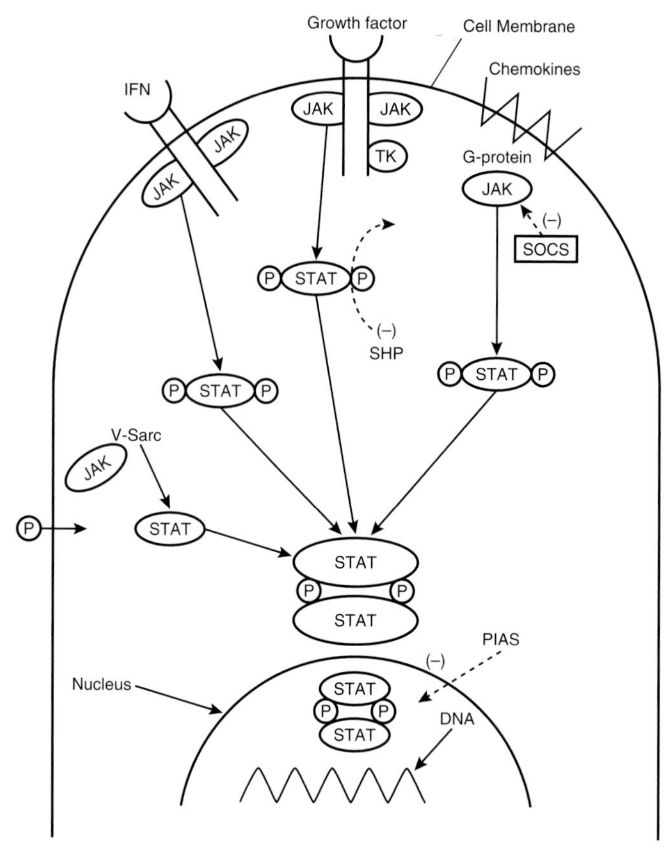

Figure 2–19. Regulation of STAT activation and signaling. Growth factors, cytokines, chemokines, and nonreceptor tyrosine kinases activate Janus kinase (JAK), which subsequently phosphorylates constitutively inactive cytoplasmic STAT molecules. STAT dimers migrate to the nucleus, bind to DNA promoter sequences, and initiate transcription. Regulation is provided by SHP, which dephosphorylates JAK, by SOCS, which blocks JAK activation, and PIAS, which blocks DNA binding.

relatively nonactivated phenotype in the hostile environment of the distal intestine.[224] Furthermore, these cells have decreased toll-like receptor (TLR4) and MD-2 expression.[225]

The c-Jun N-terminal kinase (JNK), p38 mitogen-activated protein (MAP) kinase, and JAK/STAT pathways provide alternative mechanisms to transduce proliferative, differentiation, transcriptional, and apoptotic signals from growth factors and proinflammatory cytokines such as IFNγ and IL-12 (Figs. 2–18 and 2–19). Receptor ligation with a variety of cytokines, T cell receptor complex stimulators, growth factors, and cell stressors stimulates a cascade of kinases that culminates in the activation of a family of MAP kinases, including p38, JNK, and extracellular signal related kinase (ERK) (see Fig. 2–18). p38 MAP kinase and JNK, which are activated by cytokines and stress signals, mediate cellular differentiation and apoptosis, whereas ERK is preferentially activated by growth factors and mediates proliferation.[226] Activation of these kinases leads to nuclear translocation of c-myc, c-jun activator protein-1 (AP-1), nuclear factor of activated T cells (NFAT), Activating transcription factor-2 (ATF_2), and Elk-1, which initiate transcription of a number of cytokines, including IFNγ and IL-12. An alternative pathway, the STAT transcription family, mediates activation of cytokines, such as IFNγ and IL-12, through JAKs bound to the receptors (see Fig. 2–19).[227] These kinases phosphorylate STAT molecules, which dimerize, translocate to the nucleus, and regulate transcription of a number of gene products. Regulation of STAT activation is provided by SHP, which dephosphorylates JAKs, suppressor of cytokine signaling (SOCS) proteins, which inhibit JAK activation, and protein inhibitor of activated STAT (PIAS), which blocks dimeric STAT binding to DNA. These pathways are particularly important in T cell activation and differentiation to T_{H1} versus T_{H2} phenotypes (Table 2–9). TCR-antigen binding and costimulation with IL-12 or TCR-independent pathways of environmental stressors activate JNK2 and p38 MAP kinase in T_{H1}, but not T_{H2} cells, which stimulate a pathway leading to nuclear migration of c-jun (AP-1), $NFAT_4$, and Elk-1. These transcription factors bind to specific promoter sites to induce transcription of important regulatory molecules such as IFNγ and to stimulate the growth and differentiation of T_{H1} lymphocytes.[226] Alternatively, IL-4 transcription in T_{H2} cells is negatively regulated by JNK-1, but

Table 2–9 | **Signaling Pathways for T Lymphocyte Cytokine Transcription**

T_{H1} LYMPHOCYTES		T_{H2} LYMPHOCYTES	
Stimulus	**Pathway**	**Stimulus**	**Pathway**
TCR-Ag	JNK-2, p38 MAP kinase	TCR-Ag	ERK
IL-12	JNK-2, STAT-4	IL-4, IL-13	ERK, STAT-6
IFNγ	STAT-1		
RANTES, MIP-1	STAT-1		
IL-6	STAT-3		
Inhibition	**Pathway**	**Inhibition**	**Pathway**
IL-4, IL-13	STAT-6	IL-12 IFN-γ	JNK-1, STAT-4 STAT-1

ERK, extracellular signal–related kinase; IL, interleukin; IFN-γ, interferon-γ; JNK, c-jun N-terminal kinase; MAP, mitogen-activated protein; MIP, macrophage inflammatory protein; RANTES, regulated on activation, normal T cell expressed and secreted; STAT, signal transducer and mediator of transcription; TCR-Ag, T cell receptor-antigen.

stimulated by the ERK signaling pathway. In parallel, IL-12 transcription in APC is up-regulated by p38 MAP kinase. IFNγ and IL-12 also transduce through the JAK/STAT system,[227] which also stimulates IL-18 in intestinal epithelial cells.[228] Receptor binding activates membrane-associated JAK, which phosphorylates STAT 1 (IFNγ) or STAT 4 (IL-12). Opposing signals are provided by IL-10 stimulation or STAT 3 and IL-4 and IL-13 activation of STAT 6. Important regulatory control inhibiting the JAK/STAT pathway is provided by the SOCS family, which has been shown to attenuate experimental colitis.[229]

T lymphocytes utilize a highly specialized and extremely complex signaling cascade that is initiated by antigen-MHC ligation of the TCR but mediated by the associated CD3 complex.[230] This pathway has been reviewed in considerable detail elsewhere[114] and provides an attractive target for therapeutic intervention. One important inhibitor of T cell activation and proliferation is TGF-β, which transduces signals through SMA and Mad-related protein (SMAD) isoforms.[231]

Neuroendocrine Influences

(Also see Chapter 1)

The GI tract is laced with an elaborate network of sensory and motor neurons that interact with immune cells through liberation of immunologically active neuropeptides.[232, 233] As in the other systems discussed, neuropeptides have complementary inductive and inhibitory influences on the immune system, as substance P exerts predominantly proinflammatory signals and vasoactive intestinal polypeptide (VIP) provides down-regulatory signals. Substance P, VIP, somatostatin, and neuropeptide Y induce connective tissue mast cell degranulation, although only substance P stimulates mucosal mast cells, and mast cells preferentially localize to nerve terminals.[48] An additional interactive regulatory pathway is provided by the hypothalamic-pituitary-adrenal axis. Circulating IL-1, TNF, and bacterial polymers stimulate corticotropin-releasing hormone (CRH), ultimately stimulating immune inhibitory adrenal glucocorticoids.[234] Of considerable interest, Lewis rats, in which chronic T_{H1} mediated enterocolitis develops when they are injected with bacterial cell wall polymers,[180] have a defective release of CRH when stimulated with bacterial products.[234] A key role for neuroendocrine effects in regulating immune responses is demonstrated by reactivation of chronic colitis in rats by stress; this response was shown to be T lymphocyte mediated by an elegant T cell transfer experiment.[235]

Apoptosis

Cells die by one of two routes—lysis (necrosis) or apoptosis (programmed cell death), which is a coordinated cascade of events culminating in DNA degradation at specific sites by caspases.[236] Apoptosis is induced in a variety of GI cell lineages by either TNF or Fas-mediated pathways (Fig. 2–20). Signal transduction is mediated through a number of aggregated "death domains" on scaffolding proteins that activate a cascade of caspases as well as NFκB. In most cells NFκB inhibits apoptosis,[215] providing a mechanism to prolong the survival of activated inflammatory cells. Studies in 2000 and 2001 demonstrated that intestinal epithelial cells become more sensitive to Fas-ligand mediated apoptosis as they differentiate[237] and that apoptosis of colonic epithelial cells enhances epithelial permeability.[6] Apoptosis of effector cells has profound implications for the pathogenesis and treatment of intestinal inflammation. For example, in Crohn's disease, anti-TNF monoclonal antibodies may mediate their prolonged therapeutic effects, which average 3 months after a single infusion,[140] by inducing apoptosis on monocytes or T_{H1} cells that demonstrate membrane-bound TNF (S. VanDeventer, personal communication). Supporting this concept, merely binding TNF with decoy receptors has no benefit in Crohn's disease patients.[238] Alternatively, anti-TNF antibodies have been shown to block epithelial cell apoptosis in experimental ileitis.[239] From the pathogenesis standpoint, IL-6 bound to soluble IL-6 receptor can activate T lymphocytes and prevent their apoptosis through a *trans*-activating signaling pathway requiring membrane gp 130, because T lymphocytes do not have membrane bound IL-6R.[240] Finally, the newly reported Nod-2 gene associated with Crohn's disease[58] mediates apoptotic responses to LPS, and A_{20}-deficient mice in which colitis develops have enhanced susceptibility to TNF-induced apoptosis.[216] Phagocytosis of apoptotic cells by macrophages stimulates production of TGF-β, PGE_2, and PAF, which inhibit proinflammatory cytokine production.[241] Thus, immunosuppressive cytokines synergize with apoptosis of effector cells to dampen established inflammatory responses.

Tissue Injury and Healing

Cytokines, growth factors, and soluble mediators liberated during the inflammatory response mediate tissue destruction but at the same time initiate healing responses, which when dysregulated can lead to fibrosis with attendant obstructive complication.[242, 243] TNF and IFNγ have synergistic abilities to damage epithelial cells, leading to enhanced permeability,[244] and TNF can induce apoptosis in a number of cell types, as discussed previously. Activated macrophages and eosinophils secrete reactive oxygen metabolites that injure adjacent cells,[245] and macrophages produce tissue metalloproteinases that degrade matrix constituents, thereby damaging the structural framework of the inflamed tissues. Proinflammatory cytokines, including T_{H1} products in synergy with IL-12, directly up-regulate tissue metalloproteinase transcription and secretion of collagenase and stromelysin-1 by macrophages and mesenchymal cells that account for tissue damage in in vitro inflammatory models.[246, 247] These effects are partially reversed by protective IL-10.[248] Similarly, IL-10 has been reported to preserve epithelial barrier function after in vitro challenge with proinflammatory cytokines,[249] and IL-10-deficient mice have epithelial barrier defects that appear before histologic evidence of inflammation is apparent.[250]

These studies suggest that immunosuppressive cytokines have a direct protective effect on epithelial cells that can preserve barrier function. This concept is supported by observations that IL-11 promotes mucosal integrity[251] and that TGF-β has a primary role in stimulating epithelial restitution, which is the ability of epithelial cells to repair a breach in their surface very rapidly independently of proliferation.[252] Keratinocyte growth factor was shown to enhance epithelial

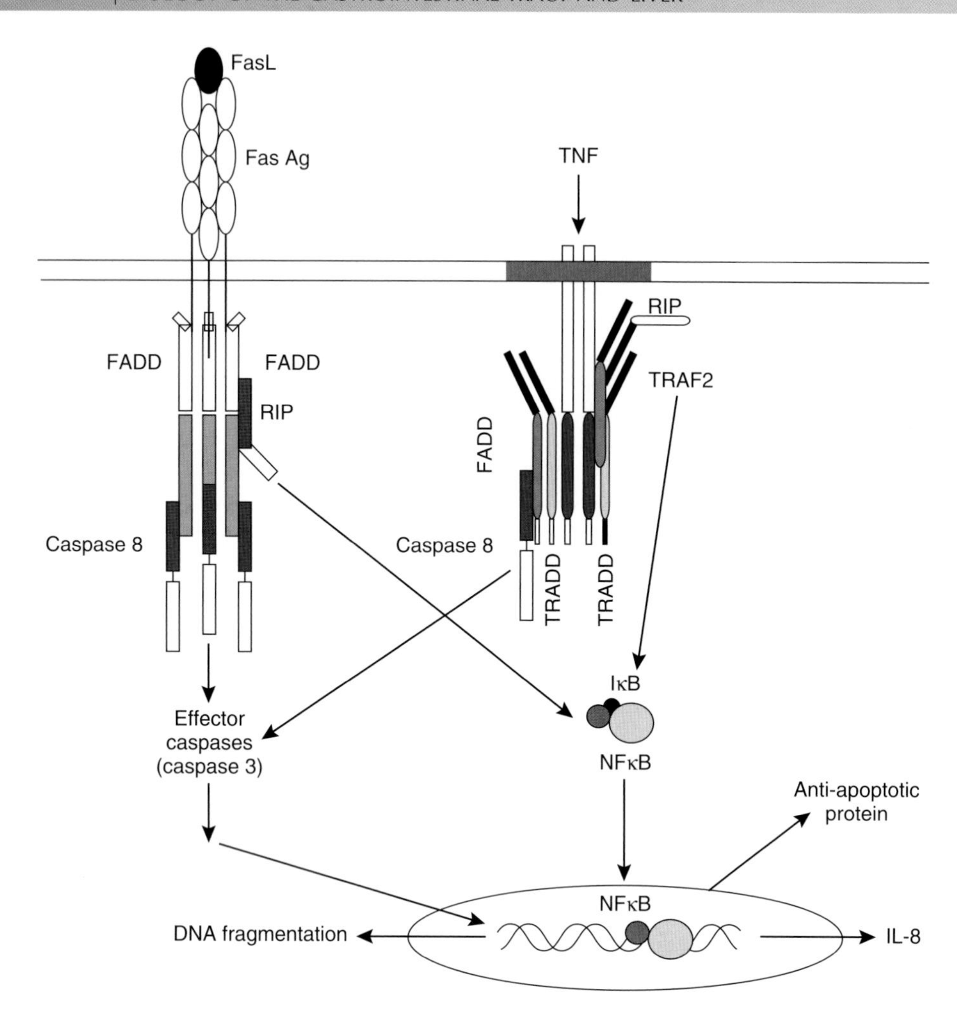

Figure 2–20. Pathways of apoptosis. Apoptosis is initiated by Fas or TNF ligation to specific receptors that stimulates a cascade of events culminating in caspase activation and DNA fragmentation. NFκB activation provides a means to inhibit apoptosis. (Courtesy of Christian Jobin, Ph.D., University of North Carolina, Chapel Hill.)

restitution,[253] possibly through its ability to induce intestinal trefoil factor.[16] Keratinocyte growth factor produced by subepithelial fibroblasts[254] and possibly intraepithelial lymphocytes has been implicated in the genesis of profound crypt hyperplasia, which is a consistent feature of T cell–mediated intestinal inflammation in both animal models and human diseases.[64]

In addition to their well-documented protective role in epithelial healing, growth factors have the capacity to stimulate matrix synthesis that contributes to healing but has the potential to lead to pathologic fibrosis if not adequately regulated.[243] Both TGF-β and insulin-like growth factor I (IGF-I) can stimulate collagen synthesis by intestinal myofibroblasts.[242, 255] An interaction between macrophages secreting proinflammatory cytokines, such as IL-1, and myofibroblasts producing IGF-I and TGF-β is suggested by their proximity by in situ staining.[256, 257] The amount of collagen accumulated in tissues is a balance between synthesis and degradation, which is determined by activity of metalloproteinases (including collagenase) and inhibitors of tissue metalloproteinases. This balance is disturbed in collagenous colitis as a result of defective inhibitors of activity.[258] These mechanisms suggest that tissue fibrosis is not a static event but under certain circumstances can be reversible. Finally, strictures in Crohn's disease have a component of hyperplasia of smooth muscle cells and myofibroblasts in addition to collagen deposition; this hyperplasia is undoubtedly secondary to growth factors liberated as a consequence of the inflammatory process.

An essential feature of healing is interruption of the inflammatory cascade by induction of protective, down-regulatory responses. In normal (resistant) hosts, proinflammatory cytokines and signal transduction pathways induce a number of protective cytokines, eicosanoids, and intracellular inhibitors (Table 2–10), which frequently selectively attenuate the molecule responsible for their induction. For example, IL-1 receptor antagonist (secreted and intracellular isoforms) is stimulated by IL-1β,[259, 260] and IκBα is induced by NFκB activation.[37] Of considerable relevance to clinical intestinal inflammation, genetically susceptible hosts can exhibit defective protective responses. For example, IBD patients exhibit disturbed balances of IL-1/IL-1RA,[261] IL-10 responses,[262] and polymorphisms in the IL-1RA[263] and IκB-like[220] genes. Finally, ingestion of dying apoptotic cells by macrophages stimulates the production of immunosuppressive molecules, including TGF-β and PGE_2.[241]

Genetic Susceptibility

Host genetic susceptibility profoundly influences intestinal inflammation through regulation of immune responses or barrier function and healing.[264] Genetically programmed regulation of APC and T cell responses may determine whether

Table 2–10 | **Induction of Protective Mediators That Downregulate (or Suppress) Inflammation**

INDUCER	SUPPRESSOR (ACTIVITY)
IL-1, TNF	IL-1 receptor antagonist (competitive inhibitor of IL-1)
IL-1, TNF	COX-2 (PGE_2, PGI_2, PGJ_2 inhibition of macrophage and T_{H1} responses)
IL-1, TNF	IL-10 (inhibition of macrophages and T_{H1} lymphocytes)
TNF	A_{20} (inhibition of NFκB activation)
IL-1, TNF, IFNγ	Heat shock protein-70 (inhibition of cell injury)
NFκB	IκBα (inhibition of NFκB activation)
Apoptotic bodies	TGF-β (inhibition of T cell proliferation and responses)
Apoptotic bodies	PGE_2 (inhibition of macrophages and T cells)

COX-2, Cyclooxygenase-2; IκBα, IL, interleukin; IFN-γ, interferon-γ; NFκB, nuclear factor κB; PG, prostaglandins; TGF-β, transforming growth factor-β; T_{H1}, T helper 1; TNF, tumor necrosis factor.

homeostasis or pathologic responses occur with exposure to commensal bacteria, pathogens, and dietary antigens. For example, HLA-DQ2 is found in 95% of patients who have celiac disease.[100] Interestingly, this same HLA haplotype is increased in patients who have microscopic colitis,[265] suggesting shared mechanisms in these two disorders. As discussed previously, 8% of Crohn's patients have a point mutation in Nod-2 on chromosome 16 that conveys defective NFκB signaling and apoptosis in response to intracellular LPS.[58, 266] Similarly, polymorphisms in the genes encoding TNF, IL-1 receptor antagonist, Mdr-1a, TAP-2, and glucocorticoid receptor 2 have been described in Crohn's disease, and HLA-DR3/DQ2, -DR103, and the IκB-like gene are related to aggressiveness of ulcerative colitis.[220, 263, 267] However, concordance rates of identical twins of 44% in Crohn's disease, 10% in ulcerative colitis, and 75% in celiac disease demonstrate the importance of environmental factors.[268] The molecular mechanisms of antigen recognition in celiac disease have been elucidated.[100] Deamination of gluten by transglutaminase exposes glutamic acid residues that selectively bind to HLA-DQ2. In rodent models of chronic intestinal inflammation, inbred strains respond differently to identical stimuli.[160, 180, 269, 270] Although genomewide searches have been performed in mouse strains demonstrating differential responses to spontaneous or induced colitis,[270, 271] the genes determining susceptibility and resistance in these models have not been identified. Lewis rats, which are susceptible to a number of chronic T cell–mediated inflammatory conditions, have abnormal hypothalamic-pituitary-adrenal axes,[234] abnormal cleavage of bradykinin,[180] and T_{H1} cytokine profiles.[188]

Inflammatory responses to transient infection or mucosal injury (NSAID, toxins, acid, etc.) in normal (genetically resistant) hosts are carefully regulated so that immunologic suppression is restored once the inciting event has been resolved (Fig. 2–21). However, in genetically susceptible individuals with either defective or overly aggressive immune responses or inefficient healing mechanisms, pathologic inflammation develops as a result of persistent or recurrent infections (in immunosuppressed individuals or those with defective barrier function) or an inappropriately aggressive immune response (in loss of tolerance) to luminal antigens from the diet (in celiac disease) or commensal bacteria (in IBD). Knowledge of key immunologic and inflammatory pathways provides novel targets for selective, relatively nontoxic therapeutic blockade of these inflammatory reactions. Finally, understanding the nuances of regulation of mucosal immune responses offers the opportunity to immunize optimally against enteric and systemic pathogens that enter through the intestine and offers mechanisms to restore inefficient protective responses in those patients afflicted with chronic inflammatory disorders or recurrent infections.

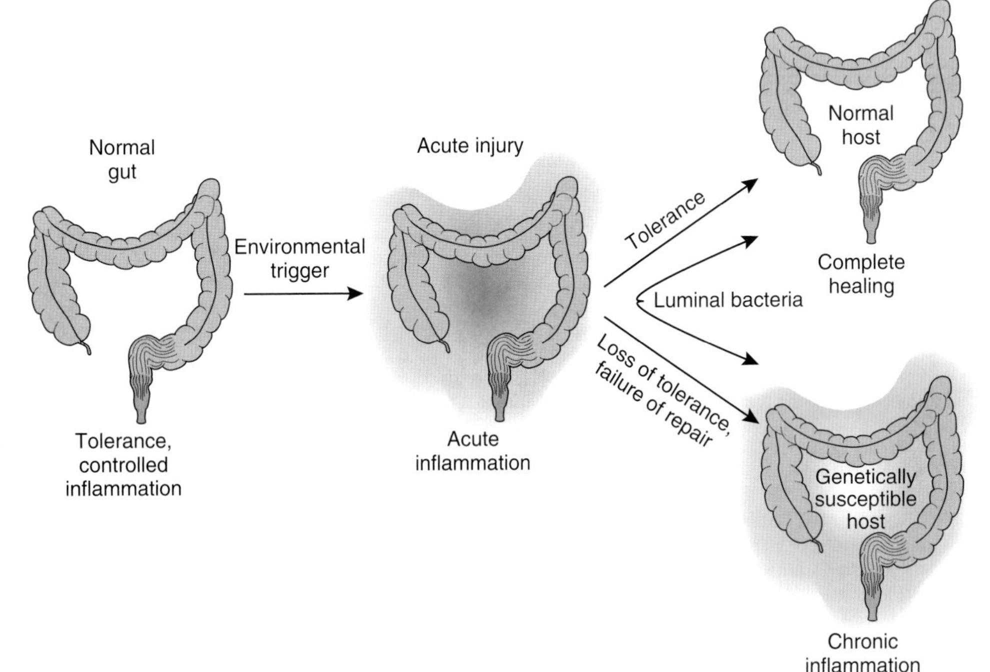

Figure 2–21. Differential responses to injury in genetically susceptible vs. resistant hosts. Nonspecific injury by environmental triggers (e.g., transient infections or NSAIDs) induce acute inflammation. Normal resistant hosts appropriately clear the offending agent and heal under the influence of regulatory T cells that prevent responses to ubiquitous luminal antigens (tolerance). The genetically susceptible host with defective immunoregulation or healing responds to ubiquitous luminal antigens (dietary or bacterial), inducing chronic inflammation. (From the American Gastroenterological Association Teaching Project, Washington, D.C., with permission.)

REFERENCES

1. Hollander D: Clinician's guide through the tight junctions. Ital J Gastroenterol Hepatol 31:435, 1999.
2. Gasbarrini G, Montalto M: Structure and function of tight junctions: Role in intestinal barrier. Ital J Gastroenterol Hepatol 31:481, 1999.
3. Itoh M, Furuse M, Morita K, et al: Direct binding of three tight junction-associated MAGUKs, ZO-1, ZO-2, and ZO-3, with the COOH termini of claudins. J Cell Biol 147:1351, 1999.
4. Itoh H, Beck PL, Inoue N, et al: A paradoxical reduction in susceptibility to colonic injury upon targeted transgenic ablation of goblet cells. J Clin Invest 104:1539, 1999.
5. Nusrat A, Parkos CA, Verkade P, et al: Tight junctions are membrane microdomains. J Cell Sci 113:1771, 2000.
6. Abreu MT, Palladino AA, Arnold ET, et al: Modulation of barrier function during Fas-mediated apoptosis in human intestinal epithelial cells. Gastroenterology 119:1524, 2000.
7. Rescigno M, Urbano M, Valzasina B, et al: Dendritic cells express tight junction proteins and penetrate gut epithelial monolayers to sample bacteria. Nat Immunol 2:361, 2001.
8. Wright NA: Interaction of trefoil family factors with mucins: Clues to their mechanism of action? Gut 48:293, 2001.
9. Van Klinken BJ, Dekker J, van Gool SA, et al: MUC5B is the prominent mucin in human gallbladder and is also expressed in a subset of colonic goblet cells. Am J Physiol 274:G871, 1998.
10. Kyo K, Muto T, Nagawa H, et al: Associations of distinct variants of the intestinal mucin gene MUC3A with ulcerative colitis and Crohn's disease. J Hum Genet 46:5, 2001.
11. Longman RJ, Douthwaite J, Sylvester PA, et al: Coordinated localisation of mucins and trefoil peptides in the ulcer associated cell lineage and the gastrointestinal mucosa. Gut 47:792, 2000.
12. Kindon H, Pothoulakis C, Thim L, et al: Trefoil peptide protection of intestinal epithelial barrier function: Cooperative interaction with mucin glycoprotein. Gastroenterology 109:516, 1995.
13. Taupin DR, Pang KC, Green SP, Giraud AS: The trefoil peptides spasmolytic polypeptide and intestinal trefoil factor are major secretory products of the rat gut. Peptides 16:1001, 1995.
14. Podolsky DK: Mechanisms of regulatory peptide action in the gastrointestinal tract: trefoil peptides. J Gastroenterol 12:69, 2000.
15. Chen YH, Lu Y, De P, et al: Transcription factor NF-kappaB signals antianoikic function of trefoil factor 3 on intestinal epithelial cells. Biochem Biophys Res Commun 274:576, 2000.
16. Iwakiri D, Podolsky DK: Keratinocyte growth factor promotes goblet cell differentiation through regulation of goblet cell silencer inhibitor. Gastroenterology 120:1372, 2001.
17. Williams KL, Fuller CR, Dieleman LA, et al: Enhanced survival and mucosal repair after dextran sodium sulfate-induced colitis in transgenic mice that overexpress growth hormone. Gastroenterology 120: 925, 2001.
18. Goldenring JR, Poulsom R, Ray GS, et al: Expression of trefoil peptides in the gastric mucosa of transgenic mice overexpressing transforming growth factor-alpha. Growth Factors 13:111, 1996.
19. Pothoulakis C, LaMont JT: Microbes and microbial toxins: Paradigms for microbial-mucosal interactions II. The integrated response of the intestine to *Clostridium difficile* toxins. Am J Physiol Gastrointest Liver Physiol 280:G178, 2001.
20. Simonovic I, Rosenberg J, Koutsouris A, Hecht G: Enteropathogenic *Escherichia coli* dephosphorylates and dissociates occludin from intestinal epithelial tight junctions. Cell Microbiol 2:305, 2000.
21. Quaroni A, Tian JQ, Goke M, Podolsky DK: Glucocorticoids have pleiotropic effects on small intestinal crypt cells. Am J Physiol 277: G1027, 1999.
22. Hermiston ML, Gordon JI: Inflammatory bowel disease and adenomas in mice expressing a dominant negative N-cadherin. Science 270:1203, 1995.
23. Mashimo H, Wu DC, Podolsky DK, Fishman MC: Impaired defense of intestinal mucosa in mice lacking intestinal trefoil factor. Science 274:262, 1996.
24. Babyatsky MW, deBeaumont M, Thim L, Podolsky DK: Oral trefoil peptides protect against ethanol- and indomethacin-induced gastric injury in rats. Gastroenterology 110:489, 1996.
25. Hecht G: Innate mechanisms of epithelial host defense: Spotlight on intestine. Am J Physiol 277:C351, 1999.
26. Cunliffe RN, Mahida YR: Antimicrobial peptides in innate intestinal host defense. Gut 47:16, 2000.
27. Kagnoff MF, Eckmann L: Epithelial cells as sensors for microbial infection. J Clin Invest 100:6, 1997.
28. Ouellette AJ, Bevins CL: Paneth cell defensins and innate immunity of the small bowel. Inflamm Bowel Dis 7:43, 2001.
29. Frye M, Bargon J, Lembcke B, et al: Differential expression of human alpha- and beta-defensins mRNA in gastrointestinal epithelia. Eur J Clin Invest 30:695, 2000.
30. Cunliffe RN, Rose FR, Keyte J, et al: Human defensin 5 is stored in precursor form in normal Paneth cells and is expressed by some villous epithelial cells and by metaplastic Paneth cells in the colon in inflammatory bowel disease. Gut 48:176, 2001.
31. Wilson CL, Ouellette AJ, Satchell DP, et al: Regulation of intestinal alpha-defensin activation by the metalloproteinase matrilysin in innate host defense. Science 286:113, 1999.
32. Qu XD, Lloyd KC, Walsh JH, Lehrer RI: Secretion of type II phospholipase A_2 and cryptdin by rat small intestinal Paneth cells. Infect Immun 64:5161, 1996.
33. O'Neil DA, Porter EM, Elewaut D, et al: Expression and regulation of the human beta-defensins hBD-1 and hBD-2 in intestinal epithelium. J Immunol 163:6718, 1999.
34. Panwala CM, Jones JC, Viney JL: A novel model of inflammatory bowel disease: Mice deficient for the multiple drug resistance gene, mdr1a, spontaneously develop colitis. J Immunol 161:5733, 1998.
35. Roediger WE, Babidge W: Human colonocyte detoxification. Gut 41: 731, 1997.
36. Jung HC, Eckmann L, Yang SK, et al: A distinct array of proinflammatory cytokines is expressed in human colon epithelial cells in response to bacterial invasion. J Clin Invest 95:55, 1995.
37. Jobin C, Sartor RB: The I kappa B/NF-kappa B system: A key determinant of mucosal inflammation and protection. Am J Physiol Cell Physiol 278:C451, 2000.
38. Dwinell MB, Lugering N, Eckmann L, Kagnoff MF: Regulated production of interferon-inducible T-cell chemoattractants by human intestinal epithelial cells. Gastroenterology 120:49, 2001.
39. Yang SK, Eckmann L, Panja A, Kagnoff MF: Differential and regulated expression of C-X-C, C-C, and C-chemokines by human colon epithelial cells. Gastroenterology 113:1214, 1997.
40. Cario E, Rosenberg IM, Brandwein SL, et al: Lipopolysaccharide activates distinct signaling pathways in intestinal epithelial cell lines expressing Toll-like receptors. J Immunol 164:966, 2000.
41. Inohara N, Koseki T, del Peso L, et al: Nod1, an Apaf-1-like activator of caspase-9 and nuclear factor-kappaB. J Biol Chem 274:14560, 1999.
42. Zhang G, Ghosh S: Toll-like receptor–mediated NF-kappaB activation: A phylogenetically conserved paradigm in innate immunity. J Clin Invest 107:13, 2001.
43. Rogler G, Andus T, Aschenbrenner E, et al: Alterations of the phenotype of colonic macrophages in inflammatory bowel disease. Eur J Gastroenterol Hepatol 9:893, 1997.
44. Grimm MC, Pavli P, Van de Pol E, Doe WF: Evidence for a CD14+ population of monocytes in inflammatory bowel disease mucosa—implications for pathogenesis. Clin Exp Immunol 100:291, 1995.
45. Rugtveit J, Nilsen EM, Bakka A, et al: Cytokine profiles differ in newly recruited and resident subsets of mucosal macrophages from inflammatory bowel disease. Gastroenterology 112:1493, 1997.
46. Rugtveit J, Haraldsen G, Hogasen AK, et al: Respiratory burst of intestinal macrophages in inflammatory bowel disease is mainly caused by CD14+L1+ monocyte derived cells. Gut 37:367, 1995.
47. Ferry DM, Butt TJ, Broom MF, et al: Bacterial chemotactic oligopeptides and the intestinal mucosal barrier. Gastroenterology 97:61, 1989.
48. Stead RH, Dixon MF, Bramwell NH, et al: Mast cells are closely apposed to nerves in the human gastrointestinal mucosa. Gastroenterology 97:575, 1989.
49. Yang PC, Berin MC, Yu L, Perdue MH: Mucosal pathophysiology and inflammatory changes in the late phase of the intestinal allergic reaction in the rat. Am J Pathol 158(2):681–690, 2001.
50. Arizono N, Kasugai T, Yamada M, et al: Infection of *Nippostrongylus brasiliensis* induces development of mucosal-type but not connective tissue-type mast cells in genetically mast cell-deficient Ws/Ws rats. Blood 81:2572, 1993.
51. Winsor GL, Waterhouse CC, MacLellan RL, Stadnyk AW: Interleukin-4 and IFN-gamma differentially stimulate macrophage chemoattractant protein-1 (MCP-1) and eotaxin production by intestinal epithelial cells. J Interferon Cytokine Res 20:299, 2000.
52. Vallance BA, Blennerhassett PA, Deng Y, et al: IL-5 contributes to

worm expulsion and muscle hypercontractility in a primary *T. spiralis* infection. Am J Physiol 277:G400, 1998.
53. Hogan SP, Mishra A, Brandt EB, et al: A critical role for eotaxin in experimental oral antigen-induced eosinophilic gastrointestinal allergy. Proc Natl Acad Sci U S A 97:6681, 2000.
54. Artis D, Humphreys NE, Potten CS, et al: Beta7 integrin-deficient mice: Delayed leukocyte recruitment and attenuated protective immunity in the small intestine during enteric helminth infection. Eur J Immunol 30:1656, 2000.
55. Hogan SP, Mishra A, Brandt EB, et al: A pathological function for eotaxin and eosinophils in eosinophilic gastrointestinal inflammation. Nat Immunol 2:353, 2001.
56. Lanier LL: On guard—activating NK cell receptors. Nat Immunol 2: 23, 2001.
57. Felstein MV, Mowat AM: Induction of proliferative and destructive graft-versus-host reactions in the small intestine. Adv Exp Med Biol 216A:653, 1987.
58. Ogura Y, Bonen DK, Inohara N, et al: A frameshift mutation in NOD2 associated with susceptibility to Crohn's disease. Nature 411: 603, 2001.
59. Farrell RJ, Murphy A, Long A, et al: High multidrug resistance (P-glycoprotein 170) expression in inflammatory bowel disease patients who fail medical therapy. Gastroenterology 118:279, 2000.
60. Jobin C, Sartor RB: NF kappa B signaling proteins as therapeutic targets for inflammatory bowel diseases. Inflamm Bowel Dis 6:206, 2000.
61. Baehner RL: Chronic granulomatous disease of childhood: Clinical, pathological, biochemical, molecular, and genetic aspects of the disease. Pediatr Pathol 10:143, 1990.
62. Korzenik JR, Dieckgraefe BK: Is Crohn's disease an immunodeficiency? A hypothesis suggesting possible early events in the pathogenesis of Crohn's disease. Dig Dis Sci 45:1121, 2000.
63. MacDonald TT, Pender SL: Lamina propria T cells. Chem Immunol 71:103, 1998.
64. MacDonald TT, Bajaj-Elliott M, Pender SL: T cells orchestrate intestinal mucosal shape and integrity. Immunol Today 20:505, 1999.
65. De Keyser F, Elewaut D, De Wever N, et al: The gut associated addressins: Lymphocyte homing in the gut. Baillieres Clin Rheumatol 10:25, 1996.
66. Howie D, Spencer J, DeLord D, et al: Extrathymic T cell differentiation in the human intestine early in life. J Immunol 161:5862, 1998.
67. Helgeland L, Brandtzaeg P, Rolstad B, Vaage JT: Sequential development of intraepithelial gamma delta and alpha beta T lymphocytes expressing CD8 alpha beta in neonatal rat intestine: Requirement for the thymus. Immunology 92:447, 1997.
68. Balk SP, Ebert EC, Blumenthal RL, et al: Oligoclonal expansion and CD1 recognition by human intestinal intraepithelial lymphocytes. Science 253:1411, 1991.
69. Christ AD, Saubermann LJ, Rousson V, et al: Oligoclonality of gastric T lymphocytes as defined by objective measure of T receptor-beta chain CDR3 size [abstract]. Gastroenterology 120:A322, 2001.
70. Suzuki H, Duncan GS, Takimoto H, Mak TW: Abnormal development of intestinal intraepithelial lymphocytes and peripheral natural killer cells in mice lacking the IL-2 receptor beta chain. J Exp Med 185: 499, 1997.
71. Jabri B, de Serre NP, Cellier C, et al: Selective expansion of intraepithelial lymphocytes expressing the HLA-E-specific natural killer receptor CD94 in celiac disease. Gastroenterology 118:867, 2000.
72. Futterer A, Mink K, Luz A, et al: The lymphotoxin beta receptor controls organogenesis and affinity maturation in peripheral lymphoid tissues. Immunity 9:59, 1998.
73. Maki K, Sunaga S, Komagata Y, et al: Interleukin 7 receptor-deficient mice lack gammadelta T cells. Proc Natl Acad Sci U S A 93:7172, 1996.
74. Boismenu R, Havran WL: Modulation of epithelial cell growth by intraepithelial gamma delta T cells. Science 266:1253, 1994.
75. Boismenu R: Function of intestinal gammadelta T cells. Immunol Res 21:123, 2000.
76. Oberhuber G, Vogelsang H, Stolte M, et al: Evidence that intestinal intraepithelial lymphocytes are activated cytotoxic T cells in celiac disease but not in giardiasis. Am J Pathol 148:1351, 1996.
77. Holtmeier W, Rowell DL, Nyberg A, Kagnoff MF: Distinct delta T cell receptor repertoires in monozygotic twins concordant for coeliac disease. Clin Exp Immunol 107:148, 1997.
78. Seki S, Habu Y, Kawamura T, et al: The liver as a crucial organ in the first line of host defense: The roles of Kupffer cells, natural killer (NK) cells and NK1.1 Ag+ T cells in T helper 1 immune responses. Immunol Rev 174:35, 2000.
79. Matsuda JL, Naidenko OV, Gapin L, et al: Tracking the response of natural killer T cells to a glycolipid antigen using CD1d tetramers. J Exp Med 192:741, 2000.
80. Wolf JL, Dambrauskas R, Sharpe AH, Trier JS: Adherence to and penetration of the intestinal epithelium by reovirus type 1 in neonatal mice. Gastroenterology 92:82, 1987.
81. Debard N, Sierro F, Browning J, Kraehenbuhl JP: Effect of mature lymphocytes and lymphotoxin on the development of the follicle-associated epithelium and M cells in mouse Peyer's patches. Gastroenterology 120:1173, 2001.
82. Kraehenbuhl JP, Neutra MR: Epithelial M cells: Differentiation and function. Annu Rev Cell Dev Biol 16:301, 2000.
83. Kerneis S, Bogdanova A, Kraehenbuhl JP, Pringault E: Conversion by Peyer's patch lymphocytes of human enterocytes into M cells that transport bacteria. Science 277:949, 1997.
84. Hashi H, Yoshida H, Honda K, et al: Compartmentalization of Peyer's patch anlagen before lymphocyte entry. J Immunol 166:3702, 2001.
85. Honda K, Nakano H, Yoshida H, et al: Molecular basis for hematopoietic/mesenchymal interaction during initiation of Peyer's patch organogenesis. J Exp Med 193:621, 2001.
86. Spahn TW, Fontana A, Faria AM, et al: Induction of oral tolerance to cellular immune responses in the absence of Peyer's patches. Eur J Immunol 31:1278, 2001.
87. Yokota Y, Mansouri A, Mori S, et al: Development of peripheral lymphoid organs and natural killer cells depends on the helix-loop-helix inhibitor Id2. Nature 397:702, 1999.
88. Matsushima A, Kaisho T, Rennert PD, et al: Essential role of nuclear factor (NF)-kappaB-inducing kinase and inhibitor of kappaB (IkappaB) kinase alpha in NF-kappaB activation through lymphotoxin beta receptor, but not through tumor necrosis factor receptor I. J Exp Med 193:631, 2001.
89. Laky K, Lefrancois L, Lingenheld EG, et al: Enterocyte expression of interleukin 7 induces development of gammadelta T cells and Peyer's patches. J Exp Med 191:1569, 2000.
90. Wagner N, Lohler J, Kunkel EJ, et al: Critical role for beta7 integrins in formation of the gut-associated lymphoid tissue. Nature 382:366, 1996.
91. Iwasaki A, Kelsall BL: Localization of distinct Peyer's patch dendritic cell subsets and their recruitment by chemokines macrophage inflammatory protein (MIP)-3alpha, MIP-3beta, and secondary lymphoid organ chemokine. J Exp Med 191:1381, 2000.
92. Varona R, Villares R, Carramolino L, et al: CCR6-deficient mice have impaired leukocyte homeostasis and altered contact hypersensitivity and delayed-type hypersensitivity responses. J Clin Invest 107:R37, 2001.
93. Hartgers FC, Figdor CG, Adema GJ: Towards a molecular understanding of dendritic cell immunobiology. Immunol Today 21:542, 2000.
94. MacPherson GG, Liu LM: Dendritic cells and Langerhans cells in the uptake of mucosal antigens. Curr Top Microbiol Immunol 236:33, 1999.
95. Kloetzel PM: Antigen processing by the proteasome. Nat Rev Mol Cell Biol 2:179, 2001.
96. Klein J, Sato A: The HLA system: First of two parts. N Engl J Med 343:702, 2000.
97. Androlewicz MJ: Peptide generation in the major histocompatibility complex class I antigen processing and presentation pathway. Curr Opin Hematol 8:12, 2001.
98. Cong Y, Weaver CT, Lazenby A, Elson CO: Colitis induced by enteric bacterial antigen-specific CD4+ T cells requires CD40-CD40 ligand interactions for a sustained increase in mucosal IL-12. J Immunol 165:2173, 2000.
99. Koppelman B, Neefjes JJ, de Vries JE, de Waal M: Interleukin 10 down-regulates MHC class II alphabeta peptide complexes at the plasma membrane of monocytes by affecting arrival and recycling. Immunity 7:861, 1997.
100. Sollid LM: Molecular basis of celiac disease. Annu Rev Immunol 18: 53, 2000.
101. Burastero SE, Rossi GA, Crimi E: Selective differences in the expression of the homing receptors of helper lymphocyte subsets. Clin Immunol Immunopathol 89:110, 1998.
102. Koizumi M, King N, Lobb R, et al: Expression of vascular adhesion molecules in inflammatory bowel disease. Gastroenterology 103:840, 1992.

103. Boyaka PN, Marinaro M, Vancott JL, et al: Strategies for mucosal vaccine development. Am J Trop Med Hyg 60:35, 1999.
104. Chen H: Recent advances in mucosal vaccine development. J Controlled Release 67:117, 2000.
105. Zabel BA, Agace WW, Campbell JJ, et al: Human G protein–coupled receptor GPR-9-6/CC chemokine receptor 9 is selectively expressed on intestinal homing T lymphocytes, mucosal lymphocytes, and thymocytes and is required for thymus-expressed chemokine-mediated chemotaxis. J Exp Med 190:1241, 1999.
106. Cepek KL, Shaw SK, Parker CM, et al: Adhesion between epithelial cells and T lymphocytes mediated by E-cadherin and the alpha E beta 7 integrin. Nature 372:190, 1994.
107. Rutgeerts P: A randomised double-blind, placebo-controlled, pan-European study of a recombinant humanised antibody to alpha 4 integrin in moderate to severely active Crohn's disease [abstract]. Gastroenterology 120:A127, 2001.
108. Coffman RL, Lebman DA, Shrader B: Transforming growth factor beta specifically enhances IgA production by lipopolysaccharide-stimulated murine B lymphocytes. J Exp Med 170:1039, 1989.
109. Schwab JH: Phlogistic properties of peptidoglycan-polysaccharide polymers from cell walls of pathogenic and normal-flora bacteria which colonize humans. Infect Immun 61:4535, 1993.
110. Mayer L, Shlien R: Evidence for function of Ia molecules on gut epithelial cells in man. J Exp Med 166:1471, 1987.
111. Bland PW, Warren LG: Antigen presentation by epithelial cells of the rat small intestine. II. Selective induction of suppressor T cells. Immunology 58:9, 1986.
112. Hershberg RM, Mayer LF: Antigen processing and presentation by intestinal epithelial cells—polarity and complexity. Immunol Today 21:123, 2000.
113. Park MS, Becker K, Mayer L: CEA (carcinoembryonic antigen) shows identity to gp180 and can modulate mucosal immune responses [abstract]. Gastroenterology 120:A60, 2001.
114. von Andrian UH, Mackay CR: T-cell function and migration: Two sides of the same coin. N Engl J Med 343:1020, 2000.
115. Targan SR, Deem RL, Liu M, et al: Definition of a lamina propria T cell responsive state: Enhanced cytokine responsiveness of T cells stimulated through the CD2 pathway. J Immunol 154:664, 1995.
116. Groux H, O'Garra A, Bigler M, et al: A CD4+ T-cell subset inhibits antigen-specific T-cell responses and prevents colitis. Nature 389:737, 1997.
117. Mason D, Powrie F: Control of immune pathology by regulatory T cells. Curr Opin Immunol 10:649, 1998.
118. Sher A, Gazzinelli RT, Oswald IP, et al: Role of T-cell derived cytokines in the downregulation of immune responses in parasitic and retroviral infection. Immunol Rev 127:183, 1992.
119. Kamradt T, Mitchison NA: Tolerance and autoimmunity. N Engl J Med 344:655, 2001.
120. Weiner HL: Oral tolerance, an active immunologic process mediated by multiple mechanisms. J Clin Invest 106:935, 2000.
121. Benson JM: T cell activation and receptor downmodulation precede deletion induced by mucosally administered antigen. J Clin Invest 106:1038, 2000.
122. Neurath MF, Fuss I, Kelsall BL, et al: Experimental granulomatous colitis in mice is abrogated by induction of TGF-beta-mediated oral tolerance. J Exp Med 183:2605, 1996.
123. Chen W, Jin W, Cook M, et al: Oral delivery of group A streptococcal cell walls augments circulating TGF-beta and suppresses streptococcal cell wall arthritis. J Immunol 161:6297, 1998.
124. Nagata S, McKenzie C, Pender SL, et al: Human Peyer's patch T cells are sensitized to dietary antigen and display a Th cell type 1 cytokine profile. J Immunol 165:5315, 2000.
125. Powrie F, Leach MW, Mauze S, et al: Phenotypically distinct subsets of CD4+ T cells induce or protect from chronic intestinal inflammation in C. B-17 scid mice. Int Immunol 5:1461, 1993.
126. Morrissey PJ, Charrier K, Braddy S, et al: CD4+ T cells that express high levels of CD45RB induce wasting disease when transferred into congenic severe combined immunodeficient mice: Disease development is prevented by cotransfer of purified CD4+ T cells. J Exp Med 178:237, 1993.
127. Thornton AM, Shevach EM: Suppressor effector function of CD4+ CD25+ immunoregulatory T cells is antigen nonspecific. J Immunol 1:190, 2000.
128. Read S, Malmstrom V, Powrie F: Cytotoxic T lymphocyte-associated antigen 4 plays an essential role in the function of CD25(+)CD4(+) regulatory cells that control intestinal inflammation. J Exp Med 192: 295, 2000.
129. Nishio A, Hosono M, Watanabe Y, et al: A conserved epitope on H+,K(+)-adenosine triphosphatase of parietal cells discerned by a murine gastritogenic T-cell clone. Gastroenterology 107:1408, 1994.
130. Nishio A, Katakai T, Oshima C, et al: A possible involvement of Fas-Fas ligand signaling in the pathogenesis of murine autoimmune gastritis. Gastroenterology 111:959, 1996.
131. Hollander GA, Simpson SJ, Mizoguchi E, et al: Severe colitis in mice with aberrant thymic selection. Immunity 3:27, 1995.
132. Veltkamp C, Tonkonogy SL, de Yong Y, et al: Continuous stimulation by normal luminal bacteria is essential for the development and perpetuation of colitis in TG epsilon 26 mice after bone marrow transplantation or adoptive transfer. Gastroenterology 120:913, 2001.
133. Garside P, Kennedy MW, Wakelin D, Lawrence CE: Immunopathology of intestinal helminth infection. Parasite Immunol 22:605, 2000.
134. Urban JFJ, Schopf L, Morris SC, et al: Stat6 signaling promotes protective immunity against *Trichinella spiralis* through a mast cell– and T cell–dependent mechanism. J Immunol 164:2046, 2000.
135. Vallance BA, Matthaei KI, Sanovic S, et al: Interleukin-5 deficient mice exhibit impaired host defence against challenge *Trichinella spiralis* infections. Parasite Immunol 22:487, 2000.
136. Hyoh Y, Nishida M, Tegoshi T, et al: Enhancement of apoptosis with loss of cellular adherence in the villus epithelium of the small intestine after infection with the nematode *Nippostrongylus brasiliensis* in rats. Parasitology 119:199, 1999.
137. Issekutz TB, Palecanda A, Kadela-Stolarz U, Marshall JS: Blockade of either alpha-4 or beta-7 integrins selectively inhibits intestinal mast cell hyperplasia and worm expulsion in response to *Nippostrongylus brasiliensis* infection. Eur J Immunol 31:860, 2001.
138. Madara JL: Review article: Pathobiology of neutrophil interactions with intestinal epithelia. Aliment Pharmacol Ther 11(suppl 3):57, 1997.
139. Neutra MR: Current concepts in mucosal immunity. V. Role of M cells in transepithelial transport of antigens and pathogens to the mucosal immune system. Am J Physiol 274:G785, 1998.
140. Targan SR, Hanauer SB, van Deventer SJ, et al: A short-term study of chimeric monoclonal antibody cA2 to tumor necrosis factor alpha for Crohn's disease: Crohn's Disease cA2 Study Group. N Engl J Med 337:1029, 1997.
141. Sachmechian A, Vasiliauskas A, Abreu MT, et al: Malignancy following Remicade therapy: Incidence and characteristics [abstract]. Gastroenterology 120:A619, 2001.
142. Sartor RB: Intestinal microflora in human and experimental inflammatory bowel disease. Curr Opin Gastroenterol 17:324, 2001.
143. Bjarnason I, Hayllar J, MacPherson AJ, Russell AS: Side effects of nonsteroidal anti-inflammatory drugs on the small and large intestine in humans. Gastroenterology 104:1832, 1993.
144. Sartor RB: Microbial factors in the pathogenesis of Crohn's disease, ulcerative colitis and experimental intestinal inflammation. In Kirsner JB (ed): Inflammatory Bowel Disease, 5th ed. Philadelphia, WB Saunders, 1999, p 153.
145. Sartor RB, Bender DE, Holt LC: Susceptibility of inbred rat strains to intestinal and extraintestinal inflammation induced by indomethacin [abstract]. Gastroenterology 102:A690, 1992.
146. Berg DJ, Weinstock JV, Lynch R: Rapid induction of inflammatory bowel disease in NSAID-treated IL-$10^{-/-}$ mice [abstract]. Gastroenterology 120:A685, 2001.
147. Asseman C, Fowler S, Powrie F: Control of experimental inflammatory bowel disease by regulatory T cells. Am J Respir Crit Care Med 162:S185, 2000.
148. Kontoyiannis D, Pasparakis M, Pizarro TT, et al: Impaired on/off regulation of TNF biosynthesis in mice lacking TNF AU-rich elements: Implications for joint and gut-associated immunopathologies. Immunity 10:387, 1999.
149. Cohn SM, Vidrich A, Summy M, et al: Emergence of perianal fistulae and ulceration in a murine model of IBD: A novel model of perianal Crohn's disease (CD) [abstract]. Gastroenterology 120:A122, 2001.
150. Neurath MF, Fuss I, Kelsall BL, et al: Antibodies to interleukin-12 abrogate established experimental colitis in mice. J Exp Med 182: 1281, 1995.
151. Kuhn R, Lohler J, Rennick D, et al: Interleukin-10-deficient mice develop chronic enterocolitis. Cell 75:263, 1993.
152. Kulkarni AB, Ward JM, Yaswen L, et al: Transforming growth factor-beta 1 null mice: An animal model for inflammatory disorders. Am J Pathol 146:264, 1995.

153. Morteau O, Morham SG, Sellon R, et al: Impaired mucosal defense to acute colonic injury in mice lacking cyclooxygenase-1 or cyclooxygenase-2. J Clin Invest 105:469, 2000.
154. Ferretti M, Casini-Raggi V, Pizarro TT, et al: Neutralization of endogenous IL-1 receptor antagonist exacerbates and prolongs inflammation in rabbit immune colitis. J Clin Invest 94:449, 1994.
155. Cohn SM, Schloemann S, Tessner T, et al: Crypt stem cell survival in the mouse intestinal epithelium is regulated by prostaglandins synthesized through cyclooxygenase-1. J Clin Invest 99:1367, 1997.
156. Kitani A, Fuss IJ, Nakamura K, et al: Treatment of experimental (trinitrobenzene sulfonic acid) colitis by intranasal administration of transforming growth factor (TGF)-beta1 plasmid: TGF-beta1-mediated suppression of T helper cell type 1 response occurs by interleukin (IL)-10 induction and IL-12 receptor beta2 chain downregulation. J Exp Med 192:41, 2000.
157. Steidler L, Hans W, Schotte L, et al: Treatment of murine colitis by *Lactococcus lactis* secreting interleukin-10. Science 289:1352, 2000.
158. Higgins LM, Frankel G, Douce G, et al: *Citrobacter rodentium* infection in mice elicits a mucosal Th1 cytokine response and lesions similar to those in murine inflammatory bowel disease. Infect Immun 67:3031, 1999.
159. Kullberg MC, Ward JM, Gorelick P, et al: *Helicobacter hepaticus* triggers colitis in specific-pathogen-free interleukin-10 (IL-10)-deficient mice through an IL-12 and gamma interferon-dependent mechanism [abstract]. Infect Immun 66:5157, 1998.
160. Smythies LE, Waites KB, Lindsey JR, et al: *Helicobacter pylori*-induced mucosal inflammation is Th1 mediated and exacerbated in IL-4, but not IFN-gamma, gene-deficient mice. J Immunol 165:1022, 2000.
161. Nilsen EM, Jahnsen FL, Lundin KE, et al: Gluten induces an intestinal cytokine response strongly dominated by interferon gamma in patients with celiac disease. Gastroenterology 115:551, 1998.
162. Monteleone G, Pender SL, Alstead E, et al: Role of interferon alpha in promoting T helper cell type 1 responses in the small intestine in coeliac disease. Gut 48:425, 2001.
163. Naluai AT, Nilsson S, Samuelsson L, et al: The CTLA4/CD28 gene region on chromosome 2q33 confers susceptibility to celiac disease in a way possibly distinct from that of type 1 diabetes and other chronic inflammatory disorders. Tissue Antigens 56:350, 2000.
164. Cong Y, Weaver CT, Lazenby A, et al: T-regulatory-1 (TR1) cells prevent colitis induced by enteric bacterial antigen-reactive pathogenic TH1 cells [abstract]. Gastroenterology 118:A683, 2000.
165. Giercksky KE, Haglund U, Rask-Madsen J: Selective inhibitors of COX-2—are they safe for the stomach? Scand J Gastroenterol 35: 1121, 2000.
166. Jobin C, Morteau O, Han DS, Sartor RB: Specific NF-kappaB blockade selectively inhibits tumour necrosis factor-alpha-induced COX-2 but not constitutive COX-1 gene expression in HT-29 cells. Immunology 95:537, 1998.
167. Tessner TG, Cohn SM, Schloemann S, Stenson WF: Prostaglandins prevent decreased epithelial cell proliferation associated with dextran sodium sulfate injury in mice. Gastroenterology 115:874, 1998.
168. Allgayer H, Deschryver K, Stenson WF: Treatment with 16,16′-dimethyl prostaglandin E2 before and after induction of colitis with trinitrobenzenesulfonic acid in rats decreases inflammation. Gastroenterology 96:1290, 1989.
169. Chang L, Karin M: Mammalian MAP kinase signalling cascades. Nature 410:37, 2001.
170. Kubes P, McCafferty DM: Nitric oxide and intestinal inflammation. Am J Med 109:150, 2000.
171. Marcinkiewicz J, Chain B, Nowak B, et al: Antimicrobial and cytotoxic activity of hypochlorous acid: Interactions with taurine and nitrite. Inflamm Res 49:280, 2000.
172. Mourelle M, Casellas F, Guarner F, et al: Induction of nitric oxide synthase in colonic smooth muscle from patients with toxic megacolon. Gastroenterology 109:1497, 1995.
173. Pizcueta P, Pique JM, Fernandez M, et al: Modulation of the hyperdynamic circulation of cirrhotic rats by nitric oxide inhibition. Gastroenterology 103:1909, 1992.
174. Salzman AL, Eaves-Pyles T, Linn SC, et al: Bacterial induction of inducible nitric oxide synthase in cultured human intestinal epithelial cells. Gastroenterology 114:93, 1998.
175. Guihot G, Guimbaud R, Bertrand V, et al: Inducible nitric oxide synthase activity in colon biopsies from inflammatory areas: Correlation with inflammation intensity in patients with ulcerative colitis but not with Crohn's disease. Amino Acids 18:229, 2000.
176. Kubes P: Inducible nitric oxide synthase: A little bit of good in all of us. Gut 47:6, 2000.
177. Colman RW, Sartor RB, Adam AA, et al: The plasma kallikrein-kinin system in sepsis, inflammatory arthritis, and enterocolitis. Clin Rev Allergy Immunol 16:365, 1998.
178. Stadnicki A, Sartor RB, Janardham R, et al: Kallikrein-kininogen system activation and bradykinin (B2) receptors in indomethacin induced enterocolitis in genetically susceptible Lewis rats. Gut 43:365, 1998.
179. Stadnicki A, Sartor RB, Janardham R, et al: Specific inhibition of plasma kallikrein modulates chronic granulomatous intestinal and systemic inflammation in genetically susceptible rats. FASEB J 12:325, 1998.
180. Sartor RB, DeLa Cadena RA, Green KD, et al: Selective kallikrein-kinin system activation in inbred rats differentially susceptible to granulomatous enterocolitis. Gastroenterology 110:1467, 1996.
181. Fiocchi C: Intestinal inflammation: A complex interplay of immune and nonimmune cell interactions. Am J Physiol 273:G769, 1997.
182. Papadakis KA, Targan SR: The role of chemokines and chemokine receptors in mucosal inflammation. Inflamm Bowel Dis 6:303, 2000.
183. MacKay CR: Chemokines: Immunology's high impact factors. Nat Immunol 2:95, 2001.
184. Prescott SM, McIntyre TM, Zimmerman GA: Events at the vascular wall: The molecular basis of inflammation. J Investig Med 49:104, 2001.
185. Issekutz AC, Rowter D, Springer TA: Role of ICAM-1 and ICAM-2 and alternate CD11/CD18 ligands in neutrophil transendothelial migration. J Leukoc Biol 65:117, 1999.
186. Sartor RB: Pathogenesis and immune mechanisms of chronic inflammatory bowel diseases. Am J Gastroenterol 92:5S, 1997.
187. Vogel JD, West GA, Sturm A, et al: Essential role of the CD40 pathway in T cell mediated induction of chemokines and cell adhesion molecules by human intestinal fibroblasts (HIF) and microvascular endothelial cells (HIMEC) [abstract]. Gastroenterology 120:A192, 2001.
188. Herfarth HH, Mohanty SP, Rath HC, et al: Interleukin 10 suppresses experimental chronic, granulomatous inflammation induced by bacterial cell wall polymers. Gut 39:836, 1996.
189. Herfarth HH, Bocker U, Janardham R, Sartor RB: Subtherapeutic corticosteroids potentiate the ability of interleukin 10 to prevent chronic inflammation in rats. Gastroenterology 115:856, 1998.
190. Roberts WG, Simon TJ, Berlin RG, et al: Leukotrienes in ulcerative colitis: Results of a multicenter trial of a leukotriene biosynthesis inhibitor, MK-591. Gastroenterology 112:725, 1997.
191. Strober W, Ludviksson BR, Fuss IJ: The pathogenesis of mucosal inflammation in murine models of inflammatory bowel disease and Crohn's disease. Ann Intern Med 128:848, 1998.
192. Mizoguchi A, Mizoguchi E, Chiba C, et al: Cytokine imbalance and autoantibody production in T cell receptor-alpha mutant mice with inflammatory bowel disease. J Exp Med 183:847, 1996.
193. Boirivant M, Fuss IJ, Chu A, Strober W: Oxazolone colitis: A murine model of T helper cell type 2 colitis treatable with antibodies to interleukin 4. J Exp Med 188:1929, 1998.
194. Davidson NJ, Judak SA, Lesley RE, et al: IL-12, but not IFN-gamma, plays a major role in sustaining the chronic phase of colitis in IL-10 deficient mice. J Immunol 161:3143, 1998.
195. Neurath MF, Fuss I, Pasparakis M, et al: Predominant pathogenic role of tumor necrosis factor in experimental colitis in mice. Eur J Immunol 27:1743, 1997.
196. Cong Y, Brandwein SL, McCabe RP, et al: CD4+ T cells reactive to enteric bacterial antigens in spontaneously colitic C3H/HeJBir mice: Increased T helper cell type 1 response and ability to transfer disease. J Exp Med 187:855, 1998.
197. Austrup F, Vestweber D, Borges E, et al: P- and E-selectin mediate recruitment of T-helper-1 but not T-helper-2 cells into inflamed tissues. Nature 385:81, 1997.
198. Xie H, Lim YC, Luscinskas FW, Lichtman AH: Acquisition of selectin binding and peripheral homing properties by CD4(+) and CD8(+) T cells. J Exp Med 189:1765, 1999.
199. Sallusto F, Lenig D, Mackay CR, Lanzavecchia A: Flexible programs of chemokine receptor expression on human polarized T helper 1 and 2 lymphocytes. J Exp Med 187:875, 1998.
200. Bonecchi R, Bianchi G, Bordignon PP, et al: Differential expression of chemokine receptors and chemotactic responsiveness of type 1 T helper cells (Th1s) and Th2s. J Exp Med 187:129, 1998.
201. Sellon RK, Tonkonogy S, Schultz M, et al: Resident enteric bacteria

are necessary for development of spontaneous colitis and immune system activation in interleukin-10-deficient mice. Infect Immun 66: 5224, 1998.
202. Mizoguchi E, Mizoguchi A, Chiba C, et al: Antineutrophil cytoplasmic antibodies in T-cell receptor alpha-deficient mice with chronic colitis. Gastroenterology 113:1828, 1997.
203. Ma A, Datta M, Margosian E, et al: T cells, but not B cells, are required for bowel inflammation in interleukin 2-deficient mice. J Exp Med 182:1567, 1995.
204. Davidson NJ, Leach MW, Fort MM, et al: T helper cell 1-type CD4+ T cells, but not B cells, mediate colitis in interleukin 10-deficient mice. J Exp Med 184:241, 1996.
205. Mizoguchi A, Mizoguchi E, Smith RN, et al: Suppressive role of B cells in chronic colitis of T cell receptor alpha mutant mice. J Exp Med 186:1749, 1997.
206. Spencer DM, Banerjee S, Levine AD: Anti-IL-12 therapy in IL-10-deficient mice prevents the onset of colitis and reverses early diseases, but is ineffective in late disease [abstract]. Gastroenterology 116: A760, 2000.
207. Dohi T, Fujihashi K, Kiyono H, et al: Mice deficient in Th1- and Th2-type cytokines develop distinct forms of hapten-induced colitis. Gastroenterology 119:724, 2000.
208. Fuss IJ, Neurath M, Boirivant M, et al: Disparate CD4+ lamina propria (LP) lymphokine secretion profiles in inflammatory bowel disease: Crohn's disease LP cells manifest increased secretion of IFN-gamma, whereas ulcerative colitis LP cells manifest increased secretion of IL-5. J Immunol 157:1261, 1996.
209. Monteleone G, Biancone L, Marasco R, et al: Interleukin 12 is expressed and actively released by Crohn's disease intestinal lamina propria mononuclear cells. Gastroenterology 112:1169, 1997.
210. Desreumaux P, Brandt E, Gambiez L, et al: Distinct cytokine patterns in early and chronic ileal lesions of Crohn's disease. Gastroenterology 113:118, 1997.
211. Kugathasan S, Binion DG, Itoh J, et al: Clonal T-cell cytokine secretion is modulated in mucosa of children with recent onset but not chronic inflammatory bowel disease [abstract]. Gastroenterology 112: A1021, 1997.
212. Ibraghimov A, Pappo J: The immune response against *Helicobacter pylori*—a direct linkage to the development of gastroduodenal disease. Microbes Infect 2:1073, 2000.
213. Kweon MN, Yamamoto M, Kajiki M, et al: Systemically derived large intestinal CD4(+) Th2 cells play a central role in STAT6-mediated allergic diarrhea. J Clin Invest 106:199, 2000.
214. Helm RM, Burks AW: Mechanisms of food allergy. Curr Opin Immunol 12:647, 2000.
215. Baldwin ASJ: Series introduction: The transcription factor NF-kappaB and human disease. J Clin Invest 107:3, 2001.
216. Lee EG, Boone DL, Chai S, et al: Failure to regulate TNF-induced NF-kappaB and cell death responses in A20-deficient mice. Science 289:2350, 2000.
217. Neurath MF, Becker C, Barbulescu K: Role of NF-kappaB in immune and inflammatory responses in the gut. Gut 43:856, 1998.
218. Neurath MF, Pettersson S, Meyer zBK, Strober W: Local administration of antisense phosphorothioate oligonucleotides to the p65 subunit of NF-kappa B abrogates established experimental colitis in mice. Nat Med 2:998, 1996.
219. Conner EM, Brand S, Davis JM, et al: Proteasome inhibition attenuates nitric oxide synthase expression, VCAM-1 transcription and the development of chronic colitis. J Pharmacol Exp Ther 282:1615, 1997.
220. de la Concha EG, Fernandez-Arquero M, Lopez-Nava G, et al: Susceptibility to severe ulcerative colitis is associated with polymorphism in the central MHC gene IKBL. Gastroenterology 119:1491, 2000.
221. Su CG, Wen X, Bailey ST, et al: A novel therapy for colitis utilizing PPAR-gamma ligands to inhibit the epithelial inflammatory response. J Clin Invest 104:383, 1999.
222. Schottelius AJ, Mayo MW, Sartor RB, Baldwin ASJ: Interleukin-10 signaling blocks inhibitor of kappaB kinase activity and nuclear factor kappaB DNA binding. J Biol Chem 274:31868, 1999.
223. Egan LJ, Mays DC, Huntoon CJ, et al: Inhibition of interleukin-1-stimulated NF-kappaB RelA/p65 phosphorylation by mesalamine is accompanied by decreased transcriptional activity. J Biol Chem 274: 26448, 1999.
224. Jobin C, Haskill S, Mayer L, et al: Evidence for altered regulation of I kappa B alpha degradation in human colonic epithelial cells. J Immunol 158:226, 1997.
225. Abreu MT, Vora P, Faure E, et al: Decreased expression of TLR-4 and MD-2 by intestinal epithelial cells (IEC) protects against dysregulated signaling and proinflammatory gene expression in response to bacterial lipopolysaccharide (LPS) [abstract]. Gastroenterology 120: A704, 2001.
226. Rincon M, Flavell RA, Davis RA: The JNK and P38 MAP kinase signaling pathways in T cell-mediated immune responses. Free Radic Biol Med 28:1328, 2000.
227. Bromberg JF: Activation of STAT proteins and growth control. Bioessays 23:161, 2001.
228. Kiessling S, Schottmann K, Falk W, et al: IFN gamma induces transcription but not secretion of IL-18 in human colonic epithelial cells [abstract]. Gastroenterology 120:A704, 2001.
229. Suzuki A, Mitsuyama K, Tomiyasu N, et al: The intrinsic inhibitors of JAK/STAT pathway: CIS3/SOCS3/SS13 and JAB/SOCS1/SS1 play a negative regulatory role in STAT3 activation and intestinal inflammation [abstract]. Gastroenterology 120:A21, 2001.
230. Delves PJ, Roitt IM: The immune system: First of two parts. N Engl J Med 343:37, 2000.
231. Wotton D, Massague J: Smad transcriptional corepressors in TGF beta family signaling. Curr Top Microbiol Immunol 254:145, 2001.
232. Furness JB, Kunze WA, Clerc N: Nutrient tasting and signaling mechanisms in the gut. II. The intestine as a sensory organ: Neural, endocrine, and immune responses. Am J Physiol 277:G922, 1999.
233. Shanahan F: Brain-gut axis and mucosal immunity: A perspective on mucosal psychoneuroimmunology. Semin Gastrointest Dis 10:8, 1999.
234. Sternberg EM, Hill JM, Chrousos GP, et al: Inflammatory mediator-induced hypothalamic-pituitary-adrenal axis activation is defective in streptococcal cell wall arthritis-susceptible Lewis rats. Proc Natl Acad Sci U S A 86:2374, 1989.
235. Qiu BS, Vallance BA, Blennerhassett PA, Collins SM: The role of CD4+ lymphocytes in the susceptibility of mice to stress-induced reactivation of experimental colitis. Nat Med 5:1178, 1999.
236. Denecker G, Vercammen D, Declercq W, Vandenabeele P: Apoptotic and necrotic cell death induced by death domain receptors. Cell Mol Life Sci 58:356, 2001.
237. Russo MP, Sartor RB, Jobin C: Flice-inhibitory protein (FLIP) inhibits NF kappa B signaling and is associated with an increased susceptibility to Fas-mediated apoptosis in differentiated HT-29 cells [abstract]. Gastroenterology 120:A696, 2001.
238. Sandborn WJ, Hanauer SB, Katz S, et al: A randomized double-blind, placebo-controlled trial of subcutaneous etanercept (p75 soluble tumor necrosis factor: Fc fusion protein) in the treatment of moderate to severe Crohn's disease [abstract]. Gastroenterology 120:A20, 2001.
239. Marini M, Rivera-Nieves J, Sicher KJ, et al: Anti-tumor necrosis factor (TNF) treatment decreased apoptosis of gut epithelial cells: A novel mechanism of anti-TNF therapy in experimental Crohn's disease (CD). Gastroenterology 120:A314, 2001.
240. Atreya R, Mudter J, Finotto S, et al: Blockade of interleukin 6 trans signaling suppresses T-cell resistance against apoptosis in chronic intestinal inflammation: Evidence in Crohn's disease and experimental colitis in vivo. Nat Med 6:583, 2000.
241. Fadok VA, Bratton DL, Konowal A, et al: Macrophages that have ingested apoptotic cells in vitro inhibit proinflammatory cytokine production through autocrine/paracrine mechanisms involving TGF-beta, PGE2, and PAF. J Clin Invest 101:890, 1998.
242. Pucilowska JB, Williams KL, Lund PK: Fibrogenesis. IV. Fibrosis and inflammatory bowel disease: Cellular mediators and animal models. Am J Physiol Gastrointest Liver Physiol 279:G653, 2000.
243. Wahl SM: TGF-beta in the evolution and resolution of inflammatory and immune processes: Introduction. Microbes Infect 1:1247, 1999.
244. Targan SR, Deem RL, Shanahan F: Role of mucosal T-cell-generated cytokines in epithelial cell injury. Immunol Res 10:472, 1991.
245. Jourd'heuil D, Morise Z, Conner EM, Grisham MB: Oxidants, transcription factors, and intestinal inflammation. J Clin Gastroenterol 25(suppl 1):S61, 1997.
246. Pender SL, Salmela MT, Monteleone G, et al: Ligation of alpha4ss1 integrin on human intestinal mucosal mesenchymal cells selectively up-regulates membrane type-1 matrix metalloproteinase and confers a migratory phenotype. Am J Pathol 157:1955, 2000.
247. Monteleone G, MacDonald TT, Wathen NC, et al: Enhancing lamina propria Th1 cell responses with interleukin 12 produces severe tissue injury. Gastroenterology 117:1069, 1999.
248. Pender SL, Breese EJ, Gunther U, et al: Suppression of T cell-mediated injury in human gut by interleukin 10: Role of matrix metalloproteinases. Gastroenterology 115:573, 1998.
249. Madsen KL, Lewis SA, Tavernini MM, et al: Interleukin 10 prevents cytokine-induced disruption of T84 monolayer barrier integrity and limits chloride secretion. Gastroenterology 113:151, 1997.

250. Madsen KL, Malfair D, Gray D, et al: Interleukin-10 gene-deficient mice develop a primary intestinal permeability defect in response to enteric microflora. Inflamm Bowel Dis 5:262, 1999.
251. Greenwood-Van MB, Tyler K, Keith JCJ: Recombinant human interleukin-11 modulates ion transport and mucosal inflammation in the small intestine and colon. Lab Invest 80:1269, 2000.
252. Podolsky DK: Mucosal immunity and inflammation. V. Innate mechanisms of mucosal defense and repair: The best offense is a good defense. Am J Physiol 277:G495, 1999.
253. Han DS, Li F, Holt LC, et al: Keratinocyte growth factor-2 (fibroblast growth factor-10) promotes healing of indomethacin-induced small intestinal ulceration in rats and stimulates epithelial cell restitution and protective molecules. Am J Physiol 279:G1011, 2000.
254. Bajaj-Elliott M, Poulsom R, Pender SL, et al: Interactions between stromal cell-derived keratinocyte growth factor and epithelial transforming growth factor in immune-mediated crypt cell hyperplasia. J Clin Invest 102:1473, 1998.
255. van Tol EA, Holt L, Li FL, et al: Bacterial cell wall polymers promote intestinal fibrosis by direct stimulation of myofibroblasts. Am J Physiol 277:G245, 1999.
256. Zimmermann EM, Sartor RB, McCall RD, et al: Insulinlike growth factor I and interleukin 1 beta messenger RNA in a rat model of granulomatous enterocolitis and hepatitis. Gastroenterology 105:399, 1993.
257. Manthey CL, Allen JB, Ellingsworth LR, Wahl SM: In situ expression of transforming growth factor beta in streptococcal cell wall-induced granulomatous inflammation and hepatic fibrosis. Growth Factors 4:17, 1990.
258. Gunther U, Schuppan D, Bauer M, et al: Fibrogenesis and fibrolysis in collagenous colitis: Patterns of procollagen types I and IV, matrix-metalloproteinase-1 and -13, and TIMP-1 gene expression. Am J Pathol 155:493, 1999.
259. Dinarello CA: The role of the interleukin-1-receptor antagonist in blocking inflammation mediated by interleukin-1. N Engl J Med 343: 732, 2000.
260. Bocker U, Damiao A, Holt L, et al: Differential expression of interleukin 1 receptor antagonist isoforms in human intestinal epithelial cells. Gastroenterology 115:1426, 1998.
261. Casini-Raggi V, Kam L, Chong YJ, et al: Mucosal imbalance of IL-1 and IL-1 receptor antagonist in inflammatory bowel disease: A novel mechanism of chronic intestinal inflammation. J Immunol 154:2434, 1995.
262. Schreiber S, Heinig T, Thiele HG, Raedler A: Immunoregulatory role of interleukin 10 in patients with inflammatory bowel disease. Gastroenterology 108:1434, 1995.
263. Tountas NA, Casini-Raggi V, Yang H, et al: Functional and ethnic association of allele 2 of the interleukin-1 receptor antagonist gene in ulcerative colitis. Gastroenterology 117:806, 1999.
264. Sartor RB, Veltkamp C: Interactions between enteric bacteria and the immune system which determine mucosal homeostasis vs. chronic intestinal inflammation: Lessons from rodent models. In Rogler G, Kullmann F, Rutgeerts P, et al (eds): IBD at the End of its Century. Amsterdam, Kluwer Academic Press, 2000, p 30.
265. Fine K, Do K, Schulte K, et al: High prevalence of celiac sprue-like HLA-DQ genes and enteropathy in patients with the microscopic colitis syndrome. Am J Gastroenterol 95:1974, 2000.
266. Hugot JP, Chamaillard M, Zouali H, et al: Association of NOD2 leucine-rich repeat variants with susceptibility to Crohn's disease. Nature 411:599, 2001.
267. Satsangi J, Parkes M, Jewell DP, Bell JI: Genetics of inflammatory bowel disease. Clin Sci 94:473, 1998.
268. Tysk C, Riedesel H, Lindberg E, et al: Colonic glycoproteins in monozygotic twins with inflammatory bowel disease. Gastroenterology 100:419, 1991.
269. Mahler M, Bristol IJ, Leiter EH, et al: Differential susceptibility of inbred mouse strains to dextran sulfate sodium-induced colitis. Am J Physiol 274:G544, 1998.
270. Bristol IJ, Farmer MA, Cong Y, et al: Heritable susceptibility for colitis in mice induced by IL-10 deficiency. Inflamm Bowel Dis 6: 290, 2000.
271. Mahler M, Bristol IJ, Sundberg JP, et al: Genetic analysis of susceptibility to dextran sulfate sodium-induced colitis in mice. Genomics 55: 147, 1999.

Chapter 3

CELLULAR GROWTH AND NEOPLASIA

Anil K. Rustgi and Daniel K. Podolsky

Neoplasms, benign and malignant, are among the most common disorders of the gastrointestinal (GI) tract. Although some features are specific to the tissue site at which a neoplasm arises, many mechanisms of oncogenesis are common to tumors throughout the GI tract. This chapter reviews mechanisms of normal cell growth and the fundamental cellular alterations that are central to the development of GI neoplasms (for a definition of terms, see Table 3–1). The common principles discussed in this chapter provide the framework for consideration of specific GI neoplasms in later chapters.

MECHANISMS OF NORMAL CELL HOMEOSTASIS: PROLIFERATION AND PROGRAMMED CELL DEATH (APOPTOSIS)

Neoplasia is the ultimate result of a disruption of the exquisite mechanisms regulating the normal cell cycle. In addition to cell proliferation, tissue growth is determined by the balance of cellular differentiation, senescence, and programmed cell death. Normal cells traverse a cycle, which includes a period of deoxyribonucleic acid (DNA) replication, designated the *S phase*. After an intervening period, designated the *G_2 phase*, actual mitosis occurs in the M phase (Fig. 3–1). After another intervening period, the G_1 phase, DNA replication can begin again.

The commitment to proceed through DNA replication and cell division occurs during the G_1 phase at the so-called start or restriction (R) point. Cells may exit this cycle of active proliferation before reaching the R point and enter a quiescent phase, G_0. Cells can subsequently re-enter the cell cycle from the G_0 state. The duration of each cell cycle phase as well as the overall length of the cycle vary among cell types.

Cell progression through the cell cycle is regulated primarily at two points: the G_2/M and G_1/S phase transitions. Regulation appears to be achieved principally by the actions of cyclins and cyclin-dependent kinases. Cyclin proteins are classified on the basis of their structural features and pattern of expression during the cell cycle (see Fig. 3–1). Cyclins A and B are expressed predominantly during the S and G_2 phases. In contrast, the cyclin D and E proteins are most active during the G_1 phase.[1] Overexpression of cyclin D1 in fibroblasts results in more rapid entry of cells into the S phase, and cyclin D1 is frequently overexpressed in a number of malignancies, including those originating from the breast, oral cavity, esophagus, and bladder.[2, 3]

Each cyclin forms a complex with a cyclin-dependent kinase (cdk) in a cell cycle–dependent fashion, and this complex may result in the acquisition of specific kinase activities. cdks physically associate with cyclins through their catalytic domains. The cyclin-cdk complexes are believed to regulate cell cycle progression through phosphorylation of key target proteins, including the retinoblastoma gene product (pRb), by cyclin D1/cdk4 or cyclin D1/cdk6,[4] and p107, a member of the pRb family, by cyclin E/cdk2.

The cell cycle is also regulated by natural cdk inhibitors.[5] Cip1 (also called WAF1 and p21) is a general inhibitor of cdks. Originally discovered to be part of a complex containing cyclin D1 and cdks, WAF1/Cip1/p21 is transcriptionally activated by the p53 tumor suppressor gene product and by cell senescence (see Fig. 3–1).[6] p53-Independent mechanisms also can activate p21. MTS-1 (also referred to as cdkN2 or p16) is another cdk inhibitor that specifically inhibits cdk4[7] and is part of a larger family of closely related inhibitors that includes p14, p15, and p18. MTS-1/cdkN2/p16 is frequently inactivated in esophageal squamous cell cancers and pancreatic ductal carcinomas, a finding that suggests that it acts as a tumor suppressor gene as well.[8–10]

Kip1 (also called p27) is another important cdk inhibitor. This inhibitor mediates arrest of the cell cycle in the G_1 phase by transforming growth factor-β (TGF-β), a key pep-

Table 3–1 | **Selected Terms**

Apoptosis: programmed cell death.
Allele: one of alternate forms of a gene occupying a locus on a chromosome.
cDNA: single-stranded DNA complementary to RNA.
Chromosome: unit of genome carrying many genes and an equal mass of proteins.
cis-Acting element: regulatory region of DNA juxtaposed to protein-encoding region of gene; *cis*- configuration indicates two sites on the same DNA molecule.
Clone: a collection of identical cells or molecules derived from a single parental cell or molecule.
Codon: nucleotide triplet corresponding to an amino acid.
Deletion: loss of a DNA sequence.
Dominant allele: allele that determines the phenotype in a heterozygote.
Gene: DNA segment encoding a peptide as well as sequences before and after coding region (leader and trailer) as well as intervening sequences (introns) between individual coding segments (exons).
Heterozygote: a person with two different alleles at a particular locus on chromosomal pairs.
Homozygote: a person with same alleles at a particular locus on chromosomal pairs.
Linkage: tendency of genes to be inherited together as a result of their proximity on a chromosome.
Locus: position on a chromosome of gene encoding a particular trait.
Mutation: any alteration in the sequence of chromosomal DNA. A germline mutation is inherited. A somatic mutation is acquired through the action of an environmental factor or failure of intrinsic cellular mechanisms of DNA replication or transcription.
Negative regulatory element: genetic element that functions by switching off transcription or translation.
Oncogene: gene whose product has the ability to transform eukaryotic cells. An oncogene carried by a retrovirus is a viral oncogene (v-onc).
Ploidy: number of copies of the chromosomes present in a cell; haploid has one copy, diploid has two copies, and so on.
Promotor: region of DNA that binds RNA polymerase to initiate transcription.
Proto-oncogene: normal counterpart in the eukaryotic genome to the oncogene carried by some retroviruses, also termed *cellular oncogenes* (c-onc).
Transformation: acquisition by normal cells (or their tissue culture equivalents) of phenotype features of malignant cells.
trans-Acting transcriptional regulatory protein: *trans*-Acting transcriptional proteins bind to *cis*-acting elements in a gene's promoter, enhancing or suppressing gene transcription.
Translocation: rearrangement in which part of a chromosome is detached by breakage and then becomes attached to another chromosome.

DNA, deoxyribonucleic acid; RNA, ribonucleic acid.

tide growth inhibiting factor (see Fig. 3–1).[11] TGF-β and cell-cell contact prevent activation of the cyclin E/cdk2 complex during the G_1 phase through activation of Kip1/p27.

DNA Ploidy

Although significant advances have been made in our understanding of the eukaryotic cell cycle, DNA ploidy (i.e., presence of a normal number of chromosomes) provides a clinically useful means to detect gross genetic alterations in GI cancers and their corresponding premalignant conditions. DNA ploidy can be determined by flow cytometry to detect whether cells within a tissue sample contain the normal diploid content (i.e., $2n$) or an aberrant amount of chromosomal DNA ($>2n$, or aneuploidy). Premalignant or malignant cells are frequently aneuploid as a result of genomic instability and clonal expansion. Studies in 1987 and 1991 demonstrated the frequent presence of aneuploid cell populations in dysplastic mucosa and superimposed cancers in patients who had Barrett's esophagus and ulcerative colitis.[12, 13] Aneuploid and hyperploid cells also have been detected in sporadic esophageal, gastric, pancreatic, colon, and hepatic cancers.

Programmed Cell Death

Apoptosis (or programmed cell death) is an important mechanism for counterbalancing cell proliferation, and escape from normal apoptotic mechanisms appears to play a critical role in oncogenesis (Fig. 3–2). Apoptosis is associated with characteristic features that include chromatin compaction, condensation of cytoplasm, and mild convolution of the nucleus and cytoplasm. These changes are followed by nuclear fragmentation and marked convolution of the cell surface. Eventually, membrane-bound apoptotic bodies that represent the cellular residue are produced and phagocytosed. Apoptosis is distinguished biochemically by cleavage of double-stranded DNA, which results in fragmented DNA.

Apoptosis is closely regulated, seemingly by a small number of specific genes. Studies of the roundworm *Caenorhabditis elegans* (*C. elegans*) led to the identification of a gene, designated *ced-9*, that protects cells from undergoing apoptosis, whereas other genes, designated *ced-3* and *ced-4*, were found to induce apoptosis.[14] The mammalian oncogene bcl-2 shares homology with ced-9 and protects lymphocytes and neurons from apoptosis[15]; bcl-2 complexes with bax, a protein that by itself contributes to apoptosis.[16] Of note, both bcl-2 and bax are part of larger gene families, and the stoichiometric relationships among different combinations of the encoded proteins may determine the balance between cell survival and cell death.[17]

Activation of caspases, which are intracellular cysteine proteases that cleave their substrates at aspartic residues, is a key step in the cellular processes that eventually lead to programmed cell death. Two well-defined activating pathways have been described in detail. One pathway is mediated through tumor necrosis factor (TNF) receptors, whereas the other involves mitochondrial changes induced by alterations in the bax-to-bcl-2 ratio. The latter pathway results in impaired mitochondrial integrity and release of cytochrome C and caspase-activating proteins, eventuating in apoptosis.

REGULATION OF NORMAL CELL PROLIFERATION: SIGNALING PATHWAYS THAT MEDIATE CELL GROWTH

Cellular proliferation is achieved through transition of cells from G_0 into the active cell cycle. Although progression through the cell cycle is controlled by the regulatory proteins described, cell proliferation is significantly modulated by external stimuli. Growth factors that bind to specific transmembrane receptors on the cell surface may be especially important. The cytoplasmic tails of these proteins produce an intracellular signal after ligand binding.

In addition to peptide growth factors, extracellular matrix

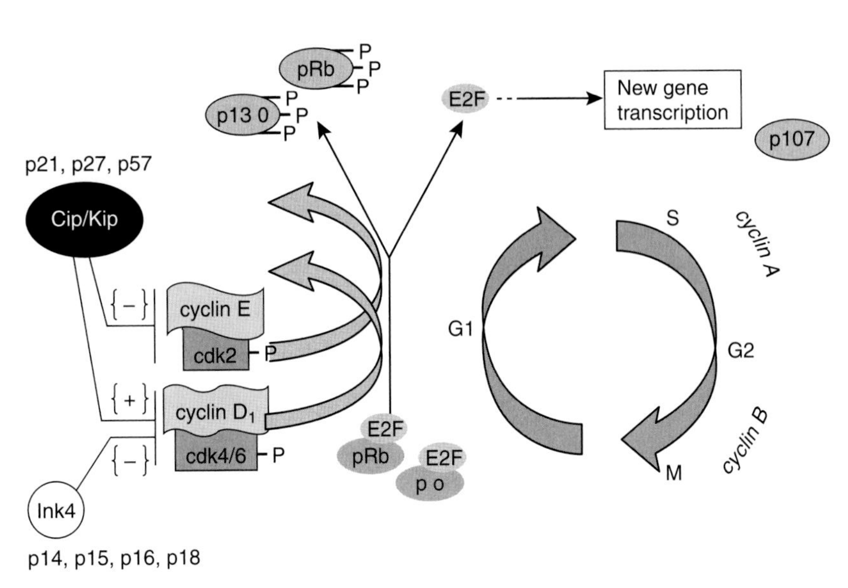

Figure 3–1. Cell cycle. In the normal cell cycle, DNA synthesis (in which chromosomal DNA is duplicated) occurs in the S phase, whereas mitosis (in which nuclei first divide to form a pair of new nuclei, followed by actual cellular division to form a pair of daughter cells) takes place in the M phase. The S phase and M phase are separated by two gap phases, the G_1 phase after mitosis and before DNA synthesis, and the G_2 phase following S phase until M phase. During these gap phases, the cell is synthesizing proteins and metabolites, increasing its mass, and preparing for the S phase and M phase. Cell cycle progression is regulated primarily at two points: the G_2/M and G_1/S boundaries, through the coordinated activities of cyclins and cyclin-dependent kinases (cdks), which, in turn, are negatively regulated by cdk inhibitors (Ink4: p14, p15, p16, and p18, as well as Cip/kip p21, p27, and p57). The mid-G_1 phase is characterized by the interaction between cyclin D1 and cdk4/6. This complex hyperphosphorylates the retinoblastoma protein (pRb) and its family members (e.g., p130). Another important complex is that among p107, cdk2, and cyclin E at the G_1/S boundary. The result is diminishing activity of pRb as a negative regulator of general transcriptional factors, e.g., E2F. In turn, E2F binds the promoters of genes that are important in DNA synthesis.

and cell-cell adhesion molecules have a significant impact on cell proliferation. Although the full spectrum of molecules that play a role in cell-matrix and cell-cell adhesion is still not defined, the spectrum is known to include integrins, cadherins, selectins, and proteoglycans. Interactions with these adhesion molecules lead to changes in the cell cytoskeleton and indirectly modulate external growth stimuli. Alterations in these matrix or cell-cell interactions are especially important in contributing to phenotypic changes that are characteristic of malignant cells (discussed later).

Interaction of ligands with their receptors at the cell surface induces intracellular signals that ultimately result in alterations in gene transcription. Four distinct pathways appear to initiate cellular signal processes through ligand-receptor interaction at the cell surface: (1) tyrosine phosphorylation, (2) serine and threonine phosphorylation, (3) cyclic nucleotide generation, and (4) calcium phosphoinositol production.

The receptors for many peptide growth factors contain intrinsic tyrosine kinase activity within the intracellular tail of the receptors. Tyrosine kinase is activated by ligand binding, thereby leading to phosphorylation of tyrosine residues in target proteins within the cell. The full spectrum of proteins phosphorylated by each tyrosine kinase remains to be determined. Most receptors also autophosphorylate tyrosine residues present in the receptors themselves, thereby frequently causing attenuation of their own activity and thus generating an intramolecular feedback regulatory mechanism.

Other receptors possess kinase activity directed toward serine or threonine rather than tyrosine. These receptors also phosphorylate a variety of cellular proteins, leading to a cascade of biologic responses. Multiple sites of serine and

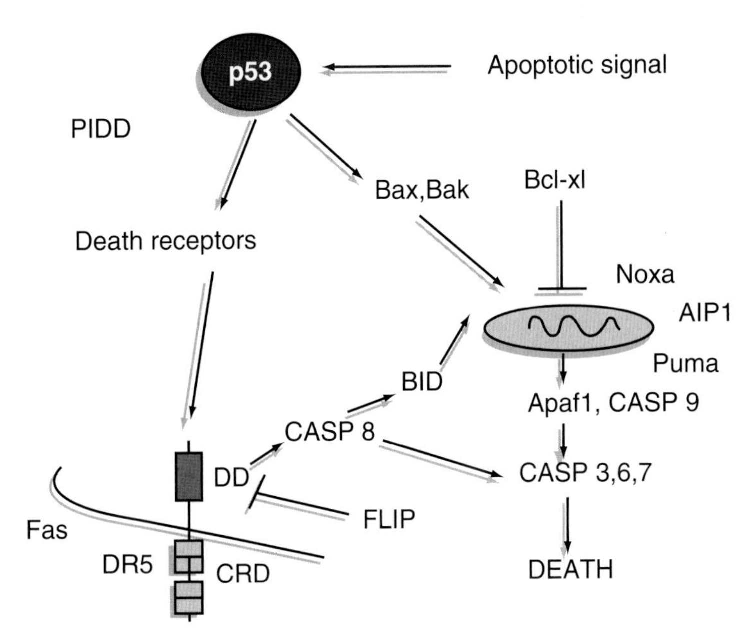

Figure 3–2. Apoptosis. There is a complex interplay of proapoptotic and antiapoptotic molecules that result in the downstream activation of signals that mediate cell death. Some of these signals are initiated through the p53 tumor suppressor gene and affect death receptors and downstream targets (DD, Bax, Bak). Activation of caspase 8 (CASP 8) influences BID. Ultimately, the complex interplay between Bax/Bak and Bcl-xl affects mitochondria and leads to activation of different caspases and cell death.

threonine phosphorylation are present on many growth factor receptors, including the tyrosine kinase receptors, suggesting the existence of significant interactions among various receptors present on a single cell.[18]

Many receptors are typically members of the so-called seven-membrane spanning receptor family. These receptors are coupled to guanosine triphosphate binding proteins, designated *G proteins*, which couple ligand binding to cellular response through modulation of the cellular concentration of cyclic nucleotides. G proteins undergo a conformational change that is dependent on the presence of guanosine phosphates.[19]

Finally, some ligand receptors exert their biologic activity through stimulation of phospholipase C at the cell membrane. This enzyme leads to generation of phosphoinositides (most importantly, inositol 1,4,5-triphosphate) as well as diacylglycerol through hydrolysis of membrane phospholipids. Both products serve as second messengers that mediate additional biochemical changes within the cell, thereby leading to coordinated changes in the intracellular flux of calcium and protein kinase C activity in the cell.[20]

Growth factor binding at the cell surface typically produces alterations in a variety of cellular functions that influence growth. These functions include ion transport (most notably of sodium and hydrogen), nutrient uptake, and protein synthesis. However, the ligand-receptor interaction must ultimately modify gene expression within the nucleus. The regulation of the content and activity of transcriptional factors within the nucleus is nearly the final step in pathways that translate an external stimulus to a change in cell proliferation. These transcriptional factors modulate expression of a cascade of genes that control cell proliferation and phenotype. Some of the most important of these genes are designated *early response genes*.

MECHANISMS OF ONCOGENESIS

Genetic and environmental factors play important roles in tumorigenesis. Both ultimately lead to expression of abnormal genes or inappropriate expression of normal genes, the products of which confer the malignant phenotype. Genetic mutation is the common denominator of agents or mechanisms that contribute to the development of neoplasia. Mutations may be inherited (germline mutation), or they may be acquired through the action of an environmental factor or failure of intrinsic cellular mechanisms of DNA replication or transcription (somatic mutation).

Somatic mutations can result from any class of carcinogen, including chemical mutagens and ionizing and ultraviolet radiation. Dietary constituents and their metabolites may act as important environmental mutagens within the GI tract. Viral agents also can lead to disruption of normal genes by entry into the host genome in a position that disrupts normal gene sequences (insertional mutagenesis) or through introduction of aberrant genes present in the virus's own genetic material. Examples of viral agents that appear to play a role in oncogenesis in the GI tract through insertional mutagenesis include human papillomavirus in squamous cell cancers of the esophagus and anus, Epstein-Barr virus in gastric lymphoepithelial malignancies, and hepatitis B virus in hepatocellular carcinoma. Ironically, many of these viral oncogenes originated as host cellular genes that were captured at some time in the past when a viral ancestor was present as a lysogen in an ancestral host genome. Transforming viruses include a wide array of DNA viruses (e.g., polyoma- and papillomaviruses) as well as the ribonucleic acid (RNA) viruses (retroviruses). Retroviruses encompass viral agents that possess reverse transcriptase, which allows the production of DNA from RNA.

The distinction between inherited and environmental factors (including viral agents, chemical carcinogens, and ionizing radiation) in tumorigenesis may be reconciled through appreciation of the multistep nature of oncogenesis and the role of clonal expansion in tumor progression. A variety of observations support the concept that malignant cells result from a series of discrete events that each may result in intermediate stages of altered biologic behavior.[21] The clinical correlate of this concept is found in the intermediate tissue alterations that are recognized as precursors to the subsequent development of cancer at various sites within the GI tract.

The multistep nature of oncogenesis is most directly illustrated by the changes that accrue in the development of colonic neoplasia (see Chapters 114 and 115). The accumulation of alterations roughly parallels the progression from normal epithelium through adenomatous polyps (or, in the case of ulcerative colitis, flat dysplastic mucosa) to frank malignant neoplasia. Studies in the molecular pathogenesis of colon cancer have served as a paradigm for the elucidation of genetic alterations in other GI cancers. For example, a similar progression is also seen in the transition from normal squamous epithelium to metaplastic mucosa (Barrett's esophagus) and subsequently through dysplasia to adenocarcinoma of the esophagus. Gastric and pancreatic oncogenesis is thought to proceed through similar multistep pathways.

Tumor Development: Multistep Formation and Clonal Expansion

Models of the multistep or "multiple hit" process of tumor formation have largely superseded earlier concepts of oncogenesis that discriminated between tumor "initiation" and subsequent "promotion."[22] Initiation was attributed to a single change in a cell that converted it from a normal to a malignant cell. Promotion reflected all the factors that acted after the initiating event to enhance tumor growth. However, oncogenesis occurs through a series of events that result in incremental changes in cell behavior until the cell eventually passes some threshold associated with the malignant phenotype. Nevertheless, there is still some merit in a more limited concept of tumor promotion. A number of factors promote the likelihood of malignant transformation through the stimulation of increased cellular turnover, which increases opportunities for somatic mutation to occur.[23] In the GI tract these factors include dietary constituents (discussed later) as well as chronic inflammation, which are associated with increased cell proliferation. Thus, a number of chronic inflammatory conditions increase the site-specific risk of cancer, for example, ulcerative colitis, chronic gastritis, chronic pancreatitis, Barrett's esophagus, and chronic hepatitis. Chronic inflammation is associated with increased rates of cell turnover in an ongoing cycle of inflammation-related epithelial destruction and regeneration.

Clonal expansion is also essential to tumor development.[24] Whereas germline mutations may lead to altered expression of a gene in all cells within a tissue, subsequent additional somatic mutations generally occur only in a small, largely random subpopulation. Clonal expansion occurs if the mutated gene results in increased growth or proliferation of the cell. A second round of clonal expansion occurs when a cell within this population sustains still another genetic alteration, which further enhances its growth properties. After several iterations, a genetic alteration eventually confers a property that, together with the preceding genetic alterations, makes a cell malignant. Clonal expansion of these cells leads to tumor formation.

The importance of clonal expansion is illustrated by the sequence of molecular events that are thought to underlie the development of colonic cancer, most notably in association with familial adenomatous polyposis (FAP). Studies described later in this chapter suggest that mutation of the FAP-associated gene leads to hyperproliferation of colonic epithelial cells. Expansion of the proliferative compartment in normal mucosa has also been thought to occur as an early event in the pathogenesis of sporadic colon cancers. Focal cancers develop through the clonal expansion of cells that undergo alteration of additional genes involved in cellular growth control.

Chemical Carcinogenesis

Metabolic activation by the host animal is a key determinant of the carcinogenic potential of many compounds. The initial compound, the procarcinogen, is changed by host enzymes to an electrophilic derivative, which then chemically modifies DNA (Fig. 3–3). Mutations result from errors that occur during DNA replication as a result of distorted base pairs. These mutations, in conjunction with other tumor-promoting factors, facilitate or cause the development of malignancy. Factors that influence the potency of any chemical carcinogen include the equilibrium between the activation of the procarcinogen or deactivation or degradation of the carcinogen.[25] Deactivation typically occurs through a conjugation reaction, usually in the liver.

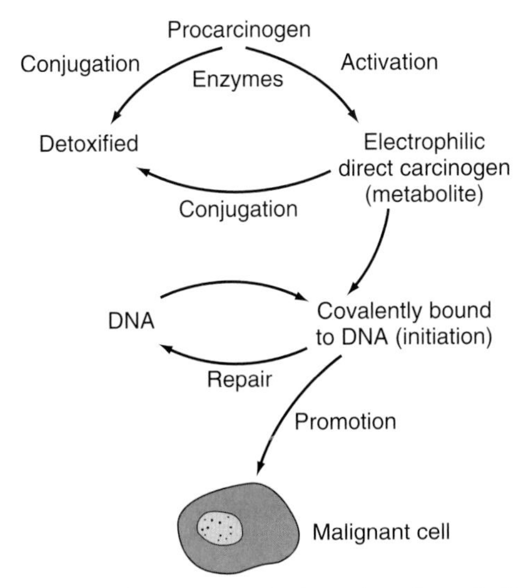

Figure 3–3. Chemical carcinogenesis. An activated metabolite modifies DNA. A procarcinogen is activated by host enzymes, most often in the liver, to yield an electrophilic carcinogen that may then bind covalently to DNA. Alternatively, the procarcinogen or carcinogen can be conjugated, resulting in detoxification. DNA bases modified by the carcinogen can also be repaired by cellular enzymes.

These principles are exemplified by experimental colonic carcinomas that arise in rodents fed cycasin, a glucosylated compound present in the cycad nut. The glucose residue of cycasin is cleaved in the rat liver by β-glucosidase to form methylazoxymethanol (MAM), which is subsequently deformylated by enzymes in the liver and colon to give rise to methyldiazonium, a carcinogen. These same metabolites are formed through hepatic enzymatic modification of the compound dimethylhydrazine and result in colon cancer in the rat.

Dietary Factors

Chemical mutagenesis may be especially important in the development of cancers within the GI tract and related organs. The mucosal surfaces from which most primary cancers in the GI tract develop are exposed to a complex mixture of dietary constituents that are potential carcinogens or procarcinogens. The ability of dietary factors to act as mutagens in humans was demonstrated directly in 1995 in some human hepatocellular carcinomas. The frequency of contamination of foodstuffs with aflatoxin, a fungal metabolite, parallels the incidence of hepatocellular carcinoma in various areas of the world.[26] Recent studies have shown that aflatoxin causes mutations in the p53 gene in hepatocellular carcinoma (discussed later).[26]

Another example of a dietary factor that may act as a procarcinogen in the GI tract is the presence of nitrates in many foods. Nitrates can be converted through bacterial action in a hypochlorhydric stomach to nitrites and subsequently to mutagenic nitrosamines.[27] These events may underlie the documented correlation between dietary intake of certain foodstuffs as well as environmental nitrate exposure and the incidence of gastric cancer among different populations.

Other dietary factors may modulate the biologic potency of dietary procarcinogens. Variations in the relative and absolute amounts of dietary fats may lead to alterations in the composition of the colonic microflora and their metabolic characteristics, resulting in modulation of the production of enzymes that convert dietary constituents into potentially mutagenic compounds. Changes in dietary fiber content can alter the transit time of luminal contents in the bowel, thereby changing the duration of exposure of the mucosa to potential mutagens.

These mechanisms could explain well-documented correlations between the intake of various dietary constituents and the incidence of colon cancer among populations. For example, populations that have a high fiber intake and resulting fast colonic transit times generally exhibit a lower incidence of colon cancer than populations with low fiber intake and delayed transit. The incidence of colon cancer among Japanese persons who immigrate to the United States and who consume a Western diet is much higher than that of native Japanese persons who consume a traditional Japanese diet.[28] These trends may reflect the different content of saturated fat and fiber of the two diets, although many other dietary and environmental factors also may play a role.

Bile salt content may be an additional luminal factor that can modulate the biologic effect of procarcinogens. Deconjugated bile salts may promote carcinogenesis through mucosal injury and enhanced epithelial proliferation. Studies have suggested a more direct role for mutagenic fecal sterols, possibly derived from bacterial metabolism of host bile salts.

NEOPLASIA-ASSOCIATED GENES

A variety of approaches have led to the identification of many genes that collectively play an important role in oncogenesis. In general, these genes lead to disruption of the orderly mechanisms of normal cell proliferation. Insofar as normal cell proliferation appears to depend on a wide variety of genes, it is not surprising that alterations in diverse genes confer part or all of the phenotypic features of transformation. Despite this diversity, all of these genes appear to belong to one of three distinct groups: oncogenes, which actively confer a growth-promoting property directly; tumor suppressor genes, the product of which normally restrains growth or proliferation; and DNA mismatch repair genes, which contribute to transformation by fostering genomic instability and facilitating mutations in other genes. Activation of oncogenes or inactivation of tumor suppressor genes and DNA mismatch repair genes can contribute to malignant transformation (Table 3–2).

Oncogenes

Typically, oncogenes are either genes that encode a normal cellular protein that is expressed at inappropriately high levels or mutated genes that produce a structurally altered protein that exhibits inappropriate function. Several genes that encode tyrosine kinase–containing growth factor receptors become oncogenes after mutations that result in unregulated tyrosine activity independent of the presence of the appropriate ligand. The normal cellular genes from which the oncogenes derive are designated *proto-oncogenes* or *cellular oncogenes*.

More than 80 oncogenes have been isolated, and additional oncogenes continue to be identified. Most of these genes are widely expressed in many different types of tumor cells. Multiple oncogenes (usually in combination with altered tumor suppressor genes) are commonly found within a single tumor. It is also apparent that no single combination of oncogenic activities is uniformly found in malignant tumor from a given tissue. Thus, various combinations of many oncogenes and tumor suppressor genes have been observed to be altered when individual GI cancers have been compared. Oncogenes encompass a range of categorically distinct genes. It is possible that any member of a group (e.g., any oncogene that encodes a protein involved in signal transduction) may be sufficient to fulfill a requirement in the multistep process of carcinogenesis for a specific tissue. Alternatively, ultimate malignant transformation in a particular tissue may result from a threshold number of events that in aggregate lead to tumor formation regardless of the specific combination.

Several mechanisms can lead to oncogene activation. These mechanisms include gene transduction or insertion, point mutation, gene rearrangement, and gene amplification. Gene transduction and insertion generally result from retroviral infection. Point mutations were recognized in a number of genes that were found to be able to confer the malignant phenotype when transfected into nontransformed cells. Many of these genes are members of the ras gene family that encode G proteins.[29] Altered ras proteins are commonly found in primary colonic and pancreatic cancers.

PRODUCTS ENCODED BY ONCOGENES: ROLE IN GASTROINTESTINAL NEOPLASIA. The proteins encoded by oncogenes comprise at least four distinct groups: peptide growth factors that may be secreted into the extracellular milieu, protein kinases, signal transducing proteins associated with the inner cell membrane surface (membrane-associated G proteins), and transcriptional regulatory proteins located in the nucleus.[30]

ONCOGENES AND GROWTH FACTORS. The transforming effects of enhanced expression of a variety of growth factors have been demonstrated both in vitro and in vivo. Several growth factor–related proteins encoded by oncogenes have now been recognized. In addition, many tumor cells exhibit enhanced production of peptide growth factors without underlying genetic mutations. It is axiomatic that cells in which the production of high levels of a growth factor results in alterations in the biologic properties of the cell must also express specific receptors that are activated by that growth factor. An autocrine growth-stimulating loop is often present in neoplasms. For example, several colon-derived cancer cell lines express TGF-α, TGF-β, and insulin-like growth factors (IGFs) I and II and their receptors. This autocrine mechanism may be contrasted with overproduction of a growth factor that exerts its influence at a remote cellular target rather than within the tumor itself, as when gastrin produced by gastrinoma cells exerts trophic effects on the gastric mucosa, which expresses receptors for this ligand, but not on the tumor itself.[31]

Several growth factors and their receptors have been found to be encoded by oncogenes in a variety of tumors. These include members of the epidermal growth factor (EGF)/TGF-α, fibroblast growth factor (FGF), IGF, and eph families.[32] Each of these factors has pro-proliferative effects in GI epithelial cell populations. The pro-proliferative factors and their receptors have been found frequently in GI tract cancers and cell lines derived from these tumors.[33] TGF-α, a protein that exhibits significant homology with EGF and binds to the same receptor, appears to promote cell proliferation in these populations.[34] This activity is counterbalanced in part by TGF-β, which is a family of proteins with no structural homology to TGF-α or EGF and inhibits epithelial cell proliferation.[35] The ubiquitiously expressed TGF-β inhibits cell proliferation primarily by binding to TGF-β type I and type II receptors.[36] Mutations in the TGF-β type II receptors that render cells incapable of transmitting a growth inhibitory signal are present in some colonic cancers and pancreatic cancers.[37, 38] Furthermore, downstream targets of this pathway (designated Smads) can be inactivated through point mutations or deletions.

Table 3–2 | **Oncogenes, Tumor Suppressor Genes, and DNA Mismatch Repair Genes Altered in Gastrointestinal Tumors***

	ESOPHAGUS	STOMACH	BILIARY TRACT	PANCREAS	COLON	LIVER
Oncogenes						
ras			+	+	+	
c-*myc*	+	+	+	+	+	+
c-*erb*-B1		+				+
c-*erb*-B2	+	+	+	+	+	+
hst-1	+	+			+	+
trk					+	
c-*raf*					+	
c-*src*	+				+	
c-*yes*						
c-*myb*		+			+	+
c-*fos*						
c-*mos*						
Tumor suppressor genes						
p53	+	+		+	+	+
DCC	+	+		+	+	
APC	+	+		+	+	
DPC4/Smad4	+				+	
DNA mismatch repair genes				+		
hMSH2, hMLH1	+	+		+	+	

*This list is not comprehensive but classifies the most important known oncogene, tumor suppressor gene, and DNA mismatch repair gene alterations in GI tumors; the frequency of cited associations varies from rare to frequent within tumor type.

APC, adenomatous polyposis coli; DCC, deleted in colon cancer; DNA, deoxyribonucleic acid; DPC-4, deleted in pancreas cancer; GI, gastrointestinal.

PROTEIN KINASE–RELATED ONCOGENES. Many oncogenes encode proteins with kinase activity. These oncogenes encompass the entire spectrum of protein kinases, including receptor and nonreceptor tyrosine kinases and cytoplasmic serine and threonine kinases. Many members of this large oncogene group are expressed within neoplasms of the GI tract.

A brief consideration of receptor protein tyrosine kinases v-erb-B and the *neu* oncogenes, both related to the EGF receptor and found in GI tract cancers, is particularly informative. The viral v-erb-b encodes a truncated form of the EGF receptor that lacks most of the external EGF-binding domain.[39] As a result, the receptor no longer requires the presence of the ligand for activation and remains continuously activated, stimulating proliferation. The *neu* oncogene in the rat is derived from a cellular oncogene in the rat closely related to the EGF receptor. The oncogene differs from its normal counterpart by a point mutation that changes a single residue (valine to glutamic acid) within the transmembrane domain, thereby causing activation of the 185-kDa tyrosine kinase protein (p185*neu*).[40] The human counterpart (c-erb-B2) of the *neu* oncogene is overexpressed or amplified in a variety of adenocarcinomas, including those arising in the stomach, breast, and prostate.[41] In addition, c-erb-B2 expression increases progressively in the transition from normal esophageal mucosa through the dysplastic state characteristic of Barrett's esophagus to esophageal adenocarcinoma.[42]

In contrast with the receptor type of tyrosine kinase that possesses intrinsic catalytic activity, many other receptors and membrane proteins lack self-contained signaling activity. Instead, they are coupled to nonreceptor tyrosine kinases on the cytoplasmic side of the plasma membrane that act as signal transducers. A number of oncogenes associated with neoplasms of the GI tract, most notably the colon, are members of the src family of nonreceptor tyrosine kinase activity. Members of the src family are approximately 60-kd phosphoproteins (pp60v-src) that possess inherent tyrosine kinase activity and associate with the inner surface of the plasma membrane. Tyrosine kinase activity is essential to the transforming activity of pp60v-src. Autophosphorylation of the normal pp60c-src leads to attenuation of its kinase activity, thereby providing inherent regulation to limit unrestrained activity.[43]

Increased levels of pp60c-src activity have been found in both colonic cancer tissue and colonic cancer–derived cell lines.[44, 45] Activation of the pp60c-src protein kinase also has been observed in colonic polyps.[46] Activation has been most consistent in large polyps that contain foci of severe atypia or cancer.

SIGNAL TRANSDUCTION–RELATED ONCOGENES (MEMBRANE-ASSOCIATED G PROTEINS). Intermediate steps that effectively translate ligand-receptor binding to an intracellular signal are essential in mediating functional responses of the cell. Mutations in genes that encode key proteins that participate in signal transduction can also lead to cellular transformation.

G proteins, which regulate the generation of cyclic nucleotides as secondary messengers, are the prototypes of a coupled signal transducer. Alterations in *ras* genes, which encode a family of proteins related to the G proteins, are among the most commonly detected oncogenes in GI tract cancers. The ras family contains three functional genes: Ha-ras, Ki-*ras*, and N-*ras*. All three encode 21-kd proteins. Post-translational modification of the carboxy-terminal end of the protein results in plasma membrane localization. Point mutations that result in amino acid substitutions at critical "hot spot" positions (residues 12, 13, 59, and 61) convert the normal gene into an oncogene.[47] These substitutions lead to alteration in the tertiary structure of the highly conserved N-terminal domain of the encoded protein. All altered *ras* genes in human tumors have been found to result from single activating point mutations.

The frequency of *ras* gene mutations varies greatly among different GI tumor types. The highest frequency is found in tumors of the exocrine pancreas; more than 90% of these tumors possess mutations in the Ki-*ras* gene.[48] *Ras* genes activated through point mutation have been identified in approximately 50% of colonic cancers as well as large benign colonic polyps.[49] In contrast, fewer than 10% of colonic adenomas less than 1 centimeter in size have *ras* mutations.

Most oncogenic mutations in *ras* cause biochemical changes that maintain p21 in the active guanosine triphosphate (GTP)–bound state by reducing guanosine triphosphatase (GTPase) activity or by destabilizing the inactive guanosine diphosphate (GDP)–bound form. However, several ras mutants retain significant GTPase activity; therefore, other mechanisms that convert *ras* to a transforming protein may be involved.[50] The GTPase-activating protein (GAP) induces a 500-fold increase in the GTPase activity of normal p21, and some mutant p21 proteins are resistant to this modifying protein.[51] In the presence of GAP, ras protein oncogenic activity correlates strongly with its reduced GTPase activity. GAP presumably maintains the normal p21 in its inactive GDP-bound state; mutant ras escapes this control and remains in the active GTP-bound state. A functional consequence of *ras* activation is the cascade phosphorylation of key serine and threonine kinases.[52]

NUCLEAR ONCOGENES. Many cellular oncogenes encode proteins that localize in the nucleus. Alteration of the level of expression of certain genes leads to enhanced cellular proliferation and suppression of normal differentiation. In essence, these nuclear oncogene products are the final mediators of the signal transduction pathways that are also affected by cytoplasmic and plasma membrane–bound oncoproteins.

In general, most nuclear oncoproteins immortalize primary cells and cooperate with other oncoproteins, especially *ras*, to cause transformation. In addition, a number of nuclear oncoproteins induce DNA synthesis in growth-arrested cells. Many nuclear oncoproteins have structural and functional properties characteristic of transcriptional factors and alter the transcription of specific target genes. Although a detailed understanding of the mechanisms through which the nuclear oncoproteins regulate transcription is still lacking, homo- and heterodimerization of these proteins through well-defined motifs is important in the process. Other domains confer DNA-binding specificity, which is critical in the regulation of genes involved in cell cycle control.

The role of nuclear oncogenes that encode transcriptional regulatory proteins and that are involved in protein-protein interaction is exemplified by the *myc* family. The c-Myc protein product is involved in critical cellular functions such as proliferation, differentiation, apoptosis, transformation, and transcriptional activation of key genes.[53] Frequently c-Myc is overexpressed in many GI cancers. The protein contains several important domains. The carboxy-terminal contains a helix-loop-helix motif that mediates binding to other proteins, such as Max.[54] These heterodimers bind DNA through the basic domain of c-Myc. The amino terminal of c-Myc contains regions that are critical for transcriptional activation of genes, transformation, and apoptosis.[55] Recently, c-Myc has been discovered to be a transcriptional target of the β-catenin/T-cell factor (TCF) complex in colon cancers, which may play a role in c-Myc overexpression in this cancer.

Tumor Suppressor Genes

The products of tumor suppressor genes prevent the acquisition of the transformed phenotype in vitro[56, 57] and appear to have similar functional properties in vivo. Mutations that disrupt the biologic function of these genes have been found in association with GI cancers. Germline mutations of this class of gene underlie all of the known inherited cancer syndromes in which a specific gene has been implicated. A number of these genes and their products have been identified and characterized (Table 3–3).

Initial recognition of the existence of tumor suppressor genes was also derived from analysis of families with a markedly increased incidence of specific tumors. Within these relatively rare kindreds, in as many as one half of first-degree relatives of a proband (and each subsequent generation) specific tumors may develop, representing as much as a several-hundred-fold greater incidence than that of the general population. These families contrast with cancer-prone kindreds in which an enhanced incidence of cancer may be observed but seldom at levels more than two- to threefold greater than that of the general population.

Virtually all types of tumors have been found to occur in an inherited form. Penetrance is variable but is often quite high (e.g., FAP and resulting colonic cancer are found in 50% of at-risk offspring). Some kindreds exhibit susceptibility to cancer at a single site, whereas others exhibit enhanced susceptibility to two or more tumor types.

Despite the variation in the type of tumor found in different inherited cancer syndromes, a number of features are common to all the syndromes. Most importantly, the marked increase in risk for a particular tumor is found in the absence of other predisposing environmental factors. In addition, in affected members multiple primary tumors often develop within the target tissue, and, as noted, those individuals are sometimes at risk for more than one type of tumor. Finally, tumors in these affected members typically arise at a younger age than they do in the general population.

Table 3–3 | **Chromosomal Localization of Key Tumor Suppressor Genes in Gastrointestinal Cancers***

CHROMOSOME	GENE
5q	APC
10p	c-ret (tyrosine kinase)
17p	p53
18q	Smad4
9p	p16
17q	Tylosis-related gene (familial esophageal squamous cancer)

*Although tumor suppressor genes have been identified through their contribution to specific familial cancer syndromes, they contribute to sporadic cancer and may play a role in tumorigenesis at more than one site. Additional tumor suppressor genes exist on the chromosomes listed.

APC, adenomatous polyposis coli.

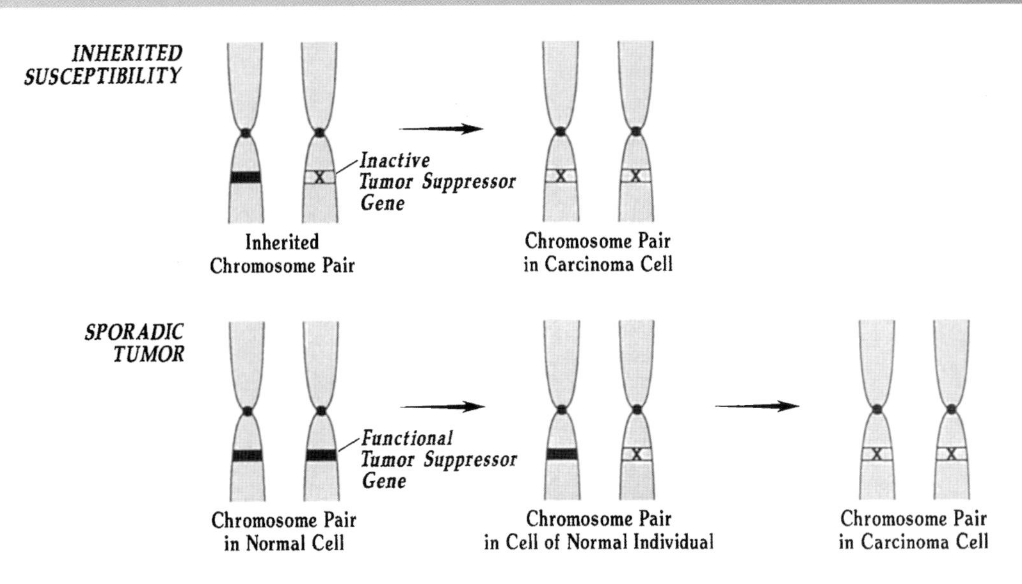

Figure 3–4. Knudson's hypothesis of tumor suppressor genes. In an inherited cancer syndrome, one chromosome has an inactive tumor suppressor gene locus because of germline mutation. The counterpart tumor suppressor gene on the remaining paired chromosome is subsequently inactivated by a somatic mutation, leading to formation of carcinoma. In contrast, in a sporadic cancer, the two alleles of the tumor-suppressor gene become inactivated through two independent somatic mutations, an unlikely event within a single cell.

These observations led Knudson to propose the hypothesis that tumors in familial cancer syndromes might derive from independent mutations in the two alleles of a specific gene (Fig. 3–4); he hypothesized that the first mutation was present in one copy of the gene inherited in the germline and therefore present in all cells in affected members of a cancer syndrome family.[58] A somatic mutation of the remaining normal allele that might occur in any cell would lead to tumor development, explaining the high incidence of cancer and multiple tumors. The same gene may play a role in the development of the same tumor type within the general population (sporadic cancer), but independent somatic mutations of each of the two alleles of the specific gene within a single cell would be required; this combination of events should be uncommon. Comings first suggested that the relevant gene in a familial cancer syndrome might encode a tumor-suppressing gene product.[59]

LOSS OF HETEROZYGOSITY AND ALLELIC DELETION. Tumor-associated genes, especially those encoding tumor suppressor genes, have also been identified through detection of regions of gene deletion in members of cancer-prone kindreds by screening of DNA with probes for markers scattered throughout the genome. In these studies, DNA of members of familial cancer kindreds was screened with a bank of probes for sequences scattered randomly throughout the genome. This approach can be combined with the technique of restriction fragment length polymorphism (RFLP) analysis (Fig. 3–5), in which the use of restriction endonucleases allows one to distinguish the two different alleles of the same genetic segment inherited from the subject's two parents. This approach provides a means of assessing whether a region of a chromosome (smaller than that necessary to be recognized by conventional karyotype techniques) might be deleted. Although these tools still detect only relatively large deletions, they have allowed the demonstration of the loss of one copy of particular areas of the genome in nontumor tissue from patients with hereditary cancer family syndromes, as predicted by Knudson and Comings. These losses, termed either *loss of heterozygosity* or *allelic deletions* (loss of an allele from one parent), affect tumor suppressor genes (see Table 3–3). This approach to identifying such genes may be superseded by analysis of single-nucleotide polymorphisms (SNPs) in the future.

Tumor suppressor genes appear to underlie all of the familial cancer family syndromes studied so far, including FAP, multiple endocrine neoplasia type II, hereditary retinoblastoma, and hereditary Wilms' tumor of the kidney. The malignancy first postulated to result from inactivation of a tumor suppressor gene was retinoblastoma, a pediatric malignant tumor of the embryonal retina. Karyotyping identified deletions in retinoblastoma cells on chromosome 13q14. RFLP analysis detected the loss of a small chromosome segment in one of the paired chromosomes in several retinoblastomas. This finding indicated that the second target gene at or near the site detected by RFLP (i.e., the gene affected by a mutation that resulted in tumor formation) was actually the second copy of the retinoblastoma (*Rb*) locus.

The *Rb* gene has been isolated, and alterations in Rb, or its 105-kd nuclear phosphoprotein product, have been found in a variety of tumors, including osteosarcoma, small cell lung carcinoma, breast carcinoma, prostate carcinoma, and leukemia, but not cancers of the GI tract. Several properties of Rb indicate that it exerts control over transcription of genes implicated in regulation of the cell cycle. Variation in Rb phosphorylation in phase-specific association with progression of the cell cycle suggests that Rb is involved in cell cycle control. Phosphorylation of Rb is in part the result of cdk kinase activity, although other molecules or cdk2-related molecules may also be involved in this phosphorylation.[60] Interestingly, it is underphosphorylated Rb found mostly in G_0 (quiescent) and G_1 cells that is "active" (i.e., the underphosphorylated protein suppresses cell proliferation).

The second gene found to encode a protein that has properties of a tumor suppressor gene was p53, which is also a nuclear phosphoprotein that appears to play a key role in cell cycle regulation.[61] The p53 protein was first detected in tumors as the product of a mutated cellular gene that was mapped to chromosome 17p, a region found to exhibit loss of heterozygosity in many tumors, suggesting that p53 might represent the product of a growth-suppressing gene. With polymerase chain reaction (PCR) methodology and DNA sequencing, point mutations in p53 have been identified in nearly 80% of sporadic colon cancers and a smaller subset

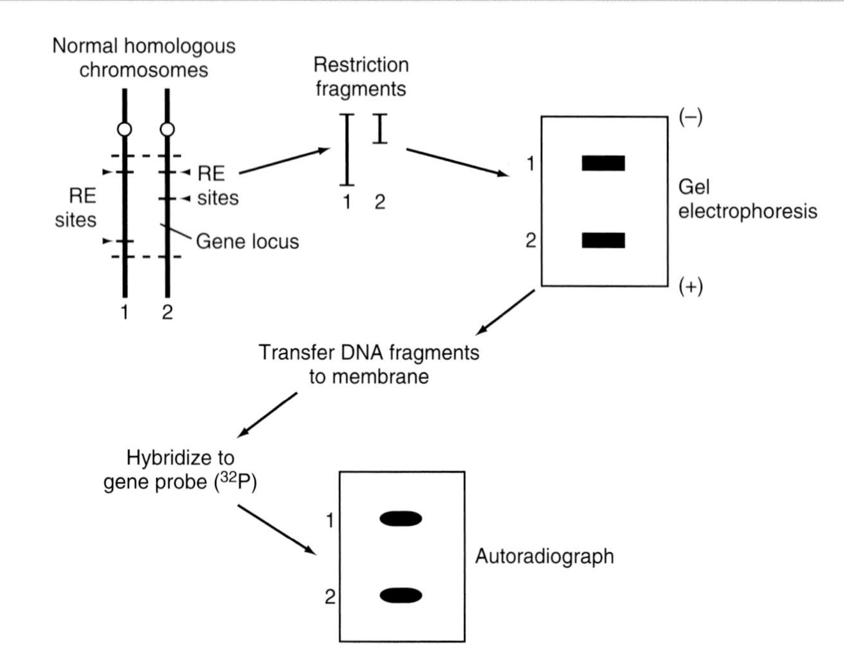

Figure 3–5. Restriction fragment length polymorphism (RFLP) analysis. Normal homologous chromosomes have sequences that can be recognized by bacterial enzymes, designated restriction endonucleases (RE). These restriction endonucleases cleave DNA at the site of these specific sequences to yield a pattern of restriction fragments. If segments of DNA inherited from the two parents differ by the presence or absence of an RE site, the RE fragments will migrate as bands of different size on gel electrophoresis. After transfer of the restriction fragments to a membrane and hybridization with a specific gene probe, different bands can be detected by autoradiography. In this manner, it can be determined whether both the paternal- and maternal-derived allele of a gene or a DNA segment are present.

of colonic adenomas as well as many other types of tumor.[62] Point mutations in p53 have also been found in esophageal squamous carcinoma and adenocarcinoma, gastric carcinoma, pancreatic adenocarcinoma, and hepatocellular carcinoma.[61] Interestingly, aflatoxin appears to induce a mutation in a single "hot spot" codon (#249) of p53 in many hepatocellular carcinomas.[63] In addition to the p53 point mutations resulting from somatic mutations in sporadic cancers, germline p53 mutations have been observed in the Li-Fraumeni syndrome, an autosomal dominant familial disorder in which a variety of tumors, including breast carcinoma, soft tissue sarcoma, osteosarcoma, leukemia, brain tumor, and adrenocortical carcinoma, can develop in affected persons.[64]

The functional importance of p53 is underscored by experiments in which wild-type p53 was reintroduced into colon cancer cells that had only mutant p53.[65] High repletion of cells with normal p53 can arrest growth in a cell cycle phase-specific manner (before the S phase). These observations are consistent with the notion that the normal function of wild-type p53 is linked to cell cycle control. It has been shown that wild-type p53 can bind DNA in a sequence-specific manner and thus may influence transcription of important genes. Mutant forms of p53 interfere with this transcriptional activation.[66]

THE ADENOMATOUS POLYPOSIS COLI GENE. The adenomatous polyposis syndromes are discussed in detail in Chapter 114. Although these syndromes are relatively rare, studies identifying genetic factors that contribute to these syndromes have shed light on mechanisms that appear to be essential to the development of common sporadic colonic cancers as well as to tumorigenesis in general[67] (Fig. 3–6).

Genetic linkage analysis revealed markers on chromosome 5q21 that were tightly linked to polyp development in affected members of kindreds with FAP and Gardner's syndrome.[68] Deletions in this region are also found in sporadic colon cancers and adenomas.[69] Further work led to the identification of the gene responsible for FAP, the adenomatous polyposis coli (APC) gene.[70] As predicted, germline mutations of APC were found in affected patients, and the germline mutations segregate with the disease within a given family pedigree.[71, 72] In addition, somatic mutations in this gene have been found in many sporadic colon polyps and cancers.[73–76]

The APC gene comprises 15 exons and encodes a predicted protein of 2843 amino acids, or approximately 310 kd. Most germline and somatic APC gene mutations result in stop codons and therefore a truncated protein product. Although mutations are most common in exon 15 of the APC gene, they may occur throughout the gene. Those occurring in the APC amino terminal are associated with a rare variant of FAP, attenuated adenomatous polyposis coli (AAPC).[77] Studies have revealed a segregation of certain APC mutations with the phenotype of congenital hypertrophy of the retinal pigment epithelium (CHRPE).[78]

APC mutations likely result in functional changes in key protein-protein interactions. Wild-type APC protein interacts with β−catenin, which is known to associate with the transmembrane E-cadherins.[79] Normally, β−catenin is degraded after association with the APC protein and glycogen synthase kinase-3 (GSK-3). However, when APC is mutated, β−catenin is stable and translocates into the nucleus in association with Tcf or Lef transcriptional factors. Members of the Tcf or Lef gene families can bind DNA to transactivate key target genes, such as c-myc and cyclin D1. In addition, targeted disruption of the APC gene in mouse embryonic stem cells through homologous recombination has facilitated study of the molecular basis of the phenotypic manifestations of FAP.

DELETED IN PANCREAS CANCER/SMAD4. Recently, a novel tumor suppressor gene, deleted in pancreas cancer (*DPC*-4), located on chromosome 18q, has been found to be deleted or mutated in most pancreatic cancers and a subset of colon cancers. This gene encodes Smad4, an essential mediator of the growth inhibitory effects of TGF-β. Mutant Smad4

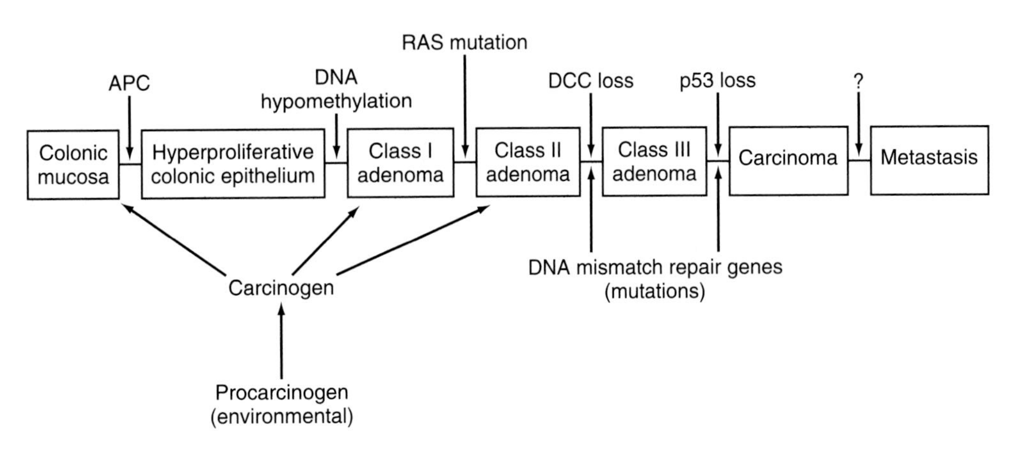

Figure 3–6. Colon cancer model: the interrelationship of genetic and environmental factors. The progression from normal colonic epithelium to carcinoma is associated with the acquisition of several genetic alterations. These alterations include the activation of oncogenes (e.g., *ras*) through a point mutation and the inactivation of tumor suppressor genes (e.g., p53, DCC, APC) through a point mutation or deletion. In addition, mutations of DNA mismatch repair genes and DNA hypomethylation may be important to the process as well. An increasing aggregate number of mutations can be correlated with progression from early benign polyp to cancer as reflected by analysis of polyps by size [class I, <1 cm (no tumor focus); class II, >1 cm (no tumor focus), and class III, >1 cm (with tumor focus)]. Various carcinogens may act at different stages of this model to cause somatic mutations that result in additional genetic alterations. Other factors ("promoters"), including dietary constituents, may enhance the likelihood of these events through stimulation of the rate of cell turnover.

blocks TGF-β-induced inhibition of proliferation. Other genes on chromosome 18q may be important in colon carcinogenesis.[80]

METHYLATION OF TUMOR SUPPRESSOR GENES. Tumor suppressor genes can be inactivated through allelic deletion and mutation. Another mechanism of inactivation is transcriptional silencing that results from methylation of CpG islands in gene promoters. Transcriptional silencing by promoter hypermethylation has been demonstrated for the gene encoding p16 in esophageal and pancreatic cancers and the gene encoding E-cadherin in gastric cancer.

DNA Mismatch Repair Genes

Cellular mechanisms have evolved to preserve fidelity of DNA replication. Errors in DNA replication result from either environmental agents (e.g., ultraviolet light, chemical carcinogens) or spontaneous mismatching of nucleotides. The latter mechanism is most likely to occur in regions of cytosine-adenosine (CA) dinucleotide repeats.[81] The DNA mismatch repair system corrects these errors. The components of this system have been studied most extensively in prokaryotes and lower eukaryotes, most notably yeast. DNA is repaired by a nucleotide excision repair system in bacteria.[81] The enzymes bind DNA, cut the damaged DNA strand, unwind the damaged DNA fragment, fill in the gap, and finally reseal the remaining nick. In eukaryotes, the nucleotide excision repair system is much more complex. The human homologs of these DNA mismatch repair genes include hMSH2, hMSH3, hMSH4, hMSH5, hMSH6, hMLH1, hMLH3, hPMS1, hPMS2, and likely others.

The genes hMSH2 and hMLH1 are the two members of the DNA mismatch repair gene family that are most frequently mutated at the germline level in hereditary nonpolyposis colorectal cancer syndromes (HNPCC).[82, 83] Mutations can lead to functional alterations that allow strand slippage during replication, and affected cells are called *replication error* (RER)*–positive*, in contrast to the RER-negative phenotype.[84, 85] DNA mismatch repair genes are mutated not only in HNPCC, but also in a subset of sporadic GI cancers, including those arising in the esophagus, stomach, pancreas, and colon. Mechanistically, the absence of DNA repair does not cause cancer directly. Rather, the absence of DNA repair permits the accumulation of mutations in a variety of other genes, such as the TGF-β type II receptor, bax, IGF type II receptor, and E2F-4.

BIOLOGIC FEATURES OF TUMOR METASTASIS

The establishment of distant metastasis requires multiple processes, many of which involve alterations in interactions between tumor cells and normal host cells. In order to metastasize, a cell or group of cells must detach from the primary tumor, gain access to the lymphatic or vascular space, adhere to the endothelial surface at a distant site and penetrate the vessel wall to invade the second tissue site, and, finally, proliferate as a second tumor focus. Angiogenesis is necessary for proliferation of both the primary tumor and tumor metastases. Tumor cells must also overcome host immune cell killing. As a result, few circulating tumor cells (less than 0.01%) successfully initiate metastatic foci. A "survival of the fittest" view of metastasis has been proposed, that is, that selective competition favors metastasis of a subpopulation of cells from the primary site.[86] Clonal expansion occurs again after initial formation of a metastatic focus.

Modulation of tumor cell interaction with the extracellular

matrix is an essential initial step leading to the formation of metastases. The basement membrane consists of a dense matrix of collagen, glycoproteins, and proteoglycans and normally does not permit passive penetration of cells. The transmigration of tumor cells through the basement membrane likely involves production of key proteolytic activities. Alternatively, the tumor cell may produce factors capable of activating proenzymes present in the extracellular matrix (e.g., the tumor may produce urokinase, itself a protease, or plasminogen activator). Once they have gained access to the interstitial stromal compartment, tumor cells can enter lymphatic and blood vessels.

Invasive carcinoma is associated with disruption of the integrity of the basement membrane, indicating that tumor cells interact with the basement membrane in a manner different from that of normal cells. The interactions of the tumor cells with the basement membrane can be subdivided into three phases: attachment, matrix dissolution, and migration (Fig. 3–7). Initially, tumor cells bind to the basement membrane through cell surface receptors of the integrin and nonintegrin families. Local matrix degradation occurs by proteases secreted from the tumor cells or tumor cell–induced protease secretion by host cells. Tumor cells traverse the stroma through mechanisms that have not been well elucidated but appear to depend on interaction between "receptor" molecules on the cell surface and "ligand" molecules in the extracellular matrix.

Angiogenesis

Angiogenesis is essential to sustain continued growth of the primary tumor. If new vessels are not developed, as the primary tumor expands, cells most distant from available vessels are deprived of an adequate source of nutrition and central necrosis occurs. Neovascularization is also an important permissive factor in facilitating metastatic dissemination of tumors.[87] A number of protein growth factors, often produced by malignant tumors, have been found to be potent stimuli of angiogenesis. Among these, basic fibroblast growth factor (bFGF) and TGF-α are especially important. Perhaps the most critical known factor is vascular endothelial growth factor (VEGF), which is up-regulated in most tumor types, including colon cancer. Multiple genetic pathways modulate VEGF expression, including mutant ras.

Angiogenesis occurs in an ordered series of events (see Fig. 3–7). Endothelial cells in the parent vessel are stimulated to degrade the endothelial basement membrane, migrate into the perivascular stroma, and initiate a capillary sprout. The sprout develops into a tubular structure that in turn develops into a capillary network. In vitro models that recapitulate the early events of angiogenesis indicate that this process involves a balance between proteases and protease inhibitors in a manner similar to that during tumor invasion. Indeed, functional parallels between tumor invasion and angiogenesis are evident in their mutual requirement for cellular motility, basement membrane proteolysis, and cell growth. The vascular endothelial cell ceases to promote angiogenesis after the angiogenic stimulus (e.g., bFGF) is removed, whereas in growing tumors these processes are unregulated.

Metastasis Genes

It is likely that properties important to the development of metastasis reflect the effects of the products of genes distinct from oncogenes involved in carcinogenesis. However, it is possible that genes for which activation or inactivation is essential to the development of metastasis are regulated by oncogenes. Although no gene specifically associated with metastasis has yet been identified, one gene, designated *nm*-23, may be a potential metastasis suppressor gene. Levels of *nm*-23 are reduced in a variety of metastatic tumors and in cell lines with high metastatic potential, compared with primary tumors and cell lines with low metastatic potential, respectively.[88] The function of *nm*-23 is uncertain but may be inferred from its high predicted amino acid homology to nucleoside diphosphate (NDP) kinases. NDP kinases are involved in microtubule assembly and signal transduction through G proteins; these functions may be important in the formation of metastases.

The CD44 transmembrane molecule, which is the receptor for hyaluronic acid, has also been implicated in tumor metastasis. This interaction may mediate cell interaction with extracellular matrix components, and alterations in CD44 may enhance malignant cell motility through the extracellular matrix. Aberrant alternative splicing of CD44 transcripts has been associated with metastatic colonic and pancreatic cancers.[89, 90]

SUMMARY OF MOLECULAR MECHANISMS OF GASTROINTESTINAL CANCERS

As the genetic basis of cancer has become better defined, common themes in the molecular pathogenesis of GI cancers have emerged. The activation of oncogenes and inactivation of tumor suppressor genes are involved in all GI cancers. Environmental-genetic interactions may also be important. The progression from normal epithelium to a premalignant stage to frank malignancy at different sites in the GI tract is associated with both common and distinctive genetic mechanisms, the paradigm for which is colon cancer (see Fig. 3–6). The temporal sequence and the accumulation of these alterations appear to be critical as well. A hypothetical schema that may provide a model for understanding the development of common GI tumors is illustrated for esophageal carcinoma in Fig. 3–8.

DIAGNOSTIC STRATEGIES: CURRENT AND FUTURE APPROACHES

DNA–Based Diagnostic Approaches: Risk Assessment, Detection, Disease Monitoring, Prediction of Response to Therapy

Progress in the identification of cancer-associated genes coupled with the inherent power of molecular biologic techniques to analyze exquisitely small amounts of DNA and

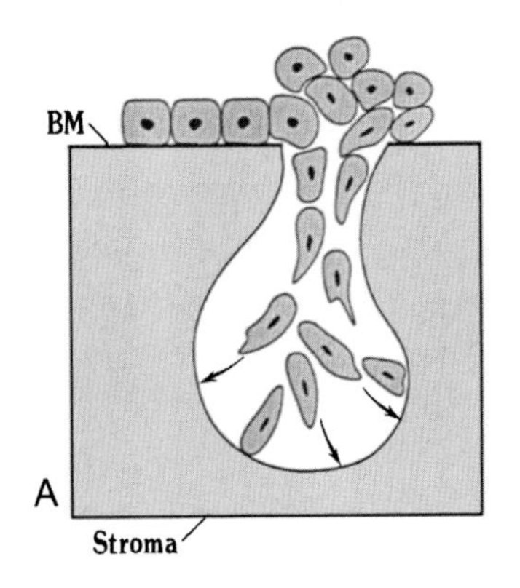

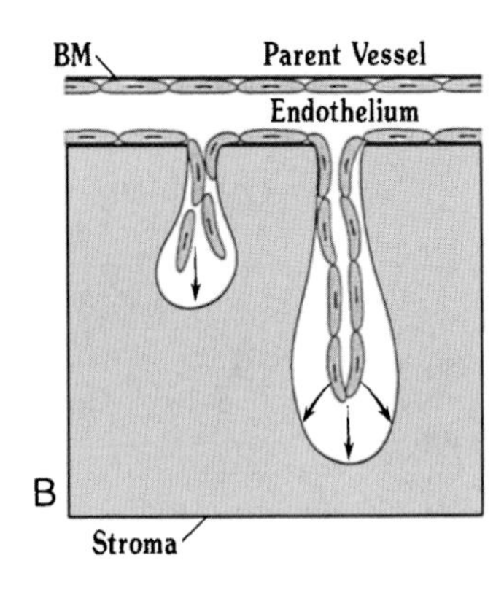

Figure 3–7. Mechanisms of tumor invasion and angiogenesis. *A,* Progression from *in situ* to invasive carcinoma involves the following sequence of events: attachment of malignant cells to the basement membrane (BM), dissolution of the basement membrane and extracellular matrix by proteases, and migration into the stroma. The malignant cells proliferate further in the stroma and invade blood and lymphatic vessels. *B,* During angiogenesis, the parent vessel basement membrane is dissolved. There is endothelial migration into the stroma toward an angiogenic stimulus (e.g., basic fibroblast growth factor). Later, proteolysis of the stroma permits expansion of the sprout diameter and formation of a lumen. (Modified from Liotta LA, Steeg P, Stetler-Stevenson WG: Cancer metastasis and angiogenesis: An imbalance of positive and negative regulation. Cell 64:327, 1991.)

protein are leading to more effective diagnostic markers (Table 3–4). The most immediate application is assessment of cancer risk in members of cancer-prone kindreds. Strategies have been developed to evaluate germline APC mutations in patients with FAP. Although DNA-based mutational analysis has proved to be labor intensive, the knowledge that APC mutations lead to truncated proteins has allowed the combined use of in vitro transcription and translation technology to distinguish wild-type from truncated APC protein with peripheral blood lymphocytes of a proband and potentially affected members within a pedigree[91] (Table 3–5). Although less than 100% sensitive, the technique illustrates the potential power of molecular diagnostics to facilitate genetic counseling and the development of new strategies for clinical screening. Familial risk assessment that is DNA based could also extend to *c-ret* mutations in MEN2, p53 mutations in the Li-Fraumeni syndrome, DNA mismatch repair mutations in HNPCC, and p16 mutations in the rare association of familial pancreatic cancer and melanoma (see Table 3–5). Application of genetic testing must take into consideration the sensitivity and specificity of the assay as well as issues of patient confidentiality and medical insurability.

Improved detection of sporadic GI cancers and their precursor lesions has also been the focus of recent research. Small numbers of shed cells obtained from colonic lavage can be assessed for the presence of specific tumor-associated oncogenes (e.g., *ras*) or allelic deletions by using the PCR methodology.[92] Pilot technology has been developed to extract DNA from stool specimens for the detection of large colonic adenomatous polyps and colorectal cancer by identification of *ras* mutations using a PCR assay.[93] In addition, a number of centers have reported the presence of *ras* mutations in DNA extracted from the pancreatic ductal fluid obtained at the time of endoscopic retrograde cholangiopancreatographic evaluation for pancreatic cancer.[94]

As tests for genetic markers become available, monitoring for disease recurrence after surgery is another important application of new insights into molecular mechanisms of tumorigenesis. Mucosal biopsy specimens, shed colonic epithelial cells, or peripheral blood may be assayed. Finally, by correlating key genetic alterations with prognosis (e.g., chro-

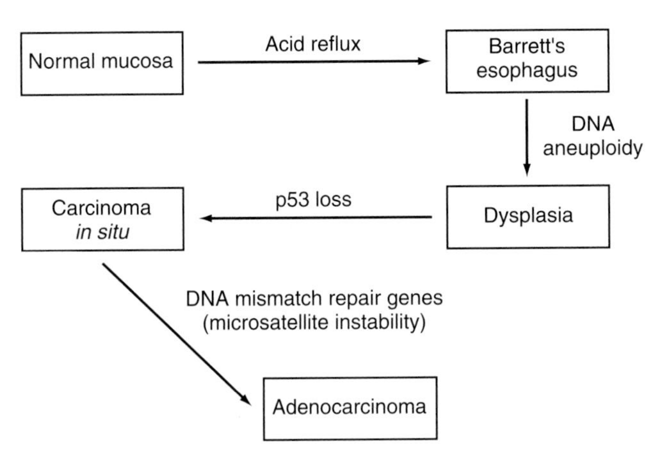

Figure 3–8. Hypothetical paradigm for multistage oncogenesis in the esophagus. These steps depict salient features but do not preclude the interaction of other environmental or genetic factors or alternative pathways. Similar paradigms can be invoked for cancers of the stomach, pancreas, and liver.

Table 3–4 | **Molecular Diagnostic Strategies for the Detection of DNA Mutations or Altered Proteins**

PCR-based strategies to detect DNA mutations	
Single-strand conformational polymorphism (SSCP)	Detection of alteration of secondary structure of single-stranded DNA due to single base mutation
Denaturing gradient gel electrophoresis (DGGE)	Detection of strand dissociation of double-stranded DNA altered by mutations
Heteroduplex analysis	Altered electrographic migration due to mutations
Heteroduplex mismatch cleavage	Chemical cleavage of mismatches in heteroduplexes
Direct DNA sequencing	Direct detection of altered DNA nucleotide sequence
PCR-based strategies to detect known mutations in genes (for example, Ki-*ras* codon 12)	
Restriction enzyme digestion	Mismatched primers followed by enzymatic cleavage
Allele-specific oligonucleotide hybridization	Hybridization of specific oligonucleotides with wild-type or mutant sequence
Protein-based strategies	
In vitro translation (IVT)	Detection of truncated protein resulting from translational terminating codon
Yeast and bacterial colorimetric assays	Altered colorimetric assay due to mutation

DNA, deoxyribonucleic acid; PCR, polymerase chain reaction.

Table 3–5 | **Applications of Molecular Diagnostics for Gastrointestinal Cancers**

DISORDER	GENE(S) DETECTED	ASSAY METHOD
Familial polyposis syndromes		
FAP	APC	IVT, DNA
HNPCC	hMSH2, hMLH1	DNA, IVT
Peutz-Jeghers syndrome	SKII	DNA
Cowden's disease	PTEN	DNA
Juvenile polyposis	PTEN, Smad4	DNA
Gastric cancer	E-cadherin	DNA
Pancreatic cancer	p16	DNA
MEN2	c-*ret*	DNA
Sporadic cancers		
Mucosal biopsies/ brushings in upper GI cancers	Yet to be defined	PCR based
Pancreatic ductal fluid in pancreas cancer	*ras*	PCR based
Bile ductal fluid in cholangiocarcinoma	*ras*, p53	PCR based
Stool in colon cancer	*ras* and others	PCR based

APC, adenomatous polyposis coli; DNA, direct deoxyribonucleic acid sequencing; FAP, familial adenomatous polyposis; GI, gastrointestinal; HNPCC, hereditary nonpolyposis colorectal cancer; IVT, in vitro translation; MEN, multiple endocrine neoplasia; PCR, polymerase chain reaction.

mosome 18q loss of heterozygosity and Dukes B colon cancer), patients may be stratified for targeted adjuvant therapeutic modalities.

Oncofetal Proteins

Characterization of malignant and transformed cells has led to the identification of markers that may be useful in the early detection and diagnosis of GI cancers. The most productive approaches have exploited the antigenicity of distinctive cell surface glycoconjugates to prepare conventional antisera or monoclonal antibodies directed against tumor-associated determinants. The first useful marker developed through this approach was the carcinoembryonic antigen (CEA), which was identified by Gold and coworkers after immunization of rabbits with colorectal cancer tissue.[95] The resulting antisera were found to recognize a determinant present in tumor tissue but largely absent from normal colonic mucosa. Further characterization proved that the same determinant was abundant in the fetal intestine, indicating that CEA was an oncofetal antigen. Most importantly, it was soon noted that the antigen recognized by the antisera was present in the sera of many patients who have colorectal cancer, generally in amounts proportional to the extent of the tumor. Subsequent characterization demonstrated that the tumor-associated determinants resided on large glycoproteins.

Study of CEA since 1978 has defined the value of this marker in the management of some patients with colorectal cancer but has also served to highlight many inherent biologic limits to the usefulness of cell surface–derived tumor markers. Further study showed that this oncofetal determinant is expressed in nonmalignant mucosa in association with increased proliferation; on a practical level the CEA concentration is "falsely" elevated in a variety of inflammatory conditions associated with increased cell turnover (e.g., ulcerative colitis). In addition, it was noted that CEA could be produced by tumors arising from many sites, particularly those elsewhere within the GI tract (e.g., gastric and pancreatic cancer). This finding underscores the relatively limited tissue specificity of transformation-associated alterations in cell surface determinants. Conversely, the determinant is not expressed by colon cancers that do not recapitulate the state of at least partial differentiation observed in the fetal colon; paradoxically the biologically most aggressive undifferentiated tumors often do not express the antigen.

Additional markers have been identified in the past several years through the production of monoclonal antibodies. Immunization with pancreatic tumor cells has led to the identification of a variety of tumor-associated glycoconjugate determinants (e.g., determinants recognized by antibodies CA19-9 and Du-Pan-2). The antigenic determinants present on tumors typically reflect modifications of blood group–related carbohydrate side chains that are present on high-molecular-weight mucin glycoproteins. Many such determinants represent distinctive forms of the Lewis blood group determinants, modified by the addition of sialic acid. As noted for CEA, the determinants recapitulate structures that are transiently expressed during fetal development. Not surprisingly, the clinical utility of each of these determinants has also been associated with limitations of specificity and sensitivity similar to those observed with CEA.

REFERENCES

1. Sherr CJ: The Pezcoller lecture: Cancer cell cycles revisited. Cancer Res 60:3689, 2000.
2. Motokura T, Bloom T, Kim H, et al: A novel cyclin encoded by a bcl1-linked candidate oncogene. Nature 350:512, 1991.
3. Nakagawa H, Zukerberg L, Togawa K, et al: Human cyclin D1 oncogene and esophageal squamous cell carcinoma. Cancer 76:541, 1995.
4. Weinberg RA: The retinoblastoma protein and cell cycle control. Cell 81:323, 1995.
5. Sherr CJ, Robert JM: Inhibitors of mammalian G_1 cyclin-dependent kinases. Genes Dev 9:1149, 1995.
6. el-Deiry WS, Tokino T, Velculescu VE, et al: WAF1, a potential mediator of p53 tumor suppression. Cell 75:817, 1993.
7. Serrano M, Hannon GJ, Beach D: A new regulatory motif in cell cycle control causing specific inhibition of cyclin D/cdk4. Nature 366:704, 1993.
8. Mori T, Miura K, Aoki T, et al: Frequent somatic mutation of the MTS1/CDK4 (multiple tumor suppressor/cyclin-dependent kinase 4 inhibitor) gene in esophageal squamous cell carcinoma. Cancer Res 54: 3396, 1994.
9. Lin Q, Yan YX, McClure M, et al: MTS-1 (CDKN2) tumor suppressor gene deletions are a frequent event in esophagus squamous cancer and pancreatic adenocarcinoma cell lines. Oncogene 10:619, 1995.
10. Caldas C, Hahn SA, da Costa LT, et al: Frequent somatic mutations and homozygous deletions of the p16 (MTS1) gene in pancreatic adenocarcinoma. Nat Genet 8:27, 1994.
11. Polyak K, Lee M, Herdjument-Bromage H, et al: Cloning of p27Kip1, a cyclin-dependent kinase inhibitor and a potential mediator of extracellular antimitogenic signals. Cell 78:59, 1994.
12. Reid BJ, Haggitt RC, Rubin CE, Rabinovitch PS: Barrett's esophagus: Flow cytometry complements histology in detection of patients at risk for adenocarcinoma. Gastroenterology 93:1, 1987.
13. Levine DS, Rabinovitch PS, Haggitt RC, et al: Distribution of aneuploid cell populations in ulcerative colitis with dysplasia or cancer. Gastroenterology 101:1198, 1991.
14. Yuan J, Shaham S, Ledoux S, et al: The *C. elegans* cell death gene

ced-3 encodes a protein similar to mammalian interleukin-1 beta converting enzyme. Cell 75:641, 1993.
15. Hengartner MO, Horvitz HR: *C. elegans* cell survival gene ced-9 encodes a functional homolog of the mammalian proto-oncogene bcl-2. Cell 76:665, 1994.
16. Oltvai ZN, Milliman CL, Korsmeyer SJ: Bcl-2 heterodimerizes in vivo with a conserved homolog, Bax, that accelerates programmed cell death. Cell 74:609, 1993.
17. Reed JC: Warner-Lambert/Parke-Davis Award Lecture: Mechanisms of apoptosis. Am J Pathol 157:1415, 2000.
18. Schlessinger J: Cell signaling by receptor tyrosine kinases. Cell 103: 211, 2000.
19. McCormick F: Signalling networks that cause cancer. Trends Cell Biol 12:M53, 1999.
20. Parekh DB, Ziegler W, Parker PJ: Multiple pathways control protein kinase C phosphorylation. EMBO J 19:496, 2000.
21. Bishop JM: Molecular themes in oncogenesis. Cell 64:235, 1991.
22. Blair DG, Oskarsson M, Wood TG, et al: Activation of the transforming potential of a normal cell sequence: A model for oncogenesis. Science 212:941, 1981.
23. Thompson TC, Southgate J, Kitchener G, Land H: Multistage carcinogenesis induced by *ras* and *myc* oncogenes in reconstituted organ. Cell 56:917, 1989.
24. Nowell P: The clonal evolution of tumor cell populations. Science 194: 23, 1976.
25. Miller EL, Miller JA: Searches for ultimate chemical carcinogens and their reactions with cellular macromolecules. Cancer 47:2327, 1981.
26. Ozturk M: p53 mutations in nonmalignant human liver: Fingerprints of aflatoxins? Hepatology 21:600, 1995.
27. Bortsch H: *N*-nitroso-compounds and human cancer: Where do we stand? IARC Sci Publ 105:1, 1991.
28. Haenszel W, Kurihara M: Studies of Japanese migrants. 1. Mortality from cancer and other diseases among Japanese in the United States. J Natl Cancer Inst 40:43, 1968.
29. Taparowsky E, Suard B, Fasano O, et al: Activation of the T24 bladder carcinoma transforming gene is linked to a single amino acid change. Nature 300:782, 1982.
30. Haubruck H, McCormick F: Ras p21: Effects and regulation. Biochim Biophys Acta 1071:215, 1991.
31. Cantley L, Auger K, Carpenter C, et al: Oncogenes and signal transduction. Cell 64:281, 1991.
32. Cross M, Dexter T: Growth factors in development, transformation, and tumorigenesis. Cell 64:271, 1991.
33. McGuigan JE: Hormones of the gastrointestinal tract. In DeGroot LR, Jameson JL, Burger H, et al (eds): Endocrinology. New York, Raven Press, 1989, p. 2741.
34. Barnard JA, Beauchamp RD, Russell WE, et al: Epidermal growth factor–related peptides and their relevance to gastrointestinal pathophysiology. Gastroenterology 108:564, 1995.
35. Massague J, Polyak K: Mammalian antiproliferative signals and their targets. Curr Opin Genet Dev 5:91, 1995.
36. Moustakas A, Lin HY, Henis YI, et al: The transforming growth factor beta receptor types I, II, and III form hetero-oligomeric complexes in the presence of ligand. J Biol Chem 268:22215, 1993.
37. Markowiltz S, Wang J, Myeroff L, et al: Inactivation of the type II TGF-β receptor in colon cancer cells with microsatellite instability. Science 268:1336, 1995.
38. Wang J, Sun L, Myderoff L, et al: Demonstration that mutation of the type II TGF-β receptor inactivates tumor suppressor activity in RER-positive colon carcinoma cells. J Biol Chem 270:22044, 1995.
39. Downward J, Yarden Y, Mayes E, et al: Close similarity of epidermal growth factor receptor and v-*erb*-B oncogene protein sequences. Nature 307:521, 1984.
40. Brandt-Rauf PW, Pincus MR, Carney WP: The c-erb B-2 protein in oncogenesis: Molecular structure to molecular epidemiology. Crit Rev Oncog 5:313, 1994.
41. Yokota J, Yamamoto T, Miyajima N, et al: Genetic alterations of the c-*erb* B-2 oncogene occur frequently in tubular adenocarcinoma of the stomach and are often accompanied by amplification of the v-*erb* A homologue. Oncogene 2:283, 1988.
42. Baggott BB, LaVolsi VA, Maguire HC, Greene MI: Increased and differential expression of the human *neu* (c-*erb*-2) oncogene product (p185*neu*) in Barrett's esophagus. Gastroenterology 98:A270, 1990.
43. Cooper JA, Gould KL, Cartwright CA, Hunter T: Tyr527 is phosphorylated in pp60c-arc: Implications for regulation. Science 31:1431, 1986.
44. Bolen JB, Veillette A, Schwartz AM, et al: Activation of pp60c-src protein kinase activity in human colon carcinoma. Proc Natl Acad Sci U S A 84: 2251, 1987.
45. Cartwright CA, Kamps MP, Meisler AI, et al: pp60c-src activation in human colon carcinoma. J Clin Investig 83:2025, 1989.
46. Cartwright C, Meisler AI, Eckhart W: Activation of the pp60c-arc protein kinase is an early event in colonic carcinogenesis. Proc Natl Acad Sci U S A 87:558, 1990.
47. Parada LF, Tabin CJ, Shih C, Weinberg RA: Human EJ bladder carcinoma oncogene is the homologue of Harvey sarcoma virus *ras* gene. Nature 297:474, 1982.
48. Sigal IS: The *ras* oncogene: Structure and some function. Nature 332: 485, 1989.
49. Bos JL, Fearon ER, Hamilton SR, et al: Prevalence of *ras* gene mutations in human colorectal cancers. Nature 237:293, 1987.
50. Bourne HR, Sanders DA, McCormick F: The GTPase superfamily. I. A conserved switch for diverse cell functions. Nature 248:125, 1990.
51. McCormick F: Activation and effectors of ras p21 proteins. Curr Opin Genet Dev 4:71, 1994.
52. Davis RJ: MAPKs: New JNKs expands the group. Trends Biochem Sci 19:470, 1994.
53. Luscher B, Eisenman RN: New light on Myc and Myb. 1. Myc. Genes Dev 4:20225, 1990.
54. Blackwood EM, Eisenman RN: Max: A helix-loop-helix zipper protein that forms a sequence-specific DNA-binding complex with Myc. Science 251:1121, 1991.
55. Evan GI, Wyllie AH, Gilbert CS, et al: Induction of apoptosis in fibroblasts by c-myc protein. Cell 69:119, 1992.
56. Harris H, Miller OJ, Klein G, et al: Suppression of malignancy by cell fusion. Nature 223:363, 1969.
57. Stanbridge EJ: Suppression of malignancy in human cells. Nature 260: 17, 1976.
58. Knudson AG: Mutation and cancer: Statistical study of retinoblastoma. Proc Natl Acad Sci U S A 68:820, 1971.
59. Comings DE: A general theory of carcinogenesis. Proc Natl Acad Sci U S A 70:3324, 1973.
60. DeCaprio JA, Ludlow JW, Lynch D, et al: The product of the retinoblastoma susceptibility gene has properties of a cell cycle regulatory element. Cell 58:1085, 1989.
61. Greenblatt MS, Bennett WP, Hoelstein M, Harris CC: Mutation in the p53 tumor suppressor gene: Clues to cancer etiology and molecular pathogenesis. Cancer Res 54:4855, 1994.
62. Nigro JM, Baker SJ, Preisinger AC, et al: Mutations in the p53 gene occur in diverse human tumour types. Nature 342:705, 1989.
63. Bressac B, Kew M, Wands J, Ozturk M: Selective G to T mutations of p53 gene in hepatocellular carcinoma from southern Africa. Nature 350:6317, 1991.
64. Malkin D, Li F, Strong L, et al: Germline p53 mutations in a familial syndrome of breast cancer, sarcomas and other neoplasms. Science 250: 1233, 1990.
65. Baker S, Markowitz K, Fearon E, et al: Suppression of a human colorectal carcinoma cell growth by wild-type p53. Science 249:1912, 1990.
66. Kern SE, Pietenpol JA, Thiagalingam S, et al: Oncogenic forms of p53 inhibit p53-regulated gene expression. Science 256:827, 1992.
67. Rustgi AK: Hereditary gastrointestinal polyposis and nonpolyposis syndromes. N Engl J Med 331:1694, 1994.
68. Leppert M, Dobbs M, Scambler P, et al: The gene for familial polyposis coli maps to the long arm of chromosome 5. Science 238:1411, 1987.
69. Solomon E, Voss R, Hall V, et al: Chromosome 5 allelic loss in human colorectal carcinomas. Nature 328:616, 1987.
70. Kinzler K, Nilbert M, Vogelstein B, et al: Identification of a gene located at chromosome 5q that is mutated in colon cancer. Science 251: 1366, 1991.
71. Groden J, Thliveris A, Samowitz W, et al: Identification and characterization of the familial adenomatous polyposis coli gene. Cell 66:589, 1991.
72. Nishisho I, Nakamura Y, Miyoshi Y, et al: Mutations of chromosome 5q21 genes in FAP and colorectal cancer patients. Science 253:665, 1991.
73. Powell SM, Zilz N, Beazer-Barclay Y, et al: APC mutations occur early during colorectal tumorigenesis. Nature 359:235, 1992.
74. Vogelstein B, Fearon ER, Kern SE, et al: Allelotype of colorectal carcinomas. Science 244:207, 1989.

75. Jessup JM, vanTuinen P, Ledbetter DH, et al: Chromosome 17 deletions and p53 gene mutations in colorectal carcinomas. Science 244: 217, 1989.
76. Fearon E, Vogelstein B: A genetic model for colorectal carcinogenesis. Cell 61:759, 1990.
77. Spirio L, Olschwang S, Groden J, et al: Alleles of the APC gene: An attenuated form of familial polyposis. Cell 75:951, 1993.
78. Olschwang S, Tiret A, Lawcent-Puig P, et al: Restriction of ocular fundus lesions to a specific subgroup of APC mutations in adenomatous polyposis coli patients. Cell 75:959, 1993.
79. Su L-K, Vogelstein B, Kinzler KW: Association of the APC tumor suppressor protein with catenins. Science 262:1734, 1993.
80. Fearon ER, Cho KR, Nigro JM, et al: Identification of a chromosome 18q gene that is altered in colorectal cancers. Science 247:49, 1990.
81. Chung DC, Rustgi AK: DNA mismatch repair and cancer. Gastroenterology 109:1685, 1995.
82. Fishel R, Lescoe NK, Rao MR, et al: The human mutator gene homolog MSH2 and its association with hereditary nonpolyposis colon cancer. Cell 75:1027, 1993.
83. Leach FS, Nicholaides NC, Papadopoulos N, et al: Mutations of a mutS homolog in hereditary nonpolyposis colorectal cancer. Cell 75:1215, 1993.
84. Parsons R, Li G-M, Longley JJ, et al: Hypermutability and mismatch repair deficiency in RER+ tumor cells. Cell 75:1227, 1993.
85. Aaltonen LA, Peltomaki P, Mecklin J-P, et al: Replication errors in benign and malignant tumors from hereditary nonpolyposis colorectal cancer patients. Cancer Res 54:1645, 1994.
86. Fidler IJ, Radinsky R: Genetic control of cancer metastasis. J Natl Cancer Inst 82:166, 1990.
87. Liotta LA, Steeg P, Stetler-Stevenson WG: Cancer metastasis and angiogenesis: An imbalance of positive and negative regulation. Cell 64:327, 1991.
88. Steeg PS, Bevilacqua G, Kopper L, et al: Evidence for a novel gene associated with low tumor metastatic potential. J Natl Cancer Inst 80: 200, 1988.
89. Tanabe KK, Ellis LM, Saya H: Expression of CD44R1 adhesion molecule in colon carcinomas and metastases. Lancet 341:725, 1993.
90. Rall CJ, N, Rustgi AK: CD44 isoform expression in primary and metastatic pancreatic adenocarcinomas. Cancer Res 55:1831, 1995.
91. Powell SM, Peterson GM, Krush AJ, et al: Molecular diagnosis of familial adenomatous polyposis. N Engl J Med 329:1982, 1993.
92. Rustgi AK: Biochemical and genetic screening of colorectal cancer. Gastroenterology 109:1003, 1995.
93. Sidransky D, Tokino T, Himilton SR, et al: Identification of rat oncogene mutations in the stool of patients with curable colorectal tumors. Science 256:102, 1992.
94. Tada M, Omata M, Kawai S, et al: Detection of ras gene mutations in pancreatic juice and peripheral blood of patients with pancreatic adenocarcinoma. Cancer Res 53:2472, 1994.
95. Gold P, Shuster J, Freedman SO: Carcinoembryonic antigen (CEA) in clinical medicine: Historical perspectives, pitfalls, and projections. Cancer 42:1399, 1978.

Section Two

APPROACH TO PATIENTS WITH SYMPTOMS AND SIGNS

Chapter 4

ABDOMINAL PAIN, INCLUDING THE ACUTE ABDOMEN

Robert E. Glasgow and Sean J. Mulvihill

Abdominal pain is an unpleasant experience commonly associated with tissue injury. The sensation of pain represents an interplay of pathophysiologic and psychosocial factors. Physiologic determinants of pain include the nature of the stimuli, the type of receptor involved, the organization of the neuroanatomic pathways from the site of injury to the central nervous system, and a complex interaction of modifying influences on the transmission, interpretation, and reaction to pain messages.[1, 2] Psychosocial factors modifying the sensation of pain include personality, ethnic and cultural background, and circumstances surrounding the injury. Thus, pain represents a complex sensation with different manifestations in different individuals. It is the clinician's responsibility to interpret the patient's complaint of pain with complete understanding of factors modifying its sensation and manifestations.

ANATOMIC BASIS OF PAIN

Sensory neuroreceptors in abdominal organs are located within the mucosa and muscularis of hollow viscera, on serosal structures such as the peritoneum, and within the mesentery.[3] In addition to nociception (the perception of noxious stimuli), sensory neuroreceptors are involved in the regulation of secretion, motility, and blood flow via local and central reflex arcs.[4] Although sensory information conveyed in this manner is usually not perceived, disordered regulation of these gastrointestinal functions can cause pain. For example, patients with irritable bowel syndrome perceive pain related to a heightened sensitivity of gut afferent neurons to normal endogenous stimuli, resulting in altered gut motility and secretion[5] (see Chapter 91).

The neuroreceptors involved in nociception are the peripheral ends of two distinct types of afferent nerve fibers: myelinated A-delta fibers and unmyelinated C fibers. A-delta fibers are distributed principally to skin and muscle and mediate the sharp, sudden, well-localized pain that follows an acute injury. These fibers convey somatoparietal pain sensations through spinal nerves. C fibers are found in muscle, periosteum, mesentery, peritoneum, and viscera. Most nociception from abdominal viscera is conveyed by this type of fiber and tends to be dull, burning, poorly localized, more gradual in onset, and longer in duration. These C fibers utilize substance P and calcitonin gene-related peptide as neurotransmitters. Stimulation of these fibers activates local regulatory reflexes mediated by the enteric nervous system and long spinal reflexes mediated by the autonomic nervous system, in addition to the transmission of pain sensation to the central nervous system.[6]

The visceral afferent fibers mediating painful stimuli from the abdominal viscera follow the distribution of the autonomic nervous system, as summarized in Figure 4–1. The cell bodies for these fibers are located in the dorsal root ganglia of spinal afferent nerves. On entering the spinal cord, these fibers branch into the dorsal horn and to Lissauer's tract cranially and caudally over several spinal segments before terminating on dorsal horn cells in laminae I and V. From the dorsal horn, second-order neurons transmit nociceptive impulses via fibers that cross through the anterior commissure and ascend the spinal cord in the contralateral spinothalamic tract. These fibers project to the thalamic nuclei and the reticular formation nuclei of the pons and medulla. The former sends third-order neurons to the somatosensory cortex, where the discriminative aspects of pain are perceived. The latter sends neurons to the limbic system and frontal cortex, where the emotional aspects of pain are interpreted.[7, 8]

Afferent pain impulses are modified by inhibitory mechanisms at the level of the spinal cord. Somatic A-delta fibers mediating touch, vibration, and proprioception from a dermatomal distribution matching the visceral innervation of the injured viscera synapse with inhibitory interneurons of the

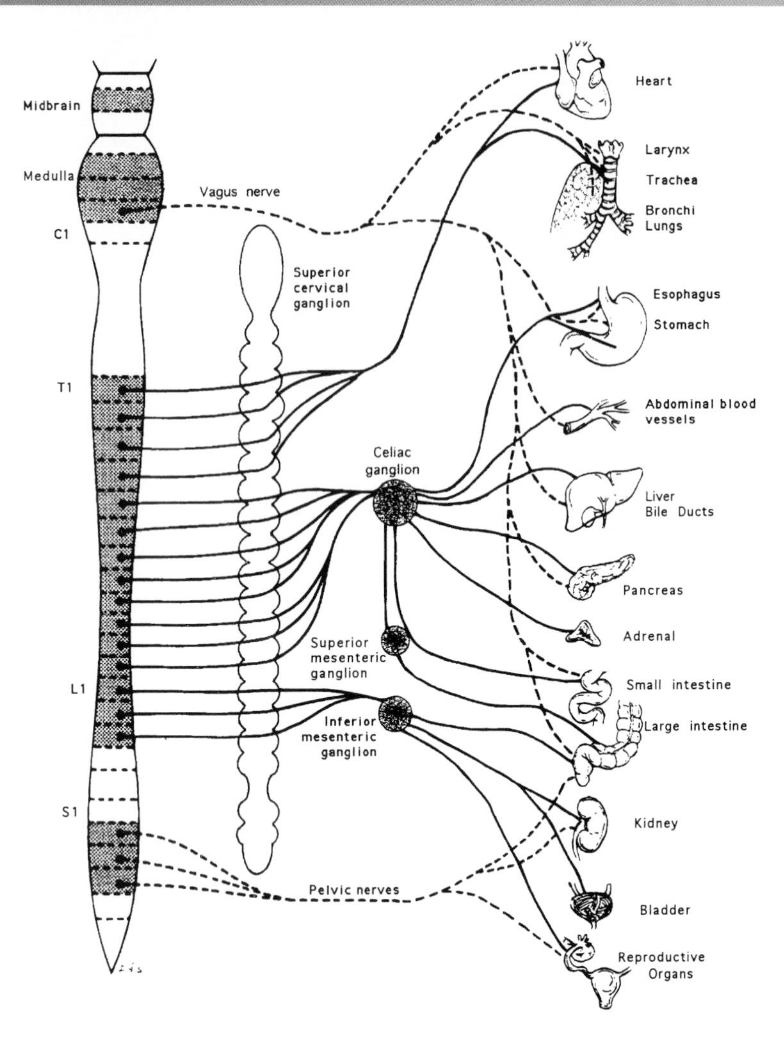

Figure 4–1. Pathways of visceral sensory innervation. The visceral afferent fibers that mediate pain travel with autonomic nerves to communicate with the central nervous system. In the abdomen, these nerves include both vagal and pelvic parasympathetic nerves and thoracolumbar sympathetic nerves. *Solid lines,* sympathetic fibers; *dashed lines,* parasympathetics.

substantia gelatinosa in the spinal cord. In addition, inhibitory neurons originating in the mesencephalon, periventricular gray matter, and caudate nucleus descend within the cord to modulate afferent pain pathways. These inhibitory mechanisms allow cerebral influences to modify afferent pain impulses.[8, 9]

STIMULANTS OF PAIN

Abdominal visceral nociceptors respond to mechanical and chemical stimuli. The principal mechanical signal to which visceral nociceptors are sensitive is stretch. Unlike for somatoparietal nociceptors, cutting, tearing, or crushing of viscera does not result in pain. Visceral stretch receptors are located in the muscular layers of the hollow viscera, between the muscularis mucosa and submucosa, in the serosa of solid organs, and in the mesentery (especially adjacent to large vessels).[3, 10] Mechanoreceptor stimulation can result from rapid distention of a hollow viscus (e.g., intestinal obstruction), forceful muscular contractions (e.g., biliary or renal colic), and rapid stretching of solid organ serosa or capsule (e.g., hepatic congestion). Similarly, torsion of the mesentery (e.g., cecal volvulus) or tension from traction on the mesentery or mesenteric vessels (e.g., retroperitoneal or pancreatic tumor) results in stimulation of mesenteric stretch receptors.

Abdominal visceral nociceptors also respond to various chemical stimuli. Chemical nociceptors are contained mainly within the mucosa and submucosa of the hollow viscera. These receptors are directly activated by substances released in response to local mechanical injury, inflammation, tissue ischemia and necrosis, and noxious thermal or radiation injury. Such substances include H^+ and K^+ ions, histamine, serotoinin, bradykinin and other vasoactive amines, substance P, calcitonin gene-related peptide, prostaglandins, and leukotrienes.[11, 12] Accumulation of nocireactive substances may change the microenvironment of the injured tissue, resulting in a reduction of the pain threshold. This increases the sensation of pain to a given stimulus and makes otherwise innocuous stimuli painful. For example, the use of chemical irritants or pressure on normal gastric mucosa is not painful, whereas the application of the same stimuli to inflamed or injured mucosa causes pain.

TYPES OF PAIN

Abdominal pain may be classified into three categories: visceral pain, somatoparietal pain, and referred pain.

Visceral pain is experienced when noxious stimuli trigger visceral nociceptors. The pain is usually dull and poorly localized in the midline epigastrium, periumbilical region, or lower midabdomen because abdominal organs transmit sensory afferents to both sides of the spinal cord (Fig. 4–2). The site where the pain is felt corresponds roughly to the dermatomes appropriate to the diseased organ's innervation.

uncommon, nor is a request of the patient for such medication during the first visit. This type of behavior reflects the patient's consideration of his or her situation as an acute condition requiring immediate symptom relief rather than as a chronic condition in which treatment must be directed toward the patient's coping and adapting to his or her situation.

Physical Examination

During the physical examination, patients with FAPS may not exhibit autonomic arousal. In fact, the presence of tachycardia, diaphoresis, and blood pressure changes suggests a more acute peripheral source for the pain. The presence of multiple surgical scars without clearly understood indications might suggest pain behaviors leading to unneeded surgical procedures. The "closed-eyes sign" may be noted.[48] When the abdomen is palpated, the patient with FAPS may wince with eyes closed, whereas those with organically caused acute abdominal pain keep their eyes open in fearful anticipation of the examination. Often the "stethescope sign," that is, gentle, distracting compression on a painful site of the abdomen with the diaphragm, elicits no response or only a minimal one and thereby affords a more accurate appraisal of the complaint. In patients with abdominal pain, which is usually but not always more acute than chronic and is associated with disease of the viscera or peritonium, compression and change in body position often increase the perceived discomfort (see Chapter 4). To try to distinguish visceral or somatic pain from central hypervigilance, Carnett's test can be performed[49]: After the site of maximal abdominal pain is identified, the subject is asked to assume a partial sitting position, thereby flexing the abdominal musculature. A positive test (i.e., increased pain) would suggest a muscle wall etiology (e.g., cutaneous nerve entrapment, hernia) or a CNS contribution to the pain (i.e., hypervigilance to body contact), whereas a negative test would be consistent with a visceral contribution to the pain.

DIAGNOSIS AND DIFFERENTIAL DIAGNOSIS

A complete history, thorough physical examination, and appropriate attention to psychosocial factors in the patient's life during the first encounter often point the physician clearly to the diagnosis of FAPS. A physical examination that does not betray evidence of other chronic intra-abdominal conditions (such as chronic pancreatitis and serious biliary tract disease), as well as a battery of routine laboratory tests (including complete blood counts, liver function tests, serum electrolytes, renal function, and examination of stools for occult blood) that are normal, rather clearly indicates that the patient's pain is not the result of a specific disease. Emphatically, these patients have the symptom criteria for FAPS (see Table 5–2), and recognition of these criteria along with the failure to find evidence of other causes for the pain listed in Table 5–1 and discussed elsewhere in this text should lead the physician to make the diagnosis (see Chapter 4). If the features of FAPS are absent or atypical, and if there are abnormalities on physical examination (e.g., abdominal mass, enlarged liver) or in screening laboratory studies (e.g., anemia, high erythrocyte sedimentation rate, low serum albumin level), another diagnosis in Table 5–2 should be strongly considered and pursued accordingly. It is also common for nonspecific abnormalities to be found (e.g., cyst in the liver, palpable lymph node, "nonspecific" bowel gas pattern), so efforts must be made to determine their relevance to the symptoms that the patient presents.

TREATMENT

Establishing a Successful Patient-Physician Relationship

Once other diagnoses have been safely ruled out and the relationship of the patient's symptoms to the possible concomitant presence of other functional gastrointestinal disorders has been taken into consideration, a successful relationship with the patient with FAPS is the most important contribution to effective management. Several factors must be immediately taken into account to help establish this relationship and to move toward successful treatment. Important among these is an accurate assessment of the patient's *psychosocial situation*. The physician must take into account the importance of the length of the history of illness, because long histories of complaints of pain and frequent visits to physicians or other health caregivers predict a poor outlook. One must determine the reason for the current visit and deal with it first. Is it because of concern for a serious illness? Is there an environmental stress? Has there been a dramatic worsening of the pain? Is the patient really seeking narcotics, a disability claim, or some other type of legitimization of illness? Has the psychiatric disturbance been exacerbated? A knowledge of prior traumatic episodes in the patient's life will be important in future treatment. Some appreciation of the degree of the patient's understanding of the illness is also important. This is particularly true for the success of a mutual treatment plan.

Answers to other questions must be sought early in the relationship, such as whether there are abnormal illness behaviors. What is the impact of the pain on the quality of life? Is there an associated psychiatric diagnosis? And finally, but extremely important, what is the role of the family or culture in the FAPS suffered by the individual? Usually family experiences with illness lead to emotional support and a focus on recovery. With dysfunctional family interactions, stresses are not well managed, and diverting attention toward illness serves to reduce family distress.[50, 51] Dysfunction is seen when spouses or parents overindulge the patient, assume undue responsibility in the management, or become the spokesperson for the patient when communicating anger. If such family dysfunction is observed, counseling should be offered as a way to help the family develop better coping strategies.

Cultural belief systems also affect how the patient is presented to the physician and how the patient responds to treatment. For example, open recognition of psychological difficulties may be a stigma for Asians, but physical symptoms may be socially sanctioned.[52] Further, patients may not comply with treatments that are not consistent with their cultural beliefs. In all of this it is important to gain a knowledge of the patient's psychosocial resources, that is, the availability of social networks such as family church, recreation clubs, and community organizations and effective coping strategies that may help to buffer the adverse effects of stress and improve the outcome.[53]

The physician should embark immediately on a course that will not only gain this information but that will also begin to establish rapport with the patient.[2, 54] *Empathy* is primary in this matter, because it acknowledges the reality and distress associated with the patient's pain.[55] It is accomplished by understanding the patient's experience while maintaining objectivity. It does not mean over-reacting to the patient's wish for rapid diagnosis and help by overmedicating or performing unneeded diagnostic studies. Diagnostic decisions are based on objective data rather than the patient's insistence that "something be done."[56]

Education of the patient to the condition is provided by eliciting his or her knowledge of the syndrome, addressing any unrealistic concerns, explaining the nature of the symptoms in a fashion that is consistent with the patient's belief system, and ensuring the patient's understanding in all matters. It helps to explain that chronic abdominal pain is a true disorder relating to abnormal sensations and/or dysregulation of neuroenteric function and that it can be modified effectively by psychopharmacologic or psychological treatments that affect the regulation of pain.

All patients need *reassurance*, because they may fear serious disease or surgery. After the evaluation is completed, the physician should respond to the patient's worries and concerns in a clear and objective manner, and then both must *negotiate the treatment*. The physician should ask about the patient's personal experience, understanding, and interests in various treatments and then provide choices rather than directives. A recommendation will be more accepted if the patient understands the reasons it is made and believes it will help. Finally, the physician in a busy practice must set *reasonable limits* in time and effort and recognize that the patient's care frequently needs to be shared with mental health professionals. Patients' demand for more time is best handled by scheduling brief, but regular, appointments of fixed duration. The key to success is to maintain an ongoing relationship and proper boundaries.

Instituting a Treatment Plan

Successful treatment rests on a plan that encompasses ongoing interviews to ensure that the patient should not expect a cure. Using an example such as arthritis, the physician can explain that a realistic treatment goal is to improve daily function. Patients must be made to increase their responsibility for the illness, and to this end they are asked to keep a diary of symptoms for a few weeks, particularly identifying the circumstances of the episodes of pain and their emotional and cognitive responses. This technique not only helps the patient to achieve insight into aggravating factors but also characterizes the patient's style of coping with the problem. Such information helps identify a strategy for behavioral treatment. Further, treatment is based on the severity of symptoms and the degree of disability and is conservative. Symptoms that are intermittent or of moderate severity, or exacerbations that are clearly linked to psychological distress, are frequently amenable to psychological treatment. However, if the pain is continuous and severe, psychoactive medications for central analgesia (e.g., tricyclic antidepressants [TCAs] such as amitriptyline or selective serotonin reuptake inhibitors [SSRIs] such as fluoxetine) may be helpful (see later).

MEDICATIONS. Most analgesics (e.g., aspirin, NSAIDs) offer little benefit, because they act peripherally. Narcotics should not be prescribed because of the potential for addiction and the narcotic bowel syndrome, where chronic use of narcotics leads to impaired motility and increased pain sensitivity.[57] Furthermore, their use subordinates the development of treatment strategies to that of providing medication. Benzodiazepines are of limited value because they can be abused and they may lower the pain threshold.[58] TCAs or SSRIs can be helpful in treating chronic pain, FAPS, and other painful functional gastrointestinal disorders.[59, 60] Because there are few data about which drug category is more effective, the choice depends on the patient's tolerance of their side effects. In general, the less expensive TCAs have been shown effective but produce more anticholinergic effects, hypotension, sedation, and cardiac arrhythmias and may require some dose adjustment to achieve an optimal effect. They can be given in doses lower than used to treat major depression (e.g., desipramine, 25 to 100 mg/day at bedtime) and to reduce side effects. However, dose ranging up to full therapeutic levels may be needed, particularly if there is psychiatric comorbidity. The SSRIs may cause agitation, sleep disturbance, vivid dreams, and diarrhea but are much safer if taken as an overdose. In most cases a single pill (e.g., 20 mg of fluoxetine, paroxetine, or citalopram or 50 mg of sertraline or fluvoxamine) will suffice. Although the efficacy of SSRIs for pain control is not well established, this class of drug has additional benefits because they are anxiolytic and are helpful for patients having other comorbid conditions, including social phobia (or agoraphobia), posttraumatic stress disorder, panic, and obsessional thoughts related to their condition.

The physician should explain that antidepressants are central analgesics, not simply drugs for psychiatric conditions, and that they effectively treat other painful medical conditions such as migraine, postherpetic neuralgia, and diabetic neuropathy. They increase the release of neurotransmitters that descend from brain centers to block pain transmission from the gut to the brain, and the dosage is usually lower than used for psychiatric disorders. The lag time for effect may take several weeks; most side effects diminish after a few days and can be reduced by temporarily lowering the dosage or implementing other strategies such as offering other medications to reduce symptoms.[61] The medication can be given for a few weeks and then the patient is reevaluated.

MENTAL HEALTH REFERRAL. Patients may be reluctant to see a psychologist or psychiatrist because they lack knowledge of the benefits of referral, feel stigmatized for possibly having a psychiatric problem, or see referral as a rejection by the medical physician. Psychological interventions are best presented as ways to help manage pain and to reduce the psychological distress of the symptoms. The medical visits should continue with the psychological treatment either regularly or occasionally for reassessment, or as needed, but with continuing availability.

SPECIFIC PSYCHOLOGICAL TREATMENTS[62]. The mental health consultant may recommend any of several types of psychological treatments for pain management. Cognitive-behavioral treatment, which identifies maladaptive thoughts, perceptions, and behaviors, is popular, and this information is used to develop new ways to increase control of the symptoms. Stress management is usually done in small groups where education and relaxation techniques are provided. Dynamic or interpersonal psychotherapy is a method that proposes psychological distress and physical symptoms are exacerbated by difficulties in interpersonal relationships. As difficulties emerge during the therapy, efforts are made to understand and address them, often improving the pain symptoms. Hypnotherapy has been investigated primarily in IBS, where the focus is on "relaxation of the gut." Relaxation training attempts to help counteract the physiologic effects of stress or anxiety.

MULTIDISCIPLINARY PAIN TREATMENT CENTERS. Multidisciplinary pain treatment centers provide comprehensive rehabilitation of patients with chronic pain. The approach is theoretically rational, and it may be the most efficient method of treating disability from refractory chronic pain symptoms.[49]

REFERENCES

1. Drossman DA, Corazziari E, Talley NJ, et al: Rome II. The Functional Gastrointestinal Disorders: Diagnosis, Pathophysiology and Treatment—a Multinational Consensus, 2nd ed. McLean, Va, Degnon Associates, 2000, 2:1–764.
2. Thompson WG, Longstreth GF, Drossman DA, et al: Functional bowel disorders and functional abdominal pain. In Drossman DA, Talley NJ, Thompson WG, et al (eds): Rome II: The Functional Gastrointestinal Disorders, 2nd ed. McLean, Va, Degnon Associates, 2000, pp 351–432.
3. Drossman DA: Patients with psychogenic abdominal pain: Six years' observation in the medical setting. Am J Psychiatry 139:1549–1557, 1982.
4. Sloth H, Jorgensen LS: Chronic nonorganic upper abdominal pain: Diagnostic safety and prognosis of gastrointestinal and nonintestinal symptoms—a 5- to 7-year follow-up study. Scand J Gastroenterol 23: 1275–1280, 1988.
5. Drossman DA: Chronic functional abdominal pain. Am J Gastroenterol 91:2270–2281, 1996.
6. Maxton DG, Whorwell PJ: Use of medical resources and attitudes to health care of patients with "chronic abdominal pain." Br J Med Econ 2:75–79, 1992.
7. Drossman DA: Diagnosing and treating patients with refractory functional gastrointestinal disorders. Ann Intern Med 123:688–697, 1995.
8. Reuler JB, Girard DE, Nardone DA: The chronic pain syndrome: Misconceptions and management. Ann Intern Med 93:588–596, 1980.
9. Woodforde JM, Merskey H: Personality traits of patients with chronic pain. J Psychosom Res 16:167–172, 1972.
10. Engel GL: The need for a new medical model: A challenge for biomedicine. Science 196:129–136, 1977.
11. Drossman DA: Presidential Address: Gastrointestinal illness and biopsychosocial model. Psychosom Med 60:258–267, 1998.
12. Drossman DA, Li Z, Andruzzi E, et al: U.S. Householder Survey of Functional Gastrointestinal Disorders: Prevalence, sociodemography, and health impact. Dig Dis Sci 38:1569–1580, 1993.
13. Casey KL: Match and mismatch: Identifying the neuronal determinants of pain. Ann Intern Med 124:995–998, 1996.
14. Melzack R, Wall P: Gate control and other mechanisms. In Melzack R, Wall P (eds): The Challenge of Pain, 2nd ed. London, Pelican Books, 1988, pp 165–193.
15. Rainville P, Duncan GH, Price DD, et al: Pain affect encoded in human anterior cingulate but not somatosensory cortex. Science 277:968–971, 1997.
16. Rosen SD, Paulesu E, Nihoyannopoulos P, et al: Silent ischemia as a central problem: Regional brain activation compared in silent and painful myocardial ischemia. Ann Intern Med 124:939–949, 1996.
17. Fields HL, Basbaum AI: Endogenous pain control mechanisms. In Wall PD, Melzack R (eds): Textbook of Pain. New York, Livingston, 1984, pp 142–152.
18. Mayer EA, Gebhart GF: Basic and clinical aspects of visceral hyperalgesia. Gastroenterology 107:271–293, 1994.
19. Coderre TJ, Katz J, Vaccarino AL, et al: Contribution of central neuroplasticity to pathological pain: Review of clinical and experimental evidence. Pain 52:259–285, 1993.
20. Ruda MA, Ling QD, Hohmann AG, et al: Altered nociceptive neuronal circuits after neonatal peripheral inflammation. Science 289:628–630, 2000.
21. Ness TJ, Metcalf AM, Gebhart GF: A psychophysiological study in humans using phasic colonic distension as a noxious visceral stimulus. Pain 43:377–386, 1990.
22. Munakata J, Naliboff B, Harraf F, et al: Repetitive sigmoid stimulation induces rectal hyperalgesia in patients with irritable bowel syndrome. Gastroenterology 112:55–63, 1997.
23. Cervero F, Janig W: Visceral nociceptors: A new world order? Trends Neurosci 15:374–378, 1992.
24. Gershon MD: Review article: Roles played by 5-hydroxytryptamine in the physiology of the bowel. Aliment Pharmacol Ther 13:15–30, 1999.
25. Bearcroft CP, Perrett D, Farthing MJG: Postprandial plasma 5-hydroxytryptamine in diarrhoea-predominant irritable bowel syndrome: A pilot study. Gut 42:42–46, 1998.
26. Camilleri M, Mayer EA, Drossman DA, et al: Improvement in pain and bowel function in female irritable bowel patients with alosetron, a 5-HT_3 receptor antagonist. Aliment Pharmacol Ther 13:1149–1159, 1999.
27. Drossman DA, Creed FH, Olden KW, et al: Psychosocial aspects of the functional gastrointestinal disorders. In Drossman DA, Corazziari E, Talley NJ, et al (eds): Rome II: The Functional Gastrointestinal Disorders: Diagnosis, Pathophysiology and Treatment—a Multinational Consensus, 2nd ed. McLean, Va, Degnon Associates, 2000, pp 157–245.
28. Drossman DA, Whitehead WE, Toner BB, et al: What determines severity among patients with painful functional bowel disorders? Am J Gastroenterol 95:974–980, 2000.
29. Drossman DA, Li Z, Leserman J, et al: Health status by gastrointestinal diagnosis and abuse history. Gastroenterology 110:999–1007, 1996.
30. Ringel Y, Drossman DA: From gut to brain and back—a new perspective into functional gastrointestinal disorders. J Psychom Res 47:205–210, 1999.
31. Gwee KA, Leong YL, Graham C, et al: The role of psychological and biological factors in postinfective gut dysfunction. Gut 44:400–406, 1999.
32. Drossman DA: Mind over matter in the postinfective irritable bowel. Gut 44:306–307, 1999.
33. Silverman DHS, Munakata JA, Ennes H, et al: Regional cerebral activity in normal and pathologic perception of visceral pain. Gastroenterology 112:64–72, 1997.
34. Ringel Y, Drossman DA, Turkington TG, et al: Dysfunction of the motivational-affective pain system in patients with IBS: PET brain imaging in response to rectal balloon distension [abstract]. Gastroenterology 118:A444, 2000.
35. Silverman DHS, Ennes H, Munakata JA, et al: Differences in thalamic activity associated with anticipation of rectal pain between IBS patients and normal subjects. Gastroenterology 108:1006, 1995.
36. Ringel Y, Drossman DA, Turkington TG, et al: Anterior cingulate cortex (ACC) dysfunction in subjects with sexual/physical abuse [abstract]. Gastroenterology 118:A444, 2000.
37. Silverman DHS, Brody AL, Saxena S, et al: Somatization in clinical depression is associated with abnormal function of a brain region active in visceral pain perception. Gastroenterology 114:A839, 1998.
38. Shin LM, McNally RJ, Kosslyn SM, et al: Regional cerebral blood flow during script-driven imagery in childhood sexual abuse-related PTSD: A PET investigation. Am J Psychiatry 156:575–584, 1999.
39. Mayberg HS, Liotti M, Brannan SK, et al: Reciprocal limbic-cortical function and negative mood: Converging PET findings in depression and normal sadness. Am J Psychiatry 156:675–682, 1999.
40. Mayberg HS, Brannan SK, Mahurin RK, et al: Cingulate function in depression: A potential predictor of treatment response. Neuroreport 8: 1057–1061, 1997.
41. Drossman DA, Talley NJ, Olden KW, et al: Sexual and physical abuse

and gastrointestinal illness: Review and recommendations. Ann Intern Med 123:782–794, 1995.
42. Blackwell B, Gutmann M: The management of chronic illness behaviour. In McHugh S, Vallis TM (eds): Illness Behavior: A Multidisciplinary Model. New York, Plenum, 1986, pp 401–408.
43. Adler RH, Zamboni P, Hofer T, et al: How not to miss a somatic needle in the haystack of chronic pain. J Psychosom Res 42:499–505, 1997.
44. Drossman DA: Psychosocial factors in the care of patients with gastrointestinal disorders. In Yamada T (ed): Textbook of Gastroenterology, 3rd ed. Philadelphia, Lippincott-Raven, 1999, pp 638–659.
45. Hislop IG: Childhood deprivation: An antecedent of the irritable bowel syndrome. Med J Aust 1:372–374, 1979.
46. Drossman DA, Leserman J, Nachman G, et al: Sexual and physical abuse in women with functional or organic gastrointestinal disorders. Ann Intern Med 113:828–833, 1990.
47. Drossman DA, Li Z, Leserman J, et al: Effects of coping on health outcome among female patients with gastrointestinal disorders. Psychosom Med 62:309–317, 2000.
48. Gray DWR, Dixon JM, Collin J: The closed-eyes sign: An aid to diagnosing nonspecific abdominal pain. BMJ 297:837, 1988.
49. McGarrity TJ, Peters DJ, Thompson C, et al: Outcome of patients with chronic abdominal pain referred to chronic pain clinic. Am J Gastroenterol 95:1812–1816, 2000.
50. Minuchin S, Rosman BL, Baker L: Psychosomatic Families: Anorexia Nervosa in Context. Cambridge, Harvard University Press, 1978.
51. Whitehead WE, Crowell MD, Heller BR, et al: Modeling and reinforcement of the sick role during childhood predicts adult illness behavior. Psychosom Med 6:541–550, 1994.
52. Kleinman A, Eisenberg L, Good B: Culture, illness, and care: Clinical lessons from anthropologic and cross-cultural research. Ann Intern Med 88:8, 1978.
53. Beckman LF, Syme SL: Social networks, host resistance, and mortality: A nine-year follow-up study of Alameda County residents. Am J Epidemiol 109:186–204, 1979.
54. Thompson WG, Longstreth GF, Drossman DA, et al: Functional bowel disorders and functional abdominal pain. Gut 45:II43–II47, 1999.
55. Zinn W: The empathic physician. Arch Intern Med 153:306–312, 1994.
56. DeVaul RA, Faillace LA: Persistent pain and illness insistence—a medical profile of proneness to surgery. Am J Surg 135:828–833, 1978.
57. Sandgren JE, McPhee MS, Greenberger NJ: Narcotic bowel syndrome treated with clonidine. Ann Intern Med 101:331–334, 1984.
58. King SA, Strain JJ: Benzodiazepines and chronic pain. Pain 41:3–4, 1990.
59. Jackson JL, O'Malley PG, Tomkins G, et al: Treatment of functional gastrointestinal disorders with antidepressants: A meta-analysis. Am J Med 108:65–72, 2000.
60. Fishbain DA, Cutler RB, Rosomoff HL, et al: Do antidepressants have an analgesic effect in psychogenic pain and somatoform pain disorder? A meta-analysis. Psychosom Med 60:503–509, 1998.
61. McElroy SL, Keck PE Jr, Friedman LM: Minimizing and managing antidepressant side effects. J Clin Psychiatry 56(suppl 2):49–55, 1995.
62. Drossman DA, Creed FH, Olden KW, et al: Psychosocial aspects of the functional gastrointestinal disorders. In Drossman DA, Corazziari E, Talley NJ, et al (eds): Rome II: The Functional Gastrointestinal Disorders: Diagnosis, Pathophysiology and Treatment—a Multinational Consensus, 2nd ed. McLean, Va, Degnon Associates, 2000, pp 157–245.

Chapter 6

Dysphagia, Odynophagia, Heartburn, and Other Esophageal Symptoms

Joel E. Richter

Occasional esophageal complaints are common and usually are not harbingers of disease. A recent survey of healthy subjects in Olmsted County, Minnesota, found that 20%, regardless of gender or age, experienced heartburn at least weekly.[1] Surely every middle-aged American adult has had one or more episodes of heartburn or chest pain and dysphagia when swallowing dry or very cold foods or beverages. Frequent or persistent *dysphagia*, *odynophagia*, or *heartburn* immediately suggests an esophageal problem that necessitates investigation and treatment. Other, less specific symptoms of possible esophageal origin include globus sensation, chest pain, belching, hiccups, rumination, and extraesophageal complaints such as wheezing, coughing, sore throat, and hoarseness, especially if other causes have been excluded. In particular, gastroesophageal reflux disease may manifest with these "atypical" complaints and should not be missed, because it is readily treatable (see Chapter 33, section on symptoms).

DYSPHAGIA

Dysphagia, from the Greek *phagia* (to eat) and *dys* (difficulty, disordered), refers to the sensation of food being hindered in its passage from the mouth to the stomach. Most patients say that food "sticks," "hangs up," or "stops" or that they feel that the food "just won't go down right." Occasionally they complain of associated pain. Dysphagia always indicates malfunction of some type in the esophagus, although associated psychiatric disorders can amplify this symptom.

Dysphagia is a common symptom, present in 12% of patients admitted to an acute care hospital and in over 50% of those in a chronic care facility.[2] An accurate, detailed history suggests its etiology and enables the physician to correctly define the cause in 80% to 85% of patients.[3, 4]

Mechanisms

Several mechanisms are responsible for dysphagia. The oropharyngeal swallowing mechanism and the primary and secondary peristaltic contractions of the esophageal body that follow usually transport solid and liquid boluses from the mouth to the stomach within 10 seconds (see Chapter 32, section on coordinated esophageal motor activity). If these orderly contractions fail to develop or progress, the accumulated bolus of food distends the lumen and causes the dull discomfort that is dysphagia. Some people fail to stimulate proximal motor activity despite adequate distention of the organ.[5] Others, particularly the elderly, generate low-amplitude primary or secondary peristaltic activity that is insufficient for clearing the esophagus.[6] A third group has primary or secondary motility disorders that grossly disturb the orderly contractions of the esophageal body. Because these motor abnormalities may not be present with every swallow, dysphagia may wax and wane (see Chapter 32, sections on achalasia and spastic disorders of the esophagus).

Mechanical narrowing of the esophageal lumen may interrupt the orderly passage of a food bolus despite adequate peristaltic contractions. Symptoms also vary with the degree of luminal obstruction, associated esophagitis, and type of food ingested. Although minimally obstructing lesions cause dysphagia only with large, poorly chewed solid boluses of such foods as meat and dry bread, lesions that totally obstruct the esophageal lumen are symptomatic for both solids and liquids. *Gastroesophageal reflux disease* may produce dysphagia by multiple mechanisms, including the syndrome of "nonobstructive" dysphagia[7] (see Chapter 33, section on symptoms). Difficulty swallowing in this situation usually results from intermittent acid-induced motility disturbances sometimes associated with mild to moderate esophageal inflammation. Finally, abnormal sensory perception within the esophagus may lead to dysphagia. Because some normal subjects experience the sensation of dysphagia when the distal esophagus is distended by a balloon, as well as by other intraluminal stimuli, an aberration in visceral perception could explain dysphagia in patients who have no definable cause.[8] This mechanism also may apply to the amplification of symptoms in patients with spastic motility disorders, among whom the prevalence of psychiatric disorders is high.[9]

Classification

Dysphagia is readily classified into two distinct types: *oropharyngeal* and *esophageal* (Table 6–1). The former is caused by abnormalities that affect the fine-tuned neuromuscular mechanism of the pharynx and upper esophageal sphincter (UES); the latter stems from one of a variety of disorders that affect the esophageal body.

Oropharyngeal Dysphagia

Neuromuscular diseases that affect the hypopharynx and upper esophagus produce a distinctive type of dysphagia. The patient is often unable to initiate swallowing and repeatedly has to attempt to swallow. A food bolus cannot be propelled successfully from the hypopharyngeal area through the UES into the esophageal body. The resulting symptom is oropharyngeal, or *transfer*, dysphagia. The patient is aware that the bolus has not left the oropharynx and specifically locates the site of symptoms to the region of the cervical esophagus. Dysphagia within 1 second of swallowing is suggestive of an oropharyngeal abnormality.[4] In this situation, a liquid bolus may enter the trachea or the nose rather than the esophagus. Some patients describe recurrent bolus impaction that requires manual dislodgment. In severe cases, saliva cannot be swallowed, and the patient drools. Coughing episodes during a meal indicate a concomitant tracheobronchial aspiration. Pain is infrequent; dysphagia predominates.

Other symptoms are less frequent and may be progressive, constant, or intermittent. Swallowing associated with a gurgling noise may suggest the presence of *Zenker diverticulum* (see Chapter 31, section on diverticula; also Chapter 20, section on diverticula of esophagus). Recurrent bouts of *pulmonary infection* may reflect spillover of food into the trachea from inadequate laryngeal protection. *Hoarseness* may result from recurrent laryngeal nerve dysfunction or intrinsic muscular disease, both of which cause ineffective vocal cord movement. Weakness of the soft palate or pharyngeal constrictors causes *dysarthria* and *nasal speech* as well as *pharyngonasal regurgitation.* Finally, *unexplained weight loss* may be the only clue to a swallowing disorder; patients avoid eating because of the difficulties encountered.

Table 6–1 | **Common Causes of Dysphagia**

OROPHARYNGEAL	ESOPHAGEAL
Neuromuscular	***Mechanical Obstruction***
Cerebrovascular accident	Benign strictures
Parkinson disease	Webs and rings (Schatzki)
Brainstem tumors	Neoplasm
Multiple sclerosis	Diverticula
Amyotrophic lateral sclerosis	Vascular anomalies
Peripheral neuropathies (i.e., poliomyelitis)	Aberrant subclavian artery (dysphagia lusoria)
Mechanical Obstruction	Enlarged aorta (dysphagia aortica)
Retropharyngeal abscess	***Motility Disorders***
Zenker diverticulum	Achalasia
Cricopharyngeal bar	Spastic motility disorders
Cervical osteophyte	Scleroderma
Thyromegaly	Chagas disease
Skeletal Muscle Disorders	Miscellaneous
Polymyositis	***Miscellaneous***
Muscular dystrophies	Diabetes
Myotonic dystrophy	Alcoholism
Oculopharyngeal dystrophy	Gastroesophageal reflux
Myasthenia gravis	
Metabolic myopathies	
Miscellaneous	
Decreased saliva	
Medications, radiation	
Sjögren syndrome	
Alzheimer disease	
Depression	

Esophageal Dysphagia

Various motility disorders or mechanical obstructing lesions can cause esophageal dysphagia. Most patients complain of difficulty "transporting" food down the esophagus, noting the sensation of food "hanging up" somewhere behind the sternum. If this symptom is localized to the lower part of the sternum, the lesion probably is in the distal esophagus; however, dysphagia frequently may be referred to the neck or substernal notch from that site in some patients.

To understand the syndrome of esophageal dysphagia, the answers to three questions are crucial:[10] (1) What type of food causes symptoms? (2) Is the dysphagia intermittent or progressive? and (3) Does the patient have heartburn? On the basis of these answers, it often is possible to distinguish the cause of dysphagia as either a mechanical or a neuromuscular defect and to accurately postulate the cause (Fig. 6–1).

Patients who report dysphagia with both solids and liquids probably have an esophageal motility disorder. When food impaction develops, it frequently can be relieved by various maneuvers, including repeated swallowing, raising the arms over the head, throwing the shoulders back, and using the Valsalva maneuver. In addition to dysphagia, most patients with *achalasia* complain of bland regurgitation of undigested food, especially at night, and of weight loss. In contrast, patients with spastic motility disorders commonly complain of chest pain and sensitivity to either hot or cold liquids. Patients with *scleroderma* of the esophagus usually have Raynaud's phenomenon and severe heartburn. In these patients, mild complaints of dysphagia can be caused by either a motility disturbance or esophageal inflammation, but severe dysphagia nearly always signals the presence of a peptic stricture (see Chapter 32, sections on achalasia, spastic disorders of esophagus, and systemic diseases of esophagus).

In patients who report dysphagia only after swallowing solid foods and never with liquids alone, a mechanical obstruction is suspected. When a luminal obstruction is of sufficiently high grade, however, it may be associated with dysphagia for both solids and liquids. If food impaction develops, the patient frequently must regurgitate for relief. Episodic and nonprogressive dysphagia without weight loss is characteristic of an *esophageal web* or a *distal esophageal ring* (i.e., Schatzki ring). The first episode typically occurs

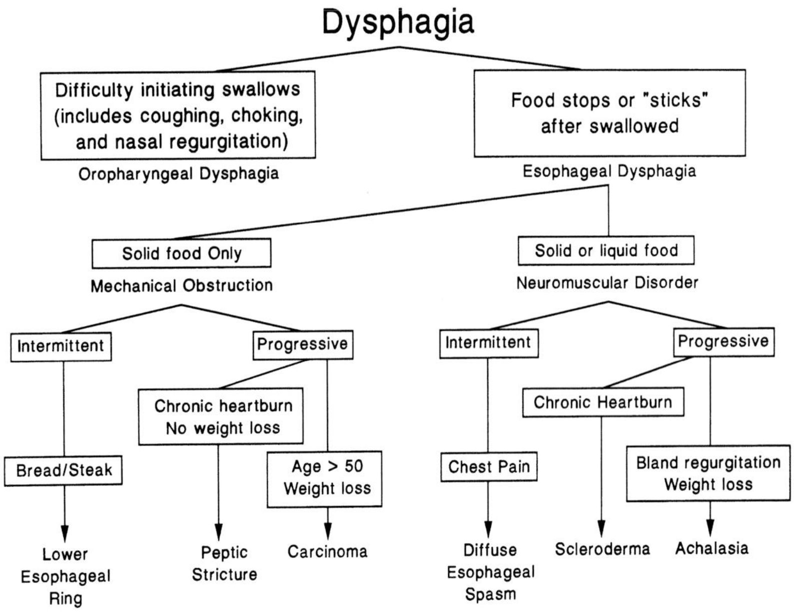

Figure 6–1. Diagnostic algorithm for the symptomatic assessment of the patient with dysphagia. Important differentiating symptoms are included within the boxes. (Modified from Castell DO, and Donner MW. Evaluation of dysphagia: A careful history is crucial. Dysphagia 2:65, 1987.)

during a hurried meal, often with alcohol. The patient notes that the bolus of food sticks in the lower esophagus; it often can be passed by drinking large quantities of liquids; after relieving the obstruction, the patient can finish the meal without difficulty. The offending food frequently is a piece of bread or steak, hence the description "steakhouse syndrome."[11] Initially, the episode may not be repeated for weeks or months, but then the episodes recur more frequently. Daily dysphagia, however, is likely not caused by a lower esophageal ring (see Chapter 31, section on rings and webs).

If solid food dysphagia is clearly progressive, the major differential diagnosis is *peptic esophageal stricture* and *carcinoma.* In about 10% of patients with gastroesophageal reflux disease, benign esophageal strictures gradually develop. Most of these patients have a long history of associated heartburn. Weight loss seldom is noticed with benign lesions because these patients have a good appetite and convert their diet to high-calorie soft and liquid foods to maintain weight. Patients with carcinoma differ from those with peptic stricture in several ways. As a group, the cancer patients are older and present with a history of rapidly progressive dysphagia. They typically do not have a history of heartburn or, if so, it is a symptom of the past but not the present. Most cancer patients have anorexia and more weight loss than the severity and duration of their dysphagia indicates (see Chapter 35, section on symptoms). True dysphagia may be seen in patients with *pill, caustic,* or *viral esophagitis;* however, the predominant complaint of patients with these acute esophageal injuries is usually odynophagia (see Chapter 23, section on caustic agents, and Chapter 34, section on infections and medications).

ODYNOPHAGIA

The second symptom specific for esophageal involvement is *odynophagia*—pain with swallowing. This symptom may range from a dull retrosternal ache on swallowing to a stabbing pain with radiation to the back so severe that patients cannot eat or even swallow their own saliva. Odynophagia usually reflects a severe inflammatory process that involves the esophageal mucosa or, in rare instances, the esophageal muscle. The most common causes of odynophagia include *caustic ingestion, pill-induced esophagitis, radiation injury,* and *infectious esophagitis* (*Candida,* herpes, and cytomegalovirus) (Table 6–2). In these diseases, dysphagia also may be present, but pain is the dominant complaint. Odynophagia is a rather infrequent complaint of patients with gastroesophageal reflux disease and, when present, usually is associated with a *severe ulcerative esophagitis.* In rare cases, a nonobstructive esophageal *carcinoma* can produce odynophagia.

HEARTBURN (PYROSIS)

Heartburn is probably the most common gastrointestinal (GI) complaint in the Western population.[1, 12, 13] This symptom reaches its maximal frequency during pregnancy, when 25% of patients may have daily heartburn.[12] It is not surprising, then, that most people do not consider heartburn a medical problem and seldom report it to their physicians.[1] They seek relief with over-the-counter antacids, accounting for most of the $1 billion-per-year sales of these nonprescription drugs. In patients who take antacids daily, this may be a dangerous habit; one study found that more than one half of these patients had endoscopic evidence of erosive esophagitis.[14]

Symptom Complex

Heartburn, the classic manifestation of gastroesophageal reflux disease, is a commonly used but frequently misunderstood word. It has many synonyms, including "indigestion," "acid regurgitation," "sour stomach," and "bitter belching." The physician should listen for these descriptors if the patient does not readily admit to the complaint of heartburn. Heartburn usually is described as a sensation of burning discomfort behind the breastbone. The description of "burn-

Table 6–2 | **Common Causes of Odynophagia**

Caustic Ingestion
Acid
Alkali (lye, Drano)
Pill-Induced Esophagitis
Antibiotics (especially doxycycline)
Potassium chloride, slow release
Quinidine
Iron sulfate
Zidovudine
NSAIDs
Radiation Esophagitis
Infectious Esophagitis
Healthy persons
  Candida albicans
  Herpes simplex
HIV patients
  Fungal (*Candida,* histoplasmosis)
  Viral (herpes simplex, cytomegalovirus, HIV, Epstein-Barr virus)
  Mycobacteria (*tuberculosis, avium*-complex)
  Protozoan (*Cryptosporidium, Pneumocystis carinii*)
  Idiopathic ulcers
Severe Ulcerative Esophagitis Secondary to GERD
Esophageal Carcinoma

NSAIDs, nonsteroidal anti-inflammatory drugs; HIV, human immunodeficiency virus; GERD, gastroesophageal reflux disease.

ing," "hot," or "acidic" sensation is typically used by patients unless the discomfort of heartburn becomes so intense that pain is experienced. In those situations, patients commonly complain of both heartburn and pain. The burning sensation often begins inferiorly and radiates up the entire retrosternal area to the neck, occasionally to the back, and rarely into the arms. The patient usually signifies the relationship with the open hand moving from the epigastrium to the neck or throat. This should be contrasted with the stationary clenched-fist gesture of the patient suffering from coronary chest pain. Heartburn caused by acid reflux is usually relieved, albeit only transiently, by the ingestion of antacids, baking soda, or milk.

Heartburn is predictably aggravated by multiple factors, particularly food (Table 6–3). Thus it is most frequently noted within 1 hour after eating, particularly after the largest meal of the day. Foods high in fats, sugars, chocolate, onions, or carminatives may aggravate heartburn by decreasing lower esophageal sphincter (LES) pressure.[15] Other foods commonly associated with heartburn, including citrus products, tomato-based foods, and spicy foods, do not affect LES pressure. They directly irritate the inflamed esophageal mucosa,[16] by pathogenetic mechanisms that include titratable acidity, low pH, or high osmolarity.[17] Many beverages, including citrus juices, soft drinks, coffee, and alcohol, also cause heartburn, by a variety of mechanisms.[15] Wine drinkers may have heartburn after hearty red wines but not after delicate white wines. Retiring, especially after a late meal or snack, brings it on within 1 to 2 hours and, in contrast to peptic ulcer disease, does not awaken the person in the early morning. Some patients say that their heartburn is more pronounced while they lie on the right side.[18]

Maneuvers that increase intra-abdominal pressure, including bending over, straining at stool, lifting heavy objects, and performing isometric exercises, may aggravate heartburn. Running also may aggravate heartburn, whereas stationary bike riding may be good exercise for those with gastroesophageal reflux disease.[19] Because nicotine lowers LES pressure and air swallowing relaxes the sphincter, *cigarette smoking* exacerbates the symptoms of reflux.[20, 21] *Emotions* such as anxiety, fear, and worry may exacerbate heartburn, probably through the amplification of symptoms rather than by increase in the amount of acid reflux.[1, 22] Some heartburn sufferers complain that certain *drugs* may initiate or exacerbate their symptoms, either by reducing LES pressure and peristaltic contractions (e.g., theophylline, calcium channel blockers) or by directly irritating the inflamed esophagus (e.g., aspirin; see Table 6–3).

Heartburn may be accompanied by the appearance of fluid in the mouth, either a bitter acidic material or a salty fluid. *Regurgitation* describes the complaint of a bitter acidic

Table 6–3 | **Aggravating Factors for Heartburn with Proposed Mechanisms**

LOW LES PRESSURE	DIRECT MUCOSAL IRRITANT	INCREASED INTRA-ABDOMINAL PRESSURE	OTHERS
Certain foods	Certain foods	Bending over	Supine position
Fats	Citrus products	Lifting	Lying on right side
Sugars	Tomato-based products	Straining at stool	Red wine
Chocolate	Spicy foods	Exercise	Emotions
Onions	Coffee		
Carminatives	Medications		
Coffee	Aspirin		
Alcohol	NSAIDs		
Cigarettes	Tetracycline		
Medications	Quinidine		
Progesterone	Potassium chloride tablets		
Theophylline	Iron salts		
Anticholinergic agents			
Adrenergic agonists			
Adrenergic antagonists			
Diazepam			
Meperidine			
Nitrates			
Calcium channel blockers			

LES, lower esophageal sphincter; NSAIDs, nonsteroidal anti-inflammatory drugs.

fluid in the mouth that is common at night or when the patient bends over. The regurgitated material comes from the stomach and is yellow or green, which suggests the presence of bile. It is important to distinguish regurgitation from vomiting, which is the primary complaint of some patients. The absence of nausea, retching, and abdominal contractions suggests regurgitation rather than vomiting. Furthermore, the regurgitation of bland material is atypical for acid reflux disease and suggests the presence of an esophageal motility disorder (i.e., achalasia) or delayed gastric emptying. In one study, the researchers found that the presence of heartburn and acid regurgitation together as dominant complaints had a sensitivity of 78% and a specificity of 60% for the presence of gastroesophageal reflux disease, as defined by prolonged esophageal pH monitoring.[23] *Water brash* is an uncommon and frequently misunderstood symptom that should be used to describe the sudden filling of the mouth with clear, slightly salty fluid. This fluid is not regurgitated material but rather secretions from the salivary glands as part of a protective, vagally mediated reflex from the distal esophagus.[24]

Mechanisms

The physiologic mechanisms that produce heartburn are, surprisingly, poorly understood. Although the reflux of gastric acid is most commonly associated with heartburn, the same symptom may be elicited by esophageal balloon distention,[25] reflux of bile salts,[26] and acid-induced motility disturbances.[27] The best evidence that the pain mechanism is probably related to the stimulation of mucosal chemoreceptors is the sensitivity of the esophagus to the presence of acid during its perfusion or by monitoring pH. The location of these receptors is not known and probably is not superficial because topical anesthetics fail to alter the pain response.[28]

The correlation of discrete episodes of acid reflux and symptoms, however, is poor. For example, postprandial gastroesophageal reflux is common in healthy people, but symptoms are rare. Intraesophageal pH monitoring of patients with endoscopic evidence of esophagitis typically shows excessive periods of acid reflux, but fewer than 20% of these reflux episodes are accompanied by complaints.[29] Moreover, one third of patients with Barrett esophagus, the most extreme form of gastroesophageal reflux disease, are acid insensitive.[30] Therefore, symptoms must require more than esophageal contact with acid. Mucosal disruption with inflammation may be a contributory factor, but on endoscopy, the esophagus appears normal in most symptomatic patients. The histologic appearance of the mucosa obtained by biopsy shows that some of these patients have polymorphonuclear leukocytes, others have only reparative changes, and many have a normal esophagus. Results of one study suggest that hydrogen ion concentration could be crucial in symptom production.[31] One group found that all 25 patients with reflux disease experienced heartburn during intraesophageal infusion of solutions having pH values of 1.0 and 1.5, but only one half had heartburn with solutions having pH values of 2.5 to 6.0. Other factors that possibly influence the report of heartburn include the acid clearance mechanism; salivary bicarbonate concentration; volume of refluxed acid, as measured by duration and proximal extent of reflux episodes; frequency of the heartburn complaints; and interaction of pepsin with acid (see Chapter 33, section on pathogenesis of gastroesophageal reflux disease).[24, 32]

GLOBUS SENSATION

Globus sensation is a feeling of a lump or tightness in the throat, unrelated to swallowing. Up to 46% of the general population have experienced the globus sensation at one time or another.[13] This particular sensation accounts for 3% of consultations to throat specialists,[33] predominantly by middle-aged women. The sensation can be described as a "lump," "tightness," "choking," or "strangling" feeling as if something is caught in the throat. The globus sensation is present between meals, and swallowing of solids or large liquid boluses may give temporary relief. Dysphagia and odynophagia are not present. Frequent dry swallowing and emotional stress may worsen the globus sensation.

Mechanisms

Evidence for physiologic and psychologic abnormalities in patients with the globus sensation has been inconsistent and controversial. Although frequently suggested, UES dysfunction has not been directly identified as the cause of the globus sensation. Modern manometric studies have consistently shown the UES to be functioning normally,[34] and the sphincter does not appear to be hyper-responsive to esophageal distention, acidification, or mental stress.[34, 35] Furthermore, esophageal distention can cause a globus sensation unrelated to the degree of rise in UES pressure,[35] and stress-induced increases in UES pressure are not associated with a globus sensation in normal subjects or in patients complaining of this symptom.[34] Heartburn has been reported in up to 90% of patients with the globus sensation.[36] Documentation of esophagitis or abnormal gastroesophageal reflux by esophageal pH monitoring, however, is found in fewer than 25% of patients.[37] Balloon distention of the esophagus produces the globus sensation at lower balloon volumes in globus sufferers than in controls, which suggests that the perception of esophageal stretch may be heightened in these patients.[35]

Psychological factors may be important in the genesis of the globus sensation. The most commonly found psychiatric diagnoses include anxiety, panic disorder, depression, hypochondriasis, somatization, and introversion.[38] Indeed, globus is the fourth most common symptom of patients with somatization disorders.[39] A combination of biologic factors, hypochondriacal traits, and learned fear after a choking episode provides a framework for misinterpretation of the symptoms and intensifies the globus symptoms or the patient's anxiety.[40]

CHEST PAIN (Table 6–4)

Recurrent chest pain of esophageal origin that mimics angina pectoris is not surprising, in view of the proximity of the two organs and their shared neural pathways. Esophageal disorders are probably the most common causes of noncardiac chest pain. Of the approximately 500,000 patients who

Table 6–4 | **Characteristics of Cardiac and Esophageal Chest Pain***

CHARACTERISTICS	DESCRIPTION	CARDIAC†		ESOPHAGEAL‡	
		N	%	*N*	%
Quality	Tight, heavy	48	92	15	83
Location	Retrosternal	51	98	18	100
Radiation	To left arm	28	38	6	33
Duration	Several hours	13	25	14	78§
	Wakens patient at night	13	25	11	61§
Provocation	Emotions	15	29	7	39
	Meals	3	6	7	39§
	Recumbency	10	19	11	61§
	Exercise	38	73	7	39
Relief	Antacids	5	10	8	44§
	Nitroglycerin	14	27	7	39
Associated gastrointestinal symptoms		24	46	15	83§

*Questionnaire results from 70 patients admitted to emergency departments with anterior chest pain of cardiac or esophageal origin.
†Total $N = 52$.
‡Total $N = 18$.
§Differences between groups significant ($P < .05$).
Modified from Davies HA, Jones DB, Rhodes J, Newcombe RG: Angina-like esophageal pain: Differentiation from cardiac pain by history. J Clin Gastroenterol 7:477, 1985.

undergo coronary angiography yearly for presumed cardiac pain, nearly 30% have normal epicardial coronary arteries; of those patients, 18% to 56% may have esophageal diseases that account for the symptoms.[41]

Intermittent anterior chest discomfort is the *sine qua non* of this syndrome. Chest pain usually is described as a squeezing or burning sensation, substernal, and radiating to the back, neck, jaw, or arms, at times indistinguishable from angina pain. Although it is not always related to swallowing, it can be triggered by ingestion of either very hot or very cold liquids. It frequently awakens the patient from sleep and may worsen during periods of emotional stress. The duration ranges from minutes to hours and may be intermittent over several days. Although the pain can be severe, causing the patient to become ashen and perspire, it often abates spontaneously and may be eased with antacids. Occasionally, its severity requires narcotics or nitroglycerin for relief. Close questioning reveals that most patients with this pain have other esophageal symptoms; however, chest pain is the only esophageal complaint in about 10%.[42]

The clinical history often does not enable the physician to distinguish between cardiac and esophageal causes of chest pain. For example, gastroesophageal reflux may be triggered by exercise[19] and cause exertional chest pain that mimics angina pectoris, even during treadmill testing.[43] Symptoms suggestive of esophageal origin include pain that continues for hours, retrosternal pain without lateral radiation, pain that interrupts sleep or is meal related, and pain that is relieved with antacid agents. The presence of other esophageal symptoms also helps in the establishment of the differential diagnosis (see Table 6–4). A serious complicating factor in diagnosis is that as many as 50% of patients with cardiac pain have one or more symptoms of esophageal pain.[44] This overlap exists because the prevalence of both cardiac and esophageal diseases—especially gastroesophageal reflux disease—increases as people grow older. Both problems not only may coexist but also may interact in producing chest pain.

Mechanisms

The specific mechanisms that produce esophageal chest pain are not well understood. Chest pain that arises from the esophagus has commonly been attributed to the stimulation of chemoreceptors (acid, pepsin, bile) or mechanoreceptors (distention, spasm), although thermoreceptors (cold) also may be involved.

Gastroesophageal reflux causes chest pain primarily through acid-sensitive esophageal chemoreceptors, as discussed earlier in the section "Heartburn (Pyrosis)." Acid-induced dysmotility was once believed to be a major cause of esophageal pain. Early studies of acid perfusion in patients with reflux demonstrated increased esophageal contraction amplitude and duration, as well as simultaneous and spontaneous contractions, while pain was produced.[45] More recently, other investigators have not been able to reproduce these observations.[46] Although diffuse esophageal spasm has been reported during spontaneous acid reflux in some patients, studies with modern equipment show that these motility changes are infrequent during acid infusion.[46] In addition, 24-hour ambulatory esophageal pH and motility monitoring[47, 48] has shown that spontaneous acid-induced chest pain is associated with esophageal motility abnormalities in fewer than 15% of patients with such discomfort.

Many patients with suspected esophageal chest pain have esophageal motility disorders characterized by high-amplitude contractions of prolonged duration or frequent simultaneous contractions.[49] One popular hypothesis is that these abnormal waveforms cause pain as high intramural esophageal tension inhibits blood flow for a critical period of time (i.e., myoischemia). Experimental studies by MacKenzie and coworkers lend support to this hypothesis.[50] They found decreased esophageal rewarming rates after cold water infusions in patients with symptomatic esophageal motility disorders in comparison with age-matched controls. Because similar studies in patients with Raynaud phenomenon are directly correlated with blood flow, the authors theorized that esophageal ischemia was the cause of the delayed rewarming rate. None of these patients, however, developed chest pain during the study. Furthermore, the extensive arterial and venous blood supply to the esophagus suggests that compromised blood flow is unlikely after even the most abnormal esophageal contractions.[51]

Complicating the relation between esophageal chest pain and abnormal esophageal contractions is the consistent observation that most of these patients are asymptomatic when the contraction abnormalities are identified.[41] These esophageal motility disorders possibly are markers for more severe esophageal disturbances during chest pain. However, the results of prolonged ambulatory esophageal motility studies confirm that this relationship is infrequent.[47, 48] In addition, amelioration of chest pain does not predictably correlate with reduction of amplitude by either pharmacotherapy[52] or surgical myotomy.[53] Results of more recent studies suggest that the motility changes may represent an epiphenomenon of a chronic pain syndrome rather than the direct cause of the complaints.[41, 48]

Other potential causes of esophageal chest pain include the excitation of temperature receptors and luminal distention. The ingestion of hot or cold liquids can produce severe chest pain. It was previously believed that this was related to esophageal spasm, but studies have shown that cold-induced pain produces esophageal aperistalsis and dilatation, which suggests that the cause of esophageal chest pain may be activation of stretch receptors by acute distention.[54] Such distention and pain are experienced with acute food impaction, the drinking of carbonated beverages (in some patients), and dysfunction of the belch reflex.[55] Another possibility is that chest pain is caused by proximal distention of the esophagus by abnormal distal contractions or by impaired LES functioning and emptying.[56] In addition, esophageal chest pain in susceptible patients can be reproduced with smaller volumes of esophageal balloon distention than the volumes that produce pain in asymptomatic patients.[57] Thus, altered pain perception may contribute to these patients' reactions to pain stimuli. Anxiolytics and antidepressants can raise pain thresholds as well as improve mood states. This may explain the mechanism by which these medications improve esophageal chest pain in the absence of manometric changes.[58, 59]

RESPIRATORY; EAR, NOSE, AND THROAT; AND CARDIAC SYMPTOMS

Extraesophageal symptoms of esophageal diseases are summarized in Table 6–5. Although these symptoms may be caused by esophageal motility disorders, they are most frequently associated with gastroesophageal reflux disease. However, the classic reflux symptoms of heartburn and regurgitation often are mild or absent.

The mechanism by which gastroesophageal reflux can cause chronic cough and other extraesophageal symptoms is probably twofold: (1) by intermittent recurrent microaspiration of gastric contents and (2) by a vagally mediated neural reflex. In animal studies, the instillation of small amounts of acid in the trachea[60] or on the vocal cords[61] can produce marked changes in airway resistance as well as vocal cord ulcers. Direct evidence for aspiration is more difficult to identify in adults, resting primarily on the presence of fat-filled macrophages in sputum,[62] radioactivity in the lungs after the tracer is placed in the stomach overnight,[63] and high esophageal or hypopharyngeal acid reflux recorded by 24-hour pH monitoring with dual probes.[64, 65] There is better evidence from both animal and human studies that a neural reflex is the pathophysiologic basis for these symptoms. Acid perfusion into the distal esophagus increases airway resistance in all subjects, but the changes are most marked in patients with asthma and heartburn.[66] Dogs do not produce this response after bilateral vagotomy[67]; nor do humans after atropine.[66] These findings suggest bronchial constriction that is vagally mediated.

Table 6–5 | **Extraesophageal Symptoms of Esophageal Diseases**

RESPIRATORY	EAR, NOSE, AND THROAT	CARDIAC
Wheezing	Chronic sore throat	Syncope
Bronchitis	Hoarseness	
Aspiration	Burning sensation in tongue	
Hemoptysis	Halitosis	
Apnea	Otalgia	
	Cervical pain	
	Globus sensation	
	Chronic cough	
	Stridor	
	Lateral neck pain	
	Dental erosion	

Abnormal amounts of acid reflux recorded by prolonged esophageal pH monitoring have been identified in 35% to 80% of asthmatic adults.[68] Symptoms that suggest *reflux-induced asthma* include the onset of wheezing at a late age without a history of allergies or asthma; nocturnal cough or wheezing; asthma worsened after meals, exercise, or the supine position; and asthma that is exacerbated by bronchodilators or that is steroid dependent. Patients who experience reflux with symptoms strongly suggestive of aspiration usually have *nocturnal cough* and *heartburn, recurrent pneumonias, unexplained fevers,* and *associated esophageal motility disorders.*[69] Ear, nose, and throat complaints associated with gastroesophageal reflux include postnasal drip, voice changes, hoarseness, sore throat, persistent cough, otalgia, halitosis, dental erosion, and excessive salivation.[70, 71] Up to 25% of patients with gastroesophageal reflux disease complain of only head and neck symptoms.[72] Examination of the vocal cords may help in suspected acid-related problems. Some patients have redness, hyperemia, and edema of the vocal cords and arytenoids. In more severe cases, vocal cord ulcers, granulomas, and even laryngeal cancer, all secondary to gastroesophageal reflux disease, have been reported. Normal results of a laryngeal examination, however, are not incompatible with acid reflux-related extraesophageal symptoms.[70] Further evidence for the connection between esophageal stimulation and vagal reflexes can be found in the syndrome of "swallow syncope." In this disorder, swallowing or pharyngeal esophageal stimulation can lead to profound, even lethal bradycardia, presumably through a vagal mechanism.[73]

REFERENCES

1. Locke GR, Talley NJ, Fett SC, et al: Prevalence of clinical spectrum of esophageal reflux: A population study in Olmsted County, Minnesota. Gastroenterology 112:1448, 1997.
2. Goker ME, Bukatman R: The prevalence of swallowing disorders in two teaching hospitals. Dysphagia 1:3, 1986.
3. Schatzki R: Panel discussion on diseases of the esophagus. Am J Gastroenterol 31:117, 1959.
4. Edwards DA: Discriminative information in the diagnosis of dysphagia. JR Coll Physicians Lond 9:257, 1975.
5. Kendall G, Thompson DG, Day S, et al: Motor responses of the esophagus to intraabdominal distension in normal subjects and patients with esophageal clearance disorders. Gut 28:272, 1987.
6. Kahrilas PJ, Dodds WJ, Hogan WJ: Effects of peristaltic dysfunction on esophageal volume clearance. Gastroenterology 91:987, 1986.
7. Triadifilopoulos G: Nonobstructive dysphagia in reflux esophagitis. Am J Gastroenterol 84:614, 1989.
8. Clouse RE, Lustman PH, McCord GS, et al: Clinical correlates of abnormal sensitivity to intraesophageal balloon distention. Dig Dis Sci 36:1040, 1991.
9. Clouse RE, Lustman PF: Psychiatric illness and contraction abnormalities of the esophagus. N Engl J Med 309:1337, 1983.
10. Castell DO, Donner MW: Evaluation of dysphagia: A careful history is crucial. Dysphagia 2:65, 1987.
11. Schatzki R, Gary JE: Dysphagia due to a diaphragm-like localized narrowing in the lower esophagus. AJR 70:911, 1953.
12. Nebel OT, Fornes MF, Castell DO: Symptomatic gastroesophageal reflux: Incidence and precipitating factors. Dig Dis Sci 21:953, 1976.
13. Thompson WA, Heaton KW: Heartburn and globus in apparently healthy people. Can Med Assoc J 126:46, 1982.
14. Graham DY, Smith JL, Patterson DJ: Why do apparently healthy people use antacid tablets? Am J Gastroenterol 78:257, 1983.
15. Feldman M, Barnett C: Relationship between acidity and osmolality of popular beverages and reported postprandial heartburn. Gastroenterology 108:125, 1995.
16. Price SF, Smithson KW, Castell DO: Food sensitivity in reflux esophagitis. Gastroenterology 75:240, 1978.
17. Lloyd DA, Borda IT: Food-induced heartburn: Effect of osmolarity. Gastroenterology 80:740, 1988.
18. Katz LC, Just R, Castell DO: Body position affects postprandial reflux. J Clin Gastroenterol 18:280, 1994.
19. Clark CS, Kraus BB, Sinclair J, et al: Gastroesophageal reflux induced by exercise in healthy volunteers. JAMA 261:3599, 1989.
20. Dennish GW, Castell DO: Inhibitory effect of smoking on the lower esophageal sphincter. N Engl J Med 284:1136, 1971.
21. Kahrilas PJ, Gupta RP: Mechanisms of acid reflux associated with cigarette smoking. Gut 31:4, 1990.
22. Bradley LA, Richter JE, Pulliam TJ, et al: Psychological factors influence the relationship between stress and reports of gastroesophageal reflux. Am J Gastroenterol 88:11, 1993.
23. Klauser AG, Schindlbeck NE, Muller-Lissner SA: Symptoms of gastroesophageal reflux disease. Lancet 335:205, 1990.
24. Helm JF, Dodds WJ, Hogan WJ: Salivary response to esophageal acid in normal subjects and patients with reflux esophagitis. Gastroenterology 93:1393, 1987.
25. Jones CM: Digestive Tract Pain. New York, Macmillan, 1958, p 12.
26. Kaye MD, Showalter JP: Pyloric incompetence in patients with symptomatic gastroesophageal reflux disease. J Lab Clin Med 83:198, 1974.
27. Swany N: Esophageal spasm. Clinical and manometric response to nitro-glycerin and long acting nitrates. Gastroenterology 72:23, 1977.
28. Hookman P, Siegel CI, Hendrix TR: Failure of oxethazaine to alter acid induced esophageal pain. Am J Dig 11:811, 1966.
29. Baldi F, Ferrarini F, Longanes A, et al: Acid gastroesophageal reflux and symptom recurrence. Analysis of some factors influencing their association. Dig Dis Sci 34:1890, 1989.
30. Johnson DA, Winters C, Spurling TJ, et al: Esophageal acid sensitivity in Barrett's esophagus. J Clin Gastroenterol 9:23, 1987.
31. Smith JL, Opekum AR, Larkai E, et al: Sensitivity of the esophageal mucosa to pH in gastroesophageal reflux disease. Gastroenterology 96: 683, 1989.
32. Weuston BLA, Akkerman LMA, vanBerge-Henegouwen GP, et al: Symptom perception in gastroesophageal reflux disease is dependent on spatiotemporal reflux characteristics. Gastroenterology 108:1739, 1995.
33. Thompson WG: Gut Reactions. New York, Plenum Press, 1989, p 93.
34. Cook IJ, Dent J, Collins SM: Upper esophageal sphincter tone and reactivity to stress in patients with a history of globus sensation. Dig Dis Sci 34:672, 1989.
35. Cook IJ, Shaker R, Dodds WJ, et al: Role of mechanical and chemical stimulation of the esophagus in globus sensation. Gastroenterology 96: 99, 1989.
36. Cherry J, Siegel CI, Marguiles SI, et al: Pharyngeal localization of symptoms of gastroesophageal reflux. Ann Otol Rhinol Laryngol 79: 912, 1970.
37. Wilson JA, Pryde A, Piris J, et al: Pharyngoesophageal dysmotility in globus sensation. Arch Otol Laryngol Head Neck Surg 115:1086, 1989.
38. Deary IJ, Wilson JA, Mitchell L, et al: Covert psychiatric disturbances in patients with globus pharyngitis. Br J Med Psychol 62:381, 1989.
39. Othmer E, DeSouza C: A screening test for somatization disorder (hysteria). Am J Psychiat 142:1146, 1985.
40. Bishop LC, Riley WT: The psychiatric management of the globus syndrome. Gen Hosp Psychiat 9:214, 1988.
41. Richter JE, Bradley LA, Castell DO: Esophageal chest pain: Current controversies in pathogenesis, diagnosis and therapy. Ann Intern Med 110:66, 1989.
42. Hewson EG, Sinclair JW, Dalton CB, et al: Twenty-four hour esophageal pH monitoring: The most useful test for evaluating noncardiac chest pain. Am J Med 90:576, 1991.
43. Schofield PM, Bennett DH, Worwell PJ, et al: Exertional gastrooesophageal reflux: A mechanism for symptoms in patients with angina pectoris and normal coronary angiograms. BMJ 294:1459, 1987.
44. Davies HA, Jones DB, Rhodes J, Newcombe RG: Angina-like esophageal pain: Differentiation from cardiac pain by history. J Clin Gastroenterol 7:477, 1985.
45. Siegel CI, Hendrix TR: Esophageal motor abnormalities induced by acid perfusion in patients with heartburn. J Clin Invest 42:686, 1963.
46. Richter JE, Johns DN, Wu WC, et al: Are esophageal motility abnormalities produced during the intraesophageal acid perfusion test? JAMA 253:1914, 1985.
47. Janssen J, Vantrappen G, Ghillibert G: 24-Hour recording of esophageal pressure and pH in patients with non-cardiac chest pain. Gastroenterology 90:1978, 1986.
48. Peters LJ, Maas LC, Petty D, et al: Spontaneous non-cardiac chest pain: Evaluation by 24-hour ambulatory esophageal motility and pH monitoring. Gastroenterology 94:876, 1988.
49. Katz PO, Dalton CB, Richter JE, et al: Esophageal testing in patients with non-cardiac chest pain and/or dysphagia. Ann Intern Med 106:593, 1987.
50. MacKenzie J, Belch J, Land D, et al: Oesophageal ischemia in motility disorders associated with chest pain. Lancet 2:592, 1988.
51. Liberman-Meffert DM, Leuscher U, Neff U, et al: Esophagectomy without thoracotomy. Is there a risk of intramediastinal bleeding? Ann Surg 206:184, 1987.
52. Richter JE, Dalton CB, Bradley LA, et al: Oral nifedipine in the treatment of non-cardiac chest pain in patients with the nutcracker esophagus. Gastroenterology 93:21, 1987.
53. Ellis FH, Crozier RE, Shea JA: Long esophagomyotomy for diffuse esophageal spasm and related disorders. In Siewert JR, Holscher AH (eds): Diseases of the Esophagus: Pathophysiology, Diagnosis, Conservative and Surgical Treatment. New York, Springer-Verlag, 1988, p 913.
54. Meyer GW, Castell DO: Human esophageal response during chest pain induced by swallowing cold liquids. JAMA 246:2057, 1981.
55. Kahrilas PJ, Dodds WJ, Hogan WJ: Dysfunction of the belch reflex. Gastroenterology 93:818, 1987.
56. Kaye MD: Anomalies of peristalsis in idiopathic diffuse oesophageal spasm. Gut 22:217, 1981.
57. Richter JE, Barish CF, Castell DO: Abnormal sensory perception in patients with esophageal chest pain. Gastroenterology 91:845, 1986.
58. Clouse RE, Lustman PJ, Eckert TC, et al: Low-dose trazodone for symptomatic patients with esophageal contraction abnormalities: A double-blind placebo controlled trial. Gastroenterology 92:1027, 1987.
59. Cannon RO, Quyyumi AA, Mincemoyer R, et al: Imipramine in patients with chest pain despite normal coronary angiogram. N Engl J Med 19:1411, 1994.
60. Tuchman DN, Boyle JT, Pack AI, et al: Comparison of airway responses following tracheal or esophageal acidification in the cat. Gastroenterology 87:872, 1984.

61. Little FB, Koufman JA, Kohut RI: Effect of gastric acid on the pathogenesis of subglottic stenosis. Ann Otol Rhinol Laryngol 94:516, 1985.
62. Crausaz FM, Favez G: Aspiration of solid food particles into lungs of patients with gastroesophageal reflux and chronic bronchial disease. Chest 93:376, 1988.
63. Chernow B, Johnson LF, Janowitz WR, et al: Pulmonary aspiration as a consequence of gastroesophageal reflux: A diagnostic approach. Dig Dis Sci 24:839, 1979.
64. Sontag SJ, O'Connell S, Khandelwal S, et al: Most asthmatics have gastroesophageal reflux with or without bronchodilator therapy. Gastroenterology 99:613, 1990.
65. Donnelly RJ, Berrisford RG, Jack CI, et al: Simultaneous tracheal and esophageal pH monitoring: Investigating reflux-associated asthma. Ann Thorac Surg 56:1029, 1993.
66. Mansfield LE, Stein MR: Gastroesophageal reflux and asthma: A possible reflex mechanism. Ann Allergy 41:224, 1978.
67. Mansfield LE, Hameister HH, Spaulding HS, et al: The role of the vagus nerve in airway narrowing caused by intraesophageal hydrochloric acid provocation and esophageal distention. Ann Allergy 47:431, 1981.
68. Harding SM, Richter JE: The role of gastroesophageal reflux in chronic cough and asthma. Chest 111:1389, 1997.
69. Pellegrini CA, DeMeester TR, Johnson LA, Skinner DB: Gastroesophageal reflux and pulmonary aspiration: Incidence, functional abnormality, and results of surgical therapy. Surgery 86:110, 1975.
70. Koufman JA: The otolaryngologic manifestations of gastroesophageal reflux disease. Laryngoscope 101(Suppl 53):1, 1991.
71. Schroeder PL, Filler SJ, Ramirez B, et al: Dental erosion and acid reflux disease. Ann Intern Med 122:809, 1995.
72. Henderson RD, Woolf C, Marryatt G: Pharyngoesophageal dysphagia and gastroesophageal reflux. Laryngoscope 86:1531, 1976.
73. Deucher DC, Trounce JR: Syncopal dysphagia. Guy's Hosp Rep 109: 29, 1960.

Chapter 7

DYSPEPSIA

Kenneth R. McQuaid

Dyspepsia affects more than one fourth of the general population in all industrialized countries and is a frequent reason for medical consultation.[1] New-onset dyspepsia occurs in up to 10% of this population each year, and up to 15% of patients with significant dyspepsia seek medical attention within a 3-month period.[2, 3] Dyspepsia accounts for up to 7% of office visits and 40% to 70% of gastrointestinal (GI) complaints in general medical practice.[4, 5] Dyspepsia appears to have a significant impact upon quality of life. It results in enormous societal costs—both direct medical costs of physician visits, diagnostic tests, and medications, and indirect costs of absenteeism from diminished productivity in the workplace.[6] In 1995, the market for prescription medications in the United States for the treatment of dyspepsia was a staggering $1.3 billion, not including nonprescription agents or drugs used in the treatment of peptic ulcer disease or gastroesophageal reflux disease.[7] The annual per person attributable costs in a health maintenance organization for peptic ulcer disease and dyspepsia have been estimated at $1183 and $431, respectively.[8]

DEFINITION

The term *dyspepsia* is used variably by health professionals to refer to a heterogeneous group of upper abdominal symptoms that may arise from numerous causes.[9] Patients seldom use the term *dyspepsia* and describe their abdominal symptoms instead in terms of discomfort, pain, aching, bloating, fullness, burning, or indigestion. The way a patient perceives and reports these symptoms is dependent upon a complex interplay of biologic variables, personality traits, social support mechanisms, coping strategies, culture, and language.

Dyspepsia is not one symptom but a constellation of symptoms—different in all patients—that arise from disparate conditions. The term generally refers to pain or discomfort centered in the upper abdomen that may also include bloating, early satiety, postprandial fullness, nausea, anorexia, heartburn, regurgitation, and burping or belching. Use of the term *dyspepsia* generally reflects the physician's interpretation that the symptoms are arising from the upper luminal GI tract. In view of its elusive definition, many primary physicians do not use the term *dyspepsia*, instead describing the quality and location of the patient's symptoms.

Even among clinical investigators, definitions of dyspepsia have varied widely, hampering research progress.[9] In 1991 an international panel of clinical investigators developed a comprehensive classification system for functional GI disorders, including dyspepsia, known as the Rome Criteria. These criteria were updated in 1999 at the Rome II consensus conference; *dyspepsia* was defined as pain or discomfort centered in the upper abdomen.[10] Discomfort may be characterized by or associated with upper abdominal fullness, early satiety, bloating, or nausea. The Rome II consensus group has attempted to distinguish patients with probable gastroesophageal reflux disorder from other patients with dyspepsia. Patients with dyspepsia may have heartburn—defined as a retrosternal burning sensation—as part of the symptom constellation. When heartburn is the dominant upper abdominal symptom, it has a high positive predictive value for the diagnosis of gastroesophageal reflux disorder. For this reason, the Rome II group concluded that dominant heartburn should not be labeled dyspepsia—even when other dyspeptic symptoms are present. Such a distinction, however, may not coincide with the conceptual framework followed by most primary care physicians in assessing a patient with upper GI symptoms.[4]

For the purposes of this chapter, it is important to distinguish the terms *dyspepsia, uninvestigated dyspepsia,* and *functional dyspepsia. Dyspepsia* encompasses all relevant upper abdominal symptoms regardless of their underlying cause. The term *uninvestigated dyspepsia* refers to new onset

Table 7–1 | **Causes of Organic Dyspepsia**

Luminal GI tract
Food intolerance
Peptic ulcer disease
Gastroesophageal reflux
Gastric or esophageal neoplasms
Gastroparesis (diabetes, postvagotomy, scleroderma, chronic intestinal pseudo-obstruction)
Infiltrative gastric disorders (Ménétrier's syndrome, Crohn's disease, eosinophilic gastroenteritis, sarcoidosis, amyloidosis)
Malabsorptive disorders (celiac sprue, lactose intolerance)
Gastric infections (CMV, fungal, TB, syphilis)
Parasites (*Giardia lamblia, Strongyloides stercoralis*)
Chronic gastric volvulus
Chronic intestinal ischemia
Irritable bowel syndrome
Medications
Ethanol
Aspirin/NSAIDs
Antibiotics (macrolides, sulfonamides, metronidazole)
Theophylline
Digitalis
Glucocorticoids
Iron, potassium chloride
Niacin, gemfibrozil
Narcotics
Colchicine
Quinidine
Estrogens
Levodopa
Nitrates
Loop diurectics
ACE inhibitors
Pancreaticobiliary disorders
Chronic pancreatitis
Pancreatic neoplasms
Biliary colic: cholelithiasis, choledocholithiasis, sphincter of Oddi dysfunction
Systemic disorders
Diabetes mellitus
Thyroid disease
Hyperparathyroidism
Adrenal insufficiency
Collagen vascular disorders
Renal insufficiency
Cardiac ischemia, congestive heart failure
Intra-abdominal malignancy
Pregnancy

ACE, angiotensin-converting enzyme; CMV, cytomegalovirus; GI, gastrointestinal; NSAIDs, nonsteroidal anti-inflammatory drugs; TB, tuberculosis.

or recurrent dyspepsia for which no diagnostic investigations yet have been performed and therefore a specific diagnosis has not been determined. In patients with uninvestigated dyspepsia, providers must decide between a course of empirical treatment versus diagnostic studies. *Functional dyspepsia* refers to persistent or recurrent dyspepsia for which diagnostic investigation (including endoscopy) has not determined an obvious organic cause of symptoms.

EPIDEMIOLOGY

Dyspepsia is extremely common among adults; the prevalence rates reported depend upon the population studied (medical patients versus the general population), the survey method used (questionnaire versus interview), the length of the observation period, and the broadness or narrowness of the definition. When symptoms of gastroesophgeal reflux (heartburn, regurgitation) are included, prevalence rates are higher than if symptoms are restricted to epigastric pain or discomfort.

On the basis of a number of population studies conducted in North America, Europe, and Australia, the annual prevalence of recurrent dyspepsia is approximately 25% (range 8% to 54%) over a 3- to 12-month period.[1, 3, 7, 11] However, if frequent heartburn is included in dyspeptic symptoms, the prevalence exceeds 40%.[2, 3, 12, 13]

Longitudinal studies suggest that dyspeptic symptoms tend to persist or recur frequently in most people. Among patients without prior dyspepsia, the incidence of new onset symptoms is as high as 10%/year; however, in one third of patients these symptoms resolve, thus maintaining an overall prevalence of dyspepsia that is fairly constant over time.[12] The prevalence of dyspepsia is modestly higher in women than in men and, surprisingly, declines slightly with age.[2, 13]

Thus, a significant proportion of the population—perhaps even the majority—experience dyspepsia, but only one half seek medical attention for these symptoms, most within 6 months of their onset.[14] Although the reason for consultation is not always clear, the severity or frequency of symptoms, fear of underlying disease (especially cancer), illness in a family member or friend, lower social class, advancing age, anxiety, psychological stress, and lack of adequate psychosocial support are all important factors affecting this decision and must be addressed.[15, 16] One fourth of patients consult nonmedical practitioners such as nutritionists, acupuncturists, and homeopaths.[14]

CAUSES OF ORGANIC DYSPEPSIA

Dyspepsia may be caused by a number of foods, medications, systemic disorders, and diseases of the luminal GI tract (Table 7–1). An organic cause is found, however, in only 40% of patients with dyspepsia, usually peptic ulcer disease, gastroesophageal reflux disease (GERD), or gastric cancer. In over half of patients, no obvious cause is found, and the dyspepsia is labeled as *idiopathic* or *functional dyspepsia*.

Food Intolerance

Contrary to common belief, overeating or ingestion of specific foods such as spices, coffee, or alcohol has never been proved by double-blind challenge to cause dyspepsia. Although avoiding certain foods on the basis of experience or advice has an enormous placebo effect, food intolerance may be due to a number of mechanisms: direct mucosal irritation or irritation of preexisting ulcer, direct stimulation of mucosal visceral afferent receptors, gastric overdistention, alterations in gastric emptying or intestinal motility, increased gas production, malabsorption, or, in rare instances, true food allergies (see Chapters 9, 89, and 101).

Specific foods are commonly implicated in dyspepsia. Although drinks with high titratable acidity (citrus) or low pH (soft drinks), coffee, wine, and other alcoholic beverages provoke heartburn, the frequency with which moderate ingestions of these substances cause dyspepsia is unknown. Coffee (including decaffeinated) commonly causes heartburn as well as dyspepsia, especially when drunk in large volumes.[17] Spicy foods, particularly red and black peppers, may cause acute mucosal injury and acute epigastric pain.[18] Alcoholic beverages in concentrations greater than 20% (40 proof) may also cause acute mucosal injury, but there is little evidence that moderate amounts cause dyspepsia.[19, 20] Heavy acute ingestion and chronic alcohol abuse both may cause dyspepsia, which is commonly worse in the morning. High-fat meals, which slow gastric emptying, may also cause dyspepsia.[21]

Lactose malabsorption may underlie dyspepsia with cramps, flatulence, and diarrhea, as well. Commonly overlooked as a cause of dyspepsia, it is implicated in up to 9% of unselected dyspepsia patients[22] (see Chapter 9).

Medication Intolerance

Medications may cause symptoms as a result of direct mucosal irritation, alterations in gastric motility, provocation of gastroesophageal reflux, or idiosyncratic mechanisms or may simply be due to concomitant ingestion of substances such as lactose or sorbitol. Both community surveys and prospective trials indicate that aspirin and other nonsteroidal anti-inflammatory drugs (NSAIDs) provoke dyspepsia in approximately 25% of patients; however, this incidence is tempered by the finding that 15% of patients treated with placebo also report symptoms.[23, 24] Among users of NSAIDS, dyspeptic symptoms are poorly correlated with the presence of peptic ulcers.[4, 25, 26] Cyclooxygenase-2 (COX-2)–selective NSAIDS have a lower associated incidence of dyspepsia.[23, 27] Other medications commonly causing dyspepsia include potassium supplements, iron, antibiotics (especially macrolides, sulfonamides, and metronidazole), digitalis, corticosteroids, niacin, gemfibrozil, narcotics, colchicines, quinidine, estrogens, theophylline, and levodopa. Review of a large prescription database also implicates nitrates, loop diuretics, and angiotensin-converting enzyme (ACE) inhibitors.[28]

Peptic Ulcer Disease

Most peptic ulcers are associated with dyspepsia, but most dyspepsia patients do *not* have peptic ulcer disease. Nevertheless, it is the first disease considered by most clinicians. The prevalence of peptic ulcers among dyspeptic patients depends upon the population studied. Among such patients selectively referred to gastroenterologists for endoscopy by their primary care physicians, the endoscopic prevalence of ulcers is approximately 12% to 25%. However, in studies of unselected dyspeptic patients who consult their primary care practitioners, the prevalence of endoscopic ulcers is approximately 13%. Finally, among subjects in the community at large invited to undergo endoscopy, the prevalence of peptic ulcers was only 8% among dyspeptics and 4% among asymptomatic adults.[7, 12] Thus, the prevalence of peptic ulcers is higher among patients referred by primary practitioners for endoscopy than among unselected patients with dyspepsia. Peptic ulcers are more common in patients who have the following characteristics: age above 40 years, *Helicobacter pylori* infection, NSAID use, night pain, relief of pain with food or antacids, prior history or family history of peptic ulcer disease, male gender, or smoking[7] (see Chapters 39 and 40).

Gastric or Esophageal Malignancy

Gastric or esophageal malignancy is present in fewer than 2% of dyspepsia patients referred for endoscopy. More than 98% of these malignancies are in patients older than 45 years. The lifetime risk of development of esophageal cancer or gastric cancer before age 45 is less than 0.1%.[4] The risk of gastric malignancy is higher among patients with a previous history of gastric surgery or a family history of gastric malignancy, in immigrants from endemic areas for gastric malignancy, and in patients with *H. pylori* infection.[29] About 95% of symptomatic adenocarcinomas are advanced, with a 5-year survival rate of 10%. Most advanced lesions are associated with at least one of the warning symptoms: persistent vomiting, GI bleeding, iron deficiency anemia, unexplained weight loss, dysphagia, or an abdominal mass. Although some early and potentially curable malignancies can exhibit symptoms indistinguishable from those of benign disease, only 1 in 10,000 dyspeptics has a potentially curable malignancy. Nevertheless, more than 40% of patients who consult physicians report concern about underlying malignancy. Although there is no evidence that endoscopy in dyspeptic patients to detect curable gastric cancer is cost-effective—especially in patients younger than 45 years or without warning symptoms—normal endoscopy findings provide reassurance for both the patient and the physician[30] (see Chapter 44).

Gastroesophageal Reflux Disease

There is a large overlap between symptoms of dyspepsia and those of gastroesophageal reflux disease (GERD), which often makes clinical distinction difficult. Among patients with upper GI symptoms, one third have heartburn (retrosternal burning sensation) with or without other dyspeptic symptoms.[3, 11, 31] Although heartburn and regurgitation are commonly viewed as the typical symptoms, over half of patients with proven GERD have dyspepsia in addition to heartburn, and up to 20% have dyspepsia alone *without* heartburn or regurgitation.

It is difficult to estimate the prevalence of GERD in dyspepsia patients. Endoscopic evidence of esophagitis is present in 15% of patients with dyspepsia (with or without heartburn), but endoscopic studies fail to detect nonerosive GERD and the true prevalence is therefore higher.[7, 12] In patients with dyspepsia alone (without heartburn) the prevalence of esophagitis is about 5%.[31] Abnormal acid reflux on esophageal pH testing is present in up to two thirds of patients with dyspepsia and dominant heartburn (sometimes called *reflux-like dyspepsia*) and up to one fourth of patients with dyspepsia with minimal or no heartburn[32] (see Chapter 33).

Thus, the accuracy of the clinical diagnosis of GERD versus dyspepsia is limited. When heartburn or regurgitation is clearly the dominant symptom—as it is in fewer than 40% of patients with proven GERD—the positive predictive value and specificity for diagnosis of GERD are 80% and 90%, respectively. However, the clinical diagnosis of GERD among all dyspepsia patients has a sensitivity of less than 80% and a specificity of only 60%.[33]

The Rome II consensus group excluded reflux-like dyspepsia (i.e., both dyspepsia and heartburn are present, but heartburn is the dominant symptom) from the dyspepsia classification system and recommended that such patients be treated as having probable GERD.[10] However, at least one third of such patients do not have increased acid reflux, do not respond to acid inhibitory therapy, and should be viewed as having functional dyspepsia.

Pancreatic and Biliary Tract Disorders

Biliary pain is characterized by discrete episodes of acute, severe upper abdominal pain that may radiate to the back or scapula. Its acute, relatively dramatic manifestation should be readily distinguished from dyspepsia in most patients. Nevertheless, diagnostic confusion may arise when an elderly or stoical patient reports biliary pain, or when a histrionic patient reports dyspepsia (see Chapter 55).

Gallstones do not cause chronic dyspepsia.[34] Despite the high incidence of both dyspepsia and gallstones in adults, results of numerous epidemiologic studies confirm that cholelithiasis does not increase the incidence of dyspepsia, and, furthermore, that patients with cholelithiasis and dyspepsia are not at a higher risk of development of acute cholecystitis.[34] Hence, investigation for cholelithiasis should not be performed routinely in dyspepsia patients, and cholecystectomy for cholelithiasis is not indicated for dyspepsia alone.

Pancreatic disorders may be manifested by symptoms that may be mistaken for those of dyspepsia. The pain of acute pancreatitis usually is severe, deep-seated, often dramatic, and accompanied by nausea and vomiting. Chronic pancreatitis is characterized by bouts of dull, steady upper abdominal pain that may radiate to the back; is aggravated by meals; and is readily confused with other causes of dyspepsia.[34] Pancreatic or ampullary cancer also may be associated with onset of symptoms that may be mistaken for dyspepsia—vague, low-grade, and nonspecific upper abdominal discomfort—but often is accompanied by weight loss, anorexia, and jaundice (see Chapters 48, 49, and 50).

Systemic Disorders

Coronary ischemia may be manifested by epigastric discomfort rather than chest pain. Pregnancy, acute or chronic renal failure, hyper- and hypothyroidism, adrenal insufficiency, and hyperparathyroidism may be accompanied by upper dyspepsia, nausea, or vomiting[4, 22] (see Chapter 29).

Uncommon Luminal Gastrointestinal Disorders

The parasites *Giardia lamblia* and *Strongyloides stercoralis* reside in the upper intestinal tract and may cause dyspepsia. Gastroparesis is manifested by nausea, early satiety, postprandial pain, and vomiting. Most cases are due to diabetes mellitus, scleroderma, vagotomy, chronic intestinal pseudo-obstruction, neurologic disorders, and gastric resection (see Chapters 29 and 37). Chronic gastric volvulus may be manifested by intermittent bouts of upper abdominal pain, bloating, belching, retching, or vomiting (see Chapter 36). Small intestinal malabsorptive disorders such as celiac sprue may be manifested by dyspepsia and flatulence (see Chapters 89 and 93). Gastric or small intestinal involvement with Crohn's disease may cause upper abdominal symptoms, as do infiltrative (lymphoma, amyloid, Ménétrier's disease), infectious (tuberculous, syphilis, fungal), and inflammatory (sarcoidosis, lymphocytic gastritis, eosinophilic gastroenteritis) disorders of the stomach, which are evident on upper endoscopy with biopsy (see Chapter 43). Chronic mesenteric ischemia may be characterized by postprandial dyspepsia rather than the classic presentation of periumbilical abdominal pain, sitophobia, and weight loss[34] (see Chapter 119).

FUNCTIONAL (NONULCER) DYSPEPSIA

Of patients with chronic dyspepsia 50% to 70% do not have a significant focal or structural lesion identified at upper endosocopy.[7, 9, 12] Although further investigation in some cases may reveal other organic causes, over half of chronic dyspepsia patients (less than 12 weeks) have no evident biochemical or organic cause or the symptoms. These patients are labeled as having *functional dyspepsia* and are an extremely difficult group to manage.[10] Functional dyspepsia is therefore a diagnosis of exclusion. A variety of terms have been used synonymously, including *nonulcer dyspepsia, nonorganic dyspepsia, idiopathic dyspepsia,* and *essential dyspepsia*; the term *functional dyspepsia* is preferred. Although symptoms remain chronic in most patients, improvement is noted in up to one half and symptom resolution in one fourth over time.[12, 35] Limited studies suggest that these chronic symptoms have a significant impact upon quality of life, interfering with daily activities, work, sleep, socializing, eating, and drinking and contributing to emotional stress.[3, 36–38]

Pathophysiology

The pathophysiologic characteristics of symptoms of functional dyspepsia are poorly understood. Dyspepsia is considered to be part of a continum of functional GI disorders that involve the entire gut. Many patients have symptoms that overlap with those of other functional GI disorders, such as functional heartburn, irritable bowel syndrome (IBS), and noncardiac chest pain (see Chapters 5, 6, and 91). More than 80% of IBS patients have dyspepsia, and one third of dyspeptics have symptoms of IBS. Additionally, patients with functional GI disorders often manifest extragut symptoms, such as migraine headaches, fibromyalgia, and disorders of urinary or gynecologic function.

Like other functional GI disorders, functional dyspepsia may be best understood in the context of the biopsychosocial model of illness in which symptoms arise out of a complex interaction between abnormal GI physiologic features (motility, visceral sensation) and psychosocial factors (personality, psychological state, social support, and coping mechanisms) that affect an individual's perception, interpretation, and response to the altered GI physiologic characteristics. Through the brain-gut axis, higher neural centers may modulate GI sensation, motility, and secretion. Individuals who have an alteration in GI physiologic attributes but no psychological abnormalities, stable social support, and good coping mechanisms either may not seek medical care or may respond readily to reassurance and life-style alterations. Patients who have similar underlying GI physiologic abnormalities who have psychological problems (anxiety, hypochondriasis), increased life stress, or poor social support may be more likely to seek medical attention; furthermore, the psychosocial factors may exacerbate the GI pathophysiologic characteristics and lead to chronic symptoms (see Chapters 5 and 122).

In evaluating the patient with functional dyspepsia, one must consider both the physiologic and the psychological factors that have given rise to the symptoms. Although pathophysiologic mechanisms may be identified in most patients with functional dyspepsia, psychosocial mechanisms are relevant to understanding why the patient is asking for medical evaluation and how the patient is adjusting to these symptoms and to planning optimal management.[39]

Abnormalities in Gastroduodenal Motility

Disorders of gastric motor function are present in up to 60% of functional dyspepsia patients (see Chapter 37). A variety of testing methods show abnormalities in gastric emptying, accommodation, and myoelectrical activity, but their role and importance in causing symptoms are debated, in part because a consistent relationship between these abnormalities and dyspeptic symptoms has not been convincingly established.

DELAYED GASTRIC EMPTYING. Delayed gastric emptying measures the integrated efficiency of gastric neuromuscular work in response to a meal. As assessed by scintigraphy, breath tests, or ultrasonography, a delay in gastric emptying of solids can be demonstrated in approximately 40% of patients with dyspepsia.[40, 41] Delayed gastric emptying may be more common in patients who report severe postprandial fullness rather than abdominal pain, vomiting, and women.[42] Therapeutic trials have shown poor correlation between improvement in symptoms and changes in the rate of gastric emptying.[41]

IMPAIRED GASTRIC ACCOMMODATION. Ultrasonography, scintigraphy, and barostats have shown that in contrast to normal subjects, whose food is initially accommodated in the fundus and body with gradual redistribution to the antrum, over 40% of patients with functional dyspepsia have impaired accommodation of the proximal stomach, which may lead to early distribution of food to the distal stomach with dilatation of the antrum.[43–45] This sudden, prolonged distention of the antrum may lead to postprandial dyspepsia. Impaired accommodation and early antral filling are associated with symptoms of early satiety or weight loss.[46] Gastric accommodation is controlled by vagal pathways that are mediated through release of nitric oxide and serotonin (5-hydroxytryptamine 1 [5-HT_1]). Accommodation is impaired in vagotomized patients, and vagal autonomic dysfunction has been demonstrated in functional dyspeptics with impaired accommodation.[43, 44, 47] Nitrates (glyceryl trinitrate); sumatriptan, a 5-HT_1 agonist; and cisapride promote gastric accommodation both in normal subjects and in patients with functional dyspepsia.[48–52]

MYOELECTRICAL ABNORMALITIES. Gastroduodenal manometry is used to assess the contractile activity in the fasting and postprandial states. Although several studies have demonstrated postprandial antral hypomotility, which may be partly attributable to early antral filling, no relationship between antral hypomotility and symptoms has been demonstrated.[41, 53] Noninvasive cutaneous electrogastrography (EGG) can measure fasting and postprandial gastric electrical activity. The basal electrical rhythm (BER) is generated by a pacemaker located in the proximal body and propagated longitudinally and circumferentially at a normal rate of 3 cycles per minute. Gastric dysrhythmias are identified by EGG in 40% of patients with functional dyspepsia but also in 20% of normal controls.[54, 55] Both slow (bradygastria, 1 to 2.4 counts per minute [cpm]) and fast (tachygastria, 3.8 to 10 cpm) dysrhythmias are detected, but the significance of these myoelectrical abnormalities is unclear. Dysrhythmias are not associated with a specific symptom profile and have a variable relation to gastric emptying abnormalities.[56, 57] One open study suggests that response of dysrhythmias to prokinetic drugs is predictive of symptom improvement.[58]

Visceral Hypersensitivity (See Chapter 5)

Afferent stimulation of gut mechanoreceptors reaches conscious perception through a three-neuron chain. Afferent fibers of the first-order neuron project from the GI tract to the prevertebral ganglia (which may reflexively affect motility and secretion) and to the cell body in the dorsal root ganglion. The second-order neuron extends from the dorsal horn via the spinothalamic and spinoreticular tracts to the thalamus and brainstem reticular formation, synapsing with neurons that project to the limbic system and cerebral cortex.[59, 60] Descending fibers from brainstem centers modulate the sensitivity of the dorsal horn neurons and control the perception of visceral sensation.

Most stimuli arising from the GI tract (accommodation, gastric emptying, distention, contractions) are not consciously perceived; however, a lowering of the perception threshold may occur in patients with functional dyspepsia, generating heightened sensitivity to normal physiologic events or minor noxious stimuli.[61] Hypersensitivity to distention of the stomach can be demonstrated in more than 50% of patients with functional dyspepsia, both those who seek medical attention and nonconsultors (Fig. 7–1).[46, 61] Using a gastric barostat, the threshold for initial perception, discomfort, or pain may be tested by altering the volume, pressure, or tension in a gastric balloon. During barostat distention, changes in blood flow distribution to brainstem and cerebral centers can be observed by means of functional magnetic resonance imaging and positron emission tomography (PET) scans in patients with functional dyspepsia.[59]

The cause of visceral hypersensitivity is not known but may be sensitization of peripheral gastric mechanoreceptors (due to inflammation, injury, or intrinsic defect), increased excitability or recruitment of spinal cord dorsal horn neurons due to repeated stimulation, dysfunction of descending spinal inhibitory systems that normally reduce visceral sensation, or altered central nervous system (CNS) processing and modulation of afferent sensation that result in increased vigilance for or amplification of visceral stimuli.[62–65] Hypersensitivity

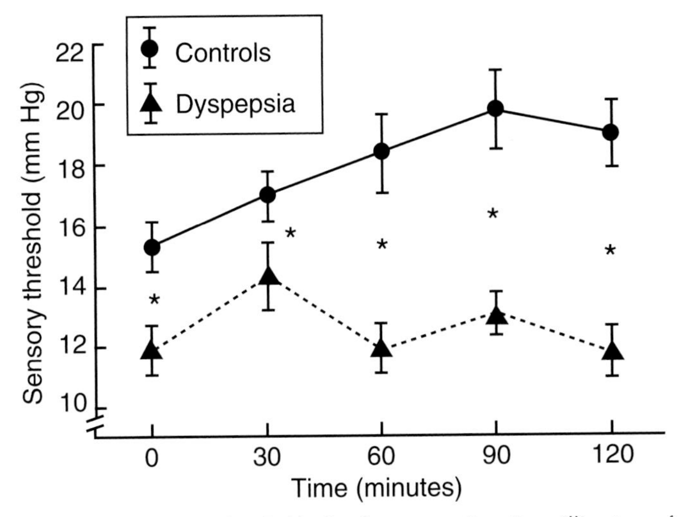

Figure 7–1. Sensory thresholds for first perception (in millimeters of mercury) of gastric barostat balloon inflated randomly to different pressures in healthy controls and subjects with chronic dyspepsia who had not sought medical attention. Distentions were repeated every half hour. Sensory threshold is lower in subjects with dyspepsia and remains lower with repeated testing compared with control subjects in whom sensory threshold actually rises with repeated testing. (From Holtmann G, Gschossmann J, Neufang-Huber J, et al: Differences in gastric mechanosensory function after repeated ramp distentions in nonconsulters with dyspepsia and healthy controls. Gut 47:332, 2000.)

does not appear to be related to abnormalities in gastric acid secretion, accommodation, compliance, or emptying,[45, 61] although it is hypothesized that individuals who have visceral hypersensitivity are more likely to experience discomfort or pain when pathophysiologic abnormalities are present.[44, 59] Heightened visceral sensitivity is demonstrated in functional dyspepsia both in patients who have consulted a physician and in those who are not health care seekers and is unrelated to the presence of psychological abnormalities.[63, 66]

At present, there are no tests available outside a clinical research setting to test for visceral hypersensitivity. A water load test, in which patients are asked to ingest water until feeling a sense of fullness, has been introduced. Compared with asymptomatic control subjects, patients with functional dyspepsia ingest approximately 300 mL less than controls; however, this difference may be attributable to impaired accommodation, visceral hypersensitivity, or psychological factors.[55]

Autonomic Neuropathy

The vagus nerve regulates gastric accommodation and emptying and exerts a visceral antinocioceptive effect.[61] As assessed by analysis of heart rate variability or plasma levels of pancreatic polypeptide in response to insulin-induced hypoglycemia, vagal efferent dysfunction can be demonstrated in a subset of patients with functional dyspepsia.[67, 68] Acute stress has also been shown to alter vagal and sympathetic autonomic function.[69] It is hypothesized that acute and chronic life stresses and psychological factors may lead to decreased vagal tone, which results in the pathophysiologic abnormalities that give rise to dyspeptic symptoms. Notwithstanding this provocative association, vagal dysfunction has not been established as the cause of dyspepsia symptoms.[47, 70]

Helicobacter pylori (See Chapter 39)

Does *H. pylori* cause functional dyspepsia? Few questions in the past decade have engendered as much controversy. Acute infection with *H. pylori* infection causes transient symptoms of nausea, vomiting, and dyspepsia. Furthermore, chronic *H. pylori* infection leads to the development of peptic ulcer disease and concomitant dyspepsia in up to 15% of patients. The high prevalence (20% to 30%) of chronic *H. pylori* infection and dyspepsia in Western countries begs the question of whether *H. pylori*–associated gastritis causes dyspepsia in some infected patients. The overwhelming available data clearly demonstrate that *H. pylori* does not play a major causal role in functional dyspepsia.

The prevalence of *H. pylori* infection in patients with functional dyspepsia is similar to that in the general population. Initial reports from case control studies of a higher prevalence of *H. pylori* infection among patients with functional dyspepsia have been refuted by better designed case control studies and cohort studies, which have controlled for confounders such as age, socioeconomic status, and prior ulcer history.[71, 72] A meta-analysis of 30 observational studies involving 3392 patients with functional dyspepsia and 11 observational studies involving 6426 people with uninvestigated dyspepsia concluded that there is no strong association between *H. pylori* infection and dyspepsia, although a weak association cannot be excluded.[73] No specific symptoms or groups of symptoms have been consistently associated with chronic *H. pylori* infection.[12, 74]

A plausible pathophysiologic mechanism by which chronic *H. pylori* infection might cause dyspepsia also has not been demonstrated. Studies have not found a consistent relationship between chronic *H. pylori* infection and other pathophysiogic abnormalities associated with functional dyspepsia. Specifically, infection by *H. pylori* does not affect gastric emptying, accommodation, or visceral sensation threshold.[74, 75]

The strongest evidence against the role of *H. pylori* in functional dyspepsia is that controlled therapeutic trials of *H. pylori* eradication demonstrate no significant long-term improvement in symptoms.[76] Three randomized, prospective, double-blind, placebo-controlled multicenter therapeutic trials involving almost 900 *H. pylori*–infected patients with functional dyspepsia did not demonstrate any significant improvement in dyspeptic symptoms 1 year after successful *H. pylori* eradication.[77–79] Symptom resolution was noted in approximately 25% of patients in both the treated and control groups (Table 7–2). A 2001 meta-analysis of seven prospective therapeutic trials of patients with functional dyspepsia reported a nonsignificant odds ratio of 1.29 (95% CI, 0.89 to 1.89) for treatment success after therapy for *H. pylori* compared with that of control groups.[76] Another meta-analysis of 12 trials detected a small but significant relative risk reduction of 9% (95% CI, 4% to 14%) resolution of symptoms among treated patients compared with controls, but some of the analyzed trials have been criticized for inclusion of patients with GERD symptoms and nonstandard symptom outcome measurements.[76, 80]

Table 7–2 | **Treatment Success in Functional Dypspepsia: Long-Term Symptom Control After *Helicobacter pylori* Treatment Compared with Control Therapy**

STUDY (REFERENCE)	*H. PYLORI* TREATMENT (N/N)	CONTROL GROUP (N/N)	DIFFERENCE (95% CI)	ODDS RATIO (95% CI)
Talley et al. (77)	24% (33/135)	22% (31/143)	2% (−8 to 12)	1.1 (0.6 to 2.0)
Blum et al. (78)	27% (45/164)	21% (34/164)	7% (−3 to 16)	1.4 (0.8 to 2.5)
Talley et al. (79)	43% (69/162)	46% (71/155)	−3% (−15 to 8)	0.9 (0.5 to 1.4)
Koelz et al. (76)	62% (55/89)	66% (61/92)	−5% (−19 to 10)	0.8 (0.2 to 4.8)
Passos et al. (76)	89% (40/45)	89% (32/36)	0% (−13 to 14)	1.0 (0.2 to 4.8)
David et al. (76)	82% (14/17)	63% (15/24)	20% (−14 to 42)	2.8 (0.5 to 16.5)
All studies				1.29 (0.89 to 1.89)

Modified from Laine L, Schoenfeld P, Fennerty B: Therapy for *Helicobacter pylori* in patients with nonulcer dyspepsia: A meta-analysis of randomized, controlled trials. Ann Intern Med 134:361, 2001.

Taken in aggregate, myriad controlled therapeutic trials provide little support for a role of *H. pylori* in functional dyspepsia. Although it is possible that a small number of infected patients (9%) derive some benefit from *H. pylori* eradication therapy, it is clear that the organism plays no pathogenetic role in most patients.

Psychosocial Factors (See Chapter 122)

The degree to which psychosocial factors are contributing and remediable should be assessed in every functional dyspepsia patient.[81] According to personality inventories, patients with functional dyspepsia are similar to patients with IBS, scoring higher than normal in areas of anxiety and neuroticism.[82] Overall, individuals who have dyspepsia do not have a unique personality profile and differ from patients with chronic pain syndromes or somatoform disorders. Patients with functional dyspepsia also have a higher incidence of psychiatric diagnoses, including depression, panic and generalized anxiety disorders, and somatoform disorders.[81]

Rather than being a cause per se of symptoms, these personality traits and psychiatric disorders appear to be important determinants of health care seeking behavior. Among community dyspeptic individuals who have not sought medical attention, the prevalence of psychological abnormalities is similar to that in the general population. By contrast, psychological factors are evident in half of dyspeptic patients seen in general medical practice and almost 90% of patients followed in a tertiary gastroenterology setting.[15, 83, 84] Psychosocial factors correlate with the number of GI symptoms and extraintestinal symptoms (e.g., headaches, fatigue). Thus, it appears that certain personality traits and psychiatric disorders are much more prevalent among patients who seek health care and those with severe or refractory symptoms.

The role of acute life stress in dyspepsia is uncertain. Although it is commonly believed that stress precipitates somatic complaints, including abdominal pain, diarrhea, fatigue, and headaches, this relationship is difficult to prove. Stress could perhaps cause symptoms by alteration of GI motility, by autonomic dysregulation, or by a reduction in visceral pain threshold, as discussed previously. Acute painful stimuli (electrical stimulation, cold immersion) or cognitive stress suppresses postprandial antral motility and induces gastric relaxation in normal subjects and patients with functional dyspepsia, but these events are not associated with symptoms.[81, 82] The relevance of these laboratory studies to acute life stresses is unknown.

The role of chronic life stress in the pathogenesis of functional dyspepsia also is controversial. Earlier studies indicated that the frequency of major life stressful events was not higher in functional dyspepsia patients than in control subjects but that patients perceived these events more negatively.[82] A recent study of patients with functional dyspepsia that used better stress assessment tools indicated that almost all patients were experiencing at least one chronic stressor (e.g., marital, employment, financial, housing, illness, death).[84] The role of life stressors in dyspeptics who do not seek medical attention is unclear. Social support and coping style affect the way a person deals with life stress and may affect reaction and adjustment to dyspeptic symptoms.

Some studies suggest that functional dyspepsia patients have impaired coping styles and less social support.[82, 85] Prior life events may also affect illness behavior, such as physical or sexual abuse, an unhappy childhood, or received positive reinforcement (parental attention, excused absence from school) for abdominal symptoms.[86] It is hypothesized that life stressors may trigger the onset of functional symptoms and the decision to seek medical attention, but psychological factors, coping strategies, and social support mechanisms determine the extent, severity, and duration of symptoms.[82–84]

For many patients with functional dyspepsia, abdominal symptoms are part of a constellation of somatic and psychological complaints. Indeed, many rank anxiety and family problems as more important than dyspepsia.[87] Patients with dyspepsia take more than twice as much sick leave, often for non-GI somatic complaints, than do nondyspeptic colleagues.[81] They tend to have more interruptions in functioning, poorer social functioning, and worse health perception than do patients with organic GI disorders.[36, 82]

APPROACH TO UNINVESTIGATED DYSPEPSIA

In evaluating patients with dyspepsia who have not previously undergone diagnostic investigation (uninvestigated dyspepsia), the physician must decide whether diagnostic studies, especially upper endoscopy, are warranted in order to distinguish organic causes of symptoms from functional dyspepsia, or whether a course of empirical treatment is the first step. Many patients exhibit mild symptoms of short duration that may resolve spontaneously.[88] The clinical history is of limited utility in distinguishing organic GI disorders from functional dyspepsia. Even experienced clinicians are correct only half the time in distinguishing peptic ulcer disease from functional dyspepsia on the basis of clinical history alone.[88] Numerous groups have suggested that classification of dyspeptic symptoms into symptom subgroups (*ulcer-like, dysmotility-like, reflux-like)* might improve diagnostic accuracy, predict underlying pathophysiologic conditions, and guide empirical treatment.[89] For example, *ulcer-like dyspepsia* (well-localized pain occurring at night or between meals and relieved by food) might predict a higher likelihood of peptic ulcer disease, whereas *dysmotility-like dyspepsia* (poorly localized discomfort aggravated by meals and accompanied by postprandial fullness, nausea, bloating, or vomiting) might be associated with gastroparesis. With the exception of *reflux-like dyspepsia*, these subgroupings have proved to have no clinical utility.[90] They do not reliably predict the presence or nature of findings on upper endoscopy nor distinguish between organic causes and functional causes of dyspepsia with sufficient accuracy.[89] Nevertheless, they remain well entrenched among clinicians.

Upper endoscopy allows direct visualization of peptic ulcers, esophagitis, and malignancy with high diagnostic accuracy. However, in many patients, findings at endoscopy, despite establishing a definitive diagnosis, may not alter the initial course of treatment.[91] Most patients, irrespective of endoscopic findings, are given a trial of therapy with an antisecretory agent, usually a proton pump inhibitor. Thus, patients found at endoscopy to have erosive GERD or peptic ulcer disease are given a course of a proton pump inhibitor, and patients with proven *H. pylori* infection are treated to eradicate it. Patients with a normal endosocopic result may have either functional dyspepsia or nonerosive GERD. Despite limited therapeutic benefit, most of such patients are given a trial of antisecretory therapy with either an H_2-receptor antagonist or a proton pump inhibitor. Thus, in patients with dyspepsia without alarm symptoms (i.e., persistent vomiting, GI bleeding, iron deficiency anemia, unexplained weight loss, dysphagia, or an abdominal mass) the advantage of upper endoscopic evaluation compared with an empirical trial of proton pump inhibitor therapy is unproved.[88] It is suggested that a normal endoscopy result may help to allay patient anxieties; however, this reassurance may be of value to only a small number of worried patients.[92]

The goal of the clinician therefore is to distinguish those patients who have a high likelihood of having a serious organic disorder warranting further diagnostic evaluation and a definitive diagnosis from the remainder of patients who may be treated initially with empirical antisecretory therapy and/or *H. pylori* eradication therapy. Noninvasive testing for *H. pylori* also can be performed and empirical anti–*H. pylori* treatment given. With empirical therapy, costly diagnostic studies may be precluded for patients with mild, self-limited symptoms. Patients with continuous or recurrent symptoms can undergo subsequent endoscopic evaluation. Although empirical therapy in a patient with undiagnosed malignancy is undesirable, malignancies are rare in dyspeptic patients without alarm symptoms, and there is no evidence that a delay in diagnosis of several weeks for a course of empirical therapy compromises outcome.

In deciding between empirical management and early endoscopy, the provider therefore must weigh several factors, including the level of patient anxiety, the patient's age, the presence of warning symptoms or signs that increase the likelihood of serious organic disease, the presence of reflux-like symptoms, and infection with *H. pylori*.[4] Such variables make a diagnostic algorithm problematic (Fig. 7–2).

Determination of Reason for Presentation

A complete history and physical examination should be performed. The reasons for medical consultation at this time should be elicited so that specific fears and concerns can be addressed. Careful inquiry into the patient's social or family history may uncover stresses that are contributing to acute symptom worsening or current concern about chronic symptoms. For symptoms that are long-standing, mild, and intermittent, reassurance and a trial of dietary and life-style modifications may be reasonable. Endoscopy may be warranted in patients with excessive concerns about underlying serious disease to allay anxiety.[4] Although it commonly is assumed that a normal endoscopy result may provide reassurance to patients and improve quality of life, the conclusions of studies of this issue are conflicting.[93, 94]

Consideration of Patient Age and/or Alarm Symptoms

The diagnosis of gastroesophageal malignancy is one of the principal justifications for early endoscopy for dyspeptic patients. Gastroesophageal malignancy, however, is extremely rare in patients younger than 45 to 50 years. Furthermore, the incidence of gastric cancer is decreasing in the industrialized world. In young patients with uncomplicated dyspepsia, the incidence of gastric malignancy is 1 per million—and the condition is usually incurable.[95] Although the likelihood of malignancy increases in patients with dyspepsia who are older than 45 years, the incidence of gastric malignancy is still less than 3%, and most of the individuals affected have at least one of several warning symptoms, such as dysphagia, severe pain, protracted vomiting, weight loss, fecal occult blood, or anemia.[7, 12, 88, 96] Therefore, numerous consensus panels have recommended that endoscopy be performed in patients with dyspepsia who are older than 45 to 50 years or have at least one alarm symptom.[4, 12, 29] Unfortunately, most cancers exhibiting alarm symptoms are advanced and incurable, and there is no evidence that early endoscopy in patients above age 45 to 50 who have uncomplicated dyspepsia leads to increased detection of early gastric cancers or improves survival rate.[4, 88] Despite these facts, current medical and legal standards of care dictate that endoscopy be performed for the evaluation of dyspepsia in older patients and patients of any age with alarm symptoms.

Evaluation for Gastroesophageal Reflux Symptoms

When heartburn or acid regurgitation is the dominant dyspeptic symptom, a presumptive diagnosis of GERD should be made because half to two thirds of patients who have

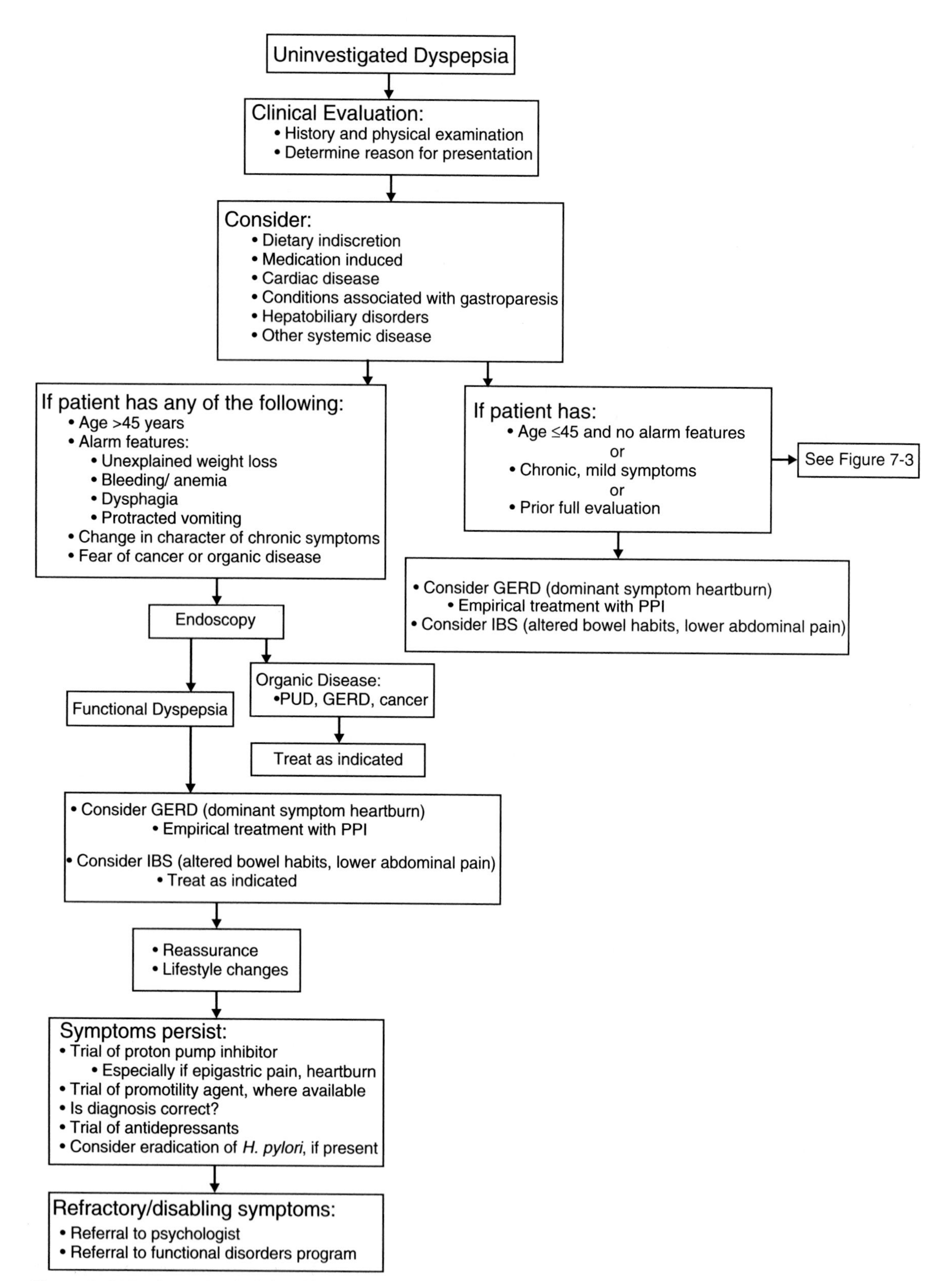

Figure 7–2. Management algorithm for patients with dyspepsia. Patients 45 years of age or younger without signs of organic disease or alarm features and without symptoms of GERD or IBS should be evaluated as per Figure 7–3. GERD, gastrointestinal reflux disease; IBS, irritable bowel syndrome; PPI, proton pump inhibitor; PUD, peptic ulcer disease.

reflux-like dyspepsia respond to antisecretory therapy.[4, 12, 97] A proton pump inhibitor (omeprazole, esomeprazole, or rabeprazole 20 mg, lansoprazole 30 mg, pantoprazole 40 mg, all given once or twice daily) should be prescribed.[4, 98] Those who do not respond to empirical treatment with a proton pump inhibitor likely do not have GERD and should be evaluated for other causes of dyspepsia.[90, 98] Endoscopy may be warranted even for patients who have longstanding reflux-like symptoms who respond to antisecretory therapy to screen for Barrett's metaplasia (see Chapter 31).[99]

Consideration of Irritable Bowel Syndrome

Dyspepsia is common in patients with irritable bowel syndrome. Patients younger than age 45 with uncomplicated dyspepsia who also have lower abdominal pain or discomfort and altered bowel habits likely have diagnosis of irritable bowel (see Chapter 91).[10]

Evaluation for Use of Offending Medications

The use of prescription and nonprescription medications should be reviewed, and medications commonly associated with dyspepsia—especially aspirin and NSAIDs—discontinued when possible. For patients in whom NSAIDs cannot be discontinued, a trial of empirical therapy with a proton pump inhibitor (omeprazole, esomeprazole, or rabeprazole 20 mg, lansoprazole 30 mg, pantoprazole 40 mg, once or twice daily) or an H_2-receptor antagonist (ranitidine or nizatidine 150 mg, famotidine 20 mg, twice daily) may improve symptoms and heal ulcers, if present. Endoscopy is warranted in NSAID users whose symptoms persist despite discontinuation of the NSAID or initiation of an antisecretory agent, and in patients who have alarm symptoms.[4, 100]

Physical Examination

A careful physical examination is mandatory to detect evidence of organic disease. Symptoms and signs of systemic disorders that may cause dyspepsia, such as cardiac disease, diabetes, and thyroid disease, should be considered. Signs such as organomegaly, abdominal mass, ascites, or positive fecal occult blood finding necessitate further evaluation. In addition, the "laying on of hands" may be therapeutic for functional patients, providing reassurance that the symptoms are being taken seriously.

Noninvasive Testing for *Helicobacter pylori* Infection

Chronic infection with *H. pylori* is associated with over 80% of peptic ulcers and over half of gastric cancers.[12, 101] In Western countries, the prevalence of *H. pylori* infection in patients with uninvestigated dyspepsia is 30% to 50% but is declining. Between 20% and 60% of patients with dyspepsia who have evidence of *H. pylori* infection based on noninvasive testing (urea breath test, serologic evaluation, fecal antigen assessment) have underlying peptic ulcer disease.[29] Most others have functional dyspepsia or GERD. In contrast, ulcers are present in less than 5% of uninfected patients with dyspepsia who are not taking NSAIDs. Empirical *H. pylori* eradication therapy of patients with dyspepsia and positive noninvasive test for *H. pylori* is expected to resolve dyspepsia in most patients who have undiagnosed peptic ulcer disease but is unlikely to have significant impact on infected patients without peptic ulcer disease.

Up to one fourth of patients with peptic ulcers continue to complain of dyspepsia even after successful *H. pylori* eradication.[29, 102] Two large prospective studies of *H. pylori*–positive patients with uninvestigated dyspepsia in a primary care setting demonstrated a significant reduction in dyspeptic symptoms after 1 to 2 years among patients treated with eradication therapy compared with those treated with a course of a proton pump inhibitor.[103, 104] Widespread screening and treatment of *H. pylori* infection in the general population also may result in a modest reduction in the prevalence of dyspepsia, presumably as a result of a reduction in peptic ulcer disease. In a large trial of *H. pylori*–positive community (nonmedical) subjects with and without dyspepsia, empirical eradication treatment of *H. pylori* infection led to a 5% reduction in the number of subjects with dyspepsia in the treatment group (28%) versus the control group (33%) but had no impact on quality of life (see Chapter 39).[105]

Laboratory and Additional Studies

After the age of 45, a complete blood count, routine electrolyte measurement, calcium level, liver chemical evaluation, and thyroid function studies may be considered; however, the cost-effectiveness of routine laboratory testing, especially in younger patients, is untested. Other studies, such as amylase level, stool evaluation for ova and parasites, and pregnancy tests, are ordered as needed.

Additional studies may be pursued in those patients whose symptoms are progressive or refractory. Gastric scintigraphy and gastroduodenal manometry should be reserved for a small minority of patients who have frequent or protracted vomiting, suggestive of gastric motility disorder. Ambulatory esophageal pH monitoring is useful to diagnose gastroesophageal reflux in patients with atypical symptoms. However, it is more cost-effective to treat such patients with an empirical trial of a proton pump inibitor because symptom improvement is highly predictive of reflux disease. Use of electrogastrography and barostat studies largely is confined to research centers. Abdominal ultrasonography and computed tomographic (CT) scanning should not be performed routinely but are indicated when symptoms or laboratory test results suggest pancreaticobiliary disease.

UNCOMPLICATED DYSPEPSIA: EMPIRICAL THERAPY VERSUS EARLY ENDOSCOPY

Should endoscopy be performed at initial presentation in all patients with dyspepsia without alarm symptoms, or should it be reserved for those who do not improve or experience relapse of symptoms after a course of empirical treatment with an antisecretory agent and/or anti–*H. pylori* therapy? Since the 1980s this question has fostered enormous debate.

Arguments in favor of empirical treatment were discussed previously. Arguments against empirical treatment are as follows: (1) Knowing which condition is being treated is beneficial to the patient and physician. A normal endoscopy finding is neither wasteful nor wasted; it reduces worry, need for symptomatic therapies, and use of the medical system. Patients without ulcers may be less preoccupied by recurrent dyspepsia, but patients with proven ulcers may be inclined to seek attention earlier for symptom relapse. In contrast, the *H. pylori*–positive patient who is empirically treated does not know whether an ulcer was present or whether therapy resulted in successful eradication; this uncertainty may cause anxiety and somatic preoccupation. (2) Most *H. pylori*–positive patients have functional dyspepsia (not ulcers), for which antibiotic therapy has no proven benefit and potential risks. Furthermore, empirical treatment sends to those with underlying functional disease the inappropriate message that the condition is caused by infection; studies to confirm eradication if symptoms persist and search for reinfection if symptoms relapse are the result. Under such circumstances, it may be difficult to persuade the patient to accept reasonable treatment goals for a functional disorder.

Several consensus panels of experts have proposed that young patients (younger than 45 to 50 years) who have uncomplicated dyspepsia be given a noninvasive test for *H. pylori* followed by empirical treatment therapy based on the results of this test[4, 12, 29] (Fig. 7–3). Testing for *H. pylori* can be performed with serologic evaluation, urea breath test, or fecal antigen test. In approximately one third of patients the result of the test for *H. pylori* is positive. Patients with positive results for *H. pylori* infection should be treated with a course of *H. pylori* eradication therapy. This strategy of empirically treating *H. pylori*–positive patients has become known as "test and treat." Of these, one third to one half have peptic ulcer disease; the remainder have functional dyspepsia or GERD. It is presumed that successful *H. pylori* eradication leads to symptom resolution in most patients with peptic ulcer disease but offers no benefit for GERD symptoms and uncertain benefit for symptoms of functional dyspepsia.[106, 107] At least two thirds of patients do not show evidence of infection with *H. pylori* and are therefore unlikely to have peptic ulcer disease. A 2- to 4-week trial of an antisecretory agent is recommended for these *H. pylori*–negative patients, virtually all of whom can be presumed to have functional dyspepsia or GERD. Endoscopy is recommended for *H. pylori*–positive or –negative patients whose symptoms persist or relapse after empirical therapy.

Because of a lack of prospective clinical trials comparing

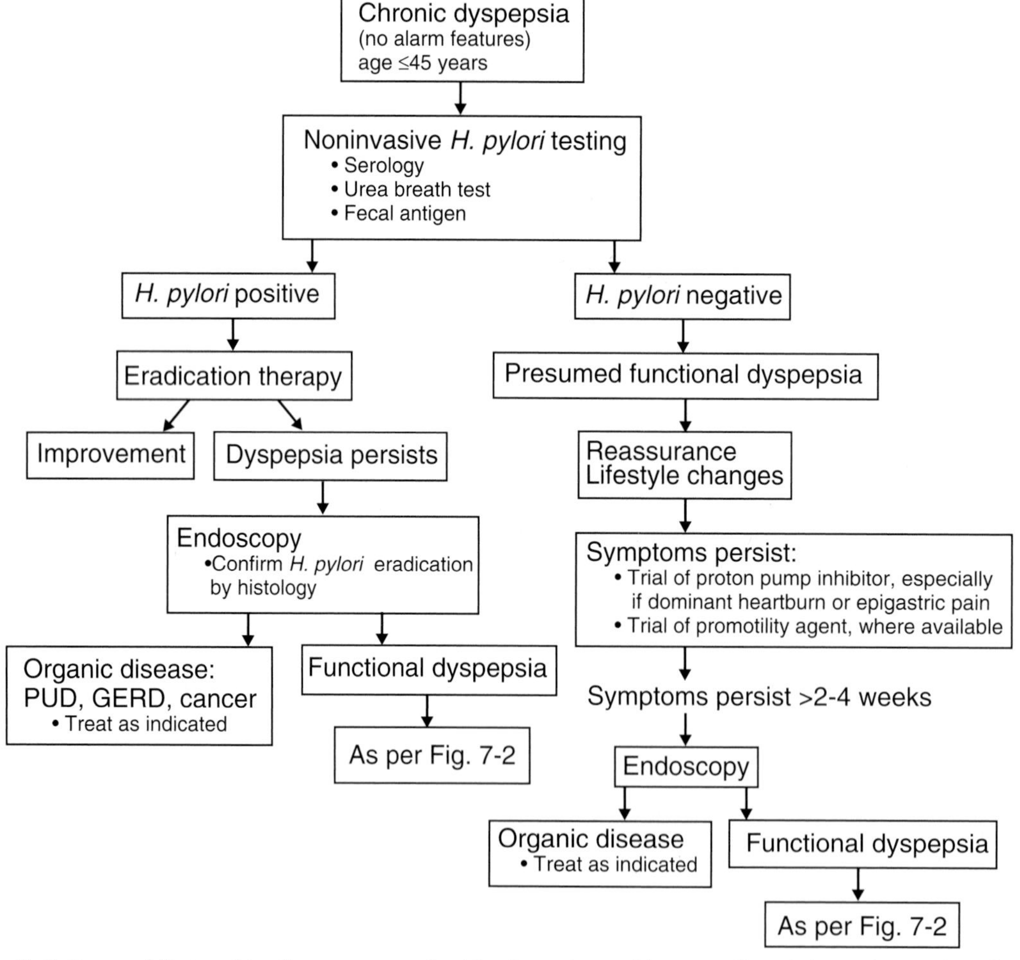

Figure 7–3. Proposed "test and treat" management algorithm for patients with uncomplicated dyspepsia (no alarm features) based on results of noninvasive testing for *H. pylori.* Although this strategy may be cost-effective in patients of any age, consensus recommendations of panels of experts endorse use of this strategy only in young patients (younger than 45 to 50 years of age). GERD, gastrointestinal reflux disease; PUD, peptic ulcer disease.

early endoscopy with empirical management strategies, the support for these expert panel recommendations is derived largely from decision analysis.[12, 30, 108] The various studies compare somewhat different strategies for uncomplicated dyspepsia, including early endoscopy for all patients, endoscopy only for patients with a positive noninvasive test result for *H. pylori* infection ("test and scope"), empirical eradication therapy for patients with positive noninvasive testing findings for *H. pylori* infection (test and treat), empirical antisecretory therapy for all patients, and empirical antisecretory therapy for patients with negative noninvasive test results for *H. pylori*.[109–113] Of note, only one of these analyses considered patient age in the model.[110]

The results of these artificial computer-aided modeling studies are difficult to compare because of their different assumptions. However, their base case assumptions suggest that either of two empirical treatment strategies—test and treat for *H. pylori* infection (with antisecretory therapy for *H. pylori*–negative patients) or empirical antisecretory therapy for all patients—is more cost-effective than strategies in which diagnostic endoscopy is performed in all patients or in patients found to be *H. pylori*–positive on noninvasive testing findings.[91] However, sensitivity analyses indicate that relative costs were influenced heavily by several factors. As the prevalence of *H. pylori* infection and peptic ulcer disease declines, the cost-effectiveness of test and treat strategies diminishes. In scenarios in which the cost of endoscopy decreases or the likelihood of dyspepsia recurrence after empirical therapy is high (requiring endoscopy), early endoscopy becomes a more cost-effective approach than empirical therapy. Furthermore, these models assumed that inexpensive, generic H_2-receptor antagonists would be used for empirical antisecretory therapy. The widespread use of the more expensive proton pump inhibitors also mitigates against the cost benefits of empirical therapy.[114] On balance, these decision analytical models, which reflect the prevailing clinical conditions of the mid-1990s, favor empirical therapy.[115] However, with the decline of *H. pylori* prevalence and the possibility of less expensive, unsedated endoscopy using small-caliber endoscopes, early endoscopy could yet prove to be a more cost-effective initial diagnostic test. Therefore, the results of these decision analyses must be viewed cautiously.[12]

The results of prospective randomized trials that compare empirical treatment with early endoscopy in patients with uninvestigated dyspepsia in a primary care setting are now becoming available.[116] In contrast to the results of the decision analysis models, these real world studies suggest that early endoscopy may be cost-neutral compared with empirical treatment strategies. In an unblinded study of 500 Danish primary care patients (mean age 45 years) with uncomplicated dyspepsia randomized to early endoscopy versus an empirical test and treat strategy for *H. pylori* infection, the number of endoscopic procedures was reduced by 60% in the empirical treatment group.[92] Yet there was no difference between the two groups after 1 year in number of dyspepsia-free days, quality of life, visits to physicians, or sick leave days. Although a formal cost analysis was not performed, these data suggest that empirical management dramatically reduces the number of endoscopic procedures without affecting overall outcome. However, 12% of patients in the empirical treatment group were dissatisfied with their care, compared with 4% in the early endoscopy group. A study in the United Kingdom randomized 762 dyspeptics to one of five strategies: immediate endoscopy for all; test and treat of *H. pylori*–positive patients and treatment with a proton pump inhibitor for *H. pylori*–negative patients; endoscopy for *H. pylori*–positive patients; or empirical proton pump inhibitor therapy for all.[117] At the end of 1 year, symptom improvement was equivalent for all groups. Although the number of endoscopic evaluations was reduced significantly in the test and treat group, 41% required endoscopy because of persistent symptoms. Furthermore, the number of medical consultations and use of antisecretory agents were higher in the empirical treatment groups; hence, the overall costs were similar across all groups. Once again, patient satisfaction with medical care was higher in the group given immediate endoscopy.

Notwithstanding the recommendations of expert panels, the optimal strategy for the approach to patients with uninvestigated dyspepsia is unclear. There are no compelling data that early endoscopy leads to improved outcomes, or that empirical test and treat strategies are cost-effective. Appropriate guidelines may vary, depending upon the prevalence of *H. pylori* infection and peptic ulcer disease, the costs of endoscopy, the costs of medical therapy, and local practice. The most appropriate approach is that with which the patient and physician are most comfortable.

TREATMENT OF FUNCTIONAL DYSPEPSIA

Most functional dyspepsia patients have intermittent, mild symptoms that respond to reassurance and life-style modifications. Refractory symptoms, however, may be difficult to manage. Lack of improvement may lead to concern that an organic cause has been overlooked and to repeated testing. Placebo treatment leads to improvement both in dyspeptic symptoms and in global health status in up to 80% as well as improvement in gastric motility. This finding strongly suggests that a positive physician-patient relationship is essential and therapeutic, potentially obviating myriad tests and pharmacologic interventions.[118] The management of functional disorders is reviewed elsewhere (see Chapters 5 and 122) and summarized as follows:[89]

- Determine reasons for consultation at this time so that specific fears or concerns can be addressed. Careful inquiry into the patient's medical, social, and family history may uncover stresses that have led to acute symptom worsening or the current concern with chronic symptoms. Rule out recent changes in diet or medications as causes for symptoms.
- Record the history and perform a physical examination in a careful, nonjudgmental manner; this action reassures the patient and promotes trust in the physician's judgment and therapeutic plan.
- Propose diagnostic evaluation that addresses the patient's concerns. Avoid overtesting, which reflects diagnostic ambivalence and erodes the patient's confidence, unless warranted by changes in symptom pattern or objective findings.
- Establish a positive diagnosis of functional dyspepsia,

stressing that it is a real disease and providing reassurance about the natural history. Discuss symptom pathophysiologic processes, including abnormalities of gut motility, heightened visceral sensation, and the importance of the "mind-gut" interaction.

- Identify dietary, emotional, and environmental factors that may trigger symptoms. A symptom and food diary may be revealing and encourages the patient to take an active role in disease management. Coffee, caffeine, and excessive alcohol should be avoided.
- Set realistic treatment goals. Because most symptoms are chronic or recurrent, the patient must adapt through lifestyle modifications and coping strategies.
- Use drugs judiciously as adjuncts for therapy, not as panaceas. Many patients do not need or want drug therapy once explanation and reassurance have been given.
- Provide suitable follow-up examination to confirm symptom response.
- Explore psychological factors. Consider referral of patients with psychological or psychiatric problems, a history of physical or sexual abuse, or refractory symptom to a psychologist or chronic pain management clinic.

Drug Therapy

Results of drug treatment for functional dyspepsia have been disappointing. Controlled clinical trials—most from single centers and with insufficient sample sizes—have yielded conflicting conclusions, and thus the efficacy of any agent remains unproved. Differences in study methodology and patient populations may partly explain these disparate results. Differences include the following: (1) various definitions of functional dyspepsia; (2) lack of uniform symptom assessment or disease specific quality of life measurement tools; (3) heterogeneous patient populations with different symptom complexes and underlying pathophysiologic processes; (4) exclusion of patients with GERD, IBS, or psychological factors in some studies but not others; (5) location of some studies in primary care settings and others in functional GI clinics; and (6) widely varying placebo response rates of 32% to 80%, which make demonstration of efficacy of active drugs very difficult and suggest either different study populations or varying impact of the physician-patient relationship.[118–120] Meta-analyses of these clinical studies have concluded that there is no unequivocal evidence of efficacy of any agent in the treatment of functional dyspepsia.[120, 121] At this time, it must be concluded that with the possible exception of proton pump inhibitors there are no currently available agents with significant efficacy for the treatment of functional dyspepsia.[121]

Antisecretory Agents

Antacids have not demonstrated efficacy in the treatment of functional dyspepsia; however, this conclusion may reflect selection bias as patients who respond to over-the-counter antacids may be less likely to seek medical attention. The utility of H_2-receptor antagonists also is questionable. Response rates in controlled clinical trials range from 35% to 80%, compared with placebo response rates of 30% to 60%. Meta-analyses of these trials suggest that H_2-receptor antagonists reduce the relative risk of dyspepsia by 30% compared with that of placebo, but the quality of these trials is poor.[120–122]

In 1998 and 2000 several large, multicenter, randomized, double-blind studies comparing proton pump inhibitors with both placebo and H_2-receptor antagonists in functional dyspepsia demonstrated only modest benefit of proton pump inhibitors in the treatment of functional dyspepsia[97, 123–125] (Table 7–3). In four multicenter trials, symptom relief was achieved in 34% to 44% of patients treated with proton pump inhibitors (omeprazole 10 to 20 mg; lansoprazole 15 to 30 mg, once daily) for 4 to 8 weeks versus 26% to 33% of those treated with placebo, but in only two of these trials was a statistically significant benefit of proton pump inhibitors demonstrated.[97, 125] In a 2-week multicenter trial, symptoms resolved in 20% more patients treated with a proton pump inhibitor than in placebo subjects, but also in 8% to 12% more patients treated with ranitidine (150 mg once daily) than in placebo subjects.[124] Subset analyses of these studies as well as other studies suggest that patients most likely to respond to proton pump inhibitors are those with reflux-like dyspepsia, that is, heartburn, and those with pre-

Table 7–3 | **Multicenter, Randomized Trials in Functional Dyspepsia Comparing Resolution of Dyspepsia in Patients Treated with Proton Pump Inhibitors, Ranitidine, or Placebo**

STUDY (REFERENCE)	TREATMENT (DOSE)	% TREATMENT SUCCESS
Talley et al.[97]		
"Bond" Study	Omeprazole (20 mg/day)	43% (93/219)*
	Omeprazole (10 mg/day)	43% (88/204)*
	Placebo	26% (57/219)
"Opera" Study	Omeprazole (20 mg/day)	34% (62/128)
	Omeprazole (10 mg/day)	30% (61/140)
	Placebo	31% (62/203)
Combined studies	Omeprazole (20 mg/day)	38% (161/421)*
	Omeprazole (10 mg/day)	36% (146/405)*
	Placebo	28% (119/422)
Peura et al.[125]		
Study 1	Lansoprazole (30 mg/day)	48% (62/128)
	Lansoprazole (15 mg/day)	44% (61/120)
	Placebo	33% (42/128)
Study 2	Lansoprazole (30 mg/day)	40% (52/130)*
	Lansoprazole (15 mg/day)	44% (57/131)*
	Placebo	26% (38/144)
Combined	Lansoprazole (30 mg/day)	44% (114/258)*
	Lansoprazole (15 mg/day)	47% (118/253)*
	Placebo	29% (80/272)
Blum et al.[124]		
	Omeprazole (20 mg/day)	
	H. pylori–positive	32% (33/103)*
	H. pylori–negative	37% (33/90)*
	Combined	34% (66/193)*
	Omeprazole (10 mg/day)	
	H. pylori–positive	24% (23/95)*
	H. pylori–negative	31% (33/107)
	Combined	28% (56/202)*
	Ranitidine (150 mg/day)	
	H. pylori–positive	19% (21/111)
	H. pylori–negative	34% (28/83)
	Combined	25% (49/194)
	Placebo	
	H. pylori–positive	11% (12/113)
	H. pylori–negative	21% (19/90)
	Combined	15% (35/203)

*$p < 0.05$ for value compared with placebo.

dominant epigastric pain and, in one study, infection with *H. pylori*.[97, 123, 124, 126, 127] Proton pump inhibitors are 30% more effective than placebo in patients with reflux-like dyspepsia and 10% more effective in patients with predominant epigastric pain.[97] Conversely, symptoms of discomfort, nausea, and bloating are not relieved with proton pump inhibitors.

In sum, antisecretory therapies—both H_2-receptor antagonists and proton pump inhibitors—are useful in a subset of patients with functional dyspepsia, primarily those with heartburn or significant epigastric pain, and an empirical trial of such agents is reasonable. It is unlikely that they afford any significant benefit to patients with other dyspeptic symptoms. In the subsets who benefit, it has not been established that proton pump inhibitors are superior to less expensive H_2-receptor antagonists.[124] It is unlikely, however, that pharmaceutical companies will sponsor such a comparative trial. Among the 30% to 50% of functional dyspepsia patients who respond to antisecretory therapies, the benefit likely represents a placebo effect in over half.

Promotility Agents

Promotility agents decrease gastroesophageal reflux, improve gastric emptying, and facilitate accommodation and might thereby be predicted to benefit some patients with functional dyspepsia.[45] Results of initial small controlled trials of promotility agents in functional dyspepsia were encouraging, indicating that treatment with cisapride (5 to 10 mg, two to three times daily) or domperidone (20 mg three times daily) achieved an impressive therapeutic gain ranging from 29% to 42% over that of placebo.[122] However, methodological flaws precluded any legitimate conclusions based upon these studies.[120] Subsequently, several large, well-designed trials comparing cisapride to placebo did not confirm significant benefit for cisapride in the treatment of functional dyspepsia.[128–130] Nevertheless, meta-analyses in 2000 and 2001 continued to suggest that both cisapride and domperidone have a significant effect upon dyspeptic symptoms.[121, 131] There are insufficient data to determine whether symptom improvement is confined to the subset of patients who have gastric emptying disorders.

At the present time, the issue of whether promotility agents benefit patients has been rendered moot by the lack of safe, available agents. Metoclopramide, the only promotility agent available in the United States, has had only limited testing for functional dyspepsia.[132] The high incidence of adverse CNS effects and extrapyramidal effects associated with metoclopramide makes it unsuitable for long-term use. Cisapride has been markedly restricted in its use by the United States Food and Drug Administration because of a low but significant risk of QT prolongation and cardiac tachyarrhythmias and should no longer be prescribed for functional dyspepsia.[132] Although domperidone, a peripherally acting dopaminergic antagonist that does not cross the CNS blood-brain barrier, is available in many countries worldwide, application for approval in the United States is not being pursued by the manufacturer.

Antidepressants

Antidepressants are increasingly used for the treatment of functional bowel disorders, including functional dyspepsia.[133] Despite a dearth of controlled clinical trials demonstrating efficacy in functional dyspepsia, some experts tout their benefit.[82] The mechanism of action by which these agents may benefit dyspepsia is unclear. Although depression is common in all functional disorders, symptom relief derived from these medications appears to be independent of the psychiatric effects of the drugs. Benefits also do not appear to be related to reduction in visceral sensitivity or improvement in sleep, and a neuromodulatory effect at the spinal cord or CNS level is hypothesized.[134] On the basis of uncontrolled experience, use of low doses of tricyclic antidepressants is favored. Experts recommend use of nortriptyline or desipramine, beginning at 10 to 25 mg/day, increasing slowly to 50 to 75 mg/day.[135] Side effects are common, and it may be necessary to try several different agents. Serotonin reuptake inhibitors may cause nausea and dyspepsia and therefore are uncommonly used.

Anti–*Helicobacter pylori* Treatment

As discussed, eradication of *H. pylori* has not been shown to improve functional dyspepsia in multicenter, randomized, placebo-controlled trials.[76] Although these trials do not exclude a small therapeutic gain (up to 9%) in *H. pylori*–positive patients with functional dyspepsia, routine screening and treating of patients are not recommended.

Miscellaneous Agents

Herbal and other nonprescription preparations are available for the treatment of dyspepsia but have had little formal testing. A combination of peppermint and caraway oil demonstrated symptom benefit in a placebo-controlled trial.[136] Bismuth subsalicylate (Pepto-Bismol) is an over-the-counter preparation commonly used for acute dyspepsia but has not been tested in patients with chronic symptoms.

Recognition of heightened visceral sensation in functional GI disorders has spawned interest in drugs that reduce gut sensation. Agents currently being investigated are $5HT_3$ serotonin receptor antagonists (which may also reduce nausea), $5\text{-}HT_4$ receptor agonists, somatostatin analogs, and kappa opioid agonists.[132] A motilin agonist was not found to benefit patients with functional dyspepsia.[137] As discussed previously, serotonin $5\text{-}HT_1$ agonists such as sumitriptan or buspirone have been shown in small studies to promote gastric accommodation and improve symptoms.[48] Further clinical study of these agents is needed before they can be recommended for treatment of functional dyspepsia.

Drug Therapy: Recommendations

Drug therapy should be reserved for patients who do not improve after reassurance and life-style changes. H_2-receptor antagonists (ranitidine or nizatidine 150 mg, cimetidine 400 mg, or famotidine 20 mg, all twice daily) or proton pump inhibitors (lansoprazole 15 to 30 mg, omeprazole, esomeprazole, or rabeprazole 20 mg, or pantoprazole 40 mg) may benefit patients with reflux-like dyspepsia or epigastric pain but should not be used for other dyspeptic symptoms. Responders should be treated with intermittent, 2- to 4-week courses for symptom episodes and the medication stopped.

Resolution of symptoms may be sustained for months.[138] Chronic antisecretory therapy should be reserved for patients with repeated symptom relapse. In patients with other dyspeptic symptoms, such as bloating, nausea, early satiety, or discomfort, the available options currently are limited. An antisecretory agent may still be tried; however, benefit is likely to be due to placebo effect. Metoclopramide can be considered, but the uncertain benefits must be weighed against potential side effects. A trial of low doses of tricyclic antidepressants may be considered even in the absence of apparent anxiety or depression.[132]

Refractory Functional Dyspepsia

A minority of patients have unresponsive symptoms that interfere with daily activities and lead to excessive use of the health care system. Referral to a mental health professional is urged for patients with obvious psychiatric disease or a history of physical or sexual abuse. Other patients may benefit from referral for stress management, relaxation training (such as yoga, meditation, or biofeedback), hypnotherapy, cognitive behavioral treatment, or psychotherapy.[82, 139, 140]

REFERENCES

1. Heading R: Prevalence of upper gastrointestinal symptoms in the general population: A systematic review. Scand J Gastroenterol 34:3, 1999.
2. Locke R III: Prevalence, incidence and natural history of dyspepsia and functional dyspepsia. Baillieres Clin Gastroenterol 12:435, 1998.
3. Frank L, Kleinman L, Ganoczy D, et al: Upper gastrointestinal symptoms in North America: Prevalence and relationship to health care utilization and quality of life. Dig Dis Sci 45:809, 2000.
4. Veldhuyzen van Zanten S, Flook N, Chiba N, et al: An evidence-based approach to the management of uninvestigated dyspepsia in the era of *Helicobacter pylori*. Can Med Assoc J 162:S3, 2000.
5. Fisher R, Parkman H: Management of nonulcer dyspepsia. N Engl J Med 339:1376, 1998.
6. Hu W, Talley N: Functional (non-ulcer) dyspepsia: Unexplained but not unmanageable. Med J Aust 168:507, 1998.
7. Rabeneck L, Wray N, Graham D: Managing dyspepsia: What do we know and what do we need to know? Am J Gastroenterol 93:920, 1998.
8. Levin T, Kunz K, Henke C, et al: Costs of acid-related disorders to a health maintenance organization. Am J Med 103:520, 1997.
9. Holtmann G, Stanghellini V, Talley N: Nomenclature of dyspepsia, dyspepsia subgroups and functional dyspepsia: Clarifying the concepts. Baillieres Clin Gastroenterol 12:417, 1998.
10. Talley N, Stanghellini V, Heading R, et al: Functional gastroduodenal disorders. Gut 45:II37, 1999.
11. Stanghellini V: Three-month prevalence rates of gastrointestinal symptoms and the influence of demographic factors: Results from the Domestic International Gastroenterology Surveillance Study (DIGEST). Scand J Gastroenterol 34:20, 1999.
12. Talley N, Silverstein M, Agreus L, et al: AGA technical review: Evaluation of dyspepsia. Gastroenterology 114:582, 1998.
13. Haque M, Wyeth J, Stace N, et al: Prevalence, severity and associated features of gastro-esophageal reflux and dyspepsia: A population-based study. N Z Med J 113:178, 2000.
14. Westbrook J, McIntosh J, Talley N: Factors associated with consulting medical or non-medical practitioners: An Australian population-based study. Aliment Pharmacol Ther 14:1581, 2000.
15. Talley N, Boyce P, Jones M: Dyspepsia and health care seeking in a community: How important are psychological factors? Dig Dis Sci 43: 1016, 1998.
16. Delaney B: Why do dyspeptic patients over age 50 consult their general practitioner? A qualitative investigation of health beliefs relating to dyspepsia. Br J Gen Pract 48:1481, 1998.
17. Boekema P, Samsom M, van Berge Henegouwen G, et al: Coffee and gastrointestinal function: Fact and fiction. Scand J Gastroenterol 34:35, 1999.
18. Lichtenberger L, Romero J, Carryl O, et al: Effect of pepper and bismuth subsalicylate on gastric pain and surface hydrophobicity. Aliment Pharmacol Ther 12:483, 1998.
19. Nankadur S, Talley N, Xia H, et al: Dyspepsia in the community is linked to smoking and aspirin but not to *Helicobacter pylori* infection. Arch Intern Med 158:1427, 1998.
20. Woodward M, Morrison C, McColl K: The prevalence of dyspepsia and use of antisecretory medication in North Glasgow: Role of *Helicobacter pylori* vs. lifestyle factors. Aliment Pharmacol Ther 13:1505, 1999.
21. Suarez F, Levitt M, Adshead J, et al: Pancreatic supplements reduce symptomatic response of healthy subjects to a high fat meal. Dig Dis Sci 44:1317, 1999.
22. Heikkinen M, Pikkarainen P, Takala J, et al: Etiology of dyspepsia: Four hundred unselected consecutive patients in general practice. Scand J Gastroenterol 30:519, 1995.
23. Peterson W, Cryer B: COX-1 sparing NSAIDs—is the enthusiasm justified? JAMA 282:1961, 1999.
24. Brun J, Jones J: Nonsteroidal anti-inflammatory drug—associated dyspepsia: The scale of the problem. Am J Med 110:12S, 2001.
25. Jones J, Raud R: Nonsteroidal anti-inflammatory drug—associated dyspepsia: Basic mechanisms and future research. Am J Med 110:14S, 2001.
26. Schoenfeld P, Kimmey M, Scheiman J, et al: Review article: nonsteroidal anti-inflammatory drug–associated gastrointestinal complications—guidelines for prevention and treatment. Aliment Pharmacol Ther 13:1273, 1999.
27. Watson D, Harper S, Zhao P, et al: Gastrointestional tolerability of the selective cyclooxygenase-2 (COX-2) inhibitor rofecoxib compared with nonselective COX-1 and COX-2 inhibitors in osteoarthritis. Arch Intern Med 160:2998, 2000.
28. Bytzer P, Hallas J: Drug-induced symptoms of functional dyspepsia and nausea: A symmetry analysis of one million prescriptions. Aliment Pharmacol Ther 14:1479, 2000.
29. Talley N, Axon A, Bytzer P, et al: Management of uninvestigated dyspepsia and functional dyspepsia: A working party report for the World Congresses of Gastroenterology 1998. Aliment Pharmacol Ther 13:1135, 1999.
30. Stanghellini V, Tosetti C, Barbara G, et al: The continuing dilemma of dyspepsia. Aliment Pharmacol Ther 14:23, 2000.
31. Talley N, Weaver A, Tesmer D, et al: Lack of discriminant value of dyspepsia subgroups in patients referred for endoscopy. Gastroenterology 105:1378, 1993.
32. Wayman J, Griffin S, Campbell F: Is functional dyspepsia largely explained by gastro-oesophageal reflux disease? Baillieres Clin Gastroenterol 12:463, 1998.
33. Klauser A, Schindlbeck N, Muller-Lissher S: Symptoms in gastro-oesophageal reflux disease. Lancet 335:205, 1990.
34. Kellow J: Organic causes of dyspepsia, and discriminating functional from organic. Baillieres Clin Gastroenterol 12:477, 1998.
35. Janssen H, Muris J, Knottnerus J: The clinical course and prognostic determinants of non-ulcer dyspepsia: A literature review. Scand J Gastroenterol 34:546, 1999.
36. Talley N, Verlinden M, Jones M: Quality of life in functional dyspepsia: Responsiveness of the Nepean Dyspepsia Index and development of a new 10-item short form. Aliment Pharmacol Ther 15:207, 2001.
37. Fass R, Fullerton S, Tung S, et al: Sleep disturbances in clinic patients with functional bowel disorders. Am J Gastroenterol 95:1195, 2000.
38. Koloski N, Talley N, Boyce P: The impact of functional gastrointestinal disorders on quality of life. Am J Gastroenterol 95:67, 2000.
39. Drossman D: The functional GI disorders and the Rome II process. In Drossman D (ed): The Functional Gastrointestinal Disorders. McLean, VA, Degnon Associates, 2000, p 1.
40. Quartero A, De Wit N, Lodder A, et al: Disturbed solid-phase gastric emptying in functional dyspepsias: A meta-analysis. Dig Dis Sci 43: 2028, 1998.
41. Stanghellini V, Corinaldesi R, Tosetti C: Relevance of gastrointestinal motor disturbances in functional dyspepsia. Baillieres Clin Gastroenterol 12:533, 1998.
42. Stanghellini V, Tosetti C, Paternico A, et al: Predominant symptoms

identify different subgroups in functional dyspepsia. Am J Gastroenterol 94:2080, 1999.
43. Berstad A, Hauken T, Gilja O, et al: Gastric accommodation in functional dyspepsia. Scand J Gastroenterol 32:193, 1997.
44. Thurmshirn M, Camilleri M, Saslow S, et al: Gastric accommodation in non-ulcer dyspepsia and the roles of *Helicobacter pylori* infection and vagal function. Gut 44:55, 1999.
45. Tack J, Piessevaux H, Coulie B, et al: Role of impaired accommodation to a meal in functional dyspepsia. Gastroenterology 115:1346, 1998.
46. Tack J: Distention in non-consulting dyspeptics: A swell idea. Gut 47: 326, 2000.
47. Tougas G: The autonomic nervous system in functional bowel disorders. Gut 47:iv78, 2000.
48. Tack J, Coulie B, Wilmer A, et al: Influence of sumitriptan on gastric fundus tone and on the perception of gastric distention in man. Gut 46:468, 2000.
49. Tack J: Receptors of the enteric nervous system: Potential targets for drug therapy. Gut 47:iv20, 2000.
50. Gilja O, Hausken T, Bang C, et al: Effect of glyceryl trinitrate on gastric accommodation and symptoms of functional dyspepsia. Dig Dis Sci 42:2124, 1997.
51. Vingerhagen S, Hausken T, Gilja O, et al: Influence of 5HT1 receptor agonist on gastric accommodation and initial transpyloric flow in healthy subjects. Neurogastroenterol Motil 12:95, 2000.
52. Tack J, Broeckaert D, Coulie B, et al: The influence of cisapride on gastric tone and the perception of gastric distention. Aliment Pharmacol Ther 12:761, 1998.
53. Bjornsson E, Abrahamsson H: Contractile patterns in patients with severe dyspepsia. Am J Gastroenterol 94:54, 1999.
54. Leahy A, Besherdas K, Clayman C, et al: Abnormalities of the electrogastrogram in functional gastrointestinal disorders. Am J Gastroenterol 94:1023, 1999.
55. Koch K, Hong S, Xu L: Reproducibility of gastric myoelectrical activity and the water load test in patients with dysmotility-like dyspepsia symptoms and in control subjects. J Clin Gastroenterol 31:125, 2000.
56. Lin Z, Eaker E, Sarosiek I, et al: Gastric myoelectrical activity and gastric emptying in patients with functional dyspepsia. Am J Gastroenterol 94:2384, 1999.
57. Parkman H, Miller M, Trate D, et al: Electrogastrography and gastric emptying scintigraphy are complementary for assessment of dyspepsia. J Clin Gastroenterol 24:214, 1997.
58. Besherdas K, Leahy A, Mason I, et al: The effect of cisapride on dyspepsia symptoms and the electrogastrogram in patients with non-ulcer dyspepsia. Aliment Pharmacol Ther 12:755, 1998.
59. Camilleri M, Coulie B, Tack J: Visceral hypersensitivity: Facts, speculations, and challenges. Gut 48:125, 2001.
60. Bueno L, Fioramonti J, Delvaux M, et al: Mediators and pharmacology of visceral sensitivity: From basic to clinical investigations. Gastroenterology 112:1714, 1997.
61. Schmulson M, Mayer E: Gastrointestinal sensory abnormalities in functional dyspepsia. Baillieres Clin Gastroenterol 12:545, 1998.
62. Kellow J, Delvaux M, Azpiroz F, et al: Principles of applied neurogastroenterology: Physiology/motility—sensation. Gut 45:II17, 1999.
63. Holtmann G, Gschossmann J, Neufang-Huber J, et al: Differences in gastric mechanosensory function after repeated ramp distentions in non-consulters with dyspepsia and healthy controls. Gut 47:332, 2000.
64. Thumshirn M, Camilleri M, Choi M, et al: Modulation of gastric sensory and motor functions by nitrergic and alpha-2 adrenergic agents in humans. Gastroenterology 116:573, 1999.
65. Distrutti E, Azpiroz F, Soldevilla A, et al: Gastric wall tension determines perception of gastric distention. Gastroenterology 116:1035, 1999.
66. Mertz H, Fullerton S, Naliboff B, et al: Symptoms and visceral perception in severe functional and organic dyspepsia. Gut 42:814, 1998.
67. Holtmann G, Goebell H, Jockenhoevel F, et al: Altered vagal and intestinal mechanosensory function in chronic unexplained dyspepsia. Gut 42:501, 1998.
68. Muth E, Koch R, Stern R: Significance of autonomic nervous system activity in functional dyspepsia. Dig Dis Sci 45:854, 2000.
69. Hveem K, Svebak S, Hausken T, et al: Effect of mental stress and cisapride on autonomic nerve functions in functional dyspepsia. Scand J Gastroenterol 33:123, 1998.
70. Berstad A: Functional dyspepsia—a conceptual framework. Gut 47: iv3, 2000.
71. Locke R III, Talley N, Nelson D, et al: *Helicobacter pylori* and dyspepsia: A population-based study of the organism and host. Am J Gastroenterol 95:1906, 2000.
72. Jaakkimainen R, Boyle E, Tudiver F: Is *Helicobacter pylori* associated with non-ulcer dyspepsia and will eradication improve symptoms? A meta-analysis. BMJ 319:1040, 1999.
73. Danesh J, Lawrence M, Murphy M, et al: Systematic review of the epidemiological evidence on *Helicobacter pylori* infection and nonulcer or uninvestigated dyspepsia. Arch Intern Med 160:1192, 2000.
74. Xia H, Talley N: *Helicobacter pylori* eradication in patients with non-ulcer dyspepsia. Drugs 58:785, 1999.
75. Rhee P, Kim Y, Son H, et al: Lack of an association of *Helicobacter pylori* infection with gastric hypersensitivity or delayed gastric emptying in functional dyspepsia. Am J Gastroenterol 94:3165, 1999.
76. Laine L, Schoenfeld P, Fennerty B: Therapy for *Helicobacter pylori* in patients with nonulcer dyspepsia: A meta-analysis of randomized, controlled trials. Ann Intern Med 134:361, 2001.
77. Talley N, Vakil N, Ballard D, et al: Absence of benefit of eradicating *Helicobacter pylori* in patients with nonulcer dyspepsia. N Engl J Med 341:1106, 1999.
78. Blum A, Talley N, O'Morain C, et al: Lack of effect of treating *Helicobacter pylori* infection in patients with nonulcer dyspepsia. N Engl J Med 339:1875, 1998.
79. Talley N, Janssens J, Lauritsen K, et al: Eradication of *Helicobacter pylori* in functional dyspepsia: Randomised double blind placebo controlled trial with 12 months' follow up. BMJ 318:833, 1999.
80. Moayyedi P, Soo S, Deeks J, et al: Systematic review and economic evaluation of *Helicobacter pylori* eradication treatment for non-ulcer dyspepsia. BMJ 321:659, 2000.
81. Drossman D, Creed F, Olden K, et al: Psychosocial aspects of functional gastrointestinal disorders. Gut 45:II25, 1999.
82. Drossman D, Creed F, Olden K, et al: Psychosocial aspects of the functional gastrointestinal disorders. In Drossman D (ed): The Functional Gastrointestinal Disorders. McLean, VA, Degnon Associates, 2000, p 157.
83. Quartero A, Post M, Numans M, et al: What makes the dyspeptic patient feel ill? A cross sectional survey of functional status, *Helicobacter pylori* infection, and psychological distress in dyspeptic patients in general practice. Gut 45:15 1999.
84. Bennett E, Piesse C, Palmer K, et al: Functional gastrointestinal disorders: Psychological, social, and somatic features. Gut 42:414, 1998.
85. Lee S, Park M, Choi S, et al: Stress, coping and depression in non-ulcer dyspepsia patients. J Psychosom Res 49:93, 2000.
86. Olden K: Are psychosocial factors of aetiological importance in functional dyspepsia? Baillieres Clin Gastroenterol 12:557, 1998.
87. Haug T, Wilhelmsen I, Ursin H, et al: What are the real problems for patients with functional dyspepsia? Scand J Gastroenterol 30:97, 1995.
88. Bytzer P: How should new-onset dyspepsia be managed in general and specialist practice? Baillieres Clin Gastroenterol 12:587, 1998.
89. Talley N, Stanghellini V, Heading R, et al: Functional gastroduodenal disorders. In Drossman D (ed): The Functional Gastrointestinal Disorders. McLean, VA, Degnon Associates, 2000, p 300.
90. Hansen J, Bytzer P, Schaffalitzky de Muckadell O: Management of dyspeptic patients in primary care: Value of the unaided clinical diagnosis and of dyspepsia subgrouping. Scand J Gastroenterol 33:799, 1998.
91. Ofman J, Rabeneck L: The effectiveness of endoscopy in the management of dyspepsia: A qualitative systematic review. Am J Med 106: 335, 1999.
92. Lassen A, Pedersen F, Bytzer P, et al: *Helicobacter pylori* test-and-eradicate versus prompt endoscopy for management of dyspeptic patients: A randomized trial: Lancet 356:455, 2000.
93. Heaney A, Collins J, Watson R, et al: A prospective randomised trial of "test and treat" policy versus endoscopy based management in young *Helicobacter pylori* positive patients with ulcer-like dyspepsia, referred to a hospital clinic. Gut 45:186, 1999.
94. Wiklund I, Glise H, Jerndal P, et al: Does endoscopy have a positive impact on quality of life in dyspepsia? Gastrointest Endosc 47:449, 1998.
95. Gillen D, McColl K: Does concern about missing malignancy justify endoscopy in uncomplicated dyspepsia in patients less than 55? Am J Gastroenterol 94:75, 1999.
96. Madsen L, Bytzer P: The value of alarm features in identifying causes of dyspepsia. Can J Gastroenterol 14:713, 2000.
97. Talley N, Meineche-Schmidt V, Pare P, et al: Efficacy of omeprazole

in functional dyspepsia: Double-blind, randomized, placebo-controlled trials (the Bond and Opera studies). Aliment Pharmacol Ther 12:1055, 1998.

98. Fass R: Empirical trials in treatment of gastroesophageal reflux disease. Dig Dis Sci 18:20, 2000.
99. Sampliner R: Practice guidelines on the diagnosis, surveillance, and therapy of Barrett's esophagus. Am J Gastroenterol 93:1028, 1998.
100. Schoenfeld P, Kimmey M, Scheiman J, et al: Nonsteroidal anti-inflammatory drug–associated gastrointestinal complications—guidelines for prevention and treatment. Aliment Pharmacol Ther 13:1273, 1999.
101. Danesh J: *Helicobacter pylori* infection and gastric cancer: Systematic review of the epidemiological studies. Aliment Pharmacol Ther 13: 851, 1999.
102. Bytzer P, Aalykke C, Rune S, et al: Eradication of *Helicobacter pylori* compared with long-term acid suppression in duodenal ulcer disease: A randomized trial with 2-year follow-up. The Danish ulcer study group. Scand J Gastroenterol 35:1023, 2000.
103. Farkilla M, Sarna S, Valtonen V, et al: "Test and treat" strategy for management of uninvestigated dyspepsia in primary health care. Gastroenterology 118:A438, 2000.
104. Chiba N, Veldhuyzen van Zanten S, Sinclair P, et al: Beneficial effect of *H. pylori* eradication therapy on long term symptom relief in primary care patients with uninvestigated dyspepsia: The Cadet-HP Study. Gastroenterology 118:A438, 2000.
105. Moayyedi P, Feltblower R, Borwn J, et al: Effect of population screening and treatment for *Helicobacter pylori* on dyspepsia and quality of life in the community: A randomised controlled trial. Lancet 355:1665, 2000.
106. Talley N: How should *Helicobacter pylori* positive dyspeptic patients be treated? Gut 45:128, 1999.
107. Stanghellini V, Tosetti C, De Giorgio R, et al: How should *Helicobacter pylori* negative patients be managed? Gut 45:132, 1999.
108. Hession P, Malagelada J: The initial management of uninvestigated dyspepsia in younger patients—the value of symptom-guided strategies should be reconsidered. Aliment Pharmacol Ther 14:379, 2000.
109. Silverstein M, Petterson T, Talley N: Initial endoscopy or empirical therapy with or without testing for *Helicobacter pylori* for dyspepsia: A decision analysis. Gastroenterology 110:72, 1996.
110. Briggs A, Logan R, Aldous J, et al: Cost effectiveness of screening for and eradication of *Helicobacter pylori* in management of dyspeptic patients under 45 years of age. BMJ 312:1321, 1996.
111. Fendrick M, Chernew M, Hirth R, et al: Alternative management strategies for patients with suspected peptic ulcer disease. Ann Intern Med 123:260, 1995.
112. Ofman J, Etchason J, Fullerton S, et al: Management strategies for *Helicobacter pylori*–seropositive patients with dyspepsia: Clinical and economic consequences. Ann Intern Med 126:280, 1997.
113. Sonnenberg A: Cost-benefit analysis of testing for *Helicobacter pylori* in dyspeptic subjects. Am J Gastroenterol 91:1773, 1996.
114. Goves J, Oldring J, Kerr D, et al: First line treatment with omeprazole provides an effective and superior alternative strategy in the management of dyspepsia compared with antacid/alginate liquid: A multicenter study in general practice. Aliment Pharmacol Ther 12:147, 1998.
115. Groeneveld P, Lieu T, Fendrick M, et al: Quality of life measurement clarifies the cost-effectiveness of *Helicobacter pylori* eradication in peptic ulcer disease and uninvestigated dyspepsia. Am J Gastroenterol 96:338, 2001.
116. Delaney B, Innes M, Deeks J, et al: Initial management strategies for dyspepsia. Cochrane Database Syst Rev CD001961, 2000.
117. Duggan A, Ellliot C, Tolley K, et al: Randomised controlled trial of four dyspepsia management strategies in primary care with 12 months follow-up. Gastroenterology 118:A438, 2000.
118. Mearin F, Balboa A, Zarate N, et al: Placebo in functional dyspepsia: Symptomatic, gastrointestinal motor, and gastric sensorial responses. Am J Gastroenterol 94:116, 1999.
119. Champion, M: Clinical trials in nonulcer dyspepsia: A cautionary note. Can J Gastroenterol 11:125, 1997.
120. Veldhuyzen van Zanten S, Cleary C, Talley N, et al: Drug treatment of functional dyspepsia: A systematic analysis of trial methodology with recommendations for design of future trials. Am J Gastroenterol 91:660, 1996.
121. Soo S, Moayyedi P, Deeks J, et al: Pharmacological interventions for non-ulcer dyspepsia. Cochrane Database Syst Rev CD001960, 2000.
122. Finney J, Kinnersley N, Hughes M, et al: Meta-analysis of antisecretory and gastrokinetic compounds in functional dyspepsia. J Clin Gastroenterol 26:312, 1998.
123. Meineche-Schmidt V, Christensen E: Which dyspepsia patients will benefit from omeprazole treatment? Am J Gastroenterol 95:2777, 2000.
124. Blum A, Arnold R, Stolte M, et al: Short course of acid suppressive treatment for patients with functional dyspepsia: Results depend on *Helicobacter pylori* status. Gut 47:473, 2000.
125. Peura D, Kovacs T, Metz D, et al: Low-dose lansoprazole: Effective for non-ulcer dyspepsia. Gastroenterology 118:A439, 2000.
126. Bytzer P, Hansen J, Rune S, et al: Identifying responders to acid suppression in dyspepsia using a random starting day trial. Aliment Pharmacol Ther 14:1485, 2000.
127. Stanghellini, V. Pain versus discomfort—is differentiation clinically useful? Aliment Pharmacol Ther 15:145, 2001.
128. Champion M, MacCannell K, Thomson A, et al: A double-blind randomized study of cisapride in the treatment of nonulcer dyspepsia. Can J Gastroenterol 11:127, 1997.
129. De Groot G, De Both P: Cisapride in functional dyspepsia in general practice: A placebo-controlled, randomized, double-blind study. Aliment Pharmacol Ther 11:193, 1997.
130. Hansen J, Bytzer P, Schaffalitzky de Muckadell O: Placebo-controlled trial of cisapride and nizatidine in unselected patients with functional dyspepsia. Am J Gastroenterol 93:368, 1998.
131. Veldhuyzen van Zanten S, Jones M, Verlinden M, et al: Efficacy of cisapride and domperidone in functional (nonulcer) dyspepsia: A meta-analysis. Am J Gastroenterol 96:689, 2001.
132. Talley N: Therapeutic options in nonulcer dyspepsia. J Clin Gastroenterol 32:286, 2001.
133. Jackson J, O'Malley P, Tomkins G, et al: Treatment of functional gastrointestinal disorders with antidepressant medications: A meta-analysis. Am J Med 108:65, 2000.
134. Mertz H, Fass R, Kodner A, et al: Effect of amitryptiline on symptoms, sleep, and visceral perception in patients with functional dyspepsia. Am J Gastroenterol 93:160, 1998.
135. Clouse R: Psychotropic medications for the treatment of functional gastrointestinal disorders. Clin Perspect Gastroenterol November/December:348, 1999.
136. May B, Kohler S, Schneider B: Efficacy and tolerability of a fixed combination of peppermint oil and caraway oil in patients suffering from functional dyspepsia. Aliment Pharmacol Ther 14:1671, 2000.
137. Talley N, Verlinden M, Snape W, et al: Failure of motilin receptor agonist (ABT-229) to relieve the symptoms of functional dyspepsia in patients with and without delayed gastric emptying: A randomized double-blind placebo-controlled trial. Aliment Pharmacol Ther 14: 1653, 2000.
138. Meineche-Schmidt V, Talley N, Pap A, et al: Impact of functional dyspepsia on quality of life and health care consumption after cessation of antisecretory treatment. Scand J Gastroenterol 34:566, 1999.
139. Heymann-Monnikes I, Arnold R, Florin I, et al: The combination of medical treatment plus multicomponent behavioral therapy is superior to medical treatment alone in the therapy of irritable bowel syndrome. Am J Gastroenterol 95:981, 2000.
140. Hamilton J, Guthrie E, Creed F, et al: A randomized controlled trial of psychotherapy in patients with functional dyspepsia. Gastroenterology 119:661, 2000.

Chapter 8

NAUSEA AND VOMITING

Makau Lee

Nausea and vomiting are clinically important for two major reasons. First, nausea and vomiting may be manifestations of a wide variety of conditions, including pregnancy, motion sickness, radiation sickness, drug toxicity, gastrointestinal obstruction, hepatitis, myocardial infarction, renal failure, increased intracranial pressure, asthma, Zollinger-Ellison syndrome, diabetes mellitus, thyrotoxicosis, and epilepsy.[1] Second, vomiting can lead to many life-threatening consequences, including aspiration pneumonia, Mallory-Weiss tears, esophageal rupture (Boerhaave's syndrome), volume and electrolyte depletion, acid-base imbalance, and malnutrition.

ACT OF VOMITING

Three components of vomiting are recognized: nausea, retching ("dry heaves"), and emesis (vomiting). Nausea may occur without retching or vomiting, and retching may occur without vomiting.[2] Characteristic but not invariable changes in gastrointestinal motility have been recognized for each of the three stages.

Nausea is a uniquely unpleasant discomfort that defies precise definition.[3] A variety of stimuli may produce nausea (e.g., labyrinthine stimulation, visceral pain, unpleasant memories). The neural pathways mediating nausea are not known, but evidence suggests that they are the same as pathways mediating vomiting. It may be that mild activation of these pathways leads to nausea, whereas more intense activation leads to retching, vomiting, or both. During nausea, gastric tone is reduced and gastric peristalsis is diminished or absent. In contrast, the tone of the duodenum and proximal jejunum tends to be increased, and reflux of duodenal contents into the stomach is frequent. Nausea is not caused by increased duodenal and jejunal tone, however, because these abnormalities are not always present in a nauseated person.

Retching consists of spasmodic and abortive respiratory movements with the glottis closed, during which time inspiratory movements of the chest wall and diaphragm are opposed by expiratory contractions of the abdominal musculature. During retching, the antrum of the stomach contracts while the fundus and cardiac relax. The mouth is closed.

Vomiting occurs as the gastric contents are forcefully brought up to and out of the mouth, which opens just before stomach evacuation. This occurs by virtue of a forceful, sustained contraction of the abdominal muscles and diaphragm at a time when the cardia of the stomach is raised and open and the pylorus is contracted.[4] Elevation of the cardia serves the purpose of eliminating the intra-abdominal portion of the esophagus, which, if present, would tend to prevent the high intragastric pressure from forcing gastric contents into the esophagus. The cardia may be so high as to cause a temporary hiatal hernia. The mechanism by which the cardia opens during vomiting is not clear.

Associated Phenomena

HYPERSALIVATION. Hypersalivation is probably due to the close proximity of the medullary vomiting and salivary centers (see section on Neural Pathways and Pathophysiology of Vomiting).

CARDIAC RHYTHM DISTURBANCES. Nausea is usually accompanied by tachycardia, and retching is accompanied by bradycardia. Cardiac arrhythmias sometimes occur in animals made to vomit, and these may be prevented by pretreatment with atropine. In humans, retching and vomiting have been associated with onset of atrial fibrillation and termination of ventricular tachyarrhythmias.[5, 6]

DEFECATION. Defecation may accompany vomiting. It has been suggested that vomiting and defecation pathways are adjacent in the area postrema of the medulla and are acted on by essentially the same kind of stimuli.[7]

NEURAL PATHWAYS AND PATHOPHYSIOLOGY OF VOMITING

The mechanism of vomiting in cats was extensively studied by Borison and colleagues.[7, 8] Although caution must be exercised in extrapolating their data to humans, the experiments can never be repeated in intact human subjects, and what little is known about the pathophysiology of vomiting in humans is compatible with experimental observations reported by Borison and colleagues[7, 8] and Baker and Bernat.[9]

A schematic of the neural pathways that mediate vomiting is depicted in Figure 8–1. The proposed neural pathways of vomiting are based on the following experimental observations[7–11]:

1. Vomiting involves a complex and reproducible set of activities that suggest some central neurologic control by a "vomiting center."
2. Animal studies performed by Borison and colleagues suggest that a vomiting center is located in the dorsal portion of the medulla and that vomiting can be induced by electrical stimulation of this area.[7, 8] However, subsequent studies have failed to locate a discrete anatomic vomiting center.[10, 11] Therefore, the current view is that the vomiting center is best regarded as a pharmacologic entity rather than an anatomic entity.[10, 11] This vomiting center is probably associated with other medullary centers controlling respiration and salivation, and integrated activities mediated by all these centers are involved in vomiting.
3. Afferent neural inputs to the vomiting center are transmitted via the vagus and sympathetic nerves.[10, 11]
4. Experimental studies suggest that there is a chemoreceptor trigger zone (CTZ) in the area postrema.[7–11] Various emetic stimuli can induce vomiting indirectly by stimulating the CTZ, which in turn activates the vomiting center. Unlike the vomiting center, the CTZ is not responsive to electrical stimulation. Instead, the CTZ is responsive to chemical stimuli in the circulation; the blood–brain barrier in the region of the CTZ is virtually nonexistent. Thus, the CTZ can be regarded as an emetic chemoreceptor, as illustrated in Figure 8–1.

Emetic stimuli generally cause vomiting by one of the following two mechanisms.[7–11] First, emetic stimuli can cause vomiting by activating afferent vagal or sympathetic neural pathways within the gastrointestinal tract that act directly on the vomiting center. For instance, orally administered copper sulfate causes vomiting by this mechanism. In experimental animals, ablation of the vagal and sympathetic pathways, as well as destruction of the reticular formation, prevents vomiting induced by orally administered copper sulfate. Although direct electrical stimulation of the vomiting center causes vomiting in experimental animals, there is no evidence that any emetic stimuli induce vomiting by direct stimulation of this center. In addition to afferent stimuli

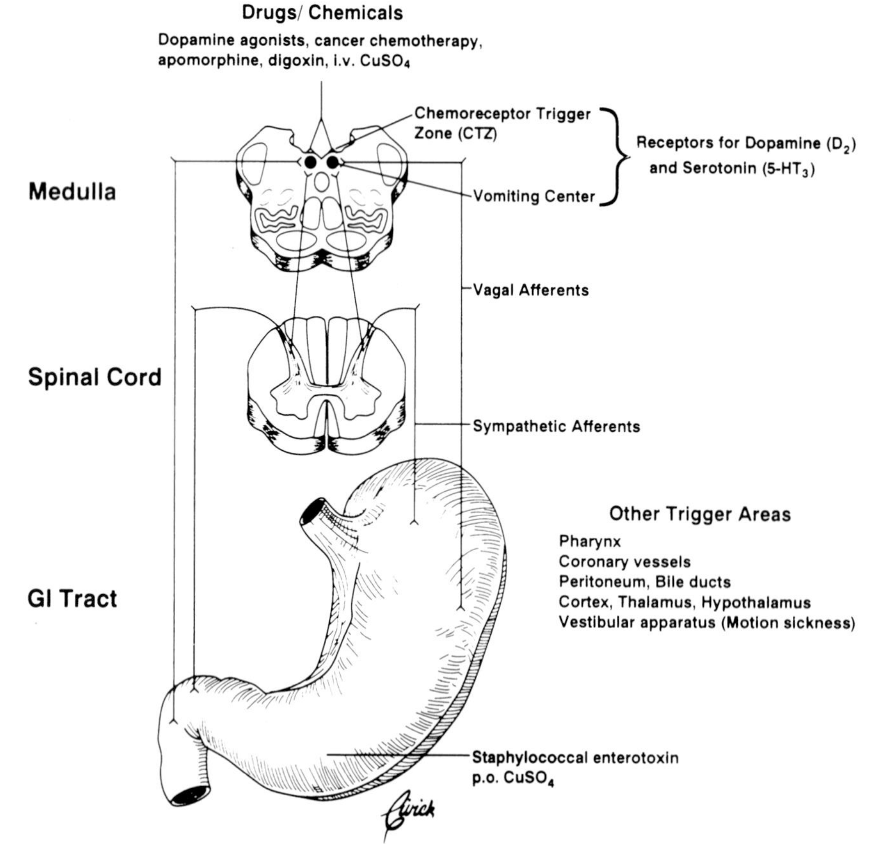

Figure 8–1. A schematic of the proposed neural pathways that mediate vomiting. GI, gastrointestinal; 5-HT, 5-hydroxytryptamine; i.v., intravenous; p.o., per os (orally).

from the gastrointestinal tract, the vomiting center can be activated by afferent impulses from the pharynx; vestibular system; heart; peritoneum; and higher central nervous system centers, such as the thalamus, hypothalamus, and cerebral cortex.

Second, other emetic stimuli can induce vomiting indirectly by stimulating the CTZ, which is located in the area postrema of the medulla in the floor of the fourth ventricle (see Fig. 8–1). For example, intravenously administered apomorphine induces vomiting by this mechanism. Although direct application of apomorphine to the area postrema causes vomiting (by acting on opiate receptors of the δ or κ subtype) in experimental animals, ablation of the area postrema or the vomiting center prevents vomiting induced by this agent.

Emetic stimuli that act on CTZ include drugs (e.g., opiates, digitalis, ergot derivatives, chemotherapy agents, emetine, salicylate, nicotine, syrup of ipecac, intravenous copper sulfate, dopamine agonists), uremia, hypoxia, diabetic ketoacidosis, enterotoxin derived from gram-positive bacteria, radiation sickness, and motion sickness.[12–14]

Although the exact neurotransmitters that are released in the CTZ and vomiting center are not known, there is strong evidence that dopamine, acting via dopamine (D_2) receptors, plays a role in mediating vomiting.[11, 12] Thus, dopamine D_2-receptor agonists, such as apomorphine, levodopa, and bromocriptine, commonly cause nausea and vomiting, whereas dopamine D_2-receptor antagonists, such as metoclopramide, domperidone, and haloperidol, are effective antiemetics.[12] In addition to dopamine, recent studies have identified numerous neurotransmitters, neuropeptides, and receptors for these ligands in mammalian CTZ. In experimental animals, serotonin, norepinephrine, glutamine, and histamine cause emesis when applied ionophoretically to the CTZ, whereas acetylcholine fails to elicit an emetic response.[11, 12]

The discovery of serotonin (5-hydroxytryptamine [5-HT]) and its receptors, specifically the 5-HT_3 receptors, in the CTZ and area postrema, as well as in the gastrointestinal tract, has led to the development of orally administered 5-HT_3 receptor antagonists, such as ondansetron and granisetron, which are effective in preventing nausea and vomiting induced by chemotherapy agents.[12, 13] Moreover, angiotensin II, neurotensin, thyrotropin-releasing hormone, vasoactive intestinal peptide, gastrin, substance P, vasopressin, and leucine-enkephalin (an opiate agonist) also induce emesis, whereas somatostatin and cholecystokinin do not.[11, 12] There is also a correlation between a neurotransmitter's ability to induce emesis and its ability to induce an increase in intracellular cyclic adenosine monophosphate level in the CTZ.[11] These findings suggest that the neurons in the CTZ contain a wide variety of receptors to enable them to respond to various chemical stimuli, endogenous neurotransmitters, and neuropeptides.

Regardless of the emetic stimulus or the mechanism by which the vomiting center is activated, the act of vomiting is initiated from the vomiting center, and efferent pathways are mainly somatic, involving the vagus, the phrenic nerves, and the spinal nerves that supply the abdominal musculature. In experimental animals, vomiting can be induced in decerebrate animals, indicating that the vomiting reflex can occur in the absence of higher cortical influences.[15]

CLINICAL APPROACH TO PATIENTS WITH NAUSEA AND VOMITING

An algorithm showing the clinical approach to patients with nausea and/or vomiting is depicted in Figure 8–2. The clinical evaluation of patients with nausea and vomiting should begin with a thorough history. Attention to the following historical aspects and characteristics of the emetic episodes facilitates differential diagnosis.[1] (See Table 8–1 for a list of differential diagnoses of nausea and vomiting in adults.)

Duration of Symptoms

Acute nausea and vomiting are usually associated with acute infection (especially of the gastrointestinal tract), ingestion of toxins (food poisoning) or a new medication, pregnancy, head trauma, or visceral pain (secondary to acute gastrointestinal obstruction, inflammation, or ischemia). On the other hand, chronic nausea and vomiting suggest partial mechanical obstruction of the gastrointestinal tract, intracranial pathology (e.g., brain tumor), motility disturbance (e.g., gastroparesis [see Chapter 37]), metabolic or endocrine etiology (see Chapter 29), or a psychogenic disturbance (see Chapter 122).

Some patients complain of chronic nausea without retching or vomiting; it is persistent or frequently recurrent over a period of months or even years. Workup of this complaint rarely, if ever, reveals a discernible organic basis, although often its onset may be dated to a particular illness in the past for which there is no evidence of organic residuum. Nausea may also be part of the symptom complex of dyspepsia (see Chapter 7). These patients, without a readily diagnosable cause for their chronic complaint, often have problems in the psychosocial aspects of their lives and must be approached as outlined in Chapter 122.

Timing of Vomiting in Relation to Meals

Vomiting during or soon after a meal is common in patients with psychogenic vomiting and occasionally occurs in pa-

Table 8–1 | **Differential Diagnosis of Nausea and Vomiting in Adults**

CAUSE	EXAMPLES
Drugs	Chemotherapy agents, antibiotics, digoxin, theophylline, alcohol
Gastrointestinal infections	Gastroenteritis, epidemic vomiting, food poisoning
Other gastrointestinal disorders	Peptic ulcer disease, gastroparesis, bowel obstruction, cholecystitis, hepatitis, pancreatitis, radiation sickness, appendicitis
Endocrine disorders	Diabetes, thyrotoxicosis, adrenal insufficiency
Central nervous system	Motion sickness, increased intracranial pressure, epilepsy, head trauma, vestibular disorders, meningitis
Psychogenic causes	Psychogenic vomiting and related disorders
Systemic illness	Myocardial infarction, renal failure, asthma, sepsis, electrolyte imbalance
Specific syndromes	Cyclic vomiting syndrome, postoperative nausea and vomiting, rumination
Miscellaneous	Pregnancy

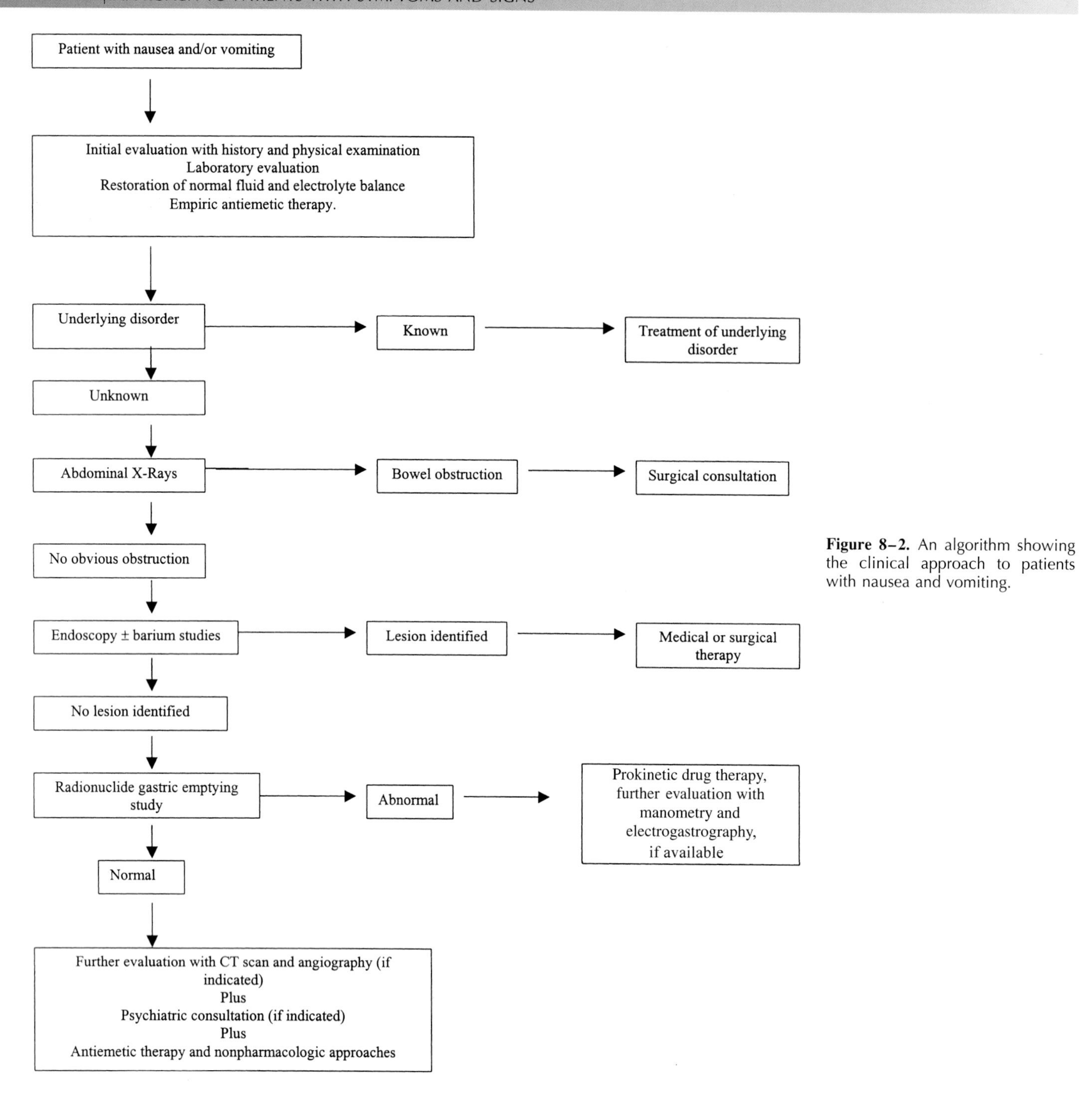

Figure 8–2. An algorithm showing the clinical approach to patients with nausea and vomiting.

tients with peptic ulcer near the pyloric channel, presumably because of pyloric irritability, edema, and spasm. Delayed vomiting (more than 1 hour after eating), especially if it occurs repeatedly, is characteristic of gastric outlet obstruction or a motility disorder of the stomach, such as diabetic or postvagotomy gastroparesis. Vomiting of material eaten 12 hours earlier is rarely, if ever, seen in patients with psychogenic vomiting and is strong evidence for gastric outlet obstruction or atony. Patients with this history often have a succussion splash over the stomach (see Chapter 40). Nausea and vomiting in the early morning, before eating, are characteristic of nausea and vomiting of pregnancy (morning sickness) and may also be seen in postgastrectomy patients with bilious vomiting as well as in individuals with uremia, alcoholism, postnasal drip, and increased intracranial pressure and in those whose symptoms have a psychogenic basis.

Relief of Pain by Vomiting

Vomiting often relieves pain due to peptic ulcer disease, occasionally due to small bowel obstruction or intestinal pseudo-obstruction, but not pain caused by pancreatitis or biliary tract disease (see Chapters 40, 48, 49, 55, 109, and 111).

Projectile Vomiting

Some use the term *projectile vomiting* to describe vomitus that is ejected forcefully from the mouth, whereas others define it as vomiting that occurs at the peak of maximum inspiration without the rhythmic hyperactivity of the respiratory muscles noted with retching. Used in the latter sense, it may be contrasted with the "dry heaves" characterized by repeated violent and explosive rhythmic respiratory activity, leading to fatigue but to little or no vomitus. The vomiting associated with raised intracranial pressure is often referred to as projectile, is said to occur without nausea or retching, and may be precipitated by exertion or stooping. However, projectile vomiting is not a specific or sensitive indicator of intracranial hypertension.

Content of the Vomitus

The significance of old food in the vomitus suggests gastric outlet obstruction, high small bowel obstruction, or a gastric motor disorder (gastroparesis). Vomiting of undigested food suggests the possibility that the "vomitus" is from the esophagus (e.g., in achalasia), from an esophageal or pharyngeal (Zenker's) diverticulum, or from the stomach if food was eaten within 20 minutes or so of the emesis. Blood or "coffee grounds" in vomitus (hematemesis) is of obvious importance (see Chapter 13). The presence of bile indicates an open connection between the proximal duodenum and stomach and generally excludes gastric outlet or proximal duodenal obstruction. Bilious vomiting is common after gastric surgery and is discussed in Chapter 42.

Odor of Vomitus

A feculent odor of vomitus suggests intestinal obstruction, peritonitis with ileus, gastrocolic fistula, ischemic injury to the gut, or long-standing gastric outlet obstruction or stasis with secondary bacterial overgrowth of the stomach. Occasionally, feculent vomiting is seen in patients with bacterial overgrowth in the proximal small bowel.

System Review, Physical Examination, and Laboratory Data

Fever, weight loss, menstrual irregularity, history of prior abdominal surgery, jaundice, headache, chest pain, and many other factors may be helpful clues in making the diagnosis.

The physical examination should be directed toward assessing the severity of the problem, as well as uncovering additional clues for the cause of the problem. Weight loss and dehydration should be documented. Abdominal examination should focus on the presence or absence of tenderness, bowel sounds, masses, succussion splash, hernia, prior surgical procedures, and stool testing for occult blood.

Finally, the choice of laboratory studies should be directed by the history and physical examination (see Fig. 8–2). Blood chemistry may reveal metabolic disturbance (usually hypokalemic, hypochloremic metabolic alkalosis), whereas flat radiographs of the abdomen may reveal mechanical obstruction. Upper gastrointestinal series or endoscopy is particularly helpful in making the diagnosis when the history and physical examination suggest that peptic ulcer disease or gastric outlet obstruction is likely. In patients with chronic nausea and vomiting who have a normal upper gastrointestinal series and endoscopy, further evaluation with a radionuclide gastric emptying study, electrogastrography, and gastrointestinal manometry should be considered[16] (see Chapter 37). In patients who have normal gastric emptying and motility studies, further evaluation with ultrasonography, computed tomography, and angiography, as well as psychiatric consultation, should be considered.

SPECIFIC SYNDROMES ASSOCIATED WITH VOMITING

Drug-Induced Nausea and Vomiting

Drugs are one of the more common causes of nausea and vomiting. As discussed already, many drugs act on the CTZ in the area postrema to induce nausea and vomiting. The major offenders in this regard are dopamine agonists (e.g., L-dopa, bromocriptine), opiate analgesics, digitalis preparations, and cancer chemotherapy agents (e.g., cisplatin).[11–13] Some drugs such as aspirin and nonsteroidal anti-inflammatory agents may induce nausea and vomiting by damaging the gastric mucosa and activating the vomiting center via ascending reflexes from the stomach. Although alcohol might induce vomiting by the same mechanism (alcoholic gastropathy), available data suggest that alcohol also may act centrally on the CTZ.[17] Before embarking on an expensive and possibly invasive workup of the patient with vomiting, the physician should elicit a careful and thorough drug history, including the use of nonprescription drugs and alcohol.

Nausea and vomiting are common in cancer patients, especially those who are terminally ill, and this can be exacerbated by cancer chemotherapy agents. Although many such agents are thought to act directly on the CTZ to induce nausea and vomiting, nausea and vomiting are usually delayed for 2 to 6 hours, and sometimes for more than 24 hours, after these agents are given, suggesting that these drugs may not act directly on the CTZ.[11, 12] Chemotherapy agents, such as cisplatin, release large amounts of serotonin from the intestine, which activates the vomiting center via vagal afferents. Chemotherapy agents may also release serotonin in the CTZ, activating 5-HT_3 receptors. Moreover, it has been suggested that susceptibility to chemotherapy-related nausea and vomiting can be predicted if the patient has a history of motion sickness.[18] A learned anticipatory nausea and vomiting syndrome may also occur in cancer patients who receive chemotherapy[19]; this psychological reaction can be treated in many instances by behavioral modification techniques.[20, 21]

Motion Sickness

Motion sickness is a common syndrome that can occur in an automobile ("car sickness"), in an airplane ("air sickness"), at sea ("sea sickness"), or even in outer space. As with drug-induced vomiting, motion sickness is readily diagnosed by history. Symptoms and signs often preceding vomiting in motion sickness include nausea, epigastric discomfort, pallor, cold sweating, headache, and hypersalivation.

In motion sickness, activation of the vestibular system leads to neural activation of the vomiting center.[14, 22] In a study using electrogastrography to evaluate gastric electrical activity in 15 subjects during experimentally induced motion sickness, 10 of the subjects developed symptoms of motion sickness and a change in gastric electrical slow-wave activity from the normal rate of 3 per minute to 4 to 9 per minute ("tachygastria").[23] The other 5 subjects did not develop motion sickness or electrogastrographic changes.[23] In healthy volunteers, the central cholinergic and α-adrenergic pathways mediate vection-evoked dysrhythmias.[24] Moreover, experimentally induced motion sickness is associated with increases in plasma vasopressin levels.[25] These findings suggest that vestibular stimulation with resultant activation of the vomiting center (and perhaps the CTZ) can secondarily affect gastric motor function. Vestibular disorders other than motion sickness (e.g., labyrinthitis, Meniere's disease) are also associated with nausea and vomiting.

Epidemic Infectious Vomiting

Epidemic infectious vomiting has many synonyms, including acute infectious nonbacterial gastroenteritis, epidemic nausea and vomiting, winter vomiting disease, and epidemic collapse. The disease is characterized by sudden and explosive outbreaks of profuse vomiting often beginning in the early hours of the morning. The urge to vomit is so intense that vomiting often occurs before the patient can get out of bed. Headache, giddiness, muscular pains, sweating, and feverishness may also occur. Diarrhea may be a feature of some outbreaks but not of the majority.

Immune electron microscopy has permitted detection of viral particles in the stool of a large percentage of patients in a given epidemic. These viruses include rotaviruses,[26] echovirus,[27] the Norwalk agent, enteric adenovirus, the Snow Mountain agent, the Hawaii agent, and human reovirus-like agent. Infection occurs in the small bowel, not the stomach. Gastric emptying may be abnormally slow during the acute phase of the illness.[28] Rapid recovery is the rule, although the disorder may last up to 10 days and relapses may occur for up to 3 weeks (see Chapter 96).

Food poisoning may cause a similar acute vomiting syndrome of epidemic proportions. In these cases, a careful history is helpful in documenting the source of contamination and the short incubation period (usually 6 to 12 hours). Organisms involved include *Staphylococcus aureus, Clostridium perfringens,* and *Bacillus cereus.*[29] Jamaican vomiting sickness is caused by ingestion of the unripe akee fruit[30] (see Chapter 96).

Cyclical Vomiting Syndrome

Cyclical vomiting syndrome is characterized by recurring attacks of severe vomiting.[31, 32] Vomiting may recur at regular intervals. Attacks may be associated with headache, abdominal pain, and fever. The onset is usually sudden, and the attack may last several hours or for up to 10 days. Recovery is usually spontaneous, although the disease can threaten life by producing profound dehydration and alkalosis. Between attacks patients are asymptomatic. The onset of the disease is usually between the ages of 3 and 7, and the episodes may end at puberty or persist into young adulthood. In some cases, episodes may begin after puberty in teenagers or young adults.[32] The frequency of attacks varies from more than one a month to three per year.

The diagnosis can usually be made from the history if numerous episodes of vomiting have occurred in the past. Radiographic studies of the gastrointestinal tract as well as careful neurologic evaluation (including computed tomography or magnetic resonance imaging) will rule out most organic lesions that may produce recurrent vomiting, such as malrotation of the midgut and intracranial tumors. It is important to reach a diagnosis early so as to avoid unnecessary surgery, such as laparotomy, which will only add to the confusion when future attacks of vomiting occur (e.g., possibility of adhesions). Recent open label studies suggest that propranolol, tricyclic antidepressants, and erythromycin are effective prophylactic agents, whereas sumatriptan and ondansetron can abort an emetic attack if taken at the onset of symptoms.[31, 32] Successful management involves a responsive, collaborative physician-patient relationship, stress management, appropriate use of various prophylactic and abortive agents mentioned earlier, and treatment of complications.[31]

Vomiting in Infants and Children

Vomiting is one of the most common problems encountered in infants and children. It may indicate anything from a minor feeding upset or a milk allergy to intestinal obstruction, and it can be a symptom of almost any disease system. A normal baby may vomit small amounts of food during or just after a meal; this may be associated with regurgitation of milk or food. Posture has a marked effect on the tendency of a baby to vomit after a meal. In the supine position, the fundus and cardia are dependent and food accumulates there, tending to result in regurgitation. In the prone position or on the right side, food tends not to regurgitate because it accumulates in the antrum. In these positions, gas rises to the cardia and burping tends to occur without food. The best way to hold the baby who regurgitates or vomits is in the right antero-oblique position.

Loss of weight, failure to gain weight, presence of bile in the vomitus, and abdominal distention in association with vomiting or regurgitation are abnormal, and their presence demands a thorough evaluation. Various congenital lesions that are incompatible with life (e.g., hypertrophic pyloric stenosis) do not necessarily give symptoms immediately after birth. A diagnosis of pneumonia, vomiting caused by feeding difficulty, gastroenteritis, or "failure to thrive" in the first week of life may well be in error, with the symptoms caused in fact by congenital defects.

If the vomiting has any suspicious features, including persistence, it is important to inquire about the passage of meconium, to perform a rectal examination, and to look carefully for evidence of abdominal distention. Repeated physical examinations are necessary to make the correct di-

Table 8–2 | **Some Serious Causes of Vomiting in Children**

CAUSE	COMMENTS
Newborn	
Tracheoesophageal fistula	Hypersalivation; cyanosis and choking with meals; abdominal distention often present
Hypertrophic pyloric stenosis	Male predominance; symptom onset before age 7 weeks but not immediately after birth; absence of bile in vomitus; palpable "olive" seldom present; high serum gastrin concentration
Duodenal atresia	Air-fluid levels in stomach and duodenum ("double-bubble")
Intestinal atresia, stenosis, diaphragms	May produce vomiting in utero with bile-stained amniotic fluid
Meconium ileus	May signify cystic fibrosis
Midgut volvulus with malrotation	Intermittent vomiting
Necrotizing enterocolitis	More common in the premature infant but can occur in full-term neonate; pneumatosis intestinalis noted on kidney-ureter-bladder film; bloody stools and thrombocytopenia may be only other findings
Intracranial hemorrhage	More common in the premature infant or child with a difficult delivery; head ultrasonogram showing blood in the ventricle may be diagnostic
Hirschsprung's disease	Delayed passage of meconium noted; absence of rectal air on a prone abdominal radiograph may be useful sign
Miscellaneous	Improper feeding; sepsis, including meningitis; adrenal insufficiency; narcotic addiction; inherited and metabolic disorders (e.g., galactosemia)
Infancy and Childhood*	
Intussusception	"Currant jelly" stool; mass; colicky pain
Appendicitis	See Chapter 107
Gastroesophageal reflux	Respiratory symptoms may be prominent; weight loss; may be associated with antral dysmotility
Reye's syndrome	Encephalopathy and microvascular steatosis of liver; association with viruses (e.g., influenza) and aspirin
Poisonings	Ipecac, alkali, theophylline, digoxin
Pancreatitis	Likely underdiagnosed in children; may be caused by a virus, cholelithiasis, or trauma
Subdural hematoma	May be related to child abuse or obvious head trauma
Esophageal foreign body	May be radiopaque
Miscellaneous	Peptic ulcer; pneumonia; viral hepatitis; intracranial tumors; cystic fibrosis; inherited and metabolic disorders (e.g., fructose intolerance)

*Although most anatomic abnormalities are manifested in early infancy, intestinal stenosis, diaphragms, malrotation with Ladd's bands or volvulus, and Hirschsprung's disease may become manifest in infancy and childhood without a significant neonatal history.

agnosis and to prevent a potentially fatal outcome. Radiographs of the abdomen and in some cases of the gastrointestinal tract are often of great value. Some of the serious causes of vomiting at different ages are listed in Table 8–2.

Nausea and Vomiting During Pregnancy

Nausea occurs in 50% to 90% of all pregnancies and vomiting in 25% to 55%.[33, 34] The onset is usually shortly after the first missed menstrual period (rarely before), and thus symptoms may begin before the woman or her physician recognizes that pregnancy has occurred. Although nausea and vomiting may rarely be caused by gallbladder disease or hepatitis, in most women the etiology is unknown. Nausea and vomiting may be more common in primigravida women, younger women, nonsmokers, obese women, women with less than 12 years of education, women who had experienced nausea and vomiting while receiving oral contraceptive medication, and women with a corpus luteum primarily on the right side of the uterus rather than on the left side.[33–35] Nausea, sometimes accompanied by vomiting, is especially prevalent in the morning, although in some cases these symptoms occur at any time of the day. The term *nausea and vomiting of pregnancy* implies that the woman has not developed fluid and electrolyte derangements or nutritional deficiency. The term *hyperemesis gravidarum* should be used if these complications are present (see later discussion).

Nausea and vomiting during early pregnancy are often associated with sleep disturbances, fatigue, and irritability. Symptoms usually disappear by the fourth month of pregnancy, although in some cases, especially those with psychological or psychiatric problems, the symptoms may persist into the third trimester.[33, 34] Women who have nausea and vomiting during a particular pregnancy are more likely to have these symptoms during subsequent pregnancies, but such recurrent symptoms are not invariable. Fetuses born to mothers with nausea and vomiting of pregnancy have birth weights similar to fetuses born to mothers without these symptoms. Furthermore, the incidence of fetal death is actually lower than normal in mothers with nausea and vomiting of pregnancy.[36] There is no evidence that the offspring of women who have nausea and vomiting of pregnancy have an increased incidence of congenital malformations.[36] Thus, the prognosis for mother and child is generally excellent.

The pathogenesis of nausea and vomiting of pregnancy is obscure. There are two leading theories: hormonal and psychological.[33, 34] Although abnormal serum levels of human chorionic gonadotropin (HCG), progesterone, and androgens have been reported in emetic subjects, results have not been consistent from study to study.[33] Psychological studies suggest that women with nausea and vomiting of pregnancy are more likely to have had an undesired pregnancy and have negative relationships with their mothers.[34] Electrogastrographic studies reveal that women with nausea and vomiting of pregnancy have more unstable electrical activities and a reduced response to food ingestion.[37] How these findings relate to nausea and vomiting is unclear.

Treatment of nausea and vomiting of pregnancy consists primarily of reassurance that the condition is quite common and temporary along with in-office supportive psychotherapy if indicated. It may be necessary to prescribe an antiemetic drug (see later discussion) if simple home remedies (e.g., drinking milk, chewing gum, or eating crackers) fail to provide relief.

HYPEREMESIS GRAVIDARUM. Hyperemesis gravidarum, also called *pernicious vomiting of pregnancy,* refers to those patients who develop fluid and electrolyte disturbances or nutritional deficiency from intractable vomiting in early pregnancy.[38, 39] As in milder cases, the onset of symptoms tends to be soon after the first missed menstrual period. Typically the vomiting disappears during the third month and rarely persists into the fourth month.[38] The reported incidence of hyperemesis gravidarum varies considerably, with an average figure of 3.5 per 1000 deliveries. The incidence is not increased by parity, race, color, or the desire for an abortion but is markedly decreased during wartime. Patients with hyperemesis gravidarum do not have an increased incidence of toxemia of pregnancy or spontaneous abortion, and their babies are not underweight or deformed.[38]

Women with twins or with molar pregnancy (hydatidiform mole) have an increased incidence of hyperemesis gravidarum. These women have elevated concentrations of HCG.[38] However, the relationship between elevated HCG and hyperemesis has not been convincingly demonstrated. Abnormalities of thyroid function tests are also common in hyperemesis gravidarum,[38] although their significance is uncertain. Because hyperthyroidism can cause vomiting per se, including during pregnancy, these observations are intriguing and deserve further study. Finally, there is still controversy about the nature of and importance of psychological derangements in the pathogenesis of this syndrome.[38]

The metabolic consequences of hyperemesis gravidarum can be severe, and the mortality rate in untreated patients is high. Salt and water depletion and potassium deficiency may be marked. Treatment of hyperemesis gravidarum is mainly directed at fluid and electrolyte replacement and supportive psychotherapy. Behavior modification techniques may also be effective.[38, 39]

ACUTE FATTY LIVER OF LATE PREGNANCY. This is a serious condition of unknown etiology, occurring in approximately 1 in 13,000 deliveries.[40] Symptoms of nausea, vomiting, headache, and malaise begin in the third trimester, usually around week 35. Features of the preeclampsia syndrome (hypertension, edema, proteinuria) may also be present. The disease often progresses to hepatic failure complicated by disseminated intravascular coagulation. If nausea and vomiting begin in the latter part of pregnancy, serum aminotransferase activity should be measured. An elevated aminotransferase level, usually 200 to 500 U/L, is an indication for liver biopsy (assuming coagulation tests permit). The characteristic finding on biopsy is microvesicular fat. Once this diagnosis is established, pregnancy termination is indicated to prevent maternal and fetal death. Differential diagnosis includes fulminant viral hepatitis and tetracycline hepatotoxicity (see Chapter 74).

Superior Mesenteric Artery Syndrome

The superior mesenteric artery (SMA) branches off the aorta at an acute angle and, traveling in the root of the mesentery, crosses over the duodenum, usually just to the right of the midline. In rare instances, the SMA may obstruct the duodenum as it crosses over it, possibly because of a more acute angle than normal between the aorta and SMA, leading to dilation of the proximal duodenum and stomach.[41–43]

Symptoms attributed to this condition include epigastric fullness and bloating after meals, bilious vomiting, and midabdominal "crampy" pain that may be relieved by the prone or knee-chest position.[41, 42] Precipitating factors include prolonged bed rest, weight loss, previous abdominal surgery, increased lordosis (including use of body casts), and loss of tone in the abdominal wall musculature. The syndrome has been reported in conjunction with pancreatitis, peptic ulcer, and other intra-abdominal inflammatory conditions. SMA syndrome with consequent megaduodenum must be differentiated from other disorders causing similar duodenal dilation, including diabetes mellitus, systemic lupus erythematosus, scleroderma, myxedema, amyloidosis, myotonic dystrophy, and chronic idiopathic intestinal pseudo-obstruction.[41–43]

Once the diagnosis of SMA syndrome is considered, confirmation usually requires a radiographic study.[41] Radiographic criteria for the diagnosis of this syndrome by upper gastrointestinal series include: (1) dilated first and second portions of the duodenum; (2) abrupt compression of the duodenal mucosal folds; (3) to-and-fro movement of barium proximal to the obstruction site; (4) delay in gastroduodenal transit of 4 to 6 hours; and (5) relief of obstruction in the left lateral decubitus, prone, or knee-chest position.[41–43] A characteristic upper gastrointestinal series showing obstruction of the duodenum by the SMA is depicted in Figure 8–3. Hypotonic duodenography may reveal the obstruction

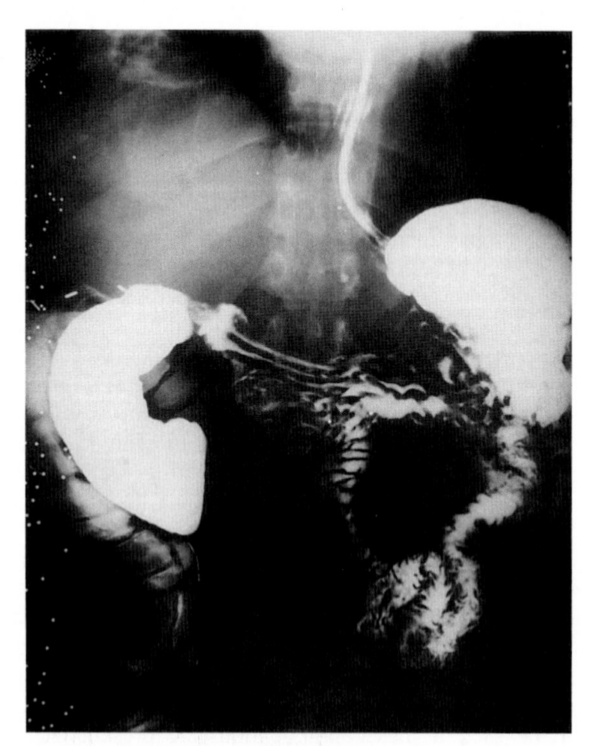

Figure 8–3. A characteristic upper gastrointestinal series showing sharp cutoff of contrast material at the third portion of the duodenum (secondary to compression by the superior mesentery artery) in a patient with the superior mesenteric artery syndrome. (Courtesy of Mark Feldman, MD.)

Table 8–3 | **Clinical Features of Psychogenic Vomiting**

- Vomiting present for years, either chronically or intermittently; history may reveal vomiting in childhood or while in high school when under emotional strain
- Family history of vomiting
- Vomiting occurs soon after the meal has begun (even after just a few bites) or just after it has been completed; delayed vomiting does not occur
- Vomiting unaccompanied by preceding nausea and may be self-induced
- Vomiting can be suppressed if necessary
- Vomiting may be of relatively little concern to the patient
- Appetite usually normal unless the patient also has a coexistent eating disorder such as anorexia nervosa and bulimia; most patients are thin, and in some, weight loss may be profound
- Vomiting may subside shortly after hospitalization

and a dilated proximal duodenum with antiperistaltic waves.[41, 43] Computed tomography represents a relatively noninvasive technique that provides an estimation of the aorta-SMA distance comparable to angiography.[43] Angiography also provides an estimation of the aortomesenteric angle and distance but is usually not necessary.[41–43] Optimal management of a patient with the SMA syndrome requires reversal or removal of the precipitating factor, decompression by nasogastric tube, and intravenous fluid and electrolyte replacement. The patient with intermittent attacks is a difficult therapeutic problem. Many surgical techniques have been employed, most often duodenojejunostomy. Gastrojejunostomy may fail because it does not adequately decompress the duodenum.

Psychogenic Vomiting

Chronic or recurrent vomiting, especially in young women, may be caused by underlying emotional disturbance.[44–46] The latter is often related to sexual and marital conflicts but may also be caused by health problems of relatives (e.g., alcoholism, aging, senility of parents), as well as by more deep-seated problems, such as loss of parental affection. Psychogenic vomiting may on rare occasions also be related to a major depression or a conversion disorder.[46] Psychogenic vomiting may be recognized by the features outlined in Table 8–3.

Although organic disease must first be ruled out by appropriate tests, the history of these patients is often so typical that the diagnosis may be strongly suspected on this basis alone. It is important that the correct diagnosis be made quickly so that the patient is not subjected to unnecessary and expensive diagnostic procedures or to abdominal surgery, which may worsen and complicate the issue. Patients with psychogenic vomiting may in time develop a second disease, and the physician should be alert for a change in the pattern of the illness.

Whether patients with psychogenic vomiting improve with antiemetic drugs has not been studied carefully. Surgery (e.g., gastroenterostomy) is of no help. It has been stated that some patients may improve with verbal catharsis and psychological support, whereas others have little insight and respond poorly to psychotherapy.[45] In one study most patients were still vomiting on follow-up approximately 1.5 years later, although to a lesser degree in many instances.[44]

Several variants of the psychogenic vomiting syndrome have been described.

SELF-INDUCED VOMITING. This is most commonly seen in young women with eating disorders such as anorexia nervosa and bulimia (see Chapter 17). These individuals may also abuse laxatives and diuretics to lose weight.[47]

CONCEALED (SURREPTITIOUS) VOMITING. One needs a high index of suspicion and some ingenuity to make and confirm this diagnosis.[48] Patients may become highly skilled in their ability to conceal vomiting. Most have no organic cause for the vomiting, although some patients with organic disease of the stomach deny vomiting, either because of secondary gain from the medical curiosity aroused by their metabolic disturbances or to prevent others from knowing of their illness. Concealed vomiting may lead to metabolic derangements, suggesting the presence of serious organic disease.

EROTIC VOMITING. In some women with underlying psychological aberrations, it has been suggested that vomiting is induced to obtain sexual gratification.[49]

Rumination

Rumination (also called *merycism*) is distinct from vomiting and consists of regurgitating food, one mouthful at a time, from the stomach to the mouth, chewing the food again, and reswallowing it.[50, 51] Regurgitation is usually involuntary, effortless, and not associated with abdominal discomfort, heartburn, or nausea. Rumination usually begins 15 to 30 minutes after a meal and lasts for about 1 hour. During this period, the patient ruminates up to 20 times. Rumination characteristically ceases when the food becomes acid to taste. It is apparently a pleasant sensation, but often embarrassing, so that patients tend to hide the fact that they reswallow their food. Rumination can be suppressed voluntarily, at least in some instances.

The cause and mechanism of rumination in adults are unknown, although almost all authors conclude that psychological factors are important.[50, 51] Recent manometric studies have demonstrated that esophageal, gastric, and upper small intestinal motility are normal.[52–54] Associated with regurgitation are spike waves corresponding to increases in intra-abdominal pressure and transient relaxation of lower esophageal sphincter.[52–54] It has been suggested that rumination is triggered by a forced inspiration against a closed glottis (Mueller maneuver).[52] Regurgitation may be associated with acid reflux, both of which may respond to biofeedback therapy.[55] Although rumination in adults is rare, it is important to be aware of this entity so that needless surgery (such as hiatal hernia repair) can be avoided.

Rumination in infants is associated with failure to thrive, marasmus, and even death, if untreated.[56, 57] Typically, previously ingested food is regurgitated and rechewed, and some is then reswallowed. The syndrome may be caused by an abnormal mother-child relationship. The mothers of these infants tend to be immature and unable to develop a close and comfortable relationship with the baby. The rumination process is interpreted as an effort to recreate the gratification of the feeding process in an emotionally deprived infant. Hospitalization often brings improvement, provided that hospital personnel can take on the role of a loving mother. Rumination is also not uncommon in mentally retarded children and may be treated successfully by various behavior modifications.[56, 57]

The differential diagnosis of rumination in infants and children includes gastroesophageal reflux, hiatal hernia, drug reaction (including drugs given to the mother), diencephalic seizures, hypothalamic tumors, milk allergy, and metabolic disorders such as fructose intolerance, as well as some of the conditions mentioned in Table 8–2.

Other Syndromes

The pathogenesis and management of idiopathic gastroparesis and nonulcer dyspepsia are discussed in Chapters 7 and 37, and the syndrome of bilious vomiting after gastric surgery is discussed in Chapter 42.

CONSEQUENCES OF VOMITING

Metabolic Derangements

Potassium deficiency results from decreased intake of potassium, from loss of potassium in the vomitus, and, most important, from renal potassium wasting due to secondary hyperaldosteronism.

Alkalosis develops because of: (1) loss of hydrogen ions in the vomitus; (2) contraction of the extracellular fluid space without a commensurate loss of extracellular bicarbonate from this compartment; (3) a shift of extracellular hydrogen ions into cells caused by cellular potassium deficiency; and (4) secondary hyperaldosteronism.

Sodium depletion develops because of loss of sodium in the vomitus and in some cases because of transient renal sodium loss in association with bicarbonate excretion (if the bicarbonate T_m* is exceeded).

Although the cause of these metabolic derangements is obvious if there is a history of vomiting, great diagnostic difficulty arises if vomiting is concealed by the patient. The differential diagnosis of unexplained hypochloremic, hypokalemic metabolic alkalosis includes concealed (surreptitious) vomiting, surreptitious diuretic use,[47] Bartter's syndrome,[58] primary hyperaldosteronism, milk-alkali syndrome, Welt's syndrome,[59] and hypokalemic periodic paralysis.

Nutritional Results

Chronic nausea and vomiting may lead to reduced caloric intake or loss of ingested calories in vomitus. Thus, regardless of etiology, nausea and vomiting may result in malnutrition and various deficiency states (see Chapter 15).

Emetic Injuries to the Esophagus and Stomach

Vomiting can lead to Mallory-Weiss lacerations and upper gastrointestinal bleeding (see Chapter 13). Vomiting can also lead to a deeper laceration involving the wall of the esophagus with a resultant confined intramural perforation or a transmural tear of the esophagus (or rarely the stomach) with free perforation (Boerhaave's syndrome). Violent vomiting can even tear the short gastric arteries and result in shock with hemoperitoneum.[60] These complications may necessitate urgent surgery and can be fatal (see Chapter 34).

Dental Disease

Chronic vomiting may result in dental erosions and caries.[61]

Purpura

Purpura, cutaneous lesions, may appear after prolonged vomiting and are acute, evanescent, pinhead-sized red macules on the face and upper neck ("mask phenomenon").[62] This eruption is probably related to a suddenly increased intrathoracic pressure.

THERAPY OF VOMITING

As shown in Figure 8–2, treatment of vomiting should begin with restoration of normal fluid and electrolyte balance. If possible, treatment of underlying disorder is warranted. When the cause of nausea and vomiting is not known or when specific treatment of the underlying disorder is not available, antiemetic agents and nonpharmacologic approaches should be employed (see later discussion).

Anticholinergic Drugs

Anticholinergic drugs (e.g., scopolamine) are effective for motion sickness.[12, 13, 63] These agents can be given as transdermal patches for prophylactic uses, and their adverse anticholinergic effects are not uncommon. Antihistamines, particularly the H_1-receptor antagonists (e.g., promethazine or meclizine) are also useful in the treatment of motion sickness and some vestibular disturbances (e.g., Meniere's disease).[12, 13, 63] For other causes of nausea and vomiting, neuroleptic agents have been shown to provide better symptomatic relief.

Neuroleptic Agents

Neuroleptic agents (e.g., prochlorperazine, chlorpromazine, and haloperidol) are effective in treating nausea and vomiting induced by drugs, radiation, or gastroenteritis.[12, 13, 63] These agents are both antihistaminic and anticholinergic, and they block dopamine D_2 receptors in CTZ and reduce afferent signals to the vomiting center. The most common side effect is sedation. Potential side effects include blood dyscrasia, jaundice, and dystonia.

Prokinetic Agents

Prokinetic agents that are useful in the treatment of nausea and vomiting include dopamine D_2-receptor antagonists, se-

*T_m, maximal tubular excretory capacity of the kidneys.

lective 5-HT_3-receptor antagonists, and motilin-receptor agonist.

Metoclopramide, a dopamine D_2-receptor antagonist, is useful in treating chemotherapy-associated emesis, gastroparesis, or pseudo-obstruction.[12, 13, 63] Its effects on the gastrointestinal tract are mediated by its central antidopaminergic effect and direct and indirect stimulation of cholinergic receptors. The use of metoclopramide is associated with numerous side effects, ranging from mild anxiety and nervousness to dystonia or tardive dyskinesia; the incidence of adverse effect is as high as 10% to 30%. Another dopamine antagonist, domperidone, which is structurally related to the phenothiazines, has therapeutic properties similar to those of metoclopramide.[64] However, domperidone does not readily cross the blood–brain barrier and causes fewer adverse effects than metoclopramide.

Selective 5-HT_3-receptor antagonists, such as ondansetron and granisetron, are effective in controlling chemotherapy-induced emesis refractory to conventional therapy with prokinetic drugs.[63, 65] The activity of these agents appears to be limited to selective inhibition of 5-HT_3 receptors in both the central nervous system and the gastrointestinal tract.[66] Adverse effects have been minimal, consisting of headache, constipation, diarrhea, and transient elevations in liver enzymes.

Erythromycin has been shown to accelerate gastric emptying in patients with diabetic gastroparesis.[67] It appears to exert its effects by interacting with motilin receptors on gastrointestinal smooth muscle membranes,[68] and this effect is unrelated to its antibiotic properties. A recent study suggests that erythromycin can also enhance gastric emptying in patients with vagotomy and antrectomy-induced gastroparesis.[69] Long-term placebo-controlled studies are needed to define the therapeutic efficacy of erythromycin in the long-term management of diabetic and nondiabetic gastroparesis.

Combinations of Drugs

Combinations of drugs are generally required to treat chemotherapy-induced emesis.[70] Most widely used combinations include phenothiazines, substituted benzamides, serotonin antagonists, benzodiazepines, adrenocorticoids, and/or cannabinoids.[65, 70] Tetrahydrocannabinol (THC), the active ingredient of marijuana, is more effective than placebo in preventing chemotherapy-induced nausea and vomiting.[63, 71] THC has been marketed as dronabinol, and its most common side effects are drowsiness, orthostatic hypotension, tachycardia, and dry mouth. Anxiety, depression, visual hallucinations, and manic psychosis may occur, especially in older individuals and patients who have never used marijuana. Although adrenocorticoids are less impressive as single agents, they are quite effective in combination with other agents, including the 5-HT_3-receptor antagonist ondansetron.[63, 65] Benzodiazepines (e.g., lorazepam) or behavior modification can be employed to reduce anticipatory nausea and vomiting that may occurs prior to chemotherapy.[20, 21] A list of cancer chemotherapy agents most likely to cause nausea (e.g., cisplatin, dacarbazine, actinomycin D) and those least likely to cause vomiting (e.g., vincristine, bleomycin, chlorambucil) has been published recently,[70] as has an algorithm for choosing antiemetic agents.[70]

Nonpharmacologic Approaches

Although drugs represent the conventional approach to the therapy of nausea and vomiting, other nonpharmacologic approaches may be efficacious in certain settings.[72] These include behavior modification treatment (e.g., in cancer chemotherapy-induced emesis[20, 21] and in idiopathic gastric stasis[73]), acupuncture or acupressure (e.g., in perioperative vomiting[72, 74]), and transcutaneous electrical nerve stimulation (e.g., in chemotherapy-induced nausea and vomiting[75]).

REFERENCES

1. Hanson JS, McCallum RW: The diagnosis and management of nausea and vomiting: A review. Am J Gastroenterol 80:210, 1985.
2. Finestone HM, Clifford JC: "Dry heaves": The sole presenting complaint in a case of ruptured abdominal aortic aneurysm. Can Med Assoc J 135:1154, 1986.
3. Melzack R, Rosberger Z, Hollingsworth ML, et al: New approaches to measuring nausea. Can Med Assoc J 133:755, 1985.
4. Johnson HD, Laws JW: The cardia in swallowing, eructation, and vomiting. Lancet 2:1268, 1966.
5. Wilson CL, Davis SJ: Recurrent atrial fibrillation with nausea and vomiting. Aviat Space Environ Med 49:624, 1978.
6. Lyon LJ, Nevins MA: Retching and termination of ventricular tachycardia. Chest 74:110, 1978.
7. Borison HL, Borison R, McCarthy LE: Role of the area postrema in vomiting and related functions. Fed Proc 43:2955, 1984.
8. Borison HL, Wang SC: Physiology and pharmacology of vomiting. Pharmacol Rev 5:193, 1953.
9. Baker PCH, Bernat JL: The neuroanatomy of vomiting in man: Association of projectile vomiting with a solitary metastasis in the lateral tegmentum of the pons and the middle cerebellar peduncle. J Neurol Neurosurg Psychiatry 48:1165, 1985.
10. Miller AD: Neuroanatomy and physiology. In Sleisenger MH (ed): The Handbook of Nausea and Vomiting. New York, Parthenon, 1993, pp 1–9.
11. Carpenter DO: Neural mechanisms of emesis. Can J Physiol Pharmacol 68:230, 1990.
12. Kovac AL: Prevention and treatment of postoperative nausea and vomiting. Drugs 59:213, 2000.
13. Haynes GR, Bailey MK: Postoperative nausea and vomiting: Review and clinical approaches. South Med J 89:940, 1996.
14. Rates BJ, Miller AD, Laced JS: Physiological basis and pharmacology of motion sickness: An update. Brain Res Bull 47:395, 1998.
15. McCarthy LE, Borison HL, Spiegel MK, et al: Vomiting: Radiographic and oscillographic correlates in the decerebrate cat. Gastroenterology 67:1126, 1974.
16. Verhagen MAMT, Samsom M, Jebbink RJA, et al: Clinical relevance of antroduodenal manometry. Eur J Gastroenterol Hepatol 11:523, 1999.
17. Shen WW: Potential link between hallucination and nausea/vomiting induced by alcohol? Psychopathology 18:212, 1985.
18. Golding JF: Motion sickness susceptibility questionnaire revised and its relationship to other forms of sickness. Brain Res Bull 47:507, 1998.
19. Redd WH, Dadds MR, Futterman AD, et al: Nausea induced by mental images of chemotherapy. Cancer 72:629, 1993.
20. Morrow GR, Morrell C: Behavioral treatment for the anticipatory nausea and vomiting induced by cancer chemotherapy. N Engl J Med 307:1476, 1982.
21. Genuis ML: The use of hypnosis in helping cancer patients control anxiety, pain, and emesis: A review of recent empirical studies. Am J Clin Hypn 37:4, 1995.
22. Takeda N, Morita M, Hasegawa S, et al: Neuropharmacology of motion sickness and emesis. Acta Otolaryngol Suppl (Stockh) 501:10, 1993.
23. Stern RM, Koch KL, Stewart WR, et al: Spectral analysis of tachygastria recorded during motion sickness. Gastroenterology 92:92, 1987.
24. Hasler W, Kim MS, Chey WD, et al: Central cholinergic and α-adrengeric mediation of gastric slow-wave dysrhythmias evoked during motion sickness. Am J Physiol 268:G539, 1995.

25. Koch KL, Summy-Long J, Bingaman S, et al: Vasopressin and oxytocin responses to illusory self-motion and nausea in man. J Clin Endocrinol Metab 71:1269, 1990.
26. Lieberman JM: Rotavirus and other viral causes of gastroenteritis. Pediatr Ann 23:529, 1994.
27. Kee F, McElroy G, Stewart D, et al: A community outbreak of echovirus infection associated with an outdoor swimming pool. J Public Health Med 16:145, 1994.
28. Meeroff JC, Schreiber DS, Trier JS, et al: Abnormal gastric motor function in viral gastroenteritis. Ann Intern Med 92:370, 1980.
29. Guerrant RL, Bobak DA: Bacterial and protozoal gastroenteritis. N Engl J Med 325:327, 1991.
30. Larson J, Vender R, Camuto P: Cholestatic jaundice due to akee fruit poisoning. Am J Gastroenterol 89:1577, 1994.
31. Li BUK, Fleisher DR: Cyclic vomiting syndrome. Dig Dis Sci 44(suppl):13S, 1999.
32. Prakash C, Clouse RE: Cyclic vomiting syndrome in adults: Clinical features and response to tricyclic antidepressants. Am J Gastroenterol 94:2855, 1999.
33. Baron T, Ramirez B, Richter JE: Gastrointestinal motility disorders during pregnancy. Ann Intern Med 118:366, 1993.
34. Deuchar N: Nausea and vomiting in pregnancy: A review of the problem with particular regard to psychological and social aspects. Br J Obstet Gynecol 102:6, 1995.
35. Samsioe G, Crona N, Enk L, et al: Does position and size of corpus luteum have any effect on nausea of pregnancy? Acta Obstet Gynecol Scand 65:427, 1986.
36. Weigel MM, Weigel RM: Nausea and vomiting of early pregnancy and pregnancy outcome: An epidemiological study. Br J Obstet Gynecol 96: 1304, 1989.
37. Riezzo G, Pezzolla F, Darconza G, et al: Gastric myoelectrical activity in the first trimester of pregnancy: A cutaneous electrogastrographic study. Am J Gastroenterol 87:702, 1992.
38. Abell TL, Riely CA: Hyperemesis gravidarum. Gastroenterol Clin North Am 21:835, 1992.
39. van Stuijvenberg ME, Schabort I, Labadarios D, et al: The nutritional status and treatment of patients with hyperemesis gravidarum. Am J Obstet Gynecol 172:1585, 1995.
40. Jwayyed SM, Blanda M, Kubina M: Acute fatty liver of pregnancy. J Emerg Med 17:673, 1999.
41. Wilson-Storey D, MacKinlay GA: The superior mesenteric artery syndrome. J R Coll Surg Edinb 31:175, 1986.
42. Hines JR, Gore RM, Ballantyne GH: Superior mesenteric artery syndrome: Diagnostic criteria and therapeutic approaches. Am J Surg 148: 630, 1984.
43. Barnes JS, Lee M: Superior mesenteric artery syndrome in an intravenous drug abuser after rapid weight loss. South Med J 89:331, 1996.
44. Rosenthal RH, Webb WL, Wruble LD: Diagnosis and management of persistent psychogenic vomiting. Psychosomatics 21:722, 1980.
45. Wruble LD, Rosenthal RH, Webb WL: Psychogenic vomiting: A review. Am J Gastroenterol 77:318, 1982.
46. Muraska M, Mine K, Matsumoto K, et al: Psychogenic vomiting: The relation between patterns of vomiting and psychiatric diagnosis. Gut 31: 526, 1990.
47. Killen JD, Taylor CB, Telch MJ, et al: Self-induced vomiting and laxative and diuretic use among teenagers: Precursors of the binge-purge syndrome? JAMA 255:1447, 1986.
48. Santangelo WC, Richey JE, Rivera L, et al: Surreptitious ipecac administration simulating intestinal pseudo-obstruction. Ann Intern Med 110: 1031, 1989.
49. Stoller RJ: Erotic vomiting. Arch Sex Behav 11:361, 1982.
50. Amarnath RP, Abell TL, Malagelada JR: The rumination syndrome in adults. Ann Intern Med 105:513, 1986.
51. O'Brien MD, Bruce BK, Camilleri M: The rumination syndrome: Clinical features rather than manometric diagnosis. Gastroenterology 108: 1024, 1995.
52. Reynolds RPE, Lloyd DA: Manometric study of a ruminator. J Clin Gastroenterol 8:127, 1986.
53. Smout AJPM, Breumelhof R: Voluntary induction of transient lower esophageal sphincter relaxation in an adult patient with the rumination syndrome. Am J Gastroenterol 85:1621, 1990.
54. Breumelhof R, Smout AJPM, Depla ACTM: The rumination syndrome in an adult patient. J Clin Gastroenterol 12:232, 1990.
55. Shay SS, Johnson LF, Wong RKH, et al: Rumination, heartburn, and daytime gastroesophageal reflux: A case study with mechanisms defined and success fully treated with biofeedback therapy. J Clin Gastroenterol 8:115, 1986.
56. Singh NN, Manning PJ, Angell MJ: Effects of an oral hygiene punishment procedure on chronic rumination and collateral behaviors in monozygous twins. J Appl Behav Anal 15:309, 1982.
57. Daniel WH: Management of chronic rumination with a contingent exercise procedure employing topographically dissimilar behavior. J Behav Exp Psychiatry 13:149, 1982.
58. Veldhuis JD, Bardin OW, Demers LM: Metabolic mimicry of Bartter's syndrome by covert vomiting: Utility of urinary chloride determinations. Am J Med 66:361, 1979.
59. Gitelman HJ, Graham JB, Welt LG: A new familial disorder characterized by hypokalemia and hypomagnesemia. Trans Assoc Am Physicians 79:221, 1966.
60. Hayes N, Waterworth PD, Griffin SM: Avulsion of short gastric arteries caused by vomiting. Gut 35:1137, 1994.
61. Kleier DJ, Aragon SB, Averbach RE: Dental management of the chronic vomiting patient. J Am Dent Assoc 108:618, 1984.
62. Alcalay J, Ingber A, Sandbank M: Mask phenomenon: Postemesis facial purpura. Cutis 38:28, 1986.
63. Wadibia EC: Antiemetics. South Med J 92:162, 1999.
64. Barone JA: Domperidone: A peripherally acting dopamine$_2$-receptor antagonist. Ann Pharmacother 33:429, 1999.
65. The Italian Group for Antiemetic Research: Dexamethasone alone or in combination with ondansetron for the prevention of delayed nausea and vomiting induced by chemotherapy. N Engl J Med 342:1554, 2000.
66. Read NW, Gwee KA: The importance of 5-hydroxytryptamine receptors in the gut. Pharmacol Ther 62:159, 1994.
67. Janssens J, Peeters TL, Vantrappen G, et al: Improvement of gastric emptying in diabetic gastroparesis by erythromycin. N Engl J Med 322: 1028, 1990.
68. Peeters T, Matthijs G, Depoortere I, et al: Erythromycin is a motilin receptor agonist. Am J Physiol 257:G470, 1989.
69. Ramirez B, Eaker EY, Drane WE, et al: Erythromycin enhances gastric emptying in patients with gastroparesis after vagotomy and antrectomy. Dig Dis Sci 39:2295, 1994.
70. Grunberg SM, Hesketh PJ: Control of chemotherapy-induced emesis. N Engl J Med 329:1790, 1993.
71. Schwartz RH, Beveridge RA: Marijuana as an antiemetic drug: How useful is it today? J Addict Dis 13:53, 1994.
72. Lee A, Done ML: The use of nonpharmacologic techniques to prevent postoperative nausea and vomiting: A meta-analysis. Anesth Analg 88: 1362, 1999.
73. Latimer PR, Malmud LS, Fisher RS: Gastric stasis and vomiting: Behavioral treatment. Gastroenterology 83:684, 1982.
74. Harmon D, Ryan M, Kelly A, et al: Acupressure and prevention of nausea and vomiting during and after spinal anaesthesia for caesarean section. Br J Anaesth 84:463, 2000.
75. Pearl ML, Fischer M, McCauley DL, et al: Transcutaneous electrical nerve stimulation as an adjunct for controlling chemotherapy-induced nausea and vomiting in gynecologic oncology patients. Cancer Nurs 22: 307, 1999.

Chapter 9

DIARRHEA

Lawrence R. Schiller and Joseph H. Sellin

Diarrhea is a universal human experience. For most individuals, episodes of diarrhea last a day or two and rapidly subside. For others, diarrhea lasts for more than a few days or is complicated by fever, prostration, or rectal bleeding. Such individuals are likely to visit their physician. Most patients can be managed successfully as outpatients; however, more than 450,000 hospital admissions each year (1.5% of adult hospitalizations) are due to gastroenteritis.[1] Over the course of a year, chronic diarrhea (liquid stools for more than 1 month) may occur in 5% of the population, making it a major cause of disability for Americans.[2]

Diarrhea is a symptom of many conditions and thus the evaluation and management of diarrhea can be complex. Research efforts over the last 40 years have uncovered some fundamental mechanisms causing diarrhea, however, and permit a rational approach to its diagnosis and management.

DEFINITION OF DIARRHEA

Most patients consider increased fluidity of stool as the essential characteristic of diarrhea.[3] Because stool consistency is difficult to quantitate, researchers also have used stool frequency or stool weight as surrogate markers of diarrhea. Three or more bowel movements per day are considered to be abnormal, and the upper limit of stool weight is generally agreed to be 200 g per day in western countries. Although stool weight often is cited as a scientific definition of diarrhea, diarrhea should not be defined solely in terms of fecal weight. Some individuals have increased fecal weight due to fiber ingestion but do not complain of diarrhea because their stool consistency is normal. Conversely, other patients have normal stool weights but complain of diarrhea because their stools are loose or watery.[4, 5]

A recent study has shed some light on objective determinants of decreased fecal consistency.[3] The ability of water-insoluble fecal solids, such as those derived from dietary fiber or bacterial cell walls, to hold or bind fecal water correlated well with fecal consistency. Too little water-holding capacity to bind all the water present resulted in loose stools, but when fecal solids had sufficient water-holding capacity to bind all the water present, stools remained thick or formed. Thus, fecal consistency correlated best with the ratio of the water-holding capacity of insoluble solids to the total water present and not to the amount of fecal water, further supporting the concept that stool weight should not be the sole criterion for diarrhea.

Fecal incontinence may be reported as "bad diarrhea" by some patients because of shame associated with this condition. Although many incontinent patients have loose stools, their major problem is with the mechanisms of continence and not with intestinal fluid or electrolyte absorption. Accordingly, all patients complaining of diarrhea should be asked about the presence of fecal incontinence. If incontinence is frequent, especially in the absence of urgency, the patient should be evaluated for incontinence and not for diarrhea (see Chapter 11).

PATHOPHYSIOLOGY AND MECHANISMS OF DIARRHEA

Diarrhea frequently represents a protective response to a variety of intestinal insults and assaults. Normally the gut secretes little fluid, and its motility provides a favorable milieu for nutrient absorption. When infectious agents, toxins, or other noxious substances are present within the gut, fluid secretion and motility are stimulated to expel the unwanted material, producing diarrhea. This protective response is valuable acutely, but, when chronic, it is inappropriate and, no longer serving an adaptive purpose, is harmful.

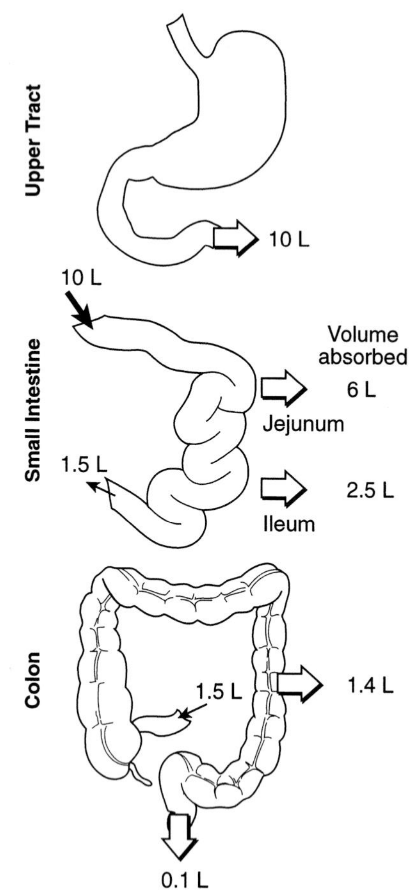

Figure 9–1. Fluid loads through the gastrointestinal tract. Each day, 9 to 10 L of fluid composed of ingested food and drink and secretions from the salivary glands, stomach, pancreas, bile duct, and duodenum pass the ligament of Treitz. The jejunum absorbs approximately 6 L and the ileum 2.5 L, leaving about 1.5 L to pass into the colon each day. The colon absorbs more than 90% of this load, leaving approximately 0.1 L in the feces. Thus, the overall absorptive efficiency for water absorption is 99%. Reduction of this efficiency by as little as 1% may lead to diarrhea. (From Schiller LR: Chronic diarrhea. In McNally P (ed): GI & Liver Secrets, 2nd ed. Philadelphia, Hanley & Belfus, 2001, pp 411–423.

Historically, diarrhea was thought to be primarily a motility disorder. An improved understanding of intestinal electrolyte transport over the last 4 decades has shifted the emphasis to epithelial function, rather than motility. It is clear, however, that both epithelial and motor function are altered in a coordinated fashion to produce it.

Diarrhea usually is due to an excess of stool water rather than a decrease in the water-holding capacity of fecal solids, implying an abnormality in water transport within the gut.[3] Normally, the small intestine and colon absorb 99% of both oral intake and endogenous secretions from the salivary glands, stomach, liver, and pancreas, a total fluid load of approximately 10 L daily (Fig. 9–1). Diarrhea results from a disruption of this normally fine-tuned mechanism; reduction of water absorption by as little as 1% can result in diarrhea. Therefore, to understand the pathogenesis of diarrhea, one needs to understand normal water absorption by the intestine and what abnormalities can impair water absorption.

Water itself is not actively transported but moves across the intestinal mucosa secondary to osmotic forces generated by the transport of solutes, that is, electrolytes and nutrients (see Chapter 87). The molecular pathways of ion and nutrient transport across the mucosa have been well characterized and are regulated by a complex communication system of extracellular and intracellular messengers that maintain fluid equilibrium throughout a wide range of physiologic conditions. Normally, whereas both absorption and secretion take place simultaneously, absorption is quantitatively greater. Either a decrease in absorption or an increase in secretion leads to additional fluid within the lumen and diarrhea. Disruption of epithelial electrolyte transport or its regulatory system by toxins, drugs, hormones, and cytokines is a major cause of diarrhea. Diarrhea due to disordered electrolyte transport is known as *secretory diarrhea*, even though it is commonly due to reduced absorption rather than to net secretion.[6] Another major cause of diarrhea is ingestion of some poorly absorbed, osmotically active substance (e.g., magnesium ion, lactulose) that osmotically retains fluid within the lumen, thereby reducing water absorption. Diarrhea due to this mechanism is known as *osmotic diarrhea* (Table 9–1).

Osmotic Diarrhea

Ingestion of poorly absorbed cations and anions or poorly absorbed sugars or sugar alcohols (e.g., mannitol, sorbitol) account for most osmotic diarrheas.[7] Ions that are poorly absorbed include magnesium, sulfate, and phosphate. These ions are transported actively by mechanisms that are saturated at low intraluminal ion concentrations and passively by mechanisms of low capacity. These processes together limit total absorption to a fraction of the amount that can be ingested. Because neither the small intestine nor colon can maintain an osmotic gradient, unabsorbed ions (and their counterions) remaining in the intestinal lumen obligate reten-

Table 9–1 | **Mechanisms of Diarrhea**

MECHANISM	CAUSES	EXAMPLES
Secretory diarrhea	Exogenous secretagogues	Enterotoxins (e.g., cholera)
	Endogenous secretagogues	Neuroendocrine tumors (e.g., carcinoid syndrome)
	Absence of ion transporter	Congenital chloridorrhea
	Loss of surface area	Intestinal resection, diffuse mucosal disease
	Ischemia	Mesenteric atherosclerosis
	Rapid transit	Intestinal hurry due to vagotomy
Osmotic diarrhea	Ingestion of poorly absorbed agent	Magnesium ingestion
	Loss of nutrient transporter	Lactase deficiency

tion of water to maintain an intraluminal osmolality equal to that of body fluids (about 290 mOsm/kg). Thus approximately 3.5 mL of water (1000 mL/kg divided by 290 mOsm/kg) are retained for every 1 mOsm of retained ions or molecules.[8, 9]

Sugars and sugar alcohols are the other category of substances causing osmotic diarrhea.[10] Monosaccharides—but not disaccharides—can be absorbed intact across the apical membrane of the intestine. When disaccharides, such as sucrose and lactose, are ingested, absence of the appropriate disaccharidase will prevent absorption. Thus, disaccharidase deficiencies can be considered to be a defect of an absorptive pathway (see Chapter 89). The most common clinical syndrome of disaccharidase deficiency is *lactase deficiency,* which accounts for lactose intolerance.[11] Lactase is present in the brush border of the small intestine of most immature mammals but disappears in adult mammals, including human beings. The main exceptions are individuals from the northern European gene pool who maintain lactase activity into adult life. Lactase activity often falls with age even in this group, and lactose malabsorption is responsible for diarrhea in some adults. Congenital deficiency of lactase is quite rare and seems to be due to a mutation in a gene distinct from that for lactase-phlorizin hydrolase.[12] Acquired deficiencies are associated with diseases of the upper small intestine (see Chapter 89). Congenital sucrase and trehalase deficiencies are rare, preventing the adequate digestion of sucrose (table sugar) and trehalose (a sugar found in mushrooms), respectively. Lactulose is a synthetic disaccharide that cannot be hydrolyzed by the human intestine and that cannot be absorbed intact in greater than trace amounts. It thereby causes an osmotic diarrhea when given in sufficient quantity to overwhelm the metabolic capacity of colonic bacteria (about 80 g/day).[10]

The essential characteristic of osmotic diarrhea is that it disappears with fasting or cessation of ingestion of the offending substance. This characteristic has been used clinically to differentiate osmotic diarrhea from secretory diarrhea that typically continues with fasting. It should also be noted that electrolyte absorption is not impaired in osmotic diarrhea; thus, electrolyte concentrations in stool water may be quite low.[8–10]

Secretory Diarrhea

Although, in contrast with osmotic diarrhea, secretory diarrhea has many causes, the driving force for this type of diarrhea is always either net secretion of chloride or bicarbonate or inhibition of net sodium absorption.[13] The stimuli for secretion most often arise from the lumen, the subepithelial space, or the systemic circulation, severely affecting the messenger system that regulates ion transport pathways. In some instances, lack of sufficient absorptive surface area limits electrolyte, particularly sodium, absorption critically; in others, congenital absence of specific transport molecules limits sodium or chloride absorption and diarrhea results.

The most common cause for secretory diarrhea is infection.[13] Enterotoxins from a host of infectious agents (primarily bacteria but also parasites and viruses) interact with receptors modulating intestinal transport and lead to increased anion secretion. Enterotoxins also may block specific absorptive pathways in addition to stimulating secretion. Most enterotoxins inhibit Na-H exchange in both the small intestine and the colon, blocking one of the significant driving forces for fluid absorption.[14, 15]

Peptides produced by endocrine tumors such as vasoactive intestinal peptide or calcitonin cause secretory diarrhea by stimulating secretion by epithelial cells, as do peptides released from subepithelial neurons and inflammatory cells (see Chapter 51).[16, 17] Neurotransmitters such as acetylcholine or serotonin (5-HT) and other modulators such as histamine and inflammatory cytokines also are potent secretory stimuli.[18, 19] Most of these endogenous regulators of intestinal transport elicit diarrhea by altering intracellular messengers, such as cyclic adenosine monophosphate (AMP), cyclic guanosine monophosphate and calcium, that control specific transport pathways.[20] In addition, peptides and other regulators may affect the synthesis, localization, and degradation of individual transport proteins.[21] Exogenous agents, such as drugs and some poisons, lead to secretory diarrhea, presumably by interacting with intracellular regulators or intracellular messengers of the enterocytes.[22]

The absence or disruption of a specific absorptive pathway may cause diarrhea. For example, there are rare congenital syndromes that are caused by the absence of a specific transport molecule, such as *congenital chloridorrhea* and *congenital sodium diarrhea.*[23] In chloridorrhea Cl-HCO_3 exchange in the ileum and colon is defective, transforming chloride into a poorly absorbed ion. Diarrhea due to chloridorrhea can be reduced by limiting chloride intake or inhibiting chloride secretion (i.e., by reducing gastric acid secretion with a proton-pump inhibitor).[24] Several transporter defects have been proposed for congenital sodium diarrhea.[23, 25]

For intestinal fluid and electrolyte absorption to be complete, the intestine must have an adequate surface area. Significant loss of surface area such as in celiac disease, inflammatory bowel disease, or after resective surgery may compromise water absorption. Even though there is a large reserve absorptive capacity in both the small intestine and the colon, sufficiently large surgical resections inevitably cause diarrhea. In some cases the problem is temporary, because over time the intestine may improve its capacity for absorption by the process of *adaptation.*[26] Such compensation, of course, is impossible following resection of certain segments of the intestine with highly specific absorptive functions that simply cannot be assumed by other segments of the gut, even over long periods. For example, ileocecal resection is followed by permanent inability to absorb sodium chloride against a concentration gradient[27] and, if sufficient ileum is resected, by failure to absorb vitamin B_{12}-intrinsic factor and/or normal amounts of conjugated bile acids (see Chapter 92).

Reduced intestinal blood flow has an important but as yet poorly defined role in diarrhea.[28] It is not clear whether ischemia has a direct effect on absorption or whether low blood flow prompts secondary responses (e.g., via cytokines or neurotransmitters) that affect fluid transport. Radiation enteritis also produces an abnormal intestinal circulation associated with persistent diarrhea that may be difficult to treat (see Chapters 102 and 119).

Secretory diarrhea may also be due to abnormal motility.[6] For fluid and electrolyte absorption to be complete, the contact time between luminal contents and the epithelium must be sufficient to permit absorption. There are some patients in whom abnormal motility produces intestinal hurry.[29] Because rapid transit prevents adequate time for absorption, diarrhea results despite intact mucosal absorptive capacity as measured by intestinal perfusion studies during which contact time is maximized by rapid infusion of fluid into the gut.[6] In some patients with intestinal hurry, oral-cecal transit time may be as short as 10 minutes.[30] Under such circumstances malabsorption of nutrients may produce an osmotic component to diarrhea. In disorders such as *diabetes mellitus* and *postvagotomy diarrhea*, intestinal hurry has been linked to abnormal enteric nervous system function.[31, 32] In other clinical settings, such as *amyloidosis, postprandial diarrhea,* and *irritable bowel syndrome*, enteric nervous system dysfunction is suspected, but unproven.[33–35] Many endocrine diarrheas, such as those due to *peptide-secreting tumors* or *hyperthyroidism*, may lead to diarrhea not only by effects on intestinal electrolyte transport but also by accelerating intestinal motility.[36]

Conversely, slow intestinal transit may lead to a secretory diarrhea by promoting bacterial overgrowth in the small intestine.[37] Excess bacteria in the small intestine disrupt digestion and may alter electrolyte transport. The best-documented example of diarrhea related to this mechanism is scleroderma.[38] Although diabetes is often suspected of causing diarrhea by slow transit and stasis as in scleroderma, such pathophysiology is not always established (see Chapter 90).[39]

Evaluation of the role of intestinal motility in the pathogenesis of diarrhea has been limited by the lack of the necessary tools to measure motility, propulsive forces, and transit time. Except for intestinal perfusion studies during which the effect of motility on electrolyte transport is eliminated, there has been no way to dissociate the effects of intestinal transport and motility on net absorption.[6] Thus, there is no clear consensus on whether too much or too little motility causes diarrhea, nor is there a firm understanding of how luminal factors may alter intestinal smooth muscle function.

Complex Diarrhea

Although classification of diarrhea as osmotic or secretory may be instructive in thinking about the pathophysiology of diarrhea, cases of pure secretory or pure osmotic diarrhea are uncommon. Most clinically significant diarrheas are complex; rather than being produced by a single pathophysiologic mechanism, they are due to several. These may include the effects of substances released by enteric endocrine cells, cytokines released by local and remote immunologically reactive cells, by the activity of the enteric nervous system, and by peripherally released peptides and hormones (paracrine, immune, neural, and endocrine systems) (see Chapter 86).

Further complicating the understanding of diarrhea is that certain mediators not only affect epithelial or muscle function, but also each other. For example, enteric nerves may stimulate mast cells and products so released from mast cells (particularly histamine) may alter enteric neuron functions.[40] A single agonist—such as prostaglandin—may have multiple, simultaneous effects on epithelial function, muscle contraction, and the paracellular pathway, leading to effects on ion transport, motility, and mucosal permeability.[41] Thus, multiple modulators and multiple effectors contribute to the final clinical picture. A full appreciation of the pathophysiology of diarrhea requires consideration of *p*aracrine, *i*mmune, *n*eural, and *e*ndocrine modulators, a regulatory system that can be abbreviated by the acronym "PINES" (Fig. 9–2).

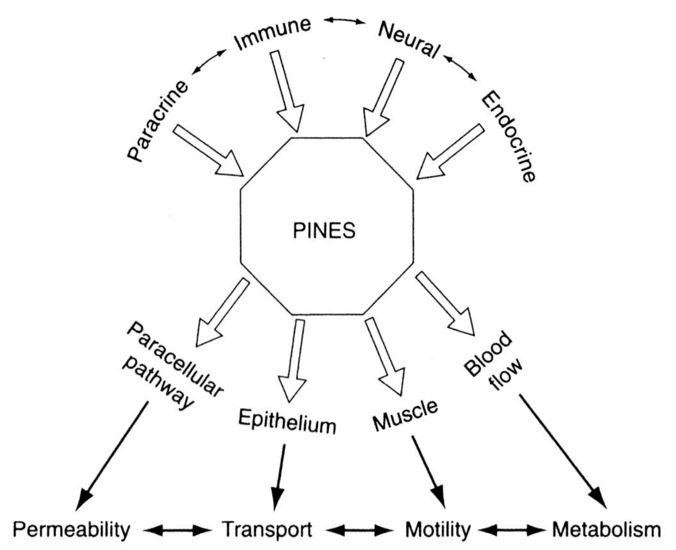

Figure 9–2. "PINES" regulatory system in the gut. The regulatory system of the gut integrates **p**aracrine, **i**mmune, **n**eural, and **e**ndocrine **s**ystems, and produces coordinated changes in mucosal and muscular function that permit adaptive responses to changing conditions. Diarrhea may be an appropriate response to acute infections. Maladaptive responses may be responsible for chronic diarrhea. (From Sellin JH: Functional anatomy, fluid and electrolyte absorption. In Feldman M, Schiller LR (eds): Gastroenterology and Hepatology. The Comprehensive Visual Reference, Vol. 7, Small Intestine. Philadelphia, Current Medicine, 1997, p 1.11.)

An example of the complexity of the pathophysiology of a diarrheal syndrome is *cholera*. Cholera is often cited as the paradigm of a pure secretory diarrhea: cholera toxin targets the epithelial cell, increases the second messenger, cyclic AMP, which opens apical chloride channels to stimulate chloride secretion, and results in diarrhea. However, the real mechanism by which cholera induces diarrhea is much more complex.[42] Cholera toxin stimulates both endocrine cells and neural elements that reinforce the direct secretory effect on enterocytes.[43] In addition, cholera toxin causes distinct changes in intestinal motility and other toxins produced by *Vibrio cholerae* target tight junctions, altering mucosal permeability (Fig. 9–3) (see Chapter 96).[44]

Another example of dysregulation of the PINES system is inflammatory bowel disease.[45] Diarrhea in inflammatory bowel disease involves more than just exudation into the lumen due to destruction of the mucosa. Intact enterocytes are barraged by multiple secretagogues released by immune cells in the intestine and by bacterial toxins that may influence enterocyte function. For example, bacterial proteins, such as flagellin, may stimulate the production of cytokines, such as interleukin-8, which further attract inflammatory cells.[46] Cytokines and immune cells also may influence enterocyte secretory and/or absorptive pathways directly.[47] Conversely, epithelial cells may secrete cytokines that enhance neutrophil function, such as interleukin-6.[48] Other factors, such as altered motility or compromised rectal reservoir

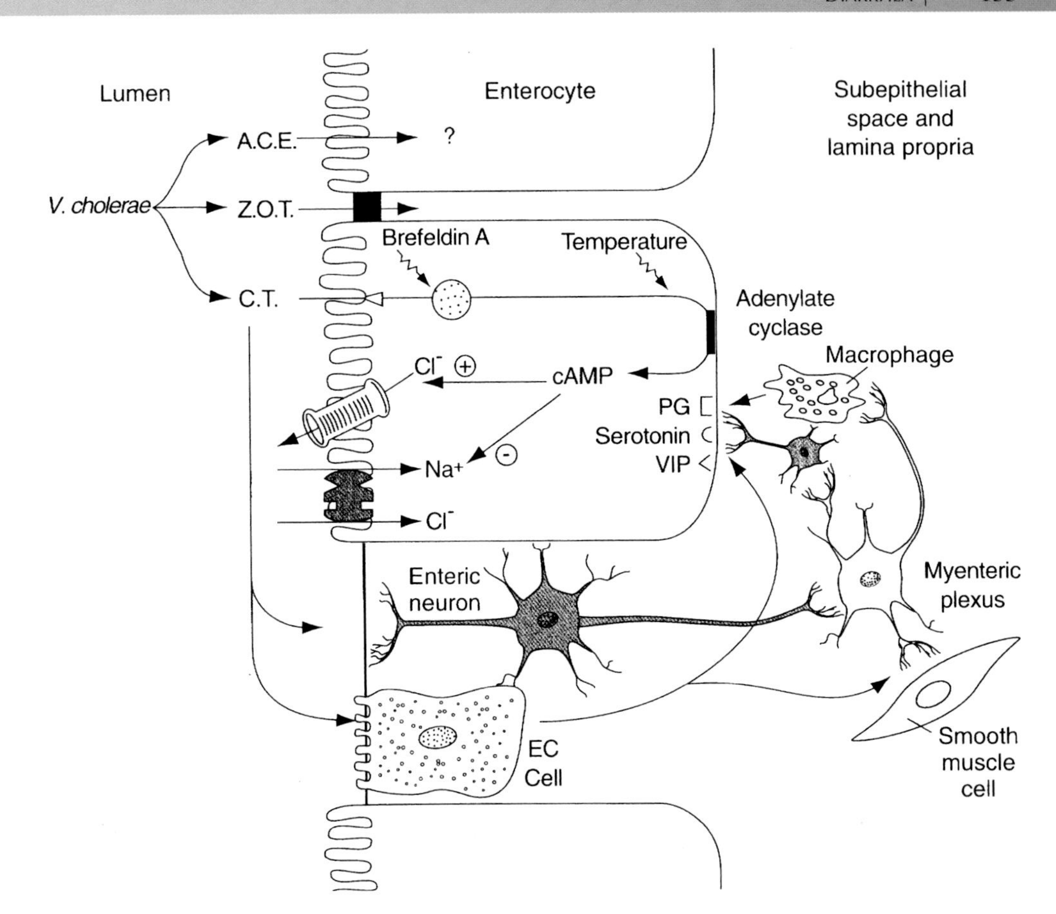

Figure 9–3. Pathophysiology of cholera. *Vibrio cholerae* produces several toxins that interact with adenylate cyclase in the enterocyte and several elements of the regulatory system of the gut, including enteric neurons and enterochromaffin cells, to produce a secretory state and voluminous diarrhea. In addition to the classic enterotoxin, cholera toxin (CT), the bacterium also produces zona occludens toxin (ZOT), which increases the permeability of the tight junction between enterocytes, and accessory cholera enterotoxin (ACE), which has unclear effects on enterocytes. In addition to cyclic adenosine monophosphate (cAMP) generated by adenylate cyclase in response to cholera toxin, secretory stimuli include prostaglandin (PG), serotonin, and vasoactive intestinal polypeptide (VIP). (From Sellin JH: Functional anatomy, fluid and electrolyte absorption. In Feldman M, Schiller LR (eds): Gastroenterology and Hepatology. The Comprehensive Visual Reference, Vol. 7, Small Intestine. Philadelphia, Current Medicine, 1997, p 1.14.)

capacity, may aggravate symptoms in inflammatory bowel diseases (see Chapters 103 and 104).

Complex pathophysiology also may be observed in *malabsorption syndromes* and *functional disorders*. Failure to absorb carbohydrates may lead to osmotic diarrhea, but failure to absorb long-chain fatty acids may complicate matters by impairing electrolyte absorption by the colon.[10, 49] Common postprandial functional diarrhea probably involves an interplay between motility and transport functions. Diarrhea due to food allergy also involves activation of immunologic, paracrine, and neural mechanisms regulating vascular permeability, electrolyte transport, and motility[50–52] (see Chapters 89 and 91).

CLINICAL CLASSIFICATION: CLUES TO DIAGNOSIS

There are several schemes for classifying diarrhea: by time course (acute vs. chronic), by volume (large vs. small), by pathophysiology (secretory vs. osmotic), by epidemiology, and by stool characteristics (watery vs. fatty vs. inflammatory). For the clinician, these classification schemes are only useful if they serve to focus the diagnostic and management approaches toward patients. In this regard, no single scheme is perfect; the experienced physician uses all of these classifications to expedite patient care.

Acute Versus Chronic

The time course of diarrhea can help direct management. Acute diarrheas (<4 weeks) usually are due to infections, most of which are self-limited or are easily treated.[1] Although there are a few infectious agents that cause prolonged diarrhea in immunocompetent individuals (such as *Giardia lamblia* or *Yersinia* spp.), chronic diarrhea is usually due to some other cause. Thus, when confronted with a patient with chronic diarrhea, the physician must generate a different differential diagnosis (see later).

Large-Volume Versus Small-Volume Stools

Differentiation of the cause of diarrhea based on the volume of individual stools (rather than total daily output) rests on the premise that the normal rectosigmoid colon functions as a storage reservoir. When that reservoir capacity is compromised by inflammatory or motility disorders involving the left colon, frequent small-volume bowel movements ensue. If the source of the diarrhea is upstream in the right colon or small bowel and if the rectosigmoid reservoir is intact, bowel movements are fewer, but larger. Thus, frequent, small, painful stools may point to a distal site of pathology, whereas painless large-volume stools suggest a right colon or small bowel source. Although it is difficult for patients to quantify volume accurately, this distinction may provide a clue for further diagnostic studies.

The daily total stool output may also provide etiologic hints. Irritable bowel syndrome often results in normal or only slightly elevated 24-hour stool weights, whereas diarrheas due to other etiologies may produce more substantial elevations of stool weight. This can be estimated by the patient's history; diarrheas that produce dehydration (in the absence of vomiting or limited oral intake) typically have stool weights greater than 1000 g and therefore are unlikely to be due to irritable bowel syndrome (see Chapter 91).

Osmotic Versus Secretory

Distinguishing between diarrheas due to malabsorption of ingested nonelectrolytes ("osmotic diarrhea") and those due to malabsorption or secretion of electrolytes ("secretory diarrhea") helps separate the small number of causes of osmotic diarrhea from the much larger number of causes of secretory diarrhea. This distinction is based on the measurement of stool electrolyte concentrations.[8] In secretory diarrheas, sodium, potassium, and accompanying anions account entirely for stool osmolality, whereas in osmotic diarrheas unabsorbable solutes within the lumen of the gut account for much of the osmotic activity of stool water (see later). Because osmotic diarrhea is due to ingestion of some poorly absorbed substance, it abates with fasting. Secretory diarrheas typically continue during fasting, although stool output may decrease somewhat due to reduced endogenous secretions.

Epidemiologic Classification

One of the most successful clinical approaches in narrowing the differential diagnosis is to relate diarrhea to its setting and, by so doing, proceed more intelligently with its evaluation. Thus, a "soccer mom" and a backpacker from Nepal conceivably could have the same etiology for diarrhea, but it is more likely to be different. Some common clinical scenarios and the diagnoses that should be considered are shown in Table 9–2.

Table 9–2 | **Likely Causes of Diarrhea in Patients with Certain Epidemiologic Characteristics**

Travelers
Bacterial infection (mostly acute)
Protozoal infections (e.g., amebiasis, giardiasis)
Tropical sprue
Epidemics/Outbreaks
Bacterial infection
Viral infection (e.g., rotavirus)
Protozoal infections (e.g., cryptosporidiosis)
Epidemic idiopathic secretory diarrhea (Brainerd diarrhea)
Diabetic Patients
Altered motility (increased or decreased)
Drugs (especially acarbose, metformin)
Associated diseases
 Celiac sprue
 Pancreatic exocrine insufficiency
 Small bowel bacterial overgrowth
AIDS Patients
Opportunistic infections (e.g., cryptosporidiosis, cytomegalovirus, herpes, *Mycobacterium avium* complex)
Drug side effect
Lymphoma
Institutionalized and Hospitalized Patients
Drug side effect
Clostridium difficile toxin-mediated colitis
Tube feeding
Ischemia
Fecal impaction with overflow diarrhea

AIDS, acquired immunodeficiency syndrome.

Watery Versus Fatty Versus Inflammatory

When diarrhea is chronic (>4 weeks), the differential diagnosis can overwhelm even the most experienced clinician. By characterizing stools as watery, fatty, or inflammatory based on simple stool tests, the further evaluation of the patient can be expedited by limiting the number of conditions that must be considered in the differential diagnosis.[2] *Watery* diarrhea implies a defect primarily in water absorption due to increased electrolyte secretion or reduced electrolyte absorption (*secretory diarrhea*) or ingestion of a poorly absorbed substance (*osmotic diarrhea*). *Fatty* diarrhea implies defective absorption of fat in the small intestine. *Inflammatory* diarrhea implies the presence of one of a limited number of inflammatory or neoplastic diseases involving the gut.

DIFFERENTIAL DIAGNOSIS OF DIARRHEA

Many gastrointestinal and systemic diseases may present with diarrhea. To facilitate the differential diagnosis, the physician should divide diarrheal diseases into acute and chronic diarrheas and further subdivide the chronic diarrheas by stool characteristics: watery, inflammatory, and fatty (Table 9–3).

Acute diarrheas are defined as less than 4 weeks, although many are shorter than 4 days,[1] and they are usually due to infectious diseases. Bacteria, viruses, protozoa, and multicellular parasites all are etiologic agents that can produce diarrhea (Table 9–4). Occasionally infections produce diarrhea over longer periods, especially if the patient is immunocompromised. Acute diarrheas also can be due to food poisoning, food allergies, and medications. Of course, diseases that lead to chronic diarrhea may present with acute onsets and therefore must be considered when acute diarrhea becomes persistent (see Chapter 96).

Chronic watery diarrhea may be due infrequently to ingestion of osmotically active substances that are poorly absorbed by the intestine (osmotic diarrhea) and, more commonly, to conditions causing secretory diarrhea. Ingestion of any of a limited number of osmotic agents—such as magnesium, phosphate, and sulfate laxatives, or poorly absorbed carbohydrates—causes the former. Chronic secretory diarrhea, in which electrolyte malabsorption leads to retention of fluid within the lumen, in contrast, is associated with a large number of clinical conditions (see Table 9–3).

Although *inflammatory bowel disease* typically produces diarrhea characterized by the presence of blood and pus, other diseases of inflammation without ulceration, such as microscopic colitis, cause diarrhea with the characteristics of a chronic secretory type. Such diarrheas are thought to be mediated by secretion of cytokines and other inflammatory mediators (see Chapters 103 and 104). Similarly *vasculitis*, in which inflammation is common without disruption of the mucosa, may produce a secretory diarrhea.

Chronic watery diarrhea can also be due to ingestion of drugs or poisons (Table 9–5).[22, 53] Identification of drugs as the cause of diarrhea depends on recognition of the coincidence of the initiation of drug ingestion and the onset of diarrhea. Such correlation, however, is not always easy and

Table 9–3 | **Differential Diagnosis of Diarrhea by Duration and Stool Characteristics**

Acute Diarrhea
- Infection
  - Bacteria
  - Virus
  - Protozoa
  - Multicellular parasites
- Food poisoning
- Food allergies
- Medication
- Initial presentation of chronic diarrhea

Chronic Diarrhea
- Watery diarrhea
  - Osmotic diarrhea
    - Osmotic laxatives (e.g., Mg^{+2}, PO_4^{-3}, SO_4^{-2})
    - Carbohydrate malabsorption
  - Secretory diarrhea
    - Congenital syndromes (e.g., congenital chloridorrhea)
    - Bacterial toxins
    - Ileal bile acid malabsorption
    - Inflammatory bowel disease
      - Ulcerative colitis
      - Crohn's disease
      - Microscopic colitis
        - Lymphocytic colitis
        - Collagenous colitis
      - Diverticulitis
    - Vasculitis
    - Drugs and poisons
    - Laxative abuse (stimulant laxatives)
    - Disordered motility/regulation
      - Postvagotomy diarrhea
      - Postsympathectomy diarrhea
      - Diabetic autonomic neuropathy
      - Irritable bowel syndrome
    - Endocrine diarrhea
      - Hyperthyroidism
      - Addison's disease
      - Gastrinoma
      - VIPoma
      - Somatostatinoma
      - Carcinoid syndrome
      - Medullary carcinoma of the thyroid
      - Mastocytosis
      - Pheochromocytoma
    - Other tumors
      - Colon carcinoma
      - Lymphoma
      - Villous adenoma
    - Idiopathic secretory diarrhea
      - Epidemic secretory (Brainerd) diarrhea
      - Sporadic idiopathic secretory diarrhea
- Inflammatory diarrhea
  - Inflammatory bowel disease
    - Ulcerative colitis
    - Crohn's disease
    - Diverticulitis
    - Ulcerative jejunoileitis
  - Infectious diseases
    - Pseudomembranous colitis
    - Invasive bacterial infections (e.g., tuberculosis, yersinosis)
    - Ulcerating viral infections (e.g., cytomegalovirus, *Herpes simplex*)
    - Invasive parasitic infections (e.g., amebiasis, strongyloides)
  - Ischemic colitis
  - Radiation colitis
  - Neoplasia
    - Colon cancer
    - Lymphoma
- Fatty diarrhea
  - Malabsorption syndromes
    - Mucosal diseases (e.g., celiac sprue, Whipple's disease)
    - Short bowel syndrome
    - Small bowel bacterial overgrowth
    - Mesenteric ischemia
  - Maldigestion
    - Pancreatic exocrine insufficiency
    - Inadequate luminal bile acid concentration

requires a detailed and careful history. The problem, of course, is more difficult in patients with surreptitious laxative abuse. These patients are deliberately deceiving the physician about the cause of their problem (see the section on factitious diarrhea).[54]

Another category of chronic watery diarrhea involves *disordered motility* or dysregulation of gut function.[29–31, 34–36] Problems such as postvagotomy diarrhea, postsympathectomy diarrhea, diabetic autonomic neuropathy, and probably diarrhea-predominant irritable bowel syndrome belong in this category. In these situations, the diarrhea has the characteristics of a secretory diarrhea, either because of primary dysregulation of electrolyte transport or because of altered motility that speeds luminal fluid past absorptive sites in the intestine (see Chapters 29, 42, and 91).

Another large category of watery diarrhea is diarrhea due

Table 9–4 | **Infections Causing Diarrhea***

Bacteria
Escherichia coli (enterotoxigenic, enteroinvasive, enterohemorrhagic)
Campylobacter spp.
Salmonella spp.
Shigella spp.
Clostridium difficile
Aeromonas spp.
Pleisiomonas spp.
Viruses
Adenovirus
Rotavirus
Norwalk agent
Parasites/Protozoa
Entamoeba histolytica
Giardia lamblia
Cryptosporidium
Microsporidium
Cyclospora

*See Chapter 96.

Table 9–5 | **Drugs and Poisons Associated with Diarrhea**

Antibiotics (most)
Antineoplastic agents (many)
Anti-inflammatory agents (e.g., NSAIDs, gold, 5-aminosalicylates)
Antiarrhythmics (e.g., quinidine)
Antihypertensives (e.g., β-adrenergic receptor blocking drugs)
Antacids (e.g., those containing magnesium)
Acid-reducing agents (e.g., H_2-receptor antagonists, proton-pump inhibitors)
Colchicine
Prostaglandin (e.g., misoprostol)
Theophylline
Vitamin and mineral supplements
Herbal products
Heavy metals

NSAIDs, nonsteroidal anti-inflammatory drugs.

to *endocrine dysfunction*.[36] Relatively common endocrine disturbances, such as hyperthyroidism and Addison's disease, can be complicated by chronic secretory diarrhea. Much rarer endocrine tumors also produce diarrhea, typically by speeding intestinal transit or by altering electrolyte absorption. The rarity of these tumors makes the pretest probability of finding these conditions very low and therefore screening tests often are falsely positive (see later, also Chapters 29 and 51).

Other tumors cause watery diarrhea either by obstructing bowel, by blocking lymphatic drainage, by interfering with absorption, or by causing electrolyte secretion. Examples of such conditions include colon carcinoma (bowel obstruction), lymphoma (lymphatic obstruction in the small bowel and mesentery), and villous adenoma of the rectum that secretes a large amount of potassium-rich gelatinous fluid into the lumen. Villous adenomas found more proximally in the colon rarely cause this type of diarrhea (see Chapters 26, 114, and 115).

The last category of chronic watery diarrhea is *idiopathic secretory diarrhea*. This rubric includes two entities: epidemic secretory diarrhea (also known as Brainerd diarrhea) and sporadic idiopathic secretory diarrhea. Both are protracted but self-limited conditions (see the section on idiopathic secretory diarrhea).[55, 56]

Chronic inflammatory diarrheas comprise a diverse group of infectious or idiopathic inflammatory and neoplastic processes. Stools are characterized by the presence of mucus and pus and are usually associated with ulceration of the mucosa. Idiopathic inflammatory bowel diseases, such as ulcerative colitis and Crohn's disease, typically produce such stools. Less commonly, other inflammatory conditions such as *diverticulitis* or *ulcerative jejunoileitis* may have blood or pus in the stool, as do infectious diseases that are invasive or ulcerating. Infections causing chronic inflammatory diarrhea include bacterial infections, such as *tuberculosis*, *yersinosis*, and *Clostridium difficile*–associated colitis; viral infections that ulcerate, such as *cytomegalovirus* and *herpes simplex*; and invasive parasitic infections, such as *strongyloidiasis*. Noninfectious diseases causing chronic inflammatory diarrhea include *ischemic colitis*, and neoplasms, such as *colon cancer* or *lymphoma*, that are complicated by ulceration of the mucosa.

Chronic fatty diarrheas are due to either malabsorption or maldigestion. Malabsorption syndromes due to mucosal diseases, such as *celiac sprue* or *Whipple's disease*, typically produce fatty diarrhea. Short bowel syndrome or postresection diarrhea can also present with this pattern, although if the resection is relatively limited, fatty diarrhea may be less likely than secretory diarrhea due to bile acid malabsorption. Small bowel bacterial overgrowth causes steatorrhea by deconjugation of bile acids. *Mesenteric ischemia* affecting the small intestine may impair absorption of fat, but weight loss is often attributed to sitophobia ("fear of eating") due to postprandial pain. Maldigestion due to *pancreatic exocrine insufficiency* or *inadequate duodenal bile acid concentration* produces steatorrhea. Although fatty, stools may not be very loose in these maldigestive conditions, because, in the absence of fat digestion, triglyceride remains intact and has little effect on colonic electrolyte absorption. In contrast, malabsorption in the presence of normal digestion may produce fairly voluminous diarrhea due to the cathartic action of free fatty acids in the colon (see Chapter 89).[49]

EVALUATION OF THE PATIENT WITH DIARRHEA

History

A careful medical history is the key to the evaluation of patients presenting with diarrhea. An essential feature is the duration of symptoms. Patients with acute diarrhea (<4 weeks' duration) should be distinguished from those patients with chronic diarrhea whose differential diagnosis is much broader. The severity of the diarrhea should be ascertained. Stool frequency is the easiest characteristic of their diarrhea for patients to define. It does not necessarily correlate with stool weight; some individuals pass small amounts of stool frequently, but others have less frequent, and more voluminous evacuations. Patients have a poor notion of stool volume, but symptoms such as dry mouth, increased thirst, decreased urine output, and weakness suggest dehydration due to higher stool outputs. Acute weight loss is also a good marker for severity.

Stool characteristics, such as the presence of blood, mucus, pus, oil droplets, or food particles, are also important. Blood in the stool signals the possibility of malignancy or inflammatory bowel disease, although it is frequently due to hemorrhoids in patients with frequent evacuations. In patients with acute infectious diarrhea, visible blood in the stool is highly specific for infection with invasive organisms.[57] Watery stools suggest an osmotic or secretory process, and the presence of oil or food particles is suggestive of malabsorption, maldigestion, or intestinal hurry. The physician should also ask about the relationship of defecation to meals or fasting, passage of stool during the day versus the night, and the presence of fecal urgency or incontinence. Urgency and incontinence are not indicative of voluminous diarrhea but suggest a problem with rectal compliance or with the muscles regulating continence. Nocturnal diarrhea that wakes the patient from sleep strongly suggests an organic cause rather than a functional problem, such as irritable bowel syndrome. Other coexisting symptoms such as abdominal pain, flatulence, bloating or gaseous distention, cramps, fever, and weight loss should be noted. Excess flatus suggests increased fermentation of carbohydrate by colonic bacteria, caused by ingestion of poorly absorbable carbohydrate or malabsorption of carbohydrate by the small intestine.

Because iatrogenic causes of diarrhea, such as drugs, previous surgery, or radiation therapy, are common, the physician should explore the history thoroughly for prior abdominal surgeries and ingestion of both prescription drugs and over-the-counter remedies including nutritional and herbal therapy. The patient's diet should be thoroughly reviewed because diarrhea may be due to ingestion of large quantities of poorly absorbable carbohydrates, such as fructose or sugar alcohols, such as sorbitol or mannitol. These may be consumed in fruit juices and soda pop (fructose and high-fructose corn syrup) or as "dietetic, sugar-free" candies and chewing gums (sorbitol and mannitol).[58] Excess coffee consumption also may be associated with diarrhea.

Epidemiologic clues also should be developed (see Table 9–2). For example, recent foreign travel—particularly to undeveloped countries—makes the diagnosis of travelers' diarrhea likely, and with the increasing globalization of commerce, has increased the incidence of once exotic infections in individuals without grossly obvious exposures.[59, 60] Identifiable foodborne illness affects at least 1 in 2000 individuals annually.[61] The physician also should take note of whether the patient's residence is rural or urban, the source of drinking water, and the patient's occupation, sexual preference, and use of alcohol or illicit drugs. Potential secondary gains from illness or a history of attempted weight loss and fixation on body image should raise the possibility of laxative abuse (see later).

History is essential in differentiating patients with *irritable bowel syndrome* from those with other functional disorders or organic conditions causing diarrhea. Current definitions of irritable bowel syndrome emphasize the presence of abdominal pain associated with defecation.[62] Painless diarrhea should no longer be considered a form of irritable bowel syndrome. Additional factors that suggest a diagnosis of irritable bowel syndrome include a long history usually extending back to adolescence or young adulthood, passage of mucus, and exacerbation of symptoms by stress. Factors that argue against a diagnosis of irritable bowel syndrome include a recent onset of diarrhea, especially in older patients; diarrhea that wakes the patient from sleep; weight loss; the presence of blood in the stool; and stool weights greater than 400 to 500 g per day. Abnormal blood tests, such as a low hemoglobin level, low serum albumin concentration or high erythrocyte sedimentation rate, also are against this diagnosis (see Chapter 91).

Physical Examination

Physical findings are usually more useful in determining the severity of diarrhea than in determining its cause. Volume status can be assessed by looking for orthostatic changes in blood pressure and pulse. Fever and other signs of toxicity should be noted. A careful abdominal examination is important, looking in particular for the presence or absence of bowel sounds, abdominal distention, localized or generalized tenderness, masses, and an enlarged liver.

On occasion physical examination may provide more direct evidence of the cause of diarrhea. Characteristic skin changes may be seen in *mastocytosis* (urticaria pigmentosa), *amyloidosis* (waxy papules, pinch purpura), *Addison's disease* (heightened pigmentation), *glucagonoma* (migratory necrotizing erythema), *carcinoid syndrome* (flushing), *Degos' disease* (malignant atrophic papulosis), and *celiac sprue* (dermatitis herpetiformis). Peripheral neuropathy and orthostatic hypotension may be the only clues to a diagnosis of amyloidosis. A thyroid nodule with cervical lymphadenopathy may be the only lead to the presence of *medullary carcinoma of the thyroid*. Tremor and other systemic signs should lead to consideration of *hyperthyroidism*. Right-sided heart murmurs may be present with *carcinoid syndrome*, as well as an enlarged, hard liver. Evidence of arthritis may be noted in *inflammatory bowel disease*, *Whipple's disease*, and some *enteric infections*. Lymphadenopathy might suggest *acquired immunodeficiency syndrome (AIDS)* or *lymphoma*. Signs of peripheral vascular disease with or without an abdominal bruit may suggest *mesenteric vascular insufficiency*. Evidence of chronic liver disease may suggest advanced *primary sclerosing cholangitis* in a patient with colitis. A careful rectal examination may disclose defective sphincter or pelvic floor muscle function that might produce fecal incontinence (see Chapter 29).

Further Evaluation of Acute Diarrhea

Most acute diarrheas are due to infectious diseases that have limited courses from a few days to a few weeks and do not require a physician's intervention unless the patient's immune system is compromised or if the patient develops complications of volume depletion or other evidence of severe toxicity, including inability to ingest fluid, frequent vomiting, and debilitating muscle or joint pain.

When these complications are present or when the diarrhea has persisted for more than a few days, a more comprehensive evaluation is warranted. In such patients a complete blood count should be done to look for anemia, hemoconcentration, or an abnormal white blood cell count. Patients with viral diarrhea usually have a normal white blood cell count differential or lymphocytosis, but those with bacterial infections, particularly with organisms that invade the mucosa, have a leukocytosis with an excess of immature white blood cells. Neutropenia, however, can occur in salmonellosis. Measurements of serum electrolyte concentrations and blood urea nitrogen and serum creatinine levels can be used to determine the extent of fluid and electrolyte depletion and its effect on renal function.

Stool samples should be examined for white blood cells to identify inflammatory diarrhea.[63] The standard method for detecting white blood cells in stool is with Wright stain and microscopy.[63] The accuracy of the test depends on the experience and skill of the observer, because both false-positive and false-negative results are common. A test for the neutrophil product, lactoferrin, is very sensitive and specific for the detection of neutrophils in stool and may be a useful alternative to microscopy.[64, 65] Studies suggest that stool cultures are unlikely to grow pathogenic bacteria in the absence of fecal leukocytes; therefore, Wright stain or a fecal lactoferrin assay can be used to decide which stool samples should be sent for bacterial culture, thereby minimizing expense.[66] This approach may be of more value in outpatients than in hospitalized patients with diarrhea, because the latter have toxicity or have failed to resolve spontaneously within a few days and hence must have stool cultures.[67] The diagnostic value of examination of stool for ova and parasites depends on the pretest probability of parasitic infections and the experience of the observer. Enzyme-linked immunosorbent assay (ELISA) for giardiasis and serologic testing for amebiasis are more accurate tests than stool microscopy and should be ordered even in the absence of fecal leukocytes.[68] Patients who have been treated with antibiotics in the preceding 3 months or those developing diarrhea in an institutional setting should be tested for *C. difficile* toxin.[69]

Abdominal radiographs should be obtained in toxic patients to assess for colitis and to look for evidence of ileus or megacolon. Proctoscopy or flexible sigmoidoscopy also should be considered in patients clearly toxic with infection, patients with blood in the stool, and those with persistent acute diarrhea. Sigmoidoscopy is probably adequate as an early investigation in such severe, acute diarrhea. In patients with AIDS-related diarrhea, colonoscopy is preferable because a substantial proportion of infections and lymphomas may be present only in the right colon,[70] although this approach has been called into question.[71] Mucosal biopsy specimens should be obtained, particularly if the mucosa appears to be grossly inflamed, because pathologists can reliably distinguish self-limited colitis from chronic ulcerative coli-

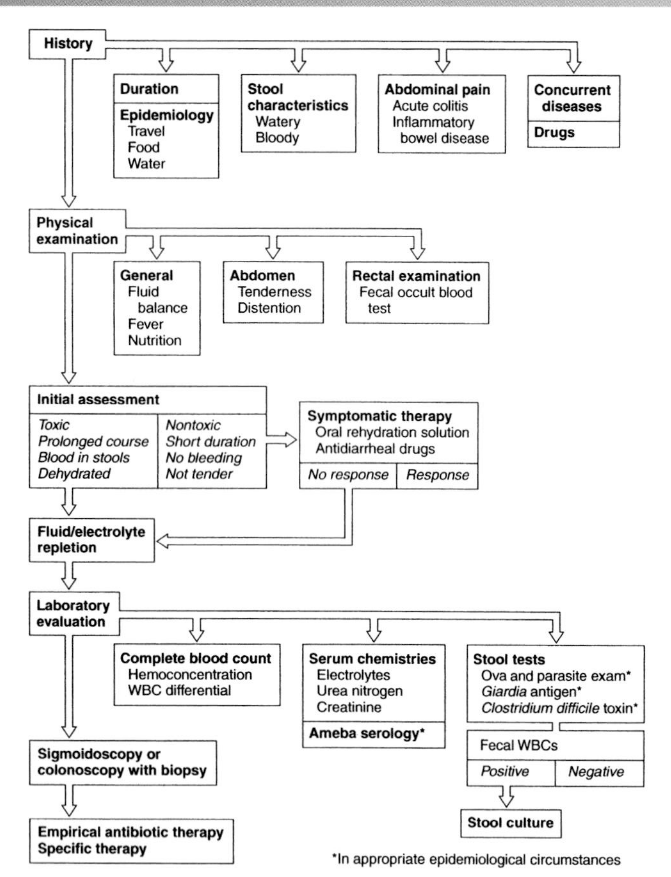

Figure 9–4. Algorithm for evaluation of patients with acute diarrhea. WBC, white blood cells. (From Schiller LR: Diarrhea. Med Clin North Am 84:1259, 2000.)

tis.[72] An algorithm for the evaluation of patients with acute diarrhea is shown in Figure 9–4.

Further Evaluation of Chronic Diarrhea

Because the differential diagnosis for chronic diarrhea is more extensive than for acute diarrhea, evaluation of these patients is more complex. Initially the physician should categorize the diarrhea as watery, inflammatory, or fatty (Fig. 9–5). In addition to the history, physical examination, and routine laboratory tests already mentioned, analysis of a stool sample can be used to categorize the diarrhea and thereby limit the number of conditions to be considered in the differential diagnosis. Stool analysis can be obtained on a random sample or a timed collection (i.e., 24- or 48-hour stool sample). The value of analyzing a timed collection is that the stool weight and hence the output of the various stool components, such as fat and electrolytes, can be more accurately measured. A daily stool weight is perhaps the best clue to the potential metabolic impact of the diarrhea. In the absence of a timed collection, however, measurements on a random sample of other stool characteristics still provide many clues to the correct diagnosis.[2] These measurements include stool sodium and potassium concentrations, pH, testing for occult blood, and searching for stool white blood cells or determining the presence of a surrogate marker, such as fecal lactoferrin.[64, 65] In appropriate circumstances, stool samples can also be analyzed for fat content and for laxatives, including magnesium, phosphate, sulfate, bisacodyl, and anthraquinones (see the section on factitious diarrhea).

Although stool collections are often viewed by patients and physicians alike as being messy and disgusting, they usually can be done easily and successfully at home or in the hospital. Perhaps the biggest hurdle is in dealing with laboratories that are inexperienced or uninterested in stool analysis. Commercially available collection units that fit into a commode and allow separation of stool and urine facilitate the collection, as does the use of preweighed plastic or metal containers and a small refrigerator or picnic cooler to keep the specimens cold. Patients should continue regular activities and should consume a regular diet, including a fat intake of 80 to 100 g of fat per day during the collection. Keeping a diary of food and liquid ingested facilitates estimation of fat and calorie intake by a dietitian. During the collection, diagnostic tests that might alter stool output or composition, such as barium radiographs, should be avoided and only essential medication should be given. Any antidiarrheal medications should be withdrawn. For most patients with diarrhea, a 48-hour collection is sufficient. Should stool output not be representative during that time, the collection can always be extended. Occasionally stool output is measured during fasting; if the diarrhea is caused by some ingested substance, fasting should abolish the diarrhea. Continuation of diarrhea during fasting is one criterion for secretory diarrhea.

Measurement of stool sodium (Na^+) and potassium (K^+) concentrations allows the physician to calculate an osmotic gap in stool water. The osmotic gap is calculated by subtracting twice the sum of the sodium and potassium concentrations from 290 mOsm/kg, the osmolality of stool within the body.[8, 73] The concentration is doubled to account for anions that accompany these cations. When the osmotic gap is small (<50 mOsm/kg), the osmolality of stool water is due mostly to incompletely absorbed electrolytes that retain excess water intraluminally. This is due to incomplete absorption or excessive secretion of electrolytes and is characteristic of secretory diarrhea (Fig. 9–6). On the other hand, when a large osmotic gap is present (>100 mOsm/kg), most of the stool osmolality is comprised of nonelectrolytes. This is characteristic of an osmotic diarrhea, usually resulting from ingestion of some poorly absorbed substance, such as magnesium salts. When, however, the sum of sodium and potassium concentrations doubled is higher than 290 mOsm/kg, ingestion of a poorly absorbed multivalent anion, such as phosphate or sulfate, is suggested.[8] This calculation of a negative osmotic gap is due to the excess cations obligated by multivalent anions. The actual measurement of stool osmolality is of value only in detecting samples that have been contaminated by the addition of water or hypotonic urine.[74] Such samples have an osmolality of less than 290 mOsm/kg. Stool osmolality tends to rise once the stool has been collected because of continuing bacterial fermentation in vitro.[10] Hence, measured osmolality should not be used to calculate the fecal osmotic gap.

The pH of stool water provides useful information about the possibility of carbohydrate malabsorption.[8] Carbohydrate reaching the colon is promptly fermented by the bacterial flora with release of gas and short-chain fatty acids. As a result of fermentation, the pH is acidic usually dropping to less than 6, a finding that indirectly indicates excess carbohydrate fermentation in the colon.

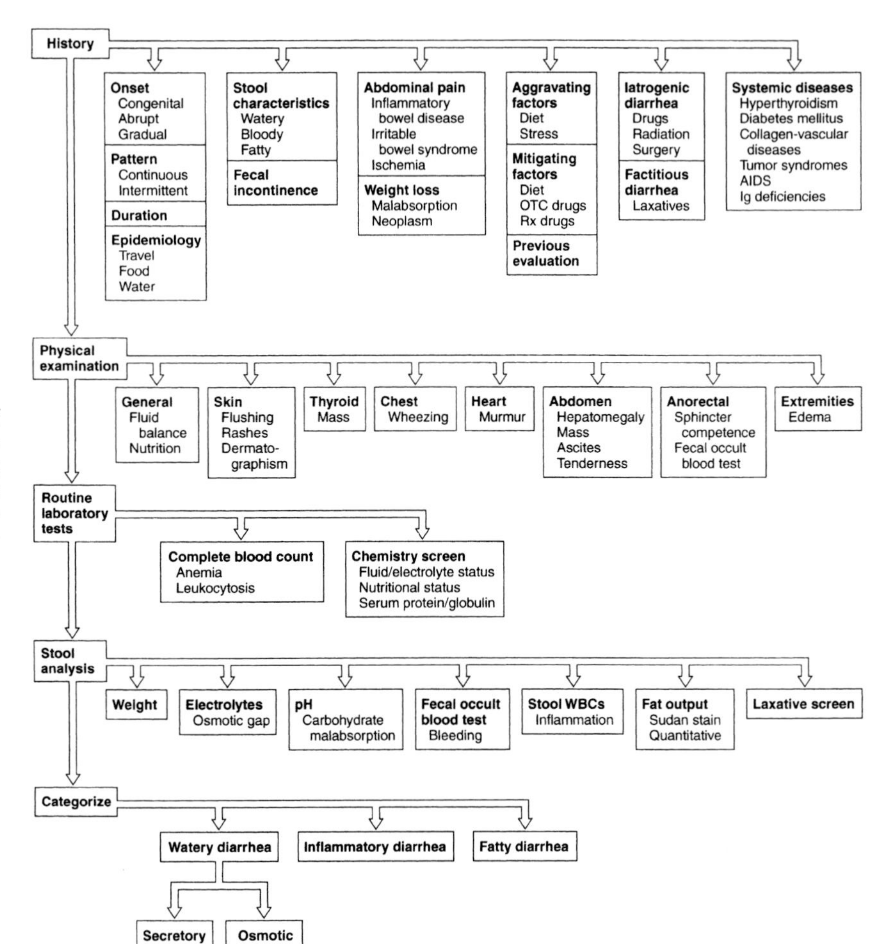

Figure 9–5. Flow chart for the initial evaluation of patients with chronic diarrhea. AIDS, acquired immunodeficiency syndrome; Ig, immunoglobulin; OTC, over-the-counter; Rx, prescription. (From Fine KD, Schiller LR: AGA technical review on the evaluation and management of chronic diarrhea. Gastroenterology 116:1464, 1999.)

Fecal occult blood testing and examination for fecal leukocytes allow one to identify inflammatory diarrheas resulting from colitis or malignancy. Other diarrheal conditions that have occult bleeding include lymphoma of the small intestine, celiac disease (positive in 50%), and refractory sprue (positive in 70%).[75]

Stool fat output can be measured quantitatively by chemical means on a timed (48- to 72-hour) collection or can be estimated qualitatively by Sudan stain on a random specimen. Steatorrhea is defined as excessive loss of fat in the stool, greater than 7 g or 9% of intake for 24 hours. This cut-off, however, may not be valid in all patients with diarrhea for the diagnosis of a disease causing fat malabsorption or maldigestion. In one study diarrhea induced with laxatives produced mild steatorrhea in 35% of normal subjects.[76] In patients with diarrhea, fat excretion in the range of 7 to 14 g per 24 hours has a low specificity for the diagnosis of defective fat absorption. However, fat excretion greater than 14 g per 24 hours strongly indicates a problem with fat absorption.[76] Fat intake during a quantitative collection should be estimated from diet diaries, because patients with diarrhea frequently have anorexia or early satiety that may reduce their fat intakes substantially, thereby reducing fat excretion. For a valid study patients should consume 70 to 100 g of fat per day for a few days before and during the timed collection. Measurement of fat excretion as a measure of malabsorption also can be compromised by ingestion of the lipase inhibitor orlistat or the fat substitute olestra.[77]

When only a random sample of stool is available, qualitative estimation of fat excretion by means of a Sudan stain of a fecal smear may be helpful.[78, 79] Semiquantitative methods can be applied to measure the number and size of fat globules, and these methods produce results that correlate well with quantitative collections[80] (see Chapter 89).

In patients who are suspected of surreptitious laxative ingestion, stool water can be analyzed for laxatives by chemical or chromatographic methods.[81] If positive, the test for the laxative should be repeated on another stool sample to confirm the finding before confronting the patient with this discovery.

Stool samples can also be tested for carbohydrate content with anthrone reagent[10] and for α_1-antitrypsin clearance for evaluation of protein-losing enteropathy.[82] These tests have limited clinical utility and should not be used routinely in the initial evaluation of a patient with chronic diarrhea unless there is a likelihood that the results will be helpful.

Once the stool analysis is completed, chronic diarrhea can be categorized as being *watery* with the subtypes of *secretory* or *osmotic* diarrhea, *inflammatory*, or *fatty*. This classification allows more direct evaluation of the cause of diarrhea.

Evaluation of Chronic Watery Diarrhea

Secretory diarrhea has a broad differential diagnosis as indicated previously (see Table 9–3) and so a wide investigative net must be cast to make a diagnosis (Fig. 9–7).

Infection should be excluded by stool culture for bacteria and special tests for other organisms. Human immunodeficiency virus (HIV) status should be clarified at this point, because patients with AIDS are more likely than others to have an infectious etiology for chronic diarrhea (see Chapter 28).[83] Although most bacteria causing diarrhea are cleared spontaneously within 4 weeks, some organisms, such as *Aeromonas* and *Pleisiomonas*, may produce chronic diarrhea.[84, 85] Special culture techniques may be needed to find these organisms. Special techniques are also required to find other pathogens. For example, coccidia and microsporidia require special microbiologic techniques for optimal detection, such as the polymerase chain reaction.[86] *Giardiasis* is sometimes difficult to diagnosis by a standard ova and parasite examination, but use of an ELISA for *Giardia* bacterial antigen has improved detection.[68] Examination of mucosal biopsy specimens with special stains or electron microscopy may be needed to find pathogens.

Small bowel bacterial overgrowth may cause secretory diarrhea, presumably due to toxins, as well as fatty diarrhea, due to bile salt deconjugation (see later). The glucose breath-hydrogen test (see later) can be used to screen for this condition, but the gold standard for diagnosis of small bowel bacterial overgrowth remains finding more than 10^6 bacteria by quantitative culture of a small bowel aspirate[87, 88] (see Chapter 90).

Structural diseases, such as *short bowel syndrome*, *gastrocolic* or *enteroenteric fistula*, *mucosal diseases*, *inflammatory bowel disease*, and *tumors* including *lymphomas* should be sought by means of radiographic and endoscopic techniques. Small bowel radiographs remain an important method for detecting structural small bowel diseases.[89] Computed tomography (CT) is of value not only for detecting small bowel and colonic diseases but also diseases extrinsic to the bowel that can cause diarrhea, such as *pancreatic tumors*.

Visualization and biopsy of the mucosa of the small bowel by endoscopy or enteroscopy can be valuable.[90–92]

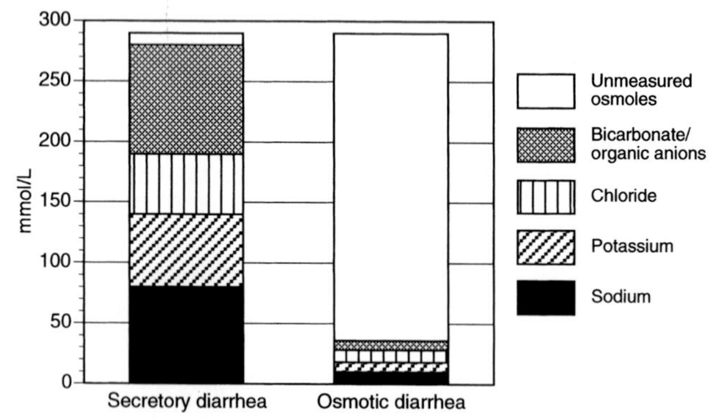

Figure 9–6. Fecal electrolytes and the fecal osmotic gap. The osmolality of colonic contents is in equilibrium with body fluids and is approximately 290 mOsm/kg. The total concentration of electrolytes, therefore, cannot exceed 290 mmol/L. In secretory diarrhea, almost all of the osmotic activity of colonic contents is due to electrolytes, and thus, the estimate of electrolyte content (2 × ($[Na^+]$ + $[K^+]$)) is almost 290 mmol/L. In osmotic diarrhea, electrolytes account for only a small part of the osmotic activity; unmeasured osmoles due to ingestion of a poorly absorbed substance account for most of the osmotic activity and so the calculated osmotic gap will be high. (From Schiller LR: Chronic diarrhea: In McNally P (ed): GI & Liver Secrets, 2nd ed. Philadelphia, Hanley & Belfus, 2001, pp 411–423.)

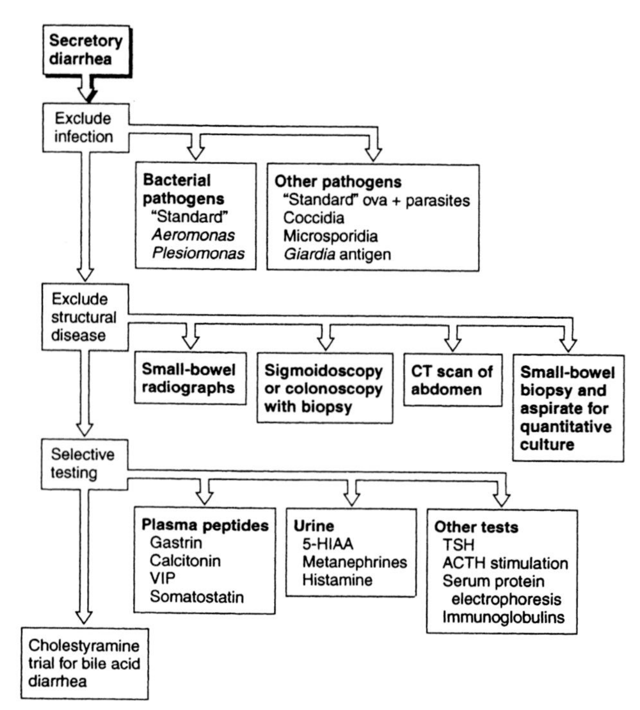

Figure 9–7. Flow chart for the evaluation of chronic secretory diarrhea. ACTH, adrenocorticotropic hormone; 5-HIAA, 5 hydroxyindole-acetic acid; TSH, thyroid-stimulating hormone; VIP, vasoactive intestinal peptide. (From Fine KD, Schiller LR: AGA technical review on the evaluation and management of chronic diarrhea. Gastroenterology 116:1464, 1999.)

Diseases that may be detected by small intestinal biopsy include *Crohn's disease*, *giardiasis*, *celiac sprue*, *intestinal lymphoma*, *eosinophilic gastroenteritis*, *tropical sprue*, *Whipple's disease*, *lymphangiectasia*, *abetalipoproteinemia*, *amyloidosis*, *mastocytosis*, and various infectious processes. Many of these disorders usually, but not always, present with steatorrhea (see Chapters 29, 89, 90, 92–100, and 103).

Sigmoidoscopy or colonoscopy can be used to visualize the colon and permit directed biopsy. Because in most patients with chronic secretory diarrhea the colonic disease is diffuse and will not lie beyond its range, sigmoidoscopy is adequate for this purpose.[93] Colonoscopy is preferable if blood is present in the stool, if there is a strong clinical suspicion of right colonic or ileal disease, or if the patient has AIDS.[70, 94, 95] Most patients with undiagnosed chronic secretory diarrhea should have mucosal biopsy specimens obtained from the colon, even when the mucosa appears normal.[2] Random biopsies should include multiple samples from several locations to give the pathologist the best chance of making a diagnosis. Chronic disorders that can be diagnosed by inspection of the colonic mucosa include *melanosis coli*, *ulceration*, *polyps*, *tumors*, *Crohn's disease*, *ulcerative colitis*, and *amebiasis*.[94] Diseases in which the colonic mucosa appears normal endoscopically, but which can be diagnosed histologically, include *microscopic colitis* (lymphocytic and collagenous colitis, see later), *amyloidosis*, *Whipple's disease*, *granulomatous infections*, and *schistosomiasis*[72, 95] (see Chapters 29, 95, 98, and 99).

The next level of investigation is selective testing for diarrhea due to peptide-secreting tumors, an intellectually interesting form of chronic watery diarrhea that is quite rare. The pretest probability of having a peptide-secreting tumor in a patient with chronic diarrhea is so low that screening these patients with a panel of serum peptide levels is far more likely to produce a false-positive than a true-positive result.[96] Testing for elevated serum peptide levels or urinary metabolites of endocrine mediators, such as 5-hydroxyindoleacetic acid (5-HIAA), metanephrines, and histamine, should be limited to those patients who have chronic diarrhea with symptoms and signs consistent with tumor syndromes, such as flushing or a big, hard liver in *carcinoid syndrome*,[97] ulcer disease suggestive of *Zollinger-Ellison syndrome*, or headache, flushing, or urticaria pigmentosa in *mastocytosis*, or those patients who have CT scans that show a tumor.[36] Scintigraphy using radiolabeled octreotide can also be used to identify peptide-secreting tumors[98] (see Chapters 41, 51, and 112).

More common endocrine diseases that cause diarrhea are *diabetes mellitus*, *hyperthyroidism*, and *Addison's disease*. In many cases, other symptoms and signs suggest the presence of these conditions, such as an enlarged thyroid or skin pigmentation characteristic of Addison's disease. It is reasonable to measure blood glucose, thyroid-stimulating hormone, and serum cortisol levels before and after injection of an adrenocorticotropic hormone analog in patients who might have these conditions. Other blood tests that may be relevant in evaluating secretory diarrhea include serum protein electrophoresis, immunoglobulin electrophoresis, and serologic tests, such as an antinuclear antibody or antibodies to HIV[2] (see Chapters 28 and 29).

Osmotic diarrhea has a much more limited differential diagnosis, and its evaluation is much simpler (Fig. 9–8).[7] For practical purposes osmotic diarrhea is due to one of three conditions: ingestion of exogenous magnesium, consumption of poorly absorbable carbohydrates, or carbohydrate malabsorption. Ingestion of other osmotically active substances is unusual. Fortunately, these conditions can be differentiated by simple stool testing.

Magnesium can be measured directly in stool water by atomic absorption spectrophotometry.[9] Excretion of more than 15 mmol (30 mEq) of magnesium daily or concentrations in stool water of more than 44 mmol/L (90 mEq/L) strongly suggests magnesium-induced diarrhea.[9] This may be intentional ingestion, as in a patient with surreptitious laxative ingestion, or accidental ingestion from the therapeutic use of magnesium-containing antacids or mineral supplements.

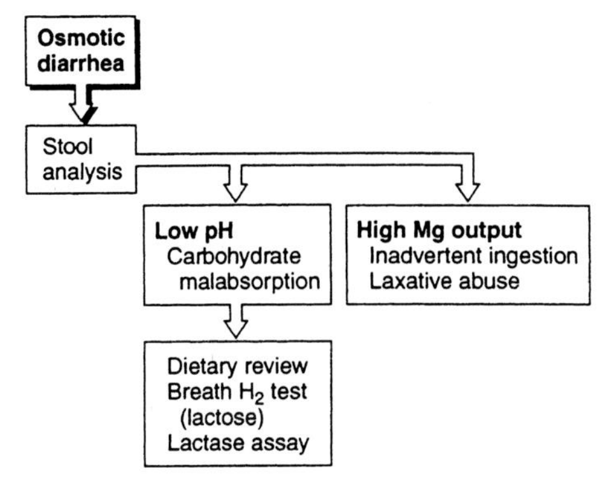

Figure 9–8. Flow chart for the evaluation of chronic osmotic diarrhea. (From Fine KD, Schiller LR: AGA technical review on the evaluation and management of chronic diarrhea. Gastroenterology 116:1464, 1999.)

Ingestion of poorly absorbed carbohydrates or carbohydrate malabsorption typically leads to a low fecal pH due to bacterial fermentation in the colon. Fecal pH of less than 6 is highly suggestive of carbohydrate malabsorption.[8, 10] More generalized malabsorption that involves fecal loss of amino acids and fatty acids in addition to carbohydrate may produce a somewhat higher pH (e.g., pH 6 to 7.5). Isolated carbohydrate malabsorption is usually due to ingestion of a poorly absorbable carbohydrate, such as lactose in someone with lactase deficiency. Other common causes include ingestion of poorly absorbed sugar alcohols that are used as artificial sweeteners, such as sorbitol or mannitol, or excessive ingestion of sugars with a limited absorption capacity, such as fructose.[58] Therapeutic use of inhibitors of carbohydrate absorption, such as acarbose, may also lead to carbohydrate malabsorption.[99] Because fermentation produces not only short-chain fatty acids that acidify the stool but also carbon dioxide and hydrogen, "gas" and bloating are clinical clues to the presence of carbohydrate malabsorption (see Chapters 10, 88, and 89).

Once the clinical picture or stool analysis suggests carbohydrate malabsorption, careful dietary review may indicate the likely source. In some individuals, a breath hydrogen test with lactose as the sugar substrate can confirm the diagnosis.[100] In this test a fasting patient is given 25 g of lactose dissolved in water, and exhaled breath is assayed for hydrogen content at baseline and at intervals for several hours. Because hydrogen is not a normal product of human metabolism, any increase in breath hydrogen concentration represents bacterial fermentation and indicates that unabsorbed lactose has reached the colon. This principle also has been applied to assessment of sucrase deficiency by administration of a sucrose load. Breath hydrogen testing has been adapted to detect small bowel bacterial overgrowth by the use of glucose that ordinarily should be completely absorbed before reaching the colon.[101] Lactulose, a nonabsorbable but easily fermented disaccharide, also has been used for detection of bacterial overgrowth and for determination of the oral-cecal transit time.[102] Breath hydrogen testing after administration of D-xylose has been advocated as a screening test for generalized intestinal malabsorption.[103] For most purposes breath hydrogen testing provides only supportive evidence when the pretest likelihood of a particular diagnosis is high.

Once a specific diagnosis has been proposed for osmotic diarrhea, therapeutic trial of an elimination diet can confirm the diagnosis.

Evaluation of Chronic Inflammatory Diarrhea

Patients with chronic diarrhea who have white blood cells or blood in the stool are classified as having *inflammatory diarrhea*. These characteristics indicate that there has been mucosal disruption and inflammation. Diagnostic considerations include *inflammatory bowel disease*, *infections*, *pseudomembranous enterocolitis*, *ischemia*, *radiation enteritis*, and *neoplasia*. Because these conditions may produce a secretory diarrhea without markers of inflammation in the stool, they must be considered in the evaluation of secretory diarrhea as well (see Chapters 96–98, 102, and 113–115).

Sigmoidoscopy or colonoscopy should be used to look

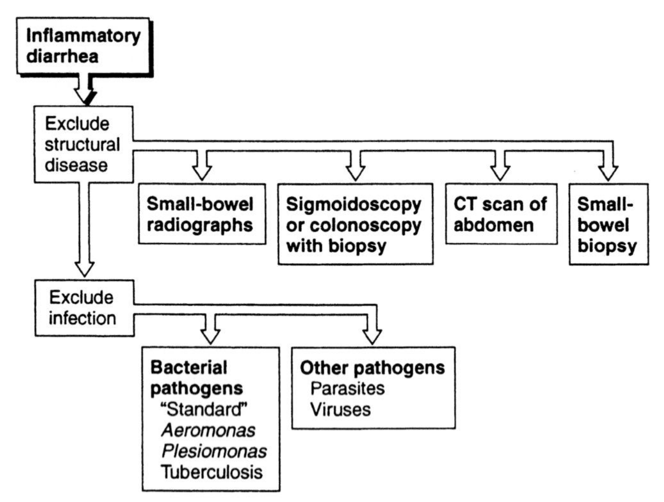

Figure 9–9. Flow chart for the evaluation of chronic inflammatory diarrhea. (From Fine KD, Schiller LR: AGA technical review on the evaluation and management of chronic diarrhea. Gastroenterology 116:1464, 1999.)

for structural changes initially, because colitis is a common cause of this type of diarrhea and neoplasm can be life threatening (Fig. 9–9). Sigmoidoscopy can detect most causes of inflammatory diarrhea.[93] Because preparation for this test is simpler than that for colonoscopy and there are fewer complications, sigmoidoscopy is preferred by some physicians. Others prefer to examine the entire colon and terminal ileum in patients with inflammatory diarrhea, especially if the fecal occult blood test is positive.[94, 95] The choice of test depends on the circumstances of the individual patient. Whichever test is selected, biopsy specimens must be obtained from the colon to aid in making the correct diagnosis.

Infection can cause a chronic inflammatory diarrhea or aggravate an existing inflammatory diarrhea due to ulcerative colitis or Crohn's disease. The most likely pathogens that might cause chronic inflammatory diarrhea are *C. difficile*, cytomegalovirus, amebiasis, and tuberculosis. In addition to biopsies, appropriate cultures and serologic tests need to be obtained to exclude these infections. They should also be sought in appropriate circumstances in patients with inflammatory bowel disease.[104]

Evaluation of Chronic Fatty Diarrhea

Steatorrhea implies the disruption of fat solubilization, digestion, or absorption in the small intestine. The evaluation of chronic fatty diarrhea is designed to distinguish between *maldigestion*—inadequate luminal breakdown of triglyceride—and *malabsorption*—inadequate mucosal transport of the products of digestion (see Chapter 89).

The major causes of maldigestion are pancreatic exocrine insufficiency (e.g., chronic pancreatitis) and lack of bile (e.g., advanced primary biliary cirrhosis). Mucosal diseases (e.g., celiac disease) are the common causes of malabsorption. Fecal fat *concentration* (grams of fat per 100 g of stool) provides a clue to the cause of steatorrhea.[105] Mucosal disease often is associated with poor fluid and electrolyte absorption, and so stool fat content is "diluted" by unabsorbed water. In addition, because fat digestion usually is intact in mucosal disease, triglycerides are broken down to fatty acids in the small intestine and pass into the colon where they inhibit electrolyte and water absorption, further diluting the fat content of stool.[49] In contrast, maldigestion due to pancreatic and biliary problems typically does not produce fatty acids and does not affect fluid and electrolyte absorption; thus, the unabsorbed fat is dispersed in a smaller stool volume. A fecal fat concentration greater than 9.5 g per 100 g in patients with suspected maldigestion strongly suggests the presence of pancreatic or biliary steatorrhea.[105]

The further evaluation of patients with chronic fatty diarrhea is relatively straightforward (Fig. 9–10). The first step is to look for structural problems involving the small bowel. This evaluation may include small bowel radiography, CT scan of the abdomen, and small bowel biopsy. When the small bowel biopsy is obtained, luminal contents should be aspirated and a sample sent for quantitative culture to exclude small bowel bacterial overgrowth. At the present time, indirect testing for small intestinal diseases, such as measuring antigluten and antiendomysial (or tissue transglutaminase) antibodies for the diagnosis of celiac disease or breath testing for bacterial overgrowth, may not be accurate enough to displace endoscopic biopsy or quantitative culture (see Chapters 90 and 93).[106, 107]

If no structural problems are discovered, abnormal pancreatic exocrine function should be considered. Available tests of pancreatic function all have limitations.

The secretin test, in which exogenous secretin is used to stimulate the gland and bicarbonate output is measured by aspiration of duodenal contents, is the most time-honored of these tests.[108] It is rarely performed because of its complexity and the limited availability of secretin for human use. The bentiromide test, in which the degree of hydrolysis of an orally administered synthetic substrate by chymotrypsin to a breakdown product is measured in a timed collection of urine, has been used widely, but, unfortunately, has limited sensitivity.[109] Direct measurement of stool chymotrypsin activity also has poor sensitivity and specificity in patients with chronic diarrhea.[110] Measurement of fecal elastase has only somewhat better reliability.[111] The best "test" for pancreatic exocrine insufficiency may be a therapeutic trial of

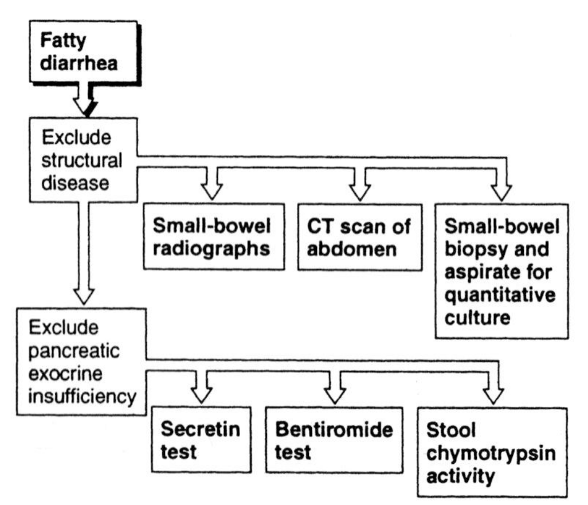

Figure 9–10. Flow chart for the evaluation of chronic fatty diarrhea. (From Fine KD, Schiller LR: AGA technical review on the evaluation and management of chronic diarrhea. Gastroenterology 116:1464, 1999.)

pancreatic enzyme supplementation. If such a trial is conducted, high doses of enzymes should be used and some objective measurement, such as fecal fat excretion or weight gain, should be monitored to assess response (see Chapter 49).

The possibility of inadequate or bile salt solubilization of dietary fat can usually be inferred from the history or physical examination, for example, a history of ileal resection or known enterocolic fistula. If proof of this mechanism is required, analysis of a postprandial duodenal aspirate can demonstrate reduced conjugated bile acid concentration.[112] This test may not be available outside specialized centers, and so a therapeutic trial may be the best way of establishing the diagnosis. Supplementation of the diet with exogenous conjugated bile acid should reduce steatorrhea, if bile acid deficiency is the problem. Such supplementation can often improve nutritional status without aggravating diarrhea.[113, 114]

NONSPECIFIC TREATMENT OF DIARRHEA

The most important treatment for diarrhea is to ensure that fluid and electrolyte deficits are replenished with intravenous fluids or oral rehydration solution. Because nutrient absorption accelerates sodium and fluid absorption in the jejunum, even when other forms of sodium absorption are impaired, saline solutions containing glucose or amino acids will be absorbed readily.[115] Although the earliest rehydration solutions used glucose to accelerate sodium absorption, cereal-based rehydration solutions are now thought to be superior.[116] Recent modifications to the formula include hypo-osmolarity and use of amylase-resistant starch to enhance colonic short-chain fatty acid and water absorption.[117, 118] Oral rehydration solutions increase fluid and electrolyte absorption; they are not designed to reduce stool output, so stool weight actually may increase with their use. Use of oral rehydration solutions is precluded in patients who are vomiting frequently. Although most sport drinks (e.g., Gatorade) are designed to replenish modest electrolyte losses from sweat, they do not have enough sodium to adequately replace losses in diarrhea. These solutions can be used if additional sources of sodium and absorbable nutrients (e.g., pretzels or crackers) are ingested concomitantly. Solutions that approximate World Health Organization oral rehydration solution more closely are available commercially (e.g., Rehydralyte, Resol, Ricalyte).

Empiric Therapy of Acute Diarrhea

Because infection is a frequent cause of acute diarrhea, empiric trials of antibiotic therapy often are considered by physicians. If the prevalence of bacterial or protozoal infection is high in a community or in a specific situation, empiric use of antibiotics is logical as in the treatment of travelers' diarrhea with a fluoroquinolone, even without bacteriologic proof of infection.[119] Empiric antibiotic therapy is often also logically used for more severely ill patients while awaiting bacterial culture results. This approach has been called into question recently with the observation that patients who develop hemolytic-uremic syndrome in response to infection with *Escherichia coli* are more likely to have received empiric antibiotic therapy.[120] Experts also advise against empiric treatment of salmonellosis unless enteric fever is present.[121]

Nonspecific antidiarrheal agents can reduce stool frequency and stool weight and can reduce coexisting symptoms, such as abdominal cramps (Table 9–6). Opiates, such as loperamide, or diphenoxylate with atropine frequently are employed.[122] Concerns about slowing the clearance of pathogens from the intestine with these antiperistaltic agents largely have not been substantiated. Intraluminal agents, such as bismuth subsalicylate (Pepto-Bismol) and adsorbents (e.g., kaolin) also may help reduce the fluidity of bowel movements.[122]

Empiric Therapy of Chronic Diarrhea

Empiric therapy is used in patients with chronic diarrhea in three situations: (1) as temporizing or initial treatment before diagnostic testing; (2) after diagnostic testing has failed to confirm a diagnosis; and (3) when a diagnosis has been made but no specific treatment is available or specific treatment has failed to produce a cure. Generally, empiric antibiotic therapy is less useful in chronic diarrhea than in acute diarrhea, because bacterial infection is far less likely as the cause. Although some clinicians try an empiric course of metronidazole or a fluoroquinolone before committing a patient to extensive diagnostic testing, this approach has no data to support it and is not recommended.

Therapeutic trials of pancreatic enzyme replacement and conjugated bile acid supplementation in unexplained steatorrhea were discussed earlier. Pancreatic enzyme supplements or bile acid–binding resins are tried empirically as well in so-called idiopathic chronic diarrhea, but satisfactory results are rare (see later).

Symptomatic treatment with opiates often is necessary in patients with chronic diarrhea because specific treatment may not be available.[122] Potent opiates such as codeine, opium, or

Table 9–6 | **Nonspecific Therapy for Chronic Diarrhea**

DRUG CLASS	AGENT	DOSE
Opiates		
μ-Opiate receptor selective	Diphenoxylate	2.5–5 mg QID
	Loperamide	2–4 mg QID
	Codeine	15–60 mg QID
	Morphine	2–20 mg QID
	Opium tincture	2–20 drops QID
Enkephalinase inhibitor (δ-opiate receptor effects)	Racecadotril (acetorphan)	1.5 mg/kg TID*
Adrenergic agonist	Clonidine	0.1–0.3 mg TID
Somatostatin analogue	Octreotide	50–250 μg TID (subcutaneously)
Bile acid–binding resin	Cholestyramine	4 g QD to QID
Fiber supplements	Psyllium	10–20 g daily
	Calcium polycarbophil	5–10 g daily

*Not yet approved in the United States.

morphine are underused in the management of these patients, largely because of fear of abuse. In fact, these agents are rarely abused by patients with chronic diarrhea, especially if a few simple measures are taken. First, the patient needs to be informed about the abuse potential of the medication and should be warned about increasing the dose without consulting the physician. Second, dosing should be started at a low level and titrated up to an effective dose. Third, use of the opiate should be monitored closely and the prescription should not be refilled until an interval appropriate with the anticipated usage has passed. New antidiarrheal drugs with effects on the δ-opiate receptor rather than the μ-opiate receptor are being studied.[123–126]

Other agents that are sometimes used as nonspecific antidiarrheal agents include octreotide and clonidine. The somatostatin analog, octreotide, has been shown to improve diarrhea in carcinoid syndrome and related endocrine diarrheas, dumping syndrome, and AIDS diarrhea.[127] It is less clear that it has much benefit in other diarrheal diseases. Clonidine, an α-adrenergic agent, has effects on both motility and intestinal transport that contribute to its antidiarrheal effect.[128] Its hypotensive effect limits its usefulness in many patients with diarrhea, but it may have a special role in diabetic diarrhea.[129] Interest has been increasing in the use of probiotics, ostensibly "good" bacteria such as certain strains of lactobacilli, as therapy for diarrhea. By modifying the colonic flora, these agents may stimulate local immunity and speed the resolution of travelers' diarrhea, antibiotic-associated diarrhea, and infantile diarrhea.[130–133] Herbal remedies for diarrhea include those containing berberine (goldenseal, barberry) and arrowroot.[134, 135]

Stool-modifying agents such as psyllium alter stool consistency but do not reduce stool weight.[136] They can be used successfully in patients with coexisting fecal incontinence and in some patients with relatively low stool weights. The change from watery to semiformed stools may be sufficient to alleviate symptoms.

HIGHLIGHTS OF SELECTED DIARRHEAL SYNDROMES

Diarrhea in Irritable Bowel Syndrome

Undoubtedly, the most common diagnosis made in patients with chronic diarrhea is *irritable bowel syndrome,* yet only a fraction of these patients actually meet the current criteria for this diagnosis, which emphasize abdominal pain as central to the diagnosis.[62] In part this reflects changing diagnostic criteria. In the past "painless diarrhea" was considered to be a subtype of irritable bowel syndrome. Such patients now would be excluded from a diagnosis of irritable bowel syndrome.

Diarrhea in irritable bowel syndrome tends to be quite variable and sometimes alternates with periods of constipation.[137] When measured, daily stool output is low, typically less than 400 g per 24 hours. Consistency varies from loose to soft and rarely is watery. Diarrhea does not wake patients from sleep. Urgency and fecal incontinence may be pronounced, especially during periods of psychological stress. Weight loss and evidence of chronic illness are uncommon (see Chapter 91).

When these features are absent, other diagnoses should be considered, the most prominent of which is carbohydrate malabsorption that can produce diarrhea of variable severity, depending on dietary intake of the malabsorbed carbohydrate, cramps, and bloating.[138] A careful dietary history and stool pH lower than 6 can distinguish this disorder from irritable bowel syndrome. Bile acid–induced diarrhea can also have variable severity, depending on the delivery of bile acid to the colon. Response to a therapeutic trial of bile acid–binding resin may be diagnostic. Most other causes of chronic diarrhea have been misdiagnosed as irritable bowel syndrome at some point before the correct diagnosis is discovered.

Microscopic Colitis Syndrome

Terminology has been a difficult issue for microscopic colitis syndrome. The term *collagenous colitis* was used to describe the histologic findings of subepithelial fibrosis and inflammation in the rectal mucosa of a woman with chronic watery diarrhea who had a normal gross appearance of the mucosa by proctoscopy.[139] Several years later the term *microscopic colitis* was introduced to describe the histologic findings of mucosal inflammation without fibrosis in patients with chronic diarrhea who had normal colonic mucosa by colonoscopy.[140] Subsequently the term *lymphocytic colitis* was coined to emphasize the presence of intraepithelial lymphocytosis in these patients.[141]

The relationship between these entities has not been clear from the start. Because their clinical presentations are so similar and their pathologic appearances differ only in the presence or absence of a thickened subepithelial collagen table, current usage now includes lymphocytic colitis and collagenous colitis as histologic subtypes of microscopic colitis syndrome. This clinical syndrome is characterized by the presence of chronic watery diarrhea, a normal or near-normal gross appearance of the colonic mucosa, and specific microscopic changes of lymphocytic-plasmacytic inflammation in the lamina propria and intraepithelial lymphocytosis with or without thickening of the subepithelial collagen table.[142, 143]

Microscopic colitis syndrome is a fairly common cause of chronic diarrhea of obscure origin at referral centers. At Baylor University Medical Center in Dallas, microscopic colitis syndrome was discovered in 10% of patients with chronic diarrhea, with an even division between lymphocytic and collagenous subtypes.[96] The keys to making this diagnosis are remembering to biopsy normal-appearing colonic mucosa in patients presenting with chronic watery diarrhea and having a skilled pathologist review the biopsy slides. Because the histologic changes in microscopic colitis are diffuse, biopsy of the mucosa of the left colon is adequate in most situations.[144]

Like idiopathic inflammatory bowel disease, the cause or causes of microscopic colitis syndrome remain unknown.[142] Bacterial antigens in the colonic lumen might play an important role. Transgenic rats genetically engineered to express human leukocyte antigen HLA-B27 routinely develop a picture identical to lymphocytic colitis, but only if the animals have bacteria in the colon.[145] Microscopic colitis in humans is not linked to HLA-B27 but has been associated with other

HLA loci. Most fascinating is the tight linkage of both lymphocytic and collagenous colitis with HLA-DQ2 and HLA-DQ1,3 (including the HLA-DQ1,3 subtypes, HLA-DQ1,7; HLA-DQ1,8; and HLA-DQ1,9) as in celiac sprue, suggesting the possibility that similar immune mechanisms are involved.[146] Gluten is almost certainly not the antigen involved, however, because many celiac patients treated with a gluten-free diet have histologic evidence of lymphocytic colitis and elimination of gluten from the diet is not effective.[147] The association of many autoimmune diseases with microscopic colitis syndrome also suggests an immune etiology.

Whatever the cause of the inflammation, it is clear that mucosal inflammation is largely responsible for the diarrhea of microscopic colitis syndrome. Colonic perfusion studies have shown that absorption of water and salt is impaired in lymphocytic colitis and collagenous colitis.[148] Colonic water absorption is inversely correlated with the cellularity of the lamina propria but not with collagen table thickness. However, net secretion of water and salt by the colon is not noted frequently.[148] Typical stool weights of 500 to 1000 g per 24 hours are consistent with little or no fluid absorption by the colon.[144]

Treatment options include anti-inflammatory drugs, such as sulfasalazine, mesalamine, and prednisone; immunosuppressive agents, such as azathioprine; and miscellaneous agents, such as bile acid binders and bismuth subsalicylate.[142] Large doses of anti-inflammatory drugs are needed to induce remission and only 30% to 50% of patients respond. No large series of patients treated with immunosuppressive drugs has been published; anecdotal evidence suggests relatively low response rates. Bile acid binders have been relatively successful in one European study.[149] The highest response rate has been reported with bismuth subsalicylate; therapy for 4 to 8 weeks resulted in symptomatic and histologic improvement in approximately 90% of patients with microscopic colitis.[150] Microscopic colitis remits in most patients with time, and so symptomatic therapy with antidiarrheal drugs may be an appropriate option.[151]

Postsurgical Diarrhea

Gastrointestinal and biliary tract surgical procedures produce a number of changes in gut function that may lead to diarrhea. Although surgery for peptic ulcer is now much less common, other current operations on the gastrointestinal and biliary tracts continue to be complicated by diarrhea.

DIARRHEA AFTER GASTRIC SURGERY. Peptic ulcer was treated surgically for many years by vagotomy with pyloroplasty or antrectomy. The introduction of highly selective vagotomy in the 1980s decreased the incidence of postoperative diarrhea. The more traditional surgeries are still done for obstructing or malignant ulcer disease.

The most common syndrome seen after gastric surgery is *dumping syndrome*, a condition characterized by flushing, hypotension, diarrhea, and hypoglycemia postprandially (see Chapter 42). This syndrome results from unregulated gastric emptying, osmotic shifts, and the rapid release of peptide hormones from the gut.[152] It can be treated successfully with a modified diet, antidiarrheal drugs, and the somatostatin analog, octreotide.[153]

Gastric surgery may also predispose patients to bacterial overgrowth in the small intestine, abnormally rapid intestinal transit, bile acid malabsorption, and pancreatic exocrine insufficiency due to poor stimulation or inadequate mixing.[152]

DIARRHEA AFTER BOWEL RESECTION. Loss of surface area promotes malabsorption of fluid, electrolytes, or nutrients, depending on the portion of the bowel resected. The bowel is endowed with an excess of surface area for absorption under ordinary circumstances. Diarrhea develops after resection of the small intestine that leaves insufficient surface area for normal absorption. The process of *intestinal adaptation* may improve intestinal electrolyte absorption with time but cannot overcome defects of specialized function.[26] For example, removal of the ileocecal area limits the ability to absorb sodium against its electrochemical gradient, a defect that cannot be compensated for elsewhere in the gut (see Chapter 92).[27] Likewise, resection of the terminal ileum results in a permanent reduction in conjugated bile acid absorption that may produce bile acid–mediated fluid and electrolyte secretion by the colon.[154]

ILEOSTOMY DIARRHEA. Normally 1 to 1.5 L enter the colon from the small intestine each day and an ileostomy will divert it from the body. Adaptation eventually results in a decrease of flow to an average of 750 mL per day provided that the patient has a sufficient length of functioning small bowel. This excess daily loss usually is readily overcome by increasing oral intake. Patients with ileostomies tolerate abnormally increased losses poorly, however, and are at risk for dehydration under such circumstances. Ileostomy diarrhea is said to be present when losses exceed 1000 mL per day (see Chapter 105).[155]

Causes of ileostomy diarrhea include stomal stenosis, partial bowel obstruction, bacterial overgrowth, recurrent disease proximal to the stoma, medication-associated diarrhea, and intraperitoneal infection. A special circumstance is in patients with ileal pouches formed to create "continent ileostomies" or as part of ileoanal anastomosis after colectomy for ulcerative colitis. These patients may develop inflammation of the pouch, so-called "pouchitis" due to bacterial overgrowth or recurrent inflammatory bowel disease.[156] This condition is treated with antibiotics, such as metronidazole, or with anti-inflammatory drugs, such as mesalamine.

Ileostomy diarrhea is treated with antidiarrheal drugs; high doses of potent agents may be necessary. If output exceeds 2000 mL per day, supplemental oral rehydration solution or intravenous fluid may have to be provided to avoid dehydration and to allow for normal urine output.

POSTCHOLECYSTECTOMY DIARRHEA. The gallbladder provides a place for bile acid to stay at night when it is not needed for digestion of fat. When the gallbladder is removed, the enterohepatic cycling of bile acid continues at night and a substantial portion of the bile acid pool is within the small bowel at all times. Every 90 minutes while fasting, the migrating myoelectric complex passes through the small intestine, sweeping intestinal contents—including much of the bile acid pool in this case—rapidly past the specialized absorptive sites in the ileum and into the colon. The local concentration of bile acid in the colon may exceed 3 to 5 mmol/L and may inhibit colonic fluid and electrolyte absorption and accelerate transit, thereby working as a laxative.[157–159]

This mechanism largely accounts for the diarrhea that occurs in up to 20% of patients after cholecystectomy, which may not begin immediately after cholecystectomy, but years later.[158, 159] Presumably this delayed onset occurs in response to some additional unknown disturbance that develops over time.

Postcholecystectomy diarrhea is best treated with bile acid binders given at bedtime and perhaps at other times during the day as well. Opiate antidiarrheals can also be helpful for refractory cases.

Diarrhea in Hospitalized Patients

Diarrhea frequently develops during hospitalization, particularly in severely ill patients hospitalized for protracted periods. Common causes for diarrhea in this setting include *medication-related diarrhea*, especially antibiotic-associated diarrhea, diarrhea associated with *tube feeding*, *intestinal ischemia*, and *fecal impaction*.

Diarrhea is a side effect of many medications, including those frequently used in hospitalized patients (see Table 9–5).[22, 53] Antibiotic therapy is particularly likely to cause diarrhea, and it does so by two main mechanisms: by impairing carbohydrate metabolism by the colonic bacterial flora and by overgrowth of *C. difficile* and production of toxins by the bacteria.[160] In some cases, the antibiotic erythromycin produces diarrhea by its motilin-like effect on gastrointestinal transit.

Carbohydrate not absorbed by the small intestine is carried to the colon where bacteria ferment it in short-chain fatty acids, hydrogen, and carbon dioxide. Under ordinary conditions all dietary fiber and about 20% of starch evades digestion and absorption and reaches the colon. The products of fermentation are absorbed and diarrhea does not result. When antibiotics kill some of the normal colonic flora, fermentation decreases and water is retained osmotically, producing diarrhea. It is conceivable that intestinal transit is modified by illness or by other drugs given concomitantly with more rapid delivery of carbohydrate to the colon, further aggravating the diarrhea. Such diarrhea should subside when the patient is fasting.

C. difficile–related diarrhea is a much more serious concern.[161] Hospitalized patients and residents of nursing homes are very likely to be colonized by this organism; indeed, approximately 20% of hospitalized patients become colonized. Physical proximity is a major factor in its spread within institutions.[162] When diarrhea develops, it can range in severity from modest to a life-threatening colitis. Patients may have severe pain, abdominal tenderness, and a marked polymorphonuclear leukocytosis with an increased percentage of immature forms. In less severely ill patients suspected of having this infection, stool must be tested for *C. difficile* toxin, and, if positive, used to guide appropriate therapy (see Chapter 97).[163] In more severely ill patients, sigmoidoscopy often identifies the characteristic findings of *pseudomembranous colitis*. Occasionally, the colitis is evident only more proximally in the colon and colonoscopy is required to confirm the diagnosis. Therapy with metronidazole or vancomycin often suppresses the diarrhea, but recurrence is common. Probiotics are being studied as a way to reduce recurrence.[164]

Diarrhea also may be a complication of enteral nutrition but is often due to coexisting problems.[165] Tube feeding, although more physiologic than parenteral nutrition, is still quite different than the normal presentation of nutrients to the intestine, and the regulatory system of the gut may not adapt to this situation. Some tube-feeding formulas are hypertonic and may induce diarrhea by a mechanism similar to that of dumping syndrome. In such cases a change of formula to an isotonic formula may be of benefit. In other cases slowing the rate of infusion and thereby decreasing the delivery of nutrients to the intestine may be helpful. This may be of limited value if nutritional needs are not being met at the slower rate of infusion, however. Addition of an antidiarrheal, such as loperamide or opium tincture, to the tube feeding may need to be considered. This approach has its limitations though, especially in patients with a tendency toward ileus (see Chapter 16).

Some patients develop intestinal ischemia during hospitalization, especially if they have hypotension or shock. They are at risk for developing bloody diarrhea due to ischemic colitis or more profound diarrhea if small bowel ischemia develops.

Fecal impaction is a risk for the elderly, patients at prolonged bowel rest, and those receiving constipating drugs. Paradoxical or "overflow" diarrhea may be the first clue to impaction. Hospitalized patients who develop diarrhea should have a digital rectal examination to exclude this possibility.

Bile Acid–Induced Diarrhea

The importance of bile acid malabsorption as a mechanism for producing chronic secretory diarrhea is controversial.[166–168] Bile acid malabsorption has been well described as the mechanism of diarrhea in ileal disease or resection that allows excessive amounts of conjugated bile acid to enter the colon.[154] Concentrations of bile acid in the colon higher than 3 to 5 mmol/L can inhibit electrolyte absorption and stimulate secretion by the colonic mucosa.[157]

It is not clear how often this mechanism produces chronic watery diarrhea when there is no overt ileal disease or resection. Studies from both Europe and the United States indicate that bile acid malabsorption is common in patients with idiopathic chronic diarrhea.[166–168] However, there is a major discrepancy in reports of the therapeutic effect of bile acid–sequestering resins in this setting. European studies often have shown that a high proportion of patients with idiopathic secretory diarrhea respond to therapeutic doses of bile acid–sequestering resins, whereas American studies have shown no consistent effect.

The clinical implications of these reports are clear. First, it is not worthwhile to do a sophisticated test for bile acid malabsorption, such as the SeHCAT retention test or fecal radiolabeled bile acid study, because diarrhea itself may make the test abnormal. Second, the test may not be predictive of successful therapy with a bile acid–sequestering resin. It therefore makes more sense to use an empiric trial of a bile acid–sequestering resin in patients with undiagnosed idiopathic diarrhea; if the medication controls the diarrhea, bile acid malabsorption may be playing a role.

Factitious Diarrhea

Laxative abusers fall into one of four categories (Table 9–7).[169] The first includes those with anorexia or bulimia who use laxatives as a way of adjusting body weight (see Chapter 17). The second comprises those who use laxative-induced illness for a secondary gain such as disability income or to generate concern in other individuals. The third consists of patients with Munchausen syndrome who feign illness to confound physicians. The fourth category includes individuals who are being poisoned with laxatives by their caregivers. Laxative abuse should be considered in an individual in whom diarrhea goes undiagnosed, especially in those who fit into one of the groups just mentioned.

Detection of laxative abuse depends on having a high index of suspicion for this diagnosis. Physicians usually assume that patients are being truthful, but up to 15% of patients being evaluated for chronic diarrhea may be abusing laxatives surreptitiously.[170, 171] Clues to laxative abuse may be found as part of the evaluation for chronic diarrhea. For example, hypokalemia may suggest ingestion of stimulant laxatives, such as senna. The finding of *melanosis coli*, a brownish pigmentation of the colonic mucosa, suggests recent, chronic ingestion of anthracene laxatives, such as senna or cascara. Presence of a large fecal osmotic gap may suggest magnesium ingestion.

In patients who may belong to one of the groups listed in Table 9–7 and in patients with diarrhea that remains undiagnosed after evaluation, stool samples should be evaluated for laxatives with standardized methods.[81] Most laxatives can be detected by spectrophotometry or chromatography. Because some patients exaggerate stool volume by adding urine or water, stool osmolality should be measured as well; values of less than 290 mOsm/kg suggest dilution of the stool with water or hypotonic urine.[74] Admixture of stool with hypertonic urine often leads to an impossibly high fecal osmolality (typically > 600 mOsm/kg) and to a negative fecal osmotic gap, because of high concentrations of sodium and potassium in urine. A negative fecal osmotic gap can also be noted when phosphate or sulfate osmotic laxatives are ingested. Unauthorized room searches for laxatives should not be conducted, given today's legal environment.

When a diagnosis of laxative abuse is made, an effort should be made to confirm the diagnosis before discussion with the patient or family. This usually involves analysis of a second stool sample. When the diagnosis is confirmed, the patient should be confronted with the findings, but not before making plans for the aftermath. Psychiatric consultation should follow the discussion with the patient because some who abuse laxatives become suicidal after being discovered and all need counseling. In cases of laxative administration by a parent or caregiver, legal proceedings should be instituted to separate the patient from the abuser.

Table 9–7 | **Groups of Patients with Laxative Abuse**

GROUP	CHARACTERISTICS
Patients with bulimia	Usually adolescent to young adult women; concerned about weight or manifesting an eating disorder
Secondary gain	May have disability claim pending; illness may induce concern or caring behavior in others
Munchausen syndrome	Peripatetic patients who relish being diagnostic challenges; may undergo extensive testing repeatedly
Polle's syndrome (Munchausen syndrome by proxy)	Dependent child or adult poisoned with laxatives by parent or caregiver to show effectiveness as caregiver; may have history of sibling who died with chronic diarrhea

Outcome studies of the effect of discovery of laxative abuse are few. One study of 11 patients seen at the Cleveland Clinic found that six patients said that they were improved and five patients claimed no benefit.[172] Four of these five patients sought further medical attention elsewhere for their problem with chronic diarrhea.

Idiopathic Secretory Diarrhea

When an exhaustive evaluation fails to reveal a cause for chronic diarrhea and stool analysis suggests a secretory diarrhea, the diagnosis of *idiopathic secretory diarrhea* is made. This condition often starts suddenly in previously healthy individuals and is differentiated from the many similar acute diarrheal illnesses by persisting beyond 4 weeks. It occurs in two forms: *epidemic* and *sporadic*.[55, 56]

The epidemic form of secretory diarrhea occurs in outbreaks seemingly linked to contaminated food or drink.[55] The initial description of this condition resulted from an outbreak in Brainerd, Minnesota, thus giving this condition its common appellation, "Brainerd diarrhea."[173] Several outbreaks have been described in the literature in different communities and even on a cruise ship.[173–175] Although such an epidemiology suggests an infectious agent, no such agent has been identified in these outbreaks.

Sporadic idiopathic secretory diarrhea affects individuals in an identical fashion but does not seem to be easily acquired by family members or others.[56] Many affected individuals give a history of travel, but this travel is not to destinations usually associated with travelers' diarrhea. Diarrhea begins abruptly and reaches its maximum intensity soon after onset. Weight loss of up to 20 pounds is characteristic, but this almost always occurs within the first few months of illness and is not progressive. Empiric trials of antibiotics and bile acid–binding resins are ineffective. Nonspecific opioid antidiarrheals may provide symptomatic improvement.

Both forms of idiopathic secretory diarrhea have self-limited courses and usually disappear within 2 years of onset.[55, 56] The offset of idiopathic secretory diarrhea occurs gradually over 2 to 3 months. This natural history can be a solace to patients who otherwise feel mired with an unending illness.

Diarrhea of Obscure Origin

Physicians sometimes fail to make a diagnosis in patients with chronic diarrhea despite an elaborate evaluation and refer such patients to centers interested in this condition. Common diagnoses resulting from re-evaluation of these patients are shown in Table 9–8.

Table 9–8 | **Frequent Diagnoses in Patients with Diarrhea of Obscure Origin**

Fecal incontinence
Functional diarrhea, irritable bowel syndrome
Iatrogenic diarrhea (drugs, surgery, radiation)
Surreptitious laxative ingestion
Microscopic colitis syndrome
Bile acid–induced diarrhea
Small bowel bacterial overgrowth
Pancreatic exocrine insufficiency
Carbohydrate malabsorption
Peptide-secreting tumors
Chronic idiopathic secretory diarrhea

While some might expect unusual or obscure conditions requiring special tests to predominate, most of the eventual diagnoses are straightforward and could have been made sooner.[96] Fecal incontinence and iatrogenic diarrhea could be recognized with a careful history. Surreptitious laxative ingestion and microscopic colitis could be diagnosed with an appropriate index of suspicion and testing (e.g., laxative screen or colonic biopsy, respectively). Bile acid–induced diarrhea, small bowel bacterial overgrowth, pancreatic exocrine insufficiency, and carbohydrate malabsorption could be discovered with a detailed history and a properly conducted therapeutic trial. Peptide-secreting tumors are rare, but serum peptide assays and scanning techniques (e.g., CT scanning and octreotide scanning) are widely available. Failure to make a diagnosis typically results from failure to appreciate the evidence at hand and to think through the differential diagnosis of chronic diarrhea.

REFERENCES

1. DuPont HL: Guidelines on acute infectious diarrhea in adults. Am J Gastroenterol 92:1962, 1997.
2. Fine KD, Schiller LR: AGA technical review on the evaluation and management of chronic diarrhea. Gastroenterology 116:1464, 1999.
3. Wenzl HH, Fine KD, Schiller LR, Fordtran JS: Determinants of decreased fecal consistency in patients with diarrhea. Gastroenterology 108:1729, 1995.
4. Talley NJ, Weaver AL, Zinsmeister AR, et al: Self-reported diarrhea: What does it mean? Am J Gastroenterol 89:1160, 1994.
5. McRorie J, Zorich N, Riccardi K, et al: Effects of olestra and sorbitol consumption on objective measures of diarrhea: Impact of stool viscosity on common gastrointestinal symptoms. Regul Toxicol Pharmacol 31:59, 2000.
6. Fordtran JS, Santa Ana CA, Morawski SG, et al: Pathophysiology of chronic diarrhoea: Insights derived from intestinal perfusion studies in 31 patients. Clin Gastroenterol 15:477, 1986.
7. Hammer HF, Santa Ana CA, Schiller LR, Fordtran JS: Studies of osmotic diarrhea induced in normal subjects by ingestion of polyethylene glycol and lactulose. J Clin Invest 84:1056, 1989.
8. Eherer AJ, Fordtran JS: Fecal osmotic gap and pH in experimental diarrhea of various causes. Gastroenterology 103:545, 1992.
9. Fine KD, Santa Ana CA, Fordtran JS: Diagnosis of magnesium-induced diarrhea. N Engl J Med 324:1012, 1991.
10. Hammer HF, Fine KD, Santa Ana CA, et al: Carbohydrate malabsorption: Its measurement and its contribution to diarrhea. J Clin Invest 86:1936, 1990.
11. Naim HY: Molecular and cellular aspects and regulation of intestinal lactase-phlorizin hydrolase. Histol Histopathol 16:553, 2001.
12. Jarvela I, Sabri Enattah N, Kokkonen J, et al: Assignment of the locus for congenital lactase deficiency to 2q21, in the vicinity of but separate from the lactase-phlorizin hydrolase gene. Am J Hum Genet 63: 1078, 1998.
13. Schiller LR: Secretory diarrhea. Curr Gastroenterol Rep 1:389, 1999.
14. Janecki AJ: Why should a clinician care about the molecular biology of transport? Curr Gastroenterol Rep 2:378, 2000.
15. Lucas ML: A reconsideration of the evidence for *Escherichia coli* Sta (heat stable) enterotoxin-driven fluid secretion: A new view of Sta action and a new paradigm for fluid absorption. J Appl Microbiol 90: 7, 2001.
16. Jensen RT: Overview of chronic diarrhea caused by functional neuroendocrine neoplasms. Semin Gastrointest Dis 10:156, 1999.
17. Smith SL, Branton SA, Avino AJ, et al: Vasoactive intestinal polypeptide secreting islet cell tumors: A 15-year experience and review of the literature. Surgery 124:1050, 1998.
18. Cooke HJ: Neurotransmitters in neuronal reflexes regulating intestinal secretion. Ann N Y Acad Sci 915:77, 2000.
19. Hansen MB, Skadhauge E: New aspects of the pathophysiology and treatment of secretory diarrhea. Physiol Res 44:61, 1995.
20. Keely SJ, Barrett KE: Regulation of chloride secretion: Novel pathways and messengers. Ann N Y Acad Sci 915:67, 2000.
21. Barrett KE, Keely SJ: Chloride secretion by the intestinal epithelium: Molecular basis and regulatory aspects. Annu Rev Physiol 62:535, 2000.
22. Chassany O, Michaux A, Bergmann JF: Drug-induced diarrhoea. Drug Saf 22:53, 2000.
23. Kere J, Hoglund P: Inherited disorders of ion transport in the intestine. Curr Opin Genet Dev 10:306, 2000.
24. Aichbichler BW, Zerr CH, Santa Ana CA, et al: Proton-pump inhibition of gastric chloride secretion in congenital chloridorrhea. N Engl J Med 336:106, 1997.
25. Muller T, Wijmenga C, Phillips AD, et al: Congenital sodium diarrhea is an autosomal recessive disorder of sodium/proton exchange but unrelated to known candidate genes. Gastroenterology 119:1506, 2000.
26. Jenkins AP, Thompson RP: Mechanisms of small intestinal adaptation. Dig Dis 12:15, 1994.
27. Arrambide KA, Santa Ana CA, Schiller LR, et al: Loss of absorptive capacity for sodium chloride as a cause of diarrhea following partial ileal and right colon resection. Dig Dis Sci 34:193, 1989.
28. Cipolla DM, Boley SJ, Luchs S, et al: Chronic mesenteric ischemia presenting as chronic diarrhea and weight loss with pneumatosis intestinalis. Gastroenterologist 4:134, 1996.
29. Read NW: Diarrhee motrice. Clin Gastroenterol 15:657, 1986.
30. Sellin JH, Hart R: Glucose malabsorption associated with rapid intestinal transit. Am J Gastroenterol 87:584, 1992.
31. Saslow SB, Camilleri M: Diabetic diarrhea. Semin Gastrointest Dis 6: 187, 1995.
32. Cullen JJ, Kelly KA: Gastric motor physiology and pathophysiology. Surg Clin North Am 73:1145, 1993.
33. Lovat LB, Pepys MB, Hawkins PN: Amyloid and the gut. Dig Dis 15: 155, 1997.
34. Quigley EM: Disturbances in small bowel motility. Baillieres Best Pract Res Clin Gastroenterol 13:385, 1999.
35. Chey WY, Jin HO, Lee MH, et al: Colonic motility abnormality in patients with irritable bowel syndrome exhibiting abdominal pain and diarrhea. Am J Gastroenterol 96:1499, 2001.
36. Alam MJ: Chronic refractory diarhoea: A manifestation of endocrine disorders. Dig Dis 12:46, 1994.
37. Riordan SM, McIver CJ, Walker BM, et al: Bacteriological method for detecting small intestinal hypomotility. Am J Gastroenterol 91: 2399, 1996.
38. Kaye SA, Lim SG, Taylor M, et al: Small bowel bacterial overgrowth in systemic sclerosis: Detection using direct and indirect methods and treatment outcome. Br J Rheumatol 34:265, 1995.
39. Virally-Monod M, Tielmans D, Kevorkian JP, et al: Chronic diarrhoea and diabetes mellitus: Prevalence of small intestinal bacterial overgrowth. Diabetes Metab 24:530, 1998.
40. Berin MC, McKay DM, Perdue MH: Immune-epithelial interactions in host defense. Am J Trop Med Hyg 60(Suppl 4):16, 1999.
41. Mohajer B, Ma TY: Eicosanoids and the small intestine. Prostaglandins Other Lipid Mediat 61:125, 2000.
42. Beubler E, Schuligoi R: Mechanisms of cholera toxin–induced diarrhea. Ann N Y Acad Sci 915:339, 2000.
43. Sellin JH: Cholera: Old story, new endings. Curr Gastroenterol Rep 1: 375, 1999.
44. Fasano A: Regulation of intercellular tight junctions by zonula occludens toxin and its eukaryotic analogue zonulin. Ann N Y Acad Sci 915:214, 2000.

45. Kolios G, Petoumenos C, Nakos A: Mediators of inflammation: Production and implication in inflammatory bowel disease. Hepatogastroenterology 45:1601, 1998.
46. Gewirtz AT, Simon PO Jr, Schmitt CK, et al: *Salmonella typhimurium* translocates flagellin across intestinal epithelia, inducing a proinflammatory response. J Clin Invest 107:99, 2001.
47. Perdue MH, McKay DM: Integrative immunophysiology in the intestinal mucosa. Am J Physiol 267:G151, 1994.
48. Sitaraman SV, Merlin D, Wang L, et al: Neutrophil-epithelial crosstalk at the intestinal luminal surface mediated by reciprocal secretion of adenosine and IL-6. J Clin Invest 107:861, 2001.
49. Ramakrishna BS, Mathan M, Mathan VI: Alteration of colonic absorption by long-chain unsaturated fatty acids: Influence of hydroxylation and degree of unsaturation. Scand J Gastroenterol 29:54, 1994.
50. Bischoff SC, Mayer JH, Manns MP: Allergy and the gut. Int Arch Allergy Immunol 121:270, 2000.
51. Savilahti E: Food-induced malabsorption syndromes. J Pediatr Gastroenterol Nutr 30(Suppl 1):S61, 2000.
52. Sicherer SH: Food protein–induced enterocolitis syndrome: Clinical perspectives. J Pediatr Gastroenterol Nutr 30(Suppl 1):S45, 2000.
53. Ratnaike RN, Jones TE: Mechanisms of drug-induced diarrhoea in the elderly. Drugs Aging 13:245, 1998.
54. Pollok RC, Banks MR, Fairclough PD, Farthing MJ: Dilutional diarrhoea: Under-diagnosed and over-investigated. Eur J Gastroenterol Hepatol 12:595, 2000.
55. Blaser MJ: Brainerd diarrhea: A newly recognized raw milk–associated enteropathy. JAMA 256:510, 1986.
56. Afzalpurkar RG, Schiller LR, Little KH, et al: The self-limited nature of chronic idiopathic diarrhea. N Engl J Med 328:1713, 1993.
57. Bardhan PK, Beltinger J, Beltinger RW, et al: Screening of patients with acute infectious diarrhoea: Evaluation of clinical features, faecal microscopy, and faecal occult blood testing. Scand J Gastroenterol 35: 54, 2000.
58. Ledochowski M, Widner B, Bair H, et al: Fructose- and sorbitol-reduced diet improves mood and gastrointestinal disturbances in fructose malabsorbers. Scand J Gastroenterol 35:1048, 2000.
59. Von Sonnenburg F, Tornieporth N, Waiyaki P, et al: Risk and aetiology of diarrhoea at various tourist destinations. Lancet 356:133, 2000.
60. Schultsz C, van Den Ende J, Cobelens F, et al: Diarrheagenic *Escherichia coli* and acute and persistent diarrhea in returned travelers. J Clin Microbiol 38:3550, 2000.
61. Wallace DJ, Van Gilder T, Shallow S, et al: Incidence of foodborne illnesses reported by the foodborne diseases active surveillance network (FoodNet)—1997. J Food Prot 63:807, 2000.
62. Thompson WG, Longstreth GF, Drossman DA, et al: Functional bowel disorders and functional abdominal pain. Gut 45(Suppl 2):43, 1999.
63. Harris JC, DuPont HL, Hornick RB: Fecal leukocytes in diarrheal illness. Ann Intern Med 76:697, 1972.
64. Guerrant RL, Araujo V, Soares E, et al: Measurement of fecal lactoferrin as a marker of fecal leukocytes. J Clin Microbiol 30:1238, 1992.
65. Fine KD, Ogunji F, George J, et al: Utility of a rapid fecal latex agglutination test detecting the neutrophil protein, lactoferrin, for diagnosing inflammatory causes of chronic diarrhea. Am J Gastroenterol 93:1300, 1998.
66. Silletti RP, Lee G, Ailey E: Role of stool screening tests in diagnosis of inflammatory bacterial enteritis and in selection of specimens likely to yield invasive enteric pathogens. J Clin Microbiol 34:1161, 1996.
67. Savola KL, Baron EJ, Tompkins LS, Passaro DJ: Fecal leukocyte stain has diagnostic value for outpatients but not inpatients. J Clin Microbiol 39:266, 2001.
68. Rosenblatt JE, Sloan LM, Schneider SK: Evaluation of an enzyme-linked immunosorbent assay for the detection of *Giardia lamblia* in stool specimens. Diagn Microbiol Infect Dis 16:337, 1993.
69. Brar HS, Surawicz CM: Pseudomembranous colitis: An update. Can J Gastroenterol 14:51, 2000.
70. Bini EJ, Cohen J: Diagnostic yield and cost-effectiveness of endoscopy in chronic human immunodeficiency virus–related diarrhea. Gastrointest Endosc 48:354, 1998.
71. Kearney DJ, Steuerwald M, Koch J, Cello JP: A prospective study of endoscopy in HIV-associated diarrhea. Am J Gastroenterol 94:596, 1999.
72. Surawicz CM, Haggitt RC, Husseman M, et al: Mucosal biopsy diagnosis of colitis: Acute self-limited colitis and idiopathic inflammatory bowel disease. Gastroenterology 107:755, 1994.
73. Duncan A, Robertson C, Russell RI: The fecal osmotic gap: Technical aspects regarding its calculation. J Lab Clin Med 119:359, 1992.
74. Topazian M, Binder HJ: Factitious diarrhea detected by measurement of stool osmolality. N Engl J Med 330:1418, 1994.
75. Fine KD: The prevalence of occult gastrointestinal bleeding in celiac sprue. N Engl J Med 334:1163, 1996.
76. Fine KD, Fordtran JS: The effect of diarrhea on fecal fat excretion. Gastroenterology 102:1936, 1992.
77. Balasekaran R, Porter JL, Santa Ana CA, et al: Positive results on tests for steatorrhea in persons consuming olestra potato chips. Ann Intern Med 132:279, 2000.
78. Khouri MR, Huang G, Shiau YF: Sudan stain of fecal fat: New insight into an old test. Gastroenterology 96:421, 1989.
79. Simko V: Fecal fat microscopy: Acceptable predictive value in screening for steatorrhea. Am J Gastroenterol 75:204, 1981.
80. Fine KD, Ogunji F: A new method of quantitative fecal fat microscopy and its correlation with chemically measured fecal fat output. Am J Clin Pathol 113:528, 2000.
81. Morton J: The detection of laxative abuse. Ann Clin Biochem 24:107, 1987.
82. Strygler B, Nicar MJ, Santangelo WC, et al: Alpha$_1$-antitrypsin excretion in stool in normal subjects and in patients with gastrointestinal disorders. Gastroenterology 99:1380, 1990.
83. Wei SC, Hung CC, Chen MY, et al: Endoscopy in acquired immunodeficiency syndrome patients with diarrhea and negative stool studies. Gastrointest Endosc 51:427, 2000.
84. Holmberg SD, Schell WL, Fanning GR, et al: *Aeromonas* intestinal infections in the United States. Ann Intern Med 105:683, 1986.
85. Penn RG, Giger DK, Knoop FC, Preheim LC: *Pleisiomonas shigelloides* overgrowth in the small intestine. J Clin Microbiol 15:869, 1982.
86. Muller A, Bialek R, Kamper A, et al: Detection of microsporidia in travelers with diarrhea. J Clin Microbiol 39:1630, 2001.
87. de Boissieu D, Chaussain M, Badoual J, et al: Small-bowel bacterial overgrowth in children with chronic diarrhea, abdominal pain, or both. J Pediatr 128:203, 1996.
88. Riordan SM, McIver CJ, Wakefield D, et al: Small intestinal bacterial overgrowth in the symptomatic elderly. Am J Gastroenterol 92:47, 1997.
89. Chatterjee H, Adhikari GN: Clinical and radiological aspects of chronic diarrhoeas. J Indian Med Assoc 82:194, 1984.
90. Gay GJ, Delmotte JS: Enteroscopy in small intestinal inflammatory diseases. Gastrointest Endosc Clin North Am 9:115, 1999.
91. Sharma BC, Bhasin DK, Makharia G, et al: Diagnostic value of push-type enteroscopy: A report from India. Am J Gastroenterol 95:137, 2000.
92. Freeman HJ: Small intestinal mucosal biopsy for investigation of diarrhea and malabsorption in adults. Gastrointest Endosc Clin North Am 10:739, 2000.
93. Fine KD, Seidel RH, Do K: The prevalence, anatomic distribution, and diagnosis of colonic causes of chronic diarrhea. Gastrointest Endosc 51:318, 2000.
94. Shah RJ, Fenoglio-Preiser C, Bleau BL, Giannella RA: Usefulness of colonoscopy with biopsy in the evaluation of patients with chronic diarrhea. Am J Gastroenterol 96:1091, 2001.
95. Bernstein CN, Riddell RH: Colonoscopy plus biopsy in the inflammatory bowel diseases. Gastrointest Endosc Clin North Am 10:755, 2000.
96. Schiller LR, Rivera LM, Santangelo W, et al: Diagnostic value of fasting plasma peptide concentrations in patients with chronic diarrhea. Dig Dis Sci 39:2216, 1994.
97. Onaitis MW, Kirshbom PM, Hayward TZ, et al: Gastrointestinal carcinoids: Characterization by site of origin and hormone production. Ann Surg 232:549, 2000.
98. Jensen RT, Gibril F, Termanini B: Definition of the role of somatostatin receptor scintigraphy in gastrointestinal neuroendocrine tumor localization. Yale J Biol Med 70:481, 1997.
99. Wolever TM, Chiasson JL, Josse RG, et al: No relationship between carbohydrate intake and effect of acarbose on HbA1c or gastrointestinal symptoms in type 2 diabetic subjects consuming 30% to 60% of energy from carbohydrate. Diabetes Care 21:1612, 1998.
100. Strocchi A, Corazza G, Ellis CJ, et al: Detection of malabsorption of low doses of carbohydrate: Accuracy of various breath H_2 criteria. Gastroenterology 105:1404, 1993.
101. Kerlin P, Wong L: Breath hydrogen testing in bacterial overgrowth of the small intestine. Gastroenterology 95:982, 1988.

102. Sarno S, Erasmus LP, Haslbeck M, Holzl R: Orocecal transit-time by the H_2 method: Effects of definitions of caecal entry and test meal. Ital J Gastroenterol 25:55, 1993.
103. Casellas F, de Torres I, Malagelada JR: Improved screening for intestinal villous atrophy by D-xylose breath test. Dig Dis Sci 45:18, 2000.
104. Miner PB Jr: Factors influencing the relapse of patients with inflammatory bowel disease. Am J Gastroenterol 92(Suppl 12):1S–4S, 1997.
105. Bo-Linn GW, Fordtran JS: Fecal fat concentration in patients with steatorrhea. Gastroenterology 87:319, 1984.
106. Valdimarsson T, Franzen L, Grodzinsky E, et al: Is small bowel biopsy necessary in adults with suspected celiac disease and IgA antiendomysium antibodies? Dig Dis Sci 41:83, 1996.
107. Corazza GR, Menozzi MG, Strocchi A, et al: The diagnosis of small bowel bacterial overgrowth: Reliability of jejunal culture and inadequacy of breath hydrogen testing. Gastroenterology 98:302, 1990.
108. Wormsley KG: Further studies of the response to secretin and pancreozymin in man. Scand J Gastroenterol 6:343, 1971.
109. Toskes PP: Bentiromide as a test of exocrine pancreatic function in adult patients with pancreatic exocrine insufficiency: Determination of appropriate dose and urinary collection interval. Gastroenterology 85: 565, 1983.
110. Stockbrugger RW, Armbrecht U, Muller E, et al: Determination of faecal chymotrypsin concentration and 72-hour faecal chymotrypsin output in the detection of pancreatic steatorrhea. Scand J Gastroenterol 26:13, 1991.
111. Loser C, Mollgaard A, Folsch UR: Faecal elastase 1: A novel, highly sensitive, and specific tubeless pancreatic function test. Gut 39:580, 1996.
112. Westergaard H: Duodenal bile acid concentrations in fat malabsorption syndromes. Scand J Gastroenterol 12:115, 1977.
113. Gruy-Kapral C, Little KH, Fordtran JS, et al: Conjugated bile acid replacement therapy for short-bowel syndrome. Gastroenterology 116: 15, 1999.
114. Little KH, Schiller LR, Bilhartz LE, Fordtran JS: Treatment of severe steatorrhea with ox bile in an ileectomy patient with residual colon. Dig Dis Sci 37:929, 1992.
115. Desjeux HL, Briend A, Butzner JD: Oral rehydration solution in the year 2000: Pathophysiology, efficacy and effectiveness. Baillieres Clin Gastroenterol 11:509, 1997.
116. Fontaine O, Gore SM, Pierce NF: Rice-based oral rehydration solution for treating diarrhoea. Cochrane Database Syst Rev 30:CD001264, 2000.
117. Dutta P, Mitra U, Dutta S, et al: Hypo-osmolar oral rehydration salts solution in dehydrating persistent diarrhoea in children: Double-blind, randomized, controlled clinical trial. Acta Paediatr 89:411, 2000.
118. Ramakrishna BS, Venkataraman S, Srinivasan P, et al: Amylase-resistant starch plus oral rehydration solution for cholera. N Engl J Med 342:308, 2000.
119. Adachi JA, Zeichner LO, DuPont HL, Ericsson CD: Empirical antimicrobial therapy for traveler's diarrhea. Clin Infect Dis 31:1079, 2000.
120. Wong CS, Jelacic S, Habeeb RL, et al: The risk of hemolytic-uremic syndrome after antibiotic treatment of *Escherichia coli* O157:H7 infections. N Engl J Med 342:1990, 2000.
121. Sirinavin S, Garner P: Antibiotics for treating salmonella gut infections. Cochrane Database Syst Rev 30:CD001167, 2000.
122. Schiller LR: Review article: Anti-diarrhoeal pharmacology and therapeutics. Aliment Pharmacol Ther 9:87, 1995.
123. Salazar-Lindo E, Santisteban-Ponce J, Chea-Woo E, Gutierrez M: Racecadotril in the treatment of acute watery diarrhea in children. N Engl J Med 343:463, 2000.
124. Lecomte JM: An overview of clinical studies with racecadotril in adults. Int J Antimicrob Agents 14:81, 2000.
125. Cezard JP, Duhamel JF, Meyer M, et al: Efficacy and tolerability of racecadotril in acute diarrhea in children. Gastroenterology 120:799, 2001.
126. Matheson AJ, Noble S: Racecadotril. Drugs 59:829, 2000.
127. Farthing MJ: The role of somatostatin analogues in the treatment of refractory diarrhoea. Digestion 57(Suppl 1):107, 1996.
128. Schiller LR, Santa Ana CA, Morawski SG, Fordtran JS: Studies of the antidiarrheal action of clonidine: Effects on motility and intestinal absorption. Gastroenterology 89:982, 1985.
129. Fedorak RN, Field M, Chang EB: Treatment of diabetic diarrhea with clonidine. Ann Intern Med 102:197, 1985.
130. Gorbach SL: Probiotics and gastrointestinal health. Am J Gastroenterol 95(Suppl 1):S2, 2000.
131. Gionchetti P, Rizzello F, Venturi A, Campieri M: Probiotics in infective diarrhoea and inflammatory bowel diseases. J Gastroenterol Hepatol 15:489, 2000.
132. De Roos NM, Katan MB: Effects of probiotic bacteria on diarrhea, lipid metabolism, and carcinogenesis: A review of papers published between 1988 and 1998. Am J Clin Nutr 71:405, 2000.
133. Roberfroid MB: Prebiotics and probiotics: Are they functional foods? Am J Clin Nutr 71(Suppl 6):1682S, 2000.
134. Anonymous: Berberine. Altern Med Rev 5:175, 2000.
135. Cooke C, Carr I, Abrams K, Mayberry J: Arrowroot as a treatment for diarrhoea in irritable bowel syndrome patients: A pilot study. Arq Gastroenterol 37:20, 2000.
136. Eherer AJ, Santa Ana CA, Porter J, Fordtran JS: Effect of psyllium, calcium polycarbophil, and wheat bran on secretory diarrhea induced by phenolphthalein. Gastroenterology 104:1007, 1993.
137. Camilleri M: Management of the irritable bowel syndrome. Gastroenterology 120:652, 2001.
138. Holtug K, Clausen MR, Hove H, et al: The colon in carbohydrate malabsorption: short-chain fatty acids, pH, and osmotic diarrhoea. Scand J Gastroenterol 27:545, 1992.
139. Lindstrom CG: "Collagenous colitis" with watery diarrhoea—a new entity? Pathol Eur 11:87, 1976.
140. Read NW, Krejs GJ, Read MG, et al: Chronic diarrhea of unknown origin. Gastroenterology 78:264, 1980.
141. Lazenby AJ, Yardley JH, Giardiello FM, et al: Lymphocytic ("microscopic") colitis: A comparative histopathologic study with particular reference to collagenous colitis. Hum Pathol 20:18, 1989.
142. Schiller LR: Microscopic colitis syndrome: Lymphocytic colitis and collagenous colitis. Semin Gastrointest Dis 10:145, 1999.
143. De La Riva S, Betes MT, Duque JM, et al: Collagenous colitis and lymphocytic colitis: Clinical and endoscopic findings. Rev Esp Enferm Dig 92:86, 2000.
144. Lee E, Schiller LR, Vendrell D, et al: Subepithelial collagen table thickness in colon specimens from patients with microscopic colitis and collagenous colitis. Gastroenterology 103:1790, 1992.
145. Taurog JD, Maika SD, Satumtira N, et al: Inflammatory disease in HLA-B27 transgenic rats. Immunol Rev 169:209, 1999.
146. Fine KD, Do K, Schulte K, et al: High prevalence of celiac sprue-like HLA-DQ genes and enteropathy in patients with the microscopic colitis syndrome. Am J Gastroenterol 95:1974, 2000.
147. Fine KD, Lee EL, Meyer RL: Colonic histopathology in untreated celiac sprue or refractory sprue: Is it lymphocytic colitis or colonic lymphocytosis? Hum Pathol 29:1433, 1998.
148. Lee E, Schiller LR, Fordtran JS: Quantification of colonic lamina propria cells by means of a morphometric point-counting method. Gastroenterology 94:409, 1988.
149. Ung KA, Gillberg R, Kilander A, Abrahamsson H: Role of bile acids and bile acid–binding agents in patients with collagenous colitis. Gut 46:170, 2000.
150. Fine KD, Lee EL: Efficacy of open-label bismuth subsalicylate for the treatment of microscopic colitis. Gastroenterology 114:29, 1998.
151. Bonner GF, Petras RE, Cheong DM, et al: Short- and long-term follow-up of treatment for lymphocytic and collagenous colitis. Inflamm Bowel Dis 6:85, 2000.
152. Carvajal SH, Mulvihill SJ: Postgastrectomy syndromes: Dumping and diarrhea. Gastroenterol Clin North Am 23:261, 1994.
153. Vecht J, Masclee AA, Lamers CB: The dumping syndrome: Current insights into pathophysiology, diagnosis, and treatment. Scand J Gastroenterol Suppl 223:21, 1997.
154. Potter GD: Bile acid diarrhea. Dig Dis 16:118, 1998.
155. Metcalf AM, Phillips SF: Ileostomy diarrhoea: Clin Gastroenterol 15: 705, 1986.
156. Heuschen UA, Autschbach F, Allemeyer EH, et al: Long-term follow-up after ileoanal pouch procedure: Algorithm for diagnosis, classification, and management of pouchitis. Dis Colon Rectum 44:487, 2001.
157. Gelbmann CM, Schteingart CD, Thompson SM, et al: Mast cells and histamine contribute to bile acid–stimulated secretion in the mouse colon. J Clin Invest 95:2831, 1995.
158. Fort JM, Azpiroz F, Casellas F, et al: Bowel habit after cholecystectomy: Physiological changes and clinical implications. Gastroenterology 111:617, 1996.
159. Arlow FL, Dekovich AA, Priest RJ, Beher WT: Bile acid–mediated postcholecystectomy diarrhea. Arch Intern Med 147:1327, 1987.
160. Hogenauer C, Hammer HF, Krejs GJ, Reisinger EC: Mechanisms and management of antibiotic-associated diarrhea. Clin Infect Dis 27:702, 1998.
161. Al-Eidan FA, McElnay JC, Scott MG, Kearney MP: *Clostridium diffi-*

cile–associated diarrhoea in hospitalized patients. J Clin Pharm Ther 25:101, 2000.
162. Chang VT, Nelson K: The role of physical proximity in nosocomial diarrhea. Clin Infect Dis 31:717, 2000.
163. El-Gammal A, Scotto V, Malik S, et al: Evaluation of the clinical usefulness of *C. difficile* toxin testing in hospitalized patients with diarrhea. Diagn Microbiol Infect Dis 36:169, 2000.
164. Pochapin M: The effect of probiotics on *Clostridium difficile* diarrhea. Am J Gastroenterol 95(Suppl 1):S11, 2000.
165. Heimburger DC, Geels VJ, Bilbrey J, et al: Effects of small-peptide and whole-protein enteral feedings on serum proteins and diarrhea in critically ill patients: A randomized trial. JPEN J Parenter Enteral Nutr 21:162, 1997.
166. Brydon WG, Nyhlin H, Eastwood MA, et al: 7α-Hydroxy-4-cholesten-3-1 and selenohomocholyltaurine (SeHCAT) whole-body retention in the assessment of bile acid–induced diarrhoea. Eur J Gastroenterol Hepatol 8:117, 1996.
167. Ung KA, Kilander AF, Lindgren A, Abrahamsson H: Impact of bile acid malabsorption on steatorrhea and symptoms in patients with chronic diarrhoea. Eur J Gastroenterol Hepatol 12:541, 2000.
168. Schiller LR, Bilhartz LE, Santa Ana CA, et al: Comparison of endogenous and radiolabeled bile acid excretion in patients with idiopathic chronic diarrhea. Gastroenterology 98:1036, 1990.
169. Ewe K, Karbach U: Factitious diarrhoea. Clin Gastroenterol 15:723, 1986.
170. Phillips SF: Surreptitious laxative abuse: Keep it in mind. Semin Gastrointest Dis 10:132, 1999.
171. Bytzer P, Stokholm M, Andersen I, et al: Prevalence of surreptitious laxative abuse in patients with diarrhoea of uncertain origin: A cost-benefit analysis of a screening procedure. Gut 30:1379, 1989.
172. Slugg PH, Carey WD: Clinical features and follow-up of surreptitious laxative users. Cleve Clin Q 51:167, 1984.
173. Osterholm MT, MacDonald KL, White KE, et al: An outbreak of a newly recognized chronic diarrhea syndrome associated with raw milk consumption. JAMA 256:484, 1986.
174. Parsonnet J, Trock SC, Bopp CA, et al: Chronic diarrhea associated with drinking untreated water. Ann Intern Med 110:985, 1989.
175. Mintz ED, Weber JT, Guris D, et al: An outbreak of Brainerd diarrhea among travelers to the Galapagos Islands. J Infect Dis 177:1041, 1998.

Chapter 10

INTESTINAL GAS

Fabrizis L. Suarez and Michael D. Levitt

Although patients frequently attribute various symptoms to excessive bowel gas, neither the volume nor the excretion rate of this gas is readily measurable. Therefore, the physician seldom has objective evidence that gas is the cause of the complaint, and treatment must be based on the patient's perception of excess gas. In reality, many symptoms arising from an irritable bowel may be incorrectly attributed to excessive gas (see Chapter 91). This chapter summarizes available data on the physiologic characteristics of intestinal gas and on the basis of these data discusses the pathogenesis, diagnosis, and treatment of problems attributed to this gas.

FACTORS INFLUENCING THE QUANTITY OF BOWEL GASES

The major sources of bowel gas are air swallowing, diffusion from the blood, bacterial production, and the reaction of bicarbonate and acid. Gas is removed from the lumen via eructation, passage per rectum, bacterial consumption, and diffusion into the blood. The net of these processes for each individual gas determines the quantity of that gas present in the gut at any moment. Figure 10–1 schematically depicts the sites of these various mechanisms.

VOLUME AND COMPOSITION OF BOWEL GAS

The volume of gas in the intestinal tract has been measured by using a body plethysmograph or a rapid intestinal infusion of argon to wash out the bowel gases.[1, 2] Both methods have indicated that the normal gut usually contains less than 200 mL of gas. The rate of gas excretion per rectum of healthy subjects was found to range from 476 to 1491 mL/day (mean of 705 mL/day).[3] Subjects ingesting their usual diet passed gas per rectum an average of 10 times per day with an upper limit of normal (mean + 2 SD) of 20 times per day.[4] Neither age nor sex significantly correlated with flatus frequency. Of the numerous foods alleged to enhance excretion of rectal gas, baked beans, and lactose are the only natural foods that have been carefully studied. A diet containing 51% of its calories as pork and beans increased flatus elimination from a basal level of 15 to 176 mL/hr.[5] Daily ingestion of 34 g of lactose (480 mL milk, 240 mL yogurt, 56 g hard cheese) by lactase maldigesters significantly increased their mean basal flatus frequency from 10 to 17 passages per day.[6]

Five gases (N_2, O_2, CO_2, H_2, and methane [CH_4]) account for more than 99% of gas passed per rectum. The composition of this gas is highly variable: N_2, 11% to 92%; O_2, 0% to 11%; CO_2, 3% to 54%; H_2, 0% to more than 86%; and CH_4, 0% to 56%.[7] In addition, many gases are present in only trace concentrations. Periods of rapid excretion of flatus are generally associated with high H_2 and CO_2 and low N_2 concentrations.[5] The composition of gas within the intestinal tract of 10 normal subjects was determined via analysis of gas washed out per rectum via a rapid infusion of argon at the ligament of Treitz.[2] Nitrogen was usually predominant; O_2 was present in very low concentrations; and the concentrations of CO_2, H_2, and CH_4 were highly variable.

SOURCES OF BOWEL GAS

Air Swallowing

The gastric bubble frequently is absent in subjects who cannot swallow air, as exemplified by patients with severe achalasia who have a liquid level in the esophagus that acts as a trap for gas. Thus, air swallowing (rather than intraluminal production) is the major source of stomach gas. Measurements obtained with ultrafast computed tomography showed that an average of 17.7 mL of gas was swallowed with each 10-mL bolus of liquid.[8] Application of these data to the daily ingestion of about 1500 mL of liquid suggests that about 2600 mL of air (2100 mL of N_2) should enter the stomach each day via this mechanism. To this volume must be added the air swallowed with food and saliva and the repetitive subconscious air swallowing carried out by some individuals. Although little, if any, N_2 is absorbed during passage through the gut, only about 500 mL of N_2 is passed in flatus each day. Thus, most swallowed air seemingly must be regurgitated, although many subjects claim to have no perception of belching.

The fraction of swallowed air passing into the duodenum is influenced by posture. When the individual is supine, eructation is difficult because gas is trapped above liquid overlying the gastroesophageal junction; thus, a large fraction of gastric air may be propelled into the small intestine.

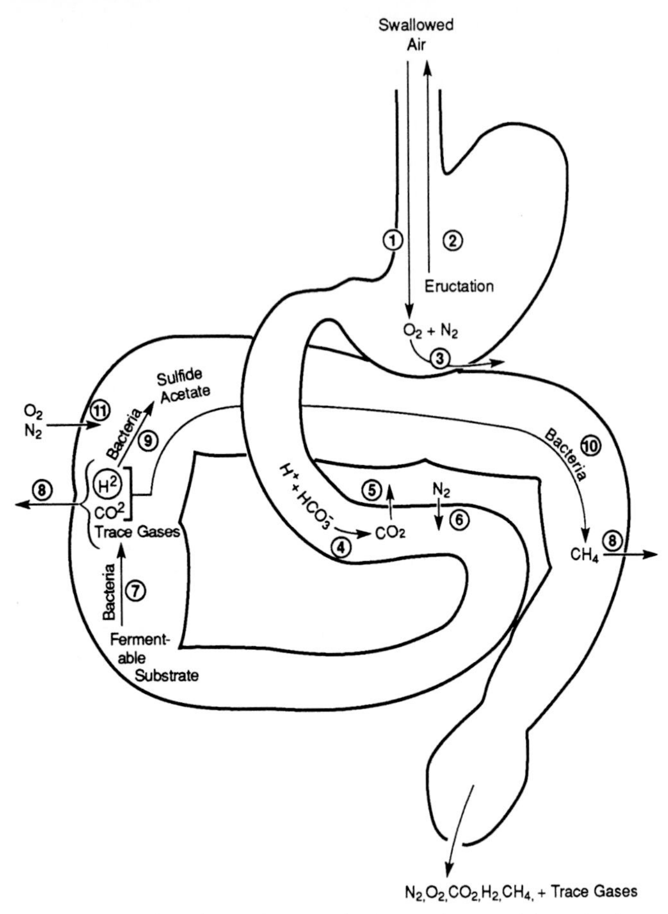

Figure 10–1. Physiology of gas production and removal from the intestinal tract. Air is swallowed (1), and a sizable fraction is then eructated (2). The O_2 of the swallowed air diffuses into the blood (3). The reaction of acid and bicarbonate in the duodenum yields CO_2 (4), which rapidly diffuses into the blood (5) while N_2 diffuses into the duodenum (6) down the gradient established by CO_2 production. In the colon, malabsorbed ingested material and mucus are fermented by bacteria releasing trace gases (some of which are odoriferous), CO_2, and H_2 (7). A fraction of the bacterial gases are absorbed into the blood perfusing the colon (8). In the right colon, H_2 is consumed by bacteria in the process of reducing sulfate to sulfide and converting CO_2 to acetate (9). In addition, H_2 is consumed in the left colon by methanogens in the process of reducing CO_2 to CH_4 (10). Nitrogen and O_2 (11) diffuse from the blood into the colonic lumen down a gradient created by the production of gas by bacteria. The net result of all of the aforementioned processes determines the composition and rate of excretion of gas per rectum.

Difficulty with eructation after fundal plication surgery may produce the "gas-bloat" syndrome (see Chapter 33).

Intraluminal Gas Production

Three gases—CO_2, H_2, and CH_4—are produced in appreciable quantity, and a variety of gases are produced in trace concentrations.

Carbon Dioxide

In the upper gut, CO_2 is liberated through the interaction of hydrogen ion and bicarbonate. The source of this acid may be gastric HCl secretion, which averages about 30 mEq/hr after meals,[9] or the fatty acids released during triglyceride digestion, which yields about 100 mEq of acid per 30 g of fat. Although bicarbonate neutralization theoretically yields 22.4 mL of CO_2 per millimole of bicarbonate, the volume of CO_2 liberated as gas may be far below this value as a result of slow decomposition of H_2CO_3 in the absence of carbonic anhydrase and the relatively high aqueous solubility of CO_2. The PCO_2 of duodenal contents after a meal averaged 300 mm Hg and 500 mm Hg in control subjects and patients with duodenal ulcers, respectively.[10] Given that pure CO_2 would have a partial pressure of 760 mm Hg, CO_2 constituted 40% and 70% of the duodenal gas of controls and ulcer patients, respectively. Because this gas is rapidly absorbed, CO_2 liberated in the upper gut contributes minimally to flatus volume. CO_2 may account for up to 60% of flatus, and such levels are usually associated with high concentrations of H_2. Because the only bowel source of H_2 is bacterial metabolism, flatus CO_2 similarly appears to be derived from fermentation reactions.

Hydrogen

HYDROGEN PRODUCTION. Germ-free rats and newborn infants produce no H_2, whereas production of this gas is detected within hours of bacterial contamination of the gut. Bacterial metabolism is therefore the sole source of H_2 in the gut. The site and rate of bacterial H_2 liberation in the normal human gut were determined by using a triple-lumen tube that had an infusion site in the jejunum and collecting sites in the proximal ileum and distal ileum.[11] During a constant infusion of N_2, negligible H_2 passed the proximal or distal ileum, both in the fasting state and after lactose instillation into the bowel. During fasting, rectal excretion of H_2 averaged only 0.23 mL/min, but it rose to 1.6 mL/min after colonic instillation of lactose. Thus, H_2-producing bacteria normally are largely limited to the colon, and these bacteria require exogenous fermentable substrate for copious H_2 production. In patients with small bowel bacterial overgrowth H_2 is produced in the small bowel as well as the colon.[11]

Intestinal bacteria liberate H_2 during fermentation of either carbohydrate or protein, although production from amino acids is appreciably less than that from sugars. In patients with malabsorption disorders, carbohydrates and proteins that are completely absorbed by the normal intestine may be malabsorbed and provide substrate for colonic H_2 production (see Chapter 89). Healthy subjects also may incompletely absorb carbohydrates (Table 10–1). Malabsorption of lactose secondary to a genetically programmed reduction in lactase synthesis is observed in most of the world's adult population (see Chapter 89). Fruits and vegetables (particularly legumes[5]) may contain high concentrations of oligosaccharides that cannot be digested by the enzymes of the normal small bowel but are fermented by the colonic bacteria with the production of gas. Hydrogen production increased in healthy subjects after ingestion of flours made from wheat, oats, potatoes, and corn, indicating that a fraction of these complex carbohydrates reached the colon.[12] In part, this malabsorption appears to reflect the presence of resistant starches: that is, starches that are present in a physical form that resists amylase digestion.[13] This amylase resistance is further enhanced when starches are refrigerated and

Table 10–1 | **Foods Containing Carbohydrates That Are Incompletely Absorbed in the Healthy Human Small Intestine and Thus Provide Substrate for Colonic Gas Production**

FOOD	MALABSORBED CARBOHYDRATE
Dairy products (milk, ice cream, cottage cheese, yogurt)	Lactose
Soft drinks, honey	Fructose
Legumes (baked beans, soy beans)	Melitose, stachyose
Dietetic candies and chewing gum	Mannitol, sorbitol, xylitol
Complex carbohydrates (wheat, corn, potatoes)	Resistant and retrograde starches
Grains, fruits, vegetables	Fiber (hemicellulose, pectin, gums, mucilage)

then reheated, a process that results in crystallization (retrogradation) of the starch.[14] White rice flour is the only complex carbohydrate that is almost totally absorbed.[12] Many soft drinks contain very large quantities of fructose, a sugar that is incompletely absorbed by a sizable fraction of the healthy population.[15] The poor absorption of sorbitol has led to its widespread use as a low-calorie sugar substitute; however, this compound is readily fermented by colonic bacteria. Although fiber is commonly assumed to generate gas production, ingestion of the usual dose of a commercial fiber preparation (psyllium) resulted in minimal increases in H_2 excretion.[4]

Fecal bacteria produce H_2 during fermentation of mucoproteins,[16] and the high fasting H_2 excretion observed in subjects with bacterial overgrowth of the small bowel or untreated celiac sprue has been attributed to increased mucus secretion (see Chapters 90 and 93).

HYDROGEN CONSUMPTION. Fecal bacteria both consume and produce H_2, and the quantity of this gas available for excretion represents the net of these two processes.[17, 18] Hydrogen is oxidized by fecal bacterial reactions that reduce CO_2 to CH_4, sulfate to sulfide, and CO_2 to acetate.[19–22] Human fecal homogenates containing high concentrations of methanogens consume H_2 far more rapidly than do non-methanogenic feces.[23] A competition for H_2 occurs in feces; thus, one of the H_2 consuming reactions tends to predominate in the feces of a given individual. Studies of fecal samples obtained from 15 healthy individuals over a 1.5- to 3-year period showed that the initial predominant H_2-consuming pathway persisted in 11 subjects, whereas an unexplained shift to a new pathway was observed in 4 subjects.[24]

The ability of bacteria to utilize H_2 is directly proportional to the H_2 tension in the feces.[18] Therefore, incubations performed at very low fecal H_2 tension (which limits consumption) permit measurement of absolute H_2 production, whereas conventional studies, in which H_2 tension is allowed to rise, measure net H_2 production. In a low–H_2 tension system, fecal samples from different individuals demonstrated relatively similar rates of absolute H_2 production during carbohydrate fermentation. In contrast, when H_2 tension was allowed to rise, marked individual differences in net H_2 production were observed as a result of individual differences in H_2 consumption.[18]

The fraction of H_2 production that escapes consumption in the feces and, therefore, is available for excretion is determined by the efficiency of fecal stirring and the quantity and type of H_2-consuming bacteria. Because hydrogen tension is maintained at a much higher level in poorly stirred feces, a greater fraction of total H_2 production is consumed in the semisolid feces of the left colon versus the liquid feces of the right colon. Consumption is markedly enhanced by the presence of methanogens, and studies with some methanogenic feces suggest that if similar concentrations of methanogens were present throughout the colon, virtually no H_2 would escape consumption. However, CH_4-producing bacteria are normally present in a high concentration only in the left colon,[25] whereas H_2 is produced throughout the colon. As a result, H_2 liberated in the right colon is not acted on by methanogens until it reaches the left colon, thus explaining the reduced but still appreciable breath H_2 excretion observed in most CH_4-producing subjects. The reported inability of some healthy subjects to increase breath H_2 excretion after carbohydrate malabsorption[26] probably reflects extremely efficient consumption of this gas. A major fermentation pathway of fecal bacteria liberates 4200 mL per 12.5 g of carbohydrate fermented.[20, 27] The actual quantity of H_2 excreted by way of breath and the anus after carbohydrate malabsorption is only a small fraction of this predicted volume,[28] suggesting that the bulk of the H_2 produced in the gut is consumed by other bacteria.

Prolonged ingestion of high doses of a malabsorbed disaccharide (lactulose by healthy controls or lactose by lactose maldigesters) has been shown to result in a markedly diminished breath H_2 response to a challenge dose of the disaccharide.[29, 30] This decline in H_2 production appears to represent an adaptation of the colonic flora to the nonabsorbed carbohydrate such that there is increased fermentation via pathways that do not yield H_2. For example, when lactose maldigesters ingested increasing quantities of lactose (maximum of 1 g/kg/day), the absolute production of H_2 by homogenates of feces obtained at the end of the period was 66% less than that of homogenates studied prior to lactose feeding.[31] Because fecal H_2 consumption did not change, lactose feeding appeared to enhance the colonic proliferation of lactose-hydrolyzing, but non–H_2-producing organisms such as bifidobacteria.

HYDROGEN BREATH TESTING. The H_2 that escapes consumption is excreted by way of the rectum or the lungs. Hydrogen is rapidly absorbed into the blood perfusing the gut. Upon arriving at the lungs, almost all H_2 is cleared during a single passage through the lungs. Thus, the rate of exhalation of H_2 equals its absorption rate. Long-term, simultaneous measurements of rectal and breath H_2 excretion have been made in adult subjects maintained in a sealed environment.[28] Over a fairly wide range of net H_2 production, breath H_2 excretion averaged about 50% of total excretion; however, at very low excretory rates, this value increased to about 65%, and at very high rates, it decreased to less than 20%. Breath H_2 excretion is equal to (alveolar ventilation) times (end-alveolar H_2 concentration). Because alveolar ventilation is relatively constant in sedentary individuals, the simple assessment of end-alveolar breath H_2 concentration can be used as an indicator of total breath H_2 excretion.[32]

In breath H_2 testing, breath H_2 concentrations are obtained before and at intervals after ingestion of a test carbohydrate.[33] An appreciable increase in H_2 concentration signifies malabsorption of carbohydrate. An early, well-designed study compared breath H_2 responses to ingestion of 50 g of lactose with lactase levels determined on intestinal biopsy specimens.[34] With hourly breath measurements over a 4-hour period, a rise in breath H_2 concentration greater than 20 parts per million (ppm) over baseline (initial sample obtained after an overnight fast) perfectly separated lactase-deficient subjects from those with normal lactase levels. This widely used 20-ppm criterion has a high specificity for carbohydrate malabsorption, although subjects with severe bacterial overgrowth of the small bowel may generate such a value in the absence of malabsorption.[35] The sensitivity of this 20-ppm criterion is very poor, however, particularly when small (<20 g) doses of the test carbohydrate are employed. False-negative results have been reported in subjects receiving antibiotics or suffering from severe diarrhea. Of more importance are reports indicating that 9% to 21% of the apparently healthy population do not produce a rise of more than 20 ppm in breath H_2 concentration, despite apparent carbohydrate malabsorption.[26] The breath H_2 response to ingestion of 10 g of lactulose was systematically studied in 55 healthy subjects.[36] When H_2 was measured hourly for 4 hours, 47% of the subjects did not increase their breath H_2 concentration by 20 ppm. A reduction of the criterion for malabsorption to an increase of 10 ppm gave much better sensitivity with only a slight reduction in specificity.

One source of error of the 20-ppm criterion for malabsorption is that subjects eating unrestricted dinners often have appreciable fasting breath H_2 concentrations the morning of the test day. With fasting, this high morning value tends to decline rapidly.[12] A rise in breath H_2 after ingestion of a test carbohydrate is superimposed on this rapidly falling basal H_2 excretion. As a result, malabsorption has to yield appreciably more than 20 ppm of breath H_2 to produce a 20-ppm increase in H_2 concentration over the initial fasting concentration. This problem can be largely eliminated if the dinner meal preceding the overnight fast contains only readily absorbed carbohydrates (i.e., rice as opposed to other complex carbohydrates[36]). Another explanation for the low sensitivity of the conventional breath H_2 test is the limitation of the test period to 4 hours. The small bowel transit time of small doses of poorly absorbed carbohydrate frequently exceeds 4 hours. Malabsorption of a 10-g dose of lactulose was detected in 53% of subjects with four hours of testing, and 76% when testing was extended to 8 hours.[36] The best sensitivity and specificity were provided by H_2 measurements obtained at 4 to 6 hours; the average breath H_2 during this period was always greater than 10 ppm following lactulose ingestion and never greater than 5 ppm after ingestion of a non-nutrient meal. Thus, new criteria based on measurements at 4 to 6 hours possibly could improve the sensitivity of breath H_2 testing. It has also been suggested that the sensitivity of the breath test will be improved if increases in breath CH_4 concentration, as well as H_2 concentration, are used as evidence of malabsorption.[37]

Breath H_2 measurements have also been used to estimate the quantity of carbohydrate malabsorbed. The rationale underlying this test was that ingestion of 5, 10, or 20 g of lactulose resulted in a relatively linear increase in breath H_2 in a given individual.[38] Because of large individual differences in H_2 excretion after ingestion of similar quantities of lactulose, the amount of carbohydrate malabsorbed was calculated from a comparison of an individual's H_2 response to an unknown carbohydrate with that after a known dose of lactulose. Although this technique provides a semiquantitative estimate of malabsorption of lactose, which is handled similarly to lactulose, there are sizable differences in the amount of H_2 released during fermentation of various carbohydrates. Breath H_2 excretion markedly underestimates malabsorption of slowly fermented, insoluble carbohydrates, such as fiber and resistant starch.[28] This underestimation results in part from the fermentation of these carbohydrates in the left colon, where efficient H_2 consumption limits the H_2 available for excretion.

Another widely used test based on breath H_2 measurements utilizes the time elapsing between the ingestion of a nonabsorbable carbohydrate and a rise in breath H_2 excretion to measure oral-cecal transit time.[39] An early rise in breath H_2 after ingestion of glucose or lactulose has been used as evidence of bacterial overgrowth of the small bowel.[35] However, a prospective comparison of breath H_2 measurements and bacterial cultures of jejunal aspirates suggested that the breath test failed to detect overgrowth in about 35% of cases.[40]

Methane

Like that of H_2, the sole source of CH_4 in humans is the metabolism of the colonic bacteria. The major methanogen in the human colon, *Methanobrevibacter smithii*, produces methane by way of the reaction $4H_2 + CO_2 \rightarrow CH_4 + 2H_2O$.[19] This reaction uses 5 mol of gas in the production of 1 mol of CH_4 and thus reduces the volume of gas that would otherwise be present in the colon. About one third of the adult population have high fecal concentrations of methanogens and excrete appreciable CH_4.[41] An individual's tendency to produce or not to produce CH_4 is usually a fairly consistent trait over a period of several years, and this tendency appears to be familial and determined by early environmental rather than genetic factors. It has been proposed that bile acids may play a role in determining an individual's methane-producing status.[42]

Subjects who produce large quantities of CH_4 have stools that consistently float in water.[43] Methane produced in the distal colon becomes trapped in the stool, reducing the fecal density to less than that of water. Whereas early reports showed a higher than expected prevalence of CH_4 production in patients with colonic cancer,[44] this finding was not observed in subsequent studies.[45]

Odoriferous Gases

None of the quantitatively important gases has an odor; thus, the unpleasant odor of feces must result from gases present in trace quantities. Although indole and skatole were implicated in early studies, a carefully performed study showed that sulfur-containing compounds such as methanethiol and dimethyldisulfide appeared to be responsible for the unpleasant odor of human feces.[46] A 1998 study of the sulfur-containing gases of flatus obtained via rectal tube from 10 healthy subjects yielded somewhat different results.[47] Blinded evaluation of the intensity of the noxious odor of flatus samples strongly correlated with the concentrations of hydrogen sulfide and methanethiol (negligible dimethyldisulfide was observed). Hydrogen sulfide is released during bacterial metabolism of a sulfate, cysteine, and mucin; thus both exogenous and endogenous compounds could supply the substrate for this reaction. Methionine appears to be the favored substrate for methanethiol production.

In addition to their noxious odor, hydrogen sulfide and methanethiol are extremely toxic, with a medium lethal dose (LD_{50}) for rodents that is comparable to that of cyanide. The colonic mucosa possesses a highly developed system that metabolizes these gases to thiosulfate,[48] and this detoxification system protects the mucosa from the damaging effects of these compounds. This pathway is so efficient that, despite the very rapid absorption of these gases, negligible quantities appear to enter the blood perfusing the colon; hence, hydrogen sulfide and methanethiol of gut origin are not excreted on the breath.[49] In contrast, a highly odoriferous sulfur-containing gas (allyl methyl sulfide) derived from garlic is not metabolized by the gut mucosa, and, thus, this gas is absorbed from the gut and excreted in expired air.[49]

Diffusion of Gas between the Lumen and the Blood

Gases passively diffuse between the lumen and the mucosal blood, and the direction of movement is determined by the partial pressure gradient. Because the luminal partial pressure of H_2 or CH_4 is always greater than that of the blood, these gases always diffuse from the lumen to blood. In contrast, the direction of diffusion of CO_2, N_2, and O_2 is variable. For example, swallowed air contains minimal CO_2, and this gas diffuses from the blood into the stomach bubble. The PCO_2 rises dramatically in the duodenum, and CO_2 now diffuses from the lumen to blood. The PN_2 of swallowed air is slightly higher than that of venous blood, and N_2 may be slowly absorbed from the stomach. In the duodenum, luminal PN_2 falls below that of the blood as a result of dilution with CO_2, and N_2 diffuses into the lumen. Similarly, the production of CO_2, H_2, and CH_4 in the colon often reduces the PN_2 of flatus to below that of blood, with a resultant movement of N_2 from the blood to the lumen. When a near maximal PN_2 difference (~1400 mm Hg) was established between the blood and the lumen, N_2 diffused across the mucosa of the entire human intestinal tract at a rate of about 100 mL/hr.[2] Because diffusion at a rate of 16 mL/hr of N_2 could account for all N_2 passed in flatus per day (400 mL), diffusion, rather than air swallowing, could be the major source of flatus N_2. The PO_2 of swallowed air is greater than that of blood, and O_2 is absorbed from the stomach. However, the low PO_2 of colonic gas results in diffusion of this gas from the blood to the lumen (see Fig. 10–1).

Propulsion of Gas through the Intestinal Tract

In a 1998 series of elegant studies, Serra and coworkers[50] constantly infused gas at varying rates into the upper small bowel of healthy human volunteers and measured the rate at which the infused gas was passed per rectum. As shown in

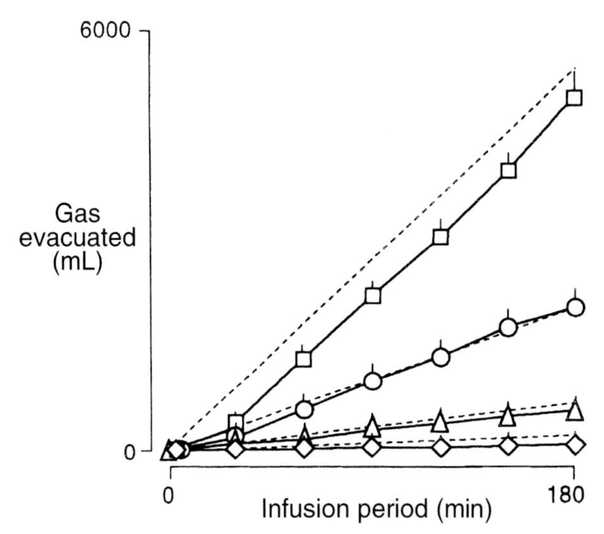

Figure 10–2. Plots of rectal gas evacuation during a 180-minute, continuous infusion of gas into the upper jejunum. Cumulative evacuation rates (*solid lines*) and cumulative infusion rates (*dotted lines*) are shown. The infusion rates were: 1 mL/min (*diamonds*); 4 mL/min (*triangles*); 12 mL/min (*circles*); 30 mL/min (*squares*). Note that the evacuation rates closely mirrored the infusion rates, indicating that only a small fraction of the infused gas was retained in the gut. (From Serra J, Aspiroz F, Malagelada JR: Intestinal gas dynamics and tolerance in humans. Gastroenterology 115:542–550, 1998.)

Figure 10–2, the cumulative passage of gas per rectum very closely mirrored the quantity infused, indicating very rapid intestinal propulsion of gas. Subjects in whom appreciable gas (>400 mL) accumulated tended to perceive more abdominal discomfort.

CLINICAL GAS PROBLEMS

Eructation

The occasional belch during or after meals expels gas swallowed in the course of ingesting food. In contrast, people who repeatedly eructate can usually be shown to aspirate air into the hypopharynx before each belch. Most of this air is noisily regurgitated and never actually enters the stomach. Patients who are under emotional stress or who have thoracic or abdominal discomfort of any cause may complain of frequent, seemingly involuntary belching. For some reason, belching appears transiently to relieve this distress. If appreciable portions of the swallowed air enter the stomach and intestines, increased discomfort could occur with the development of a vicious cycle. Unaware that they are swallowing air, patients become convinced that they have a severe digestive abnormality, and this concern further aggravates their aerophagia. Thus, chronic eructation is almost always a "functional" disorder, and an evaluation with radiographic and laboratory studies should be reserved for patients who have additional complaints suggestive of thoracic or abdominal abnormality. If no associated disease is present, counseling in which the aerophagia-belching mechanism is thoroughly explained may break the vicious cycle. Although many subjects still continue to belch, distress is diminished when the benign origin of their eructation is understood. Various maneuvers to reduce air swallowing have been recommended, including chewing rather than gulping food, eating and drinking slowly, avoiding of chewing gum, and clenching a pencil between the teeth. The effectiveness of such measures has never been demonstrated objectively.

In patients undergoing radiographic or minor surgical procedures in the supine position, diffuse distention of the entire gut often develops over a period of minutes, and this distention is aggravated by ingestion of water or soda. Such distention apparently reflects the combination of air swallowing by the nervous patient and the difficulty in eructation associated with ingestion of liquids in the supine posture. The ability of gas to pass rapidly through the gut with a mouth-to-anus transit time of 5 to 10 minutes accounts for rapid distention of the entire gut.

Abdominal Distention and Bloating

Abdominal discomfort and bloating, thought to be caused by "too much gas," are among the most frequently encountered gastrointestinal complaints. Lacking objective measurements of intestinal gas volume, physicians have accepted their patients' conviction that excessive intestinal gas is the cause of these symptoms. Understanding of the precise relationship between bloating and gas is of some importance because treatment to reduce intestinal gas volume is predicated upon the assumption that excessive gas is of etiologic importance in bloating.

Utilizing the gas washout method, a relatively crude technique, we found no significant difference in the volume of gas in the bowel of bloating subjects versus controls but did observe an increased symptomatic response to the gas infusion in the bloating subjects.[51] Subsequently, the volume of bowel gas has been estimated by summing the cross-sectional area of all gas collections visualized on abdominal radiographs. Although these measurements are highly reproducible, the volume of a spherical gas collection increases by the cube of the radius, whereas area increases by the square of the radius. Thus, to the extent that gas collections are spherical, area measurements yield an increasingly greater underestimation of volume as the area increases.

The abdominal girth and gas area of control and bloating female subjects were assessed via computed tomographic studies carried out in the morning and afternoon.[52] The anteroposterior diameter of the abdomen significantly increased between morning and evening measurements in the bloating subjects, but no significant increase in bowel gas to account for this abdominal protuberance was observed. (Controls showed no significant increase in girth nor gas during the course of the day.) In contrast, two studies using plain films of the abdomen found that subjects with irritable bowel syndrome (IBS) had significantly greater areas of gas than did controls[53, 54] (see Chapter 91). However, gas area did not significantly correlate with the complaints of bloating and distention in either of these studies. Serra and coworkers[55] observed that the retention of gas infused into the gut was much greater when lipid was simultaneously infused into the duodenum. This finding raises the possibility that food ingestion could act in concert with air swallowing to induce gaseous distention.

Although some of the preceding observations seemingly are in conflict, it seems likely that IBS subjects have disordered intestinal motility that can result in bloating or retention of gas in the abdomen. Retention of excessive gas does not appear necessary for these subjects to perceive the sensation of gut distention, but, presumably, retention of gas could aggravate these sensations. In our experience, most subjects who complain of bloating have what appear to be normal quantities of bowel gas on radiographic examination. However, the occasional distended subject has greatly increased quantities of gastric, small bowel, and colonic gas, presumably secondary to air swallowing.

Why should IBS subjects with apparently normal volumes of bowel gas sense that their gut is distended? Multiple studies have shown that the bowel of patients with IBS is unusually sensitive to balloon distention.[56] Thus, these subjects perceive distention with a volume of intestinal contents that would be well tolerated by healthy controls. The frequent claim that various foods "turn to gas" may represent the ability of foods: (1) to stimulate abnormal motility that is perceived as bloating or (2) to increase gas retention in the gut, causing sensations of bloating.

Because the primary problem of patients complaining of excessive intestinal gas seemingly represents a variant of IBS, treatment presumably should be similar to that employed for IBS. Although anticholinergic agents have been shown to induce significant benefit in some IBS subjects,[57] our experience is that these agents often aggravate bloating symptoms. In blinded, controlled trials, the prokinetic agents metoclopramide and cisapride produced a statistically significant reduction in complaints of distention when compared with placebo therapy.[58, 59] In a 2000 report, neostigmine was administered to IBS subjects who retained excessive gas during a gas infusion.[60] Unfortunately, the rapid expulsion of gas that followed neostigmine administration was associated with an increase in abdominal discomfort, suggesting that the enhanced motility induced by this drug resulted in more pain than did the gas accumulation in the gut (see Chapter 91).

Although dietary therapy to reduce "gas" production in the gut has been the mainstay of therapy for distention, such manipulations are not usually helpful, as would be predicted from the poor correlation between abdominal gas volumes and symptoms of bloating. The possibility remains that localized collections of gas could serve as a painful stimulus in appropriately reactive guts (e.g., the splenic flexure syndrome, in which patients have left upper quadrant pain, and often, chest pain relieved by flatus or bowel movements). The discomfort can be reproduced by introduction of air into the splenic flexure via a rectal tube. Often a flat film of the abdomen will show a distended flexure (gas filled) under the left side of the diaphragm. Thus, it possibly could be useful to minimize bowel gas by counseling the subject about air swallowing and dietary manipulations that reduce delivery of fermentable substrate to the colonic gas bacteria (see Table 10–1).

Although ingestion of a cup of milk by lactose maldigesters results in a readily detectable increase in breath H_2 concentration, this finding does not necessarily signify that the subject will perceive increased gases. For example, in a blinded study of subjects self-selected for severe lactose intolerance, gaseous symptoms resulting from ingestion of a cup of conventional milk with breakfast each day were no different from those reported with a cup of lactose-hydrolyzed milk.[61] A significant increase in flatulence required the daily ingestion of 34 g of lactose, the quantity present in 3 cups of milk.[6] Thus, manipulations to reduce lactose malabsorption (prehydrolyzed milk, oral lactase preparations, or the substitution of yogurt for milk) are likely to be beneficial only to subjects who are ingesting relatively large amounts of lactose.

The use of an α-D-galactosidase enzyme preparation (Beano) reduces gas production after ingestion of baked beans.[62] There is contradictory evidence concerning the ability of activated charcoal to reduce the volume of gas produced during carbohydrate fermentation. Some studies show a dramatic reduction, and other studies have shown that charcoal was not beneficial.[63, 64] Although there is limited evidence to support the efficacy of simethicone, this compound is widely used in the treatment of gaseous complaints; a well-controlled study showed that it did not alleviate the gaseous symptoms induced by lactulose.[65]

Unusually Voluminous or Odoriferous Rectal Gas

Excessive passage of gas per anus may be a source of social embarrassment or may cause the patient to suspect the existence of a serious digestive derangement. The first problem confronting the physician when treating the patient complaining of flatulence is the determination of whether the patient actually passes excessive gas. Radiographic and endoscopic studies have no value in this regard. Although it is not very precise, the frequency of gas passage may be used as a rough indicator of normality; the initial step in the workup consists of instructing the patient to keep a meticulous record of the frequency of gas passage. Healthy subjects pass gas up to 20 times per day.[4, 5] A sizable fraction of subjects with self-diagnosed excessive flatulence are found to be "normal," and hence no diagnostic nor therapeutic intervention other than reassurance is indicated.

If the patient has a flatus frequency of more than 20 times per day, gas chromatographic analysis of flatus collected via rectal tube can differentiate air swallowing (N_2 predominant) from intraluminal production (H_2, CO_2, and CH_4 predominant) as the source of the gas. In our experience, excessive flatulence usually results from excessive intraluminal gas production, although one well-documented case of severe flatulence secondary to air swallowing has been reported.[66]

Because flatus H_2 and CO_2 are largely derived from fermentation of malabsorbed carbohydrate, flatulence may be indicative of an abnormality of carbohydrate absorption due to either a generalized malabsorptive disorder or an isolated abnormality, such as lactase deficiency (see Chapters 88, 89, and 90). Much more commonly, no such absorptive problem is demonstrable, and excessive flatus appears to result from colonic fermentation of "normally" malabsorbed material plus an imbalance between gas-producing and gas-consuming bacteria. As discussed in the section on hydrogen consumption, factors that influence H_2 consumption (i.e., luminal stirring and type and location of H_2-consuming bacteria) presumably play a major role in determining the volume of gas available for excretion. A diet low in lactose, starches, and legumes reduces flatus excretion in most subjects; however, long-term adherence to such a diet is difficult.

The passage of malodorous flatus is a not uncommon complaint, which has received little scientific attention. Bacterial production of sulfur-containing gases appears to be the major cause of this malodor,[47] and presumably an overavailability of sulfur containing substrates in the colon or a flora overly proficient at sulfur gas production is responsible for excessively malodorous flatus. Although sulfur gases are very rapidly absorbed from the bowel (half-time in the rat colon of less than 1 minute[67]), rapid colonic transit could also increase rectal excretion of these gases. The importance of various sulfur-containing substrates—cruciferous vegetables or beer (sulfate), proteins (sulfur-containing amino acids), or endogenous mucin—has not been objectively assessed. Thus, dietary manipulations to reduce gas odor at present are based on anecdotal observations (e.g., avoid cabbage, beer, cheese).

A commercially produced charcoal-impregnated cushion has been touted as an aid for subjects with offensive flatus. Although it has limited practicality, sitting on this cushion was shown by objective testing to allow less than 10% sulfur gas instilled at the anus to escape into the environment.[47] Orally administered products that have been tested for their ability to reduce fecal sulfur gases include activated charcoal (eight 260 mg tablets daily), which was found to be ineffective,[68] and bismuth subsalicylate (eight 262 mg tablets daily), which almost totally eliminated hydrogen sulfide (via binding of sulfide by bismuth).[69] Unfortunately, the potential for bismuth toxicity of long-term bismuth subsalicylate ingestion probably precludes the long-term use of this compound.

Pneumatosis Cystoides Intestinalis

(see Chapter 118)

Pneumatosis cystoides intestinalis is a condition characterized by the presence of gas-filled cysts in the wall of the small bowel or colon. The cysts may be asymptomatic or associated with diarrhea, bloating, or abdominal pain. Since 1979, studies have demonstrated that almost all patients with intestinal pneumatosis have extremely high breath H_2 concentrations, a finding indicative of very high net H_2 production in the intestine.[70–72] Christl and associates found that the feces of three patients with pneumatosis of the colon had low concentrations of H_2-consuming organisms,[71] and a patient with pneumatosis limited to the small bowel was shown to have small bowel contents that produced but could not consume H_2.[72] Thus, the high net H_2 production of these subjects appears to reflect H_2 production relatively unopposed by H_2 consumption. An association between pneumatosis and chronic administration of chloral hydrate has been described, an association that appears to be explained by the ability of chloral hydrate to inhibit H_2 consumption.[73] Exactly how a high luminal H_2 tension results in pneumatosis remains controversial. It has been proposed that counterperfusion, a process responsible for tissue collections of gas in deep sea divers, could account for intestinal pneumatosis.[74] It is also possible that small intramural gas collections normally occur with some frequency but these collections are rapidly absorbed into the circulation. Very high luminal H_2

concentrations would maintain appreciable H_2 tensions in the cyst (via diffusion from the lumen). This high H_2 tension dilutes the other gases such that a gradient for the absorption of these gases cannot be established. Thus, the cyst would tend to persist indefinitely as long as H_2 was constantly "fed" to it from the lumen. The most effective treatment to eliminate the cysts consists of the administration of high concentrations of O_2 via inhalation.[75] This maneuver reduces the blood N_2 tension, and, as a result, N_2 (as well as the other gases in the cyst) diffuses into the blood. Other forms of therapy that may be effective are antibiotics that inhibit H_2 production (ciprofloxacin was used successfully in a patient with small bowel bacterial overgrowth and small bowel pneumatosis[72]) and elimination of nonabsorbable carbohydrates, such as lactose, that provide a substrate for H_2-producing reactions by the colonic bacteria.

Colonic Explosions

Two gases formed in the colon, H_2 and CH_4, are combustible and potentially explosive. Numerous explosions resulting in severe colonic trauma and perforation have been triggered by electrocautery performed through the proctosigmoidoscope.[76] The only reported explosion during electrocautery-snare polypectomy through the colonoscopy occurred in a patient who received mannitol as a purgative.[77] Mannitol serves as a substrate for H_2-producing bacteria and, therefore, is an inappropriate choice of purgative if electrocautery is contemplated. The commonly used colonic cleansing solutions contain electrolytes and polyethylene glycol, a nonabsorbable, osmotically active polymer that cannot be fermented by the colonic bacteria. After colonic cleansing with these solutions, the intracolonic concentrations of H_2 and CH_4 are well below explosive levels,[78] and we are not aware of explosions occurring in the colon adequately cleansed with these solutions.

REFERENCES

1. Bedell GN, Marshall R, Dubois AB, et al: Measurement of the volume of gas in the gastrointestinal tract. J Clin Invest 35:336, 1956.
2. Levitt MD: Volume and composition of human intestinal gas determined by means of an intestinal washout technique. N Engl J Med 284: 1394, 1971.
3. Tomlin J, Lowis C, Read NW: Investigation of normal flatus production in healthy volunteers. Gut 32:665, 1991.
4. Levitt MD, Furne J, Olsson S: Relation of passage of gas and abdominal bloating to colonic gas production. Ann Intern Med 124:422–424, 1996.
5. Steggerda FR: Gastrointestinal gas following food consumption. Ann N Y Acad Sci 150:57, 1968.
6. Suarez FL, Adshead J, Furne JF, et al: Lactose maldigestion is not an impediment to the intake of 1500 mg calcium daily as dairy products. Am J Clin Nutr 68:1118–1122, 1998.
7. Calloway DH: Gas in the alimentary canal. In Code CF (ed): Handbook of Physiology, vol 5, sec 6. Washington, DC, American Physiological Society, 1967, p 2839.
8. Pouderoux P, Ergun GA, Shezhang L, Kahrilas PJ: Esophageal bolus transit imaged by ultrafast computerized tomography. Gastroenterology 110:1422–1428, 1996.
9. Fordtran JS, Walsh JH: Gastric acid secretion rate and buffer content of the stomach after eating: Results in normal subjects and in patients with duodenal ulcer. J Clin Invest 52:645, 1973.
10. Rune SJ: Acid-base parameters of duodenal contents in man. Gastroenterology 62:533, 1972.
11. Levitt MD: Production and excretion of hydrogen gas in man. N Engl J Med 281:122, 1969.
12. Levitt MD, Hirsh P, Fetzer CA, et al: H_2 excretion after ingestion of complex carbohydrates. Gastroenterology 92:383, 1987.
13. Olesen M, Rumessen JJ, Gudmand-Hoyer E: Intestinal transport and fermentation of resistant starch evaluated by the hydrogen breath test. Eur J Clin Nutr 48:692, 1994.
14. Schepach W, Bach M, Bartram P, et al: Colonic fermentation of potato starch after a freeze-thaw cycle. Dig Dis Sci 36:1601, 1991.
15. Ravich WJ, Bayless TM, Thomas M: Fructose: Incomplete intestinal absorption in humans. Gastroenterology 84:26, 1983.
16. Perman JA, Modler S: Glycoproteins as substrates for production of hydrogen and methane by colonic bacterial flora. Gastroenterology 82: 911, 1982.
17. Levitt MD, Berggren T, Hastings J, et al: Hydrogen (H_2) catabolism in the colon of the rat. J Lab Clin Med 84:163, 1974.
18. Strocchi A, Levitt MD: Factors affecting hydrogen production and consumption by human fecal flora: The critical role of H_2 tension and methanogenesis. J Clin Invest 89:1304, 1992.
19. Gibson GR, Cummings JH, Macfarlane GT, et al: Alternative pathways for hydrogen disposal during fermentation in the human colon. Gut 31: 679, 1990.
20. Wolin MJ: Fermentation in the rumen and human large intestine. Science 213:1463, 1981.
21. Gibson GR, Macfarlane GT, Cummings JH: Occurrence of sulphate-reducing bacteria in human faeces and the relationship of dissimilatory sulphate reduction to methanogenesis in the large gut. J Appl Bacteriol 65:103, 1988.
22. Lajoie SF, Bank S, Miller TL, et al: Acetate production from hydrogen and ^{13}C carbon dioxide by the microflora of human feces. Appl Environ Microbiol 54:2723, 1988.
23. Strocchi A, Furne JK, Ellis CJ, et al: Competition for hydrogen by human fecal bacteria: Evidence for the predominance of methanobacteria. Gut 32:1498, 1992.
24. Strocchi A, Ellis CJ, Furne JK, et al: Study of constancy of hydrogen-consuming flora of human colon. Dig Dis Sci 39:494, 1994.
25. Flourie B, Etanchand F, Florent C, et al: Comparative study of hydrogen and methane production in the human colon using caecal and faecal homogenates. Gut 31:684, 1990.
26. Gilat T, Ben Hur H, Gelman-Malachi E, et al: Alterations of the colonic flora and their effect on the hydrogen breath test. Gut 19:602, 1978.
27. Grimble G: Fibre, fermentation, flora, and flatus. Gut 30:6, 1989.
28. Christl SU, Murgatroyd PR, Gibson GR, et al: Production, metabolism and excretion of hydrogen in the large intestine. Gastroenterology 102: 1269, 1992.
29. Perman JA, Modler S, Olson AC: Role of pH in production of hydrogen from carbohydrates by colonic bacterial flora. J Clin Invest 67:643, 1981.
30. Florent C, Flourie B, Leblond A, et al: Influence of chronic lactulose ingestion on the colonic metabolism of lactulose in man (an in vivo study). J Clin Invest 75:608, 1985.
31. Herztler S, Savaiano DA: Daily lactose feeding improves lactose tolerance by enhancing colonic fermentation. Gastroenterology 108(suppl): A289, 1995.
32. Metz G, Jenkins DJA, Peters TJ, et al: Breath hydrogen as a diagnostic method for hypolactasia. Lancet 1:1155, 1975.
33. Levitt MD, Donaldson RM: Use of respiratory hydrogen (H_2) excretion to detect carbohydrate malabsorption. J Lab Clin Med 75:937, 1970.
34. Newcomer AD, McGill DB, Thomas PJ, et al: Prospective comparison of indirect methods for detecting lactase deficiency. N Engl J Med 293: 1232, 1975.
35. Kerlin P, Wong L: Breath hydrogen testing in bacterial overgrowth of the small intestine. Gastroenterology 95:982, 1988.
36. Strocchi A, Corazza G, Ellis CJ, et al: Detection of malabsorption of low doses of carbohydrate: Accuracy of various breath H_2 criteria. Gastroenterology 105:1404, 1993.
37. Corazza GR, Benati G, Strocchi A, et al: The possible role of breath methane measurement in detecting carbohydrate malabsorption. J Lab Clin Med 124:695, 1994.
38. Bond JH, Levitt MD: Use of pulmonary hydrogen (H_2) measurements to quantitate carbohydrate malabsorption: Study of partially gastrectomized patients. J Clin Invest 51:1219, 1972.
39. Bond JH, Levitt MD: Investigation of small bowel transit time in man utilizing pulmonary hydrogen (H_2) measurements. J Lab Clin Med 85: 546, 1975.

40. Corazza GR, Menozzi MG, Strocchi A, et al: The diagnosis of small bowel bacterial overgrowth. Gastroenterology 98:302, 1990.
41. Bond JH, Engel RR, Levitt MD: Factors influencing pulmonary methane excretion in man. J Exp Med 133:572, 1971.
42. Florin TH, Jabbar IA: A possible role for bile acid in the control of methanogenesis and the accumulation of hydrogen gas in the human colon. J Gastroenterol Hepatol 9:112, 1994.
43. Levitt MD, Duane WC: Floating stools—flatus versus fat. N Engl J Med 286:973, 1972.
44. Haines A, Metz G, Dilawari J, et al: Breath methane in patients with cancer of the large bowel. Lancet 2:481, 1977.
45. Karlin DA, Jones RD, Stroeleim JR, et al: Breath methane excretion in patients with unresected colorectal cancer. J Natl Cancer Inst 69:573, 1982.
46. Moore JG, Jessop LD, Osborne DN: A gas chromatographic and mass spectrometric analysis of the odor of human feces. Gastroenterology 93: 1321, 1987.
47. Suarez FL, Springfield JR, Levitt MD: Identification of gases responsible for the odor of human flatus and evaluation of a device purported to reduce this odor. Gut 43:100–104, 1998.
48. Levitt MD, Furne J, Springfield J, et al: Detoxification of hydrogen sulfide and methanethiol in the cecal mucosa. J Clin Invest 104:1107–1114, 1999.
49. Suarez F, Springfield J, Furne J, et al: Differentiation of mouth versus gut as site of origin of odoriferous breath gases after garlic ingestion. Am J Physiol 39:G425–G430, 1999.
50. Serra J, Aspiroz F, Malagelada JR: Intestinal gas dynamics and tolerance in humans. Gastroenterology 115:542–550, 1998.
51. Lasser RB, Bond JH, Levitt MD: The role of intestinal gas in functional abdominal pain. N Engl J Med 293:524, 1975.
52. Maxton DG, Martin DF, Whorwell PJ, et al: Abdominal distension in female patients with irritable bowel syndrome: Exploration of possible mechanisms. Gut 32:662, 1991.
53. Chami TN, Schuster MM., Bohlman ME, et al: A simple radiologic method to estimate the quantity of bowel gas. Am J Gastroenterol 86: 599, 1991.
54. Koide A, Yamguchi T, Odaka T, et al: Quantitative analysis of bowel gas using plain abdominal radiograph in patients with irritable bowel syndrome. Am J Gastroenterol 95:1735–1741, 2000.
55. Serra J, Aspiroz F, Malagelada J: Mechanisms of postprandial symptoms. Gastroenterology 116:G4693, 1999.
56. Ritchie J: Pain from distention of pelvic colon by inflating a balloon in the irritable colon syndrome. Gut 14:125, 1973.
57. Jailwala J, Imperiale TF, Kroenke K: Pharmacologic treatment of the irritable bowel syndrome: A schematic review of randomized, controlled trials. Ann Intern Med 133:136–147, 2000.
58. Johnson AG: Controlled trial of metoclopramide in the treatment of flatulent dyspepsia. BMJ 2:25, 1971.
59. Van Outryve M, Milo R, Toussaint J, et al: "Prokinetic" treatment of constipation-predominant irritable bowel syndrome: A placebo-controlled study of cisapride. J Clin Gastroenterol 13:49, 1991.
60. Caldarella M, Serra J, Azpiroz F, et al: Stimulation of intestinal gas propulsion is the key to treat gas retention in functional patients. Gastroenterology 118:138A, 2000.
61. Suarez F, Savaiano DA, Levitt MD: A comparison of symptoms with milk or lactose-hydrolyzed milk in people with self-reported severe lactose intolerance. N Engl J Med 333:1, 1995.
62. Solomons N, Vasquez A, Grazioso C: Orally-ingested, microbial alphagalactosidases produce effective in vivo, intraintestinal digestion of the bean oligosaccharide, raffinose. Gastroenterology 100:A251, 1991.
63. Hall GH Jr, Thompson H, Strother A: Effects of orally administered activated charcoal on intestinal gas. Am J Gastroenterol 75:192, 1981.
64. Potter T, Ellis C, Levitt MD: Activated charcoal: In vivo and in vitro studies of effect on gas formation. Gastroenterology 88:620, 1985.
65. Friis H, Bode S, Rumessen JJ, et al: Effect of simethicone on lactulose-induced H_2 production and gastrointestinal symptoms. Digestion 49: 227, 1991.
66. Levitt MD, Furne JK, Aeolus MR, et al: Evaluation of an extremely flatulent patient: Case report and proposed diagnostic and therapeutic approach. Am J Gastroenterol 93:2276–2281, 1998.
67. Suarez FL, Furne JK, Springfield J, et al: Production and elimination of sulfur-containing gases in the rat colon. Am J Physiol 274:G727–G773, 1998.
68. Suarez FL, Furne JK, Springfield JR, et al: Failure of activated charcoal to reduce the release of gases produced by the colonic flora. Am J Gastroenterol 94:208–212, 1999.
69. Suarez FL, Furne JK, Springfield J, et al: Bismuth subsalicylate markedly decreases hydrogen sulfide release in the human colon. Gastroenterology 114:923–929, 1998.
70. Gillon J, Tadesse K, Logan RFA, et al: Breath hydrogen in pneumatosis cystoides intestinalis. Gut 20:1008, 1979.
71. Christl SU, Gibson GR, Murgatroyd PR, et al: Impaired hydrogen metabolism in pneumatosis cystoides intestinalis. Gastroenterology 104: 392, 1993.
72. Levitt MD, Olsson S: Pneumatosis cystoides intestinalis and high breath H_2 excretion: Insights into the role of H_2 in this condition. Gastroenterology 108:1560, 1995.
73. Florin, THJ: Alkyl halides, super hydrogen production and the pathogenesis of pneumatosis cystoides coli. Gut 41:778–784, 1997.
74. Florin TH, Hills BA: Does counter perfusion supersaturation cause gas cysts in pneumatosis cystoides coli and can breathing heliox reduce them? Lancet 345:129, 1995.
75. Forgacs P, Wright PH, Wyatt AP: Treatment of intestinal gas cysts by oxygen breathing. Lancet 1:579, 1973.
76. Carter HG: Explosions in the colon during electrodesiccation of polyps. Am J Surg 84:514, 1952.
77. Bigard MA, Gaucher P, Lassalle C: Fatal colonic explosion during colonoscopic polypectomy. Gastroenterology 77:1307, 1979.
78. Strocchi A, Bond JH, Ellis CJ, et al: Colonic concentrations of hydrogen and methane following colonoscopic preparation with an oral lavage solution. Gastrointest Endosc 36:580, 1990.

Chapter 11

FECAL INCONTINENCE

Lawrence R. Schiller

Fecal incontinence is the involuntary passage of stool through the anus. The leakage may vary in severity from causing soiling of underclothes to evacuating the rectum completely. Incontinence must be differentiated from anal discharge, which is the passage of small amounts of mucus, pus, or blood from the anus. Discharge may be a symptom of several local anorectal problems discussed in Chapter 117.

Incontinence can devastate otherwise functional persons, causing fear and anxiety and transforming them into recluses. Because of perceived shame, incontinence often is not spontaneously reported by patients, making it incumbent upon physicians to ask about it, particularly when patients report diarrhea, constipation, or other anorectal problems. It is important to do so because much can be done to alleviate this symptom.

Incontinence is not a marker of severity of diarrhea but usually represents a specific defect in neuromuscular function affecting the continence mechanisms. Although fecal incontinence is broadly viewed as a functional disorder of the anorectum,[1] it often has a distinct and demonstrable cause. Treatment is often successful in mitigating incontinence but can be costly. One study of fecal incontinence due to obstetric injuries reported that the average cost per patient for evaluation and treatment exceeded $17,000.[2] Of course, the actual monetary cost of this disorder is much higher as a result of time lost from work, and the psychological cost is incalculable in terms of its impact on self-esteem and quality of life.

PREVALENCE

One large survey of U.S. households indicates that 7.1% of the general population experiences fecal soiling and 0.7% experiences gross incontinence.[3] Half of those with gross incontinence had sought medical attention, but only one sixth of those with soiling had. Fecal soiling was equally prevalent in men and women, but gross incontinence was almost twice as common in women as in men. Persons with gross incontinence were 6.8 times more likely than those without gastrointestinal symptoms to miss work or school, averaging 50 lost days each year.

Another large community survey limited to individuals 50 years of age or older showed a prevalence of fecal incontinence of 11.1% in men and 15.2% in women.[4] In contrast, the prevalence of fecal incontinence was 18% in outpatients 50 years of age or older, but only one third of those individuals had ever discussed this problem with a physician.[5] Among acutely ill hospitalized adults, 33% had fecal incontinence; incontinence occurred more often in patients with diarrhea (43%), but even patients without diarrhea had a substantial prevalence of this symptom (27%).[6]

Noninstitutionalized elderly men and women have about the same prevalence of soiling as younger persons, but the prevalence of gross incontinence is up to five times higher in the elderly.[3, 7, 8] Incontinence is the most common reason for institutionalization of the elderly, and the prevalence of fecal and combined urinary and fecal incontinence is almost 50% in the nursing home population.[9]

Episodes of fecal incontinence develop in about 20% of elderly nursing home residents during their first year of institutionalization, usually in association with acute diarrhea or fecal impaction.[10] Five risk factors were associated with the development of incontinence: a history of urinary incontinence, neurologic disease, poor mobility, severe cognitive decline, and age older than 70 years. The development of frequent episodes of incontinence was a marker of poor health; the mortality rate over 10 months in the 7% of enrolled patients in whom persistent incontinence developed was 26%, more than three times higher than that in continent nursing home residents.[10]

MECHANISMS OF CONTINENCE AND FECAL INCONTINENCE

Continence depends on the presence of a series of anatomic barriers to the movement of feces through the anus (Fig. 11–1). These barriers include the puborectalis muscle of the pelvic floor and the internal and external anal sphincters.[11]

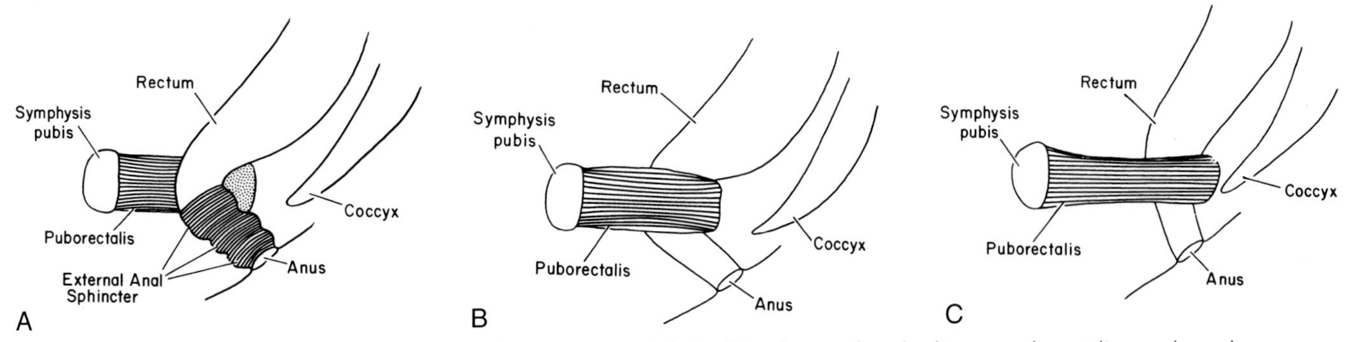

Figure 11–1. Anatomic considerations of continence. *A,* Relationship of external anal sphincter, puborectalis muscle, and rectum. *B,* Puborectalis muscle contracting to maintain continence. *C,* Puborectalis muscle relaxing to allow straightening of the rectoanal angle for defecation.

These muscles are tonically active and provide for an angulation between the axis of the rectum and the axis of the anal canal (rectoanal angle) and for occlusion of the anal canal. The rectoanal angle prevents the movement of formed and semisolid stool from the rectum into the anal canal in a fashion analogous to the way that a tractor-trailer truck cannot get around a sharp corner.[12] The anal sphincters also prevent passage of solid stool and in addition are responsible for an air- and watertight seal in the anal canal that can prevent the passage of liquid stool and gas.

Rectal distention induces relaxation of the internal anal sphincter (rectoanal relaxation reflex), which is mediated by the intrinsic nerves of the enteric nervous system. When the rectum is distended, timely external anal sphincter contraction mediated by the pudendal nerve must offset the fall in anal canal pressure if stool is to be retained in the rectum.

These barriers do not operate in isolation; normal sensation of rectal distention, intact innervation of the muscles, and adequate reservoir capacity of the rectum are necessary.[11] Although the pelvic floor muscles and external anal sphincter are tonically active, entry of stool into the rectum or upper anal canal calls for heightened contraction of these muscles to preserve continence. The sensation of a threat to continence is generated by rectal distention or by contact of stool with the very sensitive mucosa of the anal canal. The rectum is sensitive to as little as 10 mL of distention, and slightly higher volumes generate the vague sensation of a "call to stool." Contact of feces with the anal canal produces a more acute sensation of imminent defecation, which requires immediate action.[13]

If automatic defecation after rectal distention and internal anal sphincter relaxation is to be deferred, the strength of contraction of the puborectalis muscle and external anal sphincter must increase. This is mediated by the somatic innervation to these muscles from sacral levels of the spinal cord.[14] Because heightened contraction of the external sphincter can only be maintained for a minute or less, intrarectal pressure must decline if the threat to continence is to be thwarted. This is accomplished by relaxation of the rectum (rectal accommodation), which allows a larger volume to be maintained in the rectum at a lower intraluminal pressure.

When defecation is appropriate, the barriers that constitute the continence mechanism must be removed to prevent obstruction of defecation. This process is summarized in Figure 11–2.

Disorders that impair the mechanisms preserving continence can lead to incontinence (Table 11–1). In general,

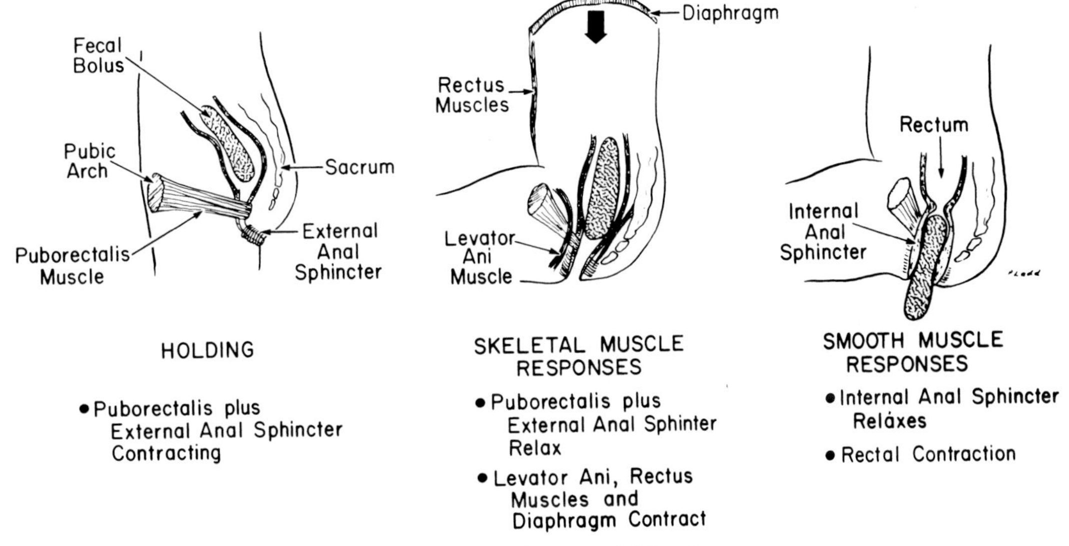

Figure 11–2. Mechanisms of defecation.

Table 11-1 | **Mechanisms of Continence and Incontinence**

MECHANISM	ROLE IN CONTINENCE	MAY BE ABNORMAL WHEN INCONTINENCE IS DUE TO
Rectal sensation	Perception of "call to stool" triggers dynamic responses to maintain continence	Diabetes mellitus, neuropathy, other diseases of the nervous system (see Table 11-2)
Internal anal sphincter tone	Maintains anal canal closure usually	Diabetes mellitus, internal sphincterotomy
External anal sphincter and puborectalis muscle tone	Maintains anorectal angle and anal closure during internal anal sphincter relaxation	Childbirth injury, pudendal neuropathy, "idiopathic" incontinence, surgical damage to external sphincter
Rectal accommodation	Allows rectal filling without high intrarectal pressures that might threaten continence	Rectal ischemia, radiation proctitis, ulcerative proctitis

there is enough redundancy that moderate impairment of any single mechanism does not cause incontinence. Most incontinent individuals have multiple abnormalities or more potent threats to continence, such as loose stools.

Diminution of rectal sensation and of the perception of a threat to continence is common in patients with incontinence.[13] In fact, dulled sensation due to dementia, spinal cord lesions, and peripheral nerve problems may underlie most complaints of fecal seepage and soiling.[15] Diarrhea itself may reduce sensory thresholds in women (but not men) and lead to internal anal sphincter relaxation at lower distention thresholds, predisposing these women to incontinence.[16] Perineal descent during straining due to weakness of the pelvic floor muscles also may cause incontinence by inducing traumatic pudendal motor neuropathy, but damage to sensory nerves may be more important.[17]

Anal sphincter weakness has long been associated with fecal incontinence. Although attention usually is focused on external sphincter weakness, dysfunction of the internal anal sphincter also contributes to incontinence.[18-20] Abnormal fibrosis, reduced elasticity, insensitivity to norepinephrine, periods of electrical silence, and more frequent spontaneous relaxations are associated with internal anal sphincter weakness.[21-24]

As noted, the functions of the external anal sphincter and puborectalis muscle are abnormal in many patients with incontinence.[24-26] Although external anal sphincter weakness may be due to traumatic damage to this muscle, pudendal motor neuropathy contributes to much of the muscle weakness in most patients. Indeed, in almost all patients with "idiopathic" incontinence pudendal neuropathy underlies the dysfunctional external anal sphincter.[27, 28] Some researchers have questioned this association[29]; this skepticism in part may be due to the variability of neural injuries seen in patients with fecal incontinence.[30, 31]

Some patients with incontinence have normal or even high anal canal pressures, raising the question of other defects in continence mechanisms. In these individuals, defects in rectal accommodation seem to be common.[32-35]

DIFFERENTIAL DIAGNOSIS OF FECAL INCONTINENCE

Diseases that compromise the neuromuscular function of the continence mechanisms cause incontinence. Prominent among these are anatomic derangements, neurologic diseases, skeletal muscle problems, and smooth muscle dysfunction (Table 11-2).

Anatomic derangements of the anus and rectum, particularly *congenital anomalies* in children, frequently cause fecal incontinence. In adults *trauma* is responsible for most fecal incontinence due to anatomic derangements, particularly an-

Table 11-2 | **Differential Diagnosis of Fecal Incontinence**

Anatomic Derangements
Congenital abnormalities of the anorectum
Fistula
Rectal prolapse
Anorectal trauma
- Injury
- Childbirth injury
- Surgery (including hemorrhoidectomy)

Sequelae of anorectal infections, Crohn's disease

Neurologic Diseases
Central nervous system processes
- Dementia, sedation, mental retardation
- Stroke, brain tumors
- Spinal cord lesions
- Multiple sclerosis
- Tabes dorsalis

Peripheral nervous system processes
- Cauda equina lesions
- Polyneuropathies
  - Diabetes mellitus
  - Shy-Drager syndrome
  - Toxic neuropathy
- Traumatic neuropathy
  - "Idiopathic" incontinence
  - Perineal descent
  - Postpartum
- Altered rectal sensation (site of lesion not known)
  - Fecal impaction
  - "Delayed sensation" syndrome

Skeletal Muscle Diseases
Myasthenia gravis
Myopathies, muscular dystrophy

Smooth Muscle Dysfunction
Abnormal rectal compliance
- Proctitis due to inflammatory bowel disease
- Radiation proctitis
- Rectal ischemia
- Fecal impaction

Internal anal sphincter weakness
- Radiation proctitis
- Diabetes mellitus
- Childhood encopresis

Miscellaneous
- Severe diarrhea
- Irritable bowel syndrome
- Idiopathic hypothyroidism
- Mastocytosis
- Acute myocardial infarction
- Splenomegaly

terior tears of the external anal sphincter in women during childbirth, which are much more common than previously thought.[36, 37] Indeed, a prospective study using ultrasonography showed that 35% of primiparous women had sphincter injury (none had demonstrated injury prepartum) and 44% of multiparous women had sphincter injury, up from 40% prepartum.[36] Symptoms of fecal urgency or incontinence were less common than ultrasonographic evidence of sphincter injury; they were present in 13% of primiparous women and in 23% of multiparous women (up from 19% prepartum). These symptoms developed within 6 weeks of delivery. Nerve injuries also are associated with vaginal deliveries and may be responsible for incontinence that develops long after delivery.[38, 39] Surgical procedures on the anus and nearby regions for anal cancer can also cause incontinence. Hemorrhoidectomy may cause fecal leakage or frank incontinence by damaging the anal cushions but is less likely to do so than anal dilation for treatment of hemorrhoids.[40, 41] Locally applied irradiation therapy can also injure the continence mechanisms.[42] Suppurative anorectal infections, x-irradiation, and Crohn's disease can cause destruction and scarring of the anal sphincter and muscles of the pelvic floor involved with continence and can result in fecal incontinence (see Chapters 102 and 103).

Neurologic diseases cause incontinence at several levels. Central nervous system processes can alter the perception of sensations required to maintain continence and can also affect motor function of the pelvic floor and anal sphincters.[43] More than one third of stroke patients have fecal incontinence on admission, and one tenth of the survivors have incontinence 6 months later.[44] *Spinal cord lesions* may also cause incontinence.[45] *Multiple sclerosis* is associated with bowel dysfunction—incontinence or constipation—in 68% of patients, and slightly more than half suffer incontinence.[46] Although both sensory and motor dysfunctions may be present in multiple sclerosis, peripheral nerve conduction is well maintained (see Chapter 29).[46, 47]

Peripheral nervous system dysfunction underlies fecal incontinence in patients with *diabetes mellitus*, the systemic disease most commonly associated with incontinence. It results from diabetic neuropathy of both sensory and motor nerves and is most often associated with internal anal sphincter dysfunction.[47–49] The most common pathogenesis for "idiopathic" incontinence is *traumatic neuropathy* resulting from obstetric injury or chronic straining during evacuation.[50] In these cases, external anal sphincter weakness, related to pudendal nerve neuropathy, is most prominent.

Skeletal muscle diseases, such as *myasthenia gravis*, *myopathies*, and *myotonic dystrophy*, can compromise continence by causing dysfunction of the puborectalis muscle or external anal sphincter.[51] Smooth muscle diseases, such as progressive systemic sclerosis, can affect continence by weakening the internal anal sphincter, particularly when the condition is complicated by diarrhea (see Chapter 29).[52, 53]

EVALUATION OF PATIENTS WITH FECAL INCONTINENCE

The goals of the evaluation of patients with fecal incontinence are: (1) to understand the severity of the problem and its impact on the patient's life, (2) to discover treatable diseases that may be responsible for incontinence, and (3) to understand the pathophysiologic characteristics of incontinence so that appropriate therapy can be instituted. These goals can be met by a careful history and physical examination and selected objective tests of the continence mechanisms.

History

An essential point is to establish that, indeed, the patient *has* incontinence. It is often difficult to do so because patients are embarrassed to volunteer this information. Accordingly, the interviewer must ask about incontinence directly, especially when patients have chronic diarrhea. A history of incontinence should also be sought when patients report fecal urgency, constipation, urinary incontinence, neuromuscular disease, and diabetes mellitus.

Once a history of incontinence is established, the physician should try to understand the severity of the problem. A key question concerns the adaptations made for this problem. These range from no change in daily activity for patients with minor leakage to life as a recluse for those with major accidents. The severity of incontinence dictates the urgency of evaluation and the intensity of management.

Questioning should be directed to the circumstances surrounding episodes of incontinence and presence of physical barriers to defecating in an appropriate place; for example, is the toilet upstairs, and does the patient require assistance to reach it? The frequency of incontinence must be judged in terms of the adaptations already made to the problem; for instance, staying within range of a bathroom may reduce the incidence of incontinence. It is essential also to know whether incontinence occurs only with loose stools, how long the patient has had incontinence, and whether it occurs only during sleep or other alterations of consciousness, such as during sedation. Additional questions include how much warning the patient has before defecation, whether defecation can be deferred for any amount of time, and whether the patient is aware that an accident is happening.

Questionnaires validated in 1996 and 2000 have been developed to screen populations and to help assess patients with fecal incontinence.[54, 55] A fecal incontinence severity index and a fecal incontinence quality of life scale also have been used to assess treatment outcomes.[56, 57]

The interviewer should then evaluate possible causes of incontinence. Questions should be directed to the many causes listed in Table 11–2. The temporal relationship between any of these predisposing factors and the onset of incontinence should be ascertained with the understanding that years may separate the inciting event from the appearance of incontinence. This is especially important if additional factors, such as the development of diarrhea or other stresses on the continence mechanisms, have led to a recent onset of incontinence.

Physical Examination

A thorough physical examination of the perineum and anus can provide important clues to the pathogenesis of fecal incontinence and can guide the selection of appropriate objective tests. The patient should be reassured and made as physically comfortable as possible in a left lateral decubitus position. The perineum and perianal area should be inspected for evidence of tumor, dermatitis, infection, fistula, scars, skin tags, hemorrhoids, and deformity of the anus. The anus and perineum should also be inspected while the patient bears down to look for rectal prolapse, leakage, and ballooning of the perineum, which suggest perineal descent due to weakness of the pelvic floor (see Chapters 117 and 118).

The next step is to stroke the perianal skin with a pin or probe to induce the cutaneoanal contractile reflex. The subcutaneous portion of the external anal sphincter should contract and produce a visible puckering at the anal margin ("anal wink"). Failure to elicit this reflex suggests a problem with either the peripheral sensory or motor nerves or the spinal cord synapses that mediate this reflex.

The gloved examining finger should be lubricated and gently inserted into the anal canal. The examiner can gain an impression of the length of the anal canal, the bulk of the perianal tissues, and the tone primarily of the internal anal sphincter. One cannot estimate anal sphincter pressure accurately in this fashion because of variation of the diameter of the examining finger from examiner to examiner and variation in the elasticity of the anal canal from patient to patient. The positive predictive value of reduced resting tone by physical examination for low basal anal sphincter pressure by manometry is only 66.7%.[58] Nevertheless, with experience one can gain an impression of the relative strength of the anal sphincter. A vague correlation between examiners' subjective opinions and objective testing has been established in one study.[59]

The anal canal should be palpated in all quadrants for the presence of fluctuance or scar. The patient should then be asked to squeeze as if trying to prevent defecation. An increase in anal canal pressure due to external sphincter contraction should be appreciated readily. The examiner should attempt to assess the relative strength of this contraction in all quadrants by rotating the examining finger in the anal canal; focal weakness can sometimes be appreciated. In one study the positive predictive value of subjective assessment of reduced voluntary contraction for external anal sphincter weakness was 80.6%.[58] The patient should then be asked to relax, and the cutaneoanal reflex should be elicited again while the examining finger is in the anal canal. A brief contraction at the external sphincter should be felt. Attention should then be shifted to the puborectalis muscle. This muscle can be palpated in the posterior midline as a transverse bar that can be followed laterally, but not anteriorly. The puborectalis muscle should then be stretched by pulling the examining finger posteriorly. Gapping of the anal canal during this maneuver indicates weakness of the skeletal muscle of the pelvic floor. The patient should then be asked to try to prevent the passage of stool again. The puborectalis muscle should contract forcefully, pulling the examining finger anteriorly. Failure to do this suggests weakness of the puborectalis muscle. The rectum should then be palpated for the presence of a rectal mass or fecal impaction.

Objective Tests

Several tests that provide generally reproducible objective data about rectoanal structure and function are increasingly available. They are most reliable, however, at centers that have technical expertise and validated normal values. Although these objective studies are complementary and, hence, are most informative in combination, they may be used selectively to evaluate patients with incontinence.[60–62] Such selection should be based on ways the results of a particular study will affect management of the patient. A list of available tests and their objectives is provided in Table 11–3.

Anal manometry provides a direct measurement of anal canal pressures at rest and during voluntary contraction of the external anal sphincter. This information is quite useful in understanding the pathophysiologic characteristics of incontinence and in designing an effective treatment regimen.[63] Anal manometry can also be used to measure the responses of the internal and external anal sphincters to rectal distention. Several systems have been devised, including perfused catheters, microtransducer arrays, and microballoon devices. Large balloons do not provide accurate pressure readings but can be used for the assessment of the rectoanal reflexes.

Anal canal pressures vary radially and longitudinally through the anal canal. With a sufficient number of recording sites, it is possible to map the three-dimensional pressure profile of the anal canal, but it is unclear whether such data are of more clinical benefit than simpler measurements of average basal and average squeeze pressures.[64] Other methods of analyzing pressure records include calculation of an anorectal manometry index,[65] measurement of a strength-duration curve,[66] determination of fatigue rate,[67] and identification of the location of the highest mean resting pressure segment,[68] but none of these has been adopted widely. Regardless of the method of analysis, pressures differ substantially between men and women, presumably as a result of anatomic differences. Anal canal pressures decrease with aging; it is unclear whether this reduction results from "normal" aging or the accumulation of subclinical pathologic damage.[69]

Table 11–3 | **Objective Tests of Rectoanal Function**

TEST	PURPOSE
Anal manometry	Measurement of basal and squeeze pressures in anal canal
Rectal balloon manometry	Measurement of rectal sensation, rectal compliance, rectoanal inhibitory reflex, and rectoanal contractile response
Electrophysiologic tests	
Electromyography	Assessment of motor nerve supply and skeletal muscle responses
Nerve conduction studies	Evaluation of motor neuropathy
Mucosal electrosensitivity	Evaluation of sensory threshold
Reflex arc stimulation	Measurement of integrated spinal reflex
Radiographic tests	Assessment of rectoanal angle, perineal descent, and puborectalis function
Defecography	
Balloon proctography	
Scintigraphy	
Anal endosonography	Evaluation of sphincter integrity
Magnetic resonance imaging	Evaluation of sphincter integrity
Objective tests of continence	Quantitative assessment of ability to maintain continence against a reproducible stress
Solid sphere	
Balloon	
Rectally infused saline	

Basal anal pressure is due largely to tonic contraction of the internal sphincter. It is well maintained even with nerve blocks that paralyze the external sphincter. The component of squeeze pressure that exceeds basal pressure is due to active contraction of the external sphincter; it is abolished by nerve blocks. Because the internal and external sphincters are coaxial over most of their lengths, anal canal pressure reflects the blended activity of both sphincters. Only at the anal verge can the pressure generated by the subcutaneous external anal sphincter be recorded by itself.

As a group, patients with fecal incontinence have significantly lower basal and squeeze pressures than age- and sex-matched controls,[69] a difference more pronounced in women than in men.[70] However, the range of pressures among incontinent patients is considerable, and many have normal sphincter pressures. Anal manometry is most valuable when it demonstrates abnormally low pressures and thus confirms the presence of a sphincter defect. An isolated decrease in basal pressure or squeeze pressure suggests a problem with internal or external anal sphincter function, respectively, but does not differentiate pathogenetically between primarily neurogenic and primarily myogenic processes.

Rectal balloon manometry can be performed with a three-balloon probe or with a balloon mounted at the end of a perfused or transducer-based anal manometry array. This study can provide information about rectal sensation, rectal compliance, the rectoanal inhibitory reflex, and the rectoanal contractile response.

Rectal sensation is assessed by inflating a rectal balloon with increasing volumes of air or water. The threshold for conscious sensation of rectal distention is the volume at which the patient first reports the sensation of something in the rectum. Most normal individuals can sense as little as 10 mL. Some incontinent patients have higher sensory thresholds, and others are unable to sense rectal distention. Some incontinent patients have delayed perception.[71] These disturbances suggest dysfunction of the afferent pathways that carry the sensation of distention to consciousness.

Measurement of rectal pressure during inflation of the rectal balloon generates a rectal compliance curve (dV/dP), corrected for the compliance properties of the balloon itself by subtraction of an extracorporeal pressure-volume curve. Patients with incontinence often have lower rectal compliance (i.e., production of higher rectal pressures by lower rectal volumes than in normal individuals) than do control patients and stress the continence mechanisms more as stool enters the rectum.[72] Conditions that are particularly likely to produce problems with rectal compliance include those that are associated with rectal fibrosis, such as rectal ischemia or radiation proctitis (see Chapters 102 and 119).

By monitoring pressure in the upper anal canal during rectal distention, reflex relaxation of the internal anal sphincter (rectoanal inhibitory reflex) can be demonstrated. This reflex is mediated by intramural neurons and probably involves nitric oxide as a neurotransmitter. The volume of distention required to achieve reflex relaxation is approximately 20 mL and usually is slightly higher than the threshold for conscious sensation. The amplitude and duration of relaxation are directly related to the distending volume. With entry of stool into the rectum, this relaxation allows stool to reach the sensitive anal canal mucosa, reinforcing rectal sensation. The rectoanal inhibitory reflex is absent in patients with Hirschsprung's disease and may be difficult to demonstrate if basal anal sphincter pressure is very low.

When the rectum is distended, pressure in the distal anal canal increases as a result of contraction of the external anal sphincter. This rectoanal contractile response is essential if automatic defecation is to be prevented. It is a learned response (probably at the time of toilet training in childhood) and is often missing in patients with fecal incontinence of a variety of causes. Absence of this response could be due to interruption of rectal sensory pathways, damage to the pudendal nerves, weakness of the external anal sphincter muscle due to injury or skeletal muscle disease, or forgetting of this learned response. Loss of this response most often correlates with pudendal neuropathy but is not diagnostic of it.[73] Relearning this response is an important objective of biofeedback training for the treatment of fecal incontinence (see later discussion).

Electrophysiologic tests can be used to assess the integrity of the sensory and motor innervation of the rectoanal region.[74–77] Electromyography (EMG) with standard concentric needles or with more sophisticated single-fiber techniques can be used to assess the viability and reactivity of skeletal muscle. Because skeletal muscle activity is dependent upon intact innervation, these tests provide information about the motor innervation of these muscles. Because these studies involve placement of needles or wires into the perineal region and have gained the reputation among patients of being unpleasant, alternative methods such as quantitative surface electromyography have been tried.[78] These methods may be more tolerable but provide less specific information than the more invasive techniques.

Information about the motor nerves innervating the external anal sphincter can be obtained by pudendal nerve terminal motor latency testing. In this test, a special glove with a stimulating electrode over the fingertip and a recording electrode at the base of the finger is worn by the examiner. The gloved finger is introduced into the anus, and the fingertip is placed between the ischial spine and the edge of the sacrum, where the pudendal nerve passes. The time for the electrically stimulated nerve impulse to travel down the pudendal nerve is prolonged in patients with pudendal neuropathy as compared with that in normal persons. Studies show that this measurement is reliable and correlates with results of anorectal manometry.[79, 80] However, in practice this test has proved to be less useful than originally anticipated.[81, 82]

Mucosal sensitivity can be assessed by gradually increasing electrical stimulation of the anal mucosa with an electrode until felt by the patient. This test is of limited value clinically since electrosensitivity diminishes with aging and is abnormal in many anorectal diseases.[83, 84]

All of these electrophysiologic tests are of most use in research settings. In clinical practice there is little to be gained by these tests unless surgery is planned and one needs to know whether denervation is so severe as to make repair of a sphincter defect unlikely to be successful.

Imaging studies allow assessment of the anatomic aspects of continence and the physiologic dynamics of defecation. These tests evaluate the rectoanal angle, quantitate perineal descent, allow diagnosis of causes of obstructed defecation, and visualize sphincter anatomic characteristics.

Defecography is the most widely available technique for evaluating the rectoanal angle, the pelvic floor muscles, and

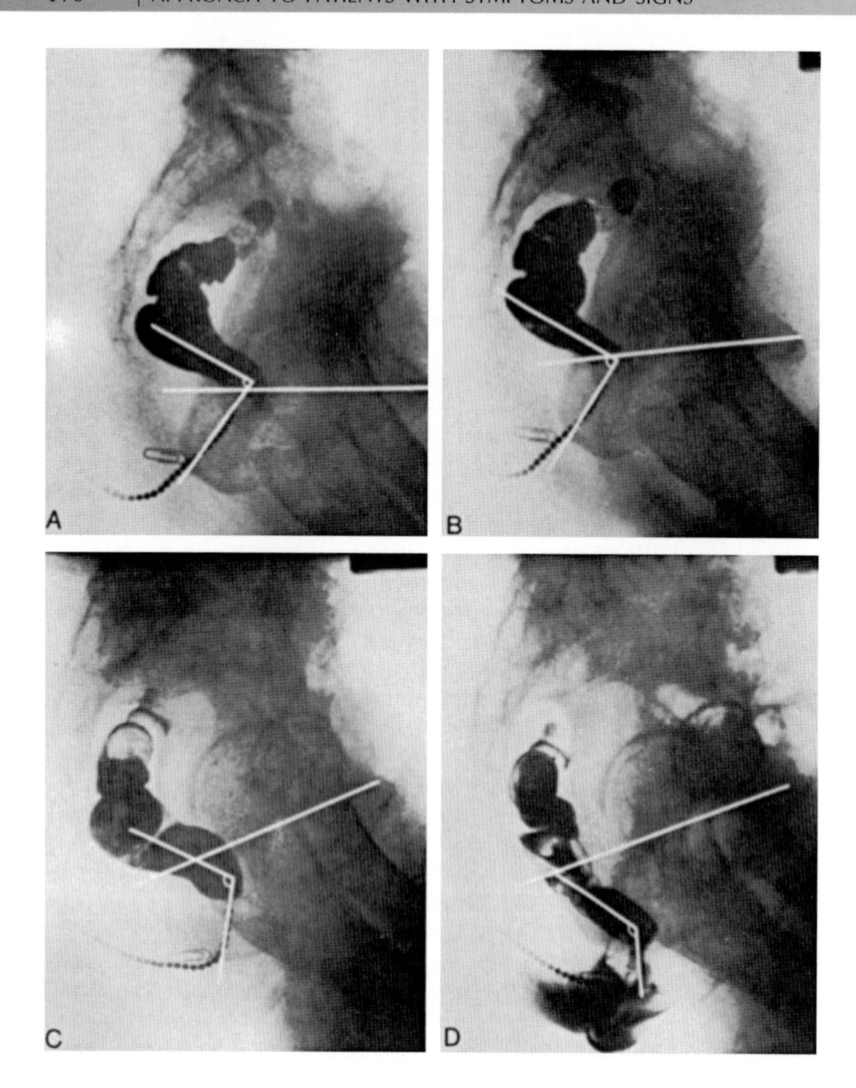

Figure 11–3. Fluoroscopic defecography is usually recorded on videotape, but contrast is too poor for photographic reproduction. These lateral radiographs of the pelvis show the relationships between the rectoanal angle and pubococcygeal line in a normal individual at rest *(A)* and during *(B)* straining. The same views are shown in a patient with perineal descent at rest *(C)* and while straining *(D)*. Note the obtuse rectoanal angle and its relation to the pubococcygeal line, a characteristic finding more common in patients with incontinence. (From Bartolo DCC, et al: Differences in anal sphincter function and clinical presentation in patients with pelvic floor descent. Gastroenterology 85:68, 1983. Copyright 1983, American Gastroenterological Association.)

the causes of obstructed defecation. A small amount of barium is injected into the rectum and the anal verge is identified with radiopaque markers. The patient is then seated on a commode, and a fluoroscopic videotape is made from the side as the patient coughs to increase abdominal pressure transiently, bears down while squeezing as if to hold onto stool, and then defecates. The angle made between the anal canal and the axis of the rectum can be measured both at rest and during straining (Fig. 11–3). Normally, this angle is maintained at about 90 degrees both at rest and during straining, but it becomes more obtuse as the puborectalis muscle weakens.

Abnormalities of the anorectal angle indicated by defecography correlate with the severity of fecal incontinence; that is, the wider the angle, the greater the severity.[85] Although defecography provides information about the status of the pelvic floor that is not obtainable through anorectal manometry, it adds relatively little clinically useful information for the assessment of incontinent patients. It may be helpful, however, in those incontinent patients who have coexisting symptoms of obstructed defecation.[86, 87]

Ultrasonography of the anal canal with an endoanal ultrasound probe is a very useful technique for demonstrating anal sphincter anatomic features. Normal findings have been well described, and sphincter defects have been demon-

Table 11–4 | **Treatment of Fecal Incontinence**

General Principles
Treatment of underlying disease
Stimulation of defecation at intervals
Treatment of diarrhea, if present
Addressing psychological problems
Continence aids
Skin care
Drug Therapy
Loperamide
? Valproate sodium
Biofeedback Training
Electrostimulation
Surgery
Sphincteroplasty
Total pelvic floor repair
Gracilis muscle transposition
Electrically stimulated muscle transposition
Anal encirclement (Thiersch procedure)
Perianal fat injection
Antegrade continence enema
Fecal diversion (ileostomy, colostomy)

strated to correlate with surgical findings.[88–90] Unusual orientations of muscle fibers can simulate sphincter defects and 5% to 25% of tests falsely identify an anterior anal sphincter defect.[91, 92] Such false-positive findings are less frequent in men and ultrasonography may be a reasonable predictor of the success of nonoperative management in men with intact sphincter anatomic features.[93] Transvaginal and perineal ultrasound examinations may also be useful in patients with incontinence.[94, 95] Use of three-dimensional endoanal ultrasonography may result in improved accuracy.[96, 97]

Magnetic resonance imaging (MRI) using an endoanal receiver coil was popularized in 1999.[98, 99] Like results of endoanal ultrasonography, MRI examination results have been compared with surgical findings. In one study, MRI correctly identified sphincter anatomic characteristics in 92% of cases.[100] Whereas some physicians believe strongly that MRI is more accurate than ultrasonography in demonstration of anal sphincter lesions,[101] others consider the two techniques equivalent in diagnosing external anal sphincter injury and believe that MRI may be inferior in diagnosing internal anal sphincter injury.[102] The high cost of MRI may limit its clinical use.

TREATMENT

General Principles

Fecal incontinence can be eliminated or minimized in most patients, including the elderly or institutionalized. A summary of available treatments is presented in Table 11–4. If a specific underlying cause is discovered, therapy directed at that cause may alleviate incontinence. For example, diabetic patients whose incontinence is caused by neuropathy may benefit from more vigorous control of hyperglycemia. In other circumstances, progressive impairment of continence may be forestalled by preventing further damage; for example, pudendal neuropathy related to perineal descent syndrome may not progress if the patient can reduce straining at stool by modifying defecation habits.

If an identifiable cause of incontinence is not found or cannot be treated, nonspecific medical therapy should be tried. One such approach is to stimulate defecation at intervals to keep the colon and rectum empty of feces. This can be of great help to institutionalized patients, especially those incontinent of solid stool. This can also help children with encopresis in whom fecal impaction and overflow incontinence may be present. Patients should be asked to set aside a regular time to have a reflex-induced bowel movement every day or every other day. The designated time should occur within 30 minutes after a meal to take advantage of the gastrocolic reflex. Initially, glycerin suppositories should be placed into the rectum at the conclusion of the meal. Glycerin draws water intraluminally by its osmotic activity, and this process results in rectal distention and reflex defecation. If glycerin suppositories do not work satisfactorily, bisacodyl suppositories or small-volume (100 mL) warm water or commercially packaged phosphate enemas can be substituted on the same schedule. Oral laxation should be held as a final option because of the unpredictability of onset of action.

One study using such a protocol in children and young adults with spina bifida showed improved continence with one or fewer episodes of incontinence each month in 79% of compliant patients.[103] Another study, of institutionalized elderly patients, indicated that complete rectal emptying results in 35% fewer episodes of fecal incontinence.[104]

Colonic irrigation, either retrograde (i.e., standard enemas) or antegrade (i.e., via a conduit into the cecum, which is discussed later), may also be helpful in some people. In one study, patients with fecal soiling or incontinence were instructed in how to use a colostomy irrigation set transanally to empty the distal part of the large bowel.[105] Most patients who were able to continue the program enjoyed a major improvement in their quality of life. Interestingly, it seemed to be more effective in those with soiling than in those with gross incontinence. In a second study, use of an enema continence catheter or antegrade continence enema delivered through a cecostomy improved incontinence in a majority of patients and led to a significant improvement in quality of life.[106]

For patients with coexisting diarrhea, intensive efforts to make a diagnosis and to treat the diarrhea may result in a solid stool that can be more readily controlled by impaired continence mechanisms. Bulking agents, such as psyllium, or nonspecific antidiarrheal drugs, such as diphenoxylate or loperamide, may produce more formed stools.

Much of the disability related to incontinence is psychological. Patients fear experiencing fecal incontinence in public, and this fear leads to reclusiveness and depression. These patients need a great deal of support from their physicians in their attempts to return to society. Patient education materials, such as the book *Keeping Control: Understanding and Overcoming Fecal Incontinence* (by Marvin M. Schuster and Jacqueline Wehmueller, Baltimore, Johns Hopkins University Press), can be of great value in helping patients deal with this problem. Advice on the use of continence aids, such as adult size training pants, can provide concrete help in relieving the fear and embarrassment of potential accidents. Studies using products that absorb leaked stool have been evaluated in a systematic review.[107] Unfortunately, existing data were of insufficient quantity and quality to provide a firm basis for a recommendation.

Breakdown of the skin of the perineum and over the buttocks is a constant threat for bed-bound incontinent patients. Attentive skin care and use of fecal incontinence pouches to direct liquid stool away from the skin can be helpful. Cleansing regimens must minimize abrasion and reduce residual soap films.[108, 109]

In addition to these general principles, four approaches are available to prevent or reduce incontinence directly: (1) drug therapy, (2) biofeedback training, (3) electrostimulation, and (4) surgery.

Drug Therapy

In theory, there are several potential sites of action for drugs in patients with fecal incontinence. These include the proximal colon, which delivers stool to the rectum; the smooth muscle of the rectum and internal anal sphincter; and the skeletal muscles of the pelvic floor and external anal sphincter. In practice, the only drugs used regularly for incontinence are opiate antidiarrheal agents that influence the delivery of stool to the rectum.

One double-blind cross-over study of 2.5 mg diphenoxylate hydrochloride with 0.025 mg atropine sulfate (Lomotil) versus placebo in ambulatory incontinent patients showed the expected reduction of stool weight and frequency with two tablets four times a day but did not show any difference in sphincter mechanics.[110] Incontinence occurred too infrequently during treatment to allow conclusions to be drawn about effects on this symptom. A similar placebo-controlled study with loperamide suggested that a dose of 4 mg three times a day significantly reduced the frequency of incontinence and urgency and increased basal anal sphincter pressure slightly.[111] In 1997, a controlled trial examined the effectiveness of loperamide oxide, a prodrug, in patients with chronic diarrhea and fecal incontinence. A dose of 4 mg twice daily reduced stool weight and increased basal sphincter pressure.[112]

For patients with chronic diarrhea and fecal incontinence, loperamide may be the nonspecific antidiarrheal agent of choice because of its additional effect on internal anal sphincter tone. It is less clear whether loperamide is effective in patients with fecal incontinence for solid stools. Intermittent use of lower doses than in diarrhea may help selected patients with incontinence for solid stools by inhibiting colonic motility and rectal filling, particularly before they leave home or attend a meeting. Patients so treated must be observed closely for the development of constipation.

New pharmacologic approaches to incontinence have been slow to develop. Because the α-adrenergic agonist phenylephrine hydrochloride produces contraction of the internal sphincter and an increase in resting pressure in the anal canal in healthy volunteers, it has been tried in patients with incontinence with internal sphincter dysfunction.[113] Unfortunately, incontinence scores or resting anal pressures were similar for the active drug and placebo, perhaps because of the inability of the damaged sphincter to respond to the drug. This approach might be more effective in patients with intact internal anal sphincter function; no data, however, are yet reported.

Biofeedback Training

Biofeedback training is a form of operant conditioning or instrumental learning in which information about a physiologic process that would otherwise be unconscious is presented to a subject with the aim of enabling the subject to modify that process. For patients with fecal incontinence, the process is external anal sphincter contraction in response to rectal distention. In a typical biofeedback treatment session, the patient uses a balloon manometry device attached to a pressure monitor and is shown how the pressure in the distal anal canal balloon can be increased by contracting the external anal sphincter. The patient is then instructed to do this every time that the rectal balloon is distended. Initially, the balloon is inflated above the sensory threshold and the patient can see his or her response by observing the pressure tracing from the anal canal. Appropriate external sphincter contraction in response to rectal distention is rewarded verbally, and the exercise is performed repeatedly. The volume distending the rectal balloon is gradually reduced as the patient is able to sense and respond to rectal distention consistently. As perception and response improve, the pressure tracing is removed from view to assess better the extent of improvement of the threshold for conscious perception of rectal distention (Fig. 11–4). Other techniques of biofeedback training for incontinence have been described, most of which use electromyography rather than pressure biofeedback as a measure of external anal sphincter contraction.[114–116]

Although a published systematic review indicated that the combination of a limited number of identified trials and methodological weaknesses would not allow reliable assessment of the role of biofeedback therapy in the management of patients with incontinence,[117] most experts believe that biofeedback training is a valuable treatment in selected patients. Reports from centers experienced with the technique suggest that about 70% of patients in whom training can be done (i.e., cooperative patients with some degree of perception of rectal distention and the ability to contract the external anal sphincter, in all perhaps two thirds of incontinent patients) experience either disappearance or substantial re-

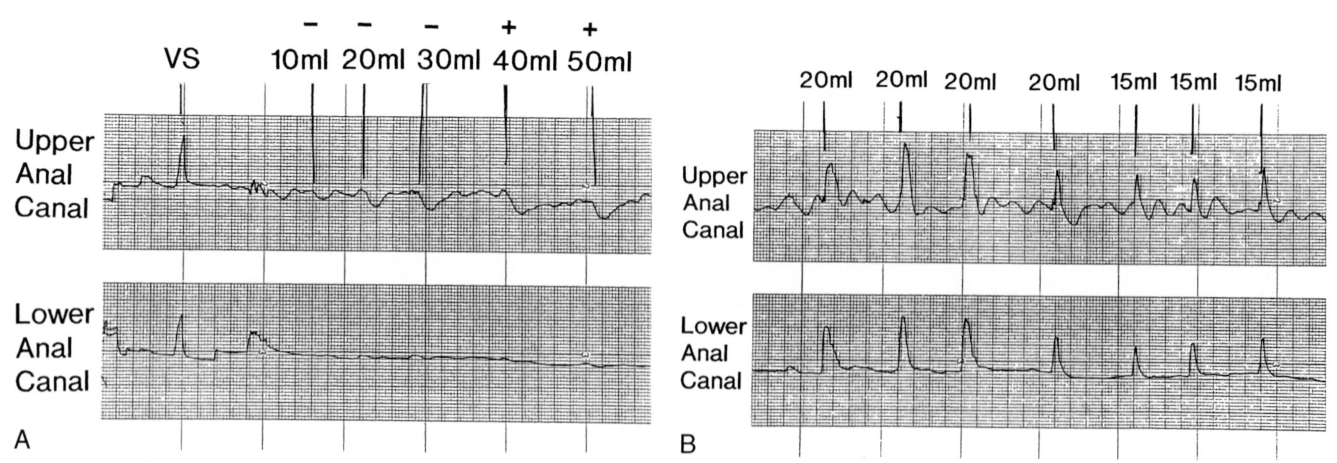

Figure 11–4. Biofeedback training. Balloon manometry before *(A)* and after *(B)* biofeedback training. The recordings from the lower anal canal balloon (lower tracing in each panel) show no lower anal canal (external anal sphincter) contraction in response to rectal distention before biofeedback training, but consistent contraction after this therapy.

duction of spontaneous incontinence.[118–124] Most patients who respond to biofeedback improve after a single session, and long-term follow-up suggests that the improvement is maintained in most.[124–126] Incontinence may not be eliminated completely in these responders, but the severity of the symptom is reduced.[125, 126] Neurogenic fecal incontinence may be less likely to respond to biofeedback training; such patients may account for the 30% in whom biofeedback fails.[127, 128]

Studies have not shown a consistent change in physiologic measurements after biofeedback training. In some studies responders have had improvement in their threshold for perception of rectal distention, whereas nonresponders had no improvement in sensation. Other studies have suggested that the ability to increase squeeze pressure may predict success of biofeedback training.[129] It is not clear which component of the biofeedback training is responsible for its beneficial results. One study suggested that either sensory training or muscle training has equivalent results.[130] A study in 1999 indicated that combination training is superior to sensory biofeedback alone.[131]

Biofeedback training is inexpensive, quick, and safe. It should be offered to all patients with fecal incontinence who are appropriate candidates. To be trainable, a patient must be able to cooperate, be well motivated, have some ability to sense rectal distention (albeit at a higher than normal volume), and have the ability to contract the external anal sphincter voluntarily. Anorectal manometry should be performed in all potential trainees to assess these criteria. Because continence is multifactorial, however, manometric findings alone do not predict the response to biofeedback training.[132]

Electrostimulation

Transanal electrostimulation has been claimed to improve continence in some incontinent patients. In this technique, electricity is applied to the anal canal by means of electrodes attached to a portable stimulator on an intermittent basis (e.g., 30 minutes daily) in an effort to stimulate muscle contraction. Results have been mixed; some studies have suggested that fewer incontinent episodes occurred after electrostimulation[133–135] and others suggested that there was no effect.[136, 137] One systematic review concluded that data are insufficient to allow reliable conclusions to be drawn and that additional studies are required.[138]

A newer form of electrical stimulation involves implanting electrodes percutaneously or operatively into the third or fourth sacral (S3 or S4) foramina and applying electrical stimulation to the sacral nerves. Preliminary studies reported from St. Mark's Hospital in London indicate that this technique can reduce incontinence.[139–141] Stimulation seemed to enhance maximal squeeze pressure and made the rectum less sensitive to distention with no change in rectal compliance.[139] Improvement was noted within a week and continued through 9 months of stimulation. Larger trials are needed to elucidate the role of this approach.

Surgery

Operative management of fecal incontinence should be considered in patients who do not respond to medical therapy or who have well-defined anatomic changes in the anorectal region. The large number of surgical procedures advocated for the relief of fecal incontinence (see Table 11–4) indicates that no single procedure is suitable for all patients. Because these procedures are technically difficult and entail complications, they should only be performed by skilled surgeons and only after meticulous preoperative evaluation to determine the best operation for each individual.[142–146]

Patients who have traumatic obstetric or iatrogenic disruption of the external sphincter usually are best treated with sphincteroplasty. This surgery involves division of scar and reapproximation of viable sphincter muscle to produce a ring of functional muscle (Fig. 11–5).[147–151] Prospective studies suggest that in approximately 75% of selected patients sphincteroplasty substantially improves continence in the short term,[147–152] but unfortunately the benefits may be short-lived.[153–155] Patients with satisfactory results have increased squeeze pressures, whereas failure to achieve this change

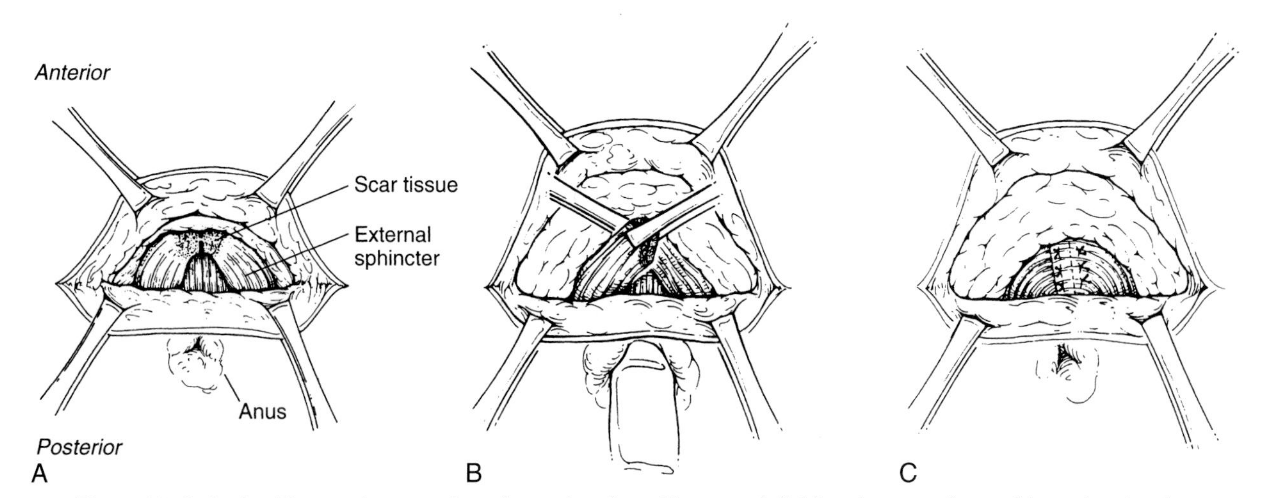

Figure 11–5. Anal sphincteroplasty consists of exposing the sphincter and dividing the area of scar *(A)*, overlapping the divided scar *(B)*, and suturing the divided sphincter to produce a complete ring of viable muscle *(C)*. (Adapted from Beart RW Jr, Block GE: Anal incontinence. In Block GE, Moosa AR [eds]: Operative Colorectal Surgery. Philadelphia, WB Saunders, 1994.)

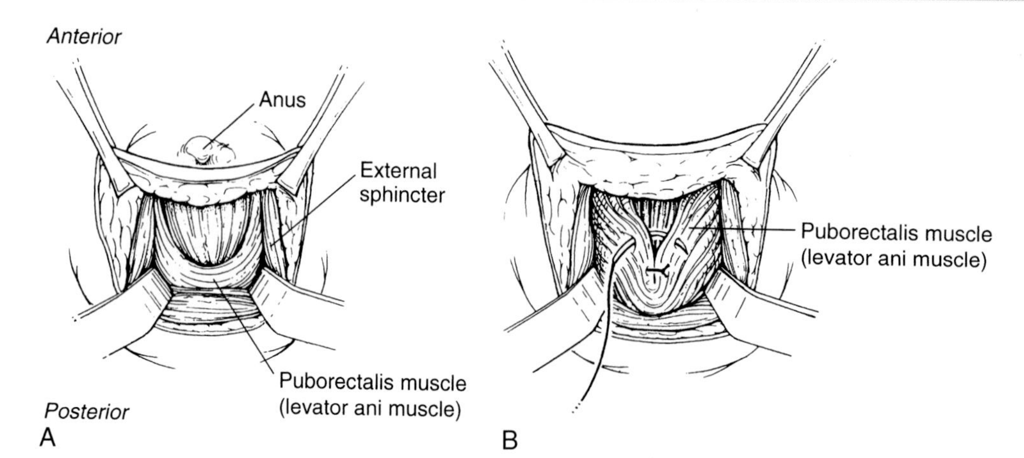

Figure 11–6. Postanal repair is part of total pelvic floor repair. In this operation, the puborectalis muscle is exposed by a dissection posterior to the anus *(A)*, and the two arms of the puborectalis muscle are plicated together to shorten their length and thus make the rectoanal angle more acute *(B)*. (Adapted from Beart RW Jr, Block GE: Anal incontinence. In Block GE, Moosa AR [eds]: Operative Colorectal Surgery. Philadelphia, WB Saunders, 1994.)

correlates with persistent external anal sphincter defects.[147, 148, 156, 157] Older individuals seem to fare as well as younger patients, but external anal sphincter atrophy, gross perineal descent, and evidence of pudendal neuropathy may lead to suboptimal results.[149, 158–163] Patients with incomplete responses may benefit from biofeedback training or a repeat repair of the anal sphincter.[164, 165] Attempts to repair internal anal sphincter defects have been less successful than repairs of external anal sphincter damage.[166–168]

Patients with neuropathic fecal incontinence have been approached surgically with total pelvic floor repair.[169–171] In this operation, the puborectalis, ischiococcygeus, and iliococcygeus muscles are sutured together, the so-called postanal repair (Fig. 11–6), and the levator muscles and external anal sphincter are plicated anteriorly. In one prospective study, complete continence was achieved with this operation in 41% and substantial improvement was noted in another 55%.[169] In another study daily incontinence persisted in 23% and only 14% of patients were rendered completely continent.[171] Alone, postanal repair or anterior levatorplasty is insufficient for most patients with neuropathic incontinence.[169, 172–175] Since these operations inconsistently improve the anatomic or physiologic characteristics of the anorectum, most of their beneficial effect may be due to creation of a local stenosis.[176]

When anal sphincter weakness is so profound that tightening of the sphincter and pelvic floor muscles is insufficient to restore continence, attempts have been made to transpose or transplant functioning skeletal muscle to create a "neosphincter." Transposition of the gracilis muscle from the thigh is most often tried (Fig. 11–7), but results have been mixed. One retrospective survey of 22 patients showed that 18 had improvement of continence 6 months after surgery, but only 1 patient was fully continent.[177] Better results have been attained by stimulating the transposed muscle with electrical current from an implanted stimulator.[178–182] In general, improved continence is seen in up to 70% of patients treated in this way. Symptomatic improvement is associated with significant increases in anal canal pressures, more normal defecographic appearances, and a better quality of life; however, most patients have complications, and 40% require one or more operations to treat them.[183] Nevertheless, the procedure appears to be cost-effective and may be useful in a subset of patients who have otherwise untreatable incontinence.[184, 185]

Another technological approach to fecal incontinence has been the development of an artificial anal sphincter. Patterned on artificial urinary sphincters, these devices involve placement of a hydraulic ring around the anal canal with a reservoir and pump device to keep the ring inflated (and the anal canal occluded) between bowel movements and to deflate it (allowing the anal canal to be opened) when defecation is desired. Results have been encouraging, but local infection remains a common complication.[186–190]

Less sophisticated surgical techniques include anal encirclement (Thiersch procedure) and injection of fat or collagen around the anal canal. Anal encirclement with nonabsorbable mesh narrows the anal canal and (ideally) increases resistance and decreases leakage without producing obstructive symptoms. Results are often less than ideal, however, and local infection remains an important complication.[191] Other approaches to increasing passive resistance in the anal canal are to inject autologous fat[192] or glutaraldehyde-treated cross-linked collagen[193] around the anal canal. These techniques may be most effective for patients with isolated internal anal sphincter dysfunction in whom the external anal sphincter remains functional.

Other surgeries can be considered when other approaches have failed or are impractical. One option is fecal diversion

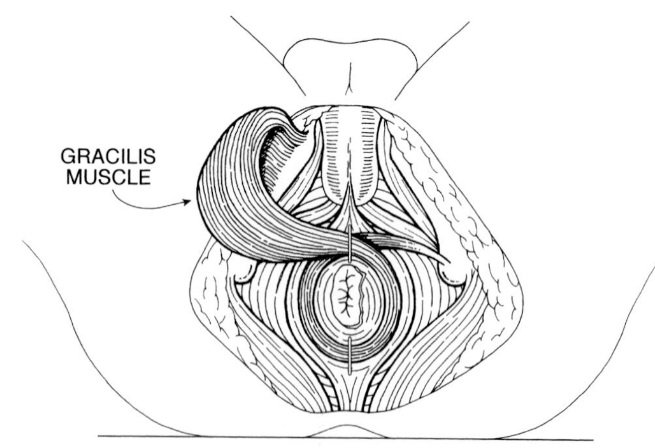

Figure 11–7. Gracilis muscle transposition involves freeing the gracilis muscle from its insertion at the knee and reflecting it back to the perineum where it is placed to encircle the anal canal. The native innervation is maintained and may be stimulated electrically by an implanted stimulator to reproduce the tonic contraction of the anal sphincter.

by means of a colostomy or ileostomy, which allows patients with devastating incontinence to achieve some measure of control over defecation. Another option is creation of an access conduit to the cecum that permits antegrade enemas to flush the colon, thus reducing the threat of fecal incontinence.[106, 194, 195] The conduit can be fashioned from a section of the cecum or from the appendix and can be intubated daily. This procedure has been used mainly for neurologically impaired children but may be applicable to some adults.

MANAGEMENT OF SPECIFIC SITUATIONS

Childhood Incontinence

Fecal incontinence is a fairly common problem among children seen by pediatric gastroenterologists; it occurs in 1% to 2% of otherwise healthy 7-year-olds. It is generally due to one of three causes: congenital anomalies, mental retardation, or childhood encopresis (functional incontinence) in which constipation and fecal incontinence coexist.

The most common congenital anomalies associated with incontinence are neural tube defects such as *myelomeningocele* or *spina bifida* and *anal atresia* (imperforate anus). Children with neural malformations can benefit from a stimulating defecation at intervals, as discussed. Anal atresia usually is treated by surgery in infancy, but approximately 20% of pull-through operations produce unsatisfactory results, often because the colon was not extended through the external anal sphincter. Reoperation then becomes necessary after electromyographic localization of this sphincter.

Mentally retarded children tend to be slow to achieve bowel control and some never do. In general, those who are more severely retarded have more problems with incontinence.

In the absence of other physical disorders, incontinence in childhood is usually part of the syndrome of *encopresis*. In affected children bowel movements are irregular, bulky, and painful. This results in fecal retention, rectal distention, and reflex internal anal sphincter relaxation, which promotes soiling.[196] Faulty toilet training may be responsible, and most of these children paradoxically contract the anal canal when attempting to defecate. The diagnosis can be made by the detection of stool in the rectum by digital examination or by plain abdominal radiography. Management consists of reversing fecal retention with a laxative program and behavioral reinforcement.[196–198] Modification of defecation dynamics by instruction or by biofeedback relaxation therapy may also help older children.

Incontinence in the Elderly

Aging compromises anal canal pressures, rectal compliance, and the reservoir capacity of the rectum.[199] The internal anal sphincter is more easily inhibited and skeletal muscle contraction may be impaired as well, particularly in older women. These physiologic changes reduce the ability to compensate for stresses on the continence mechanisms and thereby make incontinence more likely. In addition, neurologic dysfunctions, fecal impaction, medications that promote diarrhea or constipation, tube feeding, and impaired mobility may contribute to incontinence in the elderly.[200]

Many elderly patients respond to medical therapy as outlined earlier. In particular, modification of contributing disorders and drug therapy have an important role. Biofeedback training can be considered for eligible individuals. Surgery should be done only for well-defined problems.[201–203]

Diabetes Mellitus

Fecal incontinence often complicates the course of diabetes, especially once diabetic neuropathy develops. Defects in anal canal pressure and rectal sensation have been demonstrated, and incontinence usually is attributed to autonomic sensorimotor neuropathy.[47–49, 204–206] Diabetic individuals who are incontinent should undergo a diagnostic evaluation to ascertain that incontinence is not due to other causes. Diarrhea should be managed aggressively, since it frequently coexists with and aggravates fecal incontinence. If incontinence persists, biofeedback training should be tried, if possible, because results have been good in diabetics.[48] Whenever possible, surgery should not be performed, because results are uncertain and wound healing may be poor (see Chapter 29).

Postoperative Incontinence

Anorectal surgery of virtually any type may be complicated by fecal incontinence. Hemorrhoidectomy, fistulectomy, and internal sphincterotomy produced ultrasonographic evidence of anal sphincter injury in 46% of patients in one series.[207] In one third of these patients with defects, sphincter pressures were compromised and incontinence developed. In another study, 45% of patients treated with lateral internal sphincterotomy for chronic anal fissure had some degree of fecal incontinence.[208] These observations emphasize the importance of informing patients undergoing anorectal surgery of the possibility of the development of postoperative incontinence.

Obstetric Injury

Vaginal delivery often results in some damage to the pelvic floor because the diameter of the infant's head is not much smaller than the diameter of the bony pelvic outlet. When labor is prolonged, when delivery requires instrumentation, or when the infant is extremely large, damage may be extensive, including perineal rupture, sphincter disruption due to tears, or even formation of a rectovaginal fistula.[209–211] Ultrasonographic evidence of external anal sphincter injury has been reported in 9% to 30% of women who had vaginal delivery.[202, 203] Patients having forceps deliveries may have an incidence of sphincter injury as high as 83%.[210] In addition, a traumatic neuropathy can further weaken the skeletal muscles involved with continence and alter sensation.[212] However, in only about one third of patients sustaining ultrasonographic evidence of anal sphincter disruption does incontinence develop within a few months of delivery.[211] Many women experience incontinence 20 or 30 years after delivery, presumably as a result of progressive weakening of the muscles of continence.[213, 214] Because patients in whom incontinence develops after an initial vaginal delivery are at high risk for deterioration of control after a second vaginal delivery,[215] some thought should be given to elective cesarean section in these patients. Surgical sphincter repair produces symptom improvement in most women with external anal sphincter injury, even though two thirds of these women have ultrasonographic evidence of residual anal sphincter damage postoperatively.[216]

Rectal Prolapse

Rectal prolapse is an intussusception of the rectum through the anus. It is more common in women than in men and may be associated with chronic constipation with excess straining, neurologic diseases, and complicated vaginal deliveries. It is not always associated with fecal incontinence, but when it is, anal sphincter weakness is also present.[217] Children with rectal prolapse are usually managed conservatively, and adults are treated surgically with anal encirclement, proctopexy, or resection.[217, 218] Patients with less evidence of pudendal neuropathy are more likely to regain continence postoperatively.[219]

Inflammatory Bowel Disease and Ileoanal Anastomosis

Perianal *Crohn's disease* can lead to incontinence through either suppurative or iatrogenic destruction of the anal sphincters. Ulcerative colitis can alter rectal compliance and potentially predispose to fecal incontinence (see Chapters 103 and 104).

Proctocolectomy is performed to cure colitis or colonic polyposis. An increasing number of patients are opting for reconstruction by means of ileoanal anastomosis with creation of an ileal pouch. In this procedure, the voluntary muscles of continence and a cuff of smooth muscle from the distal rectum are preserved. The ileum is directed through this muscular tunnel, and thus many of the barriers to the distal movement of feces are preserved and the ileal pouch serves as a reservoir for stool. When groups of patients have been studied, anal canal and intrapouch pressures are similar to those in the normal anal canal and rectum.[220] Nevertheless, fecal incontinence, especially at night, is a recognized complication (see Chapter 105).

Manipulation of the anus during the procedure and resection of smooth muscle can weaken the continence mechanisms, and surgeons have devised modifications of the procedure to minimize this possibility.[221] The frequency of incontinence at night may be due to higher intrapouch pressure and reduced anal pressure during sleep.[222] In spite of these potential problems, patient satisfaction with this procedure is high.[223] Preoperative manometric assessment is not of proven value in selecting patients for this procedure, but most colorectal surgeons avoid ileoanal anastomosis in patients with preexisting continence defects. Functional outcome in elderly patients compares well with that in younger patients when subjects are carefully selected.[224]

REFERENCES

1. Whitehead WE, Wald A, Diamant NE, et al: Functional disorders of the anus and rectum. Gut 45(suppl 2):II55, 1999.
2. Mellgren A, Jensen LL, Zetterstrom JP, et al: Long-term cost of fecal incontinence secondary to obstetric injuries. Dis Colon Rectum 42: 857, 1999.
3. Drossman DA, Li Z, Andruzzi E, et al: U.S. householder survey of functional gastrointestinal disorders: Prevalence, sociodemography, and health impact. Dig Dis Sci 38:1569, 1993.
4. Roberts RO, Jacobsen SJ, Reilly WT, et al: Prevalence of combined fecal and urinary incontinence: A community-based study. J Am Geriatr Soc 47:837, 1999.
5. Johanson JF, Lafferty J: Epidemiology of fecal incontinence: The silent affliction. Am J Gastroenterol 91:33, 1996.
6. Bliss DZ, Johnson S, Savik K, et al: Fecal incontinence in hospitalized patients who are acutely ill. Nurs Res 49:101, 2000.
7. Talley NJ, O'Keefe EA, Zinsmeister R, Melton LJ III: Prevalence of gastrointestinal symptoms in the elderly: A population-based study. Gastroenterology 102:895, 1992.
8. Prosser S, Dobbs F: Incontinence in the over-75s. Br J Gen Pract 47: 498, 1997.
9. Borrie MJ, Davidson HA: Incontinence in institutions: Costs and contributing factors. Can Med Assoc J 147:322, 1992.
10. Chassagne P, Landrin I, Neveu C, et al: Institutionalized elderly: Incidence, risk factors, and prognosis. Am J Med 106:185, 1999.
11. Krier J: Motor function of anorectum and pelvic floor musculature. In Schultz SG, Wood JD (eds): Handbook of Physiology, vol 1. Motility and Circulation. Bethesda, Md, American Physiological Society, 1989, p 1025.
12. Hajivassiliou CA, Carter KD, Finlay IG: Anorectal angle enhances faecal continence. Br J Surg 83:53, 1996.
13. Maxwell PR, Heriot AG, Davies DC, Kumar D: Anorectal sensation and continence. Scand J Gastroenterol 34:113, 1999.
14. Uher EM, Swash M: Sacral reflexes: Physiology and clinical application. Dis Colon Rectum 41:1165, 1998.
15. Hoffman BA, Timmcke AE, Gathright JB Jr, et al: Fecal seepage and soiling: A problem of rectal sensation. Dis Colon Rectum 38:746, 1995.
16. Houghton LA, Wych J, Whorwell PJ: Acute diarrhoea induces rectal sensitivity in women but not men. Gut 37:270, 1995.
17. Gee AS, Mills A, Durdey P: What is the relationship between perineal descent and anal mucosal electrosensitivity? Dis Colon Rectum 38: 419, 1995.
18. Sangwan YP, Solla JA: Internal anal sphincter: Advances and insights. Dis Colon Rectum 41:1297, 1998.
19. Speakman CT: Pharmacology of the internal anal sphincter and abnormalities in faecal incontinence. Eur J Gastroenterol Hepatol 9:442, 1997.
20. Vaizey CJ, Kamm MA, Bartram CI: Primary degeneration of the internal anal sphincter as a cause of passive faecal incontinence. Lancet 349:612, 1997.
21. Speakman CTM, Hoyle CHV, Kamm MA, et al: Abnormal internal anal sphincter fibrosis and elasticity in fecal incontinence. Dis Colon Rectum 38:407, 1995.
22. Speakman CTM, Hoyle CHV, Kamm MA, et al: Abnormalities of innervation of internal anal sphincter in fecal incontinence. Dig Dis Sci 38:1961, 1993.
23. Farouk R, Duthie GS, MacGregor AB, Bartolo DCC: Evidence of electromechanical dissociation of the internal anal sphincter and idiopathic fecal incontinence. Dis Colon Rectum 37:595, 1994.
24. Holmberg A, Graf W, Osterberg A, Pahlman L: Anorectal manovolumetry in the diagnosis of fecal incontinence. Dis Colon Rectum 38: 502, 1995.
25. Kuijpers HC, Scheuer M: Disorders of impaired fecal control: A clinical and manometric study. Dis Colon Rectum 33:207, 1990.
26. Osterberg A, Graf W, Pahlman L: The longitudinal high-pressure zone profile in patients with fecal incontinence. Am J Gastroenterol 94: 2966, 1999.
27. Roig JV, Villoslada C, Lledo S, et al: Prevalence of pudendal neuropathy in fecal incontinence: Results of a prospective study. Dis Colon Rectum 38:952, 1995.
28. Kafka NJ, Coller JA, Barrett RC, et al: Pudendal neuropathy is the

only parameter differentiating leakage from solid stool incontinence. Dis Colon Rectum 40:1220, 1997.
29. Rasmussen OO, Christiansen J, Tetzschner T, Sorensen M: Pudendal nerve function in idiopathic fecal incontinence. Dis Colon Rectum 43: 633, 2000.
30. Sangwan YP, Coller JA, Barrett MS, et al: Unilateral pudendal neuropathy: Significance and implications. Dis Colon Rectum 39:249, 1996.
31. Sangwan YP, Coller JA, Schoetz DJ, et al: Spectrum of abnormal rectoanal reflex patterns in patients with fecal incontinence. Dis Colon Rectum 39:59, 1996.
32. Parellada CM, Miller AS, Williamson ME, Johnston D: Paradoxical high anal resting pressures in men with idiopathic fecal seepage. Dis Colon Rectum 41:593, 1998.
33. Rasmussen OO, Ronholt C, Alstrup N, Christiansen J: Anorectal pressure gradient and rectal compliance in fecal incontinence. Int J Colorectal Dis 13:157, 1998.
34. Siproudhis L, Bellissant E, Pagenault M, et al: Fecal incontinence with normal anal canal pressures: Where is the pitfall? Am J Gastroenterol 94:1556, 1999.
35. Siproudhis L, Bellissant E, Juguet F, et al: Perception of and adaptation to rectal isobaric distention in patients with faecal incontinence. Gut 44:687, 1999.
36. Sultan AH, Kamm MA, Hudson CN, et al: Anal-sphincter disruption during vaginal delivery. N Engl J Med 329:1905, 1995.
37. Kamm MA: Obstetric damage and faecal incontinence. Lancet 344: 730, 1994.
38. Snooks SJ, Henry MM, Swash M: Fecal incontinence due to external anal sphincter division in childbirth is associated with damage to the innervation of the pelvic floor musculature: A double pathology. Br J Obstet Gynecol 92:824, 1985.
39. Ismael SS, Amarenco G, Bayle B, Kerdraon J: Postpartum lumbosacral plexopathy limited to autonomic and perineal manifestations: Clinical and electrophysiological study of 19 patients. J Neurol Neurosurg Psychiatry 68:771, 2000.
40. Gibbons CP, Trowbridge EA, Bannister JJ, Read NW: Role of anal cushions in maintaining continence. Lancet 1:886, 1986.
41. Konsten J, Baeten CG: Hemorrhoidectomy vs. Lord's method: 17-Year follow-up of a prospective, randomized trial. Dis Colon Rectum 43:503, 2000.
42. Yeoh EE, Botten R, Russo A, et al: Chronic effects of therapeutic irradiation for localized prostatic carcinoma on anorectal function. Int J Radiat Oncol Biol Phys 47:915, 2000.
43. Sun WM, Read NW, Donnelly TC: Anorectal function in incontinent patients with cerebrospinal disease. Gastroenterology 99:1372, 1990.
44. Nakayama H, Jorgensen HS, Pedersen PM, et al: Prevalence and risk factors of incontinence after stroke: The Copenhagen Stroke Study. Stroke 28:58, 1997.
45. Tjandra JJ, Ooi BS, Han WR: Anorectal physiologic testing for bowel dysfunction in patients with spinal cord lesions. Dis Colon Rectum 43: 927, 2000.
46. Hinds JP, Eidelman BH, Wald A: Prevalence of bowel dysfunction in multiple sclerosis. Gastroenterology 98:1538, 1990.
47. Caruana BJ, Wald A, Hinds JP, Eidelman BH: Anorectal sensory and motor function in neurogenic fecal incontinence: Comparison between multiple sclerosis and diabetes mellitus. Gastroenterology 100:465, 1991.
48. Schiller LR, Santa Ana CA, Schmulen AC, et al: Pathogenesis of fecal incontinence in diabetes mellitus: Evidence for internal-anal sphincter dysfunction. N Engl J Med 307:1666, 1982.
49. Wald A, Tunuguntla AK: Anorectal sensorimotor dysfunction in fecal incontinence and diabetes mellitus: Modification with biofeedback therapy. N Engl J Med 310:1282, 1984.
50. Swash M: The neurogenic hypothesis of stress incontinence. Ciba Found Symp 151:156, 1990.
51. Ronnblom A, Forsberg H, Danielsson A: Gastrointestinal symptoms in myotonic dystrophy. Scand J Gastroenterol 31:654, 1996.
52. Jaffin BW, Chang P, Spiera H: Fecal incontinence in scleroderma: Clinical features, anorectal manometric findings, and their therapeutic implications. J Clin Gastroenterol 25:513, 1997.
53. Lock G, Zeuner M, Lang B, et al: Anorectal function in systemic sclerosis: Correlation with esophageal dysfunction? Dis Colon Rectum 40:1328, 1997.
54. Osterberg A, Graf W, Karlbom U, Pahlman J: Evaluation of a questionnaire in the assessment of patients with faecal incontinence and constipation. Scand J Gastroenterol 31:575, 1996.
55. Reilly WT, Talley NJ, Pemberton JH, Zinsmeister AR: Validation of a questionnaire to assess fecal incontinence and associated risk factors: Fecal Incontinence Questionnaire. Dis Colon Rectum 43:146, 2000.
56. Rockwood TH, Church JM, Fleshman JW, et al: Patient and surgeon ranking of the severity of symptoms associated with fecal incontinence: The Fecal Incontinence Severity Index. Dis Colon Rectum 42: 1525, 1999.
57. Rockwood TH, Church JM, Fleshman JW, et al: Fecal Incontinence Quality of Life Scale: Quality of life instrument for patients with fecal incontinence. Dis Colon Rectum 43:9, 2000.
58. Hill J, Corson RJ, Brandon H, et al: History and examination in the assessment of patients with idiopathic fecal incontinence. Dis Colon Rectum 37:473, 1994.
59. Buch E, Alos R, Solana A, et al: Can digital examination substitute for anorectal manometry for the evaluation of anal canal pressures? Rev Esp Enferm Dig 90:85, 1998.
60. Rao SS: Manometric evaluation of defecation disorders: Part II. Fecal incontinence. Gastroenterologist 5:99, 1997.
61. Keating JP, Stewart PJ, Eyers AA, et al: Are special investigations of value in the management of patients with fecal incontinence? Dis Colon Rectum 40:896, 1997.
62. Schafer R, Heyer T, Gantke B, et al: Anal endosonography and manometry: Comparison in patients with defecation problems. Dis Colon Rectum 40:293, 1997.
63. Rao SS, Patel RS: How useful are manometric tests of anorectal function in the management of defecation disorders? Am J Gastroenterol 92:469, 1997.
64. Braun JC, Treutner KH, Dreuw B, et al: Vectormanometry for differential diagnosis of fecal incontinence. Dis Colon Rectum 37:989, 1994.
65. Meshkinpour H, Movahedi H, Welgan P: Clinical value of anorectal manometry index in neurogenic fecal incontinence. Dis Colon Rectum 40:457, 1997.
66. Monk DN, Mills P, Jeacock J, et al: Combining the strength-duration curve of the external anal sphincter with manometry for the assessment of faecal incontinence. Br J Surg 85:1389, 1998.
67. Marcello PW, Barrett RC, Coller JA, et al: Fatigue rate index as a new measurement of external sphincter function. Dis Colon Rectum 41:336, 1998.
68. Goes RN, Simons AJ, Beart RW Jr: Level of highest mean resting pressure segment in the anal canal: A quantitative assessment of anal sphincter function. Dis Colon Rectum 39:289, 1996.
69. McHugh SM, Diamant NE: Effect of age, gender, and parity on anal canal pressures: Contribution of impaired anal sphincter function to fecal incontinence. Dig Dis Sci 32:726, 1987.
70. Mitrani C, Chun A, Desautels S, Wald A: Anorectal manometric characteristics in men and women with idiopathic fecal incontinence. J Clin Gastroenterol 26:175, 1998.
71. Sun WM, Read NW, Miner P, B: Relation between rectal sensation and anal function in normal subjects and patients with faecal incontinence. Gut 31:1056, 1990.
72. Rasmussen O, Christensen B, Sorensen M, et al: Rectal compliance in the assessment of patients with fecal incontinence. Dis Colon Rectum 33:650, 1990.
73. Sangwan YP, Coller JA, Barrett RC, et al: Distal rectoanal excitatory reflex: A reliable index of pudendal neuropathy? Dis Colon Rectum 38:916, 1995.
74. Cheong DMO, Vaccaro CA, Salanga VD, et al: Electrodiagnostic evaluation of fecal incontinence. Muscle Nerve 18:612, 1995.
75. Vernava AM, Longo WE, Daniel GL: Pudendal neuropathy and the importance of EMG evaluation of fecal incontinence. Dis Colon Rectum 36:23, 1993.
76. Vaccaro CA, Cheong DMO, Wexner SD, et al: Pudendal neuropathy in evacuatory disorders. Dis Colon Rectum 38:166, 1995.
77. Infantino A, Melega E, Negrin P, et al: Striated anal sphincter electromyography in idiopathic fecal incontinence. Dis Colon Rectum 38:27, 1995.
78. Gee AS, Jones RS, Durdey P: On-line quantitative analysis of surface electromyography of the pelvic floor in patients with faecal incontinence. Br J Surg 87:814, 2000.
79. Tetzschner T, Sorensen M, Rasmussen OO, et al: Reliability of pudendal nerve terminal motor latency. Int J Colorectal Dis 12:280, 1997.

80. Rieger NA, Sarre RG, Saccone GT, et al: Correlation of pudendal nerve terminal motor latency with the results of anal manometry. Int J Colorectal Dis 12:303, 1997.
81. Pfeifer J, Salanga VD, Agachan F, et al: Variation in pudendal nerve terminal motor latency according to disease. Dis Colon Rectum 40:79, 1997.
82. Osterberg A, Graf W, Edebol Eeg-Olofsson K, et al: Results of neurophysiologic evaluation in fecal incontinence. Dis Colon Rectum 43: 1256, 2000.
83. Ryhammer AM, Laurberg S, Bek KM: Age and anorectal sensibility in normal women. Scand J Gastroenterol 32:278, 1997.
84. Felt-Bersma RJ, Poen AC, Cuesta MA, et al: Anal sensitivity test: What does it measure and do we need it? Cause or derivative of anorectal complaints. Dis Colon Rectum 40:811, 1997.
85. Piloni V, Fioravanti P, Spazzafumo L, Rossi B: Measurement of the anorectal angle by defecography for the diagnosis of fecal incontinence. Int J Colorectal Dis 14:131, 1999.
86. Agachan F, Pfeifer J, Wexner SD: Defecography and proctography: Results of 744 patients. Dis Colon Rectum 39:899, 1996.
87. Jones HJ, Swift RI, Blake H: A prospective audit of the usefulness of evacuating proctography. Ann R Coll Surg Engl 80:40, 1998.
88. Rieger NA, Sweeney JL, Hoffman DC, et al: Investigation of fecal incontinence with endoanal ultrasound. Dis Colon Rectum 39:860, 1996.
89. Meyenberger C, Bertschinger P, Zala GF, et al: Anal sphincter defects in fecal incontinence: Correlation between endosonography and surgery. Endoscopy 28:217, 1996.
90. Romano G, Rotondano G, Esposito P, et al: External anal sphincter defects: Correlation between pre-operative anal endosonography and intraoperative findings. Br J Radiol 69:6, 1996.
91. Sentovich SM, Wong WD, Blatchford GJ: Accuracy and reliability of transanal ultrasound for anterior anal sphincter injury. Dis Colon Rectum 41:1000, 1998.
92. Karoui S, Savoye-Collet C, Koning E, et al: Prevalence of anal sphincter defects revealed by sonography in 335 incontinent patients and 115 continent patients. AJR Am J Roentgenol 173:389, 1999.
93. Chen H, Humphreys MS, Kettlewell MG, et al: Anal ultrasound predicts the response to nonoperative treatment of fecal incontinence in men. Ann Surg 229:739, 1999.
94. Stewart LK, Wilson SR: Transvaginal sonography of the anal sphincter: Reliable, or not? AJR Am J Roentgenol 173:179, 1999.
95. Peschers UM, DeLancey JO, Schaer GN, Schuessler B: Exoanal ultrasound of the anal sphincter: Normal anatomy and sphincter defects. Br J Obstet Gynaecol 104:999, 1997.
96. Gold DM, Bartram CI, Halligan S, et al: Three-dimensional endoanal sonography in assessing anal canal injury. Br J Surg 86:365, 1999.
97. Wisser J, Schar G, Kurmanavicius J, et al: Use of 3D ultrasound as a new approach to assess obstetrical trauma to the pelvic floor. Ultraschall Med 20:15, 1999.
98. deSouza NM, Williams AD, Gilderdale DJ: High-resolution magnetic resonance imaging of the anal sphincter using a dedicated endoanal receiver coil. Eur Radiol 9:436, 1999.
99. Stoker J, Rociu E: Endoluminal MR imaging of diseases of the anus and rectum. Semin Ultrasound CT MR 20:47, 1999.
100. Briel JW, Zimmerman DD, Stoker J, et al: Relationship between sphincter morphology on endoanal MRI and histopathological aspects of the external anal sphincter. Int J Colorectal Dis 15:87, 2000.
101. Rociu E, Stoker J, Eijkemans MJ, et al: Fecal incontinence: Endoanal US versus endoanal MR imaging. Radiology 212:453,1999.
102. Malouf AJ, Williams AB, Halligan S, et al: Prospective assessment of accuracy of endoanal MR imaging and endosonography in patients with fecal incontinence. AJR Am J Roentgenol 175:741, 2000.
103. King JC, Currie DM, Wright E: Bowel training in spina bifida: Importance of education, patient compliance, age, and anal reflexes. Arch Phys Med Rehabil 75:243, 1994.
104. Chassagne P, Jego A, Gloc P, et al: Does treatment of constipation improve faecal incontinence in institutionalized elderly patients? Age Ageing 29:159, 2000.
105. Briel JW, Schouten WR, Vlot EA, et al: Clinical value of colonic irrigation in patients with continence disturbances. Dis Colon Rectum 40:802, 1997.
106. Christensen P, Kvitzau B, Krogh K, et al: Neurogenic colorectal dysfunction—use of new antegrade and retrograde colonic wash-out methods. Spinal Cord 38:255, 2000.
107. Shirran E, Brazzelli M: Absorbent products for the containment of urinary and/or faecal incontinence in adults. Cochran Database Syst Rev 2:CD001406, 2000.
108. Haugen V: Perineal skin care for patients with frequent diarrhea or fecal incontinence. Gastroenterol Nurs 20:87, 1997.
109. Whittingham K, May S: Cleansing regimens for continence care. Prof Nurse 14:167, 1998.
110. Harford WV, Krejs GJ, Santa Ana CA, Fordtran JS: Acute effect of diphenoxylate with atropine (Lomotil) in patients with chronic diarrhea and fecal incontinence. Gastroenterology 78:440, 1980.
111. Read M, Read NW, Barber DC, Duthie HL: Effects of loperamide on anal sphincter function in patients complaining of chronic diarrhea with fecal incontinence and urgency. Dig Dis Sci 27:807, 1982.
112. Sun WM, Read NW, Verlinden M: Effects of loperamide oxide on gastrointestinal transit time and anorectal function in patients with chronic diarrhoea and faecal incontinence. Scand J Gastroenterol 32: 34, 1997.
113. Carapeti EA, Kamm MA, Phillips RK: Randomized controlled trial of topical phenylephrine in the treatment of faecal incontinence. Br J Surg 87:38, 2000.
114. Enck P: Biofeedback training in disordered defecation: A critical review. Dig Dis Sci 38:1953, 1993.
115. Bassotti G, Whitehead WE: Biofeedback as a treatment approach to gastrointestinal tract disorders. Am J Gastroenterol 89:158, 1994.
116. Rao SS: The technical aspects of biofeedback therapy for defecation disorders. Gastroenterologist 6:96, 1998.
117. Norton C, Hosker G, Brazzeli M: Biofeedback and/or sphincter exercises for the treatment of faecal incontinence in adults. Cochran Database Syst Rev 2:CD00211, 2000.
118. Rao SS: Can biofeedback therapy improve anorectal function in fecal incontinence? Am J Gastroenterol 91:2360, 1996.
119. Rieger NA, Wattchow DA, Sarre RG, et al: Prospective trial of pelvic floor retraining in patients with fecal incontinence. Dis Colon Rectum 40:821, 1997.
120. Patankar SK, Ferrara A, Levy JR, et al: Biofeedback in colorectal practice: A multicenter, statewide, three-year experience. Dis Colon Rectum 40:827, 1997.
121. Patankar SK, Ferrara A, Larach SW, et al: Electromyographic assessment of biofeedback training for fecal incontinence and chronic constipation. Dis Colon Rectum 40:907, 1997.
122. Glia A, Gylin M, Akerlund JE, et al: Biofeedback training in patients with fecal incontinence. Dis Colon Rectum 41:359, 1998.
123. Norton C, Kamm MA: Outcome of biofeedback for faecal incontinence. Br J Surg 86:1159, 1999.
124. Ryn AK, Morren GL, Hallbook O, Sjodahl R: Long-term results of electromyographic biofeedback training for fecal incontinence. Dis Colon Rectum 43:1262, 2000.
125. Enck P, Daublin G, Lubke HJ, Strohmeyer G: Long-term efficacy of biofeedback training for fecal incontinence. Dis Colon Rectum 37:997, 1994.
126. Guillemot F, Bouche B, Gower-Rousseau C, et al: Biofeedback for the treatment of fecal incontinence: Long-term clinical results. Dis Colon Rectum 38:393, 1995.
127. van Tets WF, Kuijpers JH, Bleijenberg G: Biofeedback treatment is ineffective in neurogenic fecal incontinence. Dis Colon Rectum 39: 992, 1996.
128. Leroi AM, Dorival MP, Lecouturier MF, et al: Pudendal neuropathy and severity of incontinence but not presence of an anal sphincter defect may determine the response to biofeedback therapy in fecal incontinence. Dis Colon Rectum 42:762, 1999.
129. Keck JO, Staniunas RJ, Coller JA, et al: Biofeedback training is useful in fecal incontinence but disappointing in constipation. Dis Colon Rectum 37:1271, 1994.
130. Latimer PR, Campbell D, Kasperski J: A components analysis of biofeedback in the treatment of fecal incontinence. Biofeedback Self Regul 9:311, 1984.
131. Fynes MM, Marshall K, Cassidy M, et al: A prospective, randomized study comparing the effect of augmented biofeedback with sensory biofeedback alone on fecal incontinence after obstetric trauma. Dis Colon Rectum 42:753, 1999.
132. Sangwan YP, Coller JA, Barrett RC, et al: Can manometric parameters predict response to biofeedback therapy in fecal incontinence? Dis Colon Rectum 38:1021, 1995.
133. Pescatori M, Pavesio R, Anatasio G, et al: Transanal electrostimulation for fecal incontinence: Clinical, psychologic, and manometric prospective study. Dis Colon Rectum 34:540, 1991.

134. Jost WH: Electrostimulation in fecal incontinence: Relevance of the sphincteric compound muscle action potential. Dis Colon Rectum 41: 590, 1998.
135. Osterberg A, Graf W, Eeg-Olofsson K, et al: Is electrostimulation of the pelvic floor an effective treatment for neurogenic faecal incontinence? Scand J Gastroenterol 34:319, 1999.
136. Scheuer M, Kuijpers HC, Bleijenberg G: Effect of electrostimulation on sphincter function in neurogenic fecal continence. Dis Colon Rectum 37:590, 1994.
137. Leroi AM, Karoui S, Touchais JY, et al: Electrostimulation is not a clinically effective treatment of anal incontinence. Eur J Gastroenterol Hepatol 11:1045, 1999.
138. Hosker G, Norton C, Brazzelli M: Electrical stimulation for faecal incontinence in adults. Cochrane Database Syst Rev 2:CD001310, 2000.
139. Vaizey CJ, Kamm MA, Turner IC, et al: Effects of short term sacral nerve stimulation on anal and rectal function in patients with anal incontinence. Gut 44:407, 1999.
140. Malouf AJ, Vaizey CJ, Nicholls RJ, Kamm MA: Permanent sacral nerve stimulation for fecal incontinence. Ann Surg 232:143, 2000.
141. Vaizey CJ, Kamm MA, Roy AJ, Nicholls RJ: Double-blind crossover study of sacral nerve stimulation for fecal incontinence. Dis Colon Rectum 43:298, 2000.
142. Nyam DC, Pemberton JH: Current advances and controversies in the surgical therapy of anorectal motility disorders. Dig Dis 15(suppl 1): 93, 1997.
143. Vaizey CJ, Kamm MA, Nicholls RJ: Recent advances in the surgical treatment of faecal incontinence. Br J Surg 85:596, 1998.
144. Christiansen J: Modern surgical treatment of anal incontinence. Ann Med 30:273, 1998.
145. Williams NS: Surgery of anorectal incontinence. Lancet 353(suppl 1): SI31, 1999.
146. Bachoo P, Brazzelli M, Grant A: Surgery for faecal incontinence in adults. Cochrane Database Syst Rev 2:CD001757, 2000.
147. Wexner SD, Marchetti F, Jagelman DG: The role of sphincteroplasty for fecal incontinence reevaluated: A prospective physiologic and functional review. Dis Colon Rectum 34:22, 1991.
148. Engel AF, Kamm MA, Sultan AH, et al: Anterior anal sphincter repair in patients with obstetric trauma. Br J Surg 81:1231, 1994.
149. Simmang C, Birnbaum EH, Kodner IJ, et al: Anal sphincter reconstruction in the elderly: Does advancing age affect outcome? Dis Colon Rectum 37:1065, 1994.
150. Sitzler PJ, Thomson JP: Overlap repair of damaged anal sphincter: A single surgeon's series. Dis Colon Rectum 39:1356, 1996.
151. Oliveria L, Pfeifer J, Wexner SD: Physiological and clinical outcome of anterior sphincteroplasty. Br J Surg 83:502, 1996.
152. Felt-Bersma RJ, Cuesta MA, Koorevaar M: Anal sphincter repair improves anorectal function and endosonographic image: A prospective clinical study. Dis Colon Rectum 39:878, 1996.
153. Malouf AJ, Norton CS, Engel AF, et al: Long-term results of overlapping anterior anal-sphincter repair for obstetric trauma. Lancet 355: 260, 2000.
154. Rothbarth J, Bemelman WA, Meijerink WJ, et al: Long-term results of anterior anal sphincter repair for fecal incontinence due to obstetric injury. Dig Surg 17:390, 2000.
155. Karoui S, Leroi AM, Koning E, et al: Results of sphincteroplasty in 86 patients with anal incontinence. Dis Colon Rectum 43:813, 2000.
156. Savoye-Collet C, Savoye G, Koning E, et al: Anal endosonography after sphincter repair. Abdom Imaging 24:569, 1999.
157. Ternent CA, Shashidharan M, Blatchford GJ, et al: Transanal ultrasound and anorectal physiology findings affecting continence after sphincteroplasty. Dis Colon Rectum 40:462, 1997.
158. Young CJ, Mathur MN, Eyers AA, Solomon MJ: Successful overlapping anal sphincter repair: Relationship to patient age, neuropathy, and colostomy formation. Dis Colon Rectum 41:344, 1998.
159. Briel JW, Stoker J, Rociu E, et al: External anal sphincter atrophy on endoanal magnetic resonance imaging adversely affects continence after sphincteroplasty. Br J Surg 86:1322, 1999.
160. Nikteas N, Korsgen S, Kumar D, Keighley MR: Audit of sphincter repair: Factors associated with poor outcome. Dis Colon Rectum 39: 1164, 1996.
161. Sangwan YP, Coller JA, Barrett RC, et al: Unilateral pudendal neuropathy: Impact on outcome of anal sphincter repair. Dis Colon Rectum 39:686, 1996.
162. Gilliland R, Altomare DF, Moreira H Jr, et al: Pudendal neuropathy is predictive of failure following anterior overlapping sphincteroplasty. Dis Colon Rectum 41:1516, 1998.
163. Chen AS, Luchtefeld MA, Senagore AJ, et al: Pudendal nerve latency: Does it predict outcome of anal sphincter repair? Dis Colon Rectum 41:1005, 1998.
164. Jensen LL, Lowry AC: Biofeedback improves functional outcome after sphincteroplasty. Dis Colon Rectum 40:197, 1997.
165. Pinedo G, Vaizey CJ, Nicholls RJ, et al: Results of repeat anal sphincter repair. Br J Surg 86:66, 1999.
166. Leroi AM, Kamm MA, Weber J, et al: Internal anal sphincter repair. Int J Colorectal Dis 12:243, 1997.
167. Morgan R, Patel B, Beynoin J, Carr ND: Surgical management of anorectal incontinence due to internal anal sphincter deficiency. Br J Surg 84:226, 1997.
168. Abou-Zeid AA: Preliminary experience in management of fecal incontinence caused by internal anal sphincter injury. Dis Colon Rectum 43:198, 2000.
169. Pinho M, Ortiz J, Oya M, et al: Total pelvic floor repair for the treatment of neuropathic fecal incontinence. Am J Surg 163:340, 1992.
170. Deen KI, Kumar D, Williams JG, et al: Randomized trial of internal anal sphincter plication with pelvic floor repair for neuropathic fecal incontinence. Dis Colon Rectum 38:14, 1995.
171. Korsgen S, Deen KI, Keighley MR: Long-term results of total pelvic floor repair for postobstetric fecal incontinence. Dis Colon Rectum 40: 835, 1997.
172. Rieger NA, Sarre RG, Saccone GT, et al: Postanal repair for faecal incontinence: Long-term follow-up. Aust N Z J Surg 67:566, 1997.
173. Matsuoka H, Mavrantonis C, Wexner SD, et al: Postanal repair for fecal incontinence—is it worthwhile? Dis Colon Rectum 43:1561, 2000.
174. Osterberg A, Graf W, Holmberg A, et al: Long-term results of anterior levatorplasty for fecal incontinence: A retrospective study. Dis Colon Rectum 39:671, 1996.
175. Aitola P, Hiltunen KM, Matikainen M: Functional results of anterior levatorplasty and external sphincter plication for faecal incontinence. Ann Chir Gynaecol 89:29, 2000.
176. van Tets WF, Kuijpers JH: Pelvic floor procedures produce no consistent changes in anatomy or physiology. Dis Colon Rectum 41:365, 1998.
177. Faucheron JL, Hannoun L, Thome C, Parc R: Is fecal continence improved by nonstimulated gracilis muscle transposition? Dis Colon Rectum 37:979, 1994.
178. Sielezneff I, Malouf AJ, Bartolo DC, et al: Dynamic graciloplasty in the treatment of patients with faecal incontinence. Br J Surg 86:61, 1999.
179. Madoff RD, Rosen HR, Baeten CG, et al: Safety and efficacy of dynamic muscle plasty for anal incontinence: Lessons from a prospective, multicenter trial. Gastroenterology 116:549, 1999.
180. Rouanet P, Senesse P, Bouamrirene D, et al: Anal sphincter reconstruction by dynamic graciloplasty after abdominoperineal resection for cancer. Dis Colon Rectum 42:451, 1999.
181. Mavrantonis C, Billotti VL, Wexner SD: Stimulated graciloplasty for treatment of intractable fecal incontinence: Critical influence of the method of stimulation. Dis Colon Rectum 42:497, 1999.
182. Mander BJ, Wexner SD, Williams NS, et al: Preliminary results of a multicentre trial of the electrically stimulated gracilis neoanal sphincter. Br J Surg 86:1543, 1999.
183. Baeten CG, Bailey HR, Bakka A, et al: Safety and efficacy of dynamic graciloplasty for fecal incontinence: Report of a prospective, multicenter trial: Dynamic Graciloplasty Therapy Study Group. Dis Colon Rectum 43:743, 2000.
184. Adang EM, Engel GL, Rutten FF, et al: Cost-effectiveness of dynamic graciloplasty in patients with fecal incontinence. Dis Colon Rectum 41:725, 1998.
185. Madoff RD, Baeten CG, Christiansen J, et al: Standards for anal sphincter replacement. Dis Colon Rectum 43:135, 2000.
186. Vaizey CJ, Kamm MA, Gold DM, et al: Clinical, physiological, and radiological study of a new purpose-designed artificial bowel sphincter. Lancet 352:105, 1998.
187. Hoogerwerf WA, Pasricha PJ: Taking control of fecal incontinence: Early results of an artificial sphincter device. Gastroenterology 116: 1005, 1999.
188. Savoye G, Leroi AM, Denis P, Michot F: Manometric assessment of an artificial bowel sphincter. Br J Surg 87:586, 2000.

189. Lehur PA, Roig JV, Duinslaeger M: Artificial anal sphincter: Prospective clinical and manometric evaluation. Dis Colon Rectum 43:1100, 2000.
190. O'Brien PE, Skinner S: Restoring control: The Acticon Neosphincter artificial bowel sphincter in the treatment of anal incontinence. Dis Colon Rectum 43:1213, 2000.
191. Sainio AP, Halme LE, Husa AI: Anal encirclement with polypropylene mesh for rectal prolapse and incontinence. Dis Colon Rectum 34: 905, 1991.
192. Shafik A: Perianal injection of autologous fat for treatment of sphincteric incontinence. Dis Colon Rectum 38:583, 1995.
193. Kumar D, Benson MJ, Bland JE: Glutaraldehyde cross-linked collagen in the treatment of faecal incontinence. Br J Surg 85:978, 1998.
194. Graf JL, Strear C, Bratton B, et al: The antegrade continence enema procedure: A review of the literature. J Pediatr Surg 33:1294, 1998.
195. Van Savage JG, Yohannes P: Laparoscopic antegrade continence enema in situ appendix procedure for refractory constipation and overflow fecal incontinence in children with spina bifida. J Urol 164:1084, 2000.
196. Loening-Baucke V: Encopresis and soiling. Pediatr Clin North Am 43: 279, 1996.
197. Loening-Baucke V: Clinical approach to fecal soiling in children. Clin Pediatr 39:603, 2000.
198. Felt B, Wise CG, Olson A, et al: Guideline for the management of pediatric idiopathic constipation and soiling. Arch Pediatr Adolesc Med 153:380, 1999.
199. Read NW, Celik AF, Katsinelos P: Constipation and incontinence in the elderly. J Clin Gastroenterol 20:61, 1995.
200. Nelson R, Furner S, Jesudason V: Fecal incontinence in Wisconsin nursing homes: Prevalence and associations. Dis Colon Rectum 41: 1226, 1998.
201. Romero Y, Evans JM, Fleming KC, et al: Constipation and fecal incontinence in the elderly population. Mayo Clin Proc 71:81, 1996.
202. Wald A: Fecal incontinence: Three steps to successful management. Geriatrics 52:44, 1997.
203. DeLillo AR, Rose S: Functional bowel disorders in the geriatric patient: Constipation, fecal impaction, and fecal incontinence. Am J Gastroenterol 95:901, 2000.
204. Camilleri M: Gastrointestinal problems in diabetes. Endocrinol Metab Clin North Am 25:361, 1996.
205. Sun WM, Katsinelos P, Horowitz M, Read NW: Disturbances in anorectal function in patients with diabetes mellitus and faecal incontinence. Eur J Gastroenterol Hepatol 8:1007, 1996.
206. Epanomeritakis E, Koutsoumbi P, Tsiaoussis I, et al: Impairment of anorectal function in diabetes mellitus parallels duration of disease. Dis Colon Rectum 42:1394, 1999.
207. Felt-Bersma RJF, van Baren R, Koorevaar M, et al: Unsuspected sphincter defects shown by anal endosonography after anorectal surgery: A prospective study. Dis Colon Rectum 38:249, 1995.
208. Nyam DC, Pemberton JH: Long-term results of lateral internal sphincterotomy for chronic anal fissure with particular reference to incidence of fecal incontinence. Dis Colon Rectum 42:1306, 1999.
209. Sultan AH, Kamm MA: Faecal incontinence after childbirth. Br J Obstet Gynaecol 104:979, 1997.
210. Varma A, Gunn J, Gardiner A, et al: Obstetric anal sphincter injury: Prospective evaluation of incidence. Dis Colon Rectum 42:1537, 1999.
211. Faltin DL, Boulvain M, Irion O, et al: Diagnosis of anal sphincter tears by postpartum endosonography to predict fecal incontinence. Obstet Gynecol 95:643, 2000.
212. Jacobs PPM, Scheuer M, Kuijpers JHC, Vingerhoets MH: Obstetric fecal incontinence: Role of pelvic floor denervation and results of delayed sphincter repair. Dis Colon Rectum 33:494, 1990.
213. Haadem K, Gudmundsson S: Can women with intrapartum rupture of anal sphincter still suffer after-effects two decades later? Acta Obstet Gynecol Scand 76:601, 1997.
214. Nygaard IE, Rao SS, Dawson JD: Anal incontinence after anal sphincter disruption: A 30-year retrospective cohort study. Obstet Gynecol 89:896, 1997.
215. Fynes M, Donnelly V, Behan M, et al: Effect of second vaginal delivery on anorectal physiology and faecal continence: A prospective study. Lancet 354:983, 1999.
216. Fitzpatrick M, Behan M, O'Connell PR, O'Herlihy C: A randomized clinical trial comparing primary overlap with approximation repair of third-degree obstetric tears. Am J Obstet Gynecol 183:1220, 2000.
217. Roig JV, Buch E, Alos R, et al: Anorectal function in patients with complete rectal prolapse: Differences between continent and incontinent individuals. Rev Esp Enferm Dig 90:794, 1998.
218. Heah SM, Hartley JE, Hurley J, et al: Laparoscopic suture rectopexy without resection is effective treatment for full-thickness rectal prolapse. Dis Colon Rectum 43:638, 2000.
219. Birnbaum EH, Stamm L, Rafferty JF, et al: Pudendal nerve terminal motor latency influences surgical outcome in treatment of rectal prolapse. Dis Colon Rectum 39:1215, 1996.
220. Gemlo BT, Belmonte C, Wiltz O, Madoff RD: Functional assessment of ileal pouch–anal anastomotic techniques. Am J Surg 169:137, 1995.
221. Becker JM, LaMorte W, St Marie G, Ferzoco S: Extent of smooth muscle resection during mucosectomy and ileal pouch–anal anastomosis affects anorectal physiology and functional outcome. Dis Colon Rectum 40:653, 1997.
222. Orkin BA, Soper NJ, Kelly KA, Dent J: Influence of sleep on anal sphincteric pressure in health and after ileal pouch-anal anastomosis. Dis Colon Rectum 35:137, 1992.
223. Fazio VW, O'Riordain MG, Lavery IC, et al: Long-term functional outcome and quality of life after stapled restorative proctocolectomy. Ann Surg 230:575, 1999.
224. Dehni N, Schlegel D, Tiret E, et al: Effects of aging on the functional outcome of coloanal anastomosis with colonic J-pouch. Am J Surg 175:209, 1998.

Chapter 12

CONSTIPATION

J. E. Lennard-Jones

Constipation, or associated symptoms, afflicts many people in the Western world; the prevalence is greatest among children and the elderly. Many people ignore the symptoms or treat themselves by dietary modification or over-the-counter remedies. Constipation is a common reason for consultation in primary care, in which its management is often simple and successful without the need for investigation or long- term use of drugs.

Only a small proportion of all patients with constipation are referred to a gastroenterologist when there has been no response to dietary or other measures. Systemic and structural gastrointestinal causes require exclusion. Psychological disturbance is common among patients with severe symptoms. Most cases represent a disorder of function involving the rate of colonic transit or difficulty in rectal expulsion, or both.

Medical treatments are reviewed, the most promising and novel of which is behavioral treatment to improve defecatory function; polyethylene glycol (PEG) solutions are a useful addition to the range of laxatives available, and new prokinetic drugs show promise. A few patients with slow colonic transit and intractable symptoms benefit from colectomy with ileorectal anastomosis; however, careful selection of such patients is necessary.

Particular clinical problems in management are constipation in childhood with soiling; slow-transit constipation in younger women; difficulty in defecation as a result of anorectal malfunction; laxative dependence; and constipation in the elderly.

PRESENTING SYMPTOMS

A person who says "I am constipated" is either conscious of an unpleasant sensation related to bowel movements or believes that bowel function is abnormal. Because the concept of constipation differs among people, it is essential to find out what each person means by the term. Often it is used to cover more than one complaint, such as those shown in Table 12–1. Difficult defecation with straining and infrequent stools is the complex of symptoms most often associated with constipation by the lay public.

Table 12–1 | **Symptoms Associated with the Term Constipation**

DEFECATION	ABDOMEN	GENERAL
Infrequent stools (may relate to concept of "normal") No urge Stools difficult to pass (small, or large, hard, much effort needed) Ineffective straining Need to digitate Sense of incomplete evacuation Anal or perineal pain Prolapse "comes down" at the anus Soiling of clothes	Bloating (distention) Discomfort or pain, related or unrelated to defecation	Bad taste in the mouth Headache Nausea Malaise

EPIDEMIOLOGY

Prevalence of Self-Regarded Constipation and Laxative Consumption in Western Societies

The prevalence of self-regarded constipation in the general population varies from country to country. For example, in a European survey[1] among approximately 2000 people in each of five countries (Table 12–2), between 6% and 23% of subjects said in response to interview that they had experienced constipation during the past 12 months, and approximately 20% of subjects had taken a laxative during the same period. At least 10% of the subjects experienced difficulty in defecation at least once a month.

All studies show that more women than men regard themselves as constipated and that the prevalence rises with increasing age (Fig. 12–1). For example, in a population study from the United States, 12.5% of subjects aged 30 to 64 years reported constipation as compared with 23% in the age group of 65 to 93 years.[2, 3]

The prevalence of laxative consumption increases with age. Among young adults in the United States 3.4% used a laxative at least once a month,[4] whereas in a population survey among people aged at least 65 years, 6.8% took 3 to 10 laxatives each week and 6.4% used enemas.[3] In a British survey, 22.6% of women and 11.6% of men in the age group 60 to 69 years reported using laxatives, though only approximately 25% of them used a laxative more than once a week.[5]

Prevalence of Bowel Symptoms and Infrequent Bowel Movements Among the General Public

Other surveys among the general population not seeking health care also reveal a surprisingly high prevalence of bowel symptoms in Western-type societies[2–4, 6–10] Table 12–3). The numbers recorded are variable, depending on the questions asked and the nature of the population. Abdominal pain relieved by defecation, hard stools, straining at defecation, a sense of incomplete evacuation, and abdominal distention each are recorded by 5% to 30% of most populations. Bowel frequency of less than three stools weekly is recorded by approximately 4% of the population and less than two stools weekly by 1% to 2%. Asked about a combination of difficult defecation and a bowel frequency of fewer than two stools weekly, a positive reply is given by fewer than 1% of subjects in most countries (see Table 12–3).

Constipation from a National Perspective

Physician visits for constipation in the United States between the years 1958 and 1986 averaged 2.5 million per year, which corresponds to a prevalence of 1.2% in the population. Twice as many visits were made by women as by men. The prevalence was about 1% among patients younger than 60 years of age, between 1% and 2% among patients 60 to 65 years of age, and between 3% and 5% among patients older than 65 years of age (see Fig. 12–1). The largest number of these patients (31%) was seen by general and family practitioners, followed by internists (20%), pediatricians (15%), surgeons (9%), and obstetricians-gynecologists (9%). Only 4% of the patients were seen by gastroenterologists, which suggests that few such patients are deemed to need specialist advice.[11]

In Britain, the prevalence of consultation for constipation in general practice was 2% to 3% of children aged 0 to 4 years, approximately 1% of women aged 15 to 64 years, 2% to 3% of both sexes aged 65 to 74 years, and 5% to 6% of patients aged 75 years and older (see Fig. 12–1). Hospital

Table 12–2 | **European Survey of Bowel Symptoms (%) in Five Countries[1]**

CHARACTERISTIC	COUNTRIES				
	France	Germany	Italy	Spain	United Kingdom
A. Self-perceived constipation	19	10	23	17	6
B. Laxative use	19	20	20	20	19
C. Difficult defecation*	13	10	16	11	13
A + B + C	7	4	8	6	2
C + <2 bowel movements weekly	0.5	0.2	1.4	0.9	0.4

*Straining and/or hard stools and/or incomplete evacuation at least once a month.

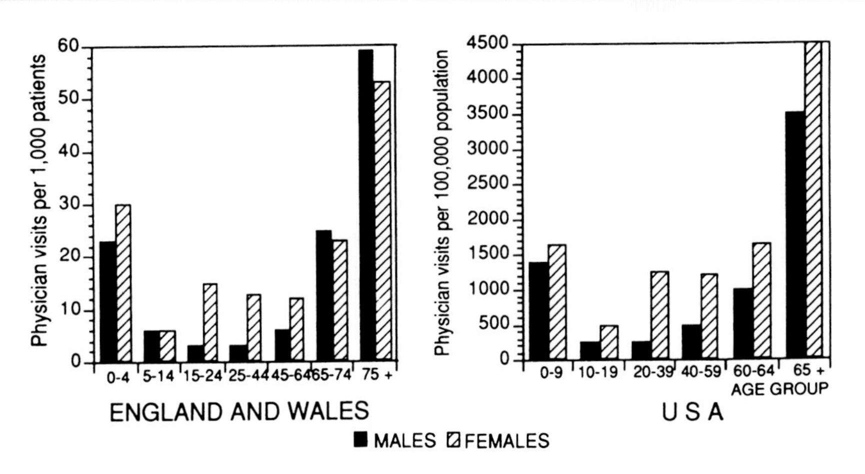

Figure 12–1. Constipation increases with age and is more common in women. The columns show annual medical consultations for constipation per 1000 of the population in England (i.e., in general practice) and the United States (i.e., all consultations). (From Johanson JF, Koch TR: Clinical epidemiology of constipation. J Clin Gastroenterol 11:525, 1989; and Sonnenberg A, Koch TR: Physician visits in the United States for constipation: 1958 to 1986. Dig Dis Sci 34:606, 1989.)

admission for constipation is unusual and of short duration; death ascribed to constipation is rare.[12]

Defecation disorder represents the chief complaint in 3% of pediatric outpatient visits and 10% to 25% of pediatric gastroenterology visits.[13] Fecal retention with the associated social problem of fecal soiling is a common cause of disability and need for medical and nursing care in childhood. The analogous situation in the elderly, especially those with mental impairment, is a major reason for nursing and residential care.

CLINICAL DEFINITION AND CLASSIFICATION

A clinical definition of constipation needs to take account of both difficult defecation and infrequent stools. According to the "Rome 2 Criteria" proposed by a working group,[14] a diagnosis of constipation requires at least 12 weeks, which need not be consecutive, during the preceding 12 months of two or more of the following symptoms listed in Table 12–4.

To qualify, a defecatory symptom should be experienced during more than one in four defecations. Abdominal discomfort or pain relieved by defecation, or with an onset associated with a change in frequency of stool, or with a change in form of stool, are features of irritable bowel syndrome. The occurrence from time to time of loose stools unrelated to laxative use suggests a diagnosis of irritable bowel syndrome. The distinction between "functional constipation" and "irritable bowel" is expedient for clinical classification of functional bowel disorders as a whole but does not exclude overlapping features in pathophysiology or symptoms. (See Chapters 5, 91, and 122 for more discussions of chronic abdominal pain, irritable bowel syndrome, and the psychosocial factors associated with abnormal bowel habit and abdominal pain.)

As later described, it is logical to consider constipation in terms of slow colonic transit leading to infrequent bowel actions and difficulty in rectal expulsion of stool leading to anorectal symptoms. It is now possible by investigation to quantitate these two physiologic functions. When this is done, constipation emerges as a heterogeneous condition and one in which symptoms correlate poorly with the results of

Table 12–3 | **Prevalence of Bowel Symptoms in Four Countries***

	COUNTRY (REFERENCE)						
VARIABLES	**U.K. (6)**	**U.K. (7,8)**	**U.S. (4)**	**U.S. (2)**	**U.S. (3)**	**Australia (9)**	**N.Z. (10)**
Size of sample	301	1896	789	690	328	202	285
Age range (years)	17–91	25–69	—	30–64	>65	>30	16–64
Abdominal pain relieved by defecation (%)	13	8	22	—	25	—	—
Straining at defecation (%)	10	4	17	18	31	5§	8
Hard stools (%)	9	—	—	23	30	—	—
Sense of incomplete emptying (%)	10	10	24	26	12§	8	—
Digitation ever (%)	—	—	11	24	—	—	—
Bloating or distention (%)	9	11	24	20	6	13	—
Stools < 3/week† (%)	—	—	4	4	—	4	—
Stools < 2/week† (%)	—	1	—	1	—	1	—
Stools < 1/week† (%)	—	—	—	—	2	—	—
Laxative use (%)	6	—	3‡	7	7	17	2‖
Painful defecation (%)	—	—	—	7	12	1	—

*Bowel symptoms among samples of the general population not seeking medical advice. All symptoms shown were recorded often or >25% of the time unless stated otherwise. Figures are percentages and are given as the nearest whole number.
†Stated bowel frequency.
‡>1 per month.
§At least once weekly.
‖>2 per week.

Table 12–4 | **Rome 2 Criteria for Diagnosis of Constipation [14,*]**

Straining
Lumpy or hard stool
Sensation of incomplete evacuation
Sensation of anorectal obstruction/blockade
Fewer than three bowel actions per week

*Based on 12 weeks (not necessarily consecutive) of two or more of the above in the preceding 12-month period.

clinical measurements. An attempt to base a definition of constipation solely on bowel transit time fails. For example, a population study in England among 731 women aged 25 to 69 years used an indirect method based on stool form to estimate intestinal transit time. Of 68 subjects with slow transit, only 28 regarded themselves as constipated, and only 11 of them fulfilled the Rome 2 criteria. Of 62 who regarded themselves as constipated, only 28 had slow transit and only 21 fulfilled the Rome criteria.[15] Among patients who were referred for investigation at a tertiary center because they complained of constipation that was resistant to treatment, 25% showed evidence of slow transit as the only abnormality of function, 21% showed evidence of anorectal dysfunction alone, 40% had evidence of both disorders, and 15% showed no demonstrable abnormality.[16] Analysis of symptoms does not enable the results of physiologic tests to be accurately predicted.[17]

This chapter describes the investigation and management of patients whose main complaint is of self-defined constipation and of those whose other complaints can be ascribed to slow bowel transit or difficulty in defecation. Patients whose main complaint is of abdominal pain or discomfort with an associated bowel irregularity, including constipation, are described in Chapters 5 and 91. Most cases of constipation reflect a disorder of bowel function rather than of structure. These disorders may be classified on the basis of symptoms, treatment, and outcome as shown in Table 12–5.

General, systemic, and psychological causes of constipation are summarized in Table 12–6 and gastrointestinal causes in Table 12–7.

PATHOPHYSIOLOGY

For simplicity of presentation, the following discussion is divided into *general factors, colonic anatomy and function, defecatory mechanism function,* and *psychological and behavioral factors,* although these overlap.

General Factors

Sex

Constipation is a greater problem for women than men[12]; individual symptoms are more frequent[2] and infrequent stools passed once or twice weekly tend to be reported almost entirely by women.[7] Observations on 220 normal subjects eating their normal diet showed that 17% of women but only 1% of the men passed less than 50 g of stool daily.[18] The reason why some women excrete such small quantities of stool is not known. Studies of circulating levels of sex and other hormones have shown no clear differences between constipated women and control subjects.[19]

Age

Among the elderly, "constipation" usually means straining during defecation rather than decreased bowel frequency. Thus in a community sample of 209 people aged 65 to 93 years, approximately one third of both men and women described themselves as constipated at least once a month. The main symptom that they used to define constipation was the need to strain to defecate; only 3% of men and 2% of women reported that their average bowel frequency was less than three per week.[20] Slow colonic transit in one study was related to psychological distress.[21] The increased prevalence of defecation straining among the elderly may be related to decreased food intake with small stools (see later), reduced mobility, weak abdominal and pelvic muscles, chronic illness, psychological factors, and medication, particularly pain-relieving drugs.[22, 23] The pronounced increase in the consumption of laxatives among the elderly may reflect not only increased difficulty with defecation but also beliefs of an earlier generation.[5]

Nationality

In the United States, constipation is 1.3 times more frequent among nonwhites than whites; both groups demonstrate similar age-specific increases in prevalence.[12] However, in Af-

Table 12–5 | **Clinical Classification of Functional Constipation**

TYPE	MAIN SYMPTOM	OTHER SYMPTOMS	DEFINING FEATURE(S)
"Simple"	Infrequent stools and/or difficult defecation	Discomfort	Reversible by diet or advice
Irritable bowel syndrome (IBS)	Abdominal pain/distention	Irregular bowels, hard or loose stools, urgency, mucus	Stools irregular in frequency and form
Slow transit	Infrequent bowel actions	Straining, pain, distention	Stools never loose; no distended gut; intractable
Outlet delay, dyssynergia, anismus	Straining	Infrequent stools, digitation	Straining; bowel frequency normal, decreased, or increased
Fecal impaction	Soiling	Fecal mass, wide distal large bowel	Relieved by emptying rectum
Pseudo-obstruction	Recurrent or constant distention	Pain, vomiting, constipation	Obstructive symptoms with gaseous distention of gut

Table 12–6 | **General, Systemic, and Psychological Causes of Constipation**

MODE OF LIFE	EXTERNAL FACTORS	ENDOCRINE/ METABOLIC FACTORS	NEUROLOGIC FACTORS	PSYCHOLOGICAL ASPECTS
Inadequate fiber Little food Repressed or ignored urge to defecate Immobility	Drugs (including opiates, anticholinergics, antidepressants, anticonvulsants, $5HT_3$ antagonists)	Hypothyroidism Hypercalcemia Porphyria	Parkinson's disease Multiple sclerosis Spinal lesions Damage to sacral parasympathetic nerves Autonomic neuropathy Autonomic failure	Depression Eating disorders (e.g., anorexia nervosa) Obsession about "inner cleanliness" Denied bowel actions

$5HT_3$, 5-hydroxytryptamine 3.

rica and India constipation appears to be rare among the native populations, whose stool weights are three to four times greater than the median of 106 g daily in Britain.[18]

Diet

Two comparisons in Europe between severely constipated and healthy subjects showed no evidence that amount of fiber intake was correlated with symptoms.[24, 25] A community study compared the diets of 18 ambulatory subjects older than 60 years of age who complained of constipation and similar control subjects without constipation. The constipated subjects reported consuming fewer meals per day ($P < .01$) and a tendency to consume fewer calories than control subjects.[21] There were no differences between groups regarding fiber or fluid intake. Thus, although differences in average stool size between countries are probably related to major differences in diet, no simple relationship between constipation and dietary fiber intake is evident within one country.

Exercise and Daily Activity

In a national survey, respondents who said that they were inactive during the day, or engaged in little recreational exercise, reported constipation more often than those who regarded themselves as active or who took moderate or much recreational exercise.[26] However, in a direct comparison patients complaining of constipation took the same amount of exercise as matched nonconstipated control subjects.[25] In healthy sedentary subjects, a 9-week program of progressively increasing exercise had no consistent effect on whole-gut transit time or stool weight.[27] The available data suggest that constipation is associated with inactivity and little exercise, but among active subjects it is unrelated to normal or vigorous amounts of exercise.

Table 12–7 | **Gastrointestinal Causes of Constipation and Related Symptoms**

GASTROINTESTINAL TRACT	ANORECTAL MALFUNCTION
Obstruction Aganglionosis (Hirschsprung's disease, Chagas' disease) Myopathy Neuropathy Systemic sclerosis Megarectum/megacolon	Anal atresia or malformation Hereditary internal anal sphincter myopathy Anal stenosis Weak pelvic floor Large rectocele Internal intussusception Anterior mucosal prolapse Prolapse Solitary rectal ulcer

Colonic Anatomy and Function

Luminal Contents

The colon contains mainly food residue, water and electrolytes, bacteria, and gas. Unabsorbed food entering the cecum contains carbohydrate resistant to digestion and absorption by the small intestine, such as resistant starch and nonstarch polysaccharides (NSPs). Some of the unabsorbed carbohydrate is susceptible to bacterial fermentation, yielding short-chain fatty acids and gas (Fig. 12–2). Availability of substrate leads to bacterial proliferation, which is favored by rapid transit through the colon.[28] The increased numbers of bacteria make an important contribution of about half the stool solids,[29] but at best this biomass does not amount to more than 30% of the carbohydrate fermented.[30] Some carbohydrate entering the cecum is fermented little, if at all, by bacterial action. This fiber can hold water within its cellular structure and adds bulk to the stool through its own residue, amounting to about 14% of stool solids.[29]

Increased bran, cabbage, or apple fiber in the diet shortens colonic transit time.[31] A meta-analysis of 20 reported studies has shown that bran decreased the transit time in each study in healthy controls, patients with irritable bowel, and those with constipation.[32] The effect may be wholly a result of increased bulk within the colonic lumen, which stimulates propulsive motor activity, but there is also a possibility that the particulate nature of some fibers may stimulate the colon. Thus, ingestion of coarse bran, 10 g twice daily, reduced colonic transit time by about a third, whereas taking the same quantity of fine bran led to no significant decrease.[33] Ingestion of inert plastic particles of the same size as coarse bran increased fecal output by almost three times their own weight and also decreased transit time[34] (see Chapter 86).

Absorption of Water and Sodium

(see Chapter 87)

The colon avidly absorbs sodium and water. Any factor that increases water absorption leads to smaller, harder stools.

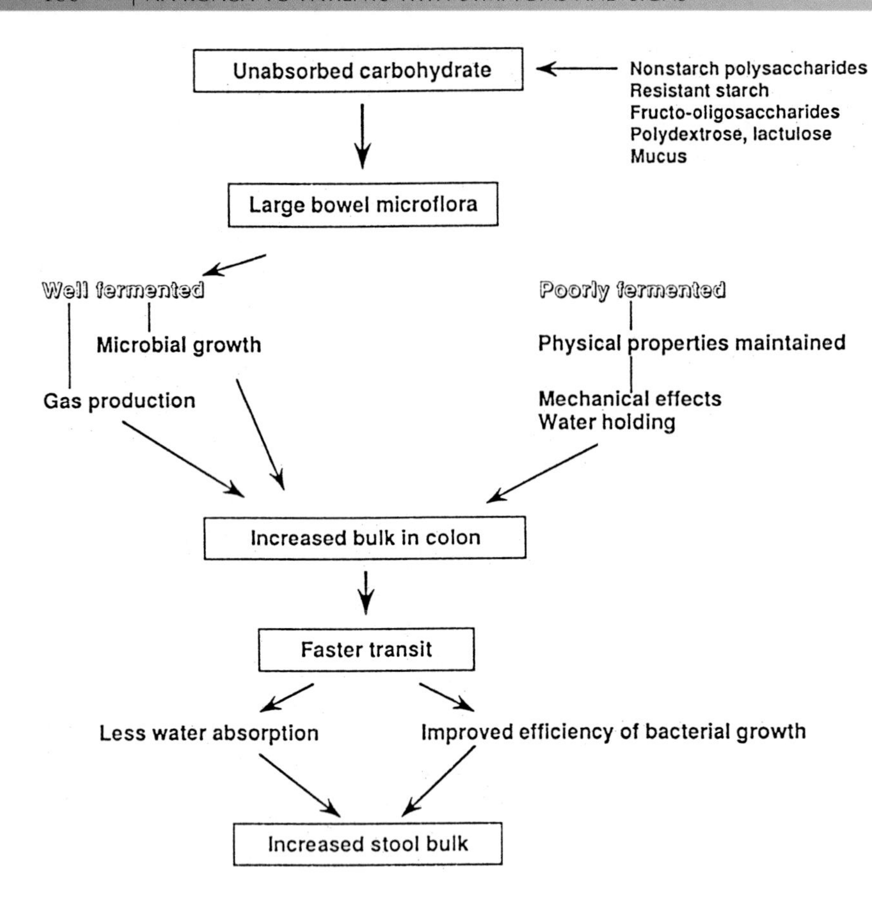

Figure 12–2. Mechanisms by which dietary unabsorbed carbohydrate may increase stool bulk. (From Cummings JH: Non-starch polysaccharides [dietary fiber] including bulk laxatives in constipation. In Kamm MA, Lennard-Jones JE [eds]: Constipation. Petersfield, England, Wrightson Biomedical Publishers, 1994.)

Theoretically, constipation could be caused by an increased rate of water and salt absorption per unit area of colonic epithelium, although this is unlikely according to experimental observations from colonic perfusion.[35] A large mucosal area and long duration of contact between stool and colonic mucosa favor increased water absorption.

Diameter and Length of the Colon

(see Chapter 84)

A wide and/or long colon is likely to lead to a slow rate of transit. The width of the colon along its length can be measured on barium enema films obtained by a standard technique. A normal range has been established for patients without constipation, and a particularly useful measurement is width of the rectosigmoid in the lateral view at the pelvic brim of less than 6.5 cm. Patients with constipation could be divided into two groups: a group with a colon of normal width, although with proven slow transit, and a group with a wide distal colon and rectum.[36]

Colonic Motor Function (see Chapter 86)

Normal colonic muscular activity and changes in constipation have been well reviewed.[37] The colonic muscle has four functions: (1) to delay passage of the luminal contents so that time is available for absorption of water; (2) to mix the contents and so allow contact with the mucosa; (3) to allow the colon to act as a storage organ between defecations; and (4) to propel the contents toward the anus. Muscle activity is affected by sleep and wakefulness, eating, emotion, the contents of the colon, and drugs. Nervous control is partly intrinsic and partly extrinsic by the sympathetic nerves and the parasympathetic sacral outflow.

The motor and corresponding electrical activity of the colon have been studied by placing (via a colonoscope) multilumen perfused tubes or electrodes throughout its length. The frequency and duration of high-pressure peristaltic colonic waves are reduced in some patients with constipation. In one study, 14 chronically constipated patients with proven slow transit of gut contents and who passed one or fewer bowel movements weekly were compared with 18 healthy subjects. Four patients had no peristaltic movement, although such movement was observed in all normal subjects during a 24-hour period. The movements in the others were fewer in number (means of 2.1 vs. 6.1; $P = .02$) and shorter in duration (means of 8.2 vs. 14.1 second; $P = .04$), and thus passed for a shorter distance along the colon in the patients than in the controls. All the healthy subjects reported abdominal discomfort or urges to defecate during peristaltic movements and two defecated, whereas only 4 of the 14 patients experienced any sensation during such movements, and none defecated.[38] Periodic motor activity in the rectum is also reduced.[39] Experimentally, it has been shown that the colonic motor response is reduced both to eating[40] and to cholinergic drug stimulation.[41]

Since the introduction of scintigraphy, it has become possible to observe transit of colonic contents over prolonged periods. Scintigraphic studies in constipated subjects have shown overall slow transit of colonic contents. In some patients the rate of movement of contents through the ascending colon and hepatic flexure was approximately normal, but it was delayed in the transverse and left colon. Other patients showed slow transit in both right and left sides of the colon.[42, 43]

INNERVATION OF COLONIC MUSCLE AND THE INTERSTITIAL CELLS OF CAJAL. A few patients with idiopathic slow-transit constipation have such severe symptoms that colectomy is advised. Routine histologic examination of the colonic muscle and nerve plexuses on transverse section reveals no abnormality, apart possibly from mucosal melanosis (see later). Special study of the myenteric plexus in the horizontal plane using a silver stain reveals, in some patients, reduced numbers of argyrophilic neurons, and the remaining ones tend to be small and irregular, with uneven staining and fewer processes than normal. Axons are also decreased in number, and there may be axonal degeneration.[44] Similar changes have been shown in the small intestine of some of these patients who suffered severe epigastric pain, nausea and vomiting, with abnormal gastroduodenal motor function.[45] A decreased number of nerve filaments has been observed by immunohistologic techniques.[46, 47] Greatly reduced volume of the interstitial cells of Cajal has also been shown in all layers of the colon in six patients with intractable constipation whose colon appeared normal on conventional histologic examination. These observations show that there is an abnormality of the myenteric plexus and interstitial cells in the colon, and possibly other parts of the gut, in some cases of very severe constipation when the colon appears otherwise normal. These changes could be secondary to long-term use of laxatives, and thus a consequence of constipation rather than its cause, though current evidence does not favor this possibility (see later).

An abnormality of parasympathetic nerve function also appears likely in some patients with slow intestinal transit. An acetylcholine spot sweat test has shown a decrease in active sweat glands on the surface of the foot in patients with severe constipation compared with control subjects.[48] Vagal cholinergic cardiac responses to deep breathing and a Valsalva maneuver were significantly different for 72 constipated patients compared with controls.[49] Measurements by laser Doppler flowmetry of rectal mucosal blood flow, which is partly determined by cholinergic extrinsic nervous activity, was less in constipated patients than in controls; in addition, the slower the transit, the more profound was the decrease in blood flow.[49] Electrophysiologic studies have shown absence or prolongation of a reflex from the dorsigenital nerve to the external anal sphincter in patients with severe idiopathic slow-transit constipation, many of whom have urologic symptoms.[50, 51] Increased bladder capacity and sensitivity of the bladder to cholinergic stimulation have also been observed.[51, 52] These findings all suggest that an abnormality of the autonomic nerve supply to the pelvic organs is present in some patients with severe constipation (see also Chapter 111 for discussion of denervation of the small and large intestine).

Defecatory Function

Normal Defecation

Normal defecation results from contraction and relaxation of both smooth and striated muscle. It takes two forms: One involves mainly the contraction of smooth muscle and may be thought of as a reflex with little voluntary effort; the other is a mechanism for emptying the rectum at will that involves mainly voluntary contraction of striated muscle.

According to experimental observations of defecation, as a propulsive peristaltic wave begins in the proximal colon and moves distally to the rectum, there is synchronous relaxation of the internal anal sphincter.[53] The proportion of the colon emptied during spontaneous defecation varies but most commonly is from the descending colon to the rectum.[54] The passage of stool is aided to a variable extent by voluntary contraction of the diaphragm and abdominal muscles. When propulsive action of smooth muscle is the major factor in passage of the stool, defecation usually requires minimal voluntary effort. However, if these colonic and rectal contraction waves are infrequent or absent, as observed in severely constipated subjects, the normal urge to defecate may be absent.[38] When a random population sample was asked "How often do you . . . hold your breath and push down in order to start passing a stool?" more than half the subjects reported never having experienced the need to strain in this way, even occasionally.[5]

The stimulus that initiates the process is related to the normal increase in activity of colonic smooth muscle that follows waking and meals. Stool is often present in the rectum before a conscious urge is felt.[54] The urge to defecate may be visceral, or tactile, arising from contact of the stool with the receptors in the upper anal canal. Retrograde movement of colonic contents has been observed when the urge to defecate is resisted,[54] and there is slowing of transit throughout the colon.[55]

Emptying of the rectum at will requires adoption of a sitting or squatting posture, often without a preliminary urge to defecate. Full flexion of the hips stretches the anal canal in an anteroposterior direction and tends to open the anorectal angle; these changes facilitate rectal emptying.[56] The intrapelvic pressure is raised by contraction of the diaphragm and abdominal musculature, while at the same time the pelvic floor is relaxed. The rectal contents are expelled by striated muscular activity with little or no assistance from colonic or rectal propulsive waves. This sequence of events may be thought of as a secondary mechanism available for use when the usual reflex mechanism fails or is inconvenient.

Failure of Relaxation of the Anal Sphincter Complex

In normal subjects passage of a stool is associated with relaxation of the smooth muscle forming the internal anal sphincter, of the striated muscles forming the puborectalis (which maintains the anorectal angle), and of the external anal sphincter.

Relaxation of the internal anal sphincter is a reflex initiated by rectal distention or by passage of a peristaltic wave down the left colon. Aganglionosis of the colon, as in Hirschsprung's disease, leads to failure of relaxation of the internal sphincter on rectal distention (see Chapter 110).

The striated muscle of the pelvic floor is tonically contracted in the resting state, and there is reflex contraction when intra-abdominal pressure rises, as during a cough. Unconscious relaxation of the striated pelvic floor muscles accompanies straining during defecation in normal subjects. However, in certain people the striated muscles of the pelvic floor contract, rather than relax, on straining; this phenomenon may also involve the gluteal muscles (Fig. 12–3). Although this phenomenon, called *anal dyssynergia* or *anismus*, occurs in some symptomless subjects, it is more common among patients who complain of difficulty in defecation.

Ineffective Straining

Some patients appear unable or unwilling to raise intrarectal pressure to a level sufficient to expel a stool, despite relaxation of the anal sphincters.[57] This phenomenon can be detected clinically by failure of the pelvic floor to descend on straining as though to defecate; it is demonstrable on defecation proctography by decreased pelvic floor descent and prolonged rectal evacuation time.[58]

Diminished Rectal Sensation

The urge to defecate is partly dependent on tension within the rectal wall, which is determined by the tone of the muscle, the rate and volume of distention, and the size of the rectum. Some patients with constipation appear to feel pain normally as the rectum is distended to the maximal tolerable volume, but they fail to experience an urge to defecate with intermediate volumes.[59, 60] It is possible that there is a neural defect, because on electrical stimulation of the mucosa, such patients require a higher than normal current to elicit pain from the rectum.[60] Others have a large, capacious rectum, and abnormally large volumes within the lumen are required to produce a defecatory urge.

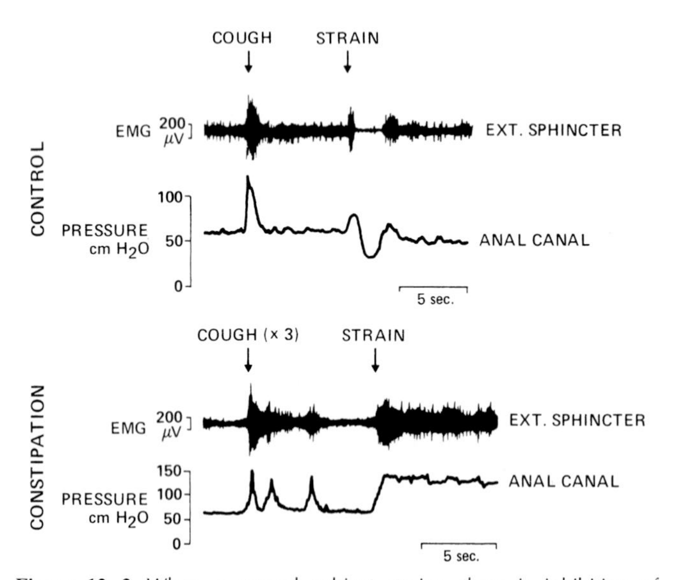

Figure 12–3. When a normal subject strains, there is inhibition of electrical activity in the external anal sphincter with a fall in pressure in the anal canal. A constipated patient fails to relax the anal sphincter on straining, and pressure within the anal canal is maintained. This paradoxical contraction has been called *anismus, anal dyssynergia,* and *spastic perineum.* (From Preston DM, Lennard-Jones JE: Anismus in chronic constipation. Dig Dis Sci 30:413,1985.)

Size and Consistency of Stool

When normal subjects were asked, in an experimental study, to expel single, hard spheres of different sizes from the rectal ampulla, the intrarectal pressure and the time needed to pass these objects varied inversely with their diameter. Small, hard stools are thus difficult to pass. When larger simulated stools were tested, a hard stool took longer to expel than a soft silicon rubber object of approximately the same shape and volume. Similarly, more of the subjects were able to expel a 50-mL water-filled compressible balloon than a hard 1.8-cm sphere.[61]

Human stools may vary in consistency from small, hard lumps to liquid, and a system of grading has been devised to permit analysis of this variation.[5] The consistency of the stool depends on its water content. Rapid transit of the fecal residue within the large bowel leads to diminished water absorption and increased bacterial content of the stool. Both factors lead to larger and softer stools because bacterial cell bodies are composed of about 80% water.[28]

A large population survey showed that minimal straining both at the start and end of defecation was associated with stools of a sausage or snake-like shape with a smooth surface. Most stools of this type were passed without conscious straining, whereas two thirds of subjects strained to initiate defecation for the passage of lumpy stools "like nuts."[5]

Psychological and Behavioral Factors

Personality affects stool size and consistency. Among 21 male volunteers selected for their normal physical health and psychological fitness and observed under closely supervised conditions for up to 6 months, the stool weight and bowel frequency correlated as closely with scores on a personality inventory as with variations in fiber intake. Heavier stools tended to be produced by people who were more socially outgoing, more energetic and optimistic, and less anxious and who described themselves in more favorable terms than the others.[62]

When the psychological profile of patients complaining of constipation is compared with a control group using various scales of measurement, sufferers as a group tend to show abnormalities. In one study of patients with functional bowel disorders, including constipation, measurements made by scintigraphy of gastric, small bowel, and colonic transit were correlated with detailed psychometric assessment. Patients with widespread delayed transit tended to be women in older age groups who contrasted with subjects showing normal transit by featuring a highly depressed mood state and frequent control of anger.[63] In another study, women with constipation scored higher on somatization and anxiety scores than healthy controls, and the psychological scores correlated inversely with rectal mucosal blood flow used as an index of innervation to the distal gut.[64] Such observations show that the gut is affected by long-standing psychological factors, just as it is by acute emotional trauma, so well shown by classic experiments on the direct effects of emotion on the rectum[65] (see Chapter 122).

Some people with bowel symptoms consult a physician, whereas others either ignore the symptoms or treat themselves. Abdominal pain, rather than infrequent stools, is the main reason for medical consultation[66] (see Chapter 5).

Apart from pain, or a definable reason, such as a recent change of symptoms, many patients seek help for problems that appear no more severe than those commonly encountered in the community. Such subjects tend also to have symptoms other than bowel complaints and to consult physicians more often for a variety of reasons.[66] This is a behavioral trait of some people who seek health care and regard symptoms more seriously than do others.

CONSTIPATION AS A MANIFESTATION OF SYSTEMIC DISORDERS

Hypothyroidism

Constipation is the most common gastrointestinal complaint in hypothyroidism. The pathologic effects are caused by an alteration of motor function and possible infiltration of the gut by myxedematous tissue. The basic electrical rhythm of the human duodenum decreases in hypothyroidism, and small bowel transit time is increased.[67] Megacolon can result from myxedematous infiltration of the muscle layers (see Chapter 110).

Diabetes Mellitus

Asymptomatic diabetic patients with cardiovascular evidence of autonomic neuropathy showed significantly ($P < 0.02$) longer whole-gut transit than a control group without evidence of neuropathy, though all results were within the normal range.[68] Studies of colonic myoelectrical and motor activity in diabetic patients with constipation showed that some with mild constipation had a delayed colonic response after a standard meal, whereas others with severe constipation had no increased activity after food. The response to neostigmine was normal in these patients, which suggests that the defect was neural rather than muscular.[69] The fact that the colonic muscle responded to a cholinergic stimulus indicates that drug therapy to potentiate cholinergic activity could be an effective treatment for constipation caused by diabetic neuropathy (see Chapter 29).

Hypercalcemia

Constipation may be a manifestation of hypercalcemia caused by conditions such as hyperparathyroidism, sarcoidosis, and malignancy involving bone (see Chapter 29).

CONSTIPATION AS A MANIFESTATION OF CENTRAL NERVOUS SYSTEM DISEASE OR EXTRINSIC NERVE SUPPLY TO THE GUT

Loss of Conscious Control

Reduction in or absence of bodily perception as a result of cerebral disability or dementia may lead to defecatory failure, possibly because of inattention.

Parkinson's Disease

Gastrointestinal dysfunction, including constipation, is well-recognized in Parkinson's disease. Physical inactivity, impaired straining as a result of an inability to raise intra-abdominal pressure, and drug side effects all may be relevant factors.

Depletion of dopamine-containing neurons in the central nervous system is a basic deficit in this disorder. Histopathologic studies of the myenteric plexus of the ascending colon in 11 patients with Parkinson's disease and constipation revealed that in 9 of the patients, the number of dopamine-positive neurons was one tenth or less that of specimens from control subjects or those with idiopathic constipation. Dopamine concentrations in the muscularis externa were significantly ($P < .01$) lower in Parkinson's disease than in controls.[70] It thus appears that the characteristic neurologic changes found in the brain are also present in the enteric nerves, where they may be related to constipation.

A further possible contributor to constipation in Parkinson's disease is the fact that some patients fail to relax the striated muscles of the pelvic floor on defecation, which is a local manifestation of the extrapyramidal motor disorder affecting all skeletal muscle[71] (see Chapter 29).

Multiple Sclerosis

Among an unselected population of 280 patients suffering from multiple sclerosis, constipation—defined in terms of diminished bowel frequency, digitation to facilitate defecation, or the use of a laxative—was experienced significantly ($P < .01$) more often than among healthy controls in all age groups. Almost 25% of the sufferers passed fewer than three stools weekly and 18% used a laxative more than once a week. All these symptoms correlated with duration of disease, although constipation preceded the diagnosis in 45% of subjects. Constipation did not correlate with immobility or the use of possibly constipating medicines.[72]

In a group of patients suffering from advanced multiple sclerosis with intermittent or chronic constipation, all had evidence of disease central to the lumbosacral spinal cord, and there was decreased compliance of the colon on infusion of fluid. Motor and electrophysiologic measurements showed that the usual increase in colonic motor activity after meals was absent.[73] Among less severely affected patients, slow colonic transit, and manometric evidence of pelvic floor muscular dysfunction have been demonstrated.[74, 75] Biofeedback treatment has been reported to help constipation, incontinence, or a combination of these symptoms, in 5 of 13 patients; limited disability and nonprogressive disease favored improvement[76] (see Chapter 11).

Spinal Cord Lesions

Lesions above the Sacral Segments

Lesions above the sacral segments lead to an upper motor neuron disorder with severe constipation. Studies of colonic transit reveal delay that affects mainly the rectosigmoid colon.[77] Abnormal colonic compliance occurs in patients with complete traumatic transection of the cord[78] with a rapid rise in pressure on instillation of relatively small volumes of fluid. No increase in motor activity is demonstrable after meals, but the colonic response to neostigmine injections is normal, which shows that the cholinergic neuromuscular junction and muscle response are intact.[78] Despite this observation, treatment with the prokinetic drug cisapride yielded inconsistent results.[77]

Studies of anorectal function in patients with traumatic complete spinal cord lesions showed that discriminant rectal sensation was abolished, although a dull pelvic sensation was experienced by some patients at maximum levels of balloon distention. Anal relaxation on rectal distention was exaggerated and occurred at a lower volume within the balloon than in normal subjects. Distention of the rectum led to a linear increase in pressure, without the plateau at intermediate values seen in normal subjects, and ended in high-pressure rectal contractions after the relatively small volume of 100 mL had entered the balloon. As expected, the rectal pressure generated by straining was less in patients than control subjects and was less in higher than in lower spinal cord lesions. Patients were unable voluntarily to contract the external anal sphincter and the sphincter did not relax on straining, which suggests that in normal subjects descending inhibitory pathways are present.[79]

These findings explain why some patients experience not only constipation but also sudden uncontrollable rectal expulsion with incontinence. Other patients cannot empty the rectum in response to laxatives or enemas, possibly related to the failure of external sphincter relaxation, and manual evacuation may be needed. The management of their constipation by patients with spinal injury is a major physical and social disability.

Electrical stimulation of anterior sacral nerve roots S2, S3, and S4 via electrodes implanted for urinary control in paraplegic patients leads to a rise in pressure within the sigmoid colon and rectum and contraction of the external anal sphincter. Contraction of the rectum and relaxation of the internal anal sphincter persist for a short time after the stimulus ceases. By appropriate adjustment of the stimulus it was possible for 5 of 12 paraplegic patients to achieve complete evacuation of feces and for most of the others to increase the frequency of defecation and reduce the time spent emptying the rectum.[80] In another series colonic transit time decreased with regular sacral nerve stimulation.[81]

Lesions of the Sacral Cord, Conus Medullaris, Cauda Equina, or Nervi Erigentes (S2 to S4)

Neural integration of anal sphincter control and rectosigmoid propulsion occurs in the sacral segments of the spinal cord. The motor neurons that supply the striated sphincter muscles are grouped in Onuf's nucleus at the level of S2. There is evidence that efferent parasympathetic nerves arising in the sacral segments enter the large intestine at the region of the rectosigmoid junction and extend distally in the intermuscular plane to reach the level of the internal sphincter and proximally to the mid-colon via the ascending colonic nerves, which retain the structure of a peripheral nerve.[82]

Damage to sacral segments of the spinal cord or to efferent nerves leads to severe constipation. Fluoroscopic studies show a loss of progression of contractions in the left colon.[83] On filling the colon with fluid, the intraluminal pressure generated is lower than normal, in contrast with the situation after higher lesions of the spinal cord. The distal colon and rectum may dilate and feces may accumulate in the distal colon.[84] Loss of sensation of the perineal skin may extend to the anal canal, and there may be diminished rectal sensation.

CONSTIPATION SECONDARY TO STRUCTURAL DISORDERS OF THE COLON, RECTUM, ANUS, AND PELVIC FLOOR

Obstruction

Anal atresia in infancy, anal stenosis developing later in life, or obstruction of the large intestine for any reason may manifest with constipation. Obstruction of the small intestine generally manifests with pain and distention, but constipation may be a feature (see Chapter 84).

Disorders of Smooth Muscle

Myopathy Affecting Colonic Muscle

Congenital or *acquired myopathy* of the colon usually manifests with pseudo-obstruction. The colon is hypotonic and inert (see Chapters 29 and 111).

Hereditary Internal Anal Sphincter Myopathy

Two families have been described in which constipation with difficulty in rectal expulsion was associated with very troublesome episodes of anorectal pain, typical of proctalgia fugax.[85, 86] Data were available for five generations in both families, and the mode of inheritance appeared to be autosomal mendelian dominance. In both families, affected members had a thickened internal anal sphincter muscle, shown by ultrasonography. The resting anal pressure was greatly increased with marked ultra-slow wave activity. In two patients, treatment with a calcium channel blocker was followed by a reduction in pain but no improvement in constipation.[86] Internal anal strip myectomy in two patients improved constipation and pain. Examination of the muscle strips showed myopathic changes with polyglycosan bodies in the smooth muscle fibers and increased endomysial fibrosis.

Systemic Sclerosis

Systemic sclerosis may be associated with replacement of intestinal smooth muscle by fibrous tissue, together with a liability to ischemia caused by blood vessel involvement. Constipation is an uncommon symptom among such patients, despite the fact that wide-mouthed diverticula or sacculations may be seen on barium enema studies and decreased colonic motor function may be demonstrable[87] (see Chapter 29).

Muscular Dystrophies

Muscular dystrophies are usually regarded as disorders of striated muscle, but visceral smooth muscle may also be abnormal.[88] In *myotonic muscular dystrophy*, a condition in which skeletal muscle fails to relax normally, megacolon may be found and abnormal function of the anal sphincters is demonstrable[89] (see Chapters 29 and 111).

Enteric Nerves

Congenital Aganglionosis or Hypoganglionosis

Congenital absence or reduction in number of ganglia in the colon leads to functional obstruction with proximal dilation, as seen in *Hirschsprung's disease* and related conditions (see Chapter 110). Hypoganglionosis is reported when small, sparse myenteric ganglia are seen. Neuronal counts can be made on full-thickness tissue specimens; in addition, baseline data for the small intestine and colon, obtained from autopsy material in childhood, have been published. Establishing the diagnosis is not easy, because of the variations of normal density.[90]

Congenital Hyperganglionosis (Intestinal Neuronal Dysplasia)

Congenital hyperganglionosis was described as a developmental defect characterized by hyperplasia of the submucosal nerve plexus. Clinical manifestation was regarded as a generalized pseudo-obstruction in childhood similar to Hirschsprung's disease or as lifelong constipation with megacolon.[91] Difficulties have been experienced in histologic definition of this condition, especially in mucosal suction biopsy specimens. A multicenter study on interobserver variation showed complete agreement in the diagnosis of Hirschsprung's disease but accord on the histologic findings in only 14% of children without aganglionosis.[92] There is concern that some of the clinical features and histologic changes previously associated with this condition in childhood may be age related and revert to normal with the passage of time.[90]

Acquired Neuropathies

Chagas' disease, which results from infection with *Trypanosoma cruzi*, is the only neuropathy in which the cause is known. The reason for neuronal degeneration is unclear but may have an immune basis.[93] Patients present with progressively worsening symptoms of constipation and abdominal distention due to a segmental megacolon, which may be complicated by sigmoid volvulus (see Chapters 29, 110, and 111).

Paraneoplastic visceral neuropathy may be associated with malignant tumors outside the gastrointestinal tract, particularly small cell carcinoma of the lung and carcinoid tumors. Pathologic examination of the affected gut reveals either neuronal degeneration or myenteric plexus inflammation.[94] An immunoglobulin reactive with myenteric neurons has been identified in some patients with this disorder[95] (see Chapters 29, 110, and 111).

Neuropathies of Unknown Cause

Severe acute neuropathies have been described that present with mainly obstructive symptoms but not principally constipation. The evidence for neuropathic features affecting the colon in some patients with severe idiopathic constipation has been presented earlier.

Disorders of the Anorectum and Pelvic Floor

Rectocele

In women, the anterior rectal wall above the anorectal junction is supported by the perineal body; a layer of fascia runs from the rectovaginal pouch of Douglas to the perineal body and adheres to the posterior vaginal wall. Above the level of the perineal body the anterior rectal wall is unsupported, and the rectovaginal septum can bulge anteriorly to form a rectocele (Fig. 12–4). Defecating proctography in symptomless healthy women shows that rectoceles are common and may protrude as much as 4 cm from the line of the anterior rectal wall without bowel symptoms, although 2 cm is the generally accepted lower limit of a rectocele that may be regarded as clinically significant.[96, 97]

The combination of features that appear to distinguish a symptomatic from a symptomless rectocele are that a woman complains she is unable to complete fecal evacuation, a lump may appear at the introitus with each straining effort, and using the thumb or fingers to support the posterior vaginal wall enables her to complete defecation.[98] Alternatively, she may use a finger to digitally evacuate the rectum. In practice, surgical repair may be considered for other symptoms such as a sense of incomplete evacuation on defecation without reference to the vagina, a sensation of local pressure or perineal pain. It is often unclear if these symptoms are related to the rectocele.

Defecating proctography can be used to demonstrate the rectocele, measure its size and show whether barium is trapped within it at the end of defecation. Correlation of radiologic findings with the results of surgical repair has not shown that the size or degree of emptying of a rectocele on defecation influences the outcome of operation.[99, 100]

Surgical repair can be performed by endorectal, transvaginal, or transperineal approaches. Other types of genital prolapse may also be present, and joint surgical and gynecologic consultation may be appropriate. For example, urinary incontinence or previous hysterectomy was more common in one series of patients with a rectocele as compared with a similar group of patients who complained of difficulty in defecation but had no demonstrable rectocele.[98] Surgical repair in carefully selected patients benefits approximately three quarters of patients,[99, 100] although in one series there

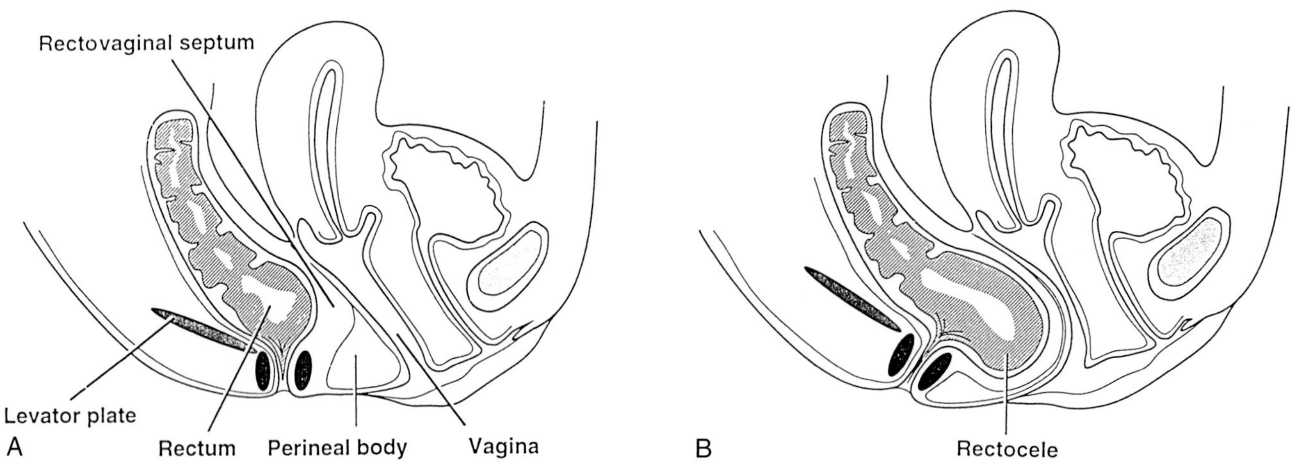

Figure 12–4. Normal anatomy (*A*) of the female pelvis. The levator plate is almost horizontal, supporting the rectum and vagina. The perineal body provides support for the lower posterior vaginal wall; above lies the rectovaginal septum. Weakness of the pelvic floor (*B*) leads to a more vertical levator plate. The perineal body is attenuated, which is favorable for the formation of a rectocele. The laxity of the pelvic floor is also favorable for mucosal prolapse. (From Loder PB, Phillips RKS: Rectocele and pelvic floor weakness. In Kamm MA, Lennard-Jones JE [eds]: Constipation. Petersfield, England, Wrightson Biomedical Publishing, 1994, p 281.)

was no clear correlation between reduction in the size of the rectocele, judged by proctography, and improvement in symptoms.[100]

Weakness of the Pelvic Floor— "Descending Perineum Syndrome"

In some patients, usually women, there is a greater descent than normal of the pelvic floor on straining during defecation associated with difficulty in rectal expulsion. Electrophysiologic changes show partial denervation of the striated muscle and prolonged latency on stimulation of the pudendal nerves, characteristic of nerve damage; histologic evidence from operative specimens confirms loss of muscle fibers.

The result of pelvic floor weakness is that the anorectal angle is widened, the rectum is more vertical than normal, the perineal body is weak (thereby facilitating formation of a rectocele), and the lax muscular support favors intrarectal mucosal intussusception or rectal prolapse. It is also possible that the pelvic floor does not provide the resistance necessary for extrusion of solid stool through the anal canal.

A common reason for pelvic floor weakness is trauma or stretching during parturition. In some cases, repeated and prolonged defecation appears to be the damaging factor.[101]

Full-Thickness Rectal Prolapse, Intrarectal Mucosal Prolapse, and Solitary Rectal Ulcer Syndrome

Some patients complain of many fruitless visits to the bathroom with prolonged straining in response to a constant desire to defecate, combined with a sense of incomplete evacuation. Time spent in the lavatory may total an hour or more daily. Infrequent passage of small, hard stools is common, as are other features of a functional bowel disorder with distention and abdominal pain. During straining efforts, mucus and blood may be passed.

Endoscopy with a proctoscope or hollow rigid sigmoidoscope shows hyperemia and edema of the anterior rectal mucosa, sometimes with ulceration or polypoid change, and prolapse into the instrument on straining. Defecating proctography may show circumferential mucosal intussusception, which enters or prolapses through the anal canal.[102] Biopsy of the mucosa reveals inflammation with characteristic extension toward the epithelium between the glands of fibers of the muscularis mucosa. Taken together, these clinical, endoscopic, and histologic features of varying degrees of rectal prolapse, inflammation, and ulceration are described as the *solitary ulcer syndrome*.[103]

Medical treatment of such patients is always difficult and entails advice to try to resist the urge to strain, along with efforts to alleviate the accompanying constipation and functional bowel symptoms. Biofeedback (see later) benefited 8 of 13 consecutive patients in one series, including 5 patients who had not been helped by surgical treatment.[104] This mode of treatment thus appears promising, and further experience with it is indicated. Surgical treatment is often required, and in one such series[105] correction of rectal prolapse gave relief to 55% to 60% of patients, and a permanent stoma was eventually constructed in approximately one third of the patients for relief of intractable symptoms unresponsive to all other measures. The results of rectal prolapse repair are variable because it may aggravate a tendency to constipation[106] (see Chapter 118).

DRUG TREATMENT THAT MAY CAUSE OR AGGRAVATE CONSTIPATION

A patient complaining of constipation must always be asked about consumption of any medication or drug. Constipation as a possible side effect of any preparation being taken long-term should be checked. Drugs commonly implicated are listed in Table 12–8. Among these are *analgesics* that often contain opiate derivatives and are taken for chronic painful conditions, such as arthritis, especially by the elderly; *anticholinergics*, including antispasmodics, some tricyclic antidepressants, phenothiazine derivatives used as long-term neuro-

Table 12–8 | **Drugs Causing or Aggravating Constipation**

Analgesics
Opiates
Anticholinergics
Antispasmodics
Tricyclic antidepressants
Phenothiazines
Antimuscarinics
Serotonin receptor antagonists
Calcium-aluminum–containing antacids

leptics, and antimuscarinic drugs used for parkinsonism; all have an anticholinergic effect; *calcium* or *aluminum-containing antacids,* now used less commonly, may have a constipating effect in some patients; and *serotonin receptor antagonists.*

PSYCHOLOGICAL DISORDERS AS CAUSES OF OR AGGRAVATING FACTORS IN CONSTIPATION

Constipation may be a symptom of psychiatric disorder or a side effect of its treatment (see Chapter 122).

Depression

For some patients, constipation can be a somatic manifestation of an affective disorder. Among patients with depression, 27% said that constipation developed or became worse at the onset of the illness.[107] Constipation can occur in the absence of other typical features of severe depression such as anorexia or psychomotor retardation with physical inactivity. Depressive features may accompany severe psychoses, and so constipation may be a feature of illnesses such as schizophrenia and delusional states.

Eating Disorders

Patients with anorexia or bulimia often complain of constipation, and prolonged whole-gut transit time has been demonstrated in both disorders.[108] Two studies in which colonic transit has been measured before and after resumption of an adequate diet have revealed that the colonic transit rate returns to normal within 3 to 4 weeks once more food is eaten.[109, 110] Pelvic floor dysfunction is found in some patients, and this does not improve with improved diet.[110]

Anorexia nervosa should be considered as a possible diagnosis particularly in any young, underweight woman who presents with constipation. Patients with eating disorders often resort to the regular use of laxatives either as treatment for constipation or in an effort to lose weight or relieve the presumed consequences of binge eating. Treatment of all such patients requires skilled psychiatric management of the eating disorder, of which constipation is but one manifestation (see Chapter 17).

Denied Bowel Movements

Patients often fail to report, and a few deny, defecation when disappearance of solid inert markers from the abdomen proves by radiologic examination that elimination has occurred. Such patients who deny that defecation has occurred despite evidence to the contrary need skilled psychiatric help.

CLINICAL ASSESSMENT

Clinical History

The *symptoms* of constipation, along with an individual complaint or complaints, as shown in Table 12–1, should be elicited. The *time course* is important to know. Is the complaint life-long, or was the onset later in life, and are the symptoms progressive? Symptoms beginning in earliest childhood suggest a congenital disorder. A recent onset of progressive symptoms in an older person should raise the suspicion of carcinoma. Drugs taken that might be constipating should be noted, as well as whether the patient has had a difficult delivery that damaged her pelvic floor.

Associated symptoms are important. Weight loss or other general symptoms encourage investigation for systemic disease. Blood in the stools is an indication for careful investigation. Colicky pain and abdominal distention, especially after meals, may indicate an obstructive lesion. The physician should take note of any possible neurologic disorder to which constipation might be secondary and should always be alert for symptoms of hypothyroidism, such as slowness, feeling cold, loss of hair, or deepening of the voice.

Social History

The physician should try to ascertain why the patient has sought help with the symptom or symptoms at the time of the visit. The physician should inquire about diet in general terms, with special reference to size of meals and their fiber content. Any recent changes in routine of life should be noted. A quick picture of the patient's background and any relevant social, behavioral, or psychological problems should be formed. The physician should be alert for manifestations of depression such as insomnia, lack of energy, loss of interest in life, loss of confidence, and a sense of hopelessness. A history of physical or sexual abuse in childhood is unlikely to emerge in the first interview but may be an important etiologic factor in severe cases of constipation. If the physician evinces no surprise at whatever is revealed, indicates that distressing events are common, and maintains a sensitive, encouraging attitude, the full story often gradually emerges at subsequent consultations, provided there is privacy, confidentiality, and adequate time (see Chapters 5, 91, and 122).

Physical Examination

The patient's general appearance or voice may point to a clinical diagnosis of *hypothyroidism, parkinsonism,* or *depression.* General physical examination should exclude major central nervous system disorders, especially spinal lesions. If spinal disease is suspected, the possibility of loss of sensation over the sacral dermatomes should be investigated.

Abdominal examination may reveal distention, hard feces in a palpable colon, or an inflammatory or neoplastic mass.

If the abdomen appears distended, a hand should be passed under the lumbar spine while the patient is lying supine to exclude anterior arching of the lumbar spine as a cause of postural bloating. While the patient lies on his or her side, the pelvic floor should be observed at rest and after the patient strains down so as to detect either absence of or excessive descent. Rectal prolapse may appear on straining or be demonstrable only on withdrawal of a proctoscope or while the patient strains in the sitting position.

Digital examination of the rectum reveals whether it is full or empty. An assessment of anal sphincter tone, both resting and on voluntary contraction, yields further information about the tone and contractile force of the external anal sphincter. A palpable abnormality of the rectum or surrounding tissues should be sought.

Endoscopy may reveal the brown or black pigmentation of melanosis coli, which may be either uniform and simulate hyperemia or patchy. Examination of the distal rectum may show evidence of anterior mucosal prolapse or a solitary rectal ulcer. The major use of endoscopy is to exclude structural disease of the large intestine.

Prospective Use of a Diary Card

Patients tend to underestimate their bowel frequency. Clinical assessment of transit rate is useful and can be judged from stool frequency and form.[5] It is useful in selected cases to provide the patient with a diary card on which to record each bowel action and the form of the stool over several days.[7]

INVESTIGATION

The high prevalence of bowel symptoms in the population implies that most are of nuisance value only and do not signify serious disease. It is, therefore, inappropriate to undertake any, or much, investigation for most patients who complain of one or more of these symptoms. This is especially true for adolescents and young adults.

Investigations may be indicated for one of two reasons: (1) to exclude as much as possible systemic illness or structural disorders of the gut as a cause of constipation and (2) to elucidate the pathophysiologic process underlying the symptoms when they are unresponsive to simple treatment.

Tests to Exclude Systemic Disease

Measurements of hemoglobin level and erythrocyte sedimentation rate and biochemical screening tests to include thyroid function, serum calcium, and other appropriate investigations are indicated if the clinical picture suggests that the symptoms result from an inflammatory, neoplastic, metabolic, or other systemic disorder.

Tests to Exclude Structural Disease of the Gut

A barium enema study reveals both the width and length of the colon and rules out any obstructing lesion severe enough to cause constipation. When fecal impaction is present, a limited enema study with water-soluble contrast material outlines the colon and fecal mass without aggravating the condition. A barium examination of the small bowel is indicated only if pseudo-obstruction or obstruction involving the small bowel is suspected (see Chapters 109 and 111).

Table 12–9 | **Criteria for Pelvic Floor Dyssynergia**[112]

Criteria for functional constipation (see Table 12–4)
Manometric, EMG, or radiologic evidence for inappropriate contraction or failure to relax pelvic floor muscles during defecation
Evidence of adequate propulsive force during attempts to defecate
Evidence of incomplete evacuation

EMG, electromyographic.

Physiologic Measurements

Much information about the physiology of defecation has been gained from a variety of tests used for research purposes. These tests are unnecessary for most patients with constipation. Some are useful in problem cases and, even then, should be kept as simple as possible. The American Gastroenterological Association Technical Review on Anorectal Testing Techniques[111] recommended the following as investigations useful in the investigation of constipation: symptom diaries (for diagnostic evaluation and monitoring treatment); colon transit studies (to confirm the patient's complaint and to assess slow transit and regional delay); anorectal manometry (to exclude Hirschsprung's disease and to support other tests of pelvic floor dysfunction); surface electromyography (EMG) (for evaluation of sphincter function and for use in biofeedback training). Tests regarded as of possible value were defecation proctography (to support the symptom of inability to defecate); balloon expulsion (to support the symptom of inability to defecate); and rectal sensory testing (to help distinguish between functional and neurologic disorders as a cause of constipation).

For a diagnosis of *pelvic floor dyssynergia*, a Rome working group[112] specified the criteria listed in Table 12–9. In patients with this disorder, constipation is established as functional and due to malfunction of the pelvic floor muscles established by physiologic tests. It is the basis for incomplete evacuation despite the presence of adequate propulsive forces.

Measurement of Whole-Gut and Colonic Transit Rate

Either whole-gut or colonic transit rate testing is needed only when objective evidence of slow transit is required, either to confirm a patient's statements or as a prelude to surgical treatment.

The simplest method of measuring whole-gut transit is to ask the patient to take 20 radiopaque solid markers enclosed in a gelatin capsule at breakfast time and perform a single radiograph of the abdomen 120 hours (5 days) later. This technique can be made somewhat more sensitive by providing markers of three different shapes (Fig. 12–5) on successive days so that a radiograph shows the position and reten-

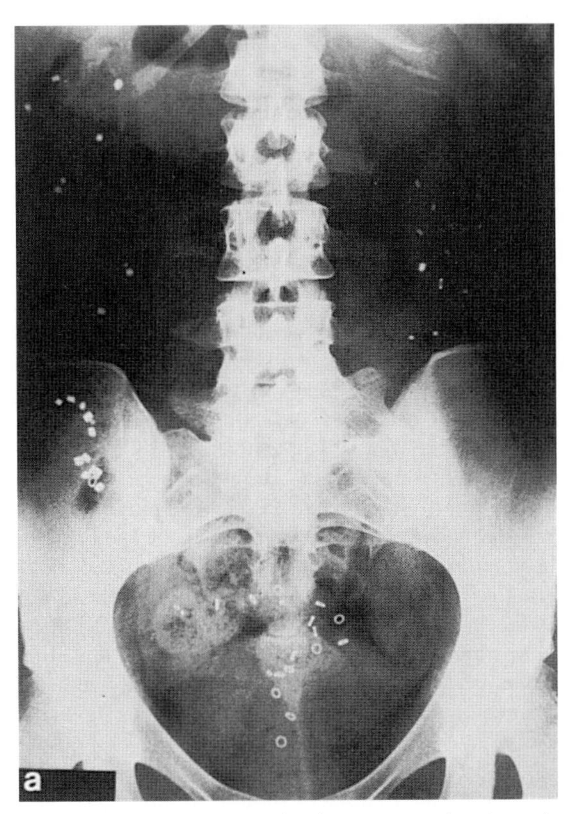

Figure 12–5. Abdominal radiograph of a constipated patient who took 20 inert ring markers 120 hours previously, 20 small cylinder markers 96 hours previously, and 20 cube-shaped markers 72 hours previously. Most of the markers are still present, showing slow whole-gut transit. See also Figure 12–6.

tion of the successive markers at 72, 96, and 120 hours after administration.[113, 114] Figure 12–6 shows the mean length of retention of markers with 95% confidence limits for both men and women.[114] Retention of four or more markers in the abdomen after 120 hours is outside the 95% confidence limit and indicates that transit is slow. Because markers are eliminated only with each defecation, the process is discontinuous; therefore, the result of a transit measurement should

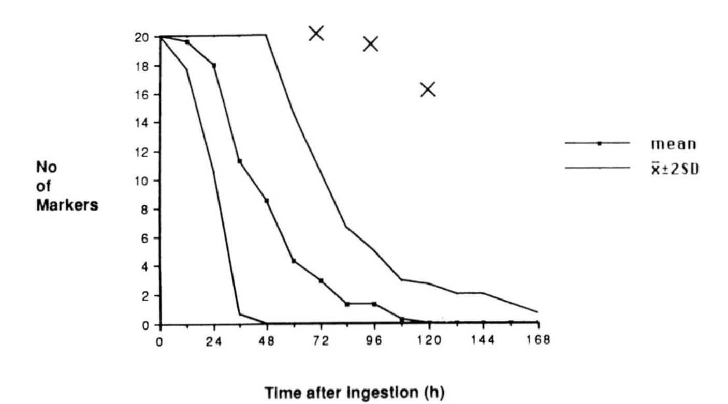

Figure 12–6. The mean plus 2 standard deviations of number of radiopaque markers remaining in the abdomen of normal subjects at various times after they ingested 20 markers at time zero. Values from the radiograph (see Fig. 12–5) are plotted (X) to illustrate the slow transit time. (From Evans RC, Kamm MA, Hinton JM, Lennard-Jones JE: The normal range and a simple diagram for recording whole-gut transit time. Int J Colorectal Dis 7:15, 1992.)

be regarded with caution, taking recent defecation into account.

Measurements of transit through different segments of the colon are of doubtful value in determining treatment. The only exception is when all the markers move rapidly to the rectum and are retained there, a situation characteristic of megarectum.

If surgical treatment for very severe constipation is being considered, sophisticated investigation to show the rates of gastric emptying, small bowel transit, and segmental colonic transit rate is valuable for confirming slow transit and correlating abnormalities with therapeutic outcome. In this circumstance, scintigraphic studies of gastrointestinal transit are indicated.[42, 43]

Physiology of Defecation (see Chapter 11)

Defecating Proctography

Defecating proctography gives information about the ability to empty the rectum, the rate of emptying, the width of the anal canal, movement of the pelvic floor, and any structural abnormalities, such as a large rectocele with trapping of barium or internal intussusception. It has the advantage of relative simplicity, but interpretation of the results must be done with caution because the normal range among symptomless subjects is wide. The most discriminating features for detection of anal dyssynergia are a reduced rate of evacuation and incomplete emptying of barium.[115] Defecography may show a narrow rectoanal angle (in contrast with the obtuse angle as in Chapter 11 [see Fig. 11–5]).

Anorectal Pressure

When the rectum is distended with a balloon, the internal anal sphincter relaxes, which is the rectoanal inhibitory reflex. The integrity of this reflex should be tested during investigation of megarectum. The reflex is absent in Hirschsprung's disease, but caution is needed in interpretation in patients with adult megacolon because a large volume in the balloon is needed to stretch the rectal wall and elicit the reflex. With the use of a variety of pressure-sensitive devices, it is possible to demonstrate paradoxical contraction of the external anal sphincter on straining during defecation (see Fig. 12–3).

EMG Testing of Striated Muscle Activity

If appropriate equipment is available, observations on external anal sphincter activity can be made by measuring electrical activity of the striated external sphincter muscle with an anal plug electrode or adhesive electrodes applied to the perianal skin.

Simulated Defecation

The ability of a patient to expel a simulated stool from the rectum can be tested using a water- or air-filled balloon for the purpose. The patients can sit on a commode in privacy.

When the patient lies in a convenient, but unphysiologic, position on their side, the test forms part of biofeedback training (see later).

Testing Rectal Sensation

Rectal sensitivity to distention can be measured by introducing successive volumes of air into a rectal balloon and recording the volume when the stimulus is first perceived, when it produces an urge to defecate, and when further additions of air can no longer be tolerated owing to discomfort. These measurements are not of value in the routine investigation of constipation, although they are of research interest. The threshold current needed to elicit sensation when the rectal mucosa is stimulated electrically by passing a current between bipolar electrodes applied to the mucosa can be used as a test of sensory nerve function, but the test is not established in general use.[60]

MEDICAL TREATMENT

General Measures

Reassurance

Some people are brought up from childhood to believe that a daily bowel action is essential for health, or they derive this opinion from advertisements, and they worry if their bowel habit is irregular or less frequent. They can be helped by information that an irregular bowel habit and other defecatory symptoms are common in the healthy general population and that their symptoms are not harmful. Such reassurance may be all they need. Other patients are concerned that their symptoms may indicate disease; they can be helped by appropriate investigation to relieve their fear.

Mode of Life

The need to set aside an unhurried and, if possible, regular time for defecation and always to respond to a defecatory urge should be stressed. If patients experience difficulty in expulsion of stool, they should be advised to place a support approximately 15 cm in height under their feet when sitting on a toilet seat so that the hips are flexed toward a squatting posture. Activity should be encouraged for those who are inactive. The use of constipating drugs requires review.

Psychological Support

Constipation may be aggravated by stress or may be a manifestation of emotional disturbance (e.g., previous sexual abuse) (see Chapter 122). For such patients, an assessment of the person's circumstances, personality, and background with supportive advice may help more than any physical measures of treatment. Behavioral treatment (described later) offers a physical approach with a psychological component, which is often acceptable and beneficial. Psychological treatment is needed only when it would be indicated in any circumstance.

Diet

When normal subjects add fiber to their diet, stool weight increases in proportion to the initial weight. It follows that when an increase in dietary fiber increases stool weight in constipated subjects who pass small stools, the resulting stool weight may still be below normal. For this reason, the therapeutic results of a high-fiber diet are often disappointing as a treatment for constipation. This is illustrated by a study of 10 constipated women who took a supplement of wheat bran, 20 g/day, which increased average daily stool weight from approximately 30 to 60 g/day, still only half the normal average weight. Their bowel frequency increased from a mean of two to three bowel actions weekly.[116] In a controlled, cross-over trial, 24 patients took 20 g of bran daily or placebo each for 4 weeks. Bran was more effective than placebo in improving bowel frequency and oroanal transit rate, but the occurrence and severity of the major symptoms of constipation experienced by the patients did not differ between the two treatment periods.[117] This result probably reflects the fact that patients mainly complain of difficulty in defecation rather than decreased frequency of bowel actions. In a series of constipated patients, about half were reported as having gained some benefit from a bran supplement of 20 g daily.[118]

Despite the fact that dietary modification may not succeed, all constipated subjects should be advised as an initial measure to increase their dietary fiber intake as the simplest, most physiologic, and cheapest form of treatment. Patients should be encouraged to take about 30 g of non-starch polysaccharides (NSPs) daily by eating whole wheat bread, unrefined breakfast and other cereals, plenty of fruit and vegetables, and, if necessary, a supplement of raw bran either with breakfast cereals or used in cooking. Specific dietary advice is often needed to achieve a satisfactory increase in dietary fiber.

Some patients, particularly women with greatly delayed colonic transit, find that bran aggravates their sense of abdominal distention[24]; this treatment may also be unhelpful in young people with megacolon and in elderly subjects, among whom it may lead to incontinence. For these patients a reduction in their fiber intake may relieve symptoms.

Fluid Intake

Dehydration or salt depletion is likely to lead to increased salt and water absorption by the large intestine, leading to the passage of small, hard small stools. Children or adults with fever, or subjects in hot environments, should therefore be advised to consume plenty of fluid.

Laxatives

Bulk Laxatives

Bulk laxatives are a concentrated form of NSPs useful for patients who cannot take adequate dietary fiber. They are based on wheat, plant seed mucilage (ispaghula), plant gums (sterculia), or synthetic methylcellulose derivatives (methylcellulose, carboxymethylcellulose). These fiber supplements are limited in therapeutic effect by the same factors as those that limit the benefit of increased dietary fiber.

WHEAT FIBER. The nearest approximation to normal dietary fiber is concentrated wheat husk, prepared as a tasteless powder containing 80% fiber that can be mixed with food. Three packets each of 3.5 g daily can double an inadequate fiber intake.

ISPAGHULA (PSYLLIUM). Ispaghula is derived from the husks of an Asian plant, has very high water-binding capacity, is fermented in the colon to a moderate extent, and increases bacterial cell mass. It is available as effervescent suspensions, as granules, and as a powder. The suspensions, which are popular, need to be drunk quickly before the husk absorbs water. The granules, which contain 90% of ispaghula husk, may be stirred briskly in half a glass of water and swallowed at once; carbonated water may be preferred. Some people like to swallow the solid granules to be followed by a glass of water.

Ispaghula (3.4 g as Metamucil) increased fecal bulk to the same extent as methylcellulose 1 to 4 g daily in constipated subjects.[119] Although both stool dry and wet weights increased, the total weekly weights remained less than those of a control group without treatment (Fig. 12–7). Similar results were obtained in another study of psyllium given to constipated patients.[120] In an observational study, 149 patients were treated with psyllium in the form of *Plantago ovata* seeds, 15 to 30 g daily, for a period of at least 6 weeks. There was a poor response to treatment among patients in whom slow colonic transit or a disorder of defecation was shown by investigation, whereas 85% of patients without a pathologic finding improved or became symptom free. The authors commented that a dietary fiber trial should be undertaken before technical investigations are undertaken.[121] These observations emphasize the heterogeneity of patients complaining of constipation, many of whom suffer from "simple" constipation (see Table 12–4), which is easily treatable by modification of fiber intake and mode of life.

Ispaghula taken by mouth can cause an acute allergic immunoglobulin E–mediated response, with facial swelling, urticaria, sensation of tightness in the throat, and cough in workers exposed to inhalation of the compound during manufacture or preparation.[122]

STERCULIA. Sterculia, a gum obtained from plants of that species, is known also as Indian tragacanth or karaya. It is sparingly soluble in water and swells to a homogeneous, adhesive, gelatinous mass. For treatment of constipation it is available as coated granules that contain 62% of the active material. The recommended daily dose is one or two heaped 5-mL spoonfuls of the granules, which are placed dry on the tongue after meals once or twice daily and swallowed immediately with plenty of liquid.

METHYLCELLULOSE. This synthetic compound varies in its chain length and the degree of methylation. The object of methylation is to reduce bacterial degradation in the colon. One study among constipated patients with an average daily fecal weight of only 35 g showed an increase in fecal solids with 1, 2, and 4 g/day, but fecal water increased only with the 4-g dose (see Fig. 12–7). The bowel frequency in this group of patients increased from an average of two to four stools weekly. However, patients did not report any marked improvement in consistency of stool or ease of passage.[119] Methylcellulose is prepared as a liquid or as 500-mg tablets; the recommended dose is up to 3 g twice daily taken with plenty of water.

CONCLUSION. Bulk laxatives have a limited role in the management of chronic constipation. They should be regarded as a long-term treatment and are not appropriate for the rapid relief of temporary constipation (Fig. 12–8). Patients should be encouraged to achieve the same result by dietary means with a supplement of natural bran. In severe constipation, neither a high-fiber diet nor a bulking agent relieves symptoms adequately. However, in mild constipation—for example, during pregnancy—a bulking agent may be a useful measure. Any of the preparations mentioned may be used, but probably the most palatable and convenient are the effervescent powders containing ispaghula (psyllium).

Unabsorbed Polyethylene Glycol Electrolyte Solution

Polyethylene glycol (PEG) is an inert polymer with a range of molecular weight. In the range of 3200 to 4000 the compound is not absorbed by the gut and is excreted unchanged in the feces; smaller molecules are absorbed by the gut and excreted unchanged by glomerular filtration in the

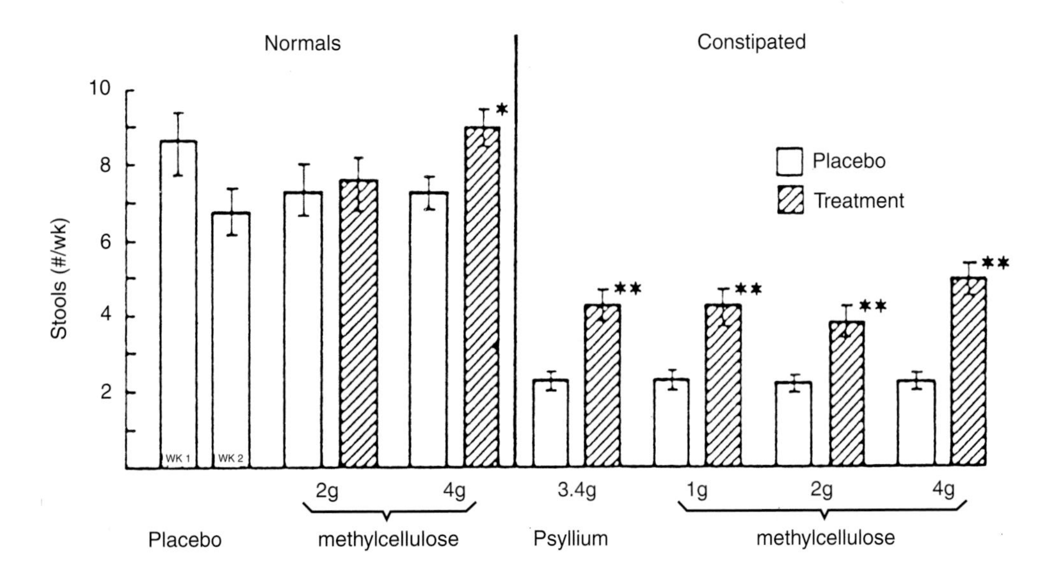

Figure 12–7. Daily weight of fecal solids in normal volunteers and constipated patients, who consumed their normal diet and a supplement of psyllium 3 to 4 g/day, or methylcellulose 1, 2, or 4 g/day. Note that the weight of fecal solids was less than normal before treatment and was still below normal while patients were taking the bulk laxative * P < 0.5 and ** P < .01 compared with placebo. (From Hamilton JW, Wagner J, Burdick BB, et al: Clinical evaluation of methylcellulose as a bulk laxative. Dig Dis Sci 33:993, 1988.)

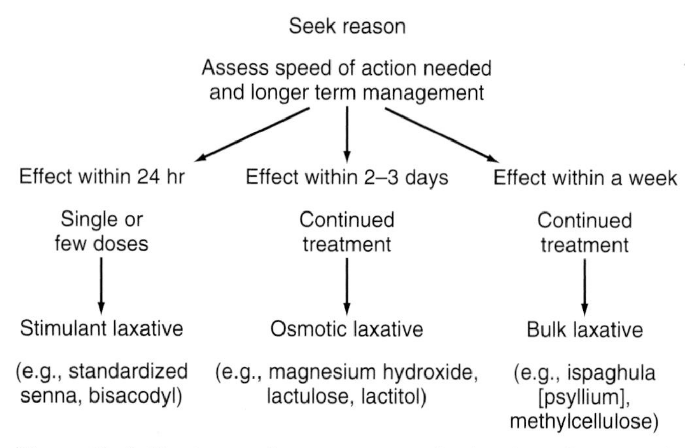

Figure 12–8. Treatment of temporary constipation (e.g., from travel, pregnancy, concurrent illness, or opiate therapy).

urine. The osmotic pressure of PEG in the colon opposes the absorption of water, with the result that the feces are softened and increased in bulk, or become liquid.

The addition of appropriate electrolytes to a PEG solution avoids the potential adverse effects of drinking a large volume of water or the passage of liquid stools, such as water intoxication, dehydration, or electrolyte imbalance. Packets are available, differing slightly in content, but all enabling a PEG-electrolyte solution to be prepared by dissolution in a measured amount of water. Such PEG-electrolyte solutions have been widely used for cleansing the colon for endoscopy.

Such solutions have been used as a short-term treatment for fecal impaction. For example, 16 severely ill patients aged from 26 to 87 years were treated who, despite treatment with various laxatives, had not had a bowel action in hospital for 5 to 23 days. All had fecal loading on clinical examination. They were advised to drink on the first day 1 L of a PEG-electrolyte solution, taken as two portions of 500 mL, each over 4 to 6 hours. The regimen was repeated on a second and third day if necessary. The full dose was taken by 12 patients on the first day and the remainder took at least half of the recommended dose; only 8 patients needed treatment on the second day and 2 on the third day. The treatment was highly effective, and after the last dose most patients were passing moderate or large volumes of soft stool with resolution of impaction. No adverse side effects, apart from abdominal rumbling, occurred, and only 1 patient, who was paraplegic, experienced incontinence.[123] Similar successful treatment has been described in patients with refractory constipation treated as outpatients,[123] in the elderly[124] and given by mouth or as a nasogastric infusion, in children with fecal impaction,[125, 126] although children found difficulty in drinking the large volume of fluid used.

Several controlled trials have now shown that repeated smaller doses of a PEG-electrolyte solution are beneficial in the treatment of severe chronic constipation. Several trials have tested the treatment for periods of a few days up to 8 weeks, all of which showed benefit compared with placebo.[127–129] A trial has now been reported of daily treatment for 6 months. During an initial period all patients were treated openly for 4 weeks with a PEG-electrolyte solution, 250 mL once or twice daily, at the end of which time bowel frequency had increased to normal, hard stools were rare, and straining on defecation was experienced by fewer than 20% of patients as compared with 80% before treatment. Patients were then randomized to continue PEG or a placebo for 20 weeks in a dose of one or two packets daily as judged to give the best result. In every parameter examined the active treatment gave significantly improved results over placebo without adverse clinical or laboratory events.[130]

Although the treatment is not recommended for children, a dose-ranging trial in children with constipation, aged between 6 months and 15 years, suggests that this is a potentially useful treatment, provided that the adult dose is reduced appropriately.[131]

A comparative trial of PEG against lactulose in 99 patients over 4 weeks showed a significantly better result for PEG as regards bowel frequency (P = .005), straining at defecation (P = .0001), and overall improvement (P < .001). There was no difference in clinical symptoms between the groups except that passage of flatus was less in the PEG group (P = .01). No clinically significant adverse events occurred in either group.[132] The successful use of PEG as compared with lactulose has also been reported in a double-blind, cross-over trial in chronic opiate-induced constipation.[133]

Saline Perfusion

Whole-gut irrigation with normal saline combined with intravenous injections of furosemide and metoclopramide has been used for treatment of fecal impaction in the elderly[134] but is likely to be superseded by PEG-electrolyte solutions.

Unabsorbed Sugars and Polyhydric Alcohols

Lactulose and lactitol are synthetic disaccharides that are not absorbed by the small bowel but are fermented in the colon to yield fatty acids, hydrogen, and carbon dioxide, with lowering of fecal pH. When normal subjects took lactulose 20 g daily, none of the sugar was detectable in the stool.[135] In larger doses, some of the sugar passes through the colon unchanged and acts as an osmotic laxative. Sorbitol and mannitol are isomers of a hexahydric alcohol. They also pass through the small intestine and are wholly or partially fermented in the colon, depending on the dose and transit rate. The presence of hydrogen in the colon is a potential danger if endoscopy with electrocautery is performed after one of these compounds has been ingested.

LACTULOSE. Lactulose is a combination of galactose and fructose, as 1,4-β-galactasidofructose. It is prepared from lactose and supplied for clinical use as a flavored syrup containing 3.3 g of lactulose per 5 mL with small amounts of galactose and lactose. The recommended dose for adults is 15 mL of the syrup twice daily, reducing as necessary. In practice, this dose often appears inadequate for treatment of severe chronic constipation. Initial recommended doses for children are 10 mL twice daily for those aged 5 to 10 years, 5 mL twice daily for those aged 1 to 5 years, and 2.5 mL twice daily for those younger than 1 year.

Its use in constipation among a group of young patients, mainly women, who passed fewer than three stools weekly has been studied by measurement of its effect in a double-blind, cross-over trial with a dose of 60 mL/day. Lactulose increased bowel frequency and percentage of stool moisture and softened the stools, in comparison with pretreatment values and with the control syrup that contained only sucrose.[136]

The effect of lactulose among elderly constipated patients has been studied in two double-blind, controlled trials against placebo. In one trial,[137] only about half the patients were found to be truly constipated; among these patients, the success rate with lactulose was 80% as opposed to 33% in the placebo (glucose) group ($P < .01$). The second trial[138] was conducted over 8 to 12 weeks among 42 elderly patients in a nursing home. The initial dose of syrup was 30 mL/day, and this could be reduced temporarily or permanently to 15 mL according to bowel frequency. Lactulose showed an advantage over the 50% glucose control syrup by an increase in the mean number of bowel movements each day and by a striking reduction in episodes of fecal impaction ($P < .015$) and the need for enemas.

Lactulose does not have an immediate laxative action, but the effect becomes evident after 2 or 3 days (see Fig. 12–8). Patients sometimes say that the preparation is effective initially but loses its effect. This is probably the result of a change in the colonic flora.[135] Some patients do not like the sweet taste, and others complain of abdominal distention or discomfort, presumably resulting from colonic gas production. In five elderly patients, the colon became distended and gas filled; the distention was more than 12 cm in diameter and attributed to gas production during treatment with lactulose.[139]

LACTITOL. Lactitol is a disaccharide derivative of galactose and sorbitol. Its effect in the colon is similar to that of lactulose. It is available as a slightly sweet-tasting white crystalline powder that can be mixed with drinks or food. The preparation has no effect on blood sugar levels and can therefore be given to diabetic patients.

A placebo-controlled, randomized, cross-over trial was conducted among institutionalized elderly but not bedridden patients.[140] The initial dose was 20 g/day of lactitol, and changes in dose by addition or subtraction of one 10-g packet daily were permitted according to the effect. Lactitol increased the average number of bowel movements from approximately four to six or seven each week ($P < .001$), with a corresponding improvement in a stool consistency score ($P < .001$). The daily dose of lactitol needed to produce soft stools was 30 to 50 g. There was no significant difference in flatulence, bloating, or abdominal cramps between the active and placebo groups.

SORBITOL. Sorbitol is widely used in the food industry as a sweetener in "sugar-free" products. Ingestion of as little as 5 g causes a rise in breath hydrogen, and 20 g produces diarrhea in about half of normal subjects.[141] Sorbitol reduces absorption of free fructose, so that its effects may be potentiated by fruits such as apples and pears.[142]

A randomized, double-blind, cross-over trial of lactulose, 20 g/day, and sorbitol, 21 g/day, in ambulant elderly men with chronic constipation showed no difference between the effect of the two compounds with regard to frequency or normality of bowel actions or patient preference.[143] Side effects were similar except that nausea was more common with lactulose. The authors of this trial, pointing out that the cost of sorbitol was one sixth or less that of lactulose, suggested that sorbitol could be used instead.

Salts

Magnesium and sulfate ions are poorly absorbed from the gut. Compounds used as laxatives include magnesium hydroxide, citrate sulfate, and sodium sulfate. Their action appears to be mainly osmotic, but other factors may also be important.[144] In mildly constipated patients, regular magnesium hydroxide 1.2 to 3.6 g/day is a useful, safe laxative.

Magnesium sulfate is a more potent laxative that tends to produce a large volume of liquid stool. The compound is not popular with patients because it often leads to a sense of distention and the sudden passage of a liquid offensive stool. The usual dose is 5 to 10 g of the crystals, which are dissolved in warm water and taken with extra fluid.

Excessive doses of magnesium salts by mouth can lead to hypermagnesemia, and medicinal doses should be used with caution in patients with renal impairment and in children. Hypermagnesemia with coma occurred in a normal 6-week old infant given 16 2-mL doses of milk of magnesia.[145] Severe toxicity with coma has also occurred in a chronically constipated child given an enema containing 32.5 mg of magnesium sulfate.[146]

Anthranoid Compounds

Anthranoid laxatives, such as senna, aloe, cascara, and frangula, are derived from plants and have many similarities. The compounds are inactive glycosides, which pass unabsorbed and unchanged through the small intestine and are hydrolyzed by bacterial glycosidases in the colon to yield the active molecules. The glycosides are thus prodrugs that have no effect on the upper gut but become active on reaching the colon.

Synthetic anthraquinones, such as 1,8-dihydroxyanthraquinone (danthron [also dantron]), are not glycosides. They are absorbed to some extent in the small bowel and have a direct action on the small intestine as well as the colon. As a result of animal carcinogenicity studies, the drug has been withdrawn by the U.S. Food and Drug Administration and its use is limited to constipation in terminally ill patients in Britain.

Active anthracene compounds have both motor and secretory effects on the colon. Animal studies suggest that the motor effect precedes the secretory effect and is the most important factor in laxative action. There is a decrease in segmenting colonic muscular activity and an increase in propulsive waves.

Senna has been shown in controlled trials to soften stools[147] and to increase not only stool frequency but also wet and dry weight.[120] The preparations available for clinical use vary from crude vegetable preparations through purified and standardized extracts to a synthetic compound. A standardized senna preparation, with total sennosides calculated as sennoside B, is available as tablets (7.5 mg), granules (5 mL containing 15 mg of sennosides), or a syrup (containing 7.5 mg per 5 mL). The tablets contain lactose, and the granules and syrup contain sucrose; diabetic patients are advised to use the tablets. These preparations are best taken in the evening or at bedtime, with the aim of producing a normal stool next morning. (see Fig. 12–8). The usual dose is 15 mg of sennosides at bedtime, but this may be decreased or increased according to the result.

POSSIBLE SIDE EFFECTS. There is controversy as to whether anthranoid laxatives, given over the long term, cause adverse functional or structural changes in the intestine. Animal studies have shown neither damage to the myenteric plexus after long-term administration of sennosides[148] nor a functional defect of motility.[149] A case control study with examination of multiple mucosal biopsy specimens showed no difference on electron microscopy in the submucous plexus between patients taking an anthranoid laxative regularly for 1 year and those not taking one of these drugs.[150]

Anthranoid laxatives appear to cause apoptosis of isolated colonic epithelial cells characterized by cytoplasmic shrinkage and by nuclear and cellular fragmentation to form rounded apoptotic bodies (Fig. 12–9). These are phagocytized by macrophages, which form a lipofuscin-like pigment[151] when anthranoid laxatives are taken, detected most sensitively by histologic analysis and sometimes on endoscopy[152] as pseudomelanosis. The proximal colon is affected more than the distal colon. If laxatives are stopped, the pigmented macrophages migrate to the lymph nodes and disappear over the course of months. Pseudomelanosis appears to be a harmless condition but is an indication of chronic laxative ingestion.

COMMENT. Anthranoid laxatives are well established and appear to be harmless if used in doses that produce normal, soft, formed stools. They act rapidly and are particularly suitable for use as single doses in temporary constipation for any reason (see Fig. 12–8). Most clinicians are cautious about recommending daily doses indefinitely for chronic constipation, and a twice-weekly regimen has been suggested.[153] Large doses produce colic and liquid stools, a situation to be avoided. There is wide variation in clinical effectiveness,[120] and some patients with severe constipation are not helped by anthranoid laxatives.

Polyphenolic (Diphenylmethane) Compounds

Polyphenolic compounds include phenolphthalein, bisacodyl, and sodium picosulfate. Phenolphthalein is best avoided because it undergoes an enterohepatic circulation and can cause a rash. Bisacodyl and sodium picosulfate are hydrolyzed to the same active metabolite, but the mode of hydrolysis differs. Bisacodyl is hydrolyzed by intestinal enzymes and thus can act on both the small and the large intestine. Sodium picosulfate is hydrolyzed by colonic bacteria. Like that of anthranoid glycosides, its action is therefore confined to the colon, but its activity is more uncertain because it depends on the bacterial flora.

The effects of bisacodyl, and presumably sodium picosulfate, on the colon are similar to those of the anthranoid laxatives. Applied to the colonic mucosa, bisacodyl induces almost immediate powerful propulsive motor activity[154] in both healthy and constipated subjects, although its effect is sometimes reduced in the latter; there is also a secretory component.

Bisacodyl is available as enteric-coated 5-mg tablets, and the recommended adult dose is 5 to 10 mg taken at night. Sodium picosulfate is available as a liquid containing 5 mg per 5 mL. The recommended adult dose is 5 to 10 mL at night.

SIDE EFFECTS. Like the anthranoid laxatives, bisacodyl leads to apoptosis of colonic epithelial cells with accumulation of phagocytic macrophages containing cellular remnants, but these are not pigmented.[151] Apart from these changes, there does not appear to be any evidence that polyphenolic laxatives cause adverse effects on long-term use.[149]

COMMENT. Bisacodyl is a useful and predictable laxative, especially suitable for single-dose use in temporary constipation (see Fig. 12–8). Its possible effect on the small bowel is a disadvantage, in comparison with that of anthranoid glycosides, but this disadvantage is not a feature of sodium picosulfate. Long-term use of bisacodyl or other of these agents is sometimes necessary in chronic severe constipation. In the doses used, some colic and liquid stools tend to

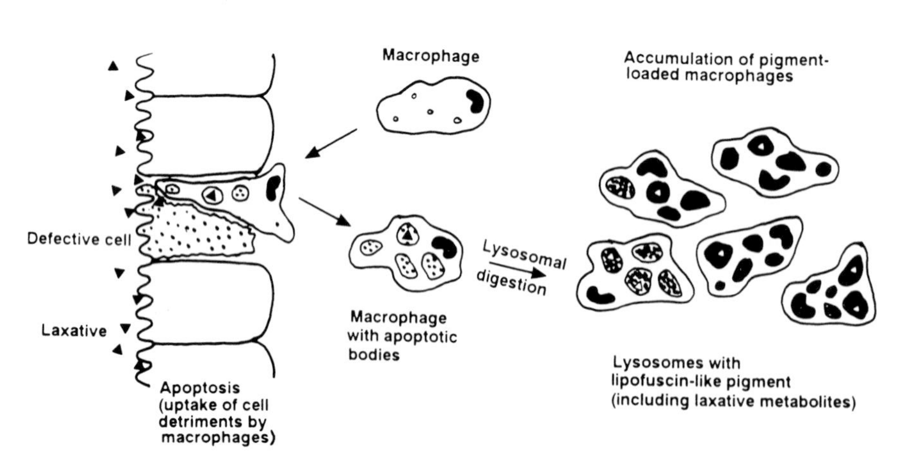

Figure 12–9. Steps in the development of pseudomelanosis coli when anthracene laxatives are taken over a long time. (From Leng-Peschlow E: Senna and its rational use. Pharmacology 44 [Suppl 1]:1, 1992.)

result. It is difficult to adjust the dose to produce soft, formed stools.

Detergents

The detergent dioctyl sodium sulfosuccinate (docusate sodium) was introduced as a stool softener, but further study of its efficacy is needed. The compound does stimulate fluid secretion by the small and large intestine,[155] but it does not increase the volume of ileostomy output or the weight of stools in normal subjects.[156] A double-blind, cross-over trial showed benefit in 5 of 15 elderly constipated subjects, as judged by patient and caregiver opinions, and a significant ($P < .01$) increase in bowel frequency.[157]

Docusate sodium is prepared as 100-mg tablets, as 250-mg capsules, as a solution containing 50 mg per 5 mL, or as a dilute solution for pediatric use containing 12.5 mg per 5 mL. The recommended adult dose is up to 500 mg/day in divided doses with water.

Liquid Paraffin

Liquid paraffin is a mineral oil that softens the stools, and emulsions are widely used. However, there are disadvantages in its use: Aspiration of the oil, causing lipoid pneumonia, can result from hold-up in the esophagus; it can cause anal seepage and a foreign body reaction if there is a break in the anorectal mucosa; and there is a theoretical risk of malabsorption of lipid-soluble vitamins.

Prokinetic Drugs

Cholinergic drugs have been used to treat constipation, but there is little published evidence of efficacy. Cisapride, a prokinetic drug, when combined with the patient's usual laxative regimen, reduced laxative consumption in one trial,[158] but the drug is no longer available. A new compound, prucalopride, a serotonin 4 (5-hydroxytryptamine 4 [5-HT_4]) agonist, which is thought to facilitate both cholinergic and nonadrenergic, noncholinergic neurotransmission, increases the rate of upper and lower gut transit in normal volunteers. Initial results of a placebo-controlled trial in treatment of patients with slow and normal transit constipation have shown increased bowel frequency ($P = .008$), decreased orocecal and whole-gut transit time ($P = .004$), improved rectal sensitivity to distention ($P < .01$), increased frequency of urge to defecate ($P = .02$), and decreased straining.[159, 160] A selective and partial 5-HT_4 receptor agonist, tegaserod, improves symptoms in constipation-predominant irritable bowel syndrome, and further trials are in progress.[161]

Compound Mixtures

Many mixtures of the compounds already described are available, for example, a bulking agent and an anthranoid laxative.[120, 162] In one trial a mixture of senna and psyllium proved more effective and cheaper than lactulose in the treatment of chronic constipation in the elderly.[162] In general it seems better to use a single compound with defined action as the first step in treatment, to substitute other compounds if the first is not satisfactory, and to use two compounds only if the combined effect is demonstrably better than that of either alone.

Alteration of Bacterial Flora

The colonic bacterial flora in some patients with constipation may digest fiber to a greater extent than usual, and so stools are small. Two groups studied the effect of vancomycin given by mouth on bowel function in severely constipated patients. In one study, most patients experienced normal bowel function during treatment with vancomycin, 250 mg three or four times daily, for 4 weeks. One of these patients who experienced relapse after treatment was given two enema infusions containing a fresh suspension of feces from her husband with the aim of altering her bowel microbial flora, after which she was well for at least 4 months.[163] Another study showed that oral vancomycin was associated with a significant improvement in stool frequency and consistency and ease of defecation in eight patients, although daily stool weight and whole-gut transit time were not significantly improved. One of the eight patients experienced complete remission of symptoms lasting at least 14 months.[164] These preliminary results encourage further research into manipulation of the colonic bacterial flora as a treatment for constipation.

Enemas and Suppositories

Compounds may be introduced into the rectum to stimulate contraction by distention or chemical action, to soften hard stools, or for both reasons. Serious damage to the rectal mucosa can result from extravasation of the enema solution into the submucosal plane. The anterior rectal mucosa is the site most vulnerable to trauma from the tip of a catheter introduced through the backward-angulated anal canal. The enema nozzle should be directed posteriorly after the anal canal has been passed.

Action Mainly by Distention of the Rectum and Softening of Feces

A saline enema or washout does no damage to the rectal mucosa[165] and may be effective. Water enemas or washouts may also be used; however, with large volumes, dangerous water intoxication can occur if the enema is retained. PEG can be incorporated in a suppository for its osmotic effect.

Action by Distention and Stimulation

Hypertonic sodium phosphate enemas are often effective. A histologic study by rectal biopsy in normal subjects showed that a single hypertonic phosphate enema caused disruption of the surface epithelium in 17 of 21 biopsies. Scanning electron microscopy showed patchy denudation of the surface epithelium with exposure of the lamina propria and absence of goblet cells. The proctoscopic appearance of the mucosa was abnormal in every case but returned to normal within a week.[165] Thus superficially damaged mucosa appears to heal rapidly. These enemas are used widely, and side effects are rarely reported.

Phosphate enema, if given to a patient who cannot evacuate it promptly, can lead to dangerous hyperphosphatemia and hypocalcemic tetany. For this reason, a patient aged 91 who was given a single phosphate enema died,[166] and coma developed in an adult who was given six of these enemas at hourly intervals without evacuation.[167] Severe metabolic disturbance has occurred in two healthy children, aged 4 months and 3 years, given a single phosphate enema.[168] The use of phosphate enemas in children 3 years of age and younger is not recommended.

Stimulant Suppositories or Enemas

Glycerin can be administered as a suppository and is often clinically effective. Its effect, if any, on the rectal mucosa is unknown. Bisacodyl (10 mg) is available as a suppository. In normal subjects a single bisacodyl suppository or an enema containing 19 mg in 100 or 200 mL produced marked changes in 23 of 25 biopsy specimens. The superficial epithelium and the epithelial cells to varying depths within the crypt were altered, and with the more concentrated enema, the surface epithelium was absent.[165] The regular use of bisacodyl suppositories thus appears unwise, though they appear clinically useful on occasion.

Oxyphenisatin (Veripaque) is a stimulant enema that is used mainly before diagnostic procedures. When given by mouth, this compound can lead to chronic hepatitis.

Fecal-Softening Agents

Enemas containing arachis oil, various wetting agents, salts, glycerol, and sorbitol in various combinations are used to soften and stimulate evacuation of stools, but their effectiveness is uncertain.

DEFECATION TRAINING, BIOFEEDBACK, AND OTHER BEHAVIORAL TREATMENTS

Role of the Trainer

Defecation training entails more than application of a mechanical or electronic technique. The personality, attitudes, and understanding of the trainer all are important. The patient usually spends between three and five treatment sessions, each lasting at least 30 minutes, with this person. Patients are encouraged to give a detailed description of their bowel symptoms, prompted by a sympathetic listener who is familiar with the full range of problems experienced by those with difficulties in defecation. This process is in itself therapeutic because it enables subsequent explanation and training to concentrate on what is really troubling the patient. Furthermore, this is probably the first time the patient has had an opportunity with adequate time to discuss symptoms hitherto regarded as a private burden. A rapport is established with the trainer that may also lead, as confidence develops, to disclosure and discussion at a subsequent session of personal problems or emotional factors that may be relevant to their bowel symptoms.

Misconceptions may be dispelled as the process of normal defecation is explained to the patient, perhaps with use of diagrams. Inquiry is made about diet, for it is possible that inadequate fiber is being taken or, conversely, that a previous overemphasis on fiber intake is aggravating symptoms such as abdominal bloating. For those with infrequent defecation, the importance of trying to develop a regular bowel habit and of not ignoring a call to defecate is emphasized. For those who spend excessive time in the bathroom with much ineffective straining, a regimen of less frequent visits to the bathroom but with effective defecation is recommended. The optimum posture for defecation, including the benefit of raising the feet above floor level when using a Western-type toilet, is described. Patients are encouraged to practice what they are taught and the fact that they may be able to help themselves often gives new self-confidence. At each visit patients are encouraged to reduce any dependence on laxatives, enemas, or suppositories. Progress in any regard is praised at successive treatment sessions.

Coordination of Abdominal and Pelvic Muscles

Although the technique of biofeedback may vary, its aims are to teach patients to relax the striated muscles of the pelvic floor during simulated defecation and to effectively raise intra-abdominal pressure.

In one successful technique,[16] the patient lies on his or her right side facing the trainer and an EMG display unit. A balloon is inserted into the rectum and inflated with 50 mL of air so that the patient has the sensation of a full rectum and thus the need to defecate. Two adherent surface electrodes are placed on the skin adjacent to the anal opening to assess external anal sphincter function. The patient is then asked to squeeze and relax the muscles of their back passage and then to cough. On the screen the patient can see first a resting trace and then a rise and fall in activity; the significance of these changes is explained. The patient is then asked to try and push out the balloon while continuing to observe the trace. At the same time, the therapist holds and exert a slight pull on the end of the tubing attached to the balloon. It is possible in this way to gauge how well the patient coordinates the defecatory muscles. If there is an increase, rather than the normal decrease, in muscular activity of the pelvic floor on defecation straining, and the balloon is not passed, the patient is encouraged to repeat the action but concentrate on the anal region and strain without any contraction of the anal sphincter. If this is successful, the balloon is passed spontaneously or can be withdrawn by exerting minimal tension on the catheter projecting from the anus. Passage of the balloon indicates the success of the maneuver. Repeated attempts may be needed until success is achieved.

Some patients fail to expel the balloon either because they fail adequately to contract their abdominal muscles or they contract them in such a way that no downward pressure is directed into the pelvis. Some perform a Valsalva maneuver with closed mouth and glottis, tightened abdominal muscles, and contracted muscles around the pelvic outlet. Patients who fail to coordinate their abdominal muscles are taught to open their mouth, brace the upper and lateral abdominal muscles (and presumably the diaphragm), yet protrude and relax the lower abdominal and pelvic muscles, so pushing downward into the pelvis with no resistance to expulsion of the stool. The situation is analogous to the abdominal muscular contractions required to push during childbirth.

Rectal Sensation

If the patient finds difficulty in sensing the presence of the inflated balloon, graded increases in distention may be used to teach the patient to sense its presence. The minimal volume detected can be improved significantly in this way, and gentle withdrawal of the balloon can make the patient aware of normal sensation during defecation.[169, 170]

Comparison of Different Methods

The original method of biofeedback training was intensive and begun during admission to hospital.[170] Subsequent experience has shown that training as an outpatient is satisfactory. A small comparative trial has shown no difference in outcome with or without use of an intrarectal balloon, or home training, or both.[171] The need for a visual display of muscular activity has been tested by randomized, controlled trial. Results were similar when training was given as described with or without access to a display.[170] In such a technique, the instructor follows the general approach outlined earlier, gives continuous information and encouragement to the patient, and observes their effect by observing how the patient strains and by sensing the effectiveness of straining through gentle tension on a rectal balloon.

Results

Some patients are unable to cope with defecation training. For example, 65 of 173 patients who completed more than one session failed to finish the course of training in one series.[172] Of those who did complete an adequate number of sessions, as judged by the therapist, ranging from 1 to 10 (median 4) in one series, 55% of patients declared that they had been helped.[16] Statistically significant improvement was shown by follow-up for at least 2 years (range 12 to 44 months; mean 23.4 months), compared with pretreatment values, in bowel frequency ($P < .001$), reduced straining episodes ($P < .01$), bloating ($P < .0001$), abdominal pain ($P < .003$), and use of laxatives ($P < .001$). Other series have shown similar symptomatic results with improved bowel frequency, decreased need to strain on defecation, and reduced use of laxatives,[172, 173] although no controlled trial against other treatments has been performed in adults. Physiologic measurements before and after treatment have shown that training results in appropriate relaxation of the puborectalis and external anal sphincter muscles,[169, 170, 173–175] increase in intrarectal pressure,[176] a widened rectoanal angle on straining during defecation, an increased rate of rectal emptying, an increased rate of colonic transit, and increased rectal mucosal blood flow.[169, 174]

Is the Outcome Dependent on Results of Physiologic and Anatomic Investigation?

Most published series have restricted this treatment to patients with demonstrable paradoxical contraction of the pelvic floor muscles. However, at one center such training appeared to benefit a high proportion of *unselected* patients with idiopathic constipation *regardless of the results of investigation of colonic transit or pelvic floor dysfunction.*[16, 174] Thus, for example, the treatment benefited patients with demonstrated slow colonic transit but no paradoxical contraction of the pelvic floor muscles. In another series[172] results of treatment did not depend on the presence or absence of a rectocele, intussusception, or perineal descent, although other investigators have shown that patients who failed to respond to the treatment had a greater degree of perineal descent than those who responded.[177] Defecation training has benefited some patients who developed constipation after hysterectomy[178] and some patients with the solitary ulcer syndrome.[104]

Comment

Defecation training is a widely applicable treatment for patients with severe idiopathic constipation of any type[172] and may also help a few patients with organic causes of defecation, such as multiple sclerosis.[76] It is labor intensive, but long-term results appear to be maintained. Long-term troublesome symptoms can be relieved, and the treatment may be cost effective, although this has not been tested, because laxatives can be stopped and surgical treatment can be avoided in some patients.

SURGICAL TREATMENT

The object of surgical treatment is to increase bowel frequency and ease of defecation; as a corollary it is hoped that operation will also relieve abdominal pain and distention. Procedures may be divided into three groups: partial or total colectomy, construction of a stoma, and anorectal operations undertaken to improve defecatory function.

Colectomy

Colectomy for constipation dates back to the early years of the 20th century, and the results of 32 published series have been reviewed.[179] There was considerable variability in patient satisfaction rates (39% to 100%) that reflected differences in the incidence of postoperative complications and in long-term functional results. For example, further surgery may be needed to correct unsatisfactory results or relieve intestinal obstruction; constipation may persist; diarrhea with possible incontinence may develop; or abdominal pain or bloating may continue, even though improved.[180, 181]

Selection of Patients

Such reports have led to a reassessment of the selection criteria for surgery and of the type of operation performed. First, it has become evident that preoperative psychological assessment is essential, because poor results are common among those who are psychologically disturbed.[182] Second, because the aim of operation is to increase bowel frequency, it is mandatory that slow colonic transit be demonstrated by an objective method. Third, it is important to assess defecatory function, inasmuch as inability to expel stools from the rectum may be a major factor in causing symptoms. Finally, it is important, as far as possible, to exclude a generalized pseudo-obstruction syndrome by appropriate radiographic study of the small intestine and, when possible, studies of gastric emptying and small bowel transit.

Series in which these steps have been taken to select a homogeneous group of patients have shown better results, although longer follow-up is awaited. For example, at one center only 74 of 1009 patients referred for possible surgical treatment of chronic constipation were operated on. Measurement of intestinal transit and tests of pelvic floor function revealed that 597 patients had no quantifiable abnormality and 249 patients had pelvic floor dysfunction without slow transit. Colectomy and ileorectal anastomosis was performed on 52 patients with demonstrable slow intestinal transit and normal defecatory function. This operation was also performed on 22 patients with both slow transit and pelvic floor dysfunction after the latter had been treated by a training program. Of the 74 patients treated surgically, 97% were satisfied with the result and 90% had a good or improved quality of life after a mean follow-up 56 months. There was no operative mortality, but 7 patients had an episode of small bowel obstruction.[183]

Type of Operation

Several series show that the results of colectomy with cecorectal or ileosigmoid anastomosis are unsatisfactory; constipation may persist or recur. Total colectomy should be performed with anastomosis of ileum to the upper rectum.[184] There have been occasional reports of proctocolectomy with ileoanal anastomosis and construction of an ileal pouch.[185] This procedure has usually followed failure of colectomy and ileorectal anastomosis. For example, in one patient ileorectal anastomosis failed because the rectum had a larger than normal capacity.[186]

Construction of a Stoma

A colostomy is occasionally performed for slow-transit constipation because it is reversible and the results of colectomy are uncertain. Most patients report subjective improvement after a colostomy performed as a primary procedure for slow-transit constipation or for neurologic disease. However, many still need to use laxatives or regular irrigation. The results of colostomy for constipation after pelvic surgery or birth trauma have been disappointing.[187]

An ileostomy is occasionally performed after failure of colectomy and ileorectal anastomosis for slow-transit constipation, either because intractable constipation persists or because of severe diarrhea and incontinence. In one series, only 5 of 10 patients felt subjectively improved; 5 continued to complain of abdominal pain, 5 of bloating, and 7 underwent further operations.[187] Patients not benefited by colectomy and ileorectal anastomosis are likely to be those with a generalized disorder of gut motility or those with psychological disturbance.

Creation of a continent catheterizable appendicostomy, through which antegrade enemas can be administered, can sometimes benefit patients with paraplegia whose disability is made worse by constipation and incontinence; such a procedure can decrease the time and medication needed for bowel care.[188, 189]

Operations for Defecatory Disorders

Operations such as puborectalis[190] or internal anal sphincter muscle division are unsuccessful in slow-transit constipation. Procedures to correct a rectocele, in carefully selected patients, may benefit local symptoms but not constipation (see earlier).

PARTICULAR CLINICAL PROBLEMS

Children and Young People

Three types of functional bowel disorder in childhood have been defined by a Rome Working Party[13]:

- Functional constipation—most stools are hard or scybalous, or firm stools are passed twice or fewer times each week. This disorder resembles that in adults and can be treated similarly.
- Functional fecal retention—large-diameter stools are passed less often than twice a week and the child appears to avoid defecation by purposefully contracting the pelvic floor and squeezing the buttocks together. The resulting fecal retention often leads to fecal soiling, abdominal cramps, and loss of appetite.
- Functional nonretentive fecal soiling—inappropriate defecation occurs in the absence of structural or inflammatory disease and in the absence of fecal retention. This inappropriate passage of normal stools into the clothes or in socially unacceptable places is usually the result of a psychological problem.

Fecal Retention with Soiling

CAUSES. If defecation is painful for any reason—for example, because of acute anal fissure—the child may try to avoid it. Stool then accumulates in the rectum and becomes hard from water absorption, with the result that the large, hard stools are even more painful to pass, thus creating a chronic problem. Finally, the internal anal sphincter becomes permanently relaxed as a result of chronic rectal distention, and semisolid stool leaks onto the perianal skin and clothing. About two thirds of children with soiling give a history of painful defecation before the age of 3 years. It is possible that some other children are born with a capacious rectum, which leads to fecal impaction and overflow incontinence. Deliberate withholding of stool to assert independence may be a factor in some instances. Psychological support may be needed if a serious behavioral disturbance develops as a result of the symptoms and/or the parents' reaction to them. Medical treatment should be directed primarily to the impacted rectum, and this topic has been well reviewed[191] (see Chapter 110).

INITIAL TREATMENT. The first essential in treatment is to gain the family's confidence and explain the mechanism of the symptoms. It is important to point out that the child cannot prevent the soiling but that it is a consequence of the full rectum. A controlled trial has shown that approximately one third of children become free of soiling if they follow a regular program of sitting on the toilet for 5 to 10 minutes within 30 minutes after each meal, combined with parental praise and reward for a successful bowel action and soiling-free days. Better results were obtained by combining such treatment with laxatives, first to empty the rectum and then to keep it empty.[192]

It can be difficult to empty the rectum, especially if the child has been frightened or experienced pain during previous anal administration of suppositories, washouts, or enemas. In these circumstances, the child vigorously resists further attempts at local treatment. Oral laxatives are often unsuccessful at removing the rectal "plug." Mineral oil in large doses has been used, and a controlled trial has compared (in children) this treatment with drinking a large volume of PEG-electrolyte solution (see earlier); children found it difficult to drink the large volume of fluid needed and vomiting proved to be a problem.[126] Success using a large volume of PEG-electrolyte solution has been reported when it was given by nasogastric tube.[125] In some severe cases, especially in adolescents with a greatly widened rectum and a distal colon full of stool, manual evacuation of the distal large bowel under anesthetic may be needed. However, it is important that the anal sphincters not be damaged by the stretching inherent in the procedure.

LONG-TERM TREATMENT. Once disimpaction has been achieved, it is essential to begin an oral daily laxative immediately and continue this treatment for months or longer if necessary (Fig. 12–10). Such children and young people need to maintain a daily semisolid bowel action; if the stools become solid, rectal impaction quickly recurs. Bulk laxatives or a high-fiber diet does not usually help these patients and may even aggravate the problem. Favored laxatives are osmotic, such as magnesium hydroxide in children, magnesium sulfate in young adults, or lactulose, and it is likely that PEG will also be used. The correct dose is that which produces a daily semiformed stool without side effects. If an osmotic laxative cannot be tolerated, a nightly dose of standardized senna may be used. It is essential that the child, the parents, and other physicians appreciate the need for regular laxatives over a prolonged period. Physicians who do not understand the problem tend to stop the laxatives, believing them to be harmful.

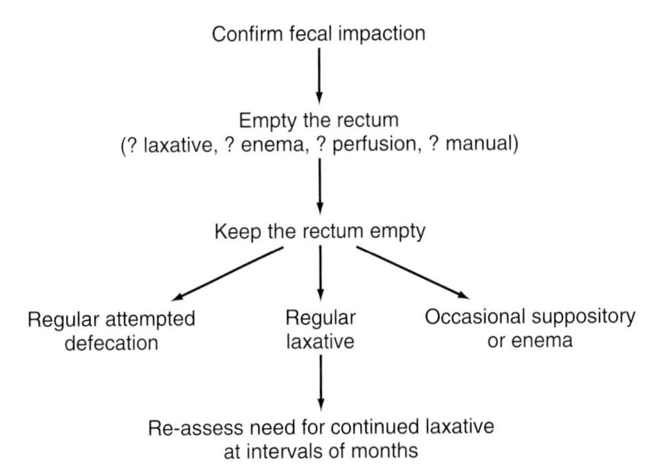

Figure 12–10. Treatment of rectal impaction with or without soiling in childhood or the elderly.

In addition, the child should continue to visit the bathroom and attempt to defecate regularly after meals. After a few months, the laxative doses can be cautiously reduced and stopped, provided that a normal bowel habit is maintained. About half of the patients can stop the laxatives within 1 year; others need to continue for longer.

BEHAVIORAL TREATMENT. The role of habit training has already been described. Biofeedback has a role in the treatment of some children with paradoxical contraction of the pelvic floor muscles on straining, a role confirmed by two controlled trials against conventional treatment.[193, 194] It is most successful if the sensory response of the rectum to distention is normal.[195]

Intractable "Slow-Transit" Constipation

Women with steadily decreasing bowel frequency and increasing abdominal symptoms present a major difficulty in treatment.[24] Figure 12–11 outlines a progressive scheme of management. Extra fiber should always be tried, but it usually fails. It often tends to aggravate the symptom of abdominal bloating without improving bowel frequency. Osmotic laxatives either are ineffective or lead to the urgent passage of a large volume of liquid stool, which is socially difficult. Stimulant laxatives are often used regularly but tend to become ineffective, so that the patient takes larger and larger doses. Such laxatives tend to cause abdominal colic and, in the doses used, to the passage of liquid stools. Regular drinks of a PEG-electrolyte solution, the volume adjusted to give a semisolid stool, may be a useful treatment. Regular enemas may also prove to be an acceptable form of treatment.

Muscular coordination training often helps these patients, even when there is no clear evidence of pelvic floor contraction on straining.[174] When available, a trial of this mode of treatment is indicated for all patients with severe symptoms. The interaction between a sympathetic, confident instructor and the patient may be an important aspect of the training program. These patients are almost all women, and many give a history of sexual abuse as a child or later. Psychological assessment and treatment are often indicated. Selected patients may benefit from colectomy (described earlier), but

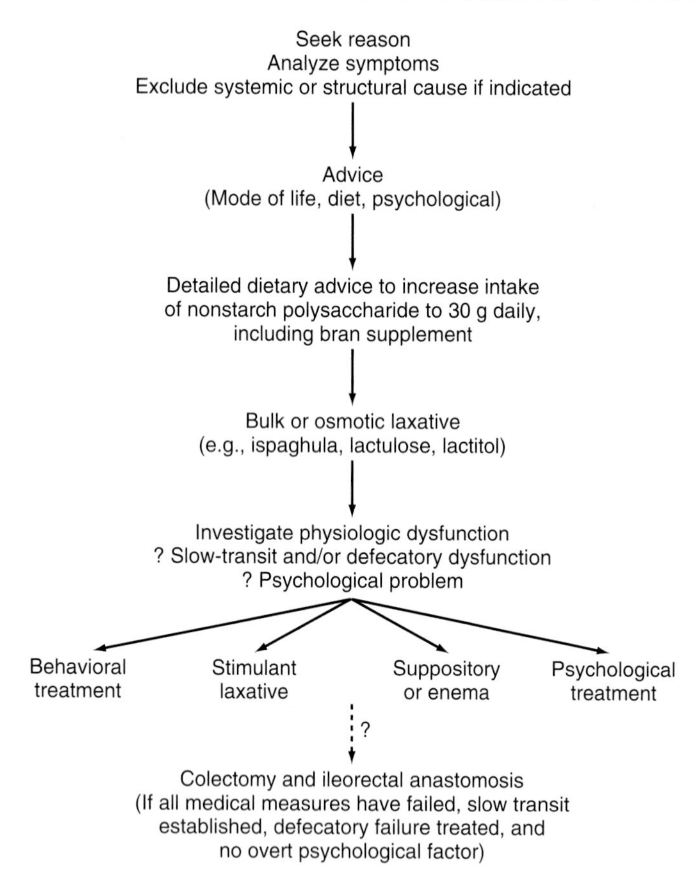

Figure 12–11. Treatment of chronic constipation. The steps shown are successive and only taken if previous measures have failed.

all possible medical measures, including biofeedback, should be tried first, and the patient should fully understand the uncertainty inherent in the procedure (see Chapter 122).

Difficult Defecation

Patients with difficult defecation, usually older women, complain of excessive and ineffective straining. Often, bowel frequency is normal or increased as a result of the ineffective passage of small stools. These patients may be helped by a high-fiber diet or laxatives to soften the stool. Muscular coordination training is often helpful. Evacuant suppositories inserted 30 minutes before attempted defecation with instruction to try to achieve evacuation without excessive or prolonged straining can help.

Pregnancy

In a British series, about 40% of women said that constipation developed at some time during pregnancy. Analysis of the symptoms in those complaining of constipation showed that hardness of the stools, rather than decreased bowel frequency, was the predominant symptom.[196] The main aim of treatment is to achieve soft stools without the use of drugs. Detailed advice to take more fiber in the diet can be effective but, during the later months of pregnancy, women find it uncomfortable to take bulky meals and prefer frequent small meals. A palatable medicinal fiber supplement may therefore be an appropriate measure.

The U.S. Food and Drug Administration (FDA) has established categories of risk for use of drugs in pregnancy.[197] Bulking agents are regarded as harmless, if taken as advised, even though they have not been tested for adverse effects. Caution is advised in the use of magnesium compounds or unabsorbed sugars, although magnesium hydroxide is widely used. Standardized senna and bisacodyl are categorized by the FDA among drugs that are generally regarded as compounds for which benefits outweigh risks. Standardized senna is the first choice when dietary measures or bulking agents are inadequate for relieving symptoms.

Most women take a dose only once a week or less frequently, and the dose should be adjusted to give a soft and formed, rather than liquid, stool.

Laxative Dependence

Patients dependent on daily laxatives are resistant to a change in this habit. If laxatives are abruptly withdrawn, there follows an inevitable interval before a stool is passed because the colon is empty. The delay before the next bowel action after laxatives are stopped should be anticipated and explained to the patient; otherwise, the patient often panics during this delay and resorts to another dose of laxative. If possible, the patient should start a palatable bulk laxative; a bran supplement may give rise to a sense of distention initially and should be avoided at this stage. The patient should also be given a small supply of evacuant suppositories or disposable enemas to use if anxiety about the need to defecate develops. A combination of a bulking supplement by mouth and the ability to use a rectal preparation to stimulate defecation may allow transition from a daily oral laxative to an occasional dose or none. The difficulties of this treatment should not be underestimated; the patient needs to be motivated and requires frequent sympathetic but firm support.

Laxative Abuse

Laxative abuse with the passage of daily liquid stools and the risk of hypokalemia is largely restricted to patients who take the drugs surreptitiously as part of an eating disorder or similar psychological disturbance (see Chapter 9). The so-called cathartic colon with lack of haustration and structural damage is now rarely seen; it was probably caused by toxic laxatives no longer used.[198] However, a blinded comparison by a radiologist of two series of barium enema radiographs, one from a group of constipated patients who took a variety of stimulant laxatives regularly and the other from constipated patients who did not take such laxatives, revealed that loss of haustral folds was a feature of the films from approximately 25% of the laxative takers but none of the control group.[199]

Elderly Patients with Overflow Incontinence

The therapeutic problem in the elderly with overflow incontinence is the same as in childhood (see Fig. 12–10). The cause is different, inasmuch as fecal impaction is often a complication of illness and immobility in the elderly, and use of pain-killing or other constipating drugs is often a factor. Furthermore, the anal sphincter tends to become weaker with age (see Chapter 11).

When an elderly patient is incontinent, it is essential to perform a digital examination of the rectum to determine whether fecal accumulation is present. The rectum is often full of soft, not hard, stool. If fecal accumulation is found, the prime aim of treatment is to empty the rectum, usually by one or more enemas administered at intervals. The use of a PEG-electrolyte solution has been described earlier. Thereafter, the aim must be to keep the rectum empty without causing incontinence. A bran supplement tends to cause bulky, semisolid stools and thus leads to incontinence in the elderly.[200] Similarly, laxatives must be used carefully.

REFERENCES

1. Stanghellini V, Reyniers G, Beerse LP: A European survey of constipation and related behavior in the general population. Gastroenterology 118:A720, 2000.
2. Talley NJ, Weaver AL, Zinsmeister AR, Melton LJ III: Functional constipation and outlet delay: A population-based study. Gastroenterology 105:781, 1993.
3. Talley NJ, O'Keefe EA, Zinsmeister AR, Melton LJ III: Prevalence of gastrointestinal symptoms in the elderly: A population-based study. Gastroenterology 102:895, 1992.
4. Sandler RS, Drossman DA: Bowel habits in young adults not seeking health care. Dig Dis Sci 32:841, 1987.
5. Heaton KW, Cripps HA: Straining at stool and laxative taking in an English population. Dig Dis Sci 38:1004, 1993.
6. Thompson WG, Heaton KW: Functional bowel disorders in apparently healthy people. Gastroenterology 79:283, 1980.
7. Heaton KW, Radvan J, Cripps H, et al: Defecation frequency and timing, and stool form in the general population: A prospective study. Gut 33:818, 1992.
8. Heaton KW, O'Donnell LJD, Braddon FEM, et al: Symptoms of irritable bowel syndrome in a British urban community: Consulters and nonconsulters. Gastroenterology 102:1962, 1992.
9. Dent OF, Goulston KJ, Zubrzycki J, Chapuis PH: Bowel symptoms in an apparently well population. Dis Colon Rectum 29:243, 1986.
10. Welch GW, Pomare EW: Functional gastrointestinal symptoms in a Wellington community sample. NZ Med J 103:418, 1990.
11. Sonnenberg A, Koch TR: Physician visits in the United States for constipation: 1958 to 1986. Dig Dis Sci 34:606, 1989.
12. Johanson JF, Sonnenberg A, Koch TR: Clinical epidemiology of chronic constipation. J Clin Gastroenterol 11:525, 1989.
13. Rasquin-Weber A, Hyman PE, Cucchiara S, et al: Childhood functional gastrointestinal disorders. Gut 45(Suppl 2):60, 1990.
14. Thompson WG, Longstreth GF, Drossman DA, et al: Functional bowel disorders and functional abdominal pain. Gut 45(Suppl 2):43, 1999.
15. Probert CSJ, Emmett PM, Cripps HA, Heaton KW: Evidence for the ambiguity of the term constipation: The role of irritable bowel syndrome. Gut 35:1455, 1994.
16. Chiotakakou-Faliakou E, Kamm MA, Roy AJ, et al: Biofeedback provides long-term benefit for patients with intractable, slow and normal transit constipation. Gut 42:517, 1998.
17. Grotz RL, Pemberton JH, Talley NJ, et al: Discriminant value of psychological distress, symptom profiles, and segmental colonic dysfunction in outpatients with severe idiopathic constipation. Gut 35:798, 1994.
18. Cummings JH, Bingham SA, Heaton KW, Eastwood MA: Fecal weight, colon cancer risk, and dietary intake of non-starch polysaccharides (dietary fiber). Gastroenterology 103:1783, 1992.
19. Kamm MA, Farthing MJG, Lennard-Jones JE, et al: Steroid hormone abnormalities in women with severe idiopathic constipation. Gut 32: 80, 1991.
20. Whitehead WE, Drinkwater D, Cheskin LJ, et al: Constipation in the elderly living at home: Definition, prevalence, and relationship to lifestyle and health status. J Am Geriatr Soc 37:423, 1989.
21. Towers AL, Burgio KL, Locher JL, et al: Constipation in the elderly: Influence of dietary, psychological, and physiological factors. J Am Geriatr Soc 42:701, 1994.
22. Merkel IS, Locher J, Burgio K, et al: Physiologic and psychologic characteristics of an elderly population with chronic constipation. Am J Gastroenterol 88:1854, 1993.
23. Read NW, Abouzekry L, Read MG, et al: Anorectal function in elderly patients with fecal impaction. Gastroenterology 89:959, 1985.
24. Preston DM, Lennard-Jones JE: Severe chronic constipation of young women: "Idiopathic slow transit constipation." Gut 27:41, 1986.
25. Klauser AG, Peyerl C, Schindlbeck NE, Müller-Lissner SA: Nutrition and physical activity in chronic constipation. Eur J Gastroenterol Hepatol 4:227, 1992.
26. Sandler RS, Jordan MC, Shelton BJ: Demographic and dietary determinants of constipation in the US population. Am J Public Health 80: 185, 1990.
27. Bingham SA, Cummings JH: Effect of exercise and physical fitness on large intestinal function. Gastroenterology 97:1389, 1989.
28. Stephen AM, Wiggins HS, Cummings JH: Effect of changing transit time on colonic microbial metabolism in man. Gut 28:601, 1987.
29. Stephen AM, Cummings JH: The microbial contribution to human faecal mass. J Med Microbiol 13:45, 1980.
30. Cummings JH: Non-starch polysaccharides (dietary fibre) including bulk laxatives in constipation. In Kamm MA, Lennard-Jones JE (eds): Constipation. Petersfield, England, Wrightson Biomedical Publishing, 1994, pp 307–314.
31. Cummings JH, Southgate DAT, Branch W, et al: Colonic response to dietary fibre from carrot, cabbage, apple, bran, and guar gum. Lancet 1:5, 1978.
32. Müller-Lissner SA: Effect of wheat bran on weight of stool and gastrointestinal transit time: A meta-analysis. BMJ 296:615, 1988.
33. Kirwan WO, Smith AN, McConnell AA, et al: Action of different bran preparations on colonic function. BMJ 4:187, 1974.
34. Tomlin J, Read NW: Laxative properties of indigestible plastic particles. BMJ 297:1175, 1988.
35. Devroede G, Soffié M: Colonic absorption in idiopathic constipation. Gastroenterology 64:552, 1973.
36. Preston DM, Lennard-Jones JE, Thomas BM: Towards a radiologic definition of idiopathic megacolon. Gastrointest Radiol 10:167, 1985.
37. Bassotti G, Iantorno G, Fiorella S, et al: Colonic motility in man: Features in normal subjects and in patients with chronic idiopathic constipation. Am J Gastroenterol 94:1760, 1999.
38. Bassotti G, Gaburri M, Imbimbo BP, et al: Colonic mass movements in idiopathic chronic constipation. Gut 29:1173, 1988.
39. Bassotti G, Betti C, Pelli MA, Morelli A: Prolonged (24-hour) manometric recording of rectal contractile activity in patients with slow transit constipation. Digestion 49:72, 1991.
40. Bassotti G, Imbimbo BP, Betti C, et al: Impaired colonic motor response to eating in patients with slow-transit constipation. Am J Gastroenterol 87:504, 1992.
41. Bassotti G, Chiarioni G, Imbimbo BP, et al: Impaired colonic motor response to cholinergic stimulation in patients with severe chronic idiopathic (slow transit type) constipation. Dig Dis Sci 38:1040, 1993.
42. Stivland T, Camilleri M, Vassallo M, et al: Scintigraphic measurement of regional gut transit in idiopathic constipation. Gastroenterology 101: 107, 1991.
43. van der Sijp JRM, Kamm MA, Nightingale JMD, et al: Radioisotope determination of regional colonic transit in severe constipation: Comparison with radiopaque markers. Gut 34:402, 1993.
44. Krishnamurthy S, Schuffler MM, Rohrmann CA, Pope ICE: Severe idiopathic constipation is associated with a distinctive abnormality of the colonic myenteric plexus. Gastroenterology 88:26, 1985.
45. Sninsky CA, Davis RH, Clench MH, et al: Severe idiopathic intestinal constipation: Comparison of histology and gastrointestinal tracing in human subjects. Gastroenterology 86:A1259, 1984.
46. Schouten WR, ten Kate FJ, de Graaf EJ, et al: Visceral neuropathy in slow transit constipation: An immunohistochemical investigation with monoclonal antibodies against neurofilament. Dis Colon Rectum 36: 1112, 1993.
47. Chong-Liang HE, Burgart L, Wang L, et al: Decreased interstitial cell of Cajal volume in patients with slow-transit constipation. Gastroenterology 118:14, 2000.
48. Altomare D, Pilot M-A, Scott M, et al: Detection of subclinical autonomic neuropathy in constipated patients using a sweat test. Gut 33: 1539, 1992.
49. Emmanuel AV, Kamm MA: Laser Doppler flowmetry as a measure of extrinsic colonic innervation in functional bowel disease. Gut 46:212, 2000.
50. Varma JS, Smith AN: Neurophysiological dysfunction in young women with intractable constipation. Gut 29:963, 1988.

51. Kerrigan DD, Lucas MG, Sun WM, et al: Idiopathic constipation associated with impaired urethrovesical and sacral reflex function. Br J Surg 76:748, 1989.
52. Watier A, Devroede G, Duranceau A, et al: Constipation with colonic inertia: A manifestation of systemic disease? Dig Dis Sci 28:1025, 1983.
53. Kamm MA, van der Sijp J, Lennard-Jones JE: Colorectal and anal motility during defaecation. Lancet 339:820, 1992.
54. Halls J: Bowel content shift during normal defaecation [summary]. Proc R Soc Med 58:859, 1965.
55. Klauser AG, Voderholzer WA, Heinrich CA, et al: Behavioral modification of colonic function: Can constipation be learned? Dig Dis Sci 35:1271, 1990.
56. Tagart REB: The anal canal and rectum: Their varying relationship and its effect on anal continence. Dis Colon Rectum 9:449, 1966.
57. Roberts JP, Womack NR, Hallan RI, et al: Evidence from dynamic integrated proctography to redefine anismus. Br J Surg 79:1213, 1992.
58. Halligan S, Thomas J, Bartram C: Intrarectal pressures and balloon expulsion related to evacuation proctography. Gut 37:100, 1995.
59. Read NW, Timms JM, Barfield LJ, et al: Impairment of defecation in young women with severe constipation. Gastroenterology 90:53, 1986.
60. Kamm MA, Lennard-Jones JE: Rectal mucosal electrosensory testing—evidence for a rectal sensory neuropathy in idiopathic constipation: Report of two cases. Dis Colon Rectum 33:419, 1990.
61. Bannister JJ, Davison P, Timms JM, et al: Effect of stool size and consistency on defecation. Gut 28:1246, 1987.
62. Tucker DM, Sandstead HH, Logan GM Jr, et al: Dietary fiber and personality factors as determinants of stool output. Gastroenterology 81:879, 1981.
63. Bennett EJ, Evans P, Scott AM, et al: Psychological and sex features of delayed gut transit in functional gastrointestinal disorders. Gut 46: 83, 2000.
64. Emmanuel AV, Mason HJ, Kamm MA: Relationship between psychological state and level of activity of extrinsic gut innervation in patients with a functional gut disorder. Gut 49:209, 2001.
65. Almy TP: Experimental studies on the irritable colon. Am J Med 9: 60, 1951.
66. Sandler RS, Drossman DA, Nathan HP, McKee DC: Symptom complaints and health care–seeking behavior in subjects with bowel dysfunction. Gastroenterology 87:314, 1984.
67. Shafer RB, Prentiss RA, Bond JH: Gastrointestinal transit in thyroid disease. Gastroenterology 86:852, 1984.
68. Werth B, Meyer-Wyss B, Spinas GA, et al: Noninvasive assessment of gastrointestinal motility disorders in diabetic patients with and without cardiovascular signs of autonomic neuropathy. Gut 33:1199, 1992.
69. Battle WM, Snape WJ Jr, Alavi A, et al: Colonic dysfunction in diabetes mellitus. Gastroenterology 79:1217, 1980.
70. Singaram C, Ashraf W, Gaumnitz EA, et al: Dopaminergic defect of enteric nervous system in Parkinson's disease patients with chronic constipation. Lancet 346:861, 1995.
71. Mathers SE, Kempster PA, Swash M, Lees AJ: Constipation and paradoxical puborectalis contraction in anismus and Parkinson's disease: A dystonic phenomenon? J Neurol Neurosurg Psychiatry 51: 1503, 1988.
72. Hinds JP, Eidelman BH, Wald A: Prevalence of bowel dysfunction in multiple sclerosis. Gastroenterology 98:1538, 1990.
73. Glick ME, Meshkinpour H, Haldeman S, et al: Colonic dysfunction in multiple sclerosis. Gastroenterology 83:1002, 1982.
74. Weber J, Grise P, Roquebert M, et al: Radiopaque markers transit and anorectal manometry in 16 patients with multiple sclerosis and urinary bladder dysfunction. Dis Colon Rectum 30:95, 1987.
75. Sørensen M, Lorentzen M, Petersen J, Christiansen J: Anorectal dysfunction in patients with urologic disturbance due to multiple sclerosis. Dis Colon Rectum 34:136, 1991.
76. Wiesel PH, Norton C, Roy AJ, et al: Gut-focused behavioural treatment (biofeedback) for constipation and faecal incontinence in multiple sclerosis. J Neurol Neurosurg Psychiatry 69:240, 2000.
77. Weber J: Constipation in spinal cord lesions, multiple sclerosis, and diabetes mellitus. In Kamm MA, Lennard-Jones JE (eds): Constipation. Petersfield, England, Wrightson Biomedical Publishing, 1994, pp 273–277.
78. Glick ME, Meshkinpour H, Haldeman S, et al: Colonic dysfunction in patients with thoracic spinal cord injury. Gastroenterology 86:287, 1984.
79. MacDonagh R, Sun WM, Thomas DG, et al: Anorectal function in patients with complete supraconal spinal cord lesions. Gut 33:1532, 1992.
80. MacDonagh RP, Sun WM, Smallwood R, et al: Control of defecation in patients with spinal injuries by stimulation of sacral anterior nerve roots. BMJ 300:1494, 1990.
81. Binnie NR, Smith AN, Creasey GH, Edmond P: Constipation associated with chronic spinal cord injury: The effect of pelvic parasympathetic stimulation by the Brindley stimulator. Paraplegia 29:463, 1991.
82. Christensen J: Morphology of the innervation of the large intestine and the neuropathology of constipation. In Kamm MA, Lennard-Jones JE (eds): Constipation. Petersfield, England, Wrightson Biomedical Publishing, 1994, pp 33–40.
83. Devroede G, Lamarche J: Functional importance of extrinsic parasympathetic innervation to the distal colon and rectum in man. Gastroenterology 66:273, 1974.
84. Devroede G, Arhan P, Duguay C, et al: Traumatic constipation. Gastroenterology 77:1258, 1979.
85. Kamm MA, Hoyle CHV, Burleigh DE, et al: Hereditary internal anal sphincter myopathy causing proctalgia fugax and constipation. Gastroenterology 100:805, 1991.
86. Celik AF, Katsinelos P, Read NW, et al: Hereditary proctalgia fugax and constipation: Report of a second family. Gut 36:581, 1995.
87. Cohen S, Laufer I, Snape WJ Jr, et al: The gastrointestinal manifestations of scleroderma: Pathogenesis and management. Gastroenterology 79:155, 1980.
88. Nowak TV, Ionasescu V, Anuras S: Gastrointestinal manifestations of the muscular dystrophies. Gastroenterology 82:800, 1982.
89. Eckardt V, Nix W: The anal sphincter in patients with myotonic muscular dystrophy. Gastroenterology 100:424, 1991.
90. Milla PJ, Smith V: Aganglionosis, hypoganglionosis, and hyperganglionosis: Clinical presentation and histopathology. In Kamm MA, Lennard-Jones JE (eds): Constipation. Petersfield, England, Wrightson Biomedical Publishing, 1994, pp 183–192.
91. Wilder-Smith CH, Meier-Ruge W, Scheurer U, et al: Colonic neuronal dysplasia: An ignored cause of constipation in adults? Eur J Gastroenterol Hepatol 4:679, 1992.
92. Koletzko S, Jesch I, Faus-Kebler T, et al: Rectal biopsy for diagnosis of intestinal neuronal dysplasia in children: A prospective multicentre study on interobserver variation and clinical outcome. Gut 44:853, 1999.
93. Miles MM: Chagas' disease and Chagasic megacolon. In Kamm MA, Lennard-Jones JE (eds): Constipation. Petersfield, England, Wrightson Biomedical Publishing, 1994, pp 205–210.
94. Chinn JS, Schuffler MD: Paraneoplastic visceral neuropathy as a cause of severe gastrointestinal motor dysfunction. Gastroenterology 95: 1279, 1988.
95. Lennon VA, Sas DF, Busk MF, et al: Enteric neuronal autoantibodies in psuedo-obstruction with small-cell lung carcinoma. Gastroenterology 100:137, 1991.
96. Bartram CI, Turnbull GK, Lennard-Jones JE: Evacuation proctography: An investigation of rectal expulsion in 20 subjects without defecatory disturbance. Gastrointest Radiol 13:72, 1988.
97. Shorvon PJ, McHugh S, Diamant NE, et al: Defecography in normal volunteers: Results and implications. Gut 30:1737, 1989.
98. Siproudhis L, Dautreme S, Ropert A, et al: Dyschezia and rectocele—a marriage of convenience? Physiologic evaluation of the rectocele in a group of 52 women complaining of difficulty in evacuation. Dis Colon Rectum 36:1030, 1993.
99. van Dam JH, Ginai AZ, Gosselink MJ, et al: Role of defecography in predicting clinical outcome of rectocele repair. Dis Colon Rectum 40: 201, 1997.
100. Van Laarhoven CJHM, Kamm MA, Bartram CI, et al: Relationship between anatomic and symptomatic long-term results after rectocele repair for impaired defecation. Dis Colon Rectum 42:204, 1999.
101. Snooks SJ, Barnes PRH, Swash M, Henry WL: Damage to the innervation of the pelvic floor musculature in chronic constipation. Gastroenterology 89:977, 1985.
102. Halligan S, Nicholls RJ, Bartram CI: Evacuation proctography in patients with solitary rectal ulcer syndrome: Anatomic abnormalities and frequency of impaired emptying and prolapse. Am J Roentgenol 164: 91, 1995.
103. Vaisey CJ, van den Bogaerde JB, Emmanuel AV, et al: Solitary ulcer syndrome. Br J Surg 85:1617, 1998.
104. Vaisey CJ, Roy AJ, Kamm MA: Prospective evaluation of the treatment of solitary rectal ulcer syndrome with biofeedback. Gut 41:817, 1997.

105. Sitzler PJ, Kamm MA, Nicholls RJ, McKee RF: Long-term clinical outcome of surgery for solitary rectal ulcer syndrome. Br J Surg 85: 1246, 1998.
106. Speakman CTM, Madden MV, Nicholls RJ, Kamm MA: Lateral ligament division during rectopexy causes constipation but prevents recurrence: Results of a prospective randomised study. Br J Surg 78:1431, 1991.
107. Garvey M, Noyes RJ, Yates W: Frequency of constipation in major depression: Relationship to other clinical variables. Psychosomatics 31:204, 1990.
108. Kamal N, Chami T, Andersen A, et al: Delayed gastrointestinal transit times in anorexia nervosa and bulimia nervosa. Gastroenterology 101: 1320, 1991.
109. Chun AB, Sokol MS, Kaye WH, et al: Colonic and anorectal function in constipated patients with anorexia nervosa. Am J Gastroenterol 92: 1879, 1997.
110. Chiarioni G, Bassotti G, Monsignori A, Menegotti M, et al: Anorectal dysfunction in constipated women with anorexia nervosa. Mayo Clin Proc 75:1015, 2000.
111. Diamant NE, Kamm MA, Wald A, Whitehead WE: American Gastroenterological Association medical position statement on anorectal testing techniques. Gastroenterology 116:732, 1999.
112. Whitehead WE, Wald A, Diamant NE, et al: Functional disorders of the anus and rectum. Gut 45(Suppl 2):55, 1999.
113. Metcalf AM, Phillips SM, Zinsmeister AR, et al: Simplified assessment of segmental colonic transit. Gastroenterology 92:40, 1987.
114. Evans RC, Kamm MA, Hinton JM, Lennard-Jones JE: The normal range and a simple diagram for recording whole-gut transit time. Int J Colorect Dis 7:15, 1992.
115. Halligan S, Bartram CI, Park HJ, Kamm MA: The proctographic features of anismus. Radiology 197:679, 1995.
116. Graham DY, Moser SE, Estes MK: The effect of bran on bowel function in constipation. Am J Gastroenterol 77:599, 1982.
117. Badiali D, Corazziari E, Habib FI, et al: Effect of wheat bran in treatment of chronic nonorganic constipation: A double-blind controlled trial. Dig Dis Sci 40:349, 1995.
118. Chaussade S, Khyari A, Roche H, et al: Determination of total and segmental colonic transit time in constipated patients: Results in 91 patients with a new simplified method. Dig Dis Sci 34:1168, 1989.
119. Hamilton JW, Wagner J, Burdick BB, Bass P: Clinical evaluation of methyl cellulose as a bulk laxative. Dig Dis Sci 33:993, 1988.
120. Marlett JA, Li BUK, Patrow CJ, Bass P: Comparative laxation of psyllium with and without senna in an ambulatory constipated population. Am J Gastroenterol 82:333, 1987.
121. Voderholzer WA, Schatke W, Muhldorfer BE, et al: Clinical response to dietary fiber treatment of chronic constipation. Am J Gastroenterol 92:95, 1997.
122. Lantner RR, Espiritu BR, Zumerchik P, Tobin MC: Anaphylaxis following ingestion of a psyllium-containing cereal. JAMA 264:2534, 1990.
123. Culbert P, Gillett H, Ferguson A: Highly effective oral therapy (polyethylene glycol/electrolyte solution) for faecal impaction and severe constipation. Clin Drug Invest 16:355, 1998.
124. Puxty JA, Fox RA: Golytely—a new approach to faecal impaction in old age. Age Ageing 15:182, 1986.
125. Ingebo KB, Heyman MB: Polyethylene glycol–electrolyte solution for intestinal clearance in children with refractory encopresis. Am J Dis Child 142:340, 1988.
126. Tolia V, Lin C, Elitsur Y: A prospective randomized study with mineral oil and oral lavage solution for treatment of faecal impaction in children. Aliment Pharmacol Ther 7:523, 1993.
127. Andorsky RI, Goldner F: Colonic lavage solution (polyethylene glycol–electrolyte lavage solution) as a treatment for chronic constipation: A double-blind, placebo-controlled study. Am J Gastroenterol 85: 261, 1990.
128. Corazziari E, Badiali D, Habib FI, et al: Small-volume isosmotic polyethylene glycol–electrolyte balanced solution (PMF-100) in treatment of chronic nonorganic constipation. Dig Dis Sci 41:1636, 1996.
129. DiPalma JA, DeRidder PH, Orlando RC, et al: A randomized, placebo-controlled, multicenter study of the safety and efficacy of a new polyethylene glycol laxative. Am J Gastroenterol 95:446, 2000.
130. Corazziari E, Badiali D, Bazzocchi G, et al: Long-term efficacy, safety, and tolerability of low daily doses of isosmotic polyethylene glycol–electrolyte balanced solution (PMF-100) in the treatment of functional chronic constipation. Gut 46:522, 2000.
131. Dupont C, Ammar F, Leluyer B, et al: Polyethylene glycol (PEG) 4000 in constipated children (6 months–15 years): A dose determination study. Gastroenterology 118:A846, 2000.
132. Attar A, Lémann M, Ferguson A, et al: Comparison of a low-dose polyethylene glycol–electrolyte solution with lactulose for treatment of chronic constipation. Gut 44:226, 1999.
133. Freedman MD, Schwartz HJ, Roby R, Fleisher S: Tolerance and efficacy of polyethylene glycol 3350/electrolyte solution versus lactulose in relieving opiate-induced constipation: A double-blinded placebo-controlled trial. J Clin Pharmacol 37:904, 1997.
134. Smith RG, Curry AE, Walls AD: Whole-gut irrigation: A new treatment for constipation. BMJ 3:396, 1978.
135. Florent C, Flourie B, Rautureau M, et al: Influence of chronic lactulose ingestion on the colonic metabolism of lactulose in man. J Clin Invest 75:608, 1985.
136. Bass P, Dennis S: The laxative effect of lactulose in normal and constipated subjects. J Clin Gastroenterol 3(Suppl 1):23, 1981.
137. Wesselius-de Casparis A, Braadbaart S, Bergh-Bohlken GE, Mimica M: Treatment of chronic constipation with lactulose syrup: Results of a double-blind study. Gut 9:84, 1968.
138. Sanders JF: Lactulose syrup assessed in a double-blind study of elderly constipated patients. J Am Geriatr Soc 26:236, 1978.
139. Wright RA: Lactulose-induced megacolon. Gastrointest Endosc 34: 489, 1988.
140. Vanderdonckt J, Coulon J, Denys W, Ravelli GP: Study of the laxative effect of lactitol (Importal) in an elderly institutionalized, but not bedridden, population suffering from chronic constipation. J Clin Exper Gerontol 12:171, 1990.
141. Hyams JS: Sorbitol intolerance: An unappreciated cause of functional gastrointestinal complaints. Gastroenterology 84:30, 1983.
142. Rumessen JJ, Gudmand-Hoyer E: Malabsorption of fructose-sorbitol mixtures: Interactions causing abdominal distress. Scand J Gastroenterol 22:431, 1987.
143. Lederle FA, Busch DL, Mattox KM, et al: Cost-effective treatment of constipation in the elderly: A randomized double-blind comparison of sorbitol and lactulose. Am J Med 89:597, 1990.
144. Donowitz M, Rood RP: Magnesium hydroxide: New insights into the mechanism of its laxative effect and the potential involvement of prostaglandin E_2. J Clin Gastroenterol 14:20, 1992.
145. Alison LH, Bulugahapitiya D: Laxative-induced magnesium poisoning in a 6-week-old infant. BMJ 300:125, 1990.
146. Ashton MR, Sutton D, Nielsen M: Severe magnesium toxicity after magnesium sulphate enema in a chronically constipated child. BMJ 300:541, 1990.
147. Exton-Smith AN, Bendall MJ, Kent F: A new technique for measuring the consistency of faeces: A report on its application to the assessment of Senokot therapy in the elderly. Age Ageing 4:58, 1975.
148. Rudolph RL, Mengs U: Electron microscopical studies on rat intestine after long-term treatment with sennosides. Pharmacology 36(Suppl 1): 188, 1988.
149. Fioramonti J, Dupuy C, Bueno L: In vivo motility of rat colon chronically pretreated with sennosides. Pharmacology 41(Suppl 1):155, 1993.
150. Riecken EO, Zeitz M, Emde C, et al: A prospective study on the effect of anthraquinone-containing laxatives on ultrastructure of colonic nerves. Gastroenterology 92:1595, 1987.
151. Mengs U, Rudolph RL: Light and electron-microscopic changes in the colon of the guinea pig after treatment with anthranoid and non-anthranoid laxatives. Pharmacology 47(Suppl 1):172, 1993.
152. Badiali D, Marcheggiano A, Pallone F, et al: Melanosis of the rectum in patients with chronic constipation. Dis Colon Rectum 28:241, 1985.
153. Whitehead WE, Chaussade S, Corazziari E, Kumar D: Report of an international workshop on management of constipation. Gastroenterol Int 4:99, 1991.
154. Kamm MA, Lennard-Jones JE, Thompson DG, et al: Dynamic scanning defines a colonic defect in severe idiopathic constipation. Gut 29: 1085, 1988.
155. Moriarty KJ, Kelly MJ, Beetham R, Clark ML: Studies on the mechanism of action of dioctyl sodium sulphosuccinate in the human jejunum. Gut 26:1008, 1985.
156. Chapman RW, Sillery J, Fontana DD, et al: Effect of oral dioctyl sodium sulfosuccinate on intake-output studies of human small and large intestine. Gastroenterology 89:489, 1985.
157. Hyland CM, Foran JD: Dioctyl sodium sulphosuccinate as a laxative in the elderly. Practitioner 200:698, 1968.
158. Müller-Lissner SA, Bavarian Constipation study group: Treatment of chronic constipation with cisapride and placebo. Gut 28:1033, 1987.

159. Emmanuel AV, Kamm MA, Roy AJ, Antonelli K: Effect of a novel prokinetic drug, R093877, on gastrointestinal transit in normal volunteers. Gut 42:511, 1998.
160. Emmanuel AV, Nicholls T, Roy AJ, et al: Prucalopride (PRU) improves colonic transit and stool frequency in patients (PTS) with slow and normal transit constipation. Gastroenterology 118:A846, 2000.
161. Prather CM, Camilleri M, Zinsmeister AR, et al: Tegaserod accelerates orocecal transit in patients with constipation-predominant irritable bowel syndrome. Gastroenterology 118:463, 2000.
162. Passmore AP, Wilson-Davies K, Stoker C, Scott ME: Chronic constipation in long-stay elderly patients: A comparison of lactulose and a senna-fibre combination. BMJ 307:769, 1993.
163. Andrews PJ, Barnes PRH, Borody TJ: Chronic constipation reversed by restoration of bowel flora: A case and a hypothesis. Eur J Gastroenterol Hepatol 4:245, 1992.
164. Celik AF, Tomlin J, Read NW: The effect of oral vancomycin on chronic idiopathic constipation. Aliment Pharmacol Ther 9:63, 1995.
165. Meisel JL, Bergman D, Graney D, et al: Human rectal mucosa: Proctoscopic and morphological changes caused by laxatives. Gastroenterology 72:1274, 1977.
166. Spinrad S, Grosskopf Y, Blum I, et al: Treating constipation with phosphate enema: An unnecessary risk. Isr J Med Sci 25:237, 1989.
167. Rohack JJ, Mehta BR, Subramanyam K: Hyperphosphatemia and hypocalcemic coma associated with phosphate enema. South Med J 78: 1241, 1985.
168. Davies RF, Eichner JM, Bleyer WA, Okamoto G: Hypocalcaemia, hyperphosphatemia, and dehydration following a single hypertonic phosphate enema. J Pediatr 90:484, 1977.
169. Koutsomanis D, Lennard-Jones JE, Roy AJ, Kamm MA: Controlled randomised trial of visual biofeedback versus muscle training without a visual display for intractable constipation. Gut 36:95, 1995.
170. Bleijenberg G, Kuijpers HC: Treatment of the spastic pelvic floor syndrome with biofeedback. Dis Colon Rectum 30:108, 1987.
171. Heymen S, Wexner SD, Vickers D, et al: Prospective, randomized trial comparing four biofeedback techniques for patients with constipation. Dis Colon Rectum 42:1388, 1999.
172. Lau CW, Heymen S, Alabaz O, et al: Prognostic significance of rectocele, intussusception, and abnormal perineal descent in biofeedback treatment for constipated patients with paradoxical puborectalis contraction. Dis Colon Rectum 43:478, 2000.
173. Papachrysostomou M, Smith AN: Effects of biofeedback on obstructive defecation—reconditioning of the defecation reflex? Gut 35:252, 1994.
174. Emmanuel AV, Kamm MA: Response to a behavioral treatment, biofeedback, in constipated patients is associated with improved gut transit and autonomic innervation. Gut 49:214, 2001.
175. Dahl J, Lindquist BL, Tysk C, et al: Behavioral medicine treatment in chronic constipation with paradoxical anal sphincter contraction. Dis Colon Rectum 34:769, 1991.
176. Rao SS, Welcher KD, Leistikow JS: Obstructive defecation: A failure of rectoanal coordination. Am J Gastroenterol 93:1042, 1998.
177. Harewood GC, Coulie B, Camilleri M, et al: Descending perineum syndrome: Audit of clinical and laboratory features and outcome of pelvic floor retraining. Am J Gastroenterol 94:126, 1999.
178. Roy AJ, Emmanuel AV, Storrie JB, et al: Behavioural treatment (biofeedback) for constipation following hysterectomy. Br J Surg 87:100, 2000.
179. Knowles CH, Scott M, Lunniss PJ: Outcome of colectomy for slow-transit constipation. Ann Surg 230:627, 1999.
180. Leon SH, Krishnamurthy S, Schuffler MD: Subtotal colectomy for severe idiopathic constipation: A follow-up study of 13 patients. Dig Dis Sci 32:1249, 1987.
181. Kamm MA, Hawley PR, Lennard-Jones JE: Outcome of colectomy for severe idiopathic constipation. Gut 29:969, 1988.
182. Fisher SE, Breckton K, Andrews HA, Keighley MRB: Psychiatric screening for patients with faecal incontinence or chronic constipation referred for surgical treatment. Br J Surg 76:352, 1989.
183. Nyam DC, Pemberton JH, Ilstrup DM, Rath DM: Long-term results of surgery for constipation. Dis Colon Rectum 40:273, 1997.
184. Pemberton JH, Rath DM, Ilstrup DM: Evaluation and surgical treatment of severe chronic constipation. Ann Surg 14:403, 1991.
185. Nicholls RJ, Kamm MA: Proctocolectomy with restorative ileoanal reservoir for severe idiopathic constipation. Dis Colon Rectum 31:968, 1988.
186. Christiansen J, Rasmussen OO: Colectomy for severe slow-transit constipation in strictly selected patients. Scand J Gastroenterol 31:770, 1996.
187. van der Sijp JR, Kamm MA, Evans RC, Lennard-Jones JE: The results of stoma formation in severe idiopathic constipation. Eur J Gastroenterol Hepatol 4:137, 1992.
188. Teichman JM, Barber DB, Rogenes VJ, Harris JM: Malone antegrade continence enemas for autonomic dysreflexia secondary to neurogenic bowel. J Spinal Cord Med 21:245, 1998.
189. Yang CC, Stiens SA: Antegrade continence enema for the treatment of neurogenic constipation and fecal incontinence after spinal cord injury. Arch Phys Med Rehabil 81:683, 2000.
190. Kamm MA, Hawley PR, Lennard-Jones JE: Lateral division of the puborectalis muscle in the management of severe constipation. Br J Surg 75:661, 1988.
191. Loening-Baucke V: Chronic constipation in children. Gastroenterology 105:1557, 1993.
192. Nolan T, Debelle G, Oberklaid F, Coffey C: Randomised trial of laxatives in treatment of childhood encopresis. Lancet 338:523, 1991.
193. Wald A, Chandra R, Gabel S, Chiponis D: Evaluation of biofeedback in childhood encopresis. J Pediatr Gastroenterol Nutr 554:558, 1987.
194. Loening-Baucke V: Modulation of abnormal defecation dynamics by biofeedback treatment in chronically constipated children with encopresis. J Pediatr 116:214, 1990.
195. Loening-Baucke V: Persistence of chronic constipation in children after biofeedback treatment. Dig Dis Sci 36:153, 1991.
196. Anderson AS: Dietary factors in the aetiology and treatment of constipation during pregnancy. Br J Obstet Gynaecol 93:245, 1986.
197. Lewis JH, Weingold AB, and Committee on FDA-Related Matters, American College of Gastroenterology: The use of gastrointestinal drugs during pregnancy and lactation. Am J Gastroenterol 80:912, 1985.
198. Müller-Lissner SA: Adverse effects of laxatives: Facts and fictions. Pharmacology 41(Suppl 1):138, 1993.
199. Joo JS, Ehrenpreis ED, Gonzalez L, et al: Alterations in colonic anatomy induced by chronic stimulant laxatives: The cathartic colon revisited. J Clin Gastroenterol 26:283, 1998.
200. Ardron ME, Main ANH: Management of constipation. BMJ 300:1400, 1990.

Chapter 13

GASTROINTESTINAL BLEEDING

Don C. Rockey

The extensive clinical spectrum of gastrointestinal bleeding may encompass many different clinical scenarios. The reason for its diversity is that bleeding can occur from multiple different lesions and sites in the gastrointestinal tract. Further, bleeding may be massive or trivial, obvious or hidden. Gastrointestinal bleeding takes one of the four following forms: (1) upper, (2) lower, (3) occult, i.e., unknown to the patient, or (4) obscure—meaning from an unknown site in the gastrointestinal tract. Patients with occult and/or evident but obscure bleeding are particularly challenging since they are unaware of bleeding, or the bleeding is difficult to diagnose accurately, or both.

Gastrointestinal bleeding results in over 300,000 hospitalizations annually in the United States.[1] Bleeding from the upper gastrointestinal tract is approximately five times more common than from the lower gastrointestinal tract.[2, 3] It is more common in men and elderly people.[2, 3]

Despite a number of recent advances in the management of patients with gastrointestinal bleeding, several fundamental clinical principles remain constant, the most important of which is immediate assessment and stabilization of the patient's hemodynamic status. Thereafter, one must (1) determine the source of bleeding, (2) stop active bleeding, (3) treat the underlying abnormality, and (4) prevent recurrent bleeding.

CLINICAL PRESENTATION

In general, the clinical signs of gastrointestinal bleeding reflect the site, etiology, and rate of bleeding. Blood loss from the gastrointestinal tract is manifest in one or more ways. *Hematemesis* is defined as the vomiting of blood and indicates an upper gastrointestinal site of bleeding, almost always proximal to the ligament of Treitz. Such blood may be either fresh, bright red blood, or it may be old and take on the appearance of coffee grounds. *Melena* is defined as passage of black, tarry, and foul-smelling stools. The black, tarry character of melena is due to degradation of blood to hematin or other hemochromes by bacteria and should not be confused with the greenish character of ingested iron or the black, nonfoul-smelling stool caused by ingestion of bismuth (i.e., in compounds such as bismuth subsalicylate [Pepto-Bismol]). *Hematochezia* refers to passage of bright red blood from the rectum that may or may not be mixed with stool. *Occult* bleeding denotes bleeding that is not apparent to the patient and results from small amounts of bleeding. Bleeding of *obscure* origin can be occult or obvious (e.g., manifest by hematemesis, melena, or hematochezia), but from a source that is difficult to pinpoint on routine examination.

Initial Patient Assessment

The first step in treating all patients with gastrointestinal bleeding is to assess the severity of bleeding. Therefore, hemodynamics is the initial focal point (Table 13–1), the basis for assessment of the patients' overall clinical condition. Not only does immediate and constant assessment of the vital signs help focus resuscitation efforts, it also provides important prognostic information and helps triage patients toward appropriate intervention. For example, patients with unstable vital signs are often bleeding from major vascular sources such as an ulcer with a visible vessel or gastroesophageal varices; moreover, the prognosis of these patients is poorer than that of those with normal vital signs.

Resuscitation

The vigor of resuscitation is proportional to the severity of bleeding. Two large-bore intravenous catheters should be

Table 13–1 | **Hemodynamics, Vital Signs, and Blood Loss**

HEMODYNAMICS (Vital Signs)	BLOOD LOSS (%) (Fraction of Intravascular Volume)	SEVERITY OF BLEED
Shock (Resting hypotension)	20–25	Massive
Postural (Orthostatic tachycardia/hypotension)	10–20	Moderate
Normal	<10	Minor

placed immediately in patients who are hemodynamically unstable. Colloid (normal saline or lactated Ringer's solution) is infused as rapidly as the patient's cardiovascular system will allow. The goal is to restore and maintain normal vital signs. Intensive care unit (ICU) monitoring is indicated in hemodynamically unstable patients. Administration of supplemental oxygen by nasal cannula or facemask is indicated in most patients. Vital signs and urine output should be monitored closely, and in selected situations (for patients with underlying cardiopulmonary disease), central venous monitoring is helpful.

The decision to transfuse the patient with gastrointestinal bleeding is often complicated and requires understanding of all aspects of the clinical situation. Virtually all patients with unstable vital signs should be transfused, and if the patient has subnormal tissue oxygenation, transfusion should be aggressive. This principle applies also to patients who are likely to have gastrointestinal lesions that bleed massively. During resuscitation, patients with continued instability in vital signs, containing bleeding, symptoms of poor tissue oxygenation, or persistently low hematocrit values (20% to 25%) likewise should be transfused continuously. The target to which the hematocrit should be raised varies; in elderly patients it should be 30%, whereas in younger, otherwise healthy patients, hematocrit values in the 20% to 25% range may be satisfactory; in those with portal hypertension, it should not be above 27% to 28%. Packed red blood cells are preferred. Whole blood transfusions are reserved for the unusual patient with rapid, high-volume blood loss who cannot be cross-matched in a timely fashion. Fresh-frozen plasma or platelets or both should be administered to patients with defects in coagulation. Patients requiring greater than 10 units of packed red blood cells should receive fresh-frozen plasma or platelets or both. Warmed blood should be administered to patients requiring massive transfusions (i.e., >3000 mL). The hematocrit should be checked after each transfusion,[4] with the knowledge that serial hematocrits are not a substitute for ongoing clinical assessment (see Laboratory Evaluation). When blood transfusion is deemed unnecessary, iron supplementation is indicated after the completion of diagnostic testing.

History, Symptoms, and Signs

As the patient's hemodynamics are being assessed and while the patient is being stabilized, the clinical history becomes important. The history helps the clinician assess the severity of bleeding and make a preliminary assessment of the site and cause (Table 13–2). Age is an important component of the history. Elderly patients may bleed from a number of diseases less common in younger persons (i.e., diverticula, ischemic colitis, cancer), whereas bleeding in younger patients is more likely from ulcer disease, esophagitis, or varices. Bleeding in patients under 30 years of age may be due to Meckel's diverticula, which is rare in older patients. Known previous gastrointestinal disease or prior bleeding focuses the differential diagnosis immediately on bleeding from a similar source (e.g., hereditary hemorrhagic telangiectasia, ulcer disease, diverticular bleeding). A history of previous surgery broadens the differential diagnosis—e.g., previous aortic surgery and aortoenteric fistula. Known liver disease raises the possibility of bleeding associated with portal hypertension. Ingestion of aspirin or other nonsteroidal anti-inflammatory drugs makes bleeding from gastric or gastroduodenal ulceration more likely. Other historical features important to ascertain include the presence of abdominal pain (peptic ulcer disease, mesenteric or colonic ischemia), retching (Mallory-Weiss tear), or change in bowel habits, anorexia, or weight loss all of which point to malignancy. Elderly patients may be less likely to report abdominal pain associated with bleeding ulcers.[5, 6] The history is also critical in ascertaining whether nongastrointestinal sources may be the cause of apparent gastrointestinal bleeding, especially from the nasopharynx.

Physical examination may reveal the presence of cutaneous signs (spider angiomata, Dupuytren's contractures) or other evidence of liver disease (splenomegaly, ascites, caput), that suggests the possibility of portal hypertension. Acanthosis nigricans may reflect underlying cancer (especially gastric cancer); cutaneous telangiectases of skin and/or mucous membranes and lips raise the possibility of hereditary hemorrhagic telangiectasia (Osler-Weber-Rendu); pigmented lip lesions are seen with Peutz-Jeghers syndrome; cutaneous tumors suggest neurofibromatosis; purpura is consistent with vascular disease (Henloch-Schönlein purpura or polyarteritis nodosa). Abdominal tenderness (peptic ulcer, pancreatitis, ischemia), abdominal masses, lymphadenopathy (malignancy), and splenomegaly (cirrhosis, splenic vein thrombosis) are all important to detect. (See chapter 18, Figs. 18–12, 18–14, 18–17, and 18–19.)

Hematemesis and *melena* are the most common symptoms and signs of gastrointestinal bleeding. Melena is caused by delivery of at least 50 mL of blood into the upper gastrointestinal tract, although volumes of up to 100 mL

Table 13–2 | **Historical Features Important in Assessing the Etiology of Gastrointestinal Bleeding**

Age
Prior bleeding
Previous gastrointestinal disease
Previous surgery
Underlying medical disorder (especially liver disease)
Nonsteroidal anti-inflammatory drugs/aspirin
Abdominal pain
Change in bowel habits
Weight loss/anorexia
History of oropharyngeal disease

may be clinically silent.[7] Vomiting of bright red blood usually indicates significant upper gastrointestinal bleeding, often from varices or an arterial lesion; however, small amounts of hematemesis are alarming. Therefore, careful inquiry about the volume of vomited blood is essential. Patients with coffee ground emesis are not usually bleeding actively but have had a recent or even remote bleed. Although hematochezia is due to bleeding from many sites in the gastrointestinal tract, bleeding is brisk and often hemodynamically significant when the source is the upper gastrointestinal tract. Chronic occult blood loss may lead to end-organ symptoms such as lightheadedness, dyspnea, angina pectoris, or even myocardial infarction.

Bedside examination of the character of the stool output provides critical information not only about the site of bleeding, but also about the acuity of bleeding. For example, patients with brown stools are unlikely to have aggressive bleeding. In contrast, patients who are actively passing stools containing red blood, maroon-colored blood, or melena—even in the absence of a positive nasogastric lavage—are likely to have active bleeding. Patients with infrequent stools are unlikely to be actively bleeding, and those with a history of coffee ground emesis only and normal-appearing stools, often positive for occult blood, have usually had a trivial bleed.

Laboratory Evaluation

It is important to understand that the hematocrit value, when determined soon after the onset of bleeding, may not reflect blood loss accurately. Because equilibration with extravascular fluid and subsequent hemodilution requires several hours, a single hematocrit level may not reflect the degree of bleeding. Thus, the severity of bleeding must not be underestimated because of a slightly depressed or even normal hematocrit. The hematocrit value falls as extravascular fluid enters the vascular space to restore volume, a process that is not complete for 24 to 72 hours[8] (Fig. 13–1).

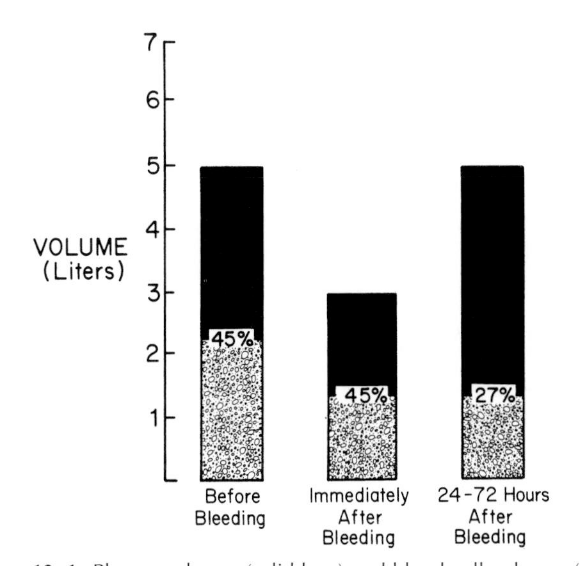

Figure 13–1. Plasma volumes (solid bars), red blood cell volumes (stippled bars), and hematocrit values (%) before bleeding and after 2 L blood loss. A baseline hematocrit value of 45% is assumed.

Patients who bleed small amounts of blood over long periods of time develop iron deficiency (see Occult Bleeding later) and despite low hematocrits may be entirely hemodynamically stable. A low mean corpuscular volume (MCV) is often an important clue in these patients, and, complemented by a low ferritin level, will make the diagnosis of iron deficiency. Importantly, the hematocrit must always be judged in the context of the patient's overall clinical state. For example, a low hematocrit may be due in part to extraintestinal bleeding. Anemia may be due to folic acid or vitamin B_{12} deficiency, depending on other associated diseases or disorders. Finally, patients with apparent gastrointestinal bleeding may bleed from other sites such as intra-abdominally or from large muscle groups.

The blood urea nitrogen (BUN) level may be mildly elevated in patients with upper GI bleeding. The elevation is typically out of proportion to elevation in the serum creatinine level,[9] due to breakdown of blood proteins to urea by intestinal bacteria and its absorption, as well as from a mild reduction in glomerular filtration rate.

Clinical Localization of Bleeding

The localization of bleeding begins with a careful history and physical examination. Hematemesis is from an upper gastrointestinal source of bleeding. Melena indicates that blood has been in the gastrointestinal tract for extended periods of time[10] and is usually the result of upper gastrointestinal bleeding, but its source may be the distal small bowel or even the ascending colon. In the latter instance, the volume of bleeding is too little to cause hematochezia but sufficiently large to provide hemoglobin for degradation. Approximately 10% of all patients with rapid bleeding from an upper source present with hematochezia.[11]

The nasogastric lavage has been used extensively to help differentiate upper from lower gastrointestinal bleeding.[12–14] A bloody aspirate confirms the upper gastrointestinal tract as the source of bleeding, since the false-positive rate is essentially nil[12] and is related to nasogastric trauma. It is important to emphasize that it may be extremely difficult to judge the acuity or activity of bleeding using nasogastric lavage; the correlation between the acuity of bleeding and the physician assessment of bleeding is weak, with a 79% sensitivity and 55% specificity for active bleeding.[14] Thus, use of the nasogastric lavage to assess bleeding activity is discouraged. It is far more effective to utilize the vital signs and other bedside diagnostic criteria. Further, a positive nasogastric lavage provides no information about the etiology of bleeding.

Although a nonbloody nasogastric aspirate suggests that bleeding is from a source other than the upper gastrointestinal tract, it is negative in up to 25% of patients with upper gastrointestinal bleeding. Even a bile-colored aspirate, which signifies sampling of the duodenum, does not exclude an upper gastrointestinal source of bleeding. If there is any question about the location of bleeding in a patient with hematochezia, especially in patients with hemodynamic instability, a nasogastric tube should be placed. Testing for occult blood in nasogastric aspirates, while commonly performed, is rarely necessary and helpful only when a coffee ground appearance of the aspirate may be caused by some foods. Although nasogastric tubes are useful to help determine the site of bleeding and to help direct further investigation, there is no evidence that their use affects the outcome.

Other clues to an upper gastrointestinal source of bleeding include hyperactive bowel sounds and an elevation in the BUN level out of proportion to creatinine. In a series of patients with gastrointestinal bleeding, the mean (± SD) BUN/creatinine ratio was significantly higher in patients with upper gastrointestinal bleeding than in those with lower gastrointestinal bleeding (22.5 ± 11.5 vs. 15.9 ± 8.2; P = .0001), although the degree of overlap indicates that it discriminates poorly.[9]

Diagnostic Tests

Diagnostic tests, of course, are important in the evaluation of patients with gastrointestinal bleeding. The major categories of tests available include: (1) endoscopy; (2) barium radiographs; (3) radionuclide imaging; (4) angiography; and (5) miscellaneous tests (abdominal computed tomographic scanning). Some help only in diagnosis; others possess therapeutic potential. Radiographic tests fall in the former category and endoscopy the latter. The importance of endoscopic therapy is emphasized by studies performed before the advent of endoscopic therapy, which demonstrated that endoscopy per se did not affect outcome for patients with upper gastrointestinal bleeding.[15]

Therapy

A major goal of treatment is to stop bleeding and prevent rebleeding. The major forms of therapy include (1) pharmacologic; (2) endoscopic; (3) angiographic; and (4) surgical. The use of each of these modalities has undergone tremendous change since the early 1980s and, in addition, each varies with the cause of bleeding. These therapeutic maneuvers are often complementary and require focused, multispecialty expertise.

ACUTE UPPER GASTROINTESTINAL BLEEDING

Upper gastrointestinal bleeding, which most commonly arises from mucosal erosive disease, has been estimated to account for up to 20,000 deaths annually in the United States. The overall incidence of acute upper gastrointestinal hemorrhage has been estimated at 50 to 100 per 100,000 patients per year, with an annual hospitalization rate of approximately 100 per 100,000 hospital admissions.[2, 16, 17] The incidence of upper gastrointestinal bleeding is increasing in elderly people; one study found that those over 65 years of age comprised over 30% of those with upper gastrointestinal bleeding.[18]

Prognosis

Patients with acute upper gastrointestinal bleeding present with a wide range of clinical severity ranging from trivial bleeds to fulminant and lethal exsanguination. The mortality rate for upper gastrointestinal bleeding has been reported to be as high as 14%, but in most studies it appears to have remained stable over the last 30 to 40 years at 8% to 10%.[2, 16] Given the aging population and the higher proportion of comorbidities in this group, the survival rate may be improving.

Many studies have addressed the factors that predict outcome in patients with upper gastrointestinal hemorrhage.[19–23] Because upper gastrointestinal bleeding is most commonly caused by ulceration, prognostic factors for it tend to reflect those for bleeding peptic ulcer. Approximately 80% of upper gastrointestinal bleeding episodes are self-limited and require only supportive therapy.[24] The two most important prognostic variables appear to be the cause of bleeding and the presence of underlying comorbidity. For example, patients with variceal hemorrhage have a mortality rate of at least 30% during their initial hospitalization, with a 1-year mortality rate approaching 60%.[25] A number of studies have identified clinical features of severe bleeding that can be recognized early in the patient's course, which predict recurrent bleeding and increased mortality (Table 13–3).[2, 20, 21, 26–29]

Several scoring systems have been designed to identify patients with a high risk of adverse outcomes; the measures have generally been ascertained from mathematical models of risk of death or rebleeding.[19, 23, 30] However, the use of such systems is not widely supported, and for the most part they have not been adopted in clinical practice. Models have also been developed to assess whether patients presenting with acute upper gastrointestinal bleeding require hospitalized management. In one study, an abbreviated "fast-track" screening score based on simple clinical features was developed.[31] This tool classified patients as at low risk of needing intervention if, at presentation, all the following were true: BUN less than 6.5 mmol/L, hemoglobin concentration greater than 130 g/L for men and 120 g/L for women, systolic blood pressure greater than 100 mm Hg, and pulse rate less than 100. Although virtually all patients who required treatment (i.e., transfusion, endoscopy) failed to meet these criteria for low risk—they had a low hemoglobin concentration, high BUN level, tachycardia, or relative systolic hypotension—this tool identified only 32% of the minor bleeds that would require no intervention.[31] A low specificity of this triage system and others like it makes the value of such scoring strategies problematic.

Approach to Diagnosis and Therapy

Following hemodynamic stabilization and thorough patient assessment, management shifts rapidly to a consideration of the cause of bleeding and the best approach to making the

Table 13–3 | **Adverse Prognostic Variables in Acute Upper Gastrointestinal Bleeding**

- Increasing age
- Increasing number of comorbid conditions
- Cause of bleeding (variceal bleeding > others)
- Red blood in the emesis and/or stool
- Shock or hypotension on presentation
- Increasing numbers of units of blood transfused
- Active bleeding at the time of endoscopy
- Bleeding from large (>2.0 cm) ulcers
- Onset of bleeding in the hospital
- Emergency surgery

diagnosis. The specific lesions that cause upper gastrointestinal bleeding are shown in Table 13–4. Since history and physical examination, although clearly important, do not uncover the precise etiology of the bleeding, diagnostic tests are necessary.

The primary diagnostic modality for evaluation of upper gastrointestinal hemorrhage is currently esophagogastroduodenoscopy. Although barium radiography can diagnose many upper gastrointestinal tract lesions accurately, it offers no therapy, and is not recommended in acute upper gastrointestinal bleeding. Endoscopy is the method of choice; however, considerable controversy remains about whether patients with hemodynamically trivial bleeding require the procedure.

For patients with significant bleeding, on the other hand, the mainstay of treatment for their bleeding lesions is endoscopic therapy. Indeed, it is the major justification for esophagogastroduodenoscopy in those with hemodynamically significant acute upper gastrointestinal bleeding, since endoscopic therapy unquestionably improves prognosis.[32] For this reason, such patients should undergo the procedure as soon as possible. In addition, the endoscopic appearance of certain lesions may help triage patients, and thereby reduce costs of hospitalization. For example, early endoscopy performed in the emergency department safely assigned 46% of patients with nonvariceal upper GI bleeding to outpatient care, significantly reducing hospital stay.[33]

However, esophagogastroduodenoscopy should be performed only when it can be accomplished safely and effectively. Patients must be adequately resuscitated prior to endoscopy, and the airway must be protected during the procedure; intubation should be performed in the setting of aggressive bleeding or altered mental status. In actively bleeding patients or those with blood obscuring the endoscopic view,[34] lavage with a large-bore orogastric tube should be performed. Appropriate endoscopic equipment is required—a therapeutic videoendoscope is mandatory; further, thermal coagulation devices and injection material must be readily available.

The approach to therapy depends largely on the specific cause of bleeding (and is discussed next under specific lesions). Besides supportive care, there is little generalized therapy to offer the patient with upper gastrointestinal bleeding. Although gastric lavage has been thought to slow or stop bleeding, a controlled study has demonstrated it to be ineffective.[35] A proposed approach to patients with upper gastrointestinal hemorrhage is shown in Figure 13–2.

Table 13–4 | **Causes of Acute Upper Gastrointestinal Bleeding**

COMMON CAUSES
Gastric ulcer
Duodenal ulcer
Esophageal varices
Mallory-Weiss tear
LESS FREQUENT CAUSES
Dieulafoy's lesions
Vascular ectasia
Portal hypertensive gastropathy
Gastric antral vascular ectasia (watermelon stomach)
Gastric varices
Neoplasia
Esophagitis
Gastric erosions
RARE CAUSES
Esophageal ulcer
Erosive duodenitis
Aortoenteric fistula
Hemobilia
Pancreatic source
Crohn's disease
No lesion identified

Specific Causes of Upper Gastrointestinal Bleeding (see Table 13–4)

Esophagitis

Significant bleeding from *esophagitis* occurs in up to 8% of patients with upper gastrointestinal hemorrhage.[2, 36–38] Bleeding from esophagitis more commonly causes occult blood loss (see later) than acute bleeding. Clinically obvious bleeding is most likely in those with extensive ulcerative disease or with an underlying coagulopathy. Specific therapy is directed at the cause of the underlying lesion (usually reflux esophagitis), and typically involves high-dose proton pump inhibitors. Endoscopic treatment of bleeding lesions may benefit patients with esophageal ulcerations and visible vessels, but because of the risk for perforation, it should be performed with caution (see Chapter 33).

Mallory-Weiss Tear

Mallory-Weiss tears are lacerations in the region of the gastroesophageal junction that typically occur in gastric mucosa, although 10% to 20% can occur in esophageal mucosa. They are an important cause of upper gastrointestinal hemorrhage and account for approximately 5% to 10% of cases of upper gastrointestinal hemorrhage.[2, 36–38] Although they are thought to be caused by retching, a history of this is obtained in only 29% of patients.[39] Bleeding from Mallory-Weiss tears stops spontaneously in 80% to 90% of patients, and less than 5% of patients rebleed[40]—most often those with an underlying bleeding diathesis.[41] Patients not bleeding during endoscopy and without other medical problems that require hospitalization are usually managed with supportive care only and can be discharged promptly. Endoscopic therapy with coagulation methods, injection, or banding effectively stops bleeding and should be performed on bleeding lesions or patients with bleeding stigmata.[42, 43] Angiographic therapy, with intra-arterial infusion of vasopressin, or embolization is successful in a high proportion of patients.[44] Surgical therapy is rarely required.

Portal Hypertension–Related Causes of Bleeding

Portal hypertension leads to bleeding from several different lesions, including esophageal varices, gastric varices, ectopic varices, and portal hypertensive gastropathy. In cohorts of patients with upper gastrointestinal bleeding, the proportion of patients with portal hypertensive bleeding varies, depending on the particular patient population. Large national surveys report that about 10% of patients with upper gastrointestinal hemorrhage bleed from varices,[37, 45] whereas in inner

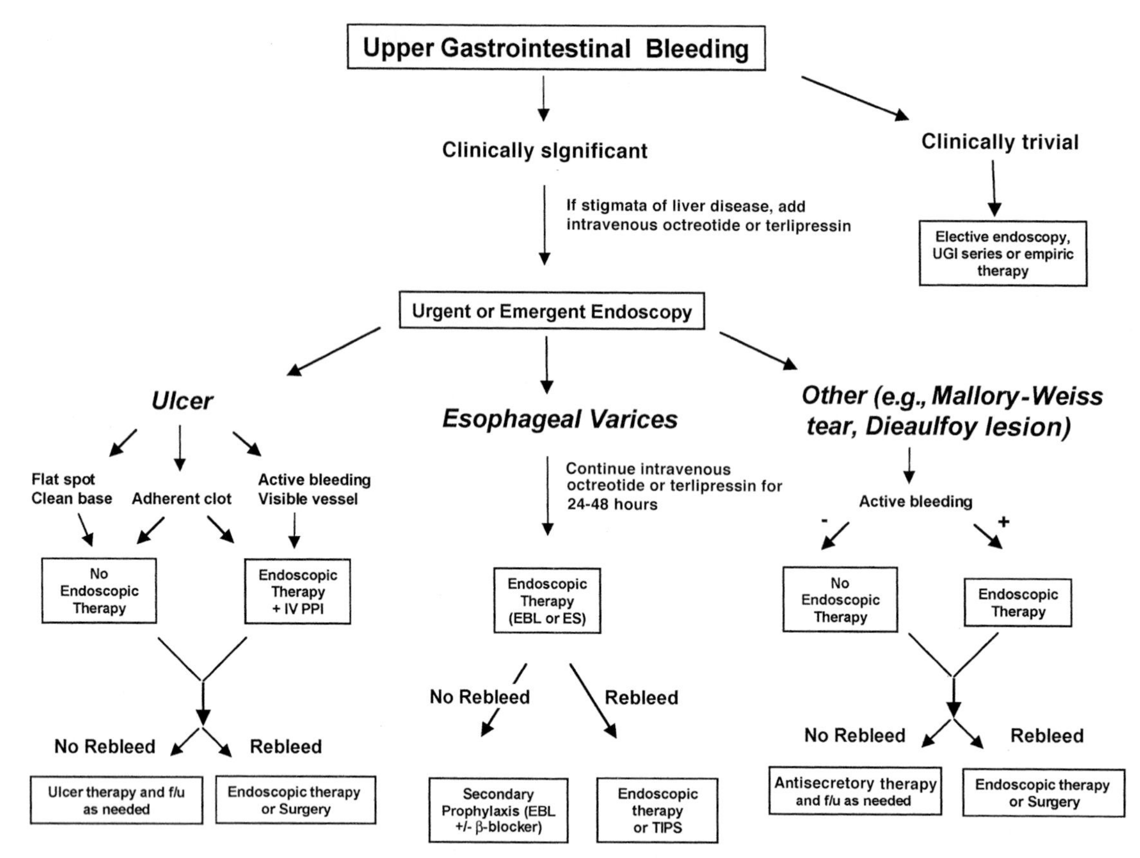

Figure 13–2. Algorithm for management of upper gastrointestinal (UGI) bleeding. (TIPS, transjugular intrahepatic portosystemic shunt; EBL, endoscopic band ligation; ES, endoscopic sclerotherapy, IV PPI, intravenous proton pump inhibitor.)

city hospital populations, approximately one third of patients bleed from varices.[36]

Bleeding from esophageal or gastric varices is often aggressive and frequently accompanied by hemodynamic instability. In contrast, bleeding from portal hypertensive gastropathy typically causes low-volume bleeding, which is often occult (see Fig. 120–10).

Patients with evidence of liver disease (by history, physical examination, or laboratory data) who have active upper gastrointestinal bleeding should begin a pharmacologic agent as soon as possible and undergo urgent endoscopy (see Fig. 13–2). Available data now clearly indicate that endoscopic therapy, preferably variceal band ligation, improves outcome in patients with variceal hemorrhage. Management of bleeding as a result of portal hypertension is discussed in Chapter 77.

Duodenal and Gastric Ulcers

Ulcer disease is the most common cause of acute upper gastrointestinal hemorrhage (see Table 13–4). As recently as 1996, it was shown that gastroduodenal ulcers were responsible for upper gastrointestinal bleeding in nearly 50% of cases.[46] The incidence of bleeding from duodenal ulcers is approximately twofold that of gastric ulcers. Given more effective medical therapy for ulcer disease, as well as the realization that predisposing factors (discussed later) can be modified, it has been predicted that the incidence of bleeding from ulcers will decline. However, the hospitalization rate for ulcer-related gastrointestinal bleeding appears to be constant at approximately 40 to 60 cases per 100,000 patients.[2, 45, 47]

Ulcers bleed when they erode into the lateral wall of a vessel. Ulcers located high on the lesser curve of the stomach or on the posteroinferior wall of the duodenal bulb are most likely to bleed (and rebleed), presumably due to the rich vascular supply in these areas. The precise pathophysiology of ulcer bleeding is unclear, but is likely to encompass factors related to the bleeding blood vessel itself (for example, an eccentric vascular branch may be important[48]), as well as factors related to the ulcer environment (see chapters 39 and 40).

Predisposing Factors for Bleeding

A number of risk factors predispose to ulcer disease and its bleeding, the most prominent being acid, *Helicobacter pylori*, and nonsteroidal anti-inflammatory drugs (NSAIDs) (see also Chapter 40). In addition, underlying medical and clinical factors predispose to ulcer disease and bleeding. In a case control study of 1122 patients and 2231 controls[49] cardiovascular and cerebrovascular disease were independent predictors of peptic ulcer–related upper gastrointestinal bleeding. Chronic pulmonary disease and cirrhosis also are associated with peptic ulcer disease. Pharmacologic agents besides aspirin and NSAIDs may predispose to ulcer disease. Glucocorticoids historically have been associated with an increased risk of peptic ulcer, although newer data raise

Table 13–5 | **Relative Risk of Acute Upper Gastrointestinal Bleeding in Persons Taking Aspirin**

STUDY	ASPIRIN DOSE	BLEEDING COMPLICATIONS		RELATIVE RISK
		Placebo	Aspirin	
AMIS* 1980[66]	1000/d	65/2257	111/2267	1.7
UK-TIA† 1988[67]	300/d	7/814	12/806	1.6
UK-TIA† 1988[67]	1200/d	7/814	19/815	2.8
PHS 1989*‡[68]	325 qod	274/11034	402/11037	1.8
SALT 1991[69]	75/d	4/684	11/676	—

The frequency of events in these studies cannot be compared because of different times of exposure.
*"Bloody stools."
†All episodes of serious gastrointestinal bleeding.
‡Melena and hematemesis combined.
AMIS, Aspirin Myocardial Infarction Study; PHS, Physicians' Health Study; SALT, Swedish Aspirin Low-dose Trial; UK-TIA, United Kingdom Transient Ischaemic Attack (trial).

doubt about this association.[50] Recent data link alendronate to the development of gastric ulcers and perhaps upper gastrointestinal bleeding.[51, 52] Also, ethanol may potentiate the damaging effects of NSAIDs in the mucosa, and, as expected, anticoagulants will facilitate bleeding.

Hospitalization appears to be an important risk factor for development of ulcer bleeding (duodenal greater than gastric).[53] Bleeding tends to occur after prolonged hospitalization and is most common in patients with severe comorbidities. Such "nosocomial" gastrointestinal bleeding is associated with poor outcome, and one study had a mortality rate of 34%.[53] Nosocomial ulcer bleeders were less likely to have a history of previous ulcer disease (13% versus 50%; $P < 0.05$), to have *H. pylori* infection (14% versus 62%; $P < 0.0001$), or to be taking NSAIDs (48% versus 68%; $P = 0.08$) than those hospitalized for ulcer bleeding.

Gastric Acid

The evidence for a role of gastric acid in peptic ulceration is overwhelming and includes the hypersecretory disorder Zollinger-Ellison syndrome, in which patients develop ulcers with high frequency (see Chapter 41).[54] The ability of antacid therapy alone to heal upper gastroduodenal tract ulceration also supports the role of acid. However, controversy exists surrounding the role of acid in inducing bleeding in non-Zollinger-Ellison ulceration. Perhaps the best evidence of a role for acid in acute upper gastrointestinal hemorrhage comes from data indicating that acid reduction by proton pump inhibitors in patients with active or recent bleeding from upper gastrointestinal ulcerative lesions reduces the risk of bleeding and rebleeding[55–59] (see Chapter 38).

Helicobacter pylori

As with acid, the link between *H. pylori* and peptic ulceration is firm. However, the role of *H. pylori* in ulcer bleeding is controversial. For example, one study revealed a decreased incidence of *H. pylori* infection in patients presenting with actively bleeding ulcers.[60] In contrast, other

Table 13–6 | **Nonsteroidal Anti-inflammatory Drug Use and Increased Incidence of Acute Upper Gastrointestinal Bleeding**

STUDY	INCIDENCE (%)		RELATIVE RISK
	NSAIDs	Control	
Griffin* 1991[71]	481/1415 (34)	918/7063 (13)	4.1
Rodriguez 1994[72]	241/1457 (17)	365/10,000 (4)	4.7
Rodriguez 1998[73]	277/1505 (18)	761/16,672 (5)	4.1
Lanas 2000[49]	520/1122 (46)	229/2231 (10)	7.4

*Outcome—all ulcer complications resulting in hospitalization or death.

studies have suggested that *H. pylori* infection increases the likelihood of hemorrhage (relative risk, approximately 1.5).[61, 62]

To complicate matters further, the role of *H. pylori* infection in causing hemorrhage of ulcers in those using NSAIDs is also controversial. On one hand, NSAID users infected with *H. pylori* had a nearly twofold risk of ulcer bleeding compared with uninfected NSAID users.[63] In contrast, other studies have suggested that *H. pylori* has little adverse effect or may even protect against NSAID–associated gastroduodenal lesions and promote ulcer healing. In a randomized study (omeprazole alone or triple therapy plus omeprazole) of 195 *H. pylori*–infected NSAID users, bleeding ulcers were healed in 86% of the omeprazole group compared with 83% of the triple therapy group ($P = 0.50$), suggesting that eradication of *H. pylori* did not affect the healing of NSAID-associated bleeding peptic ulcers (see Chapter 39).[64]

Aspirin and Nonsteroidal Anti-Inflammatory Drugs (NSAIDs)

Aspirin and NSAIDs are probably the most important predisposing factors for ulcer bleeding (see reference 65 for review). The mechanism of injury and ulceration is complex but appears to involve reduced production of cyclooxygenase-generated cytoprotective prostaglandins. Further, the risk of bleeding is increased by NSAIDs or aspirin, in part because of platelet dysfunction, as shown convincingly in a number of studies of patients taking aspirin or NSAIDs (Tables 13–5 through 13–8). For aspirin, the evidence comes largely from placebo-controlled trials (Table

Table 13–7 | **Relative Risk of Acute Upper Gastrointestinal Bleeding in Persons Taking Nonsteroidal Anti-inflammatory Drugs and COX-2 Inhibitors**

STUDY	BLEEDING COMPLICATIONS		RELATIVE RISK*
	COX-2 Inhibitor	NSAID	
Bombardier 2000[75]	14/4047	35/4029	0.40
Silverstein 2000[76]	10/3987	20/3981	0.53†

*COX-2 compared with NSAID.
†All ulcer complications.

Table 13–8 | **Relative Risk of Acute Upper Gastrointestinal Bleeding Resulting from Nonsteroidal Anti-inflammatory Compounds**

GROUP	RELATIVE RISK
Control*	1.0
COX-2 Inhibitors	1.3–1.5
ASA†	1.5–2.5
NSAIDs	4–7

The risk for gastroduodenal ulcer bleeding is approximated based on available literature.

*The rate of bleeding in untreated patients is set at 1.0.

†The risk for each ASA and NSAIDs is dose dependent, increasing with dose.

13–5).[66–70] With regard to this relationship, several important reservations must be made. Firstly, these studies were not designed to detect gastrointestinal bleeding as a primary outcome event, and thus may not have detected all cases of ulcer bleeding; secondly, bleeding from sites other than the upper gastrointestinal tract may have been attributed to gastroduodenal ulcers. In any event, the risk of gastrointestinal bleeding appears to be dose related.

The evidence for an increased risk of NSAID-induced upper gastrointestinal bleeding is derived largely from case-control studies (Table 13–6).[49, 71–73] Although these studies have inherent limitations because of their study design, they uniformly demonstrate an increased incidence of ulcers and bleeding in patients taking NSAIDs (see also reference 74 for review). Other studies have examined, on a prospective comparative basis, the risk of ulcer bleeding in patients requiring NSAIDs for underlying diseases, particularly rheumatoid arthritis or osteoarthritis.[75, 76] Although the data are not entirely consistent, the following points appear to be reliable: (1) the risk for gastric ulceration is greater than for duodenal ulceration, although both are increased; (2) the risk of bleeding varies with the individual NSAID; for example, the relative risk of bleeding is greatest with azapropazone and piroxicam, but less with ibuprofen; (3) the risk of bleeding is dose dependent; and (4) multiple cofactors contribute to NSAID risk.

Cofactors important in NSAID-induced ulceration are diverse. For example, age and previous upper gastrointestinal bleeding appear to be important predictors of NSAID-associated bleeding. One study[77] found that age greater than 75 years, history of heart disease, history of peptic ulcer, and history of previous gastrointestinal bleeding were independent predictors of NSAID-induced complications. These data are highly consistent with other data emphasizing the importance of age as an independent risk factor for NSAID ulceration.[78] In addition, *H. pylori* may be a risk factor for ulcers, although the degree of risk is controversial.[79, 80] Finally, corticosteroids,[81] the bisphosphonate alendronate,[51, 52] and ethanol[82] appear to potentiate the ulcerogenic effect of NSAIDs and may predispose to upper gastrointestinal bleeding (see Chapter 23).

Ethanol

The role of ethanol as a predisposing factor for ulcer-related acute upper gastrointestinal bleeding is difficult to assess. It is important to note that patients who ingest ethanol chronically may have alcohol-induced liver disease and secondary portal hypertension, which is an important risk factor for nonulcer upper gastrointestinal hemorrhage. Nonetheless, ethanol is well known to induce gastric mucosal injury, and thus may cause or potentiate ulcer bleeding. Deleterious effects of NSAIDs are further increased among drinkers. In a case-control study conducted in the United States and Sweden, 1224 patients hospitalized with acute upper gastrointestinal bleeding due to peptic ulcer or gastritis were compared with 2945 controls.[82] The relative risk of acute upper gastrointestinal bleeding increased with increasing alcohol consumption, rising to 2.8 among those who had 21 or more drinks per week. Among active drinkers, the relative risk of acute upper gastrointestinal bleeding due to the use of aspirin was raised at all levels of alcohol consumption; the relative risk for those taking regular aspirin at doses of over 325 mg was 7.0; for regular use at lower doses, the corresponding estimate was 2.8, and for any occasional use, it was 2.4. For those using ibuprofen regularly, the relative risk was 2.7. Thus, heavy alcohol intake independently increases the risk of upper gastrointestinal bleeding in users of aspirin or ibuprofen.

Anticoagulation Therapy

Anticoagulation increases the risk of bleeding from ulcer disease. The relative risk of hospitalization for bleeding ulcer in anticoagulated patients is about 3, and anticoagulants further increase the risk of bleeding in those taking NSAIDs.[83] Among users of oral anticoagulants, the adjusted incidence of hospitalization for bleeding peptic ulcer was 10.2 per 1000 person-years.[83] Compared with subjects who took neither anticoagulants nor NSAIDs, the relative risk of hemorrhagic peptic ulcer disease among users of both drugs was 12.7 (95% confidence interval, 6.3 to 25.7). The prevalence of NSAID use among anticoagulant users was 13.5%, similar to those not using anticoagulants. Such data emphasize the risk of anticoagulants, particularly for those who use NSAIDs.

Prognostic Factors in Ulcer Bleeding

Most ulcer bleeding is self-limited, and in these patients recovery is uneventful. However, a subset of patients have continued or recurrent bleeding, which is associated with a poorer prognosis. The prognostic factors emphasized in upper gastrointestinal bleeding (see Table 13–3) apply particularly to bleeding ulcers since they comprise the majority of upper gastrointestinal bleeding lesions. For example, old age, the presence of comorbid conditions, clinical evidence of aggressive bleeding, large ulcers (greater than 2 cm in diameter), and the onset of bleeding while hospitalized are important predictors of rebleeding and a poorer outcome.[53]

The seminal observation of Griffiths and colleagues that a visible vessel in an ulcer base was predictive of uncontrolled or recurrent bleeding established the importance of the endoscopic appearance of ulcers.[84] The most critical endoscopic features in ulcer bleeding include the following stigmata of active/recent bleeding: active arterial spurting, oozing of blood, a visible vessel, and fresh or old blood clot. Visible vessels are described endoscopically as elevated, dark red or purple lesions that protrude from the ulcer crater. A number of studies have examined endoscopic features as predictors not only of rebleeding but also of outcomes.[26, 85–88]

A critical point regarding usefulness of endoscopic findings to predict outcomes is the substantial variation in the visual appearance and interpretation of endoscopic lesions.[26, 89] This uncertainty is not surprising since endoscopic evolution of bleeding vessels within an ulcer follows a sequence from a visible vessel to a large sentinel clot that becomes darker, smaller, and flatter, which is replaced with a white plug of fibrin that disappears.[90] Thus, since patients may have endoscopy at different times after the onset of bleeding, the reported endoscopic features of ulcers after bleeding vary. Further, endoscopists disagree on the terminology for stigmata of recent hemorrhage.[91]

Despite the difficulty in assessing stigmata of ulcer bleeding, it is accepted that certain characteristics of the ulcer at the time of endoscopy provide important prognostic information. For example, increasing ulcer size (>1 cm) is associated with an increased rate of rebleeding and mortality.[92] Endoscopic hemostasis is less often successful in ulcers larger than 2 cm.[92] The appearance of the ulcer base is also important and may be one of the following: (1) a clean base only, (2) an ulcer base with a flat, pigmented spot, (3) an ulcer base with an adherent clot, (4) an ulcer base with a visible vessel (also called a pigmented protuberance or sentinel clot that appears raised and rounded and is resistant to washing); or (5) an ulcer base containing a visible vessel or an adherent clot that is actively oozing or spurting. The likelihood of rebleeding, need for surgery, and death based on the appearance of the ulcer are shown in Table 13–9.

Although there is general consensus about management of patients with active bleeding, visible vessels, flat spots, and clean bases, controversy surrounds management of adherent clots, particularly after vigorous attempts to remove the clot (see Fig. 13–2). In a study of 46 patients with adherent clots,[93] the lesion was irrigated with a 3.2-mm bipolar probe for up to 5 minutes. After irrigation, findings were adherent clot, 26 (57%); clean base, 1 (2%); flat spot, 5 (11%); nonbleeding visible vessel, 7 (13%); oozing, 6 (13%); and spurting, 1 (2%). Two of the 26 (8%) with adherent clots after washing rebled; endoscopic therapy resulted in no further bleeding. One of the 14 (7%) with active bleeding or visible vessels treated with hemostatic therapy rebled; repeat endoscopic therapy controlled the bleeding. There were no deaths during the study. These researchers concluded that vigorous irrigation was useful in this population and that endoscopic findings after washing may help triage endoscopic management at initial endoscopy.

Treatment of Peptic Ulcer Bleeding

Because bleeding from gastroduodenal ulcers remains the most common and important form of upper gastrointestinal bleeding, treatment of this problem has been studied extensively. The goals of therapy are (1) to treat the peptic ulcer, and, thus, bleeding; (2) to stop active bleeding; and (3) to prevent rebleeding.

Pharmacologic Therapy

Pharmacologic therapy for both peptic ulcer disease and bleeding has evolved enormously. A number of pharmacologic agents have been used to treat active ulcer bleeding: octreotide, somatostatin, vasopressin, secretin, H_2-receptor antagonists, proton pump inhibitors, antifibrinolytics, and prostaglandins. Although a few compounds have been marginally effective in stopping ulcer bleeding or preventing ulcer rebleeding, the only therapy for which sufficient evidence currently exists is the use of proton pump inhibitors. The greatest risk for rebleeding from ulcer disease is within the first 72 hours after the bleeding episode, so the benefit of pharmacologic therapy may be in either stopping acute bleeding or in preventing early rebleeding—most of the available literature fails to distinguish between these two events. Furthermore, most studies have examined proton pump inhibitors in the era of therapeutic endoscopy, so the effect of these agents must be considered additive to therapeutic endoscopy.

Experimental evidence indicates that acidic pH retards clotting and enhances clot dissolution by proteolytic enzymes like pepsin.[94, 95] Elevating intragastric pH may facilitate platelet aggregation.[94] Classic oral antacids do not affect the natural history of bleeding from ulcer disease. Clinical trials of H_2-receptor antagonists, including 27 randomized controlled trials of over 2500 patients, suggest that these agents may reduce the rates of rebleeding, surgery, and death by about 10%, 20%, and 30%, respectively, although these results were only marginally significant for surgery and death.[96] The effect of H_2-receptor antagonists on bleeding ulcers has thus been somewhat disappointing, presumably because these agents do not provide optimal acid inhibition. Their benefit appeared to be confined to patients with bleeding gastric ulcers. Nonetheless, because H_2-receptor antagonists are widely available, not toxic, and comparatively inexpensive, they are still used in patients with ulcer bleeding.

In contrast, proton pump inhibitors have significantly bet-

Table 13–9 | **Effect of Endoscopic Therapy on Bleeding Peptic Ulcers According to Their Appearance**

APPEARANCE	FREQUENCY	REBLEEDING RATE (%)		SURGERY RATE (%)		MORTALITY RATE (%)	
		No Rx	Rx	No Rx	Rx	No Rx	Rx
Active bleeding	18	55	20	35	7	11	<5
Visible vessel	17	43	15	34	6	11	<5
Adherent clot	15	22	5	10	2	7	<3
Flat spot	15	10	<1	6	<1	3	<1
Clean ulcer base	35	<1	—	0.5	—	2	—

Outcomes with and without endoscopic therapy are estimated based on available literature.
Adapted in part from Laine L, Peterson J: Bleeding peptic ulcer. N Engl J Med 331:717, 1994.

ter acid-reducing characteristics, particularly at high doses,[97] and they appear to be especially effective at preventing ulcer rebleeding in high-risk patients (Table 13–10).[55–59] Although the designs of these studies contained a number of variables (e.g., definition of rebleeding, doses of drug used, extent of endoscopic therapy), the trend toward reduction in rebleeding is clear.

Khuroo and coworkers demonstrated that omeprazole (40 mg given orally every 12 hours for 5 days) significantly reduced recurrent bleeding and surgery in patients with nonbleeding visible vessels or adherent clots.[57] This study was notable for the fact that endoscopic therapy was not performed as an adjunct to treatment. Another randomized study in patients with active bleeding or nonbleeding visible vessels demonstrated that omeprazole (80 mg administered intravenously after therapeutic endoscopy, followed by an infusion of 8 mg/hour for 72 hours), reduced rebleeding compared with placebo.[59] Most episodes of recurrent bleeding are in the first 3 days after initial bleeding,[58] so therapy should be initiated early in the patient's course.

These data contrast with the largest single study of a proton pump inhibitor in upper gastrointestinal hemorrhage.[98] In this double-blind placebo-controlled trial of 1147 patients, omeprazole (80 mg) was given intravenously on presentation and then for 4 days (40 mg every 12 hours). Omeprazole failed to reduce mortality, rebleeding, or transfusion requirements. However, the majority of these patients were not bleeding from ulcers, which suggests that nonpeptic ulcer causes of upper gastrointestinal hemorrhage do not benefit from proton pump inhibitor therapy; furthermore, the study did not specify the types of ulcerated lesions visualized. Other differences in the study design between this study and those shown in Table 13–10, such as the dose of omeprazole and use of endoscopic therapy, are likely to account for the beneficial effect of omeprazole in high-risk patients. Although future studies examining the cost-effectiveness of proton pump inhibitors and H_2-receptor antagonists in ulcer bleeding are necessary, it is my opinion that proton pump inhibitors (preferably given intravenously as prescribed in the studies shown in Table 13–10) should be administered in patients with high-risk ulcer bleeding.

Recent data suggest a protective role for nitric oxide (NO) in upper gastrointestinal tract ulcers and hemorrhage. In experimental studies, treatment of rats with NSAIDs that release nitric oxide but maintain anti-inflammatory properties of the original drug protected the gastrointestinal mucosa and accelerated the healing of acid-induced gastric ulcers.[99, 100] In a case control study of a cohort of patients admitted with upper gastrointestinal bleeding, the use of a nitrovasodilator (glyceryl trinitrate, isosorbide dinitrate, isosorbide mononitrate, or any dose of transdermally administered nitroglycerin) was associated with a significantly decreased risk of upper gastrointestinal tract bleeding (odds ratio, 0.6; 95% CI, interval 0.4 to 0.9).[49] Whether nitrates can or should be intentionally used to prevent or treat ulcer bleeding is currently unknown.

Endoscopic Therapy

Endoscopic treatment is widely accepted as the most effective method to control acute ulcer bleeding, and indeed, predicated on the appearance of the ulcer at the time of endoscopy, for prevention of ulcer rebleeding. Although individual studies are generally too small to show a significant effect of endoscopic therapy on mortality, meta-analysis demonstrated that endoscopic therapy prevents not only rebleeding but also death.[32] Experts and national gastroenterologic societies concur on the importance and effectiveness of endoscopic therapy for patients with high-risk ulcers (see Table 13–9).[26, 101]

Despite the data supporting the use of therapeutic endoscopy in ulcer bleeding, several important questions remain. First, lack of standardized definitions and lack of agreement about the various stigmata of recent hemorrhage[91] contribute to less than optimal understanding of the natural history of bleeding lesions. Second, therapeutic endoscopy can be dangerous, leading to further bleeding or perforation (up to 20% and 1% of patients, respectively). Finally, therapeutic endoscopy can add to the cost of treatment. Therapeutic endoscopy is clearly an important component of the management of patients with active bleeding or high-risk lesions, but it must be performed by experts in appropriate clinical settings.

Thermal Therapy

LASER. Argon and neodymium:yttrium aluminum garnet (Nd:YAG) laser therapy were the first endoscopic therapies

Table 13–10 | **Effectiveness of Omeprazole in Peptic Ulcer Bleeding***

STUDY	N	ENDOSCOPIC THERAPY	BLEEDING RATE		*P* VALUE
			Control	Omeprazole	
Hasselgren 1997[55]	322	yes†	26/163 (17%)	12/159 (8%)	N/S
Schaffalitzky de Muckadell 1997[56]	229	yes‡	37/118 (25%)	20/111 (18%)	N/S
Khuroo 1997[57]	220	no	40/110 (36%)	12/110 (11%)	<0.001
Lin 1998[58]	100	yes	8/50 (16%)||	0/50 (0%)	0.01
Lau 2000[59]	240	yes	24/120 (23%)§	5/120 (7%)	<0.001
TOTAL	1111	—	135/561 (24%)	49/550 (9%)	—

*Only large studies are included; all studies examined patients with high-risk lesions: actively bleeding ulcers, visible vessels, and/or adherent clots.
†20/322 patients (all with spurting vessels) received endoscopic therapy at index endoscopy.
‡Approximately 76% of patients underwent endoscopy (with or without therapy) prior to omeprazole.
§Bleeding at 3 days is shown.
||The control group received intravenous cimetidine followed by oral cimetidine.
N/S, not stated.

for hemostasis to be assessed in large numbers of randomized controlled trials. These trials have demonstrated that laser therapies effectively stop ulcer bleeding and reduce the risk of rebleeding.[32, 102] However, laser therapy is expensive and cumbersome and has been largely supplanted by less costly and more portable methods.

MONOPOLAR ELECTROCOAGULATION. Although effective in patients with nonbleeding visible vessels or active bleeding, it is associated with tissue adherence problems, unpredictable energy deposition, and a significant risk of tissue injury and is not recommended.

BIPOLAR OR MULTIPOLAR ELECTROCOAGULATION. The bipolar electrocoagulation device creates an electrical circuit between two electrodes on the tip of a probe; the electrical energy produced is converted to thermal energy and coagulates tissue. Bipolar and multipolar electrocoagulation are effective; parameters of important outcomes such as rebleeding rates, need for transfusion, length of stay, need for surgery, and mortality are improved with these therapies. This small mobile unit has replaced monopolar electrocoagulation. Keys to its successful use include (1) direct probe pressure to tamponade the vessel, (2) a large (3.2-mm) probe, (3) a low watt (15 to 25) setting, and (4) a prolonged period of coaptive coagulation (e.g., at least six to eight pulses of 7 to 10 seconds each.).

HEATER PROBE. The heater probe device produces thermal energy to coagulate tissue. It is effective for treatment of actively bleeding ulcers and for prevention of rebleeding of high-risk lesions. Keys to its successful use include (1) direct probe pressure to tamponade the vessel, and (2) use of a 25 to 30-J setting, and (3) repeated applications.

Injection Therapy

The major nonthermal therapy used for control and prevention of ulcer bleeding is injection. Agents that can be injected include epinephrine (1:10,000), absolute ethanol, normal saline, water, 50% dextrose in water, fibrin glue, and a number of sclerosing agents (polidocanol, sodium tetradecyl sulfate). All appear to be equally effective, and most have been shown to alter outcome significantly.[32, 103]

Newer Endoscopic Therapies

Newer therapies used to stop bleeding include metal clips, rubber band ligation, endoloops, argon plasma coagulation, and sewing devices.[104, 105] Endoscopic metal clips (hemoclips) that resemble those used in surgery appear effective for treatment of actively bleeding ulcers or visible vessels. A randomized controlled trial comparing hemoclips, hypertonic saline-epinephrine injection, and a combination of both found the three modalities to be essentially equivalent.[106] In another study of patients with high-risk stigmata of ulcer hemorrhage who were randomized to receive heater probe or hemoclip therapy, recurrent bleeding was 21% in the heater probe group compared with 1.8% in the hemoclip group ($P = 0.05$).[107] Length of stay and transfusion requirements were significantly lower in the hemoclip group. There was no evidence of clip-induced tissue injury or impaired ulcer healing. Notwithstanding these impressive results, hemoclips are limited by technical and practical considerations. They require considerable expertise, particularly in setting up the device, the need for a well-trained assistant to deploy clips, and the burden of reloading after each clip deployment. Other drawbacks include the inability to reach all lesions owing to tangential approaches and the possibility that the clips may attach improperly or fall off a fibrotic ulcer base. Finally, hemoclips may tear vessels and cause further bleeding.

A relatively new approach for treatment of bleeding from ulcers and other lesions is argon plasma coagulation, a device that allows controlled noncontact electrocoagulation by means of high-frequency energy delivered to tissue through ionized gas (argon plasma). In a prospective randomized trial of 41 patients (20 patients had heater probe therapy and 21 patients had argon plasma coagulation therapy) with active bleeding or a nonbleeding visible vessel found at the time of endoscopy, initial hemostasis (95% vs. 95.2%), recurrent bleeding (21% vs. 15%), 30-day mortality (5% vs. 4.7%), and emergency surgery (15% vs. 9.5%) were comparable in the two groups. Argon plasma coagulation provided faster hemostasis (mean 60 ± 19 vs. 115 ± 28 sec, $P < 0.05$).[104] These data suggest that argon plasma coagulation therapy is safe and effective, and that its use will expand.

Rubber band ligation and endoloops (detachable nylon snares) have been used therapeutically in ulcer bleeding. These modalities are most useful to treat varices and are difficult to apply to a fibrotic ulcer base. An endoscopic sewing device is attractive in that it may allow suture ligature of underlying vessels, but it requires substantial expertise to use.

Comparisons of Therapies

Studies comparing the various endoscopic modalities generally indicate that injection therapy, laser, and multipolar and heater probe are equivalent.[30, 106, 108, 109] The efficacy of laser and hemoclips appears to be as good as (if not better than) the other modalities. However, heater probe, bicap, and injection therapy (with virtually any substance) are favored at this time because of their simplicity and the widespread clinical experience with their use.

Combination Therapies

Combination therapy is attractive in principle; however, currently available data supporting this approach are inconsistent. In a randomized controlled trial of 276 patients with actively bleeding ulcers, Chung and coworkers compared epinephrine injection alone to epinephrine injection plus heater probe.[110] Initial hemostasis was achieved in 131 of 134 patients (98%) who received epinephrine injection alone and 135 of 136 patients (99%) who received additional heater probe treatment ($P = 0.33$). Rebleeding (12 vs. 5), requirement for emergency operation, blood transfusion, hospital stay, ulcer healing at 4 weeks, and in-hospital mortality were not significantly different in the two groups. In the subgroup of patients with spurting hemorrhage, 8 of 27 patients from the epinephrine injection alone group and 2 of

31 patients from the dual treatment group required operative intervention (relative risk in favor of dual treatment, 0.17; 0.03 to 0.87). Although these data suggest that in aggressive bleeding dual therapy may be advantageous, another study comparing hemoclip (41 patients), hypertonic saline-epinephrine (41 patients), and the two therapies combined (42 patients), reported no statistically significant differences in any outcome measured.[106]

In addition to the wide variation in injection regimens just noted, a number of studies have further addressed the use of combination injection approaches.[111, 112] One group found that addition of a sclerosant to epinephrine provided no advantage,[112] whereas another found that a combination of dilute epinephrine (1:100,000) and 600 to 1000 IU of human thrombin was superior to epinephrine alone (rebleeding occurred in 14 of 70 [20%] patients in the epinephrine group compared with 3 [4.5%] in the combination group [$P = 0.005$]) for control of bleeding in patients with active arterial bleeding or a nonbleeding visible vessel.[111] This study raised the possibility that injection using epinephrine plus a natural coagulant may be superior to injection with epinephrine alone.

Repeat Endoscopic Therapy

Since nearly 20% of patients with active bleeding or bleeding from a nonbleeding visible vessel rebleed, some investigators have proposed that "second-look" endoscopy 24 hours after the initial procedure in patients with high-risk lesions may be advantageous. A randomized trial of second-look endoscopy in 104 patients did not demonstrate a significant benefit for this strategy.[113] However, other data suggest that second-look endoscopy may be beneficial in certain subgroups; one study reported that rebleeding was reduced in high-risk patients in whom relook endoscopy had been performed.[114] Because of the high cost of endoscopic therapy in the United States, second-look endoscopy is unlikely to be cost-effective.

In patients with rebleeding after initial treatment for ulcer hemorrhage, repeat endoscopy appears to be useful. In a study of 48 patients with high-risk lesions that initially had been treated endoscopically, repeat endoscopic therapy controlled bleeding in 35 patients.[115] The presence of hypotension on initial presentation ($P = 0.01$) and an ulcer size of at least 2 cm ($P = 0.03$) were independent factors predictive of endoscopic retreatment failure.[115]

Angiographic Therapy

Angiographic therapy is rarely required in patients with ulcer bleeding but may be useful in those with severe, persistent bleeding when endoscopic therapy is unsuccessful or unavailable and surgery is too risky. Intra-arterial vasopressin (which acts by causing smooth muscle contraction and vasoconstriction) may stop ulcer bleeding in 20% to 80% of patients.[116, 117] It is most effective if infused selectively. Complications may be prominent and include bowel ischemia as well as myocardial, brain, renal, or other end-organ ischemia. Vasopressin is relatively contraindicated in those with significant coronary artery disease and is absolutely contraindicated in those with ischemic bowel. Selective occlusion of bleeding arteries with embolic agents such as gelatin sponge (Gelfoam), tissue adhesives, beads, or detachable mechanical occlusion devices (beads, clips) controls bleeding in many cases. However, rebleeding is common, and complications with these compounds can be prominent—ischemia, infarction, perforation, and abscess formation in target and nontarget organs.

Surgical Therapy

Surgery is steadily declining as an adjunct to therapy in patients with bleeding ulcers, probably as a result of acid-decreasing agents.[118] Despite a high rate of spontaneous cessation of ulcer bleeding and the added benefit of endoscopic therapy in high-risk lesions, bleeding is severe and uncontrolled in approximately 5% to 10% of patients. Once it is recognized that bleeding is unresponsive to standard therapy, surgery should be performed promptly. As expected, patients who require such operative intervention for acute hemorrhage are typically severely ill and have a mortality rate of approximately 25%, compared with 10% in unoperated patients.[119] However, such data are likely to be biased, since the sickest patients most often require surgery. Nonetheless, clinical judgment is essential in deciding on balance which patients will benefit from surgery; and in this matter, the timing of surgery requires great clinical skill and experience. Finally, the decision for surgical intervention must take into consideration local expertise in endoscopy, surgery, and intensive care. It will be chosen more often in locales lacking modern facilities and equipment for skillful endoscopy.

Given currently available treatment modalities for ulcer disease, the role of surgery has changed markedly—the primary objective of surgery is usually not to cure ulcer disease but primarily to stop hemorrhage. Surgery is indicated in patients in whom endoscopic (or angiographic in some cases) hemostasis cannot be achieved. Surgery may also be indicated in patients with massive bleeding in whom endoscopic therapy can not be performed or in those with ongoing bleeding. The type of surgery remains controversial; for example, simple oversewing can be performed quickly, and it effectively stops bleeding. However, many surgeons choose to perform an acid-reducing procedure at the same time to prevent recurrent bleeding. This decision must be individualized and depends on the underlying condition of the patient, surgical expertise, and events surrounding the bleeding episode.

Although the definition of endoscopic failure varies, surgical intervention is currently reserved primarily for patients with recurrent bleeding who have failed standard endoscopic therapy. Nonetheless, this issue has begun to be addressed; in a randomized controlled trial of 92 patients with upper gastrointestinal hemorrhage who had failed initial endoscopic therapy, 48 patients were assigned to undergo immediate endoscopic retreatment and 44 were assigned to surgery (the type of operation used was left to the surgeon).[115] Of the 48 patients who were assigned to endoscopic retreatment, 35 had long-term control of bleeding. Of the 13 patients who required salvage surgery, retreatment had failed in 11 and 2 had perforations resulting from thermocoagulation. Five patients in the endoscopy group died within 30 days, compared with eight patients in the surgery group ($P = 0.37$). Seven patients in the endoscopy group (including six who underwent salvage surgery) had complications, compared with sixteen in the surgery group ($P = 0.03$). The duration of hospitalization, the need for hospitalization in the intensive care unit and the resultant duration of that stay, and the number of blood transfusions were similar in the two groups. This study suggested that in patients with peptic ulcers and recurrent bleeding after initial endoscopic control of bleeding, endoscopic retreatment reduces the need for surgery without increasing the risk of death and is associated with fewer complications than surgery.

The role of early elective surgery for bleeding ulcer disease is controversial and has been tested in randomized studies and uncontrolled series.[115, 119–121] These studies have demonstrated that early elective surgery may be beneficial in high-risk groups and harmful in others. At this time, no data from the current endoscopic era support early surgery for bleeding ulcer.

Prevention of Recurrent Ulcer Bleeding

Prevention of recurrent ulcer disease and bleeding is critical in patients with ulcer hemorrhage. Bleeding and nonbleeding ulcers appear to have similar rates of healing with standard therapy,[122] although newer data indicate that pharmacologic therapy with proton pump inhibitors reduces the incidence of rebleeding in patients with high-risk lesions (see Table 13–10). Although its cost effectiveness is controversial, follow-up endoscopy is warranted to document healing and exclude malignancy in certain patients with gastric ulcer. Follow-up endoscopy for patients with duodenal ulcer disease in the absence of complications is not required.

The long-term management of patients after ulcer bleeding has undergone extensive refinement in the last 2 decades. It is well appreciated that patients with peptic ulcer disease are at risk for recurrent disease. Formerly, standard therapy was typically long-term treatment with H_2-receptor antagonists. This approach is supported by a study that demonstrated that ranitidine (150 mg daily) reduced the incidence of recurrent bleeding from 36% in the placebo group to 9% in the ranitidine group over a 61-week follow-up.[123] Currently, however, long-term management hinges on the etiology of the ulcer, particularly whether the ulcer developed as a result of NSAIDs or *H. pylori*.

The data linking persistent *H. pylori* with recurrent ulcer hemorrhage are compelling,[124–127] making eradication of the infection the best approach for these patients. Trials comparing *H. pylori* eradication and long-term antisecretory suppressive therapy have demonstrated slight superiority of *H. pylori* eradication in prevention of recurrent bleeding, but differences were not statistically significant[128, 129] (see Chapter 39).

Patients with bleeding gastroduodenal ulcers who are taking NSAIDs should discontinue their use. If this is not possible, treatment for peptic ulcer should be with a proton pump inhibitor because it is superior to an H_2-receptor antagonist.[130] The NSAID dosage is reduced to the minimal effective dose, and therapy with misoprostol (200 μg four times daily) should be started. For continuing prophylaxis, misoprostol and omeprazole both appear to be effective in prevention of gastroduodenal ulcers and erosions.[131, 132] In a large randomized, controlled study of patients with rheumatoid arthritis receiving NSAIDs, misoprostol led to a 35% reduction in gastrointestinal bleeding events in patients receiving misoprostol compared with placebo, although the difference did not reach statistical significance ($P = 0.06$).[77] An important problem with misoprostol is diarrhea, which can be limited by beginning therapy at 200 μg twice a day and increasing it to 200 μg four times daily as tolerated.

Long-term management of patients with bleeding ulcer is shown in Figure 13–3. For patients not taking NSAIDs, the presence of *H. pylori* should be investigated, preferably by antral biopsy or urea breath test. If present, it should be eradicated (see Chapter 39); if *H. pylori* is not present, then long-term therapy with an anti-secretory agent is indicated. For patients taking NSAIDs and in whom *H. pylori* is present, both risk factors should be eliminated if possible. Although the use of NSAIDs may not increase the risk of ulceration in patients with *H. pylori*, it may increase the risk of complications in patients with existing ulcer disease.

Summary of Therapy for Bleeding Peptic Ulcer

Therapy for bleeding ulcer disease has evolved substantially since the early 1980s. Endoscopic therapy is a cornerstone of management for acute bleeding, and should be performed

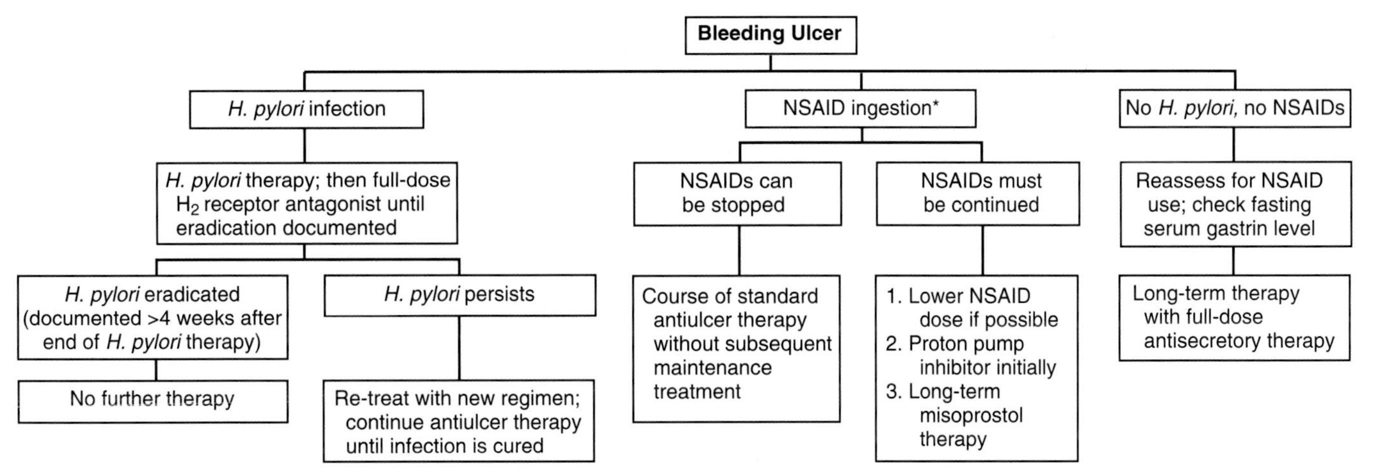

Figure 13–3. Algorithm for long-term management of patients with bleeding ulcers, based on the etiology of the ulcer. If the patient also has *Helicobacter pylori* infection, the infection should be treated and cure documented as shown.

after the patient is stabilized. Endoscopic therapy is indicated in high-risk lesions, as it significantly reduces the likelihood of rebleeding and is associated with a survival benefit. Currently available forms of endoscopic therapy, particularly injection and coagulation appear to be equally effective; the role of combined therapy remains to be defined. Current evidence suggests that an intravenous proton pump inhibitor should be used in patients with high-risk lesions and should be started immediately upon presentation; its further use should be tailored to endoscopic findings. The role of "relook" endoscopy remains controversial. Surgical therapy is an important adjunct to management and should be undertaken as soon as it is appreciated that bleeding is unresponsive to standard therapy, while angiographic therapy is reserved for patients with uncontrolled bleeding who are poor surgical candidates. Whenever possible, patients should have definitive treatment directed at the underlying cause of their ulcer disease to prevent recurrence, as just discussed in detail.

Additional Causes of Upper Gastrointestinal Bleeding

Gastric Erosions

Although hemorrhagic and erosive gastritis refer to findings at endoscopy, a definite association between gastritis and significant bleeding has not been demonstrated. Since gastritis is a histologic diagnosis, it is an inappropriate descriptor for bleeding associated with a gastric lesion. The histologic lesion is a break in the mucosa but not of the muscularis mucosae and thus not into major blood vessels. However, gastritis, most often erosive, remains a time-honored cause of upper gastrointestinal bleeding, reported by endoscopy to be the cause of bleeding in 16% of patients.[133] Such reports notwithstanding, in my experience gastritis or erosive gastric injury rarely causes hemodynamically significant bleeding. When it does, patients usually have an underlying coagulopathy.

Subepithelial erosions develop in the following clinical situations: (1) after ingestion of NSAIDs, (2) in stress-related medical illnesses, and (3) with ethanol. The most common of these is NSAID ingestion. Of patients who ingest NSAIDs chronically, 40% to 60% have erosions at any given time, and 15 to 30% have ulcers. Risk of, treatment for, and prophylaxis of NSAID-associated ulcers has been discussed.

Stress-related gastric mucosal injury occurs in extremely ill patients with serious trauma, extensive burns, major surgery, major medical illness (respiratory failure, sepsis, renal failure), and major neurologic trauma or intracranial disease. Indeed, some degree of stress-related gastric injury can be found in virtually all patients admitted to the intensive care unit, prompting the widespread use of prophylactic regimens for these patients.

Although pharmacologic prophylaxis for stress-induced gastric injury is often recommended for critically ill patients, the evidence supporting its use is mixed. Antacids, H_2-receptor antagonists, and sucralfate have all been used in an attempt to decrease bleeding from stress-related gastric lesions. However, available data suggest their indiscriminant use may not be cost effective. In one study of 2252 critically ill patients, only 1.5% of patients had clinically important bleeding.[134] A randomized controlled trial comparing placebo, intravenous cimetidine, and sucralfate in an intensive care unit revealed no difference in stress-related hemorrhage in the three groups.[135] However, a meta-analysis demonstrated that prophylaxis with H_2-receptor antagonists decreases overt gastrointestinal bleeding (odds ratio [OR], 0.58; 95% confidence interval [CI], 0.42 to 0.79) and, further, that sucralfate is associated with a reduced mortality rate (OR, 0.73; 95% CI, 0.54 to 0.97) relative to antacids and to H_2-receptor antagonists.[136] Although these later data support the use of H_2-receptor antagonists and sucralfate for prophylaxis of clinically important stress-related gastrointestinal bleeding, differences in study design and difficulty in identifying the subset of patients at greatest risk for hemorrhage make consensus difficult on an overall recommendation in this matter.

Prophylaxis for stress-induced gastric injury in specific subsets of patients is, however, warranted. Two strong independent risk factors for bleeding are respiratory failure (OR, 15.6) and coagulopathy (OR, 4.3).[134] Patients with respiratory failure on mechanical ventilation were studied in a randomized controlled trial comparing ranitidine which sucralfate.[137] Clinically significant gastrointestinal bleeding developed in 10 of 596 (1.7%) patients receiving ranitidine, compared with 23 of 604 (3.8%) of those receiving sucralfate (relative risk, 0.44; 95% CI, 0.21 to 0.92; $P = 0.02$). There was no difference in ventilator-associated pneumonia in the two groups. These data suggest that routine prophylaxis is beneficial in this population. Whether ranitidine is superior or more cost effective compared with proton pump inhibitors is unknown.

It is commonly taught that ethanol ingestion causes gastric erosions and gastrointestinal bleeding. However, support for this position is largely derived from experimental animal studies that infused extremely high concentrations of ethanol into the stomach. The term *hemorrhagic gastritis* is frequently applied to the subepithelial hemorrhages seen at endoscopy in alcoholic patients. However, histologic extravasation in such patients is typically superficial, and concomitant mucosal edema is a prominent feature in adjacent, nonhemorrhagic mucosa.[138]

Alcohol consumption is a risk factor for upper gastrointestinal hemorrhage only in those with excessive ethanol consumption (4 or more drinks per day).[139] An endoscopic study of alcoholics found that upper gastrointestinal hemorrhage in most of these patients was the result of peptic ulcer disease or disorders related to portal hypertension. Alcoholic gastric injury was considered to be the cause of bleeding in only 3 of 212 patients, and the bleeding was mild and self-limited.[140]

Endoscopic therapy is generally not useful for treatment of gastritis of any etiology, although it can be attempted if a small number of isolated erosions appear to be the source of bleeding. Selective arterial infusion of vasopressin has been reported to stop bleeding in patients with gastritis,[141] but its use requires considerable expertise, and it has not been rigorously studied. Surgical management of stress-induced gastric erosions is associated with considerable mortality and should be reserved for selected cases.

Duodenitis

Although duodenitis is often included in differential diagnosis of upper gastrointestinal hemorrhage, it is a rare cause of acute bleeding. Risk factors for severe erosive duodenitis are similar to those found in patients with bleeding peptic ulcers, like NSAIDs and *H. pylori*, and often is associated with anticoagulation therapy. The bleeding is usually self-limited and rarely requires intervention.

Malignancy

Neoplasms of the esophagus, stomach, and upper small intestine cause acute upper gastrointestinal hemorrhage infrequently. Such lesions are more often associated with occult, asymptomatic bleeding, which usually is self-limited. The majority of tumors associated with clinically significant acute upper gastrointestinal hemorrhage are malignant.[142] Of the many tumors that cause upper gastrointestinal hemorrhage, the most common is advanced gastric adenocarcinoma.[142] A small proportion of bleeding lesions have been managed with injection or coagulation therapy, and bleeding polypoid lesions can sometimes be snared,[143] but large and/or sessile bleeding lesions typically require surgical intervention. These patients with upper gastrointestinal bleeding from tumors have a 1-year survival rate of 11%.[142]

Dieulafoy's Lesion

Dieulafoy's lesion, also termed *exulceratio simplex Dieulafoy*, refers to an abnormally large artery that retains the large caliber of its feeding vessel as it approaches the mucosa.[144] This large vessel is thought to compress the mucosa and cause a small erosion with rupture of the vessel into the lumen. Dieulafoy's lesions are not uncommon, accounting for up to 6% of cases of upper gastrointestinal hemorrhage.[145] Dieulafoy's lesions are typically found in the proximal portion of the stomach, usually within 6 cm of the gastroesophageal junction, but they may be located anywhere in the gastrointestinal tract (see Fig. 120–11).

Bleeding is often massive and recurrent; it is often difficult to identify the lesion, unless it is actively bleeding or is associated endoscopically with stigmata of recent bleeding. Endosonography may be useful in the detection of Dieulafoy's disease in patients with unexplained upper gastrointestinal bleeding.[146] Therapy with injection techniques, coagulative therapy, hemoclips, and banding can all control bleeding and prevent rebleeding in over 95% of cases.[146–149] The long-term prognosis of patients with Dieulafoy's lesions, in the absence of concomitant medical illness, is excellent.

Vascular Lesions (See also Chapter 120)

Vascular Ectasia (See Figs. 120–1, 120–2, 120–3)

Vascular lesions are an uncommon, but important, cause of upper gastrointestinal tract bleeding. A number of vascular disorders can cause upper gastrointestinal hemorrhage, but the most common vascular lesions are vascular ectasias, which are most often found in the stomach or duodenum. Vascular ectasias more commonly cause lower gastrointestinal and occult bleeding (see below) than upper gastrointestinal tract bleeding.[150] They are found in a variety of conditions, including renal failure, cirrhosis, scleroderma, the CREST syndrome (Calciosis, Reynaud's phenomenon, Esophageal dysmotility, Sclerodactyly, Telangiectasis), radiation injury, collagen diseases such as pseudoxanthoma elasticum and Ehlers-Danlos syndrome, and von Willebrand's disease. Vascular ectasias appear to be most often associated with chronic renal failure. In a prospective study of upper gastrointestinal hemorrhage over a 50-month period, vascular ectasia was the etiology of upper gastrointestinal hemorrhage in 13% of patients with renal insufficiency, defined as a serum creatinine level greater than 2.0 mg/dL, and was the etiology of bleeding more often in patients with renal insufficiency than in those with normal renal function.[151] The prevalence of vascular ectasia as a cause of upper gastrointestinal bleeding was related to the duration of renal failure and the requirement for hemodialysis.

The treatment of vascular ectasias is difficult because they are rarely found in isolation. Patients with lesions that are readily identified or are actively bleeding are best treated endoscopically with laser, bipolar electrocoagulation, bicap, banding, injection therapy, or argon plasma coagulation; each technique appears to be effective and safe in this setting. Perforation of the gastrointestinal tract, however, is a risk, particularly with electrocoagulation or laser therapy. Massive bleeding may be stopped by angiographic therapy. Recurrent bleeding from a specific bleeding lesion after endoscopic or angiographic therapy is uncommon; surgical therapy is reserved for low-risk patients who have lesions that are clearly identified as the bleeding source. The use of hormonal therapy is highly controversial (see later Occult and Obscure Bleeding).

Arteriovenous Malformations

True arteriovenous malformations, which may appear as raised or nodular lesions at endoscopy, are rare. These lesions are probably congenital in origin and, in contrast to vascular ectasias, usually involve the submucosa; they may be large and involve any portion of the gut wall; the primary treatment is resection of the involved bowel (see Chapter 120).

Hereditary Hemorrhagic Telangiectasia (Osler-Weber-Rendu Disease)

Hereditary hemorrhagic telangiectasia is an autosomal dominant disorder characterized by telangiectasias of the skin, mucous membranes, and gastrointestinal tract (see Fig. 120–8). The peak incidence of bleeding is in the 6th decade of life, and can originate from any site in the gastrointestinal tract. Epistaxis is the most common manifestation which typically occurs before the 2nd decade. Approximately 80% of patients have a family history of bleeding. Lack of telangiectasias on the lips, oral and nasopharyngeal membranes, tongue, and periungual areas should cast doubt on the diagnosis. Of many forms of treatment, endoscopic therapy is most effective in stopping hemorrhage from actively bleeding lesions. Unfortunately, because of the multiplicity of lesions, bleeding often recurs. Surgical therapy is reserved for those with discrete lesions identified as the source of the bleeding. Hormonal therapy, typically with an estrogen and progesterone combination, has met with mixed results (see Chapter 120).

Hemangioma

Hemangiomas causing upper gastrointestinal hemorrhage are most commonly identified in the upper small intestine. These benign vascular tumors made up of proliferating vessels, almost all of which are cavernous hemangiomas, appear as single or multiple red, purple, or blue nodular lesions. The blue rubber nevus syndrome is characterized by cavernous hemangiomas of the skin, gastrointestinal tract, and other viscera (see Fig. 120–12). These lesions generally should not be treated endoscopically. Angiographic therapy may stop bleeding; however, the most effective treatment is surgical (see Chapter 120).

Gastric Vascular Ectasia

Gastric vascular ectasia constitutes a group of recently recognized entities that rarely cause acute upper gastrointestinal hemorrhage. This lesion is characterized by aggregates of red spots (see Chapter 120). When the aggregates are arranged in a linear pattern in the antrum of the stomach, the term *gastric antral vascular ectasia* (GAVE), or watermelon stomach, is used (see Fig. 120–9). In contrast, the ectatic red spots may be more diffuse and involve the proximal stomach, and then are termed *diffuse gastric vascular ectasia* (see Fig. 120–1). This lesion is difficult to differentiate from portal hypertensive gastropathy. Gastric vascular ectasia is most common in middle aged and elderly women who have associated achlorhydria, atrophic gastritis, and cirrhosis. Its pathogenesis is unknown.[152, 153] Although originally thought to be portal hypertensive in etiology, recent work casts doubt on this hypothesis. Indeed, 14 patients with gastric vascular ectasia had continued bleeding or no endoscopic change in their lesion after transjugular intrahepatic portosystemic shunts.[153] In comparison, approximately 75% of patients with severe portal hypertensive gastropathy ceased to bleed after transjugular intrahepatic portosystemic shunts.[153] Neither use of beta-blockers nor standard portal decompression have proved effective for treatment of gastric vascular ectasia, nor has endoscopic thermal therapy or antrectomy been effective. One small trial, ethinyl estradiol (30 μg) and norethisterone (1.5 mg) daily led to a significant decrease in transfusion requirements in the majority of patients[154]; however, these results have not been confirmed.

ACUTE LOWER GASTROINTESTINAL BLEEDING

Acute lower gastrointestinal bleeding is distinct clinically from upper gastrointestinal hemorrhage in epidemiology, prognosis, management, and outcome. Lower gastrointestinal bleeding encompasses a wide clinical spectrum ranging from trivial hematochezia to massive hemorrhage with shock, requiring emergency hospitalization. Although most instances of lower gastrointestinal bleeding are self-limited and do not require hospitalized care, approximately 21 per 100,000 adults will require hospitalization per year for severe bleeding.[3] Hospitalization rates for lower gastrointestinal bleeding are approximately one third of those for upper gastrointestinal bleeding[20] and, in a survey by the American College of Gastroenterology, accounted for 24% of all bleeding events.[37] Although lower gastrointestinal bleeding is reportedly less common than upper gastrointestinal bleeding, it is certainly underreported, as evidenced by a cross-sectional survey of American population in which 14% experienced some amount of rectal bleeding during a 12-month period, but only a fraction sought medical care.[155] Notably, the incidence of lower gastrointestinal bleeding is higher in men and increases with age, presumably due to the high incidence of diverticulosis and vascular disease in this group.

Initial management of patients with lower gastrointestinal bleeding is similar to patients with acute upper gastrointestinal hemorrhage, including assessment of the severity of bleeding, hemodynamic stabilization, and determination of prognosis. Subsequently, the clinician's attention turns to consideration of the site, potential cause(s), and specific therapy of bleeding.

Prognosis

The severity of lower gastrointestinal bleeding varies from very mild blood loss, usually manifest as intermittent hematochezia, to hemodynamically life-threatening bleeding. Compared with upper gastrointestinal hemorrhage, few data on prognostic variables for lower gastrointestinal bleeding exist. The acuity of hemorrhage in patients with lower gastrointestinal bleeding is usually less than in upper gastrointestinal hemorrhage. Orthostasis and shock were less common in patients with lower gastrointestinal hemorrhage than in those with upper gastrointestinal hemorrhage (19% vs. 35%, respectively)[37] and transfusion was more often required in upper gastrointestinal bleeders (64% vs. 36%, respectively). Nonetheless, about 50% of patients with lower gastrointestinal bleeding referred to an open-access endoscopy unit exhibited some form of hemodynamic disturbance, including 9% with cardiovascular collapse, 10% with syncope, and 30% with orthostasis.[156]

Approach to Diagnosis and Therapy

As with upper bleeding, historical information gives clues. Lower gastrointestinal bleeding in elderly patients is commonly caused by colonic *diverticula* or *vascular ectasias*, whereas in young patients, infectious or inflammatory conditions are more likely. Such bleeding in other specific subsets of the population raises the possibility of other diagnoses—e.g., the most common cause of lower gastrointestinal bleeding in HIV-infected patients is cytomegalovirus (CMV) infection.[157] NSAIDs appear to be associated with lower gastrointestinal bleeding, especially from diverticula.[158] Bleeding from diverticula or vascular ectasias is often painless; hence, the presence of abdominal pain suggests that inflammatory or ischemic colitis is more likely. A history of radiation, previous surgery, particularly vascular surgery, constipation, change in bowel habit, and anorectal disease or trauma is important to consider in making a correct diagnosis.

The evaluation should rapidly progress to an understanding of the character of the stool output. Since accounts of hematochezia vary considerably, it is important that the color of the blood first seen by the patient be ascertained. Such information appears to be the most informative.[159] Bright red blood most commonly indicates a distal source or a rapidly bleeding proximal source, whereas black stool indicates a slowly bleeding right colonic or more proximal source. Accordingly, in patients with apparent massive lower gastrointestinal bleeding, it is important to exclude upper gastrointestinal hemorrhage by examining the aspirate from a nasogastric tube.

The diagnostic approach to lower gastrointestinal bleeding is controversial and not yet standardized. Some investigators recommend urgent anoscopy and flexible sigmoidoscopy for immediate evaluation of hematochezia. I strongly encourage anoscopy in most patients as part of the initial diagnostic evaluation (Fig. 13–4). It is easily performed, inexpensive, and the best way to detect local anorectal abnormalities such as internal hemorrhoids, anal lacerations, tears, and fistulas. Flexible sigmoidoscopy may be diagnostic, following an enema preparation, for ulcerative or infectious colitis, hemorrhoids, proctitis, or solitary rectal ulcer, thus eliminating the need for emergency colonoscopy. However, this approach has not been widely studied, and sigmoidoscopy is rarely as informative as colonoscopy. Furthermore, the presence of an anal or rectal lesion does not exclude a more proximal bleeding lesion.

Few prospective data are available to judge the relative efficacy of the various diagnostic tests for lower gastrointestinal bleeding, including barium enema, colonoscopy, tagged red blood cell (RBC) scintigraphy, and visceral angiography. Barium enema is not recommended as part of the initial evaluation for acute lower gastrointestinal bleeding because it has a low diagnostic yield in this setting, and it may also interfere with subsequent performance of other tests, particularly endoscopy. RBC scintigraphy has been used extensively in patients with lower gastrointestinal hemorrhage but has no therapeutic capability. Colonoscopy, angiography, and surgery are all important diagnostic tools, and each has therapeutic potential.

Colonoscopy

Although early endoscopy for the diagnosis and treatment of upper gastrointestinal bleeding is predicated on sound data, early endoscopy for lower gastrointestinal bleeding has not been similarly adopted. Historically, colonoscopy has been used primarily for nonurgent investigation of patients with lower gastrointestinal bleeding, usually after cessation of bleeding and colonic preparation. The reluctance to perform colonoscopy acutely is due to poor visibility, potential for complications, and theoretical concern about the adverse effects of purging the colon in the setting of active gastrointestinal bleeding.[160–162]

A number of reports show that urgent colonoscopy is safe and yields a specific diagnosis in a high proportion of patients in this setting (Table 13–11).[11, 163–165] The definition of "urgent" and the timing of procedures vary greatly both in clinical practice and in published reports. The advantages of urgent colonoscopy, i.e., performed as soon as the patient has been hospitalized and prepped, include the high likelihood of detecting an actively bleeding lesion or one with stigmata of bleeding, and thereby a lesion amenable to endoscopic therapy might be discovered.

Some researchers have proposed urgent, unprepared colonoscopy for evaluation of lower gastrointestinal bleeding.[164] In one analysis of 85 consecutive patients who underwent 126 colonoscopies, a bleeding site was identified in 97%. Complications were uncommon; one patient developed asymptomatic free air after a cauterization procedure in the right colon, and two patients developed hyponatremia, possibly related to extensive irrigation of the colon.

For urgent colonoscopy, a number of bowel preparations (often polyethylene glycol–based solutions) administered by

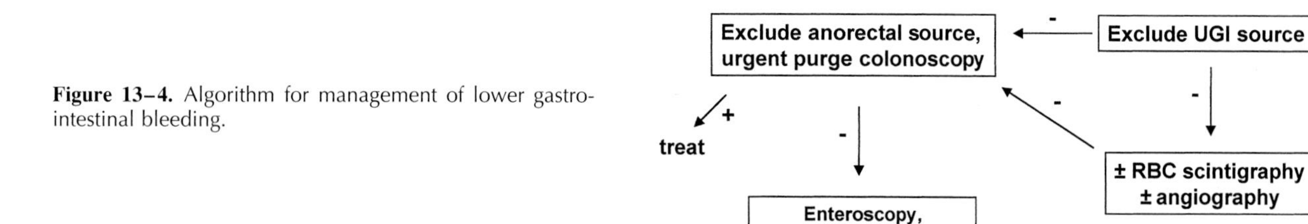

Figure 13–4. Algorithm for management of lower gastrointestinal bleeding.

Table 13–11 | **Urgent Colonoscopy for Evaluation of Lower Gastrointestinal Bleeding**

STUDY	N	BOWEL PREPARATION GIVEN %	SPECIFIC DIAGNOSIS MADE N (%)	ENDOSCOPIC THERAPY ADMINISTERED N (%)
Kok 1998[163]	190	85	148	10
Chaudry 1998[164]	85	0	82	17
Jensen 2000[165]	121	100	121	10*
TOTAL	396	—	351 (89%)	37 (9%)

*Reported only patients who received therapy specifically for diverticular lesions.

mouth or nasogastric tube have been utilized. Although bowel preparation may hinder the ability to localize fresh blood to a specific lesion, it improves visualization of the colon, substantially increases the likelihood that stigmata of definite or presumptive bleeding will be identified, and does not reactivate bleeding. The complication rate of urgent colonoscopy in this setting is low.

Based on a high diagnostic yield, low rate of complications, and theoretical therapeutic potential, national gastroenterologic societies have concluded that colonoscopy is the diagnostic procedure of choice in most patients with lower gastrointestinal bleeding.[160, 162] Whether it should be performed urgently with or without a purge preparation or can be performed expectantly is an open question at this time.

Tagged Red Blood Cell Scintigraphy

The use of scintigraphy, preferably with technetium-labeled RBC, in patients with lower gastrointestinal bleeding remains highly controversial. Although it may detect bleeding as small as 0.1 to 0.5 mL/min, the sensitivity can be decreased by bowel motility stimulated by intraluminal blood. Advantages of tagged RBC scintigraphy are (1) sensitivity to low rates of bleeding, (2) safety; (3) it is noninvasive; (4) no risk of contrast reaction, and (5) low cost. Potential disadvantages of scintigraphy include its lack of therapeutic capability and doubt about its accuracy.

A number of clinical parameters are used to predict positive RBC scintigraphy studies. If the character and color of the stool at the time of radionuclide scan indicate rapid bleeding (gross blood per rectum, frequent bloody stools, and so on), it is likely to be positive.[166] Unexpectedly, neither the number of units of blood transfused nor hemodynamics at presentation appears to predict a positive scan.[166, 167]

Perhaps the most important question surrounding RBC scintigraphy is reliability in directing specific surgical treatment. In 635 positive scans reported in the literature, the site of bleeding was correctly localized by tagged RBC scintigraphy in 343 cases, confirmed by other tests in 269 (78%).[166] One study assessing the reliability of RBC bleeding scans found that 8 of 19 (42%) patients who underwent surgery based only on a positive scan had recurrent bleeding.[168] Another study reported that of 18 patients operated on for lower gastrointestinal bleeding, 11 had negative scans for bleeding and the bleeding scan was inaccurate in the other 7 patients; thus, in no instance did the scan direct the surgical intervention.[169] Based on these data, surgical therapy is not generally recommended on the basis of tagged RBC scintigraphy alone.

Tagged RBC scintigraphy may be useful as a screening test for visceral angiography rather than as a definitive diagnostic test. A study of the utility of requiring positive tagged RBC scintigraphy prior to performing visceral angiography[170] found that it increased the yield of angiography from 22% to 53%. Furthermore, in a cost-effectiveness analysis, scintigraphic screening prior to angiography appeared to be cost saving,[171] a result contested by a study of patients who underwent both procedures, but only 33% of those with positive scintigraphy had a positive angiogram[172] and 33% of those with negative scintigraphy had a positive angiogram. The data are thus conflicting, and in the absence of randomized controlled studies, leave open the diagnostic role of RBC scintigraphy in lower gastrointestinal bleeding, particularly since accuracy depends on local expertise and experience.

Angiography

Once visceral angiography was the initial diagnostic procedure in the evaluation of acute lower gastrointestinal bleeding. Since its use is limited by visualization of active bleeding only at a rate of at least 0.5 to 1.0 mL/min, RBC scintigraphy is often used prior to angiography. Indeed, patients who develop an immediate blush on RBC scintigraphy appear to have the highest diagnostic yield at angiography.[173] The advantages of angiography are accurate localization of rapidly bleeding lesions and the potential to achieve immediate hemostasis with several therapeutic maneuvers. However, since angiography occasionally causes serious complications such as arterial thrombosis, contrast reactions, and acute renal failure, its use prior to definitive surgical therapy has been questioned.[174] Most acute lower gastrointestinal bleeding stops spontaneously; thus, it is important to use angiography specifically for those with continued bleeding in whom accurate localization and, hence, effective therapy may be life-saving.

The likelihood of a positive angiographic study in patients with lower gastrointestinal bleeding is nearly 50%,[161] a figure which may be high due to bias in reported studies[161] limiting angiography to patients with positive tagged RBC scintigraphy[170] or to those with an immediate blush on tagged RBC scintigraphy.[173] Some have proposed using vasodilators, anticoagulants, and/or thrombolytics to improve the diagnostic yield of angiography, but these methods have not been widely studied.

Comparisons of diagnostic accuracy between angiography and endoscopy in lower gastrointestinal hemorrhage are limited. In one study of 22 patients with severe hematochezia who underwent both emergency visceral angiography and endoscopy, a diagnosis was made in only 14% of patients by angiography compared with 91% of patients by endoscopy.[11] Endoscopy had no complications, but 9% of patients undergoing angiography had complications. The implementation of urgent colonoscopy may be decreasing the utilization of angiography. In one study 5 of 85 consecutive patients underwent angiography and only one had a positive study,[164] and in another, of 13 of 190 patients studied, only 4 had a positive result.[163]

Computed tomographic angiography might be useful diagnostically, particularly for colonic vascular ectasia. In a study of 28 patients with suspected bleeding from colonic vascular ectasia in whom vascular ectasias were verified by colonoscopy plus visceral angiography, a high proportion of lesions were identified by computed tomographic angiography.[175] The potential advantages of this new approach for detection of vascular ectasia are that it is noninvasive, simple to use, and less costly than conventional angiography. However, it is limited by the inability to assess active bleeding, the reliance upon indirect evidence such as dilated vessels and early venous filling to make the diagnosis, and the lack of therapeutic capability. Whether computed tomographic angiography will find a place in the diagnostic algorithm for lower gastrointestinal hemorrhage is unknown.

Specific Causes of Lower Gastrointestinal Bleeding

The two major causes of significant lower gastrointestinal bleeding are *colonic diverticula* and *vascular ectasia* (Table 13–12). Hemodynamically insignificant bleeding is frequently caused by hemorrhoids and neoplasia. Less common causes include solitary rectal ulcer, colonic varices, vasculitis, endometriosis, intussusception, and small intestinal lesions (small bowel tumors, small bowel ulceration, mesenteric vascular insufficiency, small bowel diverticula, Meckel's diverticulum, and aortoenteric fistula). Rare causes include drug-induced hemorrhagic colitis, portal colopathy, diversion colitis, and gastrointestinal bleeding in runners. The source of bleeding cannot be definitively identified in a significant number of patients.[3, 161]

Table 13–12 | **Causes of Acute Lower Gastrointestinal Bleeding**

COMMON CAUSES
Diverticula
Vascular ectasia
UNCOMMON CAUSES
Neoplasia (including postpolypectomy)
Inflammatory bowel disease
Colitis
Ischemic
Radiation
Unspecified
Hemorrhoids
Small bowel source
Upper gastrointestinal source
No lesion identified
RARE CAUSES
Dieulafoy's lesions
Colonic ulcerations
Rectal varices

Diverticula (See also Chapter 108)

Although bleeding from diverticula of the colon is infrequent, it is the most common cause of lower gastrointestinal bleeding because of its high prevalence in the Western world. Diverticula typically are located in the colonic wall at the sites of penetrating nutrient vessels. The pathogenesis of bleeding is unknown but it probably results from penetration of a colonic artery into the dome of a diverticulum, and the rupture is thought to be the result of erosion from pressure rather than infection, since evidence of concomitant diverticulitis is usually absent.

Diverticular bleeding is characterized by acute, painless hematochezia. Blood is typically bright red but may be maroon, or even melenic, depending on the site and rapidity of bleeding. Bleeding is not often hemodynamically significant, except in elderly people with comorbid conditions. Despite its frequency, the diagnosis of diverticular hemorrhage is usually made by exclusion, most often by identification of diverticula by colonoscopy or other imaging technique (usually CT), in patients with lower gastrointestinal bleeding in whom other diagnoses have been excluded. In a small proportion of patients, however, bleeding from a diverticula can be positively identified.[165, 176]

Bleeding from diverticula usually stops spontaneously and does not recur in a majority of patients.[3, 177] However, from 10% to 40% of patients will have recurrent hemorrhage.[3, 177] Of these, approximately 70% to 80% will cease bleeding spontaneously. The risk of diverticular rebleeding appears to increase with time, likely due to bleeding from another of the multiple diverticula typically present in these patients. In 83 patients whose initial diverticular bleeding episode was managed without definitive therapy, the recurrence rate (Kaplan-Meier method) was 9% at 1 year, 10% at 2 years, 19% at 3 years, and 25% at 4 years.[3] Further, the rebleeding rate for patients with diverticular hemorrhage appears to be proportional to the severity of the initial bleed. McGuire reported that only 1 of 64 (2%) patients admitted with diverticular bleeding who required 3 or fewer blood transfusions had rebleeding, whereas 25 of 42 (60%) patients who required 4 or more units rebled.[177]

When diverticular bleeding recurs, colonoscopy should be attempted at least once, preferably urgently, and after a high-quality purge preparation. The major reason for such an aggressive approach is that stigmata of bleeding may be identified in a small fraction of lesions, and, in such instances, endoscopic therapy applied to the bleeding lesion may be effective (Fig. 13–5).[165, 176, 178] Patients with recurrent bleeding usually require combinations of colonoscopic treatment, angiographic intervention, and surgical resection: Patients with aggressive re-bleeding are best treated by resection of an identified site, whereas outcomes, especially in elderly patients, are poor following blind subtotal colectomy.

Vascular Ectasia

Colonic vascular ectasias, or angiodysplasias, are a common cause of acute, chronic, and occult lower gastrointestinal bleeding. Although most common in the right colon, they have been identified in all portions of the gastrointestinal tract (see Fig. 120–3). The pathogenesis of vascular ectasias is unknown (see Chapter 120) but is probably associated

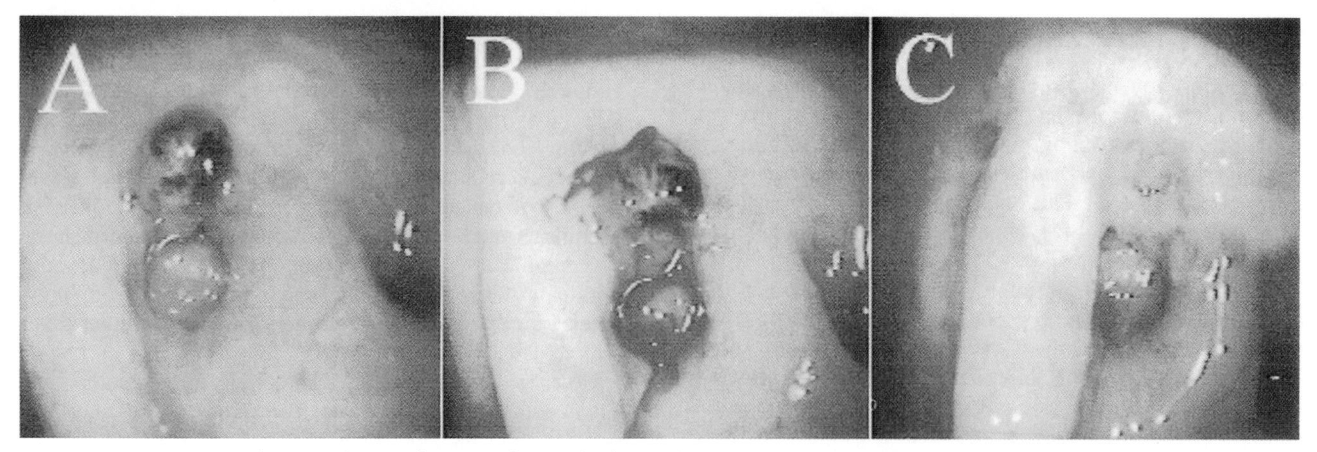

Figure 13–5. Endoscopic therapy for acute diverticular hemorrhage. *A*, Diverticular stigmata of hemorrhage, nonbleeding visible vessel. *B*, Diverticulum after circumferential injection of epinephrine (1 : 10,000) demonstrating local vasoconstriction. *C*, Elimination of bleeding site after cautery with bipolar electrocoagulation therapy. (From Bloomfeld RS, Rockey WC, Shetzline MA: Endoscopic therapy of acute diverticular hemorrhage. Am J Gastroenterol 96:2369, 2001.)

with aging. One theory suggests that repeated, partial intermittent obstruction of the submucosal veins where they pierce the muscle layers of the colon leads to dilation and tortuosity of submucosal veins. Subsequently, the arteriolar-capillary-venular unit dilates, creating a small arteriovenous communication. The predilection of the right colon for these degenerative lesions may reflect the greater tension in the cecal wall than in the rest of the colon. Vascular ectasias are most commonly identified in elderly patients; over two thirds of patients with vascular ectasias are over the age of 70 years. Colonic vascular ectasias are uncommon among healthy, asymptomatic people (prevalence, 0.83%) and when identified are typically small.[179] Patients with bleeding vascular ectasias often have chronic underlying medical conditions, renal failure in particular. An association between vascular ectasias and aortic valve disease has been proposed ("Williams syndrome")[180] but is questionable.[181]

Lower gastrointestinal bleeding caused by vascular ectasia is clinically indistinguishable from diverticular bleeding and is characterized by painless hematochezia. The character of passed blood ranges from bright red to melenic depending on the site of and rapidity of bleeding. The pace and volume of bleeding usually are less severe than with diverticular bleeding and are rarely hemodynamically significant. Patients with bleeding vascular ectasias often receive anticoagulation.[182] The diagnosis is most often made by colonoscopy or angiography. Approximately three quarters of bleeding vascular ectasias are identified in the right colon.[183] Colonoscopy most often identifies vascular ectasias without stigmata of active bleeding, making ascertainment of its role in bleeding difficult. Stigmata of bleeding in association with vascular ectasias may be found and demands immediate endoscopic therapy.

Despite the existence of few objective data, the best treatment for patients with lower gastrointestinal bleeding and colonic vascular ectasia is therapeutic endoscopy. Electrocoagulation, injection therapy, heater probe, laser, and argon plasma coagulation are all reasonably effective and safe.[166, 183, 184] The major risk of endoscopic therapy is perforation of the colon, particularly in the thin-walled right colon. Pharmacologic control of bleeding vascular ectasias (discussed later) may be effective in some patients with multiple bleeding lesions.

The role of conventional angiography in lower gastrointestinal bleeding caused by vascular ectasia is controversial, but it should be used in cases of continuing or recurrent bleeding. Angiography successfully identifies lesions in a high proportion of patients and directs therapeutic intervention with intra-arterial vasopressin or embolization, which often successfully controls the bleeding (see later).[185–190]

Most patients with a bleeding vascular ectasia can be managed without surgical intervention. However, surgical therapy is required for those with uncontrollable or recurrent bleeding, and the procedure is tailored to the specific or suspected sites of bleeding. Outcomes are best when resection is performed for a definitive, localized lesion.

Neoplasia

Acute lower gastrointestinal bleeding from colon carcinoma is uncommon. However, in one report, this diagnosis was responsible for bleeding in 36% of cases.[156, 187, 191] Bleeding, usually occult, is from mucosal defects on the luminal surface. Although colonic polyps may bleed, the bleeding is rarely aggressive, and, as with carcinomas, is generally painless, intermittent, and of small volume. Clinical features such as weight loss, intermittent hematochezia, change in caliber of stool, and evidence of chronic bleeding (i.e., iron deficiency anemia) should raise the possibility of bleeding from colonic neoplasia (see also Chapter 115).

Lower gastrointestinal bleeding after polypectomy is an uncommon but important cause of lower gastrointestinal hemorrhage,[192–194] reported as high as 3% in patients undergoing polypectomy,[166] much above more recent reports of 0.2% to 0.6%.[193, 195] Early bleeding is thought to be caused by inadequate coagulation of the blood vessel in the stalk at the time of separation of the polyp. Delayed bleeding may occur up to 3 weeks after polypectomy, and sessile cecal polyps greater than 2 cm in diameter pose the greatest risk for bleeding.[194] Most episodes usually can be managed conservatively; occasionally, endoscopic coagulation is required and is usually effective.

Hemorrhoids

Hemorrhoids are extremely common and are reported to account for 5% to 10% of acute lower gastrointestinal bleeding episodes, although a specific bleeding site is rarely identified. Hemorrhoids cause intermittent low-volume bleeding, with bright red blood seen on the toilet tissue or around, but not mixed, in the stool. Straining often exacerbates bleeding. Careful visualization of the external anal canal and anoscopy are essential for diagnosis. Since hemorrhoids are common, lower gastrointestinal hemorrhage should not be ascribed solely to hemorrhoids until other lesions have been excluded. In patients with hemorrhoids, full colonoscopic examination is given to patients over the age of 50 years, those with any risk factors for colon cancer, or those with warning symptoms of colorectal cancer such as change in bowel habit or weight loss.

Nonoperative management is usually effective in patients with bleeding hemorrhoids (sitz baths, avoidance of straining, and dietary modification). Rubber band ligation, coagulation therapy, and surgical hemorrhoidectomy are therapeutic options in patients with refractory disease[196] (see Chapter 118).

Meckel's Diverticulum

Meckel's diverticulum is a remnant of the vitelline duct present in the terminal 100 cm of the ileum in about 2% of the population. It contains gastric mucosa, which secretes acid and results in ulceration of adjacent mucosa. It bleeds most often in children, and to a lesser extent in young adults, and thus is the most common cause of gastrointestinal bleeding in patients younger than 30 years. Bleeding is often brisk and painless, the diagnosis of which is typically made by radiolabeled technetium scanning. Surgical removal is the treatment of choice in patients who have had hemorrhage.

Colitis

A number of different diseases can cause ulceration and inflammation in the colon—each is an important potential cause of lower gastrointestinal hemorrhage. The most common of the colitides to cause acute lower gastrointestinal bleeding is inflammatory bowel disease (see Chapters 103 and 104). Although *ulcerative colitis* is traditionally thought of as most likely to cause severe lower gastrointestinal bleeding, a recent report suggested that *Crohn's disease* more commonly causes lower gastrointestinal hemorrhage.[197] In this study, bleeding occurred in approximately 1% of patients admitted for inflammatory bowel disease, and the source of bleeding was most often ileocolonic or colonic, although the small intestine was the source of bleeding in some patients. Bleeding was usually self-limited and often responded to medical therapy, although acute surgical intervention was required in approximately 15% of patients. The presence of an endoscopically treatable lesion was uncommon. Recurrent hemorrhage was not rare, and for most of these patients, surgery is the most appropriate intervention.[197]

Many *infectious agents* can penetrate and injure the colonic mucosa and cause acute lower gastrointestinal bleeding. Specific diseases include the enteritides of the *Salmonella* species, *Escherichia coli* (especially the O157:H7 variant), *Shigella* species, and *Campylobacter* species (see Chapter 96). Pseudomembranous colitis (*Clostridium difficile*) and Cytomegalovirus are important causes of significant lower gastrointestinal hemorrhage; the former follows use of antibiotics, whereas the latter is prominent in immunosuppressed patients (see Chapters 28 and 97).

Radiation therapy induces inflammatory changes in the colon and can lead to radiation colitis. Radiation colitis most commonly affects the rectum and is common after pelvic radiotherapy. Steroids, hyperbaric oxygen, 5-aminosalicylic acid compounds, and sucralfate have been advocated as treatment for radiation proctitis, but few data support their effectiveness. Surgery is necessary for acute bleeding and will be successful in most cases (see Chapter 102).[198]

The incidence of *ischemic colitis*, an established cause of lower gastrointestinal hemorrhage, is unknown.[199] It is due to embolic obstruction of one of the colic arteries or to low flow due to reduced cardiac output or nonocclusive vascular disease. Bleeding from ischemic colitis is manifested by sudden, crampy abdominal pain and tenderness. Bleeding is generally not vigorous, and blood loss requiring significant transfusion is uncommon. The diagnosis of ischemic colitis is one of exclusion, being made by endoscopic identification of colonic inflammation and ulceration in a patient with advanced atherosclerosis or cardiac disease or both. Ischemic colitis is usually managed conservatively, with supportive care and correction of the underlying cardiovascular situation (see Chapter 119).

Treatment of Lower Gastrointestinal Bleeding

The majority of episodes of acute lower gastrointestinal bleeding cease spontaneously, regardless of source, but patients with continuing or recurrent bleeding require intervention. Therapy may be required to prevent rebleeding in patients at risk for serious complications of a recurrence. Therapeutic options are more limited than for upper gastrointestinal tract bleeding: endoscopic, angiographic, and surgical therapy. Currently, specific pharmacologic therapy for most patients with lower gastrointestinal bleeding is unavailable. Unfortunately, few data comparing the effectiveness of different therapeutic modalities are available at this time.

Endoscopic Therapy

Effectiveness of endoscopic therapy for lower gastrointestinal hemorrhage depends mainly on the skill and experience of the operator. Thus, in centers where urgent endoscopy is performed, abnormalities are more likely to be found during colonoscopy than when it is performed expectantly. As noted in Table 13–11, 10% to 15% of patients undergoing urgent colonoscopy had some form of endoscopic therapy.[166] Methods of hemostatic therapy include injection, laser, heater probe, monopolar and multipolar electrocoagulation, and argon plasma coagulation (see Fig. 13–5). Many abnormalities are treated; the most common are diverticula with associated active bleeding, nonbleeding visible vessels, adherent clots,[165, 176, 178] and vascular ectasias.[183, 184, 200]

Although data on the effectiveness of endoscopic therapy for lesions causing lower gastrointestinal bleeding are limited, the experience at large centers, case reports, and reported series all suggest that it may be. In the first phase of a study on endoscopic therapy in diverticular bleeding,[165] 17 patients with stigmata of such bleeding were not treated; 9 (53%) rebled, requiring surgical intervention in 6. In the second phase, 10 comparable patients underwent endoscopic therapy with epinephrine (1 : 20,000), bipolar coagulation (10 to 15 W, 1-sec pulses), or both, and no patient rebled. Not all studies, however, demonstrate such a favorable outcome after endoscopic therapy for diverticular hemorrhage. In another study of 12 patients with diverticular hemorrhage and stigmata of bleeding who underwent similar endoscopic therapy, one patient rebled early and four rebled late.[176] Endoscopic therapy for diverticular bleeding should be undertaken cautiously in the right colon because of its thin wall.

Further investigation is required to clarify which types of lesions (diverticula, vascular ectasia) and thus which patients are most likely to respond to hemostatic therapy. Also, data comparing different colonoscopic modalities of treatment, such as coagulation therapy versus injection for different lesional characteristics (active bleeding, visible vessels, or adherent clots), are not available. Further, data comparing endoscopic therapy to angiographic therapy are lacking. Finally, whether the results of treating stigmata of diverticular hemorrhage can be extrapolated to other types of bleeding colonic lesions—vascular ectasias, polypectomy sites, Dieulafoy ulcerations—is uncertain.

Angiographic Therapy

When a bleeding site is identified by angiography, hemostasis can be achieved by intra-arterial infusion of vasopressin or superselective embolization. Early studies reported a significant risk of bowel infarction, especially with embolization techniques. Various embolic agents have been used, including gelatin sponge pledglets, microcoils, and polyvinyl alcohol particles. Current techniques appear to be more effective than previous ones and have a lower risk of bowel infarction. The risk of ischemic complications is higher when angiography is performed for colonic hemorrhage than for upper tract hemorrhage owing to the comparatively sparse collateral circulation in the colon. Several recent reports emphasize the safety and efficacy of superselective embolization therapy of the lower gastrointestinal tract.[201–203] In a report of 21 patients undergoing percutaneous embolization for therapy of lower gastrointestinal bleeding,[203] hemostasis was achieved in 71%, failed in 10%, and was not technically possible in 19%. Although hemostasis was long-lasting in 48% of patients, lesions in the small bowel or cecum were more likely to rebleed than those in the more distal colon.

Angiographic therapy appears to be safe and effective, but it should be used with certain reservations. First, these procedures are technically demanding; thus local expertise will dictate their effectiveness as well as their priority among therapeutic options. Second, which patients are likely to benefit the most from angiographic intervention is unknown. Although angiographic therapy currently is most often reserved for those who are poor surgical candidates, it could find a role as an adjunct to surgery by slowing the rate of bleeding and making surgery less emergent with an attendant lower morbidity and mortality.

Surgical Therapy

Surgical therapy may be necessary for continuous or recurrent lower gastrointestinal bleeding and has been carried out in 15% to 25% of patients.[163, 190, 204] Surgical options include elective resection of a known bleeding source such as a carcinoma, Meckel's diverticulum, or rebleeding colonic diverticula; and emergency surgery for an active bleeding source localized by colonoscopy or angiography; or blind subtotal colectomy for presumed colonic hemorrhage that cannot be localized. The surgical morbidity and mortality increases with each of these surgical options.

Surgery is recommended for patients with acute lower gastrointestinal bleeding who have a high transfusion requirement (generally more than 4 units within a 24-hour period or greater than 10 units overall) and for those with recurrent bleeding. Accurate preoperative localization particularly by angiography helps minimize its morbidity and mortality. In one study, the rebleeding rate over a 1-year follow-up period was 14% after segmental colectomy directed by angiography, but 42% after blind segmental colectomy.[205]

Surgical intervention in patients with lower gastrointestinal bleeding without a clear source of bleeding requires careful consideration. This caveat is particularly true in patients with extensive diverticula in whom bleeding cannot be localized to a specific diverticulum. Blind subtotal colectomy for massive bleeding has been associated with significant morbidity and mortality in this setting[177, 206, 207] and is usually performed only as a last resort.

Summary of Lower Gastrointestinal Bleeding

Although acute lower gastrointestinal bleeding is only about one fifth as common and is usually less hemodynamically significant than upper gastrointestinal bleeding, it presents unique clinical challenges. The most common cause of significant bleeding is diverticular bleeding; that of intermittent minor hematochezia is hemorrhoidal bleeding. The best diagnostic approach for patients with active bleeding is controversial, but I advocate urgent prepped colonoscopy (see Fig. 13–4). Recent data suggest that endoscopic therapy is effective and might improve outcomes. Angiography and surgery play important roles in management of patients with lower gastrointestinal bleeding, emphasizing that successful care of patients with lower gastrointestinal hemorrhage often requires an integrated multispecialty approach.

OCCULT AND OBSCURE BLEEDING

Occult Bleeding

Occult bleeding is by far the commonest form of gastrointestinal bleeding, afflicting at least 10% of the American population. True to the definition of occult, it is bleeding of

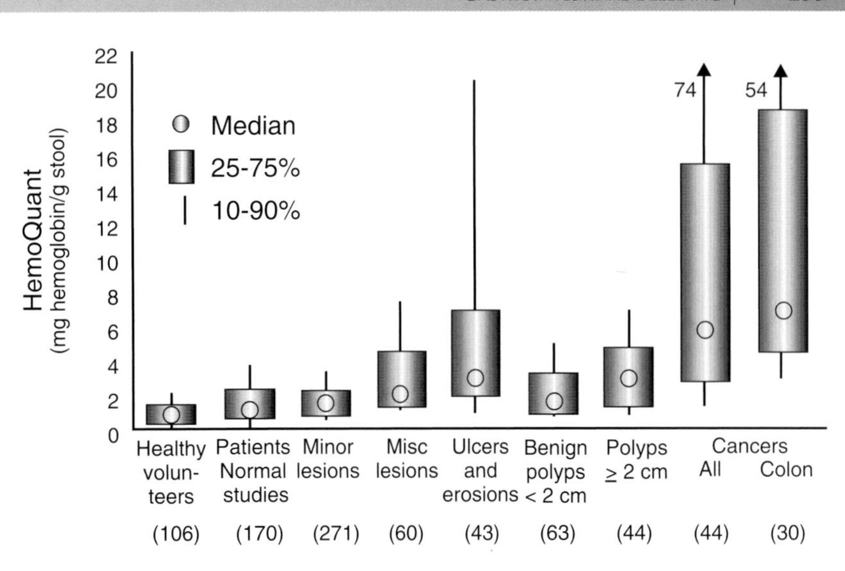

Figure 13–6. Fecal blood in healthy volunteers and patients with gastrointestinal disorders. The healthy volunteers did not ingest red meat or medication for 1 week before study. (From Ahlquist DA, McGill, DB, Schwartz S, et al: Fecal blood levels in health and disease. A study using HemoQuant. N Engl J Med. 312:1422–1428, 1985. Reprinted with permission of The New England Journal of Medicine).

which the patient is unaware, thus it is "hidden" or "concealed." The potential extent of such bleeding is emphasized by the observation that although instillation of 50 to 100 mL of blood into the stomach is required to produce melena consistently, patients losing 100 mL of blood per day may have grossly normal-appearing stools.[7, 208] Thus, occult bleeding may be accurately detected only by testing for fecal blood, or by discovery of an iron deficiency anemia if bleeding has occurred over a sufficient time period. The term *occult bleeding* also implies that it is unexplained or mysterious; hence, from an obscure source. Evident bleeding from an unidentified source and site, though much less common than detection of occult blood in the stool or iron deficiency, stall is clinically challenging.

Fecal Occult Blood

Occult gastrointestinal blood loss is most commonly identified by simple detection of blood in the stool with standard fecal occult blood tests; when such tests have been applied to large populations, 2% to 16% of subjects are positive.[209, 210] Normal fecal blood loss varies from 0.5 to 1.5 mL per day[211–213] (Fig. 13–6) and although most tests for fecal occult blood become positive when about 2 mL are lost per day, for consistent detection higher levels of fecal blood are required. Many tests are available; they are most commonly used to screen the colon for cancer[214–216] (see also Chapter 115 for review of their use for colon cancer screening), reducing mortality from colon cancer.[210, 217–219] The likelihood of detecting fecal blood depends not only on the sensitivity of a particular test but also the frequency and rate at which the causative lesion bleeds,[220] bowel motility, and the anatomic level of bleeding, all of which influence intraluminal metabolism of hemoglobin (Fig. 13–7). Fortunately, fecal occult blood tests clearly detect significant blood loss from many different lesions at many different locations in the gastrointestinal tract.

Fecal Occult Blood Tests

The prototypical fecal occult blood tests are based on the property of an organic compound, guaiac, to turn blue after oxidation by oxidants, peroxidases, or the pseudoperoxidase of hemoglobin in the presence of an oxygen donor such as hydrogen peroxide. Guaiac tests are more sensitive for detecting bleeding from the lower than upper gastrointestinal tract since hemoglobin and its pseudo-peroxidase are continuously degraded as they move down the gastrointestinal tract (see Fig. 13–6). The sensitivity of the different guaiac-based tests varies. Of the two most commonly used tests in the United States, Hemoccult II and Hemoccult II SENSA (both from SmithKline Diagnostics, Palo Alto, CA), the latter is substantially more sensitive for detecting fecal heme.[221, 222] This difference is important in screening for occult blood since increases in sensitivity result in reduced specificity (see Chapters 114 and 115).

The likelihood that a guaiac test will detect fecal blood (heme) depends critically on the quantity of hemoglobin present in the stool. In turn, the amount of hemoglobin in the stool depends on the size and location of the bleeding lesion.[223, 224] Since distal (colonic) lesions are more likely to contain undegraded heme, guaiac-based tests are best at detecting more distal lesions. The amount of undegraded heme, however, will depend on variables such as stool transit time, extent of mixing, as well as degree of intraluminal degradation of heme by bacteria. The variation in the content of fecal hemoglobin has been highlighted by Ahlquist and coworkers (Fig. 13–8).[220] Fecal hemoglobin levels must exceed 10 mg/g (10 mL daily blood loss) for 50% of Hemoccult II tests to be positive, yet stools with less than 1 mg/g of hemoglobin may be positive.[225] Such data have led many to question the effectiveness of guaiac tests for detecting colonic lesions that bleed occultly.[226, 227]

Characteristics of fecal occult blood tests are highlighted in Table 13–13. In addition to components of the diet, such as red meat and vegetables containing peroxidases, fecal rehydration markedly passes sensitivity and reduces specificity of tests for occult blood in feces.[210] Although it is commonly believed that oral iron causes positive guaiac tests, perhaps because the dark-green or black appearance of stool containing iron may be mistaken for the blue typical of a positive guaiac reaction, prospective studies have confirmed that orally administered iron, even in large amounts, does not cause guaiac to react positively.[228] Bismuth (in certain antacids and antidiarrheals) renders the stool dark but does

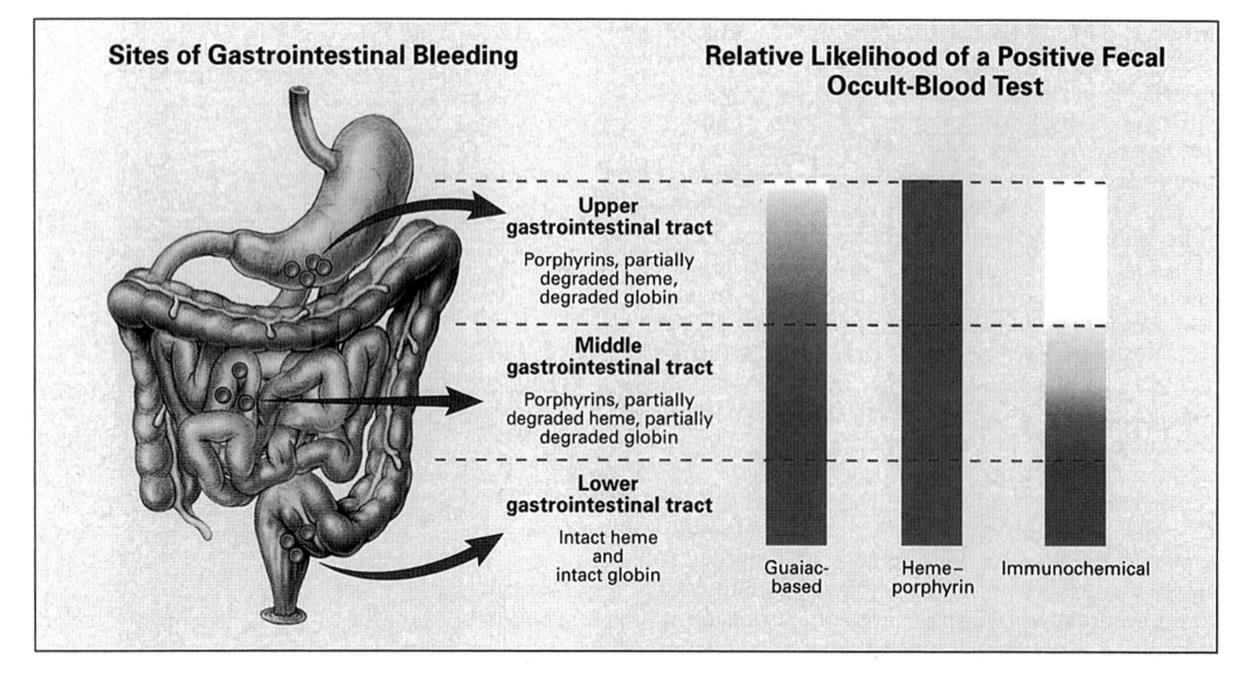

Figure 13–7. Sites of gastrointestinal bleeding, intraluminal metabolism of hemoglobin and detection of intraluminal blood by fecal occult blood tests. In the upper gastrointestinal tract, hemoglobin is cleaved to heme and globin by gastric pepsin or pancreatic proteases in the proximal small intestine. Some (generally <15%) intraluminal heme is reabsorbed in the small intestine. A portion of heme that is not absorbed is converted to porphyrins and iron through poorly understood mechanisms has been termed the intestinal converted fraction of heme. This fraction is not detected by guaiac tests but is detected by the heme-porphyrin assay (HemoQuant), which measures both heme and porphyrins, and is therefore a highly accurate indicator of bleeding, regardless of level. Globin in the upper gastrointestinal tract is digested by pepsin and pancreatic and intestinal proteases, and is thus not detected by immunochemical fecal occult blood tests. The biology of intraluminal hemoglobin degredation suggests that a combination of a guaiac-based test and an immunochemical test could theoretically help differentiate occult upper from lower gastrointestinal tract bleeding. (From Rockey DC: Occult gastrointestinal bleeding. N Engl J Med 341:38–46, 1999. Reprinted with permission of The New England Journal of Medicine).

not cause a blue guaiac reaction and should not be mistaken for blood.

Immunochemical tests use antibodies directed against human globin epitopes to detect colonic blood and are highly sensitive (as little as 0.3 mL of blood added to stool can be detected),[229] giving them a theoretical advantage in specificity over guaiac-based tests. However, they do not detect small quantities of blood from upper gastrointestinal sources (see Fig. 13–7),[222] and usefulness is limited by technical problems such as loss of hemoglobin antigenicity at room temperature and the requirement for laboratory processing. Newer slide immunochemical tests (such as FlexSure OBT, SmithKline Diagnostics, Palo Alto, CA) may help circumvent these problems.

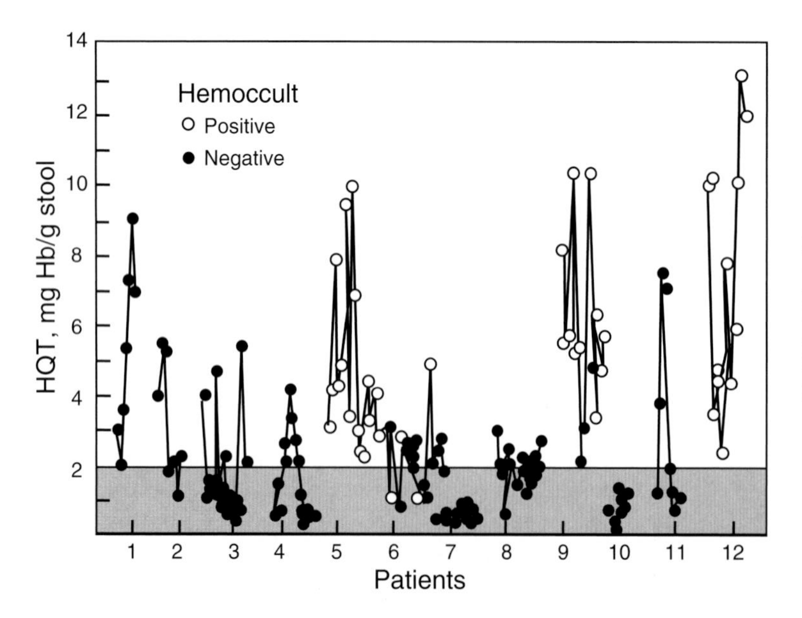

Figure 13–8. Variation in bleeding of primary colon carcinoma. Occult blood was detected using HemoQuant and hemoccult II in stools of 12 patients for 2 weeks. The shaded zone below a HemoQuant level of 2 mg Hb/g stool represents the conventional normal range. (From Ahlquist DA, McGill DB, Fleming JL, et al: Cancer 63:1826–1830, 1989. Reprinted with permission of John Wiley & Sons, Inc.).

Table 13–13 | **Characteristics of Fecal Occult Blood Tests**

VARIABLE	GUAIAC	HEME-PORPHYRIN	IMMUNO-CHEMICAL
Detection Characteristics			
Upper gastro-intestinal	+	++++	0
Small bowel	++	++++	+
Right colonic	+++	++++	+++
Left colonic	++++	++++	++++
Test Factors			
Bedside availability	++++	0	+
Time to develop	1 min	1 hr	5 min to 24 hr
Cost	$3–5	$17	$10–20
False-positives			
Animal hemoglobin	++++	++++	0
Dietary peroxidases	+++	0	0
False-negatives			
Hemoglobin degradation	++	0	++
Storage	++	++++	++
Vitamin C	++	0	0

Adapted from Rockey DC: Occult gastrointestinal bleeding. N Engl J Med 341: 38, 1999. Relative comparisons are shown on a scale of 0 to ++++, with 0 being negative and ++++ highly positive.

The heme-porphyrin test (HemoQuant, Mayo Medical Laboratories, Rochester, MN) measures porphyrin spectrofluorometrically and therefore allows precise determination of total stool hemoglobin. Substances that interfere with, or cause false-positive guaiac-based tests (e.g., vegetable peroxidases), do not affect this test. However, an important confounder of the heme-porphyrin assay is myoglobin, an important source of nonhuman heme found in red meats. This test is extremely sensitive for detecting occult blood loss, but its great sensitivity has limited its usefulness as a screening tool, primarily because of its high rate of false-positive tests.

Approach to Evaluation and Differential Diagnosis

In patients with occult bleeding the focus of the history and examination differ from that in patients with acute bleeding. Particular attention should be focused on anticoagulants and medications that can injure the gastrointestinal mucosa, including NSAIDs, alendronate, and potassium chloride. A family history suggesting a vascular anomaly (e.g., hereditary hemorrhagic telangiectasia) or a coagulopathy (e.g., von Willebrand's disease) is important. The physical examination should seek cutaneous abnormalities typical of systemic disorders that cause occult bleeding, such as dermatitis herpetiformis of celiac sprue, neurofibromas, café au lait spots, and axillary freckles of neurofibromatosis; the pigmented lip spots of the Peutz-Jeghers syndrome; osteomas and cysts of Gardner's syndrome; and the ectodermal (hair, nails) abnormalities of the Cronkite-Canada syndrome.

Lesions that bleed acutely may also bleed chronically. Therefore, virtually any gastrointestinal lesion can cause a positive fecal occult blood test, and those most often responsible for occult bleeding are highlighted in Table 13–14. The colon is the most common site of occult gastrointestinal blood due to the high prevalence of colonic adenomatous polyps greater than 2 cm and adenocarcinoma. However, the upper gastrointestinal tract is also a frequent source of bleeding from gastroduodenal ulcers, vascular ectasias, esophagitis, and gastritis. Less common but important causes of occult bleeding include small intestinal tumors and ulcers, gastric adenocarcinomas, gastric vascular ectasia, and Cameron lesions.

The finding of occult blood in the stool requires investigation initially focused on the colon. Some controversy exists with regard to which colonic imaging test is the most appropriate modality.[230–232] Colonoscopy and air contrast barium enema are the most commonly used tools. Flexible sigmoidoscopy is required for patients undergoing air contrast barium enema to evaluate fully the rectosigmoid colon.[233] Colonoscopy is generally regarded as the most accurate test and is the most widely used. Whereas some studies have demonstrated that air contrast barium enema accurately detects colonic malignancy and large adenomas,[234] others report that it is significantly less accurate than colonoscopy.[235] Nonetheless, it is important to realize that either test can miss serious neoplastic lesions.[230, 236, 237] Not only is test accuracy an issue, but also cost, patient acceptance,[238] and complication rates differ between the two modalities. Although air contrast barium enema performed by a skilled radiologist has a high likelihood of detection of large mass lesions, its sensitivity for small lesions, including adenomatous polyps, is less than for colonoscopy.[235] Initial results with computed tomographic colonography (virtual colonoscopy) are encouraging and suggest that this test may become an important tool to evaluate the colon,[239–241] but currently it is not widely available. The choice of test will vary, depending on availability, local expertise, and comfort of the patient with a specific test.

The source of bleeding in patients with fecal blood and normal colons may be in the upper gastrointestinal tract. Several studies have addressed this issue, reporting upper

Table 13–14 | **Differential Diagnosis of Occult Gastrointestinal Bleeding**

MASS LESIONS	**VASCULAR**
Carcinoma (any site)*	Vascular ectasia (any site)*
Large (>1.5 cm) adenoma (any site)	Portal hypertensive gastropathy/colopathy
INFLAMMATION	Watermelon stomach
Erosive esophagitis*	Hemangioma
Ulcer (any site)*	Dieulafoy's lesion‡
Cameron lesions†	**INFECTIOUS**
Erosive gastritis	Hookworm
Celiac sprue	Whipworm
Ulcerative colitis	Stronglyoidiasis
Crohn's disease	Ascariasis
Colitis (nonspecific)	Tuberculous enterocolitis
Idiopathic cecal ulcer	Amebiasis
MISCELLANEOUS	**SURREPTITIOUS**
Long-distance running	Hemoptysis
Factitious	Oropharyngeal (including epistaxis)
	Pancreaticobiliary source

*Most common abnormalities.
†Linear erosions within a hiatus hernia.
‡Large superficial artery underlying a mucosal defect.
Adapted from Rockey DC: Occult gastrointestinal bleeding. N Engl J Med 341: 38, 1999.
Potential lesions leading to all forms of occult gastrointestinal bleeding are shown. Some lesions that may lead to recurrent obscure bleeding are not listed (see text).

gastrointestinal tract sites in proportion equal to or greater than the lower gastrointestinal tract (Fig. 13–9).[242–247] Endoscopy of the upper gastrointestinal tract often leads to management changes in many cases. That patients with fecal occult blood have such a high number of upper gastrointestinal lesions is surprising since the guaiac-based tests that were used in these reports were thought to have a relatively low sensitivity for detecting upper gastrointestinal blood; however, guaiac-based tests clearly are capable of detecting small amounts of upper gastrointestinal tract blood.[222, 248] Furthermore, many of the lesions identified in the upper gastrointestinal tract in these reports bleed sufficiently to produce positive guaiac-based tests.[211, 222] Upper gastrointestinal tract malignancies were identified in each of these reports. An open question is whether it is cost-effective to proceed routinely with upper gastrointestinal tract investigation in patients with fecal occult blood and a normal colonic examination.

The appropriate evaluation for patients with occult blood found in stool obtained by digital rectal examination is controversial. Although anorectal trauma or dietary factors may lead to positive tests that may not reflect an underlying abnormality, nevertheless both symptomatic and asymptomatic patients with fecal blood detected by digital rectal examination harbor important lesions identified by gastrointestinal evaluation.[246, 249, 250] Available data indicate that the diagnostic yield for investigating occult blood detected by digital rectal examination is the same as for spontaneously passed stools.[246, 250] Thus, my opinion is that evaluation is warranted, and, if symptoms are present, should be directed accordingly. Whether testing stool obtained by digital rectal examination is a viable cancer screening option is currently unknown.

Occult gastrointestinal bleeding is often attributed to anticoagulant or aspirin therapy. However, fecal blood content in patients therapeutically anticoagulated have been normal,[251, 252] and low-dose aspirin alone resulted in only minimally increased fecal blood. The combination of aspirin and warfarin caused still slightly higher amounts of fecal blood.[251, 252] Neither warfarin nor low-dose aspirin alone appears to cause positive guaiac-based fecal occult blood tests.[252] Thus, a positive fecal occult blood test should not be attributed to the effect of anticoagulation or aspirin alone, but rather should lead to investigation of the gastrointestinal tract. A prospective study in anticoagulated patients with positive guaiac-based fecal occult blood tests found that 15 of 16 patients had previously undiagnosed lesions, 20% of which were malignant.[253]

Treatment

Treatment of patients with fecal occult blood depends on the underlying disorder. Most bleeding mass lesions require surgical excision. NSAIDs should be withdrawn if possible, even if clear ulcer disease cannot be identified. Particularly difficult to treat are patients with vascular ectasias, which are often multiple and bleed chronically (discussed later). The prognosis of patients with positive fecal occult blood tests but no identifiable gastrointestinal pathology appears favorable but has not been rigorously studied. It appears that only a small proportion of such patients will develop obscure bleeding or iron deficiency anemia.

Iron Deficiency Anemia

Given the normal daily blood loss of 0.5 to 1.5 mL/day, a stool weight of 150 g, and circulating hemoglobin of 15 g/dL, the usual stool hemoglobin concentration is 0.5 to 1.5 mg/g of stool. Thus, under normal circumstances, a total of 0.25 to 0.75 mg of elemental iron is lost from gastrointestinal bleeding daily. A small amount of iron is also lost in sloughed intestinal cells and from minute amounts of bleeding, making the average daily iron loss approximately 1 mg (Fig. 13–10). The absorptive capacity of the small intestine for iron can increase dramatically in response to iron depletion but normally is limited. Thus, iron deficiency results

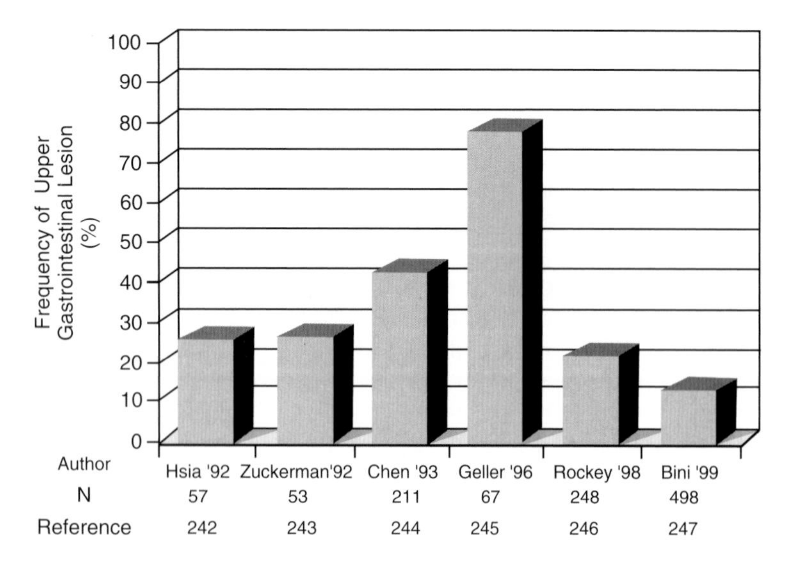

Figure 13–9. Frequency of upper gastrointestinal lesions in patients with fecal occult blood. In general, studies excluded patients with active bleeding. Variation in the criteria used to ascribe a specific lesion to the positive fecal occult blood test exists. The study by Geller and colleagues[245] included patients with small polyps detected in the colon.

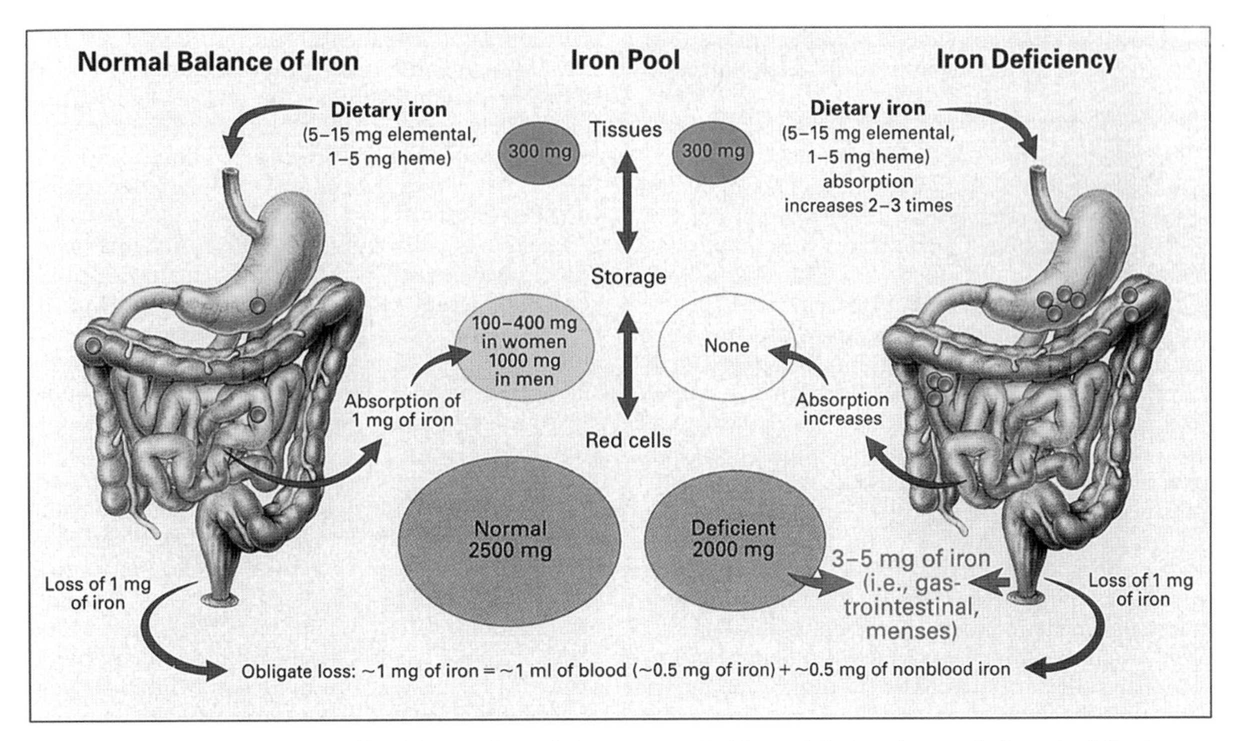

Figure 13–10. Gastrointestinal blood loss and iron balance. Normal obligate daily iron loss result from the following: (1) blood loss (presumably from gastrointestinal mucosal microerosions or microulcerations) and (2) iron in sloughed gut epithelial cells. Total daily iron loss is thus approximately 1 mg. The usual Western diet contains mostly elemental iron, of which about 10% is absorbed. Heme-iron derived primarily from myoglobin in meats is preferentially absorbed and accounts for 60% to 80% of the iron absorbed per day. Under normal circumstances, iron homeostasis is tightly regulated and daily iron loss is precisely balanced by iron absorption. Iron deficiency results only when the dynamic but limited, absorptive capacity of the small intestine is exceeded by iron loss. The time required to develop iron deficiency depends on the size of initial iron stores, the rate of bleeding and intestinal iron absorption. Iron deficiency generally occurs only with increased loss of over 5 mL of blood daily. Importantly, anemia is a late manifestation of the iron-depleted state. (From Rockey DC: occult gastrointestinal bleeding. N Engl J Med 341:38–46, 1999. Reprinted with permission of The New England Journal of Medicine).

only when iron loss exceeds absorption, usually when blood loss exceeds 5 to 10 mL/day over many weeks.

Iron deficiency anemia is the most common form of anemia worldwide. In the United States, 5% to 11% of women and 1% to 4% of men are iron deficient, and approximately 5% and 2%, respectively, have iron deficiency anemia.[254] Iron deficiency anemia is most commonly identified in women during their reproductive years because of menstrual and pregnancy-associated iron losses.[255] In groups other than premenopausal women, iron deficiency anemia traditionally has been assumed to be the result of chronic occult gastrointestinal bleeding. Thus, the standard of care for men and postmenopausal women with iron deficiency anemia is to investigate for the presence of gastrointestinal tract pathology.[208]

Approach to Evaluation and Differential Diagnosis

The history of patients with iron deficiency anemia is directed toward medications that can cause mucosal injury, symptoms of malignancy, or of other chronic diseases that may be associated with blood loss or failure to absorb iron. Again, cutaneous manifestations of gastrointestinal or systemic diseases may be present. In iron deficiency anemia, brittle, spoonlike nails suggest the presence of Plummer-Vinson syndrome (see Chapter 34).

Patients with iron deficiency anemia should be managed like those with fecal occult blood. Indeed, these two processes are very commonly linked in a continuum of diseases underlying chronic gastrointestinal bleeding. The diagnosis of iron deficiency and iron deficiency anemia is most often confirmed by a low serum ferritin level (see reference 256 for review). An accurate diagnosis of iron deficiency anemia, by serum ferritin or bone marrow examination, is critical since this diagnosis demands further evaluation. Iron deficiency without anemia also may be associated with significant gastrointestinal tract abnormalities.[257, 258]

As with all occult gastrointestinal bleeding, many lesions in the gastrointestinal tract can bleed chronically and lead to iron deficiency anemia (see Table 13–14). Although right-sided colonic cancers are considered the major source of occult bleeding and iron deficiency anemia, recent cross-sectional studies have documented prominent abnormalities in the upper gastrointestinal tract as the cause (Table 13–15). Indeed, in four series of 381 patients, upper gastrointestinal tract lesions believed to be consistent with chronic blood loss were identified more often than colonic.[259–262] Only 5% of patients had lesions capable of leading to iron deficiency in both upper and lower gastrointestinal sites.

Other research has highlighted the importance of the up-

Table 13–15 | **Major Gastrointestinal Lesions Identified in Studies of Patients with Iron Deficiency Anemia**

LESION	COOK[259]* (*n* = 100)	McINTYRE[261]* (*n* = 111)	ROCKEY[262] (*n* = 100)	KEPCZYK[260] (*n* = 70)	TOTAL (*n* = 381)
Esophagus					47
Esophagitis	14	15	6	10	
Cancer	1	NA	0	1	
Stomach					98
Ulcer	7	13	8	3	
Gastritis	14†	7	6	11	
Cancer	5	8	1	3	
Vascular ectasia	5	0	3	4	
Duodenal ulcer	1	10	11	3	25
Other upper	0	2	2	3	7
Small intestine					10
Celiac sprue‡	0	3	0	4	
Vascular ectasia	1	1	0	0	
Large intestine					85
Cancer	14	5	11	4	
Vascular ectasia	2	1	5	6	
Adenoma	6	4	5	6	
Colitis	1	2	2	1	
Other	0	3	3	4	
Upper lesion§	40 (47)	42 (51)	37	39 (43)	158 (41%)
Lower lesion	23	15	26	21	85 (22%)
Small intestine	2	4	0	4	10 (3%)
Upper + lower	7	0	1	12	20 (5%)
No GI lesion	35	50	37	6	128 (34%)

NOTE: Iron deficiency anemia was typically defined by a low hemoglobin (usually less than 12 g/dL) and a reduced ferritin level (usually less than 20 ng/mL) or absent bone marrow iron stores. Definitions of lesions varied. Hiatal hernia alone, esophageal varices alone and hemorrhoids alone were not included as sources of chronic blood loss.
n = total number of assessable patients.

*Barium enema was used to evaluate the colon in many patients.
†Duodenitis included.
‡Duodenal biopsy was not performed to evaluate for celiac sprue in all studies.
§Numbers shown represent those patients with abnormalities identified. The numbers in parentheses represent the number of reported lesions. For example, 47 lesions were identified in 40 patients by Cook et al.[259]
GI, gastrointestinal; NA, not available.

From Rockey DC: GI evaluation in iron deficiency anemia. Semin Gastroenterol 10:58, 1999.

per gastrointestinal tract in iron deficiency anemia. Pervasive occult gastrointestinal bleeding due to *Helicobacter pylori*–associated gastritis, often asymptomatic, has been reported[263] and approximately 20% of patients with iron deficiency anemia were found to have gastric achlorhydria and atrophy, implying that gastric injury in this subgroup could contribute to iron malabsorption[264] (see also Chapter 39).

In evaluating the upper gastrointestinal tract for iron deficiency anemia, one must not attribute the anemia to lesions not likely to cause significant bleeding. Clearly, mass lesions and large ulcerative upper gastrointestinal lesions lead to significant blood loss and iron deficiency (see Fig. 13–5),[211, 213] but trivial lesions such as mild inflammation and especially small adenomas do not.[211, 220] This point was emphasized by work that demonstrated that, although 67% of patients with iron deficiency anemia had gastrointestinal tract lesions, fewer than one third of these patients had elevated hemoglobin levels in gastrointestinal lavage specimens.[265] This finding may have been due to daily variability in gastrointestinal bleeding, making one-time gastrointestinal blood measurement unreliable, but nonetheless the data suggest that it is unlikely that every lesion identified is associated with occult bleeding and iron deficiency.

Some clinicians believe that gastrointestinal symptoms in patients with iron deficiency anemia help direct the gastrointestinal tract evaluation,[262, 266] whereas others have found symptoms to be unhelpful in localizing pathology.[260, 261] Directed gastrointestinal tract evaluation is desirable to minimize both risk and cost. Although many patients are entirely asymptomatic, some patients with gastrointestinal lesions will have symptoms characteristic of common diseases, such as change in bowel habit (colon cancer) or epigastric pain (peptic ulcer). It is my belief that the initial investigation should be directed toward the location of specific symptoms (Fig. 13–11). Since dual lesions are rare, identification of an abnormality consistent with bleeding, such as a mass lesion, large ulceration, or severe inflammation that is a likely cause of the symptoms, makes further evaluation unnecessary. In the absence of symptoms, particularly in elderly patients, evaluation should begin with the colon; if this examination is negative, the upper gastrointestinal tract should then be investigated.

Gastrointestinal evaluation of iron deficiency anemia in premenopausal women is controversial since it is extremely common in this population, affecting over 3 million women in the United States. A recent study found that 12% of premenopausal women with iron deficiency anemia had significant gastrointestinal tract abnormalities, half of which were malignant.[266] Moreover, lesions were as common in the upper gastrointestinal tract as in the colon.[266] Although the retrospective design of this study limits firm conclusions, it suggests that gastrointestinal investigation for most premeno-

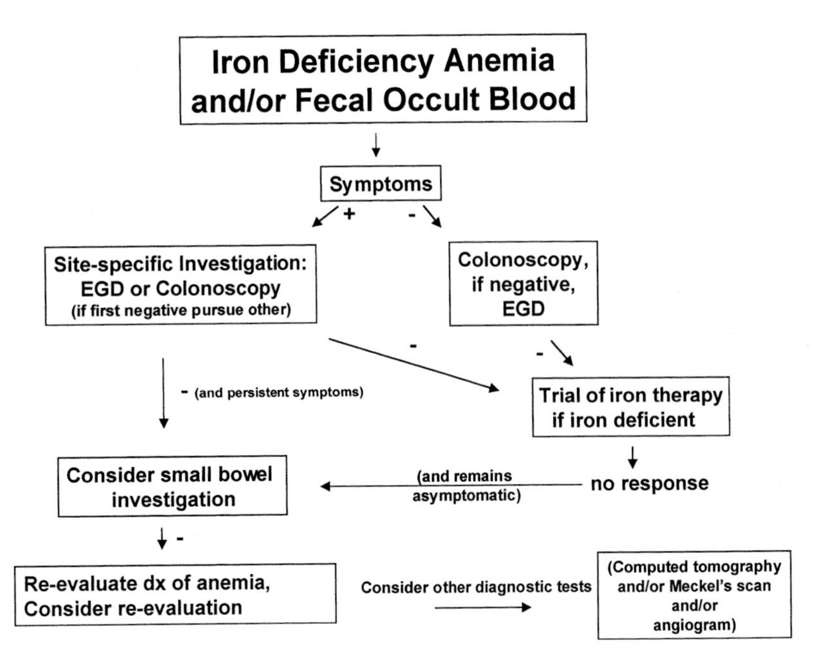

Figure 13–11. Algorithm for management of occult gastrointestinal bleeding (fecal occult blood and iron deficiency anemia).

pausal women with iron deficiency anemia is indicated but should be individualized. Certainly those with gastrointestinal symptoms, weight loss, fecal occult blood, or severe anemia must be evaluated. Gastrointestinal tract evaluation is appropriate in asymptomatic women or those with abnormal menses whose menstrual blood loss appears to be inadequate to explain the severity of their iron deficiency anemia.

The principal techniques to evaluate patients with iron deficiency anemia are endoscopic (esophagogastroduodenoscopy and colonoscopy) and radiographic (air contrast barium enema and upper gastrointestinal series). Radiographic studies are generally effective for detecting masses and large ulcerating lesions,[267] but their sensitivity for vascular ectasias and more subtle mucosal lesions such as gastritis, esophagitis, and colitis is less than with endoscopic procedures. Since patients with iron deficiency anemia have a high pretest probability of disease, much of which is mucosal, or will require biopsy, endoscopic investigation is the best first choice since many patients would require endoscopy after radiographic studies. Both lower and upper endoscopy should be performed sequentially under the same conscious sedation, a sequence that is not possible if barium studies have preceded it. Nonetheless, the cost-effectiveness of radiographic versus endoscopic studies requires further study.

The small bowel remains the potential site of bleeding in patients with negative examinations of the colon and upper gastrointestinal tract. Although tumors and vascular anomalies are the more common causes, mucosal disease must also be considered. Celiac sprue, a classic small bowel disease, not only leads to malabsorption of iron but also occult bleeding.[268] Also, mucosal ulcerative diseases should be considered in the differential diagnosis.[269] Radiographic examination of the small bowel by enteroclysis or small bowel follow-through is of limited value in this evaluation.[260, 262] Enteroscopy of the small intestine is more sensitive for detecting mucosal abnormalities and small mass lesions and is preferred in patients with negative lower and upper gastrointestinal tract evaluations. Indeed, recent studies of enteroscopy in patients with iron deficiency anemia have identified abnormalities in 6% to 27% of patients.[270, 271] Although such reports confirm that enteroscopy yields diagnoses of the source of occult bleeding and iron deficiency anemia, more investigation is required to define its role in the initial evaluation of iron deficient patients.

Many patients with iron deficiency anemia will have no identifiable gastrointestinal tract abnormality after evaluation. If such patients are refractory to empiric iron supplementation, other tests should be considered, including angiography or computed tomography. If diagnostic evaluation is unable to elucidate a gastrointestinal abnormality, explanations for iron deficiency anemia should be considered, including nongastrointestinal blood loss, misdiagnosis of the type of anemia, missed lesions, malabsorptive diseases, or nutritional deficiency.

Treatment of Iron Deficiency Anemia

When the diagnosis of iron deficiency anemia is established, iron therapy should be instituted. Oral ferrous sulfate, 325 mg two to three times daily, is recommended; it is inexpensive and effective. For those who are intolerant to ferrous sulfate, ferrous gluconate or fumarate are acceptable alternatives. Parenteral iron therapy is used only for patients with severe malabsorption or intolerance to iron supplements. The response of patients with lesions amenable to medical therapy, such as duodenal ulcer, esophagitis, and adenoma, to iron repletion is excellent. Most patients with unidentifiable gastrointestinal abnormalities generally respond to long-term iron therapy.[258, 262, 272] If patients do not respond to iron therapy, the diagnosis of iron deficiency anemia should be reassessed and repeat gastrointestinal investigation should be contemplated. Re-examination of the colon for vascular ectasias, the esophagus for Cameron lesions within hiatus hernia, the stomach for atrophic gastritis, and the small bowel for vascular ectasias or celiac sprue can be helpful. The importance of re-examination of the gastrointestinal tract is emphasized by the finding that a bleeding source is within reach of the standard upper endoscope in up to 35% of such patients.[271]

Gastrointestinal Bleeding of Obscure Origin

The source of bleeding is unidentified in about 5% of patients with gastrointestinal bleeding.[273] Whether an obscure site of bleeding may be clinically evident by obvious signs or symptoms or its occult nature is manifest only as refractory iron deficiency anemia, the diagnostic challenge is great, for readily identifiable causes of gastrointestinal bleeding have already been excluded by esophagogastroduodenoscopy and colonoscopy. Both continuing and recurrent gross or occult bleeding of unknown origin demands focus on the possible etiology and site of hemorrhage source, for only then can appropriate therapy be instituted.

Approach to Evaluation and Differential Diagnosis

Localizing the site, upper or lower, may be helped by a thorough history and physical examination. Although melena and hematochezia are usually associated with upper and lower gastrointestinal tract bleeding, respectively, patients with slow oozing from the distal small bowel or cecum may have melena and patients with aggressive bleeding from an upper gastrointestinal source may present with hematochezia. History and physical examination should focus particularly on symptoms and signs of diseases likely to be overlooked, including those reflecting small bowel disease (Table 13–16).

As with endoscopies for the initial investigation of bleeding, repeat endoscopy for bleeding of obscure origin is directed at the most likely site (Fig. 13–12), and ideally, if performed during active bleeding, a specific diagnosis may be made. In upper gastrointestinal bleeders, re-examination with a standard upper endoscope and/or enteroscope by an experienced operator will identify lesions in a substantial proportion of patients.[274–277]

If a lesion cannot be identified, further evaluation depends on the briskness of bleeding. In those with active bleeding, technetium-99 radionuclide scanning or angiography should be performed. Technetium scanning is useful only to confirm the site of bleeding, and data assessing its impact on management in patients with obscure gastrointestinal bleeding are limited. Mesenteric angiography is less sensitive than technetium-99 radionuclide scanning but reportedly more often identifies the site of bleeding,[278] perhaps because of selection bias in published studies. Other diagnostic tests such as computed tomography or Meckel's scan may be helpful in some patients.

In patients with subacute or intermittent bleeding in whom repeat endoscopy of the upper or lower gastrointestinal tract is negative, the focus of investigation should be broadened to include the small intestine (see Fig. 13–11). The lesions most commonly identified as bleeding sites in the small bowel include tumors and vascular ectasias, which vary in frequency depending on age. In patients between 30 and 50 years of age, tumors are the most common abnormalities, whereas in patients less than 25 years of age, Meckel's diverticula are the most common source of small bowel bleeding. Vascular ectasias predominate in older patients.[279]

Small bowel examination can be accomplished with standard small bowel follow-through, enteroclysis, push enteroscopy, sonde enteroscopy, or intraoperative enteroscopy. Small bowel follow-through usually is inadequate to evaluate the small intestine. Enteroclysis is capable of detecting mass lesions of the small intestine[280] but fails to detect many mucosal lesions, particularly vascular ectasias. Since vascular ectasias are often a major concern in this patient population, enteroclysis is probably best reserved for those in whom the suspicion of a mass lesion or small bowel diverticula is high or for those who have persistent bleeding and negative-push enteroscopy.

Enteroscopy, either of the "push" or Sonde variety, is important in evaluation of many patients with obscure gastrointestinal bleeding.[277] Push enteroscopy consists of peroral insertion of a specialized, long, flexible endoscope or sometimes a standard pediatric colonoscope, and it should be performed in obscure bleeders. With the patient under conscious sedation, this instrument can be passed 50 to 60 cm beyond the ligament of Treitz, allowing expeditious and thorough examination of the distal duodenum and proximal jejunum. It identifies a source in 24% to 75% of patients with obscure bleeding.[270, 274, 275, 281, 282] The major advantages of push enteroscopy are that it is readily available, relatively safe, and both biopsy and endoscopic therapy can be performed.

Sonde enteroscopy involves placement of a long, small-caliber endoscope into the proximal small bowel, with subsequent peristalsis carrying the endoscope to the more distal small intestine.[283] This procedure permits visualization of almost the entire small bowel and leads to a diagnosis in a significant number of patients.[284] Sonde enteroscopy, added to push enteroscopy, has increased the diagnostic yield.[282] Although Sonde enteroscopy is attractive diagnostically, this tedious technique requires a specialized endoscope, expertise with the procedure, and has no therapeutic capability. Although it is not widely available, its use is rapidly expanding; it probably is limited to centers of expertise in patients with negative-push enteroscopy.

Intraoperative examination with an enteroscope or standard colonoscope, permits visualization of most or all of the small intestine. Although this technique has been reported to detect abnormalities in from 70% to 100% of patients with

Table 13–16 | **Causes of Obscure Gastrointestinal Bleeding**

Vascular ectasias*
Small bowel neoplastic lesions
Hemosuccus pancreaticus
Hemobilia
Aortoenteric fistula
Dieulafoy's lesion (stomach > other sites)
Meckel's diverticulum
Extra-esophageal varices (gastric, small bowel, colonic)
Diverticula (especially small intestinal)

*Small intestinal lesions are particularly important.

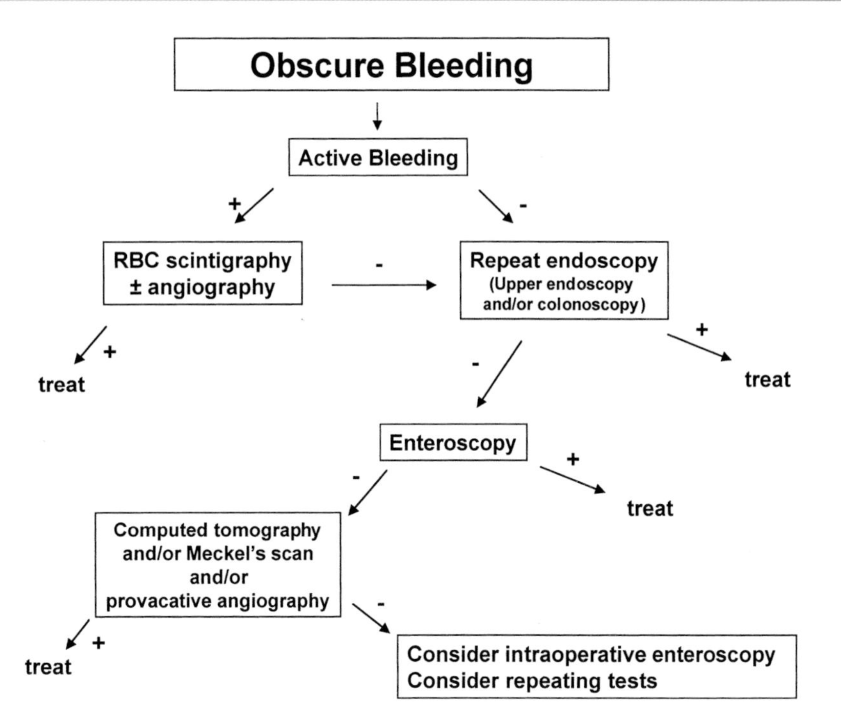

Figure 13–12. Algorithm for management of obscure gastrointestinal bleeding. Routine gastroscopy should be performed first.

obscure bleeding,[285–287] not all practitioners have been so successful.

A new, conceptually simple approach to examine the small intestine is wireless capsule endoscopy.[288, 289] In a study of canine small intestine in which radiopaque colored beads (3 to 6 mm in diameter) were randomly sewn inside 9 canine small bowels, wireless capsules identified more beads than did push enteroscopy (median, 6 [range, 2–9] vs. 3 [range, 2–6 beads]; $P < 0.001$) and, not surprisingly, more beads beyond the reach of the push enteroscope (median, 4 [range, 2–7] vs. 0; $P < 0.0001$). The capsules passed safely and caused no mucosal injury. Wireless capsule endoscopy has also been performed safely in humans.[289] A major disadvantage of such capsules is their inability to administer therapy, making investigation of small intestines in patients with obscure gastrointestinal bleeding problematic.

An alternative diagnostic approach in patients with recurrent obscure bleeding is to reactivate or augment bleeding with the use of vasodilators, anticoagulants, or thrombolytics followed by tagged RBC scintigraphy or visceral angiography. Although the literature indicates that the diagnostic yield of this procedure is on the order of 20% to 40%,[290, 291] this procedure is a highly specialized, potentially risky undertaking[292] that requires further study to clarify its role.

Specific Causes of Obscure Gastrointestinal Bleeding

Prominent among obscure lesions that bleed evidently are *vascular ectasias*, *Dieulafoy's lesion*, and *Meckel's diverticulum*. Small bowel vascular ectasias are the most commonly detected of these lesions, comprising up to 60%.[150, 293] Other sources are varices and ulcers, located at unusual sites of the gastrointestinal tract and should be considered. Rarely, patients present with factitious bleeding, having bled themselves and then ingested the blood. A high index of suspicion is necessary to make this diagnosis; it is always associated with underlying psychological illness. Other important causes of obscure bleeding are discussed next.

Small Intestinal Mass Lesions

Neoplasms of the small intestine are an uncommon, but important, cause of obscure gastrointestinal bleeding, since they may be successfully resected. Bleeding is the most common clinical manifestation of leiomyoma, the most common benign tumor, and leiomyosarcoma, a malignant stromal tumor of the small intestine.[294, 295] Benign tumors appear to bleed more commonly than malignant tumors,[295] the most common of which are adenocarcinomas, carcinoids, lymphomas, and sarcomas (see Chapter 113).

If evaluation of the small bowel as outlined as well as abdominal computed tomography does not reveal a tumor, exploratory laparotomy is required for diagnosis.[296] This search is often stimulated by symptoms that suggest partial small bowel obstruction, particularly *periumbilical* cramping pain following meals.

Aortoenteric Fistula

Aortoenteric fistulas are rare, but very serious, lesions responsible for significant gastrointestinal bleeding, and they may be obscure. They are almost always secondary to previous reconstructive aortoiliac surgery,[297] occurring with a frequency of about 0.5% following aortoiliac surgery.[298] Although these fistulas most commonly appear 3 to 5 years after graft surgery, primary aortoenteric fistulas have also been reported.[299] Aortoenteric fistulas typically involve the third portion of the duodenum but may involve other portions of the gastrointestinal tract. The usual presentation is a self-limited, so-called "herald" bleed, followed some days or even weeks later by a second, often massive and sometimes fatal bleed. Great suspicion of this lesion is, of course, provided by the history of graft surgery and an abdominal scar. Since the pathogenesis of this disease is subtle infection of the graft and perigraft area, usually with *Staphylococcus aureus* or *Escherichia coli*, low-grade fever, fatigue, weight loss, and leukocytosis in the appropriate clinical setting further raise the likelihood of this diagnosis.

All patients with previous aortic surgery and upper gastrointestinal bleeding should undergo esophagogastroduodenoscopy with particular attention to the distal duodenum and strict avoidance of biopsies. If such examination is negative, patients should undergo abdominal computed tomography, which will usually demonstrate periaortic inflammation and phlegmon, consistent with infection. Angiography is rarely helpful.

The prognosis of patients with aortoenteric fistula has been historically poor (over 50% mortality rate) but appears to be improving.[298] Definitive therapy involves extensive, arduous reconstructive surgery.

Hemobilia

Hemobilia is hemorrhage into the biliary tract. Causes of communication between the vascular and biliary tree include trauma, liver biopsy, gallstones, hepatic artery or portal vein aneurysms, liver abscesses, and neoplasia,[300] among which the most common is blunt or iatrogenic trauma. Diagnosis is always difficult, but suspicion is raised by the clinical history and is made at endoscopy by visualizing blood coming from the ampulla of Vater, or by angiography. Although both angiographic embolization[301] or surgical ligation of the hepatic feeding vessel may be successful, mortality from hemobilia is high.

Hemosuccus Pancreaticus

Hemosuccus pancreaticus is defined as bleeding from peripancreatic blood vessels into a pancreatic duct,[302] and most often results from either erosion of a pseudocyst into the splenic or peripancreatic artery or formation of an arterial aneurysm that subsequently communicates with the pancreatic duct in the course of chronic pancreatitis. The diagnosis may be made by endoscopic visualization of blood coming from the papilla. Suspicion of the diagnosis should be high in patients with this disease who have apparently obscure but clinically evident bleeding. Angiography is required to identify definitively the bleeding site. Although embolization therapy may be effective, surgery is often required to control the bleeding completely.[303]

Treatment of Obscure Bleeding

Treatment of lesions that bleed in an obscure fashion is aimed at the underlying abnormality. Thus, mass lesions are usually resected. Endoscopic or surgical therapy is often successful in patients with large, focal vascular ectasias but problematic when multiple, as is often commonly the case. For diffuse ectasias, pharmacologic therapy with estrogen/progesterone compounds[304, 305] has been tried, based on their amplification of clotting by an unknown mechanism. In a prospective longitudinal observational study of 43 patients with proven or presumed vascular ectasias treated with Ortho-Novum 1/50, containing 1 mg of norethindrone and 0.05 mg of mestranol (one tablet twice daily)[305] and followed for a mean time of 535 days (range, 25 to 1551 days), none of the 38 patients who were treated with combination hormonal therapy rebled, but the 5 patients who received estrogen alone had rebleeding episodes. Although side effects were reported as mild, other investigators have reported breast tenderness and vaginal bleeding in women and gynecomastia and loss of libido in men, necessitating cessation of therapy in a significant proportion of patients.[306] Furthermore, controlled trials using estrogen/progesterone compounds have failed to show an advantage over placebo.[306]

Octreotide has also been tried in patients with bleeding due to diffuse vascular ectasia. At a dose of 0.05 to 1 mg subcutaneously per day, this compound was reported to be effective and without side effects;[307, 308] however, no satisfactory controlled study has been done. Other agents, including aminocaproic acid, tranexamic acid, and danazol have been demonstrated in case reports to control bleeding effectively with, again, no controlled data for support.

The role of therapeutic endoscopy in patients with obscure bleeding, particularly those with vascular ectasias, also remains controversial. Enteroscopic cauterization of vascular ectasias led to an improvement in hemoglobin and a reduction in blood transfusion requirements in some studies[309, 310] but not in others.[305] Results with intraoperative enteroscopy are also inconsistent. These procedures often identify a source of bleeding, but surgical resection of these lesions does not always prevent recurrent bleeding. Although some investigators have reported rebleeding rates of as low as 20%,[287] the rebleed rate in other studies has been over 50%,[277, 286] suggesting that caution is required with this approach also, intraoperative enteroscopy and possible resection require an experienced, skilled, and dedicated team.

Summary of Occult and Obscure Gastrointestinal Bleeding

Occult gastrointestinal bleeding is the most common form of gastrointestinal bleeding and most often is manifest as occult blood in the stool. Occult gastrointestinal bleeding may also be manifest as iron deficiency anemia, often the result of chronic undetected gastrointestinal bleeding. The approach to evaluation of patients with fecal occult blood and iron deficiency anemia is similar and usually begins with investigation of the colon. Colonoscopy is preferred but flexible sigmoidoscopy plus air contrast barium enema may be an acceptable alternative. If evaluation of the colon does not reveal a bleeding site, evaluation of the upper gastrointestinal tract should be considered in all patients; in those with iron deficiency anemia, upper gastrointestinal examination is required. The role of small intestinal investigation is controversial, and is probably best reserved for patients with iron deficiency anemia and persistent gastrointestinal symptoms or those who fail to respond to appropriate therapy. Celiac sprue and other malabsorptive diseases must also be considered as a potential cause of iron deficiency anemia.

The treatment and prognosis of patients with occult blood

in the stool or iron deficiency anemia or both depends on the gastrointestinal tract abnormality(ies) identified. Those without identifiable bleeding sites generally respond to conservative management and have a favorable prognosis. Patients with refractory iron deficiency anemia or clinically apparent but obscure bleeding make up a small fraction of all patients with gastrointestinal bleeding but represent a considerable diagnostic and therapeutic challenge. They should undergo aggressive endoscopic evaluation, including small bowel investigation; in certain circumstances, other diagnostic studies are indicated (angiography, computed tomographic examination). Multiple small intestinal vascular ectasias usually cause bleeding in this subgroup of patients. Management of these patients is extremely difficult, requiring a focused and experienced team approach.

REFERENCES

1. Gilbert DA: Epidemiology of upper gastrointestinal bleeding. Gastrointest Endosc 36:S8, 1990.
2. Longstreth GF: Epidemiology of hospitalization for acute upper gastrointestinal hemorrhage: A population-based study. Am J Gastroenterol 90:206, 1995.
3. Longstreth GF: Epidemiology and outcome of patients hospitalized with acute lower gastrointestinal hemorrhage: A population-based study. Am J Gastroenterol 92:419, 1997.
4. Wiesen AR, Hospenthal DR, Byrd JC, et al: Equilibration of hemoglobin concentration after transfusion in medical inpatients not actively bleeding. Ann Intern Med 121:278, 1994.
5. Segal WN, Cello JP: Hemorrhage in the upper gastrointestinal tract in the older patient. Am J Gastroenterol 92:42, 1997.
6. Wilcox CM, Clark WS: Features associated with painless peptic ulcer bleeding. Am J Gastroenterol 92:1289, 1997.
7. Schiff L, Stevens RJ, Shapiro N, Goodman S: Observations on the oral administration of citrate blood in man. Am J Med Sci 203:409, 1942.
8. Ebert RA, Stead EA, Gibson JG: Response of normal subjects to acute blood loss. Arch Intern Med 68:578, 1940.
9. Chalasani N, Clark WS, Wilcox CM: Blood urea nitrogen to creatinine concentration in gastrointestinal bleeding: A reappraisal. Am J Gastroenterol 92:1796, 1997.
10. Hilsman JH: The color of blood-containing feces following the instillation of citrated blood at various levels of the small intestine. Gastroenterology 15:131, 1950.
11. Jensen DM, Machicado GA: Diagnosis and treatment of severe hematochezia. The role of urgent colonoscopy after purge. Gastroenterology 95:1569, 1988.
12. Luk GD, Bynum TE, Hendrix TR: Gastric aspiration in localization of gastrointestinal hemorrhage. JAMA 241:576, 1979.
13. Gilbert DA, Silverstein FE, Tedesco FJ, et al: The national ASGE survey on upper gastrointestinal bleeding. III. Endoscopy in upper gastrointestinal bleeding. Gastrointest Endosc 27:94, 1981.
14. Cuellar RE, Gavaler JS, Alexander JA, et al: Gastrointestinal tract hemorrhage. The value of a nasogastric aspirate. Arch Intern Med 150:1381, 1990.
15. Peterson WL, Barnett CC, Smith HJ, et al: Routine early endoscopy in upper-gastrointestinal-tract bleeding: A randomized, controlled trial. N Engl J Med 304:925, 1981.
16. Rockall TA, Logan RF, Devlin HB, Northfield TC: Incidence of and mortality from acute upper gastrointestinal haemorrhage in the United Kingdom. Steering Committee and members of the National Audit of Acute Upper Gastrointestinal Haemorrhage. Br Med J 311:222, 1995.
17. Vreeburg EM, Snel P, de Bruijne JW, et al: Acute upper gastrointestinal bleeding in the Amsterdam area: Incidence, diagnosis, and clinical outcome. Am J Gastroenterol 92:236, 1997.
18. Rosen AM, Fleischer DE: Upper GI bleeding in the elderly: Diagnosis and management. Geriatrics 44:26, 1989.
19. Rockall TA, Logan RF, Devlin HB, Northfield TC: Risk assessment after acute upper gastrointestinal haemorrhage. Gut 38:316, 1996.
20. Kollef MH, O'Brien JD, Zuckerman GR, Shannon W: BLEED: A classification tool to predict outcomes in patients with acute upper and lower gastrointestinal hemorrhage. Crit Care Med 25:1125, 1997.
21. Corley DA, Stefan AM, Wolf M, et al: Early indicators of prognosis in upper gastrointestinal hemorrhage. Am J Gastroenterol 93:336, 1998.
22. Thomopoulos K, Katsakoulis E, Vagianos C, et al: Causes and clinical outcome of acute upper gastrointestinal bleeding: A prospective analysis of 1534 cases. Int J Clin Pract 52:547, 1998.
23. Vreeburg EM, Terwee CB, Snel P, et al: Validation of the Rockall risk scoring system in upper gastrointestinal bleeding. Gut 44:331, 1999.
24. Fleischer D: Etiology and prevalence of severe persistent upper gastrointestinal bleeding. Gastroenterology 84:538, 1983.
25. Sharara A, Rockey DC: Esophageal variceal hemorrhage. N Engl J Med 345:669, 2001.
26. Proceedings of the Consensus Conference on Therapeutic Endoscopy in Bleeding Ulcers, March 6–8, 1989. Gastrointest Endosc 36:S1, 1990.
27. Terdiman JP, Ostroff JW: Risk of persistent or recurrent and intractable upper gastrointestinal bleeding in the era of therapeutic endoscopy. Am J Gastroenterol 92:1805, 1997.
28. Lewis JD, Shin EJ, Metz DC: Characterization of gastrointestinal bleeding in severely ill hospitalized patients. Crit Care Med 28:46, 2000.
29. Afessa B: Triage of patients with acute gastrointestinal bleeding for intensive care unit admission based on risk factors for poor outcome. J Clin Gastroenterol 30:281, 2000.
30. Saeed ZA, Winchester CB, Michaletz PA, et al: A scoring system to predict rebleeding after endoscopic therapy of nonvariceal upper gastrointestinal hemorrhage, with a comparison of heat probe and ethanol injection. Am J Gastroenterol 88:1842, 1993.
31. Blatchford O, Murray WR, Blatchford M: A risk score to predict need for treatment for upper-gastrointestinal haemorrhage. Lancet 356:1318, 2000.
32. Cook DJ, Guyatt GH, Salena BJ, Laine LA: Endoscopic therapy for acute nonvariceal upper gastrointestinal hemorrhage: A meta-analysis. Gastroenterology 102:139, 1992.
33. Lee JG, Turnipseed S, Romano PS, et al: Endoscopy-based triage significantly reduces hospitalization rates and costs of treating upper GI bleeding: A randomized controlled trial. Gastrointest Endosc 50:755, 1999.
34. Stollman NH, Putcha RV, Neustater BR, et al: The uncleared fundal pool in acute upper gastrointestinal bleeding: Implications and outcomes. Gastrointest Endosc 46:324, 1997.
35. Andrus CH, Ponsky JL: The effects of irrigant temperature in upper gastrointestinal hemorrhage: A requiem for iced saline lavage. Am J Gastroenterol 82:1062, 1987.
36. Laine L: Upper gastrointestinal tract hemorrhage. West J Med 155:274, 1991.
37. Peura DA, Lanza FL, Gostout CJ, Foutch PG: The American College of Gastroenterology Bleeding Registry: Preliminary findings. Am J Gastroenterol 92:924, 1997.
38. Wilcox CM, Clark WS: Causes and outcome of upper and lower gastrointestinal bleeding: The Grady Hospital experience. South Med J 92:44, 1999.
39. Graham DY, Schwartz JT: The spectrum of the Mallory-Weiss tear. Medicine (Baltimore) 57:307, 1978.
40. Hixson SD, Burns RP, Britt LG: Mallory-Weiss syndrome: Retrospective review of eight years' experience. South Med J 72:1249, 1979.
41. Bharucha AE, Gostout CJ, Balm RK: Clinical and endoscopic risk factors in the Mallory-Weiss syndrome. Am J Gastroenterol 92:805, 1997.
42. Bataller R, Llach J, Salmeron JM, et al: Endoscopic sclerotherapy in upper gastrointestinal bleeding due to the Mallory-Weiss syndrome [see comments]. Am J Gastroenterol 89:2147, 1994.
43. Wong RM, Ota S, Katoh A, et al: Endoscopic ligation for non-esophageal variceal upper gastrointestinal hemorrhage. Endoscopy 30:774, 1998.
44. Carsen GM, Casarella WJ, Spiegel RM: Transcatheter embolization for treatment of Mallory-Weiss tears of the esophagogastric junction. Radiology 128:309, 1978.
45. Silverstein FE, Gilbert DA, Tedesco FJ, et al: The national ASGE survey on upper gastrointestinal bleeding. II. Clinical prognostic factors. Gastrointest Endosc 27:80, 1981.
46. Skok P: The epidemiology of hemorrhage from the upper gastrointestinal tract in the mid-nineties—has anything changed? Hepatogastroenterology 45:2228, 1998.
47. Czernichow P, Hochain P, Nousbaum JB, et al: Epidemiology and course of acute upper gastro-intestinal haemorrhage in four French geographical areas. Eur J Gastroenterol Hepatol 12:175, 2000.
48. Swain CP: Pathophysiology of bleeding lesions. Gastrointest Endosc 36:S21, 1990.

49. Lanas A, Bajador E, Serrano P, et al: Nitrovasodilators, low-dose aspirin, other nonsteroidal anti-inflammatory drugs, and the risk of upper gastrointestinal bleeding. N Engl J Med 343:834, 2000.
50. Conn HO, Poynard T: Corticosteroids and peptic ulcer: Meta-analysis of adverse events during steroid therapy. J Intern Med 236:619, 1994.
51. Lanza F, Rack MF, Simon TJ, et al: Effects of alendronate on gastric and duodenal mucosa. Am J Gastroenterol 93:753, 1998.
52. Graham DY, Malaty HM: Alendronate and naproxen are synergistic for development of gastric ulcers. Arch Intern Med 161:107, 2001.
53. Terdiman JP, Ostroff JW: Gastrointestinal bleeding in the hospitalized patient: A case-control study to assess risk factors, causes, and outcome. Am J Med 104:349, 1998.
54. Roy PK, Venzon DJ, Shojamanesh H, et al: Zollinger-Ellison syndrome. Clinical presentation in 261 patients. Medicine (Baltimore) 79: 379, 2000.
55. Hasselgren G, Lind T, Lundell L, et al: Continuous intravenous infusion of omeprazole in elderly patients with peptic ulcer bleeding. Results of a placebo-controlled multicenter study. Scand J Gastroenterol 32:328, 1997.
56. Schaffalitzky de Muckadell OB, Havelund T, Harling H, et al: Effect of omeprazole on the outcome of endoscopically treated bleeding peptic ulcers. Randomized double-blind placebo-controlled multicentre study [see comments]. Scand J Gastroenterol 32:320, 1997.
57. Khuroo MS, Yattoo GN, Javid G, et al: A comparison of omeprazole and placebo for bleeding peptic ulcer. N Engl J Med 336:1054, 1997.
58. Lin HJ, Lo WC, Lee FY, et al: A prospective randomized comparative trial showing that omeprazole prevents rebleeding in patients with bleeding peptic ulcer after successful endoscopic therapy. Arch Intern Med 158:54, 1998.
59. Lau JY, Sung JJ, Lee KK, et al: Effect of intravenous omeprazole on recurrent bleeding after endoscopic treatment of bleeding peptic ulcers. N Engl J Med 343:310, 2000.
60. Hosking SW, Yung MY, Chung SC, Li AKC: Differing prevalence of *Helicobacter* in bleeding and nonbleeding ulcers. Gastroenterology 102:85, 1992.
61. Kuyvenhoven JP, Veenendaal RA, Vandenbroucke JP: Peptic ulcer bleeding: Interaction between non-steroidal anti-inflammatory drugs, *Helicobacter pylori* infection, and the ABO blood group system. Scand J Gastroenterol 34:1082, 1999.
62. Labenz J, Peitz U, Kohl H, et al: *Helicobacter pylori* increases the risk of peptic ulcer bleeding: A case control study. Ital J Gastroenterol Hepatol 31:110, 1999.
63. Hawkey CJ: Risk of ulcer bleeding in patients infected with *Helicobacter pylori* taking non-steroidal anti-inflammatory drugs. Gut 46:310, 2000.
64. Chan FK, Sung JJ, Suen R, et al: Does eradication of *Helicobacter pylori* impair healing of nonsteroidal anti-inflammatory drug–associated bleeding peptic ulcers? A prospective randomized study. Aliment Pharmacol Ther 12:1201, 1998.
65. Wallace JL: Nonsteroidal anti-inflammatory drugs and gastroenteropathy: The second hundred years. Gastroenterology 112:1000, 1997.
66. The Aspirin Myocardial Infarction Study Research Group: The aspirin myocardial infarction study: Final results. Circulation 62:V79, 1980.
67. United Kingdom transient ischaemic attack (UK-TIA) aspirin trial: Interim results. Lancet 296:316, 1988.
68. Steering Committee of the Physicians' Health Study Research Group: Final report on the aspirin component of the ongoing Physicians' Health Study. N Engl J Med 321:129, 1989.
69. The SALT Collaborative Group: Swedish Aspirin Low-Dose Trial (SALT) of 75 mg aspirin as secondary prophylaxis after cerebrovascular ischaemic events. Lancet 338:1345, 1991.
70. Roderick PJ, Wilkes HC, Meade TW: The gastrointestinal toxicity of aspirin: An overview of randomised controlled trials. Br J Clin Pharmacol 35:219, 1993.
71. Griffin MR, Piper JM, Daugherty JR, et al: Nonsteroidal anti-inflammatory drug use and increased risk for peptic ulcer disease in elderly persons. Ann Intern Med 114:257, 1991.
72. Garcia Rodriguez LA, Jick H: Risk of upper gastrointestinal bleeding and perforation associated with individual non-steroidal anti-inflammatory drugs. Lancet 343:769, 1994.
73. Garcia Rodriguez LA, Cattaruzzi C, Troncon MG, Agostinis L: Risk of hospitalization for upper gastrointestinal tract bleeding associated with ketorolac, other nonsteroidal anti-inflammatory drugs, calcium antagonists, and other antihypertensive drugs. Arch Intern Med 158:33, 1998.
74. Bjorkman DJ: Current status of nonsteroidal anti-inflammatory drug (NSAID) use in the United States: Risk factors and frequency of complications. Am J Med 107:3S, 1999. Discussion 8S.
75. Bombardier C, Laine L, Reicin A, et al: Comparison of upper gastrointestinal toxicity of rofecoxib and naproxen in patients with rheumatoid arthritis. N Engl J Med 343:1520, 2000.
76. Silverstein FE, Faich G, Goldstein JL, et al: Gastrointestinal toxicity with celecoxib vs. nonsteroidal anti-inflammatory drugs for osteoarthritis and rheumatoid arthritis; The CLASS study: A randomized controlled trial. Celecoxib Long-term Arthritis Safety Study. JAMA 284:1247, 2000.
77. Silverstein FE, Graham DY, Senior JR, et al: Misoprostol reduces serious gastrointestinal complications in patients with rheumatoid arthritis receiving nonsteroidal anti-inflammatory drugs. A randomized, double-blind, placebo-controlled trial. Ann Intern Med 123:241, 1995.
78. Soll AH, Weinstein WM, Kurata J, McCarthy D: Nonsteroidal anti-inflammatory drugs and peptic ulcer disease. Ann Intern Med 114:307, 1991.
79. Chan FK, Sung JJ, Chung SC, et al: Randomised trial of eradication of *Helicobacter pylori* before non-steroidal anti-inflammatory drug therapy to prevent peptic ulcers. Lancet 350:975, 1997.
80. Hawkey CJ, Tulassay Z, Szczepanski L, et al: Randomised controlled trial of *Helicobacter pylori* eradication in patients on non-steroidal anti-inflammatory drugs: HELP NSAIDs study. Helicobacter Eradication for Lesion Prevention. Lancet 352:1016, 1998.
81. Piper JM, Ray WA, Daugherty JR, Griffin MR: Corticosteroid use and peptic ulcer disease: Role of nonsteroidal anti-inflammatory drugs. Ann Intern Med 114:735, 1991.
82. Kaufman DW, Kelly JP, Wiholm BE, et al: The risk of acute major upper gastrointestinal bleeding among users of aspirin and ibuprofen at various levels of alcohol consumption. Am J Gastroenterol 94:3189, 1999.
83. Shorr RI, Ray WA, Daugherty JR, Griffin MR: Concurrent use of nonsteroidal anti-inflammatory drugs and oral anticoagulants places elderly persons at high risk for hemorrhagic peptic ulcer disease. Arch Intern Med 153:1665, 1993.
84. Griffiths WJ, Neumann DA, Welsh JD: The visible vessel as an indicator of uncontrolled or recurrent gastrointestinal hemorrhage. N Engl J Med 300:1411, 1979.
85. Storey DW, Bown SG, Swain CP, et al: Endoscopic prediction of recurrent bleeding in peptic ulcers. N Engl J Med 305:915, 1981.
86. Laine L: Multipolar electrocoagulation in the treatment of active upper gastrointestinal tract hemorrhage. A prospective controlled trial. N Engl J Med 316:1613, 1987.
87. Laine L: Multipolar electrocoagulation in the treatment of peptic ulcers with nonbleeding visible vessels. A prospective, controlled trial. Ann Intern Med 110:510, 1989.
88. Branicki FJ, Coleman SY, Lam TC, et al: Hypotension and endoscopic stigmata of recent haemorrhage in bleeding peptic ulcer: Risk models for rebleeding and mortality. J Gastroenterol Hepatol 7:184, 1992.
89. Lau JY, Sung JJ, Chan AC, et al: Stigmata of hemorrhage in bleeding peptic ulcers: An interobserver agreement study among international experts. Gastrointest Endosc 46:33, 1997.
90. Lau JY, Chung SC, Leung JW, et al: The evolution of stigmata of hemorrhage in bleeding peptic ulcers: A sequential endoscopic study. Endoscopy 30:513, 1998.
91. Laine L, Freeman M, Cohen H: Lack of uniformity in evaluation of endoscopic prognostic features of bleeding ulcers. Gastrointest Endosc 40:411, 1994.
92. Branicki FJ, Coleman SY, Fok PJ, et al: Bleeding peptic ulcer: A prospective evaluation of risk factors for rebleeding and mortality. World J Surg 14:262, 1990. Discussion 269.
93. Laine L, Stein C, Sharma V: A prospective outcome study of patients with clot in an ulcer and the effect of irrigation. Gastrointest Endosc 43:107, 1996.
94. Green FW, Kaplan MM, Curtis LE, Levine PH: Effect of acid and pepsin on blood coagulation and platelet aggregation. A possible contributor to prolonged gastroduodenal mucosal hemorrhage. Gastroenterology 74:38, 1978.
95. Patchett SE, Enright H, Afdhal N, et al: Clot lysis by gastric juice: An in vitro study. Gut 30:1704, 1989.
96. Collins R, Langman M: Treatment with histamine H_2-antagonists in acute upper gastrointestinal hemorrhage. Implications of randomized trials. N Engl J Med 313:660, 1985.
97. Hunt RH, Cederberg C, Dent J, et al: Optimizing acid suppression for treatment of acid-related diseases. Dig Dis Sci 40:24S, 1995.

98. Daneshmend TK, Hawkey CJ, Langman MJ, et al: Omeprazole versus placebo for acute upper gastrointestinal bleeding: Randomised double blind controlled trial. Br Med J 304:143, 1992.
99. Elliott SN, McKnight W, Cirino G, Wallace JL: A nitric oxide–releasing nonsteroidal anti-inflammatory drug accelerates gastric ulcer healing in rats. Gastroenterology 109:524, 1995.
100. Wallace JL: Mechanisms of protection and healing: Current knowledge and future research. Am J Med 110:S19, 2001.
101. Standards of Practice Committee: The role of endoscopy in the management of non-variceal acute upper gastrointestinal bleeding. Guidelines for clinical application. American Society for Gastrointestinal Endoscopy. Gastrointest Endosc 38:760, 1992.
102. Swain CP: Laser therapy for gastrointestinal bleeding. Gastrointest Endosc Clin N Am 7:611, 1997.
103. Song SY, Chung JB, Moon YM, et al: Comparison of the hemostatic effect of endoscopic injection with fibrin glue and hypertonic saline-epinephrine for peptic ulcer bleeding: A prospective randomized trial. Endoscopy 29:827, 1997.
104. Cipolletta L, Bianco MA, Rotondano G, et al: Prospective comparison of argon plasma coagulator and heater probe in the endoscopic treatment of major peptic ulcer bleeding. Gastrointest Endosc 48:191, 1998.
105. Savides TJ, Jensen DM: Therapeutic endoscopy for nonvariceal gastrointestinal bleeding. Gastroenterol Clin North Am 29:465, 2000.
106. Chung IK, Ham JS, Kim HS, et al: Comparison of the hemostatic efficacy of the endoscopic hemoclip method with hypertonic saline-epinephrine injection and a combination of the two for the management of bleeding peptic ulcers. Gastrointest Endosc 49:13, 1999.
107. Cipolletta L, Bianco MA, Marmo R, et al: Endoclips versus heater probe in preventing early recurrent bleeding from peptic ulcer: A prospective and randomized trial. Gastrointest Endosc 53:147, 2001.
108. Lin HJ, Tseng GY, Perng CL, et al: Comparison of adrenaline injection and bipolar electrocoagulation for the arrest of peptic ulcer bleeding. Gut 44:715, 1999.
109. Nagayama K, Tazawa J, Sakai Y, et al: Efficacy of endoscopic clipping for bleeding gastroduodenal ulcer: Comparison with topical ethanol injection. Am J Gastroenterol 94:2897, 1999.
110. Chung SS, Lau JY, Sung JJ, et al: Randomised comparison between adrenaline injection alone and adrenaline injection plus heat probe treatment for actively bleeding ulcers. Br Med J 314:1307, 1997.
111. Kubba AK, Murphy W, Palmer KR: Endoscopic injection for bleeding peptic ulcer: A comparison of adrenaline alone with adrenaline plus human thrombin. Gastroenterology 111:623, 1996.
112. Choudari CP, Palmer KR: Endoscopic injection therapy for bleeding peptic ulcer: A comparison of adrenaline alone with adrenaline plus ethanolamine oleate. Gut 35:608, 1994.
113. Villanueva C, Balanzo J, Torras X, et al: Value of second-look endoscopy after injection therapy for bleeding peptic ulcer: A prospective and randomized trial. Gastrointest Endosc 40:34, 1994.
114. Saeed ZA, Cole RA, Ramirez FC, et al: Endoscopic retreatment after successful initial hemostasis prevents ulcer rebleeding: A prospective randomized trial. Endoscopy 28:288, 1996.
115. Lau JY, Sung JJ, Lam YH, et al: Endoscopic retreatment compared with surgery in patients with recurrent bleeding after initial endoscopic control of bleeding ulcers. N Engl J Med 340:751, 1999.
116. Lefkovitz Z, Cappell MS, Kaplan M, et al: Radiology in the diagnosis and therapy of gastrointestinal bleeding. Gastroenterol Clin North Am 29:489, 2000.
117. Kramer SC, Gorich J, Rilinger N, et al: Embolization for gastrointestinal hemorrhages. Eur Radiol 10:802, 2000.
118. Selby NM, Kubba AK, Hawkey CJ: Acid suppression in peptic ulcer haemorrhage: A 'meta-analysis.' Aliment Pharmacol Ther 14:1119, 2000.
119. Rockall TA: Management and outcome of patients undergoing surgery after acute upper gastrointestinal haemorrhage. Steering Group for the National Audit of Acute Upper Gastrointestinal Haemorrhage. J R Soc Med 91:518, 1998.
120. Morris DL, Hawker PC, Brearley S, et al: Optimal timing of operation for bleeding peptic ulcer: Prospective randomised trial. Br Med J (Clin Res Ed) 288:1277, 1984.
121. Imhof M, Schroders C, Ohmann C, Roher H: Impact of early operation on the mortality from bleeding peptic ulcer — ten years' experience. Dig Surg 15:308, 1998.
122. Murray WR, Laferla G, Cooper G, Archibald M: Duodenal ulcer healing after presentation with haemorrhage. Gut 27:1387, 1986.
123. Jensen DM, Cheng S, Kovacs TO, et al: A controlled study of ranitidine for the prevention of recurrent hemorrhage from duodenal ulcer. N Engl J Med 330:382, 1994.
124. Graham DY, Hepps KS, Ramirez FC, et al: Treatment of *Helicobacter pylori* reduces the rate of rebleeding in peptic ulcer disease. Scand J Gastroenterol 28:939, 1993.
125. Labenz J, Borsch G: Role of *Helicobacter pylori* eradication in the prevention of peptic ulcer bleeding relapse. Digestion 55:19, 1994.
126. Rokkas T, Karameris A, Mavrogeorgis A, et al: Eradication of *Helicobacter pylori* reduces the possibility of rebleeding in peptic ulcer disease. Gastrointest Endosc 41:1, 1995.
127. Jaspersen D, Koerner T, Schorr W, et al: *Helicobacter pylori* eradication reduces the rate of rebleeding in ulcer hemorrhage. Gastrointest Endosc 41:5–9, 1995.
128. Riemann JF, Schilling D, Schauwecker P, et al: Cure with omeprazole plus amoxicillin versus long-term ranitidine therapy in *Helicobacter pylori*–associated peptic ulcer bleeding. Gastrointest Endosc 46:299, 1997.
129. Santander C, Gravalos RG, Gomez-Cedenilla A, et al: Antimicrobial therapy for *Helicobacter pylori* infection versus long-term maintenance antisecretion treatment in the prevention of recurrent hemorrhage from peptic ulcer: Prospective nonrandomized trial on 125 patients. Am J Gastroenterol 91:1549, 1996.
130. Yeomans ND, Tulassay Z, Juhasz L, et al: A comparison of omeprazole with ranitidine for ulcers associated with nonsteroidal antiinflammatory drugs. Acid Suppression Trial: Ranitidine versus Omeprazole for NSAID-associated Ulcer Treatment (ASTRONAUT) Study Group. N Engl J Med 338:719, 1998.
131. Graham DY, White RH, Moreland LW, et al: Duodenal and gastric ulcer prevention with misoprostol in arthritis patients taking NSAIDs. Misoprostol Study Group. Ann Intern Med 119:257, 1993.
132. Hawkey CJ, Karrasch JA, Szczepanski L, et al: Omeprazole compared with misoprostol for ulcers associated with nonsteroidal antiinflammatory drugs. Omeprazole versus Misoprostol for NSAID-induced Ulcer Management (OMNIUM) Study Group. N Engl J Med 338:727, 1998.
133. Laine L, Weinstein WM: Subepithelial hemorrhages and erosions of human stomach. Dig Dis Sci 33:490, 1988.
134. Cook DJ, Fuller HD, Guyatt GH, et al: Risk factors for gastrointestinal bleeding in critically ill patients. Canadian Critical Care Trials Group. N Engl J Med 330:377, 1994.
135. Ben-Menachem T, Fogel R, Patel RV, et al: Prophylaxis for stress-related gastric hemorrhage in the medical intensive care unit. A randomized, controlled, single-blind study. Ann Intern Med 121:568, 1994.
136. Cook DJ, Reeve BK, Guyatt GH, et al: Stress ulcer prophylaxis in critically ill patients. Resolving discordant meta-analyses. JAMA 275: 308, 1996.
137. Cook D, Guyatt G, Marshall J, et al: A comparison of sucralfate and ranitidine for the prevention of upper gastrointestinal bleeding in patients requiring mechanical ventilation. Canadian Critical Care Trials Group. N Engl J Med 338:791, 1998.
138. Laine L, Weinstein WM: Histology of alcoholic hemorrhagic "gastritis": a prospective evaluation. Gastroenterology 94:1254, 1988.
139. Kelly JP, Kaufman DW, Koff RS, et al: Alcohol consumption and the risk of major upper gastrointestinal bleeding. Am J Gastroenterol 90: 1058, 1995.
140. Wilcox CM, Alexander LN, Straub RF, Clark WS: A prospective endoscopic evaluation of the causes of upper GI hemorrhage in alcoholics: A focus on alcoholic gastropathy. Am J Gastroenterol 91:1343, 1996.
141. Sherman LM, Shenoy SS, Cerra FB: Selective intra-arterial vasopressin: Clinical efficacy and complications. Ann Surg 189:298, 1979.
142. Savides TJ, Jensen DM, Cohen J, et al: Severe upper gastrointestinal tumor bleeding: Endoscopic findings, treatment, and outcome. Endoscopy 28:244, 1996.
143. Lanza FL, Graham DY, Nelson RS, et al: Endoscopic upper gastrointestinal polypectomy. Report of 73 polypectomies in 63 patients. Am J Gastroenterol 75:345, 1981.
144. Fockens P, Tytgat GN: Dieulafoy's disease. Gastrointest Endosc Clin N Am 6:739, 1996.
145. Baettig B, Haecki W, Lammer F, Jost R: Dieulafoy's disease: Endoscopic treatment and follow up. Gut 34:1418, 1993.
146. Fockens P, Meenan J, van Dullemen HM, et al: Dieulafoy's disease: Endosonographic detection and endosonography-guided treatment. Gastrointest Endosc 44:437, 1996.
147. Parra-Blanco A, Takahashi H, Mendez Jerez PV, et al: Endoscopic

management of Dieulafoy lesions of the stomach: A case study of 26 patients. Endoscopy 29:834, 1997.
148. Abi-Hanna D, Williams SJ, Gillespie PE, Bourke MJ: Endoscopic band ligation for non-variceal non-ulcer gastrointestinal hemorrhage. Gastrointest Endosc 48:510, 1998.
149. Norton ID, Petersen BT, Sorbi D, et al: Management and long-term prognosis of Dieulafoy lesion. Gastrointest Endosc 50:762, 1999.
150. Foutch PG: Angiodysplasia of the gastrointestinal tract. Am J Gastroenterol 88:807, 1993.
151. Chalasani N, Cotsonis G, Wilcox CM: Upper gastrointestinal bleeding in patients with chronic renal failure: Role of vascular ectasia. Am J Gastroenterol 91:2329, 1996.
152. Spahr L, Villeneuve JP, Dufresne MP, et al: Gastric antral vascular ectasia in cirrhotic patients: Absence of relation with portal hypertension. Gut 44:739, 1999.
153. Kamath PS, Lacerda M, Ahlquist DA, et al: Gastric mucosal responses to intrahepatic portosystemic shunting in patients with cirrhosis. Gastroenterology 118:905, 2000.
154. Tran A, Villeneuve JP, Bilodeau M, et al: Treatment of chronic bleeding from gastric antral vascular ectasia (GAVE) with estrogen-progesterone in cirrhotic patients: An open pilot study. Am J Gastroenterol 94:2909, 1999.
155. Talley NJ, Jones M: Self-reported rectal bleeding in a United States community: Prevalence, risk factors, and health care seeking. Am J Gastroenterol 93:2179, 1998.
156. Bramley PN, Masson JW, McKnight G, et al: The role of an open-access bleeding unit in the management of colonic haemorrhage. A 2-year prospective study. Scand J Gastroenterol 31:764, 1996.
157. Bini EJ, Weinshel EH, Falkenstein DB: Risk factors for recurrent bleeding and mortality in human immunodeficiency virus infected patients with acute lower GI hemorrhage. Gastrointest Endosc 49:748, 1999.
158. Foutch PG: Diverticular bleeding: Are nonsteroidal anti-inflammatory drugs risk factors for hemorrhage and can colonoscopy predict outcome for patients? Am J Gastroenterol 90:1779, 1995.
159. Zuckerman GR, Trellis DR, Sherman TM, Clouse RE: An objective measure of stool color for differentiating upper from lower gastrointestinal bleeding. Dig Dis Sci 40:1614, 1995.
160. Zuccaro G: Management of the adult patient with acute lower gastrointestinal bleeding. Am J Gastroenterol 93:1202, 1998.
161. Zuckerman GR, Prakash C: Acute lower intestinal bleeding. Part I: Clinical presentation and diagnosis. Gastrointest Endosc 48:606, 1998.
162. American Society for Gastrointestinal Endoscopy: The role of endoscopy in the patient with lower gastrointestinal bleeding. Gastrointest Endosc 48:685, 1998.
163. Kok KY, Kum CK, Goh PM: Colonoscopic evaluation of severe hematochezia in an Oriental population. Endoscopy 30:675, 1998.
164. Chaudhry V, Hyser MJ, Gracias VH, Gau FC: Colonoscopy: The initial test for acute lower gastrointestinal bleeding. Am Surg 64:723, 1998.
165. Jensen DM, Machicado GA, Jutabha R, Kovacs TO: Urgent colonoscopy for the diagnosis and treatment of severe diverticular hemorrhage [see comments]. N Engl J Med 342:78, 2000.
166. Zuckerman GR, Prakash C: Acute lower intestinal bleeding. Part II: Etiology, therapy, and outcomes. Gastrointest Endosc 49:228, 1999.
167. Dusold R, Burke K, Carpentier W, Dyck WP: The accuracy of technetium-99m-labeled red cell scintigraphy in localizing gastrointestinal bleeding. Am J Gastroenterol 89:345, 1994.
168. Hunter JM, Pezim ME: Limited value of technetium 99m-labeled red cell scintigraphy in localization of lower gastrointestinal bleeding. Am J Surg 159:504, 1990.
169. Voeller GR, Bunch G, Britt LG: Use of technetium-labeled red blood cell scintigraphy in the detection and management of gastrointestinal hemorrhage. Surgery 110:799, 1991.
170. Gunderman R, Leef J, Ong K, et al: Scintigraphic screening prior to visceral arteriography in acute lower gastrointestinal bleeding. J Nucl Med 39:1081, 1998.
171. Gunderman R, Leef JA, Lipton MJ, Reba RC: Diagnostic imaging and the outcome of acute lower gastrointestinal bleeding. Acad Radiol 5:S303, 1998.
172. Pennoyer WP, Vignati PV, Cohen JL: Mesenteric angiography for lower gastrointestinal hemorrhage: Are there predictors for a positive study? Dis Colon Rectum 40:1014, 1997.
173. Ng DA, Opelka FG, Beck DE, et al: Predictive value of technetium Tc 99m-labeled red blood cell scintigraphy for positive angiogram in massive lower gastrointestinal hemorrhage. Dis Colon Rectum 40:471, 1997.
174. Cohn SM, Moller BA, Zieg PM, et al: Angiography for preoperative evaluation in patients with lower gastrointestinal bleeding: Are the benefits worth the risks? Arch Surg 133:50, 1998.
175. Junquera F, Quiroga S, Saperas E, et al: Accuracy of helical computed tomographic angiography for the diagnosis of colonic angiodysplasia. Gastroenterology 119:293, 2000.
176. Bloomfeld RS, Shetzline M, Rockey D: Urgent colonoscopy for the diagnosis and treatment of severe diverticular hemorrhage. N Engl J Med 342:1608, 2000.
177. McGuire HH: Bleeding colonic diverticula. A reappraisal of natural history and management. Ann Surg 220:653, 1994.
178. Foutch PG, Zimmerman K: Diverticular bleeding and the pigmented protuberance (sentinel clot): Clinical implications, histopathological correlation, and results of endoscopic intervention. Am J Gastroenterol 91:2589, 1996.
179. Foutch PG, Rex DK, Lieberman DA: Prevalence and natural history of colonic angiodysplasia among healthy asymptomatic people. Am J Gastroenterol 90:564, 1995.
180. Greenstein RJ, McElhinney AJ, Reuben D, Greenstein AJ: Colonic vascular ectasias and aortic stenosis: Coincidence or causal relationship? Am J Surg 151:347, 1986.
181. Imperiale TF, Ransohoff DF: Aortic stenosis, idiopathic gastrointestinal bleeding, and angiodysplasia: Is there an association? A methodologic critique of the literature. Gastroenterology 95:1670, 1988.
182. Richter JM, Christensen MR, Colditz GA, Nishioka NS: Angiodysplasia. Natural history and efficacy of therapeutic interventions. Dig Dis Sci 34:1542, 1989.
183. Gupta N, Longo WE, Vernava AM: Angiodysplasia of the lower gastrointestinal tract: An entity readily diagnosed by colonoscopy and primarily managed nonoperatively. Dis Colon Rectum 38:979, 1995.
184. Bemvenuti GA, Julich MM: Ethanolamine injection for sclerotherapy of angiodysplasia of the colon. Endoscopy 30:564, 1998.
185. Guy GE, Shetty PC, Sharma RP, et al: Acute lower gastrointestinal hemorrhage: Treatment by superselective embolization with polyvinyl alcohol particles. AJR Am J Roentgenol 159:521, 1992.
186. Zuckerman DA, Bocchini TP, Birnbaum EH: Massive hemorrhage in the lower gastrointestinal tract in adults: Diagnostic imaging and intervention. AJR Am J Roentgenol 161:703, 1993.
187. Richter JM, Christensen MR, Kaplan LM, Nishioka NS: Effectiveness of current technology in the diagnosis and management of lower gastrointestinal hemorrhage. Gastrointest Endosc 41:93, 1995.
188. Pennoyer WP, Vignati PV, Cohen JL: Management of angiogram-positive lower gastrointestinal hemorrhage: Long-term follow-up of non-operative treatments. Int J Colorectal Dis 11:279, 1996.
189. Gordon RL, Ahl KL, Kerlan RK, et al: Selective arterial embolization for the control of lower gastrointestinal bleeding. Am J Surg 174:24, 1997.
190. Vernava AM, Moore BA, Longo WE, Johnson FE: Lower gastrointestinal bleeding. Dis Colon Rectum 40:846, 1997.
191. Farrands PA, Taylor I: Management of acute lower gastrointestinal haemorrhage in a surgical unit over a 4-year period. J R Soc Med 80: 79, 1987.
192. Jentschura D, Raute M, Winter J, et al: Complications in endoscopy of the lower gastrointestinal tract. Therapy and prognosis. Surg Endosc 8:672, 1994.
193. Gibbs DH, Opelka FG, Beck DE, et al: Postpolypectomy colonic hemorrhage. Dis Colon Rectum 39:806, 1996.
194. Sorbi D, Norton I, Conio M, et al: Postpolypectomy lower GI bleeding: Descriptive analysis. Gastrointest Endosc 51:690, 2000.
195. Rosen L, Bub DS, Reed JF, Nastasee SA: Hemorrhage following colonoscopic polypectomy. Dis Colon Rectum 36:1126, 1993.
196. Randall GM, Jensen DM, Machicado GA, et al: Prospective randomized comparative study of bipolar versus direct current electrocoagulation for treatment of bleeding internal hemorrhoids. Gastrointest Endosc 40:403, 1994.
197. Pardi DS, Loftus EV, Tremaine WJ, et al: Acute major gastrointestinal hemorrhage in inflammatory bowel disease. Gastrointest Endosc 49:153, 1999.
198. Shiraishi M, Hiroyasu S, Ishimine T, et al: Radiation enterocolitis: Overview of the past 15 years. World J Surg 22:491, 1998.
199. Chou YH, Hsu SC, Wang CY, et al: Ischemic colitis as a cause of massive lower gastrointestinal bleeding and peritonitis. Report of five cases. Dis Colon Rectum 32:1065, 1989.

200. Lanthier P, d'Harveng B, Vanheuverzwyn R, et al: Colonic angiodysplasia. Follow-up of patients after endoscopic treatment for bleeding lesions. Dis Colon Rectum 32:296, 1989.
201. Ledermann HP, Schoch E, Jost R, et al: Superselective coil embolization in acute gastrointestinal hemorrhage: Personal experience in 10 patients and review of the literature. J Vasc Interv Radiol 9:753, 1998.
202. Nicholson AA, Ettles DF, Hartley JE, et al: Transcatheter coil embolotherapy: A safe and effective option for major colonic haemorrhage. Gut 43:79, 1998.
203. Peck DJ, McLoughlin RF, Hughson MN, Rankin RN: Percutaneous embolotherapy of lower gastrointestinal hemorrhage. J Vasc Interv Radiol 9:747, 1998.
204. Jensen DM, Machicado GA: Colonoscopy for diagnosis and treatment of severe lower gastrointestinal bleeding. Routine outcomes and cost analysis. Gastrointest Endosc Clin North Am 7:477, 1997.
205. Parkes BM, Obeid FN, Sorensen VJ, et al: The management of massive lower gastrointestinal bleeding. Am Surg 59:676, 1993.
206. Bender JS, Wiencek RG, Bouwman DL: Morbidity and mortality following total abdominal colectomy for massive lower gastrointestinal bleeding. 57:536, Am Surg 1991. Discussion 540.
207. Setya V, Singer JA, Minken SL: Subtotal colectomy as a last resort for unrelenting, unlocalized, lower gastrointestinal hemorrhage: Experience with 12 cases. Am Surg 58:295, 1992.
208. Rockey DC: Occult gastrointestinal bleeding. N Engl J Med 341:38, 1999.
209. Levin B, Hess K, Johnson C: Screening for colorectal cancer. A comparison of 3 fecal occult blood tests. Arch Intern Med 157:970, 1997.
210. Mandel JS, Bond JH, Church TR, et al: Reducing mortality from colorectal cancer by screening for fecal occult blood. Minnesota Colon Cancer Control Study. N Engl J Med 328:1365, 1993.
211. Ahlquist DA, McGill DB, Schwartz S, et al: Fecal blood levels in health and disease. A study using HemoQuant. N Engl J Med 312:1422, 1985.
212. Dybdahl JH, Daae LN, Larsen S: Occult faecal blood loss determined by chemical tests and a ^{51}Cr method. Scand J Gastroenterol 16:245, 1981.
213. St. John DJ, Young GP: Evaluation of radiochromium blood loss studies in unexplained iron-deficiency anaemia. Aust N Z J Med 8:121, 1978.
214. Winawer SJ, Fletcher RH, Miller L, et al: Colorectal cancer screening: Clinical guidelines and rationale. Gastroenterology 112:594, 1997.
215. Rex DK, Johnson DA, Lieberman DA, et al: Colorectal cancer prevention 2000: Screening recommendations of the American College of Gastroenterology. Am J Gastroenterol 95:868, 2000.
216. Burt RW: Colon cancer screening. Gastroenterology 119:837, 2000.
217. Kronborg O, Fenger C, Olsen J, et al: Randomised study of screening for colorectal cancer with faecal-occult-blood test. Lancet 348:1467, 1996.
218. Hardcastle JD, Chamberlain J, Robinson MHE, et al: Randomised controlled trial of faecal-occult blood screening for colorectal cancer. Lancet 348:1472, 1996.
219. Mandel JS, Church TR, Bond JH, et al: The effect of fecal occult blood screening on the incidence of colorectal cancer. N Engl J Med 343:1603, 2000.
220. Ahlquist DA, McGill DB, Fleming JL, et al: Patterns of occult bleeding in asymptomatic colorectal cancer. Cancer 63:1826, 1989.
221. Allison JE, Tekawa IS, Ransom LJ, Adrain AL: A comparison of fecal occult blood tests for colorectal cancer screening. N Engl J Med 334:155, 1996.
222. Rockey DC, Auslander A, Greenberg PD: Detection of upper gastrointestinal blood with fecal occult blood tests. Am J Gastroenterol 94:344, 1999.
223. Dybdahl JH, Daae LN, Larsen S, Myren J: Occult faecal blood loss determined by a 51Cr method and chemical tests in patients referred for colonoscopy. Scand J Gastroenterol 19:245, 1984.
224. Herzog P, Holtermuller KH, Preiss J, et al: Fecal blood loss in patients with colonic polyps: A comparison of measurements with ^{51}chromium-labeled erythrocytes and with the Haemoccult test. Gastroenterology 83:957, 1982.
225. Stroehlein JR, Fairbanks VF, McGill DB, Go VL: Hemoccult detection of fecal occult blood quantitated by radioassay. Am J Dig Dis 21:841, 1976.
226. Ahlquist DA: Occult blood screening. Obstacles to effectiveness. Cancer 70:1259, 1992.
227. Lang CA, Ransohoff DF: Fecal occult blood screening for colorectal cancer. Is mortality reduced by chance selection for screening colonoscopy? JAMA 271:1011, 1994.
228. Laine LA, Bentley E, Chandrasoma P: Effect of oral iron therapy on the upper gastrointestinal tract. A prospective evaluation. Dig Dis Sci 33:172, 1988.
229. Saito H: Screening for colorectal cancer by immunochemical fecal occult blood testing. Jpn J Cancer Res 87:1011, 1996.
230. Rex DK, Rahmani EY, Haseman JH, et al: Relative sensitivity of colonoscopy and barium enema for detection of colorectal cancer in clinical practice. Gastroenterology 112:17, 1997.
231. Ferrucci JT: Colonoscopy and barium enema: Radiologist's response. Gastroenterology 112:294, 1997.
232. Waye JD: What is a gold standard for colon polyps? Gastroenterology 112:292, 1997.
233. Kewenter J, Brevinge H, Engaras B, Haglind E: The yield of flexible sigmoidoscopy and double-contrast barium enema in the diagnosis of neoplasms in the large bowel in patients with a positive Hemoccult test. Endoscopy 27:159, 1995.
234. Ott DJ, Scharling ES, Chen YM, et al: Barium enema examination: Sensitivity in detecting colonic polyps and carcinomas. South Med J 82:197, 1989.
235. Winawer SJ, Stewart ET, Zauber AG, et al: A comparison of colonoscopy and double-contrast barium enema for surveillance after polypectomy. National Polyp Study Work Group. N Engl J Med 342:1766, 2000.
236. Haseman JH, Lemmel GT, Rahmani EY, Rex DK: Failure of colonoscopy to detect colorectal cancer: Evaluation of 47 cases in 20 hospitals [see comments]. Gastrointest Endosc 45:451, 1997.
237. Rex DK, Cutler CS, Lemmel GT, et al: Colonoscopic miss rates of adenomas determined by back-to-back colonoscopies. Gastroenterology 112:24, 1997.
238. Kim LS, Koch J, Yee J, et al: Comparison of patients' experiences during imaging tests of the colon. Gastrointest Endosc 54:67–74, 2001.
239. Hara AK, Johnson CD, Reed JE, et al: Detection of colorectal polyps by computed tomographic colography: Feasibility of a novel technique. Gastroenterology 110:284, 1996.
240. Johnson CD, Hara AK, Reed JE: Computed tomographic colonography (virtual colonoscopy): A new method for detecting colorectal neoplasms. Endoscopy 29:454, 1997.
241. Fenlon HM, Nunes DP, Schroy PC, et al: A comparison of virtual and conventional colonoscopy for the detection of colorectal polyps. N Engl J Med 341:1496, 1999.
242. Hsia PC, al-Kawas FH: Yield of upper endoscopy in the evaluation of asymptomatic patients with Hemoccult-positive stool after a negative colonoscopy. Am J Gastroenterol 87:1571, 1992.
243. Zuckerman G, Benitez J: A prospective study of bidirectional endoscopy (colonoscopy and upper endoscopy) in the evaluation of patients with occult gastrointestinal bleeding. Am J Gastroenterol 87:62, 1992.
244. Chen YK, Gladden DR, Kestenbaum DJ, Collen MJ: Is there a role for upper gastrointestinal endoscopy in the evaluation of patients with occult blood-positive stool and negative colonoscopy? Am J Gastroenterol 88:2026, 1993.
245. Geller AJ, Kolts BE, Achem SR, Wears R: The high frequency of upper gastrointestinal pathology in patients with fecal occult blood and colon polyps. Am J Gastroenterol 88:1184, 1993.
246. Rockey DC, Koch J, Cello JP, et al: Relative frequency of upper gastrointestinal and colonic lesions in patients with positive fecal occult-blood tests. N Engl J Med 339:153, 1998.
247. Bini EJ, Rajapaksa RC, Valdes MT, Weinshel EH: Is upper gastrointestinal endoscopy indicated in asymptomatic patients with a positive fecal occult blood test and negative colonoscopy? Am J Med 106:613, 1999.
248. Dybdahl JH: Occult faecal blood loss determined by a ^{51}Cr method and chemical tests in patients referred for upper gastrointestinal endoscopy. Scand J Gastroenterol 19:235, 1984.
249. Eisner MS, Lewis JH: Diagnostic yield of a positive fecal occult blood test found on digital rectal examination. Does the finger count [see comments]? Arch Intern Med 151:2180, 1991.
250. Bini EJ, Rajapaksa RC, Weinshel EH: The findings and impact of nonrehydrated guaiac examination of the rectum (FINGER) study: A comparison of 2 methods of screening for colorectal cancer in asymptomatic average-risk patients. Arch Intern Med 159:2022, 1999.
251. Blackshear JL, Baker VS, Holland A, et al: Fecal hemoglobin excre-

tion in elderly patients with atrial fibrillation: Combined aspirin and low-dose warfarin vs. conventional warfarin therapy. Arch Intern Med 156:658, 1996.
252. Greenberg PD, Cello JP, Rockey DC: Asymptomatic chronic gastrointestinal blood loss in patients taking aspirin or warfarin for cardiovascular disease. Am J Med 100:598, 1996.
253. Jaffin BW, Bliss CM, LaMont JT: Significance of occult gastrointestinal bleeding during anticoagulation therapy. Am J Med 83:269, 1987.
254. Looker AC, Dallman PR, Carroll MD, et al: Prevalence of iron deficiency in the United States. JAMA 277:973, 1997.
255. Hallberg L, Hulthen L, Bengtsson C, et al: Iron balance in menstruating women. Eur J Clin Nutr 49:200, 1995.
256. Massey AC: Microcytic anemia. Differential diagnosis and management of iron deficiency anemia. Med Clin North Am 76:549, 1992.
257. Lee JG, Sahagun G, Oehlke M, Lieberman DA: Serious gastrointestinal pathology found in patients with serum ferritin values <50 ng/ml. Am J Gastroenterol 93:772, 1998.
258. Wilcox CM, Alexander LN, Clark WS: Prospective evaluation of the gastrointestinal tract in patients with iron deficiency and no systemic or gastrointestinal symptoms or signs. Am J Med 103:405, 1997.
259. Cook IJ, Pavli P, Riley JW, et al: Gastrointestinal investigation of iron deficiency anemia. Br Med J 292:1380, 1986.
260. Kepczyk T, Kadakia SC: Prospective evaluation of gastrointestinal tract in patients with iron-deficiency anemia. Dig Dis Sci 40:1283, 1995.
261. McIntyre AS, Long RG: Prospective survey of investigations in outpatients referred with iron deficiency anaemia. Gut 34:1102, 1993.
262. Rockey DC, Cello JP: Evaluation of the gastrointestinal tract in patients with iron-deficiency anemia. N Engl J Med 329:1691, 1993.
263. Yip R, Limburg PJ, Ahlquist DA, et al: Pervasive occult gastrointestinal bleeding in an Alaska native population with prevalent iron deficiency. Role of *Helicobacter pylori* gastritis. JAMA 277:1135, 1997.
264. Dickey W, Kenny BD, McMillan SA, et al: Gastric as well as duodenal biopsies may be useful in the investigation of iron deficiency anaemia. Scand J Gastroenterol 32:469, 1997.
265. Ferguson A, Brydon WG, Brian H, et al: Use of whole gut perfusion to investigate gastrointestinal blood loss in patients with iron deficiency anaemia. Gut 38:120, 1996.
266. Bini EJ, Micale PL, Weinshel EH: Evaluation of the gastrointestinal tract in premenopausal women with iron deficiency anemia [see comments]. Am J Med 105:281, 1998.
267. Ott DJ, Gelfand DW: The future of barium radiology. Br J Radiol 70:S171, 1997.
268. Fine KD: The prevalence of occult gastrointestinal bleeding in celiac sprue [see comments]. N Engl J Med 334:1163, 1996.
269. Gostout CJ: Enteroscopy for unexplained iron-deficiency anemia: Identifying the patient with sprue. Gastrointest Endosc 39:76, 1993.
270. Landi B, Tkoub M, Gaudric M, Guimbaud R: Diagnostic yield of push-type enteroscopy in relation to indication. Gut 42:421, 1998.
271. Chak A, Cooper GS, Canto MI, et al: Enteroscopy for the initial evaluation of iron deficiency. Gastrointest Endosc 47:144, 1998.
272. Gordon S, Bensen S, Smith R: Long-term follow-up of older patients with iron deficiency anemia after a negative GI evaluation. Am J Gastroenterol 91:885, 1996.
273. Mujica VR, Barkin JS: Occult gastrointestinal bleeding. General overview and approach. Gastrointest Endosc Clin North Am 6:833, 1996.
274. Chak A, Koehler MK, Sundaram SN, et al: Diagnostic and therapeutic impact of push enteroscopy: Analysis of factors associated with positive findings. Gastrointest Endosc 47:18, 1998.
275. Zaman A, Katon RM: Push enteroscopy for obscure gastrointestinal bleeding yields a high incidence of proximal lesions within reach of a standard endoscope. Gastrointest Endosc 47:372, 1998.
276. O'Mahony S, Morris AJ, Straiton M, et al: Push enteroscopy in the investigation of small-intestinal disease. Q J Med 89:685, 1996.
277. Waye JD: Enteroscopy. Gastrointest Endosc 46:247, 1997.
278. Rollins ES, Picus D, Hicks ME, et al: Angiography is useful in detecting the source of chronic gastrointestinal bleeding of obscure origin. AJR Am J Roentgenol 156:385, 1991.
279. Lewis BS, Kornbluth A, Waye JD: Small bowel tumours: Yield of enteroscopy. Gut 32:763, 1991.
280. Rex DK, Lappas JC, Maglinte DD, et al: Enteroclysis in the evaluation of suspected small intestinal bleeding. Gastroenterology 97:58, 1989.
281. Barkin JS, Lewis BS, Reiner DK, et al: Diagnostic and therapeutic jejunoscopy with a new, longer enteroscope. Gastrointest Endosc 38:55, 1992.
282. Berner JS, Mauer K, Lewis BS: Push and sonde enteroscopy for the diagnosis of obscure gastrointestinal bleeding. Am J Gastroenterol 89:2139, 1994.
283. Gostout CJ, Schroeder KW, Burton DD: Small bowel enteroscopy: An early experience in gastrointestinal bleeding of unknown origin. Gastrointest Endosc 37:5, 1991.
284. Gostout CJ: Improving the withdrawal phase of Sonde enteroscopy with the "push-away" method. Gastrointest Endosc 39:69, 1993.
285. Lau WY, Yuen WK, Chu KW, et al: Obscure bleeding in the gastrointestinal tract originating in the small intestine. Surg Gynecol Obstet 174:119, 1992.
286. Ress AM, Benacci JC, Sarr MG: Efficacy of intraoperative enteroscopy in diagnosis and prevention of recurrent, occult gastrointestinal bleeding. Am J Surg 163:94, 1992.
287. Szold A, Katz LB, Lewis BS: Surgical approach to occult gastrointestinal bleeding. Am J Surg 163:90, 1992.
288. Appleyard M, Fireman Z, Glukhovsky A, et al: A randomized trial comparing wireless capsule endoscopy with push enteroscopy for the detection of small-bowel lesions. Gastroenterology 119:1431, 2000.
289. Iddan G, Meron G, Glukhovsky A, Swain P: Wireless capsule endoscopy. Nature 405:417, 2000.
290. Malden ES, Hicks ME, Royal HD, et al: Recurrent gastrointestinal bleeding: Use of thrombolysis with anticoagulation in diagnosis. Radiology 207:147, 1998.
291. Bloomfeld RS, Smith TP, Schneider AM, Rockey DC: Provocative angiography in patients with gastrointestinal hemorrhage of obscure origin. Am J Gastroenterol 95:2807, 2000.
292. Shetzline MA, Suhocki P, Dash R, Rockey DC: Provocative angiography in obscure gastrointestinal bleeding. South Med J 93:1205, 2000.
293. Descamps C, Schmit A, Van Gossum A: "Missed" upper gastrointestinal tract lesions may explain "occult" bleeding. Endoscopy 31:452, 1999.
294. Blanchard DK, Budde JM, Hatch GF, et al: Tumors of the small intestine. World J Surg 24:421, 2000.
295. Ciresi DL, Scholten DJ: The continuing clinical dilemma of primary tumors of the small intestine. Am Surg 61:698, 1995. Discussion 702.
296. Lewis MP, Khoo DE, Spencer J: Value of laparotomy in the diagnosis of obscure gastrointestinal haemorrhage. Gut 37:187, 1995.
297. Bastounis E, Papalambros E, Mermingas V, et al: Secondary aortoduodenal fistulae. J Cardiovasc Surg (Torino) 38:457, 1997.
298. Bergqvist D, Bjorkman H, Bolin T, et al: Secondary aortoenteric fistulae—changes from 1973 to 1993. Eur J Vasc Endovasc Surg 11:425, 1996.
299. Korkut AK, Arpinar E, Yasar T, Guney D: Primary aortoduodenal fistula complicated by abdominal aortic aneurysm. J Cardiovasc Surg (Torino) 41:113, 2000.
300. Yoshida J, Donahue PE, Nyhus LM: Hemobilia: Review of recent experience with a worldwide problem. Am J Gastroenterol 82:448, 1987.
301. Merrell SW, Schneider PD: Hemobilia—evolution of current diagnosis and treatment. West J Med 155:621, 1991.
302. Risti B, Marincek B, Jost R, et al: Hemosuccus pancreaticus as a source of obscure upper gastrointestinal bleeding: Three cases and literature review. Am J Gastroenterol 90:1878, 1995.
303. Suter M, Doenz F, Chapuis G, et al: Haemorrhage into the pancreatic duct (hemosuccus pancreaticus): Recognition and management. Eur J Surg 161:887, 1995.
304. van Cutsem E, Rutgeerts P, Vantrappen G: Treatment of bleeding gastrointestinal vascular malformations with oestrogen-progesterone. Lancet 335:953, 1990.
305. Barkin JS, Ross BS: Medical therapy for chronic gastrointestinal bleeding of obscure origin. Am J Gastroenterol 93:1250, 1998.
306. Lewis BS, Salomon P, Rivera-MacMurray S, et al: Does hormonal therapy have any benefit for bleeding angiodysplasia? J Clin Gastroenterol 15:99, 1992.
307. Rossini FP, Arrigoni A, Pennazio M: Octreotide in the treatment of bleeding due to angiodysplasia of the small intestine. Am J Gastroenterol 88:1424, 1993.
308. Nardone G, Rocco A, Balzano T, Budillon G: The efficacy of octreotide therapy in chronic bleeding due to vascular abnormalities of the gastrointestinal tract. Aliment Pharmacol Ther 13:1429, 1999.
309. Morris AJ, Mokhashi M, Straiton M, et al: Push enteroscopy and heater probe therapy for small bowel bleeding. Gastrointest Endosc 44:394, 1996.
310. Askin MP, Lewis BS: Push enteroscopic cauterization: Long-term follow-up of 83 patients with bleeding small intestinal angiodysplasia. Gastrointest Endosc 43:580, 1996.

Chapter 14

JAUNDICE

Steven D. Lidofsky

Jaundice (icterus), the most visible manifestation of liver and biliary tract disease, is a condition characterized by yellow discoloration of the skin, sclerae, and mucous membranes as a result of an elevated bilirubin concentration. Jaundice has many causes. Indeed, the optimal approach to the management of the jaundiced patient has challenged physicians for centuries.

Attempts to classify icteric syndromes appeared as early as the treatises of Hippocrates. By the time of Osler, distinctions were already made between biliary tract obstruction and nonobstructive causes of jaundice. Over the past four decades, elucidation of the mechanisms underlying bilirubin metabolism as well the development of more sophisticated biochemical and imaging techniques have made it possible to pinpoint the cause of jaundice in most patients. Powerful techniques, however, employed in an indiscriminate manner, potentially expose the patient to unnecessary risks, discomfort, and cost. Thus, an effective approach to the jaundiced patient requires selection of diagnostic and therapeutic modalities based on a careful clinical assessment of the likely underlying diseases.

This chapter covers four major areas. First, an outline of bilirubin metabolism is presented. Second, a framework for establishing a differential diagnosis is developed based on a knowledge of bilirubin metabolism as well as clues obtained from the history, physical examination, and routine biochemical tests. Third, a summary is presented of the usefulness of selected imaging studies once the differential diagnosis has been sufficiently narrowed. Fourth, a brief discussion of therapeutic options is offered.

DETERMINANTS OF SERUM BILIRUBIN CONCENTRATION

Bilirubin Metabolism

Bilirubin is a tetrapyrrole that is an end-product of heme degradation. Bilirubin metabolism has been reviewed in depth elsewhere[1] and is briefly summarized in Figure 14–1. In healthy adults, daily bilirubin production averages approximately 4 mg/kg (i.e., nearly 0.5 mmol in a 70-kg individual). Most (70% to 80%) bilirubin is derived from hemoglobin degradation from senescent erythrocytes, and a minor component arises from premature destruction of newly formed erythrocytes in the bone marrow or circulation (i.e., *ineffective erythropoiesis*). Most of the remaining 20% to 30% is formed from breakdown of nonhemoglobin hemoproteins in the liver, such as catalase and cytochrome oxidases. Although hemoproteins are also present in extrahepatic tissues, their mass is so low or their turnover rate so slow (e.g., myoglobin) that their overall contribution to bilirubin production is minimal.

The degradation of heme to bilirubin is a two-step process. First, heme is converted to *biliverdin* by the microsomal enzyme *heme oxygenase*. Second, biliverdin is rapidly converted to bilirubin by the cytosolic enzyme *biliverdin reductase*. Catabolism of erythrocyte-derived hemoglobin to bilirubin primarily takes place in macrophages in the spleen, liver, and bone marrow. By contrast, free hemoglobin, haptoglobin-bound hemoglobin, and methemalbumin are catabolized to bilirubin predominantly in hepatocytes.

Bilirubin is a hydrophobic and potentially toxic compound that circulates in plasma tightly bound to *albumin*. Elimination of bilirubin requires conversion to water-soluble conjugates by the liver and secretion into bile. Bilirubin metabolism and elimination is a multistep process for which several inherited disorders have been identified (see later).

First, bilirubin is taken up across the sinusoidal (basolateral) membrane of hepatocytes by a carrier-mediated mechanism. Bilirubin uptake is competitively inhibited by certain organic anions such as sulfobromophthalein (BSP) and indocyanine green. A candidate transport protein (organic anion transporting polypeptide-2; OATP-2) for bilirubin has been tentatively identified.[2] Second, after uptake, bilirubin is directed by cytosolic binding proteins (e.g., *ligandins, fatty acid–binding protein*) to the endoplasmic reticulum, where it is conjugated with *uridine diphosphate (UDP)-glucuronic acid* by the enzyme *bilirubin UDP-glucuronyl transferase*. Conjugation serves to convert hydrophobic bilirubin into a water-soluble form that can be readily excreted into bile. Third, conjugated bilirubin is directed toward the canalicular (apical) membrane, where it is transported into the bile canaliculus by an adenosine triphosphate (ATP)-dependent export pump. The responsible protein, multidrug resistance associated protein, or MRP2, is a member of the *ATP-binding cassette protein su-*

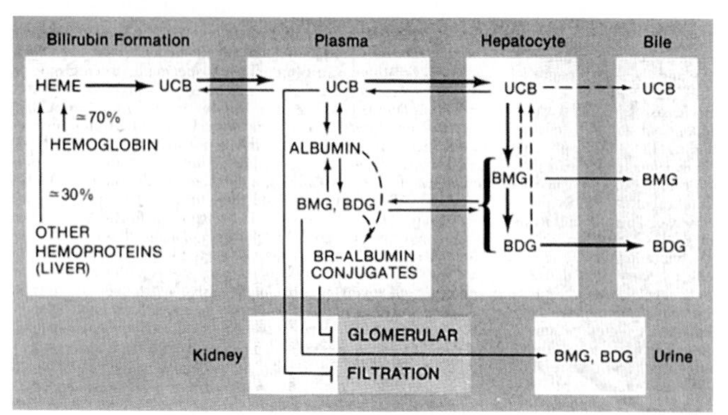

Figure 14–1. Overview of normal bilirubin metabolism and transport. Heme from hemoglobin and other hemoproteins is converted to biliverdin and then to bilirubin in extrahepatic tissue, predominantly the reticuloendothelial cells of the spleen and bone marrow. The unconjugated bilirubin (UCB) released into the plasma, which normally is tightly but reversibly bound to albumin, is taken up by hepatocytes and converted efficiently to bilirubin monoglucuronide (BMG) and bilirubin diglucuronide (BDG). Both BMG and BDG can be transported into plasma and normally account for less than 5% of total serum bilirubin. BMG in the liver is largely converted to BDG, which is then excreted in bile. Trace amounts of conjugated bilirubin are also deconjugated back to UCB. BMG and BDG in plasma also bind reversibly to albumin but less tightly than UCB. When present in abnormally high concentrations for a long time, BMG or BDG or both bind irreversibly with albumin to form BR-albumin conjugates. While UCB, BMG, BDG, and BR-albumin conjugates all enter the kidney via the bloodstream, only BMG and BDG appear in urine, presumably because they are most loosely bound to albumin and therefore most able to be filtered at the glomerulus. (From Scharschmidt, BF: Bilirubin metabolism and hyperbilirubinemia. In Wyngaarden JB, Smith LH, Jr, and Bennett JC [eds]: Cecil Textbook of Medicine, 19th ed. Philadelphia, WB Saunders, 1992, p 756.)

perfamily,[3] and it appears to function as a multispecific transporter of a variety of organic anions (including BSP but not hydrophilic bile acids).

Approximately 80% of bilirubin in human bile is in the form of diglucuronides. Almost all the rest is in the form of monoglucuronides, and only trace amounts are unconjugated. Resorption of conjugated bilirubin by the gallbladder and intestine is negligible. However, bilirubin is deconjugated by bacterial enzymes in the terminal ileum and colon and converted to colorless tetrapyrroles called *urobilinogens*. Up to 20% of urobilinogens are resorbed and ultimately excreted in bile and urine.

Measurement of Serum Bilirubin

The normal bilirubin concentration in the serum of adults is less than 1 to 1.5 mg/dL.[1] Less than 5% of circulating bilirubin is present in conjugated form. In general, jaundice is not evident until serum bilirubin concentration exceeds 3 mg/dL. Serum bilirubin is conventionally detected by the *diazo reaction* (van den Bergh reaction). With this method, bilirubin is cleaved by compounds such as diazotized sulfanilic acid to form a colored azo-dipyrole that can be assayed by spectrophotometry. Conjugated bilirubin reacts rapidly ("directly") with diazo reagents. However, unconjugated bilirubin reacts quite slowly with diazo reagents, because the site of chemical cleavage is rendered inaccessible by internal hydrogen bonding. Thus, reliable measurement of total bilirubin concentration requires the addition of an "accelerator" compound, such as ethanol or urea, which disrupts such hydrogen bonding and facilitates the reaction of unconjugated bilirubin with the diazo reagent. The concentration of the indirect bilirubin fraction is calculated by subtracting the direct bilirubin concentration (i.e., accelerator compound absent) from that of the total concentration (i.e., accelerator compound present).

Although the direct bilirubin concentration is affected by changes in conjugated bilirubin levels, the two are not equivalent. Similarly, indirect bilirubin is not equivalent to unconjugated bilirubin. In particular, reliance on direct and indirect bilirubin measurements can lead to errors in the diagnosis of isolated disorders of bilirubin metabolism (e.g., suspected Gilbert's syndrome; see later). A number of clinical laboratories have abandoned measurements of direct and indirect bilirubin and are instead using automated spectrophotometric assays that provide estimates of conjugated and unconjugated bilirubin. Although these refined assays have limitations, they are clinically useful in the management of *physiologic jaundice of the newborn* (see later), where the potential for neurotoxicity due to the passage of unconjugated bilirubin across the blood-brain barrier (kernicterus) is a clinically relevant issue. On the other hand, if an isolated disorder of bilirubin metabolism is suspected, the diagnosis may require more sophisticated chromatographic techniques that measure the concentrations of unconjugated, monoglucuronidated, and diglucuronidated bilirubin as well as conjugated bilirubin-albumin complexes.[4] However, these techniques are not widely employed. Moreover, even with such accurate techniques, measurement of conjugated and unconjugated bilirubin does not distinguish between liver disease and biliary obstruction. Thus, in most cases, these tests are of limited utility.

DIFFERENTIAL DIAGNOSIS OF JAUNDICE

Jaundice can result from either an increase in bilirubin formation or a decrease in hepatic clearance. From a practical standpoint, it is reasonable to classify conditions that produce jaundice under the broad categories of *isolated disorders of bilirubin metabolism*, *liver disease*, or *obstruction of the bile ducts* (Table 14–1).

Isolated Disorders of Bilirubin Metabolism

Unconjugated Hyperbilirubinemia

OVERVIEW. Three basic mechanisms can lead to isolated unconjugated hyperbilirubinemia: increased bilirubin production, decreased hepatocellular uptake of unconjugated bilirubin, or decreased bilirubin conjugation. In each of the following conditions, liver function is otherwise normal. In these syndromes, standard biochemical liver tests other than serum bilirubin are normal.

INCREASED BILIRUBIN PRODUCTION. Several processes can lead to excessive bilirubin production. These include hemolysis, ineffective erythropoiesis, or resorption of a hematoma.[1] Thus, jaundice may complicate the clinical course of patients with *hemolytic anemias*, either hereditary or acquired, *megaloblastic anemia* from either folate or vitamin

Table 14–1 | **Differential Diagnosis of Jaundice**

I. Isolated Disorders of Bilirubin Metabolism
- A. Unconjugated hyperbilirubinemia
  1. Increased bilirubin production
     Examples: hemolysis, ineffective erythropoiesis, blood transfusion, resorption of hematomas
  2. Decreased hepatocellular uptake
     Examples: drugs (e.g., rifampin), Gilbert's syndrome (?)
  3. Decreased conjugation
     Examples: Gilbert's syndrome, Crigler-Najjar syndrome, physiologic jaundice of the newborn
- B. Conjugated or mixed hyperbilirubinemia
  1. Dubin-Johnson syndrome
  2. Rotor's syndrome

II. Liver Disease
- A. Acute or chronic hepatocellular dysfunction
  1. Acute or subacute hepatocellular injury
     Examples: viral hepatitis, hepatotoxins (e.g., ethanol, acetaminophen, *Amanita*), drugs (e.g., isoniazid, phenytoin), ischemia (e.g., hypotension, vascular occulsion), metabolic disorders (e.g., Wilson disease, Reye's syndrome), pregnancy-related (e.g., acute fatty liver of pregnancy, preeclampsia)
  2. Chronic hepatocellular disease
     Examples: viral hepatitis, hepatotoxins (e.g., ethanol, vinylchloride, vitamin A), autoimmune hepatitis, metabolic (hemochromatosis, Wilson disease, nonalcoholic steatohepatitis, α_1-antitrypsin deficiency)
- B. Hepatic disorders with prominent cholestasis
  1. Diffuse infiltrative disorders
     Examples: granulomatous diseases (e.g., mycobacterial infections, sarcoidosis, lymphoma, drugs, Wegener's granulomatosis), amyloidosis, malignancy
  2. Inflammation of intrahepatic bile ductules and/or portal tracts
     Examples: primary biliary cirrhosis, graft-versus-host disease, drugs (e.g., chlorpromazine, erythromycin)
  3. Miscellaneous conditions
     Examples: benign recurrent intrahepatic cholestasis, drugs, estrogens, steroids, total parenteral nutrition, bacterial infections, paraneoplastic syndromes, uncommon presentations of viral or alcoholic hepatitis, intrahepatic cholestasis of pregnancy, postoperative cholestasis

III. Obstruction of the Bile Ducts
- A. Choledocholithiasis
  1. Cholesterol gallstones
  2. Pigment gallstones
- B. Diseases of the bile ducts
  1. Inflammation/infection
     Examples: primary sclerosing cholangitis, AIDS cholangiopathy, hepatic arterial chemotherapy, postsurgical strictures
  2. Neoplasms
- C. Extrinsic compression of the biliary tree
  1. Neoplasms
     Examples: pancreatic carcinoma, metastatic lymphadenopathy, hepatoma
  2. Pancreatitis
  3. Vascular enlargement (e.g., aneurysm, portal cavernoma)

AIDS, acquired immunodeficiency syndrome.

B_{12} deficiency, *iron deficiency anemia*, *sideroblastic anemia*, and *polycythemia vera*. With these disorders, bilirubin concentration does not generally exceed 4 to 5 mg/dL. Jaundice may follow *massive transfusion*, because the foreshortened lifespan of transfused erythrocytes leads to excessive bilirubin production. Patients who have suffered *major trauma* may also develop hyperbilirubinemia as a result of resorption of hematomas as well as from blood transfusions.[5] Each of these disorders involves excessive delivery of unconjugated bilirubin to the liver without intrinsic hepatic dysfunction. Consequently, other biochemical markers of liver function, including the activities in serum of alkaline phosphatase and aminotransferases, are normal.

DECREASED BILIRUBIN UPTAKE. A decrease in hepatocellular uptake of bilirubin can be seen with certain drugs. For example, the antituberculous agent *rifampin* has been shown to competitively inhibit bilirubin uptake by hepatocytes and may produce jaundice by this mechanism.[6] Decreased bilirubin uptake may also contribute to the pathogenesis of the hereditary disorder *Gilbert's syndrome*, in which the predominant abnormality is an impairment of bilirubin conjugation due to reduced bilirubin UDP-glucuronyl transferase (bilirubin UGT-1) activity.[1]

DECREASED BILIRUBIN CONJUGATION. Three familial disorders of unconjugated hyerbilirubinemia are attributable to diminished bilirubin conjugation (Table 14–2). *Gilbert's syndrome* is the most common of these, occurring in up to 10% of white populations. It is entirely benign and rarely produces clinical jaundice. Serum bilirubin may rise twofold to threefold with fasting or dehydration but is generally below 4 mg/dL. Patients with Gilbert's syndrome commonly present during or after adolescence, when isolated hyperbilirubinemia is detected as an incidental finding on routine multiphasic biochemical screening. Although the pathogenesis of Gilbert's syndrome is not entirely certain, the genetic basis has been linked to a reduction in bilirubin *UGT-1* gene (*HUG-Br1*) transcription resulting from a mutation in the promoter region (see Chapter 65).[7]

Mutations in the coding region of *HUG-Br1* appear to be responsible for *Crigler-Najjar syndrome*.[8] In type I Crigler-Najjar syndrome, bilirubin UGT-1 activity is absent, and many patients die of kernicterus in the neonatal period (see Table 14–2). Phototherapy (see later) is required to prevent this complication, but liver transplantation can be lifesaving. Patients with type II Crigler-Najjar syndrome have markedly reduced bilirubin UGT-1 activity, with serum bilirubin levels between those of Gilbert's syndrome and those of type I Crigler-Najjar syndrome (see Table 14–2). In contrast with type I Crigler-Najjar patients, patients with type II Crigler-Najjar syndrome are not ill during the neonatal period and may not be diagnosed until early childhood. Although the degree of jaundice can wax and wane, most patients with type II Crigler-Najjar syndrome experience a fall in serum bilirubin concentration to levels of 2 to 5 mg/dL with phenobarbital, which increases UGT-1 activity. Thus, such patients have normal life expectancies and do not manifest neurologic impairment (see Chapter 65).

A related disorder of bilirubin metabolism is *physiologic jaundice of the newborn*. This syndrome, which is thought to result from delayed developmental expression of bilirubin UGT-1, produces transient jaundice that generally rapidly resolves in the neonatal period. A brief course of phototherapy may be required to prevent kernicterus.

Conjugated or Mixed Hyperbilirubinemia

A selective decrease in bilirubin secretion into the bile canaliculus may produce conjugated or mixed hyperbilirubinemia. Such a defect underlies two inherited disorders: *Dubin-Johnson syndrome*, in which there is also impairment of

Table 14–2 | **Hereditary Disorders of Hepatic Bilirubin Metabolism and Transport**

	GILBERT'S SYNDROME	TYPE I CRIGLER-NAJJAR SYNDROME	TYPE II CRIGLER-NAJJAR SYNDROME	DUBIN-JOHNSON SYNDROME	ROTOR'S SYNDROME
Incidence	≤7% of population	Very rare	Uncommon	Uncommon	Rare
Inheritance	Autosomal dominant	Autosomal recessive	Autosomal dominant	Autosomal recessive	Autosomal recessive
Defect(s) in bilirubin metabolism	↓ UDP-glucuronyl transferase activity, (?) ↓ hepatic uptake	Absent UDP-glucuronyl transferase activity	↓↓ or undetectable UDP-glucuronyl transferase activity	Impaired excretion of conjugated bilirubin	Impaired excretion or storage of conjugated bilirubin
Plasma bilirubin concentration (mg/dL)	≤3 in absence of fasting or hemolysis, essentially all unconjugated	Usually > 20 (range, 17–50) all unconjugated	Usually < 20 (range, 6–45), essentially all unconjugated	Usually < 7 (range, 1–25), about half conjugated	Usually < 7, about half conjugated
Plasma sulfobromophthalein disappearance	Usually normal (<5%), mild 45-min (< 15%) retention in some patients	Normal	Normal	Slow initial disappearance (retention < 20% at 45 min) with frequent secondary rise at 1.5–2 hr	Very slow disappearance (30–50% 45-min retention) without secondary rise
Oral cholecystography	Normal	Normal	Normal	Faint or nonvisualization	Usually normal visualization
Hepatic histology	Normal, occasionally ↑ lipofuscin	Normal	Normal	Coarse pigment in centrolobular hepatocytes	Normal
Other distinguishing features	↓ Bilirubin concentration with phenobarbital	No response to phenobarbital	↓ Bilirubin concentration with phenobarbital	↑ Bilirubin concentration with estrogens, characteristic urinary coproporphyrin pattern	Sulfobromophthalein disappearance, urinary coproporphyrin pattern
Prognosis	Normal	Usually death in infancy from kernicterus	Usually normal	Normal	Normal
Treatment	None necessary	Liver transplantation; other measures not uniformly effective	Phenobarbital if bilirubin concentration markedly elevated	No specific therapy; avoid estrogens	None available

UDP, uridine diphosphate.
Adapted from Scharschmidt BF, Gollan JL: Current concepts of bilirubin metabolism and hereditary hyperbilirubinemia. In Popper H, Schaffer F (eds): Progress in Liver Diseases, vol 6. New York, Grune & Stratton, 1979, p 187.

canalicular secretion of certain organic anions such as BSP, and *Rotor's syndrome*. Each of these syndromes is associated with a benign clinical course. In Dubin-Johnson syndrome, the molecular defect has been linked to an absence of expression of the canalicular membrane multispecific organic anion transporter MRP2.[9] It has been postulated that Rotor's syndrome results from impaired vesicular targeting of MRP2 to the canalicular membrane, but the molecular basis of this disorder is currently unknown. In each of these syndromes, hepatic function is preserved. Serum bilirubin concentration is elevated, but other standard biochemical liver tests are normal.

Dubin-Johnson and Rotor's syndrome can be distinguished biochemically and histologically (see Table 14–2). In Dubin-Johnson syndrome, the liver contains a characteristic black pigment that is not seen in Rotor's syndrome. This pigment is thought to result from lysosomal deposition in hepatocytes of aromatic amino acid metabolites that are putative substrates for MRP2. However, liver biopsy is generally unnecessary in the diagnostic evaluation of patients suspected to have Dubin-Johnson or Rotor's syndrome, because neither is associated with an adverse clinical outcome.

Liver Disease

Jaundice is a common feature of *generalized hepatic dysfunction*. In contrast with isolated disorders of bilirubin metabolism, icteric liver disease is characterized by an increase in serum bilirubin concentration in association with abnormalities in other standard biochemical liver tests. The extensive differential diagnosis of icteric liver disease is briefly outlined here. In the subsequent discussion, disorders in which hyperbilirubinemia and jaundice are simply manifestations of global hepatocellular dysfunction are distinguished from those that have cholestasis as a major or predominant manifestation. The latter are often difficult to distinguish clinically from obstruction of the bile ducts.

Acute Hepatocellular Dysfunction

Generalized impairment of hepatocellular function can result from acute liver injury or chronic disease. A variety of disorders can produce acute or subacute hepatocellular injury, including viral hepatitis, exposure to hepatotoxins, hepatic ischemia, and certain metabolic derangements. *Acute viral hepatitis* is often heralded by anorexia, malaise, myalgias, or pain in the epigastrium or right upper abdominal quadrant before jaundice develops (see Chapter 68). Five major hepatitis viruses have been isolated. Hepatitis A and E viruses are transmitted enterally. Each typically produces a self-limited illness that does not progress to chronic liver disease.[10, 11] By contrast, hepatitis B, C, and D viruses are transmitted parenterally, and illness produced by these agents may be prolonged and may lead to chronic disease.[12–14] Major risk factors for hepatitis B, C, and D include intravenous drug use, exposure to blood products, and unprotected sexual intercourse. The diagnosis of each these disorders is aided by serologic testing (see later).

A number of toxins produce dose-dependent hepatocellular injury (see Chapter 73). Ingestion of significant quantities of *acetaminophen* or the mushroom *Amanita phalloides* may lead to hepatocellular necrosis and jaundice within several days after exposure.[15, 16] Toxic liver injury can have a fulminant course associated with a high mortality (see Chapter 80). Surviving patients without preexisting liver disease generally have resolution of jaundice and complete recovery of hepatic function. A variety of *drugs* can produce idiosyncratic hepatocellular injury and jaundice. Prominent agents include isoniazid, phenytoin, and propylthiouracil.[17] *Alcoholic hepatitis* should be a diagnostic consideration in the jaundiced patient with ethanol dependency, particularly when hepatomegaly and fever are present (see Chapter 71). Laboratory studies may help distinguish this entity from most acute liver diseases[18] (see later). Alcoholic hepatitis may also have an atypical cholestatic presentation that can create diagnostic confusion (see later).

Jaundice related to *hepatic ischemia* may result from hypotension, hypoxia, hyperthermia, congestive heart failure, or occlusive vascular disease (see Chapter 70). *Thrombosis of the hepatic vein* (Budd-Chiari syndrome) or *hepatic veno-occlusive disease* should be suspected in a patient who presents with rapid onset of ascites and hepatomegaly; the latter syndrome is more commonly associated with jaundice and is a complication of certain cytotoxic agents, particularly in the setting of bone marrow transplantation.[19, 20]

The inherited disorder of hepatobiliary copper secretion, *Wilson disease*, may present de novo with clinical features indistinguishable from those of acute viral hepatitis (see Chapter 67). The disease should be a diagnostic consideration in patients younger than 40 years of age, particularly when Kayser-Fleischer rings are seen on ophthalmologic examination. Coombs-negative hemolytic anemia is a part of the spectrum of Wilson disease and contributes to the disproportionate hyperbilirubinemia often present in these patients. When the clinical presentation is *fulminant*, the diagnosis of Wilson disease is suggested by a serum alkaline phosphatase/bilirubin ratio of less than 2 or a ratio of the serum aspartate aminotransferase (AST) to alanine aminotransferase (ALT) of greater than 4, particularly when the serum aminotransferase activities are less than 10-fold elevated.[21] The diagnosis of Wilson disease is confirmed by biochemical testing and liver biopsy (see later). *Reye's syndrome*, a disorder of fatty infiltration of the liver associated with impaired mitochondrial metabolism of fatty acids, may uncommonly produce jaundice.[22] It usually follows a viral illness in children and is heralded by nausea and vomiting. When jaundice is present, the patient is invariably encephalopathic, and other indices of hepatic synthetic function are generally abnormal.

Chronic Hepatocellular Dysfunction

Jaundice is a cardinal manifestation of a number of chronic hepatocellular diseases. In general, unless marked hepatic decompensation is present, the serum bilirubin concentration is lower than in the setting of acute hepatocellular injury. *Chronic viral hepatitis* should be a diagnostic consideration in patients with risk factors for exposure to causative agents (see earlier, and Chapter 68). Diagnosis is aided by serologic testing (see later). The major hepatotoxin-associated chronic hepatocellular disease is *alcoholic cirrhosis* (see Chapter 71), although cirrhosis has also been seen as a manifestation of industrial exposure to toxic compounds such as *vinylchloride* and as a consequence of chronic ingestion of significant quantities of *vitamin A*[23] (see Chapter 73). A histologic picture similar to that seen in alcoholic cirrhosis is produced in nonalcoholic steatohepatitis, a disorder that is characteristically encountered in overweight individuals and in diabetes (see Chapter 72). Certain hereditary metabolic liver diseases may progress to chronic hepatocellular injury and cirrhosis. *Hemochromatosis*, a disorder characterized by excessive intestinal iron uptake with iron accumulation and injury to the parenchymal cells of the liver, is the most common of these (see Chapter 66). Clues to the diagnosis are the presence of diabetes, arthritis, or deep pigmentation in a jaundiced individual. Confirmation of the disease is made by detection of mutations in the HFE gene or by liver biopsy. Hepatocellular copper overload in *Wilson disease* may also lead to chronic liver injury (see Chapter 67). The diagnosis should be suspected in younger individuals, and disease confirmation is made by biochemical testing and liver biopsy (see later). In a jaundiced patient with chronic obstructive pulmonary disease, α_1-antitrypsin deficiency should be suspected (see Chapter 65). In this disorder, there is impaired secretion of α_1-antitrypsin and liver injury as a result of its accumulation in the endoplasmic reticulum of hepatocytes.[24] The diagnosis of α_1-antitrypsin deficiency is confirmed by serologic testing and liver biopsy (see later). *Autoimmune hepatitis*, a disease that may be associated with systemic complaints such as malaise, fever, and arthralgia, is more commonly seen in women (see Chapter 75). The diagnosis is further aided by serologic testing and a liver biopsy (see later).

Hepatic Disorders with Prominent Cholestasis

OVERVIEW. The following icteric disorders are characterized by a predominant elevation of the serum alkaline phosphatase relative to the aminotransferases despite patent bile ducts. The clinical presentation of these disorders may mimic obstruction of the bile ducts, and it is these disorders that have the greatest potential to generate diagnostic confusion. Such disorders can be categorized histologically according to those that infiltrate the liver, those that mainly involve injury to intrahepatic bile ductules or portal triads, and those in which major histologic changes are not evident.

INFILTRATIVE DISEASES. A variety of infiltrative liver diseases are often associated with striking cholestasis. *Granulomatous diseases* of the liver include *infections*, such as tuberculosis, *Mycobacterium avium* (particularly in the immunocompromised host), leprosy, brucellosis, Q fever, syphilis, fungal diseases, parasitic diseases, mononucleosis, *toxins* (such as beryllium, quinidine, allopurinol), and sulfonamides, and *systemic disorders*, including sarcoidosis, lymphoma (in particular, Hodgkin's disease), and Wegener's granulomatosis[25] (see Chapter 69). The most common of these disorders to produce jaundice are *tuberculosis* and *sarcoidosis*. Most of these diseases are accompanied by fever (with the exception of parasitic diseases and berylliosis); other nonspecific symptoms include night sweats and weight loss. Physical examination usually reveals hepatosplenomegaly; right upper quadrant tenderness is uncommon. Lymphadenopathy is often seen in sarcoidosis and may be a clue to an infectious etiology or lymphoma, and erythema nodosum suggests either mycobacterial disease, sarcoidosis, or syphilis. The presence of eosinophilia should heighten the suspicion of sarcoidosis, parasitic disease, or drug toxicity. Radiographic chest abnormalities represent a clue to sarcoidosis or tuberculosis. Ultimately, the diagnosis may require liver biopsy if other tissue is not available.

Jaundice is an unusual manifestation of *amyloidosis*, but when present, it is invariably accompanied by marked hepatomegaly.[26] The diagnosis may be further suspected if there is clinical evidence of involvement of other organs, such as nephrotic syndrome, congestive heart failure, malabsorption, macroglossia, or peripheral neuropathy. There may be no specific biochemical clues to the presence of amyloidosis; proteinuria will be manifest if there is concomitant renal involvement. The diagnosis can usually be made on rectal valve biopsy, but if negative, liver biopsy is diagnostic. Jaundice resulting from extensive *neoplastic replacement* of hepatic parenchyma is usually heralded by anorexia and weight loss. Although signs, symptoms, and laboratory abnormalities may mimic those of biliary obstruction, the diagnosis is usually revealed by noninvasive imaging studies (see later).

DISORDERS INVOLVING BILE DUCTULES. Inflammation and loss of small intrahepatic bile ductules are characteristic of *primary biliary cirrhosis* (see Chapter 76). Such findings are also part of the spectrum of *graft-versus-host disease* encountered in organ transplant recipients (see Chapter 27). *Primary biliary cirrhosis* is a disease that occurs predominantly in women. When it manifests with jaundice, pruritus is usually present, and fatigue is common. Notably, the presence of a serum bilirubin concentration of greater than 10 mg/dL carries an extremely poor prognosis.[27] Hyperpigmented skin is often seen in primary biliary cirrhosis, and the presence of xanthelasma or xanthomata related to hypercholesterolemia is highly suggestive of the diagnosis. The diagnosis of primary biliary cirrhosis can be presumptively made serologically and confirmed by liver biopsy (see later). *Graft-versus-host disease* is a complication of transplantation of bone marrow and solid organs; hepatic involvement is rare after liver transplantation. Rash and diarrhea generally accompany jaundice in this condition.[28] Certain *drugs* can also produce cholestasis and inflammation of the portal tracts (see Chapter 73). Such agents include chlorpromazine, erythromycin (particularly the estolate salt), chlorpropamide, and methimazole.[17] Clinical features that may heighten the suspicion of drug-induced cholestasis are the presence of arthralgias, rash, or peripheral eosinophilia; cholestasis generally resolves within several months following drug discontinuation.

CHOLESTASIS WITH MINIMAL HISTOLOGIC ABNORMALITIES. Jaundice may accompany conditions characterized by minimal hepatocellular injury or histologic abnormalities. The mechanism of cholestasis in these conditions is not well understood at present and may be multifactorial. In *benign recurrent cholestasis*, an autosomal recessive disorder that has been mapped to a gene that is mutant in a distinct pediatric disorder of progressive familial cholestasis, there is a defect of biliary secretion of several classes of organic anions, including bile acids, into bile.[29] Hereditable defects in bile acid transport are discussed in Chapter 65.

Patients with benign recurrent cholestasis typically develop recurrent episodes of malaise and pruritus in association with jaundice; fever and abdominal pain are uncharacteristic findings.[30] The first episode commonly occurs before the second decade of life. During periods of jaundice, laboratory abnormalities include elevations in both serum alkaline phosphatase and aminotransferase activities, but the elevation in serum alkaline phosphatase is characteristically predominant. When performed during an icteric episode, liver biopsy findings are generally confined to centrilobular cholestasis, portal-based mononuclear infiltrates are uncommon (and, if present, are mild), and hepatocellular necrosis is not observed. Despite the recurrence of episodes over time, there is no histologic progression of disease. Cholestatic episodes may last up to several months and are separated by periods of clinical remission. Although there may be a significant impact on quality of life, liver failure does not occur, and hence the long-term clinical course is thought to be benign.

A number of drugs produce a histologically bland intrahepatic cholestasis. *Estrogens* reduce bile formation through several mechanisms. These include inhibition of the hepatocellular plasma membrane Na^+/K^+ pump, an important modulator of solute transport from blood to bile; impaired acidification of intracellular organelles, which may disrupt the targeting of organic anion transporters to their proper membrane domain; and decreased membrane fluidity, which may perturb the function of such transporters.[31] Cholestasis related to the use of *oral contraceptives* usually develops within 2 months of the initiation of therapy. Jaundice is generally accompanied by pruritus, but fever, rash, and arthralgias are absent. The syndrome promptly resolves with discontinuation of the drug. *Anabolic steroids* can produce a syndrome clinically indistinguishable from that of estrogen-induced cholestasis. The anabolic steroids methyltestosterone and norethandrolone may impair the integrity of hepatocellular microfilaments and thereby increase tight junction permeability, resulting in back-diffusion of biliary solutes into serum.[32]

The clinical features of cholestasis associated with *total parenteral nutrition* may also resemble those of estrogen and anabolic steroid–induced cholestasis.[33] It has been proposed that this syndrome is related, in part, to an altered enterohepatic circulation as well as diminished neuroendocrine stimulation of bile flow. Cholestasis and jaundice may also develop during *bacterial infections*. Although the cause is not well understood, experimental evidence has linked the cholestasis of sepsis to release of tumor necrosis factor-α by hepatic macrophages (Kupffer cells). Tumor necrosis factor-α has been shown to reduce bile flow, in part, through reduction of expression of the bile acid transporter noncholate transporting peptide, or NTCP, and by inhibiting Na^+/K^+ pump activity.[34, 35] Sepsis-related cholestasis in the critically ill patient may be extremely difficult to distinguish from obstruction of the bile ducts. Two features that aid the diagnosis are the absence of abdominal pain or pruritus with sepsis-related cholestasis. However, depending on the severity of illness and response to antibiotic therapy, imaging studies may be ultimately required to exclude the presence of intrahepatic abscesses or biliary tract obstruction.

Jaundice resulting from intrahepatic cholestasis has been reported as a paraneoplastic phenomenon (i.e., without malignant infiltration) in lymphoma and renal cell carcinoma. The latter, referred to as *Stauffer's syndrome*, is classically associated with hepatosplenomegaly.[36] Cholestasis and hepatosplenomegaly resolve after nephrectomy. Although the etiology of this disorder is uncertain, it may be related to aberrant release of cytokines (e.g., interleukin-6) by the tumor,[37] with resultant impairment of bile formation.

ATYPICAL PRESENTATIONS OF CHOLESTASIS. *Viral hepatitis* may rarely produce profound cholestasis with marked pruritus.[38] Unless the patient has risk factors for viral hepatitis (see earlier), no features reliably distinguish this disorder from those of other cholestatic syndromes or biliary tract obstruction. A high level of suspicion and appropriate serologies aid the diagnosis. When *alcoholic hepatitis* presents with fever, jaundice, abdominal pain, and leukocytosis, it too may be difficult to distinguish from obstruction of the bile ducts. Furthermore, occasionally, the increase in serum alkaline phosphatase activity is more significant than the increase in aminotransferase activity.[39] The diagnosis should be strongly considered in the jaundiced patient with ethanol dependency, especially if the activity of serum AST exceeds that of ALT. Although noninvasive (and potentially, invasive) imaging will help to assess the caliber of the biliary tree (see later), this is one setting in which urgent liver biopsy may be required to make the diagnosis.

Jaundice in Pregnancy

Several cholestatic disorders associated with pregnancy merit discussion (see Chapter 74). Jaundice may uncommonly accompany *hyperemesis gravidarum*, a generally self-limited disorder of the first trimester, but liver failure is not a feature of this illness.[40] *Intrahepatic cholestasis of pregnancy* typically occurs in the third trimester and presents with pruritus. Infrequently, it is associated with jaundice. It generally resolves within 2 weeks of delivery, tends to recur with subsequent pregnancies, and is thought to be caused by an unusual sensitivity to circulating estrogens.[41] A far more serious syndrome is *acute fatty liver of pregnancy*, which characteristically occurs in the third trimester.[42] Histologically, there is infiltration of hepatocytes with microvesicular fat that resembles *Reye's syndrome*. When jaundice is present, it is usually accompanied by nausea, abdominal pain, and encephalopathy; the disorder may be fatal unless delivery is promptly performed. *Preeclampsia*, a microvascular disorder of the third trimester heralded by hypertension and proteinuria, affects the liver in approximately 10% of cases. A particularly severe form, the syndrome of hemolysis, elevated liver function tests, and low platelet count (HELLP), requires prompt delivery.[43]

Jaundice in the Postoperative Patient

Postoperative jaundice is often multifactorial. Possible predisposing factors include inhalational anesthetic agents and a variety of other pharmacologic agents with potentially hepatotoxic effects, impaired hepatic perfusion intraoperatively or perioperatively, blood transfusions, parenteral nutrition, and occult sepsis.[44] It may be difficult to clinically distinguish disorders in which these factors predominate from *benign postoperative cholestasis*, a self-limited (less than 1 to 2 weeks) syndrome characterized by transient hyperbilirubinemia without biochemical evidence of hepatocellular injury or synthetic dysfunction.

The liver transplant recipient represents a special case,[45] in which the differential diagnosis of jaundice may not only include the disorders common to all postoperative patients but those that relate to transplantation, per se (see Chapter 83).[45] Specific diagnostic considerations include hepatocellular injury due to impaired organ preservation or hepatic arterial thrombosis (in the immediate postoperative period), graft rejection, obstruction of the bile ducts, acute viral hepatitis (e.g., cytomegalovirus), immunosuppressive drug toxicity (e.g., azathioprine), lymphoproliferative disorders, or recurrent disease (e.g., hepatitis B, hepatitis C, sclerosing cholangitis).

Obstruction of the Bile Ducts

Obstructive disorders of the biliary tree include occlusion of the bile duct lumen by gallstones, intrinsic disorders of the bile ducts, and extrinsic compression.

Choledocholithiasis

The most common cause of biliary obstruction is *choledocholithiasis*. Obstructing *cholesterol gallstones* typically originate in the gallbladder, migrate into the common bile duct, and either impact at the ampulla of Vater or produce partial obstruction in a ball-valve fashion (see Chapter 55). In patients with unconjugated hyperbilirubinemia, calcium bilirubinate stones, so-called *black pigment gallstones*, form in the gallbladder but may also form in situ at any level of the biliary tree, including the common bile duct. A distinct type of bilirubinate stone, so-called brown pigment gallstones, also forms in situ within the biliary tree. Obstruction of the bile ducts by these stones leads to repeated bouts of cholangitis (recurrent pyogenic cholangitis) in patients from certain regions in Asia (see Chapter 59) and in patients with prior biliary tract surgery.

Diseases of the Bile Ducts

Intrinsic disorders of the bile ducts may be inflammatory, infectious, or neoplastic. Congenital disorders of the bile ducts, including cysts and biliary atresia, are discussed in Chapter 52. *Primary sclerosing cholangitis*, an inflammatory disorder of the bile ducts, characterized by focal and segmental strictures, is extensively discussed in Chapter 59. Jaundice is an unusual complication of a similar picture of focal narrowing and localized obstruction of the bile ducts seen in patients infected with human immunodeficiency virus (so-called AIDS cholangiopathy[46]) (see Chapter 28). *Biliary strictures* may also follow hepatic arterial infusion of certain chemotherapeutic agents[47] or result from surgical injury to the bile duct or hepatic artery. Neoplasms of the biliary tree, including *cholangiocarcinoma*, are discussed in detail in Chapter 60.

Extrinsic Compression of the Bile Ducts

Extrinsic compression of the biliary tree may result from neoplastic involvement or inflammation of surrounding viscera. Rarely, marked enlargement of surrounding vasculature (e.g., arterial aneurysms, cavernous transformation of the portal vein) can compress the bile ducts as well (see Chapter 70).

Painless jaundice is a classic feature of carcinoma of the head of the pancreas (see Chapter 50). Occasionally, hepatoma or periportal lymph nodes enlarged by any metastatic tumor or lymphoma obstruct the extrahepatic bile ducts. Pancreatitis may also produce extrinsic biliary compression as a result of edema, pseudocyst formation, or fibrosis (see Chapters 48 and 49).

DIAGNOSTIC APPROACH TO THE PATIENT WITH JAUNDICE

A general algorithm for evaluating the patient with jaundice is depicted in Figure 14–2. The sequential approach involves (1) a careful patient history and physical examination and screening laboratory studies, (2) formulation of a working differential diagnosis, (3) selection of further specialized tests to further narrow the diagnostic possibilities, and (4) development of a strategy for treatment or further testing if unexpected diagnostic possibilities are suggested.

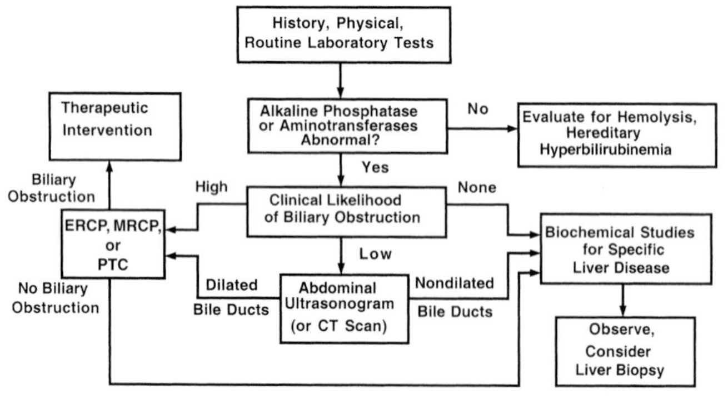

Figure 14–2. Decision tree for the evaluation and management of jaundice. CT, computed tomography; ERCP, endoscopic retrograde cholangiopancreatography; MRCP, magnetic resonance cholangiopancreatography; PTC, percutaneous transhepatic cholangiography.

History and Physical Examination

The patient history and physical examination provide important clues regarding the etiology of jaundice (Table 14–3). A history of fever, especially when accompanied by rigors, or abdominal pain, particularly in the right upper quadrant, is suggestive of cholangitis due to obstructive diseases (particularly choledocholithiasis), as does a history of prior biliary surgery. Obstructive jaundice from gallstone disease or malignant neoplasms is more common in the elderly. Symptoms compatible with a viral prodrome, such as anorexia, malaise, and myalgias, make viral hepatitis a strong possibility, as does a history of known infectious exposure, intravenous drug use, or receipt of blood products. A careful history may suggest that environmental hepatotoxins, ethanol, or medications underlie the patient's cholestatic liver disease. Finally, a family history of jaundice or liver disease suggests the possibility of a hereditary hyperbilirubinemia or genetic liver disease. All clues must be interpreted with caution, since fever and abdominal pain accompany diseases other than biliary obstruction, and patients with prior biliary surgery may fortuitously develop viral hepatitis. Conversely, anorexia and malaise are not exclusively symptoms of viral hepatitis, and patients with parenchymal liver disease frequently develop gallstones. Nonetheless, when these clues are evaluated with physical findings and routine laboratory tests, jaundice is correctly characterized as obstructive or nonobstructive in at least 75% of cases.[48]

The clues offered by the physical examination are important. High fever or abdominal tenderness (particularly right upper quadrant) suggest cholangitis, and a palpable abdominal mass, a neoplastic cause of obstructive jaundice. An abdominal scar in the midline or right upper quadrant may be the only clinical clue to prior biliary surgery (see Chapter 4, including the Acute Abdomen section). The presence of intrinsic liver disease may be suggested by evidence of portal hypertension (i.e., ascites, splenomegaly, or prominent abdominal veins) or other signs of liver disease, such as spider angiomata, gynecomastia, and asterixis. Certain physical findings may suggest particular liver diseases, such as hyperpigmentation in hemochromatosis, xanthomas in primary biliary cirrhosis, and Kayser-Fleischer rings in Wilson disease (see Chapter 67).

Initial Laboratory Studies

Essential laboratory studies include serum total bilirubin, alkaline phosphatase, aspartate and alanine aminotransferases (AST and ALT), and prothrombin time (see Chapter 64). Serum alkaline phosphatase activity reflects the presence of a number of related enzymes of overlapping substrate specificity. Alkaline phosphatase is a protein normally associated with the apical domain of the plasma membrane of hepatocytes and bile duct epithelial cells. Under physiologic condi-

Table 14–3 | **Obstructive Jaundice Versus Icteric Liver Disease**

	SUGGESTS OBSTRUCTIVE JAUNDICE	SUGGESTS ICTERIC LIVER DISEASE
History	Abdominal pain Fever, rigors Prior biliary surgery Older age	Anorexia, malaise, myalgias, suggestive of viral prodrome Known infectious exposure Receipt of blood products, use of intravenous drugs Exposure to known hepatotoxin Family history of jaundice
Physical examination	High fever Abdominal tenderness Palpable abdominal mass Abdominal scar	Ascites Stigmata of liver disease (e.g., prominent abdominal veins, gynecomastia, spider angiomata, Kayser-Fleischer rings) Asterixis, encephalopathy
Laboratory studies	Predominant elevation of serum bilirubin and alkaline phosphatase (note that dramatic increases in aminotransferases can occur with passage of common bile duct stone) Prothrombin time that is normal or normalizes with vitamin K administration Elevated serum amylase (lipase)	Predominant elevation of serum aminotransferases Prolonged prothrombin time that does not correct with vitamin K administration Blood tests indicative of specific liver disease

tions, this protein is enzymatically cleaved and released into bile, but small amounts are released into serum as well. Biliary obstruction or intrahepatic cholestasis increases both the synthesis and release of alkaline phosphatase into serum, and serum alkaline phosphatase activity increases. However, increases in activity may reflect release of alkaline phosphatase isoenzymes from extrahepatic tissues. Hence, other more specific markers, such as the serum activities of the canalicular enzymes gamma-glutamyl transpeptidase, leucine aminopeptidase, or 5′-nucleotidase are measured to confirm the hepatic origin of alkaline phosphatase. In a jaundiced patient, a predominant increase in (hepatic) alkaline phosphatase activity relative to those of serum aminotransferases suggests the possibility of biliary tract obstruction. Intrahepatic cholestatic disorders can produce an identical biochemical picture.

Cellular aminotransferases, such as AST, isozymes of which are found in both the cytosol and mitochondria of parenchymal cells of liver and several other tissues, and ALT, a cytosolic enzyme found predominantly in hepatocytes, ordinarily circulate in low concentrations only. However, liver cell damage due to ischemia, viral infection, or toxins significantly increases serum aminotransferase activity. Thus, predominant elevation of serum aminotransferase activity in comparison with alkaline phosphatase activity suggests that jaundice is due to intrinsic hepatocellular disease. A serum activity of AST that is less than 10 times the upper limits of normal and that exceeds that of ALT by at least a factor of 2 represents a clue to the diagnosis of alcoholic liver disease.[18] Acute Wilson disease may present with similar biochemical abnormalities.[21] There are exceptions to these generalizations, however, because transient biliary obstruction from choledocholithiasis associated with cholangitis may cause a brief but dramatic elevation (exceeding 10 to 20 times normal) of serum aminotransferase activity.[49]

The prothrombin time is a measure of the plasma activities of the coagulation factors I, II, V, VII, and X, each of which is synthesized in the liver. Prolongation of the prothrombin time can result from impaired hepatic synthesis of these proteins but may also reflect deficiency of vitamin K, which is required as a cofactor for essential post-translational γ-carboxylation of lysine residues of factors II, VII, IX, and X. Vitamin K absorption requires an intact enterohepatic circulation (hence an unobstructed biliary tree for intestinal absorption) of bile acids. Thus, parenteral administration of vitamin K generally normalizes a prolonged prothrombin time in patients with obstructive jaundice but not in patients with hepatocellular disease.

Decision Analysis

When taken together, history, physical examination, and laboratory studies will indicate the likelihood that obstructive jaundice is present. For example, an asymptomatic hyperbilirubinemic patient who has an unremarkable physical examination and normal levels of serum alkaline phosphatase and aminotransferases is unlikely to have liver disease or biliary obstruction. Further testing for specific disorders, such as hemolysis or isolated defects in bilirubin metabolism, is warranted (see Fig. 14–2). On the other hand, if the history, physical examination, and laboratory studies suggest the possibility of obstruction of the biliary tree, an imaging study is appropriate to either confirm the presence or absence of biliary tract obstruction. Selection of an imaging study depends on the likelihood of obstruction, diagnostic accuracy, cost, complication rate, and availability, especially if simultaneous therapeutic intervention is anticipated.

Imaging Studies

Abdominal Ultrasonography

Abdominal ultrasonography has become an accepted modality in the evaluation of hepatobiliary disease, because it determines the caliber of the extrahepatic biliary tree and reveals intrahepatic or extrahepatic mass lesions. The sensitivity of abdominal ultrasonography for the detection of biliary obstruction in jaundiced patients ranges from 55% to 91%, and the specificity ranges from 82% to 95%.[50–54] Ultrasonography can also demonstrate cholelithiasis (although common duct stones may not be well seen) and space-

Table 14–4 | **Imaging Studies for the Evaluation of Jaundice**

TEST	SENSITIVITY (%)	SPECIFICITY (%)	MORBIDITY (%)	MORTALITY (%)	COMMENTS (%)
Abdominal ultrasonogram	55–91	82–95	—	—	*Advantages:* noninvasive, portable, least expensive *Disadvantages:* bowel gas may obscure common bile duct; difficult in obese individuals
Abdominal CT	63–96	93–100	See comments	—	*Advantages:* noninvasive; higher resolution than ultrasound; not operator dependent *Disadvantages:* intravenous contrast medium required (potential nephrotoxicity)
ERCP	89–98	89–100	3	0.2	*Advantages:* provides direct imaging of bile ducts; permits direct visualization of periampullary region and acquisition of tissue distal to bifurcation of hepatic ducts; potential for simultaneous therapeutic intervention; especially useful for lesions distal to bifurcation of hepatic ducts *Disadvantages:* cannot be performed if altered anatomy precludes endoscopic access to ampulla (e.g., Roux loop)
PTC	98–100	89–100	3	0.2	*Advantages:* provides direct imaging of bile ducts; potential for simultaneous therapeutic intervention; especially useful for lesions proximal to common hepatic duct *Disadvantages:* more difficult with non-dilated intrahepatic bile ducts
MRCP	82–100	92–98	See comments	—	*Advantages:* noninvasive *Disadvantages:* requires breath holding; may miss small-caliber bile duct disease

CT, computed tomography; ERCP, endoscopic retrograde cholangiopancreatography; MRCP, magnetic resonance cholangiopancreatography; PTC, percutaneous transhepatic cholangiography.

occupying lesions greater than 1 cm in diameter. The major advantages of ultrasonography are that it is noninvasive, portable (this may be invaluable in the evaluation of the critically ill patient), and relatively inexpensive (Table 14–4). The major disadvantages are that it may be difficult to interpret in obese patients or patients with bowel gas that obscures the biliary tree. Also, dilation of the common bile duct, which usually indicates biliary tract obstruction, is common in patients who have undergone previous cholecystectomy. A final caveat is that in patients with cirrhosis and other conditions associated with poorly compliant hepatic parenchyma such as *primary sclerosing cholangitis*, intrahepatic ducts may not dilate with obstruction.

Computed Tomography of the Abdomen

Computed tomography (CT) of the abdomen with intravenous contrast is an alternative noninvasive means of evaluating the possibility of biliary tract obstruction. Abdominal CT permits accurate measurement of the caliber of the biliary tree, with a sensitivity and specificity of 63% to 96% and 93% to 100%, respectively, for detecting biliary obstruction, comparable to ultrasonography.[50–52, 54, 55] A technical refinement, spiral (helical) CT may improve the diagnostic accuracy of this method.[56] Abdominal CT also detects space-occupying lesions as small as 5 mm, is not operator dependent as in ultrasonography, and provides technically superior images in the obese and in patients in whom the biliary tree is obscured by bowel gas. The caveats that apply to the accuracy of ultrasonography for the diagnosis of biliary obstruction also apply to abdominal CT. In particular, CT it is not as accurate as ultrasonography in detecting cholelithiasis, because it images only calcified stones. Other considerations in the utilization of abdominal CT in patients with jaundice are its lack of portability, requirement for use of intravenous contrast, and expense (see Table 14–4).

Endoscopic Retrograde Cholangiopancreatography

Endoscopic retrograde cholangiopancreatography (ERCP) permits direct visualization of the biliary tree as well as the pancreatic ducts. In contrast with abdominal ultrasonography and CT, ERCP is more invasive. The procedure involves passage of an endoscope into the duodenum, introduction of a catheter into the ampulla of Vater, and injection of contrast medium into the common bile duct and/or pancreatic duct; conscious sedation is necessary. It is highly accurate in the diagnosis of biliary obstruction, with a sensitivity of 89% to 98% and specificity of 89% to 100%.[54, 57, 58] In addition to providing a radiographic image, biopsies and brushings for cytology of periampullary lesions may be taken. Moreover, if a focal cause for biliary obstruction is identified (e.g., choledocholithiasis, biliary stricture), maneuvers to relieve obstruction (e.g., sphincterotomy, stone extraction, dilation, stent placement) can be performed during the same session (see Chapter 61).

Acquisition of biopsy material and therapeutic intervention via ERCP are largely limited to lesions distal to the bifurcation of the right and left hepatic bile ducts. The technical success rate of ERCP is higher than 90%; the technique fails when the ampulla of Vater cannot be cannulated. This may be a particularly important consideration in patients with prior abdominal surgery and altered anatomy (e.g., Billroth II anastomosis with choledochojejunostomy). The morbidity and mortality associated with ERCP from untoward events such as respiratory depression, aspiration, bleeding, perforation, cholangitis, and pancreatitis, are 3% and 0.2%, respectively.[59] These rates are increased when interventional procedures are concomitantly employed.[60] A final consideration is cost, because ERCP is more expensive than noninvasive imaging procedures.

Percutaneous Transhepatic Cholangiography

Percutaneous transhepatic cholangiography (PTC) is a procedure that complements ERCP. PTC requires the passage of a needle through the skin and subcutaneous tissues into the hepatic parenchyma and advancement into a peripheral bile duct. When bile is aspirated, a catheter is introduced through the needle, and radiopaque contrast medium is injected. The sensitivity and specificity of PTC for the diagnosis of biliary tract obstruction, approximately 98% to 100% and 89% to 100%, respectively, are comparable to those of ERCP.[58, 61, 62] Like ERCP, interventional procedures, such as balloon dilation and stent placement, to relieve amenable focal obstructions of the biliary tree can be performed at the time of PTC (see Chapter 61). PTC is potentially technically advantageous under conditions in which the level of biliary obstruction is proximal to the common hepatic duct or in which altered anatomy precludes ERCP (see earlier). PTC may be technically limited in the absence of dilation of the intrahepatic bile ducts; under these conditions, multiple passes are frequently required, and cannulation of the biliary tree may be unsuccessful in up to 25% of attempts.[63] The morbidity and mortality of PTC from bleeding, perforation, and cholangitis are 3% and 0.2%, respectively.[61, 62] Like ERCP, it is more expensive than abdominal ultrasonography or CT.

Magnetic Resonance Cholangiopancreatography and Other Imaging Studies

Magnetic resonance cholangiopancreatography (MRCP) is a technical refinement of standard magnetic resonance imaging that permits rapid clear-cut delineation of the biliary tree without the requirement of intravenous contrast agents.[64] MRCP appears to be superior to conventional ultrasound or CT for detection of biliary tract obstruction. For detection of obstruction of the common bile duct, the sensitivity of MRCP is 81% to 100% and the specificity is 92% to 98%.[65–68] However, the ability of MRCP to delineate smaller intrahepatic bile ducts is less clear.[69] MRCP requires patient cooperation with breath holding. Its expense is comparable to ERCP.[64] Thus, although promising as an imaging modality, it is uncertain whether it will supplant abdominal ultrasonography or CT as an initial imaging test. Its greatest usefulness may be in circumstances in which the patient is thought to be at high risk for complications from ERCP or PTC.

Nuclear scintigraphy of the biliary tree, although helpful in the diagnosis of cholecystitis, is not sufficiently sensitive to justify its use in the diagnostic evaluation of jaundice.[51, 52] Furthermore, hepatic uptake of radiolabeled derivatives of iminodiacetic acid (e.g., HIDA) is quite limited when the serum bilirubin exceeds 7 to 10 mg/dL.[70]

Suggested Strategies for Imaging

The order of imaging studies depends largely on the clinical likelihood of obstructive jaundice (see Fig. 14–2). Several diagnostic strategies have been compared by clinical decision analysis.[71] It has been estimated that if the probability of biliary obstruction is 20%, the positive and negative predictive values of a strategy that employs ultrasonography as the initial test would be 96% and 98%, respectively, and compares favorably with a strategy that employs ERCP as the initial test. If, on the other hand, the probability of biliary obstruction is 60%, a strategy that employs ultrasonography as the first test would yield a positive predictive value of 99%, whereas the negative predictive value would fall to 89%. By contrast, when ERCP is the initial diagnostic procedure, the predictive value of a positive test would be 99% and that of a negative test would be 95%.

Stated differently, among patients in whom the probability of biliary obstruction is thought to be low but not zero, information regarding the hepatic parenchyma may be just as important as excluding the possibility of biliary obstruction. Therefore, in such patients, an abdominal ultrasonogram or CT is appropriate as an initial imaging study. If no evidence of biliary obstruction is found, the patient can be followed and undergo further evaluation for hepatic parenchymal disease as appropriate (see Fig. 14–2). Alternatively, if dilated bile ducts are visualized, then direct imaging of the biliary tree should be performed. Among patients in whom biliary obstruction is thought to be likely, ERCP (or PTC) could be considered as the initial study, because the absence of dilated ducts on abdominal ultrasound or CT does not rule out biliary obstruction. If ERCP or PTC do not show biliary obstruction, then abdominal ultrasonography or abdominal CT should be performed (if this has not been done) to image the hepatic parenchyma, and further studies, as outlined later, should be obtained. If the clinical suspicion for biliary obstruction is intermediate, and dilated bile ducts are not seen on abdominal ultrasonography or CT, MRCP is a reasonable option for imaging the biliary tree before an evaluation for hepatic parenchymal disease is undertaken.

The decision to employ ERCP versus PTC will be influenced by a variety of factors (see Table 14–4). These include the availability of each procedure at a particular facility, the presence or absence of dilated bile ducts, the suspected level of biliary obstruction, and the importance of accurately localizing the obstructing lesion (proximal with PTC, or distal with ERCP) to facilitate a plan of therapy. Under most circumstances, ERCP should be the procedure of choice, because it is comparable to PTC in availability, accuracy, technical success rate, and frequency of complications and offers a broader range of interventional options than PTC.

Further Studies

Serologic Testing

When imaging studies do not suggest biliary obstruction, evaluation for underlying liver disease is indicated in jaundiced patients with biochemical evidence of hepatocellular dysfunction or cholestasis. Appropriate screening laboratory studies would include viral serologies (including those for *hepatitis B and C*; if acute, then *hepatitis A* as well), serum levels of iron, transferrin, and ferritin (for *hemochromatosis*), ceruloplasmin (for *Wilson disease*), antimitochondrial antibodies (for *primary biliary cirrhosis*), antinuclear antibodies, anti–smooth muscle antibodies, and serum protein electrophoresis (for *autoimmune hepatitis*), and α_1-antitrypsin phenotype (for α_1-antitrypsin *deficiency*). Confirmation of these diagnoses as well as elucidation of diagnoses not revealed by serologic analysis may be made by liver biopsy.

Liver Biopsy

Liver biopsy provides precise information regarding details of hepatic lobular architecture and is most helpful in patients with undiagnosed persistent jaundice. With special histologic stains and/or quantitation of copper or iron content as appropriate, it permits the diagnosis of a number of liver diseases, including *viral hepatitis*, *alcoholic* and *nonalcoholic steatohepatitis*, *hemochromatosis*, *Wilson disease*, α_1-*antitrypsin deficiency*, *fatty liver of pregnancy*, *primary biliary cirrhosis*, *granulomatous hepatitis*, and *neoplasms*. Occasionally, it provides clues to otherwise unsuspected biliary tract obstruction, the histologic findings of which are listed in Table 14–5. However, liver histology may be entirely normal in acute biliary obstruction. Liver biopsy carries a small complication rate, predominantly from bleeding and perforation, with a morbidity of less than 0.5% and mortality of 0.1%.[72]

Table 14–5 | **Hepatic Histologic Abnormalities Associated with Biliary Obstruction**

Nonspecific findings with either extrahepatic or intrahepatic cholestasis
Canalicular bile plugs
Bile staining of parenchymal or Kupffer cells
Findings suggestive of biliary obstruction
Feathery degeneration of hepatocytes
Portal tract "edema"
Bile duct proliferation
Periductular fibrosis
Findings "diagnostic" of biliary obstruction
Bile infarct
Bile lake
Neutrophils in the wall or lumen of interlobular bile ducts (cholangitis)
Bile plugs in interlobular ducts

THERAPEUTIC OPTIONS

Biliary Obstruction

In the patient with obstruction of the bile ducts, therapy is typically directed at mechanical relief of obstruction. Interventional endoscopic or radiologic approaches available include sphincterotomy, balloon dilation of focal strictures, and placement of drains or stents. The alternatives are surgical (see Chapter 61). The therapeutic strategy chosen depends, in part, on the location and likely etiology of the obstructing lesion. Focal intrahepatic strictures may be amenable to an interventional radiologic approach, lesions distal to the bifurcation of the hepatic ducts may be more suitably managed endoscopically (notably sphincterotomy for choledocholithiasis), whereas mass lesions may require surgery.

Cholestatic Liver Disease

In cholestatic liver disease, the optimal treatment is directed toward the underlying etiology (e.g., cessation of ethanol, discontinuation of a drug, antiviral agents, phlebotomy for *hemochromatosis*, copper chelation for *Wilson disease*). Therapy for hyperbilirubinemia, per se, is not generally necessary in adults, because the neurotoxicity of bilirubin is confined to disorders characterized by extreme elevations of unconjugated bilirubin such as type I *Crigler-Najjar* syndrome.[1] In these special cases, reduction of risk for neurotoxicity can be achieved by phototherapy, in which exposure to blue or green light produces photoisomerization of bilirubin to more water-soluble enantiomers that do not require conjugation for excretion into bile.[73] In certain diseases in which bile flow is reduced (e.g., primary sclerosing cholangitis, primary biliary cirrhosis), absorption of fat-soluble vitamins (i.e., A, D, E, K) is impaired, and supplementation is recommended (see Chapters 59 and 76).

Management of Pruritus

A potentially disabling symptom of cholestatic hepatobiliary disease is pruritus. Although the chemical structure of the pruritogen awaits identification, indirect evidence suggests that it may be a bile acid or bile acid derivative, or other substances, such as endogenous opiates, that undergo enterohepatic circulation.[74] Bile acid–binding resins such as cholestyramine have been of some benefit. Phenobarbital, an inducer of xenobiotic metabolism, may relieve pruritus in individual patients, but its usefulness has not been supported in controlled trials.[75]

The choleretic bile acid ursodiol (ursodeoxycholic acid) has been studied in several cholestatic disorders.[76] It improves biochemical indices and appears to slow disease progression in *primary biliary cirrhosis* (see Chapter 76), but it has not been clearly shown to improve pruritus in this disorder.[77] Ursodiol has been shown to improve biochemical markers and pruritus in intrahepatic cholestasis of pregnancy,[78] but it does not appear to be of benefit in *primary sclerosing cholangitis*[79] (see Chapter 59).

Rifampin has been shown in some, but not all, studies to reduce pruritus in primary biliary cirrhosis and pediatric cho-

Table 14–6 | **Medical Therapy for Cholestasis-Associated Pruritus**

DRUG	REGIMEN	EFFICACY	ADVERSE EFFECTS
Antihistamines		Rarely provide significant relief apart from sedation	Drowsiness
Diphenhydramine	25–50 mg qid		
Hydroxyzine	25 mg tid		
Cholestyramine	4–6 g 30 min ac (may take double dose at breakfast and skip evening dose)	Beneficial in most patients	Fat malabsorption, decreased absorption of other medications, constipation
Phenobarbital	120 mg/day, dosage adjusted to maintain serum concentration between 10–40 μg/mL	Not superior to placebo in controlled trials	Drowsiness, potent inducer of hepatic enzymes involved in drug metabolism
Ursodiol	13–15 mg/kg/day	Beneficial in intrahepatic cholestasis of pregnancy	No major toxicity reported
Rifampin	300 mg bid	Beneficial in some but not all controlled trials	Inducer of hepatic enzymes involved in drug metabolism, potential hepatotoxicity, red-orange discoloration of secretions
Naltrexone	50 mg qd	Beneficial in small controlled trials	Opiate withdrawal symptoms transiently, rare hepatotoxicity

lestatic disorders.[80–82] Finally, the opiate receptor antagonist naltrexone has shown promise in a controlled, randomized trial, but its use may be limited by opiate withdrawal-like symptoms such as anxiety and visceral pain.[83] A small controlled trial of an oral version of the intravenous opiate receptor antagonist nalmefene has yielded similar findings.[84] In addition to these specific therapies, simple measures have been recommended. Such measures include the use of emollients and mild fragrance-free soaps (e.g., fragrance-free Dove, Basis, Aveeno), less frequent bathing, wearing light clothing, and frequent cutting of fingernails. Each of these approaches is summarized in Table 14–6.

REFERENCES

1. Berk PD, Noyer C: Bilirubin metabolism and the hereditary hyperbilirubinemias. Semin Liver Dis 14:321, 1994.
2. Konig J, Cui Y, Nies AT, Keppler D: A novel human organic anion-transporting polypeptide localized to the basolateral hepatocyte membrane. Am J Physiol 278:G156, 2000.
3. Trauner M, Meier PJ, Boyer JL: Molecular pathogenesis of cholestasis. N Engl J Med 339:1217, 1998.
4. Heirweigh KPM, Fevery J, Blanckaert N: Chromatographic analysis and structure of biliverdins and bilirubins. J Chromatogr 496:1, 1989.
5. Te Boekhorst T, Urlus M, Doesburg W, et al: Etiologic factors of jaundice in severely ill patients. J Hepatol 7:111, 1988.
6. LaPerche Y, Graillot C, Arondel J, Berthelot P: Uptake of rifampicin by isolated liver cells: Interaction with sulfobromophthalein uptake and evidence for separate carriers. Biochem Pharmacol 28:2065, 1979.
7. Borlak J, Thum T, Landt O, et al: Molecular diagnosis of a familial nonhemolytic hyperbilirubinemia (Gilbert's syndrome) in healthy subjects. Hepatology 32:792, 2000.
8. Seppen J, Bosma PJ, Goldhoorn BG, et al: Discrimination between Crigler-Najjar type I and II by expression of mutant bilirubin uridine diphosphate-glucuronosyltransferase. J Clin Invest 94:2385, 1994.
9. Tsujii H, Konig J, Rost D, et al: Exon-intron organization of the human multidrug-resistance protein 2 (MRP2) gene mutated in Dubin-Johnson syndrome. Gastroenterology 117:653, 1999.
10. Koff RS: Hepatitis A. Lancet 351:1643, 1998.
11. Mast EE, Krawczynski K: Hepatitis E: An overview. Annu Rev Med 47:257, 1996.
12. Lee WM: Hepatitis B virus infection. N Engl J Med 337:1733, 1997.
13. Liang TJ, Rehermann B, Seeff LB, Hoofnagle JH: Pathogenesis, natural history, treatment, and prevention of hepatitis C. Ann Intern Med 132:296, 2000.
14. Rosina F, Conoscitore P, Cuppone R, et al: Changing pattern of chronic hepatitis D in Southern Europe. Gastroenterology 117:161, 1999.
15. Schiodt FV, Rochling FA, Casey DL, Lee WM: Acetaminophen toxicity in an urban county hospital. N Engl J Med 337:1112, 1997.
16. Cappell MS, Hassan T: Gastrointestinal and hepatic effects of *Amanita phalloides* ingestion. J Clin Gastroenterol 15:225, 1992.
17. Lee WM: Drug-induced hepatotoxicity. N Engl J Med 333:1118, 1995.
18. Matloff DS, Selinger MJ, Kaplan MM: Hepatic transaminase activity in alcoholic liver disease. Gastroenterology 78:1389, 1980.
19. Dilawari JB, Bambery P, Chawla Y, et al: Hepatic outflow obstruction (Budd-Chiari syndrome): Experience with 177 patients and review of the literature. Medicine 73:21, 1994.
20. McDonald GB, Hinds MS, Fisher LD, et al: Veno-occlusive disease of the liver and multiorgan failure after bone marrow transplantation: A cohort study of 355 patients. Ann Intern Med 118:255, 1993.
21. Berman DH, Leventhal RI, Gavaler JS, et al: Clinical differentiation of fulminant Wilsonian hepatitis from other causes of liver failure. Gastroenterology 100:1129, 1991.
22. Treem WR: Inherited and acquired syndromes of hyperammonemia and encephalopathy in children. Semin Liver Dis 14:236, 1994.
23. Zimmerman HJ, Lewis JH: Chemical and toxin-induced hepatotoxicity. Gastroenterol Clin North Am 24:1027, 1995.
24. Perlmutter DH: Alpha$_1$-antitrypsin deficiency. Semin Liver Dis 18:217, 1998.
25. Sartin JS, Walker RC: Granulomatous hepatitis: A retrospective review of 88 cases at the Mayo Clinic. Mayo Clin Proc 66:914, 1991.
26. Peters RA, Koukolis G, Gimson A, et al: Primary amyloidosis and severe intrahepatic cholestatic jaundice. Gut 35:1322, 1994.
27. Wiesner RH, Porayko MK, Dickson ER, et al: Selection and timing of liver transplantation in primary biliary cirrhosis and primary sclerosing cholangitis. Hepatology 16:1290, 1992.
28. Ferrara JLM, Deeg HJ: Graft-versus-host disease. N Engl J Med 324:667, 1991.
29. Bull LN, van Eijk MJ, Pawlikowska L, et al: A gene encoding a P-type ATPase mutated in two forms of hereditary cholestasis. Nat Genet 18:219, 1998.
30. Brenard R, Geubel AP, Benhamou JP: Benign recurrent cholestasis: A report of 26 cases. J Clin Gastroenterol 11:546, 1989.
31. Van Dyke RW, Root KV: Ethinyl estradiol decreases acidification of rat liver endocytic vesicles. Hepatology 18:604, 1993.
32. Phillips MJ, Oda M, Fumatsu K: Evidence for microfilament involvement in norethandrolone-induced intrahepatic cholestasis. Am J Pathol 93:729, 1978.
33. Quigley EM, Marsh MN, Shaffer JL, Markin RS: Hepatobiliary complications of total parenteral nutrition. Gastroenterology 104:286, 1993.
34. Moseley RH, Wang W, Takeda H, et al: Effect of endotoxin on bile

acid transport in rat liver: A potential model for sepsis-associated cholestasis. Am J Physiol 271:G137, 1996.

35. Green RM, Beier D, Gollan JL: Regulation of hepatocyte bile salt transporters by endotoxin and inflammatory cytokines in rodents. Gastroenterology 111:193, 1996.
36. Dourakis SP, Sinani C, Deutsch M, et al: Cholestatic jaundice as a paraneoplastic manifestation of renal cell carcinoma. Eur J Gastroenterol Hepatol 9:311, 1997.
37. Walther MM, Johnson B, Culley D, et al: Serum interleukin-6 levels in metastatic renal cell carcinoma before treatment with interleukin-2 correlates with paraneoplastic syndromes but not patient survival. J Urol 159:718, 1998.
38. Gordon SC, Reddy KR, Schiff L, Schiff ER: Prolonged intrahepatic cholestasis secondary to acute hepatitis A. Ann Intern Med 101:635, 1984.
39. Perrillo RP, Griffin R, De Schryver-Kecksemeti K, et al: Alcoholic liver disease presenting with marked elevation of serum alakaline phosphatase: A combined clinical and pathological study. Am J Dig Dis 23: 1061, 1978.
40. Abell TL, Riely CA: Hyperemesis gravidarum. Gastroenterol Clin North Am 21:835, 1992.
41. Reyes H: The spectrum of liver and gastrointestinal disease seen in cholestasis of pregnancy. Gastroenterol Clin North Am 21:905, 1992.
42. Reyes H, Sandoval L, Wainstein A, et al: Acute fatty liver of pregnancy: A clinical study of 12 episodes in 11 patients. Gut 35:101, 1994.
43. Barton JR, Sibai BM: Care of the pregnancy complicated by HELLP syndrome. Gastroenterol Clin North Am 21:937, 1992.
44. Becker SD, Lamont JT: Postoperative jaundice. Semin Liver Dis 8:183, 1988.
45. Zetterman RK, McCashland TM: Long-term follow-up of the orthotopic liver transplantation patient. Semin Liver Dis 15:173, 1995.
46. Benhamou Y, Caumes E, Gerosa Y, et al: AIDS-related cholangiopathy: Critical analysis of a prospective series of 26 patients. Dig Dis Sci 38:1113, 1993.
47. Pozniak MA, Babel SG, Trump DL: Complications of hepatic arterial infusion chemotherapy. Radiographics 11:67, 1991.
48. Malchow-Møller A, Gronvall S, Hilden J, et al: Ultrasound examination in jaundiced patients: Is computer-assisted preclassification helpful? J Hepatol 12:321, 1991.
49. Anciaux ML, Pelletier G, Attali P, et al: Prospective study of clinical and biochemical features of symptomatic choledocholithiasis. Dig Dis Sci 31:449, 1986.
50. Baron RL, Stanley RJ, Lee JKT, et al: A prospective comparison of the evaluation of biliary obstruction using computed tomography and ultrasonography. Radiology 145:91, 1982.
51. Matzen P, Malchow-Møller A, Brun B, et al: Ultrasonography, computed tomography, and cholescintigraphy in suspected obstructive jaundice: A prospective comparative study. Gastroenterology 84:1492, 1983.
52. O'Connor KW, Snodgrass PJ, Swonder JE, et al: A blinded prospective study comparing four current noninvasive approaches in the differential diagnosis of medical versus surgical jaundice. Gastroenterology 84: 1498, 1983.
53. Pederson OM, Nordgard K, Kvinnsland S: Value of sonography in obstructive jaundice: Limitations of bile duct caliber as an index of obstruction. Scand J Gastroenterol 22:975, 1987.
54. Pasanen PA, Partanen KP, Pikkarainen PH, et al: A comparison of ultrasound, computed tomography, and endoscopic retrograde cholangiopancreatography in the differential diagnosis of benign and malignant jaundice and cholestasis. Eur J Surg 159:23, 1993.
55. Shimizu H, Ida M, Takayama S, et al: The diagnostic accuracy of computed tomography in obstructive biliary disease: A comparative evaluation with direct cholangiography. Radiology 138:411, 1981.
56. Zeman RK, Silverman PM, Ascher SM, et al: Helical (spiral) CT of the pancreas and biliary tract. Radiol Clin North Am 33:887, 1995.
57. Silvis SE, Rohrmann CA, Vennes JA: Diagnostic accuracy of endoscopic retrograde cholangiopancreatography in hepatic, biliary, and pancreatic malignancy. Ann Intern Med 84:438, 1976.
58. Matzen P, Haubek A, Holst-Christensen J, et al: Accuracy of cholangiography by endoscopic or transhepatic route: A prospective study. Gastroenterology 81:237, 1981.
59. Bilbao MK, Dotter CT, Lee TG, Katon RM: Complications of endoscopic retrograde cholangiopancreatography. Gastroenterology 70:314, 1976.
60. Cotton PB: Critical appraisal of therapeutic endoscopy in biliary tract disease. Annu Rev Med 41:211, 1990.
61. Pereiras R, Chiprut RO, Greenwald RA, Schiff ER: Percutaneous transhepatic cholangiography with the "skinny" needle: A rapid, simple, and accurate method in the diagnosis of cholestasis. Ann Intern Med 86: 562, 1977.
62. Gold RP, Casarella WJ, Stern G, Seaman WB: Transhepatic cholangiography: The radiological method of choice in suspected obstructive jaundice. Radiology 133:39, 1979.
63. Teplick SK, Flick P, Brandon JC: Transhepatic cholangiography in patients with suspected biliary disease and nondilated intrahepatic bile ducts. Gastrointest Radiol 16:193, 1991.
64. Barish MA, Yucel EK, Ferrucci JT: Magnetic resonance cholangiopancreatography. N Engl J Med 341:258, 1999.
65. Soto JA, Barish M, Yucel EK, et al: Magnetic resonance cholangiography: Comparison with endoscopic retrograde cholangiography. Gastroenterology 110:589, 1996.
66. Lee MG, Lee HJ, Kim MH, et al: Extrahepatic biliary diseases: 3D MR cholangiopancreatography compared with endoscopic retrograde cholangiopancreatography. Radiology 202:663, 1997.
67. Reinhold C, Taourel P, Bret PM, et al: Choledocholithiasis: Evaluation of MR cholangiography for diagnosis. Radiology 209:435, 1998.
68. Lomas DJ, Bearcroft PW, Gimson AE: MR cholangiopancreatography: Prospective comparison of a breath-hold 2D projection technique with diagnostic ERCP. Eur Radiol 9:1411, 1999.
69. Fulcher AS, Turner MA, Franklin KJ, et al: Primary sclerosing cholangitis: Evaluation with MR cholangiography—a case-control study. Radiology 215:71, 2000.
70. Krishnamurthy S, Krishnamurthy GT; Technetium-99m-iminodiacetic acid organic anions: Review of biokinetics and clinical applications in hepatology. Hepatology 9:139, 1989.
71. Richter JM, Silverstein MD, Schapiro R: Suspected obstructive jaundice: A decision analysis of diagnostic strategies. Ann Intern Med 99: 46, 1983.
72. McGill DB, Rakela J, Zinsmeister AR, Ott B: A 21-year experience with major hemorrhage after percutaneous liver biopsy. Gastroenterology 99:1396, 1990.
73. McDonough AF, Lightner DA: Phototherapy and the pathobiology of bilirubin. Semin Liver Dis 8:272, 1988.
74. Jones EA, Bergasa NV: The pruritus of cholestasis. Hepatology 29: 1003, 1999.
75. Metrau J-M, Lecompte Y, Arondel J, Dhumeaux D: Phenobarbital therapy in intrahepatic and extrahepatic cholestasis in adults. Digestion 14: 471, 1976.
76. Kowdley KV: Ursodeoxycholic acid therapy in hepatobiliary disease. Am J Med 108:481, 2000.
77. Goulis J, Leandro G, Burroughs AK: Randomised controlled trials of ursodeoxycholic acid therapy for primary biliary cirrhosis: A meta-analysis. Lancet 354:1053, 1999.
78. Palma J, Reyes H, Ribalta J, et al: Effects of ursodeoxycholic acid in patients with intrahepatic cholestasis of pregnancy. Hepatology 15: 1043, 1992.
79. Lindor KD: Ursodiol for primary sclerosing cholangitis. Mayo Primary Sclerosing Cholangitis-Ursodeoxycholic Acid Study Group. N Engl J Med 336:691, 1997.
80. Bachs L, Pares A, Elena M, et al: Effects of long-term rifampicin administration in primary biliary cirrhosis. Gastroenterology 102:2077, 1992.
81. Cynamon HA, Andres JM, Iafrate RP: Rifampin relieves pruritus in children with cholestatic liver disease. Gastroenterology 98:1013, 1990.
82. Woolf GM, Reynolds TB: Failure of rifampin to relieve pruritus in chronic liver disease. J Clin Gastroenterol 12:174, 1990.
83. Wolfhagen FH, Sternieri E, Hop WC, et al: Oral naltrexone treatment for cholestatic pruritus: A double-blind, placebo-controlled study. Gastroenterology 113:1264, 1997.
84. Bergasa NV, Alling DW, Talbot TL, et al: Oral nalmefene therapy reduces scratching activity due to the pruritus of cholestasis: A controlled study. J Am Acad Dermatol 41:431, 1999.

NUTRITION IN GASTROENTEROLOGY

Chapter 15

THE MALNOURISHED PATIENT: NUTRITIONAL ASSESSMENT AND MANAGEMENT

Samuel Klein and Khursheed N. Jeejeebhoy

Ingestion and absorption of a nutritionally adequate diet is necessary to maintain normal body composition and function. Gastrointestinal (GI) diseases can cause malnutrition by affecting nutrient intake, nutrient absorption, or nutrient requirements. Therefore, it is important for gastroenterologists to understand the principles involved in evaluating and treating malnourished patients.

BASIC NUTRITIONAL CONCEPTS

Energy Stores

Endogenous energy stores are continuously oxidized for fuel. Triglyceride present in adipose tissue is the major fuel reserve in the body and is critical for survival during periods of starvation (Table 15–1). The high energy density and hydrophobic nature of triglycerides make it a fivefold better fuel per unit mass than glycogen. Triglycerides liberate 9.3 kcal/g when oxidized and are compactly stored as an oil inside the fat cell, accounting for 85% of adipocyte weight. In comparison, glycogen produces only 4.1 kcal/g on oxidation and is stored intracellularly as a gel, containing approximately 2 g of water for every gram of glycogen. Adipose tissue is unable to provide fuel for certain tissues, such as bone marrow, erythrocytes, leukocytes, renal medulla, eye tissues, and peripheral nerves, which cannot oxidize lipids and require glucose for their energy supply. During endurance exercise, glycogen and triglycerides present within muscle tissue provide an important source of fuel for working muscles.[1]

Energy Metabolism

Energy is continuously required for normal organ function, maintenance of metabolic homeostasis, heat production, and performance of mechanical work. Total daily energy expenditure (TEE) is composed of resting energy expenditure (normally ~70% of TEE), thermic effect of feeding (normally ~10% of TEE), and energy expenditure of physical activity (normally ~20% of TEE).

Resting Energy Expenditure

Resting energy expenditure (REE) represents postabsorptive energy expenditure while a person lies quietly awake. During these conditions, approximately 1 kcal/kg body weight is consumed per hour in healthy adults. The energy requirements of specific tissues differ dramatically (Table 15–2). The liver, gut, brain, kidneys, and heart constitute approximately 10% of total body weight but account for approximately 75% of the REE. In contrast, resting skeletal muscle consumes approximately 20% of REE but represents approximately 40% of body weight, and adipose tissue consumes less than 5% of REE but usually accounts for more than 20% of body weight.

Several equations have been generated to estimate resting energy requirements[2–5] (Table 15–3). The equations for healthy subjects generate values that are usually within 10% of measured values. However, these equations are much less accurate in persons who are at extremes in weight (either very lean or obese) or who are ill because alterations in body composition and metabolic stress influence energy ex-

Table 15–1 | **Endogenous Fuel Stores in a Man Weighing 70 kg**

TISSUE	FUEL SOURCE	MASS: Grams	MASS: Kilocalories
Adipose	Triglyceride	13,000	120,000
Liver	Glycogen	100	400
	Protein	300	1200
	Triglyceride	50	450
Muscle	Protein	6000	24,000
	Glycogen	400	1600
	Triglyceride	250	2250
Blood	Glucose	3	12
	Triglyceride	4	35
	Free fatty acids	0.5	5

penditure. Malnutrition and hypocaloric feeding decrease REE to values 15% to 20% below those expected for actual body size, whereas metabolic stress, such as inflammatory diseases or trauma, often increases energy requirements. However, it is rare for most illnesses to increase REE by more than 50% of pre-illness values. For example, patients with Crohn's disease who do not have an infectious complication have normal metabolic rates[6] whereas patients with severe burns may have a 40% increase in REE.[7]

Energy Expenditure of Physical Activity

The effect of physical activity on energy expenditure depends on the intensity and duration of daily activities. Highly trained athletes can increase their TEE 10- to 20-fold during athletic events. The activity factors shown in Table 15–4, expressed as a multiple of REE, can be used to estimate TEE in active patients. The energy expended during physical activity is equal to:

$$(\text{REE}) \times (\text{activity factor}) \times (\text{duration of activity in hours}/24\text{ h}).$$

TEE represents the summation of energy expended during all daily activities, including rest periods (Table 15–5).

Thermic Effect of Feeding

Eating or infusing nutrients increases metabolic rate. Dietary protein causes the greatest stimulation of metabolic rate, followed by carbohydrate and then fat. A meal containing all these nutrients usually increases metabolic rate by 5% to 10% of ingested or infused calories.

Recommended Energy Intake in Hospitalized Patients

We developed a simple method for estimating total daily energy requirements in hospitalized patients based on body mass index (BMI)[8] (Table 15–6). In general, energy given per kilogram body weight is inversely related to BMI.

Protein

Proteins are composed of amino acids, which are nitrogen-containing compounds. Twenty different amino acids are commonly found in human proteins. Some amino acids (histidine, isoleucine, leucine, lysine, methionine, phenylalanine, threonine, tryptophan, valine, and possibly arginine) are considered essential because their carbon skeletons cannot be synthesized by the body. Other amino acids (glycine, alanine, serine, cysteine, cystine, tyrosine, glutamine, glutamic acid, asparagine, and aspartic acid) are nonessential because they can be made from endogenous precursors or essential amino acids. In disease states, nonessential amino acids may become essential. For example, it has been shown that cysteine is essential in patients with cirrhosis[9] because the transsulfuration pathway is impaired in these patients.

The body of an average 75-kg male contains approximately 12 kg of protein and 2 kg of nitrogen. In contrast to fat and carbohydrate, there is no storage depot for protein, so excess intake is catabolized and the nitrogen component is excreted. Inadequate protein intake causes net nitrogen losses, initially from organs such as the liver and then from muscle mass. Data from nitrogen balance studies suggest that the mean daily protein requirement for adults is 0.6 g/kg (with a standard deviation of 12.5%). Therefore, a protein intake of 0.75 g/kg would meet the requirements of 97% of the adult population. However, this amount is based on studies in which a reference protein containing a large proportion of essential amino acids was used. Requirements for dietary protein of lesser biologic value may be higher. Intravenously administered amino acids are as effective in maintaining nitrogen balance as oral protein of the same amino acid composition.[10]

Individual protein requirements are affected by several

Table 15–2 | **Resting Energy Requirements of a Man Weighing 70 kg**

TISSUE	TISSUE MASS: Grams	TISSUE MASS: Percentage Body Weight	ENERGY CONSUMED: Kilocalories/gram of Tissue per Day	ENERGY CONSUMED: Kilocalories/Day	ENERGY CONSUMED: Percentage REE
Liver	1550	2.2	0.28	445	19
Gut	2000	3.0	0.15	300	13
Brain	1400	2.0	0.30	420	18
Kidneys	300	0.4	1.27	360	15
Heart	300	0.4	0.80	235	10
Skeletal muscle	28,000	40.0	0.014	400	18
Adipose	15,000	21.0	0.005	80	4

REE, resting energy expenditure.

Table 15–3 | **Commonly Used Formulas for Calculating Resting Metabolic Rate**

HARRIS-BENEDICT EQUATION
Men:
66 + (13.7 × W) + (5 × H) − (6.8 × A)
Women:
665 + (9.6 × W) + (1.8 × H) − (4.7 × A)

WORLD HEALTH ORGANIZATION

Age (Years)	Male	Female
0–3	(60.9 × W) − 54	(61.0 × W) − 51
3–10	(22.7 × W) − 495	(22.5 × W) + 499
10–18	(17.5 × W) + 651	(12.2 × W) + 746
18–30	(15.3 × W) + 679	(14.7 × W) + 996
30–60	(11.2 × W) + 879	(8.7 × W) + 829
>60	(13.5 × W) + 987	(10.5 × W) + 596

OWEN ET AL.
Men:
879 + (10.2 × W)
Women:
795 + (7.18 × W)

IRETON-JONES ET AL.
Spontaneously breathing:
629 − (11 × A) + (25 × W) − (609 × Q)
Ventilator dependent:
1925 − (10 × A) + (5 × W) + (281 × G) + (292 × T) + (851 × B)

A, age in years; B, diagnosis of burn (present = 1, absent = 0); G, gender (male = 1, female = 0); H, height in centimeters; O, obesity (present = 1, absent = 0); T, diagnosis of traumas (present = 1, absent = 0); W, weight in kilograms.

factors, such as the amount of nonprotein calories provided, overall energy requirements, protein quality, and the patient's nutritional status (Table 15–7). Protein requirements increase when calorie intake does not meet energy needs. The magnitude of this increase is directly proportional to the decrease in energy supply. Conversely, at any level of suboptimal protein intake, nitrogen balance can be improved by increasing energy intake. Therefore, nitrogen balance reflects both protein intake and energy balance. Fasting animals and humans excrete nitrogen at rates that are proportional to their metabolic rates and is estimated to be approximately 2 mg N/kcal of REE.[11] Illness, by increasing catabolism and metabolic rate, also increases requirements for protein (see Table 15–7). Protein requirements are also determined by the availability of adequate amounts of essential amino acids in the protein source. Inadequate amounts of any of the essential amino acids result in inefficient utilization. In general, approximately 15% to 20% of total protein requirements should be in the form of essential amino acids in normal adults.

Table 15–4 | **Factors Used to Estimate Thermic Effect of Physical Activity**

ACTIVITY LEVEL	EXAMPLES	ACTIVITY FACTOR
Resting		1.0
Very light	Standing, driving, typing	1.1–2.0
Light	Walking 2–3 mph, shopping, light housekeeping	2.1–4.0
Moderate	Walking 3–4 mph, biking, gardening, scrubbing floors	4.1–6.0
Heavy	Running, swimming, climbing, basketball	6.1–10.0

Adapted from Alpers DA, Stenson WF, Bier DM. *Manual of Nutritional Therapeutics.* Boston: Little, Brown, 1995.

Table 15–5 | **Daily Energy Requirements in Humans**

AGE (Yr)	REE (kcal/kg)	ACTIVITY FACTOR	TEE (kcal/kg)
Male			
11–14	32.0	1.70	55
15–18	26.7	1.67	45
19–25	24.7	1.67	40
25–50	22.8	1.60	37
>51	19.8	1.50	30
Female			
11–14	28.5	1.67	47
15–18	24.9	1.60	40
19–24	23.2	1.60	38
25–50	21.9	1.55	36
>51	19.7	1.50	30

REE, resting energy expenditure; TEE, total daily energy expenditure.

Nitrogen Balance

Nitrogen balance is calculated as the difference between nitrogen intake, in the form of amino acids or protein, and nitrogen losses in urine, stool, skin, and body fluids. Nitrogen balance can be used to estimate protein balance because approximately 16% of protein consists of nitrogen and it is assumed that all body nitrogen is incorporated into protein. A positive balance (intake greater than losses) represents anabolic conditions and a net increase in total body protein, whereas a negative balance demonstrates net protein catabolism. For example, a negative nitrogen balance of 1 g/day represents a 6.25 g/day (16% of 6.25 g protein = 1 g nitrogen) loss of body protein, which is equivalent to a 30 g/day loss of hydrated lean tissue. In practice, nitrogen balance studies tend to be artificially positive because of overestimation of dietary nitrogen intake and underestimation of losses caused by incomplete urine collections and unmeasured outputs.

It is important to consider the patient's recent protein intake and nutritional status in interpreting nitrogen balance data. When a person ingesting a low-protein diet is re-fed protein, nitrogen excretion does not rise proportionately to intake and there is retention of administered nitrogen. This

Table 15–6 | **Estimated Energy Requirements for Hospitalized Patients Based on Body Mass Index**

BMI (kg/m²)	ENERGY REQUIREMENTS (kcal/kg/day)*
<15	35–40
15–19	30–35
20–29	20–25
≥30	15–20

*These values are recommended for critically ill patients and all obese patients; add 20% of total calories in estimating energy requirements in non-critically ill patients.

BMI, body mass index.

The lower range within each BMI category should be considered in insulin-resistant or critically ill patients to decrease the risk of hyperglycemia and infection associated with overfeeding.

Table 15–7 | **Recommended Daily Protein Intake**

CLINICAL CONDITION	PROTEIN REQUIREMENTS (g/kg IBW/day)
Normal	0.75
Metabolic stress	1.0–1.5
Hemodialysis	1.2–1.4
Peritoneal dialysis	1.3–1.5

IBW, ideal body weight.

Additional protein requirements are needed to compensate for excess protein loss in specific patient populations, such as patients with burn injuries, open wounds, and protein-losing enteropathy or nephropathy. Lower protein intake may be necessary in patients with chronic renal insufficiency not treated by dialysis and certain patients with liver disease and hepatic encephalopathy.

gain during early refeeding is caused by a rapid accumulation of nitrogen in the liver and, to a lesser extent, in kidneys and muscle. However, the early retention of nitrogen is not sustained and decreases markedly within 4 to 7 days. In contrast, when a person ingesting a high-protein diet decreases protein intake, the previously high urinary nitrogen loss continues for a few days despite the reduced intake, resulting in a negative nitrogen balance. Similarly, initial nitrogen loss after injury is greater in well-nourished than in malnourished patients. Therefore, a "labile" nitrogen pool of approximately 60 g contributes to short-term alterations in nitrogen balance and makes short-term nitrogen balance measurements an unreliable method for determining optimal protein intake.

Carbohydrate

Approximately 400 g of digestible carbohydrates are eaten each day in a normal diet: 60% as starch (polysaccharide made from maize, rice, wheat, and potato); 30% as sucrose (disaccharide made from sugar cane and beet sugar); and 10% as lactose (disaccharide made from milk). In addition, approximately 10 to 20 g of indigestible carbohydrate (soluble and insoluble fibers) are consumed daily. Complete digestion of the principal dietary carbohydrates generate monosaccharides (glucose, fructose, and galactose). All cells are able to generate energy (adenosine triphosphate) by metabolizing glucose to either three-carbon compounds via glycolysis or to carbon dioxide and water via glycolysis and the tricarboxylic acid cycle.

There is no dietary requirement for carbohydrate because glucose can be synthesized from endogenous amino acids and glycerol. Nevertheless, carbohydrate is an important fuel because of the interactions between carbohydrate and protein metabolism. Carbohydrate intake stimulates insulin secretion, which inhibits muscle protein breakdown,[12] stimulates muscle protein synthesis,[13] and decreases endogenous glucose production from amino acids.[14] In addition, glucose is the required or preferred fuel for red and white blood cells, the renal medulla, eye tissues, peripheral nerves, and the brain. However, once glucose requirements for these tissues (~150 g/day) are met, the protein-sparing effects of carbohydrate and fat are similar.[15, 16]

Lipids

Lipids consist of triglycerides (fat), sterols, and phospholipids. These compounds serve as sources of energy; precursors for steroid hormone, prostaglandin, thromboxane, and leukotriene synthesis; structural components of cell membranes; and carriers of essential nutrients. Dietary lipids are composed mainly of triglycerides, which contain saturated and unsaturated long-chain fatty acids of 16 to 18 carbon chains in length. The use of fat as a fuel requires the hydrolysis of endogenous or exogenous triglycerides and cellular uptake of released fatty acids. Long-chain fatty acids are delivered across the outer and inner mitochondrial membranes by a carnitine-dependent transport system.[17] Once inside the mitochondria, fatty acids are degraded by beta oxidation to acetyl coenzyme A (CoA), which then enters the tricarboxylic acid cycle. Therefore, the ability to use fat as a fuel depends on normal functioning mitochondria. A decrease in the number of mitochondria or oxidative enzymes, associated with aging or deconditioning, favors the use of carbohydrate as a fuel.[18]

Essential Fatty Acids

Most fatty acids can be synthesized by the liver, but humans lack the desaturase enzyme needed to produce the n-3 (double bond between carbons 3 and 4 counted from the methyl end) and n-6 (double bond between carbons 6 and 7) fatty acid series. Linoleic acid (C18:2, n-6) should constitute at least 2% and linolenic acid (C18:3, n-6,9,12) at least 0.5% of the daily caloric intake to prevent the occurrence of essential fatty acid deficiency (EFAD). Before the advent of parenteral nutrition, a clinical syndrome of EFAD, manifested as a rash and a specific alteration in the plasma fatty acid profile, was recognized only in infants. Adults did not seem to demonstrate this syndrome because of sufficient essential fatty acids stores in adipose tissue. The use of total parenteral nutrition given as a continuous infusion of a fat-free hypertonic glucose solution led to EFAD in adults, and the plasma pattern of EFAD was observed as early as 10 days after glucose-based total parenteral nutrition was started, before the onset of any clinically observable features.[19] The increase in plasma insulin concentrations caused by total parenteral nutrition is presumably responsible for EFAD because insulin inhibits lipolysis and, therefore, the release of endogenous essential fatty acids.

Major Minerals

Major minerals are inorganic nutrients that are required in large (>100 mg/day) quantities and are important for ionic equilibrium, water balance, and normal cell function. Malnutrition and nutritional repletion can have dramatic effects on major mineral balance. Evaluation of macromineral deficiency and recommended dietary intake for healthy adults are shown in Table 15–8.

Micronutrients

Micronutrients consist of trace elements and vitamins. Both forms of micronutrients are essential because, as constituents

Table 15–8 | **Major Mineral Requirements and Assessment of Deficiency**

MINERAL	ENTERAL	PARENTERAL	SYMPTOMS OR SIGNS OF DEFICIENCY	LABORATORY EVALUATION	
				Test	Comment
Sodium	0.5–5 g	60–150 mmol	Hypovolemia, weakness	Urinary sodium	May not reflect body stores; clinical evaluation is best
Potassium	2–5 g	60–100 mmol	Weakness, paresthesias, arrhythmias	Serum potassium	May not reflect body stores
Magnesium	300–400 mg	5–15 mmol	Weakness, twitching, tetany, arrhythmias, hypocalcemia	Serum magnesium	May not represent body stores
				Urinary magnesium	May not represent body stores
Calcium	800–1200 mg	5–15 mmol	Osteomalacia, tetany, arrhythmias	24-hr urinary calcium	Reflects recent intake
				Dual energy x-ray absorptiometry	Reflects bone calcium content
Phosphorus	800–1200 mg	20–60 mmol	Weakness, fatigue, leukocyte and platelet dysfunction, hemolytic anemia, cardiac failure, and decreased oxygenation	Plasma phosphorus	May not reflect body stores

of enzyme complexes, they regulate metabolic processes and substrate metabolism. The recommended dietary intake for trace elements and vitamins (Tables 15–9 and 15–10) is set at two standard deviations above the estimated mean so that it covers the needs of 97% of the healthy population. Therefore, the recommended dietary intake exceeds the micronutrient requirements of most persons. However, patients with disease, particularly those who have decreased GI absorptive function and increased micronutrient GI losses, may have requirements that are considerably higher than the recommended dietary intake.

Trace Elements

Trace minerals are inorganic nutrients that are required in small (<100 mg/day) quantities (see Table 15–9). Fifteen elements have been found to be essential for health in

Table 15–9 | **Trace Mineral Requirements and Assessment of Deficiency**

MINERAL	ENTERAL	PARENTERAL	SYMPTOMS OR SIGNS OF DEFICIENCY	LABORATORY EVALUATION	
				Test	Comment
Chromium	30–200 μg	10–20 μg	Glucose intolerance, peripheral neuropathy, encephalopathy	Serum	Does not reflect body stores
				Glucose tolerance test	Not specific
Copper	2 mg	0.3 mg	Anemia, neutropenia, osteoporosis, diarrhea	Serum copper	Insensitive for body stores
				Plasma ceruloplasmin	Acute phase reactant
Iodine	150 μg	70–140 μg	Hypothyroidism, goiter	Urine iodine	Reflects recent intake
				Thyroid stimulating hormone	Reflects thyroid function
Iron	10–15 mg	1–1.5 mg	Microcytic hypochromic anemia	Serum iron and total iron binding capacity	Poor measure of body stores; high specificity when levels low; poor sensitivity
Manganese	1.5 mg	0.2–0.8 mg*	Hypercholesterolemia, dementia, dermatitis	Serum manganese	Does not reflect body stores
Selenium	55 μg	20–40 μg	Cardiomyopathy (Keshan's disease), muscle weakness	Serum selenium	Insensitivity for body stores
				Blood glutathione peroxidase activity	More sensitive for body stores
Zinc	15 mg	2.5–4 mg	Growth retardation, delayed sexual maturation, hypogonadism, alopecia, acroorificial skin lesion, diarrhea, mental status changes	Plasma zinc	Poor specificity for body stores

*Recent evidence suggests that manganese toxicity, manifested as extrapyramidal and parkinsonian-like symptoms, can occur in patients with chronic liver disease or those receiving long-term parenteral nutrition. Many clinicians now limit manganese addition to parenteral nutrition solutions to < 0.1 mg/d or eliminate it entirely (see reference 21).

Table 15–10 | **Vitamin Requirements and Assessment of Deficiency**

VITAMIN	ENTERAL	PARENTERAL	SYMPTOMS OR SIGNS OF DEFICIENCY	LABORATORY EVALUATION	
				Test	Comment
A (retinol)	5000 IU	3300 IU	Night blindness, Bitot's spots, keratomalacia, follicular hyperkeratosis, xerosis	Serum retinal	Reflects recent intake and body stores
D (ergocalciferol)	400 IU	200 IU	Rickets, osteomalacia, osteoporosis, bone pain, muscle weakness, tetany	Serum 25-hydroxyvitamin D	Reflects body stores
E (alpha-tocopherol)	33 IU	33 IU	Hemolysis, retinopathy, neuropathy	Serum tocopherol	Reflects body stores
				Serum tocopherol: total lipid ratio	Ratio is preferred test
K (phylloquinone)	50–100 μg	100 μg	Easy bruising and bleeding, abnormal clotting	Prothrombin time	Not specific for vitamin 1
B_1 (thiamine)	1–1.5 mg	3 mg	Beriberi, cardiac failure, Wernicke's encephalopathy, peripheral neuropathy, fatigue, ophthalmoplegia	RBC transketolase activity	Reflects body stores
B_2 (riboflavin)	1.1–1.8 mg	3.6 mg	Cheilosis, sore tongue and mouth, eye irritation, sebhorrheic dermatitis	RBC glutathione reductase activity	Reflects body stores
B_3 (niacin)	12–20 mg	40 mg	Pellagra (dermatitis, diarrhea, dementia), sore mouth and tongue	Urinary N-methyl-nicotinamide	Reflects recent intake
B_5 (pantothenic acid)	5–10 mg	10 mg	Fatigue, weakness, paresthesias, tenderness of heels and feet	Urinary pantothenic acid	Reflects recent intake
B_6 (pyridoxine)	1–2 mg	4 mg	Sebhorrheic dermatitis, cheilosis, glossitis, peripheral neuritis, convulsions, hypochromic anemia	Plasma pyridoxal phosphate	Reflects body stores
B_7 (biotin)	100–200 μg	60 μg	Sebhorrheic dermatitis, alopecia, change in mental status, seizures, myalgia, hyperesthesia	Plasma biotin	
B_9 (folic acid)	400 μg	400 μg	Megaloblastic anemia, glossitis, diarrhea	Serum folic acid	Reflects body stores and recent intake
				RBC folic acid	Reflects body stores
B_{12} (cobalamin)	3 μg	5 μg	Megaloblastic anemia, paresthesias, decreased vibratory or position sense, ataxia, mental status changes, diarrhea	Serum cobalamin	Reflects body stores
				Serum methylmalonic acid	Tests functional block in enzyme
C (ascorbic acid)	75–90 mg (125 mg in smokers)	100 mg	Scurvy, petechia, purpura, gingival inflammation and bleeding, weakness, depression	Plasma ascorbic acid	Reflects recent intake
				Leukocyte ascorbic acid	Reflects recent stores

RBC, red blood cell.

animals: iron, zinc, copper, chromium, selenium, iodine, cobalt, manganese, nickel, molybdenum, fluorine, tin, silicon, vanadium, and arsenic. However, according to the strict criteria suggested by Cotzias,[20] only the first seven have been shown to be necessary for health in humans. Recent data suggest that the recommended daily parenteral intake for manganese may be too high in patients with chronic liver disease or those receiving long-term parenteral nutrition because of excessive manganese deposition in basal ganglia, causing extrapyramidal and Parkinson-like symptoms.[21]

Vitamins

Vitamins are organic compounds that are required in small (<100 mg/day) quantities (see Table 15–10). A negative balance between vitamin intake and vitamin utilization plus losses causes clinical symptoms of vitamin deficiency. The amount of time before the onset of clinical manifestations depends on the cumulative negative vitamin balance and the size of available vitamin stores. In general, water-soluble vitamin body stores are much smaller than fat-soluble vitamin stores, and so the onset of symptoms is more rapid for water-soluble than for fat-soluble vitamin deficiency. Blood test results usually become abnormal before the onset of clinical manifestations and can be used to assess the need for supplementation (see Table 15–10).

STARVATION

During starvation, a complex and carefully integrated series of metabolic alterations decrease metabolic rate, maintain glucose homeostasis, conserve body nitrogen, and increase the use of adipose tissue triglycerides to meet energy needs. During the first 24 hours of fasting, hepatic glucose production and oxidation decrease, whereas whole-body lipolysis and ketone body production increase.[22] The relative contribution of gluconeogenesis to hepatic glucose production increases as the rate of hepatic glycogenolysis declines; at 24 hours of fasting, only 15% of liver glycogen stores remain.[23] Glucose is oxidized predominantly by the brain and glucose-requiring tissues, accounting for approximately 20% of total energy consumption. The oxidation of fatty acids released from adipose tissue triglycerides accounts for approximately 65% of energy consumed during the first 24 hours of fasting. Approximately 15% of resting energy requirements is provided by the oxidation of protein; 70 g of amino acids are mobilized from protein stores, and 10 g of nitrogen are excreted in urine.[24]

During short-term starvation (1–14 days of fasting), the decline in plasma insulin, increase in plasma epinephrine, and increase in lipolytic sensitivity to catecholamines stimulate adipose tissue lipolysis.[25, 26] The increase in fatty acid delivery to the liver, in conjunction with an increase in the ratio of plasma glucagon:insulin concentration, enhances the production of ketone bodies by the liver.[27] A maximal rate of ketogenesis is reached by 3 days of starvation, and plasma ketone body concentration is increased 75-fold by 7 days. In contrast to fatty acids, ketone bodies can cross the blood–brain barrier and provide most of the brain's energy needs by 7 days of starvation.[28] The use of ketone bodies by the brain greatly diminishes glucose requirements and thus spares the need for muscle protein degradation to provide glucose precursors. If early protein breakdown rates were to continue throughout starvation, a potentially lethal amount of muscle protein would be catabolized in less than 3 weeks. Whole-body glucose production decreases by more than half during the first few days of fasting because of a marked reduction in hepatic glucose output. As fasting continues, the conversion of glutamine to glucose in the kidney represents almost 50% of total glucose production. Energy is conserved by a decrease in physical activity caused by fatigue and a reduction in REE caused by increased conversion of active thyroid hormone to its inactive form,[29] and suppressed sympathetic nervous system activity.[30]

During long-term starvation (14–60 days of fasting), maximal adaptation is reflected in a plateau in lipid, carbohydrate, and protein metabolism. The body relies almost entirely on adipose tissue for its fuel, which provides more than 90% of daily energy requirements. Muscle protein breakdown decreases to less than 30 g/day, causing a marked decrease in urea nitrogen production and excretion. The decrease in osmotic load diminishes urine volume to 200 mL/day, thereby limiting fluid requirements. Total glucose production decreases to approximately 75 g/day, providing fuel for glycolytic tissues (40 g/day) and the brain (35 g/day) while maintaining constant plasma glucose concentration. Energy expenditure decreases by 20% to 25% at 30 days of fasting[31] and remains relatively constant thereafter despite continued starvation.

The metabolic response to short-term and long-term starvation differs between lean and obese persons. Obesity is associated with a blunted increase in lipolysis and decrease in glucose production compared with that in lean persons.[32, 33] In addition, protein breakdown and nitrogen losses are less in obese than lean persons, thereby helping conserve muscle protein.[34]

The events that mark the terminal phase of starvation have been studied extensively in rats. Body fat mass, muscle protein, and the sizes of most organs are markedly decreased. The weight and protein content of the brain, however, remain relatively stable throughout starvation. During this final phase of starvation, body fat stores reach a critical level, energy derived from body fat decreases, and muscle protein catabolism is accelerated. Death commonly occurs when there is a 30% loss of muscle protein.[35] The mechanisms responsible for death from starvation in humans are not well understood. In general, the duration of survival during starvation depends on the amount of available body fuels and lean body mass. The possibility that there are lethal levels of body weight loss (loss of 40% of body weight),[36] of protein depletion (loss of 30%–50% of body protein),[37] of fat depletion (loss of 70%–95% of body fat stores),[38] or of body size (body mass index of 13 for men and 11 for women)[39] has been proposed. In normal-weight men, death occurs after approximately 2 months of starvation, when more than 35% (~25 kg) of body weight is lost.[38] In contrast, obese persons have undergone therapeutic fasts for more than a year without adverse consequences. The longest reported fast was that of a 207 kg man who ingested acaloric fluids, vitamins, and minerals for 382 days and lost 61% (126 kg) of his initial weight.[40]

MALNUTRITION

A normal nutritional status represents a healthy balance between nutrient intake and nutrient requirements. Malnutrition represents a continuum of events caused by nutrient disequilibrium, which alters intermediary metabolism, organ function, and finally body composition. Therefore, in a general sense, malnutrition can be defined as any metabolic, functional, or compositional alteration caused by inadequate nutrient intake. Malnutrition can be caused by specific nutrient deficiencies and a more generalized deficiency in protein and energy.

Specific Nutrient Deficiencies

A careful history and physical examination, routine blood tests, and selected laboratory tests can be used to diagnose specific macronutrient, major mineral, vitamin, and trace mineral deficiencies (see Tables 15–8 to 15–11). Replacement of the deficient nutrient usually corrects the biochemi-

Table 15–11 | **Selected Symptoms and Signs of Nutritional Deficiencies**

ORGAN SYSTEM	SYMPTOMS OR SIGNS	POSSIBLE NUTRIENT DEFICIENCY
Skin	Pallor	Iron, folate, vitamin B_{12}
	Follicular hyperkeratosis	Vitamins A and C
	Perifollicular petechiae	Vitamin C
	Dermatitis	Zinc, vitamin A, niacin, riboflavin, essential fatty acids
	Bruising, purpura	Vitamins C and K
Hair	Easily plucked, alopecia	Protein, zinc, biotin
	Corkscrew hairs, coiled hair	Vitamins A and C
Eyes	Night blindness, keratomalacia, photophobia	Vitamin A
	Conjunctival inflammation	Vitamin A and riboflavin
Mouth	Glossitis	Riboflavin, niacin, folate, vitamin B_{12}
	Bleeding or receding gums, mouth ulcers	Vitamins A, C, and K; folate
	Burning or sore mouth/tongue	Vitamins B_{12} and C; folate, niacin
	Angular stomatitis or cheilosis	Riboflavin, niacin, pyridoxin, iron
	Tetany	Calcium, magnesium
Neurologic	Paresthesias	Thiamine, pyridoxine
	Loss of reflexes, wrist drop, foot drop, loss of vibratory and position sense	Vitamins B_{12} and E
	Dementia, disorientation	Niacin, vitamin B_{12}
	Ophthalmoplegia	Thiamine

cal and physical abnormalities but may not cure the underlying cause of the problem. For example, iron therapy corrects iron deficiency anemia but not the factors responsible for the deficiency (e.g., inadequate intake, malabsorption, or iron loss).

Protein-Energy Malnutrition

The term protein-energy malnutrition (PEM) has been used to describe several nutritional deficiency syndromes, including kwashiorkor, marasmus, and nutritional dwarfism in children, and wasting associated with illness or injury in children and adults. Primary PEM is caused by inadequate nutrient intake, so the functional and structural abnormalities associated with primary PEM are often reversible with nutritional therapy. However, prolonged primary PEM can cause irreversible changes in organ function and growth. Secondary PEM is caused by illness or injury, which alter appetite, digestion, absorption, or nutrient metabolism. Wasting disorders, such as cancer, acquired immunodeficiency syndrome, and rheumatologic diseases, are characterized by involuntary loss of body weight and muscle mass in the setting of a chronic illness. These patients often experience wasting because of 1) inadequate nutrient intake caused by anorexia and possibly gastrointestinal tract dysfunction, and 2) metabolic abnormalities caused by alterations in regulatory hormones and cytokines. Alterations in metabolism cause greater loss of muscle tissue than that observed with pure starvation or semi-starvation. Restoration of muscle mass is unlikely with nutrition support unless the underlying inflammatory disease is corrected. Most of the weight that is gained after providing nutrition support is due to increases in fat mass and body water without significant increases in lean tissue.

Protein-Energy Malnutrition in Children

Undernutrition in children differs from that in adults because it affects growth and development. Much of our understanding of undernutrition in children comes from observations made in underdeveloped nations where poverty, inadequate food supply, and unsanitary conditions lead to a high prevalence of PEM. The Waterlow classification of malnutrition takes into account a child's weight-for-height (wasting) and height-for-age (stunting)[41] (Table 15–12). The characteristics of the three major clinical syndromes of PEM in children, kwashiorkor, marasmus, and nutritional dwarfism, are outlined in Table 15–13.[42] Although these three syndromes are classified separately, they may coexist in the same patient.

Marasmus

Weight loss and marked depletion of subcutaneous fat and muscle mass are characteristic features of children with marasmus. Loss of fat and muscle make ribs, joints, and facial bones prominent. The skin is thin, loose, and lies in folds.

Kwashiorkor

The word "kwashiorkor" comes from the Ga language of West Africa and can be translated as "disease of the displaced child" because it was commonly seen after weaning. The presence of peripheral edema distinguishes children with

Table 15–12 | **Waterlow Classification of Protein-Energy Malnutrition in Children**

PARAMETER	NORMAL	MILD	MODERATE	SEVERE
Weight-for-height (wasting)				
Percent of median NCHS standard	90–110	80–89	70–79	<70
Standard deviation from the NCHS median	+Z to −Z	−1.1 Z to −2 Z	−2.1 Z to −3 Z	<−3 Z
Height-for-age (stunting)				
Percent of median NCHS standard	95–105	90–94	85–89	<85
Standard deviation from the NCHS median	+Z to −Z	−1.1 Z to −2 Z	−2.1 Z to −3 Z	<−3 Z

NCHS, National Center for Health Statistics.

Table 15–13 | **Features of Protein-Energy Malnutrition Syndromes in Children**

PARAMETER	KWASHIORKOR	MARASMUS	NUTRITIONAL DWARFISM
Weight for age (% expected)	60–80	<60	<60
Weight for height	Normal or decreased	Markedly decreased	Normal
Edema	Present	Absent	Absent
Mood	Irritable when picked up, apathetic when alone	Alert	Alert
Appetite	Poor	Good	Good

kwashiorkor from those with marasmus and nutritional dwarfism. Children with kwashiorkor also have typical skin and hair changes (see sections on hair and skin changes below). The abdomen is protuberant because of weakened abdominal muscles, intestinal distension and hepatomegaly, but there is never ascites. In fact, the presence of ascites should prompt the clinician to search for liver disease or peritonitis. Children with kwashiorkor are typically lethargic and apathetic when left alone but become very irritable when held. Kwashiorkor is not caused by a relative deficiency in protein intake and, in fact, protein and energy intake are similar in children with kwashiorkor and marasmus. Kwashiorkor occurs when there is physiologic stress, such as an infection, in an already malnourished child. This explains why kwashiorkor is an acute illness compared with the chronicity of undernutrition alone and why there is overlap between marasmus and kwashiorkor. Kwashiorkor is characterized by leaky cell membranes, which permit the movement of potassium and other intracellular ions into the extracellular space. The increased osmotic load in the interstitium causes water movement and edema.

Nutritional Dwarfism

The child with failure to thrive may be of normal weight for height but has short stature and delayed sexual development. Providing appropriate feeding can stimulate catch-up growth and sexual maturation.

The diagnosis of PEM is different in adults than in children because adults do not grow in height. Therefore, undernutrition in adults causes wasting rather than stunting. In addition, although kwashiorkor and marasmus can occur in adults, most studies of adult PEM evaluated hospitalized patients who had secondary PEM and coexisting illness or injury.

Effect of Protein-Energy Malnutrition on Tissue Mass and Function

Body Composition

Although all body tissue masses are affected by undernutrition, the greatest depletion occurs in fat and muscle masses. Many patients who are malnourished also have intravascular volume depletion because of inadequate water and sodium intake, decreased plasma proteins, "leaky" capillaries, and "leaky" cells. However, the percent of body weight that is composed of water may be increased because of increased interstitial ion content and expansion of interstitial space. Therefore, malnourished patients may have diminished intravascular volume in the presence of whole-body fluid overload.

Gastrointestinal Tract

Starvation and malnutrition cause structural and functional deterioration of the intestinal tract, pancreas, and liver. The total mass and protein content of the intestinal mucosa and pancreas are markedly reduced. Mucosal epithelial cell proliferation rates decrease and the intestinal mucosa becomes atrophic with flattened villi. The synthesis of mucosal and pancreatic digestive enzyme is reduced. Intestinal transport and absorption of free amino acids are impaired, whereas hydrolysis and absorption of peptides are maintained. The abdomen may become protuberant because of hypomotility and gas distension.

Skin

The skin regenerates rapidly and it takes only 2 weeks for a basal cell of the dermis to reach the cornified layer and die. Undernutrition often causes dry, thin, and wrinkled skin with atrophy of the basal layers of the epidermis and hyperkeratosis. Severe malnutrition may cause considerable depletion of skin protein and collagen. Patients with kwashiorkor experience sequential skin changes in different locations. Hyperpigmentation occurs first, followed by cracking and stripping of superficial layers, thereby leaving behind hypopigmented, thin, and atrophic epidermis that is friable and easily macerated.

Hair

Scalp hair becomes thin, sparse, and is easily pulled out. In contrast, the eyelashes become long and luxuriant and there may be excessive lanugo hair in children. Children with kwashiorkor experience hypopigmentation with reddish-brown, gray, or blond discoloration. Adults may lose axillary and pubic hair.

Heart

Chronic undernutrition affects cardiac mass and function. Cardiac muscle mass decreases and is accompanied by fragmentation of myofibrils. Bradycardia (heart rate can decrease to less than 40 beats/min) and decreased stroke volume can cause a marked decrease in cardiac output and low blood pressure.

Lungs

Respiratory muscle function is altered by malnutrition, as evidenced by a decrease in vital capacity, tidal volume, and minute ventilation.

Kidneys

Renal mass and function are often well preserved during undernutrition, provided adequate water is consumed to prevent a severe decrease in renal perfusion and acute renal failure. However, when malnutrition is severe, there is a decrease in kidney weight, glomerular filtration rate, the ability to excrete acid, the ability to excrete sodium, and to concentrate urine. Mild proteinuria may also occur.

Bone Marrow

Severe undernutrition suppresses bone marrow red blood cell and white blood cell production, leading to anemia, leukopenia, and lymphocytopenia.

Muscle

Muscle function is impaired by malnutrition because of both a loss of muscle mass and impaired metabolism. Decreased sodium pump activity causes an increase in intracellular sodium and a decrease in intracellular potassium, which affects myocyte electrical potential and contributes to fatigue.

Immune System

Severe undernutrition causes atrophy of all lymphoid tissues, including thymus, tonsils, and lymph nodes. Cell-mediated immunity is diminished more than antibody production. Alterations in cell-mediated immunity cause impaired delayed cutaneous hypersensitivity and anergy. The ability to kill bacteria is diminished because of decreased complement and impaired neutrophil function. Gastrointestinal IgA secretion is also decreased. Malnourished patients are at increased risk for opportunistic infections and should be considered immunocompromised.

Brain

The weight and protein content of the brain remain relatively stable during prolonged malnutrition. Therefore, the integrity of the brain is preserved at the expense of other organs and tissues.

Nutritional Assessment Techniques

The current methods that are used clinically to evaluate PEM in hospitalized adult patients shifts nutritional assessment from a diagnostic to a prognostic instrument in an attempt to identify patients who can benefit from nutritional therapy. The commonly used indicators of the degree of protein-energy malnutrition, detailed below, correlate with clinical outcome. However, these indicators are always influenced by illness or injury, making it difficult to distinguish the contribution of malnutrition from the severity of illness itself on outcome. Specific features of the medical history, physical examination, and laboratory tests that emphasize the indicators which assess generalized nutritional status include the following points.

History

The patient or appropriate family members should be interviewed to provide insight into the patient's current nutritional state and future ability to consume an adequate amount of nutrients. The nutritional history should evaluate the following issues:

1. Body weight. Has the patient had mild (<5%), moderate (5%–10%), or severe (>10%) unintentional body weight loss in the last 6 months? In general, a 10% or greater unintentional loss in body weight in the previous 6 months is associated with a poor clinical outcome.[43, 44] However, it may be difficult to determine true weight loss. Morgan and coworkers[45] showed that the accuracy of determining weight loss by history was only 0.67 and the predictive power was 0.75; hence 33% of patients with weight loss would be missed, and 25% of those who have been weight-stable would have a diagnosis of weight loss. Furthermore, the nutritional significance of changes in body weight can be confounded by changes in hydration.
2. Food intake. Has there been a change in habitual diet pattern (number, size, and contents of meals)? What is the reason for altered food intake (e.g., appetite, mental status or mood, ability to prepare meals, ability to chew or swallow, gastrointestinal symptoms)?
3. Evidence of malabsorption. Does the patient have symptoms that are consistent with malabsorption?
4. Evidence of specific nutrient deficiencies. Are there symptoms of specific nutrient deficiencies, including macrominerals, micronutrients, and water (see Tables 15–8 to 15–11)?
5. Influence of disease on nutrient requirements. Does the patient's underlying illness increase nutrient needs because of high metabolic stress or nutrient losses?
6. Functional status. Has the patient's ability to function and perform normal daily activities changed?

Physical Examination

The physical examination corroborates and adds to the findings obtained by history.

1. Body mass index (BMI), which is defined as weight (in kilograms) divided by height (in square meters), can help identify patients at increased risk of an adverse clinical outcome[46, 47] (Table 15–14). Patients who are extremely underweight (BMI < 14 kg/m^2) are at high risk of death and should be considered for admission to the hospital for nutrition support.
2. Anthropometry. Triceps and subscapular skinfold thicknesses provide an index of body fat; midarm muscle circumference provides a measure of muscle mass. Although these measurements seem to be useful in population studies, their reliability in individual patients is less clear. The most commonly used standards for triceps skinfold thickness and midarm muscle circumference are those reported by Jelliffe,[48] which are based on measurements of European male military personnel and low-income American women, and those reported by Frisancho,[49] which are based on measurements of white males

Table 15–14 | **Classification of Nutritional Status by Body Mass Index in Adults**

BODY MASS INDEX (kg/m²)	NUTRITIONAL STATUS
<16.0	Severely malnourished
16.0–16.9	Moderately malnourished
17.0–18.4	Mildly malnourished
18.5–24.9	Normal
25.0–29.9	Overweight
30.0–34.9	Obese (class I)
35.0–39.9	Obese (class II)
≥40	Obese (class III)

and females participating in the 1971 to 1974 United States Health and Nutrition Survey. The use of these standards to identify malnutrition in many patients is problematic because of the restricted database and the absence of correction factors for age, hydration, and physical activity on anthropometric parameters. Several studies have demonstrated that 20% to 30% of healthy control subjects would be considered malnourished on the basis of these standards and that there is poor correlation between Jelliffe's and Frisancho's standards in classifying patients.[50, 51] Furthermore, Hall and associates[52] found considerable inconsistencies when anthropometric measurements were performed by different observers.

3. Hydration status. The patient should be evaluated for signs of dehydration (manifested by hypotension, tachycardia, postural changes, mucosal xerosis, decreased axillary sweat, and dry skin), and excess body fluid (manifested by edema or ascites).
4. Tissue depletion. A general loss of adipose tissue can be judged by clearly defined bony, muscular, and venous outlines and loose skinfolds. A fold of skin, pinched between the forefinger and thumb, can reveal the adequacy of subcutaneous fat. The presence of hollowness in the cheeks, buttocks, and perianal area suggests body fat loss. An examination of the temporalis, deltoid, and quadriceps muscles should be made to search for muscle wasting.
5. Muscle function. Strength testing of individual muscle groups should be made to evaluate for generalized and localized muscle weakness. In addition, a general evaluation of respiratory and cardiac muscle function should be made.
6. Specific nutrient deficiencies (see Tables 15–8 to 15–11). Rapidly proliferating tissues, such as oral mucosa, hair, skin, and bone marrow are often more sensitive to nutrient deficiencies than are tissues that turn over more slowly.

Laboratory Tests

Specific Nutrient Deficiencies

Suspected specific nutrient deficiencies based on history and physical examination can be further corroborated by appropriate diagnostic laboratory tests (see Tables 15–8 to 15–11).

SERUM ALBUMIN. Several studies have demonstrated that a low serum albumin concentration is correlated with an increased incidence of medical complications.[53–55] However, an understanding of albumin physiology clarifies why serum albumin concentration is correlated with disease severity in hospitalized patients, but may be inappropriate as a measure of nutritional status per se.[56] Albumin is highly water-soluble and resides in the extracellular space. The total body pool of albumin in a normal 70-kg man is approximately 300 g. Approximately one third of the total pool constitutes the intravascular compartment, and two thirds constitute the extravascular compartment.[57] The concentration of albumin in blood is greater than that in lymph or other extracellular fluids, but the ratio of intravascular to extravascular albumin concentration varies from tissue to tissue. Within 30 minutes of initiating albumin synthesis, the hepatocyte secretes albumin into the bloodstream.[58] Once albumin is released into plasma, its half-life is approximately 20 days. During steady state conditions, approximately 14 g of albumin (200 mg/kg) are produced and degraded daily. Thus, approximately 5% of the total albumin pool is degraded and replaced by newly synthesized albumin every day. Equilibration of albumin in the intravascular compartment is rapid and occurs within minutes after albumin enters the bloodstream. Equilibration between intravascular and extravascular albumin is slower. Every hour approximately 5% of the plasma albumin pool exchanges with extravascular albumin, so that the total plasma albumin mass exchanges with extravascular albumin each day.

Protein-calorie malnutrition (i.e., the state of prolonged deficient intake of protein and calories) causes a decrease in the rate of albumin synthesis. Within 24 hours of fasting, the rate of albumin synthesis decreases markedly.[59] However, a short-term reduction in albumin synthesis has little impact on albumin levels because of albumin's slow turnover rate and large pool size. Indeed, plasma albumin concentration may actually increase during short-term fasting because of reduction of intravascular water.[60] Even during chronic malnutrition, plasma albumin concentration is often maintained because of a compensatory decrease in albumin degradation and a transfer of extravascular albumin to the intravascular compartment. Prolonged protein-calorie restriction induced experimentally in human volunteers[31] or observed clinically in patients with anorexia nervosa[61] causes marked reductions in body weight but little change in plasma albumin concentration. A protein-deficient diet with adequate calories in elderly persons causes a decrease in lean body mass and muscle function without a change in plasma albumin concentration.[62]

Hospitalized patients may have low levels of plasma albumin for several reasons. Inflammatory disorders cause a decrease in albumin synthesis,[63] an increase in albumin degradation,[64] and an increase in albumin transcapillary losses.[65] Specific gastrointestinal and cardiac diseases increase albumin losses through the gut, whereas some renal diseases can cause considerable albuminuria. Wounds, burns, and peritonitis can cause albumin losses from the injured surface or damaged tissues. During serious illness, vascular permeability increases dramatically and alters albumin exchange between intravascular and extravascular compartments. Albumin losses from plasma to the extravascular space were increased twofold in patients with cancer-related cachexia and threefold in patients with septic shock. Plasma albumin levels do not increase in stressed patients until the inflammatory stress remits. For example, albumin levels fail to increase in patients with cancer after 21 days of intensive nutritional therapy.[66]

SERUM PREALBUMIN. Prealbumin is a transport protein for thyroid hormones and exists in the circulation as a retinol-binding prealbumin complex. The turnover rate of this protein is rapid, with a half-life of 2 to 3 days. It is synthesized by the liver and is catabolized partly by the kidneys. Protein-energy malnutrition reduces the levels of prealbumin, and refeeding restores levels.[67] However, prealbumin levels decrease without malnutrition in patients with infections[68] and in response to cytokine[69] and stress hormone infusion.[70] Renal failure increases levels,[71] whereas liver failure may cause a decrease in levels. The influence of disease-related factors on prealbumin concentration makes it unreliable as an index of nutritional status in hospitalized patients.

CREATININE-HEIGHT INDEX. The amount of creatinine excreted in urine provides a measure of skeletal muscle and lean body masses.[72] Approximately 2% of creatine, which is distributed mainly in muscle cells, is converted daily by an irreversible nonenzymatic reaction to creatinine, which is subsequently excreted unchanged in urine. The creatinine-height index is determined by measuring 24-hour urinary creatinine excretion in relationship to the patient's height while the patient is consuming a creatine and creatinine-free diet. However, the normal range of values was derived from healthy men and women of ideal body weight. Estimates of "ideal" muscle mass may not apply to patients whose weights do not fall within the ideal range. Furthermore, the validity of the creatinine-height index can be affected by inaccurate urine collections, alterations in protein intake, and medical variables that alter creatinine excretion, independent of muscle mass (e.g., renal failure, sepsis, trauma, exercise, and steroid therapy).

Immune Competence

Immune competence, as measured by delayed cutaneous hypersensitivity (DCH), is altered by severe malnutrition and patients suffering from severe PEM can become anergic. However, a large number of clinical factors also influence DCH, making it a poor marker of malnutrition in sick patients. The following factors alter DCH in the absence of malnutrition: 1) infection; 2) illnesses, such as uremia, cirrhosis, hepatitis, myocardial infarction, trauma, burns, and hemorrhage; 3) medications, such as steroids, immunosuppressants, cimetidine, and warfarin; and 4) medical procedures, such as anesthesia and surgery.

Discriminant Analysis

Discriminant function analysis, based on retrospective evaluation of multiple parameters, has been used to develop predictive equations of clinical outcome.[73, 74] Serum protein concentrations and DCH are important variables included in these equations. Buzby and colleagues[73] found that their predictive equation, termed the prognostic nutritional index, provided a quantitative estimate of postoperative complications when applied prospectively to patients undergoing gastrointestinal surgery.

Subjective Global Assessment

A clinical method for evaluating nutritional status, termed the subjective global assessment, encompasses historical, symptomatic, and physical parameters (Table 15–15).[75, 76] This approach defines malnourished patients as those who are at increased risk for medical complications. The purpose of this assessment is to determine whether nutrient assimilation has been restricted because of decreased food intake, maldigestion, or malabsorption; whether weight loss has occurred; whether weight loss in the previous 6 months was mild (<5%), moderate (5% to 10%), or severe (>10%); the pattern of weight loss (e.g., a patient who had recently regained weight would not be considered malnourished); whether any effects of malnutrition on organ function and body composition are present; and whether the patient's disease process influences nutrient requirements (e.g., high-stress conditions are burns, major trauma, and severe inflammation, whereas moderate-stress diseases are mild infections and limited malignant tumor).

The findings of the history and physical examination are used to categorize patients as well nourished (category A), having mild or moderate malnutrition (category B), or having severe malnutrition (category C). The rank is assigned on the basis of subjective weighting; equivocal information is given less weight than definitive data. Fluid shifts related to onset or treatment of edema or ascites must be considered in interpreting changes in body weight. In general, a patient who has experienced weight loss and muscle wasting but is currently eating well and gaining weight is classified as well nourished. A patient who has experienced moderate weight loss, continued compromised food intake, continued weight loss, progressive functional impairment, and a moderate-stress illness is classified as moderately malnourished. A patient who has experienced severe weight loss and continues to have poor nutrient intake, progressive functional impairment, and muscle wasting is classified as severely malnourished, independent of disease stress. Several studies have found that the use of subjective global assessment in evaluating hospitalized patients gives reproducible results and that there was more than 80% agreement when two blinded observers assessed the same patient.[76, 77] Detsky and colleagues[77] found that preoperative subjective global assessment was a better predictor of postoperative infectious complications than were serum albumin concentration, DCH, anthropometry, creatinine-height index, and the prognostic nutritional index.

Muscle Function

Impaired muscle function is a manifestation of malnutrition and often occurs before there are structural alterations in muscle mass. Although muscle function testing is not routinely used in nutritional assessment, it may gain greater acceptance with experience. Electrical stimulation of the ulnar nerve at the wrist permits the measurement of several involuntary muscle function parameters of the adductor pol-

Table 15–15 | **Features of Subjective Global Assessment (SGA)**

HISTORY
Weight Change
Loss in past 6 months: amount = ______ kg; % loss = ______
Change in past 2 weeks: ______ Increase ______ No change ______ Decrease.
Dietary Intake Change:
No change ______
Change ______ Duration = ______ weeks
Type:
______ Suboptimal solid diet
______ Hypocaloric liquids
______ Starvation
Gastrointestinal Symptoms (That Persisted for > 2 Weeks):
______ None ______ Nausea ______ Vomiting ______ Diarrhea ______ Anorexia
Functional Capacity
______ No dysfunction
______ Dysfunction ______ Duration = ______ weeks
Type ______ Working suboptimally
Ambulatory but not working
Bedridden
Effect of Disease on Nutritional Requirements
Primary diagnosis: ______
Metabolic Demand: ______ Low stress ______ Moderate stress ______ High stress
PHYSICAL EXAMINATION (NORMAL, MODERATE, OR SEVERE)
______ Loss of subcutaneous fat (triceps, chest)
______ Muscle wasting (quadriceps, deltoids)
______ Ankle or sacral edema
______ Ascites
SGA RATING
A = Well nourished
B = Mild or moderate malnutrition
C = Severe malnutrition

licis muscle. Studies performed during starvation and refeeding in humans suggest that muscle function testing can provide a sensitive measure of the adequacy of nutrient intake.[78–80] Short-term parenteral nutritional therapy has also been shown to improve respiratory and hand muscle function in malnourished patients with inflammatory bowel disease[81] and malnourished patients awaiting surgery.[82] Moreover, muscle function may be a better predictor of clinical outcome than other markers of nutritional status, such as arm muscle circumference, serum albumin concentration, and weight loss.[83–85]

Overview of Nutritional Assessment

At present, there is no gold standard for evaluating nutritional status, and the reliability of any nutritional assessment technique as a true measure of nutritional status has never been validated. No prospective randomized controlled clinical trials have been performed to evaluate whether providing nutrition support improves clinical outcome in patients judged to be severely malnourished compared with those who are judged to be mildly or moderately malnourished. However, a retrospective subgroup analysis of a large multicenter trial found that parenteral nutrition given preoperatively to patients with a diagnosis of severe malnutrition by subjective global assessment or a nutritional risk index (based on serum albumin and body weight change) decreased postoperative infectious complications.[86] The potential use of muscle function as a measure of nutritional status represents an exciting area for further investigation. Although there is strong evidence that muscle function provides an index of both nutritional state and the risk of medical complications, it is not clear whether the restoration of function leads to an improvement in clinical outcome. The authors recommend that nutritional assessment involve a careful nutritional history and physical examination. In addition, appropriate laboratory studies should be obtained as needed to further evaluate considerations raised during the clinical examination. The information from this evaluation should help determine the patient's current clinical condition and the anticipated duration of inadequate volitional feeding to identify patients who may require oral, enteral, or parenteral nutrition support (see Chapter 16, Enteral and Parenteral Nutrition).

REFEEDING THE MALNOURISHED PATIENT

Refeeding the severely malnourished patient is necessary to reverse the adverse effects of malnutrition and to prevent death from starvation. The goal is to inhibit mobilization of endogenous fuels and use ingested or infused nutrients to meet body nutritional requirements and rebuild lost nutrient stores.

Refeeding Syndrome

Because of the structural, functional, and metabolic alterations caused by previously inadequate food intake, injudicious nutritional therapy can have adverse clinical consequences known in part as the refeeding syndrome.[87, 88] Early evidence of the refeeding syndrome was reported at the end of World War II, when it was found that oral refeeding of chronically semistarved research volunteers and war victims caused cardiac insufficiency and neurologic complications.[89] More recently, refeeding abnormalities and serious complications have been reported after aggressive refeeding in hospitalized cachectic patients.[90, 91]

Fluid Overload

Decreased cardiac mass, stroke volume, and end-diastolic volume; bradycardia; and fragmentation of cardiac myofibrils are associated with chronic undernutrition.[92–95] In addition, carbohydrate refeeding increases the concentration of circulating insulin, which enhances sodium and water reabsorption by the renal tubule.[96] These factors put the severely malnourished patient at increased risk of fluid retention and congestive heart failure after nutritional therapy containing water, glucose, and sodium.

Mineral Depletion

Of the mineral abnormalities associated with refeeding, phosphate depletion has received the most attention. During starvation, phosphorus requirements are decreased because of the predominant use of fat as a fuel source. Serum phosphate is maintained at normal levels by mobilizing bone stores and increasing renal tubular reabsorption. Refeeding with enteral carbohydrates or glucose-based parenteral formulas stimulates insulin release and intracellular uptake of phosphate.[97] Phosphate is needed for protein synthesis and for the production of phosphorylated intermediates necessary for glucose metabolism.[98] These metabolic processes can cause extracellular phosphorus concentration to fall below 1 mg/dL within hours of initiating nutritional therapy if adequate phosphate is not given. Severe hypophosphatemia, which is associated with muscle weakness, paresthesias, seizures, coma, cardiopulmonary decompensation, and death, has occurred in patients receiving enteral or parenteral nutritional repletion.[90, 91, 99, 100] However, it is difficult to determine the contribution of hypophosphatemia to the reported clinical complications because of other coexistent medical and nutritional abnormalities.

Potassium and magnesium are the most abundant intracellular cations. Loss of body cell mass in the malnourished patient causes whole body potassium and magnesium depletion. Serum potassium and magnesium concentrations, however, remain normal or near normal during starvation because of their release from tissue and bone stores. The increases in protein synthesis rates, body cell mass, and glycogen stores during refeeding require increased intracellular potassium and magnesium. In addition, hyperinsulinemia during refeeding increases cellular uptake of potassium and can cause a rapid decline in extracellular concentrations.[101]

Glucose Intolerance

The adaptive changes during starvation enhance use of fatty acids and ketone bodies for fuel while glucose is conserved. In addition, the ability of insulin to stimulate glucose uptake and oxidation by peripheral tissues is impaired.[101] Thus, refeeding with high-carbohydrate meals or large amounts of parenteral glucose may not be well tolerated initially and may produce marked elevations in blood glucose, glucosuria, dehydration, and hyperosmolar coma.[102] Furthermore, because of the importance of thiamine in glucose metabolism, carbohydrate refeeding in patients who have thiamine depletion can precipitate Wernicke's encephalopathy.[103]

Gastrointestinal Dysfunction

Starvation and malnutrition cause structural and functional deterioration of the GI tract. The total mass and protein content of the intestinal mucosa and pancreas are markedly reduced. Mucosal epithelial cell proliferation rates, the synthesis of mucosal and pancreatic digestive enzymes, and intestinal transport and absorption of free amino acids are impaired,[104] whereas hydrolysis and absorption of peptides are better maintained.[105] These alterations limit the ability of the GI tract to digest and absorb food. When malnutrition is severe, oral refeeding has been associated with increased incidence of diarrhea and death.[106] However, most of the adverse consequences of starvation on the GI tract disappear after 1 to 2 weeks of refeeding.

Cardiac Arrhythmias

Ventricular tachyarrhythmias, which can be fatal, occur during the first week of refeeding.[107] A prolonged QT interval, often documented before death, is a contributing cause of the rhythm disturbances. It is not known whether refeeding per se or the cardiac dysfunction underlying malnutrition precipitated the terminal arrhythmias.

Clinical Recommendations

Initial Evaluation

The severity of complications during refeeding cachectic, chronically semistarved patients emphasizes the importance of a particularly cautious approach to their nutritional therapy, particularly during the first week of therapy when the risk of complications is highest. A careful search for cardiovascular and electrolyte abnormalities should be performed before refeeding. In addition, a search for infections (e.g., obtaining a white blood cell count, urine analysis and culture, blood cultures, and chest radiograph) should be considered even in the absence of physical findings, because many patients are not able to mount a normal inflammatory response.

Initial Supportive Care

Judicious resuscitation with fluids and electrolytes may be necessary before beginning feedings to prevent congestive heart failure from excessive fluid. Vitamin supplementation should be given routinely. Severely malnourished patients are poikilothermic so warm ambient temperature and warming blankets may be necessary to slowly increase core temperature. However, if warming blankets are being used, patients must be carefully monitored to avoid hyperthermia.

Feeding Regimen

Patients can be refed orally, by enteral tube feeding, by parenteral nutrition, or through a combination of these methods. Oral or enteral tube feedings are preferred over parenteral feeding because of fewer serious complications and enhanced gastrointestinal tract recovery. Isotonic feedings should be given in small amounts at frequent intervals to prevent overwhelming the body's limited capacity for nutrient processing and to prevent hypoglycemia, which can occur during brief nonfeeding intervals. Parenteral supplementation or complete parenteral nutrition may be necessary if the intestine cannot tolerate oral/enteral feeding. A combination of many nutrients, particularly nitrogen, phosphorus, potassium, magnesium, and sodium, is needed to restore lean body mass. Inadequate intake of one nutrient may impair retention of others during refeeding.

Although it is impossible to know the precise nutrient requirements of individual patients, some general guidelines are recommended for the first week of refeeding. Fluid intake should be limited to approximately 800 mL/day plus replacement for insensible losses. Adjustments in fluid intake are necessary in patients who have evidence of fluid overload or dehydration. Changes in body weight provide a useful guide for evaluating the efficacy of fluid administration. Weight gain greater than 0.25 kg/day, or 1.5 kg/week, probably represents fluid accumulation. Daily calorie intake should be approximately 15 to 20 kcal/kg, containing approximately 100 g of carbohydrate and 1.5 g of protein per kilogram body weight. Sodium should be restricted to approximately 60 mEq or 1.5 g/day, but liberal amounts of phosphorus, potassium, and magnesium should be given to patients who have normal renal function tests results. All other nutrients should be given in amounts needed to meet the recommended dietary allowance. Daily monitoring of body weight, fluid intake, urine output, and plasma glucose and electrolyte values are critical during early refeeding (first 3–7 days), so that nutritional therapy can be appropriately adjusted when necessary.

PATIENTS WITH SEVERE MALABSORPTION

Some patients become malnourished because of impaired gastrointestinal tract absorptive capacity. These patients have inadequate functional small bowel length because of intestinal resection or intestinal disease and present the most challenging nutritional management problems for the clinician. The medical management of these patients is often difficult and frustrating, but it can be made much easier by understanding the physiologic and clinical principles of treatment. Malabsorption syndromes and short bowel syndrome are discussed in greater detail in Chapters 89 and 92, respectively.

Clinical Considerations

The initial assessment of the patient with chronic malabsorption is meant to provide a logical basis for developing a treatment strategy to improve the patient's current clinical condition and prevent future complications. The therapeutic approach depends on the functioning of the intestinal tract; the presence of macronutrient, micronutrient, electrolyte, and fluid deficits; identification of risk factors for future medical complications; the presence of coexisting diseases that hamper the ability to provide nutritional therapy; and an evaluation of factors that affect the patient's daily activities.

A careful review of medical records, operative reports, and radiologic studies is needed to evaluate the absorptive capacity of the intestine by determining the length of remaining intestine, the site of intestinal disease or resection, and the presence of diseases that reduce intestinal absorption, such as pancreatic insufficiency or cholestasis. An assessment of fluid losses through diarrhea, ostomy output, and fistula volume should be made to help determine fluid requirements. Knowledge of fluid losses is also useful in calculating intestinal mineral losses by multiplying fluid loss by the estimated electrolyte concentration in intestinal fluid (Table 15–16). In patients who do not respond to treatment as predicted, dynamic studies of intestinal absorptive function may be helpful in adjusting the treatment program. Such studies include measuring fat, carbohydrate, and nitrogen balance and evaluating ostomy, fecal, or fistula mineral and fluid losses.

The urgency for medical intervention is determined by the severity of hemodynamic and nutritional abnormalities. This requires an evaluation for volume depletion, weight loss, and specific nutrient deficiencies. In addition to standard laboratory tests to evaluate for anemia (iron, folate, or vitamin B_{12} deficiency), prolonged prothrombin time (vitamin K deficiency), and electrolyte abnormalities, more sophisticated measurements to determine vitamin and trace mineral status can be obtained when deficiencies are suspected clinically. Bone mineral densitometry may be useful in many patients to establish a baseline and to screen for unrecognized bone mineral depletion. An accurate dietary history obtained by using food records is useful in evaluating nutrient requirements in nutritionally stable patients and in identifying dietary inadequacies in those with nutrient deficiencies.

Finally, it is also important to consider specific problems that interfere with the patient's quality of life. Maintaining adequate nutritional status with oral feedings at the cost of massive diarrhea and frequent bowel movements may be unacceptable to the patient with an active social or professional life outside the home. In this patient, parenteral supplementation may be necessary to improve the quality of life.

Table 15–16 | **Electrolyte Concentrations in Gastrointestinal Fluids***

LOCATION	Na (mEq/L)	K (mEq/L)	Cl (mEq/L)	HCO_3 (mEq/L)
Stomach	65	10	100	—
Bile	150	4	100	35
Pancreas	150	7	80	75
Duodenum	90	15	90	15
Mid-small bowel	140	6	100	20
Terminal ileum	140	8	60	70
Rectum	40	90	15	30

*Average values are listed; these can vary considerably from patient to patient.

Treatment

The goals of therapy are to control diarrhea; maintain fluid, electrolyte, and nutritional homeostasis; treat and prevent medical complications; and maximize the quality of life. The therapeutic approach depends on the results of the clinical evaluation. Initial therapy often requires subsequent modification using a trial-and-error approach, because of individual variability in absorptive function, continued intestinal adaptation, and the development of new medical complications or disease progression. Continued clinical monitoring is critical so that medical and nutritional therapy can be adjusted when necessary.

Control of Diarrhea

Diarrhea is often caused by a combination of factors, including increased gastrointestinal secretions, decreased intestinal transit time, and osmotic stimulation of water secretion by unabsorbed luminal contents. Therefore, therapy for diarrhea involves limiting endogenous secretions, slowing motility, and improving solute absorption.

The stomach normally produces approximately 2.5 L of fluid per day, which is absorbed by the small bowel. Gastric secretion and, in some patients, gastric hypersecretion may contribute to diarrhea. The use of H_2 receptor antagonists or proton pump inhibitors may be necessary to reduce gastric secretions. The presence of acidic jejunostomy or ileostomy contents after meals is a clear indication for acid-reduction therapy.[108] Large dosages, twice the normal amount used for the treatment of peptic ulcer disease or reflux, may be required for adequate control in certain patients because of reduced drug absorption.

The long-acting somatostatin analog, octreotide acetate (Sandostatin) can decrease small intestine secretions. Therapy with octreotide has been shown to decrease ostomy or stool volume (by 500 to 4000 g/day), decrease sodium and chloride output, and prolong small bowel transit time in patients with short bowel syndrome.[109–111] However, octreotide therapy does not improve absorption of macronutrients and other minerals. In addition, octreotide is expensive, must be given by subcutaneous injections, can decrease appetite, impair fat absorption,[112] increase the risk of gallstones,[113] and decrease the use of amino acids for splanchnic protein synthesis.[114] Nevertheless, in patients who have persistent large volume intestinal output despite standard antidiarrheal therapy, a trial of 100 μg octreotide injected subcutaneously three times a day with meals may be useful.

Opiates are the most effective means for slowing intestinal motility and act by delaying gastric emptying, decreasing peristalsis of the small and large intestine, and increasing anal sphincter tone. Loperamide (Imodium) should be tried first, because it is metabolized on first pass by the liver and does not easily cross the blood-brain barrier, thereby limiting its side effects and potential for drug dependence. If loperamide is not effective, other opiates, such as codeine or deodorized tincture of opium (10 to 25 drops every 6 hours), should be considered. In addition, the combination of an anticholinergic drug and an opiate may be beneficial. We have found that capsules containing 25 mg powdered opium and 15 mg powdered belladonna are a potent combination. However, these capsules are not commercially available and require a willing pharmacist to make them. Diphenoxylate with atropine (Lomotil) is an effective agent, but it is expensive and inconvenient if large doses are needed.

Foods and medications that cause diarrhea should be avoided. Traditionally, the recommendation has been to decrease or eliminate lactose-containing foods because of the reduction in intestinal lactase in patients who have had intestinal resection. However, patients with jejunostomies with 15 to 150 cm of jejunum remaining can tolerate 20-g lactose loads as milk or yogurt.[115] Although lactose was better absorbed from yogurt than from milk, there was no difference in clinical symptoms. Foods that have laxative effects, such as caffeine-containing drinks and diet products containing osmotically active sweeteners (sorbitol, xylitol, and mannitol), should be avoided. Medications that contain magnesium or sorbitol can also contribute to diarrhea.[116]

Enteral Feeding

The ability to use the gut to provide nutritional therapy depends on intestinal absorptive function as well as on the patient's ability to feed without producing adverse symptoms. Patients with nausea, vomiting, abdominal pain, or severe diarrhea may be unable to tolerate enteral feeding regardless of intestinal absorptive capacity. Specific foods that cause gastrointestinal complaints should be avoided. However, it is important to evaluate objectively the validity of these complaints to prevent the unnecessary withdrawal of nutritious foods. Patients with gluten-sensitive enteropathy require a strict gluten-free diet.

The goal of feeding is to provide the patient with all recommended nutritional requirements. The amount of ingested nutrients needed to reach this goal depends on the normal recommended dietary allowances modified by an estimate of absorptive function and intestinal losses. This usually requires ingestion of large amounts of fluid, calories, protein, vitamins, and minerals. Even in patients with severe short bowel syndrome, total parenteral nutrition may not be needed when vitamin and mineral supplements and large amounts of calories and protein are provided enterally.[117] Increasing the time that food is in contact with the intestine may enhance absorption in patients with limited absorptive function. For this reason, total dietary intake should be divided into at least six meals per day. If this is unsuccessful, defined liquid formulas ingested between meals or administered by continuous tube feedings at night may prevent the need for parenteral nutrition. In general, most patients with severe malabsorption must ingest 40 to 60 kcal/kg/day and 1.2 to 1.5 g of protein/kg/day. Suggested guidelines for vitamin and mineral supplementation are outlined in Table 15–17. The needs of each patient, however, can be determined only by experimentation with different dietary manipulations.

FAT INTAKE. Fat intake should not be restricted in patients with a jejunostomy or ileostomy despite the presence of steatorrhea. A high-fat, low-carbohydrate diet has been found to be comparable to a low-fat, high-carbohydrate diet with regard to total fluid, energy, nitrogen, sodium, potassium, and divalent ion absorption in patients with short bowel syndrome.[118–120] Furthermore, a high-fat diet facili-

Table 15–17 | **Guidelines for Vitamin and Mineral Supplementation in Patients with Severe Malabsorption**

SUPPLEMENT (REPRESENTATIVE PRODUCT)	DOSE	ROUTE
Prenatal multivitamin with minerals*	1 tab qd	po
Vitamin D*	50,000 U 2–3 times per week	po
Calcium*	500 mg elemental calcium tid to qid	po
Vitamin B_{12}†	1 mg qd	po
	100–500 μg q 1–2 mo	s.c.
Vitamin A†	10,000 to 50,000 U qd	po
Vitamin K†	5 mg/d	po
(Mephyton; AquaMEPHYTON)	5–10 mg/wk	s.c.
Vitamin E† (Aquasol E)	100 U/d	po
Magnesium gluconate† (Magonate) or magnesium oxide capsules (URO-MAG)	108–169 mg elemental magnesium qid	po
Magnesium sulfate†	290 mg elemental magnesium 1–3 times per wk	IM/IV
Zinc gluconate or zinc sulfate†	25 mg elemental zinc qd plus 100 mg elemental zinc/L intestinal output	po
Ferrous sulfate†	60 mg elemental iron tid	po
Iron dextran†	≤100 mg elemental iron per day based on formula or table	IV

*Recommended routinely for all patients.
†Recommended for patients with documented nutrient deficiency or malabsorption.
IM, intramuscular; IV, intravenous; po, oral; s.c., subcutaneous.

tates the ingestion of more calories. Limiting fat intake, however, may decrease gastrointestinal symptoms, colonic water secretion, hyperoxaluria, and divalent certain losses in patients who have steatorrhea and an intact colon.[121, 122]

Theoretically, medium-chain triglycerides (MCTs) are useful as a feeding supplement in patients who have impaired fat absorption, because they are rapidly hydrolyzed and do not require bile salts and micelle formation for absorption.[123] However, many patients do not find MCT oil palatable. Furthermore, MCT oil can cause nausea, vomiting, and abdominal discomfort. A dosage of 1 tablespoon (15 mL) three to four times daily, providing a total of approximately 500 kcal, is usually the maximal amount tolerated.

PREDIGESTED FORMULAS. Predigested formulas—that is; monomeric (elemental) and oligomeric formulas—have been recommended for patients with short bowel syndrome. Theoretically, these formulas, which contain nitrogen in the form of free amino acids or small peptides, are absorbed more efficiently over a shorter length of intestine than are polymeric formulas or whole food. However, the clinical efficacy of these formulas is not clear. Two prospective trials, using a randomized cross-over design, have evaluated the use of predigested formulas in patients with a jejunostomy and less than 150 cm of residual small bowel.[120, 124] McIntyre and colleagues[120] found no difference in nitrogen or total calorie absorption between a polymeric and an oligomeric diet. In contrast, Cosnes and coworkers[124] found that nitrogen absorption, but not total calorie absorption, was greater when a peptide-based diet was consumed than when a diet containing whole proteins was consumed. However, it is not known whether the increase in nitrogen absorption led to an improvement in protein metabolism or nitrogen balance, because these parameters were not measured. Blood urea nitrogen and urinary urea excretion were greater during peptide-based diet feeding than during whole protein diet ingestion, suggesting that the absorption of additional amino acids stimulated amino acid oxidation. Therefore, at present there is insufficient clinical evidence to justify the routine use of expensive predigested formulas in patients with short bowel syndrome.

ORAL REHYDRATION THERAPY. A subset of patients, usually those with 50 to 100 cm of jejunum that either ends in a jejunostomy or is anastomosed to the midtransverse or distal colon, cannot maintain fluid and electrolyte homeostasis but may be able to absorb adequate protein and calories. These patients may benefit from oral rehydration therapy that takes advantage of the sodium-glucose cotransporter present in the brush border of intestinal epithelium.[125] Frequent ingestion of small volume feedings of an isotonic glucose or starch-based electrolyte solution[126] stimulates active sodium transport across the intestine, whereas water follows passively by solvent drag.[127] Data from studies in animals and patients with short bowel syndrome suggest that sodium and water absorption is maximal from solutions containing 90 to 120 mmol/L of sodium.[128]

Unfortunately, most commercially available oral rehydration formulas and sport drinks contain lower sodium concentrations and are not optimal for patients with short bowel syndrome. However, inexpensive and more effective solutions can be made by patients at home (Table 15–18). Daily oral administration of 1 to 2 L of rehydration solutions has been successful in correcting fluid and electrolyte abnormalities and allows intravenous supplementation to be discontinued in patients who have had extensive intestinal resection.[128–131] In some patients, oral rehydration therapy has decreased ostomy output by 4 L/day.[131]

MAJOR MINERALS. Major minerals should be supplemented as needed, depending on the assessment of body content. Maintaining magnesium homeostasis is often difficult, because magnesium is poorly absorbed and enteral supplementation with magnesium salts increases diarrhea. Enteric-coated magnesium supplements should not be used, because their delayed release reduces contact with the intestine for absorption.[132]

Soluble magnesium salts, such as magnesium gluconate, are better tolerated and absorbed than are other magnesium complexes. In some patients, magnesium is best given in liquid form as magnesium gluconate (Fleming Inc., St. Louis, MO) and can be added to a oral rehydration solution in doses of 18 to 27 mmol (432 to 648 mg of elemental magnesium) per day. This solution should be sipped, not ingested as a bolus, to maximize absorption and avoid diarrhea. Normal serum magnesium levels do not exclude the possibility of magnesium deficiency. The percentage of magnesium excreted in urine after infusion may prove to be a better index of body magnesium stores; excretion of less than 80% of infused magnesium suggests whole body magnesium depletion.[133]

Table 15–18 | **Characteristics of Selected Oral Rehydration Solutions**

PRODUCT	Na mEq/L	K mEq/L	Cl mEq/L	Citrate mEq/L	Calories kcal/L	CHO g/L	Osmolarity mOsm/L
Equalyte	78m	22	68	1900 mg	100	25	305
CeraLyte 70	70	20	98	30	165	40	235
CeraLyte 90	90	20	98	30	165	40	260
Pedialyte	45	20	35	30	100	20	300
Rehydralyte	74	19	64	30	100	25	305
Gatorade	20	3	N/A	N/A	210	45	330
WHO	90	20	80	30	80	20	200
Washington University	105	0	100	10	85	20	250

Equalyte also contains fructooligosaccharides.
WHO (World Health Organization) formula: Mix 3/4 tsp sodium chloride, 1/2 tsp sodium citrate, 1/4 tsp potassium chloride, and 4 tsp glucose (dextrose) in 1 L (4 1/4 cups) of distilled water.
Washington University formula: Mix 3/4 tsp sodium chloride, 1/2 tsp sodium citrate, and 3 tbsp + 1 tsp Polycose powder in 1 L (4 1/4 cups) of distilled water.
Mix formulas with sugar-free flavorings as needed for palatability.

Supplemental calcium is given routinely because of both reduced intestinal absorption and the limited calcium content of low-lactose diets. Plasma levels of calcium are usually maintained by mobilizing bone stores unless there is concurrent magnesium or vitamin D deficiency. Therefore, urinary calcium excretion, which should be greater than 50 mg in 24 hours, is a more reliable index of calcium status. Most patients require approximately 1.5 to 2 g of elemental calcium daily. Although it has been suggested that calcium citrate is absorbed better than calcium carbonate,[134] most studies do not demonstrate any differences in calcium bioavailability from calcium ingested as carbonate, citrate, gluconate, lactate, or sulfate salt.[135, 136] However, the amount of calcium present in each calcium salt differs significantly, which influences the number of tablets needed each day.

Trace Minerals. Data regarding trace mineral requirements in patients with malabsorption disorders are limited. With the exception of zinc and iron, absorption of trace minerals from ingested foods or liquid formulas is often adequate to prevent overt deficiency syndromes. Zinc deficiency is common, and often subclinical, in patients with malabsorption. Large dosages of oral zinc supplements may become necessary, because zinc losses are often high and zinc absorption is low. Zinc gluconate is tolerated well and does not cause the gastric distress caused by zinc sulfate. Zinc should not be given with meals, because absorption is reduced by food.[137] Daily zinc supplementation of 25 mg plus an additional 100 mg/L (or 100 mg/kg) of ostomy or diarrheal output is needed to maintain zinc homeostasis.[138] Thus, many patients require approximately 150 mg of elemental zinc per day. Although zinc ingestion reduces copper absorption and can cause clinically significant copper deficiency,[139] additional copper intake usually is not needed because of the low efficiency of zinc absorption. Treating iron deficiency with oral preparations can be difficult. We recommend a liquid form of ferrous sulfate (300 mg/5 mL containing 60 mg of elemental iron) mixed in orange juice four times per day. Diluting ferrous sulfate liquid prevents staining of teeth, and the ascorbic acid present in orange juice enhances iron absorption. Some patients, however, require intermittent administration of parenteral iron.

Vitamins. Patients with malabsorption can usually absorb adequate amounts of most water-soluble vitamins from their diet, but patients with steatorrhea and bile acid depletion have difficulty absorbing fat-soluble vitamins. Vitamin K deficiency is rarely a clinical problem unless patients are receiving antibiotics. However, large doses of vitamins A, D, and E may be required to maintain normal body concentrations. Liquid vitamins present in water-miscible and water-soluble forms are more effective than are standard vitamins in pill form. An assessment of vitamin status should be used to guide therapy.

PARENTERAL FEEDING. Parenteral nutrition may be necessary to provide fluids, specific nutrients, or complete nutritional requirements in patients who cannot maintain normal hydration, electrolyte balance, or nutritional status with oral feeding. Some general guidelines are useful in deciding which patients require parenteral therapy. Patients in whom urine output is less than 1 L day are at increased risk for developing renal dysfunction and should receive intravenous fluids. Adequate levels of certain minerals—such as magnesium, potassium, and zinc—and fat-soluble vitamins are difficult to maintain with oral feedings in patients with severe steatorrhea or large intestinal fluid output and may require parenteral supplementation. Magnesium sulfate can be injected intramuscularly at a dose of 12 mmol (290 mg of elemental magnesium) one to three times per week if attempts at oral therapy are unsuccessful. Intravenous infusion of magnesium is preferred, however, because intramuscular injections are painful and can cause sterile abscesses. Monthly intramuscular injections of vitamin B_{12} (200 mg/month) are required in patients who have evidence of vitamin B_{12} malabsorption. In patients who have evidence of, or are at high risk for, vitamin K–associated hypoprothrombinemia, 5 to 10 mg of vitamin K should be given intramuscularly or intravenously each week. In some patients, total parenteral nutrition may be lifesaving or may be needed to limit diarrhea and achieve an acceptable quality of life.

REFERENCES

1. Martin WH, Klein S: Use of endogenous carbohydrate and fat as fuels during exercise. Proc Nutr Soc 57:49, 1998.
2. Harris JA, Benedict FG: Standard basal metabolism constants for physiologists and clinicians. In A Biometric Study of Basal Metabolism in Man. Publication 279, The Carnegie Institute of Washington. Philadelphia, JB Lippincott, 1919, p 223.

3. WHO (World Health Organization): Energy and Protein Requirements. Report of a joint FAO/WHO/UNU Expert Consultation Technical Report Series 724, World Health Organization, Geneva, 1985.
4. Owen OE, Kavle E, Owen RS, et al: A reappraisal of caloric requirements in healthy women. Am J Clin Nutr 44:1, 1986.
5. Ireton-Jones CS, Borman KR, Turner WW: Nutrition considerations in the management of ventilator-dependent patients. NCP 8:60, 1993.
6. Chan ATH, Fleming CR, O'Fallon WM, Huizenga KA: Estimated versus measured basal energy requirements in patients with Crohn's disease. Gastroenterology 91:75, 1986.
7. Allard JP, Jeejeebhoy KN, Whitwell J, Pashutinski L, Peters WJ: Factors influencing energy expenditure in patients with burns. J Trauma 28:199, 1988.
8. Klein S: Nutritional therapy. In Ahya S, Flood K, Paranjothi S (eds): The Washington Manual of Medical Therapeutics, 30th ed. Philadelphia: Lippincott Williams & Wilkins, 2000, pp 27–42.
9. Rudman D, Kutner M, Ansley J, Jansen R, Chipponi J, Bain RP: Hypotyrosinemia, hypocystinemia, and failure to retain nitrogen during total parenteral nutrition of cirrhotic patients. Gastroenterology 81: 1025, 1981.
10. Anderson GH, Patel DG, Jeejeebhoy KN: Design and evaluation by nitrogen balance and blood aminograms of an amino acid mixture for total parenteral nutrition of adults with gastrointestinal disease. J Clin Invest 53:904, 1974.
11. Munro HN: General aspects of the regulation of protein metabolism by diet and by hormones. In Munro HN, Allison JB (eds): Mammalian Protein Metabolism, vol 1. New York: Academic Press, 1964, pp 381–481.
12. Fukagawa NK, Minaker KL, Rowe JW, et al: Insulin-mediated reduction on whole body protein breakdown: Dose-response effects on leucine metabolism in postabsorptive men. J Clin Invest 60:648, 1985.
13. Biolo G, Fleming RYD, Wolfe RR: Physiologic hyperinsulinemia stimulates protein synthesis and enhances transport of selected amino acids in human skeletal muscle. J Clin Invest 95:811, 1995.
14. DeFronzo RA, Ferrannini E: Regulation of hepatic glucose metabolism in humans. Diabetes Dietab Rev 3:415, 1987.
15. Jeejeebhoy KN, Anderson GH, Nakhooda AF, et al: Metabolic studies in total parenteral nutrition with lipid in man: Comparison with glucose. J Clin Invest 57:125, 1976.
16. Roulet M, Detsky AS, Marliss EB, et al: A controlled trial of the effect of parenteral nutritional support on patients with respiratory failure and sepsis. Clin Nutr 2:97, 1983.
17. Coggan AR, Spina RJ, King DS, Rogers MA, Brown M, Nemeth PM, Holloszy JO: Histochemical and enzymatic comparison of the gastrocnemius muscle of young and elderly men and women. J Gerontol 47:B71, 1992.
18. Tao RC, Yoshimura NN: Carnitine metabolism and its application in parenteral nutrition. JPEN 4:469, 1980.
19. Wene JD, Connor WE, DenBesten L: The development of essential fatty acid deficiency in healthy men fed fat-free diets intravenously and orally. J Clin Invest 56:127, 1975.
20. Cotzias GC: Role and importance of trace substances in environmental health. In Hemphill DD (ed): Proceeding of the First Annual Conference on Trace Substances in Environmental Health, vol 1. Columbia, MO: University of Missouri, 1967, p 5.
21. Fitzgerald K, Mikalunas V, Rubin H, McCarthy R, Vanagunas A, Craig RM: Hypermanganesemia in patients receiving total parenteral nutrition. JPEN 23:333, 1999.
22. Romijn JA, Endert E, Sauerwein HP: Glucose and fat metabolism during short-term starvation in cirrhosis. Gastroenterology 100:731, 1991.
23. Nilsson LH, Hultman E: Liver glycogen in man—the effect of total starvation or a carbohydrate-poor diet followed by carbohydrate refeeding. Scand J Lab Clin Invest 32:325, 1973.
24. Aoki TT: Metabolic adaptations to starvation, semistarvation, and carbohydrate restriction. Nutrition in the 1980s: Constraints on our knowledge. New York: Alan R. Liss Inc., 1981, pp 161–177.
25. Klein S, Holland OB, Wolfe RR: Importance of blood glucose concentration in regulating lipolysis during fasting in humans. Am J Physiol 258:E32, 1990.
26. Klein S, Peters EJ, Holland OB, Wolfe RR: Effect of short- and long-term b-adrenergic blockade on lipolysis during fasting in humans. Am J Physiol 257:E65, 1989.
27. Foster DW: From glycogen to ketones—and back. Diabetes 33:1188, 1984.
28. Owen OE, Morgan AP, Kemp HG, Sullivan JM, Herrera MG, Cahill GF Jr: Brain metabolism during fasting. J Clin Invest 46:1589, 1967.
29. Vagenakis AG, Burger A, Portnary GI, Rudolph M, O'Brian JR, Azizi F, Arky RA, Nicod P, Ingbar SH, Braverman LE: Diversion of peripheral thyroxine metabolism from activating to inactivating pathways during complete fasting. J Clin Endocrinol Metab 41:191, 1975.
30. Young JB, Rosa RM, Landsberg L: Dissociation of sympathetic nervous system and adrenal medullary responses. Am J Physiol 247:E35, 1984.
31. Keys A, Brozek J, Henschel A, Mickelsen O, Taylor HL: The biology of human starvation. Minneapolis: University of Minnesota Press, 1950.
32. Horowitz JF, Coppack SC, Paramore D, Cryer PE, Klein S: Effect of short-term fasting on lipid kinetics in lean and obese women. Am J Physiol 276:E278, 1999.
33. Horowitz JF, Coppack SW, Klein S: Whole body and adipose tissue glucose metabolism in response to short-term fasting in lean and obese women. Am J Clin Nutr 73:517, 2001.
34. Elia M, Stubbs RJ, Henry CJK: Differences in fat, carbohydrate, and protein metabolism between lean and obsese subjects undergoing total starvation. Obesity Res 7:597, 1999.
35. Hagan SN, Scow RO: Effect of fasting on muscle proteins and fat in young rats of different ages. Am J Physiol 188:91, 1957.
36. Chossat C: Researches experimentales sur l'inanition. II. De l'alimentation insufissante. Ann Sci Nat Zool Ser 2, 20:182, 1843.
37. Montemurro DG, Stevenson JAF: Survival and body composition of normal and hypothalamic obese rats in acute starvation. Am J Physiol 198:757, 1960.
38. Leiter LA, Marliss EB: Survival during fasting may depend on fat as well as protein stores. JAMA 248:2306, 1982.
39. Henry CJ: Body mass index and the limits of human survival. Eur J Clin Nutr 44:329, 1990.
40. Stewart WK, Fleming LW: Features of a successful therapeutic fast of 382 days duration. Postgrad Med J 49:203, 1973.
41. Waterlow JC: Protein-Energy Malnutrition. London: Edward Arnold, 1992.
42. Golden MHN: Severe malnutrition. In Weatherall DJ, Ledington WGJ, Warrell DA (eds): Oxford Textbook of Medicine, 3d ed. New York: Oxford University Press, 1996, pp 1278–1296.
43. DeWys WD, Begg C, Lavin PT, et al: Prognostic effect of weight loss prior to chemotherapy in cancer patients. Am J Med 69:491, 1980.
44. Stanley KE: Prognostic factors for survival in patients with inoperable lung cancer. J Natl Cancer Inst 65:25, 1980.
45. Morgan DB, Hill GL, Burkinshaw L: The assessment of weight loss from a single measurement of body weight: The problems and limitations. Am J Clin Nutr 33:2101, 1980.
46. National Institutes of Health, National Heart, Lung, and Blood Institute: Clinical guidelines on the identification, evaluation and treatment of overweight and obesity in adults: The evidence report. Obes Res 6(S2):S53, 1998.
47. Madill J, Gutierrez C, Grossman J, Allard J, Chan C, Hutcheon M, Keshavjee AH: Nutritional assessment of the lung transplant patient: Body mass index as a predictor of 90-day mortality following transplantation. J Heart Lung Transplant 20:288, 2001.
48. Jelliffe DB: The assessment of the nutritional status of the community: With special reference to field surveys in developing regions of the world. WHO monograph. Geneva: WHO, 1966.
49. Frisancho AR: New norms of upper limb fat and muscle areas for assessment of nutritional status. Am J Clin Nutr 34:2540, 1981.
50. Harries AD, Jones LA, Heatley RV, Rhodes J: Malnutrition in inflammatory bowel disease: An anthropometric study. Hum Nutr Clin Nutr 36C:307, 1982.
51. Thuluvath PJ, Triger DR: How valid are our reference standards of nutrition? Nutrition 11:731, 1995.
52. Hall JCH, O'Quigley J, Giles GR, Appleton N, Stocks H: Upper limb anthropometry: The value of measurement variance studies. Am J Clin Nutr 33:1846, 1980.
53. Reinhardt GF, Myscofski JW, Wilkens DB, Dobrin PB, Mangan JE Jr, Stannard RT: Incidence and mortality of hypoalbuminemic patients in hospitalized veterans. JPEN 4:357, 1980.
54. Anderson CF, Wochos DN: The utility of serum albumin values in the nutritional assessment of hospitalized patients. Mayo Clin Proc 57: 181, 1982.
55. Apelgren KN, Rombeau JL, Twomey PL, Miller RA: Comparison of nutritional indices and outcome in critically ill patients. Crit Care Med 10:305, 1982.

56. Klein S: The myth of serum albumin as a measure of nutritional status. Gastroenterology 99:1845, 1990.
57. Jeejeebhoy KN: Cause of hypoalbuminaemia in patients with gastrointestinal and cardiac disease. Lancet i:343, 1962.
58. Rothschild MA, Oratz M, Schreiber SS: Albumin synthesis. N Engl J Med 286:748, 1972.
59. James WPT, Hay AM: Albumin metabolism: Effect of the nutritional state and the dietary protein intake. J Clin Invest 47:1958, 1968.
60. Broom J, Fraser MH, McKenzie K, et al: The protein metabolic response to short-term starvation in man. Clin Nutr 5:63, 1986.
61. Halmi KA, Struss AL, Owen WP, Stegink LD: Plasma and erythrocyte amino acid concentrations in anorexia nervosa. JPEN 11:458, 1987.
62. Castenada C, Charnley JM, Evans WJ, Crim MC: Elderly women accomodate to a low-protein diet with losses of body cell mass, muscle function, and immune response. Am J Clin Nutr 62:30, 1995.
63. Moshage HJ, Janssen JAM, Franssen JH, Hafkenscheid JCM, Yap SH: Study of the molecular mechanism of decreased liver synthesis of albumin in inflammation. J Clin Invest 79:1635, 1987.
64. Cohen S, Hansen JDL: Metabolism of albumin and gamma-globulin in kwashiorkor. Clin Sci 23:411, 1962.
65. Fleck A, Hawker F, Wallace PI, Raines G, Trotters J, Ledingham I, Calman KC: Increased vascular permeability: A major cause of hypoalbuminemia in disease and injury. Lancet i:781, 1985.
66. Gray GE, Meguid MM: Can total parenteral nutrition reverse hypoalbuminemia in oncology patients? Nutrition 6:225, 1990.
67. Prealbumin in Nutritional Care Consensus Group: Measurement of visceral protein status in assessing protein and energy malnutrition: Standard of care. Nutrition 11:169, 1995.
68. Hedlund JU, Hansson LO, Ortqvist AB: Hypoalbuminemia in hospitalized patients with community-acquired pneumonia. Arch Intern Med 155:1438, 1995.
69. Nieken J, Mulder NH, Buter J, Vellenga E, Limburg PC, Piers DA, de Vries EG: Recombinant human interleukin-6 induces a rapid and reversible anemia in cancer patients. Blood 86:900, 1995.
70. O'Riordain MG, Ross JA, Fearon KC, Maingay J, Farouk M, Garden OJ, Carter DC: Insulin and counterregulatory hormones influence acute-phase protein production in human hepatocytes. Am J Physiol 269:E323, 1995.
71. Cano N, Costanzo-Dufetel J, Calaf R, et al: Pre-albumin retinol-binding protein-retinol complex in hemodialysis patients. Am J Clin Nutr 47:664, 1988.
72. Forbes GF, Bruining GJ: Urinary creatinine excretion and lean body mass. Am J Clin Nutr 29:1359, 1976.
73. Buzby GP, Mullen JP, Matthews DC: Prognostic nutritional index in gastrointestinal surgery. Am J Surg 139:160, 1980.
74. Harvey KB, Moldawer LL, Bistrian BR, Blackburn GL: Biological measures for the formulation of a hospital prognostic index. Am J Clin Nutr 34:2013, 1981.
75. Detsky AS, McLaughlin JR, Baker JP, Johnston N, Whittaker S, Mendelson RA, Jeejeebhoy KN: What is subjective global assessment of nutritional status? JPEN 11:8, 1987.
76. Baker JP, Detsky AS, Wesson DE, Wolman SL, Stewart S, Whitwell J, Langer B, Jeejeebhoy KN: Nutritional assessment: A comparison of clinical judgment and objective measurements. N Engl J Med 306:969, 1982.
77. Detsky AS, Baker JP, Mendelson RA, Wolman SL, Wesson DA, Jeejeebhoy KN: Evaluating the accuracy of nutritional assessment techniques applied to hospitalized patients: Methodology and comparisons. JPEN 8:153, 1984.
78. Russell DMcR, Leiter LA, Whitwell J, Marliss EB, Jeejeebhoy KN: Skeletal muscle function during hypocaloric diets and fasting: A comparison with standard nutritional assessment parameters. Am J Clin Nutr 37:133, 1983.
79. Russell DMcR, Walker PM, Leiter LA, Sima AAF, Tanner WK, Mickle DAG, Jeejeebhoy KN: Metabolic and structural changes in muscle during hypocaloric dieting. Am J Clin Nutr 39:503, 1984.
80. Russell DMcR, Pendergast PJ, Darby PL, Garfinkel PE, Whitwell J, Jeejeebhoy KN: A comparison between muscle function and body composition in anorexia nervosa: The effect of refeeding. Am J Clin Nutr 38:229, 1983.
81. Christie PM, Hill GL: Effect of intravenous nutrition on nutrition and function in acute attacks of inflammatory bowel disease. Gastroenterology 99:730, 1990.
82. Chan STF, McLaughlin SJ, Ponting GA, Biglin J, Dudley HA: Muscle power after glucose-potassium loading in undernourished patients. Br Med J 293:1055, 1986.
83. Klidjian AM, Foster KJ, Kammerling RM, Cooper A, Karran SJ: Relation of anthropometric and dynamometric variables to serious post-operative complications. Br Med J 2:899, 1980.
84. Zeiderman MR, McMahon MJ: The role of objective measurement of skeletal muscle function in the pre-operative patient. Clin Nutr 8:161, 1989.
85. Windsor JA, Hill GL: Weight loss with physiologic impairment: A basic indicator of surgical risk. Ann Surg 207:290, 1988.
86. The Veterans Affairs Total Parenteral Nutrition Cooperative Study Group: Perioperative total parenteral nutrition in surgical patients. N Engl J Med 325:525, 1991.
87. Solomon SM, Kirby DF: The refeeding syndrome: A review. JPEN 14:90, 1990.
88. Apovian CM, McMahon MM, Bistrian BR: Guidelines for refeeding the marasmic patient. Crit Care Med 18:1030, 1990.
89. Burger GCE, Drummond JC, Sandstead HR: Malnutrition and starvation in western Netherlands, September 1944–July 1945, Parts 1 and 2. The Hague General State Printing Office, 1948.
90. Silvis SE, Paragas PD Jr: Parasthesias, weakness, seizures, and hypophosphatemia in patients receiving hyperalimentation. Gastroenterology 62:513, 1972.
91. Weinsier RL, Krumdieck CL: Death resulting from overzealous total parenteral nutrition: The refeeding syndrome revisited. Am J Clin Nutr 34:393, 1981.
92. Keys A, Henschel A, Taylor HL: The size and function of the human heart at rest in semi-starvation and in subsequent rehabilitation. Am J Physiol 50:153, 1947.
93. Garnett ES, Barnard DL, Ford J, Goodbody RA, Woodehouse MA: Gross fragmentation of cardiac myofibrils after therapeutic starvation for obesity. Lancet 1:914, 1969.
94. Heymsfield SB, Bethel RA, Ansley JD, Gibbs DM, Felner JM, Nutter DO: Cardiac abnormalities in cachectic patients before and during nutritional repletion. Am Heart J 95:584, 1978.
95. Gottdiener JS, Gross HA, Henry WL, Borer JS, Ebert MH: Effects of self-induced starvation on cardiac size and function in anorexia nervosa. Circulation 58:425, 1978.
96. DeFronzo RA, Cooke CR, Andres R, Faloona GR, Davis PJ: The effect of insulin on renal handling of sodium, potassium, calcium, and phosphate in man. J Clin Invest 55:845, 1975.
97. Corredor DG, Sabeh G, Mendelsohn LV, Wasserman RE, Sunder JH, Danowski TS: Enhanced postglucose hypophosphatemia during starvation therapy of obesity. Metabolism 18:754, 1969.
98. Rudman D, Millikan WJ, Richardson TJ, Bixler TJ 2d, Stackhouse J, McGarrity WC: Elemental balances during intravenous hyperalimentation of underweight adult subjects. J Clin Invest 55:94, 1975.
99. Silvis SE, DiBartolomeo AG, Aaker HM: Hypophosphatemia and neurological changes secondary to oral caloric intake: A variant of hyperalimentation syndrome. Am J Gastroenterol 73:215, 1980.
100. Hayek ME, Eisenberg PG: Severe hypophosphatemia following the institution of enteral feedings. Arch Surg 124:1325, 1989.
101. DeFronzo RA, Soman V, Sherwin RS, Hendler R, Felig P: Insulin binding to monocytes and insulin action in human obesity, starvation, and refeeding. J Clin Invest 62:204, 1978.
102. Wyrick WJ Jr, Rea WJ, McClelland RN: Rare complications with intravenous hyperosmotic alimentation. JAMA 211:1697, 1970.
103. Mattioli S, Miglioli M, Montagna P, Lerro MF, Pilotti V, Gozzetti G: Wernicke's encephalopathy during total parenteral nutrition: Observation in one case. JPEN 12:626, 1988.
104. Roediger WEW: Metabolic basis of starvation diarrhea: Implications for treatment. Lancet 1:1082, 1986.
105. Vazquez JA, Morse EL, Adibi SA: Effect of starvation on amino acid and peptide transport and peptide hydrolysis in humans. Am J Physiol 249:G563, 1985.
106. Behar M, Viteri F, Bressani R, Arroyave G, Squibb RL, Scrimshaw NS: Principles of treatment and prevention of severe protein malnutrition in children (Kwashiokor). Ann NY Acad Sci 69:954, 1957.
107. Isner JM, Roberts WC, Heymsfield SB, Yager J: Anorexia nervosa and sudden death. Ann Intern Med 102:49, 1985.
108. Saunders DR, Saunders MD, Sillery JK: Beneficial effects of glucose polymer and an receptor blocker in a patient with a proximal ileostomy. Am J Gastroenterol 84:192, 1989.
109. Cooper JC, Williams NS, King RF, Barker MC: Effects of long-acting somatostatin analogue in patients with severe ileostomy diarrhoea. Br J Surg 73:128, 1986.
110. Ladefoged K, Christensen KC, Hegnhj J, Jarnum S: Effect of a long-acting somatostatin analogue SMS 201–995 on jejunostomy effluents in patients with severe short bowel syndrome. Gut 30:943, 1989.

111. O'Keefe SJ, Burnes JU, Peterson ME: Octreotide in the long-term management of HPN patients with massive stomal losses of fluid and electrolytes [abstract]. Gastroenterology 100:A540, 1991.
112. Witt K, Pedersen NT: The long-acting somatostatin analogue SMS 201–995 causes malabsorption. Scand J Gastroenterol: 24:1248, 1989.
113. Fisher RS, Rock E, Levin G, Malmud L: Effect of somatostatin on gallbladder emptying. Gastroenterology 92:885, 1987.
114. O'Keefe SJ, Haymond MW, Bennet WM, et al: Long-acting somatostatin analogue therapy and protein metabolism in patients with jejunostomies. Gastroenterology 107:379, 1994.
115. Arrigoni E, Marteau P, Briet F, et al: Tolerance and absorption of lactose from milk and yogurt during short-bowel syndrome in humans. Am J Clin Nutr 60:926, 1994.
116. Edes TE, Walk BE, Austin JL: Diarrhea in tube-fed patients: Feeding formula not necessarily the cause. Am J Med 88:91, 1990.
117. Cosnes J, Gend JP, Evard D, LeQuintrec Y: Compensatory enteral hyperalimentation for management of patients with severe short bowel syndrome. Am J Clin Nutr 41:1002, 1985.
118. Woolf GM, Miller C, Kurian R, Jeejeebhoy KN: Diet for patients with a short bowel: High fat or high carbohydrate? Gastroenterology 84: 823, 1983.
119. Woolf GM, Miller C, Kurian R, Jeejeebhoy KN: Nutritional absorption in short bowel syndrome: Evaluation of fluid, caloric, and divalent cation requirements. Dig Dis Sci 32:8, 1987.
120. McIntyre PB, Fitchew M, Lennard-Jones JE: Patients with a high jejunostomy do not need a special diet. Gastroenterology 91:25, 1986.
121. Andersson H, Isaksson B, Sjogren B: FAt-reduced diet in the symptomatic treatment of small bowel disease. Gut 15:351, 1974.
122. Andersson H, Jagenburg R: Fat-reduced diet in the treatment of hyperoxaluria in patients with ileopathy. Gut 15:360, 1974.
123. Greenberger NJ, Skillman TG: Medium-chain triglycerides. N Engl J Med 280:1045, 1969.
124. Cosnes J, Evard D, Beaugerie L, et al: Improvement in protein absorption with small-peptide–based diet in patients with high jejunostomy. Nutrition 8:406, 1992.
125. Pizarro D, Posada G, Sandi L, Moran JR: Rice-based oral electrolyte solutions for the management of infantile diarrhea. N Engl J Med 324: 517, 1991.
126. Schultz SG: Sodium-coupled solute transport of small intestine: A status report. Am J Physiol 233:E249, 1977.
127. Fordtran JS: Stimulation of active and passive sodium absorption by sugars in the human jejunum. J Clin Invest 55:728, 1975.
128. Lennard-Jones JE: Oral rehydration solutions in short bowel syndrome. Clin Ther 12:129, 1990.
129. Griffin GE, Hodgson EF, Chadwick VS: Enteral therapy in the management of massive gut resection complicated by chronic floid and electrolyte depletion. Dig Dis Sci 27:902, 1991.
130. Laustsen J, Fallingborg J: Enteral glucose-polymer-electrolyte solution in the treatment of chronic fluid and electrolyte depletion in short-bowel syndrome. Acta Chir Scand 149:787, 1983.
131. MacMahon RA: The use of the World Health Organization's oral rehydration solution in patients on home parenteral nutrition. JPEN 8: 720, 1984.
132. Fine KD, Santa Ana CA, Porter JL, Fordtran JS: Intestinal absorption of magnesium from food and supplements. J Clin Invest 88:396, 1991.
133. Rude RK, Singer FR: Magnesium deficiency and excess. Annu Rev Med 32:245, 1981.
134. Nicar MJ, Pak CY: Calcium bioavailability from calcium carbonate and calcium citrate. J Clin Endocrinol Metab. 61:391, 1985.
135. Patton MB, Sutton TS: Utilization of calcium from lactate, gluconate, sulfate and carbonate salts by young college women. J Nutr 48:443, 1952.
136. Recker RR: Calcium absorption and achlorhydria. N Engl J Med 313: 70, 1985.
137. Brewer GJ, Ellis F, Bjork L: Parenteral depot method for zinc administration. Pharmacology 23:254, 1981.
138. Wohman SL, Anderson GH, Marliss EB, Jeejeebhoy KN: Zinc in total parenteral nutrition: Requirements and metabolic effects. Gastroenterology 76:458, 1979.
139. Hoffman HN, Phyliky RL, Fleming CR: Zinc-induced copper deficiency, Gastroenterology 94:508, 1988.

Chapter 16

ENTERAL AND PARENTERAL NUTRITION

Samuel Klein and Deborah C. Rubin

An understanding of the basic principles of clinical nutrition is important for the management of patients with diseases of the gastrointestinal tract. Patients who have gastrointestinal diseases are prone to develop nutritional abnormalities because the major function of the gastrointestinal tract, to process and absorb nutrients, is impaired. In addition, anorexia, dietary restrictions, medications, increased intestinal losses, and altered nutrient requirements can compromise nutritional status. Advances made during the last three decades have made it possible to feed all patients who are unable or unwilling to ingest and absorb an adequate amount of nutrients. In this chapter, the physiologic and clinical principles of providing enteral and parenteral nutrition and the clinical efficacy of nutrition support in patients with gastrointestinal diseases is reviewed.

ENTERAL NUTRITION

Principles of Enteral Feeding

It is generally accepted that, whenever possible, enteral rather than parenteral feeding should be used in patients who need nutritional support. Enteral nutrition has many advantages compared with parenteral nutrition. First, enteral nutritional therapy is probably associated with fewer serious complications. Second, enteral nutrition can supply gut-preferred fuels—glutamine, glutamate, and short-chain fatty acids—that are absent from commercially available parenteral formulations. Third, nutrients are needed in the intestinal lumen to maintain the structural and functional integrity of the gastrointestinal tract. Parenteral feeding without oral or enteral intake for more than 1 month produces mucosal atrophy.[1] Enteral feeding prevents atrophy of intestinal mucosa and the pancreas,[2, 3] maintains mucosal protein and deoxyribonucleic acid concentrations,[4] preserves mucosal[5] and pancreatic[6] digestive enzyme function, and maintains gastrointestinal IgA secretion.[7] Fourth, enteral feeding prevents cholelithiasis by stimulating gallbladder motility.[8] Finally, enteral nutrition is probably less expensive than parenteral nutrition.

In some patients, enteral feedings are either contraindicated or cannot be provided in sufficient quantities to meet nutritional requirements. The intestinal tract cannot be used effectively in some patients who have persistent nausea or vomiting, intolerable postprandial abdominal pain or diarrhea, mechanical obstruction, severe ileus, severe malabsorption, or high-output fistulas. These patients can receive adequate feeding only by parenteral nutrition. Some patients have a functional gastrointestinal tract but are unable to eat enough to meet their nutritional needs because of anorexia associated with medications, illness, or depression. These patients often can be managed with dietary modifications, appropriate liquid formula supplementation, and successful treatment of the primary disease. Another subset of patients has a functional gastrointestinal tract but cannot eat safely because of impaired consciousness or an inability to swallow. These patients may benefit from tube feedings.

Feeding Regimens

A wide variety of available feeding regimens can be tailored to each patient's clinical condition and particular nutrient requirements. These regimens can be classified into three general categories: whole food diets, defined liquid formulas, and oral rehydration therapy (see also Chapters 87 and 88).

WHOLE FOOD DIETS. Whole food diets include a standard regular diet and modified oral diets. Modified diets are altered in either consistency or nutrient content to meet specific patient requirements (Table 16–1). Diets modified in consistency include clear liquid, full liquid, purėed, and soft diets. Diets with modifications in nutrients include those with nutrient restrictions, such as low-residue, low-fat, low-sodium, and low-protein diets, and those with increased dietary components, such as a high-fiber diet.

DEFINED LIQUID FORMULAS. Defined liquid formulas are commercially made products with a known or "defined" nutrient composition. These formulas can be divided into five categories: feeding modules, monomeric formulas, oligo-

Table 16–1 | **Characteristics of Hospital Diets Modified in Nutrients and Consistency**

DIET	CHARACTERISTICS
Modified in Nutrients	
Low-fiber/residue	Contains mainly eggs, tender meats, milk, white bread or rice, strained juices, cooked vegetables, and cooked or canned fruits. No raw vegetables, nuts, seeds, or skins allowed
High-fiber	Contains total daily fiber intake of more than 20 g/day by increasing the intake of whole grains and raw fruits and vegetables. Additional fluid intake required to maintain soft stools
Low-fat	Restricts all forms of fat to < 50 g/day
Low-sodium	Restricts sodium to < 2000 mg/day
Low-protein	Restricts protein to < 60 g/day or <0.8 g/kg body weight. A low-protein diet often cannot meet all nutrient needs when protein is limited to ≤40 g/day, so vitamin and mineral supplementation is required
Modified in Consistency	
Clear liquid	Contains clear juices, broth, gelatin desserts, and popsicles
Full liquid	Contains cream soups, milk, and ice cream. This diet contains lactose and is often high in fat
Puréed	Contains foods blended to babyfood consistency. Often used for patients with dysphagia
Mechanical soft	Contains ground meat with gravy, soft-cooked vegetables, and canned fruit. Often used for patients with poor dentition
Selected soft	Contains meat, fruit, and vegetables chopped into bite-size pieces. Often used for patients with dysphagia
Soft	Contains regular textured foods, omitting fresh fruits and vegetables

meric formulas, polymeric formulas, and disease-specific formulas.

Feeding modules consist of single nutrients like protein, carbohydrate, or fat. These modules can be used as a supplement for inadequate feedings or as part of a modular enteral system, in which several nutrient modules are combined to meet specific patient needs. Protein modules contain either intact protein, hydrolyzed protein, or crystalline amino acids. The most common sources of protein are casein and whey. Carbohydrate modules usually consist of glucose polymers (also referred to as maltodextrins, oligosaccharides, and polysaccharides), which are formed by limited hydrolysis of starch. Carbohydrate modules are generally inexpensive and water soluble, readily mixing with other formulas or foods. Fat modules include formulas consisting of either long-chain triglycerides (LCTs), which contain fatty acids that are more than 12 carbons in length, or medium-chain triglycerides (MCTs), which are 6 to 12 carbons in length. The fat sources for LCTs are safflower and soybean oil, whereas MCTs are derived from coconut oil.

Medium-chain triglycerides have several advantages over LCTs.[9] The use of MCTs can be beneficial in patients who have disorders of fat digestion (e.g., pancreatic insufficiency, biliary obstruction), fat absorption (e.g., celiac sprue, short bowel syndrome), lipid transport (e.g., intestinal lymphangiectasia, abetalipoproteinemia), or in those who require a reduction in lymphatic flow (e.g., chylous ascites, thoracic duct fistula). MCTs are hydrolyzed more rapidly and more completely in the small intestine than LCTs, do not require bile acids for absorption, and can be absorbed as an intact triglyceride molecule, which is then hydrolyzed in gut epithelium. Medium-chain fatty acids are water soluble and are released into the portal vein after absorption; medium-chain fatty acids do not require reesterification, chylomicron formation, or lymphatic transport as do long-chain fatty acids. In the liver, medium-chain fatty acids can cross the mitochondrial membrane rapidly without carnitine and are readily oxidized.

MCTs also have several disadvantages.[9] The MCTs lack linoleic and linolenic acids, so that small amounts of LCTs are still needed to prevent essential fatty acid deficiency. MCTs are more ketogenic than LCTs and should not be given to patients with diabetes, ketosis, or acidosis. The use of MCTs is also contraindicated in patients with cirrhosis, particularly those with portal systemic shunts. The reduction in hepatic metabolism when functional liver mass is reduced can cause elevated serum levels of octanoate and possible neurologic toxicity.[10] Finally, MCTs can cause adverse gastrointestinal symptoms like nausea, vomiting, and diarrhea,[11] which often limit the maximum amount tolerated to approximately 500 kcal per day.

Monomeric formulas, also known as "elemental" diets, contain nitrogen in the form of free amino acids, carbohydrates as glucose polymers, and minimal amounts of fat as LCTs, usually accounting for 3% or less of total calories (Table 16–2). Because monomeric formulas require minimal digestive function for absorption, they have been recommended for use in patients who have a variety of gastrointestinal diseases. However, dipeptides and tripeptides are absorbed more efficiently than are free amino acids,[12] and balance studies have found that in the absence of pancreatic insufficiency, nutrient absorption from monomeric formulas is no better than from oligomeric or polymeric formula feedings.[13, 14] Furthermore, careful analysis of the use of "elemental" diets has refuted many of the purported clinical benefits.[15]

Monomeric formulas have several disadvantages. The presence of free amino acids and limited fat content make these preparations hyperosmolar and unpalatable. Monomeric formulas require flavoring supplements when given orally, and a feeding tube is often necessary to achieve dietary compliance. Monomeric preparations are also expensive, often more than five times the cost of polymeric formulas.

Oligomeric formulas are also known as "semi-elemental" diets (see Table 16–2). The protein present in these formulas consists of hydrolyzed casein, whey, or lactalbumin, containing different lengths of small peptides and, in some formulas, free amino acids. These formulas also include carbohydrate in the form of simple sugars, glucose polymers, or starch, and fat as either LCTs or a combination of LCTs and MCTs. The osmolality of oligomeric formulas varies considerably and is inversely related to fat content. Oligomeric formulas have been purported to be better absorbed and tolerated than are monomeric and polymeric formulas in patients who have impaired intestinal function. The theoreti-

Table 16–2 | **Composition of Selected Monomeric, Oligomeric, and Polymeric Defined Enteral Formulas**

	CALORIE CONTENT (kcal/mL)	OSMOLALITY (mOsm/kg)	PROTEIN g/L (% kcal)	CARBOHYDRATE g/L (% kcal)	FAT g/L (% kcal)	REPRESENTATIVE PRODUCTS
Monomeric formulas	1.0	550–630	21–36 (8–15)	210–230 (82–91)	2–3 (1–3)	Tolerex Vinonex T.E.N.
Oligomeric formulas	1.0–1.5	300–650	30–94 (13–25)	127–221 (36–82)	5–68 (5–39)	Alitraq Criticare HN Optimental Peptamen Reabilan Subdue Travasorb HN Travasorb STD Vital HN Vivonex Plus
Polymeric formulas:						
Blenderized	1.0–1.07	300–450	40–43 (12–25)	128–135 (48–53)	37–40 (31–40)	Compleat Modified Compleat Regular
Milk-based, breakfast	1.0–2.0	510–1130	40–110 (12–25)	87–307 (51–64)	10–50 (10–30)	Carnation Instant Forta Shake Great shakes Mighty shake Scandi shake
Lactose-free:						
Normal calorie	1.0–1.2	300–520	34–60 (13–19)	127–169 (50–57)	35–45 (29–37)	Attain Ensure Isocal Isosource Nutren 1.0 Nu Basics Boost Osmolite Resource
Normal calorie, high-nitrogen	1.0	300–610	45–63 (17–25)	113–144 (46–54)	26–45 (24–37)	Boost HP Ensure HN Isosource HN VHN NuBasics VHP Osmolite HN Promote Replete
High-calorie, high-nitrogen	1.5–2.0	430–720	53–83 (14–17)	170–250 (39–53)	50–106 (30–45)	Boost Plus Comply Ensure Plus Ensure Plus HN Isosource 1.5 Magnacal NovaSource 2.0 Nubasics Plus/2.0 Nutren 1.5/2.0 Resource Plus Sustacal Plus TwoCal HN Ultracal HN/Plus
Low-fat/fat-free	0.7–0.8	480–700	37–41 (20–25)	120–152 (73–80)	0–2 (0–2)	Citrosource Citrotein Enlive Resource
Fiber-enriched	1.0–1.2	300–520	40–54 (15–18)	127–147 (51–54)	35–42 (30–37)	Boost with fiber Ensure/fiber Fibersource/ HN Jevity/Jevity Plus Nubasics with fiber Nutren with fiber Probalance Profiber Promote with fiber Replete with fiber Sustacal with fiber Ultracal

cal advantage of oligomeric formulas is related to the absorption of dipeptides and tripeptides, which have specific transport mechanisms for their intact uptake and are absorbed more efficiently than are amino acids or whole protein. However, protein hydrolysates in currently available oligomeric formulas are made enzymatically, producing many oligopeptides that are more than 3 amino acids in length.

The potential benefits of oligomeric compared with polymeric formula feeding by improving nutrient absorption have been evaluated in several studies. Two prospective trials, using a randomized cross-over design, have evaluated the use of oligomeric formulas in patients with a jejunostomy and less than 150 cm of residual small bowel.[16, 17] McIntyre and colleagues[16] found no difference in nitrogen or total calorie absorption between polymeric and oligomeric diets. In contrast, Cosnes and coworkers[17] found that nitrogen absorption was greater when patients consumed a peptide-based diet than a diet containing whole proteins. However, it is not known whether the increase in nitrogen absorption led to an improvement in protein metabolism or nitrogen balance, because these parameters were not measured. Blood urea nitrogen and urinary urea excretion were greater during peptide-based diet feeding than during whole protein diet ingestion, suggesting that the absorption of additional amino acids stimulated amino acid oxidation. In pancreatectomized patients, nitrogen absorption was better from a hydrolyzed protein diet than from an intact protein diet.[18] However, the benefit of an oligomeric diet over the more standard practice of giving pancreatic enzymes was not evaluated. Data from several reports involving small numbers of patients have suggested that oligomeric diets may be effective in reducing diarrhea and other gastrointestinal side effects in critically ill patients[19] and in patients receiving cytotoxic therapy, such as abdominal irradiation and chemotherapy.[20, 21] Further studies are required to confirm these potential benefits.

At present, the appropriate indications for feeding with oligomeric formulas are unknown and their theoretical advantages have not been shown to be clinically important. Because they are more expensive than polymeric formulas, oligomeric formulas require further evaluation in prospective, randomized trials before precise recommendations regarding their use can be made.

Polymeric formulas contain nitrogen in the form of whole proteins, carbohydrate as glucose polymers, and lipid as LCTs or a mixture of LCTs and MCTs (see Table 16–2). These formulas can be used as a dietary supplement to increase nutrient intake, or they can meet complete calorie, protein, essential fatty acid, vitamin, and mineral requirements if given in appropriate quantities. Taste preference in patients being fed orally, individual patient requirements, and tolerance determine which formula should be used in each patient. Polymeric formulas can be categorized into three groups: blenderized food formulas, milk-based formulas, and lactose-free formulas.

Blenderized food formulas contain beef and milk as a protein source; cereal, fruits, and vegetables as a carbohydrate source; and beef purée, corn oil, and soy oil as a fat source. They help prevent constipation in patients requiring long-term enteral feeding because of their higher fiber content (4 to 8 g/L) compared with most other formulas. In patients who require tube feeding, a large-bore feeding tube is required for delivery because of poor palatability and high viscosity.

Milk-based formulas usually contain milk as a source of protein and fat, and milk with additional corn syrup solids and sucrose as a source of carbohydrate. These formulas tend to be more palatable than those of other defined diets and can be taken orally. Although milk-based formulas are not recommended for lactose-intolerant patients, they can be well tolerated when given as a continuous infusion, which diffuses the load of lactose delivered to the intestine over time. Milk-based formulas are hyperosmolar and contain a considerable amount of protein.

Lactose-free formulas, the most commonly used polymeric formulas for hospitalized patients, usually contain casein and soy as a source of protein; corn syrup solids, hydrolyzed corn starch, glucose polymers, and sucrose as a source of carbohydrate; and corn oil, soy oil, and MCT oil as a source of fat (see Table 16–2). Fiber is not present in most lactose-free formulas, but fiber-enriched products contain between 5 and 15 grams of fiber, as soy polysaccharides, per liter.

Disease-specific formulas have been designed for patients who have specific illnesses, including hepatic insufficiency, renal insufficiency, pulmonary insufficiency, diabetes, and critical illness. In general, the clinical superiority of these formulas over less expensive, standard polymeric enteral formulas remains controversial.

ORAL REHYDRATION THERAPY. The principle of oral rehydration therapy is to stimulate sodium and water absorption by taking advantage of the sodium-glucose cotransporter present in the brush border of intestinal epithelium. Glucose enhances sodium absorption by an active carrier and water absorption by solvent drag. This carrier process is often preserved during diarrheal illnesses, thereby providing a mechanism for oral sodium and fluid replacement. Oral rehydration therapy has demonstrated profound benefits in treating patients with cholera-induced diarrhea[22] and has become a life-saving measure in developing nations where children frequently die from diarrheal illnesses. Oral rehydration therapy may also aid patients with severe gastrointestinal fluid and mineral losses, such as those with high-output ostomies, short-bowel syndrome and HIV infection.[23, 24] The characteristics of selected oral rehydration solutions are shown in Table 16–3 (see also Chapter 87).

The composition of an ideal oral rehydration formula is controversial. There is debate concerning the type of carbohydrate that should be used and the appropriate concentration of sodium, potassium, chloride, and base. Glucose is the most commonly used substrate and should be provided at concentrations of between 70 and 150 mmol per liter. Higher concentrations of glucose can be deleterious because the increase in osmolality may reduce water absorption. Isotonic glucose-based oral rehydration therapy usually does not diminish the severity of diarrhea because it does not promote reabsorption of secreted fluids. Replacement of glucose with polymeric forms of carbohydrate, such as rice syrup solids, provides a hypotonic solution that is superior to a glucose-based solution in decreasing stool output.[25, 26]

The appropriate concentration of sodium depends on the clinical circumstances. A sodium concentration of 90 mmol/L

Table 16–3 | **Characteristics of Selected Oral Rehydration Solutions**

PRODUCT	Na (mEq/L)	K (mEq/L)	Cl (mEq/L)	CITRATE (mEq/L)	Calories (kcal/L)	CHO (g/L)	Osmolarity (mOsm/L)
Equalyte	78	22	68	1900 mg	100	25	305
CeraLyte 70	70	20	98	30	165	40	235
CeraLyte 90	90	20	98	30	165	40	260
Pedialyte	45	20	35	30	100	20	300
Rehydralyte	74	19	64	30	100	25	305
WHO*	90	20	80	30	80	20	200
Washington University†	105	0	100	10	85	20	250

***WHO (World Health Organization) formula:** Mix 3/4 tsp sodium chloride, 1/2 tsp sodium citrate, 1/4 tsp potassium chloride, and 4 tsp glucose (dextrose) in 1 L (4 1/4 cups) of distilled water.

†Washington University formula: Mix 3/4 tsp sodium chloride, 1/2 tsp sodium citrate, and 3 tbsp + 1 tsp Polycose powder in 1 L (4 1/4 cups) of distilled water. Mix with sugar-free flavorings as needed for palatability.

Na, sodium; K, potassium; Cl, chloride; kcal/L, kilocalories per liter; CHO, carbohydrate; mOsm/L, milliosmoles per liter.

in the World Health Organization (WHO) formula was based on balance studies in patients who had cholera. Solutions containing less than 90 mmol/L of sodium are more palatable than the WHO formula and may also be clinically effective because sodium loss in most diarrheal illnesses (~40 mmol/L during rotavirus infection)[27] is lower than in cholera (~90 mmol/L). Studies in humans have found that sodium absorption is maximal at a concentration of 120 mmol/L and it has been suggested that this higher concentration of sodium is optimal for patients who have severe short bowel syndrome and a large volume of intestinal output.[23]

The potassium concentration of most oral rehydration solutions is 20 mmol/L. This level of potassium is less than the concentrations present in the stool of many patients who have diarrhea.[27] Based on the disparity between formula and stool potassium content, it has been suggested that the concentration of potassium be increased to 30 or 35 mmol/L.[28]

Oral rehydration solutions usually contain bicarbonate or citrate because of their potential benefits in correcting metabolic acidosis and because of increased palatability compared with sodium chloride. Citrate is preferable to bicarbonate because it is more stable and equally efficacious in treating acidosis. The addition of base or base precursor is usually not necessary for managing acidosis because acidosis is often corrected by rehydration alone.

Gut-Preferred Fuels

GLUTAMINE. Glutamine, the most abundant amino acid in plasma and the intracellular amino acid pool of muscle, serves important functions in interorgan nitrogen transfer,[29] hepatic and renal glucose production,[30] and renal ammoniagenesis.[31] Glutamine is also an important metabolic substrate for rapidly replicating cells, such as gastrointestinal tract mucosa. It provides a source of nitrogen for nucleotide and protein synthesis and a source of energy for tissue oxidation.[32] The high intestinal activity of glutaminase, the enzyme necessary for glutamine metabolism, and the liver's ability to process portal vein ammonia, produced during intestinal glutamine metabolism, make the gastrointestinal tract well designed for glutamine utilization. More than half of ingested glutamine is sequestered by the splanchnic bed on the first pass.[33] Glutamine and glutamate are major intestinal fuels in the postabsorptive state. Studies performed in perfused rat intestine have found that approximately 25% of plasma glutamine is extracted with each pass, and it supplies a major portion of energy to the small intestine.[34]

Normally, glutamine accounts for approximately 8% of the amino acids present in dietary protein and in most defined liquid formulas. However, some commercially made formulas have been enriched with glutamine, and up to 30% of their amino acid content is present as free glutamine. Commercially made parenteral amino acid formulations do not contain glutamine because glutamine is a nonessential amino acid and is unstable in solution, generating ammonia and pyroglutamic acid. However, the safety of intravenously administered glutamine has been demonstrated when given as either free L-glutamine or as the more stable and soluble dipeptide form.[35] In healthy volunteers, the amount of free glutamine released by muscle exceeds the amount available from protein breakdown; glutamine produced by muscle depends largely on de novo glutamine synthesis.[36] During catabolic conditions, glutamine uptake by the intestine increases markedly, supplied in large part by an increase in glutamine release from skeletal muscle.[35] However, the rate of glutamine production by skeletal muscle cannot match the rate of glutamine uptake by the splanchnic bed, thereby causing a decrease in glutamine concentration in both plasma and muscle.[37] The close relationship between intracellular glutamine concentration and protein synthesis in skeletal muscle[38] suggests that glutamine repletion during catabolic states could increase muscle protein synthesis and nitrogen balance. In humans, postoperative intravenous glutamine supplementation has been shown to reduce the decline in plasma and skeletal muscle glutamine concentration, the decrease in muscle polyribosome content (an index of protein synthesis), and the magnitude of negative nitrogen balance.[39, 40] In contrast, a 4-hour intravenous glutamine infusion did not alter intramuscular glutamine concentrations or stimulate muscle protein synthesis in burned patients.[41] The discrepancy between studies may be related to differences in the severity of illness and the duration of glutamine administration.

The results from several studies suggest that glutamine supplementation can improve gastrointestinal tract structure and function. When plasma glutamine is experimentally reduced to undetectable levels, intestinal atrophy, ulcerations, and necrosis occur.[42] Furthermore, data from studies performed in rats suggest that intestinal atrophy and pancreatic atrophy associated with defined formula diets and total parenteral nutrition are attenuated by glutamine supplementation.[43, 44] However, other investigators were unable to demonstrate reversal of small bowel atrophy.[45, 46] In animal studies, glutamine supplementation has been found to enhance the intestinal adaptive response to massive intestinal resection[47] and decrease intestinal damage from cytotoxic therapy such as 5-fluorouracil/calcium folinate, when given parenterally,[48] methotrexate,[49] and abdominal irradiation.[50] In humans, the use of glutamine dipeptides attenuated the alterations in villus height and intestinal permeability observed after standard parenteral nutrition[51] and nonsteroidal anti-inflammatory drug therapy.[52] Parenteral nutrition supplemented with glutamine improved D-xylose absorption in critically ill patients[53] but not in stable patients receiving home parenteral nutrition.[54] The potential clinical benefits of glutamine supplementation in patients with severe metabolic stress, intestinal mucosal injury, or gastrointestinal diseases, and its potential toxicity, require further study.

Intravenous glutamine has also been used in conjunction with growth hormone and dietary manipulation to enhance intestinal adaptation in patients with short bowel syndrome. The efficacy of this treatment regimen is still unclear,[55–58] and it has been suggested that intensive dietary counseling rather than the use of glutamine and growth hormone resulted in reduction or discontinuation of parenteral nutrition in these patients.[59]

SHORT-CHAIN FATTY ACIDS. Short-chain fatty acids (SCFAs) are organic acids containing 1 to 6 carbon atoms. The predominant SCFAs in humans are acetate, propionate, and butyrate. They are produced primarily in the colon as a by-product of bacterial fermentation of undigested carbohydrates. Normally, about 90% of the 25 g of unabsorbed carbohydrates that enter the colon each day are metabolized to SCFAs and absorbed.[60] The colon can salvage as much as 500 kcal of unabsorbed carbohydrate daily by converting them to SCFAs. This process may become particularly important for recapturing lost calories in patients who have malabsorptive disorders.[61]

Short-chain fatty acids, particularly butyrate, are an important source of fuel for colonic mucosa and provide 60% to 70% of the colon's energy needs. Therefore, factors that interfere with SCFA oxidation by the colon can have adverse effects on colonic epithelial cell nutriture and function. For example, reducing fiber intake by ingesting an elemental diet causes colonic intestinal cell atrophy.[62] More extreme restrictions in SCFA metabolism by diversion of the intestinal contents from the colon or by directly inhibiting colonic SCFA oxidation, cause colitis.[63, 64] In one study, diversion colitis in humans was successfully treated by local infusion of SCFAs.[65] However, this beneficial effect could not be reproduced in subsequent studies.[66, 67]

Colonic oxidation of butyrate is decreased in patients with active ulcerative colitis.[68, 69] However, butyrate oxidation normalizes after remission is achieved, suggesting that there is no primary defect in butyrate metabolism. The use of SCFA enemas as treatment for active left-sided ulcerative colitis has been disappointing; most studies have not shown a beneficial effect or have been inconclusive.[70–73]

SCFAs that are absorbed but not oxidized by colonic epithelium enter the portal circulation and are delivered to the liver. In the liver, they can be completely oxidized for fuel, they can provide precursors for ketone bodies, glutamate, or glucose production, or they can be transported to other tissues and metabolized peripherally. Acetate, which is also produced by long-chain fatty acid oxidation in the liver, is the predominant SCFA used for interorgan energy transport; it supplies approximately 10% of daily energy needs in humans.[74]

SCFAs are also involved in regulating electrolyte and water absorption in the colon (see Chapter 87). Absorption of SCFAs is coupled with sodium-proton exchange and increases colonocyte sodium and water influx.[75] It has been hypothesized that diarrhea associated with antibiotic use[76] and abdominal surgery[77] may be related to cellular energy deficits and impaired sodium absorption caused by SCFA deficiency. The addition of fiber to liquid formula diets has been shown to restore colonic SCFA concentrations to normal and reduce the frequency of liquid stools.[78] However, excessive excretion of SCFAs can cause osmotic diarrhea with an obligatory loss of approximately 3.5 g of water for each millimole of fecal organic acid.[60]

Tube Feeding

Feeding through tubes placed in the intestine is useful for providing nutritional support in patients who cannot or will not eat but who have a functional gastrointestinal tract. Nasogastric, nasoduodenal, nasojejunal, gastrostomy, jejunostomy, pharyngostomy, and esophagostomy tubes have been used successfully for feeding. Most transnasal tubes are placed so that their tips rest either in the distal stomach or duodenum. In addition, there are surgically placed tubes that provide both gastric decompression ports and jejunum feeding channels for the patient in whom postoperative gastric stasis is suspected. The choice of access to the intestinal tract for enteral nutrition is directed by several factors, including clinical prognosis, anticipated duration of feeding, patency and motility of the gut, risk of aspirating gastric contents, and patient preference.

SHORT-TERM TUBE FEEDING. The placement of a soft, small-diameter nasogastric tube is the simplest technique for tube feeding in patients who have short-term (<4 weeks) nutritional needs. Most tubes are made of silicone or polyurethane and contain weighted tips and insertion stylets to ease placement.

LONG-TERM TUBE FEEDING. Gastrostomy tubes represent the most common method for enteral nutrition support in patients who are expected to require tube feeding for more than 4 weeks. These tubes can usually be placed radiologically or endoscopically, but they may require surgical placement in selected patients. *Percutaneous endoscopic gastrostomy* (PEG)[79] or *radiologic percutaneous gastrostomy* (RPG) has replaced surgical gastrostomy in most settings. Most candidates have permanent neurologic disease or head and neck cancers. Push (Fig. 16–1) and pull (Fig. 16–2) techniques of insertion have been successfully completed in over 90% of attempts. There is no clear advantage of one technique over the other, although the push technique can be used in the setting of a partially obstructed esophagus because it reduces trauma to the hypopharynx and esophagus.[80] Another technique for PEG placement uses a catheter that is inserted percutaneously directly into the stomach via a peel-

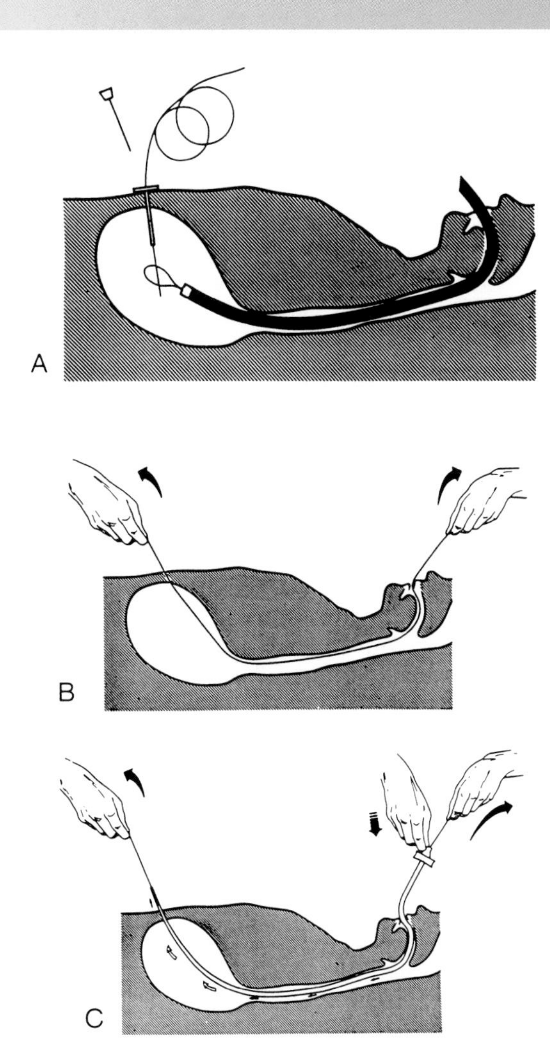

Figure 16–1. Push technique for percutaneous gastrostomy tube placement. *A,* The inner stylet is removed from a needle that was passed through the abdominal and gastric walls. A soft guidewire is threaded through the needle into the gastric lumen and grasped with an endoscopic snare. *B,* The endoscope is withdrawn, pulling the guidewire out through the patient's mouth. *C,* Tension is applied to both ends of the guidewire while the tapered introducing end of the gastrostomy tube is passed over the wire and pushed down into the stomach. The introducing end is grasped after it is pushed through the abdominal wall, and the remainder of the tube is pulled out until the inner bumper is in the appropriate position. (From Kelsey PB: Percutaneous endoscopic gastrostomy: The "push" technique. In Ponsky JL [ed]: Techniques of Percutaneous Gastrostomy. New York, Igaku-Shoin, 1988, pp 36–37.)

away sheath introduced over a previously placed J wire guide (Fig. 16–3).[81] This method requires only one passage of the endoscope. Once the gastrocutaneous fistula "matures" after PEG tube placement, a skin level "button" can replace the protruding tube. The button is easy to insert and offers greater comfort and improvement in self-image.

A review of several large series involving a total of over 1000 patients suggests that PEG tube placement is associated with mortality in 0.5%, major complications (peristomal leakage with peritonitis, necrotizing fasciitis of the anterior abdominal wall, and gastric hemorrhage) in 1%, and minor complications (minor wound infections, stomal leaks, tube extrusion or migration, aspiration, gastrocolic fistula, ileus, and fever) in 8% of patients.[82] A recent meta-analysis of seven published studies established that a single intravenous dose of a broad-spectrum antibiotic was effective in reducing the incidence of peristomal infections.[83] Gastric feeding through a PEG tube allows the option of continuous or intermittent nutrient administration because of the stomach's important function in regulating nutrient delivery to the small intestine. Conversion of PEGs to *percutaneous endoscopic gastrojejunostomies* (PEGJs) has been proposed to reduce reflux and aspiration. However, several studies have found that PEGJs are associated with higher rates of tube dysfunction (50% to 85%)[84, 85] and do not eliminate the risk of aspiration.[86, 87] In critically ill patients with major trauma, however, providing nutritional goals may be easier to achieve with PEGJ than PEG feedings.[88]

Radiologically placed percutaneous gastrostomy tubes provide an excellent alternative to PEG.[89, 90] The incidence

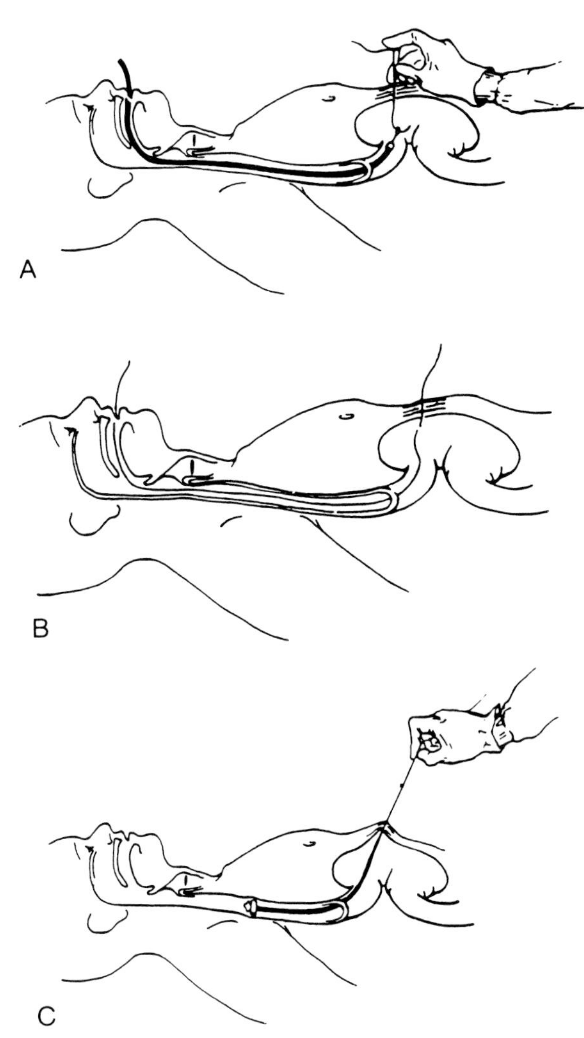

Figure 16–2. Pull technique for percutaneous gastrostomy tube placement. *A,* The inner stylet is removed from a large-bore needle catheter that was passed through the abdominal and gastric walls. A suture passed through the catheter is grasped with an endoscopic snare. *B,* The endoscope is withdrawn, pulling the suture out through the patient's mouth. *C,* The proximal end of the thread is tied to the tapered end of the gastrostomy tube. The thread and tapered end of the gastrostomy tube are then pulled through the esophagus and stomach and out the abdominal wall until the mushroom tip and crosspiece are in the appropriate position. (From Clouse RE, Rosenberg IH: Intensive nutritional support. In Sleisenger MH, Fordtran JS [eds]: Gastrointestinal Disease, 4th ed. Philadelphia, WB Saunders, 1989, p 2007.)

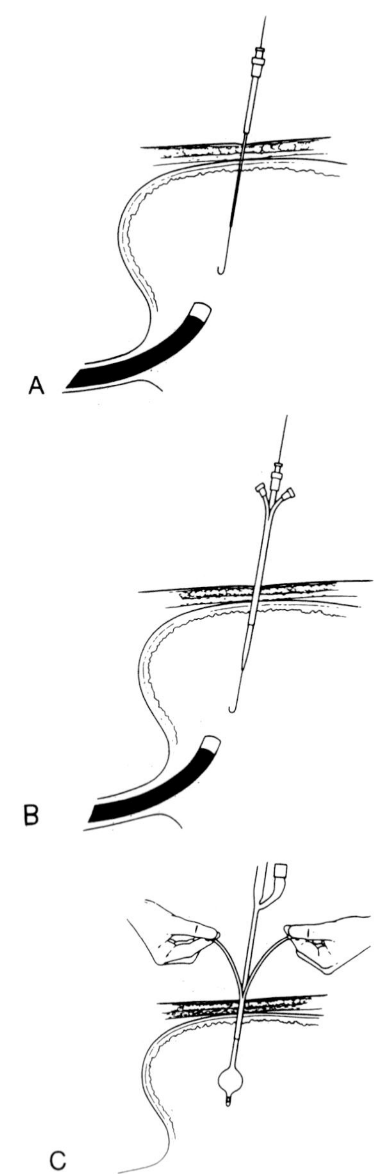

Figure 16–3. Introducer technique for percutaneous gastrostomy tube placement. *A*, A J-tipped guidewire is inserted into the gastric lumen through a needle that has been passed through the abdominal and gastric walls. *B*, The needle is removed and a peel-away introducer sheath with an inner dilator is threaded over the guidewire. *C*, The wire and dilator are removed, leaving the sheath in place. A Foley catheter is inserted through the sheath into the lumen of the stomach, and the catheter balloon is inflated with saline solution. Traction is applied until the balloon is apposed to the gastric wall, and the introducer sheath is peeled away. (From Kummer BA: Percutaneous endoscopic gastrostomy: The "Introducer" technique. In Ponsky JL [ed]: Techniques of Percutaneous Gastrostomy. New York, Igaku–Shoin, 1988, pp 42–46.)

of major and minor complications associated with RPG are similar to those of PEG. A radiologic approach for tube placement may be preferable in the presence of esophageal obstruction or other anatomic features that preclude a peroral approach. A recent comparison of RPG and PEG showed a slightly higher success rate for RPG tubes, but placement of PEG tubes was quicker, cost less, and required less tube maintenance.[84]

Other Tube Enterostomies. Surgical jejunostomies placed at the time of laparotomy consist of a subserosa tunnel (Witzel) or needle catheter jejunostomy. For the needle catheter jejunostomy, a 16-gauge polyvinyl catheter is passed through the antimesenteric border of the jejunum, 15 cm distal to the ligament of Treitz, or surgical anastomosis using techniques similar to subclavian vein catheterization.[91] A percutaneous endoscopic jejunostomy can be placed safely in patients with previous partial or total gastrotomy.[92] Laparoscopic techniques for gastrostomy and jejunostomy tube placement are available, but the optimal indication for these remains to be determined.

DELIVERY SYSTEMS. The method of nutrient delivery varies with the location of the tube. In patients with a jejunostomy, continuous feeding is preferable because bolus feeding usually creates dumping symptoms. For most patients using gastrostomies, nutritional goals can be achieved with intermittent gravity feedings. The total quantity of formula needed for a 24-hour period is divided into equal portions, and the required fractions are administered among four to six feedings. Each feeding is administered by gravity over 30 to 40 minutes. Advantages of intermittent gravity feedings include minimal equipment needs and the ability to free patients from the feedings during most of the day. Some patients with a gastrostomy experience nausea and early satiety with gravity feedings and feel better with continuous infusion of the liquid formulas at a slower rate.

COMPLICATIONS. The complications in patients receiving tube feedings can be divided into four categories: mechanical, metabolic, gastrointestinal, and pulmonary (aspiration).

Mechanical Complications. Nasogastric feeding tube misplacement occurs more commonly in unconscious than conscious patients. Intubation of the tracheobronchial tree has been reported in up to 15% of patients; intracranial placement can occur in patients with skull fractures. Erosive tissue damage can lead to nasopharyngeal erosions, pharyngitis, sinusitis, otitis media, pneumothorax, and gastrointestinal tract perforation. Tube occlusion is often caused by inspissated feedings or pulverized medications given through small-diameter (<10 French) tubes. Frequent flushing of the tube with 30 to 60 mL of water and avoiding administration of pill fragments or "thick" medications help prevent occlusion. Techniques used to unclog tubes include the use of a small-volume syringe (10 mL) to flush warm water or pancreatic enzymes (Viokase dissolved in water) through the tube. Commercially made products can be obtained that either dissolve or mechanically remove the obstruction.

Metabolic Complications. Disturbances in fluid and electrolytes are common in patients receiving tube feedings. In one study of 100 patients, 30% to 40% had at least one metabolic complication, with hypokalemia, hyponatremia, hypophosphatemia, and hyperglycemia being the most common.[93]

Gastrointestinal Complications. Gastrointestinal side effects of tube feeding include nausea and vomiting, abdominal pain, and diarrhea. Nonocclusive bowel necrosis has been reported in 0.3% of critically ill patients given tube feedings, particularly those patients receiving vasoconstrictive medications to maintain blood pressure.[94] It is likely that the increased intestinal oxygen demand induced by feeding in the presence of compromised gastrointestinal blood flow is responsible for this adverse event.[94]

Diarrhea occurs in 30% to 50% of critically ill patients receiving tube feedings and has been shown to correlate most closely with antibiotic use.[95] Antibiotics cause pseudomembranous colitis or impaired conversion of carbohydrate to SCFAs (see Chapter 97). Another common source of osmotic diarrhea in tube-fed patients is the surprisingly large dose of the nonabsorbable carbohydrate sorbitol, given through the tube with common elixirs such as acetaminophen, theophylline, and cimetidine.[96] If diarrhea from tube feeding persists after proper attention to the usual causes, trials of antidiarrheal agents such as diphenoxylate or loperamide are justified in an effort to maintain adequate delivery of nutrients (see Chapter 9, Diarrhea).

Pulmonary Complications. The etiology of pulmonary aspiration can be difficult to determine in tube-fed patients because aspiration can occur from refluxed tube feedings or oropharyngeal secretions that are unrelated to feedings. Assessing the color of respiratory secretions after adding several drops of blue food coloring to the feeding formula can help determine whether tube feedings are contributing to recovered secretions. However, case reports have documented serious and life-threatening metabolic complications associated with blue food dye administration.[97, 98] Prevention of reflux and its damage by decreasing gastric acid secretion, keeping the head of the bed elevated during feedings, and avoiding gastric feeding in high-risk patients (e.g., those with gastroparesis, gastric outlet obstruction, or frequent vomiting) is the best approach[99] (see Chapter 33). Enteric feeding administered past the ligament of Treitz should decrease the risk of aspiration by taking advantage of the barrier function of the pyloric and gastroesophageal sphincters.[100]

Refeeding Syndrome. Inappropriate feeding of the severely malnourished patient can have adverse clinical consequences known as the "refeeding syndrome." This complication and the nutritional management of the severely malnourished patient are reviewed in Chapter 15.

PARENTERAL NUTRITION

The use of the vascular system to supply nutrient requirements can be an important and even life-saving therapy. Parenteral nutrition can be administered through a central vein—central parenteral nutrition (CPN), or a peripheral vein—peripheral parenteral nutrition (PPN). The purpose of initiating parenteral nutritional therapy is to prevent or correct specific nutrient deficiencies and to prevent the adverse effects of malnutrition when the gastrointestinal tract cannot be used effectively or safely. Although these indications appear simple and straightforward, in practice it is often difficult to determine which patients should receive intravenous feedings. The reason for the confusion is that the time period at which semistarvation or complete starvation becomes clinically harmful is not known. The duration of "tolerable starvation" is different for each patient, depending upon endogenous fuel (fat) and protein (muscle) stores, underlying disease, and concomitant medical therapy. Parenteral nutrition is often recommended if enteral intake has been, or is anticipated to be, inadequate for 7 to 10 days.[101] However, there is little evidence to support the clinical efficacy of this approach, and the definition of "inadequate intake" is not clear. Continued clinical studies are needed to establish criteria that can identify which patients have a high likelihood of benefiting from parenteral nutritional therapy.

Central Parenteral Nutrition

NUTRIENT SOLUTIONS. Parenteral solutions are available to supply all basic nutrient requirements, including fluid, protein, carbohydrate, fat, minerals, trace elements, and vitamins. Typically these components are given together as an admixture, which reduces handling costs and potential breaks in sterility, or the lipid component is given separately, piggybacked to the primary nutrient mixture.

Protein. The goal of providing amino acids is to maintain nitrogen balance and replete lean tissue in cachectic patients. The amount of protein necessary to achieve these goals is affected by the amount of nonprotein calories provided and the patient's clinical condition. Insufficient nonprotein calories, catabolic illness, protein-losing enteropathy or nephropathy, hemodialysis, and peritoneal dialysis increase protein requirements. Most hospitalized patients require between 0.8 and 1.5 g of protein per kg body weight per day.

Standard commercially made solutions are composed of crystalline amino acids in concentrations of between 2.75% and 15%. These solutions usually contain 40% to 50% essential and 50% to 60% nonessential amino acids. The proportion of nitrogen consisting of essential amino acids is more than twice that required by normal adults and increases amino acid biologic availability. Each product differs in its amino acid profile and in its electrolyte and trace mineral content, but it is not known whether these variations are clinically significant. Most formulas completely lack, or have very little of, the nonessential amino acids glutamine, glutamate, aspartate, asparaginine, tyrosine, and cysteine.

Modified parenteral amino acid solutions have been developed for specific disease states and physiologic conditions. Solutions containing high concentrations of branched-chain amino acids have been advocated for use in patients who have hepatic encephalopathy. In clinical trials evaluating these solutions, the branched-chain amino acids leucine, isoleucine, and valine constitute 35% to 45% of total amino acids, whereas in standard formulas they represent only approximately 20% of the total. The results from most studies suggest that these formulas are useful in achieving higher amino acid intakes (60 to 80 g/day) with less risk of encephalopathy than that of standard formulas.[102] Solutions containing large amounts of essential amino acids have been developed for patients who have acute renal failure. Between 67% and 100% of the total amino acids in these formulas are composed of the eight essential amino acids and histidine, which is believed to be essential in patients with renal failure. However, the superiority of administering essential amino acids as the sole source of nitrogen over solutions containing a mixture of essential and nonessential amino acids has not been demonstrated in prospective randomized trials.[103]

Carbohydrate. Carbohydrate in the form of dextrose (glucose) is a vital source of fuel and has important nitrogen-sparing effects. Certain tissues, such as erythrocytes, white blood cells, bone marrow, and renal medulla, require glucose

(~40 g/day) because they lack the enzymatic machinery to oxidize fatty acids, whereas other tissues, such as the brain, prefer glucose (~120 g/day) as a fuel but can use other substrates. Providing calories as glucose stimulates insulin secretion, reduces muscle protein breakdown, and inhibits hepatic glucose output, thereby eliminating the need for skeletal muscle protein to provide amino acid precursors for gluconeogenesis. In addition, direct oxidation of glucose spares the oxidation of amino acids.

The amount of infused glucose oxidized is directly proportional to the amount of glucose administered until a threshold level is reached. Infusing more than 7 mg/kg/min (~2800 kcal/day) in stable postoperative patients does not increase glucose oxidation but could have adverse consequences by increasing lipogenesis, carbon dioxide production, and metabolic rate.[104, 105]

Dextrose is the least expensive and most commonly used intravenous energy source. Commercially made formulas are available in concentrations ranging from 5% to 70%. Most central parenteral nutrition (CPN) formulations use 50% to 70% dextrose, which is diluted to a final concentration of between 15% and 30%. The dextrose in intravenous solutions is hydrated, so each gram of dextrose monohydrate provides 3.4 kcal.

Fat. Lipid emulsions provide an intravenous source of fat calories, including the essential fatty acids linoleic and linolenic acids. These emulsions are available as a 10% (1.1 kcal/mL) or a 20% (2 kcal/mL) solution and are approximately 6 times more expensive than the equivalent glucose calories. Lipid emulsions contain soybean oil or a combination of soybean and safflower oil triglycerides, egg yolk phospholipids as an emulsifying agent, and glycerin to achieve isotonicity with plasma. The osmolarity of current formulas ranges from 270 to 340 mOsm per liter. The emulsified particles are approximately the same size and structure as chylomicrons. They consist of a hydrophobic triglyceride core surrounded by polar phospholipids. Commercially made lipid emulsions are distinct from chylomicrons in that the emulsions contain mostly essential fatty acids and are devoid of cholesterol or protein. Currently available emulsions contain approximately half to two thirds of their fatty acids as linoleic acid and approximately 5% to 10% as linolenic acid.

After infusion into the bloodstream, lipid emulsion particles rapidly acquire apolipoproteins from contact with circulating high-density lipoprotein particles and are metabolized in a fashion similar to that of nascent chylomicrons. Once sufficient amounts of glucose have been provided to meet the requirements of glucose-dependent tissues and the brain (~150 to 200 g/day glucose), lipid calories are as effective as additional glucose calories in conserving body nitrogen economy and supporting protein metabolism.[106, 107] Providing a portion of infused calories as lipid reduces plasma insulin concentration, sodium and water retention, and hepatic fat accumulation.

The optimal percentage of calories that should be infused as fat is not known. A minimum of about 5% of total calories as a lipid emulsion is necessary to prevent essential fatty acid deficiency in patients receiving continuous CPN.[108] Administering fat-free CPN can cause biochemical evidence of essential fatty acid deficiency within 2 weeks.[109] Providing daily fat calories helps maintain near-normal plasma and erythrocyte lipid concentrations[110] and reduces the potential of adverse effects of infusing excessive glucose calories. The administration of excess calories as glucose causes a marked increase in carbon dioxide production. However, increasing the glucose supply from 30% to 70% of total calories does not alter the rate of carbon dioxide production when total energy intake matches measured resting energy expenditure.[111] Since most complications associated with intravenous lipid emulsions occur when lipid calories are provided in excess of 1.0 kcal/kg/hour (0.11 g/kg/hour)[112], the rate should not exceed 0.7 kcal/kg/hour.

Lipid emulsion infusion causes an increase in plasma cholesterol, phospholipid, and concentrations of lipoprotein X. The mechanism for the alterations in plasma lipids is related to the presence in the emulsions of free phospholipid, which acquires cholesterol from red blood cell membranes and other tissues to form a cholesterol-rich lipoprotein, known as lipoprotein X. Emulsions that contain 10% lipids have greater concentrations of phospholipid and cause a greater increase in plasma cholesterol, phospholipid, and lipoprotein X than do those that contain 20% lipids. However, it seems unlikely that these alterations in plasma lipids have any adverse consequences. In fact, data from animal studies suggest that infusion of lipid emulsions may promote resorption of cholesterol from atherosclerotic plaques.[113] Rare complications of intravenous lipid emulsions include pulmonary dysfunction,[114] hepatic phospholipidosis,[115] impaired immune system function,[116] pancreatitis,[117] decreased platelet aggregation,[118] fat overload syndrome,[119] hypersensitivity reactions,[120] and delayed gastric emptying.[121]

CATHETER INSERTION. Cannulation of a large-bore, high-flow central vein, such as the superior vena cava, permits infusion of hyperosmolar (usually > 1600 mOsm/L) nutrient solutions that could not be tolerated by smaller, low-flow peripheral veins. The most common technique for catheter placement is percutaneous infraclavicular subclavian vein catheterization, with advancement of the catheter tip to the junction of the superior vena cava and right atrium. A supraclavicular approach to the subclavian vein, as well as venous access by internal jugular, basilic, saphenous, and femoral veins, has also been used. These other sites are less desirable because of decreased patient comfort or difficulty in maintaining sterility. In rare instances, when vascular access was not possible, catheters have been inserted through a thoracotomy incision directly into the right azygos vein and passed into the superior vena cava,[122] or into the right atrial appendage and advanced to the right atrium.[123]

Peripherally inserted central venous catheters (PICC) can also provide CPN. A retrospective comparison of 135 PICC lines with 135 subclavian lines used for CPN found no significant differences in the total number of catheter-related complications, even though PICC lines were in place 3 days longer than subclavian lines.[124] Considerable cost savings can be realized by using PICC lines, if inserted by allied health personnel on the hospital ward. It is important to ensure appropriate catheter tip placement, because thrombosis rates are greater when the catheter tip is in the axillosubclavian-innominate vein (60%) than when it is in the superior vena cava (25%).[125] Furthermore, catheters associated with thrombosis are more likely to become infected.

CLINICAL MANAGEMENT. Before initiating intravenous feeding, an assessment of the patient's nutrient and fluid requirements is needed. The assessment requires a careful medical examination, including history, physical examination, and laboratory studies, to evaluate for specific nutrient deficiencies and to determine nutritional needs. In particular, a complete blood count and measurement of serum glucose, electrolytes, creatinine, urea nitrogen, magnesium, phosphorus, calcium, triglycerides, and liver biochemistries should be performed before starting nutritional support. Careful monitoring is needed to ensure safety and adequate therapy. Vital signs should be checked daily. Body weight, fluid intake, and fluid output should be measured daily. Serum electrolytes, phosphorus, and glucose should be measured every 2 days until stable and then rechecked weekly. If lipid emulsions are being given, serum triglycerides should be evaluated early in the course of CPN to document adequate clearance. Triglyceride concentrations of greater than 400 mg/dL require either reduction of the rate of infusion or complete discontinuation of lipid supplementation. In patients who have abnormal glucose homeostasis, finger-stick evaluations for glucose should be performed regularly. Regular insulin can be added to the nutrient solution to maintain blood glucose concentrations between 100 and 200 mg/dL. The direct addition of insulin to the parenteral nutrient solution reduces the risk of hypoglycemia, which can occur when insulin is given subcutaneously and infusion of the CPN solution has been inadvertently or purposely stopped.

Careful attention to the catheter and catheter site is critical in preventing catheter infections. Dressings should be changed every 48 to 72 hours or when contaminated or wet. Tubing connecting the parenteral solutions with the catheter should be changed every 48 to 72 hours. A 0.22-μm filter is inserted between the intravenous tubing and the catheter when lipid-free CPN is infused, and this filter should be changed with the tubing. A 1.2-μm filter should be used when a total nutrient admixture containing a lipid emulsion is infused. When a single-lumen catheter is used to deliver CPN, the catheter should not be used to infuse other solutions or medications, with the exception of compatible antibiotics, and it should not be used to monitor central venous pressure.

The cornerstone in the management of patients receiving CPN is attention to details. Continued adjustment of the nutrient formula is often necessary because of changes in medical therapy or clinical status. The supervision of CPN by an experienced multidisciplinary nutrition support team has been demonstrated to reduce parenteral nutrition-associated complications.[126]

COMPLICATIONS. The complications associated with the use of parenteral nutrition can be divided into mechanical, vascular, infectious, metabolic, and gastrointestinal. The incidence of most complications is reduced with careful management and supervision by an experienced nutritional support team.[126]

Mechanical Complications. Central venous catheter insertion can cause damage to local structures. A misguided approach can cause pneumothorax, brachial plexus injury, subclavian and carotid artery puncture, hemothorax, thoracic duct injury, and chylothorax. Even when the subclavian vein is cannulated successfully, other mechanical complications can still occur. The catheter may be advanced upward into the internal jugular vein, or the tip can be sheared off completely if it is withdrawn back through an introducing needle.

Vascular Complications. Air embolism can occur during insertion or afterward if the connection between the catheter and intravenous tubing is not well secured. The catheter can become occluded because of thrombosis or precipitation of electrolyte salts. Subclavian vein thrombosis occurs commonly (in approximately 25% to 50% of patients), but clinically significant manifestations such as upper extremity edema, superior vena cava syndrome, or pulmonary embolism are rare during short-term CPN.[127–129] Fatal microvascular pulmonary emboli, caused by nonvisible calcium and phosphorus precipitate identified in the total nutrient admixtures, have been reported.[130, 131] The iatrogenic mortality in these patients underscores the importance of maintaining strict pharmacy standards regarding physical-chemical compatibility. Furthermore, in-line filters should be used with all parenteral nutrient solutions despite careful inspection of solutions. The smallest pulmonary capillaries are 5 μm in diameter, whereas the size limit for visually detecting microprecipitates is 50 to 100 μm.[132]

Metabolic Complications. Many metabolic complications have been observed in patients receiving parenteral nutrition. Most complications are caused by inappropriate nutrient administration, resulting in nutrient excesses or deficiencies or both. Overzealous nutrient administration may provide excess delivery of water and sodium (fluid overload), glucose (hyperglycemia, nonketotic hyperosmolar coma), amino acids (hyperammonemia, azotemia), lipids (hypertriglyceridemia, pancreatitis), and calcium (hypercalcemia, pancreatitis, renal stones).[133] Inadequate nutrient administration can cause deficiencies of glucose, electrolytes, vitamins, trace minerals, and essential fatty acids.[134]

Hyperglycemia is a common complication of parenteral nutrition that is associated with leukocyte and complement dysfunction and an increased risk of infection when blood glucose measures above 200 mg/dL. Therefore, blood glucose should be kept between 100 and 200 mg/dL initially and between 100 and 150 mg/dL when stable. Blood glucose should be kept below 120 mg/dL in pregnant patients to avoid complications of gestational diabetes and large-for-gestational-age births. A suggested management scheme for control of hyperglycemia in patients on CPN is included in Table 16–4.

Metabolic bone disease has been observed in patients receiving long-term (>3 months) CPN. The patients with clinical manifestations of bone disease range from those who are asymptomatic but have radiologic evidence of demineralization, to those who have bone pain, and ultimately to those who experience bone fracture.[135] Histologic examination has documented osteomalacia or osteopenia or both. The cause or causes of metabolic bone disease are not known, but several mechanisms have been proposed, including aluminum toxicity, vitamin D toxicity, and negative calcium balance caused by amino acid–induced hypercalciuria.

Infectious Complications. Catheter-related sepsis is the most common life-threatening complication in patients receiving CPN. The results from most studies suggest that meticulous catheter insertion and care reduce the prevalence of catheter-related infections to 3% or less.[136] Most prospective trials have demonstrated that multilumen catheters are associated

Table 16–4 | **Management of Hyperglycemia in Patients Receiving Parenteral Nutrition**

1. If blood glucose is >200 mg/dL or patient has diabetes:
   a. Obtain better control of blood glucose before starting CPN.
   b. If CPN is started: (1) limit dextrose to <200 g/day, (2) add 0.1 unit of insulin for each gram of dextrose in CPN solution (e.g., 15 units for 150 g), (3) discontinue other sources of intravenous dextrose, and (4) order subcutaneous sliding scale regular insulin with blood glucose monitoring by fingerstick every 4–6 hr or sliding scale intravenous regular insulin infusion with blood glucose monitoring by fingerstick every 1–2 hr as follows:

Blood Glucose (mg/dL)	SQ Insulin (unit) or	IV Insulin (unit/hr)
150–199	2.0	
200–249	2–3	2.5
250–300	4–6	3.0
301–350	6–8	4.0
351–400	8–12	6.0
>400		8.0

2. If blood glucose remains >200 mg/dL and patient has been receiving:
   a. *Subcutaneous insulin*: add 50% of sliding scale regular insulin given in last 24 hr to next day's CPN solution; double amount of subcutaneous insulin sliding scale dose for blood glucose values >200 mg/dL.
   b. *Intravenous insulin*: add 50% of IV insulin given in last 24 hr to next day's CPN solution; increase sliding scale IV insulin infusion rate by 50% for blood glucose values >200 mg/dL.
3. If patient's blood glucose remains >200 mg/dL, consider (1) discontinuing CPN until better glucose control can be established, (2) decreasing dextrose content in CPN, or (3) initiating insulin drip if not already started.
4. Dextrose in CPN may be increased when blood glucose control (100–150 mg/dL) is achieved. Insulin:dextrose ratio in CPN formulation should be maintained while CPN dextrose content is changed.

CPN, central parenteral nutrition.
Adapted from McMahon MM, Rizza RA: Nutrition support in hospitalized patients with diabetes mellitus. Mayo Clin Proc 71:587, 1996.

with an increased risk of infection compared with single-lumen catheters.[136] However, the need for intravenous access often makes the use of single-lumen catheters impractical. Catheter infections can be caused by entry of organisms at the catheter exit site, contamination at tubing connections, seeding from other sites of infection, and, rarely, contamination of the infusate itself.

Catheter-related sepsis in patients receiving CPN is most commonly caused by *Staphylococcus epidermidis* and *Staphylococcus* aureus. In immune-compromised patients (e.g. AIDS, immunosuppressive therapy, absolute neutrophil count <200) and those with long-term (>2 wks) CPN, *Enterococcus*, *Candida* species, *Escherichia coli*, *Pseudomonas*, *Klebsiella*, *Enterobacter*, *Acinetobacter*, *Proteus*, and *Xanthomonas* should also be considered. Table 16–5 reviews our suggested management approach for suspected catheter-related infection.

The antibiotic lock technique has also been used successfully to treat central catheter infections.[137–139] This technique involves injecting an antibiotic solution (e.g., vancomycin, 2 mg/mL) into the central catheter lumen and allowing the antibiotic to sit in the line for at least 12 hours. The catheter can be used to infuse fluids or parenteral nutritional solutions during the remaining 12 hours of the day. The catheter is periodically reinjected for a 14-day course.[138] This approach has the advantage of delivering a higher antibiotic concentration into the catheter, avoiding the side effects of systemic antibiotics, and lower cost.[137] However, this technique is not effective for treating tunnel/skin infections and is probably less efficacious in reservoir-type catheters.[137]

Gastrointestinal Complications. Hepatic abnormalities are the most common gastrointestinal complications associated with CPN. However, it is difficult to establish a true causal relationship between the use of CPN and many of the reported liver abnormalities because of the paucity of prospective randomized trials. Many of the hepatic abnormalities in patients receiving CPN might have been caused by clinical factors unrelated to the use of CPN itself. Patients who require CPN often have serious illnesses that are associated with liver disease or have received hepatotoxic therapy, which can cause liver disease.

Hepatic abnormalities are more frequent and more severe in infants receiving CPN than in adults. The first report of TPN-associated liver disease, published in 1971, was of a premature infant who developed cholestatic jaundice, bile duct proliferation, and cirrhosis after 71 days of CPN therapy.[140] Subsequent studies have shown that cholestasis is the most frequent hepatic complication in CPN-fed infants and correlates directly with decreased gestational age, decreased birth weight, and increased duration of CPN therapy.

Several hepatic abnormalities have been observed in adults receiving CPN.[141] Although these abnormalities are usually benign and transient, a small subset of patients with more serious and progressive disease has been reported.

Table 16–5 | **Management of Suspected Catheter-Related Infection**

1. Initial evaluation:
   a. Evaluate catheter insertion site and culture any drainage
   b. Obtain blood cultures from peripheral vein and central vein catheter
   c. Culture hub, skin, infusate, if clinically indicated
   d. Culture catheter tip, if removed
   e. Look for other causes of infection (e.g., urinalysis, chest radiograph, sputum, wounds)
2. Stop CPN for 48–72 hr
3. Indications for central venous catheter removal:
   a. Immediate removal
      (1) Purulent discharge or abscess at insertion site
      (2) Septic shock without another etiology for the source of infection
   b. Removal of catheters after culture results are obtained
      (1) Persistent or recurrent catheter-related bacteremia
      (2) *Candida* species or *Pseudomonas* infection
      (3) Polymicrobial infection
      (4) *Staphylococcus aureus* infection
4. Antibiotic therapy
   a. Empirical antibiotic therapy administered through central venous catheter until culture results are back:
      (1) Vancomycin, 1 g q12hr (adjust dose for creatinine/GFR)
      (2) Cefepime, 1 g q12hr (if gram-negative infection suspected)
   b. Specific antibiotic therapy administered through central venous catheter once culture results are available
   c. If a catheter is "irreplaceable," consider trial of antibiotic therapy with line in place
   d. Duration of antibiotic therapy usually ranges from 2–6 wk, depending on patient, organism, and whether central line has been left in place
5. Repeat blood cultures in 48 and 72 hr to ensure clearance of bacteremia
6. Fever should resolve within 72–96 hr if patient is given appropriate antibiotics; remove catheter if fever persists

GFR, glomerular filtration rate; CPN, central parenteral nutrition.

Most complications occur within 4 weeks of starting CPN, whereas fewer but often more severe complications occur later, usually after 16 weeks of CPN therapy. The hepatic complications include both biochemical (elevated serum aminotransferase and alkaline phosphatase) and histologic (steatosis, steatohepatitis, lipidosis and phospholipidosis, cholestasis, fibrosis, and cirrhosis) alterations. Liver biopsies have been obtained infrequently in patients receiving CPN (see Chapters 72, 73, and 82).

The mechanisms involved in the pathogenesis of hepatic complications are not well understood. Many potential contributing factors have been proposed as being responsible for CPN-associated liver disease: those associated with the patients' clinical condition or therapy, the CPN solution itself (excessive glucose calories, excessive lipid infusion, amino acid degradation products, aluminum toxicity), nutritional deficiencies (essential fatty acid deficiency, choline deficiency, carnitine deficiency), and gut factors (intestinal bacteria or endotoxin translocation, bacterial overgrowth, bacterial metabolism of bile acids).

Three types of biliary complications have been associated with the use of CPN—acalculous cholecystitis, gallbladder sludge, and cholelithiasis (see Chapters 54, 55, and 58). Biliary complications usually occur in patients receiving more prolonged (more than 4 weeks) courses of CPN. Acalculous cholecystitis has been reported to occur in about 5%,[142] cholelithiasis in about 30%,[143] and gallbladder sludge in up to 100%[8] of patients receiving prolonged CPN. The pathogenesis of acalculous cholecystitis is unclear, but it occurs in the setting of bile stasis and increased bile lithogenicity and is associated with major trauma, severe systemic illness, and major operative procedures. The pathogenesis of gallbladder sludge and stones is related to gallbladder stasis caused by the absence of enteral feeding in CPN-fed patients. Most CPN-related gallstones are pigment stones containing large amounts of calcium bilirubinate.[8, 144] The development of gallbladder sludge appears to be a prerequisite for the development of gallstones. Stimulating gallbladder contraction and emptying with either enteral feedings[145] or cholecystokinin injections[146] has been shown to reduce or completely prevent gallbladder sludge and gallstone formation.

Peripheral Vein Nutrition

Although peripheral parenteral nutrition (PPN) is often used as a temporizing maneuver to provide short-term nutritional support, the benefit of such short-term therapy is not clear. There are several alternatives once the decision has been made to use a peripheral vein for nutritional purposes. Dextrose in water, 100 to 150 g daily, with multivitamins and 20 to 30 mEq of potassium chloride/L, has been the mainstay for short-term postoperative patients for many years. This is usually given as 2 or 3 liters of 5% dextrose in water. The administration of dextrose and the stimulation of insulin secretion will decrease urinary nitrogen losses by 50% compared with the administration of saline. Amino acid infusions have been used as "protein-sparing therapy" because nitrogen balance is better with amino acids than with isocaloric dextrose.[147] The use of isotonic lipid emulsions makes it possible to infuse a considerable amount of calories through a peripheral vein. Combinations of hypotonic dextrose, amino acids, and fat emulsions can meet an average patient's basal energy and protein needs, provided that approximately half the calories are given as fat. A frequently used preparation providing a final concentration of 5% dextrose and 4.25% amino acids is shown in Table 16–6.

The major limitation in using PPN is the high incidence of thrombophlebitis.[148] The factors responsible for thrombophlebitis can be divided into four categories:

1. PPN solution (osmolality, pH, lipid content, presence of particulate matter),
2. catheter characteristics (diameter, length, and composition of the catheter),
3. infusion protocol (duration, rate, and volume of infusion), and
4. venous properties (diameter, anatomic position, and insertion technique).[149]

Modifications in the administration of PPN can increase the life of a single infusion site to more than 10 days. For example, placing a glycerol trinitrate patch over the insertion site and adding heparin (600 U/L) and hydrocortisone (6 mg/L) to a hyperosmolar (1190 mOsm/kg) formulation decreased the incidence of thrombophlebitis by 50% and doubled catheter longevity to 15 days.[150]

The following principles should be considered in all patients receiving PPN to increase catheter survival:

- Insert the catheter in as large a vein as possible in the proximal forearm using sterile technique,
- Avoid standard Teflon catheters; use a fine-bore 22- or 23-gauge polyvinyl pyrrolidine-coated polyurethane catheter,
- Place a 5-mg glycerol trinitrate ointment patch over the infusion site,
- Provide at least 50% of total energy as a lipid emulsion,
- Add 500 to 1000 U of heparin/L of PPN solution,
- Add 5 mg of hydrocortisone/L of PPN solution,
- Add sodium hydroxide if needed to buffer PPN solution to pH 7.4,
- Keep daily infused volume below 3500 mL,

Table 16–6 | **Composition of a Typical Peripheral Parenteral Nutrition Solution**

NUTRIENT	VOLUME (mL)	CALORIE CONTENT (kcal)	AMOUNT (g)	OSMOLALITY (mOsm/L)
Amino acids (8.5%)	1000	340	85	850
Dextrose (10%)	1000	340	100	505
Lipid (10%)	500	550	50	260
TOTAL	2500	1230		595

- Use an in-line 1.2-μm filter, and
- Infuse the PPN solution with a volumetric pump.

Home Parenteral Nutrition

Home parenteral nutrition (HPN) is necessary for patients who require parenteral nutrition for prolonged periods of time, such as those with gut failure. It is administered through a central catheter during an 8- to 12-hour period overnight. The distribution of calories provided in the HPN varies, depending on what and how much the patients are eating and absorbing. For patients who rely exclusively on HPN, 20% to 30% of calories are given as intravenous fat. If patients can absorb adequate dietary fat, lipid emulsions may not be necessary or can be given in limited amounts. Patients are usually given approximately 1.0 g of protein/kg/day. Vitamins, minerals, and trace elements are given in amounts adequate to maintain normal blood concentrations and body stores.

The prevalence of HPN in the United States is much higher than in other Western countries. Moreover, in the United States, HPN is often given to patients who have limited life expectancy.[151] Outcomes differ strikingly between those patients with benign diseases and those with terminal illnesses. Less than half the patients receiving HPN who had *cancer* or *AIDS* were alive at 6 months, and only 20% and 10%, respectively, were alive at 1 year. Patients who have benign diseases, such as *Crohn's disease*, *ischemic bowel*, *motility disorders*, *congenital bowel defects*, *hyperemesis gravidarum* and *chronic pancreatitis*, have a good outcome. The annual survival rate in these patients is 87%; approximately 6% of deaths have been caused by HPN-associated complications.[152] Nutrition repletion by HPN can be dramatic in patients with benign disease. Ideal body weight is achieved in almost all patients, and body composition studies have confirmed nitrogen repletion.[153] Only 5% of the total HPN days in patients with benign diseases are spent in the hospital; half the hospital time is necessary for treating HPN-associated complications and half because of disease complications.[152] Approximately 70% of patients achieve complete rehabilitation.[151]

Complications associated with HPN can be chronologically grouped. In the 1970s, most of the reported complications were micronutrient deficiencies (Table 16–7) and complications of carbohydrate overfeeding (e.g., hepatic steatosis). Since the 1980s, complications associated with increasing duration of HPN have appeared, such as venous thrombosis, chronic liver disease, cholelithiasis, and metabolic bone disease. Catheter-related septicemia is the most common major complication.

Table 16–7 | **Micronutrient Deficiencies and Clinical Presentations in Patients Receiving Parenteral Nutrition**

NUTRIENT DEFICIENCY	PRESENTATION
Vitamin A	Night blindness, reduced dark field adaptation
Vitamin E	In vitro platelet hyperaggregation, hydrogen peroxide–induced RBC hemolysis
Biotin	Dermatitis, alopecia, hypotonia
Thiamine	Wernicke's encephalopathy, refractory lactic acidosis
Copper	Neutropenia, anemia, scorbutic bone lesions, decreased plasma ceruloplasmin
Zinc	Nasolabial and perineal acrodermatitis, alopecia, decreased T cell function, decreased plasma alkaline phosphatase
Chromium	Glucose intolerance
Selenium	Myalgias, cardiomyopathy, decreased glutathione peroxidase
Molybdenum	Amino acid intolerance, tachycardia, tachypnea, central scotomas, irritability
Essential fatty acids	Eczymoid dermatitis, increased trienoic:tetraenoic plasma fatty acid ratio

CLINICAL APPLICATIONS OF NUTRITION SUPPORT

Inflammatory Bowel Disease

(See Chapters 103 and 104)

Protein-calorie malnutrition and specific nutrient deficiencies are common in patients with inflammatory bowel disease (IBD) because of decreased nutrient intake, malabsorption, drug-nutrient interactions, and protein-losing enteropathy. Therefore, nutritional therapy is an important component of the overall management of patients with IBD by preventing or correcting nutrient deficiencies. Nutritional support has also been purported to be a primary therapy for IBD, but its efficacy in this regard is more controversial.

ENTERAL NUTRITION IN CROHN'S DISEASE. Several different dietary modifications have been recommended for patients with Crohn's disease. However, no consistent data support the clinical efficacy of any specific whole food diet. Both a low-residue diet and a high-fiber diet have been recommended, but prospective randomized trials have shown that neither one is clinically beneficial.[154, 155] An exclusion diet, in which "intolerant" foods are excluded from the diet, was reported to maintain remission successfully in two prospective randomized trials.[156, 157] In contrast, another study found that alleged food sensitivities did not persist on rechallenge or could not be substantiated with a double-blinded evaluation.[158] The result of one prospective randomized trial suggests that restricting dietary fat may improve clinical outcome.[159]

The clinical efficacy of defined liquid formula diets in patients with Crohn's disease has been studied in at least 17 prospective randomized controlled trials (PCRTs).[15, 160–175] All trials evaluated the effect of short-term therapy (less than 30 days) on Crohn's disease activity as judged by a clinical index score. The trials can be divided into two general groups: studies that compared diet therapy with standard pharmacotherapy,[15, 160–167] and studies that compared one type of formula diet with another.[168–175] Most of the trials suffer from small numbers of patients, high withdrawal rates in the enterally fed groups, and heterogeneous patient populations.

Three meta-analyses of published PRCTs reviewed the

clinical efficacy of liquid formula diets versus steroids and the clinical efficacy of monomeric versus nonmonomeric liquid formula diets.[176–178] These meta-analyses pooled nearly the same studies and reached identical conclusions. Enteral nutrition was not as effective as steroid therapy in achieving clinical remission (pooled odds ratio 0.35, 95% confidence interval 0.23–0.53); overall remission rates for enteral nutrition and steroid-treated patients were 58% and 80%, respectively. Monomeric liquid formula diets were no better than nonmonomeric liquid formula diets in achieving clinical remission (pooled odds ratio 0.87, 95% confidence interval 0.41–1.83); overall remission rates for monomeric- and nonmonomeric-treated patients were 65% and 61%, respectively.

The true clinical efficacy of enteral nutritional therapy has not been evaluated because no study has compared patients receiving diet therapy with an untreated control group. However, the average remission rate reported for patients treated with enteral nutrition (approximately 60%) is higher than the remission rate reported for patients treated with placebo in other prospective randomized trials (20% to 40%)[179] and suggests that enteral nutrition may have a primary therapeutic effect on Crohn's disease. Nevertheless, the higher cost, poorer compliance, and inferior clinical efficacy of enteral nutrition compared with steroids make pharmacotherapy the treatment of choice for patients with active disease. The success most patients achieve with steroid therapy suggests that the question of whether nutrition is better than steroids is not as important as whether adjunctive enteral nutritional support can enhance remission rates or decrease steroid requirements in patients who are resistant or refractory to corticosteroids. Although this issue has not been evaluated in a PRCT, a prospective but uncontrolled trial found that a 4-week course of monomeric diet therapy was associated with clinical remission and withdrawal of steroid therapy in 10 of 16 patients with steroid-dependent or steroid-refractory disease[180] (see Chapter 103).

PARENTERAL NUTRITION IN CROHN'S DISEASE. Parenteral nutrition can be an important component of the medical management of patients with active Crohn's disease who cannot tolerate adequate oral or enteral feeding. Complete restriction of oral intake to "rest" the bowel, in conjunction with TPN to provide nutritional support, has also been proposed as a primary therapy for patients with active disease. A prospective nonrandomized trial provided 12 weeks of total parenteral nutrition via CPN and bowel rest in a final attempt to avoid surgery in 30 patients with active Crohn's disease who failed medical therapy.[181] Clinical remission was achieved and surgery was avoided in 83% of patients. However, the cumulative relapse rate was 60% after 2 years and 85% after 4 years; many of the patients required surgery for either an intestinal stricture or an intra-abdominal abscess. Subsequent PRCTs have demonstrated that bowel rest itself is not necessary for achieving clinical remission and that CPN is not more efficacious than enteral feeding.[182–185]

The clinical efficacy of parenteral nutrition in patients with Crohn's colitis has not been demonstrated. Two PCRTs[186, 187] evaluated the use of TPN in patients with Crohn's colitis. Both studies also included patients with ulcerative colitis. Patients were randomized to receive either TPN or a regular oral diet, and all patients were given oral steroid therapy. No significant differences in clinical response rates were found between the TPN and oral diet groups, but the small number of subjects studied limited the ability of these trials to detect differences between groups.

ENTERAL NUTRITION IN ULCERATIVE COLITIS. Enteral nutritional therapy in patients with active ulcerative colitis is empirical because of the absence of carefully performed clinical trials. In general, dietary management should provide adequate calories (approximately 35 kcal/kg/day) and protein (about 1.5 g/kg/day) in patients with severe exacerbations to compensate for the increase in energy expenditure, protein catabolism, and intestinal protein losses.[188] Foods that may worsen diarrhea, such as caffeine-containing drinks, should be avoided. A low-fiber diet is often recommended to reduce the frequency of bowel movements and improve patient comfort. However, the clinical efficacy of restricting dietary fiber is unproved and could have deleterious effects by limiting the production of short-chain fatty acids, which are an important colonic fuel (see Chapter 104).

PARENTERAL NUTRITION IN ULCERATIVE COLITIS. Central parenteral nutrition has not proved to be useful as primary therapy in patients with active ulcerative colitis. In three prospective randomized trials containing small numbers of patients,[186, 187, 189] the rate of clinical remission and the need for colectomy in patients treated with CPN, bowel rest, and corticosteroids were the same as in those treated with an oral or enteral diet and corticosteroids. However, patients with severe disease who cannot eat because of intestinal ileus or who might benefit from bowel rest because of severe diarrhea or anticipated surgery should be considered for CPN if more than 7 days of starvation is anticipated (see Chapter 104).

PERIOPERATIVE PARENTERAL NUTRITION. The potential usefulness of perioperative CPN in patients with IBD has not been adequately studied. A retrospective review of patients who had surgery for Crohn's disease and ulcerative colitis found that those who received 5 or more days of preoperative CPN had fewer postoperative complications than those who did not.[190] The clinical efficacy of postoperative parenteral nutrition was evaluated in 30 patients who required a proctocolectomy, half of whom had IBD.[191] Patients were randomized to receive either water and electrolytes, peripheral amino acids, or standard CPN. Perineal wound healing was more rapid in those patients receiving CPN than in the other two groups. A retrospective study examined the effect of preoperative CPN on the amount of intestine resected during either segmental small bowel resection, ileocecectomy, or colectomy for Crohn's disease.[192] Patients who received preoperative CPN had approximately 20 cm less small intestine resected during segmental small bowel resection, 11 cm less small intestine resected during ileocecectomy, and no difference in length of resection during segmental colectomy, or, of course, total colectomy. Although these studies suggest a beneficial effect of perioperative CPN, the limitations in study design and the potential for patient selection bias prevent drawing firm conclusions from these data. At present, the indications for perioperative CPN in patients with IBD do not differ from those of other patients undergoing surgery.

GROWTH FAILURE IN CHILDREN. Approximately 20% to 35% of children with Crohn's disease and 5% to 10% of children with ulcerative colitis experience impairment in linear growth at some time during their illness.[193] Growth failure may precede the onset of gastrointestinal symptoms by several months. The most important factor responsible for growth failure is prolonged insufficient dietary intake causing malnutrition and reduced circulating levels of somatomedin C, a growth-promoting peptide. Adequate nutritional supplementation alone, regardless of the form, usually stimulates growth. Increasing nutritional intake by oral supplementation,[194] nasogastric tube feeding,[195] or CPN[196] increases growth velocity and linear growth. Therefore, CPN should be considered only when attempts to feed by safer and cheaper enteral means have failed. Although corticosteroids have been implicated as a contributing factor in growth failure, medical therapy, including corticosteroids to reduce gastrointestinal symptoms, may be important so that oral intake can improve.

Gastrointestinal Fistulas

Management of gastrointestinal fistulas (see Chapter 24) depends primarily on the cause, although the number, location, and volume of drainage are other important variables. Fistulas arising from a bowel with active Crohn's disease, radiation damage, or cancer usually require surgery for definitive therapy. Even when these fistulas initially respond to medical therapy, they are unlikely to remain closed without surgery. An obstruction distal to a fistula or the presence of peritonitis requires prompt surgical intervention. Postoperative fistulas caused by anastomotic leaks in patients who do not have residual gastrointestinal disease or obstruction usually close with conservative management and do not require surgery.

Although there are no prospective randomized trials evaluating the use of nutritional support in patients with gastrointestinal fistulas, it is likely that bowel rest and nutritional therapy with CPN have contributed to the improvement in clinical outcomes observed in this patient population. Before the use of CPN, mortality in patients with gastrointestinal fistulas was from electrolyte and fluid losses, malnutrition, and generalized peritonitis.[197] A retrospective analysis of patients with small bowel fistulas found lower mortality rates (8% versus 33%), higher spontaneous fistula closures (56% versus 27%), and higher surgical closure rates (92% versus 59%) in patients who received nutritional support than in those who did not.[198] Occasionally, HPN may be useful when complicated fistulas persist after conventional inpatient CPN with bowel rest and surgical attempts at fistula closure have failed.[199]

Somatostatin and CPN may have a synergistic effect on reduction of gastrointestinal secretions and on fistula closure.[200] In 37 patients with external gastrointestinal fistulas (26 with postoperative fistulas), treatment with the combination of CPN, restriction of food intake, and somatostatin resulted in spontaneous closure in 82% of instances, with a mean time for closure of only 5 days (range, 1 to 14 days).

Acute Pancreatitis

(See Chapter 48)

Most patients with acute pancreatitis have mild or moderate disease, as defined by Ranson's criteria (see Chapter 48), and can be managed with standard supportive measures, such as analgesics and peripheral intravenous fluids. Principles used in the nutritional management of these patients include elimination of oral food intake to minimize pancreatic secretion and abdominal pain, and provision of maintenance fluids and electrolytes. Parenteral nutrition provides a mechanism for feeding patients without stimulating exocrine pancreatic secretion.[201] Recently, several studies have also demonstrated that jejunal tube feeding can be given safely to properly selected patients with pancreatitis, even those with severe disease.[202–204]

No benefit of parenteral nutrition has been demonstrated in PRCTs conducted in patients with mild or moderate pancreatitis.[202, 204–207] In fact, in one study, the use of CPN was associated with a higher prevalence of catheter-related sepsis and insulin requirements.[207] Several PRCTs have compared jejunal tube feeding with CPN.[202–204] In patients with mild or moderate pancreatitis, clinical outcome was the same in enterally fed patients and those given CPN[202] whereas in another study patients who received enteral nutrition experienced a greater reduction in levels of acute-phase response serum proteins and greater improvement in disease severity scores than those given parenteral nutrition.[203] A recent trial, conducted in patients with necrotizing pancreatitis, found patients given early enteral (within 48 hours after admission) feeding experienced fewer medical complications than those given parenteral feeding.[204] However, in all studies, it is not known whether enteral feeding was beneficial or parenteral feeding was harmful because of the absence of an unfed control group.

Providing 20% to 30% of total calories as lipid is safe in most patients and can attenuate the glucose intolerance that often accompanies protracted pancreatitis. The use of intravenous lipid emulsions in humans does not cause significant pancreatic stimulation.[208] In some patients, however, the addition of lipids to CPN has been associated with an exacerbation of pancreatitis.[209] Because of the relationship between hyperlipidemia and pancreatitis, intravenous fat emulsions should be avoided when pancreatitis is associated with significant hypertriglyceridemia (e.g., serum triglyceride concentration of 300 or more mg/dL). The ability to clear infused triglycerides should be demonstrated in all patients with pancreatitis who are given lipid emulsions because of the inhibition of lipoprotein lipase associated with pancreatitis.[210]

Cancer

During the course of their illness, patients with cancer, particularly those with cancer of the upper intestine and pancreas, usually experience significant weight loss and depletion of their body tissues. Because weight loss is an important prognosticator of survival,[211] it seems reasonable that improving nutritional status with either enteral or parenteral nutritional therapy could favorably affect the clinical outcome. Although more than 75 PRCTs have evaluated the use of nutritional support in patients with cancer, the indications for nutritional therapy in this patient population remain controversial.[212] Most studies can be criticized because of small sample size, heterogeneous patient populations, provision of excessive (and potentially harmful) calories in the nutrition-treated group, inclusion of well-nourished patients in the trial who would be less likely to benefit from nutritional therapy, and the absence of data regarding important clinical end-points, such as growth failure in children and quality of life.

CHEMOTHERAPY. In published PRCTs that evaluated the use of CPN in patients treated with chemotherapy,[212] CPN was usually given before or in conjunction with the course of chemotherapy for a period of 3 to 6 weeks. The use of CPN had no obvious overall effect on survival or hematologic and gastrointestinal toxicity. Two meta-analytic reviews found that patients receiving CPN were only two thirds as likely to achieve a complete or partial tumor response and four times more likely to develop an infection than were control patients.[213, 214] Prospective randomized studies of enteral nutrition in patients receiving chemotherapy for treatment of breast, lung, hematologic, gastrointestinal, or metastatic cancer have also failed to show clinical benefits.[214] No differences in survival or tumor response were found in patients randomized to receive enteral nutritional supplementation compared with those randomized to receive a free-choice diet.

RADIATION THERAPY. Radiation therapy itself does not cause significant metabolic stress or increase nutrient requirements unless complicated by gastrointestinal disease.[215] Neither enteral nor parenteral nutrition has been demonstrated to improve survival or tolerance to treatment in patients receiving abdominal irradiation.[212]

PERIOPERATIVE NUTRITION. Preoperative patients who are considered malnourished measured by weight loss or other commonly used indicators of nutritional status have a higher prevalence of postoperative complications and mortality than well-nourished patients.[216] This observation has led to the hypothesis that providing perioperative nutritional support to malnourished patients undergoing surgery could have beneficial therapeutic effects. However, if nutritional status is associated with the severity of disease, patients who are "malnourished" will have a poor prognosis because they are sicker than patients who are "well nourished." Therefore, nutritional therapy may not affect clinical outcome unless the presence of malnutrition itself is an independent contributor to postoperative complications.

At least 27 PRCTs have evaluated the clinical efficacy of CPN in patients with cancer who underwent surgical therapy.[212] Daily amino acids and nonprotein calories prescribed in the TPN formulations for each trial ranged from 1 to 2.5 g/day and 30 to 65 kcal/day, respectively. Patients assigned to receive CPN were not precluded from eating orally, so total protein and calorie intake for many patients may have been higher than that provided by CPN alone. Only five trials[217–221] found statistically significant differences in clinical end-points. One study[218] found that patients receiving preoperative CPN had fewer postoperative complications (abdominal abscess, peritonitis, anastomotic leakage, and ileus) and mortality. Two other trials[217, 220] found that preoperative CPN decreased postoperative complications. In contrast, the large multicenter Department of Veterans Affairs study[221] found similar rates of total major complications in both CPN and control groups but a statistically significant increase in infections in patients who received preoperative CPN. A recent meta-analysis of PRCTs, however, found that perioperative parenteral nutrition decreased postoperative complications in patients with upper gastrointestinal cancer.[221a]

Seven PRCTs evaluated the use of enteral nutrition, given either preoperatively or postoperatively, in patients treated with surgery.[212] Enteral nutrition was usually provided as a commercially prepared liquid formula diet and was infused through a nasoenteric tube or needle catheter jejunostomy. Tube feeding was associated with gastrointestinal intolerance, manifested by nausea, vomiting, abdominal pain, distention, and diarrhea in up to 50% of patients. Catheter dysfunction occurred in approximately 20% to 25% of patients fed by needle catheter jejunostomy. Perioperative mortality and the duration of hospital stay were similar in both enterally fed and control patients. The rate of perioperative complications not associated with tube feedings in the patients given enteral feedings was approximately 15% less than that of the control group. The difference in the rate of perioperative complications between groups is even greater if only studies that provided preoperative nutritional support to malnourished patients are considered.

In summary, the published data from PRCTs do not support the routine use of parenteral or enteral nutrition in patients receiving chemotherapy or radiation therapy. Therefore, the decision to initiate adjunctive nutritional therapy in these patients should be based on standard indications for nutritional support and not on the presence of cancer itself. The high rate of infection associated with parenteral feeding in patients receiving chemotherapy underscores the importance of avoiding excessive glucose and lipid calories and providing optimal catheter care. Perioperative CPN should not be given routinely to surgical patients. Parenteral nutrition, given preoperatively in patients with upper gastrointestinal cancer, may decrease postoperative complications. Severely malnourished patients, defined by percentage of body weight loss or nutrition risk index,[221] may derive greater clinical benefits from preoperative TPN, but this conclusion is based largely on retrospective analyses of prospective data. The observation that preoperative enteral feeding may be beneficial in reducing postoperative complications requires further study.

Liver Disease

The liver is a "workhorse" for metabolic activity. It is the major site for (1) the synthesis of plasma proteins, such as albumin and coagulation factors, (2) urea synthesis for normal nitrogen metabolism and ammonia clearance, (3) glucose production for maintaining euglycemia, and (4) lipid metabolism by producing lipoproteins and converting fatty acids to ketone bodies. These metabolic functions require a considerable amount of energy. The liver consumes approximately 20% of resting energy requirements while constituting only 2% of body weight. Patients who have significant liver disease demonstrate impaired hepatic metabolic function as well as extrahepatic alterations in glucose (insulin resistance and impaired glucose tolerance), lipid (increased lipolytic rates), and protein (decreased protein synthesis and increased amino acid oxidation rates) metabolism[222] (see Chapter 63).

Protein-energy malnutrition occurs commonly in patients with advanced liver disease and may be caused by several factors.[223] Decreased nutrient intake occurs because of anorexia and nausea. In patients with alcoholic liver disease, alcohol accounts for 35% to 65% of daily energy intake, and the prevalence of protein-calorie malnutrition is inversely correlated with nonalcohol calorie intake. Excessive alcohol is metabolized by the microsomal ethanol oxidizing system, which generates heat without energy production and is thus a wasteful energy cycle. Some patients with liver disease may have considerable malabsorption because of impaired bile acid secretion, pancreatic insufficiency, or direct alcohol-induced injury of the small intestine.

ALCOHOLIC HEPATITIS. The use of standard amino acids, usually given with hypotonic dextrose through a peripheral vein, has been reported in several PRCTs involving patients with alcoholic hepatitis.[224] Nutritional therapy often improved standard markers of nutritional status and liver chemistries but did not affect morbidity and mortality (see Chapter 71).

Alcoholic Cirrhosis. The results of several PRCTs evaluating oral and enteral tube feeding in patients with alcoholic cirrhosis demonstrate that aggressive feeding can be given safely and may have clinical benefits.[225–227] Oral or enteral tube feedings resulted in delivery of desired nutrient intake and often provided twice the protein and calories ingested ad lib by the control group. Feedings were usually well tolerated and did not cause major complications, such as aspiration, encephalopathy, variceal hemorrhage, or adverse gastrointestinal symptoms. Patients who received nutritional support had evidence of improvements in liver function (as assessed by hepatic function studies and liver biochemistries), hepatic encephalopathy, and Child's classification. One study[225] demonstrated improved survival in patients fed with a branched-chain enriched formula (see Chapter 71).

HEPATIC ENCEPHALOPATHY. Altering the type of dietary protein may benefit certain patients with chronic hepatic encephalopathy. Most,[228–230] but not all,[231] studies that compared vegetable with animal dietary protein found that vegetable protein diets were better tolerated than animal protein diets. Vegetable diets reduce urea production rate by increasing dietary fiber intake and increasing incorporation and elimination of nitrogen in fecal bacteria[232] (see Chapter 79).

Most patients with cirrhosis can tolerate an increasing amount of standard protein without worsening encephalopathy. The use of formulas with high concentrations of branched-chain amino acids (BCAAs) and small amounts of aromatic amino acids have been proposed for use in patients with hepatic encephalopathy, based on the observation that the ratio of plasma BCAAs to aromatic amino acids is reduced in patients who have cirrhosis. Branched-chain amino acid–enriched liquid formulas, which contain approximately 35% of total amino acids as BCAAs, may be useful in a small percentage of patients with cirrhosis who are truly intolerant of increasing dietary protein. As much as 80 g of protein given as BCAA-enriched solutions has been tolerated in patients who could not tolerate 40 g of standard dietary protein.[233] The large expense of BCAA-enriched solutions discourages their use in most settings.

The clinical efficacy of parenteral BCAA-enriched CPN solutions in patients with acute hepatic encephalopathy has been evaluated in 9 PRCTs. These trials were reviewed by using meta-analytical methodology to pool data across studies.[102] Patients who received BCAA-enriched solutions demonstrated a statistically significant improvement in mental recovery from high-grade encephalopathy during short-term (7–14 days) nutritional therapy. Considerable heterogeneity in mortality rates among studies precluded meaningful aggregation of mortality data. Although the pooled analysis of trials suggests a beneficial effect of BCAA-enriched formulas as a primary therapy in patients with acute hepatic encephalopathy, the studies have several shortcomings that limit enthusiasm for this relatively expensive therapy. The control groups usually received suboptimal, and possibly harmful, nutritional support, consisting of high-dextrose solutions without amino acids. Only one study compared BCAA-enriched CPN with a standard amino acid CPN solution. None of the studies reported on complications associated with nutritional therapy, and none evaluated whether short-term benefits of nutritional therapy led to a long-term reduction in complications (see Chapter 79).

PERIOPERATIVE NUTRITION. There is a paucity of data evaluating the usefulness of perioperative nutritional support in patients with liver disease. The results of one PRCT suggested that early postoperative enteral feeding may be beneficial in patients undergoing liver transplantation.[234] Nasojejunal tube feeding started 12 hours after transplant surgery was well tolerated and allowed increased protein and energy intake during the first 4 postoperative days. Early tube feeding was associated with a significant reduction in postoperative viral infections and a trend toward a decrease in bacterial infections. However, these results may be biased, because one third of the patients who entered the study failed to complete their assigned protocol and were not included in the final analysis. Another PRCT found that pretransplant enteral supplementation improved grip strength and other nutritional parameters but did not affect clinical outcome.[235]

One PRCT evaluated the clinical efficacy of perioperative CPN, given as a BCAA-enriched solution for 7 days before and 7 days after hepatectomy for hepatocellular carcinoma.[236] Patients randomized to receive CPN had better postoperative hepatic function and significantly fewer postoperative complications (mostly pulmonary infection and ascites).

REFERENCES

1. Macfie J: Enteral versus parenteral nutrition: The significance of bacterial translocation and gut-barrier function. Nutrition 16:606, 2000.
2. Eastwood GL: Small bowel morphology and epithelial proliferation in intravenously alimented rabbits. Surgery 82:613, 1977.
3. Hughes CA, Prince A, Dowling RH: Speed of change in pancreatic mass and in intestinal bacteriology of parenterally fed rats. Clin Sci 59:329, 1980.
4. Johnson LR, Guthrie PD: Mucosal DNA synthesis: A short-term index of the trophic action of gastrin. Gastroenterology 67:453, 1974.
5. Levine GM, Deren JJ, Steiger E, Zinno R: Role of oral intake in maintenance of gut mass and disaccharidase activity. Gastroenterology 67:975, 1974.
6. Johnson LR, Schanbacher LM, Dudrick SJ, Copeland EM: Effect of long-term parenteral feeding on pancreatic secretion and serum secretin. Am J Physiol 233(6):E524, 1977.
7. Alverdy J, Chi HS, Sheldon GF: The effect of parenteral nutrition on gastrointestinal immunity. The importance of enteral stimulation. Ann Surg 202:681, 1985.
8. Messing B, Bories C, Kunstlinger F, Bernier JJ: Does total parenteral nutrition induce gallbladder sludge formation and lithiasis? Gastroenterology 84:1012, 1983.

9. Bach AC, Babayen VK: Medium-chain triglycerides: An update. Am J Clin Nutr 36:950, 1982.
10. Linscheer WG, Blum AL, Platt RR: Transfer of medium chain fatty acids from blood to spinal fluid in patients with cirrhosis. Gastroenterology 58:509, 1970.
11. Holt PR: Medium-chain triglycerides. Gastroenterology 53:961, 1967.
12. Silk DB, Fairclough PD, Clark ML, et al: Uses of a peptide rather than free amino acid nitrogen source in chemically defined elemental diets. J Parenter Enteral Nutr 4:548, 1980.
13. Grimble GK, Silk DBA: The nitrogen source of elemental diets—an unresolved issue. Nutr Clin Pract 5:227, 1990.
14. Ford EG, Hull SF, Jennings M, Andrassy RJ: Clinical comparison of tolerance to elemental or polymeric enteral feedings in the postoperative patient. J Am Coll Nutr 11:11, 1992.
15. Gorard DA, Hunt JB, Payne-James JJ, et al: Initial response and subsequent relapse course of Crohn's disease treated with elemental diet or prednisolone. Gut 34:1198, 1993.
16. McIntyre PB, Fitchew M, Lennard-Jones JE: Patients with a high jejunostomy do not need a special diet. Gastroenterology 91:25, 1986.
17. Cosnes J, Evard D, Beaugerie L, et al: Improvement in protein absorption with a peptide-based diet in patients with high jejunostomy. Nutrition 8:406, 1992.
18. Steinhardt HJ, Wolf A, Jakober B, et al: Nitrogen absorption in pancreatectomized patients: Protein versus protein hydrolysate as substrate. J Lab Clin Med 113:162, 1989.
19. Brinson RR, Kolts BE: Diarrhea associated with severe hypoalbuminemia: A comparison of a peptide-based chemically defined diet and a standard enteral alimentation. Crit Care Med 16:130, 1988.
20. Bounous G, Le Bel E, Shuster J, et al: Dietary protection during radiation therapy. Strahlentherapie 149:476, 1975.
21. Bounous G, Gentile JM, Hugon J: Elemental diet in the management of the intestinal lesion produced by 5-fluorouracil in man. Can J Surg 14:312, 1971.
22. Nalin DR, Cash RA, Rafiqul I, et al: Oral maintenance therapy for cholera in adults. Lancet 2:370, 1968.
23. Lennard-Jones JE: Oral rehydration solutions in short bowel syndrome. Clin Ther 12(Suppl A):129, 1990.
24. Winick M: National Task Force on Nutrition in AIDS. Guidelines on nutritional support in AIDS. Nutrition 5:390, 1989.
25. Pizarro D, Posada G, Sandi L, Moran JR: Rice-based oral electrolyte solutions for the management of infantile diarrhea. N Engl J Med 324:517, 1991.
26. Dutta D, Bhattacharya MK, Deb AK, et al: Evaluation of oral hypo-osmolar glucose-based and rice-based oral rehydration solutions in the treatment of cholera in children. Acta Paediatr 89:787, 2000.
27. Molla AM, Rahman M, Sarker SA, et al: Stool electrolyte content and purging rates in diarrhea caused by rotavirus, enterotoxigenic *E. coli*, and *V. cholerae* in children. J Pediatr 98:835, 1981.
28. Nalin DR, Harland E, Ramlal A, et al: Comparison of low and high sodium and potassium content in oral rehydration solutions. J Pediatr 97:848, 1980.
29. Bulus N, Cersosimo E, Ghishan F, Abumrad NN: Physiologic importance of glutamine. Metabolism 38(Suppl 1):1, 1989.
30. Cahill GF Jr: Starvation in man. Clin Endocrinol Metab 5:397, 1976.
31. Golden MH, Jahoor P, Jackson AA: Glutamine production rate and its contribution to urinary ammonia in normal man. Clin Sci 62:299, 1982.
32. Newsholme EA, Crabtree B, Ardawi MS: The role of high rates of glycolysis and glutamine utilization in rapidly dividing cells. Biosci Rep 5:393, 1985.
33. Matthews DE, Marano MA, Campbell RG: Splanchnic bed utilization of glutamine and glutamic acid in humans. Am J Physiol 264:E848, 1993.
34. Windmueller HG, Spaeth AE: Uptake and metabolism of plasma glutamine by the small intestine. J Biol Chem 249:5070, 1974.
35. Lacey JM, Wilmore DW: Is glutamine a conditionally essential amino acid? Nutr Rev 48:297, 1990.
36. Darmaun D, Just B, Messing B, et al: Glutamine metabolism in healthy adult men: Response to enteral and intravenous feeding. Am J Clin Nutr 59:1395, 1994.
37. Askanai J, Fürst P, Michelsen CB, et al: Muscle and plasma amino acids after injury: Hypocaloric glucose vs. amino acid infusion. Ann Surg 191:465, 1980.
38. MacLennan PA, Brown RA, Rennie MJ: A positive relationship between protein synthetic rate and intracellular glutamine concentration in perfused rat skeletal muscle. FEBS Lett 215:187, 1987.
39. Stehle P, Zander J, Mertes N, et al: Effect of parenteral glutamine peptide supplements on muscle glutamine loss and nitrogen balance after major surgery. Lancet 1:231, 1989.
40. Hammarqvist F, Wernerman J, Ali R, et al: Addition of glutamine to total parenteral nutrition after elective abdominal surgery spares free glutamine in muscle, counteracts the fall in muscle protein synthesis, and improves nitrogen balance. Ann Surg 209:455, 1989.
41. Klein S, Miles J: Substrate metabolism in humans. J Parenter Enteral Nutr 20:13, 1996.
42. Baskerville A, Hambleton P, Benbough JE: Pathological features of glutaminase toxicity. Br J Exp Pathol 61:132, 1980.
43. Grant JP, Snyder PJ: Use of L-glutamine in total parenteral nutrition. J Surg Res 44:506, 1988.
44. O'Dwyer ST, Smith RJ, Hwang TL, Wilmore DW: Maintenance of small bowel mucosa with glutamine-enriched parenteral nutrition. J Parenter Enteral Nutr 13:579, 1989.
45. Bark T, Svenberg T, Theodorsson E, et al: Glutamine supplementation does not prevent small bowel mucosal atrophy after total parenteral nutrition in the rat. Clin Nutr 13:79, 1994.
46. Babst R, Horig H, Stehle P, et al: Glutamine peptide-supplemented long-term total parenteral nutrition: Effects on intracellular and extracellular amino acid patterns, nitrogen economy, and tissue morphology in growing rats. J Parenter Enteral Nutr 17:566, 1993.
47. Wang X-D, Jacobs DO, O'Dwyer ST, et al: Glutamine-enriched parenteral nutrition prevents mucosal atrophy following massive bowel resection. Surg Forum 39:44, 1988.
48. Decker-Baumann C, Buhl K, Frohmuller S, et al: Reduction of chemotherapy-induced side-effects by parenteral glutamine supplementation in patients with metastatic colorectal cancer. Eur J Cancer 35:202, 1999.
49. Fox AD, Kripke SA, DePaula J, et al: Effect of a glutamine-supplemented enteral diet on methotrexate-induced enterocolitis. J Parenter Enteral Nutr 12:325, 1988.
50. Souba WW, Klimberg VS, Hautamaki RD, et al: Oral glutamine reduces bacterial translocation following abdominal radiation. J Surg Res 48:1, 1990.
51. Van der Hulst RRWJ, von Meyenfeldt FF, van Kreel BK, et al: Glutamine and the preservation of gut integrity. Lancet 341:1363, 1993.
52. Hond ED, Peeters M, Hiele M, et al: Effect of glutamine on the intestinal permeability changes induced by indomethacin in humans. Aliment Pharmacol Ther 13:679, 1999.
53. Tremel H, Kienle B, Weilemann LS, et al: Glutamine dipeptide supplemented TPN maintains intestinal function in critically ill. Gastroenterology 107:1595, 1994.
54. Hornsby-Lewis L, Shike M, Brown P, et al: L-Glutamine supplementation in home total parenteral nutrition patients: Stability, safety, and effects on intestinal absorption. J Parenter Enteral Nutr 18:268, 1994.
55. Byrne TA, Morissey TB, Nattakom TV, et al: Growth hormone, glutamine, and a modified diet enhance nutrient absorption in patients with severe short bowel syndrome. J Parenter Enteral Nutr 19:296, 1995.
56. Byrne TA, Persinger RL, Young LS, et al: A new treatment for patients with short-bowel syndrome: Growth hormone, glutamine, and a modified diet. Ann Surg 222:243, 1995.
57. Scolapio JS, Fleming CR, Camilleri MC, et al: Effect of growth hormone, glutamine and diet in short bowel syndrome. A randomized controlled study. Gastroenterology 113:1074, 1997.
58. Szkudlarek J, Jeppesen PB, Mortensen PB: Effect of high-dose growth hormone with glutamine and no change in diet on intestinal absorption in short bowel patients: A randomized, double blind, crossover, placebo-controlled study. Gut 47:199, 2000.
59. Scolapio JS: Effect of growth hormone and glutamine on the short bowel: Five years later. Gut 47:164, 2000.
60. Hammer HF, Fine KD, Santa Ana CA, et al: Carbohydrate malabsorption: Its measurement and its contribution to diarrhea. J Clin Invest 86:1936, 1990.
61. Bond JH, Currier BE, Buchwald M, Levitt MD: Colonic conservation of malabsorbed carbohydrates. Gastroenterology 78:444, 1980.
62. Morin CL, Ling V, Bourassa D: Small intestinal and colonic changes induced by a chemically defined diet. Dig Dis Sci 25:123, 1980.
63. Roediger WE, Nance S: Metabolic induction of experimental ulcerative colitis by inhibition of fatty acid oxidation. Br J Exp Pathol 67:773, 1986.
64. Murray FE, O'Brien MJ, Birkett DH, et al: Diversion colitis: Pathologic findings in a resected sigmoid colon and rectum. Gastroenterology 93:1404, 1987.

65. Harig JM, Soergel KH, Komorowski RA, Wood CM: Treatment of diversion colitis with short-chain fatty acid irrigation. N Engl J Med 320:23, 1989.
66. Guillemot F, Colombel JF, Neut C, et al: Treatment of diversion colitis by short chain fatty acids—prospective and double-blind study. Dis Colon Rectum 34:861, 1991.
67. Schauber J, Bark T, Jaramillo E, et al: Local short-chain fatty acids supplementation without beneficial effect on inflammation in excluded rectum. Scand J Gastroenterol 35:184, 2000.
68. Den Hond E, Hiele M, Evenepoel P, et al: In vivo butyrate metabolism and colonic permeability in extensive ulcerative colitis. Gastroenterology 115:584, 1998.
69. Simpson EI, Chapman MAS, Dawson J, et al: In vivo measurement of colonic butyrate metabolism in patients with quiescent ulcerative colitis. Gut 46:73, 2000.
70. Vernia P, Marcheggiano A, Caprilli R, et al: Short chain fatty acid topical treatment in distal ulcerative colitis. Aliment Pharmacol Ther 9:309, 1995.
71. Steinhart AH, Hiruki T, Brzezinski A, Baker JP: Treatment of left-sided ulcerative colitis with butyrate enemas: A controlled trial. Aliment Pharmacol Ther 10:729, 1996.
72. Scheppach W: Treatment of distal ulcerative colitis with short chain fatty acids. A placebo-controlled trial. German-Austrian SCFA Study Group. Dig Dis Sci 41:2254, 1996.
73. Breuer RI, Soergel KH, Lashner BA, et al: Short-chain fatty acid rectal irrigation for left-sided ulcerative colitis: A randomized, placebo-controlled trial. Gut 40:485, 1997.
74. Skutches CL, Holroyde CP, Myers RN, et al: Plasma acetate turnover and oxidation. J Clin Invest 64:708, 1979.
75. Binder HJ, Mehta P: Short-chain fatty acids stimulate active sodium and chloride absorption in vitro in the rat distal colon. Gastroenterology 96:989, 1989.
76. Hoverstad T, Carlstedt-Duke B, Lingaas E, et al: Influence of ampicillin, clindamycin, and metronidazole on faecal excretion of short-chain fatty acids in healthy subjects. Scand J Gastroenterol 21:621, 1986.
77. Roediger WE: Bacterial short-chain fatty acids and mucosal diseases of the colon. Br J Surg 75:346, 1988.
78. Zimmaro DM, Rolandelli RH, Koruda MJ, et al: Isotonic tube feeding formula induces liquid stool in normal subjects: Reversal by pectin. J Parenter Enteral Nutr 13:117, 1989.
79. Nicholson FB, Korman MG, Richardson MA: Percutaneous endoscopic gastrostomy: A review of indications, complications and outcome. J Gastroenterol Hepatol 15:21, 2000.
80. Hogan RB, DeMarco DC, Hamilton JK, et al: Percutaneous endoscopic gastrostomy—to push or pull. Gastrointest Endosc 32:253, 1986.
81. Russell TR, Brotman M, Norris F: Percutaneous gastrostomy: A new, simplified and cost-effective technique. Am J Surg 184:132, 1984.
82. Klein S, Heare BR, Soloway RD: The "buried bumper" syndrome: A complication of percutaneous endoscopic gastrostomy. Am J Gastroenterol 85:448, 1990.
83. Sharma VK, Howden CW: Meta-analysis of randomized, controlled trials of antibiotic prophylaxis before percutaneous endoscopic gastrostomy. Am J Gastroenterol 95:3133, 2000.
84. Hoffer EK, Cosgrove JM, Levin DQ, et al: Radiologic gastrojejunostomy and percutaneous endoscopic gastrostomy: A prospective, randomized comparison. J Vasc Interv Radiol 10:413, 1999.
85. Simon T, Fink AS: Recent experience with percutaneous endoscopic gastrostomy/jejunostomy (PEG/J) for enteral nutrition. Surg Endosc 14:436, 2000.
86. Wolfsen HC, Kozarek RA, Ball TJ, et al: Tube dysfunction following percutaneous endoscopic gastrostomy and jejunostomy. Gastrointest Endosc 36:261, 1990.
87. DiSario JA, Foutch PG, Sanowski RA: Poor results with percutaneous endoscopic jejunostomy. Gastrointest Endosc 36:257, 1990.
88. Adams GF, Guest DP, Ciraulo DL, et al: Maximizing tolerance of enteral nutrition in severely injured trauma patients: A comparison of enteral feedings by means of percutaneous endoscopic gastrostomy vs. percutaneous endoscopic gastrojejunostomy. J Trauma 48:459, 2000.
89. Halkier BK, Ho CS, Yee AC: Percutaneous feeding gastrostomy with the Seldinger technique: Review of 252 patients. Radiology 171:359, 1989.
90. Righi PD, Reddy DK, Weisberger EC, et al: Radiologic percutaneous gastrostomy: Results in 56 patients with head and neck cancer. Laryngoscope 108:1020, 1998.
91. Sarr MG, Mayo S: Needle catheter jejunostomy: An unappreciated and misunderstood advance in the care of patients after major abdominal operations. Mayo Clin Proc 63:565, 1988.
92. Shike M, Schroy P, Ritchie MA, et al: Percutaneous endoscopic jejunostomy on cancer patients with previous gastric resection. Gastrointest Endosc 33:372, 1987.
93. Vanlandingham S, Simpson S, Daniel P, Newmark SR: Metabolic abnormalities in patients supported with enteral tube feeding. J Parenter Enteral Nutr 5:322, 1981.
94. Marvin RG, McKinley BA, McQuiggan M, et al: Nonocclusive bowel necrosis occurring in critically ill trauma patients receiving enteral nutrition manifests no reliable clinical signs for early detection. Am J Surg 179:7, 2000.
95. Guenter PA, Settle RG, Perlmutter S, et al: Tube feeding–related diarrhea in acutely ill patients. J Parenter Enteral Nutr 15:277, 1991.
96. Edes TE, Walk BE, Austin JL: Diarrhea in tube-fed patients: Feeding formula not necessarily the cause. Am J Med 88:91, 1990.
97. Bell R, Fishman S: Eosinophilia from food dye added to enteral feedings. N Engl J Med 322:1822, 1990.
98. Metheny NA, Clouse RE: Bedside methods for detecting aspiration in tube-fed patients. Chest 111:724, 1997.
99. Kirby DF, DeLegge MH, Fleming CR: American Gastroenterological Association Technical Review on Tube Feeding for Enteral Nutrition. Gastroenterology 108:1282, 1995.
100. Smith HG, Orlando R: Enteral nutrition: Should we feed the stomach? Crit Care Med 27:1652, 1999.
101. Pillar B, Perry S: Evaluating total parenteral nutrition: Final report and core statement of the technology assessment and practice guidelines forum. Program on Technology and Health Care, Department of Community and Family Medicine, Georgetown University School of Medicine, Washington, D.C., 1990, p 29.
102. Naylor CB, O'Rourke K, Detsky AS, Baker JP: Parenteral nutrition with branched-chain amino acids in hepatic encephalopathy: A meta-analysis. Gastroenterology 97:1033, 1989.
103. Kopple JD: The nutrition management of the patient with acute renal failure. J Parenter Enteral Nutr 20:3, 1996.
104. Wolfe RR, O'Donnell TF Jr, Stone MD, et al: Investigation of factors determining the optimal glucose infusion rate in total parenteral nutrition. Metabolism 29:892, 1980.
105. Covelli HD, Black JW, Olsen MS, Beckman JF: Respiratory failure precipitated by high carbohydrate loads. Ann Intern Med 95:579, 1981.
106. Smith RC, Burkinshaw L, Hill GL: Optimal energy and nitrogen intake for gastroenterological patients requiring intravenous nutrition. Gastroenterology 82:445, 1982.
107. Jeejeebhoy KN, Anderson GH, Nakhooda AF: Metabolic studies in total parenteral nutrition with lipid in man. J Clin Invest 57:125, 1976.
108. Barr LH, Dunn GD, Brennan MF: Essential fatty acid deficiency during total parenteral nutrition. Ann Surg 193:304, 1981.
109. Fleming CR, Smith LM, Hodges RE: Essential fatty acid deficiency in adults receiving total parenteral nutrition. Am J Clin Nutr 29:976, 1976.
110. Jeejeebhoy KN, Marliss EB, Anderson GH, et al: Lipid in parenteral nutrition: Studies of clinical and metabolic features. In Meng HC, Wilmore DW (eds): Fat Emulsions in Parenteral Nutrition. Chicago, American Medical Association, 1976, p 45.
111. Delafosse B, Viale JP, Tissot S, et al: Effects of glucose-to-lipid ratio and type of lipid on substrate oxidation rate in patients. Am J Physiol 267(Endocrinol Metab 30):E775, 1994.
112. Miles JM: Intravenous fat emulsions in nutritional support. Curr Opin Gastroenterol 7:306, 1991.
113. Stafford WW, Day CE: Regression of atherosclerosis effected by intravenous phospholipid. Artery 1:106, 1975.
114. Skeie B, Askanazi J, Rothkopf MM, et al: Intravenous fat emulsions and lung function: A review. Crit Care Med 16:183, 1988.
115. DeGott C, Messing B, Moreau D, et al: Liver phospholipids induced by parenteral nutrition: Histologic, histochemical, and ultrasound investigation. Gastroenterology 95:183, 1988.
116. Seidner DL, Mascioli EA, Istfan NW, et al: Effect of long-chain triglyceride emulsions on reticuloendothelial system function in humans. J Parenter Enteral Nutr 13:614, 1989.
117. Lashner BA, Kirsner JB, Hanauer SB: Acute pancreatitis associated with high-concentration lipid emulsion during total parenteral nutrition therapy for Crohn's disease. Gastroenterology 90:1039, 1986.
118. Aviram M, Deckelbaum RJ: Intralipid infusion into humans reduces in

vitro platelet aggregation and alters platelet lipid composition. Metabolism 38:343, 1989.
119. Belin RP, Bivins BA, Jona JZ, Young VL: Fat overload with a 10% soybean oil emulsion. Arch Surg 111:1391, 1976.
120. Hiyama DT, Griggs B, Mittman RJ, et al: Hypersensitivity following lipid emulsion infusion in an adult patient. J Parenter Enteral Nutr 13: 318, 1989.
121. Casaubon PR, Dahlstrom KA, Vargas J, et al: Intravenous fat emulsion (Intralipid) delays gastric emptying, but does not cause gastroesophageal reflux in healthy volunteers. J Parenter Enteral Nutr 13: 246, 1989.
122. Malt RA, Kempster M: Direct azygos vein and superior vena cava cannulation for parenteral nutrition. J Parenter Enteral Nutr 7:580, 1983.
123. Jensen GL, Bistrian BR: Techniques for administering total parenteral nutrition. J Crit Illness 4:87, 1989.
124. Alhimyary A, Fernandez C, Picard M, et al: Safety and efficacy of TPN delivered via peripherally-inserted central venous catheters. J Parenter Enteral Nutr 19:A11;165, 1995.
125. Kearns PJ, Coleman S, Wehner JH: Complications of long-arm catheters: A randomized trial of central vs. peripheral tips location. J Parenter Enteral Nutr 20:20, 1996.
126. Nehme AB: Nutritional support of the hospitalized patient: The team concept. JAMA 243:1906, 1980.
127. Bozzetti F, Scarpa D, Terno G, et al: Subclavian venous thrombosis due to indwelling catheters: A prospective study on 52 patients. J Parenter Enteral Nutr 7:560, 1981.
128. Brismar B, Hardstedt C, Jacobson S, et al: Reduction of catheter-associated thrombosis in parenteral nutrition of intravenous heparin therapy. Arch Surg 117:1196, 1982.
129. Bern MM, Lokich JJ, Wallach SR, et al: Very low-dose warfarin can prevent thrombosis. A randomized prospective trial. Ann Intern Med 112:423, 1990.
130. Hill SE, Heldman LS, Goo EDH, et al: Case Report. Fatal microvascular pulmonary emboli from precipitation of a total nutrient admixture solution. J Parenter Enteral Nutr 20:81, 1996.
131. Food and Drug Administration: Safety alert: Hazards of precipitation associated with parenteral nutrition. Am J Hosp Pharm 51:427, 1994.
132. Driscoll DF: Total nutrient admixtures: Theory and practice. Clin Nutr 10:114, 1995.
133. Daly JM, Long JM: Intravenous hyperalimentation: Techniques and potential complications. Surg Clin North Am 61:583, 1981.
134. Rudman D, Williams PJ: Nutrient deficiencies during total parenteral nutrition. Nutr Rev 43:1, 1985.
135. Klein GL, Coburn JW: Parenteral nutrition: Effect on bone and mineral homeostasis. Ann Rev Nutr 11:93, 1991.
136. Clark-Christoff N, Watters VA, Sparks W, et al: Use of triple-lumen subclavian catheters for administration of total parenteral nutrition. J Parenter Enteral Nutr 16:403, 1992.
137. Johnson DC, Johnson FL, Goldman S: Preliminary results treating persistent central venous catheter infections with the antibiotic lock technique in pediatric patients. Pediatr Infect Dis J 13:930, 1994.
138. Messing B: Catheter-sepsis during home parenteral nutrition: Use of the antibiotic-lock technique. Nutrition 14:466, 1998.
139. Carratala J, Niubo J, Fernandez-Sevilla A, et al: Randomized, double-blind trial of an antibiotic-lock technique for prevention of gram-positive central venous catheter-related infection in neutropenic patients with cancer. Antimicrob Agents Chemother 43:2200, 1999.
140. Peden VH, Witzleben CL, Skelton MA: Total parenteral nutrition. J Pediatr 78:180, 1971.
141. Klein S: Total parenteral nutrition and the liver. In Schiff L, Schiff ER (eds): Diseases of the Liver, 7th ed. Philadelphia, JB Lippincott, 1993, pp 1505–1516.
142. Roslyn JJ, Pitt HA, Mann LL, et al: Gallbladder disease in patients on long-term parenteral nutrition. Gastroenterology 84:148, 1983.
143. Pitt HA, King W, Mann L, et al: Increased risk of cholelithiasis with prolonged total parenteral nutrition. Am J Surg 145:106, 1983.
144. Pitt HA, Lewinski MA, Muller EL, et al: Ileal resection–induced gallstones: Altered bilirubin or cholesterol metabolism? Surgery 96: 154, 1984.
145. Roslyn JJ, DenBesten L, Thompson JE Jr: Effects of periodic emptying of gallbladder on gallbladder function and formation of cholesterol gallstones. Surg Forum 30:403, 1979.
146. Sitzmann JV, Pitt HA, Steinborn PA, et al: Cholecystokinin prevents parenteral nutrition–induced biliary sludge in humans. Surg Gynecol Obstet 170:25, 1990.
147. Greenberg GR, Marlis EB, Anderson H, et al: Protein-sparing therapy in postoperative patients. Effects of added hypocaloric glucose or lipid. N Engl J Med 294:1411, 1976.
148. Khawaja HT, Williams JD, Weaver PC: Transdermal glyceryl trinitrate to allow peripheral total parenteral nutrition: A double-blind placebo-controlled feasibility study. J R Soc Med 84:69, 1991.
149. Everitt NJ, McMahon MJ: Peripheral intravenous nutrition. Nutrition 10:49, 1994.
150. Tighe MJ, Wong C, Martin IG, McMahon MJ: Do heparin, hydrocortisone, and glycerol trinitrate influence thrombophlebitis during full intravenous nutrition via a peripheral vein? J Parenter Enteral Nutr 19: 507, 1995.
151. Howard L, Ament M, Fleming CR, et al: Current use and clinical outcome of home parenteral and enteral nutrition therapies in the United States. Gastroenterology 109:355, 1995.
152. Fleming CR: Comprehensive care of the patient with gut failure: Present and future. Trans Am Clin Climatol Assoc 98:197, 1986.
153. Fleming CR, Beart RW Jr, Berkner S, et al: Home parenteral nutrition for management of the severely malnourished adult patient. Gastroenterology 79:11, 1980.
154. Levenstein S, Prantera C, Luzi C, D'ubaldi A: Low residue or normal diet in Crohn's disease: A prospective controlled study in Italian patients. Gut 26:989, 1985.
155. Ritchie JK, Wadsworth J, Lennard-Jones JE, Rogers E: Controlled multicenter therapeutic trial of an unrefined carbohydrate, fibre-rich diet in Crohn's disease. Br Med J 295:517, 1987.
156. Alun Jones V, Wilson AJ, Workman E, et al: Crohn's disease: Maintenance of remission by diet. Lancet 2:177, 1985.
157. Pearson M, Tehhon K, Kevi AJ, Bjarnason I: Food intolerance in Crohn's disease. Gut 34:783, 1993.
158. Riordan AM, Hintia JO, Cowan RE, et al: Treatment of active Crohn's disease by exclusion diet: East Anglian Multicentre Controlled Trial. Lancet 342:1131, 1993.
159. Middleton SJ, Rucker JT, Kirby GA: Long-chain triglycerides reduce the efficacy of enteral feeds in patients with active Crohn's disease. Clin Nutr 14:229, 1995.
160. O'Morain C, Segal AW, Levi AJ: Elemental diets as primary treatment of acute Crohn's disease: A controlled trial. Br Med J 288:1859, 1984.
161. Saverymuttu S, Hodgson HJF, Chadwick VS: Controlled trial comparing prednisone with an elemental diet plus non-absorbable antibiotics in active Crohn's disease. Gut 26:994, 1985.
162. Malchow H, Steinhardt HJ, Lorenz-Meyer H, et al: Feasibility and effectiveness of a defined formula diet regimen in treating active Crohn's disease: European Cooperative Crohn's Disease Study III. Scand J Gastroenterol 25:235, 1990.
163. Lochs H, Steinhardt HJ, Klaus-Wentz B, et al: Comparison of enteral nutrition and drug treatment in active Crohn's disease: Results of the European Cooperative Crohn's Disease Study IV. Gastroenterology 101:881, 1991.
164. Lindor K, Fleming CR, Burnes J, et al: A randomized prospective trial comparing a defined formula diet, corticosteroids, and a defined formula diet plus corticosteroids in active Crohn's disease. Mayo Clin Proc 67:328, 1992.
165. Gonzalez-Huix F, de Leon R, Fernandez-Banares F, et al: Polymeric enteral diets as primary treatment of active Crohn's disease: A prospective steroid-controlled trial. Gut 34:778, 1993.
166. Seidman EG, Lohoues MJ, Turgeon J, et al: Elemental diet versus prednisone as initial therapy in Crohn's disease: Early and long-term results [abstract]. Gastroenterology 100:A250, 1991.
167. Seidman EG, Griffiths AM, Jones A, Issenman R: The Canadian Paediatric Crohn's Disease Study Group. Semielemental diet versus prednisone in the treatment of active Crohn's disease in children and adolescents [abstract]. Gastroenterology 104:A778, 1993.
168. Middleton SJ, Riordan AM, Hunter JO: Peptide-based diet: An alternative to elemental diet in the treatment of acute Crohn's disease [abstract]. Gut 32:A578, 1991.
169. Royall D, Jeejeebhoy KN, Baker JP, et al: Comparison of amino acid vs. peptide-based enteral diets in active Crohn's disease: Clinical and nutritional outcome. Gut 35:783, 1994.
170. Giaffer MH, North G, Holdsworth CD: Controlled trial of polymeric versus elemental diet in treatment of active Crohn's disease. Lancet 335:816, 1990.
171. Park RHR, Galloway A, Danesh BJZ, Russell RI: Double-blind trial comparing elemental and polymeric diet as primary therapy for active Crohn's disease. Eur J Gastroenterol Hepatol 3:483, 1991.

172. Raouf AH, Hildrey V, Daniel J, et al: Enteral feeding as sole treatment for Crohn's disease: Controlled trial of whole protein versus amino acid–based feed and a case study of dietary challenge. Gut 32: 702, 1991.
173. Rigaud D, Cosnes J, Le Quintrec Y, et al: Controlled trial comparing two types of enteral nutrition in treatment of active Crohn's disease: Elemental versus polymeric diet. Gut 32:1492, 1991.
174. Munkholm Larsen P, Rasmussen D, Ronn B, et al: Elemental diet: A therapeutic approach in chronic inflammatory bowel disease. J Intern Med 225:325, 1989.
175. Mansfield JC, Giaffer MH, Holdsworth CD: Amino-acid versus oligopeptide based enteral feeds in active Crohn's disease [abstract]. Gut 33 (Suppl 2):53, 1992.
176. Griffiths AM, Ohlsson A, Sherman PM, Sutherland LR: Meta-analysis of enteral nutrition as a primary treatment of active Crohn's disease. Gastroenterology 108:1056, 1995.
177. Fernandez-Banares F, Cabre E, Esteve-Comas M, Gassull MA: How effective is enteral nutrition in inducing clinical remission in active Crohn's disease? A meta-analysis of the randomized clinical trials. J Parenter Enteral Nutr 19:356, 1995.
178. Messori A, Trallori G, D'Albasio G, et al: Defined-formula diets versus steroids in the treatment of active Crohn's disease. A meta-analysis. Scand J Gastroenterol 31:267, 1996.
179. Meyers S, Janowitz HD: "Natural history" of Crohn's disease. An analytic review of the placebo lesson. Gastroenterology 87:1189, 1984.
180. O'Brien CJ, Giaffer MH, Cann PA, Holdworth CD: Elemental diet in steroid-dependent and steroid-refractory Crohn's disease. Am J Gastroenterol 86:1614, 1991.
181. Muller JM, Keller HW, Erasmi H, Pichlmaier H: Total parenteral nutrition as the sole therapy in Crohn's disease—a prospective study. Br J Surg 70:40, 1983.
182. Greenberg GR, Fleming CR, Jeejeebhoy KN, et al: Controlled trial of bowel rest and nutritional support in the management of Crohn's disease. Gut 29:1309, 1988.
183. Alun Jones V: Comparison of total parenteral nutrition and elemental diet in induction of remission in Crohn's disease. Long-term maintenance of remission by personalized food exclusion diets. Dig Dis Sci 32:1009, 1987.
184. Lochs H, Meryn S, Marosi L, et al: Has total bowel rest a beneficial effect in the treatment of Crohn's disease? Clin Nutr 2:61, 1983.
185. Wright RA, Adler EC: Peripheral parenteral nutrition is no better than enteral nutrition in acute exacerbation of Crohn's disease: A prospective trial. J Clin Gastroenterol 12:396, 1990.
186. Dickinson RJ, Ashton MG, Axon ATR, et al: Controlled trial of intravenous hyperalimentation and total bowel rest as an adjunct to the routine therapy of acute colitis. Gastroenterology 79:1199, 1980.
187. McIntyre PB, Powell-Tuck J, Wood SR, et al: Controlled trial of bowel rest in the treatment of severe acute colitis. Gut 27:481, 1986.
188. Klein S, Meyers S, O'Sullivan P, et al: The metabolic impact of active ulcerative colitis. J Clin Gastroenterol 10:34, 1988.
189. Gonzalez-Huix F, Fernandez-Banares F, Esteve-Comas M, et al: Enteral versus parenteral nutrition as adjunct therapy in acute ulcerative colitis. Am J Gastroenterol 88:227, 1993.
190. Rombeau JL, Barot LR, Williamson CE, Mullen JL: Preoperative total parenteral and surgical outcome in patients with inflammatory bowel disease. Am J Surg 143:139, 1982.
191. Collins JP, Oxby CB, Hill GL: Intravenous amino acids and intravenous hyperalimentation as protein-sparing therapy after major surgery. A controlled clinical trial. Lancet 1:788, 1978.
192. Lashner BA, Evans AA, Hanauer SB: Preoperative total parenteral nutrition for bowel resection in Crohn's disease. Dig Dis Sci 34:741, 1989.
193. Kirshner BS: Nutritional consequences of inflammatory bowel disease on growth. J Am Coll Nutr 7:301, 1988.
194. Kirshner BS, Klich JR, Kalman SS, et al: Reversal of growth retardation in Crohn's disease with therapy emphasizing oral nutrition restitution. Gastroenterology 80:10, 1981.
195. Morin CL: Continuous elemental alimentation in children with Crohn's disease and growth failure. Gastroenterology 79:1205, 1980.
196. Amarnath RP, Fleming CR, Perrault J: Home parenteral nutrition in chronic intestinal diseases: Its effect on growth and development. J Pediatr Gastroenterol Nutr 6:89, 1987.
197. Edmunds LH Jr, Williams GM, Welch CE: External fistulas arising from the gastrointestinal tract. Ann Surg 152:445, 1960.
198. Himal HS, Allard JR, Nadeau JE, et al: The importance of adequate nutrition in closure of small intestinal fistulas. Br J Surg 61:724, 1974.
199. Byrne WJ, Burke M, Fonkalsrud EW, Ament ME: Home parenteral nutrition: An alternative approach to the management of complicated gastrointestinal fistulas not responding to conventional medical or surgical therapy. J Parenter Enteral Nutr 3:355, 1979.
200. DiCostanzo J, Cano N, Martin J, et al: Treatment of external gastrointestinal fistulas by a combination of total parenteral nutrition and somatostatin. J Parenter Enteral Nutr 11:465, 1987.
201. Stabile BE, Borzatta M, Stubbs RS, DeBas HT: Intravenous mixed amino acids and fats do not stimulate exocrine pancreatic secretion. Am J Physiol 246:G274, 1984.
202. McClave SA, Greene LM, Snider HL, et al: Comparison of the safety of early enteral versus parenteral nutrition in mild acute pancreatitis. J Parenter Enteral Nutr 21:14, 1997.
203. Windsor ACJ, Kanwar S, Li AGK, et al: Compared with parenteral nutrition, enteral feeding attenuates the acute phase response and improves disease severity in acute pancreatitis. Gut 42:431, 1998.
204. Kalfarentzos F, Kehagias J, Mead N, et al: Enteral nutrition is superior to parenteral nutrition in severe acute pancreatitis: Results of a randomized prospective trial. Br J Surg 84:1665, 1997.
205. Hyde D, Floch MH: The effect of peripheral nutritional support and nitrogen balance in acute pancreatitis [abstract]. Gastroenterology 86: 1119, 1984.
206. Durr GHK, Schaefers AL, Maroske D, et al: A controlled study on the use of intravenous fat in patients suffering from acute attacks of pancreatitis. Infusionstherapie Transfusionsmed 12:128, 1985.
207. Sax HC, Warner BW, Talamini MA, et al: Early total parenteral nutrition in acute pancreatitis: Lack of beneficial effects. Am J Surg 153:117, 1987.
208. Edelman K, Valenzuela JE: Effect of intravenous lipid on human pancreatic secretion. Gastroenterology 85:1063, 1983.
209. Lashner BA, Kirsner JB, Hanauer SB: Acute pancreatitis associated with high-concentration lipid emulsion during total parenteral nutrition therapy for Crohn's disease. Gastroenterology 90:1039, 1986.
210. Kessler JI, Kniffen JC, Janowitz HD: Lipoprotein lipase inhibition in the hyperlipemia of acute alcoholic pancreatitis. N Engl J Med 269: 943, 1963.
211. Stanley KE: Prognostic factors for survival in patients with inoperable lung cancer. J Natl Cancer Inst 65:25, 1980.
212. Klein S, Koretz RL: Nutrition support in cancer: What do the data really show? Nutr Clin Prac 9:91, 1994.
213. Klein S, Simes J, Blackburn GL: Total parenteral nutrition and cancer clinical trials. Cancer 58:1378, 1986.
214. McGeer AJ, Detsky AS, O'Rourke K: Parenteral nutrition in cancer patients undergoing chemotherapy: A meta-analysis. Nutrition 6:233, 1990.
215. Klein S, Luu K, Sakurai Y, et al: Metabolic response to radiation therapy in patients with cancer. Metabolism 45:767, 1996.
216. Buzby GP, Mullen JL, Matthews DC, et al: Prognostic nutritional index in gastrointestinal surgery. Am J Surg 139:160, 1980.
217. Heatley RV, Williams RH, Lewis MH: Pre-operative intravenous feeding in a controlled trial. Postgrad Med J 55:541, 1979.
218. Muller JM, Brenner U, Dienst C, Pichlmaier H: Preoperative parenteral feeding in patients with gastrointestinal carcinoma. Lancet 1:68, 1982.
219. Askanazi J, Hensle TW, Starker PM, et al: Effect of immediate postoperative nutritional support on length of hospitalization. Ann Surg 203:236, 1986.
220. Müller JM, Keller HW, Brenner U, et al: Indications and effects of preoperative parenteral nutrition. World J Surg 10:53, 1986.
221. Veterans Affairs Total Parenteral Nutrition Cooperation Study Group: Perioperative total parenteral nutrition in surgical patients. N Engl J Med 325:525, 1991.
221a. Koretz RL, Lipman TO, Klein S: Am Gastroenterol Assoc Tech Rev: Parenteral Nutrition. Gastroenterology 2001 (in press).
222. Romijn JA, Klein S: Extrahepatic metabolic consequences of cirrhosis. Gastroenterology 102:2175, 1992.
223. McCullough AJ, Mullen KD, Smanik EJ, et al: Nutritional therapy and liver disease. Gastroenterol Clin North Am 18:619, 1989.
224. Nompleggi DJ, Bonkovsky HL: Nutritional supplementation in chronic liver disease: An analytical review. Hepatology 18:518, 1994.
225. Cabre E, Gonzalez-Heux F, Abad-Lacruz A, et al: Effect of total enteral nutrition on the short-term outcome of severely malnourished cirrhotics. Gastroenterology 98:715, 1990.

226. Kearns PJ, Young H, Garcia G: Accelerated improvement of alcoholic liver disease with enteral nutrition. Gastroenterology 102:200, 1992.
227. Hirsch S, Bunout D, Pia de la Maza R, et al: Controlled trial on nutrition supplementation in outpatients with symptomatic alcoholic cirrhosis. J Parenter Enteral Nutr 17:119, 1993.
228. Greenberger NJ, Carley J, Schenker S, et al: Effect of vegetable and animal protein diets in chronic hepatic encephalopathy. Dig Dis 22: 845, 1977.
229. Uribe M, Marquez MA, Ramos GG, et al: Treatment of chronic portal-systemic encephalopathy with vegetable and animal protein diets. Dig Dis Sci 27:1109, 1982.
230. de Bruijn KM, Blendes LM, Zilm DH, et al: Effect of dietary protein manipulations in subclinical portal-systemic encephalopathy. Gut 24: 53, 1983.
231. Shaw S, Worner TM, Lieber CS: Comparison of animal and vegetable protein sources in the dietary management of hepatic encephalopathy. Am J Clin Nutr 38:59, 1983.
232. Weber IL, Jr, Minco D, Fresard KM, Banwell JG: Effect of vegetable protein diets on nitrogen metabolism in cirrhotic subjects. Gastroenterology 89:538, 1985.
233. Horst D, Grace ND, Conn HO, et al: Comparison of dietary protein with an oral, branched chain–enriched amino acid supplement in chronic portal-systemic encephalopathy: A randomized controlled trial. Hepatology 4:279, 1984.
234. Hasse JM, Blue LS, Liepa GU, et al: Early enteral nutrition support in patients undergoing liver transplantation. J Parenter Enteral Nutr 19: 437, 1995.
235. Le Cornu KA, McKiernan FJ, Kapadia SA, Neuberger JM: A prospective randomized study of preoperative nutritional supplementation in patients awaiting elective orthotopic liver transplantation. Transplantation 69:1364, 2000.
236. Fan ST, Lo CM, Lai ECS, et al: J. Perioperative nutritional support in patients undergoing hepatectomy for hepatocellular carcinoma. N Eng J Med 331:1547, 1994.

Chapter 17

Anorexia Nervosa, Bulimia Nervosa, and Obesity

Margo A. Denke

Anorexia nervosa, bulimia nervosa, and *obesity* are three diverse disorders of energy balance. The appropriateness of body weight for height and dietary habits are key features to their diagnoses. Before a separate discussion of these disorders, the importance of body weight and its relationship to energy balance are reviewed.

IMPORTANCE OF BODY WEIGHT AS A SURROGATE FOR HEALTH

Body weight is an inexpensive predictor of morbidity and mortality. A U-shaped relationship exists, in which extremes in weight—either too lean or too heavy—are associated with higher morbidity and mortality.

The high mortality rate in persons who are starving is well established. Persons who are underweight require less energy to meet their metabolic demands than do persons whose weight is normal. The state of protein-energy malnutrition, in which nutrient intake is insufficient to maintain optimal health, begins when further reductions in marginal energy intake occur. Adaptive mechanisms aimed at weight maintenance (reduction in basal metabolic rate, reduction in spontaneous physical activity) are activated. If these adaptations are insufficient to maintain weight, energy stores in adipose tissue and protein stores in skeletal muscle are mobilized.[1] Adult humans can adapt remarkably to chronic semistarvation, surviving even when body weight is slowly reduced to half of what is desirable. Muscle mass can be reduced to 25% of its original size before more essential protein stores are depleted.[2] The survival limit is reached when further weight loss results in catabolism of essential proteins required for mediating cellular function.

Although starvation is a recognizable consequence of protein-energy malnutrition, the graded relationship between mortality and underweight suggests that even more subtle deficiencies reduce long-term survival. Underweight persons are more likely to have subclinical nutrient deficiencies because of their lower energy intakes.[3, 4] Sudden increases in metabolic demands (infection, rapid growth of cancer cells) or decreases in energy intake (anorexia, famine) lead to rapid weight loss, unmasking the underlying protein-energy malnutrition. Studies in hospitalized patients suggest that protein-energy malnutrition is common in patients who lose more than 20% of their pre-illness weight over a 6-month period.[5] In this short period of time, adaptive mechanisms sparing protein-mediated cellular functions are not fully in place. As with death from starvation, underweight persons subjected to more rapid weight loss often die from infection caused by loss of cell-mediated immunity.

The deleterious effects of excess body weight are less intuitive. Being "pleasingly plump" might provide an effective buffer against the ominous effects of rapid weight loss. The detrimental costs of higher body weight in an otherwise healthy person were not readily appreciated until the early 1900s, when actuarial data published by life insurance companies suggested that gradations of excess body weight, similar to gradations of insufficient body weight, were associated with higher mortality.[6]

The first quantitative effort to link excess body weight to mortality was the 1953 Build and Blood Pressure Study, a cooperative effort of 26 American life insurance companies. The study combined actuarial data from 4.9 million persons without heart disease, cancer, or diabetes to clarify the relationships between body build, blood pressure, and mortality.[7]

It documented that overweight persons, even those without comorbidities, suffered excess mortality similar to that of underweight persons. Based on data collected in the Build Study, in 1959 the Metropolitan Life Insurance Company began publication of desirable weight tables instead of average weight tables. Desirable weight was defined as the body weight for height, frame size, and gender associated with the lowest mortality.[8] The Metropolitan Life tables, intended for health education, spearheaded public health efforts to promote healthy weights by identifying specific weight goals for adults that were typically 5 to 10 lb less than average weights.

Healthy weight standards for adult men and women became widely adopted. Body weight was often reported as a percentage above or below ideal body weight. However, the transportability of standards defined by the Build Study cohort to other cohorts was never formally tested. The Build Study cohort was made up predominantly of white middle-class Americans. Ethnic groups with smaller frames (e.g., Asians), leaner average population weight (e.g., Africans), and greater physical activity (e.g., manual laborers) were not represented. Can an ideal weight standard be defined for the human species? Is total body weight the best measurement?

Components of Body Weight

Total body weight is the sum of weights from several distinct body components. An increase in the relative weight of a specific component is not always associated with the expected change in risk predicted by the increase in total body weight. For example, patients with kwashiorkor have an edematous form of protein-energy malnutrition. Although these individuals may have heavier total body weights than patients with marasmus (the nonedematous form of protein-energy malnutrition), they are at higher risk of death than are marasmic patients.[9] Similarly, patients who perform strength-training exercises have heavier body weights than those who are sedentary, and yet improved physical fitness is associated with lower mortality. To investigate body weight and its relationship to health more precisely, a measurement of body components is needed.

Multiple approaches have been taken to quantify the various components of total body weight. Body composition can be characterized on an anatomic level (e.g., oxygen, carbon, hydrogen), a molecular level (e.g., water, lipid, protein), a cellular level (e.g., cell mass, extracellular fluid, extracellular solids), or a tissue system level (e.g., skeletal muscle, adipose tissue, bone, blood).[10] In addition to the relative proportion of various components, body composition can be further characterized by body habitus, for example, regional body fat distribution.[11]

Each different approach relies on different techniques to measure body components, their turnover, and their metabolism. Unfortunately, each technique has its own inherent limitations that have prevented widespread use in clinical medicine. For example, counting the natural radioactive potassium isotope (^{40}K) to determine lean body mass requires a well-standardized research laboratory. Nitrogen balance and creatinine excretion to determine protein turnover appear to be straightforward techniques available in any clinical laboratory, but their measurement requires meticulous subject cooperation on a metabolic ward where dietary intake can be precisely controlled. Computed tomography (CT) or dual energy x-ray absorptiometry (DEXA) scanning to determine total body fat content requires expensive, stationary equipment and exposure of subjects to radiation. Techniques that have minimal technical requirements trade precision for feasibility. For example, bioelectrical impedance measurements to determine lean body mass are quick and require minimal equipment, but their interpretation assumes that the human body is cylindrical in shape. The least expensive measurement used to estimate body fat, skinfold thickness, is subject to substantial intraoperator variation.

The complexity of precisely determining body composition and the ability to apply that method with equal effectiveness to any situation provide a sharp contrast to the simplicity, reproducibility, and feasibility of the measurement of total body weight. Body weight usually varies less than 0.1 kg/day when measured by the most precise techniques[12]; even when equipment/observer error are added, the coefficient of variation from methodologic techniques for total body weight is small. How best to report body weight for height, gender, and frame size becomes the issue.

Concept of Body Mass Index

In the 1800s, Quetelet proposed a simple way to express relative body weight using the ratio of weight in kilograms divided by height in meters squared (kg/m^2). This ratio has been referred to as the Quetelet Index, or the body mass index (BMI).[13] BMI provides a continuous range of relative weight for height irrespective of gender and frame size. Since the 1980s, BMI has grown in popularity as a universal, simple, and inexpensive measurement of relative weight for height. For the average person, BMI is highly correlated with fat mass. In a study of over 400 women, the correlation coefficient between total weight adjusted for height squared vs. total body fat adjusted for height squared was 0.9.[12] A BMI conversion chart is provided in Table 17–1.

Clinically, BMI measurements have permitted definitions of unhealthy weights without requiring the definition of an "ideal" weight. Several national and international organizations have forwarded guidelines for classifying weight insufficiency and weight excess in adults (Table 17–2). A BMI of less than 16 kg/m^2 is diagnostic for protein-energy malnutrition in adults,[14]† and a BMI greater than 30 kg/m^2 is diagnostic for obesity.[15]

Recently published data[16] have confirmed the U-shaped curve relating BMI to all-cause mortality that had been previously described in several prospective studies of older persons.[17] The U-shaped relationship remains even when data are adjusted for smoking status or preexisting disease; the relative risk for thinness, however, is dwarfed by the higher risk for death among morbidly obese persons (Fig. 17–1). Body weight is an important vital sign that should be measured at every patient encounter.

†BMI does not adequately define the effects of protein-energy status on childhood growth requirements. In children, malnutrition is best assessed by evaluating weight for height deficits (wasting) or height for age deficits (stunting). (WHO: Measuring change in nutritional status. Geneva, World Health Organization, 1983.) Obesity in children is best assessed using age-adjusted weight for height growth curves.

Table 17–1 | **Converting Height in Feet/Inches and Weight in Pounds to Body Mass Index**

	4'10"	4'11"	5'0"	5'1"	5'2"	5'3"	5'4"	5'5"	5'6"	5'7"	5'8"	5'9"	5'10"	5'11"	6'0"	6'1"	6'2"
80	17	16	16	15	15	14	14	13	13	13	12	12	11	11	11	11	10
90	19	18	18	17	17	16	15	15	15	14	14	13	13	13	12	12	12
100	21	20	20	19	18	18	17	17	16	16	15	15	14	14	14	13	13
110	23	22	22	21	20	20	19	18	18	17	17	16	16	15	15	15	14
120	25	24	23	23	22	21	21	20	19	19	18	18	17	17	16	16	15
130	27	26	25	25	24	23	22	22	21	20	20	19	19	18	18	17	17
140	29	28	27	27	26	25	24	23	23	22	21	21	20	20	19	19	18
150	31	30	29	28	27	27	26	25	24	24	23	22	22	21	20	20	19
160	34	32	31	30	29	28	28	27	26	25	24	24	23	22	22	21	21
170	36	34	33	32	31	30	29	28	27	27	26	25	24	24	23	22	22
180	38	36	35	34	33	32	31	30	29	28	27	27	26	25	24	24	23
190	40	38	37	36	35	34	33	32	31	30	29	28	27	27	26	25	24
200	42	40	39	38	37	36	34	33	32	31	30	30	29	28	27	26	26
210	44	43	41	40	38	37	36	35	34	33	32	31	30	29	29	28	27
220	46	45	43	42	40	39	38	37	36	35	34	33	32	31	30	29	28
230	48	47	45	44	42	41	40	38	37	36	35	34	33	32	31	30	30
240	50	49	47	45	44	43	41	40	39	38	37	36	35	34	33	32	31
250	52	51	49	47	46	44	43	42	40	39	38	37	36	35	34	33	32
260	54	53	51	49	48	46	45	43	42	41	40	38	37	36	35	34	33
270	57	55	53	51	49	48	46	45	44	42	41	40	39	38	37	36	35
280	59	57	55	53	51	50	48	47	45	44	43	41	40	39	38	37	36
290	61	59	57	55	53	51	50	48	47	46	44	43	42	41	39	38	37

Table 17–2 | **Body Mass Index (BMI) Criteria for Protein-Energy Malnutrition, Normal Weight, Overweight, and Obesity**

BMI (kg/m²)	NUTRITION STATUS
<16.0	Protein energy malnutrition—severe
16.0–16.9	Protein energy malnutrition—moderate
17.0–18.4	Protein energy malnutrition—mild
18.5–24.9	Normal
25.0–29.9	Overweight
30.0–34.9	Obesity—grade I
35.0–39.9	Obesity—grade II
≥40.0	Obesity—grade III

Data from James WPT, Ferro-Luzzi A, Waterlow JC: Definition of chronic energy deficiency in adults. Report of a working party of the International Dietary Energy Consultative Group. Eur J Clin Nutr 42:969–981, 1988; and National Heart, Lung, and Blood Institute: Clinical guidelines on the identification, evaluation, and treatment of overweight and obesity in adults—the evidence report. Obes Res 6[Suppl 2]51S–209S, 1998.

Caloric Requirements to Maintain Weight, Gain Weight, or Lose Weight

Baseline Requirements

Caloric requirements can be inferred from estimates of energy expenditure. The most precise equation predicting resting caloric requirements is the Harris-Benedict equation (Table 17–3; see also Chapter 15). The equation estimates basal energy requirements of hospitalized, medically stable individuals. The key terms in the equation reflect the determinants of fat free mass, the most biologically active tissue. Women need fewer calories than men, since women have 30% less fat free mass than men. Tall persons, who have greater skeletal mass, require more calories than short persons. Heavier persons, who also have greater fat free mass, require more calories than lean persons to maintain their weight. Caloric requirements go down with age as fat free mass declines.

A simplified prediction equation for caloric requirements in outpatients has been forwarded by Owen and colleagues[18, 19] (see Table 17–3). Gender, weight, and physical activity are the only variables needed for the prediction. Minimum caloric needs are first calculated based on gender and weight; this term is then multiplied by a physical activity factor. Physical activity appropriately modifies the entire estimate, since heavier persons expend more energy during activity than lean persons.

Table 17–3 | **Equations to Predict Caloric Requirements**

Harris-Benedict Equation
Men = 66 + (13.7 × W) + (5 × H) − (6.8 × A)
Women = 655 + (9.6 × W) + (1.8 × H) − (4.7 × A)
where W = weight in kg, H = height in cm, A = age in years

Owen et al Equation
Men = [900 + 4.5 × (wt in lb)] × activity factor
Women = [800 + 3.2 × (wt in lb)] × activity factor
where activity factor low = 1.2 (e.g., sedentary job), moderate = 1.4, high = 1.6 (e.g., manual labor; daily exercise program)

Weight Gain and Loss

A weekly increase of 3700 kcal will produce on average a 1-lb gain in weight. Individual variation in weight gain is remarkable. In an 8-week overfeeding study, individuals who gained less weight had greater increases in compensatory spontaneous activity, such as fidgeting, than individuals who gained more weight.[20] The regulation of these nonessential activities is an area of investigation that may provide further clues in the pathogenesis of obesity.

A 1 lb per week weight loss occurs when a weekly deficit of 3700 kcal is achieved.

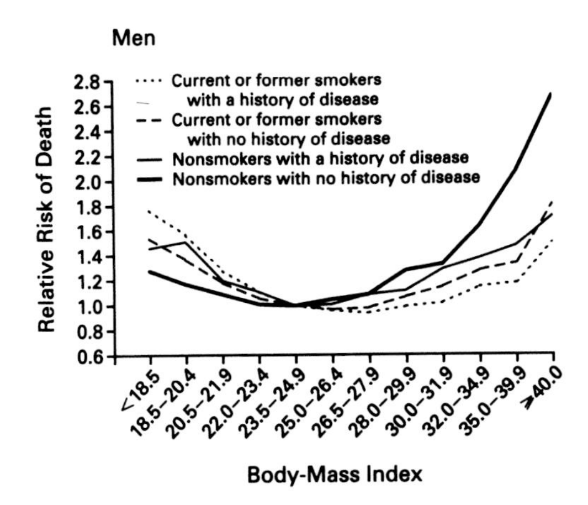

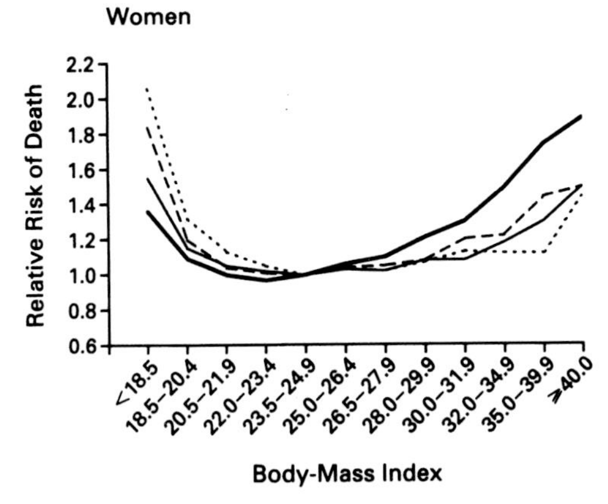

Figure 17–1. Multivariate relative risk of death from all causes among 1,184,657 men and women enrolled in the Cancer Prevention Study II according to body mass index, smoking status, and disease status. The four subgroups are mutually exclusive. Nonsmokers had never smoked. The reference category was made up of subjects with a body mass index of 23.5 to 24.9. (From Calle EE, Thun MJ, Petrelli JM, et al: Body mass index and mortality in a prospective cohort of US adults. N Engl J Med 341:1097–1105, 1999.)

Evaluating Caloric Intake/Requirements

A simple way to evaluate dietary habits and physical activity is to ask patients to describe their day chronologically. Specific questions regarding wake-up time, contents of a typical breakfast, driving time to work, physical activity in the morning, snacks and their availability, time taken for lunch, and the social environment conducive to lunchtime eating, and so forth, can often reveal opportunities for excessive dietary intake, as well as missed opportunities for exercise.

DISORDERS IN ENERGY BALANCE

Many physicians consider anorexia nervosa, bulimia nervosa, and obesity to be eating disorders, since all three diagnoses are manifestations of energy imbalance. However, eating disorders have been defined by their psychiatric, not metabolic, characteristics. The diagnosis of anorexia nervosa or bulimia nervosa is made only when patients have distinct misperceptions of body image that lead to obsessive concerns about body weight and inappropriate, unhealthy behaviors to combat weight gain. Obesity is not universally associated with psychological misconceptions in body image; therefore, obesity is not classified among the eating disorders.

ANOREXIA NERVOSA

Historical Perspective and Disease Prevalence Estimates

Anorexia nervosa is a distinct disorder first described in the 17th century by Richard Morton. A 17-year-old girl appeared "like a skeleton clad only in skin."[21] It was not named until Sir William Gull[22] collected and described three cases of weight loss in young women. Gull was struck by the patients' energetic, restless behavior despite their emaciation (nervosa) and their lack of interest in food (anorexia). Amenorrhea, bradycardia, and hypothermia were noted. Criteria for diagnosis are outlined in Table 17–4.[23] There are two distinctive subtypes of anorexia: restricting and binge eating/purging. Patients can alternate between subtypes at different periods of their illness.

The prevalence of anorexia nervosa has been estimated from a large database in Rochester, Minnesota, as 0.3% of teenage girls and 0.02% of teenage boys.[24] Lifetime prevalence has been estimated at 4% if less strict criteria are used.[25] Ninety percent of affected persons are female; most develop the disease after puberty but before age 25 years;

Table 17–4 | **Diagnostic Criteria for Anorexia Nervosa**

A. Refusal to maintain body weight at or above a minimally normal weight for age and height
B. Intense fear of gaining weight or becoming fat, even though underweight
C. Disturbance in the way in which one's body weight or shape is experienced, undue influence of body weight or shape on self-evaluation, or denial of the seriousness of the current low body weight
D. In postmenarcheal women, amenorrhea, i.e., the absence of at least three consecutive menstrual cycles. (A woman is considered to have amenorrhea if her periods occur only following hormone, e.g., estrogen, administration)

In the restricting type of anorexia nervosa, the person has not regularly engaged in binge eating or purging using self-induced vomiting, misuse of laxatives, diuretics, or enemas; in the binge-eating/purging type, the person has regularly engaged in binge-eating or purging behavior.

only rarely are women older than age 40 years newly diagnosed. Anorexia nervosa afflicts women in all socioeconomic classes and ethnicities. Women with anorexia nervosa may choose certain professions in which perfectionism and lean body weights are desired, such as ballet dancers in whom the prevalence of anorexia nervosa may be as high as 20%.[26]

Natural History

Patients with anorexia nervosa have an exaggerated fear of becoming fat. They are intensely afraid of gaining weight. This fear produces a variety of behaviors to avoid weight gain, including caloric restriction, intermittent starvation, obsessive exercise regimens,[27] and, in some patients, purging. In 5% of patients, the psychiatric issues create a vicious cycle that culminates in death from inanition, suicide, electrolyte disturbance, infection, or cardiopulmonary decompensation.[28]

The disorder may have been preceded by the initiation of a rigorous exercise program. Patients typically do not report reduced appetite. They consume food in small quantities and avoid consuming foods they believe will cause weight gain. Some prepare their own food and are reluctant to eat food in the company of others. Patients with anorexia nervosa develop protein-energy malnutrition from low-energy diets. Some preserve high dietary protein intakes by becoming nutritionally savvy, e.g., choosing low-calorie complete protein sources such as egg whites. However, regardless of food choices, the low-energy content of the diet causes an attendant low intake of micronutrients. Although overt vitamin deficiencies are rare, subclinical micronutrient deficiencies, particularly of copper and zinc, are common.[29] Theoretically, the metabolic consequences of dietary inadequacies seen in patients with anorexia nervosa should be measurable.[30]

Etiology and Psychological Aspects

The psychiatric disturbance of anorexia nervosa was not fully characterized until the 1950s. Patients share in common three cognitive disturbances: the inability to appreciate the need to be adequately nourished, a disturbance of body image perception in which the patient cannot perceive how thin she or he really is, and an intense feeling of ineffectiveness.[31] Psychodynamically, patients with anorexia nervosa have difficulty with separation and autonomy, regulation of affect, and negotiating psychosexual development.[23] Past history of sexual abuse has been reported in 20% to 50% of cases.

Clinical Features

Patients with anorexia nervosa typically come to medical evaluation because of weight loss. They often complain of epigastric discomfort, fullness following meals, and constipation. Amenorrhea is universal and may precede significant weight loss. Low levels of luteinizing hormone (LH) and loss of normal episodic variation in LH secretion, both reversible with pulsatile administration of gonadotropin-releasing hormone, point to a hypothalamic defect.[32] Despite the rigorous exercise routines, the low estradiol levels in these young women greatly diminishes bone mineral density in both cortical and trabecular bone. A history of fractures is common.[33] The height of peak bone mass is blunted, with little recovery following reversal of the amenorrhea,[34] resulting in a greater lifetime risk for fracture.[35] It is unclear whether oral contraceptive use can totally mitigate these risks.

Patients with anorexia nervosa or bulimia nervosa have a distorted importance of body weight in defining themselves and their self-worth. The distortion in the patient's body perception can be readily demonstrated by asking patients how they feel about their weight, how they would feel about gaining a small amount of weight (e.g., 2 lb) or about losing weight, what they believe their ideal weight should be, and how important body weight is compared with other areas of their life, including family, school, and work. Patients' answers to these questions may be the sole basis for the diagnosis of an eating disorder, since the physical and laboratory examinations are often normal.

Physical Examination

On physical examination, patients are thin, with depletion of subcutaneous fat. The BMI is typically less than 17.5 kg/m^2. Patients appear restless despite their emaciation. Postpubertal girls have preserved secondary sexual characteristics, with normal breast size and axillary and pubic hair. Long-standing advanced disease, however, can lead to breast atrophy. Dry skin is universally seen. To preserve thermogenic energy, 40% of patients have acrocyanosis due to selective peripheral vasoconstriction.[36] Palms and soles may be yellow-orange from hypercarotenemia. The increase in carotenoids is thought to be due to a reduction in their catabolism,[37] as well as an increase in relative intake,[38] since foods containing carotenoids have low caloric density. Seventy percent of the patients have lanugo on the trunk and limbs (Fig. 17–2); lanugo can also be prominent on the face. The extent of hypertrichosis is correlated with the existence of amenorrhea or a BMI of less than 16 kg/m^2.[39] Bradycardia and murmurs of mitral and tricuspid regurgitation are common in patients who have lost 25% of their ideal body weight. Hypotension and hypothermia may be present in severe cases.

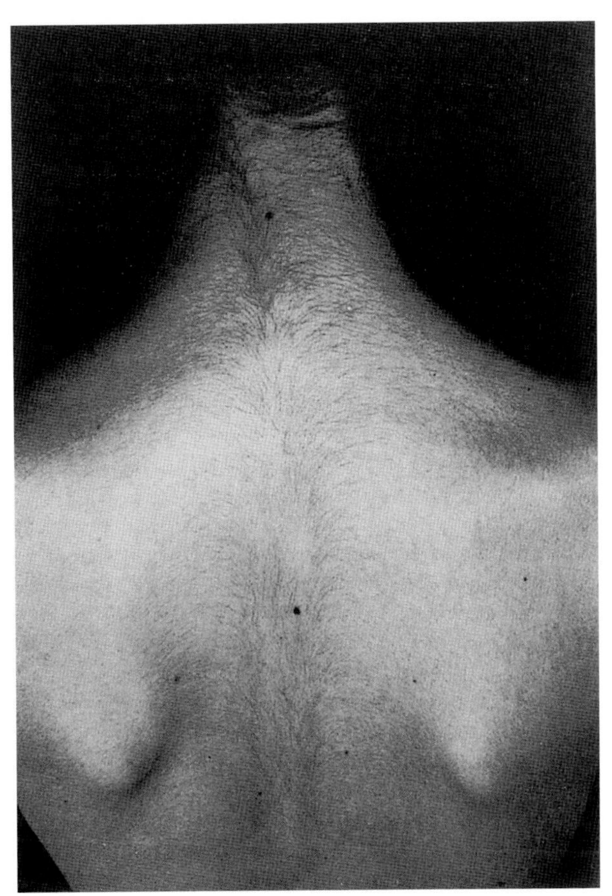

Figure 17–2. Diffuse hypertrichosis in a woman with anorexia nervosa. Note the loss of subcutaneous fat. (From Schulze UME, Pettke-Rank CV, Kreienkamp M, et al: Dermatologic findings in anorexia and bulimia nervosa of childhood and adolescence. Pediatr Dermatol 16[2]: 90–94, 1999.)

Laboratory Examination

Screening laboratory tests should include complete blood count (CBC) with white blood cell differential, serum electrolytes, calcium, magnesium, phosphorus, liver function tests, glucose, and thyroid-stimulating hormone (TSH). Hemoglobin and hematocrit are typically normal; acanthocytes are common. Iron deficiency anemia, presumably due to transient gut ischemia during rigorous exercise, has been reported in anorectic runners.[40] Electrolyte disturbances with hypokalemia and metabolic alkalosis are present in 25% of patients and usually indicate that the patient uses vomiting to purge; when present, the hypokalemia tends to be mild. Profound hypokalemia suggests a poor prognosis.[41] Hypomagnesemia, if present, suggests long-standing diuretic and purgative abuse.[42] BUN may be disproportionately high compared with creatinine, reflecting dehydration from diuretics, laxative abuse, or decreased fluid intake. Liver enzymes are abnormal in 4% of patients, typically with high alanine transaminase (ALT), aspartate transferase (AST), or alkaline phosphatase.[43] Hypercholesterolemia, thought secondary to mineral deficiency, occurs in a third of patients. TSH levels are typically normal, except in patients severely ill who have sick-euthyroid state. Growth hormone levels and serum cortisol levels may be increased. Estradiol levels are in the prepubertal range due to loss of LH pulsatility and amplitude.

In patients with hypokalemia or severe emaciation, electrocardiogram may reveal profound bradycardia, with rates as low as 35 bpm common. Ectopic ventricular beats, premature atrial beats, and paroxysmal supraventricular tachycardia can be seen. Reduced amplitude in p waves and QRS voltage can be seen. Rarely, u wave or prolonged QT interval is present, suggesting a worse prognosis.

Radiologic examination shows a diminished cardiothoracic ratio in patients with anorexia, particularly those who have lost more than 20% of their body weight.[44] Echocardiogram of the heart may show ventriculovalvular disproportion, in which the relative loss of cardiac muscle results in redundancy of the valve and a tendency to prolapse.[45] DEXA scan will show diffusely reduced bone density. Magnetic resonance imaging (MRI) may show ventricular enlargement, as evidenced by an increase in the ventricular-to-brain ratio; these changes reverse with refeeding.[46]

Differential Diagnosis

Other than a distorted body image, no specific symptoms, physical findings, or laboratory assessment make the diagnosis of anorexia nervosa. Table 17–5 lists common symptoms and the expected findings on physical examination and laboratory examination consistent with the diagnosis. In general, CBC and serum chemistries help exclude diagnoses such as malabsorption, malignancy, and psychiatric disorders associated with weight loss.

Malabsorption from celiac sprue, pancreatic insufficiency, parasitic intestinal infections, inflammatory bowel disease, or intestinal obstruction can present as weight loss and anorexia; additionally, patients complain of abdominal pain, bloating, nausea, vomiting, and diarrhea. Anemia and steatorrhea are present. In contrast to patients with anorexia nervosa, patients with malabsorption recognize their cachexia and are appropriately concerned (see Chapter 89).

Malignancy, particularly lymphoma and gastric cancer, can present with weight loss. The presence of a normal CBC and the absence of tumor mass or lymphadenopathy on physical examination will help rule out these disorders. Rarely, hypothalamic tumors can present with anorexia; patients typically complain of headaches and physical examination reveals papilledema.

Depression can present with anorexia, but the patient will be listless and withdrawn, not hyperkinetic. *Hyperthyroidism* can present with hyperactive behavior and weight loss, but the appearance of tremor and goiter, as well as elevated free T_4 estimate and suppressed TSH, will make this diagnosis. *Adrenal insufficiency* can present with weight loss; however the patient will complain of fatigue and often have a normochromic anemia (see Chapters 26, 29, and 44).

Systemic Complications

Starvation is the systemic complication of anorexia nervosa. Additional complications occur in patients who use vomiting as a means to purge. Dental erosions with loss of dental enamel, particularly of the lingual-occlusive surface of the teeth,[47] are seen in vomiters whose oral cavity is frequently

Table 17–5 | **Evaluation of Symptoms in Patients with Suspected Anorexia Nervosa**

PATIENT COMPLAINTS	FINDINGS CONSISTENT WITH THE DIAGNOSIS OF ANOREXIA NERVOSA	
	Physical Examination	**Lab and X-ray Examination**
Weakness, lassitude	Malnutrition with low BMI and loss of subcutaneous fat	Hypokalemic, hypochloremic alkalosis from vomiting; hypomagnesemia and hypophosphatemia from laxative abuse
Apathy, poor concentration	Cognitive impairment; depressed, irritable mood	CT scan: ventricular enlargement; MRI: decreased gray and white matter
Palpitations, weakness, dizziness, shortness of breath, chest pain, coldness of extremities	Irregular, weak, slow pulse; mitral and tricuspid regurgitation; mitral valve prolapse with midsystolic click; marked orthostatic blood pressure changes; acrocyanosis	Hypokalemic, hypochloremic alkalosis from vomiting; hypomagnesemia and hypophosphatemia from laxative abuse; ECG: bradycardia, arrhythmias; Q-Tc prolongation; ECHO: disproportionally large valve area for ventricular size, promoting valve prolapse
Bone pain with exercise	Point tenderness on skeletal examination; short stature	Pathologic stress fractures on plain film; reduced bone mineral, particularly in the hip and spine by DEXA
Weakness, muscle aches	Muscle wasting	Hypokalemic, hypochloremic alkalosis from vomiting; hypomagnesemia and hypophosphatemia from laxative abuse; muscle enzyme abnormalities from malnutrition, with normal or 2- to 10-fold increases in AST, ALT, and CPK possible; the possibility of chronic ipecac abuse should be investigated.
Amenorrhea	Lanugo; arrested sexual development if disorder began during puberty; normal sexual development if after completion of puberty	Hypoestrogenemia (estradiol < 20 pg/mL); prepubertal patterns of LH, FSH secretion; lack of follicular development/dominant follicle on pelvic ultrasound
Fatigue; cold intolerance; diuresis; vomiting	Hypothermia	Elevated serum cortisol; increase in reverse T_3; dehydration; electrolyte abnormalities; hypophosphatemia and hypoglycemia (rare)
Fatigue; cold intolerance	Bruises (rare)	Anemia; neutropenia with relative lymphocytosis; thrombocytopenia; low erythrocyte sedimentation rate; low fibrinogen (rare)
Vomiting; abdominal pain; bloating; obstipation; constipation	Abdominal distention with meals; succussion splash	Delayed gastric emptying; occasionally abnormal liver function test results
Painful feet	Pitting edema (rare)	Elevated BUN; low glomerular filtration rate; hypoalbuminemia (rare)
Unwanted hair growth	Lanugo	Hypoestrogenemia; prepubertal patterns of LH, FSH secretion; lack of follicular development or dominant follicle on pelvic ultrasound

ALT, alanine transferase; AST, aspartate transaminase; BMI, body mass index; BUN, blood urea nitrogen; CPK, creatine phosphokinase; CT, computed tomography; DEXA, dual-energy x-ray absorptiometry; ECG, electrocardiogram; ECHO, echocardiogram; FSH, follicle-stimulating hormone; LH, luteinizing hormone; MRI, magnetic resonance imaging; T_3, triiodothyronine.

Table 17–6 | **Indications for Hospitalization in Patients with Anorexia Nervosa or Bulimia Nervosa**

INDICATION	CLINICAL MANIFESTATIONS	THERAPEUTIC CAUTIONS
Severe malnutrition	BMI < 17 and refusal to eat; weight loss proceeding at a rapid rate	Refeeding should start at 30–40 kcal/kg with minimum of q3d laboratory monitoring of Na, K, Mg, Po'_4, daily monitoring for development of edema, congestive heart failure, arrhythmia
Volume depletion	Orthostasis with BP drop > 20 mm Hg, HR increase > 20 bpm/min standing	Patients have hyperaldosteronisim; fluid repletion > 2 L/d will cause peripheral edema; hyperaldosterone state will resolve in several weeks
Cardiac instability	HR < 40 bpm HR > 100 bpm Prolonged QT interval	Bradycardia resolves spontaneously with refeeding; patients with tachyarrhythmias and prolonged QT interval are at risk for sudden death and require cardiac monitoring
Electrolyte abnormalities	Hypokalemia, hyponatremia, hypomagnesemia or hypophosphatemia, particularly concerning patients who have had recent, rapid reductions in levels	Fluid resuscitation must take into account the hyperaldosterone state; further reductions during refeeding should be anticipated and monitored
Hypothermia	Temperature < 97°F	Sick-euthyroid state should be managed conservatively with refeeding
Psychiatric issues	Suicidal intent and plan Concurrent substance abuse Inability to gain weight or stop weight loss despite ongoing counseling and participation in a self-monitored structured plan	Requires suicide precautions More common in patients with bulimia *This is the most frequent indication for hospitalization*

BMI, body mass index; BP, blood pressure; HR, heart rate.

exposed to the low pH of gastric contents.[48] Raised callosities over the knuckles, which may be ulcerated, can appear on the hands of anorectics who manually induce vomiting using the gag reflex.[49] Benign parotid swelling and dry mouth can be seen in patients with hypokalemic alkalosis.[50] The frequency of purging behaviors and the type of purging often can explain the severity of the hypokalemia. Patients who use syrup of ipecac can consume significant quantities of the toxic alkaloid emetine. Exposure to 1250 mg of emetine (approximately forty 30-mL bottles) over a several-month period can lead to cardiomyopathy and death; left ventricular dysfunction may be reversible in some cases.[51]

The physical strain of vomiting may also have significant complications. Aspiration pneumonia in a patient with aperistaltic esophagus has been reported.[52] Pneumomediastinum following forceful vomiting has been reported, resolving spontaneously with conservative management.[53]

Gastrointestinal Complications

Symptoms due to dysfunction of the esophagus, stomach, colon, pancreas, and liver are common. All symptoms except belching improve during refeeding and rarely require drug therapy, x-ray or endoscopic evaluation.[54]

ESOPHAGEAL AND GASTRIC MOTILITY. Patients may complain of dysphagia for solids. In one series, half of patients were shown by manometry to have achalasia or nonpropulsive and repetitive contractions.[55] Whether or not the achalasia was a primary disorder or secondary to anorexia nervosa is uncertain, because both can present with vomiting and weight loss. In either case, malnutrition is the suspected underlying etiology for the dysmotility observed. Gastric motility is altered, with delayed emptying for solids but not liquids, consistent with an antral motility disturbance.[56] Gastric motility returns to normal following refeeding[57] (see Chapters 6 and 37).

SUPERIOR MESENTERIC ARTERY SYNDROME. Patients with anorexia nervosa can lose the retroperitoneal fat pad that protects the third portion of the duodenum from compression between the superior mesenteric vessels and the aorta/spine. Acute superior mesenteric artery syndrome, with severe post-prandial pain, bloating, and vomiting, has been described[58] (see Chapters 8 and 120).

ABNORMAL COLONIC MOTILITY. Patients with anorexia nervosa complain of chronic constipation. Whether or not this is due to reduction in liquid intake or is a justification for laxative abuse is unclear. Melanosis coli from laxative abuse may be seen on endoscopy. In a study of patients admitted to an inpatient unit for treatment of their anorexia nervosa, colonic transit time assessed by radiopaque markers was 86 ± 17.8 hr in those patients studied within 3 weeks of admission, compared with 34.1 ± 4.1 hr in those studied after 3 weeks of nutrition therapy and 28.0 ± 8.6 hr in controls. Slow colonic transit time was shown to improve in patients restudied following refeeding, suggesting that slow transit time was a consequence of malnutrition[59] (see Chapter 12).

HEPATIC DYSFUNCTION. Patients with anorexia nervosa may have elevations in amino transferase levels, which return to normal on refeeding.[60] A twofold to tenfold elevation in AST, with small increases in alkaline phosphatase, can be seen. One case report of a liver biopsy performed 10 days following refeeding showed periportal inflammatory infiltrates.[61] However, a more recent report failed to find inflammatory infiltrates but did show excessive accumulation of glycogenx.[62] It should be noted that AST may be of skeletal, not hepatic, origin. Skeletal muscle biopsy in patients with anorexia has shown type 2 muscle fiber atrophy and abnormal accumulation of glycogen.[63] The increased stores of hepatic and skeletal muscle glycogen may explain why hypoglycemia is a rare event in patients with anorexia nervosa.

HYPERAMYLASEMIA. Hyperamylasemia with normal imaging studies of the pancreas is common in anorexia nervosa. The source of the amylase is salivary/parotid glands.[64, 65]

PANCREATITIS. Patients with abdominal pain may have pancreatitis, as documented by increased serum amylase or increased amylase/creatinine clearance, or by ultrasound imaging of the pancreas. The pancreas can either lose its echogenicity[66] or appear grossly edematous.[67] Pancreatitis can develop following ingestion of a larger than average meal.[68] Superior mesenteric artery syndrome may be the underlying explanation for pancreatitis (see Chapters 48 and 49). No evidence of pancreatic dysfunction, such as fat malabsorption, has been observed, despite abnormal para-aminobenzoic acid (PABA) testing.[69]

Treatment

OVERVIEW OF THE PROBLEM. Patients with anorexia nervosa lack insight into their behavior and deny that being too thin is a medical problem. They may have significant underlying personal, family, and social conflicts. The fears and misconceptions regarding eating, weight gain, and body image need to be addressed in a stepwise fashion. Some patients have symptoms of depression that are secondary to malnutrition and not primary to the disorder. The majority of personality disturbances seen in the acutely anorectic patient disappear when the malnutrition is corrected.[70] (see Chapter 122). Some patients may require hospitalization (see Criteria, Table 17–6). Their clinical management typically requires the combined efforts of an internist, psychiatrist, social worker, dietitian, and recreational therapist to address all medical issues.

NUTRITIONAL SUPPORT. Nutritional support in patients with anorexia nervosa is a three-step process: cessation of weight loss, maintenance of weight, and gradual weight gain back to normal weight range. Patients with anorexia require approximately 20% fewer calories to maintain weight because of their lower basal metabolic rate. A 1 lb/wk weight gain may require only 415 kcal/day increase in dietary intake, compared with the 525 kcal/day increase required in normal persons.[71] Sudden increases in food consumption can have extreme adverse consequences. A multitude of factors can promote gastric dilatation and rupture, including long-standing hypokalemia from chronic vomiting,[72] rapid increase in osmolality of stomach contents from a large quantity of food intake,[73] gastric ulcer,[74] or gastric infarction.[75] Superior mesenteric artery syndrome has been described in a young girl forced by weakness to remain in bed during refeeding.[76] Acute pancreatitis associated with gastric dilatation following refeeding has also been described.[77] The latter is a known complication from refeeding normal persons following prolonged fasting.

Seriously malnourished patients who are medically unstable may require hospitalization to treat complications of starvation; prescriptions for forced feedings must avoid overfeeding and should consider how forced feeding may promote psychological trauma that will impair recovery.[78] In general, total parenteral nutrition or enteral nutrition support should begin at 20 to 30 kcal/kg/day and advance slowly over several weeks to no more than 70 kcal/kg/day, with the goal of a 1- to 2-lb/wk weight gain. When refeeding is initiated, the metabolic state of the patient shifts from catabolic to anabolic, and anticipatable shifts in fluids and electrolytes occur. Reductions in potassium, phosphorus, and magnesium occur when, during refeeding, these minerals leave the circulation to be incorporated into newly synthesized muscle. Every third day monitoring and aggressive repletion are usually required.

PSYCHOSOCIAL THERAPY. Psychiatric therapy is the mainstay treatment for anorexia.[23] To be effective, formal psychotherapy should begin after weight gain has started, since starvation causes reversible psychological disturbances. Until cessation of weight loss has been established, psychiatric support should focus on developing a supportive relationship. Ongoing, individualized psychotherapy is typically required for at least 1 year and may take 5 to 6 years before eventual recovery. The goals of psychiatric therapy are to establish a therapeutic alliance, to enhance the patient's motivation to cooperate in the restoration of healthy eating patterns, and to correct core dysfunctional thoughts, attitudes, and feelings related to the eating disorder. Family support and family therapy may be appropriate. Following restoration of weight, an occasional patient has benefited from antidepressant therapy.

DRUG THERAPY. Drug therapy to improve appetite and treat depression has been advocated previously. Its role today is extremely limited, because drug-induced weight gain neither shortens the duration of the illness nor improves long-term recovery.[79] Although mild cases of anorexia nervosa could be managed by a physician willing to invest the time required to administer cognitive-behavioral therapy, most patients are best managed in an outpatient setting by an experienced psychiatrist/dietitian team who will see the patient weekly, and by an experienced internist who can manage the metabolic complications of starvation, purging behaviors, and/or refeeding.

PROGNOSIS. Many patients with anorexia nervosa regain weight with cognitive therapy. In an extensive review of the subject in which weight was the sole criteria for cure, 22% to 70% of patients at follow-up were at reported normal weight, and 15% to 42% were considered underweight. Unfortunately, almost half the patients continued to follow abnormal eating patterns and purge intermittently.[80] The lifetime prevalence of obsessive-compulsive disorder may be as high as 25%.[81] Further work in the area of body dissatisfaction may help provide insights into more effective approaches to treat this devastating disorder.[82]

BULIMIA NERVOSA

Historical Perspective and Disease Prevalence Estimates

Bulimia nervosa was only recently identified as an eating disorder distinct from anorexia nervosa, by Russell in 1979.[83] The name "nervosa" identifies its similarity to anorexia nervosa. Patients share similarly distorted body image perceptions. However, only rarely do patients with bulimia nervosa present with cachexia. Typically they have a normal or slightly excessive body weight.

What primarily distinguishes patients with bulimia nervosa from those with anorexia nervosa is their binge-eating behavior. The name *bulimia* is Greek, translating literally to "ox hunger." Bulimia describes the rapid consumption of excessive calories—a behavior never observed in anorexia nervosa. Patients with bulimia nervosa report a "lack of control" regarding their eating behavior. However, their concerns regarding either the weight-gaining consequences of binge eating or the bloating/discomfort associated with bingeing promote maladaptive behaviors of purging. Purging can include measures that reduce the number of calories absorbed during a binge meal (e.g., vomiting after the binge) or measures that reduce bloating (e.g., laxative and diuretic abuse). To meet the Diagnostic and Statistical Manual (DSM) IV criteria (Table 17–7), every binge-eating episode must be followed by feelings of remorse and shame.[23]

Bulimia nervosa is more prevalent than anorexia nervosa, with estimates ranging from 1% to 2% in young adult women and 3% to 9% if broader criteria than those of the American Psychiatric Association are used.[84] The prevalence in men is 1% to 2% if broader criteria are used. In North America, there may be more men with bulimia nervosa than women with anorexia nervosa.[85] The lifetime prevalence for bulimia nervosa in women has been estimated to be as high as 5%.[23] Patients tend to be older, sexually active women in their twenties. They may be married, with children.

Table 17–7 | **Diagnostic Criteria for Bulimia Nervosa**

A. Recurrent episodes of binge eating. An episode of binge eating is characterized by both of the following:
   1. Eating, in a discrete period of time (e.g., within any 2-hr period), an amount of food that is definitely larger than most people would eat during a similar period of time and under similar circumstances
   2. A sense of lack of control over eating during the episode (e.g., a feeling that one cannot stop eating or control what or how much one is eating)

B. Recurrent inappropriate compensatory behavior in order to prevent weight gain, such as self-induced vomiting; misuse of laxatives, diuretics, enemas, or other medications; fasting; or excessive exercise.

C. The binge eating and inappropriate compensatory behaviors both occur, on average, at least twice a week for 3 months.

D. Self-evaluation is unduly influenced by body shape and weight.

E. The disturbance does not occur exclusively during episodes of anorexia nervosa.

In the purging type of bulimia nervosa, the person regularly engages in self-induced vomiting or the misuse of laxatives, diuretics, or enemas; in the nonpurging type, the person uses other inappropriate compensatory behaviors, such as fasting or excessive exercise.

From American Psychiatric Association: Practice Guideline for the Treatment of Patients with Eating Disorders, 2nd ed. Washington, DC, 2000.

Natural History

Patients with bulimia nervosa are likely to be overweight prior to their illness. Isolated episodes of dieting or purging may precede the development of the disorder.[86] Bingeing is the characteristic feature of bulimia nervosa. The food eaten during a binge is not normally part of the patient's diet and frequently consists of sweet or fatty foods. The quantity of food consumed during a binge can be astonishingly excessive (e.g., 5 lb of homemade sloppy joes). Some patients report restricted dietary patterns between infrequent binges, whereas others report daily binge-eating behavior.[87]

It is less common for patients with bulimia nervosa to participate in an excessive physical activity program, as seen in patients with anorexia nervosa.[88]

Their condition may be brought to attention because of the medical consequences of purging behavior or because of the higher prevalence of other impulsive behaviors, such as drug and alcohol abuse, theft, parasuicide, and self-mutilation.

Etiology and Psychological Aspects

Patients with bulimia nervosa may have difficulty with impulse regulation. The problem can be traced back to the lack of parental involvement during childhood growth and development. Psychodynamically, patients with bulimia nervosa may operate in a dissociated self-state, with an inability to self-regulate behavior.[23] The purging following binge eating has been described as a resentful, angry attack to meet masochistic/sadistic needs. These basic patterns may be repeated in other areas besides body image regulation. Specifically, 30% to 40% of those afflicted have a history of substance abuse.[89] A history of sexual abuse has been reported in as many as half of patients with bulimia nervosa, and these patients are more likely to have comorbid psychopathology[90] (see Chapter 122).

As with anorexia nervosa, bulimia nervosa affects men and women in all socioeconomic groups. Although all races can be affected, African American women appear more likely to develop bulimia nervosa than anorexia nervosa and are more likely to use laxatives as a purgative instead of vomiting.[91]

Clinical Features

Patients with bulimia are unlikely to come to medical attention for their energy imbalance because they feel guilty, unhappy, and ashamed of their binge behavior.[92] Patients may complain of bloating, flatulence, abdominal discomfort, constipation, and symptoms directly related to binge eating.[93] Patients who self-induce vomiting may have severe dyspeptic symptoms, as well as cough, sore throat, and odynophagia owing to the exposure of oral and esophageal cavities to gastric acid. They may have irregular menstrual cycling from polycystic ovarian disease if they are overweight; underweight bulimic patients may have amenorrhea from lack of pulsatile LH, as seen with anorexia nervosa (Table 17–8).

Physical Examination

The physical examination of patients with bulimia nervosa may be completely normal, with BMI in the normal range. Ten percent to 50% of patients may have enlargement of the parotid glands, resulting in a "chipmunk" cheek contour (Fig. 17–3).[94] Parotid swelling begins 2 to 3 days after a purging episode. Parotids may enlarge two- to fivefold, and their size indicates the frequency and duration of purging. Russell's sign (abrasions, small lacerations, and callosities on the dorsum of the hand overlying the metacarpophalangeal and interphalangeal joints) may be present (Fig. 17–4).[95] Erosions of the lingual surface of teeth (perimolysis) can be seen in up to 40% of patients (Fig. 17–5).[96] The presence of perimolysis indicates at least a 2-year duration of regular and excessive vomiting. Periorbital petechiae can occur following forceful vomiting; perioral inflammation with cheilo-

Table 17–8 | **Evaluation of Symptoms in Patients with Suspected Bulimia Nervosa**

PATIENT COMPLAINTS	FINDINGS CONSISTENT WITH THE DIAGNOSIS OF BULIMIA NERVOSA	
	Physical Examination	**Lab and X-ray Examination**
Weakness; irritability Abdominal discomfort; constipation; irritable bowel; bloating	Poor skin turgor, orthostasis Hemorrhoids; rectal prolapse	Hypokalemic, hypochloremic alkalosis from vomiting or diuretic abuse; high urine sodium and chloride levels favor diuretics, and bicarbonate levels > 38 favor vomiting as the causative agent; hypomagnesemia and hypophosphatemia from laxative abuse; ipecac abuse should be queried
Fertility problems; spotty/scanty menstrual periods	Loss of subcutaneous fat in underweight or hirsutism and male pattern baldness in overweight patients	Underweight patients: low LH, low estradiol; overweight patients: insulin resistance associated with polycystic ovarian disease; normal or increased estrogen levels
Pain in pharynx; swollen cheeks and neck	Pharyngeal erythema; enlarged salivary glands; scarring on dorsum of hand; erosion of dental enamel	Hypokalemic, hypochloremic alkalosis from vomiting; elevated serum amylase from parotid hyperplasia Dental x-rays: dental enamel erosion
Muscle weakness; palpitations	Irregular heartbeat; cardiac murmurs; limb girdle weakness	Hypokalemic, hypochloremic alkalosis from vomiting; suspect ipecac abuse as the underlying cause for skeletal pathology and cardiomyopathy

LH, luteinizing hormone.

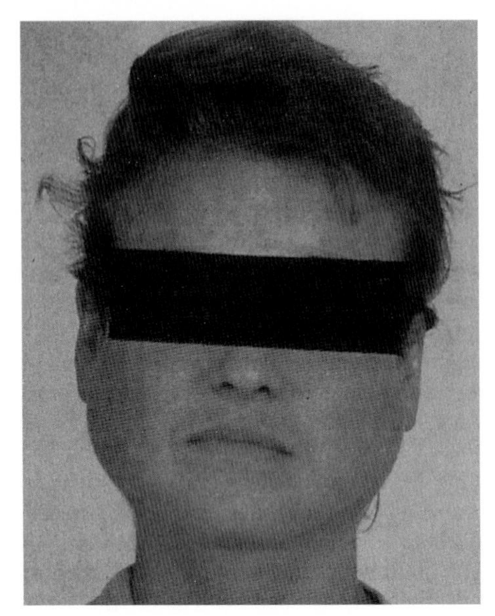

Figure 17–3. Bilateral, parotid gland enlargement associated with bulimia nervosa. (From Yanovski S: Bulimia nervosa: The role of the family physician. Am Fam Physician 44:1231–1238, 1991.)

sis can be seen in up to 10% of patients. Hemorrhoids may be seen in patients who purge by laxative abuse.

Laboratory Examination

Due to the higher prevalence of purging behaviors, metabolic disturbances are more common in patients with bulimia nervosa than in those with anorexia nervosa. Nearly one half of patients have chemical abnormalities, including elevated serum bicarbonate (27%), hypochloremia (24%), hypokalemia (14%), low serum bicarbonate (8%), and hyponatremia (5%).[97] Hypomagnesemia may be seen in patients abusing diuretics. Hyperamylasemia has been reported in 10% to 60% of patients and is usually accompanied by physical findings of parotid enlargement. Hypercholesterolemia, unlike that seen in anorexia nervosa,[98] is related to binge intake of saturated fat and cholesterol.[99] Because estrogen levels are preserved, bone mass revealed by DEXA is typically normal.[100]

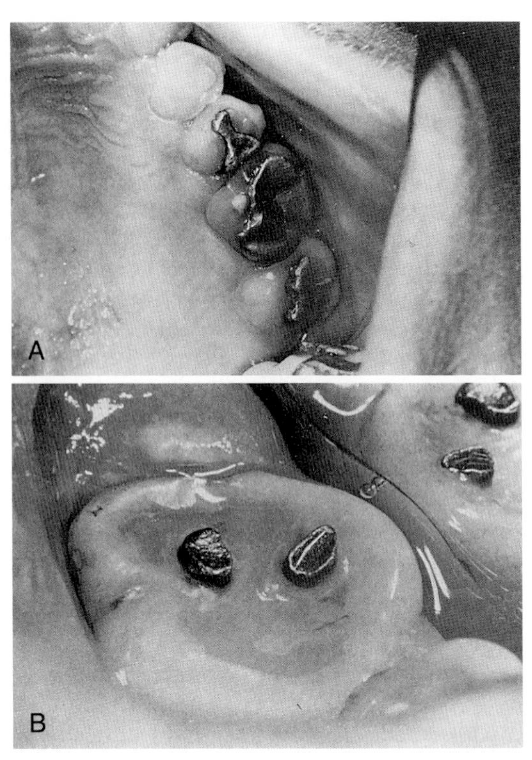

Figure 17–5. *A*, Palatal view of maxillary left posterior dentition. Marked loss of enamel creates rounding of tooth contours and exposure of the underlying dentin. The teeth appear shortened with dull surfaces. These findings are characteristic of perimolysis. *B*, Mandibular right second molar. The apparent elevation of the restorations is caused by a profound enamel decalcification from chronic acid exposure. This is a cardinal feature of perimolysis. The reflected view in the upper right-hand corner further emphasizes the vertical tooth loss. (From House RC, Grisius R, Bliziotes MM, Licht JH: Perimolysis: Unveiling the surreptitious vomiter. Oral Surg 51:152–155, 1981.)

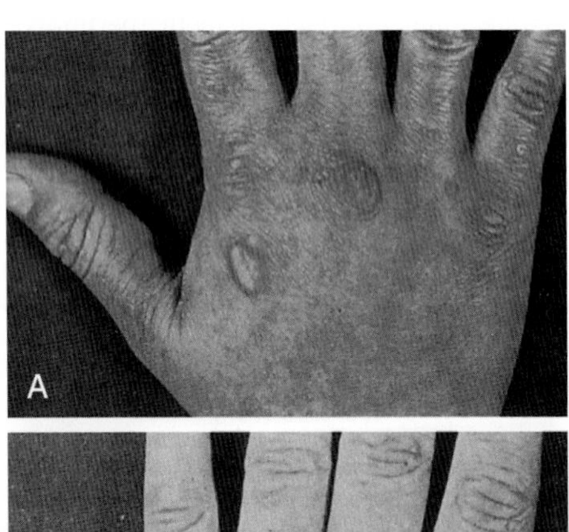

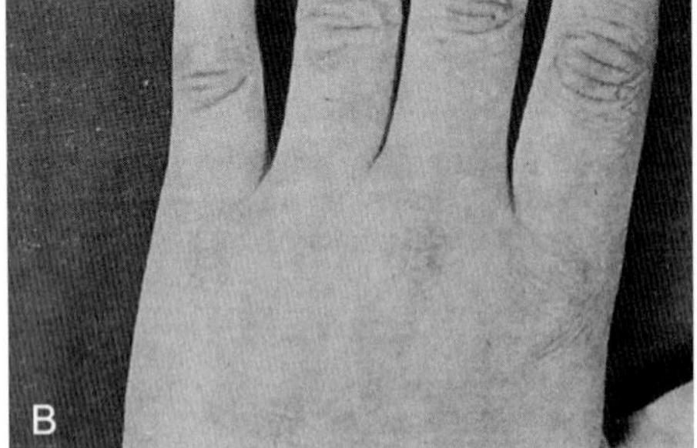

Figure 17–4. *A*, Right hand: calluses and healing ulceration of the skin. *B*, Left hand: minor ulceration of one knuckle. (From Russell G: Bulimia nervosa: An ominous variant of anorexia nervosa. Psychol Med 4:429–448, 1979.)

Differential Diagnosis

As with anorexia nervosa, no single constellation of signs or symptoms makes the diagnosis of bulimia nervosa. The only essential features are the characteristic distortion of body image and binge-eating behavior. Physical findings and laboratory and radiographic findings suggestive of bulimia nervosa are listed in Table 17–8. Scleroderma or other connective tissue disorders can reduce motility of the gastrointestinal tract and present with vomiting. Similarly, the diagnosis of peptic ulcer disease, inflammatory bowel disease, chronic pancreatitis, and Zenker's diverticulum could present with vomiting and abnormal eating patterns; the absence of binge eating by history as well as the absence of a distorted body perception will help exclude these diagnoses.

Parotid enlargement can be seen with parotid disease (duct obstruction, local infection) but usually is accompanied by pain. Sjögren's syndrome, diabetes mellitus, alcoholism, cirrhosis, hypothyroidism, and hypovitaminosis A can also cause parotid enlargement. The diagnosis should become apparent from the history.

Two specific syndromes that include bulimia as a key feature should be noted. *Kleine-Levin syndrome* affects adolescent or adult males who present with bulimia and periodic somnolence.[101] The period of somnolence lasts days to weeks, and patients, when aroused, become irritable and request to be left alone to sleep. The exact nature of the defect (psychiatric, metabolic) is uncertain: the syndrome may resolve spontaneously. *Prader-Willi syndrome* is a genetic disease that presents in childhood with hypotonia and mental retardation. The incidence is 1 in 10,000 to 20,000 births. During the toddler years, patients develop hyperphagia and intense preoccupation with food, leading to severe childhood obesity.[102] Physical dysmorphic features include narrow bitemporal diameter, almond-shaped eyes, upslanting palpebral fissures, short stature, and undescended testicles. As with other causes of bulimia per se, neither patients with Kleine-Levin syndrome nor patients with Prader-Willi syndrome have body dissatisfaction.

Systemic Complications

Ipecac cardiomyopathy for long-term heavy intake has been reported. Parotid enlargement may resolve after abstinence from vomiting. Prolonged sialadenosis may lead to chronic hypertrophy requiring parotidectomy.[103] Chronic use of diuretics and laxatives, as well as self-induced vomiting, can lead to intravascular volume depletion and orthostasis. This in turn activates the renin-angiotensin system, resulting in hyperaldosteronisim.

Gastrointestinal Complications

GASTRIC DILATATION. Gastric dilatation following an excessive binge has been reported; electrolyte disturbance from repeated vomiting/purging may have contributed.[104]

RECTAL PROLAPSE. The combination of constipation, laxative use, and increased intra-abdominal pressure from forced vomiting may result in rectal prolapse, even in young patients.[105]

Treatment

OVERVIEW OF THE PROBLEM. Patients with bulimia nervosa may have difficulty viewing their eating disorder as a primary problem and may be resistant to the continued need to self-monitor behaviors during therapy or to change their eating behaviors. Some patients can improve spontaneously if their social situation changes, highlighting the need for family and marital therapy to address underlying issues adequately. Some patients require inpatient management (see Table 17–6).

NUTRITIONAL SUPPORT. The goals of nutritional support are to reduce or eliminate binge-eating behaviors and to improve the nutritional balance during nonbinge eating. The dietitian can help the patient identify triggers that precede a binge and discuss strategies to avoid or reduce binge behavior. Counseling regarding nonbinge eating targets several issues, including minimizing food restrictions, improving the variety of foods eaten, and adopting a regular exercise program to help minimize weight surges.

PSYCHOSOCIAL THERAPY. Psychosocial therapy remains the main treatment for patients with bulimia nervosa[106]; behavior modification alone is far less effective than the combination of cognitive-behavioral therapy.[107] The goals of psychotherapy are to reduce/eliminate binge-eating behavior, improve attitudes related to the eating disorder, and address psychiatric issues that may underlie the condition, including developmental issues, identity issues, body image concerns, self-esteem in areas unrelated to body habitus, sexual and aggressive difficulties, affect regulation, gender/role expectations, family dysfunction, coping styles, and problem solving (see Chapter 122).[23]

DRUG THERAPY. Antidepressants can reduce the frequency of binge-eating episodes by 50% to 75%; their use should be combined with psychotherapy for optimum effectiveness.[108] Even patients who are not clinically depressed can reduce the frequency of binge eating with drug therapy. The severity of gastrointestinal symptoms is correlated to the severity of depressive symptoms and may improve with therapy.[109] Double-blind, placebo-controlled trials have shown efficacy with a wide variety of antidepressants, including imipramine, desipramine, fluoxitene, phenelzine, isocarboxazid, mianserin, bupropion, and trazodone—all in dosages used for depression. Fluoxitene is the only Food and Drug Administration (FDA) drug approved for use in bulimia nervosa. Bupropion may potentiate seizures in vomiters, and the MAO inhibitors phenelzine and isocarboxazid are contraindicated in patients with chaotic bingeing and purging behaviors. The side effects of fluoxitene are insomnia, nausea, and asthenia. Typical treatment doses for bulimia nervosa are 20 to 60 mg/day.

PROGNOSIS. Thirty percent of patients with bulimia nervosa diagnosed 10 years previously were found to be still engaged in recurrent binge eating or purging behaviors.[110] Although recovery rates have been reported as high as 50%,[111] it is important to note that the disorder tends to remit or relapse intermittently.[112]

OBESITY

Historical Perspective and Disease Prevalence Estimates

Human obesity can be traced back to the first recorded events of humans.[113] The depictions of obese persons in cave drawings, and later descriptions of obesity, suggested that the condition was viewed more as a curiosity than a malady.[114] Nonetheless, the medical consequences of obesity were readily apparent. Indeed, Hippocrates commented on the expected occurrence of sudden death in these persons from heart disease or suffocation.[115] Perhaps of more importance, the prevalence of morbid obesity was rare until the 20th century.

The term *obese* is derived from the Latin words *obesus* (fat) and *-esus* (devour); obesity means excess adiposity. The diagnostic criteria for obesity have been controversial because of the difficulties of quantifying total body fat and perhaps the subconscious resistance of physicians to recognize and accept their own adiposity. Delays in diagnosis were common until the release of a National Institutes of Health (NIH)-sponsored report on the identification, evaluation, and treatment of obesity.[15] Since BMI is an excellent estimate of excess adiposity,[116] BMI was identified as the sole criterion for classifying patients as either overweight (BMI, 25 to 29.9 kg/m^2) or obese (BMI, > 30 kg/m^2). The report further identified waist circumference as an additional criterion helpful in assessing a patient's risk for the medical complications of obesity (Table 17–9). Larger waists indicate central adiposity, which in turn indicates greater cardiovascular risk. The odds ratio for waist circumference identifying with the presence of at least one coronary disease risk factor has been estimated at 4.6 for men and 2.6 for women.[117]

The prevalence of obesity is tracked annually in the United States by the National Health and Nutrition Examination Survey (NHANES). In 1999, almost 27% of the American population had BMIs of greater than 30 kg/m^2. An additional 34% of Americans met the criteria for overweight, the highest percentage ever observed. The section of the American population that is experiencing the greatest exponential growth in the prevalence of obesity is children and adolescents.[118] Obesity and overweight have reached epidemic proportions, and further increases in the prevalence of obesity have been projected.

Natural History

Obesity is a direct consequence of the first law of thermodynamics. Energy that is not consumed must be stored. Obese persons become obese because of a cumulative excess in energy intake that exceeds their energy requirements.

Etiology and Psychological Aspects

Obesity is not associated with a specific personality or psychiatric profile. Obese persons do not have a higher prevalence of psychopathology, including depression, obsessive-compulsive disorders, and low self-esteem.[119] However, obese persons seeking treatment for their obesity are more likely than the general population to have psychiatric symptomatology, including depression and low self-esteem.[120]

The growing prevalence of obesity is probably the natural consequence of changes in our environment. Food is plentiful, and most Americans are sufficiently prosperous to purchase more than adequate food to meet their metabolic demands. Unfortunately, metabolic demands have declined as computer technology plus prosperity has eliminated many of the routine, day-to-day physical activities that burn energy. Leisure time, once devoted to outdoor activities, is now more commonly spent watching television or playing on the computer. If dietary intake is not reduced appropriately to meet reduced demands, weight gain will occur.

Appetite and its regulation have been a major research focus in the field of obesity. Expression of appetite is chemically coded in the hypothalamus by distinct circuitry.[121] Orexigenic signals of neuropeptide Y, galanin, endogenous opioid peptides, melanin-concentrating hormone, glutamate, and gamma-aminobutyric acid promote eating behaviors. Anorexigenic substances including an entire family of corticotropin-releasing hormone (CRH)-related peptides, neurotensin, glucagon peptide-1, melanocortin, as well as agouti-protein and cocaine promote the cessation of eating behaviors. Each is a signal with its own specific cellular receptors, occurring in high concentration in the paraventricular nucleus but also present in other areas of the brain. Feedback loops between signals have been identified, in which one signal peptide can alter the secretion of another signal peptide. No single peptide is the gatekeeper to turning on appetite; what is apparent is that an entire network of signals, their frequency, and amplitude are responsible for triggering behaviors.

The network of appetite signals accounts for the behavioral observations that appetite and food consumption patterns are dynamic and readily influenced by biologic, environmental, and psychological events.[122] Human eating behaviors are easily modified by internal clues such as habitual intake, memories of food-related activities, and anticipation of consumption. External clues, such as the appearance of food, aroma, and anticipated palatability, and the number

Table 17–9 | **Classification of Risk for Metabolic Complications of Obesity**

WAIST CIRCUMFERENCE	BMI CATEGORY* (kg/m^2)				
	18.5–24.9	25.9–29.9	30.0–34.9	35–39.9	≥40
<40″ for men <35″ for women	—	Increased	High	Very high	Extremely high
>40″ for men >35″ for women	Increased	High	Very high	Very high	Extremely high

*Waist circumference is measured midway between the lowest rib and the iliac crest; acceptable waist circumference is less than 40″ (102 cm) in a man and less than 35″ (88 cm) in a woman. From World Health Organization: Measuring obesity: Classification and description of anthropometric data. Copenhagen, WHO, 1989.

of food choices modify the perception of appetite as well as the behaviors of eating.[123]

Psychosomatic consequences of eating, such as reduction in anxiety, can exert additional influences on behavior.[124] Our understanding of eating behaviors is akin to that of memory; although memory and appetite are chemically encoded, every individual has his or her own unique circuitry underlying eating behaviors. As with memory, the circuitry can be modified over time.

A major breakthrough in the physiology of appetite regulation came with the discovery of leptin, a hormone synthesized by adipocytes. Leptin secretion increases as adipocytes enlarge and decreases during fasting. Identification of leptin receptors in the hypothalamus provided an intriguing biochemical explanation for the ability of an animal to regulate body weight tightly within a fairly narrow set-point range.[125] The leptin signal may serve as an anorexin by its ability to alter secretion of orexins and anorexins. Obese persons have appropriately elevated leptin levels, but whether this is an epiphenomenon of obesity or a clue to the pathologic cause of obesity remains unclear.

The importance of each of these anorexigenic and orexigenic signals and their receptors has been highlighted by the identification of rare families with specific genetic defects associated with childhood obesity.[126] Mutations in leptin, leptin receptor, prohormone convertase 1 (PC1), pro-opiomelanocortin (POMC), melanocortin 4 receptor (MC4-R), and peroxisome proliferator-activated receptor gamma-2 (PPAR g^2) genes have been described in patients with severe obesity.

Clinical Features

Some obese persons seek medical attention specifically to achieve weight loss. Others seek medical attention for the multiple medical complications of their excess body weight, including diabetes, hypertension, dyslipidemia, inability to walk short distances, joint pains, shortness of breath, and fatigue. Gastrointestinal complaints include gastrointestinal reflux, symptomatic gallstones, pancreatitis, liver disease, gut motility disturbances, and cancer of the colon and gallbladder.

No consistent eating behaviors underlie obesity.[127] Excessive fat intake, considered by some investigators as the cause of obesity,[128] does not account for recent increases in the population prevalence of obesity. Although the intake of simple sugars is at an all-time high, not all patients choose excessively sweet meals. Portion size may be the sole cause of caloric excess.

Taking a dietary history from an obese person is not always straightforward. Patients may not reveal their true food intake when they report compliance with a low-calorie diet that should easily result in weight loss but hasn't. The physician must shift the interview to ask about the "bad days," when either extra meals, large meals, or binge eating provides sufficient calories to obliterate the caloric deficit achieved on a good day. The chronologic recording of intake and physical activity can identify triggering events that derail dietary intentions.

Other patients, however, subconsciously do not track their eating behavior and accordingly deny their actual practices. In a study comparing self-diagnosed "diet-resistant" patients who reported an inability to lose weight on a calorically restricted diet, a systematic underreporting of caloric intake and overreporting of physical activity was observed.[129] The biologic reason for this discrepancy is uncertain. Dietary counseling is unlikely to be effective in patients who cannot recognize and report their true behaviors, making such patients candidates for psychological counseling.

It will be important to ascertain the contribution of binge-eating behavior to the clinical problem. The prevalence of binge eating coincides with the magnitude of excess body weight. In one series, 10% of women with a BMI of 25 to 28 kg/m^2 reported binge eating, compared with 40% of women with a BMI of 31 to 42 kg/m^2.[130]

Obese persons require more calories to perform routine physical activity than do lean persons,[131] since any movement requires the additional expenditure of moving excess body weight. In some patients, lower daily energy expenditure associated with reduced rates of spontaneous physical activity contributes to lifetime weight gain.[132] Anecdotally, fidgeters tend to be leaner than nonfidgeters.

Physical Examination

Obese persons have excess body fat that may be distributed in an android or gynecoid pattern. Velvety, hyperpigmented skin in the axilla, groin, and nape (acanthosis nigricans) can be seen and suggests the presence of insulin resistance. Hepatomegaly from fatty liver may be present. Although the presence of intraperitoneal fat may identify patients at higher risk for medical complications of obesity, imaging for this purpose is not recommended. Patients with headaches or visual disturbances should undergo a brain MRI to rule out hypothalamic pathology.

Laboratory Examination

Obese persons may have abnormal liver biochemical tests from fatty liver. Diabetes and glucose intolerance are more prevalent, particularly in older patients or younger patients with a family history of diabetes. TSH should be routinely measured; the high prevalence of autoimmune thyroid disease in women may contribute only marginally to weight gain (only 2 to 6 lb/yr).

Differential Diagnosis

The differential diagnosis for obesity includes rare secondary causes that can be identified by key findings on physical examination (Table 17–10). The overall distribution of fat should be noted. Obese persons may develop a buffalo hump because they have exhausted other places to store fat. Cushing's syndrome presents with a buffalo hump and central obesity; the presence of supraclavicular fat and proportionally thin extremities is a more suggestive finding of cortisol excess. Cushing's patients have thin skin due to loss of subcutaneous fat, leading to a predilection for spontaneous bruising. Hypertension and hyperglycemia are typically

Table 17–10 | **Symptoms and Signs That Suggest a Secondary Cause for Obesity**

SYMPTOM, PHYSICAL FINDING	POSSIBLE SECONDARY CAUSE OF OBESITY
Headache, papilledema	Hypothalamic tumor such as craniopharyngioma; evaluate by MRI
History of head trauma	May have hypothalamic injury of appetite center; imaging does not rule out injury
Fatigue	Serum TSH should be routinely checked on all patients; mild hypothyroidism (TSH 4–9 IU/mL) can promote 2- to 6-lb weight gain/yr
History of drug therapy with agents known to promote appetite/weight gain, including antipsychotic drugs, tricyclic and heterocyclic antidepressants, MAO inhibitors, lithium, and glucocorticoid	Focus of therapy should be prevention of additional weight gain and whether alternative regimens that do not stimulate appetite would be equally effective
Bruises, thin skin, supraclavicular fat pad, with relative wasting in extremities	Cushing's syndrome should be ruled out by a 24-hr urine measurement for urinary free cortisol
Morbid obesity since childhood; mental retardation	Prader-Willi syndrome should be suspected; patient can be referred for genetic testing; forced intervention of hyperphagia has ethical considerations. Bardet-Biedl syndrome will have polydactylism; other extremely rare genetic syndromes are listed in the online Mendelian Inheritance of Man available at http:www2.ncbi.nlm.nih.gov/omim

MAO, monoamine oxidase; MRI, magnetic resonance imaging; TSH, thyroid-stimulating hormone.

present. A 24-hour urinary free cortisol determination is the most sensitive test to rule out Cushing's; a false-positive dexamethasone suppression test can be seen in obese patients.

Several rare genetic syndromes can present with obesity in childhood, the most common being *Prader-Willi syndrome* (1:10 to 20,000 births), easily diagnosed in childhood because of the presence of mental retardation, hypotonia, hypogonadism, and short stature.[102] Tumors of the hypothalamus may lead to excessive dietary intake; patients may complain of visual defects or headaches. The reduction in basal metabolic rate from hypothyroidism leads to weight gain. Hypothyroidism leading to myxedema can be detected by doughy, dry skin, deep voice, delayed reflexes, and elevated TSH.

Systemic Complications

Most of the deleterious effects of obesity are direct consequences of excess body weight. Osteoarthritis is more common in overweight persons.[133] The prevalence of hypertension; dyslipidemia with a high total cholesterol, high triglycerides, and low HDL cholesterol levels; and diabetes increases with increasing BMI.[15] This places obese patients at high risk for the development of premature coronary disease. Besides ischemic coronary disease, overweight and obesity are independent risk factors for the development of congestive heart failure.[134] Excessive body weight predicts the severity of sleep apnea; most patients with sleep apnea have a BMI greater than 30 kg/m^2.[135]

Women, in particular, have significant hormonal consequences from excess body weight. Obese premenopausal women have high rates of menstrual irregularity and amenorrhea.[136] Polycystic ovarian disease is the most common cause[137]; because of high ovarian estrogen production levels, bone density is preserved. Excess morbidity from increased production of ovarian androgens leads to hirsutism, male pattern baldness, and acne. Obese women are prone to be infertile; if they become pregnant, greater obstetric complications ensue.[138] Weight gain in adult women increases the risk for breast cancer,[139] presumably because of the conversion of adrenal androgens to estrone by peripheral fat cells. It is speculated that the high levels of unopposed estrogens explain the increased risk for endometrial cancer.[140]

Gastrointestinal Complications

REFLUX ESOPHAGITIS/HIATAL HERNIA. It is controversial whether obesity plays a causal role in reflux esophagitis. The speculated mechanism is that increasing abdominal girth places pressure on the lower esophageal sphincter. Morbid obesity can increase intra-abdominal pressure, leading to compression of arteries and abnormal renal hemodynamics in some patients.[141] The increase in intra-abdominal pressure may be detectable only during straining.

In a study directly measuring intra-abdominal pressures in 8 obese subjects (all with a BMI of more than 35 kg/m^2) and 11 controls, straining increased intra-abdominal pressure threefold in controls, compared with a fivefold increase in obese subjects. Whether or not intermittent increases in intra-abdominal pressure increase risk for gastrosephageal reflux disease (GERD) is unknown. Verifying a true association between excess body weight and gastrointestinal reflux requires consideration of bayesian mathematics. The prevalence of GERD in the American population has been estimated at 14% to 20%.[142] Hiatal hernias detectable by computed tomography (CT) are present in 25% of men and women between ages 40 and 50 years and 75% of men and women aged 70 to 79 years.[143] Implicating a causal role based on an observed association is hazardous because both conditions are common. The relationship is further complicated by the lack of a standard definition for GERD.

In a study of 15 overweight-obese patients with obstructive sleep apnea (BMI range, 24.9–40.4 kg/m^2), when polysomnography and 24-hr esophageal pH monitoring were used to document reflux, reflux was seen in all patients during the day and in half the patients during the night; only a third reported symptoms.[144] As with normal-weight persons, not all symptomatic obese patients have evidence for reflux by endoscopy or 24-hr pH monitoring.[145]

Data against a significant association are noteworthy. In a population-based survey of 820 Swedes, self-reported symptoms of esophageal reflux were no more prevalent among those who reported ever having been overweight compared with those with normal weight.[146] A study evaluating morbidly obese subjects did not find a relationship between body weight, BMI, or ratio of waist to hip girth (WHR) to the presence of esophagitis.[145] In a randomized controlled weight loss trial in 20 obese patients with GERD diagnosed by pH monitoring and requiring drug therapy,[147] the treatment group achieved a BMI reduction of from 32.5 to 28.8, but no significant improvements were noted in symptoms, need for medication, number and duration of reflux episodes, or changes in esophageal sphincter pressures compared with controls. The control group underwent subsequent treatment with a very-low-calorie diet, reducing BMI from 30.1 to 26.6 and replicating the lack of benefit on GERD.

Proponents of the permissive nature of excess body weight on reflux esophagitis suggest that only small increases in weight increase risk. In a prospective study of 1224 patients referred for upper endoscopy, patients with grades 1 and 2 esophagitis had body weight for height 5% higher than ideal; patients with grade 3 esophagitis had BMIs in the normal range.[148] The investigators postulated that the lower weight in patients with more severe esophagitis was due to dietary restrictions imposed by the disease. In a retrospective analysis of 1389 patients undergoing upper endoscopy, excessive body weight was a significant independent risk factor for hiatal hernia, which, in turn, was a significant risk factor for esophagitis.[149] In the large NHANES database, for every 5-kg/m^2 excess BMI, a 22% increase in risk for hospitalization from gastroesophageal reflux was seen.[150] Weight loss can improve symptoms in patients with normal or grade 1 esophagitis; in a study of 34 patients whose BMI was 23.5 ± 2.3 kg/m^2, 80% improved after a 4-kg weight loss (mean BMI, 21.8 ± 1.1 kg/m^2).[151] (See Chapters 6 and 33.)

ESOPHAGEAL CARCINOMA. Obesity is a weak risk factor for the development of Barrett's esophagus and subsequent adenocarcinoma.[152] Distal esophageal carcinoma occurs in well-nourished persons[153] and may be linked to the excess saturated fat ingestion that occurs during excess caloric intake.[154] The combination of obesity and reflux appears to increase further the risk for cancer.[155] In a case control study, individuals with a BMI greater than 30 kg/m^2 had a 16-fold greater risk for esophageal adenocarcinoma and a fourfold greater risk for cardiac adenocarcinoma compared with individuals with a BMI of less than 22 kg/m^2. A weak association between BMI and esophageal squamous cell carcinoma was also seen on multivariate analysis[156] (see Chapters 33 and 35).

GALLSTONES. Gallstones are more prevalent in women, and body weight is an important risk factor that increases the risk for gallstone disease in both men and women.[157] The risk of either symptomatic gallstones or cholecystectomy is as high as 2% per year in women whose BMI is greater than 40 kg/m^2, compared with 0.3% in women whose BMI is less than 24 kg/m^2.[158] In men, the relative risk for gallstones is related to the presence of excess abdominal fat.[159]

The mechanism behind gallstone formation is multifactorial. Higher gallbladder volumes in both the fasting and postprandial state are correlated with total body weight; response to cholecystokinin is reduced.[160] In obese patients with gallstones, cholesterol secretion is elevated, resulting in a reduction in the relative percentage of bile acids and an increase in the cholesterol saturation index.[161] The cholesterol saturation index increases with BMI, independent of age, gender, or ethnicity.[162] Aggregation of phospholipids, cholesterol, and bile vesicles into crystals begins the process of gallstone formation; some have suggested that crystals in obese patients propagate more rapidly than crystals in nonobese patients[163] (see Chapter 55).

GALLBLADDER CANCER. The risk for gallbladder cancer, particularly in women, increases with increasing weight. Women who are 40% above their ideal body weight have a relative risk of gallbladder cancer of 1.53[164] (see Chapter 60).

LIVER DISEASE. The prevalence of pathologic abnormalities of the liver in obese patients is striking. In a study of 100 consecutive patients undergoing elective bariatric surgery, a wedge liver biopsy found only 2 patients to have normal liver histology.[165] Fifty-six patients had fatty infiltration, and 42 patients had hepatitis, 19 with fibrosis and 6 with cirrhosis. Similar prevalence was observed in a larger series of 528 patients—91% of men and 70% of women had fatty liver, 10% had hepatitis, 1% fibrosis, and 4% cirrhosis.[166] It has been suggested that the severity of the liver abnormalities seen with obesity is proportional to the severity of obesity,[167] but not every study has confirmed this observation.[168, 169]

The almost universal appearance of fatty change, with large-droplet accumulation in more than half of hepatocytes, suggests that fatty accumulation in the liver is a natural consequence of excess body weight.[170] Most patients are asymptomatic, and examination may show a normal liver size. The progression to the inflammatory state, nonalcoholic steatohepatitis (NASH), requires an additional insult that has yet to be defined.[171] Diabetes is a strong risk factor, and some have suggested that steatohepatitis in obese patients is a consequence of the insulin resistance syndrome.[172] However, observation that major weight loss, while improving the fatty changes and insulin resistance, increase inflammatory hepatitis is not consistent with this hypothesis.[166, 169] Autopsies of morbidly obese patients suggest the incidence of NASH to be 18%, with women and diabetic patients more likely to be affected.[173] Why 5% of morbidly obese patients progress to cirrhosis is not well understood[168, 174] (see Chapter 72).

PANCREATITIS. Obese persons are at higher risk for pancreatitis due to their higher prevalence of pancreatitis risk factors: gallstones, hypertriglyceridemia, and hypertriglyceridemia associated with diabetes. Patients with pancreatitis who are overweight[175] and obese[176] have a worse prognosis, with higher rates of pancreatic necrosis and infectious complications than normal-weight persons.

COLONIC POLYPS AND CANCER OF THE COLON. Even more than with BMI, increased waist to hip ratio is associated with the prevalence of colonic polyps seen on sigmoidoscopy.[177] Abdominal obesity is associated with higher rates of colonic polyp formation.[178] A positive relationship between body weight and risk for colon cancer has been observed in men,[179] and perhaps to a lesser extent in women.[180] Twice as many women with a BMI greater than 29 kg/m^2 had distal colon cancer, compared with women with a BMI of less than 21 kg/m^2 [177] (see Chapters 114 and 115).

Table 17–11 | **Benefits of Modest Weight Loss on Cardiovascular Risk Factors**

RISK FACTOR	5–10-LB WEIGHT LOSS	≥20-LB WEIGHT LOSS	LONG-TERM BENEFITS
Blood Pressure	Reduction in systolic pressure by 4–8 mm Hg; diastolic pressure by 4–6 mm Hg	Improvements in blood pressure can be equivalent to drug therapy	Incidence of hypertension reduced 20%–50%; patients taken off medication are less likely to return to medication if weight loss is maintained
Lipids	Reductions of 4–20 mg/dL in total cholesterol and 20–60 mg/dL in triglycerides	May allow dose reduction of lipid lowering drugs May allow patients with mixed dyslipidemia to use monotherapy	Blunts the expected rise in cholesterol (30–50 mg/dL) with age Doubles cholesterol-lowering benefits of a Step II diet
Lipoproteins	Reductions of 5–20 mg/dL in LDL; increases of 1–6 mg/dL in HDL	HDL/TG benefits are striking — no drug improves HDL to this extent	HDL is a risk factor at any age; benefits of staying lean are experienced even among older persons
Insulin resistance	18%–30% reduction in fasting insulin levels	Improvements seen in glucose tolerance testing	Over a 6-year period, individuals who lost weight and kept it off had 1/3 the incidence of diabetes than people who kept weight
Diabetes	HbA_{1c} can be reduced 0.8%–2.2%	Dosages of hypoglycemic drugs markedly reduced	Long-term glucose control has been linked to reductions in renal and retinal disease

HbA_{1c}, glycosylated hemoglobin; HDL, high-density lipoprotein; LDL, low-density lipoprotein; TG, triglyceride.

Treatment

OVERVIEW OF THE PROBLEM. The heterogeneous nature of the underlying forces that allow excess body weight to be sustained makes the treatment of obesity a clinical challenge. An effective long-term therapeutic plan that works in one patient will not work in every patient. The disheartened physician should take on at least a minimum therapeutic plan: identify for the patient the weight problem, and recommend steps to prevent further weight gain.

It is important to set goals for weight loss and to engage the patient in the goal-setting process. The goal for weight loss should include not only the amount of weight to be lost but also the time frame required for the weight loss. Many obese patients have unrealistic goals for both their target weight and the time it will take to reach that weight. Often, unrealistic expectations are the cause of "diet failures."[181] The NIH evidence-based panel recommends that a weight loss goal of 10% is achievable.[15] The striking benefit of even this small amount of weight loss on cardiovascular risk factors is outlined in Table 17–11.

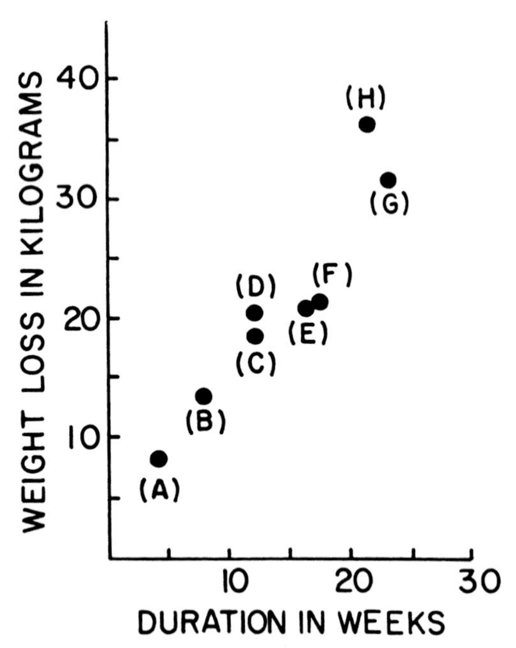

Figure 17–6. Relationship between weight loss and treatment duration in eight major studies using very low calorie diets. A to H represent individual studies. (From Wadden TA, Stunkard AJ, Brownell KD: Very low calorie diets: Their efficacy, safety, and future. Ann Intern Med 99: 675–684, 1983.)

NUTRITIONAL SUPPORT. Simplistically speaking, restriction of calories should cure every obese person. The effectiveness of diet follows a simple, straight line (Fig. 17–6),[182] showing that the magnitude of weight loss is directly proportional to the severity and duration of the caloric restriction. Two different approaches—very-low-calorie diets or low-calorie diets—can be taken. Fasting is not recommended. The long-term success of dietary therapy is enhanced when behavior modification is added to the therapy.

Very-Low-Calorie Diets. Very-low-calorie diets provide 500 to 750 kcal/day. Their macronutrient composition is designed to provide the minimum number of calories from protein to prevent negative nitrogen balance and the minimum number of calories from carbohydrate to prevent ketosis. A typical diet contains 70 g of protein, 50 g of carbohydrate, and 10 g of fat in a liquid formula to which potassium, magnesium, and other minerals are added. Some very-low-calorie diet prescriptions call for liquid intake only; others allow the addition of a single daily meal containing measured amounts of low-calorie vegetables to the liquid formula supplement. Weight loss is dramatic and predictable. Although the short-term success of these diets is impressive, in the long term these diets provide no greater weight loss at 1 year than do natural food, low-calorie diets.[183] More than 70% of patients who lose weight on these diets regain at least half of this weight within 2 years of stopping the diet.[184] The use of very-low-calorie diets is limited to patients who require immediate weight loss for treatment of a medical complication of their obesity (e.g., obstructive sleep apnea), with the caveat that these diets are only a "stopgap" measure that precedes a long-term dietary/behavior solution.[185]

Low-Calorie Diets. Low-calorie diets provide 1000 to 1500 kcal/day. The macronutrient content of these diets can be quite varied, but all must contain the same minimum grams of protein, carbohydrate, and essential fatty acids provided by the very-low-calorie diet to reduce complications of nitrogen loss and ketosis. Because the caloric content is higher, the rate of weight loss is slower than with very-low-calorie diets. The long-term success rate may be better because the diet teaches the patient to make food choices. Several free NIH web sites provide excellent materials regarding healthy diets. The web site http://www.nhlbisupport.com/chd1/lifestyles.htm discusses a Step I diet that is balanced in nutrients; more specific information regarding weight-losing diets is found at http://www.nhlbi.nih.gov. Following this by a click on "Aim for a Healthy Weight" will provide the patient a BMI calculator and a flexible low-calorie menu planner that uses the American Dietetic Exchanges.

Fad Diets. The popularity of fad weight loss diets reflects the underlying sentiment of the population—isn't there an easier way to do this? It is difficult to anticipate all the possible new twists to new diets, but fad diets usually cause weight loss by eliminating consumption of a specific food group (e.g., fruit, vegetables, meat, dairy). What makes these diets fads is their disregard for basic nutritional principles (balance, variety, moderation) that when followed assure the micro- and macronutrient sufficiency of the diet. Some diet prototypes, such as the 1990s "cabbage soup" diet, allowed participants to eat as much of the homemade cabbage soup as they wanted, but little else. If weight loss occurs, the mechanism is by lower caloric intake, not by something magical in cabbage soup.

An important note should be made of the low-carbohydrate diets (e.g., Atkins, Sugar Busters, Zone). Diets low in carbohydrates cause obligatory diuresis that takes place in the first week of the diet. The diuresis is due to mobilization of hepatic glycogen stores (and loss of hepatic water) as well as ketone body–induced diuresis at the level of the kidney. Patients develop a ketone-induced euphoria, reduced waist size, and more weight loss than can be accounted for by their caloric restriction. Half the initial weight loss is due to loss of total body water. In the long run, these diets are no more effective at reducing fat mass than traditional weight-losing diets. The mechanism of long-term weight loss is caloric restriction by elimination of carbohydrate-containing foods (breads, starches, and so on). Potentially serious long-term complications of high-protein intake make low-carbohydrate diets not recommendable.[186]

PHYSICAL ACTIVITY THERAPY. Exercise is an underutilized adjunct to dietary restriction. In a meta-analysis evaluating the benefits of exercise training, the addition of an exercise regimen reduced the percent loss of fat free mass.[187] This means that for every kilogram of weight lost, a greater percentage of weight loss was fat loss. Exercise is an impressive predictor of weight maintenance following weight loss. In an interview study comparing women who were formerly obese with normal-weight women and obese women who lost weight by dieting but regained it, 90% of women who maintained their reduced weights reported regular exercise.[188] In 102 participants of a very-low-calorie diet program, the initial weight loss of 27.2 kg diminished to an average weight loss of 11.3 kg at 2 to 3 years' follow-up. Those reporting an exercise program burning over 1000 kcal/wk maintained an average weight loss of 17.5 kg compared with those reporting no exercise, whose average weight loss was 5.6 kg.[189] Information regarding physical activity can be found on the web site: www.surgeongeneral.gov/ophs/pcpfs.htm. The amount of exercise needed to facilitate weight maintenance is not excessive. For example, walking 3 miles per day, at a leisurely pace, should burn 2000 kcal/wk.

PSYCHOSOCIAL THERAPY. The psychodynamics of excessive caloric intake are complex and highly individualized. Most obese patients are not willing to invest the time, effort, and energy to address underlying issues with a therapist. However, all patients should be enrolled in a program that includes behavioral therapy.

Behavioral therapy for obesity can be administered by a multidisciplinary team.[190] The program should

1. Teach patients to record and self-monitor dietary intake and physical activity,
2. Set realistic weight loss goals,
3. Provide nutrition education focused on balanced dietary intake,
4. Provide goals for increasing both life-style activity (e.g., taking stairs) and programmed activity (e.g., exercise routine),
5. Provide insight-oriented therapy to reduce triggers of excessive intake,
6. Provide effective problem solving to identify solutions to potential situations in which overconsumption may occur,
7. Provide cognitive restructuring, (e.g., using food as a reward) and
8. Provide patients with means to recognize relapse and ways to restart weight-losing therapies.

DRUG THERAPY. Drug therapy for obesity has undergone major changes in the past 10 years, with FDA-mandated removal of three agents from the market plus the release of two new agents. Two of the three agents removed from the market, fenfluramine and dexfenfluramine, were schedule IV drugs. These drugs were widely used as the FeN part of the Phen-FeN combination (the phentermine and fenfluramine combination was widely prescribed in the 1980s and 1990s as a drug therapy for obesity).

Both fenfluramine and dexfenfluramine reduced appetite by selectively blocking reuptake of serotonin in hypothalamic neurons; serotonin secretion was also stimulated. Both drugs were associated with the rare development of primary pulmonary hypertension; however, they were voluntarily taken off the market because of concerns that both were associated with the development of valvular heart disease.[191] The third drug taken off the market in the last 10 years, phenylpropanolamine, was an over-the-counter diet aid that reduced appetite by acting on adrenergic receptors in the paraventricular nucleus. Phenylpropanolamine had the potential to raise blood pressure; a recent large population study implicated phenylpropanolamine in hemorrhagic stroke in young women. Currently, in the United States, pharmacotherapy is essentially restricted to three drugs: phentermine, sibutramine, and orlistat (Table 17–12).

Phentermine. Phentermine hydrochloride and phentermine resin have been used extensively since the 1970s as appetite suppressants. The daily dose is typically 8 to 37.5 mg of phentermine hydrochloride or 15 to 30 mg of phentermine resin; tablets are taken first thing in the morning because of their stimulatory effect. Main side effects include dry mouth, insomnia, dizziness, depression, and bladder spasm. The majority of the weight loss occurs in the first 20 weeks of therapy; net weight loss above placebo has been shown to be 2 to 8 kg. Withdrawing the drug leads to weight regain. Intermittent phentermine can be as effective as daily phentermine.[192]

Sibutramine. Sibutramine inhibits the reuptake of both serotonin and norepinephrine. The daily dose is typically 5 to 20 mg. It can increase blood pressure, and blood pressure should be monitored during the first few months of therapy. As with phentermine, the majority of the weight loss (2 to 12 kg above placebo) is in the first few months of therapy; continuation of sibutramine therapy beyond the initial period of weight loss prevents the weight regain seen when the drug is discontinued.[193]

Orlistat. Orlistat is a selective inhibitor of pancreatic lipase; it has no effect on appetite. The inhibition of pancreatic lipase results in malabsorption of one third of dietary fat. Orlistat is taken as a 120-mg tablet with each meal; it is not systemically absorbed. The malabsorbed fat does not cause the flatulence and diarrhea associated with carbohydrate malabsorption. If fat intake is restricted to 30% of calories, most of the unabsorbed fat can be emulsified in the stool. Orlistat interferes with biliary micelle formation; fat-soluble vitamin

Table 17–12 | **Drug Therapy for Obesity**

	PHENTERMINE		SIBUTRAMINE	ORLISTAT
Site of action	CNS		CNS	Gut
Mechanism of action	Stimulates norepinephrine release		Inhibits reuptake of both serotonin and norepinephrine	Lipase inhibitor
RCCT efficacy	2–8 kg greater than placebo		2–12 kg greater than placebo	2–6 kg greater than placebo
Safety	In use since the 1970s		In use since late 1990s	In use since late 1990s; little if any systemic absorption
Major adverse events	Nervousness, irritability, headache, dry mouth, nausea, constipation, dizziness, insomnia, depression, bladder spasm		Increase in blood pressure and heart rate seen with significant increases in occasional patients; dry mouth, insomnia, constipation, headache	Nausea; oily spotting can occur 12–48 hr after high-fat meal (<30% calories from fat diet avoids this potential adverse event); vitamin E and beta-carotene absorption are reduced (daily multivitamin taken between meals is recommended)
Absolute contraindications	Patients taking MAO inhibitors		Patients taking MAO inhibitors; patients taking serotonergic drugs such as sumatriptan succinate, dihydroergotamine, dextromethorphan, meperidine, pentazocine, fentanyl, lithium, and tryptophan	Patients with bile acid deficiencies
Relative contraindications	Patients with sicca syndrome, arrhythmias, panic attacks, or hallucinations may have exacerbation of symptoms		Hypertension; use cautiously and monitor BP. Patients with coronary or cerebral atherosclerosis, CHF should be monitored for ill effects from changes in BP and HR; narrow-angle glaucoma and seizure disorder patients should be monitored for worsening disease. Use in patients taking SSRIs unproven. Metabolized by cytochrome p450 3A4	Patients with calcium oxalate nephrolithiasis may have increased risk for stone because of increased oxalate excretion; patients taking cyclosporine may have reduction in cyclosporine levels; more frequent monitoring and separation of dosing by 2 hr is recommended
Subpreparations	Hydrochloride	Resin	—	—
DEA schedule	Schedule IV	Schedule IV	Schedule IV	Not scheduled
Trade name	Fastin Phentrol Adipex-P Obermine	Ionamin	Meridia	Xenical
Generic available	Yes	Yes	No	No
Doses	8, 15, 18.75, 30, 37.5 mg	15, 30 mg	5, 10, 15 mg	120 mg

CNS, central nervous system; DEA, Drug Enforcement Agency; MAO, monoamine oxidase; RCCT, Randomized clinical control trial; SSRI, selective serotonin reuptake inhibitor.

Table 17–13 | **Criteria for Selection of Obese Patients for Surgical Treatment**

BMI > 40 kg/m²
BMI > 35 kg/m² and significant obesity comorbidity (e.g., hypertension, diabetes, sleep apnea, pickwickian syndrome, incapacitating osteoarthritis)
Documented failure to keep weight off or to prevent further weight gain using aggressive medical management that has included behavioral, pharmacologic, and low-calorie-diet components
Psychological ability to comprehend the expected changes in dietary intake necessary following surgery to achieve and sustain weight loss
Willingness to maintain continued medical management following surgery, including visits to registered dietitians, internists
Adult, nonpregnant, absence of drug addiction or chronic disease unrelated to obesity

supplements should be taken at times other than mealtimes to avoid subclinical vitamin deficiencies. Orlistat has been shown to reduce body weight an average of 2 to 6 kg; as with any drug therapy for obesity, some patients are able to achieve ideal body weight.[194]

Investigational Drugs. Human recombinant leptin has been administered to normal weight and obese patients in a 20-week trial to evaluate its use as a weight-losing therapy.[195] Those randomized to the highest dose in the trial (0.3 mg/kg/day) achieved lower caloric intakes and lost 6 kg more weight than the placebo group. The magnitude of weight loss is remarkably consistent with that achieved by the appetite-suppressant drugs currently on the market (see Table 17–12). Whether or not higher dosages of leptin will confer greater weight loss awaits results of additional clinical trials. Given our understanding of the complex network of signals altering appetite, it may be the case that any drug therapy can achieve only a certain amount of weight loss before a compensatory pathway is activated that prevents additional alterations in body weight.

BARIATRIC SURGERY. Bariatric is derived from the Greek term *baros*, meaning weight. Bariatric surgery creates an anatomic barrier preventing overconsumption and accumulation of excess calories either by restricting the gastric reservoir or by inducing malabsorption. Since these two approaches are complementary, they are frequently combined in a single operative procedure. An NIH consensus conference on the surgical treatment of obesity recommended consideration of surgery in patients with a BMI of greater than 40 kg/m² without medical complications or a BMI of greater than 35 kg/m² if a severe comorbidity were present.[196] Other factors to consider are listed in Table 17–13.

Jejunoileal Bypass. Jejunoileal bypass was one of the first surgical attempts at inducing malabsorption; the procedure completely interrupts the enterohepatic biliary circulation and creates a blind-loop type of bacterial overgrowth. In this surgery, the jejunum is transected 35 cm distal to the ligament of Treitz and anastomosed end-to-end to the ileum 10 cm proximal to the ileocecal valve (Fig. 17–7). The remaining loop of small intestine is closed proximally and anastomosed to the distal colon to drain. The surgery was extremely successful, creating dramatic weight loss of often over 100 pounds in 5 to 6 months. Due to life-threatening metabolic complications of hypokalemia, hypomagnesemia, metabolic bone disease, gallstones, renal stones, and progressive cirrhosis, this procedure was abandoned in the early 1980s. It is recommended that all patients with a jejunoileal bypass undergo surgical reversal.[197]

Biliopancreatic Bypass. In the 1970s, surgical approaches circumventing the metabolic complications of jejunoileal bypass led to the development of the biliopancreatic bypass. The rationale for biliopancreatic bypass was to induce malabsorption without interrupting enterohepatic biliary circulation or creating a blind intestinal loop. In this surgery, a two thirds distal gastrectomy is performed (an irreversible event). The proximal gastric remnant is anastomosed to the distal half of the small intestine. The first 150 cm of small bowel is then reanastomosed 50 cm proximal to the ileocecal valve (Fig. 17–8). Most patients lose weight in proportions similar to that of a jejunoileal bypass; anastomotic ulceration can occur in 11% of cases.[198] Severe metabolic complications result.[199] Vitamin supplementation is required to prevent symptomatic vitamin A deficiency, which still occurs in 3% of patients.[200]

Metabolic bone disease is a common complication that is now addressed using 2 gm/day calcium supplements plus vitamin D.[201] Anemia, mainly due to iron deficiency, was present in 40%, but the reported incidence is now 5% to 10% through use of supplemental vitamins and minerals. Protein-energy malnutrition occurs in 3% to 10%, often requiring intravenous hyperalimentation. Death from liver failure has been reported.[202] Patients require life-long follow-up and skilled management; although this operation is rarely performed in the United States today, it is still performed in

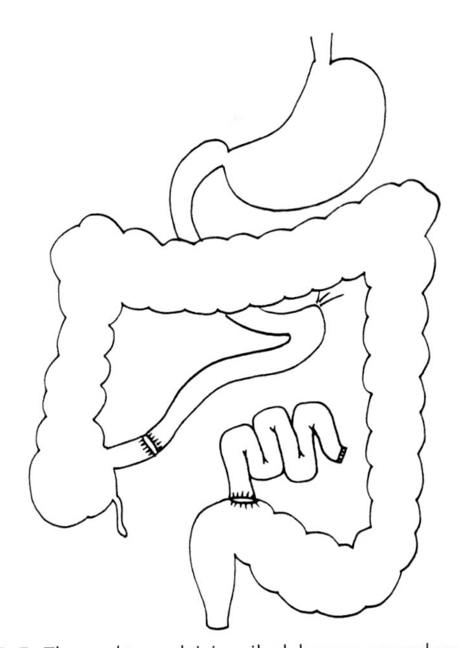

Figure 17–7. The end-to-end jejunoileal bypass procedure for severe obesity. The jejunum is transected 30 cm distal to the ligament of Treitz and is anastomosed to the distal end of the transected ileum 10 cm proximal to the ileocecal valve. The defunctionalized bypass loop of small intestine is closed proximally and drains distally into the colon. In the end-to-side variation (not shown), the transected proximal jejunum drains into the unresected distal ileum.

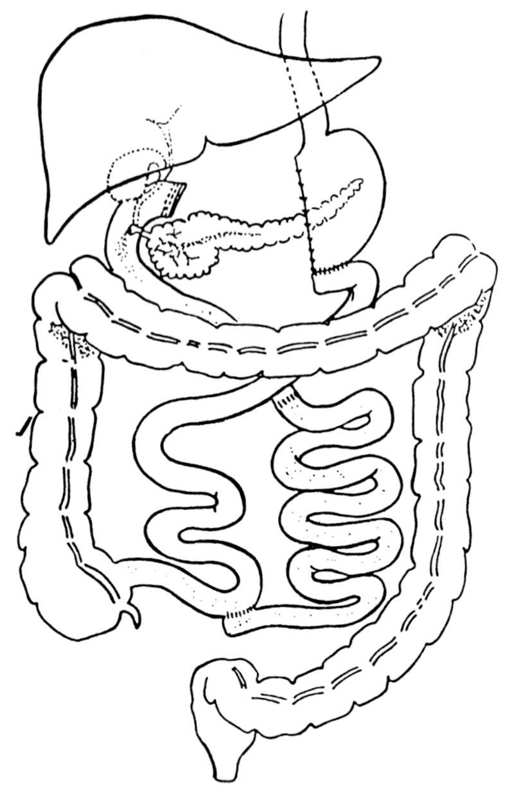

Figure 17–8. The biliopancreatic bypass procedure. After distal gastric resection, 250 cm of distal small bowel, including the ileum, is anastomosed to the remaining 200-mL gastric pouch. After cholecystectomy, the duodenum and proximal jejunum are anastomosed to the side of the terminal ileum 50 cm proximal to the ileocecal valve to create a conduit for biliopancreatic secretions. (From Tataranni PA, Mingrone G, Greco AV, et al: Glucose-induced thermogenesis in postobese women who have undergone biliopancreatic diversion. Am J Clin Nutr 60:320, 1994.)

Europe, where proponents consider that the benefits of the procedure outweigh the complications.[198]

Gastric Restriction. Gastric restriction can be achieved by several different surgical approaches. Vertical stapled gastroplasty with a banded outlet creates a small-capacity pouch that then empties into the remaining stomach. The surgery requires stapling several centimeters down the anterior stomach parallel to its hepatic border. The pouch is completed by inserting a 0.9-cm-diameter band at the bottom. The pouch capacity is only 15 to 20 mL; it empties into the remaining stomach (Fig. 17–9). Over time, excessive intake can distend and ultimately stretch the pouch.

In patients in whom stretching is a potential long-term concern, an adjustable gastric banding operation can be performed. In this operation, a gastric band is placed several centimeters beneath the esophageal-gastric junction, again creating a pouch. The inflatable gastric band is attached to a subcutaneous port that can be inflated/deflated to achieve the desired results. Complications of the adjustable gastric banding include a 5% incidence of band migrations/erosions, and a 5% incidence of gastroesophageal reflux disease (GERD).[203] In some patients, preoperative GERD symptoms improve following laproscopic adjustable esophagogastric banding.[204]

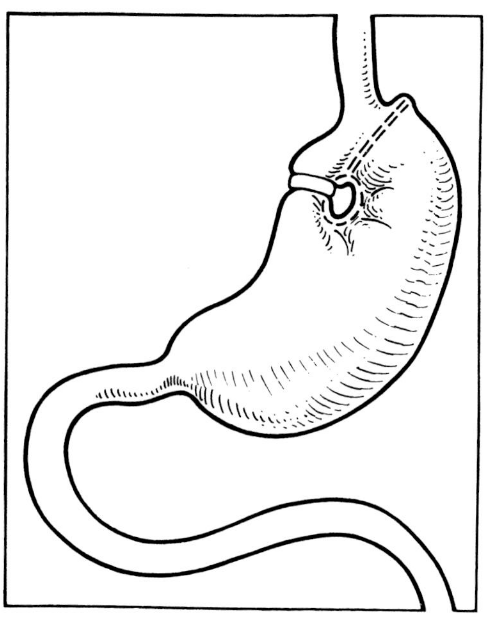

Figure 17–9. Vertical banded gastroplasty. A small 50-mL pouch with a restricted 12-mm outlet is created along the lesser curvature of the stomach with double staples and a collar of polypropylene mesh. (From Consensus Development Panel: Gastrointestinal surgery for severe obesity. Ann Intern Med 115:956, 1991.)

Gastric Bypass. The first gastric bypass surgeries for obesity were modeled after gastric resections performed for patients with recurrent ulcers or with intestinal cancers. A Roux-en-Y anastomosis was performed, with varying amounts of intestinal surface being bypassed (Fig. 17–10). Gastric bypass is the most common surgical procedure performed today for

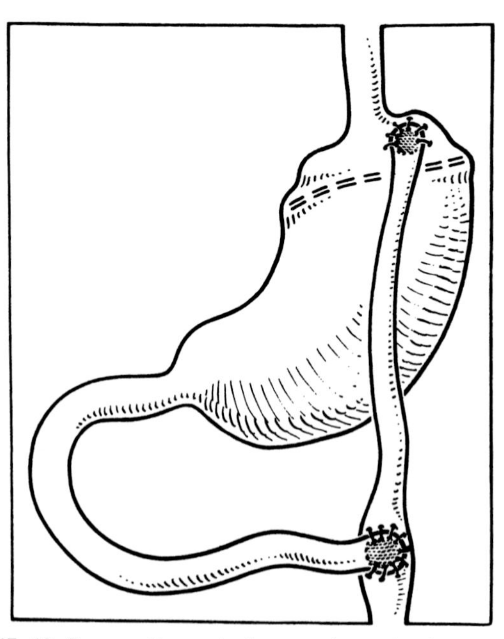

Figure 17–10. Roux-en-Y gastric bypass. A proximal 50-mL gastric pouch is created by double stapling that excludes the distal stomach. The pouch drains to the proximal small intestine through creation of a Roux-en-Y jejunal loop with anastomosis to the distal duodenum. (From Consensus Development Panel: Gastrointestinal surgery for severe obesity. Ann Intern Med 115:956, 1991.)

obesity. This surgery combines the techniques of gastric restriction with a lesser amount of intestinal bypass. A gastric pouch is created, in a similar manner to that performed in vertical stapled gastroplasty. This pouch is severed from the stomach and connected to the jejunum 50 cm from the ligament of Treitz, using a Roux-en-Y connection. Roux-en-Y gastric bypass can be an effective therapy for symptomatic GERD.[205]

Complications from Bariatric Surgery. The most immediate reported side effect of gastric restrictive or gastric bypass surgery is vomiting and regurgitation. Patients can generally control this symptom by consuming smaller meals and taking more time to consume each meal; rarely, vomiting is due to a stoma stricture that can be endoscopically dilated. Almost 70% of patients who undergo gastric bypass experience dumping, which occurs after ingestion of high-caloric, high-fat, soft foods. Patients who undergo gastric restriction do not experience dumping because the antrum is left intact. Dietary counseling can limit the severity of the dumping syndrome. Reported side effects and complications of gastric bypass surgery are listed in Table 17–14.[206]

Complications of Weight Loss from Diet/Drugs/Surgery

GALLSTONES. Weight loss from dieting or bariatric surgery further increases the risk of gallstones.[207] The incidence of new gallstones has been estimated at 12% during very-low-calorie dieting and 38% after successful gastric bypass surgery.[208] Higher initial BMI and greater absolute rate of weight loss are significant and independent predictors.[209] The mechanism is due to an increase in the cholesterol saturation index[210] and reductions in gallbladder motility.[211] Some surgeons perform a cholecystectomy at the time of gastric bypass surgery to avoid perioperative complications due to gallstone disease.[212]

Greater caloric restriction, providing faster weight loss, increases the rate of gallstone formation. In a meta-analysis of studies of weight loss in which the rate of gallstone formation was tracked by ultrasound, the prevalence of new gallstones increased from 0.5% to 3.0% per week when the magnitude of weight loss increased from 1.5 to 3 kg/wk.[213] Very-low-calorie or very-low-fat diets reduce gallbladder motility and increase the risk for gallstone formation. In a study comparing two different low-calorie diets, half the patients randomized to the 5% of calories from fat diet developed gallstones, compared with none of the subjects randomized to the 20% of calories from fat diet.[214]

Table 17–14 | **Side Effects and Complications of Gastric Bypass Surgery**

SIDE EFFECTS (%)		COMPLICATIONS (%)	
Dumping	70	B_{12} deficiency	25
Dairy intolerance	50	Abdominal pain	15
Constipation	40	Vomiting	15
Headache	40	Diarrhea	15
Hair loss	33	Incisional hernia	15
Depression	15	Anemia	15
		Arrhythmia	10
		Non-B_{12} vitamin deficiency	10

From Kral JG: Surgical treatment of obesity. In Kopelman PG, Stock MJ (eds): Clinical Obesity. Malden, MA, Oxford Press, 1998, pp 545–563.

Ursodeoxycholic acid has been used successfully to reduce the risks of gallstone formation associated with weight loss. In a randomized trial of 29 gallstone-free patients undergoing bariatric surgery, 1000 mg/day of ursodeoxycholic acid significantly prevented gallstone formation, compared with placebo (0/10 vs. 6/14).[215] The clinical significance is far greater in that two of the six placebo patients who developed gallstones required cholecystectomy. In fact, a cost savings has been estimated if ursodeoxycholic acid were provided for every obese patient who was expected to undergo rapid weight reduction.[216] Aspirin, 1300 mg/day[217] and ibuprofen, 1600 mg/day[218] have also been shown to reduce the incidence of gallstone formation in patients undergoing weight reduction.

HEPATITIS. Large and rapid weight loss has been shown to increase the prevalence of inflammatory hepatitis. One case report describes the development of occult cirrhosis in a patient whose preoperative liver biopsy was normal.[219] Two series of patients who had liver biopsies pre- and postweight reduction have been reported.

In a study of patients undergoing gastroplasty,[166] pre- and 2-year postoperative liver biopsies were performed in 69 patients. Following surgery, the mean BMI in this cohort fell from 43.9 kg/m^2 to a BMI of 31.7 kg/m^2. Although the prevalence of steatosis fell from 83% to 38%, the prevalence of steatohepatitis increased from 14% to 26%. Most of the cases were mild in severity. At the time of surgery, no biopsy specimens of the patients showed cirrhosis; a single patient had fibrosis, which was unchanged on repeat biopsy.

The increase in the prevalence of hepatitis is not due to surgical therapy. In a study of 41 patients who had liver biopsies prior to the initiation of a very-low-calorie diet and repeat liver biopsy at the time of an elective gastroplasty 4 to 20 months later,[169] a similar picture emerged. Following dietary therapy, the mean BMI fell from 43.3 to 32.9 kg/m^2. Although the prevalence of steatosis fell from 90% to 29%, the prevalence of steatohepatitis increased from 15% to 34%. On the initial biopsy, no patients showed evidence for fibrosis or cirrhosis; on repeat biopsy, fibrosis was present in five cases—two who had portal inflammation on initial biopsy, and three who had only fatty change on initial biopsy. The presence of new fibrosis was significantly associated with a higher degree of fatty change on initial biopsy; a greater reduction of fatty change on repeat biopsy, and weight loss faster than 4 lb/wk.

PROGNOSIS. Obesity is a chronic, remitting, and relapsing condition. It cannot be cured but can be modified by consistent changes in eating behaviors and physical activity. Although many obese patients complain that they have "ruined their metabolism" by intermittent attempts to lose weight using diets or drugs, basal metabolic rates of women who had repeatedly gained and lost weight were no different than those of similar weight women who had never dieted.[220] Although previous estimates suggested that only 5% to 10% of patients who participate in a clinical weight reduction program maintain their new weight for at least 3 years,[221] advances in the behavioral management of patients now suggest that 19% of patients can maintain long-term weight loss.[222]

Drug therapy and surgical therapy may be indicated in patients with significant comorbidities, since both modalities have been shown to improve risk factors. Data supporting long-term drug therapy are limited to results from trials 2 years in duration. Data from surgical therapy suggest that 25% to 40% of preoperative weight is typically achieved and maintained.[206] Using the disappearance of comorbidities as an end-point, 80% of patients receiving gastric bypass surgery improve.[223] When the encouraging preliminary data from a major Swedish surgical trial are released, the role of surgery in the management of morbid obesity may increase.[224] Although the risk for gallstone formation can be eliminated during rapid weight loss, the risk for hepatitis, and its clinical significance, remains uncertain.

At a minimum, physicians should ask patients to stop their weight gain trajectories and should recognize that some patients are in fact successful in the long term with weight reduction when all aspects of this complex disorder are optimized.

REFERENCES

1. Keys A: The Biology of Human Starvation, vols. 1 and 2. Minneapolis, University of Minnesota Press, 1950.
2. Heymsfield SB, Smith J: Muscle mass: Reliable indicator of protein-energy malnutrition severity outcome. Am J Clin Nutr 35:1192–1199, 1982.
3. Bistrian BR, Blackburn GL, Vitale J, et al: Prevalence of malnutrition in general medical patients. JAMA 235:1567–1570, 1976.
4. Bistrian BG, Blackburn GL, Hallowell E: Protein status of general surgical patients. JAMA 230:858, 1974.
5. Heymsfield SB, Baumgartner RN, Pan SF: Nutritional assessment of malnutrition by anthropometric methods. In Shils ME, Olson JA, Shike M, Ross AC (eds): Modern Nutrition in Health and Disease. Baltimore, Williams & Wilkins, 1999, pp 903–922.
6. Abraham S: Height-weight tables: Their sources and development. Clin Consult Nutr Support 3:5–8, 1983.
7. Build and Blood Pressure Study, vols. 1 and 2. Chicago, Society of Actuaries, 1959.
8. New weight standards for men and women. Statistical Bulletin of the Metropolitan Insurance Company 40:Nov-Dec, 1–4, 1959.
9. Schofield C, Ashworth A: Why have mortality rates for severe malnutrition remained so high? Bull WHO 74:223–229, 1996.
10. Wang ZM, Pierson RN, Heymsfield SB: The five-level model: A new approach to organizing body-composition research. Am J Clin Nutr 56:19–28, 1992.
11. Kissebah AH, Krakower GR: Regional adiposity and morbidity. Psychol Rev 74:761–811, 1994.
12. Heymsfield SB, Baumgartner RN, Ross R: Evaluation of total and regional body composition. In Bray GA, Bouchard C, James WPT (eds): Handbook of Obesity. New York, Marcel Dekker, 1998, pp 41–78.
13. Quetelet A: Sur l'homme et le developpement de ses facultes, ou essai de physique sociale. Paris, Bachelier, 1835.
14. James WPT, Ferro-Luzzi A, Waterlow JC: Definition of chronic energy deficiency in adults. Report of a working party of the International Dietary Energy Consultative Group. Eur J Clin Nutr 42:969–981, 1988.
15. National Heart, Lung, and Blood Institute: Clinical guidelines on the identification, evaluation, and treatment of overweight and obesity in adults—The evidence report. Obes Res 6 (Suppl2):51S–209S, 1998.
16. Calle EE, Thun MJ, Petrelli JM, et al: Body-mass index and mortality in a prospective cohort of US adults. N Engl J Med 341:1097–1105, 1999.
17. Troiano RP, Frongillo EA Jr, Sobal J, Levitsky DA: The relationship between body weight and mortality: A quantitative analysis of combined information from existing studies. Int J Obes Relat Metab Disord 20:63–75, 1996.
18. Owen OE, Kavle E, Owen RS, et al: A reappraisal of caloric requirements in healthy women. Am J Clin Nutr 44:1–19, 1986.
19. Owen OE, Holup JL, D'Alessio DA, et al: A reappraisal of the caloric requirements of men. Am J Clin Nutr 46:875–885, 1987.
20. Levine JA, Eberhardt NL, Jensen MD: Role of nonexercise activity thermogenesis in resistance to fat gain in humans. Science 283:212–214, 1999.
21. Morton R: Phthisiologia: Sue exercitationes de Phthisi. London, S. Smith, 1689.
22. Gull WW: Anorexia hysterica (apepsia hysterica). Br Med J ii,527–528, 1873.
23. American Psychiatric Association: Practice Guideline for the Treatment of Patients with Eating Disorders, 2nd ed. Washington, D.C, 2000.
24. Garfinkel PE, Line E, Goering P, et al: Should amenorrhoea be necessary for the diagnosis of anorexia nervosa? Br J Psychiatry 168:500–506, 1996.
25. Garfinkel PE, Lin E, Goering P, et al: Bulimia nervosa in a Canadian community sample: Prevalence and comparison of subgroups. Am J Psychiatry 152:1052–1058, 1995.
26. Hamilton LH, Brooks-Gunn J, Warren MP: Sociocultural influences on eating disorders in professional female ballet dancers. Int J Eat Disord 4:465–477, 1985.
27. Davis C, Kaptein S, Kaplan AS, et al: Obsessionality in anorexia nervosa: The moderating influence of exercise. Psychosom Med 60: 192–197, 1998.
28. Herzog DB, Greenwood DN, Dorer DJ, et al: Mortality in eating disorders: A descriptive study. Int J Eat Disord 28:20–26, 2000.
29. Casper RC, Kirshner B, Sandstead HH: An evaluation of trace metals, vitamins, and taste function in anorexia nervosa. Am J Clin Nutr 33: 1801–1808, 1980.
30. Marcos A: The immune system in eating disorders: An overview. Nutrition 13:853–862, 1997.
31. Bruch H: Perceptual and conceptual disturbances in anorexia nervosa. Psychosom Med 24:187–194, 1962.
32. Marshall JC, Kelch RP: Low dose pulsatile gonadotropin-releasing hormone in anorexia nervosa: A model of human pubertal development. J Clin Endocrinol Metab 49:712–718, 1986.
33. Rigotti NA, Neer RM, Skates SJ, et al: The clinical course of osteoporosis in anorexia nervosa: A longitudinal study of cortical bone mass. JAMA 265:1133–1138, 1991.
34. Bachrach LK, Katzman DK, Litt IF, et al: Recovery from osteopenia in adolescent girls with anorexia nervosa. J Clin Endocrinol Metab 72: 602–606, 1991.
35. Lucas AR, Melton LJ III, Crowson CS, O'Fallon WM: Long-term fracture risk among women with anorexia nervosa: A population-based cohort study. Mayo Clin Proc 74:972–977, 1999.
36. Freyschuss U, Fohlin L, Thoren C: Limb circulation in anorexia nervosa. Acta Paediatr Scand 67:225–228, 1978.
37. Frumar AM, Meldrum DR, Judd HL: Hypercarotenemia in hypothalamic amenorrhea. Fertil Steril 32:261–264, 1979.
38. Kemmann E, Pasquale SA, Skaf R: Amenorrhea associated with carotenemia. JAMA 249:926–929, 1983.
39. Schulze UM, Pettke-Rank CV, Kreienkamp M, et al: Dermatologic findings in anorexia and bulimia nervosa of childhood and adolescence. Pediatr Dermatol 16:90–94, 1999.
40. Ferron SM: Occult gastrointestinal bleeding with anorexia nervosa. Am J Psychiatry 156:801, 1999.
41. Wigley RD: Potassium deficiency in anorexia nervosa with reference to renal tubular vacuolation. Br Med J ii:110–113, 1960.
42. Fonseca V, Havard CWH: Electrolyte disturbances and cardiac failure with hypomagnesaemia in anorexia nervosa. Br Med J 291:1680–1682, 1985.
43. Mehler PS, Andersen AE: Eating Disorders: A Guide to Medical Care and Complications. Baltimore, John Hopkins University Press, 1999.
44. Moodie DS, Salcedo E: Cardiac function in adolescents and young adults with anorexia nervosa. J Adolesc Heath Care 4:9–14, 1983.
45. Oka Y, Ito T, Matsumoto S, et al: Mitral valve prolapse in patients with anorexia nervosa. Two-dimensional echocardiographic study. Jpn Heart J 28:873–882, 1987.
46. Golden NH, Ashtari M, Kohn MR, et al: Reversibility of cerebral ventricular enlargement in anorexia nervosa demonstrated by quantitative magnetic resonance imaging. J Pediatr 128:296–301, 1996.

47. House RC, Grisius R, Bliziotes MM, Licht JH: Perimolysis: Unveiling the surreptitious vomiter. Oral Surg 51:152–155, 1981.
48. Milosevic A, Brodie DA, Slade PD: Dental erosion, oral hygiene, and nutrition in eating disorders. Int J Eat Disord 21:195–199, 1997.
49. Russel G: Bulimia nervosa: An ominous variant of anorexia nervosa. Psychol Med 4:429–448, 1979.
50. Hasler JF: Parotid enlargement: A presenting sign in anorexia nervosa. Oral Surg 53:567–573, 1982.
51. Ho PC, Dweik R, Cohen MC: Rapidly reversible cardiomyopathy associated with chronic ipecac ingestion. Clin Cardiol 21:780–783, 1998.
52. Warren MP, Vande Wiele RL: Clinical and metabolic features of anorexia nervosa. Am J Obstet Gynecol 117:435–449, 1973.
53. Fergusson RJ, Shaw TRD, Turnbull CM: Spontaneous pneumomediastinum: A complication of anorexia nervosa. Postgrad Med J 61:815–817, 1985.
54. Waldholtz BD, Andersen AE: Gastrointestinal symptoms in anorexia nervosa. A prospective study. Gastroenterology 98:1415–1419, 1990.
55. Stacher G, Kiss A, Wiesnagrotzki S, et al: Oesophageal and gastric motility disorders in patients categorized as having primary anorexia nervosa. Gut 27:1120–1126, 1986.
56. McCallum RW, Grill BB, Lange R, et al: Definition of a gastric emptying abnormality in patients with anorexia nervosa. Dig Dis Sci 30:713–722, 1985.
57. Rigaud D, Bedig G, Merrouche M, et al: Delayed gastric emptying in anorexia nervosa is improved by completion of a renutrition program. Dig Dis Sci 33:919, 1988.
58. Burrington JD, Wayne FR: Obstruction of the duodenum by the superior mesenteric artery—does it exist in children? J Pediatr Surg 9: 733–741, 1974.
59. Chun AB, Sokol MS, Kaye WH, et al: Colonic and anorectal function in constipated patients with anorexia nervosa. Am J Gastroenterol 92: 1879–1883, 1997.
60. Bhanjji S, Mattingly D: Medical Aspects of Anorexia Nervosa. London, Butterworth, 1988.
61. Nordgren L, von Schéele C: Hepatic and pancreatic dysfunction in anorexia nervosa: A report of two cases. Biol Psychiatry 12:681–686, 1977.
62. Komuta M, Harada M, Ueno T, et al: Unusual accumulation of glycogen in liver parenchymal cells in a patient with anorexia nervosa. Intern Med 37:678–682, 1998.
63. McLoughlin DM, Wassif WS, Morton J, et al: Metabolic abnormalities associated with skeletal myopathy in severe anorexia nervosa. Nutrition 16:192–196, 2000.
64. Humphries LL, Adams LJ, Eckfeldt JH, et al: Hyperamylasemia in patients with eating disorders. Ann Intern Med 106:50, 1987.
65. Levine JM, Walton BE, Franko D, et al: Serum amylase in bulimia nervosa: Clinical status and pathophysiology. Int J Eating Disord 12: 431, 1992.
66. Cox KL, Cannon RA, Ament ME, et al: Biochemical and ultrasonic abnormalities of the pancreas in anorexia nervosa. Dig Dis Sci 28: 225–229, 1983.
67. Schoettle UC: Pancreatitis: A complication, a concomitant, or a cause of an anorexia nervosa–like syndrome. J Am Acad Child Psychiatry 18:384–390, 1979.
68. Ramping D: Acute pancreatitis in anorexia nervosa. Med J Aust 2: 194–195, 1982.
69. Lithe M, Zurbrügg RP: A puzzling triad: Anorexia nervosa, high sweat electrolytes and indication to partial exocrine pancreatic insufficiency. Helv Paediatr Acta 38:149–158, 1983.
70. Dancyger IF, Sunday SR, Eckert ED, et al: A comparative analysis of Minnesota Multiphasic Personality Inventory profiles of anorexia nervosa at hospital admission, discharge, and 10-year followup. Compr Psychiatry 38:185–191, 1997.
71. Energy and protein requirements: Report of a Joint FAO/WHO/UNU Expert Consultation. Technical report series No 724. Geneva, World Health Organization, 1985, p 185.
72. Jennings KP, Klidjian AM: Acute gastric dilatation in anorexia nervosa. Br Med J ii:477–478, 1974.
73. Browning CH: Anorexia nervosa: Complications of somatic therapy. Compr Psychiatry 18:399–403, 1977.
74. Kline CL: Anorexia nervosa: Death from complications of ruptured gastric ulcer. Can J Psychiatry 24:153–156, 1979.
75. Evans DS: Acute dilatation and spontaneous rupture of the stomach. Br J Surg 55:940–942, 1968.
76. Pentlow BD, Denkt RD: Acute vascular compression of the duodenum in anorexia nervosa. Br J Surg 68:665–666, 1981.
77. Sackettt SA: Acute pancreatitis and gastric dilatation in a patient with anorexia nervosa. Postgrad Med 61:39, 1985.
78. Wiseman CV, Harris WA, Halmi KA: Eating disorders. Med Clin North Am 82:145–159, 1998.
79. Kaye WH, Klump KL, Frank GKW, et al: Anorexia and bulimia nervosa. Annu Rev Med 51:299–313, 2000.
80. Herzog DB, Keller MB, Lavori PW: Outcome in anorexia nervosa and bulimia nervosa: A review of the literature. J Nerv Ment Dis 176: 131–142, 1988.
81. Kasvikis YG, Tsakiris F, Marks IM, et al: Past history of anorexia nervosa in women with obsessive compulsive disorder. Int J Eat Disord 5:1069–1076, 1986.
82. Thompson JK, Heinberg LJ, Altabe M, et al: Exacting Beauty: Theory, Assessment and Treatment of Body Image Disturbance. American Psychological Association, Washington, DC, 1999.
83. Russell G: Bulimia nervosa: An ominous variant of anorexia nervosa. Psychol Med 4:229–228, 1979.
84. Soundy TJ, Lucas AR, Suman VJ, et al: Bulimia nervosa in Rochester, Minnesota, from 1980–1990. Psychol Med 25:1065–1071, 1995.
85. Andersen AE: Males with Eating Disorders. New York, Brunner/ Maazel, 1990.
86. Brewerton TD, Dansky BS, Kilpatrick DG, et al: Which comes first in the pathogenesis of bulimia nervosa: Dieting or bingeing? Int J Eat Disord 28:259–264, 2000.
87. Gendall KA, Sullivan PE, Joyce PR, et al: The nutrient intake of women with bulimia nervosa. Int J Eat Disord 21:115–127, 1997.
88. Davis C, Katzman DK, Kaptein S, et al: The prevalence of high-level exercise in the eating disorders: Etiological implications. Compr Psychiatry 38:321–326, 1997.
89. Herzog DB, Keller MB, Sacks NR, et al: Psychiatric comorbidity in treatment-seeking anorexics and bulimics. J Am Acad Child Adolesc Psychiatry 31:810–818, 1992.
90. Wonderlich SA, Brewerton TD, Jocic Z, et al: Relationship of childhood sexual abuse and eating disorders. J Am Acad Child Adolesc Psychiatry 36:1107–1115, 1997.
91. Pumariega AJ, Gustavson CR, Gustavson JC: Eating attitudes in African-American women: The essence. Eat Disord J Treatment Prevention 2:5–16, 1994.
92. Hay PJ, Gilchrist PN, Ben-Tovim DI, et al: Eating disorders revisited. II: Bulimia nervosa and related syndromes. Med J Aust 169:488–491, 1998.
93. Johnson CL, Stuckey CL, Lewis LD, Schwartz DM: Bulimia: A descriptive survey of 316 cases. Int J Eat Disord 2:3–16, 1982.
94. Levin PA, Falko JM, Dixon K, et al: Benign parotid enlargement in bulimia. Ann Intern Med 93:827–889, 1980.
95. Daluiski A, Rahbar B, Meals RA: Russell's sign. Subtle hand changes in patients with bulimia nervosa. Clin Orthop 343:107–109, 1997.
96. House RC, Grisius R, Bliziotes MM, Licht JH: Perimolysis: Unveiling the surreptitious vomiter. Oral Surg 51:152–155, 1981.
97. Mitchell JE, Pomeroy C, Seppala M, et al: Pseudo-Bartter's syndrome, diuretic abuse and eating disorders. Int J Eat Disord 7:225–237, 1988.
98. Case T, Lemieux S, Kennedy SH, et al: Elevated plasma lipids in patients with binge eating disorders are found only in those who are anorexic. Int J Eat Disord 25:187–193, 1999.
99. Sullivan PF, Gendall KA, Bulik CM, et al: Elevated total cholesterol in bulimia nervosa. Int J Eat Disord 23:425–432, 1998.
100. Sundgot-Borgen J, Bahr R, Falch JA, Schneider LD: Normal bone mass in bulimic women. J Clin Endocrinol Metab 83:3144–3149, 1998.
101. Yassa R, Nair NP: The Kleine-Levin syndrome—a variant? J Clin Psychiatry 39:254–259, 1978.
102. Dimitropoulos A, Feurer ID, Roof E, et al: Appetite behavior, compulsivity, and neurochemistry in Prader-Willi syndrome. Ment Retard Dev Disabil Res Rev 6:125–130, 2000.
103. Coleman H, Altini M, Nayler S, et al: Sialadenosis: A presenting sign in bulimia. Head Neck 20:758–762, 1998.
104. Crisp AH: Some aspects of the evolution and follow-up of anorexia nervosa. Proc R Soc Med 58:814–820, 1965.
105. Malik M, Stratton J, Sweeney WB: Rectal prolapse associated with bulimia nervosa: Report of seven cases. Dis Colon Rectum 40:1382–1385, 1997.
106. Wilfley DE, Cohen LR: Psychological treatment of bulimia nervosa and binge eating disorder. Psychopharmacol Bull 33:437–454, 1997.

107. Fairburn CG, Norman PA, Welch SL, et al: A prospective study of outcome in bulimia nervosa and the long-term effects of three psychological treatments. Arch Gen Psychiatry 52:304–312, 1995.
108. Walsh BT, Wilson GT, Loeb KL, et al: Medication and psychotherapy in the treatment of bulimia nervosa. Am J Psychiatry 154:523–531, 1997.
109. Chami TN, Andersen AE, Crowell MD, et al: Gastrointestinal symptoms in bulimia nervosa: Effects of treatment. Am J Gastroenterol 90: 88–92, 1995.
110. Keel PK, Mitchell JE, Miller KB, et al: Long-term outcome of bulimia nervosa. Arch Gen Psychiatry 56:63–69, 1999.
111. Collings S, King M: Ten-year follow-up of 50 patients with bulimia nervosa. Br J Psychiatry 164:80–87, 1994.
112. Fairburn CG, Cooper Z, Doll HA, et al: The natural course of bulimia nervosa and binge eating disorder in young women. Arch Gen Psychiatry 57:659–665, 2000.
113. Bray GA: Historical framework for the development of ideas about obesity. In Bray GA, Bouchard C, James WPT (eds): Handbook of Obesity. New York, Marcel Dekker, 1998, pp 1–29.
114. Gould GM, Pyle WL: Anomalies and Curiosities of Medicine. New York, Julian Press, 1956, with original copyright 1896.
115. Wadd W: Comments on Corpulency, Lineaments of Leanness Mems on Diet and Dietetics. London, John Ebers, 1829.
116. Benn RT: Some mathematical properties of weight-for-height indices used as measures of adiposity. Br J Prev Soc Med 25:42–50, 1971.
117. Han TX, van Leer EM, Seidell JC, et al: Waist circumference action levels in the identification of cardiovascular risk factors: Prevalence study in a random sample. Br Med J 311:1401–1405, 1995.
118. Troiano RP, Flegal KM: Overweight children and adolescents: Description, epidemiology, and demographics. Pediatrics 101:497–504, 1998.
119. Wadden TA, Stunkard AJ: Psychopathology and obesity. Ann NY Acad Sci 499:55–65, 1987.
120. Williamson DA, O'Neil PM: Behavioral and psychological correlates of obesity. In Bray GA, Bouchard C, James WPT (eds): Handbook of Obesity. New York, Marcel Dekker, 1998, pp 129–142.
121. Kalra SP, Dube MG, Pu S, et al: Interacting appetite-regulating pathways in the hypothalamic regulation of body weight. Endocrinol Rev 20:68–100, 1999.
122. Rogers PJ: Eating habits and appetite control: A psychobiological perspective. Proc Nutr Soc 58:59–67, 1999.
123. Rogers PJ, Blundell JE: Psychobiological bases of food choice. Br Nutr Found Nutr Bull 15(Suppl1):31–40, 1990.
124. Robbins TW, Fray PJ: Stress-induced eating: Fact, fiction or misunderstanding? Appetite 1:103–133, 1980.
125. York DA: Peripheral and central mechanisms regulating food intake and macronutrient selection. Obes Surg 9:471–479, 1999.
126. Chen D, Garg A: Monogenic disorders of obesity and body fat distribution. J Lipid Res 40:1735–1746, 1999.
127. Spitzer L, Rodin J: Human eating behavior: A critical review of studies in normal weight and overweight individuals. Appetite 2:293–329, 1981.
128. Golay A, Bobbioni E: The role of dietary fat in obesity. Int J Obes 21(Suppl3):S2–S11, 1997.
129. Lichtman SW, Pisarska K, Berman ER, et al: Discrepancy between self-reported and actual caloric intake and exercise in obese subjects. N Engl J Med 327:1893–1898, 1992.
130. Spitzer RL, Devlin M, Walsh BT, et al: Binge eating disorder: A multisite field trial of the diagnostic criteria. Int J Eat Disord 11:191–203, 1992.
131. Welle S, Forbes GB, Statt M, et al: Energy expenditure under free-living conditions in normal weight and overweight women. Am J Clin Nut 55:14–21, 1992.
132. Zurlo F, Ferraro R, Fontvieille AM, et al: Spontaneous physical activity and obesity: Cross-section and longitudinal studies in Pima Indians. Am J Physiol 263:E296–E300, 1992.
133. Hochberg MC, Lethbridge-Cejku M, Scott WW Jr, et al: The association of body weight, body fatness and body fat distribution with osteoarthritis of the knee: Data from the Baltimore Longitudinal Study of Aging. J Rheumatol 22:488–493, 1995.
134. DiBianco R: The changing syndrome of heart failure: An annotated review as we approach the 21st century. J Hypertens 12(Suppl1):S73–S87, 1994.
135. Young T, Palta M, Dempsey J, et al: The occurrence of sleep-disordered breathing among middle-aged adults. N Engl J Med 328:1230–1235, 1993.
136. Hartz AJ, Barboriak PN, Wong A, et al: The association of obesity with infertility and related menstrual abnormalities in women. Int J Obes 3:57–73, 1979.
137. Dunaif A: Polycystic Ovary Syndrome. Boston, Blackwell Scientific Publications, 1992.
138. Johnson SR, Kolberg BH, Varner MN, et al: Maternal obesity and pregnancy. Surg Gynecol Obstet 164:431–437, 1987.
139. Huang Z, Hankinson SE, Colditz GA, et al: Dual effects of weight and weight gain on breast cancer risk. JAMA 278:1407–1411, 1997.
140. Schottenfeld D, Fraumenia JF: Cancer Epidemiology and Prevention. New York, Oxford University Press, 1996.
141. Sugerman HJ: Increased intra-abdominal pressure in obesity. Int J Obes Relat Metab Disord 22:1138, 1998.
142. Locke GR, Talley NJ, Fett SL, et al: Prevalence and clinical spectrum of gastroesophageal reflux: A population-based study in Olmsted County, Minnesota. Gastroenterology 112:1448–1456, 1997.
143. Caskey CI, Zerhouni EA, Fishman EK, et al: Aging of the diaphragm: A CT study. Radiology 171:385–389, 1989.
144. Penzel T, Becker HF, Brandenburg U, et al: Arousal in patients with gastrooesophageal reflux and sleep apnea. Eur Respir J 14:1266–1270, 1999.
145. Lundell L, Ruth M, Sandberg N, et al: Does massive obesity promote abnormal gastroesophageal reflux? Dig Dis Sci 40:1632–1635, 1995.
146. Lagergren J, Bergstrom R, Nyren O: No relation between body mass and gastro-oesophagel reflux symptoms in a Swedish population based study. Gut 47:26–29, 2000.
147. Kjellin A, Ramel S, Rossner S, Thor K: Gastroesophageal reflux in obese patients is not reduced by weight reduction. Scand J Gastroenterol 31:1047–1051, 1996.
148. Stene-Larsen G, Weberg R, Larsen I, et al: Relationship of overweight to hiatus hernia and reflux oesophagitis. Scand J Gastroenterol 23: 427–432, 1988.
149. Wilson LJ, Ma W, Hirschowitz BI: Association of obesity with hiatal hernia and esophagitis. Am J Gastroenterol 94:2840–2844, 1999.
150. Ruhl CE, Everhart JE: Overweight, but not high dietary fat intake, increases risk of gastroesophageal reflux disease hospitalization: The NHANES I Epidemiologic Followup Study. Ann Epidemiol 9:424–435, 1999.
151. Fraser-Moodie CA, Norton B, Gornall C, et al: Weight loss has an independent beneficial effect on symptoms of gastro-oesophagel reflux in patients who are overweight. Scand J Gastroenterol 34:337–340, 1999.
152. Reynolds JC, Waronker M, Pacquing MS, et al: Barrett's esophagus. Reducing the risk of progression to adenocarcinoma. Gastroenterol Clin North Am 28:917–945, 1999.
153. Pera M, Cameron AJ, Trastek VF, et al: Increasing incidence of adenocarcinoma of the esophagus and esophagogastric junction. Gastroenterology, 104:510, 1993.
154. Brown LM, Swanson CA, Gridley G, et al: Adenocarcinoma of the esophagus: Role of obesity and diet. J Natl Cancer Inst 87:104, 1995.
155. Lagergren J: Increased incidence of adenocarcinoma of the esophagus and cardia. Reflux and obesity are strong and independent risk factors according the SECC study. Lakartidningen 97:1050–1093, 2000.
156. Lagergren J, Berström R, Nyrén O: Body mass as a risk factor for esophageal and gastric cardia adenocarcinoma. Ann Intern Med 130: 883–890, 1999.
157. Khare M, Everhart JE, Maurer KR: Association of ethnicity and body mass index (BMI) with gallstone disease in the United States. Am J Epidemiol 141:S69, 1995.
158. Stampfer MJ, Maclure KM, Golditz GA, et al: Risk of symptomatic gallstones in women with severe obesity. Am J Clin Nutr 55:652–658, 1992.
159. Barbara L, Sama C, Labate AMM, et al: A population study on the prevalence of gallstone disease: The Sirmione study. Hepatology 7: 913–917, 1987.
160. Vezina WC, Paradis RL, Grace DM, et al: Increased volume and decreased emptying of the gallbladder in large (morbidly obese, tall normal, and muscular normal) people. Gastroenterology 98:1000–1007, 1990.
161. Reuben A, Maton PN, Murphy GM, et al: Bile lipid secretion in obese and non-obese individuals with and without gallstones. Clin Sci 69:71–79, 1985.
162. Grundy SM, Duane WC, Adler RD, et al: Biliary lipid outputs in young women with cholesterol gallstones. Metabolism 23:67–73, 1974.

163. Whiting MJ, Watts JM: Supersaturated bile from obese patients without gallstones supports cholesterol crystal growth but no nucleation. Gastroenterology 98:739–746, 1990.
164. Garfinkel L: Overweight and mortality. Cancer 58:1826–1829, 1986.
165. Klain J, Fraser D, Goldstein J, et al: Liver histology abnormalities in the morbidly obese. Hepatology 10:873–876, 1989.
166. Luyckx F, Desaive C, Thiry A, et al: Liver abnormalities in severely obese subjects: Effects of drastic weight loss after gastroplasty. Int J Obes 22:222–226, 1998.
167. Braillon A, Capron JP, Hervé M, et al: Liver in obesity. Gut, 26:133–139, 1985.
168. Powell E, Cooksley G, Hanson R, et al: The natural history of nonalcoholic steatohepatitis: A followup study of forty-two patients up to 21 years. Hepatology 11:74–80, 1990.
169. Andersen T, Gluud C, Franzmann M, et al: Hepatic effects of dietary weight loss in morbidly obese subjects. J Hepatol 12:224–229, 1991.
170. Clain D, Lefkowitch J: Fatty liver disease in morbid obesity. Gastroenterol Clin North Am 16:239–252, 1987.
171. Sheth SG, Gordon FO, Chopia S: Nonalcoholic steatohepatitis. Ann Intern Med 126:137–145, 1997.
172. Van Steenbergen W, Lanckmans S: Liver disturbances in obesity and diabetes mellitus. Int J Obes 19(Suppl3):S27–S37, 1995.
173. Wanless IR, Lentz JS: Fatty liver hepatitis (steatohepatitis) and obesity: An autopsy study with analysis of risk factors. Hepatology 12: 1106, 1990.
174. Buchwald H, Lober PH, Varco RL: Liver biopsy findings in 77 consecutive patients undergoing jejunoileal bypass for morbid obesity. Am J Surg 127:48, 1974.
175. Suazo-Barahona J, Carmona-Sanchez R, Robles-Diaz G, et al: Obesity: A risk factor for severe acute biliary and alcoholic pancreatitis. Am J Gastroenterol 93:1324–1328, 1998.
176. Martinez J, Sanchez-Paya J, Palazon JM, et al: Obesity: A prognostic factor of severity in acute pancreatitis. Pancreas 19:15–20, 1999.
177. Giovannucci E, Colditz GA, Stampfer MRJ, et al: Physical activity, obesity, and risk of colorectal adenoma in women (United States). Cancer Causes Control 7:253–263, 1996.
178. Kono S, Handa K, Hayabuchi H, et al: Obesity, weight gain and risk of colon adenomas in Japanese men. Jpn J Cancer Res 90:805–811, 1999.
179. Giovannucci E, Ascherio A, Rimm EB, et al: Physical activity, obesity, and risk for colon cancer and adenoma in men. Ann Intern Med 3:509–514, 1995.
180. Graham S, Marshall J, Haughey B, et al: Dietary epidemiology of cancer of the colon in western New York. Am J Epidemiol 128:490–503, 1988.
181. Bennett GA: Expectations in the treatment of obesity. Br J Clin Psychology 25:311–312, 1986.
182. Wadden TA, Stunkard AJ, Brownell KD: Very low calorie diets: Their efficacy, safety, and future. Ann Intern Med 99:675–684, 1983.
183. Wadden TA, Foster GD, Letizia KA: One-year behavioral treatment of obesity: Comparison of moderate and severe caloric restriction and the effects of weight maintenance therapy. J Consult Clin Psychol 62: 165–171, 1994.
184. Wing RR, Blair E, Marcus M, et al: Year-long weight loss treatment for obese patients with Type II diabetes: Does including an intermittent very-low-calorie diet improve outcome? Am J Med 97:354–362, 1994.
185. National Task Force on the Prevention and Treatment of Obesity: Very low caloric diets. JAMA 270:967–974, 1993.
186. Denke MA: Metabolic effects of high protein, low carbohydrate diets. Am J Cardiol 88:59–61, 2001.
187. Ballor DL, Poehlman ET: Exercise training enhances fat-free mass preservation during diet-induced weight loss: A meta-analytical finding. Int J Obes 18:35–40, 1994.
188. Kayman S, Bruvoild W, Stern JD: Maintenance and relapse after weight loss in women: Behavioral aspects. Am J Clin Nutr 52:800–807, 1990.
189. Hartman WM, Stroud M, Sweet DM, et al: Long-term maintenance of weight loss following supplemented fasting. Int J Eat Disord 14:87–93, 1993.
190. Wing RR: Behavioral approaches to the treatment of obesity. In Bray GA, Bouchard C, James WPT (eds): Handbook of Obesity. New York, Marcel Dekker, 1998, pp 855–873.
191. Poston WS, Foreyt JP: Scientific and legal issues in fenfluramine/dexfenfluramine litigation. Texas Med 96:48–56, 2000.
192. Stell JM, Munro JF, Duncan LJP: A comparative trial of different regimens of fenfluramine and phentermine in obesity. Practitioner 211: 232–236, 1973.
193. James WPT, Astrup A, Finer N, et al: Effect of sibutramine on weight maintenance after weight loss: A randomized trial. Lancet 356:2119–2125, 2000.
194. Lindgarde F: The effect of orlistat on body weight and coronary heart disease risk profile in obese patients: The Swedish Multimorbidity Study. J Intern Med 248:245–254, 2000.
195. Heymsfield SB, Greenberg AS, Fujioka K, et al: Recombinant leptin for weight loss in obese and lean adults: A randomized, controlled, dose-escalation trial. JAMA 282:1568–1575, 1999.
196. National Institutes of Health Consensus Development Conference: Gastrointestinal surgery for severe obesity. Am J Clin Nutr 55(Suppl): 487S–619S, 1992.
197. Requarth JA, Burchard KW, Colacchi TA, et al: Long-term morbidity following jejunoileal bypass: The continuing potential need for surgical reversal. Arch Surg 130:318, 1995.
198. Tottee E, Hendrickx L, van Hee R: Biliopancreatic diversion for treatment of morbid obesity: Experience of 180 consecutive cases. Obes Surg 9:161–165, 1999.
199. Scopinaro N, Gianetta E, Adami GF, et al: Biliopancreatic diversion for obesity at eighteen years. Surgery 119:261–268, 1996.
200. Smets RM, Waeben M: Unusual combination of night blindness and optic neuropathy after biliopancreatic bypass. Bull Soc Belge Ophtalmol 271:93–96, 1999.
201. Compston JE, Vedi S, Gianetta E, et al: Bone histomorphometry and vitamin D status after biliopancreatic bypass for obesity. Gastroenterology 87:350, 1984.
202. Murr MM, Balsiger BM, Kennedy FP, et al: Malabsorptive procedures for severe obesity: Comparison of pancreaticobiliary bypass and very long limb Roux-en-Y gastric bypass. J Gastrointest Surg 3:607–612, 1999.
203. Forsell P, Hallerback B, Glise H, et al: Complications following Swedish adjustable gastric banding: A long-term followup. Obes Surg 9:11–16, 1999.
204. Niville E, Vankeirsbilck J, Dams A, et al: Laparoscopic adjustable esophagogastric banding: A preliminary experience. Obes Surg 8:39–43, 1998.
205. Smith SC, Edwards CB, Goodman GN: Symptomatic and clinical improvement in morbidly obese patients with gastroesophageal reflux disease following Roux-en-Y gastric bypass. Obes Surg 7:479–484, 1997.
206. Kral JG: Surgical treatment of obesity. In Bray GA, Bouchard C, James WPT (eds): Handbook of Obesity. New York, Marcel Dekker, 1998, pp 977–993.
207. Ko CW, Lee SP: Obesity and gallbladder disease. In Bray GA, Bouchard C, James WPT (eds): Handbook of Obesity. New York, Marcel Dekker, 1998, pp 709–724.
208. Everhart JE: Contributions of obesity and weight loss to gallstone disease. Ann Intern Med 119:1029, 1993.
209. Yang H, Peterson GM, Roth MP, et al: Risk factors for gallstone formation during rapid loss of weight. Dig Dis Sci 37:912–918, 1992.
210. Shiffman ML, Sugerman HJ, Kellum JM, et al: Changes in gallbladder bile composition following gallstone formation and weight reduction. Gastroenterology 103:214–221, 1992.
211. Stone BG, Ansel HJ, Peterson FJ, et al: Gallbladder emptying stimuli in obese and normal-weight subjects. Hepatology 15:795–798, 1992.
212. Calhoun R, Willbanks O: Coexistence of gallbladder diseases and morbid obesity. Am J Surg 154:655–658, 1987.
213. Weinsier RL, Wilson LJ, Lee J: Medically safe rate of weight loss for the treatment of obesity: A guideline based on risk of gallstone formation. Am J Med 98:115, 1995.
214. Festi D, Colecchia A, Orsini M, et al: Gallbladder motility and gallstone formation in obese patients following very low calorie diets. Use it (fat) to lose it (well). Int J Obes Relat Metab Disord 22:592–600, 1998.
215. Worobetz LJ, Inglis FG, Shaffer EA: The effect of ursodeoxycholic acid therapy on gallstone formation in the morbidly obese during rapid weight loss. Am J Gastroenterol 88:1705–1710, 1993.
216. Shoheiber O, Biskupiak J, Nash DB: Estimation of the cost savings resulting from the use of ursodiol for the prevention of gallstones in obese patients undergoing rapid weight reduction. Int J Obes Relat Metab Disord 21:1038–1045, 1997.
217. Broomfield PH, Chopra R, Sheinbaum RC, et al: Effects of ursodeox-

ycholic acid and aspirin on the formation of lithogenic bile and gallstones during loss of weight. N Engl J Med 319:1567–1572, 1988.
218. Marks JW, Bonorris GG, Schoenfield LJ: Effects of ursodiol or ibuprofen on contraction of gallbladder and bile among obese patients during weight loss. Dig Dis Sci 41:242–249, 1996.
219. Drenick EJ, Simmons F, Murphy J: Effect on hepatic morphology of treatment of obesity by fasting, reducing diets, and small bowel bypass. N Engl J Med 282:829, 1970.
220. Wadden TA, Bartlett S, Letizia KA, et al: A relationship of dieting history to resting metabolic rate, body composition, eating behavior, and subsequent weight loss. Am J Clin Nutr 56S1:203S–208S, 1992.
221. Woolly SC, Garner DM: Dietary treatments of obesity are ineffective. Br Med J 309:655–656, 1994.
222. Ayyad C, Andersen T: A comprehensive literature study of long-term efficacy of dietary treatment of obesity. Int J Obes 18(Suppl C):78, 1994.
223. Pories WJ, Swanson MS, MacDonald KG, et al: Who would have thought it? An operation proves to be the most effective therapy for adult-onset diabetes mellitus. Ann Surg 222:339–352, 1995.
224. Sjostrom CD, Lissner L, Wedel H, et al: Reduction in incidence of diabetes, hypertension and lipid disturbances after intentional weight loss induced by bariatric surgery: The SOS Intervention Study. Obes Res 7:477–484, 1999.

Section Four

TOPICS INVOLVING MULTIPLE ORGANS

Chapter 18

Oral Disease and Oral-Cutaneous Manifestations of Gastrointestinal and Liver Diseases

Ginat W. Mirowski and Tsu-Yi Chuang

DISORDERS OF THE MOUTH AND TONGUE

Xerostomia (dry mouth) is a common complaint in patients with destruction or atrophy of the salivary glands as a result of autoimmune disease, after radiation therapy, or as a consequence of a variety of medications such as anticholinergics, H_1 antihistamines, tricyclic antidepressants, hypnotics, sedatives, antihypertensives, antipsychotics, antiparkinson agents and diuretics.[1, 2] *Sjögren's syndrome* is an autoimmune disease that is classified by the triad of xerostomia, keratoconjunctivitis sicca (dry eyes), and arthritis.[1] Sjögren's syndrome may be characterized as primary, when no other disorders are diagnosed, or secondary, when another connective tissue disease such as rheumatoid arthritis or systemic lupus erythematosus is present. The oral manifestations of Sjögren's syndrome are caused by the irreversible destruction of the salivary glands by a lymphocytic infiltrate that results in diminished or absent saliva. The lack of saliva is associated with difficulty chewing, painful swallowing (odynophagia), and diminished taste and smell, as well as mucosal erythema, increased incidence of dental caries, and salivary gland calculi. Sucking mints and chewing gum may help by increasing salivary flow, by improving the removal of debris, and by emitting their own flavors. Patients with xerostomia should avoid sugar-containing foods and acidic foods and beverages. Patients should be encouraged to sip water and suck ice chips frequently.[2] Antiseptic mouthwashes are also helpful. For patients with xerostomia and no salivary reserve, preparations containing 1% sodium carboxymethyl cellulose may be used to moisten the oral cavity.[2, 3] Cholinergic salivary stimulants, such as pilocarpine and bethanechol, may be helpful.[4–7] The cholinergic agonist cevilimine (Evoxac) 30 mg three times per day is approved by the U.S. Food and Drug Administration (FDA) for the treatment of dry mouth symptoms caused by Sjögren's syndrome and requires fewer doses per day than pilocarpine (5 mg three or four times per day).[8, 8a]

Glossitis, inflammation of the tongue, occurs in a heterogeneous group of disorders that includes nutritional deficiencies, chemical irritants, drug reactions, hypochromic or pernicious anemia, amyloidosis, sarcoidosis, infections (especially candidiasis), vesiculoerosive diseases (to be discussed), and systemic infections. Sometimes no underlying cause can be detected.[9] Patients complain of lingual pain (glossodynia) or burning sensation (glossopyrosis). The physical examination can show any degree of filiform depapillation ranging from mild and patchy erythema with or without erosive changes to a completely smooth, atrophic, erythematous surface (Fig. 18–1; see also Fig. 8–1). Atrophic glossitis is a sign of protein-calorie malnutrition and muscle atrophy and is commonly found in the elderly.[10] Median rhomboid glossitis can possibly present as an asymptomatic, well-defined erythematous patch in the mid-posterior dorsum of the tongue.[10]

Hypogeusia (diminished sense of taste) and dysgeusia (distortion of normal taste) are other complaints that sometimes are associated with glossitis. Hypogeusia and dysgeusia have been attributed to a variety of neurologic, nutri-

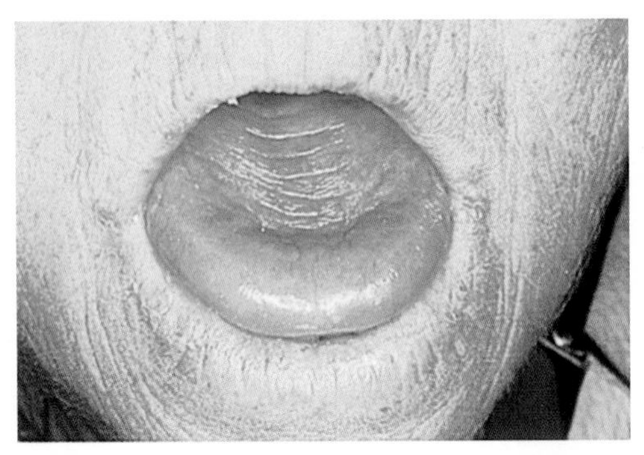

Figure 18–1. Glossitis in a patient with diabetes and malabsorption. The tongue is smooth (depapillation) and red; angular cheilitis is present.

tional, and metabolic disorders and to a large number of medications. The evidence supporting these associations is tenuous.[11, 12] How taste buds are affected by aging is not understood. Tobacco smokers, denture wearers, and patients with anxiety or other psychiatric disorders commonly complain of hypogeusia and dysgeusia. Radiation therapy to the head and neck may result in altered taste. Apparently, taste buds are extremely sensitive to irradiation. Hypogeusia after radiation therapy to the mouth is often partially reversible.[13] The therapy is empirical and includes identifying and correcting any associated condition. Patients may be treated with zinc supplementation or low-dose anxiolytic or antidepressant medication. Paradoxically, tricyclic antidepressant medications block responses to a wide range of taste stimuli and may contribute to clinical reports of hypogeusia and dysgeusia.[14]

Glossodynia (burning sensation or pain in tongue) in the absence of clinical or histologic evidence of glossitis may be associated with anxiety or depression. It is found most commonly in postmenopausal women, but hormonal therapy is of no value.[15] Hypnosis has been found to improve glossodynia when a psychogenic component or when organic disease is present.[16] Serologic evaluation for hypomagnesemia and for vitamin B_{12} and folate deficiency, as well as a complete medication history, may yield a correctable etiology.

Geographic tongue (benign migratory glossitis) is a benign, self-limited condition of unknown etiology, characterized by patchy loss of filiform papillae. Geographic tongue is reported to occur in 4% of the population. The patches form irregular, moving configurations that resemble geographic landmarks on a map. Patients may complain of pain or difficulty eating acidic, spicy, or salty foods. Recurrent episodes are common. Histologically, spongiosis and neutrophilic microabscesses are found in the epithelium with no evidence of candidiasis. Patient should be reassured that geographic tongue has no known associations with malignancy.[17]

Black hairy tongue is another common entity that results from elongation of the filiform papillae. The dorsal surface of the tongue may appear yellow, green, brown, or black due to exogenous pigment trapped within elongated keratin strands of filiform papillae.[18, 19] Acquired black hairy tongue is seen most commonly among chronic smokers and often follows a course of systemic antibiotics, the use of hydrogen peroxide, or drinking coffee or tea.[18, 20] Off-label treatment consists of 25% podophyllum or topical tretinoin (Retin-A) gel.[19]

MUCOCUTANEOUS CANDIDIASIS

Candida species (chiefly *Candida albicans)* are part of the normal flora in almost half the population. *Oral candidiasis or candidosis* (moniliasis, thrush) typically appears as white curdlike patches or as red (atrophic) or white and red friable lesions on any mucosal surface. Patients may complain of pain. Many newborns experience initial overgrowth of candida before colonization of the gastrointestinal (GI) tract. *Candidiasis* often occurs after antibiotic or glucocorticoid therapy; in denture wearers; in pregnancy; in old age; and in patients with anemia, diabetes mellitus, Hashimoto's thyroiditis, Cushing's disease, or familial hypoparathyroidism. Immunosuppression caused by human immunodeficiency virus (HIV) (discussed later), other debilitating illnesses, or cancer chemotherapy may lead to candidiasis. Oral candidiasis is also associated with xerostomia, whatever the cause.[21] Topical therapy is most effective in patients with no underlying chronic conditions and may entail the use of the following: (1) nystatin (Mycostatin), 100,000-unit vaginal tablets to be dissolved orally three to five times daily; or (2) clotrimazole (Mycelex), an oral-prepared 10-mg troche to be dissolved orally five times daily; or clotrimazole prepared as a 500-mg vaginal tablet, to be dissolved orally at bedtime.

Topical agents listed earlier and amphotericin B are effective in the absence of immunosuppression, whereas oral fluconazole is relatively effective in immunocompromised patients. In denture wearers, adjunctive measures, including regular denture cleaning, soaking in a dilute bleach solution, and use of oral antifungals, are important for clearing.[21] When dysphagia and/or upper GI bleeding accompany oral thrush, concurrent *candidal esophagitis* should be considered (see Chapter 34). Systemic candidiasis may result when normal barriers to infection, such as in neutropenic patients, are lost. Microthrombi resulting from obstruction of cutaneous and systemic vessels leads to local necrosis and manifest as small necrotic papules and ulcerations that are easily visible on the skin and mucosa.

MUCOCUTANEOUS FEATURES OF HIV INFECTION (see also Chapter 28)

Oral and cutaneous complications are common in patients with HIV infection.[22] These manifestations cause significant morbidity and can provide valuable diagnostic and prognostic information. Frequently, the first and certainly the most common HIV-associated infection of the mouth is candidiasis.[23–26] The history and physical findings usually establish the diagnosis. The presence of spores, pseudohyphae, or hyphal forms on a smear (potassium hydroxide, periodic acid–Schiff/Papanicolaou), culture, or biopsy confirms the diagnosis. Oral candidiasis in HIV should be treated systemically.[27] Systemic therapy involves the use of oral azole preparations (Fluconazole [Diflucan], 100 mg, or itraconazole [Sporanox], 100 mg). Amphotericin B (Fungizone) intravenously is also effective. Treatment for 1 to 2 weeks is usually effective, even in the late stages of HIV infection. The major problem is frequent recurrences and the need for chronic or repeated treatment. The likelihood of clinical relapse is dependent on the degree of immunosuppression and

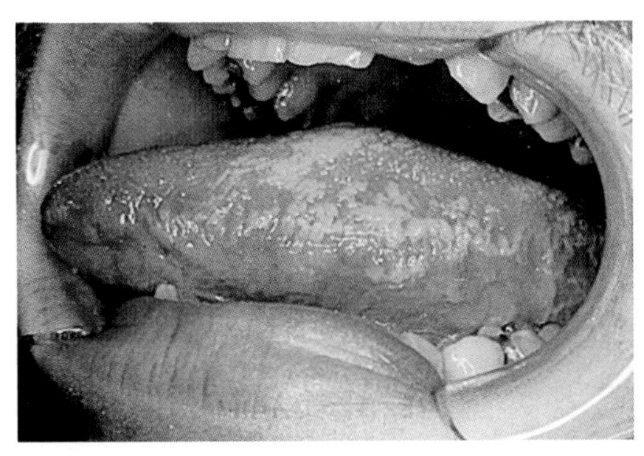

Figure 18–2. Hairy leukoplakia involving the tongue in a patient with AIDS. (Courtesy of Sol Silverman Jr, DDS, and Victor Newcomer, MD.)

the duration of therapy. As adjunctive measures, mouth rinses with chlorhexidine gluconate (Peridex), Listerine, or hydrogen peroxide–saline may be of some benefit.[28] Chronic oral candidiasis is a poor prognostic sign, reflecting profound immunosuppression.

Periodontal disease and alveolar bone loss occurs in 19% to 29% of patients with or at risk for acquired immunodeficiency syndrome (AIDS).[25]

Hairy leukoplakia (oral hairy leukoplakia [HL]) appears as corrugated white lesions (Fig. 18–2; see also Color Fig. 18–2) almost always on the lateral borders of the tongue. HL is usually asymptomatic and may be an early sign of HIV infection. The epithelium in patients with HL is infected with Epstein-Barr virus.[29, 30] The severity of HL does not correlate with the stage of HIV disease. However, the presence of HL in a HIV-infected person has been associated with the progression to AIDS. Analysis of 198 cases of HL demonstrated that the median time to onset of AIDS was 24 months, and the median time to death in the era prior to highly active antiretroviral therapy (HAART) was 41 months.[29, 31, 32] Because other mucosal white lesions, such as oral leukoplakia (Fig. 18–3; see also Color Fig. 18–3), can resemble HL lesions, biopsy confirmation should be considered if the diagnosis of HL is in doubt. HL may be confused with candidiasis (which coexists in about half the cases). A prudent first step in management is the administration of anticandidal therapy. When risk factors are apparent and the HIV status is unknown, the suspicion of HL justifies a discussion of its implications and suggestion of HIV testing (with appropriate counseling). Although HL occurs predominantly in homosexual and bisexual men, it also has been found in other HIV-infected persons and in renal and other organ transplant recipients. Because HL is usually asymptomatic, treatment is elective and empirical. HL responds to oral acyclovir, topical retinoic acid, and podophyllum. When treatment is discontinued, HL usually returns.

Kaposi's sarcoma is a common consequence of HIV infection and is associated with human herpesvirus 8. A significant decline in the incidence of Kaposi's sarcoma occurred during 1996 and 1997, which corresponds to the introduction of HAART.[33] Although Kaposi's sarcoma is usually found on the skin, more than half of patients also have intraoral lesions.[34, 35] In one study, the first sign of Kaposi's sarcoma occurred in the mouth in 22% of the patients examined, and in another 45%, Kaposi's sarcoma occurred in the mouth and skin simultaneously.[34] The cutaneous lesions of Kaposi's sarcoma appear as asymptomatic red to purple, oval macules that develop into papules, plaques, or nodules. They rarely ulcerate except on the lower extremities and genitalia. Edema often accompanies cutaneous lesions, especially on the lower extremities or on the face. Oral lesions may vary in appearance from minimal, asymptomatic, flat, purple or red macules to large nodules. The hard palate is the most frequent location, followed by the gingiva and tongue (Fig. 18–4; see also Color Fig. 18–4). The differential diagnosis includes purpura, hemangioma, coagulation defects, and bacillary angiomatosis. Diagnosis is established by biopsy.[36] Treatment approaches are mainly palliative and include radiation therapy, chemotherapy (including intralesional injections), and surgery. Patients with cutaneous Kaposi's sarcoma may have asymptomatic visceral lesions.

Lymphoma may involve the oral cavity and skin in HIV patients and rarely may be the first sign of HIV or lymphoma.[37]

Other conditions associated with HIV infection include extensive oral, genital, or cutaneous warts; recurrent aphthae; chronic mucocutaneous herpes simplex virus (HSV) infections; lymphocytic infiltrates of major salivary glands; drug reactions including drug-induced Stevens-Johnson syndrome; Bartonella infections (bacillary angiomatosis and its associated peliosis hepatis); premature and progressive periodontal disease; and acute ulcerative gingivitis.[38]

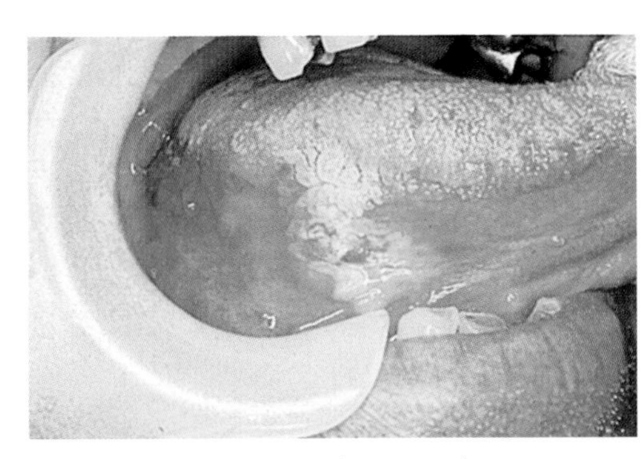

Figure 18–3. Oral leukoplakia and associated squamous carcinoma.

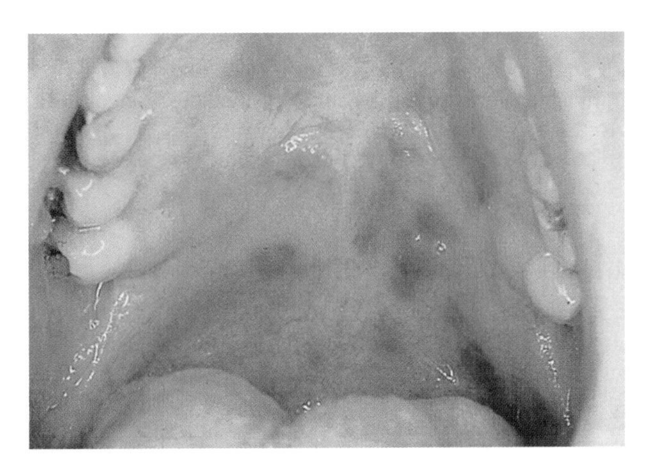

Figure 18–4. Kaposi's sarcoma involving the tongue. (Courtesy of Sol Silverman Jr, DDS, and Victor Newcomer, MD.)

MUCOCUTANEOUS ULCERATIVE DISEASES

Aphthous ulcers (canker sores) are painful, shallow ulcers often covered with a grayish-white or yellow exudate and surrounded by an erythematous margin. They appear almost exclusively on unkeratinized oral mucosal surfaces (Table 18–1). Rarely, aphthous ulcers may occur in the esophagus, upper and lower GI tracts, and anorectal epithelium. About 25% of individuals in the general population develop aphthous ulcers at some time. Aphthous ulcers recur at irregular intervals. Three clinical forms of aphthous ulcers are recognized: minor aphthae (most common), major aphthae (less common), and herpetiform aphthae (least common).[39] Minor aphthae typically are less than 5 mm in size and heal in 1 to 3 weeks (Fig. 18–5; see also Color Fig. 18–5). Major aphthae may exceed 6 mm (Fig. 18–6; see also Color Fig. 18–6) and require months to resolve. Major aphthae, when healed, often leave scars.[40, 41] Herpetiform aphthae are 1 to 3 mm in diameter, occur in clusters of tens to hundreds of ulcers and resolve quickly.[39]

A variety of conditions have been associated with aphthous ulcers, but most evidence points to an immunologic etiology.[41, 42] Frequently, the lesions are brought on or aggravated by stress. Prolonged fever or local trauma may precipitate eruptions. Patients with severe nutritional deficiencies or anemia have noted improvement after treatment with iron, folate, or vitamin B_{12},[43] but most patients with aphthous ulcers do not benefit from vitamin or mineral supplements.[44] Some patients report developing ulcers after ingesting nuts, chocolate, or citrus products. Morphologically identical lesions may be seen in *inflammatory bowel disease* (discussed later) and *Behçet's syndrome*. Gluten-sensitive enteropathy (celiac disease) is diagnosed in less than 5% of patients with recurrent aphthous ulcers. *Helicobacter pylori* has recently been found in oral lesion tissue, but the levels of serum immunoglobulin G (IgG) antibodies to *H. pylori* are not increased in patients with aphthous ulcers.[39] The workup for recurrent aphthous ulcers includes a complete blood count (CBC); erythrocyte sedimentation rate; serum iron, ferritin, folate, and B_{12} levels; KOH stain; Tzanck smear; viral culture; biopsy of skin lesions to exclude HSV; and colonoscopy. Histologically, lesional tissue shows ulcerated mucosa with chronic mixed inflammatory cells.

Management of aphthous ulcers includes palliative and curative measures. First-line therapy includes topical corticosteroids and immunosuppressive agents.[39] Aphthous ulcers can be treated effectively with a potent glucocorticoid such as fluocinonide (Lidex) or clobetasol (Temovate) gel or ointment. Analgesics and topical anesthetics such as 2% viscous lidocaine may be helpful. Second-line therapy includes colchicine 0.6 mg three times a day, cimetidine 400 to 800 mg/day, azathioprine 50 mg/day, and thalidomide (FDA approved; for HIV patients).[39] Short courses of systemic prednisone (20 to 60 mg/day) are reproducibly effective when conservative empirical approaches are not satisfactory.[45] Other topical therapies include Kaopectate and sucralfate to protect lesions and accelerate healing.[46] An elimination diet may be helpful in patients with allergic reactions to certain foods. A gluten-free diet is recommended for patients with gluten-sensitive enteropathy. Soft foods are useful in patients with oral lesions. Patients should be advised to use multivitamins with iron and avoid salty or spicy foods to minimize irritation of oral lesions.[39] The role of sodium laurel sulfate in exacerbating aphthae is controversial.[47, 48]

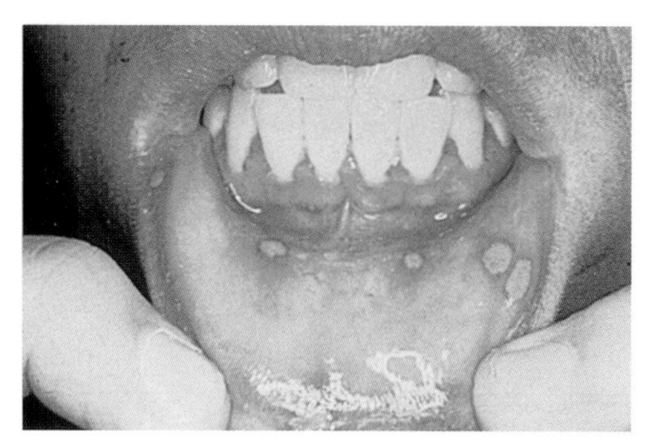

Figure 18–5. Multiple minor aphthous ulcers.

Table 18–1 | **Differential Diagnosis of Common Oral Ulcers**

MUCOSA	LOCATION	CONDITION
Unkeratinized	Lateral tongue, floor of the mouth, labial and buccal mucosa, soft palate, and pharynx	Aphthous ulcers
Keratinized	Gingiva, hard palate, dorsal tongue	Herpes simplex virus infection

Infection with the HSV commonly produces painful vesiculoulcerative lesions affecting the genitalia, eyes, lips, mouth, and skin.[49–52] *Primary herpetic gingivostomatitis* is caused by HSV type 1 (or occasionally type 2). Primary infection occurs in up to 90% of the population before puberty. The illness is often mild and mistaken for a routine upper respiratory tract infection and may include varying degrees of fever, malaise, and adenopathy, together with oral and gingival ulcers. Lesions may appear on the lips. They generally heal in 1 to 2 weeks. Management is palliative, but acyclovir, 200 mg every 4 hours while awake, may shorten the course and may reduce severity. Secondary bacterial infection is common and can be treated topically.

Recurrent orolabial herpes simplex is caused by reactiva-

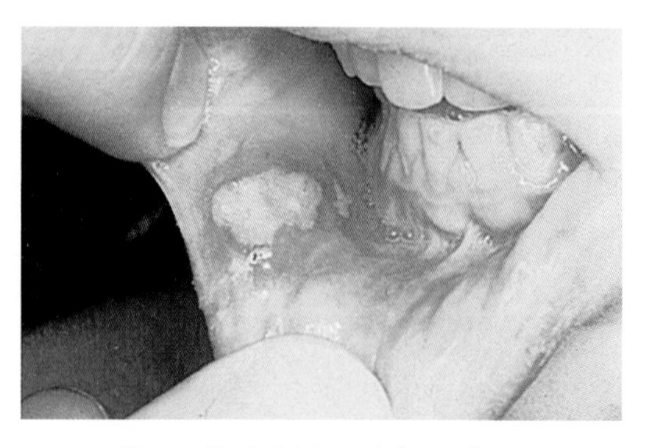

Figure 18–6. Major aphthous ulcer.

tion of HSV that has been dormant in regional ganglia, with no increase in HSV antibody titers.[51, 52] Episodes may be precipitated by fever, sunlight, and physical or emotional stress. Recurrences are variable in frequency and severity. Typically, the lesions involve the lips ("cold sores") and are preceded by several hours of prodromal symptoms such as burning sensation, tingling, or pruritus. Vesicles then appear but soon rupture, leaving small, irregular, painful ulcers. Coalescence of ulcers, crusting, and weeping of lesions are common. Intraoral recurrent herpetic ulcers occur on keratinized mucosa (i.e., hard palate or gingiva) (see Table 18–1). They appear as shallow, irregular, small ulcerations and may coalesce. Labial and oral herpetic ulcers normally heal in less than 2 weeks. Recurrent HSV is the most common cause of recurrent *erythema multiforme* (see later).[53]

In immunocompromised patients, HSV can affect any mucocutaneous surface and can appear as large, irregular, pseudomembrane-covered ulcers. This is especially true in HIV-infected persons, in whom all perineal and orolabial ulcerations should be considered manifestations of HSV until proven otherwise.

Herpes simplex is usually diagnosed from the history and clinical findings. A history of a prodrome or of vesicles, the site of lesions, and the reappearance of lesions in the same location help differentiate herpes from other ulcerative disorders. A cytologic smear (Tzanck) showing multinucleate giant cells is suggestive, although viral cultures and monoclonal antibody staining of smears are more sensitive and specific tests for diagnosing HSV infection. Topical acyclovir is of little benefit in recurrent labial herpes and of limited benefit in recurrent genital HSV. Systemic acyclovir is regularly used for treatment of primary or recurrent attacks in immunosuppressed patients (2 g orally in divided doses or 5 mg/kg intravenously three times daily until lesions heal). More recently famciclovir, 125 mg twice daily, or valacyclovir, 500 mg twice daily, has been available in the United States. Oral treatment should optimally begin within the first few hours of the prodrome. Suppression of recurrences may be accomplished with acyclovir, 200 mg orally three times daily or 400 mg twice daily. Acyclovir has been used for the prevention of recurrent oral and genital herpes associated with bone marrow transplantation.[54] Antivirals are also used to prevent recurrent herpes in other immunocompromised patients such as those with leukemia or HIV infection.[55] Care should be taken to avoid ocular autoinoculation.

Herpes zoster is caused by a reactivation of the varicella virus. The oral lesions can resemble the ulcers of aphthous stomatitis, except for the following features: the ulcers are unilateral; lip and/or skin lesions may coexist; and the onset is sudden, acutely painful, and often associated with fever. High dosages of acyclovir (4 g/day orally) or famciclovir, 500 mg every 8 hours, or valacyclovir, 1 g every 8 hours, at the onset may be helpful in accelerating healing. Herpes zoster is often the initial manifestation of HIV infection.

Cytomegalovirus affects 40% to 80% of adults, as evidenced by serologic studies. However, symptomatic disease occurs mainly after organ or bone marrow transplantation or in HIV-infected persons. Other than retinitis, mucosal ulcers are the main consequence of cytomegalovirus infection. Skin is rarely affected. Characteristic features of biopsy specimens include intranuclear and intracytoplasmic inclusions.[56]

Acute necrotizing ulcerative gingivitis is an acute inflammatory and necrotic infection affecting the interdental papillae and commonly affects healthy young adults. Treatment consists of surgical débridement, oral rinses, and systemic antibiotics.

Cutaneous amebiasis is a rare complication of amebic dysentery. Undermined ulcers of the perineum and genitalia may result from direct inoculation from the colon and rectum to the anus after contact with contaminated stool or from external inoculation after intercourse or hand (scratching) contact. Dissemination may result from invasion of the colonic mucosa with hematogenous spread to the liver and on to the lungs or chest wall.[57] When there is long-standing disease, the ulcer borders may become vegetative and proliferative and resemble a squamous cell carcinoma. Because primary carcinomas of the rectum, colon, and cervix may be secondarily colonized with *Entamoeba histolytica,* it is important that either possibility be ruled out.[58]

VESICULOBULLOUS DISEASES

Pemphigoid is a general term for heterogenous blistering disorders characterized by bullae and ulcers affecting the mucosa of the oral cavity, pharynx, esophagus, anus, conjunctiva, and skin.[59] Oral findings appear as highly inflamed (erythematous) mucosa on the buccal mucosa and gingiva. Two types of pemphigoid have been identified: *bullous pemphigoid* and *cicatricial* (mucous membrane) *pemphigoid.*[60–62] Patients with bullous pemphigoid typically have skin lesions, and about one third also have mucous membrane lesions; all patients with cicatricial pemphigoid have mucosal lesions, and about one third also have skin lesions. Ocular symblepharon (i.e., adhesion between the tarsal and bulbar conjunctiva) commonly occurs with cicatricial pemphigoid. Immunofluorescent staining of involved mucosa and skin shows linear deposition of antibody and complement in the basement membrane zone.[63] Patients with serum IgG and IgA antibodies are more likely to respond to systemic medications.[64] Serum antibodies against 230-kd and 180-kd antigens located at the squamous epithelial basement membrane have been documented. Treatment ranges from low-dose to high-dose prednisone for patients without contraindications to steroid use. Therapies for patients with contraindications or systemic toxicities to steroids include dapsone, tetracycline and nicotinamide combination, azathioprine, chlorambucil, plasma exchange, intravenous immune globulin (IVIG), cyclosporine, cyclophosphamide given orally or in a pulse-dosing format, and methotrexate.[64]

Pemphigus vulgaris differs from pemphigoid in that skin lesions are more severe (and can be life-threatening if untreated) and oral involvement can be extensive. Mucosal involvement can cause poor nutrition and severe pain.[64] Half of patients with pemphigus vulgaris present with oral lesions, and virtually 100% develop oral lesions during the illness. Autoantibodies mediate a loss of cell-to-cell adhesion. IgG antibodies and complement on the surface of squamous epithelial cells are diagnostic.[65] Indirect immunofluorescence detects circulating IgG antibodies in most patients with pemphigus vulgaris.[64] Treatment consists of various regimens of topical or systemic prednisone, sometimes supplemented with cytotoxic/immunosuppressive drugs.

Paraneoplastic pemphigus is an atypical form of pemphigus that shares features of pemphigus vulgaris and erythema multiforme.[64, 66] It is associated with a variety of malignancies, including hematologic malignancies (lymphomas and leukemias), thymomas, soft tissue sarcomas, and GI malignancies.[67, 68] Five features characterize paraneoplastic pemphigus: (1) painful mucosal erosions and a polymorphous skin eruption; (2) intraepidermal acantholysis, keratinocyte necrosis, and vacuolar interface reaction; (3) deposition of IgG and C3 intercellularly and along the epidermal basement membrane zone; (4) serum autoantibodies that bind to skin and mucosa epithelium in a pattern characteristic of pemphigus, as well as binding to simple, columnar, and transitional epithelia; and (5) immunoprecipitation of a complex of four proteins (250, 230, 210, and 190 kd) from keratinocytes by the autoantibodies.[67, 68]

The prognosis of paraneoplastic pemphigus depends on the associated underlying malignancy, and successful treatment is predicated on the successful elimination of the underlying malignancy.[64]

Epidermolysis bullosa (EB) is a heterogeneous group of rare inherited disorders of skin fragility (Fig. 18–7; see also Color Fig. 18–7). They are characterized by the formation of blisters with minimal trauma and have been divided into dystrophic (scarring), junctional, and simplex forms. Oral erosions, premature caries, and gingival involvement as well as GI disease are common in the dystrophic form but also occur in some patients with the junctional form.[69] Besides oral erosions, esophageal strictures are the most common GI complication in dystrophic EB.[69] They may be narrow or broad and most commonly occur in the upper third of the esophagus, but they also may be found in the lower third (see Chapter 34). The esophageal strictures are probably induced by repeated trauma from food and/or refluxed gastric contents. Although dilations may produce temporary improvement, they risk increasing stenosis in the long run. Therefore, strict adherence to a soft-food diet is the usual form of management. Surgical excision, feeding gastrostomy, and colonic transplantation have been effectively used in dystrophic EB patients with severe esophageal strictures. Esophageal webs in the postcricoid area have also been described. Anal stenosis and constipation with or without

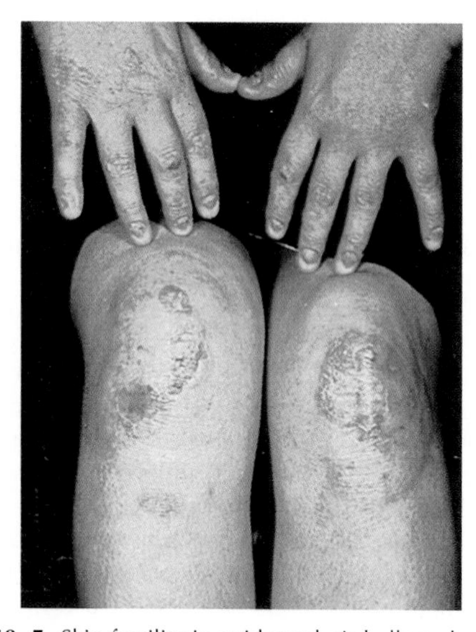

Figure 18–7. Skin fragility in epidermolysis bullosa dystrophica.

stenosis are frequent complications in patients with dystrophic EB. Junctional EB has been uniquely associated with pyloric atresia.[69] Patients with severe dystrophic and junctional EB frequently develop anemia and growth retardation, partly because of the GI and oral complications.

Patients with clinical lesions identical to the dystrophic forms of EB but with no family history and an adult onset have been identified, and their condition is called acquired EB or EB acquisita (EBA). EBA, like pemphigus and pemphigoid, is an autoimmune disease. The autoantibodies in EBA are directed against type VII collagen.[70–72] The diagnosis is established by routine histology and direct immunofluorescence examination of skin biopsy specimens. Patients may have significant mucosal involvement, like patients with cicatricial pemphigoid, especially oral and esophageal disease. Coexistent Crohn's disease has been reported in multiple patients with EBA.[72] The treatment is with immunosuppressive agents. Cyclosporine is an effective treatment.[64]

Erythema multiforme minor (EM) is an acute, benign mucocutaneous eruption that is associated with underlying infections (especially HSV). It is often preceded or accompanied by low-grade fever, malaise, and symptoms suggesting an upper respiratory tract infection. The eruption consists of alternating pink and red "target lesions" on the elbows, knees, palms, and soles and of shallow, broad oral erosions. Patients with EM may only have oral involvement.[73] Variable degrees of nonspecific erythema are found, with or without ulcers. Crusting, hemorrhagic, and moist lip ulcers may be present. Severe oral and pharyngeal pain, secondary bacterial and fungal infections, and bleeding are common complications. Herpes-associated erythema multiforme lesions are associated with expression of *pol,* an HSV gene. Some patients benefit from prophylactic therapy with acyclovir, a known *pol* inhibitor.[74] The diagnosis is made by clinical characteristics, ruling out other specifically diagnosable diseases, and by response to treatment. The biopsy reveals a nonspecific interface reaction. Oral EM can be self-limited or chronic, and often the inciting process goes unidentified. Management includes palliative measures and elimination of any offending agent. Often, glucocorticoids and/or other immunosuppressive drugs are needed.[45] Recurrences and flares have variable patterns.

Stevens-Johnson syndrome, or erythema multiforme major, is diagnosed when severe, acute EM affects the eyes, skin, and mucous membranes. Diffuse oral and pharyngeal ulceration may prevent oral intake. At endoscopy, the esophagus may show diffuse erythema, friability, and whitish plaques that can be mistaken for candidiasis. Diffuse gastric and duodenal erythema and friability may be present without esophageal involvement.[28] The colonoscopic appearance may resemble severe ulcerative or pseudomembranous colitis; however, biopsies show extensive necrosis and lymphocytic infiltration without crypt abscesses or neutrophils. This pattern is reminiscent of *graft-versus-host disease.* The mucosa of large portions of bowel may slough, accounting for reports of hematemesis, melena, and intestinal perforation in Stevens-Johnson syndrome.[75] IVIG has resulted in termination of disease progression in some patients.[76]

LICHEN PLANUS

Lichen planus is a common, chronic inflammatory disorder involving the oral mucosa and skin. The disease usually

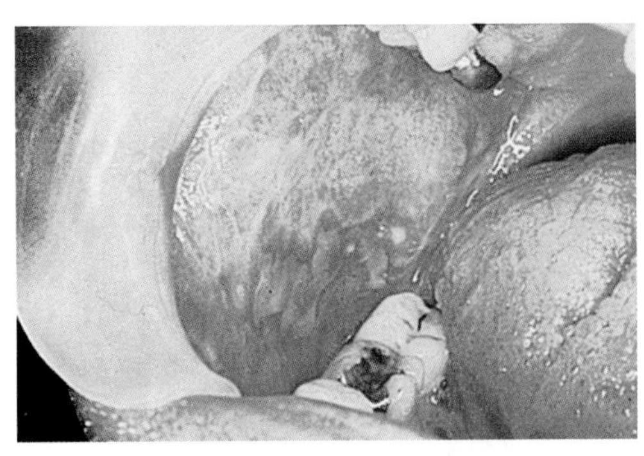

Figure 18–8. The erosive forms of oral lichen planus involving the buccal mucosa. Note the lace-like keratoses, erythema, and ulceration.

begins in adulthood, and two thirds of the patients are women.[63] Oral lesions appear as white lacelike and/or punctate patterns on any mucosal surface (Fig. 18–8; see also Color Fig. 18–8). There may be associated mucosal erythema or ulceration. An increased risk of developing *squamous carcinoma* is reported. Approximately 20% of patients with oral lichen planus also have skin lesions.[77] The lesions are small, flat-topped, pruritic, and violaceous papules. Patients with oral lesions can be asymptomatic or may develop severe oral pain. The use of topical and/or systemic glucocorticoids is effective in decreasing the signs and symptoms in almost all cases of oral and cutaneous lichen planus. In rare, refractory instances, systemic retinoids are necessary. *Esophageal involvement* with lichen planus has been reported.[78, 79] Patients developed progressive dysphagia and odynophagia after years of severe oral disease. The endoscopic findings included erythema, ulcers, or erosions throughout the esophagus. One case included a proximal esophageal web.[79] An increased prevalence of chronic liver disease, including chronic active hepatitis C and primary biliary cirrhosis, has been reported among patients with lichen planus.[80, 81]

CUTANEOUS MANIFESTATIONS OF INTESTINAL DISEASE, INCLUDING INFLAMMATORY BOWEL DISEASE

Both ulcerative colitis and Crohn's disease may be accompanied by cutaneous manifestations[82, 83] (see also Chapters 103 and 104). Skin lesions are more common (up to 44%) and often more specific in Crohn's disease than in ulcerative colitis. It is rare for cutaneous involvement by Crohn's disease to appear before symptomatic bowel disease. The most common cutaneous complications of Crohn's disease are granulomatous lesions of the perianal or perifistular skin, which occur by direct extension from underlying diseased bowel. *Metastatic Crohn's disease* refers to rare ulcerative lesions, plaques, or nodules that occur at sites distant from the bowel. Such lesions favor intertriginous areas such as the retroauricular and inframammary regions. On histologic study, both local cutaneous extension and metastatic Crohn's disease show granulomatous inflammation, and both occur with greater frequency in patients with colonic involvement by Crohn's disease.

Oral manifestations of Crohn's disease occur in 4% to 14% of patients and include aphthae (see Figs. 18–5 and 18–6), lip fissures, cobblestone plaques, cheilitis, mucosal tags, and perioral erythema. Patients may also complain of metallic dysgeusia. Aphthosis occurs in approximately 5% of patients with Crohn's disease, and the lesions are indistinguishable, clinically and histologically, from typical aphthae. *Granulomatous cheilitis* is a rare condition with recurrent lip swelling that leads to enlargement and firmness of the lips. A biopsy shows noncaseating granulomas. It may be idiopathic, a component of Melkersson-Rosenthal syndrome (scrotal tongue, lip swelling, with or without facial palsy and migraine), or in rare cases associated with Crohn's disease.[84]

Pyostomatitis vegetans (Fig. 18–9; see also Color Fig. 18–9), and its cutaneous counterpart pyoderma vegetans, is characterized by pustules, erosions, and vegetations involving the labial mucosa of the upper and lower lips, buccal mucosa, and gingival mucosa, as well as the skin of the axillae, genitalia, trunk, and scalp.[85] Both pyostomatitis vegetans and pyoderma vegetans are specific markers of inflammatory bowel disease (Crohn's and ulcerative colitis) and may precede the symptoms by months to years. Histologically, intraepithelial and subepithelial eosinophilic miliary abscesses are characteristic.[85–87] Superficial pustules coat the friable, erythematous, and eroded mucosa of the oral cavity (least commonly the floor of the mouth and tongue). Symptoms may be severe or minimal. Eosinophilia and anemia are common. Diagnosis is made from biopsy findings, and the treatment is with topical or systemic corticosteroids, dapsone, or sulfasalazine. Other cutaneous complications associated with ulcerative colitis are not specific. Aphthosis and perianal/perifistular ulcerations are not seen in ulcerative colitis.

Erythema nodosum is a common inflammatory process of the subcutaneous fat with a marked predilection for women. Lesions characteristically appear as 1 cm or larger, shiny, tender, deep, red nodules on the anterior shins. The pathogenesis is unknown. The causes of erythema nodosum are infections, especially streptococcal, systemic fungal, and tuberculous; medications (especially oral contraceptives); and leukemias. Erythema nodosum develops in 4% of patients with ulcerative colitis and 7% of patients with Crohn's disease. In addition, GI infections with *Yersinia enterocolitica*, *Shigella flexneri*, and *Campylobacter jejuni* have been associated with erythema nodosum. Treatment of the underlying disease, strict bed rest, and elevation of the legs, as well as the use of anti-inflammatory agents or potassium iodide, are effective.

Pyoderma gangrenosum is a noninfectious ulcerative cutaneous disorder of unknown pathogenesis (Fig. 18–10; see

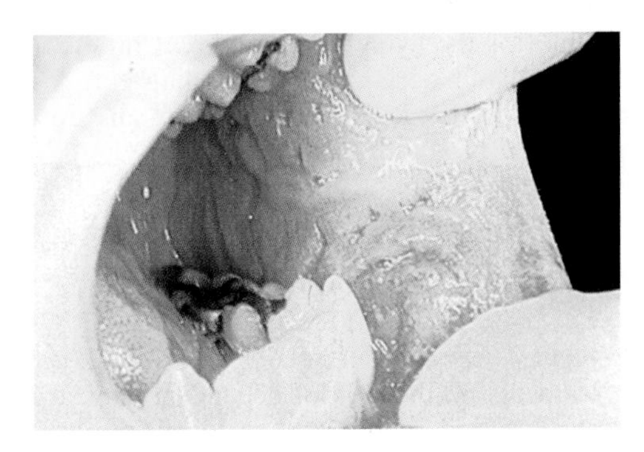

Figure 18–9. Pyostomatitis vegetans in a patient with ulcerative colitis. A biopsy revealed microabscesses.

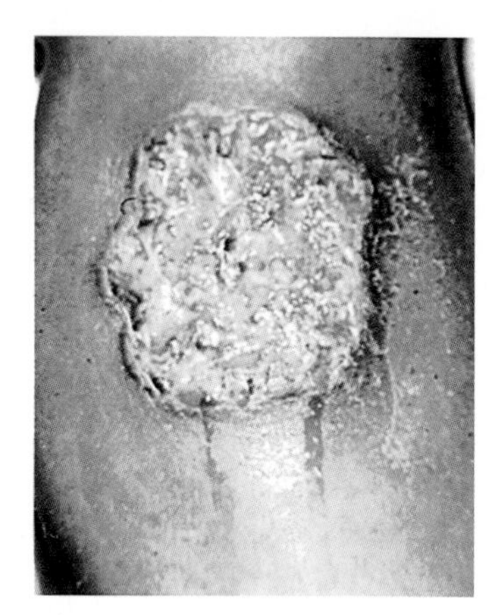

Figure 18–10. Pyoderma gangrenosum associated with ulcerative colitis.

also Color Fig. 18–10). The classic lesion is a tender or painful ulcer with an elevated, dusky purple border that is widely undermined. One or multiple lesions may occur. Lesions begin as small papulopustules that rapidly break down. Pathergy, the appearance of new ulcers at sites of minor trauma or surgery, is often present. The diagnosis is one of exclusion, inasmuch as infectious and other causes of ulceration including factitia must be ruled out. Most cases of pyoderma gangrenosum occur in patients with no underlying disease. Pyoderma gangrenosum develops in approximately 5% of patients with ulcerative colitis and 1% of patients with Crohn's disease.[82] The bowel disease may be subclinical at the time the skin lesions appear, and so bowel evaluation, especially of the distal colon, is essential in cases of pyoderma gangrenosum. If the disorder is associated with underlying bowel disease, therapy of the bowel disease may lead to improvement of the skin lesions. The usual management of pyoderma gangrenosum is systemic corticosteroids and other immunosuppressive agents.[88]

Bowel bypass syndrome is a dermatitis-arthritis syndrome that occurs in up to 50% of patients undergoing this procedure and rarely in patients with other forms of bowel disease. In addition to polyarticular arthritis, characteristic skin lesions develop in 80% of patients.[89] Erythematous macules evolve over several days to form vesiculopustular lesions on a purpuric base. A biopsy shows a perivascular and diffuse infiltrate of neutrophils. The pathogenesis of this disorder seems to be overgrowth of bacteria in a blind loop or pouch of bowel, which leads to the development of antibodies against bacterial peptidoglycans. Immune complexes are formed, sometimes in the form of cryoproteins that appear to be responsible for the symptom complex. Chronic antibiotic therapy, anti-inflammatory agents (including corticosteroids), and correction of the bowel abnormality all are variably beneficial.

VASCULAR AND CONNECTIVE TISSUE DISORDERS (see also Chapter 29)

Immune complex vasculitis of small vessels (leukocytoclastic vasculitis) appears on the skin of dependent sites as crops of *palpable purpura* and is mediated by deposition of immune complexes in postcapillary venules (Fig. 18–11; see also Color Fig. 18–11). Although GI involvement can occur in any case of small vessel vasculitis, it occurs in 50% to 75% of patients with *Henoch-Schönlein purpura* (Fig. 18–12; see also Color Fig. 18–12). Vasculitic hemorrhage, bowel wall edema, and intussusception affects the jejunum and ileum most commonly.[90] Direct immunofluorescence of early skin lesions reveals deposits of IgG in most cases of small vessel vasculitis and deposits of IgA in Henoch-Schönlein purpura.[91–93]

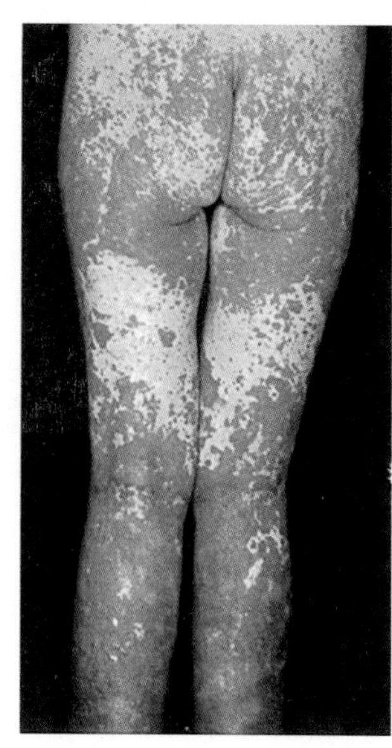

Figure 18–11. Cryoglobulinemic vasculitis caused by a drug eruption. This is also commonly seen in patients with chronic hepatitis C infection, although generally not as severe as shown here.

Polyarteritis nodosa, often associated with hepatitis B, is a vasculitis of the medium and small arteries. Arterial lesions of the abdominal viscera can lead to GI infarcts or perforation. Involvement of the appendix, gallbladder, or pancreas can simulate appendicitis, cholecystitis, or hemorrhagic pancreatitis. Cutaneous involvement occurs in 25% of cases, most typically as the development of nodules, 5 to 10 mm in size, distributed along the course of the superficial arteries. A mottled livedo vascular pattern is also frequently seen.

Malignant atrophic papulosis (Degos' disease, Köhlmeier-Degos syndrome, progressive arterial mesenterial vascular occlusive disease, or disseminated intestinal and cutaneous thromboangiitis) is a rare multisystem vasculopathy

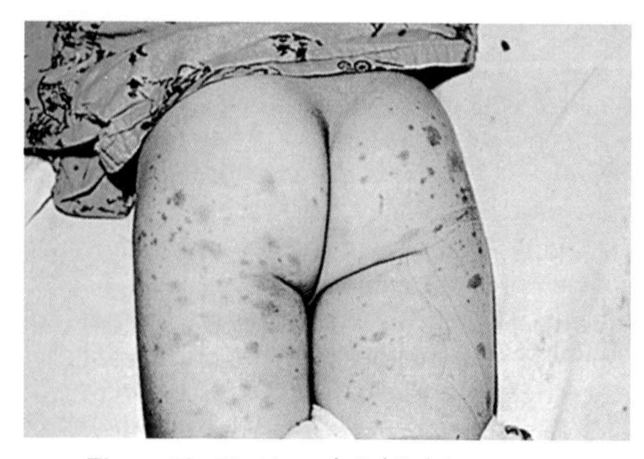

Figure 18–12. Henoch-Schönlein purpura.

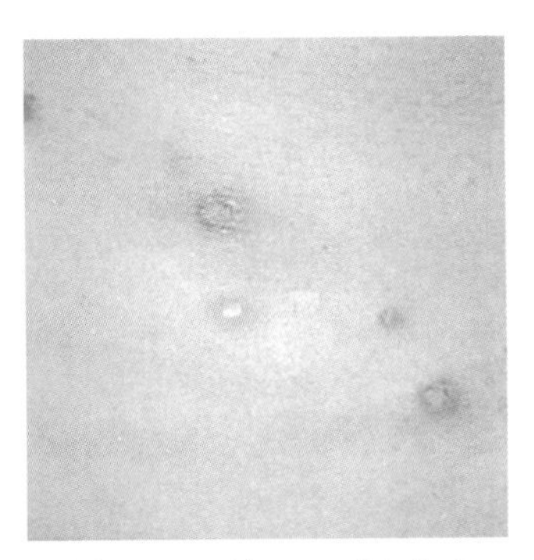

Figure 18–13. Degos' disease, with vasculitic lesions of different stages.

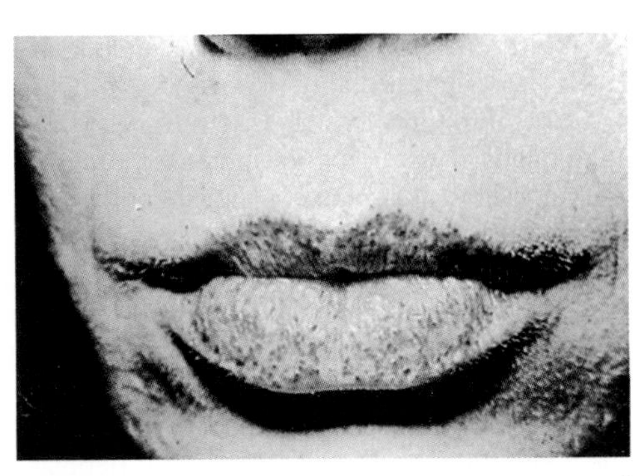

Figure 18–14. Hereditary hemorrhagic telangiectasia (Osler-Weber-Rendu disease).

disorder that is occasionally familial.[94, 95] Cutaneous lesions are the initial manifestations, appearing most commonly in early adulthood.[96] They appear as crops of asymptomatic, pink, 2- to 5-mm papules that rapidly become umbilicated and develop a characteristic atrophic, depressed, porcelain-white center (Fig. 18–13; see also Color Fig. 18–13). These lesions represent cutaneous infarcts. Similar infarcts are seen in the small bowel in virtually all cases. Although GI involvement may initially be asymptomatic or nonspecific, an acute abdominal catastrophe eventually occurs, often necessitating laparoscopy or laparotomy. Perforation of the intestine is usually found, along with multiple white, yellowish, or rose-colored flat or slightly depressed patches below an intact serosa, usually along the small intestine. The intestinal disease is recurrent and eventually it is often fatal. Approximately 20% of patients develop cerebral and peripheral nerve infarcts leading to neurologic complications that can include hemiparesis, aphasia, cranial neuropathies, monoplegia, sensory disturbances, and seizures. Histologic study reveals that the infarctive lesions of the skin, gut, and nervous system are noninflammatory thromboses. The pathogenesis of Degos' disease is unknown, but identical lesions have been reported in systemic lupus erythematosus and in a patient without systemic lupus erythematosus with anticardiolipin antibodies and a lupus anticoagulant.[97–99] Treatment has been attempted with antithrombotic agents such as aspirin, ticlopidine, and dipyridamole, with limited success.[96, 100]

Hereditary hemorrhagic telangiectasia (HHT), or Osler-Weber-Rendu syndrome, is a group of autosomal dominant disorders characterized by vascular lesions including telangiectasias, arteriovenous malformations, and aneurysms of the skin and internal organs (lung, brain, and GI tract).[101] Epistaxis and GI hemorrhage are the most common complications (see Chapter 120). In fact, the incidence of frequent epistaxis ranges from 81 to 96%.[102, 103] The skin lesions are 1- to 3-mm macular telangiectasias of the face, lips, tongue, conjunctiva, fingers, chest, and feet (Fig. 18–14; see also Color Fig. 18–14; see Fig. 120–8). Skin lesions appear later than the epistaxis, usually in the second or third decade. In the fifth to sixth decades, recurrent upper and lower GI hemorrhage may occur. Vascular malformations have been reported in the GI system (46%), the liver (26%), the pulmonary system (14%), the central nervous system (12%), the genitourinary tract (1.9%), and virtually every other organ system in the body.[102] Management of the GI bleeding may be difficult, but the use of bipolar electrocoagulation or laser techniques has been beneficial.[101] Associated von Willebrand factor deficiency may be present, and therapy with desmopressin has been successful in treating massive GI bleeding.[104] There is presently no treatment to prevent the development of telangiectatic lesions in patients with HHT.[105] Chronic therapy with estrogen and progesterone may reduce bleeding from GI telangiectasias.[106] Similar skin and oral lesions to those seen in HHT are found in some patients with the *CREST* (*c*alcinosis, *R*aynaud's phenomenon, *e*sophageal dysfunction, *s*clerodactyly, *t*elangiectasia) variant of scleroderma. The extent of cutaneous sclerosis may be limited in patients with CREST, and so differentiation by physical examination may be difficult. Epistaxis is uncommon in patients with CREST and almost universal in patients with HHT. In addition, patients with CREST have anticentromere antibodies in their serum, which are not found in patients with HHT.[107]

Blue rubber bleb nevus syndrome is a rare disorder of the skin and GI tract composed of a constellation of multiple cutaneous and GI venous malformations.[108–111] Most cases are sporadic, but there are several reports of autosomal dominant transmission. In affected patients, blue, subcutaneous, compressible nodules develop on the skin (Fig. 18–15; see also Color Fig. 18–15). GI vascular malformations are common, especially in the small intestine or colon, and bleeding is an almost universal feature. Acute GI hemorrhage, intussusception, volvulus, bowel infarction, and rectal prolapse have been described. Treatment is primarily surgical or with photocoagulation.

Primary amyloidosis commonly has prominent cutaneous and oral manifestations. Waxy papules around the eyes, nose, and central face as well as purpura involving the face,

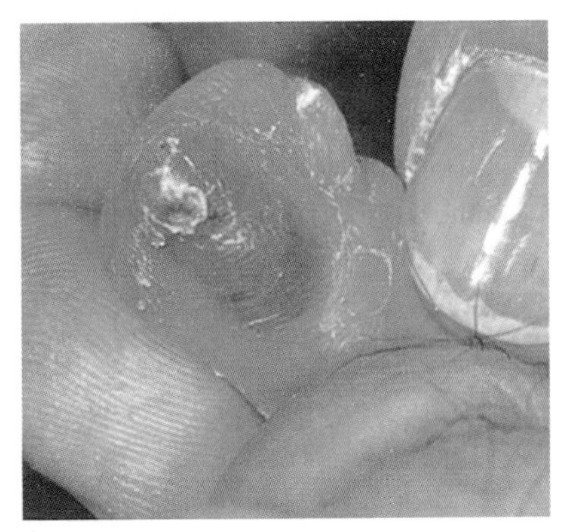

Figure 18–15. Finger tip lesion in blue rubber bleb nevus syndrome.

neck, and upper eyelids are frequently noted. If a waxy papule is pinched, hemorrhage will ensue (pinch purpura). Orbital purpura after proctoscopy, vomiting, or coughing is virtually diagnostic. Macroglossia, increased tongue firmness, enlarged submandibular structures, and indentations from the teeth occur in 20% to 50% of patients.[112] The macroglossia may interfere with eating and closing the mouth and may cause airway obstruction, especially in the reclining position. The tongue may be both enlarged and highly vascular, resulting in bleeding. Recurrent hemorrhagic bullae in the mouth are common.[113] Patients may have carpal tunnel, edema, the "shoulder pad sign" (amyloid deposits in soft tissues around shoulders), GI bleeding, peripheral neuropathies, rheumatoid arthritis–like deposits in small joints, and cardiac involvement.[114] Congestive heart failure or arrhythmias account for death in 40% of patients with systemic amyloid. Diagnosis of primary amyloidosis can be made by subcutaneous fat aspiration or by bone marrow, rectal, skin, or tongue biopsy.[112] *Secondary amyloidosis* has no cutaneous manifestations.

Pseudoxanthoma elasticum is a rare disorder characterized by aberrant calcification of mature elastic tissue. The inheritance pattern is controversial, but autosomal recessive inheritance with variable expressivity and genetic heterogeneity is favored. Skin lesions are usually the initial manifestation, appearing in the second decade as yellow to orange papules ("plucked chicken skin") on the lateral neck (Fig. 18–16; see also Color Fig. 18–16). Skin lesions may progress caudally, involving other flexural areas (axilla, groin, antecubital and popliteal fossae). Calcification of the elastic tissue of arteries leads to the major complications: retinal bleeding, intermittent claudication, premature coronary artery disease, and GI bleeding. Between 8% and 13% of patients experience GI bleeding. GI bleeding is usually from the stomach, and often no specific bleeding point is found. As opposed to the other complications of pseudoxanthoma elasticum just noted, GI bleeding tends to occur in younger patients (average age, 26 years), often occurs during pregnancy, and may be recurrent. Skin lesions may not be visible at the time of bleeding. Because apparently normal flexural or scar skin may yield diagnostic findings, a blind skin biopsy may be indicated in a young person with GI bleeding with no other explanation. Lesions identical to those seen on the skin may also be present on the lower lip and the rectal mucosa.

Two forms of *neurofibromatosis* (NF) occur: NF-I (von Recklinghausen's disease) and NF-II (bilateral acoustic neurofibromatosis). The genetic defect for NF-I has been localized to chromosome 17. The cutaneous manifestations of NF-I include six or more café au lait spots (diameter >5 mm in prepubertal persons and >15 mm in postpubertal persons); multiple soft papules (neurofibromas) (Fig. 18–17; see also Color Fig. 18–17), or a single plexiform neurofibroma; and freckling of the axillae or inguinal areas. GI involvement occurs in 10% to 15% of patients with NF-I. Intestinal neurofibromas may arise at any level of the GI tract, although small intestinal involvement is most common.[115] These tumors are generally submucosal but may extend to the serosa. Dense growths known as plexiform neurofibromatosis of the mesentery or retroperitoneal space may lead to arterial compression or nerve injury.[116] Malignant tumors may occur in neurofibromatosis. There is an increased incidence of pheochromocytoma, either with or without the multiple endocrine neoplasia type 2B syndrome.[117] Duodenal and ampullary carcinoid tumors (producing obstructive jaundice), malignant schwannomas, sarcomas, and pancreatic adenocarcinomas are seen with increased frequency. The common clinical manifestations are abdominal pain, constipation, anemia, melena, and an abdominal mass. Serious complications that have been reported include intestinal or biliary obstruction, ischemic bowel, perforation, and intussusception. Involvement of the myenteric plexus has resulted in megacolon (see Chapter 110).

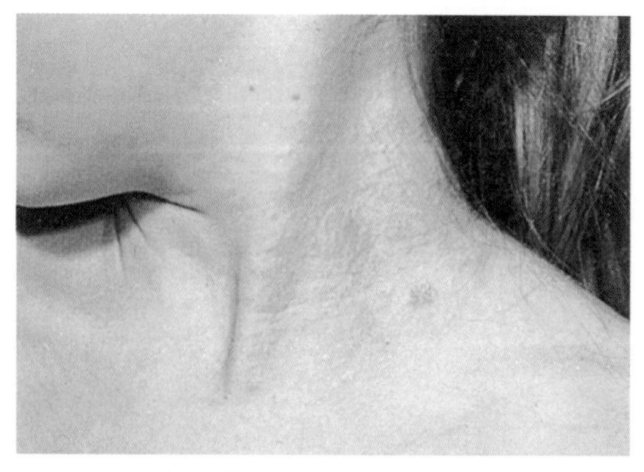

Figure 18–16. Pseudoxanthoma elasticum. (Courtesy of Victor Newcomer, MD.)

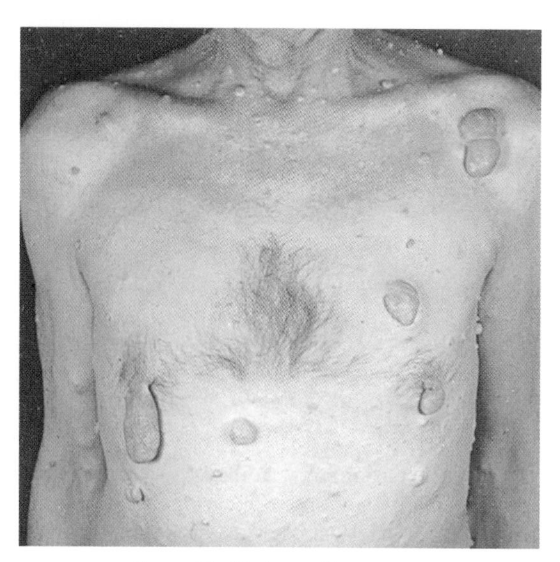

Figure 18–17. Neurofibromatosis.

Mastocytosis is characterized by mast cell infiltration of the bone marrow, skin, liver, spleen, lymph nodes, and GI tract. It occurs in both adult and pediatric patients (see Chapter 29). In children, the most common lesions consist of a large red to brown plaque (solitary mastocytoma), multiple red to brown papules or plaques (urticaria pigmentosa), or diffuse cutaneous involvement with or without flushing or blistering.[118] In adult patients most have urticaria pigmentosa type lesions (Fig. 18–18; see also Color Fig. 18–18), sometimes with prominent telangiectasia.[119] Lesions often are on the trunk. The most common GI complaint is dyspepsia and peptic ulcer disease resulting from histamine-induced gastric hypersecretion. Diarrhea and abdominal pain are also a com-

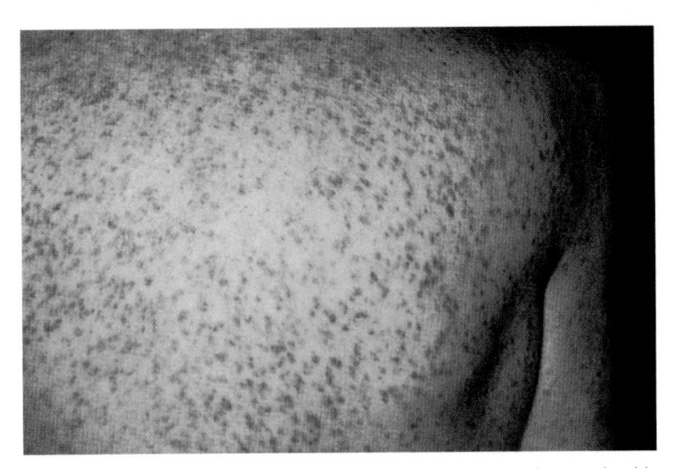

Figure 18–18. Urticaria pigmentosa in an adult. Reddish-brown freckle-like lesions are characteristic of the adult form of this disease.

mon problem and can be accompanied by malabsorption syndromes. In children, the lesions usually involute spontaneously, and systemic disease is uncommon. In adults, cutaneous lesions may resolve as well, but without improvement in systemic symptoms. In the rare pediatric case with a solitary mastocytoma and significant systemic symptoms, excision of the skin lesion may resolve the systemic complications. Extracutaneous involvement should be considered in adult patients with cutaneous mastocytosis because management of symptoms can easily be achieved.[120]

Porphyria cutanea tarda has a well-documented association with hepatitis C and is described in more detail later on. However, in nearly all of the porphyrin disorders, manifestations include some cutaneous and gastrointestinal symptoms. Skin vesicles, erosions, and bullae with hemolytic anemia and splenomegaly characterize erythropoietic porphyria. *Erythropoietic protoporphyria* patients demonstrate edematous plaques, erythema, and purpura, often with cholelithiasis and occasionally with terminal hepatic failure. *Acute intermittent porphyria* has no cutaneous manifestations but is marked by acute attacks related to the neurovisceral complex, including abdominal pain, constipation, nausea, and vomiting. *Variegate porphyria* patients have the cutaneous features of porphyria cutanea tarda and the visceral manifestations of acute intermittent porphyria. *Hereditary coproporphyria* is characterized by cutaneous blisters and similar but milder neurovisceral symptoms of acute intermittent porphyria. *Hepatoerythropoietic porphyria* is marked by occasional splenomegaly and anemia with subepidermal vesicles and blisters that often progress to scleroderma-like scarring and hyperpigmentation.

Connective tissue diseases such as systemic lupus erythematosus (SLE), dermatomyositis (DM), and progressive systemic scleroderma (PSS) all have characteristic skin and GI manifestations. SLE patients prototypically have malar erythema with photosensitivity and often erythematous raised patches with follicular plugging (discoid lupus). SLE patients can have oral ulcers, anorexia, nausea, vomiting, peritonitis with ascites, active hepatitis with hepatomegaly, and pancreatitis. DM is described in greater detail later on, but patients with DM can have proximal dysphagia and large bowel infarction from vasculopathy (especially in juvenile DM). Patients with PSS often demonstrate generalized sclerotic skin or, less commonly, morphea (sclerotic plaques with ivory-colored centers), matted telangiectasia, and Raynaud's phenomenon. Esophageal dysfunction is the most common internal symptom, although the small intestine may also be affected, producing constipation, diarrhea, and bloating.

CUTANEOUS DISORDERS ASSOCIATED WITH GASTROINTESTINAL MALIGNANCIES

Cutaneous manifestations may be of importance in recognizing individuals with cancer or from kindred with a high risk for the development of cancer. These cutaneous markers are discussed in three sections: syndromes with GI polyposis and skin findings, cutaneous markers of internal malignancy, and cutaneous manifestations of metastatic GI carcinoma.

Cancer/Polyposis Syndromes

(see also Chapter 114)

Gardner's syndrome, or familial adenomatous polyposis, is inherited as an autosomal dominant trait. The adenomatous polyposis coli (*APC*) gene on chromosome 5q21 is mutated in the germline of these patients. Adenomatous colonic polyps are the hallmark and polyps of the duodenum, especially around the ampulla of Vater, are common among affected individuals. Presentation is usually in the second or third decade, and carcinoma occurs in virtually all patients if untreated. Cutaneous features of this syndrome occur in more than 50% of the affected individuals and often appear before the polyps become symptomatic. Multiple epidermoid cysts (also called *inclusion cysts*) of the face, scalp, and extremities appear before puberty. This is in contrast with common epidermoid cysts, which usually appear on the back and occur after puberty. True sebaceous cysts (steatocystomas) are not associated with Gardner's syndrome. The oral manifestations of Gardner's syndrome include the presence of 1- to 10-mm osteomas and multiple unerupted, supernumerary teeth.

Muir-Torre syndrome is an autosomal dominant syndrome with cutaneous sebaceous neoplasms and multiple primary cancers, especially of the proximal colon.[121, 122] It is probably a part of the cancer family syndrome (CFS), or Lynch II syndrome. Review of some of the cases in the CFS kindred revealed a high prevalence of sebaceous neoplasms.[121, 122] The most prominent cutaneous manifestation is one or more sebaceous neoplasms of various degrees of differentiation from benign adenoma to aggressive sebaceous carcinoma. Because cutaneous sebaceous neoplasms are quite rare, even the presence of one lesion should prompt evaluation for this syndrome. In addition, keratoacanthomas and basal and squamous cell carcinomas of the skin develop in these patients. Multiple primary malignancies are characteristic: 40 patients in one series had a total of 106 tumors and 1 patient had 9 different primary carcinomas. The most common location for carcinomas is the GI tract (93%), especially the proximal colon. Multiple and single polyps of the intestine have been described in 38% of patients, but Lynch and colleagues believed that multiple adenomatous polyps are absent in this syndrome.[122] Urogenital carcinomas, especially

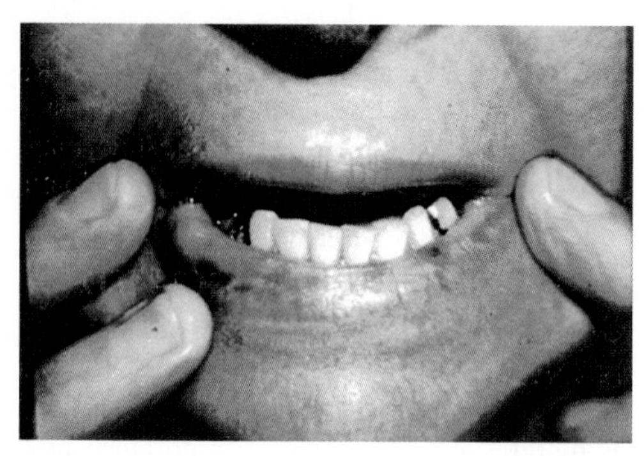

Figure 18–19. Mucocutaneous pigmentation of Peutz-Jeghers syndrome.

of the endometrium, bladder, and kidney, occur in 50% of patients. Despite the large number of primary carcinomas, patients appear to have prolonged survival.

Peutz-Jeghers syndrome is an autosomal dominant syndrome of GI hamartomas and mucocutaneous hyperpigmentation (Fig. 18–19; see also Color Fig. 18–19). The macules appear during infancy and early childhood. Mucosal lesions persist, whereas the cutaneous lesions fade over time. The hyperpigmented lesions consist of dark brown 1-mm to 1-cm macules on the lips (95%), buccal mucosa (83%), acral areas (palms, soles, digits), and around the eyes, anus, and mouth. The most common associated malignancy is duodenal carcinoma; and granulosa theca cell tumors of the ovary may be present in up to 20% of female patients. The patient with Peutz-Jeghers syndrome may carry an overall cancer relative risk of up to 18.[114a]

Cowden's syndrome, or multiple hamartoma syndrome, is an uncommon autosomal dominant syndrome with multiple mucocutaneous manifestations and an increased risk of malignancy.[123] The diagnostic skin lesions are multiple facial verrucous lesions that histologically are trichilemmomas. Oral papillomatosis is quite common. Fibrocystic disease of the breast (60% of women patients), breast carcinoma (29% of women patients), and thyroid disease (goiter, adenoma, cancer) are important components of the syndrome. GI lesions occur in at least 40% of patients and consist primarily of multiple polyps, which occur anywhere along the GI tract, most commonly the colon. These polyps are usually small and predominantly hamartomatous. Of the two patients with Cowden's syndrome who had colonic carcinomas, neither had polyps.

Cronkhite-Canada syndrome is a rare, sporadic syndrome of generalized GI polyposis, mucocutaneous hyperpigmentation, alopecia, malabsorption with malnutrition, and nail dystrophy.[124] The mean age at onset is 59 years. Diarrhea, weight loss (usually >10 kg), and abdominal pain are the most common symptoms. Nail changes (90% of patients) affect all 20 nails and consist of thinning and splitting of nails, onycholysis (separation of the nail from the nail bed), or total shedding of the nails. Alopecia (>95% of patients) is usually sudden and involves not only the scalp but also the body hair. Hyperpigmentation occurs in about 85% of patients and has been described as lentigines that may coalesce, most commonly on the upper extremities, lower extremities, palms, and soles. The cutaneous changes all resolve with treatment but may resolve spontaneously even with continued GI disease. Death occurs in about half of the patients as a result of persistent diarrhea or from malnutrition. Aggressive nutritional support in the form of total parenteral nutrition has led to complete resolution of the syndrome, suggesting that at least some of the manifestations are a complication of the metabolic abnormalities caused by the severe diarrhea.[125, 126]

Cutaneous Markers of Internal Malignancy

Dermatomyositis is manifested by a violaceous color of the eyelids, often with edema (heliotrope); keratotic papules over the knuckles (Gottron's papules) (Fig. 18–20; see also Color Fig. 18–20); a widespread erythema, often with accentuation over the elbows and knees, resembling psoriasis; photosensitivity; and nail cuticle abnormalities, including telangiectasias, thickening, roughness, overgrowth, and irregularity. About 25% of patients with dermatomyositis have internal malignancy, particularly in patients older than 50 years of age.[127–130] The type of cancer most commonly associated with dermatomyositis is gastric carcinoma. However, in Chinese, nasopharyngeal carcinoma seems to be the most common associated malignancy.[131] There does not appear to be a predilection for either sex. To detect an associated cancer, a complete medical history; physical examination, including rectal, pelvic, and breast examinations; a CBC; routine serum chemistry analysis; serum protein electrophoresis; multi-

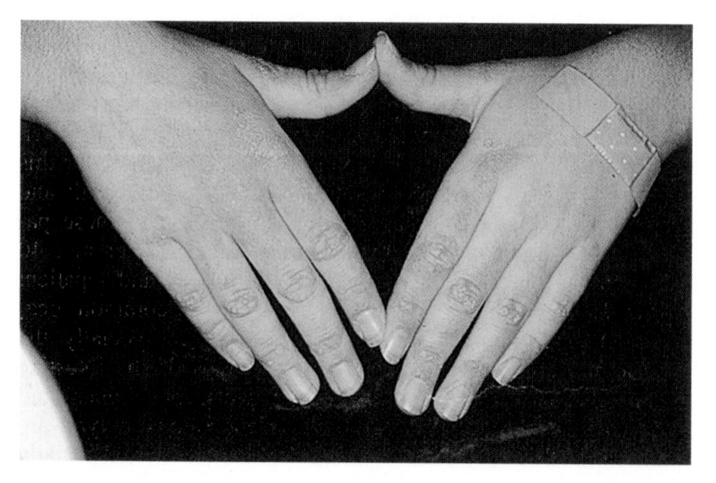

Figure 18–20. Dermatomyositis with erythematous plaques with concentration over the knuckles (Gottron's papules). (Photograph courtesy of Dr. Timothy Berger.)

ple fecal occult blood tests; a urinalysis; a chest roentgenogram; and a mammogram (in women) are recommended. Any abnormalities should be investigated further.[131, 132] Extensive blind evaluation of patients with dermatomyositis is not warranted.

Keratosis palmaris et plantaris (Howel-Evans syndrome) is an adult-onset diffuse hyperkeratosis of the palms and soles (also called *tylosis*) that has been described in association with a very high incidence of esophageal carcinoma in several kindred in Liverpool, England. The skin lesions appear during adolescence or early adulthood, and the carcinomas appear on the average at 45 years of age. Esophageal carcinoma develops in virtually all patients in these kindred with tylosis.

Tripe palms (also called acanthosis nigricans of the palms, acanthosis palmaris, pachydermatoglyphy, palmar hyperkeratosis, and palmar keratoderma) are a paraneoplastic phenomenon characterized by a mosslike or velvety texture with pronounced dermatoglyphics or by a cobbled or honeycombed surface of the palms and fingers. Of reported cases of tripe palms, 91% have occurred in association with neoplasm. Pulmonary and gastric carcinomas were the most common neoplasms, each accounting for more than 25% of all the malignancies.

Acanthosis nigricans is a cutaneous finding that presents with a velvety hyperplasia and hyperpigmentation of the skin of the neck and axillae (Fig. 18–21; see also Color Fig. 18–21), often associated with multiple skin tags. Some patients with acanthosis nigricans have internal malignancy (so-called malignant acanthosis nigricans). In these patients, the extent of involvement may be severe, including the hands, genitalia, and oral mucosa. The associated carcinoma is usually present simultaneously with the acanthosis nigricans but may not be clinically manifest. Abdominal adenocarcinomas constitute more than 85% of the associated malignancies; gastric carcinomas represent more than 60%. Survival is short, and more than 50% of patients die in less than 1 year.[133]

Bazex's syndrome (acrokeratosis paraneoplastica) is a rare but distinctive syndrome associated with either a primary malignant neoplasm of the upper aerodigestive tract or metastatic carcinoma to the lymph nodes of the neck. All of the more than 50 patients reported to date have had malignancy, including esophageal carcinoma and one gastric carcinoma with cervical metastases. The skin eruption begins acrally, as thickening of the periungual skin and marked nail dystrophy. The rash progresses proximally and also involves the tip of the nose and ears. Thickening of the palms and soles ensues initially with central sparing. This can make walking very painful. Eventually the face and scalp become involved. Treatment of the underlying carcinoma is usually associated with improvement or resolution of the skin lesions.

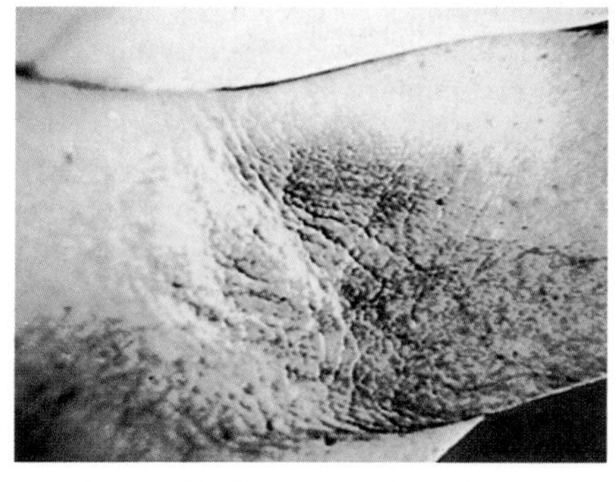

Figure 18–21. Acanthosis nigricans.

Hypertrichosis lanuginosa, another rare paraneoplastic syndrome consisting of fine, thin, downlike, unpigmented lanugo-type hair, is typically noted on the face, forehead, ears, nose, axillae, limbs, and trunk. Other manifestations include glossodynia, papillary hypertrophy of the tongue, disturbances of taste and smell, diarrhea, scleroderma, acanthosis nigricans, seborrheic keratoses, adenopathy, and weight loss. Colorectal carcinomas are second only to lung carcinoma in frequency of associated malignancies.[134]

Carcinoid tumors produce a number of vasoactive substances that can induce cutaneous flushing (see Chapter 112). However, the most common carcinoid tumors (appendix and small bowel) do not produce flushing until the vasoactive substances reach the systemic circulation. Flushing therefore generally denotes metastasis to the liver or a different primary tumor site (e.g., lung or ovary).

Glucagonoma of the pancreas often precipitates necrolytic migratory erythema of the skin.[135] The rash is common around orifices, flexural regions and the fingers. Lesions are typically papulovesicular with secondary erosions, crusting, and fissures appearing in a geographic circinate pattern. Patients can also often have weight loss, diarrhea, anemia, psychiatric disturbances, hypoaminoacidemia, and diabetes. The rash typically clears with successful removal of the tumor, which is discussed in more detail in Chapter 51.

Venous thrombosis may be associated with carcinomas of the GI tract, particularly superficial and deep venous thrombosis, and these vascular complications may be the initial manifestations of the malignancy. Up to 50% of patients with pancreatic carcinoma may suffer thromboses.[136, 137] In one series, 11 (10%) of 113 patients with a deep venous thrombosis were found to have a visceral malignancy, asymptomatic in half the cases.[138] These cancers were often intra-abdominal, leading the authors to recommend the following evaluation for patients with idiopathic deep venous thrombosis: CBC, measurements of lactate dehydrogenase and carcinoembryonic antigen, chest roentgenogram, and abdominal ultrasonography or computed tomography. Whether this approach is cost effective is unknown.

Subcutaneous fat necrosis and *polyarthralgia* could be markers for pancreatic acinar cell carcinoma. Most affected persons are men.[139] Deep, subcutaneous, erythematous nodules ranging from one to several centimeters in diameter usually appear on the legs. In uncommon instances, the nodules may break down, exuding a creamy material. Arthritis of one or several joints, especially the ankles and knees, may accompany the nodules or occur without skin lesions.[140] Abdominal pain may be absent when the skin lesions or arthritis occur. In addition to the expected elevations of amylase and lipase, eosinophilia is common. Histopathologic evaluation of skin lesions usually reveals diagnostic findings: pale staining necrotic fat cells (ghost cells) and deposits of calcium in the necrotic fat. The pathogenesis of these lesions is thought to be related to release of pancreatic enzymes into the circulation from the diseased pancreas. Lipase, phospholipase A, and trypsin levels have been found to be elevated in both the joint and skin lesions. These enzymes may lead to necrosis of fat cells and release of free fatty acids. Free fatty acids and other products of dead cells are proinflammatory and may explain perpetuation of the joint lesions once pancreatic disease is inactive. The mortality rate in cases not associated with carcinoma approaches 50%. Subcutaneous swellings, which commonly break down and drain, may also be seen in patients with *α_1-antitrypsin deficiency*. These nodules usually occur on the buttocks or proximal extremities and are often precipitated by trauma. In pancreatitis, subcutaneous nodules usually present on the anterior shins. Histologic evaluation of involved fat can differentiate pancreatitis from carcinoma. In contrast with carcinoma, pancreatic fat necrosis appears as a homogeneous, basophilic material resulting from saponification of fat by calcium salts. A bluish discoloration of the skin (ecchymosis) around the umbilicus, sometimes associated with hemorrhagic pancreatitis, is called *Cullen's sign;* when a similar process occurs in the flank, it is termed *Turner's sign*.

Some cutaneous "markers" historically thought to be associated with internal malignancies have more recently been dismissed. These include *Bowen's disease* (cutaneous squamous cell carcinoma in situ),[141, 142] *skin tags*,[143] and the *sign of Leser-Trélat* (sudden appearance of multiple seborrheic keratoses).[144–146] *Sweet's syndrome* (acute febrile neutrophilic dermatoses) might be associated with lymphoproliferative neoplasm instead of GI malignancy, if such an association truly exists.

Gastrointestinal Neoplasms Metastatic to Skin

Cutaneous metastases occur rarely with GI adenocarcinomas. They may appear anywhere on the skin and are often nonspecific, very firm, dermal or subcutaneous nodules. When metastasis to the umbilicus occurs, however, intra-abdominal GI carcinoma is found in more than half the cases and gastric carcinoma in 20%. This lesion is called *Sister Mary Joseph's nodule*.[147] Specific immunoperoxidase markers have enabled pathologists to predict the primary site of origin from biopsy specimens of metastatic nodules.

CUTANEOUS MANIFESTATIONS OF LIVER DISEASE

Besides jaundice, patients with liver disease may show vascular spiders, corkscrew scleral vessels, palmar erythema, telangiectasia, striae, and caput medusa. Patients with *hemochromatosis* often develop a generalized bronze-brown color with accentuation over sun-exposed sites. Primary biliary cirrhosis may be associated with *xanthomas* that may involve the trunk, face, and extremities. Striking plane xanthomas may develop on the palmar creases (see Chapter 76). Patients with *sarcoidosis* involving the liver or, less commonly, the GI tract may have sarcoid skin lesions (Fig. 18–22; see also Color Fig. 18–22).

Pruritus is a distressing complication of cholestatic, inflammatory, and malignant liver diseases. The itching of liver disease is not relieved by scratching, topical steroids, or ultraviolet light (which relieve other pruritic conditions, including those of renal origin) and is therefore quite difficult to manage. Amelioration of pruritus with cholestyramine or rifampin does not help in elucidating the pathogenesis of this distressing condition. Opiate antagonists, such as naloxone or oral nalmefene, may relieve pruritus, and this suggests that endogenous opioids are involved in the pathogenesis of the pruritus. The pruritus associated with metastatic disease to the liver has been successfully treated with intravenous and oral ondansetron, a serotonin receptor antagonist.[148]

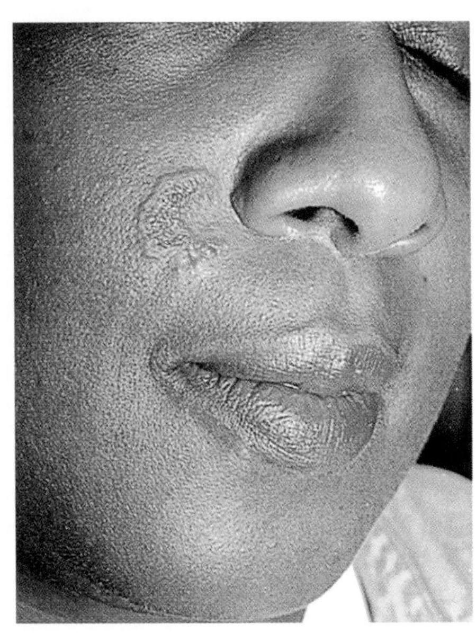

Figure 18–22. Sarcoidosis: Annular plaque of the face. (Photograph courtesy of Dr. Timothy Berger.)

Dermatologists frequently consult gastroenterologists for evaluation of patients who are being treated with *methotrexate* or *retinoids*, because these medications can cause both acute and chronic liver disease (see Chapter 73). Methotrexate is the more commonly used of these medications. It is extremely effective for severe psoriasis and psoriatic arthritis and is also used for cutaneous T-cell lymphoma, connective tissue diseases, and other dermatologic disorders. Methotrexate is usually given as a single weekly dose of 10 to 25 mg but may be used in higher dosages in selected patients. A grading system for liver biopsies has been established and is generally followed by dermatologists (Table 18–2). Current American Academy of Dermatology guidelines recommend pretreatment liver biopsies and repeated biopsies during therapy, depending on the results of regular liver function tests and other risk factors for hepatic disease (obesity with diabetes, results of prior liver biopsies, and alcohol consumption). Decisions on continuation of treatment are frequently based on the results of these biopsies.[149] An American College of Gastroenterology committee has made similar recommendations. Recommendations are summarized in Table 18–3.

Retinoids (e.g., Accutane, Acitretin), derivatives of vitamin A, are currently used for the treatment of certain forms of severe psoriasis, cystic acne, and other disorders of keratinization. Regular evaluation of liver function tests is required during this treatment. Mild elevations of alanine aminotransferase and aspartate aminotransferase levels are common (20% to 30% of patients treated),[150, 151] usually transient, or easily managed by reducing the dose. Persistent elevations may require evaluation by a gastroenterologist. Severe or even fatal hepatitis has been reported. Retinoids

Table 18–2 | **A Grading System for Liver Biopsies in Patients Taking Methotrexate**

GRADE	CRITERIA
I	Normal; fatty infiltration, mild; nuclear variability, mild; portal inflammation, mild
II	Fatty infiltration, moderate to severe; nuclear variability, moderate to severe; portal tract expansion, portal tract inflammation, and necrosis, moderate to severe
IIIA	Fibrosis, mild (portal fibrosis here denotes formation of fibrotic septa extending into the lobules; slight enlargement of portal tracts without disruption of limiting plates or septum formation does not classify the biopsy specimen as grade III)
IIIB	Fibrosis, moderate to severe
IV	Cirrhosis (regenerating nodules as well as bridging of portal tracts must be demonstrated)

From Roenigk HH Jr, Auerbach R, Maibach H, et al: Methotrexate in psoriasis: Consensus conference. J Am Acad Dermatol 38:478–485, 1998.

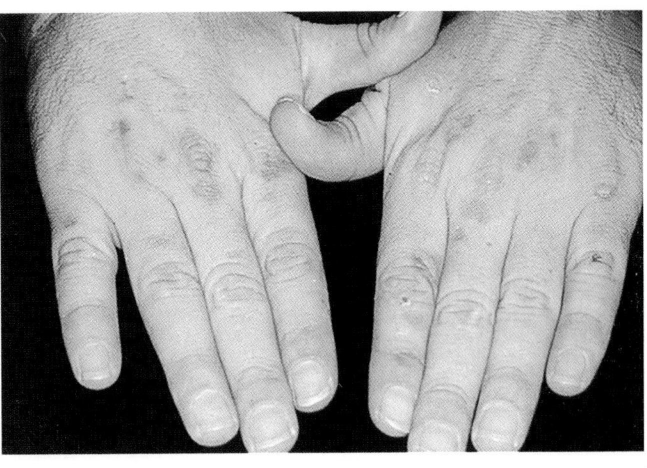

Figure 18–23. Porphyria cutanea tarda: Noninflammatory blisters and erosions of the dorsa of the hands. Patients are frequently infected with hepatitis C virus. (Photograph courtesy of Dr. Timothy Berger.)

may be used in patients with psoriasis who were previously treated with methotrexate or who have liver disease contraindicating use of methotrexate. Limited experience suggests that these patients do not suffer progression of the liver disease with such retinoid therapy. As with methotrexate, during retinoid therapy there is a poor correlation between liver function test and liver histology results. Therefore, pretreatment and intermittent liver biopsies may be requested for certain high-risk patients being treated with oral retinoids chronically.

Vitamin K is frequently administered to patients with liver disease and hypoprothrombinemia. Cutaneous reactions, although rare, may occur after subcutaneous, intramuscular, or intravenous administration. Large, erythematous, indurated, pruritic plaques occur within a few days to a few weeks.[152] These reactions may be a delayed hypersensitivity reaction, inasmuch as dermal testing can reproduce the reactions. When tested, patients have been found to be allergic to the vitamin K and not the benzoyl alcohol vehicle. Vitamin K_3 (Synkayvite), which is water soluble, has not been reported to cause similar reactions. If reactions occur after buttock injections of vitamin K, there is an almost diagnostic tendency of these plaques to spread around the waist and down the thigh, reproducing a "cowboy gun belt and holster" pattern. These reaction sites resolve over days to weeks but may persist for months to years. Either after an erythematous reaction or without prior reaction, expanding sclerotic plaques with violaceous borders similar to those of morphea have occurred months to years after injections.[153] The latter pattern usually occurs after large parenteral doses of vitamin K. In addition to these local reactions, anaphylaxis after intravenous administration has been reported.[154]

Table 18–3 | **Decisions on Continuation of Methotrexate Therapy Based on Results of Liver Biopsies**

Patients with grade I or II changes may continue to receive methotrexate therapy.
Patients with grade IIIA change(s) may continue to receive methotrexate therapy but should have a repeat liver biopsy after approximately 6 months of methotrexate therapy. Alternative therapy should be considered.
Patients with grade IIIB and IV changes should not given further methotrexate therapy. Exceptional circumstances, however, may require continued methotrexate therapy, with thorough follow-up liver biopsies.

From Roenigk HH Jr, Auerbach R, Maibach H, et al: Methotrexate in psoriasis: Consensus conference. J Am Acad Dermatol 38:478–485, 1998.

Cutaneous Complications of Viral Hepatitis (see also Chapter 68)

The association between *polyarteritis nodosa* and hepatitis B is well documented. *Urticaria* and serum sickness occur more commonly in patients with hepatitis B, although both have been reported in association with hepatitis C.[155]

Chronic hepatitis C virus is associated with a variety of cutaneous disorders. The existence of the triad of *leukocytoclastic vasculitis*, cryoglobulinemia, and chronic hepatitis C virus is well supported by multiple studies. Petechiae and palpable purpura are noted on the skin.[156]

Porphyria cutanea tarda (PCT) is a metabolic disorder characterized by skin fragility, blisters, hypertrichosis, and hyperpigmentation in sun-exposed skin (Fig. 18–23; see also Color Fig. 18–23). PCT is the most common form of porphyria and is characterized by a deficiency of uroporphyrinogen decarboxylase. Diagnosis is typically made with a 24-hour urine demonstrating elevated porphyrins, specifically uroporphyrin. Alcohol consumption, estrogens, iron, and sunlight all are known to exacerbate PCT. There is a clear and substantial link between PCT and hepatitis C.[157] The prevalence of hepatitis C in patients with PCT demonstrates regional variation, ranging from 65% in southern Europe and North America to 20% in northern Europe and Australia.[157] Treatment involves phlebotomy and antimalarials.

Lichen planus is a common, idiopathic, inflammatory disorder that can affect skin, hair, mucous membranes, and nails (see earlier). The prototypical presentation of lichen planus is violaceous, polygonal, flat-topped papules of flexural areas of the wrists, arms, and legs. The papules often have an overlying reticulated white scale known as Wickham striae. The association between lichen planus and hepatitis C is clear[158] but not as prominent as the link between PCT and HCV.

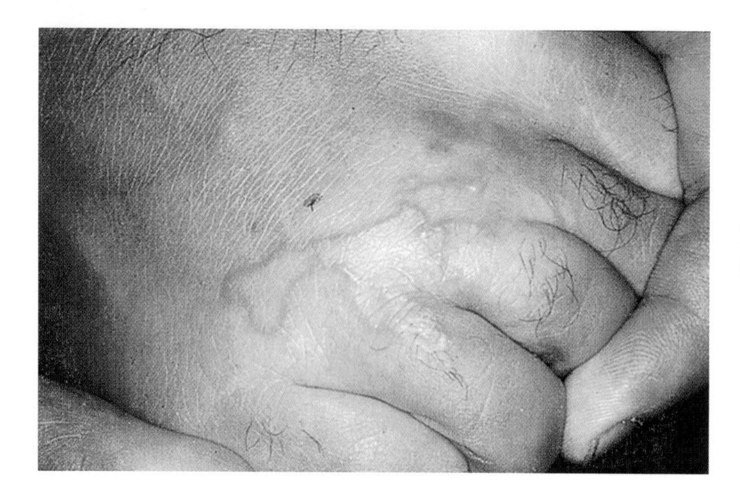

Figure 18–24. Cutaneous larva migrans: Serpiginous erythematous migratory lesion due to dog hook worms. (Photograph courtesy of Dr. Timothy Berger.)

PARASITIC DISEASES OF THE GUT AND SKIN (see also Chapter 99)

The larval forms of human and animal nematodes may cause migratory erythematous skin lesions, called *creeping eruptions*. The most common pattern is *cutaneous larva migrans*, caused by the dog and cat hookworms (Fig. 18–24; see also Color Fig. 18–24). Pruritic linear papules migrate at a rate of 1 to 2 cm daily on skin sites—usually the feet, buttocks, or back—that have come in contact with fecally contaminated soil. Lesions resolve spontaneously over weeks to months. Larva currens is caused by *Strongyloides stercoralis* larva migrating in the skin.[159] It occurs in two forms: a form localized to the perirectal skin in immunocompetent hosts and a disseminated form occurring in immunosuppressed hosts. *S. stercoralis* has the unique capacity among nematodes to develop into infective larvae within the intestine. These infective larvae may invade the perirectal skin in infected immunocompetent individuals, causing urticarial, erythematous, linear lesions that migrate up to 10 cm a day, usually within 30 cm of the anus. Skin lesions may occur very intermittently, making diagnosis difficult. In immunosuppressed hosts, repeated autoinfection through the intestine leads to a tremendous parasite burden (hyperinfection), manifested most commonly by pulmonary disease. In association, disseminated larva currens–type lesions may appear over the whole body, especially the trunk. Petechial or purpuric serpiginous lesions may also occur periumbilically.[160]

Parasitic infections are classically considered in the differential diagnosis of urticaria. Except for fascioliasis and hydatid disease, however, a direct relationship has rarely been proved. If blood eosinophilia and GI symptoms are absent, stool examination for parasites is rarely beneficial.

DERMATITIS HERPETIFORMIS AND CELIAC SPRUE

Dermatitis herpetiformis (DH) is an extremely pruritic skin disorder most commonly appearing during early adulthood. The cutaneous eruption consists of urticarial, vesicular, or bullous lesions characteristically localized to the scalp, shoulders, elbows, knees, and buttocks.[161] The disorder is so pruritic that often all the skin lesions have been excoriated, and the diagnosis must be suspected on the basis of this and the distribution (Fig. 18–25; see also Color Fig. 18–25). The diagnosis of DH is established by skin biopsy and direct immunofluorescence examination of the skin. Deposits of IgA are found in the dermal papillae at sites of itching and where vesicles are forming.[162] Patients with DH commonly have an enteropathy indistinguishable from celiac sprue (see Chapter 93). Their human leukocyte antigen (HLA) patterns (including haplotypes B8, DR3, and DQw2), abnormalities of intestinal absorption, antiendomysial and antigliadin antibodies, and bowel biopsy findings are similar to those of patients with celiac disease,[163] and yet fewer than 5% of patients with DH have symptomatic GI disease. Gluten has been shown to be the dietary trigger of DH. Patients, even those with such minimal bowel disease that the bowel biopsy finding is normal, improve on a gluten-free diet. Introduction of gluten to the diet in a symptom-free patient on a gluten-free diet leads to reappearance of pruritus and skin lesions.[164] The IgA antibodies deposited in the skin and causing the eruption have not been proved to originate in the gut. They do not seem to be directed against gluten. The pathogenesis remains unknown.

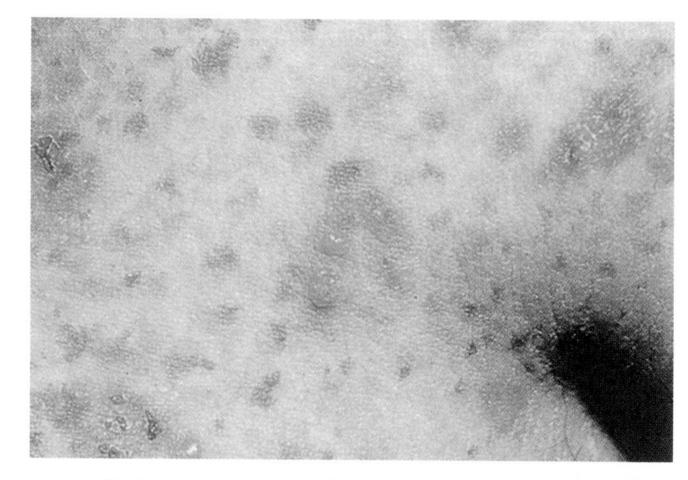

Figure 18–25. Dermatitis herpetiformis: Pruritic, urticarial papules and small blisters concentrated over the shoulders, scalp, and lumbosacral area. (Photograph courtesy of Dr. Timothy Berger.)

Because it is occasionally difficult to distinguish DH from other blistering skin diseases, a patient with an extremely pruritic eruption may be referred for endoscopy. The finding of an abnormal small intestine that is consistent with celiac sprue in a patient with a pruritic eruption would be highly suggestive of DH. The skin lesions of DH respond dramatically to sulfa drugs (dapsone or sulfapyridine), but the gut pathology and skin immunofluorescence are unchanged by sulfa drugs. Treatment with a gluten-free diet leads to gradual clearing of skin lesions, improvement of the intestinal abnormality, disappearance of the IgA from the skin, and decreased dependence on dapsone for control of the cutaneous eruption.[165]

VITAMIN DEFICIENCIES

(see also Chapter 15)

Pellagra, a deficiency of niacin, may be related to inadequate diet, medication (isoniazid), or the carcinoid syndrome.[166] The lesions appear symmetrically in sun-exposed areas as brown-red, blistering, or scaling plaques, which may become indurated. Glossodynia, atrophic glossitis, and, sometimes, ulcerative gingivostomatitis may be present. In addition to dermatitis (with or without oral lesions), diarrhea and dementia may occur (the three "Ds").

Deficiencies of zinc (acrodermatitis enteropathica), essential fatty acids, and biotin all produce a superficial scaling and an occasionally blistering eruption accentuated in the groin and periorificially. Alopecia is often present. These conditions are most common in children with congenital metabolic abnormalities, in alcoholics with cirrhosis, and in persons on hyperalimentation who have not been adequately supplemented. Replacement of the deficiency leads to rapid resolution of the dermatitis and alopecia. An entity similar to acrodermatitis enteropathica occurs in patients who are zinc deficient, including infants who are exclusively breast-fed and in patients with Crohn's disease.[167, 168]

Scurvy, or vitamin C deficiency, manifests as follicular hyperkeratosis and perifollicular hemorrhage, ecchymoses, xerosis, leg edema, poor wound healing, and/or bent or coiled body hairs.[169] Large purpuric plaques, especially on the extremities may occur. Gingivitis with gum hemorrhage occur only in dentulous patients and commonly occur in the presence of poor oral hygiene and periodontal disease.[169] Scurvy is most common in alcoholics, but it may occur with Crohn's or Whipple's disease. The focus of treatment is to correct the deficit and to replete body stores. Symptoms recede promptly and disappear within a few weeks.[169]

As discussed earlier in the chapter, patients with glucagon-secreting tumors of the pancreas frequently develop a characteristic dermatosis called *necrolytic migratory erythema*[170] (Fig. 18–26; see also Color Fig. 18–26). A skin biopsy specimen may be highly suggestive, showing psoriasiform hyperplasia, a subcorneal blister containing neutrophils, and hydropic degeneration and necrosis of the subcorneal keratinocytes. Systemic manifestations of this syndrome are discussed in Chapter 51. There are also reports of this syndrome occurring without glucagonomas, especially in the setting of cirrhosis and subtotal villous atrophy of the jejunal mucosa.[171] Glucagon is therefore probably not the cause of

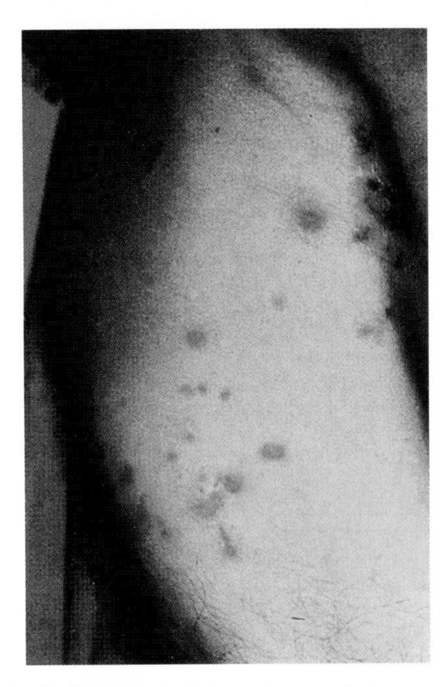

Figure 18–26. Erythema necrolytica migrans of glucagonoma demonstrating rapidly eroding superficial blisters. The eruption is usually localized to the buttocks, groin, perineum, elbows, hands, feet, and perioral area. (Courtesy Carl Grunfeld, MD, PhD.)

the eruption. Infusion of amino acids has been reported to clear the eruption despite persistently elevated glucagon levels. Zinc deficiency can cause a similar eruption (acrodermatitis enteropathica), as can biotin-responsive multiple carboxylase deficiency and essential fatty acid deficiency. The eruption therefore seems to be a cutaneous manifestation of several metabolic disorders, but the crucial pathogenic defect has not been determined.[172]

Acknowledgments

The authors and editors acknowledge the valuable assistance of Ryan Brashear, MD, and Arman David Soleymani, BS.

REFERENCES

1. Sheikh SH, Shaw-Stiffel TA: The gastrointestinal manifestations of Sjögren's syndrome. Am J Gastroenterol 90:9–14, 1995.
2. Anonymous: Treatment of xerostomia. Med Lett Drugs Ther 30:74–76, 1988.
3. Levine MJ, Aguirre A, Hatton MN, Tabak LA: Artificial salivas: Present and future. J Dent Res 66:693–698, 1987.
4. Rodriguez-Cuartero A, Garcia-Vera E, Gomez-Cerro A: Hepatitis C virus and Sjögren's syndrome. Infection 22:415–416, 1994.
5. Greenspan D, Daniels TE: Effectiveness of pilocarpine in postradiation xerostomia. Cancer 59:1123–1125, 1987.
6. Fox PC: Systemic therapy of salivary gland hypofunction. J Dent Res 66:689–692, 1987.
7. Wiseman LR, Faulds D: Oral pilocarpine: A review of its pharmacological properties and clinical potential in xerostomia. Drugs 49:143–155, 1995.
8. Cevimeline (Evoxac) for dry mouth. Med Lett Drugs Ther 42:70, 2000.

8a. Vivino FB, Al-Hashiri I, Khan Z, et al: Pilocarpine tablets for the treatment of dry mouth and dry eye symptoms in patients with Sjögren's syndrome: A radomized, placebo-controlled, fixed dose, multicenter trial. Arch Intern Med 159:174–181, 1999.

9. Dreizen S: Systemic significance of glossitis: Decoding the tongue's medical messages. Postgrad Med 75:207–215, 1984.
10. Bohmer T, Mowe M: The association between atrophic glossitis and protein-calorie malnutrition in old age. Ageing 29:47–50, 2000.
11. Schiffman SS: Taste and smell in disease: II. N Engl J Med 308: 1337–1343, 1983.
12. Schiffman SS: Taste and smell in disease: I. N Engl J Med 308:1275–1279, 1983.
13. Silverman S Jr, Thompson JS: Serum zinc and copper in oral/oropharyngeal carcinoma: A study of seventy-five patients. Oral Surg Oral Med Oral Pathol 57:34–36, 1984.
14. Schiffman SS, Zervakis J, Suggs MS, et al: Effect of tricyclic antidepressants on taste responses in humans and gerbils. Pharmacol Biochem Behav 65:599–609, 2000.
15. Gorsky M, Silverman S Jr, Chinn H: Burning mouth syndrome: A review of 98 cases. J Oral Med 42:7–9, 1987.
16. Shenefelt PD: Hypnosis in dermatology. Arch Dermatol 136:393–399, 2000.
17. Drage LA, Rogers RS III: Clinical assessment and outcome in 70 patients with complaints of burning or sore mouth symptoms. Mayo Clin Proc 74:223–228, 1999.
18. Sarti GM, Haddy RI, Schaffer D, Kihm J: Black hairy tongue. Am Fam Physician 41:1751–1755, 1990.
19. Langtry JA, Carr MM, Steele MC, Ive FA: Topical tretinoin: A new treatment for black hairy tongue (lingua villosa nigra). Clin Exp Dermatol 17:163–164, 1992.
20. Manabe M, Lim HW, Winzer M, Loomis CA: Architectural organization filiform papillae in normal and black hairy tongue epithelium: Dissection of differentiation pathways in a complex human epithelium according to their patterns of keratin expression. Arch Dermatol 135: 177–181, 1999.
21. Hay RJ: The management of superficial candidiasis. J Am Acad Dermatol 40:S35–42, 1999.
22. Mirowski GW, Greenspan D, Hilton JF, et al: Co-prevalence of cutaneous and oral diseases in HIV-positive patients. J Dent Res 75:238, 1996.
23. Melnick SL, Engel D, Truelove E, et al: Oral mucosal lesions: Association with the presence of antibodies to the human immunodeficiency virus. Oral Surg Oral Med Oral Pathol 68:37–43, 1989.
24. Phelan JA, Saltzman BR, Friedland GH, Klein RS: Oral findings in patients with acquired immunodeficiency syndrome. Oral Surg Oral Med Oral Pathol 64:50–56, 1987.
25. Silverman S Jr, Migliorati CA, Lozada-Nur F, et al: Oral findings in people with or at high risk for AIDS: A study of 375 homosexual males. J Am Dent Assoc 112:187–192, 1986.
26. Dull JS, Sen P, Raffanti S, Middleton JR: Oral candidiasis as a marker of acute retroviral illness. South Med J 84:733–735, 739, 1991.
27. Epstein JB: Antifungal therapy in oropharyngeal mycotic infections. Oral Surg Oral Med Oral Pathol 69:32–41, 1990.
28. Silverman S Jr, McKnight ML, Migliorati C, et al: Chemotherapeutic mouth rinses in immunocompromised patients. Am J Dent 2:303–307, 1989.
29. Greenspan JS, Greenspan D: Oral hairy leukoplakia: Diagnosis and management. Oral Surg Oral Med Oral Pathol 67:396–403, 1989.
30. Sciubba J, Brandsma J, Schwartz M, Barrezueta N: Hairy leukoplakia: An AIDS-associated opportunistic infection. Oral Surg Oral Med Oral Pathol 67:404–410, 1989.
31. Greenspan D, Greenspan JS: Significance of oral hairy leukoplakia. Oral Surg Oral Med Oral Pathol 73:151–154, 1992.
32. Greenspan D, Greenspan JS, Overby G, et al: Risk factors for rapid progression from hairy leukoplakia to AIDS: A nested case-control study. J. Acquir Immune Defic Syndr 4:652–658, 1991.
33. Mocroft A, Sabin CA, Youle M, et al: Changes in AIDS-defining illnesses in a London Clinic, 1987–1998. J Acquir Immune Defic Syndr 21:401–407, 1999.
34. Ficarra G, Berson AM, Silverman S Jr, et al: Kaposi's sarcoma of the oral cavity: A study of 134 patients with a review of the pathogenesis, epidemiology, clinical aspects, and treatment. Oral Surg Oral Med Oral Pathol 66:543–550, 1988.
35. Lumerman H, Freedman PD, Kerpel SM, Phelan JA: Oral Kaposi's sarcoma: A clinicopathologic study of 23 homosexual and bisexual men from the New York metropolitan area. Oral Surg Oral Med Oral Pathol 65:711–716, 1988.
36. Green TL, Beckstead JH, Lozada-Nur F, et al: Histopathologic spectrum of oral Kaposi's sarcoma. Oral Surg Oral Med Oral Pathol 58: 306–314, 1984.
37. Lowenthal DA, Straus DJ, Campbell SW, et al: AIDS-related lymphoid neoplasia: The Memorial Hospital experience. Cancer 61:2325–2337, 1988.
38. Perkocha LA, Geaghan SM, Yen TS, et al: Clinical and pathological features of bacillary peliosis hepatis in association with human immunodeficiency virus infection. N Engl J Med 323:1581–1586, 1990.
39. Rogers RS III, Hutton KP: Screening for haematinic deficiencies in patients with recurrent aphthous stomatitis. Australas J Dermatol 27: 98–103, 1986.
40. Axell T, Henricsson V: The occurrence of recurrent aphthous ulcers in an adult Swedish population. Acta Odontol Scand 43:125, 1985.
41. Olson JA, Greenspan JS, Silverman S Jr: Recurrent aphthous ulcerations. CDA J 10:53–57, 1982.
42. Savage NW, Seymour GJ, Kruger BJ: T-lymphocyte subset changes in recurrent aphthous stomatitis. Oral Surg Oral Med Oral Pathol 60: 175–181, 1985.
43. Porter SR, Scully C, Flint S: Hematologic status in recurrent aphthous stomatitis compared with other oral disease. Oral Surg Oral Med Oral Pathol 66:41–44, 1988.
44. Olson JA, Feinberg I, Silverman S Jr, et al: Serum vitamin B_{12}, folate, and iron levels in recurrent aphthous ulceration. Oral Surg Oral Med Oral Pathol 54:517–520, 1982.
45. Silverman S Jr, Lozada-Nur F, Migliorati C: Clinical efficacy of prednisone in the treatment of patients with oral inflammatory ulcerative diseases: A study of fifty-five patients. Oral Surg Oral Med Oral Pathol 59:360–363, 1985.
46. Rattan J, Schneider M, Arber N, et al: Sucralfate suspension as a treatment of recurrent aphthous stomatitis. J Intern Med 236:341–3, 1994.
47. Healy CM, Paterson M, Joyston-Bechal S, et al: The effect of a sodium lauryl sulfate–free dentifrice on patients with recurrent oral ulceration. Oral Dis 5:39–43, 1999.
48. Chahine L, Sempson N, Wagoner C: The effect of sodium lauryl sulfate on recurrent aphthous ulcers: A clinical study. Comp Contin Educat Dent (Jamesburg, NJ) 18:1238–1240, 1997.
49. Scully C: Orofacial herpes simplex virus infections: Current concepts in the epidemiology, pathogenesis, and treatment, and disorders in which the virus may be implicated. Oral Surg Oral Med Oral Pathol 68:701–710, 1989.
50. Corey L, Spear PG: Infections with herpes simplex viruses: II. N Engl J Med 314:749–757, 1986.
51. Molinari JA, Merchant VA: Herpes viruses: Manifestations and transmission. J Calif Dent Assoc 17:24–31, 1989.
52. Schubert MM, Peterson DE, Flournoy N, et al: Oral and pharyngeal herpes simplex virus infection after allogeneic bone marrow transplantation: Analysis of factors associated with infection. Oral Surg Oral Med Oral Pathol 70:286–293, 1990.
53. Huff JC, Weston WL: Recurrent erythema multiforme. Medicine (Baltimore) 68:133–140, 1989.
54. Wade JC, Newton B, Flournoy N, Meyers JD: Oral acyclovir for prevention of herpes simplex virus reactivation after marrow transplantation. Ann Intern Med 100:823–828, 1984.
55. Dan M, Siegman-Igra Y, Weinberg M, Michaeli D: Long-term suppression of recurrent herpes labialis by low-dose oral acyclovir in an immunocompromised patient. Arch Intern Med 146:1438–1440, 1986.
56. Epstein JB, Sherlock CH, Wolber RA: Oral manifestations of cytomegalovirus infection. Oral Surg Oral Med Oral Pathol 75:443–451, 1993.
57. Magana-Garcia M, Arista-Viveros A: Cutaneous amebiasis in children. Pediatr Dermatol 10:352–355, 1993.
58. Mhlanga BR, Lanoie LO, Norris HJ, et al: Amebiasis complicating carcinomas: A diagnostic dilemma. Am J Trop Med Hyg 46:759–764, 1992.
59. Silverman S Jr, Gorsky M, Lozada-Nur F, Liu A: Oral mucous membrane pemphigoid: A study of sixty-five patients. Oral Surg Oral Med Oral Pathol 61:233–237, 1986.
60. Thivolet J, Barthelemy H: Bullous pemphigoid. Semin Dermatol 7:91–103, 1988.
61. Leonard JN, Hobday CM, Haffenden GP, et al: Immunofluorescent studies in ocular cicatricial pemphigoid. Br J Dermatol 118:209–217, 1988.
62. Jordon RE, Kawana S, Fritz KA: Immunopathologic mechanisms in pemphigus and bullous pemphigoid. J Invest Dermatol 85(Suppl):72S–78S, 1985.

63. Daniels TE, Quadra-White C: Direct immunofluorescence in oral mucosal disease: A diagnostic analysis of 130 cases. Oral Surg Oral Med Oral Pathol 51:38–47, 1981.
64. Korman NJ: New and emerging therapies in the treatment of blistering diseases. Dermatol Clin North Am 18:127–137, ix–x, 2000.
65. Stanley JR: Pemphigus: Skin failure mediated by autoantibodies. JAMA 264:1714–1717, 1990.
66. Wood DR, Patterson JB, Orlando RC: Pemphigus vulgaris of the esophagus. Ann Intern Med 96:189–191, 1982.
67. Camisa C, Helm TN: Paraneoplastic pemphigus is a distinct neoplasia-induced autoimmune disease. Arch Dermatol 129:883–886, 1993.
68. Anhalt GJ, Kim SC, Stanley JR, et al: Paraneoplastic pemphigus: An autoimmune mucocutaneous disease associated with neoplasia. N Engl J Med 323:1729–1735, 1990.
69. Berger TG, Detlefs RL, Donatucci CF: Junctional epidermolysis bullosa, pyloric atresia, and genitourinary disease. Pediatr Dermatol 3: 130–134, 1986.
70. Fine-Jo D, Bauer EA, Briggaman RD: Revised clinical and laboratory criteria for subtypes of inherited epidermolysis bullosa. J Am Acad Dermatol 24:119–135, 1991.
71. Woodley DT, Briggaman RA, Gammon WT: Review and update of epidermolysis bullosa acquisita. Semin Dermatol 7:111–122, 1988.
72. Raab B, Fretzin DF, Bronson DM, et al: Epidermolysis bullosa acquisita and inflammatory bowel disease. JAMA 250:1746–1748, 1983.
73. Lozada-Nur F, Gorsky M, Silverman S Jr: Oral erythema multiforme: Clinical observations and treatment of 95 patients. Oral Surg Oral Med Oral Pathol 67:36–40, 1989.
74. Kokuba H, Imafuku S, Huang S, et al: Erythema multiforme lesions are associated with expression of a herpes simplex virus (HSV) gene and qualitative alterations in the HSV-specific T-cell response. Br J Dermatol 138:952–964, 1998.
75. Zweiban B, Cohen H, Chandrasoma P: Gastrointestinal involvement complicating Stevens-Johnson syndrome. Gastroenterology 91:469–474, 1986.
76. Viard I, Wehrli P, Bullani R, et al: Inhibition of toxic epidermal necrolysis by blockade of CD95 with human intravenous immunoglobulin. Science 282:490–493, 1998.
77. Silverman S Jr, Gorsky M, Lozada-Nur F: A prospective follow-up study of 570 patients with oral lichen planus: Persistence, remission, and malignant association. Oral Surg Oral Med Oral Pathol 60:30–34, 1985.
78. Al-Shihabi BM, Jackson JM: Dysphagia due to pharyngeal and oesophageal lichen planus. J Laryngol Otol 96:567–571, 1982.
79. Lefer LG: Lichen planus of the esophagus. Am J Dermatopathol 4: 267–269, 1982.
80. Jubert C, Pawlotsky JM, Pouget F, et al: Lichen planus and hepatitis C virus–related chronic active hepatitis. Arch Dermatol 130:73–76, 1994.
81. Mokni M, Rybojad M, Puppin D Jr, et al: Lichen planus and hepatitis C virus. J Am Acad Dermatol 24:792, 1991.
82. Greenstein AJ, Janowitz HD, Sachar DB: The extra-intestinal complications of Crohn's disease and ulcerative colitis: A study of 700 patients. Medicine 55:401–412, 1976.
83. Ploysangam T, Heubi JE, Eisen D, et al: Cutaneous Crohn's disease in children. J Am Acad Dermatol 36:697–704, 1997.
84. Brook IM, King DJ, Miller ID: Chronic granulomatous cheilitis and its relationship to Crohn's disease. Oral Surg Oral Med Oral Pathol 56:405–408, 1983.
85. Healy CM, Farthing PM, Williams DM, Thornhill MH: Pyostomatitis vegetans and associated systemic disease: A review and two case reports. Oral Surg Oral Med Oral Pathol 78:323–328, 1994.
86. Van Hale HM, Rogers RS, Zone JJ, Greipp PR: Pyostomatitis vegetans: A reactive mucosal marker for inflammatory disease of the gut. Arch Dermatol 121:94–98, 1985.
87. Philpot HC, Elewski BE, Banwell JG, Gramlich T: Pyostomatitis vegetans and primary sclerosing cholangitis: Markers of inflammatory bowel disease. Gastroenterology 103:668–674, 1992.
88. Powell FC, Schroeter AL, Su WP, Perry HO: Pyoderma gangrenosum: A review of 86 patients. Q J Med 55:173–186, 1985.
89. Drenick EJ, Ahmed AR, Greenway F, Olerud JE: Cutaneous lesions after intestinal bypass. Ann Intern Med 93:557–559, 1980.
90. Saulsbury FT: Henoch-Schonlein purpura in children: Report of 100 patients and review of the literature. Medicine 78:395–409, 1999.
91. Mills JA, Michel BA, Bloch DA, et al: The American College of Rheumatology 1990 criteria for the classification of Henoch-Schönlein purpura. Arthritis Rheum 33:1114–1121, 1990.
92. Lopez LR, Schocket AL, Stanford RE, et al: Gastrointestinal involvement in leukocytoclastic vasculitis and polyarteritis nodosa. J Rheumatol 7:677–684, 1980.
93. Saulsbury FT: Henoch-Schönlein purpura. Pediatr Dermatol 1:195–201, 1984.
94. Fruhwirth J, Mischinger HJ, Werkgartner G, et al: Köhlmeier-Degos's disease with primary intestinal manifestation. Scand J Gastroenterol 32:1066–1070, 1997.
95. Katz SK, Mudd LJ, Roenigk HH: Malignant atrophic papulosis (Degos' disease) involving three generations of a family. J Am Acad Dermatol 37:480–484, 1997.
96. Degos R: Malignant atrophic papulosis. Br J Dermatol 100:21–35, 1979.
97. Black MM, Hudson PM: Atrophie blanche lesions closely resembling malignant atrophic papulosis (Degos' disease) in systemic lupus erythematosus. Br J Dermatol 95:649–652, 1976.
98. Englert HJ, Hawkes CH, Boey ML, et al: Degos' disease: Association with anticardiolipin antibodies and the lupus anticoagulant. BMJ 289: 576, 1984.
99. Katz SK, Mudd LJ, Roenigk HH Jr: Malignant atrophic papulosis (Degos' disease) involving three generations of a family. J Am Acad Dermatol 37:480, 1997.
100. Stahl D, Thomsen K, Hou-Jensen K: Degos' disease treated with platelet-suppressive drugs. Lancet 2:46–47, 1977.
101. Guttmacher AE, Marchuk DA, White RI Jr: Hereditary hemorrhagic telangiectasia. N Engl J Med 333:918–924, 1995.
102. Planchu J, de Chedarevia J, Bideau A, et al: Age-related clinical profile of hereditary hemorrhagic telangiectasia in an epidemiologically recruited population. Am J Med Genet 32:291–297, 1989.
103. Smith CR, Bartholomew LG, Cain JC: Hereditary hemorrhagic telangiectasia and gastrointestinal hemorrhage. Gastroenterology 44:1–6, 1963.
104. Quitt M, Froom P, Veisler A, et al: The effect of desmopressin on massive gastrointestinal bleeding in hereditary telangiectasia unresponsive to treatment with cryoprecipitate. Arch Intern Med 150:1744–1746, 1990.
105. Kjeldsen AD, Vase P, Green A: Hereditary haemorrhagic telangiectasia: A population-based study of prevalence and mortality in Danish patients. J Intern Med 245:31–39, 1999.
106. Van Cutsem E, Rutgeerts P, Geboes K, et al: Estrogen-progesterone treatment of Osler-Weber-Rendu disease. J Clin Gastroenterol 10:676–679, 1988.
107. Fritzler MJ, Arlette JP, Behm AR, Kinsella TD: Hereditary hemorrhagic telangiectasia versus CREST syndrome: Can serology aid diagnosis? J Am Acad Dermatol 10:192–196, 1984.
108. Tyrrel RT, Baumgartner BR, Montemayor KA: Blue rubber bleb nevus syndrome: CT diagnosis of intussusception. AJR Am J Roentgenol 154:105–106, 1990.
109. Shahed M, Hagenmuller F, Rosch T, et al: A 19-year-old female with blue rubber bleb nevus syndrome: Endoscopic laser photocoagulation and surgical resection of gastrointestinal angiomata. Endoscopy 22: 54–56, 1990.
110. Sandhu KS, Cohen H, Radin R, Buck FS: Blue rubber bleb nevus syndrome presenting with recurrences. Dig Dis Sci 32:214–219, 1987.
111. Oranje AP: Blue rubber bleb nevus syndrome. Pediatr Dermatol 3: 304–310, 1986.
112. Kyle RA, Greipp PR: Amyloidosis (AL): Clinical and laboratory features in 229 cases. Mayo Clin Proc 58:665–683, 1983.
113. Flick WG, Lawrence FR: Oral amyloidosis as initial symptom of multiple myeloma: A case report. Oral Surg Oral Med Oral Pathol 49: 18–20, 1980.
114. Touart DM, Sau P: Cutaneous diseases: I. J Am Acad Dermatol 39: 149–123, 1998.
114a. Giardiello FM, Welsh SB, Hamilton SR, et al: Increased risk of cancer in Peutz-Jeghers syndrome. N Engl J Med 316:151, 1987.
115. Mulvihill JJ, Parry DM, Sherman JL, et al: NIH conference. Neurofibromatosis 1 (Recklinghausen disease) and neurofibromatosis 2 (bilateral acoustic neurofibromatosis): An update. Ann Intern Med 113:39–52, 1990.
116. Cameron AJ, Pairolero PC, Stanson AW, Carpenter HA: Abdominal angina and neurofibromatosis. Mayo Clin Proc 57:125–128, 1982.
117. Stamm B, Hedinger CE, Saremaslani P: Duodenal and ampullary carcinoid tumors: A report of 12 cases with pathological characteristics, polypeptide content, and relation to the MEN I syndrome and von Recklinghausen's disease (neurofibromatosis). Virchows Arch 408: 475–489, 1986.

118. Horan RF, Austen KF: Systemic mastocytosis: Retrospective review of a decade's clinical experience at the Brigham and Women's Hospital [discussion, pp 13S–14S]. J Invest Dermatol 96:5S–13S, 1991.
119. Kettelhut BV, Metcalfe DD: Pediatric mastocytosis. J Invest Dermatol 96:15S–18S, 1991.
120. Tebbe B, Stavropoulos PG, Krasagakis K, Organos CE: Cutaneous mastocytosis in adults: Evaluation of 14 patients with respect to systemic manifestations. Dermatology 197:101–108, 1998.
121. Schwartz RA, Goldberg DJ, Mahmood F, et al: The Muir-Torre syndrome: A disease of sebaceous and colonic neoplasms. Dermatologica 178:23–28, 1989.
122. Lynch HT, Lynch PM, Pester J, Fusaro RM: The cancer family syndrome: Rare cutaneous phenotypic linkage of Torre's syndrome. Arch Intern Med 141:607–611, 1981.
123. Starink TM: Cowden's disease: Analysis of fourteen new cases. J Am Acad Dermatol 11:1127–1141, 1984.
124. Daniel ES, Ludwig SL, Lewin KJ, et al: The Cronkhite-Canada syndrome: An analysis of clinical and pathologic features and therapy in 55 patients. Medicine (Baltimore) 61:293–309, 1982.
125. Russell DM, Bhathal PS, St. John DJ: Complete remission in Cronkhite-Canada syndrome. Gastroenterology 85:180–185, 1983.
126. Ferney DM, DeSchryver-Kecskemeti K, Clouse RE: Treatment of Cronkhite-Canada syndrome with home total parenteral nutrition [letter]. Ann Intern Med 104:588, 1986.
127. Bernard P, Bonnetblanc JM: Dermatomyositis and malignancy. J Invest Dermatol 100:128S–132S, 1993.
128. Zantos D, Zhang Y, Felson D: The overall and temporal association of cancer with polymyositis and dermatomyositis. J Rheumatol 21: 1855–1859, 1994.
129. Schulman P, Kerr LD, Spiera H: A reexamination of the relationship between myositis and malignancy [see comments]. J Rheumatol 18: 1689–1692, 1991.
130. Airio A, Pukkala E, Isomaki H: Elevated cancer incidence in patients with dermatomyositis: A population-based study. J Rheumatol 22: 1300–1303, 1995.
131. Chuang T-Y, Lu Y-C, Deng J-S, Hsieh T: Dermatomyositis and nasopharyngeal carcinoma. Formosan Med Assoc 73:365–373, 1974.
132. Callen JP: Relationship of cancer to inflammatory muscle diseases: Dermatomyositis, polymyositis, and inclusion body myositis. Rheum Dis Clin North Am 20:943–953, 1994.
133. Ellis DL, Kafka SP, Chow JC, et al: Melanoma, growth factors, acanthosis nigricans, the sign of Leser-Trélat, and multiple acrochordons: A possible role for α-transforming growth factor in cutaneous paraneoplastic syndromes. N Engl J Med 317:1582–1587, 1987.
134. Hovenden AL: Hypertrichosis lanuginosa acquisita associated with malignancy. Clin Dermatol 11:99–106, 1993.
135. Swenson KH, Amon RB, Hanifin JM: The glucagonoma syndrome: A distinctive cutaneous marker of systemic disease. Arch Dermatol 114: 224–228, 1978.
136. Samlaska CP, James WD: Superficial thrombophlebitis: II. Secondary hypercoagulable states. J Am Acad Dermatol 23:1–18, 1990.
137. Samlaska CP, James WD: Superficial thrombophlebitis: I. Primary hypercoagulable states. J Am Acad Dermatol 22:975–989, 1990.
138. Monreal M, Lafoz E, Casals A, et al: Occult cancer in patients with deep venous thrombosis: A systematic approach. Cancer 67:541–545, 1991.
139. Good AE, Schnitzer B, Kawanishi H, et al: Acinar pancreatic tumor with metastatic fat necrosis: Report of a case and review of rheumatic manifestations. Am J Dig Dis 21:978–987, 1976.
140. Palomo-Arellano A, Salvador-Fernandez M, Santome-Argibay F: Erythematous and tender subcutaneous nodules on lower extremities: Subcutaneous fat necrosis associated with pancreatic adenocarcinoma. Arch Dermatol 130:649, 652, 1994.
140a. Wilson HA, Askari AD, Neiderhiser DH, et al: Pancreatitis with arthropathy and subcutaneous fat necrosis: Evidence for the pathogenicity of lipolytic enzymes. Arthritis Rheum 26:121–126, 1983.
141. Chute CG, Chuang T-Y, Bergstralh EJ, Su W-PD: The subsequent risk of internal cancer with Bowen's disease: A population-based study. JAMA 266:816–819, 1991.
142. Chuang T-Y, Tse J, Reizner GT: Bowen's disease (squamous cell carcinoma in situ) as a skin marker for internal malignancy: A case-control study. Am J Prev Med 6:238–243, 1990.
143. Gould BE, Ellison RC, Greene HL, Bernhard JD: Lack of association between skin tags and colon polyps in a primary care setting. Arch Intern Med 148:1799–1800, 1988.
144. Lindelof B, Sigurgeirsson B, Melander S: Seborrheic keratoses and cancer. J Am Acad Dermatol 26:947–950, 1992.
145. Holdiness MR: The sign of Leser-Trélat. Int J Dermatol 25:564–572, 1986.
146. Cohen PR, Holder WR, Tucker SB, et al: Sweet syndrome in patients with solid tumors. Cancer 72:2723–2731, 1993.
147. Powell FC, Cooper AJ, Massa MC, et al: Sister Mary Joseph's nodule: A clinical and histologic study. J Am Acad Dermatol 10:610–615, 1984.
148. Bergasa NV, Alling DW, Talbot TL, et al: Effects of naloxone infusions in patients with the pruritus of cholestasis: A double-blind, randomized, controlled trial. Ann Intern Med 123:161–167, 1995.
149. Roenigk HH Jr, Auerbach R, Maibach H, Weinstein GD: Methotrexate in psoriasis: Revised guidelines. J Am Acad Dermatol 19:145–146, 1988.
150. David M: Adverse effects of retinoids. Med Toxicol 3:273–288, 1988.
151. Camuto P, Shupach J, Orbuch P: Long-term effects of etretinate on the liver in psoriasis. Am J Surg Pathol 11:30–37, 1987.
152. Finkelstein H, Champion MC, Adam JE: Cutaneous hypersensitivity to vitamin K_1 injection. J Am Acad Dermatol 16:540–545, 1987.
153. Brunskill NJ, Berth-Jones J, Graham-Brown RA: Pseudosclerodermatous reaction to phytomenadione injection (Texier's syndrome). Clin Exp Dermatol 13:276–278, 1988.
154. Tuppal R, Tremaine R: Cutaneous eruption from vitamin K_1 injection. J Am Acad Dermatol 27:105–106, 1992.
155. Reichel M, Mauro TM: Urticaria and hepatitis C. Lancet 336:822–823, 1990.
156. Pascual M, Perrin L, Giostra E, Schifferli JA: Hepatitis C virus in patients with cryoglobulinemia type II. J Infect Dis 162:569–577, 1990.
157. Chuang TY, Brashear R, Lewis C: Porphyria cutanea tarda and hepatitis C virus: A case-control study and meta-analysis of the literature. J Am Acad Dermatol 41:31–36, 1999.
158. Chuang TY, Stitle L, Brashear R, Lewis C: Hepatitis C virus and lichen planus: A case-control study of 340 patients. J Am Acad Dermatol 41:787–789, 1999.
159. Smith JD, Goette DK, Odom RB: Larva currens: Cutaneous strongyloidiasis. Arch Dermatol 112:1161–1163, 1976.
160. Ronan SG, Reddy RL, Manaligod JR, et al: Disseminated strongyloidiasis presenting as purpura. J Am Acad Dermatol 21:1123–1125, 1989.
161. Faure M: Dermatitis herpetiformis. Semin Dermatol 7:123–129, 1988.
162. Olbricht SM, Flotte TJ, Collins AB, et al: Dermatitis herpetiformis: Cutaneous deposition of polyclonal IgA_1. Arch Dermatol 122:418–421, 1986.
163. Hall RP, Sanders ME, Duquesnoy RJ, et al: Alterations in HLA-DP and HLA-DQ antigen frequency in patients with dermatitis herpetiformis. J Invest Dermatol 93:501–505, 1989.
164. Leonard JN, Chorzelski TP, Beutner AUUJ, et al: Gluten challenge in dermatitis herpetiformis. N Engl J Med 308:816–819, 1983.
165. van der Meer JB: Gluten-free diet and elemental diet in dermatitis herpetiformis. Int J Dermatol 29:679–692, 1990.
166. Delahoussaye AR, Jorizzo JL: Cutaneous manifestations of nutritional disorders. Dermatol Clin North Am 7:559–570, 1989.
167. Piela Z, Szuber M, Mach B, Janniger CK: Zinc deficiency in exclusively breast-fed infants. Cutis 61:197–200, 1998.
168. Myung SJ, Yang SK, Jung HY, et al: Zinc deficiency manifested by dermatitis and visual dysfunction in a patient with Crohn's disease. J Gastroenterol 33:876–879, 1998.
169. Hirschmann JV, Raugi GJ: Adult scurvy. J Am Acad Dermatol 41: 895–906, 1999.
170. Norton JA, Kahn CJ, Schiebinger R, et al: Amino acid deficiency and the skin rash associated with glucagonoma. Ann Intern Med 91:213–215, 1979.
171. Doyle JA, Schroeter AL, Rogers RS: Hyperglucagonaemia and necrolytic migratory erythema in cirrhosis—possible pseudoglucagonoma syndrome. Br J Dermatol 101:581–587, 1979.
172. Shepherd ME, Raimer SS, Tyring SK, Smith EB: Treatment of necrolytic migratory erythema in glucagonoma syndrome. J Am Acad Dermatol 25:925–928, 1991.

Chapter 19

Diverticula of the Hypopharynx, Esophagus, Stomach, Jejunum, and Ileum*

Rohan Jeyarajah and William Harford

Diverticula arise as outpouchings from tubular structures. A single outpouching is termed a *diverticulum,* whereas several outpouchings are termed *diverticula. Congenital diverticula* are present at birth, whereas *acquired diverticula* develop later in life. *True diverticula* involve all layers of the intestinal wall, whereas *false diverticula* represent herniation of the mucosa and submucosa through the muscular wall. Many diverticula contain attenuated portions of the muscular wall of the intestine and hence may be difficult to define as either true or false. True diverticula are often assumed to be congenital lesions, whereas false diverticula are assumed to be acquired. Some authors reserve the terms *false diverticula* or *pseudodiverticula* to diverticula caused by inflammatory processes. These definitions are of little clinical relevance.

ZENKER'S DIVERTICULA

Ludlow first described a patient with a hypopharyngeal diverticulum in 1764,[1] and in 1877 Zenker and Von Ziemssen reported this phenomenon in a series of 23 patients.[2] Zenker's diverticula are evident on approximately 1% of barium esophagrams.

Etiology and Pathogenesis

Normal pharyngeal swallowing involves three steps: (1) the cricopharyngeus muscle relaxes; (2) the laryngohyoid complex elevates to open the upper esophageal sphincter (UES); and (3) pharyngeal peristalsis propels the bolus through the open sphincter.

There is an area of weakness where the fibers of the cricopharyngeal sphincter meet the oblique fibers of the inferior pharyngeal constrictor muscle. This area has been named *Killian's triangle.* The primary abnormality that leads to development of Zenker's diverticula appears to be incomplete relaxation of the UES. This predisposes to herniation of the mucosa through Killian's triangle. Understanding of this pathophysiology is important because correction of the defect involves both the abnormal UES and the diverticulum.

Precise characterization of the UES with pressure transducers is difficult. The UES is asymmetric and moves with swallowing. As a consequence, validating the pathophysiology of Zenker's diverticulum has been challenging. Different investigators have found different abnormalities. Baseline UES pressures can be normal or low in patients with Zenker's diverticula,[3, 4] but several studies have shown incomplete relaxation of the UES in response to swallowing. The cross-sectional area of the UES has been found to be decreased in other studies.[5–7] Presumably, this abnormally small area persists during UES relaxation. This reduction in UES opening may be caused by scarring due the inflammation in this area, a phenomenon commonly found with Zenker's diverticula. Pharyngeal contraction against a smaller than normal UES opening leads to increased intrabolus pressures during swallowing and to herniation through Killian's triangle. An association between Zenker's diverticula and reflux disease has been suggested but not confirmed.[8, 9]

*Colonic diverticula are discussed in Chapter 108 and Meckel's diverticula are discussed in Chapter 84.

Table 19–1 | **Presenting Symptoms in Patients with Zenker's Diverticulum**

Dysphagia
Regurgitation
Cough
Aspiration pneumonia
Weight loss
Choking
Regurgitation of undigested material
Halitosis

Clinical Presentation and Diagnosis

Patients who develop Zenker's diverticula are generally in their 7th or 8th decade of life. There is a 2 : 1 male predominance.[10] Presenting symptoms are listed in Table 19–1.

Patients with symptoms of Zenker's diverticulum should be referred for a barium swallow. Failure to recognize Zenker's diverticulum can lead to serious complications, such as perforation during placement of a nasogastric tube, endoscopy, endoscopic retrograde cholangiopancreatography (ERCP), transesophageal echocardiography (TEE), or intubation for anesthesia. Perforation of Zenker's diverticula often leads to mediastinitis. Although endoscopy is not indicated for routine evaluation of Zenker's diverticula, they are sometimes encountered unexpectedly during endoscopy for dysphagia or another clinical problem. Intubation of the esophagus during endoscopy may be difficult among patients with Zenker's diverticula. Large diverticula distort hypopharyngeal anatomy. The opening of the UES is often displaced. The tip of the endoscope is often directed preferentially into the diverticulum, increasing the risk of perforation. Thus, intubation should always be done cautiously under direct vision. Safe endoscopic intubation can be accomplished by first passing a soft catheter into the esophagus under direct vision.[11] Patients known to have Zenker's diverticulum who need ERCP or TEE should first have an overtube placed with a forward-viewing endoscope. The subsequent instrument can be inserted through the overtube.[12]

Barium swallow is an excellent test for the diagnosis of Zenker's diverticulum (Fig. 19–1). Large diverticula are usually obvious even on delayed images. The opening of large Zenker's diverticula often becomes aligned with the axis of the esophagus. Thus, oral contrast medium will preferentially fill the diverticula and will empty slowly. Smaller diverticula may be difficult to visualize. Barium swallow in the lateral view using videofluoroscopy is helpful for visualizing transient filling of the diverticula. Zenker's diverticula are sometimes also encountered during endoscopy for evaluation of the symptoms listed in Table 19–1 or among patients with unrelated symptoms (Fig. 19–2).

Cancer arises rarely in Zenker's diverticula. It has been reported in 0.4% in a large series.[13] Pills may become lodged, leading to ulceration.

Treatment and Prognosis

Patients who are symptomatic or who have large diverticula should be offered treatment. The standard treatment for these diverticula is open surgical resection of the diverticulum with division of the cricopharyngeus muscle.[14, 15] Smaller diverticula may be treated with division of the cricopharyngeus muscle only. The benefit of the latter approach is that the esophageal lumen is never entered, and hence the risk of postoperative leak is low. Diverticulopexy (suspension of the diverticulum in a cranial direction) has also been used.[10, 13, 16] Most experts advocate resection of the diverticulum if possible. However, large diverticula (surface area > 10 cm^2) have a high complication rate with resection and may, in fact, do better with diverticulopexy.[14] Complications from open operation occur in less than 10% of patients but

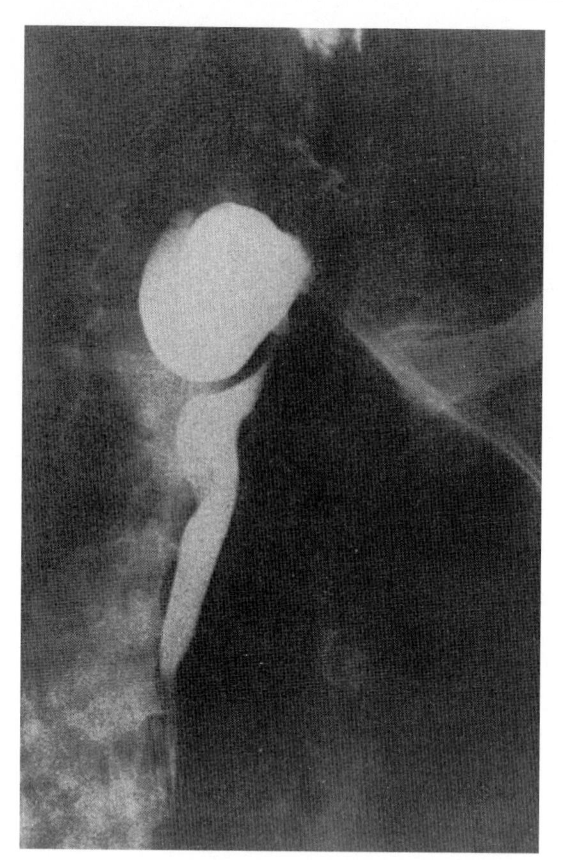

Figure 19–1. Zenker's diverticulum. This diverticulum is large enough to cause esophageal obstruction when it fills. (Courtesy of C. E. Pope, MD.)

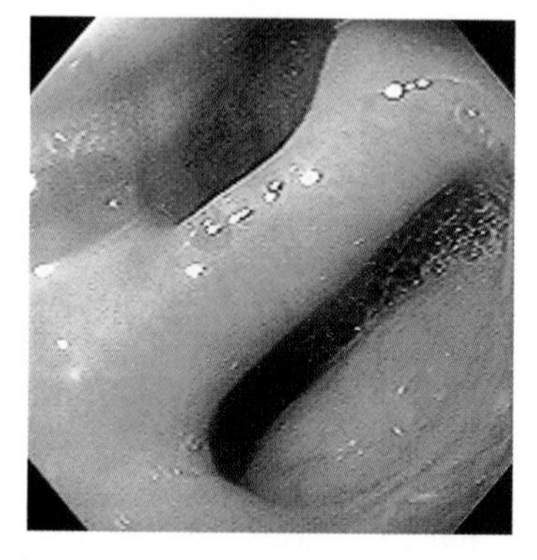

Figure 19–2. Endoscopic view of Zenker's diverticulum. It is often very difficult to distinguish the true lumen of the esophagus from that of Zenker's diverticulum. (Courtesy of D. Langdon, MD.)

can be severe. These include mediastinitis, esophagocutaneous fistula, and vocal cord paralysis from recurrent laryngeal nerve damage.

In recent years alternative techniques of endoscopic treatment of Zenker's diverticula have evolved. These include division of the wall between the diverticulum and the esophagus with CO_2 laser, electrocautery, or a stapling device.[17–21] Division of the septum between the diverticulum and the esophagus (Dohlman's procedure) can result in free perforation and mediastinitis. However, scarring and fibrosis between the two structures make this complication rare. The use of a stapling device may be the safest technique.[22–25] The septum between the diverticulum and the esophagus is stapled and divided. This septum should contain the cricopharyngeus muscle, and hence a myotomy should be performed as part of this procedure. This incorporates both components of the treatment of Zenker's diverticula. Many authors perform stapling procedures with a rigid scope and use general anesthesia.[23] Small diverticula (<2 cm in length) may not be amenable to endoscopic techniques because the myotomy may not be of adequate length.[25] Complications with the endoscopic approach have been reported to be lower than with the open approach (6% vs. 15%) in very select patient groups.[15]

The results of surgical treatment of Zenker's diverticula are excellent. More than 90% of patients become symptom free.[26, 27] Endoscopic approaches do not achieve such high rates of success but can be repeated if necessary.

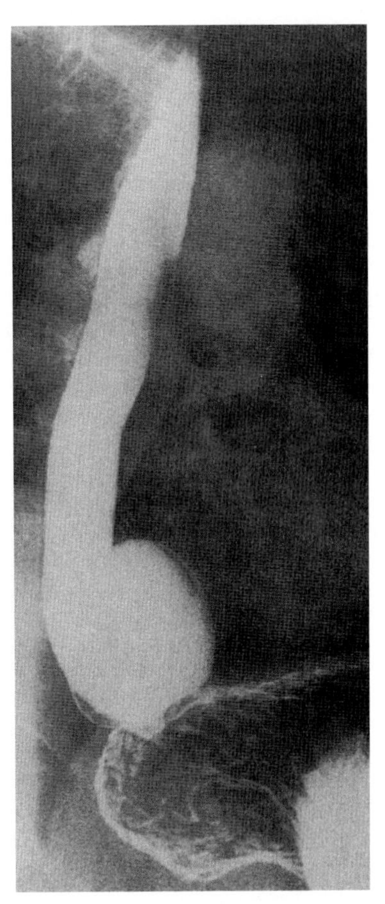

Figure 19–4. An epiphrenic diverticulum is seen immediately above the stomach. In this projection, it might be confused with a hiatus hernia. (Courtesy of C. A. Rohrmann, MD, and C. E. Pope, MD.)

DIVERTICULA OF THE ESOPHAGEAL BODY

Etiology and Pathogenesis

Diverticula of the esophagus are mainly located in the middle or lower third (Fig. 19–3). Diverticula in the lower third located near the diaphragmatic hiatus are called *epiphrenic diverticula* (Fig. 19–4). Congenital diverticula (see Chapter 31) may be associated with bronchopulmonary-foregut malformations (BPFMs), previously termed *pulmonary sequestrations*.[28] BPFMs can occur in communication with the esophagus and can present as diverticula.[29] Traction diverticula are most commonly found in developing countries. They are often related to underlying necrotic nodal infection associated with tuberculosis and histoplasmosis.[29] Centrally enlarged and necrotic mediastinal lymph nodes from lung malignancies can also result in traction diverticula.

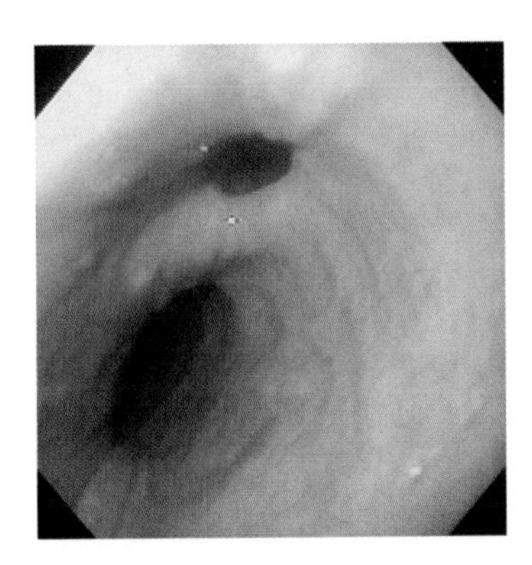

Figure 19–3. Endoscopic view of a midesophageal diverticulum. These diverticula are often most apparent when the esophagus is well insufflated.

The etiology of mid-body and distal esophageal diverticula is controversial. Many, but clearly not all, are associated with motility disorders such as diffuse esophageal spasm, hypertensive lower esophageal sphincter, or achalasia.[30–32] Many groups consider these diverticula to be false, or pseudodiverticula, but there is evidence that they may contain all layers of the intestinal wall and hence may be true diverticula.[33]

Clinical Presentation and Diagnosis

Congenital and traction diverticula are often asymptomatic. Rarely, bronchopulmonary fistulas can develop.[28] These patients present with cough, pneumonia, and recurrent bronchopulmonary infections.[29] Mid-body and distal esophageal diverticula are also usually asymptomatic. In one study 65% of patients had no related symptoms. If symptoms are not present at diagnosis, they rarely occur during follow-up.[34] The most common symptoms are dysphagia and regurgitation, although bleeding has been described.[35, 36] Dysphagia may be due either to an underlying motility disorder or to extrinsic compression of the esophagus by the fluid-filled diverticulum, which may cause obstruction.[36]

Regurgitation and aspiration during anesthesia have been reported. Perforation may occur during nasogastric intubation or upper gastrointestinal endoscopy.[35] The development of carcinoma within an epiphrenic diverticulum has been reported.[31, 33]

Chest radiograph may show an air-fluid level that may be mistaken for a diaphragmatic hernia or duplication cyst. Diagnosis is best made with a barium swallow, which serves not only to visualize the diverticulum but also to localize it more precisely than with endoscopy (Fig. 19–5; see also Fig. 19–4). Endoscopy and manometry are generally advisable if surgery is contemplated.[37] If an associated motility disorder such as diffuse spasm or achalasia is documented, surgical myotomy is an important aspect to the management of these patients. It is often difficult to pass the manometry catheter into the stomach. It has been our practice in such cases to pass a soft-tipped wire into the stomach over which the manometry catheter can be threaded.

Treatment and Prognosis

Asymptomatic diverticula of the esophagus need no treatment.[33] Only those patients with symptoms clearly related to their diverticula should be considered for therapy. The approach to surgical therapy has evolved. Currently, most surgeons advise resection of the diverticula and performance of a moderately sized myotomy of the contralateral wall of the esophagus, extended into the proximal stomach, taking care not to injure the vagus nerves.[30] This effectively releases the lower esophageal sphincter mechanism. To prevent gastroesophageal reflux, a loose, incomplete wrap (Dor or Toupet) should be added.[38]

The traditional surgical approach to esophageal diverticula has been through a left thoracotomy. Recently, however, abdominal laparoscopic techniques have allowed these procedures to be performed safely through the abdomen.[34, 35, 38, 39] Complications of the procedure include esophageal leak with mediastinitis or peritonitis, dysphagia due to a tight wrap, and reflux due to lower sphincter incompetence. Most patients are symptom free after the procedure. Hospital stay is shorter, and return to normal activities is faster with laparoscopic techniques than with open techniques. The role of balloon dilation is somewhat controversial. It is unclear if there is a higher rate of perforation when this is performed in the presence of an epiphrenic diverticulum.[40, 41]

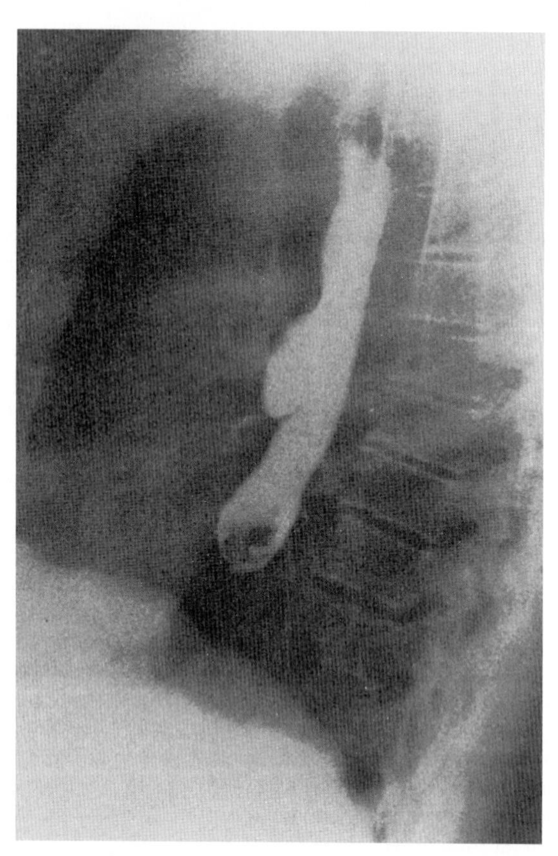

Figure 19–5. A large midesophageal diverticulum is seen in the midthoracic area. Below this is an impacted bolus of meat, causing an esophageal obstruction. After the bolus was removed, subsequent films showed no narrowing at the site where the bolus was arrested. (Courtesy of C. E. Pope, MD.)

ESOPHAGEAL INTRAMURAL PSEUDODIVERTICULA

Esophageal intramural pseudodiverticula (EIP) are multiple, small (1- to 4-mm), flasklike outpouchings involving a portion of or the entire esophagus.[42, 43] Approximately 200 cases have been reported in the literature.

Etiology and Pathogenesis

EIP are dilated submucosal esophageal glands that result in outpouchings from the main lumen[42] (Fig. 19–6*A* and *B*). There can be areas of "tracking" where communicating channels occur between EIPs, a finding that can be seen on barium swallow. The etiology of EIP is not clear. Associated conditions include a history of caustic ingestion, gastroesophageal reflux disease, esophageal dysmotility disorders, esophageal web, diabetes, candidal esophagitis, and strictures.[43–47] EIP can also be seen in patients with esophageal cancer.[48] Strictures may be related to acid reflux disease but can also involve the proximal rather than distal esophagus, which places in question the etiology of these more proximal strictures. The relationship of EIP to esophageal strictures is unclear. EIP may resolve or may persist after dilation of strictures. The finding of EIP has been demonstrated in approximately 1% of all barium swallow studies reviewed in one report.[42] However, the incidence in esophageal specimens taken at autopsy has been reported to be as high as 55%.[42]

Clinical Presentation and Diagnosis

Patients with EIP most commonly are in their 7th decade.[43] There is a male predominance. Patients are most often found to have EIP during a workup for dysphagia, odynophagia, or heartburn. Their symptoms are usually not related to the pseudodiverticula but rather to an underlying stricture or reflux disease. Pseudodiverticula resolve only rarely with treatment of stricture or acid reflux.[45] Perforation of EIP

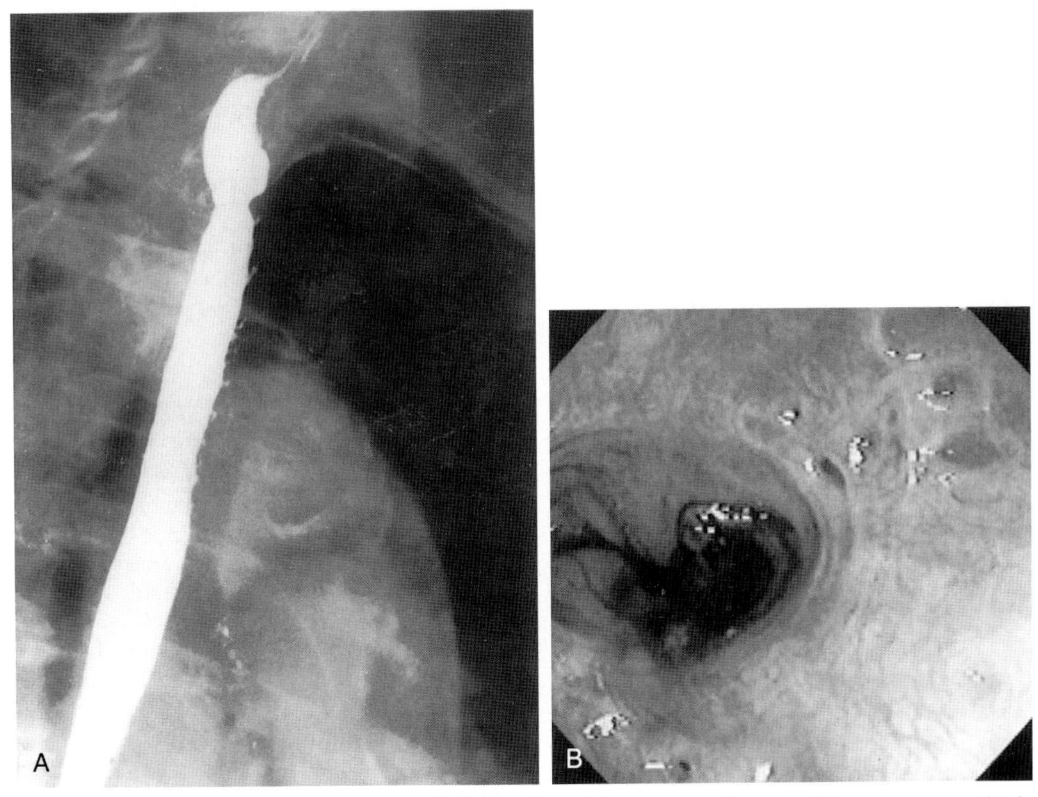

Figure 19–6. *A* and *B,* Esophageal intramural pseudodiverticula. *A,* Numerous small outpouchings are seen on this barium swallow. *B,* The small openings of the pseudodiverticula are seen on endoscopy in this patient who had a distal peptic stricture.

with mediastinitis has been reported.[44] However, these are usually microperforations that can be treated medically by placing the patient on nothing by mouth and giving antibiotics.

Diagnosis is best made with a barium swallow (see Fig. 19–6*A*). Controversy exists as to whether a single-column or double-contrast study is the preferred technique. Outpouchings (often subtle) in association with a stricture are the common features. Tracking between pseudodiverticula can be seen as columns of barium that parallel the main esophagus and represent communications between diverticula.[42] The differential diagnosis of EIP on barium swallow includes ulceration and perforation of the esophagus. Esophageal carcinoma must be ruled out in cases associated with a stricture. The endoscopic appearance of EIP is characteristic (see Fig. 19–6*B*). However, EIP may be missed on endoscopy if they are within an area of stricturing. On endoscopic ultrasound, mucosal and submucosal thickening has been reported. If no abnormality of the muscularis propria or no enlarged lymph nodes are seen, cancer is less likely.[43] Computed tomographic (CT) scan can be helpful in demonstrating mediastinal air when there has been a perforation.[44]

Treatment and Prognosis

Treatment for EIP is focused on treating the underlying disorder. For example, proton pump inhibitors can control acid reflux. Esophageal strictures can be dilated. Care must be taken to exclude cancer.[49] EIP may not resolve with treatment of the underlying disorder.

GASTRIC DIVERTICULA

Gastric diverticula are found in 0.02% of autopsy specimens.[50] Juxtacardiac diverticula make up 75% of all gastric diverticula. These are most commonly located near the gastroesophageal junction and are usually on the lesser curvature of the stomach, on the posterior aspect. These are most commonly found in middle-aged patients and measure approximately 1 to 3 cm in diameter[51, 52] (Fig. 19–7). Intramural or partial gastric diverticula are formed by projection of the mucosa of the stomach through the muscular layer. These are found more commonly in the prepyloric location and most commonly on the greater curvature of the stomach[53] (Fig. 19–8*A* and *B*). Strictures, peptic ulcer disease, and other deformities of the pylorus can look similar to prepyloric diverticula on endoscopic or barium study.

Clinical Presentation and Diagnosis

Juxtacardiac diverticula are almost always asymptomatic, although vague upper abdominal pain may occur.[53] There have been case reports of reproduction of pain by probing the diverticulum with a biopsy forceps during upper gastrointestinal endoscopy.[54] The authors concluded that reproduction of pain with manipulation indicated that symptoms were

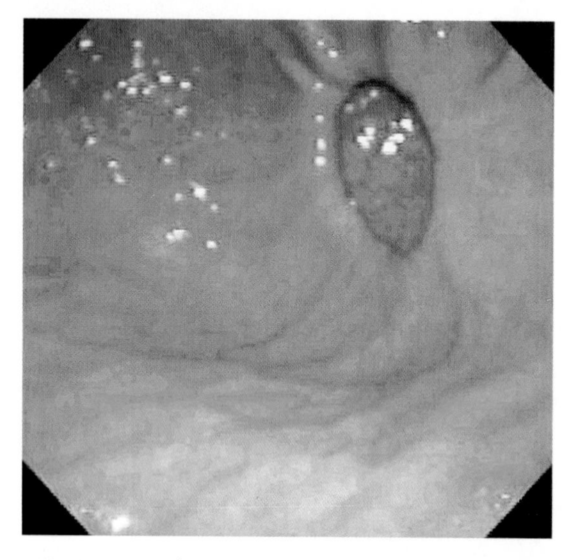

Figure 19–7. Juxtacardiac gastric diverticulum. This wide-mouthed diverticulum was noted on a retroflexed view of the cardia. The mucosa within the diverticulum is normal.

more likely to resolve with diverticulectomy. Bleeding, ulceration, and cancer formation are rare.[55, 56] Diagnosis is made by endoscopy. Juxtacardiac diverticula are best seen on retroflexed view. Juxtacardiac diverticula may be missed on barium study unless lateral views are taken. On CT scan they may appear as an air-filled or contrast-filled suprarenal mass that is not contiguous with the adrenal gland.[57]

Intramural diverticula do not usually cause symptoms. They are often mistaken for ulcers on barium studies, but movement with peristalsis should suggest the correct diagnosis.

Treatment and Prognosis

Juxtacardiac diverticula almost never need treatment. Clear association with a specific symptom complex is essential prior to resection. Bleeding, perforation, or associated cancer,[55] although rare, is treated by diverticulectomy or partial gastrectomy. Laparoscopic diverticulectomy has been reported.[55, 56] Intramural diverticula require no intervention.

DUODENAL DIVERTICULA

Duodenal diverticula can be either extraluminal or intraluminal. Extraluminal diverticula are thought to be acquired, whereas intraluminal diverticula are most likely related to congenital anomalies.

Extraluminal Duodenal Diverticula

Extraluminal duodenal diverticula are noted in up to 6% of upper gastrointestinal radiographic studies, in up to 27% of ERCPs, and in as many as 23% of autopsies.[58, 59] They are thought to be acquired. They arise in an area of the duodenal wall where a vessel penetrates or where the dorsal and ventral pancreas fuse in embryologic development. Alternative hypotheses have focused on increased intraduodenal pressure and increased levels of motilin and somatostatin.[58] Approximately 75% of these diverticula are within 2 cm of the ampulla and are termed *juxtapapillary diverticula* (JPD). When the papilla arises within the diverticulum, the term *intradiverticular papilla* (IDP) is used.[58]

Patients with extraluminal diverticula are in the 5th to 7th decade of life, and there is a slight male predominance. About 70% of JPD and IDP arise on the medial wall of the duodenum. Only 4% arise on the lateral wall.[60]

Clinical Presentation and Diagnosis

Only about 10% of extraluminal duodenal diverticula are associated with symptoms. Of these, only 1% will need any intervention.[60] Duodenal diverticulitis presents as pain in the epigastrium radiating to the back, associated with other signs

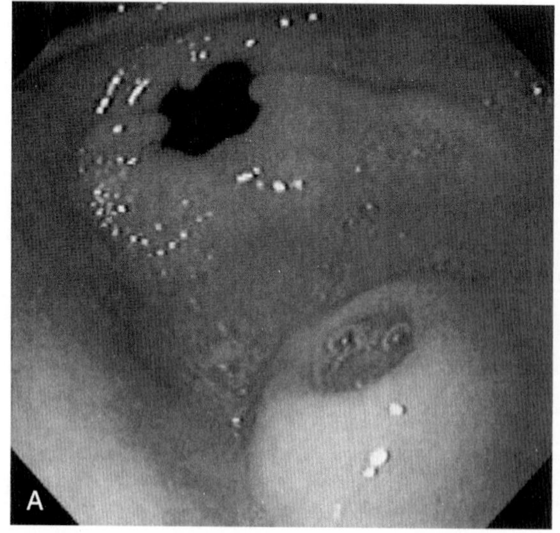

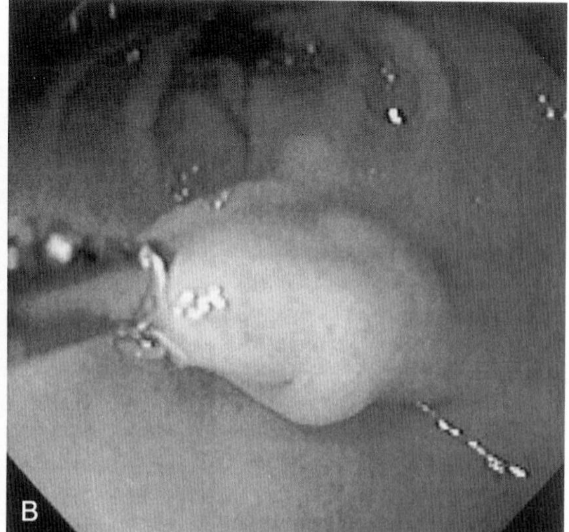

Figure 19–8. *A* and *B*, Intramural gastric diverticulum. *A*, The diverticulum protrudes into the lumen of the antrum, suggesting the possibility of a pancreatic rest or mass. *B*, However, the biopsy forceps is used to evert the mucosa, confirming that it is an intramural diverticulum.

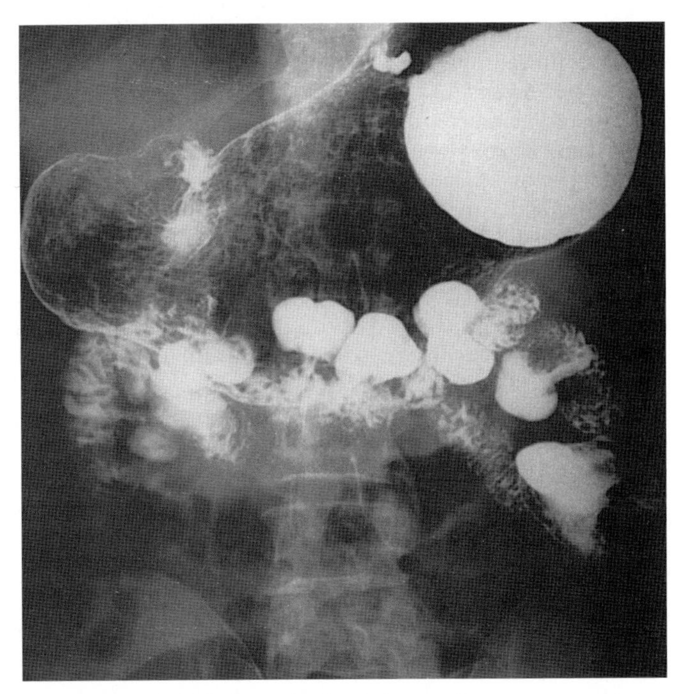

Figure 19–9. Multiple large duodenal diverticula are seen on this barium upper gastrointestinal radiograph.

and symptoms of sepsis. Plain films of the abdomen can reveal retroperitoneal air. Abdominal CT scan may reveal thickening with evidence of retroperitoneal air or phlegmon.[61] The less common lateral wall diverticula may present as free intraperitoneal rupture and acute abdomen. Rarely, bleeding from ulcerations within the diverticula can occur. Patients with multiple diverticula may develop bacterial overgrowth, with malabsorption and diarrhea (see Chapter 90).[58, 62] On ultrasound and CT the diverticulum may be mistaken for a pancreatic pseudocyst, peripancreatic fluid collection, ampullary tumor, or distal common bile duct stone.[63, 64] However, the presence of air within the structure should suggest the diagnosis of a diverticulum. Diverticula are typically diagnosed on upper gastrointestinal radiograph (Fig. 19–9). They may be missed on endoscopy, particularly if the endoscopy is done with a forward-viewing endoscope.

JPD may be associated with choledocholithiasis, cholangitis, recurrent pancreatitis, and sphincter of Oddi dysfunction. However, it has been difficult to provide a clear link between the presence of these diverticula and the development of any of these conditions.[58] Some groups now think that JPD should be ruled out in cases of otherwise idiopathic recurrent pancreatitis.[65] Stasis within these types of diverticula can result in local bacterial overgrowth, with deconjugation of bilirubin and an increased incidence of common bile duct stones.[66]

Treatment and Prognosis

Only 1% of extraluminal duodenal diverticula require intervention. Surgery should never be done for vague abdominal complaints. Bleeding and perforation are the most common problems. Endoscopic control of bleeding from diverticula has been reported, using a variety of techniques, including bipolar cautery, epinephrine injection, and application of hemoclips.[67, 68] When surgical intervention is necessary, diverticulectomy with primary closure of the duodenum or inversion of the diverticulum with duodenal reinforcement can be performed. Damage to the main pancreatic and biliary duct may occur during surgery for medial diverticula. Medial wall diverticula should be managed nonoperatively, if possible. Lateral diverticula can be treated laparoscopically.[60] Only urgent surgical intervention should be undertaken. Control of hemorrhage can be often accomplished through a lateral duodenotomy. Wide drainage of perforated medial diverticula is preferred to urgent pancreaticoduodenectomy.[69]

INTRALUMINAL DUODENAL DIVERTICULA (see Chapter 84)

Intraluminal duodenal diverticula, or windsock diverticula, are single saccular structures that usually originate in the second portion of the duodenum. They are connected either to the entire circumference or to only part of the wall of the duodenum, and they may project as far distally as the fourth part of the duodenum. There is often a second opening located eccentrically in the sac (Fig. 19–10). Both sides of the diverticulum are lined by duodenal mucosa. Fewer than 100 cases have been reported.

Etiology and Pathogenesis

During early fetal development, the duodenal lumen is occluded by proliferating epithelial cells and later recanalized. Abnormal recanalization may lead to a duodenal diaphragm or web. An incomplete or fenestrated diaphragm may not produce obstructive symptoms in childhood. However, over time, peristaltic stretching may transform the diaphragm into an intraluminal diverticulum.

Clinical Presentation and Diagnosis

Intraluminal diverticula may manifest at any age. The most common symptoms are those of incomplete duodenal obstruction.[70, 71] Plain abdominal radiograph can demonstrate findings of gastric retention or duodenal obstruction. Obstruction may be precipitated by retention of vegetable mate-

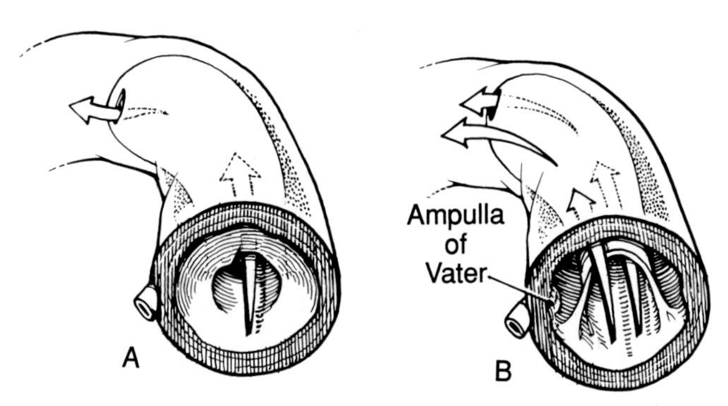

Figure 19–10. *A* and *B*, Intraluminal duodenal diverticulum (windsock diverticulum). *A*, Attachment to the entire duodenal circumference. *B*, Attachment to part of the duodenal circumference.

rial or foreign bodies. In one report, a 41-year-old man was found to have two marbles, swallowed during childhood, retained in an intraluminal diverticulum.[72] Pancreatitis and bleeding have also been reported.[73] The typical radiographic appearance is that of a barium-filled, globular structure of variable length, originating in the second portion of the duodenum with its fundus extending into the third portion, and outlined by a thin, radiolucent line. At endoscopy, an intraluminal diverticulum is seen as a saclike structure with an eccentric aperture or as a large, soft, polypoid mass, particularly if inverted orad.[74]

Treatment and Prognosis

Surgical treatment of intraluminal diverticula consists of lateral duodenotomy and excision, with care to preserve the ampulla of Vater. Fiberoptic endoscopy has been used to remove obstructing foreign bodies and to enlarge the outlet by use of needle-knife and diathermy snare. Endoscopic disruption of the weblike defects can be attempted.[74, 75]

JEJUNAL DIVERTICULA

Diverticula of the small bowel (apart from duodenal and Meckel's diverticula) are most commonly found in the proximal jejunum.[76] About 80% of jejunoileal diverticula arise in the jejunum, 15% in the ileum, and 5% in both[77] (see Chapter 90, Fig. 90–2). Small bowel diverticula were found in 0.5% to 7.1% of small bowel series and 0.3% to 4.5% of autopsies.[77, 78] These lesions are commonly multiple and can vary from millimeters to 10 cm in length. They are usually located on the mesenteric border of the small bowel. Small bowel diverticula are generally acquired in that they lack a true muscular wall.

Etiology and Pathogenesis

The etiology of jejunoileal diverticula is largely unknown. It has been suggested that chronic increase in intraluminal pressure due to underlying intestinal dysmotility can lead to herniation of layers of the bowel wall. The point of weakness tends to lie at the mesenteric border, where blood vessels penetrate the intestine.[79] This results in mesenteric diverticula, in contrast with Meckel's diverticula that occur on the antimesenteric border of the bowel (see Chapter 84). Visceral neuropathies and myopathies, including progressive systemic sclerosis (see Chapter 29), can lead to chronic atrophy and fibrosis of the intestinal wall, with resultant herniation and diverticula formation.[79]

Clinical Presentation and Diagnosis

Most jejunoileal diverticula are asymptomatic and 40% of cases are discovered incidentally.[78] In 1881, Osler wrote about a patient with jejunal diverticula who for years "had suffered much from loud rumbling noises in his belly, particularly after each meal. So loud were they that it was his habit, shortly after eating, to go out and take a walk to keep away from people, as the noises could be heard at some distance."[80] The most common symptom is abdominal pain (49%), followed by gastrointestinal bleeding (30%). Diarrhea (1.1%) and fever (3.4%) may occur.[76] Small bowel diverticula can be the cause of significant gastrointestinal bleeding. They can be extremely difficult to diagnose.[81] Pseudo-obstruction, abdominal bloating, pain, perforation, enterolith formation, and volvulus have been reported.[79, 82] Malabsorption can result from stasis and bacterial overgrowth (see Chapter 90).[83, 84] Jejunal diverticula are most efficiently diagnosed with barium contrast radiographs. Operative diagnosis can be difficult, even in experienced hands. The finding of a mesenteric inflammatory mass should raise the possibility of small bowel diverticula. The presence of simultaneous colonic and small bowel diverticula can make the localization of gastrointestinal bleeding especially difficult.

Treatment and Prognosis

Surgical resection of the section of bowel with diverticula is the treatment of choice for gastrointestinal bleeding and diverticulitis.[81, 85] Among patients with multiple small bowel diverticula and diverticulitis, the offending diverticulum can be difficult to find. These patients are often treated with antibiotics. Recurrent episodes of diverticulitis present a management problem. Repeated and extensive resection may lead to a short bowel syndrome. Surgical treatment of patients with chronic intestinal dysmotilities is fraught with complications and should be avoided. However, occasionally surgery is necessary for intestinal pseudo-obstruction.[78, 86, 87] Chronic malabsorption can be treated with oral antibiotics to decrease bacterial overgrowth (see Chapter 90).

REFERENCES

1. Ludlow AA: A case of obstructed deglutition from a preternatural dilatation of a bag formed in the pharynx. Med Observat Inquir 3:85–101, 1767.
2. Zenker FA, Von Ziemssen H: Krankheiten des oesophagus. In Von Ziemssen Heds Handbuck der Specielien: Pathologie und Therapie 7:1–87, 1877.
3. Kelly JH: Management of upper esophageal sphincter disorders: Indications and complications of myotomy. Am J Med 108:43S–46S, 2000.
4. Sideris L, Chen LQ, Ferraro P, et al: The treatment of Zenker's diverticula: A review. Semin Thorac Cardiovasc Surg 11:337–337, 1999.
5. Cook IJ, Gabb M, Panagopoulos V: Pharyngeal (Zenker's) diverticulum is a disorder of upper esophageal sphincter opening. Gastroenterology 103:1229–1235, 1992.
6. Cook IJ, Blumbergs P, Cash K: Structural abnormalities of the cricopharyngeus muscle in patients with pharyngeal (Zenker's) diverticulum. J Gastroenterol 7:556–562, 1992.
7. Lerut T, van Raemdonck D, Guelinckx P: Zenker's diverticulum: Is a myotomy of the cricopharyngeus useful? How long should it be? Hepatogastroenterology 39:127–131, 1992.
8. Resouly A, Braat J, Jackson A, et al: Pharyngeal pouch: Link with reflux and oesophageal dysmotility. Clin Otolaryngol 19:241–242, 1994.
9. Feussner H, Siewert JR: Zenker's diverticulum and reflux. Hepatogastroenterology 39:100–104, 2001.
10. Ellis FH: Pharyngoesophageal (Zenker's) diverticulum. Adv Surg 28:171–189, 1995.
11. Tsang T, Buto SK: Catheter-guided endoscopic intubation: A new technique for intubating a difficult esophagus. Gastrointest Endosc 38:49–51, 1992.
12. Dickey W, Porter KG: Duodenoscope intubation of the oesophagus in the presence of pharyngeal pouch made possible by an overtube. Endoscopy 27:212–213, 1995.

13. Payne WS: The treatment of pharyngoesophageal diverticulum: The simple and complex. Hepatogastroenterology 39:109–114, 1992.
14. Feeley M, Righi PD, Weisberger EC, et al: Zenker's diverticulum: Analysis of surgical complications from diverticulectomy and cricopharyngeal myotomy. Laryngoscope 109:858–861, 2000.
15. Zbären P, Schär P, Tschopp L, et al: Surgical treatment of Zenker's diverticulum: Transcutaneous diverticulectomy versus microendoscopic myotomy of the cricopharyngeal muscle with CO_2 laser. Otolaryngol Head Neck Surg 121:482–487, 1999.
16. Gregoire J, Duranceau A: Surgical management of Zenker's diverticulum. Hepatogastroenterology 39:132–138, 1992.
17. Hashiba K, de Paula AL, da Silva JG, et al: Endoscopic treatment of Zenker's diverticulum. Gastrointest Endosc 49:93–97, 1999.
18. Mulder CJ: Zenker's diverticulum: Treatment with a flexible endoscope. Gastrointest Endosc 50:596–597, 1999.
19. Mulder CJJ, den Hartog G, Robijn RJ, et al: Flexible endoscopic treatment of Zenker's diverticulum: A new approach. Endoscopy 27: 438–442, 1995.
20. Bremner C, DeMeester T: Endoscopic treatment of Zenker's diverticulum. Gastrointest Endosc 49:126–128, 1999.
21. Nyrop M, Svendstrup F, Jørgensen KE: Endoscopic CO_2 laser therapy of Zenker's diverticulum—experience from 61 patients. Acta Otolaryngol Suppl (Stockh) 543:232–234, 2000.
22. Luscher MS, Johansen LV: Zenker's diverticulum treated by the endoscopic stapling technique. Acta Otolaryngol (Stockh) 543:235–238, 2000.
23. Narne S, Cutrone C, Chella B, et al: Endoscopic diverticulotomy for the treatment of Zenker's diverticulum: Results in 102 patients with staple-assisted endoscopy. Ann Otol Rhinol Laryngol 108:810–815, 1999.
24. Philippsen LP, Weisberger EC, Whiteman TS, et al: Endoscopic stapled diverticulotomy: Treatment of choice for Zenker's diverticulum. Laryngoscope 110:1283–1286, 2000.
25. Omote K, Feussner H, Stein HJ, et al: Endoscopic stapling diverticulostomy for Zenker's diverticulum. Surg Endosc 13:535–538, 1999.
26. Lippert BM, Folz BJ, Rudert HH, et al: Management of Zenker's diverticulum and postlaryngectomy pseudodiverticulum with the CO_2 laser. Otolaryngol Head Neck Surg 121:809–814, 1999.
27. Peracchia A, Bonavina L, Narne S, et al: Minimally invasive surgery for Zenker diverticulum. Arch Surg 133:695–700, 1998.
28. Yoshida J, Ikeda S, Mizumachi S, et al: Epiphrenic diverticulum composed of airway components attributed to a bronchopulmonary-foregut malformation: Report of a case. Surg Today 29:663–665, 1998.
29. Reddy ER, Smith J, Clarke H: Esophageal diverticula. Can Assoc Radiol J 40:306–307, 1989.
30. Benacci JC, Deschamps C, Trastek VF: Epiphrenic diverticulum: Results of surgical treatment. Ann Thorac Surg 55:1109–1113, 1993.
31. Fekete F, Vonns C: Surgical management of esophageal thoracic diverticula. Hepatogastroenterology 39:97–99, 1992.
32. D'ugo D, Cardillo G, Granone P, et al: Esophageal diverticula: Physiopathological basis of surgical management. Eur J Cardiothorac Surg 6: 330–334, 1992.
33. Jordan PH, Kinner BM: New look at epiphrenic diverticula. World J Surg 23:147–152, 1999.
34. Myers BS, Dempsey DT: Laparoscopic resection of esophageal epiphrenic diverticulum [abstract]. J Laparoendosc Adv Surg Tech 8:201–207, 1998.
35. Tinoco RC, Tinoco AC, El-Kadre L: Perforated epiphrenic diverticulum treated by video laparoscopy. Surg Endosc 13:270–272, 1999.
36. Niv Y, Fraser G, Krugliak P: Gastroesophageal obstruction from food in an epiphrenic esophageal diverticulum. J Clin Gastroenterol 16:314–316, 1993.
37. Streitz JM Jr, Glick ME, Ellis FH: Selective use of myotomy for treatment of epiphrenic diverticula: Manometric and clinical analysis. Arch Surg 127:585–587, 1992.
38. Rosati R, Fumagalli U, Bona S, et al: Diverticulectomy, myotomy, and fundoplication through laparoscopy. Ann Surg 227:174–178, 1998.
39. Chami Z, Fabre JM, Navarro F, et al: Abdominal laparoscopic approach for thoracic epiphrenic diverticulum. Surg Endosc 13:164–165, 1999.
40. Ott DJ, Hodge RG, Chen MY: Achalasia associated with esophageal diverticula: Prevalence and potential implications. J Clin Gastroenterol 18:343–346, 1994.
41. Tarnasky PR, Brazer SR, Leung JW: Esophageal perforation during achalasia dilation complicated by esophageal diverticula. Am J Gastroenterol 89:1583–1585, 1994.
42. Canon C, Levine M, Cherukuri R, et al: Intramural tracking: A feature of esophageal intramural pseudodiverticulosis. AJR Am J Roentgenol 175:371–374, 2000.
43. Devereaux CE, Savides TJ: EUS appearance of esophageal pseudodiverticulosis. Gastrointest Endosc 51:228–231, 2000.
44. Wong J, Walton M, Issenman R: Ruptured esophageal intramural pseudodiverticulum: An unusual cause of mediastinitis in a child. Can J Surg 42:389–391, 1999.
45. Levine MS, Moolten DN, Herlinger H, et al: Esophageal intramural pseudodiverticulosis: A reevaluation. AJR Am J Roentgenol 147:1165–1170, 1986.
46. Kochhar R, Mehta SK, Nagi B, et al: Corrosive acid–induced esophageal intramural pseudodiverticulosis: A study of 14 patients. J Clin Gastroenterol 13:371–375, 1991.
47. Lingaraj K, Prabhakaran K, Quak SH: Esophageal intramural pseudodiverticulosis associated with a web in a 12-year-old boy. J Pediatr Surg 34:1573–1574, 1999.
48. Plavsic BM, Chen MYM, Gelfand DW: Intramural pseudodiverticulosis of the esophagus detected on barium esophagrams: Increased prevalence in patients with esophageal carcinoma. AJR Am J Roentgenol 165:1381–1385, 1995.
49. Castrucci G, Porziella V, Granone PL, Picciocchi A: Tailored surgery for esophageal body diverticula. Eur J Cardiothorac Surg 14:380–387, 1998.
50. Fine A: Laparoscopic resection of a large proximal gastric diverticulum. Gastrointest Endosc 48:93–95, 1998.
51. Palmer ED: Gastric diverticulosis. Am Fam Physician 7:114, 1973.
52. Fine AP: Laparoscopic resection of a gastric diverticulum [letter to the editor]. J Laparoendosc Adv Surg Tech 9:369, 1999.
53. Dickinson RJ, Freeman AH: Partial gastric diverticula: Radiologic and endoscopic features in six patients. Gut 27:954–957, 1986.
54. Anaise D, Brand DL, Smith NL, et al: Pitfalls in the diagnosis and treatment of a symptomatic gastric diverticulum. Gastrointest Endosc 30:28–30, 1984.
55. Fork FT, Toth E, Lindstrom C: Early gastric cancer in a fundic diverticulum. Endoscopy 30:S2, 1998.
56. Kim SH, Lee SW, Choi WJ, et al: Laparoscopic resection of gastric diverticulum. J Laparoendosc Adv Surg Techn 9:87–91, 1999.
57. Verbeeck N, De Geeter T: Suprarenal mass due to a gastric diverticulum. J Belge Radiol 77:119–120, 1994.
58. Lobo DN, Balfour TW, Iftikhar SY, et al: Periampullary diverticula and pancreaticobiliary disease. Br J Surg 86:588–597, 1999.
59. Lotyeit T, Skar V, Osnes M: Juxtapapillary duodenal diverticula. Endoscopy 20:175–178, 1988.
60. Coelho J, Sousa GS, Lobo DN: Laparoscopic treatment of duodenal diverticulum. Surg Laparosc Endosc 9:74–77, 1999.
61. Gore RM, Ghahremani GG, Kirsch MD: Diverticulitis of the duodenum: Clinical and radiological manifestations of seven cases. Am J Gastroenterol 86:981–985, 1991.
62. Scudmore CH, Harrison RC, White T: Management of duodenal diverticula. Can J Surg 25:311–314, 1982.
63. Stone EE, Brant WE, Smith GB: Computed tomography of duodenal diverticula. J Comput Assist Tomogr 13:61–63, 1989.
64. Levin MF, Bach DB, Vellet AD, et al: Sonolucent peripancreatic masses: Differential diagnosis and related imaging. Can Assoc Radiol J 44:168–175, 1993.
65. Uomo G, Manes G, Rafozzino A, et al: Periampullary extraluminal duodenal diverticula and acute pancreatitis: An underestimated etiological association. Am J Gastroenterol 91:1186–1188, 1996.
66. Miyazaki S, Sakamoto T, Miyata M: Function of the sphincter of Oddi in patients with juxtapapillary duodenal diverticula: Evaluation by intraoperative biliary manometry under a duodenal pressure load. World J Surg 19:307–312, 1995.
67. Dalal AA, Rogers SJ, Cello JP: Endoscopic management of hemorrhage from a duodenal diverticulum. Gastrointest Endosc 48:1–4, 1998.
68. Wu NH, Wang HP, Yang CS, et al: Endoscopic hemoclip therapy of a bleeding duodenal diverticulum. Gastrointest Endosc 51:1–4, 2000.
69. Tsukamoto T, Ohta Y, Hamba H, et al: Perforated duodenal diverticulum: Report of two cases. Hepatogastroenterology 46:1755–1758, 1998.
70. Perich Alsina J, Vilana Puig R, Maroto Genover A: Diverticulos intraduodenales: A propósito de seis observaciones. Rev Esp Enferm Dig 75:53–57, 1989.
71. Karoll MP, Ghahremani GG, Port RB, et al: Diagnosis and management of intraluminal duodenal diverticulum. Dig Dis Sci 28:411–416, 1983.

72. Abdel-Hafiz AA, Birkett DH, Ahmed MS: Congenital duodenal diverticula: A report of three cases and a review of the literature. Surgery 104:74–78, 1988.
73. Finnie IA, Ghosh P, Garvey C: Intraluminal duodenal diverticulum causing recurrent pancreatitis: Treatment by endoscopic incision. Gut 35:557–559, 1994.
74. Adams DB: Management of the intraluminal duodenal diverticulum: Endoscopy or duodenotomy? Am J Surg 151:524–526, 1986.
75. Ravi J, Joson PM, Ashok PS: Endoscopic incision of intraluminal duodenal diverticulum: Case report of a new technique. Dig Dis Sci 38: 762–766, 1993.
76. Chiu EJ, Shyr YM, Su CH, et al: Diverticular disease of the small bowel. Hepatogastroenterology 47:181–184, 2000.
77. Longo WE. Vermava AM III: Clinical implications of jejunoileal diverticular disease. Dis Colon Rectum 35:381–388, 1992.
78. Tsiotos GG, Farnell MB, Ilstrup DM: Nonmeckelian jejunalileal diverticulosis: An analysis of 112 cases. Surgery 116:726–732, 1994.
79. Krishnamurthy S, Kelly MM, Rohrmann CA, et al: Jejunal diverticulosis: A heterogeneous disorder caused by a variety abnormalities of smooth muscle or myenteric plexus. Gastroenterology 85:538–538, 1983.
80. Osler W: Notes on intestinal diverticula. Ann Anat Surg 40:202–203, 1881.
81. Hamada N, Ishizaki N, Shirahama K, et al: Multiple duodenojejunal diverticula causing massive intestinal bleeding. J Gastroenterol 35:159–162, 1999.
82. Chiu KW, Changchien CS, Chuah SK: Small-bowel diverticulum: Is it a risk for small-bowel volvulus? Gastroenterology 19:170–177, 1994.
83. Palder SB, Frey CB: Jejunal diverticulosis. Arch Surg 123:889–894, 1999.
84. Montalvo II, Cosme A, Aramburu V: Sobrecrecimiento bacteriano secundario a diverticulosis intestinal. Rev Esp Enferm Dig 87:535–537, 1995.
85. Kawamura S, Nishijima M, Yamamoto T, et al: Massive bleeding from multiple jejunal diverticula associated with an angiodysplasia: Report of a case. Surg Today 30:750–753, 2000.
86. Brown JE, Vallette R, Brown J: Recurrent jejunal diverticulosis. South Med J 78:352–353, 1985.
87. Noel RF, Schuffler MD, Helton WS: Small bowel resection for relief of chronic intestinal pseudo-obstruction. Am J Gastroenterol 90:1142–1145, 1995.

Chapter 20

Abdominal Hernias and Their Complications, Including Gastric Volvulus

William Harford and Rohan Jeyarajah

A hernia is a protrusion of an organ or structure into an opening or pouch. Abdominal wall hernias protrude through the retaining walls of the abdomen and have two parts: the orifice or defect in the aponeurotic wall of the abdomen, and the hernia sac, which consists of peritoneum and abdominal contents. Internal hernias are contained within the abdominal cavity and do not always have a hernia sac. Abdominal wall hernias are termed *external* if the sac protrudes through the abdominal wall or *interparietal* if the sac is contained within the abdominal wall. Hernias are *reducible* when the protruding organ can be returned to the abdomen and *irreducible* or *incarcerated* when it cannot. A hernia is *strangulated* when the vascular supply of the protruding organ is compromised and the organ becomes ischemic or necrotic as a consequence. In a *Richter's hernia* only one side of the bowel (usually the antimesenteric) protrudes through the hernia orifice. Thus, strangulation may occur without intestinal obstruction. Richter's hernias may occur in various locations.

DIAPHRAGMATIC HERNIAS

Diaphragmatic hernias may occur through the esophageal hiatus, through other congenital openings (such as the foramina of Bochdalek or Morgagni), or through post-traumatic defects. Most diaphragmatic hernias are sliding hernias of the stomach through the esophageal hiatus.

Etiology and Pathogenesis

Sliding hiatal hernias occur when the gastroesophageal junction and some portion of the stomach are displaced above the diaphragm. The orientation of the stomach axis is unchanged. The cause of sliding hiatal hernias is not known. The frequency of sliding hiatal hernias increases with age. The phrenoesophageal membrane anchors the gastroesophageal junction to the diaphragm. Hiatal hernias may be due to age-related deterioration of this membrane, combined with normal positive intra-abdominal pressure, and with traction of the esophagus on the stomach as the esophagus shortens during swallows.

Paraesophageal hernias occur when the stomach protrudes through the esophageal hiatus alongside the esophagus. The gastroesophageal junction may remain in a normal position at the level of the diaphragm. The entire stomach can pass into the chest (Fig. 20–1*A*). Gastric volvulus (discussed later) may result. The omentum, colon, or spleen may also enter the hernia. Patients who develop paraesophageal hernias may have a congenital defect in the diaphragmatic hiatus anterior to the esophagus. Most paraesophageal hernias contain a sliding hiatal component in addition to the paraesophageal component and are thus *mixed diaphragmatic hernias* (Fig. 20–1*B*).[1, 2]

Congenital diaphragmatic hernias result from failure of fusion of the multiple developmental components of the diaphragm (Fig. 20–2). The diaphragm is derived from the septum transversum (separating the peritoneal and pericardial spaces), the mesentery of the esophagus, the pleuroperitoneal membranes, and the muscle of the chest wall. Congenital hernias occur where fusion of these components fails. *Morgagni hernias* form at the sternocostal junctions of the diaphragm anteriorly and *Bochdalek hernias* at the lumbocostal junctions of the diaphragm posterolaterally[3] (Fig. 20–3).

Post-traumatic diaphragmatic hernias are due to blunt trauma (such as motor vehicle collisions) in about 80% of cases and to penetrating trauma (such as stab wounds or gunshots) in the remainder. During blunt trauma, abrupt changes in intra-abdominal pressure may lead to large rents in the diaphragm. Penetrating injuries often cause only small lacerations. Blunt trauma is more likely than penetrating

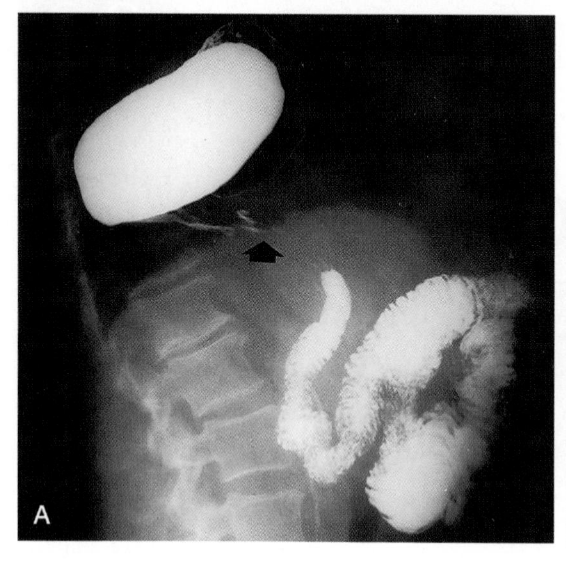

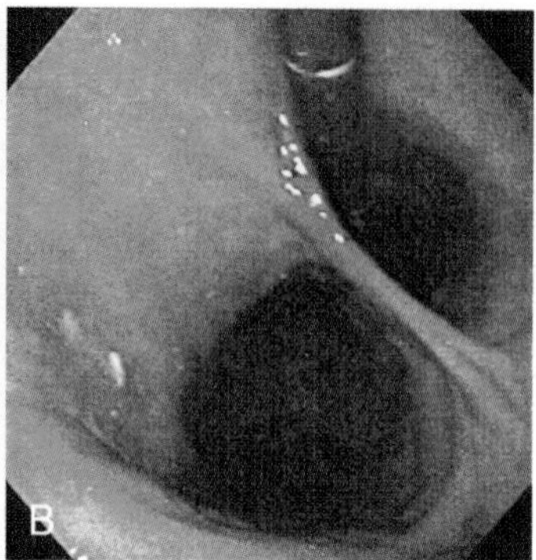

Figure 20–1. *A*, Paraesophageal hernia. A barium radiograph shows a paraesophageal hernia complicated by organoaxial volvulus of the stomach (see Fig. 20–6). The gastroesophageal junction remains in a relatively normal position below the diaphragm (*arrow*). The entire stomach has herniated into the chest, whereas the greater curvature has rotated anteriorly and superiorly. (Courtesy of H. J. Smith, MD.) *B*, Mixed hernia. In a different patient, a retroflexed endoscopic view of the proximal stomach shows the endoscope traversing a sliding hiatal hernia (right) adjacent to a large paraesophageal hernia (left).

trauma to lead to herniation of abdominal contents into the chest because the defect is usually larger. The right hemidiaphragm is somewhat protected by the liver during blunt trauma. Thus, about 70% of diaphragmatic injuries from blunt trauma occur on the left.[4–7] Diaphragmatic injury may not result in immediate herniation, but with time, normal negative intrathoracic pressure may lead to gradual enlargement of a small diaphragmatic defect and protrusion of abdominal contents through the defect. Stomach, omentum, colon, small bowel, spleen, and even kidney may be found in a post-traumatic diaphragmatic hernia.[4–6, 8]

Incidence and Prevalence

In the United States and Canada, a large proportion of adults undergoing upper gastrointestinal barium radiographs are found to have a small hiatal hernia. About 90% to 95% of hiatal hernias found by radiograph are sliding hernias, and the rest are paraesophageal or mixed.[1, 2] Most sliding hiatal hernias are small and of little clinical significance. Patients with symptomatic paraesophageal hernias are most often middle-aged to elderly.

Congenital hernias occur in about 0.1 to 0.5 per 1000 births.[9, 10] Those presenting in neonates are most often Bochdalek hernias. Only a few Bochdalek hernias are first discovered in adulthood.[9, 11, 12] Bochdalek hernias occur on the left in about 80% of cases[10] (see Fig. 20–3). Morgagni hernias make up about 2% to 3% of surgically treated diaphragmatic hernias.[9, 13, 14] Although thought to be congenital, they usually present in adults. They occur on the right side in 80% to 90% of cases.

Figure 20–2. Congenital diaphragmatic hernias. Diagram of the diaphragm from below with areas of potential herniation indicated. 1, Sternocostal foramina of Morgagni anteriorly; 2, Esophageal hiatus; 3, Lumbocostal foramina of Bochdalek posteriorly.

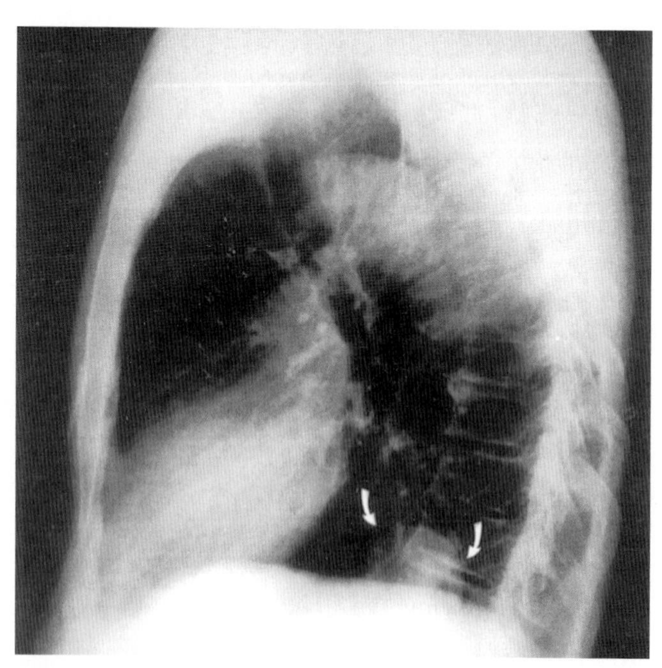

Figure 20–3. Bochdalek hernia. A plain chest radiograph in the lateral view shows a Bochdalek hernia as a small opacity in the posterior chest at the level of the diaphragm (*arrows*). (Courtesy of Nahid Eshaghi, MD.)

The incidence of post-traumatic diaphragmatic hernia is uncertain. Diaphragmatic injury occurs in about 5% of patients with multiple traumatic injuries.[7, 8]

Clinical Manifestations and Diagnosis

Many patients with small, simple *sliding hiatal hernias* are asymptomatic. The main clinical significance of the sliding hiatal hernia is its contribution to gastroesophageal reflux (see Chapter 33). In addition to heartburn and regurgitation, patients with large sliding hiatal hernias may complain of dysphagia or discomfort in the chest or upper abdomen. In a prospective, population-based study the risk of iron-deficiency anemia was found to be increased (hazard rate 2.9) in adults with hiatal hernia.[15] On chest radiograph a hiatal hernia may be noted as a soft tissue density in the retrocardiac area. Hiatal hernias are most often diagnosed on upper gastrointestinal barium radiographic studies. At endoscopy the gastroesophageal junction is noted to be proximal to the impression of the diaphragm.

Patients with sliding hiatal hernias, particularly large hernias, may develop *Cameron ulcers* or *erosions* (see Chapter 40). These mucosal lesions are usually found on the lesser curve of the stomach at the level of the diaphragmatic hiatus (Fig. 20–4). This is the location of the rigid anterior margin of the hiatus formed by the central tendon of the diaphragm. Mechanical trauma, ischemia, and peptic injury have been proposed as the etiology of these lesions. The prevalence of Cameron ulcers among patients with hiatal hernias has been reported to be about 5% of those undergoing endoscopy, with the highest prevalence in the largest hernias. Cameron ulcers may cause acute or chronic upper gastrointestinal bleeding.[16]

Patients with *paraesophageal* and *mixed hiatal hernias* are rarely completely asymptomatic if closely questioned. About half of patients with paraesophageal hernias have gastroesophageal reflux.[2, 17–19] Other symptoms include dysphagia, chest pain, vague postprandial discomfort, and shortness of breath.[1, 2, 18–20] A substantial number of patients have chronic gastrointestinal blood loss.[2, 17, 20] If the hernia is complicated by gastric volvulus, acute abdominal pain and retching will occur, often progressing rapidly to a surgical emergency (see section on Gastric Volvulus). A paraesophageal or mixed hiatal hernia may be seen on chest radiograph as an abnormal soft tissue density (often with a gas bubble) in the mediastinum. Upper gastrointestinal radiograph is the best diagnostic study (see Fig. 20–1*A*). Paraesophageal hernias are usually obvious on upper gastrointestinal endoscopy (see Fig. 20–1*B*), but the paraesophageal component of a large mixed hernia may be missed. Endoscopy may be difficult if the hernia is associated with gastric volvulus.

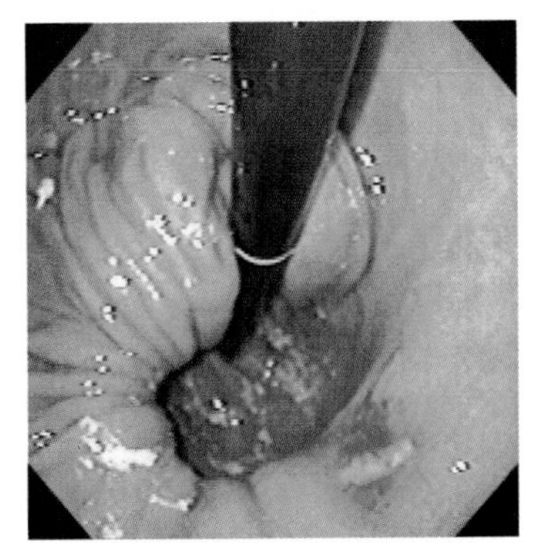

Figure 20–4. Cameron ulcer. A large hiatal hernia is seen on an endoscopic retroflex view, with a Cameron ulcer at the level of the diaphragmatic hiatus.

The presentation of *congenital diaphragmatic hernias* varies greatly, from death in the neonatal period to an asymptomatic serendipitous finding in adults. Newborns with *Bochdalek hernia* have respiratory distress, absent breath sounds on one side of the chest, and a scaphoid abdomen.[10, 21] Serious chromosomal anomalies are found in 30% to 40% of cases. The most common of these are trisomy 13, 18, and 21. Pulmonary hypoplasia occurs on the side of the hernia, but some degree of hypoplasia may also occur in the contralateral lung. Pulmonary hypertension is common. The major causes of mortality in infants with Bochdalek hernias are associated anomalies and respiratory failure. Prenatal diagnosis may be made at sonography by visualizing stomach or loops of bowel in the chest. In older children and adults, a Bochdalek hernia may present as an asymptomatic chest mass. The differential includes mediastinal or pulmonary cyst or tumor, pleural effusion, or empyema. Symptoms, when present, are due to herniation of the stomach, omentum, colon, or spleen. About half of adult patients present with acute emergencies due to incarceration. Gastric volvulus is common (see later). Other patients may have chronic intermittent symptoms, including chest discomfort, shortness of breath, dysphagia, nausea, vomiting, or constipation.[22] The diagnosis may be suspected on chest radiograph, particularly a lateral view, because Bochdalek hernias occur in the posterior chest (see Fig. 20–3). The diagnosis may be confirmed by barium upper gastrointestinal radiograph or by computed tomographic (CT) scan.[9, 12]

Morgagni hernias are most likely to present in adult life. They may contain omentum, stomach, colon, or liver. As with Bochdalek hernias, the diagnosis is often made by chest radiograph, particularly the lateral, because Morgagni hernias are anterior (Fig. 20–5*A* and *B*). The contents of the hernia can be confirmed with barium radiographs or CT scan (Fig. 20–5*C* and *D*). The differential diagnosis is similar to that of Bochdalek hernias. Many patients have no symptoms or nonspecific symptoms such as chest discomfort, cough, dyspnea, or upper abdominal distress. Gastric, omental, or intestinal incarceration with obstruction and/or ischemia may cause acute symptoms.[13, 14]

Post-traumatic diaphragmatic hernias cause either respiratory or abdominal symptoms. After serious trauma, rupture of the diaphragm is often masked by other injuries.[5] Injuries between the fourth intercostal space and the umbilicus should raise the level of suspicion. Respiratory or abdominal symptoms presenting several days to weeks after injury should suggest the possibility of diaphragmatic injury. Diaphragmatic rupture may go undetected at exploratory laparotomy. Careful examination of the chest radiograph is important but is diagnostic in only half of the cases. The use of helical CT, especially with saggital reconstruction, has facilitated the diagnosis.[4, 8] Among patients on ventilatory support after trauma, positive intrathoracic pressure may prevent herniation through a diaphragmatic tear. However, on

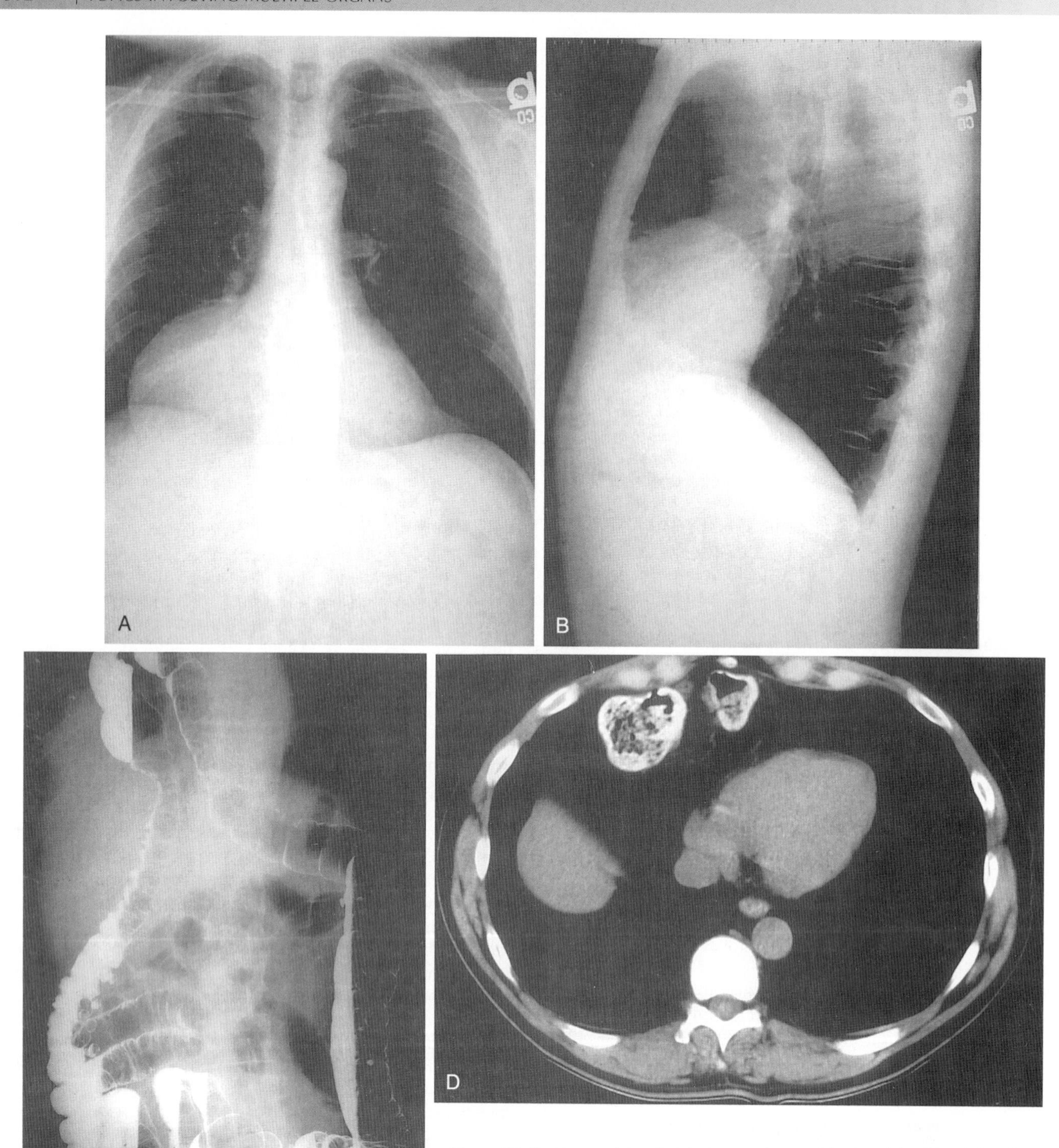

Figure 20–5. Morgagni hernia. *A,* A mass is noted in the right side of the chest on a posteroanterior view chest radiograph. *B,* A lateral chest radiograph shows that the mass is in the anterior chest. *C,* Barium enema shows that a portion of the transverse colon occupies the hernia. *D,* Computed tomography shows a contrast-filled colon in the right anterior chest.

attempted ventilator weaning, herniation may occur, causing respiratory compromise.[7] Symptoms may also present long after injury. Delays of more than 10 years are not uncommon.[6] In such cases the patient may not connect the acute illness and remote trauma.

Treatment and Prognosis

Simple *sliding hiatal hernias* do not require treatment. Patients with symptomatic *giant sliding hiatal hernias*, *paraesophageal*, and *mixed hernias* should be offered surgery.

Many experts suggest that surgery should be offered to patients with asymptomatic paraesophageal hernias, because about 30% of these patients will develop complications if left untreated.[1, 2, 20]

The extent of the preoperative evaluation needed for paraesophageal hernia repair is controversial. Many surgeons recommend routine preoperative evaluation with esophageal manometry and ambulatory esophageal pH monitoring because of the high prevalence of associated gastroesophageal reflux and esophageal motility disorders. The object of the evaluation is to determine which patients should have a fundoplication and whether to perform a complete or partial wrap. However, complete manometry is frequently not possible in these patients, and anatomic distortions may render esophageal pH monitoring unreliable.[19] Furthermore, many surgeons routinely add a fundoplication to all repairs, both to prevent postoperative reflux esophagitis and to fix the stomach in the abdomen.[18, 19, 23] Less commonly a gastrostomy is used to fix the stomach in position.[24] Patients with sliding hiatal or paraesophageal hernias may have shortening of the esophagus. This makes it difficult to restore the gastroesophageal junction below the diaphragm without tension. In such cases an extra length of neoesophagus can be constructed from the proximal stomach (Colles-Nissen procedure).[17] Paraesophageal and mixed hernias can be repaired through the chest or abdomen, with open or laparoscopic techniques.[18, 19, 23, 25] Compared with open repair, laparoscopic repair is associated with less blood loss, fewer overall complications, shorter hospital stay, and quicker return to normal activities. Long-term results are probably equal with either approach.[26] Potential surgical complications include esophageal and gastric perforation, pneumothorax, and liver laceration. Potential long-term complications may include dysphagia if the wrap is too tight or gastroesophageal reflux if the fundoplication breaks down or migrates into the chest. Recurrence rates are about 10%.[1, 27]

Like other gastric ulcers, *Cameron ulcers* or *erosions* are initially treated with antisecretory medication (see Chapter 40). However, Cameron lesions may persist or recur despite antisecretory medication in about one third of patients, in which case surgical repair of the associated hernia may be required.[16]

The first priority of treatment for infants with Bochdalek hernias is adequate ventilatory support. New techniques of ventilation, such as high-frequency oscillation and extracorporeal membrane oxygenation, are very helpful in some cases. Ventilatory support allows infants to be stabilized before diaphragmatic repair.[21] From 39% to 77% of infants survive the neonatal period after repair, but a significant number have long-term neurologic and musculoskeletal problems, and up to 50% develop gastroesophageal reflux.[10]

Laparoscopic repair of Bochdalek hernias has been reported.[11] *Morgagni hernias* have been repaired both through the chest and abdomen, using open, thoracoscopic, and/or laparoscopic techniques.[28–31]

Acute diaphragmatic ruptures may be approached from the abdomen during exploratory laparotomy or through the chest. Chronic post-traumatic diaphragmatic hernias may be associated with extensive adhesions and lack of a peritoneal hernia sac. In such cases repair is best done through the chest or by a combined thoracoscopic/abdominal approach, although laparoscopic repair has been reported.[6, 32]

GASTRIC VOLVULUS

Gastric volvulus is often associated with diaphragmatic hernia. Gastric volvulus occurs when the stomach twists on itself. The volvulus may be transient and produce few symptoms or may lead to obstruction and ischemia. Paré described the first case of gastric volvulus in 1579 in a patient who had a diaphragmatic injury from a sword wound.

Etiology and Pathogenesis

The stomach is normally fixed in position by ligamentous attachments to the duodenum, spleen, liver, and diaphragm. Laxity of these ligaments, elevation of the left hemidiaphragm, adhesions, gastric tumor, or masses in adjacent organs may predispose to volvulus. In about one third of cases the volvulus occurs below the diaphragm. In the other two thirds of cases volvulus occurs above the diaphragm in association with a diaphragmatic hernia. Sliding hiatal hernias are not associated with gastric volvulus.

Gastric volvulus may be *mesenteroaxial* or *organoaxial* (Fig. 20–6). In about 60% of cases gastric volvulus is organoaxial: the stomach twists along its long axis. This axis usually passes through the gastroesophageal and gastropyloric junctions. The antrum rotates anteriorly and superiorly, the fundus posteriorly and inferiorly, twisting the greater curvature at some point along its length (see Fig. 20–6, *3A* and *3B*). Less commonly the long axis passes through the body of the stomach itself, in which case the greater curvature of both antrum and fundus rotate anteriorly and superiorly (Fig. 20–7; see also Fig. 20–6, *2A* and *2B*). This type of volvulus is commonly associated with a diaphragmatic hernia. Organoaxial volvulus is usually an acute event. Vascular compromise and gastric infarction may occur. The other major type of gastric volvulus is mesenteroaxial, in which the stomach folds on its short axis running across from the lesser curvature to the greater curvature (see Fig. 20–6, *1A* and *1B*), and the antrum twists anteriorly and superiorly. In rare cases the antrum and pylorus rotate posteriorly. Mesenteroaxial volvulus is more likely than organoaxial volvulus to be incomplete, intermittent, and present with chronic symptoms. Mixed volvulus has been reported.[33]

Incidence and Prevalence

The incidence and prevalence of gastric volvulus are unknown. It is difficult to estimate how many cases are intermittent and undiagnosed. About 15% to 20% of cases occur in children younger than 1 year, most often in association with a congenital diaphragmatic defect. The peak incidence in adults is in the 5th decade. Men and women are equally affected.[33]

Clinical Manifestations and Diagnosis

Acute gastric volvulus causes sudden, severe pain in the upper abdomen or lower chest. Persistent, unproductive retching is common. In cases of complete volvulus, it is impossible to pass a nasogastric tube into the stomach. Hematemesis is rare but may occur owing to an esophageal tear or gastric mucosal ischemia.[34] The combination of pain, unproductive retching, and inability to pass a nasogastric tube is called *Borchardt's triad*. Symptoms of acute gastric volvulus may be mistaken for a myocardial infarction or an abdominal catastrophe such as biliary obstruction or acute pancreatitis.[33] If the volvulus is associated with a diaphragmatic hernia, physical examination may reveal evidence of the stomach in the left chest. Plain chest or abdominal films show a large gas-filled viscus in the chest. An upper gastrointestinal radiograph will confirm the diagnosis. Upper endoscopy may show twisting of the gastric folds (Fig. 20–8). However, endoscopy is not prudent if gastric ischemia is suspected.

Chronic gastric volvulus is associated with mild and nonspecific symptoms such as dysphagia, epigastric discomfort or fullness, bloating, and heartburn, particularly after meals. Symptoms may be present for months to years.[33, 35] It is likely that a substantial number of cases are unrecognized. The diagnosis should be suspected if an upper gastrointestinal radiograph shows a large diaphragmatic hernia, even if the stomach is not twisted at the time of the radiograph.

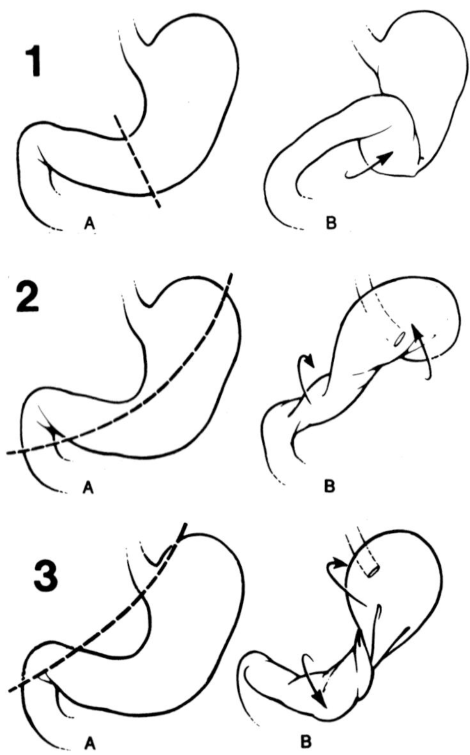

Figure 20–6. Pathogenesis of a gastric volvulus. 1A. Axis for potential mesenteroaxial volvulus bisecting the lesser and greater curvatures. 1B. Mesenteroaxial volvulus resulting from anterior rotation of the antrum along this axis. 2A. Axis for potential organoaxial volvulus passing through the body of the stomach. 2B. Organoaxial volvulus resulting from anterior, superior rotation of the antrum along this axis. 3A. Axis for potential organoaxial volvulus passing through the gastroesophageal junction and the pylorus. 3B. Organoaxial volvulus resulting from anterior superior rotation of the antrum and posterior inferior rotation of the fundus along this axis. (Redrawn from Carter R, Brewer LA, Hinshaw DB: Acute gastric volvulus. Am J Surg 140:101–102, 1980.)

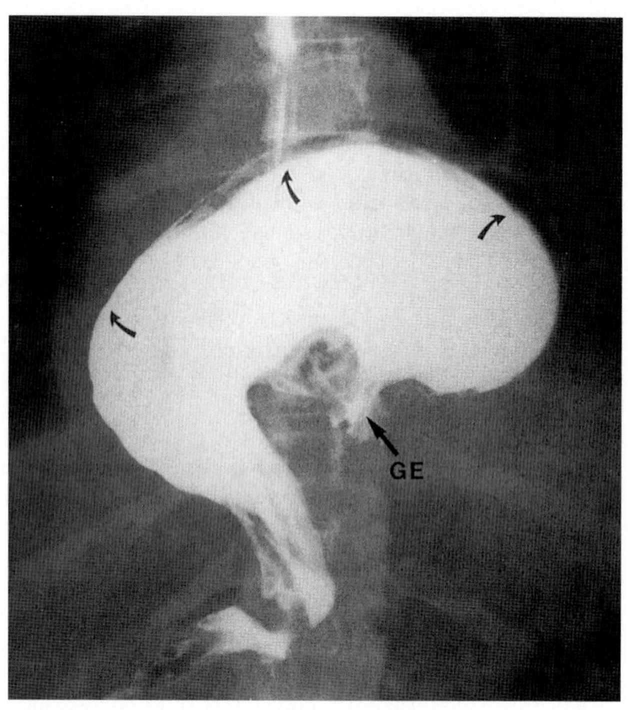

Figure 20–7. Gastric volvulus. The gastroesophageal junction (GE) is in the normal position. The stomach has herniated into a large paraesophageal hernia. The greater curvature and lesser curvature are reversed in position (upside-down stomach).

Treatment and Prognosis

Acute gastric volvulus is an emergency. Nasogastric decompression should be performed if possible. If signs of gastric infarction are not present, acute endoscopic detorsion may be considered. Using fluoroscopy, the endoscope is advanced to form an alpha loop in the proximal stomach. The tip is passed through the area of torsion into the antrum, or duodenum if possible, avoiding excess pressure. Torque may then reduce the gastric volvulus.[36, 37] The risk of gastric rupture should be weighed against the possible benefit of temporary detorsion. Surgery for gastric volvulus may be done by open or laparoscopic techniques. In recent years there has been a trend toward laparoscopic repair.[38] After the torsion is reduced the stomach is fixed by gastropexy or tube gastros-

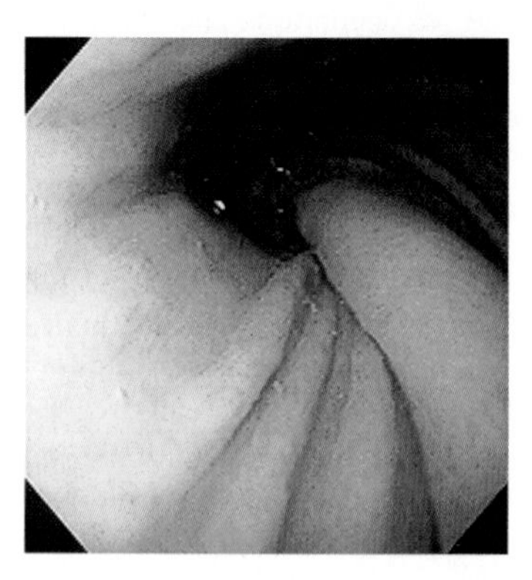

Figure 20–8. Gastric volvulus. Twisting of the gastric folds at the point of torsion is noted in this endoscopic view of a gastric volvulus.

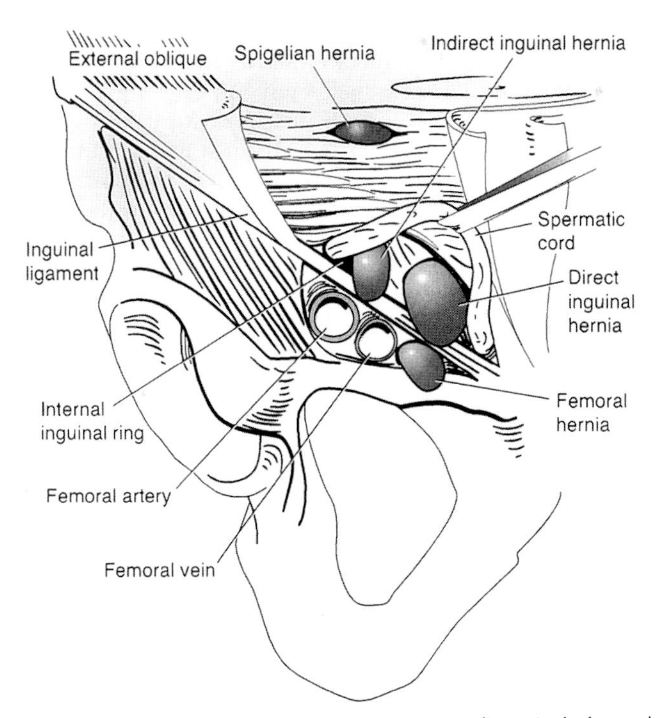

Figure 20–9. Anatomic diagram (anterior view) of inguinal, femoral, and Spigelian hernias. The external oblique muscle has been omitted, and the spermatic cord (corresponding to the round ligament in women) is retracted. Spigelian hernias occur through defects in the fused aponeurosis of the internal oblique and transverse abdominal muscles. Indirect inguinal hernias occur through the internal inguinal ring. Direct inguinal hernias occur through defects in the transversalis fascia in Hesselbach's triangle. Femoral hernias occur inferior to the inguinal ligament and medial to the femoral vein and femoral artery.

tomy. Associated diaphragmatic hernia must be repaired.[34] Combined endoscopic and laparoscopic repair or simple endoscopic gastropexy by placement of a percutaneous gastrostomy tube has been reported.[34, 39, 40] Chronic gastric volvulus is treated in the same manner as acute volvulus. Acute gastric volvulus has carried a high mortality in the past. However, in a recently reported series there were no major complications or deaths among 36 patients with gastric volvulus, including 29 who presented acutely.[34]

INGUINAL AND FEMORAL HERNIAS (GROIN HERNIAS)

Etiology and Pathogenesis

Hernias of the abdominal wall occur in areas where the fascia is devoid of the protective support of muscle. These areas may be congenital or acquired. In the groin there is such an area bounded by the rectus abdominal muscle medially, the ileopsoas muscle laterally, the pubic ramus inferiorly, and the aponeurosis of the transverse abdominal muscle superiorly. In this area the external and internal oblique muscles thin to a fascial aponeurosis only, so that there is no muscular support of the transverse abdominal fascia and the peritoneum. Upright posture causes intra-abdominal pressure to be directed to this area. During transient increases in abdominal pressure such as occur with coughing or straining, reflex abdominal muscle wall contraction narrows the myopectineal orifice and tenses the overlying fascia ("shutter mechanism").[41] For this reason, hernias are not more common in laborers than in sedentary persons. However, chronically increased intra-abdominal pressure (such as caused by obesity, pregnancy, and ascites) is associated with increased risk of hernia. Chronic muscle weakness and deterioration of connective tissue (due to aging, systemic disease, malnutrition, or smoking) promote hernia formation. During embryologic development the spermatic cord and testis in men (the round ligament in women) migrate from the retroperitoneum through the anterior abdominal wall to the inguinal canal along with a projection of peritoneum (processus vaginalis). The defect in the abdominal wall (internal inguinal ring) associated with this process represents an area of potential weakness through which an *indirect inguinal hernia* may form (Fig. 20–9). The processus vaginalis may persist in up to 20% of adults, further predisposing to hernia formation. *Direct inguinal hernias* do not pass through the internal ring but rather protrude through defects in an area called *Hesselbach's triangle,* bounded by the rectus abdominis muscle, the inferior epigastric artery, and the inguinal ligament (see Fig. 20–9). *Femoral hernias* pass through the opening associated with the femoral artery and vein. They present inferior to the inguinal ligament and medial to the femoral artery[41] (see Fig. 20–9).

Omentum, colon, small bowel, and bladder are the most common contents of groin hernias, although appendix, Meckel's diverticulum, fallopian tube, and ovary have been reported to herniate. In a *Richter's hernia* only the antimesenteric side of the bowel protrudes.

Incidence and Prevalence

The overall incidence of groin hernias in American men is 3% to 4%, if determined through interview, and about 5% if determined by physical examination. The incidence increases with age, from 1% in men younger than 45 years of age to 3% to 5% in those older than 45 years. About 750,000 groin hernia repairs are done yearly in the United States. Of these, 80% to 90% are done in men. Indirect inguinal hernias account for about 65% to 70% of groin hernias in both men and women. In men, direct inguinal hernias account for about 30% and femoral hernias for about 1.5%, whereas in women the opposite is true. Groin hernias are somewhat more common on the right than the left.[42, 43]

Clinical Manifestations and Diagnosis

Many groin hernias are asymptomatic. The most common symptom is a mass in the inguinal or femoral area that enlarges when the patient stands or strains. An incarcerated hernia may produce constant discomfort. Strangulation causes increasing pain. Symptoms of bowel obstruction or ischemia may occur. In a Richter's type hernia pain from bowel strangulation may occur without symptoms of obstruction.

On physical examination, inguinal hernias present as a soft mass in the groin. The mass may be larger on standing or straining. It may be slightly tender. It may be possible to palpate the fascial defect associated with the hernia. Direct and indirect hernias may be difficult to distinguish. Groin hernias may also be noted on a plain abdominal radiograph (Fig. 20–10), barium radiograph, sonography, or CT. Femoral hernias are more difficult to diagnose than other groin hernias. Two thirds of femoral hernias present as surgical emergencies. The correct diagnosis is often not made before surgery. The neck of femoral hernias is usually small. Even a small femoral hernia that is difficult to palpate may cause obstruction or strangulation. Richter's hernias are most common in the femoral area, further complicating the diagnosis. Femoral hernias are most common in women, in whom clinicians may have a lower level of suspicion for hernia than in men. Femoral hernias also occur in children.[44] Delay in diagnosis, strangulation, and emergency surgery are common.[45, 46] Any mass below the inguinal ligament and medial to the femoral artery should raise the suspicion of femoral hernia. Femoral hernias are commonly mistaken for adenopathy or abscess. Bedside drainage of such masses should be avoided until a hernia has been excluded. Sonography may be useful in distinguishing a hernia from adenopathy, abscess, or other mass.[47]

Treatment and Prognosis

Many surgeons recommend repair of direct and indirect inguinal hernias even if asymptomatic, but this is controversial. On the one hand, the risk of incarceration and strangulation increases with time, whereas the morbidity and mortality of elective inguinal herniorrhaphy are extremely low, even in the elderly.[48] On the other hand, many direct and indirect inguinal hernias remain small and asymptomatic indefinitely. A prospective, multicenter trial comparing early repair to watchful waiting for inguinal hernias has been undertaken by the American College of Surgeons and the Veterans Affairs Cooperative Studies Program. Femoral hernias must be repaired promptly, because the risk of strangulation is very high.[45] Groin hernias are repaired by traditional tissue-based procedures or by mesh procedures and by using either open or laparoscopic approaches.

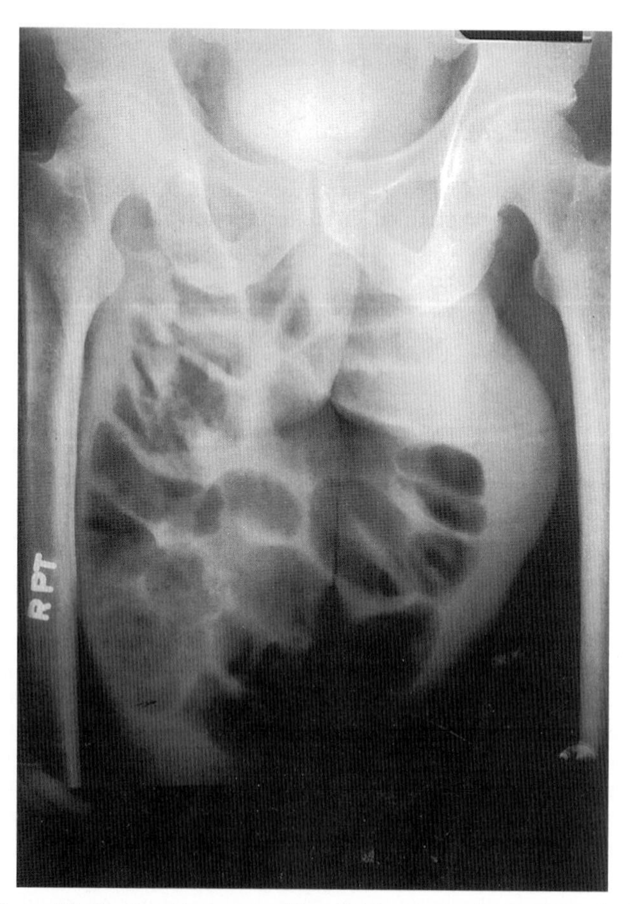

Figure 20–10. Giant incarcerated inguinal hernia. A plain radiograph of a 28-year-old man with a giant incarcerated inguinal hernia. (Courtesy of Michael J. Smerud, MD.)

The traditional tissue-based groin hernia repair involves dissection of the groin structures, excision or inversion of the hernia sac, and reinforcement of the fascial floor by suturing muscle layers over the inguinal canal and to either the inguinal ligament or to Cooper's ligament. Procedures include the Bassini, Canadian (Shouldice), and Cooper's ligament (McVay) repairs.[49–51] These procedures require considerable skill and experience to perform properly. If the repair is done with tension, the tissue may break down, leading to recurrence.

In mesh procedures the hernia defect and the transverse abdominal fascia are reinforced with a flat sheet of prosthetic mesh that is usually sutured in place. Extensive groin dissection is not required. No tension is produced, so that another term frequently used for mesh repairs is tension-free repairs. The mesh is incorporated into the abdominal wall by a fibroblastic response. Lichtenstein popularized mesh repairs.[52, 53] The mesh plug technique is a variation of mesh repair, involving the insertion of a plug of synthetic mesh into the fascial defect. The plug may be sutured in place.[54, 55] Mesh repair has the advantages of standardization and simplicity. The lack of tension in the repair reduces the risk of recurrence. Less dissection is required, making repair easier for recurrent hernias. Most inguinal hernia repairs in the United States are currently done with mesh.[42] Bilateral, very large, or complex abdominal hernias can be repaired with a large mesh that reinforces the entire ventral abdominal wall. This is called giant prosthetic reinforcement of the visceral sac, or the Stoppa procedure.[56, 57]

Repair of groin hernias may be done with open or laparoscopic techniques. Laparoscopic repair can be done from the intraperitoneal space or from a totally extraperitoneal approach (TEPA). With the TEPA, blunt dissection and gas insufflation of the preperitoneal tissues are used to expose the area of the hernia.[58, 59] Several series have compared open hernia repair to laparoscopic repair. In a multicenter, prospective, randomized study performed in the United States, open repair was compared to extraperitoneal laparoscopic repair. Open repairs were not done with mesh unless other techniques could not be used. After a follow-up of 1 to 2 years, recurrence rate after laparoscopic repair was 3% compared to 6% after open repair. Patients returned to normal activities more quickly after laparoscopic repair than after open repair.[60] In another multicenter, prospective, randomized study performed in the United Kingdom, open repair, primarily using mesh, was compared with laparoscopic repair. The recurrence rate after laparoscopic repair was 7% compared with none after open repair. As in the United States study, patients returned to normal activities more quickly after laparoscopic repair than open repair. The overall complication rate was lower after laparoscopic repair, but three serious complications occurred after laparoscopy, and none after open repair.[61] From these studies it seems reasonable to conclude that recurrence rates are low after either laparoscopic or open inguinal hernia repairs using mesh and that patients generally return to normal activities more quickly after laparoscopic repairs than after open repairs. Laparoscopic repair requires general anesthesia. Charges are usually higher for laparoscopic repair than open repair, but it is not clear which approach is more cost-effective if duration of disability is taken into account.[62]

Complications and Recurrence

Elective hernia repair has a mortality rate of less than 0.001%, and serious complications are unusual.[53, 62–64] Lacerations of the bowel, bladder, or blood vessels may occur, particularly during laparoscopic repair, and may cause serious consequences if not detected early. Damage to the bowel may also occur during reduction of an incarcerated hernia.

Minor acute complications include acute urinary retention, seroma, hematoma, and infection. Serious infection occurs in less than 1% of cases. Damage to the spermatic cord may lead to ischemic orchitis. Tissue dissection predisposes to thrombosis of the venous drainage of the testis. Symptoms are swelling and pain of the cord and testis. The condition persists for 6 to 12 weeks and may result in testicular atrophy. Fortunately, this is a rare complication, occurring after about 0.04% of tissue repairs.[65] Hydrocoele or vas deferens injury occurs in less than 1% of cases. Damage to sensory nerves is not uncommon during inguinal hernia surgery. Chronic paresthesias and pain are reported by about 10% of patients, either due to deafferentation or to a neuroma. This can often be treated by local nerve block.[62, 65, 66]

Some "recurrent" hernias are actually direct hernias missed during the first hernia repair. The risk of recurrence is related to conditions that lead to tissue deterioration, such as malnutrition, liver or renal failure, steroid therapy, and malignancies. Recurrent hernias are more common among smokers than among nonsmokers. Among patients with cirrhosis and either no ascites or moderate ascites, inguinal hernia repair is reported to be safe, although the recurrence rate is higher than in other patients.[67] Recurrence is also related to the training and experience of the surgeon, with substantially lower rates occurring in specialized centers compared with general surgery practices. Recurrence rates are higher after repair of recurrent and femoral hernias than after primary repair of inguinal hernias. Overall, recurrence rates are higher after tissue repairs than mesh repairs.[68] For inguinal hernias, the most favorable reported recurrence rates for Canadian and Cooper's ligament repairs have been about 1.5% to 2% for primary repairs and about 3% for repair of recurrent hernia. Reported recurrence rates for mesh repairs vary from none to 2% for primary repairs and none to 3.5% for repair of recurrent hernias.[50, 51, 62]

Inguinal Hernias and Colorectal Cancer Screening

Even before universal colorectal cancer screening of average-risk persons over age 50 was advocated, some practitioners recommended that patients aged 50 years or older with inguinal hernias be screened for colorectal neoplasms before hernia repair. Several prospective studies using sigmoidoscopy or barium enema to screen middle-aged or older men with inguinal hernias have reported the prevalence of polyps to be from 4% to 26% and of colorectal cancer to be from 2.5% to 5%.[69–71] In a prospective study of colonoscopy for screening of asymptomatic U.S. veterans, the prevalence of polyps was 37.5% and of colorectal cancer 1%.[72] Thus, the prevalence of colorectal neoplasms is substantial among middle-aged or older men with inguinal hernias, as it is in those without inguinal hernias. However, the presence of an inguinal hernia is not, in and of itself, an indication for screening, particularly in younger patients. Recommendations for colorectal cancer screening for patients with inguinal hernias should be based on the same criteria as those used for other patients. There is no evidence to suggest that there is an advantage to screening for colorectal cancer before hernia repair as opposed to screening after hernia repair. Large inguinal hernias, particularly incarcerated hernias, may cause difficulty during sigmoidoscopy or colonoscopy. In such patients it may be advisable to defer the examination until after the hernia repair. Incarceration of fiberoptic endoscopes within hernias has been reported.[73–76]

Inguinal Hernias and Benign Prostatic Hypertrophy

Inguinal hernia and symptomatic benign prostatic hypertrophy coincide in 9% to 25% of men. Straining to void may cause worsening of inguinal hernia. Conversely, the risk of postoperative urinary retention after hernia repair is increased by prostatic hypertrophy.[77, 78] It seems reasonable to conclude that if both elective inguinal hernia repair and transurethral prostatic resection are indicated, it would be prudent to either do the prostate surgery first or do the prostate surgery and the hernia repair at the same time.

OTHER VENTRAL HERNIAS

Patients often mistake *diastasis recti* for abdominal hernia. Diastasis recti is a separation of the rectus abdominis muscles without a defect in the abdominal fascia. This condition does not require repair. True ventral hernias include incisional, epigastric, umbilical, and spigelian hernias.

Incisional Hernias

Incisional hernias include postlaparotomy hernias, parastomal hernias, and trocar site hernias.

Etiology and Pathogenesis

Incisional hernias occur most commonly in vertical laparotomy incisions. This is the result of the tension exerted horizontally by the fibers and fascia of the abdominal wall, all of which run horizontally except for fibers of the rectus abdominis muscle. Obesity and wound infection predispose to incisional hernia. Because sternotomy incisions are usually extended to involve the subxiphoid upper abdomen, incisional hernias may occur after sternotomy as well as after laparotomy. *Parastomal hernias* are more likely to occur when a colostomy or ileostomy is placed lateral to rather than through the rectus muscle sheath. In recent years the incidence of *trocar site hernias* has increased coincident with the increase in laparoscopic surgery.

Incidence and Prevalence

Incisional hernias occur after 1% to 4% of laparotomies but in 35% to 50% of cases that are complicated by wound infection or dehiscence.[79] Up to 50% of such hernias present more than a year after surgery. Vertical incisions are more likely to be complicated by hernias than are transverse incisions. Obesity, advanced age, debility, sepsis, postoperative pulmonary complications, and corticosteroid use also increase the risk.[79–81] *Trocar site hernias* are estimated to occur after 0.5% of laparoscopic cholecystectomies.[82] They usually occur at the site of the largest trocar. *Parastomal hernias* are reported to occur after 20% of colostomies and 10% of ileostomies.[79]

Clinical Manifestations and Diagnosis

Incisional hernias cause chronic abdominal discomfort. Because the fascial defect of incisional hernias is usually large, strangulation is unusual even with incarceration. The skin over a large incisional hernia may become stretched, atrophic, or ulcerated.[83] Reduced ability to voluntarily increase intra-abdominal pressure interferes with defecation and urination. Lordosis and back pain may occur. Large incisional hernias may lead to *eventration disease*. With the loss of integrity of the abdominal wall the diaphragm cannot contract against the abdominal viscera but rather forces the viscera into the hernia. The diaphragm thus becomes inefficient. The hernia tends to enlarge. The viscera may lose the "right of domain" in the abdominal cavity. Repair of large hernias may cause a sudden increase in intra-abdominal pressure that can lead to respiratory compromise and compression of the vena cava.[79] *Trocar site hernias* cause symptoms typical of other abdominal wall hernias. Richter's hernia and small intestinal volvulus have been reported.[82, 84, 85] *Parastomal hernias* often interfere with ostomy irrigation and the fit of appliances. Incarceration and strangulation of bowel may occur.[86]

Treatment and Prognosis

Incisional hernias are best repaired with prosthetic mesh, because the recurrence rate is substantially lower than after traditional tissue repair.[80, 87] Mesh is implanted deep to the muscles of the abdominal wall but outside the peritoneum. A double-sided mesh has been developed with a Gortex-like material (expanded polytetrafluoroethylene [PTFE]) on one side. This allows the mesh to be placed directly over the abdominal contents with PTFE facing the peritoneal side.[88] If eventration disease is suspected, the abdominal wall may need to be stretched by repeated progressive pneumoperitoneum before repair. Recurrences of incisional hernia are reported in 4% to 29% of cases.[80, 87, 88] Small and minimally symptomatic *parastomal hernias* may be treated with a modified ostomy belt. If surgery is necessary, the stoma may be relocated and the original fascial defect closed. However, in some cases a suitable alternative location may not be available. In such instances the fascial defect is repaired while leaving the stoma in situ. Prosthetic mesh reinforcement is often used, particularly for recurrent hernias.[86, 89, 90] To decrease the incidence of *trocar site hernias*, it is recommended that trocar ports be removed under direct vision and the defects sutured, particularly those of the largest trocars.[82, 84]

Epigastric and Umbilical Hernias

Etiology and Pathogenesis

Epigastric hernias occur through midline defects in the aponeurosis of the rectus sheath (linea alba) between the xiphoid and the umbilicus. The defects are usually small and frequently multiple. Usually only extraperitoneal fat or omentum protrudes.[89]

Umbilical hernias in infants are congenital (see Chapter 84). They often close spontaneously. In adults umbilical hernias may develop consequent to increased intra-abdominal pressure due to ascites, pregnancy, or obesity.[91]

Incidence and Prevalence

Epigastric hernias are found in 0.5% to 10% of autopsies, but many are asymptomatic or undiagnosed during life. They generally occur in the 3rd through 5th decades. They are more common in men than in women.[92] *Umbilical hernias* occur in about 30% of African American infants and 4% of white infants at birth and are present in 13% and 2%, respectively, by 1 year of age.[91] Umbilical hernias are more common in low-birth-weight infants than in those of normal weight. Umbilical hernias occur in 20% of patients with cirrhosis and ascites.[93]

Clinical Manifestations and Diagnosis

The main symptom of *epigastric hernia* is upper abdominal pain. This pain may radiate to the chest or back. A small subcutaneous midline nodule or discrete area of tenderness may be palpable. Epigastric hernias may be multiple. Diagnosis may be difficult, particularly in obese patients. Symptoms are sometimes mistaken for peptic ulcer or biliary disease. Ultrasonography and CT may be helpful in the diagnosis.[92] *Umbilical hernias* among children are usually asymptomatic. However, incarceration and strangulation may occur both in children and adults. Spontaneous rupture of umbilical hernias may occur among patients with ascites and, rarely, in pregnant women. Cutaneous ulceration often precedes rupture. Strangulation of umbilical hernias may occasionally be precipitated by rapid removal of ascites.[93]

Treatment and Prognosis

If surgery is performed for *epigastric hernia*, the linea alba should be widely exposed because multiple defects may be found. Simple closure is adequate.[92] *Umbilical hernias* are most often left untreated in children because complications are unusual, and they usually close spontaneously if they are smaller than 1.5 cm in diameter. Repair should be considered if they are larger than 2 cm or if they are still present after 4 years of age.[91] Repair of umbilical hernias among patients with cirrhosis and ascites requires definitive control of ascites. If medical therapy is ineffective, transjugular intrahepatic portosystemic shunt or liver transplant must be considered. Pressure bandages and scrupulous local skin care may forestall rupture. Spontaneous rupture carries a mortality of 60% among patients managed medically and 14% among those managed surgically. After rupture, surgery can be delayed up to a week if the patient can be stabilized with antibiotics and sterile pressure bandages.[93]

Spigelian Hernias

Etiology and Pathogenesis

Spigelian hernias occur through defects in the fused aponeurosis of the transverse abdominal muscle and internal oblique muscle, lateral to the rectus sheath, most commonly just below the level of the umbilicus (see Fig. 20–9). At this level the fibers of the aponeurosis are parallel and relatively weak. Spigelian hernias occur deep to the external oblique muscle and are thus interparietal. Spigelian hernias are acquired.[94, 95]

Incidence and Prevalence

Spigelian hernias are rare. About 800 cases have been reported. Incidence is roughly equal in men and women. They may occur in all age groups but are most common in middle age.[94, 95]

Clinical Manifestations and Diagnosis

Spigelian hernias cause pain with localized tenderness often at the lateral edge of the rectus muscle. Frequently only omentum is present in the hernia, but large or small bowel, ovary, or fallopian tube may herniate. A Richter's hernia may occur. Palpation of the fascial defect and mass is sometimes difficult, because the defect is small and the hernia lies under the external oblique muscle. The differential diagnosis includes rectus sheath hematoma, lipoma, or sarcoma. Ultrasonography is the most useful examination for small spigelian hernias.[95, 96]

Treatment and Prognosis

Spigelian hernias may be approached by open or laparoscopic techniques. Laparoscopy allows easy identification of the defect from within the peritoneal cavity, something that may be difficult with the open technique, particularly in obese patients.[95] Mesh plugs have been used for repair.[97]

PELVIC AND PERINEAL HERNIAS

Etiology and Pathogenesis

Obturator hernias occur through the greater and lesser obturator foramina. The obturator foramen is larger in women than in men. It is ordinarily filled with fat. Marked weight loss thus predisposes to herniation.[98] *Sciatic hernias* occur through the foramina formed by the sciatic notch and the sacrospinatus or sacrotuberous ligaments. Abnormal development or atrophy of the piriform muscle may predispose to sciatic hernia. Sciatic hernias may contain ovary, ureter, bladder, or large or small bowel.[99, 100] *Perineal hernias* occur in the soft tissues of the perineum. They may be primary or postoperative. Primary perineal hernias occur anteriorly through the urogenital diaphragm or posteriorly through the levator ani muscle or between the levator ani and the coccygeus muscles. Secondary perineal hernias occur most often after surgery, such as abdominoperineal resection, pelvic exenteration, perineal prostatectomy, resection of the coccyx, or hysterectomy. Radiation therapy, wound infection, and obesity predispose to the development of secondary perineal hernias.[101–103]

Incidence and Prevalence

Pelvic hernias are rare. *Obturator hernias* typically occur in elderly cachectic women. About 600 cases have been reported.[98] In Japan, obturator hernias account for about 1% of all hernia repairs.[104] *Sciatic hernias* are less common than obturator hernias. Fewer than 100 cases have been reported. They are most common in women. *Perineal hernias* are also rare. Primary perineal hernias are most common in middle-aged women. Anterior perineal hernias do not occur in men.[101, 105, 106] Secondary perineal hernias occur after less than 3% of pelvic exenterations and less than 1% of abdominoperineal resections for rectosigmoid cancer.[105]

Clinical Presentation and Diagnosis

Obturator hernias commonly cause lower abdominal pain and symptoms of small bowel obstruction. Because the hernia orifice is small, Richter's hernia and strangulation are common. In about 50% of cases, pressure on the obturator nerve causes paresthesias and pain in the hip and inner thigh. This pain is diminished by hip flexion and increased by hip extension, adduction, or medial rotation (Howship-Romberg sign). Occasionally a mass may be palpable in the upper medial thigh or in the pelvis on pelvic or rectal examination. The diagnosis is difficult, often delayed, and usually not made preoperatively. Preoperative diagnosis is sometimes evident on ultrasonography or CT.[98, 104, 107–111] *Sciatic foramen hernias* may present as a mass or swelling in the gluteal or infragluteal area but are generally difficult to palpate, because they occur deep to the gluteal muscles. Chronic pelvic pain may occur due to incarceration of a fallopian tube and/or ovary. Impingement on the sciatic nerve may also produce pain radiating to the thigh. Intestinal or ureteral obstruction may occur. The differential diagnosis includes lipoma or other soft tissue tumor, cyst, abscess, and aneurysm. The diagnosis is often difficult and made only at laparotomy or laparoscopy.[100] In women, primary *perineal hernias* present anteriorly in the labia majora (pudendal hernia) or posteriorly in the vagina. In men they present in the ischiorectal fossa. Both primary and postoperative perineal hernias are usually soft and reducible. Most patients complain of a mass that produces discomfort on sitting. Because the orifice of the hernia is usually wide, incarceration is rare. If the bladder is involved, urinary symptoms may occur. Postoperative perineal hernias may be complicated by cutaneous ulceration. The differential diagnosis includes sciatic hernia, tumor, hematoma, cyst, abscess, and rectal or bladder prolapse.[101, 105, 112]

Treatment and Prognosis

The treatment of pelvic hernias is surgical. Laparoscopic repair of obturator and sciatic hernias has been reported.[107, 113] As mentioned earlier, obturator hernias may be difficult to diagnose and are associated with a high frequency of strangulation.

LUMBAR HERNIAS

Etiology and Pathogenesis

A *pseudohernia* may occur in the lumbar area as the result of paresis of the thoracodorsal nerves. This is due to loss of muscle control and tone, but there is no associated fascial defect. Causes include diabetic neuropathy and syringomyelia. *Incisional* and *post-traumatic hernias* also occur in the lumbar area. Incisional hernias are most common after nephrectomy. These may be true hernias or pseudohernias due to postoperative muscle paralysis. Motor vehicle collisions are the most common cause of post-traumatic lumbar hernias.[114, 115] Other lumbar hernias include *superior* and *inferior triangle lumbar hernias*. The superior triangle hernia (Grynfeltt's hernia) is bounded by the 12th rib, the internal oblique abdominal muscle, and the sacrospinalis muscle. The inferior triangle hernia (Petit's hernia) is bounded posteriorly by the latissimus dorsi, anteriorly by the external oblique muscle, and inferiorly by the iliac crest[116] (Fig. 20–11).

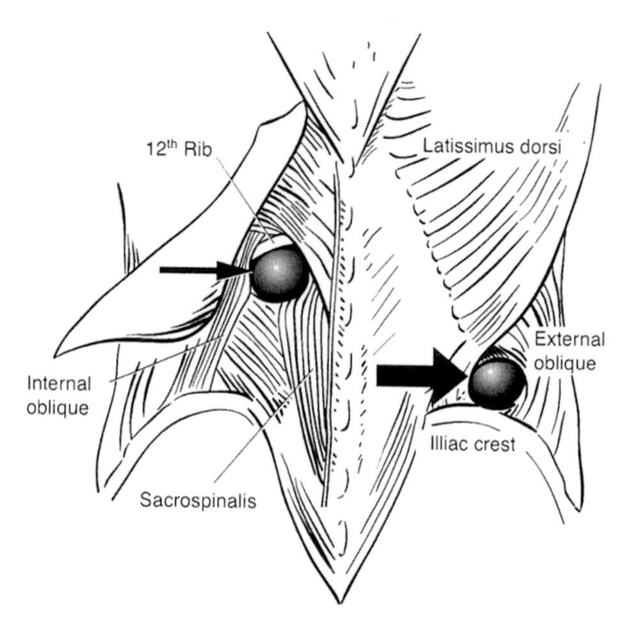

Figure 20–11. Anatomic diagram (posterior view) of Petit's and Grynfeltt's hernias. The inferior triangle hernia (i.e., Petit's hernia) (*thick arrow*) is bounded by the latissimus dorsi muscle, the external oblique muscle, and the iliac crest. The superior triangle hernia (Grynfeltt's hernia) (*thin arrow*) is bounded by the 12th rib, the internal oblique muscle, and the sacrospinalis muscle.

Incidence and Prevalence

Lumbar hernias are rare. About 300 cases have been reported.[116]

Clinical Manifestations and Diagnosis

Lumbar incisional hernias generally present as large bulges that may produce discomfort. *Inferior* and *superior lumbar triangle hernias* may occur through small defects. The differential diagnosis includes lipoma, renal tumor, abscess, and hematoma. Bowel obstruction and strangulation have been reported, but are rare because these hernias are retroperitoneal. However, bowel, mesentery, spleen, ovary, and kidney have been reported to herniate. Occasionally a small lumbar hernia may impinge on a cutaneous branch of a lumbosacral nerve, causing pain referred to the groin or thigh. CT may aid in the diagnosis of lumbar hernia.[115, 117]

Treatment and Prognosis

Large and symptomatic lumbar pseudohernias may be treated in the same manner as true lumbar hernias. Closure of large lumbar hernias as well as superior and inferior lumbar triangle hernias often requires a prosthetic mesh or aponeurotic flap. Identification of the boundaries of the defect and suture of the mesh to strong fascia are the most important elements in surgical repair.[116, 118]

INTERNAL HERNIAS

Internal hernias are protrusions into pouches or openings within the abdominal cavity rather than through the abdominal wall. Internal hernias may be the result of developmental anomalies or may be acquired.[119, 120]

Etiology and Pathogenesis

Internal hernias due to developmental anomalies include paraduodenal, foramen of Winslow, mesenteric, and supravesical hernias. During fetal development the mesentery of the duodenum, ascending colon, and descending colon becomes fixed to the posterior peritoneum. These segments of the bowel become retroperitoneal. Anomalies of mesenteric fixation may lead to abnormal openings through which internal hernias may occur. This is the likely mechanism of paraduodenal and supravesical hernias. Abnormal mesenteric fixation may lead to abnormal mobility of the small bowel and right colon, which facilitates herniation. During fetal development abnormal openings may occur in the pericecal, small bowel, transverse colon, or sigmoid mesentery, as well as the omentum, leading to mesenteric hernias.

Paraduodenal hernias are thought to occur because of anomalies in fixation of the mesentery of the ascending or descending colon. In cases of left paraduodenal hernia, an abnormal foramen (fossa of Landzert) occurs through the mesentery close to the ligament of Treitz, leading under the distal transverse and descending colon, posterior to the superior mesenteric artery. Small bowel may protrude through this fossa. The mesentery of the colon thus forms the anterior wall of a sac enclosing a portion of the small intestine. Right paraduodenal hernias occur in the same fashion through another abnormal foramen (fossa of Waldeyer), leading under the ascending colon.[121, 122]

Foramen of Winslow hernias may occur when this foramen is abnormally large, particularly if there is abnormal mesenteric fixation of the small bowel and right colon. Abnormally mobile small bowel and colon may herniate through the foramen of Winslow into the lesser sac. Symptoms of small bowel or colonic obstruction may occur. Gastric symptoms may also occur if the herniated bowel becomes distended.

Mesenteric hernias occur when a loop of intestine protrudes through an abnormal opening in the mesentery of the small bowel or colon. These mesenteric defects are thought to be developmental in origin, although they may also be acquired as a result of surgery, trauma, or infection. The most common area for such an opening is in the mesentery of the small intestine, most often near the ileocolic junction. Defects have been reported in the mesentery of the appendix and of a Meckel's diverticulum. The intestine finds its way through the defects through normal peristaltic activity. Various lengths of intestine may herniate posterior to the right colon, into the right paracolic gutter (Fig. 20–12). Compression of the loops may lead to obstruction of the herniated intestine. Strangulation may occur by compression or by torsion of the herniated segment. Obstruction may be acute, chronic, or intermittent. The herniated bowel may also compress arteries in the margins of the mesenteric defect, causing ischemia of nonherniated intestine. Similar defects may occur in the mesentery of the small bowel, transverse mesocolon, omentum, and sigmoid mesocolon. *Transmesosigmoid hernias* occur through both layers of the mesocolon, whereas *intermesosigmoid hernias* occur through only one layer of the mesocolon, so that the herniated bowel is contained within the mesocolon.[120, 123, 124]

Supravesical hernias protrude into abnormal fossae around the bladder. Some of these extend through the abdominal wall and are thus external hernias. They may be considered a variant of direct inguinal hernia. Other supravesical hernias remain within the abdominal cavity and are thus internal hernias. They may extend anterior, lateral, or posterior to the bladder. Supravesical hernias usually contain small bowel but may contain omentum, colon, ovary, or fallopian tube.[125, 126]

Acquired internal hernias may occur as a complication of surgery or trauma if abnormal spaces or mesenteric defects are created.

Retroanastomotic hernias may occur after gastrojejunostomy, colostomy or ileostomy, ileal bypass, or vascular bypass when an abnormal space is created into which small bowel, colon, or omentum may herniate. The most common retroanastomotic hernia occurs after gastrojejunostomy, usually after gastric resection with Billroth II reconstruction. The afferent loop, efferent loop, or both protrude into the space posterior to the anastomosis. Efferent loop hernias are about three times as common as afferent loop hernias. Colostomy, ileostomy, ileal bypass for obesity, and vascular bypass procedures (such as aortofemoral bypass) may also lead to the creation of a space or pouch. Renal transplant procedures are extraperitoneal, but an unrecognized inadvertent rent in the peritoneum can lead to pararenal intestinal herniation.[127–129]

Hernias may occur through the *broad ligament of the uterus*. These defects are thought to occur most commonly through tears occurring during pregnancy, because 85% oc-

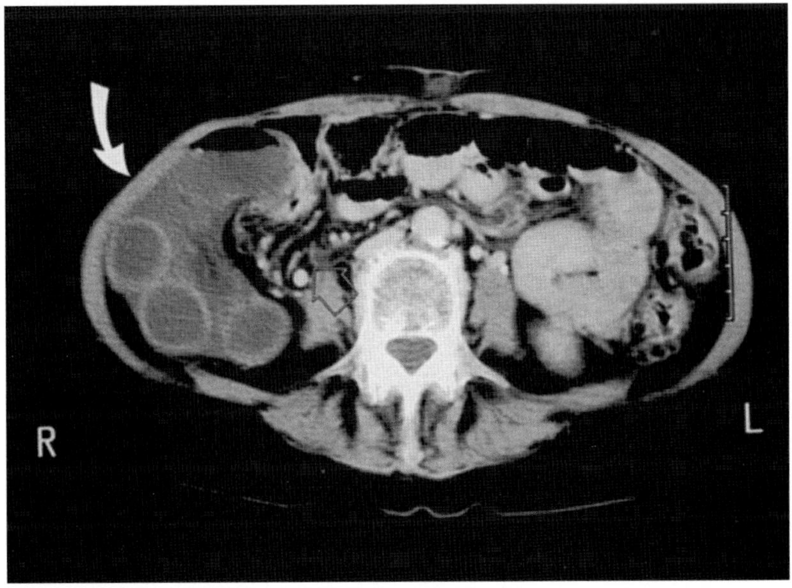

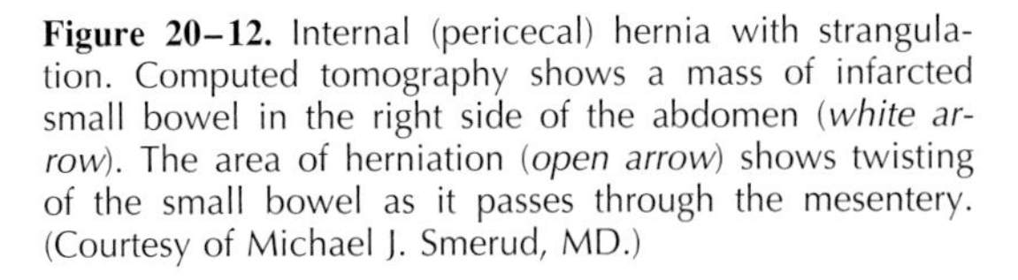
Figure 20–12. Internal (pericecal) hernia with strangulation. Computed tomography shows a mass of infarcted small bowel in the right side of the abdomen (*white arrow*). The area of herniation (*open arrow*) shows twisting of the small bowel as it passes through the mesentery. (Courtesy of Michael J. Smerud, MD.)

cur in parous women. Other cases may be developmental or due to surgery, such as uteropexy or salpingo-oophorectomy.[130, 131]

Incidence and Prevalence

Internal hernias are rare. They are found in 0.2% to 0.9% of autopsies, but a substantial proportion of these remain asymptomatic.[120] About 4% of bowel obstructions are due to internal hernias. Internal hernias occur most often in adults.

One half of developmental internal hernias are paraduodenal hernias. One percent or less of all cases of intestinal obstruction are due to paraduodenal hernias. About 500 cases have been reported. They are more common in males than females and may occur both in children and adults, but typically present between the 4th and 6th decade. Seventy-five percent of paraduodenal hernias occur on the left.[120, 122, 132, 133] Fewer than 200 cases of foramen of Winslow hernia have been reported.[134, 135] Mesenteric hernias are rare. They occur at any age.[123, 124] Fewer than 100 cases of internal supravesical hernia have been reported. They are more common in men than in women. Almost all reported cases have presented in adults, most commonly in the 6th or 7th decade.[125] Likewise, fewer than 100 cases of broad ligament hernia have been reported.[130, 131] Postgastroenterostomy internal hernias have become less common as the frequency of surgery for peptic ulcer disease has declined. Other postanastomotic internal hernias are also rare.[127]

Clinical Manifestations and Diagnosis

Any of the various forms of internal hernias may present with symptoms of acute or chronic intermittent intestinal obstruction. The diagnosis is difficult among patients with chronic symptoms and is rarely made preoperatively among patients who present with acute obstruction and strangulation.[120, 123]

About one half of patients with paraduodenal hernias develop intestinal obstruction, which may be low grade, chronic, and recurrent, or may be high grade and acute.[121, 133, 136] Barium radiographs may show the small bowel to be bunched up or agglomerated, as if it were contained in a bag, and displaced to the left or right side of the colon. Small bowel is often absent from the pelvis. The colon may be deviated by the internal hernia sac. Bowel proximal to the hernia may be dilated.[120, 121, 136] However, barium radiographs may be normal if the hernia has spontaneously reduced. Displacement of the mesenteric vessels will be noted if CT with intravenous contrast medium or arteriography is performed.[120, 137, 138]

In hernias of the foramen of Winslow small bowel herniates in about two thirds of the cases and right colon in the other one third of cases. Herniation of the gallbladder has been reported. Patients may have symptoms of gastric or proximal intestinal obstruction even in the cases of colon herniation, because of pressure of the herniated bowel on the stomach. Symptoms may be reduced by flexion of the hips and knees. Occasionally an epigastric mass is palpable. Plain abdominal radiographs may show the stomach displaced anteriorly and to the left. Contrast enema may show displacement of the cecum into the epigastrium. Ultrasonography may show a mass in the lesser sac.[120, 134, 135, 139]

Mesenteric hernias are difficult to diagnosis preoperatively. Symptoms and signs are those of acute or chronic intermittent bowel obstruction or of acute strangulation. Plain abdominal radiographs may show evidence of bowel obstruction or displacement.

Internal supravesical hernias produce symptoms of bowel obstruction. Associated symptoms of bladder compression occur in about 30% of cases. Anterior supravesical hernias may result in a suprapubic mass or tenderness. About 50% of patients also have an inguinal hernia. Barium radiographs or abdominal CT with oral contrast medium may be helpful in the diagnosis.[125, 140]

Hernias of the broad ligament of the uterus cause symptoms of bowel obstruction in about 50% of cases. Other cases are discovered incidentally at surgery. Small bowel, sigmoid colon, appendix, omentum, and ureter have been reported to herniate. CT scan may show dilation of small bowel and deviation of the uterus.[130, 131, 141]

Retroanastomotic hernias cause symptoms and signs similar to other internal hernias. Postgastrojejunostomy hernias cause symptoms of gastric outlet obstruction. The efferent loop herniates most often. Afferent loop hernias are one cause of the afferent loop syndrome (discussed in Chapter 42). About 50% of postgastrojejunostomy hernias occur within the first month after surgery, 25% occur during the first year, and the rest occur later. The physical examination is not specific. The serum amylase level is often elevated with afferent limb obstruction. Plain abdominal radiographs may show gastric distention and a fluid-filled loop. Barium upper gastrointestinal radiographs are more useful in documenting efferent limb obstruction than they are in afferent limb obstruction. Sonography or CT scan may show dilation of the afferent limb. Biliary scintigraphy shows excretion from the biliary tree but retention of the tracer in an obstructed afferent limb.[127]

Treatment and Prognosis

Symptomatic internal hernias require surgery.[121, 123, 136] Acute obstruction leads to strangulation, bowel ischemia, and death if not promptly treated. Paraduodenal hernias are usually corrected by incising the enclosing mesentery. Care must be taken to avoid injuring the superior or inferior mesenteric arteries, because they follow an abnormal course within the border of the hernia. Sometimes the small bowel can be reduced through the opening of the hernia without incising the mesentery.[121, 142]

REFERENCES

1. Oddsdóttir M: Paraesophageal hernia. Surg Clin North Am 80:1243–1252, 2000.
2. DeMeester TR, Bonavina L: Paraesophageal hiatal hernia. In Nyhus LM, Condon RE (eds): Hernia, 3rd ed. Philadelphia, JB Lippincott, 1989, pp 684–693.
3. Schumpelick V, Steinau G, Schluper I, et al: Surgical embryology and anatomy of the diaphragm with surgical applications. Surg Clin North Am 80:213–239, 2000.
4. Killeen KL, Mirvis SE, Shanmuganathan K: Helical CT of diaphragmatic rupture caused by blunt trauma. AJR Am J Roentgenol 173: 1611–1616, 1999.
5. Simpson J, Lobo DN, Shah AB, et al: Traumatic diaphragmatic rupture: Associated injuries and outcome. Ann R Coll Surg Engl 82:97–100, 2000.

6. Lin Y-K, Huang B-S, Shih C-S, et al: Traumatic diaphragmatic hernia with delayed presentation. Chin Med J (Taipei) 62:223–229, 1999.
7. Arendrup HC, Arendrup KD: Traumatic diaphragmatic hernia. In Nyhus LM, Condon RE (eds): Hernia, 3rd ed. Philadelphia, JB Lippincott, 1989, pp 708–716.
8. Shackleton KL, Stewart ET, Taylor AJ: Traumatic diaphragmatic injuries: Spectrum of radiographic findings. Radiographics 18:49–59, 1998.
9. Guttman FM, Laberge J-M: Congenital diaphragmatic hernia. In Nyhus LM, Condon RE (eds): Hernia, 3rd ed. Philadelphia, JB Lippincott, 1989, pp 694–707.
10. Langer JC: Congenital diaphragmatic hernia. Chest Surg Clin North Am 8:295–314, 1998.
11. Al-Emadi M, Helmy I, Abu Nada M, et al: Laparoscopic repair of Bochdalek hernia in an adult. Surg Laparosc Endosc Percutan Tech 9: 423–425, 1999.
12. Prieto Nieto I, Perez Robledo JP, Hardisson D, et al: Bochdalek hernia in an adult. Scand Cardiovasc J 32:113–114, 1998.
13. Lev-Chelouche D, Ravid A, Michowitz M, et al: Morgagni hernia: Unique presentations in elderly patients. J Clin Gastroenterol 28:81–82, 1999.
14. LaRosa DV Jr, Esham RH, Morgan SL, et al: Diaphragmatic hernia of Morgagni. South Med J 92:411, 1999.
15. Ruhl CE, Everhart JE: Relationship of iron-deficiency anemia with esophagitis and hiatal hernia: Hospital findings from a prospective, population-based study. Am J Gastroenterol 96:322–326, 2001.
16. Weston AP: Hiatal hernia with Cameron ulcers and erosions. Gastrointest Endosc Clin North Am 6:671–679, 1996.
17. Maziak DE, Todd TRJ, Griffith Pearson F: Massive hiatus hernia: Evaluation and surgical management. J Thorac Cardiovasc Surg 115: 53–62, 1998.
18. Perdikis G, Hinder RA, Filipi CJ, et al: Laparoscopic paraesophageal hernia repair. Arch Surg 132:586–590, 1997.
19. Gantert WA, Patti MG, Arcerito M, et al: Laparoscopic repair of paraesophageal hiatal hernias. J Am Coll Surg 186:428–433, 1998.
20. Landreneau RJ, Johnson JA, Marshall JB, et al: Clinical spectrum of paraesophageal hernia. Dig Dis Sci 37:537–544, 1992.
21. Heiss KF: Congential diaphragmatic hernia in 1994: A hard look at the need for "emergency surgery." Semin Thorac Cardiovasc Surg 6: 221–227, 1994.
22. Naunheim KS: Adult presentation of unusual diaphragmatic hernias. Chest Surg Clin North Am 8:359–369, 1998.
23. Horgan S, Eubanks TR, Jacobson G, et al: Repair of paraesophageal hernias. Am J Surg 177:354–358, 1999.
24. Agwunobi AO, Bancewicz J, Attwood SEA: Simple laparoscopic gastropexy as the initial treatment of paraoesophageal hiatal hernia. Br J Surg 85:604–606, 1998.
25. Swanstrom LL, Jobe BA, Kinzie LR, et al: Esophageal motility and outcomes following laparoscopic paraesophageal hernia repair and fundoplication. Am J Surg 177:359–363, 1999.
26. Schauer PR, Ikramuddin S, McLaughlin RH, et al: Comparison of laparoscopic versus open repair of paraesophageal hernia. Am J Surg 176:659–665, 1998.
27. Edye MB, Canin-Endres J, Gattorno F, et al: Durability of laparoscopic repair of paraesophageal hernia. Ann Surg 228:528–535, 1998.
28. Bortul M, Calligaris L, Gheller P: Laparoscopic repair of a Morgagni-Larrey hernia. J Laparoendosc Adv Surg Tech 8:309–313, 1998.
29. Nguyen T, Eubanks PJ, Nguyen D, et al: The laparoscopic approach for repair of Morgagni hernias. J Soc Laparoendosc Surg 2:85–88, 1998.
30. Vanclooster P, Lefevre A, Nijs S, et al: Laparoscopic repair of a Morgagni hernia. Acta Chir Belg 97:84–85, 1997.
31. Hussong RL Jr, Landreneau RJ, Cole FH Jr: Diagnosis and repair of a Morgagni hernia with video-assisted thoracic surgery. Ann Thorac Surg 63:1474–1475, 1997.
32. Domene CE, Volpe P, Santo MA, et al: Laparoscopic treatment of traumatic diaphragmatic hernia. J Laparoendosc Adv Surg Tech A 8:225–229, 1998.
33. Godshall D, Mossallam U, Rosenbaum R: Gastric volvulus: Case report and review of the literature. J Emerg Med 17:837–840, 1999.
34. Teague WJ, Ackroyd R, Watson DI, et al: Changing patterns in the management of gastric volvulus over 14 years. Br J Surg 87:358–361, 2000.
35. Cozart JC, Clouse RE: Gastric volvulus as a cause of intermittent dysphagia. Dig Dis Sci 43:1057–1060, 1998.
36. Tsang TK, Walker R, Yu DJ: Endoscopic reduction of gastric volvulus: The alpha-loop maneuver. Gastrointest Endosc 42:244–248, 1995.
37. Kodali VP, Maas LC: Endoscopic reduction of acute gastric volvulus. J Clin Gastroenterol 21:331–332, 1995.
38. Katkhouda N, Mavor E, Achanta K, et al: Laparoscopic repair of chronic intrathoracic gastric volvulus. Surgery 128:784–790, 2000.
39. Beqiri A, VanderKolk WE, Scheeres D: Combined endoscopic and laparoscopic management of chronic gastric volvulus. Gastrointest Endosc 46:450–452, 1997.
40. Tsang T-K, Johnson YL, Pollack J, et al: Use of single percutaneous endoscopic gastrostomy in management of gastric volvulus in three patients. Dig Dis Sci 43:2659–2665, 1998.
41. Abrahamson J: Etiology and pathophysiology of primary and recurrent groin hernia formation. Surg Clin North Am 78:953–972, 1998.
42. Rutkow IM: Epidemiologic, economic, and sociologic aspects of hernia surgery in the United States in the 1990s. Surg Clin North Am 78: 941, 1998.
43. Rutkow IM, Robbins AW: Demographic, classificatory, and socioeconomic aspects of hernia repair in the United States. Surg Clin North Am 73:413–426, 1993.
44. Ollero Fresno JC, Alvarez M, Sanchez M, et al: Femoral hernia in childhood: Review of 38 cases. Pediatr Surg Int 12:520–521, 1997.
45. Naude GP, Ocon S, Bongard F: Femoral hernia: The dire consequences of a missed diagnosis. Am J Emerg Med 15:680–682, 1997.
46. Vervest AMJS, Eeftinck Schattenkerk M, Rietberg M: Richter's femoral hernia: A clinical pitfall. Acta Chir Belg 98:87–89, 1998.
47. Loftus WK, Hewitt FM, Metreweli O: Case report: Femoral hernia causing small bowel obstruction—ultrasound diagnosis. Clin Radiol 53:618–619, 1998.
48. Gianetta E, De Cian F, Cuneo S, et al: Hernia repair in elderly patients. Br J Surg 84:983–985, 1997.
49. Wantz GE: The operation of Bassini as described by Attilo Catterina. Surg Gynecol Obstet 168:67–80, 1989.
50. Welsh DRJ, Alexander MAJ: The Shouldice repair. Surg Clin North Am 73:451–469, 1993.
51. Rutledge RH: Cooper's ligament repair: A 25-year experience with a single technique for all groin hernias in adults. Surgery 103:1–10, 1988.
52. Kurzer M, Belsham PA, Kark AE: The Lichtenstein repair. Surg Clin North Am 78:1025, 1998.
53. Shulman AG, Amid PK, Lichtenstein IL: The safety of mesh repair for primary inguinal hernias. Am Surg 58:255–257, 1992.
54. Robbins AW, Rutkow IM: Mesh plug repair and groin hernia surgery. Surg Clin North Am 78:1007, 1998.
55. Kingsnorth AN, Porter CS, Bennett DH, et al: Lichtenstein patch or Perfix plug-and-patch in inguinal hernia: A prospective double-blind randomized controlled trial of short-term outcome. Surgery 127:276–283, 2000.
56. Mathonnet M, Cubertafond P, Gainant A: Bilateral inguinal hernias: Giant prosthetic reinforcement of the visceral sac. Hernia 1:93–95, 1997.
57. Stoppa RE: The treatment of complicated groin and incisional hernias. World J Surg 13:545–554, 1989.
58. Heithold DL, Ramshaw BJ, Mason EM, et al: Five hundred total extraperitoneal approach laparoscopic herniorrhaphies: A single-institution review. Am Surg 62:69–72, 1996.
59. Crawford DL, Phillips EH: Laparoscopic repair and groin hernia surgery. Surg Clin North Am 78:1047–1062, 1998.
60. Liem MS, Van der Graaf Y, van Steensel CJ, et al: Comparison of conventional anterior surgery and laparoscopic surgery for inguinal-hernia repair. N Engl J Med 336:1541–1547, 1997.
61. The MRC Laparoscopic Hernia Trial Group: Laparoscopic versus open repair of groin hernia: A randomised comparison. Lancet 354: 185–190, 1999.
62. Bendavid R: Complications of groin hernia surgery. Surg Clin North Am 78:1089–1103, 1998.
63. MacFadyen BV Jr, Mathis CR: Inguinal herniorraphy: Complications and recurrences. Semin Laparosc Surg 1:128–140, 1994.
64. Payne JH Jr: Complications of laparoscopic inguinal herniorrhaphy. Semin Laparosc Surg 4:166–181, 1997.
65. Wantz GE: Testicular atrophy and chronic residual neuralgia as risks of inguinal hernioplasty. Surg Clin North Am 73:571–581, 1993.
66. Cunningham J, Temple WJ, Mitchell P, et al: Cooperative hernia study: Pain in the postrepair patient. Ann Surg 224:598–602, 1996.
67. Hurst RD, Butler BN, Soybel DI, et al: Management of groin hernias in patients with ascites. Ann Surg 216:696–700, 1992.
68. McGillicuddy JR: Prospective randomized comparison of the Shouldice and Lichtenstein hernia repair procedures. Arch Surg 133:978, 1998.

69. Lovett J, Kirgan D, McGregor B: Inguinal hernia justifies sigmoidoscopy. Am J Surg 158:615–616, 1989.
70. Pratt SM, Weaver FA, Potts JR III: Preoperative evaluation of patients with inguinal hernia for colorectal disease. Surg Gynecol Obstet 165: 53–56, 1987.
71. Rubin BG, Ballantyne GH, Zdon MJ, et al: The role of flexible sigmoidoscopy in the preoperative screening of patients with inguinal hernia: A high yield of neoplasms. Arch Surg 122:296–299, 1987.
72. Lieberman DA, Weiss DG, Bond JH, et al: Use of colonoscopy to screen asymptomatic adults for colorectal cancer. N Engl J Med 343: 162–168, 2000.
73. Fulp SR, Gilliam JH III: Beware the incarcerated hernia [letter]. Gastrointest Endosc 36:318–319, 1990.
74. Leichtmann GA, Feingelrent H, Pomeranz IS, et al: Colonoscopy in patients with large inguinal hernias [letter]. Gastrointest Endosc 37: 494, 1991.
75. Yamamoto K, Kadakia SC: Incarceration of a colonoscope in an inguinal hernia [letter]. Gastrointest Endosc 40:396–397, 1994.
76. Koltun WA, Coller JA: Incarceration of colonoscope in an inguinal hernia: "Pulley" technique of removal. Dis Colon Rectum 34:191–193, 1991.
77. Tundidor Bermudez AM: Hernia inguinal y prostatismo. Arch Esp Urol 47:19–21, 1994.
78. Thompson IM, Wesen CA: Prostatism and inguinal hernia. South Med J 75:1342–1344, 1982.
79. Baker RJ: Incisional hernia. In Nyhus LM, Condon RE (eds): Hernia, 3rd ed. Philadelphia, JB Lippincott, 1989, pp 321–337.
80. Anthony T, Bergen PC, Kim LT, et al: Factors affecting recurrence following incisional herniorrhaphy. World J Surg 24:95–100, 2000.
81. Carlson MA, Ludwig KA, Condon RE: Ventral hernia and other complications of 1,000 midline incisions. South Med J 88:450–453, 1995.
82. Petrakis I, Sciacca V, Chalkiadakis G, et al: A simple technique for trocar site closure after laparoscopic surgery. Surg Endosc 13:1249–1251, 1999.
83. Flament JB, Avisse C, Palot JP, et al: Trophic ulcers in giant incisional hernias—pathogenesis and treatment: A report on 33 cases. Hernia 1:71–76, 1997.
84. Stringer NH, Levy ES, Kezmoh MP, et al: New closure technique for lateral operative trocar sites: A report of 80 closures. Surg Endosc 9: 838–840, 1995.
85. Hass BE, Schrager RE: Small bowel obstruction due to Richter's hernia after laparoscopic procedures. J Laparoendosc Surg 3:421–423, 1993.
86. Leslie D: The parastomal hernia. Surg Clin North Am 64:407–415, 1984.
87. Temudom T, Siadati M, Sarr MG: Repair of complex giant or recurrent ventral hernias by using tension-free intraparietal prosthetic mesh (Stoppa technique): Lessons learned from our initial experience (fifty patients). Surgery 120:738–744, 1996.
88. Bauer JJ, Salky BA, Gelernt IM, et al: Repair of large abdominal wall defects with expanded polytetrafluoroethylene (PTFE). Ann Surg 206: 765–769, 1987.
89. Rubin MS, Schoetz DJ Jr, Matthews JB: Parastomal hernia: Is stoma relocation superior to fascial repair? Arch Surg 129:413–418, 1994.
90. Byers JM, Steinberg JB, Postier RG: Repair of parastomal hernias using polypropylene mesh. Arch Surg 127:1246–1247, 1992.
91. Harmel RP Jr: Umbilical hernia. In Nyhus LM, Condon RE (eds): Hernia, 3rd ed. Philadelphia, JB Lippincott, 1989, pp 354–356.
92. Robin AP: Epigastric hernia. In Nyhus LM, Condon RE (eds): Hernia, 3rd ed. Philadelphia, JB Lippincott, 1989, pp 360–368.
93. Belghiti J, Durand F: Abdominal wall hernias in the setting of cirrhosis. Semin Liver Dis 17:219–226, 1997.
94. Spangen L: Spigelian hernia. Surg Clin North Am 64:351–366, 1984.
95. Spangen L: Spigelian hernia. In Nyhus LM, Condon RE (eds): Hernia, 3rd ed. Philadelphia, JB Lippincott, 1989, pp 369–379.
96. Mufid MM, Abu-Yousef MM, Kakish ME, et al: Spigelian hernia: Diagnosis by high-resolution real-time sonography. J Ultrasound Med 16:183–187, 1997.
97. Sánchez-Montes I, Deysine M: Spigelian hernias: A new repair technique using preshaped polypropylene plugs. Arch Surg 133:670–672, 1998.
98. Skandalakis JE, Gray SW: Strangulated obturator hernia. In Nyhus LM, Condon RE (eds): Hernia, 3rd ed. Philadelphia, JB Lippincott, 1989, pp 416–430.
99. Epner SL, Lautin EM: Case report: Intermittent sciatic herniation of the ureter. Clin Radiol 49:832–833, 1994.
100. Black S: Sciatic hernia. In Nyhus LM, Condon RE (eds): Hernia, 3rd ed. Philadelphia, JB Lippincott, 1989, pp 432–440.
101. Pearl RK: Perineal hernia. In Nyhus LM, Condon RE (eds): Hernia, 3rd ed. Philadelphia, JB Lippincott, 1989, pp 442–446.
102. So JB, Palmer MT, Shellito PC: Postoperative perineal hernia. Dis Colon Rectum 40:954–957, 1997.
103. Candiani GB, Candiani M: Posthysterectomy Fallopian tube herniation: A report of two cases. J Reprod Med 41:915–920, 1996.
104. Yokoyama Y, Yamaguchi A, Isogai M, et al: Thirty-six cases of obturator hernia: Does computed tomography contribute to postoperative outcome? World J Surg 23:214–217, 1999.
105. Pearl RK: Perineal hernia. In Nyhus LM, Condon RE (eds): Hernia, 3rd ed. Philadelphia, JB Lippincott, 1989, pp 442–443.
106. Vorburger SA, Von Flüe M, Harder F: Pelvic floor herniation after modified York-Mason approach to the rectum: Report of a case. Dis Colon Rectum 41:389–390, 1998.
107. Naude G, Bongard F: Obturator hernia is an unsuspected diagnosis. Am J Surg 174:72–75, 1997.
108. Yokoyama T, Munakata Y, Ogiwara M, et al: Preoperative diagnosis of strangulated obturator hernia using ultrasonography. Am J Surg 174:76–78, 1997.
109. Terada R, Ito S, Kidogawa H, et al: Obturator hernia: The usefulness of emergent computed tomography for early diagnosis. J Emerg Med 17:883–886, 1999.
110. Skandalakis LJ, Androulakis J, Colborn GL, et al: Obturator hernia. Surg Clin North Am 80:71–84, 2000.
111. Green BT: Strangulated obturator hernia: Still deadly. South Med J 94:81–83, 2001.
112. Mandarano R, Giorgi G, Venturini N, et al: Perineal hernia. Minerva Chir 54:523–529, 1999.
113. Miklos JR, O'Reilly MJ, Saye WB: Sciatic hernia as a cause of chronic pelvic pain in women. Obstet Gynecol 91:998–1001, 1998.
114. Zamir G, Gross E, Simha M, et al: Incarcerated lumbar hernia-delayed consequence of a seat belt injury. Injury 7:561–563, 1998.
115. Balkan M, Kozak O, Gülec B, et al: Traumatic lumbar hernia due to seat belt injury: Case report. J Trauma 47:154–155, 1999.
116. Geis WP, Saletta JD: Lumbar hernia. In Nyhus LM, Condon RE (eds): Hernia, 3rd ed. Philadelphia, JB Lippincott, 1989, pp 401–415.
117. Hide IG, Pike EE, Uberoi R: Lumbar hernia: A rare cause of large bowel obstruction. Postgrad Med J 75:231–232, 1999.
118. Heniford BT, Iannitti DA, Gagner M: Laparoscopic inferior and superior lumbar hernia repair. Arch Surg 132:1141–1144, 1997.
119. Gullino D, Giordano O, Gullino E: Les hernies internes de l'abdomen: À propos de 14 cas. J Chir (Paris) 130:179–195, 1993.
120. Ghahremani GG: Internal abdominal hernias. Surg Clin North Am 64: 393–406, 1984.
121. Brigham RA, d'Avis JC: Paraduodenal hernia. In Nyhus LM, Condon RE (eds): Hernia, 3rd ed. Philadelphia, JB Lippincott, 1989, pp 481–486.
122. Isabel L, Birrell S, Patkin M: Paraduodenal hernia. Austral NZ J Surg 65:64–66, 1995.
123. Janin Y, Stone AM, Wise L: Mesenteric hernia. In Nyhus LM, Condon RE (eds): Hernia, 3rd ed. Philadelphia, JB Lippincott, 1989, pp 461–469.
124. Noya G, Chironi G, Niolu P, et al: L'ernia transmesenterica: Presentazione di un caso e revisione della letteratura. Minerva Chir 31:751–754, 1990.
125. Gray SW, Skandalakis JE: Supravesical hernia. In Nyhus LM, Condon RE (eds): Hernia, 3rd ed. Philadelphia, JB Lippincott, 1989, pp 388–398.
126. Abdullah TI, Pearson HJ: Strangulated internal supravesical hernia: A diagnostic problem. Eur J Surg 163:875–876, 1997.
127. Rutledge RH: Retroanastomic hernia. In Nyhus LM, Condon RE (eds): Hernia, 3rd ed. Philadelphia, JB Lippincott, 1989, pp 470–480.
128. Kawamura YJ, Sunami E, Masaki T, et al: Transmesenteric hernia after laparoscopic-assisted sigmoid colectomy. JSLS 3:79–81, 1999.
129. Serra C, Baltasar A, Bou R, et al: Internal hernias and gastric perforation after a laparoscopic gastric bypass. Obes Surg 9:546–549, 1999.
130. Slezak FA, Schlueter TM: Hernia of the broad ligament of the uterus. In Nyhus LM, Condon RE (eds): Hernia, 3rd ed. Philadelphia, JB Lippincott, 1989, pp 311–312.
131. Ishihara H, Terahara M, Kigawa J, et al: Strangulated herniation through a defect of the broad ligament of the uterus. Gynecol Obstet Invest 35:187–189, 1993.
132. McDonagh T, Jclinek GA: Two cases of paraduodenal hernia, a rare internal hernia. J Accid Emerg Med 13:64–68, 1996.
133. Pershad J, Simmons GT, Chung D, et al: Two acute pediatric abdomi-

nal catastrophes from strangulated left paraduodenal hernias. Pediatr Emerg Care 14:347–349, 1998.
134. Evrard V, Vielle G, Buyck A, et al: Herniation through the foramen of Winslow: Report of two cases. Dis Colon Rectum 39:1055–1057, 1996.
135. Sáenz Regalado D, Morales Gutiérrez C, Villeta Plaza R, et al: Hernia de ciego a través del hiato de Winslow. Rev Esp Enferm Dig 83:127–129, 1993.
136. Zimmerman LM, Laufman H: Intra-abdominal hernias due to developmental and rotational anomalies. Ann Surg 138:82–91, 1953.
137. Yeoman LJ, Patel AG, Michell MJ: Case report: Computed tomography appearances in a right paraduodenal hernia. Clin Radiol 49:898–900, 1994.
138. Schaffler GJ, Groell R, Kammerhuber F, et al: Anterior and upward displacement of the inferior mesenteric vein: A new diagnostic clue to left paraduodenal hernias? Abdom Imaging 24:29–31, 1999.
139. Panula HE, Alhava E: Internal hernia of Foramen of Winslow: A rare congenital condition. Eur J Surg 161:695–696, 1995.
140. Koksoy FN, Soybir GR, Bulut TM, et al: Internal supravesical hernia: Report of a case. Am Surg 61:1023–1024, 1995.
141. Fafet P, Souiri M, Ould Said H, et al: Hernie interne de l'intestin grêle à travers une brèche du ligament large, à propos d'une observation. J Chir (Paris) 132:314–317, 1995.
142. Uematsu T, Kitamura H, Iwase M, et al: Laparoscopic repair of a paraduodenal hernia. Surg Endosc 12:50–52, 1998.

Chapter 21

FOREIGN BODIES AND BEZOARS

Patrick R. Pfau and Gregory G. Ginsberg

Gastrointestinal foreign bodies (GIFBs) and bezoars are common. Owing to the lack of a uniform data collection mechanism, their exact incidence and related morbidity and mortality are unknown. Paralleling the development and dispersal of flexible endoscopy, numerous review articles, large case series, and case reports have addressed issues related to GIFBs and bezoars over the last 20 years. It is this body of literature that shapes our understanding of the epidemiology, pathophysiology, diagnosis, and management of GIFBs and bezoars.

FOREIGN BODIES

For the purposes of this chapter, foreign bodies include intentionally or unintentionally inserted or ingested objects, inadvertently ingested animal and fish bones, and food bolus impactions.

Epidemiology

Several patient profiles have been identified to be at above average risk for intentional or accidental foreign body ingestion. Eighty percent of cases of foreign body ingestion occur in the pediatric population, with a peak incidence between age 6 months and 3 years.[1] Ingestion by children is usually the result of natural oral curiosity, leading to inadvertent as well as intentional swallowing. The objects most frequently ingested by children are coins, followed by a variety of small objects such as keys, buttons, small toys, nails, pins, thumbtacks, and disc batteries.[2, 3]

Intentional foreign body ingestion in adults is most apt to occur among patients with psychiatric disorders and altered sensorium and those seeking some secondary gain. Among the latter are malingerers and the incarcerated. Those with psychiatric disorders commonly ingest multiple objects and on multiple occasions. One frequently cited report describes a patient with 2533 gastric foreign bodies recorded over his ingestion career.[4]

Adult patients at risk for accidental foreign object ingestion include the very elderly, the demented, and the intoxicated (Fig. 21–1). Adults with dentures and dental bridgework have an increased risk of accidental foreign body ingestion because of compromised tactile sensation during swallowing.

Foreign bodies in the rectum only rarely result from migration following oral ingestion. Rather, most are directly introduced into the anus. Rectal foreign bodies are most commonly the result of sexual activity, sexual assault, or psychiatric illness. Other causes such as packing the rectum for the smuggling of illegal drugs, inadvertent loss of objects used for relieving constipation, or even falling on objects are reported.

The most common GIFB that comes to medical attention in adults is food bolus impaction, particularly in adults older than 40 or 50 years of age. Food impaction is uncommon in children. Most patients with food bolus impactions have a predisposing factor. The incidence of esophageal pathology in patients with acute food impactions is 75% to 100%.[5–8] Benign esophageal stenoses are the most commonly observed esophageal pathology, with Schatzki's ("B") rings leading the way, followed by peptic strictures, esophageal spasm, webs, and extrinsic compression. Food bolus impactions are also encountered at surgical anastomoses, tight fundoplication wraps, and bariatric gastroplasties.[6] Esophageal cancer presenting with acute food bolus impaction is uncommon but acknowledged.[5]

Pathophysiology

It is appreciated that 80% to 90% of GIFBs pass spontaneously through the digestive tract without causing harm.[9] However, real and potential adverse outcomes are recognized. In the early part of the 20th century mortality associated with GIFBs that did not pass spontaneously was as high as 50%.[10] As late as 1977, it was estimated that up to 1500 deaths per year occurred in the United States related to GIFBs.[11]

Bowel perforation and obstruction are the most common significant complications associated with GIFBs. Other complications include bleeding, respiratory compromise, fistulization, and abscess formation (see Chapter 24). Among patients presenting with symptoms related to a GIFB, the perforation rate has been estimated to be as high as 5% (up to 35% for sharp-pointed objects).[5] Esophageal perforation is

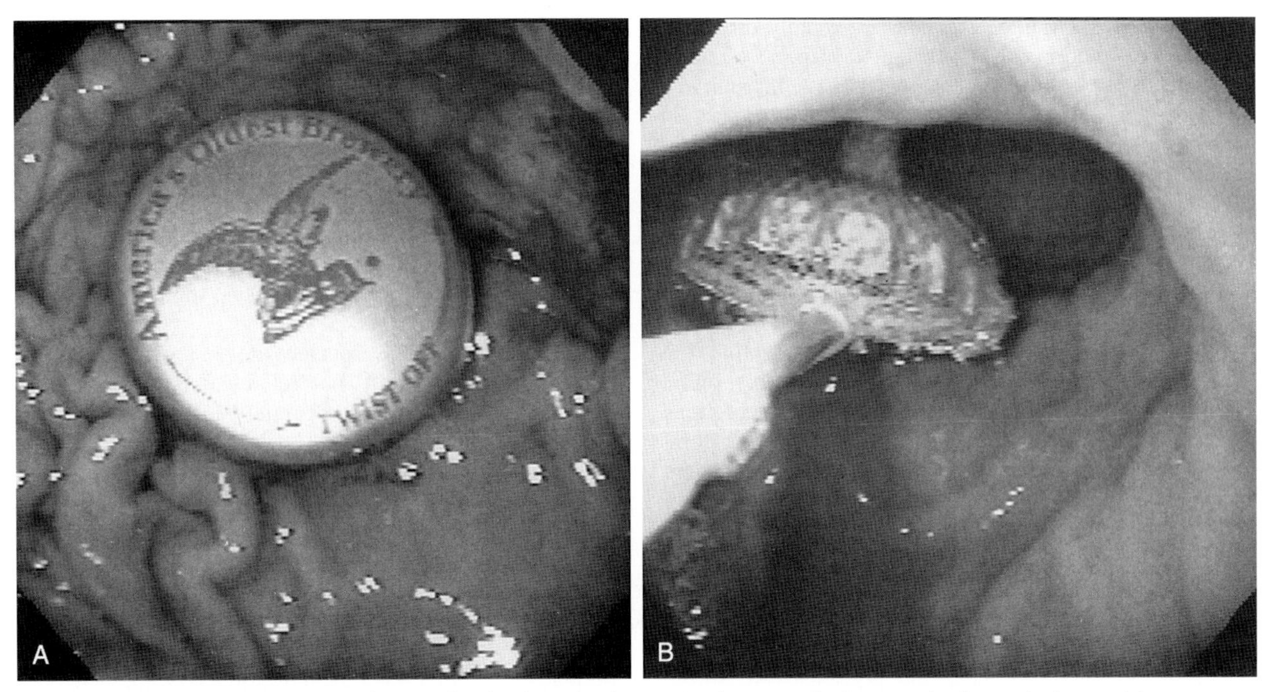

Figure 21–1. *A,* Endoscopic photograph of a beer bottle cap in the stomach that was inadvertently ingested by an intoxicated college student. *B,* The cap has been captured in a retrieval net for removal from the stomach.

associated with the greatest mortality and morbidity, including mediastinitis, lung abscess, pneumothorax, pericarditis, and cardiac tamponade.[12] Esophagorespiratory and esophagoaortic fistulas may present months to years after foreign body ingestion.[13]

Perforation and obstruction may occur anywhere in the digestive tract but are most apt to occur in locations where there is an anatomic sphincter, acute angulation, physical narrowing, prior surgery, or congenital gut malformations[14] (Fig. 21–2). Rostral to caudal, the posterior hypopharynx is the first area of the gastrointestinal tract in which a foreign body may become lodged. Sharp objects, particularly fish or chicken bones, are the most common objects to lodge in the hypopharynx and cause symptoms.[15, 16] The esophagus has four areas of physiologic narrowing where foreign bodies or food boluses are apt to become impacted. These are at the levels of the upper esophageal sphincter and cricopharyngeal muscle; the aortic arch; the crossing of the main stem bronchus; and the gastroesophageal junction. These areas have been characterized as sites of true luminal constriction with maximum normal physiologic diameters of 23 mm or less in the average adult.[17] Esophageal rings, webs, diverticula, peptic strictures, and occasionally carcinoma all further enhance foreign body entrapment in the esophagus.[16, 18] Motor disturbances such as achalasia or diffuse esophageal spasm may also predispose to entrapment of objects.[15, 18] Others have suggested that segmental variations in esophageal peristalsis and intrinsic variation in esophageal motility, rather than luminal narrowing, contribute to the occurrence and localization of impactions in the esophagus.[19]

Once in the stomach, 80% to 90% of all ingested objects pass spontaneously through the remaining digestive tract within 7 to 10 days with no complications. The relationship between the size and shape of the object to that of the pylorus determines whether the lesion is apt to pass from the

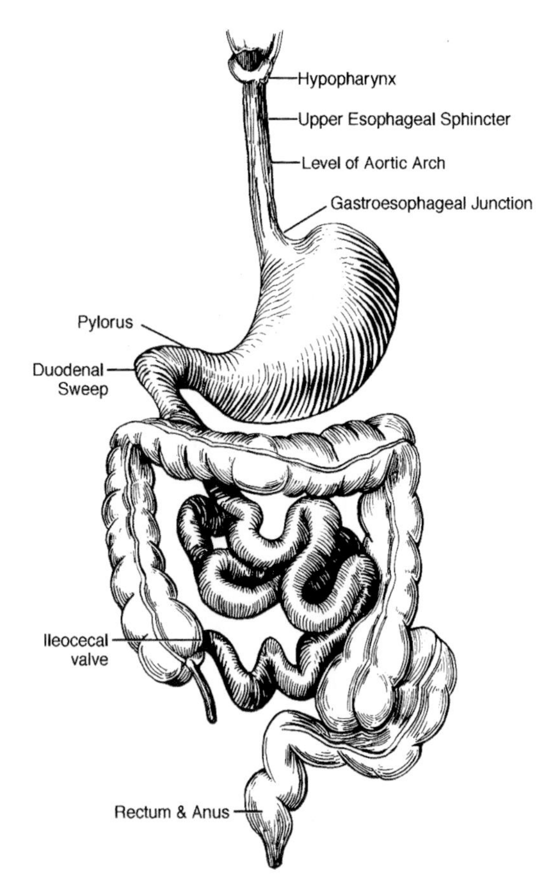

Figure 21–2. Common areas of luminal narrowing and angulation in the gastrointestinal tract leading to foreign body impaction.

stomach. Long objects (length >5 cm) are usually unable to pass through the pylorus and duodenal sweep.[14, 20] Large-diameter objects (>2 cm) are not apt to pass through the pylorus. Even smaller objects may be unable to pass in patients with pyloric stenosis, deformity due to prior ulcer disease, or history of pyloromyotomy.[15, 20] Endoscopic or surgical retrieval is indicated when these features are identified by history or on radiographic studies. Retrieval is also indicated for objects that, after observation, fail to pass in 5 to 7 days.

Points of impedance to the passage of foreign bodies in the small bowel are present proximally and distally. The duodenal sweep, because of its C-shaped turn, can prohibit the passage of long objects. Long and pointed objects tend to hang up in the duodenal sweep and can cause perforation.[8] The ligament of Treitz, due to its narrowing and angulation, is another location for foreign body obstruction. Objects that become entrapped at the ileocecal valve tend to be smaller, because they must have first passed through the pylorus, duodenal sweep, and ligament of Treitz.

However, it is rare for foreign bodies to lodge or cause complications as they course through the small bowel and colon. This is because axial flow and peristalsis are stimulated when a foreign body is encountered, which encourages the foreign body to be propelled with the blunt end leading and the sharp end trailing in the lumen.[21] Second, as the object progresses further down the gastrointestinal lumen, it tends to become centered in the lumen surrounded by stool, further protecting the bowel wall.[18]

Foreign bodies that are inserted into the rectum or are ingested and then migrate to the rectum pose the risk of serious morbidity. Patients may present with rectal bleeding, an acute abdomen, intestinal obstruction, and abscess often without a suspected or given history of foreign body ingestion or insertion.[15] The internal and external anal sphincters are natural barriers and can become tonically contracted and edematous after traumatic insertion of an object.[15] The sacral curve or ileoischial angle and valves of Houston are relatively tight anatomic areas that may prove difficult for an object to pass spontaneously after it has been pushed forcibly beyond.[18] Injury to the colon and anorectum may require primary repair or colostomy. Traumatic sphincter disruption may result in chronic dysfunction.[22]

Finally, inadvertent complications may occur related to attempts at endoscopic removal of ingested foreign bodies and food bolus impactions. Therefore, it serves the patient well for gastrointestinal endoscopists to have a thorough understanding of the principles of management of GIFBs.

Diagnosis

History and Physical Examination

In communicative adults, history of ingestion, type of ingestion, and onset of symptoms are usually reliable. Most patients who present with food bolus impactions and with animal or fish bone ingestions are symptomatic.[5] Odynophagia and a foreign body sensation often occur with sharp objects and bones, suggesting esophageal mucosal laceration. Ingestions resulting in esophageal obstruction can produce abrupt onset of substernal chest pain, inability to swallow, gagging, vomiting, or a sensation of choking.[23] Drooling and the inability to handle oral secretions suggest a more complete obstruction. Among patients with suspected foreign object ingestion, close to 80% will have a foreign body identified if dysphonia, dysphagia, or odynophagia is present. However, if the presenting symptom is retrosternal pain or pharyngeal discomfort, only 47% will have a foreign body identified.[24] Respiratory compromise may occur with aspiration of secretions or if the object is impacted at or immediately below the upper esophageal sphincter, resulting in compression of the trachea.[25]

Estimation of the suspected site or level of impaction by the patient is generally not reliable.[26] The one area where patients may be able to accurately localize the object is at the cricopharyngeal muscle, but localization becomes progressively less accurate for distally impacted foreign bodies, with an accuracy of 30% to 40% in the esophagus and close to 0% in the stomach.[26, 27]

In children and noncommunicative or mentally impaired adults, the patient history is far less reliable and symptoms are much more insidious, requiring a high level of suspicion. Children and impaired adults usually do not give a history of ingestion, but rather the ingestion is witnessed or highly suspected by a caregiver. Up to 33% of infants and children are asymptomatic after foreign body ingestion.[28] Symptoms without a history of ingestion can include choking, vomiting, blood-stained saliva, respiratory distress, and stridor.[29] Less obviously, children may simply refuse to eat or demonstrate failure to thrive.

Past medical history is important, particularly in the adult population. A careful history should be obtained documenting any prior history of dysphagia, previous food or foreign body impactions, and alcohol use. The type of meal ingested is germane for suspected food bolus impactions or animal or fish bone ingestion. The occupational history can be useful when it includes potential hazards such as tailors who hold pins and carpenters who hold nails in their mouths.

The physical examination tends to be unremarkable or nonspecific but must be carefully performed to recognize complications of GIFBs. Risk of aspiration and ventilatory and airway compromise should be determined with the consideration of establishing airway protection. Swelling, erythema, or crepitus in the neck may be present with oropharyngeal or proximal esophageal perforation. The abdominal examination should solicit signs of perforation or obstruction. Rectal examination may reveal a foreign body that is impacted.

Radiographic Studies

Patients with suspected upper gastrointestinal foreign body ingestion should have anteroposterior and lateral radiographs of the chest and abdomen to help determine the presence, type, and location of the foreign body. The plain films also aid in identifying possible complications such as aspiration, pneumoperitoneum, pleural effusion, mediastinitis, or subcutaneous emphysema.[2, 23, 30] Lateral films are needed because foreign bodies such as a bone in the cervical esophagus overlying the spine may be missed in the anteroposterior projection. Lateral films can also distinguish between coins located in the esophagus versus those in the trachea or pul-

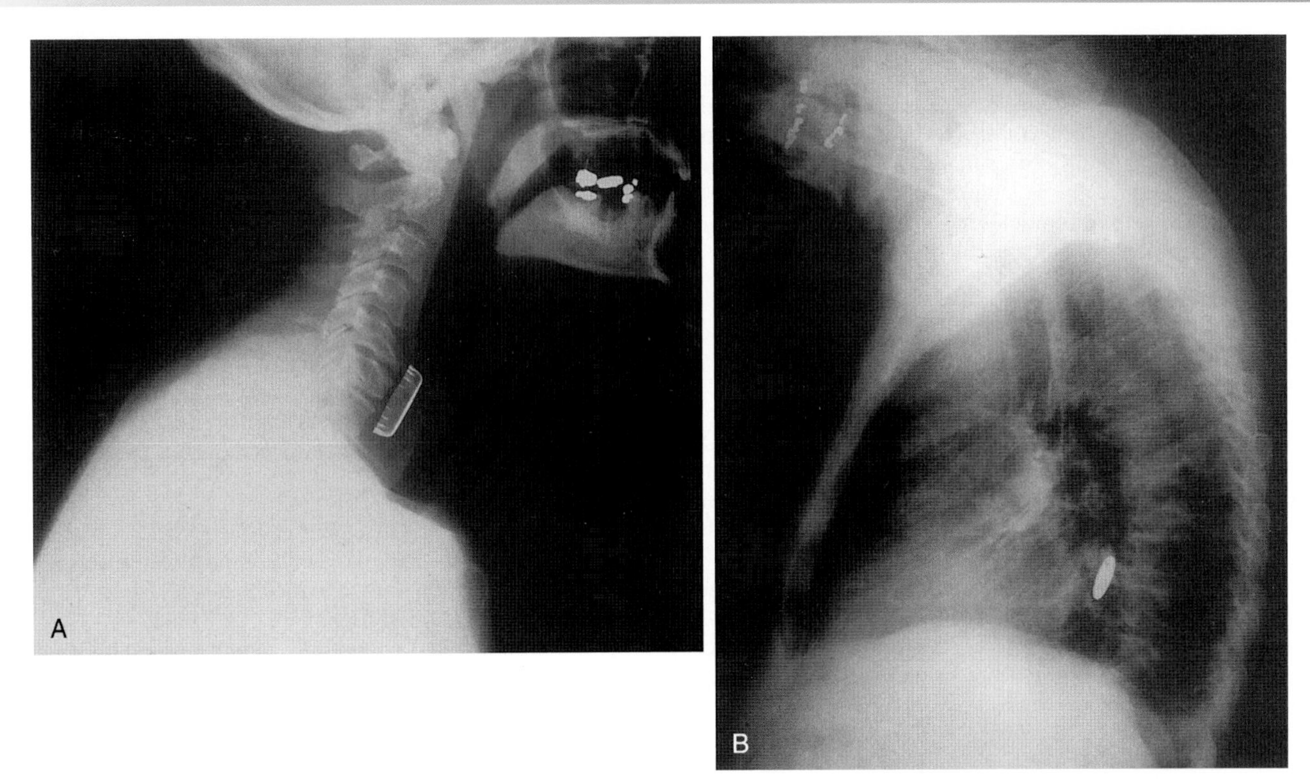

Figure 21–3. Use of lateral radiographs in foreign body ingestion. *A*, Lateral neck radiograph of an intoxicated patient who swallowed a beer cap. *B*, Lateral chest radiograph of an elderly, demented, nursing home resident who accidently swallowed a coin, mistaking it for his medication. The coin is located in the esophagus. It soon rapidly passed into the stomach and was excreted without complication.

monary tree[15, 31] (Fig. 21–3). Anteroposterior and lateral films of the neck should be obtained if there is suspicion of an object in the hypopharynx or cervical esophagus.

The diagnostic capabilities of plain film are limited by the fact that not all ingested objects are radiopaque. Most food bolus impactions, fish or chicken bones, wood, plastic, or glass are either radiolucent or not easily seen and identified on plain film. False-negative rates of radiography have been found to be as high as 47% and false-positive rates can occur in up to 20% of cases.[24, 32] An experienced radiologist should review the radiographs because 35% of films performed in the evaluation of GIFBs are misinterpreted by nonradiologists.[33]

Plain films are of equal importance in children, particularly the asymptomatic child. Mouth-to-anus screening films have been suggested as the first step in the evaluation of a child with a suspected foreign body. In an effort to limit radiation to children, other groups have advocated the use of hand-held metal detectors to establish the presence and location of foreign bodies, particularly coins. Metal detectors have been found to have a 98% sensitivity for coin detection and location.[34]

The role of contrast studies should be limited in the evaluation of foreign bodies. Barium esophagrams should not be performed if there is a suspicion of perforation because this may lead to contrast medium leaking into the pleural space or mediastinum. Barium should also be avoided in situations where complete or near-complete esophageal obstruction is suspected because barium coats the foreign body and mucosa, further occluding the lumen and making the performance of subsequent therapeutic endoscopy more difficult.[35] Transparent water-soluble contrast agents may cause less of a reaction from extravasation but can cause severe chemical pneumonitis and, rarely, death if aspirated.[12] If symptoms are unclear or nonspecific and endoscopy is relatively contraindicated, contrast radiographic studies can be useful and do give a high sensitivity and specificity for detecting most foreign bodies. However, persistent symptoms related to the esophagus should still be pursued with endoscopy, even after an apparently negative or unrevealing radiographic evaluation.[14]

Endoscopy

Endoscopy complements the findings on patient history and radiography. Endoscopy provides the highest diagnostic accuracy for the presence and location of foreign bodies and identification of coexistent gastrointestinal pathology. Moreover, endoscopy allows safe and effective therapy in most instances. Endoscopy is indicated when the history suggests a GIFB, irrespective of a negative radiograph. This approach ensures diagnosis of food impactions, nonradiopaque objects, and radiopaque objects that overlie bony structures.[14] Emergent diagnostic endoscopy is indicated when there are clinical features of high-grade esophageal obstruction and in patients with sialorrhea who are unable to manage their oral secretions. Urgent diagnostic endoscopy is indicated when an esophageal foreign object or food bolus impaction is suspected. Urgent diagnostic endoscopy is also indicated for suspected ingestion of sharp and pointed objects. Following passage or extraction of an ingested foreign object, elective diagnostic endoscopy is indicated for patients with dysphagia or persistent foreign body sensation to assess for laceration or retained foreign material. Elective diagnostic endoscopy is also indicated for patients who have had food bolus impactions to assess for underlying esophageal pathology. Endoscopy is not indicated in asymptomatic patients in whom the GIFB was a small, blunt object that has already passed into the stomach. Endoscopy is contraindicated when there is evidence of bowel perforation or small bowel obstruction beyond the ligament of Treitz.

Treatment

Indications and Timing for Therapy

Seventy-five to ninety percent of GIFBs pass spontaneously without complication.[8, 36] GIFBs that produce symptoms require therapeutic intervention. For asymptomatic patients with GIFBs, the location and characteristics of the GIFB determine the indication for and timing of intervention.

All GIFBs lodged in the esophagus should be managed on an urgent basis. An esophageal dwell time longer than 24 hours is among the most important contributors to complications from esophageal foreign object and food bolus impactions.[30]

Once an object has reached the stomach, however, the risk of complications is greatly diminished and elective management can be individualized.[37] In most cases conservative management is acceptable. For small, blunt objects, weekly radiographs should be obtained to ensure progression through the digestive tract. Patients should be advised to observe for the development of symptoms such as fever, distention, vomiting, and abdominal pain, which may signal perforation or obstruction. Endoscopic retrieval is indicated for large, long, and sharp-pointed objects and for those objects that fail to progress. Large objects (>2 cm in diameter) and long objects (>5 cm in length) should be extracted from the stomach because they are unlikely to pass the pylorus or duodenal sweep unimpeded or without incident. Sharp objects should be removed from the stomach, because their risk of perforation can be as high as 15% to 35% if they are allowed to progress.[35]

Surgery is indicated for evidence of perforation, hemorrhage, fistula formation, or small bowel and colonic obstruction secondary to a GIFB. Surgery is also indicated when GIFBs fail to progress and/or cannot be retrieved endoscopically. Finally, surgery may be considered in patients with abnormal gastrointestinal anatomy or pathology that makes uneventful passage of the GIFB unlikely.[35]

Endoscopic Management of Foreign Bodies

General Considerations

Endoscopy is the method of choice for the evaluation and management of most GIFBs and food bolus impactions. Endoscopy enables safe and effective management of foreign bodies in a controlled fashion under direct visualization. A review of the largest reports of endoscopic management of foreign bodies indicates success rates ranging from 90% to 100%, with most case series reporting success rates of greater than 95%.[5, 8, 24, 30, 31, 38–41] Endoscopic extraction failures were most often related to the number and type of object(s) ingested. Lack of patient cooperation was also a negative contributor. Given the nature of these reports, complication rates are low. Higher complication rates are observed in association with intentional as compared with accidental foreign body ingestion.

Table 21–1 | **Endoscopic Equipment for Upper GI Tract Foreign Body and Food Bolus Removal**

Endoscopes
Rigid endoscope
Flexible endoscope
Laryngoscope with a Kelly or McGill forceps
Overtubes
Standard esophageal overtube
45–60 cm length overtube
Accessory Equipment
Polypectomy snare
Dormia basket
Roth retrieval net
Foreign body rat tooth or alligator forceps
Stiegmann-Goff friction fit variceal adapter
Latex protector hood

Prior to attempted endoscopic therapy, availability of and familiarity with potential retrieval equipment should be reviewed (Table 21–1). Extracorporal practice at grasping a similar or identical object is beneficial in orchestrating a successful foreign object retrieval.[8] A retractable latex-rubber condom-type hood is effective for delivering objects across sphincters and for preventing mural injury from sharp or point-edged objects.

Overtubes are useful for removing sharp or pointed objects and for multiple foreign bodies.[5] Use of an overtube offers several advantages, including (1) airway protection during retrieval; (2) potential for multiple passes of the endoscope during removal of multiple foreign bodies or a food bolus impaction; and (3) protection of the esophageal mucosa from laceration during retrieval of sharp objects.[42] Elective endotracheal intubation is an alternative means of ensuring airway protection. General anesthesia with endotracheal intubation should be employed in small children and uncooperative patients.

Rigid and flexible endoscopic methods have equal efficacy and safety. Rigid esophagoscopy requires performance under general anesthesia and is currently used sparingly by otorhinolaryngologists for impacted cervical esophageal foreign objects that cannot be extracted by flexible endoscope. In most adult patients, flexible endoscopy using intravenous sedation is preferred because of its high success rate, thoroughness of examination, safety, availability, and affordability.[1, 14] In children, flexible endoscopy may be performed with general anesthesia rather than conscious sedation because better patient control and protection of the airway is achieved.

Small, sharp objects such as fish bones lodged at the hypopharynx may be best removed using a laryngoscope with the aid of a long Kelly or McGill forceps under direct visualization. Small-caliber, flexible nasoendoscopes have failed to demonstrate any benefit over standard per-oral flexible endoscopy.[43]

Food Bolus Impaction

Food impaction is the most common GIFB in adults.[5] The most common impacted foods are larger pieces of beef, pork, chicken, and hot dog,[5, 6] giving way to the terms "steakhouse syndrome" and "backyard barbecue syndrome." Patients present with abrupt onset of dysphagia and the sense of esophageal obstruction. Chest pain is common, owing to esophageal spasm, and may mimic angina. The patients may be dyspneic and tachypneic, but this is generally anxiety driven. Patients with food bolus impactions are able to speak, which helps discriminate this condition from true choking due to airway obstruction. Anteroposterior and lateral chest radiographs should be obtained to assess mediastinal or peritoneal free air and for bones or other radiopaque foreign material in the food bolus. Biplanar neck films should be obtained when the food impaction sensation localizes to that region.

Food bolus impactions can produce complete or only partial obstruction. Urgent management is indicated when patients are in severe distress, excessively salivating, or unable to manage their secretions. If patients are not uncomfortable and able to swallow their saliva, nonurgent endoscopy can be planned. Every effort should be made to alleviate all food bolus impactions within 12 to 24 hours of their occurrence. While endoscopy is being coordinated, food boluses may pass with intravenous glucagon (see "Nonendoscopic Therapy") and the relaxation that accompanies the reassurance of medical attention. When this is thought to have occurred, options include proceeding with endoscopy as planned versus a trial of sips of water, which if ingested successfully can precede a modified radiographic contrast study to confirm disimpaction. Otherwise, radiocontrast agents have no role in the diagnosis and management of food bolus impactions.

Endoscopy confirms the location and characteristics of food bolus impactions in the esophagus and may identify any associated esophageal pathology. Often there are nonimpacted chewed-food items lying above the source of true obstruction that need to be cleared away. Commonly, the presence of the food impaction produces esophageal muscular irritability with spastic contraction that impedes both forward and retrograde progress.

Many food boluses pass with a gentle nudge forward with the tip of the endoscope.[14, 31] This success is enhanced by esophageal muscular relaxation induced by sedation and expansion of the esophageal lumen with endoscopic air-insufflation. However, forceful blinded pushing with the endoscope is never indicated. A food bolus that fails to advance with a gentle push technique can typically be disrupted and debulked using a forceps. Once the bolus has been reduced in size, it will often pass under endoscopic visualization. In other instances, with insufflation and distention of the esophageal lumen, the endoscope can be steered around and beyond the obstructing bolus. Once this is achieved, as the endoscope has entered the stomach and assessed the luminal patency of the esophagus and gastroesophageal junction, the scope can be pulled back and used to gently push the bolus through and into the stomach. The high association of underlying esophageal pathology accompanying food bolus impactions makes the practice of forceful blind pushing with the endoscope unacceptable. Similarly, advancing retrieval devices or dilators blindly beyond the impaction invites complications.[44]

If the food impaction cannot be pushed forward into the stomach, it must be retrieved via the endoscope. Using grasping forceps (rat-toothed, or alligator type), food boluses can be removed en toto or in a piecemeal fashion. As previously stated, an overtube facilitates multiple passes of the endoscope, protects the esophageal mucosa, and minimizes the risk of aspiration. More often, meat impactions shred when grasped with forceps rather than dislodge as single or multiple large chunks. Again, once sufficiently debulked in this manner, the remaining material will pass easily into the stomach. Snares, baskets, and nets (Fig. 21–4) may be used under direct visualization, but one should avoid the tempta-

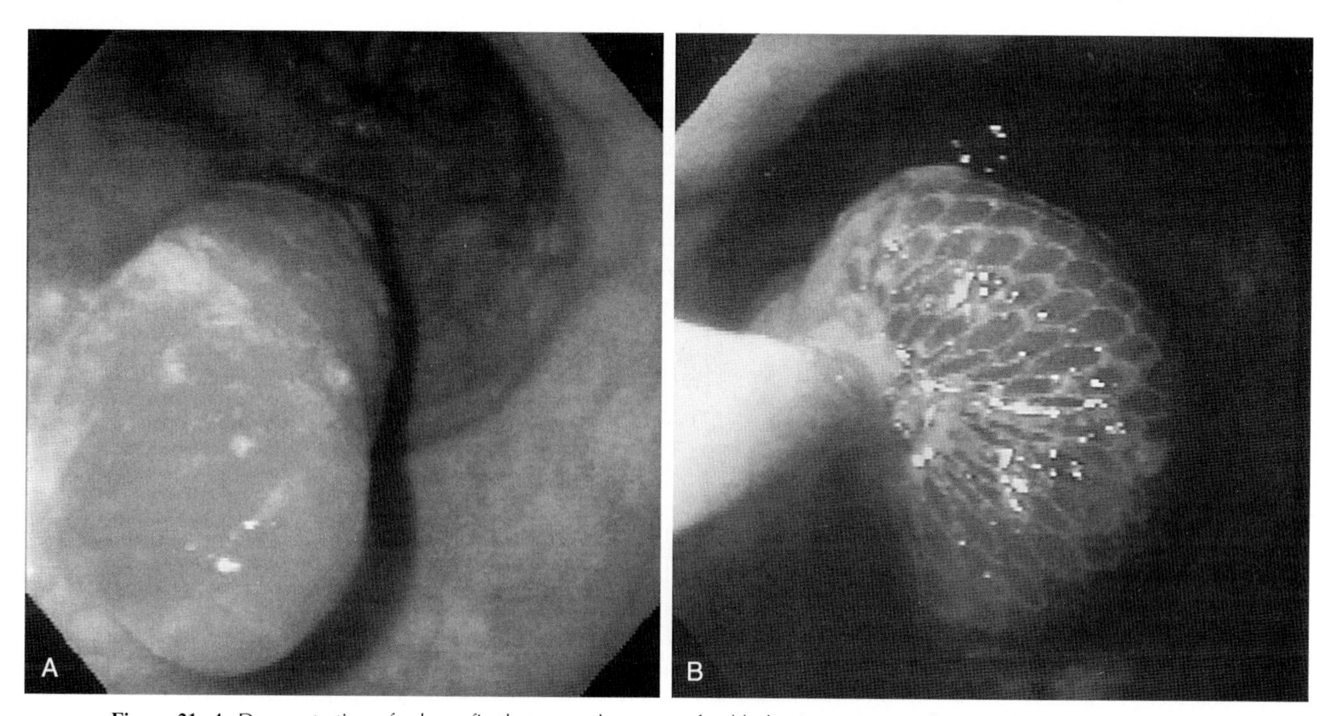

Figure 21–4. Demonstration of a large fig that caused an acute food bolus impaction *(A)* that was easily removed with the use of a Roth retrieval net *(B)*.

tion of advancing devices blindly past a food bolus impaction.

Another recommended method to treat food impactions employs the use of the transparent endoscopic cap-fitting device originally popularized for endoscopic variceal ligation and an esophageal overtube.[45] The assembly creates a direct-vision suction device to remove the impacted food. This compelling technique has been useful when attempts at grasping the impacted material prove futile. It has worked effectively for notoriously difficult items such as impacted hot dogs and chicken meat.

If a food bolus cannot be successfully removed with flexible endoscopy, options include a repeated attempt by a second endoscopist, rigid esophagoscopy, or laparotomy/thoracotomy.[40]

Once the esophageal food impaction has been cleared, the presence of underlying esophageal pathology, reported in as many as 86% to 97% of patients, should be assessed.[6–8] However, there is usually considerable mural edema and mucosal erythema and abrasion, making it difficult to discriminate an acute from a chronic process. Among patients with food bolus impactions, more than half have abnormal 24-hour esophageal pH studies and nearly half have esophageal dysmotility on manometry.[7] If a benign narrowing is observed (e.g., peptic stricture or Schatzki's ring) and there is minimal inflammation, esophageal dilatation can be performed during the same session.[6] More often, we prescribe a proton-pump inhibitor and arrange elective outpatient endoscopy with possible dilation after any acute mural inflammation has had a chance to resolve. Patients should be educated on methods of reducing further food bolus impactions. Instructions include eating more slowly, chewing foods thoroughly, and avoiding troublesome foods.

Coins and Other Small, Blunt Objects

Coins are the most common object swallowed by children and often require intervention.[3, 46] Dimes and pennies, 17 and 18 mm in diameter, respectively, usually pass spontaneously, but larger sized coins have a greater propensity to remain in the esophagus. A drinking game, "Quarters," has led to an increased incidence of coins becoming lodged in the esophagus of intoxicated adults.[47] Any blunt object lodged in the esophagus requires prompt removal. Objects left in place result in pressure necrosis and subsequent perforation or fistulization.

In very small children, removal is usually performed under general anesthesia, with endotracheal intubation protecting the airway. In larger children and adults an esophageal overtube can provide adequate airway protection if the tube is of large enough diameter to allow retrieval of the object. Endoscope device manufacturers market a variety of specialty forceps well suited for foreign body extraction. These are preferred over standard pinch biopsy forceps.[31] Another consideration is to advance the object into the stomach and then secure it for retrieval with a Roth net or Dormia-type retrieval basket. This should be done only if such advancement proceeds relatively unimpeded, assisted by luminal distention via air insufflation.

In most adults, once a coin or other small blunt object, including a disc battery has entered the stomach, conservative outpatient management with observation alone will suffice.[48] The pylorus can accept and pass objects up to 25 mm, which includes all coins except for half-dollars (30 mm) or silver dollars (38 mm). Most objects are passed within 4 to 6 days, although some may take as long as 4 weeks. While waiting for foreign bodies to pass, patients may be instructed

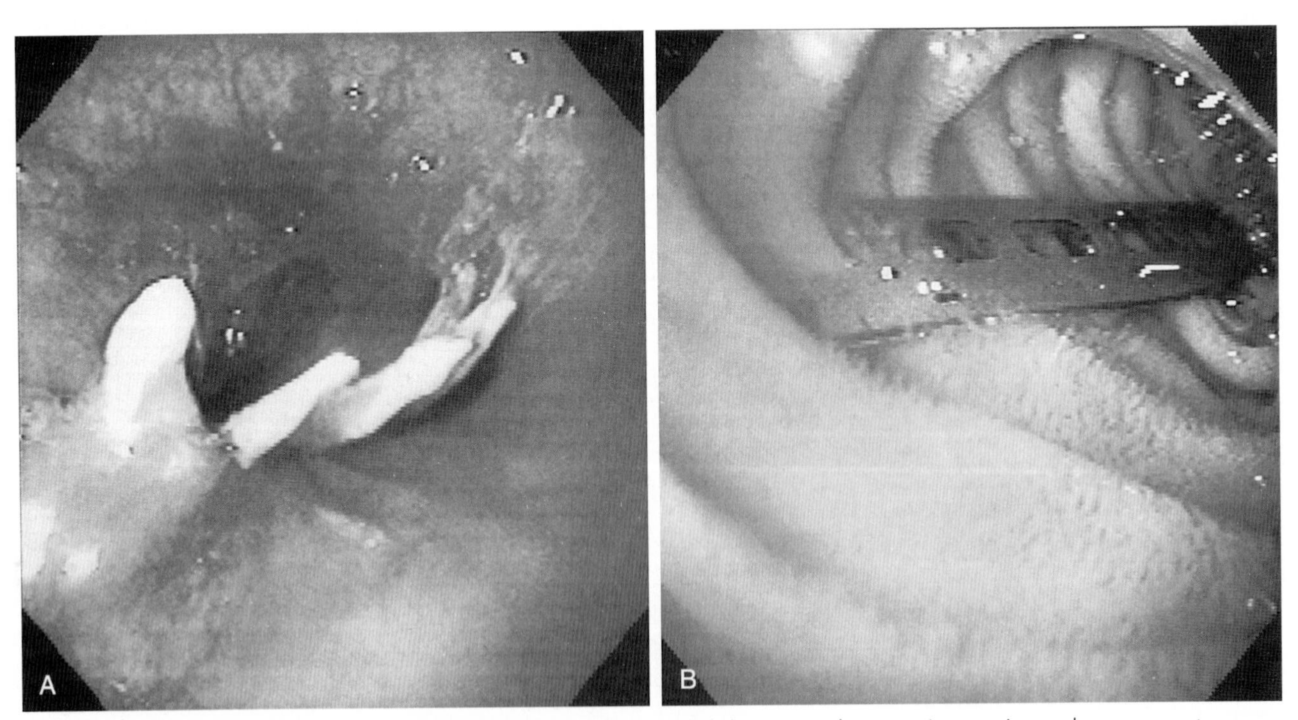

Figure 21–5. Examples of sharp foreign bodies that were ingested that required prompt intervention and management, including *(A)* a plastic fork protruding upward through the esophageal sphincter that was managed endoscopically, and *(B)* a razor blade in the jejunum that required surgical removal without complication.

to continue a regular diet and observe the stools for the ingested object. In the absence of symptoms, weekly radiographs are sufficient to follow the progression of small, blunt objects not observed to pass spontaneously. Objects that fail to leave the stomach within 3 to 4 weeks should be removed endoscopically.[49] Once past the stomach, for objects that remain in the same location for more than 1 week, surgical removal should be considered. A history of prior abdominal surgery increases the risk of complications and should prompt greater vigilance. The efficacy of laxatives to encourage the advancement of ingested foreign bodies has yet to be established. Symptoms of fever, vomiting, or abdominal pain are indications for immediate surgical evaluation.

Sharp/Pointed and Long Objects

Sharp/pointed and long foreign objects are among the most dangerous GIFBs and among the most challenging objects to remove. One third of all perforations caused by foreign bodies are caused by sharp/pointed objects, and 15% to 35% of ingested sharp/pointed objects cause a gastrointestinal perforation if untreated[49] (Fig. 21–5). Sharp/pointed and long objects in the esophagus merit urgent attention, whereas those that have passed into the stomach may be addressed with less immediacy.

Inadvertently swallowed animal bones and toothpicks are the most common GIFBs requiring surgery in this country.[31, 50] Dental bridgework is another not uncommon accidental sharp/pointed GIFB. Sharp/pointed and long objects are frequently ingested by persons with psychiatric illness, incarcerated persons seeking medical attention, and young female bulimics during ill-fated attempts at inducing emesis. Such objects include toothbrushes, dining utensils, writing instruments, cosmetic applicators, razor blades, pins, needles, nails, and metal wires.

When considering endoscopic removal of sharp/pointed objects, one should consider a paraphrase of Chevalier Jackson's axiom: "advancing points puncture, trailing points do not."[51] When attempting endoscopic extraction of a sharp or pointed object, the foreign body should be grasped and positioned axially so that the sharp/pointed end trails distally to the endoscope. An example is an open safety pin lodged in the esophagus with the open pin pointing rostrally. The safety pin should first be advanced into the stomach, reoriented and grasped at the crotch so the open pointed end is directed caudally, then withdrawn into a protective hood or overtube.

Polypectomy snares and foreign body retrieval forceps are the devices most useful for retrieving sharp/pointed objects. An esophageal overtube, if the size and configuration of the GIFB allows, should be used to protect the esophagus and oropharynx.[52] A soft latex protector hood is an alternative, effectively shielding the mucosa from the sharp edges and pointed tips[52] (Fig. 21–6). This cone-shaped hood slips over the end of the endoscope and is secured with tape or a ligature (2-0 silk suture works well). The hood is folded back on itself to give full endoscopic visualization. Once the foreign body is grasped, the scope tip is purposefully withdrawn through the lower esophageal sphincter. On doing so, the hood flips back over and the foreign body can be withdrawn into its protective cone.

Despite the increased risk of perforation with sharp objects, most still pass through the gastrointestinal tract without complications. Sharp objects that cannot be removed by endoscope should be followed with daily radiographs that document their passage, and surgical intervention should be considered if the object has failed to progress over 3 consecutive days.[1] Other indications for surgery are the acute onset of abdominal pain, fever, evidence of obstruction, and bleeding.

Long objects (particularly >10 cm) in the stomach have difficulty passing the duodenal sweep, and an attempt should be made to remove them endoscopically. Device choice for retrieval tends to be object specific. A long overtube can be most useful in removing long, pointed objects. One specific technique is described as follows. The object is grasped by a forceps or snare and withdrawn into the overtube. Then the entire assembly (i.e., foreign body, overtube, and endoscope) are withdrawn as a unit. This minimizes the risk of losing grasp of the object within the overtube and facilitates traversing of the upper esophageal sphincter and the oropharynx.[14, 53]

Narcotic Packets

Increased international drug trade has led to a GIFB requiring special attention: the narcotic packet. Two types of pa-

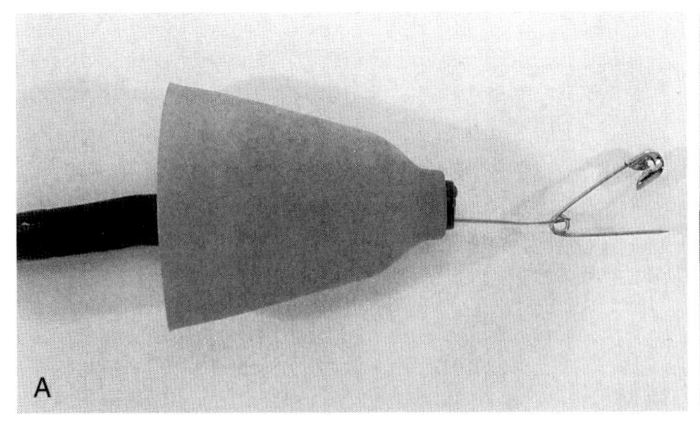

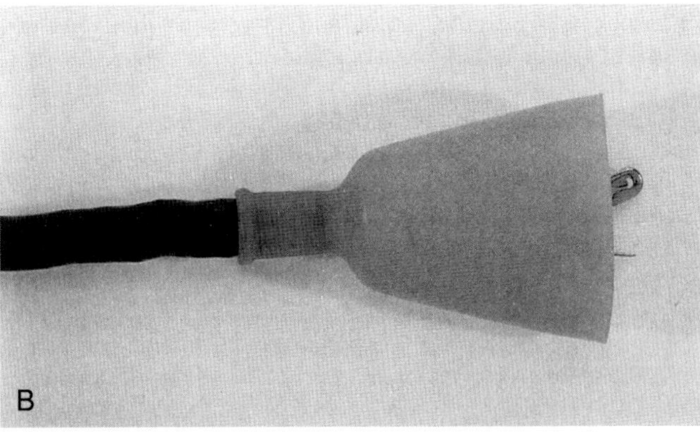

Figure 21–6. *A,* Photograph of the latex protector hood with the bell pulled back on itself providing full visualization and allowing the endoscopist to grasp the sharp object. *B,* The endoscope and hood are pulled back through the lower esophageal sphincter, flipping the hood forward and protecting the gastrointestinal mucosa from the object.

tients are encountered. One is the "body stuffer." These are typically drug users or dealers on the verge of arrest who swallow varying amounts of drugs in poorly wrapped containers. The other is the "body packer" or "mule." These are knowing or unwitting individuals who, in a smuggling attempt, ingest large amounts of carefully packaged drugs designed to withstand gastrointestinal tract transit.[54, 55] Cocaine and heroin are the most commonly trafficked.

Patients may present with an acute toxicologic emergency on bag rupture, with an intestinal obstruction, or be asymptomatic on arrest based on other suspicions. Abdominal radiographs show multiple sausage-shaped or round radiopacities in most cases (70%–90%).[55] Toxicology screens detect leakage and identify the drug, which may avail itself to a specific reversal agent.

Endoscopic removal is absolutely contraindicated to avoid inadvertent rupture of packaging.[44] If the patient is asymptomatic, inpatient observation with a clear-liquid diet is recommended. Whole-gut lavage and gentle purgatives have been described to hasten the decontamination of the gut but remain controversial because of the potential to promote package rupture.[54, 55] Surgery is the definitive therapy for signs of intestinal obstruction, failure of packets to progress, and suspected rupture.[14]

Colorectal Foreign Bodies

Colorectal foreign body impactions may result from migration of ingested objects or from direct purposeful or inadvertent insertion. Ingested objects may become lodged or impacted at the ileocecal valve, within diverticular orifices, at the sigmoid curve, and at the anorectal junction. Direct insertion occurs intentionally and unintentionally as a consequence of sexual activities, attempts at constipation relief, and criminal assault. True inadvertent rectal insertion may occur during bathing mishaps (see Chapter 116).

Foreign bodies in the rectum or colon may present with rectal or abdominal pain, hematochezia, pruritus ani, obstipation, obstruction, abscess, or peritonitis.[15, 22] The most common presentation, though, is that of an asymptomatic patient who is unable to remove an object known to have been inserted. Owing to mental or psychiatric impairment, fear of repercussions, or embarrassment, patients frequently provide only vague or fabricated histories. This can delay diagnosis and may contribute to increased risk of complications.[15, 56]

The physical examination should first focus on signs of potential complications including fever, abdominal distention, palpable mass, and peritoneal signs. The anorectum should be assessed for overt hematochezia, tears, sphincter tone, and object visibility.[22] Care should be used in performing the digital rectal examination out of respect for sharp or pointed objects. The ability to palpate the foreign body on rectal examination increases the chance of successful transanal manual removal of the object. We advise obtaining abdominal and pelvic radiographs prior to performing a digital rectal examination. Radiographs help to characterize the object(s), depict its orientation and location, and document findings of perforation or obstruction. The likelihood of the object's radiopacity needs to be considered. Computed tomographic scanning should be considered when abscess is suspected or subtle features of perforation are sought. The use of bowel contrast agents may be necessary.

In the absence of evidence for perforation or peritonitis, manual removal should be attempted when feasible. Depending on the size, shape, and location of the object, and with the aid of conscious sedation, most rectal foreign bodies can be successfully extracted manually or endoscopically through the transanal route. Blunt objects that can be grasped on two-finger digital rectal examination may be able to be withdrawn using the gloved fingers. Other blunt objects and long, sharp, or pointed objects should have removal attempted under direct visualization with a rigid proctoscope or a flexible sigmoidoscope.[22] Conscious sedation is usually sufficient. The patient should be in the left lateral-decubitus position. As in the removal of objects from the upper gastrointestinal tract, a variety of retrieval devices should be available. A latex hood attached to the sigmoidoscope can protect the mucosa from puncture or laceration when removing sharp/pointed objects (Fig. 21–7). The hood may also serve to overcome the anal sphincter's tendency to contract and grasp objects during their attempted delivery.

For larger objects and those unable to be removed using the methods described earlier, general anesthesia and sphincter dilation is required. General anesthesia allows maximum dilatation of the sphincters to facilitate instrumentation and removal of the foreign body.[57] During examination under general anesthesia, retractors, vaginal spatulas, gynecologic forceps, and suction devices all have been used for extraction with success. Hollow foreign bodies such as bottles and cups can create a suction effect in the rectum. In such instances a Foley catheter passed proximal to the foreign body is able to effectively relieve the suction phenomenon. Flexible sigmoidoscopy after removal of the object is recommended to evaluate for possible transmural injury.[57]

Surgery is generally indicated when perforation, abscess, and/or obstruction complicate foreign body impaction. Laparotomy is the last resort to remove defiant objects. Laparotomy may accompany a posterior sphincterotomy, exploratory celiotomy with milking or pushing the colorectal foreign body distally, and longitudinal colotomy followed by primary closure.[22, 32, 56] Recently, a number of case reports have described modified minimally invasive approaches using laparoscopy and "hand-port" techniques.

Nonendoscopic Therapies

A host of medical and radiologic therapies have been described for use in the management of esophageal foreign bodies. Smooth muscle relaxants such as glucagon can reduce tone in the lower esophageal sphincter.[37] Glucagon, given at 0.5 to 2 mg, has onset of action within 1 minute and duration of up to 15 minutes. The success of glucagon has been reported to range from 12% to 58% in the treatment of esophageal foreign bodies or food impactions.[58, 59] Other medications can also reduce lower esophageal sphincter pressure. Nifedipine and nitroglycerin have been described in anecdotal reports as promoting passage of the food bolus or foreign body into the stomach. However, smooth muscle relaxants do not provide definitive therapy for foreign bodies or food bolus impactions in the esophagus

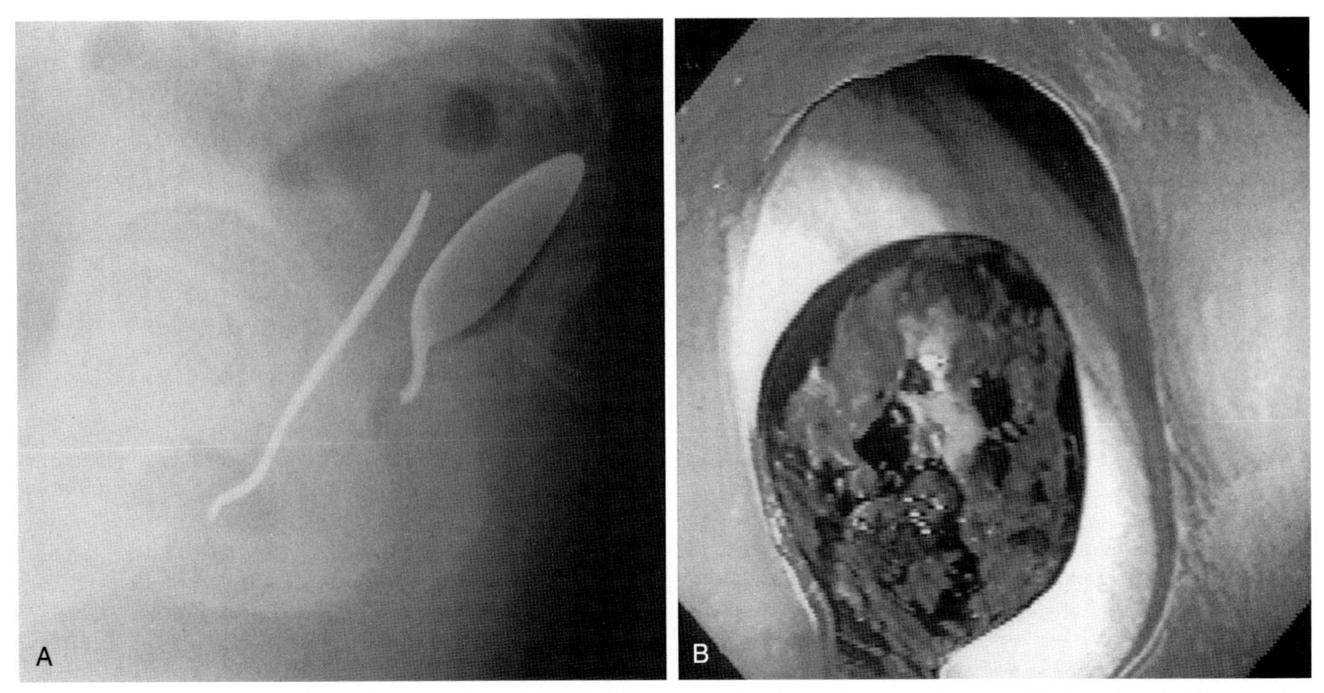

Figure 21–7. *A,* Radiograph of a broken metal spoon that was introduced into the rectum by a psychiatric patient. *B,* The spoon was visualized with the endoscope and removed with the aid of a latex protector hood.

and may produce undesired side effects, including abdominal distention, nausea with vomiting, and hypotension. Although their use is not contraindicated, it should not delay or defer definitive endoscopic inspection and therapy.

The use of gas-forming agents, either alone or in combination with a smooth muscle relaxant, has been described for the management of esophageal foreign bodies. Carbonated beverages and preparations consisting of sodium bicarbonate, citric acid, and simethicone used to release carbon dioxide gas are described. The intent is for the released gas to distend the lumen and act as a piston to push the object from the esophagus into the stomach.[60] Success rates as high as 75% to 100% have been described in small studies.[60, 61] However, esophageal rupture and perforation have also been described in association with the use of these agents.[62] Even proponents of gas-forming agents assert that they should not be used when there is a fixed rigid obstruction, when the foreign body has been in place longer than 6 hours, or when it is in the proximal third of the esophagus.[61] We do not recommend these methods under any circumstances.

Two other reported methods are mentioned for historical purposes. First, papain, an enzymatic meat tenderizer, has been used to dissolve or soften meat impactions. This may lead to esophageal necrosis and perforation and severe pulmonary complications if aspirated.[1, 18] Second, emetics have been used to promote regurgitation of a foreign body. This approach is rarely successful and risks rupture of the esophagus[63] and aspiration.

The radiology literature contains descriptions of an array of methods to extract blunt esophageal foreign bodies under fluoroscopic guidance using Fogarty (or Foley-type) balloon catheters, Dormia-type wire baskets, and suction catheters. The largest published experience has been with the use of Foley catheters. In this technique, the catheter is passed nasally or orally beyond the foreign body and the balloon is inflated. The catheter is then withdrawn to deliver the foreign body to the oropharynx.[2] In a study of 2500 patients, a success rate of 95% was achieved, with a complication rate of 0.4%. The major drawback of this method is the lack of control of the foreign body, particularly as it passes the laryngopharynx, posing a risk for aspiration. Death has been reported as a result of airway occlusion by a coin aspirated during its withdrawal using this technique.[39] Other complications include nosebleeds, dislodgment into the nose, laryngospasm, retching with vomiting, and hypoxia.[64]

The use of a magnet catheter to remove ferromagnetic metal objects such as button batteries, paper clips, and nails has been described. Paulson and Jaffe described an experience in which a magnet attached to a catheter was successful in removing 34 of 36 metallic foreign bodies.[65] Lack of control and risk of aspiration are problems, particularly because of the narrowing of the cricopharyngeal muscle and upper esophageal sphincter that may cause dislodgment.

None of these methods surpass endoscopic therapy for safety or efficacy. Generally, it is thought that techniques for removal of esophageal foreign bodies under fluoroscopic control offer little to no advantage over endoscopy and are only indicated when endoscopy is not available.[8, 14, 40] These techniques would seem to have limited appeal with the wide availability of endoscopy today.

BEZOARS

Bezoars are collections or concretions of indigestible foreign material that accumulate and coalesce in the gastrointestinal tract, usually the stomach. Bezoars can be classified into four types: phytobezoars, composed of vegetable matter;

trichobezoars, composed of hair or hairlike fibers; medication bezoars (pharmacobezoars), consisting of medications or medication vehicles; and lactobezoars, or milk curd bezoar secondary to an infant's formula.

Epidemiology

Phytobezoars are the most common type of bezoar and occur with foods such as celery, pumpkin, grape skins, prunes, raisins, leeks, beets, and, most notably, persimmon.[8, 49] These foods contain large amounts of nondigestible dietary fiber such as cellulose, hemicellulose, lignin, and fruit tannin.[66] Tannins in high concentrations form a coagulum when exposed to gastric acid. When sufficient quantity accumulates, based on rates of gastric intake and elimination, a bezoar may develop.[27]

Trichobezoars occur most frequently in children and young adult women. An associated increase is observed with conditions of mental retardation, psychiatric disorders, and pica.[67, 68] Trichobezoars result due to ingestion of large quantities of hair, carpet fiber, string, or clothing.

Medications that have resulted in bezoar formation include antacids, fiber supplements, and resin-coated extended-release products or other products that are designed to resist digestion in the stomach such as enteric-coated aspirin.[69] Medication bezoars may result in reduced medication efficacy (when the pharmacologically active agent is trapped in the bezoar and cannot be absorbed) or toxicity (when previously bound pharmacologically active agent is released in excessive concentration)[69] (Table 21–2).

Ingestion of large amounts of indigestible material is not the sole requirement for bezoar formation. The majority of patients have a predisposing factor that contributes to bezoar formation, most commonly altered gastrointestinal anatomy from previous surgery. Evidence of prior gastric surgery is present in 70% to 94% of patients with bezoars. Bezoar formation may occur in 65% to 80% of patients who have undergone vagotomy with pyloroplasty.[27, 70] Up to 20% of patients who have undergone an antrectomy may develop a gastric bezoar.[71] Bezoar formation after surgery is a result of altered gastric motility with delayed gastric emptying and a reduction of gastric accommodation, poor gastric mixing, and reduced peptic activity.[72]

Gastroparesis is commonly observed in patients with bezoars who do not have surgically altered gastric anatomy, although not all patients with bezoars have abnormal gastric emptying scans.[69, 73] Patients with comorbid illnesses such as diabetes, patients with end-stage renal disease on dialysis, or patients on mechanical ventilation have increased risk of bezoar formation.[69]

Table 21–2 | **Medications Associated with Pharmacobezoar Formation**

Nonabsorbable antacids
Bulk-forming laxatives
Cardiovascular medications
Nifedipine
Procainamide
Verapamil
Vitamins and minerals
Vitamin C tablets
Vitamin B_{12}
Lecithin
Ferrous sulfate
Miscellaneous medications
Sucralfate
Guar gum
Cholestyramine
Enteral feeding formulas
Meprobamate
Theophylline
Kayexalate resin

Clinical Presentation

Many patients with bezoars are asymptomatic or have symptoms that are indistinguishable from the underlying gastrointestinal pathology.[27] The most common presenting symptom is a vague feeling of epigastric distress, present in as many as 80% of patients with bezoars.[74] Other frequent symptoms are nausea, vomiting, anorexia, early satiety, and weight loss. Bezoars may accumulate over an extended period and grow to appreciable size. Gastric ulceration secondary to pressure necrosis is found in up to one fourth of patients with large bezoars. These ulcers may bleed or cause gastric outlet obstruction.[27, 74] As previously stated, decreased medication efficacy below that of anticipated should increase suspicion of bezoar in selected patients.

The largest series of small bowel bezoars found that most patients (78 of 87) presented with complete mechanical obstruction.[70] Small bowel bezoars as a result of "Rapunzel syndrome," where the trichobezoar extends past the pylorus into the duodenum, have caused jaundice and acute pancreatitis due to obstruction of the ampulla of Vater.[75, 76]

Diagnosis

Physical diagnosis is usually of little assistance in the diagnosis of bezoars. Occasionally a palpable mass may be felt or there may be evidence of abdominal distention. Severe halitosis may be present due to the putrefying material in the stomach.[49] With trichobezoars patchy baldness may be found if the patient suffers from trichotillomania.[77]

Plain radiographs of the abdomen may demonstrate obstruction or an outline of the bezoar. The classic radiographic finding is a gastric-filling defect on barium study[66] (Fig. 21–8). The definitive diagnosis of bezoar is established at endoscopy.[66, 74] Radiographs with or without barium may identify only one fourth of bezoars that are subsequently identified by endoscopy.[66, 74] At endoscopy, phytobezoars appear as a dark brown, green, or black mass of amorphous material in the gastric fundus, antrum, or remnant stomach. Trichobezoars often have a hard, concrete-like appearance. Enzymatic oxidation of the hair material imparts a blackened coloration.[66] In medication bezoars, whole pills or pill fragments can be seen intertwined in the bezoar.

Treatment

After diagnosis and localization of the bezoar, treatment incorporates removal and prevention of recurrence. Small bezoars may be amenable to conservative management with a

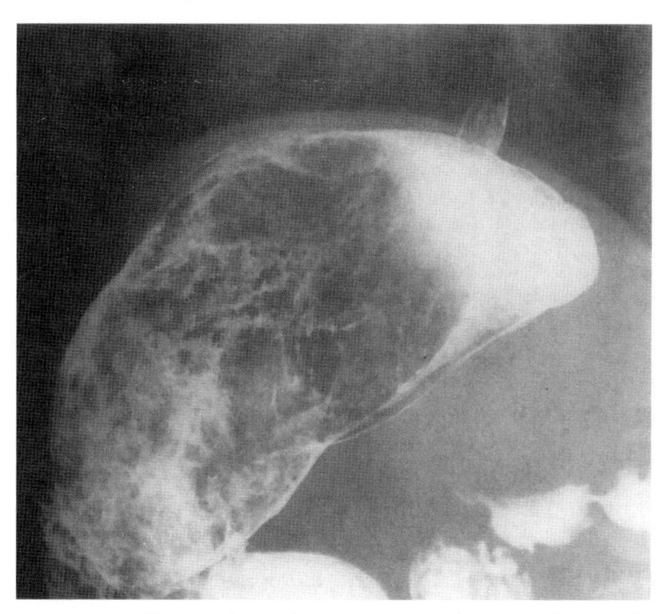

Figure 21–8. Classic radiographic appearance of a gastric bezoar displaying multiple filling defects in the stomach on a barium study. A plain radiograph would show a "bubbly" appearance to the gastric bezoar. (Courtesy of Igor Laufer, MD, Philadelphia, PA.)

clear-liquid diet and the addition of a prokinetic agent such as metoclopromide.[67] Nasogastric lavage may effectively dissolve small phytobezoars.[67] Chemical dissolution has been reported with varying degrees of success. In small case series, successful dissolution of up to 85% is reported.[27] The greatest efficacy and safety experiences have been with cellulase. Cellulase can be administered in tablet form or as a liquid instilled via a nasogastric tube or injected through an endoscope.

Most bezoars respond to endoscopic therapy with fragmentation. Reduced sized fragments may be retrieved or allowed to pass through the gut. Mechanical disruption usually can be accomplished with standard endoscopic tools such as biopsy forceps or polypectomy snares. Removal of fragmented pieces usually requires multiple passes with the endoscope. An overtube is recommended to facilitate this and to avoid aspiration of contents on withdrawal. Simple mechanical disruption and removal by endoscopy has reported successes in the range of 85% to 90%. For larger phytobezoars and trichobezoars, endoscopic removal may be more challenging. Numerous accessories have been described to accomplish this, including electrohydraulic lithotripsy, mechanical gallstone lithotripsy, pulsed water jets, Nd:YAG laser, and a needle-knife bezotome.[71, 78, 79]

Surgical removal of bezoars is occasionally required for trichobezoars. Surgery is indicated when there is a failure of endoscopic therapy and for bezoar-associated complications such as perforation, obstruction, and gastrointestinal bleeding. Gastric bezoars may be removed through a small gastrostomy.[27, 67] Small bowel bezoars typically require surgery with enterotomy. In some cases at laparotomy, the bezoar can be transmurally palpated, fragmented, and "milked" to the cecum. There exists an increased incidence of coincident gastric and small bowel bezoar formation. Thus, care should be taken to exclude multiple bezoars in other portions of the gastrointestinal tract when surgery is contemplated.

Recurrence of bezoars is common unless the underlying predisposing conditions are influenced. Avoidance of the offending agent of phytobezoar formation (i.e., persimmon, raw citrus fruit, and high-fiber foods) should be observed. Regimens of enzymatic dissolution medications, usually cellulase, can be taken as a prophylaxis added to each meal.[30] Prokinetics are helpful in some patients with motility disorders (see Chapter 37). Patients with psychiatric disorders require specific therapy to avoid recurrence.[66] Periodic endoscopy with repeated mechanical disruption is warranted in difficult recurrent cases.

REFERENCES

1. Webb WA: Management of foreign bodies of the upper gastrointestinal tract. Gastroenterology 94:204–216, 1988.
2. Shaffer HA, de lange EE: Gastrointestinal foreign bodies and strictures: Radiologic interventions. Curr Probl Diagn Radiol 23:205–249, 1994.
3. Kim JK, Kim SS, Kim JI, et al: Management of foreign bodies in the gastrointestinal tract: An analysis of 104 cases in children. Endoscopy 31:302–304, 1999.
4. Chalk SG, Faucer H: Foreign bodies in the stomach. Arch Surg 16: 494–500, 1928.
5. Vizcarrondo FJ, Brady PG, Nord HJ: Foreign bodies of the upper gastrointestinal tract. Gastrointest Endosc 29:208–210, 1983.
6. Weinstock LB, Shatz BA, Thyssen EP: Esophageal food bolus obstruction: Evaluation of extraction and modified push techniques in 75 cases. Endoscopy 31:421–425, 1999.
7. Lacy PD, Donnelly MJ, McGrath JP, et al: Acute food bolus impaction: Aetiology and management. J Laryngol Otol 111:1158–1161, 1997.
8. Webb WA: Management of foreign bodies of the upper gastrointestinal tract: Update. Gastrointest Endosc 41:39–51, 1995.
9. Schwartz GF, Polsky HS: Ingested foreign bodies of the gastrointestinal tract. Am Surg 42:236–238, 1976.
10. Terracol J: Maladies de L'esophage. Paris, Masson, 1951.
11. Devanesan J, Pisani A, Sharma P, et al: Metallic foreign bodies in the stomach. Arch Surg 112:664–665, 1977.
12. Brady P: Esophageal foreign bodies. Gastroenterol Clin North Am 20: 691–701, 1991.
13. Scher R, Tegtmeyer C, McLean W: Vascular injury following foreign body perforation of the esophagus: Review of the literature and report of a case. Ann Otol Rhinol Laryngol 99:698–702, 1990.
14. Ginsberg GG: Management of ingested foreign objects and food bolus impactions. Gastrointest Endosc 41:33–38, 1995.
15. Stack LB, Munter DW: Foreign bodies in the gastrointestinal tract. Emerg Med Clin North Am 14:493–521, 1996.
16. Quinn PG, Connors PJ: The role of gastrointestinal endoscopy in foreign body removal. Gastrointest Endosc Clin North Am 4:571–593, 1994.
17. Bloom RR, Nakano PH, Gray SW, et al: Foreign bodies of the gastrointestinal tract. Am Surg 10:618–621, 1986.
18. Lyons MF, Tsuchida AM: Foreign bodies of the gastrointestinal tract. Med Clin North Am 77:1101–1114, 1993.
19. Stein HJ, Schwizer W, DeMeester TR, et al: Foreign body entrapment in the esophagus of healthy subjects—a manometric and scintigraphic study. Dysphagia 7:220, 1992.
20. Koch H: Operative endoscopy. Gastrointest Endosc 24:65–68, 1977.
21. Davidhoff E, Towne JB: Ingested foreign bodies. NY State Med J 75: 1003–1007, 1975.
22. Cohen JS, Sackier JM: Management of colorectal foreign bodies. J R Coll Surg Edinb 41:312–315, 1996.
23. Taylor RB: Esophageal foreign bodies. Emerg Clin North Am 5:301–311, 1987.
24. Herranz-Gonzalez J, Martinez-Vidal J, Garcia-Sarandeses A, et al: Esophageal foreign bodies in adults. Otolaryngol Head Neck Surg 105: 649, 1991.
25. Yoshida C, Peura D: Foreign bodies in the esophagus. In Castell D (ed): The Esophagus. Boston, Little, Brown, 1995, pp 379–394.
26. Connolly AA, Birchall M, Walsh-Waring GP, et al: Ingested foreign bodies: Patient-guided localization is a useful clinical tool. Clin Otolaryngol 17:520–524, 1992.

27. Lee J: Bezoars and foreign bodies of the stomach. Gastrointest Endosc Clin North Am 6:605–619, 1996.
28. Classen M, Farthmann EF, Siefert E, et al: Operative and therapeutic techniques in endoscopy. Clin Gastroenterol 7:741–763, 1978.
29. Choudhurg CR, Bricknell MC, MacIver D: Oesophageal foreign body: An unusual cause of respiratory symptoms in a three-week baby. J Laryngol Otol 106:556–557, 1992.
30. Chaikhouni A, Kratz JM, Crawford FA: Foreign bodies of the esophagus. Am Surg 51:173–179, 1985.
31. Webb WA, Taylor MB: Foreign bodies of the upper gastrointestinal tract. In Taylor MB (ed): Gastrointestinal Emergencies, 2nd ed. Philadelphia, Lippincott Williams & Wilkins, 1996, pp 204–216.
32. Hodge D, Tecklenburg F, Fleischer G: Coin ingestion: Does every child need a radiograph? Ann Emerg Med 14:443–446, 1985.
33. Jones NS, Lannigan FJ, Salama NY: Foreign bodies in the throat: A prospective study of 388 cases. J Laryngol Otol 105:104, 1991.
34. Bassett KE, Schunk JE, Logan L: Localizing ingested coins with a metal detector. Am J Emerg Med 17:338–341, 1999.
35. Henderson CT, Engel J, Schlesinger P: Foreign body ingestion: Review and suggested guidelines for management. Endoscopy 19:68–71, 1987.
36. Velitchkov NG, Grigorov GI, Losanoff JE, et al: Ingested foreign bodies of the gastrointestinal tract: Retrospective analysis of 542 cases. World J Surg 20:1001–1005, 1996.
37. Jaffer SS, Makhlouf GM, Schorr BA, et al; Nature and kinetics of inhibition of lower esophageal sphincter pressure by glucagon. Gastroenterology 67:42–46, 1974.
38. Blair SR, Graeber GM, Cruzzavala, et al: Current management of esophageal impactions. Chest 104:1205–1209, 1993.
39. Hawkins DB: Removal of blunt foreign bodies from the esophagus. Ann Otol Rhinol Laryngol 99:935–940, 1990.
40. Berggreen PJ, Harrison ME, Sanowski RA, et al: Techniques and complications of esophageal foreign body extraction in children and adults. Gastrointest Endosc 39:626–630, 1993.
41. Crysdale W, Sendi K, Yoo J: Esophageal foreign bodies in children. Ann Otol Rhinol Laryngol 100:320–324, 1991.
42. Faigel DO, Stotland BR, Kochman ML, et al: Device choice and experience level in endoscopic foreign object retrieval: An in vivo study. Gastrointest Endosc 45:490–492, 1997.
43. Chu KM, Choi HK, Tuen HH, et al: A prospective randomized trial comparing the use of the flexible gastroscope versus the bronchoscope in the management of foreign body ingestion. Gastrointest Endosc 47: 23–27, 1998.
44. Guidelines for the management of ingested foreign bodies. Gastrointest Endosc 42:622–625, 1995.
45. Mamel JJ, Weiss D, Pouagare M, et al: Endoscopic suction removal of food boluses from the upper gastrointestinal tract using Stiegmann-Goff friction-fit adaptor: An improved method for removal of food impactions. Gastrointest Endosc 41:593–596, 1995.
46. Al-Quadh A, Daradkeh S, Abu-Khalaf M: Esophageal foreign bodies. Eur J Cardiothorac Surg 13:494–499, 1998.
47. Gluck M: Coin ingestion complicating a tavern game. West J Med 150: 343–344, 1989.
48. Stringer MD, Capps SN: Rationalizing the management of swallowed coins in children. BMJ 302:1321–1322, 1991.
49. Byrne WJ: Foreign bodies, bezoars, and caustic ingestion. Gastro Endosc Clin North Am 4:99–119, 1994.
50. Guber M, Suarez C, Greve J: Toothpick perforation of the intestine diagnosed by small bowel series. Am J Gastroenterol 91:789–791, 1996.
51. Jackson C, Jackson CL: Disease of the Air and Food Passages of Foreign Body Origin. Philadelphia, WB Saunders, 1937.
52. Bertoni G, Sassatelli R, Conigliaro R, et al: A simple latex protector hood for safe endoscopic removal of sharp-pointed gastroesophageal foreign bodies. Gastrointest Endosc 44:458–461, 1996.
53. Chinitz MA, Bertrand CZ: Endoscopic removal of toothbrushes. Gastrointest Endosc 36:527–530, 1990.
54. McCarron MM, Wood JD: The cocaine "body packer" syndrome: Diagnosis and treatment. JAMA 250:1417–1420, 1983.
55. Caruana DS, Weinbach B, Goerg D, et al: Cocaine packer ingestion. Ann Intern Med 100:73–74, 1984.
56. Busch DB, Starling JR: Rectal foreign bodies: Case reports and a comprehensive review of the world's literature. Surgery 100:512–519, 1986.
57. Kouraklis G, Misiakos E, Dovas N, et al: Management of foreign bodies of the rectum: Report of 21 cases. J R Coll Surg Edinb 42:246–247, 1997.
58. Ferrucci JT, Long LA: Radiologic treatment of esophageal food impaction using intravenous glucagon. Radiology 125:25–28, 1977.
59. Trenkner SW, Maglinte DT, Lehman G, et al: Esophageal food impaction: Treatment with glucagon. Radiology 149:401–403, 1983.
60. Rice BT, Spiegel PK, Dombrowski PJ: Acute esophageal food impaction treated by gas-forming agents. Radiology 146:299–301, 1983.
61. Kaszar-Seibert DJ, Korn WT, Bindman DJ, et al: Treatment of acute esophageal food impaction with a combination of glucagon, effervescent agent, and water. AJR Am J Roentgenol 154:533, 1990.
62. Smith JC, Janower ML, Geiger AH: Use of glucagon and gas-forming agents in acute esophageal food impaction. Radiology 159:567, 1986.
63. Litovitz T, Schmitz BF: Ingestion of cylindrical and button batteries: An analysis of 2382 cases. Pediatrics 89:747, 1992.
64. Schunk JE, Harrison AM, Corneli HM, et al: Fluoroscopic foley catheter removal of esophageal foreign bodies in children: Experience with 415 episodes. Pediatrics 94:709–714, 1994.
65. Paulson EK, Jaffe RB: Metallic foreign bodies in the stomach: Fluoroscopic removal with a magnetic orogastric tube. Radiology 174:191–194, 1990.
66. Andrus CH, Ponsky JL: Bezoars: Classification, pathophysiology, and treatment. Am J Gastroenterol 83:476–478, 1988.
67. Phillips MR, Zaheer S, Drugas GT: Gastric trichobezoar: Case report and literature review. Mayo Clin Proc 73:653–656, 1998.
68. Anderson JE, Akmal M, Kittur DS: Surgical complications of pica: A report of a case of intestinal obstruction and a review of the literature. Am Surg 57:663–667, 1991.
69. Taylor JR, Streetman DS, Castle SS: Medication bezoars: A literature review and a report of a case. Ann Pharmacother 32:940–946, 1998.
70. Robles R, Parrilla P, Escamilla C, et al: Gastrointestinal bezoars. Br J Surg 81:1000–1001, 1994.
71. Wang YG, Seitz U, Li L, et al: Endoscopic management of huge bezoars. Endoscopy 30:371–374, 1998.
72. Escamilla C, Robles R, Campos R, Parilla-Paricio P, et al: Intestinal obstruction and bezoars. J Am Coll Surg 179:1691–1693, 1994.
73. Tohodo H, Haruma K, Kitaldi Y, et al: Gastric emptying and bezoars in Japanese: Report of five cases. Dig Dis Sci 38:1422, 1993.
74. Dietrich NA, Gau FC: Postgastrectomy phytobezoars: Endoscopic diagnosis and treatment. Arch Surg 120:432–435, 1985.
75. Schreiber H, Filston HC: Obstructive jaundice due to gastric trichobezoar. J Pediatr Surg 11:103, 1976.
76. Shawis RN, Doig CM: Gastric trichobezoar associated with transient pancreatitis. Arch Dis Child 59:994, 1984.
77. McGehee FT, Buchanan GR: Trichophagia and trichobezoar: Etiologic role of iron deficiency. J Pediatr 97:946, 1980.
78. Kuo JY, Mo LR, Tsai CC, et al: Nonoperative treatment of gastric bezoars using electrohydraulic lithotripsy. Endoscopy 31:386–388, 1999.
79. Klamer TW, Max MH: Recurrent gastric bezoars: A new approach to treatment and prevention. Am J Surg 145:417–419, 1983.

Chapter 22

Caustic Injury to the Upper Gastrointestinal Tract

Peter M. Loeb and Michael J. Nunez

Caustic ingestion can produce a progressive and devastating injury to the esophagus and stomach.[1–3] Most patients survive the acute injury, but the reparative process can result in esophageal and/or gastric stenosis and an increased incidence of esophageal cancer (Fig. 22–1). There has been little progress in the prevention of these long-term sequelae of caustic ingestion. The most substantial gains in the prevention of these injuries have come from public education and improved product safety.

Caustic ingestion continues to be a worldwide problem, particularly among children. Most household caustic ingestions are accidental, and approximately two thirds occur in children younger than 6 years of age.[4] After the introduction of concentrated liquid alkaline products in the 1960s, the incidence of severe injury increased.[1, 5–7] The Poison Prevention Packaging Acts of 1970 and 1973, which require child-proof containers for household caustic agents with concentrations of 10% or greater and for liquid alkaline products of 2% or greater, have reduced but not eliminated severe caustic injuries in the United States.[7–9] The variety of caustic household agents has expanded; and in the 12-year period from 1988 to 2000, data from the U.S. poison control centers reveal that both the number of household ingestions and the number of related deaths have risen, despite public education efforts (Table 22–1).

CAUSTIC AGENTS

Caustic gastrointestinal injury can be caused by an alkaline or acidic agent. Commonly ingested agents are shown in Table 22–2. Concentrated acids are also found in many household cleaners. *Lye* is a broad term for a strong alkali often used in cleansing agents and can be found in granular, paste, or liquid form. Button batteries contain high concentrations of sodium and potassium hydroxide (see later). Milder injuries are usually caused by less potent agents such as sodium carbonate, ammonium hydroxide, and bleaches, although major damage can occur.[8, 10]

Pathogenesis and Pathology

The degree of injury to the gastrointestinal tract depends on the agent; its concentration, quantity, and physical state; and the duration of exposure.[11, 12] Accidental ingestions are sometimes halted by the odor of the agent or by oropharyngeal irritation. Acidic solutions usually cause immediate pain, and unless ingestion is intentional, the agent is rapidly expelled. Alkali solutions are often tasteless and odorless and may be swallowed before protective reflexes can be invoked, causing extensive contiguous damage to the entire esophagus and stomach. Caustic agents in solid or granular form adhere to mucous membranes, are more difficult to swallow, and tend to cause focal, proximal injuries.[12–14]

The primary difference between alkaline and acidic injury is the rapid tissue penetration by alkali.[1, 15] Experimental studies in cats reveal that exposure to 1 mL of 30.5% sodium hydroxide for 1 second can penetrate the full thickness of the esophagus.[1] Alkali has a potent solvent action on the lipoprotein lining, producing a *liquefaction necrosis* with saponification of the mucosa, submucosa, and muscularis of the esophagus and stomach.[1, 16, 17] Thrombosis of adjacent vessels may result in further necrosis. Sloughing of this necrotic tissue occurs 5 to 7 days after injury and is followed by intense fibroblastic activity. Ulceration may persist for months, even as collagen forms in adjacent tissue.

Studies in animals have shown that after ingestion of liquid alkali, violent regurgitation occurs into the esophagus, followed by propulsion of the alkali back into the stomach. These to-and-fro actions last for several minutes and produce extensive injury to the esophagus and stomach before eventual passage of the alkali into the duodenum.[18] The stomach is not resistant to alkali ingestion, because the neutralizing effect of gastric acid is insignificant compared with the total alkalinity of even small volumes of strong alkali.[19]

Acidic agents produce a *coagulation necrosis* that may limit penetration and injury.[7, 8, 20] Acidic agents were once thought to spare the esophagus and injure the stomach because of the alkaline environment of the oropharynx and the

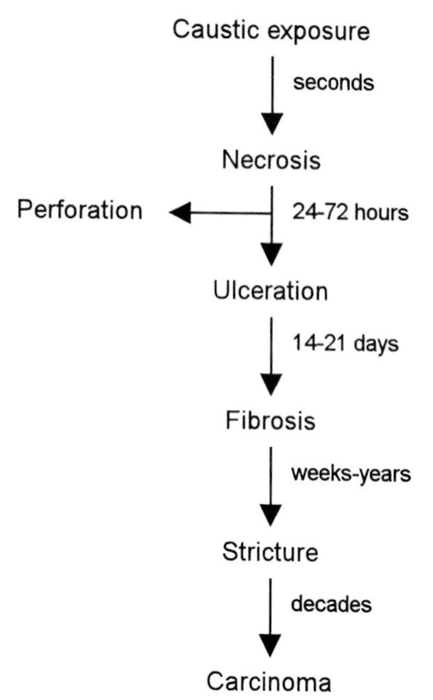

Figure 22–1. Consequences of caustic injury as a function of time after ingestion.

Table 22–2 | **Household Caustic Agents**

PRODUCT TYPE	CAUSTIC INGREDIENT(S)
Alkali Agents	
Drain openers	Sodium hydroxide, sodium hypochlorite
Oven cleaners	Sodium hydroxide
Toilet bowl cleaners	Ammonium chloride
Household cleaners	Ammonium hydroxide, ammonium chloride
Bleach products	Sodium hypochlorite, hydrogen peroxide
Dishwashing detergents	Sodium carbonate, sodium silicate
Clinitest tablets	Sodium hydroxide
Button batteries	Sodium hydroxide, potassium hydroxide
Hair wave relaxers	Calcium hydroxide, lithium hydroxide
Acidic Agents	
Toilet bowl cleaners	Hydrochloric acid, sulfuric acid, phosphoric acid
Metal cleaners	Hydrochloric acid
Pool cleaners	Hydrochloric acid
Antirust products	Hydrochloric acid, sulfuric acid, hydrofluoric acid
Battery fluids	Sulfuric acid

hydrophilic nature of acidic compounds allowing rapid transit through the esophagus. However, highly concentrated sulfuric or hydrochloric acid penetrates the esophageal mucosa and produces severe injury in approximately 50% of ingestions.[19–21] In one study, there was no difference in the rate of development of esophageal injury in patients after alkali or acid exposure.[22]

Esophageal strictures are usually located where caustic agents pool at the cricopharyngeus, the level of the aortic arch and tracheal bifurcation, and the lower esophageal sphincter. Most gastric strictures occur in the antrum of fasting patients, as opposed to the midbody in those who have recently ingested food.

Caustic injuries to the gastrointestinal tract are classified *pathologically* in the same manner as skin burns.[12]

FIRST DEGREE. This injury is superficial and produces edema and erythema of only the mucosa. The lining subsequently sloughs without scar or stricture formation.

SECOND DEGREE. Penetration occurs through the mucosa and into the submucosa and muscle layers, producing deep ulcerations and then granulation tissue. A fibroblastic reaction ensues during the second and third weeks, and over a period of weeks to months the collagen undergoes contraction. With circumferential involvement, a narrowing of the lumen of the esophagus or stomach can result.[1, 16] Scar formation appears to be complete within 8 weeks in approximately 80% of patients but can take as long as 8 months.[5]

THIRD DEGREE. This term best defines a full-thickness caustic injury.[12]

Clinical Features

EARLY MANIFESTATIONS. On presentation the patient may have visible injury to the lips, oral cavity, and pharynx with edema, ulceration, and exudate. Symptoms may include persistent salivation, vomiting, hematemesis, dysphagia, odynophagia, and chest or epigastric pain.[7, 8, 23, 24] Hoarseness and stridor indicate upper airway involvement.[25] These symptoms may develop rapidly or be delayed for several hours. Melena may occur when mucosal sloughing develops. Although most patients with esophageal or gastric injuries exhibit such signs and symptoms, many have no complaints, and examination of the mouth and pharynx may be normal in 20% to 45%.[2, 3, 25–27]

Table 22–1 | **Household Cleaning Product Ingestions in the United States**

	1988				2000			
CATEGORY	No. of Ingestions	<6 Years of Age (%)	Intentional (%)	No. of Deaths	No. of Ingestions	<6 Years of Age (%)	Intentional (%)	No. of Deaths
All cleaning products	*137,240*	*64*	*2*	*19*	*206,636*	*58*	*3*	*29*
Drain cleaners and openers	2,199	24	6	6	5,359	15	5	4
Toilet bowl cleaners	4,807	61	3	5	6,735	57	3	5
Miscellaneous acid or alkali	6,333	51	2	2	10,307	56	2	0
Rust removers	1,550	20	1	1	1,275	28	3	2
Bleaches	27,863	50	3	0	49,020	40	4	3

Data from U.S Poison Control Centers, Washington, D.C.

With third-degree burns of the esophagus, tachypnea, dyspnea, stridor, and shock may develop rapidly, and physical findings of mediastinitis may be present. Gastric perforation may result in acute peritonitis, which can be delayed for as long as 48 hours.[28]

LATE MANIFESTATIONS. Dysphagia heralds the onset of an esophageal stricture. Early satiety, weight loss, and progressive emesis suggest gastric outlet obstruction. Although the symptoms are usually progressive, they may disappear and then recur over the next 3 to 8 weeks with the development of obstruction from scar formation. Stenosis may not become apparent until 1 year after injury.[26]

MORTALITY. The mortality rate after caustic ingestion has decreased in the past 20 to 30 years from 20% to less than 1% (see Table 22–1) as a result of lower concentrations of caustic solutions, improved surgical and anesthesiologic techniques, and more effective antibiotics and nutritional support.[4, 7, 8, 28] Most deaths result from mediastinitis and peritonitis in individuals with third-degree injuries.

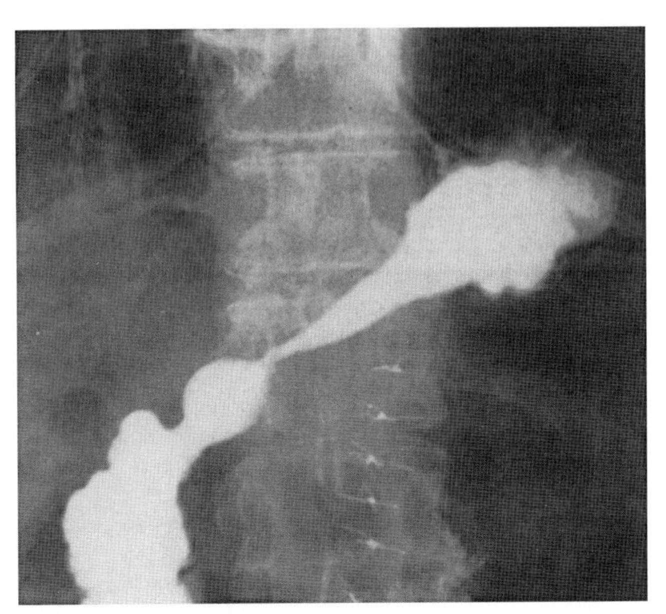

Figure 22–3. Chronic antral stricture due to caustic ingestion. (Courtesy of R. N. Berk, MD, University of California, San Diego.)

Diagnostic Studies

RADIOLOGIC STUDIES. In the acute phase of caustic injury, *upright chest* and *abdominal radiographs* may reveal evidence of perforation, such as pneumomediastinum, pneumothorax, or pneumoperitoneum.[1] If, after negative plain films, perforation is still suspected, orally administered *water-soluble contrast studies* may reveal extraluminal contrast. *Computed tomography* (CT) of the esophagus and stomach with orally administered contrast agent is the most sensitive method of detecting early perforation.

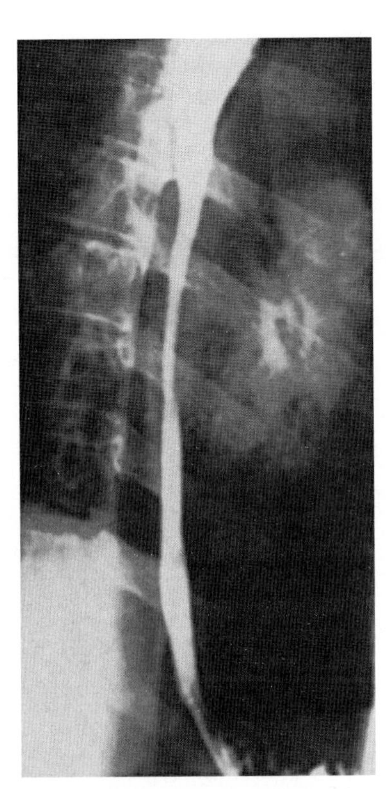

Figure 22–2. Stricture in the upper esophagus with narrowing of the midesophagus several weeks after caustic ingestion. (Courtesy of R. N. Berk, MD, University of California, San Diego.)

In the acute stages of the illness, *barium contrast films* of the esophagus and stomach are not adequately sensitive to delineate the severity and extent of injury.[26, 29, 30] Barium studies are most useful at approximately 3 weeks after injury to detect esophageal strictures or antral stenosis. Esophageal strictures can be of variable length with smooth or irregular margins (Fig. 22–2). Antral stenosis may mimic gastric cancer[31] (Fig. 22–3). The maximal wall thickness of esophageal strictures can be measured with contrast-enhanced CT scans, and this measurement correlates with resistance to esophageal dilation.[32]

ESOPHAGOGASTRODUODENOSCOPY. The reported poor correlation between signs or symptoms and the degree of injury have traditionally made it imperative that esophagogastroduodenoscopy (EGD) be performed in all patients with a history of caustic ingestion.[8, 11, 22, 27, 33] However, it has been suggested that most patients with severe injury have one or more clinical signs (e.g., oropharyngeal burns) or symptoms (e.g., drooling, dysphagia, vomiting, and abdominal pain) and that asymptomatic patients are unlikely to have lesions that progress to stricture or perforation.[34, 35] Based on these data and on the absence of proven therapy to prevent stricture (see later), it has been suggested that patients require endoscopy only if symptoms develop.[8, 36] Unfortunately, none of the studies on which these recommendations are based were controlled or prospective or had adequate follow-up.

With the use of smaller, flexible endoscopes, a complete examination of the esophageal and gastric mucosa can be safely performed.[8, 11, 13, 37] Most authors recommend performing EGD in all patients with a history of caustic ingestion as soon as the patient is stable and if there is no clinical suspicion of perforation. Kikendall, however, has suggested that the extent of damage may be better defined by waiting 48 to 72 hours.[7]

Table 22–3 | **Endoscopic Grade of Caustic Injury**

GRADE	ENDOSCOPIC FINDINGS
I	Edema and erythema
IIA	Hemorrhage, erosions, blisters, ulcers with exudate
IIB	Circumferential ulceration
III	Multiple deep ulcers with brown, black, or gray discoloration*
IV	Perforation

*See Fig. 22–4.

At endoscopy, 50% to 80% of patients with a history of caustic ingestion are found to have no injury.[3, 14, 22–24] When injury is found, endoscopic grading provides some prognostic information (Table 22–3). *Grade I injury* (superficial burn) corresponds to a first-degree burn.[3, 14, 22, 37, 38] *Grade II injury* corresponds to a second-degree burn, whereas *grade III injury* corresponds to a transmural burn and necrosis without perforation. *Grade IV injury* (perforation) is usually not encountered because clinical and radiographic suspicion of perforation precludes EGD. Zargar and associates suggested that grade II burns be labeled grade IIA if patchy or linear or grade IIB if the injury is circumferential.[37–39] The endoscopic grade is subjective, which limits its accuracy in predicting the pathologic degree of injury. Estrera and associates demonstrated that three of eight patients diagnosed endoscopically with grade IIB injuries were found at surgery to have full-thickness necrosis.[40] Grade I and grade IIA injuries (noncircumferential) rarely result in strictures, whereas 70% to 100% of grade IIB (circumferential) and grade III lesions result in strictures.[14, 23, 38]

Treatment

The goals of therapy are to prevent *perforation* and to avoid progressive *fibrosis* and *stricture*. Only emergency surgery can prevent or treat perforation. A number of *unproved* therapeutic modalities have been proposed, either alone or in combination, to prevent or treat strictures. These include caustic neutralization, corticosteroids, antibiotics, collagen synthesis inhibitors, heparin, early esophageal dilation, and esophageal stents.

EMERGENCY SURGERY. Emergency surgery is indicated in cases of esophageal or gastric perforation. With the emergence of liquid caustics as a major cause of injury, several investigators have recommended immediate surgery after either alkali or acid ingestion in patients with severe, contiguous, second-degree burns (stage IIB).[12, 28, 40, 41] Surgical exploration allows more definitive diagnosis, and gastrectomy or esophagectomy can be performed if perforation or transmural injury is found. Estrera and associates have argued that the reduced mortality achieved through early detection of impending or actual perforation outweighs the morbidity and mortality associated with surgical exploration in patients with endoscopically diagnosed second-degree burns.[40] However, early surgery has been condemned by some because the extent of the injury often cannot be delineated, anastomotic leaks frequently occur, and surgery is not needed in most patients. Although liquid caustic ingestions with severe panesophagogastric involvement are associated with a high incidence of perforation and stricture in some series, in other reports, a lower mortality rate and complete healing without immediate surgical intervention have been noted.[1, 11, 41] Most investigators admit that in selected cases early surgery would be prudent, but the criteria on which to base selection of surgical cases are not known.[19]

NEUTRALIZATION OF CAUSTICS. The manufacturers of many household alkali products recommend that neutralizers or water be given immediately after caustic ingestion. Many authors have proposed that heat produced in an exothermic neutralization reaction may increase tissue injury, based on in vitro studies.[17, 19, 42] Also, alkali injuries occur very rap-

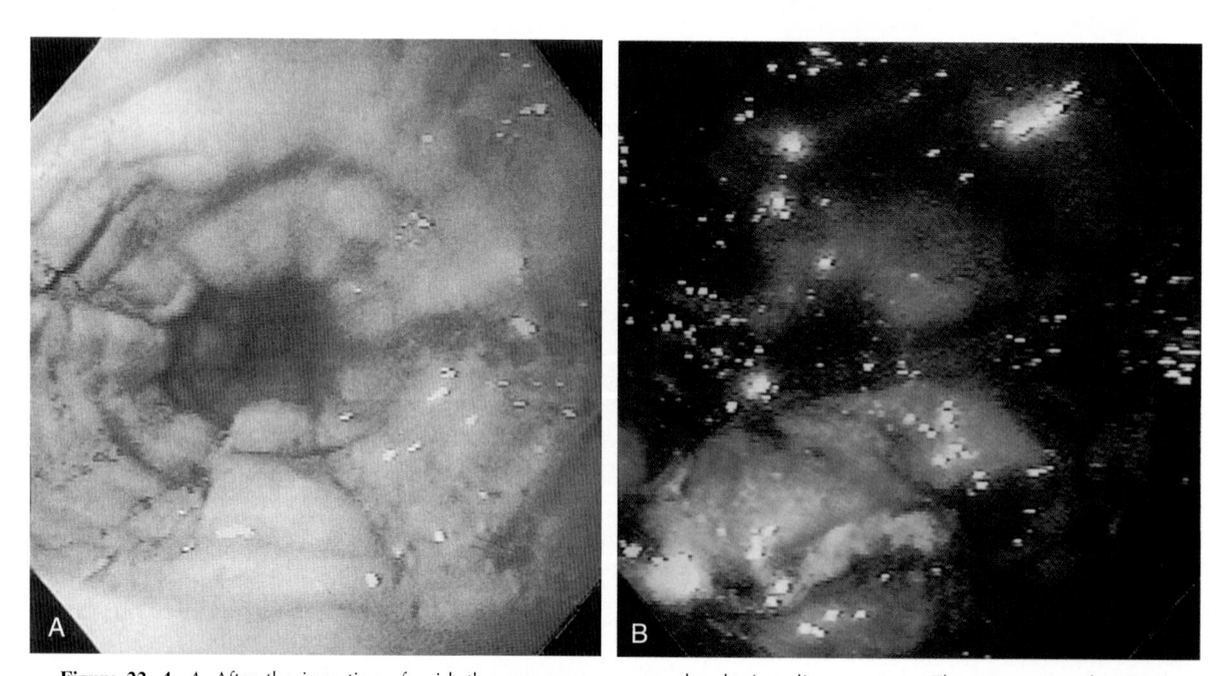

Figure 22–4. *A*, After the ingestion of acid, the squamous mucosa sloughs in a linear pattern. The mucosa is edematous and has a bluish discoloration. *B*, The gastric mucosa is hemorrhagic and edematous. (From Wilcox MC: Atlas of Clinical Gastrointestinal Endoscopy. Philadelphia, WB Saunders, 1995, p 85.)

idly, leading some to suggest that attempting neutralization is futile.[1, 20] However, a recent in vivo study using a canine model found that neutralization does not cause a rise in mucosal or intraluminal temperature.[43] Additional studies indicate that neutralization, even delayed up to 30 minutes, can reduce injury in ex vivo animal experiments.[43, 44] Despite this apparent benefit, one must weigh the risk of inducing emesis and re-exposing the esophagus and airway to the caustic agent.[19, 42, 45]

GLUCOCORTICOIDS. Studies in animals have shown that glucocorticoids given within 24 hours after alkali injury inhibit granulation and fibroblastic tissue reaction and decrease the incidence of esophageal strictures.[5, 26, 46, 47] Anecdotal clinical reports suggested that glucocorticoids reduce the incidence of strictures.[14, 15, 26, 47, 48] However, a prospective, randomized, controlled trial in children after caustic ingestion (acid and alkali) demonstrated that glucocorticoids *do not* prevent strictures.[23] In this study, strictures developed in 10 of 31 treated children and 11 of 29 control subjects. Glucocorticoids may also obscure evidence of peritonitis or mediastinitis and may increase the risk of infection and thus should not be used.[1, 12, 14, 20, 49]

ANTIBIOTICS. Controlled studies in animals reveal that if steroids are used after alkali ingestion, the marked increased incidence of local infection that develops can be prevented by the administration of broad-spectrum antibiotics.[5, 28, 46] Local infections may increase granulation response, with a resultant increase in tissue fibrosis and stricture formation. No prospective studies in humans are available. Although some experts recommend the use of prophylactic antibiotics, most assert that such therapy should be withheld until specific indications develop.[3, 7, 8, 14, 15, 20, 25, 36, 48]

NUTRITION. Parenteral nutrition has been recommended in patients with severe caustic ingestion to avoid damage to the esophagus or stomach that may occur if the patient is fed.[16, 25] There are no data to support this practice or to suggest that oral alimentation or tube feeding is injurious in acute caustic ingestion.

EARLY ESOPHAGEAL DILATION. Boyce and Palmer recommended the use of esophageal dilation immediately after injury.[50] Dilation is performed at frequent intervals until healing occurs.[51] There are no controlled data to support this approach, and others suggest that early dilation increases the risk of perforation and may accelerate fibrosis and stricture formation.[12, 14, 15, 41]

ESOPHAGEAL STENTS. Endoscopically and surgically placed intraluminal stents have been used in patients with severe injuries to prevent and treat strictures.[40, 45, 52, 53] There are no long-term, controlled data to determine the efficacy of this approach.

OTHER MODALITIES. In animals, collagen synthesis inhibitors such as β-aminoproprionitrile, penicillamine, *N*-acetylcysteine, and colchicine have been shown to prevent alkali-induced esophageal strictures.[54–56] Heparin has also been used with success in a controlled animal study to prevent stricture formation. The postulated therapeutic mechanisms include prevention of vascular thrombosis and a reduction in inflammation.[57] No human clinical studies have been performed with these agents.

Recommended Approach

If necessary, volume repletion and securing the airway should begin immediately (Fig. 22–5). When respiratory symptoms are present, direct laryngoscopy should be performed to evaluate the need for endotracheal intubation or tracheostomy. Once the patient is stable, a careful history and physical examination are performed. Some studies show a poor correlation between symptoms and endoscopic findings in cases of concentrated liquid caustic ingestion. This has led some to recommend EGD in *all* cases of caustic ingestion. However, a patient can be discharged without EGD if all the following criteria are fulfilled: (1) a detailed history can be obtained; (2) the ingestion was accidental, small in volume, and consisted of weak or low-concentration acidic or alkaline solutions; (3) the patient is asymptomatic and has no oropharyngeal injury; and (4) the patient can guarantee reliable follow-up if symptoms develop.

Otherwise, the patient is allowed nothing per mouth, and chest and abdominal radiographs are obtained. CT scan can be useful if perforation is suspected and plain radiographs are unrevealing. If there is evidence of perforation, surgery should be performed immediately.

Endoscopy is performed within 24 to 48 hours to grade the caustic injury (see Table 22–3). Endoscopy need not be performed on an emergency basis because there is no effective, urgent therapy. General anesthesia with endotracheal intubation should be used in all patients except cooperative adults without respiratory difficulties. Complete examination of the esophageal and gastric mucosa can be safely performed with low risk of perforation. Early endoscopy might be needed to avoid admitting the patient to the hospital or to facilitate discharge of the patient with suspected mild injury.

If a grade I or IIA injury is found (see Table 22–3), the patient can be started on a liquid diet and advanced to a regular diet in 24 to 48 hours. Psychiatry evaluation is required if the ingestion was intentional or the patient appears depressed.

In patients with grade IIB or III injuries, there is no

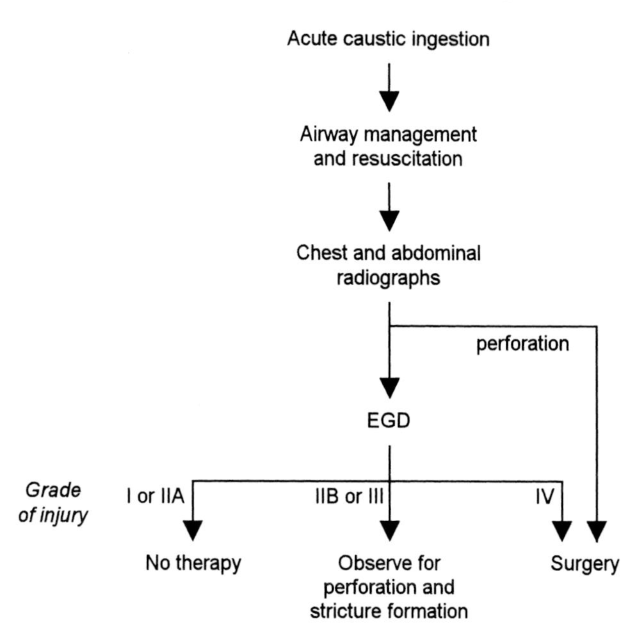

Figure 22–5. Recommended approach to acute caustic injury. EDG, esophagogastroduodenoscopy.

evidence to support the early use of antibiotics, and corticosteroids are not recommended. After 24 to 48 hours, oral liquids can be started if the patient is stable; without pain, nausea, or vomiting; and swallowing saliva without difficulty. If oral feedings are not tolerated, a nasoenteric tube can be inserted for enteral nutrition. Esophageal dilation is indicated if a stricture is identified, usually in the following 3 to 4 weeks (see Late Complications). Early dilation carries a higher risk of perforation. The use of prophylactic esophageal stents has not been proved to be effective and should be considered investigational.

Patients with grade III injuries *and* a history of ingestion of large volumes of a concentrated caustic agent are at the greatest risk for perforation in this period. When suspected, the patient must be maintained NPO, and repeat CT scan of the chest and abdomen with oral and intravenous contrast agent may be needed for early detection. If perforation is documented, exploration should be performed by an experienced surgeon.

Late Complications

ESOPHAGEAL STRICTURE. Compared with other causes, caustic esophageal strictures (see Fig. 22–2) require more numerous and more frequent dilations to achieve and maintain an adequate lumen. Care must be taken to dilate slowly and carefully. Perforation, bleeding, and sepsis may complicate dilation.[51] Minor dilation-related perforations have been successfully treated without surgery using parenteral nutrition and antibiotics, with resumption of dilation in 4 to 6 weeks.[32] Most perforations occur in long, tight, eccentric strictures that have been dilated without fluoroscopic guidance. Proton pump inhibitors should be used as an adjunct to prevent acid reflux. Intralesional steroid injections at the time of endoscopic dilation have been reported to have a beneficial effect in an uncontrolled study.[58] Rapidly developing, thick-walled strictures (as determined by CT scan) are more difficult to dilate and recur more rapidly. In 10% to 50% of patients with strictures, surgery will be necessary because the patient cannot tolerate repeat dilation, nutrition cannot be maintained, or dilation is unsuccessful.[32, 51, 59, 60] When necessary, esophageal resection is performed with esophagogastric anastomosis or colonic or jejunal interposition.

ANTRAL STENOSIS. Antral stenosis after caustic injury (see Fig. 22–3) may develop in 3 to 6 weeks or may not appear for several years.[7] Endoscopic dilation has been used successfully and should be considered as an initial maneuver in patients with antral stenosis.[61, 62] Surgery may be needed and distal gastric resection is usually recommended. Although many patients are initially achlorhydric, vagotomy is usually performed along with antrectomy because acid production may return. Pyloroplasty or gastroenterostomy have been applied successfully in a few patients. With extensive injury, subtotal or total gastrectomy or partial esophagectomy may be necessary.

CARCINOMA OF THE ESOPHAGUS. There is a strong association between caustic injury and squamous cell carcinoma of the esophagus.[63–65] Between 1% and 7% of patients with carcinoma of the esophagus have a history of caustic ingestion. It has been estimated that there is a 1000-fold to 3000-fold increase in the expected incidence of esophageal carcinoma after caustic ingestion. Such a relationship is supported by the location of the cancer at the site of the stricture (scar carcinoma) and the younger ages of patients with caustic ingestion-related carcinomas. The average interval between injury and the development of squamous cell carcinoma is 40 years. Prognosis with combined surgical and radiation therapy appears to be somewhat better than that for other squamous cell carcinomas (see Chapter 35). This may be due to younger age patients who have developed earlier symptoms due to an already compromised lumen. Furthermore, the scar tissue may limit the spread of the cancer. There are insufficient data to recommend surveillance EGD in asymptomatic patients with a history of remote caustic ingestion.

CARCINOMA OF THE STOMACH. Squamous metaplasia and carcinoma of the stomach have been reported after caustic injury.[66] These reports are isolated, and there is no reported evidence of increased risk of development of gastric carcinoma in patients with previous caustic injury.

BUTTON BATTERY INGESTION

Since the 1970s, injury to the gastrointestinal tract from button battery ingestion (see Chapter 21) has been increasingly recognized.[67–70] These batteries contain highly concentrated alkaline solutions (potassium or sodium hydroxide).[71] Ingestions occur most frequently in boys younger than 12 years of age, especially in youngsters wearing hearing aids. Fortunately, more than 90% pass through the gastrointestinal tract within 72 hours without severe consequences.[70] In the United States, more than 1800 cases were reported to poison control centers in 2000.[4] However, a 1999 review found only 17 cases of complications in the English literature (9 tracheoesophageal fistulas, 4 esophageal perforations, 3 severe burns, 1 aortoesophageal fistula) and 2 deaths.[72]

The severity of injury is influenced by the battery size, the duration of contact with mucosa, and the type of heavy metal in the battery (mercury is potentially the most toxic). Batteries larger than 15 mm in diameter are more likely to lodge in the esophagus and cause injury.[71, 73] The mucosal injury results from three effects: (1) liquefaction necrosis due to the release of highly concentrated alkali (26% to 45%); (2) local electrical current discharge; and (3) direct pressure necrosis from the foreign body. The most serious morbidities and all fatalities occur when the battery becomes lodged in the esophagus. Significant burns can occur within 4 hours, and perforation can occur within 6 hours.[70] Injury to the stomach or intestine is rare.

After ingestion, there often are no symptoms or only nonspecific complaints, such as drooling, nausea, refusal to eat, or abdominal discomfort.[70, 73] Dysphagia, odynophagia, shortness of breath, or intense abdominal pain occur infrequently. Therefore, *any* history of possible ingestion requires an immediate evaluation, even in the absence of symptoms.

The management of button battery ingestion continues to be debated.[73–75] The following approach represents a consensus of recommendations from several reviews (Fig. 22–6).[70, 73, 76, 77] Posteroanterior and lateral radiographs from mouth to anus should be obtained after physical examination.[78] If the

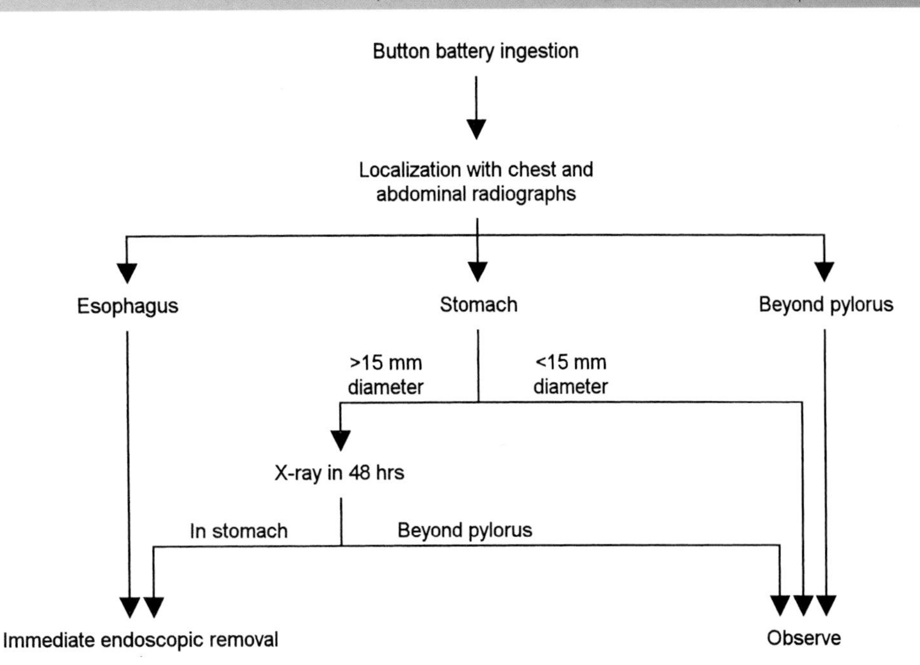

Figure 22–6. Management of button battery ingestion with esophageal battery impaction. Bronchoscopy should also be considered in selected cases (see text).

battery is lodged in the esophagus, *immediate* endoscopy with removal is performed, often with the patient under general anesthesia. The blind passage of a Foley catheter balloon or magnetic retrieval device is not recommended.[70] If the battery cannot be extracted through the mouth, it should be pushed into the stomach with the endoscope. Bronchoscopy should be performed to detect a fistula if esophageal impaction has been present for more than 4 hours or if there is endoscopic evidence of full-thickness injury, such as adherence of the battery to the esophageal wall, visible mucosal ulceration, severe edema extending from the impaction site, or bubbling within the esophagus with positive-pressure ventilation.[77] If removal is accomplished and no such endoscopic signs are present, one should still consider a barium swallow within 48 hours to rule out a fistula. A second barium examination is recommended 2 weeks later to evaluate for stricture formation.[76] Most investigators do not recommend the use of antibiotics or steroids.

If the battery is pushed into the stomach with the endoscope, removal should be attempted. If the attempt is unsuccessful or the initial radiograph shows that the battery is already in the stomach, no other invasive procedures are needed unless localized epigastric pain, coffee-ground emesis, or melena occurs or the battery does not pass the pylorus after 48 hours, is larger than 15 mm in diameter, or contains mercury.[70] Medical therapy with antacids, acid inhibitors, prokinetic agents, or laxatives has not been established as efficacious. Emetics should not be used. Once the battery is beyond the pylorus, passage should be confirmed by searching the stool for the battery. If it is not found, serial abdominal radiographs should be obtained every 4 to 7 days.[70] Although neither short- nor long-term clinical side effects have been documented with the ingestion of mercury oxide batteries,[79] blood and urine mercury levels should be monitored if the cell is observed to have split or radiographic droplets are evident.[70] Exploratory laparotomy should be performed only if signs of obstruction or peritonitis develop.

The U.S. National Button Battery Ingestion Hotline (202-625-3333) is operated from the National Capital Poison Center in Washington, DC, and is available as an emergency consultation service and case registry. Better public awareness of the potential problem of button batteries and more effective childproof devices of the products in which they are used will diminish this problem.

REFERENCES

1. Leape LL, Ashcraft KW, Carpelli DG, Holden TM: Hazard to health: Liquid lye. N Engl J Med 284:578, 1971.
2. Ray JF, Myers WO, Lawton BR, et al: The natural history of liquid lye ingestion. Arch Surg 109:436, 1974.
3. Hawkins DB, Demeter MJ, Barrett TE: Caustic ingestion: Controversies in management—a review of 214 cases. Laryngoscope 90:98, 1980.
4. Litovitz TL, Klein-Schwartz W: 2000 Annual Report of the American Association of Poison Control Centers Toxic Exposure Surveillance System. Am J Emerg Med 19:337, 2001.
5. Rosenberg N, Kunderman PJ, Vroman L, Moolten SE: Prevention of experimental lye strictures of the esophagus by cortisone. Arch Surg 63:147, 1951.
6. Muhlendahl KE, Oberdisse U, Krienke EG: Local injuries by accidental ingestion of corrosive substances by children. Arch Toxicol 39:229, 1978.
7. Kikendall JW: Caustic ingestion injuries. Gastroenterol Clin North Am 20:847, 1991.
8. Byrne WF: Foreign bodies, bezoars, and caustic ingestion. Gastroenterol Clin North Am 4:99, 1994.
9. Walton WW: An evaluation of the Poison Prevention Act. Pediatrics 69:363, 1982.
10. Lee JR, Simonowitz D, Block GE: Corrosive injury of the stomach and esophagus by non-phosphate detergents. Am J Surg 123:652, 1972.
11. Cello JP, Fogel RP, Boland R: Liquid caustic ingestion spectrum of injury. Arch Intern Med 140:501, 1980.
12. Kirsh MM, Ritter F: Caustic ingestion and subsequent damage to the oropharyngeal and digestive passages. Ann Thorac Surg 21:74, 1976.

13. Bikhazi B, Thompson ER, Shumrick DA: Caustic ingestion: Current status. Arch Otolaryngol 89:770, 1969.
14. Middlekamp JN, Ferguson TB, Roper CL, Hoffman FD: The management and problem of caustic burns in children. J Thorac Cardiovasc Surg 57:341, 1969.
15. Haller JA, Backman K: The comparative effects of current therapy on experimental caustic burns of the esophagus. Pediatrics 34:326, 1964.
16. Krey H: Treatment of corrosive lesion in the esophagus. Acta Otolaryngol Suppl 102:1, 1952.
17. Rumack BH, Burrington JD: Caustic ingestion: A rational look at diluents. Clin Toxicol 11:27, 1977.
18. Ritter FN, Newman MH, Newman DE: A clinical and experimental study of corrosive burns of the stomach. Ann Otol Rhinol Laryngol 77: 830, 1986.
19. Penner GE: Acid ingestion: Toxicity and treatment. Ann Emerg Med 9: 374, 1980.
20. Ashcraft KW, Padula R: The effect of dilute corrosives on the esophagus. Pediatrics 53:226, 1974.
21. Scher LA, Maull KI: Emergency management and sequelae of acid ingestion. JACEP 7:206, 1978.
22. Gaudreault P, Parent M, McGuigan MA, et al: Predictability of esophageal injury from signs and symptoms: A study of caustic ingestion in 378 children. Pediatrics 71:767, 1983.
23. Anderson KD, Rouse MR, Randolph JG: A controlled trial of corticosteroids in children with corrosive injury of the esophagus. N Engl J Med 323:637, 1990.
24. Bautista Casasnovas A, Esteves Martinez E, Varela Cives R, et al: A retrospective analysis of ingestion of caustic substances by children: Ten-year statistics in Galicia. Eur J Pediatr 156:410, 1997.
25. DiCostanzo J, Noirclerc M, Jouglard J, et al: New therapeutic approach to corrosive burns of the upper gastrointestinal tract. Gut 21: 370, 1982.
26. Haller JA, Andrews HG, White JJ, et al: Pathophysiology and management of acute corrosive burns of the esophagus: Results of treatment in 285 children. J Pediatr Surg 6:578, 1971.
27. Lovejoy FH, Woolf AD: Corrosive ingestions. Pediatr Rev 16:473, 1995.
28. Gago O, Ritter RN, Martel W, et al: Aggressive surgical treatment for caustic injury of the esophagus and stomach. Ann Thorac Surg 13:243, 1972.
29. Martel W: Radiologic features of esophagogastritis secondary to extremely caustic agents. Radiology 103:21, 1972.
30. Muhletaler CA, Gerlock AJ, DeSoto L, Halter SA: Gastroduodenal lesion of ingested acids: Radiologic finding. AJR Am J Roentgenol 135:1247, 1980.
31. Holzback R: Corrosive gastritis resembling carcinoma due to ingestion of acid. JAMA 205:883, 1967.
32. Lahoti D, Broor SL, Basu MD, et al: Corrosive esophageal strictures: Predictors of response to endoscopic dilation. Gastrointest Endosc 41: 196, 1995.
33. Previtera C, Guisti F, Guglielmi M: Predictive value of visible lesions (cheeks, lips, oropharynx) in suspected caustic ingestion: May endoscopy be reliably omitted in completely negative pediatric patients? Pediatr Emerg Care 6:176, 1990.
34. Gorman RL, Khin-Maung-Gyi MT, Klein-Schwartz W, et al: Initial symptoms as predictors of esophageal injury in alkaline corrosive ingestions. Am J Emerg Med 10:189, 1992.
35. Christensen HG: Predictor of complications following caustic injury in adults. Clin Otolaryngol 20:272, 1995.
36. Shaffer RT, Carrougher JG, Kadakia SC, Levine SM: Update on caustic ingestions: How therapy has changed. J Crit Illness 9:161, 1993.
37. Zargar SA, Kochhar R, Nagi B, et al: Ingestion of corrosive acids: Spectrum of injury to the upper gastrointestinal tract and natural history. Gastroenterology 97:702, 1989.
38. Zargar SA, Kochhar R, Nagi B, et al: The role of fiberoptic endoscopy in the management of corrosive ingestion and modified endoscopic classification of burns. Gastrointest Endosc 37:165, 1991.
39. Zargar SA, Kochhar R, Nagi B, et al: Ingestion of strong corrosive alkalis: Spectrum of injury to the upper gastrointestinal tract and natural history. Am J Gastroenterol 87:337, 1992.
40. Estrera A, Taylor W, Mills LJ, Platt MR: Corrosive burns of the esophagus and stomach: A recommendation for an aggressive surgical approach. Ann Thorac Surg 41:276, 1986.
41. Fell SC, Denize A, Becker NH, Hurwitt ES: The effect of intraluminal splinting in the prevention of caustic stricture of the esophagus. J Thorac Cardiovasc Surg 52:675, 1966.
42. Kirsh MM, Peterson A, Brown JW, et al: Treatment of caustic injuries of the esophagus: A ten-year experience. Ann Surg 188:675, 1978.
43. Homan CS, Singer AJ, Henry MC, et al: Thermal effects of neutralization therapy and water dilution for acute alkali exposure in canines. Acad Emerg Med 4:27, 1997.
44. Homan CS, Maitra SR, Lane BP, et al: Effective treatment for acute alkali injury to the esophagus using weak-acid neutralization therapy: An ex-vivo study. Acad Emerg Med 2:952, 1995.
45. Ray JF: Liquid caustic ingestion: A flag of caution. Arch Intern Med 140:471, 1980.
46. Spain DM, Molomut N, Habert A: The effect of cortisone on the formation of granulation tissue in mice. Am J Pathol 26:710, 1950.
47. Weiskoff A: Effects of cortisone on experimental lye burns of the esophagus. Ann Otolaryngol 61:681, 1952.
48. Knox WG, Scott JR, Zintel HA, et al: Bougienage and steroids used singly or in combination in experimental corrosive esophagitis. Ann Surg 166:930, 1967.
49. Oakes DD: Reconsidering the diagnosis and treatment of patients following ingestion of liquid lye [editorial]. J Clin Gastroenterol 21:85, 1995.
50. Boyce HW, Palmer EO: Techniques of Clinical Gastroenterology. Springfield, Ill, Charles C Thomas, 1975, p 264.
51. Broor SL, Raju GS, Bore PP, et al: Long-term results of endoscopic dilation for treatment of corrosive esophageal strictures. Gut 34:1498, 1993.
52. Coln D, Chang JH: Experience with esophageal stenting for caustic burns in children. J Pediatr Surg 21:591, 1986.
53. Mills LJ, Estrera AS, Platt MR: Avoidance of esophageal stricture following severe caustic burns by the use of an intraluminal stent. Ann Thorac Surg 28:60, 1979.
54. Butler C, Madden JW, Peacock EE: Morphologic aspects of experimental esophageal lye strictures: II. Effect of steroid hormones, bougienage, and induced lathyrism of acute lye burns. Surgery 81:431, 1977.
55. Gehanno P, Guedon C: Inhibition of experimental esophageal lye strictures by penicillamine. Arch Otolaryngol 107:145, 1981.
56. Liu AJ, Richardson MA: Effects of *N*-acetylcysteine on experimentally induced esophageal lye injury. Ann Otol Rhinol Laryngol 94:477, 1985.
57. Bingol-Kologlu M, Tanyel FC, Muftuoglu S, et al: The preventative effect of heparin on stricture formation after caustic esophageal burns. J Pediatr Surg 34:291, 1999.
58. Kochhar R, Ray J, Sriram P, et al: Intralesional steroids augment the effects of endoscopic dilation in corrosive esophageal strictures. Gastrointest Endosc 49:509, 1999.
59. Campbell GS, Burnett HF, Ransom JW, Williams D: Treatment of corrosive burns of the esophagus. Arch Surg 112:495, 1977.
60. Maull KI, Scher LA, Greenfield LJ: Surgical implications of acid ingestion. Surg Gynecol Obstet 148:895, 1979.
61. Hogan RB, Polter DE: Nonsurgical management of lye-induced antral stricture with hydrostatic balloon dilation. Gastrointest Endosc 32:228, 1986.
62. Orvar K, Fagel D, Summers RW: Savory dilation of antral strictures from lye ingestion. Gastrointest Endosc 38:512, 1992.
63. Appelqvist P, Salmo M: Lye corrosion carcinoma of the esophagus. Cancer 45:2655, 1980.
64. Hopkins RA, Postlethwait RW: Caustic burn and carcinoma of the esophagus. Ann Surg 194:146, 1981.
65. Csikos M, Horvath O, Petri A, et al: Late malignant transformation of chronic corrosive esophageal strictures. Langenbecks Arch Chir 365: 231, 1985.
66. Easton H, Tennekoon GE: Squamous carcinoma of the stomach following corrosive acid burns. Br J Surg 59:382, 1972.
67. Votteler TP, Nash JC, Rutledge JC: The hazard of ingested alkaline disk batteries in children. JAMA 249:2504, 1983.
68. Gordon AC, Gongh MH: Esophageal perforation after button battery ingestion. Ann R Coll Surg Engl 75:362, 1993.
69. Temple DM, McNeese MC: Hazards of battery ingestion. Pediatrics 71: 100, 1983.
70. Litovitz TL, Senmitz BF: Ingestion of cylindrical and button batteries: An analysis of 2382 cases. Pediatrics 89:747, 1992.
71. Thompson N, Lowe-Ponsford F, Mant TG, Volans GN: Button bat-

tery ingestion: A review. Adv Drug React Acute Poison Rev 9:157, 1990.
72. Samad L, Ali A, Ramzi H: Button battery ingestion: Hazards of esophageal impaction. J Pediatr Surg 34:1527, 1999.
73. Sheikh A: Button battery ingestions in children. Pediatr Emerg Care 9: 224, 1993.
74. Marcus SM, Honcharuk L, Ruck B, et al: Button battery recommendations questioned. Pediatrics 91:681, 1993.
75. Studley JG, Linehan IP, Ogilvie AL, Downing BL: Swallowed button batteries: Is there a consensus on management? Gut 31:867, 1990.
76. Webb W: Foreign bodies of the upper GI tract. In Taylor MB (ed): Gastrointestinal Emergencies, 5th ed. Baltimore, Williams & Wilkins, 1992, pp 1–12.
77. Sigalet D, Lees G: Tracheoesophageal injury secondary to disk battery ingestion. J Pediatr Surg 23:996, 1988.
78. Maves MD, Lloyd TV, Carithers JS: Radiographic identification of ingested disk batteries. Pediatr Radiol 16:154, 1986.
79. Bass DH, Millar AJ: Mercury absorption following button battery ingestion. J Pediatr Surg 12:1541, 1992.

Chapter 23

Nonsteroidal Anti-inflammatory Drug Injury

Byron Cryer

Nonsteroidal anti-inflammatory drugs (NSAIDs) are among the most widely used groups of drugs. They are quite effective as anti-inflammatory, antipyretic, and analgesic agents. Their widespread use is in large part attributable to the high prevalence of osteoarthritis and rheumatoid arthritis, conditions for which NSAIDs are very effective. Although these compounds represent a very effective class of drugs, their use is associated with a broad spectrum of untoward reactions especially in the gastrointestinal (GI) tract, kidney, and platelet. In some instances, however, the antiplatelet effects are beneficial, such as with aspirin for cardiovascular prophylaxis. Because the GI side effects constitute the greatest of the untoward effects of NSAIDs, there has been much recent investigation focused on improving their GI safety profile. Therefore, this chapter concentrates on the untoward effects of NSAIDs in the various regions of the GI tract.

EPIDEMIOLOGY

Worldwide, NSAIDs are prescribed more frequently than any other group of medicines. It is estimated that over the course of a year nearly one in five Americans is treated with a NSAID, either prescribed or over the counter.[1] Of individuals above the age of 65, weekly use of NSAIDs is estimated to occur in 70%.[2] In the 2001 edition of the *Physicians' Desk Reference*, there were 25 different NSAIDs available by prescription in the United States, 6 of them salicylate-based compounds and 2 of them currently classified as cyclooxgenase-2 (COX-2) specific inhibitors (Table 23–1).[3] An additional three COX-2 specific inhibitors were expected to be approved for use by 2002. All NSAIDs are currently orally administered with the exception of ketorolac, which is parenterally administered. However, it is anticipated that soon another parenterally administered NSAID, parecoxib sodium (a COX-2 specific inhibitor), will be available. Actual NSAID consumption is much greater than accounted for by the 25 prescription NSAIDs. Over-the-counter (OTC) NSAID use is estimated to be considerably higher than use of prescribed NSAIDs, including particularly high usage of nonprescription aspirin preparations. For example, whereas there are 70 million prescriptions written in the United States for NSAIDs annually, there are more than 30 billion OTC NSAID tablets sold.[4]

Unfortunately, the major adverse consequences of the widespread use of NSAIDs are significant rates of morbidity and mortality related to this class of drugs. Although the spectrum of these reactions is broad, most of the adverse effects reported after NSAID use are experienced within the GI tract. The most serious of these complications, bleeding and perforation, account for almost all NSAID-associated GI mortality and have increasing prevalence with advancing age.[5, 6] Most of what has been written concerning NSAIDs' GI effects has related to the stomach and duodenum. However, NSAIDs' effects can be found at all levels of the GI tract.

MECHANISMS OF TOXICITY OF NONSTEROIDAL ANTI-INFLAMMATORY DRUGS

Irrespective of site of GI damage, the mechanisms through which NSAIDs cause injury are similar throughout the tract. The general mechanisms can be grouped into two categories: (1) those dependent on inhibition of the enzyme cyclooxygenase and (2) those independent of cyclooxygenase inhibi-

Table 23–1 | **Nonsteroidal Anti-inflammatory Drugs**

NONSALICYLATES	SALICYLATES	COX-2 INHIBITORS
Diclofenac sodium (Voltaren)	Aspirin* (ZORprin, Easprin)	Celecoxib (Celebrex)
Diclofenac sodium plus misoprostol (Arthrotec)†	Diflunisal (Dolobid)	Rofecoxib (Vioxx)
Etodolac (Lodine)	Salsalate (Disalcid, Salflex)	Etoricoxib§
Fenoprofen calcium (Nalfon)	Choline salicylate (Trilisate)	Parecoxib sodium‡§
Flurbiprofen (Ansaid)	Magnesium salicylate (Magan)	Valdecoxib§
Ibuprofen (Motrin)*		
Indomethacin (Indocin)		
Ketoprofen (Orudis)*		
Ketorolac tromethamine (Toradol)‡		
Meclofenamate sodium		
Mefenamic acid (Ponstel)		
Meloxicam (Mobic)		
Nabumetone (Relafen)		
Naproxen (Naprosyn, Anaprox)*		
Oxaprozin (Daypro)		
Piroxicam (Feldene)		
Sulindac (Clinoril)		
Tolmetin sodium (Tolectin 200, Tolectin 600)		

*Also available as over-the-counter preparations in the United States in 2001.
†Combination tablet of NSAID/synthetic prostaglandin E.
‡Parenterally administered.
§Expected to be available in 2002.
COX-2, cyclooxygenase-2; NSAID, nonsteroidal anti-inflammatory drug.

tion. The latter category consists of local mucosal toxic processes (topical effects).

Topical Effects

Considerable evidence exists that aspirin and other NSAIDs injure the GI mucosa, in part by a direct topical effect. Within a few minutes of NSAID ingestion, denudation of surface epithelial cells and increased mucosal permeability to sodium and hydrogen ions can be observed, reflected experimentally in a decrease in transmucosal potential difference.[7] Most NSAIDs are weak organic acids that at the usual acidic gastric pHs are not ionized, thus allowing them to be freely lipid-soluble. Once they are lipid-soluble, NSAIDs diffuse across gastric mucosal epithelial cell membranes into the intracellular cytoplasm with its pH of close to 7. Intracellular NSAIDs then ionize, become water-soluble, and are trapped within the cells. Because of intracellular trapping, NSAIDs accumulate intracellularly at very high concentrations, causing local toxic effects, some dependent upon and some independent of cyclooxygenase inhibition. As is discussed later, another topical mechanism of NSAID injury is an attenuation of the phospholipid content and surface hydrophobicity of the gastric mucus gel layer.[8]

Topical effects of NSAIDs are likely the major mechanism responsible for acute hemorrhages and erosions observed acutely after NSAID challenge. Enteric coated NSAIDs produce considerably less acute topical erosive and hemorrhagic injury than plain, non–enteric-coated formulations during short-term (1 to 2 weeks) administration,[9, 10] an observation in support of a local toxic effect of NSAIDs. However, with long-term administration of enteric-coated formulations, gastric ulcers develop at rates that do not differ from those of non–enteric-coated preparations,[11] presumably as a result of the systemic mechanism of injury. Furthermore, gastric and duodenal ulcers develop after NSAIDs are administered intravenously[12] or by rectal suppository,[13] further support for a nontopical or systemic effect.

Cyclooxygenase Inhibition

The beneficial effect of NSAIDs of decreasing systemic inflammation and their deleterious effects in the GI tract are both in part related to inhibition of the enzyme cyclooxygenase. Within the GI tract, NSAID-associated reduction in gastroduodenal mucosal prostaglandin concentrations is the major contributor to NSAID mucosal toxicity. Cyclooxygenase acts upon arachidonic acid to generate prostaglandins and

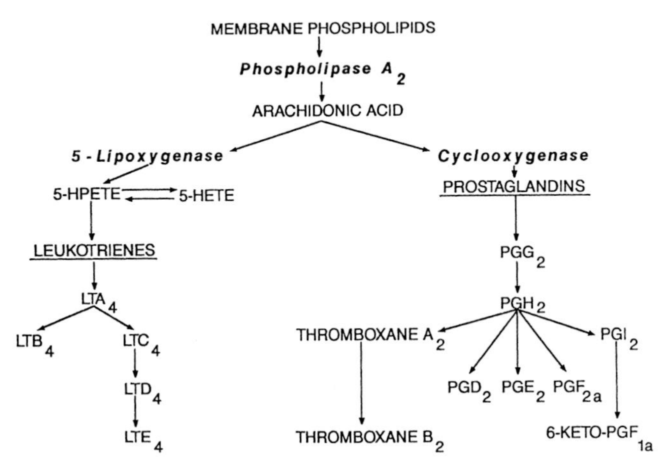

Figure 23–1. Metabolism of arachidonic acid after its release from membrane phospholipids. HPETE, hydroperoxyeicosatetraenoic acid; HETE, hydroxyeicosatetraenoic acid; LT, leukotriene; PG, prostaglandin. (From Cryer B, Feldman M: Effects of nonsteroidal anti-inflammatory drugs on endogenous gastrointestinal prostaglandins and therapeutic strategies for prevention and treatment of nonsteroidal anti-inflammatory drug-induced damage. Arch Intern Med 152:1145–1155, 1992.)

Table 23–2 | **Comparison of Cyclooxygenase-1 and Cyclooxygenase-2**

	COX-1	COX-2
Regulation	Constitutive	Inducible
Range of expression	2- to 4-fold	10- to 80-fold
Tissue expression	Most tissues, notably platelets, GI mucosa	Inflammatory sites Synoviocytes, fibroblasts, monocytes

COX-1, COX-2, cyclooxygenases 1 and 2; GI, gastrointestinal.

thromboxane (Fig. 23–1).[3] Prostaglandins are a family of related fatty acids that are found in almost all of the body's cells. In humans, prostaglandins E_2, I_2, and $F_{2\alpha}$ are the major products of arachidonic acid metabolism produced by the stomach and duodenum.[14] Prostaglandins participate in various activities, including mediation of inflammatory responses and regulation of renal blood flow. Within the GI tract, prostaglandins protect against mucosal injury. For example, if one pretreats the gastric mucosa with exogenously administered prostaglandins, protection is provided against a variety of damaging agents such as alcohol, bile salts, strong acid, hypertonic saline solution, boiling water, stress, aspirin and other NSAIDs.[15, 16] Putative mechanisms through which prostaglandins provide their mucosal protective effects include stimulation of mucosal bicarbonate secretion, stimulation of mucus secretion, increase in mucosal blood flow, prevention of disruption of the gastric mucosal barrier, acceleration of cell proliferation, stimulation of cellular ionic transport processes, stimulation of cyclic adenosine monophosphate production, promotion of formation of surface active phospholipids, maintenance of gastric mucosal sulfhydryl compounds, stabilization of cellular lysosomes, and stabilization of cell membranes.[17] Among these, maintenance of mucosal blood flow is thought to be the mechanism most responsible for the protective GI mucosal effects of prostaglandins.[17]

Cyclooxygenase, the rate limiting enzyme in prostaglandin synthesis, is inhibited by NSAIDs. With the exception of COX-2 specific inhibitors, NSAIDs inhibit cyclooxygenase, reducing gastroduodenal mucosal prostaglandin concentrations with a resulting loss of a major mechanism for protection against mucosal injury. Aspirin, by acetylation of cyclooxygenase, inhibits this enzyme irreversibly, whereas all other NSAIDs inhibit cyclooxygenase in a reversible, concentration-dependent manner. With aspirin, when cyclooxygenase is irreversibly inhibited, the capacity for prostaglandin synthesis does not return to normal for several days until new enzyme can be synthesized.[18] This may explain why aspirin, in comparison to the other NSAIDs, remains one of the most potent inhibitors of prostaglandin synthesis. A prospective evaluation of the GI effects of low doses of aspirin in humans revealed that as little as 10 mg of oral aspirin suppresses gastric prostaglandins by approximately 60% and causes gastric injury, including ulcers.[19]

In the early 1990s, two structurally related cyclooxygenase isoforms were identified in mammalian cells, cyclooxygenase-1 (COX-1) and COX-2.[20–22] As indicated by data from animal studies, COX-1 is found in most of the body's tissues, including the stomach. COX-2, by contrast, is undetectable in most tissues under normal physiologic conditions. COX-2 is inducible through the action of cytokines, growth factors, and endotoxins. Although there are many differences between the COX isoforms, one notable distinction is that COX-2 is believed to be the principal COX isoform that participates in inflammation. It is also thought that there is little COX-2 activity present in the stomach or platelet (Table 23–2). In studies of the human GI tract, little to no COX-2 protein or activity has been demonstrated, whereas abundant COX-1 protein and activity have been observed.[23]

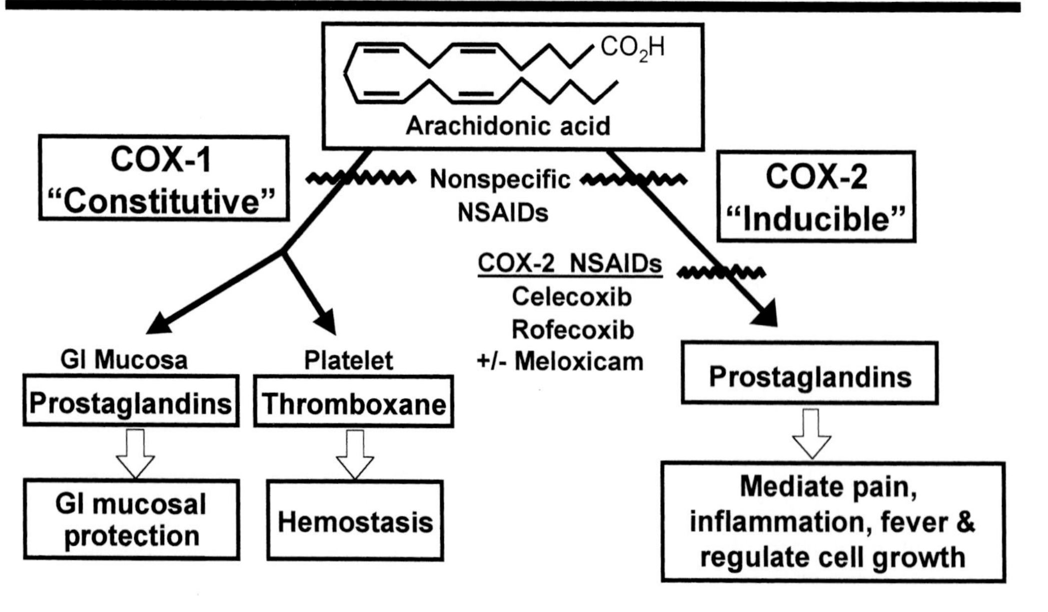

Figure 23–2. Revised concept of metabolism of arachidonic acid after its release from membrane phospholipids. Nonspecific nonsteroidal anti-inflammatory drugs (NSAIDs) inhibit both COX-1 and COX-2, whereas COX-2–specific NSAIDs inhibit only COX-2. Thus, COX-2–specific NSAIDs can be alternatively conceptualized as "COX-1 sparing."

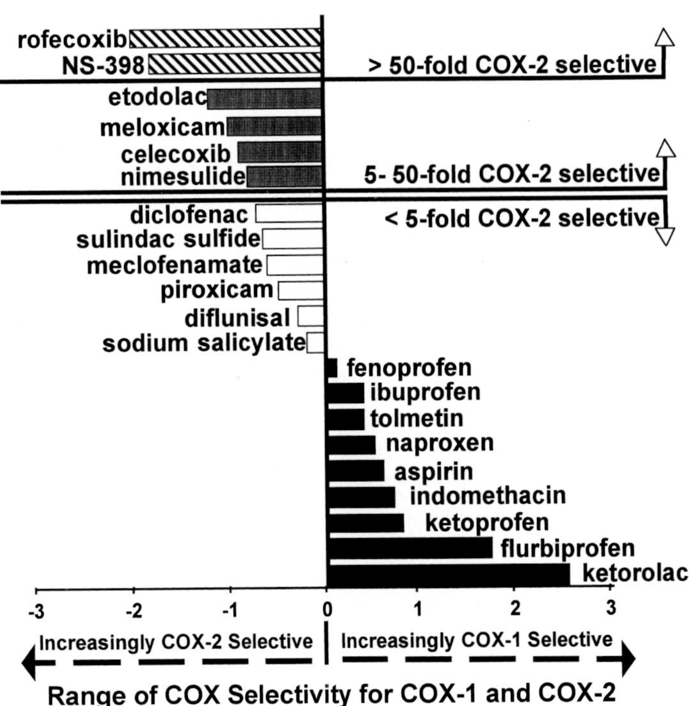

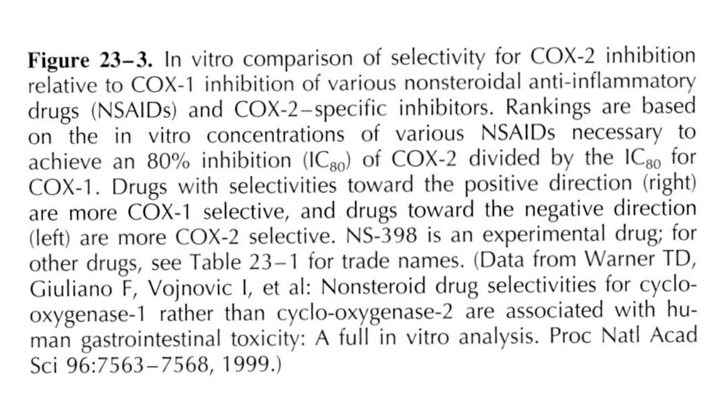

Figure 23–3. In vitro comparison of selectivity for COX-2 inhibition relative to COX-1 inhibition of various nonsteroidal anti-inflammatory drugs (NSAIDs) and COX-2–specific inhibitors. Rankings are based on the in vitro concentrations of various NSAIDs necessary to achieve an 80% inhibition (IC_{80}) of COX-2 divided by the IC_{80} for COX-1. Drugs with selectivities toward the positive direction (right) are more COX-1 selective, and drugs toward the negative direction (left) are more COX-2 selective. NS-398 is an experimental drug; for other drugs, see Table 23–1 for trade names. (Data from Warner TD, Giuliano F, Vojnovic I, et al: Nonsteroid drug selectivities for cyclo-oxygenase-1 rather than cyclo-oxygenase-2 are associated with human gastrointestinal toxicity: A full in vitro analysis. Proc Natl Acad Sci 96:7563–7568, 1999.)

In this revised hypothesis of COX inhibition (Fig. 23–2), a specific inhibitor of COX-2 should retain its anti-inflammatory properties and have reduced adverse GI and antiplatelet effects. This concept has led to development and clinical introduction of COX-2 specific NSAIDs. In 1999, two specific inhibitors of COX-2 were introduced in the United States for clinical use, celecoxib and rofecoxib (see Fig. 23–2). All NSAIDs in clinical use prior to 1999 inhibited both COX-1 and COX-2; these older NSAIDs are referred to as *nonspecific NSAIDs* (see Fig. 23–2). Animal data from 2000 indicate that for gastric ulceration to occur *both* COX-1 and COX-2 must be inhibited.[24] Interestingly, in one model selective inhibition of COX-1 alone did not cause gastric damage.[24]

Even though all nonspecific NSAIDs inhibit both COX isoforms, their selectivity for COX-1 or COX-2 widely varies. Figure 23–3 provides a comparison of relative differences in in vitro selectivity between the COX-2 NSAIDs and older NSAIDs.[25] It should be emphasized that a limitation of in vitro data is that they do not entirely parallel the in vivo effects of a given drug. For example, Figure 23–3 does not provide an indication of serum concentrations achieved with various drugs at therapeutic dosage. A better predictor of a drug's clinical GI effects is the degree to which an NSAID does (or does not) inhibit COX-1 at therapeutic dosage. Figure 23–4 provides an indication of the degree to which some selected NSAIDs at therapeutic (in vivo) dosage result in inhibition of COX-1. Only agents that do not inhibit COX-1 at therapeutic dosage should be considered as COX-2–specific NSAIDs. One NSAID, meloxicam, was approved for use in the United States in 2000, and in in vitro assays meloxicam appears relatively COX-2 selective (see Fig. 23–3). However, meloxicam's ability at therapeutic dosage to spare COX-1 is dose-related. At high (15 mg) therapeutic doses, meloxicam achieves more than 50% COX-1 inhibition, yielding a COX inhibitory profile similar to that of older, nonselective NSAIDs (see Fig. 23–4).[26] However, notwithstanding this meloxicam example or other differences between in vitro and in vivo assays for all NSAIDs, results provided by recent clinical trials of COX-2 selective inhibitors suggest that the in vitro data do indeed more or less predict clinical responses. Data from the clinical trials with

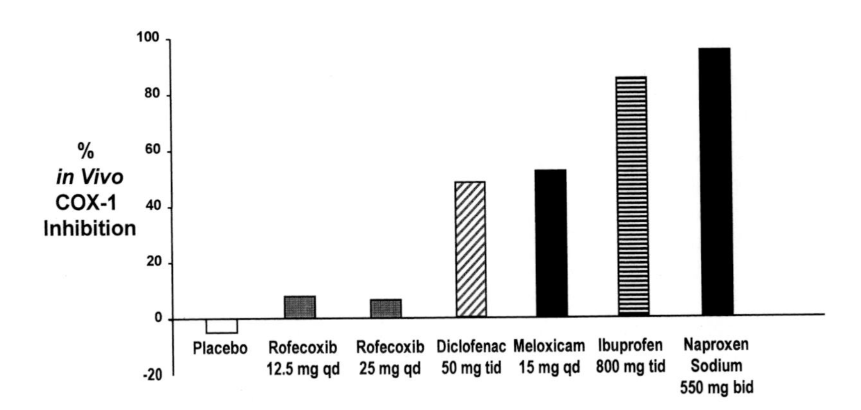

Figure 23–4. Comparison of differences in COX-1 inhibition with therapeutic (in vivo) dosing of a COX-2–specific inhibitor and with other nonsteroidal anti-inflammatory drugs (NSAIDs). (Data from Van Hecken A, Schwartz JI, Depre M, et al: Comparative inhibitory activity of rofecoxib, meloxicam, diclofenac, ibuprofen, and naproxen on COX-2 versus COX-1 in healthy volunteers. J Clin Pharmacol 40:1109–1120, 2000.)

COX-2 inhibitors are presented later in this chapter (see Nonsteroidal Anti-inflammatory Drugs with Improved Gastrointestinal Safety Profiles).

Multifactorial Mechanisms of Nonsteroidal Anti-inflammatory Drug–Induced Damage

Although inhibition of prostaglandin synthesis contributes to NSAID-induced mucosal injury, it is not settled whether prostaglandin inhibition is the primary mechanism. In some studies, there has been poor correlation between gastric mucosal injury and degree of prostaglandin suppression after NSAID administration.[15, 27] Other factors probably work in concert with prostaglandin suppression to increase the propensity for mucosal injury by NSAIDs. For example, after indomethacin administration, gastric acid secretion has been shown to increase[28] (possibly through calcium-mediated pathways[29]), gastric mucosal blood flow to decrease,[30] and duodenal bicarbonate output to decrease.[31] NSAIDs can also potentially affect mucus secretion, as they have been shown to inhibit mucus synthesis, to reduce incorporation of radiolabeled precursors into mucus glycoprotein, and to alter thickness of the mucus layer.[32] Interestingly, because prostaglandins assist in the regulation of each of the mechanisms listed, it is possible that all of the physiologic responses to NSAID administration indicated could be prostaglandin mediated.

NSAIDs may potentiate pepsinogen secretion, and, similarly to their effects on acid secretion, this effect may be regulated by calcium.[33] However, in contrast to NSAIDs' effects on gastric acid, NSAID-enhanced pepsinogen secretion is independent of endogenous prostaglandin inhibition and may act via a postreceptor mechanism.[33] Additional evidence for a role of pepsin in NSAID-induced ulceration is obtained from studies in which treatment with a pepsin inhibitor prevents NSAID-induced ulceration.[34]

The strongest argument in support of prostaglandin depletion as an essential element of NSAID-induced ulcers is that depletion of mucosal prostaglandins, by active or passive immunization with prostaglandin antibodies, leads to GI ulcers, many of which are complicated (perforated or bleeding) at the time of presentation.[35] Furthermore, NSAID-induced ulcers can be prevented by small doses of exogenous prostaglandins.[32]

It has been proposed in animal models that neutrophils contribute to the pathogenesis of NSAID-induced gastric injury. In rats, NSAID-induced gastric injury is significantly attenuated by prior induction of neutropenia.[36, 37] In response to NSAIDs, a reduction in blood flow occurs as a result of adherence of neutrophils to vascular endothelium in the gastric and mesenteric microcirculations via increased expression of intercellular adhesion molecules (ICAMs) on endothelial cells and of CD11/CD18 on leukocytes.[37] Moreover, pretreatment with monoclonal antibodies directed against these adherence sites almost completely prevents NSAID-induced injury.[37]

NSAID-induced GI injury is not entirely explained by either a topical effect or prostaglandin suppression. The more recent studies on mechanisms of NSAID-induced mucosal injury suggest that the pathophysiologic mechanisms may be more complex. Given what is currently known of mechanisms of NSAID-induced mucosal injury, it seems reasonable to conclude that even though prostaglandin suppression appears to be a prerequisite for mucosal injury, neutrophil vascular adherence and alterations in mucosal blood flow may also be necessary conditions. Furthermore, topical mucosal irritation by NSAIDs probably contributes to these other mucosal physiologic changes. Overall, our clinical observations of NSAIDs' GI manifestations likely reflect the combined effects of all of these mechanisms.

CLINICAL MANIFESTATIONS OF NONSTEROIDAL ANTI-INFLAMMATORY DRUG INJURY THROUGHOUT THE GASTROINTESTINAL TRACT

In the stomach and duodenum, the evidence for a cause and effect association between NSAID use and mucosal injury is strong, but in the other areas of the GI tract the relationships are more speculative. Most studies of NSAID injury in these other areas have been in the form of case reports or series. Nevertheless, some recurrent observations have suggested, at the least, some very strong associations between NSAID use and GI damage.

Esophagus

Ulcers

The principal toxic manifestations of NSAIDs in the esophagus are ulcers and strictures. However, esophageal ulcers are not specific to NSAIDs. Esophageal ulceration has been reported in association with at least 26 different medicines (see Chapter 34).[38, 39] Considering all of the medicines associated with esophageal ulceration, the incidence of NSAID-associated ulceration falls about in the middle of the group.

There is not a likely single unifying mechanism to explain all pill-induced esophageal ulceration because the pharmacologic properties of all of the various medicines that cause this problem are quite diverse. With aspirin, esophageal ulcers are thought to be initiated by its disruption of the esophageal mucosal barrier to hydrogen diffusion, thus rendering the underlying esophageal mucosa more susceptible to the refluxed gastric acid.[39, 40] In animals esophageal ulceration can be experimentally induced after just a few oral doses of a NSAID.[41] The one unifying mechanism in all cases of esophageal pill ulceration is prolonged mucosal contact with a medicine that has relatively caustic physical properties.

The diagnosis of NSAID-induced esophageal ulceration is a diagnosis of exclusion based first on elimination of reflux disease, cancer, or infections as possible causes in patients who are concurrently taking NSAIDs. There is no specific therapy other than to try to speed healing of the ulcer with acid suppressive therapies and to advise patients against taking their NSAIDs without food or at least 6 oz of water or before recumbency.

Strictures

Esophageal stricture as a complication of NSAID therapy has been less widely appreciated than has ulceration. The same medicines associated with pill-induced esophageal ulceration have also been associated with esophageal stricture.[39, 42] Risk factors for pill-induced stricturing are also similar; they include recumbency, pill ingestion just prior to sleep or during the postoperative period, and ingestion of sustained-release pill formulations. Esophageal strictures are most commonly caused by gastroesophageal reflux of acid and not by medications. In almost all acid-related esophageal strictures, the mucosa that lies between the stricture and the gastroesophageal junction is inflamed; thus, the diagnosis of NSAID-induced esophageal stricture is strengthened if that mucosa is endoscopically and histologically normal.

Esophagitis

The data suggesting a causal relationship between NSAID consumption and esophagitis are less strong than those for ulcer and stricture. Because gastroesophageal reflux disease (GERD) has a high prevalence in the general population, a very large study would be required to demonstrate that NSAIDs cause esophagitis independently of acid. All studies reporting NSAID-induced esophagitis have been case reports or small series.[43–45] There are no controlled, prospective well-designed trials that evaluate this potential relationship. It is of interest, however, that patients with esophagitis do have a much higher prevalence of NSAID use than control subjects.[45] The author believes that NSAIDs may exacerbate the tendency toward esophagitis in patients with GERD rather than independently cause esophageal inflammation.

Stomach and Duodenum

The stomach and duodenum are the most common and important organs damaged by NSAIDS. Much of the difficulty in attempting to quantify adverse effects attributable to NSAIDs arises from the number of ways in which NSAID-induced adverse effects can be defined. Symptoms, endoscopic mucosal lesions, and, most importantly, serious GI events have all been used to assess the magnitude of NSAIDs' toxic effects; the serious upper GI complications are the most relevant to NSAIDs' clinical morbidity. Symptomatic GI ulceration (that is, ulceration associated with pain, perforation, bleeding, or obstruction) occurs in approximately 2% to 4% of patients treated with an NSAID for 1 year.[3] When one considers the millions of people who consume NSAIDs annually, these seemingly small percentages translate into large numbers of symptomatic GI ulcers, episodes of GI bleeding, and perforations per year. However, far more common than clinically apparent NSAID-induced upper GI events are the lesser degrees of mucosal toxicity described later.

Nonsteroidal Anti-inflammatory Drug Gastropathy

Ingestion of aspirin and other NSAIDs typically produces acute gastric mucosal erosions and subepithelial hemorrhages. On microscopic evaluation of gastric biopsy specimens of patients taking NSAIDs, the occurrence of a mucosal inflammatory infiltrate is not greater than expected for age-matched controls not taking NSAIDs. Thus, NSAIDs do not actually cause a histologic gastritis. A more appropriate term for this condition is *NSAID gastropathy*. Although NSAID gastropathy can occur throughout the stomach, it has a predilection for the fundus and the body. The constellation of multiple small erosions *plus* multiple small submucosal hemorrhages throughout the stomach is very suggestive of NSAID use. These endoscopic findings, although visually disconcerting, are usually asymptomatic.

Ulcers

Prevalence

In endoscopic studies, the incidence of new gastric ulcers ranges from 10% to 40% and the incidence of duodenal ulcers ranges from 4% to 15% during the first 3 months of NSAID use.[46–50] Most are asymptomatic, however.[51, 52] The risk of clinically significant NSAID-induced ulceration is probably closer to 1% during the first 3 months of NSAID use.[3]

In a prospective endoscopic study in which ulcer patients who were taking NSAIDs were compared to ulcer patients who had not taken NSAIDs (controls), significantly fewer NSAID-using ulcer patients experienced ulcer pain than controls.[52] Asymptomatic NSAID-induced ulceration may be especially problematic in that asymptomatic patients more frequently have bleeding or perforation as their first presentation of ulcer disease.[51, 52] Among patients who have bleeding ulcers, those who have been using NSAIDs are more than twice as likely to have been asymptomatic prior to presentation than those who have no history of NSAID use.[6]

The reasons that NSAID use is associated with asymptomatic ulceration are not clear. It has been suggested that NSAIDs may induce analgesia or, alternatively, that NSAID use may exacerbate a previously existing "silent" ulcer, causing it to perforate or bleed. NSAIDs are anticoagulants as a result of their antiplatelet actions. Therefore, they can increase the tendency of an existing ulcer to bleed. Another possibility is that at initiation of NSAID therapy, many patients who are intolerant of NSAIDs because of dyspepsia discontinue the medicine. The remainder who tolerate the NSAID continue NSAID consumption and are exposed to continued risk of asymptomatic ulceration that may progress to an ulcer complication such as a bleed or perforation.

Risk Groups for Nonsteroidal Anti-inflammatory Drug–Induced Ulcers

Certain groups of NSAID users appear to be at greater risk than others for development of NSAID ulcer complications (Table 23–3) and should therefore be considered for strategies to prevent or to reduce ulceration. The most significant risk factor for a NSAID-induced complication is a history of prior peptic ulcer disease or a prior ulcer complication, factors that increase the risk for NSAID-induced GI events two- to fourfold.[53–56] It should be emphasized that a previous history of ulcer disease increases future risk of GI events in all patients, not only those who are on NSAIDs.

Advancing age is also a risk factor. Although there does not appear to be a threshold age at which risk dramatically increases, the risk increases linearly with advancing age.[53]

Table 23–3 | **Risk Factors for Nonsteroidal Anti-inflammatory Drug–Induced Ulcers**

DEFINITE	POSSIBLE
Prior peptic ulcer disease	*Helicobacter pylori*
Prior NSAID gastrointestinal complication	Smoking
Advanced age	
Concomitant use of glucocorticoids	
Concomitant use of anticoagulants	
High or multiple doses of NSAIDs	
Comorbid diseases	
Ethanol use	

NSAID, nonsteroidal anti-inflammatory drug.

Table 23–4 | **Type of Nonsteroidal Anti-inflammatory Drug and Risk of Ulcer**

RISK GROUP	DRUG	RELATIVE RISK (RANGE)
Relatively low	Ibuprofen (Motrin)	2.0 (1.4–2.8)
	Diclofenac sodium (Voltaren)	4.2 (4.2–6.8)
Medium	Naproxen (Naprosyn)	9.1 (5.5–15.1)
	Indomethacin (Indocin)	11.3 (6.3–20.3)
	Piroxicam (Feldene)	13.7 (7.1–26.3)
High	Ketoprofen (Orudis)	23.7 (7.6–74.2)
	Azapropazone (apazone)	31.5 (10.3–96.9)

Langman MJS, Weil J, Wainwright P, et al: Risks of bleeding peptic ulcer associated with individual non-steroidal anti-inflammatory drugs. Lancet 343: 1075–1078, 1994.

There have been conflicting data as to the effect of duration of NSAID exposure on the risk of NSAID-related GI events. Some case control studies have suggested that the risk of NSAID-associated GI complications is highest within the first 30 days of NSAID use.[5, 57] A potential explanation for this perceived early high-risk period could be that with continued NSAID exposure the gastric mucosa adapts to the injurious effects of NSAIDs, thus becoming more resistant later in the course of continued NSAID exposure (a phenomenon referred to as *gastric adaptation*). However, in 1995 and 2000, controlled prospective studies of arthritis patients who had long-term NSAID administration indicated that the risk of serious NSAID-induced GI complications appears to be cumulative and linear.[54–56]

It has become clear from epidemiologic studies that as the dose of an NSAID increases, the risk of ulcer complications also increases in a parallel fashion.[5, 53] This dose-response relationship is seen across all classes of NSAIDs and is also linear. Concurrent use of more than one NSAID is also a risk factor because this practice essentially increases total NSAID dose; the most common example is the combined use of prescribed NSAIDs and OTC NSAIDs or low-dose aspirin.

Other risk factors are concomitant use of glucocorticoids or anticoagulants and comorbid conditions such as significant heart disease or rheumatoid arthritis.[1, 54, 58] However, the use of glucocorticoids alone does not independently increase the risk for ulcer disease.[59]

Data from 1997 and 1999 indicate that regular alcohol consumption combined with regular NSAID use is an additive risk factor for serious upper GI adverse events.[60, 61] Interestingly, regular use of low doses of aspirin increases upper GI risk in persons frequently consuming alcohol. Among current drinkers, aspirin use at least every other day at a dose of 325 mg/day or greater is associated with a sevenfold increased risk of upper GI bleeding when compared with that in persons who do not drink or use low-dose aspirin.[61]

In the past, it was stated that the risk of peptic ulceration was equivalent for all types of NSAIDs. However, epidemiologic studies have stratified some selected older NSAIDs by risk of NSAID-induced ulcer bleeding or perforation and have ranked them as shown in Table 23–4.[51, 62] Ibuprofen is listed as an NSAID associated with a relatively low risk of ulcer complications. This characterization should be interpreted with caution because ibuprofen is frequently taken as an over-the-counter preparation, at doses that have a lower therapeutic equivalence than doses of other prescribed NSAIDs. Thus, this apparent low ranking of ibuprofen may be a reflection of dose of NSAID rather than type of NSAID. Although not evaluated in the study shown in the table, as discussed later, other NSAIDs that might be considered as posing low risk include the nonacetylated salicylates etodolac and nabumetone.

Undocumented Use and Over-the-Counter Nonsteroidal Anti-inflammatory Drugs

Precise quantification of NSAID risk is complicated by undocumented NSAID consumption. Total NSAID usage is probably underestimated, given the recent over-the-counter availability of NSAIDs. For example, Figure 23–5 shows results of a study in which the prevalence of NSAID use in patients who entered a hospital with upper GI bleeding was assessed by history.[63] In this urban population of individuals who had upper GI bleeding, 42% of the NSAIDs consumed were not prescribed (OTC). Notably, 35% of these individuals were taking some form of nonprescribed aspirin, which accounted for the overwhelming majority of NSAID use.

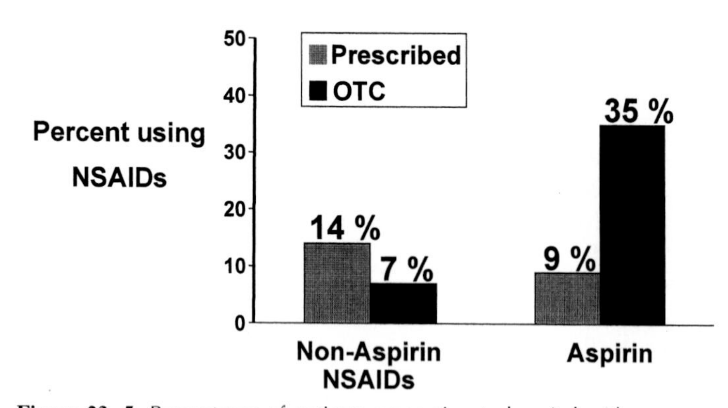

Figure 23–5. Percentages of patients presenting to hospital with upper gastrointestinal (UGI) bleeding who were using nonsteroidal anti-inflammatory drugs (NSAIDs). Use of NSAIDs was determined by taking a history. As seen in the figure, over-the-counter (OTC) use of NSAIDs was more prevalent than was prescribed NSAID usage. After adding all forms of NSAID consumption, NSAIDs were used by 65% of these patients presenting with UGI bleeding. (Data from Wilcox CM, Shalek KA, Costsonis G: Striking prevalence of over-the-counter nonsteroidal anti-inflammatory drug use in patients with upper gastrointestinal hemorrhage. Arch Intern Med 154:42–46, 1994.)

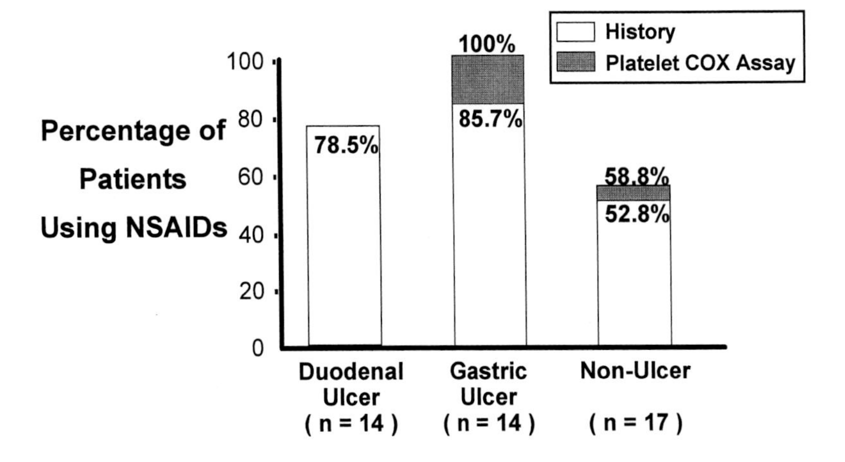

Figure 23–6. Documentation of nonsteroidal anti-inflammatory drug (NSAID) use in patients with upper gastrointestinal (UGI) bleeding. By using the thromboxane index (Tx I) in patients presenting with UGI bleeding, documentation of NSAID use was greater than documentation by history alone. (Adapted from data in Wilcox CM, Shalek KA, Costsonis G: Striking prevalence of over-the-counter nonsteroidal anti-inflammatory drug use in patients with upper gastrointestinal hemorrhage. Arch Intern Med 154:42–46, 1994.)

When all four forms of NSAID use are added together, prescribed and OTC, aspirin and nonaspirin, NSAIDs were used by 65% of these GI bleeding patients when use was assessed by history.

Numerous OTC compounds that contain aspirin or other NSAIDs are available. In the United States, aspirin, ibuprofen, naproxen, and ketoprofen are available over the counter. As suggested in Figure 23–5, OTC NSAID usage is probably more frequent than prescribed usage. Unfortunately, in many instances both the patient and the physician are unaware that such compounds are being taken.

The thromboxane index, an assay of platelet cyclooxygenase activity, is a test that has been investigationally employed to document NSAID ingestion when use is not apparent by history but is nevertheless suspected.[4, 45, 64] Because platelet cyclooxygenase is irreversibly inhibited by aspirin and variably inhibited by other NSAIDs, low serum platelet cyclooxygenase activity would suggest NSAID exposure. In a study of bleeding ulcer and nonulcer patients, the thromboxane index improved documentation of NSAID use when compared to documentation by history alone[64] (Fig. 23–6). The thromboxane index may be especially useful in patients with ulcers that are refractory to healing agents because many of these patients are chronic NSAID abusers and approximately half of them use NSAIDs surreptitiously.[65]

Low-Dose Aspirin

Low daily doses of aspirin (usually 325 mg/day or less) are very commonly prescribed for prevention of cardiovascular and cerebrovascular diseases. In controlled studies of low-dose aspirin, aspirin therapy increased the risk of GI bleeding[66] and increased the likelihood of hospitalization for ulcers.[67] Although it was suggested in many of these trials that low-dose aspirin may be associated with an increased risk of GI toxicity, there are few data reporting the degree of risk. In a case control study, aspirin use as low as 75 mg/day was associated with a greater than twofold increased risk of GI bleeding.[67] One placebo-controlled study of low-dose aspirin for prevention of cerebrovascular events reported increased rates of GI bleeding with aspirin when compared to placebo.[68] Over the course of 6 years, more than 2400 patients were randomized to placebo, aspirin 300 mg/day, or aspirin 1200 mg/day, and there was a significant dose-response relationship observed between aspirin dose and GI bleeding. The rates of upper GI bleeding in placebo and in aspirin 300 mg/day and 1200 mg/day groups were 0.1%, 0.3%, and 0.6%, respectively, an odds ratio of 3.6-fold increased risk for aspirin 300 mg/day over that of placebo[68] (Fig. 23–7). In 2000, a case control study indicated an odds ratio for upper GI bleeding for doses of aspirin of 300 mg/day or less of 2.4.[69] Buffered or enteric-coated aspirin preparations, when dosed at 325 mg/day, although probably associated with a reduced incidence of dyspepsia when compared to that of plain aspirin, have risks of upper GI bleeding that are similar to those of plain aspirin.[70] As discussed in the section on safer NSAIDs, when administered concurrently with a COX-2 specific inhibitor in a large GI outcomes trial, aspirin at a dose of 325 mg/day or less appears to eliminate the beneficial GI effects associated with celecoxib.[55] The sum of these data on risks and benefits of low daily doses of aspirin indicates that any formulation of aspirin at doses as low as 325 mg/day or less, although beneficial for vascular prophylaxis, is associated with at least a twofold and possibly as

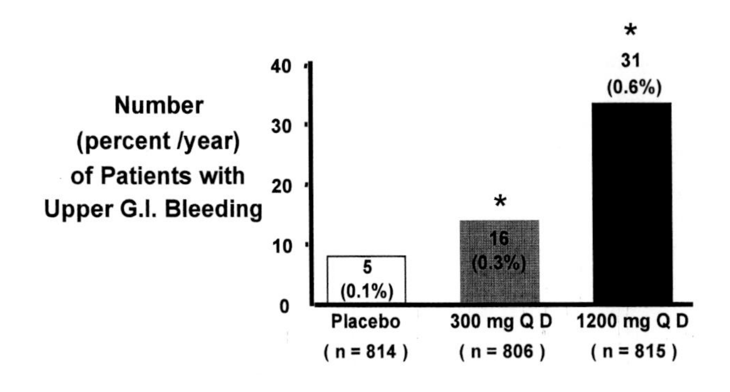

Figure 23–7. Prevalence of upper gastrointestinal (GI) bleeding with low doses of aspirin. The number of patients (and rates) of upper GI bleeding in patients taking either a placebo or aspirin (300 mg/day and 1200 mg/day) for prophylaxis against cerebrovascular vascular events are shown. As seen, even at an aspirin dose of 300 mg/day, there is a three-fold increased incidence in upper GI bleeding. *, Rates of upper GI bleeding with aspirin doses are statistically significantly higher than are rates with the placebo. (Data from Weil J, Colin-Jones DG, Langman, et al: Prophylactic aspirin and risk of peptic ulcer bleeding. BMJ 310:827–830, 1995.)

high as a fourfold increased risk of GI complications. Such conclusions have led to investigations evaluating toxicity of aspirin doses lower than 325 mg/day. In a study of low-dose aspirin administered for 3 months, 10 mg/day aspirin significantly lowered gastric mucosal prostaglandin level and caused gastric ulceration.[71] Even when administered as infrequently as 81 mg every third day, aspirin continues to suppress gastric prostaglandin level significantly for approximately 5 days after aspirin dosing.[18] Thus, it appears unlikely that there is an orally administered dose of aspirin that is efficacious for cardiovascular prophylaxis that is also without GI risks.

Helicobacter pylori and Nonsteroidal Anti-inflammatory Drugs (Also See Chapters 39 and 40)

NSAIDs and the bacterium *Helicobacter pylori* (*H. pylori*) are the two main causes of gastroduodenal ulcers. There are many characteristics of NSAID-induced ulcers and *H. pylori* related ulcers that suggest that these two types of ulceration are separate pathophysiologic entities. First, NSAID ulcers occur in individuals not infected with *H. pylori*.[72] Anatomic location, histologic characteristics, patterns of recurrence, and symptoms also distinguish the two types of ulcer. In those in whom ulcers develop in association with NSAID use, gastric ulcers are about twice as likely as duodenal and *H. pylori* related ulcers are more frequently duodenal. *H. pylori* almost always is associated with a chronic active gastritis, whereas histologic gastritis is not an expected feature of NSAID-induced ulcers.[73] Experimental administration of an NSAID does not cause a histologic gastritis.[74] Because *H. pylori* is found in up to 50% of normal subjects older than age 60, NSAID use by older individuals can be expected to result in NSAID-induced ulcers that are associated with chronic active gastritis in about half of the older ulcer patients (assuming an equivalent predisposition for ulceration in *H. pylori* infected and noninfected subjects). Indeed, in the literature about half of NSAID-associated ulcers are associated with chronic active gastritis.[73]

Another notable difference between NSAID-induced and *H. pylori* related ulcers lies in their nature or recurrence. When NSAID use is discontinued, NSAID ulcers should not recur. By contrast, to *H. pylori* related ulcers have recurrence rates of 50% to 80% by 1 year if the organism is not eradicated by antibiotics. Finally, dyspepsia is a common feature of *H. pylori* related ulcers, whereas most NSAID-induced ulcers are asymptomatic.

Because NSAIDs and *H. pylori* individually may cause ulcers, a reasonable question is whether risk for ulceration is higher for combined *H. pylori* infection and NSAID consumption than for either of those factors alone. Data on whether *H. pylori* contributes to the risk of NSAID-induced GI mucosal injury have been conflicting. For example, the results of one study indicate that in patients without a history of ulcers, eradication of *H. pylori* before use of NSAIDs markedly reduced NSAID-induced endoscopic ulcers after 8 weeks of naproxen.[75] However, the results of another study indicated that *H. pylori* eradication in patients with a history of peptic ulcer disease does not reduce endoscopic ulcers after 6 months of NSAIDs.[76] In 1998 and 1999, several other studies assessed the potential interaction between *H. pylori* and NSAIDs and provided results that were similarly discrepant.[77–79] These conflicting conclusions are probably explained by differences in patient populations, study designs, doses, duration, and types of NSAIDs evaluated throughout the various studies. The author's personal assessment of this body of literature is that with nonaspirin NSAIDs, *H. pylori* eradication probably does not reduce the incidence of NSAID-induced GI ulceration or complications. For uncertain reasons, however, there may be a synergistic injurious GI effect of aspirin and *H. pylori*.[80]

Therapy for Nonsteroidal Anti-inflammatory Drug–Induced Ulcers

Therapy for NSAID-induced ulcers needs to be tailored according to whether one is attempting to heal an already established ulcer associated with NSAIDs or attempting to prevent development of an NSAID-induced ulcer. Because therapeutic strategies differ, preventative strategies and healing strategies are discussed separately.

PREVENTION OF NONSTEROIDAL ANTI-INFLAMMATORY DRUG–INDUCED ULCERS. Prior to the clinical availability of safer classes of NSAIDs, reduction in NSAID-induced GI toxicity was primarily accomplished by prescribing drugs that when coadministered with NSAIDs would protect against mucosal ulceration. Because most patients who take NSAIDs long term never experience clinically significant ulceration, the ideal candidates for cotherapy are those considered to have high risk for NSAID-induced ulcers (see Table 23–3). Various cotherapies that have been considered are discussed in the following sections.

H_2 Receptor Antagonists. A number of studies have evaluated whether an H_2 receptor antagonist (H_2 RA), when coadministered with an NSAID, can prevent NSAID-induced ulcers.[81–83] These studies have consistently found that all four H_2 RAs, namely, cimetidine, famotidine, nizatidine, and ranitidine, at their usual ulcer-healing doses do not prevent NSAID-associated gastric ulcers. Because most NSAID-induced ulcers are gastric rather than duodenal, and because one cannot predict which type of NSAID-induced ulcer will develop, H_2 RAs are not ideal drugs for NSAID ulcer prophylaxis. However, when one of the H_2 RAs, famotidine, is administered at a high dose (40 mg twice daily) NSAID-induced duodenal and gastric ulcers are both effectively reduced.[84]

Prostaglandins. As discussed in Chapter 40, misoprostol, the synthetic prostaglandin E_1 (PGE_1) analog, reduces NSAID-induced gastric and duodenal endoscopic ulceration as well as NSAID-induced serious GI adverse events.[46, 54] The disadvantages of misoprostol are that it may cause dose-related diarrhea and is not effective in treating dyspepsia associated with NSAIDs. A combination tablet of misoprostol and the NSAID diclofenac is associated with a reduction in side effects such as diarrhea and has a favorably low ulceration rate.[85] In a 1986 direct comparison of misoprostol and ranitidine within the same study, the two drugs were equal in efficacy for prevention of NSAID-induced duodenal ulcers, whereas misoprostol was significantly more effective than ranitidine in prevention of endoscopically diagnosed gastric ulcers.[86] Even though misoprostol effectively reduces NSAID-induced GI complications, a 1997 meta-analysis estimated that 264 long-term NSAID users of average risk would need to be treated with misoprostol for 6 months to prevent one GI complication.[87] However, in high-risk NSAID users, misoprostol is more cost-effective and therefore appears more appropriate for use.[88] Thus, optimal use of cotherapies ideally should be reserved for those at high risk for NSAID-induced ulcers.

Proton Pump Inhibitors. Use of proton pump inhibitors (PPIs), omeprazole, lansoprazole, rabeprazole, pantoprazole, and esomeprazole magnesium, for prophylaxis against NSAID ulcers has become an attractive strategy for many clinicians. Support for this practice is found in two endoscopic studies demonstrating omeprazole to be more effective than ranitidine (150 mg twice a day[89]) or misoprostol (200 μg twice daily[90]) in prevention of NSAID-induced gastric and duodenal ulcers. However, there are two criticisms of the data on which the recommendation for the use of PPIs for prevention of NSAID-induced ulceration is based. First, the studies cited evaluated the ability of omeprazole to prevent *endoscopic* ulcers; there are no studies evaluating whether a PPI can prevent the *complications* of NSAID-induced ulcers. Second, the superiority of omeprazole demonstrated in the studies was to some extent attributable to the fact that the doses of its comparators (ranitidine and misoprostol) were already known to be less than ideal for prevention of NSAID-induced ulcers.[83, 91] There are no studies comparing a PPI to "high-dose" H_2 RAs or to maximum dose misoprostol for NSAID ulcer prophylaxis.

TREATMENT OF NONSTEROIDAL ANTI-INFLAMMATORY DRUG–INDUCED ULCERS. Treatment of NSAID-induced ulcers is more straightforward than prophylaxis. When attempting to treat an ulcer that has formed during NSAID use, the first step is always to stop the NSAID. Once the NSAID is stopped, rapid ulcer healing can be achieved by treatment with standard doses of H_2 RAs,[89, 92] although PPIs are also effective. When NSAIDs cannot be discontinued, use of a PPI allows ulcer healing, even while NSAID use continues.[92, 93]

Nonsteroidal Anti-inflammatory Drugs with Improved Gastrointestinal Safety Profiles

CYCLOOXGENASE-2 SPECIFIC INHIBITORS. Short-term[94] and long-term[49, 50, 95, 96] endoscopic studies of patients taking COX-2 inhibitors have demonstrated incidences of gastroduodenal endoscopic ulceration of approximately 3% to 5% (rates similar to those of placebo), which compare quite favorably to those of patients using traditional NSAIDs, which have a 20% to 40% incidence of endoscopic gastroduodenal ulcers (Fig. 23–8). However, as has been observed in a number of other NSAID studies endoscopic ulceration is generally asymptomatic and usually does not have untoward clinical consequences. Thus, the more clinically meaningful data are those that report incidences of serious GI adverse events such as ulceration associated with perforation, pain, or bleeding. In a retrospective combined analysis of eight clinical trials of patients with osteoarthritis, treatment with rofecoxib over 1 year was associated with a significantly lower incidence of serious upper GI adverse clinical events than that of treatment with comparator NSAIDs.[97] Similar retrospective observations from pooled analyses of earlier trials have also suggested that celecoxib is associated with a reduction in serious GI adverse events.[98] However, retrospective analyses are subject to biases inherent in post hoc evaluations. Thus, prospective evaluations of the GI safety of COX-2 specific inhibitors were critical in the assessment of these agents as potentially safer NSAIDs.

Prospective clinical trials designed to assess whether COX-2 inhibitors are associated with reductions in upper GI complications were completed in 2000. The acronyms for the celecoxib and rofecoxib outcome studies are *CLASS* (Celecoxib Long-term Arthritis Safety Study[55]) and *VIGOR* (Vioxx Gastrointestinal Outcomes Research[56]) trials. A comparison of the salient features of the designs of each of these outcomes trials is shown in Table 23–5.

Each trial enrolled approximately 8000 patients and was therefore sufficiently large to assess potential differences in rates of GI events between the COX-2 specific inhibitors and comparator, nonspecific NSAIDs. Celecoxib and rofecoxib were studied at doses higher than their indicated doses for osteoarthritis (OA). Thus, the rates of GI events observed in these trials are likely to fall at the higher end of the spectrum of GI toxicity found with usual clinically indicated long-term doses of these agents. The VIGOR trial exclusively enrolled rheumatoid arthritis (RA) patients, whereas the CLASS trial patient enrollment was approximately three-quarters OA and one-quarter RA patients. A very important difference between CLASS and VIGOR trials occurred in the selection of nonspecific NSAID comparators. The comparators in CLASS were diclofenac and ibuprofen; the comparator in VIGOR was naproxen. The reason that this is an

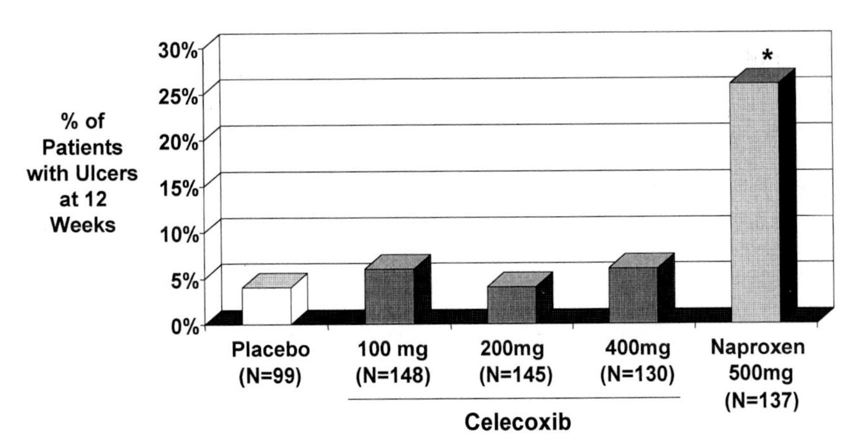

Figure 23–8. Incidence of endoscopic gastroduodenal ulcers with a COX-2 specific inhibitor. Patients with rheumatoid arthritis were treated with celecoxib (100, 200, or 400 mg twice daily), naproxen 500 mg twice daily, or a placebo for 12 weeks. Rates of gastroduodenal ulceration with naproxen were statistically higher (*, $P < .01$) than rates with celecoxib or a placebo. (Data from Simon LS, Weaver AL, Graham DY, et al: Anti-inflammatory and upper gastrointestinal effects of celecoxib in rheumatoid arthritis. JAMA 282:1921–1928, 1999.)

Table 23–5 | **Comparison of Celecoxib Long-Term Arthritis Safety Study and Vioxx Gastrointestinal Outcomes Research Trials**

STUDY DESIGNS		
	CLASS (N = 7968)	**VIGOR (N = 8076)**
Drug	Celecoxib 400 mg bid (4 × OA dose)	Rofecoxib 50 mg qd (2 × typical OA dose)
Patients	OA (72%), RA (28%)	RA
Comparator(s)	Ibuprofen 800 mg tid Diclofenac 75 mg bid	Naproxen 500 mg bid
Low-dose aspirin permitted	Yes (21%)	No
Duration of study	Median 9 months* Maximum 13 months*	Median 9 months Maximum 13 months
Primary end point	Complicated ulcers	Clinical UGI events
Secondary end point	Symptomatic ulcers	Complicated ulcers

*In the published version of the CLASS trial only 6-month data are presented.

CLASS, Celecoxib Long-Term Arthritis Safety Study; OA, osteoarthritis; RA, rheumatoid arthritis; UGI, upper gastrointestinal; VIGOR, Vioxx Gastrointestinal Outcomes Research.

CLASS data from Silverstein FE, Faich G, Goldstein JL, et al: Gastrointestinal toxicity with celecoxib vs. nonsteroidal anti-inflammatory drugs for osteoarthritis and rheumatoid arthritis: The CLASS study: A randomized controlled trial. JAMA 284:1247–1255, 2000; VIGOR data from Bombardier C, Laine L, Reicin A, et al: Rofecoxib and naproxen in patients with rheumatoid arthritis. N Engl J Med 343:1520–1528, 2000.

important difference is that historically naproxen has been associated with greater clinically relevant GI toxicity than ibuprofen or diclofenac (see Table 23–4). Thus, it is possible that some of the observed differences in these trials between the COX-2 NSAIDs and traditional NSAIDs might reflect differences in GI toxicity between the comparator NSAIDs rather than differences in GI safety between COX-2 NSAIDs.

Another important difference between CLASS and VIGOR was a difference in the use of low-dose aspirin (325 mg/day or less). Twenty-one percent of patients enrolled in CLASS were taking low-dose aspirin, whereas none of the patients enrolled in VIGOR was allowed to take low dose aspirin. Because low doses of aspirin are associated with a low, but clinically appreciable rate of GI events (see Fig. 23–7), it is likely that some of the GI events observed in the CLASS trial were attributable to low-dose aspirin. Each of the trials had a median duration of 9 months and maximum enrollments of 13 months. However, in the fully published version of CLASS, data from only the first 6 months of exposure to study drug were reported.[55] The primary end point for analysis in CLASS was complicated ulcers (upper GI bleeding, perforation, or obstruction), and the secondary end point was symptomatic ulceration (complicated ulcers *plus* noncomplicated ulcers with dyspepsia of sufficient severity to require diagnostic evaluation). The primary end point in the VIGOR trial, clinical upper GI events, can be considered to be the same as symptomatic ulceration. The VIGOR trial's secondary end point was complicated ulceration.

Overall, in the CLASS trial, there was no statistically significant difference in the incidence of complicated upper GI events between the celecoxib and NSAID groups (0.76% versus 1.45%, respectively; relative risk [RR] 0.53; 95% confidence interval [CI] 0.26 to 1.11; P = .09). However, there were statistically fewer symptomatic ulcers in the celecoxib than in the NSAID group (2.08% versus 3.54%, respectively; RR 0.59; 95% CI 0.38 to 0.94; P = .02). As 21% of patients in CLASS were taking low-dose aspirin, some of the events in the overall analysis were likely attributable to aspirin's GI toxicity rather than to GI effects of celecoxib, diclofenac, or ibuprofen. In a post hoc analysis of the 79% of patients in CLASS not taking low-dose aspirin, those taking celecoxib had statistically significantly fewer events than the NSAID group (complicated upper gastrointestinal [UGI] events; 0.44% versus 1.27%, respectively; RR 0.35; 95% CI 0.14 to 0.98; P = .04; symptomatic GI events: 1.4% versus 2.91%, respectively; RR 0.48; 95% CI 0.28 to 0.89; P = .02). However, in the 21% of patients taking low-dose aspirin along with celecoxib or with traditional NSAID comparators, there were no significant differences in either complicated UGI or symptomatic ulcers between celecoxib and traditional NSAID groups (complicated UGI, 6 events in both groups, P = .92; symptomatic ulcers, 14 events in the celecoxib versus 17 in the NSAID group, P = .49). Of note, in the CLASS trial the use of low-dose aspirin, combined with a nonselective NSAID (ibuprofen or diclofenac), did not significantly increase rates of GI ulcer

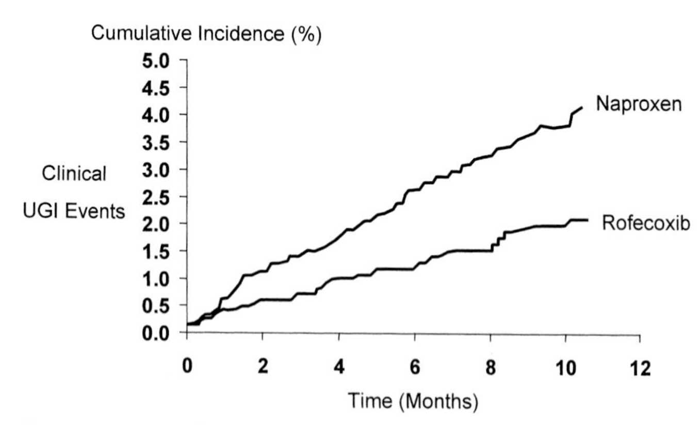

Figure 23–9. Incidence of clinical upper gastrointestinal (GI) events in an outcomes trial of patients with rheumatoid arthritis treated with a COX-2 inhibitor (rofecoxib) or naproxen. Clinical upper GI events are classified as episodes of upper GI bleeding, perforations, obstruction, and symptomatic ulceration. The relative risk for upper GI events with rofecoxib is 0.46 compared with that of naproxen (95% CI [0.33–0.64]); $P < .001$. (Data from Bombardier C, Peloso PMJ, Goldsmith CH: Salsalate-Diclofenac Study Group: Salsalate, a nonacetylated salicylate, is as efficacious as diclofenac in patients with rheumatoid arthritis. J Rheumatol 22:617–624, 1995.)

complications over those of patients receiving nonselective NSAIDs (ibuprofen or diclofenac) alone.

In the VIGOR trial, the number of confirmed upper GI events was 2.1% in the rofecoxib group and 4.5% in the naproxen group (RR 0.46; 95% CI 0.3 to 0.6; $P < .001$) (Fig. 23–9). The rate of confirmed complicated events was 0.6% with rofecoxib and 1.4% with naproxen (RR 0.4; 95% CI 0.2 to 0.8; $P = .0005$); as a result, both end points occurred significantly less often in the groups receiving rofecoxib compared to naproxen.

During the VIGOR trial, an unexpected higher rate of myocardial infarction (MI) was observed with rofecoxib than with naproxen (0.4 versus 0.1, RR 0.2; 95% CI 0.1 to 0.6). Study investigators attribute the lower risk of MI in the naproxen group to naproxen's ability to inhibit the platelet production of thromboxane (COX-1 effect [see Fig. 23–4]) and to inhibit platelet aggregation, and to maintain these effects throughout its dosing interval. Over the entire 13-month experience of the CLASS trial, rates of MI with celecoxib (0.5%) were actually higher than rates of MI with rofecoxib in the 13-month experience of the VIGOR trial (0.4%). However, rates of MI with NSAID comparators in CLASS (diclofenac and ibuprofen) were only 0.3%, a non–statistically significant difference when compared with celecoxib's rates.

Some important conclusions are derived from the CLASS and VIGOR trials. Although data are limited, it appears that the use of low-dose aspirin may reduce or eliminate any GI protective benefit of the COX-2 inhibitors. Therefore, at present, few data support the argument that patients on aspirin at any dose achieve greater GI protective benefit from the COX-2 inhibitors when compared with patients on nonselective NSAIDs. Furthermore, although rofecoxib (and possibly celecoxib) is associated with the benefit of reduced GI toxicity, when considering global (total body) safety, increased adverse events in other systems (i.e., cardiovascular events) may reduce or eliminate overall benefits of these agents compared to traditional NSAIDs, particularly in older patients who may be at risk for cardiovascular disease.

The findings of the endoscopic and outcome trials described support the contention that COX-2 specific inhibitors have better GI safety profiles than traditional NSAIDs. However, in some GI diseases (e.g., peptic ulcer that is attempting to heal) the effects of COX-2 specific inhibitors may be no better than those of traditional NSAIDs. Traditional NSAIDs delay ulcer healing; administration of specific COX-2 inhibitors to animals with experimentally induced gastric ulcers also delays ulcer healing.[99, 100] As gastric ulcers heal and repair, COX-2 messenger ribonucleic acid (mRNA) ulcer concentrations are elevated (Fig. 23–10).[101] This observation provides a mechanistic explanation for the impairment of ulcer healing that occurs with COX-2 specific NSAIDs as well as NSAIDs that inhibit both the COX-1 and -2 isoforms (traditional NSAIDs).

OLDER, SAFER NONSTEROIDAL ANTI-INFLAMMATORY DRUGS. In addition to the recently marketed COX-2 NSAIDs, several other established NSAIDs or products in development have safety profiles that indicate a documented or a potential safety advantage when compared to the NSAID class. Among the older NSAIDs, those that are clinically associated with safer GI profiles are etodolac, nabumetone, and

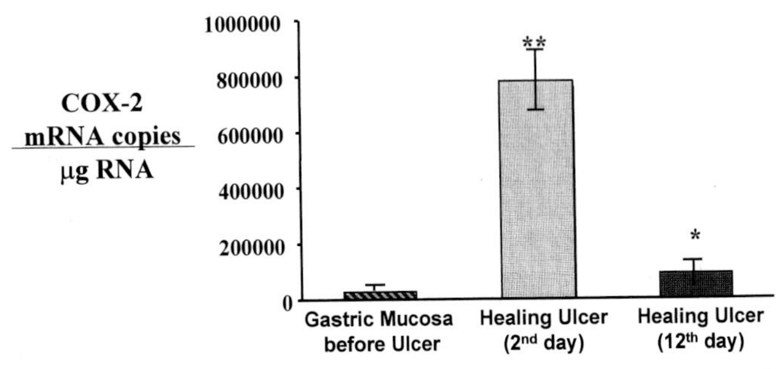

Figure 23–10. COX-2 expression in normal gastric mucosa and in healing ulcers. In rats with experimentally induced gastric ulcers, COX-2 messenger RNA expression is demonstrated before acute ulceration and during days 2 and 12 of ulcer healing. Rats express significantly higher COX-2 in day 2 ulcers than in day 12 ulcers or nonulcerated gastric mucosa. (Data from Vogiagis D, Glare EM, Misajon A, et al: Cyclooxygenase-1 and an alternatively spliced mRNA in the rat stomach: Effects of aging and ulcers. Am J Physiol 278:G820–G827, 2000.)

nonacetylated salicylates such as salsalate.[102–104] Salsalate[105] and etodolac[102, 106] have no measurable effects on gastric COX activity, and in vitro assays demonstrate that nabumetone has a moderate degree of COX-2 selectivity.[25] One possible mechanistic explanation for nabumetone's clinical GI safety profile is that in animal cell lines nabumetone selectively inhibits COX-2 while having much less of an effect on COX-1 expression.[107] However, clinically nabumetone is administered as a prodrug and its active COX inhibiting metabolite, 6-methoxy-napthyl-acetic acid (6-MNA), is a potent inhibitor of COX-1 and COX-2.[106] Thus, possible alternative explanations for nabumetone's improved safety profile may relate to its being administered as a nonacidic prodrug that has much lower gastric solubility and no enterohepatic recirculation, as do other more acidic NSAIDs.[108, 109]

Recent clinical trials have revealed that diclofenac, one of the older nonselective NSAIDs, is associated with a moderately low risk of GI ulceration. Diclofenac had rates of GI ulceration similar to those of celecoxib in a 3-month endoscopic trial[110] and in another 6-month large-scale outcomes study.[55] Although these data suggest a favorable safety profile for diclofenac, its GI risk would be best classified as low to moderate and probably not as low as that associated with nabumetone, etodoloc, and salsalate. The combination product of diclofenac sodium/misoprostol (Arthrotec) is another therapy that within one tablet combines the prophylactic component of misoprostol with an NSAID. A 1998 randomized, prospective trial of arthritis patients found that diclofenac sodium/misoprostol was associated with a lower 6-week incidence of endoscopic gastroduodenal ulcers than nabumetone.[85]

NITRIC OXIDE–RELEASING NONSTEROIDAL ANTI-INFLAMMATORY DRUGS. After conventional NSAIDs are administered, levels of mucosal prostaglandins are reduced, and, consequently, GI blood flow is lowered, a process that appears to occur because of an NSAID-induced adherence of neutrophils to vascular endothelium. Nitric oxide is now recognized as a critical mediator of GI mucosal defense, exerting many of the same actions as prostaglandins within the GI tract. In addition to other properties, nitric oxide increases mucosal blood flow and prevents neutrophil adher-

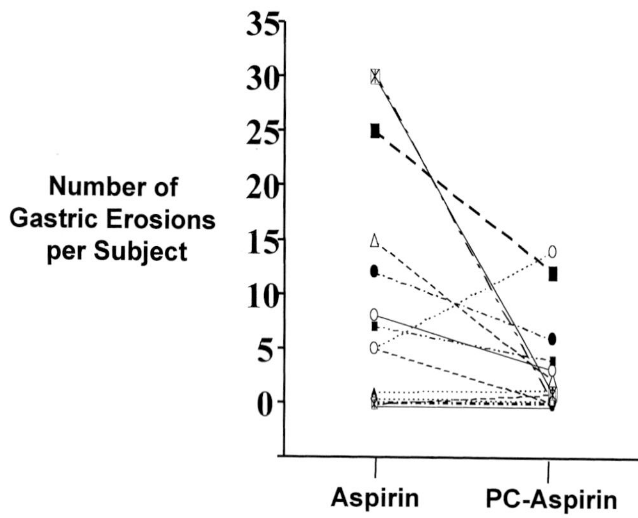

Figure 23–11. Effect of phosphatidyl choline coupled with aspirin (PC-aspirin) on gastric injury in humans. In 16 healthy humans, gastric injury after a 4-day course of aspirin (650 mg three times a day) was significantly increased compared with gastric injury after another 4-day course of an equivalent amount of PC-aspirin. (Adapted from data presented in Anand BS, Romero JJ, Sanduja SK, Lichtenberger LM: Phospholipid association reduces the gastric mucosal toxicity of aspirin in human subjects. Am J Gastroenterol 94:1818–1822, 1999.)

ence to vascular endothelium.[111] These observations have led to the development of nitric oxide (NO) releasing NSAIDs in which the native NSAID has been coupled to a nitric oxide releasing moiety. The concept is that a vasodilating component is delivered, by virtue of its attachment to the NSAID, directly to the GI mucosal location that would be potentially damaged by the NSAID component. NO-NSAIDs have been synthesized by using diclofenac, indomethacin, naproxen, flurbiprofen, and aspirin and have been demonstrated to have anti-inflammatory, antipyretic, analgesic, and antithrombotic effects comparable with those of native NSAIDs.[111, 112] However, NO-NSAIDs do not exhibit the NSAID-induced gastric[111, 112] or intestinal[113] toxicity associated with the parent compounds. Interestingly, NO-NSAIDs inhibit both COX-1 and COX-2 and reduce levels of GI prostaglandins to the same extent as native NSAIDs. However, despite the marked prostaglandin reductions achieved with NO-NSAIDs, their use is not associated with the GI toxicity seen with the parent compounds.

NO-NSAIDs have unfortunately been studied only in animal models. There are no published reports of human studies on the effects of NO-NSAIDs on the GI tract. The animal data, however, are very attractive and suggest the potential for these to be a safer class of NSAIDs that may be clinically available in the future.

PHOSPHOLIPID NONSTEROIDAL ANTI-INFLAMMATORY DRUGS. The gastric mucosa has a hydrophobic, lipid surface, mainly caused by secretion of a surfactant-like phospholipid into the gastric mucus gel layer. Gastric surface layer phospholipid content is enriched by gastroprotective agents, such as prostaglandins, and is rapidly attenuated by NSAIDs. NSAIDs reduce surface hydrophobicity by chemically associating with and destabilizing phospholipids within the mucus gel layer, in particular phosphatidylcholine.[8] Recently newer NSAIDs have been developed in which the native NSAID moiety has been coupled with synthetic phosphatidylcholine (PC). Animal studies using PC-NSAIDs indicate that these agents, when compared with the parent NSAID compounds, are associated with a reduction in GI ulceration and with faster ulcer healing in the context of continued NSAID exposure and have therapeutic activity equivalent to or better than that of the native NSAIDs.[8, 114, 115] Human studies from 1999 indicate that short-term courses of PC-aspirin are associated with reduction in acute gastric erosive injury when compared with plain aspirin courses (Fig. 23–11).[116] If subsequent clinical studies show continued safety and efficacy of this class of NSAIDs, PC-NSAIDs may be another future class of safer NSAIDs available to clinicians.

Small Intestine

The variety and magnitude of clinical consequences of NSAID use within the small intestine have, until recently, been underappreciated because the small intestine has traditionally been relatively inaccessible for investigation. For purposes of this discussion, references to the small intestine relate primarily to the jejunum and ileum.

Ulcers

It is quite common for patients to have acute or chronic GI bleeding while taking NSAIDs, yet to demonstrate no endoscopically identifiable bleeding source in the stomach, duodenum, or colon. Although the small intestine is clinically suspected as the site of blood loss, this suspicion is usually not confirmed by diagnostic studies. Endoscopic studies of the small intestine have been historically difficult because enteroscopes that allow a reasonable examination of the small intestine have, up until very recently, not been available. Radiologic studies of the small intestine have not been of great diagnostic assistance as these examinations have low sensitivity for small lesion detection.

There have been very few prospective studies evaluating the association of NSAIDs and small intestinal ulceration. One endoscopic study assessed the small intestine of rheumatoid arthritis patients who were taking NSAIDs long term and who had evidence of chronic GI blood loss. There was a 26% prevalence of small intestinal ulcers in these patients.[117] The major problem with this study, however, was that the type of endoscope used has poor sensitivity for intestinal mucosal visualization. It views about one third of the circumference of the intestinal lumen, allows very brief inspection of any particular intestinal area, and is not able to return to a suspected area for closer inspection. Newer-generation enteroscopes have since been introduced that have a more extensive field of vision and allow controlled small intestinal mucosal inspection of patients with intestinal blood loss of uncertain origin.

In addition to GI bleeding, the other life-threatening small intestinal consequence of NSAIDs is perforation. Most evidence that NSAIDs cause small intestinal perforation is from a case control study[118] and several case reports.[119–121] In a retrospective study of infants born with a patent ductus arteriosus (PDA) who were treated with indomethacin (as a prostaglandin inhibitor) or by surgical ligation of the PDA, in 10% of indomethacin-treated infants intestinal perforation developed whereas none of the surgically treated infants experienced perforations.[122] In adults, there have been a number of reports of small intestinal perforation with slow-release NSAID preparations.[119, 121] These reports suggest that a major consequence of delaying GI dissolution of an NSAID is to move the site of injury from the stomach and duodenum to more distal sites in the intestine.

More conclusive evidence for an association between NSAIDs and small intestinal ulcers was provided by an autopsy study that compared rates of ulceration in patients who had been taking NSAIDs prior to death to rates in a control group of patients who had not taken NSAIDs ante mortem.[123] This autopsy evaluation of the small intestines of NSAID users revealed small intestinal ulcers in 8.4% of the NSAID group and in only 0.6% of the control group ($P < .001$), the strongest data available to suggest NSAIDs as a cause of small intestinal ulceration. In the same autopsy study, gastric and duodenal ulcers were seen in 22% and 12%, respectively, of NSAID users.[123] However, there was no correlation between ulcers in the stomach or duodenum and ulcers in the small intestine. These data suggest that one cannot predict the absence or presence of small intestinal ulcers on the basis of endoscopic assessment of the upper GI tract. Of particular interest in this study, 25% of the NSAID users had been taking a single dose of aspirin of 300 mg per day or less. Three patients, all of whom were taking NSAIDs, died of intestinal perforation; the intestinal perforation rate related to NSAIDs was 1%.

The mechanisms for NSAID-induced small intestinal perforation are the same as those in the stomach and duodenum, that is, a local mucosal toxic effect and prostaglandin inhibition. The higher than expected rate of intestinal perforation with slow-release NSAID preparations suggests a role for a local effect.[119, 124] However, the observation that depletion of mucosal prostaglandins by immunization with antibodies directed toward prostaglandins will cause intestinal perforation in animals,[125] argues in favor of prostaglandin inhibition as the principal mechanism.

Strictures

Similarly to the effects of NSAIDs in the esophagus, NSAID use can result in strictures of the small intestine (and colon).[126–129] However, there are some unique pathologic aspects to the small intestinal strictures. Their pathologic configurations range from nonspecific broad-based strictures to intestinal diaphragms.[75–78] These diaphragms are usually multiple, thin (2 to 4 mm), concentric weblike septa, which may narrow the lumen down to the size of a pinhole (Fig. 23–12). The intestinal lumen may become so constricted that symptoms of small intestinal obstruction develop. These diaphragms are usually located in the jejunum. Their histologic appearance reveals submucosal fibrosis with normal overlying epithelium, except for the central tip of the diaphragm, which contains acute and chronic inflammatory cells. Because these intestinal diaphragms have not been associated with conditions other than use of NSAIDs, their occurrence is now thought to be pathognomonic of such use.[126] The prevalence of these diaphragms is rather low; in a retrospective review of surgically resected small intestinal specimens, diaphragms were detected in 1.5% and NSAIDs were associated with each case.[130]

Small intestinal diaphragms are particularly difficult to diagnose because no conventional diagnostic procedure is very helpful. During barium studies the strictures may mimic exaggerated plicae circulares (see Fig. 23–12). Because the diaphragms do not distort the intestinal wall, at laparotomy they are not apparent on visual inspection. During surgery it may be necessary to palpate the intestinal wall to detect the diaphragms. If the small intestine is inflated with air, they can be more easily detected.

Enteropathy

In addition to structural lesions such as ulcers, strictures, and diaphragms, NSAIDs can cause a clinical entity of diffuse intestinal inflammation and increased intestinal mucosal permeability. This so-called NSAID enteropathy may be characterized clinically by occult blood loss, iron deficiency anemia, nutrient malabsorption, and a protein losing enteropathy[126, 131–133] (Table 23–6). Of these manifestations, the blood loss is the most clinically significant. Many patients who chronically take NSAIDs have positive occult blood test result (Hemoccult-positive) stools and iron deficiency anemia and have no endoscopically identifiable source in the upper

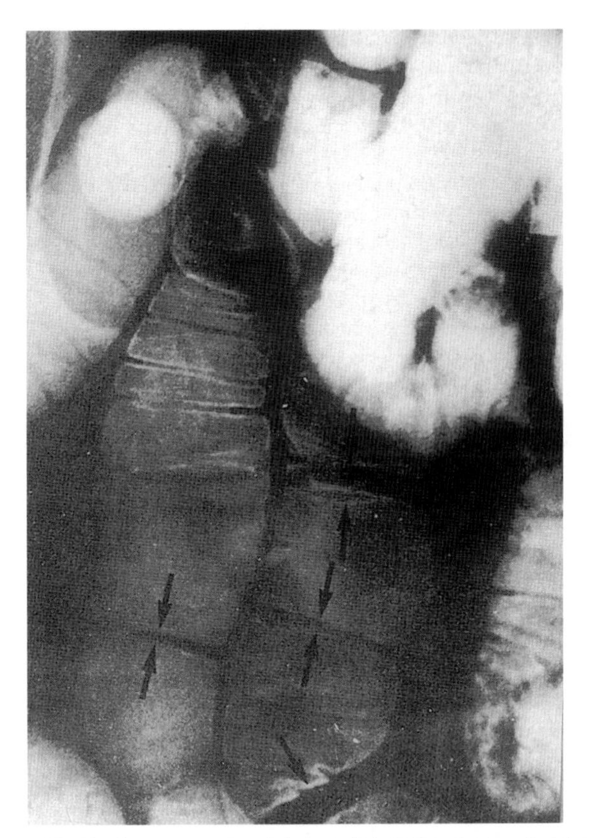

Figure 23–12. Contrast study of the small intestine (enteroclysis) in a patient on nonsteroidal anti-inflammatory drugs (NSAIDs) who at the time of surgery was found to have "diaphragm-like" intestinal strictures. The strictures (between the *arrows*) are difficult to appreciate and resemble exaggerated plica circularis. (From Bjarnason I, Hayllar J, Macpherson AJ, Russell AS: Side effects of nonsteroidal anti-inflammatory drugs on the small and large intestine in humans. Gastroenterology 104:1832–1847, 1993.)

Table 23–6 | **Nonsteroidal Anti-inflammatory Drug Enteropathy**

ABNORMALITY	CLINICAL IMPLICATION
Chronic blood loss	May contribute to iron deficiency anemia
Protein loss	May cause hypoalbuminemia
Ileal dysfunction	Asymptomatic, not clinically relevant
D-Xylose malabsorption	Mild; not clinically relevant
Steatorrhea	Mild; not clinically relevant

Adapted from Bjarnason I, Hayllar J, Macpherson AJ, Russell AS: Side effects of nonsteroidal anti-inflammatory drugs on the small and large intestine in humans. Gastroenterology 104:1832–1847, 1993.

GI tract or colon that adequately explains the bleeding.[134, 135] After blood loss, protein loss is the second most common clinical manifestation of NSAID enteropathy. Intestinal protein loss is usually mild and usually does not lead to major clinical problems. However, occasional patients with NSAID enteropathy have reported serum albumin concentrations as low as 1.7 mg/dL.[131] Ileal dysfunction may also occur but is usually asymptomatic and not clinically relevant.[133] Occasionally, diarrhea secondary to fat or bile salt malabsorption may be experienced. Laboratory detection of vitamin B_{12} deficiency is common in rheumatoid arthritis patients,[136] but clinical manifestations of B_{12} deficiency in this population are rare. D-Xylose (carbohydrate) malabsorption and fat malabsorption are also mild and usually not clinically relevant. Taking all of these various manifestations into account, it is estimated that up to 70% of patients taking NSAIDs have some component of NSAID enteropathy,[126, 131, 132] although most of these disorders are mild and are not clinically apparent.

The pathophysiologic components of NSAID enteropathy are increased intestinal permeability and intestinal inflammation. The precise mechanisms through which NSAIDs lead to these changes are uncertain. One hypothesis is that NSAIDs lead to a disruption of the small intestinal mucosal barrier that increases intestinal permeability to a variety of agents, including bacteria within the intestinal lumen.[113] Mucosal bacterial invasion induces diffuse intestinal inflammation that when combined with increased intestinal permeability may lead to the malabsorption syndrome of NSAID enteropathy.

Techniques involving radionuclide and permeability probes have been used to examine small intestinal inflammation and permeability, respectively, in patients taking NSAIDS. Each of these pathologic processes and techniques is described in more detail in the following sections.

PERMEABILITY. Intestinal permeability is assessed experimentally by measurement of urinary recovery of orally administered test probes. In the normal, intact small intestine, these test probes cannot pass from the intestinal lumen to the bloodstream. When intestinal mucosal integrity is interrupted, as with inflammation or use of NSAIDs, the probes are able to traverse the intestinal wall and appear in the systemic circulation and are excreted by the kidneys. Most studies assessing the effects of NSAIDs on small intestinal permeability have used chromium-labeled ^{51r}ethylendiaminetetraacetic acid (^{51r}EDTA).[137, 138] In arthritis patients and normal volunteers, NSAID administration results in increased urinary appearance of ^{51r}EDTA.[138] These changes are usually apparent within 12 hours of NSAID administration.[137] After cessation of NSAID therapy, intestinal permeability usually reverts to normal within 4 days.[138]

INFLAMMATION. A significant increase in intestinal inflammatory cell infiltrate occurs within 3 hours of NSAID administration.[139] Unfortunately, this assessment usually requires biopsy and histologic evaluation. A noninvasive method to assess intestinal inflammation involves intravenous injection of neutrophils labeled with indium 111 (^{111}In) followed by abdominal imaging by scintigraphy. These labeled neutrophils localize to areas of active inflammation, thus providing a means to assess the intestinal effects of NSAIDs. Approximately 50% of patients on chronic NSAID therapy have ^{111}In-labeled leukocyte scintigraphy, which demonstrates increased inflammation in an intestinal location.[126] Furthermore, over the 4 days that follow ^{111}In administration, these patients have increased ^{111}In fecal excretion. Fecal excretion of ^{111}In is quantitative and is a sensitive index of inflammation throughout the GI tract. Most patients on NSAIDs have increased ^{111}In fecal excretion.[126] Patients not treated with NSAIDs have normal ^{111}In excretion values.

Therapy

There are no therapies that have been clearly documented as effective treatments for NSAID-induced intestinal ulcers or strictures or NSAID enteropathy. Small intestinal perforation is treated surgically. Likewise, bowel obstruction secondary to NSAID-induced strictures or diaphragms may require surgery. NSAID enteropathy is usually not clinically apparent and, therefore, usually requires no therapeutic intervention. When chronic intestinal blood or protein loss produces clinical manifestations, cessation of NSAID therapy should prove therapeutic. A small retrospective study has suggested that concomitant misoprostol administration may improve anemia in NSAID enteropathy.[140] If protein malabsorption is a problem, a change of NSAID therapy to nabumetone may improve mucosal permeability[138] and consequently reduce protein loss. Coadministration of metronidazole may also reduce NSAID-induced permeability changes.[128] Improvement in NSAID-induced permeability with metronidazole may be related to its antibacterial effects; such a relationship supports the theory that increased permeability to intestinal bacteria may contribute to the pathogenesis of NSAID-induced intestinal inflammation.

Colon

As in the small intestine, most of the effects of NSAIDs in the colon are asymptomatic. A convenient way to categorize these effects is to segregate findings that occur in individuals with no prior history of colonic disease from those in which NSAIDs exacerbate preexisting colonic disorders.

Effects in Subjects with No Preexisting Colonic Disease

As in the small intestine, NSAID-induced ulceration, strictures, and diaphragms occur in the colon. In the colon,

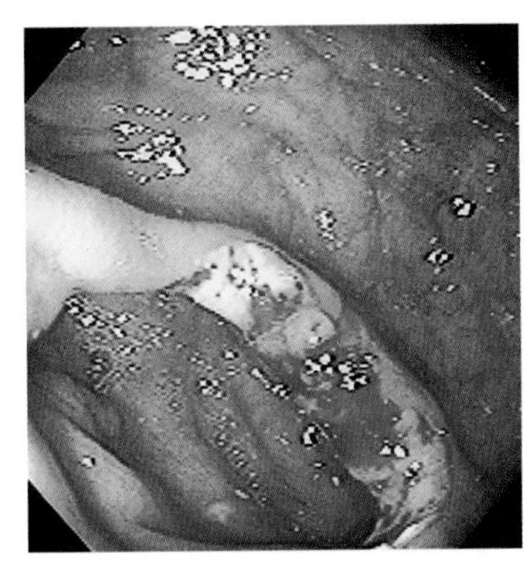

Figure 23–13. Endoscopic view of cecum showing a cecal ulcer associated with use of diclofenac (Voltaren). The patient presented with acute lower gastrointestinal bleeding. (Courtesy of Barry Sanders, MD.)

however, there are fewer reported cases. In animals with antibody-induced prostaglandin depletion far fewer ulcers develop in the colon than in the stomach or small intestine,[25] suggesting that the colon may be less vulnerable to injury. Lack of topical exposure of the colon to NSAIDs as a consequence of more proximal absorption of NSAIDs in the small intestine may also contribute to the lower toxicity.

ULCERS (Fig. 23–13). Colonic ulceration associated with NSAIDs has been reported in the cecum and transverse and sigmoid colon; the right side of the colon (especially the cecum) is the most common site of ulceration.[141–146] Ulcer histologic examination reveals nonspecific changes. All classes of NSAIDs have caused colonic ulceration, including aspirin at a dose of 325 mg/day.[143] However, diclofenac, sustained-release NSAID preparations, and NSAIDs delivered via suppositories tend to be more commonly associated with this problem. Ulceration may be complicated by bleeding[141, 144, 146] and perforation, especially in the cecum.[146] It is difficult to demonstrate a cause-and-effect relationship between NSAIDs and colonic ulceration because almost all information is obtained from case reports. However, a role for NSAIDs in colonic perforation and bleeding is supported by epidemiologic observations that patients with these complications are more than twice as likely as control subjects to have taken NSAIDs.[147] The pathogenesis of colonic ulceration induced by NSAIDs is unclear. However, it is suspected that ulceration may be the result of an inflammatory response to intraluminal NSAIDs that cause an increase in mucosal permeability.[146]

STRICTURES. Diaphragm-like strictures and broad-based strictures have also been described, again with a predilection for the cecum and right colon (see Fig. 23–13). These lesions macroscopically and microscopically resemble those in the small intestine. It has been suggested that the diaphragm-like lesions may represent a specialized mucosal response peculiar to the small and large intestine.[148] After discontinuation of NSAIDs, resolution of diaphragm-like strictures has been reported.[146]

COLITIS. NSAIDs can induce a variety of types of colitis. Cases of eosinophilic,[149] collagenous,[150] pseudomembranous,[151] and nonspecific colitis[152, 153] have been associated with NSAIDs. A disproportionately high number of cases of colitis have occurred in patients who were using mefenamic acid and flufenamic acid.[149, 152, 153] The usual symptom is watery diarrhea, which, on occasion, may be bloody. Significant weight loss may also occur. Findings of colonoscopy are usually normal, although there may be diffuse ulcerations that may mimic inflammatory bowel disease. The extent of ulceration may range from proctitis to pancolitis. Histologic examination usually reveals a nonspecific mild colitis unless one of the other variants (eosinophilic, pseudomembranous, or collagenous) is present. Because of the nonspecific histologic findings, variable presentation, and segmental distribution of NSAID-induced colitis, initial differentiation between this entity and Crohn's disease may be difficult.

ANORECTAL DISEASE. Rectal administration of NSAIDs in the form of suppositories has frequently been associated with inflammation, ulcers, and strictures of the anus and rectum.[13, 107, 146, 154, 155] Patients may complain of proctalgia, tenesmus, or watery diarrhea.[13] Bloody and mucoid stools and fecal incontinence have also been described.[155] Approximately 10% to 30% of patients receiving NSAID suppositories report a significant side effect.[146]

Effects in Subjects with Preexisting Colonic Disease

DIVERTICULAR DISEASE. (See Chapter 108.) There are individual case reports suggesting NSAIDs as the cause of colonic diverticular perforation.[118, 156] Many cases involved a sustained-release preparation of indomethacin, in which instances the perforations were attributed to a mechanical effect of the capsule's being caught in a diverticulum. In one prospective study and in another case control study, patients admitted with complications of diverticular disease had significantly greater NSAID consumption than controls.[157, 158] Overall, these studies suggest that there is a reasonable possibility that serious complications of diverticular disease may be associated with NSAIDs.

INFLAMMATORY BOWEL DISEASE. (See Chapters 103 and 104.) Not only can NSAIDs induce disease that mimics inflammatory bowel disease (IBD), they may also activate IBD that has been previously quiescent. This occurrence is more frequently observed in ulcerative colitis than in Crohn's disease. Postulated mechanisms through which NSAIDs may exacerbate colonic inflammation are inhibition of cyclooxygenase and shunting of arachidonic acid metabolism toward the proinflammatory leukotrienes. Of all patients with IBD, only a subset experience symptomatic flares when placed on an NSAID. When these patients experience relapse, they do so within a few days of receiving an NSAID.[159]

Arthritis symptoms are common extraintestinal problems in IBD patients, and several of these patients require anti-inflammatory agents to control their symptoms. Since the introduction of the COX-2 specific inhibitors, a common clinical question has been whether these newer NSAIDs would be associated with fewer intestinal problems in IBD patients than those reported with the older NSAIDs. Unfortunately there are no human data that address this question because patients with known IBD have been excluded from clinical trials of COX-2 specific inhibitors. In animal studies, however, experimental administration of a COX-2 inhibitor to mice with experimentally induced colitis results in exacerbation of the colitis as well as intestinal perforations.[160]

Therapy

All of the colonic diseases associated with NSAIDs, preexisting and de novo, should exhibit improvement with NSAID discontinuation. There is no specific treatment for colonic ulcers. They usually have significantly healed by 3 weeks after NSAID discontinuation.[141] Endoscopic balloon dilation of colonic strictures has been suggested for symptomatic patients.[148] This therapy offers an attractive alternative for those who would otherwise proceed to surgery. With use of NSAID suppositories, anorectal stenoses that occurred were sufficiently severe to warrant serial rectal dilations. Despite these treatments, in a few patients bowel obstructions requiring proctocolectomy developed.[155]

Nonsteroidal Anti-inflammatory Drug–Induced Liver Injury (see also Chapter 73)

Compared with other classes of drugs, NSAIDs have a relatively low incidence of hepatotoxicity. The prevalence of mild serum liver enzyme elevations associated with NSAID use is 1% to 15%; the effect is condidered a class effect of these agents.[3, 161] Most of these elevations are asymptomatic and without clinical symptoms, and the prevalence of clinically apparent NSAID effects is lower than the incidence of serum enzyme elevation. However, a recently introduced NSAID, bromfenac sodium (Duract), has been associated with significant hepatotoxicity. Bromfenac was a phenylacetic acid derived NSAID introduced in the United States in 1997 and withdrawn from clinical use in 1998 because of several reports of drug-induced liver injury and even fulminant hepatic failure.[162]

As most of the information regarding clinical untoward effects of NSAIDs is in the form of case reports, the true incidence of clinically significant effects is uncertain. Because use of NSAIDs is extensive, however, the relatively low incidence of clinically apparent hepatotoxicity translates into large numbers of reported cases of hepatotoxicity associated with NSAIDs. The mechanism through which almost all NSAIDs produce liver injury is an idiosyncratic reaction rather than intrinsic toxicity of the agent.[161, 163] Aspirin is an exception in that its injury appears to be dose related and reflects an intrinsic hepatotoxicity.[163] Most NSAIDs produce a hepatocellular pattern of injury, with a cholestatic or mixed pattern seen only with a minority of agents.[164] Among the various NSAIDs, diclofenac has been one of the more commonly associated with this problem.[164, 165]

Nonsteroidal Anti-inflammatory Drug–Induced Pancreatitis

Given the numerous patients who take NSAIDs, NSAID-induced pancreatitis appears to be relatively uncommon. Although there have been occasional case reports relating episodes of pancreatitis to NSAIDs, very few of these cases have met the diagnostic criteria as definite causes for pancreatitis. Criteria that should be met to prove that a drug definitely causes pancreatitis include: (1) pancreatitis that develops during treatment with the drug, (2) lack of other likely causes of pancreatitis, (3) pancreatitis that resolves with discontinuation of the drug, and (4) pancreatitis that recurs with rechallenge with the drug.[166] Sulindac is the only NSAID that has met these criteria and can, therefore, definitely be associated with pancreatitis. A number of reported cases of sulindac-associated pancreatitis recur with rechallenge.[167] Sulindac associated pancreatitis usually occurs within a few weeks or months of starting therapy; however, in one case, it occurred 5 years after use of sulindac.[167] Case reports of pancreatitis associated with NSAIDs other than sulindac are rare. Indomethacin, mefenamic acid, oxyphenbutazone, ketoprofen, and piroxicam have each been reported once to be associated with pancreatitis.[167] None of these, however, has met diagnostic criteria as the definite cause of drug-induced pancreatitis.

THERAPEUTIC EFFECTS OF NONSTEROIDAL ANTI-INFLAMMATORY DRUGS

COLORECTAL CANCER AND ADENOMATOUS POLYPS. The discussion thus far has focused on the untoward GI effects of NSAIDs. In recent years, however, chronic NSAID use has been associated with some beneficial therapeutic effects in the colon, specifically reduction of colorectal cancer[168–177] and reduction of colorectal adenomatous polyps.[168, 170, 178–182] Because these subjects are discussed in Chapters 114 and 115, only the salient features of these associations are reviewed here.

In epidemiologic studies of individuals taking long-term low doses of aspirin, there have been significant reductions in the relative risks of colorectal cancer in men[171] and women[172] when compared to risks in subjects not taking aspirin (Fig. 23–14). This relationship of a lower risk of colorectal cancer has also been observed with nonaspirin NSAIDs, although the strength of this association is less strong than that of aspirin.[173, 175, 176] Interestingly, colorectal cancer risk appears to be inversely related to aspirin dose; maximal risk reduction was observed at an aspirin dose of at least four to six tablets per week.[169]

One criticism of studies demonstrating a reduction in colorectal cancer risk in aspirin users is that the apparent benefit of decreased mortality rate attributed to aspirin may actually not have been a consequence of a therapeutic aspirin effect but, instead, due to a detection bias of increased or earlier endoscopic surveillance of long-term NSAID users in whom symptoms (i.e., GI blood loss or dyspepsia) developed. This criticism, however, has been allayed by a carefully controlled cohort study of male health professionals taking long-term aspirin. In this study, when investigators adjusted for potentially confounding factors such as screening behavior, continued strong associations between aspirin use and reduced number of colorectal adenomas and adenocarcinomas were maintained.[168]

In familial adenomatous polyposis (FAP), long-term NSAID use results in significant reductions in numbers and sizes of adenomatous polyps.[178, 182] Several of the reductions in familial adenomatous polyps have been observed for the

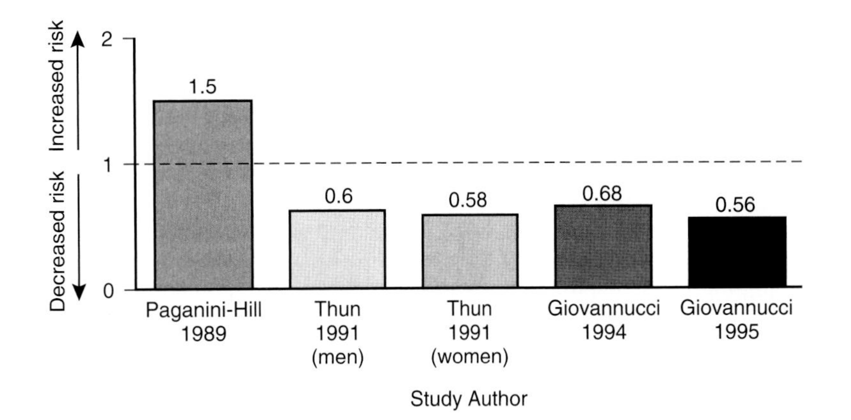

Figure 23–14. Relative risks of colorectal cancer in several studies of patients taking low doses of aspirin for vascular prophylaxis. The relative risk for colorectal cancer in users of low-dose aspirin was reduced compared with non-aspirin users in all but one comparison.

NSAID sulindac.[178, 181, 183, 184] It has been speculated that sulindac sulfide, a prodrug that is metabolized by colonic bacteria to its active metabolite sulindac sulfone, might have high concentrations of this metabolite within the colon. This would explain why this NSAID, in comparison to others, would have particularly high colonic efficacy. Although sulindac causes adenomatous polyp regression in FAP, patients generally do not have complete polyp resolution and polyps usually recur after NSAID cessation.[183, 184] In a 2000 trial of patients with FAP, a 6-month course of the COX-2 selective agent celecoxib resulted in dose-related reductions in colorectal and small intestinal adenomatous polyps (Fig. 23–15).[182] However, as with sulindac, celecoxib associated polyp regression is only partial. Because the effect of NSAIDs on polyp regression is incomplete, NSAIDs are not recommended as the sole alternative treatment to colectomy for prevention of colorectal adenocarcinoma in FAP.

Sporadic (nonhereditary) colonic adenomatous polyps (90% of all adenomatous polyps) are much more common than hereditary adenomatous polyposis syndromes such as FAP. Thus, a more clinically applicable question is whether

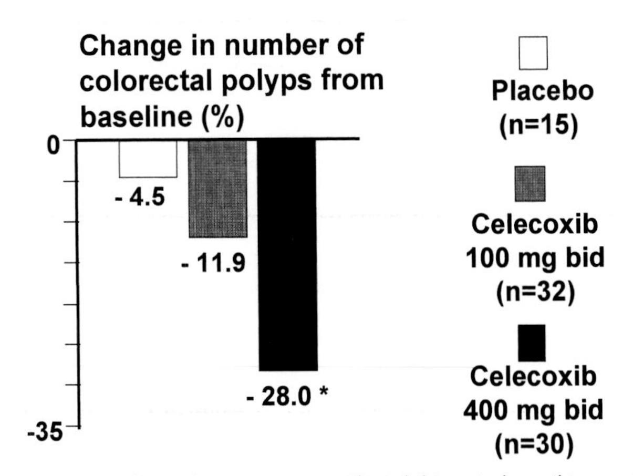

Figure 23–15. Effect of a COX-2–specific inhibitor (celecoxib) on adenomatous polyps in patients with familial adenomatous polyposis (FAP). Effects of placebo or celecoxib (100 mg twice daily) or celecoxib (400 mg twice daily) taken for 6 months on the number of polyps in patients with FAP are shown. *, Statistically significant difference of the higher dose of celecoxib versus the placebo. In the same study, celecoxib 400 mg twice a day also significantly reduced polyp size (data not shown here). (Adapted from Steinbach G, Lynch PM, Phillips RKS, et al: The effect of celecoxib, a cyclooxygenase-2 inhibitor, in familial adenomatous polyposis. N Engl J Med 342:1946–1952, 2000.)

long-term NSAID use is beneficial in individuals with sporadic colon adenomas. The answer depends on whether the intent of NSAID use is primary or secondary prevention. In case control and cohort studies of individuals taking NSAIDs long-term, there have been lower than expected prevalences of sporadic colonic adenomas in subjects taking regular doses of aspirin[168, 170, 179, 180] or nonaspirin NSAIDs.[180] This finding implies that aspirin or other NSAIDs when used for primary prevention may reduce the incidence of, but not prevent, sporadic colon adenomatous polyps. On the other hand, when NSAIDs are used for secondary prevention of sporadic colon adenomas, a similar effect has not been observed,[185, 186] suggesting that the biologic responses to NSAIDs of sporadic and hereditary adenomatous polyps may differ. Alternatively, NSAIDs may actually be effective in reducing sporadic colon polyps in secondary prophylaxis, but the duration of NSAID use or the size of study population enrolled may have to be greater than previously studied to document such efficacy. Trials of secondary prevention of the sporadic adenomas with COX-2 selective inhibitors are under way.

The mechanisms through which NSAIDs reduce colorectal neoplasia are uncertain. Colorectal adenocarcinoma is thought to arise from a progressive sequence starting with normal colonic epithelium that, after several molecular neoplastic transforming events, gives rise to adenomatous polyps that may progress to adenocarcinoma. Because patients with FAP experience hyperproliferation of the colonic mucosa, it has been speculated that NSAIDs may reduce colonic epithelial proliferation. However, after sulindac therapy adenomatous polyps regress but increased colonic mucosal proliferative rates persist.[178] Furthermore, in animal models of colon cancer, celecoxib has no effect on apoptosis, cell division, or intestinal epithelial architecture.[187] These data suggest that other mechanisms underlie NSAID-associated effects on colonic neoplasia. One alternative mechanism is that inhibition of cyclooxygenase and its metabolites (eicosanoids) by NSAIDs may attenuate polyp growth and decrease cancer risk. Data that support this hypothesis include observations that: (1) in a variety of cell types eicosanoids modulate colonic epithelial proliferation rates,[188] (2) elevated prostaglandin levels are found in colorectal adenocarcinoma tissue,[188, 189] (3) increased levels of COX-2 messenger RNA have been detected in hereditary nonpolyposis colorectal cancers[190] as well as in sporadic colon cancers,[191] and (4) rofecoxib decreases intestinal polyposis in mice[192] and celecoxib decreases polyp growth in FAP.[182] These latter observations imply that COX-2 may be a possible target for COX-2 specific NSAIDs in the prevention or treatment of colorectal adenocarcinomas. Providing evidence for this hypothesis is the observation that celecoxib reduces cancer cell growth in colon cancer cell lines.[187] However, these effects appear to be independent of its ability to inhibit COX-2 because celecoxib's cancer inhibitory capacity is observed in cancer cell lines lacking COX-2.[187] Furthermore, sulindac sulfone is able to inhibit colon cancer growth in rats without inhibiting COX,[193] providing more evidence that the antineoplastic effect of NSAIDs may be unrelated to COX-2 inhibition.

One final pertinent issue is an evaluation of the benefits of long-term NSAID use for chemoprevention of colorectal neoplasia versus the risks of NSAID-induced toxicities such as GI bleeding. The precise answer to this risk-benefit analysis is not known. None of the large epidemiologic trials of NSAID use for colorectal cancer prevention has presented data regarding NSAID-related complications. Furthermore, the risk arm of this analysis is strongly influenced by the type of NSAID used for chemoprevention.

The overall incidence of significant side effects from NSAIDs when taken at the usual therapeutic doses is 2% to 4% per year.[3] It has been estimated that use of therapeutic doses of currently available NSAIDs for chemoprevention of colorectal cancer would cause an incidence of serious toxicity that would exceed any benefit of prophylaxis.[194] Low doses of aspirin, however, as reviewed earlier in this chapter, are associated with lower incidences of GI complications than NSAIDs at therapeutic doses. Thus, the use of low-dose aspirin for colorectal cancer chemoprevention may be more justifiable, particularly in light of its known benefit in cardiovascular and cerebrovascular diseases.[194] However, we still need a better understanding of the most effective dose and duration of aspirin for prophylaxis of colorectal carcinomas. The Nurses' Health Study suggests that this dose might be four to six aspirin tablets per week for at least 10 years.[169] Unfortunately, the long-term toxicities of this aspirin schedule are unknown. Ideally future randomized aspirin intervention trials for colorectal cancer chemoprevention will focus on this risk-benefit analysis. Alternatively, if newer NSAIDs such as the COX-2 specific inhibitors are shown to have high chemopreventive efficacy, they may also have potential for long-term chemoprevention.

THERAPEUTIC EFFECTS IN OTHER GASTROINTESTINAL ORGANS. In addition to the potential beneficial consequences in colorectal diseases, NSAIDs may have beneficial effects in other GI locations. Epidemiologic studies of esophageal adenocarcinoma (see Chapter 35) indicate that individuals who take NSAIDs have a 10% to 64% lower risk for esophageal adenocarcinoma when compared to controls.[172, 195–197] A mechanism-based hypothesis for these epidemiologic observations can be derived from studies in which mucosal biopsy specimens from humans with esophageal adenocarcinoma or Barrett's esophagus have demonstrated increased COX-2 expression.[198] Moreover, this increase in COX-2 expression in these states can be attenuated by a COX-2 inhibitor.[198] Finally, NSAID exposure in hepatocellular carcinoma cell lines[199] or pancreatic adenocarcinoma cell lines[200] inhibits growth. It should be emphasized, however, that all of these data are either in vitro or in animals and to date there have been no prospective, randomized clinical studies demonstrating a conclusive benefit for in vivo administration of NSAIDs or a COX-2 inhibitor in any human GI cancer. However, several of these long-term clinical studies are currently under way, and their results are eagerly anticipated.

REFERENCES

1. Singh G, Triadafilopoulos G: Epidemiology of NSAID-induced GI complications. J Rheumatol 26(suppl 26):18–24, 1999.
2. Talley NJ, Evans JM, Fleming KC: Nonsteroidal antiinflammatory drugs and dyspepsia in the elderly. Dig Dis Sci 40:1345–1350, 1995.
3. Physicians' Desk Reference, 50th ed. Montvale, NJ, Medical Economics Data Production, 2001.
4. Lanas A, Serrano P, Bajador E: Evidence of aspirin use in both upper and lower gastrointestinal perforation. Gastroenterology 112:686–689, 1997.
5. Griffin MR, Piper JM, Daughtery JR, et al: Nonsteroidal anti-inflammatory drug use and increased risk for peptic ulcer disease in elderly persons. Ann Intern Med 114:257–263, 1991.
6. Armstrong CP, Blower AL: Non-steroidal anti-inflammatory drugs and life threatening complications of peptic ulceration. Gut 28:527–532, 1987.
7. Baskin WN, Ivey KJ, Krause WJ, et al: Aspirin-induced ultrastructural changes in human gastric mucosa: Correlation with potential difference. Ann Intern Med 85:299–303, 1976.
8. Lichtenberger LM, Wang ZM, Romero JJ: Non-steroidal anti-inflammatory drugs (NSAIDs) associate with zwitterionic phospholipids: Insight into the mechanism and reversal of NSAID-induced gastrointestinal injury. Nat Med 1:154–158, 1995.
9. Lanza FL, Royer GL, Nelson RS: Endoscopic evaluation of the effects of aspirin, buffered aspirin, and enteric-coated aspirin on gastric and duodenal mucosa. N Engl J Med 303:136–138, 1980.
10. Trondstad RI, Aadland E, Holler T, Olaussen B: Gastroscopic findings after treatment with enteric-coated and plain naproxen tablets in healthy subjects. Scand J Gastroenterol 20:239–242, 1985.
11. Silvoso GR, Ivey KJ, Butt JH, et al: Incidence of gastric lesions in patients with rheumatic diseases on chronic aspirin therapy. Ann Intern Med 91:517–520, 1979.
12. Fuller DK, Kalekas PJ: Ketorolac and gastrointestinal ulceration. Ann Pharmacother 27:978–979, 1993.
13. Hansen TM, Matzen P, Madsen P: Endoscopic evaluation of the effect of indomethacin capsules and suppositories on the gastric mucosa in rheumatic patients. J Rheumatol 11:484–487, 1984.
14. Redfern JS, Lee E, Feldman M: Effect of indomethacin on gastric mucosal prostaglandins in humans: Correlation with mucosal damage. Gastroenterology 92:969–977, 1987.
15. Whittle BJR: Mechanisms underlying gastric mucosal damage induced by indomethacin and bile salts, and the actions of prostaglandins. Br J Pharmacol 60:455–460, 1977.
16. Robert A: Cytoprotection by prostaglandins. Gastroenterology 77:761–767, 1979.
17. Gana TJ, MacPherson BR, Koo J: Gastric mucosal blood flow in misoprostol pretreated aspirin-induced ulceration. Ann Surg 327–334, 1988.
18. Feldman M, Shewmake K, Cryer B: Time course inhibition of gastric and platelet COX activity by acetylsalicylic acid in humans. Am J Physiol Gastrointest Liver Physiol 279:G1113–G1120, 2000.
19. Cryer B, Feldman M: Effects of very low dose daily, long-term aspirin therapy on gastric, duodenal and rectal prostaglandin levels and on mucosal injury. Gastroenterology 117:17–25, 1999.
20. Xie W, Chipman JG, Robertson DL, et al: Expression of a mitogen-responsive gene encoding prostaglandin synthase is regulated by mRNA splicing. Proc Natl Acad Sci U S A 88:2692–2696, 1991.
21. Kujubu DA, Fletcher BS, Varnum BC, et al: TIS10, a phorbol ester tumor promoter inducible mRNA from Swiss 3T3 cells, encodes a novel prostaglandin synthase/cyclooxygenase homologue. J Biol Chem 266:12866–12872, 1991.
22. O'Banion MK, Sadowski HB, Winn V, Young DA: A serum- and glucocorticoid-regulated 4-kilobase mRNA encodes a cyclooxygenase-related protein. J Biol Chem 266:23261–23267, 1991.

23. Kargman S, Charleson S, Cartwright M, et al: Characterization of prostaglandin G/H synthase 1 and 2 in rat, dog, monkey, and human gastrointestinal tracts. Gastroenterology 111:445–454, 1996.
24. Wallace JL, McKnight W, Reuter B, Vergnolle N: NSAID-induced gastric damage in rats: Requirement for inhibition of both cyclooxygenase 1 and 2. Gastroenterology 119:706–714, 2000.
25. Warner TD, Giuliano F, Vojnovic I, et al: Nonsteroid drug selectivities for cyclo-oxygenase-1 rather than cyclo-oxygenase-2 are associated with human gastrointestinal toxicity: A full *in vitro* analysis. Proc Natl Acad Sci U S A 96:7563–7568, 1999.
26. Van Hecken A, Schwartz JI, Depre M, et al: Comparative inhibitory activity of rofecoxib, meloxicam, diclofenac, ibuprofen, and naproxen on COX-2 versus COX-1 in healthy volunteers. J Clin Pharmacol 40: 1109–1120, 2000.
27. Ligumsky M, Golanska EM, Hansen DG, Kauffman GL: Aspirin can inhibit gastric mucosal cyclo-oxygenase without causing lesions in rat. Gastroenterology 84:756–761, 1983.
28. Feldman M, Colturi TJ: Effect of indomethacin on gastric acid and bicarbonate secretion in humans. Gastroenterology 87:1339–1343, 1984.
29. Levine RA, Nandi J, King RL: Nonsalicylate nonsteroidal antiinflammatory drugs augment pre-stimulated acid secretion in rabbit parietal cells: Investigation of the mechanisms of action. Gastroenterology 101:756–765, 1991.
30. Kauffman GL, Aures D, Grossman MI: Intravenous indomethacin and aspirin reduce basal gastric mucosal blood flow in dogs. Am J Physiol 238:G131–G134, 1980.
31. Selling JA, Hogan DL, Aly A, et al: Indomethacin inhibits duodenal mucosal bicarbonate secretion and endogenous prostaglandin E_2 output in human subjects. Ann Intern Med 106:368–371, 1987.
32. Miller TA: Protective effects of prostaglandins against gastric mucosal damage: Current knowledge and proposed mechanisms. Am J Physiol 245:601–623, 1983.
33. Lanas AI, Nerin J, Esteva F, Sainz R: Non-steroidal anti-inflammatory drugs and prostaglandin effects on pepsinogen secretion by dispersed human peptic cells. Gut 36:657–663, 1995.
34. Gaw AJ, Williams LV, Spraggs CF, Jordan CC: Role of pepsin in the development of indomethacin-induced antral ulceration in the rat. Aliment Pharmacol Ther 9:167–172, 1995.
35. Redfern JS, Lee E, Feldman M: Effect of immunization with prostaglandin metabolites on gastrointestinal ulceration. Am J Physiol 255: 723–730, 1988.
36. Lee M, Aldred K, Lee E, Feldman M: Aspirin-induced acute gastric mucosal injury is a neutrophil-dependent process in rats. Am J Physiol 263:G920–G926, 1992.
37. Wallace JL, McKnight W, Miyasaka M, et al: Role of endothelial adhesion molecules in NSAID-induced gastric mucosal injury. Am J Physiol 265:G993–G998, 1993.
38. Kikendall JW, Friedman AC, Oyewole MA, et al: Pill-induced esophageal injury: Case reports and review of the medical literature. Dig Dis Sci 28:174–181, 1983.
39. Heller SR, Fellows IW, Ogilvie AL, Atkinson M: Non-steroidal anti-inflammatory drugs and benign oesophageal stricture. BMJ 285:167–168, 1982.
40. Safaie-Shirazi S, Zike WL, Brubacher M, Den Bensten L: Effect of aspirin, alcohol, and pepsin on mucosal permeability of esophageal mucosa. Surg Forum 25:335–337, 1974.
41. Carlsby B, Densert O: Esophageal lesions caused by orally administered drugs: An experimental study in the cat. Eur Surg Res 12:270–282, 1980.
42. McCord GS, Clouse RE: Pill-induced esophageal strictures: Clinical features and risk factors for development. Am J Med 88:512–518, 1990.
43. Minocha A, Greenbaum DS: Pill-esophagitis caused by nonsteroidal antiinflammatory drugs. Am J Gastroenterol 86:1086–1089, 1991.
44. Eng J, Sabanatham S: Drug-induced esophagitis. Am J Gastroenterol 86:1127–1133, 1991.
45. Lanas A, Hirschowitz BI: Significant role of aspirin use in patients with esophagitis. J Clin Gastroenterol 13:622–627, 1991.
46. Graham DY, Agrawal NM, Roth SH: Prevention of NSAID-induced gastric ulcer with misoprostol: Multicentre, double-blind, placebo-controlled trial. Lancet 2:1277–1280, 1988.
47. Mielants H, Goemaere S, De Vos M, et al: Intestinal mucosal permeability in inflammatory rheumatic diseases. I. Role of antiinflammatory drugs. J Rheumatol 18:389–393, 1991.
48. Graham DY, White RH, Moreland LW, et al: Duodenal and gastric ulcer prevention with misoprostol in arthritis patients taking NSAIDs. Ann Intern Med 119:257–262, 1993.
49. Simon LS, Weaver AL, Graham DY, et al: Anti-inflammatory and upper gastrointestinal effects of celecoxib in rheumatoid arthritis. JAMA 282:1921–1928, 1999.
50. Laine L, Harper S, Simon T, et al: A randomized trial comparing the effect of rofecoxib, a cyclooxygenase 2–specific inhibitor, with that of ibuprofen on the gastroduodenal mucosa of patients with osteoarthritis. Gastroenterology 117:783, 1999.
51. Langman MJS, Weil J, Wainwright P, et al: Risks of bleeding peptic ulcer associated with individual non-steroidal anti-inflammatory drugs. Lancet 343:1075–1078, 1994.
52. Mellem H, Stave R, Osnes M, et al: Symptoms in patients with peptic ulcer and hematemesis and/or melena related to the use of non-steroid anti-inflammatory drugs. Scand J Gastroenterol 20:1246–1248, 1985.
53. Singh G, Ramey DR: NSAID induced gastrointestinal complications: The ARAMIS perspective. J Rheumatol 25:8–16, 1998.
54. Silverstein FE, Graham DY, Senior JR, et al: Misoprostol reduces serious gastrointestinal complications in patients with rheumatoid arthritis receiving nonsteroidal anti-inflammatory drugs: A randomized, double-blind, placebo-controlled trial. Ann Intern Med 123:241–249, 1995.
55. Silverstein FE, Faich G, Goldstein JL, et al: Gastrointestinal toxicity with celecoxib vs. nonsteroidal anti-inflammatory drugs for osteoarthritis and rheumatoid arthritis: The CLASS study: A randomized controlled trial. JAMA 284:1247–1255, 2000.
56. Bombardier C, Laine L, Reicin A, et al: Rofecoxib and naproxen in patients with rheumatoid arthritis. N Engl J Med 343:1520–1528, 2000.
57. Gabriel SE, Jaakkimainen L, Bombardier C: Risk for serious gastrointestinal complications related to use of nonsteroidal anti-inflammatory drugs. Ann Intern Med 115:787–796, 1991.
58. Rodriquez LAG, Jick H: Risk of upper gastrointestinal bleeding and perforation associated with individual non-steroidal anti-inflammatory drugs. Lancet 343:769–772, 1994.
59. Piper JM, Ray WA, Daughtery JR, Griffin MR: Corticosteroid use and peptic ulcer disease: Role of nonsteroidal anti-inflammatory drugs. Ann Intern Med 114:740, 1991.
60. Peura DA, Lanza FL, Gostout CJ: The American College of Gastroenterology Bleeding Registry: Preliminary findings. Am J Gastroenterol 92:924–928, 1997.
61. Kaufman DD, Kelly JP, Wiholm BE, et al: The risk of acute major upper gastrointestinal bleeding among users of aspirin and ibuprofen at various levels of alcohol consumption. Am J Gastroenterol 94: 3189–3196, 1999.
62. Llewellyn JG, Pritchard H: Influence of age and disease state in nonsteroidal antiinflammatory drug associated gastric bleeding. J Rheumatol 15:691–694, 1988.
63. Wilcox CM, Shalek KA, Costsonis G: Striking prevalence of over-the-counter nonsteroidal anti-inflammatory drug use in patients with upper gastrointestinal hemorrhage. Arch Intern Med 154:42–46, 1994.
64. Lanas A, Sekar MC, Hirschowitz BI: Objective evidence of aspirin use in both ulcer and nonulcer upper and lower gastrointestinal bleeding. Gastroenterology 103:862–869, 1992.
65. Lanas AI, Remacha B, Esteva F, Sainz R: Risk factors associated with refractory peptic ulcers. Gastroenterology 109:1124–1133, 1995.
66. Steering Committee of the Physician's Health Study Research Group: Final report on the aspirin component of the ongoing physician's health study. N Engl J Med 321:129–135, 1989.
67. Aspirin Myocardial Infarction Study Research Group: A randomized, controlled trial of aspirin in persons recovered from myocardial infarction. JAMA 243:661–669, 1980.
68. Slattery J, Warlow CP, Shorrock CJ, Langman MJS: Risks of gastrointestinal bleeding during secondary prevention of vascular events with aspirin—analysis of gastrointestinal bleeding during the UK-TIA trial. Gut 37:509–511, 1995.
69. Lanas A, Bajador E, Serrano P, et al: Nitrovasodilators, low-dose aspirin, other nonsteroidal antiinflammatory drugs, and the risk of upper gastrointestinal bleeding. N Engl J Med 348:834–839, 2000.
70. Kelly JP, Kaufman DW, Jurgelon JM, et al: Risk of aspirin-associated major upper-gastrointestinal bleeding with enteric-coated or buffered product. Lancet 348:1413–1416, 1996.
71. Cryer B, Luk G, Feldman M: Effects of very low doses of aspirin on gastric, duodenal and rectal prostaglandins and mucosal injury. Gastroenterology 108:A77, 1995.

72. Laine L, Marin-Sorensen M, Weinstein WM: Nonsteroidal antiinflammatory drug–associated gastric ulcers do not require *Helicobacter pylori* for their development. Am J Gastroenterol 87:1398–1402, 1992.
73. Weinstein WM: Differentiation of nonsteroidal anti-inflammatory drug associated and "ordinary" peptic ulcer. Ann Intern Med 301:301–311, 1991.
74. Laine L, Cominelli F, Sloan R, et al: Interaction of NSAIDs and *Helicobacter pylori* on gastrointestinal injury and prostaglandin production: A controlled double-blind trial. Aliment Pharmacol Ther 9: 127–135, 1995.
75. Chan FKL, Sung JY, Chung SCS: Randomized trial of eradication of *Helicobacter pylori* before non-steroidal anti-inflammatory drug therapy to prevent peptic ulcers. Lancet 350:975–979, 1997.
76. Hawkey CJ, Tullasay Z, Szczepanski L: *Helicobacter pylori* eradication in patients taking non-steroidal anti-inflammatory drugs: The HELP NSAIDs study. Lancet 352:1016–1021, 1998.
77. Aalykke C, Lauritsen JM, Hallas J, et al: *Helicobacter pylori* and risk of ulcer bleeding among users of nonsteroidal anti-inflammatory drugs: A case-control study. Gastroenterology 116:1305–1309, 1999.
78. Santolaria S, Lanas A, Benito R, et al: *Helicobacter pylori* infection is a protective factor for bleeding gastric ulcers but not for bleeding duodenal ulcers in NSAID users. Aliment Pharmacol Ther 13:1511–1518, 1999.
79. Konturek JW, Dembinski A, Konturek SJ, et al: Infection of *Helicobacter pylori* in gastric adaptation to continued administration of aspirin in humans. Gastroenterology 114:245–255, 1998.
80. Feldman M, Cryer B, Mallat D, Go MF: Role of *H. pylori* infection on gastroduodenal injury and gastric protaglandin synthesis during long-term/low dose aspirin therapy: A prospective, controlled, double-blind randomized trial. Am J Gastroenterol 96:1751–1757, 2001.
81. Levine LR, Cloud ML, Enas NH: Nizatidine prevents peptic ulceration in high-risk patients taking nonsteroidal anti-inflammatory drugs. Arch Intern Med 153:2449–2454, 1993.
82. Ten Wolde S, Dihjkmans BACJM, Hermans J, Lamers CBHW: High-dose ranitidine for the prevention of recurrent peptic ulcer disease in rheumatoid arthritis patients taking NSAIDs. Aliment Pharmacol Ther 10:347–351, 1996.
83. Robinson MG, Griffin JW, Bowers J, et al: Effect of ranitidine gastroduodenal mucosal damage induced by nonsteroidal antiinflammatory drugs. Dig Dis Sci 34:424–428, 1989.
84. Taha AS, Hundal O, Hawkey CJ: Famotidine for the prevention of gastric and duodenal ulcer caused by nonsteroidal antiinflammatory drugs. N Engl J Med 334:1435–1439, 1996.
85. Bocanegra TS, Weaver AL, Tindall EA, et al: Diclofenac/misoprostol compared with diclofenac in the treatment of osteoarthritis of the knee or hip: A randomized, placebo-controlled trial: Arthrotec Osteoarthritis Study Group. J Rheumatol 25:1602–1611, 1998.
86. Raskin JB, White RH, Jaszewski R: Misoprostol and ranitidine in the prevention of NSAID-induced ulcers: A prospective, double blind, multicenter study. Am J Gastroenterol 91:223–227, 1996.
87. Scheiman JM: Meta-analysis: Misoprostol reduced NSAID-induced gastrointestinal injury. ACP Journal Club 124:36, 1997.
88. Maetzel A, Ferraz MB, Bombardier C: The cost effectiveness of misoprostol in preventing serious gastrointestinal events associated with the use of nonsteroidal antiinflammtory drugs. Arthritis Rheum 41:16–25, 1998.
89. Yeomans ND, Tullasay Z, Juhasz L: A comparison of omeprazole with ranitidine for ulcers associated with nonsteroidal antiinflammatory drugs. N Engl J Med 338:719–726, 1998.
90. McDonald TM, Morant SV, Robinson GC: Association of upper gastrointestinal toxicity of non-steroidal anti-inflammatory drugs with continued exposure: Cohort study. BMJ 315:1333–1337, 1997.
91. Raskin JB, White RH, Jackson JE, et al: Misoprostol dosage in the prevention of nonsteroidal anti-inflammatory drug-induced gastric and duodenal ulcers: A comparison of three regimens. Ann Intern Med 123:344–350, 1995.
92. Walan A, Bader J, Classen M, et al: Effect of omeprazole and ranitidine on ulcer healing and relapse rates in patients with benign gastric ulcer. N Engl J Med 320:69–75, 1989.
93. Hawkey CJ, Karrasch JA, Szczepanski L: Omeprazole compared with misoprostol for ulcers associated with nonsteroidal antiinflammatory drugs. N Engl J Med 388:727–734, 1998.
94. Lanza FL, Rack MF, Simon TJ, et al: Specific inhibition of cyclooxygenase-2 with MK-0966 is associated with less gastroduodenal damage than either aspirin or ibuprofen. Aliment Pharmacol Ther 13:761–767, 1999.
95. Emery P, Zeidler H, Kvien TK, et al: Celecoxib versus diclofenac in long-term management of rheumatoid arthritis: Randomised double-blind comparison. Lancet 354:2106–2111, 1999.
96. Hawkey C, Laine L, Simon T, et al: Comparison of the effect of rofecoxib (a cyclooxygenase 2 inhibitor), ibuprofen, and placebo on the gastroduodenal mucosa of patients with osteoarthritis. Arthritis Rheum 43:370–377, 2000.
97. Langman MJ, Jensen DJ, Watson DJ, et al: Adverse upper gastrointestinal effects of rofecoxib compared with NSAIDs. JAMA 282:1929–1933, 1999.
98. Goldstein JL, Silverstein FE, Agrawal NM, et al: Reduced risk of upper gastrointestinal complications with celecoxib, a novel COX-2 inhibitor. Am J Gastroenterol 95:1681–1690, 2000.
99. Schmassmann A, Peskar BM, Stettler C, et al: Effects of inhibition of prostaglandin endoperoxide synthase-2 in chronic gastro-intestinal ulcer models in rats. Br J Pharmacol 123:795–804, 1998.
100. Mizuno H, Sakamoto C, Matsuda K, et al: Induction of cyclooxygenase-2 in gastric mucosal lesions and its inhibition by specific antagonists delays healing in mice. Gastroenterology 112:387–397, 1997.
101. Vogiagis D, Glare EM, Misajon A, et al: Cyclooxygenase-1 and an alternatively spliced mRNA in the rat stomach: Effects of aging and ulcers. Am J Physiol 278:G820–G827, 2000.
102. Laine L, Sloane R, Ferretti M, Cominelli F: A randomized, double-blind comparison of placebo, etodolac, and naproxen on gastrointestinal injury and prostaglandin production. Gastrointest Endosc 42:428–433, 1995.
103. Schattenkirchner M: An updated safety profile of etodolac in several thousand patients. Eur J Clin Pharmacol 10:56–65, 1990.
104. Eversmeyer W, Poland M, DeLapp RE, Jensen CP: Saftey experience with nabumetone versus naproxen, ibuprofen, and piroxicam in osteoarthritis and rheumatoid arthritis. Am J Med 95:10–18, 1993.
105. Cryer B, Goldschmiedt M, Redfern JS, Feldman M: Comparison of salsalate and aspirin on mucosal injury and gastroduodenal mucosal prostaglandins. Gastroenterology 99:1616–1621, 1990.
106. Cryer B, Feldman M: Cyclooxygenase-1 and cyclooxygenase-2 selectivity of widely used nonsteroidal anti-inflammatory drugs. Am J Med 104:413–421, 1998.
107. Meade EA, Smith WL, DeWitt DL: Differential inhibition of prostaglandin endoperoxide synthase (cyclooxygenase) isoenzymes by aspirin and other nonsteroidal anti-inflammatory drugs. J Biol Chem 268: 6610–6614, 1993.
108. Wolfe MM: Future trends in the development of safer nonsteroidal anti-inflammatory drugs. Am J Med 105:44S–52S, 1998.
109. Rothstein R: Safety profiles of leading nonsteroidal anti-inflammatory drugs. Am J Med 105:39S–43S, 1998.
110. Searle-Pfizer Pharmaceuticals: Product Information: Celebrex, celecoxib. Chicago, 1998.
111. Wallace JL, Reuter B, Cicala C, et al: Novel nonsteroidal anti-inflammatory drug derivatives with markedly reduced ulcerogenic properties in the rat. Gastroenterology 107:173–179, 1994.
112. Davies NM, Roseth AG, Appleyard CB: NO-naproxen vs naproxen: Ulcerogenic, analgesic and anti-inflammatory effects. Aliment Pharmacol Ther 11:69–79, 1997.
113. Mizogughi H, Hase S, Tanaka A, Takeuchi K: Lack of small intestinal ulcerogenicity of nitric oxide–releasing indomethacin, NCX-530, in rats. Aliment Pharmacol Ther 15:257–267, 2001.
114. Kurinets A, Lichtenberger LM: Phosphatidylcholine-associated aspirin accelerates healing of gastric ulcers in rats. Dig Dis Sci 43:786–790, 1998.
115. Lichtenberger LM, Ulloa C, Vanous AL: Zwitterionic phospholipids enhance aspirin's therapeutic activity as demonstrated in rodent model systems. J Pharmacol Exp Ther 277:1221–1227, 1996.
116. Anand BS, Romero JJ, Sanduja SK, Lichtenberger LM: Phospholipid association reduces the gastric mucosal toxicity of aspirin in human subjects. Am J Gastroenterol 94:1818–1822, 1999.
117. Morris AJ, Madhok R, Sturrock RD, et al: Enteroscopic diagnosis of small bowel ulceration in patients receiving non-steroidal anti-inflammatory drugs. Lancet 337:520, 1991.
118. Langman MJS, Morgan L, Worrall A: Use of anti-inflammatory drugs by patients admitted with small or large bowel perforations and haemorrhage. BMJ 290:347–349, 1985.
119. Day TK: Intestinal perforation associated with osmotic slow release indomethacin capsules. BMJ 287:1671–1672, 1983.

120. Madhok R, MacKenzie JA, Lee FD, et al: Small bowel ulceration in patients receiving non-steroidal anti-inflammatory drugs for rheumatoid arthritis. Q J Med 58:53–58, 1986.
121. Deakin M: Small bowel perforation associated with an excessive dose of slow release diclofenac sodium. BMJ 297:488–489, 1988.
122. Nagaraj HS, Sandhu AS, Cook LN, et al: Gastrointestinal perforation following indomethacin therapy in very low birth weight infants. J Pediatr Surg 16:1003–1007, 1981.
123. Allison MC, Howatson AG, Torrance CJ, et al: Gastrointestinal damage associated with the use of nonsteroidal antiinflammatory drugs. N Engl J Med 327:749–754, 1992.
124. Wallace JL, Tigley AW: Review article: New insights into prostaglandins and mucosal defense. Aliment Pharmacol Ther 9:227–235, 1995.
125. Redfern JS, Blair AJ, Lee E, Feldman M: Gastrointestinal ulcer formation in rabbits immunized with prostaglandin E_2. Gastroenterology 93:744–752, 1987.
126. Bjarnason I, Hayllar J, Macpherson AJ, Russell AS: Side effects of nonsteroidal anti-inflammatory drugs on the small and large intestine in humans. Gastroenterology 104:1832–1847, 1993.
127. Matsuhashi N, Yamada A, Hiraishi M, et al: Multiple strictures of the small intestine after long-term nonsteroidal anti-inflammatory drug therapy. Am J Gastroenterol 87:1183–1186, 1992.
128. Levi S, Delacy G, Price AB, et al: "Diaphragm-like" strictures of the small bowel in patients treated with non-steroidal anti-inflammatory drugs. Br J Radiol 63:186–189, 1990.
129. Bjarnason I, Zanelli G, Smethurst P, et al: Clinicopathological features of nonsteroidal antiinflammatory drug–induced small intestinal strictures. Gastroenterology 94:1070–1074, 1988.
130. Lang J, Price AB, Levi AJ, et al: Diaphragm disease: The pathology of non-steroidal anti-inflammatory drug induced small intestinal strictures. J Clin Pathol 41:516–526, 1988.
131. Bjarnason I, Prouse P, Smith T, et al: Blood and protein loss via small-intestinal inflammation induced by non-steroidal anti-inflammatory drugs. Lancet 2:711–714, 1987.
132. Bjarnason I, Zanelli G, Smith T, et al: Nonsteroidal antiinflammatory drug–induced intestinal inflammation in humans. Gastroenterology 93: 480–489, 1987.
133. Bjarnason I, Williams P, So A, et al: Intestinal permeability and inflammation in rheumatoid arthritis: Effects of non-steroidal anti-inflammatory drugs. Lancet 2:1171–1174, 1984.
134. Morris AJ, Wasson LA, MacKenzie JF: Small bowel enteroscopy in undiagnosed gastrointestinal blood loss. Gut 33:887–889, 1992.
135. Kepczyk T, Kadakia SC: Prospective evaluation of gastrointestinal tract in patients with iron-deficiency anemia. Dig Dis Sci 40:1283–1289, 1995.
136. Vreugdenhil G, Wognum AW, van Eijk HG, Swaak AJG: Anaemia in rheumatoid arthritis: The role of iron, vitamin B_{12}, and folic acid deficiency, and erythropoietin responsiveness. Ann Rheum Dis 49:93–98, 1990.
137. Bjarnason I, Williams P, Smethurst P, et al: Effect of non-steroidal anti-inflammatory drugs and prostaglandins on the permeability of the human small intestine. Gut 27:1292–1297, 1986.
138. Bjarnason I, Fehilly B, Smethurst P, et al: Importance of local versus systemic effects of non-steroidal anti-inflammatory drugs in increasing small intestinal permeability in man. Gut 32:275–277, 1991.
139. Anthony A, Dhillon AP, Nygard G, et al: Early histological features of small intestinal injury induced by indomethacin. Aliment Pharmacol Ther 7:29–40, 1993.
140. Morris AJ, Murray L, Sturrock RD, et al: Short report: The effect of misoprostol on the anaemia of NSAID enteropathy. Aliment Pharmacol Ther 8:343–346, 1994.
141. Stamm CP, Pearce WA, Larsen BA, et al: Colonic ulcerations associated with non-steroidal anti-inflammatory ingestion. Gastrointest Endosc 37:260, 1991.
142. Charuzi I, Ovnar A, Zirkin H, et al: Ibuprofen and benign cecal ulcer. J Rheumatol 12:188–189, 1985.
143. Uribe A, Johansson C, Scezak P, Rubio C: Ulceration of the colon associated with naproxen and acetylsalicylic acid treatment. Gastrointest Endosc 32:242–244, 1986.
144. Carson J, Notis WM, Orris ES: Colonic ulceration and bleeding during diclofenac therapy [letter]. N Engl J Med 323:135, 1990.
145. Gibson GR, Whitacre EB, Ricotti CA: Colitis induced by nonsteroidal anti-inflammatory drugs. Arch Intern Med 152:625–632, 1992.
146. Kurahara K, Matsumoto T, Iida M, et al: Clinical and endoscopic features of nonsteroidal anti-inflammatory drug–induced colonic ulcerations. Am J Gastroenterol 96:473–480, 2001.
147. Ravi S, Keat AC, Keat ECB: Colitis caused by NSAIDs. Postgrad Med J 62:773–776, 1986.
148. Huber T, Ruchti C, Halter F: Nonsteroidal antiinflammatory drug–induced colonic strictures: A case report. Gastroenterology 100:1119–1122, 1991.
149. Bridges AJ, Marshall JB, Diaz-Arias AA: Acute eosinophilic colitis and hypersensitivity reaction associated with naproxen therapy. Am J Med 89:526–527, 1990.
150. Giardiello FM, Hansen FC III, Lazenby AJ, et al: Collagenous colitis in setting of nonsteroidal anti-inflammatory drugs and antibiotics. Dig Dis Sci 35:257–260, 1990.
151. Bunney RG: Non-steroidal anti-inflammatory drugs and the bowel. Lancet 2:1047–1048, 1989.
152. Doman DB, Goldberg HJ: A case of meclofenamate sodium–induced colitis. Am J Gastroenterol 81:1220–1221, 1986.
153. Tanner AR, Raghunat H: Colonic inflammation and NSAID administration. Digestion 41:116–120, 1988.
154. Levy N, Gaspar E: Rectal bleeding and indomethacin suppositories. Lancet 305:577, 1975.
155. Van Gossum A, Zalcman M, Adler M, et al: Anorectal stenosis in patients with prolonged use of suppositories containing paracetamol and acetylsalicylic acid. Dig Dis Sci 38:1970–1977, 1993.
156. Coutrot S, Roland D, Barbier J, et al: Acute perforation of colonic diverticula associated with short term indomethacin. Lancet 2:1055–1056, 1978.
157. Campbell K, Steele RJC: Non-steroidal anti-inflammatory drugs and complicated diverticular disease: A case-control study. Br J Surg 78: 190–191, 1991.
158. Wilson RG, Smith AN, Macintyre IMC: Complications of diverticular disease and non-steroidal anti-inflammatory drugs: A prospective study. Br J Surg 77:1103–1104, 1990.
159. Kaufmann HJ, Taubin HL: Nonsteroidal anti-inflammatory drugs activate quiescent inflammatory bowel disease. Ann Intern Med 107:513–516, 1987.
160. Reuter BK, Asfaha S, Buret A, et al: Exacerbation of inflammation-associated colonic injury in rat through inhibition of cyclooxygenase-2. J Clin Invest 98(2076):2085, 1996.
161. Lee WM: Medical progress: Drug-induced hepatotoxicity. N Engl J Med 333:1118–1127, 1995.
162. Hunter EB, Johnston PE, Tanner G, et al: Bromfenac (Duract)–associated hepatic failure requiring liver transplantation. Am J Gastroenterol 94:2299–2301, 1999.
163. Rabinovitz M, Van Theil DH: Hepatotoxicity of nonsteroidal anti-inflammatory drugs. Am J Gastroenterol 87:1696–1704, 1992.
164. Fry SW, Seeff LB: Hepatotoxicity of analgesics and anti-inflammatory agents. In Lewis JH (ed): Gastroenterology Clinics of North America. Philadelphia, WB Saunders, 1995, pp 875–905.
165. Scully LJ, Clarke D, Barr RJ: Diclofenac induced hepatitis: 3 Cases with features of autoimmune chronic active hepatitis. Dig Dis Sci 38: 744–751, 1993.
166. Mallory A, Kern F: Drug-induced pancreatitis: A critical review. Gastroenterology 78:813–820, 1980.
167. McArthur KE: Drug-induced pancreatitis. Aliment Pharmacol Ther 10: 23–38, 1996.
168. Giovannucci E, Rimm EB, Stampfer MJ, et al: Aspirin use and the risk for colorectal cancer and adenoma in male health professionals. Ann Intern Med 121:241–246, 1994.
169. Giovannucci E, Egan KM, Hunter DJ, et al: Aspirin and the risk of colorectal cancer in women. N Engl J Med 333:609–614, 1995.
170. Suh O, Mettlin C, Petrelli NJ: Aspirin use, cancer, and polyps of the large bowel. Cancer 72:1171–1177, 1993.
171. Thun MJ, Namboodiri MM, Heath CW: Aspirin use and the reduced risk of fatal colon cancer. N Engl J Med 325:1593–1596, 1991.
172. Thun MJ, Namboodiri MM, Callee EE, et al: Aspirin use and the risk of fatal cancer. Cancer Res 53:1322–1327, 1993.
173. Kune GA, Kune S, Watson LF: Colorectal cancer risk, chronic illnesses, operation, and medications: Case-control results from the Melbourne colorectal cancer study. Cancer Res 48:4399–4404, 1988.
174. Janne PA, Mayer RJ: Chemoprevention of colorectal cancer. N Engl J Med 342:1960–1968, 2001.
175. Kauppi M, Pukkala E, Isomaki H: Low incidence of colorectal cancer in patients with rheumatoid arthritis. Clin Exp Rheumatol 14:551–553, 1996.
176. Peleg II, Lubin MF, Cotsonis GA, et al: Long-term use of nonsteroidal antiinflammatory drugs and other chemopreventers and risk of subsequent colorectal neoplasia. Dig Dis Sci 41:1319–1326, 1996.

177. Paganini-Hill A, Chao A, Ross RK, Henderson BE: Aspirin use and chronic diseases: A cohort study of the elderly. BMJ 299:1247–1250, 1989.
178. Spagnesi MT, Tonelli F, Dolara P, et al: Rectal proliferation and polyp occurrence in patients with familial adenomatous polyposis after sulindac treatment. Gastroenterology 106:362–366, 1994.
179. Greenberg ER, Baron JA, Freeman DH, et al: Reduced risk of large bowel adenomas among aspirin users. J Natl Cancer Inst 85:912–916, 1993.
180. Logan RFA, Little J, Hawtin PG, Hardcastle JD: Effect of aspirin and non-steroidal anti-inflammatory drugs on colorectal adenomas: Case-control study of subjects participating in the Nottingham faecal occult blood screening programme. BMJ 307:285–289, 1993.
181. Giardiello FM, Hamilton SR, Krush AJ, et al: Treatment of colonic and rectal adenomas with sulindac in familial adenomatous polyposis. N Engl J Med 328:1313–1316, 1993.
182. Steinbach G, Lynch PM, Phillips RKS, et al: The effect of celecoxib, a cyclooxygenase-2 inhibitor, in familial adenomatous polyposis. N Engl J Med 342:1946–1952, 2000.
183. Waddell WR, Louughry RW: Sulindac for polyposis of the colon. Am J Surg 157:175–179, 1989.
184. Rigau J, Pique JM, Rubio E, et al: Effects of long-term sulindac therapy on colonic polyposis. Ann Intern Med 115:952–954, 1991.
185. Hixson LJ, Earnest DL, Fennerty MB, Samplinger RE: NSAID effect on sporadic colon polyps. Am J Gastroenterol 88:1652–1656, 1993.
186. Ladenheim J, Garcia G, Titzer D, et al: Effect of sulindac on sporadic colonic polyps. Gastroenterology 108:1083–1087, 1995.
187. Wiliams CS, Watson AJ, Sheng H, et al: Celecoxib prevents tumor growth in vivo without toxicity to normal gut: Lack of correlation between in vitro and in vivo models. Cancer Res 60:6045–6051, 2000.
188. Eberhart CE, Dubois RN: Eicosanoids and the gastrointestinal tract. Gastroenterology 109:285–301, 1995.
189. Rigas B, Goldman IS, Levine L: Altered eicosanoid levels in human colon cancer. J Lab Clin Med 122:518–523, 1993.
190. Sinicrope FA, Lemoine M, Xi L, et al: Reduced expression of cyclooxygenase 2 proteins in hereditary nonpolyposis colorectal cancers relative to sporadic cancers. Gastroenterology 117:350–358, 1999.
191. Eberhart CE, Coffey RJ, Radhika A, et al: Up-regulation of cyclooxygenase gene expression in human colorectal adenomas and adenocarcinoma. Gastroenterology 107:1183–1188, 1994.
192. Oshima M, Murai N, Kargman S, et al: Chemoprevention of intestinal polyposis in the Apcdelta716 mouse by rofecoxib, a specific cyclooxygenase-2 inhibitor. Cancer Res 61:1733–1740, 2001.
193. Piazza GA, Alberts DS, Hixson LJ, et al: Sulindac sulfone inhibits azoxymethane-induced colon carcinogenesis in rats without reducing prostaglandin levels. Cancer Res 57:2909–2915, 1997.
194. Trujillo MA, Garewal HS, Sampliner RE: Nonsteroidal antiinflammatory agents in chemoprevention of colorectal cancer: At what cost? Dig Dis Sci 39:2260–2266, 1994.
195. Funkhouser EM, Sharp GB: Aspirin and reduced risk of esophageal carcinoma. Cancer 76:1116–1119, 1995.
196. Farrow DC, Vaughan TL, Hansten PD, et al: Use of aspirin and other nonsteroidal anti-inflammatory drugs and risk of esophageal and gastric cancer. Cancer Epidemiol Biomarkers Prev 7:97–102, 1998.
197. Langman MJ, Cheng KK, Gilman EA, Lancashire RJ: Effect of anti-inflammatory drugs on overall risk of common cancer: Case-control study in general practice research database. BMJ 320:1642–1646, 2000.
198. Shirvani VN, Ouatu-Lascar R, Kaur BS, et al: Cyclooxygenase 2 expression in Barrett's esophagus and adenocarcinoma: Ex vivo induction by bile salts and acid exposure. Gastroenterology 118:487–496, 2000.
199. Rahman MA, Dhar DK, Masunaga R, et al: Sulindac and exisulind exhibit a significant antiproliferative effect and induce apoptosis in human hepatocellular carcinoma cell lines. Cancer Res 60:2085–2089, 2000.
200. Molina MA, Sitja-Arnau M, Lemoine MG, et al: Increased cyclooxygenase-2 expression in human pancreatic carcinomas and cell lines: Growth inhibition by nonsteroidal anti-inflammatory drugs. Cancer Res 59:4356–4362, 1999.

Chapter 24

Abdominal Abscesses and Gastrointestinal Fistulas

Joseph P. Minei and Julie G. Champine

ABDOMINAL ABSCESSES

Pathophysiology

The development of an intra-abdominal abscess (IAA) occurs as a result of a host response to intra-abdominal bacterial contamination secondary to, or in conjunction with, various pathologic clinical entities. In 60% to 80% of cases intra-abdominal abscess formation is associated with perforated hollow viscera, whether secondary to inflammatory disease such as appendicitis or diverticulitis or as a consequence of penetrating or blunt trauma to the abdomen.[1–6] Other conditions associated with IAA formation include inflammatory bowel disease and complications of elective surgery (Table 24–1).[7–10] Abscesses associated with solid organs such as the pancreas or liver are discussed in Chapters 48 and 69, respectively.

There is a delicate balance of opposing forces within the peritoneal cavity between bacterial factors and the host's defense mechanisms that attempts to clear bacterial contamination and localize infection (Table 24–2). These opposing factors are often affected by the presence of adjuvant factors within the peritoneal cavity that often tip the balance toward bacterial infection with abscess formation.

Once bacteria gain access to the peritoneal cavity through perforation of the intestinal wall, several factors come into play that determine whether an active infection is initiated. The typical bacteria that make up intra-abdominal infections have the ability to adhere to peritoneal surfaces and selectively grow and utilize host nutrients. These bacteria are able to undergo metabolic processes that are adapted to the host environment (e.g., obligate anaerobic metabolism). Furthermore, these bacteria have the capacity to resist antibiotic attack. Finally, bacterial synergy plays an important role in the development of intra-abdominal infection (see "Bacteriology").[1]

The peritoneum uses a number of host defenses to combat bacterial contamination.[1, 11] The balance of host defense factors in the setting of adjuvant factors determines whether contamination continues on to infection. Lymphatic clearance of bacteria is a major defense process that is so efficient that abscess formation occurs only when adjuvant substances such as hemoglobin, barium, or necrotic tissue are present.[12] These adjuvant substances may block lymphatics (barium, fecal particulate matter), provide bacterial nutrients (iron), or impair bacterial killing. Shortly after bacterial contamination, peritoneal macrophages are the predominant phagocytic cells. These cells are also cleared by the lymphatic system. As bacteria proliferate, polymorphonuclear leukocytes invade and become more numerous. The resultant peritoneal inflammation leads to an increase in splanchnic blood flow with protein and fluid exudation into the peritoneal cavity. Procoagulatory effects of the inflammatory process and reduced levels of plasminogen activator activity enhance fibrin deposition and lead to entrapment of bacteria and localization of infection.[11]

These peritoneal defense mechanisms can have adverse effects. Lymphatic clearance of bacteria may be so brisk and effective that it results in a systemic response to bacteremia and sepsis. The exudation of fluid into the peritoneal cavity can lead to hypovolemia and shock, as well as dilute the opsonins needed in phagocytosis. Fibrin entrapment of bacteria can impair antimicrobial penetration and phagocytic migration, with the potential to localize infection and lead to abscess formation.[11] However, attempts to alter this balance of defense mechanisms are still not fully understood. In a study utilizing a rodent intraperitoneal abscess model, recombinant tissue plasminogen activator (rt-PA) was used to increase intra-abdominal fibrinolytic activity. Whereas rats treated with rt-PA had significantly lower abscess rates than controls, they had significantly higher bacteremia and mortality rates.[13] Further work in this area by the same group has utilized similar rodent models of intraperitoneal infection to study the role of a hyaluronic acid solution in abdominal adhesion and abscess formation. In bacterial peritonitis, intraperitoneal hyaluronic acid solution in the presence of antibiotics reduced the development of adhesions and abscess formation without increasing the rate of mortality.[14] Products made of hyaluronic acid suitable for clinical use are currently approved.

Table 24–1 | **Causes of Intra-abdominal Abscesses**

Crohn's disease
Abdominal trauma
Cholecystectomy
Complications of acute pancreatitis
Perforated hollow viscera
Appendicitis
Diverticulitis
Duodenal or gastric ulcer
Neoplastic disease
Ischemic colitis

Bacteriology

The bacteriologic factors associated with IAA formation are dependent on the circumstances of the initial peritoneal contamination. Patients who have abscesses that form in association with community associated peritonitis such as perforated appendicitis or as a complication of penetrating abdominal trauma often have very different microbial flora from those of the patient who has been in the intensive care unit (ICU) for a prolonged period and has been exposed to broad-spectrum antibiotics.

The typical abscess that forms as a complication of secondary bacterial peritonitis, defined as loss of integrity of the gastrointestinal (GI) tract, is a mixed aerobic and anaerobic infection. In studies of isolates from subphrenic,[15] retroperitoneal,[16] and diverticular abscesses,[17] a range of 2.9 to 3.7 bacterial isolates per abscess was recovered. The most common aerobes were *Escherichia coli* and *Enterococcus* species (range of 1.3 to 1.6 isolates per specimen). The most common anaerobes were *Bacteroides fragilis* and *Peptostreptococcus* species, which accounted for 50% to 75% of all anaerobes isolated. Other *Bacteroides* species and *Clostridium* species made up the remainder of anaerobes isolated (range of 1.7 to 2.1 isolates per specimen). In all three studies, most abscesses contained mixed aerobic and anaerobic flora (60% to 75%); the minority contained aerobic isolates only (10% to 20%) or anaerobic isolates only (15% to 20%). The number of anaerobic isolates always was greater than the number of aerobic isolates.

Bacteroides species are important microbes in the formation of IAA. A 1994 study suggested that the existence of specific repeating negatively and positively charged cell wall polysaccharides on *Bacteroides fragilis* leads to a host response that results in the formation of an IAA.[18] This host response is T cell–mediated and can be experimentally prevented by vaccination with these repeating polysaccharide units. Furthermore, this vaccination does not appear to be antigen specific in a traditional sense. Rather, the protective ability of these polysaccharides is conferred by, and perhaps specific for, a motif of oppositely charged groups.[19] Vaccination with *B. fragilis* capsular polysaccharide complex significantly reduced the mortality rate and intra-abdominal abscess formation in a rat cecal ligation and puncture model.[20] The cellular mechanism of intra-abdominal abscess formation by *B. fragilis* was elucidated in 1998.[21] *B. fragilis* capsular polysaccharide complex adheres to murine mesothelial cells (MMCs) and stimulates peritoneal macrophage tumor necrosis factor-α (TNF-α) production. This subsequently elicits significant intercellular adhesion molecule-1 (ICAM-1) expression by MMCs and enhances neutrophil attachment. Thus, the role of the capsular polysaccharide complex is to promote adhesion of *B. fragilis* to the peritoneal wall and coordinate the cellular events leading to the development of abscesses.

Table 24–2 | **Factors Influencing the Transition from Bacterial Contamination to Infection**

BACTERIAL FACTORS	ADJUVANT FACTORS	HOST DEFENSE FACTORS
Adherence capacity	Foreign material	Lymphatic clearance
Invasiveness	Fibrin	Peritoneal macrophages
Metabolic systems	Necrotic tissue	Neutrophil influx
Resistance to antibiotics	Fecal matter	Fibrin sequestration
Synergism	Blood	Lymphocyte response (omentum)

Adapted from Farthmann EH, Schoffel U: Epidemiology and pathophysiology of intraabdominal infections (IAI). Infection 26:329, 1998; and McClean KL, Sheehan GJ, Harding GK: Intraabdominal infection: A review. Clin Infect Dis 19:100, 1994.

The bacteria associated with intra-abdominal infections and abscesses in patients in the ICU who have been subjected to broad-spectrum antimicrobial selection pressure are quite different from those in patients with abscesses that result from secondary bacterial peritonitis. The microbiologic agents that cause *tertiary peritonitis*, defined as persistent intra-abdominal sepsis with or without a discrete focus of infection, generally after an operation for secondary peritonitis, are no longer *E. coli* and *B. fragilis*. Rather, nosocomial infections with resistant gram-negative organisms, *Enterococcus* species, and/or yeast are more common.[22, 23] The microbiologic analysis of abscesses in severely ill patients (Acute Physiology and Chronic Health Evaluation [APACHE] II score > 15) revealed that 38% had monomicrobial infections. The most common organisms were *Candida* (41%), *Enterococcus* (31%), and *Enterobacter* (21%) species and *Staphylococcus epidermidis* (21%); *E. coli* and *Bacteroides* species accounted for only 17% and 7%, respectively.[24]

Management

The optimal management of the patient with an IAA includes the following: (1) accurate diagnosis and localization of the collection, (2) removal or control of the source of peritoneal contamination, (3) drainage of any established collections, (4) elimination of residual contamination of the peritoneum through antimicrobial therapy, and (5) physiologic support of the patient.[11] The symptoms and signs of IAA are nonspecific, and a high level of vigilance is needed to make the diagnosis. Fever and elevated leukocyte count are common but nonspecific findings. Abdominal pain, tenderness to palpation, distention, and a palpable mass are also common findings.[25] Suspicion of the presence of an IAA warrants further diagnostic imaging.[7, 26, 27]

Diagnostic Imaging

COMPUTED TOMOGRAPHY. Computed tomography (CT) with intravenous and oral contrast medium is the imaging modality of choice for the diagnosis of most abdominal abscesses. Administration of intravenous contrast medium is useful to demonstrate the enhancing wall of an abscess and to define adjacent vascular anatomic characteristics clearly. Intravenous contrast medium is also necessary to evaluate completely for hepatic, splenic, or renal abscesses. Use of oral contrast medium is imperative to differentiate an abscess from fluid-filled unopacified bowel that may mimic an abscess. Ideally, oral contrast medium should be administered up to 2 hours prior to the study in order to opacify fully both small and large bowel. Inability to administer bowel contrast medium orally can limit the diagnostic ability of CT. If the patient is unable to drink oral contrast medium, contrast medium may be administered through a nasogastric tube or other enteric tube. Rectal contrast medium may also be administered if initial images are equivocal.

The CT diagnosis of abdominal abscess is suggested by identification of a fluid density that cannot be attributed to bowel or other known structure. Gas within an abdominal mass is highly suggestive of an abscess, although necrotic tumors and resolving hematomas may occasionally exhibit this finding. The presence of an enhancing wall and adjacent inflammatory changes is a finding that favors the likelihood of infection in fluid collections (Fig. 24–1). Any low-density fluid collection on CT should be clearly differentiated from unopacified bowel. Delayed images are often necessary to allow bowel to opacify fully and to allow the investigator to distinguish an abscess from bowel confidently. The fluid in an abscess may occasionally be higher in density when proteinaceous material is present or when the collection represents an infected hematoma. Phlegmonous inflammatory tissue does not exhibit fluid density; rather, it is solid in appearance, often with inhomogeneous enhancement.

In some cases, the CT appearance can suggest the cause of the abscess. Periappendiceal abscesses commonly have a typical location in the right lower quadrant adjacent to the cecum and often demonstrate an appendicolith (Fig. 24–2). Peridiverticular abscesses are often associated with an inflamed adjacent colon demonstrating diverticuli (Fig. 24–3).

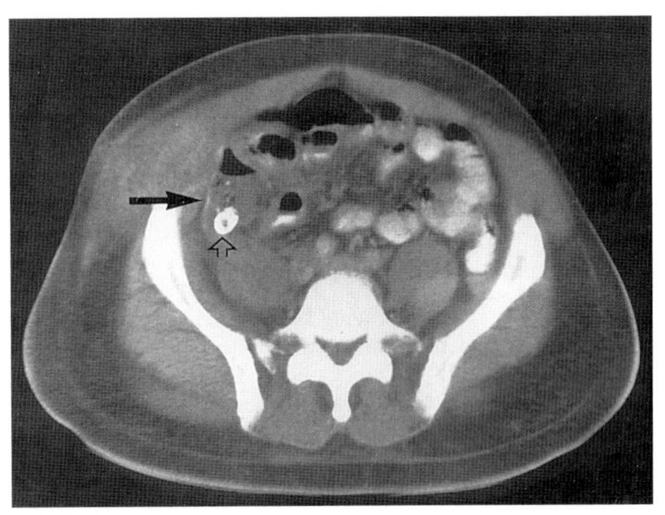

Figure 24–2. The computed tomographic scan demonstrates a right lower quadrant mass with an air fluid level *(closed arrow)* containing an appendicolith *(open arrow)* compatible with a periappendiceal abscess. Prominent inflammatory changes are noted in the adjacent right abdominal wall.

Abscesses associated with Crohn's disease may demonstrate adjacent thickened small bowel.

Although the CT appearance may strongly suggest an abscess, the diagnosis can only be made with certainty by obtaining a sample of the fluid through diagnostic aspiration. CT can be used to guide diagnostic aspiration or percutaneous abscess drainage and has advantages over other modalities in accurately identifying intervening structures.

ULTRASOUND. Ultrasound can be used to diagnose abdominal abscesses, particularly abscesses in the liver, spleen, or pelvis, because of the good visualization of these areas it provides. However, the usefulness of ultrasound can be limited in the midabdomen, where visualization is not optimal as a result of blocking of sound waves by bowel gas. Surgical dressings may also inhibit visualization by ultrasound. Unlike CT, portable ultrasonography can be performed and

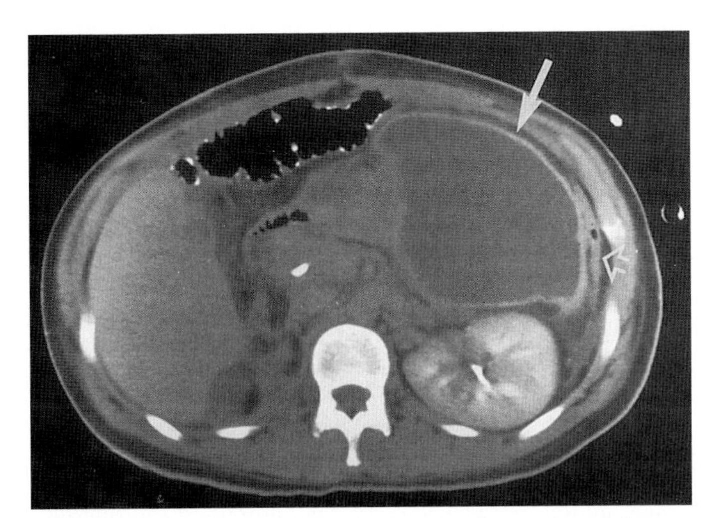

Figure 24–1. The computed tomographic scan shows a large left upper quadrant abscess *(closed arrow)* with an enhancing wall and mild adjacent inflammatory changes. The thin, collapsed bowel is noted laterally *(open arrow).*

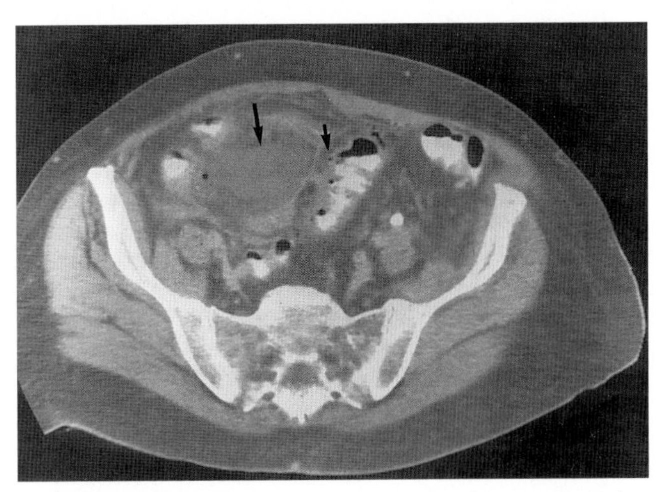

Figure 24–3. Peridiverticular abscess demonstrated by a computed tomographic scan showing a small interloop fluid collection *(long arrow)* with an adjacent thickened sigmoid colon with small diverticula *(short arrow).*

may be warranted in the initial imaging evaluation when patient condition precludes transportation.

The classic ultrasound appearance of an abscess is a localized rounded or oval area of decreased echogenicity with internal debris and a thick irregular wall (Fig. 24–4). Most abscesses exhibit fluid characteristics on ultrasound, but some may appear solid as a result of thick debris. Internal septations may be seen and are better identified by ultrasound than CT. Gas within an abscess is suggested when areas of increased echogenicity are present with posterior shadowing. The shadowing behind a gas collection tends to be less distinct than the more defined shadowing identified behind calculi on ultrasound. There is considerable overlap of the ultrasound appearance of infected and sterile fluid collections, and diagnostic aspiration is necessary to differentiate them. Ultrasound can be utilized for guidance during some percutaneous drainage procedures; however, poor visualization of intervening structures such as bowel in the midabdomen may limit its usefulness in some anatomic areas. Superficial and large abscesses tend to be more amenable to ultrasound guidance than smaller and deeper abscesses.

ABDOMINAL PLAIN FILMS. Abdominal films demonstrating nonspecific mass effect in a patient with a suspected abscess can suggest the diagnosis of an abdominal abscess. The diagnosis is further substantiated if air is visualized in an extraluminal location. A localized ileus may also be seen. The abdominal plain film is overall less sensitive than CT, and significant abscesses can be obscured by overlying normal structures.

CHEST RADIOGRAPHY. Sympathetic thoracic changes due to IAA may be demonstrated on chest radiography but are nonspecific. Abdominal abscesses can be associated with an elevated hemidiaphragm, pleural effusions, and atelectasis. Liver, splenic, and subphrenic abscesses are more likely to be associated with changes on chest radiograph than abscesses in the mid- and lower abdomen.

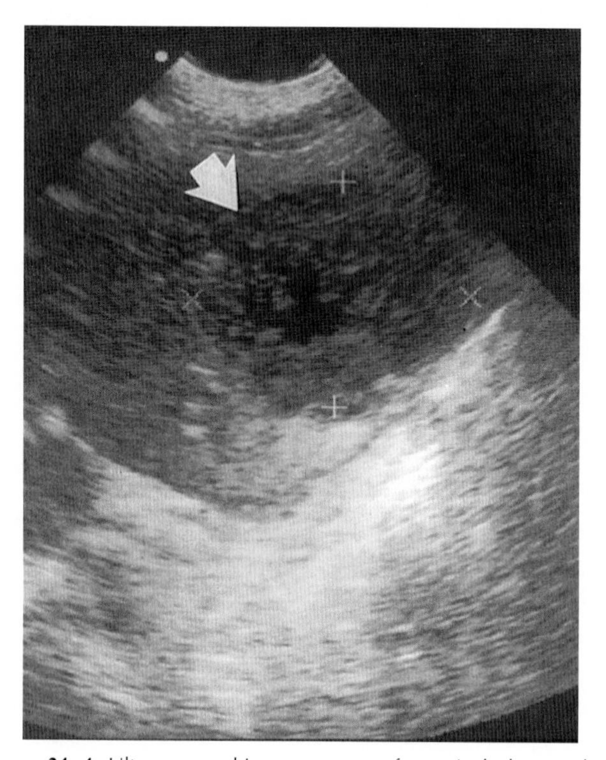

Figure 24–4. Ultrasonographic appearance of a typical abscess *(large arrow)* demonstrating central decreased echogenicity, thickened wall, and debris.

NUCLEAR IMAGING. Gallium 67 (^{67}Ga) nuclear imaging has been utilized to localize abscesses. However, uptake of ^{67}Ga is nonspecific for infection and can be demonstrated in tumors as well as within normal structures such as normal colon. Although indium 111 (^{111}In) labeled leukocyte scanning has a higher specificity for infection, the test is of limited usefulness in acute infections as a result of the time constraints of the imaging procedure. Initial images for ^{111}In–labeled leukocyte scans typically are not obtainable until 18 hours after administration of the tracer, and delayed images for up to 72 hours may be necessary to make the diagnosis. Nuclear imaging techniques are not a first-line diagnostic study for IAA but can be helpful in further clarifying equivocal findings seen on CT or ultrasound.

MAGNETIC RESONANCE IMAGING. Magnetic resonance imaging (MRI) has limited usefulness in the diagnosis of abdominal abscesses because of scan length, limited availability, cost, artifacts, and nonspecific findings. Fluid-filled bowel can be difficult to differentiate from an abscess on MRI. Oral contrast agents can be used in MRI to differentiate bowel from intra-abdominal abscess, but these agents are not widely used and are not of proven value for this application.

Mode of Drainage

Once an IAA is diagnosed and localized, a decision must be made regarding the optimal drainage technique and route. No controlled studies comparing percutaneous abscess drainage (PAD) and surgical drainage are available. For a simple, uniloculated, well-circumscribed abscess, PAD is successful 80% to 90% of the time.[28, 29] Assuming the availability of a safe route to the abscess that does not cause puncture of hollow viscera, as occurs in 85% to 90% of cases, PAD should be the drainage procedure of choice.[30] In complex, multiloculated, poorly organized abscesses, or when abscesses are multiple, interloop, or are intramesenteric, surgery should be strongly considered. This is because there is a higher failure rate with PAD techniques under these circumstances.[30] If surgery is chosen for any of the reasons indicated, an extraperitoneal approach is desirable to prevent contamination of the entire abdominal cavity.[5] In multiple abscesses or interloop abscesses, formal abdominal exploration is necessary.

PERCUTANEOUS ABSCESS DRAINAGE. Continuing advances in diagnostic imaging and percutaneous catheter development have allowed percutaneous catheter management of abdominal abscesses combined with systemic antibiotic therapy to become the standard initial treatment of abdominal abscesses in many institutions.[31, 32] The initial diagnostic imaging and the percutaneous drainage procedure can often be performed in the same session.

In order for an abdominal abscess to be amenable to PAD, careful selection criteria should be utilized. A safe percutaneous access route to the abscess cavity must be present. Bowel or adjacent organs cannot be traversed during PAD because of the risk of infecting or injuring these other structures. Major vascular structures should clearly be avoided because of the risk of hemorrhage. Coagulation studies and correction of any coagulopathy are often requested before the procedure to reduce the risk of uncontrollable hemorrhage. Although patients with multiple separate abscesses had been considered poor candidates for PAD, multiple drainage catheters are being increasingly utilized for management of multiple separate abdominal abscesses.

Some small fluid collections, typically less than 3 cm, may not accommodate a catheter. These fluid collections can be managed through percutaneous aspiration for diagnosis, followed by antibiotic therapy. One-step percutaneous needle aspiration of abdominal and pelvic abscesses combined with systemic antibiotics has also been advocated as an alternative to catheter placement in larger collections.[33] Data are limited to small series with success rates reported to vary from 60% to 90% of aspirations.[33, 34]

An inflammatory phlegmon without demonstrable fluid collection is not appropriate for percutaneous drainage. Whereas use of PAD procedures in patients with fistulas has been controversial in the past, rates of spontaneous closure up to 57% have been reported when aggressive catheter management has been combined with nutritional support.[35]

Multilocular and septated abscesses may not respond as well as unilocular collections. Urokinase has been utilized safely as an adjunct to PAD for some abscesses that are multilocular and have septa.[36]

If PAD is chosen as a drainage technique, guidance for PAD can be accomplished with several imaging modalities. The most common imaging modality utilized is CT, which more accurately demonstrates adjacent bowel and vasculature. Ultrasonography and fluoroscopy can also be utilized to guide PAD procedures in carefully selected cases, typically for larger and more superficial abscesses. The imaging modality selected is dependent on the location and size of the abscess as well as operator preference.

The imaging modality selected for guidance is utilized to identify a safe percutaneous route. Then the abscess cavity is accessed through either a trocar method or a guidewire method. The guidewire method utilizes an initial needle placement followed by a guidewire. The tract is then dilated to a diameter approximating the diameter of the planned catheter, and the catheter is placed. A sump-type double-lumen catheter is the most common catheter employed. A 12 or 14 French catheter size is generally adequate to drain most abscesses. Larger catheter size may be necessary for an abscess associated with a large amount of debris or hemorrhage.[32]

The catheter position should be confirmed by repeat imaging to ensure all catheter sideholes are within the abscess. The cavity is generally aspirated dry, followed by sterile saline solution flushing to clear any residual debris. The catheter is then placed to suction drainage. A sample of the fluid is generally saved for Gram stain and culture.

POSTCATHETERIZATION MANAGEMENT. The catheter is flushed daily with sterile saline solution to maintain patency. Catheter output and character should be documented daily. Clinical status should be monitored for adequate response by assessing temperature and by making periodic leukocyte counts.

Decisions to obtain follow-up imaging studies depend on the clinical response, catheter drainage, and presence of suspected enteric communications. If the clinical response has been satisfactory and the catheter drainage has diminished to less than 15 to 20 mL per day, the catheter can be safely removed. If clinical response is inadequate, repeat imaging is warranted. Persistently high catheter output raises suspicion of a fistula. A catheter study performed by instilling water-soluble contrast medium through the catheter under fluoroscopy is the best method to assess for an internal fistula as the cause of high drainage output. If a fistula is located, the catheter can be repositioned adjacent to the opening into the bowel for better control of bowel effluent. Poor clinical response can also be caused by catheter dislodgment from the major abscess cavity, multiple abscesses, or new abscesses. Repeat CT can evaluate for these possible causes of poor clinical response. Thick debris may occlude the catheter and inhibit daily flushing. In this circumstance, the catheter can be exchanged for a larger catheter, if warranted.[31, 32]

COMPLICATIONS OF PERCUTANEOUS ABSCESS DRAINAGE. The complication rate of PAD is close to 10%.[31] Complications include transient sepsis, organ injury, hemorrhage, pneumothorax, peritonitis, empyema, and pain.[31]

Special Considerations for Percutaneous Management of Selected Abscesses

SUBPHRENIC ABSCESSES. Subphrenic abscesses can be drained percutaneously with careful attention to technique (Fig. 24–5). Avoidance of the pleural space is optimal to prevent seeding of infection to the chest. The pleural space typically extends to the level of the eighth thoracic vertebra (T8) anteriorly, T10 laterally, and T12 posteriorly.[37] These guidelines can be utilized to prevent traversing of the pleural space. Some subphrenic fluid collections may not allow an extrapleural approach, in which case surgical alternatives should be weighed against the increased risk of transpleural drainage. The safety of a transpleural approach has been debated.[37, 38]

PELVIC ABSCESSES. Anterior access to pelvic abscesses can be limited by intervening bowel, bladder, uterus, or vascular structures. A posterior transgluteal approach through the sciatic notch with the patient in the prone position has been utilized to drain deep pelvic fluid collections that are not accessible to an anterior approach (Fig. 24–6). Care must be taken to avoid the gluteal vasculature and the sciatic nerve. Ultrasound guided transvaginal and transrectal drainage techniques have also been increasingly utilized for drainage of deep pelvic abscesses that are not accessible through other routes.[39, 40] Comparison of transrectal and transvaginal techniques has demonstrated better patient tolerance of the transrectal drainage route.[41]

APPENDICEAL ABSCESSES. Periappendiceal abscesses can often be suggested by the CT appearance. The typical appearance is a low-density fluid collection in the right lower quadrant adjacent to the cecum, often containing an appendicolith. Percutaneous abscess drainage has been increasingly

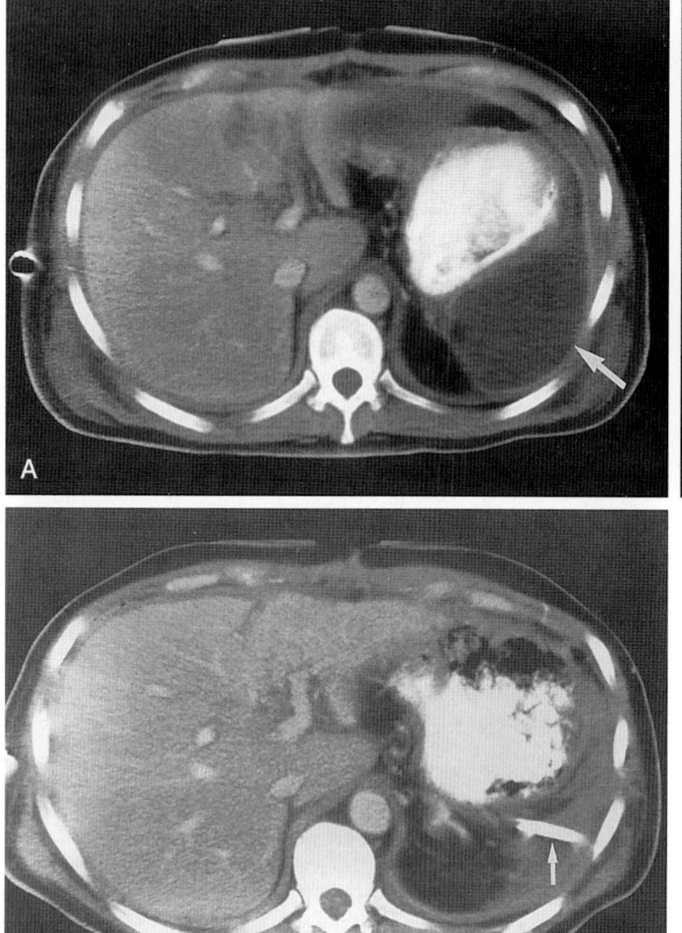

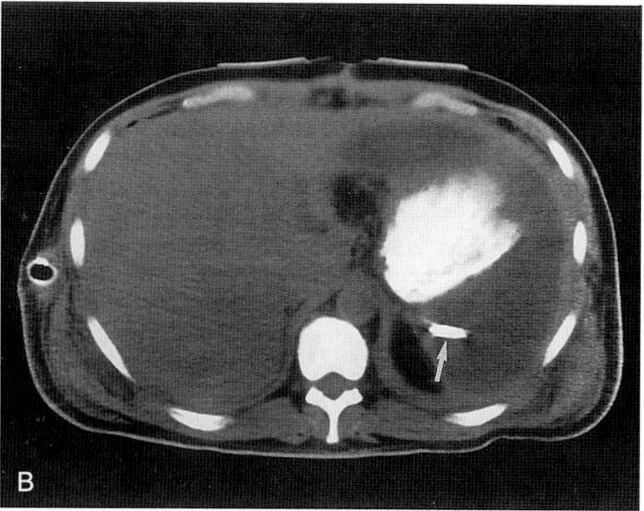

Figure 24–5. *A,* The computed tomographic (CT) scan demonstrates a left subphrenic abscess post-splenectomy *(arrow)*. *B,* A catheter is placed within the same abscess. *C,* A CT scan several days later demonstrates the catheter in the subphrenic space *(arrow)* with no residual abscess. The catheter was subsequently removed.

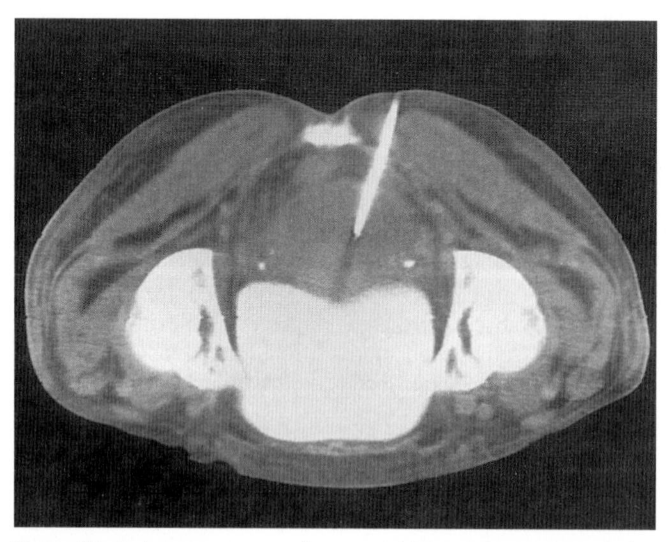

Figure 24–6. A prone computed tomographic scan demonstrates catheter placement through the sciatic notch into a deep pelvic abscess.

accepted as initial management of sepsis associated with a periappendiceal abscess, allowing the surgeon to perform a subsequent appendectomy, often laparoscopically, on an elective basis (Fig. 24–7).[32]

PERIDIVERTICULAR ABSCESSES. Percutaneous drainage of peridiverticular abscesses has also been increasingly accepted. Drainage can allow initial temporization of symptoms, followed by a one-stage surgical procedure rather than a two-stage procedure.[32]

Antibiotic Selection in Treatment of Abdominal Abscesses

Elimination of residual infection within the peritoneum is carried out by the use of antibiotics. In general, antibiotics are only effective after an abscess has been drained. This is due to a number of factors, including poor penetration of antibiotics into abscess cavities,[42, 43] very high bacterial counts within the abscess cavity ($>10^8$ colony-forming units [CFUs]/mL) that may alter bactericidal activity,[44] and the fact that pus has an acidic pH and low pO_2 from necrotic tissue and a poor blood supply[45]—all of which make use of antibiotics without abscess drainage generally ineffective.

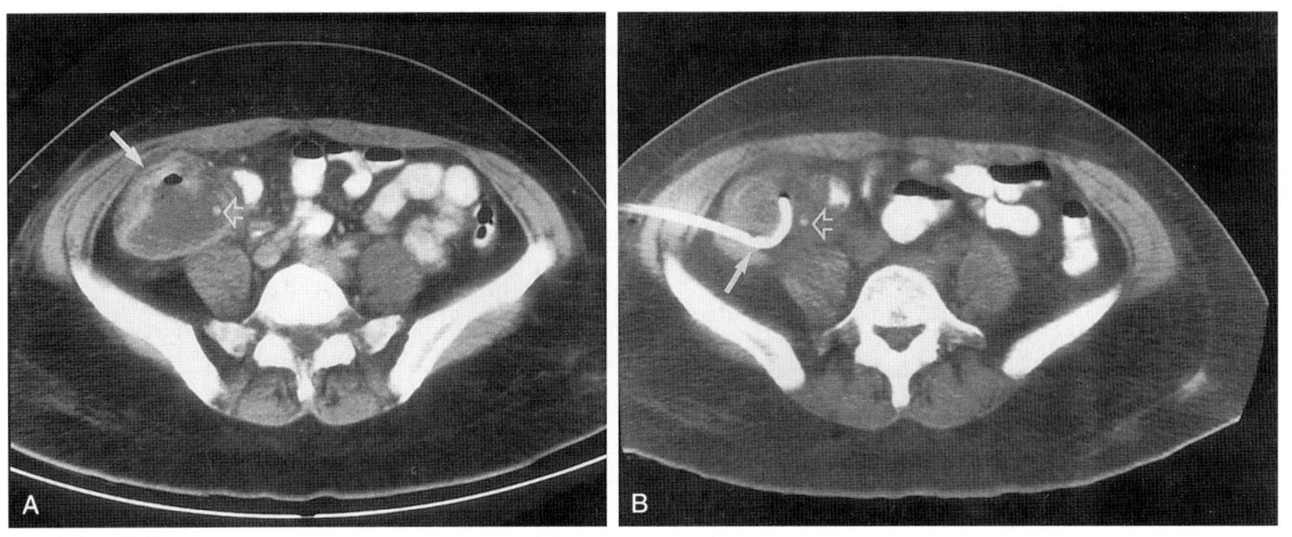

Figure 24–7. *A,* The computed tomographic scan demonstrates a right lower quadrant abscess *(closed arrow)* with a subtle appendicolith *(open arrow)* in the medial aspect. *B,* The same patient after a PAD catheter was placed *(closed arrow).* Resolution of the abscess has occurred. The appendicolith *(open arrow)* is seen medial to the catheter.

After abscess drainage, the initial choice of antibiotic should be based on the clinical picture and Gram stain findings of the abscess fluid. In an otherwise healthy individual who has a secondary bacterial peritonitis or abscess, antibiotic selection should be directed to the common organisms isolated from that type of abscess—primarily coliforms such as *E. coli* and anaerobes such as *B. fragilis*. This selection could be a second-generation cephalosporin, β-lactamase inhibitor—extended-spectrum penicillin derivative combination, or combination therapy with an aminoglycoside and antianaerobe. Because of significant resistance of *B. fragilis* to clindamycin, the antianaerobe of choice is metronidazole.[46] Studies in 1996, 1997, and 1999 documented the equivalence of broad-spectrum single-agent regimens such as carbapenems, meropenem, or imipenem/cilastatin; extended-spectrum penicillin–β-lactamase inhibitor combinations; and piperacillin/tazobactam and third-generation cephalosporin/metronidazole combinations (Table 24–3).[25, 47–49]

In a severely ill patient with postoperative tertiary peritonitis and an elevated APACHE II score, the choice of empirical therapy can be more difficult. As noted earlier, abscesses in this population are often monomicrobial. Therefore, the results of the Gram stain can be of great importance in choosing initial antibiotics. Because many of these patients have already been exposed to broad-spectrum antibiotics, antibiotic selection must be made with knowledge of previous prescriptions and information on the resistance patterns within the ICU in which the patient is housed. Attention must also be paid to the underlying organ dysfunction of any individual patient, which can also affect antibiotic selection (i.e., the use of aminoglycosides in the setting of renal dysfunction should be avoided). In renal dysfunction broad-spectrum gram-negative coverage with a desirable sensitivity pattern should be considered. This would include a choice of carbapenems, extended-spectrum penicillins, or fluoroquinolones as appropriate therapy. Combination with a β-lactamase inhibitor is desirable under these circumstances. If gram-positive organisms are found on Gram stain, vancomycin therapy should be strongly considered for the treatment of potential *Enterococcus* species or methicillin-resistant *Staphylococcus* species.

There is continued debate over the proper treatment of *Enterococcus* species isolated from IAA fluid. Although no definitive conclusions are indicated in the literature, in an otherwise healthy population with minimal comorbid condi-

Table 24–3 | **Antibiotic Choices in the Treatment of Intra-abdominal Infection**

SINGLE-AGENT THERAPY	
Second-generation cephalosporins, *Bacteroides* species–active	
Cefoxitin sodium (Mefoxin)	
Cefotetan disodium (Cefotan)	
Carbapenems	
Meropenem (Merrem)	
Imipenem/cilastatin sodium (Primaxin)	
Extended-spectrum penicillin/β-lactamase inhibitor combinations	
Ampicillin sodium/sulbactam sodium (Unasyn)	
Ticarcillin disodium/clavulanate potassium (Timentin)	
Piperacillin sodium /tazobactam sodium (Zosyn)	
COMBINATION THERAPY	
Antiaerobe	**Antianaerobe**
Aminoglycosides	Metronidazole (Flagyl)
Tobramycin (several brands)	Clindamycin phosphate (Cleocin)
Gentamicin (several brands)	
Third-generation cephalosporins	
Ceftriaxone sodium (Rocephin)	
Cefotaxime sodium (Claforan)	
Cefotaxime sodium (Cefizox)	
Ceftazidime (several brands)*	
Cefoperazone sodium (Cefobid)	
Fluoroquinolones	
Ciprofloxacin (Cipro)	
Levofloxacin (Levaquin)	
Fourth-generation cephalosporins	
Cefepime hydrochloride (Maxipime)	

*Pseudomonal coverage.

Table 24–4 | **Reasons for Treatment Failure in Intra-abdominal Abscess**

Inadequate drainage of initial collection
New intra-abdominal collection
Incorrect initial antibiotic selection and/or dosage
Development of antibiotic resistance of previous susceptible organism
New bacterial organism not initially isolated
Fungal superinfection

tions data from 1990, 1996, and 1997 support an antibiotic selection that does not specifically cover *Enterococcus* species.[25, 49, 50] This conclusion is based on the high success rate of regimens that do not have anti–*Enterococcus* species coverage, which is as high as that of regimens that do have anti-*Enterococcus* coverage. For a patient in the ICU who has an elevated APACHE II score, the isolation of *Enterococcus* species takes on a different meaning from that noted. Several studies have shown that in a population of patients with an elevated APACHE II score, comorbid conditions, and early organ dysfunction, *Enterococcus* species isolation is an independent risk factor for treatment failure.[51, 52] Here, anti–*Enterococcus* species therapy is an important part of antibiotic selection. Combination therapy with a cell wall specific antibiotic such as ampicillin in conjunction with an aminoglycoside has been shown to be synergistic as anti–*Enterococcus* species therapy.[53] Recent development of resistance to β-lactam antibiotics as well as aminoglycosides has led to increasing use of vancomycin as anti–*Enterococcus* species therapy. This use, unfortunately, has led to the development of new strains of *Enterococcus* species that carry plasmids encoding for vancomycin resistance (VRE).

Once the organism has been identified and its sensitivity pattern reported, antibiotic selection can be focused. It is important to follow the patient's response to abscess drainage and antibiotics. Continued deterioration with repeated fever and white blood cell count elevation should prompt a search for an explanation (Table 24–4). Repeat CT scanning is warranted in that situation to look for an area of undrained infection.[26, 27] A second cause of a poor response is microbial resistance to the antibiotic selection. Thought must be given to broadening the antibiotic selection further in this case. A final reason for poor response to therapy is the possibility of fungal superinfection.[54, 55] As noted earlier, *Candida* species infections constitute approximately 20% to 40% of infections in the setting of postoperative tertiary peritonitis.[23, 24] For high-risk surgical patients with intra-abdominal infections, data support the use of fluconazole prophylaxis, which prevented invasive intra-abdominal *Candida* species infections and resulting sepsis in this group of patients with complicated conditions.[56] *Candida* species are notoriously difficult to culture from blood and deep tissues. When they are isolated in this population, they should be aggressively treated with a systemic antifungal agent, either amphotericin B or fluconazole.

Duration of antibiotic therapy depends on the underlying patient condition as well as the adequacy of, and response to, invasive drainage techniques. Two studies have evaluated the risk of recurrent sepsis after the termination of antibiotics.[57, 58] In the group of patients who were afebrile with a persistent leukocytosis at the end of therapy there was a 33% recurrence rate of IAA. When both fever and leukocytosis were present, recurrent IAA occurred in 57%. However, when the patient was afebrile and had a normal leukocyte count there was no IAA recurrence.[58] These data, which were confirmed in 1998 and 1999,[59, 60] suggest that antimicrobial treatment of IAA be continued until the patient has a normal leukocyte count and is afebrile.

Outcome

Outcome after treatment of IAA is dependent on a number of factors. The mortality rate has been reported to range from less than 5% for simple secondary bacterial peritonitis to around 65% or higher for complicated tertiary peritonitis.[6, 22, 23, 36, 52, 60–62] Simple abscesses associated with perforated appendicitis that respond to surgical drainage and antibiotics have a low mortality rate. Higher mortality rates occur in elderly patients, those who have complex abscesses, those who have high APACHE II and multiple organ dysfunction (MOD) scores, and those who use steroids.[22, 23, 62] Other risk factors include multiple reoperations to control intra-abdominal sepsis, malnutrition, poor physiologic reserve, high New York Heart Association class, and multiple organ dysfunction syndrome (MODS).[61] Patients who show evidence of MODS have a particularly poor outcome, which has been thought to be secondary to inability to control intra-abdominal infection. However, a report in 1998 suggested that continued intra-abdominal infection is another manifestation of organ failure and not a cause[23]; that is, patients die *with* infection, not *of* infection. Aggressive surgical, antibiotic, and supportive care is required in this group of patients. Future treatment strategies that may include immunomodulatory therapies may be needed before significant improvements in outcome are realized for patients who have this difficult surgical problem.

GASTROINTESTINAL FISTULAS

Definitions and Classifications

The strict definition of a *fistula* is any abnormal anatomic connection between two epithelialized surfaces. This definition includes many clinical entities. Because of this fact, fistulas are generally classified by anatomic and physiologic methods.[63] Anatomic classifications rely upon sites of fistula origin and drainage point. Inherent in this anatomic classification system is whether the fistula is internal or external. Physiologic classifications rely upon fistula output in a 24-hour period (Table 24–5). Both fistula classifications are used clinically when describing a fistulous tract (e.g., a high-output enterocutaneous fistula).

Table 24–5 | **Fistula Classification**

ANATOMIC	PHYSIOLOGIC
Internal	High output
(e.g., ileocolic, colovesical)	>500 mL/day
External	Moderate output
(e.g., enterocutaneous)	200–500 mL/day
	Low output
	<200 mL/day

Compared with fistulas connected to the skin that are obvious, internal fistulas may be difficult to diagnose, depending on the organs involved. This would be the case, for example, in a cholecystoduodenal fistula, which might first be manifested by gallstone ileus. However, in a colovesical fistula the presenting signs are urinary tract infection, fecaluria, and pneumaturia. Fistulas arising in the abdomen can originate from any epithelialized surface of a hollow viscus or drainage duct within the GI or genitourinary (GU) tract, liver, or pancreas. This chapter focuses on GI fistulas; for specific discussions of fistulas arising from the biliary or pancreatic duct, see Chapters 48, 49, and 55 respectively.

Pathophysiology

GI fistulas can occur either spontaneously or postoperatively. Spontaneous fistulas account for 15% to 25% of fistulas and arise in association with inflammatory processes, cancer, and radiation treatment.[64–73] Inflammatory processes include diverticulitis, inflammatory bowel disease, peptic ulcer disease, and appendicitis. These fistulas can be internal or external and, depending on cause and anatomic variations, have different rates of spontaneous closure. The remaining 75% to 85% of fistulas are almost always postoperative, external, and iatrogenic in origin.[74–79] These fistulas occur in cancer surgery, emergency surgery in which bowel cannot be adequately prepared and cleansed, trauma surgery in which injuries may be missed, and reoperative surgery in which extensive lysis of adhesions and partial-thickness bowel injury occur. Adjuncts to formation of either spontaneous or postoperative fistulas include malnutrition, sepsis, shock/hypotension, vasopressor therapy, glucocorticoid therapy, associated disease states, and technical difficulties with a surgical anastomosis.[76, 80–83]

It is important to determine the cause of fistula formation because it often determines therapy. Fistulas that arise in inflammatory bowel disease or direct involvement of intestinal cancer are unlikely to close spontaneously and often require surgical correction. On the other hand, a postoperative low-output fistula arising from a partial anastomotic dehiscence frequently closes with appropriate conservative management. Conditions associated with nonhealing of GI fistulas are listed in Table 24–6.[35, 64, 67, 73, 80, 84–93]

Diagnosis

Once a fistula is suspected, early management should be directed to confirming the diagnosis. The anatomic site of origin and underlying cause can be determined when the

Table 24–6 | **Conditions Associated with Nonhealing Fistulas***

Foreign body within the fistula tract (see Chapter 21)
Radiation enteritis within the affected bowel (see Chapter 102)
Infection/inflammation at the fistula origin
Epithelialization of the fistula tract
Neoplasm at the fistula origin
Distal obstruction of intestine

*The acronym *FRIEND* can be used to remember these conditions.

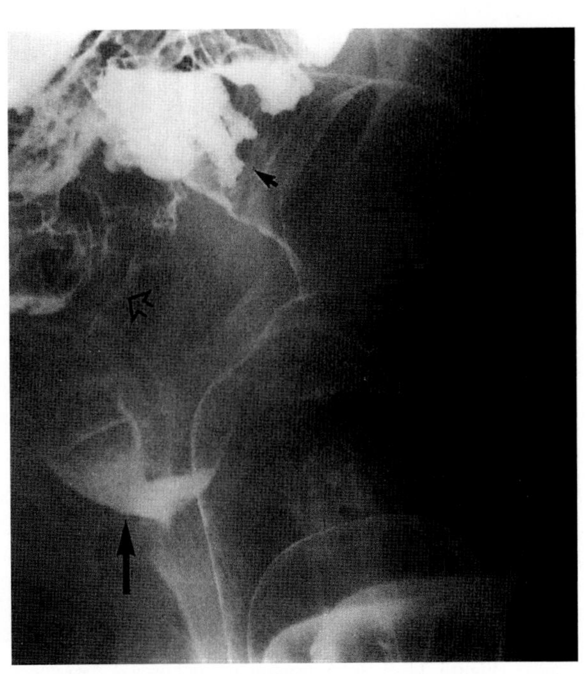

Figure 24–8. A lateral view of the rectosigmoid region on a barium enema. A colovesical fistula *(open arrow)* secondary to diverticulitis is present. Diverticular disease *(short closed arrow)* can be seen in the sigmoid colon. The bladder is shown with contrast drainage from the barium enema *(long closed arrow)*.

patient's condition is stabilized. One simple bedside maneuver to confirm the presence of an external fistula as the cause of suspicious postoperative wound drainage is to give the patient either methylene blue or charcoal orally. The fistula can then be confirmed by the presence of the dye in the suspicious drainage. Once fistula is confirmed, exact anatomic origins can be determined by radiographic dye studies. These studies can include administration of contrast medium orally or rectally (depending on the site of suspicion) to define the site of origin via the bowel lumen (Fig. 24–8). Alternatively, dye can be injected retrograde into the drainage site (fistulogram) and followed to its site of origin within the bowel (Fig. 24–9). Internal fistulas can be diagnosed by injecting contrast medium into one hollow viscus (e.g., urinary bladder) with opacification of another viscus (e.g., rectosigmoid) (Fig. 24–10).

Management

Treatment may be nonsurgical or surgical. Generally, nonsurgical treatment is the cornerstone of the early management strategy when treating GI fistulas (Table 24–7). Once a diagnosis of an enterocutaneous fistula is confirmed (e.g., with enteral charcoal), early management is directed to fluid and electrolyte replacement. This can be a daunting task if the fistula has a high output (>500 mL/day; see Table 24–5). Output in excess of 1000 mL/day is not uncommon if the fistula originates in the proximal small bowel. In order to prevent intravascular volume depletion and electrolyte imbalance, fluid and electrolyte replacement must be a first priority and should be addressed before more detailed diagnostic fistula studies are undertaken. Administration of replacement fluids should take into account the volume as well as the

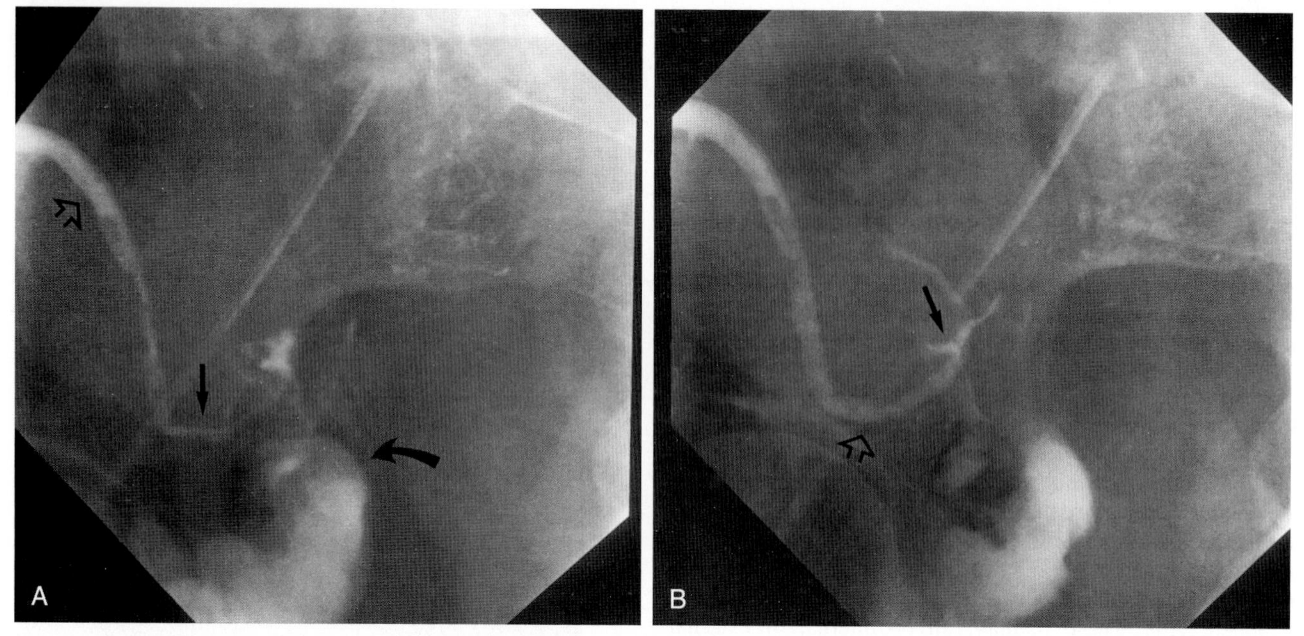

Figure 24–9. *A,* A fistulogram performed through a percutaneous catheter *(open arrow)* demonstrates a fistulous tract *(straight closed arrow)* from the small bowel *(curved closed arrow)* to the skin. *B,* The same patient with the catheter *(open arrow)* advanced near to the opening in the small bowel *(closed arrow).*

electrolyte content lost through the fistula. Generally, fistula output is iso-osmotic and high in potassium. Therefore, output should be replaced milliliter for milliliter with a balanced salt solution that contains added potassium. If difficulties are met in managing electrolyte imbalances, a sample of fistula fluid can be sent to the laboratory for electrolyte determination. Subsequent electrolyte replacement can then be formulated on the basis of laboratory results.

A second cornerstone of the early management strategy in the treatment of enterocutaneous fistulas is establishment of

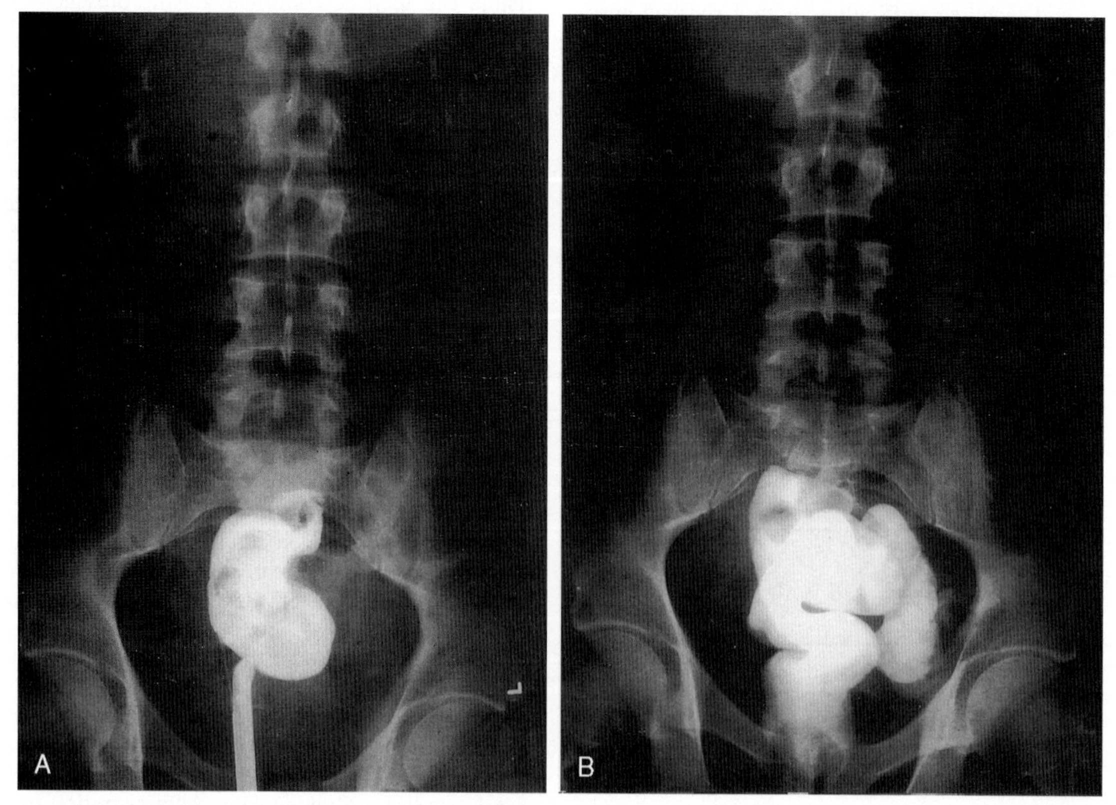

Figure 24–10. A rectovesical fistula in a patient with Crohn's disease, pneumaturia, and urinary tract infection. *A,* A catheter in the bladder with contrast beginning to fill the bowel. *B,* Contrast has filled the sigmoid colon and the rectum through the fistulous tract.

Table 24–7 | **Early Goals in the Management of New Enterocutaneous Fistulas**

Restore intravascular volume
Correct electrolyte imbalances
Correct acid-base disturbances
Initiate enterostomal therapy to protect skin
Institute bowel rest with nasogastric suction
Provide nutritional support
Control sepsis
Establish adequate drainage (percutaneous vs. surgical drainage)

adequate drainage of external fistulas. This may require minor surgical maneuvers such as opening a recent surgical incision to allow adequate drainage. As noted, percutaneous catheters are often essential in obtaining a controlled fistula. This point requires early attention because if a fistula cannot be controlled, pooling of fistula contents within the abdominal cavity can lead to infection with abscess formation and sepsis. Because most enterocutaneous fistulas occur postoperatively, some ingenuity may be required when trying to protect the skin from the caustic effects of the fistula output. Most postoperative enterocutaneous fistulas decompress through the surgical incision. As the incision shows signs of infection and drainage, it must be opened. A reopened incision that is draining intestinal contents is not amenable to simple placement of an ostomy bag to collect the drainage. An experienced enterostomal therapist should be consulted when dealing with this difficult problem.

Once the patient's condition is stabilized from the fluid and electrolyte perspective and the fistula is adequately drained, attention is turned to anatomic/diagnostic considerations to plan further therapy. Table 24–8 lists some of the prognostic factors important in determining whether the fistula has a high or low rate of spontaneous closure. Spontaneous fistula closure is more likely for low-output fistulas, fistulas secondary to surgical complications, and fistulas arising anatomically in the proximal small intestine. Well-nourished patients without infectious complications are also more likely to experience spontaneous closing.[63, 94, 95] When spontaneous closure is likely, nutritional support must be aggressively pursued. The causes of malnutrition in the patient with a GI fistula are multifactorial, including underlying disease states, lack of protein intake, protein losses through the fistula, and underlying sepsis with hypercatabolism.

Table 24–8 | **Prognostic Indicators of Successful Spontaneous Fistula Closure**

	SPONTANEOUS CLOSURE MORE LIKELY	SURGICAL CLOSURE MORE LIKELY
Output (mL/day)	<500	>500
Age (yr)	<40	>65
Site	Proximal small bowel	Distal small bowel or colon
Nutritional status	Well nourished	Malnourished
Cause	Anastomotic breakdown	Malignancy, inflammatory or infectious disease, complete anastomotic dehiscence
Anatomic characteristics	Long fistulous tract	Distal obstruction, eversion of mucosa
Duration	Acute	Chronic

Adapted from Berry SM, Fischer JE: Enterocutaneous fistulas. Curr Probl Surg 31:469, 1994; and Rombeau JL, Rolandelli RH: Enteral and parenteral nutrition in patients with enteric fistulas and short bowel syndrome. Surg Clin North Am 67: 551, 1987.

Total parenteral nutrition (TPN) seems to be the natural first choice in a patient with an enterocutaneous fistula. Soon after diagnosis aggressive caloric support must be given. Once the anatomic origin of the fistula is determined, route of feeding is considered. Data from 1989 suggest that not all patients must be placed on TPN. In a study of 335 patients with external fistulas, 85% were managed solely with enteral feedings. In a subgroup of uncomplicated fistulas, 50% healed spontaneously with this mode of nutritional therapy alone.[79] Enteral feeding has been shown to enhance mucosal proliferation of villous growth through both direct and indirect mechanisms. Nutrients in contact with the bowel mucosa provide direct stimulation to the enterocyte, and feedings high in glutamine may be particularly beneficial because glutamine is the main source of energy of the enterocyte.[96] Second, nutrients within the gut lumen release gut-derived hormones that have an indirect trophic effect on the intestinal mucosa. TPN, in contrast, has been shown to lead to gut mucosal atrophy. This may be in part due to the fact that standard TPN solutions do not contain glutamine because glutamine crystallizes out of solution. Despite the recent advances in enteral feeding of patients with GI fistulas, TPN remains the mainstay of nutritional support for most patients due to inability to absorb sufficient calories enterally.[97] In one study, Rose and associates reviewed 114 consecutive patients with GI fistulas all treated with TPN and conservative therapy.[72] They found that 61% of the fistulas closed spontaneously in an average of 26 days. The remainder continued to surgical extirpation of the fistulous tract.

The decision to support the patient with a GI fistula with enteral or parenteral nutrition has to be based on anatomic and physiologic considerations. If the fistula has a low output and is anatomically distal in the intestine, then a trial of enteral feedings should be pursued. If the fistula is in the proximal intestine and distal access to the intestine has been established, as is the case in many postoperative fistulas in which a feeding jejunostomy has been placed at the time of surgery, then enteral feeding into the distal bowel should be considered. Along with this, infusion of the proximal fistula drainage into the distal bowel should be considered. Reinfusion of succus entericus into the distal bowel has been shown to make fluid and electrolyte management easier, as well as decrease the output of the proximal fistula.[98, 99] It is not mandatory to provide full nutritional support via the enteral route to get the benefits of enteral feeding. Protein and caloric requirements can be supplemented by TPN.

Another potential adjunct to TPN in the management of the patient with a GI fistula is the use of the long-acting somatostatin analog octreotide. Octreotide has been shown to decrease fistula output by three mechanisms. First, it inhibits the release of gastrin, cholecystokinin, secretin, motilin, and other GI hormones. This inhibition decreases secretion of bicarbonate, water, and pancreatic enzymes into the intestine, subsequently decreasing intestinal volume. Second, octreotide relaxes intestinal smooth muscle, thereby allowing for a greater intestinal capacity. Third, octreotide increases intestinal water and electrolyte absorption.[100]

Initial studies evaluating the effect of octreotide on spontaneous intestinal fistula closure were either uncontrolled (or used historical controls) or unblinded.[78, 79, 101–103] These studies suggested that octreotide decreased fistula output by 55% to 94%, led to spontaneous fistula closure rates of approximately 75% to 80% of patients enrolled, decreased time to spontaneous closure to 4 to 14 days, and reduced mortality rate to 2.5% to 7%. Randomized, placebo-controlled, double-blind studies using strict entry criteria had less favorable findings for octreotide.[104–106] These studies, which had relatively small group sizes, showed no significant effects of octreotide in fistula closure rate, complication rate, or mortality rate. One study did show an improvement in healing time with octreotide.[106] At this time, the role of octreotide in the treatment of GI fistulas has not been fully defined, and octreotide cannot be recommended outside the confines of controlled studies.

Historically, conservative management of fistulas associated with Crohn's disease has been uniformly unrewarding, as most abdominal and perianal fistulas required surgical correction. However, developments in 1996 showed that production of TNF-α in the intestinal mucosa is increased in patients with Crohn's disease.[107] This finding has led to the development and clinical investigation of chimeric monoclonal antibodies against TNF-α (infliximab [Remicade]) in the

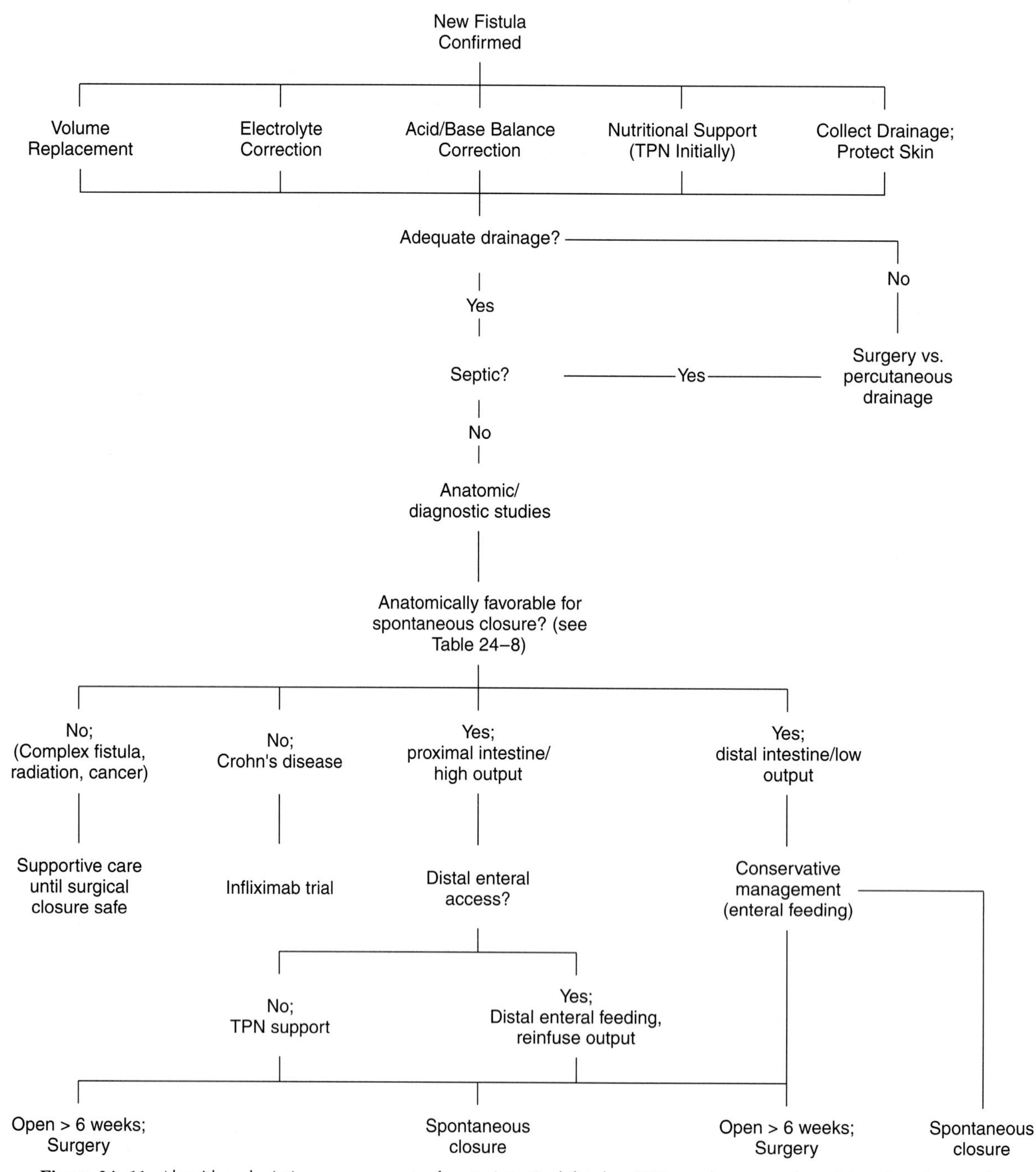

Figure 24–11. Algorithm depicting management of gastrointestinal fistulas. TPN, total parenteral nutrition. See the text for an explanation.

treatment of Crohn's disease.[108] In a randomized multicenter double-blind, placebo-controlled trial of 94 Crohn's disease patients with draining abdominal or perianal fistulas of at least 3 months' duration, 68% of patients receiving infliximab (5 mg/kg) compared with 26% of patients receiving placebo ($P = .002$) had at least a 50% reduction in draining fistulas. Furthermore, 55% of patients receiving infliximab had closure of all fistulas as compared with 13% of patients assigned to the placebo group.[109] Infliximab's salutary effects appear to be transient in most patients,[110] and infliximab's role in long-term therapy is still under investigation. In terms of these data, in the initial management of fistulas in Crohn's disease a trial of infliximab should be considered. Fistula formation in Crohn's disease is discussed in greater detail in Chapter 103.

Another nonoperative approach to the management of refractory fistulas includes the percutaneous and endoscopic use of fibrin glue and other occlusive plugs. Although reports are limited to case series at this time, a variety of techniques, including fistuloscopy, fluoroscopy, and endoscopy, have been used to cannulate fistula tracts.[111-113] Once cannulated, the tracts are débrided, then occluded with fibrin glue, collagen plugs, or gelatin sponges. Results have been encouraging in the small series evaluated, and the technique may serve as a useful adjunct for fistulas refractory to conservative management.

Surgical therapy remains the mainstay of management of the complex fistula that either is not a candidate for conservative management or has had a prolonged course of conservative management (4 to 6 weeks) without resolution of fistulous output.[91, 94] Indications for early surgery include inability to control the fistula without surgical drainage, sepsis or abscess formation, distal intestinal obstruction, bleeding, and persistence of fistulous output not responsive to conservative management. Some more complex fistulas may require surgery to remove mesh or other foreign bodies before closure can be undertaken. The goal of surgical therapy is to resect the involved bowel and restore intestinal continuity.[91] This surgery allows the patient to start eating through normal routes. Minimally invasive surgery was shown to be an option in selected patients in the surgical management of intestinal fistulas in 1997.[114]

Outcome Associated with Intestinal Fistulas

Early morbidity and mortality result from initial fluid and electrolyte derangements that are unchecked. However, the major cause of mortality in patients with GI fistulas is sepsis with multiple organ failure. The typical setting for septic complications is provided by complex fistulas for which there is inadequate or uncontrolled drainage. In this setting, pooling of enteric contents occurs within the abdominal cavity and acts as a nidus of infection. Therefore, as noted, aggressive attempts must be made to ensure that fistulous drainage is well controlled. The mortality rate from sepsis in patients with fistulas ranges from 15% to 30%.[77, 82, 86, 94, 115] Higher mortality rates are seen in those who are malnourished, have had previous irradiation therapy or have complex fistulas associated with a postoperative abdominal wall dehiscence. A second major cause of mortality in patients with GI fistulas is severe underlying disease, most often cancer. Often patients who are terminally ill secondary to malignancy forgo further operative procedures.[92]

Algorithm

GI fistulas remain a major complication of surgery. Although innovative therapy and supportive care have resulted in improving spontaneous closure rates, management of these difficult problems requires a multidisciplinary approach that includes a nutritional support service, enterostomal therapist, surgeon, invasive radiologist, and gastroenterologist. An algorithm to manage GI fistulas based on this chapter is presented in Figure 24–11.

REFERENCES

1. Farthmann EH, Schoffel U: Epidemiology and pathophysiology of intraabdominal infections (IAI). Infection 26:329, 1998.
2. Kokoska ER, Silen ML, Tracey TF Jr, et al: Perforated appendicitis in children: Risk factors for the development of complications. Surgery 124:619, 1998.
3. Reid RI, Dobbs BR, Frizelle FA: Risk factors for post-appendectomy intra-abdominal abscess. Aust N Z J Surg 69:373, 1999.
4. Stollman NH, Raskin JB: Diagnosis and management of diverticular disease of the colon in adults. Am J Gastroenterol 94:3110, 1999.
5. Fang JF, Chen RJ, Lin BC, et al: Retroperitoneal laparostomy: An effective treatment of extensive intractable retroperitoneal abscess after blunt duodenal trauma. J Trauma 46:652, 1999.
6. Abikhaled JA, Granchi TS, Wall MJ, et al: Prolonged abdominal packing for trauma is associated with increased morbidity and mortality. Am Surg 63:1109, 1997.
7. Sahai A, Belair M, Gianfelice D, et al: Percutaneous drainage of intra-abdominal abscesses in Crohn's disease: Short and long term outcome. Am J Gastroenterol 92:275, 1997.
8. Jawhari A, Kamm MA, Ong C, et al: Intra-abdominal and pelvic abscess in Crohn's disease: Results of non-invasive and surgical management. Br J Surg 85:367, 1998.
9. Memon MA, Deeik RK, Maffi TR, et al: The outcome of unretrieved gallstones in the peritoneal cavity during laparoscopic cholecystectomy. Surg Endosc 13:848, 1999.
10. Graham DJ, Stevenson JT, McHenry CR: The association of intra-abdominal infection and abdominal wall dehiscence. Am Surg 64:660, 1998.
11. McClean KL, Sheehan GJ, Harding GK: Intraabdominal infection: A review. Clin Infect Dis 19:100, 1994.
12. Dunn DL, Barke RA, Ahrenholz DH, et al: The adjuvant effect of peritoneal fluid in experimental peritonitis: Mechanism and clinical implications. Ann Surg 199:37, 1984.
13. van Goor H, de Graaf JS, Kooi K, et al: Effect of recombinant tissue plasminogen activator on intra-abdominal abscess formation in rats with generalized peritonitis. J Am Coll Surg 179:407, 1994.
14. Reijnen MMPJ, Meis JFGM, Postma VA, et al: Prevention of intra-abdominal abscesses and adhesions using hyaluronic acid solution in a rat peritonitis model. Arch Surg 134:997, 1999.
15. Brook I, Frazier EH: Microbiology of subphrenic abscesses: A 14-year experience. Am Surg 65:1049, 1999.
16. Brook I, Frazier EH: Aerobic and anaerobic microbiology of retroperitoneal abscesses. Clin Infect Dis 26:938, 1998.
17. Brook I, Frazier EH: Aerobic and anaerobic microbiology in intra-abdominal infections associated with diverticulitis. J Med Microbiol 49:827, 2000.
18. Tzianabos AO, Onderdonk AB, Rosner B, et al: Structural features of polysaccharides that induce intra-abdominal abscesses. Science 262: 416, 1993.
19. Tzianabos AO, Onderdonk AB, Zaleznik DF, et al: Structural characteristics of polysaccharides that induce protection against intra-abdominal abscess formation. Infect Immun 62:4881, 1994.
20. Tzianabos AO, Gibson FC III, Cisneros RL, et al: Protection against

experimental intraabdominal sepsis by two polysaccharide immunomodulators. J Infect Dis 178:200, 1998.
21. Gibson FC III, Onderdonk AB, Kasper DL, et al: Cellular mechanism of intraabdominal abscess formation by *Bacteroides fragilis*. J Immunol 160:5000, 1998.
22. Malangoni MA: Evaluation and management of tertiary peritonitis. Am Surg 66:157, 2000.
23. Nathens AB, Rotstein OD, Marshall JC: Tertiary peritonitis: Clinical features of a complex nosocomial infection. World J Surg 22:158, 1998.
24. Sawyer RG, Rosenlof LK, Adams RB, et al: Peritonitis into the 1990s: Changing pathogens and changing strategies in the critically ill. Am Surg 58:82, 1992.
25. Christou NV, Turgeon P, Wassef R, et al: Management of intra-abdominal infections: The case for intraoperative cultures and comprehensive broad-spectrum antibiotic coverage: The Canadian Intra-abdominal Infection Study Group. Arch Surg 131:1193, 1996.
26. Velmahos GC, Kamel E, Berne TV, et al: Abdominal computed tomography for the diagnosis of intra-abdominal sepsis in critically injured patients: Fishing in murky waters. Arch Surg 134:831, 1999.
27. Barkhausen J, Stoblen F, Dominguez-Fernandez E, et al: Impact of CT in patients with sepsis of unknown origin. Acta Radiol 40:552, 1999.
28. Gerzoff SG, Robbins AH, Johnson WC, et al: Percutaneous catheter drainage of abdominal abscesses: A five-year experience. N Engl J Med 305:653, 1981.
29. Malangoni MA, Shumate CR, Thomas HA, et al: Factors influencing the treatment of intra-abdominal abscesses. Am J Surg 159:167, 1990.
30. Gerzoff SG, Johnson WC, Robbins AH, et al: Expanded criteria for percutaneous abscess drainage. Arch Surg 120:227, 1985.
31. Lambiase RE, Deyoe L, Cronan JJ, et al: Percutaneous drainage of 335 consecutive abscesses: Results of primary drainage with 1-year follow-up. Radiology 184:167, 1992.
32. van Sonnenberg E, D'Agostino HB, Casola G, et al: Percutaneous abscess drainage: Current concepts. Radiology 181:617, 1991.
33. Wroblicka JT, Kuligowska E: One-step needle aspiration and lavage for the treatment of abdominal and pelvic abscesses. AJR Am J Roentgenol 170:1197, 1998.
34. Rajak CL, Gupta S, Jain S, et al: Percutaneous treatment of liver abscesses: Needle aspiration versus catheter drainage. AJR Am J Roentgenol 170:1035, 1998.
35. Schuster MR, Crummy AB, Wojtowycz MM, et al: Abdominal abscesses associated with enteric fistulas: Percutaneous management. J Vasc Interv Radiol 3:359, 1992.
36. Lahorra JM, Haaga JR, Stellato T, et al: Safety of intracavitary urokinase with percutaneous abscess drainage. AJR Am J Roentgenol 160: 171, 1993.
37. Neff CC, Mueller PR, Ferrucci JT Jr, et al: Serious complications following transgression of the pleural space in drainage procedures. Radiology 152:335, 1984.
38. McNicholas MM, Mueller PR, Lee MJ, et al: Percutaneous drainage of subphrenic fluid collections that occur after splenectomy: Efficacy and safety of transpleural versus extrapleural approach. AJR Am J Roentgenol 165:355, 1995.
39. Alexander AA, Eschelman DJ, Nazarian LN, et al: Transrectal sonographically guided drainage of deep pelvic abscesses. AJR Am J Roentgenol 162:1227, 1994.
40. Feld R, Eschelman DJ, Sagerman JE, et al: Treatment of pelvic abscesses and other fluid collections: Efficacy of transvaginal sonographically guided aspiration and drainage. AJR Am J Roentgenol 163: 1141, 1994.
41. Hovsepian DM, Steele JR, Skinner CS, et al: Transrectal versus transvaginal abscess drainage: Survey of patient tolerance and effect on activities of daily living. Radiology 212:159, 1999.
42. Sawyer RG, Adams RB, Pruett TL: Aztreonam vs. gentamicin in experimental peritonitis and intra-abdominal abscess formation. Am Surg 60:849, 1994.
43. Galandiuk S, Lamos J, Montgomery W, et al: Antibiotic penetration of experimental intra-abdominal abscesses. Am Surg 61:521, 1995.
44. Konig C, Simmen HP, Blaser J: Bacterial concentrations in pus and infected peritoneal fluid—implications for bactericidal activity of antibiotics. J Antimicrob Chemother 42:227, 1998.
45. Simmen HP, Blaser J: Analysis of pH and pO_2 in abscesses, peritoneal fluid, and drainage fluid in the presence or absence of bacterial infection during and after abdominal surgery. Am J Surg 166:24, 1993.
46. Betriu C, Campos E, Cabronero C, et al: Susceptibilities of species of the *Bacteroides fragilis* group to 10 antimicrobial agents. Antimicrob Agents Chemother 34:671, 1990.
47. Wilson SE: Results of a randomized, multicenter trial of meropenem versus clindamycin/tobramycin for the treatment of intra-abdominal infections. Clin Infect Dis 24(suppl 2):S197, 1997.
48. Ohlin B, Cederberg A, Forssell H, et al: Piperacillin/tazobactam compared with cefuroxime/metronidazole in the treatment of intra-abdominal infections. Eur J Surg 165:875, 1999.
49. Barie PS, Vogel SB, Dellinger EP, et al: A randomized, double-blind clinical trial comparing cefepime plus metronidazole with imipenem-cilastatin in the treatment of complicated intra-abdominal infections. Cefepime Intra-abdominal Infection Study Group. Arch Surg 132: 1294, 1997.
50. Barie PS, Christou NV, Dellinger EP, et al: Pathogenicity of the *Enterococcus* in surgical infections. Arch Surg 212:155, 1990.
51. Burnett RJ, Haverstock DC, Dellinger EP, et al: Definition of the role of enterococcus in intraabdominal infection: Analysis of a prospective randomized trial. Surgery 118:716, 1995.
52. Wacha H, Hau T, Dittmer R, et al: Risk factors associated with intraabdominal infections: A prospective multicenter study: Peritonitis Study Group. Langenbecks Arch Surg 384:24, 1999.
53. Willey SH, Hindes RG, Eliopoulos GM, et al: Effects of clindamycin and gentamicin and other antimicrobial combinations against enterococci in an experimental model of intra-abdominal abscess. Surg Gynecol Obstet 169:199, 1989.
54. Calandra T, Bille J, Schneider R, et al: Clinical significance of *Candida* isolated from peritoneum in surgical patients. Lancet 2:1437, 1989.
55. Alden SM, Frank E, Flancbaum L: Abdominal candidiasis in surgical patients. Am Surg 55:45, 1989.
56. Eggimann P, Francioli P, Bille J, et al: Fluconazole prophylaxis prevents intra-abdominal candidiasis in high risk surgical patients. Crit Care Med 27:1066, 1999.
57. Stone HH, Bourneuf AA, Stinson LD: Reliability of criteria for predicting persistent or recurrent sepsis. Arch Surg 120:17, 1985.
58. Lennard ES, Dellinger EP, Wertz MJ, et al: Implications of leukocytosis and fever at conclusion of antibiotic therapy for intraabdominal sepsis. Ann Surg 195:19, 1982.
59. Hoelzer DJ, Zabel DD, Zern JT: Determining duration of antibiotic use in children with complicated appendicitis. Pediatr Infect Dis J 18: 979, 1999.
60. Visser MR, Bosscha K, Olsman J, et al: Predictors of recurrence of fulminant bacterial peritonitis after discontinuation of antibiotics in open management of the abdomen [see comments]. Eur J Surg 164: 825, 1998.
61. Wickel DJ, Cheadle WG, Mercer-Jones MA, et al: Poor outcome from peritonitis is caused by disease acuity and organ failure, not recurrent peritoneal infection. Ann Surg 225:744, 1997.
62. Gleason TG, Crabtree TD, Pelletier SJ, et al: Prediction of poorer prognosis by infection with antibiotic-resistant gram-positive cocci than by infection with antibiotic-sensitive strains. Arch Surg 134:1033, 1999.
63. Berry SM, Fischer JE: Enterocutaneous fistulas. Curr Probl Surg 31: 469, 1994.
64. Michelassi F, Stella M, Balestracci T, et al: Incidence, diagnosis, and treatment of enteric and colorectal fistulae in patients with Crohn's disease. Ann Surg 218:660, 1993.
65. Kirsh GM, Hampel N, Shuck JM, et al: Diagnosis and management of vesicoenteric fistulas. Surg Gynecol Obstet 173:91, 1991.
66. Albu E, Gerst PH, Ene C, et al: Jejunal-rectal fistula as a complication of postoperative radiotherapy. Am Surg 56:697, 1990.
67. Yamazaki Y, Fukushima T, Sugita A, et al: The medical, nutritional and surgical treatment of fistulae in Crohn's disease. Jpn J Surg 20: 376, 1990.
68. Moss RL, Ryan JA Jr: Management of enterovesical fistulas. Am J Surg 159:514, 1990.
69. McNamara MJ, Fazio VW, Lavery IC, et al: Surgical treatment of enterovesical fistulas in Crohn's disease. Dis Colon Rectum 33:271, 1990.
70. Heyen F, Ambrose NS, Allan RN, et al: Enterovesical fistulas in Crohn's disease. Ann R Coll Surg Engl 71:101, 1989.
71. Woods RJ, Lavery IC, Fazio VW, et al: Internal fistulas in diverticular disease. Dis Colon Rectum 31:591, 1988.
72. Rose D, Yarborough MF, Canizaro PC, et al: One hundred and fourteen fistulas of the gastrointestinal tract treated with total parenteral nutrition. Surg Gynecol Obstet 163:345, 1986.
73. Jahnson S, Westerborn O, Gerdin B: Prognosis of surgically treated

radiation-induced damage to the intestine. Eur J Surg Oncol 18:487, 1992.
74. Buechter KJ, Leonovicz D, Hastings PR, et al: Enterocutaneous fistulas following laparotomy for trauma. Am Surg 57:354, 1991.
75. Schein M, Decker GA: Postoperative external alimentary tract fistulas. Am J Surg 161:435, 1991.
76. Dardai E, Pirityi S, Nagy L: Parenteral and enteral nutrition and the enterocutaneous fistula treatment. II. Factors influencing the outcome of treatment. Acta Chir Hung 32:305, 1991.
77. Rinsema W, Gouma DJ, von Meyenfeldt MF, et al: Primary conservative management of external small-bowel fistulas: Changing composition of fistula series? Acta Chir Scand 156:457, 1990.
78. Nubiola P, Badia JM, Martinez-Rodenas F, et al: Treatment of 27 postoperative enterocutaneous fistulas with the long half-life somatostatin analogue SMS 201–995 [published erratum appears in Ann Surg 211(2):246, 1990]. Ann Surg 210:56, 1989.
79. Levy E, Frileux P, Cugnenc PH, et al: High-output external fistulae of the small bowel: Management with continuous enteral nutrition. Br J Surg 76:676, 1989.
80. Spiliotis J, Briand D, Gouttebel MC, et al: Treatment of fistulas of the gastrointestinal tract with total parenteral nutrition and octreotide in patients with carcinoma. Surg Gynecol Obstet 176:575, 1993.
81. Fazio VW, Church JM, Jagelman DG, et al: Colocutaneous fistulas complicating diverticulitis. Dis Colon Rectum 30:89, 1987.
82. Kuvshinoff BW, Brodish RJ, McFadden DW, et al: Serum transferrin as a prognostic indicator of spontaneous closure and mortality in gastrointestinal cutaneous fistulas. Ann Surg 217:615, 1993.
83. Dardai E, Pirityi S, Nagy L: Parenteral and enteral nutrition and the enterocutaneous fistula treatment. I. Investigations on fistula output, nutritional status complications. Acta Chir Hung 32:287, 1991.
84. Sleeman D, Sosa JL, Gonzalez A, et al: Reclosure of the open abdomen. J Am Coll Surg 180:200, 1995.
85. Fabian TC, Croce MA, Pritchard FE, et al: Planned ventral hernia: Staged management for acute abdominal wall defects. Ann Surg 219: 643, 1994.
86. Kimose HH, Fischer L, Spjeldnaes N, et al: Late radiation injury of the colon and rectum: Surgical management and outcome. Dis Colon Rectum 32:684, 1989.
87. Galland RB, Spencer J: Surgical management of radiation enteritis. Surgery 99:133, 1986.
88. Fleshner PR, Schoetz DJ Jr, Roberts PL, et al: Anastomotic-vaginal fistula after colorectal surgery. Dis Colon Rectum 35:938, 1992.
89. Sarfeh IJ, Jakowatz JG: Surgical treatment of enteric "bud" fistulas in contaminated wounds: A riskless extraperitoneal method using split-thickness skin grafts. Arch Surg 127:1027, 1992.
90. Hugh TB, Coleman MJ, Cohen A: Persistent postoperative enterocutaneous fistula: Pathophysiology and treatment. Aust N Z J Surg 56:901, 1986.
91. Young-Fadok TM, Wolff BG, Meagher A, et al: Surgical management of ileosigmoid fistulas in Crohn's disease. Dis Colon Rectum 40:558, 1997.
92. Chamberlain RS, Kaufman HL, Danforth DN: Enterocutaneous fistula in cancer patients: Etiology, management, outcome, and impact on further treatment. Am Surg 64:1204, 1998.
93. Leber GE, Garb JL, Alexander AI, et al: Long-term complications associated with prosthetic repair of incisional hernias. Arch Surg 133: 378, 1998.
94. Campos AC, Andrade DF, Campos GM, et al: A multivariate model to determine prognostic factors in gastrointestinal fistulas. J Am Coll Surg 188:483, 1999.
95. Rombeau JL, Rolandelli RH: Enteral and parenteral nutrition in patients with enteric fistulas and short bowel syndrome. Surg Clin North Am 67:551, 1987.
96. Heys SD, Walker LG, Smith I, et al: Enteral nutritional supplementation with key nutrients in patients with critical illness and cancer: A meta-analysis of randomized controlled clinical trials. Ann Surg 229: 467, 1999.
97. Dudrick SJ, Maharaj AR, McKelvey AA: Artificial nutritional support in patients with gastrointestinal fistulas. World J Surg 23:570, 1999.
98. Prior A, Downing R: A self-regulating device for continuous reinfusion of jejunostomy effluent. J Med Eng Technol 14:21, 1990.
99. Rinsema W, Gouma DJ, von Meyenfeldt MF, et al: Reinfusion of secretions from high-output proximal stomas or fistulas. Surg Gynecol Obstet 167:372, 1988.
100. Dorta G: Role of octreotide and somatostatin in the treatment of intestinal fistulae. Digestion 60:S53, 1999.
101. Torres AJ, Landa JI, Moreno-Azcoita M, et al: Somatostatin in the management of gastrointestinal fistulas. Arch Surg 127:97, 1992.
102. Nubiola-Calonge P, Badia JM, Sancho J, et al: Blind evaluation of the effect of octreotide (SMS 201–995), a somatostatin analogue, on small-bowel fistula output. Lancet 2:672, 1987.
103. Borison DI, Bloom AD, Pritchard TJ: Treatment of enterocutaneous and colocutaneous fistulas with early surgery or somatostatin analog. Dis Colon Rectum 35:635, 1992.
104. Sancho JJ, di Costanzo J, Nubiola P, et al: Randomized double-blind placebo-controlled trial of early octreotide in patients with postoperative enterocutaneous fistula. Br J Surg 82:638, 1995.
105. Scott NA, Finnegan S, Irving MH: Octreotide and postoperative enterocutaneous fistulae: A controlled prospective study. Acta Gastroenterol Belg 56:266, 1993.
106. Hernandez-Aranda JC, Gallo-Chico B, Flores-Ramirez LA, et al: Treatment of enterocutaneous fistula with or without octreotide and parenteral nutrition. Nutr Hosp 11:226, 1996.
107. Reimund JM, Wittersheim C, Dumont S, et al: Mucosal inflammatory cytokine production by intestinal biopsies in patients with ulcerative colitis and Crohn's disease. J Clin Immunol 16:144, 1996.
108. Rutgeerts P, D'Haens G, Targan S, et al: Efficacy and safety of retreatment with anti–tumor necrosis factor antibody (infliximab) to maintain remission in Crohn's disease. Gastroenterology 117:761, 1999.
109. Present DH, Rutgeerts P, Targan S, et al: Infliximab for the treatment of fistulas in patients with Crohn's disease. N Engl J Med 340:1398, 1999.
110. Nikolaus S, Raedler A, Kuhbacher T, et al: Mechanisms in failure of infliximab for Crohn's disease. Lancet 356:1475, 2000.
111. Lomis NNT, Miller FJ, Loftus TJ, et al: Refractory abdominal-cutaneous fistulas or leaks: Percutaneous management with a collagen plug. J Am Coll Surg 190:574, 2000.
112. Wong SK, Lam YH, Lau JY, et al: Diagnostic and therapeutic fistuloscopy: An adjuvant management in postoperative fistulas and abscesses after upper gastrointestinal surgery. Endoscopy 32:311, 2000.
113. Santos F, Campos AC, Freire J, et al: Enterocutaneous fistulas: An unusual solution. Hepatogastroenterology 44:1085, 1997.
114. Joo JS, Agachan F, Wexner SD: Laparoscopic surgery for lower gastrointestinal fistulas. Surg Endosc 11:116, 1997.
115. Schein M, Decker GA: Gastrointestinal fistulas associated with large abdominal wall defects: Experience with 43 patients. Br J Surg 77:97, 1990.

Chapter 25

Protein-Losing Gastroenteropathy

Karen E. Kim

DEFINITION

Protein-losing gastroenteropathy describes a diverse group of disorders that are associated with excessive loss of serum proteins into the gastrointestinal tract. This excess serum protein loss can result in hypoproteinemia. In 1949, Albright and colleagues[1] discovered, using intravenous infusions of albumin, that excessive catabolism of albumin rather than decreased albumin synthesis was responsible for the hypoproteinemia. In 1957, Citrin and colleagues[2] were able to show that the gastrointestinal tract was the actual site of excess protein loss. These investigators demonstrated that excess serum loss of intravenously administered radioiodinated albumin could be explained by the appearance of labeled protein in the gastric secretions in patients with giant hypertrophy of the gastric mucosa (Ménétrier's disease). Subsequent research using ^{131}I-labeled polyvinylpyrrolidine, ^{51}Cr-labeled albumin, and other radiolabeled proteins, as well as immunologic methods measuring enteric loss of α_1-antitrypsin (α_1-AT), has further characterized the role of the gastrointestinal tract in the metabolism of serum proteins. These studies have shown that the gastrointestinal tract accounts for approximately 10% of the normal loss of plasma proteins, and that, in a variety of gastrointestinal disorders, this enteric protein loss can be significantly higher.[3-5]

NORMAL PHYSIOLOGY

Under physiologic conditions, most endogenous proteins found in the lumen of the gastrointestinal tract are derived from sloughed enterocytes and from pancreatic and biliary secretions.[6] Studies of gastrointestinal serum protein loss in normal subjects, measured by a variety of methods (^{67}Cu-ceruloplasmin, ^{51}Cr-albumin or α_1-AT clearance) have shown that daily enteric loss of serum proteins account for less than 1% to 2% of the serum protein pool, with enteric loss of albumin accounting for less than 10% of total albumin catabolism. In normal subjects, the total albumin pool is approximately 4 g/kg in women and 4.7 g/kg in men, with a half-life of 20 days and a rate of hepatic albumin synthesis of 0.15 g/kg per day, equaling the rate of albumin degradation.[7] Serum protein levels, therefore, reflect the balance between protein synthesis and metabolism, with gastrointestinal losses contributing only a minor proportion to total protein metabolism. However, this balance can be markedly altered in patients with protein-losing gastroenteropathy.[8, 9]

PATHOPHYSIOLOGY

Excessive plasma protein loss across the gastrointestinal epithelium can result from several pathologic alterations of the healthy mucosa. Mucosal injury can result in increased permeability to plasma proteins, mucosal erosions and ulcerations can result in the loss of an inflammatory protein-rich exudate, and lymphatic obstruction or increased lymphatic hydrostatic pressure can result in direct leakage of lymph containing plasma proteins. Changes in vascular permeability can influence the concentration of serum proteins in the interstitial fluid, thereby influencing the amount of enteric mucosal protein loss. Hypoproteinemia seen in gastrointestinal disorders can, therefore, be classified into three groups: (1) increased mucosal permeability to proteins as a result of cell damage or cell loss, (2) mucosal erosions or ulcerations, and (3) lymphatic obstruction. Diseases associated with protein-losing gastroenteropathy are listed in Table 25–1 and are discussed in more detail in other chapters of this book.

The loss of serum proteins in patients with protein-losing gastroenteropathy is independent of their molecular weights, and therefore, the fraction of the intravascular pool degraded per day remains the same for a variety of proteins, including albumin, IgG, IgA, IgM and ceruloplasmin.[8, 9] In contrast, patients with the nephrotic syndrome preferentially lose low molecular weight proteins such as albumin. Once plasma proteins pass into the gastrointestinal tract, they are degraded into their constituent amino acids by gastric, pancreatic, and small intestinal enzymes, reabsorbed by specific transporters,

Table 25–1 | **Disorders Associated with Protein-Losing Gastroenteropathy**

Mucosal Diseases without Erosions or Ulceration
AIDS-associated gastroenteropathy[11, 12]
Acute viral gastroenteritis[13]
Allergic gastritis[14]
Celiac sprue[15]
Cobalamin deficiency[16]
Collagenous colitis[17]
Eosinophilic gastroenteritis[18]
Giant hypertrophic gastropathy (Ménétrier's disease)[19, 20]
Helicobacter pylori gastritis (see text)
Henoch-Schönlein purpura[21]
Hypertrophic hypersecretory gastropathy[22]
Small intestinal bacterial overgrowth[23]
Intestinal parasitosis[24–26]
Giardiasis, schistosomiasis, nematodiasis, strongyloidiasis
Lymphocytic colitis[17]
Postmeasles diarrhea[22]
Systemic lupus erythematosus[27, 28]
Tropical sprue[30]
Vascular ectasia (gastric, colonic)[31]
Whipple's disease[32]
Mucosal Diseases with Erosions or Ulcerations
Alpha-chain disease[33]
Amyloidosis[34]
Beçhet's disease[35]
Carcinoid syndrome[36]
Crohn's disease[37, 38]
Duodenitis[39]
Erosive gastritis[39]
Gastrointestinal carcinomas[36]
Graft-versus-host disease[40]
Helicobacter pylori gastritis[41–43]
Idiopathic ulcerative jejunoileitis[44]
Infectious diarrhea
Clostridium difficile[45]
Shigella[46]
Kaposi's sarcoma[47]
Lymphoma[22]
Neurofibromatosis[48]
Ulcerative colitis[49]
Waldenström's macroglobulinemia[50]
Lymphatic Obstruction or Elevated Lymphatic Pressure
Cardiac disease[51–53]
Crohn's disease[37, 38]
Intestinal endometriosis[54]
Intestinal lymphangiectasia (congenital, acquired)[55, 56]
Lymph-enteric fistula[22]
Lymphoma[22]
Mesenteric venous thrombosis[57]
Mesenteric tuberculosis and sarcoidosis[58]
Portal hypertensive gastroenteropathy[59]
Post-transplant lymphoproliferative disease[60]
Sclerosing mesenteritis[61]
Systemic lupus erythematosus[27, 28]
Whipple's disease[32]

and recirculated. When the rate of gastroenteric protein loss exceeds the body's capacity to synthesize protein, hypoproteinemia develops.[6] Hypoalbuminemia, for example, is common in protein-losing gastroenteropathy and results when there is an imbalance between hepatic albumin synthesis, which is limited and can increase only by 25%, and albumin loss, with reductions in both the total body albumin pool and albumin half-life.[10]

Adaptive changes in endogenous protein catabolism may compensate for excessive enteric protein loss, resulting in unequal loss of specific proteins. Proteins that normally have a low fractional catabolic rate (long half-life) are, therefore, most affected by excessive enteric protein loss (i.e., albumin and most gamma globulins) compared with those with a high fractional catabolic rate (i.e., clotting factors, insulin, IgE[8, 9]). Other factors can also contribute to the excessive enteric protein loss seen in a variety of diseases. These include impaired hepatic protein synthesis, as well as increased endogenous degradation of plasma proteins.

In addition to hypoproteinemia, protein-losing gastroenteropathy can result in reduced concentrations of other serum components, such as lipids, iron, and trace metals.[8, 9] Lymphatic obstruction can result in lymphocytopenia, with alterations in cellular immunity (see later).

CLINICAL MANIFESTATIONS

As shown in Table 25–2, there is a wide spectrum in the clinical presentation of patients with protein-losing gastroenteropathy owing to the variety of gastrointestinal disorders that can manifest with excessive enteric protein loss (see Table 25–1). The most common clinical sequelae, however, is hypoproteinemia, reflected by a decrease in serum levels of albumin, gamma globulins (IgG, IgA, IgM, but not IgE), fibrinogen, lipoproteins, α_1-AT, transferrin, and ceruloplasmin.[8, 9] Dependent edema is commonly seen, secondary to diminished plasma oncotic pressure. Anasarca is rare, but unilateral edema, upper extremity edema and facial edema can be seen with lymphatic obstruction. Increased susceptibility to infections is uncommon, despite a decrease in serum gamma globulin levels, and although circulating levels of hormone-binding proteins (i.e., cortisol and thyroid-binding proteins) are decreased, free serum hormone levels are almost always within normal limits.

Several protein-losing gastroenteropathies can be associated with fat and/or carbohydrate malabsorption, resulting in diarrhea and fat-soluble vitamin deficiencies (see Chapter 89). As mentioned earlier, in patients with lymphatic obstruction, lymphocytopenia can occur, altering cellular immunity (see Table 25–2).

Table 25–2 | **Clinical Manifestations of Protein-Losing Gastroenteropathy**

Symptoms and Signs
Edema (dependent, facial, upper extremity, unilateral)
Diarrhea
Fat malabsorption
Carbohydrate malabsorption
Fat-soluble vitamin malabsorption or deficiency
Laboratory Abnormalities
Hypoproteinemia
Hypoalbuminemia
Decreased serum gamma globulins (IgG, IgA, IgM)
Decreased serum proteins: ceruloplasmin, α_1-antitrypsin, fibrinogen, transferrin, hormone-binding proteins
Decreased serum lipoproteins
Altered cellular immunity[62]
Lymphocytopenia
Decrease in serum hormone-binding proteins

DISEASES ASSOCIATED WITH PROTEIN-LOSING GASTROENTEROPATHY

As already mentioned, the diseases associated with protein-losing gastroenteropathy can be divided into three broad categories: (1) gastrointestinal mucosal damage, without ulceration or erosions, (2) gastrointestinal mucosal erosions or ulcerations, and (3) lymphatic obstruction or elevated lymphatic pressure (see Table 25–1). In some diseases, more than one of these mechanisms may be present.

Mucosal Diseases without Ulceration and Erosions

Diseases that damage the gastrointestinal epithelium can increase surface epithelial cell shedding, resulting in excess protein loss. Lesions of the small intestine that cause malabsorption are often associated with enteric leakage of plasma proteins. Infectious causes are common examples of the latter, resulting in protein leakage (i.e., viral infections, bacterial overgrowth,[23] parasitic infections[24–26]). Changes in vascular permeability due to vascular injury,[27, 28] such as with lupus vasculitis, can result in protein loss without mucosal erosions.

Ménétrier's Disease (see also Chapter 43)

Giant hypertrophic gastropathy (Ménétrier's disease[19, 20]) is the most common gastric lesion causing severe protein loss. These patients often present with weight loss, postprandial indigestion, emesis, and severe hypoproteinemia. Normal gastric glands are replaced by mucus secreting cells, reducing the number of parietal cells, resulting in hypochlorhydria or achlorhydria. An increase in intercellular permeability results in protein loss. The clinical manifestations of giant hypertrophic gastropathy can be transient in children but usually require aggressive treatment in adults. Oral administration of anticholinergic agents or histamine$_2$ (H_2) blockers can improve symptoms, but most patients improve only after subtotal or total gastrectomy.[19, 20] Recent studies have reported an association between *Helicobacter pylori* infection and Ménétrier's disease with protein-losing gastroenteropathy, both of which are reversed with eradication of the organism.[41–43]

Helicobacter pylori *Gastritis*
(see also Chapter 39)

H. pylori gastritis in the absence of Ménétrier's disease has been associated with protein-losing gastropathy, and it responds to eradication of *H. pylori* infection.[41–43] Some of these patients may have gastric erosions through which protein may be lost.

Systemic Lupus Erythematosus

Systemic lupus erythematosus (SLE) is a systemic autoimmune disease associated with protein-losing gastroenteropathy[27, 28] (Fig. 25–1). Mesenteric vasculitis can result in intestinal ischemia, edema, and altered intestinal vascular permeability. In addition, patients with SLE can develop gastritis and mucosal ulcerations, both of which may contribute to excess protein loss. Protein-losing gastroenteropathy may be the initial clinical presentation of SLE. Treat-

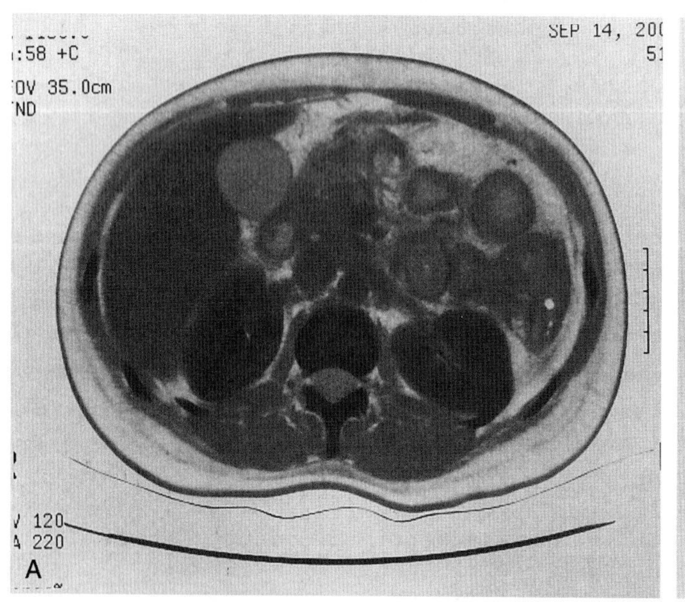

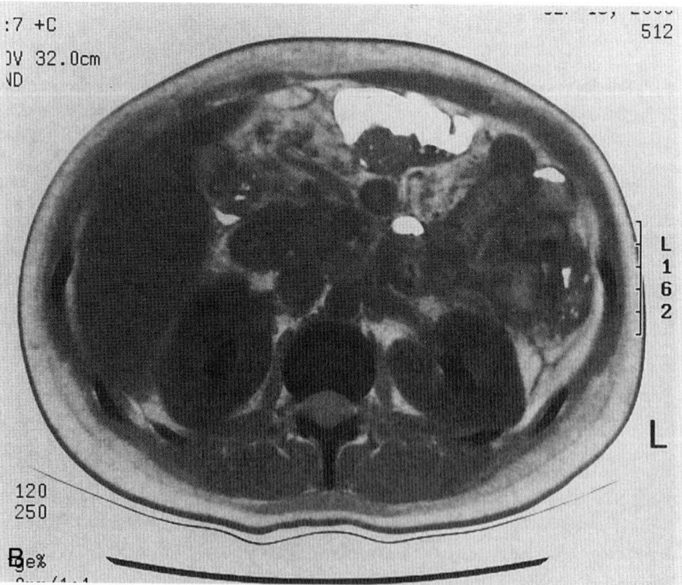

Figure 25–1. *A*, CT scan of the abdomen in a 29-year-old woman with severe watery diarrhea and diffuse, nonradiating abdominal pain. Serum albumin level was 2.9 g/dL and creatinine level was 0.6 mg/dL. Stool studies were negative for pathogens. The CT scan shows diffuse small bowel wall thickening. Her antinuclear antibody titer was 1:1280, and she was started on methylprednisolone. Her symptoms improved rapidly, with minimal diarrhea and resolution of her abdominal pain. *B*, Repeat CT scan 5 days later showed marked improvement of bowel wall thickening. Her serum albumin level was now 3.4 g/dL. Outpatient renal biopsy confirmed changes consistent with systemic lupus erythematosus.

ment with systemic steroids can lead to remission with resolution of clinical symptoms, including protein-losing gastroenteropathy.[27, 28]

Mucosal Diseases with Ulceration and Erosions

Mucosal erosions or ulcerations resulting in protein-losing enteropathy can be localized or diffuse and can be due to benign or malignant disease (see Table 25–1).[29] The severity of protein loss is dependent on the degree of cellular loss and the associated inflammation and lymphatic obstruction. Diffuse ulcerations of the small intestine or colon, as seen with Crohn's disease,[37, 38] ulcerative colitis,[49] and pseudomembranous colitis, can result in severe protein loss. Hypoalbuminemia is common in patients with gastrointestinal tract malignancies; although this is often due to a decrease in albumin synthesis, excessive enteric protein loss has been reported.[36]

Lymphatic Obstruction or Elevated Lymphatic Pressure

Lymphatic obstruction results in dilation of intestinal lymphatic channels and can result in rupture of lacteals rich in plasma proteins, chylomicrons, and lymphocytes. When central venous pressure is elevated, such as in congestive heart failure or constrictive pericarditis,[51–53] bowel wall lymphatic vessels become congested, resulting in a loss of protein-rich lymph into the gastrointestinal tract. Tortuous, dilated mucosal and submucosal lymphatic vessels are seen in patients with primary intestinal lymphangiectasias (Fig. 25–2). These patients often present by 30 years of age, with edema, hypoproteinemia, diarrhea, and lymphocytopenia, from both lymphatic leakage and rupture.[55, 56] Retroperitoneal processes, such as adenopathy, fibrosis, and pancreatitis, can also impair lymphatic drainage.

DIAGNOSIS

Laboratory Tests

The diagnosis of protein-losing gastroenteropathy should be considered in patients with unexplained hypoproteinemia in the absence of renal disease, liver disease, and malnutrition. The gold standard for diagnosing protein-losing gastroenteropathy is measuring the fecal loss of intravenously radiolabeled macromolecules, such as ^{51}Cr-albumin. Although accurate, this method of testing has major disadvantages, including radioactive exposure, expense, and the long collection period of stool and blood (6 to 10 days[63]). Alternative methods for detection of enteric protein loss have, therefore, been developed and used in the clinical setting.

α_1-AT is a useful marker of intestinal protein loss. α_1-AT is a 50,000-d glycoprotein of similar size to albumin (67,000 d) that is also synthesized in the liver. α-1 AT comprises approximately 5% of the total serum protein content. α_1-AT is resistant to proteolysis and is not actively absorbed or secreted, with low concentrations normally present in stool.[63–66] The fecal excretion of α_1-AT can, therefore, be used as an indirect measure of enteric albumin loss and has become the preferred method for measuring intestinal protein loss. Studies have shown a poor correlation between random stool α_1-AT concentrations and α_1-AT clearance measurements. Therefore, the optimal test is to measure the clearance of α_1-AT from the plasma during a 72-hour stool collection with α_1-AT plasma clearance expressed in milliliters per day. Plasma clearance of α_1-AT can also be used to monitor response to therapy.[63–66]

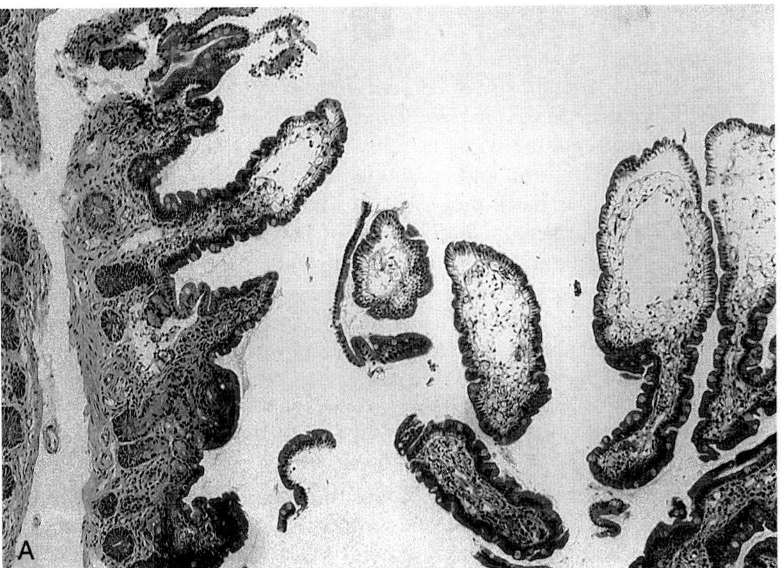

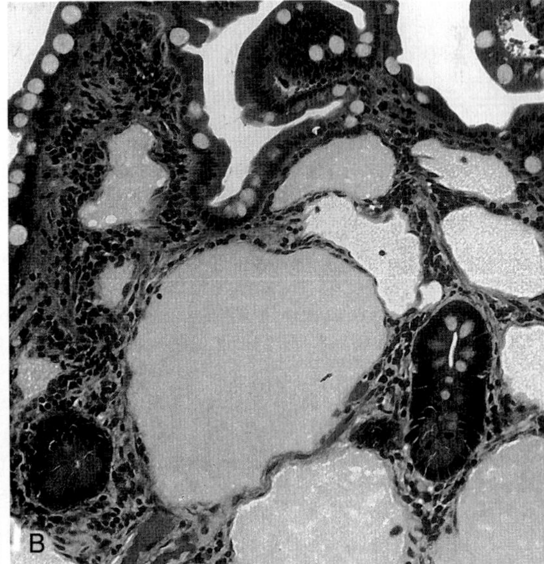

Figure 25–2. Intestinal lymphangiectasia in two patients with protein-losing enteropathy. *A,* Low-power view of small bowel biopsy showing focal lymphangiectasia (i.e., some villi are involved and others are spared), consistent with acquired (secondary) lymphangiectasia. *B,* High-power view of small bowel biopsy showing numerous dilated lymphatics consistent with diffuse lymphangiectasia, probably of the congenital type.

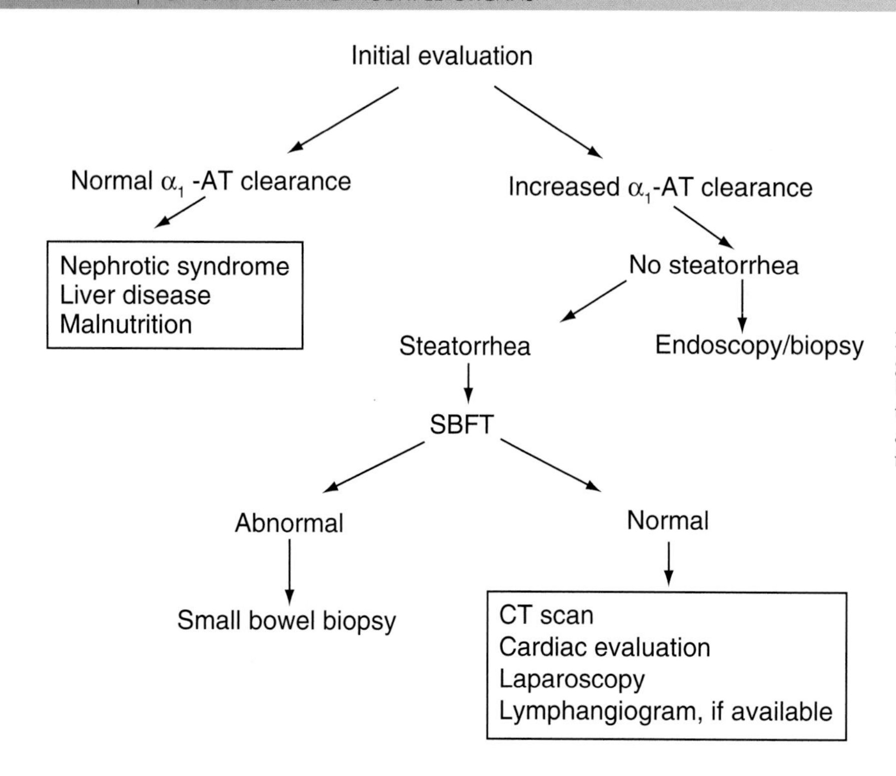

Figure 25–3. Approach to patient with protein-losing gastroenteropathy. Initial evaluation includes complete history and physical examination, laboratory evaluation (see text), and α_1-antitrypsin (α_1-AT) plasma clearance. CT, computed tomographic; SBFT, small bowel follow-through [radiograph].

Several factors can interfere with the interpretation of α_1-AT clearance from the plasma. Diarrhea can increase α_1-AT clearance and must be taken into account when reporting results. α_1-AT clearance greater than 24 mL/day in patients without diarrhea and greater than 56 mL/day in patients with diarrhea is considered abnormal. In addition, there is an inverse correlation between α_1-AT plasma clearance and the serum albumin concentration; as serum albumin levels fall below 3 g/dL, the clearance of α_1-AT exceeds 180 mL/day. In infants, meconium can interfere with testing because of the higher concentration of α_1-AT in meconium, and therefore this test should not be performed on infants suspected of having protein-losing enteropathy.[63–66] Finally, α_1-AT is degraded at a gastric pH below 3 and thus cannot be used to measure gastric protein loss. A recent study reported the use of lansoprazole to prevent the gastric degradation of α_1-AT, allowing the detection of protein-losing gastropathy.[66] In patients who test positive for fecal occult blood, interpretation of α_1-AT clearance can be difficult owing to increased clearance rates.[63–66]

Technetium 99m–labeled human serum albumin (^{99m}Tc-HSA) scintigraphy is a less sensitive test than α_1-AT to detect and monitor enteric protein loss. Studies in both children and adults have reported the use of ^{99m}Tc-HSA for detecting the specific site of gastric or enteric protein loss,[67–69] and this test can also be used to monitor response to therapy. ^{99m}Tc-HSA has a higher sensitivity in patients with lower serum albumin and total protein levels, reflecting a higher degree of enteric protein loss. This test is not widely available.

^{99m}Tc-labeled dextran lymphoscintigraphy is another method to identify and monitor enteric protein loss. ^{99m}Tc dextran is a water-soluble polysaccharide that is not bound by plasma or interstitial fluid protein and is not phagocytized in the interstitium. It has a uniform, monoexponential clearance, with a half-life of 30 minutes, and therefore reflects physiologic lymph flow. Its rapid absorption and distribution allow for both qualitative and quantitative studies of lymphatic kinetics and are useful in determining intestinal lymphangiectasia.[70] This test is also not widely available.

Currently, both of these radionuclides are in short supply or are out of production. Close consultation with the nuclear medicine department is advised.

Approach to the Patient with Suspected Protein-Losing Gastroenteropathy

(Fig. 25–3)

The diagnosis of protein-losing enteropathy can be made based on an increase in α_1-AT clearance, in the absence of confounding variables. In addition, testing with ^{99m}Tc-HSA can confirm and quantitate the extent and location of the disorder in certain patients, directing the work up to a specific organ. In the absence of labeled studies, the evaluation is methodical and should exclude potential diseases in a stepwise approach, because treatment requires identification of a specific disease process. Initial evaluation should include a thorough history and physical examination, a comprehensive metabolic panel, magnesium and calcium levels, and a complete blood count with differential and indices. Other laboratory data should include a serum protein electrophoresis and immunophoresis, C-reactive protein, prothrombin time and partial prothrombin time, iron and iron-binding capacity, thyroid function, fecal occult blood testing, and urinalysis. In those patients with diarrhea, stool should be collected for fat, ova and parasites, *Giardia* antigen, and *Clostridium difficile* toxin. In the presence of steatorrhea, diagnostic studies should concentrate on the upper gastrointestinal tract, and radiologic evaluation of the small intestine should be performed. In the absence of diarrhea, clinical work-up needs to be directed at the patient's symptoms. Often, esophagogastrodudenoscopy should be performed with random biopsies in both the stomach and small intestine. Colonoscopy with random biopsies, even with normal-appearing mucosa, should also be considered; collagenous or lymphocytic colitis can appear endoscopically normal. Retroperitoneal processes such as fibrosis, pancreatic diseases, or malignancies can be evaluated by computed tomographic scan. When these studies are inconclusive, cardiac evaluation and lymphangiogram or ^{99m}Tc-labeled dextran scintigraphy (in younger patients) should be considered. When the diagnosis remains unclear, exploratory laparotomy should be performed to exclude the possibility of occult malignancy.

TREATMENT

Treatment for protein-losing gastroenteropathy is directed at the correction of the underlying disease. For diseases affecting the stomach, such as giant hypertrophic gastropathy, gastrectomy reverses protein loss. However, an infection with *H. pylori* should be sought prior to surgical consideration and treated if present (see Chapter 39). Protein loss from the small intestine should be treated according to the individual disease process present. Diseases involving bacterial pathogens, such as Whipple's disease and small intestinal bacterial overgrowth, should be treated with antibiotic therapy (see Chapters 90 and 95), whereas inflammatory processes such as Crohn's disease require immunosuppressive therapy.[71] Colonic protein loss, as seen in ulcerative colitis and collagenous colitis, may require long-term immunosuppression, whereas infectious colitides need antibiotic treatment. Malignancy-induced enteric protein loss requires cancer-specific therapy. Enteric protein loss and lymphocytopenia seen in cardiac diseases (such as in congestive heart failure and constrictive pericarditis) can be ameliorated with medical and surgical management.

Acquired intestinal lymphangiectasia should be treated by correction of the primary disease, whereas congenital intestinal lymphangiectasia can be partially controlled with dietary restrictions. Enteric protein loss in the patients with the latter condition can be reduced by a low-fat diet enriched with medium-chain triglycerides, which do not require lymphatic transport and therefore do not stimulate lymph flow.[72]

Supportive care can reduce the incidence of secondary symptoms. Diuretics, although not tremendously useful with lymphedema, can reduce dependent edema from hypoalbuminemia, decreasing discomfort. Support stockings, if used appropriately, can reduce edema in patients with lymphedema and hypoalbuminemia. Meticulous skin care is necessary to prevent cellulitis and skin breakdown. Exercise with adequate ambulation should be encouraged to reduce the risk of venous thrombosis. Although these measures do not affect the enteric protein loss, they can minimize secondary complications.

The goal of therapy in protein-losing gastroenteropathy, therefore, is to identify the cause and direct dietary, medical, and/or surgical intervention aimed at the underlying disease.[73] With reversal or control of the primary disease, more than half of patients will have a partial or complete remission of enteric protein loss, edema, and other associated conditions.

REFERENCES

1. Albright F, Forbes AF, Barter EC, et al: Studies on fate of intravenously administered human plasma proteins in idiopathic hypoproteinemia and osteoporosis. In Youmans YB (ed): Symposia on Nutrition of the Robert Gould Research Foundation, vol 2. Springfield, Ill, Charles C Thomas, 1950, p 155.
2. Citrin Y, Sterling K, Halsted JA: Mechanisms of hypoproteinemia associated with giant hypertrophy of gastric mucosa. N Engl J Med 257: 906, 1957.
3. Gordon RS Jr: Exudative enteropathy: Abnormal permeability of gastrointestinal tract demonstrable with labeled polyvinylpyrrolidone. Lancet 1:325, 1959.
4. Schwartz M, Jarnum S: Protein-losing gastroenteropathy: Hypoproteinemia due to gastrointestinal protein loss of varying aetiology, diagnosed by means of ^{131}I-albumin. Dan Med Bull 8:1, 1961.
5. Florent C, L'Hirondel C, Dexmazures C, et al: Intestinal clearance of α_1-antitirypsin: A sensitive method for the detection of protein-losing enteropathy. Gastroenterology 81:777, 1981.
6. Freeman HJ, Kim YS, Sleisenger MH: Protein digestion and absorption in man: Normal mechanisms and protein-energy malnutrition. Am J Med 67:1036, 1979.
7. Pollak VE, Pesce AJ: Maintenance of body protein hemostasis. In Frohlich ED (ed): Pathophysiology of Altered Regulatory Mechanisms in Disease. Philadelphia, JB Lippincott, 1972, p 195.
8. Waldmann TA: Protein-losing gastroenteropathy. Gastroenterology 50: 422, 1966.
9. Waldmann TA: Protein-losing gastroenteropathies. In Haubrich WS, Kalser MA, Roth JL, Schaffner F (eds): Bockus Gastroenterology, 4th ed. Philadelphia, WB Saunders, 1985, p 1814.
10. Wochner RD, Weissman SM, Waldmann TA, et al: Direct measurement of the rates of synthesis of plasma proteins in control subjects and in patients with gastrointestinal protein loss. J Clin Invest 47:971, 1968.
11. Laine L, Garcia F, McGilligan K, et al: Protein-losing enteropathy and hypoalbuminemia in AIDS. AIDS 7:837, 1993.
12. Becker K, Linder C, Frieling T, et al: Intestinal protein leakage in the acquired immunodeficiency syndrome. J Clin Gastroenterol 25:426, 1997.
13. Schreiber DS, Blacklow NR, Trier JS: The mucosal lesion of the proximal small intestine in the acute infectious nonbacterial gastroenteritis. N Engl J Med 288:1318, 1973.
14. Waldmann TA, Wochner RD, Laster L, et al: Allergic gastroenteropathy: A cause of excessive protein loss. N Engl J Med 276:761, 1967.
15. Bai JC, Sambuelli A, Niveloni S, et al: Alpha$_1$-antitrypsin clearance as an aid in the management of patients with celiac disease. Am J Gastroenterol 86:968, 1991.
16. Ellaway CJ, Christodoulou R, Kamath K, et al: The association of protein-losing enteropathy with cobalamin C defect. J Inherit Metab Dis 21:17, 1998.
17. Stark ME, Batts KP, Alexander GL: Protein-losing enteropathy with collagenous colitis. Am J Gastroenterol 87:780, 1992.
18. Klein NC, Hargrove RL, Sleisenger MH, et al: Eosinophilic gastroenteritis. Medicine 49:299, 1970.
19. Overholt BF, Jefferies GH: Hypertrophic, hypersecretory protein-losing gastropathy. Gastroenterology 58:80, 1979.
20. Meuwissen SG, Ridwan BU, Hasper HJ, et al: Hypertrophic protein-losing gastropathy: A retrospective analysis of 40 cases in The Netherlands. The Dutch Ménétrier Study Group. Scand J Gastroenterol 194:1, 1992.
21. Reif S, Jain A, Santiago J, et al: Protein-losing enteropathy as a manifestation of Henoch-Schönlein purpura. Acta Paediatr Scand 80:482, 1991.
22. Brasitus TA, Bissonnette BM: Protein-losing gastroenteropathy. In Feldman M, Scharschmidt BF, Sleisenger MH (eds): Gastrointestinal and Liver Disease, 6th ed. Philadelphia, WB Saunders, 1998, p 369.
23. Su J, Smith M, Rerknimitr R, et al: Small intestine bacterial overgrowth presenting as protein-losing enteropathy. Dig Dis Sci 43:679, 1998.
24. Sullivan PB, Lunn PG, Northrop-Clewes CA, et al: Parasitic infection

of the gut and protein-losing enteropathy. J Pediatr Gastroenterol Nutr 15:404, 1992.
25. el Aggan HA, Marzouk S: Fecal alpha$_1$-antitrypsin concentration in patients with schistosomal hepatic fibrosis. J Egypt Soc Parasitol 22: 195, 1992.
26. Dubey R, Bavdekar S, Muranjan M, et al: Intestinal giardiasis: An unusual cause for hypoproteinemia. Indian J Gastroenterol 19:38, 2000.
27. Chung U, Oka M, Nakagawa Y, et al: A patient with protein-losing enteropathy associated with systemic lupus erythematosus. Intern Med 31:521, 1992.
28. Benner KG, Montanaro A: Protein-losing enteropathy in systemic lupus erythematosus: Diagnosis and monitoring immunosuppressive therapy by alpha$_1$-antitrypsin clearance in stool. Dig Dis Sci 34:132, 1989.
29. Landzberg BR, Pochapin MB: Protein-losing enteropathy and gastropathy. Curr Treat Options Gastroenterol 4:39, 2001.
30. Rubini ME, Sheehy TW, Meroney WH, et al: Exudative enteropathy: II. Observations in tropical sprue. J Lab Clin Med 58:902, 1961.
31. Bak YT, Kwon OS, Kim JS, et al: Protein-losing enteropathy with an endoscopic feature of "the watermelon colon." Eur J Gastroenterol Hepatol 11:565, 1999.
32. Laster L, Waldman TA, Fenster LF, et al: Reversible enteric protein loss in Whipple's disease. Gastroenterology 42:762, 1962.
33. Roth S, Havemann K, Kalbfleisch H, et al: Alpha-chain disease presenting as malabsorption syndrome with exudative enteropathy. Dtsch Med Wochenschr 101:1823, 1976.
34. Kawaguchi M, Koizumi F, Shimao M, et al: Protein-losing enteropathy due to secondary amyloidosis of the gastrointestinal tract. Acta Pathol Jpn 43:333, 1993.
35. Morita A, Asakura H, Morishita T, et al: Lymphangiographic findings in Beçhet's disease with lymphangiectasia of the small intestine. Angiology 27:622, 1976.
36. Sum PT, Hoffman MM, Webster DR: Protein-losing gastroenteropathy in patients with gastrointestinal cancer. Can J Surg 7:1, 1964.
37. Greene FE: Mechanism of hypoproteinemia in patients with regional enteritis and ulcerative colitis. Am J Med 29:405, 1961.
38. Hundegger K, Stufler M, Karbach U: Enteric protein loss as a marker of intestinal inflammatory activity in Crohn's disease: Comparability of enteric clearance and stool concentration of alpha$_1$-antitrypsin? Z Gastroenterol 30:722, 1992.
39. Murata I, Yoshikawa I, Kuroda T, et al: Varioliform gastritis and duodenitis associated with protein-losing gastroenteropathy, treated with omeprazole. J Gastroenterol 31:109, 1996.
40. Weisdorf SA, Salati LM, Longsdorf JA, et al: Graft-versus-host disease of the intestine: A protein-losing enteropathy characterized by fecal alpha$_1$-antitrypsin. Gastroenterology 85:1076, 1983.
41. Yamada M, Sumazaki R, Adachi H, et al: Resolution of protein-losing hypertrophic gastropathy by eradication of *Helicobacter pylori*. Eur J Pediatr 156:182, 1997.
42. Badov D, Lambert M, Finlay M, et al: *Helicobacter pylori* as a pathogenic factor in Ménétrier's disease. Am J Gastroenterol 93:1976, 1998.
43. Yoshikawa I, Murata I, Tamura M, et al: A case of protein-losing gastropathy caused by acute *Helicobacter pylori* infection. Gastrointest Endosc 49:2, 1999.
44. Schaad U, Zimmerman A, Gaze H, et al: Protein-losing enteropathy due to segmental erosive and ulcerative intestinal disease cured by limited resection of the bowel. Helvet Paediatr Acta 33:289, 1978.
45. Barlett JG: *Clostridium difficile* infection: Pathophysiology and diagnosis. Semin Gastrointest Dis 8:12, 1997.
46. Bennish ML, Salam MA, Wahed MA: Enteric protein loss during shigellosis. Am J Gastroenterol 88:53, 1993.
47. Laine L, Politoske EJ, Gill P: Protein-losing enteropathy in acquired immunodeficiency syndrome due to intestinal Kaposi's sarcoma. Arch Intern Med 147:1174, 1987.
48. Tatemichi M, Nagata H, Morinaga S, et al: Protein-losing enteropathy caused by mesenteric vascular involvement of neurofibromatosis. Dig Dis Sci 38:1549, 1993.
49. Anderson R, Kaariainen I, Hanauer S: Protein-losing enteropathy and massive pulmonary embolism in a patient with giant inflammatory polyposis and quiescent ulcerative colitis. Am J Med 101:323, 1996.
50. Bedine MS, Yardley JH, Elliott HL, et al: Intestinal involvement in Waldenström's macroglobulinemia. Gastroenterology 65:308, 1973.
51. Chan FK, Sung JJ, Ma KM, et al: Protein-losing enteropathy in congestive heart failure: Diagnosis by means of a simple method. Hepatogastroenterology 46:1816, 1999.
52. Wilkinson P, Pinto B, Senior JR: Reversible protein-losing enteropathy with intestinal lymphangiectasia secondary to chronic constrictive pericarditis. N Engl J Med 273:1178, 1965.
53. Bendayan I, Casaldaliga J, Castello F, et al: Heparin therapy and reversal of protein-losing enteropathy in a case with congenital heart disease. Pediatr Cardiol 21:267, 2000.
54. Henley JD, Kratzer SS, Seo IS, et al: Endometriosis of the small intestine presenting as a protein-losing enteropathy. Am J Gastroenterol 88:130, 1993.
55. Asakura H, Miura S, Morishita T, et al: Endoscopic and histopathological study on primary and secondary intestinal lymphangiectasia. Dig Dis Sci 26:312, 1981.
56. Mistilis SP, Skyring AP, Stephen DD: Intestinal lymphangiectasia: Mechanism of enteric loss of plasma protein and fat. Lancet 1:77, 1965.
57. Honbo K, Kawaji H, Tsuchimochi M, et al: Protein-losing enteropathy due to thrombophlebitis of the mesenteric vein: Report of a case. Surg Today 28:932, 1998.
58. Popovic OS, Brkic S, Bojic P, et al: Sarcoidosis and protein-losing enteropathy. Gastroenterology 78:119, 1980.
59. Conn HO: Is protein-losing enteropathy a significant complication of portal hypertension? Am J Gastroenterol 93:127, 1998.
60. Younes B, Ament M, McDiarmid S, et al: The involvement of the gastrointestinal tract in posttransplant lymphoproliferative disease in pediatric liver transplantation. J Pediatr Gastroenterol Nutr 28:380, 1999.
61. Horing E, Hingerl T, Hens K, et al: Protein-losing enteropathy: First manifestation of sclerosing mesenteritis. Eur J Gastroenterol Hepatol 7: 481, 1995.
62. Muller C, Wolf H, Gottlicher J, et al: Cellular immunodeficiency in protein-losing enteropathy: Predominant reduction of CD3+ and CD4+ lymphocytes. Dig Dis Sci 36:116, 1991.
63. Magazzu G, Jacono G, DiPasquale G, et al: Reliability and usefulness of random fecal alpha$_1$-antitrypsin concentration: Further simplification of the method. J Pediatr Gastroenterol Nutr 4:402, 1985.
64. Hill RE, Hercz A, Corey ML, et al: Fecal clearance of alpha$_1$-antitrypsin: A reliable measure of enteric protein loss in children. J Pediatr 99: 416, 1981.
65. Sharp HL: The current status of alpha$_1$-antitrypsin, a protease inhibitor, in gastrointestinal disease. Gastroenterology 70:611, 1976.
66. Takeda H, Nishise S, Furukawa M, et al: Fecal clearance of alpha$_1$-antitrypsin with lansoprazole can detect protein-losing gastropathy. Dig Dis Sci 44::2313, 1999.
67. Wang S, Tsai S, Lan J: Tc-99 albumin scintigraphy to monitor the effect of treatment in protein-losing gastroenteropathy. Clin Nucl Med 25:197, 2000.
68. Halaby H, Bakheet S, Powe J, et al: ^{99m}Tc-human serum albumin scans in children with protein-losing enteropathy. J Nucl Med 41:218, 2000.
69. Takeda H, Takahashi T, Ajitsu S, et al: Protein-losing gastroenteropathy detected by technetium-99m-labeled human serum albumin. Am J Gastroenterol 86:450, 1991.
70. Yueh T, Pui M, Zend S: Intestinal lymphangiectasia: Value of Tc-99m dextran lymphoscintigraphy. Clin Nucl Med 22:695, 1997.
71. Karbach U, Ewe K, Dehos H: Antiinflammatory treatment and intestinal alpha$_1$-antitrypsin clearance in active Crohn's disease. Dig Dis Sci 30:229, 1985.
72. Alfano V, Tritto G, Alfonsi L, et al: Stable reversal of pathologic signs of primitive intestinal lymphangiectasia with a hypolipidic, MCT-enriched diet. Nutrition 16:303, 2000.
73. Masetti PS, Marianeschi A, Capriani A, et al: Reversal of protein-losing enteropathy after ligation of systemic-pulmonary shunt. Ann Thorac Surg 67:235, 1999.

Chapter 26

Gastrointestinal Lymphomas, Including Immunoproliferative Small Intestinal Disease

Robert Collins

Lymphomas are solid malignancies of lymphoid tissue and are subdivided into Hodgkin's disease and non-Hodgkin's lymphomas (NHL).[1, 2] Hodgkin's disease rarely, if ever, involves the gastrointestinal tract, but the gastrointestinal tract is the most common site of extranodal NHL involvement.[3–5] The estimated annual incidence of NHL in the United States is 56,200[6]; lymphoma ranks as the fifth leading cause of cancer death in the United States.[6] Gastrointestinal NHL accounts for 4% to 20% of all NHL and 30% to 40% of extranodal cases.[7] Lymphomas that present predominantly in nodal areas, with the gastrointestinal tract involved as an extranodal site, are generally managed as the nodal lymphoma would be managed if extranodal disease were not present. This chapter deals with primary gastrointestinal lymphomas. Primary gastrointestinal lymphoma has been defined variously; a reasonable definition refers to it as "a lymphoma that has presented with the main bulk of disease in the gastrointestinal tract, with or without involvement of the contiguous lymph nodes, necessitating direction of treatment to that site."[3]

NON-HODGKIN'S LYMPHOMA: BACKGROUND

An understanding of the structure and function of the normal immune system (see Chapter 2) enhances understanding of lymphoma subtypes as distinct clinicopathologic entities.[8] In broad terms, the normal immune system can be thought of as a highly structured and tightly regulated interaction between primary, secondary, and tertiary lymphoid tissue, aimed at protecting the host tissue from destruction by harmful infectious agents. The primary lymphoid tissues are the sites of lymphocyte formation—the thymus for T cells and the bone marrow for B cells. Newly formed T and B cells migrate to the secondary lymphoid tissues—lymph nodes, spleen, and mucosa-associated lymphoid tissue (MALT)—where they are precisely arrayed to optimally encounter and respond to foreign antigens that pose a threat. The tertiary sites represent all other sites where antigen may be initially encountered and where specialized immune cells may ultimately have to go to eliminate harmful agents. Antigens causing tissue damage in tertiary sites activate antigen-presenting cells that then carry antigen to secondary lymphoid tissue sites for optimal presentation to the highly specialized B and T cells. Antigen-specific B and T cells then differentiate—B cells into antibody-producing plasma cells and T cells into effector T cells—which, by changes in function and homing capabilities, serve to mount an effective response to clear the threatening antigen.

Thus, in their sojourn from primary to secondary to tertiary lymphoid tissue, immune cells undergo several phenotypic and functional changes. NHL currently is best understood as a group of several distinct clinicopathologic entities, each of which is derived from malignant transformation of normal cellular counterparts at particular points of differentiation.[9] Thus, a lymphoma may be derived from a T cell or a B cell (or, more rarely, from other components of the immune system; e.g., dendritic cells or natural killer [NK] cells)[10] (Fig. 26–1). If, for example, the lymphoma is derived from a B cell, then it may be derived from any one of many putative normal counterparts, including the precursor B cell, the mantle cell, the follicle center centrocyte, the large B cell (centroblast or immunoblast), the marginal zone cell, or the plasma cell, among others. This way of conceptualizing lymphoma, along with extensive study of lymphoma in terms of clinical features, histopathology, immunophenotypic analysis, and molecular genetic analysis, has led to a lymphoma classification system, the Revised European American Lymphoma (REAL) classification, which recognizes approximately 28 distinct clinicopathologic entities.[1, 2]

Gastrointestinal Lymphoma: Overview

The lymphoid tissue of the gut is termed mucosa-associated lymphoid tissue (MALT). MALT is organized very similarly to lymph nodes and serves the same function. Just as malignant transformation of any of the immune cell types in a lymph node leads to lymphoma, malignant transformation of any of the immune cell types in gastrointestinal lymphoid tissue leads to lymphoma of this tissue. Lymphoma arising in gastrointestinal lymphoid tissue usually arises from B cells derived from the MALT marginal zone. Thus, the term MALT lymphoma has come to be synonymous with a particular lymphoma, marginal zone B cell lymphoma, which tends to have an indolent course, and in the stomach is associated with *Helicobacter pylori* infection (see Chapter 39). Lymphomas that arise from gastrointestinal lymphoid tissue but do not have marginal zone features are designated as particular clinicopathologic entities using the terminology of the REAL classification.

Gastrointestinal lymphomas most commonly involve the stomach or small intestine, although the oral pharynx, esophagus, colon, or rectum may be involved uncommonly. In developed countries, the stomach is the most common site of involvement (approximately 60% of cases) but in the Middle East, the small intestine is the most common site of gastrointestinal involvement. Table 26–1 lists the gastrointestinal lymphomas that will be discussed in this chapter. Clinicians dealing with gastrointestinal lymphoma are faced with a specific pathologic diagnosis of a lymphoma occurring in a specific site, and in some cases modified by important patient characteristics, such as human immunodeficiency virus (HIV) positivity. This chapter will encompass the main clinicopathologic entities that a clinician may encounter. Certain of these gastrointestinal lymphomas have particular features that warrant more extensive discussion; these include gastric extranodal marginal zone B cell lymphoma of MALT type, gastric diffuse large B cell lymphoma, immunoproliferative small intestinal disease (IPSID), and enteropathy-associated intestinal T cell lymphoma. The other lymphomas that may occur in the gastrointestinal tract will be covered in less detail, with the reader referred to appropriate references for additional information. Before proceeding to discussion of each entity, we will briefly review certain general principles that apply to all subtypes.[11]

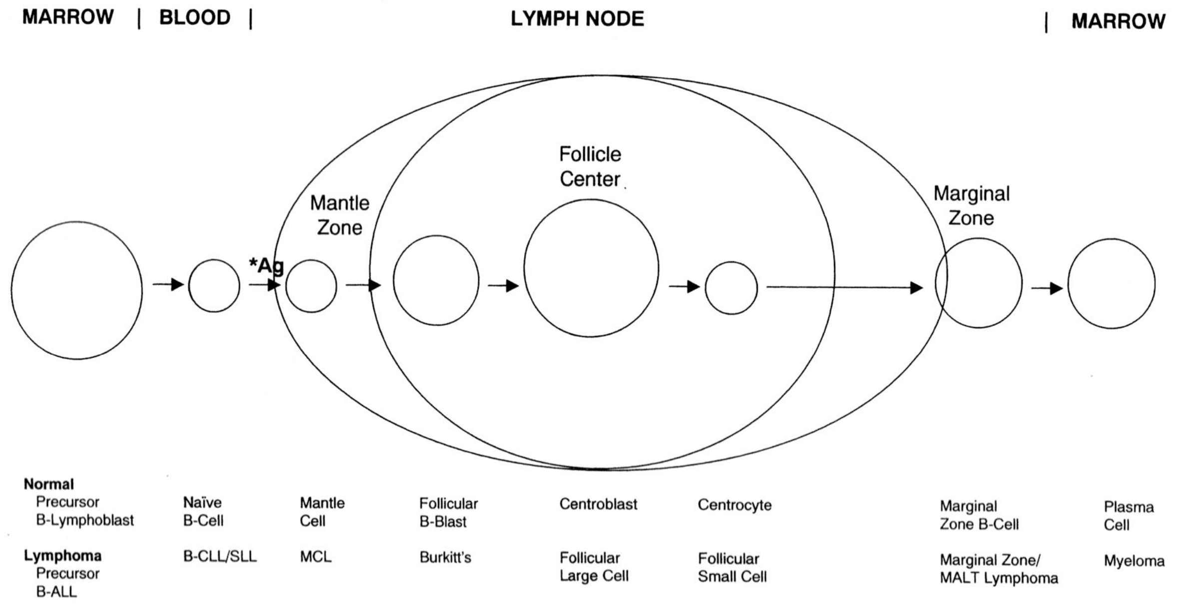

Figure 26–1. This abbreviated hypothetical scheme shows postulated developmental pathways for B-lymphocytes from bone marrow precursors through various intermediate cells to differentiated plasma cells. B cell lymphomas result from malignant transformation of normal B cells at particular points in their development. (For the sake of simplicity, an alternative B cell developmental pathway in the paracortex has been omitted.) T cells also have well-defined developmental pathways, with T cell lymphomas resulting from transformation of normal T cell counterparts. For a more thorough discussion see references 8 to 10. Ag, Antigen stimulation; B-ALL, B cell acute lymphoblastic leukemia; B CLL/SLL, B cell chronic lymphocytic leukemia/small lymphocytic leukemia; MCL, mantle cell lymphoma; MALT, mucosa-associated lymphoid tissue. (Adapted from Ferry J, Harris N: Atlas of Lymphoid Hyperplasia and Lymphoma. Philadelphia, WB Saunders, 1997.)

Table 26–1 | **Gastrointestinal Lymphomas**

Gastric lymphomas
  B cell
    Marginal zone B cell lymphoma of MALT type
    Diffuse large B cell lymphoma
  Uncommon Types
Small intestinal lymphomas
  B cell
    Non-IPSID
      Marginal zone B cell lymphoma of MALT type
      Diffuse large B cell lymphoma
      Mantle cell lymphoma (multiple lymphomatous polyposis)
      Follicular lymphoma
      Burkitt's lymphoma
    Immunoproliferative small intestinal disease (IPSID)
  T cell
    Enteropathy-associated intestinal T cell lymphoma (EATL)
    Other types not associated with enteropathy
Other sites (Waldeyer's ring, esophagus, colorectal)
Immunodeficiency-related lymphoma
  Post-transplantation
  HIV associated

GENERAL PRINCIPLES OF LYMPHOMA MANAGEMENT

Diagnosis

The diagnosis of lymphoma requires expert pathologic study (Table 26–2). Sufficient tissue should be obtained for analysis. In the gastrointestinal tract this often means multiple endoscopic biopsies; laparotomy or laparoscopy may be needed in some cases for adequate tissue specimens. Fine needle aspiration alone does not provide adequate tissue for complete classification and should be relied on only in very unusual circumstances. The minimal pathologic workup should include light microscopy and immunophenotypic analysis, either by flow cytometry or immunohistochemistry. Staining for immunoglobulin light chains assists in the documentation of monoclonality, with a clear-cut light chain restriction ($\kappa:\lambda$ ratio or $\lambda:\kappa$ ratio of 10:1 or more), strongly suggesting B cell lymphoma. Occasionally, molecular genetic analysis by Southern blot or polymerase chain reaction (PCR) is indicated, to document monoclonal immunoglobulin or T cell receptor gene rearrangements, or to assess characteristic oncogene rearrangements. The PCR test is more sensitive than Southern blotting and can be done on paraffin-embedded tissue; however, false-negative results may occur in this situation. As discussed below, microbiologic studies are indicated in certain cases. Recent studies suggest that microarray analysis of gene expression profiles may yield important prognostic information but such analyses are not yet part of the routine pathologic workup.[12]

Table 26–2 | **Pathologic Evaluation of Gastrointestinal Lymphoma**

Expert pathologist
Sufficient tissue
Light microscopy
Immunophenotypic analysis
  Flow cytometry
  Immunohistochemistry
Molecular genetic analysis (selected cases)
  Immunoglobulin or T cell receptor gene rearrangements
  Oncogene rearrangements

Table 26–3 | **Clinical Evaluation and Staging Workup of Gastrointestinal Lymphoma**

History and physical examination
Endoscopic examination
Endoscopic ultrasonography
Upper airway assessment
CT scan of the abdomen and pelvis
CT scan of the chest
Bone marrow aspiration and biopsy

Staging and Prognostic Assessment

Disease extent is assessed by careful history and physical examination; computed tomography (CT) of the chest, abdomen and pelvis; bone marrow examination; and, frequently, endoscopic ultrasonography[13] (Table 26–3; see color insert). Waldeyer's ring is often involved in gastrointestinal lymphomas; thus, examination of the upper airway is indicated. The Ann Arbor staging system, used for staging of nodal lymphomas, is deemed by many to be inadequate for staging of gastrointestinal lymphomas, and several alternative systems have been proposed, two of which are shown, along with the Ann Arbor system in Table 26–4.[14, 15]

Prognosis is assessed mainly by defining the distinct lymphoma subtype, but additional clinical features affect prognosis, including stage, age, performance status, and serum lactate dehydrogenase (LDH) level. The International Prognostic Index, originally proposed for patients with nodal diffuse large-cell lymphoma,[16] is also useful for assessing prognosis of patients with diffuse large B cell lymphoma of the stomach.[17]

Treatment

Treatment varies according to lymphoma subtype and stage, but it should be noted that the best treatment for many gastrointestinal lymphomas remains controversial. Whereas many large controlled trials have defined precisely the best treatment for many nodal lymphomas, this is not the case for gastrointestinal lymphomas. Thus, many treatment recommendations are based on small case series, extrapolation from results with nodal lymphomas, and dogmatic tradition. With this caveat in mind, we will attempt to convey as much as possible the current consensus regarding treatment of the various gastrointestinal lymphomas.

GASTRIC LYMPHOMAS

The stomach is the most common site of gastrointestinal lymphoma in developed countries. The majority of these lymphomas are classified either as marginal zone B cell lymphoma of mucosa-associated lymphoid tissue (MALT) type or as diffuse large B cell lymphoma. Other types of lymphoma involving the stomach are observed less commonly.

Table 26–4 | **Staging Systems for Gastrointestinal Lymphoma**

LUGANO STAGING SYSTEM[14]	TNM STAGING SYSTEM (MODIFIED FOR GASTRIC LYMPHOMA)[15]	ANN ARBOR STAGING SYSTEM	TUMOR INVOLVEMENT
Stage I Confined to GI tract (single primary or multiple, noncontiguous)	T1 NO MO	I_E	Mucosa, submucosa
	T2 NO MO	I_E	Muscularis propria
	T3 NO MO	I_E	Serosa
Stage II Extending into abdomen			
II_1 = local nodal involvement	T1-3 N1 MO	II_E	Perigastric lymph nodes
II_2 = distant nodal involvement	T1-3 N2 MO	II_E	More distant regional lymph nodes
Stage II_E Penetration of serosa to involve adjacent organs or tissues	T4 NO MO	I_E	Invasion of adjacent structures
Stage IV Disseminated extranodal involvement or concomitant supradiaphragmatic nodal involvement	T1-4 N3 MO	III_E	Lymph nodes on both sides of the diaphragm
	T1-4 NO-3 M1	IV_E	Distant metastases (e.g., bone marrow or additional extranodal sites)

Adapted from Zucca E, Bertoni F, Roggero E, Cavalli F: The gastric marginal zone B-cell lymphoma of MALT type. Blood 96:410–419, 2000.

Gastric Marginal Zone B Cell Lymphoma of Mucosa-Associated Lymphoid Tissue Type

Malignant transformation of B cells from the marginal zone of MALT leads to extranodal marginal zone B cell lymphoma of MALT type.[18–22] These lymphomas may arise from MALT that exists under normal physiologic circumstances (e.g., in Peyer's patches of the gut) or from MALT that has been acquired in sites of inflammation in response to infection or autoimmune processes. Gastric tissue does not normally contain MALT but may acquire it in response to chronic *H. pylori* infection.[23, 24] Malignant transformation occurs in a small percentage of patients with acquired gastric MALT and results in a lymphoma with generally indolent behavior. The malignant process appears to be driven to a large degree by chronic *H. pylori* infection, as eradication of the infection leads to regression of the lymphoma in most cases.[25, 26] However, the lymphoma sometimes behaves in a more aggressive manner, does not respond to antibiotics, and must be treated by different measures. Under the most current lymphoma classification system, this variety of NHL is termed extranodal marginal zone B cell lymphoma,[1, 2] but the disease is still commonly referred to by its prior monikers, gastric MALT lymphoma or primary low-grade gastric B cell lymphoma.

Epidemiology

Gastric marginal zone B cell lymphoma of MALT type represents approximately 40% of gastric lymphomas.[27] The incidence varies according to the incidence of *H. pylori* in the population being assessed; the incidence in northeastern Italy, where the rate of *H. pylori* infection is very high, is roughly 13 times the incidence in the United Kingdom.[28] The incidence in *H. pylori*–infected individuals is between 1:30,000 and 1:80,000.[29] The median age at diagnosis is approximately 60 years, with a wide age range. The male-to-female ratio is equal.

Etiology and Pathogenesis

Helicobacter pylori Infection

Several lines of evidence support the key role of *H. pylori* in the development of gastric MALT lymphoma (see Chapter 39). Infection by *H. pylori* is present in approximately 90% of cases of gastric MALT lymphoma examined histologically[30] and in 98% of cases with serologic studies.[31, 32] The epidemiologic studies cited previously have shown a close correlation between the prevalence of *H. pylori* infection and gastric lymphoma in a given population,[28] and case-control studies have shown an association between previous *H. pylori* infection and subsequent development of gastric lymphoma.[33] In vitro studies have shown that gastric MALT lymphoma tissue contains T cells that are specifically reactive to *H. pylori*.[34] These *H. pylori*-reactive T cells support the proliferation of neoplastic B cells.[35, 36] Lastly, many groups have documented regression of gastric MALT lymphoma in response to eradication of *H. pylori*.[15, 25, 26, 37–40]

Evidence for Antigen-Driven B Cell Proliferation

Naïve B cells contain unmutated immunoglobulin genes.[41] These genes code for immunoglobulins that are expressed on the cell surface and serve as specific receptors for particular antigens. During the T cell–dependent B cell response to antigen, the B cell immunoglobulin variable region (V) genes undergo somatic hypermutation; this leads to the production of new antigen receptors with altered antigen-binding affinity. Resultant B cell clones that express higher affinity antigen receptors have a survival advantage over B cell clones containing receptors with lower affinity. Thus, somatic mutation is a marker for antigen-driven selection of B cell clones. Sequence analysis of malignant B cells from gastric MALT lymphoma shows that the immunoglobulin genes have undergone somatic mutation.[42–44]

Helper T cells support the proliferation of various B cells through cytokines and cell-to-cell interactions.[45] These B cells may be specific for the same antigen as the T cells or may be reactive with other antigens. As noted previously, CD4+ T cells within gastric MALT lymphoma tissue are reactive with *H. pylori* antigens. The malignant B cells in gastric MALT lymphoma may be reactive with non–*H. pylori* antigens, and in fact may be self-reactive. One study showed that idiotypic immunoglobulins isolated from gastric MALT lymphoma reacted with a variety of autoantigens.[46] Another study has shown that the immunoglobulin genes from gastric MALT lymphoma are derived from germline genes commonly used for autoantibodies.[43] One study suggests the presence of selecting antigens common to different patients: analysis of the DNA and amino acid sequences of the antigen-binding region of tumor-derived immunoglobulin from two separate patients showed that although the DNA sequences differed, the resultant amino acid sequences were nearly identical.[44]

Genetic Studies

Cytogenetic studies have been limited due to small tissue samples and poor in vitro growth of tumor cells. Genes commonly rearranged in other NHLs, such as bcl-1, bcl-2, and bcl-6, have not been observed to be rearranged commonly in gastric MALT lymphoma.[47, 48] The most common genetic abnormality is the translocation t(11;18), observed in approximately 33% of cases.[49] The genes involved in this breakpoint have recently been identified (a novel gene on 18q, MLT, and the apoptosis inhibitor gene, API2).[50] Gastric MALT lymphoma with a t(11;18) translocation may be resistant to *H. pylori* treatment.[51] Translocation t(1;14) has been seen in a small percentage of cases.[52] The breakpoint involved in this translocation occurs upstream of the promoter region of a novel gene, designated bcl-10.[53, 54] The wild-type bcl-10 gene is pro-apoptotic; this activity appears to be lost in the mutated gene product[55]; however, due to conflicting studies the role of bcl-10 in lymphomagenesis is uncertain at this time.[56] Earlier studies suggesting that trisomy 3 is a frequent abnormality[57] have not been confirmed by subsequent studies.[58]

Somatic mutations of c-myc have been observed in 16% of gastric MALT lymphomas.[59] p53 serves as a tumor suppressor molecule, with loss of both copies of the allele being required for full contribution to malignant phenotype. Loss of both p53 copies by either deletion or mutation is seen in only a small percentage of low-grade gastric MALT lymphoma, but in a much higher percentage of cases of high-grade transformation.[60] p16 mutations have been reported in a small percentage of high-grade cases.[61] The replication error (RER) phenotype, which results in decreased efficiency of DNA mismatch repair, has been reported in a high percentage of cases of gastric MALT lymphomas in two studies,[62, 63] but not confirmed in another.[64] Likewise, studies regarding Fas/CD95 mutations have been conflicting.[65, 66]

A Model for Pathogenesis of Gastric MALT Lymphoma

A tentative model for the pathogenesis of gastric MALT lymphoma suggests that the evolution of the disease is a multistage process, comprising the sequential development of *H. pylori* gastritis, low-grade B cell lymphoma, and then high-grade B cell lymphoma.[20, 22] In this model, *H. pylori* infection elicits an immune response in which T cells and B cells are recruited to the gastric mucosa, where MALT is then formed. The chemokine BCA-1 and its receptor may play a key role in recruiting B cells to the gastric mucosa.[67] *H. pylori*–specific T cells promote growth of abnormal B cell clones. The abnormal B cells may not be *H. pylori* specific and may even be autoreactive; however, their continued proliferation, initially, is dependent on T cell help. The pivotal role of *H. pylori* reactive T cells in driving B cell proliferation may explain why tumor cells tend to remain localized and why the tumor regresses after eradication of *H. pylori*. However, continued B cell proliferation eventually leads to accumulation of additional genetic abnormalities, resulting in autonomous growth and more aggressive clinical behavior.

However, since lymphoma develops in only a very small percentage of *H. pylori*-infected individuals, additional environmental, microbial, or genetic factors must play a contributory role; what these factors are is unknown at this time. Particular *H. pylori* strains, expressing certain proteins, such as the CagA protein, have been suggested to play a role in development of gastric lymphoma but studies have had conflicting results.[68, 69]

Pathology

Gross Appearance and Location

Low-grade gastric MALT lymphomas are most commonly located in the antrum (41%) but may be multifocal in 33% of cases. Lesions may appear as ulcers in 47% of cases, erosions in 23%, or simply as erythema in 30%.

Histology

The key histologic feature of low-grade MALT lymphoma is the presence of lymphoepithelial lesions (Figure 26–2).[70, 71] These lesions are defined as the unequivocal invasion and partial destruction of gastric glands or crypts by tumor cell aggregates. However, these lesions can sometimes be seen in cases of florid chronic gastritis. Tumor cells are small- to medium-sized lymphocytes with irregularly shaped nuclei and moderately abundant cytoplasm. The morphology of these cells can vary, from small lymphoplasmacytoid cells to monocytoid cells that have abundant pale cytoplasm and well-defined borders. Scattered larger cells, transformed blasts, may also be seen. The lymphoma cells infiltrate the lamina propria diffusely and grow around reactive follicles; the germinal centers may be invaded, a phenomenon referred to as follicular colonization. As there is a continuous spectrum from the transition of gastritis to lymphoma, diagnosis of borderline cases can be difficult. Various parameters may assist in the distinction, such as the prominence of lymphoepithelial lesions, the degree of cytologic atypia, and the presence of neoplastic plasma cells with Dutcher bodies (intranuclear invagination of Ig-containing cytoplasm).

The presence of large cells can add further complexity to the diagnosis.[72, 73] The low-grade MALT lymphoma may have scattered large cells but is composed predominantly of

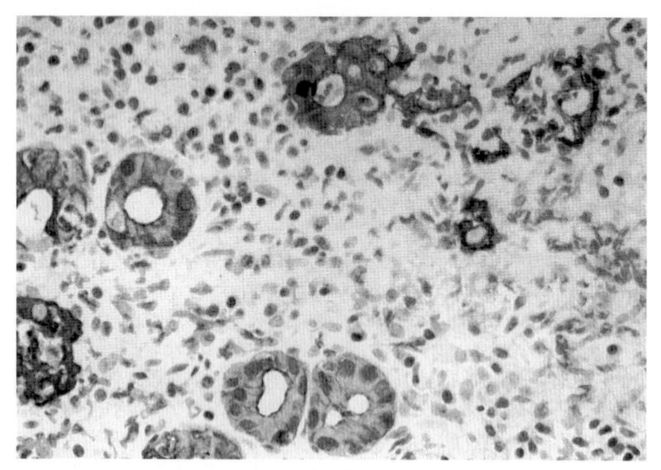

Figure 26–2. Lymphoepithelial lesion characteristic of gastric MALT lymphoma. Cytokeratin stain demonstrates invasion and destruction of some gastric glands by a monomorphic population of lymphocytes. Note for comparison the uninvolved, normal glands in the bottom, center of the photograph. Special stains demonstrated *H. pylori.*

small cells. At the other end of the spectrum, gastric lymphomas that contain only large cells or only small areas of small-cell MALT-like lymphoma should be classified as diffuse large B cell lymphomas.[1, 2] Between the ends of the spectrum are low-grade lymphomas in the process of evolving into more aggressive lymphoma, with increasing numbers of large cells being observed with transformation. Some investigators have proposed histologic grading systems to take this into account; these systems appear to facilitate prognosis based on large cell percentages and clusters but it is unclear how reproducible the systems are.[73]

Immunophenotype

Gastric MALT lymphoma cells have the typical immunophenotype of marginal zone B cells. They express pan–B cell antigens (CD19, CD20, and CD79a) and lack expression of CD5, CD10, CD23, and cyclin D1.[71] Additional immunostains in the hands of experienced pathologists can aid in identifying lymphoepithelial lesions, and in distinguishing follicular colonization from follicular lymphoma (a rare occurrence in the stomach).

Molecular Tests of Monoclonality

Southern blotting or PCR analysis of immunoglobulin heavy chain rearrangement can assist in the documentation of monoclonality.[74] B cell monoclonality may be detected in *H. pylori*–associated gastritis. Although monoclonality may predict later development of lymphoma, monoclonality alone does not allow a diagnosis of lymphoma; thus, molecular tests should always be considered in the context of histologic findings.

Clinical Features

Symptoms, Signs, and Laboratory Tests

The most common symptoms at presentation are epigastric or abdominal pain (53%) or dyspepsia (32%).[75] Nausea or evidence of gastric bleeding are unusual and B symptoms (fever, night sweats, weight loss) are distinctly unusual. Levels of serum LDH and β2-microglobulin are usually normal.

Diagnosis and Staging Studies

Patients are evaluated by esophagogastroduodenoscopy (EGD). As noted previously, findings may include erythema, erosions, or ulcers. Biopsy specimens should be taken from all abnormal areas and randomly from each area of the stomach, since disease is often multifocal. *H. pylori* infection should be established by histologic studies, breath test, or serologic studies, with serologic studies being the most sensitive test.[32] Additional staging consists of upper airway examination, CT of the abdomen and pelvis, CT of the chest or chest radiograph, bone marrow aspiration and biopsy, and measurement of serum LDH. Lastly, and very importantly, gastric endoscopic ultrasound should be performed to assess the extent of stomach wall involvement.[13, 76]

Staging System and Prognostic Assessment

Stage is assigned as outlined in Table 26–4.[14, 15] Approximately 90% of low-grade gastric MALT lymphomas are stage I at diagnosis and behave in a clinically indolent fashion; thus, prognosis is good for most patients with the diagnosis, with overall survival rates of 80% to 95% at 5 years. Prognosis is poor in the rare patients with advanced disease or with an unfavorable International Prognostic Index score.[16] Additional features that are associated with a worse prognosis are deep infiltration of the stomach wall, which is associated with a higher likelihood of regional lymph node involvement,[13] and high percentages of large cells on histologic evaluation.[73]

Treatment

Wotherspoon and associates first reported that gastric MALT lymphoma could completely regress by endoscopic, histologic, and molecular criteria after eradication of *H. pylori*.[25] Numerous studies have confirmed these observations.[15, 25, 26, 37–40] and antibiotics aimed at eradicating *H. pylori* have become the mainstay of therapy for low-grade gastric MALT lymphoma. However, it is important to recognize that the current literature in this field is less than optimal in several respects[22, 77]: older studies are limited by insufficient staging procedures and outdated classification systems; none of the reports in the literature are controlled or randomized trials; and data about long-term outcome after antibiotic treatment are still relatively scanty. Nevertheless, the current literature is sufficient to suggest to most experts in the field that early stage disease is best managed with a trial of antibiotics, reserving more toxic therapies such as radiation, chemotherapy, or surgery for more advanced disease or early stage disease that does not respond adequately to antibiotics.[20, 22]

Stage I Disease (Lugano Staging System)

Most patients with gastric MALT lymphoma have disease confined to the stomach. If endosonography confirms that disease is restricted to the mucosa or submucosa,[13] then treatment can consist of antibiotic therapy aimed at eradication of *H. pylori*. Any one of the treatment regimens discussed in Chapter 39 (see Table 39-4) is sufficient to eradicate the infection in almost all cases.[22] Follow-up endoscopy with multiple biopsies should be done 6 to 8 weeks after completion of treatment to document clearance of infection and to assess disease regression. Patients with persistence of infection should be treated with a second-line antibiotic regimen, to include a proton pump inhibitor.[78] Regression of lymphoma, but not necessarily complete regression, is usually evident at this examination. Histopathologic studies at this examination can predict ultimate response, with biopsy specimens showing only small foci of lymphoma being predictive of subsequent complete regression, and biopsy specimens showing diffuse persistent disease predicting a low likelihood of subsequent complete regression.[79] Patients are then observed with endoscopy approximately every 6 months for 2 years. Overall, approximately 70% of patients with stage I disease confined to the mucosa and submucosa will experience complete remissions. The median time to remission is 5 months but can be as long as 18 months.[75] The optimal treatment of patients with persistent disease is uncertain at this time. However, nonresponding patients may be more likely to harbor high-grade lesions, suggesting that more aggressive treatment such as chemotherapy, radiation, or surgery may be required.

Data regarding remission duration are relatively limited at this time. In one recent report remissions were durable with a median follow-up of 2 years.[39] However, late relapses have been reported, either in association with *H. pylori* reinfection or without reinfection (suggesting that malignant B cells have acquired the capability of autonomous growth). Minimal residual disease is detected by sensitive PCR techniques in about half the patients who are otherwise in complete remission; a positive PCR test may be predictive of subsequent relapse but additional study of this issue is needed.[80]

Occasional cases of gastric MALT lymphoma are *H. pylori* negative. As would be expected, these patients are much less likely to respond to antibiotic treatment[15]; however, optimal management remains undefined.

Patients with a significant component of large cells should not be treated with antibiotics alone, but will require more aggressive treatment. Exactly which management strategy should be used is uncertain but therapy should be along the lines as outlined in the section on diffuse large B cell lymphoma of the stomach (see below).

Stage I with Deep Penetration of Stomach Wall, or Stage II_E *(Lugano Staging System)*

Patients with *H. pylori* infection and more advanced stage lymphoma should be treated with antibiotics to eradicate the infection. However, antibiotics in this situation are insufficient treatment of lymphoma. The optimal management of more advanced stage gastric MALT lymphoma is uncertain at this time. Single-agent oral chemotherapy using cyclophosphamide or chlorambucil has activity with a 75% complete remission rate and a 5-year survival rate of 75% reported in 24 patients (17 patients, Ann Arbor stage I_E; and seven patients, stage IV_E) who received these drugs for a median of 18 months.[81] Radiation therapy delivered to the stomach and adjacent lymph nodes for a median total dose of 30 Gy resulted in a 100% complete remission rate and 100% event-free survival in 17 patients with stage I to II disease.[82] Surgery, alone or in combination with radiation and chemotherapy, resulted in an 82% survival rate in 21 patients with stage II_E disease.[27] Again, patients with a significant component of large cells should be treated as if they have diffuse large B cell lymphoma (see below). Unfortunately, there is currently no uniform grading system to allow a determination as to what percentage of large cells should lead to more aggressive therapy.

Stage II or IV Disease *(Lugano Staging System)*

The optimal management of low-grade gastric MALT lymphoma with spread to local or distant nodes or to bone marrow is not well defined. Therapy should probably be similar to that used in patients with marginal zone B cell lymphoma that is not associated with gastrointestinal disease.[83] Such disease is not considered curable but is often indolent and often responds to chemotherapy. Asymptomatic patients may be followed expectantly. Oral alkylating agents may be adequate for disease control in most symptomatic patients.

Table 26–5 summarizes treatment of gastric MALT lymphoma according to stage.

Diffuse Large B Cell Lymphoma of the Stomach

Epidemiology

Approximately 45% to 50% of gastric lymphomas are diffuse large B cell lymphomas. The incidence may be higher in developing nations than developed nations but clinical features appear to be similar.[84, 85] The median age is approximately 60 with a slight male predominance.

Table 26–5 | **Treatment of Gastric Marginal Zone B Cell Lymphoma of MALT Type, According to Lugano Staging System Stage**

LUGANO STAGE	TREATMENT*†
I, with disease limited to mucosa and submucosa	Antibiotics alone
I, with involvement of muscularis or serosa	Best treatment unknown at this time.
II, II_E	Reasonable options include surgery, radiation, and chemotherapy (see text).
IV	Chemotherapy for symptomatic disease. Local management with radiation or surgery may be indicated in selected cases.

*Patients with *H. pylori* infection should be treated with antibiotics to clear infection, regardless of stage.

†Patients with a high percentage of large cells should be treated as in Table 26–6 for diffuse large B-cell lymphoma. Unfortunately, current histologic grading systems are not sufficient to allow firm recommendations about what percentage of large cells should dictate aggressive management.

Etiology and Pathogenesis

The histogenesis of diffuse large B cell lymphoma of the stomach is not yet clear.[20, 86] Many large cell tumors have components of low-grade MALT tissue and are assumed to have evolved through transformation of low-grade lesions.[72, 87] However, other lesions have no evidence of associated low-grade MALT tissue; although some of these "pure" high-grade lesions may have evolved from low-grade lesions, it is unclear if all of them have. Several studies suggest that high-grade lesions with no low-grade component may have a worse prognosis but additional study will be required to resolve this issue.[88, 89]

In view of this uncertainty, it is difficult to assess the role of *H. pylori* in diffuse large B cell lymphoma of the stomach. If the large cell lesions commonly arise from progression of low-grade lesions, then *H. pylori* may have a role in the initial pathogenesis. One recent study suggested that *H. pylori* infection was more common in patients in whom large-cell lesions had a low-grade component.[88] As outlined in the previous discussion about tentative models for *H. pylori*–induced lymphoma, large-cell transformation resulting from genetic events including loss of p53 and p16 may lead to tumor cells losing their dependence on *H. pylori* for growth.[20, 22] A high incidence of somatic mutations in rearranged immunoglobulin heavy chain variable genes in one study of diffuse large B cell lymphoma of the stomach implicates antigen selection in the genesis of the lymphoma.[90] Although *H. pylori* may conceivably have a role in the early genesis of some high-grade lymphomas, it is important to emphasize that eradication of *H. pylori* by itself is not considered adequate therapy of high-grade lesions.

Pathology

Diffuse large B cell lymphoma of the stomach grossly may appear as large ulcers, protruded tumors, or multiple shallow ulcers.[91] They occur in both the body and antrum of the stomach. Tumors with a low-grade component are more likely to be multifocal than tumors with no low-grade component. Large-cell lymphomas typically invade the muscularis propria layer or more deeply.

Microscopic examination reveals compact clusters, confluent aggregates, or sheets of large cells that resemble immunoblasts or centroblasts, most often with a mixture of the two.[91] Twenty-five percent to 40% of cases show evidence of derivation from MALT, including dense infiltration of centrocyte-like cells in the lamina propria and typical lymphoepithelial lesions.[88, 92]

Immunophenotypic analysis shows expression of one or more B cell antigens (CD19, CD20, CD22, CD79a), and CD45.[93] Lesions with evidence of low-grade MALT tissue do not express CD10 (consistent with their having evolved from the CD10- marginal zone low-grade lesions). Lesions without evidence of MALT may or may not express CD10. Genetic analysis reveals monoclonal immunoglobulin gene rearrangements. Bcl-6 is frequently mutated or rearranged.[93, 94]

At this point, it is worth discussing the evolution in terminology regarding diffuse large B cell lymphoma of the stomach.[2] Many pathologists have referred to lymphomas arising in MALT lymphoma with high-grade features (with or without a component of low-grade disease) as high-grade MALT lymphoma. However, clinicians involved in the development of the REAL classification were concerned that many clinicians had come to regard the term gastric "MALT lymphoma" as synonymous with a lesion that responds to antibiotics. However, this is not the case with high-grade lesions arising in MALT. Therefore, those involved in formulating the REAL classification agreed to use the term extranodal marginal zone B cell lymphoma of MALT type for "low-grade" lesions, and the term diffuse large B cell lymphoma for "high-grade" lesions (leaving out the term "MALT").[1] Low-grade lesions involving MALT often contain varying proportions of large cells, with a worse prognosis in relation to increased percentages of large cells.[73]

Clinical Features

Patients present with epigastric or abdominal pain.[84] Large tumors may cause symptoms of obstruction. Ulcerating lesions may be associated with symptoms of gastrointestinal bleeding. B symptoms and elevated serum LDH levels are uncommon.

Staging consists of EGD, upper airway examination, CT scans of the abdomen and pelvis, CT scan of the chest or chest radiograph, bone marrow aspiration and biopsy, and measurement of LDH. In addition, gastric endoscopic ultrasonography plays an important role in assessing depth of stomach wall involvement. Lastly, *H. pylori* infection should be assessed. The majority of patients have stage I or II disease.[84] A recent study suggests that a stage-modified International Prognostic Index predicts clinical outcome of patients with localized gastric large B cell lymphoma.[17] In this study 35% of patients had two or more of the five risk factors. These patients had a significantly worse outcome than patients with no or one risk factor, with 5-year survival rates of around 40% to 60% versus 90%, respectively.

Treatment

The optimal management of diffuse large B cell lymphoma of the stomach is controversial.[4, 95, 96] The traditional approach for localized disease has been surgery alone or surgery followed by radiation or chemotherapy for patients with poor prognostic features. This approach has had the advantage of providing diagnostic and staging information and has avoided the risk of perforation or bleeding that may result from primary treatment with chemotherapy or radiation. Overall, approximately 70% of patients with stage I disease are disease-free 5 years after surgery.[97] However, several investigators have begun to question the role of surgery in the management of localized diffuse large B cell lymphoma.[4, 95] These investigators have pointed out that with the availability of endoscopy, surgery is no longer needed for diagnosis, and with the availability of CT scans and endoscopic ultrasonography, surgery is no longer needed for staging. In addition, the risk of bleeding or perforation with chemotherapy or radiation therapy appears to be less than has been thought. Several series have shown that radiation or chemotherapy can be given with only a 5% or less risk of perforation or bleeding.[98–100] On the other hand, surgery carries a 5% to 10% risk of mortality and is associated with significant morbidity.[101, 102]

Chemotherapy and radiation have been investigated as

alternatives to surgery. Radiation therapy has significant activity in gastric large B cell lymphoma. In one retrospective study, patients were treated with either radiation alone or surgery plus adjuvant radiation with no difference in 5-year survival.[103] Chemotherapy has significant activity in more advanced stage gastric large B cell lymphoma. A prospective trial of intensive anthracycline-based chemotherapy for advanced aggressive NHL included 91 patients with primary gastric lymphoma.[100] Such chemotherapy has curative potential for advanced aggressive lymphomas and the outcome in this study was no different between patients with nodal lymphomas and those with primary gastric lymphomas. Several series have suggested that chemotherapy, sometimes combined with radiation therapy, is at least as effective as surgery.[99, 102, 104–106] For example, a retrospective analysis of 59 patients with stage I or II disease treated with either anthracycline-containing chemotherapy or with surgery followed by chemotherapy showed no difference in survival between the two groups, with an overall survival rate of approximately 80%.[106] It must be emphasized, however, that none of these studies were prospective controlled trials.

It may be worth considering the question in the context of the appropriate management of stage I and II *nodal* diffuse large B cell lymphomas. In the past, radiation therapy was the standard therapy for these lymphomas when localized. However, long-term survival was impaired by distant relapses in approximately 30% to 40% of patients. Therefore, anthracycline-based chemotherapy was added to radiation therapy and shown to improve overall and disease-free survival in two large randomized controlled clinical trials.[107, 108] Thus, combined chemotherapy and radiation therapy is now the standard of care for early stage nodal diffuse large B cell lymphoma and results in cure for the majority of patients. Similarly, treatment failures in localized gastric diffuse large B cell lymphoma are usually due to distant relapse, suggesting that local treatment alone may not be adequate.[109]

Based on the above rationale, the current data, and extrapolation from results in patients with nodal disease, chemotherapy combined with radiation therapy seems a reasonable alternative to surgery, and it is reasonable for clinicians to use this practice. However, prospective controlled trials will be required to confirm the validity of this approach. Table 26–6 summarizes treatment of diffuse large B cell lymphoma by stage.

Patients with evidence of *H. pylori* infection should be treated. Interestingly, response to antibiotics in diffuse large cell lymphoma has been seen.[110] However, this certainly is not the rule, and antibiotics alone are considered inadequate treatment for diffuse large B cell lymphoma.

Table 26–6 | **Treatment of Diffuse Large B Cell Lymphoma of the Stomach According to Lugano Staging System Stage***

LUGANO STAGE	TREATMENT OPTIONS
I	1) CHOP† × 3–4 + XRT‡ 2) Surgery§ 3) Surgery + XRT
II, II_1, II_2, II_E	1) CHOP × 3–4 + XRT 2) Surgery 3) Surgery + XRT
IV	1) CHOP × 3–4 + XRT

*Optimal management of this entity is controversial (see text).
†Cyclophosphamide, doxorubicin, vincristine, prednisone for 3 to 4 cycles.
‡Radiation therapy, usually 40–50 Gy in 20–30 fractions.
§Subtotal gastrectomy with regional node resection.

Uncommon Gastric Lymphomas

B cell lymphomas other than marginal zone or diffuse large B cell may less commonly involve the stomach.[111–116] Lymphomas of T cell origin have rarely been reported.[117, 118]

Small-Bowel Lymphomas

Small intestine lymphomas may be divided into B cell tumors and T cell tumors. The B cell tumors encompass immunoproliferative small intestinal disease (IPSID) and a variety of non-IPSID subtypes, including marginal zone B cell lymphoma of MALT, diffuse large B cell lymphoma, mantle cell lymphoma, follicular lymphoma, and Burkitt's lymphoma. T cell lymphomas of the small intestine are usually enteropathy-associated intestinal T cell lymphomas; other forms of T cell lymphoma have been rarely reported.

Non-Immunoproliferative Small Intestinal Disease Lymphomas

Relatively few reports describe the non-IPSID small intestinal lymphomas, and large series have tended to group together all the lymphoma subtypes when describing manifestations and treatment outcome.[119, 120] Given the relative lack of information about these diseases with regard to their behavior in the intestine, it is probably best to consider them in light of the well-described features of their nodal counterparts. Thus, marginal zone and follicular lymphomas are regarded as indolent processes, incurable but controllable by chemotherapy, and often associated with a relatively long survival. Diffuse large-cell lymphomas and mantle cell lymphomas are more aggressive processes, which generally require chemotherapy as part of their management.

Marginal Zone B Cell Lymphoma of MALT Type

Lymphoma arising in the small intestine may have the characteristics of marginal zone B cell lymphoma, with the same histologic and immunophenotypic features described previously for gastric marginal zone B cell lymphoma.[83, 119, 120] However, an association with *H. pylori* infection has not been documented. Most cases occur in elderly patients who present with melena. The disease is usually present as a single annular or exophytic tumor, which may be present anywhere in the small intestine; disease is usually confined to the intestine or to local nodes. Treatment is usually surgical. Some patients have received chemotherapy but few data are available regarding regimens and outcome. In nodal marginal zone lymphoma, chemotherapy is usually reserved for patients with symptoms, as the disease is understood to be slow-growing and sensitive to chemotherapy but not curable by it. The 5-year survival rate is approximately 75%. As in gastric marginal zone B cell lymphoma, the small intestinal variety may have varying components of large-cell transformation. This probably confers a worse prognosis but data are scanty.

Diffuse Large B Cell Lymphoma

Diffuse large B cell lymphoma of the small intestine is similar to its gastric counterpart in histologic appearance and clinical behavior.[119, 120] Patients may present with abdominal pain, weight loss, obstruction, abdominal mass, bleeding, or perforation. Histologic findings are similar to those described previously in the section on gastric diffuse large B cell lymphoma, with some patients having a low-grade component and others having only a large-cell component. The tumor is usually an exophytic or annular lesion. Approximately half of the patients have localized disease and half have disease spread to regional or distant nodes. Surgery is usually required, and additional therapy includes anthracycline-containing chemotherapy and, in some cases, radiation therapy. Survival was reported to be approximately 40% in one series.[119] Whether this indicates a poorer prognosis for intestinal large B cell lymphoma than gastric large B cell lymphoma is uncertain; prognosis is probably dependent on disease stage and patient factors such as age and performance status.

Mantle Cell Lymphoma

Mantle cell lymphoma (multiple lymphomatous polyposis) is a relatively recently described subtype of B cell NHL.[113] Patients typically present with widespread adenopathy and frequently have bone marrow and extranodal involvement. The gastrointestinal tract is involved in 10% to 20% of patients, either at presentation or later in the course of the disease. The most common manifestation of gastrointestinal disease is multiple lymphomatous polyposis, in which multiple lymphoid polyps are present in the gastrointestinal tract (Fig. 26–3).[115, 121] The most common site of involvement is the ileocecal region (Fig. 26–4), but any other area may be involved, from the stomach to the rectum; occasional patients have involvement of all these regions. Involvement of the gastrointestinal tract may also occur without the appearance of multiple polyps. Most patients have extensive nodal and bone marrow disease at presentation although the gastrointestinal tract as the only site of involvement has been reported. Patients usually have symptoms related to the gastrointestinal involvement, which may include abdominal pain, obstruction, diarrhea, or hematochezia. It should be noted that this macroscopic presentation can also be seen with other lymphomas, especially marginal zone B cell lymphomas of MALT type and follicular lymphomas. Microscopically, mantle cell lymphoma involves the mucosa and submucosa. The malignant cells have the appearance of small atypical lymphocytes that may either surround benign-appearing germinal centers or may efface the lymphoid tissue. The tumor cells express pan-B markers and the T cell marker, CD5. The disease is characterized by a translocation, t(11;14),which results in rearrangement and overexpression of the bcl-1 gene encoding cyclin D1. Patients with obstructive tumor masses require surgical therapy, but the mainstay of treatment is chemotherapy. Although mantle cell lymphoma is initially responsive to chemotherapy, it eventually becomes refractory and the median survival is only 3 years.

Follicular Lymphoma

Follicular lymphomas of the gastrointestinal tract are rare.[114] The most common presentation is as an obstructing lesion in the terminal ileum. As noted previously, patients with this diagnosis may present with the gross appearance of multiple lymphomatous polyposis. Microscopically, most follicular lymphomas are composed of small cleaved lymphocytes (centrocytes) with a varying admixture of large cells. The

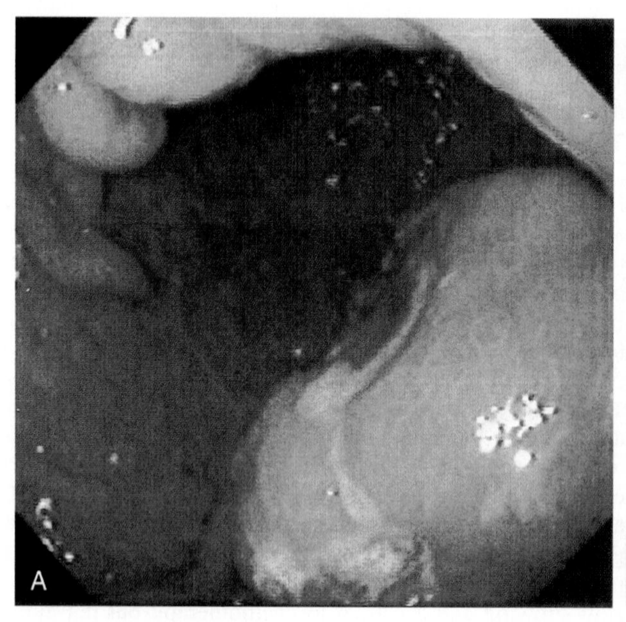

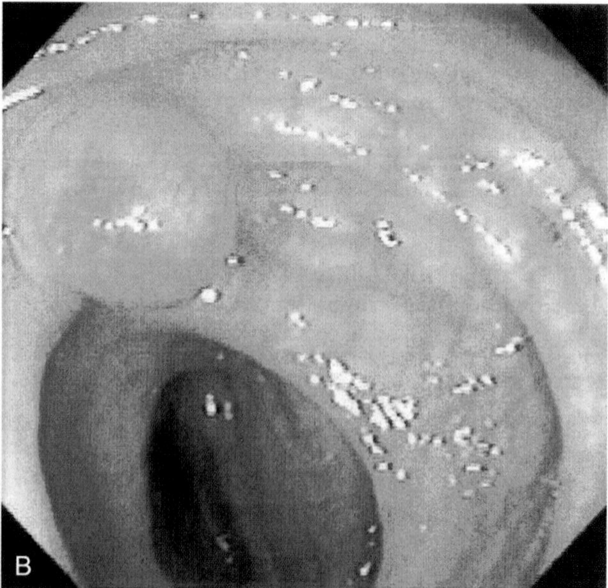

Figure 26–3. Endoscopic appearance of mantle cell lymphoma presenting as multiple lymphomatous polyposis, in the stomach (*A*) and in the colon (*B*).

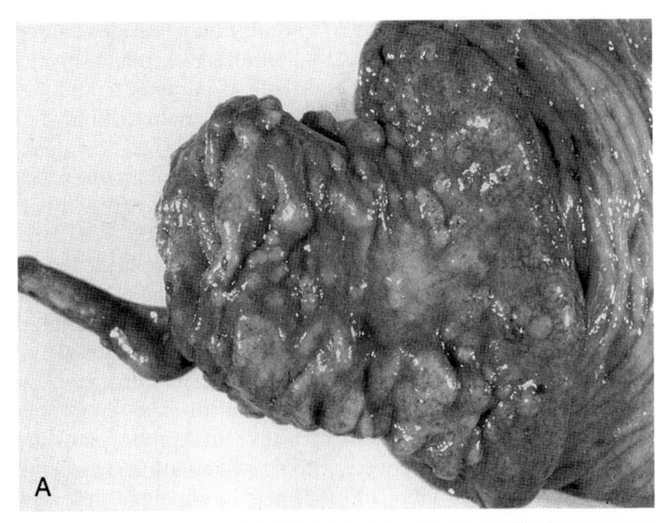

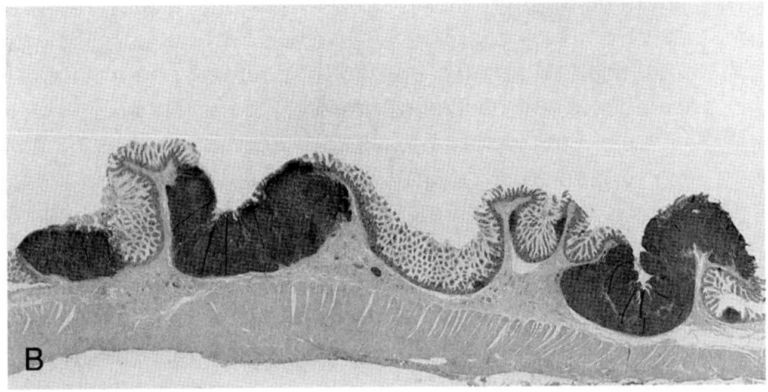

Figure 26–4. Multiple lymphomatous polyposis. *A,* Gross photograph shows numerous small polypoid lesions in the cecum. Additional synchronous and metachronous lesions were present in the ileum and the duodenum, as well as the rectum and sigmoid colon. *B,* Low-power view of ileum shows multiple discrete sites of mucosal and submucosal involvement by lymphomatous polyposis in another patient with mantle cell lymphoma.

disease is characterized by a translocation, t(14;18), which results in overexpression of the bcl-2 gene. Obstructing lesions require surgical management. Chemotherapy and radiation are sometimes indicated in management of this indolent but incurable disorder.

Burkitt's Lymphoma

Burkitt's lymphoma is a highly aggressive malignancy that, in patients infected with HIV, presents as either an endemic form, observed in Africa, or a sporadic form.[116] In the sporadic form, patients usually present with disease in the abdomen, with involvement of the distal ileum, cecum, mesentery, or both cecum and mesentery. Burkitt's tumor cells are monomorphic, medium-sized cells with round nuclei, multiple nucleoli, and basophilic cytoplasm. The involved lymphoid tissue has a starry sky appearance due to ingestion of apoptotic tumor cells by numerous benign macrophages. The tumor cells express B cell–associated antigens and surface immunoglobulin. Most cases have a rearranged c-myc gene on chromosome 8 either to the Ig heavy chain region on chromosome 14 or to one of the Ig light chain regions on chromosomes 2 or 22, resulting in a t(8;14), t(2;8), or t(8;22) translocation. Burkitt's lymphoma is rapidly fatal without treatment, but responds rapidly to institution of aggressive chemotherapy; treatment carries a high risk of tumor-lysis syndrome. Cure rates are 50% to 90%, depending on extent of the disease.

Immunoproliferative Small Intestinal Disease

Epidemiology

IPSID (alpha heavy-chain disease, Mediterranean lymphoma) is confined to certain regions of the world, especially North Africa, Israel, and surrounding Middle Eastern and Mediterranean countries.[122–126] IPSID is seen in smaller numbers in other areas, including Central and South Africa, India and East Asia, and South and Central America. A diagnosis in North America or Europe should be questioned, unless the patient has previously lived in an endemic area. The disease occurs in individuals with lower socioeconomic status who live in conditions of poor hygiene and sanitation.[127] The disease generally occurs in the second or third decade of life, although it has been observed in older individuals. The incidence in males and females is equal.

Etiology and Pathogenesis

Several observations have led to the belief that IPSID may be initiated by an infectious agent or agents: a) the association of the disease with lower socioeconomic status and poor sanitation; b) the high prevalence of intestinal microbial infestation manifested by bacterial overgrowth and parasitosis; c) a decrease in incidence when living conditions have improved in endemic areas; and d) the response of early lesions to antibiotic therapy. In addition, it is known that bowel flora stimulate IgA-producing cells, and intestinal biopsy specimens from apparently healthy individuals from endemic regions have shown an increase in lamina propria lymphocytes and plasma cells, reminiscent of findings in patients with IPSID.

As discussed in detail below, IPSID is associated with the production of an unusual IgA heavy chain protein, called α-heavy chain, which is secreted by plasma cells and is detectable in various body fluids.[128, 129] The plasma cells, which are the predominant histologic feature in the superficial mucosa, possess surface and cytoplasmic α-chain protein.[128] Centrocyte-like cells proliferating deeper in the mucosa have mainly cytoplasmic α-chain protein.[128] It is likely that these centrocyte-like cells, stimulated by microbial antigens, differentiate into the plasma cells that secrete the alpha chain protein characteristic of the disease. Genetic analyses have revealed that cellular proliferations are monoclonal even in very early lesions.[130, 131]

Thus, it can be proposed that, in a way analogous to *H. pylori*–associated gastric MALT,[20, 22] lymphocytes in intestinal MALT may be stimulated by infectious agents and proliferate in response.[126] The response becomes monoclonal and initially is dependent on the presence of antigen. However, with time, the malignant cells acquire additional genetic changes, causing them to lose their dependence on antigen persistence. This loss of antigen dependence is associated with the development of more aggressive clinical features.

Pathology

Gross lesions are generally confined to the proximal small intestine with adenopathy of adjacent mesenteric nodes.[132, 133] While some patients have thickening of mucosal folds only, others have a generalized thickening of the bowel wall, discrete masses, nodules, or polypoid lesions. Although grossly only the proximal bowel wall is involved, histologically the disease is characterized by a dense mucosal and submucosal cellular infiltrate that extends continuously throughout the length of the small intestine (Fig. 26–5).[133] A variety of pathological staging systems have been proposed (Table 26–7).[132, 134, 135] In the early stage of the disease, the cellular infiltrate is composed of benign appearing plasma cells or lymphoplasmacytic cells.[132, 134, 135] However, as noted previously, various studies assessing immunoglobulin gene rearrangements or light chain restriction have suggested that even the earliest infiltrate is monoclonal. This early infiltrate broadens villi and shortens and separates crypts, but epithelial cells remain intact. A histologic variant, the follicular lymphoid type, has been described in some patients (see Fig. 26–5).[133] This variant features a diffuse involvement of the mucosa with lymphoid follicle-like structures. As the disease progresses to intermediate and late stages, villi are further broadened and may become completely effaced, crypts are fewer, and the immunoproliferation extends more deeply. Atypical lymphoid cells infiltrate the benign-appearing plasma cells and lymphoplasmacytic cells. With time, the process evolves into overt lymphoma. Mesenteric lymph nodes are enlarged in early lesions, with preserved architecture, although follicles may be shortened by a histologically benign-appearing lymphocytic or plasmacytic infiltrate. As the disease progresses, the lymph node may acquire a more dysplastic appearance.

Clinical Features

Patients usually present with diarrhea, colicky abdominal pain, anorexia, and significant weight loss, of months' to years' duration. The diarrhea initially may be intermittent but becomes voluminous and foul-smelling as malabsorption develops (see Chapter 89). About half of patients have fever. Physical examination reveals evidence of malnutrition, digital clubbing, and peripheral edema. Late physical manifestations are ascites, hepatosplenomegaly, abdominal mass, and peripheral lymphadenopathy. Endoscopy may reveal thickened mucosal folds, nodules, ulcers, or evidence of submucosal infiltration, rendering the intestine immobile, tender, and indistensible. Small bowel barium radiographs show diffuse dilatation of the duodenum, jejunum, and proximal ileum, with thickened mucosal folds. Patients are frequently anemic due to vitamin deficiencies, and the erythrocyte sedimentation rate is increased in one third. The circulating lymphocyte count is low and measures of humoral and cellular immunity are reduced. Stool examination frequently reveals *Giardia lamblia* infestation. Serum IgG and IgM levels may be high or low; IgA levels are usually low or undetectable.

The characteristic and unique laboratory abnormality is the presence of the α-chain protein.[132, 136] This 29,000 to 34,000 molecular weight protein is a free α_1-heavy chain with an internal deletion of the variable (V_H) and C_H1 regions. It is devoid of light chains and thus corresponds to the Fc portion of the α_1 subunit of IgA. The α-chain protein amino terminal contains sequences that are not homologous to any known immunoglobulin sequence.[136] These changes are often due to insertions or deletions, usually involving the V_H-J_H and C_H2 regions,[136–138] but the source of inserted genetic material is unknown.

The α-chain protein migrates as a broad band within the $\alpha 2$ and β region on serum protein electrophoresis.[132] In addition to electrophoresis, the protein can be detected by immunoelectrophoresis[139, 140] or immunoselection (the most sensitive and specific method)[139, 141] in serum, urine, saliva, or intestinal secretions. Detection of α-chain protein from these sources is more likely in patients with early disease than in patients with more advanced disease,[135, 140, 142, 143] but, regardless of stage, α-chain protein can be detected in tissue sections in most cases of IPSID by immunofluorescence or immunoperoxidase staining of plasma cells or lymphoma cells.[136]

It has been postulated that chronic antigenic stimulation of the intestinal IgA secretory apparatus results in expansion of several plasma cell clones. Eventually a structural mutation occurs in a particular clone, resulting in an internal deletion of the α-heavy chain. This leads to an inability to make light chains and results in secretion of α-chain protein rather than intact IgA.[132, 141, 144]

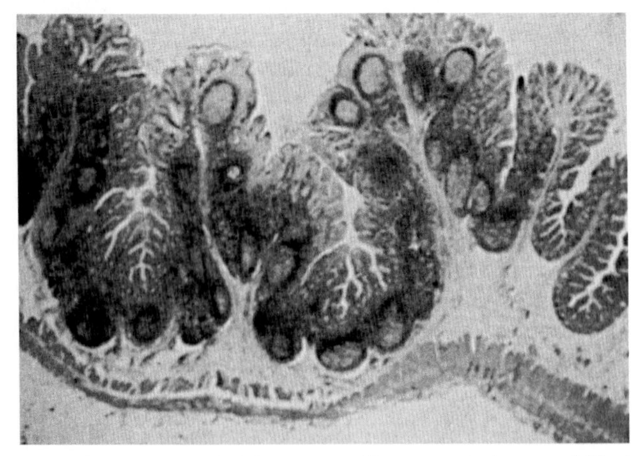

Figure 26–5. Immunoproliferative small intestinal disease: follicular lymphoid type.

Diagnosis and Staging

As the more malignant-appearing tissue may be present only in deeper layers of the intestine, endoscopic biopsy alone is often considered inadequate evaluation; staging laparotomy is therefore strongly recommended by some authors to allow full thickness intestinal biopsy and biopsy of mesenteric lymph nodes.[123, 124] However, some investigators do not routinely perform laparotomies; upper and lower endoscopy, small bowel series, bone marrow biopsies, and fine needle aspirations of enlarged lymph nodes are performed in-

Table 26–7 | **Pathologic Staging Systems for Immunoproliferative Small Intestinal Disease**

From WHO Memorandum[132]
(a) Diffuse, dense, compact, and apparently benign lymphoproliferative mucosal infiltration
(i) pure plasmacytic
(ii) mixed lymphoplasmacytic
(b) As in (a), plus circumscribed "immunoblastic" lymphoma, in either the intestine and/or mesenteric lymph nodes
(c) Diffuse "immunoblastic" lymphoma with or without demonstrable, apparently benign lymphoplasmacytic infiltration

From Salem et al.[134]
Stage
0 Benign-appearing lymphoplasmacytic mucosal infiltrate (LPI), no evidence of malignancy
I LPI and malignant lymphoma in either intestine (Ii) or mesenteric lymph nodes (In), but not both
II LPI and malignant lymphoma in both intestine and mesenteric lymph nodes
III Involvement of retroperitoneal and/or extra-abdominal lymph nodes
IV Involvement of noncontiguous nonlymphatic tissues
Unknown Inadequate staging

From Galian et al.[135]

	Small Intestine	*Mesenteric Lymph Nodes*	*Other Abdominal and Retroperitoneal Lymph Nodes*	*Other Lymph Nodes*	*Other Sites*
	Site I	Site IIa	Site IIb	Site III	Site IV
Stage A	Mature* plasmacytic or lymphoplasmacytic infiltration of mucosal lamina propria.† Inconstant and variable villous atrophy.	Mature* plasmacytic infiltration, with no or limited disorganization of general lymph node architecture.			Infiltrate cytologically similar to that in site I.
Stage B	Atypical plasmacytic or lymphoplasmacytic infiltrate, with presence of more or less atypical immunoblast-like cells, extending at least to submucosa. Subtotal or total villous atrophy.	Atypical plasmacytic or lymphoplasmacytic infiltrate, with presence of more or less atypical immunoblast-like cells. Total or subtotal obliteration of nodal architecture.‡			Infiltrate cytologically similar to that in site I.
Stage C	Lymphomatous proliferation invading the whole depth of intestinal wall.	Lymphomatous proliferation with total obliteration of nodal architecture.‡			Lymphomatous proliferation similar to that in site I.

*Rare cells may show an immature pattern.
†Limited and superficial extensions to submucosa may be observed.
‡Some sinuses, especially in the peripheral area, are usually still recognizable.
Adapted from Fine K, Stone M: α-Heavy chain disease, Mediterranean lymphoma, and immunoproliferative small intestine disease: A review of clinicopathologic features, pathogenesis, and differential diagnosis. Am J Gastroenterol 94:1139–1152, 1999.

stead.[145] One of the systems shown in Table 26–7 may then be applied to assess stage. More advanced disease, poor performance status, and comorbid illnesses portend a worse prognosis.

Treatment

Because of the relative rarity of this lymphoma, no large trials investigating therapy have been carried out.[125, 145–147] Patients often require intensive nutritional support.[148] Patients with early disease (such as Salem stage 0 disease) are generally treated with antibiotics for 6 or more months. The most commonly used regimens are tetracycline alone or a combination of metronidazole and ampicillin. Response rates have ranged from 33% to 71%[126]; in one study, the complete response rate was 71% with disease-free survival of 43% at 5 years.[145] In patients who do not significantly improve by 6 months or who do not achieve complete remission by 12 months, chemotherapy should be given.[124] Most investigators recommend anthracycline-containing regimens such as CHOP[147, 149]; for example, one investigator reports a complete response of 67% and survival of 58% at 3.5 years in patients treated with antibiotics, total parenteral nutrition, and anthracycline-based combination chemotherapy.[149] However, good results have been reported with non-anthracycline–containing regimens as well; in one report, 56% of patients with advanced disease were free of disease at 5 years.[145] Total abdominal radiation therapy has been used in a small number of patients, but, based on the current data, it is difficult to assess its proper role.[124]

Enteropathy-Associated Intestinal T Cell Lymphoma

As discussed in Chapter 93, enteropathy-associated intestinal T cell lymphoma occurs as a complication of celiac sprue.[150, 151] Malignant transformation of intraepithelial T cell leads to an aggressive and usually fatal malignancy. T cell lymphomas involving the small intestine that do not appear to have associated celiac disease have been reported rarely.[3, 152]

Epidemiology

Enteropathy-associated intestinal T cell lymphoma accounts for less than 1% of non-Hodgkin's lymphoma.[153] Celiac sprue is fairly common in Europe and the United States with an incidence in the United Kingdom of 1 in 2000 and in Ireland of 1 in 300.[151] The disease occurs worldwide but is uncommon in black Africans. In one group of celiac sprue patients, one in 20 developed lymphoma and in patients over the age of 50, the risk was one in ten.[154] The interval between diagnosis of celiac sprue and diagnosis of lymphoma is usually relatively short, with a mean interval of 3 to 5 years in two studies[155, 156]; commonly, celiac sprue is diagnosed concomitantly with lymphoma.[150, 151] Adherence to a gluten-free diet for more than 5 years appears to reduce the risk of lymphoma.[157] Males appear to be more affected than females (M:F ratio of approximately 2:1) and the median age at diagnosis is 50.[150, 151]

Etiology and Pathogenesis

Enteropathy-associated intestinal T cell lymphoma occurs in patients with adult celiac sprue.[158] As will be discussed in Chapter 93, celiac sprue is characterized by a hereditary sensitivity to gluten.[159, 160] Gluten peptides are presented by celiac sprue–specific HLA-DQ2 and HLA-DQ8 positive antigen-presenting cells and thus elicit an immune response in which gluten-specific intraepithelial lymphocytes damage intestinal epithelium. Intraepithelial T cells in celiac sprue have a normal immunophenotype (CD3+ CD8+) and are polyclonal.[161–166] Malignant transformation of intraepithelial T cells results in a monoclonal population of intraepithelial T cells that have an abnormal phenotype.[162–164, 167] Monoclonal populations of intraepithelial T cells in celiac mucosa may result in any one of several interrelated processes.[168] The first condition is called refractory celiac sprue, a condition in which patients lose responsiveness to a gluten-free diet.[161] The second condition, ulcerative jejunitis, is characterized by inflammatory jejunal ulcers and unresponsiveness to a gluten-free diet (see Chapter 106).[169, 170] The third condition is enteropathy-associated intestinal T cell lymphoma, an aggressive malignancy of the small intestine.[150, 151] In patients with any of these three conditions, uninvolved mucosa adjacent to the lesions can contain monoclonal T cells containing the same rearranged T cell receptor genes.[168, 170, 171] In addition, patients with ulcerative jejunitis can subsequently develop enteropathy-associated intestinal T cell lymphoma in which the same clone is isolated in the jejunitis and in the subsequent lymphoma. Thus, these three conditions have come to be considered to represent a spectrum of disorders mediated by monoclonal intraepithelial T cells.[168]

Pathology

Tumors typically occur in the jejunum but may occur in other sites of the small intestine. The lesions may be in single or multiple. Grossly, the lymphomas commonly appear as ulcerating lesions, with circumferential involvement of the small bowel.[150, 151] Lesions may also appear as nodules, plaques or strictures, but large masses are uncommon. Mesenteric lymph nodes are often enlarged, either due to tumor involvement or to edema and reactive changes. Distant sites, especially the bone marrow or the liver, are sometimes involved.

Histologically, the lymphoma is generally characterized by large highly pleomorphic cells with numerous bizarre, multinucleated forms.[70, 152] However, cells sometimes have a more immunoblastic, anaplastic, or, less commonly, a small-cell appearance (Fig. 26–6). Eosinophils and other inflammatory cells are often present. Histologic features often vary within the same tumor and between multiple lesions of the same patient. Uninvolved mucosa usually has the typical appearance of celiac disease with villous atrophy, crypt hyperplasia, plasmacytosis in the lamina propria, and an increase in intraepithelial lymphocytes. However, the enteropathy may be subtle in some cases, with only an increase in intraepithelial lymphocytes.

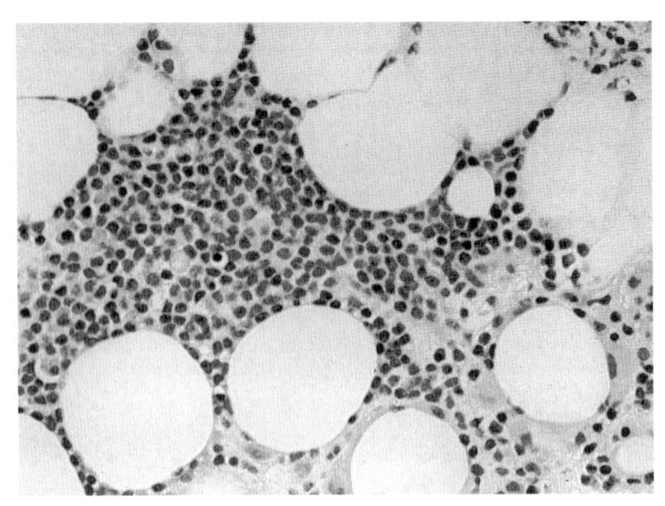

Figure 26–6. Photomicrograph of enteropathy-associated T cell lymphoma in a patient with celiac sprue. Mesenteric fat of the small bowel wall is involved with a monomorphic population of small to intermediate sized, irregular T lymphocytes. Cells were positive for CD2, CD3, CD7, and CD8, and were CD5 negative. T cell gene rearrangement studies were positive (i.e., showed a clonal band indicating a clonal T cell process).

Immunophenotyping typically shows that the malignant cells are CD3+, CD7+, CD4−, CD8−, and contain cytotoxic granules recognized by the antibody TIA-1.[164] Surface CD3 may be negative but cytoplasmic CD3ε chains will be detectable.[163] Cells are CD8+ in a minority of cases and a small percentage of cases coexpress CD8 and CD56.[172] CD103 is commonly positive. Cases with anaplastic morphology are CD30+. Genotypic studies show monoclonal T cell receptor gene rearrangements.[171, 173, 174] As noted previously, monoclonal T cell populations can also be detected in mucosa not involved by lymphoma.

Clinical Features

Patients may have a history of documented celiac sprue with the time to development of lymphoma varying widely. However, at least half the patients have celiac disease diagnosed at the same time as lymphoma.[150, 151] The most common symptoms at presentation are abdominal pain, weight loss, diarrhea, or vomiting. In one series, 23% of the patients presented with small-bowel perforation and 19% presented with small-bowel obstruction.[151] Fevers and night sweats may be present in up to one third of patients.[151] Masses are palpable in the minority of patients.[150, 151] Peripheral adenopathy is very unusual. Anemia was present in 68% and serum LDH increased in 25% of patients in one series.[151] Serum albumin is almost always decreased.

Diagnosis is usually made at laparotomy but approximately 20% of patients have been diagnosed with barium studies and small-bowel biopsies.[151] Staging consists of CT scanning and bone marrow biopsy. In the two largest recent clinical studies, 9% of the combined patients had Ann Arbor stage I_E, 62% had stage II_E, and 29% had stage IV disease.[150, 151]

Treatment

No large controlled trials of therapy for enteropathy-associated intestinal T cell lymphoma have been reported. Thus, standard treatment is not well defined. Typically, patients are treated with a combination of surgery and chemotherapy.[150, 151] Surgery involves removal of as much tumor as is feasible. Intensive chemotherapy is then administered, with the most common regimens being ones that contain anthracyclines, such as CHOP (cyclophosphamide, doxorubicin, vincristine, and prednisone). There is no evidence for superiority of any particular chemotherapy regimen. In one study in which 24 patients received chemotherapy, small-bowel perforation developed in four patients; in three of these patients, the perforation occurred soon after receiving chemotherapy and was fatal.[151] Nutritional status is commonly poor, requiring parenteral nutrition. Because of poor nutritional and performance status, fewer than 50% of patients are able to complete the prescribed treatment regimen. In one study the overall response rate to chemotherapy was 58% with a complete remission rate of 42%.[151] However, relapse occurs at a median of 6 months from diagnosis in approximately 80% of patients, usually in small bowel sites. A variety of salvage regimens have been tried for patients with relapsed disease but very few patients with relapse have survived. The actuarial 1-year and 5-year survival rates in one study were 39% and 20%, respectively, with 1- and 5-year failure-free survival rates of 19% and 3%, respectively.[151] In another study, the overall 1-year and 5-year survival rates were 31% and 11%, respectively.[150]

Thus, the prognosis for this lymphoma is very poor. Conceivably, earlier diagnosis may improve the outcome. The diagnosis should be considered in patients who present in mid-life with celiac sprue and in those who have clinical deterioration after having been stable on a gluten-free diet.

Because ulcerative jejunitis and refractory sprue may also represent related pre-neoplastic disorders that have a poor prognosis and may terminate in typical enteropathy-associated intestinal T cell lymphoma, it seems conceivable that these disorders should be treated with chemotherapy. Additional study along these lines is warranted.[161, 164]

OTHER SITES

NHL less commonly occurs in other sites of the gastrointestinal tract, including the oral pharynx,[175, 176] esophagus,[177] colon, and rectum.[178, 179] Signs and symptoms reflect the site of presentation. Because of the relative rarity of these disorders, the literature is fairly limited. Therefore, strong conclusions cannot be drawn about the optimal management of these more unusual gastrointestinal lymphomas. Standard principles of lymphoma management dictate diagnostic procedures, staging, prognostic assessment, and treatment. As is the case for all lymphomas, histologic studies and stage guide treatment.

Waldeyer's ring lymphomas are usually diffuse large-cell lymphomas but other histologic types may be present instead.[175, 176] Endoscopy and imaging of the remainder of the gastrointestinal tract should be included in the staging workup as lymphomatous involvement in other sites may accompany Waldeyer's ring involvement. Ann Arbor stage I or II diffuse large-cell lymphoma is managed with combined anthracycline-based chemotherapy and local radiation therapy.

Primary colorectal lymphomas most commonly involve the cecum,[178, 179] with high- or intermediate-grade histologic findings. Most colorectal lymphomas are Ann Arbor stage I_E or II_E. Again, therapy is dictated by histologic findings and stage. Resection is the standard therapy with adjuvant chemotherapy given for patients with aggressive histologic findings.

IMMUNODEFICIENCY-RELATED LYMPHOMAS

Post-Transplant Lymphoproliferative Disorders

Post-transplant lymphoproliferative disorders (PTLDs)[180–183] complicate 0.8% to 20% of solid organ transplants, with the incidence being highest in heart-lung transplant recipients. PTLDs are also seen in bone marrow transplant recipients, particularly in patients receiving T cell–depleted allografts. PTLD results from proliferation of Epstein-Barr virus–transformed B cell clones that have developed in part because of immunosuppression. The histologic appearance of PTLD is highly variable, with lesions being polymorphic or monomorphic; the histologic appearance may resemble infectious mononucleosis, aggressive NHL, or plasmacytoma.[182] Lesions may be polyclonal, oligoclonal, or monoclonal. The clinical presentation varies greatly, with some patients having a syndrome resembling infectious mononucleosis, and some having a more lymphoma-like presentation, with nodal or extranodal disease.[183] Involvement of extranodal areas is common, with the gastrointestinal tract being a common site. The literature regarding treatment of PTLD suffers from a lack of prospective trials and lack of standardized histologic classification. The treatment approach varies[181] but usually consists at first of withdrawal of immunosuppression, with anthracycline-based chemotherapy reserved for patients who fail to respond to this maneuver.[184] Surgical or radiation therapy may cure patients with localized disease. Other treatments have included acyclovir or ganciclovir, and interferon-alfa. Monoclonal antibodies to B cells (e.g., rituximab) have activity in this disorder,[185, 186] and donor leukocyte infusions are frequently used for patients with PTLD developing after allogeneic bone marrow transplantation.[187]

HIV-Associated Non-Hodgkin's Lymphoma

The risk of developing NHL is markedly increased in patients infected with HIV, and development of lymphoma is considered an acquired immunodeficiency disease–defining condition.[188] These malignancies are B cell neoplasms,[189, 190] with most cases having either small noncleaved cell or diffuse large cell histologic findings (see Chapter 28). Epstein-Barr virus is implicated in about half of non–central nervous system HIV-related lymphomas. HIV-associated NHL typically has an aggressive presentation, with rapidly growing disease and prominent B symptoms.[191] The gastrointestinal tract is a common site, including unusual sites such as the anus and rectum.[192] Historically, treatment has been poorly tolerated and lower dose chemotherapy regimens have been used.[193–195] Prognosis is generally poor, with 2-year survival rates of 10% to 20%. However, patients with higher CD4+ T cell counts (as is more commonly seen in view of the standard current use of highly active antiretroviral therapy) may be able to tolerate full-dose chemotherapy regimens[196] and have a better prognosis than that seen in previous studies.

Primary effusion lymphoma is a relatively recently described clinicopathologic entity that is associated with HHV-8 (Kaposi's sarcoma-associated virus).[197–199] Histologic studies show a distinctive appearance that bridges large-cell immunoblastic lymphoma and anaplastic large-cell lymphoma. Tumor cells show monoclonal immunoglobulin gene rearrangements but typically lack B cell–associated antigens. HHV-8 is detectable with PCR analysis. Patients are usually HIV positive but the syndrome has been reported in HIV-negative patients.[200] Patients present with malignant effusions in either the pleural or peritoneal cavity, which remain localized to the body cavity of origin. Disease progression is rapid with survival of only a few weeks to months. Optimal therapy has not been defined.

REFERENCES

1. Harris NL, Jaffe ES, Stein H, et al: A revised European-American classification of lymphoid neoplasms: A proposal from the International Lymphoma Study Group. Blood 84:1361–1392, 1994.
2. Harris NL, Jaffe ES, Diebold J, et al: The World Health Organization classification of neoplastic diseases of the hematopoietic and lymphoid tissues. Report of the Clinical Advisory Committee meeting, Airlie House, Virginia, November 1997. J Clin Oncol 17:3835–3849, 1999.
3. Isaacson P: Gastrointestinal lymphomas of T- and B-cell types. Mod Pathol 12:151–158, 1999.
4. Zucca E, Cavalli F: Gut lymphomas. Baillieres Clin Haematol 9:727–741, 1996.
5. Zucca E, Roggero E, Bertoni F, Cavalli F: Primary extranodal non-Hodgkin's lymphomas. Part 1: Gastrointestinal, cutaneous and genitourinary lymphomas. Ann Oncol 8:727–737, 1997.
6. Greenlee R, Hill-Harmon M, Murray T, Thun M: Cancer Statistics, 2001. CA Cancer J Clin 51:15–36, 2001.
7. D'Amore F, Brincker H, Gronbaek K, et al: Non Hodgkin's lymphoma of the gastrointestinal tract: A population-based analysis of incidence, geographic distribution, clinico-pathologic presentation features, and prognosis. J Clin Oncol 12:1673–1684, 1994.
8. Picker L, Siegelman M: Lymphoid tissues and organs. In: Fundamental Immunology, 4th ed. Philadelphia, Lippincott-Raven, 1999, pp 479–532.
9. Pugh W, McBride J: The Pathologic Basis for the Classification of Non-Hodgkin Lymphomas. Hematology: Basic Principles and Practice, 3d ed. New York, Churchill Livingstone, 2000, pp 1263–1293.
10. Ferry J, Harris N: Atlas of Lymphoid Hyperplasia and Lymphoma. Philadelphia, WB Saunders, 1997.
11. van Besien K, Cabanillas F: Clinical manifestations, staging, and treatment of non-Hodgkin lymphoma. In: Hematology: Basic Principles and Practice. New York, Churchill Livingstone, 2000, pp 1293–1339.
12. Alizadeh AA, Eisen MB, Davis RE, et al: Distinct types of diffuse large B-cell lymphoma identified by gene expression profiling. Nature 403: 503–511, 2000.
13. Sackmann M, Morgner A, Rudolph B, et al: Regression of gastric MALT lymphoma after eradication of Helicobacter pylori is predicted by endosonographic staging. MALT Lymphoma Study Group. Gastroenterology 113:1087–1090, 1997.
14. Rohatiner A, D'Amore F, Coiffier B, et al: Report on a workshop convened to discuss the pathological and staging classifications of gastrointestinal tract lymphoma. Ann Oncol 5:397–400, 1994.
15. Steinbach G, Ford R, Glober G, et al: Antibiotic treatment of gastric lymphoma of mucosa-associated lymphoid tissue: An uncontrolled trial. Ann Intern Med 131:88–95, 1999.
16. Shipp MA, Harrington DP: International non-Hodgkin's lymphoma prognostic factors project: A predictive model for aggressive non-Hodgkin's lymphoma. N Engl J Med 329:987–994, 1993.
17. Cortelazzo S, Rossi A, Roggero F, et al: Stage-modified international prognostic index effectively predicts clinical outcome of localized primary gastric diffuse large B-cell lymphoma. International extranodal lymphoma study group (IELSG). Ann Oncol 10:1433–1440, 1999.
18. Wotherspoon AC: Gastric lymphoma of mucosa-associated lymphoid tissue and *Helicobacter pylori*. Annu Rev Med 49:289–299, 1998.
19. Zucca E, Roggero E, Pileri S: B-cell lymphoma of MALT type: A review with special emphasis on diagnostic and management problems of low-grade gastric tumours. Br J Haematol 100:3–14, 1998.
20. Isaacson PG: Gastric MALT lymphoma: From concept to cure. Ann Oncol 10:637–645, 1999.
21. Isaacson PG: Mucosa-associated lymphoid tissue lymphoma. Semin Hematol 36:139–147, 1999.
22. Zucca E, Bertoni F, Roggero E, Cavalli F: The gastric marginal zone B-cell lymphoma of MALT type. Blood 96:410–419, 2000.
23. Stolte M, Eidt S: Lymphoid follicles in antral mucosa: Immune response to *Campylobacter pylori*? J Clin Pathol 42:1269–1271, 1989.
24. Genta RM, Hamner HW, Graham DY: Gastric lymphoid follicles in *Helicobacter pylori* infection: Frequency, distribution, and response to triple therapy. Hum Pathol 24:577–583, 1993.
25. Wotherspoon AC, Doglioni C, Diss TC, et al: Regression of primary low-grade B-cell gastric lymphomas of mucosa-associated lymphoid tissue to *Helicobacter pylori*. Lancet 342:575–577, 1993.
26. Savio A, Franzin G, Wotherspoon AC, et al: Diagnosis and posttreatment follow-up of *Helicobacter pylori*-positive gastric lymphoma of mucosa-associated lymphoid tissue: Histology, polymerase chain reaction, or both? Blood 87:1255–1260, 1996.
27. Cogliatti SB, Schmid U, Schumacher U, et al: Primary B-cell gastric lymphoma: A clinicopathological study of 145 patients. Gastroenterology 101:1159–1170, 1991.
28. Doglioni C, Wotherspoon AC, Moschini A, de Boni M, Isaacson PG: High incidence of primary gastric lymphoma in northeastern Italy. Lancet 339:834–835, 1992.
29. Zaki M, Schubert ML: *Helicobacter pylori* and gastric lymphoma. Gastroenterology 108:610–612, 1995.
30. Wotherspoon A, Ortiz-Hidalgo C, Falzon M, Isaacson P: *Helicobacter pylori*-associated gastritis and primary B-cell gastric lymphoma. Lancet 338:1175–1176, 1991.
31. Zucca E, Bertoni F, Roggero E, et al: Molecular analysis of the progression from *Helicobacter pylori*-associated chronic gastritis to mucosa-associated lymphoid-tissue lymphoma of the stomach. N Engl J Med 338:804–810, 1998.
32. Eck M, Greiner A, Schmausser B, et al: Evaluation of *Helicobacter pylori* in gastric MALT-type lymphoma: Differences between histologic and serologic diagnosis. Mod Pathol 12:1148–1151, 1999.
33. Parsonnet J, Hansen S, Rodriguez L, et al: *Helicobacter pylori* infection and gastric lymphoma [see comments]. N Engl J Med 330:1267–1271, 1994.
34. Hussell T, Isaacson PG, Crabtree JE, Spencer J: The response of cells from low-grade B-cell gastric lymphomas of mucosa-associated lymphoid tissue to *Helicobacter pylori*. Lancet 342:571–574, 1993.
35. Hussell T, Isaacson PG, Spencer J: Proliferation and differentiation of tumour cells from B-cell lymphoma of mucosa-associated lymphoid tissue in vitro. J Pathol 169:221–227, 1993.
36. Hussell T, Isaacson PG: *Helicobacter pylori*-specific tumour-infiltrating T cells provide contact dependent help for the growth of malignant B cells in low-grade gastric lymphoma of mucosa-associated lymphoid tissue. J Pathol 178:122–127, 1996.
37. Roggero E, Zucca E, Pinotti G, et al: Therapy outcome in primary low-grade gastric lymphoma of mucosa associated lymphoid tissue for *H. pylori* infection. Lancet 345:1591–1594, 1995.
38. Bayerdorffer E, Neubauer A, Rudolph B, et al: Regression of primary gastric lymphoma of mucosa-associated lymphoid tissue type after cure of *Helicobacter pylori* infection. MALT Lymphoma Study Group. Lancet 345:1591–1594, 1995.
39. Neubauer A, Thiede C, Morgner A, et al: Cure of *Helicobacter pylori* infection and duration of remission of low-grade gastric mucosa-asso-

ciated lymphoid tissue lymphoma. J Natl Cancer Inst 89:1350–1355, 1997.
40. Thiede C, Morgner A, Alpen B, et al: What role does *Helicobacter pylori* eradication play in gastric MALT and gastric MALT lymphoma? Gastroenterology 113:S61–S64, 1997.
41. Ghia P, Nadler LM: Recent advances in lymphoma biology. Curr Opin Oncol 9:403–412, 1997.
42. Qin Y, Greiner A, Trunk MJ, et al: Somatic hypermutation in low-grade mucosa-associated lymphoid tissue-type B-cell lymphoma. Blood 86:3528–3534, 1995.
43. Du M, Diss TC, Xie C, et al: Ongoing mutation in MALT lymphoma immunoglobulin gene suggests that antigen stimulation plays a role in the clonal expansion. Leukemia 10:1190–1197, 1996.
44. Bertoni F, Cazzaniga G, Bosshad G, et al: Immunoglobulin heavy chain diversity genes rearrangement pattern indicates that MALT-type gastric lymphoma B cells have undergone an antigen selection process. Br J Haematol 97:830–836, 1997.
45. Greiner A, Knorr C, Qin Y, et al: Low-grade B cell lymphomas of mucosa-associated lymphoid tissue (MALT-type) require CD40-mediated signaling and Th2-type cytokines for in vitro growth and differentiation. Am J Pathol 150:1583–1593, 1997.
46. Hussell T, Isaacson PG, Crabtree JE, Dogan A, Spencer J: Immunoglobulin specificity of low grade B cell gastrointestinal lymphoma of mucosa-associated lymphoid tissue (MALT) type. Am J Pathol 142: 285–292, 1993.
47. Dierlamm J, Baens M, Stefanova-Ouzounova M, et al: Detection of t(11;18q21;q21) by interphase fluorescence in situ hybridization using API2 and MLT specific probes. Blood 96:2215–2218, 2000.
48. Dierlamm J, Wlodarska I, Michaux L, et al: Genetic abnormalities in marginal zone B-cell lymphoma. Hematol Oncol 18:1–13, 2000.
49. Auer IA, Gascoyne RD, Connors SM, et al: t(11;18q21;q21) is the most common translocation in MALT lymphomas. Ann Oncol 8:979–985, 1997.
50. Dierlamm J, Baens M, Wlodarska I, et al: The apoptosis inhibitor gene API2 and a novel 18q gene, MLT, are recurrently rearranged in the t(11;18q21;q21) associated with mucosa-associated lymphoid tissue lymphomas. Blood 93:3601–3609, 1999.
51. Liu H, Ruskon-Fourmestraux A, Lavergne-Slove A, et al: Resistance of t(11;18) positive gastric mucosa-associated lymphoid tissue lymphoma to *Helicobacter pylori* eradication therapy. Lancet 357:39–40, 2001.
52. Wotherspoon AC, Pan LX, Diss TC, et al: Cytogenetic study of B-cell lymphoma of mucosa-associated lymphoid tissue. Cancer Genet Cytogenet 58:35–38, 1992.
53. Zhang Q, Siebert R, Yan M, et al: Inactivating mutations and overexpression of BCL10, a caspase recruitment domain-containing gene, in MALT lymphoma with t(1;14p22;q32). Nat Genet 22:63–68, 1999.
54. Willis TG, Jadayel DM, Du MQ, et al: Bcl 10 is involved in t(1; 14p22;q32) of MALT B cell lymphoma and mutated in multiple tumor types. Cell 96:35–45, 1999.
55. Du MQ, Pang H, Lin H, et al: BCL10 gene mutation in lymphoma. Blood 95:3885–3890, 2000.
56. Fakruddin JM, Chaganti RS, Murty VV: Lack of BCL10 mutations in germ cell tumors and B cell lymphomas. Cell 97:683–684, discussion 686–688, 1999.
57. Wotherspoon AC, Finn TM, Isaacson PG: Trisomy 3 in low-grade B-cell lymphomas of mucosa-associated lymphoid tissue. Blood 85: 2000–2004, 1995.
58. Ott G, Kalla J, Steinhoff A, et al: Trisomy 3 is not a common feature in malignant lymphomas of mucosa-associated lymphoid tissue type. Am J Pathol 153:689–694, 1998.
59. Peng H, Diss T, Isaacson PG: C-myc gene abnormalities in mucosa-associated lyphoid tissue (MALT) lymphomas. J Pathol 181:381–386, 1997.
60. Du M, Peng H, Singh N: The accumulation of p53 abnormalities is associated with progression of mucosa-associated lymphoid tissue lymphoma. Blood 86:4587–4593, 1995.
61. Neumeister P, Hoefler G, Beham Schmid C: Deletion analysis of the p16 tumor suppresser gene in gastrointestinal mucosa-associated lymphoid tissue lymphomas. Gastroenterology 112:1871–1875, 1997.
62. Chong JM, Fukayama M, Hayashi Y, et al: Microsatellite instability and loss of heterozygosity in gastric lymphoma. Lab Invest 77:639–645, 1997.
63. Peng H, Chen G, Du M, et al: Replication error phenotype and p53 gene mutation in lymphomas of mucosa-associated lymphoid tissue. Am J Pathol 148:643–648, 1996.
64. Xu WS, Chan ACL, Liang R: No evidence of replication error phenotype in primary gastric lymphoma of mucoa-associated lymphoid tissue. Int J Cancer 76:635–638, 1998.
65. Gronbaek K, Straten PT, Ralfkiaer E, et al: Somatic Fas mutations in non-Hodgkin's lymphoma: Association with extranodal disease and autoimmunity. Blood 92:3018–3024, 1998.
66. Bertoni F, Conconi A, Luminari S, et al: Lack of CD95/FAS gene somatic mutations in marginal zone B-cell lymphomas. Leukemia 3: 446–448, 2000.
67. Mazzucchelli L, Blaser A, Kappeler A, et al: BCA-1 is highly expressed in *Helicobacter pylori*-induced mucosa-associated lymphoid tissue and gastric lymphoma. J Clin Invest 104:R49–R54, 1999.
68. Peng H, Ranaldi R, Diss TC, et al: High frequency of CagA+ *Helicobacter pylori* infection in high-grade gastric MALT B-cell lymphomas. J Pathol 185:409–412, 1998.
69. de Jong D, van der Hulst RW, Pals G, et al: Gastric non-Hodgkin lymphomas of mucosa-associated lymphoid tissue are not associated with more aggressive *Helicobacter pylori* strains as identified by CagA. Am J Clin Pathol 106:670–675, 1996.
70. Isaacson PG, Norton AJ: Malignant lymphoma of the gastrointestinal tract. In: Extranodal Lymphomas. Edinburgh, Churchill Livingstone, 1994, pp 15–65.
71. Chan J: Gastrointestinal lymphomas: An overview with emphasis on new findings and diagnostic problems. Semin Diagn Pathol 13:260–296, 1996.
72. Chan JK, Ng CS, Isaacson PG: Relationship between high-grade lymphoma and low-grade B-cell mucosa-associated lymphoid tissue lymphoma (MALToma) of the stomach. Am J Pathol 136:1153–1164, 1990.
73. de Jong D, Boot H, van Heerde P, Hart GA, Taal BG: Histological grading in gastric lymphoma: Pretreatment criteria and clinical relevance. Gastroenterology 112:1466–1474, 1997.
74. Aiello A, Giardini R, Tondini C, et al: PCR-based clonality analysis: A reliable method for the diagnosis and follow-up monitoring of conservatively treated gastric B-cell MALT lymphomas? Histopathology 34:326–330, 1999.
75. Pinotti G, Zucca E, Roggero E, et al: Clinical features, treatment and outcome in a series of 93 patients with low-grade gastric MALT lymphoma. Leuk Lymphoma 26:527–537, 1997.
76. Pavlick AC, Gerdes H, Portlock CS: Endoscopic ultrasound in the evaluation of gastric small lymphocytic mucosa-associated lymphoid tumors. J Clin Oncol 15:1761–1766, 1997.
77. de Jong D, Aleman BMP, Taal BG, Boot H: Controversies and consensus in the diagnosis, work-up and treatment of gastric lymphoma: An international survey. Ann Oncol 10:275–280, 1999.
78. Hunt RH: Peptic ulcer disease: Defining the treatment strategies in the era of *Helicobacter pylori*. Am J Gastroenterol 92:S36–S40, 1997.
79. Yamashita H, Watanabe H, Ajioka Y, et al: When can complete regression of low-grade gastric lymphoma of mucosa-associated lymphoid tissue be predicted after *Helicobacter pylori* eradication? Histopathology 37:131–140, 2000.
80. Thiede C, Wundisch T, Neubauer B, et al: Eradication of *Helicobacter pylori* and stability of remissions in low-grade gastric B-cell lymphomas of the mucosa-associated lymphoid tissue: Results of an ongoing multicenter trial. Recent Results Cancer Res 156:125–133, 2000.
81. Hammel P, Haioun C, Chaumette MT, et al: Efficacy of single-agent chemotherapy in low-grade B-cell mucosa-associated lymphoid tissue lymphoma with prominent gastric expression. J Clin Oncol 13:2524–2529, 1995.
82. Schechter NR, Portlock CS, Yahalom J: Treatment of mucosa-associated lymphoid tissue lymphoma of the stomach with radiation alone. J Clin Oncol 16:1916–1921, 1998.
83. Thieblemont C, Bastion Y, Berger F, et al: Mucosa-associated lymphoid tissue gastrointestinal and nongastrointestinal lymphoma behavior: Analysis of 108 patients. J Clin Oncol 15:1624–1630, 1997.
84. Ibrahim EM, Ezzat AA, Raja MA, et al: Primary gastric non-Hodgkin's lymphoma: Clinical features, management, and prognosis of 185 patients and diffuse large B-cell lymphoma. Ann Oncol 10:1441–1449, 1999.
85. Almasri NM, al-Abbadi M, Rewaily E, Abulkhail A, Tarawneh MS: Primary gastrointestinal lymphomas in Jordan are similar to those in western countries. Mod Pathol 10:137–141, 1997.
86. De Wolf-Peeters C, Achten R: The histogenesis of large-cell gastric lymphomas. Histopathology 34:71–75, 1999.
87. Montalban C, Manzanal A, Castrillo JM, Escribano L, Bellas C: Low

grade gastric B-cell MALT lymphoma progressing into high grade lymphoma. Clonal identity of the two stages of the tumour, unusual bone involvement and leukemic dissemination. Histopathology 27:89–91, 1995.
88. Hsu C, Chen CL, Chen LT, et al: Comparison of MALT and non-MALT primary large cell lymphoma of the stomach. Cancer 91:49–56, 2001.
89. Morton JE, Leyland MJ, Vaughan Hudson G, et al: Primary gastrointestinal non-Hodgkin's lymphoma: A review of 175 British National Lymphoma Investigation cases. Br J Cancer 67:776–782, 1993.
90. Driessen A, Tirens A, Ectors N, et al: Primary diffuse large B cell lymphoma of the stomach: Analysis of somatic mutations in the rearranged immunoglobulin heavy chain variable genes indicates antigen selection. Leukemia 13:1085–1092, 1999.
91. Yoshino T, Omonishi K, Kobayashi K, et al: Clinicopathological features of gastric mucosa associated lymphoid tissue (MALT) lymphomas: High grade transformation and comparison with diffuse large B cell lymphomas without MALT lymphoma features. J Clin Pathol 53: 187–190, 2000.
92. Hsi ED, Eisbruch A, Greenson JK, et al: Classification of primary gastric lymphomas according to histologic features. Am J Surg Pathol 22:17–27, 1998.
93. Takeshita M, Inashita A, Kurihara K, et al: Histologic and immunohistologic findings and prognosis of 40 cases of gastric large B-cell lymphoma. Am J Surg Pathol 24:1641–1649, 2000.
94. Liang R, Chan WP, Kwong YL, et al: Bcl-6 gene hypermutations in diffuse large B-cell lymphoma of primary gastric origin. Br J Haematol 99:668–670, 1997.
95. Coiffier B, Salles G: Does surgery belong to medical history for gastric lymphomas? Ann Oncol 8:419–421, 1997.
96. Sheehan RG: Gastric lymphoma. Curr Treat Options Gastroenterol 2: 183–194, 1999.
97. Rossi A, Lister TA: Primary gastric non-Hodgkin's lymphoma: A therapeutic challenge. Eur J Cancer 14:1924–1926, 1993.
98. Herrmann R, Panahon AM, Barcos M: Gastrointestinal involvement in non-Hodgkin's lymphoma. Cancer 46:215–222, 1980.
99. Maor MH, Velasquez WS, Fuller LM, Silvermintz KB: Stomach conservation in stages IE and IIE gastric non-Hodgkin's lymphoma. J Clin Oncol 8:266–271, 1990.
100. Salles G, Herbrecht R, Tilly H, et al: Aggressive primary gastrointestinal lymphomas: Review of 91 patients treated with the LNH-84 regimen. A study of the Groupe d'Etude des Lymphomes Agressifs. Am J Med 90:77–84, 1991.
101. Rosen CB, van Heerden JA, Martin JK, Wold LE, Ilstrup DM: Is an aggressive surgical approach to the patient with gastric lymphoma warranted? Ann Surg 205:634–640, 1987.
102. Gobbi PG, Dionigi P, Barbieri F: The role of surgery in the multimodal treatment of primary gastric non-Hodgkin's lymphomas. A report of 76 cases and review of the literature. Cancer 65:2528–2536, 1990.
103. Taal BG, den Hartog Jager FC, Burgers JM, van Heerde P, Tio TL: Primary non-Hodgkin's lymphoma of the stomach: Changing aspects and therapeutic choices. Eur J Cancer Clin Oncol 25:439–450, 1989.
104. Tondini C, Balzarotti M, Santoro A, et al: Initial chemotherapy for primary resectable large-cell lymphoma of the stomach. Ann Oncol 8: 497–499, 1997.
105. Raderer M, Valencak J, Osterreicher C, et al: Chemotherapy for the treatment of patients with primary high grade gastric B-cell lymphoma of modified Ann Arbor Stages IE and IIE. Cancer 88:1979–1985, 2000.
106. Liu HT, Hsu C, Chen CL, et al: Chemotherapy alone versus surgery followed by chemotherapy for stage I/IIE large-cell lymphoma of the stomach. Am J Hematol 64:175–179, 2000.
107. Miller TP, Dahlberg S, Cassady TR, et al: Chemotherapy alone compared with chemotherapy plus radiotherapy for localized intermediate- and high-grade non-Hodgkin's lymphoma [see comments]. N Engl J Med 339:21–26, 1998.
108. Glick JH, Kim K, Earle J, O'Connell MJ: An ECOG randomized Phase III trial of CHOP vs CHOP + radiotherapy (XRT) for intermediate grade early stage non-Hodgkin's lymphoma (NHL) (meeting abstract). Proc Annu Meet Am Soc Clin Oncol 14:A1221, 1995.
109. Mittal B, Wasserman TH, Griffith RC: Non-Hodgkin's lymphoma of the stomach. Am J Gastroenterol 78:780-787, 1983.
110. Seymour JF, Anderson RP, Bhathal PS: Regression of gastric lymphoma with therapy for *Helicobacter pylori* infection. Ann Intern Med 127:247, 1997.
111. Aozasa K, Tsujimoto M, Inoue A, et al: Primary gastrointestinal lymphoma. A clinicopathologic study of 102 patients. Oncology 42:97–103, 1985.
112. Arends JE, Bot FJ, Gisbertz IA, Schouten HC: Expression of CD10, CD75 and CD43 in MALT lymphoma and their usefulness in discriminating MALT lymphoma from follicular lymphoma and chronic gastritis. Histopathology 35:209–215, 1999.
113. Campo E, Raffeld M, Jaffe ES: Mantle-cell lymphoma. Semin Hematol 36:115–127, 1999.
114. LeBrun DP, Kamel OW, Cleary ML, Dorfman RF, Warnke RA: Follicular lymphomas of the gastrointestinal tract. Pathologic features in 31 cases and bcl-2 oncogenic protein expression. Am J Pathol 140: 1327–1335, 1992.
115. Ruskone-Fourmestraux A, Delmer A, Lavergne A, et al: Multiple lymphomatous polyposis of the gastrointestinal tract: Prospective clinicopathologic study of 31 cases. Gastroenterology 112:7–16, 1997.
116. Bishop PC, Rao VK, Wilson WH: Burkitt's lymphoma: Molecular pathogenesis and treatment. Cancer Invest 18:574–583, 2000.
117. Itatsu T, Miwa H, Ohkura A, et al: Primary gastric T-cell lymphoma accompanied by HTLV-I, HBV and H. pylori infection. Dig Dis Sci 44:1823–1836, 1999.
118. Murata T, Nakamura S, Oka K, et al: Granzyme B-positive primary gastric T-cell lymphoma: Gastric T-cell lymphoma with the possibility of extrathymic T cell origin. Pathol Int 50:853-857, 2000.
119. Domizio P, Owen RA, Shepherd NA, Talbot IC, Norton AJ: Primary lymphoma of the small intestine. A clinicopathological study of 119 cases. Am J Surg Pathol 17:429–442, 1993.
120. Nakamura S, Matsumoto T, Takeshita M, et al: A clinicopathologic study of primary small intestine lymphoma: Prognostic significance of mucosa-associated lymphoid tissue-derived lymphoma. Cancer 88: 286–294, 2000.
121. O'Briain DS, Kennedy MJ, Daly PA, et al: Multiple lymphomatous polyposis of the gastrointestinal tract. A clinicopathologically distinctive form of non-Hodgkin's lymphoma of B-cell centrocytic type. Am J Surg Pathol 13:691–699, 1989.
122. Price SK: Immunoproliferative small intestinal disease: A study of 13 cases with alpha heavy-chain disease. Histopathology 17:7–17, 1990.
123. Martin IG, Aldoori MI: Immunoproliferative small intestinal disease: Mediterranean lymphoma and a heavy chain disease. Br J Surg 1:20–24, 1994.
124. Jones JD, Levin B, Salem P: Intestinal lymphomas, including immunoproliferative small intestinal disease. In Feldman M, Scharschmidt BF, Sleisenger MH (eds): Sleisenger and Fordtran's Gastrointestinal and Liver Disease, 6th ed. Philadelphia, WB Saunders, 1998, pp 1844–1857.
125. Malik IA, Shamsi Z, Shafquat A: Clinicopathological features and management of immunoproliferative small intestinal disease and primary small intestinal lymphoma in Pakistan. Med Pediatr Oncol 25: 400, 1995.
126. Fine K, Stone M: α-Heavy chain disease, Mediterranean lymphoma, and immunoproliferative small intestine disease: A review of clinicopathological features, pathogenesis, and differential diagnosis. Am J Gastroenterol 94:1139–1152, 1999.
127. Khojasteh A, Haghighi P: Immunoproliferative small intestinal disease: Portrait of a potentially preventable cancer from the Third World. Am J Med 89:483–490, 1990.
128. Isaacson P: Middle east lymphoma and alpha-chain disease. An immunohistochemical study. Am J Surg Pathol 3:431–441, 1979.
129. Isaacson PG, Dogan A, Price SK, Spencer J: Immunoproliferative small-intestinal disease. An immunohistochemical study. Am J Surg Pathol 13:1023–1033, 1989.
130. Smith WJ, Price SK, Isaacson PG: Immunoglobulin gene rearrangement in immunoproliferative small intestinal disease (IPSID). J Clin Pathol 40:1291–1297, 1987.
131. Isaacson PG, Price SK: Light chains in Mediterranean lymphoma. J Clin Pathol 38:601–607, 1985.
132. Alpha-chain disease and related small-intestinal lymphoma: A memorandum. Bull WHO 54:615–624, 1976.
133. Salem P, et al: Primary small intestinal lymphoma in adults. A comparative study of IPSID versus non-IPSID in the Middle East. Cancer 59:1670–1676, 1987.
134. Salem PA, Nassar VH, Shahid MJ, et al: "Mediterranean abdominal lymphoma," or immunoproliferative small intestinal disease. Part I: clinical aspects. Cancer 40:2941–2947, 1977.
135. Galian A, Lecestre MJ, Scotto J, et al: Pathological study of alpha-

chain disease, with special emphasis on evolution. Cancer 39:2081–2101, 1977.

136. Matuchansky C, Cogne M, Lemaire M, et al: Nonsecretory alpha-chain disease with immunoproliferative small-intestinal disease. N Engl J Med 320:1534–1539, 1989.
137. Banisadre M, Ala F, Modjtabai A, Dutz W, Navab F: Immunoproliferative small intestinal disease and primary small intestinal lymphoma. Relation to alpha chain protein. Cancer 56:1384–1391, 1985.
138. Cogne M, Preud'homme JL: Gene deletions force nonsecretory a-chain disease plasma cells to produce membrane-form a-chain only. J Immunol 145, 1990.
139. Seligmann M: Alpha chain disease: Immunoglobulin abnormalities, pathogenesis and current concepts. Br J Cancer 31(suppl 2):356–361, 1975.
140. Rambaud JC: Small intestinal lymphomas and alpha-chain disease. Clin Gastroenterol 12:743–766, 1983.
141. Doe WF: Alpha heavy chain disease and related small-intestinal lymphomas. In: Asequith P (ed): Immunology of the Gastrointestinal Tract. Edinburgh, Churchill Livingstone, 1979, pp 306–315.
142. Mir-Madjlessi SH, Mir-Ahmadian M: Alpha-chain disease—a report of eleven patients from Iran. J Trop Med Hygiene 82:229–236, 1979.
143. Rambaud JC, Galian A, Dannon FG, et al: Alpha-chain disease without qualitative serum IgA abnormality. Report of two cases, including a "nonsecretory" form. Cancer 51:686–693, 1983.
144. Doe WF, Danon F, Seligmann M: Immunodiagnosis of alpha chain disease. Clin Exp Immunol 36:189–197, 1979.
145. Akbulut H, Soykan I, Yakaryilmaz F, et al: Five-year results of the treatment of 23 patients with immunoproliferative small intestinal disease: A Turkish experience. Cancer 80:8–14, 1997.
146. Ben-Ayed F, Halphen M, Naijar T, et al: Treatment of alpha chain disease: Results of a prospective study in 21 Tunisian patients by the Tunisian-French intestinal lymphoma study group. Cancer 63:1251–1256, 1989.
147. Salimi M, Spinelli JJ: Chemotherapy of Mediterranean abdominal lymphoma. Retrospective comparison of chemotherapy protocols in Iranian patients. Am J Clin Oncol 19:18–22, 1996.
148. O'Keefe SJ, Winter TA, Newton KA, et al: Severe malnutrition associated with alpha-heavy chain disease: Response to tetracycline and intensive nutritional support. Am J Gastroenterol 83:995–1001, 1988.
149. El Saghir NS: Combination chemotherapy with tetracycline and aggressive supportive care for immunoproliferative small-intestinal lymphoma. J Clin Oncol 13:794, 1995.
150. Egan LJ, Walsh SV, Stevens FM, et al: Celiac-associated lymphoma. A single institution experience of 30 cases in the combination chemotherapy era. J Clin Gastroenterol 21:123–129, 1995.
151. Gale J, Simmonds PD, Mead GM, Sweetenham JW, Wright DH: Enteropathy-type intestinal T-cell lymphoma: Clinical features and treatment of 31 patients in a single center. J Clin Oncol 18:795–803, 2000.
152. Chott A, Vesely M, Simonitsch I, Mosberger I, Hanak H: Classification of intestinal T-cell neoplasms and their differential diagnosis. Am J Clin Pathol 111(suppl 1):S68–S74, 1999.
153. A clinical evaluation of the international lymphoma study group classification of non-Hodgkin's lymphoma. The non-Hodgkin's lymphoma classification project. Blood 89:3909–3918, 1997.
154. Cooper BT, Holmes GK, Cooke WT: Lymphoma risk in coeliac disease of later life. Digestion 23:89–92, 1982.
155. Cooper BT, Holmes GK, Ferguson R, Cooke WT: Celiac disease and malignancy. Medicine 59:249–261, 1980.
156. Brandt L, Hagander B, Norden A, Stenstam M: Lymphoma of the small intestine in adult coeliac disease. Acta Med Scand 204:467–470, 1978.
157. Holmes GK, Prior P, Lane MR, Pope D, Allan RN: Malignancy in coeliac disease—effect of a gluten free diet. Gut 30:333–338, 1989.
158. Isaacson PG: Intestinal lymphoma and enteropathy. J Pathol 177:111–113, 1995.
159. Trier JS: Celiac sprue. N Engl J Med 325:1709-1719, 1991.
160. Schuppan D: Current concepts of celiac disease pathogenesis. Gastroenterology 119:234–242, 2000.
161. Ryan BM, Kelleher D: Refractory celiac disease. Gastroenterology 119:243–251, 2000.
162. Carbonnel F, Grollet-Bioul L, et al: Are complicated forms of celiac disease cryptic T-cell lymphomas? Blood 92:3879–3886, 1998.
163. Cellier C, Patey N, Mauvieux, et al: Abnormal intestinal intraepithelial lymphocytes in refractory sprue. Gastroenterology 114:471–481, 1998.
164. Bagdi E, Diss TC, Munson P, Isaacson PG: Mucosal intra-epithelial lymphocytes in enteropathy-associated T-cell lymphoma, ulcerative jejunitis, and refractory celiac disease constitute a neoplastic population. Blood 94:260–264, 1999.
165. Blumberg RS, Yockey CE, Gross GG, et al: Human intestinal intraepithelial lymphocytes are derived from a limited number of T cell clones that utilize multiple V beta T cell receptor genes. J Immunol 150:5144–5153, 1993.
166. Gross GG, Schwartz VL, Stevens C, et al: Distribution of dominant T cell receptor beta chains in human intestinal mucosa. J Exp Med 180: 1337–1344, 1994.
167. Cellier C, Delabesse E, Helmer C, et al: Refractory sprue, coeliac disease, and enteropathy-associated T-cell lymphoma. French coeliac disease study group. Lancet 356:203–208, 2000.
168. Isaacson PG: Relation between cryptic intestinal lymphoma and refractory sprue. Lancet 356:178–179, 2000.
169. Jewell DP: Ulcerative enteritis. Br Med J 287:1740–1741, 1983.
170. Ashton-Key M, Diss TC, Pan L, Du MQ, Isaacson PG: Molecular analysis of T-cell clonality in ulcerative jejunitis and enteropathy-associated T-cell lymphoma. Am J Pathol 151:493–498, 1997.
171. Murray A, Cuevas EC, Jones DB, Wright DH: Study of the immunohistochemistry and T cell clonality of enteropathy-associated T cell lymphoma. Am J Pathol 146:509–519, 1995.
172. Chott A, Haedicke W, Mosberger I, et al: Most CD56+ intestinal lymphomas are CD8+CD5-T-cell lymphomas of monomorphic small to medium size histology. Am J Pathol 153:1483–1490, 1998.
173. Isaacson PG, O'Connor NT, Spencer J, et al: Malignant histiocytosis of the intestine: A T-cell lymphoma. Lancet 2:688–691, 1985.
174. Diss TC, Watts M, Pan LX; et al: The polymerase chain reaction in the demonstration of monoclonality in T cell lymphomas. J Clin Pathol 48:1045–1050, 1995.
175. Hoppe RT, Burke JS, Glatstein E, Kaplan HS: Non-Hodgkin's lymphoma: Involvement of Waldeyer's ring. Cancer 42:1096–1104, 1978.
176. Liang R, Ng RP, Todd D, et al: Management of stage I–II diffuse aggressive non-Hodgkin's lymphoma of the Waldeyer's ring: Combined modality therapy versus radiotherapy alone. Hematol Oncol 5: 223–230, 1987.
177. Okerbloom JA, Armitage JO, Zetterman R, Linder J: Esophageal involvement by non-Hodgkin's lymphoma. Am J Med 77:359–361, 1984.
178. Fan CW, Changchien CR, Wang JX, et al: Primary colorectal lymphoma. Dis Colon Rectum 43:1277–1282, 2000.
179. Doolabh N, Anthony T, Simmang C, et al: Primary colonic lymphoma. J Surg Oncol 74:257–262, 2000.
180. Opelz G, Schwarz V, Wujciak T: Analysis of non-Hodgkin's lymphomas in organ transplant recipients. Transplant Rev 9:231, 1995.
181. Paya CV, Fung JJ, Nalesnik MA, et al: Epstein-Barr virus-induced posttransplant lymphoproliferative disorders. ASTS/ASTP EBV-PTLD Task Force and The Mayo Clinic Organized International Consensus Development Meeting. Transplantation 68:1517–1525, 1999.
182. Harris NL, Ferry JA, Swerdlow SH: Posttransplant lymphoproliferative disorders: Summary of Society for Hematopathology Workshop. Semin Diagn Pathol 14:8–14, 1997.
183. Swinnen LJ: Overview of posttransplant B-cell lymphoproliferative disorders. Semin Oncol 26:21–25, 1999.
184. Swinnen LJ: Durable remission after aggressive chemotherapy for post-cardiac transplant lymphoproliferation. Leuk Lymphoma 28:89–101, 1997.
185. Benkerrou M, Jais JP, Leblond V, et al: Anti-B-cell monoclonal antibody treatment of severe posttransplant B-lymphoproliferative disorder: Prognostic factors and long-term outcome. Blood 92:3137–3147, 1998.
186. Milpied N, Vasseur B, Antoine C: Chimeric and CD20 monoclonal antibody (Rituximab) in B postransplant lympho-proliferative disorders (B PTLDs): A retrospective analysis of 32 patients (PTS). Blood 89: 631a(abst 2803), 1999.
187. Papadopoulos EB, Ladanyi M, Emanuel D, et al: Infusions of donor leukocytes to treat Epstein-Barr virus-associated lymphoproliferative disorders after allogeneic bone marrow transplantation. N Engl J Med 330:1185–1191, 1994.
188. 1993 Revised classification system for HIV infection and expanded surveillance case definition for AIDS among adolescents and adults. MMWR 41:961, 1992.
189. Gaidano G, Carbone A, Dalla-Favera R: Genetic basis of acquired immunodeficiency syndrome-related lymphomagenesis. J Natl Cancer Inst Monogr 23:95–100, 1998.

190. Kieff E: Current perspectives on the molecular pathogenesis of virus-induced cancers in human immunodeficiency virus infection and acquired immunodeficiency syndrome. J Natl Cancer Inst Monogr 23:7–14, 1998.
191. Kaplan LD: Clinical management of human immunodeficiency virus-associated non-Hodgkin's lymphoma. J Natl Cancer Inst Monogr 23: 101–105, 1998.
192. Place RJ, Huber PJ, Simmang CL: Anorectal lymphoma and AIDS: An outcome analysis. J Surg Oncol 73:1–4; discussion 4–5, 2000.
193. Kaplan LD, Strauss DJ, Testa MA, et al: Low-dose compared with standard-dose m-BACOD chemotherapy for non-Hodgkin's lymphoma associated with human immunodeficiency virus infection. National Institute of Allergy and Infectious Diseases AIDS Clinical Trials Group. N Engl J Med 336:1641–1648, 1997.
194. Remick SC, McSharry JJ, Wolf BC, et al: Novel oral combination chemotherapy in the treatment of intermediate-grade and high-grade AIDS-related non-Hodgkin's lymphoma. J Clin Oncol 11:1691–1702, 1993.
195. Sparano JA, Wiernik PH, Hu X, et al: Pilot trial of infusional cyclophosphamide, doxorubicin, and etoposide plus didanosine and filgrastim in patients with human immunodeficiency virus-associated non-Hodgkin's lymphoma. J Clin Oncol 14:3026–3035, 1996.
196. Spina M, Vaccher E, Carbone A, Tirelli U: Neoplastic complications of HIV infection. Ann Oncol 10:1271–1286, 1999.
197. Nador RG, Cesarman E, Chadburn A, et al: Primary effusion lymphoma: A distinct clinicopathologic entity associated with the Kaposi's sarcoma-associated herpes virus. Blood 88:645–656, 1996.
198. Ansari MQ, Dawson DB, Nador R, et al: Primary body cavity-based AIDS-related lymphomas. Am J Clin Pathol 105:221–229, 1996.
199. Gaidano G, Carbone A: Primary effusion lymphoma: A liquid phase lymphoma of fluid-filled body cavities. Adv Cancer Res 80:115–146, 2001.
200. Ascoli V, Scalzo CC, Danese C, et al: Human herpes virus-8 associated primary effusion lymphoma of the pleural cavity in HIV-negative elderly men. Eur Respir J 14:1231–1234, 1999.

Chapter 27

Gastrointestinal Complications of Solid Organ and Hematopoietic Cell Transplantation

Sally Weisdorf-Schindele and John R. Lake

Many gastrointestinal (GI) complications are common to all types of transplantation and can be related to immunosuppressive therapy. Infectious complications constitute a major portion of the difficulties encountered; the agents used also produce side effects that can result in GI complications. When infections occur, immunosuppression often has to be modified, putting patients at risk for either graft rejection or graft-versus-host disease (GVHD). Pneumatosis intestinalis is a common sign in patients receiving glucocorticoids or chemotherapy and in patients with ischemic changes of the intestine; it can occur after either solid organ or hematopoietic stem cell transplantation (HCT).[1] Its prevalence in any of the conditions discussed in this chapter and the lack of any specific etiology for its occurrence are indicative of the difficulties facing clinicians who deal with complications of transplantation. Clinicians need to determine whether the cause of pneumatosis is urgent and life threatening or benign. With the inflammatory response suppressed in the patient population under discussion, aggressive diagnosis and treatment are warranted.[2]

OVERVIEW OF COMPLICATIONS

Side Effects of Immunosuppressive Agents

The challenge in all types of transplantation is to modulate the immune response so that grafts are not rejected and do not react against host tissue and so that the host is not left helpless in the presence of infection. New strategies are being developed for more specific drug therapies[3, 4] and for modulation of undesired immunologic responses with specific cytokine products.[5] Two of the drugs currently being tested include mycophenolate mofetil[6, 7] and sirolimus.[8] The GI side effects and metabolic effects of these agents are yet to be fully elucidated. Agents currently used produce a variety of side effects that affect the GI system.

Prednisone

Glucocorticoids have been used for post-transplant immunosuppression since cellular and solid organ transplantations first began being performed. Glucocorticoid therapy is associated with gastric injury; prophylactic H_2-receptor antagonists or proton pump inhibitors are often used to prevent this complication. However, the loss of the gastric acid barrier to fungal infestation of the GI tract may lead to intestinal colonization and subsequent systemic infection with yeast. The hyperglycemia associated with steroid therapy also predisposes transplant patients to fungal infection.[9] The role of corticosteroids in the development of peptic ulcer disease has been long debated. In solid organ transplants, a major concern is delayed wound healing. The metabolic effects of steroid therapy can impair post-transplant healing. Glucocorticoids promote muscle breakdown and hepatic gluconeogenesis from amino acids and, thus, increase urea cycle activity to dispose of nitrogen. This alteration of energy metabolism can be clinically manifest as hyperglycemia and hypertriglyceridemia, when excess gluconeogenesis and administration of exogenous glucose leads to lipogenesis. Energy requirements then increase, and energy needed for healing of wounds and for vital vascular and visceral anastomoses is less available. An impaired healing of intestinal injury as often occurs following transplantation can lead to infection and bacterial translocation.

Azathioprine

Azathioprine (Imuran) in combination with glucocorticoids was the main immunosuppressive regimen used in solid organ transplantation up until the mid 1980s. In fact, the introduction of azathioprine into the immunosuppressive regimen was a major step in developing successful organ transplant programs. It is a derivative of 6-mercaptopurine. Its immunosuppressive effect is due to reduction in total T and B lymphocyte cell counts. Azathioprine produces two types of hepatotoxicity. First, its use has been associated with an acute hepatitis, which generally presents as a cholestatic hepatitis. Histologically, the predominant damage occurs centrizonally. The genotype for predisposition to form toxic metabolites is known and a genetic assay is commercially available, as is an assay for metabolite levels.[10] After withdrawal of azathioprine, the liver will heal completely. The second form of liver disease associated with azathioprine use is veno-occlusive disease (VOD) (see later discussion on HCT). This lesion develops slowly and insidiously. The predominant clinical manifestation is portal hypertension with either ascites formation, hypersplenism, or GI bleeding. Azathioprine use has also been reported to cause pancreatitis.

Cyclosporine

The introduction of cyclosporine (formerly called *cyclosporin A*) into immunosuppressive regimens in the early 1980s led to markedly improved solid organ transplant outcomes. As a result, the field of liver transplantation grew rapidly and was quickly followed by renewed interest in lung and heart transplantation. Cyclosporine has also been shown to be an effective drug for preventing GVHD in HCT recipients. The major toxicities of cyclosporine are renal and neurologic. Cyclosporine hepatoxicity is uncommon. The primary manifestation of cyclosporine hepatoxicity is cholestasis. It is believed to be, in part, dose dependent and rarely if ever causes serious liver disease. The predominant metabolic effects of cyclosporine include hypercholesterolemia and induction of the P-450 enzyme system,[11] which is also responsible for cyclosporine metabolism. An unanswered question is whether cyclosporine can be implicated in the increased incidence of cholelithiasis associated with elevated triglycerides seen in transplant patients.[12]

Tacrolimus (FK506)

Like cyclosporine, tacrolimus prevents T cell activation by inhibiting the calcineurin pathway.[13] It is generally used as a primary immunosuppressive agent and has been shown to be effective for liver, kidney, heart, and lung transplant recipients. Most important, it provides an alternative to cyclosporine for patients with refractory allograft rejection or cyclosporine toxicity. The introduction of tacrolimus into immunosuppressive regimens has facilitated the advancement of intestinal transplantation. In general, its side effect profile is similar to that of cyclosporine, with its major toxicities being neurotoxicity and nephrotoxicity. The main differences in the side effect profile of tacrolimus are the lack of hirsutism and gingival hypertrophy, and less hypercholesterolemia. However, diabetes has been reported to be more common with tacrolimus use and may not resolve when therapy is changed.[14] Tacrolimus is a macrolide and, as such, has GI side effects similar to those of other macrolides such as erythromycin, including diarrhea, abdominal pain, and nausea. Tacrolimus may also lead to anorexia and weight loss. These side effects tend to be dose dependent and respond to dose reduction. Questions have been raised concerning an increased incidence of post-transplant lymphoproliferative disorder (PTLD) in recipients of FK506.[15, 16]

Another GI complication that is seen both with cyclosporine and FK506 is eosinophilic colitis.[17] This results in diarrhea and is characterized by an eosinophilic colonic infiltrate. Some patients develop peripheral eosinophilia and elevated levels of serum immunoglobulin E (IgE). In some individuals, allergen-specific IgE for foods is present, which can aid in directing the therapeutic approach to this complication.

Sirolimus

Sirolimus (rapamycin) is a newer immunosuppressant that structurally resembles tacrolimus and is synergistic with cyclosporine. Its mechanism of immunosuppression, although not completely defined, is different from that of tacrolimus and cyclosporine. Rather than blocking gene transcription for interleukin-2 as do tacrolimus and cyclosporine, sirolimus blocks interleukin-2–dependent proliferation. Whereas tacrolimus and cyclosporine inhibit the enzyme serine-threonine phosphatase calcineurin, sirolimus does not. This property is thought to contribute to its varied side effect profile. Sirolimus does not cause neurotoxicity, nephrotoxicity, or diabetes but can produce the dose-dependent side effects of hyperlipidemia, thrombocytopenia, and elevations of liver aminotransferases.[18] Like tacrolimus, sirolimus is a macrolide and, as such, has GI side effects including diarrhea, abdominal pain, and nausea. These side effects may respond to dose reduction. One additional effect of sirolimus is its antiproliferative effect. On the negative side, this has led to some impaired wound healing manifested by an increased incidence of lymphoceles after kidney transplantation. On the positive side, it may lead to less post–heart transplantation coronary artery disease. Its use in liver transplantation is limited.

Mycophenolate Mofetil

Mycophenolate mofetil (MMF, Cellcept) is an immunosuppressive agent that acts as an inosine monophosphate dehydrogenase inhibitor. As such, it blocks proliferation of both T and B cells. It was originally approved for use in kidney transplant recipients in combination with cyclosporine and corticosteroids.[19] MMF also is now approved for use in liver transplant recipients. MMF also appears to have equal efficacy when combined with tacrolimus. Early in its development, use of MMF was limited by GI side effects, most notably dypepsia. Endoscopically and histologically, this was most commonly manifested as gastritis. Whether this finding translates into an increased incidence of peptic ulcer disease is unclear. This dyspepsia however, responds quite well to proton pump inhibitors. In fact, many programs automatically begin a proton pump inhibitor when patients are placed on MMF. MMF is also often dose limited by other GI side effects, notably diarrhea, which generally respond to dose reduction. Thus far, MMF has not been shown cause hepatoxicity or pancreatitis.

Antibody Therapy

ATG/OKT3. Antithymocyte globulin (ATG) and anti–T cell antibody therapy with OKT3 are generally reserved for patients with acute rejection episodes and severe acute GVHD and for those receiving hematopoietic cell grafts from unrelated donors. The major side effect is an acute flulike syndrome caused by release of cytokines when endogenous lymphocytes are lysed. Indomethacin has been shown to ameliorate this syndrome,[20] but pentoxifylline does not.[21] The abdominal pain that may accompany this syndrome can be quite severe and can present as an acute abdomen.[22] Complement activation[23] and histamine release[24] occur following OKT3 administration and may be involved in metabolic derangement.[25] However, diarrhea is the most common GI manifestation of this therapy. Diarrhea is quite predictable and generally lasts for 3 to 4 days. If this occurs, no evaluation is necessary unless the diarrhea persists.

ANTI-CD25 MONOCLONAL ANTIBODIES. Basilixamab and daclizumab are two humanized monoclonal antibodies directed against the CD25 molecule, which is a receptor for interleukin-2. These antibodies differ only in their degree of "humanization." They are used almost exclusively as part of the induction immunosuppressive regimen and have been approved for kidney transplant recipients. The antibodies are noncytolytic and as such do not produce the "cytokine release syndrome"; thus, they appear to have little, if any, GI toxicity.[26]

Infectious Complications

Bacteria

Infection remains a significant source of morbidity in both solid organ transplatation and HCT.[27] In a series from the University of Minnesota of 518 kidney, kidney-pancreas, kidney-liver, and kidney-islet transplant recipients, 65% of patients had identifiable infections and 70% of these were due to bacteria or to bacteria plus other types of organisms.[28] Antibiotic use is high in these populations for clinically diagnosed infection as well as for prophylactic bowel decontamination.[29] Accordingly, patients with symptoms of colitis need to be evaluated for *Clostridium difficile* infection as well as opportunistic infections.[30] Bacterial sepsis can have severe effects on liver function; cholestasis is commonly seen, and sepsis may precipitate multiorgan dysfunction syndrome.[31] The intestine can be a source of systemic infections from bacterial translocation.[32] Resistant enterococci are emerging as important etiologic agents in sepsis associated with an intestinal source.

Viruses

The major viral pathogen that affects the GI system in transplant patients is cytomegalovirus (CMV). CMV infection and reactivation are recognized. The incidence of active CMV disease among seropositive patients is approximately 25%. In some series, the liver is the most frequently affected organ,[33] whereas CMV gastroenteritis is more frequent in other centers.[34] CMV gastroenteritis can be diagnosed by a number of methods; a study from the Seattle HCT program has reported centrifugation culture of endoscopically obtained gastric and intestinal biopsies to be the most reliable method.[35] GI signs and symptoms of CMV infection can include hepatic enzyme level elevations, both hepatocellular and cholestatic; pneumatosis intestinalis[36]; and nausea, vomiting, and early satiety secondary to slow gastric emptying.[37] These occur in a setting of fever and decreasing peripheral white blood cell counts. CMV infection may also be present with GI bleeding. Enteritis may appear endoscopically as the typical small punched-out ulcers or may appear as much larger ulcers, typically in the right colon.

Strategies for decreasing the incidence of CMV include using CMV-negative donors for CMV-negative recipients and blood products from CMV-negative donors in CMV-negative HCT recipients. The prophylactic use of anti-CMV regimens featuring ganciclovir has decreased the risk of CMV disease. Treatment with OKT3 has been found to carry an increased risk for reactivation of CMV[38, 39] and the early use of antiviral therapy is recommended. The Pittsburgh transplantation group has found a lower incidence of CMV enteritis with immunosuppression by FK506 than by cyclosporine.[34] Other viruses that can involve the GI system include Epstein-Barr virus (EBV), herpes simplex, and varicella zoster.[40, 41] EBV-related PTLD can also affect the GI tract (see the section on neoplasia).

Hepatitis C virus (HCV) infection is problematic for transplant recipients for a variety of reasons.[42] First, the post-transplant immunosuppression produces a marked increase in HCV titers. Second, in a few cases it leads to more aggressive disease, which can progress to cirrhosis over even a 5- to 10-year time span. Third, the results of treatment with α-interferon–based regimens have generally been disappointing in immunosuppressed patients including transplant recipients. Moreover, such therapy has resulted in reactivation of chronic GVHD in HCT recipients and graft rejection in organ transplant recipients. HCV infection also seems to be immunosuppressive in that the incidence of bacterial infection is higher among HCV patients than among non–HCV-infected patients after transplantation. Nonetheless, it remains controversial whether HCV infection has a negative impact on the outcomes of kidney transplantation in the absence of cirrhosis. Most HCV-positive recipients have little or no disease activity. Strategies proposed to lessen the impact of HCV on post-transplant outcomes include limiting the use of grafts from HCV-positive donors to HCV-positive recipients or to recipients with life expectancies of less than 10 years.[43]

Hepatitis B virus (HBV) infection has been previously shown to increase the risk of death after kidney transplantation. However, the incidence of HBV infection has markedly decreased in the dialysis population owing to a variety of infection control measures, including vaccination. Although HBsAg-positive recipients may develop a flare of hepatitis B post-transplant, even developing the histologic lesion fibrosing cholestatic hepatitis, several reports have now shown that these patients may respond to lamivudine, an antiviral agent that inhibits HBV replication (see Chapter 68). As discussed in more detail in Chapter 83, liver transplantation for patients with cirrhosis from chronic hepatitis, HBV, or HCV represents another special category because of viral reinfection of the graft.[44, 45] Strategies for decreasing HBV reinfection have had some success, but these have not been effective for HCV.[46] Early graft failure may also be due to HCV recurrence.[47]

Fungi

At the University of Minnesota, 25% of liver transplant recipients had documented fungal infections.[28] *Candida* carriage in the small bowel was documented in 81% of liver transplantation candidates.[48] *Candida* overgrowth and diarrhea can easily occur when antibiotic therapy is instituted. *Aspergillus* is also an enteric pathogen in transplant recipients and can manifest with GI bleeding[49] (Figs. 27–1 and 27–2). Disseminated *Aspergillus* can invade the liver, causing cholestasis and abscess formation, as well as the GI tract.

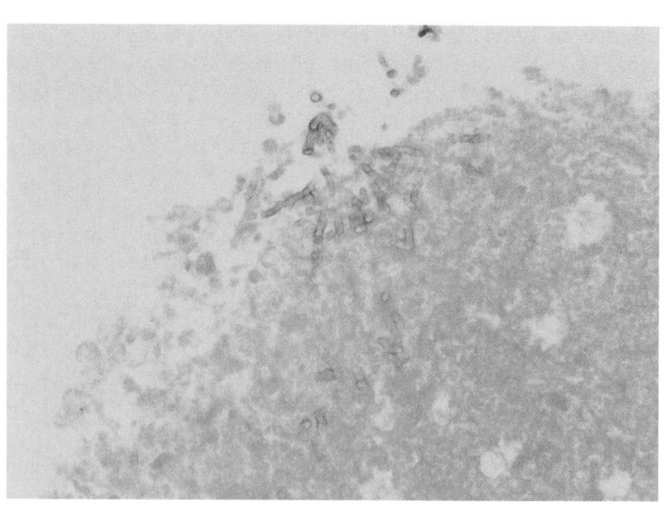

Figure 27–2. Photomicrograph of histology of aspergillosis of the gastric fundus of patient shown in Figure 27–1. (Courtesy of Jose Jessurun, MD.)

Nutritional Complications

Nutritional complications can impact any transplant recipient but are most dramatic in HCT and intestinal transplant recipients. HCT complications can represent the extreme end of the spectrum of chemotherapy and radiation effects. HCT may involve lethal chemotherapy and/or radiation therapy to achieve adequate cytoreduction for the patient to be able to engraft donor hematopoietic cells (allogeneic HCT) or to reduce the tumor burden and rescue the patient with his or her own marrow (autologous HCT).[50] Cytoreductive therapy causes painful mucositis in the oral pharynx and esophagus, altering taste sensation[51]; intestinal damage can be seen histologically up to day 21 after cytoreduction.[52] The result is typically an interval of watery diarrhea in the first week following high-dose chemotherapy or radiotherapy.[53] A prospective, randomized study of 137 recipients of bone marrow transplantation at the University of Minnesota between 1983 and 1985 showed that starting total parenteral nutrition (TPN) during cytoreduction and continuing it through the resumption of oral intake had a survival benefit.[54] In general, TPN is given to hospitalized patients for 3 to 5 weeks during the course of HCT. Resumption of oral feedings is often difficult as a result of mucositis, infections, and GVHD.[55]

In recipients awaiting solid organ transplantation, progressive organ failure produces its own unique types of nutritional debilities. Kidney transplant recipients have a unique set of nutritional complications related to the wasting that occurs during chronic dialysis[56] and chronic protein restriction.[57] Lung transplantation candidates can have severe mal-

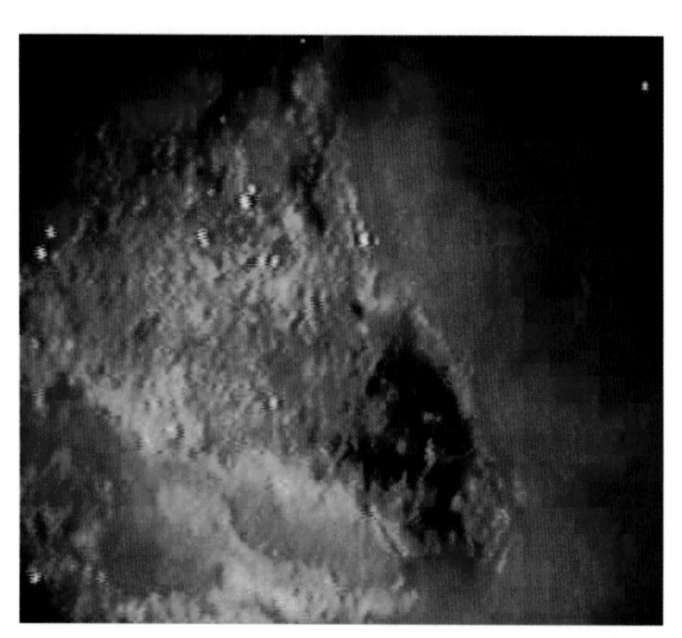

Figure 27–1. Endoscopic view of aspergillus in gastric fundus. A necrotic ulcer with clot is visible.

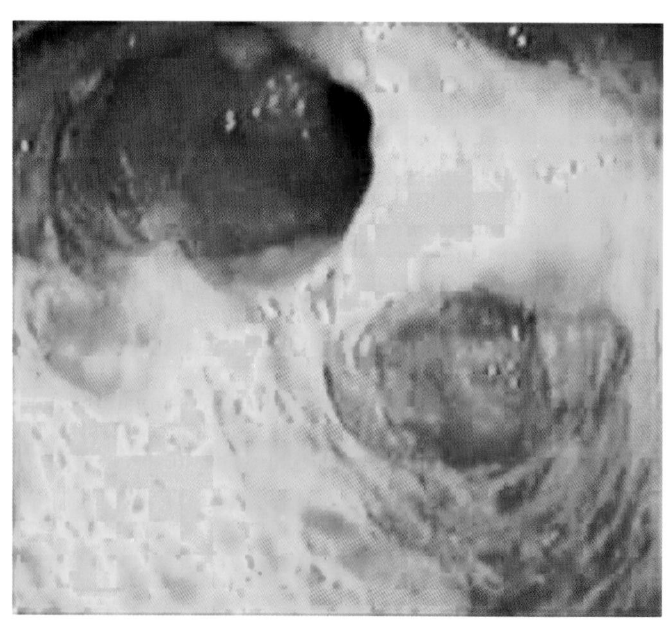

Figure 27–3. Endoscopic view of intestinal graft at the ileal-colonic anastomosis showing erythematous mucosa, which on histologic examination revealed lymphoproliferative changes (see Figure 27–4).

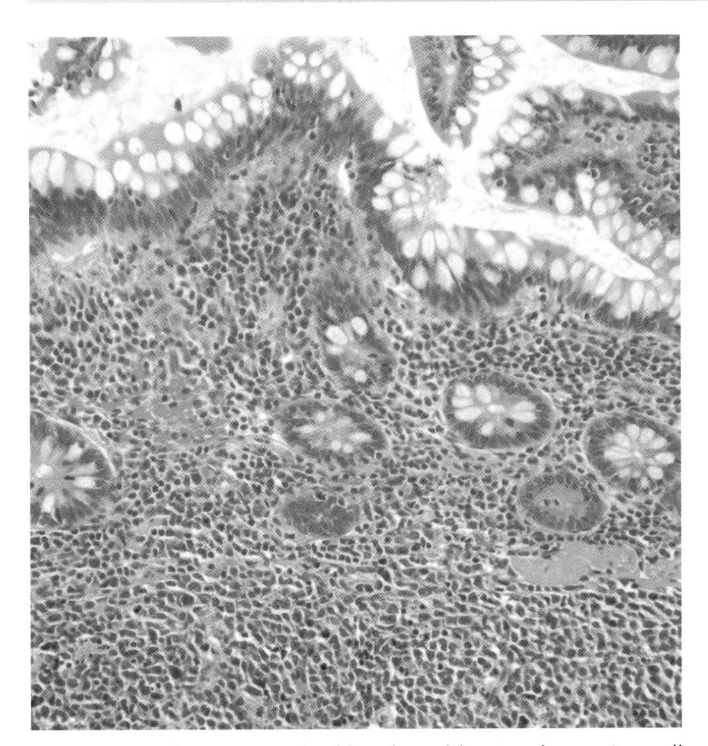

Figure 27–4. Photomicrograph of lymphoproliferative changes in small intestine. (Courtesy of Jose Jessurun, MD.)

nutrition, particularly if cystic fibrosis or emphysema is the primary disease.[58] A good response to perioperative and postoperative nutrition support in patients with cystic fibrosis who receive lung transplants has been noted to be associated with improved outcomes.[59] Short-term parenteral nutrition support has been recommended.[60] Liver failure patients can have severe nutritional deficiencies, and in children, growth failure is an indication for transplantation.[61] Nutrition assessment identified malnutrition in 17 of 20 adult liver transplantation candidates; three of these were severely malnourished.[62] It has been suggested that nutrition intervention can favorably affect graft function.[63] Pancreatic transplantation for diabetes is generally performed in conjunction with kidney transplantation. Obviously, severe nutritional depletion and metabolic derangement can occur in this setting. Intestinal transplant recipients are generally in a controlled nutrition program before transplantation and may be dependent on parenteral nutrition for a prolonged period following transplantation.[64, 65]

Neoplasia

Overall, the incidence of neoplastic disease is increased after any type of transplantation. Second malignancies can occur in patients who undergo HCT for cancer. Of particular prominence in both HCT and solid organ transplantation is PTLD, which is associated with EBV infection (see Chapter 26).[66, 67] PTLD in lymphoid tissue associated with intestinal mucosa can be diagnosed by endoscopic biopsies[68, 69] (Figs. 27–3 and 27–4). This complication has occurred with various immunosuppressive regimens, which include cyclosporine, azathioprine, and prednisone; however, in some centers an increased incidence appears to be associated with use of tacrolimus.[70] The use of OKT3 for steroid-refractory rejection is also associated with an increased risk of PTLD. It has been suggested that release of interleukin-6 by OKT3 might be involved in the pathogenesis of PTLD.[71] Various antiviral regimens have been used for prophylaxis and treatment.[72, 73] Treatment also involves lowering the amount of or even withdrawing immunosuppressant agents. For those who do not respond, chemotherapy and, more recently, immunotherapy may be effective.

Liver transplantation is a specific example of a case in which solid organ transplantation is performed with a known malignancy (such a cholangiocarcinoma or fibrolamellar carcinoma) or in which malignancy is discovered in the explant (hepatocellular carcinoma). These tumors have typical patterns of recurrence following orthotopic liver transplantation (OLT).[74] Another neoplastic complication of specific concern in liver transplantation is the development of colorectal neoplasm in patients with ulcerative colitis and primary sclerosing cholangitis for which they undergo OLT.[75] Annual surveillance colonoscopy has been recommended for these patients.[76] There has also been a recent case report of rapid progression of Barrett's esophagus without dysplasia to high-grade dysplasia in a liver transplant recipient.[77] This concern might extend to other solid organ transplant recipients.

COMPLICATIONS OF SOLID ORGAN TRANSPLANTATION

Kidney Transplantation

Complications involving the GI tract, liver, and pancreas are seen in kidney transplantation, affecting between 8% and 18% of patients. Immunosuppression and consequent infection play a major role.[78] Pancreatitis is thought to be linked to immunosuppressive medication and is reported to occur in 1% to 2% of patients. GI tract complications include peptic ulcer disease, small bowel and colon perforations, GI hemorrhage, mesenteric infarction, and infectious colitis.[79] Chylous ascites has been seen secondary to mesenteric lymphatic rupture with the transplantation of an adult organ in an infant.

Peptic ulcer disease has long been known to complicate kidney transplantation. In fact, at one time prophylactic peptic ulcer surgery was advocated. Recent reviews have shown an incidence of peptic ulcer of only 3%,[80] and that roughly half of transplant recipients have *Helicobacter pylori* infection as detected during esophagogastroduodenoscopy.[81] In one series, half of the kidney transplant patients who developed problems with ulcer disease had no previous history of acid-peptic disease.[82]

Hepatobiliary complications in renal transplant recipients primarily include viral hepatitis, as discussed earlier. In addition, cholecystitis is a common complication of kidney transplantation. A higher incidence has been reported among diabetic patients undergoing kidney or kidney-pancreas transplantation than among recipients without diabetes.[83] Cyclosporine has also been linked to a higher incidence of cholesterol gallstones. Cholecystectomy in the period immediately following kidney transplantation carries a high morbidity. Screening hepatic ultrasonography and prophylactic laparoscopic cholecystectomy for cholelithiasis have been recommended for kidney, pancreas, and heart transplantation candidates.[84] Patients undergoing transplantation for polycystic kidney disease who have associated congenital hepatic fibrosis with portal hypertension may develop worsening liver disease. This is often exacerbated when renal graft failure or cyclosporine toxicity necessitates hemodialysis. Patients undergoing renal transplantation for polycystic kidney disease need a pretransplantation evaluation for portal hypertension, in which case a combined liver-kidney transplantation procedure can be considered. Another renal condition that often necessitates combined transplants is primary oxalosis, because the renal graft is affected more quickly by the body burden of oxalate than is the native kidney. In this circumstance, the liver allograft is used for enzyme replacement therapy.

Liver Transplantation (see also Chapter 83)

The GI complications of liver transplantation that are not directly related to immunosuppression and infection are primarily complications of the surgery itself.[85] Hemorrhage, hepatic vascular compromise, biliary tract dysfunction, and bowel perforation, obstruction, and bleeding are among the described complications.[86] Pretransplantation conditions, including cirrhosis, portal hypertension, and previous surgery such as hepatoportojejunostomy, are predisposing factors.[87] In certain conditions necessitating transplantation, there is a risk for recurrence of the primary liver disease, such as with hepatitis B and C.[88, 89, 90] The noninfectious conditions in which this may apply include autoimmune hepatitis,[91, 92] primary biliary cirrhosis, and primary sclerosing cholangitis.[93]

Extensive collateralization of portal flow before transplantation from portal hypertension can predispose patients to intraoperative bleeding. Reduced size, split liver, and grafts from living related donors all result in a liver with a cut surface, which is another potential site of blood loss. Intra-abdominal hemorrhage can occur either during surgery or in the first several days after surgery. This can be caused by coagulopathy from a poorly functioning graft. Coagulopathy can be exacerbated by medications that interfere with platelet function necessary to prevent clotting of vascular anastomoses. Evacuation of peritoneal clot is important for preventing abdominal infection. If abdominal sepsis does occur, hepatic artery or portal vein rupture can result from an infected anastomosis. GI bleeding can occur after transplantation. Acute portal vein thrombosis can lead to variceal bleeding. Infectious enteritis, acid-peptic disease, and esophageal erosions have been reported to cause GI tract hemorrhage. Bleeding from a choledochojejunal biliary anastomosis can be manifest as hematochezia.

Intra-abdominal hemorrhage, hemothorax, and hemobilia may result from percutaneous liver biopsy. Most centers transfuse platelets prophylactically prior to liver biopsy if patients have platelet counts less than 80,000 to 100,000/mL, are receiving antiplatelet medications to protect vascular anastomoses from thrombotic complications or have renal insufficiency from cyclosporine or tacrolimus and resultant azotemia. Ultrasonographically guided biopsy with injection of surgical gel (Gelfoam) in the biopsy tract is also used to decrease bleeding complications, as is transjugular biopsy.

Vascular Complications

Vascular complications can involve the hepatic artery, portal vein, or, more rarely, the hepatic venous outflow tract. Hepatic artery thrombosis early in the postoperative period can be most devastating, manifesting as fulminant hepatic failure, and necessitating retransplantation.[94] The biliary anastomosis receives its blood supply from the hepatic artery, so that loss of hepatic arterial flow later in the post-transplantation course can result in bile duct necrosis and bile leakage. Bilomas and focal abscesses can result from loss of bile duct integrity.[95] A syndrome of bile duct paucity can also result from gradual loss of the hepatic arterial flow, which is histologically indistinguishable from paucity due to chronic rejection without inflammation.[96]

Portal vein thrombosis is less common than hepatic artery thrombosis. Portal vein thrombosis in the immediate postoperative period can cause severe liver dysfunction; reoperation and thrombectomy are indicated. Later in the course of transplantation, patients can develop signs of portal hypertension with variceal bleeding, splenomegaly, and ascites from either thrombosis or stenosis. Successful treatment with both operative intervention[97] and angioplasty (for stenosis) has been reported.[98] Hepatic vein thrombosis and inferior vena cava stenosis resulting in a Budd-Chiari syndrome are also rare, but the incidence is increased among patients receiving left lateral segment transplants. VOD is discussed later.

Biliary Complications

Bile leakage and biliary strictures constitute the majority of biliary complications. Current practice restricts biliary anastomosis to either a donor bile duct to recipient bile duct or a bile duct to jejunum. This practice minimizes complications such as ascending cholangitis and intrahepatic bile duct stricture formation that had been encountered with anastomoses involving the donor gallbladder, such as cholecystojejunostomy.[99] In the duct-to-duct anastomoses, a T-tube can be placed in the donor bile duct with drainage to the outside. With the duct anastomosed to a jejunal Roux-en-Y loop, a stent tube can be placed in the donor duct to drain bile to the outside.[100] The jejunal anastomosis is used in patients with prior hepatoportoenterostomy (for biliary atresia) and patients with scarring processes of their bile ducts, as in sclerosing cholangitis.[101] Bile leakage can occur at the site of the anastomosis (such as in hepatic artery insufficiency) or at the site of the T-tube exit from the donor duct in a duct-to-duct anastomosis.[102] Biliary strictures that occur within 2 to 6 months of transplantation are usually at the site of the anastomosis.[103] The placement of a T-tube across the anastomosis at the time of transplantation is intended to prevent their earlier occurrence.[104] Narrowing can occur later on and can be related to insufficient hepatic artery flow. Leaks, strictures, and other biliary problems (e.g., sphincter of Oddi dysfunction) are managed primarily with invasive radio-

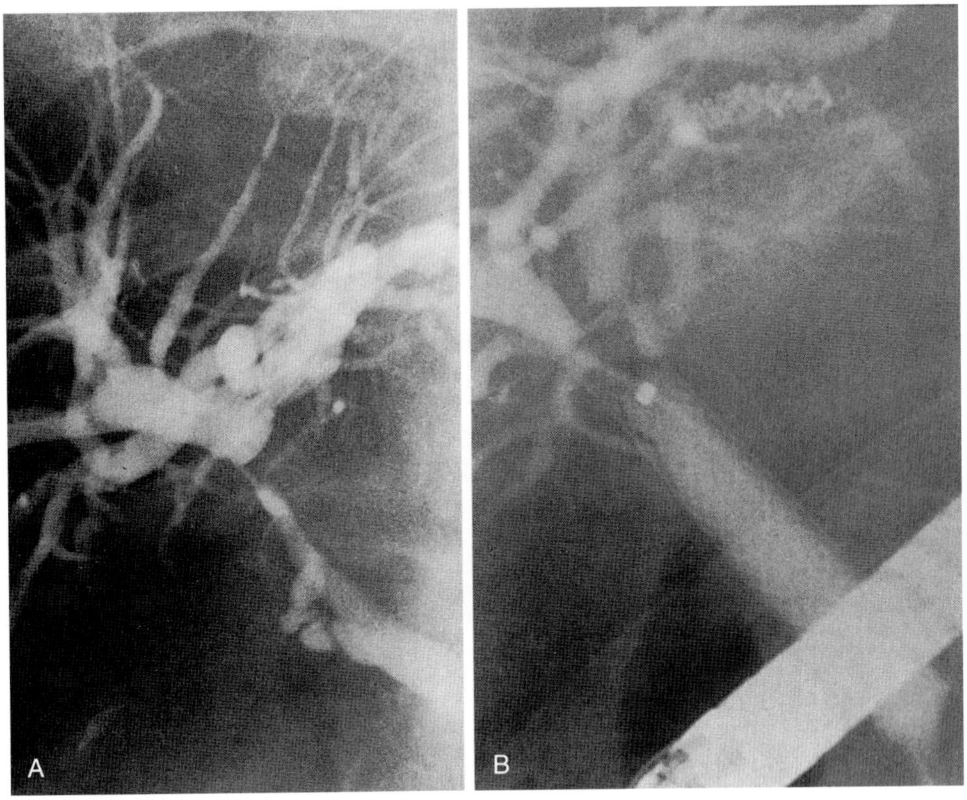

Figure 27–5. *A*, Cholangiogram of a patient who presented with jaundice 2 months following liver transplantation for hepatitis C and cirrhosis. Stricturing at the hilum and common bile duct were believed to be secondary to ischemia. *B*, A wall stent has been placed across the stricture. There was complete resolution of jaundice following stent placement. (Photographs courtesy of Jeffrey Rank, MD, and Stephen Trenkner, MD.)

logic[105] and endoscopic procedures (Figs. 27–5 and 27–6).[106] Alternatively, surgical reconstruction of a choledochojejunostomy can be used as well.[107]

Intestinal Complications

Complications involving the GI tract in liver transplantation can include hemorrhage (discussed earlier), perforation, and obstruction, as well as the infectious enteritides to which all immunosuppressed transplant patients are susceptible.[108] Anastomotic breakdown can occur at the site of jejunojejunostomy created for the formation of the Roux-en-Y loop.[85] Spontaneous bowel perforations have been reported, particularly in children with a history of previous jejunojejunostomy, 7 to 14 days after transplantation.[109, 110] Previous liver surgery[111] and steroids have been implicated in their pathogenesis.[112] The authors saw a child with gastric outlet obstruction secondary to the placement of a percutaneous transhepatic biliary drainage catheter and a drainage catheter in a biloma in addition to his original biliary stent tube. Nasojejunal feedings were successful in delivering nutrition until two of these tubes were removed. Pneumatosis intestinalis is also seen after liver transplantation; however, it may or may not be pathologic.[113] Patients receiving a liver graft for primary sclerosing cholangitis who also have ulcerative colitis may have a flare in the clinical course of their inflammatory bowel disease, particularly at the time of steroid withdrawal.[114]

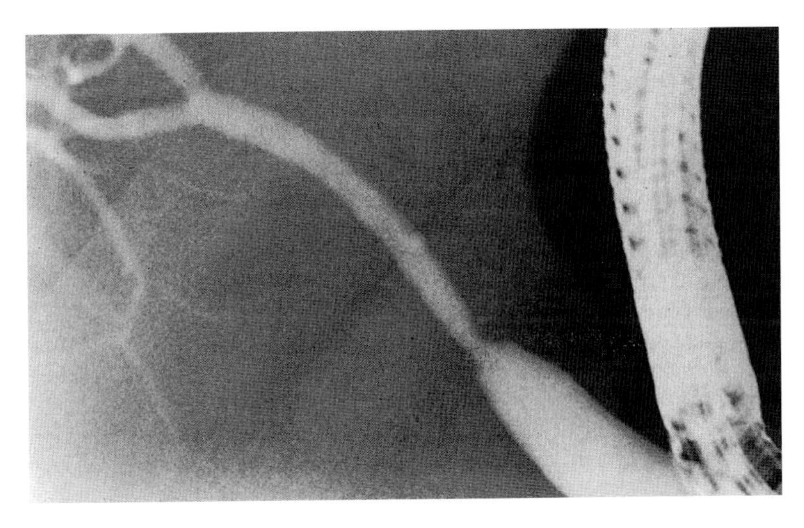

Figure 27–6. Cholangiogram of a patient 1 month following liver transplantation for hepatitis C. After transplantation, he had progressive jaundice. The native duct is dilated presumably from dysfunction of the sphincter of Oddi. Sphincterotomy was followed by resolution of jaundice. (Photographs courtesy of Jeffrey Rank, MD, and Stephen Trenkner, MD.)

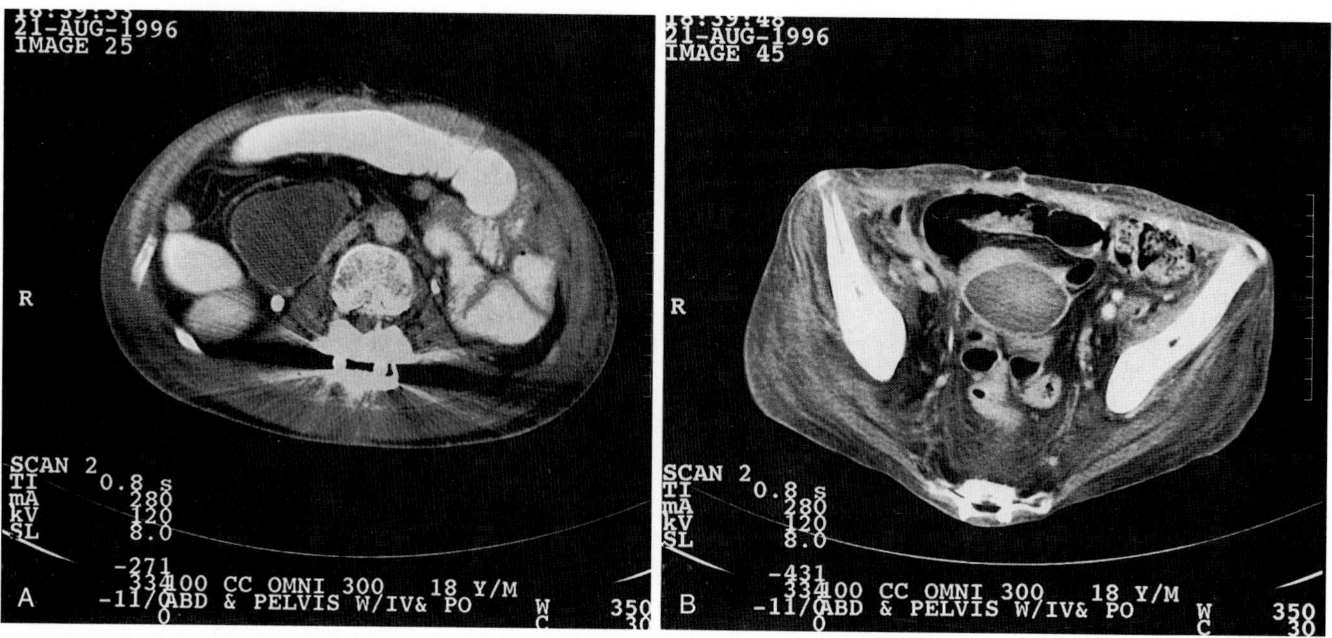

Figure 27–7. CT scan showing graft intestinal wall hematomas proximal (*A*) and distal (*B*) to ileostomy following endoscopic biopsies for rejection. The patient was asymptomatic.

Pancreas Transplantation

Other than cholecystitis (discussed earlier), most of the GI complications reported after pancreas and kidney-pancreas transplantation are those of the graft. Graft duodenitis is common, as is graft pancreatitis.[115] Graft thrombosis and duodenal leakage into the peritoneum are reported.[116] In a series of 297 pancreas and kidney-pancreas transplantations from the University of Minnesota performed with bladder drainage between 1986 and 1992, 80 patients underwent reoperation for complications, including infection, vascular graft thrombosis, bleeding, anastomotic leaks, and pancreatitis.[117] Hematuria is common after pancreas transplant with bladder drainage but can be severe, as in a case report of duodenal rupture.[118] Although the incidence of these complications is high, aggressive surgical management is associated with favorable outcomes.[119] Additional problems can be seen with slow gastric emptying and with bile reflux gastritis.

Intestine and Multivisceral En-Bloc Abdominal Transplantation

The development of tacrolimus (FK506) allowed reintroduction of intestinal transplantation and liver-intestine transplantation as feasible alternatives for patients with intestinal failure. These are patients who are dependent on, but no longer can receive, TPN because of recurrent sepsis from bowel sources, loss of all deep line sites, or end-stage cholestatic liver dysfunction. Further development is anticipated in the immunosuppression of these patients because of their prolonged requirement for intensive therapy and the high incidence (up to 20%) of EBV-associated lymphoproliferative disease.[120, 121] GVHD was theoretically a major concern; however, in practice the immunosuppression required to maintain the graft appears to be preventive in the early postoperative period, and the intestine is repopulated with lymphocytes of host origin by 2 to 4 months after transplantation.[122] With combined liver-intestine transplantation, the complications can be similar to those encountered with liver transplantation. In addition, difficulty has been reported with intestinal motility and food aversion. Frequent intestinal biopsies in these patients via their stoma can be associated with bleeding and intestinal wall hematoma formation (Fig. 27–7). In patients with Crohn's disease, anastomotic strictures in the native bowel may develop. Eosinophilic colitis (discussed earlier) was also first noted in intestinal transplant recipients.

Thoracic Transplantation (Heart, Heart-Lung, Lung)

Heart and heart-lung transplantations have a high incidence of GI complications, varying from 10% to 35% of patients.[123] Earlier reports emphasized pancreatitis and cholecystitis, which occurred in 18% and 10%, respectively, of 86 heart transplant patients at the Texas Heart Institute.[124] Half of those patients with pancreatitis had severe pancreatitis, and the mortality rate among pancreatitis patients was 40%. Other complications included CMV enteritis and perirectal abscess. A subsequent study, specifically focused on cholelithiasis, found that 3 of 74 patients developed gallstones de novo after heart transplantation and 2 required subsequent cholecystectomy. Sixteen patients had asymptomatic gallstones before transplantation, and only one of these required cholecystectomy. These authors concluded that patients with asymptomatic gallstones or sludge tend to remain asymptomatic and that prophylactic cholecystectomy is not indicated.[125] Other complications that have been reported include peptic ulceration and intestinal pseudo-obstruction,[126] intestinal perforations, GI bleeding, hepatitis, and diarrhea.[127]

The rate of GI complications in lung transplantation is similar to that in heart transplantation. The University of Minnesota lung transplantation program reported 20 such complication (11 early and 9 late) complications among 75 patients.[128] Early complications included adynamic ileus, diaphragmatic hernia, ischemic bowel, and splenic injury after colonoscopy. Late complications included colonic perforation, cholelithiasis, and mesenteric arterial pseudoaneurysm. The authors pointed out that typical symptoms may be attenuated by the anti-inflammatory therapy that patients are receiving, resulting in a delay in corrective procedures.

COMPLICATIONS OF HEMATOPOIETIC CELL TRANSPLANTATION

The GI complications seen in patients receiving hematopoietic cell transplantation (HCT) can be related to cytoreductive treatment, infection, and, for allogeneic transplantation, GVHD. As noted earlier, HCT can be viewed as the extreme case of chemotherapy-induced GI toxicity, because of the degree of cytoreduction required to eliminate the maximum tumor burden and/or allow engraftment of donor marrow. The complications with autologous hematopoietic stem cells or autologous cord blood transplantation are primarily related to the chemotherapy and/or radiation required. Allogeneic HCT, which uses related and unrelated stem cell donors and cord blood, carries the additional complications of GVHD.

Organ-Specific Complications

The infectious complications of immunosuppression as reviewed earlier (see the section on infectious complications) include those of viral, bacterial, and fungal etiologies. When increased immunosuppression is required because of acute or chronic GVHD, additional infectious risk is encountered. Noninfectious complications associated with chemotherapy and radiation can involve the liver, GI tract, and pancreas. Liver complications include VOD and hyperammonemia. Intestinal problems are primarily related to mucosal damage and disruption of the normal reparative processes of enterocytes. Pancreatitis has been described in association with cytoreductive, immunosuppressive, and antimicrobial therapies.

Liver Disorders after Hematopoietic Cell Transplantation

Veno-occlusive disease (VOD) remains a major therapeutic complication in HCT. Incidence of VOD has been reported to be as high as 54%,[129] 25% of these cases being severe. The pathophysiologic process remains poorly characterized, but VOD is described as a disorder of the hemostatic mechanism[130] with hepatic central venous hemorrhage as its major histologic feature. Clinically, VOD is defined by rising bilirubin levels and weight within 1 to 2 weeks after HCT, according to a model developed by the Seattle group to define the severity of VOD.[131] The development of VOD has been shown, also by the Seattle group, to be associated with pretransplantation elevations of serum transaminase concentrations, cytoreduction with a high-dose regimen, and persistent fever prior to transplantation during cytoreduction. VOD is most frequently diagnosed within the first 21 days after transplantation. The weight gain seen in VOD is secondary to ascites formation, because of the Budd-Chiari–like mechanism of central venous obstruction within the liver (also see Chapter 70). Renal failure is a common complication of VOD that results from a hepatorenal syndrome. The combination of hepatic venous outflow obstruction and renal failure can lead to severe fluid overload, which can then be followed by pulmonary edema and cardiac compromise. This further exacerbates the hepatic venous outflow obstruction.

Although increases in serum bilirubin level are the earliest signs of VOD, they can also be due to other causes. These include GVHD, viral infection involving the liver, the cholestasis of sepsis, cholestasis associated with TPN and lack of enteral intake, cholestasis resulting from narcotic therapy for pain, and mechanical obstruction of the bile duct with stones or sludge. Hepatic ultrasonography may be helpful in distinguishing the causes of cholestasis, as may nuclear hepatobiliary scanning. Hepatic ultrasonography with Doppler imaging can show reversal of portal vein flow early in the course of VOD. Measurement of the resistive index in the hepatic artery is also helpful, because it will increase early in the course of VOD.[132]

In addition to elevated bilirubin concentrations, VOD may result in abnormal findings on clotting studies. Protein C, but not protein S or antithrombin III, has been shown to decrease after cytoreductive therapy. Furthermore, patients who developed VOD had lower baseline protein C concentrations than patients who did not develop VOD.[131] In patients who do not produce platelets, have coagulopathy, and have increased intrahepatic pressure, percutaneous liver biopsy for confirmation of VOD is contraindicated. Transjugular biopsy can be more safely accomplished in this clinical setting.

Various therapeutic measures have been considered or attempted. Heparin and tissue plasminogen activator (tPA) infusions have achieved some success.[133] Prophylactic use of pentoxifylline has not had an impact on the development of VOD.[134] More promising results have been reported using defibrotide, a polydeoxyribonucleotide that has thrombolytic and antithrombotic properties.[135] The side effects of severe hemorrhage seen with the use of heparin and tPA do not occur with defibrotide.[136] Until such an agent becomes generally available, treatment for VOD is primarily supportive. The long-known association of VOD with malnutrition is an indication to maintain nutritional support as much as fluid restriction and renal insufficiency will allow. The use of enteral nutrition, when possible, with reduction in narcotic use decreases the contribution of extrahepatic cholestasis to the elevated serum bilirubin concentration. Careful management of fluids and electrolytes and early hemodialysis can decrease the occurrence of pulmonary complications. Ventilator support is often indicated for decreased gas exchange secondary to fluid overload. Multisystem organ failure can result from severe VOD.

Metabolic complications involving the liver include hypertriglyceridemia and hyperammonemia. Because of the damage to the GI tract from cytoreductive therapy, patients are often dependent on some form of parenteral nutritional support between the completion of cytoreduction and engraftment.[55] This generally results in dependence on TPN for at least 3 weeks. The authors' own study showed that prophylactic TPN (initiated in well-nourished patients during cytoreduction) improved long-term survival in allogeneic bone marrow recipients.[54] However, use of TPN in these stressed patients can be associated with severe metabolic derangement. Hypertriglyceridemia has been seen in association with use of cyclosporine. It is also associated with excess energy intake, resulting in lipogenesis. Glucose intolerance is frequently noted in HCT recipients receiving parenteral nutrition, resulting in exogenous insulin requirements. Poor utilization of intravenous amino acid, in addition to increased visceral and somatic protein breakdown, leads to hypoproteinemia and increased renal solute load. Many of these metabolic abnormalities are similar to those that have been described as the hypermetabolism syndrome. The hypermetabolism syndrome may result from catabolic stress such as sepsis, pancreatitis, and acute GVHD in HCT recipients.[137] The most extreme form of these metabolic derangements is the occurrence of hyperammonemia, which can manifest as an encephalopathy with altered sensorium, in patients who clinically appear to have sepsis.[138] No specific organism has been found to be associated with this syndrome, and patients generally have not been shown to have a genetic metabolic defect.

Gastrointestinal Tract Disorders

GI tract toxicity always results from pretransplantation cytoreductive therapy. Stomatitis, mucositis, and enteritis are common. Clinically detectable colitis is rarer and occurs later in the course of transplantation, usually as the result of granulocytopenia or infection. Typical cytoreduction regimens have included the combination of cyclophosphamide and busulfan and the combination of cyclophosphamide and total body irradiation. Mucositis occurs with both of these regimens; some reports suggest that radiation treatment increases the severity and duration of mucositis.[139] In a study of regimen-related toxicity of busulfan and cyclophosphamide conditioning therapy, 87% of 70 patients were reported to have stomatitis. Stomatitis or mucositis becomes most severe 10 to 14 days after transplantation and usually resolves at the same time as engraftment of the donor marrow. Mucositis also affects the small intestine, where the loss of functioning intestinal epithelium results in malabsorption and reversal of salt and water absorption. There is typically an 8- to 12-day interval of watery diarrhea after cytoreductive therapy. This is characterized by a transient increase in stool sodium to 50 to 80 mEq/L and a transient rise in exudative protein loss into the feces.[140] Protein loss is caused by mucosal disruption, and there is concomitant loss of zinc and failure to absorb minerals and vitamins (see the section on nutritional complications).

Pancreatic Disorders after Hematopoietic Cell Transplantation

Elevations of serum amylase and lipase levels can be noted in patients after HCT. One study has reported an incidence of pancreatitis of 3.5%.[141] The symptoms are similar to those seen with enteritis resulting either from chemotherapy or from GVHD (see later). Pancreatitis can result from bile duct obstruction with sludge or stone but probably more often is secondary to drug effects. Steroids, cyclosporine, sulfonamides, and cytosine arabinoside are among the drugs used in HCT that are reported to cause pancreatitis.

Multisystem Organ Failure

Multisystem organ failure, or multiple organ dysfunction syndrome, can occur as a progression from severe VOD through renal failure, pulmonary compromise, and cardiac dysfunction. It can also occur in the setting of bacterial or fungal sepsis, overwhelming viremia, or severe GVHD when intensified immunosuppression is required. It is proposed that the initiating event of multiple organ dysfunction syndrome is a perfusion defect.[142]

Graft-Versus-Host Disease

Acute Graft-Versus-Host Disease

Acute graft-versus-host disease (GVHD) is the response of donor lymphocytes to host tissue with initial T cell activation and subsequent cytokine production. The major targets of the immune response are the epithelial cells of skin, intestine, and hepatobiliary system. This response can occur in any setting in which immune surveillance is suppressed and allogeneic lymphocytes are introduced. It has been reported in intestinal transplantation, liver transplantation, and nonirradiated blood cell transfusion in immunocompromised or immunoimmature patients. Clinically, GVHD is manifested in the liver as jaundice with secondary elevations of transaminase levels. GVHD in the intestine presents as persistent vomiting or watery diarrhea in the setting of an erythematous maculopapular rash. In allogeneic HCT recipients, GVHD occurs after engraftment. With current GVHD pro-

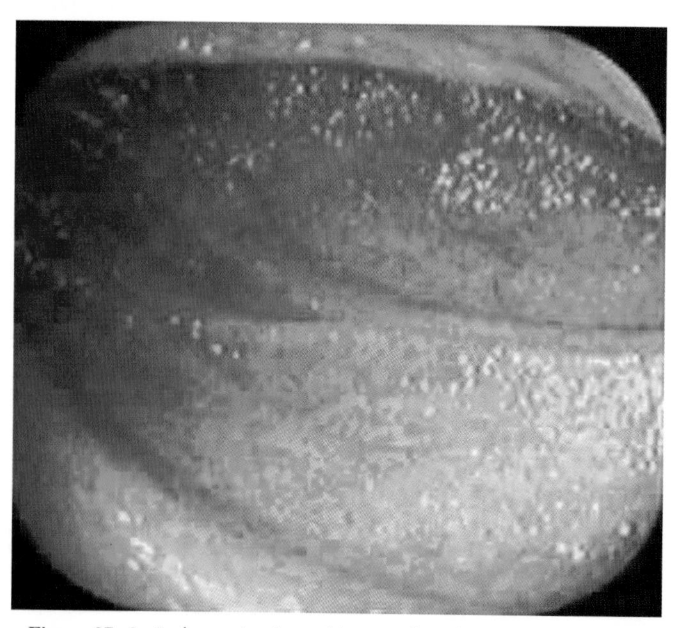

Figure 27–8. Endoscopic view of intestinal graft-versus-host disease.

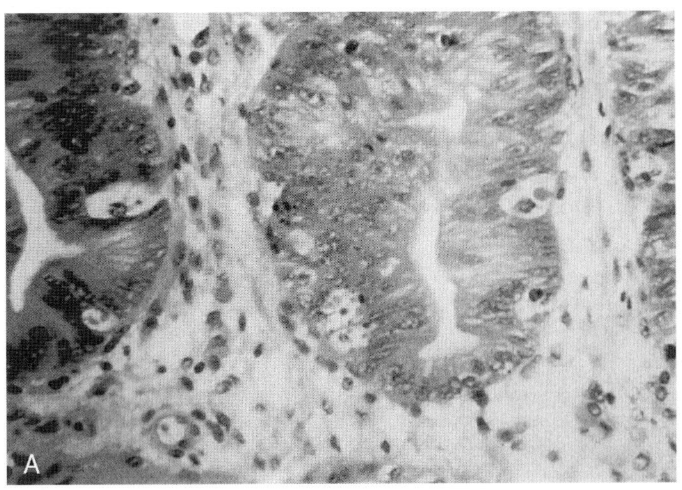

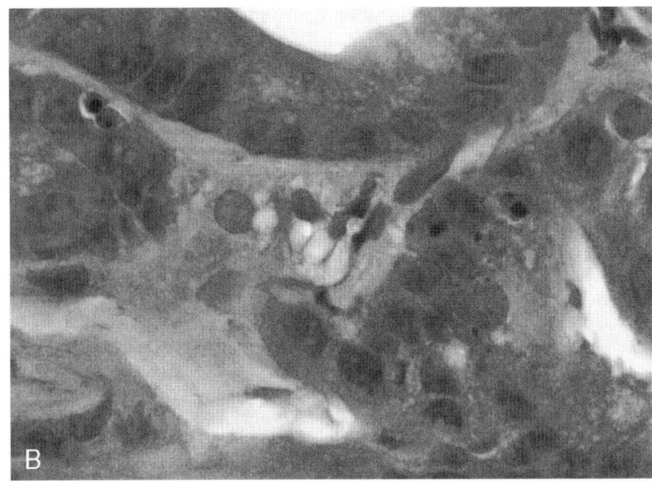

Figure 27–9. *A*, Colonic biopsy specimen from a patient with early graft-versus-host disease (GVHD). Note widely scattered apoptotic bodies. (Courtesy of Jonathan Terdiman, MD.) *B*, Photomicrograph of chronic (late) GVHD of the intestine. (Courtesy of Jose Jessurun, MD.)

phylaxis, the incidence of GVHD after fully matched, related allogeneic bone marrow transplantation (BMT) is approximately 30%. In unrelated and mismatched allogeneic HCT the incidence has been reported to be as high as 90%.[143] Any one or any combination of the three organ systems can be involved. The skin rash is often the first manifestation, and histologic confirmation can be obtained with the least morbidity from skin biopsy specimens.[52]

Intestinal tract involvement can occur at any location between the gastroesophageal junction and the rectum. Because the symptoms are nonspecific and because intestinal GVHD is difficult to distinguish from infectious enteritis, biopsy confirmation is often needed for patients both with and without a diagnostic skin biopsy. The authors' current protocol is to perform an esophagogastroduodenoscopy (EGD) and flexible sigmoidoscopy or colonoscopy when either persistent vomiting with or without nausea or watery diarrhea is present (Fig. 27–8). Patients with platelet counts lower than 40,000/mL require platelet transfusion during the endoscopic procedure(s). Prophylactic antibiotics are prescribed if the patient is not already receiving them. HCT recipients younger than 10 years of age usually require general anesthesia for EGD and for colonoscopy. Biopsy specimens are taken from the rectal mucosa, the duodenum, stomach, and esophagus and are submitted for both histologic examination and viral isolation (Fig. 27–9*A*). Histologic grading includes mild, moderate, and severe classifications. Bleeding complications after endoscopic biopsies are rare; however, duodenal hematoma can occur and results in persistent upper intestinal symptoms despite treatment. Such a hematoma can cause transient elevations of serum bilirubin and amylase levels, if the common bile duct is near the area of hematoma formation. This sequence of events may lead to further interventions with further risk. Thus, duodenal biopsy is no longer recommended to diagnose GVHD if the duodenal mucosa appears normal.

Hepatic involvement in acute GVHD is also nonspecific. Jaundice can also occur secondary to VOD, biliary obstruction, viral infection, and sepsis. GVHD of the liver without skin or intestinal involvement is, fortunately, quite rare, but it must be considered, and liver biopsy would then be necessary to diagnose hepatic GVHD. The authors' approach is to perform liver biopsy percutaneously if the platelet count can be maintained over 100,000/mL for 24 hours and if all coagulation studies are within normal limits. Otherwise, ultrasonography-guided biopsy with needle tract hemostasis, transjugular biopsy, or open liver biopsy can be considered.

Chronic Graft-Versus-Host Disease

Chronic GVHD can occur as early as 100 days after HCT and involves primarily scarring lesions of the skin (i.e., scleroderma-type lesions). In the GI tract, the esophagus is the usual site of involvement (see Chapter 34). Severe stricturing of the esophagus may occur. The intestine may become fibrotic and develop motility disorders, as in systemic sclerosis (Fig. 27–9*B*). The liver can also be involved with a disease process much like primary biliary cirrhosis or chronic liver allograft rejection with bile duct paucity. Chronic GVHD and its therapy delay the return of immunocompetence, and patients remain susceptible to bacterial, viral, and fungal infections.

REFERENCES

1. Heng Y, Schuffler MD, Haggitt RC, et al: Pneumatosis intestinalis: A review. Am J Gastroenterol 90:1747, 1995.
2. Silliman CC, Haase GM, Strain JD, et al: Indications for surgical intervention for gastrointestinal emergencies in children receiving chemotherapy. Cancer 74:203–216, 1994.
3. Allison Ad: Novel immunosuppressive and antiinflammatory drugs: A 1993 perspective. Ann N Y Acad Sci 696:xi, 1993.
4. Nevins TE: Overview of new immunosuppressive therapies. Curr Opin Pediatr 12:146–150, 2000.
5. Vose JM, Armitage JO: Clinical applications for hematopoietic growth factors. J Clin Oncol 13:1023–1035, 1995.
6. Sollinger HW: Mycophenolate mofetil. Kidney Int Suppl 52:S14, 1995.
7. Danovitch GM: Mycophenolate mofetil in renal transplantation: Results from the US randomized trials. Kidney Int Suppl 52:S93, 1995.
8. MacDonald A, Scarola J, Burke JT, Zimmerman JJ: Clinical pharma-

cokinetics and therapeutic drug monitoring of sirolimus. Clin Ther 22(Suppl B):B101–B121, 2000.
9. Verfaillie C, Weisdorf D, Haake R, et al: *Candida* infections in bone marrow transplant recipients. Bone Marrow Transplant 8:177–184, 1991.
10. Su Y, Hon YY, Chu Y, et al: Assay of 6-mercaptopurine and its metabolites in patient plasma by high-performance liquid chromatography with diode-array detection. J Chromatogr B Biomed Sci Appl 732:459–468, 1999.
11. Grahan RM: Cyclosporine: Mechanisms of action and toxicity. Cleve Clin J Med 61:308, 1994.
12. Vela CG, Cristol JP, Descomps B, Mourad G: Prospective study of lipid disorders in FK506- versus cyclosporine-treated renal transplant patients. Transplant Proc 32:398, 2000.
13. Thomson AW, Starzl TE: FK 506 and autoimmune disease: Perspective and prospects. Autoimmunity 12:303, 1992.
14. Marchetti P, Navalesi R: The metabolic effects of cyclosporine and tacrolimus. J Endocrinol Invest 23:482–490, 2000.
15. Ellis D: Clinical use of tacrolimus (FK-506) in infants and children with renal transplants. Pediatr Nephrol 9:487, 1995.
16. Shapiro R, Nalesnik M, McCauley J, et al: Posttransplant lymphoproliferative disorders in adult and pediatric renal transplant patients receiving tacrolimus-based immunosuppression. Transplantation 68: 1851–1854, 1999
17. Dhawan A, Seemayer TA, Pinsinski C, et al: Posttransplant eosinophilic gastroenteritis in children. Liver Transplant Surg 3:591–593, 1997.
18. Watson CJ, Friend PJ, Jamieson NV, et al: Sirolimus: A potent new immunosuppressant for liver transplantation. Transplantation 67:505–509, 1999.
19. Katznelson S, Cecka JM: Immunosuppressive regimens and their effects on renal allograft outcome. Clin Transplant :361–71, 1996.
20. Gaughan WJ, Francos BB, Dunn SR, et al: A retrospective analysis of the effect of indomethacin on adverse reactions to orthoclone OKT3 in the therapy of acute renal allograft rejection. Am J Kidney Dis 24: 486, 1994.
21. DeVault GA Jr, Kohan DE, Nelson EW, et al: The effects of oral pentoxifylline on the cytokine release syndrome during inductive OKT3. Transplantation 57:532, 1994.
22. Titiz MI, Turkmen F, Yegenaga I, et al: Abdominal pain that mimics acute appendicitis caused by an ATG overdose in a kidney transplant recipient. Transplant Int 7:385, 1994.
23. Parlevliet KJ, Bemelman FJ, Yong SL, et al: Toxicity of OKT3 increases with dosage: A controlled study in renal transplant recipients. Transplant Int 8:141, 1995.
24. Dykewicz MS, Rosen ST, O'Connell MM, et al: Plasma histamine but not anaphylatoxin levels correlate with anti-lymphocyte monoclonal antibodies. J Lab Clin Med 120:290, 1992.
25. Jeyarajah DR, Thistlethwaite JR Jr: General aspects of cytokine-release syndrome: Timing and incidence of symptoms. Transplant Proc 25(2 Suppl 1):16, 1993.
26. Soares MP, Latinne D, Elsen M, et al: In vivo depletion of xenoreactive natural antibodies with an anti-mu monoclonal antibody. Transplantation 56:1427–1433, 1993.
27. Boggio L, Pooley R, Roth SI, Winter JN: Typhlitis complicating autologous blood stem cell transplantation for breast cancer. Bone Marrow Transplant 25:321–326, 2000.
28. Brayman KL, Stephanian E, Matas AJ, et al: Analysis of infectious complications occurring after solid-organ transplantation. Arch Surg 127:38–47, 1992.
29. Steffen R, Reinhartz O, Blumhardt G, et al: Bacterial and fungal colonization and infections using oral selective bowel decontamination in orthotopic liver transplantations. Transplant Int 7:101–108, 1994.
30. West M, Pirenne J, Chavers B, et al: *Clostridium difficile* colitis after kidney and kidney-pancreas transplantation. Clin Transplant 13:318–323, 1999.
31. Balk RA: Pathogenesis and management of multiple organ dysfunction or failure in severe sepsis and septic shock. Crit Care Clin 16:337–352, vii, 2000.
32. Fryer JP, Kim S, Wells CL, et al: Bacterial translocation in a large-animal model of small-bowel transplantation: Portal versus systemic venous drainage and the effect of tacrolimus immunosuppression. Arch Surg 131:77, 1996.
33. Paya CV, Marin E, Keating M, et al: Solid-organ transplantation: Results and implications of acyclovir use in liver transplants. J Med Virol Suppl 1:123–127, 1993.
34. Sakr M, Hassanein T, Gavaler J, et al: Cytomegalovirus infection of the upper gastrointestinal tract following liver transplantation: Incidence, location, and severity in cyclosporine- and FK506-treated patients. Transplantation 53:786–791, 1992.
35. Hackman RC, Wolford JL, Gleaves CA, et al: Recognition and rapid diagnosis of upper gastrointestinal cytomegalovirus infection in marrow transplant recipients: A comparison of seven virologic methods. Transplantation 57:231, 1994.
36. Mannes GP, de Boer WJ, vander Jagt EJ, et al: Pneumatosis intestinalis and active cytomegaloviral infection after lung transplantation. Gronigen Lung Transplant Group. Chest 107:582–583, 1995.
37. Van Thiel DH, Gavaler JS, Schade RR, et al: Cytomegalovirus infection and gastric emptying. Transplantation 54:70–73, 1992.
38. Portela D, Patel R, Larson-Keller JJ, et al: OKT3 treatment for allograft rejection is a risk factor for cytomegalovirus disease in liver transplantation. J Infect Dis 171:1014, 1995.
39. Hooks MA, Perlino CA, Henderson JM, et al: Prevalence of invasive cytomegalovirus disease with administration of muromonab CD-3 in patients undergoing orthotopic liver transplantation. Ann Pharmacother 26:617, 1992.
40. Deen JL, Blumberg DA: Infectious disease considerations in pediatric organ transplantation. Semin Pediatr Surg 2:218, 1993.
41. Chakrabarti S, Collingham KE, Stevens RH, et al: Isolation of viruses from stools in stem cell transplant recipients: A prospective surveillance study. Bone Marrow Transplant 25:277–282, 2000.
42. Locasciulli A, Alberti A: Hepatitis B and hepatitis C virus infections in stem cell transplantation. Leuk Lymphoma 35:255–260, 1999.
43. Fishman JA, Rubin RH, Koziel MJ, et al: Hepatitis C virus and organ transplantation. Transplantation 6:147–154, 1996.
44. Villamil FG, Vierling JM: Recurrence of viral hepatitis after liver transplantation: Insights into management. Liver Transpl Surg 1(Suppl 1):89–99, 1995.
45. Marinos G, Rossol S, Carucci P, et al: Immunopathogenesis of hepatitis B virus recurrence after liver transplantation. Transplantation 69: 559–568, 2000.
46. Wright TL, Pereirat B: Liver transplantation for chronic viral hepatitis. Liver Transpl Surg 1:30–42, 1995.
47. Dickson RC, Caldwell SH, Ishtani MB, et al: Clinical and histologic patterns of early graft failure due to recurrent hepatitis C in four patients after liver transplantation. Transplantation 6:701–705, 1996.
48. Kusne S, Tobin D, Pasculle AW, et al: *Candida* carriage in the alimentary tract of liver transplant candidates. Transplantation 57:398–402, 1994.
49. Foy TM, Hawkins EP, Peters KR, et al: Colonic ulcers and lower GI bleeding due to disseminated aspergillosis. J Pediatr Gastroenterol Nephrol 18:399, 1994.
50. Blume KG, Thomas Ed: A review of autologous hematopoietic cell transplantation. Biol Blood Marrow Transplant 6:1–12, 2000.
51. Mattsson T, Arvidson K, Heimdahl A, et al: Alterations in taste acuity associated with allogeneic bone marrow transplantation. J Oral Pathol Med 21:31–37, 1992.
52. Ponec RJ, Hackman RC, McDonald GB: Endoscopic and histologic diagnosis of intestinal graft-versus-host disease after marrow transplantation. Gastrointest Endosc 49:612–621, 1999.
53. Bearman SI, Appelbaum FR, Buckner CD, et al: Regimen-related toxicity in patients undergoing bone marrow transplantation. J Clin Oncol 6:1562–1568, 1988.
54. Weisdorf SA, Lysne J, Wind D, et al: Positive effect of prophylactic total parenteral nutrition on long-term outcome of bone marrow transplantation. Transplantation 43:833–838, 1987.
55. Weisdorf S, Schwarzenberg SJ: Nutritional support of hematopoetic stem cell recipients. In Forman SJ, Thomas ED, Blume KG (eds): Hematopoietic Cell Transplantation, 2nd ed. New York, Blackwell Scientific, 1999, pp 723–732.
56. Bergstrom J: Why are dialysis patients malnourished? Am J Kidney Dis 26:229, 1995.
57. Mitch WE: Low-protein diets in the treatment of chronic renal failure. J Am Coll Nutr 14:311, 1995.
58. Madill J, Maurer JR, de Hoyos A: A comparison of preoperative and postoperative nutritional states of lung transplant recipients. Transplantation 56:347, 1993.
59. Fulton JA, Orenstein DM, Koehler AN, et al: Nutrition in the pediatric double lung transplant patient with cystic fibrosis. Nutr Clin Pract 10:67, 1995.
60. Holcombe BJ, Resler R: Nutrition support for lung transplant patients. Nutr Clin Pract 9:235, 1994.

61. Weisdorf SA: Nutrition in liver disease. In Lebenthal E (ed): Textbook of Gastroenterology and Nutrition in Early Childhood, 2nd ed. New York, Raven Press, 1989, pp 665–676.
62. Hasse J, Strong S, Gorman MA, et al: Subjective global assessment: Alternative nutrition assessment technique for liver-transplant candidates. Nutrition 9:339, 1993.
63. Driscoll DF, Palombo JD, Bistrian BR: Nutritional and metabolic considerations of the adult liver transplant candidate and organ donor. Nutrition 11:255, 1995.
64. Rovera GM, Strohm S, Bueno J, et al: Nutritional monitoring of pediatric intestinal transplant recipients. Transplant Proc 30:2519–2520, 1998.
65. Kaufman SS, Lyden ER, Brown CR, et al: Disaccharidase activities and fat assimilation in pediatric patients after intestinal transplantation. Transplantation 69:362–365, 2000.
66. Hoshino Y, Kimura H, Kuzushima K, et al: Early intervention in post-transplant lymphoproliferative disorders based on Epstein-Barr viral load. Bone Marrow Transplant 26:199–201, 2000.
67. Garnier JL, Blanc-Brunat N, Vivier G, et al: Interleukin-10 in Epstein-Barr virus–associated post-transplant lymphomas. Clin Transplant 13: 305–312, 1999.
68. Hsi ED, Singleton TP, Swinnen L, et al: Mucosa-associated lymphoid tissue–type lymphomas occurring in post-transplantation patients. Am J Surg Pathol 24:100–106, 2000.
69. Younes BS, Ament ME, McDiarmid SV, et al: The involvement of the gastrointestinal tract in posttransplant lymphoproliferative disease in pediatric liver transplantation. J Pediatr Gastroenterol Nutr 28:380–385, 1999.
70. Deschler DG, Osorio R, Ascher NL, et al: Posttransplantation lymphoproliferative disorder in patients under primary tacrolimus (FK506) immunosuppression. Arch Otolaryngol Head Neck Surg 121:1037, 1995.
71. Swinnen LJ, Fisher RI: OKT3 monoclonal antibodies induce interleukin-6 and interleukin-10: A possible cause of lymphoproliferative disorders associated with transplantation. Curr Opin Nephrol Hypertens 2:670–678, 1993.
72. Davis CL: The antiviral prophylaxis of post-transplant lymphoproliferative disorder. Semin Immunopathol 20:437–453, 1998.
73. Kuehnle I, Huls MH, Liu Z, et al: CD20 monoclonal antibody (rituximab) for therapy of Epstein-Barr virus lymphoma after hematopoietic stem-cell transplantation. Blood 95:1502–1505, 2000.
74. Schlitt HJ, Neipp M, Weimann A, et al: Recurrence patterns of hepatocellular and fibrolamellar carcinoma after liver transplantation. J Clin Oncol 17:324–331, 1999.
75. Loftus EV Jr, Aguilar HI, Sandborn WJ, et al: Risk of colorectal neoplasia in patients with primary sclerosing cholangitis and ulcerative colitis following orthotopic liver transplantation. Hepatology 27:685–690, 1998.
76. Bleday R, Lee E, Jessurun J, et al: Increased risk of early colorectal neoplasms after hepatic transplant in patients with inflammatory bowel disease. Dis Colon Rectum 36:908, 1993.
77. Trotter JF, Brazer SR: Rapid progression to high-grade dysplasia in Barrett's esophagus after liver transplantation. Liver Transpl Surg 5: 332–333, 1999.
78. Bardaxoglou E, Maddern G, Ruso L, et al: Gastrointestinal complications in renal transplantation. Transplant Int 6:45–49, 1993.
79. Soravia C, Baldi A, Kartheuser A, et al: Acute colonic complications after kidney transplantation. Acta Chir Belg 95:157–161, 1995.
80. Troppmann C, Papalois BE, Chiu A, et al: Incidence, complications, treatment, and outcome of ulcers of the upper gastrointestinal tract after renal transplantation. J Am Coll Surg 180:433–443, 1995.
81. Teenan RP, Burgoyne M, Brown IL, et al: *Helicobacter pylori* in renal transplant recipients. Transplantation 56:L56–L100, 1993.
82. Benoit G, Moukarzel M, Verdelli G, et al: Gastrointestinal complications in renal transplantation. Transplant Int 6:45–49, 1993.
83. Lowell JA, Stratta RJ, Taylor RJ, et al: Cholelithiasis in pancreas and kidney transplant recipients with diabetes. Surgery 114:858–863, 1993.
84. Graham SM, Flowers JL, Schweitzer E, et al: Opportunistic upper gastrointestinal infection in transplant recipients. Surg Endosc 9:146–150, 1995.
85. Ozaki CF, Katz SM, Monsour, et al: Surgical complications of liver transplantation. Surg Clin North Am 74:1155–1167, 1994.
86. Sze DY, Semba CP, Razavi MK, et al: Endovascular treatment of hepatic venous outflow obstruction after piggyback technique liver transplantation. Transplantation 68:446–449, 1999.
87. Clavien PA, Camargo CA Jr, Croxford R, et al: Definition and classification of negative outcomes in solid organ transplantation: Application in liver transplantation. Ann Surg 220:107–108, 1994.
88. Everhart JE, Wei Y, Eng H, et al: Recurrent and new hepatitis C virus infection after liver transplantation. Hepatology 29:1220–1226, 1999.
89. Dodson SF, Bonham CA, Geller DA, et al: Prevention of de novo hepatitis B infection in recipients of hepatic allografts from anti-HBc positive donors. Transplantation 68:1058–1061, 1999.
90. Lerut JP, Claeys N, Ciccarelli O, et al: Recurrent postinfantile syncytial giant cell hepatitis after orthotopic liver transplantation. Transplant Int 11:320–322, 1998.
91. Devlin J, Donaldson P, Portmann B, et al: Recurrence of autoimmune hepatitis followng liver transplantation. Liver Transpl Surg 1:162–165, 1995.
92. Milkiewicz P, Hubscher SG, Skiba G, et al: Recurrence of autoimmune hepatitis after liver transplantation. Transplantation 68:253–256, 1999.
93. Neuberger J: Recurrence of primary biliary cirrhosis, primary sclerosing cholangitis, and autoimmune hepatitis. Liver Transpl Surg 1(Suppl 1):109–115, 1995.
94. Tzakis AG, Gordon RD, Shaw BW Jr, et al: Clinical presentation of hepatic artery thrombosis after liver transplantation in the cyclosporine era. Transplantation 40:667–671, 1985.
95. Hesselink EJ, van Schilfgaarde R, Grand J, et al: Hepatic artery thrombosis after orthotopic liver transplantation: Clinical presentation and possible etiologic factors. Clin Transplant 2:306–311, 1988.
96. Sawyer RG, Pelletier SJ, Spencer CE, et al: Increased late hepatic artery thrombosis rate and decreased graft survival after liver transplants with zero cross-reactive group mismatches. Liver Transpl 6: 229–236, 2000.
97. Scantelbury VP, Zajko AB, Esquivel CO, et al: Successful reconstruction of late portal vein stenosis after hepatic transplantation. Arch Surg 124:503–505, 1989.
98. Funaki B, Rosenblum JD, Leef JA, et al: Percutaneous treatment of portal venous stenosis in children and adolescents with segmental hepatic transplants: Long-term results. Radiology 215:147–151, 2000.
99. Vallera RA, Cotton PB, Clavien PA: Biliary reconstruction for liver transplantation and management of biliary complications: Overview and survey of current practices in the United States. Liver Transpl Surg 1:143–152, 1995.
100. Tung BY, Kimmey MB: Biliary complications of orthotopic liver transplantation. Dig Dis 17:133–144, 1999.
101. Letourneau JG, Day DL, Hunter DW, et al: Biliary complications after liver transplantation in patients with preexisting sclerosing cholangitis. Radiology 167:349–351, 1988.
102. Tepetes K, Karavias D, Felekouras E, et al: Bile leakage following T-tube removal in orthotopic liver transplantation. Hepatogastroenterology 46:425–427, 1999.
103. Sawyer RG, Punch JD: Incidence and management of biliary complications after 291 liver transplants following the introduction of transcystic stenting. Transplantation 66:1201–1207, 1998.
104. Lake JR: Long-term management of biliary tract complications. Liver Transpl Surg 1(Suppl 1):45–54, 1995.
105. Pariente D, Bihet MH, Tammam S, et al: Biliary complications after transplantation in children: Role of imaging modalities. Pediatr Radiol 21:175–178, 1991.
106. Schwartz DA, Petersen BT, Poterucha JJ, Gostout CJ: Endoscopic therapy of anastomotic bile duct strictures occurring after liver transplantation. Gastrointest Endosc 51:169–174, 2000.
107. Davidson BR, Rai R, Nandy A, et al: Results of choledochojejunostomy in the treatment of biliary complications after liver transplantation in the era of nonsurgical therapies. Liver Transpl 6:201–206, 2000.
108. Caraceni P, Fagiuoli S, Wright HI, et al: Gastrointestinal complications of liver transplantation. Ital J Gastroenterol 27:29–39, 1995.
109. Beierle EA, Nicolette LA, Billmire DF, et al: Gastrointestinal perforation after pediatric orthotopic liver transplantation. J Pediatr Surg 33: 240–242, 1998.
110. Vilca Melendez H, Vougas V, Muiesan P, et al: Bowel perforation after paediatric orthotopic liver transplantation. Transplant Int 11:301–304, 1998.
111. Yamanaka J, Lynch SV, Ong TH, et al: Posttransplant gastrointestinal perforation in pediatric liver transplantation. J Pediatr Surg 29:635–638, 1994.
112. Soubane O, El Meteini M, Devictor D, et al: Risk and prognostic

factors of gut perforation after orthotopic liver transplantation for biliary atresia. Liver Transpl Surg 1:2–9, 1995.
113. King S, Shuckett B: Sonographic diagnosis of portal venous gas in two pediatric liver transplant patients with benign pneumatosis intestinalis: Case reports and literature review. Pediatr Radiol 22:577–578, 1992.
114. Papatheodoridis GV, Hamilton M, Mistry PK, et al: Ulcerative colitis has an aggressive course after orthotopic liver transplantation for primary sclerosing cholangitis. Gut 43:639–644, 1998.
115. Fernandez-Cruz L, Sabate L, Gilabert R, et al: Native and graft pancreatitis following combined pancreas-renal transplantation. Br J Surg 80:1429–1432, 1994.
116. Sollinger HW, Ploeg RJ, Eckhoff DE, et al: Two hundred consecutive simultaneous pancreas-kidney transplants with bladder drainage. Surgery 114:736–743; discussion 743–744, 1993.
117. Toppmann C, Dunn DL, Najarian JS, et al: Operative reintervention following early complications after pancreas transplantation. Transplant Proc 26:454, 1994.
118. Esterol RM, Stratta RJ, Taylor RJ, et al: Rejection with duodenal rupture after solitary pancreas transplantation: An unusual cause of severe hematuria. Clin Transplant 9:155–159, 1995.
119. Douzdian V, Abecassis MM, Cooper JL, et al: Incidence, management, and significance of surgical complications after pancreatic transplantation. Surg Gynecol Obstet 177:451–456, 1993.
120. Abu-Elmagd K, Todo S, Tzakis A, et al: Rejection of human intestinal allografts: Alone or in combination with the liver. Transplant Proc 26: 1430–1431, 1994.
121. Kocoshis SA: Small bowel transplantation in infants and children. Gastroenterol Clin North Am 23:727–742, 1994.
122. Todo S, Tzakis AG, Abu-Elmagd K, et al: Cadaveric small bowel and small bowel–liver transplantation in humans. Transplantation 53:369–376, 1992.
123. Cates J, Chaes M, Laks H, et al: Gastrointestinal complications after cardiac transplantation: A spectrum of diseases. Am J Gastroenterol 86:412–416, 1991.
124. Colon R, Frazier OH, Kahan BD, et al: Complications in cardiac transplant patients requiring general surgery. Surgery 1031:32–38, 1988.
125. Steck TB, Costanzo-Nordin MR, Keshavarzian A: Prevalence and management of cholelithiasis in heart transplant patients. J Heart Lung Transplant 10:1029–1032, 1991.
126. Watson CJ, Jamieson NV, Johnston PS, et al: Early abdominal complications following heart and heart-lung transplantation. Br J Surg 78: 699–704, 1992.
127. Augustine SM, Veo CJ, Buchman TG, et al: Gastrointestinal complications in heart and in heart-lung transplant patients. J Heart Lung Transplant 10:547–555, 1991.
128. Smith PC, Slaughter MS, Petty MG, et al: Abdominal complications after lung transplantation. J Heart Lung Transplant 14:44–51, 1995.
129. McDonald GB, Hinds MS, Fisher LD, et al: Veno-occlusive disease of the liver and multiorgan failure after bone marrow transplantation: A cohort study of 355 patients. Ann Intern Med 118:255, 1993.
130. Faioni EM, Krachmalmicoff A, Bearman SI, et al: Naturally occurring anticoagulants and bone marrow transplantation: Plasma protein C predicts the development of veno-occlusive disease of the liver. Blood 81:3458, 1993.
131. Bearman SI, Anderson GL, Mori M, et al: Veno-occlusive disease of the liver: Development of a model for predicting fatal outcome after marrow transplantation. J Clin Oncol 11:1729, 1993.
132. Carreras E: Veno-occlusive disease of the liver after hemopoietic cell transplantation. Eur J Haematol 64:281–291, 2000.
133. Bearman SI, Shuhart MC, Hinds MS, et al: Recombinant human tissue plasminogen activator for the treatment of established severe veno-occlusive disease of the liver after bone marrow transplantation. Blood 80:2458, 1992.
134. Clinft RA, Bianco JA, Appelbaum FR, et al: A randomized controlled trial of pentoxifylline for the prevention of regimen-related toxicities in patients undergoing allogeneic marrow transplantation. Blood 82: 2025, 1993.
135. Abecasis MM, Conceicao Silva JP, Ferreira I, et al: Defibrotide as salvage therapy for refractory veno-occlusive disease of the liver complicating allogeneic bone marrow transplantation. Bone Marrow Transplant 23:843–846, 1999.
136. Richardson PG, Elias AD, Krishnan A, et al: Treatment of severe veno-occlusive disease with defibrotide: Compassionate use results in response without significant toxicity in a high-risk population. Blood 92:737–744, 1998.
137. Weisdorf S, Schwarzenberg SJ: Cancer. In Walker WA, Watkins J (eds): Nutrition in Pediatrics, 2nd ed. New York, BC Decker, 1996, pp 572–582.
138. Mitchell RB, Wagner JE, Karp JE, et al: Syndrome of idiopathic hyperammonemia after high-dose chemotherapy: Review of nine cases. Am J Med 85:662–667, 1988.
139. Borgmann A, Emminger W, Emminger-Schmidmeier W, et al: Influence of fractionated total body irradiation on mucosal toxicity in intensified conditioning regimens for autologous bone marrow transplantation in pediatric cancer patients. Klin Padiatr 206:299, 1994.
140. Weisdorf SA, Salati LM, Longsdorf JA, et al: Graft-versus-host disease of the intestine: A protein-losing enteropathy characterized by fecal α_1-antitrypsin. Gastroenterology 85:1076–1081, 1983.
141. Werlin SL, Casper J, Antonson D, et al: Pancreatitis associated with bone marrow transplantation in children. Bone Marrow Transplant 10: 65, 1992.
142. Buchman TG: Multiple organ failure. Curr Opin Gen Surg 26–31, 1993.
143. Bron D: Graft-versus-host disease. Curr Opin Oncol 6:358, 1994.

Chapter 28

Gastrointestinal Consequences of Infection with Human Immunodeficiency Virus

C. Mel Wilcox

Since the last edition, there have been dramatic and profound changes in the management of human immunodeficiency virus (HIV) and acquired immunodeficiency syndrome (AIDS). These changes have resulted from the recent availability of potent antiretroviral therapies to treat HIV. In 1996, the protease inhibitors became widely available; when combined with other antiretroviral medications—termed *highly active antiretroviral treatment* (HAART)—these drug combinations decrease viral replication and, consequently, circulating virus. In some patients, HIV becomes undetectable in the blood.[1] Associated with a reduction in viral load, there is improvement in immune function that can be assessed by objective measures such as an increase in the CD4 lymphocyte count, and clinically by a decrease in opportunistic infections (OIs) as well as an improvement in survival.[2, 3] Many patients with CD4 counts less than 100/μL who initially receive HAART experience during long-term therapy an increase to more than 200/μL, the threshold for the development of most OIs.[4] Furthermore, both primary and secondary prophylaxis against a variety of OIs may also be discontinued in patients who respond objectively to HAART.[5, 6]

Gastrointestinal (GI) and hepatobiliary complications were previously recognized as almost universal during the course of HIV infection; however, in the era of HAART, these disorders have markedly decreased in frequency. A recent study of HIV-infected patients undergoing endoscopy for GI complaints during the period of 1995 to 1998 showed a substantial reduction in the number of opportunistic processes identified coincident with the use of HAART.[7] This reduction in opportunistic GI diseases for HIV-infected patients receiving HAART has important implications for the approach to evaluation of the symptomatic patient. Furthermore, because of the potential efficacy of these drugs in reconstituting immune function, HAART also represents a new paradigm for the management of OIs in AIDS. For example, patients may now receive HAART as "primary therapy" for OIs that are either poorly responsive to medical therapy or are untreatable; as immune function improves, the infection may resolve with HAART alone.[8] Conversely, if immune function subsequently deteriorates, recrudescence of the infection will occur.

Although substantially effective in treating (suppressing) HIV infection, these antiretroviral drugs are associated with GI and hepatic side effects that in short-term studies exceed 10%.[9] Currently, drug-induced side effects and other nonopportunistic diseases are among the most common causes of GI symptoms in those receiving these combination drug therapies.[7, 10]

Because patients are generally approached based on clinical presentation, accordingly, this chapter is organized primarily around symptom diagnosis (diarrhea, odynophagia and dysphagia, anorectal disease, abdominal pain, GI bleeding, jaundice, and hepatomegaly). Specific HIV-related disorders and their treatments are presented within the context of their most common associated symptoms. In addition, the relevant impact of HAART in relation to these symptom complexes and diseases are discussed.

EVALUATION AND MANAGEMENT OF GASTROINTESTINAL AND HEPATOBILIARY SYMPTOMS IN AIDS

Although HAART has dramatically altered the occurrence of GI complications, many of the same principles of management established pre-HAART remain applicable. Several general points must be considered when evaluating GI symptoms in AIDS:

1. Clinical signs and symptoms infrequently suggest a specific diagnosis.
2. GI symptoms in a patient on HAART are most often drug induced or nonopportunistic in etiology.
3. Likely diagnoses may be predicted based on the extent of immunocompromise, that is, CD4 count greater than 200/μL—common bacteria and other nonopportunistic diseases; CD4 count les than 100/μL—cytomegalovirus (CMV), fungi, *Mycobacterium avium* complex (MAC), unusual protozoa.
4. In AIDS, GI pathogens are usually part of a systemic infection (e.g., CMV, MAC). Thus, identification of a pathogen outside the gut in the appropriate clinical setting may negate GI evaluation.
5. Evaluation should proceed from less invasive to more invasive and should be dictated by the severity and acuity of symptoms.
6. Multiple infections are common.
7. Evidence of tissue invasion should be sought as a hallmark of pathogenicity.
8. Without improvement of immune function (HAART), recurrence of OIs is almost uniform, necessitating maintenance antimicrobial therapy.
9. Treatment of all opportunistic disorders should include HAART. The natural history of opportunistic diseases can be favorably altered by HAART.

In general, the approach to investigating GI symptoms in the patient with AIDS should not be markedly different than non–HIV-infected patients. As with any patient, the clinician must weigh the discomfort, invasiveness, and cost of additional procedures against the severity of the patient's complaints, and the likelihood of the procedure identifying a disorder that will either alter medical therapy or change management. Noninvasive methods of diagnosis such as stool collection should be employed first.

DIARRHEA

Differential Diagnosis and Specific Therapies (Tables 28–1 and 28–2)

Studies pre-HAART demonstrated that diarrhea occurred in up to 90% of patients during the course of HIV disease, especially those from developing countries. Recent reports suggest that diarrhea remains a frequent complaint but etiologically is now most often drug-induced (antiretroviral therapy) or is caused by disorders unrelated to HIV infection.[10] Alterations in the mucosal immune system in AIDS predispose to intestinal infections, may lead to untreatable infection by organisms that typically cause self-limited infection

Table 28–1 | **Differential Diagnosis of Diarrhea in AIDS**

Protozoa	**Fungi**
Toxoplasma	*Histoplasmosis*
*Microsporidium**	*Coccidioidomycosis*
*Cryptosporidium**	*Cryptococcosis*
Isospora belli	*Candida albicans*
Giardia lamblia	**Gut Neoplasms**
Entamoeba histolytica	Lymphoma
Leishmania donovani	Kaposi's sarcoma
Blastocystis hominis	**Idiopathic**
Cyclospora sp.	"AIDS enteropathy"
Pneumocystis carinii	**Drug-Induced**
Bacteria	HIV protease inhibitors
Clostridium difficile	Other drugs
*Salmonella**	**Pancreatic Insufficiency**
*Shigella**	Chronic pancreatitis
*Campylobacter**	Infectious pancreatitis (CMV, MAC)
MAC	Drug-induced pancreatitis (pentamidine)
Mycobacterium tuberculosis	Tumor invasion (lymphoma, Kaposi's sarcoma)
Small bowel bacterial overgrowth	
Vibrio sp.	
Viruses	
*Cytomegalovirus**	
Herpes simplex	
Adenovirus	
Rotavirus	
Norwalk	
HIV?	

*More frequent.
AIDS, acquired immunodeficiency syndrome; CMV, cytomegalovirus; MAC, *Mycobacterium avium* complex.

in healthy hosts (e.g., *Cryptosporidium*) and may contribute to a more virulent clinical course of otherwise common enteric infections (e.g., *Salmonella, Shigella, Campylobacter*). Despite the vast spectrum of protozoal, viral, bacterial, and fungal organisms that cause diarrhea in the patient with AIDS, a differential diagnosis can be developed based on the clinical presentation and degree of immunodeficiency.

Protozoa are the most prevalent class of diarrheal pathogens in most series,[11, 12] largely because many of these infections can lead to chronic diarrhea and are refractory to treatment (see Chapter 98). *Cryptosporidium,* a member of the sporozoa class, causes self-limited diarrhea in healthy hosts.[13] In HIV-infected patients, *Cryptosporidium* is the most frequent protozoa identified[11, 12, 14] and its presentation and outcome are related to the degree of immunocompromise; for those with a normal CD4 count or those less immunocompromised, the illness may be transient or fluctuate, whereas chronic severe diarrhea with shortened survival characterizes the disease in severely immunocompromised patients.[15, 16] The small bowel is the most common site of infection, although the organisms can be recovered in all regions of the gut, as well as in biliary and respiratory epithelium. As such, epigastric or mid-abdominal discomfort or borborygmi are commonly reported; right upper quadrant pain suggests biliary tract involvement (see later). The pathogenesis of this infection is uncertain; the organism rests on the surface of the enterocyte, where it is enveloped by the host cell membrane, and generally incites only modest if any inflammatory response and cell injury. However, in some patients, the inflammatory response may be severe, usually in association with a high-parasite burden.[17] The diagnosis of intestinal cryptosporidiosis is most often made by acid-fast stain of the stool, where the organisms appear

Table 28–2 | **Specific Treatment of Diarrhea in AIDS**

	TREATMENT	DURATION (DAYS)*
Bacteria		
Salmonella, Shigella, Campylobacter	Ciprofloxacin 500 mg q12 hr	10–14*
Clostridium difficile	Vancomycin, metronidazole	10–14
Small bowel overgrowth	Metronidazole, ciprofloxacin	10–14
Mycobacteria		
Mycobacterium tuberculosis	Isoniazid, rifampin, pyrazinamide, ethambutol	9–12 months*
Mycobacterium avium complex	Multidrug regimens for symptomatic infection (see text)	9–12 months*
Viruses		
Cytomegalovirus	Ganciclovir 5 mg/kg IV q12hr	14–28*
	Foscarnet 60 mg/kg IV over 1 hr q8hr	14–28*
Herpes simplex	Acyclovir 200 mg 5 times/day (oral)	5–10*
Fungi		
Histoplasmosis	Amphotericin B 0.6 mg/kg/d; then itraconazole	28
Coccidioidomycosis	Amphotericin B 0.6 mg/kg/d; then fluconazole	28
Cryptococcus	Amphotericin B 0.6 mg/kg/d; then fluconazole	28
Protozoa		
Cryptosporidia	Paromomycin	14–28
Cyclospora	Trimethoprim-sulfamethoxazole or ciprofloxacin	14–28
Isospora belli	Trimethoprim-sulfamethoxazole or ciprofloxacin or pyramethamine	14–28
Microsporidia	Albendazole (*Encephalitozoon intestinalis*);	14–28
	Metronidazole, atovaquone (*Enterocytozoon bienusi*)	14–28

AIDS, acquired immunodeficiency syndrome.
*Duration of therapy dictated by immune reconstitution with HAART.

as bright red spherules, similar in size to red blood cells. Examination of multiple stools may be required for diagnosis. The sensitivity of stool testing depends on the burden of organisms, character of the stool (formed vs. liquid), and primary site of infection.[18] Not infrequently, cryptosporidia may be identified in small bowel or rectal biopsies even when the stool examination is negative.[11, 19]

Specific antimicrobial treatment of cryptosporidial infection remains disappointing. Numerous antimicrobial agents have been tested most without significant effect. The agent that has shown the most efficacy, albeit modest, is paromomycin, an oral aminoglycoside.[20] The somatostatin analog octreotide has not been consistently effective.[21] Although not pathogen specific, currently, the most effective therapy for cryptosporidia is HAART. In a study of four patients, the institution of HAART resulted in a clinical remission of diarrhea and clearance of cryptosporidia from the stool as well as on small bowel biopsy.[8] For patients failing HAART and/or in whom antimicrobial therapy is ineffective, symptomatic treatment should include fluid support and antidiarrheal agents as required. Patients with severe diarrhea may benefit from narcotics to control the diarrhea and tincture of opium can be particularly effective in these patients.

Cyclospora, organisms similar to cryptosporidia,[22] are an uncommon cause of diarrheal disease both in immunocompetent and immunodeficient patients. These pathogens appear similar, although larger in size (8 to 10 μm in diameter) than *Cryptosporidium.* Acid-fast stool staining may establish the diagnosis. Small bowel biopsy with electron microscopy may also be diagnostic. Trimethoprim-sulfamethoxazole and ciprofloxacin have shown efficacy in controlled trials.[23]

Isospora belli is a sporozoan, which, like *Cryptosporidium,* causes self-limited diarrhea in healthy hosts but may result in chronic diarrhea in untreated patients with HIV infection. The disease is rare in the United States but it is more frequent and endemic in developing countries such as Haiti. The organism may be identified by acid-fast stain of the stool or duodenal secretions or on mucosal biopsy. Like other protozoa, multiple stool specimens may occasionally be required before the organism is recovered. Unlike *Cryptosporidium,* however, this infection can be effectively treated with antibiotics, specifically sulfonamides, pyrimethamine, and ciprofloxacin.[24] The widespread use of trimethoprim-sulfamethoxazole for *Pneumocystis carinii* prophylaxis may be one explanation for the low prevalence of *Isospora* in the United States.

Microsporidium has emerged as one of the most common intestinal infections in AIDS. Intestinal and hepatobiliary disease may be caused by two species—*Enterocytozoon bienusi* and *Encephalitozoon intestinalis.* In a large U.S. study of 141 AIDS patients with diarrhea, microsporidia were the most commonly identified pathogen, found in 39%.[25] Other studies have found microsporidia ranging in frequency from less than 15%[12, 14] to greater than 30%,[26, 27] suggesting potential geographic differences in prevalence. Typical symptoms include watery nonbloody diarrhea of mild to moderate severity usually without associated crampy abdominal pain. Weight loss is common, although not to the degree observed with *Cryptosporidium.* Infection is associated with severe immunodeficiency with median CD4 counts of infected individuals of less than 100/μL.[12, 14] Persistent infection does not invariably lead to mucosal injury or development of diarrhea.[28] This extremely small organism may be seen by electron microscopy at the luminal enterocyte surface where the typical merozoite vacuole is identified intracellularly near the enterocyte nucleus. The organism incites little tissue inflammation and is rarely associated with villous atrophy and cell degeneration.[29] No pathogenetic mechanism has been proposed. Transmission has been most associated with water exposure.[30] Microsporidia can also be discerned by light microscopy when tissue is embedded in plastic or paraffin. (Fig. 28–1). Staining of embedded muco-

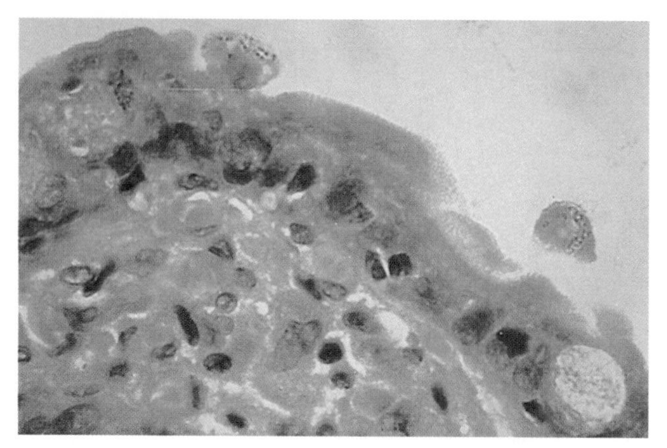

Figure 28–1. Endoscopic biopsy specimen of small bowel microsporidiosis. This thin plastic section demonstrates shedding of an epithelial cell containing microsporidial oocysts. (From Gazzard BG: Diarrhea in human immunodeficiency virus antibody-positive patients. Semin Gastroenterol 2:3, 1991.)

sal biopsies with Brown-Brenn, Gram stain, or modified trichrome is superior to routine hematoxylin and eosin staining.[31] *E. intestinalis* can usually be differentiated from *E. bienusi* by its larger size and infection of lamina propria macrophages; electron microscopy is definitive. Stool staining techniques are available with the modified trichrome stain used most frequently.[32] The sensitivity of these stool stains is only modest, whereas polymerase chain reaction (PCR) of stool is highly accurate but currently only available as a research tool.[33]

Effective therapies for microsporidia have not been fully defined. Symptomatic improvement has been shown with metronidazole and atovaquone, although the organism is not eradicated. Albendazole is effective for *E. intestinalis* but not for *E. bienusi*.[34] Like cryptosporidia, institution of HAART in infected individuals may result in resolution of diarrhea with loss of this pathogen from stool and on small bowel biopsy.[8]

For unclear reasons, infections by the protozoa *Giardia lamblia* and *Entamoeba histolytica* are not uniformly seen with increased frequency or virulence in AIDS.[35] However, in a study from Taiwan where this pathogen is endemic, amebic colitis was identified as a common cause of diarrhea.[36, 37] The nonpathogenic *Entamoeba dispar* is morphologically similar to *E. histolytica* and can only be distinguished by more specific stool or enzyme-linked immunosorbent assay tests.[38] *Blastocytis hominis, Endolimax nana,* and *Entamoeba coli* are nonpathogenic protozoa that are more common in homosexual men than other risk groups and are often found in association with other protozoal parasites.

Rare cases of enteric leishmaniasis have been described, with either small or large bowel infiltration.[39] *Pneumocystis carinii* and toxoplasmosis have also been reported as causes of colitis and diarrhea.[39]

Helminths, particularly *Ancylostoma duodenale* and *Strongyloides stercoralis,* have occasionally been described in large series.[40] Patients may present with abdominal pain, diarrhea, and eosinophilia. The clinical syndrome and recurrence rate associated with these parasites do not appear to be altered in the setting of HIV infection (see Chapter 99).

Viral infection of the large bowel, and rarely the small bowel, may account for diarrhea. CMV is the most common viral cause of diarrhea and the most frequent cause of chronic diarrhea in patients with AIDS and multiple negative stool tests.[41, 42] This infection characteristically occurs late in the course of HIV infection when the CD4 lymphocyte count falls below 100/μL.[41–43] Infection is most common in the colon, but concomitant disease in the esophagus, stomach, or small bowel may be observed. Isolated small bowel disease typically results in abdominal pain and rarely a predominantly diarrheal illness. The pathogenesis has not been totally elucidated. Infection of vascular endothelial cells is common, suggesting a role for mucosal ischemia; true histopathologic evidence of vasculitis is rare. An important role for local proinflammatory cytokine activation has been suggested.[44]

The clinical manifestations of enteric CMV infection vary greatly and include asymptomatic carriage, nonspecific symptoms of weight loss and fevers, and focal enteritis/colitis including appendicitis or diffuse ulcerating hemorrhagic involvement with bleeding or perforation. As a result, patients can present with one of several constellations of symptoms, including abdominal pain, peritonitis, watery nonbloody diarrhea, or hematochezia.[43, 45] The most common presentation, however, is abdominal pain associated with chronic diarrhea. Although the endoscopic spectrum is variable, the hallmark of CMV enteritis/colitis is subepithelial hemorrhage and mucosal ulceration.[43]

The diagnosis of GI CMV infection is best established by demonstrating viral cytopathic effect in tissue specimens.[46] The inclusions may be quite atypical in appearance or few in number, requiring immunostaining and/or in situ hybridization for confirmation.[47] Cultures for CMV are usually positive when inclusions are present, but they are less sensitive and specific than histopathologic identification.[46] If inclusions are demonstrable in tissue that appears macroscopically normal and are very few in number, the patient should be considered to have CMV infection (colonization) rather than true disease.[48]

A number of effective therapies are available for the treatment of CMV. The most commonly used agent is ganciclovir, an acyclovir derivative, which is effective in approximately 75% of cases.[49] Ganciclovir requires daily intravenous administration for several weeks, depending on the location and severity of disease. The oral form has some efficacy for retinitis,[50] but because of limited absorption, its use for the treatment of GI disease is not appropriate. An alternative to ganciclovir is foscarnet,[51] a pyrophosphate analog that inhibits viral replication. In contrast to ganciclovir, it has the advantage of being less marrow suppressive, although renal insufficiency and electrolyte disturbances (hypocalcemia, hypomagnesemia, hypophosphatemia) are frequent and it tends to be less well tolerated than ganciclovir. A randomized trial comparing ganciclovir to foscarnet for CMV GI disease in AIDS found similar efficacy.[52] Combination therapy of foscarnet with ganciclovir has been used with some success.[53] Cidofovir is the newest agent. Like ganciclovir and foscarnet, it must be given intravenously, and similar efficacy rates have been reported for retinal disease[54]; anecdotal experience suggests it to be effective for GI disease. Because of its long half-life (2 weeks), it can be given once weekly, which may be particularly advantageous for some patients. The main side effect is nephrotoxicity that may be irreversible. No randomized studies have compared cidofovir to either ganciclovir or foscarnet. Because of the severe immunodeficiency required for the development of CMV disease, recurrences are common following withdrawal of therapy unless long-term maintenance therapy is given or HAART is instituted.[55, 56] Nevertheless, despite maintenance therapy for CMV, relapse is almost uniform if severe immunodeficiency persists.

A reasonable approach to treating enteric CMV infection is to administer ganciclovir for 2 to 4 weeks for patients with documented, symptomatic infection. Cidofovir may be an option for those in whom daily intravenous drug administration is not feasible. Maintenance therapy should be considered if the patient subsequently develops a documented recurrence and severe immune dysfunction persists. If immune function can be improved and sustained with HAART, maintenance therapy may not be required. At the time of diagnosis, all patients should have ophthalmologic examination to exclude retinitis, because this site of infection requires close follow-up to ensure remission, thereby preventing blindness. The role of CMV antigenemia or DNA concentrations to predict subsequent disease and guide the use of preemptive therapy remains undefined.[57]

A number of other viruses (e.g., Norwalk, adenovirus) as well as novel enteric viruses (astrovirus, picobirnavirus) have been identified in both symptomatic and asymptomatic patients, but their overall contribution to diarrheal disease in AIDS is small.[58, 59] There are, however, occasional cases of well-documented hemorrhagic colitis from adenovirus infection.[60]

The role of HIV itself as a diarrheal pathogen remains controversial. Investigators have identified HIV within gut tissue in up to 40% of patients with AIDS,[61, 62] where the virus was confined to lamina propria macrophages and enterochromaffin cells, and not epithelial cells. In culture, HIV can infect colon cell lines[63]; however, the origins of these cell lines and their relevance to epithelial infection by HIV in vivo are not established. A more plausible potential mode of enteric HIV infection may be via viral uptake by M cells, which are abundant in rectal mucosa.[64] These specialized cells are capable of binding HIV and could directly transport the virus to lymphoid cells in the lamina propria.[64]

An *idiopathic AIDS enteropathy* has been proposed to account for the diarrhea in AIDS patients who lack an identifiable pathogen and may reflect indirect effects of HIV on enteric homeostasis. Although the precise features of this syndrome are not agreed on, the term implies a chronic diarrheal illness in patients with AIDS, where no cause can be identified despite an extensive evaluation; the inclusion of mucosal hypoproliferation as a defining feature has been advocated. With improvements in diagnostic techniques, greater awareness of the spectrum of diarrheal pathogens in AIDS and use of panendoscopy with biopsy for patients with negative stool tests, a diminishing fraction of patients have truly "idiopathic diarrhea." It has been suggested that in these patients enteric HIV infection leads to mucosal atrophy, which in turn might impair small bowel absorption, causing diarrhea and weight loss.[65] Even in patients with minimal morphologic changes and no detectable infection, malabsorption and altered intestinal permeability can be detected, suggesting cellular dysfunction.[66, 67] The basis for mucosal atrophy is not established but has been proposed to result from diminished numbers of activated lymphocytes expressing the interleukin-2 receptor (CD25 cells),[65] leading to a reduced mucosal responsiveness to this trophic lymphokine.

HIV infection of the gut is also associated with a diminished ratio of CD4/CD8 intestinal lymphocytes,[68, 69] much as systemic HIV results in reduced ratios of circulating lymphocytes. Reduced total intestinal CD4 cells have also been reported,[68] which may predispose to intestinal infection. The effects of intestinal HIV infection on local humoral immunity are not thoroughly elucidated. Moreover, the importance of altered secretory immunity to the frequency of GI infections in AIDS is not known. Reduced numbers of IgA plasma cells have been reported in intestinal mucosa of AIDS patients in association with increased IgM plasma cells[70]; however, it is not known whether these changes result directly from local HIV infection. In addition, increased concentration of serum IgG and IgA have been found in duodenal fluid, suggesting exudation of serum immunoglobulins into the intestine.[70]

Another mechanism of AIDS enteropathy may be via the effects of enteric HIV on autonomic nerves. Degeneration of nerve axons has been demonstrated in several patients with HIV infection,[71] implying that these patients may be at risk for motility disturbances, including intestinal pseudo-obstruction.[72] It is uncertain how prevalent these neural changes are, how often they are symptomatic, and whether they are a direct or indirect consequence of mucosal HIV infection.

The management of diarrhea in patients with idiopathic diarrhea parallels that of any other patient and should include bulking agents, antidiarrheal agents such as loperamide, and tincture of opium for more severe diarrhea (see Table 28–2). Institution of protease inhibitors has been shown to improve chronic unexplained diarrhea.[73, 74]

Infections by enteric bacteria are more frequent and more virulent in HIV-infected individuals compared with healthy hosts. *Salmonella, Shigella,* and *Campylobacter* all have higher rates of both bacteremia and antibiotic resistance.[75] Recurrent *Salmonella* bacteremia establishes the diagnosis of AIDS in an HIV-infected patient. There is no clear explanation for these frequent recurrences, but they could result from impaired reticuloendothelial cell clearance owing to HIV infection of splenic or hepatic macrophages (Kupffer cells). Patients with HIV infection are also particularly susceptible to food-borne enteric infections (especially *Salmonella, Campylobacter,* and *Listeria*) and should be cautioned against eating raw or undercooked seafood, shellfish, poultry, meat or dairy products, as well as unpasteurized milk or milk products.

Diagnosis of *Shigella* or *Salmonella* is straightforward, because the organisms usually can be grown from stool samples. Conversely, *Campylobacter* is more difficult to grow; thus, patients may be stool-culture negative, with the organisms found only by culturing tissue biopsy specimens.[76] These enteric infections typically present with high fever, abdominal pain, and diarrhea that may be bloody. Abdominal pain can be severe mimicking an acute abdomen. As noted, bacteremia is common, and parenteral antibiotics should be administered empirically in severely ill patients when these infections are suspected pending results of stool and blood culture evaluations. Low-dose antibiotic prophylaxis has been recommended if a recurrence is documented following successful initial therapy. The choice of antibiotic is determined by culture and sensitivity results; ciprofloxacin may be a particularly attractive choice for empirical therapy and if organisms are multiply resistant.[77]

Diarrhea due to *Clostridium difficile* is common in AIDS patients, not because it is an OI but rather because antibiotic use is far greater and hospitalization more frequent in this population than in healthy hosts. The clinical presentation, response to therapy, and relapse rate are no different than in immunocompetent patients.[78] Diagnosis rests on standard assays of stool for *C. difficile* enterotoxin. Treatment with metronidazole or vancomycin is generally effective.

Small bowel bacterial overgrowth (see Chapter 90) is uncommon in AIDS patients,[79] and its role in causing diarrhea appears limited. Overgrowth is believed to result from the increased prevalence in AIDS of gastric achlorhydria,[80] resulting in failure of gastric acid to neutralize ingested bacteria. Impaired motility due to HIV-induced autonomic neuropathy could also lead to small bowel colonization.

Mycobacterial involvement of the bowel either by *Mycobacterium tuberculosis* or MAC may lead to diarrhea, abdominal pain, and, rarely, obstruction or bleeding. In some series, MAC is the most commonly identified organism in patients with chronic diarrhea and low CD4 lymphocyte counts.[81] Although *M. tuberculosis* infection appears to be symptomatic in all cases, a large number of patients with MAC have asymptomatic infection of the small bowel. Duodenal involvement is most common and may be suspected at endoscopy by the presence of yellow mucosal nodules, often in association with malabsorption, bacteremia, and systemic infection.[82]

Diagnosis of GI MAC infection is best made by endoscopic biopsy; fecal smear is much less sensitive than culture. The organism is readily seen on biopsy specimens with acid-fast staining, and the number of organisms is often striking.[82] Blood culture positivity may suggest the diagnosis. Affected patients have severe malabsorption and weight loss in association with villous blunting and suffusion of macrophages with mycobacteria. As is typical of MAC infection in AIDS, there is a poorly formed inflammatory response, and granulomas are rarely present. Response to antibiotic therapy is variable and depends in part on the extent of immunocompromise; however, eradication is rarely achieved. Multidrug regimens including amikacin, ethambutol, rifampin, clarithromycin, and ciprofloxacin can reduce, but not eradicate, MAC organisms.[83] As with other OIs, institution of HAART in these patients may improve immune function, hasten clinical resolution of the infection, and prevent relapse.[6, 84]

Although extrapulmonary *M. tuberculosis* in AIDS is common, luminal GI tract involvement remains infrequent but, when present, usually involves the ileocecal region or colon.[39] Fistula formation, intussusception, and perforation, as well as peritoneal and rectal involvement have also been reported.[85] Tuberculosis involvement of the gut in HIV is most commonly found in developing countries.[86] In contrast with MAC, *M. tuberculosis* infections in AIDS generally respond to multidrug antituberculous therapy with clinical and microbiologic cure.

Fungal infections of the gut have been recognized in AIDS. GI *histoplasmosis* has been most commonly described and occurs in the setting of systemic infection, often in association with pulmonary and hepatic disease. It may manifest as a diffuse colitis with large ulcerations and diarrhea, as a mass, or as serosal disease in association with peritonitis.[87, 88] The diagnosis is established by fungal smear and culture of infected tissue or blood; histoplasmosis antigen assay may provide supportive evidence.[88] The infection is often managed initially by amphotericin B administration. Long-term suppressive therapy with itraconazole has been used successfully; ketoconazole is ineffective. *Coccidioidomycosis* of the gut is rare and, like histoplasmosis, occurs in the context of systemic infection. Liver involvement appears to be more common than luminal disease. Treatment with amphotericin B is indicated following diagnosis by fungal smear and culture. Rare cases of systemic *cryptococcosis* with gut involvement have also been described.[89] A peculiar fungal infection due to *Penicillium marneffei* has been reported from Southeast Asia that can cause colitis and chronic diarrhea.[37]

With the advent of HAART, *drug-induced diarrhea* is becoming increasingly important. The most common agents associated with diarrhea are the protease inhibitors, with nelfinavir having the highest rate, approaching 20%.[90] In general, the diarrhea is mild to moderate in severity and is not associated with weight loss. The mechanism(s) for diarrhea due to these agents is poorly understood. Symptomatic therapies are generally effective.

Evaluation (Table 28–3)

Prior to extensive evaluation of diarrhea, a careful history should be obtained, primarily to exclude lactose or food intolerance, as well as to suggest whether GI symptoms might be part of a systemic infection. Unfortunately, the clinical history is not likely to establish a specific diagnosis in most patients, because the symptom is usually due to infection, possibly by more than one organism concurrently. Chronic diarrhea associated with weight loss strongly suggests an underlying OI. A careful history can often aid in localizing the segment of luminal GI tract most severely involved. For example, symptoms of periumbilical cramps, bloating, and nausea suggest gastric or small bowel involvement or both, raising the possibility of infection with *Cryp-*

Table 28–3 | **Evaluation of Diarrhea in AIDS**

In all patients
- Stool specimen for
  - Bacterial culture: *Salmonella, Shigella, Campylobacter*
  - Stool smear
    - Fecal leukocytes
    - Ova and parasite examination (at least 3–6 specimens)
    - Acid-fast stain
    - *Clostridium difficile* toxin

If patient has rectal bleeding, tenesmus, or fecal leukocytes
- Flexible sigmoidoscopy with
  - Biopsy of mucosa for pathology, viruses, protozoa
  - Cultures of rectal tissue for bacteria (especially *Campylobacter*), viruses (optional)

If diarrhea and weight loss persist in an otherwise active patient
- Upper endoscopy with
  - Small bowel mucosal biopsy; electron microscopy if available

AIDS, acquired immunodeficiency syndrome.

tosporidium, I. belli, or *Giardia.* Severe watery diarrhea that occurs while fasting resulting in dehydration, electrolyte disturbances, and weight loss suggests intestinal cryptosporidiosis. Hematochezia usually implies colitis most frequently resulting from colonic infection by CMV, *Shigella,* or *Campylobacter.* As discussed later in this chapter, unprotected receptive anal intercourse followed by severe tenesmus, dyschezia, and urgency suggests acute anorectal infection with herpes simplex, gonococci, or *Chlamydia.*

The physical examination generally provides few diagnostic clues in the evaluation of diarrhea in AIDS. Fever and cachexia are common with MAC infection. Abdominal tenderness is more typical for CMV and bacterial colitis but may be observed with other disorders, thus limiting specificity.

As stated earlier, the most important goal of evaluating diarrhea in HIV infection is to identify a treatable cause with the minimum workup necessary (see Table 28–3). Studies have shown that up to 65% of patients with chronic diarrhea in whom no diagnosis has been made by multiple stool tests may have a diagnosis established by colonoscopy and/or upper endoscopy with biopsy.[91] If both upper and lower endoscopy are performed in addition to stool tests in all patients with uninvestigated chronic diarrhea, the diagnostic yield may be as high as 85%.[11] Most studies have found a higher prevalence of colonic than small bowel disease. Patients with a low CD4 count ($<100/\mu L$) are most likely to have a diagnosis established by endoscopy with biopsy.[91]

Initial evaluations should include no less than three stools for ova and parasite examination, including acid-fast smear, as well as culture for enteric bacterial pathogens. Patients with acute severe illness may require earlier endoscopic evaluation if the initial stool studies are negative. If a diagnosis is not reached following careful stool analyses, sigmoidoscopy is appropriate, with biopsies obtained from any abnormal regions, or randomly from rectal mucosa if no abnormalities are apparent. Colonoscopy has been advocated instead of sigmoidoscopy to diagnose isolated right-sided colonic CMV infection[45] which has been variably reported in 0% to 30%.[91] If lower tract evaluation is negative, upper endoscopy may occasionally uncover proximal small bowel infection by *Cryptosporidium, Microsporidium,* or MAC. Jejunal biopsies may be superior to duodenal biopsies, primarily for identifying microsporidia.[92] However, ileal biopsy performed at the time of colonoscopy may negate the need for upper endoscopy with biopsy.[42] In a study evaluating duodenal and ileal biopsies, the yield for *Cryptosporidium* and *Microsporidium* was equal.[42] Duodenal fluid can also be aspirated during endoscopy to evaluate for protozoal infection or small bowel bacterial overgrowth, although this approach is not recommended given the low yield. The diagnostic value of radiographic contrast studies for evaluating diarrhea is very low because most disorders require mucosal biopsy for diagnosis. If required for other reasons, radiographic studies should be obtained after all stools are collected because barium interferes with microscopic stool examination for ova and parasites. For the patient presenting with concomitant severe abdominal pain, computed tomographic (CT) scan may be the initial test; colonic wall thickening suggests bacterial or CMV colitis.

The role of an empirical antibiotic trial for the patient in whom stool evaluations and flexible sigmoidoscopy are nondiagnostic is unknown. This approach may be rational for areas with high prevalence rates of giardiasis or possibly to treat culture-negative *Campylobacter,* bacterial overgrowth, or enteroaggregative *Escherichia coli.*[93] For these purposes, a quinolone antibiotic and/or metronidazole can be particularly efficacious. The decision to undertake this approach, however, should be made in the appropriate clinical context. For example, a patient with severe symptoms and associated fever or abdominal pain should be more vigorously investigated than one whose symptoms interfere minimally with daily activities. In addition, no studies have critically evaluated this strategy. Furthermore, some studies have shown spontaneous resolution or improvement of chronic diarrhea in up to 38% of patients.[41] Consideration must always be given to a drug-induced cause for diarrhea in the patient with negative stool tests. A drug holiday can help establish a drug-induced cause of symptoms, especially when reinstitution results in recurrent diarrhea.

In summary, diarrhea remains a frequent source of morbidity in the HIV-infected population. Although HAART has not markedly altered the overall frequency of diarrhea, it has changed the etiologic spectrum, reduced the number of patients with severe diarrhea, and enhanced our treatment of OIs that cause diarrhea.

ODYNOPHAGIA AND DYSPHAGIA

Differential Diagnosis (Table 28–4)

Before the era of HAART, esophageal complaints *(dysphagia* and *odynophagia)* were common, reported to occur in at least one third of patients during the course of HIV disease,[94] and the incidence increased with disease progression, given the many esophageal pathogens that complicate severe immunodeficiency. Because of HAART, the incidence of esophageal disease has fallen, and the number of patients with diseases not unique to AIDS, such as gastroesophageal reflux, is rising.[7]

Candida albicans is the most frequent esophageal infection in AIDS. Prospective endoscopic studies of symptomatic patients have found *Candida* esophagitis in up to 64%,[95, 96] and *Candida* also frequently coexists with other disorders.[94, 97] Although most cases of *Candida* occur in the setting of AIDS, *Candida* esophagitis may occur during primary HIV

Table 28–4 | **Differential Diagnosis of Dysphagia and Odynophagia in AIDS**

*Candida albicans**
Cytomegalovirus*
Idiopathic ulcerations*
Herpes simplex
Histoplasma capsulatum
Mycobacterium avium complex
Cryptosporidium
Neoplasm: Kaposi's sarcoma, lymphoma, squamous cell carcinoma, adenocarcinoma
Non-AIDS esophageal disease
Gastroesophageal reflux
Pill-induced esophagitis

*More common.
AIDS, acquired immunodeficiency syndrome.

infection as a result of transient immunosuppression.[98] Oral thrush often predicts concurrent esophagitis; however, the absence of thrush does not exclude the possibility of esophageal candidiasis. Overall, the positive and negative predictive values of thrush for *Candida* esophagitis are 90% and 82%, respectively.[99]

Patients with esophageal candidiasis generally complain of substernal dysphagia; odynophagia, when present, is usually not severe. Definitive diagnosis is established by upper endoscopy, which reveals either focal or diffuse plaques in association with mucosal hyperemia and friability; well-circumscribed ulcer(s) suggests an additional process (Fig. 28–2). Biopsies show desquamated epithelial cells with typical-appearing yeast forms; fungal invasion is usually present only in the superficial epithelium.[100] Positive brushings for *Candida* display evidence of pseudomycelia.

Although CMV is the most commonly identified pathogen in AIDS, its association with esophageal disease is less frequent than *Candida*. As with other patients with esophageal ulcers, patients with CMV esophagitis complain of odynophagia or substernal chest pain, characteristically severe.[101] Dysphagia is much less common than in patients with *Candida* esophagitis and is rarely the primary complaint. Fever may be reported. Generally, upper endoscopy reveals extensive ulcerations that are large and deep, although the endoscopic pattern is variable (Fig. 28–3).[102] Associated candidal infection is common. Mucosal biopsies characteristically demonstrate viral cytopathic effect in mesenchymal and/or endothelial cells in the granulation tissue. As is typical for gut involvement with CMV, characteristic inclusions may be absent, necessitating confirmation by immunohistochemical stains.[47] Biopsy of granulation tissue in the ulcer base provides the highest yield for viral cytopathic effect;

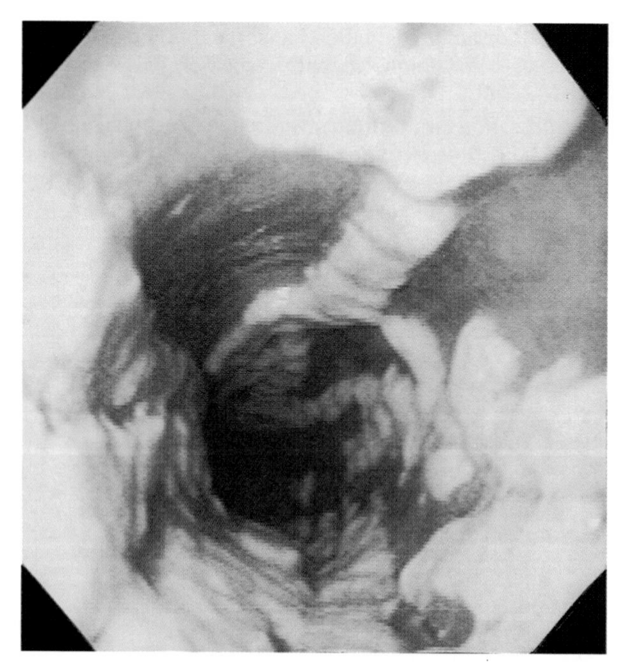

Figure 28–2. *Candida* esophagitis. Typical-appearing raised, confluent yellow plaques. The yellow plaques assume a linear pattern in some areas, with normal intervening mucosa. (From Wilcox CM: Atlas of Clinical Gastrointestinal Endoscopy. Philadelphia, WB Saunders, 1995, p 23.)

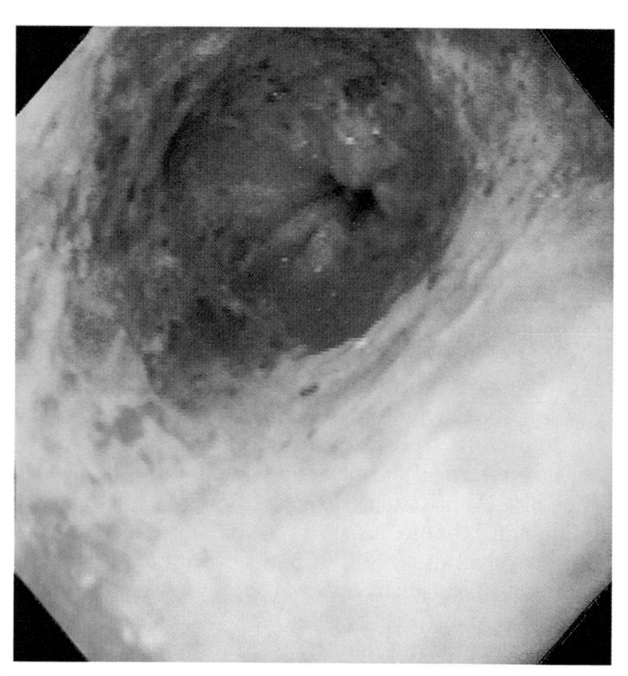

Figure 28–3. Cytomegalovirus and herpes simplex virus esophagitis. Diffuse circumferential ulceration. The gastrointestinal junction is seen in the distance. In patients with AIDS, multiplicity of pathogens is frequent. (From Wilcox CM: Atlas of Clinical Gastrointestinal Endoscopy. Philadelphia, WB Saunders, 1995, p 28.)

viral culture of biopsy specimens is usually positive, whereas cytologic brushings are unhelpful.

A syndrome of nonspecific (idiopathic, aphthous) esophageal ulceration is common[101] (Fig. 28–4). Like patients with CMV, the presentation is that of severe odynophagia or chest pain with endoscopic evidence of deep, large ulcerations.[103] In fact, the endoscopic appearance of these idiopathic ulcers is indistinguishable from the well-circumscribed ulcers caused by CMV. Criteria for diagnosis of idiopathic ulcers include the following: (1) endoscopic and histopathologic ulcer; (2) no evidence of viral cytopathic effect by both routine histology and immunohistochemical studies; and (3) no clinical or endoscopic evidence of reflux disease or pill-induced esophagitis. As with CMV, these ulcers occur in late-stage disease, with most patients having a CD4 count less than 50/μL. The pathogenesis of these ulcers remains unknown. Although HIV has been identified in these lesions by in situ hybridization,[104] a causative role is unlikely, because HIV can be found with a similar prevalence in other causes of esophageal disease in AIDS.[104, 105] In addition, HIV has been seen only in inflammatory cells in ulcer tissue rather than in squamous epithelial cells.[105]

The idiopathic ulcer syndrome may occur coincident with acute HIV seroconversion. In these patients the ulcers are usually multiple and small.[106] There may be an associated maculopapular skin rash and oral ulcers.[107] In some patients electron microscopy demonstrated retroviral-like particles at the ulcer site but no CMV or herpes inclusions.[106]

In contrast with other immunocompromised hosts, herpes simplex virus esophagitis is infrequent in AIDS.[101] In healthy patients, esophagitis is usually due to herpes simplex type I; however, AIDS patients may have esophagitis due to either type I or type II herpes. The disease is similar to herpetic infections of other mucous membranes in that the pathogenetic features follow a predictable sequence: discrete vesicles form, then shallow ulcers, which finally coalesce into regions of diffuse shallow ulceration. It is during this late stage of diffuse esophagitis that most patients with herpes are evaluated. In contrast with CMV esophagitis and idiopathic ulcer, these ulcers tend to be shallow; large, deep ulcers are rare (Fig. 28–5).[108] Biopsies and cytologic brushings taken from the margin of the ulcers (the sites of active viral replication) are most likely to show epithelial cell invasion and nuclear changes typical of herpes infections. Viral cultures of biopsy specimens are usually positive.

Esophageal neoplasms have also been described in AIDS patients, including non-Hodgkin's lymphoma, Kaposi's sarcoma, squamous cell carcinoma, and adenocarcinoma.[94, 109]

Isolated cases of esophagitis/ulcerations in AIDS owing to pills (zidovudine [AZT], didanosine [ddc]), bacteria (actinomycosis, MAC), fungi (*Histoplasma, Mucormycosis, Torulopsis, Pneumocystis*) and parasites (*Leishmania*, cryptosporidiosis) all have been reported.[94, 110]

Evaluation

There is no way to definitely identify the specific cause of esophageal complaints in the AIDS patient based on symptoms or physical examination alone. However, a few generalizations may be made. The presence of oral thrush associated with mild to moderate dysphagia without odynophagia is likely due to *Candida* esophagitis. In contrast, the patient with severe odynophagia without dysphagia or thrush is more likely to have ulcerative esophagitis (viral, idiopathic). The patient complaining of substernal burning and regurgitation is most likely to have gastroesophageal reflux disease. Endoscopy with biopsy is the only means of establishing a specific etiology for the cause of dysphagia and odynophagia.

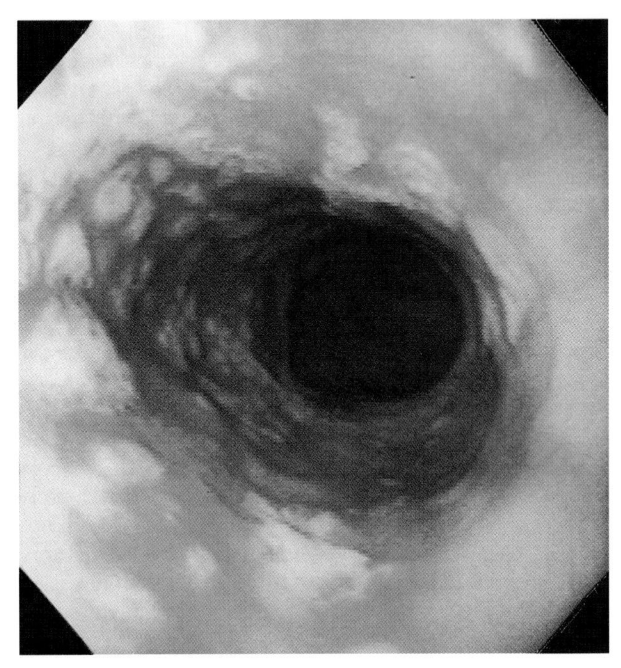

Figure 28–5. Herpes simplex virus esophagitis manifested by multiple whitish plaques. Diffuse erythema surrounds the plaques, representing shallow ulceration. Islands of normal-appearing esophageal mucosa are still present.

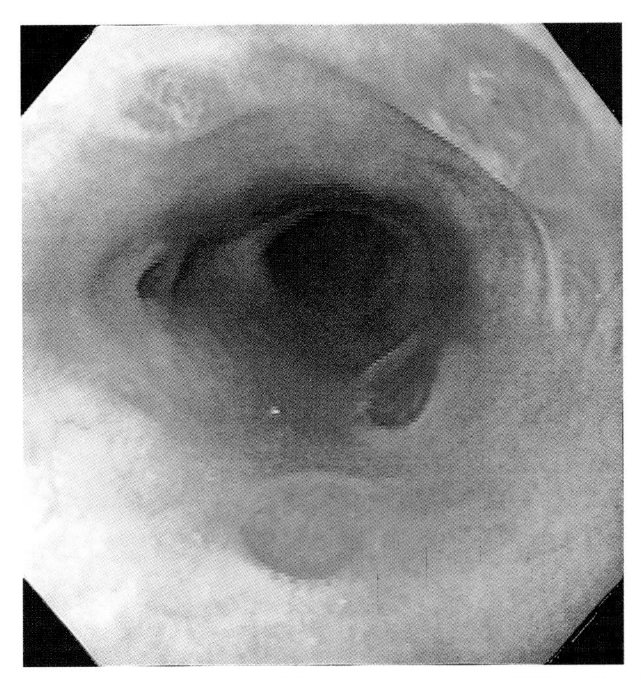

Figure 28–4. Human immunodeficiency virus–associated idiopathic ulcer. Multiple well-circumscribed ulcerations throughout the esophagus. The ulcers have a punched-out appearance, with normal-appearing intervening mucosa. The ulcers seem to be raised above the normal level of the esophageal wall, resulting in this heaped-up appearance. (From Wilcox CM: Atlas of Clinical Gastrointestinal Endoscopy. Philadelphia, WB Saunders, 1995, p 75.)

In general, cultures of esophageal biopsies for fungi and viruses are less useful than is histology, because cultures alone do not distinguish between true pathogens and secondary colonizers, are less sensitive, and take several days to become positive. Conventional barium swallow radiography in the patient with esophageal complaints is not worthwhile, although it may reveal typical features of *Candida*, CMV, or herpes.[108] A randomized trial comparing barium esophagography to endoscopy for symptomatic HIV-infected patients found endoscopy to be much more sensitive.[111] In addition, the radiographic appearance of an esophageal ulcer cannot adequately distinguish etiology, thus mandating subsequent endoscopy and biopsy for a definitive diagnosis.

Treatment

Given the preponderance of *Candida* infection, an empirical approach to the management of esophageal symptoms is reasonable in most patients with AIDS. Patients with dysphagia and/or odynophagia who also have oral thrush should be treated empirically with fluconazole 100 mg per day after a 200-mg loading dose.[112] Itraconazole or fluconazole suspensions are also effective.[113, 114] Despite the additional expense, we prefer fluconazole over ketoconazole, given its superior efficacy.[115] The absorption of ketoconazole, and less so with itraconazole, is highly pH dependent,[116] whereas fluconazole absorption is not pH dependent.[117] If symptoms persist despite a 1-week empirical trial, endoscopy with biopsy should be performed in preference to the initiation of other empirical trials or escalation of the dose of fluconazole.[118] Narcotics are appropriate for the patient with severe pain until specific treatment for the underlying cause can be initiated. Relapse of *Candida* esophagitis almost invariably occurs[94] unless immune function is improved with antiretroviral treatment. Despite chronic prophylaxis, relapse frequently occurs often due to antifungal resistance.[119] This is much less of a problem now that patients are receiving HAART.[120]

Documented infections with CMV generally respond to a 2- to 3-week course of intravenous ganciclovir; relapses may require an additional course of therapy and/or a maintenance regimen.[121] Effective alternative therapies include foscarnet and cidofovir.

Idiopathic ulcers respond in more than 90% of patients to oral corticosteroids (40 mg per day, tapered over 4 weeks).[122] Intralesional steroid injections have also been used but not compared with oral therapy or used in refractory ulcers. The basis for corticosteroid efficacy is unknown; infectious causes should be assiduously excluded before administering steroids in this setting. Thalidomide is also highly effective and may be effective when prednisone fails.[123] The main side effects of thalidomide are somnolence, rash, and neuropathy. The devastating teratogenic effects mandate its use to be limited to men.

Herpes simplex esophagitis responds to acyclovir and related agents, including valacyclovir; however, relapses may occur. Rare instances of acyclovir-resistant herpes have been reported in AIDS; such patients may respond to foscarnet.[51]

Before the era of HAART, the long-term survival for patients with esophageal infections was poor despite effective therapies, reflecting the severe immunodeficiency of these patients. For example, the median survival for patients with CMV esophagitis was 7.6 months and somewhat longer for patients with idiopathic ulcers.[101] Survival has been improved in these patients with HAART.[124]

ABDOMINAL PAIN

Differential Diagnosis (Table 28–5)

The exact frequency of abdominal pain in patients with AIDS is unknown, but like other GI complications of AIDS, the prevalence and etiology have been altered by HAART. In most patients with AIDS, abdominal pain, when severe, is directly related to HIV and its consequences.[125] However, the physician must consider not only the manifestations of OIs and neoplasms but also the more common causes of abdominal pain in the general population. Many studies have been published specifically addressing the evaluation of abdominal pain in AIDS; all underscore the broad spectrum of potential causes for abdominal pain in this population.[125, 126]

The differential diagnosis of abdominal pain in AIDS, presented in Table 28–5, is organized by the site of origin of the pain. For each organ system, a list of potential complications with their likely causes is offered. In some instances causes are listed because of their known ability to produce symptoms by involving a particular organ. The Table does not include non–AIDS-specific diagnoses that are assuming more importance in the era of HAART. Table 28–6 defines abdominal pain in terms of the four most common pain syndromes, their most likely causes, and the diagnostic methods indicated. Generally, the duration and severity of symptoms dictate the urgency of evaluation.

Table 28–5 | **Differential Diagnosis of Abdominal Pain in AIDS**

ORGAN	CAUSES
Stomach	
Gastritis	CMV,* *Cryptosporidium, Helicobacter pylori*
Focal ulcer	CMV,* acid-peptic
Outlet obstruction	*Cryptosporidium,** CMV, lymphoma
Mass	Lymphoma, KS, CMV
Small bowel	
Enteritis	*Cryptosporidium,** CMV, MAC
Obstruction	Lymphoma,* KS
Perforation	CMV,* lymphoma
Colon	
Colitis	CMV, enteric bacteria,* HSV
Obstruction	Lymphoma,* KS, intussusception
Perforation	CMV,* lymphoma, HSV
Appendicitis	KS,* *Cryptosporidium,* CMV
Anorectum	
Proctitis	HSV,* bacteria, CMV
Tumor	KS, lymphoma, condyloma
Liver, spleen	
Infiltration	Lymphoma,* CMV, MAC
Biliary tract	
Cholecystitis	CMV,* *Cryptosporidium,** *Microsporidium*
Papillary stenosis	CMV,* *Cryptosporidium,** KS, cholangitis, CMV*
Pancreas	
Inflammation	CMV,* KS, pentamidine, dDI
Tumor	Lymphoma, KS
Mesentery, peritoneum	
Infiltration	MAC,* *Cryptococcus,* KS, lymphoma, histoplasmosis, tuberculosis, coccidioidomycosis, toxoplasmosis

*More frequent.

KS, Kaposi's sarcoma; CMV, cytomegalovirus; MAC, *Mycobacterium avium* complex; HSV, herpes simplex virus; dDI, didanosine; AIDS, acquired immunodeficiency syndrome.

Evaluation (see Table 28–6)

The history is helpful in localizing the origin of abdominal pain. Associated symptoms and signs should suggest the

Table 28–6 | **Evaluation of Abdominal Pain Syndromes in AIDS**

SYNDROME	SUSPECTED DIAGNOSIS	DIAGNOSTIC METHOD
Dull pain, diarrhea, mild nausea, vomiting	Infectious enteritis	Stool cultures, ova and parasites, sigmoidoscopy
Acute, severe pain, with peritoneal irritation	Perforation, infectious peritonitis	Abdominal plain films, surgical consultation; ultrasound or CT; paracentesis if ascites present; laparoscopy
Right upper quadrant pain, abnormal liver biochemical tests	Cholecystitis, cholangitis, hepatic infiltrates, cholangiopathy	CT/ultrasound, ERCP, liver biopsy
Subacute pain, severe nausea and vomiting	Obstruction	Barium small bowel series, barium enema, endoscopy

AIDS, acquired immunodeficiency syndrome; CT, computed tomography; ERCP, endoscopic retrograde cholangiopancreatography.

particular organ involved, and the quality and duration of the abdominal pain may implicate specific diseases. Generally, the same workup as for a patient without AIDS should be initiated. Abdominal ultrasonography and CT scanning are useful early in the assessment of abdominal pain and may highlight regions of disease not suspected clinically.

In general, *perforation* results most often from CMV infection, frequently in the distal small bowel or colon, and is the most common cause of the acute abdomen in AIDS. *Obstruction* is most likely to develop from an intestinal neoplasm. Intussusception may be one unusual form of lymphomatous obstruction, or it may be caused by an infection.[47] *Infectious enteritis* may lead to dull, intermittent abdominal pain or acute, severe pain in the absence of obstruction or perforation; diarrhea is usually present but may not be prominent. The site of involvement (large vs. small bowel) dictates the specific symptoms and signs.

Infectious or *nonspecific peritonitis* in the absence of bowel perforation has been well documented. Infectious etiologies include histoplasmosis, tuberculosis, MAC, *Vibrio vulnificus,* toxoplasmosis, and cryptococcosis. In the patient with ascites, paracentesis is safe and can uncover bacterial or fungal infection or lymphoma.[127] High-protein ascites of uncertain etiology has also been reported, and may necessitate laparoscopy in hopes of identifying a cause.[128]

Pancreatitis is a frequent cause of abdominal pain in AIDS patients and may arise from a variety of causes, most prominently drug induced and infectious.[129] Its presentation and prognosis are similar to patients without HIV disease.[129–131] Serum amylase elevations in the absence of pancreatic disease may indicate macroamylasemia, which has been observed in AIDS.[132]

The most common cause of pancreatitis in AIDS is drug-induced disease, most frequently dideoxyinosine (ddI) or pentamidine.[133] A 5% incidence of symptomatic pancreatitis has been reported in trials of ddI, with increasing rates at higher doses. Pentamidine-induced pancreatitis may develop following either inhaled or parenteral administration and is often accompanied by abnormalities in glucose metabolism. Occasional cases of drug-induced pancreatitis have also been seen following use of trimethoprim-sulfamethoxazole. Antiretroviral drugs may also cause hyperlipidemia leading to acute pancreatitis.

Potential infectious causes of pancreatitis in AIDS are multiple and include CMV, mycobacteria, *Cryptococcus,* and herpes simplex.[134] Infectious pancreatitis may not always be clinically obvious and should be suspected in any AIDS patient with abdominal pain and elevated serum amylase level.[135] A definitive diagnosis is difficult given the infrequency of pancreatic biopsy.

Pancreatic infiltration by lymphoma or Kaposi's sarcoma may occasionally occur, manifested either by mass effect on adjacent duodenum, exocrine insufficiency if the pancreatic duct is obstructed, or acute pancreatitis.

Management

Management of abdominal pain falls broadly into surgical versus nonsurgical options. Indications for surgical intervention in AIDS patients are the same as for patients without AIDS. All tissue specimens must be submitted for viral and fungal culture and for pathologic examination, and mesenteric nodes should undergo biopsy. Laparoscopic surgery may provide a less invasive alternative to laparotomy in selected patients such as those with acute cholecystitis.

The morbidity and mortality in early reports of surgical procedures in patients with AIDS were exceedingly high.[136, 137] In part, this is likely attributable to the poor underlying health of AIDS patients requiring laparotomy; most had CMV infection, which tends to occur in patients with late-stage AIDS. Complications and mortality are likely to be far less common for patients with asymptomatic HIV infection and those who have responded to HAART. Indeed, in stable patients with AIDS undergoing elective surgery, mortality rates have been much lower.[137]

The nonsurgical management of abdominal pain is determined by the clinical evaluation. Treatable *infections* contributing to the symptoms should be managed with appropriate antimicrobial agents. Symptoms due to lymphoma or Kaposi's sarcoma may respond to chemotherapy or radiation therapy. Symptomatic treatment with analgesics may be indicated in addition to specific antimicrobial or antineoplastic drug regimens. Perioperative nutritional support is an important component of the care plan and may require parenteral supplementation for a limited period. Pancreatitis should be treated similarly to the non–HIV-infected patient with careful attention to excluding drugs and hyperlipidemia as causes.

ANORECTAL DISEASE

Differential Diagnosis (Table 28–7)

The frequency of anorectal disease among homosexual AIDS patients is quite high. Common findings in HIV-infected patients include perirectal abscesses, anal fistulas, idiopathic ulcerations and infectious proctitis, but lymphoma, ulcerations due to CMV, tuberculosis, and histoplasmosis may also be seen (see Table 28–7).

Anorectal carcinomas are more common in homosexual men than in other members of the population, and the risk increases with HIV infection. A prospective cohort study of 158 HIV-seropositive and 147 HIV-seronegative homosexual men without anal dysplasia found high-grade anal squamous

Table 28–7 | **Differential Diagnosis of Anorectal Disease in AIDS**

Infections	**Neoplasms**
Bacteria	Lymphoma*
*Chlamydia trachomatis**	Kaposi's sarcoma
Lymphogranuloma venereum	Squamous cell carcinoma
*Neisseria gonorrhoeae**	Cloacogenic carcinoma
Shigella flexneri	Condyloma acuminatum
Mycobacterium tuberculosis	**Other**
Protozoa	Idiopathic ulcers*
Entamoeba histolytica	Perirectal abscess, fistula*
Leishmania donovani	
Viruses	
Herpes simplex*	
Cytomegalovirus*	
Fungi	
Candida albicans	
Histoplasma capsulatum	

*More frequent.
AIDS, acquired immunodeficiency virus.

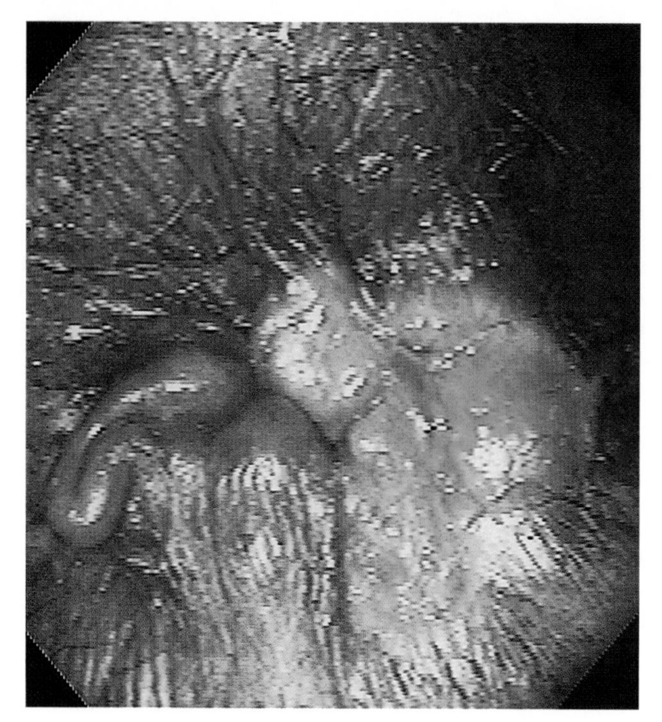

Figure 28–6. Perianal herpes simplex virus. Shallow perianal ulcer anteriorly suggests herpes simplex virus disease. Two thrombosed external hemorrhoids are present posteriorly. (From Wilcox CM: Atlas of Clinical Gastrointestinal Endoscopy: Companion to Sleisenger and Fordtran's Gastrointestinal Disease. Philadelphia, WB Saunders, 1995.)

intraepithelial neoplasia after a mean follow-up of 21 months[138] in 15.2% and 5.4%, respectively. These neoplasms appear to result from human papillomavirus (HPV) infections acquired through sexual contact, particularly HPV types 16 and 18.[138] Morphologic studies have documented histologic progression, often in the same lesion, from a benign lesion, condyloma acuminatum to marked anal dysplasia, or anal squamous cell carcinoma. No increased incidence of anorectal carcinoma has been recognized in HIV-infected subgroups other than homosexual men. Cytologic specimens of the anal canal, similar to Papanicolaou smears, are sensitive means to detect dysplasia.[138]

Approach to Anorectal Symptoms (see also Chapter 117)

A careful history of the HIV-infected homosexual patient with anorectal symptoms who does not have AIDS may uncover symptoms of advancing HIV disease. Weight loss, fever, fatigue, and night sweats all raise the possibility of neoplasm or anorectal OI.

GI herpes simplex virus infections in AIDS patients occur most frequently in the perianal area that may involve the distal rectum (Fig. 28–6) and occasionally the esophagus (see Fig. 28–5). Mucosal involvement typically is focal, with painful ulcerations, tenesmus, and occasional bleeding. There may be associated bladder or bowel dysfunction. The infection can be diagnosed by the appearance of typical vesicles or ulcers in affected tissue, with evidence of epithelial cell inclusions in biopsy samples. Most herpes infections respond to acyclovir or famciclovir although acyclovir-resistant strains are being increasingly encountered; foscarnet may be a suitable alternative in this situation.[51]

In HIV-infected patients and patients with AIDS, physical examination should include careful inspection of the skin and mucous membranes as well as palpation of the lymph nodes. Visual inspection of the anus for fissures and masses should precede digital examination. Palpation of the perianal area and buttocks for abscess should be performed. The presence of severe pain on rectal examination strongly suggests ulcerative disease, hemorrhoids, or neoplasms. Palpation of the anal canal may reveal masses or fissures not otherwise evident. All patients with anorectal symptoms should have anoscopy and sigmoidoscopy (rigid or flexible) with mucosal biopsy. Evaluation may be necessary under general anesthesia when pain is severe. Specimens should be evaluated for evidence of neoplasm or infection; when appropriate, they should be examined with bacterial (including gonococcal and chlamydial), viral, and fungal cultures. CT scan may define the extent of disease if a neoplasm is identified.

Healing of anorectal disease following surgical or nonsurgical therapy may largely be determined by the stage of HIV infection. HIV-positive patients without AIDS have favorable outcomes following anorectal surgery with acceptable wound healing, whereas patients with AIDS are more likely to have a poor outcome.[139]

GASTROINTESTINAL BLEEDING

GI bleeding complicates AIDS in less than 1% of patients but may pose difficult diagnostic and therapeutic challenges when occurring in the patient with HIV infection. Moreover, in the absence of HAART, the presence of GI bleeding is independently associated with reduced survival.[140]

Differential Diagnosis (Table 28–8)

GI bleeding in AIDS is as likely to arise from sources not unique to AIDS as from OIs or neoplasms. Infections and neoplasms seen exclusively with AIDS can rarely cause GI

Table 28–8 | **Differential Diagnosis of Gastrointestinal Bleeding in AIDS (Excluding Non-AIDS Specific Diagnoses)**

Upper Gastrointestinal Tract	Lower Gastrointestinal Tract
Esophagus	Cytomegalovirus*
*Candida**	*Entamoeba histolytica*
Cytomegalovirus*	*Campylobacter*
Herpes simplex	*Clostridium difficile*
Idiopathic ulcer	*Shigella* sp.
Stomach	Idiopathic ulcerations
Cryptosporidiosis	Kaposi's sarcoma*
Cytomegalovirus*	Lymphoma
Kaposi's sarcoma*	
Lymphoma	
Small intestine	
Kaposi's sarcoma*	
Lymphoma*	
Cytomegalovirus	
Salmonella sp.	
Cryptosporidium	

*More frequent.
AIDS, acquired immunodeficiency syndrome.

bleeding and are listed in Table 28–8. Studies have found that the causes of upper GI bleeding are most frequently due to disorders not linked to AIDS, including peptic ulcer,[141] whereas in contrast, the most common cause of lower GI bleeding is CMV colitis.[142, 143]

CMV involvement of the GI tract causes bleeding by mucosal ulceration in involved tissue. In some patients, ischemia, infarction, or both, most commonly in the colon or distal small bowel, may present with bleeding. CMV ulcers of the esophagus and stomach can also cause frank bleeding. Hemorrhage from colonic infection may be due to either focal or diffuse inflammation, usually with well-defined ulcers. Like CMV, herpes simplex virus esophagitis may be complicated by bleeding but is less common than CMV, probably because mucosal disease is more superficial.

C. albicans infection has been reported to induce esophageal hemorrhage via direct fungal invasion, causing a severe erosive esophagitis, often occurring in the setting of a coagulopathy.

Enteric pathogens including *Campylobacter, Shigella, Salmonella, E. histolytica,* and *Chlamydia* may cause rectal bleeding. Other pathogens such as MAC, microsporidia, and cryptosporidia almost never cause bleeding, because mucosal infection does not typically result in ulceration.

Enteric Kaposi's sarcoma lesions may ulcerate and bleed spontaneously, although most enteric Kaposi's sarcoma lesions are asymptomatic.

Evaluation

The evaluation of GI bleeding in a patient with AIDS parallels the approach taken in otherwise healthy patients (see Chapter 13). In patients with upper GI bleeding and severe immunodeficiency, endoscopy is preferred over barium studies, given the likelihood of opportunistic diseases that generally require mucosal biopsy for diagnosis. Patients with one or more concurrent major illnesses have a poorer outcome from GI bleeding and may benefit from earlier endoscopy. Less invasive diagnostic methods, including stool examination and culture, are indicated if blood loss is not severe enough to require endoscopic examination and an infectious colitis is suspected.

Treatment

Appropriate initial management of severe GI bleeding due to AIDS-related diseases does not require a specific diagnosis. Treatment consists of blood product support, and, if necessary, surgery. Nonsurgical endoscopic means of hemostasis should be employed wherever possible. Selective embolization of bleeding sites can be used in cases of isolated small bowel hemorrhage. Specific therapies for the underlying disease necessarily depend on the results of mucosal biopsy and/or microbiologic studies.

HEPATOMEGALY AND JAUNDICE

Hepatomegaly, with or without *jaundice,* is a frequent finding in AIDS. Hepatomegaly may be detected on examination in most patients.[144] Hepatomegaly is usually associated with one or more liver chemistry test abnormalities, although significant jaundice due to parenchymal disease is uncommon.[145] As with other organ systems, the spectrum of hepatic infections in patients with HIV evolves as immunocompromise advances. Clinical manifestations of hepatobiliary disease can vary from no symptoms to liver failure.

Differential Diagnosis (Table 28–9)

Conditions associated with HIV infection or its treatment account for most cases of liver disease. No single feature or combination of findings are common to all patients with hepatic disease in AIDS.[146, 147] Hepatobiliary disease can be broadly classified into either hepatic parenchymal abnormalities, biliary abnormalities, or a combination of the two. Currently, parenchymal abnormalities are most often related to viral hepatitis and drug-induced disease; however, neoplasms, in particular non-Hodgkin's lymphoma, and OIs are not infrequent.

Drug-induced liver injury has emerged as the most prevalent cause of liver test abnormalities and is related to the increasing array of antiretroviral medications. Use of prescription or nonprescription drugs as well as herbal remedies should also be considered a cause of abnormal liver test results in the HIV-infected patient. Before HAART, drug hepatotoxicity was most commonly due to sulfonamides, and the increased frequency of adverse reactions to these medications is well recognized in AIDS. Recent studies have found protease inhibitors to be the most common causes of abnormal liver tests.[148, 149] Although idiosyncratic reactions are the most common mechanism for liver injury, exacerbation of underlying viral hepatitis due to immune reconstitution from HAART is responsible in some patients (see later). In contrast to hepatotoxicity from sulfonamides, where liver biopsy typically shows evidence of granulomas containing eosinophils,[150] the histologic findings of drug-induced injury from these newer antiretroviral agents has not been well

Table 28–9 | **Differential Diagnosis of Jaundice/Hepatomegaly in AIDS**

Hepatic Parenchymal Disease
Infection
Mycobacterium avium complex
Cytomegalovirus
Hepatitis C
Bacillary peliosis hepatis
Mycobacterium tuberculosis
Cryptococcus
Hepatitis B, D
Pneumocystis carinii
Microsporidium
Drug-induced, especially sulfa, zidovudine (AZT)
Neoplasm
Lymphoma
Kaposi's sarcoma
Biliary Disease
Cholangitis
Cytomegalovirus
Cryptosporidium
Microsporidium
Neoplasm
Lymphoma
Kaposi's sarcoma

AIDS, acquired immunodeficiency syndrome.

characterized. The liver test abnormalities usually follow a hepatocellular pattern; jaundice is uncommon but has been observed most frequently with indinavir.

A newly described syndrome characterized by marked hepatomegaly, steatosis, lactic acidosis, and liver failure has been increasingly recognized.[151, 152] The pathogenesis of the syndrome is due to impaired mitochondrial DNA synthesis usually from the nucleoside reverse transcriptase inhibitors such as zidovudine, ddI, and stavudine.[151, 152] An associated myopathy, peripheral neuropathy, and pancreatitis may occur as well. The liver tests typically show a hepatocellular pattern but can be normal. Hepatic steatosis is usually evident on imaging of the liver. Although reversal has occurred in some patients following drug withdrawal, most patients have worsening disease and death. Liver transplantation is curative.

MAC is consistently the most frequent specific hepatic finding in AIDS, documented in up to 46% of patients in late-stage HIV disease.[153] The pathologic hallmark of the infection is the presence of poorly formed granulomas containing acid-fast bacilli within foamy histiocytes. Organisms may be observed in the absence of granulomas and can be cultured from liver biopsy in the absence of infected histiocytes.

M. tuberculosis, in contrast to MAC, may occur before HIV-infected patients are profoundly immunocompromised. Extrapulmonary tuberculosis is common in patients with HIV infection, especially in patients with prior OIs and those whose risk behavior is injection drug use. Hepatic disease as part of miliary tuberculosis has been noted. Rarer manifestations include tuberculous abscesses and bile duct tuberculomas.[154] The diagnosis of hepatic tuberculosis is made by culture of the organism from liver tissue obtained by percutaneous or laparoscopic biopsy. PCR may allow earlier diagnosis. As with MAC, typical appearing mycobacteria can be seen by appropriate staining of biopsy specimens.

CMV is the most frequent infectious pathogen in AIDS, and the liver is involved in 5% to 25% of liver biopsies.[144] However, its discovery in the liver antemortem is extremely unusual. Typical viral inclusions are usually identified in Kupffer cells but can sometimes be seen in hepatocytes or sinusoidal endothelial cells[144] or in association with granulomas.[146] Mononuclear cell infiltration is a common finding. Monoclonal antibody staining or in situ hybridization can be used to confirm or identify the virus in liver.

Clinical manifestations and histologic features of *viral hepatitis* from HBV, HCV, or hepatitis D virus are altered in the presence of HIV coinfection but in remarkably different ways for each virus.

Clinical and autopsy studies in AIDS patients have reported up to a 90% seroprevalence of hepatitis B markers indicating past or present infection.[144, 155, 156] There have been no recent studies to evaluate for reductions in seroprevalence with the adoption of safer sex practices, particularly in homosexual men. Concurrent HIV and HBV infections lead to alterations of HBV antigen-antibody display, viral replication, and clinical consequences. Several reports have described reappearance of hepatitis B surface antigen (HBsAg) in HIV-infected patients previously thought to be immune to hepatitis B virus as indicated by the presence of anti-HBs.[157] Recurrence of HBsAg may arise from either reinfection or reactivation with advanced immunodeficiency.[157] In addition, there is an accelerated loss of naturally acquired anti-HBs even in those patients who remain HBsAg negative.[158] With loss or reduction in immunity to HBV, there is an increased prevalence of hepatitis B e antigen expression, elevated mean levels of DNA polymerase, and increased titers of anti–hepatitis B core antigen.[159, 160] Acquisition of the chronic carrier state is also much more likely in the HIV-infected patient, especially if infection occurs when immunodeficiency is more advanced. Thus, a larger proportion of patients with HIV and hepatitis B infections have a chronic carrier state, with highly infectious serum and body fluids, compared with those who are HIV negative.

Although HIV infection leads to more prevalent chronic HBV carriage, it appears to attenuate the severity of biochemical and histologic liver disease in most,[159, 160] but not all[161] patients. In one study, the mean alanine aminotransferase (ALT) level correlated with CD4 lymphocyte count.[162] The mechanism for reduced hepatitis B virus–related liver injury following HIV infection is not certain but has been attributed to a diminution in lymphocyte-mediated hepatocellular injury as a result of HIV effects on lymphocytes. In those patients without serologic evidence of past or present hepatitis B virus and HIV infection, vaccination appears to be ineffective, regardless of the stage of immunocompromise.[163] HBV has no independent effect on survival for patients with HIV.[164]

Conversely, the institution of HAART in a chronic carrier of hepatitis B virus can have catastrophic consequences. Patients may develop an acute flare of hepatitis that can be severe leading to fulminant hepatic failure. However, the proportion of coinfected patients who develop an acute hepatitis B flare following use of HAART is unknown. In a retrospective study of coinfected patients, acute hepatitis was not observed, whereas seroconversion occurred in 1 of the 24 patients.[165] It is believed that reconstitution of immune function with HAART leads to production of antibody that is directed to infected hepatocytes as in the normal host. Inclusion of lamivudine, which has potent antiviral effects on hepatitis B virus, in the HAART regimen may reduce the likelihood of acute hepatitis B. These observations suggest that all patients who are to receive HAART therapy should be screened for active or past HBV infection.

The consequences of HIV infection on delta hepatitis appear similar to those of HBV, although far fewer patients have been studied. HIV does not directly affect the prevalence of delta hepatitis in HIV, which ranges from 0% to 15% in the United States,[166] and delta infection is more closely correlated with geographic location, and sexual and drug use habits. In small series, however, HIV coinfection was associated with enhanced delta virus replication without increased liver disease,[167] and in a single patient, reactivation of delta hepatitis was ascribed to acute HIV infection.[168]

The prevalence of HCV in those with HIV infection depends on the risk group evaluated and the assay used. Prevalence is highest in injection drug users (52% to 89%) and hemophiliac patients with HIV,[169] whereas in military populations and non–drug users, the prevalence is much lower, ranging from 1% to 11%.[170] Assaying antibodies to hepatitis C virus alone, rather than hepatitis C virus RNA, may underestimate the true prevalence, because loss of antibody may occur with progression of immunodeficiency.[171]

Unlike hepatitis B virus, the clinical course of hepatitis C virus appears to worsen as HIV-related immunocompromise advances. This has been best documented in HIV-infected hemophiliac patients. Studies in large cohorts of hemophiliac patients have demonstrated dramatic increases in hepatitis C virus RNA levels with progressive HIV disease, associated with aspartate aminotransferase (AST) elevations and hepatomegaly.[166, 172, 173] Coinfected patients also have a higher rate of active cirrhosis on biopsy and an accelerated course to clinical cirrhosis and liver failure. The mechanism for this more rapid disease course is unknown but has been similarly recognized in other immunocompromised patients. Because patients with late-stage HIV often have multiple life-threatening infections, HCV alone is not an independent determinant of mortality.[170] However, as HIV-infected patients are living longer owing to HAART, hepatitis C virus–induced liver disease and its consequences (e.g., hepatocellular cancer) are assuming more clinical relevance. Like hepatitis B, hepatitis C virus does not cause progression of HIV disease.[174]

The effect of HAART on hepatitis C viral dynamics and liver injury is variable. Some studies have found attenuation of disease,[175] whereas others had documented exacerbations reflected by increases in serum transaminases.[176] Hepatitis C viral load has also been variably affected.

The role of interferon therapy for HIV/HCV coinfected patients remains unsettled. α-Interferon is less effective for treating hepatitis C virus liver disease in coinfected patients than in otherwise healthy individuals, particularly if the CD4 count is very low ($<200/mm^3$).[177] More recently, combination therapy of interferon and ribavirin has shown promise. In a study of 20 patients, combination therapy was effective in 50% of cases in clearing serum hepatitis C virus RNA.[178] As in the non–HIV-infected patient, hepatitis C virus genotype I was associated with a low response rate.

Fungal infections of the liver are not unusual when immunocompromise is advanced. *Histoplasmosis* of the liver may be seen in patients with disseminated fungal disease, predominantly but not exclusively in regions of high prevalence of the organism.[88] Biopsies of the liver may also show caseating granulomas containing fungal organisms. Culture of hepatic tissue, blood, or bone marrow can confirm the diagnosis, but several weeks may be required for the organism to grow in culture. Pulmonary disease is seen in most patients at diagnosis. *Cryptococcus* may infect the liver in the setting of disseminated infection.[144] Typically the organism is found in the sinusoids and is associated with a poor inflammatory response. Similarly, coccidioidomycosis can involve the liver as part of a systemic infection, especially in endemic regions.[179] The organisms appear as spherules within a fibrosing granulomata. *Candida* infection of the liver is rare, in contrast to its high prevalence in mucosal sites. Hepatic microabscesses or macroabscesses are most likely to occur if the patient is neutropenic, especially following chemotherapy for non-Hodgkin's lymphoma.

Kaposi's sarcoma, which is caused by infection with human herpesvirus 8 (HHV-8) has a predilection for periportal regions of the liver and is seen in 10% to 15% of liver biopsies.[144] Tumor nodules appear grossly as violaceous or hemorrhagic masses within hepatic parenchyma. Microscopically, the characteristic spindle cells and vascular slits of Kaposi's sarcoma usually directly abut normal-appearing liver tissue. Most often, evidence of hepatic Kaposi's sarcoma is found at postmortem or incidentally at liver biopsy but may occasionally cause aminotransferase elevations or jaundice.[180] The cell of origin of Kaposi's sarcoma is the lymphatic endothelial cell,[181] which may explain its extensive nature.

Hepatic involvement by *non-Hodgkin's lymphoma* may be the index manifestation of AIDS in homosexual men and may be the primary site of the neoplasm. The lesions are usually focal and may be large. In addition, Hodgkin's disease in the AIDS patient tends to be more aggressive histologically and clinically, spreading rapidly to extranodal sites, making liver involvement more likely. The prognosis is determined largely by the extent of underlying immunocompromise and Karnofsky performance score rather than the lymphoma itself.[182]

Isolated cases of *P. carinii* pneumonia (PCP) hepatitis have been described and are attributable to the use of inhaled pentamidine, which fails to protect extrapulmonic sites from PCP.[183] In addition to PCP, the liver may be the site of infection by the protozoa *Cryptosporidium, Microsporidium,* or *Dicrocoelium dentriticum* or by other multicellular organisms.

Bacillary peliosis hepatis, caused by either *Bartonella henselae* or *Bartonella quintana,*[184] is a systemic infection that may be associated with fever, skin lesions, abdominal pain, and lytic bone lesions.[185] Liver tests usually show a disproportionate elevation of the alkaline phosphatase. Liver biopsies demonstrate regions of a myxoid stroma in association with granular purple material, which with Warthin-Starry stain or electron microscopy reveals clumps of organisms.[184] Treatment with either erythromycin (orally, or in severe cases, intravenously), tetracycline, minocycline, or a cephalosporin are reportedly effective, although prolonged or lifelong therapy is necessary.

The significance of a number of the nonspecific findings in the liver are uncertain. In particular, granulomas in the absence of fungal or mycobacterial organisms are common, often prompting concern for tuberculosis.[185] Microvesicular and macrovesicular steatosis is one of the most common nonspecific findings, possibly owing to malnutrition, because the findings are similar to those seen in patients with kwashiorkor. Massive steatosis has also been observed from antiretroviral drug use (see earlier).

Biliary tract involvement in AIDS may result in marked liver test abnormalities and right upper quadrant symptoms; jaundice is unusual. A syndrome resembling sclerosing cholangitis with papillary stenosis is well recognized and has been termed *AIDS cholangiopathy* (Fig. 28–7). Patients characteristically develop significant upper abdominal pain in association with marked elevation of alkaline phosphatase, and minimal elevations of bilirubin, AST, and ALT. Rarely, the liver tests are normal. Currently, biliary tract disease is as frequent from non–HIV-related diseases (e.g., common bile duct stones) as those linked to AIDS.

Ductular changes may consist of either papillary stenosis alone, sclerosing cholangitis–like lesions alone, a combination of the two, or long extrahepatic strictures. Most series have found papillary stenosis with intrahepatic disease as the most common findings. Ultrasonography or CT detects ductular abnormalities in 77% of those with cholangiographically proven disease, implying that a negative imaging study does not definitively exclude the diagnosis.[186] The etiology in most cases is infectious because *Cryptosporidium,* CMV, or *Microsporidium* may be found in bile, duodenal, or bili-

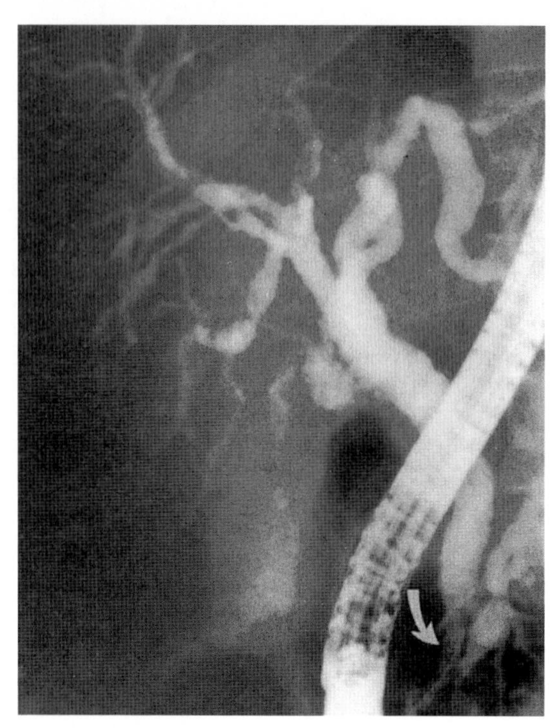

Figure 28–7. ERCP in AIDS cholangiopathy. Papillary stenosis was present (*arrow*).

ary epithelium.[187–189] For patients with predominantly papillary stenosis, sphincterotomy results in a symptomatic improvement in most patients[189]; alkaline phosphatase may continue to rise, however, probably reflecting progression of associated intrahepatic disease.[190] AIDS cholangiopathy is not associated with a shortened survival.[189]

Other less common causes of biliary tract disease in AIDS include primary bile duct lymphoma, epithelial angiomatosis, lymphomatous nodal obstruction, Kaposi's sarcoma, and biloma. In addition, chronic pancreatitis or choledocholithiasis may lead to biliary obstruction, although their incidence is not clearly increased in HIV infection.

Acalculous cholecystitis has also been described in AIDS patients,[191] presenting as severe abdominal pain and, occasionally, peritonitis. This syndrome is usually caused by a specific infection, most frequently CMV.[191] Cholecystitis has also been reported from microsporidia, cryptosporidia, and *I. belli*.

Evaluation

The initial decision in evaluating the AIDS patient with jaundice, hepatomegaly, or both, is to determine whether the findings are due to intrahepatic or extrahepatic disease. Simultaneous disease in both sites must also be considered. A history of mild jaundice, often in association with fever and constitutional symptoms, is more consistent with intrahepatic disease, whereas symptoms of deep jaundice associated with pain of relatively acute onset suggest extrahepatic disease. Careful review of medications, both prescription and nonprescription, is essential.

Because the clinical history and the finding of symptomatic hepatomegaly are nonspecific, further evaluation is always necessary. Elevations of ALT or AST or both, are common, but neither the pattern nor the extent of elevation of these tests appears to correlate with specific findings in the liver.[186] Nevertheless, some generalization can be made. Significant elevation of the transaminases favors a drug-induced or viral cause. In contrast, marked elevation of alkaline phosphatase correlates statistically with the presence of MAC infection in the liver in AIDS when extrahepatic obstruction is absent.[188] CT scan and ultrasonography should be employed early because they are especially useful in identifying ductal dilation, gallbladder pathology, and focal hepatic lesions. There may be a role for MR cholangiography in selected cases, but this has not yet been adequately explored in AIDS.

The indications for liver biopsy for the patient in whom intrahepatic disease is suspected are not well defined. Biopsy is appropriate when symptomatic, treatable disease of the liver is suspected and when a specific diagnosis of hepatic disease is needed. Although a specific diagnosis is likely in most patients, the impact on patient management is difficult to measure. Biopsy findings are abnormal in 90% to 100% of patients with AIDS[147, 186] and yield diagnostic information in up to 64%[147]; however, in one retrospective review, liver biopsy identified a previously undiagnosed infection or neoplasm in only 2 of 26 patients, suggesting that the liver is rarely the site of disease not manifest elsewhere.[186] This observation underscores the importance of reserving liver biopsy for those circumstances where less invasive diagnostic methods such as blood cultures and bone marrow biopsy have not yielded a diagnosis. Focal lesions identified by abdominal imaging can be sampled under ultrasonography or CT guidance. Specific infections or neoplasms are usually evident on tissue sections of appropriately stained biopsy material. *MAC* is almost always present within hepatic granulomas, although it may occasionally be detectable only after culture of biopsy material for acid-fast bacilli or seen by routine staining techniques. *Cryptococcus* and *Histoplasma* are also associated with granulomas.[88] CMV nuclear inclusions can be localized within Kupffer cells or hepatocytes.[88] *Kaposi's sarcoma* and *lymphomas* are easily identified by their homogeneous neoplastic appearance. When lymphoma is suspected, material should be fixed in paraformaldehyde to allow for thin plastic sections to define the histologic type. Drug-induced hepatitis may be recognized on occasion by the presence of eosinophils within granulomas.[150]

An extrahepatic cause for jaundice is suggested on CT or ultrasonography by the presence of dilated ducts or other biliary and/or pancreatic abnormalities. Once extrahepatic obstruction is recognized, the possibility of papillary stenosis associated with AIDS cholangiopathy must be considered as well as the possibility of choledocholithiasis or other disorders, depending on the imaging studies. Further evaluation, when indicated, may include endoscopic retrograde cholangiopancreatography (ERCP) if CT or ultrasonography demonstrates extrahepatic biliary ductal dilation. Ampullary and duodenal biopsy specimens or bile and/or biliary cytology (with appropriate staining) collected during ERCP can be examined for the presence of viruses, protozoa, or neoplastic cells.

Management

Therapy of intrahepatic disease is dictated either by the history (i.e., use of potentially hepatotoxic drugs, especially sulfonamides) or the findings on skinny needle aspirate, liver biopsy, or nonliver studies that suggest that the liver disease is part of a systemic process. Thus, treatment often includes antimicrobials or chemotherapy for a specific infection or neoplasm, respectively.

Biliary obstruction may respond to endoscopic sphincterotomy if papillary stenosis or tumor is present at the ampulla of Vater or bile duct stones are identified. Neoplastic extrahepatic obstruction not amenable to papillotomy can usually be treated by endoscopic stent placement. Surgery is indicated for patients with clinical evidence of cholecystitis, preferably with a laparoscopic approach.[192]

REFERENCES

1. Lederman MM, Valdez H: Immune restoration with antiretroviral therapies. JAMA 284:223, 2000.
2. Mocroft A, Katlama C, Johnsom AM, et al: AIDS across Europe, 1994–98: The EuroSIDA Study. Lancet 356:291, 2000.
3. Kaplan JE, Hanson D, Dworkin MS, et al: Epidemiology of human immunodeficiency virus–associated opportunistic infections in the United States in the era of highly active antiretroviral therapy. Clin Infect Dis 30:S5, 2000.
4. Kauffmann GR, Bloch M, Zaunders JJ, et al: Long-term immunological response in HIV-1-infected subjects receiving potent antiretroviral therapy. AIDS 14:959, 2000.
5. Kovacs JA, Masur H: Prophylaxis against opportunistic infections in patients with human immunodeficiency virus infection. N Engl J Med 342:1416, 2000.
6. Currier JS, Williams, PL, Koletar SL, et al: Discontinuation of *Mycobacterium avium* complex prophylaxis in patients with antiretroviral therapy–induced increased in CD4 cell count. Ann Intern Med 133: 493, 2000.
7. Monkemuller KE, Call SA, Lazenby AJ, et al: Declining prevalence of opportunistic gastrointestinal disease in the era of combination antiretroviral therapy. Am J Gastroenterol 95:547, 2000.
8. Carr A, Marriott D, Field A, et al: Treatment of HIV-1 associated microsporidiosis and cryptosporidiosis with combination antiretroviral therapy. Lancet 351:228, 1998.
9. Bonfanti P, Valsecchi L, Parazzini F, et al: Incidence of adverse reactions in HIV patients treated with protease inhibitors: A cohort study. J Acquir Immune Defic Syndr Hum Retrovirol 23:236, 2000.
10. Call SA, Heudebert G, Saag M, et al: The changing etiology of chronic diarrhea in HIV-infected patients wth CD4 cell counts less than 200 cells/mm^3. Am J Gastroenterol 95:3142, 2000.
11. Blanshard C, Francis N, Gazzard BG: Investigation of chronic diarrhea in acquired immunodeficiency syndrome: A prospective study of 155 patients. Gut 39:824, 1996.
12. Weber R, Ledergerber B, Zbinden R, et al: Enteric infections and diarrhea in human immunodeficiency virus–infected persons: Prospective community-based cohort study. Arch Intern Med 159:1473, 1999.
13. DuPont HL, Chappell CL, Sterling CR, et al: The infectivity of *Cryptosporidium parvum* in healthy volunteers. N Engl J Med 332:855, 1995.
14. Navin TR, Weber R, Vugia DJ, et al: Declining CD4 T-lymphocyte counts are associated with increased risk of enteric parasitosis and chronic diarrhea: Results on a 3-year longitudinal study. J Acquir Immune Defic Syndr Hum Retrovirol 20:154, 1999.
15. Pozio E, Rezza G, Boschini A, et al: Clinical cryptosporidiosis and human immunodeficiency virus (HIV)-induced immunosuppression: Findings from a longitudinal study of HIV-positive and HIV-negative former injection drug users. J Infect Dis 176:969, 1997.
16. Manabe YC, Clark DP, Moore RD, et al: Cryptosporidiosis in patients with AIDS: Correlates of disease and survival. Clin Infect Dis 27:536, 1998.
17. Goodgame RW, Kimball K, Ou CN, et al: Intestinal function and injury in acquired immunodeficiency syndrome–related cryptosporidiosis. Gastroenterology 108:1075, 1995.
18. Weber R, Bryan RT, Bishop HS, et al: Threshold of detection of *Cryptosporidium* oocysts in human stool specimens: Evidence for low sensitivity of current diagnostic methods. J Clin Microbiol 29:1323, 1991.
19. Greenberg PD, Koch J, Cello JP: Diagnosis of *Cryptosporidium parvum* in patients with severe diarrhea and AIDS. Dig Dis Sci 41:2286, 1996.
20. White AC, Chappell CL, Hayat CS, et al: Paromomycin for cryptosporidiosis in AIDS: A prospective, double-blind trial. J Infect Dis 170:419, 1994.
21. Simon DM, Cello JP, Valenzuela J, et al: Multicenter trial of octreotide in patients with refractory acquired immunodeficiency syndrome–associated diarrhea. Gastroenterology 108:1753, 1995.
22. Curry A, Smith HV: Emerging pathogens: *Isospora,* cyclospora, and microsporidia. Parasitology 117:S143, 1998.
23. Verdier RI, Fitzgerald DW, Johnson WD, et al: Trimethoprim-sulfamethoxazole compared with ciprofloxacin for treatment and prophylaxis of *Isospora belli* and *Cyclospora cayetanensis* infection in HIV-infected patients. Ann Intern Med 132:885, 2000.
24. Pape JW, Verdier R-I, Johnson WD, et al: Treatment and prophylaxis of *Isospora belli* infection in patients with the acquired immunodeficiency syndrome. N Engl J Med 320:1044, 1989.
25. Kotler DP, Orenstein JM: Prevalence of intestinal microsporidiosis in HIV-infected individuals referred for gastroenterological evaluation. Am J Gastroenterol 89:1998, 1994.
26. Wanachiwanawin D, Manatsathit S, Lertlaituan P, et al: Intestinal microsporidiosis in HIV-infected patients with chronic diarrhea in Thailand. Southeast Asian J Trop Med Public Health 29:767, 1998.
27. Gumbo T, Sarbah S, Gangaidzo IT, et al: Intestinal parasites in patients with diarrhea and human immunodeficiency virus infection in Zimbabwe. AIDS 13:819, 1999.
28. Rabeneck L, Genta RM, Gyorkey F, et al: Observations on the pathological spectrum and clinical course of microsporidiosis in men infected with the human immunodeficiency virus: Follow-up study. Clin Infect Dis 20:1229, 1995.
29. Goodgame R, Stager C, Marcantel B, et al: Intensity of infection in AIDS-related intestinal microsporidiosis. J Infect Dis 180:661, 1985.
30. Dascomb K, Frazer T, Clark RA, et al: Microsporidiosis and HIV. J Acquir Immune Defic Syndr Hum Retrovirol 24:290, 2000.
31. Kotler DP, Giang TT, Garro ML, et al: Light microscopic diagnosis of microsporidiosis in patients with AIDS. Am J Gastroenterol 89:540, 1994.
32. Weber R, Bryan RT, Owen RL, et al: Improved light-microscopical detection of microsporidia spores in stool and duodenal aspirates. N Engl J Med 326:161, 1992.
33. Carville A, Mansfield K, Widmer G, et al: Development and application of genetic probes for detection of *Enterocytozoon bieneusi* in formalin-fixed stools and in intestinal biopsy specimens from infected patients. Clin Diagn Lab Immunol 4:405, 1997.
34. Dore GJ, Marriott DJ, Hing MC, et al: Disseminated microsporidiosis due to *Septata intestinalis* in nine patients infected with the human immunodeficiency virus: Response to therapy with albendazole. Clin Infect Dis 21:70, 1995.
35. Jessurun J, Barron-Rodriguez LP, Fernandez-Tinoco G, et al: The prevalence of invasive amebiasis is not increased in patients with AIDS. AIDS 6:307, 1992.
36. Hung CC, Chen PJ, Hsieh SM, et al: Invasive ameobiasis: An emerging parasitic disease in patients infected with HIV in an area endemic for amoebic infection. AIDS 13:2421, 1999.
37. Wei SC, Hung CC, Chen MY, et al: Endoscopy in acquired immunodeficiency syndrome patients with diarrhea and negative stool studies. Gastrointest Endosc 51:427, 2000.
38. Bhargava A, San P, Swaminathan A, et al: *Entamoeba histolytica-Entamoeba dispar* infections in human immunodeficiency virus–infected patients in the United States. Clin Infect Dis 30:955, 2000.
39. Monkemuller KE, Wilcox CM: Diagnosis and treatment of colonic disease in AIDS. Gastointest Endosc Clin North Am 8:889, 1998.
40. Cimerman S, Cimerman B, Lewi DS: Prevalence of intestinal parasitic infections in patients with acquired immunodeficiency syndrome in Brazil. Int J Infect Dis 3:203, 1999.
41. Wilcox CM, Schwartz DA, Cotsonis GA, et al: Evaluation of chronic unexplained diarrhea in human immunodeficiency virus infection: Determination of the best diagnostic approach. Gastroenterology 110:30, 1996.
42. Kearney DJ, Steuerwald M, Koch J, et al: A prospective study of endoscopy in HIV-associated diarrhea. Am J Gastroenterol 94:596, 1999.
43. Wilcox CM, Chalasani N, Lazenby A, et al: Cytomegalovirus colitis in AIDS: An endoscopic and clinical study. Gastrointest Endosc 48: 58, 1998.
44. Smith PD, Saini SS, Raffeld M, et al: Cytomegalovirus induction of

tumor necrosis factor-α by human monocytes and mucosal macrophages. J Clin Invest 90:1642, 1992.
45. Dieterich DT, Rahmin M: Cytomegalovirus colitis in AIDS: Presentation in 44 patients and a review of the literature. J Acquir Immune Defic Syndr Hum Retrovirol 4:S29, 1991.
46. Goodgame RW: Gastrointestinal cytomegalovirus disease. Ann Intern Med 119:924, 1993.
47. Monkemuller KE, Bussian AH, Lazenby AJ, et al: Special histologic stains are rarely beneficial for the evaluation of HIV-related gastrointestinal infections. Am J Clin Pathol 114:387, 2000.
48. Beaugerie L, Cywiner-Golenzer C, Monfort L, et al: Definition and diagnosis of cytomegalovirus colitis in patients infected by human immunodeficiency virus. J Acquir Immune Defic Syndr Hum Retrovirol 14:423, 1997.
49. Markham A, Faulds D: Ganciclovir: An update of its therapeutic use in cytomegalovirus infection. Drugs 3:455, 1994.
50. Drew WL, Ives D, Lalezari JP, et al: Oral ganciclovir as maintenance treatment for cytomegalovirus retinitis. N Engl J Med 333:615, 1995.
51. Wagstaff AJ, Bryson HM: Foscarnet: A reappraisal of its antiviral activity, pharmacokinetic properties, and therapeutic use in immunocompromised patients with viral infections. Drugs 48:199, 1994.
52. Blanshard C, Benhamou Y, Dohin E, et al: Treatment of AIDS-associated gastrointestinal cytomegalovirus infection with foscarnet and ganciclovir: A randomized comparison. J Infect Dis 172:622, 1995.
53. Dieterich DT, Poles MA, Dicker M, et al: Foscarnet treatment of cytomegalovirus gastrointestinal infections in acquired immunodeficiency syndrome patients who have failed ganciclovir induction. Am J Gastroenterol 88:542, 1993.
54. Plosker GL, Noble S: Cidofovir: A review of its use in cytomegalovirus retinitis in patients with AIDS. Drugs 58:325, 1999.
55. Macdonald JC, Torriani FJ, Morse LS, et al: Lack of reactivation of cytomegalovirus (CMV) retinitis after stopping CMV maintenance therapy in AIDS patients with sustained elevations in CD4 T cells in response to highly active antiretroviral therapy. J Infect Dis 177:1182, 1998.
56. Bini EJ, Gorelick SM, Weinshel EH: Outcome of AIDS-associated cytomegalovirus colitis in the era of potent antiretroviral therapy. J Clin Gastroenterol 30:414, 2000.
57. Salmon-Ceron D, Mazeron MC, Chaput S, et al: Plasma cytomegalovirus DNA, pp65 antigenaemia, and a low CD4 cell count remain risk factors for cytomegalovirus disease in patients receiving highly active antiretroviral therapy. AIDS 14:1041, 2000.
58. Gonzalez GG, Pujol FH, Liprandi F, et al: Prevalence of enteric viruses in human immunodeficiency virus seropositive patients in Venezuela. J Med Virol 55:288, 1998.
59. Grohmann GS, Glass RI, Pereira GH, et al: Enteric viruses and diarrhea in HIV-infected patients. N Engl J Med 329:14, 1993.
60. Khoo SH, Bailey AS, deJong JC, et al: Adenovirus infections in human immunodeficiency virus–positive patients: Clinical features and molecular epidemiology. J Infect Dis 172:629, 1995.
61. Ullrich R, Zeitz M, Heise W, et al: Small intestinal structure and function in patients infected with human immunodeficiency virus (HIV): Evidence for HIV-induced enteropathy. Ann Intern Med 111: 15, 1989.
62. Fox CH, Kotler D, Tierney A, et al: Detection of HIV-1 RNA in the lamina propria of patients with AIDS and gastrointestinal disease. J Infect Dis 159:467, 1989.
63. Moyer MP, Gendelman HE: HIV replication and persistence in human gastrointestinal cells cultured in vitro. J Leukoc Biol 49:93, 1991.
64. Amerongen HM, Weltzin R, Farnet CM, et al: Transepithelial transport of HIV-1 by intestinal M cells: A mechanism for transmission of AIDS. J Acquir Immune Defic Syndr Hum Retrovirol 4:760, 1991.
65. Zeitz M, Ullrich R, Schneider T, et al: Cell differentiation and proliferation in the gastrointestinal tract with respect to the local immune system. Ann N Y Acad Sci 733:75, 1994.
66. Keating J, Bjarnason I, Somasundaram S, et al: Intestinal absorptive capacity, intestinal permeability, and jejunal histology in HIV and their relation to diarrhoea. Gut 37:623, 1995.
67. Batman PA, Kapembwa MS, Miller ARO, et al: HIV enteropathy: Comparative morphometry of the jejunal mucosa of HIV-infected patients resident in the United Kingdom and Uganda. Gut 43:350, 1998.
68. Rodgers VD, Fassett R, Kagnoff MF, et al: Abnormalities in intestinal mucosal T cells in homosexual populations including those with the lymphadenopathy syndrome and acquired immunodeficiency syndrome. Gastroenterology 90:552, 1986.
69. Schneider T, Ullrich R, Bergs C, et al: Abnormalities in subset distribution, activation, and differentiation of T cells isolated from large intestine biopsies in HIV infection. Clin Exp Immunol 95:430, 1994.
70. Janoff EN, Jackson S, Wahl SM, et al: Intestinal mucosal immunoglobulins during human immunodeficiency virus type I infection. J Infect Dis 170:299, 1994.
71. Griffin GE, Miller A, Batman P, et al: Damage to jejunal intrinsic autonomic nerves in HIV infection. AIDS 2:379, 1988.
72. Victorino R, MM Lucan, M Neto, et al: HIV infection and intestinal pseudo-obstruction. AIDS 4:599, 1990.
73. Foudraine NA, Weverling GJ, van Gool T, et al: Improvement of chronic diarrhea in patients with advanced HIV-1 infection during potent antiretroviral therapy. AIDS 12:35, 1998.
74. Bini EJ, Cohen J: Impact of protease inhibitors on the outcome of human immunodeficiency virus–infected patients with chronic diarrhea. Am J Gastroenterol 94:3553, 1999.
75. Molina JM, Casin I, Hausfater P, et al: *Campylobacter* infections in HIV-infected patients: Clinical and bacteriological features. AIDS 9: 881, 1995.
76. Perlman DM, Ampel NM, Schifman RB, et al: Persistent *Campylobacter jejuni* infections in patients infected with human immunodeficiency virus (HIV). Ann Intern Med 108:540, 1998.
77. Jacobson MA, Hahn S, M Gerberding, et al: Ciprofloxacin for *Salmonella* bacteremia in the acquired immunodeficiency syndrome (AIDS). Ann Intern Med 110:1027, 1989.
78. Lu SS, Schwartz JM, Simon DM, et al: *Clostridium difficile*–associated diarrhea in patients with HIV positivity and AIDS: A prospective controlled study. Am J Gastroenterol 89:1226, 1994.
79. Wilcox CM, Waites KB, Smith PD: No relationship between gastric pH, small bowel bacterial colonisation, and diarrhea in HIV-1 infected patients. Gut 44:1201, 1999.
80. Belitsos PC, Greenson JK, Yardley JH, et al: Association of gastric hypoacidity with opportunistic enteric infections in patients with AIDS. J Infect Dis 166:277, 1992.
81. Antony MA, Brandt LJ, Klein RS, et al: Infectious diarrhea in patients with AIDS. Dig Dis Sci 33:1141, 1988.
82. Poorman JC, Katon RM: Small bowel involvement by *Mycobacterium avium* complex in a patient with AIDS: Endoscopic, histologic, and radiographic similarities to Whipple's disease. Gastrointest Endosc 40: 753, 1994.
83. Chaisson RE, Benson CA, Dube MP, et al: Clarithromycin therapy for bacteremic *Mycobacterium avium* complex disease. Ann Intern Med 121:905, 1994.
84. Furrer J, Telenti AM, Rossi M, et al: Discontinuing or withholding primary prophylaxis against *Mycobacterium avium* in patients on successful antiretroviral combination therapy. The Swiss HIV Cohort Study. AIDS 14:1409, 2000.
85. Wood BJ, Kumar PN, Cooper C, et al: AIDS-associated intussusception in young adults. J Clin Gastroenterol 21:158, 1995.
86. Lanjewaar DN, Anand BS, Genta G, et al: Major differences in the spectrum of gastrointestinal infection associated with AIDS in India versus the west: An autopsy study. Clin Infect Dis 23:482, 1996.
87. Balthazar EJ, Megibow AJ, Barry M, et al: Histoplasmosis of the colon in patients with AIDS: Imaging findings in four cases. AJR Am J Roentgenol 161:585, 1993.
88. Wheat LJ, Connolly-Stringfield PA, Baker RL, et al: Disseminated histoplasmosis in the acquired immune deficiency syndrome: Clinical findings, diagnosis, and treatment, and review of the literature. Medicine 69:361, 1990.
89. Chalasani LN, Wilcox CM, Hunter HT, Schwartz DA: Endoscopic features of gastrointestinal cryptococcosis in AIDS. Gastrointest Endosc 45:315, 1997.
90. Markowitz M, Conant M, Hurley A: A preliminary evaluation of nelfinavir mesylate, an inhibitor of human immunodeficiency virus (HIV)-1 protease, to treat HIV infection. J Infect Dis 177:1533, 1998.
91. Wilcox CM, Rabeneck L, Friedman S: AGA Technical review: Malnutrition and cachexia, chronic diarrhea, and hepatobiliary disease in patients with human immunodeficiency virus infection. Gastroenterology 111:1724, 1996.
92. Bini EJ, Weinshel EH, Gamagaris Z: Comparison of duodenal with jejunal biopsy and aspirate in chronic human immunodeficiency virus–related diarrhea. Am J Gastroenterol 93:1837, 1998.
93. Wanke CA, Gerrior J, Blais V, et al: Successful treatment of diarrheal disease associated with enteroaggregative *Escherichia coli* in adults infected with human immunodeficiency virus. J Infect Dis 178:1369, 1998.

94. Wilcox CM, Monkemuller KE: Diagnosis and management of esophageal disease in the acquired immunodeficiency syndrome. South Med J 91:1002, 1998.
95. Connolly GM, Hawkins D, Harcourt-Webster JN, et al: Oesophageal symptoms, their causes, treatment, and prognosis in patients with the acquired immunodeficiency syndrome. Gut 30:1033, 1989.
96. Bonacini M, Young T, Laine L: The causes of esophageal symptoms in human immunodeficiency virus infection: A prospective study of 110 patients. Arch Intern Med 151:1567, 1991.
97. Wilcox CM: Evaluation of a technique to evaluate the underlying mucosa in patients with AIDS and severe *Candida* esophagitis. Gastrointest Endosc 42:360, 1995.
98. Pena M, Martinez-Lopez MA, Arnalich F, et al: Esophageal candidiasis associated with acute infection due to human immunodeficiency virus: Case report and review. Rev Infect Dis 13:872, 1991.
99. Wilcox CM, Straub RF, Clark WS: Prospective evaluation of oropharyngeal findings in human immunodeficiency virus–infected patients with esophageal ulceration. Am J Gastroenterol 90:1938, 1995.
100. Wilcox CM, Schwartz DA: Endoscopic-pathologic correlates of *Candida* esophagitis in acquired immunodeficiency syndrome. Dig Dis Sci 41:1337, 1996.
101. Wilcox CM, Schwartz DA, Clark WS: Esophageal ulceration in human immunodeficiency virus infection: Etiology, response to therapy, and long-term outcome. Ann Intern Med 123:143, 1995.
102. Wilcox CM, Straub RF, Schwartz DA: Prospective endoscopic characterization of cytomegalovirus esophageal ulceration in patients with AIDS. Gastrointest Endosc 40:481, 1994.
103. Wilcox CM, Schwartz DA: Endoscopic characterization of idiopathic esophageal ulceration associated with human immunodeficiency virus infection. J Clin Gastroenterol 16:251, 1993.
104. Smith PD, Eisner MS, Manischewitz JF, et al: Esophageal disease in AIDS is associated with pathologic processes rather than mucosal human immunodeficiency virus type 1. J Infect Dis 167:547, 1993.
105. Wilcox CM, Zaki SR, Coffield LM, et al: Evaluation of idiopathic esophageal ulcer for human immunodeficiency virus. Mod Pathol 8: 568, 1995.
106. Rabeneck L, Boyko WJ, McLean DM, et al: Unusual esophageal ulcers containing enveloped virus-like particles in homosexual men. Gastroenterology 90:1882, 1986.
107. Schacker T, Collier AC, Hughes J, et al: Clinical and epidemiologic features of primary HIV infection. Ann Intern Med 125:257, 1996.
108. Baehr PH, McDonald GB: Esophageal infections: Risk factors, presentation, diagnosis, and treatment. Gastroenterology 106:509, 1994.
109. Chalasani N, Parker K, Wilcox CM: Barrett's adenocarcinoma in a patient with acquired immunodeficiency syndrome. J Clin Gastroenterol 24:184, 1997.
110. Kikendall JW: Pill esophagitis. J Clin Gastroenterol 28:298, 1999.
111. Connolly GM, Forbes A, Gleeson JA, et al: Investigation of upper gastrointestinal symptoms in patients with AIDS. AIDS 3:453, 1989.
112. Wilcox CM, Alexander LN, Clark WS, et al: Fluconazole compared with endoscopy for human immunodeficiency virus–infected patients with esophageal symptoms. Gastroenterology 110:1803, 1996.
113. Wilcox CM, Darouiche RO, Laine L, et al: A randomized double-blind comparison of itraconazole oral solution and fluconazole tablets in the treatment of *Candida* esophagitis. J Infect Dis 176:227, 1997.
114. Barbaro G, Barbarini G, Calderon W, et al: Fluconazole versus intraconazole for *Candida* esophagitis in acquired immunodeficiency syndrome. Gastroenterology 111:1169, 1996.
115. Laine L, Dretler RH, Conteas CN, et al: Fluconazole compared with ketoconazole for the treatment of *Candida* esophagitis in AIDS: A randomized trial. Ann Intern Med 117:655, 1992.
116. Blum RA, D'Andrea DT, Florentin BM, et al: Increased gastric pH and the bioavailability of fluconazole and ketoconazole. Ann Intern Med 114:755, 1991.
117. Lim SG, Sawyer AM, Hudson M, et al: The absorption of fluconazole and itraconazole under conditions of low intragastric acidity. Aliment Pharmacol Ther 7:317, 1993.
118. Wilcox CM, Straub RF, Alexander LN, et al: Etiology of esophageal disease in human immunodeficiency virus–infected patients who fail antifungal therapy. Am J Med 101:599, 1996.
119. Fichtenbaum CJ, Koletar S, Yiannoutsos C, et al: Refractory mucosal candidiasis in advanced human immunodeficiency virus infection. Clin Infect Dis 30:749, 2000.
120. Arribas JR, Hernandez-Albujar S, Gonzalez-Garcia JJ, et al: Impact of protease inhibitor therapy on HIV-related orpharyngeal candidiasis. AIDS 14:979, 2000.
121. Wilcox CM, Straub RF, Schwartz DA: Cytomegalovirus esophagitis in AIDS: A prospective evaluation of response to ganciclovir therapy, relapse rate, and long-term outcome. Am J Med 98:169, 1995.
122. Wilcox CM, Schwartz DA: Comparison of two corticosteroid regimens for the treatment of HIV-associated idiopathic esophageal ulcer. Am J Gastroenterol 89:2163, 1994.
123. Alexander LN, Wilcox CM: A prospective trial of thalidomide for the treatment of HIV-associated idiopathic esophageal ulcers. AIDS Res Hum Retrovirus 13:301, 1997.
124. Bini EJ, Micale PL, Wenshel EH: Natural history of HIV-associated esophageal disease in the era of protease inhibitor therapy. Dig Dis Sci 45:1301, 2000.
125. Parente F, Cernuschi M, Antinori S, et al: Severe abdominal pain in patients with AIDS: Frequency, clinical aspects, causes and outcome. Scand J Gastroenterol 29:511, 1994.
126. O'Keefe EA, Wood R, Van Zyl A, et al: Human immunodeficiency virus–related abdominal pain in South Africa: Aetiology, diagnosis, and survival. Scand J Gastroenterol 33:212, 1998.
127. Cappell MS, Shetty V: A multicenter, case-controlled study of the clinical presentation and etiology of ascites and of the safety and clinical efficacy of diagnostic abdominal paracentesis in HIV seropositive patients. Am J Gastroenterol 89:2172, 1994.
128. Wilcox CM, Forsmark CE, Darragh J, et al: High-protein ascites in patients with acquired immunodeficiency syndrome. Gastroenterology 100:745, 1991.
129. Cappell MS, Marks M: Acute pancreatitis in HIV-seropositive patients: A case control study of 44 patients. Am J Med 3:243, 1995.
130. Dutta SK, Ting CD, Lai LL: Study of prevalence, severity, and etiological factors associated with acute pancreatitis in patients infected with human immunodeficiency virus. Am J Gastroenterol 92:2044, 1997.
131. Manocha AP, Sossenheimer M, Martin SP, et al: Prevalence and predictors of severe acute pancreatitis in patients with acquired immune deficiency syndrome. Am J Gastroenterol 94:784, 1999.
132. Foo Y, Konecny P: Hyperamylasemia in asymptomatic HIV patients. Ann Clin Biochem 34:259, 1997.
133. Schindzielorz A, Pike A, Daniels M, et al: Rates and risk factors for adverse events associated with didanosine in the expanded access program. Clin Infect Dis 19:1076, 1994.
134. Chehter EZ, Longo MA, Laudanna AA, et al: Involvement of the pancreas in AIDS: A prospective study of 109 post mortems. AIDS 14:1879, 2000.
135. Wilcox CM, Forsmark CE, Grendell JH, et al: Cytomegalovirus-associated acute pancreatic disease in patients with acquired immunodeficiency syndrome. Gastroenterology 99:263, 1990.
136. Albaran RG, Webber J, Steffes CP: CD4 cell counts as a prognostic factor of major abdominal surgery in patients infected with the human immunodeficiency virus. Arch Surg 133:626, 1998.
137. Emparan C, Iturburu IM, Ortiz J, et al: Infective complications after abdominal surgery in patients infected with human immunodeficiency virus: Role of CD4+ lymphocytes in prognosis. World J Surg 22:778, 1998.
138. Critchlow CW, Surawicz CM, Holmes KK, et al: Prospective study of high-grade anal squamous intraepithelial neoplasia in a cohort of homosexual men: Influence of HIV infection, immunosuppression and human papillomavirus infection. AIDS 9:1255, 1995.
139. Lord RV: Anorectal surgery in patients infected with human immunodeficiency virus: Factors associated with delayed wound healing. Ann Surg 226:92, 1997.
140. Parente F, Cernuschi M, Valsecchi L, et al: Acute upper gastrointestinal bleeding in patients with AIDS: A relatively uncommon condition associated with reduced survival. Gut 32:987, 1990.
141. Bini EJ, Micale PL, Weinshel EH: Risk factors for rebleeding and mortality from acute upper gastointestinal hemorrhage in human immunodeficiency virus infection. Am J Gastroenterol 94:358, 1999.
142. Chalasani N, Wilcox CM: Etiology and outcome of lower gastrointestinal bleeding in patients with AIDS. Am J Gastroenterol 93:175, 1998.
143. Bini EJ, Weinshel EH, Falkenstein DB: Risk factors for recurrent bleeding and mortality in human immunodeficiency virus–infected patients with acute lower GI hemorrhage. Gastointest Endosc 49:748, 1999.
144. Glasgow BJ, Anders K, Layfield LJ: Clinical and pathologic findings of the liver in the acquired immunodeficiency syndrome (AIDS). Am J Clin Pathol 83:582, 1985.

145. Chalasani N, Wilcox CM: Etiology, evaluation, and outcome of jaundice in patients with acquired immunodeficiency syndrome. Hepatology 110:30, 1996.
146. Wilkins MJ, Lindley R, Dourakis SP, et al: Surgical pathology of the liver in HIV infection. Histopathology 18:459, 1991.
147. Dieterich DT, Poles MA, Schwart ED, et al: Liver biopsy findings in 501 patients infected with HIV. J AIDS 11:170, 1996.
148. Saves M, Vandentorren S, Daucourt V, et al: Severe hepatic cytolysis: Incidence and risk factors in patients treated by antiretroviral combinations Aquitaine Cohort, France, 1996–1998. AIDS 13:F115, 1999.
149. Sulkowski MS, Thomas DL, Chaisson RE, et al: Hepatotoxicity associated with antiretroviral therapy in adults infected with human immunodeficiency virus and the role of hepatitis C and B virus infection. JAMA 283:74, 2000.
150. Lebovics E, Thung SN, Schaffner F, et al: The liver in the acquired immunodeficiency syndrome: A clinical and histologic study. Hepatology 5:293, 1985.
151. Miller KD, Cameron M, Wood LV, et al: Lactic acidosis and hepatic steatosis associated with use of stavudine: Report of four cases. Ann Intern Med 133:192, 2000.
152. Carr A, Miller J, Law M, et al: A syndrome of lipoatrophy, lactic acidaemia, and liver dysfunction association with HIV nucleoside analogue therapy: Contribution to protease inhibitor-related lipodystrophy syndrome. AIDS 14:F25, 2000.
153. Horsburgh CR, Mason VG, Farhi DC, et al: Disseminated infections with *Mycobacterium avium-intracellulare*: A report of 13 cases and review of the literature. Medicine (Baltimore) 64:36, 1985.
154. Cappell MS: Hepatobiliary manifestations of the acquired immune deficiency syndrome. Am J Gastroenterol 86:1, 1991.
155. Rustgi VK, Hoofnagle JH, Gerin JL: Hepatitis B virus infection in the acquired immunodeficiency syndrome. Ann Intern Med 101:795, 1986.
156. Rodriguez-Mendez ML, Gonzalez-Quintela A, Aguilera A, et al: Prevalence, patterns, and course of past hepatitis B virus infection in intravenous drug users with HIV-1 infection. Am J Gasteroenterol 95: 1316, 2000.
157. Waite J, Gilson RJC, Weller IVD, et al: Hepatitis B virus reactivation or reinfection associated with HIV-1 infection. AIDS 2:443, 1988.
158. Laukamm-Josten U, Muller O, Bienzle U, et al: Decline of naturally acquired antibodies to hepatitis B surface antigen in HIV-1 infected homosexual men. AIDS 2:400, 1988.
159. Perrillo RP, Regenstein FG, Roodman ST, et al: Chronic hepatitis B in asymptomatic homosexual men with antibody to the human immunodeficiency virus. Ann Intern Med 105:382, 1986.
160. Krogsgaard K, Lindhart BO, Nielsen JO, et al: The influence of HTLV III infection on the natural history of hepatitis B virus infection in male homosexual HBsAg carriers. Hepatology 7:37, 1987.
161. Housset C, Pol S, Carnot F, et al: Interactions between human immunodeficiency virus-1, hepatitis delta virus, and hepatitis B virus infections in 260 chronic carriers of hepatitis B virus. Hepatology 15:578, 1992.
162. Bodsworth N, Donovan B, Nightingale BN: The effect of concurrent human immunodeficiency virus infection on chronic hepatitis B: A study of 150 homosexual men. J Infect Dis 160:577, 1989.
163. Collier AC, Corey L, Murphy VL, et al: Antibody to human immunodeficiency virus (HIV) and suboptimal response to hepatitis B vaccination. Ann Intern Med 109:101, 1988.
164. Scharschmidt BF, Held MJ, Hollander HH, et al: Hepatitis B in patients with HIV infection: Relation of AIDS and patient survival. Ann Intern Med 117:837, 1992.
165. Piroth LA, Ngui SL, Kaur S, et al: Reactivation of hepatitis B in patients with human immunodeficiency virus infection treated with combination antiretroviral therapy. Am J Med 108:249, 2000.
166. Solomon RE, Kaslow RA, Phair JP, et al: Human immunodeficiency virus and hepatitis delta virus in homosexual men. Ann Intern Med 108:5, 1988.
167. Buti M, Esteban R, Espanol MT, et al: Influence of human immunodeficiency virus infection on cell-mediated immunity in chronic D hepatitis. J Infect Dis 163:1351, 1991.
168. Shattock AG, Finlay H, Hillary IB: Possible reactivation of hepatitis D with chronic gamma antigenaemia by human immunodeficiency virus. BMJ 294:1656, 187.
169. Eyster ME, Diamondstone LS, Lien J, et al: Natural history of hepatitis C virus infection in multitransfused hemophiliacs: Effect of coinfection with human immunodeficiency virus. J Acquir Immune Defic Syndr Hum Retrovirol 6:602, 1993.
170. Wright TL, Hollander H, Pu X, et al: Hepatitis C in HIV-infected patients with and without AIDS: Prevalence and relationship to patient survival. Hepatology 20:1152, 1994.
171. Cribier B, Rey D, Schmitt C, et al: High hepatitis C viraemia and impaired antibody response in patients coinfected with HIV. AIDS 9: 1131, 1995.
172. Telfer P, Sabin C, Devereux H, et al: The progression of HCV-associated liver disease in a cohort of haemophilic patients. B J Haematol 87:555, 1994.
173. Thomas DL, Astemborski J, Vlahov D, et al: Determinants of the quantity of hepatitis C virus RNA. J Infect Dis 181:844, 2000.
174. Dorrucci M, Pezzotti P, Phillips AN, et al: Coinfection of hepatitis C virus with human immunodeficiency virus and progression to AIDS. J Infect Dis 172:1503, 1995.
175. Pouti M, Gargiulo F, Roldan EQ, et al: Liver damage and kinetics of hepatitis C virus and human immunodeficiency virus replication during the early phases of combination antiretroviral treatment. J Infect Dis 181:2033, 2000.
176. Gavazzi G, Bouchard O, Leclercq P, et al: Change in transaminases in hepatitis C virus and HIV coinfected patients after highly active antiretroviral therapy: Differences between complete and partial virologic responders? AIDS Res Hum Retrovir 16:1021, 2000.
177. Dieterich DT, Purow JM, Rajapaska R: Activity of combination therapy with interferon alfa-2b plus ribavirin in chronic hepatitis C patients coinfected with HIV. Semin Liver Dis 19:87, 1999.
178. Landau A, Batisse D, Van Huyen JPD, et al: Efficacy and safety of combination therapy with interferon-2b and ribavirin for chronic hepatitis C in HIV-infected patients. AIDS 14:839, 2000.
179. Bronnimann DA, Adam RD, Galgiani JN, et al: Coccidioidomycosis in the acquired immunodeficiency syndrome. Ann Intern Med 106: 372, 1987.
180. Hasan FA, Jeffers LJ, Welsh SW, et al: Hepatic involvement as the primary manifestation of Kaposi's sarcoma in the acquired immune deficiency syndrome. Am J Gastroenterol 84:1449, 1989.
181. Boshoff C, Schulz TF, Kennedy MM, et al: Kaposi's sarcoma–associated herpesvirus infects endothelial and spindle cells. Nat Med 1:1274, 1995.
182. Tirelli U, Spina M, Gaidano G, et al: Epidemiological, biological, and clinical features of HIV-related lymphomas in the era of highly active antiretroviral therapy. AIDS 14:1675, 2000.
183. Rockley PF, Wilcox CM, Moynihan M, et al: Splenic infection simulating lymphoma: An unusual presentation of disseminated *Pneumocystis carinii* infection. South Med J 87:530, 1994.
184. Gasquet S, Maurin M, Brouqui B, et al: Bacillary angiomatosis in immunocompromised patients. AIDS 12:1793, 1998.
185. Schwartzman WA: Infections due to *Rochalimaea*: The expanding clinical spectrum. Clin Infect Dis 15:893, 1992.
186. Schneiderman DJ, Arenson DM, Cello JP, et al: Hepatic disease in patients with the acquired immune deficiency syndrome (AIDS). Hepatology 7:925, 1987.
187. Benhamou Y, Caumes E, Gerosa Y, et al: AIDS-related cholangiopathy: Critical analysis of a prospective series of 26 patients. Dig Dis Sci 38:1113, 1993.
188. Pol S, Romana CA, Richard S, Amouyal P, et al: Microsporidia infection in patients with the human immunodeficiency virus and unexplained cholangitis. N Engl J Med 328:95, 1993.
189. Ducreux M, Buffet C, Lamy P, et al: Diagnosis and prognosis of AIDS-related cholangitis. AIDS 9:875, 1995.
190. Cello JP, Chan MF: Long-term follow-up of endoscopic retrograde cholangiopancreatography sphincterotomy for patients with acquired immune deficiency syndrome papillary stenosis. Am J Med 99:600, 1995.
191. Wilcox CM, Monkemuller KE: Hepatobiliary disease in patients with AIDS: Focus on AIDS cholangiopathy. Dig Dis 16:205, 1998.
192. Tanner AG, Hartley JE, Darzi A, et al: Laparoscopic surgery in patients with human immunodeficiency virus. Br J Surg 81:1647, 1994.

Chapter 29

GASTROINTESTINAL MANIFESTATIONS OF SYSTEMIC DISEASES

David D. Kim and James C. Ryan

Numerous systemic and extraintestinal diseases have gastrointestinal manifestations. Because it is impossible to discuss each entity in great detail in a single chapter, we endeavor here to emphasize frequently encountered diseases and those that may be of particular interest to the reader because of recent developments. For the sake of clarity, some diseases that result in similar manifestations are presented in tabular form. Some topics are taken up in detail in other chapters. The reader is referred to these chapters for a more complete discussion. Chapter 82 deals with hepatic manifestations of systemic disease in more detail than presented here.

RHEUMATOLOGIC AND COLLAGEN DISEASES

Rheumatologic diseases encompass a wide variety of clinical syndromes and are frequently associated with gastrointestinal abnormalities (Table 29–1). In addition, the medications used to treat these diseases often produce gastrointestinal toxicity. This section focuses on the more common abnormalities that may be encountered by the gastroenterologist.

Rheumatoid Arthritis

With chronic *rheumatoid arthritis* (RA), temporomandibular arthritis resulting in tenderness, swelling, and crepitance may impair mastication.[1] Esophageal dysmotility, common in RA, is characterized by low-amplitude peristaltic waves in the middle and lower esophagus and reduced lower esophageal sphincter (LES) pressure.[1] Despite these abnormalities, heartburn and dysphagia are unusual. *Rheumatoid vasculitis* is a serious complication, affecting 1% of patients.[2] It appears in the setting of severe arthritis, rheumatoid nodules, and high titers of rheumatoid factor. Often these patients display signs of cutaneous vasculitis as well as peripheral neuritis. In 10% of these cases the vasculitis may involve the gastrointestinal tract. Patients may develop ischemic cholecystitis or appendicitis, ulceration, pancolitis, infarction, or intra-abdominal hemorrhage due to a ruptured visceral aneurysm.[3, 4] Cyto-

Table 29–1 | **Gastrointestinal Manifestations of Rheumatologic Diseases**

DISEASE	ABNORMALITY/ASSOCIATION	MANIFESTATIONS
Rheumatoid arthritis	Temporomandibular arthritis	Impaired mastication
	Esophageal dysmotility	Dysphagia, reflux esophagitis
	Visceral vasculitis	Abdominal pain, cholecystitis, bowel ulceration and infarction
	Amyloidosis	Pseudo-obstruction, malabsorption, protein-losing enteropathy, intestinal ulceration and infarction, gastric outlet obstruction
	Portal hypertension (Felty's syndrome)	Variceal hemorrhage
	Gold enterocolitis	Enteritis, diarrhea, fever, eosinophilia, megacolon
Scleroderma	Esophageal dysmotility	Dysphagia, reflux esophagitis, strictures, Barrett's metaplasia
	Gastroparesis	Gastric retention, gastroesophageal reflux
	Intestinal fibrosis and dysmotility	Constipation, pseudo-obstruction, malabsorption, intussusception, volvulus, pneumatosis intestinalis
	Pseudodiverticula	Hemorrhage, stasis, bacterial overgrowth
	Arteritis (rare)	Intestinal thrombosis, infarction, pancreatic necrosis
	Pancreatitis	Calcific pancreatitis, exocrine insufficiency
SLE	Esophageal dysmotility	Dysphagia, reflux
	Mesenteric vasculitis (2%)	GI ulceration, intestinal infarction, intussusception, pancreatitis, pneumatosis intestinalis
Sjögren's syndrome	Dessication of membranes	Oral fissures, oropharyngeal dysphagia
	Esophageal webs	Dysphagia
	Gastric infiltrates	Gastric masses
	Pancreatitis	Abdominal pain, exocrine insufficiency
	Primary biliary cirrhosis	Jaundice, hepatic failure, variceal hemorrhage
Polymyositis-dermatomyositis	Skeletal muscle dysfunction	Aspiration, impaired glutition
	Dysmotility	Dysphagia, reflux, gastroparesis, constipation, diverticula
	Mesenteric vasculitis (rare)	GI ulceration, perforation, pneumatosis intestinalis
MCTD	Dysmotility	Dysphagia, reflux, stricture, gastroparesis, bezoars, pseudo-obstruction
	Mesenteric vasculitis (rare)	Ulceration, perforation, pancreatitis
PAN	Mesenteric vasculitis (80%)	Cholecystitis (17%), appendicitis, bowel infarction, pancreatitis, perforation, strictures, mucosal hemorrhage, submucosal hematomas
CSS	Mesenteric vasculitis (42%)	Hemorrhage, ulceration, infarction, perforation
	Eosinophilic gastritis	Gastric masses
Henoch-Schönlein purpura	Mesenteric vasculitis (68%)	Intussusception, ulcers, cholecystitis, hemorrhage, infarction, appendicitis, perforation
Kohlmeier-Degos disease	Mesenteric vasculitis	Hemorrhage, ulceration, infarction, malabsorption
Cogan's syndrome	Mesenteric vasculitis (infrequent)	Hemorrhage, ulceration, infarction, intussusception
	Crohn's disease (infrequent)	Bloody diarrhea, abdominal pain, fissures, fistulas
Wegener's granulomatosis	Mesenteric vasculitis (5%)	Cholecystitis, appendicitis, ileocolitis, infarction
Cryoglobulinemia	Mesenteric vasculitis (rare)	Infarction, ischemia
Behçet's syndrome	Mucosal ulcerations	Hemorrhage, perforation, pyloric stenosis
		Complications as above (see Rheumatoid Arthritis)
Reactive arthritis	Ileocolonic inflammation	Usually asymptomatic
Familial Mediterranean fever	Serositis/peritonitis, amyloidosis, PAN (1%), Henoch-Schönlein purpura (5–7%)	Abdominal pain, fever, dysmotility
Marfan/Ehlers-Danlos syndrome	Defective collagen	Megaesophagus, hypomotility, diverticula, megacolon, malabsorption, perforation, arterial rupture

CSS, Churg-Strauss syndrome; GI, gastrointestinal; MCTD, mixed connective tissue disease; PAN, polyarteritis nodosa; SLE, systemic lupus erythematosus.

toxic agents may be more effective therapy than corticosteroids.[5] Other gastrointestinal complications of RA include *amyloidosis* and *malabsorption. Felty's syndrome*—RA, splenomegaly, and leukopenia (see Chapter 82) has been associated with severe infections, portal hypertension, and variceal hemorrhage.[5]

The most common gastrointestinal problems encountered in patients with RA are due to drug therapy aimed at the disease. Gastroduodenal damage can be seen on endoscopy in 20% to 40% of patients who take nonsteroidal anti-inflammatory drugs (NSAIDs), and high-dose therapy produces more lesions. Several risk factors for serious upper gastrointestinal events in patients with RA include age older than 60 years, history of peptic ulcer disease, use of corticosteroids, and the presence of extra-articular manifestations.[6] In patients with RA, the use of selective cyclooxygenase-2 inhibitors results in a lower incidence of gastrointestinal complications than that seen with nonselective NSAIDs.[7] *Helicobacter pylori* and NSAIDs are independent (and possibly synergistic) risk factors for peptic ulceration. As such, chronic NSAID users with a high risk of developing ulcers who are infected with *H. pylori* should be considered for *H. pylori* testing and eradication.[8] Although hypergastrinemia has been reported in patients with RA,[9] the incidence of peptic ulcers is no greater than that seen in patients with osteoarthritis.[9]

The optimal strategy to prevent NSAID-induced gastrointestinal complications continues to evolve (see Chapter 23). Although misoprostol and high-dose H_2-blockers can prevent NSAID-associated gastric and duodenal ulcers,[10–16] proton pump inhibitors may be even more efficacious. In addition, proton pump inhibitors are better tolerated than misoprostol, whose use is limited by its gastrointestinal side effects and its abortifacient action in women of childbearing age. Once identified, ulcers may be treated successfully using proton pump inhibitors despite continued NSAID therapy. The cost-effectiveness of selective cyclooxygenase-2 inhibitors as compared with combination therapy with antiulcer prophylaxis and traditional NSAIDs is the subject of continuing debate.

Historically, disease-modifying agents such as gold have been used to treat RA. Treatment with colloidal gold has been associated with gastrointestinal complications, most notably mild diarrhea.[17] Rarely, serious colitis may complicate chrysotherapy.[18] The onset of *gold colitis* usually occurs within several weeks after the start of therapy and is manifest by nausea, vomiting, diarrhea, and fever.[17] The severity ranges from limited ileal involvement to fulminant pancolitis, toxic megacolon, and death. Although the colon is most commonly involved, gold-induced gastrointestinal toxicity may affect the esophagus, stomach, and small bowel.[18] Twenty-five percent of patients have peripheral eosinophilia. The cause of this condition remains obscure. Treatment includes discontinuation of the drug and administration of corticosteroids, cromolyn sodium, or the chelating agent dimercaprol.

The use of colloidal gold in the treatment of RA has been largely abandoned in favor of newer disease-modifying agents such as infliximab, etanercept, and antimetabolites. The antimetabolites methotrexate and leflunomide can cause acute liver injury and transaminase elevations. Methotrexate in large cumulative doses (1.5 to 2 g total) can also cause hepatic fibrosis. Routine liver biopsy is not currently recommended in RA patients on methotrexate, but liver biopsy may be considered in patients with suspected liver injury in the setting of significant methotrexate exposure or confounding preexisting liver disease (see Chapters 18 and 73).[19]

Adult-onset Still's disease, the adult form of juvenile RA, often has gastrointestinal manifestations such as weight loss (76%), sore throat (92%), hepatomegaly (44%) with elevated liver chemistries (76%), and abdominal pain (48%), in addition to fever.[20] Severe liver failure in adult Still's disease may be associated with aspirin or NSAID therapy, and close monitoring of liver tests in adult Still's disease patients treated with these agents is recommended.[20]

Progressive Systemic Sclerosis

Progressive systemic sclerosis (PSS, scleroderma) is a multisystem disorder characterized by obliterative small vessel vasculitis and proliferation of connective tissue with fibrosis of multiple organs. Patients with limited cutaneous involvement frequently display findings of the CREST syndrome (*c*alcinosis, *R*aynaud's phenomenon, *e*sophageal dysmotility, *s*clerodactyly, and *t*elangiectasias).

Gastrointestinal manifestations of PSS are found in 82% of patients.[21] Gastrointestinal tract involvement can occur from the mouth to the anus. Atrophy and fibrosis of the perioral skin may limit mandibular motion. The periodontal ligament may become hypertrophic, and the gingivae, tongue papillae, and buccal mucosa may become friable and atrophic, resulting in impaired sensation and taste.

Esophageal involvement occurs in most patients with PSS. Dysphagia, due to impaired esophageal motility, and gastroesophageal reflux disease (GERD), due to hypotensive LES pressures, are the major problems. The incidence of esophagitis approaches 100% in patients with severe cutaneous involvement.[22] The extent of hypomotility varies from occasional uncoordinated contractions to complete paralysis.[23] *Stricture formation* from GERD may contribute to dysphagia, affecting approximately 8% of patients.[24] Esophageal ulcerations may cause bleeding, or rarely, esophageoatrial fistulas.[25] Severe *esophagitis* typically responds to proton pump inhibitors but may require higher doses for maximal effects.[26] A neuropathic, achalasia-like syndrome has also been reported.[27] Although one study reported that 38% of symptomatic patients with PSS have *Barrett's metaplasia* of the esophagus,[28] a definitive increase in the incidence of adenocarcinoma of the esophagus has not been reported.[29] Delayed gastric emptying is frequently associated with esophageal transit disorders in patients with PSS and may be an important factor in the development of GERD.[30, 31] Metoclopramide may increase LES pressures and improve gastric emptying in some patients with PSS. Erythromycin may also accelerate gastric emptying in PSS.[32]

The pathologic changes in the small bowel of PSS patients consist of smooth muscle atrophy and deposition of collagen in submucosal, muscular, and serosal layers. Small bowel hypomotility is present in as many as 88% of cases.[33] In the early stages of the disease, this is due to neuropathic involvement, which may be more responsive to prokinetic agents. In advanced cases, hypomotility is more likely due to "myopathic" and "fibrotic" changes.[34] The interdigestive migrating motor complex (IMMC) is frequently absent or markedly diminished in amplitude in PSS patients with symptoms of intestinal dysmotility.[35] Small bowel radiographic abnormalities are present in about 60% of PSS patients, but they may not correlate with symptoms. The duodenum is often dilated, especially in the second and third portions, often with prolonged retention of barium.[36] Typically, the jejunum is dilated and foreshortened owing to mural fibrosis, but valvulae conniventes of normal thickness give rise to an "accordion-like" appearance. *Pneumatosis cystoides intestinalis, pseudo-obstruction, pseudodiverticula, sacculations, intussusception, acquired intestinal lymphangiectasia*, and *small bowel volvulus* have been noted.[37–39]

Symptoms of small intestinal PSS include bloating, borborygmi, anorexia, nausea, and vomiting. Rarely, thrombosis of large mesenteric arteries with extensive bowel necrosis may occur.[40] *Malabsorption* with steatorrhea is present in as many as a third of PSS patients[33] and is due to bacterial overgrowth (see Chapters 89 and 90). Although antibiotic therapy is effective in these patients, D-xylose malabsorption is often incompletely reversed, suggesting that collagen deposition in PSS may also contribute to malabsorption.[41] Although often disappointing, the use of prokinetic agents such as metoclopramide may be effective in some cases. Octreotide in low doses and erythromycin may also provide sustained relief from nausea, abdominal pain, and bloating in some patients with pseudo-obstruction.[42] Delayed colonic transit and impaired anal sphincter function are frequently found in constipated patients with PSS.[43] Colonic and anorectal motility abnormalities are usually associated with motility disturbances elsewhere in the gastrointestinal tract.[44] Mucosal telangiectasias may be a source of hemorrhage.[45] Wide-necked pseudodiverticula can be seen, especially in the antimesenteric border of the transverse and descending colon. Finally, rectal prolapse worsens anal sphincter function, aggravating fecal incontinence in patients with PSS.[46]

Pancreatic exocrine secretion is depressed in a third of patients with PSS, and idiopathic calcific *pancreatitis* has been reported.[47] In addition, arteritis, leading to pancreatic necrosis has been described in patients with PSS.[48, 49]

Systemic Lupus Erythematosus

Systemic lupus erythematosus (SLE) is a multisystem disease characterized by immune system abnormalities and the production of autoantibodies with tissue damage. Gastrointestinal symptoms are common in patients with active SLE. Nausea, anorexia, or vomiting affects 50% of patients.[49] Esophageal dysmotility results in heartburn and dysphagia. Malabsorption of D-xylose, steatorrhea, and protein-losing enteropathy have been described (see Chapter 25, Fig. 25–1; the latter can be steroid responsive.[50] Ascites can be due to peritoneal or mesenteric vasculitis, pancreatitis, nephrotic syndrome, serositis, or cardiac failure. Patients with ascites taking corticosteroids may develop spontaneous bacterial peritonitis. Lupus peritonitis is a diagnosis that can be made only after other causes have been carefully excluded. *Pneumatosis cystoides intestinalis* may be an isolated benign condition or may accompany lupus vasculitis or necrotizing enterocolitis.[51, 52]

One of the most devastating complications of lupus is gastrointestinal vasculitis. Affecting only 2% of patients, it has a fatality rate of more than 50%.[53] Common sequelae include ulceration, hemorrhage, perforation, and infarction.[54–56] Pancreatitis,[57, 58] gastritis, hemorrhagic ileocolitis resembling inflammatory bowel disease (Fig. 29–1), and intussusception have also been reported. Changes of lupus mesenteric vasculitis usually affect the bowel supplied by the superior mesenteric artery and rarely involve the distal transverse or left colon.[59] Although occasional case reports have documented polyarteritis-like changes on visceral arteriograms (described later), the typical pathologic changes are seen in the small vessels of the bowel wall rather than the medium-sized vessels of the bowel wall.[51] Because visceral angiography routinely is not helpful, the diagnosis is difficult to establish. The roles of endoscopy, computed tomography (CT), or of upper gastrointestinal series in the diagnosis of lupus vasculitis are not well defined. The diagnosis currently rests on clinical judgment, inferences from nonspecific findings on CT scans, and occasionally from surgical specimens when exploratory laparotomy is undertaken to rule out acute surgical emergencies.[59] Treatment of abdominal lupus-induced vasculitis with corticosteroids has been largely unsatisfactory. Although a controlled clinical trial comparing cyclophosphamide with corticosteroids has not been performed, anecdotal reports of dramatic responses to intravenous cyclophosphamide are promising.[51] Some investigators have suggested that cyclophosphamide be considered early in patients who have not shown significant improvement shortly after high-dose corticosteroids are started. The association between SLE and autoimmune hepatitis is discussed in Chapter 75.

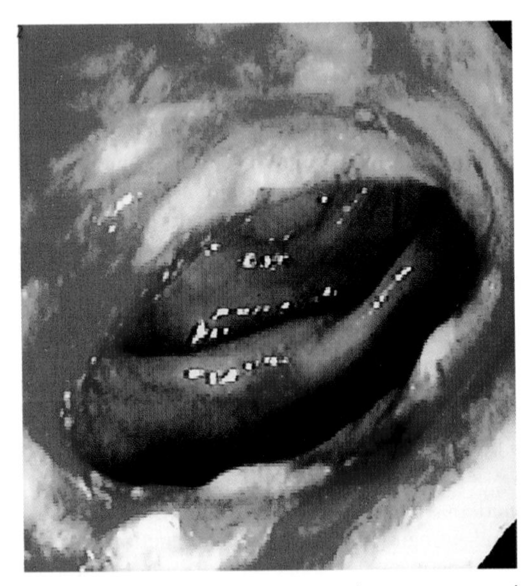

Figure 29–1. Sigmoidoscopic examination of an intravenous drug user with a footdrop and guaiac-positive stool. There is a focal area of circumferential ulceration and partial stricturing in the rectosigmoid, with entirely normal mucosa in the rectum and in the proximal sigmoid colon. A sural nerve biopsy confirmed the diagnosis of polyarteritis nodosa.

Polymyositis and Dermatomyositis

Polymyositis is a syndrome characterized by weakness, high serum levels of striated muscle enzymes (creatine kinase, aldolase), and electromyographic (EMG) or biopsy evidence of an inflammatory myopathy. When accompanied by a characteristic violaceous rash on the extensor surfaces of the hands and periorbital regions, the disease is termed *dermatomyositis* (see Fig. 29–1). The primary gastrointestinal symptoms are due to involvement of the cricopharyngeus, resulting in nasal regurgitation, tracheal aspiration, and impaired deglutition.[60] Involvement is not limited to skeletal muscle fibers. Disordered esophageal motility, impaired gastric emptying, and poorly coordinated small intestinal peristalsis have been noted. Pathologically, edema of the bowel wall, muscle atrophy, fibrosis, and mucosal ulcerations or perforation due to vasculitis may be seen at any level of the gut. Symptoms include heartburn, bloating, constipation, and gastrointestinal hemorrhage. Pneumoperitoneum, pneumatosis intestinalis, colonic dilation, and pseudodiverticula may also be seen. Perforations of the esophagus and of duodenal diverticula have been described as rare complications.[61, 62]

In adults, certain subgroups of patients with dermatomyositis have been reported to have an increased prevalence (5% to 8%) of malignancy.[63] The possibility that gastrointestinal symptoms may be due to an underlying malignancy should be considered when evaluating these patients.

Mixed Connective Tissue Disease

Mixed connective tissue disease (MCTD) is a syndrome having overlapping features of PSS, polymyositis, and SLE, often in the presence of high levels of antibody directed against ribonucleoprotein. Upper gastrointestinal symptoms are seen in most patients.[64] Abnormalities include diminished esophageal peristalsis (48%), esophageal stricture (6%), abnormal gastric emptying (6%), and gastric bezoar (2%).[64]

Small intestinal and colonic involvement includes dilation of proximal bowel, slow transit, intestinal pseudo-obstruction, diverticulosis, and, rarely, intestinal vasculitis. Pancreatitis has also been reported.[64] Unlike PSS, the esophageal motility disturbances seen in MCTD appear to improve with the administration of corticosteroids.

Sjögren's Syndrome

Sjögren's syndrome (SS) is characterized by lymphocytic tissue infiltration of lacrimal and salivary glands with the clinical findings of keratoconjunctivitis sicca and xerostomia (see Chapter 18). Excessive dryness of the mouth and pharynx leads to fissuring and ulceration of the lips and oral mucous membranes. Dysphagia, reported by up to three fourths of patients with SS, can result from a lack of saliva but may also result from connective tissue abnormalities of the esophagus.[65] Upper esophageal webs occur in as many as 10%, and motility disturbances have been reported in 36% of patients.[66] The most common associated gastrointestinal abnormality is chronic atrophic gastritis, which can occasionally give the appearance of gastric carcinoma on barium study.[67] There have been reports of acute and chronic pancreatitis complicating SS. Chronic pancreatitis may coexist with sclerosing cholangitis.[49, 68] Pancreatic exocrine function is frequently impaired. Primary biliary cirrhosis is more common in patients with SS as well (see Chapter 76).[65] These associated conditions have led some to speculate that some patients with SS exhibit an "autoimmune exocrinopathy," comprised of sialoadenitis, pancreatitis, and primary biliary cirrhosis.[69]

Polyarteritis Nodosa and Other Arteritides

Polyarteritis nodosa (PAN) is a necrotizing vasculitis of small- and medium-sized muscular arteries, frequently with visceral involvement.[70] A characteristic feature of this condition is the finding of aneurysmal dilatations up to 1 cm in size seen on visceral angiography (Fig. 29–2). Abdominal symptoms occur in 44% of patients, abdominal pain being the most common symptom.[71] Other signs and symptoms include fever, hypertension, arthralgia and arthritis, peripheral and central nervous system (CNS) dysfunction, and glomerulonephritis.[70, 71] Gastrointestinal tract involvement is a serious prognostic factor.[72] Mesenteric visceral arteriograms are estimated to be abnormal in up to 80% of patients.[73] Organ damage resulting from ischemia frequently underlies symptoms. Gastrointestinal hemorrhage from intestinal ischemic lesions is seen in roughly 6% of cases, bowel perforation in 5%, and bowel infarction in 1.4%.[73] *Acalculous cholecystitis* results from direct vasculitic involvement of the gallbladder in 17% of patients.[71] *Pancreatitis*,[74] *appendicitis*,[75] and solitary *biliary strictures*[76] have also been reported to complicate PAN. In addition, a chronic wasting syndrome resembling tuberculous enteritis or neoplasm may be the primary manifestation of vasculitis.[71] Mesenteric angiography may establish the diagnosis in these patients and should be considered when the initial workup of a patient with chronic wasting has been unrevealing, particularly if fever is present. Hepatitis B–related PAN is an acute disease that clinically is indistinguishable from classic PAN and occurs shortly

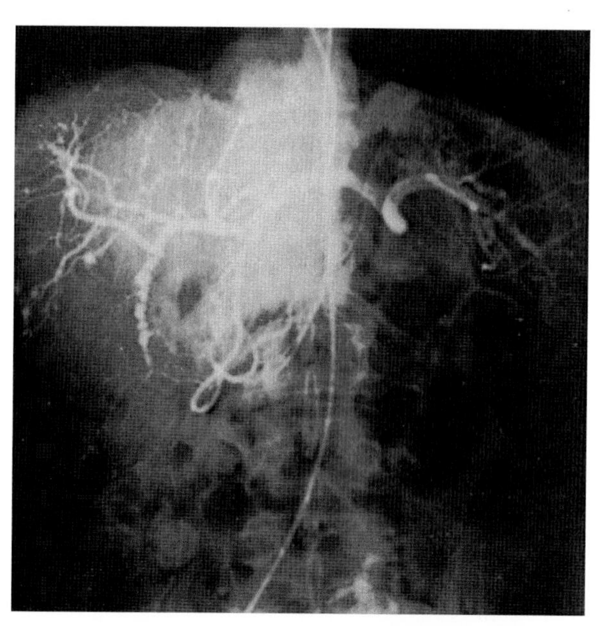

Figure 29–2. Celiac arteriogram in a patient with polyarteritis nodosa and hepatitis B surface antigenemia. Multiple saccular and fusiform aneurysms as well as arterial tapering and beading are seen throughout the celiac axis. (Courtesy of Connie Wofsy, M.D.)

after infection. Although available data are limited, successful treatment of the hepatitis B virus infection with interferon and lamivudine (plus prednisone) may lead to regression of PAN.[77]

Churg-Strauss syndrome (CSS) is a variant of visceral arteritis characterized by asthma, hypereosinophilia, necrotizing vasculitis, and extravascular granulomas. Gastrointestinal symptoms are seen in most patients with CSS, including abdominal pain (59%), diarrhea (33%), and bloody stool (18%).[78] Gastrointestinal involvement includes eosinophilic infiltration of the stomach and duodenum resembling eosinophilic gastroenteritis,[79] as well as multiple gastric, small intestinal, and colonic ulcerations.[80, 81] Although visceral angiograms may be abnormal, many cases are not diagnosed until surgery or death.[82]

Henoch-Schönlein purpura (HSP) is a clinical syndrome characterized by nonthrombocytopenic purpura, arthralgias, renal disease, and colicky abdominal pain. Although the disease is frequently seen in children, adults of any age may be affected. Abdominal symptoms are usually the result of vasculitis and have been reported in as many as 68% of patients.[71] Symptoms include abdominal pain, nausea, and vomiting. Gastrointestinal bleeding occurs in roughly 40% of patients.[71] Colonoscopic and endoscopic findings in bleeding patients include erosive duodenitis, small aphthous ulcerations, and petechial colonic lesions.[83] Less common but serious abdominal complications include intramural hematomas, intussusception,[84] infarction,[84] perforation,[85] appendicitis,[86] and cholecystitis.[87]

Malignant atrophic papulosis (Kohlmeier-Degos disease) is a rare vasculitis that causes malabsorption, bowel ischemia, and perforation. Scattered on the skin are red papules that become hypopigmented, atrophic scars (see Fig. 18–18).

Cogan's syndrome is characterized by nonsyphilitic interstitial keratitis, audiovestibular symptoms, and large-vessel

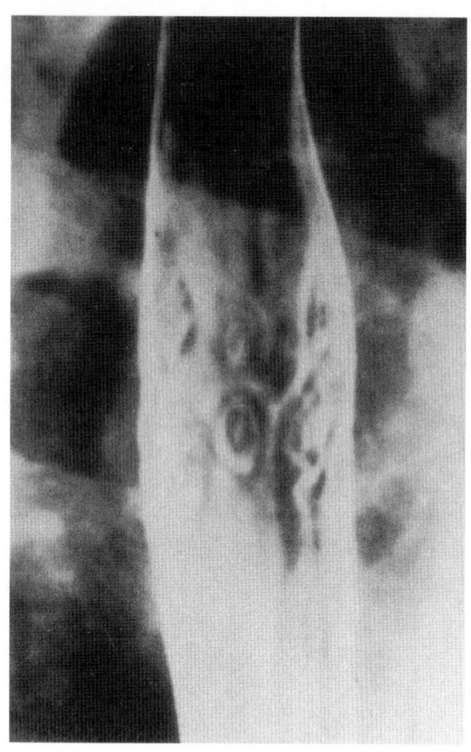

Figure 29–3. Esophageal ulcerations in Behçet's disease. (Courtesy of the Radiology Learning Center, University of California School of Medicine, San Francisco.)

vasculitis that may involve the gut. *Crohn's disease* has been reported in association with this rare condition.[88]

Wegener's granulomatosis, a systemic vasculitis characterized by pulmonary, sinus, and renal involvement, less commonly affects the gut.[89] Inflammatory ileocolitis with hemorrhage,[90] cholecystitis,[91] and bowel infarction all have been reported.[92]

Mixed IgG-IgM cryoglobulinemia may complicate chronic hepatitis C infection (see Chapters 18 and 68) and a variety of immune diseases, including inflammatory bowel disease, celiac disease,[93] and postintestinal bypass syndrome. Cryoglobulinemia may cause severe vasculitis with large and small bowel ischemia.[94, 95] Successful therapy of hepatitis C can lead to amelioration of cryoglobulinemia.[96] Hepatosplenomegaly and lymphoid hyperplasia of the terminal ileum may be seen.

Drug-induced vasculitis has been associated with the use of prescription medications as well as recreational drugs. Prescription drugs, including antihypertensives (hydrochlorothiazide, hydralazine, spironolactone), antibiotics (penicillins, tetracyclines, sulfonamides), oral hypoglycemics such as chlorpropamide, and agents to treat gout (allopurinol, colchicine) all have been implicated in hypersensitivity vasculitis.[97] The use of the newer biologic agents—interferon-α, -β, and -γ as well as granulocyte colony-stimulating factor (G-CSF)—has also been associated with hypersensitivity vasculitis.[98] Hypersensitivity vasculitis primarily involves the skin but on rare occasions involves the viscera. Case reports describing CNS and mesenteric vasculitis in association with recreational methamphetamine use have been described.[99] Cerebral vasculitis has been rarely described with cocaine use, but cocaine-induced mesenteric ischemia is most commonly caused by the vasoconstrictive effects of cocaine itself.[100, 101]

Behçet's Syndrome

Behçet's syndrome is a chronic relapsing multisystem disease characterized by oral ulceration, genital ulceration, and uveitis. In addition to Behçet's triad, features of this syndrome also include synovitis, cutaneous vasculitis resembling erythema nodosum, meningoencephalitis, large artery aneurysms, phlebitis, and discrete ulcers of the gut. Involvement of the esophagus includes ulcers (Fig. 29–3), varices, and perforation.[102] The typical intestinal involvement in Behçet's syndrome includes "punched-out" ileocecal ulcerations.[103] The rate of postoperative recurrence of these ulcers is high.[104] Anal ulceration,[105] peritonitis,[106] pyloric stenosis,[107] and secondary amyloidosis have also been reported.[108] Intestinal ulcerations may perforate and bleed. In clinical presentation as well as pathologic and endoscopic appearance, ulcers can be strikingly similar to Crohn's disease,[109] and most large series of Behçet's disease contain a few patients who have or will develop Crohn's disease. Although some lesions respond to corticosteroid therapy, the effects are often transient and inconsistent.

Seronegative Spondyloarthropathies (Reactive Arthritides)

The term *seronegative spondyloarthropathy* is used to describe an interrelated group of inflammatory disorders that include *ankylosing spondylitis*, *Reiter's syndrome*, and *psoriatic arthritis*. The term has also been used to describe the enteropathic spondylitis associated with *Crohn's disease* and *ulcerative colitis*.[110] These disorders are characterized by arthritis accompanying inflammation of various extra-articular sites and are distinguished from each other on clinical and radiographic grounds. There is a high prevalence of clinically silent inflammatory colon lesions in patients with these seronegative spondyloarthropathies.[111] Frank inflammatory bowel disease can occasionally be seen complicating psoriatic arthritis.[110] Although infliximab has recently been shown to induce remissions in some patients with ankylosing spondylitis as well as in Crohn's disease, the effect of infliximab on gastrointestinal inflammatory lesions in typical seronegative spondyloarthropathies has not yet been studied.[112]

Marfan's and Ehlers-Danlos Syndromes

Owing to defective collagen synthesis, patients with Marfan's or Ehlers-Danlos syndrome develop skin fragility, megaesophagus, small intestine hypomotility, giant jejunal diverticula, bacterial overgrowth, and megacolon.[113] Mesenteric arterial rupture and intestinal perforation can also occur.[114]

Familial Mediterranean Fever

Familial Mediterranean fever (FMF) is an autosomal recessive inherited disease characterized by recurrent self-limiting attacks of fever, joint pain, and abdominal pain. Acute attacks typically last 3 to 5 days and may be alleviated with colchicine therapy. In refractory cases, corticosteroids may be useful.[115] FMF typically affects those of Jewish, Turkish, Arabic, and Armenian ancestry, although FMF patients of northern European, Irish, and Cuban descent have been identified. The gene responsible for FMF in Mediterranean patients, designated *MEFV*, was recently identified on chromosome 16.[116] The gene product is a 781-amino acid protein called *pyrin* or *marenostrin*, with structural features of a nuclear transcription factor.[117, 118] It is speculated that pyrin/marenostrin is a neutrophil-specific transcription factor that likely regulates the expression of target genes involved in the suppression of serosal and synovial inflammation.[117]

Gastrointestinal symptoms typically manifest as abdominal pain, which may be the presenting symptom in as many as 50% of cases. Abdominal pain may be diffuse or localized and may range from mild bloating to acute *peritonitis* with boardlike rigidity, rebound tenderness, and air-fluid levels on upright radiographs. The presentation may be confused with acute appendicitis, especially because most patients with FMF present before the age of 20 years. Relapsing and remitting attacks of abdominal pain may also be confused with other diseases such as porphyrias, which can be distinguished by laboratory evaluations during acute attacks. Intra-abdominal adhesions caused by recurrent episodes of sterile peritonitis or due to previous exploratory surgeries may result in *small bowel obstruction* in 3% of cases. In patients with obstruction due to adhesions, abdominal attacks without other typical symptoms (arthralgias, fever) should tip off the clinician to consider an obstruction.[116] Although the inflammatory attacks that characterize the disease may sometimes be debilitating, secondary *amyloidosis* may be the most serious manifestation of FMF. In approximately 25% of patients, a renal form of amyloidosis (AA type) progresses over many years leading to renal failure. Prophylactic colchicine has been shown to reduce the frequency of attacks, prevent amyloidosis, and avoid renal failure.[119] Additional conditions associated with FMF include certain forms of vasculitis that may affect the gastrointestinal tract. *HSP* has been reported in 5% to 7% of children with FMF, whereas *PAN*, which itself may cause fever and abdominal pain, occurs in approximately 1% of patients with FMF.[116]

NEOPLASTIC DISEASES

Metastasis to the gut can occur by direct invasion from adjacent organs, by intraperitoneal seeding, or by hematogenous or lymphatic spread. About 20% of all patients with nongastrointestinal malignancies have metastases to the gastrointestinal tract, among which breast, lung, and ovarian cancers and melanoma (Fig. 29–4) are the most common.[120] Patterns of metastases are not random but reflect the location and histologic type of the primary tumor. The esophagus is most frequently affected by direct extension from tumors arising from adjacent structures (chest and stomach). The stomach is a particularly common site of breast cancer metastases, and the intestine can be involved by tumor extension from the stomach, pancreas, biliary system, kidney, or retroperitoneum. The ileum may be affected by cancers arising in the colon or pelvis. Metastases to the gut typically develop in the serosa or submucosa and produce intraluminal lesions that can lead to obstruction, ulcerated mucosal lesions, or submucosal polypoid masses that can result in intussusception. The most common presenting clinical condition in patients with metastatic lesions to the gut is small bowel obstruction. In addition, pain, fever, ascites, bleeding, and perforation all have been described.

Metastases to the gastrointestinal tract may be difficult to diagnose. Barium contrast studies may reveal extramural masses, mucosal ulcerations, or a stomach with the appearance of linitis plastica. CT may be helpful in determining the primary tumor, in tumor staging, and in detecting large serosal implants. Small bowel metastases, however, are detectable radiographically in only 50% of cases.[121]

When feasible, surgical resection should be used to treat gastrointestinal metastases that result in obstruction, perforation, or significant hemorrhage. If a solitary bowel metastasis is the only evident site of disseminated malignancy, segmental bowel resection should be performed, offering a small chance for cure. In aggressive resections of melanoma me-

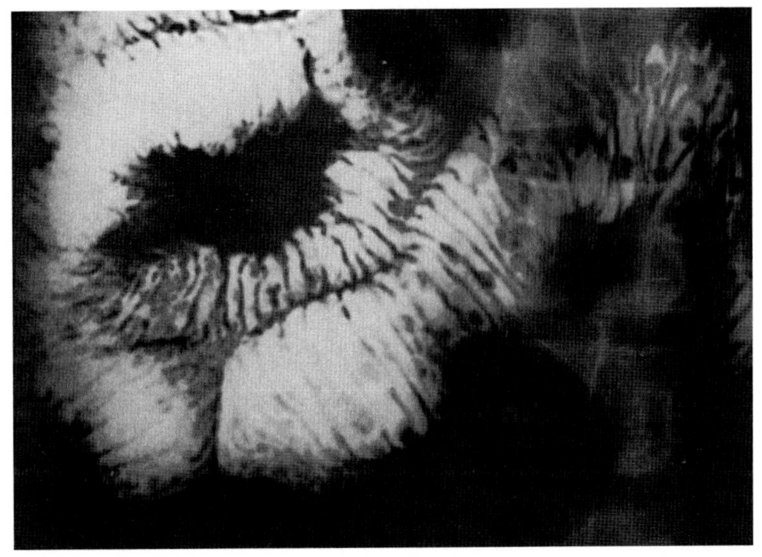

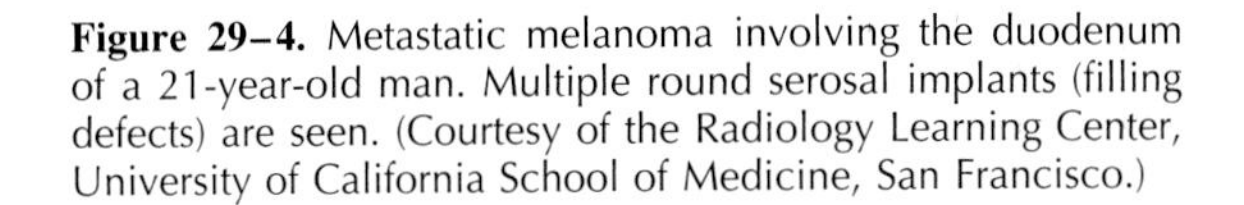

Figure 29–4. Metastatic melanoma involving the duodenum of a 21-year-old man. Multiple round serosal implants (filling defects) are seen. (Courtesy of the Radiology Learning Center, University of California School of Medicine, San Francisco.)

tastases, the mesenteric nodes draining the involved segment of bowel should be resected, because they frequently contain tumors.[122]

Paraneoplastic syndromes affecting the gut include the hormonal effects of carcinoid tumors, VIPomas, gastrinomas, and somatostatinomas (see Chapter 51), as well as the gastrointestinal effects of hypercalcemia (constipation, nausea, and vomiting). A watery diarrhea syndrome with elevated serum immunoreactive vasoactive intestinal polypeptide (VIP) has been described accompanying squamous cell carcinomas of the lung and pheochromocytomas.[123] Elevated serum levels of somatostatin, calcitonin, gastrin, and corticotropin have also been reported in pheochromocytoma.[124]

Paraneoplastic hepatic dysfunction in the absence of hepatic metastases, *Stauffer's syndrome*, is commonly seen in renal cell carcinoma. Stauffer's syndrome manifests as hepatomegaly with elevated alkaline phosphatase levels and prolongation of the prothrombin time.[125] Frank jaundice has also been reported as a reversible complication of Stauffer's syndrome.[125] Liver biopsy typically reveals hepatic sinusoidal dilation.[126] The etiology of this syndrome remains obscure, but complete resolution of hepatic abnormalities after removal of the primary tumor has been described.[125]

A striking paraneoplastic syndrome affecting the gastrointestinal tract is disordered motility with *intestinal pseudo-obstruction* (see Chapter 111). This rare condition is most frequently associated with small cell carcinoma of the lung but has been described with other tumors such as squamous cell lung carcinoma, lymphoma, melanoma, and cancers of the kidney, breast, and prostate.[127–129] Patients with paraneoplastic intestinal pseudo-obstruction characteristically suffer from constipation and obstipation and from symptoms of intestinal obstruction. In addition, dysphagia (from achalasia and esophageal spasm), bladder dysfunction, autonomic insufficiency, and peripheral neuropathy have been described.[130] The onset of symptoms may precede the discovery of the primary tumor by several years. The gastrointestinal pathology in this syndrome is confined to the myenteric plexus, where an inflammatory lymphocytic infiltrate is variably seen accompanying neuronal degeneration.[131] Cross-reacting autoantibodies found in the sera of these patients bind to the primary tumor cells and to neural cells in the myenteric plexus, resulting in inflammation and destruction of the myenteric plexus.[132] The detection of circulating anti-neuronal nuclear antibodies (ANNA-1) in the sera of these patients may aid in the diagnosis.[129] Although the symptoms of paraneoplastic pseudo-obstruction may resolve with successful treatment of the primary tumor, persistence of gastrointestinal symptoms despite effective anticancer treatment is more common. Attempts to alleviate the symptoms of pseudo-obstruction with prokinetic agents have been disappointing.

HEMATOLOGIC DISEASES

Lymphoma (see Chapters 26 and 28)

Lymphoma involves the gastrointestinal tract either as the primary site or secondarily from systemic lymphomas. Lymphomas may affect any organ and must be included in the differential diagnosis of any gastrointestinal symptom, especially in patients with advanced acquired immunodeficiency syndrome.

Leukemia

Approximately 10% of patients with leukemia suffer significant gastrointestinal complications, either from the leukemia itself or as the result of chemotherapy (Table 29–2).[133] Examination of autopsy specimens reveals gastrointestinal involvement in almost half of all patients with leukemia.[134] Acute myelogenous leukemia is the type most likely to affect the gut. Lesions result from four major causes: leukemia cell infiltration, immunodeficiency, coagulation disorders, and drug toxicities. Radiologically, leukemic lesions assume many forms. Infiltration of the bowel may produce polypoid masses, plaquelike thickenings, ulcers, and diffuse masses. Esophageal filling defects with clot and debris have been described.[135] Gastric mucosal folds can assume a "brainlike," deeply convoluted appearance resembling adenocarcinoma. Diffuse intestinal leukemoid polyposis may produce obstruction, hemorrhage, or intussusception.

Immunodeficiency and immunocytopenia may lead to agranulocytic ulcers with bacterial invasion and bleeding. Coagulation defects can produce intramural hematomas and hemorrhagic necrosis of the bowel. Clinical syndromes are myriad. Common oral symptoms (see Chapter 18) are gingi-

Table 29–2 | **Gastrointestinal Complications of Leukemia**

Leukemic Invasion of the Bowel and Related Structures
Mechanical obstruction
Adynamic ileus, intussusception
Mucosal ulceration
Perforation, hemorrhage
Hepatosplenomegaly
Splenic infarction, rupture
Portal hypertension
Ascites, variceal hemorrhage, portosystemic encephalopathy
Biliary and pancreatic duct obstruction
Protein-losing enteropathy
Pneumatosis intestinalis
Immunodeficiency
Necrotizing enterocolitis (typhlitis)
Increased susceptibility to common infections
Appendicitis, wound infections, perirectal abscess, sepsis
Opportunistic infections
Esophageal or hepatic candidiasis, mucositis
Herpes infection (HSV < CMV); protozoa
Pseudomembranous colitis
Coagulation Defects
Intramural hemorrhage
Hemorrhagic necrosis, obstruction
GI hemorrhage
Drug Toxicity
Oral mucositis
Nausea and vomiting
Ileus, megacolon
Bowel necrosis
Hemorrhagic colitis
Pancreatitis
Complications Peculiar to BMT (see Chapter 27)
VOD of the liver
Ascites, encephalopathy, hepatic failure
Graft-versus-host disease
Hemorrhage, malabsorption, strictures, webs
Cholestatic liver disease, protein-losing enteropathy
Lymphoproliferative syndromes
EBV-associated B cell proliferative disease
B cell lymphoma

HSV, herpes simplex virus; CMV, cytomegalovirus; GI, gastrointestinal; BMT, bone marrow transplantation; VOD, veno-occlusive disease; EBV, Epstein-Barr virus.

val bleeding, hypertrophy, inflammation, and focal ulcerations. Oral mucositis (stomatitis) is a severe inflammatory condition seen in the setting of recent chemotherapy, radiation therapy, or bone marrow transplantation. Treatment consists of appropriate antifungal, antiviral, or antibacterial therapy as well as viscous lidocaine and systemic analgesia. Esophageal lesions, usually caused by candidiasis or herpes viruses, may cause odynophagia, dysphagia, or bleeding (see Chapter 34). Peptic ulcers have been reported in a patient with hyperhistaminemia secondary to basophilic granulocytic leukemia.[136] Massive gastrointestinal hemorrhage may result from infectious lesions, agranulocytic ulcers, or primary leukemic lesions of the gastrointestinal tract. The treatment of bleeding gastric and colonic leukemic lesions with radiation therapy has occasionally met with success and has been advocated by some investigators.[137]

A dire complication, seen in 5% of patients with acute leukemia and 3% of those with chronic leukemia, is the development of an acute abdomen. Acute appendicitis, abdominal abscesses, and perforation are noted with increased frequency. *Necrotizing ileocecal enterocolitis* and leukemic *typhlitis* are relatively infrequent but life-threatening problems in neutropenic leukemia patients. Typhlitis complicates 6.5% of cases of acute myeloid leukemia and 4.6% of cases of acute lymphoblastic leukemia.[138] Typhlitis typically manifests after antineoplastic therapy and is usually associated with neutropenia.[139, 138] Although the cause of this condition is not entirely clear, the invasion of neutropenic ulcers by bacteria, most commonly by *Clostridium septicum*, has been implicated in its pathogenesis.[140] Cecal superinfection with fungi and with cytomegalovirus has also been associated with typhlitis. Patients usually present with fever, severe right lower quadrant pain, and occasionally with an acute abdomen. Bloody diarrhea accompanies typhlitis in 35% of patients.[141] The diagnosis can be inferred indirectly by the finding of symmetric cecal thickening on abdominal ultrasonography or CT.[142] Most patients with leukemic typhlitis can be managed conservatively with the administration of intravenous fluids, packed red blood cells, and, as needed, G-CSF, platelets, and broad-spectrum antibiotics. On rare occasions, surgery may be required if dire complications arise. Pseudomembranous colitis may complicate leukemia even in the absence of antibiotic therapy.[143] Other rare complications are listed in Table 29–2. Proctologic problems can include stercoral ulcers, neutropenic ulcers, and perirectal abscesses. The latter lesions occasionally have been managed successfully with broad-spectrum antibiotics in lieu of surgery for these acutely ill patients.[144]

Bone Marrow Transplantation

For discussion of bone marrow transplantation, see Chapter 27.[145–148]

Myeloproliferative Syndromes
(see also Chapter 82)

Agnogenic myelofibrosis and myeloid metaplasia (AMM) are myeloproliferative diseases characterized by hepatosplenomegaly, a leukoerythroblastic blood picture, and fibrotic marrow.[149] *Portal hypertension*, which occurs in 7% of patients with AMM, results from increased portal venous flow and from infiltration of the liver by foci of extramedullary hematopoiesis. Massive gastrointestinal hemorrhage complicates 5% of cases and most often is due to bleeding esophageal varices. Small intestinal hemorrhage from submucosal sites of extramedullary hematopoiesis has also been reported.[150] Increased thrombotic complications have been associated with AMM, polycythemia vera, and essential thrombocythemia.[151] As many as 42% of patients with hepatic vein thrombosis, or the *Budd-Chiari syndrome*, have an overt myelodysplastic syndrome, and one study[152] suggests that 80% of patients with hepatic vein thrombosis may have latent myeloproliferative abnormalities without overt disease (see Chapter 70).

Dysproteinemias

Multiple myeloma or plasma cell tumors may directly involve the gastrointestinal tract with *amyloidosis* or with local infiltration by *plasmacytomas*. Twenty-one percent of patients with amyloidosis have multiple myeloma.[153] As with gastrointestinal involvement by amyloidosis from other causes (see later), bowel wall infiltration and dysmotility underlie most clinical symptoms. Only about 5% of patients with malignant plasma cell disorders have plasmacytomas of the gut.[154] They can occur throughout the gastrointestinal tract from the oral cavity to the rectum and are associated with multiple myeloma in 25% of patients.[155] The tumors may be asymptomatic or may cause anorexia, vomiting, abdominal pain, or bleeding.

Gastrointestinal infiltration is found in patients with *Waldenström's macroglobulinemia*. Extracellular IgM is deposited in the lamina propria and in the mesenteric nodes; lacteals are dilated.[156] Small intestinal mucosal IgM deposits may stain weakly with periodic acid–Schiff, simulating the microscopic appearance of Whipple's disease. Lymphocytoid plasma cells also infiltrate the small intestine, and thickened folds, luminal dilation, and filling defects are noted on small bowel radiologic studies. Symptoms may include diarrhea, abdominal pain, flatulence, and weight loss. Coagulopathy may produce retroperitoneal or gastrointestinal hemorrhage.[157] Steatorrhea, decreased D-xylose and vitamin B_{12} absorption, and intestinal protein loss all have been recorded.[158]

The rare plasma cell proliferative disorder, gamma heavy-chain disease, has been associated with abdominal pain, weight loss, and gastric infiltration from malignant plasma cells.[159] Alpha heavy-chain disease is an immunoproliferative disorder of the secretory IgA system associated with poor sanitary conditions.[160] This disorder is characterized by plasma cell infiltration of the small intestinal lamina propria resulting in malabsorption (see Chapter 26).

Coagulation Disorders

Twenty percent of bleeding episodes in patients with hemophilia may originate in the gastrointestinal tract.[161] *von Willebrand's disease*, heparin or warfarin therapy, hepatic failure, qualitative or quantitative platelet defects, and other bleeding diatheses may also result in gastrointestinal hemorrhage or intramural bowel hematomas (Table 29–3). Radiologically, intramural bleeding can be recognized by thick-

Table 29–3 | **Causes of Intramural Bowel Hematomas**

Platelet Deficiency	**Pharmacotherapy**
Idiopathic thrombocytopenia	Heparin
Thrombotic thrombocytopenic purpura	Warfarin (Coumadin)
Hemolytic-uremic syndrome	Streptokinase/urokinase
Leukemia (see Table 29–2)	Tissue plasminogen activator
Hypersplenism (massive)	**Trauma**
Platelet Dysfunction	Blunt abdominal trauma
Glanzmann's thrombasthenia	Endoscopic manipulation
Bernard-Soulier syndrome	Forceful vomiting (esophagus)
Coagulation Defects	**Vasculitis**
Hemophilia	Polyarteritis nodosa
von Willebrand's disease	Henoch-Schönlein purpura
Dysfibrinogemia	Ehlers-Danlos syndrome
Disseminated intravascular coagulation	
Hepatic failure	

ened mucosal folds, rigidity, luminal narrowing (Fig. 29–5), and intragastric masses. Intestinal obstruction and intussusception may result.

Hemolytic-uremic syndrome (HUS) consists of a triad of acute renal failure, microangiopathic hemolytic anemia, and thrombocytopenia without the consumption of humoral clotting factors through defibrination. In children, idiopathic, sporadic, and epidemic cases have variously been described. In adults, HUS occurs in conjunction with complications during childbirth[162] or with various soft tissue tumors, especially after chemotherapy with mitomycin C or bleomycin.[163] More commonly, adult HUS is preceded by a mild prodromal illness, and approximately 90% of these prodromes have gastrointestinal symptoms.[164] Enteric pathogens associated with the HUS prodrome ("HUS colitis") include *Shigella, Salmonella, Yersinia, Campylobacter,* and the "hemorrhagic" 0157:H7 strain of *Escherichia coli* (see Chapter 96).[164–168] One recent prospective study demonstrated that antibiotic therapy of *E. coli* 0157:H7 with antibiotics increases the risk of development of HUS in children, presumably through the antibiotic-induced release of preformed bacterial toxins.[169] Once HUS appears, colonic involvement is common owing to microangiopathic thrombosis of submucosal vessels and intramural hemorrhage.[170] Pancreatitis has also been described.[171] Radiographic abnormalities include mucosal irregularities, intestinal dilation, filling defects, bowel wall edema, and findings that may resemble those of idiopathic ulcerative colitis, or vasculitis.[172] Because HUS is usually self-limited, therapy consists of hemodialysis and supportive gastrointestinal care. Severe complications may include toxic megacolon, rectal prolapse, transmural necrosis with perforation, or colonic stricture.[173]

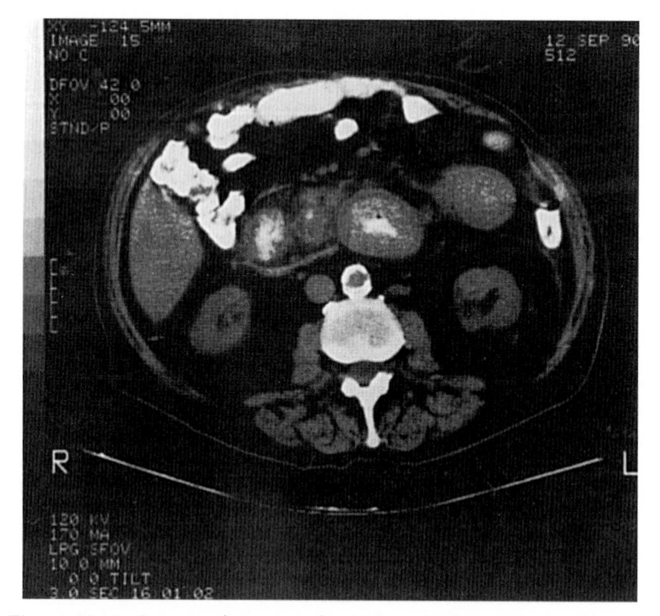

Figure 29–5. Computed tomographic (CT) scan demonstrating an intramural hematoma of the third portion of the duodenum in a patient treated with warfarin (Coumadin). The contrast-filled duodenal lumen is circumferentially narrowed by a submucosal infiltrate with the same CT density as that of blood. The hematoma resolved with conservative measures and with a reduction in warfarin dosage. (Courtesy of J.C. Ryan, M.D.)

Thrombotic thrombocytopenic purpura (TTP) is an idiopathic disorder consisting of thrombocytopenia, microangiopathic hemolytic anemia (without significant consumption of clotting factors), fever, renal insufficiency, and profound neurologic dysfunction. Compared with HUS, CNS symptoms predominate in TTP. Twenty percent of patients have nonspecific abdominal complaints. The bleeding diathesis of TTP can lead to gastrointestinal hemorrhage, but TTP may also cause thrombosis of intestinal vessels that resembles HUS, both clinically and pathologically. *Acute colitis, cholecystitis,* and *pancreatitis* all have been described.[174, 175] Therapy of the TTP-HUS syndrome using plasma exchange, with or without prednisone, antiplatelet agents, or IgG infusion is successful in the treatment of this condition in more than 90% of cases.[176, 177]

Red Blood Cell Dyscrasias

Sickle cell anemia is an autosomal recessive disorder of hemoglobin synthesis. Eight percent of African Americans are heterozygous for the hemoglobin S trait and homozygotes comprise 0.2% of African Americans. Patients with *sickle cell anemia* and other hemoglobinopathies may develop splenic infarction and liver disease, likely from ischemic injury due to sickling and hypercoagulation from the relative protein C and S deficiencies seen in patients with sickle cell anemia (see Chapter 82). Chronic anemia due to hemolysis is typically present and predisposes to bilirubin elevation and to the formation of pigmented gallstones. Sickle crisis, an acute manifestation of this disease, is characterized by severe skeletal pain and fever. Abdominal pain is also commonly present, and it is important to distinguish vaso-occlusive crises from surgical conditions such as cholecystitis, bowel infarction, and appendicitis. Abdominal pain from vaso-occlusive crises tends to be more diffuse and associated with remote pain such as limb and chest pain. The pain of vaso-occlusive crises is typically relieved with hydration and oxygen within 48 hours.[178]

Patients with *thalassemia* typically develop hepatomegaly from extramedullary hematopoiesis. These patients can also develop iron overload due to multiple transfusions, with the resulting end-organ dysfunction in the liver, gonads, and pancreas. The early parenteral use of the iron-chelating agent desferoxamine, in an amount proportional to the iron load, has been shown to be effective in halting the progression of fibrosis in patients with thalassemia major.[179] However, deferiprone, an orally acting iron-chelating agent, has not been as effective in reducing the body iron burden and may worsen the fibrosis.[180] Further studies are needed to better define the role of orally active iron chelators in thalassemic patients with iron overload. Patients with hereditary defects in red blood cell cytoskeletal proteins causing *hereditary spherocytosis* and *hereditary elliptocytosis* have diminished red blood cell survival, leading to an increased incidence of pigmented gallstones.

ENDOCRINE DISEASES (Table 29–4)

Diabetes Mellitus

GENERAL CONSIDERATIONS. Many patients with diabetes mellitus develop autonomic nervous system dysfunction and *diabetic autonomic neuropathy* (DAN). This syndrome is caused by one or more metabolic abnormalities that result from prolonged hyperglycemia. Clinical symptoms of enteric DAN are more common in older patients with long-standing insulin-dependent diabetes, poor glucose control, and symptoms of cardiovascular or peripheral neuropathy. Symptoms include constipation, abdominal pain, nausea, vomiting, dysphagia, diarrhea, and fecal incontinence. Although motility disturbances are common in these patients, they do not correlate well with the presence or severity of symptoms. This suggests that other manifestations of DAN may play a role in the development of symptoms.

In experimental animals, enteric DAN primarily affects the sympathetic innervation of the small intestine and proximal colon. Classic experiments in diabetic animals have demonstrated axonal neuropathic changes in the sympathetic nerves supplying the gut. Damage to the vagus nerve seems not to be as profound as damage to the sympathetic ganglia, postganglionic sympathetic nerves, and intramural adrenergic plexuses.[181] Thus, diminished motility seen in DAN may be due to cholinergic denervation and alteration of sympathetic nerve function. Injury to the sympathetic ganglia and nerves may also explain the attenuated response to α_2-adrenoreceptor agonists, which normally stimulate intestinal fluid and electrolyte absorption.[182] Abnormalities in gut motility may also be due to relative deficiencies of stimulatory neurotransmitters, such as neuropeptide Y and MET-enkephalin.[183, 184]

ESOPHAGEAL DYSFUNCTION. Motor activity of the esophagus is abnormal in most diabetics, particularly those with gastroparesis.[185] Abnormal esophageal motor activity is so common in patients with DAN that its absence in persons with gastrointestinal symptoms should cast doubt on the diagnosis of diabetic gastroenteropathy.[186] These abnormal motor findings include the absence of coordinated peristaltic activity and the presence of many low-amplitude, double-peaked, and tertiary contractions.[187] Such esophageal disturbances are frequently asymptomatic, although dysphagia can be seen in as many as one third of patients. Diminished resting pressure of the LES may be responsible for occasional complaints of heartburn.[188] The absence of symptoms in many patients with abnormal manometric studies may be due to sensory diabetic neuropathy.

GASTRIC DYSFUNCTION. Abnormal gastric motility (see also Chapters 8 and 37) results in disordered gastric emptying, or gastroparesis diabeticorum (GD), which affects as many as 58% of diabetic patients.[189] In this disorder, the normal physiology of gastric emptying, largely under the control of the vagus nerve, is grossly disturbed. Liquid emptying may be normal, but solid emptying is frequently delayed. There is an increased frequency of postcibal antral dysrhythmias such as antral tachygastria. Phase 3 contractions of the IMMC, which normally stimulate antral contractions, are frequently absent, resulting in poor antral grinding. Furthermore, maintenance of the gastroduodenal pressure gradient, as well as receptive relaxation of the stomach, is abnormal.[190] Prolonged pyloric contractions (pylorospasm) may cause functional resistance to gastric outflow.[191] The pathophysiology of these motor disturbances is unclear. Experimentally induced acute hyperglycemia can cause delayed gastric emptying in diabetic patients as well as in normal volunteers.[192] As noted earlier, vagal parasympathetic function, which is involved in gastric emptying, may not be entirely normal. High plasma levels of the gut peptide motilin are reported in patients with GD.[192] Because motilin stimulates the initiation of phase 3 activity, the elevation of this peptide in diabetic patients with GD may, in part, be compensatory. This is consistent with the observation that the treatment of GD with prokinetic agents is associated with a fall in plasma motilin levels.[192]

Symptoms of GD include epigastric distress, nausea, bloating, postprandial vomiting, and early satiety. Markedly delayed gastric emptying may make the regulation of blood glucose levels difficult. Hyperglycemia further impairs gastric emptying and may accelerate the onset of diabetic ketoacidosis, particularly when it is associated with severe vomiting. GD may also lead to the formation of bezoars. Although many diabetics have abnormal gastric emptying, few develop overt clinical symptoms. Furthermore, an occasional patient may have symptoms but little or no delay in gastric emptying.

The diagnosis of GD should be strongly suspected from the history. Physical examination may reveal gastric dilation with a succussion splash. A saline load test is not a sensitive test in GD, because liquid emptying is frequently normal. The usual method for diagnosis is exclusion of structural lesions by esophagogastroduodenoscopy or by standard barium radiographic examination. Such studies should be followed by more quantitative measurements of the degree of delay. Radiolabeled scintigraphy is the preferred way to confirm the diagnosis and to quantify the response to therapy.[190] When interpreting these studies, it should be noted that anticholinergics, tricyclic antidepressants, benzodiazepines, and ganglionic-blocking agents all may contribute to delayed emptying in these patients.

The management of GD is complex. Improvement in the control of blood glucose levels may accelerate emptying. Antinausea drugs are not usually effective. Indeed, they may have adverse effects because of the anticholinergic side effects of most phenothiazine preparations. Prokinetic agents, which increase gastric motor activity, are frequently used to treat GD. Metoclopramide (10 mg, 30 minutes before each meal and at bedtime) is a dopamine antagonist that also stimulates acetylcholine release in the myenteric plexus. Domperidone (10 to 20 mg four times a day), which is not

Table 29–4 | **Effects of Endocrine Diseases on the Gastrointestinal System**

DISEASE	ABNORMALITY/ASSOCIATION	GASTROINTESTINAL MANIFESTATION
Hyperthyroidism	Round cell mucosal infiltrate	Superficial gastritis, steatorrhea
	Accelerated intestinal transit	Diarrhea
	Ulcerative colitis (3.8%)	Bloody diarrhea
	Minor histologic changes: liver	Transaminase elevation, mild indirect hyperbilirubinemia
	Rare chronic hepatitis (with thyroiditis)	Increased ALP, transaminases
Hypothyroidism	Impaired LES function	Reflux esophagitis
	Gastric hypomotility	Bezoars
	Decreased intestinal transit	Constipation, fecal impaction, volvulus, pseudo-obstruction, rectal prolapse, diarrhea, steatorrhea (bacterial overgrowth)
	Liver test abnormalities (50%)	Normal histology
	Primary biliary cirrhosis	Hepatic cirrhosis
	Canada-Cronkhite syndrome	Intestinal polyps (see Chapter 114)
	Celiac sprue	Diarrhea, steatorrhea
	Familial polyendocrine failure	Esophageal candidiasis, adrenal insufficiency, hypogonadism, diabetes, hypothyroidism
MCT	Increased calcitonin	Watery diarrhea (increased intestinal secretion due to calcitonin?)
	MEN 2A, 2B	Pheochromocytoma (see below), mucosal neuromas, ileus, megacolon
Adrenal insufficiency	Corticosteroid deficiency	Nausea, vomiting, anorexia, diarrhea, malabsorption
	Familial polyendocrine failure	Esophageal candidiasis, hypothyroidism, hypogonadism, diabetes, hypoparathyroidism
Pheochromocytomas	Increased catecholamines	Paralytic ileus, megacolon
	Cholelithiasis	Biliary colic, cholecystitis
	MEN 2A	MCT (see above)
Hypercortisolism (Cushing's disease)	Increased pituitary ACTH	Gastric ulceration
Acromegaly	Increased pituitary GH	Colorectal polyps
Panhypopituitarism	Adrenal insufficiency	As for adrenal insufficiency
Hyperparathyroidism	Increased serum calcium	Constipation, nausea, vomiting
	Peptic ulceration (5–15%)	Bleeding, abdominal pain, perforation
	Pancreatitis (1–2%)	Acute pancreatitis
	MEN-1	Gastrinoma, VIPoma, etc. (see Chapter 51)
Hypoparathyroidism	Familial polyendocrine failure	Esophageal candidiasis, hypothyroidism, hypogonadism, diabetes, adrenal insufficiency
	Malabsorption (4–29%)	Diarrhea, steatorrhea
	Intestinal lymphangiectasia	Protein-losing enteropathy
Diabetes mellitus	Esophageal dysmotility	Dysphagia, reflux esophagitis
	Esophageal candidiasis	Odynophagia, dysphagia
	Gastroparesis/gastritis	Nausea, vomiting, gastric outlet obstruction, bezoars
	Small intestinal dysmotility	Bacterial overgrowth, malabsorption, diarrhea
	Impaired intestinal fluid reabsorption	"Diabetic" diarrhea
	Colonic dysmotility	Constipation, megacolon, fecal incontinence
	Intestinal ischemia	Ischemic colitis, bowel infarction
	Pancreatic disease	Acute pancreatitis, pancreatic carcinoma
	Cholelithiasis	Biliary sepsis
	Sclerosing cholangitis	Biliary obstruction, sepsis
	Hepatic steatonecrosis	Abnormal liver tests, hepatic fibrosis
	Hepatocellular carcinoma	2.5-fold increased risk
	Diabetic radiculopathy	Unexplained abdominal pain
	Familial polyendocrine failure	Candidiasis, hypothyroidism, hypogonadism, hypoparathyroidism, adrenal insufficiency
	Celiac sprue	Diarrhea, steatorrhea

ACTH, adrenocorticotropic hormone; ALP, alkaline phosphatase; GH, growth hormone; LES, lower esophageal sphincter; MCT, medullary carcinoma of the thyroid; MEN, multiple endocrine neoplasia; VIP, vasoactive intestinal polypeptide.

available in the United States, has a similar mechanism of action.[193] These agents increase gastric tone and accelerate gastric emptying in GD, coordinating these effects with pyloric relaxation and duodenal peristalsis.[194] The beneficial effects of these agents may diminish after 4 to 6 weeks, although patients may continue to be symptom free.[195] Metoclopramide has a central effect on vagal function that promotes emptying. It suppresses the vomiting center as well. Metoclopramide should be prescribed in courses of 4 to 12 weeks, and intravenous use should be limited to 1 or 2 days because of adverse CNS effects, including drowsiness, restlessness, and, rarely, symptoms and signs of parkinsonism. Domperidone does not cross the blood-brain barrier in appreciable amounts and has fewer CNS side effects. In some patients, treatment with either agent leads to increased prolactin secretion, breast tenderness, and galactorrhea. Metoclopramide may lower the seizure threshold in persons with epilepsy, and the intravenous (but not oral) administration of domperidone may cause cardiac arrhythmias.[194] A third prokinetic drug is cisapride which, although efficacious in GD, has recently been restricted due to life-threatening proarrhythmic cardiac side effects.

The antibiotic erythromycin, a motilin agonist, has been found to be effective in accelerating gastric emptying in GD.[196] Intravenous infusion of erythromycin (200 mg over 5 to 10 minutes every 8 hours) is effective in the acute setting.[190] A recent meta-analysis suggests that the beneficial effects of oral erythromycin on gastric emptying and on symptoms are superior to those seen with either metaclopramide, domperidine, or cisapride.[197] Unfortunately, tachyphylaxis to the effects of erythromycin remains a significant problem and remains the object of pharmacologic research.

Acute erosive *gastritis* is common in diabetic ketoacidosis and is frequently accompanied by bleeding. The incidence of *H. pylori* infection may be increased in diabetic patients, but the association between diabetes and *H. pylori* has recently been called into question.[198, 199] The incidence of duodenal ulcer in diabetes, however, is lower than expected. *Autoimmune chronic gastritis* and *gastric atrophy* may also be seen with long-standing diabetes. These conditions are often associated with significant titers of circulating anti–parietal cell and antithyroid antibodies explaining the higher rates of pernicious anemia and hypothyroidism in diabetic patients.

DIABETIC DIARRHEA. Diarrhea is a common symptom of autonomic neuropathy, affecting 3.7% of diabetic patients, predominantly affecting type 1 diabetics (see also Chapter 9).[200] A common cause of diarrhea in diabetic patients is drug therapy with metformin, but diarrhea or increased stool frequency due to celiac sprue, bacterial overgrowth, or fecal incontinence can be seen in up to half of patients in tertiary referral diabetes practices.[200, 201] True diabetic diarrhea frequently affects patients with dyspeptic symptoms and GD, and it appears to be more common in men than in women. It may be particularly troublesome at night. Diabetic diarrhea occurs mostly in patients with poorly controlled insulin-dependent diabetes who also have evidence of diabetic peripheral and autonomic neuropathy. Associated steatorrhea is common and does not necessarily imply a concomitant gastrointestinal disease. The diarrhea is often intermittent and painless, and it may alternate with periods of normal bowel movement or with constipation.

The pathogenesis of diabetic diarrhea is unclear. Marked abnormalities are found in the motor pattern of the small intestine. Phase 3 contractions are shorter, and phase 2 activity of the stomach and upper small intestine is abnormal. No significant differences between diabetic patients and control subjects, however, can be observed in mouth-to-cecum or whole-gut transit times. In patients treated with prokinetic agents, fasting IMMC and fed motor patterns in the small intestine may be normalized, but the symptomatic improvement of diarrhea is no better than with placebo.[202] As discussed earlier, sympathetic denervation of the gut is common in diabetic patients with autonomic neuropathy. Because adrenergic nerves normally stimulate intestinal reabsorption of fluids and electrolytes, decreased intestinal resorption, rather than intestinal dysmotility, may underlie the pathogenesis of diabetic diarrhea.

The management of diabetic diarrhea is difficult, but strict control of blood glucose levels may help. Because gastrointestinal adrenergic function is impaired in autonomic neuropathy, adrenergic agonists may stimulate intestinal absorption of fluids and electrolytes. In addition, they may partially correct the motility disturbances of DAN. The α_2-adrenergic agonist clonidine (0.1 to 0.6 mg twice daily) may be successful in the therapy of diabetic diarrhea, presumably by reversing the peripheral adrenergic resorptive abnormalities. Because the antihypertensive effects of clonidine are mediated through the CNS, diabetic patients with severe autonomic neuropathy may not necessarily experience worsening of preexisting postural hypotension during therapy. Clonidine does not alter diabetic control or renal function. If the medication needs to be withdrawn, it should be done slowly to avoid "rebound" hypertension.

The long-acting somatostatin analog octreotide (50 to 75 μg subcutaneously, twice daily) may be used in the treatment of refractory diabetic diarrhea.[203, 204] It may, however, predispose to intestinal bacterial overgrowth owing to decreased small bowel transit time, and it may aggravate steatorrhea by inhibiting pancreatic exocrine function. Symptomatic measures that may be employed include the prescription of codeine sulfate (30 mg every 6 to 8 hours), diphenoxylate with atropine (Lomotil), or loperamide. In some patients, psyllium hydrophilic mucilloid (Metamucil) may be helpful.

FECAL INCONTINENCE. A troublesome symptom of DAN is fecal incontinence (see Chapter 11). Incontinence often coincides with the onset of diabetic diarrhea, but in most cases the total stool volume is normal. Steatorrhea is present in as many as 30% of cases.[205] Autonomic dysfunction is thought to be responsible for the impairment of both normal sphincter resting tone and reflexive internal sphincter relaxation during defecation. Management is empiric and includes biofeedback training and antidiarrheal therapy.[206] In some patients incontinence remits spontaneously.

CONSTIPATION AND MEGACOLON. The colon is frequently involved in diabetes mellitus. The most common gastrointestinal complaint of diabetics is constipation, related in some cases to autonomic neuropathy.[207–209] Occasionally, severe constipation with megacolon may be encountered. Rarely, chronic intestinal pseudo-obstruction may result.[209] High-fiber diets have not proved to be of great benefit, and anorectal myectomy has not been adequately evaluated. Complications of severe constipation include stercoral ulcer, perforation volvulus, anal overflow diarrhea. Treatment is aimed at symptomatic relief with enemas, laxatives, and cathartics.

UNEXPLAINED ABDOMINAL PAIN. Diabetic *radiculopathy* or diabetic plexus neuropathy of thoracic nerve roots may cause otherwise unexplained upper abdominal pain in patients with diabetic neuropathy. Pain may be associated with anorexia and weight loss, at times suggesting intra-abdominal malignancy. The diagnosis may be strengthened by an abnormal EMG of the anterior abdominal wall muscles when compared with an EMG of thoracic paraspinal muscles.[210]

LIVER AND BILIARY TREE. Lithogenic bile composition and stasis of bile in the gallbladder may contribute to stone formation in patients with diabetes, and it is generally thought that diabetics have an increased incidence of *cholelithiasis*. As with infections in general, hepatobiliary sepsis tends to be more severe in diabetic patients. In addition to severe bouts of cholecystitis and ascending cholangitis, unusual infections with gas-producing organisms and rare abscesses due to *Yersinia enterocolitica* have been reported.[211, 212] An increased incidence of *sclerosing cholangitis* has also been reported in diabetic patients.[213] Despite the increased severity of cholecystitis and cholangitis in diabetic patients, however, it is not recommended that diabetic patients with asymptomatic gallstones undergo "prophylactic" cholecystectomy.

The most prominent abnormality of the liver in diabetes mellitus is *steatosis*. It is present in as many as 78% of patients. When present, it reflects poor long-term glucose control. With increasing amounts of fat, nonalcoholic steatohepatitis can be seen, with Mallory's hyaline, increased numbers of glycogen nuclei, and fibrosis (see Chapter 72). In unusual cases of steatonecrosis, patients may be jaundiced and have severe hepatic damage. An association has been described between steatonecrosis and type 5 hyperlipoproteinemia in insulin-dependent diabetes.[214] *Hepatocellular carcinoma* is 2.5 times more frequent in diabetic patients.

PANCREATIC DISEASE. The prevalence of pancreatic disease (see Chapter 49) and pancreatic insufficiency is increased in patients with diabetes. *Acute pancreatitis* is twice as frequent in young, type 1 diabetics. Acute pancreatitis causing ketoacidosis has a particularly serious prognosis, with a high mortality rate.[215, 216] The incidence of clinically apparent chronic pancreatitis, however, is not increased. Adenocarcinoma of the pancreas is two to four times more common in diabetic alcoholics than in the general population.[217] In some cases, it is difficult to determine whether the diabetes antedates or is caused by the malignancy, and recent data suggest that the relationship between pancreatic cancer and diabetes may be an epiphenomenon and that diabetes is not a risk factor for pancreatic malignancy.[218]

Thyroid Disease

HYPERTHYROIDISM. Hyperthyroidism may underlie a number of important gastrointestinal symptoms, owing to its own effects on almost all organs of the gastrointestinal system. In addition, these symptoms sometimes occur in the absence of the cardinal features of hyperthyroidism ("apathetic" hyperthyroidism). Apathetic thyrotoxicosis may present with protracted abdominal pain, recurrent vomiting, marked weight loss, and altered bowel habits. Patients affected by thyroid storm may display a constellation of symptoms involving high fever, marked tachycardia, agitation, and delirium along with intestinal manifestations that include acute abdominal pain, vomiting, jaundice and severe diarrhea.

Hyperthyroidism clearly affects gastrointestinal motility. Excess thyroid hormone may cause myopathy, resulting in dysfunction of the striated muscles of the pharynx and the cervical esophagus. This is a potential mechanism that may explain dysphagia.[219] Dysphagia is a rare manifestation of hyperthyroidism and can be readily reversible with correction of the thyrotoxic state.[220]

More than 25% of hyperthyroid patients have mild to moderate diarrhea. Intestinal transit time inversely correlates with thyroid hormone levels,[221] whereas gastric emptying is not significantly increased with the hyperthyroid state.[221, 222] Although hypermotility is the most likely explanation for diarrhea, thyroid hormone itself can induce secretory diarrhea by increasing intracellular cyclic adenosine monophosphate, akin to the actions of cholera toxin and VIP. Hyperthyroid-associated diarrhea (and steatorrhea, when present) readily responds to treatment with propylthiouracil. Treatment with propylthiouracil can lead to a euthyroid state with concomitant normalization of orocecal transit times and relief of gastrointestinal symptoms.[223]

Infrequently, hyperthyroidism may coexist with *ulcerative colitis*. Hyperthyroidism may intensify the symptoms of ulcerative colitis, and it may impair the response to therapy.[224] Hyperthyroidism is often associated with minor histologic changes in the liver.[225] Mild elevation of liver enzymes are frequently observed, especially alkaline phosphatase (40% of patients).[226, 227] Less commonly, transaminase elevations are present. Mild elevations of liver enzymes can also commonly be observed with propylthiouracil therapy. These effects are often transient and subclinical. It appears that propylthiouracil may be continued with caution unless overt hepatitis develops.[228]

HYPOTHYROIDISM. *Hypothyroidism* is most commonly caused by an autoimmune mechanism or as a consequence of therapy for hyperthyroidism. It is occasionally seen in association with other diseases such as *ulcerative colitis*,[224] *pernicious anemia*,[229] and *primary biliary cirrhosis*.[230] Hypothyroidism is seen in approximately 20% of patients with primary biliary cirrhosis.[231] Rarely, *celiac disease* or *diabetes mellitus* is also associated with *autoimmune thyroiditis*.

Hypothyroidism is associated with hypomotility of the gastrointestinal tract. Disturbances of esophageal peristalsis and gastroesophageal sphincter function resulting in reflux and esophagitis may be seen with severe hypothyroidism. Replacement therapy can normalize sphincter tone and restore peristalsis. Hypothyroidism also may result in gastric and intestinal hypomotility. In rare instances, phytobezoars may form and result in gastrointestinal obstructions.[232] Severely impaired colonic motility may manifest with constipation, obstipation, sigmoid volvulus, rectal prolapse, fecal impaction, and rarely megacolon. Hypothyroidism can be a cause of ileus and should be considered as an etiology of pseudo-obstruction.[233] Diarrhea, although rare in hypothyroidism, may be due to bacterial overgrowth from bowel hypomotility. Antibiotic treatment can result in resolution of diarrheal symptoms.[234] Routine liver function tests are mildly abnormal in approximately 50% of hypothyroid patients, whereas liver histology is usually normal. Hypothyroidism may cause ascites with high serum-to-ascites albumin gradients (SAAG $>$ 1.1 g/dL) and high-protein content.[235] Interferon-α treatment for chronic hepatitis C may induce autoimmune thyroiditis with hypothyroidism or hyperthyroidism, especially in predisposed patients.[236] Myxedema has also been found in association with *Cronkhite-Canada syndrome* (see Chapter 114).[237]

MEDULLARY CARCINOMA OF THE THYROID. *Medullary carcinoma of the thyroid* (MCT) is a calcitonin-producing tumor of the C cells of the thyroid gland. Diarrhea is seen in one third of patients with MCT. Diarrhea may occur presumably due to the effects of high circulating calcitonin on the gut.[238] MCT may also produce VIP and prostaglandins, which contribute to diarrhea. Decreased colonic transit time due to as yet unknown humoral agents may also underlie the diarrhea of MCT.[239] MCT is also associated with multiple endocrine neoplasia (MEN) syndromes 2A and 2B. These syndromes can be complicated by hyperparathyroidism and pheochromocytomas and in MEN 2B with mucosal neuromas.

Adrenal Disease

Adrenal insufficiency, or Addison's disease, is associated with gastrointestinal symptoms and/or pathology in more than half of cases. A constellation of symptoms including anorexia, weight loss, nausea, vomiting, diarrhea, and abdominal pain may be present. Cyclical vomiting in children may rarely be due to adrenal insufficiency.[240] Malabsorption and diarrhea seen in some patients with Addison's disease are apparently due to functional defects in enterocytes that can be readily reversed with the administration of corticosteroids. *Atrophic gastritis, achlorhydria*, and *pernicious anemia* may be present in association with autoimmune Addison's disease.

Pheochromocytomas are tumors arising from the adrenal medulla and chromaffin tissue that secrete high levels of catecholamines. The humoral effects of high circulating levels of catecholamines may result in ileus or pseudo-obstruction.[241] Gastrointestinal manifestations of pheochromocytoma also include ischemic colitis, diarrhea, acute abdominal pain, and, rarely, gastrointestinal bleeding.[242] For unclear reasons, pheochromocytoma is associated with an increased incidence of cholelithiasis. Some patients also have MEN 2A or 2B syndrome (see earlier).

Pituitary Disease

Pituitary disorders infrequently affect the gastrointestinal tract, except in association with MEN 1 syndrome. *Hypercortisolism*, caused by the inappropriate secretion of corticotropin in Cushing's disease, may be associated with an increased incidence of gastric ulceration when concomitant NSAIDs are used.[243] *Panhypopituitarism* may present with addisonian crisis, with hypotension, nausea, vomiting, abdominal pain, and diarrhea. The excessive secretion of pituitary growth hormone results in *acromegaly*. The incidence of adenomatous colonic polyps may be increased in patients with acromegaly.[244] One study showed that patients with acromegaly also present with proximal colonic polyps at a younger age, and this increased incidence of colonic polyps appeared to affect only male patients with acromegaly.[245] Although a more recent prospective study did not show a significantly increased incidence of colonic neoplasia in patients with acromegaly, more right-sided polyps and polyps with advanced histology were found in these patients.[246]

Parathyroid Disease

HYPERPARATHYROIDISM. Gastrointestinal problems are common in patients with *hyperparathyroidism*.[247] Most common complaints are constipation, diffuse abdominal discomfort, or nausea and vomiting. A minority (5% to 15%) have peptic ulcer disease, and a small percentage (1% to 2%) develop pancreatitis. An association between pancreatitis and hyperparathyroidism has been reported with subsequent remission of pancreatitis after parathyroidectomy.[248] Severe pancreatitis may also occur immediately following parathyroidectomy.[249] Gastrointestinal symptoms associated with hypercalcemia include nausea, vomiting, anorexia, and abdominal pain. Some patients with hyperparathyroidism have MEN 1 or 2 syndrome (see earlier).

HYPOPARATHYROIDISM. *Hypoparathyroidism* with hypocalcemia may be associated with malabsorption and mild to moderate steatorrhea. Constipation, and in rare instances, even pseudo-obstruction may be important gastrointestinal disturbances in this disease. In the *familial polyendocrine failure syndrome* (candidiasis endocrinopathy, or polyendocrine autoimmune disease, type 1), patients have hypoparathyroidism, adrenal insufficiency, hypogonadism, and, in many cases, diabetes mellitus. From 4% to 29% also have malabsorption. Varying degrees of gastric atrophy with anti–parietal cell antibodies, hypochlorhydria, hepatitis, dental enamel hypoplasia, and severe oral and esophageal candidiasis are also seen.[250] *Intestinal lymphangiectasia* with *protein-losing enteropathy* has also been reported in association with malabsorption and hypoparathyroidism.[251] Idiopathic hypoparathyroidism may also coexist with *celiac disease* likely due to autoimmune reactivity. When this occurs, a gluten-free diet may lead to the disappearance of parathyroid immunoreactivity.[252]

RENAL DISEASES

Renal Failure

Upper gastrointestinal tract symptoms are common in patients with chronic renal failure (CRF). Anorexia, singultus, nausea, vomiting, epigastric pain, and heartburn are common manifestations of azotemia. Although prior studies showed that patients who receive hemodialysis have no demonstrable abnormality in gastric emptying, whether symptomatic or not, a recent study demonstrated a significant decrease in gastric emptying in dyspeptic patients compared with non-dyspeptic patients.[253] Although the prevalence of peptic ulcer is only 2%, which is not significantly different from that in the general population,[254] gastritis, duodenitis, and mucosal erosions are commonly seen.[254] A variety of data suggests that hyperacidity, hypergastrinemia, and *H. pylori* play no major roles in the pathogenesis of uremic gastritis, although these data have recently been called into question.[255] Impaired mucosal cytoprotection has been postulated but not proved. Also seen on esophagogastroduodenoscopy are esophagitis, Brunner's gland hyperplasia, gastric fold thickening, and nodular duodenitis (which resolves after transplantation) and angiodysplasia.[256–258]

It is possible that angiodysplastic lesions in the upper and lower gastrointestinal tract are no more common in patients with CRF than in the general population but are discovered more frequently because of their greater tendency to bleed. Three mechanisms by which renal failure may contribute to the generation of these lesions include (1) functional failure of the precapillary sphincter secondary to volume overload and submucosal venous obstruction, leading to vascular ectasia; (2) a low-flow state related to dialysis followed by reactive hyperemia, resulting in eventual angiodysplasia[259]; and (3) potassium- or gastrin-mediated reduction of precapillary arteriolar tone, causing pathologic arteriolar dilation.[260, 261] Clinically, upper gastrointestinal tract bleeding is a common cause of death in dialysis patients.[262] Angiodysplastic lesions are much more likely to bleed in patients with CRF than in patients with normal renal function,[263] perhaps because of uremic platelet dysfunction. In a recent series of CRF patients with upper gastrointestinal hemorrhage, gastric ulcer (37%) and duodenal ulcer (23%) were the two most common bleeding lesions, but angiodysplasia of the upper gastrointestinal tract was the cause of bleeding in 13% of patients.[264] In contrast, angiodysplasia was only responsible for 1.3% of upper intestinal tract bleeding in control patients.[264] In CRF patients with recurrent hemorrhage, angiodysplasia was the most frequent cause of bleeding.[264] Angiodysplasia as a cause of bleeding was most closely associated with the duration of renal failure and the need for hemodialysis in patients with CRF.[264] In CRF, peptic lesions may be managed successfully with standard medical treatments in appropriate doses (see Chapter 40), and angiodysplasia may be treated with laser, electrocoagulation, or surgery (see Chapter 120). Small intestinal complications of CRF include ileus, ulceration, and nonocclusive ischemic bowel disease.[265–267] Malabsorption has been reported in uremic patients and may result from bacterial overgrowth.[267] In addition, exocrine pancreatic insufficiency has been documented in a number of hemodialysis patients.[268] The cause of the condition is not known, but patients may improve clinically with pancreatic enzyme replacement.

Patients with CRF appear more likely to develop colonic perforation from ruptured diverticula, fecalomas (secondary to the use of aluminum-containing antacids or barium), or cecal ulcers that may bleed profusely.[269] Life-threatening hemorrhage from rectal ulcers has also been reported.[270] Colonic intussusception and ileus are also encountered in CRF. The diarrhea experienced by some patients with CRF appears to be related to abnormal bile acid metabolism.[271] Duodenal and fecal levels of deoxycholate are decreased; those of ursodeoxycholate are increased. It appears that uremia impairs bile acid deconjugation and dehydroxylation by normal intestinal flora, decreasing deoxycholate levels. Low ileal deoxycholate content may promote ileal bacterial overgrowth with anaerobes and colonic organisms. These species generate increased levels of unusual bile acids such as ursodeoxycholate, which correlate with the presence of diarrhea in patients with CRF.[271]

Nephrotic syndrome can produce a low-protein ascites with a low SAAG. Because nephrotic syndrome is associated with the renal loss of IgG, patients with nephrosis have a propensity toward infections with encapsulated organisms. Although patients with spontaneous bacterial peritonitis are typically infected with gram-negative coliforms, pediatric patients with nephrotic syndrome and ascites may have an increased incidence of bacterial peritonitis owing to encapsulated organisms such *Pneumococcus*.[272]

Nephrogenic ascites is an entity that manifests as refractory ascites with end-stage renal disease where nephrotic syndrome, portal hypertension, infectious causes and malignant processes have been excluded (see Chapter 78). Most patients with nephrogenic ascites are undergoing hemodialysis. The ascites typically has a high-protein content and a low SAAG, suggesting that altered peritoneal membrane permeability or impaired fluid resorption may underlie the pathogenesis of this condition.[273] Treatment of nephrogenic ascites includes aggressive (daily) hemodialysis, which alleviates the condition in up to 75% of patients within 3 weeks.[273] The institution of peritoneal dialysis can successfully treat refractory cases, but renal transplantation is the definitive treatment of nephrogenic ascites. In patients with a long history of peritoneal dialysis, chronic peritonitis has been implicated as a cause of ascites.[274] Total nephrectomy and surgical removal of diseased peritoneal tissue, as well as peritoneovenous shunts, have been used successfully to reduce excess fluid.[275]

Renal Transplantation

See Chapter 27 for a complete discussion of renal transplantation.

NEUROLOGIC DISEASES

Neurologic diseases are frequently associated with gastrointestinal symptoms. Some of the more common disorders affecting the CNS, spinal cord, cranial nerves, autonomic nervous system, neuromuscular junction, and musculature are presented in Table 29–5 and in the following sections.

Neurogenic Abdominal Pain

Neurogenic causes of abdominal pain originate in either the CNS or peripheral nervous system. Central neurogenic abdominal pain can result from *abdominal migraines*. Although classic migraine headaches are often associated with nausea and vomiting, abdominal migraine is a migraine variant characterized by recurrent gastrointestinal symptoms, including vomiting and epigastric pain.[276] It is often seen in children and is not always associated with headache. The pathophysiology of the gastrointestinal symptoms is unclear, and some have questioned the validity of this controversial diagnosis. In one Greek study, most pediatric patients with abdominal migraine had evidence of esophagitis, gastritis, or duodenitis at endoscopy.[277] A more recent study of 53 children with abdominal migraine and no underlying gastrointestinal pathology demonstrated symptomatic improvement or successful prophylaxis using standard antimigraine therapies such as propranolol or cyproheptadine.[278] Adults with migraine do not tend to report abdominal pain,[279] although some investigators believe that a subset of adult patients with recurrent nonorganic abdominal pain may suffer from abdominal migraine. Unfortunately, the lack of a precise definition of abdominal migraine has made research in this area difficult.

Abdominal epilepsy is an uncommon cause of central neurogenic abdominal pain. One retrospective study describes the spectrum and clinical course of 10 patients with abdominal epilepsy.[280] These patients, each with temporal lobe electroencephalographic (EEG) abnormalities, experi-

Table 29–5 | **Gastrointestinal Manifestations of Neurologic Diseases**

DISEASE	GASTROINTESTINAL MANIFESTATION
Cerebrum/Cerebellum	
Cerebrovascular accident	Oropharyngeal dysphagia, gastroparesis, constipation, peptic ulceration, anorectal dysfunction
Multiple sclerosis	Oropharyngeal dysphagia, gastroparesis, constipation, anorectal dysfunction
Cerebral palsy	Oropharyngeal dysphagia
Migraine headache	Nausea, vomiting, abdominal pain (abdominal migraine), peptic ulceration
"Abdominal epilepsy"/viscerosensory auras	Abdominal pain, bloating, diarrhea
Pseudotumor cerebri	Nausea, vomiting
Brainstem/Cranial Nerve	
Cerebrovascular accident, other brainstem disorders	Oropharyngeal dysphagia, dysgeusia
Multiple sclerosis	Oropharyngeal dysphagia, dysgeusia
Pseudobulbar palsy	Oropharyngeal dysphagia
Diphtheria	Oropharyngeal dysphagia
Spinal Cord/Peripheral Nerve	
Spinal cord injury/transection	Gastroparesis, constipation, incontinence, megacolon, ileus, autonomic dysreflexia
Amyotrophic lateral sclerosis	Oropharyngeal dysphagia, ileus
Charcot-Marie-Tooth syndrome	Oropharyngeal dysphagia, delayed gastric emptying
Tabes dorsalis	Abdominal crises, diarrhea
Poliomyelitis	Ileus, gastric atony, megacolon
Alcoholic and amyloid neuropathy	Esophageal and gastrointestinal dysmotility
Extrapyramidal/Autonomic	
Parkinson's disease	Oropharyngeal dysphagia, constipation, fecal incontinence
Huntington's chorea	Oropharyngeal dysphagia, gastroparesis, constipation
Familial dysautonomia (Riley-Day syndrome)	Esophageal dysmotility, vomiting crises, gastric atony, (rare) diarrhea, megacolon
Shy-Drager syndrome	Postprandial orthostatic hypotension, esophageal dysmotility, achlorhydria, constipation
Chagas' disease	Achalasia, megaesophagus, megaduodenum, megacolon
Paraneoplastic neuropathy	Achalasia, megacolon, pseudo-obstruction
Ganglioneuromatosis	Constipation, megacolon
Diabetic neuropathy	See Table 29–4
Neuromuscular Junction	
Myasthenia gravis	Oropharyngeal dysphagia, autoimmune hepatitis, primary biliary cirrhosis
Muscle Disease	
Stiff-man syndrome	Oropharyngeal dysphagia
Oculopharyngeal muscular dystrophy	Oropharyngeal dysphagia
Mitochondrial neurogastrointestinal encephalomyopathy	Dysmotility, achalasia, malabsorption, pseudo-obstruction, diarrhea
Duchenne's muscular dystrophy	Oropharyngeal dysphagia, gastric atony, malabsorption, megacolon, pseudo-obstruction
Familial visceral myopathy	Dysphagia, pseudo-obstruction (see Chapter 111)
Myotonic dystrophy	Oropharyngeal dysphagia, esophageal dysmotility, gastric atony, megacolon, pseudo-obstruction, volvulus, gallbladder dysfunction
Polymyositis/dermatomyositis	See Table 29–1

enced a variety of paroxysmal gastrointestinal symptoms that included periumbilical and right upper quadrant pain, bloating, and diarrhea. All of the patients also experienced CNS symptoms such as headaches, confusion, dizziness, syncope, or blindness, occurring daily in association with the gastrointestinal complaints. Anticonvulsant therapy resulted in resolution of both gastrointestinal and CNS disturbances. Even patients with classic epileptic seizure disorders may experience viscerosensory auras (vague epigastric sensations and nausea). Although they can occur in patients with temporal lobe mass lesions, epigastric auras are more frequently associated with hippocampal sclerosis. These epigastric auras can be unpleasant or even debilitating. Unfortunately, 25% of patients who are rendered seizure free after anteromedial temporal lobe resection continue to have persistent epigastric auras.[281] Although epilepsy with gastrointestinal symptoms is uncommon, an EEG should be considered in the diagnostic workup of patients with unexplained paroxysmal gastrointestinal complaints associated with CNS symptoms.

Peripheral neurogenic abdominal pain emanating from peripheral nerves or spinal nerve roots is usually intermittent and sharp. It is not associated with food intake or abdominal distention and is usually easy to diagnose. Possible causes include infections such as herpes zoster (pain may precede the rash), and syphilis (gastric crisis in tabes dorsalis); inflammatory conditions such as PAN; metabolic disturbances such as diabetic neuropathy (see earlier); toxic ingestions such as lead poisoning; and nerve root impingement due to osteoarthritis, tumors, or herniated discs.

Gastrointestinal Complications of Acute Head Injury and Cerebrovascular Accidents

Increased intracranial pressure from any cause may lead to episodic projectile vomiting, which may precede other signs. In addition to direct effects of CNS injury on the control of oropharyngeal muscle movement during swallowing, acute head trauma and stroke (cerebrovascular accidents) are associated with a high incidence of upper gastrointestinal tract pathology.[282] In one prospective study, acute gastrointestinal erosive lesions were found at endoscopy in 75% of patients.[283] Erosive gastritis was seen in 69% of cases, gastric ulcer in 23%, esophagitis in 11%, and duodenal inflammation in 8%.[283] Most lesions were present within a week of injury. There was no correlation between steroid administration in these patients and the development of upper gastrointestinal tract lesions. Although these lesions fall within the spectrum of stress gastritis (see Chapters 40 and 43), an additional pathogenetic mechanism may play a role in their development. Serum gastrin levels are elevated in patients with head injury,[284] presumably through a direct neurogenic reflex, and gastric hypersecretion has been reported.[285] Unlike typical stress-related ulcerations and erosions, these lesions may perforate.[286] Because these injuries are largely preventable, patients with acute neurologic injury due to trauma, severe strokes, neurosurgery, or some other condition should receive prophylactic antiulcer therapy.

Gastrointestinal Problems after Spinal Cord Injury

The effect of spinal cord injuries on the gastrointestinal tract depends on the level of the lesion. Delayed gastric emptying is seen in patients with cervical spinal cord injuries.[287] In the early postinjury period, severe gastric stasis, gastric dilation, and ileus are often present.[288] Nasogastric suction is frequently required. Promotility agents such as metoclopramide can be effective because the enteric nervous system and smooth muscle layers are intact. A frequent problem in the first weeks after injury is peptic ulceration. Upper gastrointestinal hemorrhage is more common with cervical cord injuries, with the use of oral anticoagulants, or when there is respiratory distress.[289] Ulcer perforation and peritonitis may not be detected initially because of myelopathy involving sensory fibers or because of concomitant corticosteroid therapy. When ulcer surgery is required, gastric resection or simple closure of the perforation is sufficient; truncal vagotomy is not performed because of the risk of severe gastric retention.[290] *Pancreatitis*, another early complication of spinal injuries, may also be related to the effects of steroids.[288, 291] *Autonomic dysreflexia*, a life-threatening condition, sometimes affects patients whose lesion lies above the fifth thoracic root, the upper level of greater splanchnic flow. The pathophysiology involves an abnormal autonomic reflex that is initiated by fecal impaction or bladder distention and leads to severe hypertension and tachycardia.[292] If untreated, seizures, subarachnoid hemorrhage, and stroke may result. Routine bladder catheterization and avoidance of constipation are preventive.

Patients often face a different set of problems in the months to years following permanent spinal cord damage. With chronic loss of function, patients with quadriplegia are more likely to have gut complications than are patients with paraplegia. The incidence of gastroesophageal reflux is increased.[288] There may be decreased bioavailability of orally administered drugs owing to impaired gastric emptying.[293] Secondary *amyloidosis* involving the gastrointestinal tract is more common, especially when chronic pyelonephritis and renal failure complicate spinal cord disease.[288, 294] Other complications include *cholelithiasis*, the *superior mesenteric artery syndrome* (see Chapter 8), hemorrhage due to *solitary colonic ulcer*, and the precocious appearance of *diverticulosis*.[288, 295] Many patients with spinal cord injury have marked impairment of their bowel function. Fecal incontinence and urgency can have a significant impact on quality of life.[296]

Chronic constipation plagues many patients with spinal cord injury. Damage to neurons in the spinal cord eliminates both the sensation of rectal fullness and the voluntary control of defecation. There may be decreased splanchnic outflow, impairing the coordination of intestinal and colonic motility. Recordings of myoelectric activity in these patients show high levels of basal spike activity[297] and diminished colonic compliance.[298] These findings suggest that the spinal cord exerts an inhibitory influence on basal colon motility. Further, the gastrocolic reflex after feeding is often absent.[297] Fortunately, the lower motor neurons of the second, third, and fourth sacral roots, which provide the sensory and motor fibers for the defecation reflex, are usually intact.

Rehabilitation of bowel function is individualized to each patient's disability. Physical exercise, adequate fluid intake, and stool softeners are prescribed, as for constipation of any origin. Most patients can learn to distend the rectum digitally on a regular schedule to initiate the defecation reflex. Stimulatory laxatives such as bisacodyl suppositories occasionally are necessary. It is not clear which patients, if any, may benefit from promotility agents. Patients with spinal cord injuries often have subtle symptoms and signs of colorectal emergencies that may lead to a delayed diagnosis and increased morbidity and mortality.[299]

Diseases of the Autonomic Nervous System

Congenital and neurodegenerative diseases of the autonomic nervous system all may affect the gastrointestinal tract and are listed in Table 29–5. These include *familial dysautonomia*, or the *Riley-Day syndrome*. Patients present at birth with feeding difficulties, poor temperature control, and motor incoordination. Common gastrointestinal symptoms include dysphagia, gastroesophageal reflux, and abnormal swallowing reflexes. A large percentage of patients require feeding gastrostomy or fundoplication. Lower gastrointestinal tract symptoms are less common, but patients may develop diarrhea due to decreased motility and bacterial overgrowth.[300]

Idiopathic autonomic neuropathy is a relatively uncommon acquired cause of autonomic neuropathy.[300] It can affect both sympathetic and parasympathetic function (pandysautonomia), or it may be limited to a parasympathetic deficit (cholinergic dysautonomia). The onset of symptoms can be acute or subacute. Cholinergic dysautonomia usually affects patients in their teens, whereas pandysautonomia manifests in early middle age.[301] The etiology of this condition is unknown, but most cases develop after nonspecific viral infections. The syndrome has also been seen in association with mononucleosis,[302] Stevens-Johnson syndrome,[303] and herpes zoster[304] or herpes simplex infections.[304] In close to 70% of cases, the initial manifestation of the disease is in the gastrointestinal tract. The most common symptoms are due to excessive cholinergic activity, such as diarrhea, hyperhidrosis, and hypersalivation. Although a large proportion of these patients have manometric abnormalities, complications of motility disorders such as bacterial overgrowth are usually not seen.[300]

A poorly understood autonomic condition is *postprandial*

orthostatic hypotension, which occurs commonly in the elderly and in patients with autonomic dysfunction. Direct gastrointestinal symptoms are infrequent, but abdominal pain and nausea may occur after meals. Other clinical manifestations include postprandial presyncope and syncope. Diagnosis is established with the demonstration of orthostatic hypotension with postprandial tilt testing. Fludrocortisone may dramatically improve these symptoms.[305]

Secondary causes of autonomic neuropathy include the *porphyrias* (variegate, acute intermittent, hereditary coproporphyria), *diabetes mellitus*, *paraneoplastic autonomic neuropathy*, *amyloidosis*, and *Chagas' disease*.

Extrapyramidal Disorders

Huntington's chorea is a hereditary neurodegenerative basal ganglia disease characterized by chorea, dementia, and emotional changes. Dysphagia is a common symptom that may potentially lead to fatal complications from aspiration pneumonia.[306] Gastroparesis and constipation have also been reported.

Parkinson's disease is frequently associated with gastrointestinal symptoms. Oropharyngeal dysphagia and drooling can be particularly distressing. Abnormalities are found in the oral, pharyngeal, and esophageal stages of deglutition. Poor voluntary control of the tongue results in lingual hesitancy, poor bolus formation, and delayed transit into the pharynx. This defect in bolus propulsion persists in the poorly contracting pharynx. Food is often retained in the valleculae, and tracheal aspiration frequently occurs even in asymptomatic patients. Although most patients localize their symptoms to the oropharynx, many patients with Parkinson's disease have disordered motility of the esophageal body that can be associated with *Candida* esophagitis.[307] Manometric studies suggest that more than 60% of patients have abnormal esophageal function, including aperistalsis, simultaneous waves, and ineffective waves, but only 33% of patients have both symptoms and manometric abnormalities.[308] Furthermore, there is evidence to suggest incomplete relaxation of the lower and upper esophageal sphincters in some patients. Treatment of swallowing difficulties in patients with Parkinson's disease should include optimization of therapy directed at the tremor and associated depression and treatment of underlying gastroesophageal reflux if it exists. Levodopa has beneficial effects on the oral and pharyngeal aspects of swallowing and should be taken at mealtimes. Anticholinergics may impair esophageal motility, and excessive dosing of levodopa itself may cause nausea. Constipation due to delayed colonic transit and external sphincter dysfunction can be seen in Parkinson's disease.[307, 309] Finally, smaller and more frequent meals of soft food and posterior spoon placement may help in the oral phase of swallowing. An excellent review that summarizes the available scientific data, pathophysiology, and treatment recommendations for patients suffering from the swallowing disorder seen in Parkinson's disease has been published.[310]

Multiple Sclerosis

Multiple sclerosis (MS) is frequently associated with bowel dysfunction, even in mild cases. Fecal incontinence and constipation are two common problems (see Chapters 11 and 12). One study showed that 43% of MS patients experienced constipation and 53% experienced incontinence.[311] Impaired external and internal anal sphincter function contributes to fecal incontinence in MS.[312] Defecography in patients with intractable constipation can demonstrate rectal intussusception, rectal outlet obstruction, and failure of the puborectalis and anal sphincter muscles to relax appropriately.[311, 313] Cranial nerve involvement may also lead to oropharyngeal dysphagia.

Neuromuscular Disorders and Muscular Diseases

Degenerative diseases of peripheral motor neurons can present with gastrointestinal symptoms. *Amyotrophic lateral sclerosis* ultimately leads to dysphagia due to the impaired coordination of pharyngeal and upper esophageal swallowing mechanisms.[314] *Charcot-Marie-Tooth* degenerative peripheral neuropathy has also been reported to cause pharyngeal dysphagia and abnormal gastrointestinal motility with delayed gastric emptying and disordered motility of the esophageal body.[315]

Motor end-plate disorders such as *myasthenia gravis*, an autoimmune disorder of the neuromuscular junction, are frequently associated with oropharyngeal dysphagia. *Autoimmune hepatitis* and *primary biliary cirrhosis* may also be associated with myasthenia gravis.[316, 317]

Inherited muscular dystrophies, including myotonic dystrophies, are generally believed to involve only skeletal muscles. However, several muscular (and neuromuscular) disorders have been associated with motor disturbances of the gastrointestinal system. *Duchenne's muscular dystrophy* is an X-linked recessive disease that is the most common neuromuscular disease of childhood. Patients with Duchenne's muscular dystrophy may experience nausea and vomiting, as well as abdominal distention, constipation, pseudo-obstruction, and gastric dilation. Even when gastrointestinal symptoms are absent, dysfunction of smooth muscle in the upper gastrointestinal tract is detectable.[318] Patients with Duchenne's muscular dystrophy as well as those with *oculopharyngeal muscular dystrophy* may experience cervical dysphagia.

Mitochondrial neurogastrointestinal encephalomyopathy (MNGIE) is a rare autosomal recessive mitochondrial myopathy defined by the constellation of peripheral neuropathy, opthalmoparesis, and gastrointestinal dysmotility; muscle biopsy reveals histologic features of a mitochondrial myopathy.[319] Gastrointestinal symptoms include dysmotility, diarrhea, pseudo-obstruction, achalasia, and malabsorption. A possible variant of MNGIE may be the "3-A" syndrome of familial *a*chalasia, *a*lacrima, and *A*CTH (corticotropin) sensitivity, characterized by postural hypotension, achalasia, decreased sweating and tears, and denervation hypersensitivity of the pupils.[320]

Stiff-man syndrome manifests as symmetrical stiffness and painful spasm of the axial musculature. Dysphagia, perhaps due to spasm of the cricopharyngeus and upper esophagus, has been reported. *Myotonic dystrophy*, an autosomal dominant disease of both striated and smooth muscle is considered a rare cause of gastrointestinal dilation and abnormal peristalsis. A fairly recent study, however, has shown that many patients with myotonic dystrophy list gastrointestinal problems as the most disabling consequences of the disease. Gastrointestinal symptoms include abdominal pain (55%), dysphagia (45%), emesis (35%), diarrhea (33%), and fecal incontinence (30%).[321]

PULMONARY DISEASES/ICU PATIENTS

Chronic obstructive pulmonary disease is associated with peptic ulcers. The etiology of peptic ulceration remains obscure, but the risk appears to increase with the amount of cigarettes smoked per day.[322] Patients with chronic lung disease secondary to α_1-antitrypsin deficiency also appear to be at increased risk for peptic ulceration.[323] Hepatic complications of α_1-antitrypsin deficiency are discussed in Chapter 65.

Mechanical ventilation in the intensive care unit (ICU) is associated with significant gastrointestinal and hepatobiliary complications. Acute *stress-induced gastritis* is a common finding in ICU patients (see Chapters 40 and 43), and the propensity for clinically significant hemorrhage is increased in patients on mechanical ventilation and in those with significant coagulopathies.[324] The successful prophylaxis of stress gastritis in the ICU setting is discussed in Chapter 40. *Ischemic colitis* may be seen following cardiac arrest or hypotensive episodes. *Acalculous cholecystitis* is also commonly seen in severely ill ICU patients and manifests as acute abdominal pain or abdominal sepsis. The diagnosis and therapy of acalculous cholecystitis are discussed in Chapter 58.

CARDIAC DISEASES

Congestive heart failure, cor pulmonale, or constrictive pericarditis can result in intestinal *malabsorption* (see Chapter 89) or *protein-losing enteropathy* (see Chapter 25). *Cardiac ascites* can also complicate congestive heart failure. Many patients have high SAAG with high-protein content as a consequence of the high systemic venous pressures of the liver and peritoneal cavity (see Chapter 78). Ischemic "low-flow" hepatopathy may also result (see Chapter 70). Mucosal hypoxemia in patients with reduced cardiac outputs may cause stress ulcers or *ischemic colitis*.

It is commonly believed that bleeding from colonic *angiodysplasia* (discussed in Chapter 120) is associated with valvular aortic stenosis. There are even scattered reports that aortic valve replacement in these patients prevents further hemorrhage, prompting some practitioners to suggest that intestinal bleeding from angiodysplasia in the setting of aortic stenosis (Heyde's syndrome) is an indication for valve replacement.[325]

INFILTRATIVE DISEASES

Amyloidosis

The diffuse extracellular tissue deposition of amyloid results in systemic *amyloidosis*. Amyloid is an insoluble, eosinophilic complex glycoprotein that demonstrates green birefringence under polarized light after Congo red staining. Amyloidosis has been subclassified according to clinical and biochemical criteria, but all types can involve the gastrointestinal tract.[153, 326] The chief sites of intestinal amyloid deposition are the blood vessel walls (producing ischemia and infarction), the muscle layers of the intestine (causing dysmotility), and the muscularis mucosa (impairing absorption).[326] The mucosa is infiltrated only with massive deposition. Direct-pressure damage to cells in the myenteric plexus and visceral nerve trunks has also been demonstrated.[327]

Amyloidosis may cause gastrointestinal symptoms extending from the mouth to the anus, although intestinal amyloidosis can be asymptomatic. Macroglossia and temporomandibular arthritis may cause drooling and difficulties with mastication.[328] Intestinal dysmotility can result in diarrhea, constipation, megacolon, fecal incontinence, or rectal prolapse.[153, 329] An esophageal motility disturbance similar to achalasia may cause dysphagia. Dysmotility may cause intestinal *pseudo-obstruction*, although mechanical obstruction due to amyloid infiltration of the mesentery has also been reported.[330] *Malabsorption*, found in about 5% of cases, may be due to bacterial overgrowth, mucosal ischemia, exocrine pancreatic insufficiency, or submucosal amyloid deposition that creates a physical barrier to absorption. Functional or mechanical *gastric outlet obstruction* may be due to dysmotility or to the presence of an antral amyloidoma.[331] Gastrointestinal bleeding (presumably from increased capillary fragility),[332] *intestinal infarction* (secondary to massive amyloid deposition in blood vessels),[333] and *protein-losing enteropathy*[334] have also been seen. A third of patients presents with hepatosplenomegaly or ascites.[153]

Radiographic abnormalities include esophageal dysmotility and the appearance of diminished or rigid gastric rugal folds on upper gastrointestinal tract series. Small intestinal radiographs are often the first tests to suggest amyloidosis. The most common findings are sharply demarcated thickening of the valvulae conniventes (Fig. 29–6), dilation of the bowel due to replacement of the muscular layers, and the presence of multiple nodular lesions.[335] Colonic imaging studies may show multiple filling defects, ulceration due to ischemia, or narrowing and rigidity, especially in the sigmoid colon and the rectum.

Diagnosis is established by histologic demonstration of amyloid protein in involved tissues. Although rectal biopsy establishes the diagnosis in as many as 80% of cases, more recent data suggest that duodenal biopsies may be positive in 100% of cases.[326, 336] Ligamentous biopsy at the time of carpal tunnel release is also reported to be 100% sensitive.[153] Finally, abdominal fat pad biopsy is safe and often diagnostic, but false-negative results are not uncommon.

There is no specific therapy for primary amyloidosis. Amyloidosis secondary to FMF is treated with colchicine,[337] and amyloidosis secondary to a plasma cell disorder such as multiple myeloma may be partially alleviated by therapy of the underlying dyscrasia.[338] Surgical decompression has been used for intractable colorectal symptoms.[339] The use of prokinetic agents may result in marginal symptomatic improvement in amyloidosis due to multiple myeloma.[340]

Systemic Mastocytosis

Systemic mastocytosis is characterized by mast cell proliferation in skin, bones, lymph nodes, and parenchymal organs.

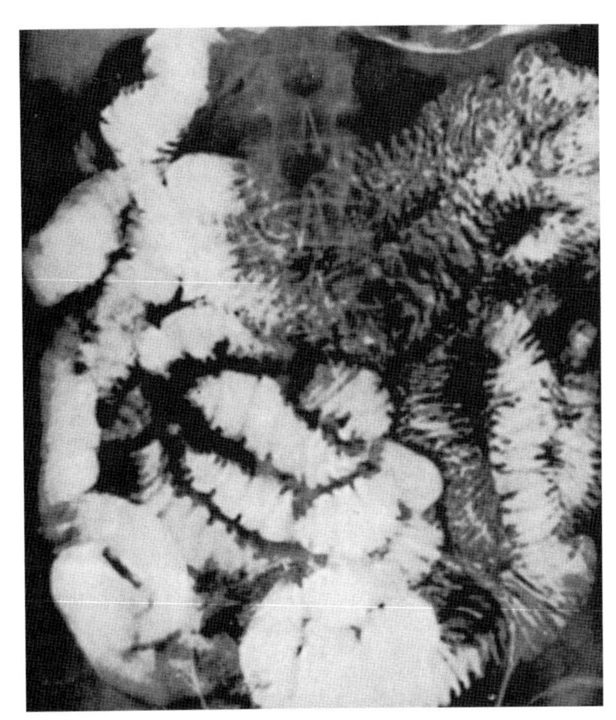

Figure 29–6. Symmetrical, sharply demarcated thickening of the valvulae conniventes throughout the small intestine, producing a uniform appearance characteristic of amyloidosis. (Courtesy of R.H. Marshak, M.D.)

The classic dermatologic finding of *urticaria pigmentosa* may be seen with or without systemic involvement (see Chapter 18). The typical symptoms of mastocytosis (pruritus, flushing, tachycardia, asthma, headache) are believed to result from the release of histamine and prostaglandins from mast cells.[341–343] Heparin is also released from mast cells and may contribute to a bleeding diathesis.[344] Eighty percent of patients have gastrointestinal symptoms,[345] which include nausea, vomiting, diarrhea, and abdominal pain.[341] Hepatomegaly, portal hypertension, splenomegaly, and ascites may occur frequently.[342] These symptoms often are provoked by the ingestion of small amounts of alcohol.[341] Hyperhistaminemia produces gastric hypersecretion in more than 40% of cases,[345] and secretion may be as marked as in Zollinger-Ellison syndrome.[346] Gastric acidity correlates with the degree of histaminemia and with the presence of acid-peptic disease.[345, 346] Duodenal ulceration or duodenitis has been reported in more than 40% of cases.[345] Gastrointestinal hemorrhage from peptic ulcers and from bleeding esophageal varices has been reported.[341, 346] Diarrhea has been reported in as many as 60% of cases, and minimal fat malabsorption occurs in some cases.[344, 345] Decreased absorption of D-xylose and of vitamin B_{12} is also found in patients with mastocytosis.[345] The cause of diarrhea is unclear. Some diarrheal symptoms (but not malabsorption) respond to H_2-receptor antagonists, but there is no clear correlation between stool output and the degree of plasma histaminemia or gastric acidity.[345] It is presumed that diarrhea and malabsorption are the result of morphologic changes in the absorptive mucosa. Jejunal biopsy specimens may show large numbers of mast cells in the lamina propria, muscularis mucosa, and submucosa, with normal villi or mild villous atrophy.[347] Endoscopy may reveal urticaria-like mucosal lesions,[348] and small bowel radiographic abnormalities include bull's eye lesions resembling metastases, edema, thickened folds, and a nodular mucosal pattern.[349] Diffuse colonic involvement with acute inflammatory infiltrates and mucosal edema have been reported.[350] H_1-receptor and H_2-receptor antagonists, anticholinergics, oral disodium cromoglycate, and, rarely, corticosteroids with or without cyclophosphamide have been used successfully to relieve the diarrhea and abdominal pain of mastocytosis.[345, 351, 352]

Sarcoidosis

Clinical manifestations of gastrointestinal involvement in *sarcoidosis* are unusual. When present, symptoms result from granulomatous infiltration of the affected organ. Hilar and mediastinal lymph node enlargement may cause dysphagia.[353] The most common luminal gastrointestinal site affected by sarcoidosis is the stomach. Histologic differentiation from Crohn's disease, tuberculosis, or secondary syphilis can be difficult. There may be diffuse ulceration and antral narrowing, or the disease can resemble linitis plastica or Ménétrier's disease.[353] Seventy-five percent of patients with gastric sarcoidosis present with pain and 25% present with bleeding. Gastric outlet obstruction may occur. Half of patients require surgery for bleeding or suspected malignancy; two of three patients improve symptomatically with corticosteroid therapy.[353] The healing of a sarcoid ulcer with antacids has been reported.[353, 354] The small intestine may be involved indirectly in sarcoidosis via mesenteric lymph node enlargement. Dilated lacteals seen on a small intestine biopsy specimen are evidence of possible lymphatic obstruction. *Malabsorption* and *protein-losing enteropathy* have been reported.[355, 256] Colonic sarcoidosis is rare. The sole proctoscopic finding may be friable mucosa,[357] a pattern of nodular hyperplasia,[358] or a constricting lesion resembling carcinoma.[358, 359] *Granulomatous hepatitis* is extremely common is sarcoidosis (see Chapter 82). Other rare hepatobiliary complications of sarcoidosis are Budd-Chiari syndrome and obstructive jaundice caused by hepatic hilar lymphadenopathy or strictures of the bile ducts.[360] Sarcoidosis involving the pancreas appears to be rare. The clinical presentation may be similar to that of pancreatic cancer or acute pancreatitis.[361, 362] Pancreatic insufficiency in sarcoidosis has been reported.[363]

Other Infiltrative Disorders

Eosinophilic infiltration of the gastrointestinal mucosa characterizes *eosinophilic gastroenteritis* (see Chapter 100), the *hypereosinophilic syndrome*, *CSS*, systemic gold toxicity, and *PAN*. Langerhans' cell granulomatosis (histiocytosis X, eosinophilic granuloma) may also infiltrate the gastrointestinal tract.

Small vessel hyalinosis is a rare familial syndrome consisting of diarrhea, rectal bleeding, malabsorption, and protein-losing enteropathy, combined with poikiloderma, hair graying, and cerebrovascular calcifications.[364] Pathologically, basement membrane–like deposits can be seen in the subepithelial space of intestinal capillaries arterioles and small veins.

DISORDERS OF LIPID METABOLISM

Hyperlipoproteinemia

In familial hyperchylomicronemia (type I phenotype), the plasma is lactescent, with marked elevation of chylomicrons and triglycerides due to a deficiency of lipoprotein lipase. Manifestations can appear early in life and include recurrent episodes of abdominal pain, fever, peritonitis, and pancreatitis (see Chapter 47). In most patients the cause of recurrent attacks of pain is not known.[365] Patients with familial hyperbetalipoproteinemia (type IV phenotype) suffer from premature atherosclerosis, hyperuricemia, and attacks of pancreatitis that generally occur when plasma triglyceride values are above 2000 mg/dL.[366] The hyperlipidemia may mask elevated plasma amylase values. The patients also have an increased incidence of cholelithiasis and cholecystitis.[367] Patients with familial hyperlipoproteinemia (type V phenotype) are prone to bouts of abdominal pain, with or without pancreatitis. Exacerbation of endogenous hypertriglyceridemia by diabetes, diet, alcohol, or medications can also cause pancreatitis.[366]

Fabry's Disease

Fabry's disease is an X-linked disorder of glycolipid metabolism due to the deficiency or absence of the enzyme α-galactosidase A, resulting in sphingolipid deposition in all tissues and subsequent organ dysfunction. Impaired motility is the prominent gastrointestinal abnormality.[368] Electron microsopic examination of biopsy specimens from the small intestine and rectum reveals large sphingolipid-filled vacuoles in the ganglion cells of Meissner's plexus within smooth muscle cells of the muscularis mucosa and within endothelial cells lining the blood vessels. Mucosal enterocytes are normal.[368] Patients complain of recurrent episodes of crampy abdominal pain with frequent watery stools. Delayed gastric emptying, bacterial overgrowth, increased fecal bile acid loss, and cholelithiasis have been documented. Successful treatment of the gastrointestinal component of this disorder with metoclopramide and tetracycline has been reported. Glycolipid deposition in small vessels can induce severe vasculitis and thrombosis, resulting in ischemic bowel lesions. Ileal perforation has also been reported.[369]

Abetalipoproteinemia

Abetalipoproteinemia is an autosomal-recessive disorder characterized by acanthotic erythrocytes, serum lipid abnormalities, ataxia, atypical retinitis pigmentosa, and steatorrhea.[370] The typical laboratory feature is complete absence in plasma of all lipoproteins containing apolipoprotein B (chylomicrons, low-density lipoprotein, and very-low-density lipoprotein). The histologic appearance of the small intestine after an overnight fast is marked by mucosal epithelial cells loaded with lipid droplets (Fig. 29–7).[371] By contrast, the submucosa and lamina propria show practically no lipid, and the lymphatics are empty. The villi are normal in length and configuration. Mild steatorrhea with onset during the first 2 years of life is seen (see Chapter 89). Cholesterol malabsorption with increased endogenous cholesterol synthesis has also been reported.[372] The intestinal mucosa may appear yellowish on endoscopy, reflecting the presence of mucosal lipid.[373] Therapy consists of substituting medium-chain for long-chain triglycerides.

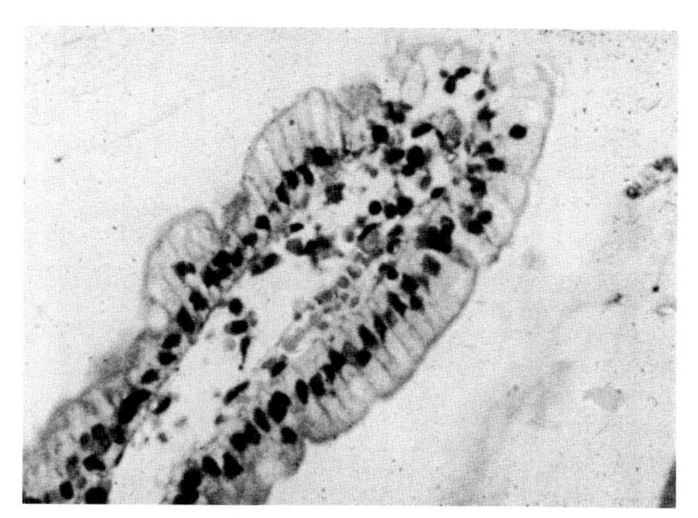

Figure 29–7. Small intestinal biopsy of a patient with abetalipoproteinemia. The biopsy is notable for the accumulation of lipid droplets within the intestinal epithelial cells. (Courtesy of Dr. Carolyn Montgomery.)

Gaucher's Disease

Gaucher's disease is a rare autosomal-recessive deficiency of the enzyme β-glucocerebrosidase resulting in the deposition of glucosylceramide in the cells of the reticuloendothelial system, including the liver and spleen. In the adult form of the disease gastrointestinal complications predominate, including hepatosplenomegaly, hepatic cirrhosis, ascites, and esophageal variceal hemorrhage.[374, 375]

Niemann-Pick Disease

Niemann-Pick disease is a rare autosomal-recessive disease with a predilection for Ashkenazi Jewish people. Types A and B result from defects in acid sphingomyelinase. In type C Niemann-Pick disease, mutation in Niemann-Pick protein C results in defective transport of cholesterol across the lysosomal membrane.[376] Sphingomyelinase deficiency results in the deposition of sphingomyelin and cholesterol in the liver and spleen, the CNS, and the lungs and skin. Gastrointestinal complications include hepatosplenomegaly and liver failure.[377] Rare adult survivors of Niemann-Pick disease have been reported.[377]

Tangier Disease

Tangier disease is an autosomal-recessive disorder characterized by accumulation of cholesterol esters in macrophages in tonsils, thymus, lymph nodes, marrow, liver, and the gut. Tangier disease is caused by a mutation in the adenosine triphosphate–binding cassette protein, ABCA1, which mediates the efflux of excess cellular sterol to apolipoprotein A-I, a step leading to the formation of beneficial high-density lipoprotein (HDL).[378] These patients have very low levels of plasma cholesterol and HDLs, owing to a lack of apolipoprotein A-I. The gene encoding apolipoprotein A-I is normal in Tangier disease, but a defect in post-translational processing results in its rapid degradation.[378] The striking clinical findings include yellow-orange "streaked" tonsils in 80% of cases, hepatosplenomegaly, and peripheral neuropathy. Patients may have diarrhea without steatorrhea. Colonoscopy reveals orange-brown mucosal "spots" throughout the colon and rectum, and laparoscopy reveals similar yellow patches on the surface of the liver due to cholesterol esters in hepatic reticuloendothelial cells.[379]

PREGNANCY

As many as 20% of pregnant women with medical complaints severe enough to seek medical attention have primarily gastrointestinal symptoms. Although the most severe gastrointestinal complications of pregnancy are hepatic,[380] as discussed in Chapter 74, conditions affecting the esophagus, stomach, and intestine are much more common. Pregnancy alters the motility of the esophagus, stomach, small intestine, and biliary tree,[381] accounting for most gastrointestinal symptoms.[382] Pregnancy also displaces the stomach, small intestine, and mobile portions of the colon (including the appendix) from their customary anatomic positions. In addition, it attenuates the body's response to intra-abdominal crises such as inflammation, perforation, and obstruction.[383] As a result, history and physical examination findings of the gravid patient may be misleading, and standard laboratory indicators of inflammation may be of little clinical value. Moreover, concern for the fetus may restrain the clinician from pursuing a thorough diagnostic workup, including radiographic and endoscopic studies. Even if the correct diagnosis is made, therapy is often limited by considerations for the well-being of the fetus.

Nausea and Vomiting (see also Chapter 8)

The majority of pregnancy-related gastrointestinal symptoms are due to altered gut motility. Nausea, with or without vomiting, is a common self-limited symptom of early pregnancy. Nausea may occur as early as 3 weeks after the last menstrual period, and it may persist beyond 20 weeks in a small percentage of patients. The designation *hyperemesis gravidarum*[384] is reserved for first-trimester patients with persistent, severe nausea and vomiting that lead to a reduction of 5% or more in body weight and disturbed fluid and electrolyte balance. Abnormal antral motility has been described in nauseated pregnant patients, and recent reports suggest strong association between *H. pylori* infection and hyperemesis gravidarum.[385, 386] Although generally benign, nausea and vomiting may result in gastrointestinal hemorrhage from Mallory-Weiss esophageal tears, the most common cause of upper gastrointestinal tract hemorrhage during pregnancy.[384]

Before initiating therapy, other causes of nausea and vomiting must be ruled out, such as urinary tract infections, gastroenteritis, hepatitis, or biliary tract disease. Peptic ulcer disease is uncommon during pregnancy. The treatment of nausea and vomiting during pregnancy is conservative. Frequent, small meals and reassurance are often successful in mild cases. Severe cases are treated with intravenous fluid and electrolyte repletion and the judicious use of antiemetics. Although the safety of prochlorperazine or metoclopramide has not been definitively established in pregnant patients, these agents have been used in severe cases of hyperemesis with the appropriate informed consent. The role of *H. pylori* eradication in the treatment of hyperemesis gravidarum has not been fully investigated.

The prognosis for mother and child is generally good. Several large series have demonstrated lower perinatal mortality for babies whose mothers had mild first-trimester nausea and vomiting, suggesting that nausea and vomiting may be signs of a healthy pregnancy.[387] These studies support previous observations that women likely to abort tend to have less nausea and vomiting than those who do not. Women with extreme vomiting and loss of more than 5% of their prepregnancy weight, however, have higher incidences of low-birth weight infants.[384]

Gastroesophageal Reflux

(see also Chapter 33)

Many women suffer from symptomatic *gastroesophageal reflux* during pregnancy. Onset is usually in the second trimester, and reflux usually worsens as pregnancy progresses. Basal LES pressures decrease throughout pregnancy, reaching a nadir immediately before delivery when estrogen and progesterone levels peak.[388, 389] Although gastroesophageal reflux is common, it is rarely serious. Erosive esophagitis may be a significant cause of upper gastrointestinal hemorrhage during pregnancy, but overall it is quite rare, considering the number of patients with symptomatic reflux.

Treatment is aimed at reducing reflux or neutralizing gastric contents. Avoiding recumbency after meals, eliminating certain foods, elevating the head of the bed, and using antacids usually bring relief. First-line therapy in these patients should be limited to antireflux precautions, antacids, and sucralfate. H_2-blockers and proton pump inhibitors cannot be formally recommended during pregnancy and should be reserved for extreme, refractory cases. Nevertheless, safe and effective use of proton pump inhibitors and H_2-blockers has been reported during pregnancy.[390, 391] The H_2-blockers ranitidine and cimetidine, which are category B drugs (unproved safety in pregnancy), are preferable to nizatadine, which is teratogenic in laboratory animals (category C). By the same token, the proton pump inhibitor lansoprazole (category B) is preferable to omeprazole (category C).

Constipation

Constipation is common during pregnancy, perhaps owing to progesterone-induced smooth muscle inhibition. Infrequent reports suggest that the prevalence of constipation in pregnant women varies greatly, from 11 % to 38%.[392] Constipation, and the hemorrhoids that frequently accompany it, usually respond to nonabsorbable stool softeners and to dietary fiber supplements.

Pancreaticobiliary Manifestations

Gallbladder emptying is inhibited by progesterone, and bile acid output is decreased by estrogens.[393] These factors may account for the increased incidence of *cholelithiasis* in pregnant women. The incidence of cholecystitis, however, is not increased. *Pancreatitis* occurs infrequently during pregnancy but carries a high risk of maternal and fetal mortality. Although usually associated with choledocholithiasis, pancreatitis in pregnancy may also be caused by the hypertriglyceridemic effects of estrogens on underlying lipoprotein disorders[394] or as a postoperative complication.[383] As in nonpregnant patients, attacks of gallstone pancreatitis frequently subside with conservative measures, allowing the postponement of definitive therapy until after delivery. Safe and successful management of refractory, severe gallstone pancreatitis has been reported using endoscopic papillotomy with stone extraction or using open or laparoscopic cholecystectomy with common bile duct exploration.[395–397]

Appendicitis

Appendicitis is the most common gastrointestinal condition requiring surgery during pregnancy (incidence approximately 1 in 2000 pregnancies).[398] Diagnosis may be difficult in view of the abnormal location of the appendix in the gravid abdomen. Because the enlarging uterus displaces the cecum and appendix cephalad, the site of maximal tenderness may be above the umbilicus or even beneath the right costal margin. Graded-compression sonography appears to be the preferred procedure for detecting acute appendicitis during pregnancy, especially in the first and second trimesters.[399, 400] Early surgery is indicated because the development of peritonitis has led to increased maternal and fetal morbidity and mortality in the past. More recent studies suggest that modern supportive care can effectively prevent fetal loss in the setting of perforated appendicitis.[401] If a normal appendix is discovered, it was previously suggested that its removal should be avoided, because this practice increased the rate of fetal loss.[402] More recent studies, however, suggest that a normal appendix discovered during exploratory laparotomy should be removed in pregnant as well as in nonpregnant patients.[403] A recent review showed that laparascopic appendectomy can be safely performed in pregnant patients in the first and second trimesters. The increased size of a gravid uterus that interferes with visualization and instrumentation may be a relative contraindication in third-trimester pregnancy.[404]

Miscellaneous Conditions

A rare and unexplained cause of acute volume loss, with or without abdominal pain, during pregnancy with high maternal and fetal mortality rates is ruptured *splenic artery aneurysm*.[406] The cause of this condition remains obscure. The diagnosis should be suspected in pregnant women with acute abdominal distress and hypotension and is made angiographically. Surgery is indicated even for asymptomatic aneurysms, because their natural course is to rupture. *Acute granulomatous peritonitis* has been described in women with abdominal pain during pregnancy and following cesarean section.[406, 407] It appears to result from the rupture of fetal contents into the peritoneum or meconium spillage during cesarean section.

REFERENCES

1. Sun DC, et al: Upper gastrointestinal disease in rheumatoid arthritis. Am J Dig Dis 19:405–410, 1974.
2. Scott DG, Bacon PA, Tribe CR: Systemic rheumatoid vasculitis: A clinical and laboratory study of 50 cases. Medicine (Baltimore). 60: 288–297, 1981.
3. Achkar AA, et al: Rheumatoid vasculitis manifesting as intra-abdominal hemorrhage. Mayo Clin Proc 70:565–569, 1995.
4. Burt RW, et al: Rheumatoid vasculitis of the colon presenting as pancolitis. Dig Dis Sci 28:183–188, 1983.
5. Nakad A, et al: Nodular regenerative hyperplasia of the liver and esophageal varices in Felty's syndrome: A clinicopathologic case report with review of the literature. Acta Clin Belg 43:45–50, 1988.
6. Voskuyl AE, et al: Extra-articular manifestations of rheumatoid arthritis: Risk factors for serious gastrointestinal events. Ann Rheum Dis 52:771–775, 1993.
7. Bombardier C, et al: Comparison of upper gastrointestinal toxicity of rofecoxib and naproxen in patients with rheumatoid arthritis. N Engl J Med 343:1520–1528, 2000.
8. Sung J, et al: Nonsteroidal anti-inflammatory drug toxicity in the upper gastrointestinal tract. J Gastroenterol Hepatol 15(Suppl):G58–G68, 2000.
9. Wolfe F, Hawley DJ: The comparative risk and predictors of adverse gastrointestinal events in rheumatoid arthritis and osteoarthritis: A prospective 13-year study of 2131 patients. J Rheumatol 27:1668–1673, 2000.
10. Graham DY, Agrawal NM, Roth SH: Prevention of NSAID-induced gastric ulcer with misoprostol: Multicentre, double-blind, placebo-controlled trial. Lancet 2:1277–1280, 1988.
11. Bardhan KD, et al: The prevention and healing of acute nonsteroidal anti-inflammatory drug-associated gastroduodenal mucosal damage by misoprostol. Br J Rheumatol 32:990–995, 1993.
12. Graham DY, et al: Duodenal and gastric ulcer prevention with misoprostol in arthritis patients taking NSAIDs. Misoprostol Study Group (see comments). Ann Intern Med 119:257–262, 1993.
13. Silverstein FE, et al: Misoprostol reduces serious gastrointestinal complications in patients with rheumatoid arthritis receiving nonsteroidal anti-inflammatory drugs: A randomized, double-blind, placebo-controlled trial (see comments). Ann Intern Med 123:241–249, 1995.
14. Taha AS, et al: Famotidine for the prevention of gastric and duodenal ulcers caused by nonsteroidal antiinflammatory drugs (see comments). N Engl J Med 334:1435–1439, 1996.
15. Yeomans ND, et al: A comparison of omeprazole with ranitidine for ulcers associated with nonsteroidal antiinflammatory drugs. Acid Suppression Trial: Ranitidine versus Omeprazole for NSAID-associated Ulcer Treatment (ASTRONAUT) Study Group (see comments). N Engl J Med 338:719–726, 1998.
16. Hawkey CJ, et al: Omeprazole compared with misoprostol for ulcers associated with nonsteroidal antiinflammatory drugs. Omeprazole versus Misoprostol for NSAID-induced Ulcer Management (OMNIUM) Study Group (see comments). N Engl J Med 338:727–734, 1998.
17. Heuer MA, et al: An analysis of worldwide safety experience with auranofin. J Rheumatol 12:695–699, 1985.
18. Michet CJ Jr, Rakela J, Luthra HS: Auranofin-associated colitis and eosinophilia. Mayo Clin Proc 62:142–144, 1987.
19. Kremer JM, et al: Methotrexate for rheumatoid arthritis: Suggested guidelines for monitoring liver toxicity. American College of Rheumatology (see comments). Arthritis Rheum 37:316–328, 1994.
20. Pouchot J, et al: Adult Still's disease: Manifestations, disease course, and outcome in 62 patients. Medicine (Baltimore). 70:118–136, 1991.
21. Abu-Shakra M, Guillemin F, Lee P: Gastrointestinal manifestations of systemic sclerosis. Semin Arthritis Rheum 24:29–39, 1994.
22. Bassotti G, et al: Esophageal dysfunction in scleroderma: Relationship with disease subsets. Arthritis Rheum 40:2252–2259, 1997.
23. Garrett JM, et al: Esophageal deterioration in scleroderma. Mayo Clin Proc 46:92–96, 1971.
24. Lock G, et al: Gastrointestinal manifestations of progressive systemic sclerosis. Am J Gastroenterol 92:763–771, 1997.
25. Lambert DR, et al: Esophageal-atrial fistula. J Clin Gastroenterol 9: 345–349, 1987.
26. Hendel L, et al: Omeprazole in the long-term treatment of severe gastro-oesophageal reflux disease in patients with systemic sclerosis. Aliment Pharmacol Ther 6:565–577, 1992.
27. Park RH, et al: Achalasia-like syndrome in systemic sclerosis. Br J Surg 77:46–49, 1990.

28. Katzka DA, et al: Barrett's metaplasia and adenocarcinoma of the esophagus in scleroderma. Am J Med 82:46–52, 1987.
29. Segel MC, et al: Systemic sclerosis (scleroderma) and esophageal adenocarcinoma: Is increased patient screening necessary? Gastroenterology 89:485–488, 1985.
30. Wegener M, et al: Gastrointestinal transit through esophagus, stomach, small and large intestine in patients with progressive systemic sclerosis. Dig Dis Sci 39:2209–2215, 1994.
31. Maddern GJ, et al: Abnormalities of esophageal and gastric emptying in progressive systemic sclerosis. Gastroenterology 87:922–926, 1984.
32. Fiorucci S, et al: Effect of erythromycin administration on upper gastrointestinal motility in scleroderma patients. Scand J Gastroenterol 29:807–813, 1994.
33. Greydanus MP, Camilleri M: Abnormal postcibal antral and small bowel motility due to neuropathy or myopathy in systemic sclerosis. Gastroenterology 96:110–115, 1989.
34. Lock G, Holstege A, Lang B, et al: Gastrointestinal manifestations of progressive systemic sclerosis. Am J Gastroenterol 92:763–771, 1997.
35. Rees WD, et al: Interdigestive motor activity in patients with systemic sclerosis. Gastroenterology 83:575–580, 1982.
36. Horowitz AL, Meyers MA: The "hide-bound" small bowel of scleroderma: Characteristic mucosal fold pattern. AJR Am J Roentgenol 119:332–334, 1973.
37. Rohrmann CA Jr, et al: Radiologic and histologic differentiation of neuromuscular disorders of the gastrointestinal tract: Visceral myopathies, visceral neuropathies, and progressive systemic sclerosis. AJR Am J Roentgenol 143:933–941, 1984.
38. Netscher DT, Richardson JD: Complications requiring operative intervention in scleroderma. Surg Gynecol Obstet 158:507–512, 1984.
39. van Tilburg AJ, van Blankenstein M, Verschoor L: Intestinal lymphangiectasia in systemic sclerosis. Am J Gastroenterol 83:1418–1419, 1988.
40. Akesson A, et al: Gastrointestinal function in patients with progressive systemic sclerosis. Clin Rheumatol 4:441–448, 1985.
41. Kahn IJ, Jeffries GH, Sleisenger MH: Malabsorption in intestinal scleroderma: Correction by antibiotics. N Engl J Med 274:1339–1344, 1966.
42. Verne GN, et al: Effect of octreotide and erythromycin on idiopathic and scleroderma-associated intestinal pseudo-obstruction. Dig Dis Sci 40:1892–1901, 1995.
43. Basilisco G, et al: Anorectal dysfunction and delayed colonic transit in patients with progressive systemic sclerosis. Dig Dis Sci 38:1525–1529, 1993.
44. Hamel-Roy J, et al: Comparative esophageal and anorectal motility in scleroderma. Gastroenterology 88:1–7, 1985.
45. Baron M, Srolovitz H: Colonic telangiectasias in a patient with progressive systemic sclerosis. Arthritis Rheum 29:282–285, 1986.
46. Leighton JA, et al: Anorectal dysfunction and rectal prolapse in progressive systemic sclerosis. Dis Colon Rectum 36:182–185, 1993.
47. Greif JM, Wolff WI: Idiopathic calcific pancreatitis, CRST syndrome, and progressive systemic sclerosis. Am J Gastroenterol 71:177–182, 1979.
48. Abraham AA, Joos A: Pancreatic necrosis in progressive systemic sclerosis. Ann Rheum Dis 39:396–398, 1980.
49. Dreiling DA, Soto MJ: The pancreatic involvement in disseminated "collagen" disorders: Studies of pancreatic secretion in patients with scleroderma and Sjögren's "disease." Am J Gastroenterol 66:546–553, 1976.
50. Edmunds SE, et al: Protein-losing enteropathy in systemic lupus erythematosus. Aust N Z J Med 18:868–871, 1988.
51. Laing TJ: Gastrointestinal vasculitis and pneumatosis intestinalis due to systemic lupus erythematosus: Successful treatment with pulse intravenous cyclophosphamide. Am J Med 85:555–558, 1988.
52. Kleinman P, et al: Necrotizing enterocolitis with pneumatosis intestinalis in systemic lupus erythematosus and polyarteritis. Radiology 121: 595–598, 1976.
53. Zizic TM, Classen JN, Stevens MB: Acute abdominal complications of systemic lupus erythematosus and polyarteritis nodosa. Am J Med 73:525–531, 1982.
54. Gore RM, et al: Ischemic colitis associated with systemic lupus erythematosus. Dis Colon Rectum 26:449–451, 1983.
55. Helliwell TR, et al: Arteritis and venulitis in systemic lupus erythematosus resulting in massive lower intestinal haemorrhage. Histopathology 9:1103–1113, 1985.
56. Zizic TM, Shulman LE, Stevens MB: Colonic perforations in systemic lupus erythematosus. Medicine (Baltimore) 54:411–426, 1975.
57. Mekori YA, et al: Pancreatitis in systemic lupus erythematosus—a case report and review of the literature. Postgrad Med J 56:145–147, 1980.
58. Borum M, et al: Chronic pancreatitis: A complication of systemic lupus erythematosus. Gastroenterology 104:613–615, 1993.
59. Shapeero LG, et al: Acute reversible lupus vasculitis of the gastrointestinal tract. Radiology 112:569–574, 1974.
60. de Merieux P, et al: Esophageal abnormalities and dysphagia in polymyositis and dermatomyositis. Arthritis Rheum 26:961–968, 1983.
61. Thompson JW: Spontaneous perforation of the esophagus as a manifestation of dermatomyositis. Ann Otol Rhinol Laryngol 93:464–467, 1984.
62. Kaplinsky N, et al: Spontaneous duodenal perforation during fulminant dermatomyositis. J Am Med Womens Assoc 33:213–214, 1978.
63. Bohan A, et al: Computer-assisted analysis of 153 patients with polymyositis and dermatomyositis. Medicine (Baltimore) 56:255–286, 1977.
64. Marshall JB, et al: Gastrointestinal manifestations of mixed connective tissue disease. Gastroenterology 98:1232–1238, 1990.
65. Sheikh SH, Shaw-Stiffel TA: The gastrointestinal manifestations of Sjögren's syndrome. Am J Gastroenterol 90:9–14, 1995.
66. Kjellen G, et al: Esophageal function, radiography, and dysphagia in Sjögren's syndrome. Dig Dis Sci 31:225–229, 1986.
67. Takasugi M, et al: Gastric involvement in Sjögren's syndrome simulating early gastric carcinoma. Endoscopy 11:263–266, 1979.
68. Versapuech JM, et al: Sclerosing cholangitis, chronic pancreatitis and Sjögren's syndrome. Ann Med Interne 137:147–151, 1986.
69. Nishimori I, et al: Pancreatic involvement in patients with Sjögren's syndrome and primary biliary cirrhosis. Int J Pancreatol 17:47–54, 1995.
70. Guillevin L, et al: Gastrointestinal tract involvement in polyarteritis nodosa and Churg-Strauss syndrome. Ann Med Interne 146:260–267, 1995.
71. Fauci AS: Vasculitis. J Allergy Clin Immunol 72:211–223, 1983.
72. Guillevin L, et al: Prognostic factors in polyarteritis nodosa and Churg-Strauss syndrome: A prospective study in 342 patients. Medicine (Baltimore) 75:17–28, 1996.
73. Cupps TR, Fauci AS: The vasculitides. Major Probl Intern Med 21:1–211, 1981.
74. Bocanegra T, et al: Pancreatic pseudocyst: A complication of necrotizing vasculitis (polyarteritis nodosa). Arch Intern Med 140:1359–1361, 1980.
75. McCauley RL, Johnston MR, Fauci AS: Surgical aspects of systemic necrotizing vasculitis. Surgery 97:104–110, 1985.
76. Barquist ES, Goldstein N, Zinner MJ: Polyarteritis nodosa presenting as a biliary stricture. Surgery 109:16–19, 1991.
77. Erhardt A, et al: Successful treatment of hepatitis B virus–associated polyarteritis nodosa with a combination of prednisolone, alpha-interferon, and lamivudine. J Hepatol 33:677–683, 2000.
78. Lanham JG, et al: Systemic vasculitis with asthma and eosinophilia: A clinical approach to the Churg-Strauss syndrome. Medicine (Baltimore) 63:65–81, 1984.
79. Abell MR, et al: Allergic granulomatosis with massive gastric involvement. N Engl J Med 282:665–668, 1970.
80. Kimura T, et al: Churg-Strauss syndrome diagnosed and followed with gastrointestinal fiberscopic studies and electroneuromyography. Intern Med 37:646–650, 1998.
81. Shimamoto C, et al: Churg-Strauss syndrome (allergic granulomatous angiitis) with peculiar multiple colonic ulcers. Am J Gastroenterol 85: 316–319, 1990.
82. Chumbley LC, Harrison EG Jr, DeRemee RA: Allergic granulomatosis and angiitis (Churg-Strauss syndrome): Report and analysis of 30 cases. Mayo Clin Proc 52:477–484, 1977.
83. Cappell MS, Gupta AM: Colonic lesions associated with Henoch-Schönlein purpura. Am J Gastroenterol 85:1186–1188, 1990.
84. Martinez-Frontanilla LA, et al: Surgical complications in Henoch-Schönlein purpura. J Pediatr Surg 19:434–436, 1984.
85. Smith HJ, Krupski WC: Spontaneous intestinal perforation in Schönlein-Henoch purpura. South Med J 73:603–606, 610, 1980.
86. Mohammed R: Acute appendicitis: A complication of Henoch-Schönlein purpura. J R Coll Surg Edinb 27:367, 1982.
87. Kumon Y, et al: A case of vasculitic cholecystitis associated with Schönlein-Henoch purpura in an adult. Gastroenterol Jpn 23:68–72, 1988.
88. Froehlich F, et al: Association of Crohn's disease and Cogan's syndrome. Dig Dis Sci 39:1134–1137, 1994.

89. Camilleri M, et al: Gastrointestinal manifestations of systemic vasculitis. Q J Med 52:141–149, 1983.
90. Haworth SJ, Pusey CD: Severe intestinal involvement in Wegener's granulomatosis. Gut 25:1296–1300, 1984.
91. Fauci AS, et al: Wegener's granulomatosis: Prospective clinical and therapeutic experience with 85 patients for 21 years. Ann Intern Med 98:76–85, 1983.
92. McNabb WR, Lennox MS, Wedzicha JA: Small intestinal perforation in Wegener's granulomatosis. Postgrad Med J 58:123–125, 1982.
93. Doe WF, et al: Coeliac disease, vasculitis, and cryoglobulinaemia. Gut 13:112–123, 1972.
94. Speiser JC, Moore TL, Zuckner J: Ulcerative colitis with arthritis and vasculitis. Clin Rheumatol 4:343–347, 1985.
95. Laurence J, Nachman R: Cryoglobulinemia. Dis Mon 27:1–48, 1981.
96. Misiani R, et al: Interferon alfa-2a therapy in cryoglobulinemia associated with hepatitis C virus (see comments). N Engl J Med 330:751–756, 1994.
97. Mullick FG, et al: Drug-related vasculitis: Clinicopathologic correlations in 30 patients. Hum Pathol 10:313–325, 1979.
98. Merkel PA: Drugs associated with vasculitis. Curr Opin Rheumatol 10:45–50, 1998.
99. Sigal LH: The neurologic presentation of vasculitic and rheumatologic syndromes: A review. Medicine (Baltimore) 66:157–180, 1987.
100. Merkel PA, et al: Cocaine-associated cerebral vasculitis. Semin Arthritis Rheum 25:172–183, 1995.
101. Sudhakar CB, et al: Mesenteric ischemia secondary to cocaine abuse: Case reports and literature review. Am J Gastroenterol 92:1053–1054, 1997.
102. Yashiro K, et al: Esophageal lesions in intestinal Behçet's disease. Endoscopy 18:57–60, 1986.
103. Masugi J, et al: A case of Behçet's disease with multiple longitudinal ulcers all over the colon. Am J Gastroenterol 89:778–780, 1994.
104. Iida M, et al: Postoperative recurrence in patients with intestinal Behçet's disease. Dis Colon Rectum 37:16–21, 1994.
105. Iwama T, Utzunomiya J: Anal complication in Behçet's syndrome. Jpn J Surg 7:114–117, 1977.
106. Griffin JW Jr, et al: Behçet's disease with multiple sites of gastrointestinal involvement. South Med J 75:1405–1408, 1982.
107. Satake K, et al: Pyloric stenosis: An unusual complication of Behçet's disease. Am J Gastroenterol 81:816–818, 1986.
108. Hamza M, et al: Intestinal amyloidosis: An unusual complication of Behçet's disease [letter]. Am J Gastroenterol 83:793–794, 1988.
109. Tolia V, et al: A case of Behçet's disease with intestinal involvement due to Crohn's disease. Am J Gastroenterol 84:322–325, 1989.
110. Moll JM, et al: Associations between ankylosing spondylitis, psoriatic arthritis, Reiter's disease, the intestinal arthropathies, and Behçet's syndrome. Medicine (Baltimore) 53:343–364, 1974.
111. Altomonte L, et al: Clinically silent inflammatory gut lesions in undifferentiated spondyloarthropathies. Clin Rheumatol 13:565–570, 1994.
112. Brandt J, et al: Successful treatment of active ankylosing spondylitis with the anti-tumor necrosis factor alpha monoclonal antibody infliximab. Arthritis Rheum 43:1346–1352, 2000.
113. McLean AM, et al: Malabsorption in Marfan (Ehlers-Danlos) syndrome. J Clin Gastroenterol 7:304–308, 1985.
114. Stillman AE, Painter R, Hollister DW: Ehlers-Danlos syndrome type IV: Diagnosis and therapy of associated bowel perforation. Am J Gastroenterol 86:360–362, 1991.
115. Odabas AR, et al: Severe and prolonged febrile myalgia in familial Mediterranean fever. Scand J Rheumatol 29:394–395, 2000.
116. Samuels J, et al: Familial Mediterranean fever at the millennium: Clinical spectrum, ancient mutations, and a survey of 100 American referrals to the National Institutes of Health. Medicine (Baltimore) 77: 268–297, 1998.
117. Ancient missense mutations in a new member of the RoRet gene family are likely to cause familial Mediterranean fever. The International FMF Consortium. Cell 90:797–807, 1997.
118. A candidate gene for familial Mediterranean fever. The French FMF Consortium. Nat Genet 17:25–31, 1997.
119. Goldfinger SE: Colchicine for familial Mediterranean fever. N Engl J Med 287:1302, 1972.
120. Abrams HL, Spiro R, Goldstein N: Metastases in carcinoma: Analysis of 1000 autopsied cases. Cancer 3:74–85, 1950.
121. Herbsman H, et al: Tumors of the small intestine. Curr Probl Surg 17: 121–182, 1980.
122. Das Gupta TK, Brasfield RD: Metastatic melanoma of the gastrointestinal tract. Arch Surg 88:969–973, 1964.
123. Said SI, Faloona GR: Elevated plasma and tissue levels of vasoactive intestinal polypeptide in the watery-diarrhea syndrome due to pancreatic, bronchogenic, and other tumors. N Engl J Med 293:155–160, 1975.
124. Viale G, et al: Vasoactive intestinal polypeptide–, somatostatin-, and calcitonin-producing adrenal pheochromocytoma associated with the watery diarrhea (WDHH) syndrome: First case report with immunohistochemical findings. Cancer 55:1099–1106, 1985.
125. Dourakis SP, et al: Cholestatic jaundice as a paraneoplastic manifestation of renal cell carcinoma. Eur J Gastroenterol Hepatol 9:311–314, 1985.
126. Aoyagi T, et al: Sinusoidal dilatation of the liver as a paraneoplastic manifestation of renal cell carcinoma. Hum Pathol 20:1193–1197, 1989.
127. Sodhi N, et al: Autonomic function and motility in intestinal pseudo-obstruction caused by paraneoplastic syndrome. Dig Dis Sci 34:1937–1942, 1989.
128. Schuffler MD, et al: Intestinal pseudo-obstruction as the presenting manifestation of small-cell carcinoma of the lung: A paraneoplastic neuropathy of the gastrointestinal tract. Ann Intern Med 98:129–134, 1983.
129. Lucchinetti CF, Kimmel DW, Lennon VA: Paraneoplastic and oncologic profiles of patients seropositive for type 1 antineuronal nuclear autoantibodies. Neurology 50:652–657, 1998.
130. Chinn JS, Schuffler MD: Paraneoplastic visceral neuropathy as a cause of severe gastrointestinal motor dysfunction. Gastroenterology 95: 1279–1286, 1988.
131. Lhermitte F, et al: Paralysis of digestive tract with lesions of myenteric plexuses: A new paraneoplastic syndrome (author's transl). Rev Neurol 136:825–836, 1980.
132. Lennon VA, et al: Enteric neuronal autoantibodies in pseudo-obstruction with small-cell lung carcinoma (see comments). Gastroenterology 100:137–142, 1991.
133. Hunter TB, Bjelland JC: Gastrointestinal complications of leukemia and its treatment. AJR Am J Roentgenol 142:513–518, 1984.
134. Leukaemia and the bowel [editorial]. Med J Aust 1:89–90, 1975.
135. Stratemeier PH: Massive esophageal hemorrhage in leukemia. AJR Am J Roentgenol 129:1106–1107, 1977.
136. Anderson W, Helman CA, Hirschowitz BI: Basophilic leukemia and the hypersecretion of gastric acid and pepsin. Gastroenterology 95: 195–198, 1988.
137. Kothur R, et al: Endoscopic leukemic polyposis. Am J Gastroenterol 85:884–886, 1990.
138. Buyukasik Y, et al: Neutropenic enterocolitis in adult leukemias. Int J Hematol 66:47–55, 1997.
139. Kunkel JM, Rosenthal D: Management of the ileocecal syndrome: Neutropenic enterocolitis. Dis Colon Rectum 29:196–199, 1986.
140. Yeong ML, Nicholson GI: *Clostridium septicum* infection in neutropenic enterocolitis. Pathology 20:194–197, 1988.
141. Katz JA, et al: Typhlitis: An 18-year experience and postmortem review. Cancer 65:1041–1047, 1990.
142. Merine DS, et al: Right lower quadrant pain in the immunocompromised patient: CT findings in 10 cases. AJR Am J Roentgenol 149: 1177–1179, 1987.
143. Fainstein V, Bodey GP, Fekety R: Relapsing pseudomembranous colitis associated with cancer chemotherapy. J Infect Dis 143:865, 1981.
144. Sehdev MK, et al: Perianal and anorectal complications in leukemia. Cancer 31:149–152, 1973.
145. Iqbal N, et al: Diagnosis of gastrointestinal graft-versus-host disease. Am J Gastroenterol 95:3034–3038, 2000.
146. Kaur S, et al: Incidence and outcome of overt gastrointestinal bleeding in patients undergoing bone marrow transplantation. Dig Dis Sci 41: 598–603, 1996.
147. Chirletti P, et al: Gastrointestinal emergencies in patients with acute intestinal graft-versus-host disease. Leuk Lymphoma 29:129–137, 1998.
148. Terdiman JP, et al: The role of endoscopic evaluation in patients with suspected intestinal graft-versus-host disease after allogeneic bone-marrow transplantation. Endoscopy 28:680–685, 1996.
149. Silverstein MN, Wollaeger EE, Baggenstoss AH: Gastrointestinal and abdominal manifestations of agnogenic myeloid metaplasia. Arch Intern Med 131:532–537, 1973.
150. Schreibman D, et al: Small intestinal myeloid metaplasia. JAMA 259: 2580–2582, 1988.
151. Buss DH, Stuart JJ, Lipscomb GE: The incidence of thrombotic and hemorrhagic disorders in association with extreme thrombocytosis: An analysis of 129 cases. Am J Hematol 20:365–372, 1985.
152. Valla D, et al: Primary myeloproliferative disorder and hepatic vein

thrombosis: A prospective study of erythroid colony formation in vitro in 20 patients with Budd-Chiari syndrome. Ann Intern Med 103:329–334, 1985.

153. Kyle RA, Greipp PR: Amyloidosis (AL): Clinical and laboratory features in 229 cases. Mayo Clin Proc 58:665–683, 1983.
154. Gradishar W, Recant W, Shapiro C: Obstructing plasmacytoma of the duodenum: First manifestation of relapsed multiple myeloma. Am J Gastroenterol 83:77–79, 1988.
155. Rao KG, Yaghmai I: Plasmacytoma of the large bowel: A review of the literature and a case report of multiple myeloma involving the rectosigmoid. Gastrointest Radiol 3:225–228, 1978.
156. Mattila J, et al: Macroglobulinemia with abdominal symptoms caused by intestinal extracellular macroglobulin. Virchows Arch 389:241–251, 1980.
157. Bohus R, et al: Retroperitoneal haemorrhage with abscess formation complicating Waldenström's macroglobulinaemia. Int Urol Nephrol 17:255–259, 1985.
158. Brandt LJ, et al: Small intestine involvement in Waldenström's macroglobulinemia: Case report and review of the literature. Dig Dis Sci 26: 174–180, 1981.
159. Kyle RA, Greipp PR, Banks PM: The diverse picture of gamma heavy-chain disease: Report of seven cases and review of literature. Mayo Clin Proc 56:439–451, 1981.
160. Ryan JC: Premalignant conditions of the small intestine. Semin Gastrointest Dis 7:88–93, 1996.
161. Dodds WJ, Spitzer RM, Friedland GW: Gastrointestinal roentgenographic manifestations of hemophilia. AJR Am J Roentgenol 110: 413–416, 1970.
162. Miller JM Jr, Pastorek JG: Thrombotic thrombocytopenic purpura and hemolytic-uremic syndrome in pregnancy. Clin Obstet Gynecol 34:64–71, 1991.
163. Lesesne JB, et al: Cancer-associated hemolytic-uremic syndrome: Analysis of 85 cases from a national registry. J Clin Oncol 7:781–789, 1989.
164. Neill MA, Agosti J, Rosen H: Hemorrhagic colitis with *Escherichia coli* 0157:H7 preceding adult hemolytic-uremic syndrome. Arch Intern Med 145:2215–2217, 1985.
165. Koster F, et al: Hemolytic-uremic syndrome after shigellosis: Relation to endotoxemia and circulating immune complexes. N Engl J Med 298:927–933, 1978.
166. Baker NM, et al: Haemolytic-uraemic syndrome in typhoid fever. BMJ 2:84–87, 1974.
167. Prober CG, Tune B, Hoder L: *Yersinia* pseudotuberculosis septicemia. Am J Dis Child 133:623–624, 1979.
168. Chamovitz BN, et al: *Campylobacter jejuni*–associated hemolytic-uremic syndrome in a mother and daughter. Pediatrics 71:253–256, 1983.
169. Wong CS, et al: The risk of the hemolytic-uremic syndrome after antibiotic treatment of *Escherichia coli* O157:H7 infections. N Engl J Med 342:1930–1936, 2000.
170. Sun CC, Hill JL, Combs JW: Hemolytic-uremic syndrome: Initial presentation mimicking intestinal intussusception. Pediatr Pathol 1: 415–422, 1983.
171. Grodinsky S, et al: Gastrointestinal manifestations of hemolytic-uremic syndrome: Recognition of pancreatitis. J Pediatr Gastroenterol Nutr 11:518–524, 1990.
172. Yates RS, Osterholm RK: Hemolytic-uremic syndrome colitis. J Clin Gastroenterol 2:359–363, 1980.
173. Wallon P, et al: Pseudo-surgical aspects of hemolytic-uremic syndrome in childhood. Chir Pediatr 22:255–259, 1981.
174. Lichtin AE, Silberstein LE, Schreiber AD: Thrombotic thrombocytopenic purpura with colitis in an elderly woman [letter]. JAMA 255: 1435–1436, 1986.
175. Jacobs WA: Acute thrombotic thrombocytopenic purpura and cholecystitis. J Emerg Med 2:265–269, 1985.
176. Bell WR, et al: Improved survival in thrombotic thrombocytopenic purpura/hemolytic-uremic syndrome: Clinical experience in 108 patients. N Engl J Med 325:398–403, 1991.
177. Dervenoulas J, et al: Thrombotic thrombocytopenic purpura/hemolytic-uremic syndrome (TTP/HUS): Treatment outcome, relapses, prognostic factors—a single-center experience of 48 cases. Ann Hematol 79:66–72, 2000.
178. Baumgartner F, Klein S: The presentation and management of the acute abdomen in the patient with sickle-cell anemia. Am Surg 55: 660–664, 1989.
179. Brittenham GM, et al: Efficacy of deferoxamine in preventing complications of iron overload in patients with thalassemia major. N Engl J Med 331:567–573, 1994.
180. Olivieri NF, et al: Long-term safety and effectiveness of iron-chelation therapy with deferiprone for thalassemia major. N Engl J Med 339: 417–423, 1998.
181. Schmidt RE, et al: Ultrastructural and immunohistochemical characterization of autonomic neuropathy in genetically diabetic Chinese hamsters. Lab Invest 61:77–92, 1989.
182. Ramabadran K, et al: Streptozotocin-diabetes attenuates alpha$_2$-adrenoceptor agonist–induced delay in small intestinal transit in mice. J Auton Pharmacol 10:163–171, 1990.
183. Lucas PD, Sardar AM: Effects of diabetes on cholinergic transmission in two rat gut preparations. Gastroenterology 100:123–128, 1991.
184. Di Giulio AM, et al: Denervation and hyperinnervation in the nervous system of diabetic animals: I. The autonomic neuronal dystrophy of the gut. J Neurosci Res 24:355–361, 1989.
185. Sundkvist G, et al: Esophageal motor function evaluated by scintigraphy, video-radiography, and manometry in diabetic patients. Acta Radiol 30:17–19, 1989.
186. Pozzi M, et al: Upper gastrointestinal involvement in diabetes mellitus: Study of esophagogastric function. Acta Diabetol Lat 25:333–341, 1988.
187. Holloway RH, et al: Relationship between esophageal motility and transit in patients with type I diabetes mellitus. Am J Gastroenterol 94:3150–3157, 1999.
188. Murray FE, et al: Esophageal function in diabetes mellitus with special reference to acid studies and relationship to peripheral neuropathy. Am J Gastroenterol 82:840–843, 1987.
189. Horowitz M, et al: Disordered gastric motor function in diabetes mellitus: Recent insights into prevalence, pathophysiology, clinical relevance, and treatment. Scand J Gastroenterol 26:673–684, 1991.
190. Malagelada JR: Diabetic gastroparesis. Semin Gastrointest Dis 6:181–186, 1995.
191. Mearin F, Camilleri M, Malagelada JR: Pyloric dysfunction in diabetics with recurrent nausea and vomiting. Gastroenterology 90:1919–1925, 1986.
192. Achem-Karam SR, et al: Plasma motilin concentration and interdigestive migrating motor complex in diabetic gastroparesis: Effect of metoclopramide. Gastroenterology 88:492–499, 1985.
193. Patterson D, et al: A double-blind multicenter comparison of domperidone and metoclopramide in the treatment of diabetic patients with symptoms of gastroparesis. Am J Gastroenterol 94:1230–1234, 1999.
194. Brown CK, Khanderia U: Use of metoclopramide, domperidone, and cisapride in the management of diabetic gastroparesis. Clin Pharmacol 9:357–365, 1990.
195. Horowitz M, et al: Acute and chronic effects of domperidone on gastric emptying in diabetic autonomic neuropathy. Dig Dis Sci 30:1–9, 1985.
196. Janssens J, et al: Improvement of gastric emptying in diabetic gastroparesis by erythromycin: Preliminary studies. N Engl J Med 322: 1028–1031, 1990.
197. Sturm A, et al: Prokinetics in patients with gastroparesis: A systematic analysis. Digestion 60:422–427, 1999.
198. Oldenburg B, Diepersloot RJ, Hoekstra JB: High seroprevalence of *Helicobacter pylori* in diabetes mellitus patients. Dig Dis Sci 41:458–461, 1996.
199. Dore MP, et al: Diabetes mellitus and *Helicobacter pylori* infection. Nutrition 16:407–410, 2000.
200. Lysy J, Israeli E, Goldin E: The prevalence of chronic diarrhea among diabetic patients. Am J Gastroenterol 94:2165–2170, 1999.
201. Valdovinos MA, Camilleri M, Zimmerman BR: Chronic diarrhea in diabetes mellitus: Mechanisms and an approach to diagnosis and treatment. Mayo Clin Proc 68:691–702, 1993.
202. Camilleri M, et al: Effect of six weeks of treatment with cisapride in gastroparesis and intestinal pseudo-obstruction. Gastroenterology 96: 704–712, 1989.
203. Tsai ST, Vinik AI, Brunner JF: Diabetic diarrhea and somatostatin [letter]. Ann Intern Med 104:894, 1986.
204. von der Ohe MR, et al: Differential regional effects of octreotide on human gastrointestinal motor function. Gut 36:743–748, 1995.
205. Schiller LR, et al: Pathogenesis of fecal incontinence in diabetes mellitus: Evidence for internal anal sphincter dysfunction. N Engl J Med 307:1666–1671, 1982.
206. Marzuk PM: Biofeedback for gastrointestinal disorders: A review of the literature. Ann Intern Med 103:240–244, 1985.
207. Atkinson M, Hosking DJ: Gastrointestinal complications of diabetes mellitus. Clin Gastroenterol 12:633–650, 1983.
208. Battle WM, Cohen JD, Snape WJ Jr: Disorders of colonic motility in patients with diabetes mellitus. Yale J Biol Med 56:277–283, 1983.

209. Anuras S, Shirazi SS: Colonic pseudo-obstruction. Am J Gastroenterol 79:525–532, 1984.
210. Streib EW, et al: Diabetic thoracic radiculopathy: Electrodiagnostic study. Muscle Nerve 9:548–553, 1986.
211. Hayashi Y, et al: Gas-containing pyogenic liver abscess—a case report and review of the literature. Jpn J Surg 19:74–77, 1989.
212. Watson JA, Windsor JA, Wynne-Jones G: Conservative management of a *Yersinia enterocolitica* hepatic abscess. Aust N Z J Surg 59:353–354, 1989.
213. Lillemoe KD, Pitt HA, Cameron JL: Sclerosing cholangitis. Adv Surg 21:65–92, 1988.
214. Lenaerts J, et al: Fatty liver hepatitis and type 5 hyperlipoproteinemia in juvenile diabetes mellitus: Case report and review of the literature. J Clin Gastroenterol 12:93–97, 1990.
215. Malone JI: Juvenile diabetes and acute pancreatitis. J Pediatr 85:825–827, 1974.
216. Renner IG, et al: Death due to acute pancreatitis: A retrospective analysis of 405 autopsy cases. Dig Dis Sci 30:1005–1018, 1985.
217. Cuzick J, Babiker AG: Pancreatic cancer, alcohol, diabetes mellitus, and gallbladder disease. Int J Cancer 43:415–421, 1989.
218. Frye JN, et al: Pancreatic cancer and diabetes: Is there a relationship? A case-controlled study. Aust N Z J Surg 70:722–724, 2000.
219. Meshkinpour H, Afrasiabi MA, Valenta LJ: Esophageal motor function in Graves' disease. Dig Dis Sci 24:159–161, 1979.
220. Noto H, et al: Hyperthyroidism presenting as dysphagia. Intern Med 39:472–473, 2000.
221. Wegener M, et al: Effect of hyperthyroidism on the transit of a caloric solid-liquid meal through the stomach, the small intestine, and the colon in man. J Clin Endocrinol Metab 75:745–749, 1992.
222. Jonderko K, et al: Gastric emptying in hyperthyroidism. Am J Gastroenterol 92:835–838, 1997.
223. Papa A, et al: Effects of propylthiouracil on intestinal transit time and symptoms in hyperthyroid patients. Hepatogastroenterology 44:426–429, 1997.
224. Modebe O: Autoimmune thyroid disease with ulcerative colitis. Postgrad Med J 62:475–476, 1986.
225. Huang MJ, Liaw YF: Clinical associations between thyroid and liver diseases. J Gastroenterol Hepatol 10:344–350, 1995.
226. Biscoveanu M, Hasinski S: Abnormal results of liver function tests in patients with Graves' disease. Endocr Pract 6:367–369, 2000.
227. Gurlek A, Cobankara V, Bayraktar M: Liver tests in hyperthyroidism: Effect of antithyroid therapy. J Clin Gastroenterol 24:180–183, 1997.
228. Liaw YF, et al: Hepatic injury during propylthiouracil therapy in patients with hyperthyroidism: A cohort study. Ann Intern Med 118: 424–428, 1993.
229. Uibo R, et al: Relation of parietal cell and thyroid antibodies to the state of gastric mucosa and basal serum gastrin levels during a 6-year follow up. Clin Exp Immunol 77:202–205, 1989.
230. Crowe JP, et al: Primary biliary cirrhosis: The prevalence of hypothyroidism and its relationship to thyroid autoantibodies and sicca syndrome. Gastroenterology 78:1437–1441, 1980.
231. Elta GH, et al: Increased incidence of hypothyroidism in primary biliary cirrhosis. Dig Dis Sci 28:971–975, 1983.
232. Mangold D, Woolam GL, Garcia-Rinaldi R: Intestinal obstruction due to phytobezoars: Observations in two patients with hypothyroidism and previous gastric surgery. Arch Surg 113:1001–1003, 1978.
233. Bassotti G, et al: Intestinal pseudo-obstruction secondary to hypothyroidism: Importance of small bowel manometry. J Clin Gastroenterol 14:56–58, 1992.
234. Goldin E, Wengrower D: Diarrhea in hypothyroidism: Bacterial overgrowth as a possible etiology. J Clin Gastroenterol 12:98–99, 1990.
235. Desrame J, et al: Isolated ascites revealing a hypothyroidism: Study of 2 cases. Gastroenterol Clin Biol 22:732–735, 1998.
236. Dusheiko G: Side effects of alpha interferon in chronic hepatitis C. Hepatology 26:112S–121S, 1997.
237. Storset O, et al: A patient with Cronkhite-Canada syndrome, myxedema, and muscle atrophy. Acta Med Scand 205:343–346, 1979.
238. Cox TM, et al: Role of calcitonin in diarrhoea associated with medullary carcinoma of the thyroid. Gut 20:629–633, 1979.
239. Rambaud JC, et al: Pathophysiological study of diarrhoea in a patient with medullary thyroid carcinoma: Evidence against a secretory mechanism and for the role of shortened colonic transit time. Gut 29:537–543, 1988.
240. Li BU, et al: Heterogeneity of diagnoses presenting as cyclic vomiting. Pediatrics 102:583–587, 1998.
241. Khafagi FA, Lloyd HM, Gough IR: Intestinal pseudo-obstruction in pheochromocytoma. Aust N Z J Med 17:246–248, 1987.
242. Vazquez-Quintana E, et al: Pheochromocytoma and gastrointestinal bleeding. Am Surg 61:937–939, 1995.
243. Guslandi M, Tittobello A: Steroid ulcers: A myth revisited [editorial]. BMJ 304:655–666, 1992.
244. Terzolo M, et al: High prevalence of colonic polyps in patients with acromegaly: Influence of sex and age. Arch Intern Med 154:1272–1276, 1994.
245. Delhougne B, et al: The prevalence of colonic polyps in acromegaly: A colonoscopic and pathological study in 103 patients. J Clin Endocrinol Metab 80:3223–3226, 1995.
246. Renehan AG, et al: The prevalence and characteristics of colorectal neoplasia in acromegaly. J Clin Endocrinol Metab 85:3417–3424, 2000.
247. Su AY, Bilhartz LE: Endocrine-related gut dysfunction. Semin Gastrointest Dis 6:217–227, 1995.
248. Smith MD, et al: Hyperparathyroidism and chronic pancreatitis. S Afr J Surg 37:12–14, 1999.
249. Mjaland O, Normann E: Severe pancreatitis after parathyroidectomy. Scand J Gastroenterol 35:446–448, 2000.
250. Ahonen P, et al: Clinical variation of autoimmune polyendocrinopathy-candidiasis-ectodermal dystrophy (APECED) in a series of 68 patients. N Engl J Med 322:1829–1836, 1990.
251. O'Donnell D, Myers AM: Intestinal lymphangiectasia with protein-losing enteropathy, toxic copper accumulation, and hypoparathyroidism. Aust N Z J Med 20:167–169, 1990.
252. Wortsman J, Kumar V: Idiopathic hypoparathyroidism coexisting with celiac disease: Immunologic studies. Am J Med Sci 307:420–427, 1994.
253. Van Vlem B, Schoonjans R, Vanholder R, et al: Delayed gastric emptying in dyspeptic chronic hemodialysis patients. Am J Kidney Dis 36:962–968, 2000.
254. Kang JY, et al: Prevalence of peptic ulcer in patients undergoing maintenance hemodialysis. Dig Dis Sci 33:774–778, 1988.
255. Moustafa FE, et al: *Helicobacter pylori* and uremic gastritis: A histopathologic study and a correlation with endoscopic and bacteriologic findings. Am J Nephrol 17:165–171, 1997.
256. Musola R, et al: Prevalence of gastroduodenal lesions in uremic patients undergoing dialysis and after renal transplantation. Gastrointest Endosc 30:343–346, 1984.
257. Zuckerman GR, et al: Upper gastrointestinal bleeding in patients with chronic renal failure. Ann Intern Med 102:588–592, 1985.
258. Paimela H, et al: Relation between serum group II pepsinogen concentration and the degree of Brunner's gland hyperplasia in patients with chronic renal failure. Gut 26:198–202, 1985.
259. Selkurt EE, Rothe CF, Richardson D: Characteristics of reactive hyperemia in the canine intestine. Circ Res 15:532, 1964.
260. Kiel JW, Riedel GL, Shepherd AP: Local control of canine gastric mucosal blood flow. Gastroenterology 93:1041–1053, 1987.
261. Texter EC Jr, et al: Effects of major cations on gastric and mesenteric vascular resistances. Am J Physiol 212:569–573, 1967.
262. Hida M, et al: Clinical report on hemodialysis in the Department of Transplantation, Tokai University School of Medicine. Tokai J Exp Clin Med 6:247–257, 1981.
263. Navab F, et al: Angiodysplasia in patients with renal insufficiency. Am J Gastroenterol 84:1297–1301, 1989.
264. Chalasani N, Cotsonis G, Wilcox CM: Upper gastrointestinal bleeding in patients with chronic renal failure: Role of vascular ectasia. Am J Gastroenterol 91:2329–2332, 1996.
265. Rubenstein RB, et al: Uremic ileus: Uremia presenting colonic obstruction. N Y State J Med 79:248–249, 1979.
266. Cooney DR, et al: Small bowel obstruction and ileal perforation: Complications of uremia. J Indiana State Med Assoc 69:781–784, 1976.
267. Mitch WE: Effects of intestinal flora on nitrogen metabolism in patients with chronic renal failure. Am J Clin Nutr 31:1594–1600, 1978.
268. Sachs EF, et al: Pancreatic exocrine hypofunction in the wasting syndrome of end-stage renal disease. Am J Gastroenterol 78:170–173, 1983.
269. Bischel MD, Reese T, Engel J: Spontaneous perforation of the colon in a hemodialysis patient. Am J Gastroenterol 74:182–184, 1980.
270. Goldberg M, Hoffman GC, Wombolt DG: Massive hemorrhage from rectal ulcers in chronic renal failure. Ann Intern Med 100:397, 1984.
271. Gordon SJ, et al: Abnormal intestinal bile acid distribution in azo-

taemic man: A possible role in the pathogenesis of uraemic diarrhoea. Gut 17:58–67, 1976.
272. Milner LS, et al: Penicillin-resistant pneumococcal peritonitis in nephrotic syndrome. Arch Dis Child 62:964–965, 1987.
273. Han SH, Reynolds TB, Fong TL: Nephrogenic ascites: Analysis of 16 cases and review of the literature. Medicine (Baltimore) 77:233–245, 1998.
274. Rodriguez HJ, et al: Recurrent ascites following peritoneal dialysis: A new syndrome? Arch Intern Med 134:283–287, 1974.
275. Yen MC, Stewart EH: Peritoneovenous shunt for ascites associated with maintenance dialysis. Clin Nephrol 8:446–448, 1977.
276. Silberstein SD: Migraine symptoms: Results of a survey of self-reported migraineurs. Headache 35:387–396, 1995.
277. Mavromichalis I, Zaramboukas T, Giala MM: Migraine of gastrointestinal origin. Eur J Pediatr 154:406–410, 1995.
278. Worawattanakul M, et al: Abdominal migraine: Prophylactic treatment and follow-up. J Pediatr Gastroenterol Nutr 28:37–40, 1999.
279. Blau JN, MacGregor EA: Is abdominal pain a feature of adult migraine? Headache 35:207–209, 1995.
280. Peppercorn MA, Herzog AG: The spectrum of abdominal epilepsy in adults. Am J Gastroenterol 84:1294–1296, 1989.
281. Fried I, Spencer DD, Spencer SS: The anatomy of epileptic auras: Focal pathology and surgical outcome. J Neurosurg 83:60–66, 1995.
282. Ullman T, Reding M: Gastrointestinal dysfunction in stroke. Semin Neurol 16:269–275, 1996.
283. Kamada T, et al: Acute gastroduodenal lesions in head injury: An endoscopic study. Am J Gastroenterol 68:249–253, 1977.
284. Bowen JC, Fleming WH, Thompson JC: Increased gastrin release following penetrating central nervous system injury. Surgery 75:720–724, 1974.
285. Idjadi F, et al: Prospective study of gastric secretion in stressed patients with intracranial injury. J Trauma 11:681–688, 1971.
286. Cushing H: Peptic ulcers and interbrain. Surg Gynecol Obstet 55:1–34, 1932.
287. Segal JL, Milne N, Brunnemann SR: Gastric emptying is impaired in patients with spinal cord injury. Am J Gastroenterol 90:466–470, 1995.
288. Gore RM, Mintzer RA, Calenoff L: Gastrointestinal complications of spinal cord injury. Spine 6:538–544, 1981.
289. Kiwerski J: Bleeding from the alimentary canal during the management of spinal cord injury patients. Paraplegia 24:92–96, 1986.
290. Osteen RT, Barsamian EM: Delayed gastric emptying after vagotomy and drainage in the spinal cord injury patient. Paraplegia 19:46–49, 1981.
291. Berlly MH, Wilmot CB: Acute abdominal emergencies during the first four weeks after spinal cord injury. Arch Phys Med Rehabil 65:687–690, 1984.
292. McGuire TJ, Kumar VN: Autonomic dysreflexia in the spinal cord-injured: What the physician should know about this medical emergency. Postgrad Med 80:81–84, 89, 1986.
293. Halstead LS, et al: Drug absorption in spinal cord injury. Arch Phys Med Rehabil 66:298–301, 1985.
294. Meshkinpour H, Vaziri N, Gordon S: Gastrointestinal pathology in patients with chronic renal failure associated with spinal cord injury. Am J Gastroenterol 77:562–564, 1982.
295. Bernstein L, Joseph R, Staas WE Jr: Solitary colonic ulcer in a spinal cord–injured patient. Arch Phys Med Rehabil 67:194–195, 1986.
296. Lynch AC, Wong C, Anthony A, et al: Bowel dysfunction following spinal cord injury: A description of bowel function in a spinal cord–injured population and comparison with age- and gender-matched controls. Spinal Cord 38:717–723, 2000.
297. Aaronson MJ, Freed MM, Burakoff R: Colonic myoelectric activity in persons with spinal cord injury. Dig Dis Sci 30:295–300, 1985.
298. Meshkinpour H, Nowroozi F, Glick ME: Colonic compliance in patients with spinal cord injury. Arch Phys Med Rehabil 64:111–112, 1983.
299. Longo WE, Ballantyne GH, Modlin IM: Colorectal disease in spinal cord patients: An occult diagnosis. Dis Colon Rectum 33:131–134, 1990.
300. Chelimsky G, Wszolek Z, Chelimsky TC: Gastrointestinal dysfunction in autonomic neuropathy. Semin Neurol 16:259–268, 1996.
301. Hart RG, Kanter MC: Acute autonomic neuropathy: Two cases and a clinical review. Arch Intern Med 150:2373–2376, 1990.
302. Vassallo M, et al: Gastrointestinal motor dysfunction in acquired selective cholinergic dysautonomia associated with infectious mononucleosis. Gastroenterology 100:252–258, 1991.
303. Suarez GA, et al: Idiopathic autonomic neuropathy: Clinical, neurophysiologic, and follow-up studies on 27 patients. Neurology 44: 1675–1682, 1994.
304. Neville BG, Sladen GE: Acute autonomic neuropathy following primary herpes simplex infection. J Neurol Neurosurg Psychiatry 47: 648–650, 1984.
305. Jansen RW, et al: Postprandial hypotension in elderly patients with unexplained syncope. Arch Intern Med 155:945–952, 1995.
306. Kagel MC, Leopold NA: Dysphagia in Huntington's disease: A 16-year retrospective. Dysphagia 7:106–114, 1992.
307. Byrne KG, Pfeiffer R, Quigley EM: Gastrointestinal dysfunction in Parkinson's disease: A report of clinical experience at a single center. J Clin Gastroenterol 19:11–16, 1994.
308. Bassotti G, et al: Esophageal manometric abnormalities in Parkinson's disease. Dysphagia 13:28–31, 1998.
309. Pfeiffer RF: Gastrointestinal dysfunction in Parkinson's disease. Clin Neurosci 5:136–146, 1998.
310. Johnston BT, et al: Swallowing and esophageal function in Parkinson's disease. Am J Gastroenterol 90:1741–1746, 1995.
311. Fowler CJ, Henry MM: Gastrointestinal dysfunction in multiple sclerosis. Semin Neurol 16:277–279, 1996.
312. Caruana BJ, et al: Anorectal sensory and motor function in neurogenic fecal incontinence: Comparison between multiple sclerosis and diabetes mellitus. Gastroenterology 100:465–470, 1991.
313. Gill KP, et al: Defecography in multiple sclerosis patients with severe constipation. Radiology 191:553–556, 1994.
314. Strand EA, et al: Management of oral-pharyngeal dysphagia symptoms in amyotrophic lateral sclerosis. Dysphagia 11:129–139, 1996.
315. Garcia CA: A clinical review of Charcot-Marie-Tooth. Ann N Y Acad Sci 883:69–76, 1999.
316. Han YS, et al: Autoimmune hepatitis in a patient with myasthenia gravis and thymoma—a report on the first case in Korea. Korean J Intern Med 15:151–155, 2000.
317. Horigome H, et al: Coexistence of primary biliary cirrhosis and myasthenia gravis: A case study. Hepatogastroenterology 47:125–127, 2000.
318. Staiano A, et al: Upper gastrointestinal tract motility in children with progressive muscular dystrophy. J Pediatr 121:720–724, 1992.
319. Hirano M, et al: Mitochondrial neurogastrointestinal encephalomyopathy (MNGIE): Clinical, biochemical, and genetic features of an autosomal recessive mitochondrial disorder. Neurology 44:721–727, 1994.
320. Allgrove J, et al: Familial glucocorticoid deficiency with achalasia of the cardia and deficient tear production. Lancet 1:1284–1286, 1978.
321. Ronnblom A, Forsberg H, Danielsson A: Gastrointestinal symptoms in myotonic dystrophy. Scand J Gastroenterol 31:654–657, 1996.
322. Wakabayashi O, et al: The etiology of peptic ulceration in patients with chronic pulmonary emphysema. Nippon Shokakibyo Gakkai Zasshi 91:2174–2182, 1994.
323. Rotter JI: The genetics of peptic ulcer: More than one gene, more than one disease. Prog Med Genet 4:1–58, 1980.
324. Cook DJ, et al: Risk factors for gastrointestinal bleeding in critically ill patients. Canadian Critical Care Trials Group. N Engl J Med 330: 377–381, 1994.
325. Knobloch W, et al: Calcifying aortic valve stenosis and occult gastrointestinal hemorrhage (Heyde syndrome): description of 2 cases. Z Kardiol 88:448–453, 1999.
326. Yamada M, Hatakeyama S, Tsukagoshi H: Gastrointestinal amyloid deposition in AL (primary or myeloma-associated) and AA (secondary) amyloidosis: Diagnostic value of gastric biopsy. Hum Pathol 16: 1206–1211, 1985.
327. Gilat T, Spiro HM: Amyloidosis and the gut. Am J Dig Dis 13:619–633, 1968.
328. Schwartz Y, et al: An unusual case of temporomandibular joint arthropathy in systemic primary amyloidosis. J Oral Med 34:40–44, 1979.
329. Case records of the Massachusetts General Hospital. Case 43–1985. N Engl J Med 313:1070, 1985.
330. Raffi F, et al: Peritoneal amyloidosis in Waldenström's macroglobulinemia: X-ray computed tomographic aspects. J Radiol 66:735–738, 1985.
331. Dastur KJ, Ward JF: Amyloidoma of the stomach. Gastrointest Radiol 5:17–20, 1980.
332. Levy DJ, Franklin GO, Rosenthal WS: Gastrointestinal bleeding and amyloidosis. Am J Gastroenterol 77:422–426, 1982.
333. Choi HS, et al: Infarction of intestine with massive amyloid deposition

in two patients on long-term hemodialysis. Gastroenterology 96:230–234, 1989.
334. Hunter AM, et al: Protein-losing enteropathy due to gastrointestinal amyloidosis. Postgrad Med J 55:822–823, 1979.
335. Seliger G, et al: The spectrum of roentgen appearance in amyloidosis of the small and large bowel: Radiologic-pathologic correlation. Radiology 100:63–70, 1971.
336. Tada S, et al: Endoscopic and biopsy findings of the upper digestive tract in patients with amyloidosis. Gastrointest Endosc 36:10–14, 1990.
337. Zemer D, et al: Colchicine in the prevention and treatment of the amyloidosis of familial Mediterranean fever. N Engl J Med 314:1001–1005, 1986.
338. Buxbaum JN, et al: Amyloidosis of the AL type: Clinical, morphologic, and biochemical aspects of the response to therapy with alkylating agents and prednisone. Am J Med 67:867–878, 1979.
339. Ek BO, et al: Enterostomy in patients with primary neuropathic amyloidosis. Am J Gastroenterol 70:365–370, 1978.
340. Fraser AG, Arthur JF, Hamilton I: Intestinal pseudo-obstruction secondary to amyloidosis responsive to cisapride. Dig Dis Sci 36:532–535, 1991.
341. Fishman RS, Fleming CR, Li CY: Systemic mastocytosis with review of gastrointestinal manifestations. Mayo Clin Proc 54:51–54, 1979.
342. Jensen RT: Gastrointestinal abnormalities and involvement in systemic mastocytosis. Hematol Oncol Clin North Am 14:579–623, 2000.
343. Horan RF, Austen KF: Systemic mastocytosis: Retrospective review of a decade's clinical experience at the Brigham and Women's Hospital. J Invest Dermatol 96:5S–13S; discussion 13S–14S, 1991.
344. Adler SN, Klein RA, Lyon DT: Bleeding after liver biopsy in a patient with systemic mastocytosis and malabsorption. J Clin Gastroenterol 7:350–353, 1985.
345. Cherner JA, et al: Gastrointestinal dysfunction in systemic mastocytosis: A prospective study. Gastroenterology 95:657–667, 1988.
346. Keller RT, Roth HP: Hyperchlorhydria and hyperhistaminemia in a patient with systemic mastocytosis. N Engl J Med 283:1449–1450, 1970.
347. Jarnum S, Zachariae H: Mastocytosis (urticaria pigmentosa) of skin, stomach, and gut with malabsorption. Gut 8:64–68, 1967.
348. Borda F, Uribarrena R, Rivero-Puente A: Gastroscopic findings in systemic mastocytosis. Endoscopy 15:342–343, 1983.
349. Quinn SF, et al: Bull's-eye lesions: A new gastrointestinal presentation of mastocytosis. Gastrointest Radiol 9:13–15, 1984.
350. Legman P, et al: Colonic involvement in systemic mastocytosis. Semin Hop 58:1460–1463, 1982.
351. Frieri M, Alling DW, Metcalfe DD: Comparison of the therapeutic efficacy of cromolyn sodium with that of combined chlorpheniramine and cimetidine in systemic mastocytosis: Results of a double-blind clinical trial. Am J Med 78:9–14, 1985.
352. Soter NA, Austen KF, Wasserman SI: Oral disodium cromoglycate in the treatment of systemic mastocytosis. N Engl J Med 301:465–469, 1979.
353. Chinitz MA, et al: Symptomatic sarcoidosis of the stomach. Dig Dis Sci 30:682–688, 1985.
354. Ona FV: Gastric sarcoid: Unusual cause of upper gastrointestinal hemorrhage. Am J Gastroenterol 75:286–288, 1981.
355. Popovic OS, et al: Sarcoidosis and protein-losing enteropathy. Gastroenterology 78:119–125, 1980.
356. Sprague R, et al: Disseminated gastrointestinal sarcoidosis: Case report and review of the literature. Gastroenterology 87:421–425, 1984.
357. Mora RG, Gullung WH: Sarcoidosis: A case with unusual manifestations. South Med J 73:1063–1065, 1980.
358. Ell SR, Frank PH: Spectrum of lymphoid hyperplasia: Colonic manifestations of sarcoidosis, infectious mononucleosis, and Crohn's disease. Gastrointest Radiol 6:329–332, 1981.
359. Kohn NN: Sarcoidosis of the colon. J Med Soc N J 77:517–518, 1980.
360. Ishak KG: Sarcoidosis of the liver and bile ducts. Mayo Clin Proc 73: 467–472, 1998.
361. Bacal D, et al: Sarcoidosis of the pancreas: Case report and review of the literature. Am Surg 66:675–678, 2000.
362. Lazaro Asegurado L, et al: Acute pancreatitis and sarcoidosis: A case report and review of the literature. Arch Bronconeumol 31:290–292, 1995.
363. Chaun H, et al: Sarcoidosis of the pancreas. Am J Dig Dis 17:725–730, 1972.
364. Rambaud JC, et al: Digestive tract and renal small vessel hyalinosis, idiopathic nonarteriosclerotic intracerebral calcifications, retinal ischemic syndrome, and phenotypic abnormalities: A new familial syndrome. Gastroenterology 90:930–938, 1986.
365. Brunzell JD, Bierman EL: Chylomicronemia syndrome: Interaction of genetic and acquired hypertriglyceridemia. Med Clin North Am 66: 455–468, 1982.
366. Ohmoto K, et al: Severe acute pancreatitis associated with hyperlipidemia: report of two cases and review of the literature in Japan. Hepatogastroenterology 46:2986–2990, 1999. Review.
367. Ahlberg J, et al: Prevalence of gallbladder disease in hyperlipoproteinemia. Dig Dis Sci 24:459–464, 1979.
368. O'Brien BD, et al: Pathophysiologic and ultrastructural basis for intestinal symptoms in Fabry's disease. Gastroenterology 82:957–962, 1982.
369. Bryan A, Knauft RF, Burns WA: Small bowel perforation in Fabry's disease [letter]. Ann Intern Med 86:315–316, 1977.
370. Isselbacher KJ, Scheig R, Plotkin GR: Congenital B-lipoprotein deficiency: An hereditary disorder involving a defect in the absorption and transport of lipids. Medicine (Baltimore) 43:347, 1964.
371. Glickman RM, et al: Immunofluorescence studies of apolipoprotein B in intestinal mucosa: Absence in abetalipoproteinemia. Gastroenterology 76:288–292, 1979.
372. Illingworth DR, et al: Lipid metabolism in abetalipoproteinemia: A study of cholesterol absorption and sterol balance in two patients. Gastroenterology 78:68–75, 1980.
373. Delpre G, et al: Endoscopic assessment in abetalipoproteinemia (Bassen-Kornzweig-syndrome). Endoscopy 10:59–62, 1978.
374. Beutler E: Gaucher disease. Blood Rev 2:59–70, 1988.
375. Aderka D, et al: Fatal bleeding from esophageal varices in a patient with Gaucher's disease. Am J Gastroenterol 77:838–839, 1982.
376. Liscum L: Niemann-Pick type C mutations cause lipid traffic jam. Traffic 1:218–225, 2000.
377. Tassoni JP Jr, Fawaz KA, Johnston DE: Cirrhosis and portal hypertension in a patient with adult Niemann-Pick disease. Gastroenterology 100:567–569, 1991.
378. Bodzioch M, Orso E, Klucken J, et al: The gene encoding ATP-binding cassette transporter 1 is mutated in Tangier disease. Nat Genet 22:316–318, 1999.
379. Tarao K, et al: Japanese adult siblings with Tangier disease and statistical analysis of reported cases. Tokai J Exp Clin Med 9:379–387, 1984.
380. Kaplan MM: Acute fatty liver of pregnancy. N Engl J Med 313:367–370, 1985.
381. Torbey CF, Richter JE: Gastrointestinal motility disorders in pregnancy. Semin Gastrointest Dis 6:203–216, 1995.
382. Baron TH, Ramirez B, Richter JE: Gastrointestinal motility disorders during pregnancy. Ann Intern Med 118:366–375, 1993.
383. Bynum TE: Hepatic and gastrointestinal disorders in pregnancy. Med Clin North Am 61:129–138, 1977.
384. Gross S, Librach C, Cecutti A: Maternal weight loss associated with hyperemesis gravidarum: A predictor of fetal outcome. Am J Obstet Gynecol 160:906–909, 1989.
385. Kocak I, et al: *Helicobacter pylori* seropositivity in patients with hyperemesis gravidarum. Int J Gynaecol Obstet 66:251–254, 1999.
386. Hayakawa S, et al: Frequent presence of *Helicobacter pylori* genome in the saliva of patients with hyperemesis gravidarum. Am J Perinatol 17:243–247, 2000.
387. Brandes JM: First-trimester nausea and vomiting as related to outcome of pregnancy. Obstet Gynecol 30:427–431, 1967.
388. Brock-Utne JG, et al: Gastric and lower oesophageal sphincter (LOS) pressures in early pregnancy. Br J Anaesth 53:381–384, 1981.
389. Bainbridge ET, et al: Gastro-oesophageal reflux in pregnancy: Altered function of the barrier to reflux in asymptomatic women during early pregnancy. Scand J Gastroenterol 19:85–89, 1984.
390. Larson JD, et al: Double-blind, placebo-controlled study of ranitidine for gastroesophageal reflux symptoms during pregnancy. Obstet Gynecol 90:83–87, 1997.
391. Brunner G, Meyer H, Athmann C: Omeprazole for peptic ulcer disease in pregnancy. Digestion 59:651–654, 1998.
392. Anderson AS, Whichelow MJ: Constipation during pregnancy: Dietary fibre intake and the effect of fibre supplementation. Hum Nutr Appl Nutr 39:202–207, 1985.
393. Shaffer EA, et al: The effect of a progestin on gallbladder function in young women. Am J Obstet Gynecol 148:504–507, 1984.

394. Weinberg RB, et al: Treatment of hyperlipidemic pancreatitis in pregnancy with total parenteral nutrition. Gastroenterology 83:1300–1305, 1982.
395. Block P, Kelly TR: Management of gallstone pancreatitis during pregnancy and the postpartum period. Surg Gynecol Obstet 168:426–428, 1989.
396. Jamidar PA, et al: Endoscopic retrograde cholangiopancreatography in pregnancy. Am J Gastroenterol 90:1263–1267, 1995.
397. Binmoeller KF, Katon RM: Needle knife papillotomy for an impacted common bile duct stone during pregnancy. Gastrointest Endosc 36: 607–609, 1990.
398. Horowitz MD, et al: Acute appendicitis during pregnancy: Diagnosis and management. Arch Surg 120:1362–1367, 1985.
399. Lim HK, Bae SH, Seo GS: Diagnosis of acute appendicitis in pregnant women: Value of sonography. AJR Am J Roentgenol 159:539–542, 1992.
400. Barloon TJ, et al: Sonography of acute appendicitis in pregnancy. Abdom Imaging 20:149–151, 1995.
401. Tracey M, Fletcher HS: Appendicitis in pregnancy. Am Surg 66:555–559; discussion 559–560, 2000.
402. Punnonen R, et al: Appendicectomy during pregnancy. Acta Chir Scand 145:555–558, 1979.
403. Mayer IE, Hussain H: Abdominal pain during pregnancy. Gastroenterol Clin North Am 27:1–36, 1998.
404. DePerrot M, Jenny A, Morales M, et al: Laparoscopic appendectomy during pregnancy. Surg Laparosc Endosc Percutan Tech 10:368–371, 2000.
405. Trastek VF, et al: Splenic artery aneurysms. Surgery 91:694–699, 1982.
406. Bokhari SI, et al: Maternal meconium granulomatous peritonitis. Arch Intern Med 141:658–659, 1981.
407. Schwartz IS, et al: Maternal vernix caseosa peritonitis following premature rupture of fetal membranes. JAMA 254:948–950, 1985.

Chapter 30

Complications of Gastrointestinal Endoscopy

Marta L. Davila and Emmet B. Keeffe

Complications of gastrointestinal endoscopy are remarkably uncommon, in spite of the striking increase in the number and diversity of procedures performed since the 1970s.[1, 2] In this chapter, the complications of diagnostic and therapeutic endoscopy of the upper and lower gastrointestinal tract in adults are discussed, with emphasis on the more commonly performed procedures. The indications and contraindications for endoscopic procedures, and all aspects of endoscopic retrograde cholangiopancreatography (ERCP), percutaneous gastroscopy, and laparoscopy are considered in other chapters.

Informed consent is an important risk management technique and should be obtained before every endoscopy. The key element of informed consent is disclosure—that is, the nature of the proposed procedure, the reason for performing endoscopy, the benefits of the procedure, the risks and complications, and the alternatives to the procedure.[3, 4] Analysis of the database files of the Physicians Insurers Association of America reveals that malpractice claims and suits related to endoscopic procedures were distributed as follows: (1) upper endoscopy, including esophageal dilation (39%); (2) colonoscopy and related procedures (34%); (3) sigmoidoscopy, including rigid and flexible (25%); and (4) ERCP (2%).[5] Iatrogenic injury claims were almost entirely limited to perforation. "Improper performance" was the most frequent allegation, cited in 55% of claims; "diagnostic error" was next in frequency, alleged in 25% of claims.[5] The most frequent associated issue in the claims reviewed were problems with informed consent (44% of cases).[5] Complications and the possibility of being sued for medical malpractice are unavoidable risks of performing endoscopy; there are no "routine" procedures, and proper informed consent with emphasis on the risk of perforation is important for every case.

Gastrointestinal endoscopy fortunately has maintained a remarkably good overall safety record, as documented by large retrospective surveys documenting low complication rates.[6–17] Estimated average complication rates of upper and lower diagnostic and therapeutic procedures are shown in Table 30–1. Reported complication rates of endoscopic procedures vary substantially because of several factors. The definition of what constitutes a complication and how to grade its severity has not been uniform, making it difficult to assess average complication rates accurately. Much of the information on complications was compiled from the early developmental phase of endoscopy and may not be representative of current endoscopic practice. Reports of complication rates from institutions with extensive experience are likely to be lower than rates found in general endoscopic practice. Finally, complication rates that are derived from retrospective surveys may suffer from underreporting—that is, immediate complications are typically recorded whereas late complications may not be included.

In a prospective analysis of complications after outpatient upper endoscopy, in which a complication was defined as any deviation from the optimal course after the procedure, ten complications (2.1%) were documented early after endoscopy.[18] Eighty-six additional complications were discovered by telephone follow-up 30 days after the procedure (18.2%). The majority of these late complications were oropharyngeal or abdominal discomfort; however, 10 of the 86 patients required an emergency department or physician visit, and 3 patients were hospitalized.[18] In a similar study reviewing complications 30 days after outpatient colonoscopy, significantly more complications were identified with later follow-up.[19]

Every attempt should be made to limit the total number of complications of endoscopy by paying attention to all aspects of procedural safety[20] (Table 30–2). Some determinants of safety are more fixed (e.g., the type of procedure or the medical condition of the patient), whereas other determinants are more variable (e.g., use of conscious sedation, monitoring practices, training and competence of the endoscopist, and how the recovery period is managed). An individual procedure may have its own "inherent" complication rates (e.g., a higher incidence of complications from therapeutic versus diagnostic procedures). Adherence to all safety

Table 30–1 | **Complications of Upper Endoscopy and Colonoscopy***

PROCEDURE	MAJOR COMPLICATION (%)	DEATH (%)
Upper endoscopy		
Diagnostic	0.2	0.01
Esophageal dilation†	0.5	0.01
Variceal sclerotherapy	8.0	1.5
Colonoscopy		
Diagnostic	0.4	0.02
Polypectomy	2.0	0.05

*Estimated average figures from large retrospective reviews.[6–17]
†Mercury bougies or metal olives; pneumatic dilation excluded.

issues, particularly sedation and monitoring, and the standardization of endoscopic training and practice may lower the complication rate of endoscopy and improve the already good safety record.

GENERAL COMPLICATIONS

Adverse Effects of Medications

Medications administered to facilitate endoscopy may cause complications from allergic reactions or, more importantly, from doses that prove excessive for certain individuals.[21, 22] The major adverse effect of sedative medications is respiratory depression,[6–11, 23, 24] and serious cardiorespiratory events may complicate as many as 0.5% of procedures.[25] More than 50% of deaths associated with endoscopy are related to cardiopulmonary complications.[22]

MEDICATIONS USED FOR CONSCIOUS SEDATION. Endoscopy, particularly diagnostic upper endoscopy[26, 27] but also colonoscopy,[28] can be performed without conscious sedation, but surveys from the United States[29] and United Kingdom[30] indicate that both endoscopists and patients prefer some form of premedication. It is possible but unproven that the performance of endoscopic procedures without sedation will lower complications, particularly cardiopulmonary events. The usual premedications used for endoscopy are intravenous benzodiazepines, such as diazepam or midazolam, either alone or with a narcotic, such as meperidine or fentanyl.[21, 22] The combination of a benzodiazepine and narcotic can achieve sedation more smoothly, but the incidence of respiratory depression is significantly increased.[22, 31] The technique and sequence of administration of drugs used for conscious sedation are important safety issues (e.g., bolus administration of midazolam is associated with greater oxygen desaturation than a slow, titrated injection).[32] Arterial oxygen desaturation, which is occasionally severe, occurs in the majority of patients undergoing either upper endoscopy or colonoscopy.[33, 34] A benzodiazepine antagonist, flumazenil, can reverse all the behavioral effects of diazepam or midazolam, can dramatically shorten the recovery period following conscious sedation, and may find future use for managing oversedation or even for routine reversal.[35]

Side effects of benzodiazepines, other than respiratory depression, include occasional paradoxical excitement and phlebitis, the latter occurring more often with diazepam than with midazolam.[21, 22] Droperidol, a neuroleptic, is a useful adjunctive agent in selected patients (e.g., those with active alcohol abuse or withdrawal, who are at risk for paradoxical agitation with benzodiazepines and/or narcotics).[36] Other side effects of narcotics include nausea, vomiting, hypotension, and rare allergic reactions. Naloxone is a readily available antagonist of the narcotic effects of meperidine and reverses respiratory depression, sedation, and hypotension in 1 to 2 minutes.

MISCELLANEOUS MEDICATIONS. Anaphylactoid reactions and systemic toxicity to topical anesthetics for upper endoscopy are rare but potentially lethal.[37] An unusual complication of local anesthesia is benzocaine-induced methemoglobinemia in genetically predisposed individuals.[38] A link between the use of local anesthetic sprays and the development of pneumonia after upper endoscopy may exist.[10] The need for pharyngeal anesthesia during endoscopy is debatable, and not all endoscopists use these agents.[21, 22]

Inhibition of motor and secretory activity of the intestinal tract can be achieved with atropine, dicyclomine hydrochloride, and glucagon. Complications of atropine include increased intraocular pressure in patients with narrow-angle glaucoma, bradycardia, tachycardia, and atrioventricular block. Most endoscopists no longer employ these drugs routinely for upper endoscopy, but glucagon is occasionally used during colonoscopy.

Table 30–2 | **Potential Determinants of Endoscopic Procedural Safety**

WHAT
- Procedure is performed?
  - diagnostic vs. therapeutic
- Conscious sedation or anesthesia is used?
  - benzodiazepine alone vs. with narcotic
  - bolus vs. titration
- Level of monitoring is employed?
  - personnel (GI nurse) assisting
  - electronic equipment (oximetry, ECG) used
  - resuscitation equipment available

WHO
- Undergoes endoscopy?
  - young vs. elderly
  - medically fit vs. unfit
  - full consultation vs. brief "checklist"
- Performs endoscopy?
  - training and experience
  - competence and judgment

WHY
- Endoscopy is performed?
  - indicated vs. contraindicated

WHERE
- Endoscopy is performed?
  - fully staffed hospital endoscopy unit vs. small hospital vs. clinic or office
  - elective (endoscopy unit) vs. emergency (ICU or other hospital ward)

HOW
- The patient's recovery is monitored?
- The outpatient is discharged?

Modified from Keeffe EB: Endoscopic procedural safety. In McCloy R (ed): Quality Control in Endoscopy/An International Forum, Berlin, Springer Verlag, 1991, p 33.

Cardiopulmonary Problems

ASPIRATION. Sedation, pharyngeal anesthesia, and supine positioning during upper endoscopy contribute to development of bronchopulmonary aspiration and its sequelae. A full stomach, active bleeding, and retained GI secretions due to obstructive lesions are additional risk factors. Elderly and other patients who have depressed cough and gag reflexes must be handled with special care. The incidence of aspiration is 0.08%, but the mortality rate of this complication may reach 10%.[9] The likelihood of aspiration is minimized by turning patients and encouraging them to cough immediately after endoscopy.[39]

HYPOXEMIA. Changes in oxygenation that occur during gastrointestinal endoscopy have been extensively studied.[31] A number of conclusions can be derived from analysis of these reports: (1) oxygen saturation decreases during both upper and lower endoscopy; (2) there is no consistent correlation between the fall in oxygen saturation and the type or dose of medication and the age or sex of the patient; (3) data are conflicting regarding whether the length of the procedure or use of sedation has an impact on oxygen saturation; and (4) fall in oxygen saturation is related to the use of larger diameter endoscopes for upper endoscopy, the additive effect of a narcotic with a benzodiazepine, and the presence of preexisting pulmonary disease.[31] In view of the frequency of oxygen desaturation during upper and lower endoscopy, some endoscopists recommend the use of supplemental oxygen in high-risk patients as a strategy preferable to treatment of hypoxemia after it occurs.[32]

CARDIAC EVENTS. Disturbances of cardiac rhythm during endoscopy are most frequently seen in patients with underlying chronic heart or lung disease,[40] but medications and hypoxemia are contributing factors.[6, 31] Electrocardiographic changes that are seen frequently in monitoring studies include sinus tachycardia, premature ventricular contractions, and ST segment changes.[2, 22, 33]

CARDIOPULMONARY MONITORING DURING ENDOSCOPY. The excellent safety record of endoscopy has been dependent, in large part, on the clinical monitoring of patients by gastrointestinal nurses who regularly determine vital signs and assess the patient's tolerance for the procedure. Therapeutic procedures often require two nurses, one to monitor the patient and one to assist the endoscopist. The availability of electronic equipment, such as pulse oximetry and continuous electrocardiographic and blood pressure monitoring devices, has led to their widespread use by endoscopists,[31] even though uncertainty remains regarding the role of additional monitoring in reducing cardiopulmonary complications.[41] A published guideline regarding monitoring practices emphasizes the importance of clinical assessment during endoscopy and states that oximetry and electrocardiographic monitoring may be beneficial for certain high-risk patients and/or procedures.[42] However, the likelihood that further monitoring will enhance the safety of conscious sedation, as well as medicolegal considerations, is leading to the routine rather than selective use of electronic monitoring devices in the United States, as is officially recommended in the United Kingdom.[43]

Infections Complications

TRANSMISSION OF INFECTION. Spread of infection from one patient to another, or to endoscopic personnel, is a source of great concern. Fortunately, documented instances of this complication are extremely rare.[44, 45] A crude estimate of the incidence of infection transmitted by endoscopy is 1 per 1.8 million procedures. *Salmonella* and *Pseudomonas* transmission have been reported,[46, 47] and other organisms reported to have spread include *Escherichia coli, Enterobacter cloacae, Staphylococcus* epidermidis, *Klebsiella, Serratia marcescens, Clostridium difficile,* and *Helicobacter pylori.*[45, 48] Among the viruses, hepatitis B and C and human immunodeficiency virus (HIV) are the main causes for worry, but fears have not been realized to date; endoscopic hepatitis B transmission is very rare, and HIV cross-infection by endoscopy has not been reported.[49, 50] Universal precautions against contact with patients' blood or body fluids should be employed routinely by endoscopists during the performance of all procedures.[51]

Disinfection of endoscopes and accessories is the main preventive measure. Mechanical cleansing with water and detergent, immersion in 2% glutaraldehyde solution for 10 to 30 minutes, rinsing, and air drying are the usual steps employed.[48, 52] It is important that disinfection of instruments be carried out by experienced personnel according to strict protocols.[53, 54] Another approach to prevent transmission of infectious agents during endoscopy is to use disposable equipment. However, there are only limited data on the efficacy and cost-effectiveness of this approach.[55, 56]

BACTEREMIA AND ANTIBIOTIC PROPHYLAXIS. The frequency of bacteremia during endoscopy varies with the type of procedure and is highest following esophageal dilation and variceal sclerotherapy[57, 58] (Table 30–3). Therapeutic endoscopy, including procedures listed in Table 30–3, and others, such as laser treatment, endoscopic mucosal resection (EMR), and colonoscopic polypectomy, are associated with higher rates of bacteremia than are seen with diagnostic endoscopy.[57–61]

In normal individuals, bacteremia is transient (typically less than 15 minutes), and bacteria are cleared without complication. Susceptible patients, however, may develop serious infection; use of prophylactic antibiotics is therefore a logical strategy to prevent serious infectious complication related to endoscopy. However, very few conclusive data demonstrating the efficacy of prophylactic antibiotic are available.

Table 30–3 | **Frequency of Bacteremia with Endoscopic Procedures**

PROCEDURE	MEAN INCIDENCE (%)	RANGE (%)
Esophageal dilation	45	0–54
Variceal sclerotherapy	18	5–52
Upper endoscopy	4	0–11
Colonoscopy	3	0–27
Sigmoidoscopy	3	0–9

Modified from Neu HC, Fleischer D: Controversies, dilemmas, and dialogues. Recommendations for antibiotic prophylaxis before endoscopy. Am J Gastroenterol 84:1488, 1989.

Table 30–4 | **ASGE–Recommended Antibiotic Prophylaxis for Endoscopic Procedures**[60]

PATIENT CONDITION	PROCEDURE CONTEMPLATED	ANTIBIOTIC PROPHYLAXIS	COMMENTS
Prosthetic valve History of endocarditis Systemic-pulmonary shunt Synthetic vascular graft (<1 yr old)	Stricture dilation; varix sclerosis ERCP/obstructed biliary tree	Recommended	High-risk conditions for development of infectious complication; procedures are associated with relatively high bacteremia rates
	Other endoscopic procedures, including EGD and colonoscopy (with or without biopsy/polypectomy), variceal ligation	Insufficient data to make firm recommendation; endoscopists may choose on case-by-case basis	Although conditions are high risk, procedures are associated with low rates of bacteremia
Rheumatic valvular dysfunction Mitral valve prolapse with insufficiency Hypertrophic cardiomyopathy Most congenital cardiac malformations	Stricture dilation, varix sclerosis ERCP/obstructed biliary tree	Insufficient data to make firm recommendation; endoscopists may choose on case-by-case basis	Conditions pose lesser risk for infectious complications than prosthetic valve, and so on
	Other endoscopic procedures, including EGD and colonoscopy (with or without biopsy/polypectomy), variceal ligation	Not recommended	Procedures are associated with relatively low bacteremia rates
Other cardiac conditions (including CABG, pacemakers, implantable defibrillators)	All endoscopic procedures	Not recommended	Conditions are low risk for infectious complications from endoscopic procedures
Obstructed bile duct Pancreatic pseudocyst	ERCP	Recommended	Prudent, but no substitute for definitive drainage
Cirrhosis and ascites Immunocompromised patient	Stricture dilation, varix sclerosis ERCP/obstructed biliary tree	Insufficient data to make firm recommendation; endoscopists may choose on case-by-case basis	Risk for infectious complications related to endoscopic procedures not established
	Other endoscopic procedures, including EGD and colonoscopy (with or without biopsy/polypectomy), variceal ligation	Not recommended	Procedures are associated with relatively low bacteremia rates
All patients	Endoscopic feeding tube placement	Recommended	May decrease risk of soft tissue infection
Prosthetic joints	Any endoscopic procedure	Not recommended	No literature to support infectious risk from endoscopic procedures

CABG, Coronary artery bypass graft; EGD, esophagogastroduodenoscopy; ERCP, endoscopic retrograde cholangiopancreatography.

Based on the limited and sometimes conflicting data, differences in opinion regarding the use of prophylactic antibiotic exist.[60, 62] However, in up to 15% of patients undergoing endoscopy, a decision regarding whether to administer prophylactic antibiotic has to be made.[63] Table 30–4 summarizes the latest recommendation proposed by the American Society for Gastrointestinal Endoscopy (ASGE).[60]

The most feared infectious complication associated with endoscopy is bacterial endocarditis. Fortunately, only a few cases of bacterial endocarditis as a complication of endoscopy have been documented.[57] Cardiac conditions at high risk for the development of endocarditis include prosthetic heart valves, previous bacterial endocarditis, and surgically constructed systemic-pulmonary shunts.[60] Endocarditis prophylaxis is recommended for these patients when they undergo endoscopic procedures with a high risk of bacteremia (esophageal dilatation and sclerotherapy). The use of antibiotic prophylaxis is optional for these patients when they undergo endoscopic procedures with a low infection risk (upper and lower endoscopy, with or without biopsy). For patients with an intermediate risk for endocarditis (rheumatic valvular dysfunction, mitral valve prolapse with insufficiency, hypertrophic cardiomyopathy, and most congenital cardiac malformations), antibiotic prophylaxis is optional for high-risk procedures and is not recommended for low-risk procedures. Endocarditis prophylaxis prior to endoscopy is not recommended for patients with cardiac lesions that do not confer an increased risk of endocarditis (coronary artery bypass, pacemaker, implanted defibrillators, mitral valve prolapse, or previous rheumatic fever without valvular dysfunction or regurgitation).

The risk of infection in a synthetic vascular graft is highest prior to complete pseudointimal coverage of the graft. For the first year after placement of a synthetic vascular graft, antibiotic prophylaxis is indicated for patients undergoing an endoscopic procedure with a high risk of bacteremia. There is theoretical concern regarding infection in patients with implanted orthopedic prostheses or peritoneal shunts and in patients who are immunosuppressed following solid organ transplantation, but the necessity for antibiotic prophylaxis during endoscopy has not been established in these patients.[57, 58] However, a study of bone marrow transplant recipients documented a 19% incidence of clinically relevant bacteremia following upper endoscopy, leading to a recommendation for antibiotic prophylaxis.[64] The current regimens recommended by the American Heart Association for antibiotic prophylaxis of patients with high-risk cardiac conditions undergoing esophageal and gastrointestinal procedures are listed in Table 30–5 and Table 30–6 respectively.

Electrosurgical Hazards

Complications from the use of electrosurgical devices during endoscopy include explosion, perforation, and bleeding. Burns and cardiac arrhythmias are other accidents that may be avoided by knowledge of the principles of electrosurgery.[65] At the low power typically used for polypectomy, burns to the patient or endoscopist are rare and, when they do occur, trivial.[39, 65] Although most modern pacemakers are unaffected, a patient may develop cardiac arrhythmias if monopolar current passes through the pacemaker or the heart; bipolar electrosurgery is safer. However, pacemaker malfunction with the use of electrocautery during endoscopy has not been reported.[66]

Abdominal Distention

Abdominal distention from insufflated gas is seldom a major problem during routine upper endoscopy, but laser therapy and sclerotherapy can create troublesome distention because they are of longer duration and more gas insufflation is required to maintain clear visibility. Colonic distention by gas during colonoscopy can cause marked discomfort and may also impair mucosal blood flow.[67] Carbon dioxide rather than air insufflation during colonoscopy may offer some advantages: it is absorbed from the colon; it is nonexplosive; and mucosal blood flow is less affected, with a reduced chance of colonic ischemia.[67, 68]

Table 30–5 | **Prophylactic Regimens for Esophageal Procedures**

SITUATION	AGENT	REGIMEN
Standard general prophylaxis	Amoxicillin	Adults: 2.0 g; children: 50 mg/kg orally 1 h before procedure
Unable to take oral medications	Ampicillin	Adults: 2.0 g IM or IV; children: 50 mg/kg IM or IV within 30 min before procedure
Allergic to penicillin	Clindamycin or	Adults: 600 mg; children: 20 mg/kg orally 1 h before procedure
	Cephalexin* or cefadroxil* or	Adults: 2.0 g; children: 50 mg/kg orally 1 h before procedure
	Azithromycin or clarithromycin	Adults: 500 mg; children: 15 mg/kg orally 1 h before procedure
Allergic to penicillin and unable to take oral medications	Clindamycin or Cefazolin*	Adults: 600 mg; children: 20 mg/kg IV within 30 min before procedure Adults: 1.0 g; children: 25 mg/kg IM or IV within 30 min before procedure

IM, intramuscularly; IV, intravenously. From Dajani AS, Taubert KA, Wilson W, et al: Prevention of bacterial endocarditis: Recommendations by the American Heart Association. JAMA 277:1794–1801.

*Cephalosporins should not be used in individuals with immediate-type hypersensitivity reaction (urticaria, angioedema, anaphylaxis) to penicillins.

Table 30–6 | **Prophylactic Regimens for Gastrointestinal Procedures**

SITUATION	AGENTS	REGIMEN
High-risk patients	Ampicillin plus gentamicin	Adults: ampicillin 2.0 g IM or IV plus gentamicin 1.5 mg/kg (not to exceed 120 mg) within 30 min of starting procedure; 6 h later, ampicillin 1 g IM/IV or amoxicillin 1 g orally Children: ampicillin 50 mg/kg IM or IV (not to exceed 2.0 g) plus gentamicin 1.5 mg/kg within 30 min of starting the procedure; 6 h later, ampicillin 25 mg/kg IM/IV or amoxicillin 25 mg/kg orally
High-risk patients allergic to ampicillin/amoxicillin	Vancomycin plus gentamicin	Adults: vancomycin 1.0 g IV over 1–2 h plus gentamicin 1.5 mg/kg IV/IM (not to exceed 120 mg); complete injection/infusion within 30 min of starting procedure Children: vancomycin 20 mg/kg IV over 1–2 h plus gentamicin 1.5 mg/kg IV/IM; complete injection/infusion within 30 min of starting procedure
Moderate-risk patients	Amoxicillin or ampicillin	Adults: amoxicillin 2.0 g orally 1 h before procedure, or ampicillin 2.0 g IM/IV within 30 min of starting procedure Children: amoxicillin 50 mg/kg orally 1 hr before procedure, or ampicillin 50 mg/kg IM/IV wihin 30 min of starting procedure
Moderate-risk patients allergic to ampicillin/amoxicillin	Vancomycin	Adults: vancomycin 1.0 g IV over 1–2 h complete infusion within 30 min of starting procedure Children: vancomycin 20 mg/kg IV over 1–2 h; complete infusion within 30 min of starting procedure

IM, intramuscularly; IV, intravenously. From Dajani AS, Taubert KA, Wilson W, et al: Prevention of bacterial endocarditis: Recommendations by the American Heart Association. JAMA 277:1794–1801.

COMPLICATIONS OF UPPER ENDOSCOPY

Perforation

The esophagus or stomach is perforated during diagnostic upper endoscopy in 0.03% to 0.1% of procedures.[6, 24] Perforation occurs most commonly when the endoscope is passed blindly (e.g., the pharynx and upper esophagus), and the esophagus is perforated more commonly than the stomach.[39] Osteoarthritic spurs on the cervical spine, Zenker's diverticulum, anastomoses, strictures, and weakening of the wall of the esophagus or stomach from inflammation, neoplasm, or caustic ingestion are predisposing factors. Perforation of the midesophagus usually results from biopsy of a carcinoma.[6] Perforation of the duodenum during diagnostic upper endoscopy is extremely rare.[69] This complication is more often seen during endoscopic sphincterotomy of the ampulla.[70]

Therapeutic endoscopy carries an increased risk of perforation (see Table 30–1). Dilation of esophageal strictures may lead to perforation at or proximal to the narrowing. Hydrostatic balloon dilation of benign esophageal stenosis is complicated by perforation in 0.4% of procedures.[71] The incidence of perforation from endoscopic balloon dilation of strictures at some other sites is as follows: pyloric stenosis, 0.5%; gastroenterostomy, 2.2%; and gastric staple line, 0.8%.[71] Other causes of luminal narrowing and other methods of dilation yield different statistics.

With sclerotherapy, complications develop in 20% to 40% of cases, and the death rate is 1% to 2%.[12] Esophageal complications are discussed in more detail in Chapter 34 and include ulceration (25% to 75%), stricture (2% to 31%), and perforation (1% to 3%). Sclerotherapy ulcers may heal more rapidly with control of acid-pepsin reflux (e.g., with omeprazole),[72] and rebleeding during long-term sclerotherapy may be reduced with the use of sucralfate.[73] Some other complications of sclerotherapy include chest pain, pneumonitis, pleural effusions, fever, and bacteremia. In contrast, variceal band ligation is associated with a lower complication rate of 2% to 3%. However, esophageal laceration and perforation due to passage of the overtube have been reported. The incidence of this complication is unknown.[12] Endoscopic therapy of nonvariceal bleeding sites in the upper tract by laser, multipolar coagulation, heater probe, or injection is quite safe, and the perforation rate is less than 1%.[74–77]

Palliation of esophageal carcinoma by laser or bipolar coagulation leads to perforation or tracheoesophageal fistula in at least 5% of patients.[77] It is sometimes difficult to determine whether the complication is attributable to the carcinoma, laser treatment, other treatment (e.g., radiation), or a combination of factors.[78, 79] Gastric polypectomy may result in perforation or hemorrhage; significant bleeding requiring surgical intervention occurred in 2 of 45 patients (4%) in one series.[80]

The preferred treatment for early cancer of the esophagus and stomach in Japan is now endoscopic mucosal resection (EMR), and this procedure is increasingly being performed in the United States. The basic technique involves the injection of saline into the submucosa to create a bleb that separates the mucosal lesion from the muscularis propria. A snare is placed over the base of the raised area, and the mucosa is resected with electrocautery. The main complication of EMR is perforation, which fortunately is a rare event. The reported perforation rate is 0.7% to 2.5% with removal of esophageal cancers.[81, 82] After EMR of gastric cancers, the perforation rate is 0.06% to 2.4%.[83, 84]

Push enteroscopy is being used with increased frequency for the diagnosis and treatment of small bowel lesions. Complications of enteroscopy have not been well defined, but it is clear that enteroscopy is not merely an extended upper endoscopy but a procedure with its own risks and technical difficulties. A duodenal perforation due to overtube insertion[85] and two gastric lacerations due to pinching of the mucosa between the overtube and the endoscope[86] have been described. A new, painless method of imaging the entire small bowel, wireless capsule endoscopy, was recently compared with push enteroscopy in a randomized trial in an animal model and found to detect more small bowel abnormalities.[87] If confirmed in human studies, capsule endoscopy could replace push enteroscopy as a safer and painless alternative procedure.

Endoscopic perforation of the esophagus or stomach may be obvious immediately or within a few hours. Cervical pain, subcutaneous emphysema, fever, tachycardia, and characteristic radiographic appearances make the diagnosis easy, but some distal esophageal injuries are more subtle.[39] An immediate esophagogram should be obtained if perforation is suspected. A major leak, or one that occurred through a tumor or an ulcer, requires urgent operation.[39, 88] Limited or absent extravasation on x-ray study allows treatment by intravenous antibiotics and close observation.

A small perforation of the duodenum may not be recognized until a few hours after the procedure, when the patient develops abdominal pain, fever, and leukocytosis. X-ray films may show retroperitoneal air. Computed tomography may be needed to confirm the diagnosis. A large perforation will lead to obvious subcutaneous emphysema. Retroperitoneal air may travel via the pararenal fascial plane across the diaphragmatic hiatus into the mediastinum, resulting in pneumomediastinum, pneumothorax, and cervical subcutaneous emphysema. Most of the patients with duodenal perforation can be managed initially by conservative therapy with nasogastric suction and intravenous antibiotics. Surgery will be needed if the patient's clinical status continues to deteriorate.[69, 70] However, some workers advocate early surgical intervention.[89]

Bleeding

Bleeding from diagnostic endoscopy, even with biopsy, is rare (about 0.03% of procedures),[6] and coagulopathy likely increases this risk. The bleeding site is more often gastric than esophageal. A Mallory-Weiss tear has been reported as a complication of endoscopy.[90] Therapeutic procedures such as sclerotherapy, polypectomy, endoscopic mucosal resection, laser destruction of tumors, and dilation of strictures cause bleeding more frequently.

Miscellaneous Complications

Rare complications of upper endoscopy include parotid gland enlargement, temporomandibular joint dislocation, and impaction of the endoscope in the distal esophagus or in a hiatal hernia.[1, 6, 69]

COMPLICATIONS OF SIGMOIDOSCOPY AND COLONOSCOPY

Perforation

The incidence of bowel perforation with rigid sigmoidoscopy ranges from 0.002% to 0.02% of procedures.[91] Less experience has been reported with flexible sigmoidoscopy, but perforation appears also to be very rare, even when examinations are performed by primary care physicians (0.01% perforation rate).[92] The incidence of perforation with colonoscopy is 0.2% to 0.4% following diagnostic procedures, and 0.3% to 1% with polypectomy.[6, 14, 93] Hydrostatic balloon dilation of colonic anastomotic strictures is associated with a high rate of perforation (4.6%).[71]

Mechanical perforation by the tip of the instrument occurs at sites of weakness of the colonic wall (e.g., diverticula, inflammation, radiation injury, or ischemia) and distal to obstructing points (e.g., neoplasms, strictures, flexures, or kinks). The shaft of the endoscope may act as a lead point if the instrument is flexed sharply, and perforation can develop as shown in Figure 30–1. Fixation of the sigmoid colon in the pelvis by diverticular disease or previous pelvic surgery predisposes to this mechanism.

Pneumatic perforation of the colon or the ileum results from distention by insufflated air.[94–96] If the ileocecal valve is competent to retrograde flow and the colonoscope obstructs the lumen distally, the colon forms a closed loop, and the pressure in the cecum may become extreme.[94, 95]

Perforation from colonoscopic polypectomy is an electrosurgical injury, either an immediate full-thickness cut through the wall by a snare or hot biopsy forceps or a delayed rupture of necrotic tissue.[16, 97–99] The risk of perforation when using the hot biopsy forceps in the cecum and ascending colon was 0.3% in a survey of endoscopists.[100] The postpolypectomy coagulation syndrome of pain, peritoneal irritation, and fever may represent a microperforation.

The possibility of perforation is greater in the presence of a poor bowel preparation, acute bleeding, or an uncooperative patient.[39] A biopsy forceps, brush, dilator, or other accessory may perforate the colon. Perforation of the cecum during colonoscopic decompression of nonobstructive colonic dilation has also been noted.[101]

Free perforation into the peritoneal cavity may be recognized during the procedure if abdominal viscera are seen. In other situations, marked persistent abdominal distention and pain prompt the ordering of radiographs, which may reveal pneumoperitoneum. Symptoms of perforation may be delayed for several days if the leak is tiny and well localized.

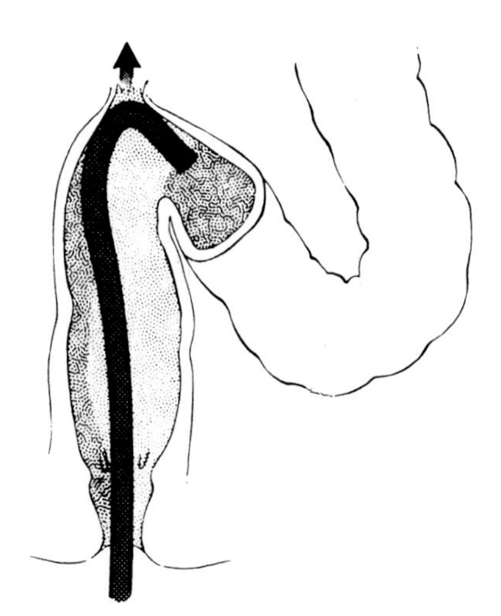

Figure 30–1. Perforation by the shaft of a sharply flexed colonoscope or sigmoidoscope. (From Katon RM, Keeffe EB, Melnyk CS: Flexible Sigmoidoscopy. Orlando, Grune & Stratton, 1985.)

Retroperitoneal perforation, usually a pneumatic injury, gives rise to subcutaneous emphysema. X-ray studies reveal subcutaneous, retroperitoneal, and mediastinal air. Rarely, pneumothorax may develop.[102] Fever and leukocytosis may develop eventually in any of these varieties of perforation.

Large lacerations seen directly through the colonoscope demand immediate operation.[39, 103] If no defect is observed endoscopically and plain abdominal radiographs show pneumoperitoneum, a water-soluble contrast enema x-ray study should be obtained.[98] Gross extravasation requires operation, but in the absence of leakage or clinical evidence of peritoneal irritation, treatment with intravenous antibiotics and close observation may be considered.[104] Benign pneumoperitoneum is manifested by relatively asymptomatic abdominal distention and responds well to antibiotics.[105] Most retroperitoneal perforations and those associated with the postpolypectomy coagulation syndrome also do not require operation initially.[94, 99, 103]

Bleeding

Clinically significant bleeding from biopsy sites or mucosal tears during diagnostic colonoscopy or sigmoidoscopy is rare. The incidence of hemorrhage after colonoscopic polypectomy is 0.7% to 2.5%.[93, 106] Hemorrhage following use of the hot biopsy forceps is 0.4%.[100] Postpolypectomy bleeding may occur immediately, but in 30% to 50% of cases, it is delayed for 2 days to a week, when the eschar sloughs.[20] Sessile polyps, large thick stalks, equipment failure, and faulty technique account for some of the bleeding associated with polypectomy. Prevention depends on recognition of potential problems and expertise in performing the procedures. Immediate bleeding can be treated by resnaring the remaining stalk and tightening the snare for 10 to 15 minutes, usually without further electrocoagulation.[39] Injection of 5 to 10 mL of 1:10,000 epinephrine solution into the stalk or submucosally also may be helpful. Bleeding may also be stopped by a variceal band ligator.[107] Interventional angiography with selective infusion of pitressin or embolization and even laparotomy are necessary occasionally. Delayed bleeding usually stops spontaneously, although transfusions and endoscopic therapy may be required.[39]

Miscellaneous Complications

Potentially explosive concentrations of combustible gases, mostly hydrogen but also methane in some patients, can be avoided by preparing the colon with electrolyte solution containing sodium sulfate and polyethylene glycol.[108, 109] Bacteria produce hydrogen from mannitol, and although antibiotics suppress the responsible fecal flora, there is little reason to incur even the small risk of *explosion* associated with this cathartic.[110–112] Carbon dioxide insufflation during colonoscopy is an additional safety precaution, but it has not been widely adopted.[67, 68]

Preparation of the colon with laxatives and enemas can lead to *dehydration*, but sodium sulfate–polyethylene glycol lavage seems to avoid these problems.[108, 109] However, a number of *aspiration events* followed by the adult respiratory distress syndrome (ARDS) have been reported secondary to the nasogastric administration of polyethylene glycol–electrolyte solutions. Certain patient populations are potentially at higher risk, including patients with neurologic disorders, confused patients, and perhaps patients with delayed gastric emptying. These patients thus require close observation if a nasogastric tube is used for administration of the lavage solution.[113, 114]

An *acute, self-limited colitis* following sigmoidoscopy or colonoscopy has been linked to endoscopes that had been previously submerged in glutaraldehyde as part of the cleaning process.[115] The spleen is normally tethered to the colon, and *splenic injury or rupture* may result from traction on the splenic flexure during colonoscopy.[116, 117] Vascular complications with ischemia resulting from colonoscopy are very rare. Risk factors for *mesenteric vascular thrombosis* include acute occlusive events and low-flow states.[118] Patients with connective tissue disease and severe atherosclerotic disease are at highest risk for ischemia. The pathogenesis proposed involves compromise of small vessel circulation by air distention and trauma during colonoscopy.[118, 119]

Endoscopic tattooing with India ink is the most common method used for marking colonic lesions. A number of complications have been reported with tattooing, including abdominal pain, fever, leukocytosis, and abscess formation. Potential pathogenetic mechanisms include a hypersensitivity reaction caused by any of the components of the ink, an infection from unsterilized ink, or the passage of gastrointestinal bacteria by needle injection.[120]

Volvulus of the colon or the ileum is a rare complication of colonoscopy.[121] Finally, the colonoscope or flexible sigmoidoscope can become incarcerated in an inguinal hernia[122, 123] or in a diaphragmatic hernia.[124]

REFERENCES

1. Habr-Gama A, Waye JD: Complications and hazards of gastrointestinal endoscopy. World J Surg 13:193, 1989.
2. Hart R, Classen M: Complications of diagnostic gastrointestinal endoscopy. Endoscopy 22:229, 1990.
3. Standards of Training and Practice Committee: American Society for Gastrointestinal Endoscopy: Informed consent for gastrointestinal endoscopy. Gastrointest Endosc 34:26S, 1988.
4. Ad Hoc Committee on Risk Management, American Society for Gastrointestinal Endoscopy: Risk Management. An Information Resource Manual. Manchester, MA, American Society for Gastrointestinal Endoscopy, 1990.
5. Gerstenberger PD, Plumeri PA: Malpractice claims and suits in gastrointestinal endoscopy: Analysis of an insurance industry database. Gastrointest Endosc 39:132, 1993.
6. Shahmir M, Schuman BM: Complications of fiberoptic endoscopy. Gastrointest Endosc 26:86, 1980.
7. Mandelstam P, Sugawa C, Silvis SE et al: Complications associated with esophagogastroduodenoscopy and with esophageal dilation. An analysis of the 1974 A/S/G/E survey. Gastrointest Endosc 23:16, 1976.
8. Andersen KE, and Clausen N: Outpatient gastroscopy risks. Endoscopy 10:180, 1978.
9. Schiller KFR, Cotton PB, Salmon PR: The hazards of digestive fibre-endoscopy: A survey of British experience [abstract]. Gut 13:1027, 1972.
10. Quine MA, Bell GD, McCloy RF, et al: Prospective audit of upper gastrointestinal endoscopy in two regions of England: Safety, staffing and sedation method. Gut 36:462, 1995.
11. Newcomer MK, Brazer SR: Complications of upper gastrointestinal endoscopy and their management. Gastrointest Endosc Clin North Am 4:551, 1994.
12. Young HS, Matsui SM, Gregory PB: Endoscopic control of upper gastrointestinal variceal bleeding. In Yamada T, Alpers DH Owyang C, et al: (eds): Textbook of Gastroenterology, 2nd ed. Philadelphia, JB Lippincott, 1995, p 2969.
13. Waye JD, Lewis BS, Yessayan S: Colonoscopy: A prospective report of complications. J Clin Gastoenterol 15:347, 1992.
14. Rogers BHG, Silvis SE, Nebel OT, et al: Complications of flexible fiberoptic colonoscopy and polypectomy. An analysis of the 1974 A/S/G/E survey. Gastrointest Endosc 22:73, 1975.
15. Gilbert DA, Hallstrom AP, Shaneyfelt SL, et al: The national ASGE colonoscopy survey—complications of colonoscopy [abstract]. Gastrointest Endosc 30:156, 1984.
16. Smith LE: Fiberoptic colonoscopy. Complications of colonoscopy and polypectomy. Dis Colon Rectum 19:407, 1976.
17. Macrae FA, Tan KG, Williams CB: Towards safer colonoscopy: A report on the complications of 5000 diagnostic or therapeutic colonoscopies. Gut 24:376, 1983.
18. Zubarik R, Eisen G, Mastropietro C, et al: Prospective analysis of complications 30 days after outpatient upper endoscopy. Am J Gastroenterol 94:1539, 1999.
19. Zubarik R, Fleischer DE, Mastropietro C, et al: Prospective analysis of complications 30 days after outpatient colonoscopy. Gastrointest Endosc 50:322, 1999.
20. Keeffe EB: Endoscopic procedural safety. In McCloy R (ed): Quality Control in Endoscopy/An International Forum. Berlin, Springer Verlag, 1991, p 33.
21. Ross WA: Premedication for upper gastrointestinal endoscopy. Gastrointest Endosc 35:120, 1989.
22. Bell GD: Review article: Premedication and intravenous sedation for upper gastrointestinal endoscopy. Aliment Pharmacol Therap 4:103, 1990.
23. Gilbert DA, Silverstein FE, Tedesco FJ: National ASGE survey on upper gastrointestinal bleeding. Complications of endoscopy. Dig Dis Sci 26:55s, 1981.
24. Silvis SE, Nebel O, Rogers G, et al: Endoscopic complications. Results of the 1974 American Society for Gastrointestinal Endoscopy survey. JAMA 235:928, 1976.
25. Arrowsmith JB, Gerstman BB, Fleischer DE, et al: Results from the American Society for Gastrointestinal Endoscopy/U.S. Food and Drug Administration collaborative study on complication rates and drug use during gastrointestinal endoscopy. Gastrointest Endosc 37:421, 1991.
26. Al-Atrakchi HA: Upper gastrointestinal endoscopy without sedation: A prospective study of 2000 examinations. Gastrointest Endosc 35:79, 1989.
27. Ladas SD, Giorgiotis C, Pipis P, et al: Sedation for upper gastrointestinal endoscopy: Time for reappraisal? Gastrointest Endosc 36:417, 1990.
28. Herman FN: Avoidance of sedation during total colonoscopy. Dis Colon Rectum 33:70, 1990.
29. Keeffe EB, O'Connor KW: 1989 A/S/G/E survey of endoscopic sedation and monitoring practices. Gastrointest Endosc 36:S13, 1990.
30. Daneshmend TK, Bell GD, Logan RFA: Sedation for upper gastrointestinal endoscopy: Results of a nationwide survey. Gut 32:12, 1991.
31. Fleischer D: Monitoring the patient receiving conscious sedation for gastrointestinal endoscopy: Issues and guidelines. Gastrointest Endosc 35:262, 1989.
32. Bell GD, Antrobus JHL, Lee J, et al: Bolus or slow titrated injection of midazolam prior to upper gastrointestinal endoscopy? Relative effect on oxygen saturation and prophylactic value of supplemental oxygen. Aliment Pharmacol Therap 4:393, 1990.
33. Dark DS, Campbell DR, Wesselius LJ: Arterial oxygen desaturation during gastrointestinal endoscopy. Am J Gastroenterol 85:1317, 1990.
34. Fennerty MB, Earnest DL, Hudson PB, et al: Physiologic changes during colonoscopy. Gastrointest Endosc 36:22, 1990.
35. Rosario MT, Costa NF: Combination of midazolam and flumazenil in upper gastrointestinal endoscopy: A double-blind randomized study. Gastrointest Endosc 36:30, 1990.
36. Wilcox CM, Forsmark CE, Cello JP: Utility of droperidol for conscious sedation in gastrointestinal endoscopic procedures. Gastrointest Endosc 36:112, 1990.
37. Patel D, Chopra S, Berman MD: Serious systemic toxicity resulting from use of tetracaine for pharyngeal anesthesia in upper endoscopic procedures. Dig Dis Sci 34:882, 1989.
38. Collins JF: Methemoglobulinemia as a complication of 20% benzocaine spray for endoscopy. Gastroenterology 98:211, 1990.
39. Cotton PB, Williams CB: Practical Gastrointestinal Endoscopy, 3rd ed. Oxford, England, Blackwell Scientific Publications, 1990.
40. Lee JG, Leung JW, Cotton PB: Acute cardiovascular complications of endoscopy: Prevalence and clinical characteristics. Dig Dis 13:130, 1995.
41. Froehlich F, Gonvers JJ, Fried M: Conscious sedation, clinically rele-

vant complications and monitoring of endoscopy: Result of a nationwide survey in Switzerland. Endoscopy 1994; 26:231.
42. Standards of Practice Committee, American Society for Gastrointestinal Endoscopy: Sedation and monitoring of patients undergoing gastrointestinal endoscopic procedures. Gastrointest Endosc 42:626, 1995.
43. Bell GD, McCloy RF, Charlton JE, et al: Recommendations for standards of sedation and patient monitoring during gastrointestinal endoscopy. Gut 32:823, 1991.
44. Technology Assessment Committee: Transmission of infection by gastrointestinal endoscopy. Gastrointest Endosc 39:885, 1993.
45. Spach DH, Silverstein FE, Stamm WE: Transmission of infection by gastrointestinal endoscopy and bronchoscopy. Ann Intern Med 118: 117, 1993.
46. O'Connor BH, Bennett JR, Alexander JG, et al: Salmonellosis infection transmitted by fiberoptic endoscopes. Lancet 2:864, 1982.
47. Doherty DE, Falko JM, Lefkovitz N, et al: *Pseudomonas aeruginosa* sepsis following retrograde cholangiopancreatography. Dig Dis Sci 27: 169, 1982.
48. Hughes CE, Gebhard RL, Peterson LR, et al: Efficacy of routine fiberoptic endoscope cleaning and disinfection for killing *Clostridium difficile*. Gastrointest Endosc 32:7, 1986.
49. Villa E, Pasquinelli C, Rigo G, et al: Gastrointestinal endoscopy and HBV infection: No evidence for a causal relationship. A prospective controlled study. Gastrointest Endosc 30:15, 1984.
50. Hanson PJ: AIDS: Practising safe endoscopy. Clin Gastroenterol 4: 477, 1990.
51. Centers for Disease Control: Guidelines for prevention of transmission of human immunodeficiency virus and hepatitis B virus to health-care and public-safety workers. MMWR 38:1, 1989.
52. Gerding DN, Peterson LR, Vennes JA: Cleaning and disinfection of fiberoptic endoscopes: Evaluation of glutaraldehyde exposure time and forced-air drying. Gastroenterology 83:613, 1982.
53. Standards of Practice Committee, American Society for Gastrointestinal Endoscopy: Infection control during gastrointestinal endoscopy. Gastrointest Endosc 49:836, 1999.
54. Society of Gastroenterology Nurses and Associates: Recommended Guidelines for Infection Control in Gastrointestinal Endoscopy Settings. Monograph Series-1. Chicago, Society of Gastrointestinal Nurses and Associates, 1990.
55. Axon AT: Disinfection and endoscopy: Summary and recommendations. Working party report to the World Congresses of Gastroenterology, Sydney, 1990. J Gastroenterol Hepatol 6:23, 1991.
56. Technology Assessment Committee, American Society for Gastrointestinal Endoscopy: Disposable endoscopic accessories. Gastrointest Endosc 42:618, 1995.
57. Botoman VA, Surawicz CM: Bacteremia with gastrointestinal endoscopic procedures. Gastrointest Endosc 32:342, 1986.
58. Neu HC, Fleischer D: Controversies, dilemmas, and dialogues. Recommendations for antibiotic prophylaxis before endoscopy. Am J Gastroenterol 84:1488, 1989.
59. Wolf D, Fleischer D, Sivak MV Jr: Incidence of bacteremia with elective upper gastrointestinal endoscopy laser therapy. Gastrointest Endosc 31:247, 1985.
60. Standard of Practice Committee, American Society for Gastrointestinal Endoscopy: Antibiotic prophylaxis for gastrointestinal endoscopy. Gastrointest Endosc 42:630, 1995.
61. Lee T, Hsueh P, Yeh W, et al: Low frequency of bacteremia after endoscopic mucosal resection. Gastrointest Endosc 52:223, 2000.
62. Dajani AS, Bisno AL, Chung KJ et al: Prevention of endocarditis. Recommendations by the American Heart Association. JAMA 264: 2919, 1990.
63. Zuckerman GR, O'Brien J, Halstead R: Antibiotic prophylaxis in patients with infectious risk factors undergoing gastrointestinal endoscopic procedures. Gastrointest Endosc 40:538, 1994.
64. Bianco JA, Pepe MS, Higano C, et al: Prevalence of clinically relevant bacteremia after upper gastrointestinal endoscopy in bone marrow transplant recipients. Am J Med 89:134, 1990.
65. Barlow DE: Endoscopic applications of electrosurgery. A review of basic principles. Gastrointest Endosc 28:73, 1982.
66. Technology Assesment Committee, American Society for Gastrointestinal Endoscopy: Electrocautery use in patients with implanted cardiac devices. Gastrointest Endosc 40:794, 1994.
67. Brandt LJ, Boley SJ, Sammartano R: Carbon dioxide and room air insulation of the colon. Effects on colonic blood flow and intraluminal pressure in the dog. Gastrointest Endosc 32:324, 1986.
68. Williams CB: Who's for CO_2 [editorial]? Gastrointest Endosc 32:365, 1986.
69. Girardi A, Pizza I, Guinta G, et al: Retroperitoneal, mediastinal, and subcutaneous emphysema as a complication of routine upper gastrointestional endoscopy. Endoscopy 22:83, 1990.
70. Savides T, Sherman S, Kadell B, et al: Bilateral pneumothoraces and subcutaneous emphysema after endoscopic sphincterotomy. Gastrointest Endosc 39:814, 1993.
71. Kozarek RA: Hydrostatic balloon dilation of gastrointestinal stenoses: A national survey. Gastrointest Endosc 32:15, 1986.
72. Gimson A, Polson R, Westaby D, et al: Omeprazole in the management of intractable esophageal ulceration following injection sclerotherapy. Gastroenterology 99:1829, 1990.
73. Polson RJ, Westaby D, Gimson AES, et al: Sucralfate for the prevention of early rebleeding following injection sclerotherapy for esophageal varices. Hepatology 10:279, 1989.
74. Matthewson K, Swain CP, Bland M, et al: Randomized comparison of Nd:YAG laser, heater probe, and no endoscopic therapy for bleeding peptic ulcers. Gastroenterology 98:1239, 1990.
75. Laine L: Multipolar electrocoagulation versus injection therapy in the treatment of bleeding peptic ulcer. A prospective, randomized trial. Gastroenterology 99:1303, 1990.
76. Chung SCS, Leung JWC, Sung JY, et al: Injection or heat probe for bleeding ulcer. Gastroenterology 100:33, 1991.
77. Fleischer D, Sivak MV Jr: Endoscopic Nd:YAG laser therapy as palliation for esophagogastric cancer. Parameters affecting initial outcome. Gastroenterology 89:827, 1985.
78. Cello JP, Gerstenberger PD, Wright T, et al: Endoscopic neodymium YAG laser palliation of nonresectable esophageal malignancy. Ann Intern Med 102:610, 1985.
79. Ell CH, Rieman JF, Lux G, et al: Palliative laser treatment of malignant stenoses in the upper gastrointestinal tract. Endoscopy 18(Suppl 1):21, 1986.
80. Hughes RW: Gastric polyps and polypectomy: Rationale, technique and complications. Gastrointest Endosc 30:101, 1984.
81. Inoue H, Tani M, Nagai K, et al: Treatment of esophageal and gastric tumors. Endoscopy 31:47, 1999.
82. Kodama M, Kakegawa T: Treatment of superficial cancer of the esophagus: A summary of responses to a questionnaire on superficial cancer of the esophagus in Japan. Surgery 123:432, 1998.
83. Makuuchi H, Kise Y, Shimada H, et al: Endoscopic mucosal resection for early gastric cancer. Semin Surg Oncol 17:108, 1999.
84. Chonan A, Mochizuki F, Ando M, et al: Endoscopic mucosal resection of early gastric cancer—usefulness of aspiration EMR using capfitted scope. Dig Endosc 10:31, 1998.
85. Landi B, Cellier C, Fayenmendy L, et al: Duodenal perforation occurring during push enteroscopy. Gastrointest Endosc 43:631, 1996.
86. Yang R, Laine L: Mucosal stripping: A complication of push enteroscopy. Gastrointest Endosc 41:156, 1995.
87. Appleyard M, Fireman Z, Glukhovsky A, et al: A randomized trial comparing wireless capsule endoscopy with push enteroscopy for the detection of small-bowel lesions. Gastroenterology 119:1431, 2000.
88. Chung R: Dilation of strictures of the upper gastrointestinal tract: In Dent TL, Strodel WE, Turcotte JG, Harper ML (eds): Surgical Endoscopy. Chicago, Year Book Medical Publishers, 1985, p 123.
89. Bell RWC, Stiegmann GV, Goff J, et al: Decision for surgical management of perforation following endoscopic sphincterotomy. Am Surg 57:237, 1991.
90. Watts HD: Mallory-Weiss syndrome occurring as a complication of endoscopy. Gastrointest Endosc 22:171, 1976.
91. Selby JV, Friedman GD: Sigmoidoscopy in the periodic health examination of asymptomatic adults. JAMA 261:595, 1989.
92. Groveman HD, Sanowski RA, Klauber MR: Training primary care physicians in flexible sigmoidoscopy—performance evaluation of 17,167 procedures. West J Med 148:221, 1988.
93. Muhldorfer AM, Kekos G, Hahn EG, et al: Complications of therapeutic gastrointestinal endoscopy. Endoscopy 24:276, 1992.
94. Katon RM, Keeffe EB, Melnyk CS: Flexible Sigmoidoscopy. Orlando, FL, Grune & Stratton, 1985.
95. Kozarek RA, Earnest DL, Silverstein ME, et al: Air-pressure-induced colon injury during diagnostic colonoscopy. Gastroenterology 78:7, 1980.
96. Razzak LA, Millan J, Schuster MM: Pneumatic ileal performation: An unusual complication of colonoscopy. Gastroenterology 70:268, 1976.
97. Nivatvongs S: Complications in colonoscopic polypectomy: Lessons to learn from an experience with 1576 polyps. Am Surg 54:61, 1988.
98. Berei G, Panish JF, Schapiro M, et al: Complications of colonoscopy and polypectomy: Report of the Southern California Society for Gastrointestinal Endoscopy. Gastroenterology 67:584, 1974.

99. Schrock TR: Colonoscopic polypectomy. In Dent TL, Strodel WE, Turcotte JG, Harper ML, (eds): Surgical Endoscopy. Chicago, Year Book Medical Publishers, 1985, p 233.
100. Wadas DD, Sanowski RA: Complications of the hot biopsy forceps technique. Gastrointest Endosc 34:32, 1988.
101. Bode, WE, Beart RW Jr, Spencer RJ, et al: Colonoscopic decompression for acute pseudo-obstruction of the colon (Ogilvie's syndrome). Report of 22 cases and review of the literature. Am J Surg 147:243, 1984.
102. Schmidt G, Borsch G, Wegener M: Subcutaneous emphysema and pneumothorax complicating diagnostic colonoscopy. Dig Colon Rectum 29:136, 1986.
103. Carpio G, Albu E, Gumbs MA, et al: Management of colonic perforation after colonoscopy. Report of three cases. Dis Colon Rectum 32: 624, 1989.
104. Farley DR, Bannon MP, Zietlow SP, et al: Management of colonoscopic perforations. Mayo Clin Proc 72:729, 1997.
105. Ecker MD, Goldstein M, Hoexter B, et al: Benign pneumoperitoneum after fiberoptic colonoscopy. A prospective study of 100 patients. Gastroenterology 73:226, 1977.
106. Rex DK, Lewis BS, Waye JD: Colonoscopy and endoscopic therapy for delayed post-polypectomy hemorrhage. Gastrointest Endosc 1992: 38:127.
107. Slivka A, Parsons WG, Carr-Locke DL: Endoscopic band ligation for treatment of post-polypectomy hemorrhage. Gastrointest Endosc 1994: 40:230.
108. Davis GR, Santa Ana CA, Morawski SG, et al: Development of a lavage solution associated with minimal water and electrolyte absorption or secretion. Gastroenterology 78:991, 1980.
109. Goldman J, Reichelderfer M: Evaluation of rapid colonoscopy preparation using a new gut lavage solution. Gastrointest Endosc 28:9, 1982.
110. Bond JH, Jr, Levitt MD: Factors affecting the concentration of combustible gases in the colon during colonoscopy. Gastroenterology 68: 1445, 1975.
111. Taylor EW, Bentley S, Young D, et al: Bowel preparation and the safety of colonoscopic polypectomy. Gastroenterology 81:1, 1981.
112. La Brooy SJ, Avgerinos A, Fendick CL, et al: Potentially explosive colonic concentrations of hydrogen after bowel preparation with mannitol. Lancet 1:634, 1981.
113. Marschall H, Bartels F: Life-threatening complications of nasogastric administration of polyethylene glycol-electrolyte solutions (GoLYTELY) for bowel cleansing. Gastrointest Endosc 47:408, 1998.
114. Gabel A, Muller S: Aspiration: A possible severe complication in colonoscopy preparation of elderly people by orthograde intestine lavage. Digestion 60:284, 1999.
115. Caprilli R, Viscido A, Frieri G, et al: Acute colitis following colonoscopy. Endoscopy 30:428, 1998.
116. Gores PF, Simso LA: Splenic injury during colonoscopy. Arch Surg 124:1342, 1989.
117. Ahmed A, Eller PM, Schiffman FJ: Splenic rupture: An unusual complication of colonoscopy. Am J Gastroenterol 92:1201, 1997.
118. Rice E, DiBaise JK, Quigley EM: Superior mesenteric artery thrombosis after colonoscopy. Gastrointest Endosc 50:706, 1999.
119. McGovern RP, Franco RA: Acute mesenteric ischemia after colonoscopy. Am J Gastroenterol 90:170, 1995.
120. Dell'Abate P, Iosca A, Galimberti A, et al: Endoscopic preoperative colonic tattooing: A clinical and surgical complication. Endoscopy 31: 271, 1999.
121. Keeffe EB: Ileal volvulus following colonoscopy. Gastrointest Endosc 31:228, 1985.
122. Williard W, Satava R: Inguinal hernia complicating flexible sigmoidoscopy. Am Surg 56:800, 1990.
123. Koltun WA, Coller JA: Incarceration of colonoscope in an inguinal hernia. "Pulley" technique of removal. Dis Colon Rectum 334:191, 1991.
124. Baumann UA, Mettler M: Diagnosis and hazards of unexpected diaphragmatic hernias during colonoscopy: Report of two cases. Endoscopy 31:274, 1999.

Section Five

ESOPHAGUS

Chapter 31

Anatomy, Histology, Embryology, and Developmental Anomalies of the Esophagus

John D. Long and Roy C. Orlando

ANATOMY AND HISTOLOGY

The esophagus acts as a conduit for the transport of food from the oral cavity to the stomach. To carry out this task safely and effectively, the esophagus is an 18- to 26-cm hollow muscular tube with an inner skinlike lining of stratified squamous epithelium (Fig. 31–1). Between swallows, the esophagus is collapsed, but the lumen distends up to 2 cm anteroposteriorly and 3 cm laterally to accommodate a swallowed bolus.[1] Structurally, the esophageal wall is composed of four layers: innermost mucosa, submucosa, muscularis propria, and outermost adventitia; unlike the remainder of the gastrointestinal tract, the esophagus has no serosa. These layers are depicted anatomically as viewed with endoscopic ultrasonography in Figure 31–2.

Musculature

The muscularis propria is responsible for carrying out transport function. The upper 5% to 33% are composed exclusively of skeletal muscle, and the distal 33% are composed of smooth muscle. In between is a mixture of both types.[2] Proximally the esophagus begins where the inferior pharyngeal constrictor merges with the cricopharyngeus, an area of skeletal muscle known functionally as the upper esophageal sphincter (UES) (Fig. 31–3*A*). The UES is contracted at rest and thereby creates high pressure, which prevents inspired air from entering the esophagus. Below the UES, the esophageal wall separates into inner circular and outer longitudinal layers of muscle (see Fig. 31–2*A*). The esophageal body lies within the posterior mediastinum behind the trachea and left mainstem bronchus and swings leftward to pass behind the heart and in front of the aorta.[1] At the T10 vertebral level, the esophageal body leaves the thorax through a hiatus located within the right crus of the diaphragm. Within the diaphragmatic hiatus, the esophageal body ends in a 2- to 4-cm long, asymmetrically thickened circular smooth muscle known as the lower esophageal sphincter (LES) (see Fig. 31–3*B*).[3] The phrenicoesophageal ligament, which originates from the diaphragm's transversalis fascia and inserts on the lower esophagus, contributes to fixation of the LES within the diaphragmatic hiatus. This positioning is beneficial because it enables diaphragmatic contractions to assist the LES in maintenance of a high-pressure zone during exercise. The LES is contracted at rest, creating a high-pressure zone that prevents gastric contents from entering the esophagus. During swallowing, the LES relaxes to permit the swallowed bolus to be pushed by peristalsis from the esophagus into the stomach (see Chapter 32).

Innervation

The smooth muscle portion of the esophageal wall is innervated by both parasympathetic and sympathetic nerves; the parasympathetic nerves regulate peristalsis through the vagus nerve (Fig. 31–4). The cell bodies of the motor neurons of the vagus nerves originate in the medulla. Those located within the nucleus ambiguus control skeletal muscle, and those of the dorsal motor nucleus control smooth muscle. The former medullary vagal efferent nerves terminate directly on the motor end plate of the skeletal muscle of the upper esophagus, whereas the latter vagal preganglionic efferent nerves to the smooth muscle of the distal esophagus terminate on neurons within Auerbach's (myenteric) plexus, located between the circular and longitudinal muscle layers (see Fig. 31–4).[4] A second neuronal sensory network, Meissner's plexus, located within the submucosa, is the site of afferent impulses within the esophageal wall. These are

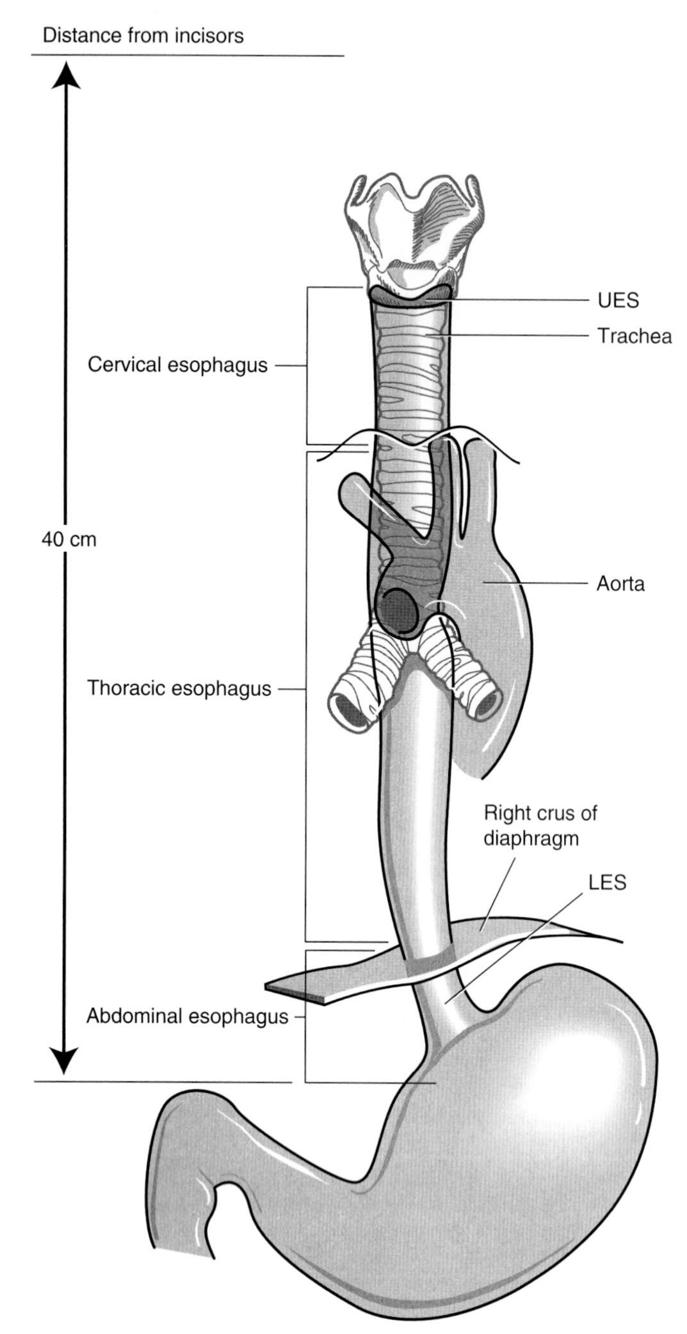

Figure 31–1. Anterior view of the esophagus. The esophagus, which is 18 to 26 cm in length, originates in the neck at the level of the cricoid cartilage, passes through the chest, and ends after passage through the hiatus in the right crus of the diaphragm by joining the stomach below. On barium esophagogram, adjacent structures may indent the esophageal wall, including the aortic arch, left mainstem bronchus, left atrium, and diaphragm. UES and LES, upper and lower esophageal sphincters. (Adapted from Liebermann-Meffert, D: Anatomy, embryology, and histology. In Pearson FG, Deslauriers J, Ginsberg RJ, et al [eds]: Esophageal Surgery. New York, Churchill Livingstone, 1995, p 2.)

transmitted to the central nervous system through both vagal parasympathetic and thoracic sympathetic nerves. Sensory signals transmitted via vagal afferent pathways travel to the nucleus tractus solitarius within the central nervous system; from there, nerves pass to the nucleus ambiguus and dorsal motor nucleus of the vagus nerve where their signals may influence motor function.[5]

Circulation

The arterial and venous blood supply to the esophagus is segmental. The upper esophagus is supplied by branches of the superior and inferior thyroid arteries; the midesophagus by branches of the bronchial and right intercostal arteries and descending aorta; and the distal esophagus by branches of the left gastric, left inferior phrenic, and splenic arteries.[6] These vessels anastomose to create a dense network within the submucosa that probably accounts for the rarity of esophageal infarction. The venous drainage of the upper esophagus is through the superior vena cava, the midesopha-

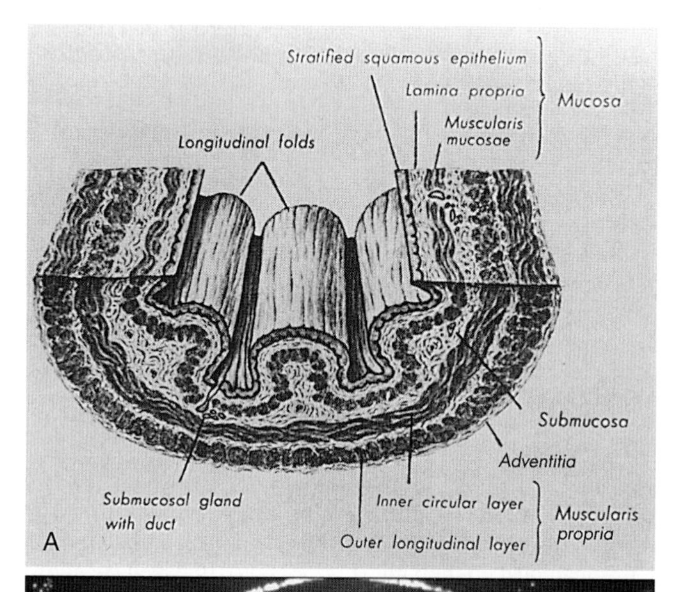

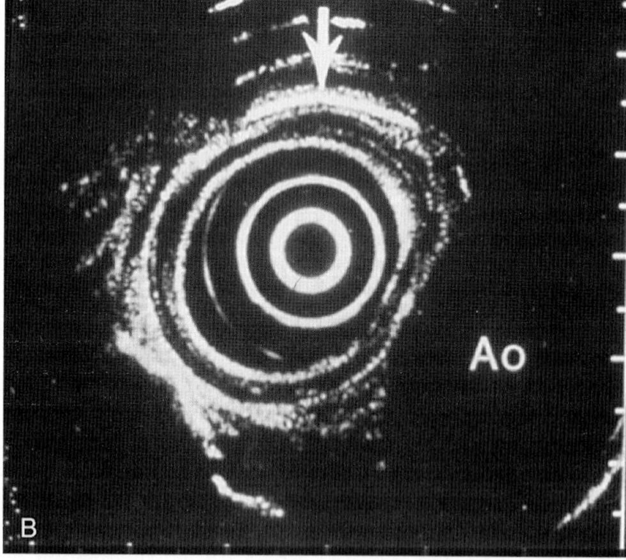

Figure 31–2. Cross-sectional and endoscopic ultrasonographic anatomy of the esophagus. *A*, The anatomic layers within the wall of the esophagus are depicted. (From Neutra MR, Padykula HA: The gastrointestinal tract. In Weiss L [ed]: Histology, Cell and Tissue Biology, 5th ed. New York, Elsevier Science Publishing Company, 1983, p 664.) *B*, An endoscopic ultrasonographic image depicting the pattern of light and dark rings created by echos from the different layers. (From American Gastroenterological Association Clinical Teaching Project: Esophageal disorders: Endoscopic ultrasonography of the normal esophagus, slide 11. Washington, D.C., American Gastroenterological Association, 1995.)

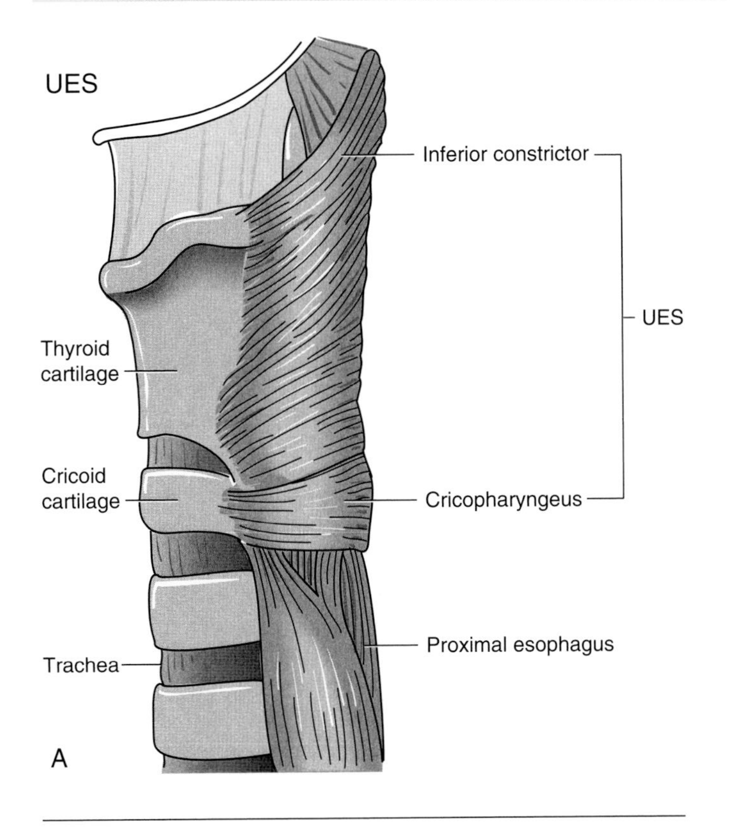

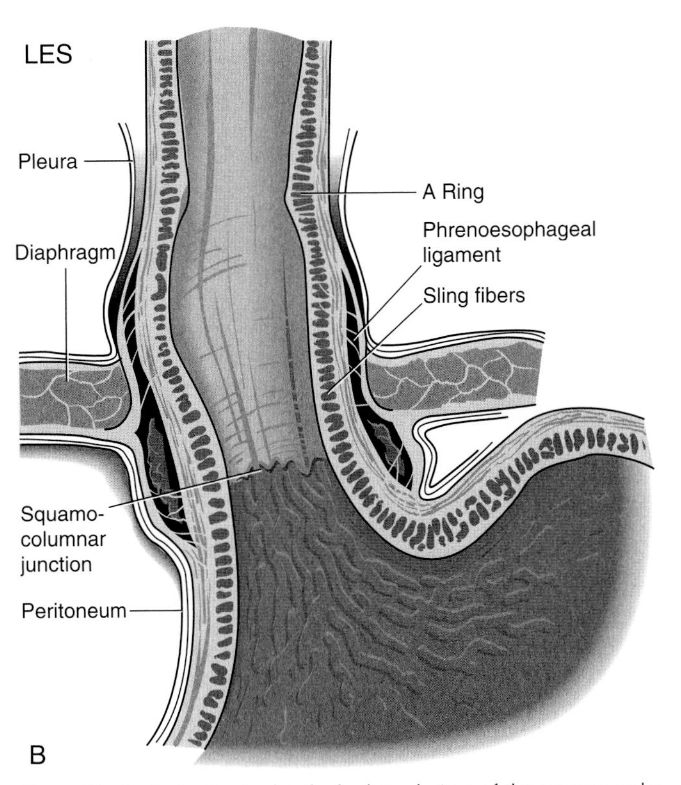

Figure 31–3. *A,* Anatomic detail of a lateral view of the upper esophageal sphincter (UES) and its relationship to adjacent structures. (Adapted from American Gastroenterological Association Clinical Teaching Project: Esophageal disorders: Upper esophageal sphincter anatomy, slide 14. Washington, D.C., American Gastroenterological Association, 1995.) *B,* Anatomic detail of the lower esophageal sphincter region and its relationship to the diaphragm, phrenoesophageal ligament, and squamocolumnar junction. (Adapted from Kerr RM: Hiatal hernia and mucosal prolapse. In Castell DO [ed]: The Esophagus. Boston, Little, Brown & Company, 1992, p 763.)

gus through the azygous veins, and the distal esophagus through the portal vein by means of the left and short gastric veins. The submucosal venous anastomotic network is also important because it is where esophageal varices occur in patients with portal hypertension.[7] The lymphatic system of the esophagus also appears segmental; the upper esophagus drains to the deep cervical nodes, the midesophagus to the mediastinal nodes, and the distal esophagus to the celiac and gastric nodes. However, these lymphatic systems are also interconnected by numerous channels, accounting for the spread of most esophageal cancers beyond the region at discovery.

Mucosa

On endoscopy, the esophageal mucosa appears smooth and pink. The esophagogastric junction can be recognized by the presence of an irregular white Z line (ora serrata), demarcating the interface between the light esophageal and the red gastric mucosae. On a biopsy specimen, histologic study shows the mucosa lined by nonkeratinized stratified squamous epithelium (Fig. 31–5). This multilayered epithelium consists of three functionally distinct layers: stratum corneum, stratum spinosum, and stratum germinativum. The most lumen-oriented stratum corneum acts as a permeability barrier between luminal content and blood by having layers of pancake-shaped glycogen-rich cells connected laterally to each other by tight junctions and having their intercellular spaces filled with a dense matrix of glycoconjugate material.[8] The middle layer of stratum spinosum contains metabolically active cells with a spiny shape.[9] The spiny shape is due to the numerous desmosomes connecting cells throughout the layer. Furthermore, this same desmosomal network maintains the structural integrity of the tissue. The basal layers of stratum germinativum contain cuboidal cells that occupy 10% to 15% of the epithelium's thickness and are uniquely capable of replication.[9] Consequently, basal cell hyperplasia, defined as basal cells occupying more than 15% of epithelial thickness, is common in gastroesophageal reflux disease, reflecting an increased rate of tissue repair.[9] The esophageal epithelium contains a small number of other cell types including argyrophilic endocrine cells, melanocytes, lymphocytes, Langerhans cells (macrophages), and eosinophils. Neutrophils are not present in healthy epithelium.

Below the epithelium is the lamina propria, a loose network of connective tissue within which are blood vessels and scattered lymphocytes, macrophages, and plasma cells (see Fig. 31–5). The lamina propria protrudes at intervals into the epithelium to form rete pegs or dermal papillae. Normally, these protrude to less than 50% of the epithelium's thickness; when greater, it is a recognized marker of gastroesophageal reflux disease (see Chapter 33).[9] The muscularis mucosae is a thin layer of smooth muscle that separates the lamina propria above from the submucosa (see Fig. 31–2*A*). Its functions are unclear.

Submucosa

The submucosa comprises a dense network of connective tissue within which are blood vessels, lymphatic channels, neurons of Meissner's plexus, and esophageal glands (see

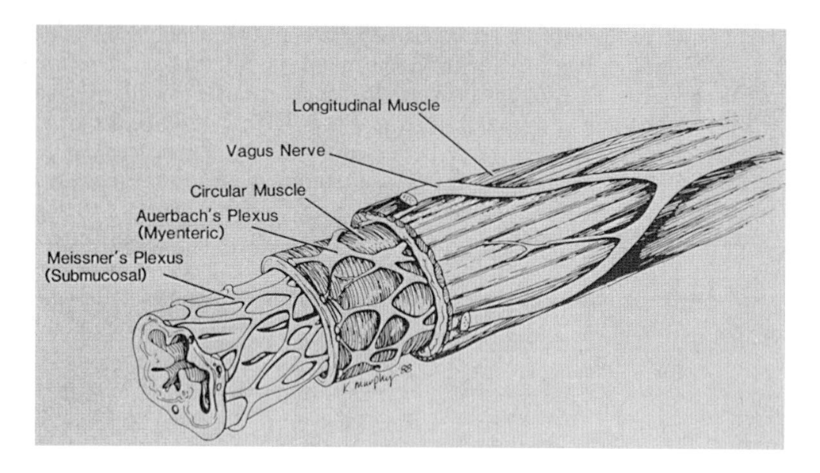

Figure 31–4. Neuromuscular anatomy of the esophagus. Extrinsic innervation is provided principally by the vagus nerve. Between the inner circular and outer longitudinal muscle bundles lies Auerbach's myenteric plexus for coordination of peristalsis, and between the mucosa and the circular muscle layer is Meissner's submucosal plexus for reception of sensory input from different layers within the esophageal wall. (From Kahrilas, PJ: The anatomy and physiology of dysphagia. In Gelfand DW, Richter JE [eds]: Dysphagia: Diagnosis and Treatment. New York, Igaku-Shoin, 1989, p 15.)

Fig. 31–2*A*). These glands, which vary as to number and distribution along the esophagus, consist of cuboidal cells organized as acini.[10] They produce and secrete a lubricant, mucus, and factors such as bicarbonate and epidermal growth factor that are important for epithelial defense and repair. The secretions from these glands pass into tortuous collecting ducts that deliver them to the esophageal lumen (see Fig. 31–2*A*).

EMBRYOLOGY

A brief review of the embryology of the upper digestive system is presented as a guide to understanding the origin of many of the developmental anomalies discussed in this chapter. In the developing fetus, the oropharynx and esophageal components of the gastrointestinal tract and the larynx, trachea, bronchi, and lungs of the respiratory tract develop from a common tube.[11] By gestational week 4, this tube, composed of endoderm, develops a diverticulum on its ventral surface that is destined to become the epithelium and glands of the respiratory tract (Fig. 31–6*A* and *B*). This diverticulum subsequently elongates, becomes enveloped by splanchnic mesenchyme (future cartilage, connective tissue, and smooth muscle), and buds off to become the primitive respiratory tract (Fig. 31–6*C* and *D*). Concomitantly, the lumen of the dorsal tube, the primitive foregut, fills with proliferating (ciliated columnar) epithelium. By week 10, vacuoles appear and subsequently coalesce within the primitive foregut to reestablish the lumen. By week 16, the columnar epithelium lining the primitive foregut and future esophagus is replaced by stratified squamous epithelium, a process that is complete by birth.

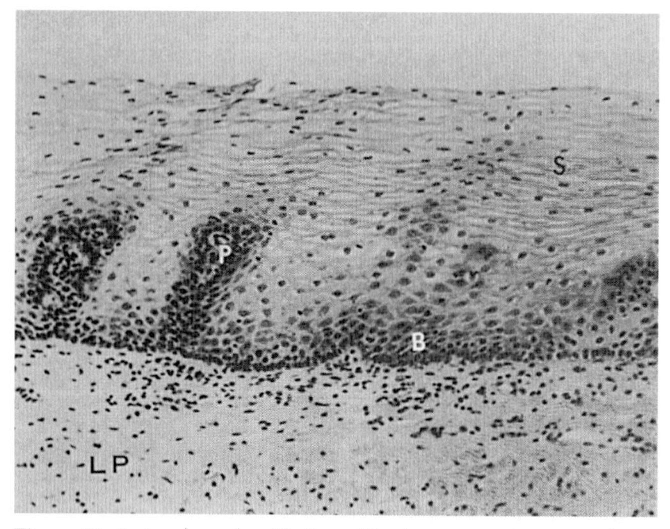

Figure 31–5. Esophageal epithelium. The human esophagus as shown on biopsy is lined by nonkeratinized stratified squamous epithelium (S). The cells of the surface are long and flat and have a small nuclear-to-cytoplasmic ratio that contrasts to the cells of the basal layer (B), whose density, cuboidal shape, and large nuclear-to-cytoplasmic ratio account for their prominence. Rete pegs, or dermal papillae (P) containing elements of lamina propria (LP), extend into the epithelium normally less than half the distance to the lumen.

DEVELOPMENTAL ANOMALIES

Congenital anomalies of the esophagus are relatively common (1 in 3000 to 1 in 4500 live births) and are due to either genetic defects or intrauterine stress that impedes fetal maturation.[11, 12] Esophageal anomalies are common in premature infants and 50% have other anomalies, reflected by the term VACTERL (formerly VATER), a mnemonic for the association of anomalies of the Vertebral, Anal, Cardiac, Tracheal, Esophageal, Renal, and Limb systems.[12, 13] Common associated defects include patent ductus arteriosus, cardiac septal deformity, and imperforate anus.[11, 13]

Esophageal Atresia and Tracheoesophageal Fistula

Esophageal atresia and tracheoesophageal fistulas are the most common and most important developmental anomalies of the esophagus (Fig. 31–7). The former results from failure of the primitive foregut to recanalize; the latter results from failure of the lung bud to separate completely from the foregut.

Esophageal atresia occurs as an isolated anomaly in only 7% of cases; the remaining 93% are accompanied by a form of tracheoesophageal fistula.[14] In isolated atresia the upper esophagus ends in a blind pouch and the lower esophagus connects to the stomach (see Fig. 31–7*A*). The condition is suspected prenatally by the development of polyhydramnios (due to the inability of the fetus to swallow and so absorb

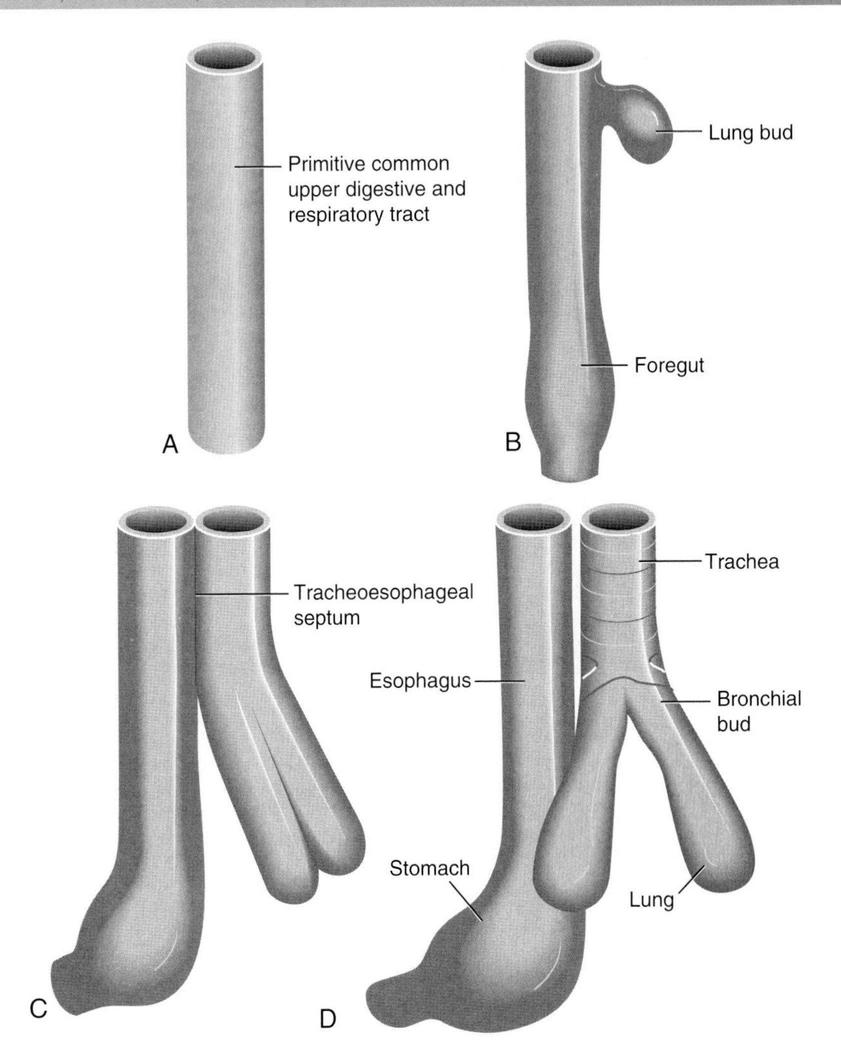

Figure 31–6. Developmental stages in the formation of separate respiratory and digestive systems. These systems are shown to be derived from a common tube of endoderm during embryogenesis. *A,* Single primitive tube. *B,* Formation of lung bud in the 4th week. *C,* Elongation of dorsal tube (primitive foregut) and lung bud, and formation of tracheoesophageal septum by 4 to 6 weeks. *D,* Separation of primitive foregut from the tracheobronchial tree at 6 weeks.

amniotic fluid) or at birth by the regurgitation of saliva and a scaphoid (gasless) abdomen. Furthermore, and as an indicator of high gastrointestinal obstruction, esophageal atresia results in the rapid onset of choking, coughing, and regurgitation on first feeding (Table 31–1). Once suspected, the diagnosis can be confirmed by failure to pass a nasogastric tube into the stomach and by a concurrent chest radiograph with air contrast in the upper esophageal segment (the air being introduced through a catheter positioned within the upper esophageal segment). In some instances, injection of 1 mL of barium into the obstructed segment helps with the diagnosis.

Esophageal atresia usually (93% of cases) is associated with a tracheoesophageal fistula, and in 86% of cases, it is the distal type (see Fig. 31–7*B*). Thus, the atretic upper esophagus ends in a blind pouch and the trachea communicates with the distal esophageal segment. The clinical presentation with this configuration is usually similar to that of isolated esophageal atresia with the additional risk of aspiration pneumonia from refluxed gastric contents entering the trachea through the fistula (see Table 31–1). Nonetheless, distinction between an isolated atresia and one associated with a distal tracheoesophageal fistula is straightforward because the communication between the trachea and the esophagus results in a gas-filled abdomen, as shown on plain radiographs. Isolated atresia without a distal tracheoesophageal fistula results in a gasless abdomen because no pathways exist for inspired or swallowed air to enter the bowel. In some instances, confirmation of the type of configuration is obtained by esophagography with or without bronchoscopy.[1]

The three less common types of tracheoesophageal fistula are when (1) the atretic upper esophagus communicates with the trachea, (2) both upper and lower segments of the atretic esophagus communicate with the trachea, and (3) a nonatretic esophagus communicates with the trachea in an H-type configuration (see Figs. 31–7*C* to *E*). Because these types have in common the communication between upper esophagus and trachea, they all present clinically with signs and symptoms of recurrent (aspiration) pneumonia (see Table 31–1). Distinguishing among types, however, should not be difficult. Esophageal atresia accompanied by proximal tracheoesophageal fistula presents in infancy as recurrent pneumonia, and the presence or absence of bowel gas on a plain radiograph indicates whether an accompanying distal tracheoesophageal fistula exists. In contrast, in those with an H-type tracheoesophageal fistula without esophageal atresia, the diagnosis can be delayed until childhood or, at times, adulthood.[15] Diagnosis of a suspected H-type fistula is usually made by esophagography,[15] but this may be difficult because

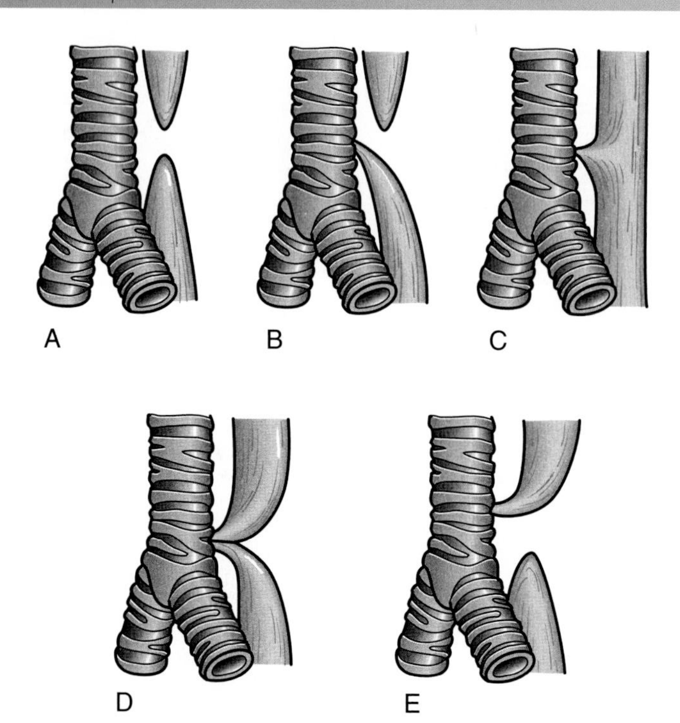

Figure 31–7. Esophageal atresia and tracheoesophageal fistulas. Esophageal atresia (*A*) and tracheoesophageal fistulas (*B* through *E*) are the most common developmental anomalies of the esophagus. The most common tracheoesophageal fistula is that in which the trachea communicates with the distal segment of the atretic esophagus (*B*). The next most common is the H-type tracheoesophageal fistula, in which the trachea communicates with an otherwise normal esophagus (*C*). The tracheoesophageal fistulas in which the trachea communicates with both upper and lower segments of an atretic esophagus (*D*) or only the upper segment of an atretic esophagus (*E*) are rare. (Adapted from Lewin KJ, Riddell RH, Weinstein WM [eds]: Gastrointestinal Pathology and its Clinical Implications. New York, Igaku-Shoin, 1992, p 383.)

of the small size of some communications. In such cases, detection may be improved by ingestion of methylene blue and searching by bronchoscopy for the stained fistula site.

Treatment of esophageal atresia and tracheoesophageal fistulas is surgical, and the choice of procedure depends on the distance between the upper and lower esophageal segments. Short gaps permit end-to-end anastomosis, as do some long gaps after lengthening of the upper segment by either bougienage or intraoperative myotomy.[14] If approximation of the two segments is not possible, the colon is interposed. The results of surgical correction of esophageal atresia are excellent when it exists as an isolated anomaly, with survival rates of 90%.[13] Overall outcome is determined by the gravity of accompanying genetic anomalies and by the birth weight of the infant.[14]

Patients who survive for many years after successful repair of esophageal atresia are at increased risk for the development of gastroesophageal reflux disease.[16, 17] These patients have higher rates of reflux symptoms, endoscopic and histologic esophagitis, and Barrett's metaplasia compared to the normal population. This increased risk is due to abnormalities of esophageal motility and impaired esophageal luminal acid clearance.[18] After esophageal atresia repair, approximately 6% to 45% of patients are treated for gastroesophageal reflux disease by surgical fundoplication; however, 15% to 30% of Nissen operations fail, usually resulting in reoperation.[19]

Congenital Stenosis

Esophageal stenosis is a rare anomaly, occurring in only 1 in every 25,000 live births.[20] The stenotic segment varies from 2 to 20 cm in length and is usually located within the middle or lower third of the esophagus (Fig. 31–8). The precise cause of congenital stenoses is not entirely clear. When resected, many stenotic walls contain sequestered res-

Table 31–1 | **Clinical Aspects of Esophageal Developmental Anomalies**

ANOMALY	AGE AT PRESENTATION	PREDOMINANT SYMPTOMS	DIAGNOSIS	TREATMENT
Atresia alone	Newborns	Regurgitation of feedings Aspiration	Esophagogram* Radiograph—gasless abdomen	Surgery
Atresia + distal fistula	Newborns	Regurgitation of feedings Aspiration	Esophagogram* Radiograph—gas-filled abdomen	Surgery
H-type fistula	Infants to adults	Recurrent aspiration pneumonia Bronchiectasis	Esophagogram* Bronchoscopy	Surgery
Esophageal stenosis	Infants to adults	Dysphagia Food impaction	Esophagogram* Endoscopy†	Bougienage‡ Surgery§
Duplication cysts	Infants to adults	Dyspnea, stridor, cough (infants) Dysphagia, chest pain (adults)	EUS* MRI/CT† Esophagogram	Surgery
Vascular anomalies	Infants to adults	Dyspnea, stridor, cough (infants) Dysphagia (adults)	Esophagogram* Angiography† MRI/CT/EUS	Diet modification‡ Surgery§
Esophageal rings	Children to adults	Dysphagia Food impaction	Esophagogram* Endoscopy†	Bougienage
Esophageal webs	Children to adults	Dysphagia	Esophagogram* Endoscopy†	Bougienage

*Diagnostic test of choice.
†Confirmatory test.
‡Primary therapeutic approach.
§Secondary therapeutic approach.
CT, computed tomography; EUS, endoscopic ultrasonography; MRI, magnetic resonance imaging.

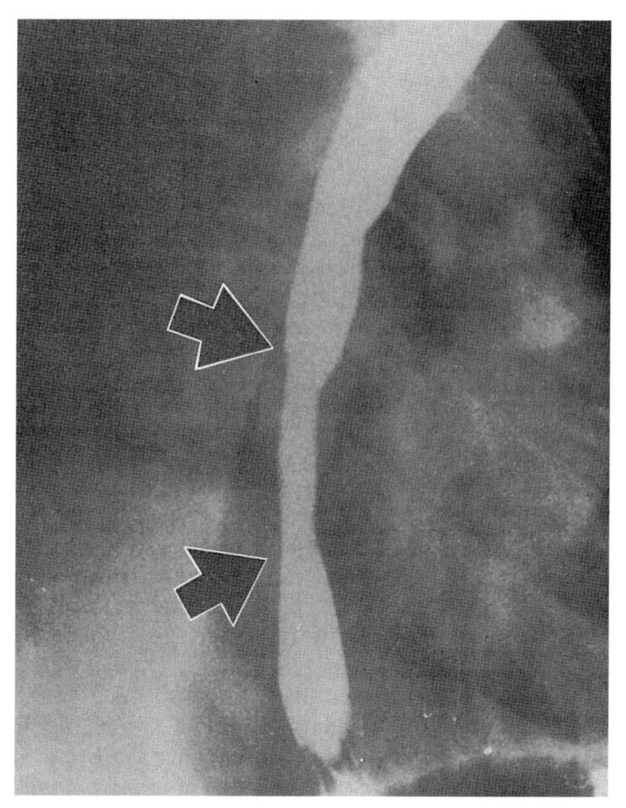

Figure 31–8. Congenital esophageal stenosis. A barium esophagogram shows a 5-cm long, symmetric narrowing at the juncture of the middle and distal thirds of the esophagus (*arrows*). (From McNally PR, Lemon JC, Goff JS, et al: Congenital esophageal stenosis presenting as noncardiac, esophageal chest pain. Dig Dis Sci 38:370, 1993.)

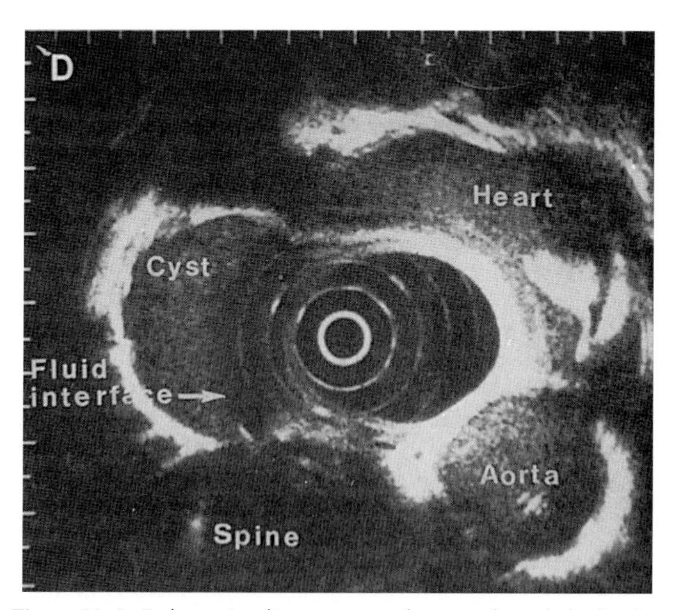

Figure 31–9. Endoscopic ultrasonogram of an esophageal duplication cyst. The distortion of the esophageal wall by the hypoechoic area created by the cyst is indicated, as is the cyst's relationship to other hypoechoic areas created by the heart, aorta, and spine. (From Geller A, Wang KK, DiMagno EP: Diagnosis of foregut duplication cysts by endoscopic ultrasonography. Gastroenterology 109:839, 1995.)

piratory tissue (hyaline cartilage, respiratory epithelium), suggesting its origin is incomplete separation of lung bud from primitive foregut. In other cases, stenosis results from fibromuscular hypertrophy or from damage to the myenteric plexus with loss of the muscle-relaxing nitric oxide–producing neural elements.[21]

Although tight stenoses are symptomatic in infancy, most patients present with dysphagia and regurgitation in childhood when more solid food is ingested (see Table 31–1). Patients with mild symptoms may go undetected until adulthood. Nine of ten cases are males and most have longstanding dysphagia (years). A history of food impaction is common.[20] The stenosis is best demonstrated by esophagography, which in some cases reveals a characteristic pattern of ringlike submucosal structures in the region of the stenosis. Endoscopy may be of value in some cases to demonstrate normal mucosa in the stenotic region, and endoscopic ultrasound may show thickening of single or multiple layers of the esophageal wall.[20] Treatment varies; some patients improve after endoscopic-guided bougienage, whereas others with problematic stenoses require surgical resection of the involved segment. Endoscopists are advised to approach esophageal dilation carefully in these patients because chest pain and mucosal tears are commonly reported.[20]

Esophageal Duplications

Congenital duplications of the esophagus occur in 1 in 8000 live births.[22] They arise as epithelial-lined outpouchings off the primitive foregut and evolve to produce either cystic or tubular structures that do not communicate with the esophageal lumen. Cysts account for 80% of the duplications and are usually single, fluid-filled structures (Fig. 31–9).[22] They may be found attached to the esophagus or to the tracheobronchial tree within the posterior mediastinum. Some cysts are discovered while asymptomatic, presenting as a mediastinal mass on a chest radiograph or submucosal lesion on an esophagogram. Others present with symptoms from compression of structures adjacent to the tracheobronchial tree (coughing, stridor, tachypnea, cyanosis, wheezing, or chest pain) and of structures adjacent to the esophageal wall (dysphagia, chest pain, or regurgitation) (see Table 31–1).[22]

The diagnosis of an esophageal duplication cyst is supported by the demonstration of a cystic mass on computed axial tomography, magnetic resonance imaging, or endoscopic ultrasonography.[23] However, only surgical excision for pathologic assessment can exclude a cystic neoplasm. Surgical excision is also favored because it has low morbidity.[24] Rarely, large duplication cysts present as acute life-threatening respiratory symptoms. In this circumstance, decompression can be afforded emergently by radiologic or endoscopically guided needle aspiration or by internal marsupialization.[25]

The tubular esophageal duplication is far less common than its cystic counterpart. It is usually located within the esophageal wall, parallels the true esophageal lumen, and, unlike duplication cysts, communicates with the true lumen at either or both ends of the tube.[26] Tubular duplications usually cause chest pain, dysphagia, or regurgitation in infancy, and the diagnosis is established by esophagography or endoscopy. Reconstructive surgery is indicated for those patients who are symptomatic.[24]

Vascular Anomalies

Intrathoracic vascular anomalies are present in 2% to 3% of the population. Only rarely do they produce symptoms of esophageal obstruction despite evident vascular compression on an esophagogram.[27] Most infants with intrathoracic vascular anomalies present with respiratory symptoms from compression of the tracheobronchial tree.[27] Later in childhood or adulthood, however, these same abnormalities can produce dysphagia and regurgitation, owing to esophageal compression (see Table 31–1).

Dysphagia lusoria is the term given for symptoms arising from vascular compression of the esophagus by an aberrant right subclavian artery (Fig. 31–10).[28] The right subclavian artery in this circumstance arises from the left side of the aortic arch and courses from the lower left to the upper right side posterior to the esophagus. In 20% of cases, the artery courses anterior to the esophagus.[29] It is estimated that dysphagia lusoria is present in 0.7% of the general population based on autopsy studies.[28] Typically the diagnosis is established by barium esophagogram, which shows the characteristic pencil-like indentation at the level of the fourth thoracic vertebrae.[28] Confirmation is provided by computed tomography, magnetic resonance imaging, arteriography, or endoscopic ultrasonography.[29] Given the frequency with which such lesions are asymptomatic, endoscopy or esophageal manometry may be desirable to exclude other causes of dysphagia. During endoscopy, the right radial pulse may diminish or disappear from instrumental compression of the right subclavian artery.[27] Manometry has demonstrated a high-pressure zone at the location of the aberrant artery.[30] Symptoms usually respond to simple modification of the diet to meals of soft consistency and small size. When necessary, surgery relieves the obstruction by reanastomosing the aberrant artery to the ascending aorta.[31]

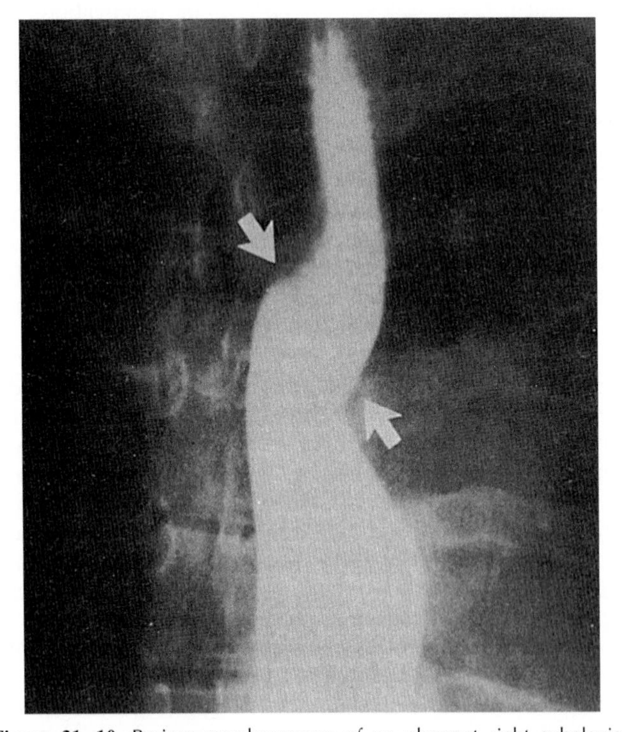

Figure 31–10. Barium esophagogram of an aberrant right subclavian artery. There is an oblique indentation of the esophageal wall (*arrows*) produced by the aberrant artery as it courses behind the esophagus from the aortic arch toward the right shoulder. The phenomenon of dysphagia in association with such aberrant vasculature is known as dysphagia lusoria. (From Van Son JAM, Julsrud PR, Hagler DJ, et al: Surgical treatment of vascular rings: The Mayo Clinic experience. Mayo Clin Proc 68:1060, 1993.)

Heterotopic Gastric Mucosa

Heterotopic gastric mucosa (the inlet patch) refers to the appearance on endoscopy of a small (0.5–2 cm) distinctive, velvety red island amid a pink-colored squamous mucosa generally localized immediately below the upper esophageal sphincter. When sought, an inlet patch is found in 3% to 10% of endoscopies,[32, 33] and biopsy specimens reveal gastric oxyntic- (fundic-) or antral- (pyloric-)type mucosa. The oxyntic-type mucosa contains chief and parietal cells and thus in some specimens retains the capacity for acid secretion.[34] Similar to gastric mucosa elsewhere in the stomach, the inlet patch may be infected with *Helicobacter pylori*.[35] However, inlet patches are usually asymptomatic and unassociated with disease and thus require no treatment. In rare instances, however, an inlet patch is found in association with an esophageal web, stricture, or ulcer, the latter resulting in bleeding or perforation.[36] In addition, a total of 15 cases of adenocarcinoma arising in an inlet patch have been reported in the literature.[37]

Esophageal Rings

The distal esophagus contains two "rings," the A and B (Schatzki) rings, that demarcate anatomically the proximal and distal borders of the esophageal vestibule (Fig. 31–11).[38] The A (muscular) ring is located at the proximal border. It is a broad (4–5 mm) symmetric band of hypertrophied muscle that constricts the tubular esophageal lumen at its junction with the vestibule. In this location the A ring, which is covered by squamous epithelium, corresponds to the upper end of the lower esophageal sphincter.[39] The A ring is rare, and because it varies in caliber on the esophagogram, depending on the degree of esophageal distension, it is generally asymptomatic. Occasionally, a ring is found in association with dysphagia for solids and liquids (see Table 31–1).[39] Symptomatic A rings can be treated by passage of a 50-F mercury-weighted esophageal dilator or by injection of botulinum toxin.[39]

The B ring, otherwise known as the mucosal or Schatzki ring, is very common and found in 6% to 14% of subjects who undergo a routine upper gastrointestinal series.[38] On barium-enhanced studies, the B ring is always found in association with a hiatal hernia and is recognized as a thin (2 mm) membrane that constricts the esophageal lumen at the junction of vestibule and the gastric cardia (see Fig. 31–11). The Schatzki ring has squamous epithelium on its upper surface and columnar epithelium on its lower surface and so demarcates the squamocolumnar junction.[38] The ring itself is composed of only mucosa and submucosa; there is no muscularis propria. Schatzki rings are probably congenital in origin, although a relationship to gastroesophageal reflux disease has been proposed.[38] Most are asymptomatic; however, when the diameter of the esophageal lumen is narrowed to less than or equal to 13 mm, rings are a common cause of dysphagia for solids and acute solid-food impactions (see

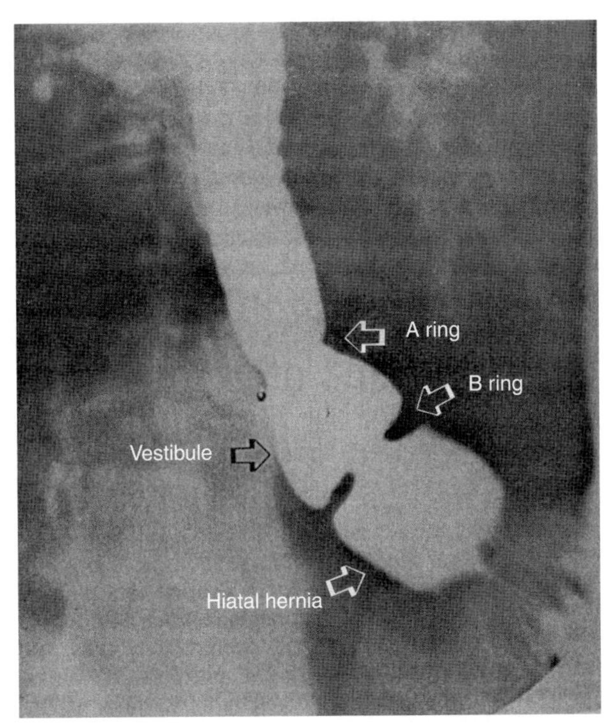

Figure 31–11. Barium esophagogram of the lower esophageal A and B rings. The proximal A ring is hypertrophied muscle whereas the distal B or Schatzki ring is a ring of mucosa localized to the squamocolumnar junction. The A and B rings circumscribe the esophageal vestibule, whereas below the vestibule is a hiatal hernia. The hernia is visualized as a small sac between the B ring above and diaphragm below. (From Marshall JB, Kretschmar, JM, Diaz-Arias AA: et al: Gastroesophageal reflux as a pathogenetic factor in the development of symptomatic lower esophageal rings. Arch Intern Med 150:1670, 1990. Copyright 1990, American Medical Association.)

Table 31–1).[38] Identification of symptomatic rings on esophagography or endoscopy is generally not difficult (see Fig. 31–11), although care should be taken to adequately distend the distal esophagus.[40] In some instances, the obstructing ring is best demonstrated radiographically by its ability to trap a swallowed marshmallow or barium tablet. Asymptomatic rings require no treatment, and those producing dysphagia are effectively treated by passage of either a single, large (50-F), mercury-weighted dilator or a series of such dilators of progressively larger diameter.[41] Repeat dilatations are required in most patients because 90% of patients have recurrence of dysphagia by three years.[41] The benefit of acid-reducing drugs such as proton pump inhibitors to reduce recurrence of Schatzki rings is uncertain. Symptomatic rings that are refractory to dilatation have been treated by endoscopic rupture using either electrocautery or four-quadrant biopsies.[42]

Esophageal Webs

Esophageal webs are congenital anomalies characterized by one or more thin horizontal membranes of stratified squamous epithelium within the upper esophagus and midesophagus. Unlike rings, these anomalies rarely encircle the lumen but instead protrude from the anterior wall, extending laterally but not to the posterior wall (Fig. 31–12). Webs are common in the cervical esophagus and are best demonstrated on an esophagogram with the lateral view.[38] In up to 5% of cases they are identified in an asymptomatic state, but when they are symptomatic they cause dysphagia for solids (see Table 31–1).[38] Webs are fragile membranes and so respond well to esophageal bougienage with mercury-weighted dilators.

An association between cervical esophageal webs, dysphagia, and iron deficiency anemia in adults (particularly women) has been described as the Plummer-Vinson or Paterson-Kelly syndrome.[43] Recent reports have shown an association between Plummer-Vinson syndrome and celiac sprue.[44] It is an uncommon but important syndrome because it identifies a group of patients at increased risk for squamous carcinoma of the pharynx and esophagus.[43] Correction of iron deficiency in Plummer-Vinson syndrome may result in resolution of the associated dysphagia as well as disappearance of the web.[45] The pathogenesis of the syndrome is unclear.

Finally a syndrome in which multiple esophageal webs are found has been described.[46] The majority (90%) of patients are males and typically they report long-standing dysphagia to solids (often since childhood). Patients lack any history of acquired causes of esophageal webs such as skin diseases, caustic ingestion, nonsteroidal anti-inflammatory drugs, and gastroesophageal reflux disease. Some authorities consider this entity a form of congenital esophageal stenosis. However, patients with multiple webs do not have an obvious stricture on barium esophagogram, although on endoscopy it is often difficult to pass the endoscope through the esophagus.[46] Esophageal dilatation is necessary to relieve dysphagia but these patients are prone to significant mucosal tears from bougienage; therefore, careful dilatation is suggested.

The term "corrugated ringed esophagus" is often used interchangeably for "multiple esophageal webs," although rings and webs differ histopathologically in that the former has a muscular component and the latter consists of mucosa

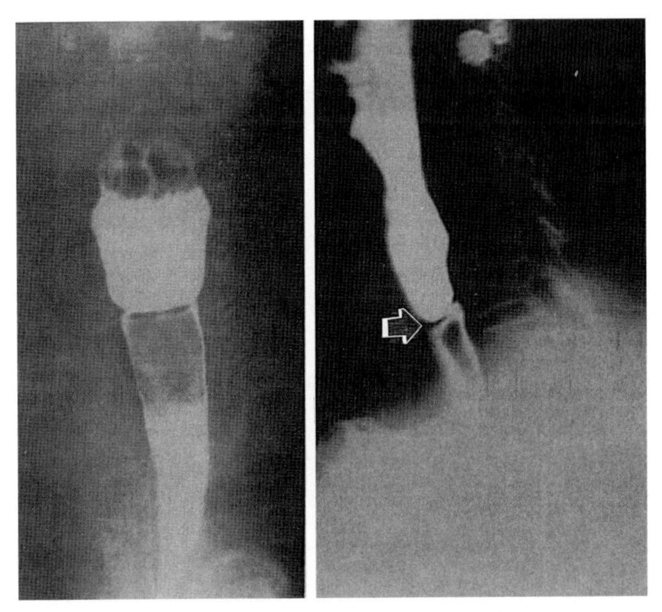

Figure 31–12. Barium esophagogram of a cervical web. *A*, AP view. *B*, Lateral view. The web is seen on the lateral view as a thin membrane protruding from the anterior esophageal wall. Webs, unlike rings, often incompletely encircle the esophageal lumen (*arrow*). (Courtesy of F.E. Templeton, M.D.)

and submucosa only. When specifically referred to, corrugated ringed esophagus generally implies a condition in which the muscular rings are concentric and evenly spaced over a long segment of esophagus, usually starting proximally and extending, in many instances, the entire length of the organ. These rings are usually not apparent on barium studies but on endoscopy persist despite maximal air insufflation. Another defining characteristic of the corrugated ringed esophagus is that dilatation is difficult, so mucosal tears and perforations are common. For this reason, it is recommended that dilatation be limited in patients with solid food dysphagia to a maximum diameter of a 40-F bougie. Finally, support for the corrugated ringed esophagus being a developmental anomaly is based on the large male predominance (56 of 63 reported cases) and history of solid food dysphagia, often with impactions, beginning in early childhood.[46] It recently was proposed that some cases may be the result of gastroesophageal reflux and that antisecretory therapy with a proton pump inhibitor may be beneficial.[47]

REFERENCES

1. Pope CE 2nd: Normal anatomy and developmental anomalies. In Sleisenger MH, Fordtran JS (eds): Gastrointestinal Disease, 5th ed. Philadelphia, WB Saunders, 1993, pp 311–318.
2. Meyer GW, Austin RM, Brady CE, et al: Muscle anatomy of the human esophagus. J Clin Gastroenterol 8:131, 1986.
3. Mittal RK, Balaban DH: The esophagogastric junction. N Engl J Med 336:924, 1997.
4. Cunningham ET, Sawchenko PE: Central neural control of esophageal motility: A review. Dysphagia 5:35, 1990.
5. Hornby PJ, Abrahams TP: Central control of lower esophageal sphincter relaxation. Am J Med 108(suppl. 4A):90S, 2000.
6. Liebermann-Meffert D, Luescher U, Neff U, et al: Esophagectomy without thoracotomy: Is there a risk of intramediastinal bleeding ? Ann Surg 206:184, 1987.
7. Vianna A, Hayes PC, Moscoso G, et al: Normal venous circulation of the gastroesophageal junction: A route to understanding varices. Gastroenterology 93:876, 1987.
8. Orlando RC: Pathophysiology of gastroesophageal reflux disease: Esophageal epithelial resistance. In Castell DO, Richter JE (eds): The Esophagus, 3rd ed. Philadelphia, Lippincott Williams & Wilkins, 1999, pp 409–419.
9. DeNardi FG, Riddell RH: The normal esophagus. Am J Surg Pathol 15:296, 1991.
10. Long JD, Orlando RC: Esophageal submucosal glands: Structure and function. Am J Gastroenterol 94:2818, 1999.
11. Yazbeck S: Gastrointestinal emergencies of the neonate. In Roy CC, Siverman A, Alagille D (eds): Pediatric Clinical Gastroenterology, 4th ed. St. Louis, Mosby–Year Book, 1995, p 53.
12. Depaepe A, Dolk H, Lechat MF, and a Eurocat Working Group: The epidemiology of tracheoesophageal fistula and oesophageal atresia in Europe. Arch Dis Child 68:743, 1993.
13. Spitz L, Kiely EM, Morecroft JA, et al: Oesophageal atresia: At-risk groups for the 1990s. J Pediatr Surg 29:723, 1994.
14. Spitz L: Esophageal atresia: Past, present, and future. J Pediatr Surg 31: 19, 1996.
15. Danton MHD, McMahon J, McGiugan J, et al: Congenital oesophageal respiratory tract fistula presenting in adult life. Eur Respir J 6:1412, 1993.
16. Lindahl H, Rintala R, Sariola H: Chronic esophagitis and gastric metaplasia are frequent late complications of esophageal atresia. J Pediatr Surg 28:1178, 1993.
17. Krug E, Bergmeijer JHLJ, Dees J, et al: Gastroesophageal reflux and Barrett's esophagus in adults born with esophageal atresia. Am J Gastroenterol 94:2825, 1999.
18. Tovar JA, Diez Pardo JA, Murcia J, et al: Ambulatory 24-hour manometric and pH metric evidence of permanent impairment of clearance capacity in patients with esophageal atresia. J Pediatr Surg 30:1224, 1995.
19. Bergmeijer JHLJ, Tibboel D, Hazebroek FWJ: Nissen fundoplication in the management of gastroesophageal reflux occurring after repair of esophageal atresia. J Pediatr Surg 35:573, 2000.
20. Katzka DA, Levine MS, Ginsberg GG, et al: Congenital esophageal stenosis in adults. Am J Gastroenterol 95:32, 2000.
21. Singaram C, Sweet MA, Gaumitz EA, et al: Peptidergic and nitrinergic denervation in congenital esophageal stenosis. Gastroenterology 109: 275, 1995.
22. Arbona JL, Figueroa Fazzi JG, Mayoral J: Congenital esophageal cysts: Case report and review of the literature. Am J Gastroenterol 79:177, 1984.
23. Geller A, Wang KK, DiMagno EP: Diagnosis of foregut duplication cysts by endoscopic ultrasonography. Gastroenterology 109:838, 1995.
24. Cioffi U, Bonavina L, De Simone M, et al: Presentation and surgical management of bronchogenic and esophageal duplication cysts in adults. Chest 113:1492, 1998.
25. Van Dam J, Rice TW, Sivak MV: Endoscopic ultrasonography and endoscopically guided needle aspiration for the diagnosis of upper gastrointestinal tract foregut cysts. Am J Gastroenterol 87:762, 1992.
26. Ratan ML, Anand R, Mittal SK, et al: Communicating oesophageal duplication: A report of two cases. Gut 29:254, 1988.
27. Boyce GA, Boyce HW Jr: Esophagus: Anatomy and structural anomalies. In Yamada T, Alpers DH, Owyang C, et al (eds): Textbook of Gastroenterology, 2nd ed. Philadelphia, JB Lippincott, 1995, p 1156.
28. Janssen M, Baggen MGA, Veen HF, et al: Dysphagia lusoria: Clinical aspects, manometric findings, diagnosis, and therapy. Am J Gastroenterol 95:1411, 2000.
29. De Luca L, Bergman JGHM, Tytgat GNJ, et al: EUS imaging of the arteria lusoria: Case series and review. Gastrointest Endosc 52:670, 2000.
30. Nguyen P, Gideon RM, Castell DO: Dysphagia lusoria in the adult: Associated esophageal manometric findings and diagnostic use of scanning techniques. Am J Gastroenterol 89:620, 1994.
31. Van Son JAM, Julsrud PR, Hagler DJ, et al: Surgical treatment of vascular rings: The Mayo Clinic experience. Mayo Clin Proc 68:1056, 1993.
32. Jabbari M, Goresky CA, Lough J, et al: The inlet patch: Heterotopic gastric mucosa in the upper esophagus. Gastroenterology 89:352, 1985.
33. Borhan-Manesh F, Farnum JB: Incidence of heterotopic gastric mucosa in the upper esophagus. Gut 32:968, 1991.
34. Galan AR, Katzka DA, Castell DO: Acid secretion from an esophageal inlet patch demonstrated by ambulatory pH monitoring. Gastroenterology 115:1574, 1998.
35. Borhan-Manesh F, Farnum JB: Study of *Helicobacter pylori* colonization of patches of heterotopic gastric mucosa (HGM) at the upper esophagus. Dig Dis Sci 38:142, 1993.
36. Sanchez-Pernaute A, Hernando F, Diez-Valladares L, et al: Heterotopic gastric mucosa in the upper esophagus ("inlet patch"): A rare cause of esophageal perforation. Am J Gastroenterol 94:3047, 1999.
37. Lauwers GY, Scott GV, Vauthey JN: Adenocarcinoma of the upper esophagus arising in cervical ectopic gastric mucosa. Dig Dis Sci 43: 901, 1998.
38. Tobin RW: Esophageal rings, webs, and diverticula. J Clin Gastroenterol 27:285, 1998.
39. Hirano I, Gilliam J, Goyal RK: Clinical and manometric features of the lower esophageal muscular ring. Am J Gastroenterol 95:43, 2000.
40. Ott DJ, Chen YM, Wu WC, et al: Radiographic and endoscopic sensitivity in detecting lower esophageal mucosal ring. AJR Am J Roentgenol 147:261, 1986.
41. Eckardt VF, Kanzler G, Willems D: Single dilatation of symptomatic Schatzki rings. Dig Dis Sci 37:577, 1992.
42. Chotiprasidhi P, Minocha A: Effectiveness of single dilation with Maloney dilator versus endoscopic rupture of Schatzki's ring using biopsy forceps. Dig Dis Sci 45:281, 2000.
43. Hoffman RM, Jaffe PE: Plummer-Vinson syndrome: A case report and literature review. Arch Intern Med 155:2008, 1995.
44. Dickey W, McConnell B: Celiac disease presenting as the Paterson-Brown-Kelly (Plummer-Vinson) syndrome. Am J Gastroenterol 94:527, 1999.
45. Dantas RO, Villanova MG: Esophageal motility impairment in Plummer-Vinson syndrome. Correction by iron treatment. Dig Dis Sci 38: 968, 1993.
46. Longstreth GF, Sitzer ME: Multiple esophageal webs: Treatment and follow-up of seven patients. J Clin Gastroenterol 24:199, 1997.
47. Morrow JB, Vargo JJ, Goldblum JR, Richter JE: The ringed esophagus: histologic features of GERD. Am J Gastroenterol 96:984, 2001.

Chapter 32

ESOPHAGEAL MOTOR AND SENSORY FUNCTION AND MOTOR DISORDERS OF THE ESOPHAGUS

Ray E. Clouse and Nicholas E. Diamant

Normal esophageal function is the result of numerous interacting control mechanisms that not only regulate activities arising from esophageal continuity with the rest of the gut but also tie the esophagus intimately to other systems and organs, such as the central nervous system, the heart, and the lungs.[1–6] Esophageal motor abnormalities can be explained on the basis of an exaggeration of normal physiologic mechanisms or interference with these mechanisms at one or more levels of control. In some instances, well-defined nerve or muscle diseases interfere with esophageal function. In other situations, the motor disorders appear to result from dysfunction of the neuromuscular apparatus that may even normalize over time, possibly without intervention. With their variety of causes, esophageal motor disorders are common and important considerations in clinical practice, the manifestations ranging from intermittent inconvenience to a severely disabling process.

This chapter describes the elements involved in normal esophageal motor function and the basic types of dysfunction responsible for motor disorders. It also focuses on the manifestation, diagnosis, and management of disorders involving the upper esophageal sphincter (UES) and the cervical esophageal body, the remaining upper portion of the tubular esophagus, and the lower esophageal sphincter (LES). Although of importance in the causation of dysphagia, the oropharyngeal stage of swallowing and its disorders will be considered in less detail. From an overview standpoint, normal control of the human esophagus should be considered with the following, more general functional characteristics in mind.

1. Functionally, the esophagus can be divided into three zones: the UES, the esophageal body, and the LES. The function of the esophageal sphincters is coordinated not only with the activity of the esophageal body but also with the activity in the oropharynx and stomach, which abut the UES and LES, respectively.
2. A number of mechanisms for initiation and control of esophageal motor activity are located at different levels within the central nervous system as well as peripherally within the intramural nerves and muscles. This redundancy has implications for operation of reserve mechanisms when a primary control mechanism is damaged or dysfunctional.
3. Within the swallowing process, voluntary and involuntary control mechanisms act together. Deglutition, or the act of swallowing, is the primary initiator of integrated esophageal activity. During the oropharyngeal phase of swallowing, the bolus is moved voluntarily into the pharynx. Thereafter, the process becomes involuntary.
4. In the esophagus, the activity of two types of muscle is intimately coordinated. Five percent of the upper esopha-

geal body, including the UES along with the muscles involved in the oropharyngeal phase of swallowing, is entirely striated muscle. About 50% to 60% of the distal esophagus, including the LES, is entirely smooth muscle, the circular muscle layer extending more proximally than the longitudinal layer. The transition zone of striated and smooth muscle includes up to 40% of the esophageal length in between.[7] This distribution of two muscle types has functional significance because most esophageal motor abnormalities involve the smooth muscle portion.
5. Between swallows, the esophageal body and its sphincters are not entirely passive but serve other functions. Tone in the UES and LES serves as a protective barrier to esophagopharyngeal and gastroesophageal reflux respectively, and within the esophageal body, peristaltic or nonperistaltic esophageal contractions can arise independently of swallowing, following such events as gastroesophageal reflux and stress.[8, 9]
6. In the human, normal activity of the esophagus is programmed to proceed in the aboral direction, although there is provision for necessary retrograde activity, such as a belch or vomiting.

MOTOR AND SENSORY INNERVATION

Extrinsic Innervation

Swallowing Center

Extrinsic control for esophageal motor function resides in a brainstem "swallowing center" (Fig. 32–1).[1–3, 10] This center, composed of two intimately connected half centers, is located in the medulla and pons and has three functional components: an afferent reception system; an efferent system of motor neurons; and a complex organizing, or internuncial, system of neurons. Although voluntary initiation of swallowing occurs through activation of frontal cortical centers, the reflex onset of the process in the pharynx and its progression into the esophageal phase is highly dependent on peripheral sensory input from oropharyngeal structures.

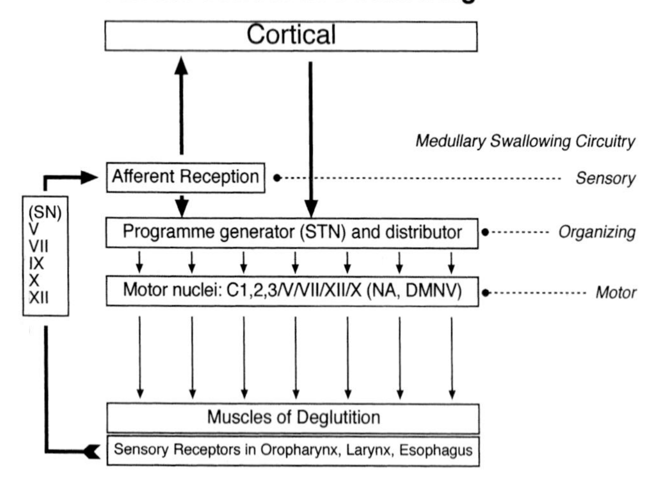

Figure 32–1. Central organization of swallowing: STN, solitary tract nucleus; SN, sensory nucleus; NA, nucleus ambiguus; DMNV, dorsal motor nucleus of the vagus; C, cervical. The mylohyoid locus is predominantly in the primary motor cortex, with extension into the inferior frontal region, while the pharyngeal and esophageal loci are more anterior and medial predominantly in the premotor cortex (see Fig. 32–2).

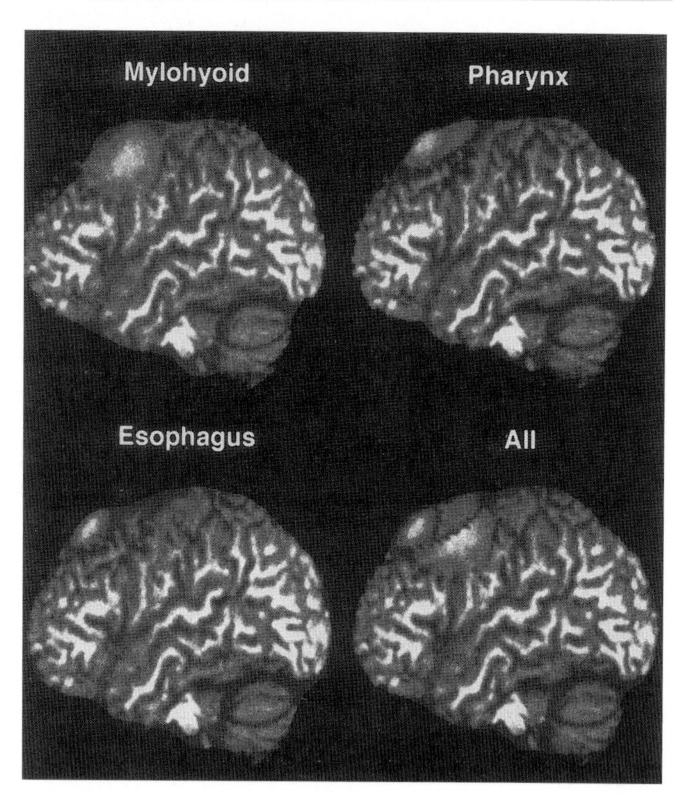

Figure 32–2. Cortical localization of areas responding to transcutaneous magnetic stimulation of the cortex with production of an electromyographic response in the mylohyoid muscle and the muscles of the pharynx and upper striated muscle of the esophagus of a human subject. (From Hamdy S, Aziz Q, Rothwell JC, et al.: The cortical topography of human swallowing musculature in health and disease. Nat Med 2:1217, 1996.)

Cortical Input

Recent studies have provided a clearer picture of the location of some cortical sites connected to the muscles of deglutition. Using transcutaneous magnetic stimulation of the cerebral cortex and recording the electromyographic responses in muscles of the mandible, pharynx, and upper esophagus, the cortical sites for these muscles are shown to have a somatotopic organization and to be bilaterally represented with one side dominant (Fig. 32–2).[11] Furthermore, peripheral electrical stimulation of the pharynx and esophagus can have an impact on the cortex to enhance the cortical representation.[12] It is not clear how these corticofugal pathways interact with the swallowing center to initiate swallowing since the strength of the stimulus is insufficient to do so in humans,[13] although a single cortical stimulus can initiate swallowing in awake or lightly sedated animals.[14, 15] However, these findings have important implications in patients with infarcts (e.g., due to a cortical stroke). Dysphagia is associated with damage to the dominant "swallowing" cortex, and recovery from dysphagia coincides with enlargement of the representation on the non-dominant side.[16] The prospects of facilitating recovery of functional swallowing by enhancing the cortical sites for the initiation of deglutition are now foreseeable.

Afferent Reception

Afferent information from the periphery ultimately enters the solitary tract nucleus, the afferent reception portal of the swallowing center. This sensory information can a) initiate deglutition and the swallowing sequence; b) alter previously initiated activity in the swallowing center and therefore modify ongoing motor activity; or c) function within reflexes, affecting the esophageal body and its sphincters independently of swallowing. Sensory information from the oropharyngeal area and other information that is involved with this stage of the swallowing mechanism enter through non-vagal cranial nerve (trigeminal, facial, hypoglossal, and glossopharyngeal) and vagal nerve pathways.[17, 18] Sensory information from the entire esophagus, including the sphincters, is carried in the vagus nerve with the cell bodies in the nodose ganglion. This sensory pathway is considered important for monitoring and modulating esophageal motor activity, although it may also have a role in modifying cognitive sensation through central descending pathways.[19] Sensory information also passes by way of the sympathetics to the spinal cord segments C1 to L3.[20, 21] Among the functions of this sensory sympathetic pathway is its concern with cognitive sensation and appreciation of symptoms such as chest pain and heartburn. Its role in modulating esophageal motor activity is not clear.

Coordinating Region

The portion of the swallowing center that programs the entire swallowing sequence is located in the solitary tract nucleus (NTS) and the neighboring reticular substance.[2, 22] It is best described functionally as a central pattern generator (CPG). One level of integration (dorsal) within this center is involved in the initiation of swallowing and the organization of the entire swallowing sequence, whereas a second level of organization (ventral) appears to serve primarily as a connecting pathway to the various motor pools involved in the swallowing sequence. The latter may also include some programming function and would include integration of the swallowing sequence with the activity in other medullary centers, such as the respiratory center. Of particular interest in this regard is the effect of swallowing on the perihiatal diaphragm, which serves an antireflux function at the gastroesophageal junction (see Chapter 33) and relaxes during LES relaxation.[23, 24]

Present concepts picture the CPG for swallowing and activation of the muscles of deglutition as a serial network of linked neurons within the NTS and neighboring reticular formation. Once activated, its rostrocaudal organization produces sequential excitation of motor neurons serving muscles along the deglutition pathway.[2, 25] At least two subnetworks are considered present, one for the oropharyngeal phase and the other for the esophageal phase of swallowing.[26, 27] Even segmental subcircuits have been suggested for the striated muscle portion.[28] Within the dorsal level there is a particular subnucleus, the central nucleus, that serves to control the striated muscle esophagus via its connections to the nucleus ambiguus. Presumably, a similar subnucleus subserves the smooth muscle esophagus via the dorsal motor nucleus of the vagus (DMNV). Within the serial network of the CPG, sensory input from the periphery starts the program at about the same level (or just above) where the original sensory input arose.[29, 31] Stimuli arising from the pharynx elicit a pharyngeal swallow that begins in the posterior tongue and pharynx and proceeds through the esophagus. Stimuli such as retained esophageal contents or refluxed acid induce the process such that it begins in the esophagus from about the point of stimulation downward; this is secondary peristalsis.

For the striated muscle esophagus of the rat and rabbit, premotor neurons of that part of the subnucleus centralis of the NTS that receive esophageal afferent input also receive input from pharyngeal premotor neurons in the intermediate and interstitial subnuclei of the NTS, and connect with third-order esophageal neurons in multiple nuclei of the reticular formation.[27] Knowledge of this connectivity along the NTS makes it possible to correlate structure and function in the human where the UES and upper esophageal body are altered by brainstem strokes.[32]

Finally, a number of neurotransmitters are found in the brainstem and have been implicated in various functions of the swallowing control mechanism. Nitric oxide (NO) is involved in the initiation of oropharyngeal swallowing and the initiation and programming of peristalsis in the smooth muscle portion of the esophagus. Muscarinic cholinergic excitation facilitates the initiation of peristalsis in the striated muscle portion of the rat esophagus whether centrally or peripherally induced, although excitatory amino acids appear to be most important.[26, 34, 35] Nicotinic stimulation initiates esophageal peristalsis in the cat.[36] On the other hand, activation of gamma-amino butyric acid (GABA) receptors inhibits the oropharyngeal-esophageal linkage and initiation of esophageal peristalsis in the rat.[37] Other neurotransmitters are also likely playing an important role, and include the excitatory amino acids (EAA) activating both N-methyl-D-aspartate (NMDA) and non-NMDA receptors,[26, 38, 39] somatostatin,[40, 41] as well as catecholamines, serotonin, thyrotropin-releasing hormone, vasopressin, and oxytocin.[26] The potential therefore exists to utilize pharmacotherapy that acts centrally to deal with swallowing disorders and some esophageal motor disorders.

Efferent Output

Motor neurons involved in the swallowing sequence lie mainly in the trigeminal, facial, and hypoglossal nuclei, the nucleus ambiguus of the vagus (for esophageal striated muscle), and the DMNV (for esophageal smooth muscle with some input for striated muscle).[17, 18, 42] The vagus nerve receives efferent fibers from both the nucleus ambiguus and the DMNV, innervating the striated and smooth muscle portions of the esophagus, respectively, including the sphincters. For the LES, two motor neuron pools have been identified within the DMNV, one producing contraction, the other relaxation of the sphincter.[43] For the smooth muscle of the esophageal body, tracing studies have also shown two neuron pools, but the functional role of these has not been established.[44]

Sympathetic

The efferent sympathetic connections to the esophagus and its sphincters arise in the cervical ganglia, celiac ganglion, and ganglia of the paravertebral chains (T4 to L2) and reach the esophagus by way of the vascular supply and, to a lesser extent, through connections to the vagus nerves.[1, 45] The location of the preganglionic cell bodies within the spinal cord reflects the distribution of postganglionic neurons in the sympathetic ganglia. In humans, sympathetic innervation to the LES and lower esophagus probably also occurs by way of splanchnic nerves, as in the cat.[46–48]

Intramural Innervation

A myenteric nerve plexus is found in both the striated and the smooth muscle segments of the esophagus; this is less well developed in the striated muscle portion (see Chapter 31). The submucosal plexus is present but also sparse.[49] For sensory reception, free nerve endings are present in the mucosa and submucosa, whereas unusual laminar nerve endings, which may serve as mechanoreceptors, have been described within the myenteric ganglia.[50]

Striated Muscle

The efferent vagal fibers, mainly in the recurrent laryngeal nerve, make contact with nicotinic cholinergic endplates on the muscle fibers.[51, 52] The nerve fibers contain both acetylcholine (ACh) and calcitonin gene-related peptide (CGRP), the role of the latter being unknown. Some neurons in the myenteric plexus contain nitric oxide synthase (NOS) and vasoactive intestinal polypeptide (VIP) and can send terminals to the motor endplates.[53–56] It is not known if these connections can modulate motor activity in the striated muscle portion. Therefore in the striated muscle, the plexuses presumably serve mainly a sensory role, although an inhibitory pathway to the LES also may exist therein.[57, 58]

Smooth Muscle

The efferent preganglionic vagal fibers synapse predominantly on myenteric neurons. In the smooth muscle segment, the relations between morphology and function of the nerve plexuses are yet to be determined.[49, 59–61] There are two important types of effector neurons that innervate the smooth muscle body and the LES. One is capable of mediating cholinergic excitation of both longitudinal and circular layers of smooth muscle, predominantly through M_3 receptors; the other is capable of mediating nonadrenergic, noncholinergic (NANC) inhibition mainly of the circular muscle layer.[1, 62–67] Nitric oxide (NO) or a similar nitroso compound appears to be the agent primarily responsible for the inhibition.[68–70] Both types of neuron are excited by cholinergic input from preganglionic vagal fibers and intramural interneurons. Cholinergic excitation of the excitatory neuron is nicotinic, whereas that of the NANC neuron can be muscarinic (M_1 receptors) as well. Other neuropeptides are also present in the myenteric neurons.[55, 61, 71, 72] Therefore, purine nucleotides and peptide hormones, such as vasoactive intestinal polypeptide, have been among other substances proposed as active neurotransmitters or modulators.[73, 74]

Identification of various peptides, including opiates within the esophageal neural tissues, has raised questions as to the functional importance of these peptides.[75] Furthermore, it is apparent both in vivo and in vitro that the smooth muscle esophagus, especially in the region of the LES, is sensitive to the action of most peptide hormones and drugs, as well as to the action of other substances, such as histamine, prostaglandins, dopamine, GABA, and serotonin.[1, 76] Most of these agents can act on muscle, nerve, or both, and there are significant variations among species. Their importance awaits further study, but their presence provides future targets for therapy. Until then, it is reasonable to consider that the cholinergic excitatory neuron and the NANC inhibitory neuron represent the basic effector machinery of the smooth muscle esophagus.

Interstitial Cells of Cajal

Another group of cells, the interstitial cells of Cajal (ICCs), are probably of major functional importance. These "intermediate" cells are embryologically similar to muscle cells[77] and are found inserted between nerves and smooth muscle cells, forming intimate gap junction contact with both.[78–81] ICCs throughout the gastrointestinal tract also contain neuropeptides. It is proposed that through the close contacts and the intrinsic electrical activity and peptide content of the ICCs, these special cells act as transducers or modulators of the nerve-smooth muscle interaction and muscle-muscle conduction pathways, and as regulators of the muscle behavior.[82, 83] If this is true, dysfunction of the ICCs would probably result in esophageal motor disorder, and the ICCs could serve as targets for pharmacologic intervention.[84]

Sympathetic

Sympathetic nerves also are present within the myenteric plexus of the striated and smooth muscle portions of the esophagus. There is no reason to suspect a motor function for this innervation in the striated muscle portion. In the smooth muscle portion, most sympathetic nerves terminate in the myenteric plexus and serve mainly to modulate the activity of other neurons and the release of their respective neurotransmitters, thereby modulating features such as contraction amplitude and velocity and LES tone.[46, 85, 86] Beta-adrenergic effect is inhibitory,[86] and alpha-adrenergic effect is excitatory.[46] The sensory function of the sympathetic nerves has already been noted and is discussed below.

Esophageal Sensation

Although the symptoms of dysphagia and heartburn are identified with an esophageal source, the esophagus is often also suspected or implicated as the cause of noncardiac chest pain. This fact, coupled with recent attention to brain-gut interactions in the functional gastrointestinal disorders, has fostered a renewed interest in the neural pathways and mechanisms involved with visceral sensation, the esophagus being no exception.[87–89]

Intramural Sensory Apparatus

Free vagal and spinal afferent nerve endings are found in the submucosa and intraepithelial regions of the esophagus, while within the myenteric ganglia, intraganglionic laminar structures are also seen.[50, 61, 90–92] The latter appear to be vagal in origin[50] and are assumed to be mechanoreceptors. Presumably, mechanoreceptors function through sensory-motor interaction to modulate contractile activity and perhaps mediate non-noxious sensation such as satiety. For this role, they are characterized by their maximum discharge rate reached in the non-noxious distention range, their low threshold of activation, and their slow adaptation nature. These "pure" mechanoreceptors are found only in the vagal pathway, but other slowly adapting mechanoreceptors with a relatively low threshold and with a wide dynamic range of response that does not saturate are seen within the spinal afferent pathway. The latter have been labeled mechanonociceptors.[20] Furthermore, spinal afferents can have nerve endings within the circular muscle layer.[92] Therefore it is likely that some spinal afferents contribute to the modulation of motor activity, acting centrally or via connections to the prevertebral ganglia as elsewhere in the gut.[88, 93] Noxious stimuli are thought to be carried almost exclusively in the spinal afferents and primarily through the response of high threshold, rapidly adapting nociceptors, with a contribution from the wide-range mechanonociceptors.[20] However, it is clear that vagal afferents can also modulate spinal afferent information and therefore have an impact on sensation.[19, 94–96] Therefore, in considering the relationship between motor activity and sensation, it is necessary to factor in the potential dual role of both the vagal and spinal afferent pathways. In addition, within the vagal afferent receptors in the esophagus there is evidence for regional organization that may coincide with the presence of separate neuromuscular units and the central subunits of neural control within the NTS noted previously.[61, 97]

Central Processing

The vagal afferents with their cell bodies in the nodose ganglion terminate in the NTS. However, their influence passes to higher brain regions including the thalamus and limbic and insular cortical structures, predominantly via the parabrachial nucleus. In this way, these afferents serve in autonomic, neuroendocrine, and behavioral functions in addition to their sensory-motor functions.[88, 98] The modulation of nociception involves the locus ceruleus and the nucleus raphe magnus.[87, 94]

The spinal afferents with their cell bodies in the dorsal root ganglia pass centrally by a number of routes, predominantly in the spinothalamic tracts and dorsal columns. At the spinal level there is a wide distribution of the afferents from each esophageal region,[99] which also overlaps with the innervation from other organs such as the heart.[100] With convergence of sensory input from different organs on spinal neurons, the referral pattern of symptoms such as pain may be similar for different organs,[101] the esophagus for example producing the same spectrum of referral as the heart.

More centrally, the medial spinothalamic neurons, through many connections of the cingulate cortex to the prefrontal, frontal, and other regions, are primarily concerned with cognitive, affective, and motivational aspects of pain, while the lateral spinothalamic neurons mediate stimulus localization through connections to the sensory cortex. The latter also may involve the cingulate cortex. The insular cortex is involved in affective processing, learning, and memory as well as autonomic function such as swallowing[102] and receives inputs from the spinothalamic tracts. The role of the dorsal column tracts in esophageal sensation is still unknown.

Clinical Implications

A number of techniques are now being used to assess sensory-motor pathways, central processing, and the relationship of these aspects to esophageal symptoms and motor function in health and disease.[88] These techniques include positron emission tomography, functional magnetic resonance imaging, sensory cortical-evoked potential recording, transcutaneous magnetic stimulation, magnetoencephalography, and the study of neurocardiac reflexes induced by esophageal stimulation. Derived information points to the value of these techniques regarding brain loci that process esophageal sensation induced by electrical or mechanical stimulation of the esophagus[102, 103]; brain loci activated by swallowing; cortical representation of motor cortex for swallowing musculature, its alteration in stroke and recovery from stroke, and its modulation by sensory stimulation[11, 12, 16]; modulation of neurocardiac function by esophageal stimulation and the use of this phenomenon to assess patients with noncardiac chest pain[104, 108]; and the effects of drugs on cortical-evoked potentials and sensory thresholds.[106] Further use of these techniques in combination with motility and pH recording methods should help with assessment and management of conditions wherein sensation and motor function are altered by disease, as with the functional gastrointestinal disorders wherein visceral hypersensitivity is prominent.[87]

COORDINATED ESOPHAGEAL MOTOR ACTIVITY

The classic coordinated motor pattern of the esophagus, initiated by the act of swallowing, is called *primary peristalsis* (Fig. 32–3). A rapidly progressing pharyngeal contraction transfers the bolus through the relaxed UES into the esophagus. As the UES closes, a progressive circular contraction begins in the upper esophagus and proceeds distally along the esophageal body to propel the bolus through the relaxed LES. The LES subsequently closes with a prolonged contraction.

Secondary peristalsis is a progressive contraction in the esophageal body that is induced not by a swallow but rather by stimulation of sensory receptors in the esophageal body. Usually attributed to distention by a bolus, such as food not completely cleared by a primary swallow or refluxed gastric contents, secondary peristalsis occurs only in the esophagus. It usually begins at or above a level corresponding to the location of the stimulus, and it closely resembles the peristalsis induced by a swallow.

In the absence of connections to the swallowing center, a local intramural mechanism can at times take over as a

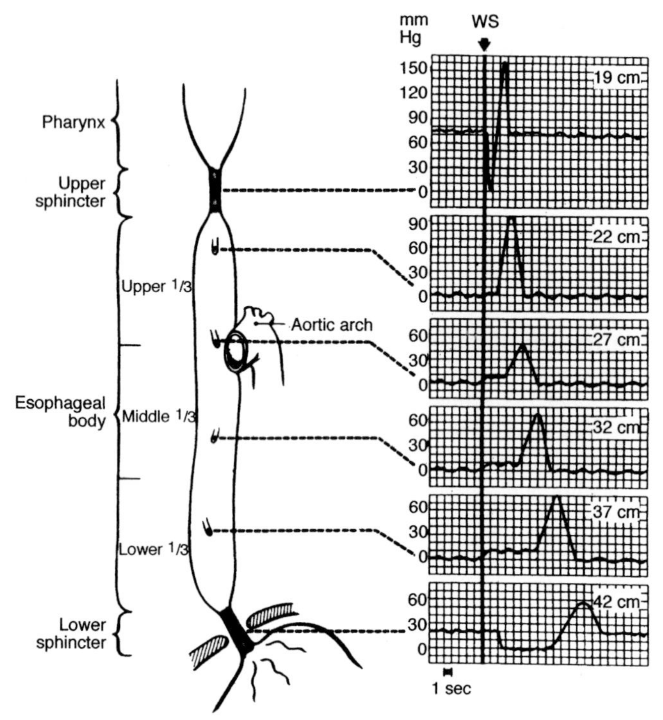

Figure 32–3. Manometric pressure changes with a swallow of an 8-mL bolus (WS). Distance (centimeters) from nares is shown on tracings. Proximal and distal tracings are from the upper (UES) and lower (LES) esophageal sphincters, respectively. Immediately after a swallow, UES pressure falls transiently. Shortly thereafter, LES pressure falls and remains low until the peristaltic contraction passing aborally through the UES and the esophageal body closes the LES. (From Dodds WJ: In Margulis AR, Burhenne HJ [eds]. Alimentary Tract Radiology, 3rd ed, Vol. 1. St. Louis, CV, Mosby Co, 1983, pp 529–603.)

reserve mechanism to produce peristalsis in the smooth muscle segment of the esophagus. This has been called tertiary peristalsis,[107] and the term should not be confused with tertiary contractions, which are uncoordinated or simultaneous contractions in the esophageal body.[108]

Upper Esophageal Sphincter

At rest, the UES is tonically closed as a result of continuous neural excitation; in addition, there is a small passive component to the tone.[109] The neural discharge essentially ceases during sleep or general anesthesia and UES pressure falls to approximately 10 mm Hg.[110] Pressures are higher anteriorly and posteriorly,[111] and this asymmetry has made definition of normal pressures highly dependent on the method that is used.[112–115] Excitatory discharge to the UES and UES pressure increase with each inspiration, and slow distention and acid in the upper esophagus cause a reflex increase in UES pressure,[116, 117] as do a Valsalva maneuver, gagging, and secondary peristalsis.[1] Some of the excitatory reflex mechanisms may explain the globus sensation in certain patients (see Chapter 6). On the other hand, belching, vomiting, and abrupt esophageal distention are associated with a decrease in UES pressure to permit release of esophageal contents and decompression of the esophagus.[118]

Within 0.2 to 0.3 seconds after a swallow, central excitatory discharge to the UES ceases transiently in exquisite coordination with the rapid sequence of muscle activity in the oropharyngeal phase of swallowing. Cessation of neural excitation to the UES and elevation and forward movement of the larynx act together to decrease UES resting pressure for less than 1 second and to open the sphincter on swallowing.[119] A short burst of excitation and contraction follows. The upward and forward movement of the larynx also serves to close the entrance to the airway and produce a uniform funnel for direction of the bolus to the UES.

Esophageal Body

As the peristaltic contraction passes through the esophagus, the amplitude of the waves varies. Contraction waves of low pressure are seen in short segments, 4 to 6 cm below the UES and as peristalsis reaches the LES. The former is a region in which striated and smooth muscle portions are about equal in amount, and where vagal innervation changes from the recurrent laryngeal nerve proximally to the short direct branches from the vagus distally. Using multiple recording sites at short intervals along the esophagus and a method to produce a topographic plot of the contractions in time and space, an additional amplitude trough can be detected that roughly divides the smooth muscle region in half (Fig. 32–4).[120] This division may represent the transition of excitatory cholinergic dominance to prominent inhibitory NANC innervation. Further observations using these techniques suggest the presence of separate neuromuscular units, perhaps in some way related to the central subunits of neural control within the NTS or perhaps related to the intramural neural gradients described below.[26–28, 121] If the former is at least partially correct, central control may be grouped into three larger segments, UES with the upper striated muscle esophagus, proximal smooth muscle esophageal body, and distal smooth muscle body with LES.

The duration of normal contractions is usually less than 7 seconds, and normal contraction amplitudes seldom exceed 200 mm Hg.[122] It takes 6 to 8 seconds for peristalsis to proceed through the esophagus with an average velocity of 3 to 4 cm/sec. Propagation velocity varies through the striated and smooth muscle regions in a bimodal fashion (Fig. 32–5).[123]

Striated Muscle

The contraction of the striated muscles is directed and coordinated by sequential excitation through vagal fibers programmed by the central control mechanism.[42, 124, 125] Afferent information from the esophagus and elsewhere has a significant effect on the central program to alter the force and velocity of the peristaltic contraction in both the striated and the smooth muscle segments of the esophagus (see the section "Smooth Muscle, Central Control Mechanisms"). It is not known whether connections from the myenteric plexus to the motor end plates modulates this activity.[53–55]

Smooth Muscle

The control mechanisms that direct and modulate peristalsis in the smooth muscle esophagus have generated considerable

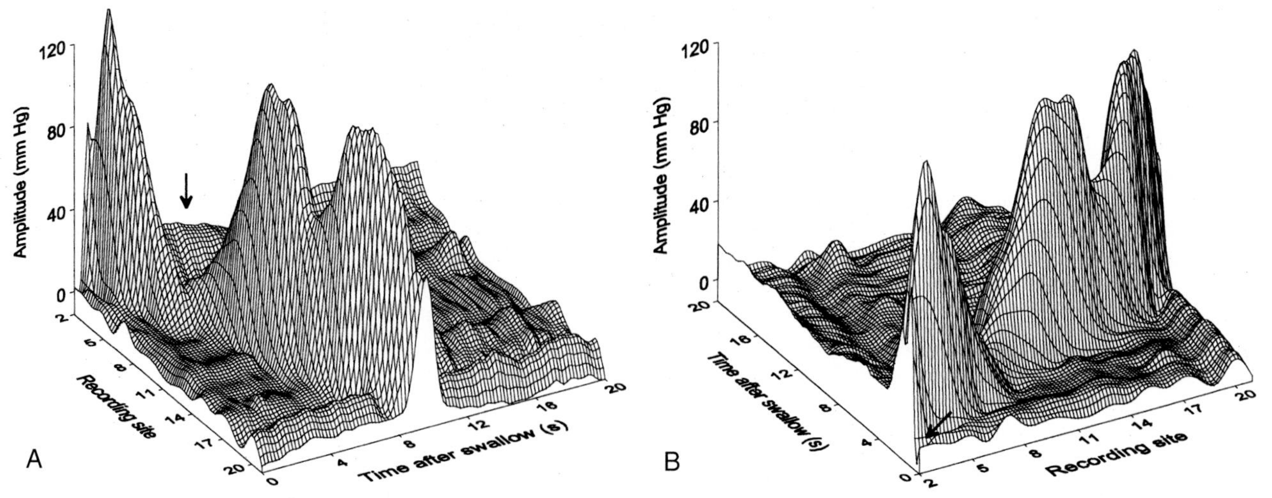

Figure 32–4. Topographic surface plots of esophageal peristalsis using high-resolution manometric methods. Two perspectives of the same swallow are shown, with the most proximal recording port placed in the region of the upper esophageal sphincter. *A,* A view from the distal esophagus showing the decay in peristaltic amplitude at the junction of smooth and skeletal muscle esophageal regions (*arrow*). *B,* The plot is rotated counterclockwise 90 degrees to view the same swallow from the vantage point of the upper sphincter, the drop in sphincter pressure occurring with swallowing (*arrow*). A second pressure trough dividing the smooth muscle region into two equal-sized segments is apparent in both panels. (From Clouse RE, Staiano A, Alrakawi A: Development of a topographic analysis system for manometric studies in the gastrointestinal tract. Gastrointest Endosc 48:395–401, 1998.)

controversy. There are three main potential levels of control for the production of peristalsis in the smooth muscle esophagus[2, 26, 34, 99, 126–132]: (1) Stimuli from the central program cause different efferent motor fibers to fire sequentially during both primary and secondary peristalsis in the smooth as well as the striated muscle esophagus[124, 125, 133]; (2) there is an intramural neural mechanism that can be excited to produce peristalsis near the onset of vagal stimulation or intraluminal balloon distension (an "on-response" or "A wave") or after the vagal or balloon stimulus is terminated (an "off-response" or "B wave")[63, 64, 66, 67]; and (3) some type of mechanism exists for myogenic propagation of a contraction.[134–136] Under normal circumstances, all three levels of control must successfully integrate their different mechanisms for regulation of peristalsis and its characteristics.

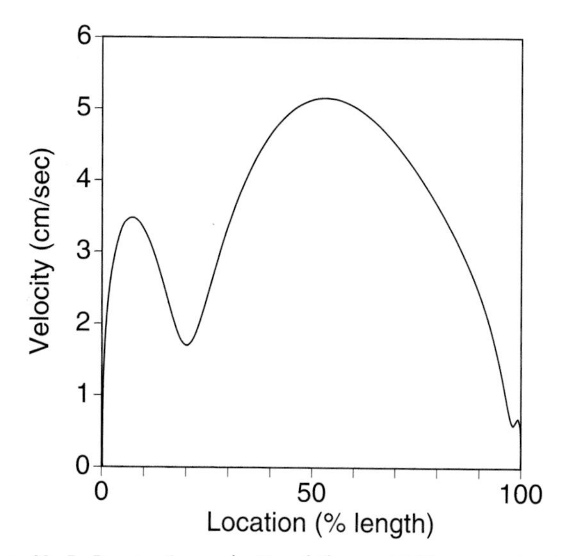

Figure 32–5. Propagation velocity of the peristaltic wave front as it traverses the esophageal body from just distal to the upper sphincter to 100% of esophageal length. The bimodal wave represents the rates of propagation through the proximal, striated muscle and distal, smooth muscle regions with deceleration near the LES. (From Clouse RE, Staiano A, Bickston SJ, Cohn SM: Characteristics of the propagating pressure wave in the esophagus. Dig Dis Sci 41:2369–2376, 1996.)

In the human, monkey, and especially the cat, swallow-induced peristalsis is highly atropine-sensitive,[137–139] while peristalsis can be augmented by cholinergic agonists or by inhibition of the enzyme acetylcholinesterase.[140, 141] Therefore, in these species, direct smooth muscle excitation by the intramural cholinergic neurons is the predominant mechanism for induction of the muscle contraction and regulation of its amplitude during normal peristalsis. Two related questions then arise: (1) What mechanism or mechanisms determine the direction and velocity of the peristaltic wave? and (2) How does the centrally programmed sequential vagal discharge interact with the local neural and muscle control mechanisms to produce normal primary and secondary peristalsis? These questions are still not fully answered. This derives from the fact that in some species, such as the opossum and cat, the intramural mechanism is capable of producing neurally mediated peristalsis on its own either in the absence of extrinsic vagal innervation or with experimental vagal stimulation that does not incorporate sequential excitation.[63, 64, 67] How muscle properties contribute to peristalsis directed by either central or intramural neural mechanisms is not clear.

Intramural Neural Control Mechanisms

Dodds and coworkers, using vagal stimulation with selected parameters, characterized two intramural neural mechanisms for control of peristalsis in the opossum and cat.[63, 64, 67] The on-contraction (A wave) has an apparent propagation velocity that resembles that of swallow-induced peristalsis, is atropine-sensitive, and is induced by low-frequency stimulation. The off-contraction (B wave) has a much more rapid propagation similar to that of the off-response delays of serial muscle strips in vitro, is atropine-resistant, and occurs at higher stimulation frequencies. The on-contraction mechanism is attributed to the activation of the excitatory cholinergic neurons, although the nature of the circuitry dictating the progressive distal delays is not known.[62] The off-contraction mechanism has been attributed to muscle depolarization with an associated contraction, events following initial muscle hyperpolarization from activation of the NANC inhibitory neurons. As previously noted, the inhibitory neurotransmitter is nitric oxide or a similar nitroso compound. The membrane depolarization is perceived as being caused by passive rebound of the membrane potential as well as some type of active excitation.[142, 146] This presupposes that the onset of NANC inhibition is almost simultaneous at all levels and that regional differences in the muscle and neural properties produce a delay to onset of contraction, the delay becoming progressively longer distally.

There is increasing evidence that the excitatory cholinergic influence is most prominent proximally and decreases distally, while the inhibitory influence is most active distally, these neural gradients in influence affecting both contraction amplitude and the direction and velocity of propagation (Fig. 32–6).[66–68, 70, 137, 138, 144–154] In terms of amplitude, contractions are more atropine-sensitive proximally. Any NANC inhibitory influence contributing to contraction amplitude appears to have a more prominent effect distally, as a reduction in amplitude is usually seen only in the very distal segment when the NANC system is blocked. This effect may be controlled centrally rather than by the enteric nervous system.[33]

Therefore, independent of sequential excitation, differences in the cholinergic and NANC inhibitory influence along the esophagus can have an effect on timing of the contraction. Cholinergic influence tends to decrease the delay to onset of a contraction when a stimulus is given, while the NANC inhibitory influence increases the delay. If the excitatory cholinergic influence is most prominent proximally, and the inhibitory influence is most prominent distally, the balance of neural influence would therefore be programmed to produce a progressive delay in the contractions along the esophagus and provide one mechanism for regulation of the direction and velocity of the peristaltic wave. As shown in Figure 32–6, blockade of either the cholinergic or nitrinergic innervation could result in an increase in peristaltic velocity, cholinergic blockade shifting the wave to a later time,[66, 137] while NANC blockade would result in an earlier wave.[153] In the opossum, different frequencies of vagal stimulation can alter and shift the neural influence from one to the other and change either the propagation velocity or even the direction of peristalsis.[66] In these contexts, alterations in the balance could potentially result in motor disorders of the esophagus. There are many peptides within the myenteric neurons.[55, 60, 71, 77] Although those investigated may have effects to modulate the esophageal contractions,[155–157] they do not seem to play a primary role.

Intramural Muscle Control Mechanisms

The myogenic control system in most of the mammalian gut is manifest by two fundamental characteristics: (a) electrical oscillations of the smooth muscle cells called the electrical control activity, slow wave type action potentials, or slow waves; and (b) the ability of the smooth muscle cells to communicate with each other (coupling) so the whole tissue can operate as a functional unit.[158, 159] Both of these phenomena have been demonstrated in the esophagus and both require adequate excitation such as with cholinergic stimulation to become manifest.[134, 136, 160, 161] Furthermore, the ICCs as transducers for nerve to muscle signaling, as pacemakers for the smooth muscles themselves, and as conduction paths for muscle to muscle communication are likely integral components of any myogenic control system. Therefore, the potential exists for esophageal peristalsis to occur based on myogenic properties as long as adequate excitation is present.

Central Control Mechanisms

As with the striated muscle esophagus,[2, 18] there is likely a set of programmed neurons in the swallowing center con-

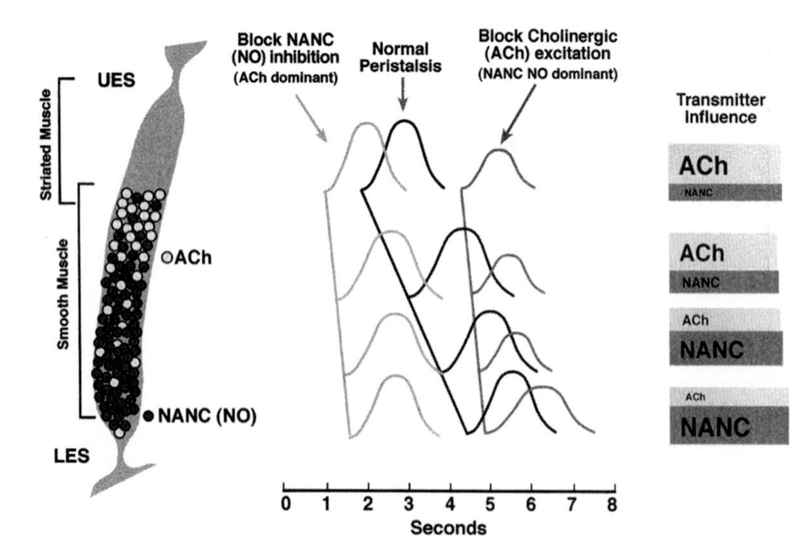

Figure 32–6. Cholinergic (ACh, O) and noncholinergic (NANC, ●) influences in the smooth muscle esophagus and the potential interplay of two intramural neural mechanisms in the production of peristalsis. Cholinergic influence is most prominent proximally and decreases distally; the reverse is true for the noncholinergic influence. Proximally, where the cholinergic influence is dominant, the contraction is more atropine sensitive and tends to occur earlier. More distally, where the noncholinergic influence is dominant, the contraction is delayed. Blockade of either the cholinergic or nitrergic innervation could result in an increase in peristaltic velocity (as depicted by a steeper slope in the lines), NANC blockade resulting in an earlier wave, and cholinergic blockade in a later wave. (From Crist J, Gidda JS, Goyal RK: Intramural mechanism of esophageal peristalsis: Roles of cholinergic and noncholinergic nerves. Proc Natl Acad Sci 81:3595, 1984; and Gilbert RJ, Dodds WJ: Effect of selective muscarinic antagonists on peristaltic contractions in opossum smooth muscle. Am J Physiol 250: G50, 1986.)

cerned with smooth muscle peristalsis, but this has not yet been demonstrated. However, in both the baboon and the opossum, different vagal fibers discharge with a timing corresponding to the peristaltic contractions in both striated and smooth muscle sections.[124, 125] The mechanism whereby this central discharge integrates with the peripheral neural and muscle control mechanisms in the smooth muscle esophagus is not yet clarified.

Nevertheless, afferent stimulation acting centrally has a major effect on peristalsis. An esophageal bolus increases the duration and frequency of the efferent vagal discharges to the esophagus in animals,[124] and in humans, the amplitude and duration of the contraction increases and the peristalsis velocity decreases.[162] A similar effect of sensory feedback also occurs from stimuli not originating in the esophagus, such as increased intra-abdominal pressure.[163] This latter sensory effect presumably acts through the central level of control. Additionally, stroke can be associated with peristaltic and LES dysfunction.[164–166]

Integration of Central and Peripheral Mechanisms

It is clear that both central and peripheral levels of control are highly integrated. Studies to date have not established how this integration occurs, nor which level of control of peristalsis is normally dominant. With a swallow the process is obviously started and proceeds through the oropharyngeal stage and the upper striated muscle esophagus under central control. For initiation of a contraction and regulation of its amplitude in the smooth muscle portion, the major focus of neural integration is probably the excitatory cholinergic neuron. Whether this neuron reaches threshold and discharges sufficiently to induce a contraction would be determined by excitatory and inhibitory input, both central and peripheral. In species and circumstances where the NANC inhibitory neuron also is present and active, adequate excitation of the muscle for induction of a contraction will depend on the amount and timing of the release of acetylcholine and the inhibitory neurotransmitter.[67] As previously noted, the direction and velocity of the peristaltic contraction appear to depend at least on the balance between excitatory and inhibitory neural influences along the esophagus. Presumably, sequential activation of excitatory or inhibitory neurons is also involved through central and perhaps peripheral neural inputs.

If the final propagation of the peristaltic wave also involves a myogenic contribution, the neural mechanisms, either extrinsic or intramural, would need to provide controlled activation of the muscle in such a way as to permit passage of a single contraction aborally along the esophagus. Fortunately, the myogenic system is intrinsically set to operate in a period similar to normal swallow-induced activity,[136] a characteristic feature of linked control systems serving a common function. Therefore, the relationship of the neural and myogenic mechanisms could include the following: (a) the myogenic system plays no significant role, with peristaltic contraction controlled entirely by the timing and balance of the excitatory and inhibitory innervation; (b) the myogenic control system serves as the primary mediator of the peristaltic contraction, with nerves regulating the coupling, the excitability, and the oscillatory characteristics, thus modulating the direction, velocity, and amplitude of the contraction while ensuring the occurrence of a single contraction; and (c) regional differences in muscle properties along the length of the esophagus permit different muscle responses (e.g., timing, duration of muscle contraction) to the innervation. A corollary of the multiple levels of control is that it is possible to conceive of a local intramural mechanism for peristalsis operating independently if central mechanisms are defective or absent.

Deglutitive Inhibition

Deglutitive inhibition in the esophagus is primarily a function of the swallowing center. A second swallow, initiated when the previous swallow is in the striated muscle segment of the esophagus, causes inhibition of contractile activity induced by the first swallow and with LES relaxation. This results from cessation of excitatory discharges from the central program, and specific vagal activation of the NANC inhibitory neurons may also be operative in production of the quiescence in the smooth muscle portion of the esophagus.[167–169] With a series of swallows at short intervals, the esophagus remains inhibited and quiescent, and the LES is relaxed. After the last swallow in the series, a normal peristaltic wave occurs.

A recent swallow or the presence of a swallow wave within the esophagus can alter the nature of a subsequent swallow wave dramatically, decreasing its amplitude, either increasing or decreasing its velocity, and at times rendering it nonperistaltic.[167, 170] These effects can mimic a motor disorder and last for 20 to 30 seconds. Therefore, routine clinical studies of esophageal motility should include at least this interval between swallows.

Lower Esophageal Sphincter

The LES in the human is composed of at least two muscle clasp fibers that partially encircle the distal esophagus medially, and the gastric sling fibers laterally on the left.[171] The clasp fibers have significant myogenic tone but are less responsive to cholinergic stimulation, while the sling fibers have little resting tone but contract vigorously to cholinergic stimulation.[172] Radial asymmetry in recorded LES pressures is less marked than that in the UES. The higher pressures are in the left lateral portion of the sphincter and appear to relate to the presence of the cholinergic gastric sling fibers in this portion of the sphincter.[173] The diaphragm also impinges on the left lateral side and may contribute to the proximal part.[174] Therefore, it is likely that the sling, in addition to the clasp, is an integral and important physical and physiologic contributor to the LES. For this reason, Schneider and associates have suggested importance to regional LES differences in patients with achalasia,[175] and similar attention has been paid to the two muscle regions and their potential role in the pathogenesis of gastroesophageal reflux disease.[176]

The LES is tonically closed at rest, maintaining an average pressure of about 20 mm Hg. The resting tone is determined by a combination of myogenic properties and active tonic neural excitation, modulated by a complex interaction of numerous other neural and hormonal factors. The majority of studies of the LES muscle properties have not differentiated between sling and clasp fibers and appear to involve predominantly the clasp fibers or its equivalent circular muscle in other species.[177] The myogenic component of tone is calcium dependent, and calcium blocking agents reduce LES pressure, a potentially useful therapeutic effect in patients with achalasia.[178] Other studies of the properties of the muscle have revealed insight into the nature of the ionic channels, the metabolic and biochemical nature of the contractile machinery, and the cellular messenger systems involved with contraction and relaxation, but as yet they have not led to significant therapeutic advances.[177, 179–186]

In the human, as well as in the cat, dog, and monkey but not the opossum, the resting tone in vivo is variably atropine sensitive or significantly reduced by vagal interruption.[137, 187] Therefore, part of the tone is due to the release of acetylcholine from excitatory neurons. Some of this release probably is a result of tonically firing vagal fibers, as in the dog,[188] and perhaps there is some adrenergic release of acetylcholine, as in the cat.[46, 58] Although nitric oxide is the neurotransmitter primarily responsible for active inhibition of the LES,[189–191] there is little effect of nitric oxide synthase blockade on LES resting tone in the human and cat,[153–154] whereas LES tone increases after such blockade in the dog.[184] Therefore, depending on the species, resting myogenic tone is regulated by a balance between excitatory and inhibitory neural influences. Both are strongly centrally mediated.

A number of reflex mechanisms, physiologic alterations, and ingested substances can markedly alter resting LES tone. Every 1.5 to 2 hours, LES pressure fluctuates with the migrating motor complex; pressures are highest in association with the intense phase III motor activity in the stomach.[192] LES pressure also increases after a meal, as the result of both neural and hormonal influences, and with increased intra-abdominal pressure caused by an excitatory cholinergic reflex whose afferent pathway is probably in the vagus nerves.[193] On the other hand, transient LES relaxation (TLESR) occurs independently of swallowing, and this relaxation frequently is associated with gastroesophageal reflux in normal subjects and in patients with esophagitis.[9, 194] TLESR is neurally mediated by a vagal reflex pathway and at least is a response to intraesophageal and intragastric stimuli.[195, 196]

A large number of factors may influence LES pressure.[1] Many of these have obvious clinical and therapeutic implications. For example, factors that decrease sphincter pressure would tend to produce or aggravate gastroesophageal reflux, on one hand, or they could be used to treat conditions such as achalasia, on the other hand. Factors that increase sphincter pressure would have the opposite clinical and therapeutic implications.

On swallowing, LES pressure falls within 1.5 to 2.5 seconds and remains low for 6 to 8 seconds as the peristaltic contraction traverses the esophageal body. The LES relaxes with virtually 100% of swallows, even though the swallow may not induce esophageal body motor activity. In humans, as in other species, the swallow-induced LES inhibition probably includes both active inhibition of the muscle by activation of the NANC inhibitory neurons and cessation of tonic neural excitation to the sphincter.[169, 188] In the dog and cat, and probably in most other species, there is provision for central participation in control of this LES relaxation. Intramural pathways within at least the smooth muscle segments of the esophageal body also can inhibit the LES.[57, 58] There is reason to believe that efferent vagal fibers serving both LES excitation and relaxation enter the esophagus at some point well above the LES. Truncal vagotomy[197] and selective vagotomy,[198] which may separate the vagus nerves from up to 9 cm of the lower esophagus, have virtually no affect on LES tone, relaxation, or responsiveness to cholinergic stimulation.

PATHOGENESIS AND CATEGORIZATION OF MOTOR DISORDERS

Upper Esophageal Sphincter and Cervical Esophageal Region

Motor disorders in this region arise primarily from failed sequential excitation through extrinsic innervation or from striated muscle disease. The complete dependence on extrinsic neural input leads to an important mechanistic differentiation of motor disorders in this region from the more distal disorders.

Distal Esophageal Body and Lower Esophageal Sphincter Region

Despite the host of possibilities for motor dysfunction based on the types and levels of control, motor disorders in this region typically fall into two broad categories (Fig. 32–7).[199, 200] The groups necessarily are heterogeneous in their representation of underlying mechanistic abnormalities, but clinical outcomes and management approaches favor a reductionistic scheme. The first is characterized by *hypomotility*, in which decreased amplitude of contractions or the absence of a contraction in all or part of this region is noted with a swallow. In the second group, *hypermotility* is predominant. Swallow-induced waves may be of high amplitude, prolonged, or repetitive; spontaneous contractions may be frequent; and intraesophageal pressure may be increased. A similar clinical categorization applies to the LES. Hypomotility is characterized by low resting pressure, feeble contraction following relaxation, and perhaps increased inhibition as with the TLESR. Hypermotility may manifest as a hypertensive sphincter or poor relaxation with a swallow. The pattern of coordination can be altered in either group, although increased propagation velocity and non-progressive contractions most often accompany the hypermotility disorders.

It is possible to imagine that when hypomotility exists, at least three mechanisms can be responsible. Either the muscle is abnormal and unable to expand to excitation (e.g., as in advanced scleroderma[201]), excitation to the muscle is diminished (e.g., as in early scleroderma or esophagitis[201–203]), or the muscle is suppressed by excessive or unopposed inhibition, such as through activity of the NANC inhibitory neuron (e.g., as with TLESRs in gastroesophageal reflux disease, and with esophagitis).[194, 202] If the final common pathway for excitation of the smooth muscle primarily is via

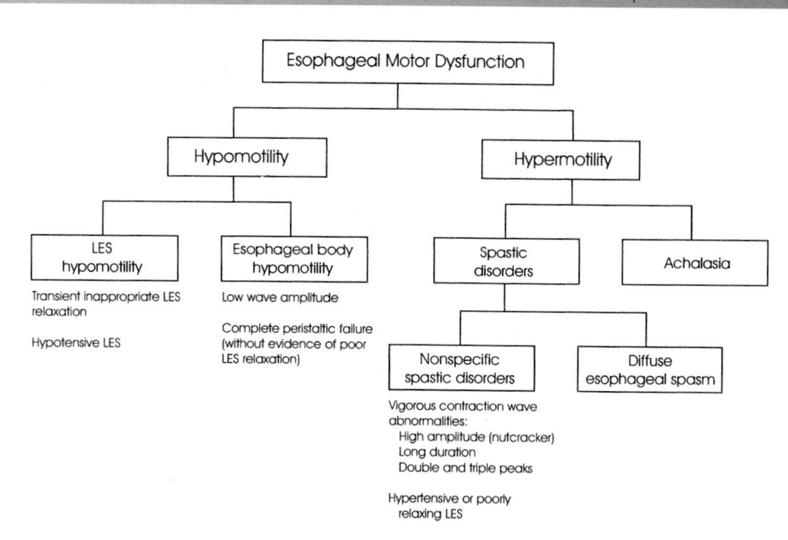

Figure 32–7. A method for categorizing motor disorders of the distal esophagus and lower esophageal sphincter (LES) based on principal type of motor dysfunction. Some patients have a mixture of hypomotility and hypermotility features and cannot be classified solely into one branch. Hypermotility typically is associated with hypersensitivity to endogenous, intraluminal, and chemical stimuli, whereas hypomotility is associated with hyposensitivity. (From Clouse RE: Spastic disorders of the esophagus. Gastroenterologist 5:112–127, 1997.)

the excitatory cholinergic neuron, diminished activity of this neuron could occur if the neuron was abnormal, if it failed to receive adequate excitatory input from central or intramural pathways, or if it was actively inhibited. In the LES, hypotension has been attributed to a number of potential disturbances, including abnormality of the muscle, lack of normal cholinergic excitation, decreased reflex excitation, decreased stimulation through low levels or poor responsiveness to circulating substances such as gastrin, and active inhibition.[204, 205]

The hypermotility disorders can be viewed from the same perspective. The muscle may be abnormal (e.g., thickened in some patients with idiopathic diffuse esophageal spasm[206]) or hyperresponsive to excitatory neurotransmitters or circulating hormones. Alternatively, neural excitation to the muscle may be increased. Potential mechanisms producing this effect include excessive cholinergic drive from a hyperactive central program, overactive afferent reflex pathways working centrally or peripherally, or reduced inhibition of the cholinergic neuron. Perhaps the spastic disorders represent a mixture of these explanations, all resulting in an imbalance between inhibition and contraction.[207] In contrast, the hypermotility seen in achalasia and closely related variants may be exclusively related to loss of inhibitory regulation. Abnormalities of the inhibitory mechanism could readily explain most of the observed hypermotility in the esophageal body and LES, including failure of LES relaxation on swallowing, an appealing and unifying explanation for hypermotility disorders in general.[62, 207] Likewise, if the NANC neurons are important in determining progressive delays in the peripheral control mechanisms for peristalsis,[68, 70] their dysfunction or absence could be responsible for intermittently rapid and non-progressive responses in the spastic disorders and render the esophagus aperistaltic in achalasia. As presently perceived, the mechanisms behind hypermotility and hypomotility are not mutually exclusive. Indeed, some patients may exhibit a combination of findings.

Sensory abnormalities accompanying motor disorders have been underappreciated, yet this aspect of neuromuscular dysfunction may contribute importantly to the symptom presentation. In general, sensory abnormalities parallel motor abnormalities. Processes causing hypermotility typically produce hypersensitivity to chemically excitatory or intraluminal stimuli, and processes causing hypomotility produce hyposensitivity. Examples of the former include exaggerated reaction (both motility and pain) to cholinergic stimulation in achalasia, and pain with low-volume balloon distention, intraluminal acid perfusion, and cholinergic and alpha-adrenergic provocation in the spastic disorders.[200] Hypomotility accompanies aging, diabetes mellitus, connective tissue disease, and Barrett's esophagus, processes associated with reduced sensitivity to electrical stimulation or intraluminal acid perfusion.[208–210] As for the broad categories of motor dysfunction, the location of sensory dysfunction may vary—increased perception of esophageal signals representing either peripheral hypersensitivity or abnormal central processing, for example.[211]

DIAGNOSING MOTOR DISORDERS

Clinical History

Distinguishing proximal, oropharyngeal symptoms from a distal, esophageal syndrome is the first important step when taking a clinical history. Characteristics more typical of oropharyngeal dysphagia are described in the section on "Disorders of the UES and Cervical Esophageal Region, Clinical Manifestations." Dysphagia is the dominant symptom in the proximal syndromes. Symptoms of both disordered transit (e.g., dysphagia, regurgitation) and pain typify distal motor disorders, although their relative presence is highly variable. Pain and other chest discomforts (such as a burning sensation) are not specific for esophageal disease. Similar symptoms occur with a host of disorders ranging from cardiac angina to diseases involving the chest wall, pulmonary processes, and even intra-abdominal pathologic conditions. Transit symptoms are more typical of esophageal disease but are not specific for the motor disorders; they also result from other intrinsic or extrinsic lesions (e.g., inflammatory or neoplastic diseases).

When interviewing the patient with a suspected motor disorder, several aspects of the history can be useful in improving its diagnostic value. First, transit symptoms should be sought in the patient who complains primarily of chest discomfort. For example, episodic chest pain may be the primary and most bothersome symptom, but a detailed history may reveal concurrent dysphagia. Waxing and waning of symptoms over a relatively long period is characteristic of the distal motor disorders and may accompany even the more severe forms. An intermittent character to the symptoms and presence of dysphagia for liquids as well as for solid foods are the two features that most strongly suggest a motor disturbance.[212]

A more detailed inquiry into individual symptoms also can have discriminatory value. Provocation of dysphagia by ingestion of cold liquids or foods and improvement of symptoms with warm or hot liquids or foods is an observation that has some specificity for motor disturbances.[213] Patients with achalasia and related disorders with poor esophageal emptying may report alleviation of dysphagia with physical maneuvers that increase intraesophageal pressure, such as straightening of the back or raising the arms above the head. Other symptoms of motor dysfunction include tracheobronchial aspiration, chronic cough or recurring aspiration pneumonia, and, on occasion, weight loss. Additional historical features of value in specific motor disorders are described subsequently in this chapter. Systemic symptoms are rarely present with uncomplicated motor disorders unless the neuromuscular derangement is a component of multisystem disease. Unfortunately, cardiac angina and pain of esophageal disease are sufficiently similar that differentiation on a historical basis alone often is not possible.

Diagnostic Tests

Radiologic and Radionuclide Imaging

A radiologic evaluation is commonly included in the investigation of esophageal symptoms. The evaluation is less informative if the history has not distinguished oropharyngeal symptoms from esophageal symptoms or if the radiologist has not been informed of intermittent symptoms or of symptoms precipitated by specific types of foods. A combination of radiologic techniques may be needed, including full-column or double-contrast esophagograms, motion recording during fluoroscopy of swallows, and specialized supplemental examinations.[214] The latter may include iced or acidified barium suspensions or radiopaque solids.

Complete radiologic evaluation of the oropharyngeal phase of swallowing mandates motion-recording techniques (e.g., videofluoroscopy) because of the rapid sequence of motor events in this region.[215] Morphologic abnormalities are determined from spot radiographs taken in posteroanterior and lateral views.[216] The evaluation can be purely diagnostic or can be used to establish an individualized swallowing technique that prevents tracheobronchial aspiration in patients with oropharyngeal swallowing disorders. The latter "modified" barium swallow study is conventionally performed by a radiologist and a speech pathologist working together. The examination is in part tailored to the individual and commonly involves various head and body positions, different consistencies of barium, and barium mixed with foods.[216] Although several techniques have been reported for assessing oropharyngeal swallowing, the modified barium swallow with videofluoroscopy demonstrates more aspects of this phase of swallowing than does any other technique and has helped in the development of compensatory strategies for eliminating symptoms.[217] Interpretation of the videofluoroscopic abnormalities in the oropharyngeal region remains less uniform than interpretation of esophageal abnormalities and is dependent on the experience of the radiologist.

Radiologic evaluation of the esophageal body detects and diagnoses the majority of severe distal motor disturbances.[214] Double-contrast or mucosal detail techniques improve the sensitivity of the screening esophagogram for other esophageal diseases responsible for the symptoms, but fluoroscopic observation without motion-recording devices may be sufficient for evaluating motor disorders in this region. Several limitations interfere with diagnostic accuracy. First, the test is evaluated subjectively, because transit cannot be quantitated readily. Second, only a small number of swallows can be evaluated because of radiation exposure. This imposes a significant limitation, in view of the interswallow variability in normal persons and because major derangements may be intermittent. Third, techniques for taking swallows during radiologic examinations have been less standardized than for other, more quantitative diagnostic tests, which is an important limitation in view of the impact that such variables as bolus size, bolus temperature, and time delay between swallows have on normal peristalsis.[170, 218–220] Finally, radiologic studies cannot provide information on contraction alterations that have little or no impact on bolus transit. These limitations interfere in a lesser way with the diagnosis of more severe motor derangements.

Radionuclide studies examine bolus transit throughout the esophageal body and add a quantitative capability not possible with conventional radiographic studies.[221] A supine patient is given an oral liquid bolus labeled with technetium-99m. Radioactivity within the esophageal body and stomach is measured with a gamma camera positioned over the patient. Transit studies are easy to perform, are well tolerated by patients, and produce minimal radiation exposure. Recognition of severe motor derangements through this technique exceeds that by conventional radiographic studies,[222, 223] but technical factors can produce false-positive results of radionuclide transit studies in some situations.[224] The primary utility of radionuclide studies remains as a research tool for quantification of transit, but this noninvasive alternative to manometry may be useful for clarifying the type of motor dysfunction in some clinical settings.

Transnasal or Transoral Videoendoscopy

Endoscopy typically has been used to detect structural lesions responsible for symptoms that might mimic a motor disorder. However, a growing body of literature supports the use of videoendoscopic methods for evaluating the functional swallow. Small caliber endoscopes passed transnally or transorally can detect tracheobronchial aspiration in neurogenic dysphagia and have the added benefit of demonstrating aspiration of saliva, a clinically relevant event.[225] The addition of sensory testing at the time of endoscopy determines laryngopharyngeal sensory discrimination thresholds to assist in estimating the risk for tracheobronchial aspiration.[226, 227] This is accomplished with an endoscopically delivered pulse of air to stimulate the mucosa innervated by the superior laryngeal nerve. Outcomes, as measured by the incidence of aspiration pneumonia and pneumonia-free interval, were similar when endoscopic evaluation with sensory testing or modified barium swallow with videofluoroscopy was used to guide dietary and behavioral management.[227] Thus, the two tests may be equivalent in assessing risk of aspiration. The portable, bedside characteristics of the former make it appealing as a diagnostic test.

Manometry

Intraluminal manometry is important for diagnosing esophageal motor disorders, disorders categorized and defined by muscle contraction characteristics. These characteristics can be indirectly identified by positioning a recording probe that is sensitive to pressures generated primarily by the circular muscle layer. Intraluminal manometers measure both the hydrodynamic pressure within the fluid bolus and the contact or squeeze pressure of the wall on the manometric probe.[228] Normal or abnormal sphincter function can be identified. Several types of recording devices have satisfactory fidelity for measuring esophageal contraction. One technique involves a catheter containing multiple, small-caliber lumens. Each lumen is perfused with water from a low-compliance perfusion device. Nonperfused systems with transducers embedded directly into the probe have excellent recording fidelity and are tolerated well by patients, but the number of recording sites is limited. Detailed descriptions of manometric technique can be found in monographs on this topic.[229] Normal manometric values for distal esophageal parameters are listed in Table 32–1. The reference ranges reflect physiologic variables as well as variations in manometric technique.[230–232]

Manometry has advantages in its quantitative approach and is the standard for diagnosis of motor disorders of the esophageal body and LES. Disorders of the UES are defined more satisfactorily with radiography. Systematic characterization of four aspects of the swallow is sufficient to diagnose the majority of disorders encountered in clinical practice: 1) peristaltic performance (percentage of swallows with progressive contraction sequences), 2) contraction wave configuration (e.g., amplitude, duration), 3) LES basal pressure, and 4) LES relaxation with swallowing.[233] From these characteristics, the pattern of motor dysfunction can be established (see Fig. 32–7). The limitations of manometry are primarily technical. Because sedating medications are not used, the study may be poorly tolerated by some patients. In addition, the manometry probe cannot take into account alterations in longitudinal muscle contraction after the swallow. Resultant axial displacement is not detected by the rigid probes and may produce artifactual results.[234, 235] Also, the hydrodynamic pressures created within the fluid bolus and direct squeeze pressures created by the esophageal wall cannot be differentiated confidently by examining the resultant waves alone,[228, 236] and nonocclusive contractions may remain undetected. Finally, manometry measures only the final step in the sequence of events leading to muscle contraction. Two distinct disorders, such as one affecting intramural nerves and one affecting muscle cells, could result in hypomotility and yet produce identical manometric diagnoses. Despite these limitations, manometry provides sufficient information to be used as a principal diagnostic tool.

Limitations are reduced by increasing the number and density of pressure recording sites.[121, 237] Because of the

Table 32–1 | **Normal Esophageal Manometric Values**

PARAMETER	CLOUSE AND STAIANO (1983)*	RICHTER ET AL. (1987)†	BASSOTTI ET AL. (1988)‡	ALIPERTI AND CLOUSE (1991)§
N	40	95	34	20
Mean age (years)	40	43	44	27
Peristaltic sequences (% of swallows)	100%	>95%	—	—
Contraction wave parameters				
Amplitude (mm Hg)	>34, <135‖	<180¶	<167¶	—
Duration (seconds)	<5.6	<5.8	—	—
Double-peaked waves** (% of swallows)	<10%	<50%††	—	—
Triple-peaked waves (% of swallows)	0	0	—	—
LES basal pressure (mm Hg)	10–37 (RPT)	5–53 (RPT) ≤ 37 (SPT)	—	—
LES relaxation (residual pressure; mm Hg)	—	—		Two of the following: Mean for all leads <2.6; Mean for one lead <4; All observations <8

RPT, rapid pull-through technique; SPT, station pull-through technique, end-expiration.
*Mapping technique; values derived from 95% confidence intervals; see reference 230.
†Stationary technique; values derived from mean ± 2 SD; see reference 122.
‡Stationary technique; values derived from mean ± 2 SD; see reference 231.
§See reference 232.
‖Contraction wave parameters taken from a zone 2–7 cm above the lower esophageal sphincter (LES).
¶Average values from two sites, 3 and 8 cm above the LES.
**Differences may be related to stationary versus mapping techniques.
††Cannot be accurately calculated from the data reported.
Values are highly dependent on manometric technique. See Kahrilas, P. J., Clouse, R. E., and Hogan, W. J. American Gastroenterological Association technical review on the clinical use of esophageal manometry. Gastroenterology *107*:1865, 1994.
Adapted from Clouse RE: Motor disorders of the esophagus. In Snape WJ Jr (ed): Consultations in Gastroenterology. Philadelphia: WB Saunders, 1996.

amount of data generated, three-dimensional, topographic plots have been used to display the swallows. Interpolation across recording sites allows visualization of the propagating wave as it traverses the esophageal body and sphincters. The high resolution afforded by this approach appears to increase the accuracy of manometric diagnosis compared with conventional techniques using considerably fewer recording sites and overcomes problems generated by axial esophageal movement.[238] Widespread use of topographic methods remains limited by the technical demands inherent in the catheter and perfusion requirements, but the approach is likely to unify manometric technique and interpretation.

DISORDERS OF THE UES AND CERVICAL ESOPHAGEAL REGION

Clinical Manifestations

Diseases affecting this region produce a distinct type of dysphagia: Patients truly have difficulty swallowing. The food bolus cannot be propelled successfully from the pharynx and hypopharynx, through the UES, and into the esophageal body. The resultant symptom complex is termed *oropharyngeal dysphagia.* The bolus fails to enter the esophagus, even with repeated efforts; tracheobronchial aspiration or nasopharyngeal regurgitation are potential outcomes. Although a sense that food is lodging in the more proximal esophagus is reported frequently by patients with the distal motor disorders, only occasionally is the symptom complex so localized or complete as to be confused with the causes of oropharyngeal dysphagia (Table 32–2). The motor disorders are often representative of central nervous system disease or of striated muscle diseases with diffuse muscle involvement, and clinical manifestations that accompany such diseases should be sought.

The described features of oropharyngeal dysphagia differ from the globus sensation. This sensation of cervical fullness, a "lump in the throat," or a lodged foreign body is not accompanied by true dysphagia. Bolus transfer into the esophagus is normal without aspiration or nasopharyngeal regurgitation, and indeed the sensation often improves or abates during swallowing. The globus sensation can accompany gastroesophageal reflux disease and some distal motor disorders, such as achalasia, but most commonly is an idiopathic symptom.[239] In the latter case, the symptom is no longer considered psychogenic; rather, it is believed to represent esophageal sensory or motor dysfunction as occurs in other functional esophageal disorders. Because of this, the simple term globus is preferred over the original term, *globus hystericus*, for the functional disorder. Some evidence that alterations in the cricopharyngeus muscle participate in producing this sensation has been obtained from observations in gastroesophageal reflux. An experimental correlate is the increase in UES pressure produced by perfusing the distal esophagus with acid or distending it with a balloon.[240] Despite this indirect mechanistic evidence, studies in patients with globus have not convincingly demonstrated any evidence of motor dysfunction in the UES region.[241] The symptom can be induced more easily with a balloon distention stimulus in patients than in asymptomatic subjects, supporting the presence of a visceral sensory abnormality.[242] Studies continue to show that psychological abnormalities are more common in patients with globus than in suitable control subjects,[243] but the relationship of these findings to symptoms remains unclear (see Chapter 6).

Table 32–2 | **Causes of Oropharyngeal Dysphagia***

STRUCTURAL PHARYNGOESOPHAGEAL LESIONS
Intrinsic Lesions
Oropharyngeal carcinoma
Esophageal carcinoma
Benign esophageal tumor
Esophageal web
Zenker's diverticulum
High esophageal stricture
Inflammatory disease (e.g., pharyngitis, tonsillar abscess)
Postsurgical change
Foreign body
Extrinsic Lesions
Thyroid enlargement or tumor
Vertebral spur
Cervical lymphadenopathy
Vascular anomalies
NEUROMUSCULAR DISEASES
Central Nervous System Diseases
Cerebrovascular accident
Parkinson's disease
Brainstem tumor
Amyotrophic lateral sclerosis
Other motor neuron diseases
Huntington's chorea
Tabes dorsalis
Poliomyelitis
Spinocerebellar degeneration
Syringobulbia
Progressive bulbar paralysis
Other congenital or degenerative disorders
Cranial Nerve Diseases
Diabetes mellitus
Recurrent laryngeal nerve palsy (e.g., mediastinal tumor, postsurgical)
Transection or injury
Diphtheria
Rabies
Lead poisoning
Other neurotoxins
Skeletal Muscle Disease
Inflammatory myopathies
Polymyositis
Dermatomyositis
Scleroderma
Mixed connective tissue disease
Inclusion body myositis
Muscular dystrophies
Oculopharyngeal muscular dystrophy
Myotonia dystrophica
Hyperthyroidism
Myxedema
Stiff-man syndrome
Other muscle disorders
Cricopharyngeal Dysfunction
Other Neuromuscular Disorders
Myasthenia gravis
Amyloidosis
Botulism

*The most common conditions in each category are listed first.

Neurologic Diseases

Cerebrovascular Accidents

Oropharyngeal dysphagia can result from cerebrovascular accidents that damage the swallowing center or motor nuclei controlling striated muscles of the hypopharynx and upper esophageal region.[244] Lesions involving the vertebrobasilar arteries or the posterior inferior cerebellar artery may result in oropharyngeal motor dysfunction. Severe bulbar involvement with evidence of bilateral disease is most likely to be associated with measurable motor abnormalities. Bilateral hemispheric cerebrovascular accidents also interfere with swallowing because of the disruption of cortical input to the swallowing centers (as in pseudobulbar palsy).[245] Some evidence of oropharyngeal motor dysfunction can be detected from unilateral hemispheric infarcts,[246] but few patients with these lesions have oropharyngeal dysphagia. The onset of oropharyngeal dysphagia caused by cerebrovascular accidents is often abrupt. Other evidence of neurologic damage is generally present, particularly in the distribution of cranial nerves.

Parkinson's Disease

This degenerative lesion can affect the swallowing center. Stasis in the hypopharynx with associated UES dysfunction is a prevalent finding in untreated patients.[247] Failure of UES opening is thought to result from an imbalance of dopaminergic and cholinergic ganglia in the brainstem region. Despite the prevalence of these demonstrable abnormalities, many patients remain relatively asymptomatic.[248] The disease not only affects the UES but also influences how the patient is able to manipulate and form the bolus in the mouth. Patients with oropharyngeal dysphagia from Parkinson's disease have a better prognosis than do patients with many other neurologic causes, because the condition may improve with conventional therapy for Parkinson's disease.[249]

Other Neurologic Causes

Although cerebrovascular accidents and Parkinson's disease are the most common neurologic causes of oropharyngeal dysphagia, this symptom and proximal esophageal dysfunction are associated with a variety of other central and peripheral neurologic diseases as well (see Table 32–2). Oropharyngeal dysphagia is encountered infrequently in patients with multiple sclerosis, and UES dysfunction has been observed.[250] Plaque-like lesions may possibly be detected in the brainstem by magnetic resonance imaging in such patients. As would be expected, other neurologic diseases involving the brainstem, such as amyotrophic lateral sclerosis, Huntington's chorea, brainstem tumors, and poliomyelitis, potentially result in proximal esophageal dysfunction.[247, 251, 252] Attention has been given to dysphagia from the post-polio syndrome, which appears decades after the initial attack.[253] Overwork of the surviving motor neurons with their accelerated aging and deterioration is presumably responsible for the progressive symptoms. Amyotrophic lateral sclerosis is relentless in denervation of striated muscle, and progressive dysphagia is common. These patients often require measures to improve swallowing and, later in their course, tube or gastrostomy feedings (see Chapter 16).

Diseases of the cranial nerves and their branches also may produce similar findings. Although poor UES opening and oropharyngeal dysphagia do not consistently result from unilateral disease, UES dysfunction has been reported to occur after unilateral sectioning of the cranial nerves to this region. The recurrent laryngeal branches of the vagus nerve innervate the upper esophagus and cricopharyngeus muscle (not the hypopharynx). Unilateral damage to these nerve branches from malignancy or accidental injury during neck surgery can produce vocal cord paralysis and oropharyngeal dysphagia simultaneously in some patients.[254] Other diseases of the cranial nerves that uncommonly produce this syndrome include focal cranial neuropathies (e.g., diphtheria, diabetes mellitus, tetanus) and more generalized peripheral neuropathies.[255] Abnormalities in oropharyngeal motor function may be more prevalent among diabetic patients with other evidence of peripheral or autonomic neuropathy than is clinically appreciated (see Chapter 29).

Striated Muscle Disorders

Inflammatory Myopathies

The inflammation of skeletal musculature observed in dermatomyositis and polymyositis involves striated muscle of the esophagus (see Chapter 29). About 10% to 15% of patients with these myopathies have dysphagia, usually in association with severe disease and a poor prognosis. As would be expected, poor contraction of the pharyngeal constrictors, pooling and retention of barium in the valleculae, and nasal regurgitation of the bolus are radiographic observations.[256] Manometric studies can identify decreased contractions in the pharynx with a reduction in UES resting tone; contraction waves in the proximal esophageal body are also of low amplitude. Similar findings can be observed in some patients with scleroderma or mixed connective tissue disease. Corticosteroid therapy often improves peripheral muscle function in patients with polymyositis and dermatomyositis and has been found to improve esophageal motor function in some symptomatic patients.[257]

Inclusion body myositis is an adult-onset disorder of skeletal muscle. The inflammatory myopathy is chronic and painless and is usually resistant to immunosuppressive therapy. Limb involvement is well described, and a few patients with swallowing difficulties have been reported.[258] Decreased pharyngeal peristalsis is observed as with the other myopathies. Treatment strategies such as those for other forms of oropharyngeal dysphagia should be used (discussed below), but cricopharyngeal myotomy may be required.

Muscular Dystrophies

Two uncommon forms of muscular dystrophy involve the striated muscles of the pharyngoesophageal region, and dysphagia with tracheobronchial aspiration is commonly encountered in both syndromes. Myotonia dystrophica is a familial disease characterized by myopathic facies, myotonia, swan neck, muscle wasting, frontal baldness, testicular atrophy, and cataracts. Decreased contraction pressures in the pharynx and upper esophagus, as well as decreased resting pressure of the UES, have been reported in these patients.[259] Similar manometric features in the proximal esophagus are noted in patients with oculopharyngeal dystrophy.[260] This syndrome appears later in life with ptosis and dysphagia as presenting features (the dysphagia usually preceding the ptosis) and has a dominant pattern of inheritance.

Other Muscle Diseases

Oropharyngeal dysphagia is caused by other diseases that can affect the striated musculature. The symptoms may be associated with both hyperthyroidism and hypothyroidism. Improvement in symptoms and restoration of normal swallowing function have been observed after treatment of myxedema.[261] Esophageal involvement has also been reported in the stiff-man syndrome, a diffuse striated muscle disease resulting from uninhibited muscle stimulation by the anterior horn cells in the spinal cord.[262]

Myasthenia Gravis

Myasthenia gravis, a disorder of the motor end plate, affects striated esophageal musculature and has clinical manifestations that resemble the myopathies and dystrophic diseases involving the same region. Characteristic of the fatiguing effect of repeated effort on other skeletal muscles in this disorder, successive pharyngoesophageal transfer worsens with repeated swallows or as a meal progresses.[247, 251, 263] Resting to allow reaccumulation of acetylcholine in nerve endings or administration of an anticholinesterase (edrophonium chloride) improves pharyngoesophageal functions and symptoms simultaneously.[263]

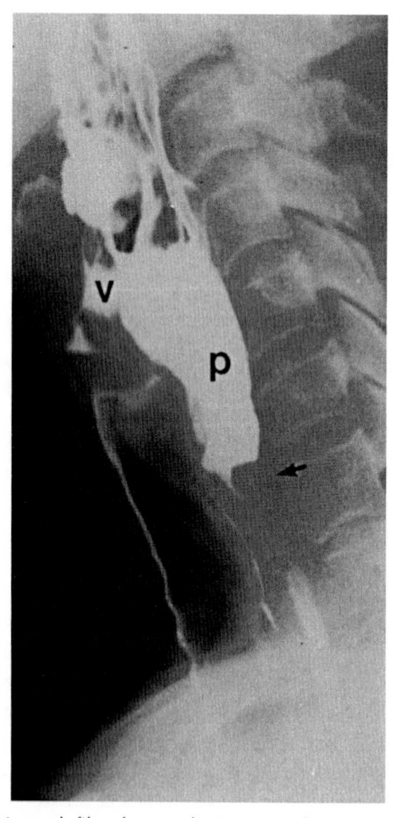

Figure 32–8. Lateral film from a barium esophagogram in an elderly patient with oropharyngeal dysphagia and cricopharyngeal dysfunction. The film demonstrates a prominent indentation by the cricopharyngeus muscle (*arrow*). Dilatation of the piriform sinuses (p) is present, and aspiration of barium into the laryngeal vestibule (v) and trachea is well demonstrated on this film.

Table 32–3 | **Guidelines for the Evaluation and Management of Oropharyngeal Dysphagia**

- Perform careful history and physical examination to determine if oropharyngeal dysphagia is likely and to identify the potential etiologies
- Identify structural etiologies of oropharyngeal dysfunction (e.g., osteophytes, cricopharyngeal bars, Zenker's diverticulum) and explore potential surgical or endoscopic therapies
- Determine the functional integrity of the swallow mechanism, using tests like videofluoroscopy, nasoendoscopy of the oropharynx, and esophageal manometry
- Evaluate the risk of aspiration pneumonitis, typically by using videofluoroscopy
- Determine if the pattern of dysphagia is amenable to therapy

From American Gastroenterological Association: AGA medical position statement on management of oropharyngeal dysphagia. Gastroenterology 116:452–454, 1999.

Cricopharyngeal Dysfunction

Dysfunction of the cricopharyngeus muscle may be present without other evidence of neurologic or muscle disease. This presumably primary disorder produces obstructive symptoms in the region of the UES. Radiographic studies reveal more than simply a prominence of the normal cricopharyngeal indentation. Barium passes the cricopharyngeus muscle slowly, and the muscle appears to relax poorly during swallowing. Ballooning of the pharynx may be noted, and evidence of aspiration can be apparent (Fig. 32–8). *Spasm of the cricopharyngeus* and *cricopharyngeal achalasia* are terms that have been applied to these phenomena.

Diagnosis rests on radiography, and the best evaluation is by videofluoroscopy. Peculiarities in the radiographs should be clarified with direct visualization with endoscopy because proximal esophageal neoplasms can produce similar clinical and radiographic features. Affected patients are frequently considered for cricopharyngeal myotomy because no pharmacologic therapy is available. Simpler measures, such as bougienage, generally have little lasting effect. Relief of dysphagia in the majority of patients follows myotomy (described below).[264] An increased amount of fibrous tissue has been detected in sections of the cricopharyngeus muscle obtained surgically.[265] Other myopathic features have been detected in some patients. A fibrotic process that gradually restricts the maximum luminal opening of the relaxed UES would be compatible with the clinical picture in many patients.

Treatment

Management of disorders involving the UES and cervical esophageal region can be difficult and frustrating. Many of the neurologic disorders affecting motor function are progressive and untreatable. In general, the management approach is aimed at provision of adequate nutrition and development of a safe swallow without tracheobronchial aspiration. Consensus guidelines have been developed that guide a logical evaluation approach leading up to treatment (Table 32–3).[266, 267] Three categories of treatment are available for improving swallowing function[217]: *Compensatory strategies* eliminate symptoms but do not directly change swallowing physiology; these strategies include adjustments of head and body and alterations of food consistency, volume, and delivery rate.[267, 268] *Indirect therapies* are designed to improve neuromuscular controls necessary for swallowing without actually producing a swallow; exercise programs for tongue coordination and chewing are examples. *Direct therapies* are intended to actually change swallow physiology; medical treatments of primary diseases, maxillofacial prosthetics, and cricopharyngeal myotomy are direct therapies that are effective in some instances. Swallow maneuvers (e.g., the supraglottic swallow) also change swallow physiology and can be used in patients without cognitive or language deficits who can follow the instructions.

If there is no direct therapy for the primary illness that readily alleviates symptoms, management must begin with a careful bedside and radiologic assessment so that treatment can be individualized.[269] The modified barium swallow study is performed jointly by a radiologist and a speech pathologist. From this assessment, a variety of specific recommendations can be made.[217] During evaluation and initiation of the management plan, consideration must be given to the nutritional state of the patient; a temporary or permanent feeding gastrostomy may be required.[270] Correct application of the strategies listed previously, however, can allow reversion to oral feeding, removal of gastrostomy feeding tubes, and a cost-effective improvement in quality of life for many patients initially offered gastrostomy without attempts to improve swallowing function.[271]

The role of cricopharyngeal myotomy in the management of oropharyngeal dysphagia disorders is changing. Movement of the hyolaryngeal complex upward and forward is responsible for opening of the UES once it has relaxed.[272] In some instances of neuromuscular disease involving the region, reduced laryngeal movement is the actual abnormality responsible for poor opening of the UES and can be corrected by a specific swallow maneuver.[217] Thus, a careful assessment that considers all management options (including the likelihood of spontaneous recovery, as in some patients with cerebrovascular accidents) should be undertaken before myotomy is performed. Despite its probably imperfect use in many situations, myotomy has been at least moderately effective in a wide variety of neuromuscular disorders causing swallow dysfunction.[272, 273] The combination of defective UES opening and increased intrabolus pressure is predictive of good surgical outcome, findings typical of primary cricopharyngeus dysfunction.[274] Although cricopharyngeal myotomy significantly reduces UES basal pressure, it may not pose the dangerous risk of esophagopharyngeal reflux as presumed in the past.[275, 276] Alternatives to surgical myotomy have been introduced recently, including botulinum toxin injection in the UES and endoscopic myotomy.[277]

ACHALASIA

Achalasia is the most recognized motor disorder of the esophagus and is the hallmark example of hypermotility mechanisms. The term achalasia means "failure to relax" and describes a cardinal feature of this disorder: a poorly relaxing LES. Thus the sphincter produces a functional obstruction of the esophagus and the expected symptoms of dysphagia, regurgitation, chest discomfort, and, eventually, weight loss. Transit from esophagus to stomach is further impaired by a defect involving the esophageal body that results in aperistalsis. The symptom history, which resembles that of a progressively serious and ultimately fatal disease, and radiographs, which demonstrate a grossly contorted and dilated esophagus, together produce a dramatic clinical presentation.

Cause

The cause of achalasia, a disease with only esophageal manifestations, remains unknown. Although a viral cause has been postulated, electron microscopic examination of the vagus nerve and intramural plexus has not revealed viral particles; viral genomic products are not consistently identified in the plexuses; and epidemiologic features do not suggest an infectious cause.[278, 279] Genetic influences also appear to have limited contribution unless achalasia is related to a multisystem disorder,[280] although associations with HLA loci have been described.[281–283] Data suggest that antibodies to myenteric neurons are present in as many as half of patients with achalasia, which raises the possibility of an autoimmune process.[284]

Pathology and Pathophysiology

Abnormalities in both muscle and nerve components can be detected in this disease, although the neural lesion is thought to be of primary importance. Careful examination of the intramural esophageal nerve plexus has demonstrated reduction in number of NANC inhibitory ganglion cells,[285, 286] presumably the most important pathophysiologic defect. An activated T-cell lymphocytic infiltrate surrounds the remaining degenerating nerve fibers,[287, 288] and the loss of inhibitory ganglia extends into the proximal stomach.[289] In addition, electron microscopic examination of the esophageal vagal branches reveals degeneration of myelin sheaths and disruption of axonal membranes, the wallerian degenerative changes typical of experimental nerve transection.[290] Degenerative changes, including fragmentation and dissolution of nuclear material, have also been reported in ganglia of the vagal dorsal motor nucleus.[285] These extraesophageal neuropathic changes have been demonstrated in only small numbers of achalasia patients. Nevertheless, lesions of the vagus nerve or its motor nuclei are plausible in this disease, inasmuch as bilateral lesions in the feline dorsal motor nuclei of the vagus can produce dysfunction resembling achalasia.[291] The interrelationship of ganglion cell loss from the esophageal wall and the vagal and brainstem lesions is not fully understood. A disorder affecting both intrinsic and extrinsic sites could be operational; on the contrary, some degree of vagal degeneration could result secondarily from ganglion cell disease. The circular muscle of the lower esophagus is thickened, but muscular changes are thought to be secondary to underlying neuropathology.

Physiologic studies have confirmed the presence of denervation of the smooth muscle segment of the esophagus in patients with achalasia. First, muscle strips from the esophageal body contract in response to direct stimulation (acetylcholine) but not in response to ganglionic stimulation (nicotine).[292] Similarly, strips from the region of the LES do not relax in response to ganglionic stimulation in patients with achalasia, in contrast to normal controls.[292] Second, exaggerated contractions in the esophageal body and sphincter can be measured when patients with achalasia are given parenteral injection of the acetylcholine analog acetyl-beta-methacholine (Mecholyl).[293] This response is thought to be indicative of denervation hypersensitivity. Third, cholecystokinin octapeptide (CCK-8) produces an unexpected increase in LES pressure in the achalasia patient. This effect may represent loss of inhibitory neurons in the LES region, inasmuch as these neurons normally produce the predominant response to CCK-8 stimulation.[294] All these observations are evidence of functional impairment of intramural ganglion cells in the esophageal body and LES region. Only meager physiologic evidence of vagal dysfunction (primarily inhibitory) exists despite neurohistologic observations.[295]

Anatomic and physiologic observations are adequate for explaining the manifestations of this disease. A loss of ganglion cells in the region of the LES, particularly if the loss is predominantly of inhibitory neurons, would result in an increased basal pressure and poor relaxation under normal circumstances. Vagal changes, whether primary or secondary, could also predominantly affect inhibitory stimulation to sphincter muscle, further compounding this problem. Degeneration of ganglion cells in the esophageal body itself would eventually lead to permanent aperistalsis and allow for esophageal dilatation. The lesion in the LES region may be the earliest finding, and the aperistalsis of some early nondilated cases may be related to esophageal obstruction at the level of the sphincter. In these patients, occasional peristalsis may be observed at least temporarily after reduction in LES pressure with pneumatic dilation or myotomy.

Clinical Manifestations

The annual incidence of achalasia is approximately 1 to 2 per 200,000 population.[296] The disease affects both sexes equally and can occur at any age. Onset is usually in the third to fifth decades, and fewer than 5% of patients have symptoms before adolescence. Symptoms rather than physical findings are the hallmarks of this disease. The duration of symptoms at presentation averages 2 years, although a wide variation is seen.[297] Dysphagia is almost uniformly the predominant symptom.[297] Dysphagia for solid foods is present in nearly all patients; dysphagia for liquids is reported by at least two thirds. The combination of dysphagia for both liquids and solid foods has some utility in suggesting achalasia over obstructive strictures or tumors.[212] The severity of dysphagia fluctuates, but for many it reaches a plateau and does not worsen with time. For others, the sense of obstruction is so severe that weight loss is pronounced. Patients may report the use of postural changes, such as raising the arms above the head, straightening the back, or standing at very erect posture, to increase intraesophageal pressure and improve emptying. Slow, deliberate swallowing during a meal seems to alleviate retrosternal fullness in some patients. It has been suggested that this maneuver takes advantage of the 10- to 20-mm Hg increment in intraesophageal pressure produced by swallowing a food or liquid bolus, an increment that could encourage esophageal emptying.

Chest pain is reported by one third to one half of patients with achalasia and tends to improve with the course of the disease.[297, 298] The pain is retrosternal and typical of other forms of esophageal pain. Chest pain is often precipitated by eating and is the cause of decreased intake and weight loss in some patients. Interestingly, chest pain is sufficiently dissociated from dysphagia in this disorder that treatments successfully improving dysphagia and esophageal emptying may have little impact on pain.[298] Sixty percent to 90% of patients regurgitate undigested foods during or shortly after a meal, and the regurgitation is often active and unprovoked. Some patients induce regurgitation to relieve the uncomfortable feeling of fullness in the retrosternal region after a meal. These symptoms may be confused with those of eating disorders, and achalasia may be mistaken for anorexia nervosa or bulimia.[299] Weight loss is common, and when significant, it usually represents advanced disease with marked retention of food and liquid. Pulmonary symptoms indicate aspiration of esophageal contents. In one large series, 30% of patients reported nocturnal coughing spells, and nearly 10% had significant bronchopulmonary complications.[300]

Diagnosis

The disease is suspected from a compatible clinical history, and diagnosis is usually easily accomplished. Early cases may be misdiagnosed if screening radiographs fail to reveal the esophageal dilatation and distortion seen in more advanced cases. Some symptoms of this disease, notably chest pain and active regurgitation, may be most pronounced early in the course, before the esophagus overtly dilates.

Radiographic Studies

A barium swallow study with fluoroscopy is an appropriate screening test in a patient with esophageal dysphagia when achalasia is suspected because the study can streamline further testing and therapy.[301] In the recumbent patient with achalasia, peristalsis fails to clear the barium bolus from the esophagus. Contrast material may be moved up and down the esophageal body by nonpropulsive, tertiary contraction or may simply lie in the atonic organ. The LES opens intermittently, allowing contrast material to escape in small quantities from the esophagus. Relaxation does not appear to be associated temporally with swallowing. Plain radiographs of the chest may show absence of a gastric bubble and, in advanced disease, a dilated esophagus.

Once enough barium is swallowed to fill the esophagus, other typical features are seen (Fig. 32–9). The esophageal body is dilated, and dilatation is greatest in the distal esophagus. The barium column terminates in a tapered point, the location of the tight, nonrelaxing sphincter. This smoothly tapered projection is commonly called a "bird's beak," because the silhouette of this projection in conjunction with the dilated distal esophagus resembles the beaks of common North American songbirds. Because the skeletal muscle portion of the esophagus is least involved, the proximal esophagus may have a normal contour.

In cases with relatively short histories of symptoms, the esophageal body may be only slightly or not dilated, and radiographic diagnosis may be incorrect if fluoroscopy is not used. In fact, the diagnosis of achalasia is either overlooked

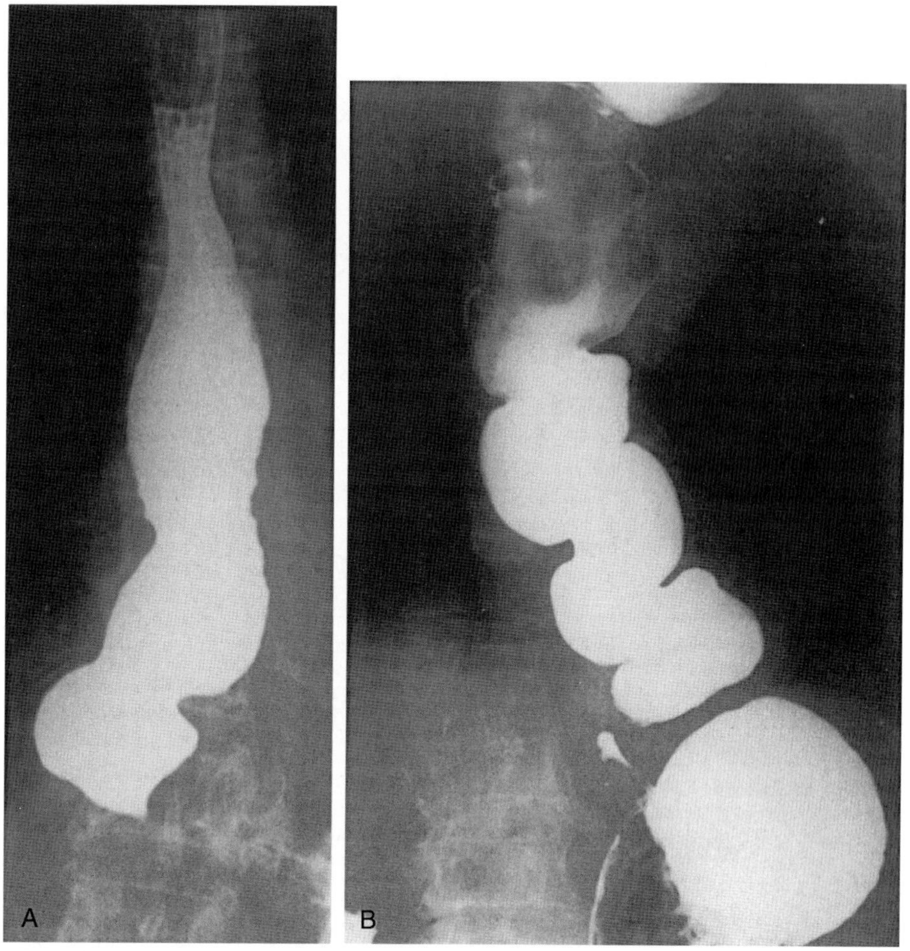

Figure 32–9. *A,* Typical barium esophagogram from a patient with achalasia. The dilated esophagus ends in a so-called pointed bird's beak that represents the nonrelaxing lower esophageal sphincter. Fluoroscopy during the swallow revealed no meaningful peristalsis in the esophageal body. *B,* Achalasia of the esophagus with marked distortion of the esophageal body. The esophagus itself resembles colon.

or not established with barium radiography in at least one third of patients outside of the research setting.[302, 303] Upright radiographs showing barium retention with an air-fluid level in the esophagus are helpful in revealing poor emptying in unclear instances. Epiphrenic diverticula arising immediately proximal to the region of the LES can be seen in this disease. Diverticula can be massive, interfering significantly with other diagnostic tests and therapeutic maneuvers.

Endoscopy

Endoscopy is an important diagnostic tool in the patient with symptoms of achalasia and should be performed even if radiographic evaluation findings are typical. The purpose of endoscopy is twofold: (1) to rule out several of the diseases that mimic achalasia, and (2) to evaluate the esophageal mucosa before therapeutic manipulations. Typical endoscopic findings include dilatation and atony of the esophageal body and a puckered, closed LES that does not open during the procedure. The instrument passes through the sphincter and into the stomach with gentle pressure. Absence of a stricture or constricting mass is best established if an endoscope of relatively large caliber is used. The esophagogastric junction must be examined carefully for any evidence of neoplasm; unfortunately, a reasonable number of tumors that mimic achalasia are infiltrative and not detectable by this means.[304, 305] Because adenocarcinoma of the stomach is the most common neoplasm associated with an achalasia-like presentation, examination of the gastric cardia and fundus by retroflexion is essential. Inflammatory changes of the esophageal mucosa can be related to stasis of esophageal contents, caustic damage from medications, or *Candida albicans* infection. If a mucosal biopsy specimen reveals evidence of *C. albicans* infection, antifungal therapy before treatment is recommended as prophylaxis against mediastinal contamination in case of perforation or soiling.

Manometry

Manometry confirms or establishes the diagnosis of achalasia and is particularly important when radiographs are reportedly normal or inconclusive. The test contributes less in advanced cases with classic radiographic findings and endoscopic appearance. Several features of manometry are typical of achalasia. First, sequentially propagated waves traversing the distal esophageal body are absent. Contraction waves that are measured are generally of low amplitude and are simultaneous in onset (Fig. 32–10). The pressure tracings from different parts of the esophageal body show remarkable similarity, which indicates that the recording ports on the manometry probe are detecting isobaric pressure changes within a closed chamber: the dilated esophageal body with closed sphincters at each end. Only occasional peristaltic sequences return after successful reduction in LES pressure with pneu-

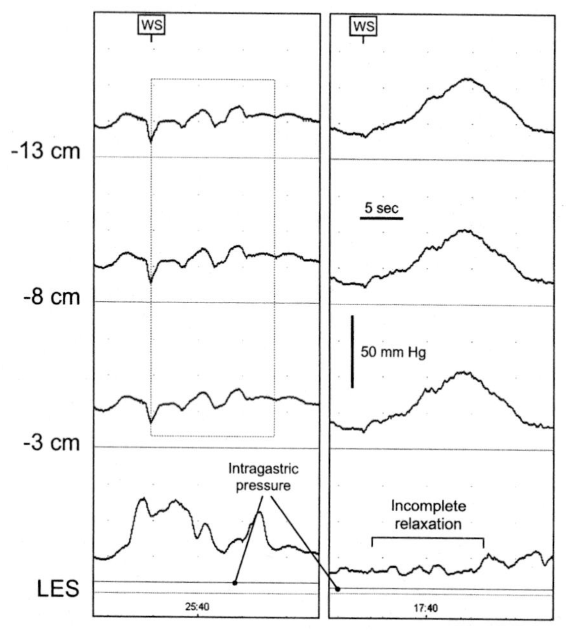

Figure 32–10. Mamometric findings recorded from the lower esophageal sphincter (LES) and three sites in the smooth muscle esophageal body in two patients with idiopathic achalasia. Responses noted in the esophageal body are identical on the three leads (box), indicating a closed chamber with isobaric measurements across sites. The LES does not show meaningful relaxation to the level of intragastric pressure in response to a wet swallow (WS) in either case. Broad pressure response following one swallow (*right panel*) is not progressive through the esophageal body; progressive responses did not follow any swallow in either patient. The combination of aperistalsis and incomplete LES relaxation typifies this disorder.

matic dilation or myotomy, which indicates the degree of damage to normal peristaltic mechanisms by the disease process.[306]

Intraesophageal resting pressure is often higher than intragastric resting pressure, a reverse of the normal pattern. The intraesophageal pressure increment appears to be attributable to retained food and secretions within the esophagus, inasmuch as it can be eliminated with esophageal evacuation. A further increase in esophageal baseline pressure, as well as the occurrence of high-amplitude, repetitive contractions in the esophageal body, is observed with administration of methacholine chloride (Mecholyl).[307] It does not provoke any meaningful peristalsis. This pharmacologic agent has been administered to patients with achalasia to add support to the diagnosis. However, the pain and unpleasant cholinergic side effects produced do not justify its routine use, in view of the scant additional information gained.

LES characteristics are important for manometric diagnosis. An elevated resting pressure is detected in 55% to 90% of untreated patients.[308] (Pressure values vary considerably, depending on measurement and analysis technique, making interstudy comparison of absolute pressure values difficult.) The high-pressure zone is also longer than that seen in normal persons. More important to the diagnosis of achalasia than resting sphincter characteristics, however, is the demonstration of incomplete sphincter relaxation after a swallow (see Fig. 32–10). This manometric finding distinguishes the achalasia pattern from hypomotility disorders with aperistalsis. Some degree of relaxation may be observed intermittently, but this finding is largely a recording artifact.[309–311] In most cases, sphincter pressure drops by only approximately 30% of its increase over gastric baseline, leaving an abnormally high residual pressure at the relaxation nadir.[311, 312] Of all the manometric findings in this disorder, the combination of aperistalsis with incomplete LES relaxation (with or without an increase in resting sphincter pressure) most importantly typifies achalasia. It does not differentiate idiopathic achalasia from disorders that can closely mimic this disease (discussed below). A subset of achalasia patients with higher amplitude contractions in the esophageal body has been identified as having vigorous achalasia, but the distinction is apparently without clinical importance.[313–315] A short, aperistaltic segment also has been reported in an occasional patient with otherwise typical achalasia.[315]

Table 32–4 | **Disorders with Manometric and Radiologic Features that Mimic Idiopathic Achalasia**

DISORDER	REFERENCE NO.
Malignancy	316
Chronic idiopathic intestinal pseudo-obstruction	317
Amyloidosis	318
Sarcoidosis	319
Chagas' disease	320
Postvagotomy disturbance	321
Pancreatic pseudocyst	322
Von Recklinghausen's neurofibromatosis	323
Anderson-Fabry's disease	324
Familial glucocorticoid deficiency syndrome	325
Multiple endocrine neoplasia, type IIb	326
Juvenile Sjögren's syndrome with achalasia and gastric hypersecretion	327

Differential Diagnosis

A group of disorders that either mimic idiopathic achalasia or include an achalasia-like component in a multisystem disease must be considered in making a diagnosis (Table 32–4). These diseases may resemble idiopathic achalasia so closely that results of conventional diagnostic tests are misleading.[316–327] The most alarming pretenders are the malignant neoplasms, and a variety of tumors have been reported (Table 32–5). The tumors mimic the esophageal manifesta-

Table 32–5 | **Malignancies Associated with Features Resembling Achalasia**

Gastric adenocarcinoma*
Esophageal squamous cell carcinoma
Lymphoma
Lung carcinoma (squamous cell, small-cell [oat cell], adenocarcinoma)
Pancreatic carcinoma
Prostatic carcinoma
Hepatocellular carcinoma
Anaplastic carcinoma
Colon carcinoma
Esophageal lymphangioma
Primary esophageal small-cell carcinoma
Pleural mesothelioma

*Represents over 65% of reported cases.

Table 32–6 | **Comparison of Primary Treatments for Idiopathic Achalasia**

COMPARATIVE FEATURE	SMOOTH MUSCLE RELAXANTS	BOTULINUM TOXIN INJECTION	PNEUMATIC DILATION	SURGICAL MYOTOMY	
				Open Technique	Minimally Invasive Technique*
Response					
Initial	50%–70%	90% at 1 mo	60%–90% at 1 yr	>90% at 1 yr	>90% at 1 year
Later	<50% at 1 yr	60% at 1 yr	60% at 5 yrs	75% at 20 yrs	85% at 5 years
Morbidity					
Minor	30% (headache, hypotension)	20% (rash, transient chest pain)	Rare technique-related complications	<10% at 1 yr (symptomatic reflux)	10% (symptomatic reflux)
Serious	Not reported	Not reported	3%–5% (perforation)	10% dysphagia, <2% mortality	Not available
Advantage(s)	Rapidly initiated; well accepted	Low morbidity; modest response durability; well accepted	Good response durability	Best response rate and durability	Avoids thoracotomy; likely equivalent response to open technique
Disadvantage(s)	Inconvenient side effects; tachyphylaxis; poor effect on esophageal emptying	Repeat injection often required within 1 yr; fibroinflammatory reaction at LES	Perforation rate low but of concern to patient and physician	Thoracotomy required; more common and severe reflux may develop	Long-term outcome remains unknown, conversion to open procedure in very small percentage

*Includes thoracoscopic and laparoscopic methods.
LES, lower esophageal sphincter.

tions of achalasia primarily by one of two mechanisms: (1) The tumor mass encircles or compresses the at least 50% of the circumference of the distal esophagus, producing a constricting segment, or (2) malignant cells infiltrate the esophageal neural plexus, impairing postganglionic LES innervation.[328] In rare instances, tumors interfere with the myenteric plexus without direct infiltration,[308] and achalasia has been associated with type 1 antineuronal (anti-Hu) nuclear autoantibodies.[329] Certain historical features can help the clinician suspect a malignancy.[304, 330] A short duration of symptoms (less than 6 months), presentation later in life (over age 50 to 60 years), and rapid weight loss are all more typical of malignancy than of idiopathic achalasia, although these have relatively poor specificity. An achalasia-like picture following fundoplication is being reported with increasing frequency related to the escalating use of antireflux surgery.[331, 332] A poorly constructed fundus wrap is most often responsible for this outcome.

Manometry cannot discriminate patients with neoplasms from patients with idiopathic achalasia.[304, 316] Even methacholine may, as in achalasia, induce a marked increase in intraesophageal pressure. Apparent ulceration in the narrowed segment may suggest a tumor on barium studies, particularly when the narrowed segment is long with an abrupt proximal margin, but irregularities in this region have also been noted in patients with idiopathic achalasia.[300, 333] Amyl nitrite administration during the barium study improves the accuracy of this radiologic technique for differentiating achalasia from malignancy. The reduction in LES pressure after amyl nitrite administration in patients with idiopathic achalasia is not observed in patients with malignancies that are behaving as distal strictures.[304, 316] Likewise, response to botulinum toxin injection may provide some useful information.[334] Although frequently performed, computed tomography is of limited value in accurately detecting these tumors, as are endoscopy and endoscopic ultrasonography.[335] The tumors are often infiltrative and can be identified only after repeated evaluations, including endoscopic biopsies, in patients having suspicious clinical histories (see Chapters 35 and 44).[305]

Treatment

The degenerative neural lesion of this disease cannot be corrected. Treatment is directed at palliation of symptoms and prevention of complications. Although aggressive therapy is not necessary for a patient who has few symptoms and minimal esophageal dilatation, it is required for those with dilatation and food retention to prevent serious pulmonary complications. Development of carcinoma in achalasia, although uncommon, may also be related to dilatation and chronic mucosal irritation from stasis. (Further observations regarding these complications are discussed later in this chapter.) Effective peristalsis is rarely restored with successful treatment, but improvement in esophageal emptying and reduction in the esophageal diameter are generally expected.

Four palliative treatments are available: pharmacotherapy, botulinum toxin injection, dilation, and myotomy. All are intended to reduce LES pressure and improve emptying by gravity. Symptomatic improvement, however, is not always accompanied by these benefits. Each treatment has its place in the management of achalasia, and a comparative overview of the approaches is shown in Table 32–6. Pneumatic dilation and surgical myotomy offer long-lasting benefits for both symptoms and esophageal emptying and are considered optimal treatments for this disease.[336]

Pharmacotherapy

Agents that have a direct relaxant effect on smooth muscle fibers of the LES alleviate symptoms in up to 70% of patients.[337] Nitrites have this effect, and the acute administration of amyl nitrite can rapidly enhance esophageal emptying.[338] Sublingual isosorbide dinitrate (Isordil), 5 to 10 mg before meals, improves symptoms in the majority of treated patients.[339] Typical adverse effects of nitrates, particularly headache, prevent continued use of the drug in up to one third of patients. Substitution of the oral formulation reduces the likelihood of adverse effects but may have a less dependable onset of action because of esophageal retention.

Calcium channel blockers (diltiazem, nifedipine, verapamil) also have recognized relaxant effects on LES muscle. These drugs interfere with calcium uptake by smooth muscle cells, cells that are dependent on intracellular calcium for contraction. In isolated cases, the LES in achalasia relaxes within 15 minutes in response to 10 to 20 mg nifedipine.[340] Placebo-controlled trials of calcium channel blockers have not demonstrated consistent clinical benefits,[341] but selected patients appear to have a reduction in symptoms. To attain maximal benefits from a therapeutic trial, these agents should be given immediately before a meal in a sublingual, short-acting form. The response may be best in patients with minimal esophageal dilatation (< 5 cm).[342]

The role of pharmacologic agents in the long-term management of achalasia is limited, primarily because of their unsatisfactory effect on esophageal emptying. Even for symptomatic responders, it is unlikely that continued use will prevent esophageal dilatation and complications. Patients with medical conditions that interfere with pneumatic dilation or myotomy are certainly candidates. In addition, normal nutritional status can potentially be re-established for patients with severe weight loss, rendering them better candidates for other forms of treatment.

Botulinum Toxin Injection

Botulinum toxin type A is derived from the controlled fermentation of *Clostridium botulinum*. Direct injection of this agent into skeletal muscle bodies has been used extensively in neurologic practice for treatment of focal involuntary muscle overactivity, particularly focal dystonias.[343] The toxin binds to presynaptic cholinergic neuronal receptors, is internalized, and irreversibly interferes with acetylcholine release, presumably by blocking the ability of the neurotransmitter vesicle to dock and fuse with the axonal membrane.[354] Paralysis occurs over several days, but axonal sprouts soon appear and allow for gradual return of neuromuscular function. Evidence of distant paralysis is not seen when the injections are used for neurologic indications wherein findings at other sites are limited to minor electromyographic abnormalities.

Pasricha and colleagues first demonstrated the ability of botulinum toxin to reduce LES basal tone and improve symptoms in patients with achalasia.[345] An initial beneficial response to 80 U injected circumferentially during endoscopy at the level of the LES occurs in 60% to 75% of patients, but symptoms reappear within a year in the majority of these patients.[346–349] Repeat injection is effective for a reasonable subset, so that the overall treatment benefit of as-needed injections can approach that of a single pneumatic dilation for up to 2 years, but this approach generally is not cost-effective[350–352] (Fig. 32–11). Similar to pharmacologic treatment of achalasia, botulinum toxin injection has a greater effect on symptoms than on esophageal emptying.[348, 353, 354] Side effects from treatment are rare and include chest

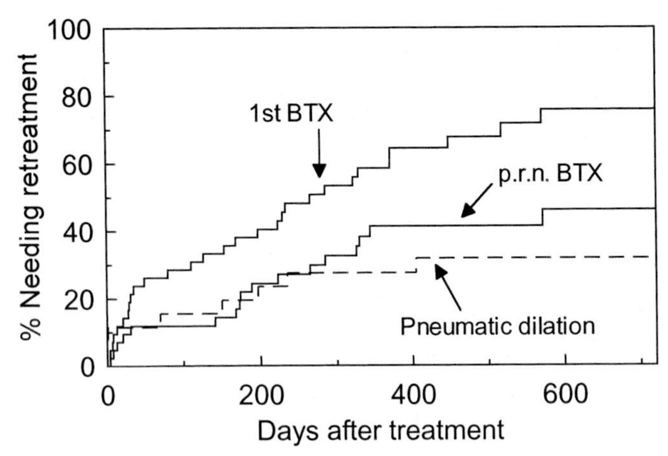

Figure 32–11. Kaplan-Meier plots of the percentage of achalasia subjects requiring retreatment of any type following initial treatment with botulinum toxin injection (first BTX) or pneumatic dilation. Data are also shown for subjects treated with botulinum toxin alone, repeated as needed (prn BTX), who ultimately required retreatment with pneumatic dilation, esophagomyotomy, or feeding tube placement. (Adapted from Prakash C, Freedland KE, Chan MF, Clouse RE: Botulinum toxin injections for achalasia symptoms can approximate the short-term efficacy of a single pneumatic dilation. A survival analysis approach. Am J Gastroenterol 94:328–333, 1999.)

discomfort for several days after injection and occasional rash. An inflammatory reaction at the site of the injection leads to local fibrosis. This reaction can interfere in a limited way with surgical intervention, if needed for subsequent management.[355, 356] Consequently, botulinum toxin injection appears best suited for those who would benefit from its short-term effects or who would not tolerate treatments producing a more durable response.

Dilation

Bougienage with large-caliber dilators (50 F or larger) produces transient improvement for several days at most. Forceful dilation to a diameter of approximately 3 cm is necessary to tear the circular muscle and to effect lasting reduction in LES pressure. Of the various types of dilators developed for this purpose, the pneumatic dilators are conventionally used today.[297] The technique of pneumatic dilation, including inflation pressure and duration of inflation, varies considerably from author to author. Data are insufficient as to whether one technique is superior to another, but the efficacy of pneumatic dilation may have improved in general with the development of more rigid balloons that retain their shape once the required inflation pressure has been attained.[336, 357] The trend is to begin with smaller diameter balloons and shorter dilation times.[358]

After dilation, a small amount of water-soluble contrast material (such as Hypaque) is given cautiously by mouth through a small-caliber nasal tube that has been carefully placed into the midesophagus or through the central lumen of a polyvinyl dilator that has been withdrawn into the esophagus. The purpose of the test is to detect distal esophageal leaks near the region of the esophagogastric junction, not to determine the adequacy of dilation.[359] If no leakage is seen, the patient is observed carefully over the subsequent 6 hours, and then the diet is gradually resumed. Because perforation may be delayed and there may be no evidence of this complication on the immediate contrast study, a period of close observation after the procedure is essential. The patient with a small contained perforation, in which contrast material extends beyond the normal esophageal lumen, can be treated conservatively.[360] Such patients exhibit no evidence of shock, sepsis, or hemorrhage; no radiographic evidence of communication of the perforated area with either the pleural or peritoneal spaces; and evidence that the perforation cavity freely communicates with the esophageal lumen. Administration of broad-spectrum antibiotics that cover oral flora including anaerobes should be initiated, as should close observation for signs of infection, such as worsening pain and fever. Surgical consultation is undertaken as soon as perforation is evident. Clinical deterioration or the presence of free-flowing barium into the mediastinum mandates immediate thoracotomy and repair. If the tear is small, the repair and myotomy can be performed in the same operation.

With the exception of dilator diameter, the influence of most technical variables on outcome is minimal. At least 60% of patients have a good response,[361] and success rates exceeding 95% have been reported. Unlike pharmacologic treatment or botulinum toxin injection, symptomatic outcome is much more dependent on a satisfactory reduction in LES pressure and improvement in esophageal emptying.[362, 363] The response rate varies with patient age (younger patients do not do as well as older patients[364]) and duration of symptoms (those with a shorter history do not respond as well), but it does not seem to be related to the degree of esophageal dilatation or tortuosity.[365] Efficacy of this procedure is reduced by as much as half for subsequent dilations (Fig. 32–12). Thus, patients who have a poor initial result or rapid recurrence of symptoms have a lesser likelihood of responding to additional dilations. The likelihood of response to myotomy is not conclusively reduced by a previous dilation. Morbidity is mostly related to esophageal perforation, a complication in approximately 3% of patients,[336, 357, 361] but surgical repair has been required in less than half of the recognized cases. Mortality from pneumatic dilation has rarely been reported. Perforation may be more likely in severely malnourished patients, which raises the possibility that nutritional restitution could favorably affect the complication rate from dilation.[366]

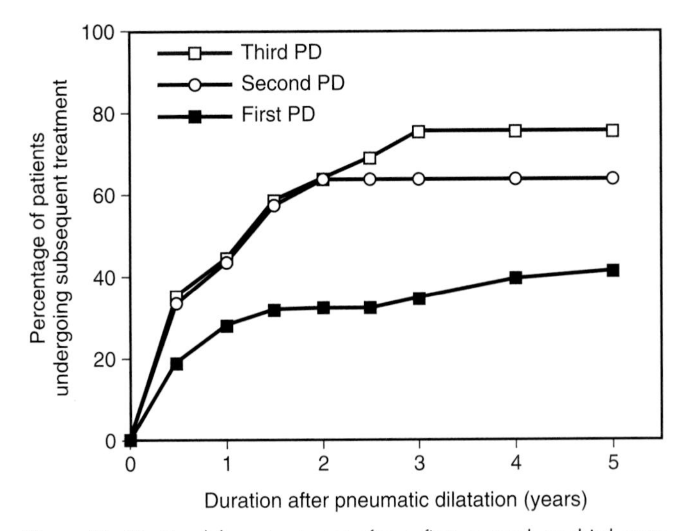

Figure 32–12. Need for retreatment after a first, second, or third pneumatic dilation (PD). Data presented as a 5-year life-table analysis. (From Parkman HP, Reynolds JC, Ouyang A, et al: Pneumatic dilatation or esophagomyotomy treatment for idiopathic achalasia: Clinical outcomes and cost analysis. Dig Dis Sci 38:75, 1993.)

Pneumatic dilation has a durable treatment response not afforded by pharmacotherapy or botulinum toxin injection. Advantages of pneumatic dilation over myotomy are the brief period of discomfort, very short hospital stay, and consequent low expense. The disadvantages are lesser efficacy in comparison with myotomy and the risk, albeit small, of serious complications. It seems unlikely that further refinements in dilation technique will reduce the perforation rate much below its current level. The authors recommend that when conventional treatments are being contemplated at institutions where skilled personnel are available for both procedures, both options should be explained to the patient and pneumatic dilation encouraged on the basis of the low likelihood of an adverse outcome.

Esophagomyotomy

The goal of surgical therapy in achalasia is to reduce LES resting pressure without completely compromising its competency against gastroesophageal reflux. Complete disruption of the sphincter, as with cardioplasty, rapidly relieves dysphagia but predisposes to severe esophagitis and stricturing, negating the utility of the operation. The open Heller procedure was described in 1913, and a modification of this procedure is used most commonly in the open surgical management of achalasia.[367, 368] An anterior myotomy is performed by dividing the circular muscle fibers down to the level of the mucosa. The myotomy extends less than 1 cm onto the stomach and to several centimeters above the palpated region of the LES. For the open procedure, a transthoracic approach is preferred because it allows for careful palpation and inspection of the esophagus, helps confirm the diagnosis, and permits extension of the myotomy proximally as far as necessary by palpation.

Good results from open myotomy occur in 80% to 90% or more of patients.[300, 369] Myotomy reduces LES pressure more dependably than does pneumatic dilation, accounting for its greater efficacy.[357, 370] The most significant complication is gastroesophageal reflux. The modified Heller procedure does not completely destroy sphincter competency if extension of the myotomy onto the stomach is not excessive. Thus, the incidence of symptomatic reflux is less than 10%, although higher rates have been noted and symptoms worsen one to two decades after treatment.[371] Severe dysphagia persists in fewer than 10% of patients treated surgically, but the functional improvement also appears to decay over time.[372] Consequently, even this management option with the best available long-term results does not promise lifelong palliation of symptoms. Completion esophagectomy may be required and is associated with very good outcome despite its seemingly radical nature.[373]

Although long-term outcome data remain limited, the minimally invasive approaches to myotomy have rapidly become the surgical procedures of choice for achalasia.[336, 374] The procedures are as effective as their open counterparts yet have the advantages of shorter hospital stays, less time absent from work, less blood loss during surgery, less parenteral narcotic use, and less incisional morbidity.[375, 376] A thoracoscopic myotomy is performed without an antireflux procedure. Very good to excellent initial treatment response benefits 85% to 90% of patients, and conversion to the open procedure is uncommon for surgeons with technical experience.[377] The laparoscopic approach may be associated with a shorter hospital stay, better initial outcome, and lower incidence of postoperative dysphagia and reflux,[378, 379] and this approach has taken the lead over the thoracoscopic operation. A floppy Toupet fundoplication is attached to the sides of the myotomy in most laparoscopic procedures, as increased mobilization of the gastroesophageal junction appears to enhance reflux potential. Follow-up of the minimally invasive procedures exceeding several years is becoming available, and the results appear as durable as those for the open operations.[378] Life-table analyses predict sustained benefits at 5 years.[380] Despite the technical disadvantages of prior botulinum toxin injection or pneumatic dilation on the surgical procedure itself, neither is a contraindication to minimally invasive myotomy nor significantly influences outcome.[353, 356, 381–383]

Evaluation of recurrent dysphagia following myotomy should include barium radiography and endoscopy. These two studies demonstrate the luminal caliber at the LES, the presence of esophagitis or stricture, and change in the retention of a barium column. A standardized method of measuring the barium column 1 and 5 minutes after ingestion has been recommended for assessing the success of either surgery or dilation for achalasia.[363] Gastroesophageal reflux is an important consideration in most patients, as the correlation between typical reflux symptoms (e.g., heartburn) and measurable reflux is poor in this patient group.[379, 384] Fundoplications that are too tight can result in severe dysphagia, a complication responding to pneumatic dilation in the majority and necessitating additional surgical intervention in the remainder.[332] The rate of mortality from surgery is less than 2%.[374, 378, 385, 386]

Complications of Achalasia

The complications of achalasia are related to retention and stasis in the esophagus. Irritation of the mucosal lining results in an endoscopically evident esophagitis. Symptoms or complications of esophagitis (e.g., stricture formation or hemorrhage) are not recognized. A more serious complication is the aspiration of esophageal contents. As many as 30% of patients report nocturnal coughing spells[300]; fewer develop pulmonary infiltrates from aspiration, but this complication may be severe. Severity is increased by the fact that retained esophageal contents harbor many bacteria (see Chapter 6).

As discussed in Chapter 35, esophageal carcinoma has been reported in association with achalasia with rates as high as 20%, but such series were contaminated by patients with primary tumors that mimicked achalasia.[316] Even with more careful exclusion of patients with this presentation, the prevalence of carcinoma is higher in patients with achalasia than should be observed, rates ranging from 2% to 7% in the larger case series.[387, 388] It is now accepted that achalasia is a risk factor for the development of squamous carcinoma,[389] the complication possibly being more likely in patients who have had unsatisfactory or no treatment. This latter observation suggests that stasis and mucosal irritation may be precipitating factors for this complication, as well.[390] The tumors often arise in a greatly dilated esophagus, symptoms can be quite delayed, and neoplasms can be large and advanced when detected, even in patients who have had regular medical attention. A regular surveillance program presently is not the standard of practice, although recommendations for periodic endoscopy are appearing.[391] Other factors (e.g., tobacco or alcohol use) may contribute to risk of carcinoma, mandating surveillance of such higher risk subgroups.

OTHER HYPERMOTILITY DISORDERS OF THE DISTAL ESOPHAGUS AND LES (SPASTIC DISORDERS)

Definition

A spectrum of non-achalasic disorders with hypermotility features is encountered in clinical practice. At one extreme are minor deviations from normal manometric values; at the other are severe derangements with manometric and radiologic manifestations closely resembling those of achalasia. The spectrum of disorders, also called spastic disorders, unquestionably represents multiple underlying processes manifesting the hypermotility mechanisms previously described (see the section "Pathogenesis and Categorization of Motor Disorders"). In nearly all cases, the etiology is unknown. Symptoms can be produced from functional obstruction, but identical motility patterns can be found in both symptomatic and asymptomatic patients. The clinician must scrutinize each presentation to determine whether the symptoms and motor dysfunction can be linked before treating the motor dysfunction aggressively.

Diagnosis and classification within the group is accomplished primarily by manometry (see Fig. 32–7). Diffuse esophageal spasm is segregated from the remainder because of non-peristaltic responses to swallows, and the diagnosis may actually represent achalasia or a closely related pathologic process in some instances. However, overlap with the remaining nonspecific spastic disorders is great.[200] The authors have chosen to discuss these disorders together because the clinical presentations of patients are quite similar within the entire group, a pathologic basis has been determined for none, management approaches are similar for all, and an outcome that appears specific to any one subset is not recognized.

Pathology and Pathophysiology

The esophageal muscles and neural plexuses are not readily accessible for routine biopsy. This inaccessibility, in conjunction with the nonfatal character of these motor disorders, has resulted in little material for pathologic examination. Diffuse muscular thickening in the distal esophagus has been found in some but not all patients with more severe manometric abnormalities.[392] This inconsistent finding is not thought to be a primary abnormality. In contrast to achalasia, little specific evidence of neuropathology has been reported. Loss of ganglion cells in the intramural plexuses has not been demonstrated. Changes in vagal fibers have been found inconsistently by electron microscopy[392, 393]; some of these changes resemble wallerian degeneration. In contrast to achalasia, however, these hypermotility disorders rarely entail a progression in disease severity, as might be expected from a degenerative neural process. Deterioration from more severe abnormalities to achalasia has been reported,[394] but these are exceptional cases. Hypermotility contraction wave abnormalities are prevalent among alcoholic patients and diabetic patients with peripheral neuropathy, but the manometric findings appear to be independent of neuropathy.[395]

Physiologic studies suggest a neural defect. The esophagus in these disorders is particularly sensitive to cholinergic stimulation. Cholinergic agonists produce an exaggeration of abnormal manometric findings in many patients.[396, 397] Edrophonium chloride, a cholinesterase inhibitor, produces similar results. An exaggerated response also follows parenteral injection of ergonovine maleate.[398] As with cholinergic stimulation, responses to this alpha-adrenergic agent are seen in some control subjects, responses are more exaggerated in patients with hypermotility disorders, and not all patients show a worsening of manometric findings. These physiologic studies do not add sufficient information to localize the pathologic process or processes. Some evidence indicates that central nervous system disease could participate in producing the manometric abnormalities. In normal persons, central nervous system stimulation with psychological stress produces repetitive waves that resemble the described contraction abnormalities. Likewise, loud noise or stressful mental tasks performed during manometry increase contraction wave amplitude in the distal esophagus, although the magnitude of change is small.[399]

Results from provocative testing provide the best evidence that a sensory abnormality at least partially independent of motor dysfunction is also active in many symptomatic patients found to have these motor disorders (Fig. 32–13). In the previously mentioned studies, some degree of differential stimulation to either the motor or sensory component has been observed. Cholinergic stimulation frequently precipitates motility change (with or without pain), but pain provocation may be an independent event. Balloon distention reproduces pain at low distending volumes without an abnormal increment in wall tension.[400] This provocative test precipitates pain in some patients who have no abnormality or mild findings on baseline manometry and who have no dysphagia. In such patients, a sensory disorder may be the predominant finding, and treatment efforts aimed at altering motility may have little impact. Acid instillation stimulates sensitive neural receptors that produce discomfort independent of motor events. As suggested in Figure 32–13, psychiatric illness may produce its effect by altering sensory perception; this concept has been promoted for some other chronic pain and functional gastrointestinal disorders, but an association of psychiatric illness with hypermotility is better established.[401] The physiologic heterogeneity of the population of patients with spastic disorders was well demonstrated in a study using a combination of neurophysiologic techniques.[402] The disorders were represented by variable abnormalities in receptor sensitivity, central processing, and sensory neuropathy, and there was no correlation between manometric diagnosis and abnormal neurophysiology.

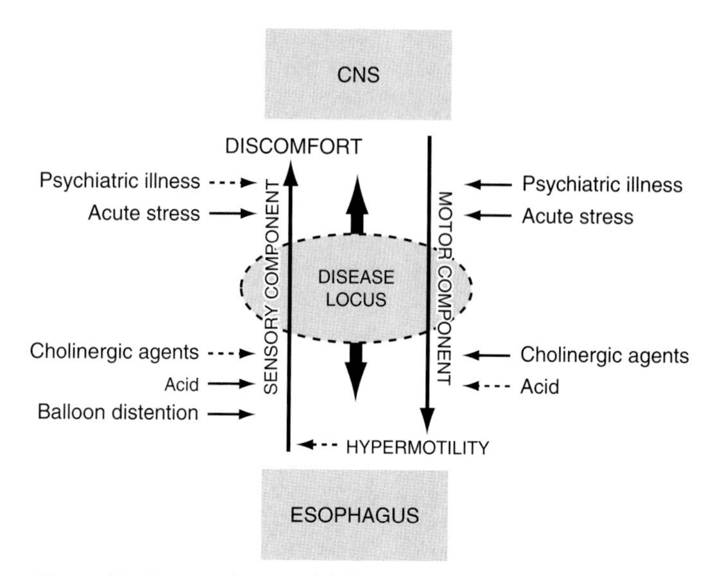

Figure 32–13. A working model displaying types of dysfunction found in patients with chest symptoms and spastic disorders. The location of pathology in these disorders (disease locus) is not known and may vary within the brain-gut axis from patient to patient. Both motor and sensory components are identified, and the two processes may not be involved equally in all cases. A variety of stimuli or provoking situations are associated with (—) or suspected of affecting (---) the sensory and motor limbs of this model. Esophageal hypermotility may produce symptoms directly, possibly further activate the sensory limb, or be just a marker for the underlying process. CNS, central nervous system.

Clinical Manifestations (see also Chapter 6)

While these motility disorders have been detected in all age groups, the mean age at presentation is approximately 40 years. A female predominance exists among patients with hypermotility contraction wave abnormalities as the sole findings.[403] Of patients presenting for manometric evaluation and subsequently diagnosed with a spastic disorder, chest pain is reported by 80% to 90%. The pain generally is retrosternal, may radiate directly into the back, and often is more severe than the recurrent pain characteristic of coronary artery disease. A dull residual discomfort persisting after the severe episode abates helps differentiate the pain from angina. Pain episodes may last from minutes to hours, and swallowing generally is not impaired during the episodes. Dysphagia is reported by 30% to 60% of patients with spastic findings.[403, 404] This symptom is intermittent, varying on a daily basis from mild to very severe. It does not usually have a direct relationship to chest pain, but it is often more severe during periods when pain is more frequent or severe. Regurgitation of a food or liquid bolus into the mouth or nasopharynx may accompany dysphagia but is infrequent in comparison with achalasia. In addition, in contrast to achalasia, dysphagia generally is neither progressive nor severe enough to cause weight loss. Heartburn is a component of the syndrome in as many as 20% of patients.[403]

The disparity between symptoms and manometric findings is pronounced. Mechanisms other than motor dysfunction contribute to the clinical presentation and complicate attempts at a concise clinical description. In fact, the chest pain reported by patients with spastic disorders may not only be unrelated to motor dysfunction, it may be originating from non-esophageal sites—further adding to the vague clinical picture. Other gastrointestinal symptoms typical of functional bowel disorders are reported with relatively high prevalence. Symptoms of psychological dysfunction, particularly those of anxiety and depression, are also common.[401]

Diagnosis

These diagnoses are commonly encountered when dysphagia, chest pain, or both are reported with the vague and inconsistent history outlined previously. Because of the poor specificity of manometric findings for an esophageal source of chest pain, esophageal testing has not alleviated the need for careful consideration and exclusion of potentially coexisting disorders. The pain can mimic coronary artery disease sufficiently that extensive cardiac evaluation is commonly required (see Chapter 6).

Radiologic Findings

A barium study of the esophagus with fluoroscopy can reveal abnormalities consistent with these diagnoses and at times can demonstrate the direct association of faulty transit with symptoms. This demonstration has important treatment implications. Frequent, nonpropulsive contractions may indent the barium column in the smooth muscle portion of the esophagus. These indentations are produced by dysfunctional circular muscle contractions that, in extreme situations, trap barium between powerfully contracted segments. Transit of barium from the esophagus may be markedly delayed as the contractions produce a kneading effect. This distorted radiographic appearance has been described as a "corkscrew esophagus," a "rosary bead esophagus," or as esophageal "curling" (Fig. 32–14) and is associated with more severe manometric abnormalities. Few radiographic findings are present during fluoroscopy in patients with nutcracker esophagus or related nonspecific spastic disorders. In all cases, uncoordinated postswallow contractions are intermixed with swallows that have a normal appearance. Sliding hiatal hernias appear to be more frequent in patients with the spastic disorders, possibly because of esophageal shortening during intense muscle contraction.[405]

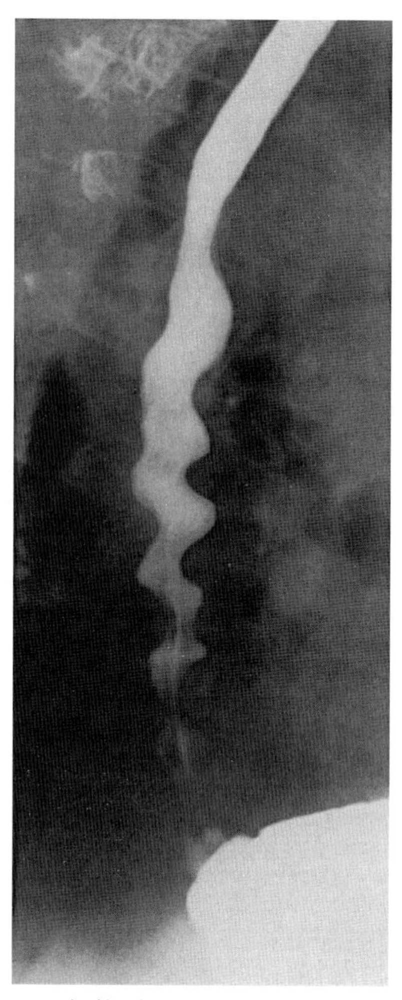

Figure 32–14. A single film from an esophagogram demonstrates broad muscular indentations, producing the configuration of "corkscrew esophagus." This patient was asymptomatic despite the fact that this configuration was observed on multiple swallows.

Endoscopy

No features are typical of these disorders, and the endoscopic appearance is normal. The test may detect alternative explanations for symptoms, such as esophagitis or stricture.

Manometric Features

Manometric findings are restricted to the smooth muscle portion of the esophagus and are most pronounced in its distal half and at the LES. High-resolution, topographic manometry demonstrates their focus on the segment within the esophageal body having greatest inhibitory nerve influence.[406] Several types of abnormalities have been described, and each may have a different underlying mechanism. These findings are (1) nonperistaltic (simultaneous) contractions after many or most swallows, (2) abnormalities of the contraction wave characteristics (e.g., increased amplitude or duration and frequency of multipeaked waveforms), and (3) hypertension or poor relaxation of the LES.[200] Sporadic, long periods of intense or repetitive contractions, at times associated with baseline pressure elevations, may also fit into this category but are infrequently detected.

The first of these findings is the most consistent criterion in the various definitions of diffuse esophageal spasm. Although the simultaneous contraction sequences are often without contraction wave abnormalities,[407] multipeaked or repetitive contractions follow the initial nonperistaltic contraction response in more exaggerated forms (Fig. 32–15). Swallows with normal propagation are also seen during the study, differentiating the tracing from aperistalsis, as in achalasia. When at least 10% of wet swallows are followed by nonperistaltic sequences, some degree of abnormal motor function is present.[122, 230] The diagnosis of diffuse esophageal spasm is often reserved for patients who have nonperistaltic responses after 30% or more of the swallows. This threshold is arbitrary, however. Studies with concurrent ma-

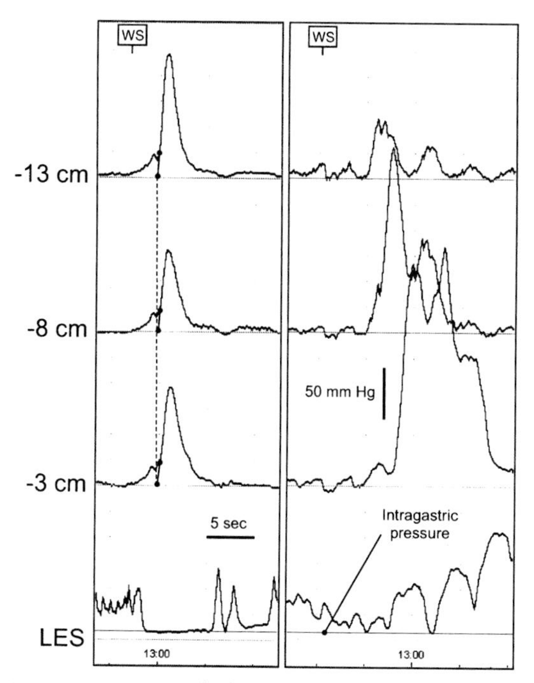

Figure 32–15. Manometric findings recorded from the lower esophageal sphincter (LES) and three sites in the smooth muscle esophageal body in two patients with spastic disorders. A swallow demonstrating a nonperistaltic response with simultaneous contraction onset across several recording sites is shown in the left panel. This is the defining abnormality in diffuse esophageal spasm. Contraction onset is measured from the extrapolated start of the rapid upstroke for each wave. In the right panel, a swallow is followed by vigorous contraction wave abnormalities typical of nonspecific spastic disorders. The waves in the distal esophagus are of high amplitude with broad duration and have multipeaked configuration. LES relaxation is also abnormal qualitatively. WS, wet swallow.

nometry and videofluoroscopy show that a propagation velocity exceeding 6.25 cm/sec is sufficient to produce abnormal bolus transit[408]; on the contrary, some apparently simultaneous sequences are not representative of abnormal bolus transit.[236]

The remainder of the hypermotility disorders collectively can be termed nonspecific spastic disorders, although not all authorities have agreed on this nosology (see Fig. 32–7).[200] Many patients with the clinical features described have only the second type of abnormality that involves the contraction wave configuration.[230, 409] These contraction wave abnormalities are most severe near the LES, are not observed in the skeletal muscle portion of the esophagus, and are defined as exceeding normal limits established from asymptomatic control populations.[308] Increased wave amplitude, increased wave duration, and presence of triple-peaked contraction waves are interrelated findings in this category.[308] Excessive occurrence of double-peaked contraction waves is also represented in the contraction wave abnormalities, but some double-peaked waves are detected in normal persons.[230, 231, 406] The measured waves may be mildly distorted, or they may have all features to an exaggerated degree. All combinations of these contraction wave abnormalities are found in patients referred for manometry, but symptoms correlate poorly with manometric findings. The term *nutcracker esophagus* has been applied to the subgroup with a marked increase in contraction amplitude.[409] Long-term manometry and repeat manometric evaluations show that this pattern of contraction wave abnormalities and the pattern of diffuse esophageal spasm have some interconvertability.[410] Cluster analysis of a large number of patient tracings does not segregate the nonspecific spastic disorders from diffuse esophageal spasm, further supporting their similarities.[233]

Hypermotility characteristics of the LES commonly coexist with spastic abnormalities in the esophageal body. An elevation in resting LES pressure is seen in at least one third of patients with more severe derangements.[308, 411] Poor relaxation of the LES has been detected in some patients,[230, 412] but this is a less common feature. Both findings may occur without other hypermotility characteristics and have been associated with the symptomatic state.[308, 413] Incomplete LES relaxation without aperistalsis can be an early feature of achalasia, although very few progress to manifest this disease. This finding is also present in some patients with Chagas' disease and very occasionally after vagotomy.[414]

Other Tests

Tests to provoke chest pain have not helped in determining whether the spastic disorders are actually responsible for the symptoms. Three provocative tests are most commonly used: (1) intraluminal hydrochloric acid, (2) intravenous edrophonium chloride (most typically 80 μg/kg), and (3) esophageal balloon distention. The provocation of pain is too independent of motor events to clarify the role of hypermotility in symptom production[415] (see Chapter 6). Radionuclide transit studies may demonstrate disorganized bolus transit in some patients, but the test has not contributed sufficiently to diagnosis for routine use in these patients. Ambulatory motility monitoring has been used primarily for chest pain evaluation and demonstrates an association of motility events with chest pain in a small number of patients.[416, 417] Disagreement regarding the correct way to analyze the tracings persists, and this type of study remains investigational.

Treatment

Except in rare cases, these disorders are not progressive or fatal, and treatment is directed at symptom reduction. Because of the difficulties in establishing the direct role of the motor abnormalities in producing symptoms, it behooves the clinician to thoroughly consider other potential diagnoses (e.g., cardiac disease) and to refrain from overly aggressive management tactics. If the symptoms are primarily those of abnormal transit (dysphagia, regurgitation), treatments similar to those used for achalasia may be of benefit. This is particularly true if delayed bolus or barium-pill transit is demonstrated on radiographic studies, if the defect is primarily at the level of the LES, and/or if incomplete LES relaxation is detected on manometric evaluation. Of course, careful exclusion of other mechanical obstructive processes must be performed. Pharmacotherapy with smooth muscle relaxants may be particularly helpful in these cases, whereas this approach is of inconsistent benefit for other patients with unexplained symptoms and these motor disorders. Ingestion of warm liquids with meals may be helpful for some, as might simple bougienage.[213, 418]

Unfortunately, the principal symptom encountered is otherwise unexplained pain, and establishing a direct relationship of the motor disorder to the pain is only occasionally possible. In these patients, a systematic exclusion of other potentially relevant processes, including reflux disease, is a priority and often helpful (see Chapters 6 and 33). For those whose symptoms remain unexplained, a series of therapeutic trials may be worthwhile. In uncontrolled trials, short- and long-acting nitrate preparations have reduced pain and improved manometric or radiographic patterns in some patients.[419, 420] Isosorbide dinitrate, 5 to 10 mg sublingually, can be tried. These medications are thought to be beneficial because of their relaxant effects on smooth muscle, although the effects on manometric parameters may actually be minimal. Anecdotal reports also support trying a calcium channel blocker as an alternative smooth muscle relaxant. A controlled trial in patients with high-amplitude contractions, however, did not support a benefit of nifedipine over placebo in reduction of chest pain (their major presenting symptom) despite significant effects on motility.[421]

Antidepressant regimens are of proven benefit in patients with unexplained chest pain, with or without hypermotility findings. The severity of manometric abnormality does not appear to predict response. A double-blind, controlled trial with trazodone hydrochloride at 100 to 150 mg/day produced global improvement and reduced distress from esophageal symptoms in patients with nonspecific spastic disorders.[422] The overall improvement was not dependent on any change in manometric pattern during the course of the study. Imipramine at a bedtime dose of 50 mg was superior to placebo in two separate studies,[423, 424] the benefit being unrelated to the presence of or change in manometric findings when examined.[423] Although most experience has involved tricyclic antidepressants, a recent report demonstrated utility of a contemporary antidepressant, sertraline, on chest pain.[425] Esophageal motility abnormalities, if present, were not described in that study. Symptoms in patients with diffuse esophageal spasm who fail other treatment efforts also may respond to antidepressant regimens, open-label response being reported for clomipramine and trazodone.[426] Tricyclic antidepressants, in particular, have many effects that might be useful in pain management,[427] but the benefits do not appear related to improved mood in the reported studies that typically have used low daily dosages. Prolonged symptomatic remissions can be achieved in more than three-quarters of patients with initially favorable responses to these drugs.[428] Transcutaneous electrical nerve stimulation, another approach used for chronic pain syndromes, may have a role in some patients.[429]

At present, it is unknown which patients might be better candidates for one type of treatment (e.g., calcium channel blockers) or another (e.g., antidepressants). If several different medications fail, more aggressive treatment can be considered but at a minimum should be reserved for patients with refractory symptoms. Bougienage generally is ineffective. Pneumatic dilation of the LES reportedly helps 40% of patients with severe manometric abnormalities, its greatest effect being, not surprisingly, on dysphagia.[430] As for the management of transit symptoms, pneumatic dilation is more appropriate for pain patients having incomplete relaxation of the LES.[412] This subgroup may be more closely related to achalasia,[394] and there is no evidence that the complications of pneumatic dilation are more common in these patients than in those with achalasia. Nevertheless, the trend is to try medical management, such as antidepressants, before resorting to mechanical treatments. Long esophagomyotomy extending above the level of muscular thickening (usually to the level of the aortic arch) reportedly has been successful in severe cases and even when manometry has revealed only nonspecific spastic disorders.[431] Success rates exceeding 50% have been described, but the long-term surgical results for pain management are not good.[432] Myotomy for pain with spastic disorders should certainly be reserved for patients in whom manometry or radiography has convincingly and reliably linked pain to abnormal motor activity.

ESOPHAGEAL HYPOMOTILITY

Esophageal Hypomotility Associated with Systemic Disease

Scleroderma and Other Connective Tissue Diseases

Scleroderma frequently involves the esophagus (see Chapter 29).[433] As many as 74% of patients with typical skin manifestations will have evidence of esophageal involvement at autopsy, and clinical involvement may exceed this rate.[258] Light microscopy demonstrates muscle atrophy and fibrosis that affect predominantly the smooth muscle region of the esophagus. The end result is severe hypomotility: failure of muscle contraction in the distal esophagus and incompetency of the LES. In some patients with this connective tissue disease, the esophageal muscle may still be sensitive to cholinergic stimulation, which suggests that neural dysfunction might have preceded muscle atrophy and fibrosis.[435] Similarly, normal reactivity of smooth muscle but impaired neural responses has been demonstrated in both the small and large intestine in early cases of scleroderma. Despite additional evidence in the esophagus that physiologic motor disturbances precede histologic change, a distinct neuropathologic lesion has not been described in the esophagus or other parts of the gut. Inflammatory infiltrates composed of mast cells and eosinophils are found in skin lesions early in the course of this disease and have been detected in close association with intestinal neural plexuses[436]; this finding may have relevance to physiologic observations.

Clinical features of esophageal involvement by scleroderma include symptoms of heartburn and dysphagia. Although the degree of motor dysfunction is often profound, these symptoms are reported by less than half of patients and typically do not surface for at least 5 years following diagnosis of the connective tissue disease.[437] Esophageal hyposensitivity accompanying the hypomotility likely is responsible. Gastroesophageal reflux is pronounced because of loss of LES competency in conjunction with poor esophageal clearance. Evidence of esophageal involvement may actually be present on plain films of the chest. Dysphagia may result from the motor disturbance itself or from a stricture complicating reflux.[437] Barium studies further clarify the loss of normal motility (Fig. 32–16) and also may provide evidence of esophagitis or stricture. A barium swallow with videofluoroscopy has high accuracy in differentiating the motor dysfunction of severe hypomotility from other advanced motor disorders, such as achalasia—at least in the research setting.[438]

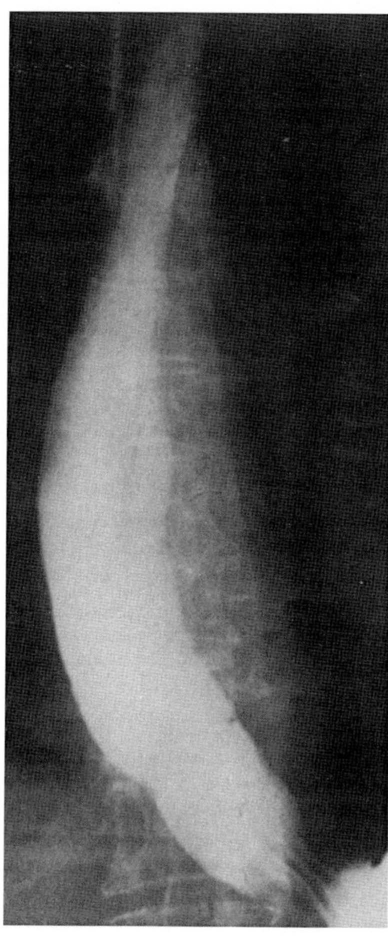

Figure 32–16. An atonic esophagus with wide patency of the lower esophageal sphincter region in a patient with scleroderma and esophageal involvement. Free reflux to the thoracic inlet was readily demonstrated, as was complete absence of a primary peristaltic stripping wave.

Manometry in the patient with scleroderma will show abnormalities both in the smooth muscle portion of the esophageal body and in the LES (Fig. 32–17). Dysfunction in the esophageal body becomes evident before the loss of LES tone, and reduction in contraction strength precedes the aperistalsis of advanced involvement. The combination of aperistalsis in the smooth muscle region of the esophageal body with hypotension of the LES is so typical that it has been labeled scleroderma esophagus.[230] From a diagnostic standpoint, the pattern is not specific as fewer than 40% of patients identified at a motility laboratory with these findings have any evidence of connective tissue disease.[439] Radionuclide transit studies correlate well with manometry in scleroderma, and these well-tolerated tests may have some utility in staging the disease.

Treatment cannot reverse the esophageal motor abnormalities in scleroderma and is directed toward gastroesophageal reflux and its complications. Dysphagia without stricture may also improve with treatment of reflux esophagitis. Conventional antireflux therapy should be used, and typical medical maneuvers are beneficial (see Chapter 33). Management should be aggressive, in view of the predisposition of this group to serious complications. Stricture formation also seems to be more insidious in scleroderma patients than in others with gastroesophageal reflux and may occur without a history of significant heartburn. Antireflux surgery has been discouraged because it potentially may worsen the dysphagia. Despite this concern, good results have been reported, and such management could be considered in exceptionally refractory cases (see Chapter 33).[440]

Esophageal features similar to those described for scleroderma have been seen in other connective tissue diseases, especially those that overlap with typical scleroderma (CREST syndrome [calcinosis, Raynaud's phenomenon, esophageal motility disorders, sclerodactyly, and telangiectasia], polymyositis, dermatomyositis, mixed connective tissue disease).[441, 442] Esophageal motor abnormalities are most likely when Raynaud's phenomenon is a component of the connective tissue disease manifestations, but primary Raynaud's disease is less likely to influence motility and esophageal emptying times than scleroderma.[435, 443]

Diabetes Mellitus (see also Chapter 29)

Abnormalities in esophageal motility are frequently detected in patients with diabetes mellitus when they are studied with either radiography or manometry (see Chapter 29).[395] The direct relation of these abnormalities to the metabolic disease remains uncertain. More than 60% of diabetic persons with evidence of peripheral or autonomic neuropathy may have disordered motility, but symptoms are reported by a minority of these patients. Radiographic studies reveal failure of the

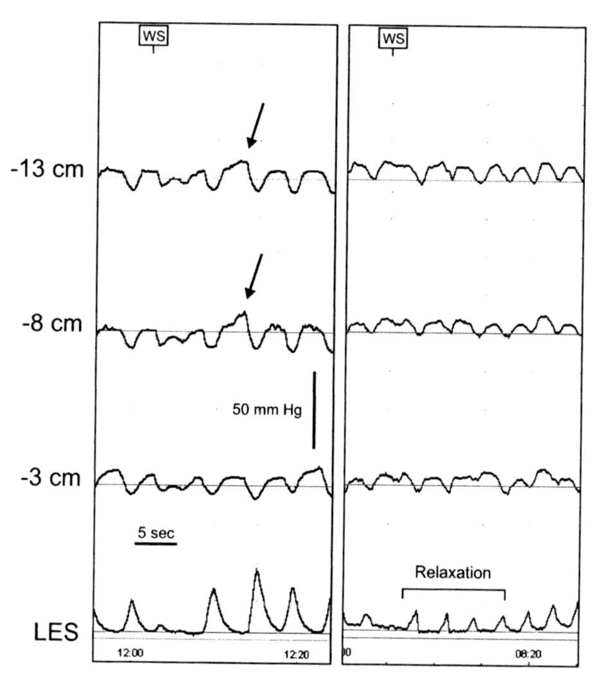

Figure 32–17. Manometric tracings from patients with severe esophageal hypomotility, one with scleroderma (*right panel*) and one idiopathic (*left panel*). The catheter is recording from the level of the lower esophageal sphincter (LES) and three proximal sites in the smooth muscle region. Minimal contractile response superimposed on respiratory variation is appreciated in one swallow (*arrows*), but its progressive nature cannot be determined. Crural diaphragmatic indentations are superimposed on very low (*right panel*) or absent (*left panel*) resting LES pressure preceding the swallow, but end-expiratory sphincter pressure reaches or remains at gastric baseline pressure with swallowing in each instance. WS, wet swallow.

stripping wave in some cases and yield findings suggestive of a hypermotility disorder in others. Manometry also has demonstrated failed contraction sequences[444] as well as the contraction abnormalities seen with the hypermotility disorders.[395, 445] Vagal neuropathy has been proposed as the cause of these findings, but histologic evidence is meager. Although features of both hypermotility and hypomotility have been observed in diabetic patients, reductions in contraction amplitude and duration appear to have the most significant independent association with advancing diabetes.[395]

Other Diseases

Disordered esophageal motility has been described in association with a variety of diseases that are not restricted to the esophagus. A direct relationship between the motor abnormalities and the systemic disease is often incompletely proved. A reduction in distal contraction amplitudes can be observed with hypothyroidism, chronic alcoholism, amyloidosis, and chronic idiopathic intestinal pseudo-obstruction. The defect can be severe enough that no measurable waves can be detected in some of these disorders (see Chapters 29 and 111). In addition to the disorders known to produce oropharyngeal dysphagia, steroid myopathy and alcoholic myopathy may interfere with function of the striated muscle portion of the esophagus.[446, 447]

Idiopathic Hypomotility

The contraction strength in the distal esophageal body gradually decays with aging.[448] However, most of the clinically relevant hypomotility is encountered in the symptomatic gastroesophageal reflux population.[449] Varying degrees of hypomotility in the esophageal body and LES are common in this group that has no evidence of systemic illness to explain the findings (see Chapter 33). Low distal wave amplitudes (<30 mm Hg) or nontransmitted contractions after at least 30% of wet swallows are the most common indicators of hypomotility in the esophageal body and have been labeled ineffective esophageal motility by some investigators.[450] These hypomotility features occur more often in patients with atypical reflux manifestations (e.g., cough, asthma) than in patients with heartburn,[450] a finding reflecting the association of hypomotility with hyposensitivity. Hypomotility accompanying reflux disease typically is fixed and does not normalize with effective antireflux treatment. Some degree of peristaltic improvement occurs following antireflux surgery, a finding resulting from mechanical effects of the obstructing fundoplication rather than healing of esophagitis.[451] Segregating patients by degree of hypomotility in the esophageal body has been used by some to tailor antireflux surgery. The need for this remains controversial, as several case series suggest that dysphagia following fundoplication is not dependent on this preoperative measurement.[452]

The principal outcome of hypomotility is gastroesophageal reflux disease, but similar processes in the esophageal body may contribute to food bolus impaction and promote other consequences of poor esophageal transit—such as pill-induced caustic damage (see Chapter 34).[453–455] The unsuspected presence of esophageal hypomotility may help explain the limited value of intravenous glucagon in resolution of food bolus impactions. The reduction in LES pressure produced by glucagon is accompanied by reduction of contractile strength in the esophageal body, potentially countering positive benefits.[456]

REFERENCES

1. Goyal RK, Sivarao DV: Functional anatomy and physiology of swallowing and esophageal motility. In Castell DO, Richter JE (eds): The Esophagus, 3rd ed. Philadelphia: Lippincott Williams & Wilkins, 1999, p 31.
2. Jean A: Brain stem control of swallowing: Neuronal network and cellular mechanisms. Physiol Rev 81:929, 2001.
3. Carpenter DO: Central nervous system mechanisms in deglutition and emesis. In Schultz SG, Wood JD, Rauner BB (eds): Handbook of Physiology. Section 6: The Gastrointestinal System. Bethesda, Md: American Physiological Society, 1989, p 685.
4. Bieger D: Central nervous system control of swallowing: A neuropharmacological perspective. Dysphagia 8:308, 1993.
5. Diamant NE: Regulation and dysregulation of esophageal motor function. In Janssens J (ed): Progress in Understanding and Management of Gastrointestinal Motility Disorders. Belgium: University of Leuven, 1993, p 85.
6. Jean A: Brainstem control of swallowing: Localization and organization of the central pattern generator for swallowing. In Taylor A (ed): Neurophysiology of the Jaws and Teeth. New York: Mc Millan Press, 1990, p 294.
7. Meyer GW, Austin RM, Brady CE, et al: Muscle anatomy of the human esophagus. J Clin Gastroenterol 8:131, 1986.
8. Stacher G, Schmierer G, Landgraf M: Tertiary esophageal contractions evoked by acoustical stimuli. Gastroenterology 77:49, 1979.
9. Dent J, Dodds WJ, Friedman RH, et al: Mechanism of gastroesophageal reflux in recumbent asymptomatic human subjects. J Clin Invest 65:256, 1980.
10. Sumi T: Role of the pontine reticular formation in the neural organization of deglutition. Jpn J Physiol 22:295, 1972.
11. Hamdy S, Aziz Q, Rothwell JC, et al: The cortical topography of human swallowing musculature in health and disease. Nature 2:1217, 1996.
12. Hamdy S, Rothwell JC, Aziz O, et al: Long-term reorganization of human motor cortex driven by short-term sensory stimulation. Nat Neurosci 1:64, 1998.
13. Diamant NE: Firing up the swallowing mechanism. Nat Med 2:1190, 1996.
14. Valdez DT, Salapatek AM, Niznik G, et al: Swallowing and upper esophageal sphincter contraction with transcranial magnetic-induced electrical stimulation. Am J Physiol 264:G213, 1993.
15. Hamdy S, Xue S, Valdez D, et al: Induction of cortical swallowing activity by transcranial magnetic stimulation in the anaesthetized cat. Neurogastroenterol Motil 13:65, 2001.
16. Hamdy S, Aziz Q, Rothwell JC, et al: Recovery of swallowing after dysphagic stroke relates to functional reorganization in the intact motor complex. Gastroenterology 115:1104, 1998.
17. Carpenter DO: Central nervous system mechanisms in deglutition and emesis. In Schultz SG, Wood JD, Rauner BB (eds): Handbook of Physiology. The Gastrointestinal System 1. Baltimore: Waverly Press, 1989, p 685.
18. Doty RW: Neural organization of deglutition. In Code CF (ed): Handbook of Physiology. Section 6: Alimentary Canal. Washington, DC: American Physiological Society, 1968, p 1861.
19. Randich A, Gebhart GF: Vagal afferent modulation of nociception. Brain Res Brain Res Rev 17:77, 1992.
20. Sengupta JN, Saha JK, Goyal RK: Stimulus-response function studies of esophageal mechanosensitive nociceptors in sympathetic afferents of opossum. J Neurophysiol 64:796, 1990.
21. Collman PI, Tremblay L, Diamant NE: Distribution of vagal and spinal sensory neurons to the esophagus of the cat. Gastroenterology 100:A432, 1991.
22. Jean A: Brainstem organization of the swallowing network. Brain Behav Evol 25:109, 1984.
23. Salducci J, Naudy B: Dissociation between the electrical activity of the diaphragmatic dome and crura muscular fibers during esophageal distension, vomiting and eructation. J Physiol (Paris) 74:541, 1978.

24. Mittal RK, Fisher MJ: Electrical and mechanical inhibition of the crural diaphragm during transient relaxation of the lower esophageal sphincter. Gastroenterology 99:1265, 1990.
25. Jean A: Localization and activity of medullary swallowing neurones. J Physiol (Paris) 64:227, 1972.
26. Bieger D: Neuropharmacologic correlates of deglutition: Lessons from fictive swallowing. Dysphagia 6:147, 1991.
27. Broussard DL, Lynn RB, Wiedner EB, et al: Solitarial premotor neuron projections to the rat esophagus and pharynx: Implications for control of swallowing. Gastroenterology 114:1268, 1998.
28. Lu WY, Bieger D: Vagovagal reflex motility patterns of the rat esophagus. Am J Physiol 274:R1425, 1998.
29. Kessler JP, Jean A: Identification of the medullary swallowing regions in the rat. Exp Brain Res 57:256, 1985.
30. Jean A: Control of the central swallowing program by inputs from the peripheral receptors. A review. J Auton Nerv Syst 10:225, 1984.
31. Shaker R, Ren J, Zamir Z, et al: Effect of aging, position, and temperature on the threshold volume triggering pharyngeal swallows. Gastroenterology 107:396, 1994.
32. Martino R: Dysphagia in a patient with lateral medullary syndrome: Insight into the central control of swallowing. Gastroenterology (in press), 2001.
33. Beyak MJ, Xue S, Collman PI, et al: Central nervous system nitric oxide induces oropharyngeal swallowing and esophageal peristalsis in the cat. Gastroenterology 119:377, 2000.
34. Bieger D: Muscarinic activation of rhombencephalic neurones controlling oesophageal peristalsis in the rat. Neuropharmacology 23:1451, 1984.
35. Lu WY, Bieger D: Vagal afferent transmission in the NTS mediating reflex responses of the rat esophagus. Am J Physiol 274:R1436, 1998.
36. Greenwood B, Blank E, Dodds WJ: Nicotine stimulates esophageal peristaltic contractions in cats by a central mechanism. Am J Physiol 262:G567, 1992.
37. Wang YT, Bieger D: Role of solitarial GABAergic mechanisms in control of swallowing. Am J Physiol 261:R639, 1991.
38. Kessler JP, Cherkaoui N, Catalin D, et al: Swallowing responses induced by microinjection of glutamate and glutamate agonists into the nucleus tractus solitarius of ketamine-anesthetized rats. Exp Brain Res 83:151, 1990.
39. Kessler JP, Jean A: Evidence that activation of N-methyl-D-aspartate (NMDA) and non-NMDA receptors within the nucleus tractus solitarii triggers swallowing. Eur J Pharmacol 201:59, 1991.
40. Broussard DL, Bao X, Altschuler SM: Somatostatin immunoreactivity in esophageal premotor neurons of the rat. Neurosci Lett 250:201, 1998.
41. Cunningham ET Jr, Sawchenko PE: A circumscribed projection from the nucleus of the solitary tract to the nucleus ambiguus in the rat: Anatomical evidence for somatostatin-28-immunoreactive interneurons subserving reflex control of esophageal motility. J Neurosci 9:1668, 1989.
42. Roman C, Gonella J: Extrinsic control of digestive tract motility. In Johnson LR (ed): Physiology of the gastrointestinal tract. New York: Raven, 1987, p 507.
43. Rossiter CD, Norman WP, Jain M, et al: Control of lower esophageal sphincter pressure by two sites in dorsal motor nucleus of the vagus. Am J Physiol 259:G899, 1990.
44. Collman PI, Tremblay L, Diamant NE: The central vagal efferent supply to the esophagus and lower esophageal sphincter of the cat. Gastroenterology 104:1430, 1993.
45. Collman PI, Tremblay L, Diamant NE: Distribution of sympathetic neurons innervating the striated, smooth muscle and LES regions of the cat esophagus. Gastroenterology 99:1209, 1990.
46. Gonella J, Niel JP, Roman C: Sympathetic control of lower oesophageal sphincter motility in the cat. J Physiol London 287:177, 1979.
47. Gonella J, Niel JP, Roman C: Mechanism of the noradrenergic motor control on the lower oesophageal sphincter in the cat. J Physiol London 306:251, 1980.
48. Baumgarten HG, Lange W: Adrenergic innervation of the oesophagus in the cat (Felis domestica) and Rhesus monkey (Macacus rhesus). Z Zellforsch Mikrosk Anat 95:529, 1995.
49. Christensen J: The oesophagus. In Christensen J, Wingate DL (eds): A Guide to Gastrointestinal Motility. London: Wright PSG, 1983, p 75.
50. Rodrigo J, Hernandez CJ, Vidal MA, et al: Vegetative innervation of the esophagus. II. Intraganglionic laminar endings. Acta Anat (Basel) 92:79, 1975.
51. Toyama T, Yokoyama I, Nishi K: Effects of hexamethonium and other ganglionic blocking agents on electrical activity of the esophagus induced by vagal stimulation in the dog. Eur J Pharmacol 31:63, 1975.
52. Zhou DS, Desaki J, Komuro T: Neuro-muscular junctions of longitudinal and circular muscle fibers of the guinea-pig esophagus and their relation to myenteric plexus. J Auton Nerv Syst 58:63, 1996.
53. Sang Q, Young HM: Development of nicotinic receptor clusters and innervation accompanying the change in muscle phenotype in the mouse esophagus. J Compar Neurol 386:119, 1997.
54. Neuhuber WL, Worl J, Berthoud HR, et al: NADPH-diaphorase-positive nerve fibers associated with motor endplates in the rat esophagus: New evidence for co-innervation of striated muscle by enteric neurons. Cell Tiss Res 276:23, 1994.
55. Singaram C, Sengupta A, Sweet MA, et al: Nitrinergic and peptidergic innervation of the human oesophagus. Gut 35:1690, 1994.
56. Morikawa S, Komuro T: Distribution of myenteric NO neurons along the guinea-pig esophagus. J Auton Nerv Syst 74:91, 1998.
57. Mann CV, Code CF, Schlegel JF, et al: Intrinsic mechanisms controlling the mammalian gastro-oesophageal sphincter deprived of extrinsic nerve supply. Thorax 23:634, 1968.
58. Reynolds RPE, El-Sharkawy TY, Diamant NE: Lower esophageal sphincter function in the cat: Role of central innervation assessed by transient vagal blockade. Am J Physiol 246:G666, 1984.
59. Yamamoto T: Histological studies on the innervation of the esophagus in Formosan macaque. Arch Histol Jpn 18:545, 1960.
60. Seelig LL Jr, Doody P, Brainard L, et al: Acetylcholinesterase and choline acetyltransferase staining of neurons in the opossum esophagus. Anat Rec 209:125, 1984.
61. Kressel M, Radespiel-Troger M: Anterograde tracing and immunohistochemical characterization of potentially mechanosensitive vagal afferents in the esophagus. J Comp Neurol 412:161, 1999.
62. Diamant NE, El-Sharkawy TY: Neural control of esophageal peristalsis. A conceptual analysis. Gastroenterology 72:546, 1977.
63. Dodds WJ, Stef JJ, Stewart ET, et al: Responses of feline esophagus to cervical vagal stimulation. Am J Physiol 235:E63, 1978.
64. Dodds WJ, Christensen J, Dent J, et al: Esophageal contractions induced by vagal stimulation in the opossum. Am J Physiol 235:E392, 1978.
65. Gilbert R, Rattan S, Goyal RK: Pharmacologic identification, activation and antagonism of two muscarine receptor subtypes in the lower esophageal sphincter. J Pharmacol Exp Ther 230:284, 1984.
66. Crist J, Gidda JS, Goyal RK: Intramural mechanism of esophageal peristalsis: Roles of cholinergic and noncholinergic nerves. Proc Natl Acad Sci USA 81:3595, 1984.
67. Gilbert RJ, Dodds WJ: Effect of selective muscarinic antagonists on peristaltic contractions in opossum smooth muscle. Am J Physiol 250: G50, 1986.
68. Yamato S, Spechler SJ, Goyal RK: Role of nitric oxide in esophageal peristalsis in the opossum. Gastroenterology 103:197, 1992.
69. Tottrup A, Svane D, Forman A: Nitric oxide mediating NANC inhibition in opossum lower esophageal sphincter. Am J Physiol 260:G385, 1991.
70. Anand N, Paterson WG: Role of nitric oxide in esophageal peristalsis. Am J Physiol 266:G123, 1994.
71. Singaram C, Sengupta A, Sugarbaker DJ, et al: Peptidergic innervation of the human esophageal smooth muscle. Gastroenterology 101: 1256, 1991.
72. Wattchow DA, Furness JB, Costa M, et al: Distributions of neuropeptides in the human esophagus. Gastroenterology 93:1363, 1987.
73. Goyal RK, Rattan S: Neurohumoral, hormonal, and drug receptors for the lower esophageal sphincter. Gastroenterology 74:598, 1978.
74. Goyal RK, Rattan S, Said SI: VIP as a possible neurotransmitter of non-cholinergic non-adrenergic inhibitory neurones. Nature 288:378, 1980.
75. Aggestrup S, Uddman R, Jensen SL, et al: Regulatory peptides in the lower esophageal sphincter of man. Regul Pept 10:167, 1985.
76. Blackshaw LA, Staunton E, Lehmann A, et al: Inhibition of transient LES relaxations and reflux in ferrets by GABA receptor agonists. Am J Physiol 277:G867, 1999.
77. Lecoin L, Gabella G, LeDouarin N: Origin of the c-kit-positive interstitial cells in the avian bowel. Development 122:725, 1996.
78. Daniel EE, Posey-Daniel V: Neuromuscular structures in opossum esophagus: Role of interstitial cells of Cajal. Am J Physiol 246:G305, 1984.

79. Berezin I, Daniel EE, Huizinga JD: Ultrastructure of interstitial cells of cajal in the canine distal esophagus. Can J Physiol Pharmacol 72: 1049, 1993.
80. Christensen J, Rick GA, Soll DJ: Intramural nerves and interstitial cells revealed by the Champy-Maillet stain in the opossum esophagus. J Auton Nerv Syst 19:137, 1987.
81. Faussone-Pellegrini MS, Cortesini C: Ultrastructural features and localization of the interstitial cells of cajal in the smooth muscle coat of human esophagus. J Submicrosc Cytol 17:187, 1985.
82. Daniel EE, Berezin I: Interstitial cells of cajal. Are the major players in control of gastrointestinal motility? J Gastrointest Motil 4:1, 1992.
83. Sanders KM: A case for interstitial cells of cajal as pacemakers and mediators of neurotransmission in the gastrointestinal tract. Gastroenterology 111:492, 1996
84. Huizinga JD, Thuneberg L, Vanderwinden J-M, et al: Interstitial cells of cajal as targets for pharmacological intervention in gastrointestinal motor disorders. Trends Pharmacol Sci 18:393, 1997.
85. Jacobowitz DA-N P Jr: The autonomic innervation of the esophagus of the dog. J Thorac Cardiovasc Surg 58:678, 1969.
86. Lyrenas E, Abrahamsson H: Beta adrenergic influence on oesophageal peristalsis in man. Gut 27:260, 1986.
87. Mayer EA, Gebhart GF: Basic and clinical aspects of visceral hyperalgesia. Gastroenterology 107:271, 1994.
88. Aziz Q, Thompson DG: Brain-gut axis in health and disease. Gastroenterology 114:559, 1998.
89. Gebhart GF: Pathobiology of visceral pain: Molecular mechanisms and therapeutic implications IV. Visceral afferent contributions to the pathobiology of visceral pain. Am J Physiol 278:G834, 2000.
90. Rodrigo J, Hernandez CJ, Vidal MA, et al: Vegetative innervation of the esophagus. III. Intraepithelial endings. Acta Anat (Basel) 92:242, 1975.
91. Clerc N, Condamin M: Selective labeling of vagal sensory nerve fibers in the lower esophageal sphincter with anterogradely transported WGA-HRP. Brain Res 424:216, 1987.
92. Mazzia C, Clerc N: Ultrastructural analysis of spinal primary afferent fibers within the circular muscle of the cat lower esophageal sphincter. Histochem Cell Biol 113:235, 2000.
93. Kreulen DL, Szurszewski JH: Reflex pathways in the abdominal prevertebral ganglia: Evidence for a colo-colonic inhibitory reflex. J Physiol London 295:21, 1979.
94. Janig W, Khasa SG, Levine JD, et al: The role of vagal visceral afferents in the control of nociception. In Mayer EA, Saper CB (eds): The Biological Basis for Mind Body Interactions. Amsterdam: Elsevier, 2000, p 273.
95. Janig W, Habler H-J: Specificity in the organization of the autonomic nervous system: A basis for precise neural regulation of homeostatic and protective body functions. In Mayer EA, Saper CB (eds): The Biological Basis for Mind Body Interactions. Amsterdam: Elsevier, 2000, p 351.
96. Renehan WE, Zhang X, Beierwaltes WH, et al: Neurons in the dorsal motor nucleus of the vagus may integrate vagal and spinal information from the GI tract. Am J Physiol 268:G780, 1995.
97. Mei N: Gastrointestinal vagal mechanoreceptors in the cat. Exp. Brain Res 11:502, 1970.
98. Saper CB: Pain as a visceral sensation. In Mayer EA, Saper CB (eds): The Biological Basis for Mind Body Interactions. Amsterdam: Elsevier, 2000, p 237.
99. Collman PI, Tremblay L, Diamant NE: The distribution of spinal and vagal sensory neurons that innervate the esophagus of the cat. Gastroenterology 103:817, 1992.
100. Cervero F, Connell LA, Lawson SN: Somatic and visceral primary afferents in the lower thoracic dorsal root ganglia of the cat. J Comp Neurol 228:422, 1984.
101. Cervero F, Tattersall JEH: Cutaneous receptive fields of somatic and viscerosomatic neruones in the thoracic spinal cord of the cat. J Comp Neurol 237:325, 1985.
102. Aziz Q, Andersson JLR, Valind S, et al: Identification of human brain loci processing esophageal sensation using positron emission tomography. Gastroenterology 113:50, 1997.
103. Hobson AR, Sarkar S, Furlong PL, et al: A cortical evoked potential study of afferents mediating human esophageal sensation. Am J Physiol 279:G139, 2000.
104. Hollerbach S, Bulat R, May A, et al: Abnormal cerebral processing of oesophageal stimuli in patients with noncardiac chest pain (NCCP). Neurogastroenterol Motil 12:555, 2000.
105. Tougas G, Kamath M, Watteel G, et al: Modulation of neurocardiac function by oesophageal stimulation in humans. Clin Sci 92:167, 1997.
106. Johnston BT, Shils J, Leite LP, et al: Effects of octreotide on esophageal visceral perception and cerebral evoked potentials induced by balloon distension. Am J Gastroenterol 94:65, 1999.
107. Roman C, Tieffenbach L: Electrical activity of esophageal smooth muscle in vagotomized and anesthetized cats. J Physiol (Paris) 63:733, 1971.
108. Meyer GW, Castell DO: Anatomy and physiology of the esophageal body. In Castell DO, Johnson LF (eds): Esophageal Function in Health and Disease. New York: Elsevier Biomedical, 1983, p 1.
109. Asoh R, Goyal RK: Manometry and electromyography of the upper esophageal sphincter in the opossum. Gastroenterology 74:514, 1978.
110. Kahrilas PJ, Dodds WJ, Dent J, et al: Effect of sleep, spontaneous gastroesophageal reflux, and a meal on upper esophageal sphincter pressure in normal human volunteers. Gastroenterology 92:466, 1987.
111. Winans CS: The pharyngoesophageal closure mechanism: A manometric study. Gastroenterology 63:768, 1972.
112. Castell JA, Dalton CB, Castell DO: Pharyngeal and upper esophageal sphincter manometry in humans. Am J Physiol 258:G173, 1990.
113. Cook IJ, Dent J, Shannon S, et al: Measurement of upper esophageal sphincter pressure. Effect of acute emotional stress. Gastroenterology 93:526, 1987.
114. Cardoso PFG, Miller L, Diamant NE: The effect of catheter diameter on upper esophageal sphincter pressure measurement in normal subjects. Gullet 2:145, 1992.
115. Kahrilas PJ, Dodds WJ, Dent J, et al: Upper esophageal sphincter function during deglutition. Gastroenterology 95:52, 1988.
116. Preiksaitis HG, Diamant NE: The physiology of swallowing: Pharyngeal and cricopharyngeal mechanisms. In Pearson FG, Deslauriers J, Ginsberg RJ, et al (eds): Esophageal Surgery. New York: Churchill Livingstone, 1995.
117. Freiman JM, El-Sharkawy TY, Diamant NE: Effect of bilateral vagosympathetic nerve blockade on response of the dog upper esophageal sphincter (UES) to intraesophageal distention and acid. Gastroenterology 81:78, 1981.
118. Kahrilas PJ, Dodds WJ, Dent J, et al: Upper esophageal sphincter function during belching. Gastroenterology 91:133, 1986.
119. Jacob P, Kahrilas PJ, Logemann JA, et al: Upper esophageal sphincter opening and modulation during swallowing. Gastroenterology 97:1469, 1989.
120. Clouse RE, Alrakawi A, Staiano A: Intersubject and interswallow variability in topography of esophageal motility. Dig Dis Sci 43:1978, 1998.
121. Clouse RE, Prakash C: Topographic esophageal manometry: An emerging clinical and investigative approach. Dig Dis 18:64, 2000.
122. Richter JE, Wu WC, Johns DN, et al: Esophageal manometry in 95 healthy adult volunteers. Variability of pressures with age and frequency of "abnormal" contractions. Dig Dis Sci 32:583, 1987.
123. Clouse RE, Staiano A, Bickston SJ, Cohn SM: Characteristics of the propagating pressure wave in the esophagus. Dig Dis Sci 41:2369, 1996
124. Roman C, Tieffenbach L: Recording the unit activity of vagal motor fibers innervating the baboon esophagus. J Physiol (Paris) 64:479, 1972.
125. Gidda JS, Goyal RK: Swallow-evoked action potentials in vagal preganglionic efferents. J Neurophysiol 52:1169, 1984.
126. Amri M, Car A: Pontine deglutition neurons in sheep. II. Effects of stimulation of peripheral afferents and the fronto-orbital cortex. Exp Brain Res 48:355, 1982.
127. Amri M, Car A, Jean A: Medullary control of the pontine swallowing neurones in sheep. Exp Brain Res 55:105, 1984.
128. Barone FC, Lombardi DM, Ormsbee HS: Effects of hindbrain stimulation on lower esophageal sphincter pressure in the cat. Am J Physiol 247:G70, 1984.
129. Barrett RT, Bao X, Miselis RR, et al: Brain stem localization of rodent esophageal premotor neurons revealed by transneuronal passage of pseudorabies virus. Gastroenterology 107:728, 1994.
130. Bennett JA, Goodchild CS, Kidd C, et al: Neurones in the brain stem of the cat excited by vagal afferent fibres from the heart and lungs. J Physiol London 369:1, 1985.
131. Car A: Cortical control of deglutition. 2. Medullary impact of corticofugal swallowing pathways. J Physiol (Paris) 66:553, 1973.
132. Car A, Amri M: Pontine deglutition neurons in sheep. I. Activity and localization. Exp Brain Res 48:345, 1982.

133. Tieffenbach L, Roman C: The role of extrinsic vagal innervation in the motility of the smooth-musculed portion of the esophagus: Electromyographic study in the cat and the baboon. J Physiol (Paris) 64:193, 1972.
134. Sarna SK, Daniel EE, Waterfall WE: Myogenic and neural control systems for esophageal motility. Gastroenterology 73:1345, 1977.
135. Helm JF, Bro SL, Dodds WJ, et al: Myogenic mechanism for peristalsis in opossum smooth muscle esophagus. Am J Physiol 263:G953, 1992.
136. Preiksaitis HG, Diamant NE: Myogenic mechanism for peristalsis in the cat esophagus. Am J Physiol 277:G306, 1999.
137. Dodds WJ, Dent J, Hogan WJ, et al: Effect of atropine on esophageal motor function in humans. Am J Physiol 240:G290, 1981.
138. Paterson WG, Hynna-Liepert TT, Selucky M: Comparison of primary and secondary esophageal peristalsis in humans: Effect of atropine. Am J Physiol 260:G52, 1991.
139. Blank EL, Greenwood B, Dodds WJ: Cholinergic control of smooth muscle peristalsis in the cat esophagus. Am J Physiol 257:G517, 1989.
140. Hollis JB, Castell DO: Effects of cholinergic stimulation on human esophageal peristalsis. J Appl Physiol Washington 40:40, 1976.
141. Humphries TJ, Castell DO: Effect of oral bethanechol on parameters of esophageal peristalsis. Dig Dis Sci 26:129, 1981.
142. Chan WW-L, Diamant NE: Electrical off response of cat esophageal smooth muscle: An analog simulation. Am J Physiol 230:233, 1976.
143. Diamant NE: Physiology of esophageal motor function. Gastroenterol Clin North Am 18:179, 1989.
144. Crist J, Kauvar D, Goyal RK: Gradient of cholinergic innervation in opossum esophageal circular smooth muscle. Gullet 1:92, 1991.
145. Crist J, Gidda JS, Goyal RK: Characteristics of "on" and "off" contractions in esophageal circular muscle in vitro. Am J Physiol 246: G137, 1984.
146. Serio R, Daniel EE: Electrophysiological analysis of responses to intrinsic nerves in circular muscle of opossum esophageal muscle. Am J Physiol 254:G107, 1988.
147. Dodds WJ, Christensen J, Dent J, et al: Pharmacologic investigation of primary peristalsis in smooth muscle portion of opossum esophagus. Am J Physiol 237:E561, 1979.
148. Sifrim D, Janssens J: Inhibitory and excitatory mechanisms in the control of esophageal peristalsis in cats. Gastroenterology 108:A691, 1995.
149. Conklin JL, Murray J, Ledlow A, et al: Effects of recombinant human hemoglobin on motor functions of the opossum esophagus. J Pharmacol Exp Ther 273:762, 1995.
150. Knudsen MA, Frobert O, Tottrup A: The role of the L-arginine-nitric oxide pathway for peristalsis in the opossum oesophageal body. Scand J Gastroenterol 29:1083, 1994.
151. Chakder S, Rosenthal GJ, Rattan S: In vivo and in vitro influence of human recombinant hemoglobin on esophageal function. Am J Physiol 268:G443, 1995.
152. Murray JA, Ledlow A, Launspach J, et al: The effects of recombinant human hemoglobin on esophageal motor function in humans. Gastroenterology 109:1241, 1995.
153. Xue S, Valdez DT, Collman PI, et al: Effects of nitric oxide synthase blockade on esophageal peristalsis and the lower esophageal sphincter in the cat. Can J Physiol Pharmacol 74:1249, 1996.
154. Hirsch DP, Holloway RH, Tytgat GNJ, et al: Involvement of nitric oxide in human transient lower esophageal sphincter relaxations and esophageal primary peristalsis. Gastroenterology 115:1374, 1998.
155. Foster JM, Houghton LA, Whorwell PJ, et al: Altered oesophageal motility following the administration of the 5-HT1 agonist, sumatriptan. Aliment Pharmacol Ther 13:927, 1999.
156. Masclee AA, Lam WF, Lamers CB: Effect of bombesin on esophageal motility in humans. Dis Esophagus 12:54, 1999.
157. Penagini R, Picone A, Bianchi PA: Effect of morphine and naloxone on motor response of the human esophagus to swallowing and distension. Am J Physiol 271:G675, 1996.
158. Bardakjian BL, Diamant NE: Electronic models of oscillator-to-oscillator communications. In Sperelakis N, Cole W (eds): Cell Interactions and Gap Junctions. Boca Raton, Fla: CRC Press, 1989, p 211.
159. Daniel EE, Bardakjian BL, Huizinga JD, et al: Relaxation oscillators and core conductor models are needed for understanding of GI electrical activities. Am J Physiol 266:G339, 1994.
160. Kannan MS, Jager LP, Daniel EE: Electrical properties of smooth muscle cell membrane of opossum esophagus. Am J Physiol 248: G342, 1985.
161. Crist J, Surprenant A, Goyal RK: Intracellular studies of electrical membrane properties of opossum esophageal circular smooth muscle. Gastroenterology 92:987, 1987.
162. Dodds WJ, Hogan WJ, Reid DP, et al: A comparison between primary esophageal peristalsis following wet and dry swallows. J Appl Physiol Washington 35:851, 1973.
163. Dodds WJ, Hogan WJ, Stewart ET, et al: Effects of increased intra-abdominal pressure on esophageal peristalsis. J Appl Physiol Washington 37:378, 1974.
164. Aithal GP, Nylander D, Dwarakanath AD, et al: Subclinical esophageal peristaltic dysfunction during the early phase following a stroke. Dig Dis Sci 44:274, 1999.
165. Weber J, Roman C, Hannequin D, et al: Esophageal manometry in patients with unilateral hemispheric cerebrovascular accidents or idiopathic parkinsonism. J Gastrointest Motil 3:98, 1991.
166. Lucas CE, Yu P, Vlahos A, et al: Lower esophageal sphincter dysfunction often precludes safe gastric feeding in stroke patients. Arch Surg 134:55, 1999.
167. Vanek AW, Diamant NE: Responses of the human esophagus to paired swallows. Gastroenterology 92:643, 1987.
168. Hellemans J, Vantrappen G, Janssens J: Electromyography of the esophagus. 4. The deglutitive inhibition. In Vantrappen G, Hellemans J (eds): Diseases of the Esophagus. New York: Springer-Verlag, 1974, p 280.
169. Hornby PJ, Abrahams TP. Central control of lower esophageal sphincter relaxation. Am J Med 108(suppl 4a):90S, 2000.
170. Meyer GW, Gerhardt DC, Castell DO: Human esophageal response to rapid swallowing: Muscle refractory period or neural inhibition? Am J Physiol 241:G129, 1981.
171. Liebermann-Meffert D, Allgower M, Schmid P, et al: Muscular equivalent of the lower esophageal sphincter. Gastroenterology 76:31, 1979.
172. Preiksaitis HG, Diamant NE: Regional differences in the cholinergic activity of muscle fibers from the human gastroesophageal junction. Am J Physiol 272:G1324, 1997.
173. Richardson BJ, Welch RW: Differential effect of atropine on rightward and leftward lower esophageal sphincter pressure. Gastroenterology 81:85, 1981.
174. Heine KJ, Dent J, Mittal RK: Anatomical relationship between crural diaphragm and lower oesophageal sphincter: An electrophysiological study. J Gastrointest Motil 5:89, 1993.
175. Schneider JH, Grund KE, Becker H-D: Lower esophageal sphincter measurements in four different quadrants in normals and patients with achalasia. Dis Esophagus 11:120, 1998.
176. Stein HJ, Liebermann-Meffert D, DeMeester TR, et al: Three-dimensional pressure image and muscular structure of the human lower esophageal sphincter. Surgery 117:692, 1995.
177. Daniel EE: Lower esophagus: Structure and function. In Daniel EE, Tomita T, Tsuchida S, Watanabe M (eds): Sphincters: Normal Function—Change in Diseases. Boca Raton, Fla: CRC Press, 1992, p 49.
178. Bortolotti M, Labo G: Clinical and manometric effects of nifedipine in patients with esophageal achalasia. Gastroenterology 80:39, 1981.
179. Harnett KM, Cao W, Kim N, et al: Signal transduction in esophageal and LES circular muscle contraction. Yale J Biol Med 72:153, 1999.
180. Szymanski PT, Chacko TK, Rovner AS, et al: Differences in contractile protein content and isoforms in phasic and tonic smooth muscle. Am J Physiol 275:C684, 1998.
181. Murphy RA: Myosin phosphorylation and contraction of feline esophageal smooth muscle. Am J Physiol 249:C9, 1985.
182. Tottrup A, Forman A, Uldbjerg, N, et al: Mechanical properties of isolated human esophageal smooth muscle. Am J Physiol 258:G338, 1990.
183. Biancani P, Zabinski M, Kerstein M, et al: Lower esophageal sphincter mechanics: Anatomic and physiologic relationships of the esophagogastric junction of cat. Gastroenterology 82:468, 1982.
184. Salapatek AMF, Daniel EE: Modulation of canine LES tone by nitric oxide synthase in muscle. Gastroenterology 108:A681, 1995.
185. Cao WB, Harnett KM, Chen Q, et al: Group I secreted PLA2 and arachidonic acid metabolites in the maintenance of cat LES tone. Am J Physiol 277:G585, 1999.
186. Zhang Y, Miller DV, Paterson WG: Opposing roles of K(+) and Cl(-) channels in maintenance of opossum lower esophageal sphincter tone. Am J Physiol 279:G1226, 2000.
187. Price LM, El-Sharkawy TY, Mui HY, et al: Effect of bilateral cervical vagotomy on balloon-induced lower esophageal sphincter relaxation in the dog. Gastroenterology 77:324, 1979.

188. Miolan JP, Roman C: Activity of vagal efferent fibres innervating the smooth muscle of the dog's cardia. J Physiol (Paris) 74:709, 1978.
189. Paterson WG, Anderson MA, Anand N: Pharmacological characterization of lower esophageal sphincter relaxation induced by swallowing, vagal efferent nerve stimulation, and esophageal distention. Can J Physiol Pharmacol 70:1011, 1992.
190. Murray JA, Du C, Ledlow A: Is nitric oxide the noncholinergic, nonadrenergic neurotransmitter responsible for lower esophageal sphincter relaxation? Am J Physiol 263:G97, 1992.
191. McKirdy HC, McKirdy ML, Lewis MJ, et al: Evidence for involvement of nitric oxide in the non-adrenergic non-cholinergic (NANC) relaxation of human lower oesophageal sphincter muscle strips. Exp Physiol 77:509, 1992.
192. Dent J, Dodds WJ, Sekiguchi T, et al: Interdigestive phasic contractions of the human lower esophageal sphincter. Gastroenterology 84: 453, 1983.
193. Crispin JS, McIver DK, Lind JF: Manometric study of the effect of vagotomy on the gastroesophageal sphincter. Can J Surg 10:299, 1967.
194. Dodds WJ, Dent J, Hogan WJ, et al: Mechanisms of gastroesophageal reflux in patients with reflux esophagitis. N Engl J Med 307:1547, 1982.
195. Paterson WG, Rattan S, Goyal RK: Experimental induction of isolated lower esophageal sphincter relaxation in anesthetized opossums. J Clin Invest 77:1187, 1986.
196. Holloway RH, Blank E, Takahashi I, et al: Variability of lower esophageal sphincter pressure in the fasted unanesthetized opossum. Am J Physiol 248:G398, 1985.
197. Higgs RH, Castell DO: The effect of truncal vagotomy on lower esophageal sphincter pressure and response to cholinergic stimulation. Proc Soc Exp Biol Med 153:379, 1976.
198. Temple JG, Goodall RJ, Hay DJ, et al: Effect of highly selective vagotomy upon the lower oesophageal sphincter. Gut 22:368, 1981.
199. Alrakawi A, Clouse RE: The changing use of esophageal manometry in clinical practice. Am J Gastroenterol 93:2359, 1998.
200. Clouse RE: Spastic disorders of the esophagus. Gastroenterologist 5: 112, 1997.
201. Cohen S, Fisher R, Lipshutz W, et al: The pathogenesis of esophageal dysfunction in scleroderma and Raynaud's disease. J Clin Invest 51: 2663, 1972.
202. Salapatek AMF, Diamant NE: Assessment of neural inhibition of the lower esophageal sphincter in cats with esophagitis. Gastroenterology 104:810, 1993.
203. Higgs RH, Castell DO, Eastwood GL: Studies on the mechanism of esophagitis-induced lower esophageal sphincter hypotension in cats. Gastroenterology 71:51, 1976.
204. Dodds WJ, Hogan WJ, Helm JF, et al: Pathogenesis of reflux esophagitis. Gastroenterology 81:376, 1981.
205. Halter F, Scheurer U: Motility abnormalities of the lower esophageal sphincter (LES) in reflux esophagitis. In Vantrappen G (ed): Proceedings of the 5th International Symposium on GI Motility. Herentals, Belgium: Typoff Press, 1975, p 349.
206. Henderson RD: Primary disordered motor activity of the esophagus ("diffuse spasm"). In Henderson RD, Godden JO (eds): Motor Disorders of the Esophagus. Baltimore: Williams & Wilkins, 1976, p 146.
207. Sifrim D, Janssens J, Vantrappen G: Failing deglutitive inhibition in primary esophageal motility disorders. Gastroenterology. 106:875, 1994.
208. Fass R, Pulliam G, Johnson C, Garewal HS, Sampliner RE: Symptom severity and oesophageal chemosensitivity to acid in old and young patients with gastro-oesophageal reflux. Age Ageing 29:125, 2000.
209. Johnson DA, Winters C, Spurling TJ, et al: Esophageal acid sensitivity in Barrett's esophagus. J Clin Gastroenterol 9:23, 1987.
210. Trimble KC, Pryde A, Heading RC: Lowered esophageal sensory threshold in patients with symptomatic but not excess gastroesophageal reflux disease: Evidence for a spectrum of visceral sensitivity in GERD. Gut 37:7, 1995.
211. Kamath MV, May A, Hollerbach S, et al: Effects of esophageal stimulation in patients with functional disorders of the gastrointestinal tract. Crit Rev Biomed Engl 28:87, 2000.
212. Cattau EL Jr, Castell DO: Symptoms of esophageal dysfunction. In Castell DO, Johnson LF (eds): Esophageal Function in Health and Disease. New York: Elsevier Biomedical, 1983, pp 31–46.
213. Triadafilopoulos G, Tsang HP, Segall GM: Hot water swallows improve symptoms and accelerate esophageal clearance in esophageal motility disorders. J Clin Gastroenterol 26:239, 1998.
214. Ott DJ: Radiologic evaluation of esophageal dysphagia. Curr Probl Diagn Radiol 17:1, 1988.
215. Dodds WJ, Stewart ET, Logemann JA: Physiology and radiology of the normal oral and pharyngeal phases of swallowing [review]. AJR 154:953, 1990.
216. Jones BJ, Donner MW: How I do it. Examination of the patient with dysphagia. Radiology 167:319, 1988.
217. Logemann JA: Approaches to management of disordered swallowing. Bailliere's Clin Gastroenterol 5:269, 1991.
218. Hollis JB, Castell DO: Effect of dry swallows and wet swallows of different volumes on esophageal peristalsis. J Appl Physiol 38:1161, 1975.
219. Weihrauch TR: Esophageal Manometry. Methods and Clinical Practice. Baltimore: Urban & Schwarzenberg, 1981, pp 38–63.
220. Vanek AW, Diamant NE: Responses of the human esophagus to paired swallows. Gastroenterology 92:643, 1987.
221. Bartlett RJV: Scintigraphy of the oesophagus. In Robinson, PJA (ed): Nuclear Gastroenterology. Edinburgh: Churchill Livingstone, 1986.
222. DeCaestecker JS, Blackwell JN, Adam RD, et al: Clinical value of radionuclide oesophageal transit measurement. Gut 27:659, 1986.
223. Holloway RH, Lange RC, Plankey MW, McCallum RW: Detection of esophageal motor disorders by radionuclide transit studies. A reappraisal. Dig Dis Sci 34:905, 1989.
224. Blackwell JN, Richter JE, Wu WC, et al: Esophageal radionuclide transit tests: Potential false positive results. Clin Nucl Med 9:679, 1984.
225. Schroter-Morasch H, Bartolome G, Troppmann N, Ziegler W: Values and limitations of pharyngolaryngoscopy (transnasal, transoral) in patients with dysphagia. Folia Phoniatr Logop 51:172, 1999.
226. Aviv JE, Kaplan ST, Thomson JE, Spitzer J, Diamond B, Close LG: The safety of flexible endoscopic evaluation of swallowing with sensory testing (FEESST): An analysis of 500 consecutive evaluations. Dysphagia 15:39, 2000.
227. Aviv JE: Prospective, randomized outcome study of endoscopy versus modified barium swallow in patients with dysphagia. Laryngoscope 110:563, 2000.
228. Brasseur JG, Dodds WJ: Interpretation of intraluminal manometric measurements in terms of swallowing mechanics. Dysphagia 6:100, 1991.
229. Castell DO, Castell JA (eds): Esophageal Motility Testing, 2nd ed. Norwalk, Conn: Appleton & Lange, 1994.
230. Clouse RE, Staiano A: Contraction abnormalities of the esophageal body in patients referred for manometry. A new approach to manometric classification. Dig Dis Sci 28:784, 1983.
231. Bassotti G, Bacci G, Biagini D, et al: Manometric investigation of the entire esophagus in healthy subjects and patients with high-amplitude peristaltic contractions. Dysphagia 3:93, 1988.
232. Aliperti G, Clouse RE: Incomplete lower esophageal sphincter relaxation in subjects with peristalsis: Prevalence and clinical outcome. Am J Gastroenterol 86:609, 1991.
233. Clouse RE, Staiano A: Manometric patterns using esophageal body and lower sphincter characteristics: Findings in 1013 patients. Dig Dis Sci 37:289, 1992.
234. Dodds WJ, Stewart ET, Hogan WJ, et al: Effect of esophageal movement on intraluminal esophageal pressure recording. Gastroenterology 67:592, 1974.
235. Edmundowicz SA, Clouse RE: Shortening of the human esophagus in response to swallowing. Am J Physiol 260:G512, 1991.
236. Massey BT, Dodds WJ, Hogan WJ, et al: Abnormal esophageal motility. An analysis of concurrent radiographic and manometric findings. Gastroenterology 101:344, 1991.
237. Clouse RE, Staiano A, Alrakawi A: Development of a topographic analysis system for manometric studies in the gastrointestinal tract. Gastrointest Endosc 48:395, 1998.
238. Clouse RE, Staiano A, Alrakawi A, Haroian L: Application of topographic methods to clinical esophageal manometry. Am J Gastroenterol 95:2720, 2000.
239. Moser G, Wenzel-Abatzi TA, Stelzeneder M, et al: Globus sensation: Pharyngoesophageal function, psychometric and psychiatric findings, and follow-up in 88 patients. Arch Intern Med 158:1365, 1998.
240. Gerhardt DC, Shuck TJ, Bordeaux RA, Winship DH: Human upper esophageal sphincter. Response to volume, osmotic, and acid stimuli. Gastroenterology 75:268, 1978.
241. Cook IJ, Dent J, Collins SM: Upper esophageal sphincter tone and reactivity to stress in patients with a history of globus sensation. Dig Dis Sci 34:672, 1989.

242. Cook IJ, Shaker R, Doods WJ, et al: Role of mechanical and chemical stimulation of the esophagus in globus sensation. Gastroenterology 96: A99, 1989.
243. Drossman DA, Corazziari E, Talley NJ, Thompson WG, Whitehead WE (eds): Rome II: The Functional Gastrointestinal Disorders, 2nd ed. McLean, Va: Degnon Associates, 2000.
244. Mann G, Hankey GJ, Cameron D: Swallowing disorders following acute stroke: Prevalence and diagnostic accuracy. Cerebrovasc Dis 10: 380, 2000.
245. Kirshner HS: Causes of neurogenic dysphagia. Dysphagia 3:184, 1989.
246. Weber J, Roman C, Hannequin D, et al: Esophageal manometry in patients with unilateral hemispheric cerebrovascular accidents or idiopathic parkinsonism. Gastrointest Motil 3:98, 1991.
247. Silbiger MI, Pikielney R, Donner MW: Neuromuscular disorders affecting the pharynx: Cineradiographic analysis. Invest Radiol 2:442, 1967.
248. Calne DB, Shaw DG, Spiers ASD, Sterne GM: Swallowing in parkinsonism. Br J Radiol 43:456, 1970.
249. Nowack WJ, Hatelid JM, Sohn RS: Dysphagia in parkinsonism. Arch Neurol 34:320, 1977.
250. Daly DD, Code CF, Andersen HA: Disturbances of swallowing and esophageal motility in patients with multiple sclerosis. Neurology 12: 250, 1962.
251. Fischer RA, Ellison GW, Thayer WR, et al: Esophageal motility in neuromuscular disorders. Ann Intern Med 63:229, 1965.
252. Bosma JF: Residual disability of pharyngeal area resulting from poliomyelitis. JAMA 165:216, 1957.
253. Sonies BC, Dalakas MC: Dysphagia in patients with the post-polio syndrome. N Engl J Med 324:1162, 1991.
254. Henderson RD, Boszko A, VanNostrand AWP: Pharyngoesophageal dysphagia and recurrent laryngeal nerve palsy. J Thorac Cardiovasc Surg 68:507, 1974.
255. Lathrop DL, Griebel M, Horner J: Case report. Dysphagia in tetanus: Evaluation and outcome. Dysphagia 4:173, 1989.
256. Kagen LJ, Hochman RB, Strong EW: Cricopharyngeal obstruction in inflammatory myopathy (polymyositis/dermatomyositis). Report of three cases and review of the literature. Arthritis Rheum 28:630, 1985.
257. Pearson CM, Currie S: Polymyositis and related disorders. In Walton JN (ed): Disorders of Voluntary Muscle, 3rd ed. Edinburgh: Churchill Livingstone, 1974, p 614.
258. Wintzen AR, Bots GT, de Bakker HM, et al: Dysphagia in inclusion body myositis. J Neurol Neurosurg Psychiatry 51:1542, 1988.
259. Eckardt VF, Nix W, Kraus W, Bohl J: Esophageal motor function in patients with muscular dystrophy. Gastroenterology 90:628, 1986.
260. Duranceau AC, Beauchamp G, Jamieson GG, Barbeau A: Oropharyngeal dysphagia and oculopharyngeal muscular dystrophy. Surg Clin North Am 63:825, 1983.
261. Wright RA, Penner DB: Myxedema and upper esophageal dysmotility. Dig Dis Sci 26:376, 1981.
262. Sulway MJ, Baume PE, Davis E: Stiff-man syndrome presenting with complete esophageal obstruction. Am J Dig Dis 15:79, 1970.
263. Kilman WJ, Goyal RK: Disorders of pharyngeal and upper esophageal sphincter motor function. Arch Intern Med 136:592, 1976.
264. Duranceau A, Lafontaine ER, Taillefer R, Jamieson GG: Oropharyngeal dysphagia and operations on the upper esophageal sphincter. Surg Annu 19:317, 1987.
265. Cruse JP, Edwards DAW, Smith JF, Wyllie JH: The pathology of cricopharyngeal dysphagia. Histopathology 3:223, 1979.
266. American Gastroenterological Association: AGA medical position statement on management of oropharyngeal dysphagia. Gastroenterology 116:452, 1999.
267. Cook IJ, Kahrilas PJ: AGA technical review on management of oropharyngeal dysphagia. Gastroenterology 116:455, 1999.
268. Ohmae Y, Ogura M, Kitahara S, Karaho T, Inouye T: Effects of head rotation on pharyngeal function during normal swallow. Ann Otol Rhinol Laryngol 107:344, 1998.
269. Sorin R, Somers S, Austin W, Bester S: The influence of videofluoroscopy on the management of the dysphagic patient. Dysphagia 2: 127, 1988.
270. Bath PM, Bath FJ, Smithard DG: Interventions for dysphagia in acute stroke. Cochrane Database Syst Rev 2:CD000323, 2000.
271. Klor BM, Mikianti FJ: Rehabilitation of neurogenic dysphagia with percutaneous endoscopic gastrostomy. Dysphagia 14:162, 1999.
272. Dodds WJ, Man KM, Cook IJ, et al: Quantification of swallow-induced hyoid movement. AJR 150:1307, 1988.
273. Bonavina L, Khan NA, DeMeester TR: Pharyngoesophageal dysfunctions. The role of cricopharyngeal myotomy. Arch Surg 120:541, 1985.
274. Mason RJ, Bremner CG, DeMeester TR, et al: Pharyngeal swallowing disorders: Selection for and outcome after myotomy. Ann Surg 228: 598, 1998.
275. Williams RB, Ali GN, Hunt DR, Wallace KL, Cook IJ: Cricopharyngeal myotomy does not increase the risk of esophagopharyngeal acid regurgitation. Am J Gastroenterol 94:3448, 1999.
276. Williams RB, Ali GN, Hunt DR, Wallace KL, Cook IJ: Cricopharyngeal myotomy does not increase the risk of esophagopharyngeal acid regurgitation. Am J Gastroenterol 94:3448, 1999.
277. Kelly JH: Management of upper esophageal sphincter disorders: Indications and complications of myotomy. Am J Med 108(suppl 4a):43S, 2000.
278. Niwamoto H, Okamoto E, Fujimoto J, et al: Are human herpes viruses or measles virus associated with esophageal achalasia? Dig Dis Sci 40:859, 1995.
279. Robertson CS, Martin BAB, Atkinson M: Varicella-zoster virus DNA in the oesophageal myenteric plexus in achalasia. Gut 34:299, 1993.
280. Mullaney PB, Weatherhead R, Millar R, et al: Keratoconjunctivitis sicca associated with achalasia of the cardia, adrenocortical insufficiency and lacrimal gland degeneration: Keratoconjunctivitis sicca secondary to lacrimal gland degeneration may parallel degenerative changes in esophageal and adrenocortical function. Ophthalmology 105:643, 1998.
281. Eckrich JD, Winans CS: Discordance for achalasia in identical twins. Dig Dis Sci 24:221, 1979.
282. De la Concha EG, Fernandez-Arquero M, Mendoza JL, et al: Contribution of HLA class II genes to susceptibility in achalasia. Tissue Antigens 52:381, 1998.
283. Verne GN, Hahn AB, Pineau BC, Hoffman BJ, Wojciechowski BW, Wu WC: Association of HLA-DR and -DQ alleles with idiopathic achalasia. Gastroenterology 117:26, 1999.
284. Verne GN, Sallustio JE, Eaker EY: Anti-myenteric neuronal antibodies in patients with achalasia: A prospective study. Gastroenterology 108:A705, 1995.
285. Cassella RR, Brown AL Jr, Sayre GP, Ellis FH Jr: Achalasia of the esophagus: Pathologic and etiologic considerations. Ann Surg 160:474, 1964.
286. Csendes A, Smok G, Braghetto I, et al: Gastroesophageal sphincter pressure and histological changes in distal esophagus in patients with achalasia of the esophagus. Dig Dis Sci 30:941, 1985.
287. Raymond L, Lach B, Shamji FM: Inflammatory aetiology of primary oesophageal achalasia: An immunohistochemical and ultrastructural study of Auerbach's plexus. Histopathology 35:445, 1999.
288. Clark SB, Rice TW, Tubbs RR, Richter JE, Goldblum JR: The nature of the myenteric infiltrate in achalasia: An immunohistochemical analysis. Am J Surg Pathol 24:1153, 2000.
289. De Giorgio R, Di Simone MP, Stanghellini V, et al: Esophageal and gastric nitric oxide synthesizing innervation in primary achalasia. Am J Gastroenterol 94:2357, 1999.
290. Cassella RR, Ellis FH Jr, Brown AL Jr: Fine-structure changes in achalasia of the esophagus: I. Vagus nerves. Am J Pathol 46:279, 1965.
291. Higgs B, Kerr FWL, Ellis FH Jr: The experimental production of esophageal achalasia by electrolytic lesions in the medulla. J Thorac Cardiovasc Surg 50:613, 1965.
292. Misiewicz JJ, Waller SL, Anthony PP, Gummer JW: Achalasia of the cardia: Pharmacology and histopathology of isolated cardiac sphincteric muscle from patients with and without achalasia. Q J Med 38:17, 1969.
293. Heitmann P, Espinoza J, Csendes A: Physiology of the distal esophagus in achalasia. Scand J Gastroenterol 4:1, 1969.
294. Dodds WJ, Dent J, Hogan WJ, et al: Paradoxical lower esophageal sphincter contraction induced by cholecystokinin-octapeptide in patients with achalasia. Gastroenterology 80:327, 1981.
295. Eckardt VF, Krause J, Bolle D: Gastrointestinal transit and gastric acid secretion in patients with achalasia. Dig Dis Sci 34:665, 1989.
296. Mayberry JF, Atkinson M: Studies of incidence and prevalence of achalasia in the Nottingham area. Q J Med 56:451, 1985.
297. Wong RKH, Johnson LF: Achalasia. In Castell DO, Johnson LF (eds): Esophageal Function in Health and Disease. New York: Elsevier, 1983, pp 99–123.
298. Eckardt VF, Stauf B, Bernhard G: Chest pain in achalasia: Patient characteristics and clinical course. Gastroenterology 116:1300, 1999.

299. Stacher G, Kiss A, Wiesnagrotzki S, et al: Oesophageal and gastric motility disorders in patients categorized as having primary anorexia nervosa. Gut 27:1120, 1986.
300. Vantrappen G, Hellemans J, Deloof W, et al: Treatment of achalasia with pneumatic dilatations. Gut 12:268, 1971.
301. Spechler SJ: AGA medical position statement on treatment of patients with dysphagia caused by benign disorders of the distal esophagus. Gastroenterology 117:229, 1999.
302. Schima W, Ryan JM, Harisinghani M, et al: Radiologic detection of achalasia: Diagnostic accuracy of videofluoroscopy. Clin Radiol 53: 372, 1998.
303. Howard PJ, Maher L, Pryde A, Cameron EW, Heading RC: Five year prospective study of the incidence, clinical features, and diagnosis of achalasia in Edinburgh. Gut 33:1011,1992.
304. Tucker HJ, Snape WJ Jr, Cohen S: Achalasia secondary to carcinoma: Manometric and clinical features. Ann Intern Med 89:315, 1978.
305. Tracey JP, Traube M: Difficulties in the diagnosis of pseudoachalasia. Am J Gastroenterol 89:2014, 1994.
306. Bianco A, Cagossi M, Scrimieri D, Greco AV: Appearance of esophageal peristalsis in treated idiopathic achalasia. Dig Dis Sci 31:40, 1986.
307. Kramer P, Ingelfinger FJ: Esophageal sensitivity to mecholyl in cardiospasm. Gastroenterology 19:242, 1951.
308. McCord GS, Staiano A, Clouse RE: Achalasia, diffuse spasm and non-specific motor disorders. Bailliere's Clin Gastroenterol 5:307, 1991.
309. Katz PO, Richter JE, Cowan R, Castell DO: Apparent complete lower esophageal sphincter relaxation in achalasia. Gastroenterology 90:978, 1986.
310. Mearin F, Malagelada JR: Complete lower esophageal sphincter relaxation observed in some achalasia patients is functionally inadequate. Am J Physiol 278:G376, 2000.
311. Staiano A, Clouse RE: Detection of incomplete lower esophageal sphincter relaxation using point pressure sensors. Am J Gastroenterol (in press), 2001.
312. Cohen S, Lipshutz W: Lower esophageal sphincter dysfunction in achalasia. Gastroenterology 61:814, 1971.
313. Todorczuk JR, Aliperti G, Staiano A, Clouse RE: Reevaluation of manometric criteria for vigorous achalasia. Is this a distinct clinical disorder? Dig Dis Sci 36:274, 1991.
314. Goldenberg SP, Burrell M, Fette GG, et al: Classic and vigorous achalasia: A comparison of manometric, radiographic, and clinical findings. Gastroenterology 101:743, 1991.
315. Hirano I, Tatum RP, Shi G, Sang Q, Joehl RJ, Kahrilas PJ: Manometric heterogeneity in patients with idiopathic achalasia. Gastroenterology 120:789, 2001.
316. Kahrilas PJ, Kishk SM, Helm JF, et al: Comparison of pseudoachalasia and achalasia. Am J Med 82:439, 1987.
317. Schuffler MD: Chronic intestinal pseudo-obstruction syndromes. Med Clin North Am 65:1331, 1981.
318. Costigan DJ, Clouse RE: Achalasia-like esophagus from amyloidosis: Successful treatment with pneumatic bag dilatation. Dig Dis Sci 28: 763, 1983.
319. Dulfresne CR, Jeyasingham K, Baker RR: Achalasia f the cardia associated with pulmonary sarcoidosis. Surgery 94:32, 1983.
320. Koberle F: Chagas' disease and Chagas' syndrome: The pathology of American trypanosomiasis. Adv Parasitol 6:63, 1968.
321. Greatorex RA, Thorpe JA: Achalasia-like disturbance of oesophageal motility following truncal vagotomy and antrectomy. Postgrad Med J 59:100, 1983.
322. Woods CA, Foutch PG, Waring JP, Sanowski RA: Pancreatic pseudocyst as a cause for secondary achalasia. Gastroenterology 96:235, 1989.
323. Foster PN, Stewart M, Lowe JS, Atkinson M: Achalasia like disorder of the oesophagus in von Recklinghausen's neurofibromatosis. Gut 28: 1522, 1987.
324. Roberts DH, Gilmore IT: Achalasia in Anderson-Fabry's disease. J R Soc Med 77:430, 1984.
325. Stuckey BG, Mastaglia FL, Reed WD, Pullan PT: Glucocorticoid insufficiency, achalasia, alacrima with autonomic and motor neuropathy. Ann Intern Med 106:62, 1987.
326. Cuthbert JA, Gallagher ND, Turtle JR: Colonic and oesophageal disturbance in a patient with multiple endocrine neoplasia, type 2b. Aust N Z J Med 8:518, 1978.
327. Similä S, Kokkonen J, Kaski M: Achalasia sicca—juvenile Sjögren's syndrome with achalasia and gastric hyposecretion. Eur J Pediatr 129: 175, 1978.
328. Song CW, Chun HJ, Kim CD, Ryu HS, Hyun JH, Kahrilas PJ: Association of pseudoachalasia with advancing cancer of the gastric cardia. Gastrointest Endosc 50:486, 1999.
329. Lucchinetti CF, Kimmel DW, Lennon VA: Paraneoplastic and oncologic profiles of patients seropositive for type 1 antineuronal nuclear autoantibodies. Neurology 50:652,1998.
330. Moonka R, Patti MG, Feo CV, et al: Clinical presentation and evaluation of malignant pseudoachalasia. J Gastrointest Surg 3:456, 1999.
331. Floch NR, Hinder RA, Klingler PJ, et al: Is laparoscopic reoperation for failed antireflux surgery feasible? Arch Surg 134:733, 1999.
332. Gaudric M, Sabate JM, Artru P, Chaussade S, Couturier D: Results of pneumatic dilatation in patients with dysphagia after antireflux surgery. Br J Surg 86:1088, 1999.
333. Woodfield CA, Levine MS, Rubesin SE, Langlotz CP, Laufer I: Diagnosis of primary versus secondary achalasia: Reassessment of clinical and radiographic criteria. AJR 175:727, 2000.
334. Katzka DA, Castell DO: Use of botulinum toxin as a diagnostic/therapeutic trial to help clarify an indication for definitive therapy in patients with achalasia. Am J Gastroenterol 94:637, 1999.
335. Van Dam J: Endosonographic evaluation of the patient with achalasia. Endoscopy 30:A48, 1998.
336. Vaezi MF, Richter JE: Current therapies for achalasia: Comparison and efficacy. J Clin Gastroenterol 27:21, 1998.
337. Bassotti G, Annese V: Review article: Pharmacological options in achalasia. Aliment Pharmacol Ther 13:1391, 1999.
338. Dodds WJ, Stewart ET, Kishk SM, et al: Radiologic amyl nitrite test for distinguishing pseudoachalasia from idiopathic achalasia. AJR 146: 21, 1986.
339. Gelfond M, Rozen P, Gilat T: Isosorbide dinitrate and nifedipine treatment of achalasia: A clinical manometric and radionuclide evaluation. Gastroenterology 83:963, 1982.
340. Berger K, McCallum RW: Nifedipine in the treatment of achalasia. Ann Intern Med 96:61, 1982.
341. Short TP, Thomas E: An overview of the role of calcium antagonists in the treatment of achalasia and diffuse oesophageal spasm. Drugs 43:177, 1992.
342. Bortolotti M: Medical therapy of achalasia: A benefit reserved for few. Digestion 60:11, 1999.
343. Hughes AJ: Botulinum toxin in clinical practice. Drugs 48:888, 1994.
344. Jankovic J: Botulinum toxin in movement disorders. Curr Opin Neurol 7:358, 1994.
345. Pasricha PJ, Ravich WJ, Hendrix TR, et al: Intrasphincteric botulinum toxin for the treatment of achalasia. N Engl J Med 322:774, 1995.
346. Pasricha PJ, Rai R, Ravich WJ, et al: Botulinum toxin for achalasia: Long-term outcome and predictors of response. Gastroenterology 110: 1410, 1996.
347. Prakash C, Freedland KE, Chan MF, Clouse RE: Botulinum toxin injections for achalasia symptoms can approximate the short term efficacy of a single pneumatic dilation: A survival analysis approach. Am J Gastroenterol 94:328, 1999.
348. Vaezi MF, Richter JE, Wilcox CM, et al: Botulinum toxin versus pneumatic dilatation in the treatment of achalasia: A randomized trial. Gut 44:231, 1999.
349. Muehldorfer SM, Schneider TH, Hochberger J, Martus P, Hahn EG, Ell C: Esophageal achalasia: intrasphincteric injection of botulinum toxin A versus balloon dilation. Endoscopy 31:517, 1999.
350. Annese V, Basciani M, Borrelli O, Leandro G, Simone P, Andriulli A: Intrasphincteric injection of botulinum toxin is effective in long-term treatment of esophageal achalasia. Muscle Nerve 21:1540, 1998.
351. Panaccione R, Gregor JC, Reynolds RP, Preiksaitis HG: Intrasphincteric botulinum toxin versus pneumatic dilatation for achalasia: A cost minimization analysis. Gastrointest Endosc 50:492, 1999.
352. Annese V, Bassotti G, Coccia G, et al: A multicentre randomized study of intrasphincteric botulinum toxin in patients with oesophageal achalasia. GISMAD achalasia study group. Gut 46:597, 2000.
353. Andrews SE, Anvari M, Dobranowski J: Laparoscopic Heller's myotomy or botulinum toxin injection for management of esophageal achalasia. Patient choice and treatment outcomes. Surg Endosc 13:742, 1999.
354. Greaves RR, Mulcahy HE, Patchett SE, et al: Early experience with intrasphincteric botulinum toxin in the treatment of achalasia. Aliment Pharmacol Ther 13:1221, 1999.
355. Horgan S, Hudda K, Eubanks T, McAllister J, Pellegrini CA: Does

botulinum toxin injection make esophagomyotomy a more difficult operation? Surg Endosc 13:576, 1999.
356. Patti MG, Feo CV, Arcerito M, et al: Effects of previous treatment on results of laparoscopic Heller myotomy for achalasia. Dig Dis Sci 44: 2270,1999.
357. Spiess AE, Kahrilas PJ: Treating achalasia: From whalebone to laparoscope. JAMA 280:638, 1998.
358. Gideon RM, Castell DO, Yarze J: Prospective randomized comparison of pneumatic dilatation technique in patients with idiopathic achalasia. Dig Dis Sci 44:1853, 1999.
359. Ott DJ, Richter JE, Wu WC, et al: Radiographic evaluation of esophagus immediately after pneumatic dilatation for achalasia. Dig Dis Sci 32:962, 1987.
360. Swedlund A, Traube M, Siskind BN, McCallum RW: Nonsurgical management of esophageal perforation from pneumatic dilatation in achalasia. Dig Dis Sci 34:379, 1989.
361. Reynolds JC, Parkman HP: Achalasia. Gastroenterol Clin North Am 18:223, 1989.
362. Alonso P, Gonzalez-Conde B, Macenlle R, et al: Achalasia: The usefulness of manometry for evaluation of treatment. Dig Dis Sci 44:536, 1999.
363. Vaezi MF, Baker ME, Richter JE: Assessment of esophageal emptying post-pneumatic dilation: Use of the timed barium esophagram. Am J Gastroenterol 94:1802, 1999.
364. Clouse RE, Abramson BK, Todorczuk JR: Achalasia in the elderly: Effects of aging on clinical presentation and outcome. Dig Dis Sci 36: 225, 1991.
365. Khan AA, Shah SW, Alam A, et al: Massively dilated esophagus in achalasia: Response to pneumatic balloon dilation. Am J Gastroenterol 94:2363, 1999.
366. Fennerty MB: Esophageal perforation during pneumatic dilatation for achalasia: A possible association with malnutrition. Dysphagia 5:227, 1990.
367. Scott HW Jr, DeLozier JB III, Sawyers JL, Adkins RB Jr: Surgical management of esophageal achalasia. South Med J 78:1309, 1985.
368. Pai GP, Ellison RG, Rubin JW, Moore HV: Two decades of experience with modified Heller's myotomy for achalasia. Ann Thorac Surg 38:201, 1984.
369. Vantrappen G, Hellemans J: Treatment of achalasia and related motor disorders. Gastroenterology 79:144, 1980.
370. Csendes A, Velasco N, Braghetto I, Henriquez A: A prospective randomized study comparing forceful dilatation and esophagomyotomy in patients with achalasia of the esophagus. Gastroenterology 80:789, 1981.
371. Ellis FH Jr, Watkins E Jr, Gibb SP, Heatley GJ: Ten- to 20-year clinical results after short esophagomyotomy without an antireflux procedure (modified Heller operation) for esophageal achalasia. Eur J Cardiol Thorac Surg 6:86, 1992.
372. Malthaner RA, Todd TR, Miller L, Pearson FG: Long-term results in surgically managed esophageal achalasia. Ann Thorac Surg 58:1343, 1994.
373. Banbury MK, Rice TW, Goldblum JR, et al: Esophagectomy with gastric reconstruction for achalasia. J Thorac Cardiovasc Surg 117: 1077, 1999.
374. Patti MG, Tamburini A, Pellegrini CA: Cardiomyotomy. Semin Laparosc Surg 6:186, 1999.
375. Dempsey DT, Kalan M, Gerson RS, Parkman HP, Maier WP: Comparison of outcomes following open and laparoscopic esophagomyotomy for achalasia. Surg Endosc 13:747, 1999.
376. Richardson WS, Bowen JC: Minimally invasive esophageal surgery. Surg Clin North Am 78:795, 1998.
377. Pellegrini C, Wetter LA, Patti M, et al: Thoracoscopic esophagomyotomy: Initial experience with a new approach for the treatment of achalasia. Ann Surg 216:291, 1992.
378. Patti MG, Pellegrini CA, Horgan S, et al: Minimally invasive surgery for achalasia: An 8-year experience with 168 patients. Ann Surg 230: 587, 1999.
379. Champion JK, Delisle N, Hunt T: Comparison of thoracoscopic and laparoscopic esophagomyotomy with fundoplication for primary motility disorders. Eur J Cardiothorac Surg 16(suppl 1):S34, 1999.
380. Zaninotto G, Costantini M, Molena D, et al: Treatment of esophageal achalasia with laparoscopic Heller myotomy and Dor partial anterior fundoplication: Prospective evaluation of 100 consecutive patients. J Gastrointest Surg 4:282, 2000.
381. Bonavina L, Incarbone R, Antoniazzi L, et al: Previous endoscopic treatment does not affect complication rate and outcome of laparoscopic Heller myotomy and anterior fundoplication for oesophageal achalasia. Ital J Gastroenterol Hepatol 31:827, 1999.
382. Ponce J, Juan M, Garrigues V, Pascual S, Berenguer J: Efficacy and safety of cardiomyotomy in patients with achalasia after failure of pneumatic dilatation. Dig Dis Sci 44:2277, 1999.
383. Beckingham IJ, Callanan M, Louw JA, Bornman PC: Laparoscopic cardiomyotomy for achalasia after failed balloon dilatation. Surg Endosc 13:493, 1999.
384. Wang PC, Sharp KW, Holzman MD, et al: The outcome of laparoscopic Heller myotomy without antireflux procedure in patients with achalasia. Am Surg 64:515, 1998.
385. Okike N, Payne WS, Neufeld DM, et al: Esophagomyotomy versus forceful dilation for achalasia of the esophagus: Results in 899 patients. Ann Thorac Surg 28:119, 1979.
386. Jara FM, Toledo-Pereyra LH, Lewis JW, Magilligan DJ Jr: Long-term results of esophagomyotomy for achalasia of esophagus. Arch Surg 114:935, 1979.
387. Lortat-Jacob JL, Richard CA, Fekete F, Testart J: Cardiospasm and esophageal carcinoma: Report of 24 cases. Surgery 66:969, 1969.
388. Wychulis AR, Woolam GL, Andersen HA, Ellis FH Jr: Achalasia and carcinoma of the esophagus. JAMA 125:1638, 1981.
389. Streitz JM Jr, Ellis FH Jr, Gibb SP, Heatley GM: Achalasia and squamous cell carcinoma of the esophagus: Analysis of 241 patients. Ann Thorac Surg 59:1604, 1995.
390. Loviscek LF, Cenoz MC, Badaloni AE, Agarinakazato O: Early cancer in achalasia. Dis Esophagus 11:239, 1998.
391. Dunaway CP, Wong CR: Risk and surveillance intervals for squamous cell carcinoma in achalasia. Gastrointest Endosc Clin North Am 11: 425, 2001.
392. Gillies M, Nicks R, Skyring A: Clinical, manometric and pathological studies in diffuse oesophageal spasm. BMJ 2:527, 1967.
393. Cassella RR, Ellis FH Jr, Brown AL: Diffuse spasm of the lower part of the esophagus. Fine structure of esophageal smooth muscle and nerve. JAMA 191:379, 1965.
394. Vantrappen G, Janssens J, Hellemans J, Coremans G: Achalasia, diffuse esophageal spasm, and related motility disorders. Gastroenterology 76:450, 1979.
395. Clouse RE, Lustman PJ, Reidel WL: Correlation of esophageal motility abnormalities with neuropsychiatric status in diabetics. Gastroenterology 90:1146, 1986.
396. Kramer P, Fleshler B, McNally E, Harris LD: Oesophageal sensitivity to Mecholyl in symptomatic diffuse spasm. Gut 8:120, 1967.
397. Nostrant TT, Sams J, Huber T: Bethanechol increases the diagnostic yield in patients with esophageal chest pain. Gastroenterology 91: 1141, 1986.
398. London RL, Ouyang A, Snape WJ Jr, et al: Provocation of esophageal pain by ergonovine or edrophonium. Gastroenterology 81:10, 1981.
399. Richter JE, Dalton CB, Katz PO, et al: Stress: A modulator of esophageal contractions. Gastroenterology 90:1603, 1986.
400. Richter JE, Barish CF, Castell DO: Abnormal sensory perception in patients with esophageal chest pain. Gastroenterology 91:845, 1986.
401. Clouse RE, Lustman PJ: Psychiatric illness and contraction abnormalities of the esophagus. N Engl J Med 309:1337, 1983.
402. Rate AJ, Hobson AR, Barlow J, Bancewicz J: Abnormal neurophysiology in patients with oesophageal motility disorders. Br J Surg 86: 1202, 1999.
403. Reidel WL, Clouse RE: Variations in clinical presentation of patients with esophageal contraction abnormalities. Dig Dis Sci 30:1065, 1985.
404. Ellis FH Jr, Olsen AM, Schlegel JF, Code CF: Surgical treatment of esophageal hypermotility disturbances. JAMA 188:862, 1964.
405. Clouse RE, Eckert TC, Staiano A: Hiatus hernia and esophageal contraction abnormalities. Am J Med 81:447, 1986.
406. Clouse RE, Staiano A, Alrakawi A: Topographic analysis of esophageal double-peaked waves. Gastroenterology 118:469, 2000.
407. Dalton CB, Castell DO, Hewson EG, et al: Diffuse esophageal spasm. A rare motility disorder not characterized by high-amplitude contractions. Dig Dis Sci 36:1025, 1991.
408. Hewson EG, Ott DJ, Dalton CB, et al: Manometry and radiology. Complementary studies in the assessment of esophageal motility disorders. Gastroenterology 98:3, 1990.
409. Benjamin SB, Gerhardt DC, Castell DO: High amplitude, peristaltic esophageal contractions associated with chest pain and/or dysphagia. Gastroenterology 77:478, 1979.
410. Eypasch EP, Stein HJ, DeMeester TR, et al: A new technique to

define and clarify esophageal motor disorders. Am J Surg 159:144, 1990.
411. DiMarino AJ Jr, Cohen S: Characteristics of lower esophageal sphincter function in symptomatic diffuse esophageal spasm. Gastroenterology 66:1, 1974.
412. Ebert EC, Ouyang A, Wright SH, et al: Pneumatic dilatation in patients with symptomatic diffuse esophageal spasm and lower esophageal sphincter dysfunction. Dig Dis Sci 28:481, 1983.
413. Katz PO, Dalton CB, Richter JE, et al: Esophageal testing of patients with noncardiac chest pain or dysphagia. Ann Intern Med 106:593, 1987.
414. Guelrud M, Zambrano-Rincones V, Simon C, et al: Dysphagia and lower esophageal sphincter abnormalities after proximal gastric vagotomy. Am J Surg 149:232, 1985.
415. Kahrilas PJ, Clouse RE, Hogan WJ: American Gastroenterological Association technical review on the clinical use of esophageal manometry. Gastroenterology 107:1865, 1994.
416. Breumelhof R, Nadorp JHSM, Akkermans LMA, Smout AJPM: Analysis of 24-hour esophageal pressure and pH data in unselected patients with noncardiac chest pain. Gastroenterology 99:1257, 1990.
417. Peters L, Maas L, Petty D, et al: Spontaneous non-cardiac chest pain: Evaluation by 24-hour ambulatory esophageal motility and pH monitoring. Gastroenterology 94:878, 1988.
418. Colon VJ, Young MA, Ramirez FC: The short- and long-term efficacy of empirical esophageal dilation in patients with nonobstructive dysphagia: A prospective, randomized study. Am J Gastroenterol 95:910, 2000.
419. Parker WA, MacKinnon GL: Nitrites in the treatment of diffuse esophageal spasm. Drug Intell Clin Pharm 15:806, 1981.
420. Mellow MH: Effect of isosorbide and hydralazine in painful primary esophageal motility disorders. Gastroenterology 83:364, 1982.
421. Richter JE, Dalton CB, Bradley LA, Castell DO: Oral nifedipine in the treatment of noncardiac chest pain in patients with the nutcracker esophagus. Gastroenterology 93:21, 1987.
422. Clouse RE, Lustman PJ, Eckert TC et al: Low-dose trazodone for symptomatic patients with esophageal contraction abnormalities: A double-blind, placebo-controlled trial. Gastroenterology 92:1027, 1987.
423. Cannon RO, Quyyumi AA, Mincemoyer R, et al: Imipramine in patients with chest pain despite normal coronary angiograms. N Engl J Med 330:1411, 1994.
424. Cox ID, Hann CM, Kaski JC: Low dose imipramine improves chest pain but not quality of life in patients with angina and normal coronary angiograms. Eur Heart J 19:250, 1998.
425. Varia I, Logue E, O'Connor C, et al: Randomized trial of sertraline in patients with unexplained chest pain of noncardiac origin. Am Heart J 140:367, 2000.
426. Handa M, Mine K, Yamamoto H, Hayashi H, Tsuchida O, Kanazawa F, Kubo C: Antidepressant treatment of patients with diffuse esophageal spasm. A psychosomatic approach. J Clin Gastroenterol 28:228, 1999.
427. Clouse RE: Antidepressants for functional gastrointestinal syndromes. Dig Dis Sci 39:2352, 1994.
428. Prakash C, Clouse RE: Long-term outcome from tricyclic antidepressant treatment of functional chest pain. Dig Dis Sci 44:2373, 1999.
429. Borjesson M, Pilhall M, Eliasson T, Norssell H, Mannheimer C, Rolny P: Esophageal visceral pain sensitivity: Effects of TENS and correlation with manometric findings. Dig Dis Sci 43:1621, 1998.
430. Vantrappen G, Janssens J: To dilate or to operate? That is the question. Gut 24:1013, 1983.
431. Horton ML, Goff JS: Surgical treatment of nutcracker esophagus. Dig Dis Sci 31:878, 1986.
432. Ellis FH Jr: Long esophagomyotomy for diffuse esophageal spasm and related disorders: An historical overview. Dis Esophagus 11:210, 1998.
433. Generini S, Fiori G, Pignone AM, et al: Systemic sclerosis. A clinical overview. Adv Exp Med Biol 455:73, 1998.
434. Rodnan GP, Medsger TA Jr, Buckingham RB: Progressive systemic sclerosis-CREST syndrome: Observations on natural history and late complications in 90 patients. Arthritis Rheum 18:423, 1975.
435. Cohen S, Fisher R, Lipshutz W, et al: The pathogenesis of esophageal dysfunction in scleroderma and Raynaud's disease. J Clin Invest 51: 2663, 1972.
436. DeSchryver-Kecskemeti K, Clouse RE: Gastrointestinal neuropathic changes in a group of patients with systemic connective tissue disease. Dig Dis Sci 29:549, 1984.
437. Weston S, Thumshirn M, Wiste J, Camilleri M: Clinical and upper gastrointestinal motility features in systemic sclerosis and related disorders. Am J Gastroenterol 93:1085, 1998.
438. Fuller L, Huprich JE, Theisen J, et al: Abnormal esophageal body function: Radiographic manometric correlation. Am Surg 65:911, 1999.
439. Schneider HA, Yonker RA, Longley S, et al: Scleroderma esophagus: A nonspecific entity. Ann Intern Med 100:848, 1984.
440. Orringer MB: Surgical management of scleroderma reflux esophagitis. Surg Clin North Am 63:859, 1983.
441. Tatelman M, Keech MK: Esophageal motility in systemic lupus erythematosus, rheumatoid arthritis and scleroderma. Radiology 86:1041, 1966.
442. Sharp GC, Irvin WS, Tan EM, et al: Mixed connective tissue disease: An apparently distinct rheumatic disease syndrome associated with a specific antibody to an extractable nuclear antigen (ENA). Am J Med 52:148, 1972.
443. Bestetti A, Carola F, Conciato L, Marasini B, Tarolo GL: Esophageal scintigraphy with a semisolid meal to evaluate esophageal dysmotility in systemic sclerosis and Raynaud's phenomenon. J Nucl Med 40:77, 1999.
444. Hollis JB, Castell DO, Braddom RL: Esophageal function in diabetes mellitus and its relation to peripheral neuropathy. Gastroenterology 73: 1098, 1977.
445. Loo FD, Dodds WJ, Soergel KH, et al: Multipeaked esophageal peristaltic pressure waves in patients with diabetic neuropathy. Gastroenterology 88:485, 1985.
446. Cohen S: Motor disorders of the esophagus. N Engl J Med 301:184, 1979.
447. Weber LD, Nashel DJ, Mellow MH: Pharyngeal dysphagia in alcoholic myopathy. Ann Intern Med 95:189, 1981.
448. Grande L, Lacima G, Ros E, et al: Deterioration of esophageal motility with age: A manometric study of 79 healthy subjects. Am J Gastroenterol 94:1795, 1999.
449. Galmiche JP, Janssens J: The pathophysiology of gastro-oesophageal reflux disease: An overview. Scand J Gastroenterol 30(suppl 211):7, 1995.
450. Fouad YM, Katz PO, Katlebakk JG, Castell DO: Ineffective esophageal motility: The most common motility abnormality in patients with GERD-associated respiratory symptoms. Am J Gastroenterol 94:1464, 1999.
451. Hunter JG, Trus TL, Branum GD, et al: A physiologic approach to laparoscopic fundoplication for gastroesophageal reflux disease. Ann Surg 223:673, 1996.
452. Farrell TM, Archer SB, Galloway KD, et al: Heartburn is more likely to recur after Toupet fundoplication than Nissen fundoplication. Am Surg 66:229, 2000.
453. Mazzadi S, Salis GB, Garcia A, et al: Foreign body impaction in the esophagus: Are there underlying motor disorders? Dis Esophagus 11: 51, 1998.
454. Lacy PD, Donnelly MJ, McGrath JP, et al: Acute food bolus impaction: Aetiology and management. J Laryngol Otol 111:1158, 1997.
455. Jaspersen D: Drug-induced oesophageal disorders: Pathogenesis, incidence, prevention and management. Drug Saf 22:237, 2000.
456. Colon V, Grade A, Pulliam G, et al: Effect of doses of glucagon used to treat food impaction on esophageal motor function in normal subjects. Dysphagia 14:27, 1999.

Chapter 33

Gastroesophageal Reflux Disease and Its Complications, Including Barrett's Metaplasia

Peter J. Kahrilas and John E. Pandolfino

DEFINITIONS AND EPIDEMIOLOGY

The term *gastroesophageal reflux disease* (GERD) describes any symptomatic condition or histopathologic alteration resulting from episodes of gastroesophageal reflux. Reflux esophagitis is a condition experienced by a subset of GERD patients with endoscopically evident lesions in the esophageal mucosa. However, gastroesophageal reflux often causes symptoms in the absence of esophagitis, and 24-hour esophageal pH monitoring can be helpful in identifying this subset of GERD patients. Nonerosive, or endoscopy-negative, GERD patients have reflux symptoms and abnormal esophageal acid exposure during ambulatory 24-hour pH monitoring, but no endoscopic evidence of esophagitis. The acid sensitive esophagus patient is in a subset of the endoscopy-negative GERD population characterized by normal esophageal acid exposure but nonetheless a strong correlation between reflux symptoms and gastroesophageal reflux events.[1]

Although GERD is widely reported to be one of the most prevalent clinical conditions afflicting the gastrointestinal tract, incidence and prevalence figures are based more on estimates than on actual data. This difficulty occurs partly because GERD and esophagitis cannot be differentiated by a clinical history and partly because there is no gold standard for the recognition or exclusion of GERD. Thus, epidemiologic estimates regarding GERD must make assumptions; the most obvious is that heartburn is an indicator of GERD. A cross-sectional study surveying hospital employees in the United States in the 1970s found that 7% of individuals experienced heartburn daily, 14% weekly, and 15% monthly.[2] With respect to esophagitis, even though endoscopic changes in the esophageal mucosa are accepted as a standard for diagnosis, its prevalence is difficult to ascertain in the absence of population based studies. Early reports using ambulatory esophageal pH monitoring to define GERD found that 48% to 79% of patients with pathologic acid exposure had esophagitis.[3, 4] A review from 1999, perhaps less subject to selection bias, has suggested that the prevalence of esophagitis among the GERD population is lower, in that 55% to 81% of patients have endoscopy-negative disease.[5] Similar to that of esophagitis, the prevalence of Barrett's metaplasia is difficult to determine in the absence of a characteristic symptom profile or population studies. As an illustration, an autopsy study suggested that fewer than one in six patients with Barrett's metaplasia was recognized clinically prior to death.[6]

GERD is equally prevalent among men and women, but there is a male preponderance of esophagitis (2 : 1 to 3 : 1) and of Barrett's metaplasia (10 : 1).[7] Pregnancy is associated with the highest incidence of GERD: 48% to 79% of pregnant women complain of heartburn.[8] All forms of GERD affect whites more frequently than members of other races. There is substantial geographic variation in prevalence with very low rates in Africa and Asia and high rates in North America and Europe.[9] The pathogenic role of medications in GERD has focused on agents that decrease lower esophageal

*This work was supported by grant RO1 DC00646 (PJK) from the Public Health Service.

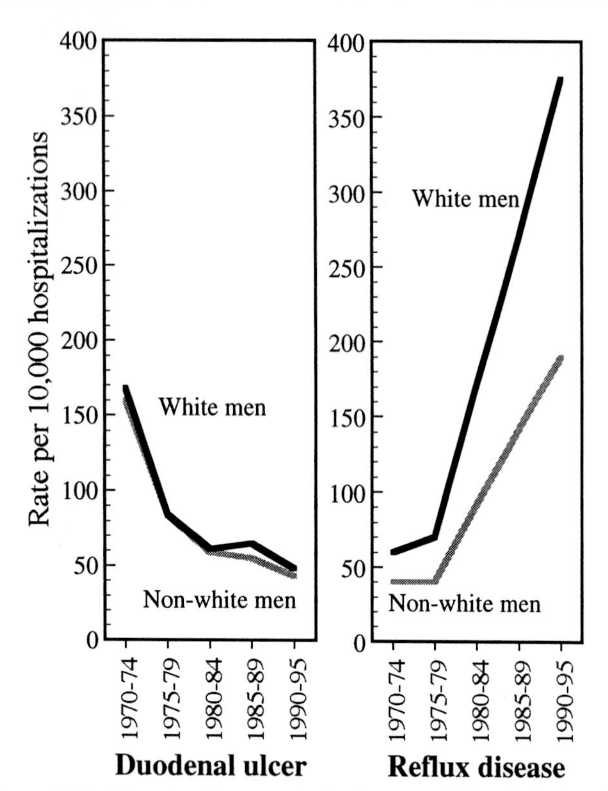

Figure 33–1. Opposing time trends in the rates of hospitalization for duodenal ulcer and gastroesophageal reflux disease. Hospitalization rates were analyzed using the computerized database from the U.S. Department of Veteran Affairs. (Modified from El-Serag HB, Sonnenberg A: Opposing time trends of peptic ulcer and reflux disease. Gut 43:327, 1998.)

sphincter (LES) pressure and on nonsteroidal anti-inflammatory drugs (NSAIDs). A study conducted in 2000 reported that 33% of patients who chronically used LES relaxing medications experienced reflux symptoms compared with 16% of control patients.[10] The relationship between NSAIDs and GERD is controversial. Studies suggest that NSAIDs may be associated with peptic strictures.[11] El-Serag reported a small but significant odds ratio of 1.4 for reflux esophagitis in a large veteran population using NSAIDs.[12]

The role of *Helicobacter pylori* in GERD deserves special attention given the striking inverse time trends in the prevalence of GERD and *H. pylori*–related peptic ulcer disease[13] (Fig. 33–1). Epidemiologic data reveal that GERD patients with esophagitis are less likely to have *H. pylori* infection.[14] *H. pylori* infection is also associated with a decreased prevalence of Barrett's metaplasia.[15] Further supporting the protective role of *H. pylori* infection are two studies suggesting an increased incidence of esophagitis[16] and pathologic gastroesophageal reflux[17] after antibiotic eradication of *H. pylori*. Additional data suggest that *H. pylori* infection improves the efficacy of antisecretory therapy in healing esophagitis and maintaining remission.[18, 19] These epidemiologic data have led some to believe that *H. pylori* should not be eradicated in patients with GERD. However, *H. pylori* is a risk factor for the development of peptic ulcer and gastric cancer, causing many practitioners to be uncomfortable with that recommendation. Currently, this issue is not resolved.

HISTOPATHOLOGY OF GASTROESOPHAGEAL REFLUX DISEASE

The esophagus is lined with noncornified stratified squamous epithelium (see Chapter 31). The basal cell layer predominantly contains cells with a high nuclear-to-cytoplasm ratio and is the site of cellular proliferation, generally accounting for less than 15% of the total thickness of the epithelium. At the squamocolumnar junction, the basal cell layer is in continuity with the columnar cells of the stomach.[20] Toward the luminal surface of the squamous epithelium, the basal cell layer blends abruptly with the stratified squamous cells. The prickle cell layer, adjacent to the basal cell layer, has prominent intercellular bridges. The squamous cells show progressive flattening and nuclear elongation as they migrate toward

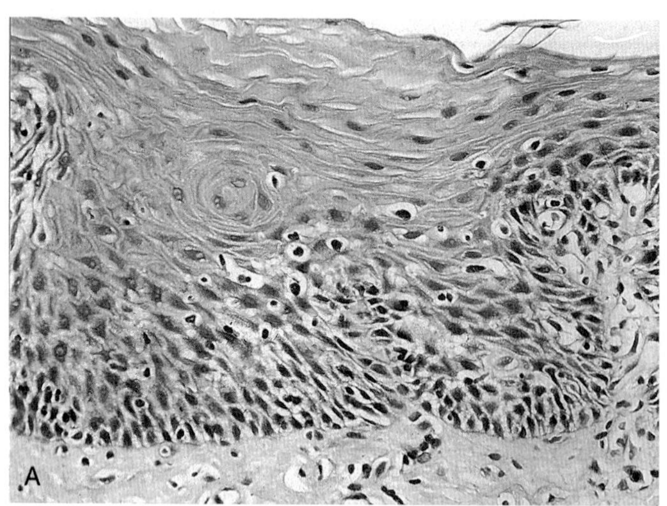

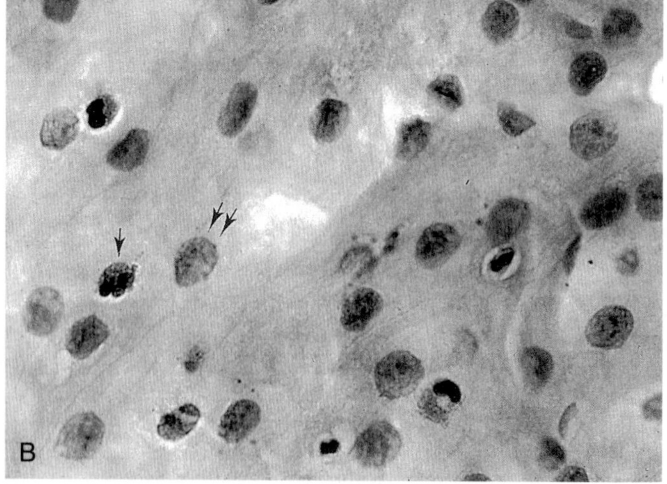

Figure 33–2. Histopathology of gastroesophageal reflux disease. *A*, Esophageal biopsy slows basal cell hyperplasia, papillary hyperplasia, and numerous intramucosal inflammatory cells. *B*, Higher power shows intramucosal inflammatory cells with multiple-lobed nuclei and a granular cytoplasm representing predominantly eosinophils (*single arrow*). Compare these cells with the nuclei of the normal squamous epithelium (*double arrow*). (Courtesy of Edward Lee, MD, and Mark Feldman, MD.)

the surface. Papillae containing thin walled blood vessels (analogous to the dermal pegs of the skin) indent the overlying squamous mucosa. The length of these papillae is normally less than two thirds of the overall thickness of the epithelium.

GERD can cause histopathologic changes to the esophageal epithelium even without endoscopically evident esophagitis (Fig. 33–2). These are reactive epithelial changes, as opposed to the inflammatory cell infiltration that occurs with esophagitis. Reactive epithelial changes cause hyperplasia of the basal zone and elongation of the papillae such that they extend more than two thirds of the way to the surface.[21] In addition, there may be increased mitotic figures, vascularization of the epithelium with dilated vessels at the apices of the papillae, increased papillae, loss of longitudinal orientation of the surface epithelium, and balloon cells.

When mucosal erosions are evident endoscopically, histopathologic findings include severe epithelial injury usually accompanied by neutrophilic or eosinophilic infiltration. These changes are typically confined to the mucosa, lamina propria, and muscularis mucosa. The potential complications of esophagitis—peptic stricture, pseudodiverticula, Barrett's metaplasia (discussed later), inflammatory polyps, and reactive changes that can mimic dysplasia—are all consequences of the repair process.[22, 23] Perforation and fistulization are rare complications.

PATHOGENESIS

The fundamental abnormality in GERD is exposure of esophageal or supraesophageal epithelium to gastric secretions that results in either histopathologic injury or elicitation of symptoms. Some degree of gastroesophageal reflux is considered normal, but symptoms occur when the tolerance of the epithelium is exceeded. This can occur for many reasons, including an excessive number of reflux events, prolonged acid clearance, impaired mucosal resistance, or an interaction between some degree of reflux and dietary, behavioral, or emotional cofactors. The intermittent nature of symptoms in many individuals with GERD suggests that the injurious and restorative processes are part of a delicately balanced system that is susceptible to perturbation. Potential symptoms that might then ensue include heartburn, regurgitation, chest pain, dysphagia, and laryngitis (see Chapter 6).

Mechanisms of Reflux

A prerequisite for GERD is gastroesophageal reflux, an event normally prevented by a competent esophagogastric junction. The functional integrity of the esophagogastric junction has been attributed to numerous anatomic and physiologic mechanisms including intrinsic LES pressure, extrinsic compression of the LES by the crural diaphragm, the intra-abdominal location of the LES, integrity of the phrenoesophageal ligament, and maintenance of the acute angle of His between the distal esophagus and proximal stomach with its flap valve function. Quite possibly, the competence of the antireflux barrier is the sum of its parts and incompetence becomes increasingly severe as successive components are compromised. Furthermore, the dominant mechanism protecting against reflux may vary with physiologic circumstance. For example, the intra-abdominal segment of the LES may be important in preventing reflux associated with swallowing, the diaphragmatic crus may be of cardinal importance during episodes of increased intra-abdominal pressure, and the basal LES pressure may be of primary importance during restful recumbency. As these protective mechanisms are compromised the effect is additive, resulting in increasingly abnormal esophageal acid exposure.

Investigations have focused on three dominant mechanisms of esophagogastric junction incompetence: (1) transient LES relaxations without anatomic abnormality, (2) LES hypotension without anatomic abnormality, and (3) anatomic distortion of the esophagogastric junction inclusive of, but not limited to, hiatal hernia. The latter category may affect both the frequency of transient LES relaxation and the pressure topographic characteristics of the LES.[24] Individual patients can be found exemplifying each of these pathogenic mechanisms; however, the portion of the entire GERD population that can be assigned to each category remains controversial. Evidence from 1988 and 1995 suggests that the dominant mechanism may vary with disease severity with transient LES relaxations dominant in mild disease and mechanisms associated with hiatal hernia and/or a weak sphincter dominant in more severe disease.[25–27]

Transient Lower Esophageal Sphincter Relaxation

There is compelling evidence that transient LES relaxations are the most frequent mechanism for reflux in patients who have normal LES pressure (>10 mm Hg) just prior to the episode of reflux. Figure 33–3 highlights the differences between transient LES relaxation and swallow-induced LES relaxation. Transient LES relaxations occur independently of swallowing, are not accompanied by peristalsis, are accompanied by diaphragmatic inhibition, and persist for longer periods (>10 seconds) than do swallow-induced LES relaxations.[27, 28] Prolonged manometric recordings have not demonstrated an increased frequency of transient LES relaxations in GERD patients compared with normal control patients.[29] However, the frequency of acid reflux (as opposed to gas reflux) during transient LES relaxations has been reported to be higher in GERD patients.[29] Identifying risk factors for this predisposition to acid reflux is the subject of ongoing investigation.

Recognizing the importance of transient LES relaxations in promoting reflux, investigators have attempted to define this reflex by using physiologic and pharmacologic manipulations. The dominant stimulus for transient LES relaxation is distention of the proximal stomach, which is not surprising given that transient LES relaxation is the physiologic mechanism for belching.[30, 31] Transient LES relaxation can be elicited experimentally either by gaseous distention of the stomach or by distention of the proximal stomach with a barostat bag. Gastric distention activates vagal afferent mechanoreceptors in the gastric cardia that project to the nucleus tractus solitarii in the brainstem and subsequently to the dorsal motor nucleus of the vagus. The transient LES relaxation reflex is abolished by vagotomy.[27] Several pharmacologic agents have been reported to inhibit transient LES relaxations, although none of these agents has been shown

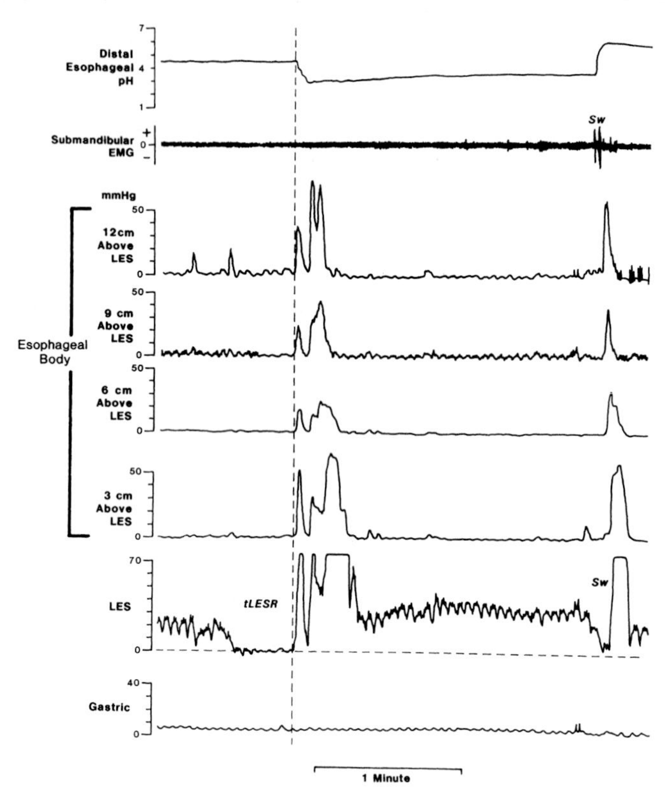

Figure 33–3. Example of a transient lower esophageal sphincter (LES) relaxation (LLESR). LES pressure is referenced to gastric pressure, which is indicated by the *horizontal dotted line.* Note that the transient LES relaxation persisted for almost 30 seconds, whereas the swallow-induced LES relaxation to the right (Sw) persisted for only 5 seconds. Also note the absence of a submandibular electromyographic (EMG) signal during the transient LES relaxation, which indicates absence of a pharyngeal swallow. Finally, the associated esophageal motor activity is different in the two types of LES relaxation: the swallow-induced relaxation is associated with primary peristalsis, whereas the transient LES relaxation is associated with a vigorous, repetitive "off contraction" throughout the esophageal body. (From Kahrilas PJ, Gupta RR: Mechanisms of reflux of acid associated with cigarette smoking. Gut 31:4, 1990.)

clinically useful in this capacity (Table 33–1). Further work along this line may eventually provide another treatment modality for GERD.

Hypotensive Lower Esophageal Sphincter

Physiologically, the LES is a 3- to 4-cm segment of tonically contracted smooth muscle at the esophagogastric junction. Resting tone of the LES varies among normal individuals from 10 to 30 mm Hg relative to intragastric pressure. Continuous LES pressure monitoring reveals considerable temporal variation. Large increases in LES pressure occur with the migrating motor complex; during phase III LES pressure may exceed 80 mm Hg. Lesser fluctuations occur throughout the day with pressure decreasing in the postcibal state and increasing during sleep.[32] Intra-abdominal pressure, gastric distention, peptides, hormones, various foods, and many medications affect resting LES pressure (see Table 33–1). The genesis of LES tone is a property of both the muscle itself and its extrinsic innervation. The myogenic component is calcium dependent[33] and persists after treatment with the neurotoxin tetrodotoxin.[34] Extrinsic neurogenic control of LES tonic contraction is mainly vagal and is cholinergic (atropine sensitive).[35]

Gastroesophageal reflux disease can occur in the context of LES pressure diminished by either strain-induced or free reflux. Strain-induced reflux occurs when a hypotensive LES is overcome and blown open by an abrupt increase of intra-abdominal pressure (Fig. 33–4). Manometric data suggest that this type of reflux rarely occurs when the LES pressure is greater than 10 mm Hg.[36] Free reflux is characterized by a fall in intraesophageal pH without an identifiable change in either intragastric pressure or LES pressure. Episodes of free reflux are observed only when the LES pressure is within 0 to 4 mm Hg of intragastric pressure.

A puzzling clinical observation, and one that supports the importance of transient LES relaxations, is that only a minority of patients with GERD have a resting LES pressure of less than 10 mm Hg.[37, 38] This observation can be partially reconciled when one considers the dynamic nature of LES pressure (see Table 33–1). The isolated resting measurement of LES pressure under fasting conditions is probably useful only for identifying patients with a grossly hypotensive sphincter; such individuals are constantly susceptible

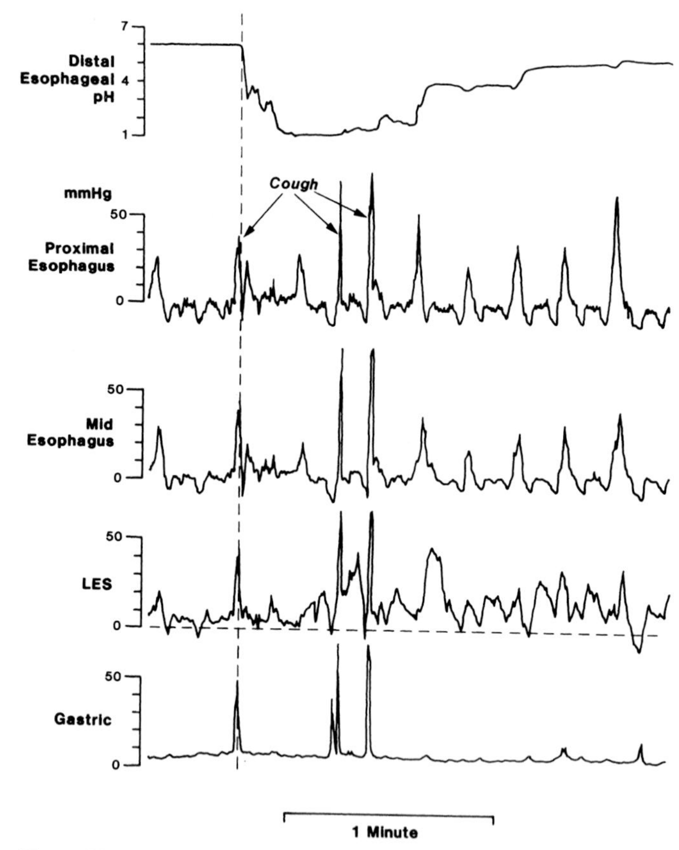

Figure 33–4. Gastroesophageal acid reflux event occurring in a smoker with reflux disease during the smoking period. Coughing (*arrows*) was associated with abrupt increases in intra-abdominal (*bottom tracing*) and intrathoracic pressure. As was typical of manometric records obtained during smoking, there were wide intrathoracic and lower esophageal sphincter (LES) pressure fluctuations with somewhat labored respiration. The swallow frequency was often three to four per minute, which was considerably higher than normal. The lower esophageal sphincter (LES) pressure value immediately before reflux was 5 mm Hg and was apparently overcome by the abdominal strain associated with coughing resulting in acid reflux. (From Kahrilas PJ, Gupta RR: Mechanisms of reflux of acid associated with cigarette smoking. Gut 31:4, 1990.)

Table 33–1 | **Substances That Modulate Lower Esophageal Sphincter Contractility**

	RESTING LES PRESSURE		TRANSIENT LES RELAXATION FREQUENCY	
	Increased	**Decreased**	**Increased**	**Decreased**
Hormones	Gastrin Motilin Substance P	Secretin Cholecystokinin Glucagon Gastric inhibitory polypeptide Vasoactive intestinal polypeptide Progesterone	Cholecystokinin	
Neural agents	α-Adrenergic agonists β-Adrenergic antagonists Cholinergic agonists	α-Adrenergic antagonists β-Adrenergic agonists Cholinergic antagonists Serotonin	L-Arginine	L-NAME* Serotonin
Medications	Metoclopramide Domperidone Prostaglandin $F_{2\alpha}$ Cisapride	Nitrates Calcium channel blockers Theophylline Morphine Meperidine Diazepam Barbiturates	Sumatriptan	Atropine Morphine Loxiglumide Baclofen
Foods	Protein	Fat Chocolate Ethanol Peppermint	Fat	

*Inhibitor of nitric oxide synthase.
LES, lower esophageal sphincter.

to stress and free reflux. However, there is probably a larger population of patients susceptible to strain-induced or free reflux when their LES pressure periodically decreases as a result of specific foods, drugs, or habits.[39]

Diaphragmatic Sphincter, Hiatal Hernia, and Other Anatomic Variables

Physiologic investigations in 1982 and 1985 advanced the two-sphincter hypothesis for maintenance of esophagogastric junction competence, suggesting that both the intrinsic smooth muscle LES and the extrinsic crural diaphragm serve a sphincteric function. Independent control of the crural diaphragm can be demonstrated during esophageal distention, vomiting, and belching when electrical activity in the crural diaphragm is selectively inhibited despite continued respiration.[40, 41] This reflex inhibition of crural activity is eliminated with vagotomy.[40] On the other hand, crural diaphragmatic contraction is augmented during abdominal compression, straining, or coughing.[42] Additional evidence of the sphincteric function of the hiatus derives from manometric data from patients after distal esophagectomy.[43] These patients still exhibited a pressure of about 6 mm Hg within the hiatal canal despite the removal of the smooth muscle LES.

The clinical significance of esophagogastric junction pressure attributed to the crural diaphragm and hiatal canal pertains to a condition potentially associated with its anatomic disruption: hiatal hernia. The impact of hiatal hernia was demonstrated in studies in which the susceptibility to gastroesophageal reflux elicited by straining maneuvers was tested in individuals with and without hiatal hernia. Of several physiologic and anatomic variables tested, the size of hiatal hernia was reported to have the highest correlation with the susceptibility to strain-induced reflux (Fig. 33–5). The implication of this observation is that hiatal hernia patients exhibit progressive impairment of the diaphragmatic component of the esophagogastric junction proportional to the extent of axial herniation.[44]

Another effect of hiatal hernia on the antireflux barrier is diminution of the intraluminal pressure within the esophago-

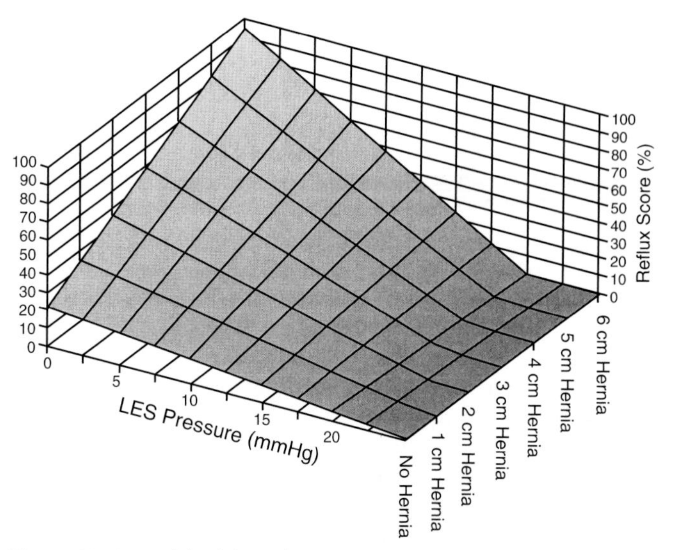

Figure 33–5. Model of the relationship between the lower esophageal sphincter (LES) pressure, the size of hiatal hernia, and the susceptibility to gastroesophageal reflux induced by provocative maneuvers as reflected by the reflux score on the vertical axis. The overall equation of the model is: reflux score = 22.64 + 12.05 (hernia size) − 0.83 (LES pressure) − 0.65 (LES pressure × hernia size). The multiple correlation coefficient of this equation for the 50 subject data set was 0.86. Thus, the susceptibility to stress reflux is dependent upon the interaction of the instantaneous value of LES pressure and the size of the hiatal hernia. (From Sloan S, Rademaker AW, Kahrilas PJ: Determinants of gastroesophageal junction incompetence: Hiatus hernia, lower esophageal sphincter, or both? Ann Intern Med 117:977, 1992.)

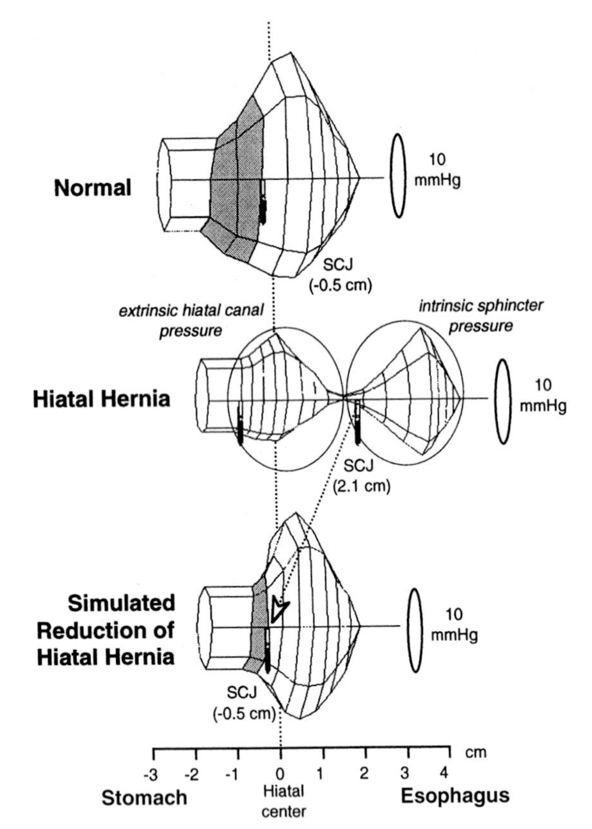

Figure 33–6. Axial pressure topography of the gastroesophageal junction of normal subjects (top) and hiatal hernia patients (middle). Position zero on the axial scale is the midpoint of the diaphragmatic hiatus. The wireframe representations are rotated such that the right anterior pressure is at the top and left posterior pressure is at the bottom, thus accentuating the radial pressure asymmetry. The proximal clip indicates the median position of the squamocolumnar junction (SCJ), and the distal clip marks the median position of the intragastric aspect of the gastroesophageal junction as imaged endoscopically. All values of length and pressure are the medians for the subject groups. The lower figure is a simulation of reducing the hiatal hernia by algebraically repositioning the pressure values of the intrinsic LES (pressure peak proximal to the squamocolumnar junction) to within the extrinsically determined pressure of the hiatal canal. For each subject the positioning of the proximal high pressure zone was such that the squamocolumnar junction mucosal clip attained the median normal position, 0.5 cm distal to the hiatus. The *shaded area* indicates the portion of the sphincter segment distal to the squamocolumnar junction in the normals and in the transposed panels. (From Kahrilas PJ, Lin S, Chen J, Manka M: The effect of hiatus hernia on gastroesophageal junction pressure. Gut 44:476, 1999.)

gastric junction. Relevant animal experiments revealed that simulating the effect of hiatal hernia by severing the phrenoesophageal ligament reduced the LES pressure and that the subsequent repair of the ligament restored the LES pressure to levels similar to baseline.[45] Similarly, manometric studies in humans using a topographic representation of the esophagogastric junction high-pressure zone of hiatal hernia patients revealed distinct intrinsic sphincter and hiatal canal pressure components, each of which was of lower magnitude than the esophagogastric junction pressure of a comparator group of normal control patients.[46] However, simulating reduction of the hernia by arithmetically repositioning the intrinsic sphincter back within the hiatal canal resulted in calculated esophagogastric junction pressures that were practically indistinguishable from those of the control subjects (Fig. 33–6). Along with previous investigations these data also demonstrated that hiatal hernia reduced the length of the esophagogastric junction high-pressure zone attributable to the intrinsic LES.[44] This effect is likely due to disruption of the LES segment distal to the squamocolumnar junction that is attributable to the opposing sling and clasp fibers of the gastric cardia.[47]

In addition to its deleterious effect on the basal LES pressure and prevention of strain-induced reflux, hiatal hernia may also predispose to gastroesophageal reflux by augmenting the frequency of transient LES relaxations and the associated acid reflux. This was reported in a 2000 investigation that used a potent stimulus for transient LES relaxations, intragastric air infusion.[24] The frequency of transient LES relaxation elicited by this stimulus was found to be directly proportional to the extent of axial herniation (Fig. 33–7). Another observation in that study was that swallow-induced relaxation, which was an unusual mechanism of reflux in both normal and nonhernia GERD patients, accounted for about 50% of reflux events in hernia patients. This distinction was even more evident in a 2000 investigation that used ambulatory 24-hour manometry and pH recording to compare the mechanisms of reflux in GERD patients with and without hernias.[48] Although transient lower esophageal sphinchter relaxations (tLESRs) were slightly more frequent in the patients with hiatal hernia, the dominant factors accounting for the increased acid exposure in the hernia patients were reflux during swallow-induced LES relaxation and reflux during periods of LES hypotension, with or without abdominal straining.

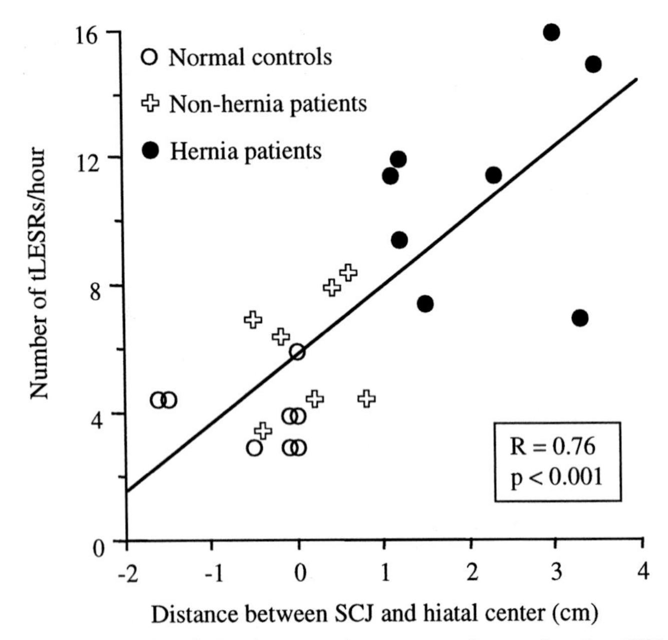

Figure 33–7. Correlation between the squamocolumnar junction (SCJ) to hiatal center separation and the number of transient lower esophageal sphincter relaxations (tLESRs) elicited per hour during a period of intragastric air infusion. Note that the sensitivity to distension-induced tLESRs is directly related to the size of hiatal hernia. (From Kahrilas PJ, Shi G, Manka M, Joehl RJ: Increased frequency of transient lower esophageal sphincter relaxation induced by gastric distention in reflux patients with hiatal hernia. Gastroenterology 118:688, 2000.)

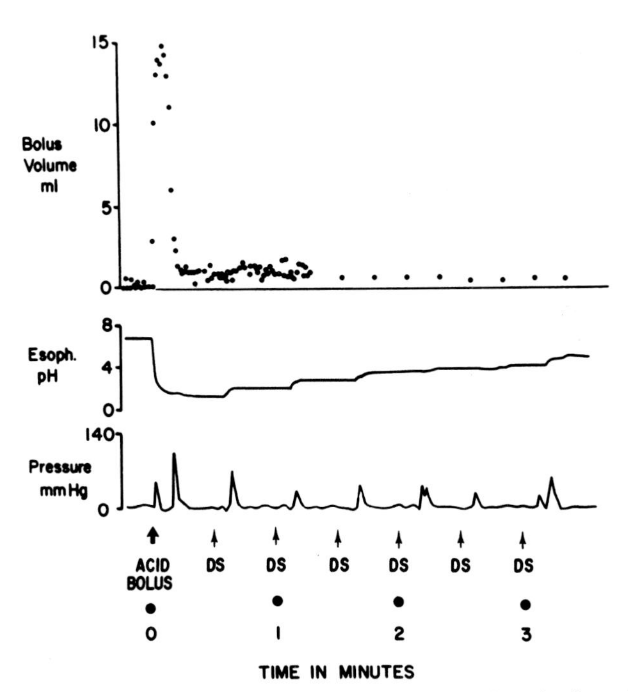

Figure 33–8. Relationship between esophageal peristalsis, distal esophageal pH, esophageal emptying, and esophageal acid clearance during an acid clearance test done with radiolabeled 0.1 N hydrochloric acid. Bolus volumes within the esophagus are derived from scintiscanning over the chest. Note that, although all but 1 mL of the infused fluid is cleared from the esophagus by the first peristaltic contraction, the distal esophageal pH remains unchanged. Stepwise increases in distal esophageal pH occur with subsequent swallows. DS, dry swallow. (From Helm JF, Dodds WJ, Pelc LR, et al: Effect of esophageal emptying and saliva on clearance of acid from the esophagus. N Engl J Med 310:284, 1984.)

Delayed Gastric Emptying

Delayed gastric emptying may exacerbate GERD because the associated gastric distention has several potentially deleterious effects: (1) increasing the gastroesophageal pressure gradient, (2) increasing gastric volume and hence volume of potential refluxate, (3) increasing tLESR frequency, and (4) increasing gastric acid secretion.[49] This potential has led some investigators to hypothesize that delayed gastric emptying was important in the pathogenesis of GERD. However, available clinical data do not support this conclusion. An extensive review of 30 published studies on the subject concluded that only a fraction of GERD patients have significantly delayed gastric emptying and others actually have accelerated emptying.[50] This finding, along with the observation that most patients with functional gastroparesis do not have concomitant esophagitis, makes it more likely that delayed gastric emptying is a potential cofactor exacerbating GERD rather than a cause of GERD per se.

Esophageal Acid Clearance

After an acid reflux event, the duration of time that the esophageal mucosa remains acidified to a pH of less than 4 is termed the *esophageal acid clearance time*. Acid clearance begins with peristalsis, which empties the refluxed fluid from the esophagus and is completed by titration of the residual acid by swallowed saliva. This process was demonstrated in an elegant study using radiolabeled 0.1 N hydrochloric acid[51] (Fig. 33–8). Aspirating saliva from the mouth prolonged acid clearance, suggesting that it was the swallowed saliva rather than peristalsis that restored esophageal pH. Approximately 7 mL of saliva is required to neutralize 1 mL of 0.1 N hydrochloric acid; 50% of this neutralizing capacity is attributable to bicarbonate. The typical rate of salivation is 0.5 mL/minute.[51] Thus, in individuals with normal esophageal emptying, substances that increase salivation such as oral lozenges, chewing gum, or bethanechol chloride hasten acid clearance, whereas hyposalivation or replacement of saliva with equal parts of water prolongs acid clearance. Of note, although salivation virtually ceases during sleep,[52] some acid clearance, attributable to bicarbonate secretion from esophageal submucosal glands, is still achieved.[53]

Prolongation of esophageal acid clearance among patients with esophagitis was demonstrated along with the initial description of an acid clearance test.[54] Subsequent investigations have demonstrated heterogeneity within the patient population such that about half of the GERD patients had normal clearance values and the other half had prolonged values.[55, 56] Ambulatory pH monitoring studies suggest that this heterogeneity is at least partially attributable to hiatal hernia, as this subset of individuals tended to have the most prolonged supine acid clearance.[57] Clinical data also suggest that prolonged acid clearance correlates with both the severity of esophagitis and the presence of Barrett's metaplasia.[58–60] From what we know of the mechanisms of acid clearance, the two main potential causes of prolonged esophageal acid clearance are impaired esophageal emptying and impaired salivary function.

Impairments of Esophageal Emptying

Impaired esophageal emptying in reflux disease has been inferred from the observation that symptoms of gastroesophageal reflux improve with change to an upright posture, a maneuver that allows gravity to augment fluid emptying. Two mechanisms of impaired esophageal emptying have been identified: peristaltic dysfunction and re-reflux associated with nonreducing hiatal hernias. Peristaltic dysfunction in esophagitis has been described by a number of investigators. Of particular significance are failed peristalsis and hypotensive peristaltic contractions (<30 mm Hg), which result in incomplete emptying.[61] As esophagitis increases in severity, so does incidence of peristaltic dysfunction.[38] A 1997 investigation of peristaltic function labeled this mechanism *ineffective esophageal motility*, defined by the occurrence of more than 30% hypotensive or failed contractions.[62] With respect to the reversibility of peristaltic dysfunction, studies from 1994 and 1997 showed no improvement after healing of esophagitis by acid inhibition[63] or by antireflux surgery.[64] Most likely, the acute dysfunction associated with active esophagitis is partially reversible, but that associated with stricturing or extensive fibrosis is not.

Hiatal hernia also can impair esophageal emptying. Concurrent pH recording and scintigraphy above the esophagogastric junction showed that impaired clearance was caused by reflux of fluid from the hernia sac during swallowing.[65] This observation was subsequently confirmed radiographically in an analysis of esophageal emptying in patients with reducing and nonreducing hiatal hernias.[66] The efficacy of emptying was significantly diminished in both hernia groups when compared with that in normal control subjects. Emptying was particularly impaired in the nonreducing hiatal hernia patients, who exhibited complete emptying with only one third of test swallows (Fig. 33–9). The patients with nonreducing hernias were the only group who exhibited retrograde flow of fluid from the hernia during deglutitive relaxation, consistent with the scintigraphic studies just discussed.[65]

Salivary Function

The final phase of esophageal acid clearance depends on salivation. Just as impaired esophageal emptying prolongs acid clearance, so does diminished salivary neutralizing capacity. Diminished salivation during sleep, for instance, is the reason that reflux events during sleep or immediately before sleep are associated with markedly prolonged acid clearance times. Similarly, chronic xerostomia is associated with prolonged esophageal acid exposure and esophagitis.[67] However, no systematic difference has been found in the salivary function of GERD patients compared with that in control subjects. One group of subjects shown to have prolonged esophageal acid clearance times attributable to hyposalivation are cigarette smokers. Even those without symptoms of reflux disease exhibited acid clearance times 50% longer than those of nonsmokers, and the salivary titratable base content was only 60% of that of the age matched nonsmokers.[68]

In addition to bicarbonate, saliva contains growth factors that have the potential to enhance mucosal repair. Epidermal

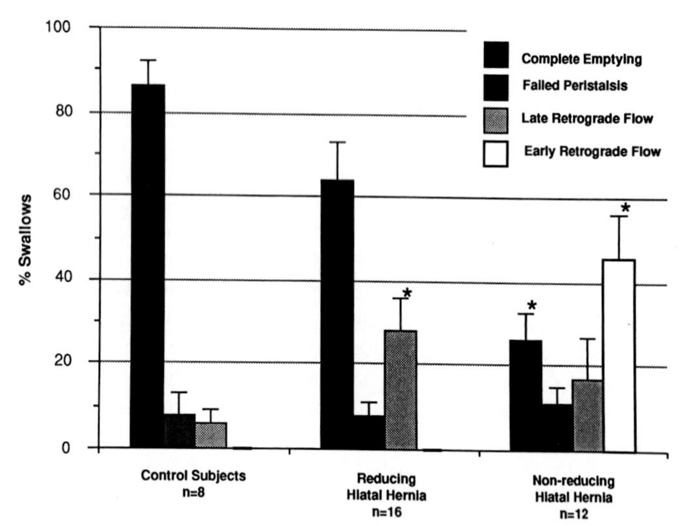

Figure 33–9. The effect of hiatal hernia on the efficacy of esophageal emptying. Control subjects had complete esophageal emptying without retrograde flow in 86 ± 6% of test swallows compared to 61 ± 9% in the reducing hernia group and 31 ± 8% in the non-reducing hernia group ($P < .05$ versus controls). The reducing hernia group exhibited significantly more late retrograde flow ($P < .05$ versus controls), and the non-reducing hernia group consisted of the only individuals to exhibit early retrograde flow ($P < .01$ versus other groups). (From Sloan S, Kahrilas PJ: Impairment of esophageal emptying with hiatal hernia. Gastroenterology 100:596, 1991.)

growth factor (EGF), produced in submaxillary ductal cells and duodenal Brunner's glands, has been extensively studied.[69] In animal models, EGF has been shown to provide cytoprotection against irritants, enhance healing of gastroduodenal ulceration, and decrease permeability of the esophageal mucosa to hydrogen ions.[69–71] However, because studies have not shown consistent differences in EGF concentration in esophagitis or Barrett's metaplasia patients,[72, 73] one cannot conclude that perturbations of growth factor secretion are important in the pathogenesis of gastroesophageal reflux disease.

Tissue Resistance and Mediators of Tissue Injury

The esophageal mucosa possesses several morphologic and physiologic defenses against cellular acidification; taken together, these are referred to as *tissue resistance*. Conceptually, tissue resistance can be subdivided into pre-epithelial, epithelial, and postepithelial.[74] Preepithelial defense, although important in the stomach and small intestine, has a minimal role in the esophagus.[75] Thus the burden of defense shifts to the integrity of the epithelium itself. As reviewed in Chapter 31, the esophageal epithelium is a 25- to 30-cell layer thick, nonkeratinized squamous epithelium divided into a proliferating basal cell layer (stratum basale), a midzone layer of metabolically active squamous cells (stratum spinosum epidermis), and a 5- to 10-cell-thick layer of dead squamous cells (stratum corneum epidermis). The epithelium also contains sparse submucosal glands that secrete bicarbonate into the submucosa, mucosa, and lumen.[76] The epithelium both provides a structural barrier retarding acid diffusion and exhibits metabolic specialization whereby hydrogen ions are neutralized within the intercellular space and cytoplasm. The esophageal epithelium is a tight epithelium composed of cell membranes, tight junctions, and an intercellular glycoprotein matrix that retard diffusion of acid and pepsin through the apical cell membrane and intercellular space.[77] Proteins, phosphates, and bicarbonate ions within this intercellular matrix may buffer hydrogen ions that penetrate the surface. When the cytosolic buffering capacity is overwhelmed, basolateral membrane transporters act to extrude hydrogen ion from epithelial cells and preserve intracellular pH.[78–80] Postepithelial defenses, mainly increased vascular perfusion, interact with epithelial defense mechanisms by providing nutrients and bicarbonate and removing hydrogen ion.[81] The mediator of this increased perfusion appears to involve the release of nitric oxide and histamine.[82]

Luminal acid attacks the esophageal epithelium by damaging the intercellular junctions and allowing hydrogen ion penetration, which eventually leads to acidification of the intercellular space. Evidence of this increased permeability is indicated by transmission electron microscopic findings that reveal dilated intercellular spaces. Eventually, the buffering capacity of the intercellular space is overwhelmed, leading to acidification of the cell cytosol via the basolateral membrane. Acidification of the cytosol is the crucial event leading to cell edema (balloon cells) and death.

Although most of what we know about GERD suggests that it is primarily a motility disorder, implicit in the pathogenic model is that gastric contents are damaging to the esophageal mucosa and that the more prolonged the contact, the more severe the injury. However, this effect is not due to a qualitative or quantitative abnormality of gastric secretion. Although the extreme subgroup of patients with acid hypersecretion due to Zollinger-Ellison syndrome are prone to esophagitis (see Chapter 41), those data cannot be generalized to typical GERD patients.[83] Supporting this contention is a report comparing gastric secretion in 115 patients with esophagitis with that in 508 age and disease matched controls.[84] Fasting, basal, and maximal secretion of both acid and pepsin were similar in both groups, and on a case by case basis, the severity of esophagitis was not related to any of these secretion parameters.

Although the eventual mediator of epithelial cell injury is probably the hydrogen ion, gastroesophageal refluxate is a heterogeneous mixture; pepsin, bile acids, trypsin, lysolecithin, and food hyperosmolarity can all facilitate esophageal mucosal injury. Pepsin, a normal component of gastric juice, probably plays a very significant role in esophageal injury. A proteolytic enzyme, pepsin has optimal activity at pH 1.3 to 3.3 and is denatured at pH 7.0. Therefore, there is some degree of peptic activity in the pH range of 1.3 to 6.9.[85] The addition of pepsin to pH 1.3 to 3.5 HCl increases esophageal injury in animal models. The mechanism whereby pepsin facilitates esophageal injury may be disruption of the tight junctions between epithelial cells, which allows acid access to the intercellular space, or digestion of collagen in the basement membrane.

The role of duodenal contents in esophageal injury seems minimal with the possible exception of patients who have had partial gastrectomy. Bile salt concentrations measured in the refluxate of GERD patients are noncytotoxic, and the epithelial injury pattern observed in esophagitis is consistent with an acid peptic attack rather than that resultant from a detergent as might be expected with bile salts. Nonetheless, studies using a fiberoptic spectrophotometer (Bilitec 2000, Synectics, Irving, TX), which utilizes the optical properties of bilirubin to document duodenogastroesophageal reflux, suggest that mucosal injury is more likely to occur when acid reflux is combined with duodenogastric reflux.[86] Thus, a synergy between acid and bile salts similar to the relationship between acid and pepsin may exist.

CLINICAL PRESENTATION AND NATURAL HISTORY

Although reflux disease is widely accepted as one of the most prevalent gastrointestinal disorders, there is remarkably little agreement on what constitutes typical reflux disease or on the natural history of the disorder. This difficulty stems from the heterogeneity of symptoms attributable to GERD and the lack of a universally accepted definition. As discussed earlier, GERD may be defined as any symptom or clinical condition that results from exposure of the esophageal and supraesophageal epithelia to gastric juice. However, without peptic esophagitis, there is no standard for the definition. Ambulatory pH monitoring is helpful in documenting abnormal acid reflux, but patients differ widely in esophageal sensitivity to acid and can have reflux disease in the context of seemingly normal acid reflux. Given these limitations, one must use the patient symptom profile to define the disease.

Typical Symptoms

The most common symptoms of GERD are heartburn, acid regurgitation, and dysphagia (see Chapter 6). Heartburn (pyrosis) is characterized by a discomfort or burning sensation behind the sternum that arises from the epigastrium and may radiate toward the neck. Heartburn is an intermittent symptom, most commonly experienced within 60 minutes of eating, during exercise, and while lying recumbent. The discomfort is relieved by drinking water or using antacid but can occur frequently and interfere with normal activities. Heartburn that occurs three or more times a week has been shown to impair an individual's perceived quality of life.[87] Although there is some correlation between frequency of heartburn, degree of esophageal acid exposure, and presence or extent of mucosal injury,[88] this correlation is far from perfect.[89] Some patients with severe esophagitis or Barrett's metaplasia do not report having any heartburn.[90]

Regurgitation is the effortless return of esophageal or gastric contents into the pharynx without nausea or retching. Patients note the presence of a sour or burning fluid in the throat or mouth that may also contain undigested food particles. Bending, belching, or moving in a manner that increases intra-abdominal pressure can provoke regurgitiation.

Some degree of dysphagia is reported by more than 30% of individuals with GERD.[91] It can be caused by peptic stricture, a Schatzki ring (B ring), peristaltic dysfunction, or simple mucosal inflammation. Dysphagia also occurs in the absence of any identifiable abnormality, in which case it is likely the result of abnormal sensitivity to bolus movement during peristalsis.

Other, less common symptoms of reflux disease include water brash, globus sensation, and odynophagia. Water brash is excessive salivation resulting from a vagal reflex triggered by esophageal acidification. Globus sensation is the perception of a lump or fullness in the throat that is felt irrespective of swallowing. Odynophagia is more common with pill or infectious esophagitis than with reflux esophagitis and should prompt a search for these causes. When odynophagia does occur in GERD it is likely related to an esophageal ulcer or deep erosion.

Atypical Symptoms

Posterior Laryngitis

In 1968, Cherry first indicated that reflux was a predisposing factor in laryngeal mucosal breakdown,[92] with a disease spectrum encompassing chronic hoarseness, posterior laryngeal erythema and edema, contact ulceration of the vocal folds, and vocal fold granulomata. Since then, other reports have supported this contention. It is currently estimated that 4% to 10% of patients evaluated by otolaryngologists have reflux-related disease[93] and that patients who have esophagitis are twice as likely to have laryngitis as those who do not.[94] Experimental pH monitoring studies using multiple pH recording sites suggest that otolaryngologic manifestations of GERD are caused by refluxed acid that reaches the proximal esophagus and subsequent regurgitation into the hypopharynx.[95–97]

Asthma

The relationship between asthma and GERD was first suggested by Osler's observation in 1892 that stomach distention aggravated wheezing. Epidemiologic studies subsequently confirmed this association. A case control questionnaire based survey of a large group of asthmatic and control subjects found that 77% of asthmatic subjects reported heartburn and 55% reported regurgitation, significantly more than the controls.[98] Although the association is clear, it is less clear whether GERD causes asthma. Theories have proposed both reflex and aspiration mechanisms, both of which can be demonstrated experimentally. In a unique investigation in which tracheal and esophageal pH were monitored in four patients with severe asthma, peak expiratory flow rates decreased by 16 L/minute when esophageal and tracheal acid were simultaneously present compared with 4 L/minute when only the esophagus was acidified.[99] Abundant 24-hour esophageal pH data demonstrate that distal acid exposure is prevalent in asthmatic individuals.[100, 101] However, the data regarding the effects of simulated and real gastroesophageal reflux on pulmonary function have been conflicting. In a critical review of the literature Field and Sutherland concluded that the effect of esophageal acid perfusion on pulmonary function is minimal.[102] Despite the minimal changes in pulmonary function, clinical data suggest that treatment of GERD in asthma patients usually improves respiratory symptoms.[103, 104]

Cough

Chronic cough is associated with a variety of disorders of which postnasal drip, asthma, and GERD constitute an estimated 80% to 90% of cases.[105] Estimates of the prevalence of GERD-associated cough range from 10% to 40%, depending on whether symptoms or pH monitoring is used as the diagnostic criterion for GERD.[106] Because 50% to 75% of these patients do not report reflux symptoms, the association is often unrecognized. The pathogenesis of GERD-associated cough is believed to be secondary to acid stimulation of nerve endings in the esophagus which then activate the cough center.[107] Dual probe pH studies and esophageal perfusion studies support this hypothesis. Two pH monitoring studies demonstrated a high correlation between reflux and coughing in chronic cough patients.[108, 109] Ing and associates examined the response characteristics of afferent receptors in 22 GERD patients with chronic cough by alternately challenging them with acid and saline solution perfusion of the esophagus.[110] Cough frequency was significantly increased with acid infusion compared with saline solution infusion. Furthermore, lidocaine, acting as a topical anesthetic, blocked acid-induced cough. On the other hand, ipratropium bromide, a muscarinic blocker, had no effect when instilled in the esophagus but blocked acid-induced cough when inhaled, presumably by preventing activation of the efferent limb of the reflex. These functional studies strongly support the presence of a vagally mediated esophagotracheobronchial reflex activated by stimulation of the esophageal mucosa.

Noncardiac Chest Pain (Also see Chapter 6)

Approximately 30% of patients who have coronary angiography for chest pain have normal coronary arteries. Once cardiac ischemia is ruled out, the cause of chest pain in these individuals can be difficult to establish and the esophagus is often implicated. Initially investigators focused on esophageal motor abnormalities, such as diffuse esophageal spasm or nutcracker esophagus, as potential causes of chest pain. However, most of these patients had normal manometric study findings[111] and the correlation between abnormal contractions and symptoms was poor.[112] Given these observations and the clinical availability of potent inhibitors of acid secretion, the focus has shifted to acid reflux as a cause. Esophageal pH monitoring studies reported that abnormal acid exposure was often present in patients who had noncardiac chest pain and, more importantly, that episodes of chest pain were often associated with reflux.[113, 114] This causal relationship was further strengthened by a prospective double-blind placebo-controlled study using intensive acid inhibition in a group of 36 patients with angina-like chest pain and GERD.[115] Significant clinical improvement was demonstrated in the proton pump inhibitor arm with a reduction in chest pain score of 81% compared with a reduction of 44% in the placebo arm. The mechanism by which reflux of acid induces chest pain is unclear, but an abundance of evidence suggests that esophageal afferent nerves discriminate poorly among stimuli such that both distention and reflux may be perceived as either chest pain or heartburn.

Natural History

Patients seeking medical attention for GERD typically report having had symptoms for 1 to 3 years prior to seeking medical attention.[116] Beyond that, little information exists on the natural history of GERD. Reports in 1997 and 1999 suggest no consistent disease progression or relationship between disease severity and duration of GERD symptoms.[9, 117] With respect to esophagitis, especially severe esophagitis, it is clear that most cases are chronic and relapsing. Although most patients with erosive esophagitis may be healed with adequate medical therapy, recurrence can be anticipated in approximately 80% of patients, most within 3 months of discontinuation of therapy.[118] Even so, mortality associated with GERD (other than adenocarcinoma) is minimal; estimates of 0.1 per 100,000 are typical.[116] The prevalence of peptic stricture in patients with esophagitis ranges from 8% to 20% and that of ulceration is 5%.[119] However, data from 1989 suggest that these complication rates are decreasing, most likely because of widespread use of proton pump inhibitors. Similarly, significant bleeding is uncommon, occurring in less than 2% of patients, and perforation is extremely rare.[7]

Differential Diagnosis

Although generally quite characteristic, symptoms of GERD must be distinguished from symptoms related to infectious esophagitis, pill esophagitis, peptic ulcer disease, dyspepsia, biliary colic, coronary artery disease, and esophageal motor disorders. It is especially important that coronary artery disease be given early consideration because of its potentially lethal implications. Patients whose gastrointestinal symptoms are accompanied by unexplained chest pain should have cardiography and exercise stress testing before a gastrointestinal evaluation. Furthermore, because patients with inferior myocardial ischemia may experience only gastrointestinal symptoms, those without chest pain but with dyspnea, diaphoresis, fatigue, or significant cardiac risk factors should also be evaluated for coronary artery disease before gastrointestinal evaluation.

The remaining elements of the differential diagnosis mentioned earlier can be addressed by endoscopy, upper gastrointestinal series, or biliary tract ultrasonography, as appropriate. The distinction between peptic esophagitis and either infectious esophagitis or pill esophagitis is usually easily made by endoscopy. Aside from their distinct appearance, both infectious and pill esophagitis are accompanied by substantial odynophagia, which is rare in esophagitis. In terms of endoscopic appearance, infectious esophagitis is diffuse and tends to involve the proximal esophagus far more frequently than does reflux esophagitis. In candidal esophagitis, the esophagus classically has a diffuse, heavy, curdlike exudate, in contrast with the linear streaks emerging from the esophagogastric junction typical of peptic esophagitis (see Fig. 28–2). The ulcerations seen in peptic esophagitis are usually large, solitary, and distal, whereas infectious ulcerations are punctate and diffuse. Esophageal ulceration caused by oral medications such as potassium chloride, quinidine, tetracycline, or NSAIDs is usually singular and deep at points of narrowing, especially near the carina, with sparing of the distal esophagus.

Associated Conditions

Pregnancy is by far the most common condition predisposing to GERD; approximately 50% to 80% of pregnant patients report heartburn.[8] As the uterus enlarges, the pressure gradient promoting reflux increases. In addition to this anatomic change, LES pressure decreases and gastric emptying is slowed. These motility effects are likely due to increases in progesterone levels, explaining why reflux begins early in the first trimester.

Scleroderma is associated with impaired esophageal function in about 90% of patients. Characteristic abnormalities are diminished peristaltic amplitude in the smooth muscle segment of the esophagus and diminished or absent LES pressure. Although most frequently associated with scleroderma, these esophageal changes are nonspecific and may occur with any of the mixed connective tissue disorders. Sjögren's syndrome, which disrupts normal salivary secretion and interferes with esophageal acid clearance, also increases risk for reflux esophagitis. Changes in gastric emptying associated with diabetic gastroparesis, intestinal pseudo-obstruction, and collagen vascular disorders may also predispose to GERD.

Most of the conditions predisposing to the development of GERD are associated with abnormalities of the antireflux barrier and/or esophageal acid clearance. One exception is Zollinger-Ellison syndrome, in which the quality and quantity of the refluxate are the primary abnormalities. An analysis of 122 Zollinger-Ellison syndrome patients found that 42% had endoscopic evidence of esophagitis.[83] Patients with Zollinger-Ellison do not exhibit any abnormalities of esophageal motility compared with normal control subjects.[120]

MANAGEMENT

It is neither practical nor necessary to embark on a diagnostic evaluation of every patient who experiences only heartburn. The primary goal of therapy in these patients is symptom relief. Diagnostic evaluation can, however, be useful in selected GERD patients to confirm the diagnosis, direct therapy, or identify complications. Regardless of whether diagnostic tests are used, the therapy of GERD need not necessarily progress in a stepwise fashion, beginning with the most conservative treatments. In some patients, such as those with severe or atypical symptoms, intensive medical therapy is appropriate as the initial treatment plan and may in fact help establish the diagnosis of GERD.

Diagnostic Evaluation

The history is usually sufficient to confirm the diagnosis of GERD and to warrant appropriate treatment. However, GERD patients can also have atypical symptoms, leaving one to rely on diagnostic studies to confirm that abnormal acid reflux is occurring and potentially responsible for the syndrome in question. Diagnostic studies are also indicated for a GERD patient when heartburn is extremely chronic (raising the possibility of Barrett's metaplasia), refractory to treatment, or accompanied by the so-called warning signs of dysphagia, odynophagia, gastrointestinal bleeding, or weight loss.

Endoscopy should be used as the first diagnostic test of suspected GERD because it provides a means for both detecting and managing complications of GERD as well as excluding other diseases. A double-contrast barium swallow may be useful in identifying strictures and esophageal ulcers but fails to detect most cases of esophagitis and Barrett's metaplasia. Endoscopy is diagnostic of GERD if erosive esophagitis is present, with a specificity of 90% to 95%; most false-positive results are attributable to either infectious or pill-induced mucosal injury. However, because only 30% to 40% of patients with GERD have esophagitis indicated by endoscopy,[121, 122] its sensitivity is poor.[123, 124] It is also now generally accepted that endoscopically defined minimal changes, such as edema, friability, and an irregular Z line, are poorly reproducible observations that should not be interpreted as esophagitis.[4, 125] Furthermore, because of the multitude of classification schemes proposed for esophagitis (generally ranging from grade 1 to 4 or 5), their interpretation can be confusing. The most thoroughly evaluated classification scheme for esophagitis is the Los Angeles system, which categorizes mucosal injury as grade A, B, C, or D (Table 33–2).[126] However, it is important to note that the Los Angeles system does not consider strictures, hiatal hernia, or Barrett's metaplasia; the endoscopist is required to describe these separately.

In atypical or complicated GERD cases, diagnostic tests

Table 33–2 | **Los Angeles Endoscopic Grading Scheme for Esophagitis Severity**

Grade A	One (or more) mucosal breaks no longer than 5 mm that do not extend between the tops of two mucosal folds.
Grade B	One (or more) mucosal breaks more than 5 mm long that do not extend between the tops of two mucosal folds.
Grade C	One (or more) mucosal breaks that are continuous between the tops of two or more mucosal folds but involve <75% of the circumference.
Grade D	One (or more) mucosal breaks that involve at least 75% of the esophageal circumference.

From Lundell LR, Dent J, Bennett JR, et al: Endoscopic assessment of oesophagitis: Clinical and functional correlates and further validation of the Los Angeles classification. Gut 45:172, 1999.

other than endoscopy may be useful. In particular, two dilemmas may arise: (1) determining whether a patient's atypical symptoms are related to GERD and (2) identifying why GERD therapy has failed in a patient. In attempting to determine whether symptoms are related to GERD, the Bernstein test was devised to reproduce symptoms by perfusing the esophagus with 0.1 N HCl. If symptoms occur during acid perfusion, but not during saline solution infusion, the test result is considered positive. The sensitivity of this test for typical symptoms ranges from 42% to 100%, and specificity ranges from 50% to 100%.[127] However, in the evaluation of atypical symptoms the sensitivity decreases to 7% to 27%, although high specificity is maintained.[111, 128] Similarly to endoscopy, this test is fairly reliable with a positive result, but a negative test result does not rule out GERD.

Ambulatory 24-hour pH monitoring is the most widely used test to establish the presence of excessive gastroesophageal reflux and to correlate symptoms temporally with reflux. The test is performed by transnasally positioning a thin pH probe 5 cm above the proximal margin of the LES as determined manometrically. The patient then conducts normal daily activities while recording symptoms, meals, and sleep in a diary. Esophageal acid exposure is defined as the percentage of the recording time that the pH is less than 4; values greater than 3.5% are considered abnormal.[129] An important limitation of pH monitoring is that there exists no absolute threshold value that reliably identifies GERD patients. Investigators evaluating the sensitivity of pH monitoring report obtaining normal esophageal acid exposure in 25% of patients with reflux esophagitis and about 30% of patients with nonerosive reflux disease.[130–132] This lack of high sensitivity is likely due to the multifactorial origin of reflux symptoms. Symptoms are dependent on mucosal resistance and acid sensitivity as well as esophageal acid exposure; therefore, it is overly simplistic to equate any specific duration and quantity of acid exposure with the presence or absence of GERD. Despite this limitation, ambulatory pH monitoring is still the best available test for quantifying esophageal acid exposure. The principal indication for ambulatory esophageal pH monitoring is a need to document excessive acid reflux in patients without endoscopic esophagitis or to evaluate the efficacy of medical or surgical treatment. Paradoxically, minimal data have been obtained on the sensitivity or specificity of the test in this latter application. An alternative way of interpreting ambulatory pH monitoring studies is to correlate symptoms reported by the patient and reflux events. Unfortunately, not all reflux events are associated with symptoms, and vice versa. The best available method for establishing a statistically significant correlation between reflux events and symptoms is the symptom association probablility (SAP).[133] It is important to note, however, that this scheme has yet to be prospectively evaluated.

An alternative management strategy for a patient with suspected GERD is an empirical trial of potent antisecretory therapy. Several investigators have demonstrated that 1- to 2-week therapeutic trials with proton pump inhibitors identify most individuals likely to respond to prolonged therapy, including a substantial fraction of individuals judged not to have reflux on the basis of ambulatory pH monitoring studies.[134, 135] Although this is a very pragmatic approach to identifying patients with acid-related symptoms, attaching a sensitivity or specificity to such a strategy is impossible in the absence of a standard for the diagnosis of GERD. Furthermore, it must be recognized that empirical treatment may be associated with false-positive results by masking the symptoms of peptic ulcer disease or malignancy and that this pragmatic approach does not allow the physician to diagnose Barrett's metaplasia if present.

In summary, GERD patients are usually well managed by using a careful medical history and empirical trials of antireflux therapy. Patients with long-standing symptoms or warning signs may benefit from endoscopic evaluation. Ambulatory pH monitoring is unnecessary in most patients but can be of value for patients refractory to antireflux therapy or for documentation of abnormal acid reflux in an individual who is being evaluated for antireflux therapy. Patients with atypical symptoms who do not respond to empirical therapy may also benefit from ambulatory pH monitoring. Esophageal manometry is of minimal use in diagnosing or managing GERD, with the exceptions of detecting major motor disorders or evaluating peristaltic function prior to antireflux surgery.

Nonprescription Therapy

Epidemiologic studies suggest that more than 36% of the U.S. population suffers from heartburn at least once a month.[2] Few of these patients seek medical care for their condition, instead choosing to treat themselves or to ignore their symptoms. Consequently, as many as 27% of adult Americans take antacids more than twice a month, and the preponderance of these are reflux sufferers.[136] Along with antacids, nonprescription therapy for GERD often includes life-style modifications and on-demand use of over-the-counter histamine-2 (H_2) receptor antagonists. Life-style modifications include head of the bed elevation, avoidance of tight fitting garments, weight loss, dietary modification, restriction of alcohol use and elimination of smoking. These interventions are aimed at enhancing esophageal acid clearance, minimizing the occurrence of acid reflux, or doing both. Head of the bed elevation is achieved by putting 6- to 8-inch blocks under the legs at the head of the bed or putting a polystyrene plastic (Styrofoam) wedge under the mattress and has been shown to improve esophageal acid clearance.[137] The relevance of this maneuver is, however, limited to the patient who has nighttime reflux. Smoking should be eliminated because it prolongs acid clearance by decreasing salivation and increases the frequency of reflux events through its synergistic actions of decreasing LES pressure and increasing the number of straining events such as coughing and deep inspiration.[39, 68] Strain-induced reflux can also be minimized by avoiding tight-fitting garments and losing weight. Dietary modifications affecting GERD may be related to the type of food, the timing of meals, and the size of meals. Many foods have been shown to decrease LES pressure (see Table 33–1), and these should be avoided in individuals in whom they cause heartburn. Patients should also avoid assuming a supine position after meals and should not eat within 3 hours of bedtime. An additional treatment for mild heartburn is the augmentation of salivation by either chewing gum or using oral lozenges. In general, because minimal data related to the efficacy of these nonpharmacologic therapies for GERD have been published,[138] it is unlikely that they will suffice except in mild GERD cases.

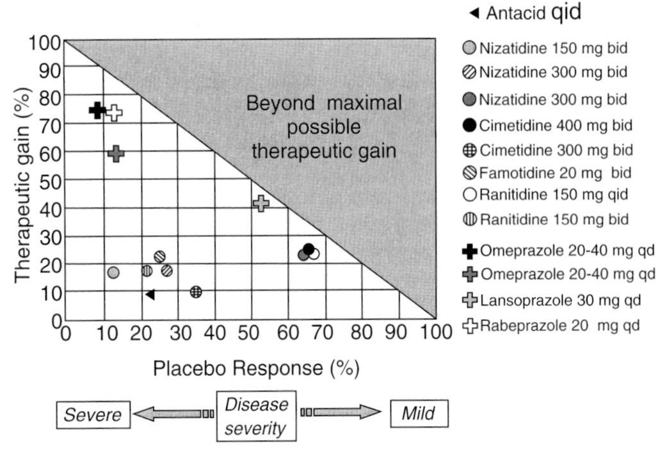

Figure 33–10. Efficacy of acid inhibitors and antacids in the therapy of esophagitis plotted in terms of therapeutic gain versus a placebo. Each placebo-controlled trial involved at least 50 subjects with a period of therapy ranging from 8 to 12 weeks. Trials are stratified by the placebo response rate as an indicator of severity of esophagitis. Note that the therapeutic gain of the histamine-2 receptor antagonists is almost constant regardless of the placebo healing rate, thus making these therapies ineffective for severe esophagitis. Proton pump inhibitors exhibit increasing therapeutic gain with increased disease severity. (Modified from Kahrilas PJ: Gastroesophageal reflux disease. JAMA 276:983, 1996.)

Acid Suppressive Medications

Although hypersecretion of acid is rare in GERD, the most common and effective treatment of GERD is suppression of acid secretion by either H_2 receptor antagonists or proton pump inhibitors. The object of these therapies is to raise the intragastric pH above 4 during the periods of the day that reflux is likely to occur. The more extreme an individual's esophageal acid exposure, the greater the degree of acid suppression required. Consistent with this principle, a meta-analysis of the therapeutic literature suggests that the likelihood of healing erosive esophagitis with a particular regimen is proportional to the fraction of the day that regimen maintains the intragastric pH above 4.[139]

There are four H_2 receptor antagonists (cimetidine, ranitidine, famotidine, and nizatidine) and five proton pump inhibitors (omeprazole, lansoprazole, rabeprazole, pantoprazole, and esomeprazole magnesium) currently in clinical use (see Chapter 38). H_2 receptor antagonists suppress gastric acid secretion most effectively during fasting and during sleep. Their efficacy is limited by the rapid development of tachyphylaxis and the inability to suppress meal related acid secretion effectively.[140] Proton pump inhibitors suppress acid much more effectively than any H_2 receptor antagonist dosage because they act on the final common pathway of acid secretion rather than on one of the three classes of membrane receptors (histamine, acetylcholine, gastrin), as do the H_2 receptor antagonists. Because proton pump inhibitors can only act on membrane bound activated H^+,K^+-adenosine triphosphatase (H^+,K^+-ATPase) molecules, they should be administered about 30 minutes before meals for optimal acid suppression.[141] Omeprazole, 20 to 30 mg/day for 1 week, reduces gastric acid secretion by more than 90% compared with 50% for cimetidine, 1000 mg/day, and 70% for ranitidine, 300 mg/day.[142, 143]

Controlled studies evaluating the effectiveness of acid suppressive medications have yielded variable results, largely because the efficacy of therapy in GERD is dependent on disease severity and neither disease severity nor the definition of esophagitis is constant among the studies. One way of comparing data among studies is to consider the placebo response rate as an indicator of esophagitis severity and therapeutic gain relative to placebo as an indicator of drug efficacy. This is done in Figure 33–10. Note that all of the H_2 receptor antagonists demonstrate a therapeutic gain of only 10% to 24% relative to placebo for healing esophagitis regardless of esophagitis severity or the dose of H_2 receptor antagonist used. The proton pump inhibitors, on the other hand, demonstrate increasing therapeutic gain with increasing esophagitis severity. Furthermore, unlike that of the H_2 receptor antagonists, the efficacy of the proton pump inhibitors increases with increasing dosage and/or potency. In a major trial from the Netherlands in which patients with severe esophagitis resistant to prolonged therapy with H_2 receptor antagonist were treated with proton pump inhibitors, 100% of refractory esophagitis patients were healed during 20 weeks of therapy with omeprazole in a dose of 40 or 60 mg/day. Similarly, comparison of the most potent proton pump inhibitor, esomeprazole magnesium, with omeprazole demonstrated significantly higher healing rates for esophagitis of all severities.[144]

Despite their clinical superiority when compared with H_2 receptor antagonists, proton pump inhibitors are not perfect in their ability to suppress acid secretion. Although proton pump inhibitors do not exhibit tachyphylaxis,[145] rebound hypersecretion occurs with discontinuation of the medication as a result of secondary hypergastrinemia. Proton pump inhibitors also exhibit considerable interindividual variation in the degree of suppression of acid secretion. This is evident in gastric pH monitoring studies analyzed for the fraction of a 24-hour period that the intragastric pH is maintained above pH 4. Data from one such cross-over study are shown in Figure 33–11.[146] Fifty-five percent of patients taking omeprazole 20 mg/day and 46% of patients taking esomeprazole 20 mg/day did not maintain intragastric pH greater than 4 for 12 hours or longer, whereas only 8% of patients taking esomeprazole 40 mg/day did not maintain intragastric pH above 4 for 12 hours. The fraction of individuals achieving

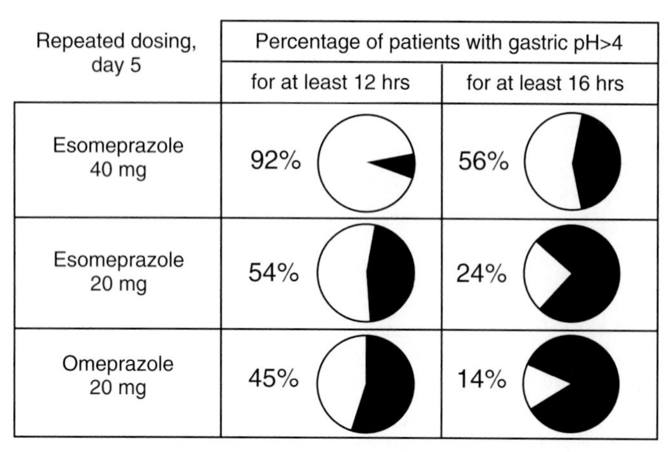

Figure 33–11. A crossover study showing the relative efficacy of three proton pump inhibitor regimens in inhibiting gastric acid secretion after 5 days of treatment. In each case, the percentage of patients maintaining intragastric pH > 4 for at least 12 and 16 hours is shown. The efficacy of therapy in gastroesophageal reflux disease is directly related to the percentage of the day that the intragastric pH is maintained above 4. (Modified from Lind T, Rydberg A, Jonsson T, et al: Esomeprazole provides improved acid control vs. omeprazole in patients with symptoms of gastro-oesophageal reflux disease. Aliment Pharmacol Ther 14:861, 2000.)

pH control for 16 hours was proportionately lower for all three regimens. The clinical implications of these data are the following: (1) more potent or higher doses of proton pump inhibitors are more likely to be effective, and (2) there is a solid rationale for using proton pump inhibitors in a twice a day regimen should a once a day regimen prove ineffective.

The observed intersubject variability in response to proton pump inhibitors is likely multifactorial. *Helicobacter pylori* infection has been shown to enhance the acid suppression achieved, possibly because of gastric atrophy.[18, 19, 147, 148] Another relevant factor involves genetic polymorphism of the cytochrome P-450 enzyme (Cyp2C19), a major metabolic pathway of proton pump inhibitors. Overexpression of Cyp2C19 would be expected to reduce the efficacy of proton pump inhibitors, although deficiencies would lead to an enhanced effect. A 2000 report confirmed that the efficacy of omeprazole and lansoprazole in increasing intragastric pH correlated with Cyp2C19 status.[149, 150]

Prokinetic Drugs

Gastroesophageal reflux disease is characterized by incompetence of the antireflux barrier, impaired esophageal acid clearance, and delayed gastric emptying. Thus, an ideal therapy would be to target these pathophysiologic abnormalities, obviating the need for acid suppression. Most recently, metoclopramide and cisapride have been used, but unfortunately these agents have minimal effect on relevant motor function and are associated with significant side effects.

Metoclopramide is an antidopaminergic agent that also acts as a 5-hydroxytryptamine (5-HT_3) antagonist, a 5-HT_4 agonist, and a cholinomimetic. Although earlier studies reported mild symptom improvement in GERD symptoms, a 1983 study comparing metoclopramide to H_2 receptor antagonists, alone or as a combination therapy, reported marginal to no benefit.[151] Furthermore, metoclopramide has a significant side effect profile, as up to 25% of patients experience central nervous system side effects such as tremor, parkinsonism, depression, and tardive dyskinesia.[152] Cisapride is also a mixed serotoninergic agent with 5-HT_3 antagonist and 5-HT_4 agonist activity. It acts by enhancing release of acetylcholine from postganglionic nerve endings of the myenteric plexus. Controlled trials report that cisapride, 10 mg four times per day, was as efficacious as standard H_2 receptor antagonist therapy in controlling symptoms and healing grade 1 to 2 esophagitis.[153] However, the clinical use of cisapride has been curtailed as a result of its cardiotoxic effects, especially when used in combination with agents that are metabolized by the cytochrome P-450 system. Prolongation of the QT interval, ventricular arrhythmia, and death have been reported.[154] Despite these setbacks, there is still great interest in developing other serotoninergic agents similar to cisapride, given its established activity profile.

Because transient LES relaxations are the dominant mechanism of gastroesophageal reflux, they represent an attractive target in GERD treatment (see Table 33–1). Our current understanding is that transient LES relaxation is a vagovagal reflex initiated by gastric distention that activates mechanoreceptors in the subcardiac region of the stomach. The first medications reported to decrease the frequency of transient LES relaxations in patients with GERD were morphine and atropine.[155, 156] Although these agents are not appropriate for clinical use, these observations sparked interest in devising pharmacologic therapy targeting transient LES relaxations, and new experimental agents with more specific activity are emerging. The cholecystokinin A (CCK_A) antagonist loxiglumide decreases transient LES relaxations stimulated by gastric distention.[157] N^G-monomethyl-L-arginine, a nitric oxide (NO) synthase inhibitor, has also been found to decrease the frequency of transient LES relaxations that occur in response to gastric distention.[158] Although the mechanism by which these agents affect transient LES relaxations is unknown, it is likely related to changes in gastric tone and relaxation. L-Baclofen, a γ-aminobutyric acid B ($GABA_B$) receptor agonist, is yet another agent reported to decrease transient LES relaxations in humans.[159] Its mechanism of action is also unknown, but it is likely mediated by its agonist action on both peripheral and central $GABA_B$ receptors. L-Baclofen will likely be the first agent targeting transient LES relaxations to be tested clinically; it is already approved for the treatment of spastic disorders and chronic hiccups.

Maintenance Therapy

The development and use of proton pump inhibitors enhanced the understanding of the natural history and varied manifestations of GERD. Although almost all severe esophagitis could be healed with proton pump inhibitor therapy, recurrence occurred in approximately 80% of patients within 6 months of discontinuation of therapy,[118] and the likelihood of recurrence was related to the initial severity of esophagitis.

Because esophagitis relapses, maintenance medical therapy is usually necessary. Current evidence suggests that maintenance therapy with either H_2 receptor antagonists or cisapride is significantly less effective than therapy with proton pump inhibitors.[160] Vigneri and associates reported a randomized prospective study of 175 patients with esophagitis healed with omeprazole 40 mg/day and then randomized to one of five maintenance regimens.[161] Remission was maintained for 12 months in 49% of the ranitidine group, 54% of patients in the cisapride group, 66% in the ranitidine plus cisapride group, 80% of the omeprazole group, and 89% in the cisapride plus omeprazole group. Omeprazole was significantly more effective than either ranitidine or cisapride alone, and the combination of omeprazole and cisapride was more effective than the combination of ranitidine and cisapride.

Very few data support the use of step-down therapy for maintenance treatment in esophagitis initially shown to require proton pump inhibitor therapy. In 2000, Klinkenberg-Knol and associates reported data from patients with refractory esophagitis who were receiving maintenance therapy with omeprazole for a mean period of 6.5 years.[162] In 230 patients followed there were 158 relapses of esophagitis over 1490 treatment years (1 per 9.4 treatment years). Despite sporadic increases and decreases in the omeprazole dose for individual patients, the median dose required to maintain remission was at or near the dose required for healing esophagitis (Fig. 33–12).

As maintenance therapy has become the rule, rather than the exception in patients with esophagitis and moderate to severe symptoms, drug safety becomes an important issue. For short-term use, proton pump inhibitors have proved quite safe, although they stimulate the cytochrome P-450 system in the liver, sometimes necessitating dosage adjustment of warfarin, phenytoin, and diazepam. Side effects with these medications include headache ($<5\%$) and diarrhea ($<5\%$), both of which are reversible with cessation of therapy. Two safety issues have been raised regarding long-term treatment with proton pump inhibitors: (1) induction of hypergastrinemia along with the potential occurrence of gastric carcinoid tumors and (2) occurrence of gastric atrophy associated with concomitant *H. pylori* infection.

The initial approval of omeprazole for the treatment of esophagitis was delayed for several years after it was observed that in laboratory rats fed lifelong high doses of the drug, hypergastrinemia and gastric carcinoid tumors developed. It was subsequently shown that chronic ranitidine therapy and subtotal resection of the gastric fundus were also associated with hypergastrinemia, and all had the same potential as omeprazole to induce gastric carcinoids in rats. However, the relevance of these data to humans has always been dubious,[163] and critical evaluation of the relevant data suggests that these concerns remain entirely theoretical.[164, 165] Furthermore, although patients treated with omeprazole therapy for up to 11 years have shown increased corpus gastritis and argyrophil cell hyperplasia, no dysplasia or neoplastic change has been observed.[162]

Another concern regarding maintenance therapy is the propensity to development of atrophic gastritis among omeprazole-treated patients while on therapy. Long-term treatment with proton pump inhibitors changes the pattern of *H. pylori* gastritis from the duodenal ulcer type with antral predominance to the gastric cancer type with predominant corpus gastritis.[166–168] Whether antisecretory therapy accelerates the development of preneoplastic lesions in patients infected with *H. pylori* remains unclear. In 1996, Kuipers and coworkers reported that in more than 30% of *H. pylori* infected patients treated with omeprazole for 5 years atrophy developed, but not in *H. pylori*–negative patients.[169] Despite criticism regarding the definition of atrophy and comparison to an inappropriate control group, these data caused concern regarding the long-term safety of omeprazole therapy. However, a subsequent study comparing patients on maintenance omeprazole therapy to a control group who underwent fundoplication did not confirm these findings. There was no difference between the groups in terms of gastric glandular atrophy, nor in the occurrence of intestinal metaplasia in *H. pylori* infected GERD patients.[170] In addition, the longest-duration follow-up data that exist for continuous proton pump inhibitor therapy for up to 11 years revealed no significant difference in mucosal histologic characteristics in patients with and without *H. pylori* gastritis.[162]

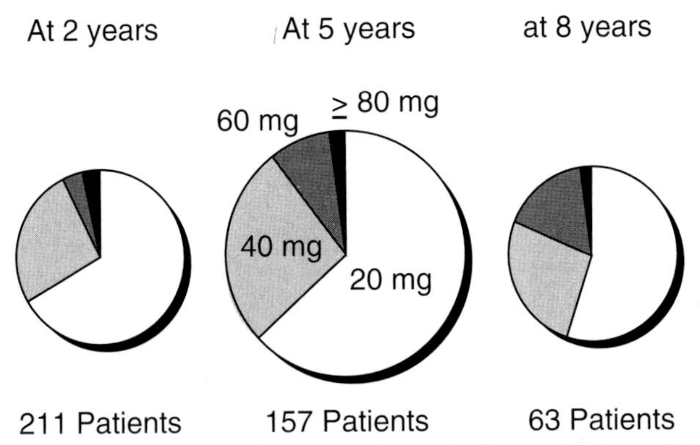

Figure 33–12. The dose of omeprazole required to maintain remission in patients with refractory esophagitis. For a mean period of 6.5 years (range, 1.4 to 11.2 years), 230 patients were monitored. There were 158 relapses of esophagitis over 1490 treatment years (1 per 9.4 treatment years). Despite sporadic increases and decreases in the omeprazole dose for individual patients, the median dose required to maintain remission was at or near the dose required for healing esophagitis. (Holloway RH [ed]: Reflux Disease. Baillieres Clin Gastroenterol 14[5]: 811, 2000.)

Nonerosive Gastroesophageal Reflux Disease

In contrast to the multitude of treatment trials of patients with esophagitis, there are relatively few studies assessing the efficacy of antireflux therapy in patients with nonerosive GERD. Given that endoscopic healing is not an applicable end point for evaluating nonerosive GERD patients, symptom response becomes the primary outcome variable. The current available studies' evaluation of symptom control in nonerosive GERD reveal a hierarchy of efficacy from either H_2 receptor antagonists or cisapride to proton pump inhibitors, similar to that seen in erosive GERD.[160] In these studies complete relief of heartburn was obtained in 35% to 57% of patients on omeprazole 20 mg/day. From these data, it appears that elimination of heartburn proves to be a more difficult therapeutic end point to achieve than esophagitis healing. Thus, the data do not support the viewpoint that nonerosive GERD is more responsive to therapy than erosive esophagitis and, hence, easily treated with less potent antisecretory therapy.

Contrary to the observations on severe esophagitis, data on less severe esophagitis and endoscopy-negative GERD support a less aggressive therapeutic approach to maintain remission. Studies from 1999 suggest that intermittent or on-demand therapy may be adequate for symptom control in endoscopy-negative GERD. Defining remission as the absence of symptomatic recurrence, Bardhan and associates prospectively evaluated 526 patients with nonerosive GERD and erosive GERD treated with either H_2 receptor antagonists or proton pump inhibitors on an as-needed basis.[171] Approximately 50% of patients did not take any acid suppressing medication for at least 6 of the 12 months, and this proportion was similar in all treatment groups, regardless of whether low-grade esophagitis was initially present. In another study, 424 patients with nonerosive GERD were randomized to on-demand therapy with omeprazole 10 mg, omeprazole 20 mg, or placebo.[172] At 6 months, remission was maintained in 83% of patients with omeprazole 20 mg, 69% with omeprazole 10 mg, and 56% with placebo. Given these observations, it is evident that over half the patients with nonerosive GERD did not require maintenance therapy and that on-demand therapy is a viable option to maintain symptom relief in nonerosive GERD.

Antireflux Surgery

Although many operations have been devised to control reflux disease, most are of historical interest only. Before the explosion of laparoscopic surgery the three most commonly performed operations were the Nissen fundoplication, the Belsey Mark IV repair, and the Hill posterior gastropexy. Currently, the two most popular procedures are the laparoscopic Nissen (360-degree) fundoplication and the Toupet (270-degree) fundoplication. Regardless of whether the procedures are done in an open or laparoscopic fashion they likely work similarly. Unlike medical therapy, fundoplication, via both mechanical and physiologic modifications, attempts to correct the underlying abnormalities associated with GERD. The essential procedure of fundoplication is to mobilize the lower esophagus, reduce the associated hiatal hernia, and wrap the gastric fundus either partially or totally around the esophagus. The operation reestablishes competence of the antireflux barrier by repairing the hiatal hernia and increasing resting LES pressure.[173] It may also reduce reflux by decreasing the frequency and/or effectiveness of transient LES relaxations.[174]

Antireflux surgery can produce excellent results when performed by expert surgeons. Unfortunately, although modern technique and careful patient selection have minimized risk, the nature of surgical intervention is such that it will always be associated with a finite mortality rate. Perdikis and colleagues pooled reports on laproscopic Nissen fundoplication published between 1991 and 1995 and arrived at a mortality rate of 0.2% among 2453 patients.[175] In addition to the mortality rate associated with antireflux surgery, fundoplication has the potential to produce clinically significant dysphagia, gas bloating, and flatulence. Estimates of the frequency with which these complications occur vary among series, most of which are uncontrolled. A controlled comparison in 2000 of the outcome of laparoscopic versus conventional fundoplication was terminated after the 1-year interim analysis revealed that 7 of the 57 patients who had had laparoscopic Nissen fundoplication had persistent dysphagia that was severe enough to require reoperation in 4.[176]

Whether antireflux surgery is as good as or superior to modern medical therapy is difficult to ascertain. Currently there are no valid data comparing laparoscopic antireflux therapy to long-term proton pump inhibitor therapy. Thus, the decision to pursue medical or surgical therapy ultimately depends on a risk-to-benefit analysis. The previous reservations aside, an argument for antireflux surgery can be made in the following circumstances: (1) failed medical therapy, with persistent symptomatic esophagitis; (2) medical success in a young healthy patient unwilling to take, or intolerant of, long-term proton pump inhibitor therapy; and (3) persistent symptoms due to regurgitation (laryngitis, asthma, bronchiectasis). A strong argument against antireflux surgery can be made for the following individuals: (1) elderly patients with concomitant disease and high surgical risk, (2) patients with continued symptoms but without quantifiable abnormal reflux, (3) patients with concomitant bloating or functional symptoms likely to be made worse by fundoplication, and (4) patients with poor or absent peristaltic function who are at risk of development of severe dysphagia after fundoplication. There are no credible data that fundoplication reduces the risk of death of esophageal cancer. In fact, a decision analysis based on U.S. epidemiologic data suggests that even among highly symptomatic white men (who have the greatest risk of esophageal adenocarcinoma), the risk of death due to a fundoplication procedure exceeds the risk of death due to esophageal adenocarcinoma.[177]

Peptic Strictures

In esophagitis patients, prevalence of peptic stricture ranges from 8% to 20%.[7] The natural history of peptic strictures is similar to that of erosive esophagitis in that the most severe grade is reached at the onset of disease.[9] This prevalence of strictures, however, appears to be decreasing in response to the widespread use of proton pump inhibitors. Factors that predispose one esophagitis patient to formation of strictures and another to healing without complication are unclear. However, it does appear that patients in whom strictures develop have a more profound disruption of the antireflux barrier than typical GERD patients.[65, 178] Presumably, the heightened acid exposure leads to ulceration and reactive fibrosis that result in a fixed stricture that is not altered by antisecretory therapy.

The treatment of peptic strictures focuses on restoring lumen patency, healing esophagitis, and preventing recurrence. Dilation with mercury-filled tapered dilators may achieve dramatic relief of dysphagia. However, these dilators are inadequate when the stricture is unyielding, tortuous, or associated with either extreme luminal narrowing or pseudodiverticula. In such instances, an endoscopically placed balloon dilator or dilator employing a metal guidewire is desirable. The two most commonly used over-the-wire dilators are the Savary-Gilliard and the American Dilation System. Through-the-scope pneumatic balloon dilators, such as those used to treat vascular stenosis, have also been adapted for treatment of peptic strictures. These two modalities appear to be equally effective and safe.[179, 180]

Successful dilation of peptic strictures to a lumen diameter of 15 mm (45 French) generally relieves dysphagia. The schedule for serial dilations should be based on the type of stricture, its response to initial and subsequent dilation, and the patient's tolerance of the procedure. Although never subjected to a controlled study, dilations are typically performed at 1- to 2-week intervals with no more than three successive dilator size increases in a single session.[181] The main risks of esophageal dilation are perforation, bleeding, and bacteremia. Esophageal perforation is the most severe complication of esophageal dilation and is reported to occur in fewer than 4 of 1000 procedures.[182, 183] Bleeding that requires blood transfusion occurs in fewer than 5 of 1000 procedures. Transient bacteremia may occur during dilation therapy, and prophylactic antibiotics are generally administered to patients at risk for bacterial endocarditis.[184] Given the effectiveness of long-term conservative management, surgery is rarely required in the treatment of peptic strictures.

Most studies report that more than 50% of patients with peptic strictures require repeat dilation.[185, 186] Risk factors predicting the likelihood of future stricturing are the number of previous recurrences and persistent reflux esophagitis. Data from 1999 suggest that adjunct therapy with proton pump inhibitors decreases the need for recurrent dilation.[187] Maintenance therapy with proton pump inhibitors should be continued indefinitely and has been shown to be cost-effective as a result of decreased frequency of future dilations and complications.[188]

BARRETT'S METAPLASIA, DYSPLASIA, AND ADENOCARCINOMA

The most serious histologic consequence of GERD is Barrett's metaplasia with the associated risk of esophageal adenocarcinoma. The epithelial type responsible for this malignant potential is specialized intestinal metaplasia.[189, 190] Histolopathologically, specialized intestinal metaplasia exhibits a villous architecture containing goblet cells (Fig. 33–13A). Intestinal metaplasia is divided into four subtypes, three of which are relevant to Barrett's metaplasia. In type I, or complete intestinal, metaplasia there is a complete brush border with mature goblet cells and Paneth cells are usually seen in the crypt bases. Types II and III are defined as incomplete intestinal metaplasia because the columnar cells lack the intestinal absorptive ability or ultrastructural characteristics of true intestinal cells.[191] Any of these three types of metaplastic epithelium can become dysplastic and potentially malignant (see Fig. 33–13*B*). Dysplastic alterations in Barrett's metaplasia have been classified as low grade or high grade, depending on the degree of nuclear pleomorphism, hyperchromatism, and altered nuclear polarity. High-grade dysplasia is an ominous finding that is often associated with carcinoma.

Barrett's metaplasia is generally believed to be an intermediate step in the development of esophageal adenocarcinoma (see Chapter 35). Although this is an uncommon cancer, the incidence is rapidly increasing in the United States and is greatest among white men. A 1999 nationwide population based case control study attempted to define the risk factors for development of esophageal adenocarcinoma reported from Sweden.[192] Findings from that study revealed a strong relationship between reflux symptoms and esophageal adenocarcinoma. The adjusted odds ratio for adenocarcinoma was 7.7 (95% confidence interval [CI], 5.3 to 11.4) in patients with recurrent reflux symptoms and 43.5 (95% CI, 18.3 to 103.5) in patients with severe symptoms for more than 20 years when compared with asymptomatic control subjects. Interestingly, only 62% of the resected esophagi showed areas of concomitant Barrett's metaplasia. The most likely explanation for this is that small areas of metaplasia were overgrown by the tumor and, hence, undetectable by the time of resection. In addition to reflux symptoms, obesity was found to be an independent risk factor for esophageal adenocarcinoma.[193] When both reflux symptoms and increased body mass index were present, the associated relative risk was 180 compared with that of persons with neither reflux nor obesity. However, even though these risk ratios appear alarming, the absolute risk of adenocarcinoma is actually still quite small because of its low incidence. In fact, these investigators calculated that even among the highest

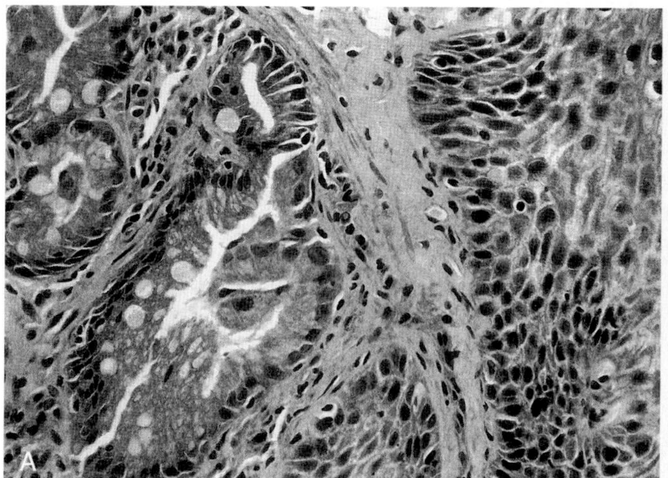

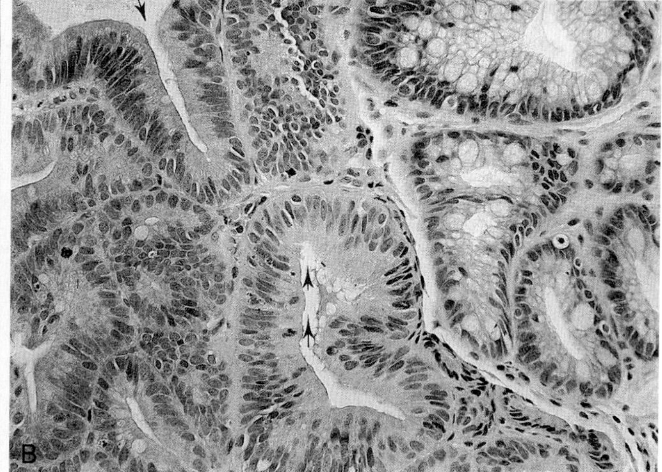

Figure 33–13. Histopathology of Barrett's metaplasia of the esophagus. *A,* Metaplasia showing glands lined by columnar epithelial cells with several goblet cells visible. Note an area of inflamed squamous epithelium to the right. *B,* Esophageal biopsy obtained from a patient with Barrett's metaplasia during surveillance. A *single arrow* near the top of the figure points to a gland showing low-grade dysplasia. The *double arrow* in the center of the figure points to an adjacent gland showing high-grade dysplasia. Note on the right an area of metaplasia without dysplasia. (Courtesy of Edward Lee, MD.)

risk group, obese white men with severe reflux symptoms, 2189 screening endoscopic examinations would be required to detect one case of adenocarcinoma.[194]

Definition and Epidemiology

Originally described in 1950 by Sir Norman Barrett as columnar lined esophagus, *Barrett's esophagus* has been redefined more times than we care to recount. The underlying significance of Barrett's metaplasia is its predisposition to development into adenocarcinoma of the esophagus. Subsequently, it was recognized that the epithelial type responsible for this malignant potential is specialized intestinal metaplasia. Demonstrating this form of metaplasia became a required feature of Barrett's metaplasia.[189, 190] However, the factor that most complicated the definition of Barrett's metaplasia was the recognition that specialized intestinal metaplasia is a relatively common finding and may occur in three distinct settings: (1) classic long segment Barrett's metaplasia in which salmon colored epithelium extends at least 3 cm proximally from the esophagogastric junction; (2) short segment Barrett's metaplasia, which is similarly endoscopically evident, but in which the metaplastic epithelium projects less than 3 cm from the esophagogastric junction; and (3) gastric cardia intestinal metaplasia, in which no metaplastic tongues are evident projecting from the esophagogastric junction, but biopsy specimens taken distal to the squamocolumnar junction nonetheless demonstrate specialized intestinal metaplasia.

The prevalence of long segment Barrett's metaplasia in patients who have upper gastrointestinal endoscopy is approximately 1%[6, 195] and increases with increasing severity of GERD.[196] The average age of affected patients ranges from 55 to 65 years with a male-to-female ratio of 10 : 1[7] and a white–to–African American ratio of 10 : 1.[197] Although the annual incidence of adenocarcinoma in long segment Barrett's metaplasia has been reported to be as high as 1.5%,[198] an analysis in 2000 suggested that this risk is overestimated because of publication bias and that the actual incidence is probably closer to 0.5% per year.[199] Short segment Barrett's metaplasia is clearly more prevalent than long segment Barrett's metaplasia but the precise incidence is difficult to define because published reports do not distinguish it from gastric cardia intestinal metaplasia. Although dysplasia and adenocarcinoma have been reported in short segment Barrett's metaplasia,[200] the magnitude of this risk is unknown; reports attempting to quantify it concluded that the malignant potential of short segment Barrett's metaplasia was much lower than that of long segment Barrett's metaplasia.[201–203]

Although there is general agreement that both long segment and short segment Barrett's metaplasia are associated with GERD and adenocarcinoma, the cause and natural history of gastric cardia intestinal metaplasia remain controversial. Gastric cardia intestinal metaplasia has been linked to both GERD and *H. pylori* gastritis.[203–207] Differentiating features of gastric cardia intestinal metaplasia compared with long or short segment Barrett's metaplasia are that the former is commonly associated with an *H. pylori* infection and is predominantly complete intestinal metaplasia (type I), whereas the incomplete types (II and III) are observed with long or short segment Barrett's metaplasia.[191] This distinction suggests that gastric cardia intestinal metaplasia is attributable to *H. pylori* gastritis rather than GERD. However, there is also evidence that intestinal metaplasia and inflammation of the gastric cardia can occur without an *H. pylori* infection, in which case they are presumed to be associated with chronic reflux.[204] The likelihood of detecting either gastric cardia intestinal metaplasia or short segment Barrett's metaplasia is estimated to be 18% to 33% in patients who have upper endoscopy.[195, 208] Fortunately, the incidence of dysplasia is low in gastric cardia intestinal metaplasia, estimated at 1.4% per year.[209]

Pathophysiology

Although the cause of Barrett's metaplasia is uncertain, it is clearly associated with GERD and believed to occur as a consequence of excessive esophageal acid exposure.[210] Ambulatory pH studies have demonstrated that Barrett's metaplasia patients have an increased number of reflux events and prolonged esophageal acid exposure compared with both normal and GERD patients.[58, 211, 212] This increased acid exposure may be related to a number of motor abnormalities associated with severe esophagitis. Most patients with severe esophagitis have a hiatal hernia; consequently there is a high prevalence of hiatal hernia in Barrett's metaplasia. Cameron reported finding a hernia greater than 2 cm in 96% of patients with long segment Barrett's metaplasia and 72% of patients with short segment Barrett's metaplasia.[213] In addition, manometric studies in long segment Barrett's metaplasia reveal decreased LES pressure and peristaltic dysfunction similar to that seen in severe esophagitis. Why Barrett's metaplasia develops in some patients with severe esophagitis and not in others remains to be determined. It is typically found at the onset of disease, and the epidemiologic literature suggests a potential genetic predisposition. Other factors, such as the role of duodenogastroesophageal reflux, are also being explored.

Management

Management of patients with Barrett's metaplasia has two aspects: treating the underlying GERD and managing the risk of adenocarcinoma of the esophagus. The principles for treating peptic esophagitis and controlling symptoms in Barrett's metaplasia are the same as for uncomplicated GERD with the proviso that because it is associated with extreme esophageal acid exposure, it will likely require more intensive treatment. In general, mucosal damage and symptoms can be controlled with proton pump inhibitor therapy, but surgery may be needed, or even desirable, in refractory cases.

On the basis of in vitro and in vivo cell proliferation studies reporting increased cell proliferation and decreased differentiation in tissue exposed to acid, some authorities believe that complete acid suppression is desirable in therapy for Barrett's metaplasia.[214, 215] However, there is no clinical evidence that aggressive antisecretory therapy or antireflux surgery prevents the occurrence of adenocarcinoma or causes regression of intestinal metaplasia. Proton pump inhibitor therapy has proved to be of no avail in reversing metaplasia or preventing adenocarcinoma.[216–218] Thus, the available data support titrating therapy to control symptoms and treat esophagitis, irrespective of the presence of Barrett's metaplasia.

Given that at present there is no known way of modifying risk of Barrett's metaplasia, we are left with attempting to minimize the cancer risk. This is done with periodic endoscopic biopsy examination of the metaplastic tissue, searching for dysplasia. The accepted regimen of histologic sampling is to obtain biopsy samples from each quadrant every 2 cm axially within the metaplastic tissue.[219] The rationale for this regimen is that dysplasia within Barrett's metaplasia is often multifocal and obtaining fewer samples increases the likelihood of overlooking dysplastic areas. All patients with proven Barrett's metaplasia should have the surveillance protocol to detect dysplasia. The importance of detecting high-grade dysplasia is emphasized by the observation that in 25% of high-grade dysplasia patients adenocarcinoma developed during 46-month follow-up.[220]

The optimal surveillance interval for a patient with Barrett's metaplasia is a function of histologic severity. For patients without dysplasia the previous recommendations were for surveillance at 2- to 3-year intervals.[219] A study in 2000 challenged this surveillance interval on the basis of compelling evidence that the cancer risk in Barrett's metaplasia has been overestimated and that in fact it is closer to 0.5% per year than the previously held 1% per year.[199] Although this difference may seem trivial, it is important to recognize that the modeled cost-effectiveness of surveillance endoscopy is marginal compared with that of other cancer preventing measures.[221] Such modeling suggests that if the cancer incidence were 0.5% per year, the cost per quality-adjusted year of life gained might well exceed the $100,000 value often viewed as the limit of what society is willing to pay.

If dysplasia is found in Barrett's metaplasia, the finding should be reviewed and confirmed by an expert pathologist. Patients found to have low-grade dysplasia should be given a 12-week course of high-dose antisecretory therapy with proton pump inhibitors to eliminate the confounding effect of inflammation, followed by repeat biopsy. If low-grade dysplasia persists, the current recommendation is that the patient have endoscopy every 6 months for 1 year, then yearly if no high-grade dysplasia is noted.[219] The finding of high-grade dysplasia has enormous ramifications given the high risk of development of adenocarcinoma. Focal high-grade dysplasia is defined as having a single focus (fewer than five dysplastic glands) of high-grade dysplasia on a single biopsy specimen. Although focal high-grade dysplasia patients have a lower risk of progression to adenocarcinoma than multifocal high-grade dysplasia patients, the risk is still significant; one study reported progression to cancer in 27% of patients over a mean of 3 years of surveillance.[222] In addition to the high rate of progression to adenocarcinoma, there is a high prevalence of unexpected coexisting cancer in patients who have high-grade dysplasia. Review of the English literature between 1990 and 1997 reveals that 47% of patients who undergo esophagectomy for high-grade dysplasia harbored an unexpected adenocarcinoma in the resected specimen.[223]

Although the preceding evidence supports a significant prevalence of adenocarcinoma and a high rate of progression from high-grade dysplasia to cancer, controversy regarding the treatment of patients with high-grade dysplasia remains. Esophagectomy, intensive endoscopic surveillance, and mucosal ablation have all been advocated. Currently, most experts advocate esophagectomy when high-grade dysplasia is discovered in an otherwise healthy patient with minimal surgical risk. However, esophagectomy has a reported operative mortality rates ranging from 3% to 10% and a substantial short-term morbidity rate.[224] Given these data, alternative management therapies have been proposed. Two prospective studies evaluating aggressive endoscopic surveillance in the management of high-grade dysplasia have been published. Levine and coworkers followed 29 patients with high-grade dysplasia for a 2- to 46-month period and found progression to intramucosal carcinoma in 24%.[220] Of the remainder, 27% were down-graded to a less severe histologic diagnosis and around half remained stable. Schnell and colleagues reported similar results from a prospective study of 72 patients with high-grade dysplasia for up to 17 years.[225] During this study adenocarcinoma developed in 11 patients (15%). Of these 11 patients, 10 had surgically curable disease and underwent esophagectomy. The one patient who died of esophageal cancer was lost to surveillance for a prolonged period and returned with an unresectable tumor. These data suggest that intensive endoscopic surveillance, rather than immediate esophagectomy, may have a role in the management of high-grade dysplasia.

Given the risks of esophagectomy, endoscopic ablative therapy has been proposed as an alternative treatment of high-grade dysplasia. Endoscopic therapy can be performed by using thermal, chemical, or mechanical methods. In each case, the principle is that removing the metaplastic tissue or dysplastic epithelium in the setting of intense acid inhibition results in regeneration of squamous epithelium. Thermal ablation can be achieved with either multipolar electrocoagulation, argon beam plasma coagulation, or laser coagulation. Multiple treatments are required, and perforation is a reported complication.[223] Currently, the more widely used alternative ablative method is photodynamic therapy, a technique utilizing the interaction between a photosensitizer that accumulates in the tissue and laser light of appropriate wavelength. The photosensitizer absorbs light energy and transfers it to oxygen, thus creating a high-energy oxygen radical that then causes tissue necrosis. Similarly to thermal methods, photodynamic therapy is associated with side effects including chest pain, nausea, and the development of esophageal strictures. In addition, patients need to be warned about limiting sun exposure secondary to skin photosensitivity. Although long-term results are not available, photodynamic therapy results in a downgrading of dysplasia status in 90% of treated patients. Residual Barrett's metaplasia has been reported in 58% of patients undergoing photodynamic therapy after 2 to 62 months of follow-up,[223] and there are reports of development of adenocarcinoma after therapy. Mechanical ablative techniques differ from both thermal and chemical methods in that they use localized endoscopic mucosal resection therapy addressing raised lesions within Barrett's metaplasia. Early esophageal cancer has been treated by this technique in patients not fit for surgery.[226] Although all of these ablative therapies have been shown to have some efficacy in modifying Barrett's metaplasia, presently there are no prospective randomized controlled trials available to advocate ablative therapy outside established research protocols.

REFERENCES

1. Shi G, Bruley des Varannes S, Scarpignato C, et al: Reflux related symptoms in patients with normal oesophageal exposure to acid. Gut 37:457, 1995.
2. Nebel OT, Fornes MF, Castell DO: Symptomatic gastroesophageal reflux: Incidence and precipitating factors. Am J Dig Dis 21:953, 1976.
3. DeMeester TR, Wang CI, Wernly JA, et al: Technique, indications, and clinical use of 24-hour esophageal pH monitoring. J Thorac Cardiovasc Surg 79:656, 1980.
4. Johnsson F, Joelsson B, Gudmundsson K, Greiff L: Symptoms and endoscopic findings in the diagnosis of gastroesophageal reflux disease. Scand J Gastroenterol 22:714, 1987.
5. Achem SR: Endoscopy-negative gastroesophageal reflux disease: The hypersensitive esophagus. Gastroenterol Clin North Am 28:893, 1999.
6. Cameron AJ, Zinsmeister AR, Ballard DJ, Carney JA: Prevalence of columnar-lined (Barrett's) esophagus: Comparison of population-based clinical and autopsy findings. Gastroenterology 99:918, 1990.
7. Wienbeck M, Barnert J: Epidemiology of reflux disease and reflux esophagitis. Scand J Gastroenterol Suppl 156:7, 1989.
8. Bainbridge ET, Temple JG, Nicholas SP, et al: Symptomatic gastro-oesophageal reflux in pregnancy: A comparative study of white Europeans and Asians in Birmingham. Br J Clin Pract 37:53, 1983.
9. Sonnenberg A, El-Serag HB: Clinical epidemiology and natural history of gastroesophageal reflux disease. Yale J Biol Med 72:81, 1999.
10. Lagergren J, Bergstrom R, Adami HO, Nyren O: Association between medications that relax the lower esophageal sphincter and risk for esophageal adenocarcinoma. Ann Intern Med 133:165, 2000.
11. Kim SL, Hunter JG, Wo JM, et al: NSAIDs, aspirin, and esophageal strictures: Are over-the-counter medications harmful to the esophagus? J Clin Gastroenterol 29:32, 1999.
12. El-Serag HB, Sonnenberg A: Associations between different forms of gastro-oesophageal reflux disease. Gut 41:594, 1997.
13. El-Serag HB, Sonnenberg A: Opposing time trends of peptic ulcer and reflux disease. Gut 43:327, 1998.
14. El-Serag HB, Sonnenberg A, Jamal MM, et al: Corpus gastritis is protective against reflux oesophagitis. Gut 45:181, 1999.
15. Wu JC, Sung JJ, Chan FK, et al: *Helicobacter pylori* infection is associated with milder gastro-oesophageal reflux disease. Aliment Pharmacol Ther 14:427, 2000.
16. Labenz J, Blum AL, Bayerdorffer E, et al: Curing *Helicobacter pylori* infection in patients with duodenal ulcer may provoke reflux esophagitis. Gastroenterology 112:1442, 1997.
17. Feldman M, Cryer B, Sammer D, et al: Influence of *H. pylori* infection on meal-stimulated gastric acid secretion and gastroesophageal acid reflux. Am J Physiol 277:G1159, 1999.
18. Verdu EF, Armstrong D, Idstrom JP, et al: Effect of curing *Helicobacter pylori* infection on intragastric pH during treatment with omeprazole. Gut 37:743, 1995.
19. Labenz J, Tillenburg B, Peitz U, et al: *Helicobacter pylori* augments the pH-increasing effect of omeprazole in patients with duodenal ulcer. Gastroenterology 110:725, 1996.
20. Hamilton SR: Reflux esophagitis and Barrett esophagus. Monogr Pathol 31:11, 1990.
21. Ismail-Beigi F, Horton PF, Pope CE: Histopathologic consequences of gastroesophageal reflux in man. Gastroenterology 58:163, 1970.
22. Rabin MS, Bremner CG, Botha JR: The reflux gastroesophageal polyp. Am J Gastroenterol 73:451, 1980.
23. Jacob P, Kahrilas PJ, Desai T, et al: Natural history and significance of esophageal squamous cell dysplasia. Cancer 65:2731, 1990.
24. Kahrilas PJ, Shi G, Manka M, Joehl RJ: Increased frequency of transient lower esophageal sphincter relaxation induced by gastric distention in reflux patients with hiatal hernia. Gastroenterology 118:688, 2000.
25. Barham CP, Gotley DC, Mills A, Alderson D: Precipitating causes of acid reflux episodes in ambulant patients with gastro-oesophageal reflux disease. Gut 36:505, 1995.
26. Dent J, Holloway RH, Toouli J, Dodds WJ: Mechanisms of lower oesophageal sphincter incompetence in patients with symptomatic gastrooesophageal reflux. Gut 29:1020, 1988.
27. Mittal RK, Holloway RH, Penagini R, et al: Transient lower esophageal sphincter relaxation. Gastroenterology 109:601, 1995.
28. Holloway RH, Penagini R, Ireland AC: Criteria for objective definition of transient lower esophageal sphincter relaxation. Am J Physiol 268:G128, 1995.
29. Sifrim D, Tack J, Lerut T, Janssens J: Transient lower esophageal sphincter relaxations and esophageal body muscular contractile response in reflux esophagitis. Dig Dis Sci 45:1293, 2000.
30. Wyman JB, Dent J, Heddle R, et al: Control of belching by the lower oesophageal sphincter. Gut 31:639, 1990.
31. Kahrilas PJ, Dodds WJ, Dent J, et al: Upper esophageal sphincter function during belching. Gastroenterology 91:133, 1986.
32. Dent J, Dodds WJ, Friedman RH, et al: Mechanism of gastroesophageal reflux in recumbent asymptomatic human subjects. J Clin Invest 65:256, 1980.
33. Biancani P, Hillemeier C, Bitar KN, Makhlouf GM: Contraction mediated by Ca^{2+} influx in esophageal muscle and by Ca^{2+} release in the LES. Am J Physiol 253:G760, 1987.
34. Goyal RK, Rattan S: Genesis of basal sphincter pressure: Effect of tetrodotoxin on lower esophageal sphincter pressure in opossum in vivo. Gastroenterology 71:62, 1976.
35. Dodds WJ, Dent J, Hogan WJ, Arndorfer RC: Effect of atropine on esophageal motor function in humans. Am J Physiol 240:G290, 1981.
36. Dent J, Dodds WJ, Hogan WJ, Toouli J: Factors that influence induction of gastroesophageal reflux in normal human subjects. Dig Dis Sci 33:270, 1988.
37. Behar J, Biancani P, Sheahan DG: Evaluation of esophageal tests in the diagnosis of reflux esophagitis. Gastroenterology 71:9, 1976.
38. Kahrilas PJ, Dodds WJ, Hogan WJ, et al: Esophageal peristaltic dysfunction in peptic esophagitis. Gastroenterology 91:897, 1986.
39. Kahrilas PJ, Gupta RR: Mechanisms of acid reflux associated with cigarette smoking. Gut 31:4, 1990.
40. De Troyer AJR: Reflex inhibition of the diaphragm by esophageal afferents. Neurosci Lett 30:43, 1982.
41. Altschuler SM, Boyle JT, Nixon TE, et al: Simultaneous reflex inhibition of lower esophageal sphincter and crural diaphragm in cats. Am J Physiol 249:G586, 1985.
42. Mittal RK, Fisher M, McCallum RW, et al: Human lower esophageal sphincter pressure response to increased intra-abdominal pressure. Am J Physiol 258:G624, 1990.
43. Klein WA, Parkman HP, Dempsey DT, Fisher RS: Sphincterlike thoracoabdominal high pressure zone after esophagogastrectomy. Gastroenterology 105:1362, 1993.
44. Kahrilas PJ: The role of hiatus hernia in GERD. Yale J Biol Med 72:101, 1999.
45. Michelson E, Siegel C: The role of the phrenico-esophageal ligament in the lower esophageal sphincter. Surg Gynecol Obstet 118:1291, 1964.
46. Kahrilas PJ, Lin S, Manka M, et al: Esophagogastric junction pressure topography after fundoplication. Surgery 127:200, 2000.
47. Liebermann-Meffert D, Allgower M, Schmid P, Blum AL: Muscular equivalent of the lower esophageal sphincter. Gastroenterology 76:31, 1979.
48. Van Herwaarden MA, Samsom M, Smout AJ: Excess gastroesophageal reflux in patients with hiatus hernia is caused by mechanisms other than transient LES relaxations. Gastroenterology 119:1439, 2000.
49. Holloway RH, Hongo M, Berger K, McCallum RW: Gastric distention: A mechanism for postprandial gastroesophageal reflux. Gastroenterology 89:779, 1985.
50. Scarpignato C: Gastric emptying in gastroesophageal reflux disease and other functional esophageal disorders. In Scarpignato C, Galmiche JP (eds): Functional Investigation in Esophageal Disease. Basel, Karger, 1994, pp 223–259.
51. Helm JF: Role of saliva in esophageal function and disease. Dysphagia 4:76, 1989.
52. Schneyer LH, Pigman W, Hannahan L, Gilmore RW: Rate and flow of human parotid, sublingual, and submaxillary secretions during sleep. J Dent Res 35:109, 1956.
53. Singh S, Bradley LA, Richter JE: Determinants of oesophageal "alkaline" pH environment in controls and patients with gastro-oesophageal reflux disease. Gut 34:309, 1993.
54. Booth DJ, Kemmemer WT, Skinner DB: Acid clearing from the distal esophagus. Arch Surg 96:731, 1968.
55. Stanciu C, Bennett JR: Oesophageal acid clearing: One factor in production of reflux esophagitis. Gut 15:852, 1974.

56. Dodds WP, Kahrilas PJ, Dent J, et al: Analysis of spontaneous gastroesophageal reflux and esophageal acid clearance in patients with reflux esophagitis. J Gastrointest Motil 2:79, 1990.
57. Johnson LF: 24-Hour pH monitoring in the study of gastroesophageal reflux. J Clin Gastroenterol 2:387, 1980.
58. Gillen P, Keeling P, Byrne PJ, Hennessy TP: Barrett's oesophagus: pH Profile. Br J Surg 74:774, 1987.
59. Karvelis KC, Drane WE, Johnson DA, Silverman ED: Barrett esophagus: Decreased esophageal clearance shown by radionuclide esophageal scintigraphy. Radiology 162:97, 1987.
60. Singh P, Adamopoulos A, Taylor RH, Colin-Jones DG: Oesophageal motor function before and after healing of oesophagitis. Gut 33:1590, 1992.
61. Kahrilas PJ, Dodds WJ, Hogan WJ: Effect of peristaltic dysfunction on esophageal volume clearance. Gastroenterology 94:73, 1988.
62. Leite LP, Johnston BT, Barrett J, et al: Ineffective esophageal motility (IEM): The primary finding in patients with nonspecific esophageal motility disorder. Dig Dis Sci 42:1859, 1997.
63. Timmer R, Breumelhof R, Nadorp JH, Smout AJ: Oesophageal motility and gastro-oesophageal reflux before and after healing of reflux oesophagitis: A study using 24-hour ambulatory pH and pressure monitoring. Gut 35:1519, 1994.
64. Rydberg L, Ruth M, Lundell L: Does oesophageal motor function improve with time after successful antireflux surgery? Results of a prospective, randomised clinical study. Gut 41:82, 1997.
65. Mittal RK, Lange RC, McCallum RW: Identification and mechanism of delayed esophageal acid clearance in subjects with hiatus hernia. Gastroenterology 92:130, 1987.
66. Sloan S, Kahrilas PJ: Impairment of esophageal emptying with hiatal hernia. Gastroenterology 100:596, 1991.
67. Korsten MA, Rosman AS, Fishbein S, et al: Chronic xerostomia increases esophageal acid exposure and is associated with esophageal injury. Am J Med 90:701, 1991.
68. Kahrilas PJ, Gupta RR: The effect of cigarette smoking on salivation and esophageal acid clearance. J Lab Clin Med 114:431, 1989.
69. Konturek JW, Bielanski W, Konturek SJ, et al: Distribution and release of epidermal growth factor in man. Gut 30:1194, 1989.
70. Skov Olsen P, Poulsen SS, Therkelsen K, Nexo E: Oral administration of synthetic human urogastrone promotes healing of chronic duodenal ulcers in rats. Gastroenterology 90:911, 1986.
71. Sarosiek J, Feng T, McCallum RW: The interrelationship between salivary epidermal growth factor and the functional integrity of the esophageal mucosal barrier in the rat. Am J Med Sci 302:359, 1991.
72. Maccini DM, Veit BC: Salivary epidermal growth factor in patients with and without acid peptic disease. Am J Gastroenterol 85:1102, 1990.
73. Rourk RM, Namiot Z, Sarosiek J, et al: Impairment of salivary epidermal growth factor secretory response to esophageal mechanical and chemical stimulation in patients with reflux esophagitis. Am J Gastroenterol 89:237, 1994.
74. Orlando RC: Esophageal epithelial defenses against acid injury. Am J Gastroenterol 89:S48, 1994.
75. Quigley EM, Turnberg LA: pH of the microclimate lining human gastric and duodenal mucosa in vivo: Studies in control subjects and in duodenal ulcer patients. Gastroenterology 92:1876, 1987.
76. Meyers RL, Orlando RC: In vivo bicarbonate secretion by human esophagus. Gastroenterology 103:1174, 1992.
77. Orlando RC: The pathogenesis of gastroesophageal reflux disease: The relationship between epithelial defense, dysmotility, and acid exposure. Am J Gastroenterol 92:3S, 1997.
78. Tobey NA, Reddy SP, Keku TO, et al: Studies of pH in rabbit esophageal basal and squamous epithelial cells in culture. Gastroenterology 103:830, 1992.
79. Tobey NA, Reddy SP, Khalbuss WE, et al: Na^+-dependent and -independent Cl^-/HCO_3^- exchangers in cultured rabbit esophageal epithelial cells [published erratum appears in Gastroenterology 105(2): 649, 1993]. Gastroenterology 104:185, 1993.
80. Laycock WS, Oddsdottir M, Franco A, et al: Laparoscopic Nissen fundoplication is less expensive than open Belsey Mark IV. Surg Endosc 9:426, 1995.
81. Hollwarth ME, Smith M, Kvietys PR, Granger DN: Esophageal blood flow in the cat: Normal distribution and effects of acid perfusion. Gastroenterology 90:622, 1986.
82. Feldman MJ, Morris GP, Dinda PK, Paterson WG: Mast cells mediate acid induced augmentation of opossum esophageal blood flow via histamine and nitric oxide. Gastroenterology 110:121, 1996.
83. Miller LS, Vinayek R, Frucht H, et al: Reflux esophagitis in patients with Zollinger-Ellison syndrome. Gastroenterology 98:341, 1990.
84. Hirschowitz BI: A critical analysis, with appropriate controls, of gastric acid and pepsin secretion in clinical esophagitis. Gastroenterology 101:1149, 1991.
85. Hirschowitz BI: Pepsin and the esophagus. Yale J Biol Med 72:133, 1999.
86. Sears RJ, Champion GL, Richter JE: Characteristics of distal partial gastrectomy patients with esophageal symptoms of duodenogastric reflux. Am J Gastroenterol 90:211, 1995.
87. Carlsson R, Dent J, Bolling-Sternevald E, et al: The usefulness of a structured questionnaire in the assessment of symptomatic gastroesophageal reflux disease. Scand J Gastroenterol 33:1023, 1998.
88. Joelsson B, Johnsson F: Heartburn—the acid test. Gut 30:1523, 1989.
89. Berstad A, Hatlebakk JG: The predictive value of symptoms in gastro-oesophageal reflux disease. Scand J Gastroenterol Suppl 211:1, 1995.
90. Cooper BT, Barbezat GO: Barrett's esophagus: A clinical study of 52 patients. Q J Med 238:97, 1987.
91. Jacob P, Kahrilas PJ, Vanagunas A: Peristaltic dysfunction associated with nonobstructive dysphagia in reflux disease. Dig Dis Sci 35:939, 1990.
92. Cherry JMS: Contact ulcer of the larynx. Laryngoscope 78:1937, 1968.
93. Ormseth EJ, Wong RK: Reflux laryngitis: Pathophysiology, diagnosis, and management. Am J Gastroenterol 94:2812, 1999.
94. El-Serag HB, Sonnenberg A: Comorbid occurrence of laryngeal or pulmonary disease with esophagitis in United States military veterans. Gastroenterology 113:755, 1997.
95. Jacob P, Kahrilas PJ, Herzon G: Proximal esophageal pH-metry in patients with "reflux laryngitis." Gastroenterology 100:305, 1991.
96. Katz PO: Ambulatory esophageal and hypopharyngeal pH monitoring in patients with hoarseness. Am J Gastroenterol 85:38, 1990.
97. Shaker R, Milbrath M, Ren J, et al: Esophagopharyngeal distribution of refluxed gastric acid in patients with reflux laryngitis. Gastroenterology 109:1575, 1995.
98. Field SK, Underwood M, Brant R, Cowie RL: Prevalence of gastroesophageal reflux symptoms in asthma. Chest 109:316, 1996.
99. Jack CI, Calverley PM, Donnelly RJ, et al: Simultaneous tracheal and oesophageal pH measurements in asthmatic patients with gastro-oesophageal reflux. Thorax 50:201, 1995.
100. Gastal OL, Castell JA, Castell DO: Frequency and site of gastroesophageal reflux in patients with chest symptoms: Studies using proximal and distal pH monitoring. Chest 106:1793, 1994.
101. Harding SM, Guzzo MR, Richter JE: 24-h Esophageal pH testing in asthmatics: Respiratory symptom correlation with esophageal acid events. Chest 115:654, 1999.
102. Field SK: A critical review of the studies of the effects of simulated or real gastroesophageal reflux on pulmonary function in asthmatic adults. Chest 115:848, 1999.
103. Field SK, Sutherland LR: Does medical antireflux therapy improve asthma in asthmatics with gastroesophageal reflux? A critical review of the literature. Chest 114:275, 1998.
104. Field SK, Gelfand GA, McFadden SD: The effects of antireflux surgery on asthmatics with gastroesophageal reflux. Chest 116:766, 1999.
105. Yu ML, Ryu JH: Assessment of the patient with chronic cough. Mayo Clin Proc 72:957, 1997.
106. Harding SM, Richter JE: The role of gastroesophageal reflux in chronic cough and asthma. Chest 111:1389, 1997.
107. Ing AJ: Cough and gastroesophageal reflux. Am J Med 103:91S, 1997.
108. Irwin RS, Zawacki JK, Curley FJ, et al: Chronic cough as the sole presenting manifestation of gastroesophageal reflux. Am Rev Respir Dis 140:1294, 1989.
109. Ing AJ, Ngu MC, Breslin AB: Chronic persistent cough and gastro-oesophageal reflux. Thorax 46:479, 1991.
110. Ing AJ, Ngu MC, Breslin AB: Pathogenesis of chronic persistent cough associated with gastroesophageal reflux. Am J Respir Crit Care Med 149:160, 1994.
111. Katz PO, Dalton CB, Richter JE, et al: Esophageal testing of patients with noncardiac chest pain or dysphagia: Results of three years' experience with 1161 patients. Ann Intern Med 106:593, 1987.
112. Achem SR, Crittenden J, Kolts B, Burton L: Long-term clinical and manometric follow-up of patients with nonspecific esophageal motor disorders. Am J Gastroenterol 87:825, 1992.
113. DeMeester TR, O'Sullivan GC, Bermudez G, et al: Esophageal func-

tion in patients with angina-type chest pain and normal coronary angiograms. Ann Surg 196:488, 1982.
114. Hewson EG, Dalton CB, Richter JE: Comparison of esophageal manometry, provocative testing, and ambulatory monitoring in patients with unexplained chest pain. Dig Dis Sci 35:302, 1990.
115. Achem SR, Kolts BE, MacMath T, et al: Effects of omeprazole versus placebo in treatment of noncardiac chest pain and gastroesophageal reflux. Dig Dis Sci 42:2138, 1997.
116. Brunnen PL, Karmody AM, Needham CD: Severe peptic oesophagitis. Gut 10:831, 1969.
117. Isolauri J, Luostarinen M, Isolauri E, et al: Natural course of gastroesophageal reflux disease: 17–22 Year follow-up of 60 patients. Am J Gastroenterol 92:37, 1997.
118. Hetzel DJ, Dent J, Reed WD, et al: Healing and relapse of severe peptic esophagitis after treatment with omeprazole. Gastroenterology 95:903, 1988.
119. Weihrauch TR, Ewe K, Forster CF, et al: Action of domperidone on the lower esophageal sphincter: A double-blind cross-over study. Verh Dtsch Ges Inn Med 83:417, 1977.
120. Strader DB, Benjamin SB, Orbuch M, et al: Esophageal function and occurrence of Barrett's esophagus in Zollinger-Ellison syndrome. Digestion 56:347, 1995.
121. Venables TL, Newland RD, Patel AC, et al: Omeprazole 10 milligrams once daily, omeprazole 20 milligrams once daily, or ranitidine 150 milligrams twice daily, evaluated as initial therapy for the relief of symptoms of gastro-oesophageal reflux disease in general practice. Scand J Gastroenterol 32:965, 1997.
122. Armstrong D: Endoscopic evaluation of gastro-esophageal reflux disease. Yale J Biol Med 72:93, 1999.
123. Richter JE: Severe reflux esophagitis. Gastrointest Endosc Clin North Am 4:677, 1994.
124. Richter JE, Castell DO: Gastroesophageal reflux: Pathogenesis, diagnosis, and therapy. Ann Intern Med 97:93, 1982.
125. Gustavsson S, Bergstrom R, Erwall C, et al: Reflux esophagitis: Assessment of therapy effects and observer variation by video documentation of endoscopy findings. Scand J Gastroenterol 22:585, 1987.
126. Lundell LR, Dent J, Bennett JR, et al: Endoscopic assessment of oesophagitis: Clinical and functional correlates and further validation of the Los Angeles classification. Gut 45:172, 1999.
127. Richter J: Disorders of Esophageal Function. New York, Academy Professional Informational Services, 1998.
128. Richter JE, Hewson EG, Sinclair JW, Dalton CB: Acid perfusion test and 24-hour esophageal pH monitoring with symptom index: Comparison of tests for esophageal acid sensitivity. Dig Dis Sci 36:565, 1991.
129. Kahrilas PJ, Quigley EM: Clinical esophageal pH recording: A technical review for practice guideline development. Gastroenterology 110:1982, 1996.
130. Johnsson F, Joelsson B: Reproducibility of ambulatory oesophageal pH monitoring. Gut 29:886, 1988.
131. Wiener GJ, Morgan TM, Copper JB, et al: Ambulatory 24-hour esophageal pH monitoring: Reproducibility and variability of pH parameters. Dig Dis Sci 33:1127, 1988.
132. Younes Z, Johnson DA: Diagnostic evaluation in gastroesophageal reflux disease. Gastroenterol Clin North Am 28:809, 1999.
133. Weusten BL, Roelofs JM, Akkermans LM, et al: The symptom-association probability: An improved method for symptom analysis of 24-hour esophageal pH data. Gastroenterology 107:1741, 1994.
134. Schindlbeck NE, Klauser AG, Voderholzer WA, Muller-Lissner SA: Empiric therapy for gastroesophageal reflux disease. Arch Intern Med 155:1808, 1995.
135. Schenk BE, Kuipers EJ, Klinkenberg-Knol EC, et al: Omeprazole as a diagnostic tool in gastroesophageal reflux disease. Am J Gastroenterol 92:1997, 1997.
136. Graham DY, Smith JL, Patterson DJ: Why do apparently healthy people use antacid tablets? Am J Gastroenterol 78:257, 1983.
137. Johnson LF, DeMeester TR: Evaluation of elevation of the head of the bed, bethanechol, and antacid formula tablets on gastroesophageal reflux. Dig Dis Sci 26:673, 1981.
138. Meining A, Classen M: The role of diet and lifestyle measures in the pathogenesis and treatment of gastroesophageal reflux disease. Am J Gastroenterol 95:2692, 2000.
139. Chiba N, De Gara CJ, Wilkinson JM, Hunt RH: Speed of healing and symptom relief in grade II to IV gastroesophageal reflux disease: A meta-analysis. Gastroenterology 112:1798, 1997.
140. Jones DB, Howden CW, Burget DW, et al: Alteration of H_2 receptor sensitivity in duodenal ulcer patients after maintenance treatment with an H_2 receptor antagonist. Gut 29:890, 1988.
141. Hatlebakk JG, Katz PO, Camacho-Lobato L, Castell DO: Proton pump inhibitors: Better acid suppression when taken before a meal than without a meal. Aliment Pharmacol Ther 14:1267, 2000.
142. Walt RP, Male PJ, Rawlings J, et al: Comparison of the effects of ranitidine, cimetidine and placebo on the 24-hour intragastric acidity and nocturnal acid secretion in patients with duodenal ulcer. Gut 22:49, 1981.
143. Sharma BK, Walt RP, Pounder RE, et al: Optimal dose of oral omeprazole for maximal 24-hour decrease of intragastric acidity. Gut 25:957, 1984.
144. Kahrilas PJ, Falk GW, Johnson DA, et al: Esomeprazole improves healing and symptom resolution as compared with omeprazole in reflux oesophagitis patients: A randomized controlled trial. Aliment Pharmacol Ther 14:1249, 2000.
145. Merki HS, Witzel L, Walt RP, et al: Double blind comparison of the effects of cimetidine, ranitidine, famotidine, and placebo on intragastric acidity in 30 normal volunteers. Gut 29:81, 1988.
146. Lind T, Rydberg L, Kyleback A, et al: Esomeprazole provides improved acid control vs. omeprazole in patients with symptoms of gastro-oesophageal reflux disease. Aliment Pharmacol Ther 14:861, 2000.
147. Verdu EF, Armstrong D, Idstrom JP, et al: Intragastric pH during treatment with omeprazole: Role of *Helicobacter pylori* and *H. pylori*–associated gastritis. Scand J Gastroenterol 31:1151, 1996.
148. Labenz J, Tillenburg B, Peitz U, et al: Efficacy of omeprazole one year after cure of *Helicobacter pylori* infection in duodenal ulcer patients. Am J Gastroenterol 92:576, 1997.
149. Sagar M, Tybring G, Dahl ML, Bertilsson L, Seensalu R: Effects of omeprazole on intragastric pH and plasma gastrin are dependent on the *Cyp*2C19 polymorphism. Gastroenterology 119:670, 2000.
150. Adachi K, Katsube T, Kawamura A, et al: *Cyp*2C19 genotype status and intragastric pH during dosing with lansoprazole or rabeprazole. Aliment Pharmacol Ther 14:1259, 2000.
151. Temple JG, Bradby GV, O'Connor FO, et al: Cimetidine and metoclopramide in oesophageal reflux disease. BMJ 286:1863, 1983.
152. McCallum RW: Clinical pharmacology forum: Motility agents and the gastrointestinal tract. Am J Med Sci 312:19, 1996.
153. Sontag SJ: The medical management of reflux esophagitis: Role of antacids and acid inhibition. Gastroenterol Clin North Am 19:683, 1990.
154. DeVault KR, Castell DO: Updated guidelines for the diagnosis and treatment of gastroesophageal reflux disease: The Practice Parameters Committee of the American College of Gastroenterology. Am J Gastroenterol 94:1434, 1999.
155. Penagini R, Bianchi PA: Effect of morphine on gastroesophageal reflux and transient lower esophageal sphincter relaxation. Gastroenterology 113:409, 1997.
156. Mittal RK, Holloway R, Dent J: Effect of atropine on the frequency of reflux and transient lower esophageal sphincter relaxation in normal subjects. Gastroenterology 109:1547, 1995.
157. Boeckxstaens GE, Hirsch DP, Fakhry N, et al: Involvement of cholecystokinin A receptors in transient lower esophageal sphincter relaxations triggered by gastric distention. Am J Gastroenterol 93:1823, 1998.
158. Hirsch DP, Holloway RH, Tytgat GN, Boeckxstaens GE: Involvement of nitric oxide in human transient lower esophageal sphincter relaxations and esophageal primary peristalsis. Gastroenterology 115:1374, 1998.
159. Lidums I, Lehmann A, Checklin H, et al: Control of transient lower esophageal sphincter relaxations and reflux by the GABA(B) agonist baclofen in normal subjects. Gastroenterology 118:7, 2000.
160. An evidence-based appraisal of reflux disease management—the Genval Workshop Report. Gut 44(suppl 2):S1, 1999.
161. Vigneri S, Termini R, Leandro G, et al: A comparison of five maintenance therapies for reflux esophagitis. N Engl J Med 333:1106, 1995.
162. Klinkenberg-Knol EC, Nelis F, Dent J, et al: Long-term omeprazole treatment in resistant gastroesophageal reflux disease: Efficacy, safety, and influence on gastric mucosa. Gastroenterology 118:661, 2000.
163. Freston JW: Omeprazole, hypergastrinemia, and gastric carcinoid tumors [editorial]. Ann Intern Med 121:232, 1994.
164. Yeomans ND, Dent J: Personal review: Alarmism or legitimate concerns about long-term suppression of gastric acid secretion? Aliment Pharmacol Ther 14:267, 2000.

165. Laine L, Ahnen D, McClain C, et al: Review article: Potential gastrointestinal effects of long-term acid suppression with proton pump inhibitors. Aliment Pharmacol Ther 14:651, 2000.
166. Kuipers EJ, Uyterlinde AM, Pena AS, et al: Increase of *Helicobacter pylori*–associated corpus gastritis during acid suppressive therapy: Implications for long-term safety. Am J Gastroenterol 90:1401, 1995.
167. Logan RP, Walker MM, Misiewicz JJ, et al: Changes in the intragastric distribution of *Helicobacter pylori* during treatment with omeprazole. Gut 36:12, 1995.
168. Stolte M, Meining A, Schmitz JM, et al: Changes in *Helicobacter pylori* induced gastritis in the antrum and corpus during 12 months of treatment with omeprazole and lansoprazole in patients with gastro-oesophageal reflux disease. Aliment Pharmacol Ther 12:247, 1998.
169. Kuipers EJ, Lundell L, Klinkenberg-Knol EC, et al: Atrophic gastritis and *Helicobacter pylori* infection in patients with reflux esophagitis treated with omeprazole or fundoplication. N Engl J Med 334:1018, 1996.
170. Lundell L, Miettinen P, Myrvold HE, et al: Lack of effect of acid suppression therapy on gastric atrophy: Nordic GERD Study Group. Gastroenterology 117:319, 1999.
171. Bardhan KD, Muller-Lissner S, Bigard MA, et al: Symptomatic gastro-oesophageal reflux disease: Double blind controlled study of intermittent treatment with omeprazole or ranitidine: The European Study Group. BMJ 318:502, 1999.
172. Lind T, Havelund T, Lundell L, et al: On demand therapy with omeprazole for the long-term management of patients with heartburn without oesophagitis—a placebo-controlled randomized trial. Aliment Pharmacol Ther 13:907, 1999.
173. Rydberg L, Ruth M, Lundell L: Mechanism of action of antireflux procedures. Br J Surg 86:405, 1999.
174. Johnsson F, Holloway RH, Ireland AC, et al: Effect of fundoplication on transient lower oesophageal sphincter relaxation and gas reflux. Br J Surg 84:686, 1997.
175. Perdikis G, Hinder RA, Lund RJ, et al: Laparoscopic Nissen fundoplication: Where do we stand? Surg Laparosc Endosc 7:17, 1997.
176. Bais JE, Bartelsman JF, Bonjer HJ, et al: Laparoscopic or conventional Nissen fundoplication for gastro-oesophageal reflux disease: Randomised clinical trial: The Netherlands Antireflux Surgery Study Group. Lancet 355:170, 2000.
177. Spechler SJ: Barrett's esophagus: An overrated cancer risk factor [editorial]. Gastroenterology 119:587, 2000.
178. Parkman HP, Fisher RS: Contributing role of motility abnormalities in the pathogenesis of gastroesophageal reflux disease. Dig Dis 15:40, 1997.
179. Saeed ZA, Winchester CB, Ferro PS, et al: Prospective randomized comparison of polyvinyl bougies and through-the-scope balloons for dilation of peptic strictures of the esophagus. Gastrointest Endosc 41:189, 1995.
180. Cox JG, Winter RK, Maslin SC, et al: Balloon or bougie for dilatation of benign esophageal stricture? Dig Dis Sci 39:776, 1994.
181. Spechler SJ: AGA technical review on treatment of patients with dysphagia caused by benign disorders of the distal esophagus. Gastroenterology 117:233, 1999.
182. Marks RD, Richter JE: Peptic strictures of the esophagus. Am J Gastroenterol 88:1160, 1993.
183. Marshall JB, Afridi SA, King PD, et al: Esophageal dilation with polyvinyl (American) dilators over a marked guidewire: Practice and safety at one center over a 5-yr period. Am J Gastroenterol 91:1503, 1996.
184. Nelson DB, Sanderson SJ, Azar MM: Bacteremia with esophageal dilation. Gastrointest Endosc 48:563, 1998.
185. Patterson DJ, Graham DY, Smith JL, et al: Natural history of benign esophageal stricture treated by dilatation. Gastroenterology 85:346, 1983.
186. Glick ME: Clinical course of esophageal stricture managed by bougienage. Dig Dis Sci 27:884, 1982.
187. Richter JE: Peptic strictures of the esophagus. Gastroenterol Clin North Am 28:875, 1999.
188. Marks RD, Richter JE, Rizzo J, et al: Omeprazole versus H_2 receptor antagonists in treating patients with peptic stricture and esophagitis. Gastroenterology 106:907, 1994.
189. Spechler SJ, Goyal RK: The columnar-lined esophagus, intestinal metaplasia, and Norman Barrett. Gastroenterology 110:614, 1996.
190. Reid BJ, Weinstein WM: Barrett's esophagus and adenocarcinoma. Annu Rev Med 38:477, 1987.
191. Spechler SJ: The role of gastric carditis in metaplasia and neoplasia at the gastroesophageal junction. Gastroenterology 117:218, 1999.
192. Lagergren J, Bergstrom R, Lindgren A, Nyren O: Symptomatic gastroesophageal reflux as a risk factor for esophageal adenocarcinoma. N Engl J Med 340:825, 1999.
193. Lagergren J: Increased incidence of adenocarcinoma of the esophagus and cardia: Reflux and obesity are strong and independent risk factors according to the SECC study. Lakartidningen 97:1950, 2000.
194. Lagergren J, Ye W, Bergstrom R, Nyren O: Utility of endoscopic screening for upper gastrointestinal adenocarcinoma [letter]. JAMA 284:961, 2000.
195. Spechler SJ, Zeroogian JM, Antonioli DA, et al: Prevalence of metaplasia at the gastro-oesophageal junction. Lancet 344:1533, 1994.
196. Winters C Jr, Spurling TJ, Chobanian SJ, et al: Barrett's esophagus: A prevalent, occult complication of gastroesophageal reflux disease. Gastroenterology 92:118, 1987.
197. Spechler SJ: Epidemiology and natural history of gastro-oesophageal reflux disease. Digestion 51:24, 1992.
198. Drewitz DJ, Sampliner RE, Garewal HS: The incidence of adenocarcinoma in Barrett's esophagus: A prospective study of 170 patients followed 4.8 years. Am J Gastroenterol 92:212, 1997.
199. Shaheen NJ, Crosby MA, Bozymski EM, Sandler RS: Is there publication bias in the reporting of cancer risk in Barrett's esophagus? Gastroenterology 119:333, 2000.
200. Schnell TG, Sontag SJ, Chejfec G: Adenocarcinomas arising in tongues or short segments of Barrett's esophagus. Dig Dis Sci 37:137, 1992.
201. Sharma P, Morales TG, Sampliner RE: Short segment Barrett's esophagus—the need for standardization of the definition and of endoscopic criteria. Am J Gastroenterol 93:1033, 1998.
202. Weston AP, Krmpotich PT, Cherian R, et al: Prospective long-term endoscopic and histological follow-up of short segment Barrett's esophagus: Comparison with traditional long segment Barrett's esophagus. Am J Gastroenterol 92:407, 1997.
203. Hirota WK, Loughney TM, Lazas DJ, et al: Specialized intestinal metaplasia, dysplasia, and cancer of the esophagus and esophagogastric junction: Prevalence and clinical data. Gastroenterology 116:277, 1999.
204. Oberg S, Peters JH, DeMeester TR, et al: Inflammation and specialized intestinal metaplasia of cardiac mucosa is a manifestation of gastroesophageal reflux disease. Ann Surg 226:522, 1997.
205. Csendes A, Smok G, Sagastume H, Rojas J: Biopsy and endoscopic prospective study of the prevalence of intestinal metaplasia in the gastroesophageal junction in controls and in patients with gastroesophageal reflux (see comments). Rev Med Chil 126:155, 1998.
206. Goldblum JR, Vicari JJ, Falk GW, et al: Inflammation and intestinal metaplasia of the gastric cardia: The role of gastroesophageal reflux and *H. pylori* infection. Gastroenterology 114:633, 1998.
207. Chen YY, Antonioli DA, Spechler SJ, et al: Gastroesophageal reflux disease versus *Helicobacter pylori* infection as the cause of gastric carditis. Mod Pathol 11:950, 1998.
208. Nandurkar S, Talley NJ, Martin CJ, et al: Short segment Barrett's oesophagus: Prevalence, diagnosis and associations. Gut 40:710, 1997.
209. Morales TG, Camargo E, Bhattacharyya A, Sampliner RE: Long-term follow-up of intestinal metaplasia of the gastric cardia. Am J Gastroenterol 95:1677, 2000.
210. Lidums I, Holloway R: Motility abnormalities in the columnar-lined esophagus. Gastroenterol Clin North Am 26:519, 1997.
211. Iascone C, DeMeester TR, Little AG, Skinner DB: Barrett's esophagus: Functional assessment, proposed pathogenesis, and surgical therapy. Arch Surg 118:543, 1983.
212. Singh P, Taylor RH, Colin-Jones DG: Esophageal motor dysfunction and acid exposure in reflux esophagitis are more severe if Barrett's metaplasia is present. Am J Gastroenterol 89:349, 1994.
213. Cameron AJ: Barrett's esophagus: Prevalence and size of hiatal hernia. Am J Gastroenterol 94:2054, 1999.
214. Fitzgerald RC, Omary MB, Triadafilopoulos G: Dynamic effects of acid on Barrett's esophagus: An ex vivo proliferation and differentiation model. J Clin Invest 98:2120, 1996.
215. Ouatu-Lascar R, Fitzgerald RC, Triadafilopoulos G: Differentiation and proliferation in Barrett's esophagus and the effects of acid suppression. Gastroenterology 117:327, 1999.
216. Sharma P, Sampliner RE, Camargo E: Normalization of esophageal pH with high-dose proton pump inhibitor therapy does not result in regression of Barrett's esophagus. Am J Gastroenterol 92:582, 1997.

217. Cooper BT, Neumann CS, Cox MA, Iqbal TH: Continuous treatment with omeprazole 20 mg daily for up to 6 years in Barrett's oesophagus. Aliment Pharmacol Ther 12:893, 1998.
218. Sampliner RE: New treatments for Barrett's esophagus. Semin Gastrointest Dis 8:68, 1997.
219. Sampliner RE: Practice guidelines on the diagnosis, surveillance, and therapy of Barrett's esophagus: The Practice Parameters Committee of the American College of Gastroenterology. Am J Gastroenterol 93: 1028, 1998.
220. Levine DS, Haggitt RC, Blount PL, et al: An endoscopic biopsy protocol can differentiate high-grade dysplasia from early adenocarcinoma in Barrett's esophagus. Gastroenterology 105:40, 1993.
221. Provenzale D, Schmitt C, Wong JB: Barrett's esophagus: A new look at surveillance based on emerging estimates of cancer risk. Am J Gastroenterol 94:2043, 1999.
222. Weston AP, Sharma P, Topalovski M, et al: Long-term follow-up of Barrett's high-grade dysplasia. Am J Gastroenterol 95:1888, 2000.
223. van den Boogert J, van Hillegersberg R, Siersema PD, et al: Endoscopic ablation therapy for Barrett's esophagus with high-grade dysplasia: A review. Am J Gastroenterol 94:1153, 1999.
224. Orringer M: Current status of nshiatal esophagectomy. Adv Surg 34:193, 2000.
225. Schnell T, Sontag S, Chejfec G, et al: High grade dysplasia still is not an indication for surgery in patients with Barrett's esophagus: An update. Gastroenterology 114:AG1149, 1998.
226. Ell C, May A, Gossner L, et al: Endoscopic mucosal resection of early cancer and high-grade dysplasia in Barrett's esophagus. Gastroenterology 118:670, 2000.

Chapter 34

Esophageal Disorders Caused by Infection, Systemic Illness, Medications, Radiation, and Trauma

David J. Kearney and George B. McDonald

INFECTIONS

Most patients who experience infections of the esophagus have impaired host defenses. Those with more subtle immunologic deficiencies typically become infected with *Candida albicans*, although profound and persistent defects in immunity may lead to a variety of fungal, viral, parasitic, and bacterial infections. In immunosuppressed patients, clinical presentations can be deceptive; heartburn, nausea, fever, or bleeding may be the only manifestation of infection in patients with human immunodeficiency virus (HIV) infection (see Chapter 28) and in transplant recipients.[1] Hence, the rigor of the diagnostic approach should depend upon the nature and severity of defects in host defenses. Most esophageal infections respond readily to specific treatment.

Fungal Infections

Colonization and Infection by Candida Species

Candida albicans, a yeast found in normal oral flora, is the predominant cause of fungal esophagitis. Non–*Candida* albicans fungal species (*Candida tropicalis, C. Krusei, C. parapsilosis, C. glabrata*, for example) are also human commensal organisms but are less numerous in human flora, less adherent to mucosal surfaces, and only occasionally pathogenic. *Candida* species are oval dimorphic yeasts that reproduce by budding. Tissue invasion is characterized by an advancing margin of hyphae and pseudohyphae. Mucosal infection by *Candida* species is viewed as a two-step process. The first pathologic step, colonization, entails superficial adherence and proliferation. Defenses against *Candida* colonization of the esophagus include host factors such as salivation, motility, acid reflux events, healthy epithelia, and the normal competitive balance among bacterial and fungal flora. This competitive balance can be disturbed by antibiotic therapy, permitting overgrowth of *Candida albicans*. The only population-based study of *Candida* colonization of the esophagus in healthy ambulatory adults reported a prevalence of approximately 20%.[2] The second step of *Candida albicans* infection, invasion into the epithelial layer, usually requires a defect in cellular immunity. In clinical practice, the differentiation between colonization and infection is usually based on the gross appearance of lesions at endoscopy and the microscopic appearance of tissue and exudate obtained by brush or biopsy. Because hyphae and masses of budding yeast are rarely seen with colonization alone, these findings on brushings of esophageal lesions are consistent with invasive infection. Also characteristic of *Candida* infection are firmly adherent plaques that, when removed, reveal a raw and friable surface. Swallowed clumps of tenacious material containing fungi (from oral thrush or poorly cleaned dentures, for example) may resemble esophageal plaques; however, because they are easily washed away, they do not represent fungal esophagitis. In some cases the mucosal injury due to *Candida* infection may penetrate below the epithelial layer and lead to ulceration of the mucosa. Only rarely do *Candida* ulcers result in esophageal desquamation or perforation into the mediastinum.

*Infection by Non–*Candida *Species Fungi*

Other fungi (*Aspergillus, Histoplasma, Cryptococcus, Blastomyces* species) and some plant molds are acquired from the environment rather than from the endogenous flora. Primary esophageal infection with these organisms is seen only in severely immunosuppressed patients. *Aspergillus* species, primarily *A. fumigatus* and *A. flavus,* infect the sinuses, lungs, and adjacent organs with disregard for tissue planes. Although most reported *Aspergillus* esophagitis is a result of direct extension from mediastinal structures, primary esophageal *Aspergillus* infection has been described. The esophagus may also become secondarily infected from pulmonary or mediastinal foci of *Histoplasma* or *Blastomyces* species. Invasive esophagitis caused by dematiaceous fungi such as *Cladophialophora* species has been described in organ transplant recipients; these infections may be more amenable to antifungal therapy than are *Aspergillus* infections.[3] A fatal case of necrotizing esophagitis caused by *Penicillium chrysogenum* has been reported in a patient with acquired immunodeficiency syndrome (AIDS).[4]

Prevalence and Predisposing Factors

The prevalence of symptomatic fungal infection of the esophagus is high in patients with AIDS who are not receiving protease inhibitors and in patients with leukemia and lymphoma (particularly after chemotherapy) and is low (<5%) in a population of general medical patients with intestinal complaints. HIV infection is currently the most significant risk factor for the development of esophageal candidiasis, which typically occurs among HIV-infected persons with persistently low CD4 lymphocyte counts (see Chapter 28). However, in some individuals recently infected with HIV *Candida* esophagitis develops during the transient phase of lymphocyte dysfunction characteristic of HIV seroconversion syndrome. When chronic HIV infection leads to immunodeficiency, the risk of *Candida* species infections rises in proportion to the severity of immunodeficiency. Effective treatment of HIV with protease inhibitors has resulted in a decreased prevalence of serious esophageal infection as long as CD4 lymphocyte counts are maintained above the level of 100 to 200/μL.[5] Patients with hematologic malignancies also have a high prevalence of esophageal fungal infections because of T cell defects. In addition, aggressive irradiation and chemotherapeutic protocols further impair immune surveillance and disrupt host epithelial integrity. Because effective antifungal prophylaxis is widely employed, transplant patients have a low prevalence of symptomatic fungal esophagitis despite immunosuppressive medications.

Other medical illnesses that predispose to fungal esophagitis via impaired immune surveillance include diabetes mellitus, adrenal dysfunction, alcoholism, and advanced age.[1] Interestingly, of the many congenital immunodeficiency syndromes, only chronic mucocutaneous candidiasis is associated with *Candida* esophagitis with any significant frequency. In this disease there is defective chemotaxis of leukocytes leading to chronic *Candida* infections of the skin and mucous membranes. Illnesses that interfere with esophageal peristalsis (such as achalasia, progressive systemic sclerosis, and esophageal neoplasia) contribute to esophageal fungal colonization, with resultant overgrowth and infection in many affected patients.

Glucocorticoids contribute to fungal infection through suppression of both lymphocyte and granulocyte function. Even topical glucocorticoids (contained in inhalers for treatment of asthma) have led to oropharyngeal and esophageal candidiasis in otherwise healthy adults.[6] Less commonly used immunosuppressive agents such as cyclophosphamide, azathioprine, chlorambucil, and methotrexate are seldom associated with esophageal infection. Hypochlorhydria caused by acid suppressive medications or gastric surgery or associated with AIDS predisposes to fungal esophagitis by removing the cleansing effect of normal periodic acid reflux events. This effect is most noticeable in patients who also have impaired esophageal peristalsis, as in systemic sclerosis. Among 66 patients with systemic sclerosis, the prevalence of *Candida* esophagitis was 44% (21 of 48 patients) for those on no acid suppression, compared with 89% (16 of 18 patients) among those on potent acid suppressive therapy.[7]

Clinical Presentation

Acute onset of difficult or painful swallowing is the most frequent presenting symptom of fungal esophagitis. Additional complaints include retrosternal discomfort, heartburn, and nausea. The intensity of these symptoms often correlates with the severity of impaired host defenses. Even in advanced AIDS, infection is typically limited to the epithelium and subepithelial space as granulocyte function is relatively spared. However, in a granulocytopenic patient, *Candida* species esophagitis may be accompanied by fever, sepsis, and abdominal pain caused by hepatic (see Chapter 69), splenic, or renal fungal abscesses.

Oral thrush, a frequent finding among patients with esophageal infection, is often an indicator of the underlying pathologic esophageal process. In three series totaling 133 patients with AIDS, the presence of both esophageal symptoms and oral candidiasis had a positive predictive value for *Candida* esophagitis ranging from 71% to 100%.[8–10] Oral thrush, however, is absent in approximately 25% of *Candida* esophagitis cases.[1] Furthermore, oral thrush may occur when an organism other than *Candida* infects the esophagus. To illustrate, oral thrush was reported in 7 of 14 patients with herpes simplex virus esophagitis and in 2 of 10 patients with HIV-associated idiopathic ulcers of the esophagus.[11, 12]

Candida species esophagitis may be asymptomatic, particularly when patients have subtle immune deficiencies with few adherent plaques in the esophagus. Among 3501 patients who had routine upper endoscopy, 41 cases of *Candida* species esophagitis were diagnosed, of which 27 (67%) had no esophageal symptoms.[13] A high prevalence of asymptomatic *Candida* esophagitis is also seen in patients with AIDS.

Diagnosis

The advent of highly active antiretroviral therapy (HAART) has altered the diagnostic evaluation and management of HIV-infected subjects. If a patient at risk for HIV infection is not receiving antiretroviral therapy and exhibits painful or difficult swallowing, *Candida* esophagitis should be suspected. If physical examination reveals oral candidiasis, many physicians treat the patient with a systemic antifungal medication such as fluconazole, reserving further diagnostic study for patients in whom a second esophageal infection is more likely and for patients who do not respond to empirical therapy within 3 to 5 days.[14] When persistent nausea and vomiting, abdominal pain, intestinal bleeding, fever, cough, or diarrhea is present in addition to esophageal symptoms, *Candida* is unlikely to be the only infecting organism in the esophagus.[1, 15] These patients should receive further diagnostic evaluation.

The optimal method for formulating an accurate diagnosis of fungal esophagitis employs endoscopically directed brushing and biopsy specimens. Endoscopic appearance alone is insufficient for diagnosis of fungal esophagitis (see Fig. 28–2). Plaquelike material resembling *Candida* infection may be found in severe reflux esophagitis, herpes simplex virus infection, cytomegalovirus infection, pill esophagitis, and swallowed oropharyngeal debris. Furthermore, adherent fungal plaques are not always present in fungal esophagitis. An advantage of the endoscopic approach to diagnosis is that biopsies and brushings can be visually directed and the severity of esophagitis can be assessed. Candidal plaques are typically creamy white or pale yellow and, if successfully dislodged, reveal a raw mucosal surface. Brushings from exudative surfaces and ulcer craters should be obtained with a sheathed cytology brush, spread onto slides, and submitted for periodic acid–Schiff (PAS), silver, or Gram staining. The presence of mycelial forms and masses of budding yeast is consistent with *Candida* infection. Obtaining cultures for fungus is seldom indicated as *Candida* species are commensal organisms and cultures cannot reliably differentiate among normal flora, colonization, and infection. However, cultures are useful if an unusual pathogen such as an azole-resistant *Candida* species, *Aspergillus* species, dematiaceous fungi, *Mycobacterium tuberculosis,* or bacterial esophagitis is suspected on clinical or endoscopic grounds. Finally, viral cultures are more accurate than histologic examination for the diagnosis of herpesvirus infections and should be routinely obtained when viral esophagitis is included in the differential diagnosis, even when *Candida* esophagitis is obvious.

Blind brush cytology is an alternative, seldom-used method of obtaining samples from the esophagus. A sheathed brush is advanced through the nose or mouth into the esophagus, exposed, moved to and fro, resheathed, and removed. Smears from blind brushing have a sensitivity of 88% to 96% for *Candida* species esophagitis and a specificity of 85%. The sensitivity of blind brush methods appears better than the presence of oral thrush in predicting *Candida* esophagitis in patients with AIDS and approaches that of endoscopy.

Radiographic studies are of limited value in establishing an accurate diagnosis of esophageal infection, as abnormalities are often nonspecific and concurrent infections are likely to be missed. The classic appearance of *Candida* esophagitis on double-contrast esophagogram is that of discrete plaque-like lesions oriented longitudinally, with linear or irregular filling defects with distinct margins produced by trapped barium. Severe *Candida* esophagitis may produce coalescing plaques and debris that form a grossly abnormal shaggy appearance, whereas mild *Candida* esophagitis can produce a subtle granular appearance. Pseudoulcerations simulating ulcerations of viral esophagitis have also been described in patients with *Candida* esophagitis. Other nonspecific abnormalities seen in *Candida* esophagitis include tumor-like masses, strictures, and fistulas. Because of their limited diagnostic accuracy and the ready availability of endoscopy, radiologic contrast studies of the esophagus are rarely used, especially if endoscopy is planned, regardless of the radiographic findings. Radiographic examination is useful when endoscopy is not available, when endoscopic biopsy is precluded by thrombocytopenia, when perforation is suspected, or when the upper esophagus is severely strictured.

Treatment

There are three general classes of drugs used to treat esophageal fungal infections: (1) topically active, poorly absorbable agents such as nystatin, clotrimazole, and oral amphotericin B; (2) orally administered absorbable agents such as fluconazole, itraconazole, and voriconazole; and (3) parenterally administered agents such as amphotericin B (including liposomal formulations), fluconazole, itraconazole, voriconazole, and caspofungin. The choice of treatment of fungal esophagitis is determined by the degree of host defense impairment and the severity of infection.[1, 16]

Most patients with minimal immunologic deficiencies who have fungal esophagitis can be treated with oral fluconazole or topical antifungal agent. Fluconazole pills (100 to 200 mg/day) are commonly used because they are more convenient than topical therapy. The advantage of nonabsorbable agents is that they are virtually devoid of adverse effects and drug-drug interactions. Clotrimazole, a nonabsorbable imidazole, is well tolerated when delivered as a 10-mg buccal troche dissolved in the mouth five times daily for 1 week. Nystatin, a nonabsorbable polyene with a different mechanism of action and less palatability than clotrimazole, is also effective when used at a dose of one or two troches (each containing 200,000 units) four or five times daily for up to 14 days.

Patients with moderately impaired host defenses, such as those with AIDS who have low CD4 counts, suffer more extensive infections and deeper invasion than patients with minimal impairment and should be treated more aggressively.[17] Orally administered, absorbable agents such as fluconazole, 100 to 200 mg orally per day for 10 to 14 days, is our treatment of choice for this group of patients. Patients who do not improve within 3 to 5 days of starting fluconazole should have an endoscopic evaluation. Some patients with AIDS have candidal infections that persist despite treatment with azoles. There are several reasons for this resistance to treatment, including *Candida albicans* isolates that are resistant to fluconazole, poor drug absorption, and unremitting severe immune deficiency.[18–20] Resistant candidal isolates can be identified by using new standardized in vitro antifungal susceptibility tests that have been shown to correlate well with in vivo responses to azole therapy.[21] Itraconazole 200 mg/day is an alternative effective therapy for HIV-related esophageal candidiasis, particularly when given as a liquid formulation.[22] Nonabsorbable agents can also be effective, but at a higher dose and for a longer duration than in minimally immune deficient patients. Clotrimazole 100 mg vaginal tablets dissolved in the mouth three times daily effectively cleared esophageal symptoms and endoscopic findings of *Candida* esophagitis in 25 of 25 AIDS patients.[23] Oral amphotericin B suspension (500 mg four times daily for 2 weeks) was effective in 40% of AIDS patients who had candidal lesions refractory to fluconazole.[24] Miconazole, although seldom used for this indication in developed countries, has been cost-effective for treatment of AIDS-related esophageal candidiasis in less developed areas.[25]

Fungal esophagitis in granulocytopenic patients should be treated with intravenous amphotericin B as these patients are at risk for disseminated fungal disease. The standard dose of amphotericin for patients who are known to be infected with *Candida albicans,* who are febrile, and who have evidence of disseminated infection is 0.5 mg/kg/day; the duration of therapy is dependent on the degree and duration of granulocytopenia. Liposomal formulations of amphotericin at 3–5 mg/kg/day are effective against *C. albicans* infection and produce fewer systemic and renal side effects than standard amphotericin B. When there is clinical evidence of disseminated infection with candidal organisms that are likely to be non–*C. albicans* species (for example, *C. glabrata* or *C. krusei*), higher-dose amphotericin (1 mg/kg/day) should be given.[16] Disseminated *Candida* infection in a persistently granulocytopenic patient is generally treated with a cumulative amphotericin dose of 1500 to 2000 mg over 6 to 12 weeks. Less aggressive dosing of amphotericin B (e.g., 0.3 mg/kg/day for 7 to 10 days) is usually effective in granulocytopenic patients who have no evidence of infection beyond epithelial tissues. Those patients in whom granulocyte counts increase and fevers and esophageal symptoms resolve can often be switched from intravenous amphotericin B to oral fluconazole or caspofungin for a 10- to 14-day course of antifungal therapy. There is an emerging role for newer antifungal drugs as initial therapy for candidal infection in patients who are granulocytopenic. For example, fluconazole as primary treatment for oropharyngeal and esophageal candidiasis in granulocytopenic cancer patients achieved a clinical cure in 82% of patients.[26] Other drugs shown to be useful for these patients are liquid itraconazole, voriconazole, and caspofungin. Marrow colony-stimulating factors may help restore granulocyte counts in some granulocytopenic patients.

A lipid formulation of intravenous amphotericin B (5 mg/kg/day) is the recommended treatment for *Aspergillus* esophagitis; newer agents such as voriconazole and caspofungin also have activity against these fungi. Although complications of *Histoplasma* infection involving the esophagus, such as fistula or obstruction, have traditionally been treated with surgery, amphotericin B has cured extrinsic compression, abscess, and fistula. Orally administered azole antifungal agents such as itraconazole are also effective against *Histoplasma* and may be used by patients with uncomplicated disease.[27]

At the time fungal esophagitis is diagnosed, risk factors for fungal infection should be sought and eliminated whenever possible. When risk factors cannot be eliminated, fungal esophagitis is likely to recur. HIV-infected patients in whom *Candida* esophagitis recurs are candidates for prophylaxis against fungal infection. The goal of such therapy is to suppress the number of fungal organisms in host flora, thereby reducing the risk of colonization and invasion. Among patients with AIDS, fluconazole or itraconazole is effective in reducing the risk of oropharyngeal or esophageal *Candida* recurrences,[22] but at the risk of making a subsequent candidal infection less responsive to azole therapy.[19] A more effective strategy employs antiretroviral therapy and elevation of CD4 counts to more than 200/μL.[5] Among patients who are in intensive care units or who have hematologic disorders, prophylactic fluconazole or oral amphotericin B therapy reduces the incidence of *Candida* esophagitis. One must strike a balance, however, between clinical effectiveness and adverse effects, including drug toxicity and the development of resistant infections with *Candida* and non–*Candida* organisms such as *Aspergillus*.

Viral Infections

Herpes Simplex Virus

Herpes simplex virus (HSV), a large, enveloped, double-stranded deoxyribonucleic acid (DNA) virus, causes painful vesicles with erythematous bases in the squamous epithelium of skin, mouth, and esophagus. Resolution of acute HSV infection is followed by latency in the roots and ganglia of nerves supplying the affected regions. Although HSV esophagitis may be primary, it most often results from reactivation of latent virus in the distribution of the laryngeal, superior cervical, and vagus nerves.[28] Healthy individuals often have relatively mild reactivation episodes due to partial immunity, whereas immunocompromised patients suffer more frequent and severe reactivation episodes.[1] If the host's response to HSV infection is profoundly compromised, primary infection or reactivation may disseminate to the liver, lungs, and central nervous system.

Immunocompetent patients with HSV esophagitis typically experience acutely painful and difficult swallowing.[28, 29] Other frequently reported symptoms include constant retrosternal discomfort, nausea, vomiting, and, occasionally, hematemesis. Immunocompromised individuals such as hematopoietic stem cell transplant recipients may experience persistent nausea and vomiting as their only symptoms. Intra-abdominal and systemic symptoms are not common in HSV infection. About 25% of HSV esophagitis cases have evidence of either HSV or *Candida* infection in the oropharyngeal or genital area.[1]

On occasion, a diagnosis of HSV esophagitis in an immunocompetent person can be made on clinical grounds. For example, a previously healthy patient with a history of recurrent cold sores who experiences concurrent onset of nasolabial herpetic lesions and esophageal symptoms is likely to have HSV esophagitis. The course of esophageal symptoms in this patient closely follows that of the nasolabial lesions, with spontaneous resolution of symptoms in a few days. Provided the diagnosis can be made soon after onset of symptoms, recovery may be hastened by early initiation of antiviral therapy. A randomized, double-blind trial of high-dose oral acyclovir in the treatment of 174 nonimmunocompromised patients with recurrent labial HSV found that early initiation of acyclovir (within 1 hour of the first sign or symptom) hastened time to lesion resolution by 27% and time to pain resolution by 36%.

The diagnosis of HSV esophagitis is usually made at endoscopy (see Fig. 34–1; see also Fig. 28–5). The earliest esophageal lesions are rounded 1- to 3-mm vesicles in the mid- to distal esophagus, the centers of which slough to form discrete circumscribed ulcers with raised edges. These "volcano" lesions are responsible for the classic appearance of HSV esophagitis on double-contrast esophagogram. Plaques, cobblestoning, or a shaggy ulcerative appearance indistinguishable from that of *Candida* esophagitis may be present in advanced HSV esophagitis. As often as not, radiographic findings are nonspecific in HSV esophagitis and endoscopy is necessary to provide the diagnosis. The discrete ulcerations seen at early endoscopic or radiologic examination can coalesce into very large ulcers. As HSV preferentially infects epithelial cells, achieving an accurate histologic or culture diagnosis can be difficult when there is near-total denudement of esophageal epithelium. The endoscopist must attempt to identify ulcer margins or islands of squamous mucosa from which to obtain samples. Samples from epithelial margins should be submitted in transport media for HSV culture as well as for routine histologic examination. Tissue specimens from the base of esophageal ulcers are devoid of epithelial cells and are inadequate to exclude the diagnosis of HSV (Fig. 34–1). Results of HSV cultures are often available within 24 hours when immunologic staining of centrifugation cultures is done. Viral culture methods are more sensitive than routine histologic examination of brush and biopsy specimens. Histologic stains of HSV infected epithelial cells demonstrate multinucleated giant cells, ballooning degeneration, "ground glass" intranuclear Cowdry type A inclusion bodies, and margination of chromatin. Immunohistologic stains using monoclonal antibodies to HSV antigens or in situ hybridization techniques may improve the diagnostic yield in difficult cases by identifying infected cells that lack characteristic morphologic changes.

HSV esophagitis is treated initially with intravenous acyclovir, 250 mg/m^2 every 8 hours, changing to oral therapy with valacyclovir, 1000 mg three times daily, when swallowing allows, for a total of 7 to 10 days of therapy. Strains of HSV resistant to acyclovir have emerged via mutations in viral DNA polymerase and thymidine kinase. Although many of these strains have attenuated virulence, clinical dis-

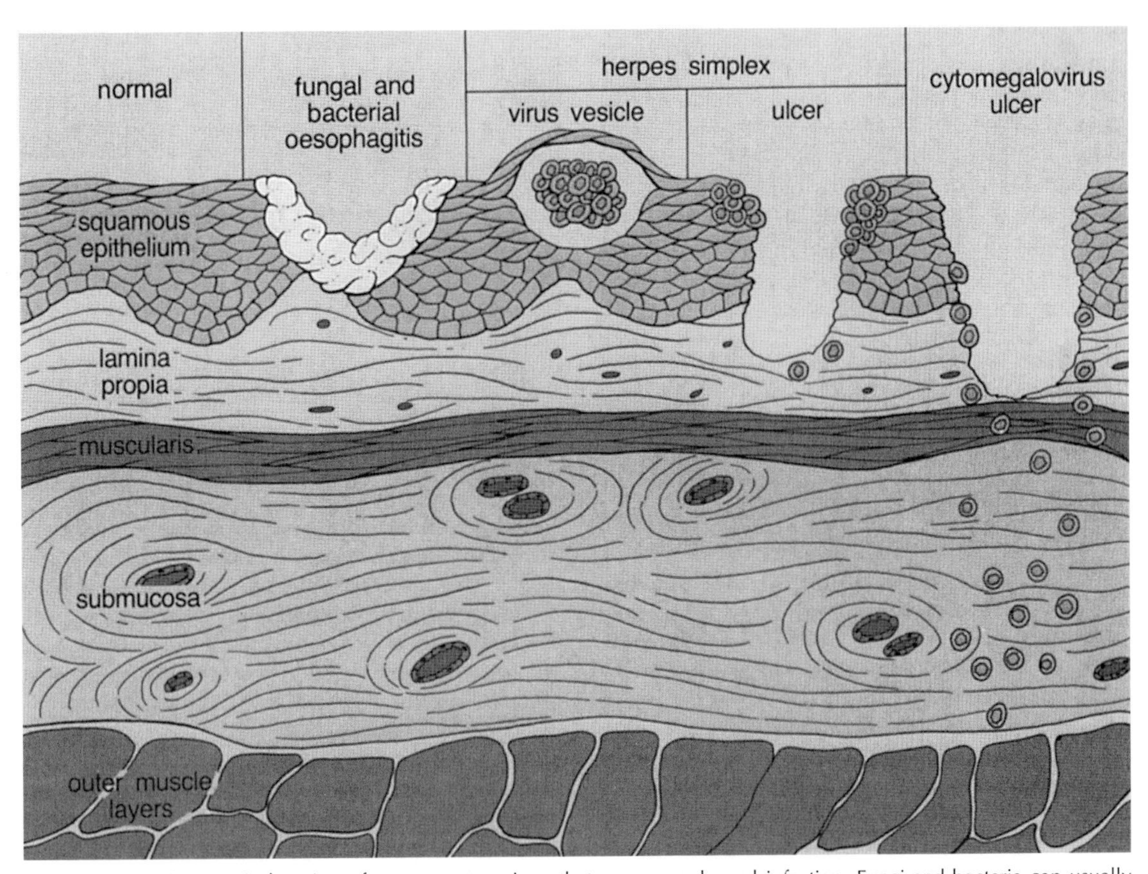

Figure 34–1. Microscopic location of common organisms that cause esophageal infection. Fungi and bacteria can usually be recovered from the surface layers of esophageal erosions and ulcers. Herpes simplex virus (HSV) is seen in epithelial cells but rarely in nonepithelial cells in the base of an ulcer. Cytomegalovirus (CMV), in contrast to HSV, is never found in squamous epithelial cells but only in subepithelial cells such as fibroblasts and endothelial cells in the base of ulcers. Detection of these herpesviruses in biopsy specimens may require immunohistologic methods if viral culture is not available. (From Silverstein FE, Tytgat GNJ: Atlas of Gastrointestinal Endoscopy, 2nd ed. New York, Gower Medical Publishing, 1991.)

ease in immunocompromised patients may progress. Foscarnet at a dose of 40 mg/kg three times daily is effective in treating most strains of acyclovir-resistant HSV, although some isolates have resistance to both foscarnet and acyclovir. Foscarnet is more expensive and less well tolerated than acyclovir; complications include nephrotoxicity, nausea, vomiting, seizures, and electrolyte disturbances. HSV prophylaxis with oral acyclovir or valacyclovir is indicated for immunosuppressed patients who are at high risk for reactivation of HSV infection, that is, HSV-seropositive transplant recipients and AIDS patients who have recurrent herpetic infections. Complications of unresponsive or untreated HSV esophagitis in immunosuppressed patients include extensive mucosal necrosis, superinfection, Boerhaave's syndrome, hemorrhage, strictures, HSV pneumonia, tracheoesophageal fistula formation, and disseminated HSV infection.[1, 30]

Cytomegalovirus

Cytomegalovirus (CMV) is a ubiquitous herpesvirus that infects most of the world's adult population. In healthy individuals with latent infection, CMV DNA can be found in many tissues of the body, including leukocytes. Latent infection is responsible for the high incidence of CMV transmission through transfusion or transplantation from CMV-seropositive donors into CMV-seronegative recipients. CMV disease in immunosuppressed patients either is newly acquired or is due to reactivation of latent infection. In CMV esophagitis the virus does not infect the squamous epithelium but instead infects submucosal fibroblasts and endothelial cells of the esophagus, usually as part of a widespread infectious process (see Fig. 34–1). The onset of symptoms in CMV disease is typically more gradual than in HSV or *Candida* esophagitis. Painful or difficult swallowing is less prominent than nausea, vomiting, fever, epigastric pain, and weight loss. Abdominal symptoms reflect the fact that CMV infection typically involves multiple organs, as well as the esophagus.[1]

The diagnosis of CMV esophagitis depends upon endoscopic biopsy, as neither clinical assessment, radiography, nor endoscopic appearance (see Fig. 28–3) is sufficiently accurate to warrant antiviral therapy. Esophageal radiographs may demonstrate discrete small superficial ulcerative lesions indistinguishable from lesions of HSV esophagitis, but in some patients radiographs may reveal large, flat elongated ulcers similar to those seen in patients with HIV-associated idiopathic esophageal ulcers. The characteristic endoscopic appearance of CMV esophagitis includes superficial erosions with serpiginous nonraised borders in the mid- to distal esophagus. As the infection progresses, shallow ulcerations may deepen, extend for 10 to 15 cm, and even become strictured. Tissue specimens are needed to confirm CMV infection and to allow evaluation for concurrent fungal, viral, parasitic, or bacterial pathogens. Multiple biopsy specimens should be obtained from the bases of the esophageal ulcers, where CMV infected subepithelial fibroblasts and endothelial cells reside (see Fig. 34–1).[31] Superficial brushings of ulcers for cytologic examination do little to increase the diagnostic yield for CMV infection, but brushings may be the only safe method in patients who have very low platelet counts. Histologic specimens that contain only squamous epithelium are not evaluable for CMV and should not be reported as "negative" for CMV findings but as inadequate specimens. CMV is capable of infecting both epithelial and lamina propria cells of the stomach and intestines. In patients in whom CMV infection is suspected, biopsy specimens of abnormal mucosa in these areas should also be sent for histologic evaluation and viral cultures.

CMV infected cells in the subepithelial layer are large, with amphophilic intranuclear inclusions and a halo surrounding the nucleus. Unlike HSV and varicella-zoster virus (VZV), small cytoplasmic inclusions are also present. Immunohistochemical staining for early, intermediate, and late antigens and in situ hybridization can confirm the diagnosis of CMV infection when infected cells are neither "megaloid" nor inclusion bearing. In a study of HIV infected patients, however, immunohistochemical stains were not cost effective, compared with routine stains.[32] These histologic and immunohistological methods, however, are only about half as sensitive as modern viral culture methods.[31] For this reason, we suggest that the biopsy specimen obtained from the ulcer base be sent for viral culture. Polymerase chain reaction (PCR) for CMV DNA is the most sensitive test, but interpretation of a positive result can be problematic, as latent CMV infection can yield a positive PCR result.

Ganciclovir and foscarnet are both effective antiviral drugs in the treatment of CMV infection. Intravenous ganciclovir therapy, 5 mg/kg every 12 hours for 2 weeks is highly effective in eliminating CMV from esophageal ulcers, when compared with placebo.[33] Several uncontrolled studies in organ transplant recipients and AIDS patients report clinical improvement in symptoms of enteric CMV infection after ganciclovir therapy. However, esophageal symptoms, along with nausea, anorexia, and vomiting, are slow to respond, and large ulcers are slow to heal.[33] Furthermore, in the absence of immune reconstitution, recurrence of disease is common after short courses of therapy. Accordingly, full dose antiviral therapy should be administered for 2 to 3 weeks, until there is a documented decline in viral load in the bloodstream, followed by maintenance therapy for several additional weeks or until immunosuppression resolves. HIV infected patients with a history of recurrent CMV infection may remain on indefinite maintenance therapy with ganciclovir. The adverse effects of ganciclovir therapy include bone marrow toxicity, which can be severe, especially when ganciclovir is administered concurrently with other marrow toxic agents, such as zidovudine (AZT), or when opportunistic marrow infection is present. Long-term therapy with ganciclovir has been accompanied by emergence of ganciclovir-resistant strains of CMV. These strains are usually sensitive to foscarnet, at least initially. Foscarnet therapy for CMV disease is typically 90 mg/kg intravenously every 12 hours for 2 to 3 weeks followed by maintenance therapy of 90 to 120 mg/kg/day. Patients on foscarnet should be monitored carefully for the adverse effects of therapy. As with ganciclovir, treatment with foscarnet has been accompanied by the emergence of foscarnet-resistant strains of CMV, some of which are also resistant to ganciclovir. Another alternative drug, cidofovir, has been shown to be effective when CMV infection did not respond to ganciclovir, but at the cost of renal toxicity.[34]

Prevention of CMV disease is a cornerstone of modern transplant programs. Studies have demonstrated that careful screening of all donor blood products for CMV antibodies has significantly decreased the morbidity and mortality rates of primary CMV infection among CMV-naive transplant recipients. Organ transplant recipients who are CMV-seropositive or who receive organs from CMV-seropositive donors may receive antiviral prophylaxis to prevent CMV infection and disease. Ganciclovir is effective whether administered when CMV is first detected in circulating leukocytes, or at the first excretion of virus, or as prophylaxis.[35]

Varicella-zoster Virus

VZV is a DNA virus that causes chickenpox and herpes zoster. Although oropharyngeal VZV lesions are common in normal children with chickenpox, symptomatic esophageal involvement is uncommon, and it is even more rare among adults with zoster.[36] However, VZV can cause severe esophagitis in profoundly immunocompromised individuals.[37] The esophageal component of VZV infection may be relatively minor in comparison with other manifestations of disseminated infection such as varicella encephalitis, pneumonitis, and fulminant hepatitis. As in HSV esophagitis, patients experience acutely painful or difficult swallowing. The key to the diagnosis of VZV esophagitis is the finding of concurrent dermatologic VZV lesions, for only rarely does HSV infection cause a varicelliform or zosteriform eruption. VZV can be distinguished from HSV by culture or immunostaining of fluid from fresh vesicles. The endoscopic appearance of VZV ranges from occasional vesicles to discrete ulcerative lesions to confluence of ulcerations with necrosis. Such lesions should be biopsied and brushed thoroughly for histologic and cytologic evaluation and for viral culture. The characteristic histologic features of epithelial cells infected with VZV are edema, ballooning degeneration, and presence of multinucleated giant cells with intranuclear eosinophilic inclusion bodies. Immunohistochemical staining using monoclonal antibodies to VZV antigens is helpful in differentiating VZV from HSV infection. Routine viral culture techniques are of limited clinical utility as VZV is more difficult to isolate than HSV, and development of cytopathic changes may take more than 1 week. Drug therapy for VZV infection initially employs intravenous acyclovir, which is followed by oral therapy with valacyclovir when swallowing permits. Foscarnet appears to be a viable alternate therapy for treatment of acyclovir resistant VZV infection among adult AIDS patients who have recurrent VZV eruptions.

Epstein-Barr Virus

Reports of esophageal manifestations of Epstein-Barr virus (EBV) in healthy subjects are rare, although in infectious mononucleosis a sore throat is a nearly universal symptom. Odynophagia and hematemesis due to esophageal ulceration can complicate infectious mononucleosis in an immunocompetent person.[38] Three HIV-infected patients with dysphagia and discrete esophageal ulcers were found to have Epstein-Barr virus at the ulcer bases by in situ hybridization.[39] The histologic features of these esophageal lesions were similar to those of oral hairy leukoplakia caused by EBV in patients with AIDS. Because oral hairy leukoplakia lesions have been effectively cleared with oral acyclovir in some patients, it is reasonable therapy for these esophageal lesions.[39] The response of oral hairy leukoplakia to oral acyclovir is dependent on continuing presence of the drug; reappearance follows drug withdrawal. Therefore, successful treatment of symptomatic esophageal EBV lesions may require long-term maintenance acyclovir therapy. EBV-infected T lymphocytes may involve the esophagus as part of a lymphomatous process.[40] Some authors have described a relationship between EBV and esophageal squamous cell carcinoma.[41]

Human Immunodeficiency Virus

(See Chapter 28)

HIV infection can lead to esophageal ulcerations in the absence of any identifiable pathogens. These lesions, referred to as *HIV-associated idiopathic esophageal ulcers,* appear as multiple small aphthoid lesions during the transient fever, chills, malaise, and skin rash of early HIV infection and later in the course of HIV infection as giant, deep ulcers extending up to several centimeters (see Fig. 28–4). The larger ulcers may become complicated by fistula formation, perforation, hemorrhage, superinfection, or stricture formation.[42] HIV can be detected in ulcerative lesions, but the pathogenesis of ulcers is not well understood. A study in 1997 suggested that squamous epithelial cells in the esophagus undergo apoptosis as an "innocent bystander" effect of nearby HIV-related T cell activity.[43] These ulcers do not respond to empirical antiviral or antifungal therapies but do respond to immunosuppressive drugs, supporting the hypothesis that they are immunologically mediated. There are differences of opinion about the optimal first-line therapy for HIV-associated ulcers. Clinical experience suggests that more than 90% of patients respond to prednisone (40 mg/day for 2 weeks, then tapered over a month).[44] Others favor thalidomide 200 mg/day for 4 weeks, shown in a randomized, placebo-controlled trial to effect healing of HIV-associated ulcers in 73% of patients, compared with 23% of patients taking placebo.[45] Thalidomide in low, intermittent doses, however, is ineffective in preventing recurrent HIV-associated ulcers.[46] Both glucocorticoid and thalidomide therapy present some risk, for example, opportunistic infections related to depression of granulocyte function with prednisone[44] and sedation, skin rash, neuropathy, and birth defects with thalidomide.[45]

Human Papillomavirus

Human papillomavirus (HPV) is a small, double-stranded DNA virus that infects squamous epithelium of healthy individuals, producing warts and condylomata. The virus is sexually transmitted; HIV infection is a risk factor for esophageal HPV infection.[47] Esophageal infections with HPV are typically asymptomatic. HPV lesions are most frequently found in the mid- to distal esophagus as erythematous macules, white plaques, nodules, or exuberant frondlike lesions.[48] In one patient a papilloma developed at a sclerotherapy injection site.[49] The diagnosis is made by histologic demonstration of koilocytosis (an atypical nucleus surrounded by a ring), giant cells, or immunohistochemical stains. Treatment is often not necessary, although large lesions have required endoscopic removal. Other treatments such as those employing systemic interferon-α (IFN-α), bleomycin, and etoposide have yielded varying results.[50] One patient had numerous lesions in the esophagus and upper airway that were unresponsive to all forms of therapy and eventually fatal.[51]

HPV has been implicated as a pathogenetic factor in squamous cell carcinoma, particularly cervical carcinoma. An association between HPV and squamous cell carcinoma of the esophagus has been demonstrated by polymerase chain reaction or in situ DNA hybridization in esophageal specimens from South Africa, northern China, and Alaska.[52] In contrast, HPV DNA was not found in or near esophageal squamous cell carcinomas from the continental United States, Europe, Japan, or Hong Kong.[53, 54]

Poliovirus

Dysphagia is part of the syndrome of acute bulbar poliomyelitis. There is also a late postpolio syndrome in which dysphagia has been described.[55] Neuromuscular control of swallowing is abnormal in these patients, leading to transfer dysphagia.

Bacterial Infections

Bacterial Esophagitis Caused by the Normal Flora

Bacterial infections of the esophagus are infrequently reported, although autopsy series of immunocompromised patients suggest that they are often unrecognized.[56] The most significant risk factors are granulocytopenia and use of acid suppressive medications, particularly proton pump inhibitors.[57, 58] The overall risk for bacterial infection in the AIDS population is much lower than in patients receiving chemotherapy for malignancy, as a result of relative sparing of granulocytes in AIDS. Symptoms of bacterial esophagitis include painful, difficult swallowing and retrosternal pain. Fever is reported in a minority of cases. Findings at endoscopy include nonspecific mucosal friability, plaques, pseudomembranes, and ulcerations.[56] Gram stain of biopsy specimens can identify bacteria more readily than can hematoxylin and eosin stains. The diagnosis of bacterial esophagitis is established when sheets or masses of confluent bacteria invade subepithelial tissues with little inflammatory reaction. Bacterial cultures of endoscopic biopsy specimens are rarely performed because of the infrequency of invasive bacterial esophagitis and unavoidable bacterial contamination of the endoscope. When cultures are performed, they typically confirm infection with organisms found in normal flora of the mouth and upper respiratory tract, such as *Staphylococcus aureus* or *Staphylococcus epidermidis, Streptococcus viridans,* and *Bacillus* species. Infection is often polymicrobial. Subsequent adjustments of antimicrobial therapy depend upon clinical response and culture results. The same organisms are responsible for retropharyngeal abscesses, which may cause dysphagia.

Mycobacterial Infections

There are more than 90 reports of esophageal *Mycobacterium tuberculosis* infections in recent literature; most cases are from areas of endemic tuberculosis. The AIDS epidemic has also increased the prevalence of active tuberculosis through reactivation of latent mycobacterial infections.[59] Esophageal manifestations of tuberculosis are almost exclusively a result of direct extension from adjacent mediastinal structures, but there are well-documented cases of primary esophageal tuberculosis[60, 61] The clinical presentation of secondary esophageal tuberculosis is quite different from that of most other causes of infectious esophagitis: that is, dysphagia is often accompanied by weight loss, cough, chest pain, and fever. Subsequent complications include bleeding, perforation, and fistula formation[59, 61] Choking upon swallowing may be indicative of an underlying fistula between the esophagus and respiratory tract. Other radiographic findings include displacement of the esophagus by mediastinal lymph nodes and sinus tracts extending into the mediastinum. Endoscopy is often necessary to confirm active tuberculosis; caution is advised to prevent infection of medical staff by aerosolized tubercle bacilli. Endoscopic findings include shallow ulcers, heaped up lesions mimicking neoplasia, and extrinsic compression of the esophagus.[62] Lesions should be biopsied and brushed thoroughly, and specimens should be obtained for acid-fast stain, mycobacterial culture, and PCR, in addition to routine studies. When extrinsic compression is the only esophageal manifestation of tuberculosis, then the diagnosis must be confirmed by bronchoscopy, mediastinoscopy, or transesophageal fine-needle aspiration cytologic evaluation.[63] Surgery is sometimes required to repair fistulas, perforations, and bleeding ulcers.[61]

Infection with *Mycobacterium avium* complex bacteria is commonly reported in patients with advanced AIDS. Although the disease may be widespread, esophageal involvement (ulcerations, fistulas, mediastinal adenopathy) is rare.[64]

Other Infections: Syphilis, Diphtheria, Tetanus, Nocardiosis, Actinomycosis

Syphilis, which became increasingly prevalent in the United States in the 1990s, can cause esophageal disease in immunocompetent individuals. Earlier literature described gummas, diffuse ulceration, and strictures of the esophagus in tertiary syphilis.[65] The diagnosis of syphilitic esophagus should be considered when a patient has an inflammatory stricture and other evidence of tertiary syphilis. Histologic evaluation may show perivascular lymphocytic infiltration; however, specific immunostaining should be done if this diagnosis is a possibility. Diphtheria is a disease marked by severe mucosal inflammation with thick exudative membranes of the pharynx, throat, nose, and occasionally the tracheobronchial tree. The esophagus may become involved through direct extension of inflammatory membranes from the oropharynx. Tetanus is remarkable for painful tonic contractions caused by action of the neurotropic toxin of *Clostridium tetani* on the central nervous system. Dysphagia may be the presenting symptom in rare instances.[66] The AIDS epidemic has resulted in novel cases in which *Nocardia* infection caused an esophageal ulcer (which doxycycline healed completely) and actinomycosis formed sinus tracts from the mediastinum to the esophagus.[67, 68] Esophageal infection with *Actinomyces* also has been described as an infection complicating preexisting CMV esophagitis in AIDS; treatment with penicillin G healed the ulcers and resolved symptoms.[69]

Helicobacter Pylori

In Barrett's esophagus patients who have gastric *Helicobacter pylori* infection, this bacterium can be in the mucus layer of the esophagus and adherent to areas of gastric metaplasia.[70] *H. pylori* may also be associated with heterotopic gastric epithelium in an inlet patch of the esophagus (see Chapter 31). There may be an association between esophageal *H. pylori* infection and mucosa-associated lymphoid tissue (MALT) in Barrett's esophagus,[71] but there is no association with adenocarcinoma of the esophagus.[72] In fact, studies suggest that *H. pylori* gastritis protects against the development of reflux esophagitis, Barrett's esophagus, and adenocarcinoma (see Chapters 33, 35, and 39).[73] In contrast, inflammation and intestinal metaplasia just below the ora serrata, in the gastric cardia, are highly correlated with *H. pylori* infection.[74]

Parasitic Infections

Chagas' Disease

Chagas' disease is the result of progressive destruction of mesenchymal tissues and nerve ganglion cells throughout the body by *Trypanosoma cruzi,* a parasite endemic to South America. Abnormalities of the heart, esophagus, gallbladder, and intestines are the clinical consequence. Esophageal manifestations may appear 10 to 30 years after the acute infection and typically include symptoms of difficulty in swallowing, chest pain, cough, and regurgitation. Nocturnal aspiration is common. Manometric recordings from the esophageal body are identical to findings in achalasia, although the LES pressure is lower in Chagas' disease.[75] Manometric abnormalities of the esophagus can also be found in asymptomatic seropositive patients.[76] A chagasic esophagus may be responsive to nitrates, balloon dilation, or, ultimately, myectomy at the gastroesophageal junction.[77] Patients who have intractable symptoms or pulmonary complications secondary to megaesophagus may be candidates for esophagectomy.[78] Those with long-standing stasis due to Chagas' disease often have hyperplasia of esophageal squamous epithelia and are at increased risk for esophageal cancer (see Chapters 32 and 98).

Other Parasites

Infections with *Cryptosporidium, Pneumocystis carinii, Leishmania donovani,* and *Trichimonas* have been reported in patients with AIDS, associated with nonspecific inflammation in the distal esophagus.[79–83] Esophageal involvement due to adjacent amebic liver abscess, echinococcal cyst, and nematode infestations has also been described.

SYSTEMIC ILLNESS

Skin Disorders (See Chapter 18)

Epidermolysis Bullosa

Epidermolysis bullosa encompasses several rare disorders characterized by blister formation that follows minor trauma. There are several subtypes. Dystrophic epidermolysis bullosa is an inherited disorder in which trauma to the skin and mucous membranes causes bullae and scarring.[84] Esophageal involvement is more common in the recessive than the dominant or junctional form of the disease.[84] In most patients bullae of the skin, mouth, and esophagus develop in childhood. Esophageal bullae develop at sites of trauma by food at the proximal and distal esophagus and at the level of the carina, leading to dysphagia, poor oral intake, and malnutrition.[84] Both the skin and mucosal lesions heal by fibrosis, leading to mummification of the extremities, constriction of the mouth, and recurrent esophageal strictures.[84] Pain and dysphagia result from strictures, the bullae themselves, and impacted food. Because the skin manifestations of the disease are so striking, the diagnosis of esophageal involvement is usually an obvious one on esophagrams. Endoscopy is relatively contraindicated because it may cause bullae to form. Medical management includes intake of soft foods, glucocorticoids, phenytoin, and careful dilation of strictures.[84] Although dilation may carry a high risk of perforation in this disease, successful dilation with either standard bougies or balloons has been described.[84] Total parenteral nutrition may be needed to sustain life when caloric intake is limited. Some patients require esophageal resection and replacement, usually with colon interposition.[84]

Epidermolysis bullosa acquisita is a rare acquired blistering disorder associated with autoimmunity to type VII collagen. Esophageal involvement is rarely reported.[85] An association with Crohn's disease has been described.[86]

Pemphigus Vulgaris

Pemphigus vulgaris is an autoimmune disease that affects the skin, mouth, and other mucous membranes with intraepidermal bullous lesions. The underlying abnormality is the presence of autoantibodies to the cell adhesion molecule desmoglein 3 that is strongly expressed in stratified squamous epithelia.[87] Most patients initially report mouth lesions, typically in the fourth to fifth decade of life. Any mucosal surface lined by stratified squamous epithelium may be affected. Typical esophageal lesions include bullae, exfoliative erosions, and ulcers. Like the oropharynx, the esophagus can be involved without causing symptoms. Several endoscopic series have confirmed esophageal involvement in the majority of patients.[88, 89] The esophagus may rarely be severely involved with only minimal oral involvement.[90] The diagnosis is based on four criteria: typical clinical findings, histologic evidence of intraepithelial acantholysis, presence of immunoglobulin G (IgG) autoantibodies on the affected epithelium indicated by direct immunofluorescence, and evidence of circulating autoantibodies.[91] Glucocorticoid treatment is highly effective, but esophageal involvement may cause bleeding, strictures, and formation of casts from epithelial sloughing despite therapy.

Bullous Pemphigoid

Bullous pemphigoid is the most common bullous skin disease and typically occurs in elderly patients. The skin lesions are initially intensely pruritic plaques that evolve into tense, pruritic bullae.[91] Oral lesions are uncommon and are usually transient.[92] Esophageal bullae are rare and may slough as casts. Most patients have no symptoms, but some have bleeding and dysphagia. The diagnosis is made by endoscopic findings, presence of circulating antibodies to basement membrane, histologic evidence of subepidermal bullae, and immunohistologic findings of IgG and complement deposition along basement membranes. Glucocorticoid treatment is effective. Bullous pemphigoid may predispose to esophageal carcinoma.[93]

Cicatricial Pemphigoid

Also known as *benign mucous membrane pemphigoid,* cicatricial pemphigoid is a rare chronic vesiculobullous disease involving mucosal surfaces of the eyes, the mouth, and occasionally the pharynx, nasal mucosa, genital mucosa, rectum, and esophagus. The bullous lesions heal with scarring. Cutaneous lesions are minimal or absent. It involves the esophagus in less than 5% of cases, but the course is more troublesome than in bullous pemphigoid.[94] Radiologic and endoscopic findings include bullae, webs, and dense strictures, usually of the upper esophagus.[94] Rarely, endoscopy may cause bullae to form, as in epidermolysis bullosa. Histologic findings are relatively nonspecific: inflammation and bullae in the subepithelium and basement membrane deposition of IgG and complement. Patients with cicatricial pemphigoid have been shown to have significant IgA in addition to IgG circulating antibasement membrane antibodies.[95] Repeated dilations may be needed to relieve dysphagia.[96] Glucocorticoids and dapsone may be effective. An association between cicatricial pemphigoid and esophageal carcinoma has been reported.[97]

Drug-Induced Skin Diseases

Drug-induced skin diseases (erythema multiforme, Stevens-Johnson syndrome, toxic epidermal necrolysis) may rarely affect the esophagus with a blistering process and desquamation of large areas of epithelium. Both focal and long strictures and webs may result, requiring dilation.

Other Skin Diseases

Lichen planus has esophageal involvement in approximately 25% of patients and may result in strictures and dysphagia.[98] *Psoriasis* has been associated with esophageal webs and dysphagia.[99] *Acanthosis nigricans* appears as granular nodules in the esophagus in patients who have carcinoma elsewhere, usually in the gastrointestinal tract.[100] *Leukoplakia* and similar lesions of the oral cavity can be seen in the esophagus.[101, 102] Hyperkeratotic papules may stud the esophagus in *Darier's disease.* Squamous papillomas of the esophagus have been described in patients with *focal dermal hypoplasia.*[103] *Tylosis* (diffuse palmoplantar keratoderma) is a rare hereditary skin disease that predisposes to bronchial, laryngeal, and esophageal cancer (see Chapters 18 and 35).[104]

Behçet's Disease

Behçet's disease is a multisystem inflammatory process characterized by oral aphthous ulcers, genital ulcers, uveitis that may cause blindness, and pustular skin lesions that can be induced by needlesticks (termed the *pathergy test*).[105] The cause is unknown. An infectious cause has been postulated; herpes simplex virus DNA has been reported in increased frequency in some studies, whereas other studies have shown a higher than expected prevalence of serum antibodies against *Streptococcus sanguis.*[106] The underlying pathologic process is a vasculitis that results in aneurysms in the arterial and pulmonary circulation, phlebitis of both large and small veins, and discrete intestinal ulcerations. The mucosal lesions are oval, white ulcerations with a red rim. They recur in crops and heal without scars. Behçet's disease is most common and most severe in countries of the eastern Mediterranean and Asia, whereas intestinal involvement varies among countries, being common in Japan and rare in Turkey. North American and British patients of Celtic origin have different clinical features and human leukocyte antigen (HLA) haplotypes.[105]

In the intestine, the ileum and colon are most commonly involved, and the lesions may be difficult to distinguish from those in inflammatory bowel disease (see Chapter 29). The esophagus is estimated to be affected in 2% to 11% of cases.[107] Esophageal lesions include oval ulcerations similar to the mouth lesions, deep ulcers or fistulas that may communicate with adjacent organs, luminal strictures, pseudomembranes, and esophageal varices that may be associated with either superior vena cava obstruction or portal vein thrombosis.[107] Barium studies may show well-demarcated ulcers or fistulas. Esophageal biopsy reveals nonspecific inflammation and rarely vasculitis. Gastrointestinal lesions of Behçet's disease are treated with the same medications that have shown to be useful for the treatment of inflammatory bowel disease, principally sulfasalazine, cyclosporine, and glucocorticoids.[108, 109] Thalidomide has also been shown to be effective for severe colitic lesions.[106] Mucosal ulcerations may wax and wane without treatment. Esophageal strictures may require dilation or, in the case of fistulas or perforation, surgery.

Graft-versus-Host Disease (See Chapter 27)

In patients who have received allogeneic hematopoietic stem cell transplantation, graft-versus-host disease (GVHD), an immunologic reaction against host tissues by donor lymphoid cells, may develop. Histologic changes of acute GVHD can be found in esophageal squamous epithelium and in extreme cases can lead to mucosal sloughing and ulceration.[110] Particularly severe acute GVHD can occur after mismatched allogeneic transplantation, or after discontinuation of prophylactic drugs such as cyclosporine and tacrolimus, or after allogeneic donor lymphocyte infusion. Chronic GVHD may also damage the esophagus, but its presentation is more subtle that that of acute GVHD. Chronic GVHD involves the skin, eyes, mucous membranes, and liver as part of a systemic disease of the immune system. Esophageal symptoms include dysphagia, retrosternal pain, and aspiration.[111, 112] Barium contrast radiography may reveal webs, rings, and tight strictures in the upper esophagus and mid-esophagus but often fail to show the generalized desquamation and bullous lesions apparent on endoscopy.[112–114] There may be poor acid clearing caused by salivary gland involvement as well as motor abnormalities. Dilations and antireflux measures are usually successful in relieving symptoms, but there is an increased risk of esophageal perforation during dilation.[111] However, unless the immunologic abnormalities underlying esophageal mucosal injury and submucosal fibrosis are controlled, strictures and webs usually recur. Prednisone, cyclosporine, tacrolimus, and thalidomide are the immunosuppressive drugs most commonly used to treat chronic GVHD. Early treatment for chronic GVHD prevents esophageal involvement.

Nontransplantation patients in whom sudden fever, erythroderma, liver dysfunction, leukopenia, and thrombocytopenia develop after blood transfusions may have acute GVHD. In two fatal cases, basal cell necrosis of the esophageal epithelium was found, consistent with acute GVHD of the esophagus.[115]

Inflammatory Bowel Disease

Esophageal involvement in patients with *Crohn's disease* is uncommon. Most patients have concomitant ileocolonic disease but rarely is the esophagus the only organ affected. The prevalence of esophageal involvement appears to be higher in children than in adults, particularly when there is both ileal and colonic involvement (see Chapter 103).[116, 117] The patient with acute Crohn's esophagitis exhibits painful swallowing caused by aphthous ulcers in the esophagus.[118] Aphthous lesions of the mouth, hypopharynx, and cricopharyngeal area may also be present.[117] Glucocorticoid therapy may effect healing of these ulcers, but some cases progress to a chronic illness in which transmural inflammation and strictures lead to dysphagia, odynophagia, nausea, and weight loss.[118] Fistulas to adjacent organs may occur.[119] Radiographic and endoscopic examination of the esophagus show aphthous ulcers, inflammatory strictures, sinus tracts, filiform polyps, and fistulas to adjacent viscera. Histologic evaluation reveals diffuse and nodular lymphoid aggregates; noncaseating granulomas can be found in 50% of endoscopic biopsy specimens.[118] Inflammatory lesions respond to glucocorticoid therapy, whereas strictures, fissures, sinus tracts, and fistulas mirror the course of recurrent Crohn's disease in the intestine.[118] A case of severe esophageal fistulous disease has been reported to respond to a single infusion of infliximab (Remicade).[120] Strictures can be successfully dilated, but surgical resection of strictures and fistulas may be necessary.

Earlier literature described an association between ulcerative colitis and inflammatory esophagitis, but infectious causes were not excluded in these cases. Of children with newly diagnosed ulcerative colitis, 13 of 40 had nonspecific esophageal inflammation, 1 of whom had an ulcer.[116] One of 10 ulcerative colitis patients has aphthous ulcers of the mouth, which also may be seen in the esophagus, all of which may be confused with herpes simplex virus lesions.

Sarcoidosis

The esophagus in patients who have generalized sarcoidosis may have transmural granulomatous inflammation with dysphagia due to strictures or dysmotility. These lesions may also affect muscle and vagal nerves.[121] Symptoms and manometric abnormalities have been reported to normalize after treatment with glucocorticoids.[122] Enlarged mediastinal nodes may also compress the esophagus. It may be difficult to distinguish esophageal Crohn's disease from sarcoidosis. Dilation is used to treat strictures; surgical interposition may rarely be needed (see Chapter 29).

Chronic Granulomatous Disease

Chronic granulomatous disease is an inherited disorder, usually X-linked, in which granulocytes and monocyte/macrophages do not generate reactive oxygen species in response to ingested bacteria (see Chapter 2). Severe recurrent infections of the skin, lymph nodes, lungs, liver, and bones develop. Children (usually boys) with chronic granulomatous disease have experienced dysphagia and vomiting due to inflammatory lesions in the distal esophagus.[123] No microorganisms were found in the reported cases, and glucocorticoid therapy effected resolution of esophageal symptoms. Other effective therapies include cyclosporine and interferon-γ (IFN-γ).[124]

Metastatic Cancer

The most common tumors that metastasize to the upper gastrointestinal tract are melanoma, lung cancer, and breast cancer.[125] Other tumors that metastasize to the foregut include renal cell carcinoma, colon cancer, osteogenic sarcoma, Merkel cell carcinoma of the skin, prostate cancer, and germ cell tumors.[125, 126] Leukemic and lymphomatous infiltrates can be found in the esophagus in patients who have disseminated soft tissue infiltration.[127] The diagnosis is best made by barium contrast radiography and computed tomography (CT).[128] Endoscopy can exclude primary esophageal lesions but may fail to obtain a tissue diagnosis of cancer unless there is transmural infiltration.[129] Treatment with radiation therapy or placement of an endoprosthesis may provide palliation.[130] Successful, curative resection of metastatic breast cancer involving the esophagus has been reported.[131]

Esophageal involvement with lymphoma, Kaposi's sarcoma, and squamous cell carcinoma has been recognized in AIDS patients.[132, 133] These tumors may coexist with viral and fungal infections of the esophagus (see Chapter 28).

Collagen Vascular Diseases

Motility disorders of the esophagus can be seen with progressive systemic sclerosis, mixed connective tissue disease, polymyositis-dermatomyositis, Sjögren's syndrome, systemic lupus erythematosus, and Raynaud's phenomenon (see Chapter 29). Epithelial damage occurs when there is poor clearing of acid due to salivary disease, poor esophageal peristalsis, and weakness of the lower esophageal sphincter; immune suppression leading to esophageal infection (see earlier discussion); or retention of pills that causes esophagitis (discussed later).

Vascular disease may rarely affect the esophagus. Esophageal ulceration related to vasculitis has been described in a patient with Wegener's granulomatosis.[134] A hypercoagulable state seen in the anticardiolipin antibody syndrome may lead to focal ischemia, esophageal necrosis, and perforation.[135]

MEDICATIONS AND RADIATION INJURY

Pill Esophagitis

Pills that have been reported to cause esophageal mucosal injury are listed in Table 34–1.[136] Antibiotics, antiviral drugs, potassium chloride, iron-containing pills, nonsteroidal anti-inflammatory drugs, quinidine, and bisphosphonate medications for osteoporosis account for 90% of the reported cases. A long list of other drugs, many described in single case reports, constitute the other 10%.

Table 34–1 | **Pills That Have Been Reported to Cause Esophageal Mucosal Injury**

NSAIDS	**CARDIOVASCULAR MEDICATIONS**
Aspirin containing pills	Quinidine
Naproxen	Nifedipine
Ibuprofen	Verapamil
Indomethacin	Captopril
Piroxicam	Alprenolol
Others	
ANTIBIOTICS AND ANTIVIRALS	**OTHER COMMONLY PRESCRIBED MEDICATIONS**
Tetracyclines, including doxycycline	Alendronate sodium, pamidronate disodium, etidronate sodium (bisphosphonates)
Pivmecillinam	Theophylline
Other penicillins	Phenytoin
Clindamycin	Glucocorticoids
Antivirals such as AZT, ddC, and foscarnet	Ascorbic acid
	13-*cis*-Retinoic acid
	Oral contraceptives
IRON AND POTASSIUM FORMULATIONS	**LESS COMMONLY PRESCRIBED MEDICATIONS**
Ferrous sulfate or succinate	Emepronium bromide
Potassium chloride	Thiazinium
	Naftidrofuryl

AZT, zidovudine; ddC, zalcitabine; NSAIDs, nonsteriodal anti-inflammatory drugs. Adapted from Kikendall JW: Pill esophagitis. J Clin Gastroenterol 28:298, 1999.

Risk Factors for Esophageal Injury

Properties of pills that cause esophageal injury include the chemical nature of the drug, its solubility, and its contact time with the mucosa. Although many of the drugs in Table 34–1 cause damage because they are acidic in solution (for example, iron salts, tetracycline, aspirin), other medications that produce alkaline solutions (phenytoin) or neutral pH (quinidine) can also cause severe injury. Contact time is related to the size, shape, and coating of the pill in addition to vagaries of anatomy and the behavior of patients who swallow the pills. Small, oval, heavier tablets are easier to swallow than those that are larger, round, and lighter.[137] Some pills appear to cause proximal esophagitis because of their large size (doxycycline, quinidine gluconate). Pills coated with gelatinous material invariably stick in the esophagus, especially when taken with insufficient water.[137] Even in normal subjects, swallowed pills remain in the esophagus for 5 minutes or longer, delayed at the level of the aortic arch, a common site of injury, and above the lower esophageal sphincter.[137] Sustained release formulations (ferrous sulfate, naproxen, bisphosphonates) appear to cause more severe esophageal injury. Most of the cases of KCl esophagitis and many of the reported fatalities are due to a wax matrix form of the drug.[138] Cellulose fiber and guar gum pills may swell and lodge in the esophagus, causing complete obstruction. When papain solutions are placed in the esophagus to dissolve meat boluses, they may cause esophagitis, particularly in previously damaged mucosa.

Most pill esophagitis occurs in patients who do not have preexisting swallowing problems or anatomic abnormalities.[136] However, narrowings of the esophagus caused by disease and abnormal peristalsis, for example, left atrial enlargement and prior cardiac surgery, may predispose patients to pill damage.[136, 138] Patients who have preexisting esophageal strictures, tumors, achalasia, scleroderma, and other conditions that can delay esophageal emptying should swallow the pills listed in Table 34–1 in the upright position with adequate (6 to 8 ounces) water or, preferably, substitute liquid formulations. Bedtime pill taking may contribute to esophageal injury because the supine position and decreased salivation and swallowing during sleep favor pill retention in the esophagus. For certain drugs (e.g., alendronate sodium, patients should be instructed not to lie down for at least 30 minutes after ingestion.

Injury Caused by Specific Pills

(See Table 34–1)

NONSTEROIDAL ANTI-INFLAMMATORY DRUGS. Nonprescription drugs such as aspirin, aspirin-containing pills, naproxen, and ibuprofen account for most of the reported cases of esophageal injury due to nonsteroidal anti-inflammatory drugs (NSAIDs).[136] Bleeding is a common feature in these reports, and perforation and strictures have developed in some patients. However, severe esophagitis must be an uncommon complication of NSAID use, in view of their widespread use. A more subtle form of injury by NSAIDs involves the distal esophagus. Several epidemiologic studies have noted a higher prevalence of distal esophageal ulcers and strictures among NSAID users than among control subjects, suggesting that mucosal damage caused by pills contributes to what would otherwise be called peptic esophagitis.[139, 140]

ANTIMICROBIAL AGENTS. Tetracyclines are the most common antibiotics that cause esophagitis, and doxycycline is most frequently cited.[136] Sudden onset of painful swallowing and retrosternal pain are common, but symptoms usually resolve after pills are discontinued. Because tetracyclines are often prescribed for acne and malaria prophylaxis, patients who have this form of esophagitis tend to be young. HIV-infected patients taking protease inhibitors commonly complain of difficulty in swallowing, but there are few reported cases of severe esophageal injury.

BISPHOSPHONATES (ALENDRONATE SODIUM, PAMIDRONATE DISODIUM, ETIDRONATE SODIUM). Bisphosphonate medications are the most frequently cited cause of pill esophagitis in the recent literature.[136] Discomfort is often noted with ingestion of the first pill in a prescription, and most affected patients report severe esophageal pain within a week. Biopsies show an intense inflammatory exudate and granulation tissue that may contain polarizable crystals and multinucleated giant cells.[141] The frequency of bleeding and perforation appears to be high, compared with antibiotic-related esophageal injury, for example. The population at greatest risk are older women, who may not swallow pills with enough water or stay upright before going to bed.

CARDIOVASCULAR MEDICATIONS. Several medications in common use in treating cardiovascular disease have been reported as causes of esophagitis, for example, captopril, nifedipine, verapamil, alprenolol, and especially quinidine.[136] Quinidine deserves special mention because it has been reported to lead to intense, exudative injury and strictures, with less pain than is seen in other causes of pill esophagitis.[136] Quinidine cannot be discontinued as readily as other drugs because of the risk of recurrent arrhythmias, and this characteristic may account for its prolonged use despite symptoms of esophageal injury.

IRON AND POTASSIUM MEDICATIONS. Ferrous salts and potassium chloride, particularly when formulated as sustained release pills, are notable for their propensity to cause severe esophageal injury, including perforation and dysphagia.[136] Diagnosis of pill esophagitis may be delayed because of the lack of pain associated with pill taking and the development of dysphagia that is slowly progressive.

Diagnosis

A careful history and a high index of suspicion should suffice to make the diagnosis in most cases. The most common symptom is retrosternal pain that develops after hours, days, or weeks of pill taking.[136] Pain is usually continuous but may become worse upon swallowing food or more pills, limiting oral intake. Dysphagia suggests a stricture or large inflammatory mass. Inflammatory strictures are far more commonly associated with potassium chloride, bisphosphonates, or quinidine than with other drugs in Table 34–1.[136, 138] Bleeding, perforation, stricture formation, and intramural hematomas are more commonly associated with pills containing potassium chloride, iron, bisphosphonates, and quinidine than with pills such as antibiotics that are usually taken for shorter periods. The diagnosis of pill esophagitis in AIDS patients may be especially difficult, as ulcerations from commonly used medications such as protease inhibitors and foscarnet may resemble ulcers caused by infection.

The diagnosis can also be suggested by a double-contrast barium x-rays of the esophagus that show ulcers, a stricture, or a mass. The mass lesions, particularly in the mid- and upper esophagus, may resemble carcinomas. Endoscopy is invariably abnormal, ranging from reddened, edematous mucosa to small superficial ulcers to large ulcers with heaped up, inflamed margins, often with profuse exudate, resembling carcinoma.[136] Pill fragments may be seen. Biopsy may show nonspecific inflammatory changes in addition to crystalline material and giant cells,[141] but cytologic results should be interpreted cautiously, as hyperplastic cells resulting from inflammation can be mistaken for carcinoma.

Treatment

In uncomplicated cases caused by antibiotics and other drugs, symptoms and epithelial inflammation resolve 1 to 6 weeks after pills are stopped.[136] Control of acid peptic reflux may allow faster healing. Continuation of offending pills, especially potassium chloride, bisphosphonates, and quinidine, may lead to strictures and perforation. Strictures may require repeated dilation, which can be difficult but generally successful if injury to the epithelium ceases. Some patients, however, require surgery for strictures. Patients who have esophageal obstruction caused by ingestion of guar gum pills may require endoscopic removal of tenacious material.

Chemotherapy Esophagitis

Dactinomycin, bleomycin, cytarabine, daunorubicin, 5-fluorouracil, methotrexate, vincristine, and chemotherapy regimens used in hematopoietic stem cell transplantation may cause severe dysphagia as a result of oropharyngeal mucositis, a process that can also involve the esophageal mucosa.[142] Esophageal damage is unusual in the absence of oral changes. Although mucositis is self-limited in most cases, some patients have oral and esophageal damage that persists for weeks to months. Chemotherapy that is given months after thoracic irradiation to the esophagus, particularly doxorubicin, may cause a "recall" esophagitis. Vinca alkaloid drugs are neurotoxic; colonic dilatation is the most common manifestation, but dysphagia may also complicate vincristine therapy.[143] Chemotherapy-induced vomiting may lead to Mallory-Weiss tear, intramural hematoma, and esophageal perforation, all potentially lethal in patients with low platelet counts and immunodeficiency. Perforations and fistulas may also develop when cytoreductive therapy results in necrosis of tumors involving the esophageal wall.

Radiation and Chemoradiation Esophagitis

Acute radiation injury to the esophagus is very common but usually self-limited.[144, 145] The late effects of radiation injury, although less common, can be debilitating. Radiation therapy greater than 30 Gy to the mediastinum causes acute retrosternal burning and painful swallowing, usually mild and limited to the duration of therapy. A third of patients undergoing thoracic irradiation for carcinoma of the lung with these symptoms had normal appearing esophageal mucosa, but as the dose of radiation approached 40 Gy, mucosal redness and edema became more frequent.[146] Histologically, acute radiation esophagitis is characterized by basal cell necrosis, submucosal edema, capillary dilatation, and swollen endothelial cells. About 2 weeks after the initial dose, superficial erosions develop; they resolve within 3 to 4 weeks after the last dose.[147] The most common abnormalities seen by barium-contrast radiography in symptomatic patients are failure to generate complete peristaltic waves, granular appearance of the mucosa, and focal narrowing, suggesting that acute symptoms may be related to both neuromuscular damage and mucosal injury.[148] If radiation ports include the oropharynx, salivary flow may be markedly diminished, removing a barrier to acid damage.[149] The incidence and severity of esophageal damage rise with twice-daily doses of radiation greater than 45 Gy.[150] Esophageal injury is also related to the manner of delivery: that is, more injury is seen with accelerated fractionation schedules.[145] There is also clinical evidence of enhanced radiation sensitivity in patients with certain diseases, including collagen vascular diseases and AIDS.[151-153]

More severe acute esophageal damage may develop in patients who receive certain chemotherapeutic drugs concomitantly with thoracic irradiation.[154-156] Chemotherapy potentiates radiation injury in the esophagus, such that damage can be seen with radiation doses below 25 Gy. This effect is particularly common with doxorubicin but has also been described with bleomycin, dactinomycin, cyclophosphamide, fluorouracil, etoposide, methotrexate, cisplatin, paclitaxel, and carboplatin. Severe esophageal toxicity can be lessened by separating chemotherapy and radiation doses and by administering irradiation once daily instead of twice daily.[155] However, the current practice of some radiation oncologists is to administer twice-daily irradiation and accept a temporary inability to swallow solid food in exchange for improved long-term survival.[155]

There are no proven means to prevent or effectively treat acute radiation esophagitis. It is common practice to prescribe antacids, H_2 receptor antagonists, proton pump inhibitors, topical anesthetics, and drugs that improve motility for symptomatic relief of acute radiation esophagitis, but there are no controlled studies of these modalities. Randomized trials have shown that both sucralfate and naproxen are ineffective. The radioprotectant amifostine has been reported to be protective in uncontrolled trials.[157]

Several months after high-dose radiation therapy, the epithelium regenerates and the submucosa heals by fibrosis, but esophageal smooth muscle may remain strikingly abnormal in some patients. Late effects of esophageal radiation include motor dysfunction as well as tapering strictures due to subepithelial fibrosis.[158, 159] The interval from irradiation to stricture formation varies from 3 months to many years.[160] Patients with HIV infection who receive thoracic irradiation may develop strictures more rapidly.[153] Esophageal perforation and tracheoesophageal fistulas may appear years after irradiation, probably as a result of radiation vasculitis. Squamous cell carcinomas have also been described as sequelae of radiation esophagitis.[161] The frequency of late radiation injury is difficult to assess, as the high mortality rate of underlying malignancy precludes lengthy follow-up of many patients. One study that focused on esophageal toxicity reported an 18% incidence of late radiation injury.[145] The risk of late toxicity is largely related to dosimetry, that is, the extent of the length and circumference of the esophagus that is irradiated.[145]

Band Ligation and Sclerotherapy for Varices

Esophageal injury can result from both endoscopic sclerotherapy and band ligation of varices; the frequency of complications is far lower after banding.[162] Band ligation leads to superficial ulcers that occur where the bands are placed, but the frequency of deep esophageal injury is low. However, fatal transmural necrosis has been reported after band ligation in patients administered glucocorticoids. There is debate whether the combination of endoscopic sclerotherapy and band ligation results in a higher rate of complications than banding alone; there appears to be no clinical advantage in performing both modalities.[163, 164]

Injection of sclerosant into and around varices causes necrosis of esophageal tissues and mucosal ulcers. Small ulcers appear within the first few days after sclerotherapy in virtually all patients; larger ulcers develop in roughly half of patients. However, the endoscopic appearance of the esophagus after sclerotherapy grossly underestimates the extent of the inflammatory process in the esophageal wall and mediastinum. In a prospective study of 17 patients, CT before and within 48 hours after intravariceal sclerotherapy showed that after sclerotherapy the size of the esophageal wall doubled, mediastinal changes developed in all cases, and pleural effusions were noted in 84%.[165] The nonsterile nature of sclerotherapy and the extent of the inflammatory process it incites explain the reports of almost every imaginable complication, but fortunately the frequency of serious complications is small (2% to 10%) (see Chapters 13 and 77).

Clinical Manifestations of Esophageal Injury

Many patients have transient retrosternal discomfort, dysphagia, or odynophagia after band ligation or sclerotherapy. With banding, the frequency of these symptoms appears to increase with placement of more than six bands.[166] Although the ulcerations produced by banding are not as deep as with sclerotherapy (involving only the mucosa and submucosa), significant bleeding may occasionally occur at the sites of banding. Complications may also result from the placement of an overtube that is required for variceal ligation when using a single-band ligator. A prospective study of 50 patients who had endoscopic variceal ligation revealed mucosal injury related to the overtube in 72% of sessions.[167] Severe bleeding and esophageal perforation have also been reported.[168, 169] Modification of the overtube used in single-band ligation appears to have decreased the frequency of such injuries. The introduction of the multiband ligator has obviated the need for passage of an overtube in most cases in which variceal ligation is performed. After sclerotherapy, symptoms correlate with the size of esophageal ulcers. Large volumes of sclerosant and repeated injections over a short time are the most important determinants of large ulcers. Symptoms of pain and dysphagia disappear in 3 to 5 days, but large ulcers persist, often without symptoms, for 2 to 4 weeks before healing. The problems associated with large ulcers are bleeding, delays in further sclerotherapy sessions to eradicate varices, and development of strictures.

An autopsy study of 32 patients who died shortly after sclerotherapy showed perforation in 5 patients (of a total population of 170 patients sclerosed).[170] Perforation was related to sclerotherapy during active bleeding, extravariceal injection, and formation of microabscesses, all in patients with advanced liver disease. These patients lacked the typical signs and symptoms of perforation; their condition slowly deteriorated and they died 1 to 3 weeks later. The larger sclerosant volume used at the time of active bleeding has been shown to produce more complications than the volume used during elective sclerotherapy. Other unusual manifestations of deep needle penetration include pericarditis, esophageal-pleural fistula, and intramural hematoma.[171] Pericardial injection may also result in constrictive pericarditis and cardiac tamponade that appear months after sclerotherapy. The incidence of perforation is probably considerably higher than patient signs and symptoms would indicate.

Vagal dysfunction has been demonstrated after esophageal variceal sclerotherapy.[172] Several dysmotility patterns have been described, including decreases in the amplitude of peristaltic waves, prominent simultaneous contractions in the lower esophagus, and increased reflux.[173, 174] Although these conditions usually revert to normal 4 weeks after completion of sclerotherapy, manometric motility abnormalities in the lower esophagus are still more common 60 days post sclerotherapy than in cirrhotic control subjects.[173] Strictures may develop weeks to months after sclerotherapy. As with ulcers, the reported incidence of symptomatic strictures varies from series to series, ranging from 2% to 13%.[162] The major risk factor for stricture formation is persistent, large esophageal ulcers. Poor acid clearing may contribute to stricture formation, but intensity of submucosal fibrosis is probably more important.

An association between sclerotherapy and development of esophageal carcinoma has been reported.[175] Because most reported cases are squamous cell carcinoma and many cirrhotic individuals have risk factors for esophageal carcinoma (alcoholism and smoking), causality is tenuous. A prospective study found no cases of carcinoma among 68 patients who had endoscopy 3 years after sclerotherapy.[176] Regardless, nonhealing ulcers, persistent strictures, and mass lesions after sclerotherapy require biopsy to exclude carcinoma.

Treatment and Prevention

Because the development of ulcers is related to the placement of bands or injection of sclerosant and its attendant inflammation, one can lessen the initial tissue damage only by using fewer bands and less sclerosant. Control of gastric acid secretion after sclerotherapy with either ranitidine or omeprazole did not reduce the incidence of large ulcers (compared with that of placebo) in 105 patients.[177, 178] A trial that randomized 52 patients with postsclerotherapy ulcers to receive sucralfate suspension or antacids has shown significantly faster ulcer healing for patients receiving sucralfate.[179] Odynophagia after band ligation may be relieved with a 1:1 mixture of antacid and 2% lidocaine taken before meals.[166]

The role of acid peptic reflux in postsclerotherapy stricture formation has been investigated. A small series of patients studied with 24-hour pH probe monitoring showed that 7 of 12 sclerotherapy patients had persistent reflux, but that strictures formed equally in patients with and without reflux. A randomized trial compared postsclerotherapy treatment of antacids, cimetidine, and sucralfate with no therapy; symptomatic strictures developed in 3 of 31 treated patients, compared with 12 of 31 untreated patients ($p < .01$).[180] A trial that randomized 47 patients to omeprazole or placebo showed no effect on stricture formation but was too small to exclude a beneficial effect.[178] Postsclerotherapy treatment with omeprazole or sucralfate is a reasonable option, particularly for patients who have had high-volume, repeated injections, but its efficacy in preventing large ulcers and strictures remains unproven.

Most patients who have symptomatic postbanding or postsclerotherapy strictures can have successful dilation with either wire-guided Savary or balloon dilators. Mild dysphagia may persist after successful dilation because of motility disorders caused by sclerotherapy. Manometric studies carried out 6 to 17 months after sclerotherapy show decreased amplitude of peristaltic waves and increased tertiary contractions in the distal esophagus. No effective therapy for this motility disorder has been reported.

TRAUMA

Perforation

Causes (Table 34–2)

The most common causes of esophageal perforation are medical tubes and instruments, blunt trauma, and forceful vomiting (Boerhaave's syndrome).[181, 182] Medical procedures now cause more than half of all perforations, a significant change during the 1990s. It is clear that any medical instrument introduced into the esophagus may cause perforation (see Table 34–2).[181] Diagnostic upper endoscopy carries a risk of perforating the normal esophagus of lower than 1 in 1000, but the risk rises when therapeutic techniques such as dilation, stent placement, sclerotherapy, foreign body removal, placement of an endoprosthesis for esophageal cancer, electrocautery, overtube placement, and laser therapy are performed (see Chapter 30).[181, 183] An increasingly frequent cause of hypopharyngeal and cervical esophageal perforation is attempted endotracheal intubation, especially during resuscitation outside the hospital.[184] Placement of both nasogastric and orogastric tubes may result in esophageal perforation.[185] Surgical instruments can perforate during mediastinoscopy, vagotomy, hiatal hernia repair, or any periesophageal procedure. Esophageal perforation may follow anterior cervical spine surgery (usually done for stabilization of fractures) and may present in the early postoperative period or months later.[186] Hyperextension of the neck during accidents or cervical manipulation can also cause perforation of the cervical esophagus. Gunshot and stab wounds to the chest and neck may injure the esophagus.

Table 34–2 | **Causes of Esophageal Perforation**

OUT OF HOSPITAL CAUSES	MEDICAL AND SURGICAL INJURY
Spontaneous	**Instrumentation**
• Vomiting (Boerhaave's syndrome)	• Endoscopic sclerotherapy
• Caustic ingestion (Chapter 22)	• Band ligation of varices
• Infectious ulcers in immunosuppressed hosts	• Overtube placement for foreign body removal or banding
• Pill esophagitis (KCl, quinidine, bisphosphonates)	• Hemostasis devices (cautery, heater probe, epinephrine injection, laser therapy)
• Barrett's associated ulcer	• Dilation of stricture, cancer
• Peptic esophagitis (gastrinoma)	• Guidewire placement
• Heterotopic gastric mucosa	• Balloon dilation (achalasia)
• Webs, rings	• Rigid esophagoscopy
Traumatic	• Flexible esophagoscopy
• Foreign body or food impaction	• Naso- or orogastric tube
• Blunt trauma (falls, collisions, fights, child abuse, etc.)	• Endotracheal intubation attempt
• Penetrating trauma (bullet, knife, etc.)	• Stent placement for cancer
• Barotrauma (blast injury)	• Radiation or chemoradiation therapy
• Hyperextension of the neck	**Paraesophageal Surgery**
• Cervical spine manipulation	• Anterior cervical spine surgery
• Spinal cord injury	• Operations near the esophagus
	• Thoracostomy tube
	• Surgical anastomoses

Very forceful retching and vomiting may lead to spontaneous perforation of the esophagus (Boerhaave's syndrome). Retching and vomiting may also result in less severe mucosal injury, including Mallory-Weiss tears and intramural hematomas (see Chapter 8). Delays in the diagnosis of Boerhaave's syndrome are common because the traumatic episode may occur during an alcoholic stupor or the patient's signs and symptoms are considered nonspecific. Common mistaken diagnoses in patients proved to have Boerhaave's syndrome include myocardial infarction, tension pneumothorax, lung abscess, empyema, pancreatitis, and pericarditis. If the diagnosis of spontaneous esophageal perforation is a consideration, even if physical findings are absent, contrast radiography studies of the esophagus and a CT scan must be obtained promptly to allow an early diagnosis. A similar approach is appropriate for patients who have suffered blunt trauma to the thorax and neck, especially after auto accidents. The site of perforation in these cases is usually the cervical and upper thoracic esophagus, in contrast to that in distal perforations in cases of Boerhaave's syndrome, but problems of early recognition are similar.[187]

Not all spontaneous esophageal perforations are due to forceful vomiting (see Table 34–2). Perforation by foreign bodies is more often caused by slow pressure necrosis than by transmural laceration by a sharp edge; therefore, the clinical picture differs from that of Boerhaave's syndrome (see Chapters 21 and 22).[188] Food impaction may also lead to esophageal perforation.[189]

Several medical conditions may exhibit spontaneous perforation (see Table 34–2). Although the first priority in these cases is to treat the perforation and its consequences, identification of the underlying cause of the perforation may indicate a different therapeutic approach, for example, control of acid peptic secretion for a patient who has a perforated Barrett's ulcer or gastrinoma and treatment of an infection or placement of a stent in a patient with AIDS.[190–192]

Diagnosis

HISTORY AND PHYSICAL EXAMINATION. The characteristic features of esophageal perforation are the triad of pain, fever, and subcutaneous or mediastinal air.[181] The pain is usually localized to the site of perforation; the pain is in the neck for cervical perforations and substernal for thoracic perforations. Air dissects along tissue planes and manifests as crunching or crepitus (Hamman's sign) in the neck for cervical perforations and as mediastinal air for thoracic perforations. With cervical perforations, crepitus can be detected in 60% of patients by palpation and in 95% by radiographs. Many of these findings are not apparent in the first few hours after a perforation but reflect continuing leak and inflammation. Every large series has patients whose perforation was not apparent upon admission to the hospital, usually because typical symptoms were absent or because perforation was not an initial diagnosis. Glucocorticoids may mask the signs of perforation. Routine radiography after medical instrumentation reveals that occasionally asymptomatic patients have been perforated. Perforation may be apparent only at autopsy in some patients.

RADIOLOGY. Chest and upright abdominal radiographs should be obtained in cases of suspected esophageal perforation. Although plain radiographs indicate abnormal findings in up to 90% of esophageal perforations, findings may be normal soon after perforation, because the common abnormalities appear only after hours to days have passed.[193] Films may reveal subcutaneous emphysema, pneumomediastinum, mediastinal air-fluid levels, mediastinal widening, pneumothorax, hydrothorax, pleural effusion, or pulmonary infiltrates.[183] Chest radiographs taken shortly after instrumental perforation revealed pneumomediastinum or a density in the left cardiophrenic angle in 12 of 15 patients.[194] After perforation of the cervical esophagus, plain radiographs of the neck usually show air in the soft tissues and prevertebral space. Projections with the neck hyperextended allow better views of the esophageal inlet. Extraesophageal air and periesophageal fluid can be more clearly seen on CT scans than plain radiographs.[193] A CT scan alone is not adequate to exclude perforation; contrast studies of the esophagus are required to identify the location and size of the perforation fully. Perforations of the posterior wall of the cervical esophagus may reach the retropharyngeal space and extend into the mediastinum. Surgery may necessarily involve both neck and mediastinum if so indicated by CT.

The proximal portion of the thoracic esophagus lies just beneath the right pleura. Perforations there lead to air, fluid, and pus collections in the mediastinum and right pleural space. A CT scan can be useful to define mediastinal abnormalities, especially when the perforation site has sealed over. In contrast, perforations of the distal esophagus usually lead to leaking of air and fluid into the left pleural space, mediastinum, or abdomen. Perforation into the abdomen can also involve the retroperitoneal space and lesser sac.

Contrast radiographic studies should be performed in cases of clinically suspected esophageal perforation. Water-soluble contrast medium should be used in small boluses at first to prevent aspiration because of this agent's pulmonary toxicity.[195] Although barium contrast material clearly is superior in demonstrating small perforations, it causes an in-

Table 34–3 | **Guidelines for Medical and Surgical Management of Esophageal Perforation**

MEDICAL (NONOPERATIVE) MANAGEMENT	SURGICAL MANAGEMENT
• Patients who are clinically stable (minimal pain, normotension, minimal fever, mild leukocytosis) • Instrumental perforations of patient on NPO status and perforation detected within 2 hours • Perforations with a long delay in diagnosis such that the patient has already demonstrated a tolerance for the perforation • Perforations that are well contained and drain into the esophageal lumen (i.e., no crepitus, pneumothorax, pneumoperitoneum, or leak into the abdominal cavity)	• Boerhaave's syndrome • Patients who are clinically unstable (sepsis, respiratory failure, hypotension) • Noncontained perforations with contamination of the mediastinum or pleural space • Perforation of the intra-abdominal esophagus • Associated pneumothorax • Perforations with retained foreign bodies • Perforations from esophageal diseases for which elective surgery would be considered in the absence of a perforation (achalasia, stricture, carcinoma)

NPO, nothing by mouth.
Data from Pashricha PJ, Fleischer DE, Kalloo AN: Endoscopic perforations of the upper digestive tract: A review of their pathogenesis, prevention and management. Gastroenterology 106:787, 1994; Younes Z, Johnson DA: The spectrum of spontaneous and iatrogenic esophageal injury: Perforations, Mallory-Weiss tears, and hematomas. J Clin Gastroenterol 29:306, 1999; Bufkin BL, Miller JI Jr, Mansour KA: Esophageal perforation: Emphasis on management. Ann Thorac Surg 61:1447, 1996; Altorjay A, Kiss J, Voros A, et al: The role of esophagectomy in the management of esophageal perforations. Ann Thorac Surg 65:1433, 1998.

flammatory response in the mediastinal, pleural, and peritoneal cavities.[195] However, barium is the preferred contrast agent in cases of suspected tracheoesophageal fistula. When examination with a water-soluble contrast agent fails to show an esophageal perforation, barium esophagraphy should be performed immediately as a second study and may reveal a previously unsuspected esophageal perforation in up to 22% of cases.[196] One form of incomplete perforation is the double-barreled esophagus, in which the mucosa is dissected off the muscular layer to form two channels.[197]

ENDOSCOPY. Endoscopy has a limited role in the diagnosis of esophageal perforation, particularly that caused by medical instruments.[181] An exception may be patients with possible trauma to the esophagus from penetrating wounds, in whom endoscopic evaluation can be useful.[198] Endoscopes usually perforate the esophagus during intubation of the esophagus or during attempts to pass the instrument forcefully through narrowings. Insufflation of the esophagus during endoscopy may result in a high-pressure perforation and may also extend a preexisting incomplete perforation.[199, 200] For this reason radiologic studies, not endoscopy, are the tests of choice in evaluating a patient with a possible perforation.

Treatment

NONOPERATIVE MANAGEMENT. Esophageal perforation is a highly lethal complication that demands early surgical consultation. Nonoperative approaches apply only to very specific situations (Table 34–3). Patients whose perforation was iatrogenic and discovered early are the best candidates for nonoperative management.[201] Individuals who have perforations caused by forceful vomiting, foreign bodies, nasogastric and endotracheal tubes, and blunt trauma are not optimal candidates for medical management as these cases are seldom recognized promptly and may have been grossly contaminated. Perforations into the abdominal or pleural cavity require immediate surgical repair.

PATIENTS WITH ESOPHAGEAL CANCER. Perforation of esophageal cancer during endoscopy, dilation, or placement of an endoprosthesis is a difficult problem. Most of these perforations happen in inoperable cancer patients during attempts at palliative treatment.[181, 202] Endoscopic stenting, administration of antibiotics, and transcatheter pleural drainage (if needed) constitute the preferred treatment. The nonoperative management of perforation in esophageal cancer patients has been described in a series of 35 consecutive patients, all treated with antibiotics, nutritional support, and protection of the perforation site.[201] In 10 patients, the site was sealed off by immediate placement of an endoprosthesis; mediastinitis developed in only 1 patient. In 24 patients, nonoperative treatment was followed by placement of an endoprosthesis within 1 week, and no deaths related to perforation occurred.[201] The highest mortality rates have been reported in series in which endoprostheses were not used to seal perforations,[203] and generally favorable results have been reported in case series in which endoprostheses are used to seal cancer-related fistulas and perforations.[202, 204, 205] Attempts at a resection of the cancer or esophagus after the cancer has been perforated have usually been unsuccessful, but this remains an option for some patients.[181, 206]

PATIENTS WITH UPPER ESOPHAGEAL PERFORATIONS. Perforations in the hypopharynx and cervical esophagus contained within the soft tissues can usually be managed without surgery unless there is mediastinal involvement.[182, 207, 208] In newborn infants, endotracheal and nasogastric tubes are the cause of most cervical perforations, which usually can be managed without surgical repair. When upper esophageal perforations are caused by retained foreign bodies rather than medical instruments or tubes, the extent of contamination can be high and surgery is indicated.

PATIENTS WITH PERFORATIONS OF THE THORACIC ESOPHAGUS. When the thoracic esophagus has been perforated, deciding between operative and nonoperative management is not easy, as even small perforations can lead to sepsis, mediastinitis, and pleural contamination. Nonoperative treatment can be considered for patients who have minimal signs and symptoms and drainage of the leak back into the esophagus. These contained perforations are more likely in patients with esophageal cancer or previous inflammation or irradiation than in those with normal mediastinal anatomy. Nineteen consecutive instrumental perforations in patients without malignancy have been reported from Amsterdam.[201] Most were due to dilation of strictures and were recognized within 2 hours. Fourteen patients recovered after 1 week of nonoperative management with intravenous broad-spectrum antibiotics, parenteral or enteral nutrition, and protection of the perforation site by a nasoesophageal tube whose side holes straddled the leak. Five patients were treated surgically by primary closure and drainage because of either intra-abdominal perforation or suspected gross contamination. All patients recovered. Another study of 12 patients with early, contained leaks without clinical sepsis reported a 100% survival rate with nonoperative management.[209] These series, which took an aggressive approach to early diagnosis of perforation, contrast with a British report of 12 patients who were perforated during dilation for strictures and who were managed conservatively. Ten of these patients died.[210] In order to achieve the good results of reported series of nonoperative management, one clearly must follow the selection criteria and techniques for nonoperative management and must be prepared to operate if a seemingly localized perforation progresses to cause mediastinitis and sepsis. Case reports have described successful nonoperative management after immediate placement of a coated stent to seal the site of perforation.[211, 212] Surgical management is indicated for patients with uncontained esophageal perforations or clinical evidence of sepsis or shock (see Table 34–3).

Perforation after pneumatic balloon dilation for achalasia is frequently nontransmural and can be managed nonoperatively.[213] Complete rupture of the esophagus into the abdominal cavity or mediastinum after pneumatic dilation for achalasia requires surgery.[214, 215] Successful laparoscopic repair of perforation after pneumatic dilation for achalasia has been reported.[215] All patients managed conservatively should be watched closely for abscess formation, continued leak, and mediastinal extension of the suppurative process.

There is evidence to support the placement of drainage catheters as an important adjunct in the nonoperative management of esophageal perforations. Two groups have reported successful management of 14 patients with esophageal perforations by placing drainage catheters into sites of contamination under fluoroscopic guidance.[216, 217] While further leakage was minimized by use of large bore sump tubes in the lumen of the esophagus, mediastinal abscesses were drained via tubes placed either transesophageally through the perforation or percutaneously, and pleural abscesses were drained percutaneously. Surgeons have used a similar approach for high-risk patients with delayed presentation or failure of primary repair, in whom a sump tube is placed through the esophageal mucosal defect into the abscess cavity under endoscopic guidance.[218, 219] These methods should be undertaken only with the advice and consent of an experienced surgeon and are an option for patients unable to withstand general anesthesia and thoracotomy.

SURGICAL MANAGEMENT. Surgery is necessary for suspected contamination of a perforation site, obvious infection, sepsis, pleural or peritoneal perforation, respiratory failure, and failure of nonoperative treatment (abscess formation, failure of perforation site to close) (see Table 34–3).[209, 220] Some surgeons, however, believe that all patients with a hole in the esophageal wall should undergo an operation. For cervical perforations, primary closure and drainage of surrounding tissue are optimal, and for small leaks drainage alone is sufficient.[182, 208, 209] For perforations of the thoracic esophagus, the defect should be closed if possible and supported with a local tissue flap when primary closing is not possible. The importance of a tissue flap has been repeatedly emphasized in reviews of surgical technique.[220, 221] If there is gross contamination of the mediastinum at the time of surgery, primary repair is generally not performed. The options are resection of the esophagus, T tube placement in the esophagus to divert all secretions, or an exclusion and diversion procedure with later esophageal reconstruction.[209] When a stricture is present distal to a thoracic esophageal perforation, many surgeons recommend a one- or two-stage resection and reconstruction.[210, 222] These operations may be the only way to control persistent mediastinal and pleural infection; the mortality rate in this group of patients is high. Several reviews supply details of current surgical approaches to this difficult problem.[181, 220, 223]

Intramural Hematoma

Bleeding into the wall of the esophagus is a rare complication that may develop in association with all conditions that cause perforation, including sclerotherapy, foreign body or pill ingestion, vomiting, and use of esophageal dilators.[224] Intramural hematomas also may occur spontaneously, particularly in patients who are using aspirin or warfarin or have disorders of hemostasis.[225] Some patients who have spontaneous intramural hematomas have a history of retching, but many do not. A female preponderance has been reported. It has been suggested that spontaneous intramural hematoma of the esophagus may represent an intermediate stage in the spectrum from Mallory-Weiss tear to Boerhaave's syndrome, although a mucosal tear is not always seen and the clinical presentation varies, in that many patients who have an intramural hematoma have no history of vomiting and symptoms often appear during eating or drinking.[224, 226] Patients with normal hemostasis are more likely to have a distal esophageal hematoma, whereas those with impaired hemostasis are more likely to have a proximal hematoma.[227] Some large hematomas dissect the entire length of the esophagus and may cause esophageal obstruction. Typical symptoms include chest pain, dysphagia, and hematemesis. Such sudden onset of severe retrosternal pain in an adult patient usually suggests myocardial infarction, dissecting aortic aneurysm, or pulmonary embolism, but dysphagia and hematemesis should direct attention to the esophagus. The diagnosis is made by contrast radiography, which often reveals a "double barrel" of contrast material that represents flow of contrast material into the dissected tissue planes of the wall of the esophagus. Luminal narrowing may also be seen. CT and magnetic resonance imaging (MRI) can accurately define the extent of intramural dissection and determine whether a perforation has occurred. Endoscopy is not necessary if the clinical and radiographic findings are consistent. Endoscopy should be pursued with caution, as many intramural hematomas are contained perforations. Because the esophagus lacks a serosal layer, insufflation of air may convert a contained perforation into a free perforation.[200] Most hematomas resolve spontaneously over 7 to 14 days. Some patients may require surgery for control of bleeding.[228]

Chronic Nasogastric Tube Injury

Until the 1970s, esophageal strictures were a recognized complication of nasogastric tubes that were in place for a long time.[229] Strictures that developed (usually discovered only after the tube was pulled) involved the length of the esophagus and proved difficult to dilate. This complication has disappeared, probably because modern plastic tubes are

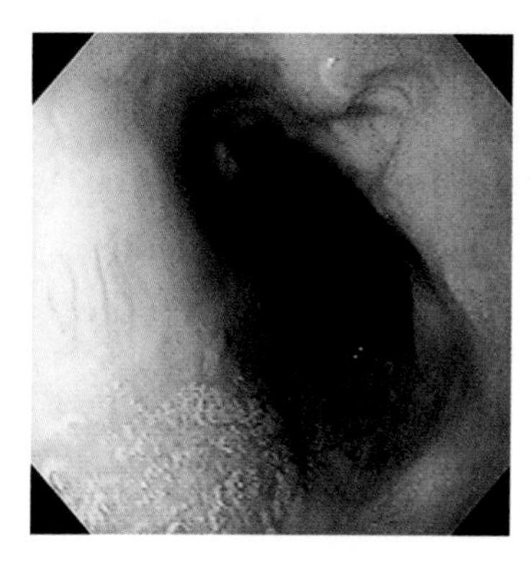

Figure 34–2. Endoscopic view of the distal esophagus showing a deep, notch-like ulcer at 1 o'clock, secondary to an indwelling plastic nasogastric tube.

less irritating. A randomized trial of cimetidine plus antacid to reduce acid secretion versus no agents in patients with nasogastric tubes showed the same degree of esophageal damage in both groups,[230] suggesting that even plastic tubes, rather than acid, cause local irritation (Fig. 34–2). Nasogastric tubes in place for prolonged periods may also erode into adjacent structures, including major vessels and congenital vascular rings.[231, 232]

Vascular-Esophageal Fistula

Aortoesophageal fistula is a rare cause of gastrointestinal bleeding that is usually catastrophic and fatal. The causes of aortoesophageal fistulas include thoracic aortic aneurysms, esophageal or bronchial malignancies, erosion of a prior aneurysm repair site, and foreign bodies (especially those with sharp projections such as bones, dentures, and pins). Aortoesophageal fistulas in children are frequently caused by foreign body ingestion.[232] Fistulization from the left subclavian artery to the esophagus has also been described after ingestion of fish bones.[233, 234] Patients with AIDS and infectious esophagitis due to mycobacterial infection may exhibit bleeding from fistulas to the blood vessels in the mediastinum.[235]

Patients typically have midthoracic pain or dysphagia followed by a "herald" hemorrhage that may be followed by fatal exsanguination.[236, 237] As with many aortoenteric fistulas, the diagnosis can be difficult, even with endoscopy and angiography. Endoscopy typically reveals a pulsatile mass that may contain an overlying blood clot located 20 to 30 cm from the incisors.[238, 239] Biopsy should not be performed. Other endoscopic findings may include bluish gray discoloration of the esophageal mucosa due to hematoma, an esophageal ulcer, esophagitis, or rarely a fistula opening.[236] CT is useful to identify an aneurysm or other abnormality such as an abscess or neoplasm. Angiography may not demonstrate the fistula if there is no active bleeding at the time of the study. If there is strong clinical suspicion of an aortoesophageal fistula based on the clinical presentation and imaging studies, emergency surgery is indicated. Bleeding is usually fatal, but a small number of patients have survived after emergency thoracotomy.[238, 240] Esophageal tamponade with a balloon has been used to stabilize patient status before thoracotomy.[241] Successful embolization of an aortoesophageal fistula has been described.[242]

REFERENCES

1. Baehr PH, McDonald GB: Esophageal infections: Risk factors, presentation, diagnosis, and treatment. Gastroenterology 106:509, 1994.
2. Anderson LI, Frederiksen HJ, Appleyard M: Prevalence of esophageal *Candida* colonization in a Danish population, with special reference to esophageal symptoms, benign esophageal disorders, and pulmonary disease. J Infect Dis 165:389, 1992.
3. Singh N, Chang FY, Gayowski T, et al: Infections due to dematiaceous fungi in organ transplant recipients: Case report and review. Clin Infect Dis 24:369, 1997.
4. Hoffman M, Bash E, Berger SA: Fatal necrotizing esophagitis due to *Penicillium chrysogenum* in a patient with acquired immunodeficiency syndrome. Eur J Clin Microbiol Infect Dis 11:1158, 1992.
5. Bini EJ, Micale PL, Weinshel EH: Natural history of HIV-associated esophageal disease in the era of protease inhibitor therapy. Dig Dis Sci 45:1301, 2000.
6. Simon MR, Houser WL, Smith KA, et al: Esophageal candidiasis as a complication of inhaled corticosteroids. Ann Allergy Asthma Immunol 79:333, 1997.
7. Hendel L, Svejgaard E, Walsoe I, et al: Esophaeal candidosis in progressive systemic sclerosis: Occurrence, significance, and treatment with fluconazole. Scand J Gastroenterol 23:1182, 1988.
8. Porro GB, Parente F, Cerunushi M: The diagnosis of esophageal candidiasis in patients with acquired immunodeficiency syndrome: Is endoscopy always necessary? Am J Gastroenterol 84:143, 1989.
9. Bonacini M, Laine L, Gal AA, et al: Prospective evaluation of blind brushing of the esophagus for *Candida* esophagitis in patients with human immunodeficiency virus infection. Am J Gastroenterol 85:385, 1990.
10. Tavitian A, Raugman JP, Rosenthal LE: Oral candidiasis as a marker for esophageal candidiasis in the acquired immunodeficiency syndrome. Ann Intern Med 104:54, 1986.
11. Levine MS, Loevner LA, Saul SH: Herpes esophagitis: Sensitivity of double contrast esophagography. AJR Am J Roentgenol 151:57, 1988.
12. Levine MS, Loercher G, Katzka DA: Giant, human immunodeficiency virus–related ulcers in the esophagus. Radiology 180:323, 1991.
13. Naito Y, Yoshikawa T, Oyamada H, et al: Esophageal candidiasis. Gastroenterol Jpn 23:363, 1988.
14. Wilcox CM, Alexander LN, Clark WS: Fluconazole compared with endoscopy for human immunodeficiency virus–infected patients with esophageal symptoms. Gastroenterology 110:1803, 1996.
15. Monkemuller KE, Wilcox CM: Diagnosis of esophageal ulcers in acquired immunodeficiency syndrome. Semin Gastrointest Dis 10:85, 1999.
16. Rex JH, Walsh TJ, Sobel JD, et al: Practice guidelines for the treatment of candidiasis. Clin Infect Dis 30:662, 2000.
17. Dietrich DT, Wilcox CM: Diagnosis and treatment of esophageal diseases associated with HIV infection. Gastroenterology 91:2265, 1996.
18. Cartledge JD, Midgley J, Petrou M, et al: Unresponsive HIV-related oro-oesophageal candidosis—an evaluation of two new in-vitro azole susceptibility tests. J Antimicrob Chemother 40:517, 1997.
19. Laing RB, Brettle RP, Leen CL: Clinical predictors of azole resistance, outcome and survival from oesophageal candidiasis in AIDS patients. Int J STD AIDS 9:16, 1998.
20. Hood SV, Hollis S, Percy M, et al: Assessment of therapeutic response of oropharyngeal and esophageal candidiasis in AIDS with use of a new clinical scoring system: Studies with D0870. Clin Infect Dis 28:587, 1999.
21. Walsh TJ, Gonzalez CE, Piscitelli S, et al: Correlation between in vitro and in vivo antifungal activities in experimental fluconazole-resistant oropharyngeal and esophageal candidiasis. J Clin Microbiol 38:2369, 2000.
22. Smith D, Midgley J, Gazzard B: A randomised, double-blind study of itraconazole versus placebo in the treatment and prevention of oral or oesophageal candidosis in patients with HIV infection. Int J Clin Pract 53:349, 1999.
23. Lalor E, Rabeneck L: Esophageal candidiasis in AIDS: Successful

therapy with clotrimazole vaginal tablets taken by mouth. Dig Dis Sci 36:279, 1991.
24. Fichtenbaum CJ, Zackin R, Rajicic N, et al: Amphotericin B oral suspension for fluconazole-refractory oral candidiasis in persons with HIV infection. AIDS 14:845, 2000.
25. Ravera M, Reggiori A, Agliata AM, et al: Evaluating diagnosis and treatment of oral and esophageal candidiasis in Ugandan AIDS patients. Emerg Infect Dis 5:274, 1999.
26. Akova M, Akalin HE, Uzun O: Efficacy of fluconazole in the treatment of upper gastrointestinal candidiasis in neutropenic patients with cancer: Factors influencing the outcome. Clin Infect Dis 18:298, 1994.
27. Wheat J: Histoplasmosis: Recognition and treatment. Clin Infect Dis 19(suppl):S19, 1994.
28. Ramanathan J, Rammouni M, Baran J Jr, et al: Herpes simplex virus esophagitis in the immunocompetent host: An overview. Am J Gastroenterol 95:2171, 2000.
29. Wishingrad M: Sexually transmitted esophagitis: Primary herpes simplex virus type 2 infection in a healthy man. Gastrointest Endosc 50: 845, 1999.
30. Dieckhaus KD, Hill DR: Boerhaave's syndrome due to herpes simplex virus type 1 esophagitis in a patient with AIDS. Clin Infect Dis 26: 1244, 1998.
31. Hackman RC, Wolford JL, Gleaves CA, et al: Recognition and rapid diagnosis of upper gastrointestinal cytomegalovirus infection in marrow transplant recipients: A comparison of seven virologic methods. Transplantation 57:231, 1994.
32. Monkemuller KE, Bussian AH, Lazenby AJ, et al: Special histologic stains are rarely beneficial for the evaluation of HIV-related gastrointestinal infections. Am J Clin Pathol 114:387, 2000.
33. Reed EC, Wolford JL, Kopecky KJ, et al: Ganciclovir for the treatment of cytomegalovirus gastroenteritis in bone marrow transplant patients: A randomized, placebo-controlled trial. Ann Intern Med 112: 505, 1990.
34. Ljungman P, Deliliers GL, Platzbecker U, et al: Cidofovir for cytomegalovirus infection and disease in allogeneic stem cell transplant recipients. Blood 97:388, 2001.
35. Boeckh M, Bowden RA, Gooley T, et al: Successful modification of a pp65 antigenemia-based early treatment strategy for prevention of CMV disease in allogeneic marrow transplant recipients [letter]. Blood 93:1781, 1999.
36. Maillot C, Riachi G, Francois A, et al: Digestive manifestations in an immunocompetent adult with varicella. Am J Gastroenterol 92:1361, 1997.
37. Sherman RA, Silva J, Gandour-Edwards R: Fatal varicella in an adult: Case report and review of the gastrointestinal complications of chickenpox. Rev Infect Dis 13:424, 1991.
38. Tilbe KS, Lloyd DA: A case of viral esophagitis. J Clin Gastroenterol 8:494, 1986.
39. Kitchen VS, Helbert M, Francis ND: Epstein-Barr virus associated oesophageal ulcers in AIDS. Gut 31:1223, 1990.
40. Abe Y, Muta K, Ohshima K, et al: Cytotoxic T-cell lymphoma diffusely involving the entire gastrointestinal tract associated with Epstein-Barr virus and tubercle bacilli infection. Int J Hematol 71:379, 2000.
41. Wang LS, Chow KC, Wu YC, et al: Detection of Epstein-Barr virus in esophageal squamous cell carcinoma in Taiwan. Am J Gastroenterol 94:2834, 1999.
42. Borum ML, Marks ZH: Esophageal stricture from idiopathic ulcers in an AIDS patient: A case report and review of the literature. J Clin Gastroenterol 28:260, 1999.
43. Houghton JM, Korah RM, Kim KH, et al: A role for apoptosis in the pathogenesis of AIDS-related idiopathic esophageal ulcers. J Infect Dis 175:1216, 1997.
44. Wilcox CM, Schwartz DA: Comparison of two corticosteroid regimens for the treatment of HIV-associated idiopathic esophageal ulcer. Am J Gastroenterol 89:2163, 1994.
45. Jacobson JM, Spritzler J, Fox L, et al: Thalidomide for the treatment of esophageal aphthous ulcers in patients with human immunodeficiency virus infection. J Infect Dis 180:61, 1999.
46. Jacobson JM, Greenspan JS, Spritzler J, et al: Thalidomide in low intermittent doses does not prevent recurrence of human immunodeficiency virus–associated aphthous ulcers. J Infect Dis 183:343, 2001.
47. Trottier AM, Coutlee F, Leduc R, et al: Human immunodeficiency virus infection is a major risk factor for detection of human papillomavirus DNA in esophageal brushings. Clin Infect Dis 24:565, 1997.
48. Ravakhah K, Midamba F, West BC: Esophageal papillomatosis from human papilloma virus proven by polymerase chain reaction. Am J Med Sci 316:285, 1998.
49. Yamada Y, Ninomiya M, Kato T, et al: Human papillomavirus type 16–positive esophageal papilloma at an endoscopic injection sclerotherapy site. Gastroenterology 108:550, 1995.
50. Leventhal BG, Kashima HK, Mounts P: Long-term response of recurrent respiratory papillomatosis to treatment with lymphoblastoid interferon-alfa-n1. N Engl J Med 325:613, 1991.
51. Hording M, Hording U, Daugaard S: Human papilloma virus type 11 in a fatal case of esophageal and bronchial papillomatosis. Scand J Infect Dis 21:229, 1989.
52. Sur M, Cooper K: The role of the human papilloma virus in esophageal cancer. Pathology 30:348, 1998.
53. Poljak M, Cerar A, Seme K: Human papillomavirus infection in esophageal carcinomas: A study of 121 lesions using multiple broad-spectrum polymerase chain reactions and literature review. Hum Pathol 29:266, 1998.
54. Saegusa M, Hashimura M, Takano Y, et al: Absence of human papillomavirus genomic sequences detected by the polymerase chain reaction in oesophageal and gastric carcinomas in Japan. Mol Pathol 50: 101, 1997.
55. Silbergleit AK, Waring WP, Sullivan MJ, et al: Evaluation, treatment and follow-up results of post polio patients with dysphagia. Otolaryngol Head Neck Surg 104:333, 1991.
56. Walsh TJ, Belitsos NJ, Hamilton SR: Bacterial esophagitis in immunocompromised patients. Arch Intern Med 146:1345, 1986.
57. Yeomans ND, Brimblecone RW, Elder J, et al: Effects of acid suppression on microbial flora of upper gut. Dig Dis Sci 40:81S, 1995.
58. Larner AJ, Hamilton MIR: Review article: Infective complications of therapeutic gastric acid inhibition. Aliment Pharmacol Ther 8:579, 1994.
59. Ravera M: Tuberculous bronchoesophageal fistula in a patient infected with the HIV virus. Endoscopy 29:146, 1997.
60. Jain S, Kumar N, Das DK, et al: Esophageal tuberculosis: Endoscopic cytology as a diagnostic tool. Acta Cytol 43:1085, 1999.
61. Fang HY, Lin TS, Cheng CY, et al: Esophageal tuberculosis: A rare presentation with massive hematemesis. Ann Thorac Surg 68:2344, 1999.
62. Perdomo JA, Naomoto Y, Haisa M, et al: Tuberculosis of the esophagus. Dis Esophagus 11:72, 1998.
63. Kochhar R, Sriram PV, Rajwanshi A, et al: Transesophageal endoscopic fine-needle aspiration cytology in mediastinal tuberculosis. Gastrointest Endosc 50:271, 1999.
64. Calore EE, Cavaliere JM, Perez NM, et al: Esophageal ulcers in AIDS. Pathologica 89:155, 1997.
65. Stone J, Friedberg SA: Obstructive syphilitic esophagitis. JAMA 177: 711, 1961.
66. Scholz DG, Olson JM, Thurber DL, et al: Tetanus: An uncommon cause of dysphagia. Mayo Clin Proc 64:335, 1989.
67. Kim J, Minamoto GY, Grieco MH: *Nocardia* infection as a complication of AIDS: Report of six cases and review. Rev Infect Dis 13:624, 1991.
68. Dux M, Gehling U, Schmitteckert H, et al: Mediastinal actinomycosis with formation of an esophagotracheal fistula: A case report. Radiologe 34:537, 1994.
69. Poles MA, McMeeking AA, Scholes JV, et al: *Actinomyces* infection of a cytomegalovirus esophageal ulcer in two patients with acquired immunodeficiency syndrome. Am J Gastroenterol 89:1569, 1994.
70. Sharma VK, Demian SE, Taillon D, et al: Examination of tissue distribution of *Helicobacter pylori* within columnarlined esophagus. Dig Dis Sci 44:1165, 1999.
71. Weston AP, Cherian R, Horvat RT, et al: Mucosa-associated lymphoid tissue (MALT) in Barrett's esophagus: Prospective evaluation and association with gastric MALT, MALT lymphoma, and *Helicobacter pylori*. Am J Gastroenterol 92:800, 1997.
72. Weston AP, Badr AS, Topalovski M, et al: Prospective evaluation of the prevalence of gastric *Helicobacter pylori* infection in patients with GERD, Barrett's esophagus, Barrett's dysplasia, and Barrett's adenocarcinoma. Am J Gastroenterol 95:387, 2000.
73. Vaezi MF, Falk GW, Peek RM, et al: CagA-positive strains of *Helicobacter pylori* may protect against Barrett's esophagus. Am J Gastroenterol 95:2206, 2000.

74. Voutilainen M, Farkkila M, Mecklin JP, et al: Chronic inflammation at the gastroesophageal junction (carditis) appears to be a specific finding related to *Helicobacter pylori* infection and gastroesophageal reflux disease. Am J Gastroenterol 94:3175, 1999.
75. Dantas RO, Godoy RA, de Oliveria RB: Lower esophageal sphincter pressure in Chagas' disease. Dig Dis Sci 35:508, 1990.
76. Dantas RO, Deghaide NH, Donadi EA: Esophageal manometric and radiologic findings in asymptomatic subjects with Chagas' disease. J Clin Gastroenterol 28:245, 1999.
77. Herbella FA, Del Grande JC, Lourenco LG, et al: Late results of Heller operation and fundoplication for the treatment of the megaesophagus: Analysis of 83 cases [in Portuguese]. Rev Assoc Med Bras 45:317, 1999.
78. Pinotti HW, Felix VN, Zilberstein B, et al: Surgical complications of Chagas' disease: Megaesophagus, achalasia of the pylorus, and cholelithiasis. World J Surg 15:198, 1991.
79. Kazlow PG, Shah K, Benkov KJ, et al: Esophageal cryptosporidiosis in a child with acquired immune deficiency syndrome. Gastroenterology 91:1301, 1986.
80. Grimes MM, LaPook JD, Bar MH, et al: Disseminated *Pneumocytis carinii* infection in a patient with acquired immunodeficiency syndrome. Hum Pathol 18:307, 1987.
81. Trevenzoli M, Lanzafame M, Lazzarini L, et al: Esophageal cryptococcosis in a patient with AIDS [letter]. Am J Gastroenterol 94:1981, 1999.
82. Borczuk AC, Hagan R, Chipty F, et al: Cytologic detection of *Trichomonas* esophagitis in a patient with acquired immunodeficiency syndrome. Diagn Cytopathol 19:313, 1998.
83. Villanueva JL, Torre-Cisneros J, Jurado R, et al: *Leishmania* esophagitis in an AIDS patient: An unusual form of visceral leishmaniasis. Am J Gastroenterol 89:273, 1994.
84. Travis SPL, McGrath JA, Turnbull AJ, et al: Oral and gastrointestinal manifestations of epidermolysis bullosa. Lancet 340:1505, 1992.
85. Tokuda Y, Amagai M, Yaoita H, et al: A case of an inflammatory variant of epidermolysis bullosa acquisita: Chronic bullous dermatosis associated with nonscarring mucosal blisters and circulating IgG anti–type-VII-collagen antibody. Dermatology 197:58, 1998.
86. Schattenkirchner S, Lemann M, Prost C, et al: Localized epidermolysis bullosa acquisita of the esophagus in a patient with Crohn's disease. Am J Gastroenterol 91:1657, 1996.
87. Shirakata Y, Amagai M, Hanakawa Y, et al: Lack of mucosal involvement in pemphigus foliaceus may be due to low expression of desmoglein 1. J Invest Dermatol 110:76, 1998.
88. Gomi H, Akiyama M, Yakabi K, et al: Oesophageal involvement in pemphigus vulgaris [letter]. Lancet 354:1794, 1999.
89. Mignogna MD, Lo Muzio L, Galloro G, et al: Oral pemphigus: Clinical significance of esophageal involvement: Report of eight cases. Oral Surg Oral Med Oral Pathol Oral Radiol Endod 84:179, 1997.
90. Schissel DJ, David-Bajar K: Esophagitis dissecans superficialis associated with pemphigus vulgaris. Cutis 63:157, 1999.
91. Nousari HC, Anhalt GJ: Pemphigus and bullous pemphigoid. Lancet 354:667, 1999.
92. Korman NJ: Bullous pemphigoid: The latest in diagnosis, prognosis, and therapy. Arch Dermatol 134:1137, 1998.
93. Yamamota T, Tanaka A, Furuse Y: Bullous pemphigoid with esophageal cancer. J Dermatol 21:283, 1994.
94. Naylor MF, MacCarty RL, Rogers RS: Barium studies in esophageal cicatricial pemphigoid. Abdom Imaging 20:97, 1995.
95. Egan CA, Hanif N, Taylor TB, et al: Characterization of the antibody response in oesophageal cicatricial pemphigoid. Br J Dermatol 140: 859, 1999.
96. Watkinson AF, Vretenar DF, Morrison MD, et al: Benign mucous membrane pemphigoid: Treatment of esophageal stricture. Can Assoc Radiol J 45:140, 1994.
97. Austey A, Wojnarowska F, Whitehead P, et al: Oesophageal webs preceding carcinoma and rupture of the oesophagus in cicatricial pemphigoid. Clin Exp Dermatol 16:395, 1991.
98. Kirsch M: Esophageal lichen planus: A forgotten diagnosis. J Clin Gastroenterol 20:145, 1995.
99. Harty RF, Boharski MG, Harned RK, et al: Psoriasis, dysphagia, and esophageal webs or rings. Dysphagia 2:136, 1988.
100. Kozlowski LM, Nigra TP: Esophageal acanthosis nigricans in association with adenocarcinoma from an unknown primary site. J Am Acad Dermatol 26:348, 1992.
101. Kaye MD: Esophageal leukoplakia. Gastrointest Endosc 33:254, 1987.
102. Lam TS, Lack E, Benjamin SB: Compact parakeratosis of esophageal mucosa: A non-specific lesion mimicking "leukoplakia." Gastrointest Endosc 36:379, 1990.
103. Brinson RR, Schuman BM, Mills LR, et al: Multiple squamous papillomas of the esophagus associated with Goltz syndrome. Am J Gastroenterol 82:1177, 1987.
104. Ellis A, Field JK, Field EA, et al: Tylosis associated with carcinoma of the oesophagus and oral leukoplakia in a large Liverpool family—a review of six generations. Eur J Cancer 30B:102, 1994.
105. O'Duffy JD: Behçet's disease. Curr Opin Rheumatol 6:39, 1994.
106. Kaklamani VG, Vaiopoulos G, Kaklamanis PG: Behçet's disease. Semin Arthritis Rheum 27:197, 1998.
107. Bayraktar Y, Ozaslan E, Van Thiel DH: Gastrointestinal manifestations of Behçet's disease. J Clin Gastroenterol 30:144, 2000.
108. Sakane T, Takeno M, Suzuki N, et al: Behçet's disease. N Engl J Med 341:1284, 1999.
109. Ikezawa K, Kashimura H, Hassan M, et al: A case of Behçet's syndrome with esophageal involvement treated with salicylazosulfapyridine and prednisolone. Endoscopy 30:S52, 1998.
110. Otero Lopez-Cubero S, Sale GE, McDonald GB: Acute graft-versus-host disease of the esophagus. Endoscopy 29:S35, 1997.
111. McDonald GB, Sullivan KM, Schuffler MD, et al: Esophageal abnormalities in chronic graft-versus-host disease in humans. Gastroenterology 80:914, 1981.
112. Minocha A, Mandanas RA, Kida M, et al: Bullous esophagitis due to chronic graft-versus-host disease. Am J Gastroenterol 92:529, 1997.
113. McDonald GB, Sullivan KM, Plumley TF: Radiographic features of esophageal involvement in chronic graft-versus-host disease. AJR Am J Roentgenol 142:501, 1984.
114. Schima W, Pokieser P, Forstinger C, et al: Videofluoroscopy of the pharynx and esophagus in chronic graft-versus-host disease. Abdom Imaging 19:191, 1994.
115. Iwakuma A, Matsuyoshi T, Arikado T, et al: Two cases of postoperative erythroderma—clinical and pathological investigation. J Jpn Assoc Thorac Surg 39:209, 1991.
116. Ruuska T, Vaajalahti P, Arajarvi P, et al: Prospective evaluation of upper gastrointestinal mucosal lesions in children with ulcerative colitis and Crohn's disease. J Pediatr Gastroenterol Nutr 19:181, 1994.
117. Lenaerts C, Roy CC, Vaillancourt M, et al: High incidence of upper gastrointestinal tract involvement in children with Crohn disease. Pediatrics 83:777, 1989.
118. D'Haens G, Rutgeerts P, Geboes K, et al: The natural history of esophageal Crohn's disease: Three patterns of evolution. Gastrointest Endosc 296:300, 1994.
119. Rholl JC, Yavorski RT, Cheney CP, et al: Esophagogastric fistula: A complication of Crohn's disease—case report and review of the literature. Am J Gastroenterol 93:1381, 1998.
120. Heller T, James SP, Drachenberg C, et al: Treatment of severe esophageal Crohn's disease with infliximab. Inflamm Bowel Dis 5:279, 1999.
121. Davies RJ: Dysphagia, abdominal pain, and sarcoid granulomata. BMJ 3:564, 1972.
122. Geissinger BW, Sharkey MF, Criss DG, et al: Reversible esophageal motility disorder in a patient with sarcoidosis. Am J Gastroenterol 91: 1423, 1996.
123. Hiller N, Fisher D, Abrahamov A, et al: Esophageal involvement in chronic granulomatous disease. Pediatr Radiol 25:308, 1995.
124. Rosh JR, Tang HB, Mayer L, et al: Treatment of intractable gastrointestinal manifestations of chronic granulomatous disease with cyclosporine. J Pediatr 126:143, 1995.
125. Hsu CC, Chen JJ, Changchien CS: Endoscopic features of metastatic tumors in the upper gastrointestinal tract. Endoscopy 28:249, 1996.
126. Nakamura T, Mohri H, Shimazaki M, et al: Esophageal metastasis from prostate cancer: Diagnostic use of reverse transcriptase–polymerase chain reaction for prostate-specific antigen. J Gastroenterol 32:236, 1997.
127. Fulp SR, Nestok BR, Powell BL, et al: Leukemic infiltration of the esophagus. Cancer 71:112, 1993.
128. Heater K, MacMahon H, Vyborny CJ: Occult lung carcinoma presenting with dysphagia: The value of computed tomography. Clin Imaging 13:122, 1989.
129. Kadakia SC, Parker A, Canales L: Metastatic tumors to the upper gastrointestinal tract: Endoscopic experience. Am J Gastroenterol 87: 1418, 1992.
130. Redleaf MI, Moran WJ, Gruber B: Mycosis fungoides involving the cervical esophagus. Arch Otolaryngol Head Neck Surg 119:690, 1993.

131. Shimada Y, Imamura M, Tobe T: Successful esophagectomy for metastatic carcinoma of the esophagus from breast cancer—a case report. Jpn J Surg 19:82, 1989.
132. Frager DH, Wolf EL, Competiello LS, et al: Squamous cell carcinoma of the esophagus in patients with acquired immunodeficiency syndrome. Gastrointest Radiol 13:358, 1988.
133. Chow DC, Bleikh SH, Eickhoff L, et al: Primary esophageal lymphoma in AIDS presenting as a nonhealing esophageal ulcer. Am J Gastroenterol 91:602, 1996.
134. Fallows GA, Hamilton SF, Taylor DS, et al: Esophageal involvement in Wegener's granulomatosis: A case report and review of the literature. Can J Gastroenterol 14:449, 2000.
135. Cappell MS: Esophageal necrosis and perforation associated with the anticardiolipin antibody syndrome. Am J Gastroenterol 89:1241, 1994.
136. Kikendall JW: Pill esophagitis. J Clin Gastroenterol 28:298, 1999.
137. Hey H, Jorgensen F, Sorensen K, et al: Oesophageal transit of six commonly used tablets and capsules. BMJ 285:1717, 1982.
138. McCord GS, Clouse RE: Pill-induced esophageal strictures: Clinical features and risk factors for development. Am J Med 88:512, 1990.
139. El-Serag HB, Sonnenberg A: Association of esophagitis and esophageal strictures with diseases treated with nonsteroidal anti-inflammatory drugs. Am J Gastroenterol 92:52, 1997.
140. Sopena F, Lanas A, Sainz R: Esophageal motility and intraesophageal pH patterns in patients with esophagitis and chronic nonsteroidal antiinflammatory drug use. J Clin Gastroenterol 27:316, 1998.
141. Abraham SC, Cruz-Correa M, Lee LA, et al: Alendronate-associated esophageal injury: Pathologic and endoscopic features. Mod Pathol 12: 1152, 1999.
142. Shubert MM, Peterson DE, Lloid ME: Oral complications. In Thomas ED, Blume KG, Forman SJ, et al (eds): Hematopoietic Cell Transplantation, 2nd ed. Cambridge, Mass, Blackwell Science, 1999, p 751.
143. Wang WS, Chiou TJ, Liu JH, et al: Vincristine-induced dysphagia suggesting esophageal motor dysfunction: A case report. Jpn J Clin Oncol 30:515, 2000.
144. Choy H, LaPorte K, Knill-Selby E, et al: Esophagitis in combined modality therapy for locally advanced non–small cell lung cancer. Semin Radiat Oncol 9:90, 1999.
145. Maguire PD, Sibley GS, Zhou SM, et al: Clinical and dosimetric predictors of radiation-induced esophageal toxicity. Int J Radiat Oncol Phys 45:97, 1999.
146. Mascarenhas F, Silvestre ME, Sa da Costa M: Acute secondary effects in the esophagus in patients undergoing radiotherapy for carcinoma of the lung. Am J Clin Oncol 12:34, 1989.
147. Berthong M: Pathologic changes secondary to radiation. World J Surg 10:155, 1986.
148. Collazzo LA, Levine MS, Rubesin SE, et al: Acute radiation esophagitis: Radiographic findings. AJR Am J Roentgenol 169:1067, 1997.
149. Korsten MA, Rosman AS, Fishbein S: Chronic xerostomia increases esophageal acid exposure and is associated with esophageal injury. Am J Med 90:701, 1991.
150. Choi NC, Herndon JE II, Rosenman J, et al: Phase I study to determine the maximum-tolerated dose of radiation in standard daily and hyperfractionated-accelerated twice-daily radiation schedules with concurrent chemotherapy for limited-stage small-cell lung cancer. J Clin Oncol 16:3528, 1998.
151. Coia LR, Myerson RJ, Tepper JE: Late effects of radiation therapy on the gastrointestinal tract. Int J Radiat Oncol Biol Phys 31:1213, 1995.
152. Costleigh BJ, Miyamoto CT, Micaily B, et al: Heightened sensitivity of the esophagus to radiation in a patient with AIDS. Am J Gastroenterol 90:812, 1995.
153. Leigh BR, Lau DH: Severe esophageal toxicity after thoracic radiation therapy for lung cancer associated with the human immunodeficiency virus: A case report and review of the literature. Am J Clin Oncol 21: 479, 1998.
154. Werner-Wasik M, Scott C, Graham ML, et al: Interfraction interval does not affect survival of patients with non–small cell lung cancer treated with chemotherapy and/or hyperfractionated radiotherapy: A multivariate analysis of 1076 RTOG patients. Int J Radiat Oncol Phys 44:327, 1999.
155. Turrisi AT III, Kim K, Blum R, et al: Twice-daily compared with once-daily thoracic radiotherapy in limited small-cell lung cancer treated concurrently with cisplatin and etoposide. N Engl J Med 340: 265, 1999.
156. Byhardt RW, Scott C, Sause WT, et al: Response, toxicity, failure patterns, and survival in five Radiation Therapy Oncology Group (RTOG) trials of sequential and/or concurrent chemotherapy and radiotherapy for locally advanced non-small-cell carcinoma of the lung. Int J Radiat Oncol Phys 42:469, 1998.
157. Tannehill SP, Mehta MP, Larson M, et al: Effect of amifostine on toxicities associated with sequential chemotherapy and radiation therapy for unresectable non-small-cell lung cancer: Results of a phase II trial. J Clin Oncol 15:2850, 1997.
158. Seeman H, Gates JA, Traube M: Esophageal motor dysfunction years after radiation therapy. Dig Dis Sci 37:303, 1992.
159. Silvain C, Barrioz T, Babin P, et al: Treatment and long-term outcome of chronic radiation esophagitis after radiation therapy for head and neck tumors: A report of 13 cases. Dig Dis Sci 38:927, 1993.
160. Mahboubi S, Silber JH: Radiation-induced esophageal strictures in children with cancer. Eur Radiol 7:119, 1997.
161. Shimizu T, Matsui T, Kimura O: Radiation-induced esophageal cancer: A case report and review of the literature. Jpn J Surg 20:97, 1990.
162. Laine L, Cook D: Endoscopic ligation compared with sclerotherapy for treatment of esophageal variceal bleeding. Ann Intern Med 123: 280, 1995.
163. Argonz J, Kravetz D, Suarez A, et al: Variceal band ligation and variceal band ligation plus sclerotherapy in the prevention of recurrent variceal bleeding in cirrhotic patients: A randomized, prospective and controlled trial. Gastrointest Endosc 51:157, 2000.
164. Saeed ZA, Stiegmann GV, Ramirez FC, et al: Endoscopic variceal ligation is superior to combined ligation and sclerotherapy for esophageal varices: A multicenter prospective randomized trial. Hepatology 25:71, 1997.
165. Shiozaki H, Yano T, Imanoto H: Changes in the chest on CT examinations after endoscopic intravascular sclerotherapy of the esophageal varices. J Jpn Surg Soc 89:516, 1988.
166. Ahmad N, Ginsberg GG: Variceal ligation with bands and clips. Gastrointest Endosc Clin N Am 9:207, 1999.
167. Dennert B, Ramirez FC, Sanowski RA: A prospective evaluation of the endoscopic spectrum of overtube-related esophageal mucosal injury. Gastrointest Endosc 45:134, 1997.
168. Minoli G: Esophageal perforation and variceal banding. Endoscopy 26:633, 1994.
169. Saltzman JR, Arora S: Complications of esophageal variceal band ligation. Gastrointest Endosc 39:203, 1993.
170. Korula J, Pandya K, Yamada S: Perforation of esophagus after endoscopic variceal sclerotherapy: Incidence and clues to pathogenesis. Dig Dis Sci 34:324, 1989.
171. Chen TA, Lo GH, Lai KH: Spontaneous rupture of iatrogenic intramural hematoma of esophagus during endoscopic sclerotherapy. Gastrointest Endosc 50:850, 1999.
172. Mistry FP, Sreenivasa D, Narawane NM, et al: Vagal dysfunction following endoscopic variceal sclerotherapy. Indian J Gastroenterol 17: 22, 1998.
173. Grande L, Planas R, Lacima G, et al: Sequential esophageal motility studies after endoscopic injection sclerotherapy: A prospective investigation. Am J Gastroenterol 86:36, 1991.
174. Sidhu SS, Bal C, Karak P, et al: Effect of endoscopic variceal sclerotherapy on esophageal motor functions and gastroesophageal reflux. J Nucl Med 36:1363, 1995.
175. Sakata K, Ishida M, Hiraishi H, et al: Adenosquamous carcinoma of the esophagus after endoscopic variceal sclerotherapy: A case report and review of the literature. Gastrointest Endosc 47:294, 1998.
176. Dina R, Cassisa A, Baroncini D, et al: Role of esophageal brushing cytology in monitoring patients treated with sclerotherapy for esophageal varices. Acta Cytol 36:477, 1992.
177. Pulanic R, Vrhovac B, Jokic N, et al: Prophylactic administration of ranitidine after sclerotherapy of esophageal varices. Int J Clin Pharmacol Ther Toxicol 29:347, 1991.
178. Garg PK, Sidhu SS, Bhargava DK: Role of omeprazole in prevention and treatment of postendoscopic variceal sclerotherapy esophageal complications: Double-blind randomized study. Dig Dis Sci 40:1569, 1995.
179. Yang WG, Hou MC, Lin HC, et al: Effect of sucralfate granules in suspension on endoscopic variceal sclerotherapy induced ulcer: Analysis of the factors determining ulcer healing. J Gastroenterol Hepatol 13:225, 1998.
180. Snady H, Rosman AS, Korsten MA: Prevention of stricture formation

after endoscopic sclerotherapy of esophageal varices. Gastrointest Endosc 35:377, 1989.
181. Pasricha PJ, Fleischer DE, Kalloo AN: Endoscopic perforations of the upper digestive tract: A review of their pathogenesis, prevention and management. Gastroenterology 106:787, 1994.
182. Tilanus HW, Bossuyt P, Schattenkerk ME, et al: Treatment of oesophageal perforation: A multivariate analysis. Br J Surg 78:582, 1991.
183. Younes Z, Johnson DA: The spectrum of spontaneous and iatrogenic esophageal injury: Perforations, Mallory-Weiss tears, and hematomas. J Clin Gastroenterol 29:306, 1999.
184. Ku PK, Tong MC, Ho KM, et al: Traumatic esophageal perforation resulting from endotracheal intubation. Anesth Analg 87:730, 1998.
185. Gruen R, Cade R, Vellar D: Perforation during nasogastric and orogastric tube insertion. Aust N Z J Surg 68:809, 1998.
186. Gaudinez RF, English GM, Gebhard JS, et al: Esophageal perforations after anterior cervical surgery. J Spinal Disord 13:77, 2000.
187. Niezgoda JA, McMenamin P, Graeber GM: Pharyngoesophageal perforation after blunt neck trauma. Ann Thorac Surg 50:615, 1990.
188. Samad L, Ali M, Ramzi H: Button battery ingestion: Hazards of esophageal impaction. J Pediatr Surg 34:1527, 1999.
189. Gougoutas C, Levine MS, Laufer I: Esophageal food impaction with early perforation. AJR Am J Roentgenol 171:427, 1998.
190. Serna DL, Vovan TT, Roum JH, et al: Successful nonoperative management of delayed spontaneous esophageal perforation in patients with human immunodeficiency virus. Crit Care Med 28:2634, 2000.
191. Guillem PG, Porte HL, Saudemont A, et al: Perforation of Barrett's ulcer: A challenge in esophageal surgery. Ann Thorac Surg 69:1707, 2000.
192. Bondeson AG, Bondeson L, Thompson NW: Stricture and perforation of the esophagus: Overlooked threats in the Zollinger-Ellison syndrome. World J Surg 14:361, 1990.
193. Mizutani K, Makuuchi H, Tajima T, et al: The diagnosis and treatment of esophageal perforations resulting from nonmalignant causes. Surg Today 27:793, 1997.
194. Panzini L, Burrell MI, Traube M: Instrumental esophageal perforation: Chest film findings. Am J Gastroenterol 89:367, 1994.
195. Dodds WJ, Stewart ET, Vlymen WJ: Appropriate contrast media for evaluation of esophageal disruption. Radiology 144:439, 1982.
196. Buecker A, Wein BB, Neuerburg JM, et al: Esophageal perforation: Comparison of use of aqueous and barium-containing contrast media. Radiology 202:683, 1997.
197. Low DE, Patterson DJ: Complete esophageal obstruction secondary to dissecting intramural hematoma after endoscopic variceal sclerotherapy. Am J Gastroenterol 83:435, 1988.
198. Horwitz B, Krevsky B, Buckman RF, et al: Endoscopic evaluation of penetrating esophageal injuries. Am J Gastroenterol 88:1249, 1993.
199. Gubbins GP, Nensey YM, Schubert TT, et al: Barogenic perforation of the esophagus distal to a stricture after endoscopy. J Clin Gastroenterol 12:310, 1990.
200. Skillington PD, Matar KS, Gardner MA, et al: Intramural haematoma of the oesophagus complicated by perforation. Aust N Z J Surg 59: 430, 1989.
201. Wesdorp IC, Bartelsman JF, Huibregtse K, et al: Treatment of instrumental oesophageal perforation. Gut 25:398, 1984.
202. Morgan RA, Ellul JP, Denton ER, et al: Malignant esophageal fistulas and perforations: Management with plastic-covered metallic endoprostheses. Radiology 204:527, 1997.
203. Bisgaard T, Wojdemann M, Heindorff H, et al: Nonsurgical treatment of esophageal perforations after endoscopic palliation in advanced esophageal cancer. Endoscopy 29:155, 1997.
204. Watkinson A, Ellul JP, Entwistle K, et al: Plastic-covered metallic endoprostheses in the management of oesophageal perforation in patients with oesophageal carcinoma. 50:304, 1995.
205. Nicholson AA, Royston CM, Wedgewood K, et al: Palliation of malignant oesophageal perforation and proximal oesophageal malignant dysphagia with covered metal stents. Clin Radiol 50:11, 1995.
206. Adam DJ, Thompson AM, Walker WS, et al: Oesophagogastrectomy for iatrogenic perforation of oesophageal and cardia carcinoma. Br J Surg 83:1429, 1996.
207. Hine KR, Atkinson M: The diagnosis and management of perforations of esophagus and pharynx sustained during intubation of neoplastic esophageal strictures. Dig Dis Sci 31:571, 1986.
208. Dolgin SR, Wykoff TW, Kumar NR, et al: Conservative medical management of traumatic pharyngoesophageal perforations. Ann Otol Rhinol Laryngol 101:209, 1992.
209. Bufkin BL, Miller JI Jr, Mansour KA: Esophageal perforation: Emphasis on management. Ann Thorac Surg 61:1447, 1996.
210. Moghissi K, Pender D: Instrumental perforations of the oesophagus and their management. Thorax 43:642, 1988.
211. Pajarinen J, Ristkari SK, Mokka RE: A report of three cases with an oesophageal perforation treated with a coated self-expanding stent. Ann Chir Gynaecol 88:332, 1999.
212. Segalin A, Bonavina L, Lazzerini M, et al: Endoscopic management of inveterate esophageal perforations and leaks. Surg Endosc 10:928, 1996.
213. Molina EG, Stollman N, Grauer L, et al: Conservative management of esophageal nontransmural tears after pneumatic dilation for achalasia. Am J Gastroenterol 91:15, 1996.
214. Metman EH, Lagasse JP, d'Alteroche L, et al: Risk factors for immediate complications after progressive pneumatic dilation for achalasia. Am J Gastroenterol 94:1179, 1999.
215. Bell RC: Laparoscopic closure of esophageal perforation following pneumatic dilatation for achalasia: Report of two cases. Surg Endosc 11:476, 1997.
216. Meranze SG, LeVeen RF, Burke DR, et al: Transesophageal drainage of mediastinal abscesses. Radiology 165:395, 1987.
217. Maroney TP, Ring EJ, Gordon RL, et al: Role of interventional radiology in the management of major esophageal leaks. Radiology 170: 1055, 1989.
218. Jorgensen JO, Hunt DR: Endoscopic drainage of esophageal suture line leaks. Am J Surg 165:362, 1993.
219. Larsson S, Pettersson G, Lepore V: Esophagocutaneous drainage to treat late and complicated esophageal perforation. Eur J Cardiothorac Surg 5:579, 1991.
220. Wright CD, Mathisen DJ, Wain JC, et al: Reinforced primary repair of thoracic esophageal perforation. Ann Thorac Surg 60:245, 1995.
221. Kotsis L, Kostic S, Zubovits K: Multimodality treatment of esophageal disruptions. Chest 112:1304, 1997.
222. Gupta NM: Emergency transhiatal oesophagectomy for instrumental perforation of an obstructed thoracic oesophagus. Br J Surg 83:1007, 1996.
223. Altorjay A, Kiss J, Voros A, et al: The role of esophagectomy in the management of esophageal perforations. Ann Thorac Surg 65:1433, 1998.
224. Hiller N, Zagal I, Hadas-Halpern I: Spontaneous intramural hematoma of the esophagus. Am J Gastroenterol 94:2282, 1999.
225. Geller A, Gostout CJ: Esophagogastric hematoma mimicking a malignant neoplasm: Clinical manifestations, diagnosis, and treatment. Mayo Clin Proc 73:342, 1998.
226. Van Laethem JL, Deviere J, Cremer M: Serial endoscopic findings of spontaneous intramural hematoma of the esophagus. Endoscopy 29:44, 1997.
227. Sanaka M, Kuyama Y, Hirama S, et al: Spontaneous intramural hematoma localized in the proximal esophagus: Truly "spontaneous." J Clin Gastroenterol 27:265, 1998.
228. Folan RD, Smith RE, Head JM: Esophageal hematoma and tear requiring emergency surgical intervention: A case report and literature review. Dig Dis Sci 37:1918, 1992.
229. Douglas WK: Oesophageal stricture associated with gastroduodenal intubation. Br J Surg 43:404, 1956.
230. Buchman AL, Waring JP: Mucosal bridge formation in the esophagus caused by injury from a nasoenteric feeding tube. J Parenter Enteral Nutr 18:278, 1994.
231. McKeating J, Smith S, Kochanck P, et al: Fatal aortoesophageal fistula due to double aortic arch: An unusual complication of prolonged nasogastric intubation. J Pediatr Surg 25:1298, 1990.
232. Sigalet DL, Laberge JM, DiLorenzo M, et al: Aortoesophageal fistula: Congenital and acquired causes. J Pediatr Surg 29:1212, 1994.
233. Leow CK: Subclavian arterio-esophageal fistula secondary to fish bone impaction: Report of a case. Surg Today 28:409, 1998.
234. Ohta N, Koshiji T, Imamura M, et al: Aortoesophageal fistula caused by foreign body. Jpn J Thorac Cardiovasc Surg 8:184, 2000.
235. O'Leary M, Nollet DJ, Blomberg DJ: Rupture of a tuberculous pseudoaneurysm of the innominate artery into the trachea and esophagus: Report of a case and review of the literature. Hum Pathol 8:458, 1977.
236. Amin S, Luketich J, Wald A: Aortoesophageal fistula: Case report and review of the literature. Dig Dis Sci 43:1665, 1998.
237. Heckstall RL, Hollander JE: Aortoesophageal fistula: Recognition and diagnosis in the emergency department. Ann Emerg Med 32:502, 1998.

238. Da Silva ES, Tozzi FL, Otochi JP, et al: Aortoesophageal fistula caused by aneurysm of the thoracic aorta: Successful surgical treatment, case report, and literature review. J Vasc Surg 30:1150, 1999.
239. Reardon MJ, Brewer RJ, LeMaire SA, et al: Surgical management of primary aortoesophageal fistula secondary to thoracic aneurysm. Ann Thorac Surg 69:967, 2000.
240. Luketich JD, Sommers KE, Griffith BP, et al: Successful management of secondary aortoesophageal fistula. Ann Thorac Surg 62:1852, 1996.
241. Wu MH, Lai WW: Aortoesophageal fistula induced by foreign bodies. Ann Thorac Surg 54:155, 1992.
242. Reedy FM: Embolization of aortoesophageal fistula: A new therapeutic approach [letter]. J Vasc Surg 8:349, 1988.

Chapter 35

ESOPHAGEAL TUMORS

Gregory G. Ginsberg and David E. Fleischer

This chapter reviews the epithelial and nonepithelial tumors of the esophagus. From among the epithelial tumors, the balance of the chapter focuses upon primary esophageal neoplasms, specifically squamous cell carcinoma of the esophagus, adenocarcinoma of the esophagus, and adenocarcinoma of the esophagogastric (EG) junction. The epidemiologic, biologic, and genetic characteristics; clinical presentation; diagnosis; staging; and treatment options are detailed. There is an expanded section on endoscopic palliation of malignant dysphagia. Other malignant and benign epithelial and nonepithelial tumors are covered in the remainder of the chapter.

MALIGNANT EPITHELIAL TUMORS

Malignant epithelial tumors of the esophagus, for the most part, comprise primary esophageal carcinomas. Generically, esophageal cancer comprises squamous cell carcinoma and adenocarcinoma of the esophagus and the EG junction. Worldwide, esophageal cancer ranks fifth in mortality rate among tumor sites.[1] In the United States, esophageal cancer has a frequency of 3.3 per 100,000 population for squamous cell and adenocarcinoma subtypes combined. Annually, approximately 12,300 Americans are diagnosed with esophageal cancer, and 12,100 die of this malignancy.[2] Of the new cases, 9200 occur in men and 3100 occur in women. In the United States, the median age of patients who contract esophageal cancer is 67 years.[3]

Worldwide, squamous cell carcinoma remains the most common type. However, cancer incidence trends show an overall decrease in squamous cell carcinoma since the early 1970s. In contrast, the incidence of esophageal adenocarcinoma has increased rapidly in the United States and Europe, where the incidence of adenocarcinoma of the esophagus and EG junction has risen fivefold. This rate of increase has exceeded that of any other cancer. Adenocarcinoma has now surpassed squamous cell carcinoma as the predominant cell type of esophageal cancer in the United States.[4, 5] Although these two tumor types vary in epidemiologic features, their biologic behavior, diagnosis, staging, and treatment options are sufficiently similar to allow a uniform handling of these topic areas. Aspects unique to one particular tumor type are discriminated as necessary.

Epidemiology

Squamous Cell Carcinoma

Squamous cell carcinoma (SCCA) of the esophagus arises from malignant conversion of the squamous mucosal surface of the esophagus. This process is thought to result in many, if not all, cases from a progression through degrees of cellular dysplasia that may be detected histologically. Epidemiologically, striking regional variations of SCCA of the esophagus have been observed. Markedly high incidences of esophageal SCCA have been observed in discrete regions of China, northern Iran, southern Turkey, and northern Africa. Linxian Province in China is one such highly endemic region. In the 1980s the incidence of esophageal cancer in China was approximately 32 per 100,000, whereas in Linxian the incidence was greater than 700 per 100,000.[6] In the United States, a high prevalence of SCCA has been concentrated in urban regions.[6a]

A number of theories have been proposed with varying levels of support to explain these geographic and regional differences. These have included genetic predisposition, dietary habits, environmental exposures, and alcohol and tobacco use. There is a male predominance, and most patients seek treatment in the 6th or 7th decade of life. In the ethnically diverse United States, the incidence among black men is higher than that of any other ethnic group.

DIET AND NUTRITION. Dietary habits and nutritional deficits have been associated with SCCA of the esophagus. SCCA appears more prevalent in populations in whom the staple food diets are deficient in vitamins and minerals, although no single nutrient deficiency or group deficiency has been identified as a specific cause. Nitrosamines may be concentrated in diets as a result of food selections, methods of preparation, and methods of storage. Nitrosamines have been linked to SCCA in Linxian Province, China. Fungi present in the soil, grains and cereals in that region are thought to catalyze the reduction of nitrates to nitrosamines. Some new evidence[6b] suggests that polyaromatic hydrocarbons given off from coal that is used to cook in unventilated kitchen areas may pose a risk and may explain the high cancer incidence in women in this area who do not smoke cigarettes. Links have been drawn to the development of SCCA of the esophagus in humans and pharyngeal SCCA in domestic fowl in these regions.[7, 8] Other causes proposed for the populations of Iran and Turkey include the drinking of very hot tea or coffee and chewing of sunflower seeds. Finally, chewing of "betel quid," popular among millions of Southeast Asians, has similarly had an associated risk suggested.[9]

ALCOHOL AND TOBACCO. Alcohol and tobacco, alone or in combination, are linked to SCCA. With respect to alcohol the risk is directly related to the quantity and type consumed. Distilled spirits are associated with the highest risk. Paradoxically, wine is the preferred alcoholic beverage in the high-incidence regions in Italy and France. France has the highest per capita consumption of alcohol in the Western world, as well as the highest incidence of SCCA. Similarly, states and regions in the United States that have high alcohol use have a high prevalence of SCCA. The causal relationship is unclear. Nitrosamines are found in alcohol. Beer has the highest concentrations, yet its link to SCCA is weakest. Nutritional deficiencies associated with chronic alcohol abuse have been given strong consideration. Although a poor diet may increase the alcohol-associated risk, a good diet may not reduce or eliminate it.[10, 11]

The use of tobacco in all forms, including cigarettes,

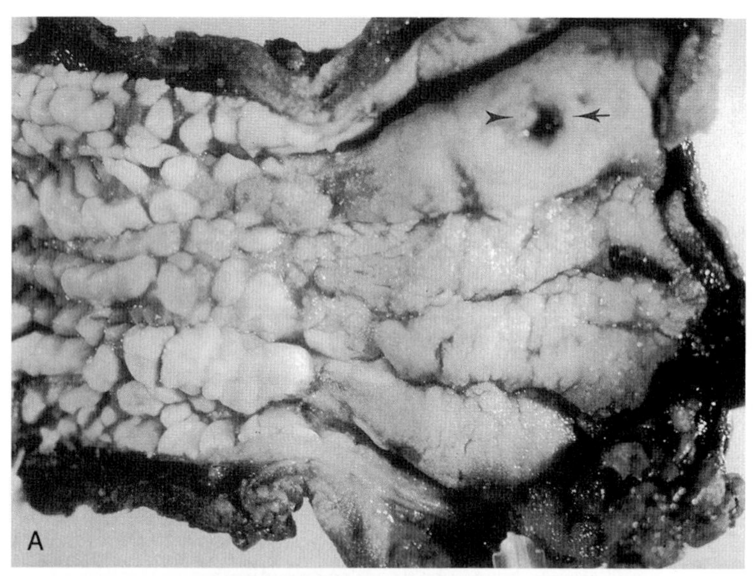

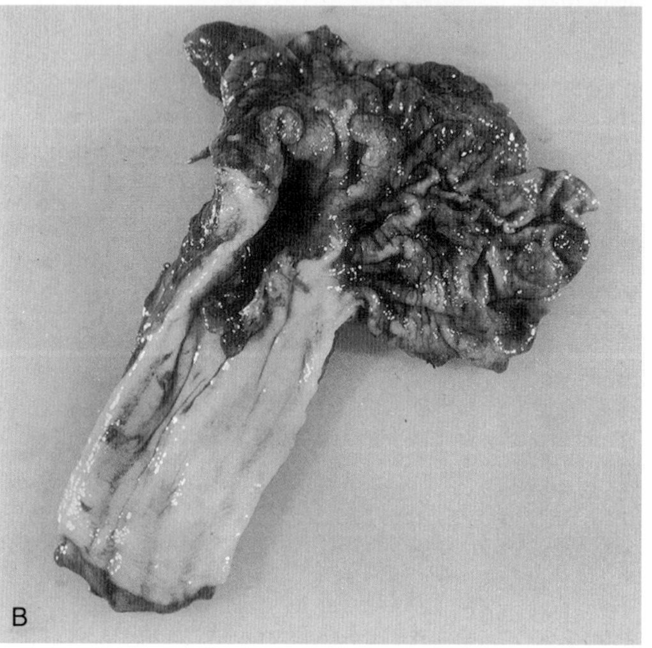

Figure 35–1. *A,* Gross photograph of a distal esophagectomy specimen. The normal white squamous epithelium, shown on the left, has been replaced by metaplastic Barrett's epithelium on the right. Note the small, irregular ulcer (*arrows*), which represents a focus of adenocarcinoma. *B,* Resected specimen of distal esophagus and proximal stomach in a patient with Barrett's esophagus. Note the large, irregular, ulcerating adenocarcinoma, which involves a small portion of proximal stomach.

pipes, cigars, and chewing tobacco, is associated with increased risk of SCCA. Nitrosamines concentrated in tobacco products have also been implicated.[12]

HIGH-RISK DISEASES. There are a number of conditions that appear to increase the risk of SCCA of the esophagus. Patients who have long-standing achalasia appear to be at increased risk of development of SCCA of the esophagus (see Chapter 32). A 20-year interval from the time of diagnosis of achalasia to the development of SCCA has been reported for both treated and untreated achalasia. The time lag from diagnosis to cancer was the same for those treated with pneumatic dilation and surgical myotomy. The incidence of SCCA in achalasia patients has been estimated at 340 per 100,000, which is significantly greater than that expected among the general population.[13] Another study reported a 16-fold greater risk of development of SCCA among achalasia patients compared with the general population.[14] Periodic endoscopic surveillance should be considered for patients who have long-standing achalasia, though the cost effectiveness of such measures is questionable. It is hypothesized that stasis due to aperistalsis and hypertensive lower esophageal sphincter leads to prolonged contact of noxious substances with the epithelial surface of the esophagus. No discrete biochemical promoter has been identified.

Patients with long-standing caustic strictures due to lye ingestion appear at increased risk of development of SCCA (see Chapter 34) 4 to 5 decades after the initial injury.[15] In addition to the food stasis that such chronic strictures are likely to promote, chronic inflammation and epithelial hyperplasia associated with the initial injury may contribute as well. Surveillance may be considered in selected patients, but its efficacy is unproved.

A syndrome linking esophageal webs and iron deficiency anemia along with a variety of other epithelial lesions is called the *Plummer-Vinson syndrome* in the United States and *Patterson-Kelly syndrome* in the United Kingdom.[16] The associated epithelial findings include spoon shaped or concave fingernails and angular stomatitis. It has been suggested that patients with this rare syndrome are at increased risk of development of SCCA of the esophagus. The iron deficiency anemia appears unrelated to the malignancy.

Tylosis, a rare autosomal dominant disease marked by hyperkeratosis of the palms of the hands and the soles of the feet (see Chapter 18), is associated with a high incidence of SCCA.[17] In up to 95% of tylosis patients squamous cell carcinoma of the esophagus develops by age 65. In addition to screening of patients by periodic endoscopy other members of the kindred may also benefit from endoscopic surveillance.

Historically, 0.7% to 10.4% of SCCA patients have had previous partial gastrectomy.[18] It is difficult to separate out confounding factors of nutritional deficiencies and cigarette smoking. There are no established recommendations for surveillance for SCCA of the esophagus among patients who have undergone partial gastrectomy.

A history or concurrent diagnosis of squamous cell carcinoma in the head or neck region is highly associated with SCCA of the esophagus. Patients in whom a laryngo-oropharyngeal tumor is diagnosed, particularly those with a history of alcohol and tobacco use, should have endoscopy in order to screen for early esophageal SCCA.

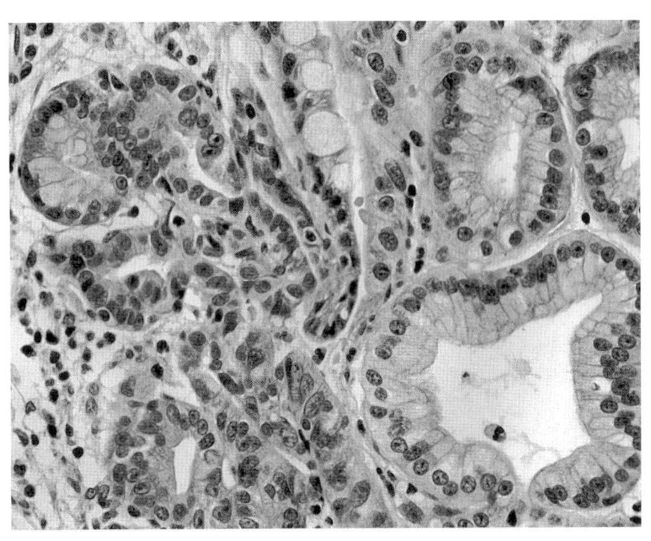

Figure 35–2. Histopathology of adenocarcinoma arising in Barrett's epithelium. Photograph shows a moderately differentiated adenocarcinoma. Note the small focus of specialized columnar epithelium characterized by globlet cells. Note also three non-metaplastic glands on the right, which probably represent normal cardiac glands.

Esophageal dysplasia and SCCA have been associated with the human papillomavirus (HPV). The virus has been observed to affect the squamous epithelial cells with subsequent replication and production of oncogene proteins that contribute to malignant transformation.[19] The same process has been observed to a lesser degree with Epstein-Barr virus.[20]

In contrast to adenocarcinoma of the esophagus, no relationship appears to exist between SCCA of the esophagus and gastroesophageal reflux, Barrett's esophagus, body mass index, or *Helicobacter pylori* infection.

Adenocarcinoma of the Esophagus and Esophagogastric Junction

(Figs. 35–1 and 35–2)

In Western societies, SCCA of the esophagus occurs more commonly in blacks, and adenocarcinoma (AdenoCA) of the esophagus and EG junction occurs predominantly in white men. In another contrast to SCCA of the esophagus, AdenoCA of the esophagus does not appear to be related to alcohol use, and studies on smoking have yielded conflicting results.[21–24]

GASTROESOPHAGEAL REFLUX. In response to mucosal injury, predominantly due to acid reflux, the normal squamous epithelium of the esophagus may be replaced by columnar epithelium of the specialized intestinal type, as reviewed in Chapter 33. Most if not all AdenoCA of the esophagus and EG junction arises from specialized intestinal metaplasia. Not surprisingly then, a history of gastroesophageal reflux is associated with AdenoCA of the esophagus and EG junction.[25] The results of a population based, case controlled study from Sweden strongly suggest that symptomatic gastroesophageal reflux is a risk factor for esophageal AdenoCA. The frequency, severity, and duration of reflux symptoms have been correlated with increased risk of esophageal AdenoCA.[25]

BARRETT'S ESOPHAGUS. Recent investigations[25a] in the United States have suggested that the annual incidence of cancer in Barrett's esophagus is 0.5% to 0.8% (one case/100 to 200 patient-years). This represents a 30- to 60-fold increased risk when compared with that of the general population. Barrett's esophagus has been stratified into three categories. *Long-segment Barrett's* esophagus arbitrarily designates those patients in whom the histologic squamocolumnar junction extends 3 cm or more above the anatomic EG junction determined endoscopically. *Short-segment Barrett's* designates those patients with less than 3 cm of specialized intestinal metaplasia extending above the gastroesophageal junction. When the EG junction and squamocolumnar junction are in the same location (that is, no endoscopically recognizable Barrett's) and specialized intestinal metaplasia is detected on biopsy specimens taken from or just below the squamocolumnar junction, this entity represents *specialized intestinal metaplasia of the EG junction* (see Chapter 33).

Barrett's esophagus is present in approximately 5% to 15% of persons who have elective upper endoscopy for any clinical indication. Short-segment Barrett's esophagus and specialized intestinal metaplasia at the EG junction are much more prevalent than long-segment Barrett's esophagus. Studies show that there is an increased risk, albeit small, of neoplastic progression with increasing Barrett's segment length.[26] Nonetheless, the risk for esophageal AdenoCA is present in patients with short-segment Barrett's at a risk level not substantially lower than that for patients with longer segments. Although the likelihood of dysplasia and cancer associated with specialized intestinal metaplasia at the EG junction is low, the overall prevalence of specialized intestinal metaplasia at the EG junction is high. The total of patients with short-segment Barrett's esophagus and those with specialized intestinal metaplasia at the EG junction is much greater than the total number of long-segment Barrett's esophagus patients (conservatively, seven times greater). These figures may help to explain the rising prevalence and incidence of AdenoCA at the EG junction.

In addition to segment length, other features associated with an increased risk of development of AdenoCA arising from Barrett's esophagus include the presence of a hiatal hernia, increased body mass index, and perhaps the use of drugs that as a secondary effect contribute to lower esophageal sphincter relaxation.[27–30]

HELICOBACTER PYLORI. An inverse relationship between *Helicobacter pylori* infection, or conversely its eradication, and the risk for development of AdenoCA of the esophagus in the EG junction has been described. This relationship suggests that *H. pylori* infection may be protective against Barrett's esophagus and its associated AdenoCA. The prevalence of the more virulent cagA+ strain of *H. pylori* was decreased in patients with more severe complications of gastroesophageal reflux disease (GERD).[31] In addition, the odds of having Barrett's esophagus complicated by dysplasia or cancer were reduced more than twofold in patients infected with a cagA+ strain compared with other groups. The protective effect of cagA+ strain has been demonstrated to be maintained irrespective of Barrett's esophagus segment length.[32, 33]

Biology and Genetics

The progression from basal cell hyperplasia and varying degrees of dysplasia to the development of invasive SCCA is variable and may be of long duration, as early premalignant stages may persist for 20 years or more. Regression from severe to mild dysplasia or no dysplasia may be seen. However, progression to carcinoma is more likely. The rate of progression may vary as a result of tissue sampling limitations and environmental and genetic factors. Similarly the progression from specialized intestinal metaplasia, to varying grades of dysplasia, and finally to invasive AdenoCA is variable.

As in other cancers of the digestive tract, SCCA of the esophagus is thought to be due in part to the accumulation of alterations in oncogenes, tumor suppressor genes, and deoxyribonucleic acid (DNA) mismatch repair genes. Certainly environmental factors play a role in mitigating the genetic alterations. Cyclin D1, the oncogene most closely associated with esophageal SCCA pathogenesis, is one of a family of cell cycle regulatory proteins. Cyclin D1 is overexpressed in cancers, especially those of squamous epithelial origin, and is overexpressed in up to 50% of esophageal SCCA and associated with a poor prognosis.[34, 35] A knowledge of the association of cyclin D1 with esophageal cancer has been used to develop a transgenic mouse model.[36]

Knowledge of the progression from intestinal metaplasia to AdenoCA has similarly benefitted from valuable information about tumor initiation extrapolated from rare inherited syndromes of familial gastrointestinal (GI) and specifically gastroesophageal cancers.[37] The p53 gene is a key tumor suppressor gene important to cell cycle regulation. The gene is mutated up to 70% of esophageal cancers.[38] The E-cadherin molecule also plays a role as a tumor suppressor gene. Inherited germline mutations of the E-cadherin gene lead to loss of E-cadherin expression. Loss of the adhesion molecules on the surface membranes of cancer cells makes them far more likely to have invasive properties. Furthermore, when E-cadherin expression is reduced, there is increased activation of target oncogenes such as cyclooxygenase-2 (COX-2) and c-myc that may induce proliferation.[39]

Abnormal variants of the interleukin-1 gene are associated with an increased risk of development of cancer in the gastric cardia.[40] It has been hypothesized that identification of E-cadherin mutations and interleukin-1 polymorphisms may make possible screening of individuals with intestinal metaplasia in whom invasive carcinoma is more likely to develop.[41] Furthermore, this association has led to speculation that anti-inflammatory drugs such as cyclooxygenase inhibitors may provide a means of medical intervention.[41]

Clinical Presentation

SCCA occurs predominantly in the middle and upper thirds of the esophagus. AdenoCA occurs predominantly in the distal third of the esophagus and at the EG junction. There is no clear-cut separation between AdenoCA of the distal esophagus and AdenoCA of the EG junction. In many instances it is difficult or impossible to categorize tumors in this region as primary gastric cardia cancers extending proximally versus true EG junction carcinomas versus lower esophageal carcinomas extending distally.

Dysphagia is the most common symptom (90%), followed by odynophagia (50%). Up to 75% of patients have experienced anorexia and weight loss when they seek medical attention. In part as a result of luminal compromise, most patients have altered their diets considerably during the months before consulting a physician. The presence of odynophagia coincides with an ulcerated tumor. Chest pain or pain radiating to the back is a particularly sinister symptom, in that it implies invasion into neuromediastinal structures.

Advanced lesions typically appear endophytic as polypoid, fungating, or ulcerated masses. Lesions may be eccentric or circumferential. Both tumor types may also exhibit an infiltrative submucosal spreading process with no appreciable intraluminal mass. Tumors that show these characteristics may defy a histologic diagnosis by endoscopic biopsy forceps tissue sampling. When this process occurs at the EG junction, it may mimic achalasia and is therefore termed *pseudoachalasia* (see Chapter 37).

SCCA of the esophagus is an aggressively invasive tumor. Vocal cord paralysis accompanies recurrent laryngeal nerve invasion. Cough or recurrent pneumonia may indicate chronic aspiration as a result of esophageal obstruction or esophagorespiratory fistula due to direct tumor extension. Esophagorespiratory fistulas occur in 5% of patients. The development of an esophagorespiratory fistula confers a particularly poor prognosis with a median survival time of 1.5 to 4 months.[42] Pulmonary, hepatic, bone, and brain metastasis may all be observed at presentation or during tumor progression. Hematemesis may be due to tumor ulceration. Exsanguinating bleeds occur with the development of an aortaesophageal fistula. AdenoCAs are not similarly locally invasive, and esophagorespiratory fistulas are uncommon in AdenoCA. Lymphangitic and hematogenous metastases, however, do occur early to regional and distant lymph nodes and to the liver. Patients with advanced esophageal carcinoma succumb to widespread metastases and direct complications of bleeding and respiratory compromise.

Most patients have advanced disease at the time of symptom presentation because the esophagus has a rich lymphovascular supply and lacks a serosal lining. The absence of a serosa enables tumors to expand into surrounding tissue before luminal stenosis becomes symptomatic. Lymph node metastasis occurs early and almost uniformly. The rich lymphovascular network promotes lymphovascular metastases even among tumors confined to the esophageal wall. Tumors limited to the mucosa have lymph node metastases in approximately 3% of cases. However, once the tumor has penetrated the muscularis mucosa and invaded the submucosa, lymph node metastases are documented in 30% of cases, and when into the muscularis propria, in 60% of cases. Most patients have tumors that have invaded through the muscularis propria into the periesophageal fat (T3), wherein the rate of lymph node metastasis is considered nearly universal (see Table 35–1). Micrometastases are detectable in bone marrow from resected rib segments in almost 90% of patients with EG carcinoma selected for curative esophagectomy.[43] When present, this feature best predicted prognosis by multivariate analysis. These findings help to explain the high rate of recurrent disease even among those patients in whom no lymph node metastases are detected at the time of esophageal resection.

Table 35–1 | **Tumor, Node, Metastasis Definitions Used to Stage Cancer of the Esophagus***

Primary tumor (T)
TX: Primary tumor cannot be assessed
T0: No evidence of primary tumor
Tis: Carcinoma is situ
T1: Tumor invades lamina propria (T1a) or submucosa (T1b)
T2: Tumor invades muscularis propria
T3: Tumor invades adventitia
T4: Tumor invades adjacent structures
Regional lymph nodes (N)
NX: Regional lymph nodes cannot be assessed
N0: No regional lymph node metastasis
N1: Regional lymph node metastasis
Distant metastasis (M)
MX: Distant metastasis cannot be assessed
M0: No distant metastasis
M1: Distant metastasis
Tumors of the lower thoracic esophagus
M1a: Metastasis in celiac lymph nodes
M1b: Other distant metastasis
Tumors of the midthoracic esophagus
M1a: Not applicable
M1b: Nonregional lymph nodes and/or other distant metastasis
Tumors of the upper thoracic esophagus
M1a: Metastasis in cervical nodes
M1b: Other distant metastasis

*The American Joint Committee on Cancer (AJCC) staging system is based on the tumor, node, metastasis (TNM) classification shown in Table 35–2.

From American Joint Committee on Cancer: Esophagus. In AJCC Cancer Staging Manual, 5th ed. Philadelphia, Lippincott-Raven, 1997, p 65.

Diagnosis

Patients who exhibit symptoms suggestive of esophageal carcinoma may appear chronically ill with weight loss and loss of muscle mass. Otherwise there are no specific physical findings. Palpable peripheral lymph nodes are uncommon. Hepatomegaly may be appreciated when multiple hepatic metastases are present. Laboratory results may indicate hypoalbuminemia and anemia secondary to bleeding or chronic disease. Hypercalcemia due to bony metastases or circulating humoral factors such as parathyroid hormone (PTH)-related peptide in SCCA has been reported in 15% to 30% of patients.[44] Liver-associated enzymes, including alkaline phosphatase, and the prothrombin time may be elevated in the setting of hepatic metastases. There are no specific serologic markers that correlate with esophageal carcinoma.

Radiography

Posteroanterior (PA) and lateral chest radiography is indicated in patients with chronic cough and abnormal findings of auscultative examination of the chest to demonstrate pulmonary metastases and/or infiltrates suggestive of aspiration or esophagorespiratory fistula. Findings may also include lateral deviation of the mediastinal contents, widening of the mediastinum, and esophageal air-fluid levels.

Contrast esophagography is indicated in selected patients. Barium swallow radiography details high-grade stenoses, complete obstruction, and fistulas. As endoscopy is generally indicated irrespective of radiographic findings in patients who are suspected of having esophageal carcinoma, esophagography should be limited to those patients in whom findings are likely to affect management. Contrast radiographic studies should be used to confirm or refute suspected esophagorespiratory fistula and complete obstruction (Fig. 35–3). In this context, barium is generally the preferred contrast agent, as opposed to diatrizoate meglumine (gastrografin), which may cause pulmonary inflammation or edema if aspirated. Computed tomographic (CT) scanning of the chest and upper abdomen is indicated to assess for lymph node, pulmonary, and hepatic metastases. The primary tumor is seen as a low-density soft tissue mass arising in the region of the esophagus. The length and direct extent of the tumor may be assessed as well.

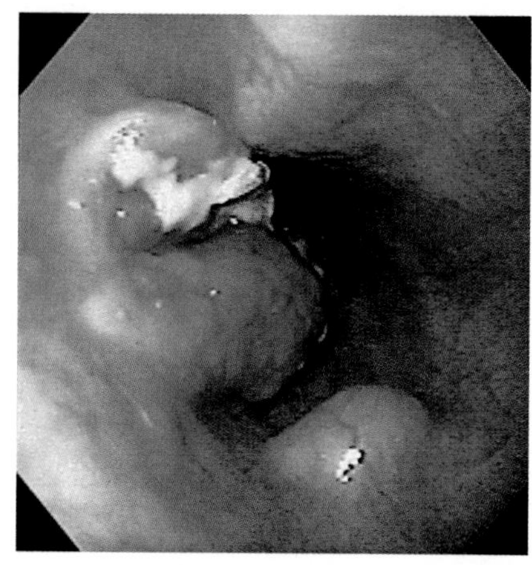

Figure 35–4. Squamous cell carcinoma of the esophagus. (From Wilcox CM: Atlas of Clinical Gastrointestinal Endoscopy. Philadelphia, WB Saunders, 1995, p 39.)

Endoscopy

Flexible endoscopy is indicated in suspected esophageal carcinoma. Endoscopy allows direct visualization of the esophagus as well as tissue sampling to confirm the diagnosis. Endoscopy allows accurate characterization of the tumor's configuration, length, and localization (Fig. 35–4). Endoscopy also allows initial relief of dysphagia in that dilation can be performed at the time of diagnosis.

Standard endoscopic forceps biopsy typically yields a diagnosis. Brush cytology may be used as a complementary technique to enhance the yield in establishing a diagnosis. Biopsy procedures should be directed at non-necrotic areas. At least six biopsy samples should be obtained to yield an accuracy approaching 100%.[45] Occasionally submucosal spreading tumors require endoscopic ultrasound (EUS)-guided fine-needle aspiration for histologic diagnosis when standard forceps biopsies fail. (The role of EUS for staging esophogeal cancers is discussed later.)

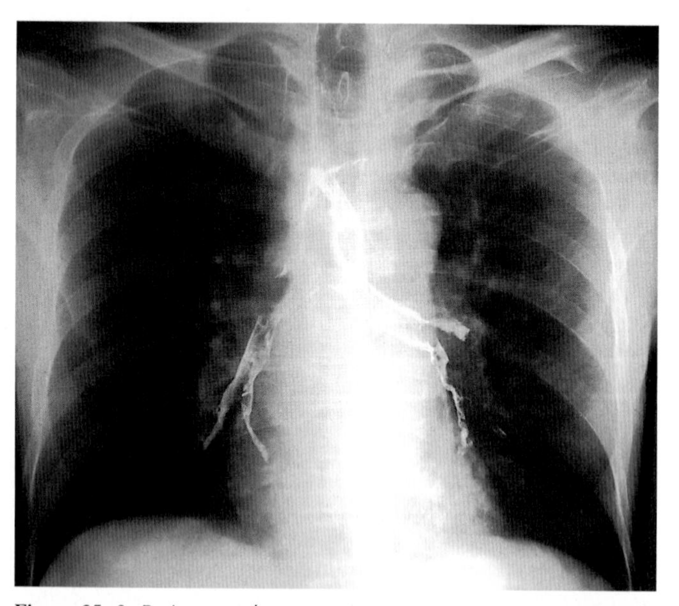

Figure 35–3. Barium esophagogram in a patient complaining of cough and dysphagia demonstrates complete esophageal obstruction and an esophagotracheal fistula. Note the presence of ingested barium seen in bilateral airways.

Screening

There is no evidence to establish that screening would result in a decrease in the mortality rate from esophageal cancer in the U.S. population. However, surveillance of high-risk groups is appealing because of the overall poor prognosis of esophageal cancer that presents with symptoms. Early lesions are more likely to be asymptomatic. They may be identified during endoscopic evaluation for unrelated or vague symptoms or as part of a surveillance program in patients with high-risk conditions. Early lesions may demonstrate only mild irregularity of the normal esophagus (in the case of SCCA) or of Barrett's esophageal mucosa (in the case of AdenoCA), including focal erythema, nodularity, elevation, or ulceration.

Early detection of SCCA or dysplastic squamous epithelium may be enhanced with vital staining. Diluted Lugol's solution delivered endoscopically through a spray catheter has been most widely used.[46] Lugol's solution is rapidly taken up by normal squamous mucosa, in contrast with dysplastic squamous epithelium, which remains unstained (Fig. 35–5). This technique may also be applied to detect the extent of mucosal surface involvement when endoscopic therapy is being contemplated for macroscopically recognized lesions. Tissue sampling from the unstained areas confirms the presence and extent of mucosal involvement.[47]

Endoscopic surveillance is recommended in patients with Barrett's esophagus in an effort to identify early carcinoma. The outcomes of patients diagnosed with cancer associated with Barrett's esophagus who were undergoing endoscopic surveillance were markedly improved compared with those of patients who had no surveillance.[48] Improved survival rates can be attributed to a shift in the diagnosis of the disease to an earlier stage. Specific recommendations for endoscopic surveillance for patients with Barrett's esophagus are covered elsewhere (see Chapter 33).

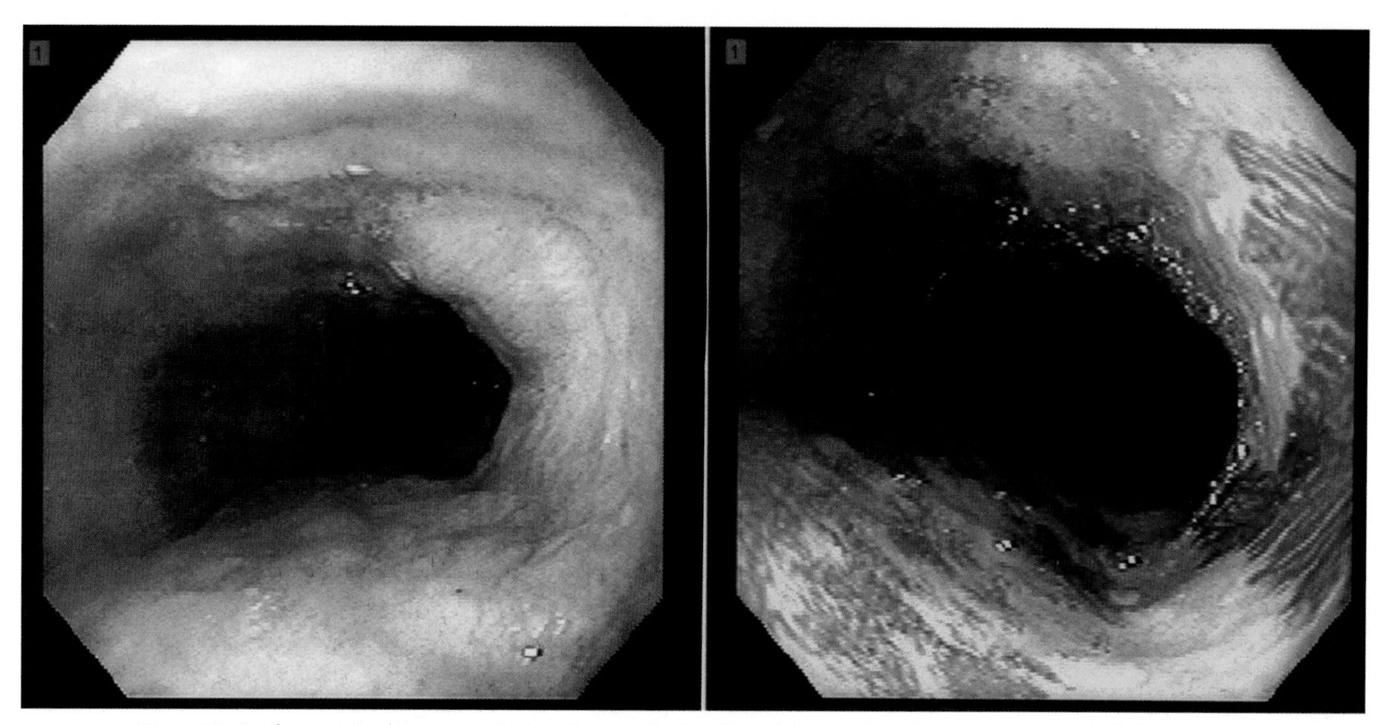

Figure 35–5. The unstained image on the left shows only slightly nodular esophageal mucosa. Biopsies had demonstrated squamous cell carcinoma in situ. After Lugol's staining, the image on the right demonstrates broad areas of unstained mucosa, allowing targeted sampling or therapy of dysplastic epithlium.

Attempts to apply vital staining and chromoendoscopic techniques to distinguish focal high-grade dysplasia (HGD) or invasive carcinoma within fields of Barrett's esophagus have been less rewarding. Methylene blue dye staining has been demonstrated to be useful in the detection of specialized columnar epithelium, but its accuracy in detecting neoplastic changes has not been confirmed consistently.[49]

Nonendoscopic balloon cytologic evaluation is an attractive alternative to endoscopic surveillance in high-risk groups because it may reduce surveillance costs many times. Nonendoscopic balloon cytologic evaluation has been used with success in populations with a high risk of SCCA of the esophagus in China. By using a latex balloon covered with nylon mesh advanced into the cardia and withdrawn through the esophagus, squamous cells are retrieved for cytologic analysis (Fig. 35–6). Among 500,000 Chinese who had balloon cytologic screening, this technique had 90% accuracy in detection of cancer. Among lesions detected, 70% to 80% were early lesions.[50] However, widespread balloon screening has not been demonstrated to be effective in other populations and does not appear feasible even in high-risk U.S. populations because the rarity of the disease and high rate of false-positive findings contribute to its lack of cost-effectiveness.

Nonendoscopic balloon cytologic examination in Barrett's esophagus has been evaluated. When balloon cytologic examination was compared with endoscopic brush cytologic evaluation, adequate columnar epithelium was obtained in 52 of 63 (83%) patients by balloon cytologic evaluation and 59 of 61 (97%) by brush cytologic evaluation.[51] Balloon cytologic evaluation yielded abnormal cells in six of eight patients with AdenoCA, two of two patients with HGD, and two of eight patients with low-grade dysplasia. Sensitivity of balloon cytologic evaluation for HGD or carcinoma was 80% but only 25% for low-grade dysplasia. No patients without dysplasia or carcinoma had abnormal cells. Findings of brush cytologic evaluation were abnormal in all 11 patients with HGD or carcinoma but in only 2 of 9 patients with low-grade dysplasia (sensitivity, 22%). Two of 39 patients without dysplasia had abnormal cells (specificity, 95%). Balloon cytologic evaluation was six times less costly than endoscopy with biopsy. The potential cost savings of balloon cytologic evaluation compared with endoscopic can-

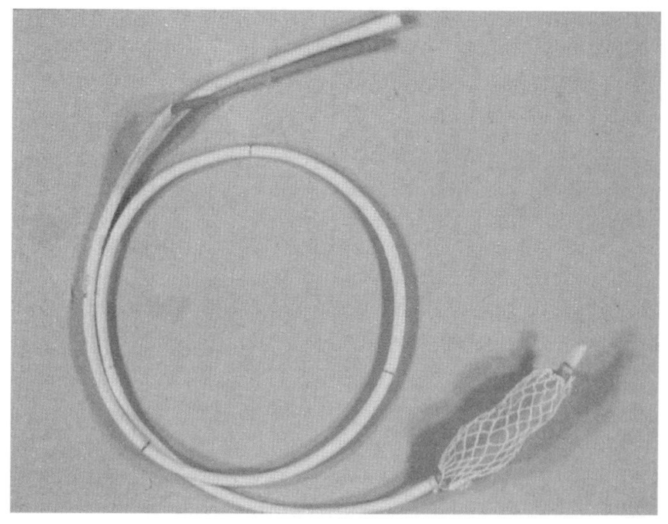

Figure 35–6. Cytology balloon used for mass screening in China.

Table 35–2 | **Recommendations for Therapy of Esophageal Cancer Based on Stage**

AJCC STAGE GROUPINGS	THERAPIES
Stage 0 Tis, N0, M0	Surgery Endoscopic mucosal resection* Photodynamic therapy*
Stage I T1, N0, M0	Surgery Endoscopic mucosal resection* Photodynamic therapy*
Stage IIA T2, N0, M0 T3, N0, M0	Surgery Chemotherapy plus radiation therapy with or without subsequent surgery
Stage IIB T1, N1, M0 T2, N1, M0	Surgery Chemotherapy plus radiation therapy with or without subsequent surgery
Stage III T3, N1, M0 T4, any N, M0	Surgical resection of T3 lesions Chemotherapy plus radiation therapy with or without subsequent surgery Palliation†
Stage IV Any T, any N, M1	Palliation†
Stage IVA Any T, any N, M1a	Palliation†
Stage IVB Any T, any N, M1b	Palliation†

*Under clinical evaluation.
†May include external beam radiation therapy, brachytherapy, systemic chemotherapy, combination radiation therapy and chemotherapy, and endoscopic dilation, intubation, photodynamic therapy, and laser, contact thermal, and injection ablative therapies.
From Esophageal Cancer (PDQ) Treatment—Health Professionals, CancerNet: National Cancer Institute's Comprehensive Cancer Database. Available at http://cancernet.nci.nih.gov/pdqfull.html

cer surveillance in Barrett's esophagus support further studies of this technique.

Staging of Esophageal Cancers

Outcome and treatment options are largely stage dependent. Therefore, accurate staging at the time of diagnosis is important to prediction of prognosis and critical to selection from among treatment options in the individualization of management. Tumor stage determines whether the intent of therapy is curative or palliative (see Tables 35–1 and 35–2). Patients who have stage T1 or T2, TN0, TM0, or lower-stage tumors have acceptable surgical cure rates. Patients with more advanced tumors (T3 or N1) are still potentially curable but do poorly with surgery alone. These patients may benefit from multimodality therapy. Patients with local invasion into surrounding vital structures (aorta, airway, pleura, and spine) and those with evidence of hematogenous metastatic spread should be treated with palliation alone.

The American Joint Committee on Cancer (AJCC) has designated staging by tumor, node, metastasis (TNM) classification (see Table 35–1).[52] The extent of tumor invasion has substantial impact on the 5-year survival rate: T1 = 46%; T2 = 30%; T3 = 22%; T4 = 7%.[53] Among patients with surgically resectable tumors, the 5-year survival rate is 40% for node-negative status compared with only 17% for N1 status. Among patients with metastasis to distant lymph nodes and solid organs, the 5-year survival rates are 5.2% and 3%, respectively. Among patients with complete surgical pathologic staging, 5-year survival rates for stages I, II, III, and IV are 60%, 31%, 20%, and 4%, respectively.

The current staging system for esophageal cancer is based largely on retrospective data from the Japanese Committee for Registration of Esophageal Carcinoma.[54] The system is most applicable to patients with SCCA of the upper and middle thirds of the esophagus, as opposed to the increasingly common distal esophageal and EG junction AdenoCA.[55] In particular, the classification of involved abdominal lymph nodes as M1 disease has been criticized. For tumors of midthoracic esophagus the M1b designation should be used only, because these tumors with metastasis to nonregional lymph nodes have a poor prognosis equal to that of those with metastasis in other distant sites. The presence of positive abdominal lymph node findings does not appear to carry as grave a prognosis as metastases to distant organs.[56] Patients with regional and/or celiac axis lymphadenopathy should not necessarily be considered to have unresectable disease as a result of metastases as occasionally long-term survival is evidenced. Complete resection of the primary tumor and appropriate lymphadenectomy should be considered in suitable operative candidates.

Cross-Sectional Imaging Studies

CT and magnetic resonance imaging (MRI) are highly effective in identifying solid organ metastases when these lesions are larger than 5 to 10 mm. The accuracy of CT detection of liver metastases is as high as 94%. Although CT can recognize soft tissue abnormalities (Fig. 35–7), it is less accurate in the cervical and lower esophageal regions than in the middle portion of the esophagus.[57] CT is much less accurate in detecting lymph node metastases and is more accurate for subdiaphragmatic lymph nodes than for mediastinal ones. MRI can assess mediastinal invasion and liver metastasis as

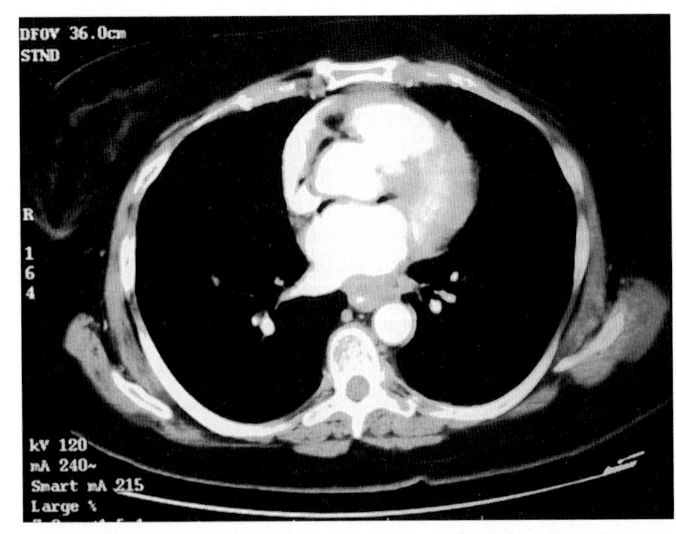

Figure 35–7. CT scan in a patient with a distal esophageal tumor demonstrates soft tissue thickening at the tumor location. While CT scanning is effective for detection of distant metastasis, it does not allow accurate local tumor staging.

well as CT can but has not demonstrated any significant advantages. Because of accessibility and its lower cost, CT is preferred.

Positron Emission Tomography

Positron emission tomography (PET) holds promise as a staging tool in esophageal cancer patients. Whole-body PET scan, acquired after injection of fludeoxyglucose F 18 and evaluated for areas of increased focal uptake, has been compared with surgical staging of patients with potentially resectable esophageal cancer.[58] For distant metastases, the sensitivity was 88%, the specificity was 93%, and the accuracy was 91% (Fig. 35–8). However, for local-regional nodal metastases, the sensitivity was 45%, the specificity was 100%, and the accuracy was 48%. In another study that compared PET with CT and EUS for local lymph node (LN), the sensitivity of PET was lower than that of EUS (33% vs. 81%), but the specificity may have been higher (89% vs. 67%).[59] PET did not detect four T1 cancers. For the assessment of regional and distant LN involvement, compared with the combined use of CT and EUS, PET had a higher specificity (90% vs. 98%, respectively) and a similar sensitivity (46% vs. 43%). PET significantly improves the detection of stage IV disease in esophageal cancer when compared with the conventional staging modalities and may improve the diagnostic specificity for LN staging. However, because PET is not yet widely available and is not routinely reimbursed by third party payers, its use in staging esophageal cancer has not become standard practice.

Endoscopic Ultrasonography

Endoscopic ultrasonography (EUS) staging of esophageal cancer has compared favorably with cross-sectional imaging modalities and is considered the most accurate tool for tumor staging. Most published series have used radial scanning echoendoscopes with 7.5- and 12-MHz-frequency transducers. A limited number of studies using linear array echoendoscopes have demonstrated comparable results.[60] Numerous studies have demonstrated the accuracy of EUS for local tumor and regional lymph node staging of esophageal cancer.[61] The overall accuracy for T stage is approximately 75% to 85% and for N stage 65% to 75% (Fig. 35–9). T stage accuracy is equivalent for both AdenoCA and SCCA.

EUS is most accurate in identifying T3 or T4 stage (Table 35–3). The designation of T2 stage is the least accurate: equal numbers of lesions are understaged and overstaged. EUS is the only staging modality effective in assessing T1 tumor stage. The most frequent contributors to inaccurate T staging are microscopic tumor invasion, peritumorous inflammatory changes, luminal stenosis, and oblique scanning artifacts. Obstructing tumors can be dilated to allow passage of the echoendoscope for complete EUS staging.[62, 63]

Overall EUS nodal staging is less accurate. EUS accuracy is best for periesophageal lymph nodes in the mediastinum and varies inversely with the axial distance of the nodes from the esophageal axis.[64] Efforts to develop objective criteria to distinguish malignant from benign lymph nodes seen by EUS have been disappointing. Features that have been associated with malignancy have included size greater than 1 cm, hypoechogenicity, distinct margins, and round shape.

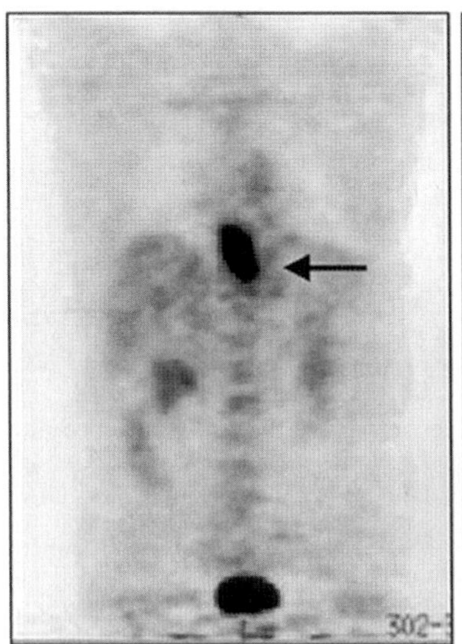

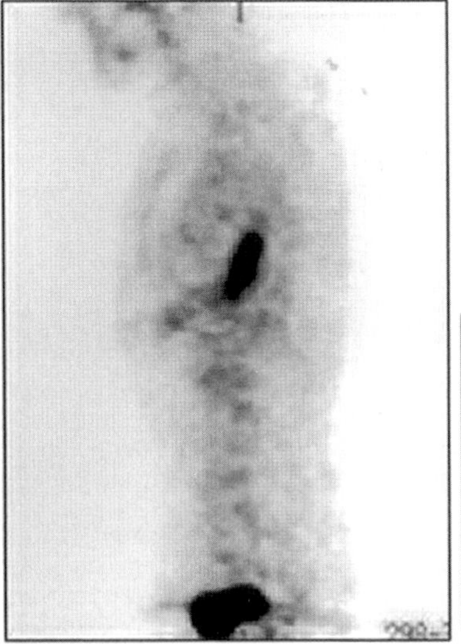

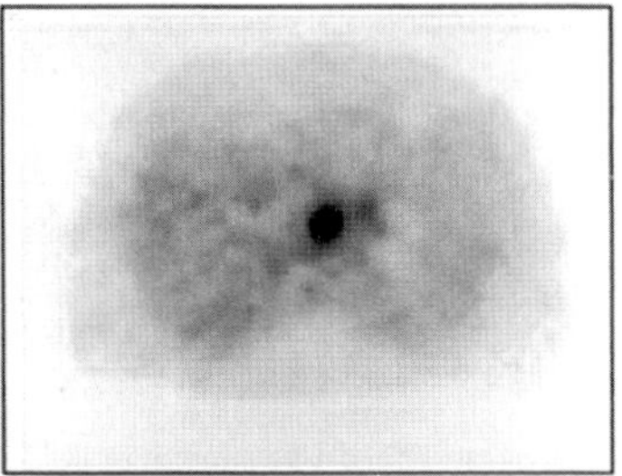

Figure 35–8. PET scan in patient with a distal esophageal carcinoma. The primary lesion is readily identified by focal uptake. There are no areas of focal uptake in the liver, but a small focus of increased uptake is seen adjacent to the primary tumor in the third panel, correlating with a regional lymph node metastasis. (Courtesy of Abas Alavi, M.D., Department of Nuclear Medicine, University of Pennsylvania Medical Center, Philadelphia.)

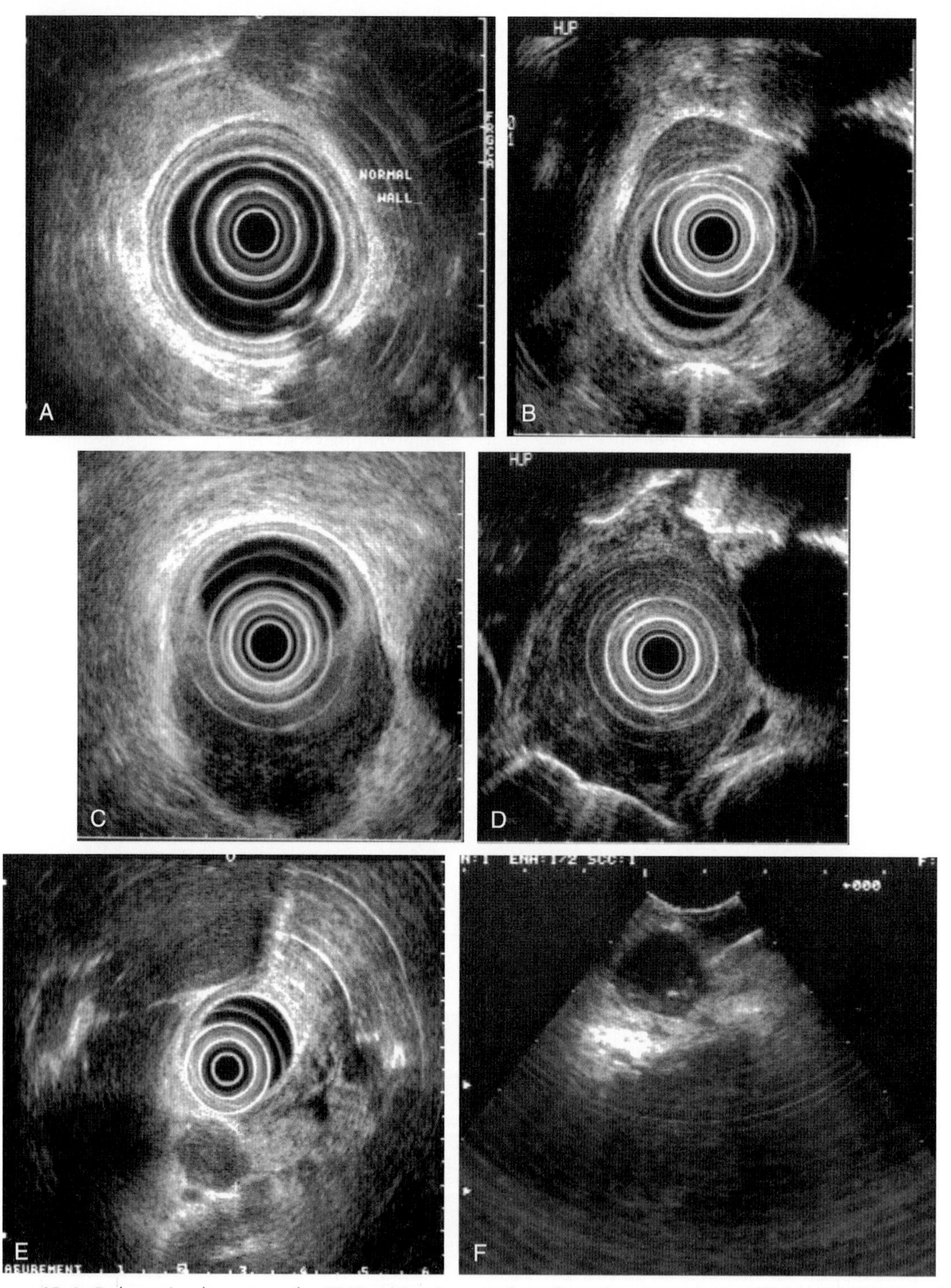

Figure 35–9. Endoscopic ultrasonography (EUS) staging images of esophageal tumors using a radial scanning echoendoscope: *A,* A T1 lesion is observed as a hypoechoic thickening of the mucosal layer adjacent to the normal-appearing wall pattern; *B,* a T2 lesion is seen as a hypoechoic mass invading into but not through the muscularis propria; *C,* a T3 lesion is seen as a hypoechoic mass (inferior) with an irregular margin extending into the periesophageal fat tissue and disrupting the normal wall layer pattern seen, in contrast, at the top of the image; *D,* the T4 lesion seen here is a circumferential hypoechoic mass with direct extension in the wall of the thoracic aorta (2 to 3 o'clock) and the right mainstem bronchus (6 to 8 o'clock), conferring unresectability; *E,* a typical malignant-appearing lymph node is greater than 1 cm in diameter, hypoechoic, and round, and has sharply demarcated borders. *F,* EUS-guided fine-needle aspiration performed using a linear array echoendoscope allows cytopathologic sampling to confirm lymph node metastases.

Table 35–3 | **Accuracy of Endoscopic Ultrasonography in the Local Tumor and Regional Lymph Node Staging of Esophageal Cancer, by Histopathologic Stage**

HISTOPATHOLOGIC STAGE	NUMBER	ACCURACY (%)
T1	185	81
T2	153	76
T3	419	92
T4	153	86
N0	231	69
N1	343	89

Adapted from Rosch T: Endosonographic staging of esophageal cancer: A review of the literature results. Gastrointest Endosc Clin N Am 5(3):537–548, 1995.

In a study by Bhutani and associates, no single feature independently predicted malignant status.[65] When all four features were present, the accuracy in predicting malignancy was 80%. However, these combined features were present in only 25% of the malignant lymph nodes observed.

EUS guided fine needle aspiration (FNA) has significantly improved the ability to confirm malignant adenopathy. The procedure has been demonstrated to be safe and effective for puncturing periesophageal mediastinal nodes as well as celiac lymph nodes.[66] High gastric lymph nodes are less commonly identified and are less accessible to the EUS guided FNA technique. When present, celiac lymph nodes are generally easily identified. For primary esophageal carcinoma, EUS guided FNA of periesophageal mediastinal nodes is curtailed by the focal presence of tumor. Only those lymph nodes to which the path of the needle avoids the primary tumor are suitable for FNA, as the passage of the needle through primary tumor en route to lymph node may contribute to false-positive sampling results. A meticulous evaluation of the false negative rate for this technique in esophageal carcinoma has not yet been reported.

IMPACT OF ENDOSCOPIC ULTRASOUND STAGING ON PATIENT OUTCOMES. In a retrospective multicenter analysis, the outcome of 79 patients with esophageal cancers staged as T4 by EUS was reported.[67] Two groups were distinguished, representing those who had operative or nonoperative therapy. Among those patients who had surgery, EUS was much more accurate than CT scanning in identifying tumor invasion (88% vs. 44%). The overall mortality rate was not significantly different in the operative and nonoperative groups: 60% of the surgical group and 65% of the nonsurgical group at the time of follow-up. This study supported the notion that EUS accurately identifies patients with advanced T4 tumors who have a poor prognosis and that prognosis is independent of mode of therapy. It should be noted that the operative group was significantly younger and had more distal esophageal AdenoCA than the nonoperative group.

Among patients who had locally or regionally advanced disease (T3 and/or N1) and for those with tumors limited to the wall (T1 to T2 and N0), the survival rate for patients in whom EUS was performed, in addition to other standard staging tests preoperatively, was higher than for patients who did not have EUS.[68] Among patients with tumors limited to the wall, EUS did not affect survival rates. Five-year survival rate was 60% in the EUS group and 70% in the non-EUS group. In patients with locally or regionally advanced disease, however, the EUS group had a significantly improved survival rate of 22% versus 10%. Patients who had undergone EUS as part of their preoperative staging were more likely to have received preoperative chemoradiotherapy and to have had negative surgical margins compared with the non-EUS group. Multivariate analysis identified preoperative chemoradiotherapy and negative surgical margins as predictors of improved survival rate.

In a prospective study of 204 consecutive patients, pretreatment EUS predicted long-term survival accurately on the basis of initial T stage and the presence of lymphadenopathy.[69] These findings did not vary with patient's age, gender, or histologic characteristics of tumor. The absence of detectable lymphadenopathy was the most important predictor of survival. Studies such as this highlight the value of including EUS in pretreatment staging of patients enrolled in clinical trials assessing multimodality therapy for esophageal cancer.

ENDOSCOPIC ULTRASOUND FOR RESTAGING AFTER NEOADJUVANT THERAPY. Although the broad application of neoadjuvant chemoradiotherapy for patients with esophageal cancer remains controversial, studies to date indicate that patients who demonstrate response with significant shrinkage or elimination of the primary tumor are more likely to have improved outcome and long-term survival. Isenberg and colleagues reaffirmed preliminary reports by others that accuracy of T staging by conventional criteria is poor (43%).[70] However, as a means of assessing response to therapy on the basis of reduction of maximal cross-sectional tumor area by 50%, responders could be discriminated from nonresponders. Further, 10 of 13 patients with at least a 50% reduction in maximal cross-sectional area had T0, T1 or T2 tumors at surgery, whereas 9 of 10 nonresponders had T3 or T4 tumors at surgery. These data support the role of EUS in the evaluation and management of patients who have multimodality therapy, particularly those enrolled in clinical trials. Assessment of response can be used to determine which patients are most likely to benefit from surgery versus a consideration of additional nonoperative therapy.

ENDOSCOPIC ULTRASOUND AS A PREDICTOR OF EARLY CANCERS. Promotion of endoscopic treatments for tumors limited to the mucosa, such as endoscopic mucosal resection and photodynamic therapy, has heightened the importance of accurate staging in candidate patients. For T1 esophageal lesions, EUS staging is particularly attractive. As esophageal lesions that have penetrated only into the submucosa still have malignant lymphadenopathy in up to 30% of cases, the challenge is to identify accurately those patients with lesions limited to the mucosal and submucosal layers who have node-negative results. It is critical, therefore, to be able to discern T1a from T1b tumors (see Table 35–1). The accuracy of EUS in predicting early stage esophageal cancer may be greater for AdenoCA than for SCCA.[71, 72]

As patients who have Barrett's esophagus and HGD may have unrecognized early carcinoma, EUS takes on an important role. The value of EUS for such patients has been controversial. A 1994 study by Falk and colleagues showed poor accuracy, including both overstaging and understaging.[73] However, we have demonstrated a high sensitivity, accuracy, and most importantly negative predictive value for submucosal invasion of esophageal cancer in the setting of Barrett's esophagus with HGD or intramucosal carcinoma.[74] These findings are most applicable for patients with macroscopically recognizable nodules in the Barrett's esophagus involved segment.

High-frequency (15-, 20-, and 30-MHz) catheter ultrasound miniprobes can be passed through the endoscope and placed over a small lesion under endoscopic guidance. These high-resolution images are likely to improve staging accuracy of superficial esophageal carcinoma.

Other Staging Modalities

Improved nodal staging accuracy has been demonstrated with the addition of laparoscopy and thoracoscopy for the identification of abdominal peritoneal lymph nodes and mediastinal lymph nodes[75] and of transcutaneous ultrasonography for the identification of cervical lymphadenopathy.[76]

Therapy

Outcome is tied to stage, and, therefore, treatment options are largely stage dependent (see Table35–2). Esophageal cancer is a treatable disease that is rarely curable. The overall 5-year survival rate in patients amenable to surgery ranges from 5% to 20%. The occasional patient with early disease has a better chance of survival. Patients with HGD in esophageal Barrett's mucosa often have coincident in situ cancer. After resection, these patients usually have an excellent prognosis.

Primary treatment modalities include surgery alone or chemotherapy with radiation therapy. Combined modality therapy (chemotherapy plus surgery, or chemotherapy and radiation therapy plus surgery) is under clinical evaluation. Endoscopic mucosal resection[77] and/or photodynamic therapy[78] in selected patients with superficial carcinoma is also under clinical evaluation. Effective palliation may be obtained in individual cases with various combinations of surgery, chemotherapy, radiation therapy, and endoscopic therapy.

Primary Therapy

SURGERY, RADIATION, AND CHEMOTHERAPIES. Surgery is the treatment of choice for early (superficial) tumors. Asymptomatic small tumors confined to the esophageal mucosa or submucosa are detected by chance or by surveillance of high-risk patients.[79] Endoscopic surveillance of patients with Barrett's esophagus may detect AdenoCA at an earlier stage more amenable to curative resection.[80] Stage 0 to Stage I esophageal SCCA is not usually seen in the United States. Surgery for these stages of cancer is used successfully in Asia. Once symptoms (dysphagia, in most cases) are present, esophageal cancers have usually invaded the muscularis propria or beyond and may have metastasized to lymph nodes or other organs.

Surgical treatment of resectable esophageal cancers results in 5-year survival rates of 5% to 20%; higher survival rates occur in patients with early stage cancers. This rate is associated with a 3% to 10% operative mortality rate.[81] Operative morbidity includes anastomotic leaks and strictures (~20%), and cardiopulmonary complications. There is controversy as to the optimal surgical procedure. One approach advocates transhiatal esophagectomy with anastomosis of the stomach to the cervical esophagus. A second approach advocates abdominal mobilization of the stomach and transthoracic excision of the esophagus with anastomosis of the stomach to the upper thoracic esophagus or the cervical esophagus. Combined thoracoscopic and laparoscopic esophagectomy techniques are under evaluation as means to decrease the trauma of surgery.

As an alternative to surgery, definitive radiation therapy in combination with chemotherapy has been studied. One series, evaluating radiation therapy and chemotherapy with fluorouracil and mitomycin, produced a 75% local control rate, associated with improved swallowing, and a 30% actuarial disease-free survival rate (18% overall survival) at 5 years for stage I and stage II patients.[82] A randomized trial of chemotherapy and radiation therapy versus radiation therapy alone showed an improvement in 5-year survival rate for the combined modality group (26% vs. 0%).[83] However, the morbidity rate was quite high in the combination therapy group. An Eastern Cooperative Oncology Group trial of 135 patients showed similar results, in that chemotherapy plus radiation yielded a better 2-year survival rate than radiation therapy alone.[84]

Neoadjuvant therapy is under evaluation as a means to increase operative resectability and improve long-term postoperative survival. A number of phase II studies have suggested an improved survival rate for induction chemoradiotherapy followed by resection when compared with that for surgery only historical controls.[84–90] Approximately 25% of patients have a complete response with no histologic evidence of cancer in the resected specimen, albeit in some series at the cost of increased postoperative morbidity and mortality rates. A multicenter prospective randomized trial compared preoperative combined chemotherapy (cisplatin) and radiation therapy (3700 cGy in 370-cGy fractions) followed by surgery with surgery alone in patients with SCCA and found no improvement in overall survival rate and a significantly higher postoperative mortality rate (12% vs. 4%) in the combined modality arm.[91] In patients with AdenoCA of the esophagus, a single-institution phase III trial demonstrated a modest survival benefit (16 months vs. 11 months) for patients treated with induction chemoradiotherapy consisting of 5-fluorouracil, cisplatin, and 4000 cGy (267-cGy fractions) plus surgery as opposed to treatment with resection alone.[92] The small sample size, short follow-up, early ending based on interim analysis, disproportionate number of patients withdrawn from the combined modality arm, and lack of stratification based on pretreatment stage are some of the concerns regarding this trial. Therefore, the role of combined modality therapy remains unproved. The results of a national study showed no statistically significant difference in disease-free or overall survival rate for preoperative and postoperative chemotherapy alone versus surgery alone for AdenoCA or SCCA of the esophagus.[93] A summary of trials comparing combined chemoradiotherapy plus surgery with surgery alone is displayed in Table 35–4. The use of pretreatment EUS for staging was limited or absent in these studies, so the impact of staging inaccuracy is uncer-

Table 35–4 | **Neoadjuvant Therapy for Esophageal Cancer**

RANDOMIZED TRIALS OF NEOADJUVANT PREOPERATIVE (COMBINATION) THERAPY VERSUS SURGERY ALONE					
Author	**Year**	**n: C/S**	**Type**	**Regimen**	**Survival**
Nygaard et al.[93a]	1992	47/41	SCCa	P, B, 35 Gy	NS
Le Prise et al.[93b]	1994	41/45	SCCa	P, F, 20 Gy	NS
Apinop et al.[93c]	1994	35/34	SCCa	P, F, 40 Gy	NS
Urba et al.[88]	1995	50/50	SC & AdCa	P, F, V, 45 Gy	NS
Walsh et al.[92]	1996	48/54	AdCa	P, F, 40 Gy	$P = .01$
Bosset et al.[91]	1997	143/139	SCCa	P, 18.5 Gy	NS
Kelsen et al.[93]	1998	213/227	SC & AdCa	P, F (p&p)	NS

AdCa, adenocarcinoma; B, bleomycin; C, combination therapy; F, 5-fluorouracil; P, cisplatin; p & p, preoperative and postoperative; S, surgery alone; SCCa, squamous cell carcinoma; V, vinblastine.

tain. Most clinical studies have dealt with SCCA. There has been no positive trial of postsurgical adjuvant therapy.

Further progress in clinical management awaits studies in patients with AdenoCa of the esophagus and EG junction and studies comparing definitive radiation therapy with surgery for patients who have responded to initial chemotherapy. All newly diagnosed patients should be considered candidates for new therapies and clinical trials comparing various treatment modalities.

ENDOSCOPIC THERAPY FOR SUPERFICIAL CARCINOMA. Endoscopic mucosectomy (EM) is a potential alternative to esophagectomy for macroscopically recognizable focal cancer limited to the mucosa. "Lift and cut" methods of EM have used submucosal saline solution injections and jumbo biopsy forceps.[94] A transparent suction cap, fitted to the end of the endoscope, has been used after submucosal injection to create a pseudopolyp that is resected by snare polypectomy[95] (Fig. 35–10). Among 37 patients with early squamous cell esophageal cancer, all had a complete (i.e., curative) mucosal resection. There were no local recurrences, and 92.5% of patients survived 5 years. Among 64 patients with superficial adenocarcinoma or HGD associated with Barrett's esophagus, complete resection was achieved in 78%.[96] Only short-term follow-up findings are available at this time. Procedure-related risks include bleeding and perforation.

Photodynamic therapy (discussed in more detail in "Palliative Therapy") has been reported to be successful in about 80% of patients with superficial squamous cell carcinomas of the esophagus,[97] and in patients with Barrett's esophagus with HGD and/or superficial AdenoCA (Fig. 35–11).[98] However, instances of residual dysplastic epithelium and significant complications are reported.

As surgery is curative for most patients with superficial carcinoma of the esophagus, endoscopic therapies should be reserved for those patients unfit for or unwilling to have operative therapy and for clinical trials.

Palliative Therapy

Most patients with esophageal cancer have advanced disease at the time of initial medical consultation, and less than 20%

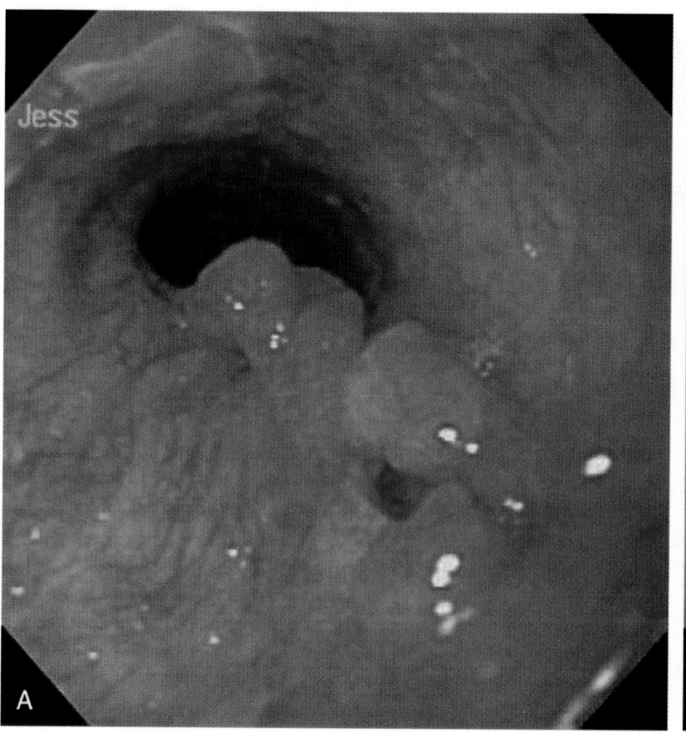

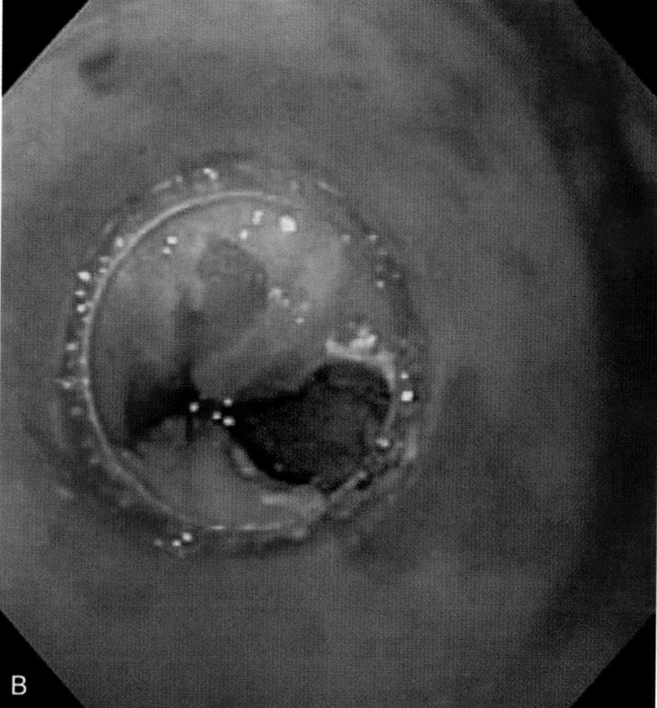

Figure 35–10. Endoscopic mucosal resection of esophageal cancer: *A*, A macroscopically recognizable superficial carcinoma is seen arising within short-segment Barrett's esophagus. The lesion was resected following injection of methylene blue–stained saline solution using a cap-assisted electrocautery snare technique. *B*, The transparent cap remains affixed to the tip of the endoscope.

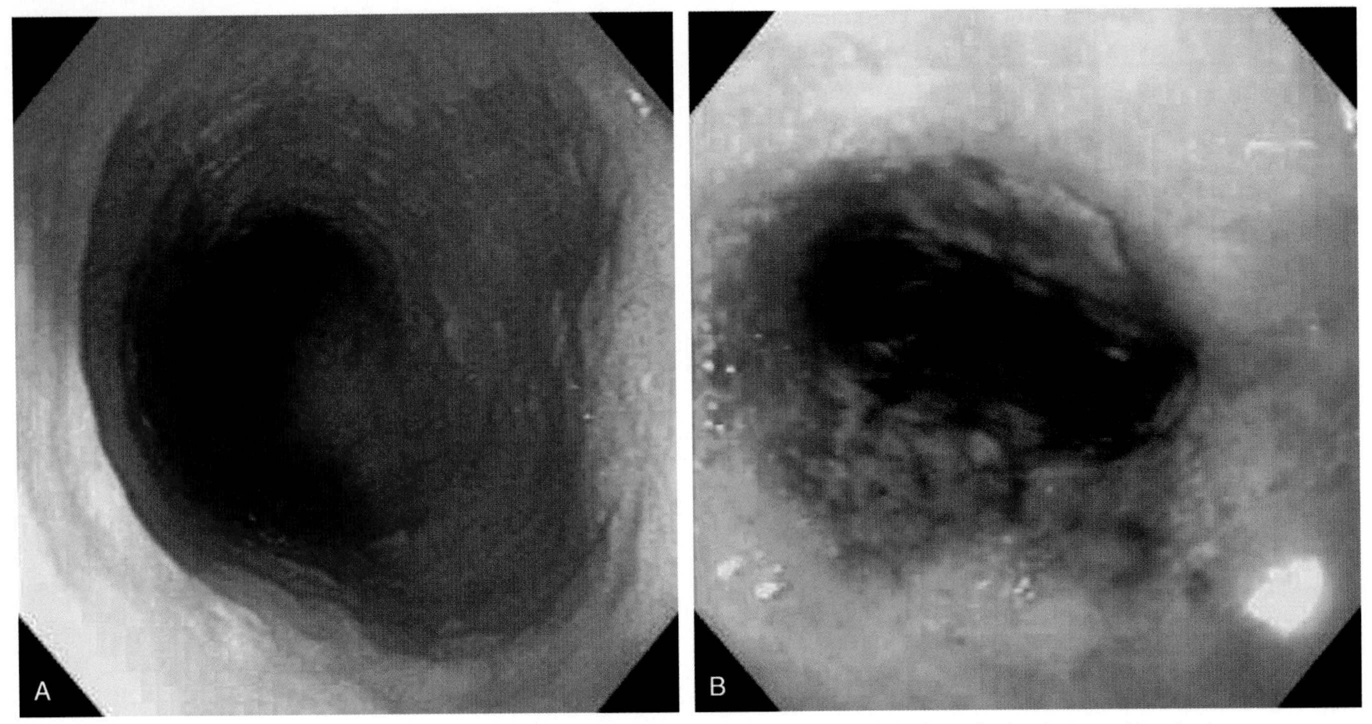

Figure 35–11. *A*, Photodynamic therapy of dysplasia in Barrett's esophagus with high-grade dysplasia on biopsies in a patient who was not a candidate for esophagectomy. *B*, Forty-eight hours after photodynamic therapy, there is an intense circumferential superficial tissue destruction with sharply demarcated borders delineating the proximal extent of laser light exposure.

survive 1 year after the time of diagnosis. At diagnosis, approximately 50% of patients with esophageal cancer have metastatic disease and are candidates for palliative therapy. Standard palliative treatment options may include radiation therapy, intraluminal brachytherapy,[99] chemotherapy, and endoscopic therapies. All of the preceding modalities may be offered in combination with endoscopic tumor dilation, intubation, or ablation. Chemotherapy has yielded partial responses among patients with metastatic distal esophageal AdenoCA.[100] Many chemotherapeutic agents are active in esophageal cancer. Objective response rates of 30% to 50% are commonly reported with platinum based combination regimens with fluorouracil, a taxane, or a topoisomerase inhibitor.[101] All recurrent esophageal cancer patients present difficult problems in palliation. Treatment consists of palliative use of any of the standard therapies, including supportive care.

In the presence of complete esophageal obstruction without clinical evidence of systemic metastasis, surgical excision of the tumor with mobilization of the stomach to replace the esophagus has been the traditional means of relieving the dysphagia. Surgical esophagectomy has a 3% to 10% mortality rate and a significant morbidity rate. As the median age of esophageal cancer patients is 67 years, many patients are of advanced age and/or have comorbid diseases that make operative resection a less compelling option. For all these reasons, endoscopic palliative therapy plays a critical role in the management of patients with esophageal cancer. No significant differences are observed in effectiveness of endoscopic palliation of SCCA versus AdenoCa of the esophagus.

The main goal of endoscopic therapy is to palliation of dysphagia, which contributes to improved nutritional status and quality of life. Endoscopic palliative therapies can be divided into those methods that displace (dilation, stenting) and those that ablate tissue. Ablative therapies destroy tissue by using contact thermal, noncontact thermal, cytotoxic injection, and photodynamic therapies. Bleeding and esophagorespiratory fistulas are other complications that can be managed with endoscopic therapy, but symptoms of pain and anorexia cannot be managed. Esophagorespiratory fistulas, which are a dire complication of SCCA of the esophagus as well as primary pulmonary malignancies that invade the esophagus, are particularly well managed with esophageal stent placement.

In considering options for palliative therapy, endoscopy serves to establish or confirm the diagnosis of cancer with tissue biopsy by allowing direct evaluation of the lesion's location, length, configuration, luminal diameter, and relationship to the upper esophageal sphincter and the EG junction. A contrast radiographic swallowing study may be used adjunctively to delineate the location, extent, and configuration of the tumor and its luminal stenosis. Contrast radiography is particularly useful when an esophagorespiratory fistula is suspected (see Fig. 35–3). A cross-sectional imaging study should be performed to assess for metastases to other organs.

DILATION THERAPY. Dilation achieves tumor displacement by the use of lateral shearing forces to stretch and tear the stenotic tissue. Dilation may be performed as primary palliative therapy or adjunctively to facilitate longer lasting thermal or stent therapy. Dilation is generally an effective means of providing temporary relief of dysphagia in patients with esophageal cancer. There are two types of commonly used dilators: polyvinyl dilators (Savary-Guilliard or American type) and hydrostatic through the scope (TTS) balloons.

Advantages of dilation include simplicity, low cost, wide availability, short procedure time and relative safety. Most patients derive initial benefit from dilation therapy. However, initial dilation of a tight stenosis may require sequential sessions before dysphagia is relieved. The main disadvantage of dilation therapy is that its relief is often short-lived, and as the disease progresses, symptom-free intervals decrease in duration, requiring more frequent sessions.[102] Dilation therapy alone is inadequate for satisfactory palliation in most patients.

CONTACT THERMAL THERAPY. Electrosurgical tumor probe therapy is a contact thermal ablation technique used primarily in the palliation of circumferential esophageal malignancies. The tumor probe (BICAP tumor probe, ACMI Circon, Santa Barbara, Calif) has electrical plates arranged circumferentially around an olive-shaped metal cylinder attached to a flexible shaft fashioned with scored 1-cm distance markers. A flexible spring tip obturator screws into the electrically active multipolar probe. The assembled apparatus has a central lumen that enables the system to be passed over a guidewire. The probes have electrical contact plates arranged circumferentially, allowing a 360-degree radius of coagulation. The contact portions of the probes vary in diameter. The shaft is connected to an electrical power source that allows the generation of an electrosurgical current, which is then delivered from the probe. Although the depth of coagulation effect varies with the power settings and the duration of application, the tumor probe produces a predictable depth of injury because contact with nondesiccated tissue is required to complete the circuit.

The procedure is performed under combined endoscopic and fluoroscopic guidance. In the recommended retrograde approach, the tumor probe is passed over a guidewire and through the area of luminal narrowing. Under fluoroscopic guidance the probe is then pulled back in retrograde fashion so that the electrosurgical component of the tumor probe is in contact with the malignant tissue. The active electrode is 1.5 cm in length, so by withdrawing the tumor probe at 1-cm intervals, a small amount of overlap is achieved and uniform tissue injury is delivered to the treatment zone, extending 1 to 2 mm circumferentially. Power of 50 W is generally applied for 15 seconds' duration at each station. The probe is segmentally withdrawn and applied sequentially until the entire tumor is treated. Short segments may be treated in the antegrade fashion under endoscopic guidance with a small-diameter endoscope placed alongside the flexible shaft. At follow-up endoscopy 48 hours post procedure, necrotic debris is removed and additional therapy applied on the basis of clinical results.

Technical success with increased luminal diameter and significant improvement in dysphagia grade in post-treatment assessment has been consistently reported for 80% to 90% of patients.[103–106] Generally, one or two treatment sessions achieved a mean duration of palliation of 7.6 weeks. However, major complications of tracheoesophageal fistula and delayed hemorrhage occurred in up to 20%.

The BICAP tumor probe is best suited for bulky or infiltrating symmetrical circumferential tumors. It is ill suited for asymmetrical tumors, tortuous segments, and tightly stenotic tumors. Advantages are its relative low cost and its ability to treat a large extent of tumor in a single setting. Inadvertent treatment of opposing or marginal nonmalignant tissue may result in pain and stricture. Although this modality may be well suited for a minority of patients, most authorities have abandoned its use in favor of other means of endoscopic palliation.

ENDOSCOPIC LASER PHOTOABLATION. Endoscopic laser therapy (ELT) is a noncontact means of thermal ablation. Laser photoablation has been used extensively in the palliation of malignant dysphagia associated with esophageal cancers. Thermal lasers deliver energy focused in a beam of light transmitted through a flexible glass fiber that can be passed through the accessory channel of an endoscope. Tissue effects vary with the distinctive characteristics of the tissue-wavelength interaction of the laser in use. Neodymium:yttrium-aluminum-garnet (Nd:YAG), potassium titanyl phosphate (KTP), and argon lasers have been used for thermal therapy of GI malignancies. The greatest experience and success have been attained with the Nd:YAG wavelength in the noncontact mode. Laser therapy has the capacity to vaporize tissue in addition to producing coagulation necrosis. Large areas of tumor can be treated in a single session. The noncontact mode prevents the problem of tissue's sticking to the device.

ELT may be performed using the Nd:YAG laser at high power settings (40 to 100 W) in 1-second pulsed or continuous mode. With the laser fiber distanced approximately 1 cm from the target tissue, a combination of vaporization and coagulation necrosis occurs. When feasible, the retrograde method is preferred.[107, 108] The endoscope is passed beyond the malignant stricture. Laser treatment is begun at the distal tumor margin and proceeds cephalad until the most proximal margin is treated. For annular lesions, circumferential treatment should be applied at each level (Fig. 35–12). ELT, in addition to tumor ablation and coagulation necrosis, often produces some tissue edema and swelling, which may result in transient luminal narrowing. When complete luminal obstruction is present, ELT in antegrade fashion is necessary. When using coaxial gas, distention of the stomach may occur, producing patient discomfort. This problem is overcome by using a large channel or double-channel therapeutic endoscope that allows adequate suction while the laser fiber is in place.

Patients are routinely evaluated 48 hours later and retreated until maximal luminal patency is achieved. It is uncommon to require more than three sessions to achieve satisfactory luminal patency. The occasional patient may experience chest pain and odynophagia briefly after the procedure. A low-grade fever and mild elevation of the leukocyte count can be expected. Once the desired extent of luminal patency has been attained, follow-up endoscopy should be carried out in 3 to 4 weeks to assess the need for repeat ELT. A contrast barium swallow may be considered after completion of ELT to document the effects of therapy. The diet should include liquid nutritional supplements. Patients are instructed to chew foods well, to avoid stringy foods, and to drink large amounts of liquids after eating solid foods.

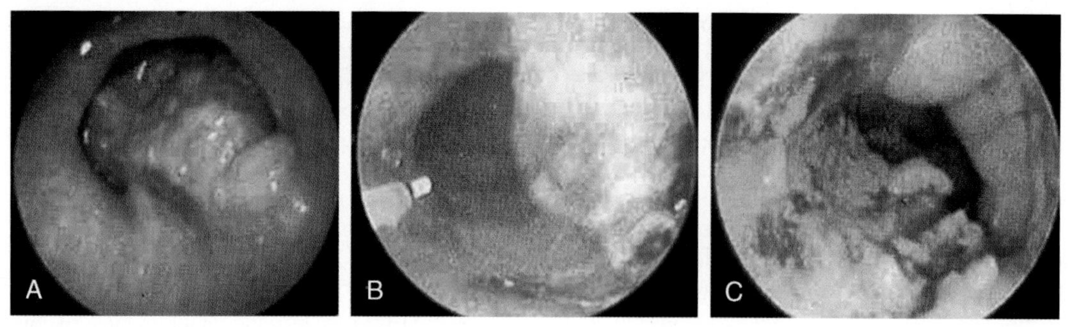

Figure 35–12. Laser therapy of esophageal cancer. A focal fungating adenocarcinoma (*A*) can be debulked for palliation of dysphagia with a noncontact laser (*B*), resulting in tumor coagulative necrosis and vaporization, with reconstitution of the esophageal lumen (*C*).

The success of ELT in palliation of esophageal malignancy is well documented.[109–116] ELT achieves technical success with luminal patency in 97% of cases, although functional success defined by relief of dysphagia occurs in only 70% to 85%. Sixty to seventy percent of patients remain free of dysphagia for 3 to 6 weeks. Only 20% to 25% of patients treated remain symptom-free for 3 months or more. In one study,[117] after initial successful therapy, repeat ELT was performed on the basis of monthly endoscopic findings. With this approach symptom relief persisted for a mean of 4.2 months and 76% of patients experienced palliation of symptoms until death. Studies have demonstrated that laser therapy improved patients' quality of life by allowing them to eat and improved their performance status, but increased survival rate was not proved.[118]

Overall complications occurred in 4.1% of cases in a survey of 1359 cases.[119] Perforation occurred in only 2%; the procedure-related mortality rate was 1%; the incidence of fistula or hemorrhage was 1%; and sepsis occurred in 0.5% to 1%. Perforations are more likely to occur in patients who have had prior radiation therapy. Although initial equipment costs are high and repair costs can be considerable, once a laser is in place and operational, its use is not much more costly than other treatment modalities.

Favorable and unfavorable characteristics of endoscopic laser therapy have been identified.[120] Characteristics that favor successful ELT include a mucosal, exophytic, or polypoid endoscopic appearance of the tumor. These characteristics allow better distinction between normal and abnormal tissue, more precise aiming of the laser beam, and alignment of the laser beam in the axis of the lumen, reducing the risk of perforation. Examples include asymmetrical, noncircumferential tumors; polypoid masses; soft fleshy lesions; recurrences at surgical resection sites; and tumor overgrowth of endoprostheses. Lesions that cause complete luminal obstruction may also be treated with ELT. Submucosal or extrinsic lesions are less amenable to ELT because the extent of tumor is difficult to appreciate endoscopically, and because overlying normal mucosa must be treated, pain and increased risk of perforation result. Straight segments are more easily treated and have better outcomes than angulated segments. Short tumor segments, less than 6 cm, are more effectively treated than more extensive ones. Lesions that occur in close proximity to the upper esophageal sphincter are difficult to treat because aiming the laser beam is more difficult in this location. Likewise, lesions at the EG junction that are horizontal in orientation are more difficult to treat because of difficulty in aiming.

ARGON PLASMA BEAM COAGULATION. The argon plasma beam coagulator delivers monopolar electrocoagulation by using a stream of ionized argon gas ignited by a high voltage discharged at the tip of a flexible catheter probe. Application and control are easier than in use of noncontact free beam lasers. The depth of treatment is uniform and consistent, although it is superficial. Although argon plasma beam coagulation is emerging as an alternative to laser photocoagulation for ablation of superficial luminal digestive tract lesions, it produces a depth of tissue injury that is insufficient to effect relief of dysphagia associated with esophageal carcinoma.[121]

CYTOTOXIC INJECTION THERAPY. Chemical injection therapy is theoretically attractive in that it is cheap, simple, and readily available. A variety of chemical agents have been used for palliation of esophageal cancers, both by debulking tumors and by controlling bleeding.[122–124] Injectates have included chemotherapeutic agents and chemical sclerosants such as polidocanol, ethanol, and sodium morrhuate. Tissue destruction is brought about by chemical necrolysis. Hemostasis is achieved by the combination of edema, vasoconstriction, and thrombosis. Disadvantages are the inability to control the depth of tissue injury and the lack of immediately visible tissue effects. Only small numbers of patients have been treated, and the technique has not been standardized or compared with other ablative methods of palliation.[122–124]

PHOTODYNAMIC THERAPY. The biologic effects of photodynamic therapy (PDT) are photochemical, as cytotoxicity is induced by nonthermal laser light energy. A photosensitizing agent is administered and is selectively retained in tumor cells. The photosensitizing agent is then activated by low-dose, wavelength-specific laser light delivered in close proximity to the lesion. Activation by light produces a local cytotoxic effect mediated by singlet oxygen. The extent of necrosis is dependent on tissue concentration of the photosensitizing agent and the light dose given (see Fig. 35–11).

PDT using a hematoporphyrin derivative has received Food and Drug Administration (FDA) approval for the palliation of malignant dysphagia associated with esophageal cancer. Two randomized comparative trials reported that PDT provides palliation equivalent to that of Nd:YAG laser

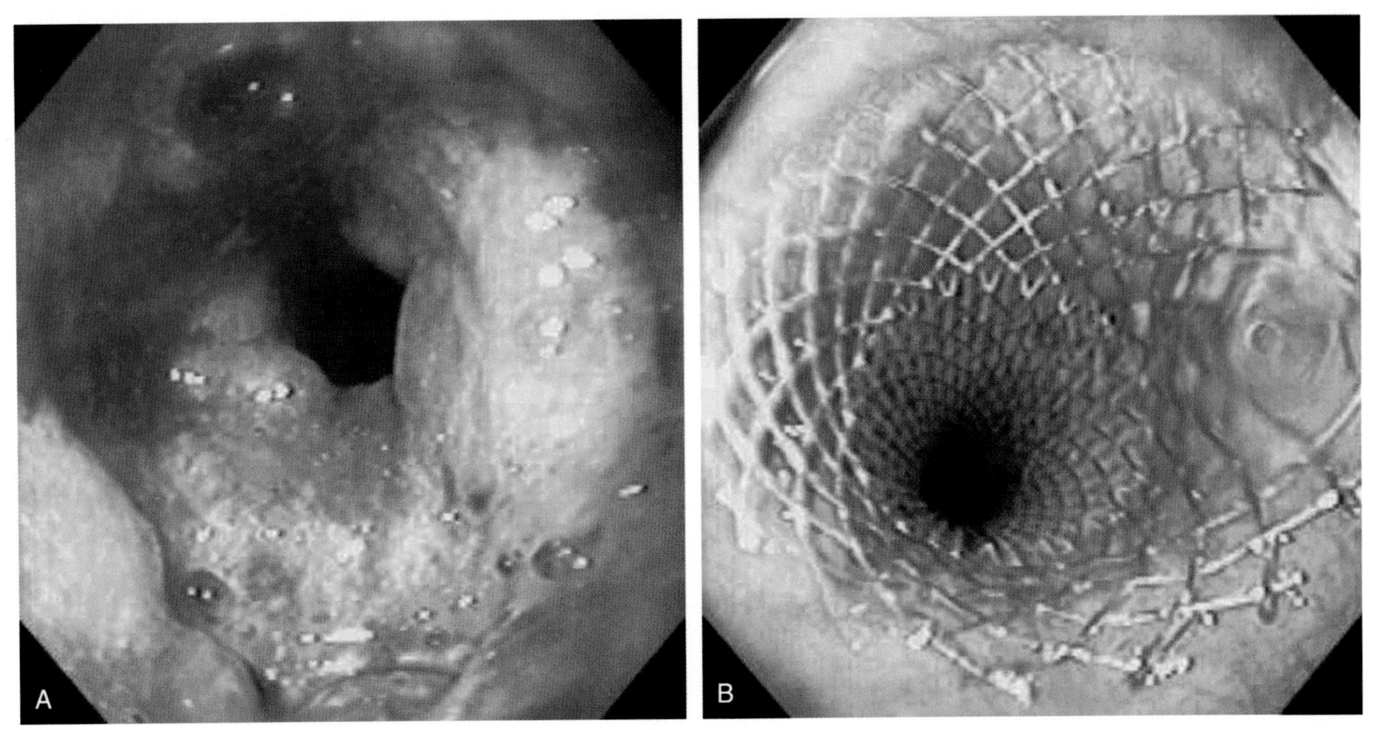

Figure 35–13. Stent therapy of esophageal fistula. *A,* This patient with a circumferential esophageal carcinoma, previously treated with chemoradiotherapy, developed an esophagomediastinal fistula, seen inferiorly. *B,* Placement of a covered self-expanding metallic stent achieved long-term palliation of the patient's dysphagia and fistula.

therapy.[125, 126] The reported clinical experience indicates that PDT achieves and maintains significant palliation of dysphagia in about 75% of patients 1 month after treatment.[127] PDT has also been effective in reestablishing the lumen in completely obstructing esophageal tumors. The PDT protocol used in these studies consisted of intravenous administration of 2 mg/kg of hematoporphyrin derivative, followed 48 hours later by 300 J/cm of 630-nm light from a tunable argon pumped dye laser delivered endoscopically through a 2.5-cm-length cylindrical diffusing tip of a glass laser fiber. The light dose is typically repeated during a second session 48 hours after the first.

A major advantage of PDT is that large areas may be treated during a single session. Complications and adverse events associated with PDT include skin photosensitivity, chest pain, atrial fibrillation, odynophagia, and stricture formation. There are considerable costs of the photosensitizing agent (~$2000 per patient), cylindrical diffusion fibers, and start-up laser cost. Occasional complete responses, reported in earlier series, suggest that PDT may be better suited for the eradication of early tumors rather than advanced ones.[128]

ESOPHAGEAL STENT THERAPY. Expandable metallic esophageal stents are indicated for the palliation of luminal stenosis due to esophageal cancer and for the management of esophagorespiratory fistulas. Self-expanding metallic stents (SEMSs) have replaced their semirigid plastic predecessors because they are easier to place, achieve more effective palliation, and are associated with fewer complications. SEMSs compare favorably with other palliative modalities because they provide immediate and long-lasting relief of obstructive symptoms. Typically they can be placed in an outpatient endoscopic procedure performed with conscious sedation. Covered or coated SEMSs are the most effective means of palliating esophagorespiratory fistula (Fig. 35–13).

For SEMS placement, the patient assumes a left lateral decubitus or supine position. Sedation and monitoring practices should be optimized. The risk of aspiration of oropharyngeal secretions and enteric contents requires particular vigilance. Accurate tumor length measurement is critical to successful SEMS deployment. Recording the length of scope insertion at the bite block as it is withdrawn from the distal to the proximal tumor margins effectively measures tumor length. Prior radiographic contrast swallowing studies may be helpful to characterize a tortuous stenosis or an esophagorespiratory fistula. Although the technique is not unanimously accepted, most practitioners use combined endoscopic and fluoroscopic guidance for stent placement and deployment. The type, length, and diameter of stent selected are individualized to the specific patient's condition and the operator's experience.

Gradual dilation to 12 to 15 mm has been a common practice but may not be routinely necessary or beneficial. Dilation is necessary, however, when luminal obstruction does not permit the endoscope to pass. Accurate tumor margin marking is critical to effective stent placement. One or more marking techniques may be used. Externally affixed radiopaque markers become less useful if the patient moves during delivery device insertion. Simply marking the proximal and distal tumor margins, as measured endoscopically, on the delivery device is sufficient in many cases. More precise marking of the tumor margins or center point can be achieved by submucosal injection of a radiocontrast agent using a sclerotherapy needle or endoscopic placement of metallic mucosal clips. Familiarity with the specific stent delivery apparatus, the significance of its radiopaque markings, and the degree of anticipated foreshortening is critical. Communication and mutually understood terminology of the endoscopist and the GI assistants are necessary to ensure the best results.

Post procedure, patients who have stents placed across the EG junction should have head-of-bed elevation greater than 30 degrees at all times. A decision to obtain a post–stent placement radiograph or contrast study is individualized. However, the latter should be obtained routinely when a stent is placed to seal an esophagorespiratory fistula. Antiemetics and antitussives should be used when retching, coughing, or hiccuping is significant early on to prevent stent dislodgment. Clear liquids may be initiated on the same or the following day and the diet advanced as tolerated. Dietary recommendations should be individualized. Patients are advised to chew food well; avoid stringy meats, fruits, and vegetables; flush the esophagus frequently with liquids during meals; and contact the physician should symptoms of stent occlusion or food impaction develop.

There are a variety of esophageal SEMSs commercially available. Initial-generation uncovered SEMSs have largely been replaced by covered versions. The Wallstent (formerly Schneider, Minneapolis, Minn; now Microvasive, Boston Scientific, Inc., Natick, Mass) consists of a bilayer stainless steel tubular mesh coated with a polyurethane sleeve between two mesh tubes. It is available in a variety of lengths and maximal luminal diameters. In one version the stent can be recaptured and repositioned when up to 50% has been deployed. The Wallstent is delivered on an introducer catheter over a previously placed guidewire and deployed by withdrawing a translucent outer sheath under fluoroscopic guidance.

The Ultraflex stent (Microvasive, Boston Scientific, Inc., Natick, Mass) consists of a knitted nitinol wire tube. The stent is constrained on the introducer catheter by a spiral retention suture. Unraveling the suture deploys the stent. One unique advantage of this stent is that models with distal or proximal release systems can be selected. The latter offers a considerable advantage when precise placement in required. It is available in a variety of lengths and maximal luminal diameters. The delivery device is 5 to 7 mm in diameter and allows insertion of the endoscope alongside the stent delivery device for concomitant endoscopic and fluoroscopic imaging during placement and deployment.

The "Z"-stent (Cook Medical, Inc., Winston Salem, NC) is made of stainless steel wires shaped in a Z configuration. Initial versions were fully covered to prevent tumor ingrowth and excessive granulation tissue reaction around the stent struts. Unfortunately, this feature contributed to an increase in stent migration. The most recent version has uncovered segments in the proximal and distal sections that have reduced this risk. The stent releases without shortening to a diameter of 18 mm. A model designed with a latex "windsock" extending from the distal opening of the stent and intended to prevent gastroesophageal reflux has been marketed for EG junction and distal esophageal cancers for which the stent must bridge the EG junction.

The Esophacoil (Instent, Minneapolis, Minn) is constructed from a single ribbon of nitinol wire tightly wound onto the delivery device. It is tethered at the distal, proximal, and medial aspects by sutures. On release of the stent, the length shortens as the coils expand. The stent diameters are 16 to 18 mm in the shaft and 21 to 25 mm at the ends. It has the greatest expansile force among the available SEMSs, although it is more rigid and has considerable foreshortening. Moreover, it is rather unforgiving with respect to position adjustment once deployment has been initiated. At the time of this writing, the Esophacoil stent had been withdrawn from the U.S. market.

Knyrim and coworkers reported a randomized trial comparing the results of palliation of malignant dysphagia with an uncovered Wallstent (postdeployment diameter of 16 mm) versus a 16-mm-diameter plastic prosthesis.[129] Palliation was equal in both groups. However, there were fewer complications, and no fatal complications, in the Wallstent group. The reduction in complications resulted in decreased hospital stay and translated into lower costs. Tumor ingrowth or overgrowth was the most common cause of recurrent dysphagia in the uncovered Wallstent group (24%) and was managed effectively with endoscopic laser therapy.

Although there are few comparative trials, prospective series have reported uniformly good results for palliation of dysphagia as well as esophagorespiratory fistulas.[130–135] Proper stent positioning and deployment are achieved in 90% to 100% of cases. Dysphagia scores decrease by one to two grades. Complications occur in 30% to 40% of patients during follow-up after SEMS placement, but most are minor and few are procedure-related. The mortality rate is minimal. Esophagorespiratory fistula, a devastating complication, occurs in 5% to 15% of patients with mediastinal tumors. Covered SEMSs were effective in palliating fistulas in 70% to 100% of cases. There are no published large prospective, randomized trials comparing different types of SEMSs, SEMSs with other endoscopic therapies, or SEMSs alone or in combination with nonendoscopic palliative therapies.

The selection of a stent for palliation of dysphagia associated with esophageal cancer must be individualized and take into account the tumor length, location, and configuration; the patient's performance status and prognosis; and local or regional expertise. Lesions that prove challenging to the technical and functional success of SEMS include tumors in the high cervical esophagus, and the EG junction and those without a ledge to anchor the stent in place. Prior or pending chemoradiotherapy may increase the risk of complications, but this possibility remains controversial and is under evaluation.

Potential complications of SEMS placement may include tumor ingrowth or tumor overgrowth (5% to 20%), stent migration (10%), and chest pain. Laser or contact thermal therapy is effective for ablation of tumor overgrowth of previously placed stents. Other complications may include procedure-related perforation, food bolus impaction, bleeding, foreign body sensation, and reflux esophagitis. Enterorespiratory aspiration is of particular concern among patients in whom the stent crosses the EG junction. Patient instruction about food selections, eating habits, and body positioning is intended to prevent complications of food impaction and enterorespiratory reflux, but its effectiveness is unproved. Although the material costs of SEMSs are high, they are likely to be cost effective when they successfully minimize subsequent health care expenditures as they promote improved quality of life.

Enteral Nutrition and Analgesic Therapy

Most patients with advanced esophageal cancer have compromised nutritional status at their initial medical consultation. When feasible, enteral is preferred to parenteral nutrition support. Enteral nutrition support may be indicated in an attempt to improve functional status before and after surgery, during chemoradiotherapy, and as an adjunct to other palliative measures. As functional success does not always match technical success in the palliation of malignant dysphagia, enteral access may effectively supplement oral intake. In many cases, endoscopic palliative therapies are effective in allowing patients to swallow their own secretions but anorexia, gastric dysmotility, and generalized debilitation preclude restoration of nutritional status by the oral route alone. Enteral access can be achieved surgically, radiographically, or endoscopically. A surgical jejunostomy should routinely be created at the time of esophageal resection. Percutaneous endoscopic gastrostomy (PEG) is safe and effective for nonoperative candidates. PEG placement is not appropriate for candidates for subsequent esophagectomy with gastric pull-up. Direct gastric feeding may be contraindicated in patients with SEMSs that extend beyond the EG junction and in postesophagectomy patients because of its increased risk of gastrorespiratory reflux and aspiration. Poor gastric emptying is observed in many patients who have EG junction carcinomas that extend into the gastric cardia and fundus. In these patients, endoscopic enteral access can be achieved by creating a direct percutaneous endoscopic jejunostomy or a PEG with a jejunal feeding tube extension.[136]

Pain due to tumor ulceration and neural invasion is observed in patients with advanced esophageal cancer. Pain may be significant in some patients after stent insertion, as a result of radial expansion. This pain generally lasts 1 to 2 weeks. Esophageal cancer pain should be managed with narcotic analgesia. Long-acting sustained release preparations maybe supplemented with shorter-acting agents. Parenteral applications, such as transdermal patches, have obvious appeal for use in patients with dysphagia. Consultation with a pain specialist may be helpful to minimize sedation and maximize functional ability.

OTHER MALIGNANT EPITHELIAL TUMORS (see Table 35–5)

Squamous Cell Carcinoma Variants

An uncommon variant of SCCA, verrucous carcinoma, is characterized by an exophytic papillary growth. Microscopically verrucous carcinomas are composed of moderately differentiated squamous cells amid a fibrous stroma. These tend to be slow growing and have low metastatic potential and an accompanying more favorable prognosis.[137]

SCCAs mixed with spindle cell elements is uncommon. They are thought to arise from mesenchymal metaplasia of malignant squamous cells. These carcinosarcomas may be solitary or multiple. They are often large polypoid lesions. They occur more commonly in men, appearing in middle or advanced age. When dysphagia due to luminal obstruction occurs, the large size usually implies esophageal wall invasion and lymph node involvement. Management and prognosis are similar to those for typical SCCA.[138]

Table 35–5 | **Classification of Esophageal Tumors**

EPITHELIAL TUMORS	NONEPITHELIAL TUMORS
Malignant	Malignant
Squamous cell carcinoma	Lymphoma
Adenocarcinoma of the esophagus	Sarcomas
Adenocarcinoma of the esophagogastric junction	Metastatic carcinoma
Verrucous carcinoma	Benign
Carcinosarcoma	Leiomyoma
Small cell carcinoma	Granular cell tumor
Malignant melanoma	Fibrovascular tumor
Benign	Hemangioma
Squamous papilloma	Hamartoma
Adenoma	Lipoma
Inflammatory fibroid polyps	

Small Cell Carcinoma

The esophagus is the most common extrapulmonary site of small cell carcinoma. Primary small cell carcinomas of the esophagus account for 0.8% to 4.7% of all esophageal neoplasms.[139] Like SCCA, small cell tumors metastasize early, most commonly to periesophageal, mediastinal lymph nodes and the liver, and are highly lethal. The 1-year survival rate is 10%. Surgical resection is appropriate if preoperative evaluation rules out extranodal metastasis.

Malignant Melanoma

Primary esophageal melanoma is rare and is estimated to account for 0.1% of esophageal tumors.[140, 141] It is suspected when primary skin, ocular, and anal melanoma are ruled out. Primary esophageal melanomas begin as polypoid tumors. When they grow large and ulcerate, bleeding and odynophagia are the presenting symptoms. Early metastasis to lymphatics, liver, and lung are common, conferring a generally poor survival rate. Surgery offers the best chance for long-term survival.

BENIGN EPITHELIAL TUMORS OF THE ESOPHAGUS

Squamous Papilloma

Squamous cell papillomas are usually small, white or pink, sessile or polypoid benign tumors that are histologically composed of finger-like projections of lamina propria covered by hyperplastic squamous epithelium. Mucosal biopsy or polypectomy is safe and usually is diagnostic. Their pathogenesis is not known; however, both gastroesophageal reflux disease (GERD) and human papillomavirus (HPV) infection have been implicated.[142] Malignant transformation of a squamous papilloma is very rare. Recent data linking HPV with dysplasia and squamous cell carcinoma in the anogenital region should prompt further investigation into the possible association of HPV, squamous cell papilloma, and squamous cell carcinoma.

Adenoma

True adenomatous polyps, arising within segments of Barrett's esophagus, are observed rarely. They are benign but are considered dysplastic with malignant potential similar to that of adenomas elsewhere in the digestive tract, such as dysplasia-associated lesion or masses (DALMs) in the colon in ulcerative colitis. They may be sessile or pedunculated. Endoscopic management using standard snare or mucosectomy techniques may be curative.

Inflammatory Fibroid Polyps

Inflammatory fibroid polyps are rare in the esophagus—incidence is 1 in more than 300,000 surgical specimens.[143] These non-neoplastic polyps are also called *inflammatory pseudopolyps* and *eosinophilic granulomas*. Chronic inflammation from GERD is thought to have a causal role. Inflammatory fibroid polyps are the most common incidental finding on endoscopy performed in the evaluation of GERD symptoms. They occur in the distal esophagus or at the EG junction. Endoscopic resection yields diagnosis and cure.

MALIGNANT NONEPITHELIAL TUMORS

(see Table 35–5)

Lymphoma (See Chapter 26)

Lymphomatous involvement of the esophagus is generally due to extrinsic compression or direct invasion from mediastinal lymph nodes. Except in patients with acquired immunodeficiency syndrome (AIDS), the esophagus is rarely the primary site of extranodal lymphoma.[144] B cell lymphoma is most common. Dysphagia and weight loss are the symptoms at initial medical consultation. Esophageal fistulas are common. Therapy is dependent on symptoms, disease stage, and patient performance status. Chemoradiotherapy generally provides remission.

Sarcoma

Malignant mesenchymal esophageal tumors are rare.[145] About 5% of all GI sarcomas occur in the esophagus.[146] Leiomyosarcomas are the most common and can be difficult to distinguish from leiomyomas (see later). Other sarcomas include rhabdomyosarcoma, fibrosarcoma, fibrous histiocytoma, and choriocarcinoma.[147] Tumor characteristics include spindle shaped smooth muscle cells, high mitotic rates, local invasion, and, infrequently, distant metastasis. Most patients exhibit dysphagia. Endoscopic biopsy specimens are typically nondiagnostic, although the bite-on-bite technique may improve yield. EUS with EUS-guided FNA may contribute to diagnosis.[148] Cytologic needle aspiration specimens, however, cannot reliably exclude malignancy. Operative resection followed by radiotherapy optimizes cure and/or long-term survival.[149]

Kaposi's sarcoma (KS), a rare mesenchymal tumor before the AIDS epidemic, has been reported in the esophagus. Esophageal involvement is typically seen with concomitant oral and skin lesions.[150] Esophageal lesions are found incidentally or during evaluation of dysphagia or odynophagia. In symptomatic patients, endoscopic laser ablation or injection sclerotherapy may be attempted for hemorrhage or obstruction.

Metastatic Carcinoma

Metastatic carcinoma to the esophagus is unusual. Melanoma and breast cancer are the malignancies that most frequently metastasize to the esophagus. Few patients have lesions that allow clinical evaluation. Those who have dysphagia due to tumor infiltration or extrinsic compression present at a mean interval of 8 years and as late as 22 years after initial diagnosis of breast cancer.[151] Radiographic and endoscopic studies typically demonstrate compression without disruption of the mucosa. EUS is useful in distinguishing extrinsic and intrinsic involvement and in detecting lymphadenopathy. EUS guided FNA has proved useful in confirming the suspected diagnosis. Periodic dilation or SEMSs are used for palliation of dysphagia.

BENIGN NONEPITHELIAL TUMORS

(see Table 35–5)

Leiomyoma

Leiomyomas are the most common benign tumors of the esophagus (Fig. 35–14). In an autopsy series review, 161 esophageal leiomyomas were identified in 180,222 autopsies (1 per 1119).[152] Leiomyomas may occur in all parts of the esophagus; however, most (90%) are in the distal third. Most patients have a single tumor, though multiple leiomyomas may occur.

Leiomyomas arise from smooth muscle cells or their precursors in the muscularis propria or less commonly in the muscularis mucosa. Previously classified as smooth muscle tumors, they rarely express a typical smooth muscle cell immunophenotype.[153] Over the past few years the term *gastrointestinal stromal tumor* (GIST) has been introduced to classify mesenchymal tumors arising in the luminal tract. Histopathologic evaluation reveals that leiomyomas are firm, round, gray or yellow, unencapsulated, and composed of spindle shaped smooth muscle cells with cigar-shaped elongated nuclei. The risk of malignant transformation of esophageal leiomyomas to sarcomas is unknown. Some GIST tumors that have mutations of c-*kit* respond to the tyrosine kinase inhibitor imatinib mesylate (Gleevac).

Approximately one half of patients exhibit symptoms, which may include dysphagia (50%), retrosternal pain (50%), pyrosis, cough, odynophagia, weight loss, and rarely bleeding.[154] Most leiomyomas are endocentric (intraluminal polypoid growth). Barium swallow shows a smooth crescent shaped defect in the contour of the esophageal lumen with-

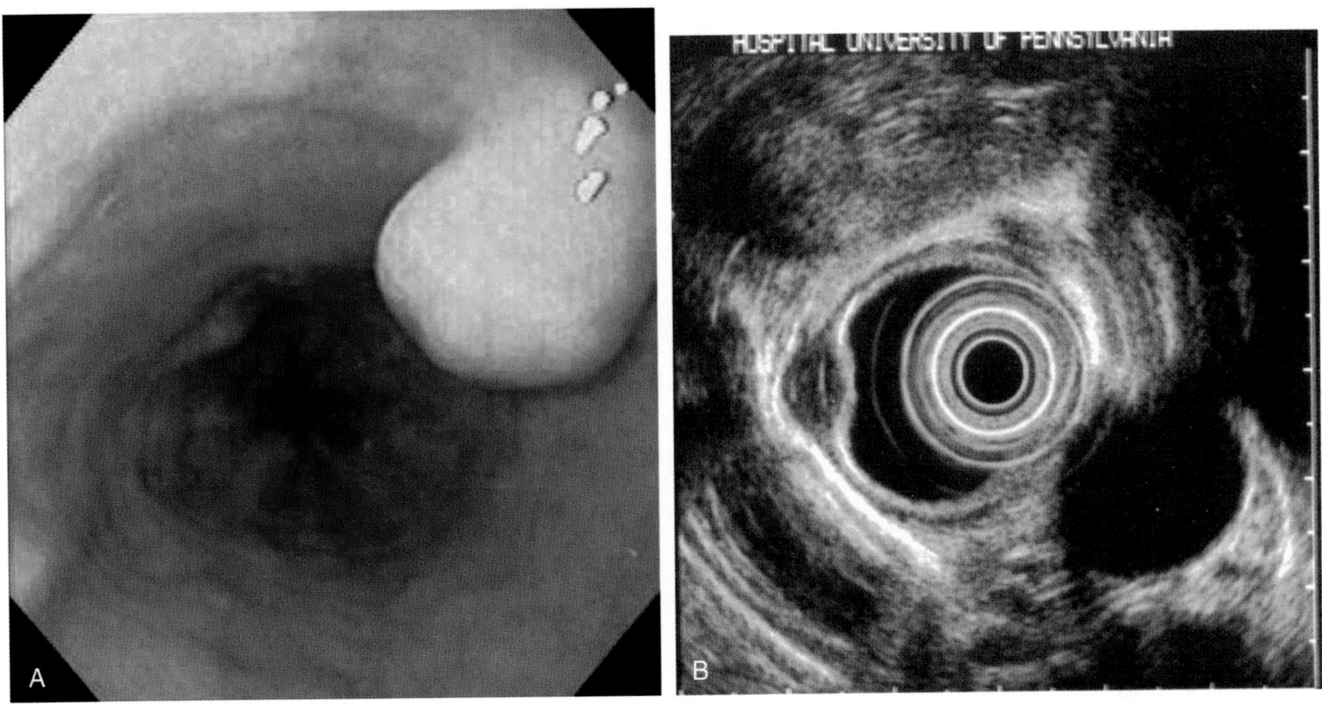

Figure 35–14. Esophageal leiomyoma. *A*, Endoscopic image of a submucosal esophageal mass. *B*, EUS demonstrates the lesion to represent a hypoechoic mass arising from the muscularis propria layer. These features are compatible with a leiomyoma.

out mucosal abnormality.[155] On endoscopy the mucosa is usually intact and the mass appears as a rounded, smooth raised lesion protruding into the esophageal lumen. Rarely, there may be central umbilication or ulceration. Palpation with a closed tip of a biopsy forceps reveals a firm but pliable lesion. Forceps biopsies typically are nondiagnostic revealing only normal surface epithelium.

EUS is the most accurate tool for diagnosing leiomyomas and distinguishing them from other submucosal lesions.[156, 157] EUS evaluation reveals that leiomyomas typically arise from the fourth wall layer (the muscularis propria) and are hypoechoic and homogeneous and have sharply demarcated margins. Less commonly leiomyomas arise from the muscularis mucosa within the deep mucosa, the second wall layer as seen on EUS examination. Leiomyomas arising from this layer may be amenable to endoscopic excision.

Management is dependent on the presence of symptoms and the prospect of unrecognized malignancy. Most small asymptomatic lesions that have characteristics of a leiomyoma can be followed. Continuing growth and the possibility of malignant transformation often require intervention. Neither EUS nor needle aspiration cytologic examination accurately distinguishes benign from malignant smooth muscle tumors preoperatively. Surgery should be considered in symptomatic patients, in those in whom the diagnosis is uncertain, and in those in whom there is suspicion of malignant transformation. Surgical excision or enucleation is performed via right thoracotomy or by a transhiatal approach for tumors of the lower third of the esophagus. Laparoscopic and thoracoscopic options were successfully applied, minimizing the trauma of surgery and shortening recovery time.[158] Palliative options for nonsurgical candidates include thermal laser ablation and tissue desiccation by alcohol injection.

Granular Cell Tumor

Granular cell tumors are submucosal neoplasms that are thought to originate from cells of neural origin because they stain for S100 protein and resemble Schwann cells on electron microscopy.[159] Approximately 10% of granular cell tumors involve the GI tract; the esophagus is the most frequent site, and most occur in the lower third.[160] Endoscopically, they appear broad based, with normal overlying mucosa, pinkish tan in color, and rubbery in consistency. On EUS, they are hypo- to isoechoic and arise within the submucosal layer. Diagnostic tissue can usually be confirmed with endoscopic biopsy samples obtained by the bite-on-bite technique. Management options include observation, ELT, polypectomy, and surgery. When small asymptomatic tumors are detected incidentally, conservative management is suggested. Granular cell tumors larger than 4 cm in size or those that exhibit growth should be considered potentially malignant.[161] For large symptomatic lesions, surgical excision is the preferred approach.

Fibrovascular Tumor

Large benign fibrovascular polyps occur most commonly on the upper third of the esophagus, near the cricopharyngeus muscle. They may contain a mixture of fibrovascular tissue, adipose cells, and stroma but are uniformly covered by squamous epithelium.[162] Although most are asymptomatic, bizarre symptoms of polyp regurgitation and asphyxiation are reported.[163] Barium esophagography and endoscopy are usually sufficient for diagnosis, but MRI can help to determine the origin of these polyps and to plan for surgery. The latter is recommended for polyps larger than 2 cm, but endoscopic snare resection of giant fibrovascular polyps can safely be done if EUS detects no large feeding vessels in the polyp stalk.

Hamartoma

Hamartomas of the esophagus are uncommon. They are frequently included in the category of fibrovascular polyps. As in other locations in the body, esophageal hamartomas are benign developmental tumors consisting of disorganized and excessive focal growth of mature normal cells.[164] On pathologic examination, the mass can contain various elements, including cartilage, bone and bone marrow, adipose and fibrous tissue, and smooth and skeletal muscle.[165]

Esophageal hamartomas may grow to large size as long pedunculated polyps. Most occur in the upper esophagus and show obstructive symptoms and, less commonly, hematemesis. Surgical or endoscopic excision is required for symptomatic lesions.[166]

Hemangioma

Hemangiomas represent 2% to 3% of benign esophageal tumors. Twenty-nine case reports have been published.[167] Two types have been described: cavernous hemangiomas, which are the vast majority, and capillary hemangiomas. Hemangiomas appear nodular, are blue to red, and are soft and pliable when probed with a closed biopsy forceps. Classically, pressure from the forceps causes the lesion to blanch. Common symptoms are hemorrhage and dysphagia. Differential diagnosis should consider Kaposi's sarcoma. Therapy has traditionally been surgery, but endoscopic therapies may be considered on an individualized basis.

Lipoma

Lipomas may occur anywhere in the GI tract, with increasing frequency from the esophagus down to the colon. They are encapsulated tumors composed of well-differentiated adipose tissue generally arising in the submucosa. Esophageal lipomas are rare.[168] Of those reported, most are intraluminal and pseudopedunculated, exhibiting obstructive symptoms. Lipomas with long pedicles produce laryngeal obstruction and asphyxiation.[169]

Barium studies are typically nondiagnostic, and the mass can be mistaken for a foreign body. On endoscopy, lipomas classically have smooth and normal appearing overlying mucosa and a yellowish tint. Occasionally there is central ulceration. When grasped with biopsy forceps, these lesions tend to "tent." When palpated with a closed biopsy forceps, they indent or "cushion." Biopsy specimens are usually nondiagnostic. EUS classically reveals a homogeneous hyperechoic lesion with smooth outer margins, arising in the third wall layer (corresponding to the submucosa).[170] Rarely, they may be located in the subadventitia. Because most other tumors that arise in the submucosa are hypoechoic, the EUS appearance is virtually diagnostic, provided that there are no features suggesting invasion or metastases, as in the exceedingly uncommon liposarcoma.

REFERENCES

1. The World Health Report 1997. Geneva, World Health Organization, 1997.
2. Greenlee RT, Murray T, Bolden S, et al: Cancer statistics, 2000. CA Cancer J Clin 50(1):7–33, 2000.
3. Ginsberg RJ: Cancer treatment in the elderly. J Am Coll Surg 187(4): 427–428, 1998.
4. Pera M, Cameron AJ, Trastek VF, et al: Increasing incidence of adenocarcinoma of the esophagus and esophago-gastric junction. Gastroenterology 104:510–513, 1993.
5. Devesa SS, Blot WJ, Fraumeni JF Jr: Changing patterns in the incidence of esophageal and gastric cardia cancer in the United States. Cancer 83:2049–2043, 1998.
6. Parkin DM, Laara E, Muir CS: Estimates of the worldwide frequency of 16 major cancers in 1980. Int J Cancer 41:184, 1988.

6a. Yang PC, Davis S: Incidence of cancer of the esophagus in the U.S. by histologic type. Cancer 61:612–617, 1988.

6b. Roth MJ, Strickland KL, Wang GQ, et al: High levels of carcinogenic polycyclic aromatic hydrocarbons present within food from Linxian, China, may contribute to that region's high incidence of esophageal cancer. Eur J Canc 34:757, 1998.

7. Van Rensburg SJ: Epidemiologic and dietary evidence for a specific nutritional pre-disposition to esophageal cancer. J Natl Cancer Inst 67: 643, 1981.
8. Dutta SK, Fleisher AS, Silverstein RJ, et al: Effects of beta carotene supplementation on nitrosamine induced squamous cell carcinoma of the esophagus in rats. Gastroenterology 108:A462, 1995.
9. Blot WJ: Esophageal cancer trends and risk factors. Semin Oncol 21: 403, 1994.
10. Rothman KJ: The proportion of cancer attributable to alcohol consumption. Prev Med 9:174, 1980.
11. Pottern LM, Morris LE, Blot J, et al: Esophageal cancer in black men in Washington D.C.: Alcohol, tobacco and other risk factors. J Natl Cancer Inst 67:777, 1981.
12. Franceschi S, Talamini R, Barra S, et al: Smoking and drinking in relation to cancers of the orocavity, pharynx, larynx and esophagus in Northern Italy. Cancer Res 50:6502, 1990.
13. Meijssen MA, Tilanus HW, Van Blankenstein M, et al: A prospective study of esophageal squamous cell carcinoma in achalasia. Gut 33: 155, 1992.
14. Sandler RS, Nyrien O, Ekbom A, et al: The risk of esophageal cancer in patients with achalasia: A population based study. Gastroenterology 108:A533, 1995.
15. Appelquist P, Salmo M: Lye corrosion carcinoma of the esophagus: A review of 63 cases. Cancer 45:2655, 1980.
16. Larsson LG, Sandstrom A, Westling P: Relationship of Plummer-Vinson disease to cancer of the upper alimentary tract in Sweden. Cancer Res 35:3308, 1975.
17. Harper PS, Harper RMJ, Howell-Evans AW: Carcinoma of the esophagus with tylosis. Q J Med 39:317, 1970.
18. Tachibana M, Abe S, Yoshimura H, et al: Squamous cell carcinoma of the esophagus after partial gastrectomy. Dysphagia 10:49, 1995.
19. Bogawa K, Rustgi AK: A novel human papilloma virus sequence based on L-1 general primers. Virus Res 36:293, 1995.
20. Jenkins TD, Nakagawa H, Rustgi AK: The association of Epstein-Barr virus BAM, H-1W, fragment repair genomic sequences with esophageal squamous cell carcinoma. Oncogene 13:1809, 1995.
21. Gammon MD, Schonenberg JB, Ashan H, et al: Tobacco, alcohol and socioeconomic status and adenocarcinomas of the esophagus and gastric cardia. J Natl Cancer Inst 89:1277–1284, 1997.
22. Vaughan T, Davis S, Kristen D, et al: Obesity, alcohol and tobacco as risk factors for cancers of the esophagus and gastric cardia: Adenocarcinoma vs. squamous cell carcinoma. Cancer Epidemiol Biomarkers Prev 5:761–768, 1996.
23. Zhang ZF, Kurtz RC, Sun M, et al: Adenocarcinoma of the esophagus and gastric cardia: Medical conditions, tobacco, alcohol and socioeconomic factors. Cancer Epidemiol Biomarkers Prev 4:85–92, 1995.

24. Brown LM, Silverman DT, Pottern LM, et al: Adenocarcinoma of the esophagus and esophago-gastric junction in white men in the United States: Alcohol, tobacco and socio-economic factors. Cancer Causes Control 5:333–340, 1994.
25. Lagergren J, Bergstrom R, Lingren A, Nyren O: Symptomatic gastroesophageal reflux as a risk factor for esophageal adenocarcinoma. N Engl J Med 340:825–831, 1999.
25a. Drewitz DJ, Sampliner GE, Garewal HS: The incidence of adenocarcinoma in Barrett's esophagus: A prospective study of 170 patients followed 4.8 years. Am J Gastroenterol 92:212, 1997.
26. Rudolph RE, Vaughan TL, Storer BE, et al: Effect of segment length on risk for neoplastic progression in patients with Barrett's esophagus. Ann Intern Med 132:612–620, 2000.
27. Farrow DC, Vaughan TL, Hansten PD, et al: Use of aspirin and other non-steroidal anti-inflammatory drugs and risk of esophageal and gastric cardia. Cancer Epidemiol Biomarkers Prev 7:97–102, 1998.
28. Lagergren J, Bergstrom R, Adami HO, Nyren O: Association between medications that relax the lower esophageal sphincter and risk for esophageal adenocarcinoma. Ann Intern Med 133:165–167, 2000.
29. Lagergren J, Bergstrom R, Nyren O: Association between body mass and adenocarcinoma of the esophagus and gastric cardia. Ann Intern Med 130:883–890, 1999.
30. Vaughan TL, Farrow DC, Hansten PD, et al: Risk of esophageal and gastric adenocarcinoma in relation to the use of calcium channel blockers, asthma drugs, and other medications that promote gastroesophageal reflux. Cancer Epidemiol Biomarkers Prev 7:749–756, 1998.
31. Vicari J, Peek RM, Faulk GW, et al: The sero prevalence of cagA+ *H. pylori* strains in the spectrum of gastroesophageal reflux disease. Gastroenterology 115:50–57, 1998.
32. El-Serag HB, Sonnenberg A: Opposing time trends of peptic ulcer and reflux disease. Gut 143:327–333, 1998.
33. Chow WH, Blaser MJ, Blot WJ, et al: An inverse relation between cagA+ strains of *Helicobacter pylori* infection and risk of esophageal and gastric cardia adenocarcinoma. Cancer Res 58:589–590, 1998.
34. Jiang W, Kahn SM, Tomita N, et al: Amplification and expression of the human cyclin D gene in esophageal cancer. Cancer Res 52:2980, 1992.
35. Nakagawa H, Zukerberg L, Togawa K, et al: Cyclin D-1 oncogene in esophageal squamous cell carcinoma. Cancer 76:541, 1995.
36. Mueller A, Odze R, Jenkins TD, et al: A transgenic mouth model with cyclin D-1 over-expression results in cell cycle, epidermal growth factor receptor and P-53 abnormalities. Cancer Res 57:5542, 1997.
37. Richards FM, McKee SA, Rajpar MH, et al: Germ Line E-cadherin gene (CDH-1) mutations pre-disposed to familial gastric and colorectal cancer. Hum Mol Genet 4:607–610, 1999.
38. Bennett WP, Hollstein MC, Metcalf RA, et al: p53 Mutation and protein accumulation during multi-stage human esophageal carcinogenesis. Cancer Res 52:6092, 1992.
39. Eastman Q, Grosschedl R: Regulation of LEF-1/TCF transcription fractures by WNT and other signals. Curr Opin Cell Biol 11:233–240, 1999.
40. El-Omar EM, Carrington M, Chow W, et al: Interleukin 1 polymorphisms associated with increased risk of gastric cancer. Nature 404: 398–402, 2000.
41. Jankowski JA, Perry I, Harrison RF: Gastroesophageal cancer: Death at the junction: Understanding changes at molecular level could lead to screening opportunities. BMJ 321:463–464, 2000.
42. Altorki NK, Migliore M, Skinner DB: Esophageal carcinoma and air way invasion: Evolution and choices of therapy. Chest 104:742, 1994.
43. O'Sullivan G, Sheahan D, Clarke A, et al: Micrometastases in esophagogastric cancer: High detectiom rate in resected rib segments. Gastroenterology 116:543–548, 1999.
44. Kuwano H, Baba H, Matsuda H, et al: Hypercalcemia related to poor prognosis in patients with squamous cell carcinoma of the esophagus. J Surg Oncol 42:229, 1989.
45. Graham DY, Schwartz JT, Cain GD, et al: Prospective evaluation of biopsy number in the diagnosis of esophageal and gastric carcinoma. Gastroenterology 82:228, 1982.
46. Shiozkai H, Tahara H, Kobayashi K, et al: Endoscopic screening of early esophageal cancer with the Lugol's dye method in patients with head and neck cancer. Cancer 66:2068, 1990.
47. Mori M, Adachi Y, Matsushima T, et al: Lugol staining pattern and histology of esophageal lesions. Am J Gastroenterol 88:701, 1993.
48. van Sandick JW, van Lanschot JJ, Kuiken BW, et al: Impact of endoscopic biopsy surveillance of Barrett's oesophagus on pathological stage and clinical outcome of Barrett's carcinoma. Gut 43(2):216–222, 1998.
49. Kesslich R, Hahn M, Herrmann G, Jung M: Screening for specialized columnar epithelium with methylene blue: Chromoendoscopy in patients with Barrett's esophagus and a normal control group. Gastrointest Endosc 53:47–52, 2001.
50. Shen Q, Wang TQ: Cytologic screening for carcinoma and dysplasia of the esophagus in the Peoples Republic of China. In Delarue N, Wilkins EW, Wong J (eds): International Trends in General Thoracic Surgery: Esophageal Cancer, vol 4. St. Louis, CV Mosby, 1988, p 25.
51. Falk GW, Chittajallu R, Goldblum JR, et al: Surveillance of patients with Barrett's esophagus for dysplasia and cancer with balloon cytology [see comments]. Gastroenterology 112(6):1787–1797, 1997.
52. American Joint Committee on Cancer: Esophagus. In AJCC Cancer Staging Manual, 5th ed. Philadelphia, Lippincott-Raven, 1997, pp 65–69.
53. American Joint Committee on Cancer: Esophagus. In Beahrs OH, Hansen DE, Hutter RVP, et al (eds): Manual for Staging of Cancer, 4th ed. Philadelphia, JB Lippincott, 1992, p 57.
54. Esophageal Cancer (PDQ) Treatment—Health Professionals, CancerNet: National Cancer Institute's Comprehensive Cancer Database. Available at http://cancernet.nci.nih.gov/pdqfull.html
55. Japanese Committee for Registration of Esophageal Carcinoma Cases: Parameters linked to ten-year survival in Japan of resected esophageal carcinoma. Chest 96(5):1005–1011, 1989.
56. Korst RJ, Rusch VW, Venkatraman E, et al: Proposed revision of the staging classification for esophageal cancer. J Thorac Cardiovasc Surg 115(3):660–670, 1998.
57. Thompson WM, Halvorsen RA: Staging esophageal carcinoma. II. CT and MRI. Semin Oncol 21:447, 1994.
58. Luketich JD, Schauer PR, Meltzer CC, et al: Role of positron emission tomography in staging esophageal cancer. Ann Thorac Surg 64(3):765–769, 1997.
59. Flamen P, Lerut A, Van Cutsem E, et al: Utility of positron emission tomography for the staging of patients with potentially operable esophageal carcinoma. J Clin Oncol 18(18):3202–3210, 2000.
60. Vilmann P, Khattar S, Hancke S: Endoscopic ultrasound examination of the upper gastrointestinal tract using a curved array transducer: A preliminary report. Surg Endosc 5:79–82, 1991.
61. Rosch T: Endosonographic staging of esophageal cancer: A review of the literature results. Gastrointest Endosc Clin N Am 5(3):537–548, 1995.
62. Kallimanis GE, Gupta PK, Al-Kawas FH, et al: Endoscopic ultrasound for staging esophageal cancer, with or without dilation, is clinically important and safe. Gastrointest Endosc 41:540–546, 1995.
63. Pfau PR, Ginsberg GG, Lew RJ, et al: Esophageal dilation for endosonographic evaluation of malignant esophageal strictures is safe and effective. Am J Gastroenterol 95(10):2813–2815, 2000.
64. Chandawarkar RY, Kakegawa T, Fujita H, et al: Endosonography for pre-operative staging of specific nodal groups associated with esophageal cancer. World J Surg 20(6):700–702, 1996.
65. Bhutani MS, Hawes RH, Hoffman BJ: A comparison of the accuracy of echo features during endoscopic ultrasound and EUS guided fine needle aspiration for diagnosis of malignant lymph node invasion. Gastrointest Endosc 45(6):474–479, 1997.
66. Bentz JS, Kochman ML, Faigel DO, et al: Endoscopic ultrasound-guided realtime fine needle aspiration: Clinicopathologic features of 60 patients. Diagn Cytopathol 18:98–109, 1998.
67. Chak A, Canto M, Gerdes H, et al: Prognosis of esophageal cancers preoperatively staged to be locally invasive (T4) by endoscopic ultrasound (EUS): A multicenter retrospective cohort study. Gastrointest Endosc 42:501–506, 1995.
68. Zuccaro G, Rice TW, Vargo JJ, et al: EUS directed therapy improves survival of patients with locoregionally advanced esophageal cancer. Gastrointest Endosc 47:AB157, 1998.
69. Pfau PR, Ginsberg GG, Lew RJ, et al: Endoscopic ultrasound predictors of long term survival in esophageal carcinoma. Gastrointest Endosc 54:414–416, 2001.
70. Isenberg G, Chak A, Canto MI, et al: Endoscopic ultrasound in restaging of esophageal cancer after neoadjuvant chemoradiation. Gastrointest Endosc 48:158–163, 1998.
71. Rosch T, Lorenz R, Zenker K, et al: Local staging and assessment of resectability in carcinoma of the esophagus, stomach and duodenum

by endoscopic ultrasonography. Gastrointest Endosc 38:460–467, 1992.
72. Dittler HJ, Siewert JR: Role of endoscopic ultrasonography in esophageal carcinoma. Endoscopy 25:156–161, 1993.
73. Falk GW, Catalano MF, Sivak MV, et al: Endosonography in the evaluation of patients with Barrett's esophagus and high grade dysplasia. Gastrointest Endosc 40:207–212, 1994.
74. Scotiniotis IA, Kochman ML, Lewis JD, et al: Accuracy of EUS in the evaluation of Barrett's esophagus and HGD or intramucosal carcinoma. Gastrointest Endosc 54:689–696, 2001.
75. Luketich JD, Schauer P, Landreneau R, et al: Minimally invasive surgical staging is superior to endoscopic ultrasound for detecting lymph node metastasis and esophageal cancer. J Thorac Cardiovasc Surg, 114(5):817–821, 1997.
76. Natsugoe S, Yoshinaka H, Morinaga T, et al: Ultrasonographic detection of lymph-node metastasis in superficial carcinoma of the esophagus. Endoscopy 28(8):674–679, 1996.
77. Ell C, May A, Gossner L, et al: Endoscopic mucosal resection of early cancer and high-grade dysplasia in Barrett's esophagus. Gastroenterology 118:67–70, 2000.
78. Overholt BF, Panjehpour Mhaydek JM: Photodynamic therapy for Barrett's esophagus: Follow up in 100 patients. Gastrointest Endosc 49:1–6, 1999.
79. Farrow PC, Vaughn PL: Determinants of survival following the diagnosis of esophageal adenocarcinoma (US). Cancer Causes Control 7: 322–327, 1996.
80. Lerut T, Coosemans W, Van Raemdonck D, et al: Surgical treatment of Barrett's carcinoma: Correlations between morphologic findings and prognosis. J Thorac Cardiovasc Surg 107(4):1059–1066, 1994.
81. Kelsen DP, Bains M, Burt M: Neoadjuvant chemotherapy and surgery of cancer of the esophagus. Semin Surg Oncol 6(5):268–273, 1990.
82. Coia LR, Engstrom PF, Paul AR, et al: Long-term results of infusional 5-FU, mitomycin-C, and radiation as primary management of esophageal carcinoma. Int J Radiat Oncol Biol Phys 20(1):29–36, 1991.
83. Cooper JS, Guo MD, Herskovic A, et al: Chemoradiotherapy of locally advanced esophageal cancer: Long-term follow-up of a prospective randomized trial (RTOG-85-01). JAMA 281(17):1623–1627, 1999.
84. Smith TJ, Ryan LM, Douglass HO Jr, et al: Combined chemoradiotherapy vs. radiotherapy alone for early stage squamous cell carcinoma of the esophagus: A study of the Eastern Cooperative Oncology Group. Int J Radiat Oncol Biol Phys 42(2):269–276, 1998.
85. Forastiere AA, Orringer MB, Perez-Tamayo C, et al: Preoperative chemoradiation followed by transhiatal esophagectomy for carcinoma of the esophagus: Final report. J Clin Oncol 11(6):1118–1123, 1993.
86. Poplin E, Fleming T, Leichman L, et al: Combined therapies for squamous cell carcinoma of the esophagus, a Southwest Oncology Group Study (SWOG-8037). J Clin Oncol 5(4):622–628, 1987.
87. Stewart JR, Hoff SJ, Johnson DH, et al: Improved survival with neoadjuvant therapy and resection for adenocarcinoma of the esophagus. Ann Surg 218(4):571–578, 1993.
88. Urba SG, Orringer MB, Perez-Tamayo C, et al: Concurrent preoperative chemotherapy and radiation therapy in localized esophageal adenocarcinoma. Cancer 69(2):285–291, 1992.
89. Stahl M, Wilke H, Fink U, et al: Combined preoperative chemotherapy and radiotherapy in patients with locally advanced esophageal cancer: Interim analysis of a phase II trial. J Clin Oncol 14(3):829–837, 1996.
90. Bates BA, Detterbeck FC, Bernard SA, et al: Concurrent radiation therapy and chemotherapy followed by esophagectomy for localized esophageal carcinoma. J Clin Oncol 14(1):156–163, 1996.
91. Bosset JF, Gignoux M, Triboulet JP, et al: Chemoradiotherapy followed by surgery compared with surgery alone in squamous-cell cancer of the esophagus. N Engl J Med 337(3):161–167, 1997.
92. Walsh TN, Noonan N, Hollywood D, et al: A comparison of multimodal therapy and surgery for esophageal adenocarcinoma. N Engl J Med 335(7):462–467, 1996.
93. Kelsen DP, Ginsberg R, Pajak TF, et al: Chemotherapy followed by surgery compared with surgery alone for localized esophageal cancer. N Engl J Med 339(27):1979–1984, 1998.
93a. Nygaard K, Hagen S, Hansen HS, et al: Pre-operative radiotherapy prolongs survival in operable esophageal carcinoma: A randomized, multicenter study of pre-operative radiotherapy and chemotherapy: The second Scandinavian trial in esophageal cancer. World J Surg 16: 1104–1110, 1992.
93b. Le Prise E, Etienne PL, Meunier B, et al: A randomized study of chemotherapy, radiation therapy, and surgery versus surgery for localized squamous cell carcinoma of the esophagus. Cancer 73:1779–1784, 1994.
93c. Apinop C, Puttisak P, Preecha N: A prospective study of combined therapy in esophageal cancer. Hepato-Gastroenterology 41(4):391–393, 1994.
94. Narahara H, Iishi H, Tatsuta M, et al: Effectiveness of endoscopic mucosal resection with submucosal saline injection technique for superficial squamous carcinomas of the esophagus. Gastrointest Endosc 52:730–734, 2000.
95. Inoue H, Takeshita K, Hori H, et al: Endoscopic mucosal resection with a cap-fitted panendoscope for esophagus, stomach, and colon mucosal lesions. Gastrointest Endosc 39:58, 1993.
96. Ell C, May A, Gossner L, et al: Endoscopic mucosal resection of early cancers and high-grade dysplasia in Barrett's esophagus. Gastroenterology 118:670–677, 2000.
97. Radu A, Wagnieres G, van den Bergh H, Monnier P: Photodynamic therapy of early squamous cell cancers of the esophagus. Gastrointest Endosc Clinics N Am 10(3):439–460, 2000.
98. Wang KK: Photodynamic therapy of Barrett's esophagus. Gastrointest Endosc Clinics N Am 10(3):409–419, 2000.
99. Sur RK, Donde B, Levin VC, et al: Fractionated high dose rate intraluminal brachytherapy in palliation of advanced esophageal cancer. Int J Radiat Oncol Biol Phys 40(2):447–453, 1998.
100. Waters JS, Norman A, Cunningham D, et al: Long-term survival after epirubicin, cisplatin and fluorouracil for gastric cancer: Results of a randomized trial. Br J Cancer 80(1/2):269–272, 1999.
101. Enzinger PC, Ilson DH, Kelsen DP: Chemotherapy in esophageal cancer. Semin Oncol 26(suppl 15):12–20, 1999.
102. Tytgat G, den Hartog Jager F: To dilate or intubate? Gastrointest Endosc 29:58–59, 1983.
103. Johnston J, Fleischer D, Petrini J, et al: Palliative bipolar electrocoagulation therapy of obstructing esophageal cancer. Gastrointest Endosc 33:349–353, 1987.
104. Fleischer D, Ranard R, Kanath R, et al: Stricture formation following BICAP tumor probe therapy for esophageal cancer. Gastrointest Endosc 33:183(A), 1987.
105. Jensen D, Macchicado G, Randall G, et al: Comparison of low-power YAG laser and BICAP tumor probe for palliation for esophageal cancer stricture. Gastroenterology 94:1263–1270, 1988.
106. Maunoury V, Brunetaud J, Cochelard et al: Endoscopic palliation for inoperable malignant dysphagia: Long term follow up. Gut 33:1602–1607, 1992.
107. Pietraffitta J, Dwyer R: New laser technique for the treatment of malignant esophageal obstruction. J Surg Oncol 35:157–162, 1987.
108. Pietraffitta J, Bowers G, Dwyer R: Prograde versus retrograde endoscopic laser therapy for the treatment of malignant esophageal obstruction: A comparison of techniques. Lasers Surg Med 8:288–293, 1988.
109. Fleischer D, Kessler F: Endoscopic Nd:YAG laser therapy for carcinoma of the esophagus: A new form of palliative treatment. Gastroenterology 85:600–606, 1983.
110. Mellow M, Pinkas H: Endoscopic therapy for esophageal carcinoma with Nd:YAG laser: Prospective evaluation of efficacy, complications and survival. Gastrointest Endosc 30:334–339, 1984.
111. Cello J, Gerstenberger P, Wright T, et al: Endoscopic neodymium-YAG laser palliation of non-resectable esophageal malignancy. Ann Intern Med 102:610–612, 1985.
112. Pietrafitta J, Dwyer R: Endoscopic laser therapy of malignant esophageal obstruction. Arch Surg 121:395–400, 1986.
113. Bown S, Hawes R, Mattewson K, et al: Endoscopic laser palliation for advanced malignant dysphagia. Gut 28:799–807, 1987.
114. Buset M, des Marez B, Baize M, et al: Palliative endoscopic management of obstructive esophagogastric cancer: Laser for prosthesis? Gastrointest Endosc 33:357–361, 1987.
115. Krasner N, Barr H, Skidmore C, et al: Palliative laser therapy for malignant dysphagia. Gut 28:792–798, 1987.
116. Richter J, Hilgenberg A, Chistensen M, et al: Endoscopic palliation of obstructive esophagogastric malignancy. Gastrointest Endosc 34:454–458, 1988.
117. Maunoury V, Brunetaud J, Cochelard et al: Endoscopic palliation for inoperable malignant dysphagia: Long term follow up. Gut 33:1602–1607, 1992.
118. Stange E, Dyalla J, Fleig W: Laser treatment of upper gastrointestinal tract carcinoma: Determinants of survival. Endoscopy 21:254–257, 1989.

119. Ell C, Demling L: Laser therapy of tumor stenosis in the upper gastrointestinal tract: An international inquiry. Lasers Surg Med 7: 491–494, 1987.
120. Fleischer D, Sivak M. Endoscopic Nd:YAG laser therapy as palliation for esophagogastric cancer: Parameters affecting initial outcome. Gastroenterology 89:827–831, 1985.
121. Gosner L, Ell d: Malignant stricture: Thermal treatment. Gastrointest Endosc Clin N Am 1998:8(2):493–501.
122. Chong SC, Leong HT, Choi CY, et al: Palliation of malignant esophageal obstruction by endoscopic alcohol injection. Endoscopy 26:275–280, 1994.
123. Nwokolo CO, Payne-James JJ, Silk DB, et al: Palliation of malignant dysphagia by ethanol induced tumor necrosis. Gut 35:299–301, 1994.
124. Monga SP, Wadleigh R, Sharma A, et al: Intratumoral therapy of cisplatin/epinephrine injectable gel for palliation in patients with obstructive esophageal cancer. Am J Clin Oncol 23(4):386–392, 2000.
125. Lightdale CJ, Heier SK, Marcon NE, et al: PDT with porfimer sodium versus thermal ablative therapy with Nd:YAG laser for palliation of esophageal cancer: A multicenter randomized trial. Gastrointest Endosc 1995:42:507–512.
126. Heier SK, Rothman KA, Heir LM, et al: Photodynamic therapy for obstruction esophageal cancer: Light dosimetry and randomized comparison with Nd:YAG laser therapy. Gastroenterology 109:63, 1995.
127. Saidi RF, Marcon NE: Nonthermal ablation of malignaat esophageal strictures: Photodynamic therapy, endoscopic intratumoral injection, and novel modalities. Gastrointest Endosc Clin of N Am 8(2):465–491, 1998.
128. Overholt BF, Panjehpour M: Photodynamic therapy for Barrett's esophagus. Gastrointest Endosc Clin N Am 7:207–220, 1997.
129. Knyrim K, Wagner H, Bethge N, et al: A controlled trial of an expansile metal stent for palliation of esophageal obstruction due to inoperable cancer. N Engl J Med 329:1302–1307, 1993.
130. Raijman I, Siddique I, Ajani J, Lynch: Palliation of malignant dysphagia and fistulae with coated expandable metal stents: Experience with 101 patients. Gastrointest Endosc 48:172–179, 1998.
131. Bethge N, Sommer A, Vakil N: Palliation of malignant obstruction due to intrinsic and extrinsic lesions with expandable mental stents. Am J Gastroenterol 93:1829–1832, 1998.
132. May A, Ell d: Palliative treatment of malignant esophagorespiratory fistula with Gianturco-Z stents: A prospective clinical trial and review of the literature on covered metal stents. Am J Gastroenterol 93:532–535, 1998.
133. Raijman I: Endoscopic management of esophagorespiratory fistulas: Expanding our options with expandable stents. Am J Gastroenterol 93: 496–499, 1998.
134. Neuhaus H: The use of stents in the management of malignant esophageal strictures. Gastrointest Endosc Clin N Am 8(2):503–519, 1998.
135. Carr-Locke D (ed): Expandable metal stents. Gastrointest Endosc Clin N Am 9(3):1–544, 1999.
136. Ginsberg GG: Direct percutaneous endoscopic jejunostomy. Tech Gastrointest Endosc 3(1):42–49, 2001.
137. Agha FP, Weatherbee L, Sama JS: Verrucous carcinoma of the esophagus. Am J Gastroenterol 79:844, 1984.
138. Gal AA, Martin SE, Kernen JA, Patterson MJ: Esophageal carcinoma with prominent spindle cells. Cancer 60:2244, 1987.
139. Craig SR, Carey FA, Walker WS, et al: Primary small-cell cancer of the esophagus. J Thorac Cardiovasc Surg 109:284–288, 1995.
140. Mikami T, Fukuda S, Shimoyama T, et al: A case of early stage primary malignant melanoma of the esophagus. Gastrointest Endosc 53:365–367, 2001.
141. Schneider A, Martini N, Burt ME: Malignant melanoma metastatic to the esophagus. Ann Thorac Surg 55:516–519, 1993.
142. Politoske E: Squamous papilloma of the esophagus associated with the human papillomavirus. Gastroenterology 102:668–671, 1992.
143. LiVolsi V, Perzin K: Inflammatory pseudotumors (inflammatory fibrous polyps) of the esophagus: A clinicopathologic study. Dig Dis 20:475–479, 1975.
144. Orvidas LJ, McCaffrey TV, Kurtin PJ, et al: Lymphoma involving the esophagus. Ann Otol Rhinol Laryngol 103:843–847, 1994.
145. Perch SJ, Soffen EM, Whittington R, Brooks JJ: Esophageal sarcomas. J Surg Oncol 48:194–198, 1991.
146. McGrath PC, Neifeld JP, Lawrence W, et al: Gastrointestinal sarcomas. Ann Surg 206:706–710, 1987.
147. Aagaard MT, Kristensen IB, Lund O, et al: Primary malignant nonepithelial tumors of the thoracic oesophagus and cardia in a 25 year surgical material. Scand J Gastroenterol 25:875–882, 1990.
148. Tio TL, Tytgat GNJ: Endoscopic ultrasound in analyzing periintestinal lymph node abnormality. Scand J Gastroenterol 21(suppl 123):158–163, 1986.
149. Pesarini AC, Ernst H, Ell C, et al: Leiomyosarcoma of the esophagus: Clinical aspects, diagnosis and therapy based on an individual case (clinical conference). Med Klin 92(4):234–240, 1997.
150. Connolly GM, Hawkins D, Harcourt-Webster JN, et al: Oesophageal symptoms, their causes, treatment, and prognosis in patients with the acquired immunodeficiency syndrome. Gut 30:1033–1038, 1989.
151. Goldberg RI, Ranis H, Stone B, et al: Dysphagia as the presenting symptoms of recurrent breast carcinoma. Cancer 135:1243–1245, 1987.
152. Seremetis MG, Lyons WS, DeGuzman VC, Peabody JW: Leiomyomata of the esophagus. Cancer 38:2166–2177, 1976.
153. Wisecarver JL: Getting to the GIST of it. Am J Gastroenterol 96:644–645, 2001.
154. Solomon MP, Rosenblum H, Rosato FE: Leiomyoma of the esophagus. Ann Surg 80:246–248, 1984.
155. Gallinger S, Steinhardt MI, Goldberg M: Giant leiomyoma of the esophagus. Am J Gastroenterol 78:708–711, 1983.
156. Yasuda K, Nakajima M, Kawai K: Diagnosis of submucosal lesions of the upper gastrointestinal tract by endoscopic ultrasound. Gastrointest Endosc 36:S17, 1990.
157. Boyce GA, Sivak MV, Rosch T, et al: Evaluation of submucosal upper gastrointestinal tract lesions by endoscopic ultrasound. Gastrointest Endosc 37:449, 1991.
158. Schorlemmer GR, Battaglini JW, Murray GF: The cervical approach to esophageal leiomyomas. Ann Thorac Surg 35:469–471, 1983.
159. Stefansson K, Wollman R: S100 protein in granular cell tumors (granular cell myoblastoma). Cancer 49:1834, 1982.
160. Orlowska J, Pachlewski J, Gugulski A, Butruk E: A conservative approach to granular cell tumors of the esophagus: Four case reports and literature review. Am J Gastroenterol 88:311–315, 1993.
161. Vuyk H, Snow G, Tiwari R, et al: Granular cell tumor of the proximal esophagus, a rare disease. Cancer 55:445–449, 1985.
162. Avezzano EA, Fleischer DE, Merida MA, et al: Giant fibrovascular polyps of the esophagus. Am J Gastroenterol 85:299–301, 1990.
163. Owens JL, Donovan DT, Alford EL, et al: Life-threatening presentations of fibrovascular esophageal and hypopharyngeal polyps. Ann Otol Rhinol Laryngol 103:838–842, 1994.
164. Beckerman RC, Taussig LM, Froede RC, et al: Fibromuscular hamartoma of the esophagus in an infant. Am J Dis Child 134:153–155, 1980.
165. Saitch U, Inomata Y, Tadaki N, Mimaki S: Pedunculated intraluminal osteochondromatous hamartoma of the esophagus. J Otolaryngol 19: 339–342, 1990.
166. Halfhide BC, Ginai AZ, Spoejstra HAA, et al: Case report: A hamartoma presenting as a giant oesophageal polyp. Br J Radiol 68:85–88, 1995.
167. Cantero D, Yoshida T, Ito T, et al: Esophageal hemangioma: Endoscopic diagnosis and treatment. Endoscopy 26:250–253, 1994.
168. Bernatz PE, Smith JL, Ellis FH, et al: Benign, pedunculated, intraluminal tumors of the esophagus. J Thorac Surg 35:503–512, 1958.
169. Cochet B, Hohl P, Sans M, Cox JN: Asphyxia caused by laryngeal impaction of an esophageal polyp. Arch Otolaryngol Head Neck Surg 106:176–178, 1988.
170. Yoshikane H, Tsukamoto Y, Niwa Y, et al: The coexistence of esophageal submucosal tumor and carcinoma. Endoscopy 27:119–123, 1995.

Section Six

STOMACH AND DUODENUM

Chapter 36

ANATOMY, HISTOLOGY, EMBRYOLOGY, AND DEVELOPMENTAL ANOMALIES OF THE STOMACH AND DUODENUM

Carol A. Redel

This chapter will focus on the anatomy and associated anomalies of the stomach and duodenum, and updates an earlier version[1] published in the sixth edition of the text.

ANATOMY OF THE STOMACH

General Considerations

The stomach, as a J-shaped dilation of the alimentary canal, is continuous with the esophagus proximally and the duodenum distally. It functions primarily as a reservoir to store large quantities of recently ingested food, thus allowing intermittent feedings, initiating the digestive process, and releasing its contents in a controlled fashion downstream to accommodate the much smaller capacity of the duodenum. The stomach volume ranges from about 30 mL in a neonate to 1.5 to 2 L in adulthood.

The stomach is recognizable in the fourth week of gestation as a dilation of the distal foregut (Fig. 36–1).[2] As the stomach enlarges, the dorsal aspect grows more rapidly than the ventral aspect, thus forming the greater curvature. Additionally, during the enlargement process, the stomach rotates 90 degrees around its longitudinal axis, orienting the greater curvature (the dorsal aspect) to the left and the lesser curvature (ventral aspect) to the right. The combined effects of rotation and ongoing differential growth result in the stomach lying transversely in the mid and left upper abdomen. The events also explain the vagal innervation of the stomach: the right vagus nerve innervating the posterior stomach wall (the primordial right side) and the left vagus nerve innervating the anterior wall (the primordial left side).

The final location of the stomach is variable owing in part to its two-point fixation at the gastroesophageal and gastroduodenal junctions, allowing for considerable mobility. The gastroesophageal junction generally lies to the left of the 10th thoracic vertebral body, 1 to 2 cm below the diaphragmatic hiatus. The gastroduodenal junction lies at L1 and generally to the right of the midline in the recumbent fasted individual. The gastroduodenal junction of a distended upright adult may be considerably lower. The left-sided and caudal greater curvature may extend below the umbilicus depending on the degree of distention, position, and gastric peristaltic phase.

The greater curvature forms the left lower stomach border, whereas the lesser curvature forms the right upper border. Posteriorly, portions of the pancreas, transverse colon, diaphragm, spleen, and apex of the left kidney and suprarenal gland bound the stomach. The posterior wall of the stomach actually comprises the anterior wall of the omental bursa, or lesser peritoneal sac. Anteriorly, the liver bounds the stomach, whereas the inner aspect of the anterior abdominal wall bounds the anterior left lower aspect.

The stomach is completely invested by peritoneum, excepting a small bare area at the gastroesophageal junction. This peritoneum passes as a double layer from the lesser curvature to the liver as the gastrohepatic portion of the lesser omentum and then hangs down from the fundus and greater curvature as the greater omentum, extending to the transverse colon (as the gastrocolic ligament), spleen (as the gastrosplenic ligament), and diaphragm (as the gastrophrenic ligament).

The stomach is divided into four regions, which can be defined by anatomic or histologic landmarks (Fig. 36–2).[3]

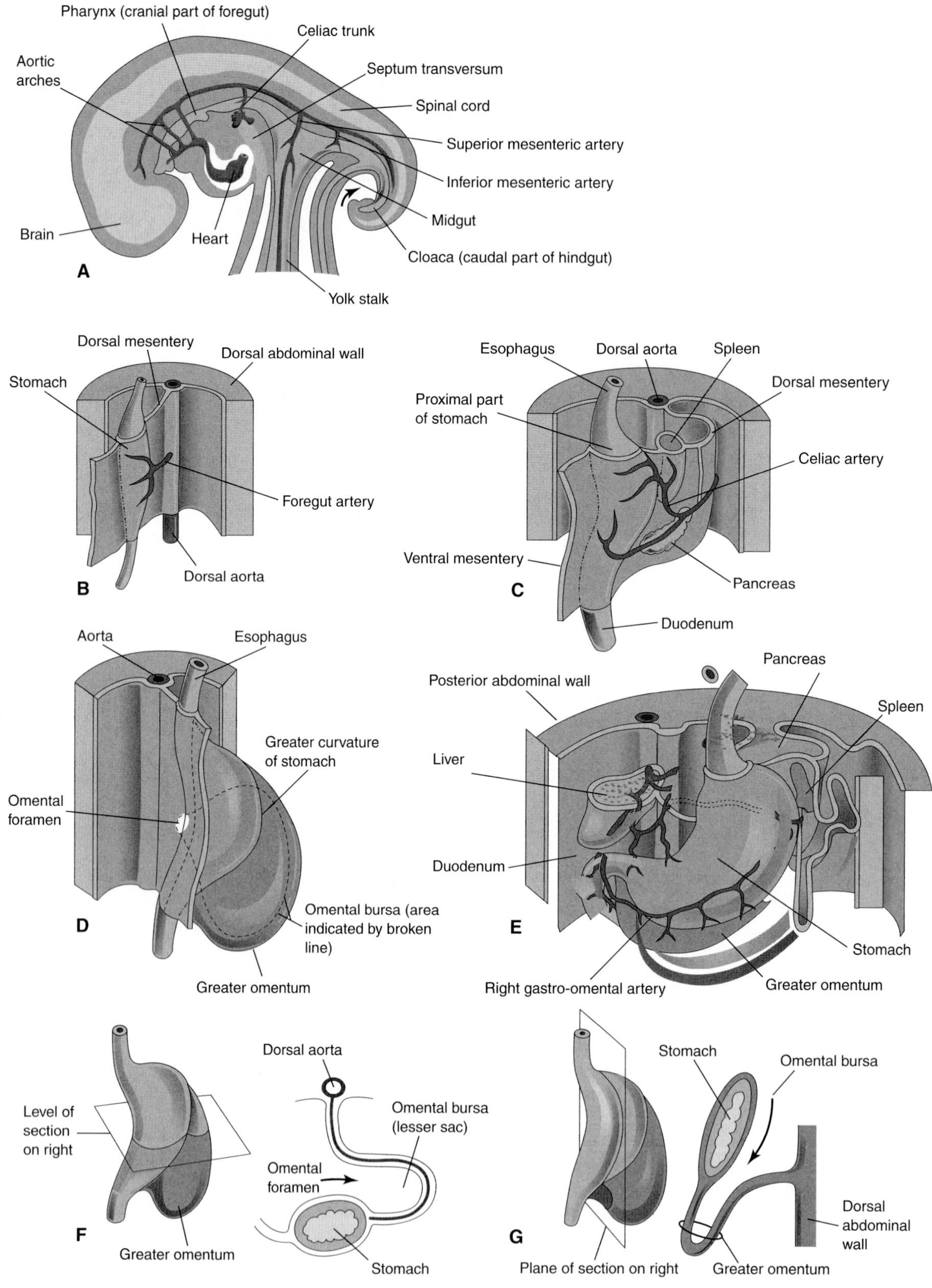

Figure 36–1. Development and rotation of the stomach and formation of the omental bursa (i.e., the lesser sac) and the greater omentum. *A,* 28 days. *B,* Anterolateral view, 28 days. *C,* 35 days. *D,* 40 days. *E,* 48 days. *F,* Lateral view, 52 days. Transverse section of the omental foramen and the omental bursa. *G,* Sagittal section of the omental bursa and the greater omentum. (From Moore KL, Persaud TVN: The Developing Human, 6th ed. Philadelphia, WB Saunders, 1998, p 274.)

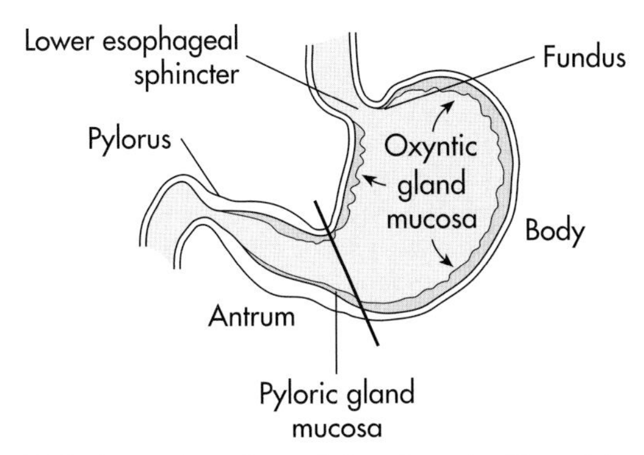

Figure 36–2. Anatomic regions of the stomach. (From Johnson, LR: Gastrointestinal Physiology, 6th ed. St. Louis, CV Mosby, 2001, p 76.)

The *cardia* is the small, ill-defined area of the stomach immediately adjacent to its junction with the esophagus and is located slightly left of the midline. The cardia is the most fixed portion of the stomach. The *fundus* projects upward, above the cardia and gastroesophageal junction. This dome-shaped area of the stomach is its most superior portion and is in contact above with the left hemidiaphragm and to the left with the spleen. The *body,* or corpus, the largest portion of the stomach, is located immediately below and continuous with the fundus. The *incisura angularis,* a fixed, sharp indentation two thirds of the distance down the lesser curvature, marks the caudal aspect of the gastric body (Fig. 36–3). The gastric *antrum* extends from its indistinct border with the body to the junction of the pylorus with the duodenum. These gross anatomic landmarks correspond roughly with the mucosal histology, because antral mucosa actually extends from an area on the lesser curvature somewhat above the incisura. The *pylorus* (pyloric channel) is a tubular structure joining the duodenum to the stomach and contains the palpable circular muscle, the pyloric sphincter. The pylorus is somewhat mobile owing to its enclosure between the peritoneum of the greater and lesser omenta but is generally located 2 cm to the right of midline at L1.

Vascular Supply and Drainage; Lymphatic Drainage

The arterial blood supply to the stomach is derived from branches of the celiac artery—common hepatic, left gastric, and splenic arteries—that form two arterial arcades situated along the lesser curvature and the lower two thirds of the greater curvature. The lesser curvature is supplied from above by the left gastric artery and from below by the right gastric artery, a branch of the common hepatic artery or gastroduodenal artery (which is a branch of the common hepatic artery). The greater curvature below the fundus is supplied from above by the left gastroepiploic artery (a branch of the splenic artery) and from below by the right gastroepiploic artery (a branch of the gastroduodenal artery). The right and left gastroepiploic arteries usually terminate by anastomosing, thus completing the greater curvature arterial arcade; occasionally they end without anastomosis. The arterial supply to the gastric fundus and left upper aspect of the greater curvature is via the short gastric arteries, which arise from the splenic artery.

The venous drainage of the stomach generally accompanies the arterial supply, emptying into the portal vein or one of its tributaries, the splenic or superior mesenteric veins. The left and right gastric veins drain the lesser curvature of the stomach. The left gastric vein is also known as the *coronary vein.* The right and left gastroepiploic veins drain the inferior aspect and a portion of the greater curvature of the stomach. The right gastroepiploic vein, with several more distal veins, becomes the gastrocolic veins, eventually terminating in the superior mesenteric vein. There is no gastroduodenal vein. The left gastroepiploic vein becomes the splenic vein and later receives the short gastric veins, thus draining the fundus and upper great curvature of the stomach.

Most of the lymphatic drainage of the stomach eventually reaches the celiac nodes after passing through intermediary lymph nodes. Lymphatic channels anastomose freely in the gastric wall, with lymphatic flow directed through one-way valves into one of four groups of nodes. The inferior gastric region drains into subpyloric and omental nodes, then the hepatic nodes, and finally terminates in the celiac nodes. The splenic or superior aspect of the greater curvature lymph initially drains into pancreaticosplenic nodes and then into celiac nodes. The superior gastric or lesser curvature region lymph drains into the left and right gastric nodes adjacent to their respective vessels and terminates in the celiac nodes. The hepatic or pyloric portion of the lesser curvature lymph drains into the suprapyloric nodes, then the hepatic nodes, and finally, into the celiac nodes.

Gastric Innervation

The autonomic innervation of the stomach stems from both the sympathetic and parasympathetic nervous systems deliv-

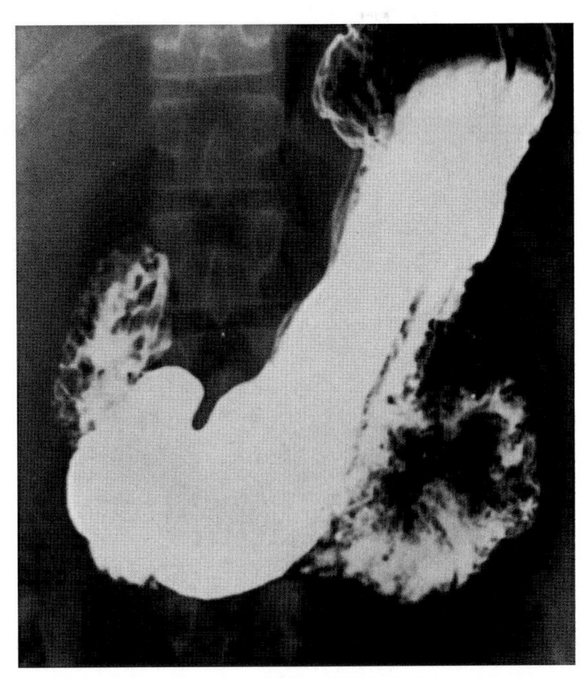

Figure 36–3. Upper gastrointestinal radiograph demonstrating the incisura angularis on the distal lesser curvature. (Courtesy of James W. Weaver, MD.)

ered via a complex tangle of nerves coursing along the visceral arteries.

The gastric sympathetic innervation is derived from preganglionic fibers arising predominantly from T6 to T8 spinal nerves, which synapse within the bilateral celiac ganglia to neurons whose postganglionic fibers course through the celiac plexus along the vascular supply of the stomach. Accompanying these sympathetic nerves are afferent pain-transmitting fibers from the stomach and motor fibers to the pyloric sphincter.

The parasympathetic innervation is via the right and left vagus nerves, which form the distal esophageal plexus, which gives rise to the posterior and anterior vagal trunks near the gastric cardia. The trunks contain preganglionic parasympathetic fibers as well as afferent fibers from the viscera. Both trunks give rise to celiac and hepatic branches before continuing on within the lesser omentum slightly to the right of the lesser curvature as the anterior nerve of Latarjet and the posterior nerve of Latarjet. These nerves give rise to multiple gastric branches to the stomach wall, where the preganglionic fibers synapse with the ganglion cells in the submucosal (Meissner's) and myenteric (Auerbach's) plexuses. From these plexuses, postganglionic fibers are distributed to secretory components, including cells and glands, and to motor components, such as muscle.

Tissue Layers of the Stomach

The luminal surface of the gastric wall forms thick, longitudinally oriented folds or rugae, which flatten with distention. Four layers make up the gastric wall: mucosa, submucosa, muscularis propria, and serosa. Mucosa lines the gastric lumen, appearing as a smooth, velvety, blood-filled lining. The mucosa of the cardia, antrum, and pylorus is somewhat paler than that of the fundus and body. It is within the gastric mucosa that most of the functional secretory elements of the stomach are located (see Chapter 38). The submucosa, immediately deep to the mucosa, provides the dense connective tissue skeleton of collagen and elastin fibers. Lymphocytes, plasma cells, arterioles, venules, lymphatics, and the submucosal plexus are also contained within the submucosa. The third tissue layer, the muscularis propria, is a combination of three muscle layers: inner oblique, middle circular and outer longitudinal. The inner oblique muscle fibers course over the gastric fundus, covering the anterior and posterior aspects of the stomach wall. The middle circular fibers encircle the body of the stomach, thickening distally to become the pyloric sphincter. The outer longitudinal muscle fibers course primarily along the greater and lesser curvatures of the stomach. The final layer of the stomach is the transparent serosa, a continuation of the visceral peritoneum.

Microscopic Anatomy

The gastric mucosal surface is composed primarily of a simple layer of columnar epithelial cells 20 to 40 μm in height. These surface mucous cells (Fig. 36–4), which are similar throughout the stomach, contain basally located nuclei, prominent Golgi stacks, and dense cytoplasm with especially apically dense mucin-containing membrane-bound

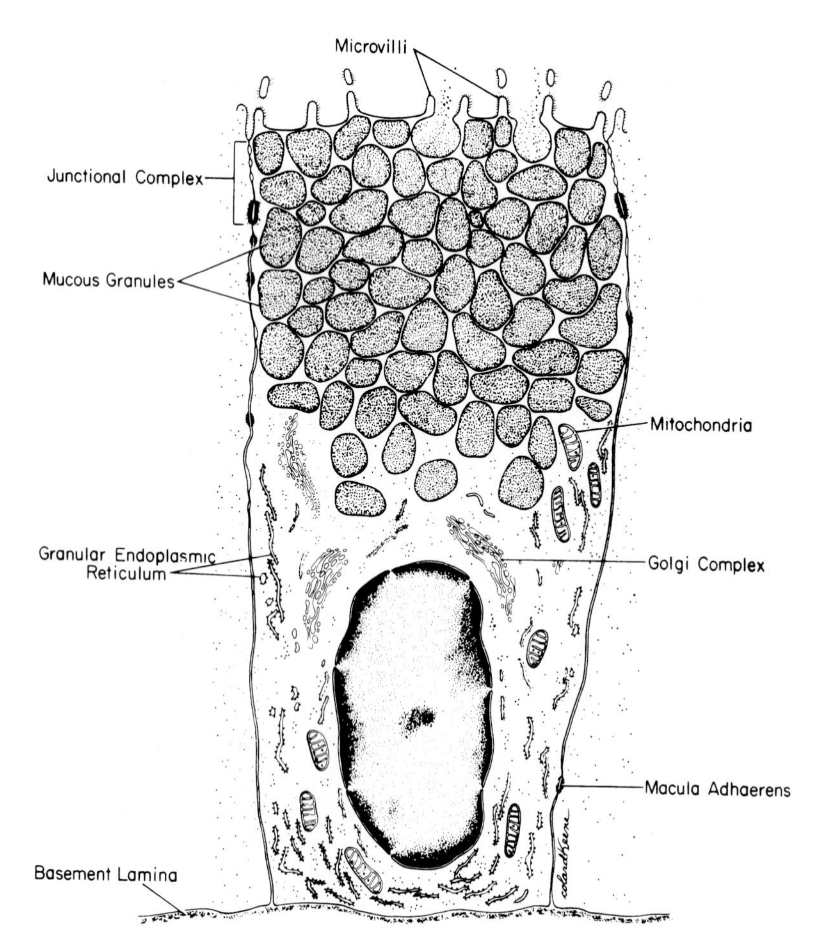

Figure 36–4. Surface mucous cell.

granules. The cells secrete mucus in granules, which are released via exocytosis, apical expulsion, and cell exfoliation. The primary role of mucus, along with bicarbonate, is luminal cytoprotection from "the elements": acid, pepsin, ingested substances, and pathogens. Cellular renewal time for a gastric surface mucous cell is approximately 3 days.

The surface epithelial lining is invaginated by gastric pits, or foveolae, which provide the gastric glands access to the gastric lumen, with a ratio of one pit to four or five gastric glands. The gastric glands of different anatomic regions of the stomach are lined with different types of specialized epithelial cells, allowing for differentiation of these regions by type of gastric gland (see Fig. 36–2). The first region, the cardia, is a small (1.5 to 3 cm) transition zone from esophageal squamous epithelium to gastric columnar epithelium. The cardiac glands have a branched and tortuous configuration and are populated by mucous, endocrine, and undifferentiated cells. There is a gradual transition from cardiac glands to the second region, the acid-secreting segment of the stomach. This region encompasses the gastric fundus and body and contains the oxyntic (or parietal or fundic) glands. Parietal, chief (also known as peptic), endocrine, mucous neck, and undifferentiated cells compose the oxyntic glands. The final region, corresponding to the antrum and pylorus, contains the pyloric glands, composed of endocrine, mucous, and gastrin-producing G cells.

By far the most numerous and distinctive gastric glands are the oxyntic glands (Fig. 36–5), responsible for the secretion of acid, intrinsic factor, and most gastric enzymes. These fairly straight and simple tubular glands are closely associated in the areas of gastric fundus and body. A typical gland is subdivided into three areas: the isthmus (where oxyntic and surface mucous cells predominate), the neck (where oxyntic and mucous neck cells predominate), and the base (primarily chief cells, plus some oxyntic and mucous neck cells). Therefore, parietal cells are predominantly in the isthmus and neck regions, whereas chief cells predominate in the base. Endocrine cells, somatostatin-containing D cells, and histamine-secreting enterochromaffin-like (ECL) cells—are scattered throughout the oxyntic epithelium.

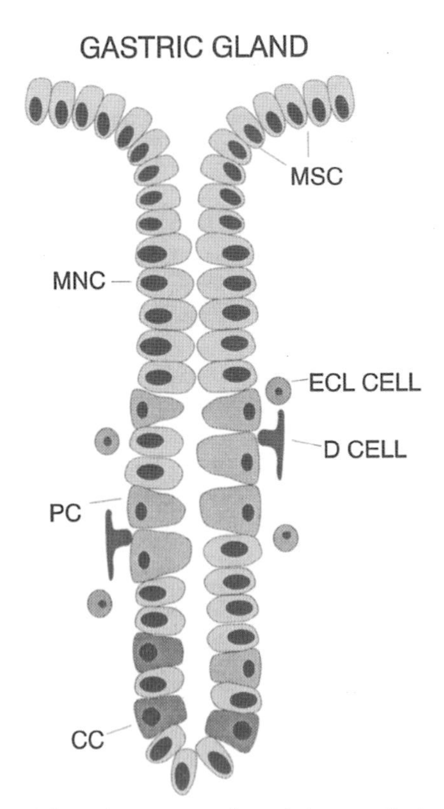

Figure 36–5. Schematic representation of the oxyntic (gastric) gland, with mucous surface cells (MSC), mucous neck cells (MNC), enterochromaffin-like (ECL) cells, somatostatin containing D cells (D CELL), parietal cells (PC), and chief cells (CC). (From Lloyd KCK, Debas, T: The peripheral regulation of gastric acid secretion. In Johnson LR, et al [eds]: Physiology of the Gastrointestinal Tract, vol 2, 3rd ed. New York, Lippincott-Raven, 1994.)

The principal cell type of the oxyntic gland is the parietal cell (Fig. 36–6), responsible for the oxyntic mucosal secretion of 3×10^6 hydrogen ions per second, at a final HCl concentration of around 150 mmol/L. Parietal cells bulge into the lumina of the oxyntic glands, and, as the primary hydrogen secretors, have ultrastructural characteristics different from other gastric cells: large mitochondria, microvilli lacking in glycocalyx, and a cytoplasmic canaliculi system in contact with the lumen. In the nonsecreting parietal cell, a cytoplasmic tubulovesicular system predominates, and short microvilli line the apical canaliculus. In the secreting state, the tubulovesicular system disappears, leaving an extensive system of intracellular canaliculi containing long microvilli. Mitochondria occupy approximately 30% to 40% of the secreting parietal cell volume, providing energy required for acid secretion across apical microvilli (see Fig. 36–6). The so-called proton pump—the H^+/K^+-ATPase—resides in the apical microvillus membrane, as does carbonic anhydrase. The apical H^+/K^+-ATPase functions as the proton translocator in gastric acid secretion (see Chapter 38). Acid secretion begins within 5 to 10 minutes of stimulation. Additionally, parietal cells are the site of intrinsic factor secretion via membrane-associated vesicle transport.

Closely associated with parietal cells are mucous neck cells, which appear singly close to parietal cells, or in groups of two or three in the oxyntic gland neck or isthmus. Mucous neck cells differ from their surface counterparts in their synthesis of acidic, sulfated mucus rather than the neutral mucus secreted by the surface mucous cells. Additionally, mucous neck cells have basal nuclei and larger mucous granules around the nucleus rather than apically located granules. Function of the two cell types appears different, in that surface mucous cells are cytoprotective, whereas the mucous neck cell functions as a stem cell precursor for surface mucous, parietal, chief, and endocrine cells.

Chief cells, also known as *zymogen cells,* predominate in deeper layers of the oxyntic glands. These pyramid-shaped cells play a role in synthesis and secretion of pepsinogens I and II. The cytoplasm of chief cells has prominent basophilic staining owing to abundance of ribosomes; these ribosomes are either free in cytoplasm or in association with an extensive endoplasmic reticulum system. Zymogen granules lie in the apical cytoplasm; their cytoplasm is released into the gastric lumen following fusion of the limiting membrane of the granule with the luminal membrane. Once in the lumen, pepsinogens are converted to pepsin.

A variety of endocrine, or enteroendocrine, cells are scattered among the cells of the oxyntic glands. These cells vary in location, being either open or closed relative to the gastric lumen. Open endocrine cells have apical membranes containing receptors; these open cells discharge their contents by

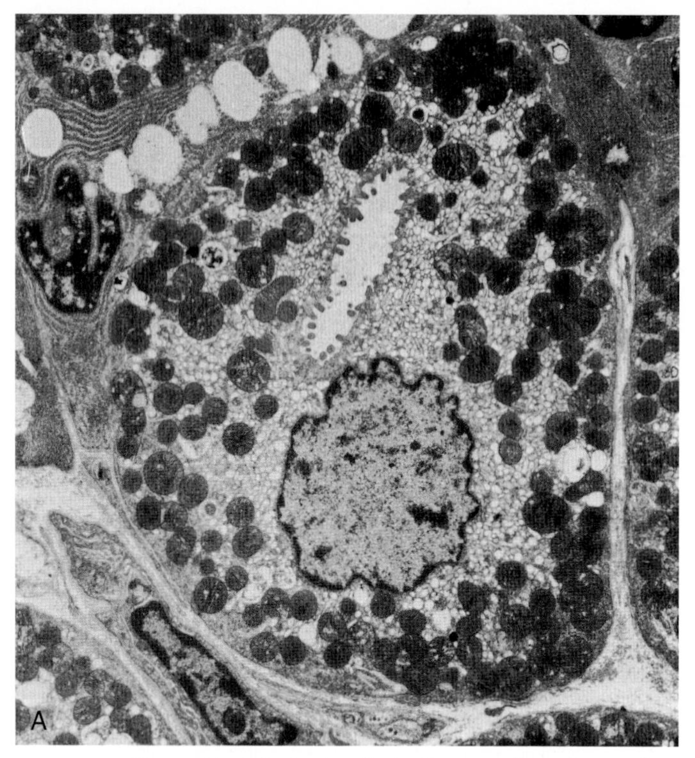

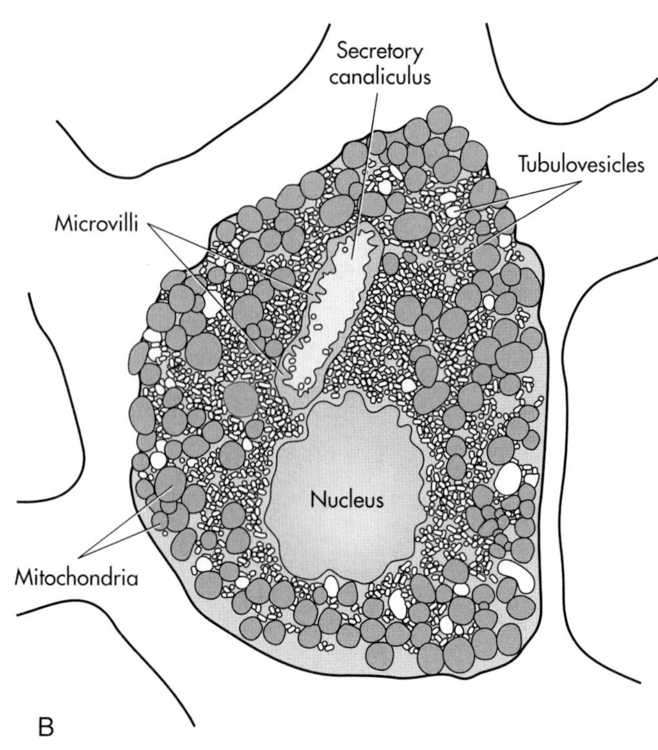

Figure 36–6. Parietal cell. *A,* Electron photomicrograph. *B,* Schematic. (*A* and *B,* From Johnson LR: Gastrointestinal Physiology, 6th ed. St. Louis, CV Mosby, 2001, pp 78 and 79.)

basilar exocytosis into the bloodstream, thus exerting an endocrine effect. The closed endocrine cells contain several processes that terminate near its target cells, constituting the so-called paracrine effect. The oxyntic gland model of the closed cell is the D cell, which secretes somatostatin via long processes reaching ECL, parietal, and chief cells.

Enteroendocrine cell types have also been classified by their granular staining with silver or chromium. Those cells containing granules that reduce silver without pretreatment are called *argentaffin cells.* Argentaffin cells, which stain with potassium dichromate, are termed *enterochromaffin (EC) cells*; most of these contain serotonin. Cells with granules staining with silver only in the presence of a reducing agent are called *argyrophilic,* or ECL cells. Located primarily in the oxyntic glands, ECL cells are the only enteroendocrine cells containing histamine.

The final region of the stomach encompasses the antrum and pylorus and contains extensively coiled antral glands composed of endocrine and epithelial cells. The epithelial cells are predominantly mucous cells, and there are small numbers of pepsinogen II–secreting oxyntic cells. Although also small in number, gastrin-secreting (G) cells play a vital physiologic role and are the prototype of the open enteroendocrine cell. These cells, which occur either singly or in small clusters in the mid to deep sections of antral glands, contain a basilar cytoplasm densely packed with gastrin-containing secretory granules (Fig. 36–7). Gastrin release is stimulated by gastric distention, vagal stimulation, dietary amino acids, and peptide, with rapid appearance of the hormone into the bloodstream in the postprandial period (see Chapter 38). The apical or luminal surface of the G cell is narrowed into small microvilli thought to contain receptors responsible for amino acid and peptide stimulation of gastrin release. Significant quantities of gastrin are also secreted into the gastric lumen, but its physiologic fate remains unknown. Recent evidence suggests that gastrin itself may function in precursor cell differentiation to parietal, chief, and ECL cell lines.[4, 5] Antral enteroendocrine D cells found in close association with G cells manufacture somatostatin, a potent inhibitor of gastrin secretion. These D cells are also present in small numbers in oxyntic glands. Somatostatin is thought to inhibit acid secretion through paracrine (direct action on ECL and perhaps parietal cells or indirect action on G cells) or endocrine effects (direct action on parietal cells).

Immediately deep to the basement membrane of the gastric mucosa epithelial layer lies the lamina propria, which contains a variety of leukocytes (polymorphonuclear leukocytes, plasma cells, lymphocytes, eosinophils), mast cells, fibroblasts, and endocrine-like cells. A few lymphatic channels course through the lamina propria. Additionally, the mucosal capillary plexus lies in the lamina propria and forms a venule plexus, which communicates with the venules in the muscularis mucosa. These venules eventually empty into veins of the submucosa.

ANATOMY OF THE DUODENUM

General Considerations

The duodenum is the most proximal of the four sections of the small intestine and is continuous proximally with the pylorus and distally with the jejunum. It forms a C-shaped loop around the head of the pancreas. In the adult, the

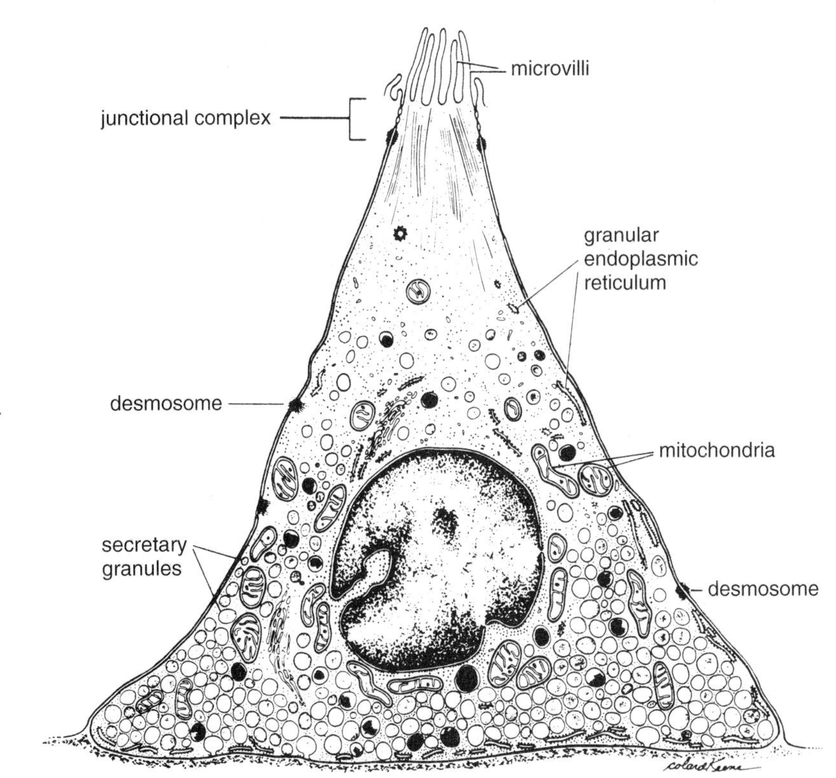

Figure 36–7. G cell from the pyloric gland.

length of the duodenum is approximately 30 cm (12 inches, hence its name *duodenum*), and is subdivided into four sections (commonly termed the first, second, third, and fourth parts), whose borders are delineated by angular course changes.

The first part of the duodenum is about 5 cm in length and courses rightward, upward, and backward from the pylorus. Loosely attached to the liver by the hepatoduodenal portion of the lesser omentum, the first part moves in response to movement by the pylorus. The gastroduodenal artery, the common bile duct, and the portal vein are located posterior, while the gallbladder lies anterior to the first part of the duodenum. The proximal portion of the first part of the duodenum is also referred to as the *duodenal bulb* or *cap*. The second part of the duodenum is 7 to 10 cm in length, coursing downward parallel and in front of the hilum of the right kidney and to the right in contact with the pancreatic head. Slightly inferior to the midpoint of the second part of the duodenum on the posteromedial wall, the nipple-like major duodenal papilla marks the location of the *ampulla of Vater*, through which the pancreaticobiliary ducts empty into the duodenum. On the same wall 2 cm proximal to the major papilla, there may be a minor duodenal papilla that forms the opening for the accessory pancreatic duct. The third part of the duodenum is about 10 cm in length and courses transversely from right to left crossing the midline anterior to the spine, aorta, and inferior vena cava. The superior mesenteric artery and vein course anterior to the third part of the duodenum generally to the right of midline. The fourth and final section of the duodenum is 5 cm long and courses upward to the left of the aorta to reach the inferior border of the pancreas. The junction between the duodenum and the jejunum (*duodenojejunal flexure*) is fixed posteriorly by the *ligament of Treitz*.

The duodenal wall is composed of outer longitudinal and inner circular muscle layers. As is the case with the remainder of the small intestine, the luminal surface is lined with mucosa, forming circular folds known as the *plicae circulares* or *valvulae conniventes*. An exception to this is the duodenal bulb, distinguished radiographically and endoscopically by its smooth, featureless mucosa.

The first few centimeters of the duodenum are shrouded by anterior and posterior elements of the peritoneum. The remainder of the duodenum lies posterior to the peritoneum and thus is retroperitoneal.

The duodenum develops during the fourth week of gestation from the distal foregut, proximal midgut, and the adjacent splanchnic mesenchyme. The junction of the foregut and midgut occurs in the second part of the duodenum, slightly distal to the major papilla. As the stomach rotates, so too does the duodenum, thus developing a C-shaped configuration. During weeks 5 and 6 of embryologic development, the duodenal lumen is temporarily obliterated owing to proliferation of its mucosal lining. During the following weeks, luminal vacuolization and degeneration of some of the proliferating cells result in recanalization of the duodenal lumen. Epithelium and glands develop from embryonic endoderm, whereas connective tissue, muscle, and serosa are derived from mesoderm.

Vascular, Lymphatic, and Nerve Supply

The arterial supply to the duodenum is based on its embryonic origin in that branches of the celiac trunk (as derived from foregut) supply the proximal duodenum, whereas the distal duodenum (as derived from midgut) is supplied by branches of the *superior mesenteric artery*. From the celiac trunk arises the hepatic artery, from which arises the *gastroduodenal artery*. The gastroduodenal artery in turn branches into the superior *pancreaticoduodenal artery*, which gives off anterior and posterior branches to the duodenum. These branches anastomose with analogous branches of the inferior pancreaticoduodenal artery, a branch of the superior mesenteric artery.

The venous drainage corresponds to the arterial supply, with the superior pancreaticoduodenal veins coursing between the duodenum and pancreatic head to enter the portal vein. Likewise, both anterior and posterior inferior pancreaticoduodenal veins empty into either a *jejunal vein* or directly into the *superior mesenteric vein*.

The duodenal lymphatic drainage also corresponds to the vascular supply. Small anterior and posterior duodenal lymph channels drain into the *pancreaticoduodenal nodes*. From these nodes, lymph drains superiorly into the hepatic nodes, or inferiorly into superior mesenteric nodes located at the origin of the superior mesenteric artery.

As in the case in the stomach, duodenal innervation is provided by both sympathetic and parasympathetic nervous systems. The preganglionic sympathetic nerves course through the celiac and superior mesenteric ganglia, with postganglionic neurons entering the duodenal intramural plexuses. Afferent fibers accompany the sympathetic neurons, primarily carrying fibers for visceral pain sensation. Parasympathetic fibers, supplied by the hepatic branch of the anterior vagus nerve and the mesenteric nerves, synapse with Meissner's and Auerbach's plexuses in the duodenal wall.

Microscopic Anatomy

Microscopically, the duodenum differs dramatically from the gastric mucosa with the change from gastric glands and pits to a mucosa lined with villi surrounded by *crypts of Lieberkühn* and submucosa with characteristic *Brunner's glands*. A single layer of epithelial cells provides the interface between the duodenal lumen and mucosa in the areas of both villi and crypts. Deep to this epithelial layer are contained absorptive cells, Paneth cells (which secrete lysozyme and other host defense factors), mucous cells, and endocrine cells.

The villi in the proximal duodenum have distorted appearance thought related to gastric acid. In contrast, the villi of the distal duodenum are tall, slender, and very regular, similar to those in the jejunum. The ratio of villi to crypts in the distal duodenum is 4 : 1 or 5 : 1, again similar to the ratio in the jejunum. Within the submucosa of the duodenum are located the branched Brunner's glands, which secrete an alkaline and clear mucus–containing bicarbonate, epidermal growth factor, and pepsinogen II. Brunner's glands are most numerous in the proximal duodenum and decrease in number distally. Rather than emptying into the duodenum through their own duct system, Brunner's glands empty into the duodenum through adjacent intestinal glands.

CONGENITAL ANOMALIES OF THE STOMACH AND DUODENUM

The congenital anomalies of the stomach and duodenum are summarized in Table 36–1.

Gastric Anomalies

Congenital anomalies of the stomach are among the least frequently encountered malformations of the gastrointestinal tract. These lesions may present during the neonatal period or later in life, depending on the degree of gastric outlet obstruction.

Gastric Atresia

Gastric atresias generally occur in the antrum or pylorus in one of three forms: complete segmental defect, segmental defect bridged by a remnant of a fibrous cord, or a membrane (also called a *web, diaphragm,* or *septum*). These lesions are uncommon, with a reported incidence of 1 to 3/100,000; membranes comprise the majority. Membranes consist of gastric mucosa, submucosa, and muscularis mucosa. In contrast, the fibrous cord generally lacks mucosal elements but contains normal serosal and muscular layers. Membranes may be complete (totally obstructive), or incomplete (perforate). For the sake of clarity, incomplete gastric membranes, which are by definition not atresias, are also considered here.

Pathogenesis

The cause of these lesions remains unknown, but the timing of a contrary developmental event may determine the type of atresia. For example, if there is fusion of redundant endoderm prior to 8 weeks' gestation (prior to muscle layer development), then discontinuity of gastric wall musculature would result in a segmental defect with or without a fibrous cord. On the other hand, if redundancy occurs after 8 weeks' gestation, when muscle layers are complete, a simple membrane develops. An alternative mechanism—focal ischemia at a critical time in development—has been proposed. Finally, failure of recanalization of the gastric lumen following temporary obstruction from mucosal proliferation has been proposed as a cause but is not a viable explanation because obstruction/recanalization does not occur in the stomach (unlike the esophagus and duodenum).[6] Recently, total epithelial detachment of gastric mucosa, associated with $\alpha_6\beta_4$ integrin expression deficiency at the junction of epithelial cells and lamina propria, has been noted in a child with pyloric atresia.[7]

Genetic factors are also important because there is a familial form (autosomal recessive). Also, both Down's syndrome and junctional epidermolysis bullosa are associated with an increased incidence of gastric atresia. In the case of epidermolysis bullosa–pyloric atresia–obstructive uropathy association, mutations in the α_6 and β_4 integrin subunits of the hemidesmosome have been noted.[8, 9] Other associated anomalies are malrotation, atrial septal defect, absent gallbladder, tracheoesophageal fistula, vaginal atresia, and absent extrahepatic portal vein.[10]

Chemical Presentation and Diagnosis

In proximal gastrointestinal obstruction polyhydramnios is commonly noted during pregnancy. Newborn infants with any variant of gastric atresia have signs of gastric outlet

Table 36–1 | **Anomalies of the Stomach and Duodenum**

ANOMALY	INCIDENCE	AGE AT PRESENTATION	SYMPTOMS AND SIGNS	THERAPY
Gastric, antral, or pyloric atresia	3:100,000, when combined with webs	Infancy	Nonbilious emesis	Gastroduodenostomy, gastrojejunostomy
Pyloric or antral membrane	As above	Any age	Failure to thrive, emesis	Incision or excision, pyloroplasty
Microgastria	Rare	Infancy	Emesis, malnutrition	Continuous-drip feedings or jejunal reservoir pouch
Pyloric stenosis	United States, 3:1,000 (regional, 1:1,000–8:1,000) male/female, 4:1	Infancy	Nonbilious emesis	Pyloromyotomy
Gastric duplication	Rare male/female, 1:2	Any age	Abdominal mass, emesis, hematemesis; peritonitis if ruptured	Excision or partial gastrectomy
Gastric diverticulum	Rare	Any age	Usually asymptomatic	Usually unnecessary
Gastric teratoma	Rare	Any age	Upper abdominal mass	Resection
Gastric volvulus	Rare	Any age	Emesis, feeding refusal	Reduction of volvulus, anterior gastropexy
Duodenal atresia or stenosis	1:20,000	Newborn	Bilious emesis, upper abdominal distention	Duodenojejunostomy or gastrojejunostomy
Annular pancreas	1:10,000	Any age	Bilious emesis, failure to thrive	Duodenojejunostomy
Duodenal duplication	Rare	Any age	Gastrointestinal bleeding, pain	Excision
Malrotation and midgut volvulus	Rare	Any age	Bilious emesis, upper abdominal distention	Reduction, division of bands, possibly resection

obstruction including onset of forceful, nonbilious emesis following the first feeding. There may be drooling and respiratory distress. The abdomen is generally scaphoid unless gastric distention is present. When diagnosis is delayed, severe metabolic acidosis, dehydration, and shock occur; prolonged gastric distention may result in perforation. Abdominal radiographs demonstrate gaseous distention of the stomach and a gasless intestine. Upper gastrointestinal contrast study shows complete obstruction of the stomach, generally at the level of the antrum or pylorus. The type of lesion (such as a membrane) can be determined only via surgical exploration.

In the usual case of incomplete antral and pyloric membranes, the age of presentation depends on the degree of obstruction; symptoms may therefore develop at any age from infancy to adulthood. These lesions, except for the presence of membrane perforations, are identical to the membranes of gastric atresia. Luminal narrowing occurs secondary to the malformation itself and also from inflammation and edema in the membrane itself. The primary symptom is vomiting, which in the case of the infant or child may result in failure to establish normal weight gain. In older children and adults, the symptoms may mimic those of peptic ulcer disease with nausea, epigastric pain, and weight loss. Diarrhea has been observed, but its physiologic basis is unknown. The abdominal radiograph is typically normal, although gastric distention may be noted. Occasionally the diagnosis may be suggested by prenatal ultrasonographic findings of dilated stomach without polyhydramnios. Definitive diagnosis is established by contrast radiography, ultrasonography, or upper endoscopy. Contrast radiography demonstrates the membrane as a thin, circumferential filling defect in the antrum or pylorus. Careful observation shows contrast material with delayed passage through a central defect in the membrane; overall gastric emptying is delayed. Ultrasonography may demonstrate segmentation of the antrum, whereas on upper endoscopy a small, fixed opening in the antrum or pylorus may be evident, surrounded by a mucosa free of folds.

Treatment

Following patient stabilization with fluids and gastric decompression, definitive treatment is surgical. Complete or incomplete antral membranes are treated by simple excision. Pyloric membranes require pyloroplasty. The presence of a concomitant duodenal atresia has been described (also known as *windsock diaphragm*), and its presence or absence is verified by passage of a catheter distally into the duodenum intraoperatively. Endoscopic resection using snare, papillotome, laser, or dilation via balloon has also been described. In cases involving atretic gap, gastroduodenostomy is considered curative. An alternative approach is pyloric sphincter reconstruction via longitudinal pyloromyotomy followed by end-to-end anastomosis of cul-de-sacs of gastric and duodenal mucosa.[11] Gastrojejunostomy is not recommended in children because of the risk of marginal ulcer.

Microgastria

Microgastria is an extremely rare congenital anomaly of the caudal part of the foregut. There is a small, tubular or saccular, incompletely rotated stomach associated with a megaesophagus. Varying degrees of the anomaly occur owing to arrested development during the fifth week of gestation in differentiation of the greater curvature of the stomach; neither rotation nor fusiform dilation of the stomach occurs.[12] Fortunately, normal histology is preserved. Microgastria may occur as an isolated anomaly or in association with duodenal atresia; nonrotation of the midgut; hepatic symmetry; ileal duplication; hiatal hernia; asplenia; partial situs inversus; or renal, upper limb, cardiac, pulmonary, skeletal, or spinal anomalies. In isolation, microgastria is not lethal, but other associated anomalies may be. Familial occurrence has not been described; chromosome analysis is normal. The etiology is unknown.

Clinical Presentation and Diagnosis

The infant typically presents with postprandial vomiting and malnutrition. There may also be diarrhea (a result of rapid gastric emptying), dumping syndrome, respiratory distress at birth, or aspiration. Anemia may occur owing to iron deficiency, because decreased gastric acid secretion precludes adequate iron absorption, and cobalamin (vitamin B_{12}) deficiency due to hyposecretion of intrinsic factor. Prenatal ultrasonography may detect a small stomach and polyhydramnios. Contrast radiography shows the megaesophagus and tubular or small stomach. The lower esophageal sphincter is poorly defined, and gastroesophageal reflux is usually severe.

Treatment

The conservative management of microgastria includes frequent, small-volume feedings or continuous-drip feedings into the stomach. An alternative feeding is nocturnal drip feedings via jejunostomy to supplement oral intake.[13] The creation of a double-lumen Roux-en-Y pouch anastomosed to the greater curvature of the stomach has been described. This Hunt-Lawrence jejunal pouch has allowed normal growth and development and prevented reflux and dumping syndrome.[14]

Gastric Diverticulum (see also Chapter 19)

A gastric diverticulum is the rarest type of gastrointestinal diverticulum. The true congenital diverticulum contains all gastric tissue layers and is located on the posterior wall of the cardia. The intramural (or partial) diverticulum projects into but not through the muscular layer, most commonly located along the greater curvature of the antrum. The false (or pseudo-) diverticulum is formed by mucosal and submucosal herniation through a defect in the muscular wall and lacks muscularis propria. Familial occurrence has not been described for any of these lesions.

Clinical Presentation and Diagnosis

Most congenital gastric diverticula are asymptomatic and are incidental findings on radiography or endoscopy, or at autopsy (see Chapter 19). Size varies from 1 to 11 cm. Contrast radiography shows a rounded, well-delineated mobile pouch often with an air-fluid level. Emptying of the diverticulum may be delayed. On endoscopy, the diverticulum is seen as a well-delineated opening. Symptoms, when present, may be epigastric or lower chest pain,[15] indigestion, or nonbilious emesis. The differential diagnosis includes an acquired gastric diverticulum secondary to trauma, ulcer disease, or malignancy. Hiatal hernia and hypertrophic gastric folds may mimic a diverticulum on contrast studies. Radiology cannot distinguish between congenital and acquired diverticula.

Treatment

In the case of an incidentally discovered proximal gastric diverticulum, treatment is unnecessary. If symptoms are thought to be consistent with the diagnosis, the diverticulum may be amputated or invaginated. Because of the risk of malignancy associated with distal gastric diverticula, surgical treatment by amputation, invagination, or segmental resection has been recommended. Laparoscopic resection following gastroscopic localization has been described.[16, 17]

Gastric Duplication

Approximately 20% of all gastrointestinal duplications are gastric. Duplication of the stomach can occur in isolation, as a triplication (two gastric duplications in one individual), or with duplications of other structures in the gastrointestinal tract, such as the esophagus or duodenum. Location is generally along the greater curvature or posterior wall and contains all layers of the gastric wall. Because the duplication rarely communicates with the stomach, a tubular, fusiform, or spherical cystic mass develops. Infrequently there may be a connection to the colon,[18] pancreas, or pancreatic duplication[19]; communication may be the result of an acquired fistula from a penetrating peptic ulcer within the duplication. Several embryologic defects have been proposed as etiologies for duplications, including errors in separation of notochord and endoderm, persistence of embryonic diverticula, and persistence of vacuoles within the epithelium of the primitive foregut.[6] Most duplications occur in females (65%) and are detected during infancy or childhood (80%). Carcinomas arising in congenital duplications have been described in adults.

Clinical Presentation and Diagnosis

The clinical presentation of gastric duplication depends on factors such as size, location, and communicating structure (if any). Symptoms and signs vary and may include abdominal mass; epigastric pain; failure to gain appropriate weight; vomiting; occult or frank upper or lower gastrointestinal bleeding secondary to peptic ulceration, the latter occurring via erosion into colon[18]; hematobilia in a communication with intrahepatic bile duct[20]; hemoptysis (perforated cyst fistulized to lung); pyloric obstruction; peritonitis secondary to rupture; pancreatitis; pancreatic pseudocyst; and acute abdomen. In early infancy symptoms may mimic those of hypertrophic pyloric stenosis. Diagnosis is suggested by an abdominal radiograph showing displacement and extrinsic compression of gastric lumen. Contrast radiography may demonstrate the duplication via mass effect on the stomach, or the cyst may be imaged directly when there is communication with the gastrointestinal tract. Ultrasound, including prenatal ultrasound,[21] computed tomographic (CT) scan, and endoscopy, may also demonstrate the lesion.

Treatment

Surgical excision is considered optimal therapy. When complete excision is not possible, as may be the case when cyst and viscus have a common muscle layer, debulking, cyst-gastrostomy, or partial gastrectomy may be necessary.

Gastric Teratoma

Gastric teratomas are benign neoplasms of the stomach, which occur almost exclusively in males. Gastric teratomas are rare, comprising only 1% of all childhood teratomas. These tumors may have their origins in pluripotential cells and contain all three embryonic germ cell layers. They are almost always diagnosed during infancy owing to their large size. Most are located along the greater curvature of the stomach and are extragastric, although intramural extension has been reported.[22] The immature type (containing yolk cell tumor, germinoma, and embryonal carcinoma) may infiltrate regional structures—omentum, regional lymph nodes, left lobe of the liver—whereas the mature tissue form does not.

Clinical Presentation and Diagnosis

The typical patient is a male infant with an abdominal mass; mean age at presentation is 3.2 months.[23] Vomiting may be present from intrinsic compression and gastrointestinal bleeding due to transmural growth and disruption of gastric mucosa. The newborn infant with a teratoma may be delivered prematurely or have respiratory distress on the basis of increased abdominal pressure. Delivery may be difficult, putting the infant at risk for injuries such as shoulder dystocia.

Noncontrast radiography demonstrates calcifications typical of the lesion. Ultrasonography demonstrates solid and cystic areas, and CT or magnetic resonance (MR) imaging confirms the diagnosis and evaluates for regional infiltration.[23]

Treatment

Tumor excision with primary gastric repair is the procedure of choice and is curative. Partial or total gastrectomy is required for intramural tumor extension. Malignant transformation to adenocarcinoma has been reported,[24] as well as premalignant changes,[25] and peritoneal gliomatosis has been observed.

Gastric Volvulus

Gastric volvulus is discussed in Chapter 20.

Infantile Hypertrophic Pyloric Stenosis

Infantile hypertrophic pyloric stenosis (IHPS) is a form of gastric outlet obstruction caused by hypertrophy of circular muscle surrounding the pyloric channel. Correction of IHPS is the most common abdominal operative procedure during the first 6 months of life. Because the muscular hypertrophy and obstruction develop during the postnatal period, IHPS is not a true congenital defect.

The etiology of IHPS remains the subject of speculation. A localized lack of nitric oxide synthase, or abnormal neuronal innervation associated with decreased muscle neurofilaments, nerve terminals, synaptic vesicle protein, and neural cell adhesion molecule[26] have been implicated, but anatomic studies cannot determine whether nitric oxide synthase deficiency is a primary or secondary event.[27] Pacemaker cells in the regulation of gastrointestinal motility, the interstitial cell of Cajal, are observed only near the submucosa in IHPS instead of throughout the pylorus.[28, 29] Epidermal growth factor (EGF), EGF receptor, and heparin binding EGF-like growth factor are markedly increased in smooth muscle cells in IHPS,[30] but their triggers are unknown.

The incidence of IHPS in the United States is approximately 3 in 1000 live births but varies among ethnic groups and regions from 1 to 8 in 1000 live births. Incidence is highest among whites (especially northern Europeans), whereas incidence is lower among African Americans, Africans, and is lowest among Asians. Males outnumber females by a ratio of 4:1 or 5:1.

Familial clustering of IHPS is widely recognized, but the disorder does not follow mendelian inheritance patterns. Approximately 50% of identical twins are affected, leading credence to the roles of both genetic and environmental factors. Male relatives of affected females are more likely to develop IHPS, such that siblings and offspring of affected females are more likely to develop IHPS than relatives of affected males are. Other infants with increased risk are first-born males, especially those with high birthweights or born to professional parents. IHPS also occurs in association with Turner's syndrome, trisomy 18, Cornelia de Lange syndrome, esophageal atresia, Hirschsprung's disease, phenylketonuria, and congenital rubella syndrome. In addition, neonates receiving erythromycin for pertussis prophylaxis have increased risk of developing IHPS.[31]

Clinical Presentation and Diagnosis

Infants with IHPS were typically asymptomatic until 3 to 4 weeks of age, although a small number may present as early as the first week of life. Initially infants present with mild spitting, which progresses to projectile vomiting following feedings. Vomiting may be so forceful as to exit through the nostrils as well as the mouth. Emesis may contain coffee-ground material or small amounts of frank blood but is rarely bilious. Early in the course, the infant remains hungry following vomiting episodes, but with time, loses interest in feeding and may present wasted and severely dehydrated. Decreased urinary and stool output accompanies dehydration. Marked metabolic alkalosis develops secondary to chloride loss in the vomitus. Infants may be misdiagnosed with formula allergy or gastroesophageal reflux.

On physical examination, the infant with IHPS may appear wasted and dehydrated, but the extent is variable and related to severity and duration of symptoms. The classic physical signs are a palpable pyloric mass and visible peristaltic waves. The palpable "olive" is most easily felt in a wasted patient, immediately following emesis or aspiration of the stomach. The location of the olive varies from the level of the umbilicus to near the epigastrium. The pyloric mass is palpable in 70% to 90% of affected infants, depending on the experience and patience of the examiner. Peristaltic waves are best observed during feeding of the naked infant, while the infant is cradled in the mother's left arm.

Many infants appear jaundiced due to an indirect hyperbilirubinemia related to dehydration and perhaps malnutrition.

When the presentation is typical and the olive palpated, no other studies are necessary. However, in the minority of infants with projectile vomiting, definitive diagnosis requires radiologic studies. Noncontrast radiography demonstrates a distended stomach with paucity of gas beyond the stomach. Diagnosis is confirmed by ultrasonography of the pylorus, which has supplanted contrast radiography as the diagnostic study of choice for IHPS. On ultrasonogram, the hypertrophied circular muscle thickness is greater than 3 mm and appears as a characteristic sonolucent "donut" (Fig. 36–8). Also, the length of the pyloric channel measures greater than 1.5 cm. However, when the differential diagnosis includes IHPS, reflux, or other upper gastrointestinal disorders, contrast radiography may be the appropriate first test. Contrast radiography must be done carefully, because gastric contents should first be aspirated. The infant is given barium by nipple and imaged in a semiprone position. Characteristic findings include an elongated narrow pylorus with the appearance of a "double channel." There is also indentation of the adjacent antrum and duodenum by the pyloric mass producing the so-called shoulders (Fig. 36–9). Diagnosis of IHPS by endoscopy has been described: the pylorus appears as a cauliflower-like narrowing, through which a 7.8-mm (external diameter) endoscope cannot be passed.[32] Another report on endoscopic diagnosis has refuted these claims,[33] so the benefits of endoscopic diagnosis are uncertain.

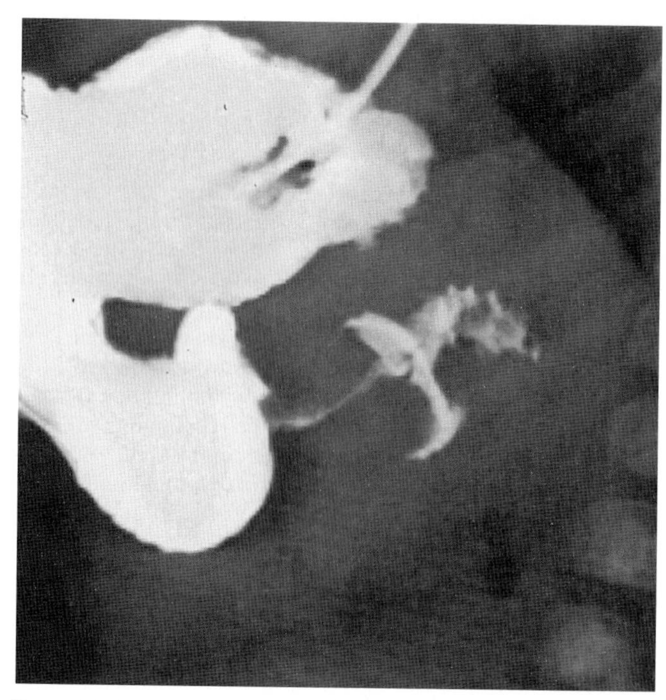

Figure 36–9. Upper gastrointestinal contrast radiograph in a 1 month old with idiopathic hypertrophic pyloric stenosis demonstrating elongated pylorus and antral and duodenal "shoulders" secondary to a mass effect. (Courtesy of Marcia Pritchard, MD.)

Treatment

The initial therapy for IHPS is fluid and electrolyte replacement to correct dehydration and hypochloremic metabolic alkalosis. Depending on severity, fluid and electrolyte repletion can usually be accomplished within 24 hours. Definitive therapy is the Ramstedt pyloromyotomy, which entails a longitudinal incision through the hypertrophied pyloric muscle down to the submucosa on the anterior surface of the pylorus. After spreading the muscle, the intact mucosa bulges through the incision to the level of the incised muscle. Infants may vomit for the first few days postoperatively, but persistent vomiting is suggestive of inadequate surgery.

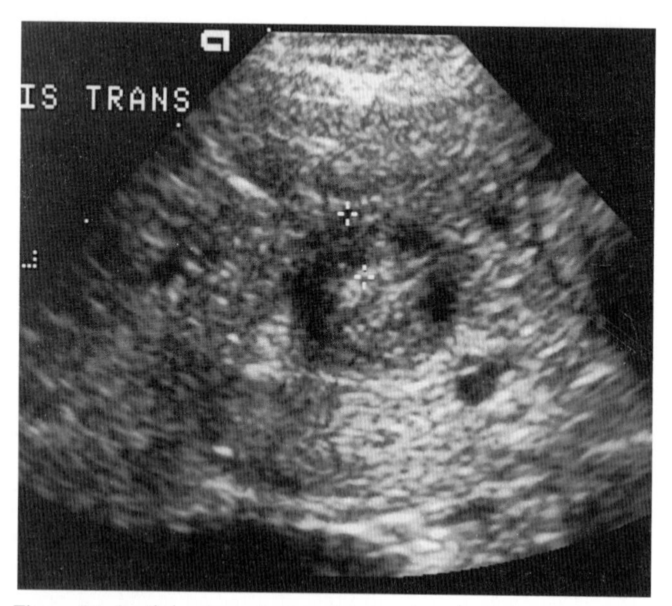

Figure 36–8. Abdominal ultrasound in a 1-month-old infant with idiopathic hypertrophic pyloric stenosis demonstrating the sonolucent "donut" of pyloric hypertrophy on cross-section. (Courtesy of Marcia Pritchard, MD.)

Nonoperative therapy consists of the use of atropine-like medications and paste-consistency feedings until such time that the muscle hypertrophy resolves.[34] Because of the high failure rate, the prolonged recovery period (compared with surgery), and the low risk of pyloromyotomy, the nonoperative approach is rarely used in the United States.

The prognosis following surgery is excellent. The infant resumes normal growth and development. Although divergent gastric emptying rates have been observed many years following treatment of IHPS, a recent study of gastric emptying by scintigraphy found no differences in emptying rates for liquids or solids between patients treated surgically or conservatively, or controls.[32]

Adult Hypertrophic Pyloric Stenosis

Hypertrophic pyloric stenosis rarely occurs in adults. When HPS occurs in adults, its anatomic features are identical to the infantile type. In adults, pyloric hypertrophy is generally associated with peptic ulcer disease or carcinoma. In a few cases, no etiology is determined; it is therefore unknown whether these are missed infantile cases or whether the hypertrophy occurred later in life. There is a family history of IHPS in some cases of adult HPS, thus again suggesting a role for genetic predisposition. In addition, 80% of adult HPS occurs in men. The resected pylorus demonstrates normal mucosa and marked circumferential thickening of the muscularis propria.[35]

Clinical Presentation and Diagnosis

Symptoms of adult HPS are similar to those observed in infancy: nausea, mild vomiting, early satiety, and epigastric pain, especially after eating. In contrast with the infantile form, the physical examination may not be helpful, because the adult pyloric mass is difficult to palpate. On contrast radiography, the elongated narrow pylorus is again apparent; gastric emptying is delayed, and the stomach may be dilated. Ultrasonography is the screening procedure of choice, whereas upper endoscopy is indicated to differentiate idiopathic HPS from carcinoma or chronic peptic ulcer disease.

Treatment

Traditionally, surgical pyloromyotomy or resection of the involved region has been considered the procedure of choice. Because of the risk of a small focus of carcinoma, surgical resection of the pylorus has been recommended. Endoscopic balloon dilation has also been efficacious in the management of HPS, but a high postprocedure recurrence rate—80% within the first 6 months—has been reported.[36]

Duodenal Anomalies

Duodenal Atresia or Stenosis

Duodenal atresia and stenosis are congenital defects characterized by complete and partial obstruction of the duodenum, respectively. Atresias occur in various anatomic configurations, including a blind-ending pouch with no connection to the distal duodenum (least common), a pouch with a fibrous cord connecting to the distal duodenum, or a complete membrane obstructing the lumen (most common). Perforate membranes are also a cause of duodenal stenosis. All three lesions occur with greatest frequency near the ampulla of Vater, with most lesions (80%) occurring distal to this landmark. The overall incidence of the three anomalies combined is about 1 per 200,000 live births. The etiology of these lesions may relate to failure to recanalize the duodenal lumen by vacuolization at 8 to 10 weeks' gestation. Alternatively, the etiology may be local ischemia. Recently, duodenal stenosis has been observed in *sonic hedgehog* (*shh*) mutant mice, thus adding to our understanding that mutations in signaling pathways may play a role in this malformation.[37]

In two recent series of more than 100 cases,[38, 39] more than 50% of affected patients had associated congenital defects, including pancreatic defects, intestinal malrotation with congenital bands, esophageal atresia, Meckel's diverticulum, imperforate anus, congenital heart disease, central nervous system lesions, renal anomalies, and, rarely, biliary tract anomalies. Trisomy 21 is strongly associated with duodenal atresia/stenosis/web in that 25% to more than 50% of cases are in infants and children with this chromosomal anomaly. Familial occurrence is rare. A report of father and son with periampullary obstruction due to duodenal stenosis and annular pancreas (in the father) and segmental duodenal atresia (in the son) serves as a reminder that with increased survival of affected infants, a genetic basis may be realized in the future.[40]

Clinical Presentation and Diagnosis

The diagnosis of duodenal atresia may be suspected prenatally when ultrasonography demonstrates gastric and proximal duodenal dilation and polyhydramnios. Polyhydramnios is present in 33% to 50% of cases of duodenal atresia. The absence of gastric and proximal duodenal dilation in the presence of polyhydramnios does not exclude the diagnosis, because intrauterine emesis may limit preobstructive dilation. High-frequency transvaginal transducers used in ultrasonography may overdiagnose intestinal dilation, so longer scanning is recommended once obstruction is suspected.[41]

The infant with duodenal atresia is often born preterm and has early feeding intolerance characterized by vomiting and upper abdominal distention. Emesis is usually bilious because most lesions occur distal to the entry of the bile duct into the duodenum. Nonbilious emesis is seen in 15% to 20% of cases secondary to more proximal obstruction. Any child with trisomy 21 and vomiting (especially bile stained) requires further evaluation. Duodenal stenosis or a partial membrane may present at any age, depending on degree of obstruction. Infants and children present with vomiting, failure to gain weight adequately, and/or aspiration. Vomiting may be intermittent and of variable severity such that symptomatic lesions may remain undiagnosed for months to years. Occasionally, diagnosis is delayed until adulthood.

Noncontrast radiographs of the infant with duodenal obstruction classically demonstrate the presence of air in the stomach and in the first portion of the duodenum—the "double-bubble" sign (Fig. 36–10). The absence of air beyond the second bubble should be interpreted as probable duodenal atresia. Contrast radiography is generally effective in demonstrating atresias, stenosis, membranes, and other anomalies resulting in external compression of the duodenum (Fig. 36–11). In addition, normal or abnormal rotation and fixation of the bowel can be assessed. Occasionally, upper endoscopy is useful in diagnosing or defining a duodenal stenosis or membrane.

Treatment

A newborn infant suspected of duodenal obstruction should have a nasogastric tube placed for decompression, and correction of fluid and electrolyte abnormalities should be instituted. The surgical approach was duodenojejunostomy in the past, but now duodenoduodenostomy is preferred with diamond-shaped anastomosis.[39] Associated malrotation is corrected with a Ladd procedure. Passage of a catheter into the distal duodenum is done to investigate for a second obstruction, which occurs in about 3% of cases. Membranes may be excised without anastomosis if the membrane was an isolated finding. Endoscopic laser resection of a membrane has been reported[42]; unfortunately, the presence of an undiagnosed annular pancreas in this case eventually necessitated laparotomy. Late complications continue to plague patients even following surgical repair: motility problems, megaduo-

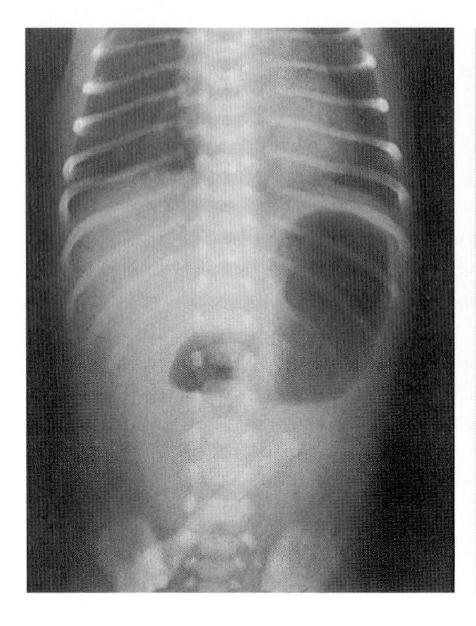
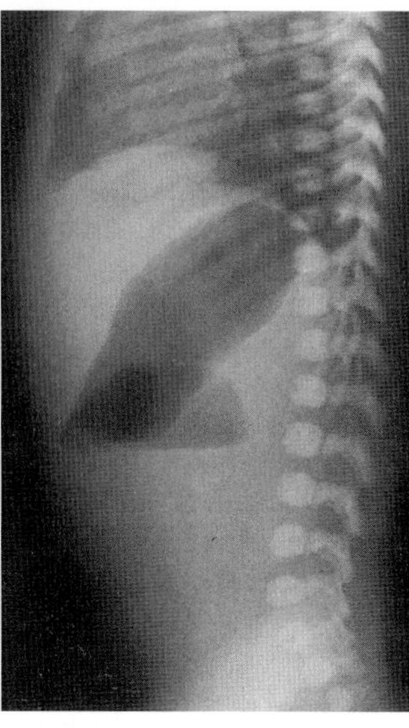

Figure 36–10. Anteroposterior and lateral noncontrast radiographs of an infant with duodenal atresia, demonstrating the "double-bubble" sign. (Courtesy of Marcia Pritchard, MD.)

denum, gastroesophageal reflux unresponsive to medications, gastritis, and peptic ulcer disease occur months to years following primary repair.[39] Two teenagers have presented with choledochal cyst.[38] Megaduodenum proximal to the obstruction, with abnormal peristalsis, is a common long-term issue, but most patients are asymptomatic. For symptomatic patients with megaduodenum, bowel plication may be indicated.[43, 44]

Annular Pancreas

Annular pancreas is an unusual congenital malformation characterized by a thin ring of pancreatic tissue encircling the second portion of the duodenum, resulting in variable degrees of obstruction (see Chapter 45). The lesion may present in the neonatal period, in childhood, or adulthood. Some cases remain asymptomatic and are discovered as an incidental finding during endoscopic retrograde cholangiopancreatography (ERCP) or at autopsy. The anomalous tissue is histologically normal and contains a moderately sized pancreatic duct. The pancreatic tissue may penetrate the muscularis of the duodenal wall or remain distinct from the duodenum.

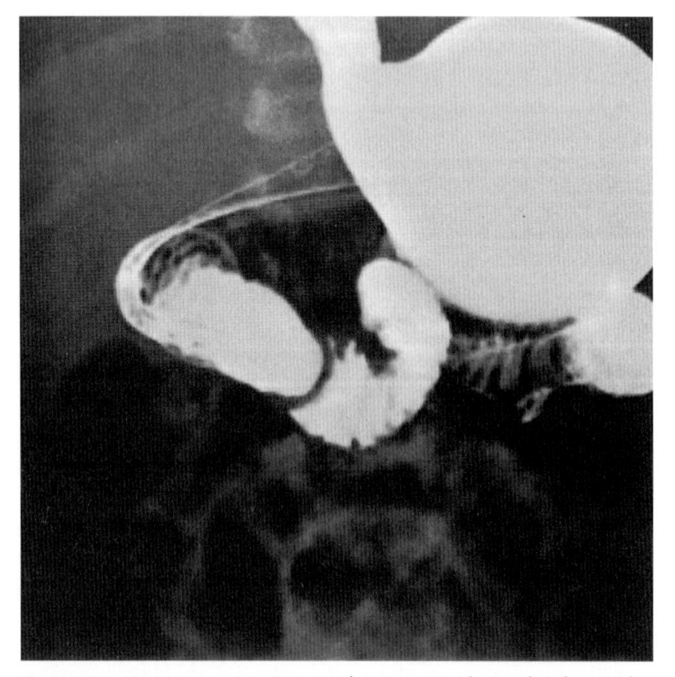

Figure 36–11. Upper gastrointestinal contrast radiograph of an infant with a duodenal membrane, demonstrating a pinched appearance at the site of the membrane. (Courtesy of Marcia Pritchard, MD.)

Several hypotheses exist regarding embryologic origin of annular pancreas. Evidence appears to favor Lecco's 1910 hypothesis that the ventral pancreatic anlage becomes fixed to the duodenal wall prior to rotation during the fifth week of gestation. With subsequent growth and fusion of the dorsal and ventral anlagen, a partial (75%) or complete (25%) ring of pancreatic tissue is formed.[6]

Incidence of the disorder is approximately 1 in 100,000 live births, but this figure does not account for cases found during adulthood, during ERCP (where it is usually noted as an incidental finding), or at autopsy. The true incidence may be as high as 1 per 250 living births. In infancy the incidence is equal in males and females. In adulthood males outnumber females by 2:1. Infant and childhood cases are associated with other congenital anomalies in an estimated 40% to 70% of cases, including trisomy 21, duodenal atresia, cardiac defects, anorectal malformations, Meckel's diverticulum, and tracheoesophageal fistula. These associations are not noted among adult cases. Familial occurrence has not been reported.

Clinical Presentation and Diagnosis

Annular pancreas produces symptoms when the tissue obstructs the duodenum or biliary tree. Infants may present with high-grade obstructive symptoms indistinguishable from duodenal atresia or malrotation with mid-gut volvulus: bilious emesis and upper abdominal distention. During childhood, intermittent bilious emesis and failure to thrive are common presenting symptoms, whereas during adulthood, the most common symptom is abdominal pain. Other symptoms and signs in adults include nausea, vomiting, gastric outlet obstruction, pancreatitis, pancreatolithiasis,[45] pancreas divisum, pancreatic mass, gastric or duodenal ulcer, or biliary obstruction resulting in jaundice. In the adult development of symptoms peaks in the third to fifth decades.

Noncontrast radiography of the infant may demonstrate the double-bubble sign identical to that seen in duodenal atresia (see Fig. 36–10). Contrast radiography should be done to ensure that the obstruction is not due to mid-gut volvulus, a surgical emergency. In adults, transabdominal ultrasound, endoscopic ultrasound, CT scan, or MR pancreatography may diagnose annular pancreas. ERCP may demonstrate ductular structures consistent with annular pancreas, but in some cases it may not be technically feasible owing to duodenal obstruction proximal to the major ampulla. Endoscopic ultrasonography is especially useful when prior gastric resection or duodenal obstruction precludes ERCP; in addition, a mass may be staged or undergo fine-needle aspiration at the time of endoscopic ultrasound.[46] The ability to evaluate for mass is a new consideration, given reports of ampullary carcinoma in association with annular pancreas; hence, jaundice should not be attributed to annular pancreas until carcinoma is ruled out.[47] MR pancreatography, which allows spacial resolution of the entire pancreaticobiliary tree, can identify the annulus and the duct within that surrounds the duodenum.[48] Finally, intraoperative diagnosis at laparotomy is not unusual.

Treatment

The preferred operative therapy for annular pancreas includes duodenostomy or duodenojejunostomy. Prognosis postoperatively is excellent with either, and postoperative deaths among infants are generally due to associated anomalies. Division or dissection of the pancreatic tissue is not recommended owing to the high risk of complications, including pancreatitis, pancreatic fistula, and incomplete relief of symptoms. Recently, an annular pancreas identified at the time of organ procurement was transplanted along with a long segment of duodenum with good results, so that annular pancreas can be considered suitable for transplantation.[49]

Duodenal Duplication Cysts

Duodenal duplication cysts are a rare anomaly, totaling only 7% of gastrointestinal duplications. Most commonly located posterior to the first or second portion of the duodenum, these spherical or tubular cysts generally do not communicate with the duodenal lumen but do share blood supply with the duodenum. There are three histologic criteria for duodenal duplication cysts: gastrointestinal mucosa, a smooth muscle layer in the wall, and an association with the duodenal wall. The mucosa is typically duodenal, but in 15% of cases there is gastric mucosa, and very rarely, pancreatic tissue is found. Male incidence equals that of females.

Clinical Presentation and Diagnosis

Presenting signs and symptoms of these cysts include vomiting, decreased oral intake, periumbilical tenderness, and abdominal distention. Also, the cyst mucosa may ulcerate so that gastrointestinal bleeding may be the initial presentation. In the neonate duodenal obstruction due to a large duplication cyst has been reported. Infected duodenal duplication cyst has been noted as well.[50] Recurrent pancreatitis may occur if the cyst compresses or is in communication with the pancreatic duct. Finally, jaundice and duodenojejunal intussusception resulting in small bowel obstruction have been reported.[51]

Noncontrast as well as contrast radiography may demonstrate obstruction or compression effect, but in general, findings are nonspecific and only suggestive. Abdominal ultrasonograms may show unilocular cystic structure with echogenic mucosa surrounded by thin hypoechoic halo of muscle layer.[50] Also, peristaltic waves through the cyst may be evident on ultrasound. CT scan may demonstrate an encapsulated, noncommunicating cyst posterior to the duodenum. On ERCP, a compressible periampullary mass may be seen.

Treatment

Surgical therapy should be individualized in accordance with the anatomy of the cyst. Bergman and Jacir have recommended mucosal stripping of the common muscular wall and resection coupled with removal of free walls.[52] Endoscopic drainage has been successful in adult and pediatric cases. Recently, invasive carcinoma has been reported in an adult with duodenal duplication cyst, so that endoscopic drainage without resection may require reconsideration.

Malrotation and Midgut Volvulus

The entity of malrotation and volvulus are described in detail in Chapters 20 and 84. Refer to Table 36–1 and the aforementioned chapters for additional information.

REFERENCES

1. Redel CA, Zwiener RJ: Anatomy and anomalies of the stomach and duodenum. In Feldman M, Scharschmidt BF, Schleisenger MH (eds): Gastrointestinal Disease, 6th ed. Philadelphia, WB Saunders, 1996, pp 557–571.
2. Moore KL, Persaud TVN: The Developing Human, 6th ed. Philadelphia, WB Saunders, 1998, pp 271–278.
3. Johnson LR: Gastrointestinal Physiology, 6th ed. St. Louis, CV Mosby, 2001, pp 75–94.
4. Koh TJ, Goldenring JR, Ito S, et al: Gastrin deficiency results in altered gastric differentiation and decreased colonic proliferation in mice. Gastroenterology 113:1015, 1997.
5. Langerhans N, Rindi G, Chiu M, et al: Abnormal gastric histology and decreased acid production in cholecystokinin-B/gastrin receptor–deficient mice. Gastroenterology 112:280, 1997.
6. Skandalakis JE, Gray SW, Ricketts R: The stomach. In Skandalakis JE, Gray SW (eds): Embryology for Surgeons, 2nd ed. Baltimore, Williams & Wilkins, 1994, pp 150–183.
7. Lachaux A, Bouvier R, Loras-Duclaux I, et al: Isolated deficient $\alpha_6\beta_4$ integrin expression in the gut associated with intractible diarrhea. J Pediatr Gastroenterol Nutr 29:395, 1999.
8. Sonnenberg A, Calafat J, Janssen H, et al: Integrin α_6/β_4 complex is located in hemidesmosomes, suggesting a major role in epidermal cell–basement membrane adhesion. J Cell Biol 113:907, 1997.
9. Wallerstein R, Klein ML, Genieser N, et al: Epidermolysis bullosa, pylotic atresia, and obstructive uropathy: A report of two case reports with molecular correlation and clinical management. Pediatr Dermatol 17:286, 2000.
10. Okoye BO, Parikh DH, Buick RG, et al: Pyloric atresia: Five new

cases, a new association, and a review of the literature with guidelines. J Pediatr Surg 36:1242, 2000.
11. Dessant A, Iannuccelli M, Dore A, et al: Pyloric atresia: An attempt at anatomic pyloric sphincter reconstruction. J Pediatr Surg 35:1372, 2000.
12. Hernaiz Driever P, Gohlich-Ratmann G, Konig R, et al: Congenital microgastria, growth hormone deficiency, and diabetes insipidus. Eur J Pediatr 156:37, 1997.
13. Murray KF, Lillehei CW, Duggan C: Congenital mocrogastria: Treatment with transient jejunal feedings. J Pediatr Gastroenterol Nutr 28: 343, 1999.
14. Kroes EJ, Festen C: Congenital microgastria: A case report and review of literature. Pediatr Surg Int 13:416, 1998.
15. Ciftci AO, Tanyei FC, Hicsonmez A: Gastric diverticulum: An uncommon cause of abdominal pain in a 12 year old. J Pediatr Surg 33:529, 1998.
16. Fine A: Laparoscopic resection of a large proximal gastric diverticulum. Gastrointestinal Endosc 48:93, 1998.
17. Vogt DM, Curet MJ, Zucker KA: Laparoscopic management of gastric diverticula. J Laparoendosc Surg 9:405, 1999.
18. Mahnovski V, Mahour GH, Rowland JM: Gastric duplication–colonic fistula with colonic ulceration and bleeding. J Pediatr Surg 33:1815, 1998.
19. Materne R, Clapuyt P, Saint-Martin C, et al: Gastric cystic duplication communicating with a bifid pancreas: A rare cause of recurrent pancreatitis. J Pediatr Gastroenterol Nutr 27:102, 1998.
20. Kaneko K, Ando H, Watanabe Y, et al: Gastric duplication communicating with the left hepatic duct: A rare cause of recurrent hemobilia in a child. J Pediatr Surg 34:1536, 1999.
21. Correia-Pinto J, Tavares ML, Monteiro J, et al: Prenatal diagnosis of abdominal enteric duplications. Prenat Diagn 20:163, 2000.
22. Dunlap JP, James CA, Maxson RT, et al: Gastric teratoma with intramural extension. Pediatr Radiol 25:383, 1995.
23. Gupta DK, Srinivas M, Dave S, et al: Gastric teratoma in children. Pediatr Surg Int 16:329, 2000.
24. Matsukuma S, Wada R, Daibou M, et al: Adenocarcinoma arising from gastric immature teratoma. Cancer 75:2663, 1995.
25. Bourke CJ, Mackay AJ, Payton D: Malignant gastric teratoma: Case report. Pediatr Surg Int 12:192, 1997.
26. Kobayashi H, O'Brian S, Puri P: Immunochemical characterization of neural cell adhesion molecule (NCAM), nitric oxide synthase, and neurofilament protein expression in pyloric muscle of patients with pyloric stenosis. J Pediatr Gastroenterol Nutr 20:319, 1995.
27. Abel RA: The ontogeny of the peptide innervation of the human pylorus with special reference to understanding the aetiology and pathogenesis of infantile hypertrophic pyloric stenosis. Ann R Coll Surg Engl 82:371, 2000.
28. Vanderwinden JM, Liu H, de Laet MH, et al: Study of the interstitial cells of Cajal in infantile pyloric stenosis. Gastroenterology. 111:279, 1996.
29. Vanderwinden JM, Rumessen JJ: Interstitial cells of Cajal in human gut and gastrointestinal disease. Microsc Res Tech 47:344, 1999.
30. Shima H, Ohshiro K, Puri P: Increased local synthesis of epidermal growth factors in infantile hypertrophic pyloric stenosis. Pediatr Res 47: 201, 2000.
31. Honein MA, Paulozzi LJ, Himelright IM, et al: Infantile hypertrophic pyloric stenosis after pertussis prophylaxis with erythromycin: A case review and cohort study. Lancet 354:2101, 1999.
32. De Baker A, Bove T, Vandenplas Y, et al: Contribution of endoscopy to early diagnosis of hypertrophic pyloric stenosis. J Pediatr Gastroenterol Nutr 18:78, 1994.
33. Michaud L, Gottrand F, Ategbo S, et al: Pitfalls of endoscopy for diagnosis of pyloric stenosis. J Pediatr Gastroenterol Nutr 21:483, 1995.
34. Yamataka A, Tsukada K, Yokoyama-Laws Y, et al: Pyloromyotomy versus atropine sulfate for infantile hypertrophic pyloric stenosis. J Pediatr Surg 35:338, 2000.
35. Graadt van Roggen JF, van Krieken JHJM: Adult hypertrophic pyloric stenosis: Case report and review. J Clin Pathol 51:479, 1998.
36. Kuwada SK, Alexander GL: Long-term outcome of endoscopic dilation of nonmalignant pyloric stenosis. Gastrointest Endosc 41:15, 1995.
37. Ramalho-Santos M, Melton DA, McMahon AP: Hedgehog signals regulate multiple aspects of gastrointestinal development. Development 127:2763, 2000.
38. Dalla Vecchia LK, Grosfeld JL, West KW, et al: Intestinal atresia and stenosis. Arch Surg 133:490, 1999.
39. Murshed R, Nicholls G, Spitz L: Intrinsic duodenal obstruction: Trends in management and outcome over 45 years (1951–1995) with relevance to prenatal counselling. Br J Obstet Gynaecol 106:1197, 1999.
40. Mitchell CE, Marshall DG, Reid WD: Preampullary duodenal obstruction in a father and son. J Pediatr Surg 29:1582, 1993.
41. Zimmer EZ, Bronshtein M: Early diagnosis of duodenal atresia and possible sonographic pitfalls. Prenat Diag 16:564, 1996.
42. Ziegler K, Schier F, Waldschmidt J: Endoscopic laser resection of a duodenal membrane. J Pediatr Surg 27:1582, 1992.
43. Takahashi A, Tomomasa T, Suzuki N, et al: The relationship between disturbed transit and dilated bowel, and manometric findings of a dilated bowel in patients with duodenal atresia and stenosis. J Pediatr Surg 32:1157, 1997.
44. Ein SH, Kim PCW, Miller HAB: The late nonfunctioning duodenal atresia repair—a second look. J Pediatr Surg 35:690, 2000.
45. Yogi Y, Kpsai S, Higasi S, et al: Annular pancreas associated with pancreatolithiasis. Hepatogastroenterology 46:527, 1999.
46. Gress F, Yiengpruksawan A, Sherman S, et al: Diagnosis of annular pancreas by endoscopic ultrasound. Gastrointest Endosc 44:485, 1996.
47. Benger JR, Thompson MH: Annular pancreas and obstructive jaundice. Am J Gastroenterol 92:713, 1997.
48. Fulcher AS, Turner MA: MR pancreatography: A useful tool for evaluating pancreatic disorders. Radiographics 19:5, 1999.
49. Romagnoli J, Papalois VE, Hakim NS: Transplantation of an annular pancreas with enteric drainage. Int Surg 83:36, 1998.
50. Oshima K, Suzuki N, Ikeda H, et al: Infected duodenal duplication with unusual clinical and radiological manifestations: A case report. Pediatr Radiol 28:518, 1998.
51. Zamir G, Gross E, Shmushkevich A, et al: Duodenal duplication cyst manifested by duodenojejunal intussusception and hyperbilirubinemia. J Pediatr Surg 34:1297, 1999.
52. Bergman KS, Jacir NN: Cystic duodenal duplication-staged management in a premature infant. J Pediatr Surg 28:1584, 1993.

Chapter 37

Gastric Motor and Sensory Function, and Motor Disorders of the Stomach

Eamonn M.M. Quigley

GASTRIC MOTOR PHYSIOLOGY

The main functions of gastric motility are to accommodate and store the ingested meal, grind down or "triturate" solid particles, and then empty all of the constituents of the meal in a carefully controlled and regulated fashion into the duodenum. Specialized muscle of the lower esophageal and pyloric sphincters regulates transit across these regions and prevents orad reflux. Recent evidence suggests an active role for the stomach in the generation of satiety and, perhaps, in the regulation of food intake.

To subserve these functions the stomach demonstrates a degree of regional specialization; in functional terms, the stomach can be divided into three distinct regions:- proximal stomach (incorporating the cardia, fundus, and proximal corpus), distal stomach (distal corpus and antrum), and pylorus. To subserve its role in optimizing the digestion of food delivered to the intestine, gastric motor function is regulated by feedback from the small intestine. Through yet another reflex arc, the stomach also plays a crucial role in the regulation of lower esophageal sphincter patency.

Electrophysiologic Basis of Gastric Motor Activity

Contractile activity at any level in the gastrointestinal tract is based on fundamental electrophysiologic properties.[1] A consistent feature of extracellular recordings of gastrointestinal myoelectric activity is an omnipresent, highly regular and recurring electrical pattern called the *slow wave* (Fig. 37–1). Slow waves do not usually lead to contractions; these are related to the occurrence of spike potentials. As spikes usually occur on the crest of slow waves, the frequency of spikes and, therefore, contractions are phase locked to slow waves. In this manner, the maximal frequency of contractile activity at a given site is directly related to the slow wave frequency in that region. In the stomach, slow waves occur at a frequency of three cycles per minute; the maximal frequency of phasic contractions is, therefore, three cycles per minute. Gastric slow waves are thought to originate at a site along the greater curvature in the proximal to middle corpus; from this location, referred to as the *gastric pacemaker*, slow waves migrate in both circumferential and longitudinal directions. Longitudinal migration proceeds in an aborad direction, thereby setting the stage for coordinated,

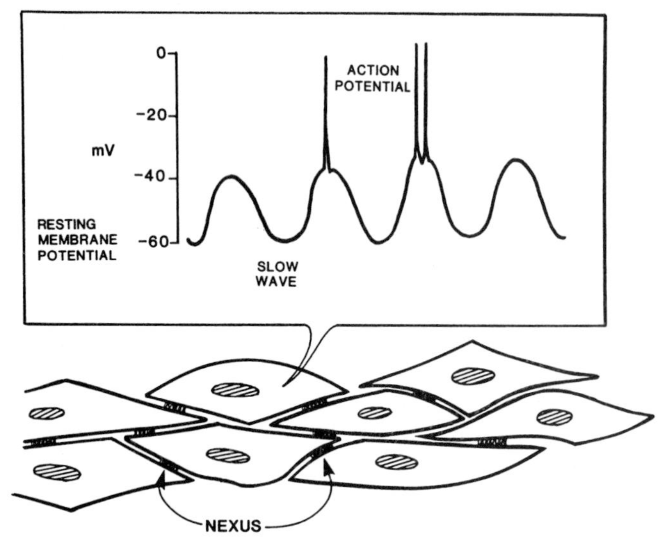

Figure 37–1. The basic concepts of the generation and organization of electrical activity in gastric smooth muscle cells. Inset represents recording of intracellular electrical activity from a smooth muscle cell in the pacemaker region of the stomach. *Note:* Resting membrane potential of −60 mV, which regularly undergoes spontaneous depolarization to −40 mV to produce rhythmic slow waves. Action potentials, which occur only on the summit of slow waves, result in muscular contraction. Areas of close contact, nexus, permit propagation of electrical signals between individual cells. (From Quigley EM: Small intestinal motor activity—its role in gut homeostasis in health and disease. Q J Med, 65:799, 1987.)

propulsive peristaltic activity. Electrical signals do not, for the most part, traverse the pylorus, ensuring separation between gastric and duodenal slow waves; the latter occur at a much higher frequency of 11 to 12 cycles per minute. In clinical manometric studies, this separation permits a clear differentiation between rhythmic antral and duodenal contractions.[2]

Intracellular recordings from smooth muscle cells throughout the stomach have provided a more fundamental electrophysiologic basis for the myogenic contribution to the motor functions of the stomach's respective regions (Fig. 37–2).[1] In interpreting these recordings attention is focused on several features: the resting membrane potential (which varies from −48 to −75 mV), the mechanical threshold (−52 to −40 mV), the presence or absence of a pacemaker potential, the configuration of the spontaneous action potential (if present), and the presence or absence of superimposed spike potentials or oscillations. An important principle is that once the muscle cell depolarizes to a level above the mechanical threshold, a contraction occurs.

In electrophysiologic terms, fundic smooth muscle cells are unique, in the stomach, in being electrically silent. Their resting membrane potential (−48 mV) normally lies at or above the mechanical threshold, thereby promoting sustained tonic contraction. Excitatory or inhibitory neural input to the region increases or decreases this tone; the magnitude and duration of the response are directly related to the intensity and duration of the neural discharge.

Intracellular recordings from the midcorpus, the "pacemaker" region, reveal a resting membrane potential of −61 mV and a spontaneous and complex action potential. Spontaneous action potentials in the corpus, antrum, and pylorus begin with a sharp upstroke, which is due to rapid depolarization. This upstroke is terminated by a rapid, but partial depolarization and followed by a sustained positive potential that later slowly drifts back to the resting potential; these latter phases are collectively referred to as the *plateau potential.* In the midcorpus alone, the resting membrane potential does not remain stable thereafter but slowly drifts toward a less negative value until the critical threshold is reached and another action potential is generated. This slow potential is referred to as the *pacemaker potential.*

In the corpus and antrum, the initial rapid depolarization

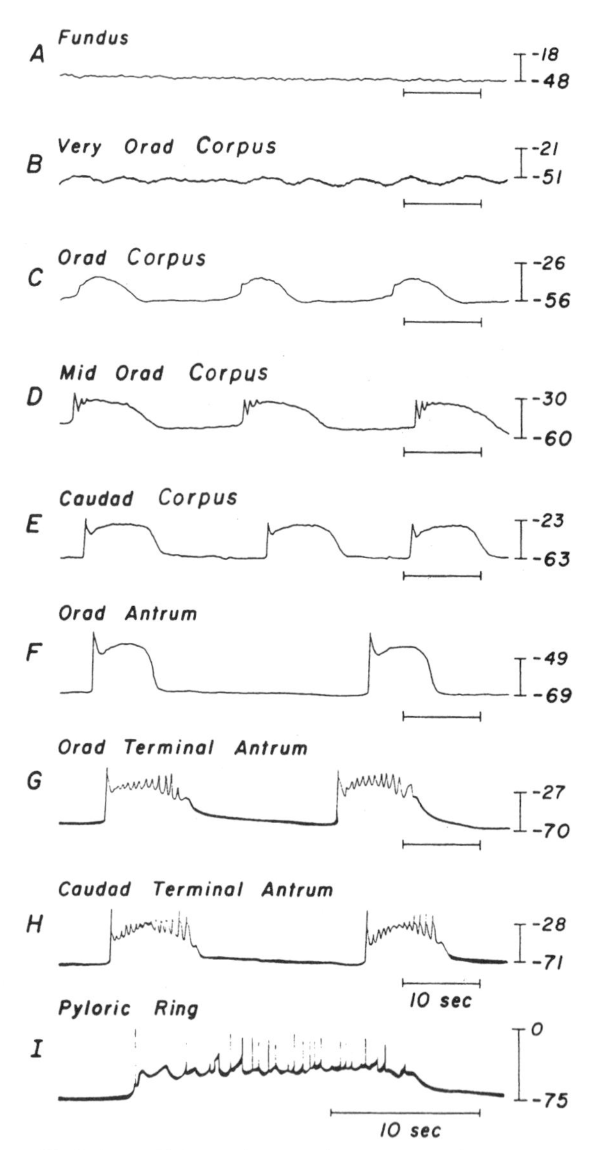

Figure 37–2. Intracellular resting membrane potential and spontaneous action potentials recorded from various parts of the stomach, from the fundus to the pyloric ring. *Note:* (1) Resting membrane potential becomes progressively more negative as one moves in a caudad direction along the stomach; (2) no spontaneous activity in the fundus; (3) the remainder of the stomach generates a spontaneous action potential of varying contour, (4) pacemaker potential in the orad corpus; (5) action potential in the corpus and antrum features a rapid initial depolarisation followed by plateau potential; (6) prominent, superimposed oscillations in the antrum and pylorus. (From Szurszewski JH: Electrophysiological basis of gastrointestinal motility. In Johnson LR [ed]: Physiology of the Gastrointestinal Tract, 2nd ed. New York, Raven Press, 1986, p 383.)

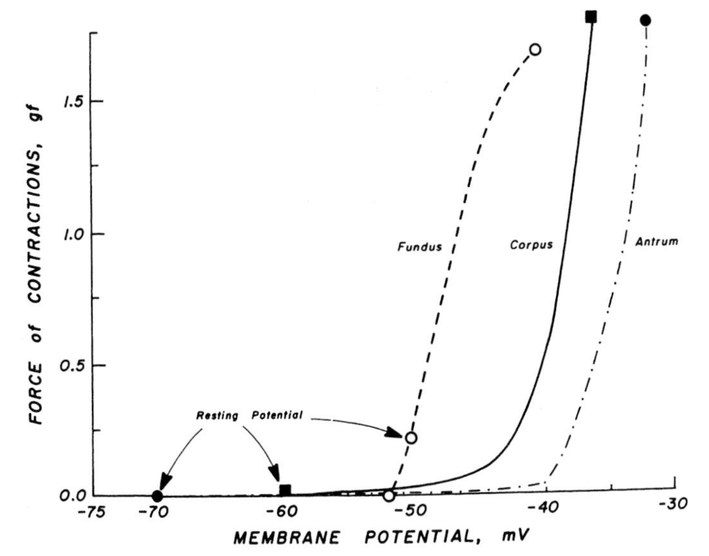

Figure 37–3. Voltage-tension curves for the fundus, corpus, and antrum. *Note:* (1) Relationships between resting membrane potential and threshold for contraction in each location. Thus, in the fundus, the resting membrane potential is already above the threshold, thereby generating tone; in contrast, in the antrum, the resting membrane potential lies 30 mV below threshold (−70 versus −40 mV); (2) steep slope of voltage-tension curve above threshold. (From Szurszewski JH: Electrophysiological basis of gastrointestinal motility. In Johnson LR (ed): Physiology of the Gastrointestinal Tract, 2nd ed. New York, Raven Press, 1986, p 383.)

crosses the threshold for depolarization and results in a transient but usually imperceptible contraction (referred to as the *first contraction*). In these regions of the stomach, the plateau potential also exceeds the mechanical threshold to produce the second or peristaltic contraction. In this manner, gastric peristalsis owes its genesis to events related to the plateau potential. Extrinsic stimuli that increase the amplitude and duration of the plateau potential result in a sustained contraction. In the distal antrum, spikes or oscillations superimposed on the plateau potential result in peristalsis. At the pylorus, the plateau potential is very prolonged in duration and constantly superimposed with spike potentials, which, in turn, promote closure of this area.

Szurszewski has provided an elegant electrophysiologic explanation, based on voltage-tension curves, for the differing contractile behavior of the various parts of the stomach (Fig. 37–3).[1] In the fundus, the resting membrane potential is already above the mechanical threshold and also located on the steep portion of the voltage-tension curve, thereby generating tone and rendering fundic tone exquisitely sensitive to excitatory and inhibitory stimuli. Action potentials are not generated, and neural and hormonal input modulates tone rather than generating peristaltic contractions. In this manner, brief inhibition produces receptive relaxation, and sustained inhibition, the accommodation response. In the corpus, the resting membrane potential lies 10 mV below the mechanical threshold; both the initial rapid depolarization and the plateau potential traverse the threshold, result in contractions (the first and second contractions described), and move the potential on to the steep portion of the voltage-tension curve. Given that the plateau potential remains at a level less negative than the mechanical threshold for a more prolonged period than the brief initial depolarization, the former produces the greater contraction. In the antrum, the resting membrane potential lies 30 mV below mechanical threshold, a gap that cannot be overcome by physiologic stimulation. However, during the action potential, the initial rapid depolarization wave traverses the mechanical threshold; stimulation applied during the plateau potential may also lead it to cross this critical threshold; first and second contractions then ensue. Although the initial, or first, contraction is of little mechanical consequence in the corpus and antrum, it does play a crucial role in the pylorus, an area whose luminal diameter is already considerably smaller than that of the rest of the stomach. Here the first contraction, initiated by the initial rapid depolarization phase of the pyloric action potential, "clicks" the pylorus closed ahead of the peristaltic wave generated by the antral plateau potential. In this way the contour of the action potential, including the time lag between its associated first and second contractions, promotes the trituration and sieving functions of the antrum and pylorus.

The recognition of the distinctive morphologic, electrophysiologic, and biochemical properties of the interstitial Cajal cells (ICCs) has prompted a reevaluation of the primacy of smooth muscle cells as the originators of gastric slow wave activity.[3] In the stomach, ICCs located in the myenteric plexus (IC-MY) are responsible for the generation of slow wave activity; these cells are electrically coupled to smooth muscle cells via gap junctions. There is now convincing evidence that the slow wave mechanism is an exclusive feature of the ICCs and that the active propagation of slow waves occurs through the interstitial cell network.[3] Slow waves are then electronically conducted into and depolarize smooth muscle cells. The pacemaking role of a certain region of the stomach may well, therefore, be based on the electrophysiologic properties of its interstitial cells rather than those of adjacent smooth muscle cells. Another group of ICCs, located within the muscular layers (IC-IM), lie in close proximity to enteric nerves within the stomach. These ICCs receive more neural input than the adjacent muscle; through these neural synapses and by virtue of gap junctions with smooth muscle cells, IC-IMs play a central role in neuromuscular interactions (Fig. 37–4).[4, 5] Throughout the gut, ICC density closely parallels that of inhibitory innervation; in the gastric fundus ICCs are heavily innervated by inhibitory neurons and may serve as the conduit for the transmission of those inhibitory signals that regulate tone in

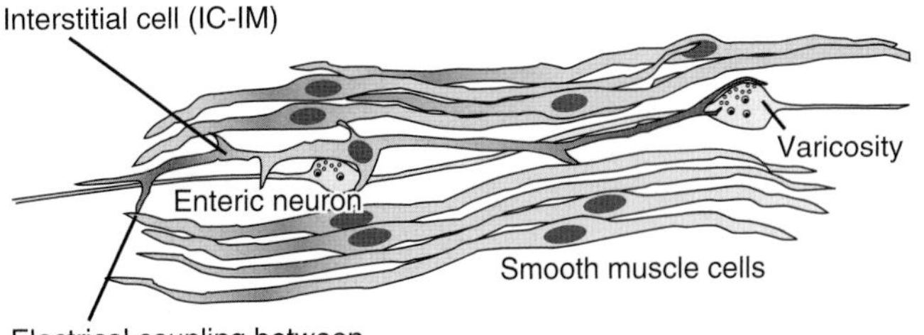

Figure 37–4. Relationships between intramuscular interstitial cells of Cajal (IC-IM) and enteric neurons. According to this concept, IC-IM and enteric neurons are intimately related, permitting the interstitial cells of Cajal (ICCs) to play a key role in neurotransmission. (With permission, from the Annual Reviews of Physiology, Volume 61 © 1999 by Annual Reviews www.AnnualReviews.org.)

this part of the organ. At the pylorus, loss of ICCs and the associated loss of inhibitory neural input may contribute to the development of infantile pyloric stenosis.[6]

Patterns of Gastric Contractile Activity

The Fasted Stomach

Along the length of the gut, patterns of motor activity during fasting and after food intake differ fundamentally. In the fasted state, motor activity is highly organized into a distinct and cyclically recurring sequence of events known as the *migrating motor complex* (MMC).[7]

As is discussed in more detail in Chapter 85, the MMC consists of three distinct phases of motor activity that occur in sequence and migrate slowly along the length of the small intestine (Fig. 37–5). Each sequence begins with a period of motor quiescence (phase I), is followed by a period of apparently random and irregular contractions (phase II), and culminates in a burst of uninterrupted phasic contractions (phase III, or the activity front). Individual cycles (i.e., phases I to III) last between 1 and 2 hours, originate in the proximal small intestine, and migrate aborally; the velocity of propagation slows as the activity front progresses distally. Related cyclical motor activity has been identified in the stomach, lower esophageal sphincter, gallbladder, and sphincter of Oddi.

In the stomach, patterns of MMC activity tend to commence and end simultaneously at all sites rather than propagate, as occurs in the small bowel.[7] As phase III develops in the proximal duodenum, several associated motor events occur in the stomach and esophagus. Basal tone in the lower esophageal sphincter is increased and exhibits superimposed phasic contractions, thereby preventing reflux of gastric contents during this time of intense gastric contractile activity. Tone increases in the proximal stomach, and superimposed phasic waves can be identified. At the same time, one-cycle-per-minute high-amplitude waves develop in the body of the stomach. True rhythmic activity occurs only in the distal antrum, where contractions at three to five cycles per minute may be seen at the end of phase III. As phase III approaches and develops, antropyloroduodenal coordination increases and high-amplitude contractions propagate through the antrum across the pylorus into the proximal duodenum, where they are associated with brief clusters of phasic contractions (Fig. 37–6).

Although the integration of gastric events with the MMC remains incompletely understood, it appears that both extrinsic nerves (especially the vagus) and hormonal factors (motilin, in particular) are involved. In the stomach, phase III activity appears independent of extrinsic innervation but is abolished by the administration of a motilin neutralizing antibody, suggesting that the gastric component of phase III may be induced by motilin, released from the proximal duodenum during the intense contractile activity associated with the activity front. In contrast, phase II of the MMC during fasting and the conversion, on eating, to the fed pattern (discussed later) are, in large part, mediated through the vagus.

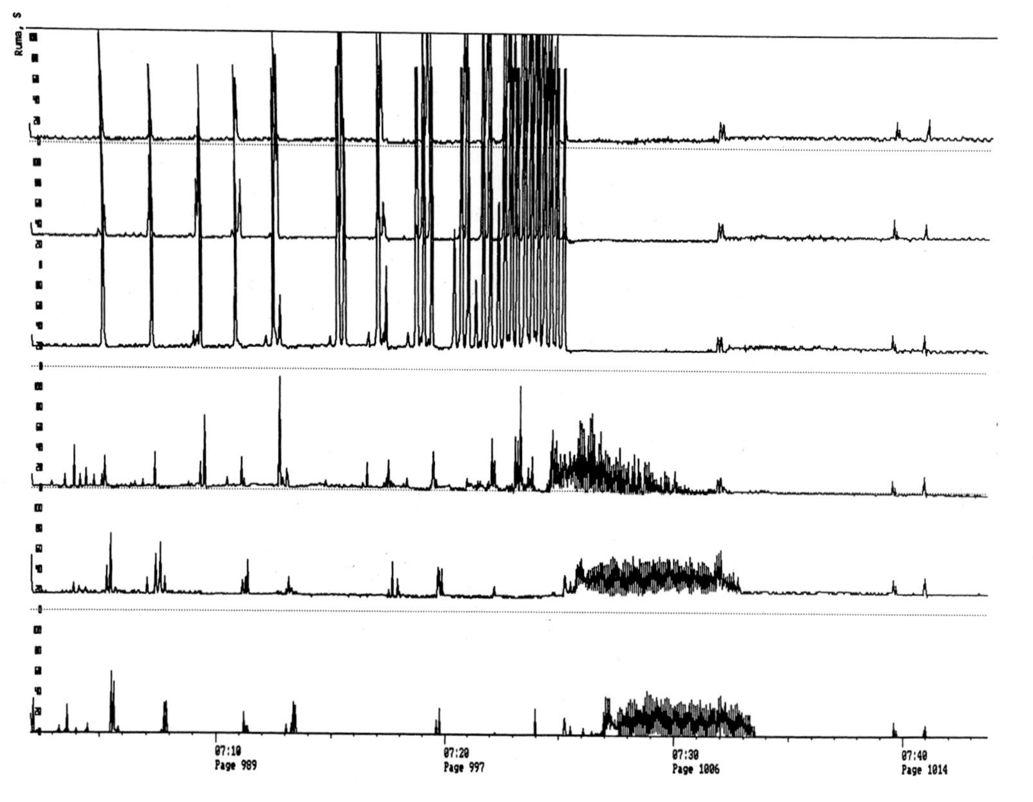

Figure 37–5. Fasting motor activity—the migrating motor complex. Simultaneous recordings of motor activity from the antrum (top three recording sites) and duodenum (bottom three recording sites) demonstrate the three phases of the migrating motor complex, in sequence, beginning on the extreme left: Phase 1, motor quiescence; Phase 2, regular activity; and Phase 3, a band of uninterrupted rhythm contractions which migrates in an aboral direction. *Note:* differences in amplitude and frequency of antral and duodenal contractions.

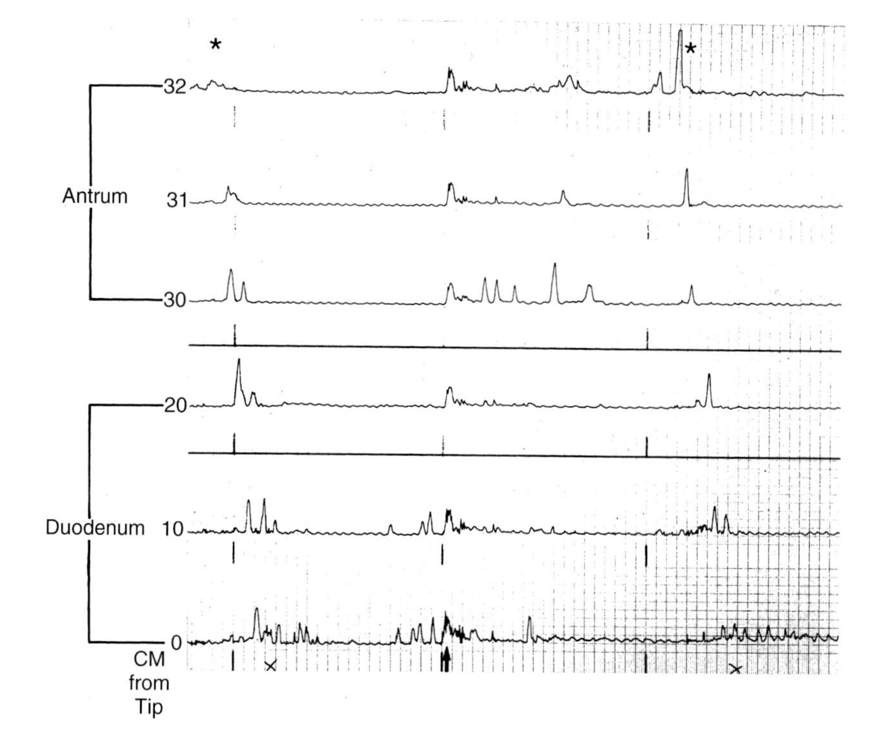

Figure 37–6. Antropyloroduodenal coordination. Simultaneous recording of antral and duodenal motor activity (antral activity in recording sites 32, 31, and 30 cm from the catheter tip, duodenal activity in recording sites at 20, 10, and 0 cm from the catheter tip). *Note:* Individual antral waves (*) migrate across the antrum and are associated with a brief, "cluster" of phasic contractions in the duodenum. Arrow indicates an artifact.

Motor Response to a Meal

Receptive Relaxation and Accommodation

On initiation of a swallow sequence, the gastric fundus undergoes vagally mediated receptive relaxation. As the meal enters the stomach, tone and phasic contractions in the proximal stomach are inhibited, leading to accommodation. Accommodation results in a dramatic two- to threefold increase in gastric volume,[8] leading to the retention of food in the stomach until it may be distributed to the antrum (Fig. 37–7). Fundic tone reflects a balance between cholinergic (excitatory) and nitrergic (inhibitory) input; during fasting, cholinergic input dominates. On meal ingestion, the accommodation response is triggered by distention-induced stimulation of mechanoreceptors. Mediated by a vagovagal reflex that relays in the nucleus of the tractus solitarius and effected through projections to the dorsal motor nucleus (DMN) of the vagus, fundic relaxation may be induced, in the DMN, either by the activation of inhibitory or the inhibition of excitatory vagal efferents to the fundus.[9] On the efferent side, the primary inhibitory neurotransmitter is nitric oxide (NO); vasoactive inhibitory peptide (VIP) may also play a role. Serotoninergic (5-hydroxytryptamine 1 [5-HT_1]) receptors on nitrergic neurons are also involved in the inhibitory pathway (Fig. 37–8).[10]

Several other factors have been shown to modulate fundic tone. Relaxation is induced by antral distention (a gastrogastric reflex), duodenal acidification,[11] distention and intraluminal perfusion with lipid and protein (a duodenogastric reflex), and colonic distention (a cologastric reflex). These

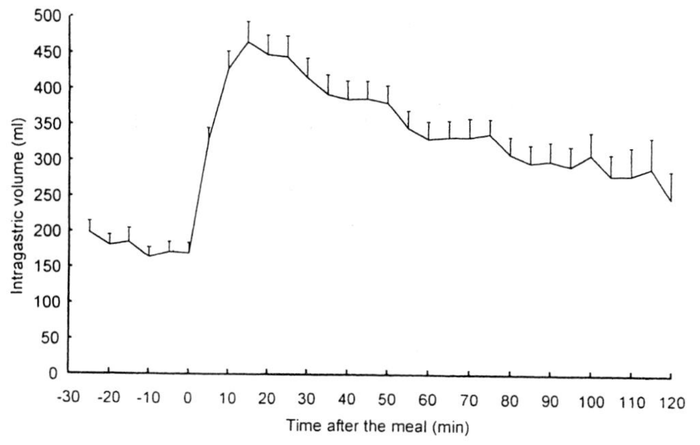

Figure 37–7. Normal accommodation response, as recorded from a barostat, a balloon placed in the upper stomach, in healthy volunteers. Meal ingested at time zero; note dramatic increase in volume of the upper stomach on meal ingestion. (From Tack J, Piessevuax H, Coulie B, et al: Role of impaired gastric accommodation to a meal in functional dyspepsia. Gastroenterology 115:1346, 1998.)

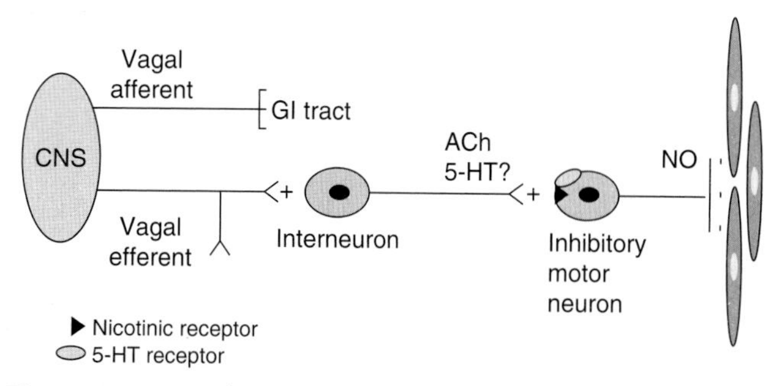

Figure 37–8. Neural pathways proposed to mediate the accommodation response. Both arms of the arc are mediated by the vagus nerve; relaxation is effected through stimulation of an inhibitory, nitrergic neuron. ACh, acetylcholine; 5-HT, 5-hydroxytryptamine (serotonin); NO, nitric oxide. (From Tack J: Receptors of the enteric nervous system: Potential targets for drug therapy. Gut 47 [suppl IV]:IV20, 2000.)

reflexes are in large part neurally mediated. For example, the gastrogastric reflex is effected through an arc initiated by capsaicin-sensitive afferent vagal fibers and mediated by 5-HT_3, gastrin-releasing peptide (GRP), and cholecystokinin A (CCK_A) receptors.[12]

Under experimental circumstances the fundus can be induced to relax by the administration of CCK, secretin,[11] VIP, gastrin, somatostatin, dopamine, gastin-releasing peptide, glucagon, and bombesin. With the exception of CCK and VIP, a role for many of these peptides in fundic motor physiologic processes remains to be defined.

The Abolition of the Migrating Motor Complex

Food ingestion also results in the abolition of the cyclical pattern of the MMC and its replacement by a band of random contractions called the *fed pattern* (Fig. 37–9), which may last from 2.5 to 8 hours, at which time the fasted pattern resumes, assuming that no more food has been ingested.[13] In the stomach, the duration of the fed pattern is related to the nature and caloric content of the meal.

Intragastric Meal Distribution, Trituration, and Emptying

Gastric emptying of liquids and solids, suspended in the liquid phase, is ultimately dependent on the interplay between the propulsive force generated by tonic contractions of the proximal stomach and the resistance presented by the antrum, pylorus, and duodenum. A fundamental property of the stomach is its ability to differentiate among different types of meals and the components of individual meals.

Liquids rapidly disperse throughout the stomach (Fig. 37–10) and begin to empty without a lag period. For non-nutrient liquids, emptying is rapid; nutrient-containing liquids, such as dextrose, are retained for longer periods in the antrum and emptied more slowly[14] (see Fig. 37–10). Emptying of liquids follows a simple, exponential pattern (see Fig. 37–10), and its rate is influenced by the volume ingested, as well as the nutrient content and osmolarity of the liquid. Carbonation further delays gastric emptying of liquids.[15] The rate of emptying of liquid meals is largely determined by the interaction between gastric volume, on the one hand, and duodenal feedback mechanisms, on the other.[16] In the past fundic tone was regarded as the primary regulator of liquid emptying; in 1995 its primacy was challenged.[17] Studies employing high-resolution manometry concluded that an antroduodenal pressure gradient (perhaps generated by gastric tone), and not antral peristalsis, was the primary factor generating liquid emptying, with pyloric opening exerting a modulatory role.[18]

Solids empty in two phases: an initial lag phase, during which little emptying occurs, followed by a linear emptying phase (Fig. 37–11). The solid component is first retained in the proximal stomach; as liquids empty, the solid component moves to the antrum during the lag phase and is subsequently emptied in a linear fashion. Redistribution is thus a major component of the lag phase.[13] An essential component of the normal response to a solid meal is the ability of the antropyloric region to discriminate solid particles by size and to restrict emptying of particles greater than 1 mm in diameter. The antropyloric mill grinds down, or triturates, larger particles into smaller ones, which are then emptied, in a linear fashion, with the liquid phase to promote optimal digestion. While trituration proceeds, solid emptying does not occur, thus giving rise to the lag phase; duration of the lag phase is directly related to the size and consistency of the solid component of the meal. After a typical solid-liquid meal, the lag phase lasts approximately 60 minutes. Trituration is a function of coordinated high-amplitude waves that originate in the proximal antrum and are propagated to the pylorus. As these contractions traverse the midantrum, the pylorus is open and duodenal contractions are inhibited, permitting transpyloric flow of liquids and suspended or liquefied solid particles. When liquids and solids reach the distal

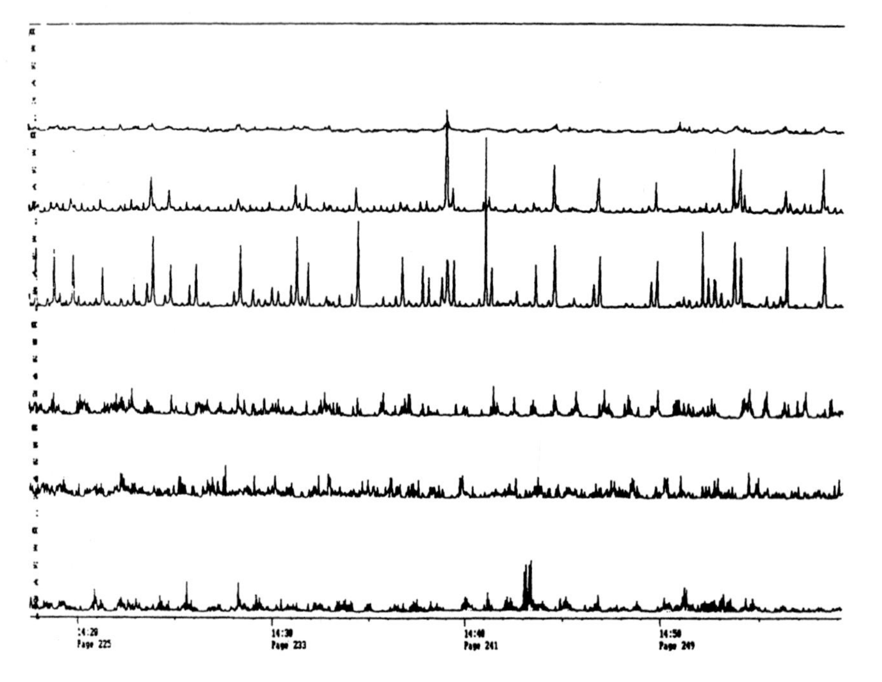

Figure 37–9. Fed motility. Simultaneous recordings from the antrum (top three channels) and the duodenum (lower three channels) demonstrating the intense, uncoordinated activity typical of the normal motor response to meals. (From Quigley EM: Gastric and small intestinal motility in health and disease. Gastroenterol Clin North Am 25:113, 1996).

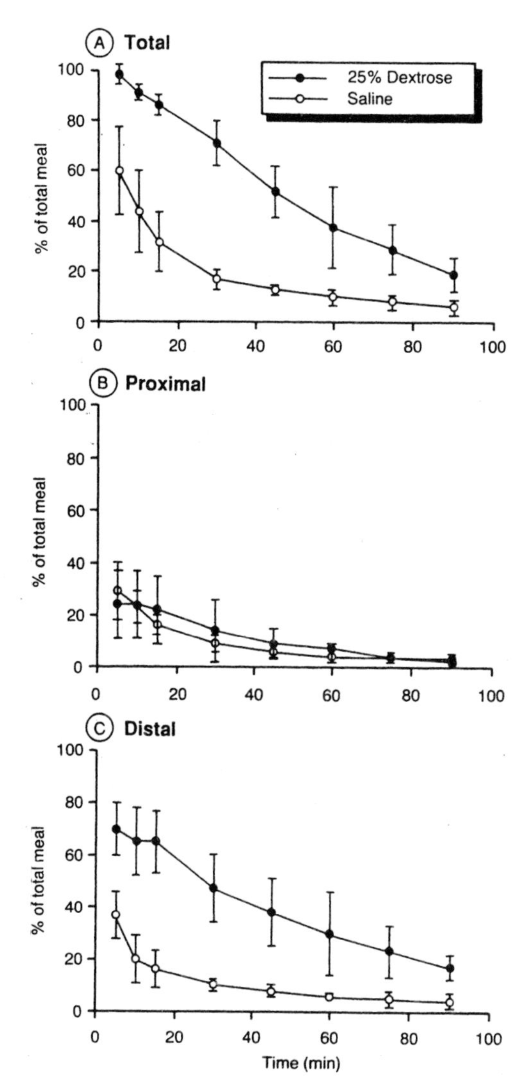

Figure 37–10. Total *(A)*, proximal *(B)*, and distal *(C)* gastric emptying curves for the liquid component of a mixed solid/liquid meal. Liquid component was either saline *(open circles)* or 25% dextrose *(closed circles)*. Each curve describes the disappearance of radioactivity from the stomach over time, as detected by scintigraphy. *Note:* (1) Liquid component disperses rapidly throughout the stomach; (2) emptying is slower for the dextrose-containing meal owing to greater retention in the distal stomach. (From Collins PJ, Houghton LA, Read NW, et al: Role of the proximal and distal stomach in mixed solid and liquid meal emptying. Gut 32:615, 1991.)

antrum, the terminal antral contraction (the aforementioned first contraction) closes the pylorus, promoting retropulsion of particles that are too large to have exited throughout the pylorus (Fig. 37–12). In this manner, solid food particles continue to move in and out of the antrum until they are small enough to exit the pylorus.

The pylorus regulates the egress of material from the stomach through several mechanisms, which include a relatively narrowed and fixed lumen, the maintenance of pyloric tone, and the generation of isolated pyloric pressure waves. The latter are associated, one assumes, with the repetitive spike discharges recorded from pyloric smooth muscle cells superimposed on the plateau potential. Of these mechanisms, pyloric tone has been an inconsistent feature in human recordings, and more emphasis is placed on the participation of the pylorus in coordinated antropyloroduodenal activity. Antropyloroduodenal coordination is suppressed during the lag phase, and isolated pyloric contractile waves are prominent, perhaps serving to maintain solid particles in the stomach until trituration has occurred. Once emptying begins, the incidence of antropyloroduodenal coordinated activity again increases, and that of isolated pyloric waves diminishes. The emptying of solids is thus influenced by several factors. Of major importance is particle size; under normal circumstances only particles less than 1 mm in diameter exit through the pylorus; larger particles must remain in the stomach until they have been ground down to this size by repetitive exposure to the forces of antral peristalsis. Solid emptying is also influenced by meal volume, caloric density, and content.

Fatty foods present a unique challenge to the stomach. At body temperature fats become liquid and by virtue of their

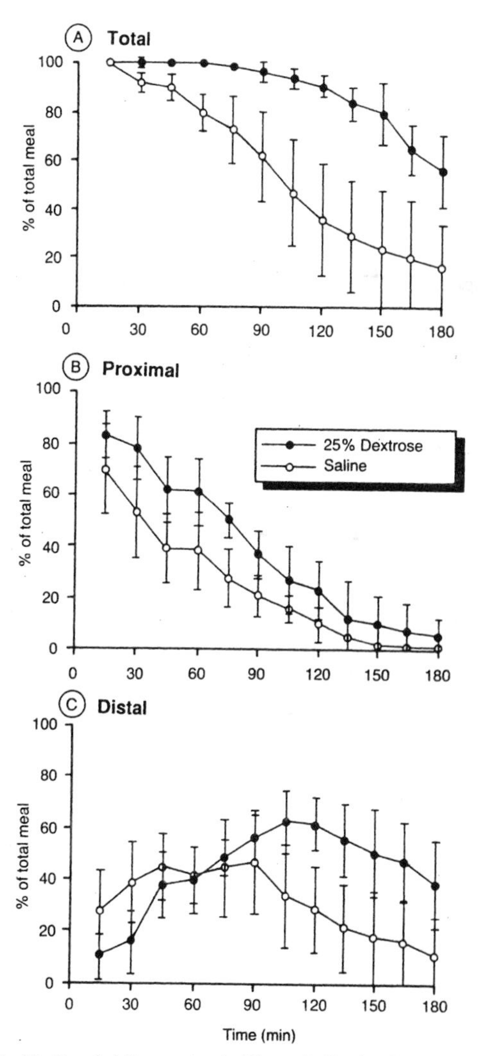

Figure 37–11. Total *(A)*, proximal *(B)*, and distal *(C)* gastric emptying curves for the solid component of a mixed solid/liquid meal (liquid = 25% dextrose or saline). *Note:* (1) Initial lag phase for total solid emptying, after which solids empty in a similar fashion to liquids; (2) solids initially retained in the proximal stomach; (3) solids later redistribute to the distal stomach meal; (4) dextrose delays solid emptying. (From Collins PJ, Houghton LA, Read NW, et al: Role of the proximal and distal stomach in mixed solid and liquid meal emptying. Gut 32:615, 1991.)

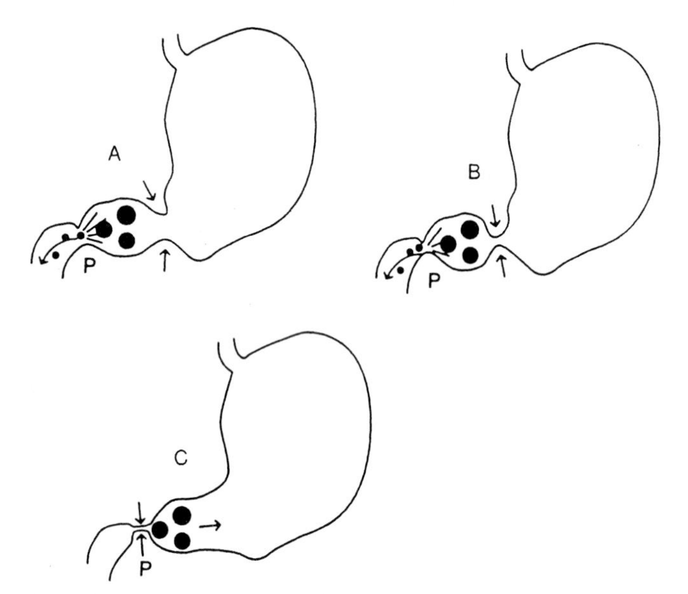

Figure 37–12. Interrelationships between antral peristalsis and pyloric patency: the role of antropyloric motility in gastric emptying of solids and liquids. *A* and *B*, Antral contractions *(arrows)* propel the food bolus from the corpus through the antrum toward the pylorus (P). Liquids and tiny particles are allowed to pass through the gastroduodenal junction into the duodenum, whereas large solid particles are retained. *C*, As the contraction wave reaches the terminal antrum *(arrows)*, the pylorus closes, trapping remaining liquids and solids in the terminal antrum. Peristalsis forcefully compresses the antral content, grinding (triturating) the solids. Because they are unable to pass forward, the antral contents are retropelled in a retrograde fashion from the terminal antrum back into the corpus. (Reproduced with permission from Quigley EMM: Gastric and small intestinal motility in health and disease. Gastroenterol Clin North Am 25:113, 1996.)

lower density tend to float on the liquid layer but are emptied more slowly than other liquids. Being poorly water-soluble, fats tend to coalesce into large globules that are not dispersed into fine particles by antral contractions. Magnetic resonance imaging studies of the gastric response to fat confirm a retarding effect on gastric emptying but also reveal a stimulation of to-and-fro movements in the antrum, perhaps representing the attempts of the antrum to disrupt the globules. Furthermore, products of fat digestion in the duodenum are among the most potent inhibitors of gastric motor events and gastric emptying.

Indigestible solids provide an even greater challenge and are not emptied in the immediate postprandial period but must await the return of MMC activity, when they are swept out of the stomach, through an open pylorus, during phase III.

Regulation of Gastric Emptying and Related Motor Activity

Extrinsic neural input to the stomach is provided by the vagus and splanchnic nerves. Tracer studies in 2000 indicated that, unlike the small intestine and colon, virtually all myenteric ganglia in the stomach receive direct vagal input.[19] In the stomach, again in contrast to the small intestine, myenteric ganglia are smaller and less numerous and submucosal ganglia are scarce or absent.[20] Taken together, these findings support a greater degree of extrinsic vagal influence in the stomach than in the small intestine, in accord with both results of physiologic studies and the clinical consequences of vagotomy. Most vagal efferents to the stomach are spontaneously active; this activity, generated in large part by mechanosensitive input from vagal afferents, produces vagal tone.

Whereas the vagus contains both excitatory and inhibitory fibers, sympathetic input to the stomach is primarily inhibitory. Postganglionic neurons in the splanchnic nerves terminate, for the most part, in the ganglia of the enteric nervous system; occasional neurons terminate directly on the smooth muscle.

The role of higher centers in the regulation of gastric motor function is most vividly manifested by the effects of certain stressors. A variety of acute and chronic stressors, such as labyrinthine stimulation and cold-induced pain, produce a dramatic inhibition of gastric emptying and antral motility and may disrupt the fed motor response and induce phase III–type activity in the postprandial period. Corticotropin-releasing factor (CRF) plays a central role in the mediation of stress-related gastric dysfunction.[21] CRF effects are in turn mediated through central dopaminergic (DA1 and DA2) and arginine vasopressin (AVP) pathways in the paraventricular nucleus and are subject to modulation by CCK.

A variety of peptides, including pituitary adenylate cyclase-activating peptide (PACAP),[22] glucagon-like peptide-1 (GLP1),[23] and gastrin-releasing peptide (GRP),[24] have also been shown to influence gastric motor function; their role in the physiologic regulation of gastric motility is not known.

Many of the factors that modulate gastric emptying rate (Table 37–1) exert their influence via a duodenal feedback control mechanism. Duodenal distention, acidification, or perfusion with fat and protein suppresses antral contractions and inhibits transpyloric flow through an inhibition of antropyloroduodenal coordination and a stimulation of isolated pyloric pressure waves and pyloric tone. These feedback control mechanisms are usually mediated by enterogastric neural reflexes and often involve the release of the hormone CCK, which binds to CCK_A receptors on gastric afferents. It is important to recognize that fat- and other nutrient-induced delays of gastric emptying are mediated by the products of their digestion; these "brakes" are not, therefore, operable in conditions of impaired digestion, such as pancreatic insufficiency.[25, 26]

On the efferent side of these reflex arcs, nitric oxide (NO) appears to be an important inhibitory mediator throughout the stomach. Nitrergic pathways figure prominently in the regulation of the various phenomena that con-

Table 37–1 | **Factors That May Modulate the Rate of Gastric Emptying**

Meal Factors	
Volume	Emptying rate proportional to volume
Acidity	Slowing of emptying
Osmolarity	Slower emptying of hypertonic meals
Nutrient density	Emptying rate inversely proportional to nutrient density
Fat	Slowing of emptying
Certain amino acids (e.g., L-tryptophan)	Slowing of emptying
Other Factors	
Ileal fat	Slowing of emptying (ileal "brake")
Rectal/colonic distention	Slowing of emptying
Pregnancy	Slowing of emptying

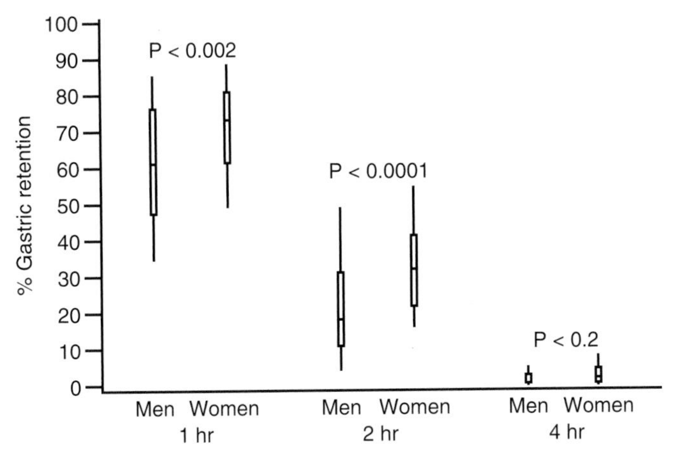

Figure 37–13. Gender differences in gastric emptying rate. Gastric retention (%) of a standardized low-fat meal at 1, 2, and 4 hours in 63 normal men and 60 normal women. Each box represents the median and the first and third quartile; the vertical lines (the whiskers) represent the 10th and 90th percentiles. *Note:* (1) Wide variation in gastric emptying rate for normal individuals; (2) slower emptying in women at 1 and 2 hours. (From Tougas G, Eaker EY, Abell TL, et al: Assessment of gastric emptying using a low fat meal: establishment of international control values. Am J Gastroenterol 95:1456, 2000.)

tribute to transpyloric flow, antral motility, pyloric contractions, and pyloric tone.

The rate of gastric emptying, especially that of solids, is slower in women[27–29] (Fig. 37–13). Although this relative delay in women is assumed to be hormonal in origin, not all studies have documented a relationship between gastric emptying rate and phase of the menstrual cycle, or cyclical variations in estradiol and progesterone concentrations.[30]

Gastric Sensation

Physiologic Characteristics of Gastric Sensation

Specialized sensory receptors are not a feature of the gastric mucosa; free nerve endings act as polymodal receptors that respond to touch, acid, and other chemical stimuli. Sensory information is conveyed from receptors in one of three types of primary afferent neurons: intrinsic primary afferent neurons (IPANs), whose cell bodies lie in the submucous or myenteric plexus; vagal afferents, which have cell bodies that lie in the nodose ganglion and which provide input primarily to the nucleus of the tractus solitarius; and splanchnic or spinal primary afferents, whose cell bodies lie in the dorsal horn of the spinal cord and synapse with second-order neurons that ascend in the spinothalamic and spinoreticular tracts and the dorsal columns. Visceral sensory axons are almost exclusively thin myelinated A-delta or unmyelinated C fibers (Fig. 37–14).

IPANs provide the sensory arm of intrinsic enteric reflexes; vagal and splanchnic afferents facilitate vagovagal and spinal reflexes and transmission of visceral sensory input to the higher centers. IPANs are present in both myenteric and submucosal ganglia and respond to luminal chemical stimuli, mechanical deformation of the mucosa, and muscle stretch and tension.[31] IPANs may also be activated by serotonin released from local enterochromaffin cells.

Spinal afferents include a population of capsaicin-sensitive unmyelinated C fibers that contain neuropeptides such as calcitonin gene-related peptide (CGRP), VIP, somatostatin, dynorphin, substance P, and neurokinin A. These fibers are the primary route for the transmission of a variety of nocicepitve stimuli from the gut. They respond to a variety of inflammatory mediators, stimuli that also awaken silent nociceptor fibers.[31–33]

Vagal afferent axons ramify extensively in the enteric plexus and infiltrate muscle sheets, where they course with ICCs.[19] Vagal afferents include mucosal chemosensitive and mechanosensitive neurons as well as neurons conveying input from tension receptors in the muscle layers. Mucosal receptors on vagal afferents are primarily activated by "physiologic" mechanical and chemical stimuli; their proximity to enterochromaffin and mast cells suggests that they may also be activated by serotonin (e.g., in the induction of nausea and vomiting) and other neuropeptides. These afferents mediate the sensory response to intraluminal acid; several mediators may be involved, including CCK, secretin, CGRP, and somatostatin, as well as a direct action of acid on sensory nerve endings.[34, 35] Although vagal afferents are viewed as being predominantly involved in the transmission of non-noxious stimuli, they should not be considered irrelevant to nociception. Indeed, vagal fibers may not only directly transmit nociceptive input but also play an important role in the modulation of nociceptive information traversing other pathways through the activation of antinociceptive descending spinal pathways.

The Origins of Gastric Sensations in Humans

The study of gastric sensations in humans is in its infancy. In an attempt to understand the pathogenesis of dyspeptic symptoms (see Chapter 7), emphasis to date has been placed

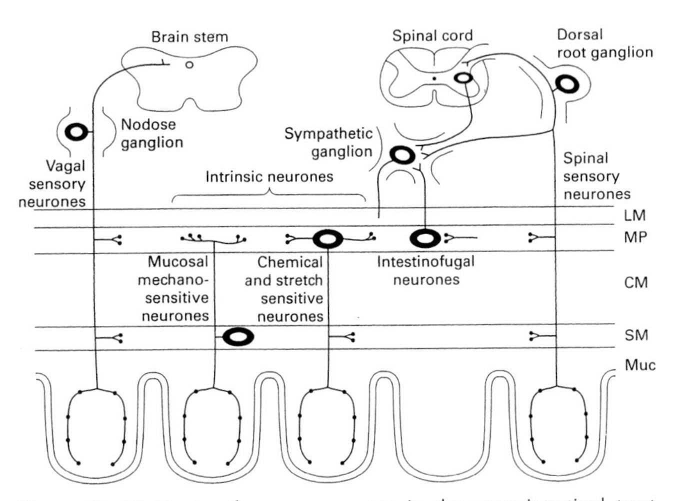

Figure 37–14. Types of sensory neurons in the gastrointestinal tract. *Note:* (1) Vagal and spinal sensory neurons, the location of their cell bodies, and their central connections are shown on the extreme left and right, respectively; (2) two types of intrinsic primary afferent neurons (IPANs) are represented in the center. Their cell bodies lie either in the submucosal (SM) plexus or myenteric plexus (MP). (CM, circular muscle; LM, longitudinal muscle; MP, myenteric plexus; Muc, mucosa.) (From Furness JB, Clerc N, Kunze WAA: Memory in the enteric nervous system. Gut 47 (Suppl IV):IV60, 2000, with permission.)

on attempts to relate sensations to stimuli applied to various parts of the stomach. Observations made by noninvasive methods reveal that the expansion in antral diameter induced by meal ingestion correlates directly with the development of a "normal" sensation of fullness, but not of satiety.[36] Fundic expansion, in contrast, is associated with the development of bloating.[37] When these different parts of the stomach are distended with balloons, both fundic and antral distention induces bloating at low levels of distention and pain at higher volumes, and antral distention alone induces nausea.[38] Interestingly, both bloating and pain develop at lower volumes of distention in the antrum than in the fundus. These findings suggest that the antrum, rather than the fundus, may be the prime source of postprandial sensations and symptoms.

The interpretation of all these studies is complicated by the interactions between sensation and motor activity both within and outside the stomach. Factors that may influence the response to distention include gastric wall tension[39] and the presence of nutrients and lipid, particularly in the duodenum.[40]

Role of the Stomach in the Regulation of Digestion and Food Intake

Several factors contribute to the role of the stomach in the maintenance of intestinal homeostasis. These include the feedback mechanisms already described, whereby nutrients and fat, in particular, delay gastric emptying, inhibit antral motility, and relax the fundus. In this manner, the delivery of the ingested meal to the small intestine is appropriately retarded. Enterogastric reflexes originating at more distal sites may play a similar role. One of the best described is the so-called ileal brake, whereby the instillation of nutrients into the ileum delays gastric emptying.[41] This mechanism may fulfill an important homeostatic role in conditions in which absorption and digestion have not been optimal and nutrients may be lost. The degree of enteric inhibition of gastric emptying is related to the length of intestine exposed to the nutrient.[42] The mediation of these reflexes remains uncertain; whereas peptide YY (PYY) was formerly regarded as the hormonal mediator of the ileal brake, evidence generated over the past several years tends to implicate CCK.[25, 26] Studies of the response to a liquid meal indicate an interaction between gastric and orosensory factors. Whereas direct infusion of nutrient into the duodenum induces neither fullness nor satiety, direct infusion of the same nutrient into the stomach provokes appetite suppression. However, the greatest suppression of appetite occurs when the nutrient is taken orally; this mechanism suggests roles for central, oral, and gastric factors in the induction of satiety.[43]

CCK, by virtue of its release by nutrients, its known interaction with gastric sensory receptors, its effects in the central nervous system, and its proposed effects on a variety of gastric motor phenomena, has become the prime canididate to serve as the crucial link among food intake, gastric motor function, and conscious response to a meal (fullness, satiety). Furthermore, CCK receptors are widely distributed throughout the stomach, where CCK_A receptor immunoreactivity has been identified in neurons in the myenteric plexus and in nerve fibers in the muscle layers and the mucosa. These neurons often colocalize with other inhibitory and excitatory neurotransmitters, supporting the suggestion that CCK_A activation may generate responses mediated by other peptides.[44]

The role of CCK in the physiologic regulation of gastric emptying and motor activity remains unclear. Studies employing physiologic doses of CCK suggested an ability to inhibit liquid emptying. The response to selective CCK_A antagonists has been inconsistent; some, but not all, induce an acceleration of emptying. On the other hand, CCK does appear to be an important mediator of gastric sensations through an action on CCK_A receptors. According to this hypothesis, CCK released in response to luminal contents activates CCK_A receptors on vagal primary afferent neurons that synapse in the nucleus of the tractus solitarius, which sends both ascending neurons to the paraventricular nucleus, inducing satiation and a decrease in food intake, and also sends descending vagal inhibitory neurons, which inhibit gastric emptying and promote fundic relaxation.

In 1998 leptin was isolated from the rat stomach, and some researchers have suggested that leptin may be involved in an early, CCK-mediated response to food intake.[45] Leptin also exerts effects on gastric motor function. When administered directly into the central nervous system (CNS), leptin delays gastric emptying and reduces food intake.[46] Peripheral effects of leptin are also important; acting on its gastric receptor, leptin can modulate neuronal activity in the brainstem through a mechanism that suggests a possible role in sensing meal intake.[47] Other factors may also exert parallel effects on gastric emptying and food intake and are, therefore, candidates for a role in satiety. For example, urocortin, a corticotropin-releasing R2 (CRF-R2) agonist, has been shown to reduce food intake and delay gastric emptying in both lean and obese mice.[48]

The brain and the stomach appear to be inextricably linked in the regulation of food intake.[49] The potential clinical impact of this integration has been illustrated by a study of 114 children of varying body habitus, in which a close correlation between body weight and fasting antral area, but not gastric emptying rate, was noted.[50]

Development of Gastric Motor Activity

Gastric peristalsis appears between the gestational ages of 14 and 23 weeks; by 24 weeks, grouped or clustered peristaltic waves are evident.[51] Electrophysiologic parameters demonstrate a similar maturational pattern; electrogastrographic (EGG) recordings obtained from preterm infants delivered at 35 weeks are similar to those recorded in full-term infants.[52] EGG parameters mature further over the first 6 to 24 months of life and remain stable thereafter.[53, 54]

At a molecular level, glial-derived neurotrophic factor (GD) and its receptors are essential to the development of the enteric nervous system in the stomach and, especially, in its very early development as it migrates from the neural crest to the gut.[55] The factors that regulate the later development of enteric neurons and their differentiation into specific neuronal types are not known.

Studies of ICC development have been greatly facilitated by the development of labels for the receptor tyrosine kinase, *kit,* and by the availability of knockout models. Interstitial cells of Cajal demonstrate differential development: *kit*-expressing ICCs, such as IC-MY, develop before birth, and interstitial cells in the deep muscular plexus (IC-DMP) develop after birth. The observation that neural and ICC networks are not fully developed and that ICCs and smooth muscle cells are poorly coupled at birth[3] may well explain the progressive perinatal development of gastric rhythmicity and contractility.

CLINICAL ASSESSMENT OF GASTRIC MOTOR FUNCTION AND DYSFUNCTION

Assessment of Gastric Emptying by Scintigraphy

Noninvasive scintigraphic techniques have almost entirely replaced perfusion methods requiring intubation and have become the mainstay of the assessment of gastric function in clinical practice.[56, 57] Various meals and isotopes are used; the important principle is that the isotope should remain totally bound with the meal during emptying. A solid phase marker isotope should not leech into the liquid phase, and a liquid phase marker isotope should not be absorbed into the solid phase. To achieve standardized results, meals should always be consumed in the same position. Correction for movement of the meal in three dimensions within the stomach can be made by using anterior and posterior cameras and calculating a geometric mean. Typically, indium 111–diethylenetriaminepentaacetic acid (^{111}In-DTPA) labeled water and technetium 99m (^{99m}Tc)-labeled scrambled eggs are employed as markers for the liquid and solid phases of a meal, respectively. From these curves, various parameters can be calculated to describe emptying and permit comparisons of groups of subjects and to relate the result in a given individual to a normal range. For solid emptying, the duration of the lag phase and the slope of the linear phase can be computed. For both solids and liquids, the time for half of the meal to empty ($t_{1/2}$) is a frequently used parameter.

Comparisons of gastric emptying results at different centers have been hampered by variations in test substance and methods of scanning and calculation. However, by using a standardized meal and adhering to a strict protocol, reproducible results can be obtained. In a multicenter protocol based on a low-fat, egg substitute–based meal reported in 2000, scanning was performed, without loss of accuracy, on only four occasions: at 0, 60, 120, and 240 minutes.[29] Median values (and their 95th percentile) for percentage of meal remaining in the stomach at 60, 120, and 240 minutes were 69% (90%), 24% (60%), and 1.2% (10%), respectively (see Fig. 37–13).

In the interpretation of gastric emptying studies, one needs to be aware not only of the physiologic factors that may influence emptying rate (see Table 37–1), but also of the many medications that can affect gastric emptying (Table 37–2).

The sensitivity of an emptying study in detecting gastroparesis is in part related to the nature of the test material: indigestible solids provide the greatest sensitivity and liquids the least. In practice, a conventional solid phase meal may provide useful clinical information.

Alternatives to Scintigraphy

Because of radiation exposure, problems in standardization, and limitations in terms of correlation with symptoms and therapeutic outcome, efforts continue to develop less invasive, less expensive, and more reproducible alternatives to scintigraphy. One of the earliest of these inexpensive and reproducible alternatives was the radiographic assessment of the gastric emptying of indigestible solids by using radiopaque markers. Although the emptying of markers and radiolabeled eggs has been shown to be correlated in both

Table 37–2 | **Representative Medications and Their Effect on Gastric Emptying**

MEDICATION	THERAPEUTIC USE	GE	MODE OF ACTION
Cardiovascular			
Potassium	Electrolyte balance	Delay	Not known
Dopamine	Vasopressor	Delay	Via dopamine receptor
Nifedipine, diltiazem, verapamil, others	Antihypertensive, antianginal	Delay or no effect	Calcium channel blocker
Respiratory			
Isoproterenol	Asthma, COPD	Delay	β-Adrenergic
Theophylline	Asthma, COPD	Not known	Smooth muscle relaxant
Gastrointestinal			
Sucralfate	Peptic ulcer	Delay or no effect	Mucosal coating and antacid
Aluminum hydroxide	Dyspepsia, heartburn	Delay	Antacid
Bulk laxatives	Constipation	Acceleration	Gastric distention
Opiates	Diarrhea	Delay	Increased smooth muscle tone
Psychiatric/Neurologic			
Tricyclics	Depression	Delay	Anticholinergic, norepinephrine-enhancing
Phenothiazines	Psychosis, antiemetic	Delay	Anticholinergic
Diazepam	Anxiety	Acceleration	Spasmolytic
L-Dopa	Parkinson's disease	Delay	Via dopamine receptor
Hormonal			
Synthetic estrogen	Hormonal therapy	Delay	? Gastric sex hormone receptors

COPD, chronic obstructive pulmonary disease; GE, gastric emptying; L-dopa, levodopa.
Adapted from Chaudhuri TK, Fink S: Update: Pharmaceuticals and gastric emptying. Am J Gastroenterol 85:223, 1990.

healthy control subjects and patients with gastroparesis, the role of the radiopaque marker test in clinical practice remains unclear.[58, 59] The acetaminophen-paracetamol absorption test has been employed as a measure of gastric emptying in research studies but also does not have an established role in clinical practice.[60]

Both ^{13}C octanoic acid[61] and ^{13}C acetate[62] breath tests have been developed to measure solid and liquid emptying, respectively. The ^{13}C octanoic acid breath test has received more attention. In the test a test meal containing radiolabeled octanoic acid is given. After emptying from the stomach, octanoic acid is absorbed in the small intestine and oxidized to CO_2, which is then excreted in the lungs, where it can be detected in breath samples. For optimal results breath sampling should be continued for 6 hours. With this protocol, the test is reproducible, although comparisons with scintigraphy have revealed variable results.[63, 64]

Ultrasonography

Ultrasonography is a noninvasive process that can provide a detailed but short-term evaluation of antropyloric function and yields considerable information regarding relationships among pyloric patency, transpyloric flow, and antral and duodenal contractions.[65, 66] Ultrasonography has also been advocated as a noninvasive test of gastric emptying and has been shown to be equivalent to scintigraphy[66–68]; in this respect three-dimensional ultrasound appears superior and has the added advantage of permitting an evaluation of the intragastric distribution of the meal.[69] Its widespread clinical application has been limited by the high level of expertise required to perform and interpret these studies, by the short observation time feasible, and by a paucity of data from studies in disease states.

Magnetic Resonance Imaging

In the early 1990s, magnetic resonance imaging (MRI) techniques were employed to measure gastric emptying and demonstrate intragastric distribution of a meal.[70, 71] This noninvasive, very expensive, methodology offers considerable promise for the detailed evaluation of the gastric motor response to a meal. It is capable of measuring total and regional emptying, regional distribution of the meal within the stomach, and even antral contractions.[72–74] Its potential role in clinical practice has yet to be determined but is likely to be limited by its cost and by lack of accessibility.

Electrical Impedance Methods

Because liquids and solids impede electrical current passed across the abdominal wall, electrical impedance methods have been used to evaluate gastric emptying in humans.[75, 76] Although good correlations have been demonstrated between impedance and standard scintigraphic techniques, impedance studies of both liquid and solid emptying remain subject to considerable "noise" despite the use of multiple electrode pairs.

Electrogastrography

Until the early 1980s technical problems limited the usefulness of EGG, a relatively simple and noninvasive technique.[77] Using modern electronic equipment, several centers have reported the consistent and reliable recording of gastric electric activity from surface electrodes.[78] Reports of abnormal gastric electrical rhythms, associated with delayed emptying and certain symptom patterns, have appeared over the past several years.

Because of interference from a multitude of artifacts, as well as competing biologic signals, the raw EGG signal is difficult to decipher, and its analysis depends on such computer based methods as Fourier transformation and running spectral analysis.[79] These applications are also problematic in that they may lead to erroneous diagnoses of bradygastria and tachygastria as a result of the inadvertent inclusion, in the computerized analysis, of any number of artifacts.[80] Previously confined to research laboratories, EGG systems are now commercially available. Though ambulatory systems are also available, optimal EGG recordings are really feasible only with the patient at rest; even in this position slight movement may contribute troublesome artifact. Nevertheless, the gastric slow wave can be readily and reliably recorded in fasting conditions, and this technique can also detect changes in slow wave frequency in response to environmental and pharmacologic manipulations as well as in disease states.[79] The physiologic significance of the amplitude (or power) of the EGG signal is less certain. The correlation between EGG power and the strength of gastric contractions is subject to question.[81] The concept of the power ratio (i.e., the change in power related to meal ingestion) also remains in doubt, as postprandial signal changes may be related more to alterations in the spatial relationship between the surface electrode (s) and the gastric antrum than to a real increase in the electrical signal.[81–83]

Because EGG is noninvasive, it is attractive for use in such conditions as pregnancy, but the clinical role of EGG remains to be established. Very few studies have critically evaluated the role of the EGG in clinical diagnosis. Published comparisons with scintigraphy[84] and manometry[85] suggest that broader clinical application of the EGG will require further improvements.

Barostat Systems

In the proximal stomach, where changes in tone and nonoccluding phasic contractions predominate, conventional manometric systems are not useful. To monitor changes in tone in this region, a barostat system has been developed.[86] Although this development has provided important insights into the physiologic characteristics of this region, clinical utility of this invasive methodology remains to be defined.

A noninvasive method for the assessment of gastric accommodation was described in 1999.[87] ^{99m}Tc pertechnetate is injected intravenously to outline the gastric wall, and changes in gastric volume are then monitored over time by single photon emission computed tomography (SPECT) after the ingestion of a meal. An accommodation response similar in magnitude to that recorded by a barostat was identified. Studies in disease states are eagerly awaited.

Antroduodenal Manometry

The direct measurement of pressure activity in the antrum, duodenum, and small intestine has now entered clinical practice, though it remains confined to specialized centers.[56, 57, 78, 88] In most institutions, a multilumen perfused catheter assembly is employed and the assembly customized according to the site in the intestine in which recordings are planned. Thus, in the antroduodenal region, where recordings from the distal antrum and pylorus are sought, the assembly should straddle the pylorus with either an array of closely spaced sensors or a sleeve system. To define relationships between gastric and small intestinal activity these assemblies also include recording sites, spaced at greater distances, in the duodenum and proximal jejunum. To provide constant monitoring of assembly position and detect sensor migration, some assemblies incorporate transmucosal potential difference (TMPD) electrodes at each end of the pyloric recording sites; maintenance of the assembly in the desired position is supported by the detection of the expected TMPD difference between the stomach and the duodenum. These assemblies are placed under fluoroscopic guidance and recordings typically performed for several hours during fasting and after the ingestion of a standardized liquid-solid meal. Recordings are analyzed for the various phases of the MMC, for the presence and nature of the "fed" motor response to the meal, and for abnormal patterns.

Ambulatory systems that combine either solid state miniaturized strain gauges[2, 89] or a miniaturized multiple perfused catheter system[90] with a data logger and appropriate computer software have been developed. Such systems permit prolonged (typically 24-hour) ambulatory recordings of motor activity from antrum, duodenum, and jejunum and can be used in the patient's home environment. In this way several cycles of the MMC may be recorded, diurnal variations appreciated, and response to a number of meals assessed. In theory, these prolonged recordings should reduce the inter- and intraindividual variability noted in more short-term stationary recordings, but an advantage of ambulatory systems over the well-established stationary perfusion system in clinical practice has yet to be demonstrated. Furthermore, problems with ensuring maintenance of sensors within the antrum throughout prolonged ambulant recordings, and especially in the immediate postprandial period, limit the usefulness of solid state systems for the assessment of antral motor activity.[89] Initial results obtained from an ambulatory perfusion system suggest that they may not be affected by this problem.[90] However, even a standard multilumen stationary system may fail to detect all antral conractile activity.[91]

Separate assessments of stationary and ambulatory protocols attest to the ability of each methodology to detect significant neuropathic or myopathic disorders.[92, 93] However, it must be emphasized that such evaluations rarely involve a pathologic confirmation of the final diagnosis.

Gastrointestinal Neuropathology

Clinical-pathologic correlation is rare in gastrointestinal (GI) motor disorders and has, to date, been possible only after gastric or intestinal resection.[94] Progress in understanding the pathophysiologic characteristics of these frustrating disorders has, accordingly, been considerably hampered. Researchers in 1994 advocated use of laparoscopic full-thickness intestinal biopsy,[95] but the clinical impact of this increasingly available technique has not, as yet, been defined.

Current Status of Gastric Motility Testing

Where are we, therefore, in the evaluation of gastric motor activity in clinical practice? For the moment, tests of gastric emptying will remain at the forefront of clinical practice. The ^{13}octanoic acid breath test offers considerable promise as a noninvasive, accessible test and could emerge as a widely available and acceptable screening test for gastric motor dysfunction. A major question that continues to plague all tests of gastric emptying is clinical relevance. As discussed later, gastric emptying rate does not appear to correlate well with symptoms and is poorly predictive of therapeutic response to available therapeutic prokinetic agents. The EGG has had major technical progress and is now a clinical reality, but its role in the evaluation of symptoms and dysfunction has not been established. Antroduodenal manometry has become considerably standardized in terms of protocol and interpretation but remains invasive and available only at a few referral centers. Its main utility is in excluding diffuse motor dysfunction in those rare instances in which substantial doubt lingers.

GASTRIC MOTOR DISORDERS

Symptoms, Gastric Emptying, and Motor Function

Given that the primary motor function of the stomach is to generate emptying, its motor disorders have traditionally been classified according to their effects on emptying;[96] gastroparesis, or delayed emptying, is the more common clinical entity (Table 37–3). Symptoms typically associated with gastroparesis include postprandial fullness, bloating, abdominal distention, nausea, and vomiting. In contrast, late postprandial vomiting of undigested food, if present, is more truly suggestive of gastroparesis. In some instances, pain related to gastric distention may be an important component of the clinical picture.[97] In diabetics, disruption of diabetic control and a tendency to hypoglycemia, in particular, may be the first indications of a gastric motility problem.[98]

The appropriateness of this division of gastric motor disorders according to gastric emptying rate may be questioned. First, as described later, in relation to both diabetic and idiopathic gastroparesis, symptoms often correlate poorly

Table 37–3 | **Causes of Gastroparesis***

Acid-peptic disease
Gastroesophageal reflux
Gastric ulcer disease
Gastritis
Atrophic gastritis ± pernicious anemia
Viral gastroenteritis (e.g., CMV)
Metabolic and endocrine
Diabetic ketoacidosis (acute)
Diabetic gastroparesis (chronic)*
Hypothyroidism
Pregnancy
Uremia
Liver disease
Collagen vascular disease
Scleroderma
Pseudo-obstruction
Idiopathic
Secondary (e.g., scleroderma, amyloidosis, muscular dystrophies, Parkinson's disease)
Postgastric surgery*
Vagotomy
Roux-en-Y syndrome
Medications (see Table 37–2)
Psychogenic
Anorexia nervosa
Stress
Trauma
Head injury
Spinal cord injury
Idiopathic*

CMV, cytomegalovirus.
*Among the most common disorders.

with a demonstrated abnormality on a gastric emptying study. Second, the same pathologic process may lead to either accelerated or delayed emptying. Thus, some of the components of the same surgical procedure may serve to accelerate emptying and others may promote gastric stasis. Similarly, in diabetes mellitus, accelerated and delayed emptying may represent separate events in the evolution of the same disease process. Finally, a narrow focus on gastric emptying may lead us to ignore other important phenomena such as altered gastric tone, small intestinal dysmotility, and abnormalities in visceral sensation and perception that may well prove to be important components of an individual disease process. Wherever possible, therefore, gastric motor disorders should be classified according to pathophysiologic characteristics; when this is not feasible, the temptation to classify what remains poorly understood according to gastric emptying study results should be resisted.

Postsurgical Syndromes

Vagotomy (also see Chapter 42)

The effects of vagotomy on gastric motor function are complex. Receptive relaxation, a vagally mediated reflex, is impaired. As a consequence, the early phase of liquid emptying is accelerated. This acceleration causes rapid emptying of hyperosmolar solutions into the proximal small intestine and may result in the early dumping syndrome. In contrast, and as a consequence of impaired antropyloric function, the later phases of liquid and solid emptying are prolonged by vagotomy. Other motor effects of vagotomy include an impairment of the motor response to feeding (which contributes to the pathophysiologic mechanisms of postvagotomy diarrhea) and a suppression of the antral component of the MMC.[99] The latter phenomenon is particularly prevalent among individuals who have symptomatic postvagotomy gastroparesis.

The now standard addition of a drainage procedure, such as a pyloroplasty or gastroenterostomy, has tended to negate the effects of vagotomy alone. In most patients, the net result of the combined procedure is little alteration in the gastric emptying of liquids or solids. Thus, prolonged postoperative gastroparesis (i.e., lasting longer than 3 to 4 weeks) is, in fact, rare (<2.5% of patients after either vagotomy and pyloroplasty or vagotomy and antrectomy) (see Chapter 42). Significant postoperative gastroparesis may occur, however, in patients who have a prior history of prolonged gastric outlet obstruction. In this circumstance, normal gastric emptying may not return for several weeks.

Longitudinal studies suggest that vagotomy-related gastroparesis tends to resolve over time. Indeed, a 1999 study suggested that gastric emptying rates in those who had undergone either a truncal or a highly selective vagotomy were similar by 12 months after the procedure.[100]

Persisting postsurgical gastric motor dysfunction often presents a formidable management challenge. Therapeutic responses to prokinetic agents have proved particularly disappointing in this group. In these resistant cases a completion gastrectomy may be the best alternative. It should be noted, however, that in one large series this course was deemed successful in only 43%.[101]

Gastrectomy (also see Chapter 42)

Antral resection, by removing the antral mill, renders the stomach incontinent to solids and leads to accelerated emptying. The symptomatic "dumping" that may result has been described in up to 50% of patients after Billroth I or II gastrectomy.[102] Symptoms are usually mild but occasionally prove incapacitating. Early dumping symptoms, occurring within 10 to 20 minutes of meal ingestion, include weakness, nausea, borborygmi, urgency, diarrhea, and diaphoresis. Late dumping symptoms occur 90 to 120 minutes after a meal and are a consequence of reactive hypoglycemia.

Treatment is based on dietary manipulation, with emphasis on preventing rapid delivery of hyperosmolar solutions to the small intestine. Pharmaceutical interventions, with the possible exception of use of octreotide, have proved largely unsuccessful. Surgery, in the form of a Roux-en-Y anastomosis, conversion of Billroth I to II, and pyloric reconstruction, is rarely indicated and, even then, successful in only 50% of cases.

Delayed gastric emptying sometimes results from a Billroth II gastrectomy as a result of a large atonic gastric remnant.[102]

Roux-en-Y Syndrome

The creation of a Roux-en-Y gastroenterostomy may be associated with a specific clinical entity, Roux syndrome.[103] Severe symptoms of postprandial abdominal pain, bloating, and nausea many develop. Studies have variably described impaired gastric motor function[104] and a "functional" obstruction within the duodenal Roux limb due to motor asynchrony.[103, 105] Whereas the latter can be revealed by manometry, the status of these motility patterns in the pathophysiologic processes of this syndrome remains unclear.[106]

Pyloromyotomy

Although pyloromyotomy is not associated with any long-term effect on gastric emptying rate, it augments pyloric tone and increases the number but reduces the amplitude of pyloric pressure waves.[107]

Pancreatectomy

Pancreatectomy and the pylorus preserving pancreaticoduodenectomy in particular have been associated with a high incidence of postoperative gastric stasis. The principal predictor of gastric emptying delay after these operations is the occurrence of other postoperative complications.[108, 109] Operative technique appears, in general, to be of less importance, though there is a suggestion that an antecolic anastomosis may be associated with less emptying delay.

Antireflux Operations

The performance of a laparoscopic Nissen fundoplication has in a few patients been associated with the development of dyspeptic symptoms and gastric motor dysfunction, including gastric emptying delay. The pathophysiologic process in these occurrences is unclear. In some, postsurgical gastroparesis may represent the overt appearance of an unrecognized preoperative disorder; in others there is compelling evidence to incriminate vagal injury. In prospective studies, fundoplication has been shown to decrease the compliance of the proximal stomach and impair the postprandial relaxation response; those changes can induce dyspeptic symptoms, especially in predisposed individuals.[110] In these same studies, however, fundoplication was shown to accelerate, and not delay, gastric emptying.[110]

Diabetic Gastroenteropathy

(also see Chapter 29)

Gastroparesis as a specific complication of diabetes does not appear to increase mortality rate,[111] but it can represent a major challenge for the patient and physician. It should also be stressed that the spectrum of gastric motor abnormalities among diabetics extends to include both accelerated and delayed emptying, as well as abnormalities in proximal gastric function. In describing this range of GI motor abnormalities that may accompany diabetes, the term *diabetic gastroenteropathy* is preferred to the more limited term *gastroparesis*.

Surveys performed in diabetic clinics suggest that GI symptoms are very common, but there are few data on the community prevalence of either GI symptoms or associated functional abnormalities among diabetics. Not surprisingly, prevalence rates for manifestations of gastroenteropathy such as gastroparesis, for example, have varied widely, depending on patient population studied and methodology employed.[112–115]

Prominent symptoms among diabetics who have gastroparesis include early satiety, postprandial distress, constipation, diarrhea, fecal incontinence, and dysphagia. Prospective studies of gastric emptying in patients with long-standing diabetes mellitus have demonstrated that disordered emptying of solids and especially indigestible solids is common and frequently asymptomatic.[116, 117] Furthermore, even among symptomatic patients, this disease frequently runs a fluctuating course of episodes of pronounced symptoms interspersed with relatively symptom-free intervals. Disordered gastric motor function is important not only because of its associated symptoms but also because of its effects on nutrient delivery to the small intestine and resultant fluctuations in blood glucose levels.[118] Accelerated emptying is especially common in type 2 diabetes, in which it may be an early manifestation of gastric motor dysfunction;[115, 116, 119] its occurrence appears unrelated to the rate of solid emptying, the duration of diabetes, or the presence of autonomic neuropathy.[120]

Several motor abnormalities have been documented in diabetics with symptomatic gastroparesis. These have included abnormal intragastric distribution of food,[121] a reduced incidence of the antral component of the MMC, antral dilatation and fasting and postprandial hypomotility,[118] and electrical dysrhythmias.[122] The loss of antral phase III provides a physiologic basis for the occurrence of bezoars in these patients. Pyloric dysfunction (pylorospasm) was documented in one study[123] but not confirmed in another, which employed a more accurate methodology for the assessment of pyloric function.[124] Fundic tone is reduced and the accommodation response impaired.[37] Many of these features are consistent with extrinsic autonomic denervation. Furthermore, autonomic function testing in affected diabetic patients frequently demonstrates evidence of autonomic denervation in other organs. It should be noted, however, that studies defining autonomic neuropathologic changes have been relatively few in number and far from unanimous in their conclusions.[125–127] In addition, several recently developed lines of evidence, as well as prior clinical observations,[118] indicate that a number of other factors may be relevant to the pathophysiologic mechanisms of GI symptoms in the diabetic. First, hyperglycemia per se can modulate a variety of GI functions.[128] Hyperglycemia can delay gastric emptying,[129–132] induce antral hypomotility,[133] promote isolated pyloric contractions,[134] and provoke gastric electrical dysrhythmias.[135] It is important to emphasize that relatively minor elevations in blood sugar level, even within the physiologic range, can delay emptying in both normal volunteers and diabetics. However, the magnitude of the delay is small and of questionable clinical significance.[132] Fasting hyperglycemia, induced by raising blood glucose to a level that mimics that of physiologic postprandial hyperglycemia, can induce fullness, impair antral contractility, blunt the pyloric response to intraduodenal lipid infusion,[136] and modify sensory responses.[137]

Other evidence suggests the direct involvement of the enteric nervous system in diabetes.[138, 139] This includes reports of pathologic abnormalities in both the myenteric and submucosal plexus in diabetic patients.[139] It is unclear whether these and other abnormalities in enteric and autonomic neural function reflect the acute effects of hyperglycemia, the long-term consequences of poor metabolic control, or other factors. As there is considerable evidence that chronic hyperglycemia is one of the important factors in the pathophysiologic processes of diabetic peripheral neuropathy, it seems not unreasonable to suggest that hyperglycemia, whether acute or sustained, can induce similar biochemical and/or morphologic changes in autonomic and enteric neurons to those described in peripheral neurons. Indeed, variations in motor function related to fluctuations in blood sugar level may explain the clinical observation that symptoms and gastric emptying pattern can fluctuate considerably in a given patient. Will strict blood sugar level control prevent or reverse these GI problems? Few studies have addressed this issue. Holzapfel and colleagues studied gastric emptying in a group of type 2 diabetics before and after readjustment of diabetic control and documented no relationship between blood glucose concentration and gastric emptying rate,[140] despite improving control.

Idiopathic Gastroparesis, Nonulcer Dyspepsia, and Dysmotility

Idiopathic Gastroparesis

Several studies conducted since 1985 have described a group of patients with postprandial fullness, nausea, and bloating in association with delayed gastric emptying in whom no primary abnormality can be identified.[141–145] As a consequence, the term *idiopathic gastroparesis* has been added to the gastroenterologist's lexicon. This term is used to describe patients (almost exclusively young women) who experience intractable "functional" symptoms and are found to have delayed gastric emptying on formal testing. Their symptoms vary and in some studies at least pain is a very prominent feature. A 1998 study delineated some of the prognostic factors for this group and suggested that those whose illness began with a viral prodrome are more likely to do well in the long term and to respond to prokinetic agents in the short term.[146] Some of these patients go on to require supplemental nutrition, gastrostomy, and jejunostomy and some have had gastric electrical stimulation and surgical procedures. In most of these patients, there is no histologic confirmation of a diffuse motor disorder. Although it is certainly plausible, and indeed likely, that some do suffer from a severe disorder of gastric emptying, we need to be most cautious in our approach. In the absence of defined abnormality, it could be argued that these symptoms represent no more than the severe end of the spectrum of functional dyspepsia.

This issue may not be restricted to individuals who have "functional" disorders. There is no reason why patients with diabetes mellitus, for example, should be immune to functional dyspepsia. Indeed, a 1998 multicenter study that evaluated the response to a prokinetic agent in diabetes found little correlation between therapeutic response and gastric emptying rate. There was similar improvement in those with and without pretherapy gastroparesis.[147]

Gastric Motor Dysfunction in Functional Dyspepsia (also see Chapter 7)

Of the various parameters of motor function that have been studied in patients with dyspepsia, gastric emptying has received most attention. Delayed gastric emptying has been demonstrated, on average, in 40% of patients with functional dyspepsia. However, emptying was delayed, on average, by a factor of only 1½ times the normal rate.[148, 149] Of patients with functional dyspepsia delayed gastric emptying is most likely among women who have predominant motility-type symptoms (such as fullness) and low body weight.[150] In any event, even with the most rigorous approach to patient selection, relationships among symptoms, gastric emptying delay, and therapeutic response to prokinetics in dyspepsia are far from perfect. It must also be remembered that delayed gastric emptying could well be an epiphenomenon in these patients, representing either a response to symptoms themselves or the influence of factors such as stress and psychopathologic conditions on gastric motor activity. EGG studies have reported a rather similar prevalence of dysrhythmias among patients with dyspepsia.[84]

A 1996 study focused attention on more subtle abnormalities of gastric function.[151] This emphasis first received attention in a 1994 study that demonstrated regional abnormalities in the distribution of a meal within the stomach among patients with dyspepsia whose total rate of gastric emptying was normal.[152] The more recent Quigley study in 1996 with a fair degree of consistency showed that the fundus is less likely to relax completely after meal ingestion in dyspeptics and causes premature and inappropriate distribution of the meal to the antrum, which, in turn, may become distended or dilated.[151] Of particular relevance to these observations has been the demonstration that both impaired fundic accommodation[8] and antral dilatation[36] are associated with the precipitation of symptoms. In one study impaired accommodation was observed in 42% of patients in association with the presence of early satiety and weight loss.[8] It is also plausible that antral dilatation may, in turn, explain the antral hypomotility recorded on manometric studies by several authors.[141–143, 145]

The other line of investigation that has been eagerly pursued is that of visceral hypersensitivity.[153–155] This phenomenon appears to be ubiquitous among patients with functional GI disorders, and it has been clearly demonstrated that patients with functional dyspepsia are more sensitive to a variety of intragastric stimuli. The extent to which this hypersensitivity is, in turn, determined by alterations in tone in the proximal stomach is unclear. There is also some, but not consistent[156] evidence to suggest that *Helicobacter pylori*–related inflammation may lower thresholds for sensation in functional dyspepsia.[157]

Other Functional Disorders

In the evaluation of the patient with unexplained nausea and vomiting the clinician must give special attention to the patient's history.[158] Three particular entities are likely to cause diagnostic confusion: rumination, the cyclical vomiting syndrome (Chapter 8), and anorexia nervosa and related eating disorders (Chapter 17).

Delayed gastric emptying and EGG abnormalities appear to be common in cyclical vomiters.[159] There is also an increased prevalence of delayed gastric emptying in anorexia nervosa and bulimia,[160, 161] which may also pose diagnostic challenges.

The diagnosis of rumination can be established on clinical grounds alone in most patients.[162] Manometry should be reserved for those situations in which the history is not typical and other disorders need to be considered.[163] More detailed motility studies have revealed a high prevalence of gastric motor and sensory dysfunction in ruminators, as 50% demonstrate impaired gastric accommodation. Other abnormalities include gastric hypersensitivity and a more sensitive lower esophageal relaxatory response to gastric distention.[164] Rumination was formerly recognized primarily among children with neurodevelopmental disorders. It is now evident that rumination is common among apparently healthy adolescents and young adults. Formal testing may uncover a primary psychological disturbance, and therapy is based on behavioral approaches.

Gastric Motor Function in Acid Peptic Disease

Gastric ulcer disease is associated with impaired antropyloric motor function, but it remains to be established whether this abnormality is indicative of a primary motor disorder or is simply a consequence of the ulcer process.[165]

Although it has often been postulated that delayed clearance of acid from the duodenal bulb could contribute to slow healing of duodenal ulcers, conclusive evidence in support of this hypothesis has been lacking. Of interest, patients with functional dyspepsia (discussed previously and in Chapter 7) clear infused acid more slowly than normal individuals from the duodenal bulb. This delay is associated with both an impaired motor response to acid and the onset of nausea.[166] In a detailed manometric study, a striking disruption of antropyloroduodenal motor coordination was noted in relation to both active and healed duodenal ulcers.[167] Accelerated gastric emptying has been described in association with the Zollinger-Ellison syndrome[168] and duodenal ulcer disease.[169] *Helicobacter pylori* infection does not influence either gastric emptying or gastric motor activity[144, 170, 171] but may be associated with abnormal gastric myoelectrical activity (on EGG) that is reversible after eradication of infection.[171]

Apart from instances of reflux secondary to overt gastric outlet obstruction or severe established gastroparesis, the role of delayed gastric emptying in the pathophysiologic processes of gastroesophageal reflux disease (GERD) remains uncertain (see Chapter 33). Available evidence suggests a relatively minor role.[172]

Given the role of the proximal stomach in the initiation of transient lower esophageal sphincter relaxations (tLESRs), it should be no surprise that this relationship has been an area of active inquiry. Fundic function is abnormal in GERD. In response to a meal, the fundus becomes more relaxed in GERD, and this relaxation lasts longer.[173, 174] GERD patients also demonstrate decreased sensory thresholds and increased retention of solids and liquids in the proximal stomach. These abnormalities may facilitate the induction of tLESRs.

Gastrointestinal Motor Dysfunction Related to Viral Illness

Clinicians have recognized for some time that many acute illnesses, including viral infections, may be associated with the development of symptoms suggestive of gastric motor dysfunction. Among patients with functional dyspepsia and delayed gastric emptying, those with a history of a viral prodrome have an excellent prognosis.[146, 175, 176] In some instances, viral infections of the gastric mucosa have been directly linked with disturbed emptying.[177] Examples include cytomegalovirus (CMV) and herpes simplex virus (HSV) gastritis, which may occur in immunocompromised patients.[177] Case studies in 1977 and 1986 reported GI motor dysfunction in relation to viral infections in immunocompetent patients. Although the evidence for such an association is somewhat inconclusive and a direct cause and effect relation remains to be established, the suggestion that common viruses, such as members of the herpes simplex virus family, might evoke in certain individuals dysmotility through effects on the CNS, autonomic supply, or the motor apparatus of the gut[178, 179] is intriguing and deserving of further study.

Gastric Motor Function in Autonomic Neuropathy, Pseudo-obstruction Syndromes, and Systemic Diseases

Gastroparesis and related symptoms may be prominent features of any disorder associated with autonomic neuropathy (see Chapter 29) and may also be components of both primary and secondary intestinal pseudo-obstruction syndromes (see Chapter 111). In scleroderma, one of the most common causes of pseudo-obstruction, gastroparesis is common and gastric involvement tends to parallel that of the esophagus (see Chapter 29). Gastric motor dysfunction has also been described in achalasia and may be prominent in Chagas' disease (see Chapter 98).

As discussed in Chapter 29, gastric motor dysfunction has been described in a variety of neurologic diseases, including spinal cord[180, 181] and head injuries,[182] amyotrophic lateral sclerosis,[183] and Parkinson's disease.[184] Delayed emptying occurs in 50% of patients with spinal cord injury[181]; risk factors for gastroparesis include female gender and a high level of injury. Other diseases and conditions associated with gastric motor dysfunction and gastroparesis include cirrhosis,[185] chronic renal failure,[186] endotoxemia, acute pancreatitis, and the Rett syndrome (lack of development, autistic behavior, ataxia, and dementia in young girls). Delayed gastric emptying is common among cancer patients and is multifactorial in origin.[187] Pathogenetic factors may include the local and systemic effects of the cancer per se, paraneoplastic neuropathic syndromes, as well as the effects of cytotoxic chemotherapy and radiation.[188] Gastroparesis is often overlooked in many of these ill patients and its impact on nutrition and its associated risk for aspiration ignored.

THERAPY

Gastric dysmotility continues to pose a significant therapeutic challenge. Recent concerns regarding safety of cisapride led to severe restrictions on its use in the United States. Moreover, the unavailability of a dopamine antagonist besides metoclopramide complicates matters further.

Available Compounds

Cholinergic Agonists

Cholinergic agonists, the original promotility agents, stimulate muscarinic M_2-type receptors on the smooth muscle cell. Recently, anticholinesterases have also been used to a limited extent. Evidence for their effectiveness in motility disorders is inconsistent. Although bethanechol had been used for reflux and gastroparesis,[189] its use for these indications has virtually disappeared with the introduction of newer agents.

Dopamine Antagonists

Until recently, the most widely used prokinetic agent was metoclopramide, a dopamine antagonist with central and peripheral effects. Domperidone, a dopamine antagonist that does not cross the blood-brain barrier and operates primarily through peripheral (DA_2) receptors, is available for use throughout Europe, Canada, and South America but not in the United States.[190, 191] The efficacy of metoclopramide in motility disorders has been far from consistent, and its long-term use has been complicated by a trend toward tolerance and a troubling incidence of CNS side effects.[192, 193] Up to 25% of patients may experience side effects, the most troubling of which are extrapyramidal reactions.[194] Both metoclopramide and domperidone may elevate serum prolactin levels and cause gynecomastia and galactorrhea. These dopamine antagonists are primarily effective in the foregut and have shown efficacy in gastroparesis, GERD, and dyspepsia.[147, 192–195] An important advantage of these agents is that both also act as central antiemetics, by virtue of the fact that the vomiting center lies on the blood side of the blood-brain barrier. Furthermore, metoclopramide is available for both oral and parenteral use and in a generic form. Levosulpiride, a DA_2 antagonist in development, has been shown to accelerate gastric emptying in diabetics and to improve glycemic control over a 6-month period.[196] Levosulpiride also appears effective in dyspepsia,[197] perhaps via acceleration of gastric emptying.

Substituted Benzamides

In the substituted benzamide group of prokinetics, cisapride is the prototype. It facilitates acetylcholine release from myenteric neurons through a 5-HT_4 receptor–mediated effect. Cisapride has been shown to promote esophageal peristalsis, augment lower esophageal sphincter pressure, and accelerate gastric emptying. Of the commonly available oral agents, cisapride appears to have the most diffuse GI effects. Several studies have demonstrated benefit in both short- and long-term therapy of gastroparesis and dyspepsia.[198–202] Interestingly, there has been a poor relationship between symptomatic improvement and acceleration of gastric emptying.[200] Studies to date suggest that tolerance may be less of a problem than for metoclopramide.[198] There have been reports of serious cardiac arrhythmias with cisapride related to QT interval prolongation.[203–205] Most of these instances have occurred in the context of concomitant use of drugs that either inhibit cisapride metabolism or prolong the QT interval or in individuals who had a history of prolonged QT interval or related arrhythmias, renal failure, ischemic heart disease, congestive heart failure, hypokalemia, hypomagnesemia, or respiratory failure. These concerns led in 1998 to the imposition of severe restrictions on its use in the United States and have spurred on interest in the development of alternative 5-HT_4 agonists. One of these, prucalopride, has been studied primarily for its effect on the colon,[206] and another, tegaserod (an aminoguanidine indole and not a substituted benzamide), has been shown to accelerate intestinal transit and reduce esophageal acid exposure.[207]

Macrolides

It has been known for some time that erythromycin is a motilin agonist. Evidence for therapeutic efficacy in gastroparesis is more recent. In a comprehensive review, Camilleri concluded that erythromycin is most useful in acute gastroparesis and recommended a regimen that begins with intravenous erythromycin lactobionate (3 mg/kg every 8 hours) and continues with oral administration (250 mg three times a day) for 5 to 7 days.[208] Efficacy with long-term oral administration has been less obvious and may be complicated by the risks associated with long-term antibiotic use.[209] There is also evidence that the salutory response to erythromycin may be blunted by hyperglycemia.[210, 211] Other modes of administration are under evaluation,[212, 213] but even more promising may be the development of a macrolide motilin agonist with minimal antibiotic activity and predictable pharmacokinetic characteristics and devoid of tolerance.[214]

Treatment of the Patient with Established Gastroparesis

Dehydration and electrolyte abnormalities should be corrected by oral or intravenous routes, as appropriate. Gastric decompression by nasogastric suction remains an important component of management in the acute stage. Malnutrition develops in many patients who have chronic, established gastroparesis as a result of inadequate oral intake and vomiting. Therefore, attention to diet and nutrition remains of paramount importance. When oral intake fails, jejunostomy feeding may be considered. Percutaneous or, preferably, surgical placement of a combined gastrostomy-jejunostomy tube simultaneously decompresses the stomach and permits enteral nutrition. Although the real clinical impact of chronic hyperglycemia on motility is unclear, it seems reasonable to advise that diabetic control should be optimized.

In terms of pharmacologic therapy, cisapride (where available), metoclopramide or domperidone (where available), and erythromycin have the best evidence for efficacy in gastroparesis. Whereas erythromycin should probably be reserved for intravenous use in the acutely ill patient, either cisapride or metoclopramide may be used for long-term oral therapy. Both have significant side effect issues, of which the prescribing clinician must be fully apprised.

Nausea may be a significant problem for many of these patients and may respond to concomitant administration of an antiemetic. In these latter circumstances, an antiemetic such as a phenothiazine derivative or a 5-HT_3 antagonist should be employed and can often be used successfully as circumstances may require. In choosing a particular antiemetic, attention should be paid to the appropriateness of available formulations, duration of action, and cost.

In 1998 gastric stimulation was proposed as an alternative for individuals with intractable gastroparesis.[215] Although the precise mode of action of gastric stimulation remains uncertain and may be independent of an acceleration of gastric emptying,[216] the results of two pilot studies[215, 217] were impressive, and this approach deserves further study. In a small number of patients, usually those with long-standing, complicated type 1 diabetes, severely symptomatic and apparently intractable gastroparesis develops. Near-total gastrectomy with Roux-en-Y anastomosis has been performed for such patients and good results have been reported, albeit in small series.[218]

Motility Issues in Dyspepsia

Prokinetic agents, such as metoclopramide, domperidone, and cisapride, have been widely used and studied among patients with functional dyspepsia. Their use has been based on the assumption that dysmotility is a factor in the pathogenesis of this disorder. Meta-analyses in 1989 and 1998 suggested that domperidone and cisapride have modest efficacy in dyspepsia, but attempts to relate this response to a correction of motor dysfunction have not produced convincing results.[219, 220] Indeed, it remains unresolved whether their use should be restricted to patients with dysmotility. Several other factors, such as a central antiemetic effect in the case of domperidone, correction of gastric dysrhythmias, or a modulation of gastric tone or visceral sensation, could explain their ability to resolve symptoms in some patients. At present, there is considerable interest in novel pharmacologic approaches to correct abnormalities in tone, sensation, and accommodation that may induce dyspeptic symptoms that formerly were considered a reflection of gastroparesis. Reports of efficacy in addressing these other motor abnormalities in functional dyspepsia are beginning to emerge (see Chapter 7). In initial studies, 5-HT_1 agonists,[221] nitrate donors, and clonidine[222] have been shown to relax the fundus.

REFERENCES

1. Szurszewski JH: Electrophysiological basis of gastrointestinal motility. In Johnson LR (ed): Physiology of the Gastrointestinal Tract, 2nd ed. New York, Raven Press, 1986, p 383.
2. Wilson P, Perdikis G, Redmond EJ, et al: Prolonged ambulatory antroduodenal manometry in humans. Am J Gastroenterol 89:1489, 1994.
3. Horowitz B, Ward SM, Sanders KM: Cellular and molecular basis for electrical rhythmicity in gastrointestinal muscles. Annu Rev Physiol 61:19, 1999.
4. Sanders KM: Postjunctional electrical mechanisms of enteric neurotransmission. Gut 47 (suppl IV):iv23, 2000.
5. Ward SM: Interstitial cells of Cajal in enteric neurotransmission. Gut 47 (suppl IV):iv40, 2000.
6. Vanderwinden J-M, Liu H, De Laet M-H, Vanderhaegen J-J: Study of the interstitial cells of Cajal in infantile hypertrophic pyloric stenosis. Gastroenterology 111:279, 1996.
7. Kellow JE, Borody TJ, Phillips SF, et al: Human interdigestive motility: Variations in patterns from esophagus to colon. Gastroenterology 91:386, 1986.
8. Tack J, Piessevaux H, Coulie B, et al: Role of impaired gastric accommodation to a meal in functional dyspepsia. Gastroenterology 115:1346, 1998.
9. Rogers RC, Hermann GE, Travagli RA: Brainstem pathways responsible for oesophageal control of gastric motility and tone in the rat. J Physiol (Lond) 514:369, 1999.
10. Tack J: Receptors of the enteric nervous system: Potential targets for drug therapy. Gut 47 (suppl IV):iv20, 2000.
11. Lu YX, Owyang C: Duodenal acid-induced gastric relaxation is mediated by multiple pathways. Am J Physiol 276:G1501, 1999.
12. Bozkurt A, Oktar BK, Kurtel H, et al: Capsaicin-sensitive vagal fibres and 5-HT3-, gastrin releasing peptide- and cholecystokinin A-receptors are involved in distension-induced inhibition of gastric emptying in the rat. Regul Pept 83:81, 1999.
13. Malagelada J-R, Azpiroz F: Determinants of gastric emptying and transit in the small intestine. In Schultz SG, Wood JD, Rauner BB (eds): The Gastrointestinal System: Motility and Circulation. Handbook of Physiology, sec 6, vol 1, part 2. Bethesda, Md, American Physiology Society, 1989, p 909.
14. Collins PJ, Houghton LA, Read NW, et al: Role of the proximal and distal stomach in mixed solid and liquid meal emptying. Gut 32:615, 1991.
15. Ploutz-Snyder L, Foley J, Ploutz-Snyder R, et al: Gastric gas and fluid emptying assessed by magnetic resonance imaging. Eur J Appl Physiol 78:212, 1999.
16. Moran TH, Wirth JB, Schwartz GJ, et al: Interactions between gastric volume and duodenal nutrients in the control of liquid gastric emptying. Am J Physiol 276:R997, 1999.
17. Hasler WL: The physiology of gastric motility and gastric emptying. In Yamada T (ed): Textbook of Gastroenterology, 2nd ed. Philadelphia, JB Lippincott, 1995, p 188.
18. Indireshkumar K, Brasseur JG, Fass H, et al: Relative contributions of "pressure pump" and "peristaltic pump" to gastric emptying. Am J Physiol 278:G604, 2000.
19. Powley T: Vagal input to the enteric nervous system. Gut 47 (suppl IV):iv30, 2000.
20. Grundy D, Schemann M: The interface between the enteric and central nervous system. In Tache Y, Wingate DL, Burks TF (eds): Innervation of the Gut, Pathophysiological Implications. Boca Raton, Fla, CRC Press, 1994, p 157.
21. Gue M: Neuromodulation of corticotrophin releasing factor–induced gastrointestinal motility alterations. In Tache Y, Wingate DL, Burks TF (eds): Innervation of the Gut, Pathophysiological Implications. Boca Raton, Fla, CRC Press, 1994, p 15.
22. Krowicki ZK, Arimura A, Nathan NA, et al: Hindbrain effects of PACAP on gastric motor function in the rat. Am J Physiol 272: G1221, 1997.
23. Imeryuz N, Yegen BC, Bozkurt A, et al: Glucagon-like peptide-1 inhibits gastric emptying via vagal afferent–mediated central mechanisms. Am J Physiol 272:G920, 1997.
24. Bozkurt A, Oktar BK, Kurtel H, et al: Capsaicin-sensitive vagal fibres and 5-HT3-, gastrin releasing peptide- and cholecystokinin A-receptors are involved in distension-induced inhibition of gastric emptying in the rat. Regul Pept 83:81, 1999.
25. Raybould HE, Meyer JH, Tabrizi Y, et al: Inhibition of gastric emptying in response to intestinal lipid is dependent on chylomicron formation. Am J Physiol 274:R1834, 1998.
26. McLaughlin JT, Luca MG, Jones MN, et al: Fatty acid chain length determines cholecystokinin secretion and effect on gastric motility. Gastroenterology 116:46, 1999.

27. Teff KL, Alavi A, Chen J, et al: Muscarinic blockade inhibits gastric emptying of mixed-nutrient meal: Effects of weight and gender. Am J Physiol 276:R707, 1999.
28. Bennink R, Peeters M, Van Den Maegdenbergh V, et al: Comparison of total and compartmental gastric emptying and antral motility between healthy men and women. Eur J Nucl Med 25:1293, 1998.
29. Tougas G, Eaker EY, Abell TL, et al: Assessment of gastric emptying using a low fat meal: Establishment of international control values. Am J Gastroenterol 95:1456, 2000.
30. Caballero-Plasencia AM, Valenzuela-Barranco M, Martin-Ruiz JL, et al: Are there changes in gastric emptying during the menstrual cycle? Scand J Gastroenterol 34:772, 1999.
31. Costa M, Brookes SJH, Hennig GW: Anatomy and physiology of the enteric nervous system. Gut 47 (suppl IV):iv15, 2000.
32. Holzer P: Spinal afferent nerves: Sensory, afferent, and effector functions. In Tache Y, Wingate DL, Burks TF (eds): Innervation of the Gut: Pathophysiological Implications. Boca Raton, Fla, CRC Press, 1994, p 123.
33. Gebhard GF: Visceral pain—peripheral sensitisation. Gut 47 (suppl IV):iv54, 2000.
34. Schuligoi R, Jocic M, Heinemann A, et al: Gastric acid–evoked cfos messenger RNA expression in the rat brainstem is signalled by capsaicin-resistant vagal afferents. Gastroenterology 115:649, 1998.
35. Yuan-Xu L, Owyang C: Duodenal acid–induced gastric relaxation is mediated by multiple pathways. Am J Physiol 276:G1501, 1999.
36. Jones KL, Doran SM, Hveem K, et al: Relation between postprandial satiation and antral area in normal subjects. Am J Clin Nutr 66:127, 1997.
37. Samson M, Roelofs JMM, Akkermans LMA, et al: Proximal gastric motor activity in response to a liquid meal in type 1 diabetes with autonomic neuropathy. Dig Dis Sci 43:491, 1998.
38. Ladabaum U, Koshy SS, Woods ML, et al: Differential symptomatic and electrogastrographic effects of distal and proximal human gastric distension. Am J Physiol 275:G418, 1998.
39. Distrutti F, Azpiroz F, Soldevilla A, et al: Gastric wall tension determines perception of gastric distension. Gastroenterology 116:1035, 1999.
40. Ladabaum U, Brown MB, Pan W, et al: Effects of nutrients and serotonin 5-HT_3 antagonism on symptoms evoked by distal gastric distension in humans. Am J Physiol 280:G201, 2001.
41. Lin HC, Kim BH, Elashoff JD, et al: Gastric emptying of solid food is most potently inhibited by carbohydrate in the canine distal ileum. Gastroenterology 102:793, 1992.
42. Meyer JH, Tabrizi Y, DiMaso N, et al: Length of intestinal contact on nutrient-driven satiety. Am J Physiol 275:R1308, 1998.
43. Cecil JE, Francis J, Read NW: Relative contributions of intestinal, gastric, oro-sensory influences and information to changes in appetite induced by the same liquid meal. Appetite 31:377, 1998.
44. Sternini C, Wong H, Pham T, et al: Expression of cholecystokinin A receptors in neurons innervating the cat stomach and intestine. Gastroenterology 117:1136, 1999.
45. Bado A, Levasseur S, Attoub S, et al: The stomach as a source of leptin. Nature 394:790, 1998.
46. Martinez V, Barrachina MD, Wang L, et al: Intracerebroventricular leptin inhibits gastric emptying of a solid nutrient meal in rats. Neuroreport 10:3217, 1999.
47. Yuan C-S, Attele AS, Wu JA, et al: Peripheral gastric leptin modulates brain stem neuronal activity in neonates. Am J Physiol 277: G626, 1999.
48. Asakawa A, Inui A, Ueno N, et al: Urocortin reduces food intake and gastric emptying in lean and ob/ob obese mice. Gastroenterology 116: 1287, 1999.
49. Taylor IL: Of mice and men—the control of food intake and body weight. Gastroenterology 116:1487, 1999.
50. Chiloiro M, Caroli M, Guerra V, et al: Gastric emptying in normal weight and obese children—an ultrasound study. Int J Obes Relat Metab Disord 23:1303, 1999.
51. Sase M, Tamura H, Ueda K, et al: Sonographic evaluation of antepartum development of fetal gastric motility. Ultrasound Obstet Gynecol 13:323, 1999.
52. Cucchiara S, Salvia G, Scarcella A, et al: Gestational maturation of electrical activity of the stomach. Dig Dis Sci 44:2008, 1999.
53. Chen JDZ, Co E, Liang J, et al: Patterns of gastric myoelectrical activity in human subjects of different ages. Am J Physiol 272:G1022, 1997.
54. Patterson M, Rintala R, Lloyd DA: A longitudinal study of electrogastrography in normal neonates. J Pediatr Surg 35:59, 2000.
55. Young HM, Hearn CJ, Newgreen DF: Embryology and development of the enteric nervous system. Gut 47 (suppl IV):iv12, 2000.
56. Camilleri M, Hasler WL, Parkman HP, et al: Measurement of gastrointestinal motility in the GI laboratory. Gastroenterology 115:747, 1998.
57. Kellow JE, Delvaux M, Azpiroz F, et al: Principles of applied neurogastroenterology: Physiology—motility—sensation. Gut 45 (suppl 1): 17, 1999.
58. Stotzer PO, Fjalling M, Gretarsdottir J, et al: Assessment of gastric emptying: Comparison of solid scintigraphic emptying and emptying of radiopaque markers in patients and healthy subjects. Dig Dis Sci 44:729, 1999.
59. Poitras P, Picard M, Dery R, et al: Evaluation of gastric emptying in clinical practice. Dig Dis Sci 42:2183, 1997.
60. Spiller RC: Chemical detection of transit. In Kumar D, Wingate D (eds): An Illustrated Guide to Gastrointestinal Motiltity, 2nd ed. Edinburgh, Churchill Livingstone, 1993, p 308.
61. Maes BD, Ghoos YF, Rutgeerts PJ, et al: *C octanoic acid breath test to measure gastric emptying rate of solids. Dig Dis Sci 39 (suppl): 1045, 1994.
62. Mossi S, Meyer-Wyss B, Beglinger C, et al: Gastric emptying of liquid meals measured non-invasively in humans with ^{13}C acetate breath test. Dig Dis Sci 39 (suppl):1075, 1994.
63. Choi M-G, Camilleri M, Burton DD, et al: Octanoic acid breath test for gastric emptying of solids: Accuracy, reproducibility, and comparison with scintigraphy. Gastroenterology 112:1155, 1997.
64. Choi M-G, Camilleri M, Burton DD, et al: Reproducibility and simplification of the 1 octanoic acid breath test for gastric emptying of solids. Am J Gastroenterol 93:92, 1998.
65. Hausken T, Odegaard S, Berstad A: Antroduodenal motility studied by real-time ultrasound. Gastroenterology 100:59, 1991.
66. Bolondi L, Bortolotti M, Santi V, et al: Measurement of gastric emptying time by real time ultrasound. Gastroenterology 89:752, 1985.
67. Benini L, Sembenini C, Heading RC, et al: Simultaneous measurement of gastric emptying of a solid meal by ultrasound and by scintigraphy. Am J Gastroenterol 94:2861, 1999.
68. Darwiche G, Almer LO, Bjorgell O, et al: Measurement of gastric emptying by standardized real-time ultrasonography in healthy subjects and diabetic patients. J Ultrasound Med 18:673, 1999.
69. Gilja OH, Detmer PR, Jong JM, et al: Intragastric distribution and gastric emptying assessed by three-dimensional ultrasonography. Gastroenterology 113:38, 1997.
70. Evans DF, Lamont G, Stehling MK: Prolonged monitoring of the upper gastrointestinal tract using echo planar magnetic resonance imaging. Gut 34:848, 1993.
71. Schwizer W, Meecke H, Fried M: Measurement of gastric emptying by magnetic resonance imaging in humans. Gastroenterology 103:369, 1992.
72. Sica GT: MR imaging for assessment of gastric motility: Has its time come? Radiology 207:9, 1998.
73. Younes Z, Regan F, Schuster MM: Functional MRI for the assessment of gastric motility—a better test? Am J Gastroenterol 94:851, 1999.
74. Knuz P, Crelier GR, Schwizer W, et al: Gastric emptying and motility assessment with MR imaging—preliminary observations. Radiology 207:33, 1998.
75. Avill R, Mangnall YF, Bird NC, et al: Applied potential tomography: A new noninvasive technique for measuring gastric emptying. Gastroenterology 92:1019, 1987.
76. Mangnall YF, Kerrigan DD, Johnson AG, et al: Applied potential tomography: Noninvasive method for measuring gastric empyting of a solid test meal. Dig Dis Sci 36:1680, 1991.
77. Smout AJPM, Van Der Schee EJ, Grashuis JL: What is measured in electrogastrography? Dig Dis Sci 25:179, 1980.
78. Parkman HP, Harris AD, Krevsky B, et al: Gastroduodenal motility and dysmotility: An update on techniques available for evaluation. Am J Gastroenterol 90:869, 1995.
79. Chen JDZ, McCallum RW: Clinical applications of electrogastrography. Am J Gastroenterol 88:1324, 1993.
80. Verhagen MA, Van Schelvan LJ, et al: Pitfalls in the analysis of electrogastrographic recordings. Gastroenterology 117:453, 1999.
81. Mintchev MP, Kingma YJ, Bowes KL: Accuracy of cutaneous recordings of gastric electrical activity. Gastroenterology 104:1273, 1993.
82. Levanon D, Zhang M, Orr WC, et al: Effects of meal volume and

composition on gastric myoelectrical activity. Am J Physiol 274:G430, 1998.
83. Levanon D, Zhang M, Chen JD: Efficiency and efficacy of the electrogastrogram. Dig Dis Sci 43:1023, 1998.
84. Chen JDZ, Lin Z, Pan J, McCallum RW: Abnormal gastric myoelectrical activity and delayed gastric emptying in patients with symptoms suggestive of gastroparesis. Dig Dis Sci 41:1538, 1996.
85. Di Lorenzo C, Reddy SN, Flores AF, et al: Is electrogastrography a substitute for manometric studies in children with functional gastrointestinal disorders? Dig Dis Sci 42:2310, 1997.
86. Azpiroz F, Malagelada J-R: Perception and reflex relaxation of the stomach in response to gut distension. Gastroenterology 98:1193, 1990.
87. Kuiken SD, Samsom M, Camilleri M, et al: Development of a test to measure gastric accommodation in humans. Am J Physiol 277:G1217, 1999.
88. Quigley EMM: Intestinal manometry—technical advances: Clinical limitations. Dig Dis Sci 37:10, 1992.
89. Holland R, Gallagher MD, Quigley EMM: An evaluation of an ambulatory manometry system in the assessment of antroduodenal motor activity. Dig Dis Sci 41:1531, 1996.
90. Samsom M, Smout AJPM, Hebbard G, et al: A novel portable perfused manometric system for recording of small intestinal motility. Neurogastroenterol Motil 10:139, 1998.
91. Wright J, Evans D, Gowland P, Mansfield P: Validation of antroduodenal motility measurements made by echo-planar magnetic resonance imaging. Neurogastroenterol Motil 11:19, 1999.
92. Thumshirn M, Bruninga K, Camilleri M: Simplifying the evaluation of postprandial antral motor function in patients with suspected gastroparesis. Am J Gastroenterol 92:1496, 1997.
93. Quigley EMM, Deprez PH, Hellstrom P, et al: Ambulatory intestinal manometry: A consensus report on its clinical role. Dig Dis Sci 42: 1618, 1997.
94. Quigley EMM: Enteric neuropathology—recent advances and implications for clinical practice. Gastroenterologist 5:233, 1997.
95. Familoni BO, Abell TL, Voeller G: Measurement of gastric and small bowel electrical activity at laparoscopy. J Laparoendosc Surg 4:325, 1994.
96. Minami H, McCallum RW: The physiology and pathophysiology of gastric empyting in humans. Gastroenterology 86:1592, 1989.
97. Hoogerwerf WA, Pasricha PJ, Kalloo AN, et al: Pain: The overlooked symptom in gastroparesis. Am J Gastroenterol 94:1029, 1999.
98. Tio TL, Sie LH, Tytgat GNJ: Reduced postprandial blood glucose levels in recently diagnosed non–insulin dependent diabetics secondary to pharmacologically induced delayed gastric emptying. Dig Dis Sci 38:51, 1993.
99. Fich A, Neri M, Camilleri M, et al: Stasis syndromes following gastric surgery: Clinical and motility features of sixty symptomatic patients. J Clin Gastroenteral 12:505, 1990.
100. Chang TM, Chen TH, Tsou SS, et al: Differences in gastric emptying between highly selective vagotomy and posterior truncal vagotomy combined with anterior seromyotomy. J Gastrointest Surg 3:533, 1999.
101. Forstner-Barthell AW, Murr MM, Nitecki S, et al: Near-total completion gastrectomy for severe postvagotomy gastric stasis: Analysis of early and long-term results in 62 patients. J Gastrointest Surg 3:15, 1999.
102. Akkermans LMA, Hendrikse CA: Post-gastrectomy problems. Dig Liver Dis 32 (suppl 3):S263, 2000.
103. Mathias JR, Fernandez A, Sninsky CA, et al: Nausea, vomiting and abdominal pain after Roux-en-Y anastomosis: Motility of the jejunal limb. Gastroenterology 88:101, 1985.
104. Hinder RA, Esser MB, DeMeester TR: Management of gastric emptying disorders following the Roux-en-Y procedure. Surgery 104:765, 1988.
105. Vantrappen G, Coremans G, Janssens J, et al: Inversion of the slow wave frequency gradient in symptomatic patients with Roux-en-Y anastomosis. Gastroenterology 101:1282, 1991.
106. Miedema BW, Kelly KA, Camilleri M, et al: Human gastric and jejunal transit and motility after Roux gastrojejunostomy. Gastroenterology 103:1133, 1992.
107. Sun WM, Doran SM, Jones KL, et al: Long-term effects of pyloromyotomy on pyloric motility and gastric emptying in humans. Am J Gastroenterol 95:92, 2000.
108. Fabre JM, Burgel JS, Navarro F, et al: Delayed gastric emptying after pancreaticoduodenectomy and pancreaticogastrostomy. Eur J Surg 165: 560, 1999.
109. Horstmann O, Becker H, Post S, et al: Is delayed gastric emptying following pancreaticoduodenectomy related to pylorus preservation? Langenbecks Arch Surg 384:354, 1999.
110. Vu MK, Straathof JW, van der Schaar PJ, et al: Motor and sensory function of the proximal stomach in reflux disease and after laparoscopic Nissen fundoplication. Am J Gastroenterol 94:1481, 1999.
111. Kong MF, Horowitz M, Jones KL, et al: Natural history of diabetic gastroparesis. Diabetes Care 22:503, 1999.
112. Feldman M, Schiller LR: Disorders of gastrointestinal motility associated with diabetes mellitus. Ann Intern Med 98:378, 1983.
113. Loo FD, Palmer DW: Gastric emptying in patients with diabetes mellitus. Gastroenterology 86:485, 1984.
114. Keshavarzian A, Iber FL, Vaeth J: Gastric emptying in patients with insulin-requiring diabetes mellitus. Am J Gastroenterol 82:29, 1987.
115. Horowitz M, Harding PE, Maddox AF, et al: Gastric and oesophageal emptying in insulin-dependent diabetes mellitus. J Gastroenterol Hepatol 1:97, 1991.
116. Annese V, Bassotti G, Caruso N, et al: Gastrointestinal motor dysfunction, symptoms, and neuropathy in non-insulin-dependent (type 2) diabetes mellitus. J Clin Gastroenterol 29:171, 1999.
117. Iber FL, Parveen S, Van Drunen M, et al: Relation of symptoms to impaired stomach, small bowel and colon motility in long-standing diabetes. Dig Dis Sci 38:45, 1993.
118. Samson M, Smout AJPM: Abnormal gastric and small intestinal motor function in diabetes mellitus. Dig Dis 15:263, 1995.
119. Phillips WT, Schwartz JG, McMahon CA: Rapid gastric emptying of an oral glucose solution in type 2 diabetic patients. J Nucl Med 33: 1490, 1992.
120. Weytjens C, Keymeulen B, Van Haleweyn C, et al: Rapid gastric empyting of a liquid meal in long-term type 2 diabetes mellitus. Diabet Med 15:1022, 1998.
121. Troncon LEA, Rosa-Silva L, Oliveira RB, et al: Abnormal intragastric distribution of a liquid nutrient meal in patients with diabetes mellitus. Dig Dis Sci 43:1421, 1998.
122. Soykan I, Lin Z, Sarosiek I, McCallum RW: Gastric myoelectrical activity, gastric emptying, and correlations with symptoms and fasting blood glucose levels in diabetic patients. Am J Med Sci 317:226, 1999.
123. Mearin F, Camilleri M, Malagelada J-R: Pyloric dysfunction in diabetics with recurrent nausea and vomiting. Gastroenterology 90:1919, 1986.
124. Fraser R, Horowitz M, Maddox A, et al: Organization of antral, pyloric and duodenal motility in patients with gastroparesis. J Gastrointest Motil 5:167, 1993.
125. Kristensson K, Nordborg C, Olsson Y, Sourander P: Changes in the vagus nerve in diabetes mellitus. Acta Pathol Microbiol Scand 79:684, 1971.
126. Smith B: Neuropathology of the oesophagus in diabetes mellitus. J Neurol Neurosurg Psychiatry 37:1151, 1974.
127. Rathmann W, Enck P, Frieling T, et al: Visceral afferent neuropathy in diabetic gastroparesis. Diabetes Care 14:108, 1991.
128. Kong MF, Horowitz M: Gastric emptying in diabetes mellitus: Relationship to blood-glucose control. Clin Geriatr Med 15:321, 1999.
129. Fraser R, Horowitz M, Maddox AF, et al: Hyperglycemia slows gastric emptying in type 1 (insulin dependent) diabetes mellitus. Diabetologia 33:675, 1990.
130. Aylett P: Gastric emptying and change of blood glucose level as affected by glucagon and insulin. Clin Sci 22:171, 1962.
131. MacGregor IL, Guellar R, Watts HD, et al: The effect of acute hyperglycemia on gastric emptying in man. Gastroenterology 78:286, 1976.
132. Schvarcz E, Plamar M, Aman J, et al: Physiological hyperglycemia slows gastric emptying in normal subjects and patients with insulin-dependent diabetes mellitus. Gastroenterology 113:60, 1997.
133. Barnett JL, Owyang C: Serum glucose concentration as a modulator of interdigestive gastric motility. Gastroenterology 94:739, 1988.
134. Fraser R, Horowitz M, Dent J: Hyperglycemia stimulates pyloric motility in normal subjects. Gut 32:475, 1991.
135. Jebbink RJA, Samsom M, Bruijs PPM, et al: Hyperglycemia induces abnormalities of gastric myoelectrical activity in patients with type 1 diabetes mellitus. Gastroenterology 107:1390, 1994.
136. Andrews JM, Rayner CK, Doran S, et al: Physiological changes in blood glucose affect appetite and pyloric motility during intraduodenal lipid infusion. Am J Physiol 275:G797, 1998.
137. Lingenfelser T, Sun W-M, Hebbard GS, et al: Effects of duodenal

distension on antropyloroduodenal pressures and perception are modified by hyperglycemia. Am J Physiol 276:G711, 1999.

138. Takahashi T, Nakamura K, Itoh H, et al: Impaired expression of nitric oxide synthase in the gastric myenteric plexus of spontaneously diabetic rats. Gastroenterology 113:1535, 1997.
139. Quigley EMM: The pathophysiology of diabetic gastroenteropathy: More vague than vagal. Gastroenterology 113:1790, 1997.
140. Holzapfel A, Festa A, Stacher-Janotta G, et al: Gastric emptying in type II (non-insulin-dependent) diabetes mellitus before and after therapy readjustment: No influence of actual blood glucose concentration. Diabetologia 42:1410, 1999.
141. Malagelada J-R, Stanghellini V: Manometric evaluation of functional upper gut symptoms. Gastroenterology 88:1223, 1985.
142. Labo G, Bortolotti M, Vezzadini P, et al: Interdigestive gastroduodenal motility and serum motilin levels in patients with idiopathic delay in gastric emptying. Gastroenterology 90:20, 1986.
143. Kerlin P: Post-prandial antral hypomotility in patients with idiopathic nausea and vomiting. Gut 30:54, 1989.
144. Scott AM, Kellow JE, Shuter B, et al: Intragastric distribution and gastric emptying of solids and liquids in functional dyspepsia: Lack of influence of symptom subgroups and *Helicobacter pylori* infection. Dig Dis Sci 38:2247, 1993.
145. Waldron B, Cullen PT, Kumar R, et al: Evidence for hypomotility in non-ulcer dyspepsia: A prospective multifactorial study. Gut 32:246, 1991.
146. Soykan I, Sivri B, Sarosiek I, et al: Demography, clinical characteristics, psychological and abuse profiles, treatment and long-term follow-up of patients with gastroparesis. Dig Dis Sci 43:2398, 1998.
147. Silvers D, Kipnes M, Broadstone V: The DOM-USA-5 study group: Domperidone in the management of symptoms of diabetic gastroparesis: Efficacy, safety and quality-of-life outcomes in a multicenter controlled trial. Clin Ther 20:438, 1998.
148. Quartero AO, De Wit NJ, Lodder AC, et al: Disturbed solid-phase gastric emptying in functional dyspepsia. Dig Dis Sci 43:2028, 1998.
149. Maes BD, Ghoos YF, Hiele MI, et al: Gastric emptying rate of solids in patients with nonulcer dyspepsia. Dig Dis Sci 42:1158, 1997.
150. Stanghellini V, Tosetti C, Paternico A, et al: Predominant symptoms identify different subgroups in functional dyspepsia. Am J Gastroenterol 94:2080, 1999.
151. Quigley EMM: Symptoms and gastric function in dyspepsia—goodbye to gastroparesis? Neurogastroenterol Motil 8:273, 1996.
152. Troncon LEA, Bennett RJM, Ahluwahlia NK, et al: Abnormal distribution of food during gastric emptying in functional dyspepsia patients. Gut 35:327, 1994.
153. Mearin F, Cucala M, Azpiroz F, et al: The origin of symptoms on the brain-gut axis in functional dyspepsia. Gastroenterology 101:996, 1991.
154. Coffin B, Azpiroz F, Guarner F, et al: Selective gastric hypersensitivity and reflex hyporeactivity in functional dyspepsia. Gastroenterology 107:1345, 1994.
155. Lemann M, Dederding JP, Flourie B, et al: Abnormal perception of visceral pain in response to gastric distention in chronic idiopathic dyspepsia: The irritable stomach. Dig Dis Sci 36:1249, 1991.
156. Marzio L, Falucci M, Grossi L, et al: Proximal and distal gastric distension in normal subjects and *H. pylori*–positive and -negative dyspeptic patients and correlation with symptoms. Dig Dis Sci 43: 2757, 1998.
157. Thumshirn M, Camilleri M, Saslow SB, et al: Gastric accommodation in non-ulcer dyspepsia and the roles of *Helicobacter pylori* infection and vagal function. Gut 44:55, 1999.
158. Quigley EMM, Hasler WL, Parkman HP: AGA technical review on nausea and vomiting. Gastroenterology 120:263, 2001.
159. Chong SK: Electrogastrography in cyclic vomiting syndrome. Dig Dis Sci 44(suppl):64S, 1999.
160. Kamar N, Chami T, Andersen A, et al: Delayed gastrointestinal transit times in anorexia nervosa and bulimia nervosa. Gastroenterology 101: 1320, 1991.
161. Abell TL, Malagelada J-R, Lucas AR, et al: Gastric electromechanical and neurohormonal function in anorexia nervosa. Gastroenterology 93: 958, 1987.
162. Amarnath RP, Abell TL, Malagelada J-R: The rumination syndrome in adults. Ann Intern Med 105:513, 1986.
163. O'Brien MD, Bruce BK, Camilleri M: The rumination syndrome: Clinical features rather than manometric diagnosis. Gastroenterology 108:1024, 1995.
164. Thumshirn M, Camilleri M, Hanson RB, et al: Gastric mechanosensory and lower esophageal sphincter function in the rumination syndrome. Am J Physiol 275:G314, 1998.
165. Lu CC, Schultze-Delrieu K: Pyloric deformation from peptic disease: Radiographic evidence for incompetence rather than obstruction. Dig Dis Sci 35:1459, 1990.
166. Samsom M, Verhagen MAMT, vanBerge Henegouwen GP, et al: Abnormal clearance of exogenous acid and increased acid sensitivity of the proximal duodenum in dyspeptic patients. Gastroenterology 116:515, 1999.
167. Kerrigan DD, Read NW, Houghton LA, et al: Disturbed gastroduodenal motility in patients with active and healed duodenal ulceration. Gastroenterology 100:892, 1991.
168. DuBois A, Van Eerdewegh P, Gardner JD: Gastric emptying and secretion in Zollinger-Ellison syndrome. J Clin Invest 59:255, 1977.
169. Williams NS, Elashoff J, Meyer JH: Gastric emptying of liquids in normal subjects and patients with healed duodenal ulcer disease. Dig Dis Sci 31:943, 1986.
170. Testoni PA, Bagnoli F, Masci E, et al: Different interdigestive antroduodenal motility patterns in chronic antral gastritis with and without *Helicobacter pylori* infection. Dig Dis Sci 38:2255, 1993.
171. Lin Z, Chen JDZ, Parolisi S, et al: Prevalence of gastric myoelectrical abnormalities in patients with nonulcer dyspepsia and *H. pylori* infection. Dig Dis Sci 46(4):739, 2001.
172. Quigley EMM: Gastroesophageal reflux disease: The roles of motility in pathophysiology and therapy. Am J Gastroenterol 88:1649, 1993.
173. Zerbib F, des Varannes SB, Ropert A, et al: Proximal gastric tone in gastro-oesophageal reflux disease. Eur J Gasteroenterol Hepatol 11: 511, 1999.
174. Penagini R, Hebbard G, Horowitz M, et al: Motor functions of the proximal stomach and visceral perception in gastroesophageal reflux disease. Gut 42:251, 1998.
175. Bityutskiy LP, Soykan I, McCallum RW: Viral gastroparesis: A subgroup of idiopathic gastroparesis—clinical observations and long-term outcomes. Am J Gastroenterol 92:1501, 1997.
176. Oh JJ, Kim CH: Gastroparesis after a presumed viral illness: Clinical and laboratory features and natural history. Mayo Clin Proc 65:636, 1990.
177. MacGilchrist AJ, Quigley EMM: Transplantation. In: Shearman D, Finlayson NDC, Carter D, Camilleri M (eds): Diseases of the GI Tract and Liver, 2nd ed. London, Churchill Livingstone, 1995, p 1151.
178. Bortolotti M, Mattioli S, Alampi G, et al: Brainstem viral-like encephalitis as a possible cause of a gastroduodenal motility disorder: A case report. J Gastrointest Motil 1:99, 1989.
179. Vassalo M, Camilleri M, Caron BL, et al: Gastrointestinal motor dysfunction in acquired selective cholinergic dysautonomia associated with infectious mononucleosis. Gastroenterology 100:252, 1991.
180. Kao CH, Ho YJ, Changlai SP, et al: Gastric emptying in spinal cord injury patients. Dig Dis Sci 44:1512, 1999.
181. Kao CH, ChangLai S-P, Chieng P-U, et al: Gastric emptying in male neurologic trauma. J Nucl Med 39:1798, 1998.
182. Kao CH, ChangLai S-P, Chieng P-U, Yen T-C: Gastric emptying in head-injured patients. Am J Gastroenterol 93:1108, 1998.
183. Toepfer M, Folwaczny C, Lochmuller H, et al: Non-invasive ^{13}C-octanoic acid breath test shows delayed gastric emptying in patients with amyotrophic lateral sclerosis. Digestion 60:567, 1999.
184. Soykan I, Lin Z, McCallum RW: Gastric myoelectrical activity in patients with Parkinson's disease: Evidence of a primary gastric abnormality. Dig Dis Sci 44:927, 1999.
185. Galati JS, Holdeman KP, Dalrymple GV, et al: Delayed gastric emptying of both the liquid and solid components of a meal in chronic liver disease. Am J Gastroenterol 89:708, 1994.
186. Ko CW, Chang CS, Lien HC, et al: Gastric dysrhythmia in uremic patients on maintenance hemodialysis. Scand J Gastroenterol 33:1047, 1998.
187. DiBaise JK, Quigley EMM: Tumor-related dysmotility: Gastrointestinal dysmotility syndromes associated with tumors. Dig Dis Sci 43: 1369, 1998.
188. Brand RE, DiBaise JK, Quigley EMM, et al: Gastroparesis as a cause of nausea and vomiting after high-dose chemotherapy and hemopoietic stem-cell transplantation. Lancet 352:1985, 1998.
189. Malagelada J-R, Rees WDW, Mazzotta LJ: Gastric motor abnormalities in diabetic and post-vagotomy gastroparesis: Effect of metoclopramide and bethanechol. Gastroenterology 78:286, 1980.
190. Barone JA: Domperidone: A peripherally acting dopamine 2-receptor antagonist. Ann Pharmacol 33:429, 1999.

191. Champion MC, Hartnett M, Yen M: Domperidone, a new dopamine antagonist. Can Med Assoc J 135:457, 1986.
192. Pinder RN, Brogden RN, Sawyer PR, et al: Metoclopramide: A review of its pharmacological properties and clinical use. Drugs 12:81, 1976.
193. Albibi R, McCallum RW: Metoclopramide: Pharmacology and clinical application. Ann Intern Med 98:86, 1983.
194. Ganzini L, Casey DE, Haffman WF, et al: The prevalence of metoclopramide-induced tardive dyskinesia and acute extrapyramidal movements. Arch Intern Med 153:1469, 1993.
195. Horowitz M, Harding PE, Chatterton BE, et al: Acute and chronic effects of domperidone on gastric emptying in diabetic autonomic neuropathy. Dig Dis Sci 30:1, 1985.
196. Melga P, Mansi C, Ciuchi E, et al: Chronic administration of levosulpiride and glycemic control in IDDM patients with gastroparesis. Diabetes Care 20:55, 1997.
197. Corazza GR, Biagi F, Albano O, et al: Levosulpiride in functional dyspepsia: A multicentric, double-blind, controlled trial. Ital J Gastroenterol 28:317, 1996.
198. Abell TL, Camilleri M, DiMagno EP, et al: Long-term efficacy of oral cisapride in symptomatic upper gut dysmotility. Dig Dis Sci 36:621, 1991.
199. Wehrmann T, Lembecke B, Caspary WF: Influence of cisapride on antroduodenal motor function in healthy subjects and diabetics with autonomic neuropathy. Aliment Pharmacol Ther 5:599, 1991.
200. Camilleri M, Malagelada J-R, Abell TL, et al: Effect of six weeks of treatment with cisapride in gastroparesis and intestinal pseudo-obstruction. Gastroenterology 96:705, 1989.
201. McHugh S, Lico S, Diamant NE: Cisapride versus metoclopramide: An acute study in diabetic gastroparesis. Dig Dis Sci 37:997, 1992.
202. Richards RD, Valenzuela JA, Davenport KS, et al: Objective and subjective results of a randomized, double-blind, placebo-controlled trial using cisapride to treat gastroparesis. Dig Dis Sci 38:811, 1993.
203. Bedford TA, Rowbotham DJ: Cisapride: Drug interactions of clinical significance. Drug Saf 15:167, 1996.
204. Nightingale SL: New warnings added to cisapride labeling. JAMA 280:410, 1998.
205. Vitola J, Vukanovic J, Roden DM: Cisapride-induced torsades de pointes. J Cardiovasc Electrophysiol 9:1109, 1998.
206. Bouras EP, Camilleri M, Burton DD, et al: Selective stimulation of colonic transit by the benzofuran 5-HT4 agonist, prucalopride, in healthy humans. Gut 44:682, 1999.
207. Kahrilas PJ, Quigley EMM, Castell DO, et al: The effects of tegaserod (HFT 919) on oesophageal acid exposure in gastro-oesophageal reflux disease. Aliment Pharmacol Ther 14:1503, 2000.
208. Camilleri M: The current role of erythromycin in the clinical management of gastric emptying disorders. Am J Gastroenterol 88:169, 1993.
209. Richards RD, Davenport K, McCallum RW: The treatment of idiopathic and diabetic gastroparesis with acute intravenous and chronic oral erythromycin. Am J Gastroenterol 88:203, 1993.
210. Jones KL, Berry M, Kong MF, et al: Hyperglycemia attenuates the gastrokinetic effect of erythromycin and affects the perception of postprandial hunger in normal subjects. Diabetes Care 22:339, 1999.
211. Petrakis IE, Vrachassotakis N, Sciacca V, et al: Hyperglycemia attenuates erythromycin-induced acceleration of solid-phase gastric emptying in idiopathic and diabetic gastroparesis. Scand J Gastroenterol 34:396, 1999.
212. Brand RM, Lof J, Quigley EMM: Transdermal delivery of erythromcyin lactobionate—implications for the therapy of gastroparesis. Aliment Pharmacol Ther 11:589, 1997.
213. DiBiase JK, Quigley EMM: Efficacy of long-term intravenous erythromycin in the treatment of severe gastroparesis: One center's experience. J Clin Gastroenterol 28:131, 1999.
214. Tanaka T, Mizumoto A, Mochiki E, et al: Effects of EM 574 and cisapride on gastric contractile and emptying activity in normal and drug-induced gastroparesis in dogs. J Pharmacol Exp Ther 287:712, 1998.
215. McCallum RW, Chen JDZ, Lin Z, et al: Gastric pacing improves emptying and symptoms in patients with gastroparesis. Gastroenterology 114:456, 1998.
216. Tougas G, Huizinga JD: Gastric pacing as a treatment for intractable gastroparesis—shocking news? Gastroenterology 114:598, 1998.
217. FamiloniBO, Abell TL, Voeller G, et al: Electrical stimulation at a frequency higher than basal rate in human stomach. Dig Dis Sci 42: 885, 1997.
218. Ejskjaer NT, Bradley JL, Buxton-Thomas MS, et al: Novel surgical treatment and gastric pathology in diabetic gastroparesis. Diabet Med 16:488, 1999.
219. Dobrilla G, Comberlato N, Steela A, Vallaperta P: Drug treatment of functional dyspepsia: Meta-analysis of randomised controlled clinical trials. J Clin Gastroenterol 11:169, 1989.
220. Finney JS, Kinnersley N, Hughes M, et al: Meta-analysis of antisecretory and gastrokinetic compounds in functional dyspepsia. Clin Gastroenterol 26:312, 1998.
221. Tack J, Coulie B, Wilmer A, et al: Influence of sumatriptan on gastric fundus tone and on the perception of gastric distension in man. Gut 46:468, 2000.
222. Thumshirn M, Camilleri M, Choi MG, et al: Modulation of gastric sensory and motor functions by nitrergic and α-2-adrenergic agents in humans. Gastroenterology 116:573, 1999.

Chapter 38

GASTRIC SECRETION

Mark Feldman

PHYSIOLOGY

The stomach secretes water, electrolytes (H^+, K^+, Na^+, Cl^-, HCO_3^-), enzymes with activity at acid pH (pepsins, lipase), and glycoproteins (intrinsic factor, mucins). Gastric juice also contains small amounts of calcium and magnesium, as well as zinc and iron in trace amounts.[1] The physiologic functions of these various secretions are summarized in Table 38–1.

Much of our knowledge regarding gastric secretion derives from in vivo studies in animals (dogs, rabbits, rats, mice, cats) or in vitro experiments using cells or glands derived from these animals.[2] Because of considerable species-to-species differences, extrapolations of such results to humans should be made cautiously. This chapter focuses on gastric secretion in humans whenever possible. Several types of cells participate in gastric secretion or regulate the output of the secretory cells, as discussed in the following sections.

Exocrine Epithelial Cells (Table 38–2)

Gastric exocrine cells originate from stem cells located in the mid-region (neck) of gastric glands. Upward flow of neck cells toward the surface is a rapid process (<1 week), whereas downward flow of neck cells into gastric glands may require several weeks, as undifferentiated cells mature into more specialized cells such as *parietal cells* and *chief cells* (see Chapter 36). Columnar cells lining the gastric surface and its pits (*surface cells*) secrete Na^+ in exchange for H^+, HCO_3^-, mucins, and phospholipids, all of which help protect the gastric mucosa from damage by luminal acid-pepsin and ingested toxins. Mucus cells in more deeply situated gastric glands secrete mucins and group II pepsinogens (PGII). Furthermore, oxyntic glands that occupy most of the stomach also contain parietal cells, which secrete hydrochloric acid (HCl) and intrinsic factor (IF), and chief cells, which secrete PGI. Recently, chief cells have been reported to contain IF (see later) and also leptin, a hormone normally found in adipocytes.[3] Leptin receptors are also present on gastric surface cells,[3] but the role of leptin in gastric secretion, if any, is not yet known.

Endocrine, Endocrine-Like, and Neural Regulatory Cells

Gastric glands contain numerous types of endocrine and endocrine-like cells, many of which are intimately involved in the regulation of gastric exocrine secretion. The relative distribution of endocrine and endocrine-like cells in human oxyntic and pyloric glands is shown in Figure 38–1.[4]

Somatostatin-secreting *D cells* and serotonin-secreting enterochromaffin *(EC)* cells are present in all types of gastric glands, although the role of the latter in gastric secretion is not established. Histamine-secreting enterochromaffin-like cells *(ECL cells)* are restricted to oxyntic glands, in close relation to parietal cells (see Chapter 36). Like ECL cells, mast cells in the lamina propria of the gastric mucosa contain histamine, and they actually outnumber ECL cells in the human stomach. However, their physiologic role in stimulating gastric acid secretion is uncertain. Gastrin cells (*G cells*) are found only in pyloric glands, in close relation to D cells. G cells release gastrin directly into the circulation (*endocrine secretion*), whereas D cells and ECL cells secrete their products primarily into the extracellular fluid to exert their effects on neighboring exocrine or endocrine cells (*paracrine secretion*). Gastric neurons that release acetylcholine and neuropeptides also play a major role in gastric secretion (*neurocrine secretion*). Neuropeptides that may affect gastric secretion include gastrin-releasing peptide (GRP)—the mammalian analog of the amphibian peptide bombesin, calcitonin gene–related peptide (CGRP), and pituitary adenylate cyclase–activating polypeptide (PACAP), as discussed later.

Two approaches have been used to establish whether an endocrine, paracrine, or neurocrine product plays a physio-

Table 38–1 | **Physiologic Functions of Gastric Exocrine Secretions**

PRODUCT	FUNCTION
Hydrochloric acid	Provides optimal pH for pepsin and gastric lipase (see below) Facilitates duodenal inorganic iron absorption Negative feedback of gastrin release Stimulation of pancreatic HCO_3^- secretion Suppression of ingested microorganisms
Pepsins	Early hydrolysis of dietary proteins Liberation of vitamin B_{12} from dietary protein
Gastric lipase	Early hydrolysis of dietary triglyceride
Intrinsic factor	Binding of vitamin B_{12} for subsequent ileal absorption
Mucin/HCO_3^-	Protection against noxious agents

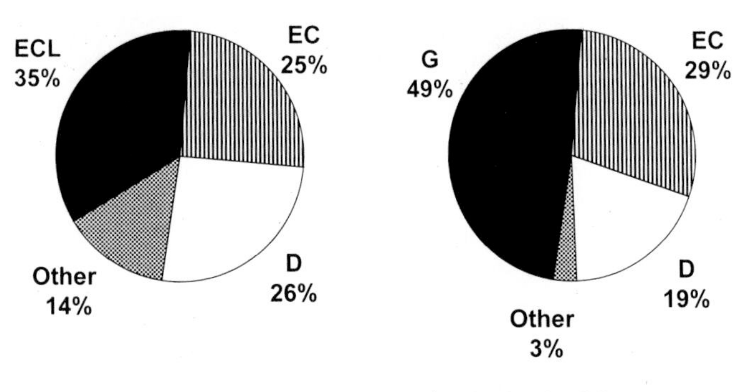

Figure 38–1. Distribution of human gastric endocrine cells in glands from the oxyntic mucosa (left) and pyloric mucosa (right). ECL, enterochromaffin-like (histamine); EC, enterochromaffin (serotonin); D (somatostatin); G (gastrin).

logic role in regulating gastric secretion. In the first approach, gastric secretion is measured after the substance in question is infused into the circulation to achieve a "physiologic" concentration (e.g., the concentration achieved after a meal). This method is applicable to endocrine mediators but not to paracrine or neurocrine substances. In the second approach, a specific or highly selective antagonist or antibody to the substance in question is administered, or the gene coding for the protein product is knocked out or disrupted. This second approach has been used in humans in a limited way, because few specific and safe antagonists are available and because infusion of antibodies and gene knockout experiments are not applicable. Recently, studies with a new antagonist to GRP-preferring bombesin receptors[5] and with new antagonists to cholecystokinin A (CCK_A) and to CCK_B/gastrin receptors[6] have improved our understanding of the physiologic role of GRP, CCK, and gastrin in gastric secretion (see later).

Table 38–2 | **Exocrine Cells within Gastric Glands and Their Secretory Products*,†**

GLAND AREA (% OF TOTAL)	ANATOMIC COUNTERPART	EXOCRINE CELLS WITHIN GLANDS	SECRETORY PRODUCTS
Cardiac (<5%)	Proximal stomach just below esophagogastric junction	Mucus neck	Mucin, PGII
Oxyntic (75%)	Fundus and body	Mucus neck	Mucin, PGI and PGII‡
		Chief	PGI and PGII,‡ leptin
		Parietal	HCl, intrinsic factor§
Pyloric (~25%)	Antrum and pylorus	Mucus neck	Mucin, PGII

*Pepsinogen I (PGI), includes Pg1–5; PGII includes Pg6 and Pg7.
†Endocrine cells are also present within glands (see Fig. 38–1).
‡PGI and PGII are colocalized in zymogen granules and are secreted concurrently.
§Some intrinsic factor may also be produced in chief cells and endocrine cells.[112]

Active H^+ Transport via H^+,K^+-ATPase (the Proton Pump)

When gastric HCl secretion is stimulated, there is a dramatic morphologic transformation of the membrane of the parietal cell[7] (see Chapter 36). Tubulovesicular membranes, which are prominent in the cytoplasm of the resting cell, diminish in concert with a 6-fold to 10-fold increase in an apical canalicular membrane and the appearance of long apical microvilli. The tubulovesicular membranes appear to fuse with the apical plasma membrane. There is evidence that the enzyme H^+,K^+-ATPase (the proton pump) as well as K^+ and Cl^- transporters ("symporters") are translocated from the tubulovesicles to the secretory canaliculus just before initiation of H^+ secretion,[8] perhaps with the aid of the phosphorylated cytoskeletal protein ezrin.[9]

The proton pumps of parietal cells[10] secrete protons (H^+), or more likely hydronium (H_3O^+) ions, against a concentration gradient higher than 10^6. Chloride ions accompanying hydrogen ions are secreted against both a parietal cell-to-lumen concentration gradient and an electrical gradient. Thus, HCl secretion by parietal cells is an active, energy-dependent process. Parietal cells contain abundant mitochondria to accomplish this active H^+ transport.

Adenosine triphosphate (ATP) provides the energy necessary for the active pumping of protons by the H^+,K^+-ATPase.[10] This magnesium-dependent enzyme is found only on secretory membranes of parietal cells (apical plasma membrane, tubulovesicular membrane). The adenosine triphosphatase (ATPase) is phosphorylated and dephosphorylated sequentially, resulting in H^+ (or H_3O^+) secretion in exchange for recycled K^+ (Fig. 38–2).

Acid is generated within the parietal cell from the dissociation of two molecules of H_2O to form H_3O^+ and OH^- (see Fig. 38–2). The H_3O^+ is secreted by the proton pump in exchange for K^+, whereas the corresponding OH^- combines in the cell with CO_2 to form HCO_3^-, a reaction catalyzed by carbonic anhydrase II. Intracellular HCO_3^- ions thus formed during H^+ secretion are rapidly exchanged for Cl^- ions at the basolateral membrane of the parietal cell, so that intracellular pH remains only slightly alkaline ($\approx$ 7.5) during H^+ secretion.[11] Rapid entry of HCO_3^- from parietal

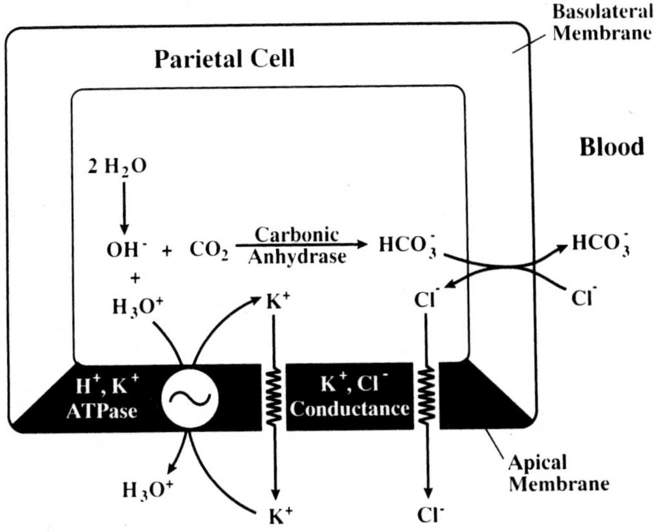

Figure 38–2. Model of gastric acid secretion by the parietal cell. Hydrogen or hydronium (H_3O^+) ions are exchanged for K^+ by the proton pump, the H^+,K^+-ATPase. Closely associated with the proton pump is a conductance pathway for K^+ and Cl^-. K^+ is largely recycled, whereas Cl^- is secreted with acid. OH^- that remains after H_3O^+ is pumped is converted to HCO_3^-, aided by carbonic anhydrase II, and is exchanged for Cl^- at the basolateral membrane. There is probably also an HCO_3^-/Na^+ cotransporter that is present at the basolateral membrane (not shown) and that unloads the parietal cell of excessive HCO_3^-. HCO_3^- from the parietal cell then enters the blood either to be secreted by surface epithelial cells or returned to the circulation (i.e., alkaline tide).

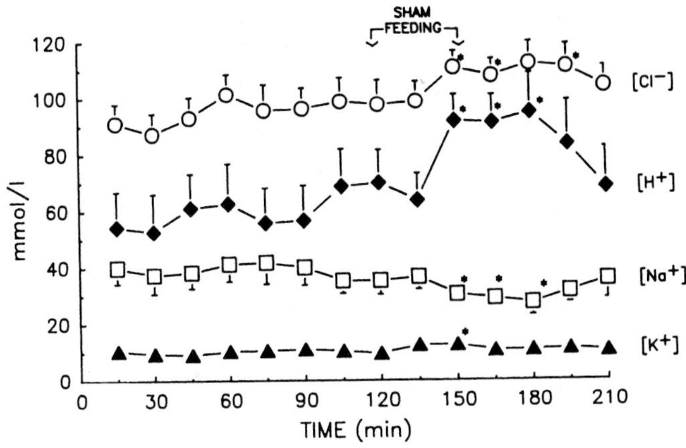

Figure 38–3. Mean (± standard error) gastric juice concentrations of Cl^-, Na^+, H^+, and K^+ for a 2-hour period of fasting and then following vagal stimulation induced by 30 minutes of sham feeding in nine healthy volunteers. Significant changes from fasting period are shown as asterisks. (From Feldman M, Goldschmiedt M: Gastric HCO_3^- secretion: Relationship with Na^+ secretion and effect of acetazolamide in humans. Am J Physiol 261:G320, 1991.)

cells into blood has been referred to as the "alkaline tide," and some of this HCO_3^- may be secreted by surface cells (see later). Cl^- that entered the parietal cell from the blood in exchange for HCO_3^- is transported into the secretory canaliculus of the stimulated cell via a conductance pathway closely associated with a K^+ conductance (KCl symporter) and with the H^+,K^+-ATPase. The net result is parietal cell secretion of H^+ and Cl^- at concentrations of ≈ 160 mM, whereas K^+ ions are primarily recycled. Water molecules probably follow HCl secretion passively. Even though aquaporin-4 is present in the basolateral membrane of the human parietal cell,[12] knockout of its gene in mice does not affect H^+ secretion.[13] At very high rates of H^+ secretion, H_2O cannot diffuse into gastric juice as rapidly as H^+, and gastric juice becomes hypertonic to plasma (~ 320 mOsm/kg).

The basal and stimulated concentration of H^+ in human gastric juice is typically much less than its secreted concentration of 160 mM (pH 0.8).[14] This difference occurs even though the apical membranes of gastric epithelial cells are quite impermeable to H^+ and Cl^- and allow little HCl secreted by parietal cells to diffuse back into the healthy mucosa. The concentration of H^+ in gastric juice is closer to 50 to 100 mM (Fig. 38–3), because secreted H^+ is diluted by fluid from other nonparietal gastric secretory cells and some H^+ is neutralized by gastric HCO_3^- (see later).

The proton pump is a heterodimer composed of two polypeptide subunits, a larger α catalytic subunit that reacts with ATP and a smaller heavily glycosylated β subunit that appears to play a key role in the function of the proton pump and in the development of the oxyntic mucosa.[10, 15] The α subunit crosses the apical membrane 10 times, whereas the β subunit crosses it only once (Fig. 38–4).[10] The α chain is inhibited by covalent antagonists such as the substituted benzimidazoles omeprazole, its *S*-isomer esomeprazole, lansoprazole, pantoprazole, and rabeprazole (proton pump inhibitors [PPIs]). The α chain also can be inhibited by K^+-competitive antagonists.[10] The cytoplasmic tail of the β subunit contains a tetrapeptide motif that is probably important in recycling the pump from the "active" secretory cana-

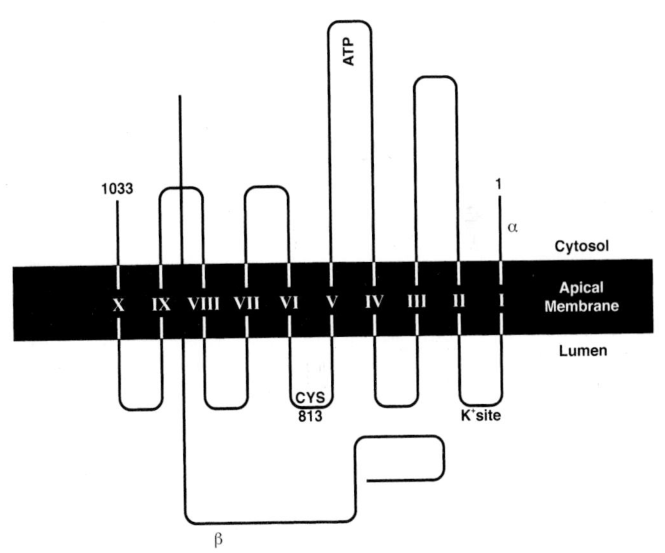

Figure 38–4. Two-dimensional model of the parietal cell's proton pump, with its a and β subunits. The α chain has 10 transmembrane domains (I to X). The luminal K^+-binding site is located between domains I and II. The cytosolic adenosine triphosphate–binding site is located between domains IV and V. The luminal cystine (CYS) target of acid-activated proton pump inhibitors (PPIs) such as omeprazole is shown at position 813 between domains V and VI. Certain PPIs also inhibit cystines at position 321 or 822 (not shown). The β chain crosses the apical membrane only once between domains VIII and IX and stabilizes the α chain. (Adapted from Munson K, Lambrecht N, Shin JM, et al: Analysis of the membrane domain of the gastric H^+/K^+-ATPase. J Exp Biol 203:161, 2000.)

liculi back to the tubulovesicular membranes when the cell reverts to a "resting" state. (A similar tetrapeptide motif is present in the transferrin receptor that is endocytosed to move Fe^{2+} into cells.) Mutation of this motif in mice leads to overactivity of the H^+,K^+-ATPase, increased acid secretion by glands isolated from these mice, oxyntic mucosal hypertrophy, and gastric ulcers, resembling a hypertrophic, hypersecretory gastropathy.[16]

Benzimidazole PPIs are weak bases (pKa 4 to 5) that concentrate in secretory canaliculi of the parietal cells (pH < 1). In the canaliculi (or perhaps in acid compartments within the parietal cell), these sulfoxide prodrugs are protonated to their "active" ionized forms (PPI^+), namely sulfonamides (Fig. 38–5). Sulfonamides bond covalently with sulfhydryl groups on cystine residues within the luminal (canalicular) domain of the α subunit of H^+,K^+-ATPase,[10] most critically with cystine residue 813, but also with other luminal-domain cystines, depending on the PPI. As a result of the formation of cystinyl sulfonamides, ion channels involved in expulsion of H^+ (H_3O^+) from the cell and retrieval of K^+ are blocked. Because activation of H^+,K^+-ATPase is the terminal step in the acid secretory process, PPIs inhibit H^+ secretion following all known stimuli in humans.[17–21]

When H^+ secretion decreases after a PPI in administered, intragastric pH rises, in turn increasing serum gastrin concentration because of loss of negative feedback by H^+ (see later). Gastrin acts via CCK_B/gastrin receptors on ECL cells to increase histidine decarboxylase activity, increasing histamine production. Histamine then acts on the histamine$_2$ (H_2) receptor of the parietal cell to increase messenger RNA for H^+,K^+-ATPase.[22] This process represents an unsuccessful attempt by the parietal cell to restore (up-regulate) acid secretion after a PPI is administered.

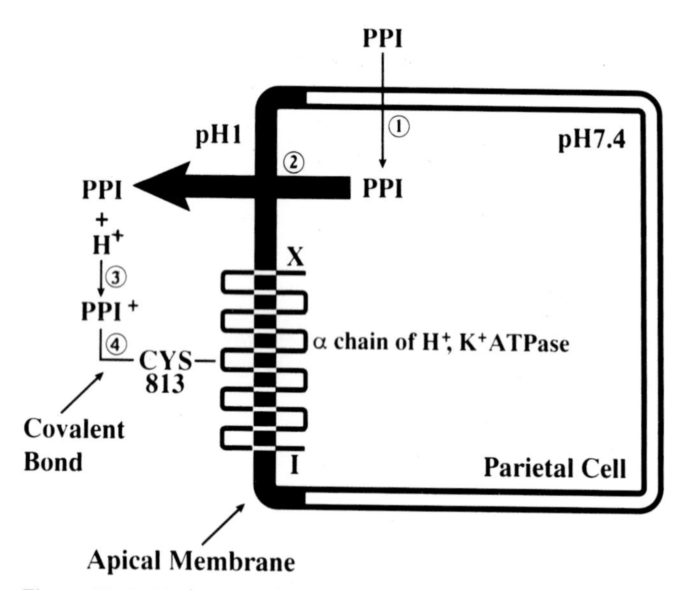

Figure 38–5. Mechanism of action of benzimadazole proton pump inhibitors (PPIs) on parietal cell H^+,K^+-ATPase. PPIs (i.e., omeprazole, esomeprazole, lansoprazole, rabeprazole, and pantoprazole) are weak bases (pKa ~4–5) and are taken up into all cells, including the parietal cell (step 1). The PPI then crosses the apical membrane and enters the secretary canaliculus of the parietal cell, where the pH is 1 or less (step 2). At this point the weak base accepts a proton and ionizes to a cationic sulfenamide (PPI^+; step 3). Ionization to PPI^+ "traps" the drug and concentrates it. The PPI^+ then forms a covalent bond with the cystine (CYS) in position 813 of the α chain of the proton pump, thus forming a cystinylsulfonamide (step 4). (PPIs bind to other cystines in the pump, but Cys 813 seems to be critical.) The cystinylsulfonamide blocks proton pumping until new α subunits can be synthesized and inserted into the apical membrane.

Parietal Cell Secretagogues

Regulation of H^+ secretion by parietal cells is complex and incompletely understood. A working model is proposed in Figure 38–6, with emphasis on human parietal cell regulation. Secretagogues are reviewed first; then inhibitors are discussed.

GASTRIN. Gastrin is the most potent endogenous stimulant of gastric acid secretion. Gastrin is not a single peptide but a family of peptides of varying lengths processed from a larger precursor of 101 amino acids (preprogastrin). The carboxyl-terminal tetrapeptide, G-4, is necessary for the biologic activity of gastrin. Fragments longer than G-4, such as G-6, G-14, G-17, G-34, G-52, and (probably) G-71 all stimulate acid secretion. G-17, G-34, and G-52 are nearly equipotent.[23]

The major stimulant of G cells in pyloric (and duodenal) glands is luminal amino acids, especially the aromatic amino acids phenylalanine and tyrosine derived from peptic hydrolysis of dietary proteins. Pepsin preferentially hydrolyzes dietary proteins at peptide bonds containing aromatic amino acids (see later). Amino acids released by peptic activity are decarboxylated to amines, which are taken up passively by G cells and which induce gastrin release into the blood. The major target for circulating gastrin appears to be fundic ECL cells (see later). ECL cells release histamine, which acts on H_2 receptors to increase H^+ secretion from the parietal cell.

When the pH in the gastric lumen falls below 3 as a result of gastrin-mediated H^+ secretion, gastrin release is inhibited by negative feedback. H^+ ions within the lumen protonate (and hence ionize) amines derived from dietary amino acids, thereby reducing their passive uptake by G cells.[24] Moreover, luminal H^+ appears to activate sensory nerve endings that, via CGRP, enhance somatostatin release from pyloric D cells, thereby suppressing the release of gastrin from adjacent G cells.[25, 26] A direct topical effect of H^+ on antral G cells (inhibitory) or D cells (stimulatory) has not been excluded. Release of gastrin is also inhibited indirectly by CCK released into the circulation by amino acids and fatty acids in the duodenum. This inhibition is mediated by a stimulatory CCK_A receptor located on the pyloric D cell. Thus, CCK_A-receptor antagonists such as loxiglumide block the postprandial release of pyloric somatostatin and markedly augment the release of gastrin stimulated by food.[27–29]

During the cephalic-vagal stimulation that occurs during eating, stimulatory and inhibitory neural pathways to the G cell are active. The inhibitory pathway to the human G cell is cholinergic-muscarinic (i.e., it is blocked by small amounts of atropine).[30] The stimulatory neurotransmitter responsible for gastrin release during vagal stimulation is uncertain. It does not appear to be GRP, because a specific GRP inhibitor does not block vagally mediated gastrin release in humans.[5] Although cholinergic nerves inhibit pyloric D cells and thus may enhance gastrin release indirectly by suppressing somatostatin release,[2] cholinergic neurons appear

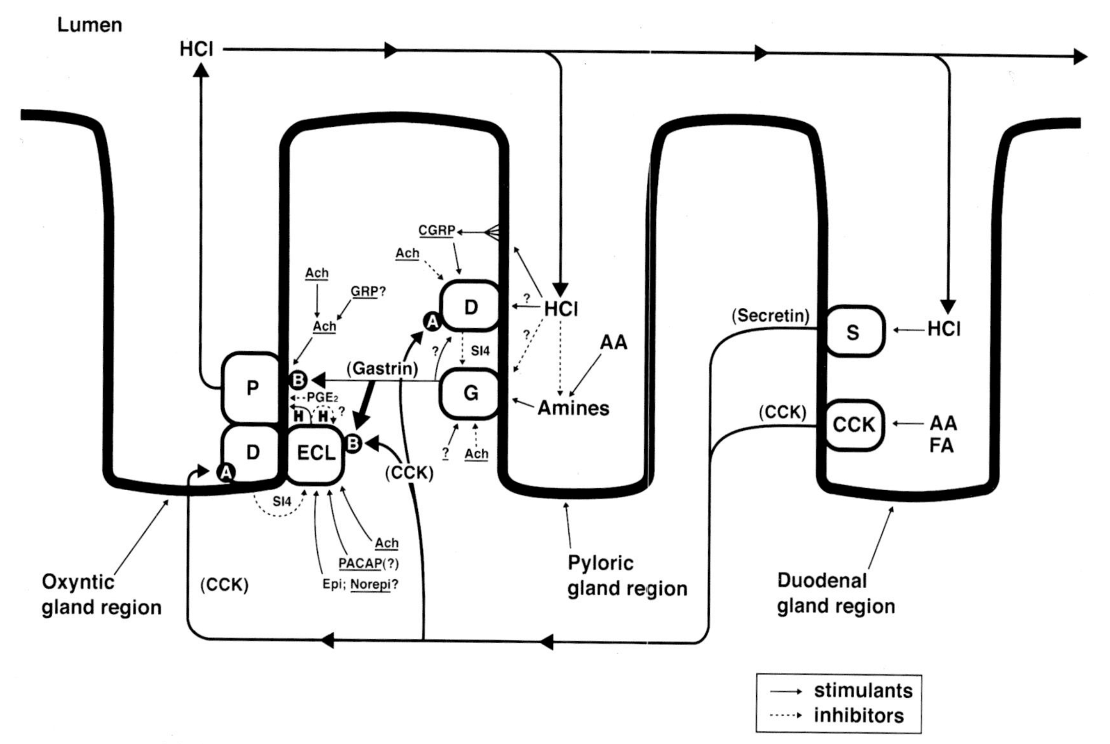

Figure 38–6. Model for regulation of hydrochloric acid (HCl) secretion by the parietal cell (P). Neurotransmitters are underlined, and circulating (humoral) mediators are shown in parentheses. Stimulants are shown as *solid lines*; inhibitors are indicated by *dashed lines*. Parietal cells located in the oxyntic gland area have stimulatory receptors for histamine (H) from oxyntic ECL cells (H_2 receptor), for circulating gastrin and cholecystokinin (CCK) (CCK_B receptor, shown as B), and for acetylcholine from neurons (M_3 receptor). Oxyntic and pyloric D cells are stimulated by circulating CCK via CCK_A receptors (shown as A), which have a 1000-fold more affinity for CCK than for gastrin. AA, dietary amino acids; FA, dietary fatty acids; CGRP, calcitonin gene-related peptide; S14, somatostatin 14; GRP, gastrin-releasing peptide; PGE_2, prostaglandin E_2; PACAP, pituitary adenylate cyclase activated peptide; Epi, epinephrine. See the text for more details.

to have a net inhibitory effect on G cells in humans.[30] The small amount of gastrin released during cephalic-vagal stimulation appears to contribute in a major way to the cephalic phase of gastric acid secretion.[6, 31]

ACETYLCHOLINE, GRP, AND OTHER NEUROTRANSMITTERS. Acetylcholine released from postganglionic nerves whose cell bodies are located primarily in the submucosal (Meissner's) plexus acts on parietal cell muscarinic (M_3) receptors. Cell bodies of these cholinergic neurons are innervated by long, preganglionic vagal fibers and by other enteric neurons involved in local reflexes, such as those activated by gastric distention. One chemical activator of these short, postganglionic cholinergic neurons appears to be acetylcholine itself, which acts via M_1 receptors. Atropine nonselectively blocks parietal cell M_3 receptors and ganglionic M_1 receptors and reduces H^+ secretion. However, atropine and related drugs are not especially useful acid antisecretory agents, because more potent agents are available and muscarinic blockade causes adverse effects in other tissues. M_1-selective antimuscarinic agents have fewer side effects than those of atropine and reduce gastric acid secretion to a modest degree, probably by acting on submucosal postganglionic neurons.

The neuropeptide GRP may be an important neurotransmitter in the vagal-cholinergic pathway to the parietal cell. The specific GRP antagonist BIM26226 blocks vagally mediated acid secretion in humans in a manner similar to that of atropine.[5]

Many other peptide and nonpeptide neurotransmitters are being investigated for a possible role in the regulation of gastric acid secretion. These neuropeptides include CGRP[25, 26] and PACAP,[32, 33] and the nonpeptides include nitric oxide[34] and norepinephrine (perhaps via β_3-adrenoreceptors).[35, 36] In rats, PACAP acts on both ECL cells to release histamine and fundic D cells to release somatostatin.[32, 33] PACAP may be yet another postganglionic neurotransmitter (in addition to acetylcholine and GRP) released by gastric nerves during the cephalic phase of gastric acid secretion.[37]

HISTAMINE. ECL cells constitute fewer than 1% of cells in the human oxyntic mucosa but play a key role in gastric acid secretion.[38, 39] ECL cells are localized to the base of oxyntic glands and are "closed" to the lumen. They are small (8 to 10 μm in diameter) and synthesize histamine from histidine via the enzyme histidine decarboxylase. ECL cells, which can be detected by silver stains, have long cytoplasmic extensions suggesting that the cells function via a paracrine mechanism. Stimulants of oxyntic ECL cells include gastrin, CCK, and acetylcholine, all of which increase the concentration of Ca^{2+} in ECL cells. PACAP may act on ECL cells to increase cyclic adenosine monophosphate (cAMP).[32] The most important inhibitor of the ECL cell is somatostatin from oxyntic D cells, which lowers ECL cell cAMP. In animals, histamine secreted by the ECL cell may act on an H_3 receptor on the ECL cell membrane to inhibit secretion of histamine (autocrine inhibition).[2, 40, 41]

Unlike parietal and chief cells, which have a limited capacity to divide, ECL cells can divide under the influence of gastrin, acting via the CCK_B/gastrin receptor. Hyperplasia of ECL cells occurs in certain pathologic conditions associated with hypergastrinemia (e.g., gastrinoma with multiple endocrine neoplasia type 1 [MEN-1] syndrome, chronic atrophic gastritis [CAG] with pernicious anemia), with an associated increase in the incidence of gastric carcinoid tumors (ECLomas) (see Chapters 41 and 112).

Unlike ECL cells, there is no relationship between serum gastrin levels and the density of gastric mast cells, nor is there convincing evidence that gastrin stimulates histamine release from mast cells. It has been speculated that mast cells play a role in gastric inflammatory conditions[38] but not in the regulation of gastric secretion. Histamine in the pyloric mucosa may release gastrin indirectly via an inhibitory H_3 receptor on the D cell. Conversely, somatostatin in the pyloric mucosa suppresses the release of both gastrin and histamine.[2, 40]

Receptors, Receptor-Coupled G Proteins, and Intracellular Stimulatory Messengers

The basolateral membrane of parietal cells has receptors for the three endogenous stimulants just discussed: an *M_3 receptor* for acetylcholine; an *H_2 receptor* for histamine; and a *CCK_B receptor* for gastrin. Each of these receptors has seven transmembrane-spanning domains typical of G protein–binding receptors.[42–44]

When the *M_3 receptor* on the parietal cell is occupied by its ligand, acetylcholine, the intracellular concentration of calcium increases. One Ca^{2+} signal is generated by a high-affinity M_3 receptor linked to a G protein, which increases Ca^{2+} conductance from extracellular fluid to cytosol. A second Ca^{2+} signal is generated by a low-affinity M_3 receptor linked to an apparently different G protein that activates phospholipase C, which in turn converts phosphatidylinositol 4,5-bisphosphate in the cell membrane to diacylglycerol and inositol trisphosphate (IP_3). IP_3 then releases Ca^{2+} from stores within the endoplasmic reticulum. The increase in acid secretion following M_3 stimulation appears to depend more on Ca^{2+} entry than on IP_3-mediated release of intracellular Ca^{2+}.[43] Although acetylcholine can release histamine from ECL cells, acetylcholine remains a potent stimulant of the parietal cell even when parietal cell H_2 receptors are blocked and ECL cell histamine is depleted,[39] indicating that acetylchloline has an important direct action on the parietal cell M_3 receptor.

The *H_2 receptor* for histamine on the parietal cell is linked via a G protein to membrane-bound adenylate cyclase, which converts cytosolic ATP to cAMP. The steps between elevation of cAMP and stimulation of the proton pump have not been clarified, although the enzyme protein kinase A is undoubtedly involved. Histamine also elicits an IP_3-mediated Ca^{2+} signal in the parietal cell.[45] Studies suggest that the H_2 receptor is linked to both cAMP and Ca^{2+} signal mechanisms, possibly via the same G protein.[42] Certain H_2 receptor antagonists, such as cimetidine and ranitidine, up-regulate H_2 receptors that cannot be down-regulated by histamine, a property that is referred to as *inverse agonism*[46] and may explain the development of tolerance to H_2-receptor blockers.[47]

Occupation of the *CCK_B/gastrin receptor* of the parietal cell by gastrin or CCK also increases intracellular Ca^{2+} via IP_3. This increase is blocked not only by CCK_B/gastrin receptor antagonists but also by H_2-receptor antagonists. The Ca^{2+} signal to gastrin in the presence of an H_2-receptor antagonist can be restored by cAMP.[48] This finding may explain why isolated parietal cells respond poorly to gastrin in the absence of histamine or cAMP. CCK_B/gastrin receptors are also present on ECL cells. These latter CCK_B/gastrin receptors appear to be much more important than the parietal cells' CCK_B/gastrin receptors in stimulating H^+ secretion. For example, blockade of the parietal cell H_2 receptor or depletion of ECL cell histamine[39] virtually abolishes gastrin-mediated gastric H^+ secretion, even though gastrin can still bind to the parietal cell CCK_B/gastrin receptor. Antagonists of the CCK_B/gastrin receptor markedly reduce gastrin-stimulated or food-stimulated gastric acid secretion.[6, 49]

Parietal Cell Inhibitors

SOMATOSTATIN. The somatostatin gene encodes a preprosomatostatin peptide that is processed to prosomatostatin and then to S-28 and S-14 (see Chapter 1). Most of the somatostatin in the stomach is S-14 and acts via a paracrine mechanism, whereas the somatostatin entering the circulation after a meal is mostly the S-28 peptide derived from the small intestine. S-28 has not been proven conclusively to be a circulating hormone that regulates gastric acid secretion or gastrin release.[50]

Oxyntic and pyloric somatostatin-secreting D cells are stimulated by circulating CCK via a CCK_A receptor. Whether or not somatostatin inhibits human parietal cells directly is unknown; most of its effects on H^+ secretion appear to be mediated via the inhibitory effect of somatostatin on oxyntic ECL cells and pyloric G cells. The pyloric D cell is stimulated by luminal acid (perhaps indirectly via CGRP neurons)[25, 26] and (possibly) by gastrin released into extracellular fluid, allowing for negative feedback of G cells by D cells. In certain animal models, the pyloric D cell is inhibited by cholinergic neurons and by histamine via an H_3 receptor.[2, 40]

CHOLECYSTOKININ. CCK is released from duodenal endocrine cells in response to dietary fatty acids and amino acids (see Chapter 88). CCK and gastrin share an identical carboxyl-terminal pentapeptide (G-5) and are equally potent in stimulating highly purified preparations of parietal cells in vitro. In vivo, however, gastrin is a potent stimulant of gastric acid secretion in humans, whereas CCK is a weak stimulant at best. This apparent paradox is explained by the finding that, at physiologic concentrations, CCK (but not gastrin) stimulates not only CCK_B/gastrin receptors but also CCK_A receptors on oxyntic and pyloric D cells. When these CCK_A receptors on D cells are occupied by CCK, they release S-14, which inhibits acid secretion from oxyntic glands (by suppressing histamine release from ECL cells) and inhibits release of gastrin from pyloric G cells.[25–27, 51–53] If CCK is infused intravenously into humans together with a CCK_A receptor antagonist such as loxiglumide, CCK will act exclusively on CCK_B/gastrin receptors and stimulate gastric acid secretion nearly as well as gastrin.[51]

SECRETIN AND RELATED PEPTIDES. Secretin is released into the circulation from duodenal S cells in response to the entry of H^+ into the duodenum from the stomach (see Chapter 46). Not only does the release of duodenal secretin elicit pancreatic HCO_3^- secretion to help neutralize H^+ in the proximal small intestine but it also inhibits further gastric H^+ secretion. Inhibition of gastric acid secretion by secretin is blocked by indomethacin,[54] suggesting indirect mediation by prostaglandins.

Peptides with amino acid homologies to secretin also inhibit gastric H^+ secretion when administered exogenously, although their physiologic roles are unclear. Such peptides include two glucose-dependent insulinotropic hormones, glucagon-like peptide-1 (GLP-1) and gastric inhibitory peptide (GIP),[55, 56] as well as the neuropeptides PACAP and vasoactive intestinal peptide (VIP).[33, 57]

OTHER GASTROINTESTINAL PEPTIDES. Many other gastrointestinal peptides can inhibit gastric acid secretion, but their physiologic roles are also unclear. These include GLP-2 and peptide YY, which (with GLP-1) are colocalized to ileocolonic L cells[58]; neurotensin from ileal N cells; the neuropeptides NPY and CGRP[25, 26]; and the epidermal growth factor (EGF) family, which includes EGF, transforming growth factor-α (TGF-α), and amphiregulin.[59, 60]

PROSTAGLANDIN E_2. Prostaglandin E analogs, such as misoprostol (Cytotec), reduce gastric acid secretion to approximately the same extent as H_2-receptor antagonists. There appear to be prostaglandin E_2 receptors on parietal cells that have effects opposite to those of the H_2 receptors; that is, they reduce adenylate cyclase activity, intracellular cAMP, and protein kinase A. However, the physiologic effect of prostaglandin E_2 and other endogenous prostaglandins on gastric secretion is less clear. Some (but not all) agents that block prostaglandin synthesis, such as the cyclooxygenase inhibitor indomethacin, increase basal gastric acid secretion,[61] but the effect is modest. Moreover, the stomachs of mice deficient in cyclooxygenase-1, the rate-limiting enzyme for prostaglandin synthesis in the stomach, produce normal amounts of HCl.[62]

QUANTITATIVE ASPECTS OF ACID SECRETION IN HUMANS

Development

Parietal cells and their H^+,K^+-ATPase can be demonstrated in the fetal human oxyntic and pyloric gland areas by the end of the first trimester, but parietal cells are restricted to the oxyntic gland region by the time of birth.[63] Gastrin appears to play a critical role in the development of parietal cells and their proton pumps, as well as ECL cells. In mice with a targeted disruption of the gastrin gene, basal acid secretion is absent, and there is no acid secretory response to gastrin, histamine, or carbachol (a cholinergic-muscarinic agonist). In such mice, parietal cells are hypoplastic and lack protein pumps, and ECL cells have deficient levels of histidine decarboxylase, the rate-limited enzymes in histamine synthesis. Proton pump activity and acid secretion can be partially restored by postpartum administration of gastrin.[64]

In preterm infants as young as 24 weeks' gestation, gastric acid secretion is present on the first day of life and increases as the infants become more mature.[65] The peak acid output (PAO) is lower in infants than adults, but by the age of 2 years, the PAO is similar to that of adults, when corrected for body weight.[66] Gastric acid secretion rates reach adult levels by the latter part of the second decade of life.

Aging

Gastric acid secretion rates remain nearly constant throughout adulthood. There is a decline in acid secretion in the elderly, but this can be attributed to their increased prevalence of chronic gastritis (see Chapter 43).[67, 68] In Norway, where CAG is common, the fasting gastric juice pH is lower than 3 in only 20% of elderly people in their 9th or 10th decade of life.[69] However, in populations in which CAG is uncommon, little or no decline in gastric acid secretion occurs with aging. For example, most healthy American subjects in their 9th or 10th decades of life studied in the author's laboratory had a fasting gastric pH lower than 3.[68] Likewise, the median gastric pH in elderly British subjects was 2.[70]

Measurement of Acid Secretion

Indications for Secretory Testing

Measurements of gastric acid secretion can assist in the clinical diagnosis and management of patients with gastrinoma and other acid hypersecretory states (see Chapter 41) and in the diagnosis of an incomplete vagotomy in patients with postoperative recurrent peptic ulcer (see Chapter 42). Furthermore, demonstrating fasting acid secretion (or an acidic fasting gastric pH) excludes achlorhydria as a cause of a markedly elevated fasting serum gastrin concentration (see Chapter 41). Patients should to be taken off gastric antisecretory drugs before such fasting acid secretory measurements are made (2 or 3 days for H_2-receptor blockers; 5 to 7 days for PPIs).

Methodology

The aspirating ports of a gastric tube are positioned by fluoroscopy in the most dependent portion of the stomach. Gastric juice is collected by manual suction or by a suction machine. When the tube is carefully positioned, only 5% to 10% of gastric juice escapes collection and enters the duodenum. Neutralization by HCO_3^- and diffusion of tiny amounts of secreted H^+ back into the mucosa result in a small underestimation of the true rate of gastric acid secretion.

The H^+ concentration in a sample of gastric juice can be determined by one of two methods. First, the specimen can be titrated in vitro with a base (e.g., NaOH). The millimoles of base needed to titrate a volume of gastric juice to an arbitrary pH endpoint (e.g., 7.0) represent the "titratable" acidity (in millimoles per liter) of the sample. A second (and simpler) method is to measure the pH of the sample with an electrode. Because pH electrodes measure H^+ activity and not concentration, it is necessary to convert activity to concentration using a table of activity coefficients for H^+ in gastric juice.[71] Once the H^+ concentration of the sample in millimoles per liter is determined by either of these two methods, it is multiplied by the volume of the sample in liters to determine the *acid output* during the collection period (e.g., millimoles per hour or millimoles per kilogram of body weight per hour).

BASAL ACID OUTPUT (BAO). The BAO represents gastric acid secreted in the absence of intentional and avoidable stimulation. Approximately two of three normal people secrete some gastric acid under basal conditions. The upper limit of normal for BAO is about 10.0 mmol per hour in men and 5 mmol per hour in women. BAO fluctuates from hour to hour in the same person. The lowest BAO occurs between 5 and 11 AM, and the highest occurs between 2 and 11 PM. Variation in BAO is also related to cyclic gastric motor activity, probably because of fluctuations in cholinergic tone. In one study of 11 people, BAO increased from about 40 μmol per minute (2.4 mmol per hour) in gastric phases I and II to nearly 150 μmol per minute (9 mmol per hour) in late gastric phase III (migrating motor complex), with a return to 40 μmol per minute at the beginning of the next cycle.[72]

MAXIMAL ACID OUTPUT (MAO) AND PEAK ACID OUTPUT (PAO). The maximal secretory capacity of the stomach can be estimated by determining the MAO or PAO following parenteral administration of a maximally effective dose of pentagastrin or histamine. The PAO in 800 consecutive healthy subjects in our laboratory ranged from 0.0 to 99.6 mmol per hour; only 20 subjects (2.5%) had a PAO of zero. The MAO and PAO are higher in men than in women and in smokers than in nonsmokers.[68, 73] Neither pentagastrin nor histamine is currently available in the United States. Fortunately, measurement of MAO or PAO adds relatively little to the BAO in most patients.[74]

MEAL-STIMULATED ACID SECRETION. The most common method to measure acid secretion with food in the stomach, in vivo intragastric titration, is primarily a research tool.[75] Rates of gastric acid secretion after eating increase rapidly and approach the PAO (Fig. 38–7*A*). Despite this, the pH in the stomach actually increases, because most foods have a pH that is higher than that of gastric juice and because the proteins in food buffer secreted acid (Fig. 38–7*B*). Postprandial intragastric pH eventually decreases below the basal pH as gastric acid secretion continues at a high rate and as food buffers are used or emptied from the stomach.

Two major mechanisms contribute to the stimulation of gastric acid secretion after a meal: cephalic-vagal stimulation and interactions of the meal with the gastrointestinal tract. The former accounts for about one third and the latter for about two thirds of the acid secreted.

Cephalic-Vagal Stimulation. The smell, sight, and thought of appetizing food sends signals from the cerebral cortex and lateral hypothalamus downward through the brainstem to the medulla oblongata, specifically the dorsal motor nuclei of the vagus nerves (DMN-10) (Fig. 38–8). The taste of appetizing food is carried through cranial nerves VII to IX to the nucleus tractus solitarius (NTS) in the medulla, which then stimulates the DMN-10. The DMN-10 contribute long, preganglionic neurons that travel to the wall of the stomach, where their axons terminate near short, postganglionic neu-

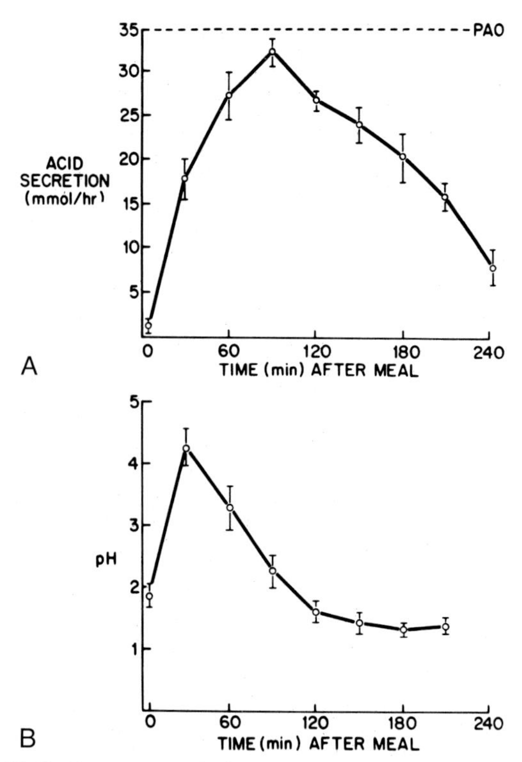

Figure 38–7. Mean (± standard error) acid secretion (*A*) and intragastric pH (*B*) after eating a sirloin steak meal. Acid secretion was measured by in vivo intragastric titration to a pH of 5.5 in six subjects. Intragastric pH was allowed to seek its natural level on another day in 10 subjects. The basal acid secretion rate (top) and the basal pH (bottom) before the meal are shown at 0 min. Peak acid output (PAO) is also indicated.

rons that innervate target cells (e.g., parietal, chief, and ECL cells in oxyntic glands; G and D cells in pyloric glands).

The vagal neurotransmitter that activates the postganglionic gastric neuron has been believed to be acetylcholine (acting on a nicotinic or an M_1 receptor on postganglionic neurons). However, a recent study has suggested a role for GRP at this synapse.[5] Once activated, the postganglionic neuron releases acetylcholine, which then acts on M_3 receptors located on the basolateral membranes of the parietal cell and the ECL cell. PACAP may also play a role as a postganglionic transmitter.[37] The noncholinergic, non-GRP neurotransmitter that releases gastrin during the cephalic phase of gastric acid secretion in humans is unknown.

Cephalic-vagal stimulation of gastric acid secretion in humans is usually studied by sham feeding, in which subjects see, smell, and taste appetizing food without actually swallowing it. Sham feeding causes a large increase in gastric acid output above the BAO, with a peak response of 50% to 60% of the PAO. Thought and taste appear to play more important roles than sight and smell.[76] Atropine abolishes cephalic-vagal stimulation of acid secretion,[28] suggesting that central or peripheral cholinergic neural pathways, or both, are critical. A specific GRP antagonist also abolishes sham feeding-stimulated gastric acid secretion, perhaps by acting at the level of the submucosal ganglion.[5] Several other central nervous system peptides affect gastric acid secretion via vagal pathways in animals, including corticotropin-releasing hormone, thyrotropin-releasing hormone, CGRP, and endor-

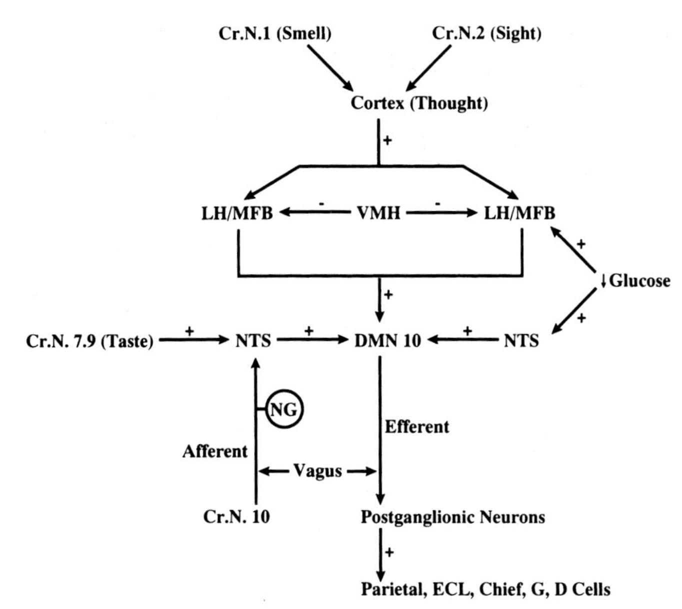

Figure 38–8. Cephalic-vagal stimulation of gastric acid secretion. All stimuli (i.e., smell, sight, thought, taste) ultimately activate the dorsal motor nuclei of the vagus nerves (DMN 10), which send long preganglionic efferents to the stomach where they synapse with short postganglionic neurons near target cells. DMN 10 can also be activated by the nucleus tractus solitarius (NTS), either as a consequence of low blood glucose or afferent vagal stimulation (e.g., induced by gastric distention). The lateral hypothalamus (LH) and the median forebrain bundle (MFB) are involved in stimulation of acid secretion, whereas the ventromedial hypothalamus (VMH) inhibits acid secretion. Cr.N, cranial nerve; NG, nodose ganglion of the vagus nerve. (Modified from Hersey SJ, Sachs G: Gastric acid secretion. Physiol Rev 75:155, 1995.)

phins/enkephalins. The role of these peptides and PACAP, as well as other substances such as nitric oxide and serotonin, in the cephalic-vagal stimulation of gastric acid secretion in humans is unknown.

Interactions of the Meal with the Gastrointestinal Tract. Mechanical distention of the stomach by a meal stimulates gastric acid secretion by activating reflexes. Vagal *afferents* with their nuclei in the nodose (inferior) ganglion and vagal *efferents* with their nuclei in DMN-10 play a major role in eliciting this acid secretion (see Fig. 38–8). Studies using gastric balloons have shown that distention of the gastric body elicits more acid secretion than does distention of the antrum. Gastric distention releases a relatively small amount of gastrin, probably because distention simultaneously activates noncholinergic (possibly adrenergic) stimulatory and cholinergic inhibitory pathways to the G cell.[77]

The gastric acid secretory response to a liquid meal is much greater than the response to distention with the same amount of inert fluid. The secretory response to food is the result of chemical reactions of food with the gastrointestinal mucosa. The stomach has a stimulatory role, whereas the intestine has an inhibitory effect. *Proteins* and products of peptic digestion are potent stimulants of acid secretion. Amino acids, especially aromatic amino acids (phenylalanine and tryptophan), stimulate gastric acid secretion mainly by releasing gastrin. Amino acids are decarboxylated to amines, which stimulate G cells to release gastrin into the circulation.[24] Amino acids also can release gastrin by a mechanism independent of amine precursor uptake and decarboxylation.[78] Moreover, amino acids can stimulate gastric acid secretion via the circulation following intestinal absorption.[79] *Carbohydrates* inhibit gastric acid secretion, but the mechanism is uncertain. *Triglycerides* are strong inhibitors of acid secretion, and omega-3 fatty acids (fish oils) may be especially potent inhibitors.[80] Several gut peptides, including CCK, secretin, GIP, neurotensin, GLP-1 and GLP-2, VIP, and peptide YY, are released into the circulation by meals containing fat. With the exception of CCK, it has not been proven that release of any of these peptides is sufficient to account for the observed inhibition of gastric acid secretion.

Coffee (caffeinated or decaffeinated), *tea, milk,* and *soft drinks* increase gastric acid secretion.[81] *Wine* and *beer* (both fermented alcoholic beverages), but not whiskey, gin, or cognac, are potent stimulants of gastric acid secretion.[81, 82] The stimulant of acid secretion in wine and beer appears to be two dicarboxylic acid fermentation products, maleic acid and succinic acid, acting through a nongastrin pathway.[83] *Capsaicin* (an extract of cayenne peppers) reduces gastric acid secretion, presumably by activating sensory afferent neurons.[84] Even vigorous exercise does not affect postprandial gastric acidity.[85]

MUCUS/BICARBONATE SECRETION

Mucus and Mucins

A highly viscous gel-like layer of mucus 0.2- to 0.6-mm thick covers the gastric epithelium (surface and glands).[86] The mucus gel consists of approximately 95% water and 5% mucin glycoprotein that is rich in threonine and serine residues. Surface cells secrete both highly sulfated, acidic mucins that can be stained by Alcian blue and neutral mucins that can be stained with periodic acid–Schiff. Mucous neck cells in gastric glands secrete predominantly neutral mucins. Gastric-type mucin is also expressed in the gallbladder, terminal ileum, and right colon.[87]

The intact mucin glycoprotein is a tetramer with a molecular weight of about 2000 kd (>80% of which is carbohydrate). Each subunit of the tetramer consists of carbohydrate side chains (≈15 sugars long) attached to threonine and serine residues of the protein core. The main sugars include galactose, fucose, *N*-acetylgalactosamine, *N*-acetylglucosamine, and sialic acids. The sialic acid content decreases with aging.[88] Differences in the terminal sugar sequences of the side chains impart antigenic differences between gastric mucins in gastric juice. Persons secrete mucins with antigenic determinants for blood group A, B, or H (O) corresponding to the person's blood type.

The four subunits of the intact glycoprotein are joined by disulfide bridges connecting cystine residues in the central, nonglycosylated parts of the protein core. If disulfide bridges are broken by pepsin or reduced by *N*-acetyl-L-cysteine (Mucomist), the glycoprotein is degraded into its four subunits, loses its gel-forming and viscous properties, and becomes solubilized (Fig. 38–9). Thus, the mucus gel occurs in two physical forms: a thin layer of highly viscous mucin firmly adherent to the gastroduodenal mucosal surface (adherent mucus), and mucin that mixes with luminal fluid and can be washed from the mucosal surface (soluble mucus). Under normal conditions in vivo, the adherent mucus gel is

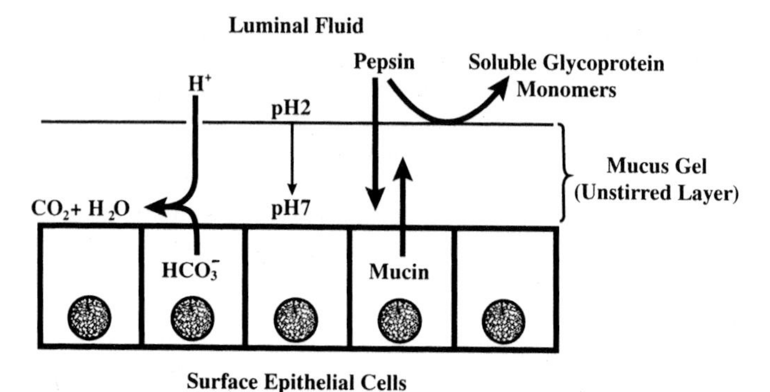

Figure 38–9. Model for surface neutralization of H^+ by HCO_3^- within the unstirred (adherent) layer of gastric mucus gel. HCO_3^- secretion into the gel by surface epithelial cells keeps pH near the mucosal surface close to 7. Although HCO_3^- may be generated within surface epithelial cells by the action of carbonic anhydrase II, the source of some of the secreted HCO_3^- may actually be parietal cells, with HCO_3^- from H^+-secreting parietal cells entering capillaries that perfuse surface epithelial cells. Mucin glycoprotein tetramers are secreted continuously into the mucus gel by surface epithelial cells, and the gel is digested continuously into soluble glycoprotein monomers by luminal pepsin acting at an acidic pH (~2). Mucus and HCO_3^- are stimulated by prostaglandins in the stomach.[89, 90]

secreted continuously by gastric epithelial cells and degraded by pepsin. Gastric mucin provides surface lubrication and an unstirred water layer that slows inward diffusion of H^+ toward the mucosa. The mucus barrier to H^+, in combination with secretion of HCO_3^- into the gel by surface epithelial cells, serves to protect the surface epithelium against injury from luminal acid and pepsin (see Fig. 38–9). Secretion of phospholipids into the gel makes the gastric surface hydrophobic, retarding the uptake of water-soluble materials.

There has been considerable investigation into how acid from parietal cells located in the neck and base of oxyntic glands crosses the mucus gel layer and enters the gastric lumen to carry out its physiologic functions (see Table 38–1). Recently, an animal model using microelectrodes showed a pH gradient within the mucus gel from 3.0 adjacent to parietal cells to 4.6 to 5.0 adjacent to the gland outlet and near the gastric surface, suggesting that H^+ is transported toward the surface simultaneously with secreted mucins.[11] Acid secreted by parietal cells may penetrate this gel and flow into the gastric lumen by a physical process called *viscous fingering*.[91] Once in the lumen, H^+ presumably is retarded from diffusing back toward the cell surface by the highly viscous gel.

Bicarbonate

HCO_3^- is secreted by surface cells that are rich in carbonic anhydrase II.[90] Because these cells also secrete mucin, a mucus gel with a high pH blankets the gastric epithelium.[86] Once in the lumen, H^+ diffuses very slowly back through the mucus gel toward the surface epithelium and, as it does, H^+ is neutralized by secreted HCO_3^-. Furthermore, as pepsin diffuses through the mucus gel toward the mucosa, its activity declines rapidly as the pH in the microenvironment near the surface of the mucosa increases above 5 (see Fig. 38–9).

Under most conditions, secreted HCO_3^- reaching the lumen is overwhelmed by luminal H^+ and converted to CO_2. Therefore, HCO_3^- is not ordinarily present in gastric juice, and measurement of gastric HCO_3^- secretion is difficult and indirect.[92] With the use of a potent acid antisecretory drug, it is possible to measure gastric HCO_3^- secretion by in vitro titration of an acidic gastric juice with HCl. One method measures gastric HCO_3^- secretion without inhibiting H^+ secretion and is based on the observation that HCO_3^- neutralizes an equimolar amount of H^+, with disappearance of HCO_3^- (as CO_2 and H_2O are formed) and a proportionate fall in gastric juice acidity and osmolality.[93]

Gastric HCO_3^- secretion is an energy-dependent, metabolic process, although the exact mechanism by which gastric HCO_3^- is secreted is unclear. That there is virtually no change in gastric electrical potential difference during stimulation of HCO_3^- secretion suggests that HCO_3^- transport may take place via an electroneutral ion exchange mechanism, possibly an exchange of HCO_3^- for Cl^- at the luminal surface. It also is possible that electroneutral HCO_3^- secretion is coupled 1:1 with secretion of a cation, such as Na^+ (see later). The source of some of the bicarbonate secreted during H^+ secretion may actually be acid-secreting parietal cells ("alkaline tide") rather than surface cells. HCO_3^- from H^+-secreting parietal cells may alkalinize the blood that perfuses the surface epithelial cells and then may be secreted by surface cells to protect the cells from the acid that has been secreted.[94] However, marked inhibition of gastric H^+ secretion by the PPI omeprazole does not significantly affect gastric HCO_3^- secretion in patients with duodenal ulcer.[95]

Vagal stimulation increases gastric HCO_3^- secretion by a cholinergically mediated mechanism.[96] Prostaglandin E_2 analogs also stimulate gastric HCO_3^- secretion,[93] and some studies, but not others, have found that blockade of endogenous prostaglandin synthesis reduces gastric HCO_3^- secretion.[61, 97] Gastric HCO_3^- secretion declines with age.[98] Gastric mucosal prostaglandin synthesis also declines in the elderly,[99] and lower gastric HCO_3^- secretion could be a consequence of reduced prostaglandin synthesis. There are also racial differences in gastric HCO_3^- secretion, with higher rates in African Americans than in whites.[100]

SECRETION OF OTHER ELECTROLYTES (K^+, Na^+, Cl^-)

In addition to H^+, the two other major cations in gastric juice are K^+ and Na^+. The K^+ concentration in gastric juice exceeds plasma K^+ by 2.5-fold to 4-fold. Although some K^+ derives from nonparietal secretion, most arises from acid-secreting parietal cells. The gastric juice concentration of Na^+ is, in general, inversely proportional to that of H^+. Because Na^+ is not secreted by parietal cells, it is an excellent marker of nonparietal gastric secretion. When acid secretion is stimulated, the concentrations of H^+, K^+, and Cl^- increase, whereas the concentration of Na^+ actually decreases (see Fig. 38–3). Cl^- originates from parietal and nonparietal cells, and during stimulation of H^+ secretion, the concentration of Cl^- in gastric juice often exceeds that of plasma Cl^-, reflecting active Cl^- secretion by parietal cells.

PEPSINOGENS AND OTHER GASTRIC ASPARTIC PROTEASES

Pepsinogens (PGs), which belong to a family of enzymes called *gastric aspartic proteases,* are polypeptide proenzymes known as *zymogens.* PGs are converted in the gastric lumen by gastric acid to pepsins, which contain two active-site aspartate residues.[101] Once this reaction begins, pepsins can convert PGs to pepsins autocatalytically. Using electrophoresis, several proteolytic enzymes in extracts from gastric mucosa are detectable. Five isozymogens (Pg1 to Pg5) that migrate toward the anode most rapidly are similar immunologically and are referred to as *PGI* (also called *PGA*). PGI is expressed only in chief and mucous cells of the oxyntic mucosa.[102] Pg3 is the most abundant PGI. Migrating slightly behind the PGIs are two immunologically similar isozymogens (Pg6 and Pg7), the PGII (also called *Pg3* or *progastricsin*). PGII is secreted by cardiac, oxyntic, pyloric, and duodenal (Brunner's) glands. PGII (gastricsin) represents approximately 20% of the total pepsin content in gastric juice.[103] Both pepsin I and II are optimally active at pH of 1.8 to 3.5. Pepsins are reversibly inactivated around pH 5.0 and are irreversibly denaturated at pH 7 to 8. Pepsins preferentially cleave peptide bonds formed by the aromatic amino acids phenylalanine and tyrosine, thereby exposing the most potent amino acids with respect to stimulating the release of gastrin. Furthermore, gastric acid not only provides an optimal pH for peptic activity but also denatures dietary protein, making it more susceptible to peptic hydrolysis. Thus, acid and pepsin work in concert to facilitate peptic digestion of dietary protein in the stomach.

PGI and PGII are also detected in the blood, and PGI is detected in urine. PGII is present in semen.

Two gastric aspartic proteases distinct from PGI and PGII have activity at acidic pH. These glycoproteins include an electrophoretically slow-moving protease—cathepsin E, and a lysosomal enzyme found in cells throughout the body—cathepsin D. The role of gastric cathepsins D and E in protein digestion, if any, is not known.

In vitro studies using chief cells or gastric glands have identified factors that regulate PG secretion.[104–107] cAMP analogs and agents that increase cAMP in the chief cell (e.g., secretin, VIP, forskolin, prostaglandin E_2, and isoproterenol) augment PG secretion. The secretion of PG is also stimulated in vitro by agents that increase intracellular Ca^{2+} (e.g., acetylcholine analogs, CCK, leukotriene B_4, GRP, and the calcium ionophore A23187). Ca^{2+}-mediated agents also stimulate nitric oxide synthase, thereby increasing nitric oxide and cyclic guanosine monophosphate, which amplifies the stimulatory effect of Ca^{2+}. Aquaporin-4, a water channel protein, is expressed in human chief cells,[12] but its role in the secretion of pepsin is unknown.

Human chief cells have been isolated from endoscopic biopsies.[106] The major stimulants of pepsin secretion in vitro are acetylcholine via a muscarinic receptor (probably M_3), CCK (CCK_A receptor), and histamine (H_2 receptor). The growth factors EGF and TGF-α also stimulate PG secretion in vitro using tyrosine kinase. In vivo, PG secretion is stimulated by acetylcholine analogs, histamine, gastrin, and secretin and inhibited by somatostatin. Gastrin is a weak stimulant of PG secretion from isolated chief cells in vitro but a strong stimulant in vivo, probably because in vivo gastrin releases histamine from ECL cells via CCK_B/gastrin receptors. Recently, the cytokine interleukin-1β has been shown to reduce PG secretion in response to cAMP and histamine but not to other stimuli.[107]

HUMAN GASTRIC LIPASE

In addition to proteolytic enzymes discussed earlier, an enzyme that initiates digestion of dietary triglycerides (human gastric lipase [HGL]) is secreted into gastric juice.[108] This highly glycosylated lipolytic enzyme contains 379 amino acids; an *N*-glycosylated asparagine at residue 308 protects the enzyme from peptic proteolysis and is important for the enzymatic activity of HGL.[109] HGL has properties that are quite distinct from those of human pancreatic lipase (HPL).[110] HGL has a pH optimum of 4.5 to 5.5, compared with 6.5 to 7.5 for HPL. Unlike HPL, HGL is inhibited by bile acid micelles and does not require colipase for activity. The stimulation and inhibition of HGL secretion occur under conditions similar to those for PG secretion. The amount of HGL secreted after a meal is small relative to the amount of HPL. However, the specific activity of HGL is equal to or greater than that of HPL, and HGL is capable of considerable lipolysis in the absence of HPL. Although secretion of HGL does not increase when HPL secretion is reduced, HGL contributes importantly to fat absorption in patients with pancreatic insufficiency (see Chapter 49).[110] Thus, HGL, pepsins, and salivary amylase initiate digestion of dietary triacylglycerols, proteins, and polysaccharides, respectively, before entry of chyme into the duodenum. Fat in the small intestine inhibits HGL secretion by a humoral mechanism, with GLP-1 considered a candidate mediator.[111]

INTRINSIC FACTOR

Intrinsic factor (IF) is a 50-kd glycoprotein secreted by human parietal cells and, to a lesser degree, chief cells and endocrine cells.[112] All stimulants and inhibitors of gastric acid secretion discussed earlier have similar effects on gastric IF secretion, although the duration of the IF secretory response is briefer than the duration of the acid secretory response. IF binds cobalamin (Cbl) (vitamin B_{12}) to facilitate its absorption and has structural homologies to another Cbl-binding protein, transcobalamin II (TCB-II).[113]

The role of IF in Cbl absorption is summarized in Figure 38–10. Cbl is released from dietary protein by pepsin in the acidic stomach.[114] Two Cbl-binding proteins are secreted into gastric juice: IF and R binder.[115] R binder has rapid migration during electrophoresis and is also secreted in saliva and bile. R binds Cbl more efficiently than IF in the acidic stomach and, therefore, most Cbl initially becomes attached to R binder. In the upper small intestine, R-Cbl complexes are cleaved by pancreatic trypsin, and the freed Cbl binds to IF. IF-Cbl complexes are resistant to pancreatic proteolysis and eventually attach to a specific receptor on

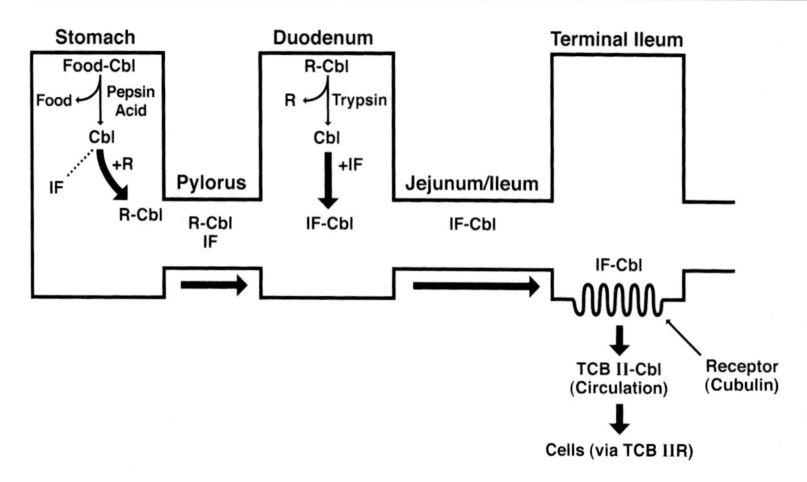

Figure 38–10. Steps in the absorption of cobalamin (Cbl) from food protein. Cbl moves from food protein to R binder, to intrinsic factor (IF), to cubulin (IF-Cbl receptor), and finally to transcobalamin II (TCB II). Gastric pepsin, gastric acid, and pancreatic trypsin all play a role in Cbl absorption. The ileal receptor for the IF-Cbl complex, cubulin, takes up IF-Cbl by endocytosis. TCB II, which has homologies with IF, transports Cbl to tissues for uptake by a TCB II receptor (TCB IIR) or to the liver for storage. (There is another mechanism for passive Cbl absorption that does not require IF or ileal receptors, but this mechanism is not shown here.) Thus, very high oral doses of Cbl (e.g., 2 mg/day) can reliably correct a Cbl deficiency. (From Kuzminski A, Del Giacco EJ, Allen RH, et al: Effective treatment of cobalamin deficiency with oral cobalamin. Blood 92:1191, 1998.)

ileal mucosa. This receptor, cubulin, is expressed in clefts between microvilli of the ileal apical brush border and mediates endocytosis of the IF-Cbl complex.[116] An autosomal recessive mutation of the cubulin receptor can lead to IF-B_{12} malabsorption and juvenile megaloblastic anemia, also referred to as *Imerslund-Graesbeck syndrome*.[117, 118] Once within the ileal enterocyte, Cbl is exported from the basal side of the cell bound to TCB-II, which then transports Cbl to tissues for uptake via a TCB-II receptor. Cells convert Cbl to its active forms, methylcobalamin and 5-deoxyadenosyl Cbl.

When radiolabelled Cbl is administered orally and a large dose of nonradioactive Cbl is given parenterally, patients with IF deficiency excrete much lower amounts of radioactive Cbl in a 24-hour urine collection than do normal people (Schilling test, part I). If IF is administered orally together with radioactive Cbl to IF-deficient patients, urinary radioactive Cbl excretion normalizes (Schilling test, part II). In addition to IF deficiency, Cbl malabsorption may result from achlorhydria or hypochlorhydria (reduced peptic hydrolysis of Cbl from food protein),[119] bacterial overgrowth[120] (Cbl competed for by bacteria; see Chapter 90), pancreatic insufficiency[115] (impaired tryptic cleavage of R-Cbl complex), ileal receptor defect (cubulin mutation),[117, 118] or ileal disease (see Chapter 103) or resection (see Chapter 92) (absent Cbl absorptive site).

Secretion of IF far exceeds the amount necessary for Cbl absorption. In most patients with hypochlorhydria, continued IF secretion in low amounts is sufficient to prevent Cbl deficiency and pernicious anemia. PPIs do not reduce IF secretion by parietal cells, although they may impair peptic release of Cbl from food-Cbl.[121] H_2-receptor blockers reduce IF secretion,[122] but resulting Cbl deficiency is extremely rare, if it occurs at all.

Circulating antibodies to IF are found in many patients with pernicious anemia[123] and in some patients with CAG (see Chapter 43). These autoantibodies may play a role in the pathogenesis of these disorders.[124] In rare patients, IF secretion is absent despite normal gastric acid secretion. This usually occurs in children (congenital or juvenile pernicious anemia), although cases in adults have been reported.[125] In even rarer cases, juvenile pernicious anemia may result from secretion of an abnormal IF molecule sensitive to proteolysis by acid-pepsin[126] or from an intracellular block in the secretion of IF.[127]

GASTRIC SECRETION IN DISEASE

Diseases Associated with Increased Gastric Secretion

DUODENAL ULCER. Gastric acid secretion is increased in approximately 30% to 50% of patients with duodenal ulcer. Whether gastric acid hypersecretion is a consequence of *Helicobacter pylori* infection is controversial (see Chapters 39 and 40).[128, 129] It has been hypothesized that *H. pylori* contains arginine decarboxylase that converts arginine to agmatine, which may increase gastric acid secretion.[130] However, one year after *H. pylori* eradication in patients with a duodenal ulcer, 24-hour gastric pH is unchanged (1.7 before, 1.6 after eradication).[128] Patients with duodenal ulcer have, on the average, a larger parietal cell mass and higher PAO than nonulcer controls, possibly because of the trophic effect of a somewhat higher serum gastrin level on parietal cells and possibly because of more frequent cigarette smoking.

ZOLLINGER-ELLISON SYNDROME (GASTRINOMA). In patients with the Zollinger-Ellison syndrome, serum gastrin concentrations and basal gastric acid secretion are elevated as a result of a gastrin-producing tumor of the pancreas or duodenum (see Chapter 41). The BAO is almost always higher than 15 mmol per hour and sometimes as high as 150 mmol per hour. The BAO/PAO ratio is often 0.6 or greater. One of four patients with this syndrome has MEN-1 syndrome (see Chapters 29, 41, and 51).

RETAINED ANTRUM SYNDROME. This extremely rare syndrome can develop after an antrectomy and Billroth II gastrojejunostomy if the most distal antral and pyloric glands are not resected (see Chapter 42). Because of their location at the end of the afferent loop, the retained pyloric glands are bathed continually in alkaline secretions and release gastrin into the circulation. The consequence is gastrin-driven acid hypersecretion from remaining parietal cells, and this may result in recurrent peptic ulceration.

OTHER HYPERSECRETORY CONDITIONS. Uncommon causes

of gastric acid hypersecretion include extensive small bowel resection, increased intracranial pressure, antral G cell hyperplasia (see Chapter 41), and foregut carcinoid tumors with overproduction of histamine (see Chapter 112). Histamine overproduction also occurs in some patients with systemic mastocytosis (see Chapter 29) or basophilic leukemia. In hyperparathyroidism, increased acid secretion and peptic ulcer disease are usually caused by a coexisting gastrinoma (MEN-1 syndrome) (see Chapter 29). There is no conclusive evidence that increased acid secretion occurs in patients with hyperparathyroidism without gastrinoma or with chronic hypercalcemia of other causes.[131] In some patients, acid hypersecretion has no known cause ("idiopathic basal hypersecretion").

CONSEQUENCES. Acid hypersecretion can result not only in acid-peptic disorders of the esophagus, stomach, duodenum, or even jejunum but also in chronic diarrhea, with or without malabsorption and vomiting, with hypokalemic, hypochloremic metabolic alkalosis.

Diseases Associated with Decreased Gastric Secretion

CHRONIC ATROPHIC GASTRITIS. In CAG involving the oxyntic mucosa, inflammation destroys parietal and chief cells, resulting in a marked reduction in the secretion of gastric acid and pepsin. Severe CAG is caused by autoimmune (type A) gastritis, with or without pernicious anemia (see later), and, less commonly, is a consequence of chronic *H. pylori* gastritis (see Chapter 39).[132] Certain IgG molecules synthesized by plasma cells in CAG may be directed against parietal cell antigens or even components of the proton pump and reduce secretion of HCl.[124] In patients with CAG associated with *H. pylori* infection, acid hyposecretion is potentially reversible.[133] The decline in gastric acid secretion seen in the elderly is explained by their higher prevalence of CAG of the oxyntic mucosa (and of chronic active superficial gastritis; see later) rather than aging, per se.[48, 67] CAG of the pyloric mucosa is usually a consequence of *H. pylori* infection (see Chapter 39).

CHRONIC ACTIVE SUPERFICIAL GASTRITIS. Chronic active superficial gastritis (CASG) is almost always caused by infection with *H. pylori* (see Chapters 39 and 43). CASG tends to be more severe in the pyloric than the oxyntic mucosa. Despite the mild hypergastrinemia that results from CASG of the pyloric mucosa, which may be cytokine mediated, gastric acid secretion in *H. pylori*–related CASG is normal or only slightly reduced. The severity of CASG in the oxyntic mucosa correlates with the degree to which gastric acid output is reduced.[68] The decline in gastric acid output with CASG also is probably cytokine mediated, because parietal cells are intact and acid output often increases after elimination of *H. pylori*–associated CASG with antibiotics.[133, 134] Candidate cytokines are interleukin-1β and TGF-α.[135] Recent studies from the author's laboratory have demonstrated that gastric acid secretion is unaffected by *H. pylori*–related CASG but that alkaline (nonparietal) secretion is increased. These findings may explain the reductions in gastric acidity and gastric acid output in the face of preserved H^+ secretion.[134]

HUMAN IMMUNODEFICIENCY VIRUS. Hyposecretion of gastric acid and IF has been reported in some patients with acquired immunodeficiency syndrome (AIDS).[136] However, human immunodeficiency virus infection without AIDS is typically associated with normal rates of secretion[137] (see Chapter 28).

OTHER HYPOSECRETORY CONDITIONS. Reduced gastric acid secretion occurs in some patients with gastric ulcer, gastric polyps, and gastric cancer, most of whom also have CAG or CASG. On rare occasions, islet cell tumors produce hormones, such as VIP or somatostatin, that inhibit acid secretion (see Chapter 51). Persons with severe hypocalcemia (e.g., from hypoparathyroidism) are often achlorhydric, and gastric acid secretion increases when serum calcium concentrations are normalized. Patients with leprosy also have modestly reduced gastric acid secretion rates.[138] Partial gastric resection and vagotomy reduce acid secretion as well (see Chapter 42).

CONSEQUENCES. A marked reduction in gastric exocrine secretion of any cause interferes with normal gastric physiology (see Table 38–1) and may contribute to protein or lipid maldigestion and malabsorption; Cbl malabsorption (see Chapter 89); an increased risk of enteric infections (see Chapter 96); iron deficiency anemia (see Chapter 42); and hypergastrinemia, with its potential for hyperplasia and neoplasia of ECL cells (gastric carcinoids, see Chapter 44). It also may cause small bowel bacterial overgrowth, but usually this is of little consequence to the patient.[70]

Diseases Associated with Heterotopic Gastric Acid Secretion

Parietal cells may be present in unusual (heterotopic) locations and cause acid-related disease. Examples include an inlet patch of the upper esophagus (see Chapter 31),[139] Barrett's esophagus, (see Chapter 33), Meckel's diverticulum, and intestinal duplication (see Chapter 84).

Normosecretory Acid-Related Disorders

Patients with many disorders associated with quantitatively normal rates of gastric acid secretion nevertheless benefit from the pharmacologic reduction in gastric secretion, including gastroesophageal reflux disease and its sequelae (see Chapter 33), gastric and duodenal ulcers associated with *H. pylori* (see Chapters 39 and 40) or nonsteroidal anti-inflammatory drugs (see Chapters 23 and 40), and stress-induced ulcers (see Chapter 40). Table 38–3 summarizes the drugs, including PPIs, H_2-receptor antagonists, and prostaglandins that are currently used to reduce gastric acid secretion in humans.

Acknowledgments
The author thanks Jim Hardy for help with illustrations and Vicky Robertson for help with preparation of the chapter.

Table 38–3 | **Drugs that Reduce Gastric Acid Secretion in Humans**

DRUG CATEGORY	EXAMPLE (U.S. TRADE NAME)	DAILY DOSE (U.S.)†	ROUTE
Proton pump inhibitors‖	Omeprazole§ (Prilosec)	20–40 mg	Oral
	Esomeprazole (Nexium)	20–80 mg	Oral
	Lansoprazole (Prevacid)	15–30 mg	Oral
	Pantoprazole (Protonix)	40–80 mg	Oral, injection
	Rabeprazole (Aciphex)	20–40 mg	Oral
Receptor antagonists			
Histamine$_2$¶	Cimetidine (Tagamet)	800 mg	Oral, injection
	Ranitidine (Zantac)	300 mg	Oral, injection
	Nizatidine (Axid)	300 mg	Oral
	Famotidine (Pepcid)	40 mg	Oral, injection
Muscarinic$_3$	Atropine/related drugs	Varies with drug	Oral, injection
Muscarinic$_1$	Pirenzepine*	—	Oral
Cholecystokinin-B	L 365,260*/ spiroglumide*	—	Oral
Receptor agonists			
Prostaglandin E	Misoprostol (Cytotec)	400–800 μg	Oral
Somatostatin	Octreotide (Sandostatin)	≥100 μg	Injection

*Not available in the United States as of 2001.
†Higher doses may be necessary in certain patients (e.g., in Zollinger-Ellison syndrome).
§The *S*-isomer of omeprazole, esomeprazole, is somewhat more active than omeprazole and is being tested in clinical trials.[21]
‖Data on proton pump inhibitors largely taken from References 17, 18, and 21.
¶Data on histamine$_2$ receptor antagonists largely taken from Reference 140.

REFERENCES

1. Powell JJ, Greenfield SM, Thompson RPH: Concentrations of metals in gastric juice in health and peptic ulcer disease. Gut 33:1617, 1992.
2. Schubert ML: Regulation of gastric acid secretion. Curr Opin Gastroenterol 14:425, 1998.
3. Sobhani I, Bado A, Vissuzaine C, et al: Leptin secretion and leptin receptor in the human stomach. Gut 47:178, 2000.
4. Simonsson M, Eriksson S, Håkanson R, et al: Endocrine cells in the human oxyntic mucosa: A histochemical study. Scand J Gastroenterol 23:1089, 1988.
5. Hildebrand P, Lehmann FS, Ketterer S, et al: Regulation of gastric function by endogenous gastrin-releasing peptide in humans: Studies with a specific gastric-releasing peptide receptor antagonist. Gut 49:23, 2001.
6. Beltinger J, Hildebrand P, Drewe J, et al: Effects of spiroglumide, a gastrin receptor antagonist, on acid secretion in humans. Eur J Clin Invest 29:153, 1999.
7. Helander HF: Parietal cell structure during inhibition of acid secretion. Scand J Gastroenterol 19(Suppl 101):21, 1984.
8. Hersey SJ, Sachs G: Gastric acid secretion. Physiol Rev 75:155, 1995.
9. Hanzel D, Reggio H, Bretscher A, et al: The secretion-stimulated 80K phosphoprotein of parietal cells is ezrin, and has properties of a membrane cytoskeletal linker in the induced apical microvilli. EMBO J 10:2363, 1991.
10. Munson K, Lambrecht N, Shin JM, et al: Analysis of the membrane domain of the gastric H^+/K^+-ATPase. J Exp Biol 203:161, 2000.
11. Schreiber S, Nguyen TH, Stüben M, et al: Demonstration of a pH gradient in the gastric gland of the acid-secreting guinea pig mucosa. Am J Physiol Gastrointest Liver Physiol 279:G597, 2000.
12. Misaka T, Abe K, Iwabuchi K, et al: A water channel closely related to rat brain aquaporin 4 is expressed in acid- and pepsinogen-secretory cells of human stomach. FEBS Lett 381:208, 1996.
13. Wang KS, Komar AR, Ma T, et al: Gastric acid secretion in aquaporin-4 knockout mice. Am J Physiol Gastrointest Liver Physiol 279: G448, 2000.
14. Feldman M, Goldschmiedt M: Gastric HCO_3^- secretion: Relationship with Na^+ secretion and effect of acetazolamide in humans. Am J Physiol 261:G320, 1991.
15. Scarff KL, Judd LM, Toh BH, et al: Gastric H^+,K^+-adenosine triphosphatase β subunit is required for normal function, development, and membrane structure of mouse parietal cells. Gastroenterology 117:605, 1999.
16. Courtois-Coutry N, Roush D, Rajendran V, et al: A tyrosine-based signal targets H/K-ATPase to a regulated compartment and is required for the cessation of gastric acid secretion. Cell 90:501, 1997.
17. Stedman CAM, Barclay ML: Comparison of the pharmacokinetics, acid suppression, and efficacy of proton pump inhibitors. Aliment Pharmacol Ther 14:963, 2000.
18. Welage LS, Berardi RR: Evaluation of omeprazole, lansoprazole, pantoprazole, and rabeprazole in the treatment of acid-related diseases. J Am Pharm Assoc 40:52, 2000.
19. Metz DC, Pratha V, Martin P, et al: Oral and intravenous dosage forms of pantoprazole are equivalent in their ability to suppress gastric acid secretion in patients with gastroesophageal reflux disease. Am J Gastroenterol 95:626, 2000.
20. Dammann HG, Burkhardt F: Pantoprazole versus omeprazole: Influence on meal-stimulated gastric acid secretion. Eur J Gastroenterol Hepatol 11:1277, 1999.
21. Kahrilas PJ, Falk GW, Johnson DA, et al: Esomeprazole improves healing and symptom resolution as compared with omeprazole in reflux oesophagitis patients: A randomized controlled trial. Aliment Pharmacol Ther 14:1249, 2000.
22. Tari A, Yamamoto G, Sumii K, et al: Role of histamine$_2$ receptor in increased expression of rat gastric H^+-K^+-ATPase α-subunit induced by omeprazole. Am J Physiol 265:G752, 1993.
23. Hansen CP, Stadil F, Rehfeld JF: Metabolism and influence of gastrin-52 on gastric acid secretion in humans. Am J Physiol 269:G600, 1995.
24. Lichtenberger LM, Nelson AA, Graziani LA, et al: Amine trapping: Physical explanation for the inhibitory effect of gastric acidity on the postprandial release of gastrin. Studies on rats and dogs. Gastroenterology 90:1223, 1986.
25. Manela FD, Ren J, Gao J, et al: Calcitonin gene–related peptide modulates acid-mediated regulation of somatostatin and gastrin release from rat antrum. Gastroenterology 109:701, 1995.
26. Ren J, Dunn ST, Tang Y, et al: Effects of calcitonin gene–related peptide on somatostatin and gastrin gene expression in rat antrum. Regul Pept 73:75, 1998.
27. Schmidt WE, Schenk S, Nustede R, et al: Cholecystokinin is a negative regulator of gastric acid secretion and postprandial release of gastrin in humans. Gastroenterology 107:1610, 1994.
28. Jebbink MCW, Lamers CBHW, Mooy DM, et al: Effect of loxiglumide on basal and gastrin- and bombesin-stimulated gastric acid and serum gastrin levels. Gastroenterology 103:1215, 1992.
29. Beglinger C, Hildebrand P, Meier R, et al: A physiological role for cholecystokinin as a regulator of gastrin secretion. Gastroenterology 103:490, 1992.
30. Feldman M, Richardson CT, Taylor IL, et al: Effect of atropine on vagal release of gastrin and pancreatic polypeptide. J Clin Invest 63: 294, 1979.
31. Feldman M, Richardson CT: "Partial" sham feeding releases gastrin in normal human subjects. Scand J Gastroenterol 16:13, 1981.
32. Zeng N, Athmann C, Kang T, et al: PACAP type I receptor activation regulates ECL cells and gastric acid secretion. J Clin Invest 104:1383, 1999.
33. Li P, Chang TM, Coy D, et al: Inhibition of gastric acid secretion in rat stomach by PACAP is mediated by secretin, somatostatin, and PGE_2. Am J Physiol Gastrointest Liver Physiol 278:G121, 2000.

34. Konturek JW, Fischer H, Gromotka PM, et al: Endogenous nitric oxide in the regulation of gastric secretory and motor activity in humans. Aliment Pharmacol Ther 13:1683, 1999.
35. Levasseur S, Bado A, Laigneau JP, et al: Characterization of a β_3-adrenoceptor stimulating gastrin and somatostatin secretions in rat antrum. Am J Physiol Gastrointest Liver Physiol 35:G1000, 1997.
36. Coruzzi G, Bertaccini G: The β_3-adrenoceptor agonist SR58611A inhibits gastric acid secretion in the conscious cat. Naunyn-Schmiedebergs Arch Pharmacol 356:263, 1997.
37. Wank SA: PACAP upsets stomach theory. J Clin Invest 104:1341, 1999.
38. Bechi P, Romagnoli P, Panula P, et al: Gastric mucosal histamine storing cells: Evidence for different roles of mast cells and enterochromaffin-like cells in humans. Dig Dis Sci 40:2207, 1995.
39. Andersson K, Cabero JL, Mattsson H, et al: Gastric acid secretion after depletion of enterochromaffin-like cell histamine: A study with α-fluoromethylhistidine in rats. Scand J Gastroenterol 31:24, 1996.
40. Vuyyuru L, Schubert ML, Harrington L, et al: Dual inhibitory pathways link antral somatostatin and histamine secretion in human, dog, and rat stomach. Gastroenterology 109:1566, 1995.
41. Soldani G, Bertini S, Rouleau A, et al: Gastric antisecretory effects of compound BP 2-94—a histamine H_3-receptor agonist prodrug. Dig Dis Sci 44:2380, 1999.
42. DelValle J, Wang L, Gantz I, et al: Characterization of H_2 histamine receptor: Linkage to both adenylate cyclase and $[Ca^{2+}]_i$ signaling systems. Am J Physiol 263:G967, 1992.
43. Kijimura M, Reuben MA, Sachs G: The muscarinic receptor gene expressed in rabbit parietal cells is the M_3 subtype. Gastroenterology 103:870, 1992.
44. Kopin AS, Lee YM, McBridge EW, et al: Expression cloning and characterization of the canine parietal cell gastrin receptor. Proc Natl Acad Sci 89:3605, 1992.
45. Chew CS: Cholecystokinin, carbachol, gastrin, histamine, and forskolin increase $[Ca^{2+}]_i$ in gastric glands. Am J Physiol 250:G814, 1986.
46. Smit MJ, Leurs R, Alewijnse AE, et al: Inverse agonism of histamine H_2 antagonists accounts for upregulation of spontaneously active histamine H_2 receptors. Proc Natl Acad Sci 93:6802, 1996.
47. Lachman L, Howden CW: Twenty-four-hour intragastric pH: Tolerance within 5 days of continuous ranitidine administration. Am J Gastroenterol 95:57, 2000.
48. Geibel J, Abraham R, Modlin I, et al: Gastrin-stimulated changes in Ca^{2+} concentration in parietal cells depends on adenosine 3′,5′-cyclic monophosphate levels. Gastroenterology 109:1060, 1995.
49. Murphy MG, Sytnik B, Kovacs TOG, et al: The gastrin-receptor antagonist L-365,260 inhibits stimulated acid secretion in humans. Clin Pharmacol Ther 54:533, 1993.
50. Hildebrand P, Ensinck JW, Buettiker J, et al: Circulating somatostatin-28 is not a physiologic regulator of gastric acid production in man. Eur J Clin Invest 24:50, 1994.
51. Verhulst ML, Gielkens HAJ, Hopman WPM, et al: Loxiglumide inhibits cholecystokinin-stimulated somatostatin secretion and simultaneously enhances gastric acid secretion in humans. Regul Pept 53:185, 1994.
52. Burckhardt B, Delco F, Ensinck JW, et al: Cholecystokinin is a physiological regulator of gastric acid secretion in man. Eur J Clin Invest 24:370, 1994.
53. Konturek JW, Stoll R, Konturek SJ, et al: Cholecystokinin in the control of gastric acid secretion in man. Gut 34:321, 1993.
54. Taylor SD, Soudah HC, Chey WY, et al: Duodenal acidification and secretin, but not intraduodenal fat, inhibit human gastric acid secretion via prostaglandins. Gastroenterology 107:1680, 1994.
55. Wettergren A, Petersen H, Orskov C, et al: Glucagon-like peptide-1 7–36 amide and peptide YY from the L-cell of the ileal mucosa are potent inhibitors of vagally induced gastric acid secretion in man. Scand J Gastroenterol 29:591, 1994.
56. Wettergren A, Maina P, Boesby S, et al: Glucagon-like peptide-1 7–36 amide and peptide YY have additive inhibitory effect on gastric acid secretion in man. Scand J Gastroenterol 32:552, 1997.
57. Zimmerman RP, Gates TS, Mantyh CR, et al: Vasoactive intestinal peptide (VIP) receptors in the canine gastrointestinal tract. Peptides 9: 1241, 1989.
58. Wøjdemann M, Wettergren A, Hartmann B, et al: Inhibition of sham feeding–stimulated human gastric acid secretion by glucagon-like peptide-2. J Clin Endocrinol Metab 84:2513, 1999.
59. Joshi V, Ray GS, Goldenring JR: Inhibition of parietal cell secretion is mediated by the classical epidermal growth factor receptor. Dig Dis Sci 42:1194, 1997.
60. Abe S, Sasano H, Katoh K, et al: Immunohistochemical studies on EGF family growth factors in normal and ulcerated human gastric mucosa. Dig Dis Sci 42:1199, 1997.
61. Feldman M, Colturi TJ: Effect of indomethacin on gastric acid and bicarbonate secretion in humans. Gastroenterology 87:1339, 1984.
62. Borrelli F, Welsh NJ, Sigthorsson G, et al: Gastric acid secretion in cyclooxygenase-1 deficient mice. Aliment Pharmacol Ther 14:1365, 2000.
63. Kelly EJ, Brownlee KG: When is the fetus first capable of gastric acid, intrinsic factor, and gastrin secretion? Biol Neonate 63:153, 1993.
64. Friis-Hansen L, Sundler F, Li Y, et al: Impaired gastric acid secretion in gastrin-deficient mice. Am J Physiol Gastrointest Liver Physiol 274: G561, 1998.
65. Kelly EJ, Newell SJ, Brownlee KG, et al: Gastric acid secretion in preterm infants. Early Human Dev 35:215, 1993.
66. Agunod M, Yamaguchi N, Lopez R, et al: Correlative study of hydrochloric acid, pepsin, and intrinsic factor secretion in newborns and infants. Am J Dig Dis 14:400, 1969.
67. Kekki M, Samloff IM, Ihamaki T, et al: Age- and sex-related behaviour of gastric acid secretion at the population level. Scand J Gastroenterol 17:737, 1982.
68. Feldman M, Cryer B: Effects of aging and gastritis on gastric acid and pepsin secretion in humans: A prospective study. Gastroenterology 110:1043, 1996.
69. Husebye E, Skar V, Hoverstad T, et al: Fasting hypochlorhydria with gram-positive gastric flora is highly prevalent in healthy old people. Gut 33:1331, 1992.
70. Pereira SP, Gainsborough N, Dowling RH: Drug-induced hypochlorhydria causes high duodenal bacterial counts in the elderly. Aliment Pharmacol Ther 12:99, 1998.
71. Moore EW, Scarlata RW: The determination of gastric acidity by the glass electrode. Gastroenterology 49:178, 1965.
72. Dalenbäck J, Fändriks L, Olbe L, et al: Mechanisms behind changes in gastric acid and bicarbonate outputs during the human interdigestive motility cycle. Am J Physiol Gastrointest Liver Physiol 270:G113, 1996.
73. Lanas A, Hirschowitz BI: Influence of smoking on basal and on vagally and maximally stimulated gastric acid and pepsin secretion. Scand J Gastroenterol 27:208, 1992.
74. Metz DC, Starr JA: A retrospective study of the usefulness of acid secretory testing. Aliment Pharmacol Ther 14:103, 2000.
75. Feldman M: Comparison of the effects of over-the-counter famotidine and calcium carbonate antacid on postprandial gastric acid: A randomized controlled trial. JAMA 275:1428, 1996.
76. Feldman M, Richardson CT: Role of thought, sight, smell, and taste of food in the cephalic phase of gastric acid secretion in man. Gastroenterology 90:428, 1986.
77. Schiller LR, Walsh JH, Feldman M: Distention-induced gastrin release: Effects of luminal acidification and intravenous atropine. Gastroenterology 78:912, 1980.
78. DelValle J, Yamada T: Amino acids and amines stimulate gastrin release from canine antral G-cells via different pathways. J Clin Invest 85:139, 1990.
79. Isenberg JI, Maxwell V: Intravenous infusion of amino acids stimulates gastric acid secretion in man. N Engl J Med 298:27, 1978.
80. Riber C, Wøjdemann M, Bisgaard T, et al: Fish oil reduces gastric acid secretion. Scand J Gastroenterol 34:845, 1999.
81. McArthur K, Hogan D, Isenberg JI: Relative stimulatory effects of commonly ingested beverages on gastric acid secretion in humans. Gastroenterology 83:199, 1982.
82. Chari S, Teyssen S, Singer MV: Alcohol and gastric acid secretion in humans. Gut 34:843, 1993.
83. Teyssen S, González-Calero G, Schimiczek M, et al: Maleic acid and succinic acid in fermented alcoholic beverages are the stimulants of gastric acid secretion. J Clin Invest 103:707, 1999.
84. Mózsik G, Debreceni A, Abdel-Salam OME, et al: Small doses of capsaicin given intragastrically inhibit gastric basal acid secretion in healthy human subjects. J Physiol 93:433, 1999.

85. van Nieuwenhoven MA, Brouns F, Brummer RJ: The effect of physical exercise on parameters of gastrointestinal function. Neurogastroenterol Motil 11:431, 1999.
86. Engel E, Guth PH, Nishizaki Y, et al: Barrier function of the gastric mucus gel. Am J Physiol 269:G994, 1995.
87. Toribara NW, Roberton AM, Ho SB, et al: Human gastric mucin: Identification of a unique species by expression cloning. J Biol Chem 268:5879, 1993.
88. Corfield AP, Wagner SA, Safe A, et al: Sialic acids in human gastric aspirates: Detection of 9-O-lactyl- and 9-O-acetyl-*N*-acetylneuraminic acids and a decrease in total sialic acid concentration with age. Clin Sci 84:573, 1993.
89. Johansson C, Kollberg B: Stimulation by intragastrically administered E_2 prostaglandins of human gastric mucus output. Eur J Clin Invest 9: 229, 1979.
90. Feldman M: Gastric bicarbonate secretion in humans: Effect of pentagastrin, bethanechol, and 11,16,16-trimethyl prostaglandin E_2. J Clin Invest 72:295, 1983.
91. Bhaskar KR, Garik P, Turner BS, et al: Viscous fingering of HCl through gastric mucin. Nature 360:458, 1992.
92. Parkkila S: Carbonic anhydrase in the alimentary tract. Scand J Gastroenterol 31:305, 1996.
93. Odes HS, Hogan DL, Steinbach JH, et al: Measurement of gastric bicarbonate secretion in the human stomach: Different methods produce discordant results. Scand J Gastroenterol 27:829, 1992.
94. de Beus AM, Fabry TL, Lacker HM: A gastric acid secretion model. Biophys J 65:362, 1993.
95. Singh K, Nain CK, Singh V: Effect of omeprazole on gastric bicarbonate secretion in patients with duodenal ulcer. Indian J Gastroenterol 17:136, 1998.
96. Konturek SJ, Kwicien N, Obtulowicz W, et al: Vagal cholinergic control of gastric alkaline secretion in normal subjects and duodenal ulcer patients. Gut 28:739, 1987.
97. Mertz-Nielsen A, Hillingso J, Bukhave K, et al: Indomethacin decreases gastroduodenal mucosal bicarbonate secretion in humans. Scand J Gastroenterol 30:1160, 1995.
98. Feldman M, Cryer B: Effects of age on gastric alkaline and nonparietal fluid secretion in humans. Gerontology 44:222, 1998.
99. Cryer B, Redfern JS, Goldschmiedt M, et al: Effect of aging on gastric and duodenal mucosal prostaglandin concentrations in humans. Gastroenterology 102:1118, 1992.
100. Cryer B, Feldman M: Racial differences in gastric function among African Americans and Caucasian Americans: Secretion, serum gastrin, and histology. Proc Assoc Am Physicians 108:481, 1996.
101. Richter C, Tanaka T, Yada RY: Mechanism of activation of the gastric aspartic proteinases: Pepsinogen, progastricsin, and prochymosin. Biochem J 335:481, 1998.
102. Samloff IM: Peptic ulcer: The many proteinases of aggression. Gastroenterology 96:586, 1989.
103. Jones AT, Balan KK, Jenkins SA, et al: Assay of gastricsin and individual pepsins in human gastric juice. J Clin Pathol 46:254, 1993.
104. Fiorucci S, Santucci L, Gresele P, et al: Effect of NSAIDs on pepsinogen secretion and calcium mobilization in isolated chief cells. Am J Physiol 268:G968, 1995.
105. Fiorucci S, Distrutti E, Chiorean M, et al: Nitric oxide modulates pepsinogen secretion induced by calcium-mediated agonist in guinea pig gastric chief cells. Gastroenterology 109:1214, 1995.
106. Lanas AI, Anderson JW, Uemura N, et al: Effects of cholinergic, histaminergic, and peptidergic stimulation on pepsinogen secretion by isolated human peptic cells. Scand J Gastroenterol 29:678, 1994.
107. Serrano MT, Lanas AI, Lorente S, et al: Cytokine effects on pepsinogen secretion from human peptic cells. Gut 40:42, 1997.
108. Aoubala M, Douchet I, Laugier R, et al: Purification of human gastric lipase by immunoaffinity and quantification of this enzyme in the duodenal contents using a new ELISA procedure. Biochim Biophys Acta 1169:183, 1993.
109. Wicker-Planquart C, Canaan S, Riviere M, et al: Site-directed removal of *N*-glycosylation sites in human gastric lipase. Eur J Biochem 262: 644, 1999.
110. Carrière F, Renou C, Lopez V, et al: The specific activities of human digestive lipases measured from the in vivo and in vitro lipolysis of test meals. Gastroenterology 119:949, 2000.
111. Wøjdemann M, Riber C, Bisgaard T, et al: Inhibition of human gastric lipase by intraduodenal fat involves glucagon-like peptide-1 and cholecystokinin. Regul Pept 80:101, 1999.
112. Howard TA, Misra DN, Grove M, et al: Human gastric intrinsic factor expression is not restricted to parietal cells. J Anat 189:303, 1996.
113. Seetharam B, Bose S, Ni N: Cellular import of cobalamin (vitamin B_{12}). J Nutr 129:1761, 1999.
114. Carmel R: In vitro studies of gastric juice in patients with food-cobalamin malabsorption. Dig Dis Sci 39:2516, 1994.
115. Gueant JL, Djalali M, Aouadj R, et al: In vitro and in vivo evidences that the malabsorption of cobalamin is related to its binding on haptocorrin (R binder) in chronic pancreatitis. Am J Clin Nutr 44:265, 1986.
116. Xu D, Fyfe JC: Cubilin expression and posttranslational modification in the canine gatrointestinal tract. Am J Physiol Gastrointest Liver Physiol 279:G748, 2000.
117. Kristiansen M, Aminoff M, Jacobsen C, et al: Cubilin P1297L mutation associated with hereditary megaloblastic anemia 1 causes impaired recognition of intrinsic factor–vitamin B (12) by cubilin. Blood 96:405, 2000.
118. Aminoff M, Carter JE, Chadwick RB, et al: Mutations in CUBN, encoding the intrinsic factor-vitamin B_{12} receptor, cubilin, cause hereditary megaloblastic anaemia 1. Nat Genet 21:309, 1999.
119. Aimone-Gastin I, Pierson H, Jeandel C, et al: Prospective evaluation of protein bound vitamin B_{12} (cobalamin) malabsorption in the elderly using trout flesh labelled in vivo with 57Co-cobalamin. Gut 41:475, 1997.
120. Sutter PM, Golner BB, Goldin BR, et al: Reversal of protein-bound vitamin B_{12} malabsorption with antibiotics in atrophic gastritis. Gastroenterology 101:1039, 1991.
121. Kittang E, Aadland E, Schjonsby H: Effect of omeprazole on the secretion of intrinsic factor, gastric acid, and pepsin in man. Gut 26: 594, 1985.
122. Binder HJ, Donaldson RM: Effect of cimetidine on intrinsic factor and pepsin secretion in man. Gastroenterology 74:371, 1978.
123. Gueant JL, Safi A, Aimone-Gastin I, et al: Autoantibodies in pernicious anemia type I patients recognize sequence 251–256 in human intrinsic factor. Proc Assoc Am Physicians 109:462, 1997.
124. Burman P, Karlsson FA, Loof L, et al: H^+,K^+-ATPase antibodies in autoimmune gastritis: Observations on the development of pernicious anemia. Scand J Gastroenterol 26:207, 1991.
125. Carmel R: Gastric juice in congenital pernicious anemia contains no immunoreactive intrinsic factor molecule: Study of three kindreds with variable ages at presentation, including a patient first diagnosed in adulthood. Am J Hum Genet 35:67, 1983.
126. Yang Y, Ducos R, Rosenberg AJ, et al: Cobalamin malabsorption in three siblings due to an abnormal intrinsic factor that is markedly susceptible to acid and proteolysis. J Clin Invest 76:2057, 1985.
127. Levine JS, Allen RH: Intrinsic factor within parietal cells of patients with juvenile pernicious anemia: A retrospective immunohistochemical study. Gastroenterology 88:1132, 1985.
128. Savarino V, Mela GS, Zentilin P, et al: Effect of *Helicobacter pylori* eradication on 24-hour gastric pH and duodenal gastric metaplasia. Dig Dis Sci 45:1315, 2000.
129. Iijima K, Ohara S, Sekine H, et al: Changes in gastric acid secretion assayed by endoscopic gastrin test before and after *Helicobacter pylori* eradication. Gut 46:20, 2000.
130. Molderings GJ, Burian M, Homann J, et al: Potential relevance of agmatine as a virulence factor of *Helicobacter pylori*. Dig Dis Sci 44: 2397, 1999.
131. Corleto VD, Minisola S, Moretti A, et al: Prevalence and causes of hypergastrinemia in primary hyperparathyroidism: A prospective study. J Clin Endocrinol Metab 84:4554, 1999.
132. Oksanen A, Sipponen P, Karttunen R, et al: Atrophic gastritis and *Helicobacter pylori* infection in outpatients referred for gastroscopy. Gut 46:460, 2000.
133. Haruma K, Mihara M, Okamoto E, et al: Eradication of *Helicobacter pylori* increases gastric acidity in patients with atrophic gastritis of the corpus—evaluation of 24-h pH monitoring. Aliment Pharmacol Ther 13:155, 1999.
134. Feldman M, Cryer B, Lee E: Effects of *Helicobacter pylori* gastritis on gastric secretion in normal human beings. Am J Physiol Gastrointest Liver Physiol 274:G1011, 1998.
135. Saperas E, Cominelli F, Taché Y: Potent inhibition of gastric acid

secretion by intravenous interleukin-1β and -1α in rats. Peptides 13: 221, 1992.
136. Herzlich BC, Schiano TD, Moussa Z, et al: Decreased intrinsic factor secretion in AIDS: Relation to parietal cell acid secretory capacity and vitamin B_{12} malabsorption. Am J Gastroenterol 87:1781, 1992.
137. Shaffer RT, LaHatte LJ, Kelly JW, et al: Gastric acid secretion in HIV-1 infection. Am J Gastroenterol 87:1777, 1992.
138. Eisig JN, Zaterka S, Boyd HK, et al: Hansen's disease and the digestive system: Clinical symptoms and gastric secretory profile at baseline conditions and following maximum stimulation with pentagastrin. Acta Leprol 11:99, 1999.
139. Nakajima H, Munakata A, Sasaki Y, Yoshida Y: pH profile of esophagus in patients with inlet patch of heterotopic gastric mucosa after tetragastrin stimulation: An endoscopic approach. Dig Dis Sci 38: 1915, 1993.
140. Feldman M, Burton ME: Histamine$_2$-receptor antagonists: Standard therapy for acid-peptic diseases. N Engl J Med 323:1672, 1749, 1990.

Chapter

39 HELICOBACTER PYLORI

Walter L. Peterson and David Y. Graham

Helicobacter pylori was brought to the world's attention in 1983 when Warren and Marshall, two Australian investigators, reported isolation of spiral organisms from mucosal biopsies of patients with chronic active gastritis.[1] First named *Campylobacter* ("curved rod") *pyloridis*, its name was changed to *Helicobacter pylori* when biochemical and genetic characterization of the organism showed that it was not a member of the *Campylobacter* genus. Microbiologists, particularly those working in the area of *Campylobacter*, took up the challenge, and there was an almost immediate outpouring of scientific papers that confirmed and extended the original observation. The gastroenterology community was slower to accept the hypothesis that a bacterium might be the cause of peptic ulcer disease. Proof was eventually forthcoming, and it is now acknowledged that *H. pylori* gastritis is the one of the most common human bacterial infectious diseases and is causally linked with gastritis, peptic ulcer disease, gastric adenocarcinoma, and gastric B-cell lymphoma.

H. pylori is a slow-growing, microaerophilic, highly motile, gram-negative spiral organism whose most striking biochemical characteristic is the abundant production of urease. This enzyme is one of several factors important for colonization and is an important indirect marker of the organism's presence, because it is the basis of biopsy rapid urease tests, the urea breath test, and as an antigen for serologic detection. *H. pylori* is tropic for gastric epithelium (i.e., stomach and areas of gastric metaplasia outside the stomach). A very small proportion of organisms can be found intracellularly, but the significance of this in relation to the inflammatory response and evasion of antimicrobial therapy is unclear. *H. pylori* infection elicits robust inflammatory and immune responses that are life-long unless the infection is cured.

EPIDEMIOLOGY

Prevalence in Healthy Individuals

The prevalence of *H. pylori* in otherwise healthy individuals varies depending on age, socioeconomic class, and country of origin (Fig. 39–1). The infection is usually acquired in childhood. In developing countries, children are typically infected by age 10 years, whereas in developed countries there is an age-related increase in prevalence. This represents a cohort phenomenon reflecting the steadily falling rate of acquisition of the infection during childhood as well as loss of the infection possibly owing to the widespread use of antibiotics.[2, 3] The prevalence of *H. pylori* in the United States has decreased in the white middle and upper class population 50 years of age or younger to approximately 10%, but the infection is still common among the socially disadvantaged and in the large immigrant population.[4] In developed countries, prevalence may vary among different ethnic groups of similar socioeconomic status (Fig. 39–2).[5] The explanation for these observations has both environmental and host genetic components.

Environmental Factors

Acquisition of *H. pylori* infection occurs primarily during childhood, with acquisition during adulthood occurring at a rate of only 0.3% to 0.5% a year. In developed countries the rate of loss of infection in any age group is equal to or greater than the rate of acquisition, leading to a decline in overall prevalence.[6–8] The major risk factor for infection is the socioeconomic status of the family during childhood (Fig. 39–3), as reflected in the number of persons in a household, sharing a bed, and absence of a fixed hot water supply, all of which probably are markers for the level of sanitation and household hygiene.[9–11] As the socioeconomic status of individuals and countries has risen, the prevalence in younger generations has declined.[12] The age-related apparent increase in the prevalence of the infection in developed countries (see Fig. 39–1) can best be explained by the "birth cohort effect." As successive generations have been less likely to become infected as children, these cohorts show a lower frequency of infection as adults. Improvement in socioeconomic status among blacks and Hispanics in the United States has lagged behind other groups and is one explanation why the overall prevalence of *H. pylori* in these

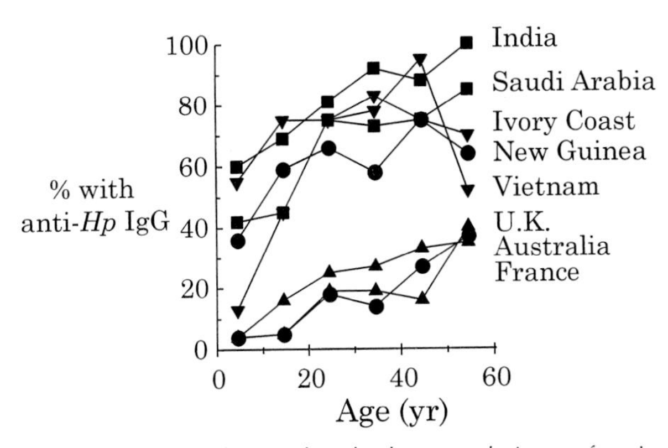

Figure 39–1. Seroprevalence of *Helicobacter pylori* as a function of age in developing countries (India, Saudi Arabia, Ivory Coast, New Guinea, Vietnam) and developed countries (United Kingdom, Australia, France). (Data from Graham DY, Adam E, Reddy GT, et al: Seroepidemiology of *Helicobacter pylori* infection in India: Comparison of developing and developed countries. Dig Dis Sci 36:1084–1088, 1991.)

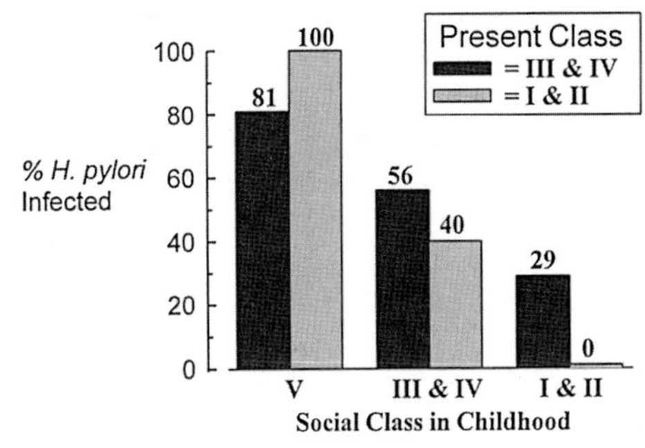

Figure 39–3. Seroprevalence of *Helicobacter pylori* in the United States as a function of social class during childhood and at the present. Income is highest in class I and lowest in class V. (From Malaty HM, Graham DY: Effect of childhood socioeconomic status on the current prevalence of *Helicobacter pylori* infection. Gut 35:742–745, 1994.)

groups is higher (see Fig. 39–2). Socioeconomic and sanitary conditions have improved even more slowly in developing countries, which is thought to account for the continuing high rates of infection in young people.

Genetic Factors

Genetic susceptibility to infection has been confirmed in studies showing that monozygotic twins reared apart or together had a higher rate of concordance of infection than did age-matched dizygotic twins.[13] This study confirmed older data showing a genetic effect in the *H. pylori*–related disease, peptic ulcer disease.[14]

Transmission of Infection

Evidence of *H. pylori* has been found in water using the polymerase chain reaction (PCR),[15] and there is strong epidemiologic evidence of waterborne transmission in Peru and Colombia. In countries where water treatment is advanced, this association has not been found despite studies that suggest the presence of *H. pylori* in groundwater, well water, or untreated wastewater in the United States, Canada, Japan, or Sweden.[16–19] With regard to a possible animal reservoir, the organism has been cultured from a colony of research cats[20] but has not been found in stray cats.[21] Sardinian shepherds were found to have a higher prevalence of *H. pylori* than their siblings despite living within the same household.[22] *H. pylori* was subsequently cultured from the milk and stomach of sheep in Sardinia.[23] Regardless of whether sheep are the ancestral host of *H. pylori*, the preponderance of data is consistent with the notion that the primary mode of transmission is person to person. Support for this concept comes from studies of children in institutions of custodial care, where prevalence is higher than expected[24] and from studies of families in which there is at least one infected child.[25, 26] Whether an infected child[25] or parent[26] is considered the index case, other family members are substantially more likely to be infected than family members of an uninfected person (Fig. 39–4).

The means by which *H. pylori* is transmitted among individuals is uncertain, and arguments can be made for and against each possibility. The possibility of fecal-oral transmission is supported by the detection of *H. pylori* in the stool by PCR[27] and culture[28, 29]; shedding of bacteria into the stool may be enhanced by diarrhea[30] or drugs that raise gastric pH.[31] Unfortunately, culture of *H. pylori* from stool

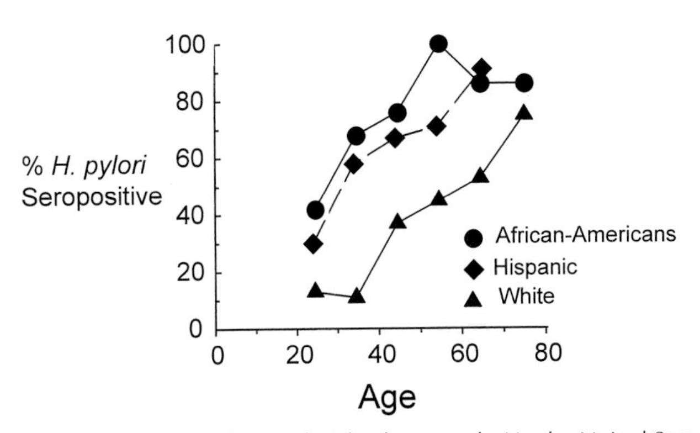

Figure 39–2. Seroprevalence of *Helicobacter pylori* in the United States as a function of age in asymptomatic African-Americans, Hispanics, and whites. (From Malaty HM, Evans DG, Evans DJJ, Graham DY: *Helicobacter pylori* in Hispanics: Comparison with blacks and whites of similar age and socioeconomic class. Gastroenterology 103:813–816, 1992.)

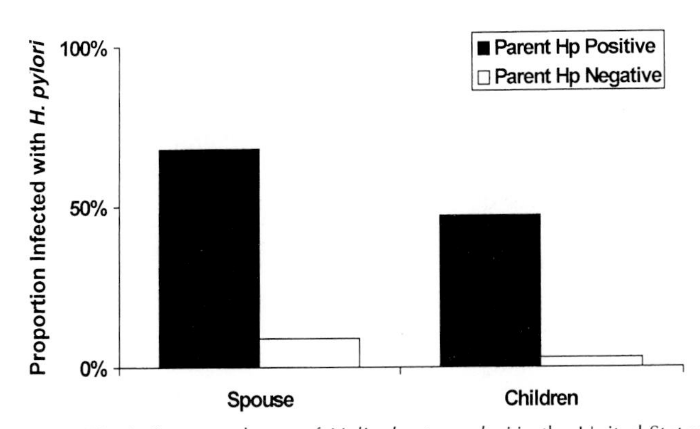

Figure 39–4. Seroprevalence of *Helicobacter pylori* in the United States in spouses and children of parents who are seropositive or seronegative for *H. pylori* infection. (From Malaty HM, Graham DY, Evans DG, et al: Transmission of *Helicobacter pylori* infection. Studies in families of healthy individuals. Scand J Gastroenterol 26:927–932, 1991.)

has proven difficult. A second possibility is oral-oral transmission. *H. pylori* has been found by culture and PCR in dental plaque and saliva.[32–34] Evidence against oral-oral transmission is that couples without children have a low prevalence of concordance of *H. pylori* infection[35] and that dentists and dental staff are not at increased risk of infection.[36]

A third potential means of transmission is gastro-oral.[37] Evidence to support such a model include well-described epidemics of *H. pylori* gastritis in volunteers undergoing gastric intubation experiments,[38, 39] transmission of infection from one patient to another by inadequately disinfected endoscopes,[40] and possibly a higher-than-expected prevalence of *H. pylori* infection in gastroenterologists, especially those who had not worn gloves in the past.[41] One means by which gastro-oral transmission could occur from child to child or child to parent in a natural setting is through contact with the vomitus, or a "spitting up," of an infected child.[28, 42] Although more work is needed to sort out this aspect of *H. pylori* epidemiology, it appears *H. pylori* is primarily an opportunist, such that any method by which *H. pylori* can obtain access to the stomach can potentially serve as a means of transmission. For prevention of transmission we need better understanding of the most common modes of transmission in children as well as identification of weak links in the transmission chain.

VIRULENCE FACTORS

Virulence factors of *H. pylori* may be divided into colonization factors and factors that are responsible for tissue injury (Table 39–1).

Colonization Factors

Colonization factors are those attributes of *H. pylori* that allow it to establish its presence in the stomach and to persist despite the body's attempts to rid itself of infection. These factors permit *H. pylori* to thrive in a niche that is inhospitable to virtually every other enteric organism.

Motility via Flagella

H. pylori possesses unipolar, sheathed flagella that, with its spiral shape, allow the organism to move quickly from the lumen of the stomach, where pH is low, through the mucus layer to an area where pH is near neutral to permit optimal growth. Mutant strains of *H. pylori* that are nonmotile will not colonize the gnotobiotic piglet, a well-described animal model for *H. pylori* infection.[43]

Table 39–1 | **Virulence Factors of *Helicobacter pylori* that Promote Colonization and Induce Tissue Injury**

Promote Colonization
Flagella (for motility)
Urease*
Adherence factors
Induce Tissue Injury
Lipopolysaccharide
Leukocyte recruitment and activating factors
Vacuolating cytotoxin (VacA)
Cytotoxin-associated antigen (CagA)
Outer membrane inflammatory protein (OipA)
Heat shock proteins (HspA, HspB)

*Not essential for colonization.

Urease

H. pylori is a more powerful producer of urease than almost any other bacterial species. This enzyme is not essential for colonization because urease-negative *H. pylori* have been cultured from patients with duodenal ulcer disease and have been used to successfully infect experimental animals. *H. pylori* can survive in acidic nutrient media without urea, suggesting that it has multiple mechanisms for survival in acid and that production of ammonia via urease is only one.[44] Other roles for urease may be by providing an essential nitrogen source for *H. pylori* protein synthesis (via urea hydrolysis). It has recently been learned that the activity of intrabacterial urease increases as the ambient pH is lowered, probably through a change in membrane permeability at lower pH levels that allows urea access to urease. The critical factor underlying this phenomenon is believed to be UreI, a 21-kd membrane protein that functions as a proton gated urea channel.[45, 46]

Adherence Factors

The ability of *H. pylori* to bind specifically to gastric-type epithelium is termed *tissue tropism,* a property that prevents the organism from being shed during cell and mucus turnover.[47] Adherence may also be important in targeting toxins and leukocyte recruitment factors in host epithelium.[47, 48] An *N*-acetylneuraminyllactose-binding fibrillar hemagglutinin has been described for *H. pylori,* as has a specific gastric glycerolipid receptor on gastric mucosal cells.[49, 50] Tight attachment of the fibrillar adhesin on the bacterium to the carbohydrate receptor on the mucosal cell results in the formation of an attaching-effacing lesion (adherence pedestal), which in turn leads to actin polymerization and possibly epithelial cell disruption.[51–53] Failure of adherence results in less epithelial cell injury.[54] As with most pathogens, there are a number of adhesins, and the redundancy of the system has prevented the strategy of using antiadhesins for successful therapy. Differences in the availability of specific receptors has been suggested as one means to explain genetic differences in susceptibility to infection with *H. pylori.*[55]

Factors Mediating Tissue Injury

(see Chapter 2)

Lipopolysaccharide

Lipopolysaccharides are a family of glycolipids found in the cell envelope of gram-negative bacteria, including *H. pylori.*[56] Because they are bound to the bacterium, they are also called *endotoxins.* Lipopolysaccharides, primarily through the lipid A component, stimulate the release of cytokines and possess endotoxic properties. Other actions of lipopolysaccharides include interference with the gastric epithelial cell–laminin interaction, which may lead to loss of mucosal integrity; inhibition of mucin synthesis; and stimulation of pepsinogen secretion.[56] Despite the general toxicity of endotoxins, the lipid A of *H. pylori* is substantially less potent than the lipid A of *Escherichia coli*, which may account for the organism's adaptation for long-term residence in the stomach.

Other Leukocyte Recruitment and Activating Factors

H. pylori elaborates a number of lipopolysaccharide-independent soluble surface proteins with chemotactic properties to recruit monocytes and neutrophils to the lamina propria and to activate these inflammatory cells.[57–60] These include *H. pylori* neutrophil-activating protein,[60] expressed by the *nap A* gene, and the immunologically active porins.[59]

Vacuolating Cytotoxin (VacA)

Approximately 50% of *H. pylori* strains produce a substance that induces vacuole formation in eukaryotic cells.[61] The protein responsible for vacuolation (VacA) has been purified and the gene encoding the toxin (*vacA*) has been cloned.[62] This gene encodes a 140,000 molecular weight protein that is processed to a mature toxin of 90 kd. All strains of *H. pylori* possess the *vacA* gene, but only about 50% express the mature toxin. Studies in mice have demonstrated that supernatants from *H. pylori* strains expressing the toxin, but not those without, cause severe acute superficial mucosal injury.[63] No clinical correlation with this observation has yet been described.

The *vacA* gene has been further characterized.[64] The gene has two families of alleles of the middle region (m1,m2) and at least three families of alleles of the signal sequence (s1a,s1b,s2). Strains with the s2m2 genotype produce little or no toxin.[62, 65] The vacA genotype s1 is strongly, but not exclusively, associated with the presence of *cagA* (see later). Overall, studies with more than 1500 strains have not supported the notion of an important role for vacA genotyping in relation to cytotoxin activity, virulence, histologic findings, or risk of a particular *H. pylori* disease.[65]

Cytotoxin-Associated Antigen (CagA)

CagA, a 120- to 140-kd molecular weight highly antigenic protein, is encoded by the *cagA* gene that is part of the *cag* pathogenicity island.[66] In Western countries 60% to 80% of *H. pylori* have an intact *cag* pathogenicity island, whereas in Asia, more than 90% of isolates express CagA.[65] The presence of the *cag* pathogenicity island is associated with a more prominent inflammatory tissue response than is seen with strains lacking this virulence factor.[64] The increase in inflammation is associated with an increased risk of developing a symptomatic outcome of the infection such as peptic ulcer disease, and adenocarcinoma.[67] Nonetheless, *H. pylori* without the *cag* pathogenicity island have been isolated from patients with peptic ulcer and with gastric cancer showing that increased risk is not the same as being able to predict outcome. For example, in Japan approximately 95% of strains express CagA regardless of whether the presentation is asymptomatic gastritis or one of the symptomatic diseases associated with *H. pylori*.[65, 68] The *cag* pathogenicity island is now known to be a type IV secretory apparatus that actually injects CagA into mammalian cells.[69] CagA undergoes phosphorylation and is responsible for the changes in actin polymerization seen in the infected cell. Knockout of CagA prevents the cytoskeletal changes but not the enhanced inflammatory response that is mediated through NF-κB. Attachment is required for *cag* pathogenicity island positive *H. pylori* to elicit an interleukin-8 (IL-8) response from cell lines in vitro.

Outer Membrane Inflammatory Protein (OipA)

OipA is a 34-kd outer membrane protein that along with the *cag* pathogenicity island is associated with an enhanced inflammatory response in the mucosa.[70] The presence of the *cag* pathogenicity island and OipA leads to a more marked inflammatory response than does either alone. The molecular mechanism of this interaction is as yet unknown. In Japan OipA is almost universally present in strains with the *cag* pathogenicity island, whereas in Western strains, especially those from patients with latent and asymptomatic gastritis, it is present in less than one half of cases.[70]

Heat Shock Proteins

H. pylori expresses two heat shock proteins (HspA and HspB).[71] They are highly antigenic, but their role in the pathogenesis of infection remains unknown. HspA binds nickel ions and is a chaperonin.

In summary, gastric inflammation is present whenever *H. pylori* is present. No putative virulence factor has demonstrated an all-or-none or even a tight association with any of the different diseases etiologically associated with the infection. The differences described to date have been in degree. The fact that in populations the prevalence of symptomatic outcomes such as gastric cancer has declined, whereas the prevalence of the *cag* pathogenicity island has not, suggests that the host, environment, and bacterium all interact to produce clinical disease. *H. pylori* research is still in the information-gathering and hypothesis-generating phase. Although no clear breakthroughs are evident, it is recognized that cure of the infection results in healing of gastritis and cure of peptic ulcer disease.

ACUTE INFECTION

Acute infection with *H. pylori* has been observed in a number of individuals.[72–75] In two cases, investigators themselves knowingly ingested a culture of *H. pylori* after endoscopic biopsy had confirmed absence of preexisting infection.[72–74] Both subjects developed a neutrophilic gastritis and, in one, fasting gastric pH was above 7.0 from days 8 to 39 after ingestion. Another individual, a clinical investigator working with gastric juice, developed an illness characterized by epigastric pain and nausea. On the fifth day of illness an endoscopic biopsy disclosed a neutrophilic gastritis and culture grew *H. pylori*.[75] Although this individual did not have a baseline endoscopic examination, seroconversion occurred between days 14 and 74. Fasting gastric pH was above 7.0

on days 14 and 37 but fell to 2.0 on day 74. The earliest effect of the infection appears to be an increase in basal acid secretion that is followed by reduction in acid secretion.[76] It appears likely that the fall in acid secretion correlates best with the degree of inflammation in the corpus of the stomach.

The neutrophilic gastritis with transient hypochlorhydria observed in these subjects is reminiscent of cases noted in several research laboratories during the 1970s and 1980s.[38, 77] In one of these outbreaks, 17 of 37 healthy volunteers participating in acid secretory studies and 1 patient with Zollinger-Ellison syndrome became rapidly and profoundly hypochlorhydric.[77] Nine of the 17 volunteers who became hypochlorhydric had noted a 1- to 4-day illness consisting of mild to moderate epigastric pain accompanied by nausea in 4 and vomiting in 2. Biopsies of the gastric body in 12 of the hypochlorhydric subjects invariably revealed severe neutrophilic gastritis. Short-term follow-up showed lessening of the severity of gastritis and return of acid secretion to near baseline levels in 14 of the 17 hypochlorhydric volunteers within a mean of 4 months. Despite an intensive search for an etiologic agent, none was found at the time.

Following the recognition of *H. pylori*, the investigators involved reviewed the original biopsy material and found *H. pylori* organisms in 7 of 12 subjects. Additionally, serum samples stored from before, during, and after hypochlorhydria were tested for IgG and IgM antibodies to *H. pylori*.[39] Data from these studies strongly suggest that, in retrospect, these cases of acute gastritis with hypochlorhydria were temporally related to acute infection with *H. pylori*. Biopsies in 5 of the 12 subjects showed intense gastritis but no evidence of *H. pylori*. In four of these, convalescent biopsies were positive for *H. pylori* or IgG seroconversion occurred. It may well be that the intensity of the inflammatory reaction and/or the hypochlorhydria led to temporary suppression of the organisms. As the host and the organism reached a state of equilibrium, the intensity of inflammation decreased and acid secretion returned.

CHRONIC INFECTION

It is not known how often acute infection with *H. pylori* spontaneously clears. Studies in children suggest that spontaneous loss of infection may be common.[4] Infection in adults appears to be typically long lived and is probably life-long.[39] Most infected individuals have chronic active, nonatrophic, superficial gastritis (Fig. 39–5). This histologic form of *H. pylori* gastritis is usually asymptomatic but may be associated with duodenal ulcer disease (see Chapter 40) and a number of other putative abnormalities. Chronic atrophic gastritis (see Chapter 43), gastric adenocarcinoma (see Chapter 44), or gastric lymphoma (see Chapters 26 and 44) are less frequent outcomes of the infection.

Chronic Nonatrophic (Superficial) Gastritis

(see also Chapter 43)

Histologic Manifestations

Antral biopsies of individuals infected with *H. pylori* show focal epithelial cell damage as well as an inflammatory infiltrate in the lamina propria[78] (see Fig. 43–3). This infiltrate consists of polymorphonuclear leukocytes, eosinophils, and mononuclear cells. The latter include B and T lymphocytes and typically includes development of lymphoid follicles,[80] monocytes, and plasma cells. The lymphocytic component of the inflammatory response is referred to as mucosa-associated lymphoid tissue. Although biopsies from individuals not infected with *H. pylori* have occasional aggregates of lymphocytes at the junction of the glandular mucosa and the muscularis mucosa, lymphoid follicles are rarely, if ever, found.[79] Biopsies from the gastric body also usually demonstrate inflammation but typically the inflammation is somewhat less severe than in the antrum. In patients with duodenal ulcer the gastritis is typically severe in the antrum and moderate, mild, or even absent in the corpus.[80, 81]

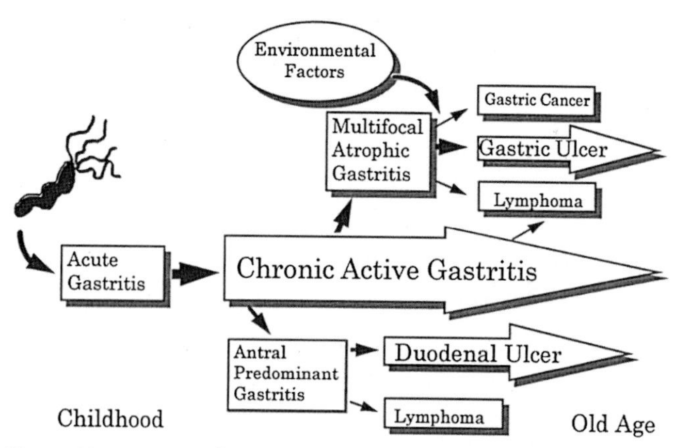

Figure 39–5. Proposed natural history of *Helicobacter pylori* infection in humans.

Pathogenesis of Inflammation

H. pylori stimulates the release of a variety of inflammatory mediators both directly by bacterial products such as vacuolating cytotoxin, lipopolysaccharide, neutrophil-activating factor, and porins and indirectly as a result of interaction with gastric epithelial cells.[48, 82] In general, the inflammatory response requires attachment of the bacteria to host epithelium. Most recent research has focused on the release of the inflammatory cytokine, IL-8, and the recruitment and activation of neutrophils. In addition there is the generation of reactive oxygen metabolites and the up-regulation of neutrophil expression of CD11b/CD18.[48] The latter enhances CAM-1-dependent neutrophil adherence. With neutrophil adhesion comes changes in microvascular permeability and mast cell degranulation. This rich mixture of cytokines may also play a role in down-regulating somatostatin, thereby leading to enhanced gastrin release (see later). Conceptually and practically, *H. pylori* infection is a chronic bacterial infection on a mucosal surface.

Physiologic Manifestations of Inflammation

Numerous studies have consistently shown that mean fasting serum gastrin levels are 35% to 45% higher in normal subjects infected with *H. pylori* than in uninfected controls.[83–85] The gastrin response to meals in healthy subjects has been studied using in vivo intragastric titration.[83, 84] When intragastric pH was maintained by titration at pH 5.0 or 7.0, there were substantially and significantly higher mean postprandial gastrin responses to the meals in *H. pylori*–infected subjects than in negative controls. When the intragastric titration pH was lowered to 2.5, as would occur in the natural state as acid is secreted in response to a meal, there was almost complete (95%) suppression of meal-stimulated gastrin release in uninfected subjects.[84] By contrast, infected subjects exhibited only a 52% suppression of gastrin release at pH 2.5, significantly less than the uninfected subjects.

Infusion of gastrin-releasing peptide (GRP), the mammalian analog of bombesin, activates many of the stimulatory (and inhibitory) mechanisms elicited by meals and has been used by some investigators as a surrogate for meal studies.[86] As gastrin is released and acid is secreted, gastric pH falls. It, therefore, accomplishes in a less cumbersome manner what is achieved by changing the intragastric titration pH of a meal from 7.0 to 2.5.[84] In one study, the median plasma gastrin concentration after GRP infusion in *H. pylori*–infected normal subjects was more than three times that which occurred in noninfected controls.[85] Elimination of *H. pylori* restored fasting and GRP-stimulated serum gastrin to levels found in noninfected subjects.[85] Gastrin and somatostatin are regulated in opposite directions. *H. pylori* enhances gastrin release and reduces somatostatin release. These phenomena appear to be related to the presence of the inflammatory response, although the exact details are still lacking.

The pattern of acid secretion in response to a meal or to GRP mirrors that of the gastrin response. When meal-stimulated acid secretion is measured by in vivo titration at a high pH (5.0 to 7.0), no differences are seen between infected and noninfected normal subjects.[83, 84] However, when carried out at a pH of 2.5, infected subjects have a significantly higher acid response to the meal than noninfected controls.[84] This reflects a failure of normal inhibition of acid output at low pH in *H. pylori*–infected subjects, a situation analogous to that with serum gastrin (see earlier). Similar results have been noted using GRP[85]; the median acid output to 40 pmol/kg per hour GRP was three times greater in *H. pylori*–infected normal subjects. Because gastric pH falls in response to GRP-stimulated acid output, this may again reflect impairment by *H. pylori* of "normal" inhibition of acid output at low pH. Differences between the groups remain when GRP is given in doses high enough to elicit maximum acid output (MAO).[85] The findings with GRP and bombesin are related to an upward shift in the dose response to these stimuli. *H. pylori*–infected individuals produce approximately 90% of their MAO compared with about 30% in those without *H. pylori* infection. Following cure of the infection, both duodenal ulcer patients and those with *H. pylori* infection but without ulcer disease return to the normal pattern of GRP-stimulated acid secretion (about 30% of MAO).[85] *H. pylori*–infected patients with duodenal ulcer (see Chapter 40) have fasting and GRP-stimulated gastrin levels similar to normal subjects infected with the organism.[85] Acid secretory values, on the other hand, are different. Compared with *H. pylori*–infected normal subjects, *H. pylori*–infected patients with duodenal ulcer have significantly higher basal acid output (BAO), peak acid output (PAO), and GRP-stimulated acid secretion.[85] When measured 1 year after successful therapy of the infection, basal and GRP-stimulated acid secretion had normalized. Whether PAO falls after cure of *H. pylori* infection remains an area of controversy, but it seems that in most successfully treated patients, there is either no change or a minor fall, suggesting that the abnormality possibly predated the infection or that increases in parietal cell mass are not reversible.

Although abnormalities have been noted in meal- or GRP-stimulated acid secretion, BAO in *H. pylori*–infected normal subjects has been reported to be not significantly different from uninfected subjects in one series,[87] significantly higher in another[85] and somewhat lower in two other series.[83, 84] PAO or MAO to exogenous gastrin or pentagastrin is not significantly different in normal subjects infected with *H. pylori* compared with uninfected controls.[83–85, 87] One variable that must be considered in interpreting studies of acid secretion in normal subjects infected with *H. pylori* is the degree of corpus inflammation. The effect of gastritis on gastric secretion was studied repeatedly from the mid-1950s through the early 1970s. Although the studies were often hampered by the inability to obtain gastric mucosal biopsies from precise gastric locations, the results consistently showed that gastric secretion was inversely related to the presence and severity of corpus gastritis[88] and demonstrated an inverse relationship between MAO and the degree of corpus damage. A number of recent studies have confirmed the older observations and have shown that cure of the *H. pylori* infection and resolution in gastric inflammation are associated with a marked increase in acid secretion.[89] This is in contrast with patients with antral predominant gastritis and duodenal ulcer, where stimulated acid secretion either does not change or decreases slightly after cure of the infection. It has become evident that interpretation of the effect of *H. pylori* on gastric secretory physiology requires simultaneous assessment of the pattern and severity of gastritis.

Clinical Conditions Associated with Chronic, Nonatrophic Gastritis

The most readily accepted condition associated with chronic active, nonatrophic gastritis is duodenal ulcer disease (see Chapter 40). However, there have been a number of other conditions suggested as causally related to *H. pylori* gastritis (Table 39–2). A careful review of the data supporting these associations has recently been published.[90] In virtually every instance, such data are weak, having been obtained in uncontrolled, nonrandomized studies that did not control for factors that might be common to both *H. pylori* infection and the disease of interest. Many of these associations are suggested to be related to effects of *H. pylori* on coagulation

Table 39–2 | **Nongastrointestinal Tract Diseases Possibly Associated with *Helicobacter pylori* Infection**

Iron deficiency anemia	Autoimmune thrombocytopenic purpura
Coronary artery disease	Hyperammonemia
Cerebrovascular disease	Sudden infant death syndrome
Hypertension	Growth retardation
Raynaud phenomenon	Anorexia of aging
Migraine headaches	Rosacea
Vomiting of pregnancy	Chronic urticaria

From Leontiadis GI, Sharma VK, Howden CW: Non-gastrointestinal tract associations of *Helicobacter pylori* infection. Arch Intern Med 159:925–940, 1999.

and markers of systemic inflammation, although data to support even these physiologic manifestations are weak. In other instances a plausible biologic rationale is absent. Finally, treatment trials, especially randomized, controlled trials, are unavailable. One condition that has been assessed by a treatment trial, albeit uncontrolled, is iron deficiency.[91] Twenty-four patients with long-standing iron deficiency anemia were successfully treated for *H. pylori* and at 12 months' follow-up. Most (92%) were found to have resolved their anemia without further iron supplementation.

Chronic Atrophic Gastritis

(see also Chapter 43)

In some individuals, chronic superficial *H. pylori* gastritis progresses over time to atrophic gastritis (see Fig. 43–3), with an annual increase in prevalence among otherwise normal subjects of 1% to 3%.[92–95] Such progression leads to three patterns of atrophic gastritis: body predominant (diffuse corporal atrophic gastritis), antral predominant atrophic gastritis, and both body and antrum atrophy (multifocal atrophic gastritis). In one study, the relative proportions of these patterns was 31%, 45%, and 24%.[96] The pattern of development of chronic atrophic gastritis correlates well with the pattern of superficial gastritis (i.e., antral-predominant superficial gastritis progresses to antral-predominant atrophic gastritis). As the degree of atrophy progresses, the presence of active *H. pylori* infection appears to decrease, probably related to the transformation of the stomach lining from the *H. pylori*–friendly normal superficial epithelial cells to intestinal metaplasia on which *H. pylori* are infrequently found. Hypochlorhydria may also create an uninviting milieu for the organism because in the absence of acid, other organisms can survive in the stomach and provide competition. Because *H. pylori* has been found in stomachs with achlorhydria, it is unlikely that decreased acid secretion alone is the critical variable. Although the ability to detect *H. pylori* histologically is impaired in these patients, antibodies to *H. pylori* are often present and the titer may decline after empiric treatment, suggesting that *H. pylori* may actually still be present in low numbers.

The mechanism by which the gastric mucosal damage progresses from superficial gastritis to atrophy is unclear and is probably multifactorial. The major factor may be environmental because the proportion of the infected population varies remarkably in different geographic areas (e.g., Peru vs. United States). The environmental factor may also be differences in characteristics of the primary type of *H. pylori* circulating in the region. Another possibility is the presence of *H. pylori* antibodies that cross-react with gastric autoantigens.[97] Because cure of the infection results in healing of the gastritis, the presence of autoantibodies cannot explain the whole process.

The speed with which chronic superficial gastritis progresses to atrophic gastritis of the body and fundus varies with different clinical situations. Patients with duodenal ulcer virtually never develop body atrophic gastritis and, as a result, maintain robust acid secretion.[98–101] On the other hand, patients with gastric ulcer,[99, 102] duodenal ulcer patients after vagotomy,[103, 104] and perhaps patients on long-term proton pump inhibitors (PPIs)[105] exhibit more rapid progression. Other investigators have reported that although PPIs increase the degree of gastritis, at least in the short term they do not lead to actual atrophy.[106–109] A unifying hypothesis for this phenomenon is based on the observation that *H. pylori* has impaired ability to cause inflammation in regions of the stomach where gastric secretion is high.[110–112] This is consistent with older observations that individuals with robust acid secretion have relative sparing of the proximal stomach and slow or absent progression to corpus atrophy.[113] The hypothesis also suggests that long-term antisecretory therapy would allow the development of corpus gastritis to proceed at the normal or an accelerated rate. Progression of gastritis from the antrum to the corpus leads to a reduction in acid output, and if this occurs naturally or in association with antisecretory drug therapy, one would expect that an increasing percentage of duodenal ulcers would "burn out" when the ability to secrete acid fell below the critical level required to sustain the ulcer. This burn-out of duodenal ulcers has been reported but is unlikely to be common. Because of the data suggesting an increase in the degree of body atrophic gastritis, a risk factor for gastric adenocarcinoma, in *H. pylori*–infected individuals who are receiving long-term acid-suppressive therapy (e.g., for severe gastroesophageal reflux disease), it has been suggested that such patients be tested for *H. pylori* and treated if tests are positive.[114, 115]

Body-predominant atrophic gastritis is associated with pernicious anemia. Such patients have antibodies directed against the proton pump and pepsinogen.[116] In these patients, loss of secretory function begins with acid, followed by pepsinogen, and, finally, intrinsic factor. Pernicious anemia is thus a marker for the most severe, end-stage form of diffuse corporal atrophic gastritis. There has been a long-held belief that the pathogenesis of chronic atrophic gastritis associated with pernicious anemia is "autoimmune," because (1) there are antibodies to the secretory elements and (2) pernicious anemia is associated with other autoimmune diseases. Furthermore, the prevalence of *H. pylori* is low by both tissue staining and serum antibodies, suggesting not even a remote infection with the organism.[117] Although the concept is now being challenged, the marked regional variation in the prevalence of pernicious anemia suggests that the genetics of the host play a critical role. Pernicious anemia is also found in areas where *H. pylori* is uncommon (e.g., near Rochester, Minnesota). Nevertheless, pernicious anemia can occur as a consequence of chronic *H. pylori* infection. *H. pylori*–related pernicious anemia is typically associated with multifocal atrophic gastritis and thus differs from typical autoimmune pernicious anemia in which the antral mucosa is normal.[118]

DIAGNOSIS

Diagnostic tests for *H. pylori* may be divided into those that do and those that do not require samples of gastric mucosa. Although tissue is generally obtained by endoscopic biopsy, modestly less invasive methods are available such as the use of a small bowel biopsy tube or capsule, or a biopsy forceps can be passed directly through a modified nasogastric tube positioned either in the gastric body or antrum to obtain a specimen.[119] Generally, biopsy is unnecessary unless one wishes to isolate the organism for antibiotic sensitivity testing. Successful culture requires an experienced laboratory.

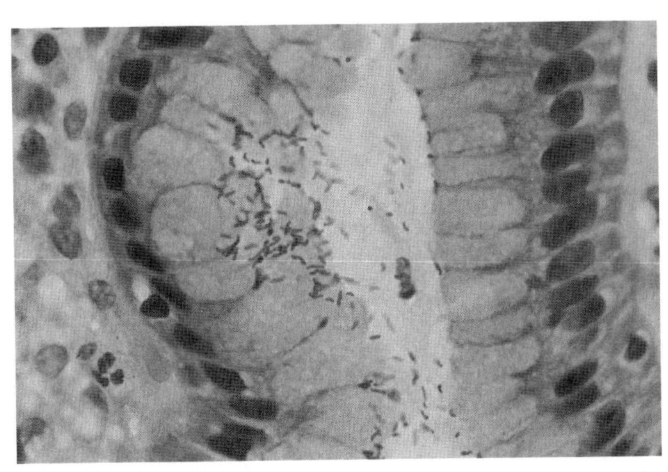

Figure 39–6. Photomicrographs of biopsy specimen, stained with the Genta stain, from a patient with *Helicobacter pylori* gastritis. The bacteria are well seen. (Courtesy of Dr. Robert Genta, Baylor College of Medicine, Houston, TX.)

Mucosal biopsy and histologic examination of the specimen for the presence of *H. pylori* and/or gastritis has been the diagnostic method of choice until recently. Recommendations to maximize diagnostic yield include the use of large-cup biopsy forceps, obtaining at least three samples (from the lesser curve angularis, the greater curve prepyloric antrum, and the greater curve body), proper mounting and preparation of the samples, and use of an appropriate stain.[120] The standard hematoxylin and eosin (H&E) stain is excellent to determine histologic chronic or chronic active inflammation (gastritis) and demonstrates *H. pylori* if large numbers of organisms are present. A special stain (e.g., silver stain) is better at detecting the organism if small numbers of bacteria are present but does not show tissue histology to advantage. Attributes of both the H&E and a special stain are found in the Genta and El-Zimaity "triple" stains, which combine the H&E stain, *H. pylori* selective stains, and Alcian blue (Fig. 39–6).[121] The El-Zimaity stain and the El-Zimaity modifications of the Genta stain can be performed on an autostainer and are thus practical for the routine laboratory. One of these two triple stains is recommended when there is a low density of bacteria, a small biopsy specimen, abundant debris or mucus on the gastric surface and pits, or extensive intestinal metaplasia. The alternative is to use two different stains; a combination of an H&E and a Diff-Quik is probably the best alternative.

Mucosal biopsies may also be tested for the presence of urease by agar gel slide tests, such as the CLOtest or *hp*fast, or by the membrane test, PyloriTek. Rapid urease tests consist of a urea-rich medium with a pH-sensitive dye. If urease is present in the mucosal biopsy, it catalyzes the hydrolysis of urea into ammonia and carbon dioxide.[122] The resultant increase in pH of the medium from ammonia generation changes the color of the indicator. Recommendations to maximize the rapidity and sensitivity of rapid urease tests are to warm the slide and to use two regular or one jumbo biopsy specimen(s). Although the PyloriTek test should be read no later than 2 hours after placement of the biopsy on the membrane, the agar gel tests may take up to 24 hours to turn positive, particularly in the presence of a low bacterial density. Recent use of antibiotics, bismuth, or PPIs may render rapid urease tests falsely negative. The relative accuracy of acute or chronic inflammation on histology, the Warthin-Starry silver stain, and the CLO test in the diagnosis of *H. pylori* infection is compared in Table 39–3.[123] The silver stain had the best combination of sensitivity and specificity. Rapid urease tests have specificity and sensitivity of greater than 90% but false-positive results do occur. Rapid urease testing is the least expensive, an excellent screening test, and the diagnostic test of first choice when an ulcer is present. Mucosal biopsies can be saved and, if the rapid urease test is negative, sent the next day for histologic assessment. Because of the excellent results of rapid urease testing, one can use the results as a rough guide of the accuracy of the pathologist. If there are many discrepancies, it behooves one to meet with his or her pathologist and resolve why.

Many endoscopists erroneously believe that a diagnosis of *H. pylori* gastritis can be made by the gross appearance of the gastric mucosa at endoscopy. Results of the one study that has examined this hypothesis critically suggest that antral nodularity has a positive predictive value of 90% but a sensitivity of only 32%.[124] The best endoscopic predictor is the presence of an ulcer, but as there are other causes of ulcer disease, a diagnostic test for *H. pylori* should always be employed.

Tests that do not require a mucosal biopsy include serologic tests, urea breath tests, and the stool antigen test. Chronic *H. pylori* infection elicits a circulating IgG antibody response that can be quantitatively measured by enzyme-linked immunosorbent assay (ELISA) tests.[125–127] Tests for IgA or IgM antibodies are unreliable, so only IgG antibodies should be determined. Serologic tests are as sensitive and specific as biopsy-based methods (see Table 39–3) and have been adapted for rapid use in the office. In-the-office tests are also available that use whole blood instead of serum.[128] Although it is possible to detect antibodies to *H. pylori* in saliva, gingival transudate, and urine, no reliable tests are yet commercially available in the United States.

Serologic tests are useful for the initial diagnosis of *H. pylori* infection but are less useful to confirm cure after antimicrobial therapy. Although it has been reported that a fall in antibody titers of 20% or more 6 months after completion of therapy may be sensitive in confirming cure of the infection,[129] it is not a practical method. Paired specimens are required (i.e., "before" serum specimens must be frozen

Table 39–3 | **Accuracy of Diagnostic Tests for *Helicobacter pylori***

PARAMETER	PERCENTAGES			
	Sens.	Spec.	PPV	NPV
Chronic inflammation	100	66	84	100
Acute inflammation	87	94	96	80
Warthin-Starry silver stain	93	99	99	89
Rapid urease test	90	100	100	84
Serum IgG antibody	91	97	95	85
Urea breath test	90	96	98	84

Sens., sensitivity; Spec., specificity; PPV, positive predictive value; NPV, negative predictive value; IgG, immunoglobulin G.

From Cutler AF, Havstad S, Ma CK, et al: Accuracy of invasive and noninvasive tests to diagnose *Helicobacter pylori* infection. Gastroenterology 109:136–141, 1995.

and stored to be run at the same time as "after" specimens), and testing must be delayed at least 6 months after therapy. A negative ELISA test, if performed at least 18 months after eradication therapy, has been reported to be 60% sensitive and 100% specific for successful eradication.[130] This may be of use if a patient reports taking a course of antimicrobial therapy in the distant past and the physician wishes to determine if *H. pylori* infection has been cured.

Urea breath tests use urea labeled with either ^{13}C or ^{14}C that is ingested.[131] If urease is present in the stomach as a consequence of *H. pylori* infection, labeled carbon dioxide will be split off and absorbed into the circulation where its presence can be determined by analysis of expired breath (Fig. 39–7). This test is quite accurate, although small numbers of organisms may not produce enough urease to be detected by the urea breath test (i.e., a false-negative result). ^{13}C-labeled urea has the advantage of not being radioactive but requires a mass spectrometer for analysis. ^{14}C-labeled urea can be measured with a scintillation counter but does expose the individual to a small, long-lasting dose of radioactivity. These tests are the preferred means of evaluating the success of antimicrobial therapy in clinical practice, although the test should not be conducted unless the patient has been off PPIs for at least 7 days. If not, one third of patients infected with *H. pylori* will have false-negative tests.[132] A ^{13}C-urea blood test provides diagnostic accuracy comparable with a ^{13}C-urea breath test.[133, 134]

Another new, noninvasive diagnostic test is a stool antigen test (HpSA test). Overall, studies using pretreatment *H. pylori* stool antigen tests have shown that the sensitivity and specificity of the test were comparable to histology or urea breath testing.[135] Other studies have reported less satisfactory results, and the optimum cut-off values for optical density have varied among studies. It has become evident that there may be considerable lot-to-lot variation in the stool antigen tests. The most likely explanation is that the polyclonal sera used to capture antibody is obtained from rabbits and thus difficult to standardize. Stool antigen testing has proven to be less reliable when used soon after the end of therapy, and it is now generally recommended that one must wait longer (e.g., up to 12 weeks) to reliably confirm eradication.[136] The concept of a stool antigen test is a good one, and several companies have tests in trial that use monoclonal antibodies. This test is susceptible to inaccuracy during concomitant administration of PPIs.[137–139]

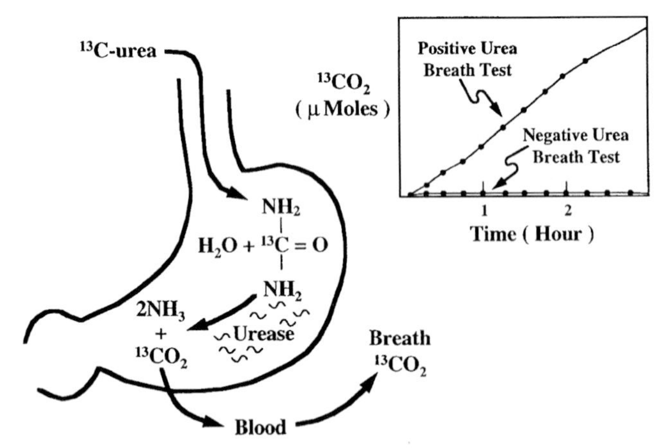

Figure 39–7. The urea breath test. (Reprinted with permission of the *New England Journal of Medicine* and the Massachusetts Medical Society, from Walsh JH, Peterson WL: Drug therapy: The treatment of *Helicobacter pylori* infection in the management of peptic ulcer disease. N Engl J Med 333:984–991, 1995. All rights reserved.)

Diagnostic Strategy

The selection of the appropriate test for a given patient depends on the clinical situation. The basic premise is that the diagnosis of an active *H. pylori* infection should be followed by therapy. For patients in whom an endoscopy is clinically indicated to diagnose or treat a peptic ulcer, it is reasonable at the same time to obtain mucosal biopsies for a rapid urease test and, if necessary, histology. A rapid urease test is the least expensive of the biopsy tests and should be performed first; extra biopsies from normal-appearing mucosa should be taken and can be held for submission for histologic examination if the rapid urease test is negative. Culturing for antibiotic susceptibility testing is not currently widely available but may become necessary if the frequency of resistance to metronidazole or clarithromycin increases and to select the appropriate therapy for those who fail therapy.

For patients in whom endoscopy is not indicated for other clinical reasons, endoscopy should not be performed solely to diagnose infection with *H. pylori*. Serologic tests are quick, inexpensive, and reliable; they are the initial screening test of choice. If concern remains that a positive serologic test may be only a "scar" from prior infection and does not accurately reflect the current status, a urea breath test or stool antigen can document the presence of active infection. Currently, screening of asymptomatic individuals is only recommended by the authors for first-degree relatives of patients with gastric cancer or peptic ulcer disease. If the pretest probability of *H. pylori* infection is high (e.g., a patient with a peptic ulcer), false-positive tests are rare, but if the pretest probability is low (e.g., an asymptomatic population in a developed country), false-positive tests are more likely.[140] False-negative results are rare. Therefore, when screening for latent *H. pylori* infection in an asymptomatic population, positive tests should be confirmed (e.g., urea breath test or stool antigen) before starting therapy.

TREATMENT

Cure of *H. pylori* infection is not easy and requires combinations of antibiotics often with additional nonantibiotic adjunctive agents; single agents are ineffective. In some settings cure rates in the range of 95% to 100% have been achieved. Therefore, *H. pylori* infection should be thought of in the same light as other serious, but curable, bacterial infections such as tuberculosis. The general rule for such infections is that one expects a cure rate of greater than 95% when treating antibiotic-susceptible organisms. Research into the antibiotic therapy of *H. pylori* infection has largely been done by gastroenterologists. The difficulty in identifying a truly successful regimen resulted in acceptance of cure rates that are much lower than desired. For example, a number of recent meta-analyses have shown that the most commonly used therapies produce cure rates in the range of 80%.[141–143] One of the problems has been that pretreatment antibiotic susceptibility testing has not been routinely performed and, therefore, the proportion of failures due to resistant organisms is unknown. In addition, there are few head-to-head studies of antibiotic dose or duration of therapy such that the parameters required for a truly successful therapy remain unknown. Observations that have emerged from the treatment trials include the following:

1. Results from different studies of what outwardly appears to the same drug combination can vary enormously. Only regimens that give consistent results from country to country and study to study should be used.
2. Successful cure of infection requires at least two antimicrobial agents.
3. The duration of therapy required to yield a high cure rate is unknown. Generally, 1 week of therapy is less effective than longer durations.[144]
4. Antibiotic resistance leads to reduced efficacy with that antibiotic.
5. Compliance is important for successful cure of the infection. Thus, regimens should be designed so that side effects that may reduce compliance are minimized.

Antibiotics Used in Regimens to Eradicate *Helicobacter pylori*

AMOXICILLIN. *H. pylori* is very sensitive in vitro to this antibiotic, but gastric antisecretory cotherapy is required for any meaningful effectiveness. Resistance to amoxicillin is rare. The most common side effects are skin rash, candidiasis, and diarrhea.

TETRACYCLINE HCl. Tetracycline is effective in vitro against *H. pylori* and is active at low pH. Resistance is rare in Western countries but has been seen in up to 6% of isolates in Japan and Korea.[145] Tetracycline is quite useful and is probably underused in anti–*H. pylori* therapies. It is contraindicated in children because of the staining of teeth.

METRONIDAZOLE. *H. pylori* ordinarily is highly sensitive to metronidazole, which is actively secreted into gastric juice and saliva and whose activity is independent of pH. Primary resistance of *H. pylori* to metronidazole is common and is generally associated with a reduction in cure rates with regimens that include this antimicrobial.[146–149] The frequency of primary resistance to metronidazole varies substantially throughout the world. On the other hand, metronidazole resistance can apparently be overcome by increasing the dosage (e.g., from 250 mg three or four times daily to 500 mg three times daily).[150] Metronidazole is a prodrug that must undergo activation by bacterial nitroreductases. There are a number of *H. pylori* enzymes with the potential to reduce metronidazole, and it is possible that the increased dosage and resulting very high concentrations in the stomach allow sufficient drug to become activated to kill the organism. Side effects of metronidazole include a metallic taste, diarrhea, and nausea, the latter occurring primarily at doses higher than 1 g per day. Some individuals may experience a disulfiram (Antabuse)-like effect with ingestion of alcoholic beverages. Tinidazole, a nitroimidazole not available in the United States, gives results that are comparable to metronidazole.

CLARITHROMYCIN. This antibiotic is a macrolide with an antibacterial spectrum similar to erythromycin but that is more acid stable, better absorbed, and more active against *H. pylori*. When given in a high dose as monotherapy, clarithromycin cures *H. pylori* infection in up to 54%.[151] As with metronidazole, *H. pylori* can become resistant to clarithromycin, the level of resistance in a population being related to the use of the antibiotic for other conditions. In the United States the level of resistance appears to be stable and less than 15%.[152] Unlike metronidazole, there is no evidence that increasing the dosage will overcome resistance. Clarithromycin requires binding to the bacteria's ribosome, and resistance is associated with loss of that binding. Side effects include taste perversion in most patients.

BISMUTH. Bismuth compounds are topical antimicrobials that act directly on bacterial cell walls to disrupt their integrity by accumulating in periplasmic space and along membranes. Bismuth is most widely available in the United States as bismuth subsalicylate (Pepto-Bismol). Bismuth subcitrate is available in other parts of the world as a single agent and has been tested much more fully than bismuth subsalicylate. Although equivalence of activity of these two forms of bismuth has not been tested critically, bismuth subsalicylate has proven active in "triple therapy" regimens. Bismuth subcitrate is also available as a component of ranitidine bismuth citrate. Antibacterial concentrations of bismuth are achieved in antral mucus for about 2 hours after dosing. Side effects with these two bismuth compounds are minimal, although blackening of the stool may occur.

FURAZOLIDONE. Furazolidone, a nitrofuran antibiotic, has broad antibacterial activity based on interference with bacterial enzymes. It has been used empirically to treat peptic ulcer disease in China for more than 20 years with reported good results. Furazolidone is a monoamine oxidase inhibitor and, as such, can interact with a number of foods and other drugs. It is currently not considered a first-line antibiotic.

Adjunctive Agents Used in Regimens to Eradicate *Helicobacter pylori*

HISTAMINE$_2$ RECEPTOR ANTAGONIST (H_2RA). This class of drugs has long been used to promote healing of peptic ulcers. The agents have no effect by themselves against *H. pylori* but are useful to reduce acidity and make the acid-sensitive drugs, clarithromycin and amoxicillin, more effective. In general, the cure rates with H_2RAs as adjuvants are approximately the same or slightly less as with PPIs.

H^+,K^+-ATPase (PROTON PUMP) INHIBITORS. Omeprazole, the first of the substituted benzimidazoles, may be used as a model for all PPIs (see Chapter 38). In vitro, omeprazole inhibits the growth of *H. pylori* and, to a lesser extent other bacteria, at pH below 7[110]; omeprazole inhibits the growth of *H. pylori* at a pH of 7 only in its active sulfonamide form.[110] Omeprazole's mechanism of action on *H. pylori* is not through inhibition of urease, because the effect is seen with a urease-deficient strain of *H. pylori* or in the absence of urea in the medium. When omeprazole and other PPIs are employed as single agents in vivo, *H. pylori* infection is suppressed.[153] This effect is likely minor in relation to *H. pylori* eradication because the H_2RAs are approximately as effective as adjuvant therapy and have no effect on *H. pylori* in vivo. The importance of the anti–*H. pylori* effect of PPIs relates to the effect they have on the accuracy of tests that require the presence of relatively large numbers of *H. pylori* such as histology and urea breath and stool antigen tests (see section on Diagnosis). PPIs have proven to be especially useful as part of combination therapy with antimicrobial agents to cure *H. pylori* infection. The major activities are related to increasing intragastric pH, which may enhance the effectiveness of the local immune response, reduce the washout of antibiotics from the mucosa, and lower the minimal inhibitory concentrations of pH sensitive antibacterial agents. The decreased gastric juice volume that results from these antisecretory drugs may also increase intragastric concentrations of antibacterial agents.

RANITIDINE BISMUTH CITRATE (RBC). This is a novel compound with characteristics of both ranitidine (antisecretory) and bismuth. RBC is useful when combined with antibiotics and the combination of RBC with antibiotics has proven to be as good as, and possibly superior to, the same combination with a PPI.[141, 154] This should not be surprising in that RBC provides a H_2RA and the antimicrobial, bismuth, to the regimen. Side effects are minimal. The drug is no longer available in the United States.

Therapeutic Regimens to Treat *Helicobacter pylori* Infection

Regimens to treat *H. pylori* may be classified by the number of antibiotics and adjunctive agents employed.

ONE ANTIBIOTIC PLUS ONE ADJUNCTIVE AGENT. Dual therapies were the first therapies introduced for *H. pylori* therapy. Dual therapies with a PPI and clarithromycin or amoxicillin, or RBC with clarithromycin are no longer recommended because of low cure rates and a high frequency of clarithromycin resistance among the treatment failures.

TWO ANTIBIOTICS PLUS ONE ADJUNCTIVE AGENT (TRIPLE THERAPY). Triple therapy with either bismuth or a PPI combined with two antibiotics is now the most widely used regimen. Ranitidine bismuth citrate may be substituted for bismuth or a PPI but is no longer marketed in the United States. Therapy with metronidazole, tetracycline, and bismuth ("traditional" triple therapy) produces very good cure rates, especially with organisms sensitive to metronidazole.[146, 155, 156] Substitution of clarithromycin for metronidazole gives similar results.[157] Amoxicillin should be substituted for tetracycline in children to avoid staining of teeth. The most popular PPI triple therapy combines the PPI with any two of amoxicillin, metronidazole, and clarithromycin.

TWO ANTIBIOTICS PLUS TWO ADJUNCTIVE AGENTS (QUADRUPLE THERAPY). The triple therapy described above is quite good unless the organism being treated is resistant to clarithromycin or metronidazole. One regimen that provides effective eradication of *H. pylori* in either instance is high-dose, quadruple therapy. This consists of metronidazole, tetracycline, bismuth subsalicylate, and a PPI twice daily. Although it is intuitive that this regimen would be effective against strains resistant to clarithromycin, it has also been shown to be effective against strains resistant to metronidazole.[150]

Therapeutic Strategy

The most effective regimens to cure *H. pylori* infection are combinations of two antibiotics and one or two adjunctive agents taken for 7 to 14 days (Table 39–4). Although regimens composed of two antibiotics with a PPI are expensive, they are easy to take and have few major side effects. Unless a patient has taken clarithromycin previously, one of the two regimens containing this antibiotic, or traditional bismuth therapy plus a PPI is recommended. If metronidazole resistance is likely, we recommend either the PPI plus amoxicillin and clarithromycin or quadruple therapy. Overall, the clinical trials suggest that longer durations of therapy provide better results. The minimum duration is 7 days, but we recommend that therapy be continued for 10 to 14 days.[144] Head-to-head treatment trials of duration of therapy are needed, with the goal of being able to consistently cure more than 90% of cases.

Definition of Cure

It has become clear that failure to detect *H. pylori* immediately after a course of antimicrobial therapy does not mean that the infection has been cured. In many instances the infection has only been suppressed, with follow-up studies performed several weeks later readily disclosing its presence. *H. pylori* may occupy "sanctuary sites" that preclude cure but from which it ultimately emerges to regain its foothold. Thus, cure of infection is defined as absence of the organism by tests performed no sooner than 4 weeks after cessation of antimicrobial therapy. Because PPIs alone can suppress the infection, PPI therapy should be discontinued for at least 1 week before evaluation of effectiveness of therapy. Reinfection is rare. In one study, 173 patients whose infection was "cured" were followed for a mean of 5.1 years.[158] Re-

Table 39–4 | **Recommended Regimens to Treat *Helicobacter pylori****

Recommended Regimens
Bismuth Triple Therapy
Bismuth, 2 tablets four times daily
+
Metronidazole, 250 mg three times daily
+
Tetracycline, 500 mg four times daily
PPI Triple Therapy
PPI twice daily
+
Amoxicillin, 1000 mg two times daily
+
Clarithromycin, 500 mg two times daily
OR
Metronidazole, 500 mg two times daily
Quadruple Therapy
PPI twice daily
+
Bismuth, 2 tablets four times daily
+
Metronidazole, 250 mg three times daily
+
Tetracycline, 500 mg four times daily

*Treatment for 10–14 days is recommended.
PPI, proton pump inhibitor.

current infection was diagnosed in 9 (5.2%) after a mean of 8.7 months. It was possible to compare the initial and recurrent isolates in 8 of the 9 patients. In 3, the second isolate was different from the original isolate but identical to that of the patient endoscoped immediately before (i.e., endoscopic transmission). In the other 5, the original and second isolates were identical, suggesting the infection had been suppressed but not eradicated. Thus, there were no apparent cases of community acquired reinfection with *H. pylori*.

Follow-up of Patients after Antimicrobial Therapy

The first decision to be made following therapy is whether a follow-up test is required. On the one hand, a cure rate of 80% to 90% argues against the routine confirmation of therapy as does the fact that one must wait at least 4 weeks following cessation of therapy before confirming eradication. On the other hand, rates of cure in the community are lower than those obtained in controlled trials. Additionally, failed therapy in an ulcer patient almost uniformly is associated with recurrence of the ulcer, with ulcer symptoms and the potential for an ulcer complication. Recurrent ulcer is associated with additional visits to the health care provider, additional tests, and medications, as well as time lost from work. The widespread availability of simple noninvasive methods such as the urea breath and stool antigen tests make it feasible to confirm the results of therapy in every patient. For patients with a history of bleeding or perforated ulcer associated with *H. pylori*, it is critical to document cure of the infection before maintenance H_2RA or PPI therapy is stopped. If endoscopy is required, mucosal biopsies can be taken; otherwise, a urea breath test can be used.

Treatment of Patients Whose Initial Course of Therapy Failed

If antibiotic susceptibility results are available, the choice of a regimen will be determined by the antibiotics to which the organism is sensitive. If susceptibility results are unavailable, one may select a regimen containing antibiotics not used initially (e.g., metronidazole for clarithromycin or vice versa). The best results are obtained with bismuth-based quadruple therapy or with furazolidone-based quadruple therapy.

IMMUNIZATION

A long-term, worldwide solution to *H. pylori*–related disease can be effected only by prevention of acquisition of the infection. One method is to develop a successful preventive vaccine. Antimicrobial therapy is cumbersome, expensive, and ineffective in countries where reinfection rates are high, and when given to adults, perhaps too late to reverse significant pathology or prevent transmission to children. Animal models are being used to develop vaccines by defining appropriate antigens to use (e.g., adhesins, urease, heat shock proteins, and vacA) and to find effective and safe adjuvants.[159] Vaccination also offers the possibility of treating patients with established *H. pylori* infection.[160] It seems that the naturally infected stomach does not mount an effective secretory IgA response to the infection. Vaccination reverses this and an effective mucosal immune response to one of the surface proteins of *H. pylori* leads to both prevention of infection as well as cure of ongoing infections. Whether the encouraging results from animal experimentation will be applicable to humans remains to be evaluated.

REFERENCES

1. Marshall B: Unidentified curved bacilli on gastric epithelium in active chronic gastritis [letter]. Lancet 1:1273–1274, 1983.
2. Graham DY, Malaty HM, Evans DG, et al: Epidemiology of *Helicobacter pylori* in an asymptomatic population in the United States. Gastroenterology 100:1495–1501, 1991.
3. Megraud F: Epidemiology of *Helicobacter pylori* infection. Gastroenterol Clinic North Am 22:73–88, 1993.
4. Everhart JE: Recent developments in the epidemiology of *Helicobacter pylori*. Gastroenterol Clin North Am 29:559–578, 2000.
5. Malaty HM, Evans DG, Evans DJJ, Graham DY: *Helicobacter pylori* in Hispanics: Comparison with blacks and whites of similar age and socioeconomic class. Gastroenterology 103:813–816, 1992.
6. Parsonnet J, Blaser MJ, Perez-Perez GI, et al: Symptoms and risk factors of *Helicobacter pylori* infection in a cohort of epidemiologists. Gastroenterology 102:41–46, 1992.
7. Kuipers EJ, Pena AS, van Kamp G, et al: Seroconversion for *Helicobacter pylori*. Lancet 342:328–331, 1993.
8. Cullen DJE, Collins BJ, Christiansen KJ, et al: When is *H. pylori* infection acquired? Gut 34:1681–1682, 1993.
9. Mendall MA, Goggin PM, Molineaux N, et al: Childhood living conditions and *Helicobacter pylori* seropositivity in adult life. Lancet 339:896–897, 1992.
10. Malaty HM, Graham DY: Effect of childhood socioeconomic status on the current prevalence of *Helicobacter pylori* infection. Gut 35: 742–745, 1994.
11. Webb PM, Knight T, Greaves S, et al: Relation between infection with *Helicobacter pylori* and living conditions in childhood: Evidence for person-to-person transmission in early life. BMJ 308:750–753, 1994.
12. Haruma K, Okamoto S, Kawaguchi H, et al: Reduced incidence of *Helicobacter pylori* infection in young Japanese persons between the 1970s and the 1990s. J Clin Gastroenterol 25:583–586, 1997.
13. Malaty HM, Engstrand L, Pedersen NL, Graham DY: *Helicobacter pylori* infection: Genetic and environmental influences. A study of twins. Ann Intern Med 120:982–986, 1994.
14. Malaty HM, Graham DY, Isaksson I, et al: Are genetic influences on peptic ulcer dependent or independent of genetic influences for *Helicobacter pylori?* Arch Intern Med 160:105–109, 2000.
15. Hulten K, Han SW, Enroth H, et al: *Helicobacter pylori* in the drinking water of Peru. Gastroenterology 110:1031–1035, 1996.
16. Fiedorek SC, Malaty HM, Evans DG, et al: Factors influencing the epidemiology of *Helicobacter pylori* infection in children. Pediatrics 88:578–582, 1991.
17. McKeown I, Orr P, MacDonald S, et al: *Helicobacter pylori* in the Canadian arctic: Seroprevalence and detection in community water samples. Am J Gastroenterol 94:1823–1829, 1999.
18. Sasaki K, Tajiri Y, Sata M, et al: *Helicobacter pylori* in the natural environment. Scand J Infect Dis 31:275–279, 1999.
19. Hulten K, Enroth H, Nystrom T, Engstrand L: Presence of *Helicobacter* species DNA in Swedish water. J Appl Microbiol 85:282–286, 1998.
20. Handt LK, Fox JG, Dewhirst FE, et al: *Helicobacter pylori* isolated from the domestic cat: Public health implications. Infect Immun 62: 2367–2674, 1994.
21. El-Zaatari FA, Woo JS, Badr A, et al: Failure to isolate *Helicobacter pylori* from stray cats indicates that *H. pylori* in cats may be an anthroponosis—an animal infection with a human pathogen. J Med Microbiol 46:372–376, 1997.
22. Dore MP, Bilotta M, Vaira D, et al: High prevalence of *Helicobacter pylori* infection in shepherds. Dig Dis Sci 44:1161–1164, 1999.
23. Dore MP, Sepulveda AR, Osato MS, et al: *Helicobacter pylori* in sheep milk. Lancet 354:132, 1999.

24. Vincent P, Gottrand F, Pernes P, et al: High prevalence of *Helicobacter pylori* infection in cohabiting children: Epidemiology of a cluster, with special emphasis on molecular typing. Gut 35:313–316, 1994.
25. Drumm B, Perez-Perez GI, Blaser MJ, Sherman PM: Intrafamilial clustering of *Helicobacter pylori* infection. N Engl J Med 322:359–363, 1990.
26. Malaty HM, Graham DY, Evans DG, et al: Transmission of *Helicobacter pylori* infection: Studies in families of healthy individuals. Scand J Gastroenterol 26:927–932, 1991.
27. Mapstone NP, Lynch DAF, Lewis FA, et al: PCR identification of *Helicobacter pylori* in faeces from gastritis patients. Lancet 342:1419–1420, 1993.
28. Parsonnet J, Shmuely H, Haggerty T: Fecal and oral shedding of *Helicobacter pylori* from healthy infected adults. JAMA 282:2240–2245, 1999.
29. Dore MP, Osato MS, Malaty HM, Graham DY: Characterization of a culture method to recover *Helicobacter pylori* from the feces of infected patients. Helicobacter 5:165–168, 2000.
30. Thomas JE, Gibson GR, Darboe MK, et al: Isolation of *Helicobacter pylori* from human faeces. Lancet 340:1194–1195, 1992.
31. Fox JG, Blanco MC, Yan L, et al: Role of gastric pH in isolation of *Helicobacter mustelae* from the feces of ferrets. Gastroenterology 104:86–92, 1993.
32. Krajden S, Fuksa M, Anderson J, et al: Examination of human stomach biopsies, saliva, and dental plaque for *Campylobacter pylori.* J Clin Microbiol 27:1397–1398, 1989.
33. Ferguson DA, Li C, Patel NR, et al: Isolation of *Helicobacter pylori* from saliva. J Clin Microbiol 31:2802–2804, 1993.
34. Nguyen AH, Engstrand L, Genta RM, et al: Detection of *Helicobacter pylori* in dental plaque by reverse transcription-polymerase chain reaction. J Clin Microbiol 31:783–787, 1993.
35. Perez-Perez GI, Witkin SS, Decker MD, Blaser MJ: Seroprevalence of *Helicobacter pylori* infection in couples. J Clin Microbiol 29:642–644, 1991.
36. Malaty HM, Evans DJ, Afranoritch K, et al: *Helicobacter pylori* infection in dental workers: A seroepidemiology study. Am J Gastroenterol 87:1728–1731, 1992.
37. Axon ATR: Is *Helicobacter pylori* transmitted by the gastro-oral route? Aliment Pharmacol Ther 9:585–588, 1995.
38. Gledhill T, Leicester RJ, Addis B, et al: Epidemic hypochlorhydria. BMJ 76:1449–1457, 1985.
39. Harford WV, Barnett C, Lee E, et al: Acute gastritis with hypochlorhydria: Report of 35 cases with long-term follow-up. Gut 47:467–472, 2000.
40. Langenberg W, Rauws EAJ, Oudbier JH, Tytgat GNJ: Patient-to-patient-transmission of *Campylobacter pylori* infection by fiberoptic gastroduodenoscopy and biopsy. J Infect Dis 161:507–511, 1990.
41. Mitchell HM, Lee A, Carrick J: Increased incidence of *Campylobacter pylori* infection in gastroenterologists: Further evidence to support person-to-person transmission of *C. pylori.* Scand J Gastroenterol 24:396–400, 1989.
42. Leung W, Siu KLK, Kwok CKL, et al: Isolation of *Helicobacter pylori* from vomitus in children and its implication in gastro-oral transmission. Am J Gastroenterol 94:2881–2884, 1999.
43. Eaton KA, Morgan DR, Krakowka S: *Campylobacter pylori* virulence factors in gnotobiotic piglets. Infect Immun 57:1119–1125, 1989.
44. Itoh T, Yanagawa Y, Shingaki M, et al: Isolation of *Campylobacter pyloridis* from human gastric mucosa and characterization of the isolates. Microbiol Immunol 31:603–614, 1987.
45. Skouloubris S, Thiberge JM, Labigne A, deReuse H: The *Helicobacter pylori* UreI protein is not involved in urease activity but is essential for infection and acid survival in vivo. Infect Immun 66:4517–4521, 1998.
46. Scott DR, Marcus EA, Weeks DL, et al: Expression of the *Helicobacter pylori* UreI gene is required for acidic pH activation of cytoplasmic urease. Infect Immun 68:470–477, 2000.
47. Logan RPH: Adherence and *Helicobacter pylori.* Aliment Pharmacol Ther 10:3–15, 1996.
48. Crowe SE, Alvarez L, Dytoc M, et al: Expression of interleukin 8 and CD54 by human gastric epithelium after *Helicobacter pylori* infection in vitro. Gastroenterology 108:65–74, 1995.
49. Evans DG, Evans DJ, Moulds JJ, Graham DY: *N*-acetylneuraminyllactose-binding fibrillar hemagglutinin of *Campylobacter pylori*: A putative colonization factor antigen. Infect Immun 56:2896–2906, 1988.
50. Gold BD, Dytoc M, Huesca M, et al: Comparison of *Helicobacter mustelae* and *Helicobacter pylori* adhesion to eukaryotic cells in vitro. Gastroenterology 109:692–700, 1995.
51. El Shoura SM: *Helicobacter pylori*: I. Ultrastructural sequences of adherence, attachment, and penetration into the gastric mucosa. Ultrastruct Pathol 19:323–333, 1995.
52. Smoot DT, Resau JH, Naab T, et al: Adherence of *Helicobacter pylori* to cultured human gastric epithelial cells. Infect Immun 61:350–355, 1993.
53. Dytoc M, Gold BD, Louie M, et al: Comparison of *Helicobacter pylori* and attaching-effacing *Escherichia coli* adhesion to eukaryotic cells. Infect Immun 61:448–456, 1993.
54. Hessey SJ, Spencer J, Wyatt JI, et al: Bacterial adhesion and disease activity in *Helicobacter*-associated chronic gastritis. Gut 31:134–138, 1990.
55. Boren T, Falk P, Roth KA, et al: Attachment of *Helicobacter pylori* to human gastric epithelium mediated by blood group antigens. Science 262:1892–1895, 1993.
56. Moran AP: The role of lipopolysaccharide in *Helicobacter pylori* pathogenesis. Aliment Pharmacol Ther 10:39–50, 1996.
57. Mai UEH, Perez-Perez GI, Wahl LM, et al: Soluble surface proteins from *Helicobacter pylori* activate monocytes/macrophages by lipopolysaccharide-independent mechanism. J Clin Invest 87:894–900, 1991.
58. Neilsen H, Andersen LP: Chemotactic activity of *Helicobacter pylori* sonicate for human polymorphonuclear leukocytes and monocytes. Gut 33:738–742, 1992.
59. Tufano MA, Rossano F, Catalanotti P, et al: Immunobiological activities of *Helicobacter pylori* porins. Infect Immun 62:1392–1399, 1994.
60. Evans DJ, Evans DG, Takemura T, et al: Characterization of a *Helicobacter pylori* neutrophil-activating protein. Infect Immun 63:2213–2220, 1995.
61. Leunk RD, Johnson PT, David BC, et al: Cytotoxic activity in broth-culture filtrates of *Campylobacter pylori.* J Med Microbiol 26:93–99, 1988.
62. Blaser MJ: Role of *vac A* and the *cag A* locus of *Helicobacter pylori* in human disease. Aliment Pharmacol Ther 10:73–77, 1996.
63. Telford JL, Ghiara P, Dell'Orco M, et al: Gene structure of the *Helicobacter pylori* cytotoxin and evidence of its key role in gastric disease. J Exp Med 179:1653–1658, 1994.
64. Atherton JC, Cao P, Peek RM, et al: Mosaicism in vacuolating cytotoxin alleles of *Helicobacter pylori:* Association of specific *vac A* types with cytotoxin production and peptic ulceration. J Biol Chem 270:17771–17777, 1995.
65. Yamaoka Y, Kodama T, Kita M, et al: Relationship of vacA genotypes of *Helicobacter pylori* to cagA status, cytotoxin production, and clinical outcome. Helicobacter 3:241–253, 1998.
66. Atherton JC: CagA: A role at last. Gut 47:330–331, 2000.
67. Spechler SJ, Fischbach L, Feldman M: Clinical aspects of genetic variability in *Helicobacter pylori.* JAMA 283:1264–1266, 2000.
68. Graham DY, Yamaoka Y: Disease-specific *Helicobacter pylori* virulence factors—the unfulfilled promise. Helicobacter 5:3–9, 2000.
69. Covacci A, Rappuoli R: Tyrosine-phosphorylated bacterial proteins: Trojan horse for the host cell [comment]. J Exp Med 191:587–592, 2000.
70. Yamaoka Y, Kwon DH, Graham DY: A M(r) 34,000 proinflammatory outer membrane protein (oipA) of *Helicobacter pylori.* Proc Natl Acad Sci U S A 97:7533–7538, 2000.
71. Kansau I, Labigne A: Heat shock proteins of *Helicobacter pylori.* Aliment Pharmacol Ther 10:51–56, 1996.
72. Marshall BJ, Armstrong JA, McGechie DB, Glancy RJ: Attempt to fulfill Koch's postulates for pyloric *Campylobacter.* Med J Aust 142:436–439, 1985.
73. Morris A, Nicholson G: Ingestion of *Campylobacter pyloridis* causes gastritis and raised fasting gastric pH. Am J Gastroenterol 82:192–199, 1987.
74. Morris AJ, Ali MR, Nicholson GI, et al: Long-term follow-up of voluntary ingestion of *Helicobacter pylori.* Ann Intern Med 114:662–663, 1991.
75. Sobala GM, Crabtree JE, Dixon MF, et al: Acute *Helicobacter pylori* infection: Clinical features, local and systemic immune response, gastric mucosal histology, and gastric juice ascorbic acid concentrations. Gut 32:1415–1418, 1991.
76. Graham DY, Alpert LC, Smith JL, Yoshimura HH: Iatrogenic *Campylobacter pylori* infection is a cause of epidemic achlorhydria. Am J Gastroenterol 83:974–980, 1988.

77. Ramsey EJ, Carey KV, Peterson WL, et al: Epidemic gastritis with hypochlorhydria. Gastroenterology 76:1449–1457, 1979.
78. Peterson WL, Lee E, Feldman M: Relationship between *Campylobacter pylori* and gastritis in healthy humans after administration of placebo or indomethacin. Gastroenterology 95:1185–1197, 1988.
79. Genta RM, Hamner HW, Graham DY: Gastric lymphoid follicles in *Helicobacter pylori* infection: Frequency, distribution, and response to triple therapy. Hum Pathol 24:577–583, 1993.
80. Bayerdorffer E, Lehn N, Hatz R, et al: Difference in expression of *Helicobacter pylori* gastritis in antrum and body. Gastroenterology 102:1575–1582, 1992.
81. Feldman M, Cryer B, Lee E: Effects of *Helicobacter pylori* gastritis on gastric secretion in healthy human beings. Am J Physiol 274: G1011–G1017, 1998.
82. Crabtree JE: Gastric mucosal inflammatory responses to *Helicobacter pylori*. Aliment Pharmacol Ther 10:29–37, 1996.
83. Peterson WL, Barnett C, Evans DJ, et al: Acid secretion and serum gastrin in normal subjects and patients with duodenal ulcer: The role of *Helicobacter pylori*. Am J Gastroenterol 88:2038–2043, 1993.
84. Tarnasky PR, Kovacs TOG, Syntik B, Walsh JH: Asymptomatic *Helicobacter pylori* infection impairs pH inhibition of gastrin and acid secretion during second hour of peptone meal stimulation. Dig Dis Sci 38:1681–1687, 1993.
85. El-Omar EM, Penman ID, Ardill JES, et al: *Helicobacter pylori* infection and abnormalities of acid secretion in patients with duodenal ulcer disease. Gastroenterology 109:681–691, 1995.
86. McColl KEL, El-Omar EM: Gastrin-releasing peptide and its value in assessing gastric secretory function [review]. Aliment Pharmacol Ther 9:341–348, 1995.
87. Katelaris PH, Seow F, Lin BPC, et al: Effect of age, *Helicobacter pylori* infection, and gastritis with atrophy on serum gastrin and gastric acid secretion in healthy men. Gut 34:1032–1037, 1993.
88. Gutierrez O, Melo M, Segura AM, et al: Cure of *Helicobacter pylori* infection improves gastric acid secretion in patients with corpus gastritis. Scand J Gastroenterol 32:664–668, 1997.
89. Dore MP, Graham DY: Pathogenesis of duodenal ulcer disease: The rest of the story. Baillieres Clin Gastroenterol 14:97–107, 2000.
90. Leontiadis GI, Sharma VK, Howden CW: Non-gastrointestinal tract associations of *Helicobacter pylori* infection. Arch Intern Med 159: 925–940, 1999.
91. Annibale B, Marignani M, Monarca B, et al: Reversal of iron deficiency anemia after *Helicobacter pylori* eradication in patients with asymptomatic gastritis. Ann Intern Med 131:668–672, 1999.
92. Corea P, Haenszel W, Cuello C, et al: Gastric precancerous process in a high-risk population: Cohort follow-up. Cancer Res 50:4737–4740, 1990.
93. Villako K, Kekki M, Maaroos H, et al: Chronic gastritis: Progression of inflammation and atrophy in a six-year endoscopic follow-up of a random sample of 142 Estonian urban subjects. Scand J Gastroenterol 26(Suppl 186):135–141, 1991.
94. Kuipers EJ, Uyterlinde AM, Pena AS, et al: Long-term sequelae of *Helicobacter pylori* gastritis. Lancet 345:1525–1528, 1995.
95. Ihamaki T, Kekki M, Sipponen P, Siurala M: The sequelae and course of chronic gastritis during a 30–40-year bioptic follow-up study. Scand J Gastroenterol 20:485–491, 1985.
96. Karnes WE, Samloff IM, Siurala M, et al: Positive serum antibody and negative tissue staining for *Helicobacter pylori* in subjects with atrophic body gastritis. Gastroenterology 101:167–174, 1991.
97. Negrini R, Lisato L, Zanelli I, et al: *Helicobacter pylori* infection induces antibodies cross-reacting with human gastric mucosa. Gastroenterology 101:437–445, 1991.
98. Louw JA, Falck V, Varenburg C, et al: Distribution of *Helicobacter pylori* colonisation and associated gastric inflammatory changes—differences between patients with duodenal and gastric ulcers. J Clin Pathol 46:745–756, 1993.
99. Kekki M, Sipponen P, Siurala M, Laszewich W: Peptic ulcer and chronic gastritis: Their relation to age, sex, and to location of ulcer and gastritis. Gastroenterol Clin Biol 14:217–223, 1990.
100. Fiocca R, Villani L, Luinetti O, et al: *Helicobacter* colonisation and histopathological profile of chronic gastritis in patients with or without dyspepsia, mucosal erosion, and peptic ulcer—a morphological approach to the study of ulcerogenesis in man. Virchows Arch A Pathol Anat 19:489–498, 1992.
101. Kekki M, Sipponen P, Siurala M: Progression of antral and body gastritis in patients with active and healed duodenal ulcer and duodenitis. Scand J Gastroenterol 19:328–388, 1984.
102. Maaroos H, Salupere V, Uibo R, et al: Seven-year follow-up study of chronic gastritis in gastric ulcer patients. Scand J Gastroenterol 20: 198–204, 1985.
103. Jonsson KA, Strom M, Bodemar G, Norrby K: Histologic changes in the gastro-duodenal mucosa after long-term medical treatment with cimetidine or parietal cell vagotomy in patients with juxtopyloric ulcer disease. Scand J Gastroenterol 23:433–441, 1988.
104. Peetsalu A, Maaroos H, Sipponen P, Peetsalu M: Long-term effect of vagotomy on gastric mucosa and *Helicobacter pylori* in duodenal ulcer patients. Scand J Gastroenterol 26(Suppl 186):77–83, 1991.
105. Kuipers EJ, Lundell L, Klinkenberg-Knol EC, et al: Atrophic gastritis and *Helicobacter pylori* in patients with reflux esophagitis treated with omeprazole of fundoplication. N Engl J Med 334:1018–1022, 1996.
106. Lundell L, Miettinen P, Myyvold HE, et al: Lack of effect of acid suppression therapy on gastric atrophy. Gastroenterology 117:319–326, 2000.
107. Stolte M, Meining A, Schmitz JM, et al: Changes in *Helicobacter pylori*–induced gastritis in the antrum and corpus during 12 months of treatment with omeprazole and lansoprazole in patients with gastro-oesophageal reflux disease. Aliment Pharmacol Ther 12:247–253, 2000.
108. Meining A, Kiel G, Stolte M: Changes in *Helicobacter pylori*–induced gastritis in the antrum and corpus during and after 12 months of treatment with ranitidine and lansoprazole in patients with duodenal ulcer disease. Aliment Pharmacol Ther 12:735–740, 2000.
109. Uemara N, Okamoto S, Yamamoto S, et al: Changes in *Helicobacter pylori*–induced gastritis in the antrum and corpus during long-term acid-suppressive treatment in Japan. Aliment Pharmacol Ther 14: 1345–1352, 2000.
110. McGowan CC, Cover TL, Blaser MJ: The proton pump inhibitor omeprazole inhibits acid survival of *Helicobacter pylori* by a urease-independent mechanism. Gastroenterology 107:1573–1578, 1994.
111. Lee A, Dixon MF, Danon SJ, et al: Local acid production and *Helicobacter pylori*: A unifying hypothesis of gastroduodenal disease. Eur J Gastroenterol Hepatol 7:461–465, 1995.
112. Graham DY: *Campylobacter pylori* and peptic ulcer disease. Gastroenterology 96:615–625, 1989.
113. Tarpila S, Kekki M, Samloff IM, et al: Morphology and dynamics of the gastric mucosa in duodenal ulcer patients and their first-degree relatives. Hepatogastroenterology 30:198–201, 1983.
114. Kuipers EJ, Uyterlinde AM, Pena AS, et al: Increase of *Helicobacter pylori*–associated corpus gastritis during acid-suppressive therapy: Implications for long-term safety. Am J Gastroenterol 90:1401–1406, 1995.
115. Kuipers EJ, Lee A, Klinkenberg-Knol EC, Meuwissen SGM: The development of atrophic gastritis—*Helicobacter pylori* and the effects of acid-suppressive therapy [review]. Aliment Pharmacol Ther 9:331–340, 1995.
116. Mardh S, Song Y: Characterization of antigenic structures in autoimmune atrophic gastritis with pernicious anemia. Acta Physiol Scand 136:581–587, 1989.
117. Haruma K, Komoto K, Kawaguchi H, et al: Pernicious anemia and *Helicobacter pylori* infection in Japan: Evaluation in a country with a high prevalence of infection. Am J Gastroenterol 90:1107–1110, 1995.
118. Annibale B, Marignani M, Azzoni C, et al: Atrophic body gastritis: Distinct features associated with *Helicobacter pylori* infection. Helicobacter 2:57–64, 1997.
119. Cryer B, Lee E, Feldman M: Gastric mucosal biopsy via a nasogastric tube: A nonendoscopic method for diagnosing fundic and antral mucosal gastritis and *Helicobacter pylori* infection in man. Gastrointest Endosc 44:317–323, 1996.
120. Genta RM, Graham DY: Comparison of biopsy sites for the histopathologic diagnosis of *Helicobacter pylori*: A topographic study of *H. pylori* density and distribution. Gastrointest Endosc 40:342–345, 1994.
121. Genta RM, Robason GO, Graham DY: Simultaneous visualization of *Helicobacter pylori* and gastric morphology: A new stain. Hum Pathol 25:221–226, 1994.
122. Mobley HLT: The role of *Helicobacter pylori* urease in the pathogenesis of gastritis and peptic ulceration. Aliment Pharmacol Ther 10(Supp 1):57–64, 1996.
123. Cutler AF, Havstad S, Ma CK, et al: Accuracy of invasive and noninvasive tests to diagnose *Helicobacter pylori* infection. Gastroenterology 109:136–141, 1995,
124. Laine L, Cohen H, Sloane R, et al: Interobserver agreement and

predictive value of endoscopic findings for *Helicobacter pylori* and gastritis in normal volunteers. Gastrointest Endosc 42:420–423, 1995.
125. Perez-Perez GI, Dworkin BM, Chodos JE, Blaser MJ: *Campylobacter pylori* antibodies in humans. Ann Intern Med 109:11–17, 1988.
126. Evans DJJ, Graham DY, Klein PD: A sensitive and specific serologic test for detection of *Campylobacter pylori* infection. Gastroenterology 96:1004–1008, 1989.
127. Talley N, Newell DG, Ormand JE, et al: Serodiagnosis of *Helicobacter pylori*: Comparison of enzyme-linked immunosorbent assays. J Clin Microbiol 29:1635–1639, 1991.
128. Rose S, Johnson C, Crowe H, et al: Evaluation of a physician's office rapid serology test which detects *Helicobacter pylori* IgG antibodies with whole blood samples [abstract]. Gut 37(Suppl 1):A15, 1995.
129. Cutler AF, Prasad VM: Long-term follow-up of *Helicobacter pylori* serology after successful eradication. Am J Gastroenterol 91:85–88, 1996.
130. Feldman M, Cryer B, Lee E, Peterson WL: Role of seroconversion in confirming cure of *Helicobacter pylori* infection. JAMA 280:363–365, 1998.
131. Graham DY, Klein PD: What you should know about the methods, problems, interpretations, and uses of urea breath tests. Am J Gastroenterol 86:1118–1122, 1991.
132. Laine L, Estrada R, Trujillo M, et al: Effect of proton-pump inhibitor therapy on diagnostic testing for *Helicobacter pylori*. Ann Intern Med 129:547–550, 1998.
133. Chey WD, Murthy U, Toskes P, et al: The ^{13}C-urea blood test accurately detects active *Helicobacter pylori* infection: A United States multicenter trial. Am J Gastroenterol 94:1522–1524, 1999.
134. Cutler AF, Toskes P: Comparison of [^{13}C]urea blood test to [^{13}C]urea breath test for the diagnosis of *Helicobacter pylori*. Am J Gastroenterol 94:959–961, 1999.
135. Vaira D, Malfertheiner P, Megraud F, et al: Diagnosis of *Helicobacter pylori* infection with a new non-invasive antigen-based assay. Lancet 354:30–33, 1999.
136. Makristathis A, Pasching E, Schutze K, et al: Detection of *Helicobacter pylori* in stool specimens by PCR and antigen enzyme immunoassay. J Clin Microbiol 36:2772–2774, 1998.
137. Vakil N, Affi A, Robinson J, et al: Prospective blinded trial of a fecal antigen test for the detection of *Helicobacter pylori* infection. Am J Gastroenterol 95:1699–1701, 2000.
138. Vaira D, Malfertheiner P, Megraud F, et al: Noninvasive antigen-based assay for assessing *Helicobacter pylori* eradication: A European multicenter study. Am J Gastroenterol 95:925–929, 2000.
139. Manes G, Balzano A, Iaquinto G, et al: Accuracy of the stool antigen test in the diagnosis of *Helicobacter pylori* infection before treatment and in patients on omeprazole therapy. Aliment Pharmacol Ther 15: 73–79, 2001.
140. Loy CT, Irwig LM, Katelaris PH, Talley NJ: Do commercial serological kits for *Helicobacter pylori* infection differ in accuracy? A meta-analysis. Am J Gastroenterol 91:1138–1144, 1996.
141. Gisbert JP, Gonzalez L, Calvet X, et al: *Helicobacter pylori* eradication: Proton pump inhibitor vs. ranitidine bismuth citrate plus two antibiotics for 1 week—a meta-analysis of efficacy. Aliment Pharmacol Ther 14:1141–1150, 2000.
142. Gisbert JP, Gonzalez L, Calvet X, et al: Proton pump inhibitor, clarithromycin and either amoxycillin or nitroimidazole: A meta-analysis of eradication of *Helicobacter pylori*. Aliment Pharmacol Ther 14: 1319–1328, 2000.
143. Laheij RJF, VanRossum LGM, Jansen JBMJ, et al: Evaluation of treatment regimens to cure *Helicobacter pylori* infection—a meta-analysis. Aliment Pharmacol Ther 13:857–864, 1999.
144. Calvet X, Garcia N, Lopez T, et al: A meta-analysis of short versus long therapy with a proton pump inhibitor, clarithromycin, and either metronidazole or amoxycillin for treating *Helicobacter pylori* infection. Aliment Pharmacol Ther 14:603–609, 2000.
145. Kwon DH, Kim JJ, Lee M, et al: Isolation and characterization of tetracycline-resistant clinical isolates of *Helicobacter pylori*. Antimicrob Agents Chemother 44:3203–3205, 2000.
146. Pentson JG: *Helicobacter pylori* eradication—understandable caution but no excuse for inertia [review]. Aliment Pharmacol Ther 8:369–390, 1994.
147. Houben MHMG, Van De Beek D, Hensen EF, et al: A systematic review of *Helicobacter pylori* eradication therapy—the impact of antimicrobial resistance on eradication rates. Aliment Pharmacol Ther 13: 1047–1055, 1999.
148. Dore MP, Leandro G, Realdi G, et al: Effect of pretreatment antibiotic resistance to metronidazole and clarithromycin on outcome of *Helicobacter pylori* therapy—a meta-analytical approach. Dig Dis Sci 45: 68–70, 2000.
149. van der Wouden EJ, Thijs JC, van Zwet AA, et al: The influence of in vitro resistance on the efficacy of nitroimidazole-containing anti–*Helicobacter pylori* regimens: A meta-analysis. Am J Gastroenterol 94:1751–1759, 1999.
150. Graham DY, Osato MS, Hoffman J, et al: Metronidazole-containing quadruple therapy for infection with metronidazole-resistant *Helicobacter pylori*: A prospective study. Aliment Pharmacol Ther 14:745–750, 2000.
151. Peterson WL, Graham DY, Marshall B, et al: Clarithromycin as monotherapy for eradication of *Helicobacter pylori:* A randomized, double-blinded trial. Am J Gastroenterol 88:1860–1864, 1993.
152. Osato MS, Reddy R, Reddy SG, et al: Pattern of primary resistance of *Helicobacter pylori* to metronidazole or clarithromycin in the United States. Arch Intern Med 161:1217, 1220, 2001.
153. Weil J, Bell GD, Powell K, et al: Omeprazole and *Helicobacter pylori:* Temporary suppression rather than true eradication. Aliment Pharmacol Ther 5:309–313, 1991.
154. Van Oijen AH, Verbeek AL, Jansen JB, de Boer WA: Treatment of *Helicobacter pylori* infection with ranitidine bismuth citrate– or proton pump inhibitor–based triple therapies [review]. Aliment Pharmacol Ther 14:991–999, 2000.
155. Tytgat GNJ: Treatments that impact favourably upon the eradication of *Helicobacter pylori* and ulcer recurrence [review]. Aliment Pharmacol Ther 8:359–368, 1994.
156. Graham DY, Lew GM, Malaty HM, et al: Factors influencing the eradication of *Helicobacter pylori* with triple therapy. Gastroenterology 102:493–496, 1992.
157. Al-Assi MT, Ramirez FC, Lew GM, et al: Clarithromycin, tetracycline, and bismuth: A new non-metronidazole therapy for *Helicobacter pylori* infection. Am J Gastroenterol 89:1203–1205, 1994.
158. van der Hulst RWM, Koycu B, Keller JJ, et al: *H. pylori* reinfection after successful eradication analyzed by RAPD or RFLP [abstract]. Gastroenterology 110:A284, 1996.
159. Lee A, Buck F: Vaccination and mucosal responses to *Helicobacter pylori* infection. Aliment Pharmacol Ther 10:129–138, 1996.
160. Corthesy-Theulaz I, Porta N, Glauser M, et al: Oral immunization with *Helicobacter pylori* urease B subunit as a treatment against *Helicobacter* infection in mice. Gastroenterology 109:115–121, 1995.

Chapter 40

Peptic Ulcer Disease and its Complications

Stuart Jon Spechler

Peptic ulcerations are excavated defects (holes) in the gastrointestinal mucosa that result when epithelial cells succumb to the caustic effects of acid and pepsin in the lumen (Fig. 40–1*A*). The term *peptic ulcer disease* commonly is used to refer to ulcerations of the stomach, duodenum, or both, but peptic ulcers can develop in any portion of the gastrointestinal tract that is exposed to acid and pepsin in sufficient concentration and duration. For example, gastroesophageal reflux disease (GERD) can be complicated by peptic ulcerations in the esophagus (see Chapter 33), or a Meckel's diverticulum can be lined by an acid-secreting, gastric-type mucosa that causes peptic ulceration in the distal ileum (see Chapter 84). In this chapter, unless otherwise specified, the term *peptic ulcer disease* refers to gastric and duodenal ulcers that are caused by acid-peptic injury.

Ulcers have been defined histologically as necrotic mucosal defects that extend through the muscularis mucosae and into the submucosa or deeper layers (Fig. 40–1*B*), whereas more superficial necrotic defects are considered erosions.[1] This histologic definition has little practical value to the clinician, however, because peptic ulcers usually are identified on the basis of gross endoscopic or radiographic features. In practice, clinicians seldom have histologic confirmation that the lesions they call "peptic ulcers" in fact have breached the muscularis mucosae, or that lesions deemed "erosions" indeed have spared the muscularis mucosae.

In the early part of the 20th century, stress and diet were judged to be important pathogenetic factors for peptic ulceration. Consequently, patients with peptic ulcers were treated with hospitalization, bed rest, and the prescription of "bland" diets. By the 1950s, when investigators and clinicians had focused their attention primarily on the pathogenetic role of gastric acid, antacid therapy had become the treatment of choice for peptic ulcer disease. When histamine H_2 receptor antagonists became available for clinical use in the 1970s, acid suppression with antisecretory therapy rapidly emerged as the treatment of choice for patients with peptic ulcer disease. With the advent of proton pump inhibitors (PPIs) in the 1980s, even more potent acid suppression and higher rates of ulcer healing could be achieved. Although numerous investigations showed that most acute peptic ulcerations healed with acid suppression therapy, most patients experienced recurrences within 1 year of discontinuing treatment with antacids or antisecretory agents alone.[2] For most of the 20th century, therefore, peptic ulcer disease was considered a chronic, incurable disorder characterized by frequent exacerbations and remissions.

During the 1980s, investigators learned that most peptic ulcerations were associated either with gastric infection by the bacterium *Helicobacter pylori*, or with the ingestion of nonsteroidal anti-inflammatory drugs (NSAIDs) (Fig. 40–2).[3] Furthermore, numerous studies showed that if *H. pylori* infection and NSAID use could be eliminated, then peptic ulceration recurred infrequently. These observations have revolutionized the therapeutic approach to peptic ulcer disease, and a search for these "curable" causes of peptic ulceration has become a key component of modern patient management. Moreover, it appears that a number of peculiar epidemiologic features of peptic ulcer disease that had puzzled early investigators can be explained by considering the

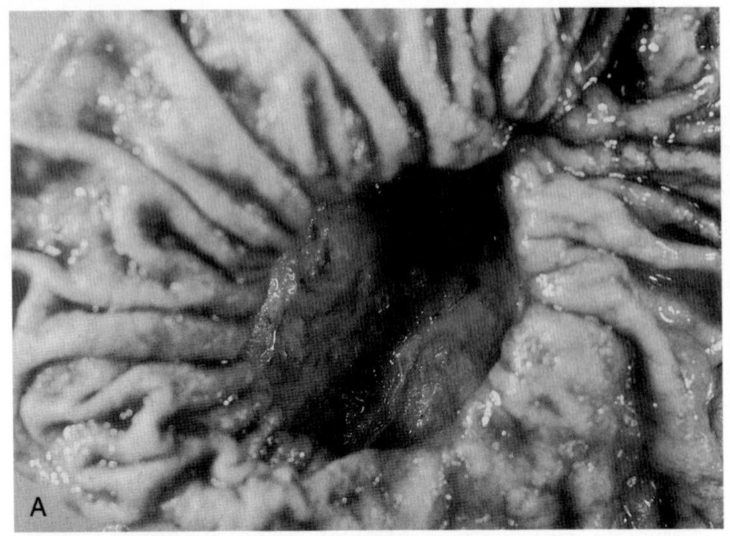

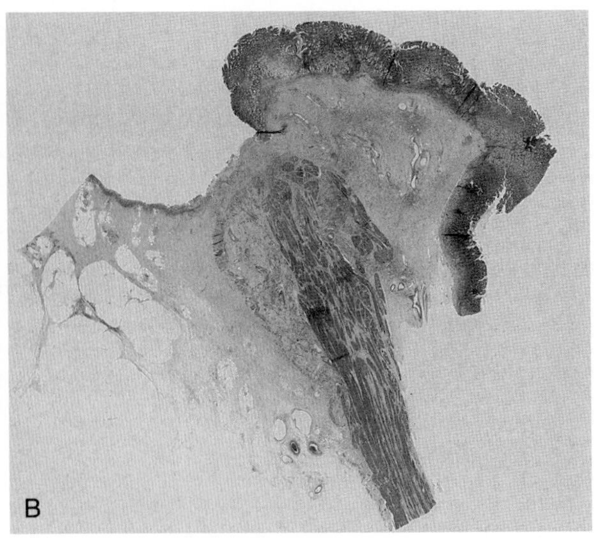

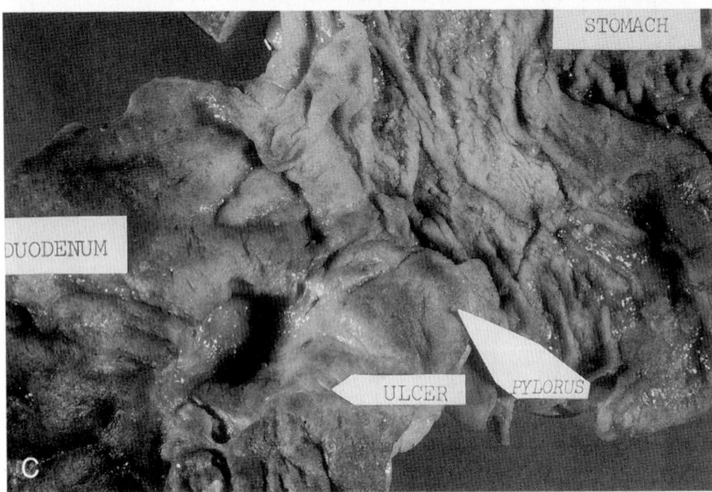

Figure 40–1. *A*, Gross pathology specimen showing a large, deep benign ulcer in the body of the stomach. *B*, Photomicrograph of the gastric ulcer, which has penetrated through the muscularis mucosae, the submucosa, and the muscularis propria. *C*, Autopsy specimen showing a large deep benign ulcer in the first portion of the duodenum.

epidemiology of *H. pylori* infection and NSAID use (see later). Nevertheless, there remains a substantial minority of patients with peptic ulcerations who have no apparent predisposing factor.[4]

PATHOPHYSIOLOGY OF PEPTIC ULCERATION

Epithelial Defense Mechanisms

Ultimately, peptic ulceration results when the caustic effects of acid and pepsin in the gastrointestinal lumen overwhelm the ability of the mucosa to resist those effects. The gastroduodenal mucosa is exposed to acid and pepsin continuously, yet ulceration is an abnormal event. The mechanisms that normally enable the mucosa to resist acid-peptic attack can be divided into three major components—pre-epithelial, epithelial, and postepithelial defense mechanisms.

Pre-epithelial Defense Mechanisms

The pre-epithelial defense mechanisms are features that impede contact between epithelial cells and noxious agents in the gastrointestinal lumen. As described in Chapters 38 and 87, gastric and duodenal epithelial cells normally are shielded from acid-peptic attack by a prominent coat of mucus and by a layer of unstirred water that is rich in bicarbonate.[5, 6] Both mucus and bicarbonate are secreted into the lumen by gastric epithelial cells and by Brunner's glands in the duodenum. Bicarbonate from the blood also enters the unstirred water layer through the process of paracellular diffusion. Within the mucus layer, glycoproteins form a physical barrier to the diffusion of pepsin, and the bicarbonate ions that accompany the glycoproteins can neutralize acid. Mucus also contains substantial quantities of surface-active phospholipids that are secreted by epithelial cells.[7] These phospholipids may protect the mucosa by forming a hydrophobic layer that repels acid at the luminal surface of the mucus gel. As a result of these pre-epithelial defense mechanisms, the pH on the surface of the gastroduodenal epithelial cell normally can be maintained in the neutral range, even when pH in the lumen falls below 2.0 (see Fig. 38–9 in Chapter 38).[8] Finally, acid-peptic injury to the gastroduodenal mucosa results in an outpouring of mucus, fibrin, and cellular debris that forms a protective cap that clings to the injured epithelium and impedes further contact with acid.[9] Abnormalities in these pre-epithelial defense mechanisms may contribute to peptic ulcer disease. For example, *H. pylori* infection can be associated with abnormalities in gastrointestinal mucus and in duodenal bicarbonate secretion that predispose to peptic ulceration (see later).[10, 11]

Epithelial Defense Mechanisms

When acid and pepsin breach the pre-epithelial defenses, there are epithelial mechanisms that can prevent or minimize acid-peptic injury. The apical cell membranes and the tight junctional complexes between the surface cells are barriers that limit the diffusion of hydrogen ions into the mucosa. Exposure of the apical membranes to dilute acid causes an increase in resistance to the passage of hydrogen ions through the tight junctions, whereas exposure to concentrated acid ($pH < 2.5$) induces injury that allows hydrogen ions to leak through this paracellular pathway.[12] Excess hydrogen ions that enter the epithelial cells can be removed by ion pumps in the basolateral cell membrane that include a Na^+/H^+ exchanger and a Cl^-/HCO_3^- exchanger.[13] Duodenal epithelial cells also have a Na^+/HCO_3^- cotransporter that helps to regulate intracellular pH.[14] When these defense mechanisms are overwhelmed and cells succumb to acid-peptic injury, superficial mucosal defects can be sealed quickly through a process called *rapid restitution* in which healthy cells in the mucous neck region of the gland migrate along the basement membrane to close the mucosal gap.[15] This process is regulated in part by growth factors such as epidermal growth factor and fibroblast growth factor.[16] Rapid restitution merely involves cell migration, not cell division, and the wandering cells can seal only minor mucosal defects. The healing of large peptic lesions is effected through regeneration, a process in which new cells are created by cell division.[17] Regeneration also is regulated by growth factors.[16–18]

Postepithelial Defense Mechanism

Mucosal blood flow comprises the postepithelial defense mechanism. Blood flow provides much of the energy and the substrates necessary both for maintaining epithelial cell integrity and for effecting protective epithelial cell functions such as mucus production and bicarbonate secretion. Blood flow also removes acid that diffuses through an injured mucosa. During gastric acid secretion, HCO_3^- transported across the parietal cell basolateral membrane produces an "alkaline tide" in the submucosa (see Chapter 38). Blood flow transports the HCO_3^- of this alkaline tide to the surface epithelial cells, a process that appears to protect against acid-peptic injury during acid secretion by the stomach.[19]

Peptic ulceration results when the caustic effects of acid and pepsin in the gastrointestinal lumen overwhelm all three components of epithelial defense.

Abnormalities in Gastric Acid Secretion, Acid Homeostasis, and Gastroduodenal Motility

The presence of acid is a sine qua non for peptic ulceration, a concept proposed by Schwarz in 1910 with his famous dictum, "no acid, no ulcer."[20] Benign ulcerations have been described rarely in the upper gastrointestinal tract of patients with achlorhydria, but such ulcerations are not, by definition, peptic lesions.[21] In the era just before the discovery of *H. pylori*, when peptic ulceration was regarded primarily as a disorder of gastric acid homeostasis, numerous studies on peptic ulcer disease focused on identifying abnormalities in gastric acid secretion for patients with duodenal and gastric ulcers. Modern studies have shown that some of these abnormalities (e.g., increased basal and gastrin-releasing peptide (GRP)-stimulated acid output, and elevated fasting and meal-stimulated gastrin levels in duodenal ulcer patients) may not be primary defects but reversible consequences of infection with *H. pylori*.[22]

Reported abnormalities in gastric acid secretion, acid homeostasis, and gastroduodenal motility that are associated with peptic ulcer disease are reviewed in this section (Table 40–1). While considering this section, the reader should bear in mind that the association between peptic ulcer disease and *H. pylori* infection was not known before publication of the landmark report on this issue by Marshall and Warren in 1984.[23] Consequently, clinical investigations on peptic ulcer conducted before 1984 do not even consider the *H. pylori* status of the study population. Although this infection is found in more than 80% of patients with duodenal ulcer and in more than 60% of patients with gastric ulcer,[3] the precise contribution of *H. pylori* to a number of the physiologic abnormalities described in peptic ulcer disease remains unclear. For a detailed discussion of the physiology of gastric acid secretion and the influence of *H. pylori* infec-

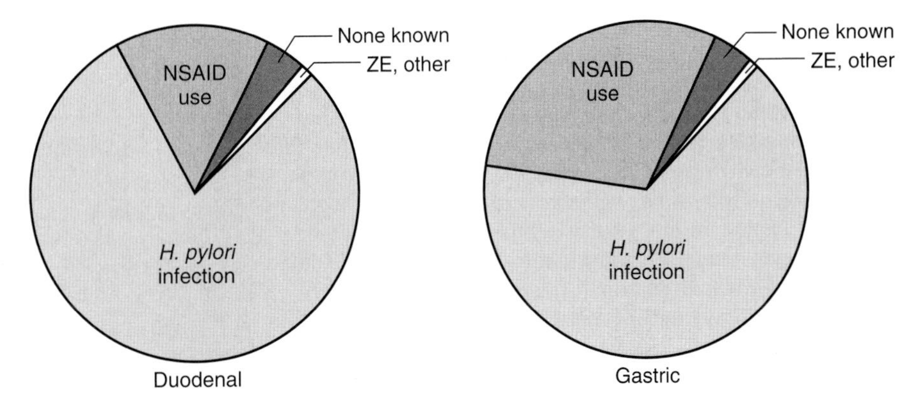

Figure 40–2. Pie charts depicting conditions associated with peptic ulcer disease. The percentages shown are rough approximations based on studies from Western countries. The relative contributions of *Helicobacter pylori* infection and NSAID use to peptic ulcer vary considerably among different populations and, within populations, vary with age and socioeconomic status. Also, the separation depicted in this figure is somewhat artificial, because NSAID use and *H. pylori* infection often coexist. (ZE, Zollinger-Ellison syndrome and other rare disorders.)

Table 40–1 | **Reported Abnormalities in Gastric Acid Secretion and Acid Homeostasis in Peptic Ulcer Disease**

Duodenal Ulcer
Increased
Mass of gastric parietal cells
Maximal acid output
Peak acid output stimulated by meals*
Duration of meal-stimulated acid secretion
Basal acid output*
Daytime acid output
Nocturnal acid output
Fasting serum gastrin levels*
Meal- and GRP-stimulated gastrin levels*
Serum concentrations of pepsinogen I*
Rate of gastric emptying for liquids
Decreased
Bicarbonate production by the proximal duodenum
Gastric Ulcer
Increased
Serum levels of pepsinogen II
Duodenogastric reflux
Decreased
Mass of gastric parietal cells
Maximal acid output

*Evidence suggests that this abnormality may be a reversible consequence of *Helicobacter pylori* infection.
GRP, gastrin-releasing peptide.

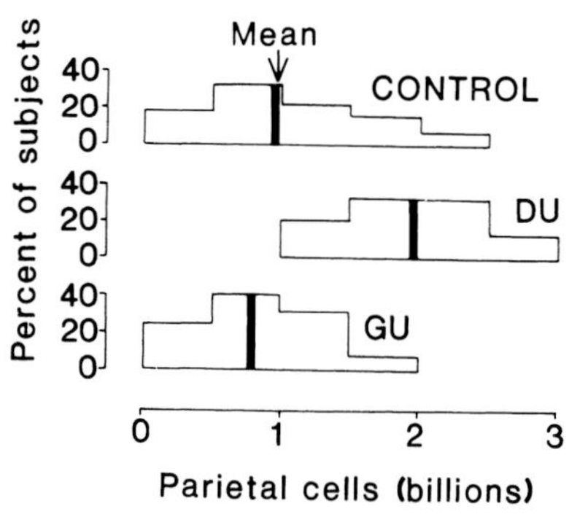

Figure 40–3. Mean number of parietal cells in healthy control subjects, patients with duodenal ulcer (DU), and patients with gastric ulcer (GU). (Data from Cox AJ: Stomach size and its relation to chronic peptic ulcer. Arch Pathol 54:407, 1952.)

tion on secretory status, the reader is referred to Chapters 38 and 39.

Abnormalities Associated with Duodenal Ulcer

Numerous studies have concluded that patients with duodenal ulcer disease tend to be hypersecretors of gastric acid. Autopsy studies have shown that groups of duodenal ulcer patients have greater mean numbers of gastric parietal cells than groups of control subjects without peptic ulcers, although much overlap is observed between these groups (Fig. 40–3).[24] The average maximal acid output (which correlates with parietal cell mass), the mean peak acid output, and the mean duration of meal-stimulated acid secretion also are greater in patients with duodenal ulcer than in control subjects, again with considerable overlap among individuals within the groups.[25–27] Similarly, basal acid output, daytime acid output, and nocturnal acid output are, on average, increased in patients with duodenal ulcer compared with control subjects without peptic ulcer disease (Fig. 40–4).[26, 28–30] The abnormality in nocturnal gastric acid secretion may be particularly important because during sleep, when there is no food in the stomach to buffer gastric acid, the gastroduodenal mucosa may be especially susceptible to peptic injury.

Abnormalities in the homeostatic mechanisms that regulate gastric acid output may contribute to the acid hypersecretion found in some patients with duodenal ulcer. For example, fasting serum gastrin levels are higher in duodenal ulcer patients than in normal control subjects.[22, 31–34] Meal- and GRP-stimulated gastrin levels also are higher in *H. pylori*–infected duodenal ulcer patients than in uninfected normal control subjects, but these levels in ulcer patients are no higher than those of control subjects with *H. pylori* infection

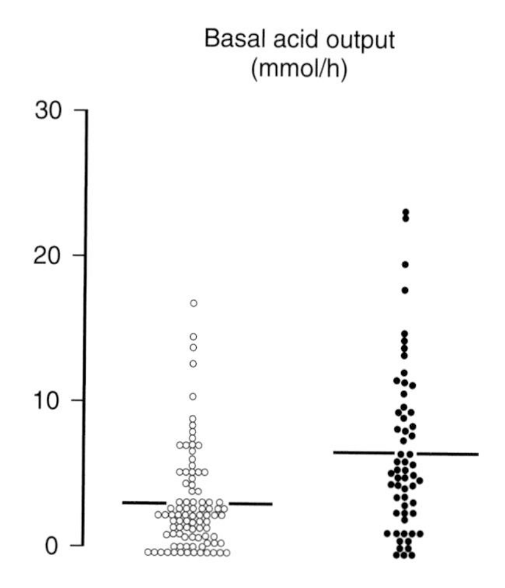

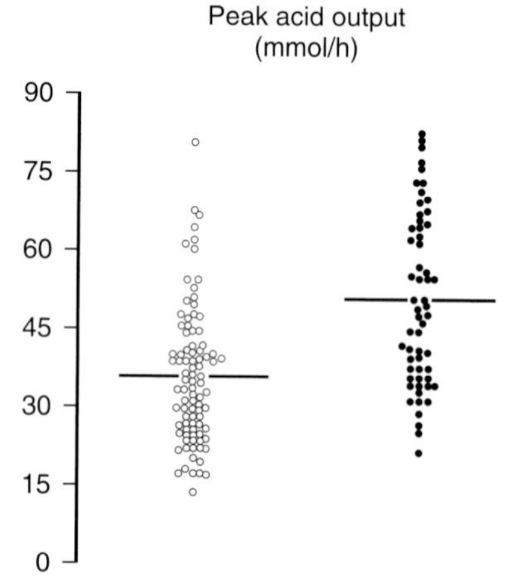

Figure 40–4. Basal and peak acid outputs in response to pentagastrin stimulation in normal subjects (*open circles, left*) and in patients with duodenal ulcer (*closed circles, right*). Note the substantial overlap in values among individual patients in the groups. Horizontal lines indicate mean values. (From Blair AJ III, Feldman M, Barnett C, et al: Detailed comparison of basal and food-stimulated gastric acid secretion rates and serum gastrin concentrations in duodenal ulcer patients and normal subjects. J Clin Invest 79:582–587,1987.)

who are otherwise normal.[22, 34] In some instances, the gastrin abnormalities associated with duodenal ulcer are reversible with eradication of *H. pylori* infection.[22, 34] The precise mechanisms underlying the aberrant gastrin secretion found in duodenal ulcer disease are not clear but may involve *H. pylori*–induced increases in cytokines that stimulate gastrin release from G cells (e.g., tumor necrosis factor-α), and *H. pylori*–mediated decreases in the mucosal expression of somatostatin, a peptide that normally suppresses gastrin release.[35] This decrease in mucosal somatostatin may underlie the impaired inhibition of acid secretion in response to antral distention and antral acidification that has been described in some patients with duodenal ulcer disease.[36]

Serum concentrations of pepsinogen I, a protease made by chief and mucous neck cells in the gastric oxyntic mucosa, are elevated in as many as 50% of patients with duodenal ulcers.[37–39] This phenomenon may reflect the increased gastric secretory mass of patients who have duodenal ulcers. Although once regarded as a genetic marker for duodenal ulcer disease, hyperpepsinogenemia I appears to be another reversible consequence of *H. pylori* infection of the stomach.[40, 41]

Abnormalities in the vagal control of acid secretion have been postulated in some duodenal ulcer patients. These patients exhibit a dramatic decrease in acid secretion after vagotomy or atropine administration.[42] In some patients who have basal acid hypersecretion, sham feeding (which activates vagal efferent pathways to the stomach) does not cause a further increase in acid output.[43] In these patients, the basal acid hypersecretion appears to be driven by increased basal vagal tone that cannot be augmented by sham feeding. One report has suggested that the vagus nerves even may be larger in duodenal ulcer patients than in control subjects without ulcers.[44]

An increased rate of gastric emptying for liquids has been described in some patients with duodenal ulcer disease.[45, 46] Conceivably, rapid emptying of gastric acid into a vulnerable duodenum might predispose to ulceration. Compared with normal individuals, furthermore, patients with active duodenal ulcer exhibit a significant decrease in bicarbonate production by the proximal duodenum.[47] This phenomenon also might predispose to acid-peptic injury in the duodenum. Foci of gastric metaplasia are found in the duodenal bulb of most patients with duodenal ulcer.[48–50] Whereas *H. pylori* can infect gastric, but not intestinal mucosa, it has been proposed that these islands of infected gastric tissue in the duodenal bulb may be especially susceptible to peptic ulceration. Some investigators have found a higher prevalence of gastric metaplasia in the proximal duodenum of patients with duodenal ulcer disease compared with healthy control subjects,[22] whereas others have failed to confirm an association between duodenal gastric metaplasia and duodenal ulceration.[51, 52] Consequently, the role of duodenal gastric metaplasia in duodenal ulcer disease remains unclear.

An increased acid load in the duodenum may predispose to ulceration directly, through the caustic effects of acid on the duodenal epithelium, and, indirectly, through mechanisms involving *H. pylori*. The growth of *H. pylori* is inhibited by bile acids that are present in duodenal juice.[53] Acid can precipitate bile acids,[54] an effect that might allow *H. pylori* to proliferate and contribute to ulceration in the duodenum.

Abnormalities Associated with Gastric Ulcer

The gastric antrum normally is lined by a columnar epithelium that does not secrete acid, whereas an acid-secreting (oxyntic) mucosa with abundant parietal cells lines the gastric body and fundus. Most gastric ulcers occur in the non–acid-secreting epithelium at or near its junction with oxyntic mucosa, a phenomenon suggesting that the non–acid-secreting epithelium is inherently more susceptible to peptic ulceration.[1] Long-standing gastritis, as occurs in *H. pylori* infection, can cause atrophy of the oxyntic mucosa, with the development of intestinal metaplasia and the extension of a non–acid-secreting type of epithelium into the proximal stomach.[55] Patients who have ulcers located in the proximal stomach usually have chronic gastritis and substantial gastric atrophy. Not surprisingly, therefore, peptic ulcer disease that involves only the body and fundus of the stomach (type I gastric ulceration) has been found to be associated with hyposecretion of gastric acid, with a low-normal parietal cell mass and a decreased maximal acid output.[24, 56] Serum levels of pepsinogen II, a protease found in antral as well as oxyntic mucosa, are elevated in patients with type I gastric ulcers.[37] In contrast, patients who have concomitant ulcers of the gastric body and the duodenum (type II gastric ulceration) and patients who have gastric ulcers confined to the prepyloric antrum (type III gastric ulceration) have abnormalities in gastric acid homeostasis similar to those of patients with duodenal ulcer disease, often with elevated levels of pepsinogen I.

It has been proposed that the reflux of noxious material from the duodenum into the stomach may contribute to gastric ulceration in some patients. Potentially damaging agents in duodenal juice include bile salts and lysolecithin, and increased amounts of these agents have been found in the stomachs of patients with gastric ulcers.[57] Decreased pyloric sphincter pressures have been found in patients with gastric ulcer, a phenomenon that might predispose to duodenogastric reflux.[58] Antral motility abnormalities and abnormalities in the gastric emptying of solids also have been associated with gastric ulceration in some patients.[59, 60] The importance of any of these abnormalities in the pathogenesis of peptic ulcers remains unclear, and it is not known whether the observed motility abnormalities are primary defects or secondary effects of gastric ulceration.

Helicobacter pylori

This section deals only with some fundamental features of *H. pylori* infection that are essential for an understanding of peptic ulcer disease. For a detailed discussion of *H. pylori* and its effects on the gastrointestinal tract, the reader is referred to Chapter 39.

H. pylori is a gram-negative, spiral, flagellated bacterium. With its large, circular chromosome comprising more than 1400 genes, *H. pylori* is one of the most genetically diverse of all bacterial species.[61, 62] The organism is uniquely adapted for survival in the hostile environment of the stomach. For example, *H. pylori* produces large amounts of urease, an enzyme that catalyzes the breakdown of urea to alkaline ammonia and carbon dioxide.[63] Through this reaction, the bacterium may protect itself from acid injury by surrounding itself with alkaline material. The spiral structure and the flagella enable the organism to burrow through the gastric mucus layer.[64] After penetrating the mucus layer, *H. pylori* is able to attach itself to carbohydrates and sphingolipids on the luminal surface of the gastric epithelial cell.

It has been estimated that more than one half of the world's population is infected with *H. pylori*.[65] The infection appears to be spread from person to person, probably by the fecal-oral route. Within populations, rates of gastric infection with *H. pylori* are inversely proportional to socioeconomic status, and the prevalence of infection increases with age. In developing countries, children between 2 and 8 years of age acquire *H. pylori* infection at the rate of approximately 10% per annum.[3] Consequently, most adolescents and adults in developing countries are infected with *H. pylori*.[66] In Western countries, evidence of *H. pylori* infection can be found in approximately 20% of individuals younger than 40 years of age and in approximately 50% of those older than 60 years of age.[67, 68] In the United States, the frequency of infection in African Americans is approximately twice that of whites.[68]

Inflammation of the stomach (gastritis) is found in virtually all patients infected with *H. pylori*. Without treatment, *H. pylori* gastritis persists for decades and can lead to gastric atrophy with intestinal metaplasia.[55] With antibiotic therapy that eradicates the infection, however, the gastric inflammation disappears. Proof that *H. pylori* infection causes chronic gastritis was provided by several investigators who intentionally ingested the organism.[69] These investigators developed a chronic, superficial gastritis that abated when the infection was eradicated with antibiotic therapy.

H. pylori infection is strongly associated with peptic ulceration of the duodenum and stomach. Indeed, early studies suggested that almost all duodenal ulcers, and most gastric ulcers, were associated with *H. pylori* infection.[3] More recent studies suggest that these early estimates were somewhat exaggerated.[70] In the United States, perhaps 80% of patients who have duodenal ulcers are infected with the organism, as are more than 60% of those with gastric ulcers. Although the strong association between *H. pylori* and peptic ulcer disease is indisputable, the mechanisms whereby this infection predisposes to ulceration are incompletely understood. It has been estimated that fewer than 20% of individuals who are chronically infected with *H. pylori* ever develop a peptic ulcer.[71] This suggests that the development of peptic ulcer disease in infected individuals involves complex and poorly understood interactions among a number of factors, including the susceptibility of the host and the virulence of the infecting strains. Regardless of the mechanisms involved in ulcer pathogenesis, a number of long-term studies have shown that eradication of *H. pylori* with antibiotics dramatically decreases the ulcer recurrence rate to well below 10% in 1 year (Fig. 40–5).[2, 72]

In a number of bacterial species, virulence is associated with the presence of unique, lengthy DNA sequences known as *pathogenicity islands*. Some strains of *H. pylori* have a *cag* pathogenicity island, a 40-kb-pair segment of DNA comprising a collection of approximately 30 genes that may be involved in bacterial virulence.[73] The *cag*A gene, located at one end of the pathogenicity island, encodes for the CagA

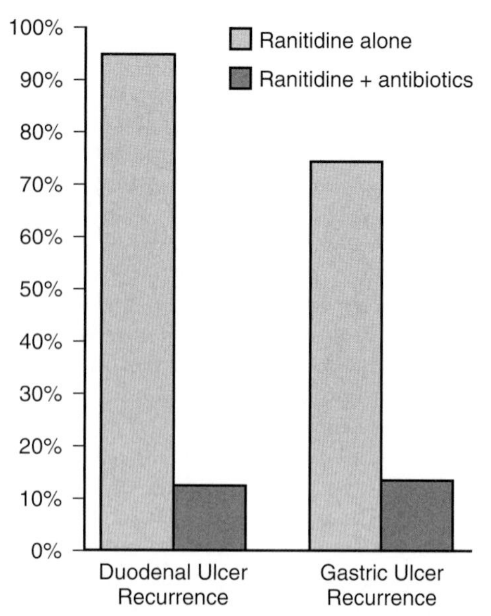

Figure 40–5. Recurrence of duodenal or gastric ulcer within 2 years in patients treated with a short course of either ranitidine alone to heal the ulcer, or a combination of ranitidine plus antibiotics designed also to eradicate *Helicobacter pylori* infection. (Data from Graham DY, Lew GM, Klein PD, et al: Effect of treatment of *Helicobacter pylori* infection on the long-term recurrence of gastric or duodenal ulcer. A randomized, controlled study. Ann Intern Med 116:705–708, 1992.)

protein.[74] Individuals infected with such strains develop circulating antibodies to CagA and, consequently, serologic tests can be used to diagnose *cag*A-positive infections. *cag*A positivity appears to be associated with an elevated risk for peptic ulcer disease (compared with *cag*A negativity).[75] However, testing for CagA status presently is not yet recommended for clinical purposes.

It seems paradoxical that *H. pylori* infection promotes acid hypersecretion and duodenal ulceration in some patients, whereas others develop gastric atrophy, intestinal metaplasia, and cancer.[76] One popular hypothesis relates the outcome of *H. pylori* infection to the severity and pattern of gastritis that it induces.[77] According to this hypothesis, *H. pylori* infection that involves the antrum predominantly, while relatively sparing the acid-secreting portion of the stomach, will predispose to duodenal ulceration. In contrast, *H. pylori* infection that causes intense inflammation in the oxyntic mucosa will result in gastric atrophy with a decreased acid output and a predisposition to gastric ulceration and cancer. The severity and pattern of gastritis induced by *H. pylori* may be determined by the virulence of the infecting organism, by host factors, by the age of the host at the time the infection is acquired, and by environmental influences. Although this hypothesis is conceptually appealing, it is based largely on circumstantial evidence and speculation. Proof of this hypothesis will require substantial further investigation.

A number of tests (discussed in Chapter 39) are available to establish the diagnosis of *H. pylori* infection.[78] Any of the diagnostic tests can be repeated after treatment to establish that the organism has been eradicated, but serologic tests have limited usefulness in this regard because antibody levels may fall slowly after *H. pylori* eradication.[79]

Nonsteroidal Anti-inflammatory Drugs

This section deals only with the fundamental features of NSAIDs that are essential for an understanding of peptic ulcer disease. For a detailed discussion of NSAIDs and their effects on the gastrointestinal tract, the reader is referred to Chapter 23.

NSAIDs can injure the gastroduodenal mucosa through both topical and systemic effects.[80] In acidic gastric juice, weakly acidic NSAIDs such as aspirin are in an un-ionized form in which they can freely penetrate gastric cells. In the neutral pH environment within the cell, H^+ ions dissociate, and the resulting negatively charged NSAID molecule cannot cross the cell membrane. In this manner, potentially injurious NSAIDs rapidly become concentrated within the mucosal cells. Hence, superficial injury (e.g., petechiae, erosions) can occur within minutes of ingesting NSAIDs. Some NSAID metabolites that are excreted in bile also can cause topical injury to the gastrointestinal mucosa.[81]

Superficial NSAID injury of the stomach can be lessened with the use of enteric-coated preparations or administration of the NSAIDs through the parenteral or rectal routes.[82–84] However, these preparations do not appear to reduce the risk of gastroduodenal ulceration.[85] These and other observations suggest that ulceration is due to the systemic, rather than topical, effects of NSAIDs.[86, 87] Presumably, ulceration is a consequence of the reduced mucosal prostaglandin synthesis that accompanies NSAID-induced inhibition of cyclooxygenase. Inhibition of prostaglandin synthesis can result in decreased epithelial secretion of mucus and bicarbonate, diminished mucosal blood flow, reduced mucosal proliferation, and impaired resistance to peptic injury.[80, 81, 86, 88]

Superficial gastric lesions such as petechiae and erosions are found in approximately 50% of individuals who chronically consume NSAIDs, but these lesions appear to have little clinical importance. Ulcerations can be documented endoscopically in 15% to 30% of patients on chronic NSAID therapy.[89–91] Indeed, most peptic ulcerations that are not associated with *H. pylori* infection are associated with NSAID ingestion.[3] NSAIDs clearly increase the risk of ulcer complications such as bleeding and perforation.[92] However, only a small minority of patients who take NSAIDs develop ulcers that are symptomatic or complicated. For patients who have no risk factors for NSAID complications (see later), several studies suggest that the incidence of developing a serious complication such as bleeding or perforation from chronic NSAID use is approximately 0.5% per year, and only approximately 1% of these average-risk patients will develop an uncomplicated ulcer that causes symptoms.[93–95]

The concomitant use of corticosteroids and NSAIDs appears to increase the incidence of complicated peptic ulcer disease above that of NSAID ingestion alone.[96] Although some data have suggested an association between peptic ulceration and the use of corticosteroids (without NSAIDs) in high dosages, most studies on this issue have not found an increased risk for peptic ulceration in patients taking steroids unless the steroids were used together with NSAIDs. In addition to the concomitant use of corticosteroids, the following are well-established risk factors for NSAID-induced ulcerations and complications: (1) history of previous peptic ulceration or gastrointestinal bleeding, (2) advanced age, and (3) serious systemic disorders. The use of NSAIDs in high doses, multiple different NSAIDs, and the concomitant administration of anticoagulants also increase the risk for NSAID-associated gastrointestinal events.[91, 97, 98]

NSAID use and *H. pylori* infection are generally regarded as independent risk factors for peptic ulcer disease.[99] When an *H. pylori*–infected patient who uses NSAIDs develops a peptic ulcer, however, it is difficult to determine the contribution of each factor to the peptic lesion. Some data suggest that active *H. pylori* infection increases the risk for peptic ulceration during NSAID therapy. In a study of patients in Hong Kong who were treated with naproxen for 8 weeks, for example, endoscopic examination at 8 weeks revealed peptic ulcers in only 3% of those whose *H. pylori* infections were eradicated at the start of naproxen therapy, whereas ulcers were found in 26% of patients with untreated *H. pylori* infection.[100] A recent case-control study has suggested that NSAID users infected with *H. pylori* have an almost twofold increased risk for developing bleeding peptic ulcers compared with uninfected NSAID users.[101] Another recent study has shown that low-dose aspirin causes more gastric injury in *H. pylori*–infected subjects than in uninfected individuals.[102] Thus, evidence is accumulating that *H. pylori* infection and NSAID use may be more than just additive risk factors for ulcer disease, but these issues require further investigation.

Other Ulcerogenic Drugs

There are a number of drugs, other than NSAIDs, that appear to predispose to peptic injury. For example, cancer chemotherapy with hepatic arterial infusion of 5-fluorouracil has been associated with gastric and duodenal ulcers.[103] Solid preparations of potassium chloride also can cause gastrointestinal ulcerations. The use of crack cocaine has been associated with ulcers of the prepyloric antrum that are complicated by perforation.[104] Much recent attention has focused on the ulcerogenic potential of the bisphosphonates.

Two bisphosphonates, alendronate and risedronate, are used widely for the treatment or prevention of osteoporosis.[105] Although early, premarketing studies revealed no important gastrointestinal toxicity for the bisphosphonates, numerous postmarketing reports have described esophageal and gastric ulcerations associated with the use of these agents.[106, 107] In a recent blinded, crossover study in which healthy volunteers were randomly assigned to receive either alendronate 10 mg daily or placebo, endoscopic examination after 2 weeks of treatment revealed antral ulcers or large antral erosions in 6 of 24 subjects taking alendronate (25%), and in none of those taking placebo.[108] In a study in which healthy, postmenopausal women were treated with either risedronate 5 mg daily or alendronate 10 mg daily for 2 weeks,[109] gastric ulcers were seen in 4% of patients in the risedronate group and in 13% of the alendronate group; duodenal ulcers were uncommon (<1% of both groups). Although the precise mechanism by which these agents cause gastrointestinal injury is not clear, it has been suggested that the bisphosphonate molecules disrupt the surface phospholipid layer that protects the epithelial cells.[109] Alendronate has a primary amino side chain, whereas risedronate has a pyridinyl side chain. The primary amino side chain of alendronate may be the molecular feature that predisposes to this gastrointestinal toxicity.[108] It is not yet known whether infection with *H. pylori* or the concomitant use of NSAIDs potentiates the ulcerogenic effects of the bisphosphonates.

Hypersecretory Conditions

As discussed earlier, most peptic ulcer disease is the result of defects in epithelial defenses and acid homeostasis that are caused by *H. pylori* infection or by NSAID ingestion (see Fig. 40–2). Rarely, peptic ulcer disease results from disorders that cause the stomach to secrete gastric acid in quantities so large that they overwhelm the normal epithelial defense mechanisms. In addition to causing peptic ulceration, the copious amounts of gastric acid dumped into the duodenum in these hypsersecretory conditions can denature pancreatic digestive enzymes and cause malabsorption with diarrhea (see Chapter 89). Hypersecretory conditions should be considered in any patient who has peptic ulcer disease in the absence of *H. pylori* infection or NSAID use, especially if there is associated diarrhea and if the ulcer disease is severe, complicated, or involves the postbulbar duodenum.

Gastrinoma

A syndrome of severe peptic ulcer disease associated with extreme hypersecretion of gastric acid and non-beta islet cell tumors of the pancreas was described by Zollinger and Ellison in 1955, and is discussed in Chapter 41.

Systemic Mastocytosis and Myeloproliferative Disorders with Basophilia

Systemic mastocytosis is a rare disorder characterized by mast cell infiltration of a number of organs.[110] The mast cells release histamine, the agent principally responsible for most of the symptoms of systemic mastocytosis that include flushing, tachycardia, asthma, pruritus, and headache. The elevated serum levels of histamine appear to cause the profound gastric acid hypersecretion that has been documented in some patients. Duodenal ulceration occurs in approximately 40% of cases. Like mast cells, basophils also contain histamine. Occasionally, myeloproliferative disorders associated with basophilia (e.g., polycythemia vera, basophilic chronic myelogenous leukemia) have been accompanied by gastric acid hypersecretion and peptic ulcer disease.[111]

Antral G Cell Hyperfunction

In the era before the discovery of *H. pylori*, a rare syndrome characterized by gastric acid hypersecretion associated with elevated fasting serum gastrin levels and marked postprandial hypergastrinemia was described.[112] It was proposed that this syndrome was due to hyperfunction of the antral G cells. It now appears that this syndrome is a consequence of *H. pylori* infection in most cases, although there may be a rare, primary form of antral G cell hyperfunction that is not associated with *H. pylori*.[113]

EPIDEMIOLOGY

Trends in the Frequency of Peptic Ulcer Disease

It has been estimated that there are approximately 500,000 new cases and 4 million recurrences of peptic ulcers in the United States each year[114, 115] and that approximately 10% of individuals in Western countries will develop a peptic ulcer at some point during their lifetimes.[116]

Peptic ulcer disease appears to have been a rare disorder before the 19th century.[117] Early in that century, cases of perforated peptic ulcerations of the stomach were first described in young women. Over the ensuing decades, peptic ulcer disease became more frequent in men and, by the end of the 19th century, duodenal ulcer disease had surpassed gastric ulcer disease in frequency. The incidence of peptic ulceration rose dramatically through the first half of the 20th century. However, late in the 1960s, the overall incidence of peptic ulcer disease began to decline.[118] This trend has continued and has been accompanied by a decreasing frequency of hospitalizations (Fig. 40–6) and physician visits for peptic ulcer disease (especially for uncomplicated duodenal ulcer), and by declining rates of operations for and deaths from peptic ulceration.[117, 119, 120]

The temporal trends in the frequency of peptic ulcer disease perhaps are best appreciated by evaluating birth cohorts (groups of subjects born during the same time period) rather than by evaluating the frequency of ulcer events in a given time period. In Western countries and in Japan, the risk of developing peptic ulcer disease rose in birth cohorts born before the turn of the 20th century and then declined in subsequent generations.[118, 121, 125] The peak mortality rates for gastric ulcer occurred in individuals born between 1870 and 1890, whereas the peak mortality rates for duodenal ulcer were found in birth cohorts born between 1880 and 1900 (Fig. 40–7).

If a disease exhibits a birth-cohort phenomenon, it implies that the disease was influenced importantly by exposure to exogenous risk factors early in life. The declining incidence of peptic ulcer disease in birth cohorts born during the last century suggests that the childhood exposures responsible for ulcerations in adults have been decreasing for almost 100 years. Much evidence suggests that the declining prevalence of *H. pylori* infection in individuals born after the turn of the 20th century underlies, at least in part, the declining frequency of peptic ulcer in birth cohorts.[126] However, it is likely that factors other than *H. pylori* infection also have influenced the trends of peptic ulcer occurrence.

In contrast to the profound decline in the frequency of uncomplicated peptic ulcer disease, the rate of hospitalization for ulcer complications including hemorrhage and perforation has not decreased substantially in the past few decades. Indeed, the rate of these complications in elderly individuals appears to be increasing, especially for gastric ulcers.[127, 128] Available evidence suggests that the rising rate of peptic ulcer complications in the elderly may be due, at

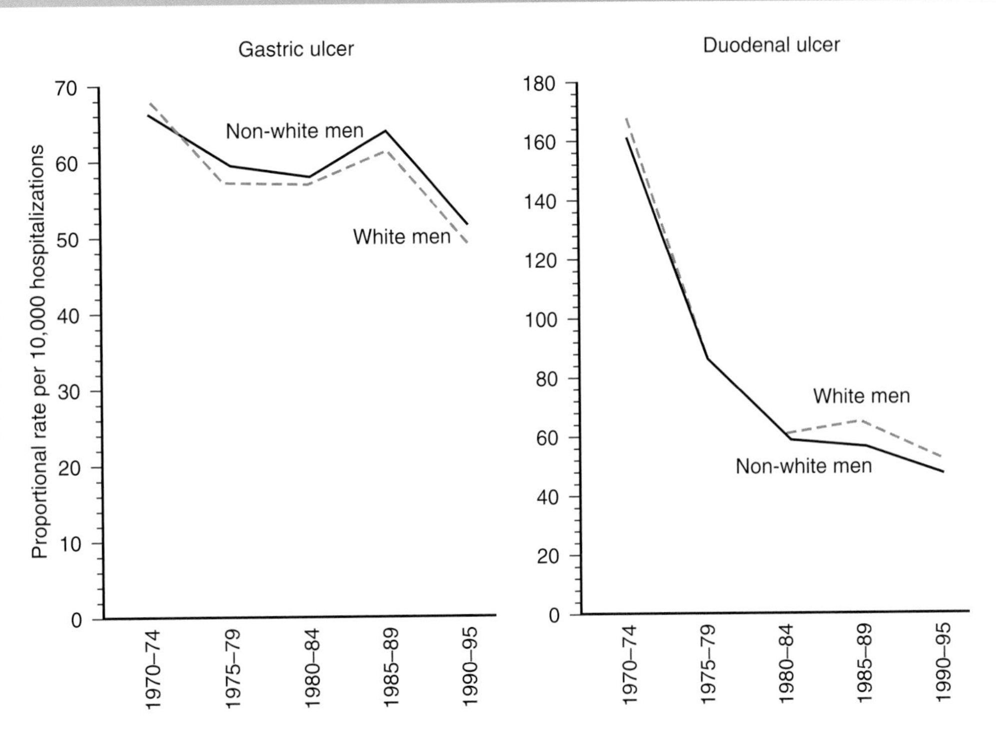

Figure 40–6. Time trends of hospitalization for gastric and duodenal ulcer among male veterans in the United States. Note different vertical scales for gastric and duodenal ulcers. (Adapted from El-Serag HB, Sonnenberg A: Opposing time trends of peptic ulcer and reflux disease. Gut 43:327–333, 1998.)

least in part, to their increased usage of NSAIDs that predispose to ulcer perforation and bleeding.[128–130]

Cigarette Smoking

Cigarette smoking is a risk factor for peptic ulcer disease and its complications.[4, 131–133] Furthermore, cigarette smoking may adversely affect the healing of peptic ulcerations and, in the absence of treatment for *H. pylori*, may predispose to relapses.[134] Cigarette smoking does not appear to influence the relapse rate for peptic ulceration when *H. pylori* has been eradicated,[135] however, and at least one study has disputed the association between smoking and peptic ulcer disease.[136] Cigarette smokers have been found to have decreased prostaglandin concentrations in their gastric and duodenal mucosae,[137] and smoking has been shown to inhibit acid-stimulated duodenal mucosal bicarbonate secretion.[138] Other proposed mechanisms whereby smoking might promote peptic ulceration include increased gastric acidity[139] and *H. pylori* proliferation.[140] It is not clear which, if any, of these proposed mechanisms contributes to peptic ulceration in cigarette smokers.

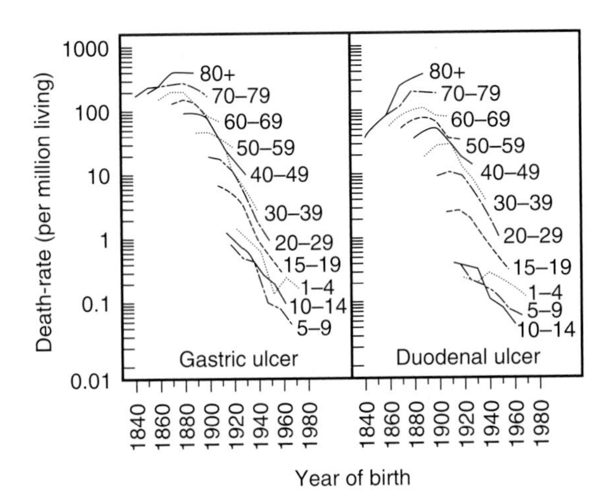

Figure 40–7. Age-specific death rates from peptic ulcer according to year of birth. The curves are the weighted average of data from 10 countries. (From Sonnenberg A: Temporal trends and geographical variations of peptic ulcer disease. Aliment Pharmacol Ther 9(Suppl 2):3–12, 1995.)

Alcohol

There is a common misconception among clinicians that alcohol ingestion is a strong risk factor for peptic ulcer disease. In fact, few published data support this notion. Wine and beer are potent gastric acid secretagogues, but the importance of this phenomenon in the pathogenesis of peptic ulceration is dubious.[141, 142] Although absolute ethanol (200 proof) has been shown to damage the gastrointestinal mucosa of experimental animals,[143] ethanol in the concentrations ordinarily found in alcoholic beverages has been found to cause only superficial mucosal injury of unclear importance in humans.[144] The prevalence of ulcer disease appears to be increased for patients with alcoholic cirrhosis,[145] but no such association has been established for drinkers without cirrhosis. Indeed, one retrospective study suggested that modest alcohol consumption might even protect against peptic ulceration.[146]

Diet

No study has established a convincing link between diet and peptic ulcer disease. Patients often describe dyspepsia associated with the ingestion of certain foods (e.g., spicy foods), but the evidence that such foods cause ulceration is virtually nonexistent. Coffee, tea, and colas are potent gastric acid secretagogues,[141, 147] but epidemiologic studies have not established an association between these beverages and peptic ulcer disease. Of note, both caffeinated and decaffeinated coffee appear to be equal in their ability to stimulate gastric acid secretion.[141] Although it was once traditional to prescribe a bland diet for patients with peptic ulcers, such diets have been found to be quite stimulating to the parietal cell. Bland diets have not been shown to have any benefit in preventing or treating peptic ulcer disease.

Diseases Associated with Peptic Ulcer

A number of chronic illnesses have been associated with peptic ulcer disease. For example, peptic ulcerations have been found in up to 30% of patients with chronic pulmonary disease.[148–150] The mechanisms responsible for this association are not clear, although cigarette smoking may underlie both conditions. Patients with cirrhosis appear to have an increased risk of developing peptic ulceration and its complications.[151, 152] Chronic renal failure has been proposed as a risk factor for peptic ulcer disease, but studies on this issue are contradictory.[153] Other disorders allegedly associated with peptic ulceration, but for which firm evidence is lacking, include Cushing's disease, hyperparathyroidism, and coronary artery disease.[1] The frequency of *H. pylori* infection among patients with these chronic disorders is not yet clear, and the possible contribution of *H. pylori* to the association of these conditions with peptic ulceration has not yet been explored adequately.

Emotional Stress

A number of reports have suggested that emotional stress might cause or exacerbate peptic ulceration.[154, 155] During the bombing of London in World War II, for example, British physicians observed a substantial increase in the incidence of perforated peptic ulcers.[156, 157] The lay public has long embraced the concept that emotional stress and peptic ulcers go hand in hand. Since the recognition of the importance of *H. pylori* in the pathogenesis of peptic ulcer, however, physician interest in the association between emotional stress and ulcer disease has waned. Emotional stress alone does not appear to be sufficient to cause ulcers in most patients, because eradication of *H. pylori* and elimination of NSAIDs generally prevents ulcer recurrence irrespective of emotional factors. Nevertheless, some modern studies still suggest that stress contributes to peptic ulcer disease.[158] After the devastating earthquake that killed thousands in the Hanshin-Awaji region of Japan, for example, investigators observed an increased frequency of bleeding gastric ulcers.[159] Furthermore, it is not known why only a few individuals who take NSAIDs or who are infected with *H. pylori* develop peptic ulcers, and emotional stress may well be a risk factor in these susceptible subjects.

Genetics

Genetic factors appear to predispose to ulcer disease. For example, the concordance for peptic ulcer among identical twins has been found to be higher than for nonidentical twins, and first-degree relatives of ulcer patients have been shown to be at high risk for developing peptic ulcers.[1] The genes responsible for this apparent ulcer predisposition are not known. Furthermore, it now appears that some of this familial clustering of ulcer disease is the result of a high rate of *H. pylori* infection in family members rather than a consequence of genetic factors predisposing to ulcer disease per se. An elevated level of serum pepsinogen I, initially thought to be a genetic marker for ulcer disease,[160] also appears to be a reversible consequence of *H. pylori* infection.[40, 41] Other proposed genetic markers for ulcer disease include blood group O antigen, the lack of secretion of blood group antigens in the saliva, and the presence of certain HLA subtypes.[161] The association of certain blood group antigens with peptic ulcer may be explicable, at least in part, by the fact that these antigens may affect an individual's susceptibility to *H. pylori* infection. For example, Lewis blood group antigens have been shown to mediate *H. pylori* attachment to the human gastric mucosa.[162] In a large study of Danish men, Hein and associates found that Lewis phenotype Le (a^+b^-) and the ABH nonsecretor trait were markers for ulcer disease.[163] The investigators suggested that these traits might confer a genetic susceptibility to *H. pylori* infection rather than a specific susceptibility to peptic ulceration.

CLINICAL FEATURES OF UNCOMPLICATED PEPTIC ULCERS

Abdominal pain is the cardinal symptom of peptic ulcer disease. However, the mechanism whereby peptic ulceration causes pain is not clear. Traditionally, physicians have attributed the pain of ulcers to episodes of acid exposure that stimulate nociceptors exposed by the peptic injury.[164] This concept clearly is too simplistic, however. Endoscopic studies have shown that peptic ulcerations are often asymptomatic and, in one study, duodenal acid perfusion in patients with active peptic ulceration produced pain in only 16 of 40 cases.[165] Conversely, pain syndromes indistinguishable from those of classic peptic ulcer disease occur frequently in patients who have no demonstrable ulcer craters,[166] and patients who have healed their peptic ulcers nevertheless may experience ulcer-type pain.[167]

The pain of duodenal ulceration often is described as burning or gnawing in character and usually is located in the epigastrium. Characteristically, the pain occurs 2 to 3 hours after a meal, and the discomfort is relieved by the ingestion of food or antacids. Approximately two thirds of patients describe pain that awakens them in the middle of the night, but pain on awakening in the morning is unusual.[168] Some patients describe pain episodes that occur in clusters of days to weeks, followed by longer pain-free intervals. Anorexia and weight loss occur infrequently in uncomplicated duodenal ulcer. Indeed, patients often describe hyperphagia and weight gain, perhaps because eating typically relieves the pain of duodenal ulceration.

Patients with gastric ulcers also describe burning or gnawing pain in the epigastrium that may be indistinguishable from that of duodenal ulcer disease. The pain of gastric ulcer tends to occur sooner after meals than duodenal ulcer pain, however, and relief by food and antacids may not occur as reliably. Indeed, eating may precipitate pain immediately in some patients. Only approximately one third of patients with gastric ulcers describe pain that awakens them from sleep.[168] Anorexia and weight loss may occur in up to one half of patients. These symptoms may be a consequence of the delayed gastric emptying that can accompany ulceration of the stomach, even in the absence of mechanical gastric outlet obstruction. Consequently, benign and malignant gastric ulcers are not distinguished reliably by history alone, because both may present with similar degrees of pain, anorexia, and weight loss.

Many patients who present to the hospital with life-threatening complications of peptic ulceration, such as hemorrhage and perforation, have no previous symptoms of ulcer disease.[169] Often, these complications occur in elderly patients who are taking NSAIDs. In addition to their role in promoting peptic ulceration, it has been proposed that NSAIDs may mask the pain of peptic ulcer disease.

Reliance on symptoms is neither a sensitive nor specific means to diagnose peptic ulcer disease. Neoplasms involving the stomach and pancreas may cause pain similar to that of peptic ulceration. Pancreatitis and cholecystitis can cause epigastric pain, sometimes with characteristics of peptic ulcer disease. The pyrosis of acid reflux disease can be referred to the epigastrium, as can pain due to Crohn's disease that involves the upper gastrointestinal tract. Mesenteric vascular insufficiency can cause postprandial pain mimicking that of peptic ulcer disease. For a complete discussion of the broad differential diagnosis of acute and chronic abdominal pain, the reader is referred to Chapters 4 and 5. If peptic ulcer disease is suspected on the basis of symptoms, objective tests are necessary to confirm the diagnosis.

DIAGNOSTIC TESTS

Radiography and Endoscopy

For decades before flexible endoscopy became widely available, barium contrast examination of the upper gastrointestinal tract was the standard test for establishing the presence of peptic ulcer disease. Since the introduction of flexible endoscopy into clinical practice in the 1960s, however, radiography has assumed a much lesser role in the evaluation of peptic ulcers, largely for two reasons: (1) The barium contrast examination is substantially less sensitive than endoscopy for identifying peptic ulcerations and other mucosal lesions of the upper gastrointestinal tract, and (2) unlike endoscopy, barium studies do not allow the opportunity to obtain biopsy specimens from suspicious lesions. The demonstration of lesions suspicious for cancer on barium contrast examination often will require endoscopic evaluation for confirmation and biopsy sampling. Consequently, endoscopy has become the recommended first test for confirming the presence of peptic ulceration in patients with dyspeptic symptoms.[170, 171] After the endoscopic demonstration of a peptic ulcer, radiography will not be needed at all in most patients. For selected patients with complicated ulcer disease, however, barium contrast radiography occasionally may provide important information about gastroduodenal anatomy that cannot be ascertained by endoscopic examination alone.

A number of studies have compared the accuracy of upper gastrointestinal radiology and upper gastrointestinal endoscopy for diagnosing peptic ulcer disease. For double-contrast barium studies, the reported accuracy for identifying peptic ulcerations (compared with endoscopy) is approximately 80% to 90%, whereas single-contrast barium studies have only a 60% to 80% rate of accuracy.[172, 173] Although few would dispute that endoscopy is more accurate than radiography as a diagnostic test for peptic ulceration, the clinician should appreciate that studies comparing radiography and endoscopy generally have been biased in favor of endoscopy. This is because endoscopy usually has been used as the gold standard for establishing the presence of mucosal disease. In this situation, the diagnostic accuracy of radiology at best can only equal, and can never exceed, that of endoscopy. A mucosal lesion missed by the gold standard endoscopic examination would either be missed or dismissed as a spurious finding on the barium contrast study.

Peptic ulcers can involve any part of the stomach, but more than 80% are located on the lesser curvature within 90 mm of the pylorus.[174] Peptic ulcerations are inflammatory lesions that burrow into the wall of the involved organ. Benign gastric ulcers reflect this basic pathophysiology by displaying the following radiographic features:

1. The ulcer appears to project outside the lumen of the stomach (i.e., into the wall of the stomach).
2. There are thickened, smooth, symmetrical (inflammatory) folds that radiate to the ulcer crater.
3. There is an incisura (indentation) on the wall of the stomach opposite the ulcer crater (a consequence of the thick, inflammatory folds).
4. There may be a smooth, radiolucent band or collar at the neck of the ulcer caused by the intense inflammation and accompanying edema.
5. There may be a thin, radiolucent line (Hampton line) at the rim of the ulcer crater where the mucosa has been undermined by the inflammatory process.

An example of a radiologically benign gastric ulcer is shown in Figure 40–8. In contrast to benign peptic ulcers, malignant ulcerations are necrotic lesions that develop in neoplastic tissue, often when portions of the tumor have outgrown their blood supply. Radiographically, these ulcerated neoplasms appear as irregular collections of barium within an intraluminal mass (the ulcer does not project outside the lumen of the stomach). There may be thickened folds surrounding the ulcer crater but, because the folds represent neoplastic infiltration rather than inflammation, they are usually not smooth and symmetrically distributed. The radiographic demonstration of ulcer healing with treatment is regarded as a sign of benignity, but complete healing of malignant ulcerations has been documented occasionally.

Malignant gastric ulcers clearly can appear benign by radiographic criteria. Older studies suggest that the risk of cancer in a radiographically benign gastric ulceration is approximately 3% to 5%.[175] Consequently, gastric ulcers found by barium studies require endoscopic evaluation and biopsy sampling to exclude malignancy. Ulcerations of the duodenal bulb are rarely neoplastic, in contrast, and endoscopic evaluation to exclude cancer is not recommended routinely for patients who have barium studies that demonstrate uncomplicated duodenal ulcerations.

Endoscopically, peptic ulcers typically appear as discrete, excavated lesions with a whitish base (Fig. 40–9; see also Color Fig. 40–9). The edges of benign ulcers usually are smooth and regular, and symmetrically thickened (inflammatory) folds typically radiate to the ulcer base. In contrast, malignant ulcers characteristically have irregular edges, and the surrounding, asymmetrical folds do not radiate to the base of the ulcer. Such folds may appear nodular or clubbed. Often, there is an obvious mass surrounding the malignant ulcer. Endoscopic appearance alone is an imperfect index for malignancy, however. In one series of 87 gastric ulcerations that eventually proved to be benign, the endoscopic appearance was deemed benign in only 73 cases (84%), malignant in 4 cases (5%), and indeterminate in 10 cases (11%).[176] Conversely, among 20 proven gastric malignancies, the endoscopic appearance was deemed benign in 6 cases (30%), malignant in 12 cases (60%), and indeterminate in 2 cases (10%).

During endoscopic evaluation, biopsy samples are not obtained routinely from duodenal ulcers because these ulcers are so rarely malignant. In contrast, multiple biopsy specimens must be taken to distinguish benign from malignant gastric ulcerations (see Chapter 44). Biopsy specimens should be taken primarily from the mucosa at the edges of the gastric ulceration, because specimens obtained from the ulcer crater often show only necrotic debris and granulation tissue. The optimum number of biopsy specimens to take at the initial endoscopic evaluation of a gastric ulcer is disputed, but a number of studies on this issue suggest that approximately 98% of all gastric cancers will be found if at least six biopsy specimens are obtained.[176–179] With the addition of brush cytology to this biopsy regimen, the accuracy for diagnosing gastric cancer on initial evaluation approaches 100%.[180]

In the era before the widespread availability of flexible endoscopy, when biopsy sampling of radiographically demonstrated gastric ulcerations was not performed routinely, a key component of patient management was the documentation (with follow-up barium studies) that the gastric ulcers healed with medical therapy. This practice evolved because of the substantial inaccuracy of radiography for excluding malignancy in gastric ulcers, and clinicians believed that a demonstration of healing was required to establish that an ulceration was benign. Follow-up barium contrast examinations were performed routinely in patients who had medical treatment for gastric ulcers, and surgery was recommended for those whose ulcers did not heal completely after an appropriate interval (e.g., 12 weeks). As discussed earlier, initial endoscopic evaluation of gastric ulcers now can identify malignant gastric ulcers with an accuracy of more than 98%. Nevertheless, the traditional practice of requiring a demonstration of ulcer healing to exclude cancer has carried over into the endoscopic era. Recent studies have found that this practice detects few additional cancers, and the authors of these reports discourage routine follow-up endoscopy for gastric ulcers.[181, 182] Some authorities have suggested that after an initial endoscopic evaluation of gastric ulcer that includes brush cytology and at least six biopsy specimens, repeat endoscopy to document healing should not be performed routinely if the ulcer is benign by endoscopic, histologic, and cytologic criteria.[180] Follow-up endoscopy is recommended only if any of these tests suggest malignancy.

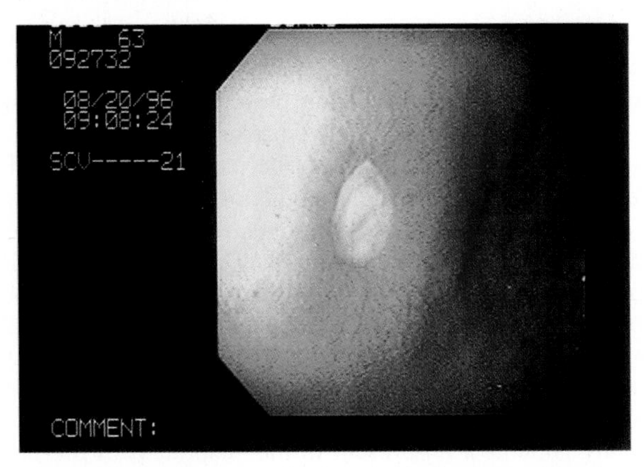

Figure 40–9. Endoscopic photograph of a benign gastric ulcer.

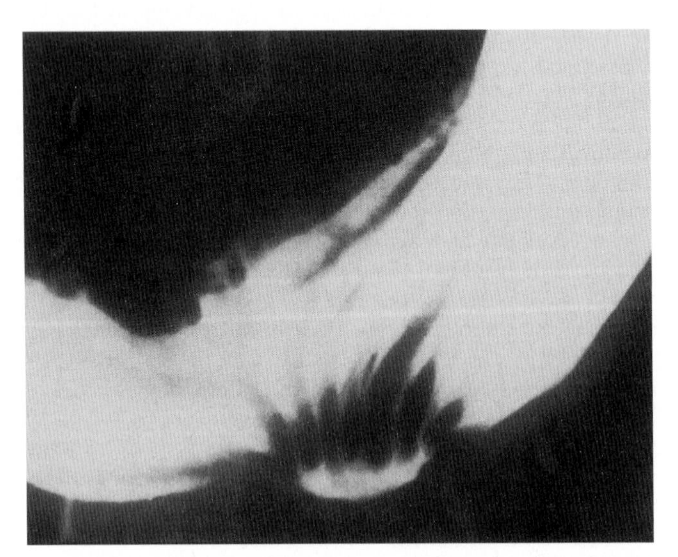

Figure 40–8. Barium contrast examination showing a benign gastric ulcer. Note the smooth, symmetric folds radiating to the ulcer crater that appears to project outside the lumen of the stomach.

TREATMENTS FOR PEPTIC ULCER DISEASE

Patients found to have peptic ulcers should be tested for *H. pylori* infection and should be questioned carefully regarding the use of NSAIDs. If *H. pylori* infection is documented, patients should be treated with one of the regimens recommended in Chapter 39, irrespective of whether there is a history of NSAID use. If possible, NSAID therapy should be stopped. Specific therapies for peptic ulcer are discussed in the following sections.

Histamine H_2 Receptor Antagonists

Currently, four histamine H_2 receptor antagonists are used widely as antisecretory agents—cimetidine (Tagamet), ranitidine (Zantac), famotidine (Pepcid), and nizatidine (Axid). All four agents are available without a prescription (over the counter) in the United States. The histamine H_2 receptor antagonists inhibit acid secretion by blocking histamine H_2 receptors on the gastric parietal cell.

The histamine H_2 receptor antagonists are well absorbed after oral dosing, and absorption is not affected by food. The concomitant administration of antacids and sucralfate can decrease absorption by 10% to 20%, however. Peak blood levels are achieved within 1 to 3 hours after an oral dose. These drugs are well distributed throughout the body, and all cross the blood-brain barrier and the placenta.[183, 184] After oral administration, cimetidine, ranitidine, and famotidine undergo first-pass hepatic metabolism that reduces their bioavailability by 35% to 60%. In contrast, nizatidine does not undergo first-pass metabolism, and its bioavailability approaches 100% with oral dosing. With intravenous administration, the bioavailability of all four agents is close to 100%.[185–192]

All four histamine H_2 receptor antagonists are eliminated by a combination of renal excretion and hepatic metabolism. The renal excretion is accomplished both by glomerular filtration and by tubular secretion of the agents. Sixty percent to 80% of orally administered cimetidine, ranitidine, and famotidine is cleared by the liver, whereas the elimination of oral nizatidine is accomplished primarily through renal excretion. After intravenous administration, in contrast, all four agents are eliminated principally through renal excretion. Dose reductions are recommended for patients with renal insufficiency (Table 40–2). Dialysis does not remove substantial amounts of the histamine H_2 receptor antagonists, and so dose adjustments for dialysis are not necessary. Liver failure has been found to prolong the half-life of cimetidine, but dose reductions generally are not needed for patients with hepatic failure unless it is accompanied by renal insufficiency.[185]

The histamine H_2 receptor antagonists are competitive inhibitors of histamine-stimulated acid secretion, although famotidine appears to have some component of noncompetitive inhibition as well.[186] In addition to blocking histamine-stimulated gastric acid secretion, all four agents suppress basal acid output and acid output stimulated by meals. When administered in the evening, the drugs are especially effective in suppressing basal acid output at night.[193] This effect appears to be particularly important, because the healing rate for peptic ulcers with antisecretory therapy correlates strongly with the degree of reduction in nocturnal gastric acidity.[194]

Early experience with the histamine H_2 receptor antagonists in peptic ulcer disease involved multiple-dose regimens (e.g., cimetidine 300 mg four times a day). With the recognition that control of nocturnal gastric acidity plays a key role in the healing of peptic ulcers, subsequent investigations demonstrated that single-evening-dose regimens, with the drug administered between the evening meal and bedtime, were at least as effective as multiple-dose regimens for hastening the healing of peptic ulcerations. Using the single-evening-dose regimens summarized in Table 40–2 for 4 to 6 weeks, healing rates for duodenal ulcer of 70% to 80% can be achieved. Healing rates for gastric ulcer at 4 to 6 weeks appear to be somewhat lower, in the range of 55% to 65%. All four agents achieve comparable healing rates, and no agent has been shown to be clearly superior to the others in healing efficacy.

The histamine H_2 receptor antagonists are a remarkably safe and well-tolerated group of agents. The overall incidence of side effects is less than 4%, and serious side effects are decidedly uncommon. One meta-analysis of randomized clinical trials concluded that the overall rate of adverse effects reported for the H_2 blockers did not differ significantly from that for placebo.[195] Nevertheless, a number of untoward effects have been described, primarily in anecdotal reports and uncontrolled series. Most attention regarding adverse events has focused on cimetidine, probably because it was the first histamine H_2 receptor antagonist released for clinical use and because it has undergone the most extensive post-marketing surveillance. Although the potential for drug interactions may be highest for cimetidine (see later), no clear-cut safety advantage has been established for any one of the four histamine H_2 receptor antagonists.

Some of the putative side effects of the histamine H_2 receptor antagonists may result from the inhibition of H_2 receptors in organs other than the stomach. There are histamine H_2 receptors in the heart that mediate inotropic and chronotropic effects, for example, and the use of histamine H_2 receptor antagonists (particularly by the intravenous route) rarely has been associated with bradyarrhythmias and tachyarrhythmias, atrioventricular conduction abnormalities, hypotension, and cardiac arrest.[185, 196] These effects have been observed predominantly in patients who were seriously ill, some of whom received the drugs in a rapid intravenous bolus injection. If these agents are to be used intravenously, it seems prudent to avoid rapid bolus injection.

There are histamine H_2 receptors on suppressor T lymphocytes. It has been proposed that blockade of these immune cell receptors with histamine H_2 receptor antagonists might enhance cell-mediated immunity.[197, 198] In addition, some authorities have suggested that cimetidine may have immunomodulatory actions independent of its H_2 receptor–

Table 40–2 | **Histamine H_2 Receptor Antagonists**

	CIMETIDINE	RANITIDINE	NIZATIDINE	FAMOTIDINE
Serum $T_{1/2}$ (hours)	1.5–2.3	1.6–2.4	1. 1–1.6	2.5–4
Biological $T_{1/2}$ (hours)	6	8	8	12
Dose (mg/day)				
Creatinine clearance >75 mL/min	800	300	300	40
Creatinine clearance 30–75 mL/min	800	225	225	30
Creatinine clearance 15–30 mL/min	600	150	150	20
Creatinine clearance <15 mL/min	400	75	75	10

Data from Wolfe MM, Sachs G: Acid suppression: Optimizing therapy for gastroduodenal ulcer healing, gastroesophageal reflux disease, and stress-related erosive syndrome. Gastroenterology 118:S9–S31, 2000.

blocking effects.[198] If the histamine H_2 receptor antagonists indeed enhance cell-mediated immunity, then patients with organ transplants who are treated with these drugs might exhibit an increased incidence of transplant rejection. Most studies on this issue have not found such an increased rate of transplant rejection in patients taking histamine H_2 receptor antagonists, however.[199]

Cimetidine has weak antiandrogenic activity that occasionally can cause gynecomastia and impotence.[200] With short-term, conventional-dose therapy, these effects are rare. Among patients with hypersecretory conditions who are treated chronically with high-dose cimetidine, however, almost one half have experienced substantial antiandrogenic effects.[200–202] This antiandrogenic activity appears to be specific to cimetidine and is not observed with the other histamine H_2 receptor antagonists. The intravenous administration of cimetidine or ranitidine can stimulate prolactin release, and the chronic oral administration of cimetidine rarely has resulted in galactorrhea.[203] This effect presumably is mediated through the blockade of histamine H_2 receptors in the anterior pituitary.

A variety of central nervous system (CNS) symptoms have been reported in patients taking histamine H_2 receptor antagonists, including headaches, restlessness, somnolence, dizziness, depression, memory problems, confusion, psychosis, and hallucinations.[204] In outpatients, CNS symptoms attributable to histamine H_2 receptor antagonists are rare. The serious CNS problems that have been attributed to H_2 blockers have occurred predominantly in elderly patients who were hospitalized, often in an intensive care unit. CNS problems are common in this setting, irrespective of H_2 blocker therapy, and the contribution of the drugs to the observed CNS disorders is difficult to establish. The precise frequency with which these agents cause CNS problems is not known, but clearly the frequency is low. Even with the intravenous administration of histamine H_2 receptor antagonists, the incidence of CNS side effects is less than 1%.[183, 205]

Myelosuppression is an uncommon, presumably idiosyncratic side effect of the histamine H_2 receptor antagonists. Cases of leukopenia, anemia, thrombocytopenia, and pancytopenia have been described with a frequency of substantially less than 1%.[206] In one large series of patients with bone marrow transplants, however, ranitidine was implicated as a possible cause of myelosuppression in 5%.[207] The contribution of ranitidine to the bone marrow suppression in these patients is not clear, but, pending further data, it seems prudent to avoid histamine H_2 receptor antagonists in bone marrow transplant recipients.

The histamine H_2 receptor antagonists can cause mild, asymptomatic elevations in the serum levels of hepatic aminotransferases (up to a three-fold increase), especially when the agents are administered intravenously.[208] These mild laboratory abnormalities may resolve spontaneously, even if the H_2 blocker therapy is continued. Rare cases of hepatitis have been described, sometimes associated with fever and eosinophilia.[208, 209] In all reports, the hepatitis has resolved with discontinuation of the drug. Whereas important hepatic injury due to H_2 blocker therapy is rare, routine monitoring of liver enzymes is not recommended for most patients treated with these agents. The histamine H_2 receptor antagonists also can cause a mild elevation (up to a 15% increase) in the serum creatinine level because these agents compete with creatinine for secretion by the renal tubule.[185] The glomerular filtration rate is not affected, and the mild elevation of serum creatinine has no clinical importance.

Potentially important drug interactions have been described for cimetidine and, to a lesser extent, for ranitidine.[210, 211] Both of these agents bind to the hepatic cytochrome P450 mixed-function oxidase system, and this binding can inhibit the elimination of other drugs that are metabolized through the same system, including theophylline, phenytoin, lidocaine, quinidine, and warfarin. Consequently, toxic blood levels of these drugs could result from the coadministration of cimetidine or ranitidine. Famotidine and nizatidine have no significant avidity for the cytochrome P450 system, and these agents do not appear to have any important drug interactions. Even with cimetidine, the agent with the highest affinity for cytochrome P450, important drug interactions are uncommon. Nevertheless, if a histamine H_2 receptor antagonist is needed for a patient who is taking theophylline, phenytoin, lidocaine, quinidine, or warfarin, it seems prudent to use either famotidine or nizatidine.

Finally, three of the four histamine H_2 receptor antagonists (cimetidine, ranitidine, and nizatidine) have been shown to inhibit gastric alcohol dehydrogenase, an enzyme that plays a minor role in the metabolism of ingested ethanol.[212, 213] Although some data suggest that these drugs may contribute to an elevation in serum alcohol levels during moderate ethanol ingestion, the effect appears to be small and of little clinical importance.

Tolerance to the antisecretory effects of histamine H_2 receptor antagonists appears to develop quickly and frequently. In one study of 12 healthy volunteers given intravenous infusions of ranitidine for 72 hours, for example, gastric pH exceeded 4 for 67% of day 1 compared with only 43% of day 3.[214] This tolerance could not be overcome by increasing the infusion of ranitidine, even to doses higher than 500 mg per 24 hours. During the third day of treatment, the gastric pH was less than 4 for more than 12 hours in 9 of the 12 volunteers despite attempts to titrate the ranitidine dose to elevate the gastric pH. A similar development of tolerance has been observed with the use of orally administered histamine H_2 receptor antagonists.[215] The mechanisms that mediate tolerance to the antisecretory effects of histamine H_2 receptor antagonists are not entirely clear, but some data suggest that this tolerance is associated with the up-regulation of enterochromaffin-like (ECL) cell activity that accompanies the hypergastrinemia induced by antisecretory therapy (see the section on PPIs). Because the histamine H_2 receptor antagonists are competitive inhibitors of the histamine H_2 receptor, their antisecretory effects can be diminished by an increased release of histamine from ECL cells. This phenomenon might explain the rapid development of tolerance to histamine H_2 receptor antagonism.

Rebound hypersecretion of gastric acid has been reported after discontinuation of histamine H_2 receptor antagonist therapy,[216, 217] although studies on this issue have yielded contradictory results.[218–220] Some of the studies that failed to show rebound hypersecretion were flawed because they measured acid secretion too soon after treatment was stopped (i.e., while the drug may still have been exerting antisecretory effects) or too late after treatment was discontinued (i.e., weeks later, when rebound acid secretion may have waned). Furthermore, some studies measured effects on maximal acid output, whereas rebound hypersecretion after H_2 receptor blocker therapy is best appreciated by measuring nocturnal gastric acid output. The rebound elevation in nocturnal gastric acid output is short-lived, disappearing by 9 days after the termination of treatment.[221] The mechanism is not known, but the hypersecretion may be a manifestation of transiently up-regulated ECL cell activity.

Proton Pump Inhibitors (see also Chapter 38)

The PPIs are a class of drugs that decrease gastric acid secretion through inhibition of H^+,K^+ATPase, the proton pump of the parietal cell. Presently, five PPIs are used widely as antisecretory agents—omeprazole (Prilosec), esomeprazole (Nexium, the S optical isomer of omeprazole), lansoprazole (Prevacid), pantoprazole (Protonix), and rabeprazole (Aciphex). The PPIs are clearly the most effective inhibitors of gastric acid secretion available. The PPIs all are substituted benzimidazoles. These agents are prodrugs that must be activated by acid to effect inhibition of H^+,K^+ATPase. Ironically, however, the prodrugs are acid-labile compounds that must be protected from degradation by stomach acid during oral administration.[222–224] Consequently, the agents are enteric coated and administered in delayed-release capsules.

The PPIs are weak bases, with a pKa of approximately 4.0 for omeprazole, lansoprazole, and pantoprazole, and a pKa of approximately 5.0 for rabeprazole. The agents are well absorbed after oral dosing, and the simultaneous administration of antacids does not appear to affect their bioavailability. Food may delay the absorption of lansoprazole, pantoprazole, and rabeprazole,[223, 225] but this delay does not alter the area under the plasma concentration-time curve, which is a key factor in achieving clinical efficacy for these agents.[224] Absorption of the enteric-coated agents may be erratic, and peak serum concentrations are not achieved until 2 to 5 hours after oral administration. The bioavailability of omeprazole appears to increase with multiple dosing, rising from 35% for a first dose to 60% after repeated dosing.[226, 227] The explanation for this phenomenon is not clear, but it may be that the antisecretory effects of the early doses result in decreased degradation of the acid-labile drug in the stomach or proximal small bowel. It is also possible that hepatic enzymes may become saturated with omeprazole, thus decreasing the first-pass metabolism of subsequent doses.[228] In contrast, the bioavailability of rabeprazole does not appear to change appreciably with multiple dosing.[225] This can result in greater antisecretory effects for rabeprazole during the first day of therapy, but the clinical importance of this phenomenon in the treatment of peptic ulcer disease is minimal.

The PPIs are metabolized in the liver by the cytochrome P450 enzyme system (especially CYP2C19), and the inactive products of this metabolism are excreted in the urine.[226, 229–234] Hepatic metabolism of the S optical isomer of omeprazole is slower than that of the R isomer. Consequently, esomeprazole (the S isomer) is metabolized more slowly than omeprazole (contains equal quantities of S and R isomers), and this may result in greater acid inhibition for esomeprazole.[234a] It is not clear that this effect confers any clinical advantage to esomeprazole over omeprazole for the healing of gastric and duodenal ulcers, however. Liver failure can delay PPI clearance, but clearance is not affected importantly by renal insufficiency because the metabolites that are excreted in the urine are not active agents.[231, 235] Even with liver failure, however, PPI dose adjustments generally are not necessary because of the wide safety margins of the agents. Approximately 3% of whites and 15% of Asians are deficient in the cytochrome P450 enzyme CYP2C19, and these individuals exhibit elevations in the maximum plasma concentrations and areas under the plasma concentration-time curve.[236–239] Although the plasma half-life of the PPIs is short (<2 hours), the duration of acid inhibition is long (>24 hours) as a result of covalent binding to the H^+,K^+ATPase enzyme (see Chapter 38).

As a result of their requirement for concentration and activation in acidic compartments, the PPIs bind predominantly to those proton pumps that are actively secreting acid. Thus, the efficacy of the PPIs for inhibiting acid secretion is limited if they are administered during the fasting state, when only approximately 5% of the stomach's proton pumps are active. With meal stimulation, in contrast, 60% to 70% of the proton pumps actively secrete acid. Thus, the PPIs are most effective if they are administered immediately before meals. For once-daily dosing, it is recommended that the PPIs should be taken immediately before breakfast.[240] When given in this fashion, the PPIs are remarkably effective inhibitors of gastric acid secretion. After 1 week of conventional-dose therapy, the PPIs inhibit basal and pentagastrin-stimulated acid secretion by more than 98%.[222, 241] Eradication of *H. pylori* infection has been found to render PPIs somewhat less effective in elevating the gastric pH in patients with duodenal ulcer.[242] The mechanism by which *H. pylori* infection augments the pH-elevating effect of the PPIs is not clear. Conceivably, this phenomenon might be a consequence of alkaline ammonia produced from urea by the organism or, more likely, due to the increased gastric bicarbonate secretion[243] and decreased gastric acid secretion associated with ongoing infection.

Recent studies using prolonged intragastric pH monitoring have shown that approximately 70% of individuals who take a PPI twice a day experience nocturnal gastric acid breakthrough, a phenomenon defined as a nocturnal gastric pH less than 4 for more than 1 hour.[244] In normal volunteers, nocturnal acid breakthrough can be abolished (at least in the short term) by adding a histamine H_2 receptor blocker at bedtime (Fig. 40–10).[245] It seems unlikely that nocturnal acid breakthrough interferes substantially with the healing of peptic ulcers in the stomach and duodenum, but a role for this phenomenon has been proposed for patients who have refractory symptoms of GERD (see Chapter 33).[246]

Using PPIs in the once-daily dose regimens summarized in Chapter 38, healing rates for duodenal ulcer of 80% to 100% can be achieved after 4 to 8 weeks of therapy. Healing rates for gastric ulcer at 4 to 8 weeks appear to be somewhat lower, in the range of 70% to 85%. No single PPI has been shown to be clearly superior to the others in healing efficacy. The healing of peptic ulcers appears to be effected more rapidly and frequently with PPIs than with histamine H_2 receptor antagonists (Fig. 40–11).[247–250] For peptic ulcers that are not associated with NSAIDs (see later), however, it is not clear that the modest increase in healing rates afforded by the PPIs justifies their higher cost compared to other available agents.

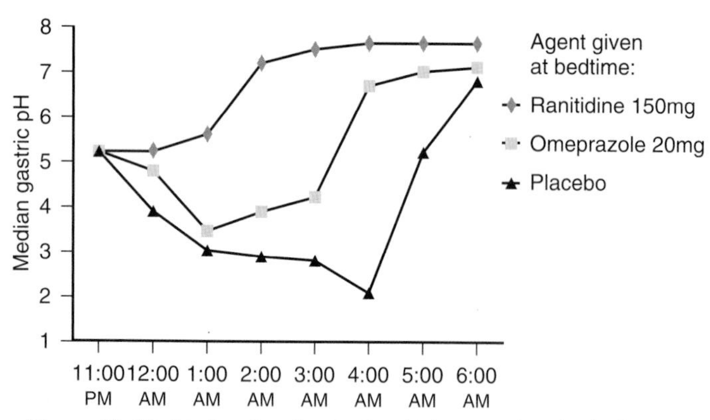

Figure 40–10. Median hourly gastric pH in normal individuals taking omeprazole 20 mg twice a day who were given a bedtime dose of either placebo, omeprazole 20 mg, or ranitidine 150 mg. Note that ranitidine controlled nocturnal gastric acid breakthrough better than another dose of omeprazole. (Adapted from Peghini PL, Katz PO, Castell DO: Ranitidine controls nocturnal gastric acid breakthrough on omeprazole: A controlled study in normal subjects. Gastroenterology 115:1335–1339, 1998.)

The PPIs are a remarkably safe and well-tolerated group of agents. The most frequently reported side effects are headache and diarrhea, and the rate with which patients develop these symptoms does not differ significantly from that for patients treated with placebo.[228, 251–253] Serious side effects of PPI therapy are rare.

The elevation of gastric pH induced by the PPIs can affect the absorption of a number of medications. However, this antisecretory action rarely has clinically important effects on drug pharmacokinetics, except when the PPIs are given with ketoconazole or digoxin.[224] Ketoconazole requires stomach acid for absorption, and this drug may not be absorbed effectively after PPIs have inhibited gastric acid secretion. Conversely, an elevated gastric pH facilitates the absorption of digoxin, resulting in increased plasma levels of this agent. If a patient requires both PPI and antifungal therapy, it is recommended that an agent other than ketoconazole be chosen. For patients treated concomitantly with PPIs and digoxin, clinicians should consider monitoring plasma digoxin levels.

Because the PPIs are metabolized by the cytochrome P450 system, there is potential for them to alter the metabolism of other drugs that are eliminated by cytochrome P450 enzymes.[254] Among the available PPIs, omeprazole appears to have the greatest potential for such drug interactions, and omeprazole has been shown to delay the clearance of warfarin, diazepam, and phenytoin.[222, 255, 256] Lansoprazole, pantoprazole, and rabeprazole appear to interact with the cytochrome P450 system to a lesser degree. Even with omeprazole, however, clinically important drug interactions are uncommon.[257]

For most patients with peptic ulcers who are treated with PPIs, only short-term therapy (4 to 8 weeks) is required because eradication of *H. pylori* or elimination of NSAIDs will prevent ulcer recurrences in most cases. However, long-term PPI therapy may be necessary for patients with peptic ulcerations associated with hypersecretory conditions, for patients who cannot discontinue NSAIDs, and for selected patients with complicated peptic ulcer disease. With long-term use, the profound suppression of gastric acid secretion effected by the PPIs creates the potential for a number of gastrointestinal problems, including (1) adverse effects of PPI-induced hypergastrinemia; (2) hastening gastric atrophy in patients infected with *H. pylori;* (3) problems associated with bacterial overgrowth in the stomach; (4) increased risk of enteric infections; and (5) effects on the absorption of nutrients.[258]

Potential for Adverse Effects of PPI-Induced Hypergastrinemia

Gastrin, released from antral G cells in response to meals and other stimuli, causes gastric parietal cells to secrete acid.

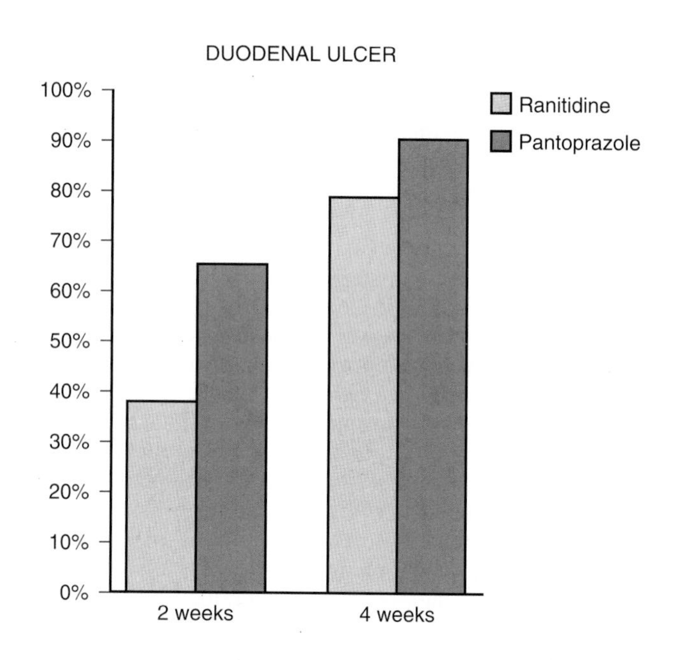

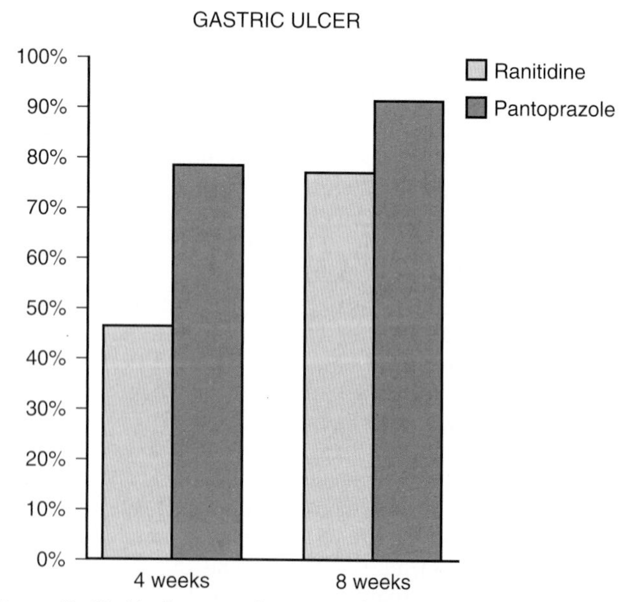

Figure 40–11. Healing rates for peptic ulcers treated with either ranitidine 300 mg/day or pantoprazole 40 mg/day. (Data from Bader JP, Delchier JC: Clinical efficacy of pantoprazole compared with ranitidine. Aliment Pharmacol Ther 8(Suppl 1): 47–52, 1994.)

This acid in the gastric lumen stimulates D cells in the antrum to release somatostatin, which, in turn, inhibits the further release of gastrin from antral G cells (see Chapter 38). Thus, in a negative-feedback loop, gastrin release stimulates acid secretion that then prevents further gastrin release. By inhibiting gastric acid secretion, PPIs and other antisecretory agents can interrupt this negative-feedback loop and cause hypergastrinemia. The rise in serum gastrin levels induced by PPI therapy usually is modest. Although most patients exhibit a twofold to fourfold elevation in the fasting serum gastrin level within 2 weeks, these gastrin elevations exceed the upper limit of normal (>100 pg/mL) in only approximately 10% of cases during short-term therapy.[259, 260] After 1 year of PPI therapy, as many as 23% of patients may have fasting serum gastrin levels higher than 100 pg/mL.[261] Profound elevations of the serum gastrin level (>400 pg/mL) can be found in approximately 5% of patients on chronic PPI therapy.[262–264] The elevated gastrin levels return to normal within 4 weeks of discontinuing the PPIs. Treatment with histamine H_2 receptor antagonists also can elevate serum gastrin levels, but generally to a lesser extent than the PPIs.[259, 260]

In addition to stimulating acid secretion, gastrin has been shown to have trophic effects on the gastrointestinal mucosa. In the stomach, these trophic effects are manifested predominantly in the ECL cells. Patients who have had prolonged, severe hypergastrinemia associated with either atrophic gastritis or Zollinger-Ellison syndrome (with multiple endocrine neoplasia type 1 [MEN 1]) have developed ECL cell hyperplasia and, uncommonly, gastric carcinoid tumors.[265, 266] Female rats that have had protracted hypergastrinemia induced by treatment with PPIs, histamine H_2 receptor antagonists, partial gastric fundectomy, or repeated infusions of gastrin also have developed ECL cell hyperplasia and gastric carcinoid tumors.[267–270] In these rat models, the ECL cell hyperplasia and carcinoid tumor formation can be prevented by antrectomy (which prevents the hypergastrinemia induced by gastric acid suppression),[271] and can be reduced by the infusion of proglumide, a gastrin receptor antagonist.[272, 273] These observations all support the hypothesis that hypergastrinemia can cause ECL cell hyperplasia that can lead to the development of carcinoid tumors. Indeed, early concerns regarding hypergastrinemia and carcinoid tumor formation delayed the release of omeprazole in the United States.

A number of observations suggest that antisecretory therapy poses little risk for promoting carcinoid tumor formation in humans. Although ECL cell hyperplasia has been observed in a number of different species treated long-term with antisecretory agents, there is substantial variation among the species in their propensity to develop carcinoid tumors. As many as 40% of female rats develop carcinoid tumors during long-term treatment with PPIs that are administered in high dosage,[273] but these tumors have not been seen in mice, guinea pigs, chickens, hamsters, and dogs treated with PPIs in similar dosage and duration.[268, 274–276] Patients with atrophic gastritis and Zollinger-Ellison syndrome with MEN 1 who have developed carcinoid tumors have had serum gastrin levels that are far higher than the modest gastrin elevations typical of patients on PPI therapy.[277, 278] A number of studies have shown that long-term PPI therapy can cause ECL cell hyperplasia in humans, especially in patients who are infected with *H. pylori*.[262, 279–281] However, none of these studies have found ECL cell neoplasms in any patient and, to date, there are no reports of gastric carcinoid tumors attributable to antisecretory therapy in humans. Even in patients with Zollinger-Ellison syndrome who have severe hypergastrinemia, carcinoid tumors are uncommon and occur predominantly in patients with MEN.[282] This observation suggests that a genetic abnormality may be necessary to develop an ECL cell neoplasm in patients who have elevated serum gastrin levels. Hypergastrinemia alone (i.e., without atrophic gastritis or a genetic abnormality) has not been documented to promote carcinoid tumor formation in humans.[258] Thus, PPI therapy does not appear to be a risk factor for gastric carcinoid tumors.

Some patients treated chronically with PPIs have developed gastric fundic gland polyps and hyperplastic gastric polyps. Although it has been proposed that these polyps may be a consequence of PPI-induced hypergastrinemia, this has not yet been established. In one retrospective study, gastric polyps were found in 7% of 231 patients after a mean duration of PPI therapy of 32.5 months.[283] The polyps were typically small (<1 cm in diameter), sessile, multiple, and located in the proximal stomach. Disappearance of gastric polyps was documented in one patient when PPI therapy was discontinued. Hyperplastic and gastric fundic gland polyps generally are considered to have little neoplastic potential, but the natural history of such polyps in the setting of chronic PPI use has not been evaluated.

Some animal studies have suggested that gastrin also might have trophic effects on the colonic mucosa.[284–286] These observations have raised the possibility that the hypergastrinemia induced by PPI therapy might predispose to colorectal cancer. Studies on the association of hypergastrinemia and colonic neoplasia are contradictory and inconclusive, however.[287–292] Investigations on the development of colon cancer in patients with hypergastrinemia due to pernicious anemia, vagotomy, gastric surgery, and Zollinger-Ellison syndrome generally have not found a significantly increased incidence of colonic neoplasms.[287, 293–297] Few data are available on the effect of PPI therapy on the development of colonic malignancies in humans, but available evidence has not implicated these agents as a risk factor for colorectal cancer.

Potential for Hastening Gastric Atrophy in Patients Infected with Helicobacter pylori

Some data suggest that the chronic administration of PPIs to patients who are infected with *H. pylori* might accelerate the development of atrophic gastritis. *H. pylori* infection is the major cause of chronic active gastritis, a condition that can lead to gastric atrophy, intestinal metaplasia, and adenocarcinoma of the stomach. In Western patients who are not taking antisecretory agents, the highest concentrations of *H. pylori* and the most intense inflammatory changes generally are found in the gastric antrum. Studies have shown that PPI therapy can alter this pattern so that the most intense inflammatory changes involve the gastric body and fundus.[298] In one study, investigators took gastric biopsy specimens from 50 patients at baseline and after 8 weeks of treatment with omeprazole.[299] Seventeen of the 50 patients had no evidence of *H. pylori* infection by culture and histology, and none of these subjects had gastritis either before or after treatment with the PPI. In contrast, all of the 33 *H. pylori*–positive patients had gastritis that involved the antrum predominantly before treatment. After 8 weeks of PPI therapy, however, inflammation and bacterial concentration in the antral biopsy specimens decreased to the point that the organism could no longer be found by histologic examination in 45% of the infected patients. In contrast, the inflammatory changes increased significantly in the gastric body. In theory, this shift from antral-predominant to gastric body–predominant inflammation induced by PPI therapy might cause atrophy of the acid-producing portion of the stomach.

A well-publicized study, conducted in the Netherlands and in Sweden, explored the development of atrophic gastritis in patients with severe GERD treated with either chronic omeprazole therapy or with antireflux surgery (fundoplication).[300] There were 105 Dutch patients (mean age, 62 years) in the chronic omeprazole therapy group, 59 of whom were infected with *H. pylori*. At baseline, none of the 59 infected patients had atrophic gastritis. After a mean period of 5 years on PPI therapy, however, 31% of the *H. pylori*–positive patients had developed atrophic gastritis. In contrast, none of the 72 Swedish patients (mean age, 53 years) who were treated with fundoplication, including 31 who had *H. pylori* infection, developed atrophic gastritis during a similar period of follow-up. This study has been criticized for a number of deficiencies. The investigation was not a randomized, controlled trial but rather a comparison of two different cohorts, with different mean ages, treated in different countries. Authorities have questioned the validity and importance of the histologic criteria used by the study pathologists for grading atrophic gastritis, and none of the patients in either group developed intestinal metaplasia, the lesion thought to be the precursor of gastric adenocarcinoma. Nevertheless, as a result of this publication, the U.S. Food and Drug Administration (FDA) convened a Gastrointestinal Advisory Committee meeting to address the issue of whether PPIs accelerate the development of atrophic gastritis in patients with *H. pylori* infection. The Committee concluded that the available data did not establish such an effect, and the members did not recommend routine treatment of *H. pylori* before starting PPI therapy. The Committee did feel that further studies were needed to investigate this issue. A recent, large Scandinavian study has found no difference in the development of gastric atrophy between GERD patients treated for 3 years with either chronic PPI therapy or antireflux surgery.[301] Nevertheless, this issue remains unsettled. Presently, it is not recommended that patients who are candidates for chronic PPI therapy have routine testing and treatment for *H. pylori* infection solely to prevent the development of atrophic gastritis.

Potential for Problems Associated with Bacterial Overgrowth in the Stomach

Gastric acid is bactericidal and helps prevent colonization of the proximal gastrointestinal tract by ingested microbes. Except for *H. pylori*, which is uniquely adapted for survival in the hostile environment of the stomach, the gastric juice of healthy individuals is virtually devoid of bacteria.[302] Gastric and duodenal juice sampled from individuals treated with PPIs or histamine H_2 receptor antagonists has been found to have increased concentrations of bacteria, however.[302–308] These bacteria have included strains that can convert dietary nitrates to potentially carcinogenic *N*-nitroso compounds.[309] Furthermore, bacteria in the stomach can deconjugate bile acids in gastric juice, and it has been proposed that these deconjugated bile acids might be particularly harmful to the gastrointestinal mucosa, especially when gastric acidity has been reduced by antisecretory agents.[309–311] These observations have prompted speculation that protracted use of antisecretory agents might promote the development of gastric cancers. However, no study has established an association between gastric cancer and the use of antisecretory agents.[274]

Potential for Increased Risk of Enteric Infections

As discussed earlier, gastric acid can kill ingested bacteria. If pathogenic microbes that can cause enteric infections are ingested, therefore, it is conceivable that acid suppression might facilitate infection. In support of this hypothesis, hypochlorhydria has been established as a risk factor for infection by a number of enteric pathogens, including *Salmonella, Shigella,* and *Vibrio cholerae*.[312–317] At least one study has documented a small increased risk for acquiring enteric infections in patients taking short-term PPI therapy but not in patients who had been taking PPIs for more than 1 year.[318] Evidence to date suggests that if there is any increased risk for acquiring enteric infections for patients taking antisecretory medications, the increase is small. Individuals who travel to developing countries where enteric infections are endemic should take precautions to prevent these infections, whether or not they are taking antisecretory medicines.

Potential Effects on the Absorption of Nutrients

Gastric acid is known to promote the release of certain minerals from organic food matrices and to facilitate the maintenance of metal ions (e.g., iron) in soluble forms that can be absorbed. Therefore, it is conceivable that acid suppression might decrease mineral absorption. The limited studies that are available on this issue suggest that short-term PPI therapy does not affect the absorption of magnesium, calcium, phosphorus, or zinc[319] and that long-term PPI therapy does not alter serum iron and ferritin concentrations.[320]

Several studies have shown that antisecretory therapy decreases the absorption of protein-bound cobalamin (vitamin B_{12}).[321–323] The absorption of unbound cobalamin appears to be unaffected by antisecretory therapy, suggesting that the reduced absorption of the protein-bound vitamin is the result of decreased peptic activity rather than a proposed decrease in intrinsic factor secretion.[324] Despite the effect on cobalamin absorption, most available studies have found that serum cobalamin levels are largely unaffected by long-term antisecretory therapy.[320, 321, 322] However, one study has documented the development of subnormal serum cobalamin levels in 8 of 131 patients with Zollinger-Ellison syndrome who were treated long-term with antisecretory agents in high dosage.[325] The risk of developing cobalamin deficiency for patients without Zollinger-Ellison syndrome who are treated with antisecretory drugs in conventional dosage appears to be minimal, and the agents do not appear to promote the development of pernicious anemia.[326]

Tolerance and Rebound Acid Hypersecretion

Tolerance to the antisecretory effects of PPI therapy has not been seen during short-term investigations.[327] As discussed earlier, such tolerance develops frequently in patients taking histamine H_2 receptor antagonists, presumably as a result of hypergastrinemia that up-regulates ECL cell activity. Although PPI use also results in hypergastrinemia and up-regulation of ECL cell activity, the PPIs bind irreversibly to the proton pump. This irreversible inhibition of the final step in acid secretion will not be overcome by increased release of histamine from ECL cells.

Early studies looking for rebound acid hypersecretion after termination of PPI therapy found no such effect.[221, 328] However, the duration of PPI therapy in these studies was short (14 to 25 days). In a more recent investigation in which 9 patients were treated with omeprazole 40 mg daily for 90 days, basal and pentagastrin-stimulated acid secretion were found to be increased significantly above baseline at 14 days after the termination of PPI therapy.[329] These patients also had developed elevated serum levels of chromogranin A, an index of ECL cell mass, during their treatment with the PPI. The authors concluded that termination of protracted therapy with a PPI can result in rebound acid hypersecretion, possibly as a result of increased ECL cell mass. Further studies on this issue are needed to confirm these results and to determine the frequency and duration of rebound hypersecretion when PPI therapy is stopped. Also, the clinical importance of rebound hyperacidity after antisecretory therapy is not clear.

Antacids

Although antacids were the mainstay of ulcer therapy for decades before the advent of antisecretory agents, the first large, controlled study to document that antacids indeed hastened the healing of peptic ulcers was not published until 1977.[330] Compared with antisecretory therapy, the treatment of peptic ulcer disease with antacids generally is less convenient, less palatable, and less effective for the long-term control of gastric acidity. Furthermore, antacids are more likely than antisecretory agents to cause unpleasant side effects such as diarrhea or constipation (see later). Consequently, few modern physicians prescribe antacids as first-line therapy for peptic ulcer disease. Nevertheless, a number of antacid preparations are available over the counter, and they are used widely by patients to treat a variety of dyspeptic symptoms.

Although physicians logically have assumed that antacids promote ulcer healing by neutralizing gastric acid, recent studies suggest that the therapeutic efficacy of these agents cannot be attributed solely to acid neutralization. In 1977, Peterson and coworkers showed that a liquid antacid preparation of magnesium-aluminum hydroxide, administered in a dosage of 30 mL 1 and 3 hours after meals and at bedtime (approximately 1000 mmol neutralizing capacity per day), was more effective than placebo for hastening the healing of duodenal ulcer.[330] This inconvenient dosing schedule, which often caused diarrhea, was designed to have maximal efficacy for elevating the gastric pH based on the physiology of gastric acid secretion and the effects of food on gastric acidity. Later studies showed that far smaller doses of antacids (as low as 120 mmol per day) had virtually identical efficacy for healing peptic ulcerations.[331] The precise mechanisms by which antacids hasten the healing of peptic ulcerations are not clear, but a variety of cytoprotective effects have been proposed for these agents, especially for those that contain aluminum.[332, 333] For example, aluminum hydroxide antacids have been reported to bind epidermal growth factor, and it has been suggested that this may result in increased delivery of the growth factor to the injured mucosa. Other proposed beneficial effects of antacids include enhancement of mucosal prostaglandin levels, stimulation of mucus and bicarbonate secretion, inhibition of pepsin activity, binding of bile salts, and promotion of angiogenesis.[332–335]

A number of proprietary antacid preparations are available that differ in their chemical composition, acid-neutralizing capacity, taste, form (liquid or tablet), and cost. The most widely used formulations are those containing a combination of magnesium and aluminum hydroxide (e.g. Maalox, Mylanta) and those that contain calcium carbonate (e.g. TUMS, Rolaids). The proprietary antacids generally are well tolerated by patients who have normal renal function. For the magnesium-containing agents, the most common side effect is diarrhea. In contrast, antacids that contain aluminum hydroxide primarily, or those that contain calcium, may cause constipation. Although calcium carbonate has substantial acid-neutralizing capacity, the calcium can stimulate gastrin release and acid secretion, a phenomenon sometimes called *acid rebound.* It is not clear whether this acid rebound has any adverse consequences for patients with peptic ulcer disease. Some individuals still use baking soda (sodium bicarbonate) as an antacid, but the use of this agent should be discouraged because of its propensity for causing fluid overload (due to sodium retention) and alkalosis in susceptible patients (e.g., those with renal insufficiency). All of the antacids must be used with caution, if at all, in patients who have renal insufficiency. In such patients, magnesium-containing agents can cause hypermagnesemia, and the use of calcium carbonate can cause hypercalcemia, alkalosis, and further renal impairment (milk-alkali syndrome). Studies have documented increased plasma concentrations of aluminum in patients with chronic renal insufficiency who were treated with aluminum hydroxide antacids, and it has been proposed that the chronic use of such agents could cause aluminum neurotoxicity in this setting.[336, 337]

Sucralfate

Sucralfate (Carafate) is a complex metal salt of sulfated sucrose.[338] Although the sucralfate molecule contains aluminum hydroxide, the agent has little acid-neutralizing capac-

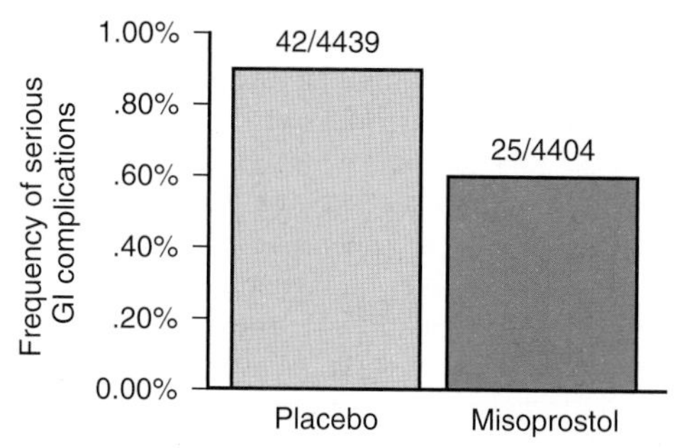

Figure 40–12. Results of a 6-month trial of misoprostol versus placebo for 8843 patients with rheumatoid arthritis who were taking NSAIDs. Although the relative risk reduction for gastrointestinal complications was approximately 40%, the absolute risk reduction was only approximately 0.4%. (Data from Silverstein FE, Graham DY, Senior JR, et al: Misoprostol reduces serious gastrointestinal complications in patients with rheumatoid arthritis receiving nonsteroidal anti-inflammatory drugs. A randomized, double-blind, placebo-controlled trial. Ann Intern Med 123:241–249, 1995.)

ity. When exposed to gastric acid, the aluminum hydroxide dissociates, leaving sulfate anions that can bind electrostatically to positively charged proteins in damaged tissue. In this fashion, sucralfate adheres to ulcer craters, where it appears to form a protective barrier that may prevent further acid-peptic attack. Other proposed beneficial effects of sucralfate include enhancement of mucosal prostaglandin levels, stimulation of mucus and bicarbonate secretion, binding of bile salts, binding of epidermal growth factors, and promotion of angiogenesis.[339, 340]

Although the precise mechanisms of action of sucralfate are not clear, the drug has demonstrated efficacy (similar to that of the histamine H_2 receptor antagonists) in healing duodenal ulcer when given in a dose of 1 g four times daily.[339] The drug has demonstrated efficacy in the treatment of gastric ulcer as well, but sucralfate has not been approved by the FDA for this indication. Compared with the histamine H_2 receptor antagonists and the PPIs, however, there is much less published experience with sucralfate. Less than 5% of the sucralfate administered is absorbed, and the drug appears to have no systemic toxicity.[338, 339] Gastric bezoar formation has been reported uncommonly. Concern has been raised about the potential for aluminum neurotoxicity in patients with chronic renal failure who are treated with sucralfate, and the drug perhaps is best avoided in this population. Sucralfate can bind to a number of medications, including phenytoin and warfarin. Important drug interactions appear to be rare, however, and can be avoided entirely if sucralfate is administered separately from other medications.[338] Despite the great safety and demonstrated efficacy of sucralfate in the treatment of duodenal ulcer, the drug has never achieved great popularity among prescribing physicians. Perhaps physicians feel that the four-times-daily dosing is inconvenient, that the mechanism of action is not well defined, or that the published experience with sucralfate is too limited.

Miscellaneous Antiulcer Medications

Bismuth

Bismuth preparations such as bismuth subsalicylate (e.g., Pepto-Bismol) and colloidal bismuth subcitrate (e.g., De-Nol) are used widely to treat diarrhea and a variety of dyspeptic symptoms. These agents have some demonstrated efficacy in healing peptic ulcers, but the mechanisms underlying this therapeutic effect are not clear.[341–343] The bismuth forms complexes with mucus that appears to coat ulcer craters, perhaps affording protection from acid-peptic attack. Effects on increasing mucosal prostaglandin synthesis and bicarbonate secretion also have been proposed, and bismuth has documented antimicrobial actions against *H. pylori*. There is the potential for bismuth neurotoxicity if the agents are given for extended periods in high dosage, especially in patients with renal failure,[344] but there appears to be little risk of toxicity with short-term, conventional-dose therapy. Although there is little role for bismuth preparations as antiulcer agents per se, they are occasionally used in combination with other antibiotics for the treatment of *H. pylori* infection in patients with peptic ulcer disease.

Prostaglandin Analogs

Prostaglandins have a number of effects that should be beneficial for patients with peptic ulcer disease (see Chapter 23). For example, prostaglandins inhibit gastric acid secretion, stimulate mucus and bicarbonate secretion from the gastrointestinal mucosa, and increase mucosal blood flow.[345–350] In the late 1970s and early 1980s, there was a flurry of interest in developing prostaglandin analogs for ulcer therapy, and a number of agents were tested. These efforts have been largely abandoned because of problems with prostaglandin side effects (e.g., frequent diarrhea, abortifacient actions), recognition of the role of *H. pylori* in peptic ulcer disease, and the development of safe and highly effective antisecretory agents. Misoprostol (Cytotec) is the only prostaglandin analog that has been approved by the FDA for clinical use in peptic ulcer disease, and only for the prevention of NSAID-induced gastric ulcers in patients at high risk for complications (Fig. 40–12). Although the drug is not approved for the treatment of active ulcers, misoprostol does appear to have efficacy comparable to that of omeprazole for healing NSAID-induced ulcers.[351] The use of this agent is discussed in Chapter 23.

Anticholinergics

Anticholinergic medications inhibit basal and meal-stimulated gastric acid secretion, but generally by less than 50%.[352, 353] Thus, they are substantially less effective antisecretory agents than the histamine H_2 receptor antagonists and the PPIs. For antiulcer therapy, the nonselective anticholinergic agents like atropine have prohibitive systemic side effects such as blurred vision and urinary retention. Side effects are less common with the use of selective anticholinergic medications such as pirenzepine, but these agents have limited efficacy and essentially no role in the treatment of peptic ulcer disease.

Surgery

The need for elective surgery to reduce gastric acid secretion as a means for treating peptic ulcer disease has been virtually abolished by the development of safe and highly effective antisecretory medications and by the recognition that ulcers recur uncommonly if *H. pylori* infection and NSAID use are eliminated. As discussed later in this chapter, surgery may be necessary for patients who have bleeding from peptic ulceration that does not respond to endoscopic therapy, for patients with perforated peptic ulcers, and for patients with ulcers that have caused gastric outlet obstruction that cannot be relieved with endoscopic dilation treatments. Surgical therapy of peptic ulcer disease is discussed in detail in Chapter 42.

Treatment of Peptic Ulcers Associated with NSAID Therapy (see also Chapter 23)

For patients who develop peptic ulcerations associated with the use of NSAIDs, it is recommended that the NSAID therapy should be discontinued if possible.[354] For patients with severe arthritis, however, interruption of NSAID therapy may result in disabling symptoms. A number of studies have shown that NSAID-associated peptic ulcers can heal with antisecretory therapy even if NSAID treatment continues, but that healing is delayed in this setting.[355–360]

As is the case for peptic ulcerations that are not associated with NSAIDs, the healing rate for ulcers in patients who use NSAIDs varies with ulcer size. In one study, 90% of aspirin-associated gastric ulcers less than 0.5 cm in diameter healed within 8 weeks of treatment with cimetidine and antacids despite the continued use of aspirin, whereas only 25% of gastric ulcers with diameters greater than 0.5 cm healed in this same setting.[357] In a large study of patients with NSAID-associated ulcers who continued to take NSAIDs, PPI therapy resulted in healing rates at 8 weeks of more than 80%.[351] During 6 months of maintenance treatment for the patients whose ulcers had healed, 61% of patients given a PPI remained in remission compared to only 27% of those given a placebo. Moreover, PPIs have been shown to be clearly superior to the histamine H_2 receptor antagonists for the healing and maintenance therapy of peptic ulcers in patients who continue to use NSAIDs. In a recent large, randomized trial of antisecretory therapies for patients with NSAID-associated gastric and duodenal ulcers who continued NSAID treatment, ulcer healing at 8 weeks was found in 80% of patients given omeprazole 20 mg daily but in only 63% of those given ranitidine 150 mg twice daily.[361] When the patients whose ulcers had healed were randomly assigned to maintenance therapy with either omeprazole or ranitidine while they continued NSAID use, furthermore, the estimated proportion of patients in remission at the end of 6 months was 72% in the omeprazole group and 59% in the ranitidine group. In another study of 350 patients with NSAID-associated gastric ulcers who continued to use NSAIDs, ulcer healing at 8 weeks was found in 69% of patients given lansoprazole 15 mg daily, in 73% of those given lansoprazole 30 mg daily, but in only 53% of those given ranitidine 150 mg twice daily.[362]

Studies have shown that ranitidine given in a conventional dose (150 mg twice daily) has some efficacy in preventing duodenal but not gastric ulcers in patients who take NSAIDs chronically for arthritis.[363, 364] High-dose famotidine (40 mg twice daily) has been found to prevent both gastric and duodenal ulcers during 24 weeks of NSAID therapy in patients with arthritis.[365] As discussed in detail in Chapter 23, misoprostol has been shown to prevent both gastric and duodenal ulcers and their complications in patients who take NSAIDs (see Fig. 40–12).[366–369] The demonstrated efficacy of PPIs in preventing both gastric and duodenal ulcers during NSAID therapy, their ease of administration, infrequent side effects, and excellent safety profile all have made the PPIs a popular choice for ulcer prophylaxis in high-risk patients who take NSAIDs. However, large-scale studies necessary to demonstrate that PPIs protect against peptic ulcer complications have not yet been done.

In a recent review, Laine[91] recommended the following approach for patients who have had peptic ulcers and who require analgesic or anti-inflammatory therapy:

1. Consider using non-NSAID analgesics such as acetaminophen.
2. If an NSAID is required, use the drug in the lowest effective dose.
3. If nonselective NSAIDs are to be used, consider using those with potentially lower risk of ulcerogenesis such as etodolac or the nonacetylated salicylates.
4. Consider using a cyclooxygenase-2 selective agent (e.g., celecoxib, rofecoxib).
5. Consider using cotherapy with misoprostol or a PPI.

Treatment of Refractory Peptic Ulcers

As discussed earlier, most peptic ulcerations heal within 8 weeks of initiating antisecretory therapy. Nevertheless, there is a small, but considerable, minority of patients whose ulcers persist despite conventional treatment. Such ulcers can be considered "refractory." There is no standardized definition for a refractory peptic ulcer, however, and different investigators have used different criteria for the diagnosis. A number of variables must be considered before declaring an ulcer refractory to medical treatment, including (1) type of therapy (e.g., should an ulcer be considered refractory if it fails to heal with antacids, sucralfate, or histamine H_2 receptor antagonists, or is it only refractory if it fails to heal with PPI therapy?); (2) duration of therapy (e.g., is an ulcer refractory if it fails to heal within 6 weeks, 8 weeks, 12 weeks, and so forth?); (3) treatment for *H. pylori* infection (e.g., is an ulcer refractory if it fails to heal in the presence of persistent *H. pylori* infection, or only after the infection has been eradicated?); (4) ongoing NSAID use (e.g., should an ulcer be considered refractory if it fails to heal while the patient continues to use NSAIDs, or only after NSAIDs have been stopped?).

The lack of a standardized definition for refractory peptic ulcer makes comparisons among studies difficult. In one recent study, 80 patients with resistant peptic ulcers (defined as duodenal ulcers that failed to heal after more than 6 weeks of treatment with either a histamine H_2 receptor antagonist or a PPI, or gastric ulcers that failed to heal after 8 to 12 weeks of antisecretory therapy) were followed prospectively for a mean duration of 40 months.[370] NSAID use (with or without *H. pylori* infection) was identified in 24 cases, *H. pylori* infection alone was found in 44, and 12 patients had neither of these factors associated with the peptic ulceration. Among the 24 patients found to be using NSAIDs, the use of these agents was surreptitious in 9 (i.e., they denied using NSAIDs, but a blood test for platelet cyclooxygenase activity was abnormal). Among the 12 patients without NSAID use or *H. pylori* infection, gastric secretory studies did not reveal hypersecretory conditions. Indeed, basal acid output was below normal in this group for reasons that were not clear. Eight of the 12 patients were cigarette smokers, a factor known to be associated with poor healing in patients treated with histamine H_2 receptor antagonists.[371] The ulcers eventually healed with PPI therapy in 9 of the 12 patients, and 5 of those patients required maintenance antisecretory therapy to remain in remission. Others also have found that most peptic ulcers refractory to treatment with histamine H_2 receptor antagonists will eventually heal with PPI therapy.[372, 373]

For the patients whose peptic ulcer does not heal despite a trial of conventional therapy, the clinician should consider the following:

1. Has there been compliance with the prescribed treatment? Testing to evaluate a cause for drug resistance is not warranted for patients who merely have not taken their prescribed medications. Such patients can be counseled regarding the importance of compliance with medical therapy and given another trial of conventional treatment.
2. Is there *H. pylori* infection? If antibiotic therapy already has been prescribed, the patient should be tested to confirm that the infection indeed has been eradicated. Antibiotic regimens for patients with resistant infections are discussed in Chapter 39. If there has been no attempt to seek and eradicate *H. pylori* infection, this should be done.
3. Is there ongoing NSAID use? As discussed earlier, NSAID use may be surreptitious. A careful history regarding the use of NSAIDs should be obtained, and NSAIDs should be stopped if possible.
4. Is there cigarette smoking? If so, the patient should be counseled strongly to discontinue cigarettes, at least during the period of ulcer treatment.
5. Has the duration of ulcer treatment been adequate? As discussed, large ulcerations require a longer duration of therapy than small ulcers to effect complete healing. A large ulceration (e.g., >2 cm) probably should not be considered refractory until it has persisted beyond 12 weeks of antisecretory therapy.
6. Has PPI therapy been used? If not, a trial of PPI treatment can be initiated.
7. Is there evidence for a hypersecretory condition? A family history of gastrinoma or MEN 1, a history of chronic diarrhea, hypercalcemia due to hyperparathyroidism, or ulcers involving the postbulbar duodenum all suggest a diagnosis of Zollinger-Ellison syndrome (see Chapter 41). Although patients with this syndrome clearly can have peptic ulcers that are resistant to antisecretory agents administered in conventional doses, an unrecognized hypersecretory condition nevertheless is an uncommon cause of refractory peptic ulcer.
8. Is the ulcer indeed peptic? Primary or metastatic neoplasms, infections (e.g., cytomegalovirus), cocaine use, and nonpeptic inflammatory bowel diseases (e.g., Crohn's disease) can cause ulcerations of the stomach and duodenum that can mimic peptic ulcers. These disorders should be considered and excluded appropriately.

SPECIFIC MANAGEMENT RECOMMENDATIONS

As mentioned earlier, all patients found to have peptic ulcers should be tested for *H. pylori* infection and should be questioned carefully regarding the use of NSAIDs. Whenever possible, *H. pylori* infection should be treated, and NSAID therapy should be stopped. The following management recommendations are based on the review of the literature on peptic ulcer disease presented earlier and, where conclusive studies are not available, on the opinion of the author.

Duodenal Ulcer

If a clear-cut diagnosis of duodenal ulcer is made by barium contrast examination, endoscopic evaluation generally is not necessary. If the diagnosis is made endoscopically, biopsy samples are not obtained routinely from duodenal ulcers because they are so rarely malignant. Gastric biopsy specimens should be taken to seek *H. pylori* infection. Alternatively, serologic, breath, or stool tests for *H. pylori* infection can be used (see Chapter 39). If *H. pylori* infection is documented, the patient should be treated with one of the regimens recommended in Chapter 39, irrespective of whether there is a history of NSAID use. All these regimens involve the use of an antisecretory agent for approximately 2 weeks. Although a number of recent studies suggest that this 2-week course of antibiotic/antisecretory therapy might be sufficient to heal duodenal ulcers in the majority of cases,[373a,b] far more data are available regarding the efficacy of antisecretory agents given for at least 4 weeks in duodenal ulcer disease. Pending further studies, therefore, at the end of the course of therapy for *H. pylori*, the same antisecretory agent should be continued, in the dosage outlined in Table 38–3, until the patient has received a total of 4 weeks of antisecretory therapy.

If there is no *H. pylori* infection, ongoing NSAID use, or obvious hypersecretory condition, then reasonable choices for medical therapy include a histamine H_2 receptor antagonist (see Table 40–2 for dosing), a PPI (see Table 38–3 for dosing), or, perhaps, sucralfate in a dose of 1 g four times daily for 4 weeks. Although healing rates are somewhat higher and faster for PPIs compared to the H_2 receptor antagonists (and probably to sucralfate), the clinical importance of these differences in duodenal ulcer disease appears to be small. Present data do not clearly favor the use of PPIs over the other therapies for uncomplicated duodenal ulcers in patients who are not taking NSAIDs.

Follow-up endoscopic examination to ensure healing and testing to document *H. pylori* eradication after antibiotic therapy are not recommended routinely for patients with uncomplicated duodenal ulcers whose symptoms resolve completely with therapy. Such testing should be considered, however, for patients with persistent or recurrent symptoms or for patients with duodenal ulcers complicated by bleeding or perforation (see later).

Gastric Ulcer

If a diagnosis of gastric ulcer is made by barium contrast examination, endoscopic evaluation always is necessary to exclude malignancy. During endoscopy, at least six biopsy specimens should be taken from the mucosa at the edges of the ulceration. The role of brush cytology in the evaluation of gastric ulcerations is disputed, and it is not clear that this test adds sufficient information to justify the additional expense of cytologic evaluation. Gastric biopsy specimens remote from the ulcer can be taken to seek *H. pylori* infection. Alternatively, serologic, breath, or stool tests for *H. pylori* infection can be used (see Chapter 39). If *H. pylori* infection is documented, the patient should be treated with one of the regimens recommended in Chapter 39 that includes a PPI, irrespective of whether there is a history of NSAID use. At the end of the course of therapy for *H. pylori*, the same PPI should be continued, in the dosage outlined in Table 38–3, until the patient has received a total of 8 weeks of antisecretory therapy.

If there is no *H. pylori* infection, then any PPI listed in Table 38–3 can be used for 8 weeks of therapy. Compared with duodenal ulcers, gastric ulcers are larger, have slower healing rates, and have less reliable responses to antisecretory therapy. Furthermore, healing rates for patients treated with a PPI are higher than for those treated with a histamine H_2 receptor antagonist at 4 and 8 weeks.[359, 374–378] These features probably justify the routine use of a PPI rather than a histamine H_2 receptor antagonist for patients with gastric ulcer. Follow-up endoscopy to document healing is not performed routinely if the ulcer appears clearly benign by endoscopic and histologic criteria.

Follow-up endoscopy after 8 weeks of therapy is recommended if any of the tests are equivocal or suggestive of malignancy, if symptoms do not resolve entirely with therapy, or if the ulcer was complicated by bleeding or perforation (see later). Follow-up testing to ensure eradication of *H. pylori* should be considered for complicated ulcers as well.

Maintenance Therapy

After eradication of *H. pylori* infection and elimination of NSAIDs, maintenance therapy with antisecretory agents is not recommended routinely for patients with uncomplicated peptic ulcers. Even patients who have had complicated ulcers may not require maintenance therapy if the predisposing factor (*H. pylori* or NSAIDs) clearly has been eliminated.[379, 380] However, studies on maintenance therapy for complicated ulcers are limited, and this issue remains disputed. Pending further data, one reasonable approach is to consider maintenance therapy with a PPI taken once a day for patients with complicated ulcers for whom an ulcer recurrence would have a high risk of dire consequences (e.g., very elderly patients or those with severe comorbidities).

COMPLICATIONS OF PEPTIC ULCER DISEASE

Hemorrhage

Peptic ulcerations that burrow into arterial vessels can result in life-threatening hemorrhage. It has been estimated that peptic ulceration is responsible for nearly 50% of all cases of acute hemorrhage from the upper gastrointestinal tract (see Chapter 13). There are approximately 150,000 hospitalizations for bleeding peptic ulcers each year in the United States.[381] NSAID use is strongly associated with ulcer hemorrhage, presumably because these agents both predispose to ulceration and inhibit platelet function.[382–389] Although corticosteroid use alone does not appear to increase the risk for bleeding ulcer substantially, the combined use of corticosteroids and NSAIDs may increase the risk of this complication by nearly 10-fold.[96, 390] Approximately 20% of patients with bleeding peptic ulcers present with melena and 30% present with hematemesis, whereas 50% have both melena and hematemesis on initial presentation.[391] As many as 5% of patients have bleeding that is brisk enough to cause hematochezia.[392]

The rationale for aggressive antisecretory therapy in patients with peptic ulcers seems reasonable: Pepsin is inactive when the gastric pH rises above 4, and therefore antisecretory therapy should prevent further peptic damage to the injured blood vessels. Furthermore, antisecretory therapy should enhance hemostasis by preventing peptic digestion of blood clots and by improving platelet function which is impaired by acid.[393, 394] Unfortunately, numerous studies on histamine H_2-blocker therapy for patients with bleeding ulcers showed no definitive benefit in controlling hemorrhage.[395–397] Some early studies on the role of PPIs for bleeding peptic ulceration found no benefits,[398] whereas others suggested that such treatment might have had beneficial effects, especially when the PPIs were administered intravenously.[399–402] Definitive conclusions could not be drawn from these methodologically flawed investigations, however. Also, by the time the PPIs became available in the late 1980s, therapeutic endoscopy had become the standard of care for patients with ulcer hemorrhage (see Chapter 13). These endoscopic techniques are highly effective for achieving hemostasis. With endoscopic methods that can control bleeding in nearly 90% of cases, it is difficult to demonstrate any added benefit from a medical intervention.

Two recent reports strongly suggest that PPI treatment indeed might be beneficial for the acute management of bleeding ulcers.[403, 404] One report described a prospective, randomized, placebo-controlled, trial of PPI therapy that was conducted at a hospital in India where therapeutic endoscopy was not available.[403] In this study, 220 patients who had bleeding peptic ulcers with endoscopic stigmata of hemorrhage were randomly assigned to receive either oral omeprazole (40 mg twice daily) or placebo for 5 days. The patients treated with omeprazole were found to have significantly less recurrent bleeding, fewer blood transfusions, and shorter hospital stays than the patients who received placebo. It is not clear that these results are applicable to Western patients, however. Indians have fewer gastric parietal cells than Western individuals, and so it may be easier to control their gastric acid output with antisecretory agents. Also the patients in this study were somewhat younger and healthier than most patients with bleeding peptic ulcers in Western hospitals.

In a more recent study from Hong Kong, 240 Chinese patients with bleeding peptic ulcers had endoscopic treatment with epinephrine injection and thermocoagulation that stopped the acute hemorrhage.[404] Patients then were randomly assigned to receive either intravenous omeprazole (80 mg bolus followed by infusion of 8 mg per hour for 72 hours) or placebo. After the infusion, all patients were given oral omeprazole (20 mg daily) for 8 weeks. As in the aforementioned study, the patients who received intravenous omeprazole were found to have significantly less recurrent bleeding, fewer blood transfusions, and shorter hospital stays than the patients who received placebo. Again, it is not clear that these results are applicable to Western patients and, at this time, intravenous preparations of PPIs only recently have become available for clinical use in the United States. Nevertheless, it seems likely that this therapy will be used routinely as an adjunct to endoscopic treatment for bleeding peptic ulcers.

Perforation

Free perforation of a duodenal or gastric ulcer into the peritoneal cavity can be a catastrophic, life-threatening event. Most patients with this complication are elderly, and the perforations are associated with NSAID use in up to one half of cases.[405, 406] Smoking is also associated with perforated peptic ulcer and, in patients younger than 75 years of age, smoking appears to be a stronger risk factor for perforation than NSAIDs.[407, 408] The use of crack cocaine has been associated with perforated ulcers of the prepyloric antrum, perhaps a result of cocaine-induced vasoconstriction and ischemia.[104] There is no prior history of peptic ulcer symptoms in 10% to 25% of patients who present with perforated peptic ulcer. In up to 10% of patients, the perforation is accompanied by hemorrhage. Duodenal ulcers that perforate involve the anterior wall of the duodenal bulb in most cases. Perforated gastric ulcers usually involve the lesser curvature.

Classically, there are three clinical stages of free perforation: The initial symptoms are caused by the sudden outpouring of caustic gastric juice into the peritoneal cavity, an event heralded by the abrupt onset of intense abdominal pain that is often accompanied by shock. This stage lasts from minutes to hours, depending on the size of the perforation and the extent to which the peritoneal cavity is flooded by gastric juice. During the next clinical stage, the patient often begins to look and feel better, perhaps because fluid that pours out of the injured tissue buffers and dilutes the caustic gastric juice. The improvement in symptoms belies the severity of the insult, however, and the inexperienced clinician who evaluates the patient during this stage might mistakenly assume that the problem no longer requires emergent attention. Despite the apparent clinical improvement, however, physical examination usually will reveal signs of peritonitis even during this latent period. The latent period is followed by a stage of frank peritonitis during which pain and signs of a systemic inflammatory response intensify. Death ensues without appropriate therapy, which should be initiated well before the stage of frank peritonitis.

Evidence of free air within the abdominal cavity may be seen on a plain or upright radiograph of the abdomen and chest in approximately 70% of cases.[409] Endoscopy should be avoided when perforated ulcer is suspected, because the air infused to distend the stomach during this procedure could open a perforation that has sealed and could extend the peritoneal soiling (at least in theory). In equivocal cases, an upper gastrointestinal series using a water-soluble contrast agent (e.g., Gastrografin) can reveal the site of the perforation.

In addition to resuscitation and the intravenous administration of broad-spectrum antibiotics, surgery to close the perforation and irrigate the peritoneal cavity is the traditional therapy for perforated peptic ulcer (see Chapter 42).[408] For patients who develop perforations in the setting of *H. pylori* infection, eradication of the infection may prevent ulcer recurrence after simple surgical closure.[408, 410] In highly selected patients (e.g., those who are tolerating the insult well and in whom the perforation seems to have sealed), nonoperative therapy may be appropriate.[411, 412] However, the decision to pursue nonoperative therapy for perforated peptic ulcer is a difficult one that should be made only after evaluation by and close consultation with an experienced surgeon. If nonoperative treatment is chosen, then the patient will require frequent clinical evaluation so that operative therapy can be initiated at the first sign of clinical deterioration.

Penetration

Penetration occurs when a peptic ulcer burrows through the wall of the stomach or duodenum but, instead of perforating freely into the peritoneal cavity, the crater bores into an adjacent organ.[413] Duodenal ulcers that involve the posterior wall of the bulb can penetrate into the pancreas. Penetrating gastric ulcers often involve the left lobe of the liver. Rarely, penetrating peptic ulcers can result in the development of fistulas between the duodenum and the common bile duct (choledochoduodenal fistula) or between the stomach and the colon (gastrocolic fistula). There is little recent literature dealing with penetrating peptic ulcers. Older surgical series suggest that evidence of penetration could be found in as many as 20% of ulcers at the time of operation, but only infrequently was the penetration associated with any symptoms other than those typical of peptic ulcer disease.[413] Penetration can be associated with a change in the typical pattern of ulcer symptoms, however. For example, patients may complain of an increasing intensity or longer duration of pain, or they may notice that the pain radiates into the back or that eating no longer relieves the discomfort. Presently, the finding of penetration, per se, appears to have little therapeutic implication for the treatment of peptic ulcer. Indeed, since proof of penetration usually requires surgery or imaging procedures such as computed tomography that are seldom indicated for the evaluation of peptic ulcer disease, clinicians rarely have confirmation that they are dealing with an ulcer that has penetrated. In rare cases of peptic ulcers that have penetrated into the biliary tree or colon, surgery may be required to close the fistulas.

Obstruction

Peptic ulcerations of the antrum, pylorus, and duodenum can obstruct the gastric outlet as a result of the swelling and edema that accompanies the active ulceration or as a consequence of the cicatrization that can attend ulcer healing. Until the 1970s, peptic ulcer disease was the most common cause of gastric outlet obstruction.[414] For the past several decades, however, the frequency of obstruction due to peptic ulceration has declined, and malignancy is now the leading cause of gastric outlet obstruction.[415, 416] Patients with an obstructed gastric outlet typically complain of epigastric pain, bloating, early satiety, nausea, and vomiting that occur during or shortly after a meal. Vomiting may relieve the discomfort temporarily. Weight loss can be profound, and dehydration with electrolyte disturbances can develop with high-grade obstruction. Physical examination may reveal a succussion splash (an audible splash of gastric contents produced by shaking the patient's torso) in approximately one third of cases.

Aspiration of gastric contents through a nasogastric tube often reveals substantial quantities of retained fluid in patients with gastric outlet obstruction. A gastric aspirate volume of more than 300 mL at 4 hours after a meal or more than 200 mL after an overnight fast is evidence of delayed gastric emptying.[417] Mechanical obstruction of the gastric outlet can be confirmed by endoscopy or by barium contrast examination. Endoscopy generally is preferred because retained gastric material interferes with the interpretation of the barium study, and it may not be possible to make a specific diagnosis of the lesion causing the obstruction. Before the procedure, the gastric contents can be evacuated using a large-bore nasogastric tube (e.g., an Ewald tube) to facilitate the endoscopic examination. The functional obstruction to gastric emptying can be confirmed with a saline load test in which 750 mL of saline is placed in the stomach through a nasogastric tube, and the gastric contents are aspirated 30 minutes later.[418] Recovery of more than 300 mL of the saline is considered evidence of delayed gastric emptying. Although this test was once used to aid the clinician in choosing between operative and nonoperative therapy for gastric outlet obstruction,[419] today the saline load test is used infrequently.

Surgical management principles for gastric outlet obstruction were established in an era when this peptic complication was common, when recurrence was likely without definitive surgical therapy, when potent antisecretory therapy and endoscopic dilation techniques were not available, and when parenteral nutrition options were limited. Whereas patients often presented with substantial debility due to profound weight loss and electrolyte disturbances, expectant medical management of the outlet obstruction ran the risk of dangerously delaying surgery while the malnutrition progressed. Consequently, early operation often was advised. Today, gastric outlet obstruction from peptic ulcer disease is uncommon, ulcer recurrence is unlikely when *H. pylori* and NSAIDs are eliminated, there is excellent antisecretory therapy, there are a number of endoscopic techniques for dilating stenoses, and total parenteral nutrition is widely available. Therefore, an immediate decision regarding the need for surgery generally is not necessary for a patient who presents with gastric outlet obstruction. The problem can be managed with medical and endoscopic means in approximately 70% of cases, and only 30% will eventually require an operation to bypass the gastric outlet obstruction.[420, 421] Surgical approaches are discussed in Chapter 42.

PHYSIOLOGIC STRESS AND PEPTIC INJURY

Severe physiologic stress (e.g., that caused by major trauma, burns, sepsis, multisystem organ failure) often is associated with peptic injury of the upper gastrointestinal tract.[422] Typically, this injury is manifested as multiple, superficial erosions that involve the oxyntic mucosa of the stomach. In contrast with chronic peptic ulcerations associated with *H. pylori* infection, these acute, superficial stress lesions are accompanied by little inflammatory reaction in the surrounding mucosa. However, a spectrum of peptic lesions can accompany severe physiologic stress, ranging from the typical, asymptomatic gastric erosions to deep ulcerations of the stomach and duodenum that can be complicated by life-threatening hemorrhage and perforation. Consequently, a number of terms have been used to describe stress-related peptic injury, including *stress erosion, stress gastritis, stress ulcer,* and *stress-related erosive syndrome.*[423] Acute peptic ulcers that occur in patients with severe burns are called *Curling's ulcers.* Peptic ulcers that occur in patients with acute head injuries are called *Cushing's ulcers.* Cushing's ulcers are associated with hypergastrinemia and hypersecretion of gastric acid and, in this regard, they differ from other stress-related peptic injuries that are not accompanied by excess secretion of gastrin or acid.[424, 425]

Severe physiologic stress results in impaired mucosal resistance to peptic injury. This breakdown in epithelial defense appears to be largely a consequence of decreased mucosal blood flow.[426] Poor blood flow causes mucosal ischemia, which can lead to local acidosis, free radical formation, diminished acid-buffering capacity, decreased mucosal secretion of mucus and bicarbonate, and impaired rapid restitution.[427–430] These effects allow acid in the lumen to reenter the mucosa (so-called acid "back-diffusion") and cause further injury.

Studies in which endoscopic examinations were performed on severely ill patients in intensive care units have found gastroduodenal mucosal lesions in more than 75% of cases.[431–433] In some older series, furthermore, these stress-related lesions caused substantial morbidity and mortality. In one study of patients with extensive burns, for example, 30% developed major hemorrhage or perforation from acute ulcerations.[432] However, the frequency with which stress-related mucosal lesions cause clinically important consequences appears to have declined substantially since the 1970s, perhaps as a result of advances in the medical management of critically ill patients.[423] In a recent, prospective study of more than 2000 patients admitted to intensive care units, only 1.5% developed clinically important bleeding.[434] The investigators found that respiratory failure and coagulopathy were strong, independent risk factors for stress-related hemorrhage. Important bleeding occurred in 3.7% of the 847 patients who had one or both of these risk factors, whereas only 0.1% of 1405 patients without respiratory failure or coagulopathy factors experienced such bleeding. Other proposed risk factors for important stress-related mucosal lesions include shock, sepsis, head injury, severe burns, multiorgan failure, acute renal failure, cirrhosis, and quadriplegia due to acute cervical spine injury.[435, 436]

Clinicians have attempted to prevent stress-related mucosal injury by the prophylactic administration of antacids, sucralfate, and antisecretory medications to severely ill patients. By the 1980s, such "stress ulcer prophylaxis" had become established as routine in many intensive care units throughout the world.[436] Unfortunately, the literature dealing with stress ulcer prophylaxis is confusing and often contradictory. Even meta-analyses of these studies have yielded disparate conclusions.[437–442] Comparisons among studies can be difficult because of major differences in patient populations and in the criteria used to establish the presence of bleeding. One recent, and especially rigorous, meta-analysis of meaningful studies on stress ulcer prophylaxis for critically ill patients concluded that prophylaxis with histamine H_2 receptor antagonists clearly decreased the incidence of clinically important gastrointestinal bleeding (odds ratio, 0.44; 95% confidence interval, 0.22 to 0.88).[442] These investigators identified a trend favoring histamine H_2 receptor antagonists over antacids in the prevention of clinically important bleeding, whereas the histamine H_2 receptor antagonists did not clearly differ from sucralfate in their ability to prevent important bleeding. However, the use of sucralfate for stress ulcer prophylaxis was associated with a lower mortality rate than either histamine H_2 receptor antagonists or antacids. To date, there are no large, randomized trials of PPIs for stress ulcer prophylaxis, but the limited studies available suggest a beneficial effect for these agents.[443, 444]

As mentioned, critically ill patients who received stress ulcer prophylaxis with sucralfate appeared to have a lower overall mortality rate than those given antacids or antisecretory agents for prophylaxis. The explanation for this proposed benefit is not clear but might be related to the lower rate of nosocomial pneumonia in patients treated with sucralfate. By raising the gastric pH, antacids and antisecretory agents predispose to the growth of gram-negative bacteria in the stomach.[445] Aspiration of these bacteria into the airway of severely ill patients might cause pneumonia, and the large volume of antacids used for stress ulcer prophylaxis might predispose to gastroesophageal reflux and pulmonary aspiration. In contrast, sucralfate has little effect on gastric pH and volume, and its use would not be expected to increase the rate of aspiration pneumonia. Studies on this issue are not definitive, however, and authorities still dispute the contribution of stress ulcer prophylaxis to nosocomial pneumonia in critically ill patients.

Although the indications and optimal choice of agents for stress ulcer prophylaxis of critically ill patients remain disputed, Tryba and Cook[435] suggested the following guidelines based on their extensive experience and review of available literature:

1. Stress ulcer prophylaxis is not required for all patients in an intensive care setting but should be considered strongly for those with respiratory failure, coagulopathy, sepsis, shock, trauma, quadriplegia, extensive burns, or head trauma and after neurosurgery. Prophylaxis also should be considered for patients who have a history of peptic ulcer disease, cirrhosis, and acute renal failure.
2. Sucralfate should be used for stress ulcer prophylaxis whenever enteral administration is possible.
3. If parenteral stress prophylaxis is the only reasonable choice, then histamine H_2 receptor antagonists should be used. Tryba and Cook[435] suggested that the dose of these agents should be titrated so as to achieve a gastric pH in the 3 to 4 range.

CAMERON ULCERS (LINEAR GASTRIC EROSIONS IN HIATAL HERNIAS)

There are numerous older reports of unexplained anemia and chronic gastrointestinal blood loss in patients who had large hiatal hernias.[446] Surgical repair of the hernias often corrected the anemia in these patients.[447] In 1986, Cameron and Higgins reported the results of a prospective, endoscopic study of 109 elderly patients who had large hiatal hernias.[448] Fifty-five of the patients were anemic, and 54 were not. In 23 of the anemic patients, linear gastric erosions were seen on the crests of mucosal folds located at or near the level of the diaphragm. Similar lesions were found in 13 of the 54 patients who were not anemic. In most patients, the anemia responded well to therapy with oral iron. The cause of the characteristic linear, gastric erosions was not clear, but the authors speculated that they were caused by the mechanical trauma of diaphragmatic contraction. These lesions have come to be called *Cameron ulcers*.

A recent review estimates that Cameron ulcers can be found in 5% of all patients with hiatal hernias who have endoscopic examinations[449] (see Fig. 20–4 in Chapter 20). The incidence increases with the size of the hernia. The lesions are multiple in approximately two thirds of cases. Although Cameron ulcers can cause anemia and even life-threatening hemorrhage, these lesions often are found incidentally during endoscopic evaluation for unrelated causes. The cause of Cameron ulcers remains unclear, but it is likely that mechanical trauma and, perhaps, ischemia play a primary role in their pathogenesis. Acid-peptic attack may extend the injury, but it seems unlikely that these are primarily peptic lesions. The response to antisecretory therapy is variable, supporting the notion that Cameron ulcers are not primarily peptic lesions. Treatment is empirical and includes antisecretory therapy and supplemental iron. Uncommonly, surgery to repair the hiatal hernia may be required for patients who do not respond to medical therapy.

REFERENCES

1. Grossman MI (ed): Peptic Ulcer: A Guide for the Practicing Physician. Chicago, Year Book, 1981.
2. Graham DY, Lew GM, Klein PD, et al: Effect of treatment of *Helicobacter pylori* infection on the long-term recurrence of gastric or duodenal ulcer: A randomized, controlled study. Ann Intern Med 116:705–708, 1992.
3. Marshall BJ: *Helicobacter pylori.* Am J Gastroenterol 89(Suppl):S116–S128, 1994.
4. Kurata JH, Nogawa AN: Meta-analysis of risk factors for peptic ulcers: Nonsteroidal anti-inflammatory drugs, *Helicobacter pylori,* and smoking. J Clin Gastroenterol 24:2–17, 1997.
5. Flemstrom G, Garner A: Gastroduodenal HCO_3 transport: Characteristics and proposed role in acidity regulation and mucosal protection. Am J Physiol 242:G183–G193, 1982.
6. Allen A, Garner A: Mucus and bicarbonate secretion in the stomach and their possible role in mucosal protection. Gut 21:249–262, 1980.
7. Scheiman JM, Kraus ER, Boland CR: Regulation of canine gastric mucin synthesis and phospholipid secretion by acid secretagogues. Gastroenterology 103:1842–1850, 1992.
8. Quigley EMM, Turnberg LA: pH of the microclimate lining human gastric and duodenal mucosa in vivo: Studies in control subjects and in duodenal ulcer patients. Gastroenterology 92:1876–1884, 1987.
9. Wallace JL, McKnight GW: The mucoid cap over superficial gastric damage in the rat: A high-pH microenvironment dissipated by nonsteroidal anti-inflammatory drugs and endothelin. Gastroenterology 99:295–304, 1990.
10. Sarosiek J, Marshall BJ, Peura DA, et al: Gastroduodenal mucus gel thickness in patients with *Helicobacter pylori*: A method for assessment of biopsy specimens. Am J Gastroenterol 86:729–734, 1991.
11. Hogan DL, Rapier RC, Dreilinger A, et al: Duodenal bicarbonate secretion: Eradication of *Helicobacter pylori* and duodenal structure and function in humans. Gastroenterology 110:705–716, 1996.

12. Chen MC, Chang A, Buhl T, et al: Apical acidification induces paracellular injury in canine gastric mucosal monolayers. Am J Physiol 267:G1012–G1020, 1994.
13. Kaneko K, Guth PH, Kaunitz JD: Na^+/H^+ exchange regulates intracellular pH of rat gastric surface cells in vivo. Pflugers Arch 421:322–328, 1992.
14. Isenberg JI, Ljungstrom M, Safsten B, Flemstrom G: Proximal duodenal enterocyte transport: Evidence for Na^+/H^+ and Cl^-/HCO_3^- exchange and $NaHCO_3$ cotransport. Am J Physiol 265:G677–G685, 1993.
15. Feil W, Klimesch S, Karner P, et al: Importance of an alkaline microenvironment for rapid restitution of the rabbit duodenal mucosa in vitro. Gastroenterology 97:112–122, 1989.
16. Kato K, Chen MC, Nguyen M, et al: Effects of growth factors and trefoil peptides on migration and replication in primary oxyntic cultures. Am J Physiol 276:G1105–G1116, 1999.
17. Barnard JA, Beauchamp RD, Russell WE, et al: Epidermal growth factor–related peptides and their relevance to gastrointestinal pathophysiology. Gastroenterology 108:564–580, 1995.
18. Folkman J: Seminars in medicine of the Beth Israel Hospital, Boston: Clinical applications of research on angiogenesis. N Engl J Med 28: 1757–1763, 1995.
19. Kivilaakso E, Fromm D, Silen W: Effect of the acid secretory state on intramural pH of rabbit gastric mucosa. Gastroenterology 75:641–648, 1978.
20. Schwarz K: Uber penetrierende magen- und jejunalgeschwure. Beitr Klin Chirurgie 5:96–128, 1910.
21. Goldschmiedt M, Peterson WL, Vuitch F, Feldman M: Postbulbar duodenal ulcer in a patient with pentagastrin-fast achlorhydria. Gastroenterology 97:771–774, 1989.
22. El-Omar EM, Penman ID, Ardill JE, et al: *Helicobacter pylori* infection and abnormalities of acid secretion in patients with duodenal ulcer disease. Gastroenterology 109:681–691, 1995.
23. Marshall BJ, Warren JR: Unidentified curved bacilli in the stomach of patients with gastritis and peptic ulceration. Lancet 1:1311–1315, 1984.
24. Cox AJ: Stomach size and its relation to chronic peptic ulcer. Arch Pathol 54:407–422, 1952.
25. Lam SK: Pathogenesis and pathophysiology of duodenal ulcer. Clin Gastroenterol 13:447–472, 1984.
26. Blair AJ III, Feldman M, Barnett C, et al: Detailed comparison of basal and food-stimulated gastric acid secretion rates and serum gastrin concentrations in duodenal ulcer patients and normal subjects. J Clin Invest 79:582–587, 1987.
27. Malagelada JR, Longstreth GF, et al: Gastric secretion and emptying after ordinary meals in duodenal ulcer. Gastroenterology 73:989–994, 1997.
28. Merki HS, Fimmel CJ, Walt RP, et al: Pattern of 24-hour intragastric acidity in active duodenal ulcer disease and in healthy controls. Gut 29:1583–1587, 1988.
29. Moore JG, Halberg F: Circadian rhythm of gastric acid secretion in men with active duodenal ulcer. Dig Dis Sci 31:1185–1191, 1986.
30. Feldman M, Richardson CT: Total 24-hour gastric acid secretion in patients with duodenal ulcer: Comparison with normal subjects and effects of cimetidine and parietal cell vagotomy. Gastroenterology 90: 540–544, 1986.
31. Peterson W, Barnett C, Evans DJ, et al: Acid secretion and serum gastrin in normal subjects and patients with duodenal ulcer: The role of *Helicobacter pylori*. Am J Gastroenterol 88:2038–2043, 1993.
32. Mossi S, Meyer-Wyss B, Renner EL, et al: Influence of *Helicobacter pylori*, sex, and age on serum gastrin and pepsinogen concentrations in subjects without symptoms and patients with duodenal ulcers. Gut 34:752–756, 1993.
33. Wagner S, Haruma K, Gladziwa U, et al: *Helicobacter pylori* infection and serum pepsinogen A, pepsinogen C, and gastrin in gastritis and peptic ulcer: Significance of inflammation and effect of bacterial eradication. Am J Gastroenterol 89:1211–1218, 1994.
34. Beardshall K, Moss S, Levi S, et al: Suppression of *Helicobacter pylori* reduces gastrin releasing peptide stimulated gastrin release in duodenal ulcer patients. Gut 33:601–603, 1992.
35. Calam J, Gibbons A, Healey ZV, et al: How does *Helicobacter pylori* cause mucosal damage? Its effect on acid and gastrin physiology. Gastroenterology 113(6 Suppl):S43–S49, 1997.
36. Olbe L, Hamlet A, Dalenback J, Fandriks L: A mechanism by which *Helicobacter pylori* infection of the antrum contributes to the development of duodenal ulcer. Gastroenterology 110:1386–1394, 1996.
37. Samloff IM, Stemmermann GN, Neilbrun LK, Nomura A: Elevated serum pepsinogen I and II levels differ as risk factors for duodenal ulcer and gastric ulcer. Gastroenterology 90:570–576, 1986.
38. Samloff IM: Peptic ulcer: The many proteinases of aggression. Gastroenterology 96:586–589, 1989.
39. Sumii K, Kimura M, Morkawa A, et al: Recurrence of duodenal ulcer and elevated serum pepsinogen I levels in smokers and nonsmokers. Am J Gastroenterol 85:1493–1497, 1990.
40. Asaka M, Kimura T, Kudo M, et al: Relationship of *Helicobacter pylori* to serum pepsinogens in an asymptomatic Japanese population. Gastroenterology 102:760–766, 1992.
41. Parente F, Maconi G, Sngaletti O, et al: Behaviour of acid secretion, gastrin release, serum pepsinogen I, and gastric emptying of liquids over six months from eradication of Helicobacter pylori in duodenal ulcer patients: A controlled study. Gut 37:210–215, 1995.
42. Kirkpatrick PM Jr, Hirschowitz BI: Duodenal ulcer with unexplained marked basal gastric acid hypersecretion. Gastroenterology 79:4–10, 1980.
43. Feldman M, Richardson CT, Fordtran JS: Effect of sham feeding on gastric acid secretion in healthy subjects and duodenal ulcer patients: Evidence for increased basal vagal tone in some ulcer patients. Gastroenterology 79:796–800, 1980.
44. Gravgaard E: A study of the vagus nerves at the lower end of the esophagus, with special reference to duodenal ulcer and acute gastroduodenal ulcerations. Scand J Gastroent 3:327–333, 1968.
45. Howlett PJ, Sheiner HJ, Barber DC, et al: Gastric emptying in control subjects and patients with duodenal ulcer before and after vagotomy. Gut 17:542–550, 1976.
46. Lam SK, Isenberg JI, Grossman MI, et al: Rapid gastric emptying in duodenal ulcer patients. Dig Dis Sci 27:598–604, 1982.
47. Isenberg JI, Selling JA, Hogan DL, Koss MA: Impaired proximal duodenal mucosal bicarbonate secretion in patients with duodenal ulcer. N Engl J Med 316:374–379, 1987.
48. Wyatt JI, Rathbone BJ, Dixon MF, Heatley RV: *Campylobacter pyloridis* and acid-induced gastric metaplasia in the pathogenesis of duodenitis. J Clin Pathol 40:841–848, 1987.
49. Hui WM, Lam SK, Chau PY, et al: Persistence of *Campylobacter pyloridis* despite healing of duodenal ulcer and improvement of accompanying duodenitis and gastritis. Dig Dis Sci 32:1255–1260, 1987.
50. Blanco M, Pajares JM, Jimenez ML, Lopez-Brea M: Effect of acid inhibition on *Campylobacter pylori*. Scand J Gastroenterol 142:107–109, 1988.
51. Hogan DL, Rapier RC, Dreilinger A, et al: Duodenal bicarbonate secretion: Eradication of *Helicobacter pylori* and duodenal structure and function in humans. Gastroenterology 110:705–716, 1996.
52. Savarino V, Mela GS, Zentilin P, et al: Twenty-four-hour gastric pH and extent of duodenal gastric metaplasia in *Helicobacter pylori*–positive patients. Gastroenterology 113:741–745, 1997.
53. Graham DY: *Helicobacter pylori* infection in the pathogenesis of duodenal ulcer and gastric cancer: A model. Gastroenterology 113:1983–1991, 1997.
54. Hofmann AF, Mysels KJ: Bile acid solubility and precipitation in vitro and in vivo: The role of conjugation, pH, and Ca^{2+} ions. J Lipid Res 33:617–626, 1992.
55. Stemmermann GN: Intestinal metaplasia of the stomach: A status report. Cancer 74:556–564, 1994.
56. Grossman MI, Kirsner JB, Gillespie IE: Basal and histalog-stimulated gastric secretion in control subjects and in patients with peptic ulcer or gastric cancer. Gastroenterology 45:14, 1963.
57. Johnson AG, McDermott SJ: Lysolecithin: A factor in the pathogenesis of gastric ulceration? Gut 15:710–713, 1974.
58. Fisher RS, Cohen S: Pyloric-sphincter dysfunction in patients with gastric ulcer. N Engl J Med 288:273–276, 1973.
59. Miller LJ, Malagelada JR, Longstreth GF, Go VL: Dysfunctions of the stomach with gastric ulceration. Dig Dis Sci 25:857, 1980.
60. Garrett JM, Summerskill WH, Code F: Antral motility in patients with gastric ulcer. Am J Dig Dis 11:780, 1966.
61. Suerbaum S, Smith JM, Bapumia K, et al: Free recombination within *Helicobacter pylori*. Proc Natl Acad Sci 95:12619–12624, 1998.
62. Alm RA, Ling LSL, Moir DT, et al: Genomic-sequence comparison of two unrelated isolates of the human gastric pathogen *Helicobacter pylori*. Nature 397:176–180, 1999.
63. Mobley HL, Cortesia MJ, Rosenthal LE, Jones BD: Characterization of urease from *Campylobacter pylori*. J Clin Microbiol 26:831–836, 1988.
64. Goodwin CS, Worsley BW: Microbiology of *Helicobacter pylori*. Gastroenterol Clin North Am 22:5–19, 1993.

65. The EUROGAST Study Group. Epidemiology of, and risk factors for, *Helicobacter pylori* infection among 3194 asymptomatic subjects in 17 populations. Gut 34:1672–1676, 1993.
66. Dwyer B, Kaldor J, Tee W, et al: Antibody response to *Campylobacter pylori* in diverse ethnic groups. Scand J Infect Dis 20:349–450, 1988.
67. Graham DY, Klein PD, Opekun AR, Boutton TW: Effect of age on the frequency of active *Campylobacter pylori* infection diagnosed by the ^{13C}urea breath test in normal subjects and patients with peptic ulcer disease. J Infect Dis 157:777–780, 1988.
68. Graham DY, Malaty HM, Evans DG, et al: Epidemiology of *Helicobacter pylori* in an asymptomatic population in the United States: Effect of age, race, and socioeconomic status. Gastroenterology 100: 1495–1501, 1991.
69. Marshall BJ: *Helicobacter pylori* in peptic ulcer: Have Koch's postulates been fulfilled? Ann Med 27:565–568, 1995.
70. Ciociola AA, McSorley DJ, Turner K, et al: *Helicobacter pylori* infection rates in duodenal ulcer patients in the United States may be lower than previously estimated. Am J Gastroenterol 94:1834–1840, 1999.
71. Blaser MJ: Not all *Helicobacter pylori* strains are created equal: Should all be eliminated? Lancet 349:1020–1022, 1997.
72. Hopkins RJ, Girardi LS, Turney EA: Relationship between *Helicobacter pylori* eradication and reduced duodenal and gastric ulcer recurrence: A review. Gastroenterology 110:1244–1252, 1996.
73. Atherton JC: CagA, the *cag* pathogenicity island and *Helicobacter pylori* virulence. Gut 44:307–308, 1999.
74. Blaser MJ: Role of vacA and cagA locus of *Helicobacter pylori* in human disease. Aliment Pharmacol Ther 10(Suppl 1):73–77, 1996.
75. Spechler SJ, Fischbach L, Feldman M: Clinical aspects of genetic variability in *Helicobacter pylori*. JAMA 283:1264–1266, 2000.
76. Hansson LE, Nyren O, Hsing AW, et al: The risk of stomach cancer in patients with gastric or duodenal ulcer disease. N Engl J Med 335: 242–249, 1996.
77. Graham DY, Yamaoka Y: *H. pylori* and *cagA*: Relationships with gastric cancer, duodenal ulcer, and reflux esophagitis and its complications. Helicobacter 3:145–151, 1998.
78. Cutler AF: Diagnostic tests for *Helicobacter pylori* infection. Gastroenterologist 5:202–212, 1997.
79. Feldman M, Cryer B, Lee E, Peterson WL: Role of seroconversion in confirming cure of *Helicobacter pylori* infection. JAMA 280:363–365, 1998.
80. Schoen RT, Vender RJ: Mechanisms of nonsteroidal anti-inflammatory drug-induced gastric damage. Am J Med 86:449–458, 1989.
81. Wolfe MM, Lichtenstein DR, Singh G: Gastrointestinal toxicity of nonsteroidal antiinflammatory drugs. N Engl J Med 340:1888–1899, 1999.
82. Lanza FL, Royer GL, Nelson RS: Endoscopic evaluation of the effects of aspirin, buffered aspirin, and enteric-coated aspirin on gastric and duodenal mucosa. N Engl J Med 303:136–138, 1980.
83. Henry D, Dobson A, Turner C: Variability in the risk of major gastrointestinal complications from nonaspirin nonsteroidal anti-inflammatory drugs. Gastroenterology 105:1078–1088, 1993.
84. Maliekal J, Elboim CM: Gastrointestinal complications associated with intramuscular ketorolac tromethamine therapy in the elderly. Ann Pharmacother 29:698–701, 1995.
85. Kelly JP, Kaufman DW, Jurgelon JM, et al: Risk of aspirin-associated major upper-gastrointestinal bleeding with enteric-coated or buffered product. Lancet 348:1413–1416, 1996.
86. Rich M, Scheiman JM: Nonsteroidal anti-inflammatory drug gastropathy at the new millennium: Mechanisms and prevention. Semin Arthritis Rheum 30:167–179, 2000.
87. Cryer B, Kliewer D, Sie H, et al: Effects of cutaneous aspirin on the human stomach and duodenum. Proc Am Assoc Physicians 111:448–456, 1999.
88. Whittle BJR: Mechanisms underlying gastric mucosal damage induced by indomethacin and bile salts, and the actions of prostaglandins. Br J Pharmacol 60:455–460, 1977.
89. Larkai EN, Smith JL, Lidsky MD, Graham DY: Gastroduodenal mucosa and dyspeptic symptoms in arthritic patients during chronic nonsteroidal anti-inflammatory drug use. Am J Gastroenterol 82:1153–1158, 1987.
90. Graham DY, Agrawal NM, Roth SH: Prevention of NSAID-induced gastric ulcer with misoprostol: Multicentre, double-blind, placebo-controlled trial. Lancet 2:1277–1280, 1988.
91. Laine L: Approaches to nonsteroidal anti-inflammatory drug use in the high-risk patient. Gastroenterology 120:594–606, 2001.
92. Allison MC, Howatson AG, Torrance CJ, et al: Gastrointestinal damage associated with the use of nonsteroidal antiinflammatory drugs. N Engl J Med 327:749–754, 1992.
93. Gabriel SE, Jaakkimainen L, Bombardier C: Risk for serious gastrointestinal complications related to use of nonsteroidal anti-inflammatory drugs: A meta-analysis. Ann Intern Med 115:787–796, 1991.
94. Singh G, Triadafilopoulos G: Epidemiology of NSAID-induced gastrointestinal complications. J Rheumatol 26:18–24, 1999.
95. Silverstein FE, Graham DY, Senior JR, et al: Misoprostol reduces serious gastrointestinal complications in patients with rheumatoid arthritis receiving nonsteroidal anti-inflammatory drugs: A randomized, double-blind, placebo-controlled trial. Ann Intern Med 123:241–249, 1995.
96. Piper JM, Ray WA, Daugherty JR, Griffin MR: Corticosteroid use and peptic ulcer disease: Role of nonsteroidal anti-inflammatory drugs. Ann Intern Med 114:735–740, 1991.
97. Garcia-Rodriguez LA, Jick H: Risk of upper gastrointestinal bleeding and perforation associated with individual nonsteroidal anti-inflammatory drugs. Lancet 343:769–772, 1994.
98. Cappell MS, Schein JR: Diagnosis and treatment of nonsteroidal anti-inflammatory drug-associated upper gastrointestinal toxicity. Gastroenterol Clin North Am 29:97–124, 2000.
99. Graham DY, Lidsky MD, Cox AM, et al: Long-term nonsteroidal antiinflammatory drug use and *Helicobacter pylori* infection. Gastroenterology 100:1653–1657, 1991.
100. Chan FK, Sung JJ, Chung SC, et al: Randomised trial of eradication of *Helicobacter pylori* before nonsteroidal anti-inflammatory drug therapy to prevent peptic ulcers. Lancet 350:975–979, 1997.
101. Aalykke C, Lauritsen JM, Hallas J, et al: *Helicobacter pylori* and risk of ulcer bleeding among users of nonsteroidal anti-inflammatory drugs: A case-control study. Gastroenterology 116:1305–1309, 1999.
102. Feldman M, Cryer B, Mallat D, Go MF: Role of *Helicobacter pylori* infection on gastroduodenal injury and gastric prostaglandin synthesis during long-term/low-dose aspirin therapy: A prospective placebo-controlled, double-blinded randomized trial. Am J Gastroenterol 96:1751–1757, 2001.
103. Shike M, Gillin JS, Kemeny N, et al: Severe gastroduodenal ulcerations complicating hepatic artery infusion chemotherapy for metastatic colon cancer. Am J Gastroenterol 81:176–179, 1986.
104. Feliciano DV, Ojukwu JC, Rozycki GS, et al: The epidemic of cocaine-related juxtapyloric perforations: With a comment on the importance of testing for *Helicobacter pylori*. Ann Surg 229:801–804, 1999.
105. Leder BZ, Kronenberg HM: Gastroenterologists and choosing the right bisphosphonate. Gastroenterology 119:866–871, 2000.
106. De Groen PC, Lubbe DF, Hisrsch LJ, et al: Esophagitis associated with the use of alendronate. N Engl J Med 335:1016–1021, 1996.
107. Lowe CE, Depew WT, Vanner SJ, et al: Upper gastrointestinal toxicity of alendronate. Am J Gastroenterol 95:634–640, 2000.
108. Graham DY, Malaty HM: Alendronate gastric ulcers. Aliment Pharmacol Ther 13:513–519, 1999.
109. Lanza FL, Hunt RH, Thomson ABR, et al: Endoscopic comparison of esophageal and gastroduodenal effects of risedronate and alendronate in postmenopausal women. Gastroenterology 119:631–638, 2000.
110. Cherner JA, Jensen RT, Dubois A, et al: Gastrointestinal dysfunction in systemic mastocytosis: A prospective study. Gastroenterology 95: 657–667, 1988.
111. Anderson W, Helman CA, Hirschowitz BI: Basophilic leukemia and the hypersecretion of gastric acid and pepsin. Gastroenterology 95: 195–198, 1988.
112. Cooper RG, Dockray GJ, Calam J, Walker R: Acid and gastrin responses during intragastric titration in normal subjects and duodenal ulcer patients with G-cell hyperfunction. Gut 26:232–236, 1985.
113. Annibale B, de Magistris L, Corleto V, et al: Zollinger-Ellison syndrome and antral G-cell hyperfunction in patients with resistant duodenal ulcer disease. Aliment Pharmacol Ther 8:87–93, 1994.
114. Kurata JH: Ulcer epidemiology: An overview and proposed research framework. Gastroenterology 96:569–580, 1989.
115. Munnangi S, Sonnenberg A: Time trends of physician visits and treatment patterns of peptic ulcer disease in the United States. Arch Intern Med 157:1489–1494, 1997.
116. Rosenstock SJ, Jorgensen T: Prevalence and incidence of peptic ulcer disease in a Danish County—a prospective cohort study. Gut 36:819–824, 1995.
117. Jennings D: Perforated peptic ulcer: Changes in age-incidence and

sex-distribution in the last 150 years. Lancet 1:395–398, 444–447, 1940.
118. Sonnenberg A: Temporal trends and geographical variations of peptic ulcer disease. Aliment Pharmacol Ther 9(Suppl 2):3–12, 1995.
119. El-Serag HB, Sonnenberg A: Opposing time trends of peptic ulcer and reflux disease. Gut 43:327–333, 1998.
120. Bloom BS: Cross-national changes in the effects of peptic ulcer disease. Ann Intern Med 114:558–562, 1991.
121. Susser M, Stein Z: Civilization and peptic ulcer. Lancet 1:115–119, 1962.
122. Susser M: Period effects, generation effects, and age effects in peptic ulcer mortality. J Chron Dis 35:29–40, 1982.
123. Sonnenberg A, Muller H, Pace F: Birth-cohort analysis of peptic ulcer mortality in Europe. J Chron Dis 38:309–317, 1985.
124. Sonnenberg A: Causative factors in the etiology of peptic ulcer disease become effective before the age of 15 years. J Chron Dis 38: 309–317, 1985.
125. Westbrook JI, Rushworth RL: The epidemiology of peptic ulcer mortality 1952–1989: A birth-cohort analysis. Int J Epidemiol 22:1085–1092, 1993.
126. Parsonnet J: The incidence of *Helicobacter pylori* infection. Aliment Pharmacol Ther 9(Suppl 2):45–51, 1995.
127. Walt R, Katschinski B, Logan R, et al: Rising frequency of ulcer perforation in elderly people in the United Kingdom. Lancet 1:489–492, 1986.
128. Jolobe OM, Montgomery RD: Changing clinical pattern of gastric ulcer: Are anti-inflammatory drugs involved? Digestion 29:164–170, 1984.
129. Henry D, Robertson J: Nonsteroidal anti-inflammatory drugs and peptic ulcer hospitalization rates in New South Wales. Gastroenterology 104:1083–1091, 1993.
130. Hernandez-Diaz S, Rodriguez LA: Association between nonsteroidal anti-inflammatory drugs and upper gastrointestinal tract bleeding/perforation: An overview of epidemiologic studies published in the 1990s. Arch Intern Med 160:2093–2099, 2000.
131. Piper DW, Nasiry R, McIntosh J, et al: Smoking, alcohol, analgesics, and chronic duodenal ulcer: A controlled study of habits before the first symptoms and before diagnosis. Scand J Gastroenterol 19:1015–1021, 1984.
132. Rogot E, Murray JL: Smoking and causes of death among US veterans: Sixteen years of observation. Public Health Rep 95:213–222, 1980.
133. Svanes C, Soreide JA, Skarstein A, et al: Smoking and ulcer perforation. Gut 2:177–180, 1997.
134. Sonnenberg A, Muller-Lissner A, Vogel E, et al: Predictors of duodenal ulcer healing and relapse. Gastroenterology 81:1061–1067, 1981.
135. Chan F, Sung J, Lee YT, et al: Does smoking predispose to peptic ulcer relapse after eradication of *Helicobacter pylori?* Am J Gastroenterol 92:442–445, 1997.
136. Aldoori WH, Giovannucci EL, Stampfer MJ, et al: A prospective study of alcohol, smoking, caffeine, and the risk of duodenal ulcer in men. Epidemiology 4:420, 1997.
137. Cryer B, Lee E, Feldman M: Factors influencing gastroduodenal mucosal prostaglandin concentrations: Roles of smoking and aging. Ann Intern Med 116:636–640, 1992.
138. Ainsworth MA, Hogan DL, Koss MA, Isenberg JI: Cigarette smoking inhibits acid-stimulated duodenal mucosal bicarbonate secretion. Ann Intern Med 119:882–886, 1993.
139. Bauerfeind P, Cilluffo T, Fimmel CJ, et al: Does smoking interfere with the effect of histamine H_2-receptor antagonists on intragastric acidity in man? Gut 28:549–556, 1987.
140. Bateson MC: Cigarette smoking and *Helicobacter pylori* infection. Postgrad Med J 69:41–44, 1993.
141. McArthur K, Hogan D, Isenberg JI: Relative stimulatory effects of commonly ingested beverages on gastric acid secretion in humans. Gastroenterology 83:199–203, 1982.
142. Peterson WL, Barnett C, Walsh JH: Effect of intragastric infusions of ethanol and wine on serum gastrin concentration and gastric acid secretion. Gastroenterology 91:1390–1395, 1986.
143. Tarnawski A, Brzozowski T, Sarfeh IJ, et al: Prostaglandin protection of human isolated gastric glands against indomethacin and ethanol injury: Evidence for direct cellular action of prostaglandin. J Clin Invest 81:1081–1089, 1988.
144. Stern AI, Hogan DL, Isenberg JI: A new method for quantitation of ion fluxes across in vivo human gastric mucosa: Effect of aspirin, acetaminophen, ethanol, and hyperosmolar solutions. Gastroenterology 86:60–70, 1984.
145. Bonnevie O: Causes of death in duodenal and gastric ulcer. Gastroenterology 73:1000–1004, 1977.
146. Friedman GD, Siegelaub AB, Seltzer CC: Cigarettes, alcohol, coffee, and peptic ulcer. N Engl J Med 290:469–473, 1974.
147. Cohen S, Booth GH: Gastric acid secretion and lower esophageal sphincter pressure in response to coffee and caffeine. N Engl J Med 293:897–899, 1975.
148. Langman MJ, Cooke AR: Gastric and duodenal ulcer and their associated diseases. Lancet 1:680–683, 1976.
149. Kellow JE, Tao Z, Piper DW: Ventilatory function in chronic peptic ulcer; A controlled study of ventilatory function in patients with gastric and duodenal ulcer. Gastroenterology 91:590–595, 1986.
150. Stemmermann GN, Marcus EB, Buist AS, MacLean CJ: Relative impact of smoking and reduced pulmonary function on peptic ulcer risk. Gastroenterology 96:1419–1424, 1989.
151. Kirk AP, Dooley JS, Hunt RH: Peptic ulceration in patients with chronic liver disease. Dig Dis Sci 25:756–760, 1980.
152. Siringo S, Burroughs AK, Bolondi L, et al: Peptic ulcer and its course in cirrhosis: An endoscopic and clinical prospective study. J Hepatol 22:633–641, 1995.
153. Kang JY, Wu AY, Sutherland IH, Vathsala A: Prevalence of peptic ulcer in patients undergoing maintenance hemodialysis. Dig Dis Sci 33:774–778, 1988.
154. Peters MN, Richardson CT: Stressful life events, acid hypersecretion, and ulcer disease. Gastroenterology 84:114–119, 1983.
155. Walker P, Feldman M: Psychosomatic aspects of peptic ulcer disease: A multifactorial model of stress. Gastroenterol Int 5:33–47, 1992.
156. Stewart DN, Winser DM: Incidence of perforated peptic ulcer: Effect of heavy air raids. Lancet 2:259–261, 1942.
157. Spicer CC, Stewart DN, Winser DM: Perforated peptic ulcer during the period of heavy air raids. Lancet 1:14, 1944.
158. Feldman M: Mental stress and peptic ulcers: An earthshaking association. Am J Gastroenterol 93:291–292, 1998.
159. Aoyama N, Kinoshita Y, Fujimoto S, et al: Peptic ulcers after the Hanshin-Awaji earthquake: Increased incidence of bleeding gastric ulcers. Am J Gastroenterol 93:311–316, 1998.
160. Rotter JI, Sones JQ, Samloff IM, et al: Duodenal ulcer disease associated with elevated serum pepsinogen I: An inherited autosomal dominant disorder. N Engl J Med 300:63–66, 1979.
161. Rotter JI: Peptic ulcer. In Emery AEH, Rimoin DL (eds): The Principles and Practice of Medical Genetics. New York, Churchill Livingstone, 1983, pp 863–878.
162. Boren T, Falk P, Roth KA, et al: Attachment of *Helicobacter pylori* to human gastric epithelium mediated by blood group antigens. Science 262:1892–1895, 1993.
163. Hein HO, Suadicani P, Gyntelberg F: Genetic markers for peptic ulcer: A study of 3387 men aged 54 to 74 years. The Copenhagen Male Study. Scand J Gastroenterol 32:16–21, 1997.
164. Palmer WL: The "acid test" in gastric and duodenal ulcer. JAMA 88: 1778, 1927.
165. Kang JY, Yap I, Guan R, Tay HH: Acid perfusion of duodenal ulcer craters and ulcer pain: A controlled double-blind study. Gut 27:942–945, 1986.
166. DeLuca VA, Winnan GG, Sheahan DG, et al: Is gastroduodenitis part of the spectrum of peptic ulcer disease? J Clin Gastroenterol 3(Suppl 2):17–22, 1981.
167. Isenberg JI, Peterson WL, Elashoff JD, et al: Healing of benign gastric ulcer with low-dose antacid or cimetidine: A double-blind, randomized, placebo-controlled trial. N Engl J Med 308:1319–1324, 1983.
168. Horrocks JC, De Dombal FT: Clinical presentation of patients with "dyspepsia": Detailed symptomatic study of 360 patients. Gut 19:19–26, 1978.
169. Pounder R: Silent peptic ulceration: Deadly silence or golden silence. Gastroenterology 96:626–631, 1989.
170. Health and Public Policy Committee, American College of Physicians: Endoscopy in the evaluation of dyspepsia. Ann Intern Med 102:266–269, 1985.
171. Committee on Endoscopic Utilization, American Society for Gastrointestinal Endoscopy: Appropriate use of gastrointestinal endoscopy. August 1992.
172. Levine MS: Role of the double-contrast upper gastrointestinal series in the 1990s. Gastroenterol Clin North Am 24:289–308, 1995.

173. Glick SN: Duodenal ulcer. Radiol Clin North Am 32:1259–1274, 1994.
174. Sun DCH, Stempien SJ: Site and size of the ulcer as determinants of outcome. Gastroenterology 61:576–584, 1971.
175. Grossman MI: Resume and comment: The Veterans Administration Cooperative Study on Gastric Ulcer. Gastroenterology 61:635–640, 1971.
176. Graham DY, Schwartz JT, Cain D, Gyorkey F: Prospective evaluation of biopsy number in the diagnosis of esophageal and gastric carcinoma. Gastroenterology 82:228–231, 1982.
177. Witzel L, Halter F, Gretillat PA, et al: Evaluation of specific value of endoscopic biopsies and brush cytology for malignancies of the oesophagus and stomach. Gut 17:375–377, 1976.
178. Dekker W, Tytgat GN: Diagnostic accuracy of fiber endoscopy in the detection of upper intestinal malignancy. Gastroenterology 73:710–714, 1977.
179. Llanos O, Guzman S, Duarte I: Accuracy of the first endoscopic procedure in the differential diagnosis of gastric lesions. Ann Surg 195:224–226, 1982.
180. Kochman ML, Elta GH: Gastric ulcers—when is enough enough? Gastroenterology 105:1582–1584, 1993.
181. Bytzer P: Endoscopic follow-up study of gastric ulcer to detect malignancy: Is it worthwhile? Scan J Gastroenterol 26:1193–1199, 1991.
182. Pruitt RE, Truss CD: Endoscopy, gastric ulcer, and gastric cancer: Follow-up endoscopy for all gastric ulcers? Dig Dis Sci 38:284–288, 1993.
183. Cantu TG, Korek JS: Central nervous system reactions to histamine$_2$-receptor blockers. Ann Intern Med 114:1027–1034, 1991.
184. Michaletz-Onody PA: Peptic ulcer disease in pregnancy. Gastroenterol Clin North Am 21:817–826, 1992.
185. Feldman M, Burton ME: Histamine$_2$-receptor antagonists: Standard therapy for acid-peptic diseases. N Engl J Med 323:1672–1680; 1749–1755, 1990.
186. Langtry HD, Grant SM, Goa KL: Famotidine: An updated review of its pharmacodynamic and pharmacokinetic properties, and therapeutic use in peptic ulcer disease and other allied diseases. Drugs 38:551–590, 1989.
187. Price AH, Brogden RN: Nizatidine: A preliminary review of its pharmacodynamic and pharmacokinetic properties, and its therapeutic use in peptic ulcer disease. Drugs 36:521–539, 1988.
188. Grant SM, Langtry HD, Brogden RN: Ranitidine: An updated review of its pharmacodynamic and pharmacokinetic properties and therapeutic use in peptic ulcer disease and other allied diseases. Drugs 37: 801–870, 1989.
189. Brogden RN, Heel RC, Speight TM, Avery GS. Cimetidine: A review of its pharmacological properties and therapeutic efficacy in peptic ulcer disease. Drugs 15:93–131, 1978.
190. Abate MA, Hyneck ML, Cohen IA, Berardi RR: Cimetidine pharmacokinetics. Clin Pharmacol 1:225–233, 1982.
191. Echizen H, Ishizaki T: Clinical pharmacokinetics of famotidine. Clin Pharmacokinet 21:178–194, 1991.
192. Lin JH: Pharmacokinetic and pharmacodynamic properties of histamine H$_2$-receptor antagonists: Relationship between intrinsic potency and effective plasma concentrations. Clin Pharmacokinet 20:218–236, 1991.
193. Patel N, Ward U, Rogers MJ, Primrose JN: Night-time or morning dosing with H$_2$-receptor antagonists: Studies on acid inhibition in normal subjects. Aliment Pharmacol Ther 6:381–387, 1992.
194. Jones DB, Howden SW, Burget DW, et al: Acid suppression in duodenal ulcer: A meta-analysis to define optimal dosing with antisecretory drugs. Gut 28:1120–1127, 1987.
195. Richter JM, Colditz GA, Huse DM, et al: Cimetidine and adverse reactions: A meta-analysis of randomized clinical trials of short-term therapy. Am J Med 87:278–284, 1989.
196. Hughes DG, Dowling EA, De Meersman RE, et al: Cardiovascular effects of H$_2$-receptor antagonists. J Clin Pharmacol 29:472–477, 1989.
197. Jurlander J, de Nully Brown P, Skov PS, et al: Improved vaccination response during ranitidine treatment, and increased plasma histamine concentrations, in patients with B cell chronic lymphocytic leukemia. Leukemia 9:1902–1909, 1995.
198. Kumar A: Cimetidine: An immunomodulator. DICP 24:289–295, 1990.
199. Burgess E, Muruve D: Renal effects of peptic ulcer therapy. Drug Saf 7:282–291, 1992.
200. Jensen RT, Collen MJ, Pandol SJ, et al: Cimetidine-induced impotence and breast changes in patients with gastric hypersecretory states. N Engl J Med 308:883–887, 1983.
201. Sax MJ: Clinically important adverse effects and drug interactions with H$_2$-receptor antagonists: An update. Pharmacotherapy 7:110S–115S, 1987.
202. Galbraith RA, Michnovicz JJ: The effects of cimetidine on the oxidative metabolism of estradiol. N Engl J Med 321:269–274, 1989.
203. Ehrinpreis MN, Dhar R, Narula A: Cimetidine-induced galactorrhea. Am J Gastroenterol 8:563–565, 1989.
204. Lipsy RJ, Fennerty B, Fagan TC: Clinical review of histamine$_2$ receptor antagonists. Arch Intern Med 150:745–751, 1990.
205. Porter JB, Beard K, Walker AM, et al: Intensive hospital monitoring study of intravenous cimetidine. Arch Intern Med 146:2237–2239, 1986.
206. Aymard JP, Aymard B, Netter P, et al: Haematological adverse effects of histamine H$_2$-receptor antagonists. Med Toxicol Adverse Drug Exp 3:430–448, 1988.
207. Agura ED, Vila E, Petersen FB, et al: The use of ranitidine in bone marrow transplantation: A review of 223 cases. Transplantation 46: 53–56, 1988.
208. Lewis JH: Hepatic effects of drugs used in the treatment of peptic ulcer disease. Am J Gastroenterol 82:987–1003, 1987.
209. Black M: Hepatotoxic and hepatoprotective potential of histamine (H$_2$)-receptor antagonists. Am J Med 83:68–75, 1987.
210. Hansten PD: Drug interactions with antisecretory agents. Aliment Pharmacol Ther 5(Suppl 1):121–128, 1991.
211. Smith SR, Kendall MJ: Ranitidine versus cimetidine: A comparison of their potential to cause clinically important drug interactions. Clin Pharmacokinet 15:44–56, 1988.
212. Miller TA, Robinson M: H$_2$-receptor antagonists and blood alcohol levels. Gastroenterology 103:1102–1104, 1992.
213. Raufman JP, Notar-Francesco V, Raffaniello RD, Straus EW: Histamine$_2$ receptor antagonists do not alter serum ethanol levels in fed, nonalcoholic men. Ann Intern Med 118:488–494, 1993.
214. Merki HS, Wilder-Smith CH: Do continuous infusions of omeprazole and ranitidine retain their effect with prolonged dosing? Gastroenterology 106:60–64, 1994.
215. Wilder-Smith CH, Ernst T, Genonni M, et al: Tolerance to oral H$_2$-receptor antagonists. Dig Dis Sci 8:976–983, 1990.
216. Fullarton GM, McLaughlin G, MacDonald A, et al: Rebound nocturnal hypersecretion after four weeks treatment with an H$_2$-receptor antagonist. Gut 30:449–454, 1989.
217. Nwokolo CU, Smith JTL, Sawyerr AM, et al: Rebound intragastric hyperacidity after abrupt withdrawal of histamine H$_2$-receptor blockade. Gut 32:1455–1460, 1991.
218. Saunders JHB, Wormsley KG: Long-term effects and after-effects of treatment of duodenal ulcer. Lancet 1:765–767, 1977.
219. Binder HJ, Cocco A, Crossley RJ, et al: Cimetidine versus intensive antacid therapy for duodenal ulcer: A multicenter trial. Gastroenterology 74(Suppl):389–392, 1978.
220. Sewing KF, Hagie L, Ippoliti AF, et al: Effect of one-month treatment with cimetidine on gastric secretion and serum gastrin and pepsinogen levels. Gastroenterology 74(Suppl):376–379, 1978.
221. Prewett EJ, Hudson M, Nwokolo CU, et al: Nocturnal intragastric acidity during and after a period of dosing with either ranitidine or omeprazole. Gastroenterology 100:873–877, 1991.
222. Howden CW: Clinical pharmacology of omeprazole. Clin Pharmacokinet 20:38–49, 1991.
223. Anersson T: Pharmacokinetics, metabolism, and interactions of acid pump inhibitors: Focus on omeprazole, lansoprazole, and pantoprazole. Clin Pharmacokinet 31:9–28, 1996.
224. Lew EA: Pharmacokinetic concerns in the selection of anti-ulcer therapy. Aliment Pharmacol Ther 13(Suppl 5):11–16, 1999.
225. Yasuda S, Ohnishi A, Ogawa T, et al: Pharmacokinetic properties of E3810, a new proton pump inhibitor, in healthy male volunteers. Int J Clin Pharmacol Ther 32:466–473, 1994.
226. Cederberg C, Andersson T, Skanberg I: Omeprazole: Pharmacokinetics and metabolism in man. Scand J Gastroenterol Suppl 166:33–40, 1989.
227. Andersson T, Andren K, Cederberg C, et al: Pharmacokinetics and bioavailability of omeprazole after single and repeated oral administration in healthy subjects. Br J Clin Pharmacol 29:557–563, 1990.
228. Clissold SP, Campoli-Richards DM: Omeprazole: A preliminary review of its pharmacodynamic and pharmacokinetic properties, and

therapeutic potential in peptic ulcer disease and Zollinger-Ellison syndrome. Drugs 32:15–47, 1986.
229. Landes BD, Petite JP, Flouvat B: Clinical pharmacokinetics of lansoprazole. Clin Pharmacokinet 8:458–470, 1995.
230. Huber R, Kohl B, Sachs G, et al: The continuing development of proton pump inhibitors with particular reference to pantoprazole. Aliment Pharmacol Ther 9:363–378, 1995.
231. Andersson T: Pharmacokinetics, metabolism, and interactions of acid pump inhibitors: Focus on omeprazole, lansoprazole, and pantoprazole. Clin Pharmacokinet 3:9–28, 1996.
232. Petersen KU: Omeprazole and the cytochrome P450 system. Aliment Pharmacol Ther 9:1–9, 1995.
233. Bertilsson L: Geographical/interracial differences in polymorphic drug oxidation: Current state of knowledge of cytochromes P450 (CYP) 2D6 and 2C19. Clin Pharmacokinet 9:192–209, 1995.
234. Pichard L, Curi-Pedrosa R, Bonfils C, et al: Oxidative metabolism of lansoprazole by human liver cytochromes P450. Mol Pharmacol 47: 410–418, 1995.
234a. Andersson T, Rohss K, Bredberg E, Hassan-Alin M: Pharmacokinetics and pharmacodynamics of esomeprazole, the S-isomer of omeprazole. Aliment Pharmacol Ther 15:1563–1569, 2001.
235. Hoyumpa AM, Trevino-Alanis H, Grimes I, Humphries TJ: Rabeprazole: Pharmacokinetics in patients with stable, compensated cirrhosis. Clin Ther 21:691–701, 1999.
236. Ferguson RJ, De Morais SM, Benhamou S, et al: A new genetic defect in human CYP2C19: Mutation of the initiation codon is responsible for poor metabolism of *S*-mephenytoin. J Pharmacol Exp Ther 284:356–361, 1998.
237. Andersson T, Regardh CG, Lou YC, et al: Polymorphic hydroxylation of *S*-mephenytoin and omeprazole metabolism in Caucasian and Chinese subjects. Pharmacogenetics 2:25–31, 1992.
238. Sohn DR, Kobayashi K, Chiba K, et al: Disposition kinetics and metabolism of omeprazole in extensive and poor metabolizers of *S*-mephenytoin 4′-hydroxylation recruited from an Oriental population. J Pharmacol Exp Ther 262:1195–1202, 1992.
239. Ishizaki T, Sohn DR, Kobayashi K, et al: Interethnic differences in omeprazole metabolism in the two *S*-mephenytoin hydroxylation phenotypes studied in Caucasians and Orientals. Ther Drug Monit Apr 16:214–215, 1994.
240. Wolfe MM, Sachs G: Acid suppression: Optimizing therapy for gastroduodenal ulcer healing, gastroesophageal reflux disease, and stress-related erosive syndrome. Gastroenterology 118:S9–S31, 2000.
241. Sachs G, Munson K, Hall K, Hersey SJ: Gastric H^+,K^+-ATPase as a therapeutic target in peptic ulcer disease. Dig Dis Sci 35:1537–1544, 1990.
242. Labenz J, Tillenburg B, Peitz U, et al: *Helicobacter pylori* augments the pH-increasing effect of omeprazole in patients with duodenal ulcer. Gastroenterology 110:725–732, 1996.
243. Feldman M, Cryer B, Sammer D, et al: Influence of *H. pylori* infection on meal-stimulated gastric acid secretion and gastroesophageal acid reflux. Am J Physiol 277:G1159–G1164, 1999.
244. Peghini PL, Katz PO, Bracy NA, Castell DO: Nocturnal recovery of gastric acid secretion with twice-daily dosing of proton pump inhibitors. Am J Gastroenterol 93:763–767, 1998.
245. Peghini PL, Katz PO, Castell DO: Ranitidine controls nocturnal gastric acid breakthrough on omeprazole: A controlled study in normal subjects. Gastroenterology 115:1335–1339, 1998.
246. Katz PO, Anderson C, Khoury R, Castell DO: Gastro-oesophageal reflux associated with nocturnal gastric acid breakthrough on proton pump inhibitors. Aliment Pharmacol Ther 12:1231–1234, 1998.
247. Holt S, Howden CW: Omeprazole: Overview and opinion. Dig Dis Sci 36:385–393, 1991.
248. Poynard T, Lemaire M, Agostini H: Meta-analysis of randomized clinical trials comparing lansoprazole with ranitidine or famotidine in the treatment of acute duodenal ulcer. Eur J Gastroenterol Hepatol 7: 661–665, 1995.
249. Dekkers CP, Beker JA, Thjodleifsson B, et al: Comparison of rabeprazole 20 mg versus omeprazole 20 mg in the treatment of active duodenal ulcer: A European multicentre study. Aliment Pharmacol Ther 13:179–186, 1999.
250. Bader JP, Delchier JC: Clinical efficacy of pantoprazole compared with ranitidine. Aliment Pharmacol Ther 8(Suppl 1):47–52, 1994.
251. Colin-Jones D: Safety of lansoprazole and omeprazole. Lancet 343: 1369, 1994.
252. Solvell L: The clinical safety of omeprazole. Digestion 47(Suppl 1): 59–63, 1990.
253. Nelis GF: Safety profile of omeprazole: Adverse events with short-term treatment. Digestion 44(Suppl 1):68–76, 1989.
254. Van den Branden M, Ring BJ, Binkley SN, Wrighton SA: Interaction of human liver cytochromes P450 in vitro with LY307640, a gastric proton pump inhibitor. Pharmacogenetics 6:81–91, 1996.
255. Gugler R, Jensen JC: Omeprazole inhibits oxidative drug metabolism: Studies with diazepam and phenytoin in vivo and 7-ethoxycoumarin in vitro. Gastroenterology. 89:1235–1241, 1985.
256. Humphries TJ: Clinical implications of drug interactions with the cytochrome P-450 enzyme system associated with omeprazole. Dig Dis Sci 36:1665–1669, 1991.
257. Humphries TJ, Merritt GJ: Drug interactions with agents used to treat acid-related diseases. Aliment Pharmacol Ther 13(Sppl 3):18–26, 1999.
258. Laine L, Ahnen D, McClain C, et al: Potential gastrointestinal effects of long-term acid suppression with proton pump inhibitors. Aliment Pharmacol Ther 14:651–658, 2000.
259. McQuaid KR: Much ado about gastrin. J Clin Gastroenterol 13:239–254, 1991.
260. Pounder R, Smith J: Drug-induced changes in plasma gastrin concentration. Gastroenterol Clin North Am 19:141–153, 1990.
261. Koop H, Arnold R: Long-term maintenance treatment of reflux esophagitis with omeprazole: Prospective study in patients with H_2-blocker–resistant esophagitis. Dig Dis Sci 36:552–557, 1991.
262. Lamberts R, Creutzfeldt W, Struber HG, et al: Long-term omeprazole therapy in peptic ulcer disease: Gastrin, endocrine cell growth, and gastritis. Gastroenterology 104:1356–1370, 1993.
263. Kuipers EJ, Meuwissen SG: The efficacy and safety of long-term omeprazole treatment for gastroesophageal reflux disease. Gastroenterology 118:795–798, 2000.
264. Klinkenberg-Knol EC, Nelis F, Dent J, et al, and Long-Term Study Group: Long-term omeprazole treatment in resistant gastroesophageal reflux disease: Efficacy, safety, and influence on gastric mucosa. Gastroenterology 118:661–669, 2000.
265. Hirschowitz BI, Griffith J, Pellegrin D, Cummings OW: Rapid regression of enterochromaffin-like cell gastric carcinoids in pernicious anemia after antrectomy. Gastroenterology 102:1409–1418, 1992.
266. Cadiot G, Laurent-Puig P, Thuille B, et al: Is the multiple endocrine neoplasia type 1 gene a suppressor for fundic argyrophil tumors in the Zollinger-Ellison syndrome? Gastroenterology 105:579–582, 1993.
267. Mattsson H, Havu N, Brautigam J, et al: Partial gastric corpectomy results in hypergastrinemia and development of gastric enterochromaffinlike-cell carcinoids in the rat. Gastroenterology 100:311–319, 1991.
268. Havu N: Enterochromaffin-like cell carcinoids of gastric mucosa in rats after life-long inhibition of gastric secretion. Digestion 35(Suppl 1):42–55, 1986.
269. Havu N, Mattsson H, Ekman L, Carlsson E: Enterochromaffin-like cell carcinoids in the rat gastric mucosa following long-term administration of ranitidine. Digestion 45:189–195, 1990.
270. Ryberg B, Axelson J, Hakanson R, et al: Trophic effects of continuous infusion of [Leu15]-gastrin-17 in the rat. Gastroenterology 98:33–38, 1990.
271. Larsson H, Carlsson E, Hakanson R, et al: Time-course of development and reversal of gastric endocrine cell hyperplasia after inhibition of acid secretion: Studies with omeprazole and ranitidine in intact and antrectomized rats. Gastroenterology 95:1477–1486, 1988.
272. Delwaide J, Latour P, Gast P, et al: Effects of proglumide and enprostil on omeprazole-induced fundic endocrine cell hyperplasia in rats. Gastroenterol Clin Biol 17:792–796, 1993.
273. Carlsson E, Larsson H, Mattsson H, et al: Pharmacology and toxicology of omeprazole—with special reference to the effects on the gastric mucosa. Scand J Gastroenterol Suppl 118:31–38, 1986.
274. Freston JW: Clinical significance of hypergastrinaemia: Relevance to gastrin monitoring during omeprazole therapy. Digestion 51(Suppl 1): 102–114, 1992.
275. Ekman L, Hansson E, Havu N, et al: Toxicological studies on omeprazole. Scand J Gastroenterol Suppl 108:53–69, 1985.
276. Axelson J, Hakanson R, Rosengren E, Sundler F: Hypergastrinaemia induced by acid blockade evokes enterochromaffin-like (ECL) cell hyperplasia in chicken, hamster, and guinea-pig stomach. Cell Tissue Res 254:511–516, 1988.
277. Borch K, Renvall H, Liedberg G: Gastric endocrine cell hyperplasia and carcinoid tumors in pernicious anemia. Gastroenterology 88:638–648, 1985.
278. Maton PN, Lack EE, Collen MJ, et al: The effect of Zollinger-Ellison

syndrome and omeprazole therapy on gastric oxyntic endocrine cells. Gastroenterology 99:943–950, 1990.
279. Klinkenberg-Knol EC, Festen HPM, Jansen JBMJ, et al: Long-term treatment with omeprazole for refractory reflux esophagitis: Efficacy and safety. Ann Intern Med 121:161–167, 1994.
280. Eissele R, Brunner G, Simon B, et al: Gastric mucosa during treatment with lansoprazole: *Helicobacter pylori* is a risk factor for argyrophil cell hyperplasia. Gastroenterology 112:707–717, 1997.
281. Solcia E, Fiocca R, Havu N, et al: Gastric endocrine cells and gastritis in patients receiving long-term omeprazole treatment. Digestion 51(Suppl 1):82–92, 1992.
282. Solcia E, Capella C, Fiocca R, et al: Gastric argyrophil carcinoidosis in patients with Zollinger-Ellison syndrome due to type 1 multiple endocrine neoplasia: A newly recognized association. Am J Surg Pathol 4:503–513, 1990.
283. Choudhry U, Boyce HW Jr, Coppola D: Proton pump inhibitor–associated gastric polyps: A retrospective analysis of their frequency, and endoscopic, histologic, and ultrastructural characteristics. Am J Clin Pathol 110:615–621, 1998.
284. Johnson LR, Lichtenberger LM, Copeland EM, et al: Action of gastrin on gastrointestinal structure and function. Gastroenterology 68:1184–1192, 1975.
285. Dembinski AB, Johnson LR: Growth of pancreas and gastrointestinal mucosa in antrectomized and gastrin-treated rats. Endocrinology 105: 769–773, 1979.
286. Johnson LR, Guthrie PD: Proglumide inhibition of trophic action of pentagastrin. Am J Physiol 246:G62–G66, 1984.
287. Creutzfeldt W, Lamberts R: Is hypergastrinaemia dangerous to man? Scand J Gastroenterol Suppl 180:179–191, 1991.
288. Smith JP, Wood JG, Solomon TE: Elevated gastrin levels in patients with colon cancer or adenomatous polyps. Dig Dis Sci 34:171–174, 1989.
289. Seitz JF, Giovannini M, Gouvernet J, Gauthier AP: Elevated serum gastrin levels in patients with colorectal neoplasia. J Clin Gastroenterol 13:541–545, 1991.
290. Ciccotosto GD, McLeish A, Hardy KJ, Shulkes A: Expression, processing, and secretion of gastrin in patients with colorectal carcinoma. Gastroenterology 109:1142–1153, 1995.
291. Suzuki H, Matsumoto K, Terashima H: Serum levels of gastrin in patients with colorectal neoplasia. Dis Colon Rectum 31:716–717, 1988.
292. Yapp R, Modlin IM, Kumar RR, et al: Gastrin and colorectal cancer: Evidence against an association. Dig Dis Sci 37:481–484, 1992.
293. Sobhani I, Lehy T, Laurent-Puig P, et al: Chronic endogenous hypergastrinemia in humans: Evidence for a mitogenic effect on the colonic mucosa. Gastroenterology 105:22–30, 1993.
294. Talley NJ, Chute CG, Larson DE, et al: Risk for colorectal adenocarcinoma in pernicious anemia: A population-based cohort study. Ann Intern Med 111:738–742, 1989.
295. Mellemkjaer L, Gridley G, Moller H, et al: Pernicious anaemia and cancer risk in Denmark. Br J Cancer 73:998–1000, 1996.
296. Thiruvengadam R, Hench V, Melton LJ, DiMagno EP: Cancer of the nongastric hollow organs of the gastrointestinal tract after gastric surgery. Arch Intern Med 148:405–407, 1988.
297. Siurala M, Lehtola J, Ihamaki T: Atrophic gastritis and its sequelae: Results of 19–23 years' follow-up examinations. Scand J Gastroenterol 9:441–446, 1974.
298. Solcia E, Villani L, Fiocca R, et al: Effects of eradication of *Helicobacter pylori* on gastritis in duodenal ulcer patients. Scand J Gastroenterol Suppl 201:28–34, 1994.
299. Kuipers EJ, Uyterlinde AM, Peña AS, et al: Increase of *Helicobacter pylori*–associated corpus gastritis during acid suppressive therapy: Implications for long-term safety. Am J Gastroenterol 90:1401–1406, 1995.
300. Kuipers EJ, Lundell L, Klinkenberg-Knol EC, et al: Atrophic gastritis and *Helicobacter pylori* infection in patients with reflux esophagitis treated with omeprazole or fundoplication. N Engl J Med 334:1018–1022, 1996.
301. Lundell L, Miettinen P, Myrvold HE, et al, and the Nordic GERD Study Group: Lack of effect of acid suppression therapy on gastric atrophy. Gastroenterology 117:319–326, 1999.
302. Fried M, Siegrist H, Frei R, et al: Duodenal bacterial overgrowth during treatment in outpatients with omeprazole. Gut 35:23–26, 1994.
303. Sharma BK, Santana IA, Wood EC, et al: Intragastric bacterial activity and nitrosation before, during, and after treatment with omeprazole. BMJ 289:717–719, 1984.
304. Verdu E, Viani F, Armstrong D, et al: Effect of omeprazole on intragastric bacterial counts, nitrates, nitrites, and *N*-nitroso compounds. Gut 35:455–460, 1994.
305. Stockbrugger RW, Cotton PB, Eugenides N, et al: Intragastric nitrites, nitrosamines, and bacterial overgrowth during cimetidine treatment. Gut 23:1048–1054, 1982.
306. Howden CW, Hunt RH: Relationship between gastric secretion and infection. Gut 28:96–107, 1987.
307. Gray JD, Shiner M: Influence of gastric pH on gastric and jejunal flora. Gut 8:74–81, 1967.
308. Yeomans ND, Brimblecombe RW, Elder J, et al: Effects of acid suppression on microbial flora of upper gut. Dig Dis Sci 40(2 Suppl): 81S–95S, 1995.
309. Theisen J, Nehra D, Citron D, et al: Suppression of gastric acid secretion in patients with gastroesophageal reflux disease results in gastric bacterial overgrowth and deconjugation of bile acids. J Gastrointest Surg 4:50–54, 2000.
310. Kauer WKH, Peters JH, DeMeester TR, et al: Mixed reflux of gastric and duodenal juices is more harmful to the esophagus than gastric juice alone: The need for surgical therapy re-emphasized. Ann Surg 222:525–533, 1995.
311. Wetscher GJ, Hinder RA, Smyrk T, et al: Gastric acid blockade with omeprazole promotes gastric carcinogenesis induced by duodenogastric reflux. Dig Dis Sci 44:1132–1135, 1999.
312. Giannella RA, Broitman SA, Zamcheck N: *Salmonella* enteritis: I. Role of reduced gastric secretion in pathogenesis. Am J Dig Dis 16: 1000–1006, 1971.
313. Giannella RA, Broitman SA, Zamcheck N: Influence of gastric acidity on bacterial and parasitic enteric infections: A perspective. Ann Intern Med 78:271–276, 1973.
314. DuPont HL, Hornick RB, Snyder MJ, et al: Immunity in shigellosis: I. Response of man to attenuated strains of *Shigella*. J Infect Dis 125:5–11, 1972.
315. Cash RA, Music SI, Libonati JP, et al: Response of man to infection with Vibrio cholerae: I. Clinical, serologic, and bacteriologic responses to a known inoculum. J Infect Dis 129:45–52, 1974.
316. Nalin DR, Levine RJ, Levine MM, et al: Cholera, non-vibrio cholera, and stomach acid. Lancet 2:856–859, 1978.
317. Wingate DL: Acid reduction and recurrent enteritis. Lancet 335:222, 1990.
318. Garcia Rodriguez LA, Ruigomez A: Gastric acid, acid-suppressing drugs, and bacterial gastroenteritis: How much of a risk? Epidemiology 8:571–574, 1997.
319. Serfaty-Lacrosniere C, Wood RJ, Voytko D, et al: Hypochlorhydria from short-term omeprazole treatment does not inhibit intestinal absorption of calcium, phosphorus, magnesium, or zinc from food in humans. J Am Coll Nutr 14:364–368, 1995.
320. Koop H, Bachem MG: Serum iron, ferritin, and vitamin B_{12} during prolonged omeprazole therapy. J Clin Gastroenterol 14:288–292, 1992.
321. Schenk BE, Festen HPM, Kuipers EJ, et al: Effect of short- and long-term treatment with omeprazole on the absorption and serum levels of cobalamin. Aliment Pharmacol Ther 10:541–545, 1996.
322. Steinberg WM, King CE, Toskes PP: Malabsorption of protein-bound cobalamin but not unbound cobalamin during cimetidine administration. Dig Dis Sci 25:188–191, 1980.
323. Marcuard SP, Albernaz L, Khazanie PG: Omeprazole therapy causes malabsorption of cyanocobalamin (vitamin B_{12}). Ann Intern Med 120: 211–215, 1994.
324. Binder HJ, Donaldson RM Jr: Effect of cimetidine on intrinsic factor and pepsin secretion. Gastroenterology 74:371–375, 1978.
325. Termanini B, Gibril F, Sutliff VE, et al: Effect of long-term gastric acid suppressive therapy on serum vitamin B_{12} levels in patients with Zollinger-Ellison syndrome. Am J Med 104:422–430, 1998.
326. Howden CW: Vitamin B_{12} levels during prolonged treatment with proton pump inhibitors. J Clin Gastroenterol 30:29–33, 2000.
327. Sandvik AK, Brenna E, Waldum HL: The pharmacological inhibition of gastric acid secretion—tolerance and rebound. Aliment Pharmacol Ther 11:1013–1018, 1997.
328. Sharma B, Axelson M, Pounder RP, et al: Acid secretory capacity and plasma gastrin concentration after administration of omeprazole to normal subjects. Aliment Pharmacol Ther 1:67–76, 1987.
329. Waldum HL, Arnestad JS, Brenna E, et al: Marked increase in gastric acid secretory capacity after omeprazole treatment. Gut 39:649–653, 1996.
330. Peterson WL, Sturdevant RAL, Frankl HD, et al: Healing of duodenal ulcer with an antacid regimen. N Engl J Med 297:341–345, 1977.
331. Rydning A, Weberg R, Lange O, Berstad A: Healing of benign gastric

ulcer with low-dose antacids and fiber diet. Gastroenterology 91:56–61, 1986.
332. Konturek SJ: New aspects of clinical pharmacology of antacids. J Physiol Pharmacol 44(Suppl 1):5–21, 1993.
333. Nicklas W: Aluminum salts. Res Immunol 143:489–494, 1992.
334. Gasbarrini G, Andreone P, Baraldini M, et al: Antacids in gastric ulcer treatment: Evidence of cytoprotection. Scand J Gastroenterol Suppl 174:44–47, 1990.
335. Tarnawski A, Hollander D, Gergely H: Antacids: New perspectives in cytoprotection. Scand J Gastroenterol Suppl 174:9–14, 1990.
336. Haram EM, Weberg R, Berstad A: Urinary excretion of aluminum after ingestion of sucralfate and an aluminum-containing antacid in man. Scand J Gastroenterol 22:615–618, 1987.
337. Sherrard DJ: Aluminum—much ado about something. N Engl J Med 324:558–559, 1991.
338. Brogden RN, Heel RC, Speight TM, Avery GS: Sucralfate: A review of its pharmacodynamic properties and therapeutic use in peptic ulcer disease. Drugs 27:194–209, 1984.
339. McCarthy DM: Sucralfate. N Engl J Med 325:1017–1025, 1991.
340. Rees WD: Mechanisms of gastroduodenal protection by sucralfate. Am J Med 91:58S–63S, 1991.
341. Wagstaff AJ, Benfield P, Monk JP: Colloidal bismuth subcitrate: A review of its pharmacodynamic and pharmacokinetic properties, and its therapeutic use in peptic ulcer disease. Drugs 36:132–157, 1988.
342. Hall DW: Review of the modes of action of colloidal bismuth subcitrate. Scand J Gastroenterol Suppl 157:3–6, 1989.
343. Konturek SJ, Dembinski A, Warzecha Z, et al: Epidermal growth factor (EGF) in the gastroprotective and ulcer healing actions of colloidal bismuth subcitrate (De-Nol) in rats. Gut 29:894–902, 1988.
344. Gladziwa U, Koltz U: Pharmacokinetic optimisation of the treatment of peptic ulcer in patients with renal failure. Clin Pharmacokinet 27: 393–408, 1994.
345. Walt RP: Misoprostol for the treatment of peptic ulcer and antiinflammatory-drug-induced gastroduodenal ulceration. N Engl J Med 327: 1575–1580, 1992.
346. Chen MC, Amirian DA, Toomey M, et al: Prostanoid inhibition of canine parietal cells: Mediation by the inhibitory guanosine triphosphate–binding protein of adenylate cyclase. Gastroenterology 94: 1121–1129, 1988.
347. Wilson DE: Antisecretory and mucosal protective actions of misoprostol: Potential role in the treatment of peptic ulcer disease. Am J Med 83:2–8, 1987.
348. Davis GR, Fordtran JS, Dajani EZ: Dose-response, meal-stimulated gastric antisecretory study of prostaglandin E_1 analog, misoprostol, in man. Dig Dis Sci 33:298–302, 1988.
349. Isenberg JI, Hogan DL, Koss MA, Selling JA: Human duodenal mucosal bicarbonate secretion: Evidence for basal secretion and stimulation by hydrochloric acid and a synthetic prostaglandin E_1 analogue. Gastroenterology 91:370–378, 1986.
350. Leung FW, Miller JC, Guth PH: Dissociated effects of misoprostol on gastric acid secretion and mucosal blood flow. Dig Dis Sci 31(2 Suppl):86S–90S, 1986.
351. Hawkey CJ, Karrasch JA, Szezepanski L, et al: Omeprazole compared with misoprostol for ulcers associated with nonsteroidal antiinflammatory drugs: Omeprazole versus Misoprostol for NSAID-induced Ulcer Management (OMNIUM) Study Group. N Engl J Med 338:727–734, 1998.
352. Feldman M, Richardson CT, Peterson WL, et al: Effect of low-dose propantheline on food-stimulated gastric acid secretion: Comparison with an "optimal effective dose" and interaction with cimetidine. N Engl J Med 297:1427–1430, 1977.
353. Texter EC, Reilly PA: The efficacy and selectivity of pirenzepine: Review and commentary. Scand J Gastroenterol Suppl 72:237–246, 1982.
354. Soll AH: Medical treatment of peptic ulcer disease: Practice guidelines. Practice Parameters Committee of the American College of Gastroenterology. JAMA 275:622–629, 1996.
355. Croker JR, Cotton PB, Boyle AC, Kinsella P: Cimetidine for peptic ulcer in patients with arthritis. Ann Rheum Dis 39:275–278, 1980.
356. Davies J, Collins AJ, Dixon SA: The influence of cimetidine on peptic ulcer in patients with arthritis taking anti-inflammatory drugs. Br J Rheumatol 25:54–58, 1986.
357. O'Laughlin JC, Silvoso GK, Ivey KJ: Resistance to medical therapy of gastric ulcers in rheumatic disease patients taking aspirin: A double-blind study with cimetidine and follow-up. Dig Dis Sci 27:976–980, 1982.
358. Lancaster-Smith MJ, Jaderberg ME, Jackson DA: Ranitidine in the treatment of nonsteroidal anti-inflammatory drug associated gastric and duodenal ulcers. Gut 32:252–255, 1991.
359. Walan A, Bader JP, Classen M, et al: Effect of omeprazole and ranitidine on ulcer healing and relapse rates in patients with benign gastric ulcer. N Engl J Med 320:69–75, 1989.
360. Langman MJ, Brooks P, Hawkey CJ, et al: Nonsteroidal anti-inflammatory drug associated ulcer: Epidemiology, causation, and treatment. J Gastroenterol Hepatol 6:442–449, 1991.
361. Yeomans ND, Tulassay Z, Juhasz L, et al: A comparison of omeprazole with ranitidine for ulcers associated with nonsteroidal antiinflammatory drugs. Acid Suppression Trial: Ranitidine Versus Omeprazole for NSAID-Associated Ulcer Treatment (ASTRONAUT) Study Group. N Engl J Med 338:719–726, 1998.
362. Agrawal NM, Campbell DR, Safdi MA, et al: Superiority of lansoprazole versus ranitidine in healing nonsteroidal antiinflammatory drug-associated gastric ulcers: Results of a double-blind, randomized, multicenter study. NSAID-Associated Gastric Ulcer Study Group. Arch Intern Med 160:1455–1461, 2000.
363. Robinson MG, Griffin JW, Bowers J, et al: Effect of ranitidine on gastroduodenal mucosal damage induced by nonsteroidal antiinflammatory drugs. Dig Dis Sci 34:424–428, 1989.
364. Ehsanullah RS, Page MC, Tildesley G, Wood JR: Prevention of gastroduodenal damage induced by nonsteroidal anti-inflammatory drugs: Controlled trial of ranitidine. BMJ 297:1017–1021, 1988.
365. Taha AS, Hudson N, Hawkey CJ, et al: Famotidine for the prevention of gastric and duodenal ulcers caused by nonsteroidal antiinflammatory drugs. N Engl J Med 334:1435–1439, 1996.
366. Graham DY, Agrawal NM, Roth SH: Prevention of NSAID-induced gastric ulcer with misoprostol: Multicentre, double-blind, placebo-controlled trial. Lancet 2:1277–1280, 1988.
367. Graham DY, White RH, Moreland LW, et al: Duodenal and gastric ulcer prevention with misoprostol in arthritis patients taking NSAIDs. Misoprostol Study Group. Ann Intern Med 119:257–262, 1993.
368. Raskin JB, White RH, Jackson JE, et al: Misoprostol dosage in the prevention of nonsteroidal anti-inflammatory drug-induced gastric and duodenal ulcers: A comparison of three regimens. Ann Intern Med 123:344–350, 1995.
369. Silverstein FE, Graham DY, Senior JR, et al: Misoprostol reduces serious gastrointestinal complications in patients with rheumatoid arthritis receiving nonsteroidal anti-inflammatory drugs: A randomized, double-blind, placebo-controlled trial. Ann Intern Med 123:241–249, 1995.
370. Lanas A, Remacha B, Sainz R, Hirschowitz BI: Study of outcome after targeted intervention for peptic ulcer resistant to acid suppression therapy. Am J Gastroenterol 95:513–519, 2000.
371. Armstrong D, Arnold R, Classen M, et al: Prospective multicentre study of risk factors associated with delayed healing of recurrent duodenal ulcers (RUDER). RUDER Study Group. Gut 34:1319–1326, 1993.
372. Bardhan KD: Is there any acid peptic disease that is refractory to proton pump inhibitors? Aliment Pharmacol Ther 7(Suppl 1):13–24, 1993.
373. Van Rensburg CJ, Louw JA, Girdwood AH, et al: A trial of lansoprazole in refractory gastric ulcer. Aliment Pharmacol Ther 10:381–386, 1996.
373a. Lai KC, Hui WM, Wong BC, et al: Ulcer-healing drugs are required after eradication of *Helicobacter pylori* in patients with gastric ulcer but not duodenal ulcer haemorrhage. Aliment Pharmacol Ther 14: 1071–1076, 2001.
373b. Ge ZZ, Zhang DA, Xiao SD, et al: Does eradication of *Helicobacter pylori* alone heal duodenal ulcers? Aliment Pharmacol Ther 14:53–58, 2000.
374. Howden CW, Hunt RH: The relationship between suppression of acidity and gastric ulcer healing rates. Aliment Pharmacol Ther 4:25–33, 1990.
375. Lauritsen K, Rune SJ, Wulff HR, et al: Effect of omeprazole and cimetidine on prepyloric gastric ulcer: Double-blind comparative trial. Gut 29:249–253, 1988.
376. Schepp W, Classen M: Omeprazole in the acute treatment of gastric ulcer. Scand J Gastroenterol Suppl 166:58–62, 1989.
377. Bate CM, Wilkinson SP, Bradby GV, et al: Randomised, double-blind comparison of omeprazole and cimetidine in the treatment of symptomatic gastric ulcer. Gut 30:1323–1328, 1989.
378. Omeprazole and cimetidine in the treatment of ulcers of the body of the stomach: A double-blind comparative trial. Danish Omeprazole Study Group. BMJ 298:645–647, 1989.
379. Rokkas T, Karameris A, Mavrogeorgis A, et al: Eradication of *Helico-*

bacter pylori reduces the possibility of rebleeding in peptic ulcer disease. Gastrointest Endosc 41:1–4, 1995.
380. Jaspersen D, Koerner T, Schorr W, et al: *Helicobacter pylori* eradication reduces the rate of rebleeding in ulcer hemorrhage. Gastrointest Endosc 41:5–7, 1995.
381. Laine L, Peterson WL: Bleeding peptic ulcer. N Engl J Med 331:717–727, 1994.
382. Somerville K, Faulkner G, Langman M: Non-steroidal anti-inflammatory drugs and bleeding peptic ulcer. Lancet 1:462–464, 1986.
383. Griffin MR, Ray WA, Schaffner W: Nonsteroidal anti-inflammatory drug use and death from peptic ulcer in elderly persons. Ann Intern Med 109:359–363, 1988.
384. Holvoet J, Terriere L, Van Hee W, et al: Relation of upper gastrointestinal bleeding to nonsteroidal anti-inflammatory drugs and aspirin: A case-control study. Gut 32:730–734, 1991.
385. Laporte JR, Carne X, Vidal X, et al: Upper gastrointestinal bleeding in relation to previous use of analgesics and nonsteroidal anti-inflammatory drugs. Catalan Countries Study on Upper Gastrointestinal Bleeding. Lancet 337:85–89, 1991.
386. Griffin MR, Piper JM, Daugherty JR, et al: Nonsteroidal anti-inflammatory drug use and increased risk for peptic ulcer disease in elderly persons. Ann Intern Med 114:257–263, 1991.
387. Carson JL, Strom BL, Soper KA, et al: The association of nonsteroidal anti-inflammatory drugs with upper gastrointestinal tract bleeding. Arch Intern Med 147:85–88, 1987.
388. Bloom BS: Risk and cost of gastrointestinal side effects associated with nonsteroidal anti-inflammatory drugs. Arch Intern Med 149: 1019–1022, 1989.
389. Laszlo A, Kelly JP, Kaufman DE, et al: Clinical aspects of upper gastrointestinal bleeding associated with the use of nonsteroidal antiinflammatory drugs. Am J Gastroenterol 93:721–725, 1998.
390. Gabriel SE, Jaakkimainen L, Bombardier C: Risk for serious gastrointestinal complications related to use of nonsteroidal anti-inflammatory drugs: A meta-analysis. Ann Intern Med 115:787–796, 1991.
391. Wara P, Stodkilde H: Bleeding pattern before admission as guideline for emergency endoscopy. Scand J Gastroenterol 20:72–78, 1985.
392. Jensen DM, Machicado GA: Diagnosis and treatment of severe hematochezia: The role of urgent colonoscopy after purge. Gastroenterology 95:1569–1574, 1988.
393. Green FW, Kaplan MM, Curtis LE, Levine PH: Effect of acid and pepsin on blood coagulation and platelet aggregation: A possible contributor to prolonged gastroduodenal mucosal hemorrhage. Gastroenterology 74:38–43, 1978.
394. Patchett SE, Enright H, Afdhal N, et al: Clot lysis by gastric juice: An in vitro study. Gut 30:1704–1707, 1989.
395. Walt RP, Cottrell J, Mann SG, et al: Continuous intravenous famotidine for haemorrhage from peptic ulcer. Lancet 340:1058–1062, 1992.
396. Zuckerman G, Welch R, Douglas A, et al: Controlled trial of medical therapy for active upper gastrointestinal bleeding and prevention of rebleeding. Am J Med 76:361–366, 1984.
397. Collins R, Langman M: Treatment with histamine H_2 antagonists in acute upper gastrointestinal hemorrhage: Implications of randomized trials. N Engl J Med 313:660–666, 1985.
398. Villanueva C, Balanzo J, Torras X, et al: Omeprazole versus ranitidine as adjunct therapy to endoscopic injection in actively bleeding ulcers: A prospective and randomized study. Endoscopy 27:308–312, 1995.
399. Lanas A, Artal A, Blas JM, et al: Effect of parenteral omeprazole and ranitidine on gastric pH and the outcome of bleeding peptic ulcer. J Clin Gastroenterol 21:103–106, 1995.
400. Lin HJ, Lo WC, Lee FY, et al: A prospective randomized comparative trial showing that omeprazole prevents rebleeding in patients with bleeding peptic ulcer after successful endoscopic therapy. Arch Intern Med 158:54–58, 1998.
401. Schaffalitzky de Muckadell OB, Havelund T, et al: Effect of omeprazole on the outcome of endoscopically treated bleeding peptic ulcers: Randomized double-blind placebo-controlled multicentre study. Scand J Gastroenterol 32:320–327, 1997.
402. Hasselgren G, Lind T, Lundell L, et al: Continuous intravenous infusion of omeprazole in elderly patients with peptic ulcer bleeding: Results of a placebo-controlled multicentre study. Scand J Gastroenterol 32:328–333, 1997.
403. Khuroo MS, Yattoo GN, Javid G, et al: A comparison of omeprazole and placebo for bleeding peptic ulcer. N Engl J Med 336:1054–1058, 1997.
404. Lau JYW, Sung JJY, Lee KKC, et al: Effect of intravenous omeprazole on recurrent bleeding after endoscopic treatment of bleeding peptic ulcers. N Engl J Med 343:310–316, 2000.
405. Gunshefski L, Flancbaum L, Brolin RE, Frankel A: Changing patterns in perforated peptic ulcer disease. Am Surg 56:270–274, 1990.
406. Collier DS, Pain JA: Nonsteroidal anti-inflammatory drugs and peptic ulcer perforation. Gut 26:359–363, 1985.
407. Svanes C, Soreide JA, Skarstein A, et al: Smoking and ulcer perforation. Gut 41:177, 1997.
408. Svanes C: Trends in perforated peptic ulcer: Incidence, etiology, treatment, and prognosis. World J Surg 24:277–283, 2000.
409. Shaffer HA: Perforation and obstruction of the gastrointestinal tract: Assessment by conventional radiology. Radiol Clin North Am 30: 405–426, 1992.
410. Ng EKW, Lam YH, Sung JJY, et al: Eradication of *Helicobacter pylori* prevents recurrence of ulcer after simple closure of duodenal ulcer perforation: Randomized controlled trial. Ann Surg 231:153–158, 2000.
411. Crofts TJ, Park KG, Steele RJ, et al: A randomized trial of nonoperative treatment for perforated peptic ulcer. N Engl J Med 320:970–3,
412. Rigg KM, Stuart RC, Rosenberg IL: Conservative management of perforated peptic ulcer. Lancet. 1989. 2:1429–30,
413. Norris JR, Haubrich WS: The incidence and clinical features of penetration in peptic ulceration. JAMA 1961. 178:386,
414. Ellis H: The diagnosis of benign and malignant pyloric obstruction. Clin Oncol 1976. 2:11–5,
415. Johnson CD, Ellis H: Gastric outlet obstruction now predicts malignancy. Br J Surg 1990. 77:1023–4,
416. Quigley RL, Pruitt SK, Pappas TN, Akwari O: Primary hypertrophic pyloric stenosis in the adult. Arch Surg 1990. 125:1219–21,
417. Walker CO: Complications of peptic ulcer disease and indications for surgery. In: Sleisenger MH, Fordtran JS (eds). Gastrointestinal Disease. Pathophysiology, Diagnosis, Management, 2nd ed. Philadelphia, WB Saunders, 1978, pp 914–932,
418. Goldstein H, Boyle JD: The saline load test—a bedside evaluation of gastric retention. Gastroenterology 1965. 49:375–380, 1989.
419. Boyle JD, Goldstein H: Management of pyloric obstruction. Med Clin North Am 52:1329–1337, 1968.
420. Zittel TT, Jehle EC, Becker HD: Surgical management of peptic ulcer disease today—indication, technique, and outcome. Langenbecks Arch Surg 385:84–96, 2000.
421. Khullar SK, DiSario JA: Gastric outlet obstruction. Gastrointest Endosc Clin North Am 6:585–603, 1996.
422. Haglund U: Stress ulcers. Scand J Gastroenterol 25(Suppl 175):27–33, 1990.
423. Beejay U, Wolfe MM: Acute gastrointestinal bleeding in the intensive care unit. Gastroenterol Clin North Am 29:309–336, 2000.
424. Norton L, Greer J, Eiseman B: Gastric secretory response to head injury. Arch Surg 101:200–204, 1970.
425. Bowen JC, Fleming WH, Thompson JC: Increased gastrin release following penetrating central nervous system injury. Surgery 75:720–724, 1974.
426. Cheung LY, Ashley SW: Gastric blood flow and mucosal defense mechanisms. Clin Invest Med 10:201–208, 1987.
427. Flynn R, Stuart RC, Gorey TF, et al: Stress ulceration and gastric mucosal cell kinetics: The influence of prophylaxis against acute stress ulceration. J Surg Res 55:188–192, 1993.
428. Marrone GC, Silen W: Pathogenesis, diagnosis, and treatment of acute gastric mucosal lesions. Clin Gastroenterol 13:635–650, 1984.
429. Smith P, O'Brien P, Fromm D, Silen W: Secretory state of gastric mucosa and resistance to injury by exogenous acid. Am J Surg 133: 81–85, 1977.
430. Szabo S: Gastroduodenal mucosal injury—acute and chronic: Pathways, mediators, and mechanisms. J Clin Gastroenterol 13(Suppl 1): S1–S8, 1991.
431. Peura DA, Johnson LF: Cimetidine for prevention and treatment of gastroduodenal mucosal lesions in patients in an intensive care unit. Ann Intern Med 103:173–177, 1985.
432. Czaja AJ, McAlhany JC, Pruitt BA Jr: Acute gastroduodenal disease after thermal injury: An endoscopic evaluation of incidence and natural history. N Engl J Med 291:925–929, 1974.
433. Lucas CE, Sugawa C, Riddle J, et al: Natural history and surgical dilemma of "stress" gastric bleeding. Arch Surg 102:266–273, 1971.
434. Cook DJ, Fuller HD, Guyatt GH, et al: Risk factors for gastrointestinal bleeding in critically ill patients. Canadian Critical Care Trials Group. N Engl J Med 330:377–381, 1994.
435. Tryba M, Cook D: Current guidelines on stress ulcer prophylaxis. Drugs 54:581–596, 1997.
436. Soderstrom CA, Ducker TB: Increased susceptibility of patients with

cervical cord lesions to peptic gastrointestinal complications. J Trauma 25:1030–1038, 1985.
437. Shuman RB, Schuster DP, Zuckerman GR: Prophylactic therapy for stress ulcer bleeding: A reappraisal. Ann Intern Med 106:562–567, 1987.
438. Lacroix J, Infante-Rivard C, Jenicek M, Gauthier M: Prophylaxis of upper gastrointestinal bleeding in intensive care units: A meta-analysis. Crit Care Med 17:862–869, 1989.
439. Cook DJ, Witt LG, Cook RJ, Guyatt GH: Stress ulcer prophylaxis in the critically ill: A meta-analysis. Am J Med 9:519–527, 1991.
440. Tryba M: Prophylaxis of stress ulcer bleeding: A meta-analysis. J Clin Gastroenterol 13(Suppl 2):S44–S55, 1991.
441. Cook DJ, Laine LA, Guyatt GH, Raffin TA: Nosocomial pneumonia and the role of gastric pH: A meta-analysis. Chest 100:7–13, 1991.
442. Cook DJ, Reeve BK, Guyatt GH, et al: Stress ulcer prophylaxis in critically ill patients. JAMA 275:308–314, 1996.
443. Otani Y, Kitajima M, Sugiyama M, et al: Inhibitory effects of intravenous lansoprazole on gastric acid hypersecretion in patients with postoperative stress. J Clin Gastroenterol 20 Suppl 2:S22–S26, 1995.
444. Levy MJ, Seelig CB, Robinson NJ, Ranney JE: Comparison of omeprazole and ranitidine for stress ulcer prophylaxis. Dig Dis Sci 42: 1255–1259, 1997.
445. du Moulin GC, Paterson DG, Hedley-Whyte J, Lisbon A: Aspiration of gastric bacteria in antacid-treated patients: A frequent cause of postoperative colonisation of the airway. Lancet 1:242–245, 1982.
446. Bock AV, Dulin JW, Brooke PA: Diaphragmatic hernia and secondary anemia: Ten cases. N Engl J Med 209:615–625, 1933.
447. Johns TNP, Clements EL: The relief of anemia by repair of hiatus hernia. J Thorac Cardiovasc Surg 41:737–747, 1961.
448. Cameron AJ, Higgins JA: Linear gastric erosion: A lesion associated with large diaphragmatic hernia and chronic blood loss. Gastroenterology 91:338–342, 1986.
449. Weston AP: Hiatal hernia with Cameron ulcers and erosions. Gastrointest Endosc Clin North Am 6:671–679, 1996.

Chapter 41

Zollinger-Ellison Syndrome and Other Hypersecretory States

Joseph R. Pisegna

ZOLLINGER-ELLISON SYNDROME

Historical Aspects

In 1955, Zollinger and Ellison described a syndrome with recurrent and often fatal gastrointestinal bleeding from peptic ulcers, proposing that this syndrome was a result of a pancreatic endocrine tumor. Nearly a decade later, it became feasible to measure serum levels of the hormone gastrin, and this hormone was soon shown to be secreted by pancreatic endocrine tumors in patients with the syndrome described by Zollinger and Ellison. The triad of severe peptic ulcer disease, gastric acid hypersecretion, and nonbeta cell gastrin-producing tumor of the pancreas is now referred to as the Zollinger-Ellison syndrome (ZES). (Other types of islet cell tumors of the pancreas are discussed in Chapter 51.) Release of gastrin into the circulation by these tumors is a paradigm for the study of endocrine tumors of the pancreas. This is because gastrin is one of the prominent gastrointestinal hormones whose pathobiology has been extensively characterized (Chapters 1 and 38). The description of ZES provided an impetus for the discovery of syndromes associated with hypersecretion of other gastrointestinal hormones and has permitted the discovery of physiologic mechanisms involved in hormonal control of secretion, motility, and tumor growth.

When ZES was discovered, a poor understanding of the physiologic and pharmacologic control of acid secretion existed. Consequently, the major form of therapy for this condition was surgical intervention; often total gastrectomy, because lesser ulcer operations failed to control ulcer complications. In the subsequent decades, understanding and control of gastric acid secretion improved dramatically and the focus of ZES management shifted to localization and treatment of the gastrinoma. Moreover, as improved pharmacologic control of gastric acid secretion led to prolonged survival, genetic disorders such as the multiple endocrine neoplasm type I syndrome (MEN I; Wermer's syndrome) were recognized to be associated with a sizable minority of patients with ZES. In addition, there were refinements in the radiologic and surgical detection of gastrinomas, leading to the possibility of a cure for ZES in some patients. Recently, we have also witnessed improvements in detecting gastrinomas, using radiolabeled somatostatin analogs, that have incorporated an understanding of the presence of somatostatin receptors on these tumors, and these agents may also have therapeutic value.

Despite these many accomplishments, the treatment of metastatic tumors remains a daunting challenge.

Physiology of Gastrin and Pathophysiologic Effects

Five years following the original description of ZES, Gregory and colleagues reported that extracts from pancreatic islet cell tumors from patients with this clinical syndrome could stimulate gastric acid secretion.[1] In 1968, McGuigan and Trudeau showed, by radioimmunoassay, that sera from patients with ZES contained elevated gastrin levels.[2] The same year, Gregory and Grossman and their associates identified two forms of gastrin that are elevated in the circulation of patients with ZES, a 17- and a 34-amino acid form (G17 and G34).[3] Gastrin is synthesized as a pre-prohormone that is processed to a prohormone and later into both sulfated and nonsulfated G17 and G34 forms.[4,5] Patients with gastrinoma also have elevated serum levels of progastrin.[6]

In addition to its potent effects on gastric acid secretion, gastrin is able to stimulate growth of the gastric mucosa. Gastric trophic effects of gastrin have been demonstrated in hypergastrinemic mice, in which gastrin stimulates the growth of enterochromaffin-like (ECL) and parietal cells.[7] ECL and parietal cell hyperplasia also occurs in patients with ZES.[8] At the other extreme, the gastric epithelium of animals with a targeted disruption of the gastrin gene is underdeveloped at birth.[9]

The hyperproliferation of ECL cells in patients with ZES is similar to that observed in hypergastrinemic pernicious anemia patients with atrophic gastritis and achlorhydria.[10] Moreover, patients with ZES (especially those with MEN I) and pernicious anemia are more likely to develop gastric carcinoid tumors than are people without either condition (see Chapter 44). Extensive biopsy sampling of both the greater and lesser curve of the stomach may help detect changes of ECL cell hyperplasia or early carcinoid tumor formation in ZES.[11] In one study, loss of heterozygosity (LOH) was observed at a locus on chromosome 11 (11q13), the MEN I gene, in 75% of carcinoid tumors identified from patients with ZES and MEN I syndrome, compared with a 16% frequency of LOH in gastric carcinoids from patients with chronic atrophic gastritis.[12] The data suggest that the inactivation of the MEN I gene may be important in the genesis of the carcinoid tumors in some patients with ZES. Gastric carcinoid tumors are discussed further in Chapters 44 and 112.

Pathology

Gastrinomas belong to a larger group of tumors within the neuroendocrine tumor (NET) family. NETs as a whole appear under the light microscope as monotonous sheets of cells with small nuclei and prominent nucleoli (Fig. 41–1). These cells typically stain positive for chromogranins, as well as for neuron-specific enolase and synaptophysins.[13, 14] Gastrinomas can be distinguished from other NETs with light microscopy by means of specific immunostaining and with electron microscopy by the distinct granule morphology of gastrin (G) cells. Although gastrin is the most prominent hormone expressed by gastrinomas, other hormones can be produced as well.[14] Telomerase, a marker for malignancy, is also up-regulated in some neuroendocrine tumors.[15]

The majority of gastrinomas occur in the "gastrinoma

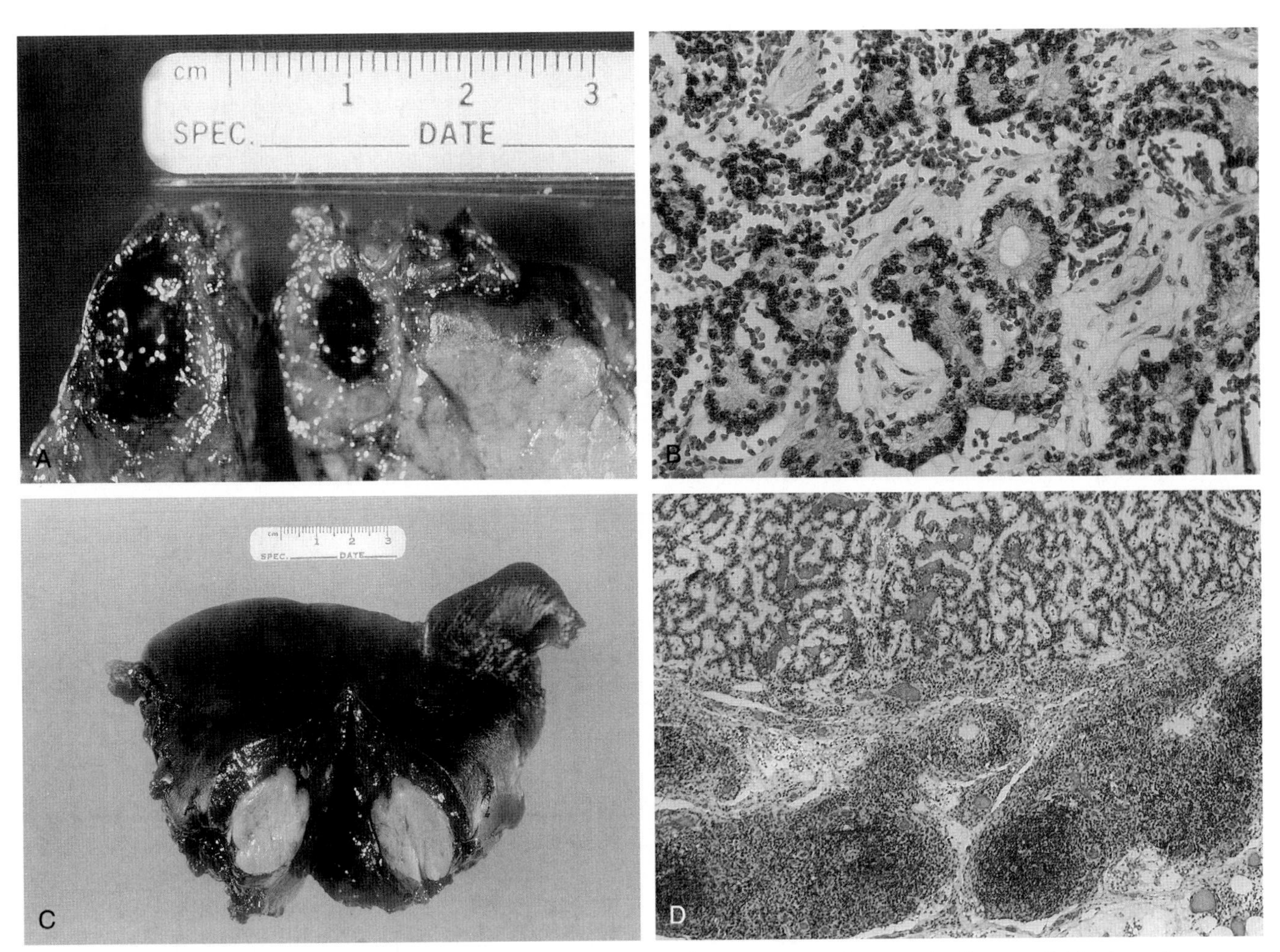

Figure 41–1. *A*, Hemorrhagic and cystic gastrinoma in the tail of pancreas measuring 2 cm in diameter. *B*, Histology of pancreatic gastrinoma, which is similar to that of other islet cell tumors. The highly vascular tumor is composed of tubules lined by bland endocrine cells. Note the vascularity of the tumor. *C*, Hepatic gastrinoma resected, with long-term cure. Note the well-circumscribed gray-white neoplasm that measures 3 cm in diameter. *D*, Histology of gastrinoma in a lymph node. At the top, a vascular endocrine neoplasm is visible, forming a cord and tubules, whereas at the bottom, there is normal lymphoid tissue. In some cases, removal of such a lymph node has led to cure.

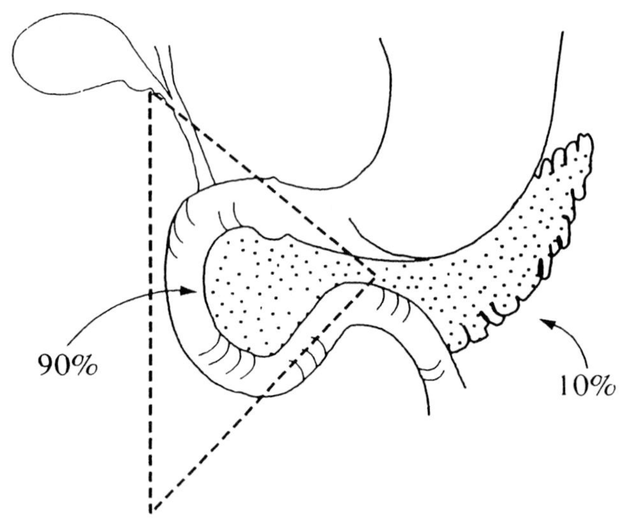

Figure 41–2. Gastrinoma triangle; more than 90% of gastrinomas are found within the limits of this anatomic triangle (From Stabile B, Morrow D, Passaro E: The gastrinoma triangle: Operative indications. Am J Surg 14:725, 1984).

triangle" (Fig. 41–2). This anatomic region is defined, superiorly, by the confluence of the cystic and common bile duct; inferiorly, by the junction of the second and third portions of the duodenum; and medially, by the junction of the neck and body of the pancreas. An equal number of gastrinomas occur in the pancreas and duodenum.

Duodenal and pancreatic gastrinomas are compared in Table 41–1. The majority of duodenal gastrinomas are small (<2 cm in size) and localized to the submucosa; this makes attempts at endoscopic removal dangerous.[16] More than 90% of duodenal gastrinomas occur in the first or second portion of the duodenum, and about 50% of them are solitary.[17] In contrast to duodenal gastrinomas, the majority of the pancreatic and peripancreatic tumors are greater than 2 cm in size (see Fig. 41–1*A*). The larger the gastrinoma, the more likely there will be metachronous liver metastases.[18]

There has been a growing recognition of extrapancreatic islet cell tumors occurring in peripancreatic lymph nodes (see Fig. 41–1*D*), although it is unclear whether the site of origin of these tumors is the lymph node itself or whether the node represents a site of local spread from a tiny primary focus in the pancreas.[19]

Ectopic gastrinomas occur outside the classic "gastrinoma triangle," or the body and tail of the pancreas, arising in such distant sites as the ovary.[20] In one series, an ectopic localization was identified in 5.6% of ZES patients.[21] Ectopic sites (besides the ovary) include the liver, common bile duct, omentum, and pylorus.[21–23] It is unclear whether ectopic tumors are more aggressive than those identified in the duodenum or pancreas. Rarely, a mixed epithelial (ductal) endocrine pancreatic neoplasm may produce ZES.[24] Gastrinomas metastasize to the liver, lymph nodes, and bone and rarely elsewhere, such as to the heart.[25]

Epidemiology

The exact incidence and prevalence of ZES are difficult to ascertain. With the increasing use of potent antisecretory medications like proton pump inhibitors, symptoms of gastric hypersecretion may be masked, leading to underdiagnosis. Indeed, the majority of patients with ZES today do not present with multiple and severe peptic ulcerations, as originally described by Zollinger and Ellison. ZES has an estimated incidence of 0.1 to 3 patients per million population.[26] The mean age at the time of diagnosis is 50 years, although patients may present at much younger or older ages. Men and women are affected equally. Gastrinomas are among the commonest of the islet cell tumors, second only to insulinomas in frequency.[27] However, unlike insulinomas, the majority of gastrinomas are malignant.

MEN I syndrome is present in nearly one third of ZES patients.[28–30] The remaining cases represent so-called sporadic ZES. The presence of MEN I has important ramifications with regard to prognosis and treatment and reflects different biologies for the tumors (Table 41–2). Genetic and clinical aspects of MEN I are discussed later in this chapter.

Table 41–1 | **Comparison of Duodenal and Pancreatic Gastrinomas**

	DUODENAL	PANCREATIC*
Frequency	~50%	~50%
Size of tumor	Small (<2 cm)	Large (>2 cm)
Metastatic potential	Lower	Higher
Site of metastases	Node > liver	Node = liver
Resectability (intraoperative test)	Yes (endoscopic transillumination)	Yes (ultrasound)
Surgical cure rate	50%	60%

*Includes gastrinomas in peripancreatic lymph nodes.

Clinical Presentation

The majority of ZES patients, nowadays, present with epigastric discomfort, a complication of peptic ulceration (e.g., bleeding), and/or chronic diarrhea. Diarrhea occurs in ZES patients because of malabsorption that results from large volumes of gastric acid entering the small intestine, leading to a destruction of pancreatic enzymes and damage to the intestinal mucosa (Chapter 89). Diarrhea appears to be less frequent in ZES patients with MEN I syndrome than in sporadic ZES.[31] Any patient presenting with chronic watery diarrhea in whom a diagnosis cannot be easily established

Table 41–2 | **Comparison of the Clinical Characteristics of Sporadic Zollinger-Ellison Syndrome (ZES) and MEN I–Associated ZES**

	SPORADIC ZES	MEN I ZES
Frequency	65%–75%	25%–35%
Genetic locus	Unknown	Chromosome 11q13
Tumor location	Pancreas > duodenum	Duodenum ≥ pancreas
Number of tumors	Solitary (usually)	Multifocal (usually)
Size of tumor(s)	Large (>2 cm)	Small (<2 cm)
Metastatic potential	Higher	Lower
20-Year survival	<70%	>90%
Surgery for cure	Possible	Uncommon
Association with gastric carcinoid tumors	No	Yes

MEN I, multiple endocrine neoplasia, type I.

should be evaluated for ZES.[32] ZES needs to be distinguished from other potential causes of abdominal pain and malabsorption. In one series of five cases, ZES was found to be associated with pancreatitis despite no evidence that the gastrinoma obstructed the pancreatic duct.[33] Erosive esophagitis also can occur and can be difficult to treat in ZES.[34, 35] Salivary secretion of epidermal growth factor (EGF) is higher in ZES patients than in patients with nonulcer dyspepsia, possibly affording some protection against esophagitis.[35] The clinical presentation of ZES can be elusive, and consequently ZES is frequently misdiagnosed. Some clinical features that should raise suspicion for ZES are listed in Table 41–3.

Diagnosis

In a patient suspected clinically of having ZES, based on one or more of the features in Table 41–3, a fasting gastrin level should be measured; a markedly elevated serum gastrin level (>1000 pg/mL) should be considered specific for the diagnosis but not highly sensitive. Thus, a fasting serum gastrin level of greater than 1000 pg/mL outside the setting of chronic atrophic gastritis is virtually diagnostic of ZES. However, relying on serum gastrin measurements alone (i.e., without a gastric analysis to rule out atrophic gastritis) is not an accurate way to diagnose ZES. In one study, 16 of 35 patients (46%) had hypergastrinemia because of gastric hypo- or achlorhydria.[36] Therefore, gastric analysis is useful to confirm the presence of gastric acid hypersecretion and to exclude the presence of achlorhydria secondary to chronic atrophic gastritis or severe *H. pylori*–associated chronic gastritis (see Chapter 38). An elevated serum gastrin level in the setting of achlorhydria makes a diagnosis of ZES extremely unlikely. In patients with ZES, basal acid output (BAO) generally is greater than 10 mEq/hr and averages around 40 mEq/hr. Gastric analysis is useful not only for making the diagnosis of ZES but also in monitoring the degree of control of gastric acid secretion with antisecretory medications (discussed later).

A diagnosis of ZES is easily made in a patient with a markedly elevated fasting serum gastrin level combined with gastric acid hypersecretion.[37] Many patients with gastrinoma, however, have fasting gastrin levels below 1000 pg/mL, and there are other causes of elevated serum gastrin levels in this range. With the increasing use of potent inhibitors of gastric acid secretion, such as *proton pump inhibitors*, there can be false-positive gastrin results. Patients taking these drugs should have them discontinued for at least 1 week, if possible, before the fasting gastrin level is remeasured. *Vagotomy* without gastric resection also can raise the fasting gastrin level,[38] as well as *small bowel resection*, albeit transiently.[39] Patients with *renal failure* have reduced clearance of gastrin, thereby resulting in elevated serum gastrin levels.[40] It is interesting that patients with renal failure do not typically develop gastric acid hypersecretion, as one would expect with the increase in circulating gastrin. Gastrin also has been reported to be increased in patients with *primary hyperparathyroidism*,[41] although some of these patients could have occult MEN-I and gastrinoma(s). Finally, the presence of *hyperlipidemia* may falsely elevate the reported level of serum gastrin by interfering with the gastrin radioimmunoassay in vitro.[42]

The secretin provocative test is a useful way to confirm the diagnosis of ZES when the fasting serum gastrin level is only modestly elevated and the diagnosis is in doubt.[43] After measuring the fasting serum gastrin level once or twice, secretin (2 U/kg) is rapidly injected intravenously. (The current scarcity of secretin should be remedied by the time of publication of this text by the availability of synthetic secretin.[44]) After secretin injection, the serum gastrin level is remeasured after 2, 5, and 10 minutes. In ZES patients, the rise in gastrin occurs rapidly, generally within 5 minutes, thereby obviating the need for collection of additional samples at 15, 20, or 30 minutes. A positive secretin test is defined by an elevation of gastrin of at least 200 pg/mL above the basal level. The secretin test has a sensitivity of about 90% for making the diagnosis of ZES. The test may be less sensitive for the diagnosis of small duodenal gastrinomas.[45] Because peptide receptors of several types have been identified on gastrinomas, including receptors for secretin,[46] it is possible that these latter receptors are involved in the stimulation of gastrin released from gastrinomas in response to a secretin challenge. However, one study using gastrinoma tissue in vitro failed to demonstrate an effect of exogenously administered secretin on adenylyl cyclase activity.[47] Intravenous injection of secretin has also been performed during surgery to help localize small ("micro") gastrinomas, but larger studies are necessary to assess the positive predictive value and practicality of this intraoperative test.[48]

Table 41–3 | **Clinical Features Suspicious for Zollinger-Ellison Syndrome**

• Postbulbar duodenal ulcer	• History of PUD and nephrolithiasis
• Multiple duodenal and/or jejunal ulcers	• Recurrent PUD in the absence of *Helicobacter pylori* or NSAID usage
• PUD in association with chronic diarrhea	• Family history of PUD and hypercalcemia
• PUD refractory to medical therapy	

NSAID, nonsteroidal anti-inflammatory drug; PUD, peptic ulcer disease.

Differential Diagnosis

The differential diagnosis of gastrinoma includes the hypergastrinemic and pseudohypergastrinemic conditions discussed earlier, as well as other islet cell tumors of the pancreas that can occur either concurrently with gastrinoma or as a separate tumor mass.[49, 50] Concurrent islet cell tumors may occur in the setting of MEN I syndrome (see Chapter 51). A high index of suspicion and the use of radioimmunoassay are required to evaluate for coexistence of islet cell tumors and gastrinoma. The differential diagnosis of acid hypersecretory states (with or without hypergastrinemia) is discussed at the end of this chapter.

Multiple Endocrine Neoplasia Type I

MEN I syndrome is an autosomal, dominantly inherited syndrome characterized by tumors in multiple endocrine organs, especially the parathyroid, pituitary, and pancreas (the three "Ps"). In 1988, the genetic locus for MEN I was ascribed to a segment of the long arm of chromosome 11 (11q13) and, with the observation of losses of heterozygosity at this locus in several kindreds, the MEN I gene was identified.[51] The gene encodes for a nuclear protein named menin, which may be an endocrine tumor suppression gene.[52, 53] Although the exact function of menin is unknown, research is in progress to identify its function.[54–56] Conservation of the MEN I gene has been demonstrated among different species, suggesting similarities in the genesis of these tumors across different species.[57, 58]

Familial clustering of MEN I syndrome was previously recognized in a family in the Bruin Peninsula/Fortune Bay area of Newfoundland (MEN I bruin), where patients would develop pituitary tumors (prolactinomas), parathyroid tumors, and intestinal carcinoids.[59] A germline MEN I gene mutation was identified in the majority of patients with this syndrome. Studies from a large family from Tasmania identified over 150 individuals affected with MEN 1.[60] Of the affected individuals, hyperparathyroidism was the most common abnormality, usually developing by age 30 years. Gastrinomas occurred in up to 60% of the affected Tasmanian patients.

Some of the clinical features of MEN I syndrome are listed in Table 41–4. MEN I syndrome should be suspected in any ZES patient who has hypercalcemia or complications of hypercalcemia, such as renal stones.[61] The majority of endocrine tumors in MEN I are benign, although the foregut carcinoid tumors and the pancreatic islet cell tumors may be malignant.[62] Atypical manifestations of MEN I include pheochromocytoma, which is more commonly seen in MEN II syndrome.[63]

Hyperparathyroidism occurs in 90% to 100% of patients with MEN I syndrome. One or two parathyroid adenomas are typically present.[64] Pituitary gland adenomas also develop in nearly all MEN I patients, whereas gastrinomas develop in about 60% of patients. In some cases of MEN I associated with ZES, gastric acid hypersecretion and serum gastrin levels can be substantially reduced after parathyroidectomy.[65, 66] The recent cloning of the heptahelical calcium-sensing receptor and its expression on rat and human gastric glands and on human antral G cells indicate a possibly novel mechanism for the regulation of gastrin release from the gastric mucosa in response to elevations in intragastric or serum calcium.[67–70]

Given the 60% prevalence of gastrinomas in patients with MEN I, it is recommended that all MEN I-positive patients be screened for the presence of ZES with fasting gastrin measurement, with or without secretin testing. Also, given the increased risk of developing gastric and duodenal carcinoid tumors, a careful upper endoscopic examination should be performed at the time of diagnosis of MEN I and probably periodically thereafter.[71, 72] The incidence of carcinoids in the thymus also may be increased in MEN I patients.[73] A curious combination of dermatologic features, referred to as the Carney complex, is also now known to be specific for MEN I.[74] Furthermore, up to two thirds of patients with MEN I develop lipomas, cutaneous angiofibromas, and/or collagenomas.[75] The relationship between lipomas, which are commonly seen in patients with MEN I, and LOH on chromosome 11q13 is debated, suggesting that perhaps another genetic abnormality may account for lipomas in patients with MEN I.[76]

The overall prognosis of patients affected with MEN I is controversial.[77] The biologic behaviors of tumors are diverse, with the majority being asymptomatic. There are frequently multiple small tumors throughout the pancreas. In general, the risk of metastasis from an islet cell tumor in MEN I is low, compared with patients with sporadic ZES, and this probably in part is related to the tumor size (see Table 41–2). In one study of 59 MEN I patients, 27 (46%) died from illnesses directly attributable to MEN I: islet cell tumor in 12, carcinoid tumor in 6, peptic ulcer complication in 6, and hypercalcemia in 3. Nine other patients died from nonendocrine malignancy.[78]

Given the recent advances in the molecular diagnosis of MEN I, mutational analysis of the MEN I locus (11q13) can be considered for patients with a known risk of MEN I. This would include patients with ZES or another islet cell tumor, as well as asymptomatic first-degree relatives of MEN I patients. Although a single report indicated that MEN I gene mutations can also occur in patients with sporadic ZES, a routine genetic testing is probably not yet indicated unless there is a MEN I phenotype.[79] In individuals with a MEN I phenotype, additional testing of serum calcium, intact parathyroid hormone, and prolactin is indicated.[80] If the patient has any symptom compatible with pituitary involvement, pituitary magnetic resonance imaging should be performed and the pancreas imaged (discussed later).[81] Although phenotype screening based on symptoms of MEN I is useful (see Table 41–4), confirmatory genetic testing is advised. In one study involving 152 members of a large MEN I family, 10% of patients who met clinical characteristics of MEN I were discovered to be genetically normal at the MEN I locus.[82]

The medical management of ZES occurring in the setting of MEN I is similar to the management of patients with sporadic ZES (described later). On the other hand, the surgical management of patients with MEN I and ZES may differ from that for sporadic ZES, because it is difficult to achieve cure following gastrinoma resection in MEN I (see Table 42–2; discussed later also).[83]

In 31% of patients with sporadic ZES, mutations of the MEN I gene have been identified.[84] Likewise, in gastrinomas removed from patients with sporadic ZES, LOH has been identified in up to 44% of the tumors.[85] There was no correlation with the presence of such mutations and either tumor extent, location of the gastrinoma, or aggressive behavior of the tumor. Another study involving eight gastrinoma patients identified rearrangements on chromosome 1 in more aggressive tumors, suggesting that there may be additional genetic abnormalities in patients with ZES that are not explained solely by LOH of the MEN I gene.[86] Another tumor suppressor gene, located at 3p25, has been suggested

Table 41–4 | **Clinical Features of MEN I Syndrome**

• Nephrolithiasis	• Acromegaly
• Skin lesions*	• Galactorrhea
• Peptic ulcer disease	• Amenorrhea
• Hypoglycemia	• Cushing's syndrome
• Headache	• Islet cell tumors of the pancreas
• Visual field defects	• Carcinoid tumors of the stomach and duodenum
• Carcinoid tumors of the stomach and duodenum	
• Hypopituitarism	

*Lipomas, collagenomas, angiofibromas, Carney complex.[74]
MEN I, multiple endocrine neoplasia, type I.

like the MEN-1 locus at 11q13 to be implicated in the genesis of sporadically occurring pancreatic neuroendocrine tumors.[87] Somatic point mutations of the menin gene have also been shown to be associated with the development of sporadic parathyroid adenomas, insulinomas, and VIPomas (vasoactive intestinal polypeptide-secreting tumors).[88–93] An additional tumor suppressor gene at the 11q13 locus may be involved in sporadic pituitary tumors.[94]

Prognostic Factors in ZES

By far the most important predictor of long-term survival in ZES is the presence or absence of liver metastasis at the time of diagnosis. A diagnosis of MEN I may be associated with lower cure rates, whereas gender and age at the time of diagnosis do not appear to affect disease course. In patients with sporadic ZES, Cushing's syndrome caused by the ectopic release of ACTH from the gastrinoma is generally associated with a more aggressive disease course.[95] Of note, Cushing's syndrome also may occur in about 20% of patients with the MEN I syndrome and is usually caused by the overproduction of ACTH by a pituitary adenoma.

After resection of a gastrinoma for attempted cure, an immediate postoperative normalization in the serum gastrin level or a negative (i.e., normal) secretin stimulation test has a high predictive value for cure.[96] Conversely, autoantibodies directed against the tumor suppressor protein p53 have been suggested to be a predictor of poor survival, but more data are needed.[97] High serum chromogranin A levels may predict disease progression,[98] but further studies are needed.

Overview of Management of ZES

Once a diagnosis of ZES is suspected, based on clinical features (see Table 41–3) and confirmed by serum gastrin testing and gastric analysis, the first step in the management of ZES is to control gastric acid secretion with a proton pump inhibitor (see Fig. 41–3).[81] Following adequate control of gastric acid secretion, imaging studies should be performed to locate the tumor and to stage the disease. Imaging studies include endoscopic ultrasound (EUS),[99] magnetic resonance imaging (MRI), spiral (helical) computed tomography (CT), and somatostatin receptor scintigraphy (SRS; OctreoScan). If metastatic lesions are imaged (see Fig. 41–2), management should shift to palliative antitumor therapy with a combination of chemotherapy, hormonal therapy with a somatostatin analog, or surgical debulking. In some cases, a biopsy may be required to confirm metastases (e.g., liver biopsy). In patients without liver metastases on imaging studies, a determination should be made as to whether the patient is a surgical candidate and whether he or she has sporadic ZES or ZES associated with MEN I syndrome (see Table 41–2). In patients with nonmetastatic, sporadic ZES, surgical exploration should be performed with the goal of tumor extirpation to effect cure.[100] The role of surgical exploration and gastrinoma resection in patients with ZES and MEN I is more controversial.

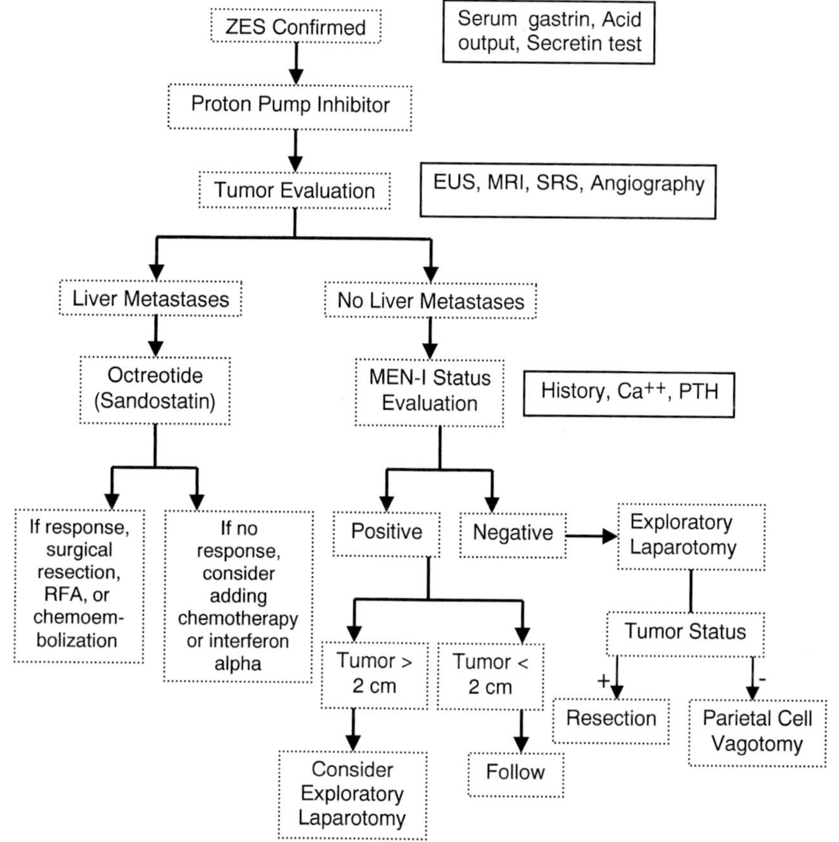

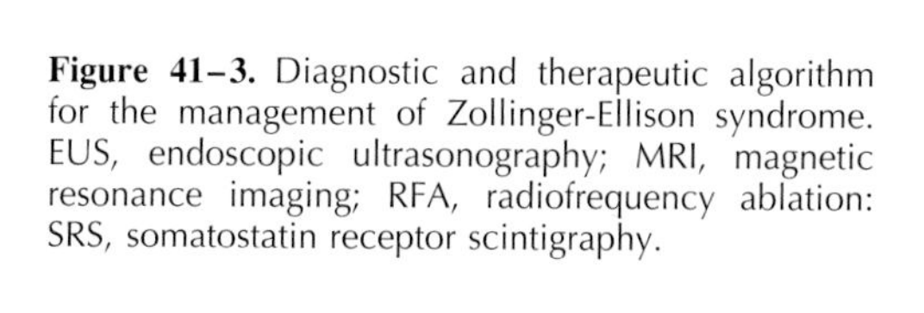

Figure 41–3. Diagnostic and therapeutic algorithm for the management of Zollinger-Ellison syndrome. EUS, endoscopic ultrasonography; MRI, magnetic resonance imaging; RFA, radiofrequency ablation: SRS, somatostatin receptor scintigraphy.

Control of Gastric Acid Hypersecretion

The control of gastric acid secretion in ZES is crucial because of the risks of peptic ulcer complications and other acid-peptic disease (e.g., esophagitis). In one study involving 21 ZES patients, the mean basal acid output was 48 mEq/hr in sporadic cases and 24 mEq/hr in patients with MEN I (normal, <10 mEq/hr), indicating the need for aggressive control of gastric acid secretion.[101]

Proton pump inhibitors (PPIs) are the most effective drugs in controlling gastric acid hypersecretion in patients with ZES, although receptor antagonists are also effective. The exact medication and dose should be adjusted to maintain the basal acid output at less than 10 mEq/hr (<5 mEq/hr in patients with previous acid-reducing gastric surgery). If basal acid output prior to the next scheduled dose is zero, the dose can be carefully reduced, if desired. Median daily doses of PPIs or histamine$_2$-receptor antagonists to control acid secretion in ZES are given in Table 41–5.[100] Even ZES patients who have undergone a successful gastrinoma resection and have biochemical evidence of cure usually continue to require long-term control of gastric acid secretion with antisecretory drugs.[102] This is because of the expansion in the parietal cell mass that occurs following long-term hypergastrinemia. The safety of PPIs in pregnancy has not been tested, and the Food and Drug Administration lists the majority of these agents as Category B. In patients who are pregnant, it is recommended to use the lowest possible dose of histamine$_2$-receptor antagonist.[103]

Once acid secretion in a patient with ZES is well controlled with a PPI, the dose can be safely reduced over time to approximately half the starting dose. Dose reductions should be made more cautiously in patients with MEN I, patients with prior gastric surgery (especially partial gastrectomy), and patients with severe gastroesophageal reflux disease (GERD).[104] A careful endoscopic examination of the esophagus, stomach, and as much of the duodenum as possible should be performed periodically to ensure that no active ulcerations are present and that medications are working.

Of the four PPIs currently available, long-term treatment studies in ZES have been performed with omeprazole, lansoprazole and pantoprazole.[105, 106] These PPIs differ with regard to their bioavailability, absorption, and drug interaction profiles. Long-term safety studies of the newest PPIs, pantoprazole and rabeprazole, indicate similarities to omeprazole and lansoprazole.[106] The most recently studied of the PPIs is pantoprazole (Protonix). In an ongoing long-term treatment study of 20 ZES patients, the average daily dose of pantoprazole required to control gastric acid secretion is 80 mg. As shown previously with omeprazole (Prilosec), it is likely that this dose can ultimately be reduced by 50%.

In ZES patients admitted to the hospital to undergo a gastrinoma resection or to receive chemotherapy, uninterrupted control of gastric acid secretion is important to prevent complications of peptic ulcer disease. Previously, IV ranitidine was used for short-term control of gastric acid secretion in these patients, usually at an intravenous dose of 1 mg/kg/hr. Although useful, tachyphylaxis to ranitidine occurred, with a consequent decrease in its efficacy.[107] Pantoprazole is available as an intravenous formulation. Intravenous pantoprazole has been shown to control gastric acid secretion effectively and safely in ZES patients, with onset of control within 1 hour. The duration of effect of IV pantoprazole in ZES is usually 12 hours or longer (Table 41–6).[101] In one study, IV pantoprazole was shown to be particularly useful for inpatient management of ZES patients, and switching back and forth between oral PPI and IV pantoprazole was performed without a loss in efficacy.[101]

PPIs are very safe in ZES, even in high doses, although such high doses are quite expensive. In the 1980s, there was significant concern over the development of gastric carcinoid tumors in rodents given PPIs.[108] The pathophysiologic basis for the development of these tumors was achlorhydria-related hypergastrinemia, leading to enterochromaffin-like (ECL) hyperplasia and tumors. In a comprehensive study of hypergastrinemic ZES patients also taking high doses of PPIs (omeprazole, 80 to 160 mg/day), successive gastric biopsy samples failed to reveal significant morphometric changes in the ECL cells of the gastric mucosa.[109] The effects of gastrin on gastric mucosal ECL cells is greater in women than men and is greater in MEN I patients with ZES than in patients with sporadic ZES, indicating that genetic

Table 41–5 | **Median Doses of Antisecretory Agents Used to Control Gastric Acid Hypersecretion in ZES**

AGENT	MEDIAN DOSE (RANGE)
Proton Pump Inhibitors	
Omeprazole (Prilosec)	80 mg/d (20–60 mg bid)
Lansoprazole (Prevacid)	60 mg/d (30–60 mg bid)
Pantoprazole (Protonix)	80 mg/d (40–80 mg bid)
Histamine$_2$-Receptor Antagonists	
Cimetidine (Tagamet)	3.6 g/d (1.2–12.6)
Ranitidine (Zantac)	1.2 g/d (0.45–6)
Famotidine (Pepcid)	0.25 g/d (0.05–0.8)

From Pisegna JR: The effect of Zollinger-Ellison syndrome and neuropeptide-secreting tumors on the stomach. Curr Gastroenterol Rep 1:511, 1999.

Table 41–6 | **Onset and Duration of Action of IV Pantoprazole (Protonix) at a Dose of 80 mg in 21 Patients with ZES, Either Sporadic or Associated with MEN I**

	SPORADIC ZES (n = 14)	MEN I ZES (n = 7)	ALL (n = 21)
Onset of action (n)			
15 min	1	0	1
30 min	5	3	8
45 min	10	7	17
60 min	14	7	21
Duration of effect (n)			
6 hr	13	6	19
8 hr	13	6	19
10 hr	13	5	18
12 hr	12	5	17

Approximately 80% of ZES patients can be controlled with this dose of IV pantoprazole. The onset of action is rapid, and the duration of action is prolonged. The mean basal acid output in these patients was nearly 40 mEq/hr before the proton pump inhibitor was given.

Adapted from Lew EA, Pisegna JR, Starr JA, et al: Intravenous pantoprazole is a novel proton pump inhibitor that rapidly and effectively controls gastric acid hypersecretion in patients with Zollinger-Ellison syndrome. Gastroenterology 118: 696, 2000.

factors are important determinants for the promotion of gastric carcinoids in ZES.[110]

Long-term treatment with PPIs leads to a reduction in serum cobalamin (vitamin B_{12}) levels (but not in serum folate levels), as a result of a reduction in cobalamin absorption from dietary sources.[111] However, chronic usage of PPIs does not lead to the development of cobalamin deficiency.[112] Nevertheless, patients with ZES being controlled with long-term PPI therapy should undergo periodic measurement of serum cobalamin levels. There appears to be no disturbances in the absorption of iron in patients with ZES treated with long-term antisecretory medications.[113]

Localization of Gastrinomas

Following successful control of gastric acid hypersecretion, the next objective in patient management is the accurate localization of the gastrinoma (see Fig. 41–3). In addition, it is critical to determine whether metastases are present in the liver, lymph nodes, or other sites, such as bones. There have been significant advances in imaging studies for the detection of gastrinoma.[114] These imaging studies have focused primarily on the detection of tumor in the pancreas and liver.[115]

Over the past decade, percutaneous ultrasonography (US), endoscopic ultrasonography (EUS), computed tomography (CT), angiography (ANGIO), and magnetic resonance imaging (MRI) have all been investigated. Figure 41–4 illustrates a CT and MRI in a patient with ZES. In one study, MRI was shown to have the highest sensitivity (83%) for the detection of hepatic metastases, compared with ANGIO (61%), CT (56%), and US (50%).[115] However, MRI was less sensitive for detection of primary pancreatic tumors. Novel MRI techniques may be useful for the detection of duodenal gastrinomas, but they are experimental at the present time.[116]

ANGIO is quite sensitive for the detection of primary pancreatic tumors, but as mentioned is less sensitive than MRI for detecting hepatic metastases. Used in conjunction with selective intra-arterial contrast, the sensitivity of ANGIO for detecting gastrinomas may be increased.[117] Helical CT imaging is also quite sensitive for the detection of primary pancreatic tumors, and it detects hepatic metastases almost as well as MRI does. By ANGIO, gastrinomas are identified as diffusely enhancing lesions. Selective ANGIO has sensitivity ranging from 50% to 75%; however, considerable skill is required in performing the study.[118] Selective ANGIO can be performed with selective venous sampling for gastrin measurement both basally and following injection of secretin.[119] Selective ANGIO can identify the site of tumor in up to 75% of cases[120] but has been largely supplanted by the combination of OctreoScan, EUS, and helical (spiral) CT.[121] Although portal venous sampling may yield similar rates for tumor detection, there is a higher rate of complications than with less invasive imaging modalities.[122]

EUS has been shown to be very sensitive (80% to 90%) for the detection of pancreatic islet cell tumors. With placement of the ultrasonic transducer in the gastric antrum, the body and tail of the pancreas can be imaged almost entirely. Pancreatic gastrinomas on EUS typically appear as round, homogeneous, and hypoechoic masses (Fig. 41–5).[123] One of every two gastrinomas is located in the duodenal wall and escapes detection by EUS. In these cases, the tumor usually can be localized intraoperatively by means of duodenal transillumination with an endoscope.[100] Fine-needle aspiration of a submucosal duodenal tumor may then be possible under either endoscopic or EUS guidance. Because the tumors are submucosal, the cytologic yield can be enhanced with the injection of saline and aspiration with a large caliber needle.[124]

More recently, it was discovered that gastrinomas have somatostatin type 2 receptors; consequently, somatostatin receptor scintigraphy (SRS) using ^{111}indium-labeled octreotide (OctreoScan), a somatostatin analog, is useful for detection of primary pancreatic and duodenal gastrinomas, as well as metastases.[125, 126] ^{111}Indium-labeled octreotide, followed by whole-body gamma camera scintigraphy, localizes islet cell tumors (Fig. 41–6), with a sensitivity of 71% to 75% and a specificity of 86% to 100%, with a positive predictive value of 63% and an 82% overall accuracy.[126, 127] In comparative studies, SRS was found to be superior for the detection of

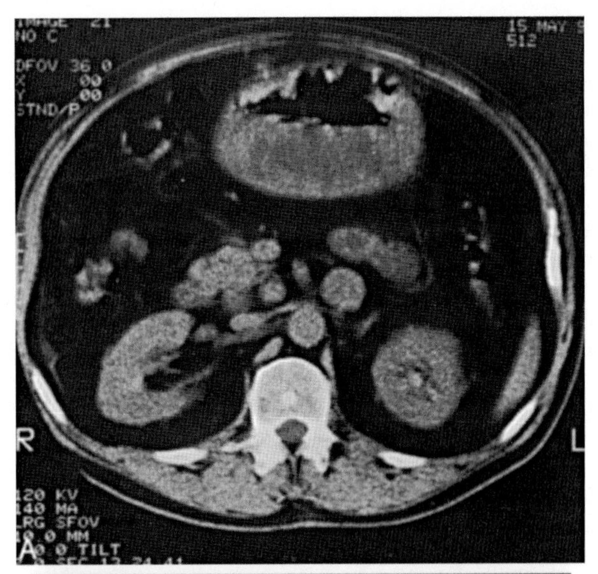

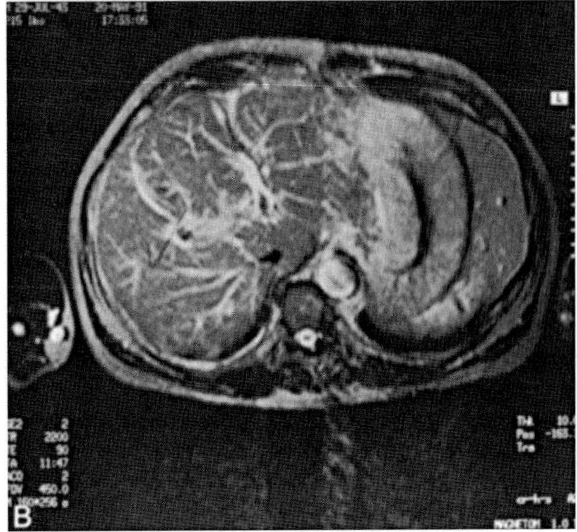

Figure 41–4. *A,* CT scan demonstrating thickened gastric folds and increased secretions in the stomach (supine position). Gastrinoma is seen anterior and to the left of the aorta. *B,* MRI study demonstrating enormously thickened gastric wall in the same patient.

extrahepatic and lymph node involvement, compared with CT and MRI.[126] In one study, SRS was found to be more sensitive than conventional bone scan for detection of bony metastases, which can occur in up to 30% of patients with hepatic metastases.[127] However, other studies found that SRS and bone scan had similar abilities to detect bony metastases.[128, 129] SRS has also proved useful for distinguishing hepatic hemangiomas (a common hepatic tumor) from metastatic gastrinomas in ZES patients who are shown to have hepatic masses on US, CT, or MRI.[130] Furthermore, in patients with MEN I and ZES, SRS may also detect coexisting gastric carcinoids, which easily can be confused with a gastrinoma.[131] The use of gastroscopy and CT may help discriminate between a gastric carcinoid and a pancreatic endocrine tumor in such patients. Unfortunately, the use of SRS changes the overall management in less than 50% of ZES cases.[132]

The sensitivity of positron emission tomography (PET) for the detection of primary and metastatic islet cell tumors is currently under investigation.

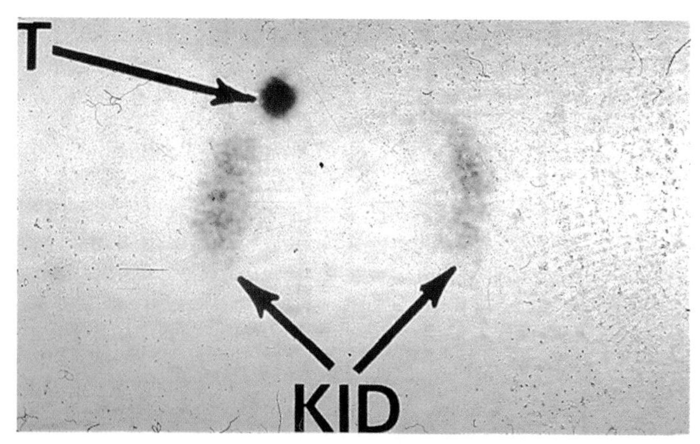

Figure 41–6. Somatostatin receptor scintigraphy (SRS) localization of a gastrinoma in the pancreatic head area in a patient with Zollinger-Ellison syndrome. This figure shows the localization of the tumor (T) using SRS with [^{111}In-DTPA-DPhe^{1}]-octreotide. The isotope is primarily excreted by the kidneys (KID).

Surgical Management of Gastrinomas

Fortunately, the recent advances in the pharmacologic management of gastric acid secretion, discussed earlier, have largely eliminated the need for acid-reducing operations such as total gastrectomy.[133, 134] Surgical management is directed at resection of gastrinoma to achieve cure.[133] If preoperative imaging studies have clearly identified the location of the primary tumor, extirpation should be attempted if there is no evidence of metastases.[135] If preoperative imaging studies are negative or equivocal, intraoperative exploration to locate the tumor is mandatory. In general, all patients who have sporadic ZES and who are good surgical candidates should undergo laparotomy in order to try to achieve cure.[136]

As mentioned earlier, the resection of the primary tumor for cure in patients with ZES and MEN I syndrome is controversial.[137, 138] For tumors less than 2 cm in size, which is the rule, I do not recommend resection. On the other hand, surgery should be considered for tumors larger than 2 cm in patients with ZES and MEN I syndrome.[83] In one study, only 5% of ZES patients with MEN I syndrome were cured by surgery, based on normalization of the fasting serum gastrin level or a negative secretin stimulation test after tumor resection.[96] Surgical resection of symptomatic pituitary or parathyroid adenomas in MEN I should be attempted.[139] In another large series, gastrinoma resection in ZES and MEN I patients did not appear to effect cure or prevent the spread of tumor to either lymph nodes or the liver.[31]

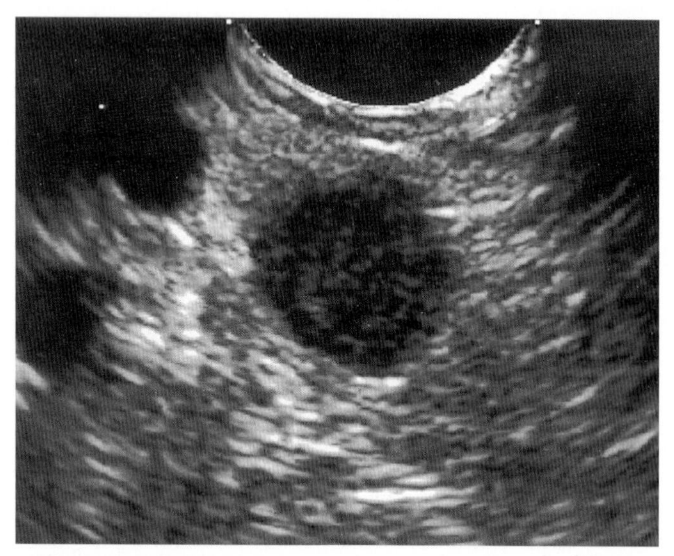
Figure 41–5. Gastrinoma (7 mm in size) in the neck of the pancreas as visualized by linear endoscopic ultrasound (EUS).

At surgery for cure, pancreatic gastrinomas should be enucleated, if possible. The majority (90%) of tumors arising in the pancreatic head can be resected by enucleation.[140] A pancreaticoduodenectomy (Whipple procedure) should be performed only when either the size of the pancreatic tumor or the proximity of it to the pancreatic duct prevents a simpler enucleation.[141] Intraoperative US may be useful to ascertain the proximity of the pancreatic tumor to the pancreatic duct. One study employed intraoperative secretin (IOS) testing to predict curability of gastrinoma resection and concluded that IOS was clinically useful.[48]

The great majority of gastrinomas will be found in the "gastrinoma triangle" (see Fig. 41–2). However, if preoperative imaging studies of this region are negative or equivocal, intraoperative endoscopy is required in order to transilluminate the duodenal wall. Since nearly 50% of gastrinomas are located in the wall of the duodenum (second and third portion), duodenal transillumination at exploratory laparotomy has permitted the detection and resection of many of the previously elusive gastrinomas.[142] The use of selective arterial secretin injection (SASI) testing to detect duodenal gastrinomas is currently under investigation and may prove useful for the detection of tumor as small as 1.5 cm.[143] Curative resection often can be achieved with the detection and removal of a duodenal gastrinoma.[144] Surgery also may play a role in patients with localized hepatic tumor (see Fig. 41–1*C*). In one study of 69 ZES patients who underwent either hepatic lobectomy or hepatic wedge resection, the 5-year survival was 85%, although the cure rate was less than 30%.[145]

In patients undergoing exploratory surgery, in which a primary gastrinoma cannot be identified, a search for ectopic tumor should be made as this occurs in about 1 in 20 ZES patients.[21] The most common sites for ectopic tumors are liver, bile duct, jejunum, omentum, pylorus, and ovary. Some tumors may be located in the pancreas but are too tiny to feel. Intraoperative US has been used to help localize pancreatic endocrine tumors that cannot be seen or palpated.[146] Intraoperative US also may assist the surgeon in deciding whether simple enucleation is feasible and whether lymph nodes are involved. However, the sensitivity and specificity of intraoperative US are quite operator dependent.

In about 30% of patients, a gastrinoma cannot be identified at laparotomy, even using duodenal transillumination and intraoperative US of the pancreas. If a gastrinoma is not identified, the use of parietal cell vagotomy (highly selective vagotomy) should be considered as a method of control of gastric acid hypersecretion postoperatively.[147] In patients with ZES who are anticipating pregnancy, an elective parietal cell vagotomy also should be considered as a means of reducing the need for high doses of antisecretory medications during pregnancy, and at other times as well.[147]

An assessment of cure should be established soon after surgery by performing a fasting serum gastrin measurement or a secretin infusion test. The use of SRS postoperatively also has been suggested.[148] In patients who are not cured following the initial surgery, the role of a second-look operation is questionable. In the only study that reports on the role of reoperation for gastrinoma patients, the researchers concluded that reoperation is indicated only when tumor is imaged before the reoperation.[149]

Surgical Management of Metastatic Gastrinoma to the Liver

As noted, a localized hepatic tumor can be resected with good survival and a 30% cure rate. Several studies are under way to investigate the effectiveness of intraoperative radiofrequency ablation (RFA) and cryosurgery for hepatic metastases. A role for hepatic transplantation for patients with widely metastatic tumor in the liver is also under study. Hepatic transplantation should be considered only if the primary tumor already has been resected. The long-term survival in these patients is unknown. At several large centers, transplantation has been performed for patients with metastatic hepatic tumors, but the outcome has yet to be evaluated. The use of SRS to help evaluate patients for suitability for hepatic transplantation has been recommended.[150]

Nonsurgical Management of Metastatic Gastrinoma

RADIATION THERAPY. The majority of neuroendocrine tumors are relatively resistant to the effects of ionizing radiation. Therefore, radiation therapy is limited to the management of symptomatic bony metastases. Radiation therapy in this group of patients will provide relief of bone-associated pain, although patients with bony metastases have a poor prognosis.[151] The use of ionizing radiation for the treatment of metastatic hepatic gastrinomas has not been proved very useful. In rare cases, some efficacy has been observed with 40 Gy of external beam radiation.[152]

Because [^{111}In] DTPA-D-Phe-octreotide has been proved useful for imaging gastrinomas, recently higher doses of this radiopharmaceutical have been used for treating some of these tumors. Although clinical trials are currently being conducted, response rates as high as 50% have been reported (L. Anthony, Louisiana State University, personal communication, 2001). The major side effect of this therapy is renal toxicity.

CHEMOTHERAPY. Several chemotherapy protocols have been investigated for the treatment of metastatic gastrinomas. In general, these agents are not highly efficacious against islet cell tumors because these tumors are slow growing. Response rates as high as 40% have been observed, but the duration of response is poor. At our institution, chemotherapy is generally reserved for rapidly growing tumors that have failed to respond to the other modalities discussed later. The most efficacious of the chemotherapy agents are streptozotocin, 5-fluorouracil, doxorubicin (Adriamycin), and tubericidin. Combination therapy with these agents leads to the best results.[153, 154] One study found that the use of three chemotherapy agents resulted in a short-lasting response, but significant toxicity was noted.[155]

INTERFERON THERAPY. Interferons possess antitumor activity by a direct antiproliferative action against certain tumors, as well as through modulation of the host immune response. Interferons are thought to up-regulate the host's T cytotoxic and natural killer cell activity directed against the tumor. Human recombinant interferon has been reported effective in patients with a variety of metastatic neuroendocrine tumors, although responses have been variable.[156] In one study, 17 of 22 patients, including 3 of 4 patients with metastatic gastrinoma, had an objective tumor response, which was defined as a 50% or greater reduction in tumor mass or as a 50% or greater reduction in serum hormone or tumor marker levels.[157] In another study, interferon reduced growth of gastrinomas in 40% of patients, although the response was short-lived.[158] In a third study, a partial response to interferon plus doxorubicin was observed in 18% of patients with advanced islet cell and carcinoid tumors.[159]

HORMONAL THERAPY. Since pancreatic islet cell tumors express somatostatin type-2 receptors (SST2), somatostatin analogs such as octreotide (Sandostatin) might be able to inhibit their growth. A reduction in tumor growth has been demonstrated both in vitro and in vivo in animals.[160, 161] Moreover, two large phase II trials demonstrated that octreotide significantly inhibited tumor growth in 37% to 50% of patients with advanced islet cell tumors, but this effect was short lasting.[162, 163] The long-acting synthetic analog of somatostatin is not yet approved for the management of metastatic gastrinoma.

Although somatostatin analogs and interferon may have some modest efficacy when used as monotherapy, they appear to have greater efficacy when used in combination. In small open studies, treatment with the combination of octreotide and alpha interferon had a synergistic antiproliferative effect among patients unresponsive to octreotide alone.[164, 165] In one European study, 6 of 14 patients (42%)

with metastatic islet cell tumor treated with a combination of octreotide (200 μg subcutaneously three times daily) and human recombinant alpha interferon (Intron A), at a dose of 5 million IU subcutaneously three times a week, had an objective tumor response. One of the six had partial tumor regression and five had stable disease for up to 34 months.[164] In another European study, 22 patients with islet cell tumors (4 with gastrinomas) were treated with a combination of the same doses of octreotide and alpha interferon; CT scan was used to assess the tumor response at 3-month intervals.[165] Twelve patients had stable disease and one patient had a 25% or greater reduction in tumor size, for an overall response rate of 59%. Of the four patients with gastrinomas, two had stable disease and two had a biochemical response with a greater than 50% reduction in gastrin levels following treatment. The regimen was generally well tolerated. Side effects included fever, weight loss, and diarrhea. This combination treatment strategy is particularly important given the lack of other currently available treatment for patients with metastatic islet cell tumors. Since there is some evidence for efficacy and a relatively low risk of serious adverse events, it would be reasonable to try this approach first before using more toxic chemotherapy. A prospective study using a combination of long-acting octreotide (Sandostatin LAR Depot) and interferon (Infergen) in patients with metastatic neuroendocrine tumors is currently under way at our institution. A preliminary analysis of the data indicates that 40% of the patients had a complete response with disappearance of their tumor, 40% had stable metastatic disease, and 20% showed no response.[166] In another study, cytoreductive surgery followed by adjuvant treatment with octreotide was shown to palliate the symptoms associated with hepatic metastases.[167]

CHEMOEMBOLIZATION. Chemoembolization[168] using the hepatic artery can be considered for the management of metastatic tumors to the liver. Chemoembolization involves an invasive radiologic technique to isolate a feeding arterial supply to the tumor and the injection of glass beads, or Gelfoam, that will result in necrosis of the tumor supplied by the injected vessel. The effectiveness of this therapy depends on the radiologic technique used and varies widely from institution to institution. It is preferable if the lesions are isolated and few. The disadvantages with this method, besides side effects (pain, fever, and infection), are the inability to embolize tumors that are not readily visualized. There are no prospective studies comparing this technique with other techniques for the treatment of metastatic islet cell tumors.

OTHER GASTRIC HYPERSECRETORY STATES

In addition to ZES, at least five uncommon disorders are associated with marked gastric acid hypersecretion. Furthermore, in some patients, no cause for gastric acid hypersecretion is found, and it is considered idiopathic.

Systemic Mastocytosis

In this disease, histamine-producing mast cells infiltrate the gastrointestinal tract, skin, liver, and bone marrow. Excessive release of histamine results in gastric acid hypersecretion, as well as vasoactive systemic responses such as flushing and wheezing. Urticarial skin lesions may occur (urticaria pigmentosa) and be the first sign of this disorder. Patients with this disease may have a basal acid output greater than 15 mEq/hr. In patients suspected of having mastocytosis, biopsies of the gastric or intestinal mucosa may reveal a significant increase in infiltrating mast cells. Treatment consists of a histamine$_2$-receptor antagonist, which will block the gastric secretory effects of histamine as well as its systemic effects. In addition, a histamine$_1$-receptor antagonist (e.g., Claritin) may help treat the other systemic manifestations such as flushing, wheezing, and urticaria. *Basophilic leukemia* may produce a similar syndrome.

Massive Resection of the Small Bowel

(see Chapter 92)

In patients who have undergone a massive resection of the small bowel (e.g., for bowel infarction), gastric acid hypersecretion may develop, last for months or longer, and lead to peptic ulcers with upper GI bleeding. Although the exact mechanism responsible for this syndrome is unknown, it may be related to removal of intestinal peptides that normally inhibit gastric acid secretion and/or gastrin release.[39] The management of gastric acid hypersecretion in these patients is particularly challenging because absorption of orally administered histamine$_2$-receptor antagonists or proton pump inhibitors may be impaired. In one patient treated at our institution, IV pantoprazole was used effectively for nearly a year to control postresection gastric acid hypersecretion and its complications.[168] In these complex patients, a recommended starting dose of IV pantoprazole is 80 mg twice a day.

Antral G Cell Hyperfunction and Hyperplasia

Patients with antral G cell hyperfunction, or hyperplasia, develop exaggerated serum gastrin concentrations in response to food, with resultant postprandial acid hypersecretion. These patients are at risk for the development of peptic ulcer disease and can be confused with ZES patients. The major difference is the existence of a gastrin-releasing tumor in the ZES patient. Furthermore, intravenous secretin testing is typically positive in ZES (gastrin increase $>$ 200 pg/mL above basal) and negative in antral G cell hyperfunction. Many patients with *H. pylori* infection develop an exaggerated serum gastrin response to food, which disappears after *H. pylori* eradication. The complex effects of *H. pylori* infection on gastrin release and gastric secretion are discussed in Chapters 38 and 39.

REFERENCES

1. Gregory RA, Tracy HJ, French JM, Sircus W: Extraction of gastrin-like substance from a pancreatic tumour in a case of Zollinger-Ellison syndrome. Lancet 1:1045, 1960.
2. McGuigan JE, Trudeau WL: Immunochemical measurement of elevated levels of gastrin in the serum of patients with pancreatic tumors of the Zollinger-Ellison variety. N Engl J Med 278:1308, 1968.

3. Gregory RA, Grossman MI, Tracey HJ, Bentley PH: Amino acid constitution of two gastrins isolated from Zollinger-Ellsion variety. N Engl J Med 278:1308, 1968.
4. Rehfield JF, Stadil F, Vikelsoe J: Immunoreactive gastric components in human serum. Gut 15:102, 1974.
5. Dockray GJ, Walsh JH: Amino terminal gastrin fragment in serum of Zollinger-Ellison syndrome patients. Gastroenterology 68:222, 1975.
6. Bardram L: Gastrin in non-neoplastic pancreatic tissue from patients with and without gastrinomas. Scand J Gastroenterol 25:945, 1990.
7. Cattan D, Roucayrol AM, Launay JM, et al: Circulating gastrin, endocrine cells, histamine content and histidine decarboxylase activity in atrophic gastritis. Gastroenterology 97:586, 1989.
8. Helander HF, Rutgersson K, Helander KG, et al: Stereologic investigations of human gastric mucosa, oxynic mucosa from patients with Zollinger-Ellison syndrome. Scand J Gastroenterol 27:875, 1992.
9. Chen D, Zhao CM, Dockray GJ, et al: Glycine-extended gastrin synergizes with gastrin 17 to stimulate acid secretion in gastrin-deficient mice. Gastroenterology 119:756, 2000.
10. Lehy T, Roucayrol AM, Mignon M: Histomorphological characteristics of gastric mucosa in patients with Zollinger-Ellison syndrome or autoimmune gastric atrophy: Role of gastrin and atrophying gastritis. Microsc Res Tech 48:327, 2000.
11. Bordi C, Azzoni C, Ferraro G, et al: Sampling strategies for analysis of enterochromaffin-like cell changes in Zollinger-Ellison syndrome Am J Clin Pathol 114:419, 2000.
12. Debelenko LV, Emmert-Buck MR, Zhuang Z, et al: The multiple endocrine neoplasia type I gene locus is involved in the pathogenesis of type II gastric carcinoids. Gastroenterology 113:773, 1997.
13. O'Conner DT, Deftos LJ: Secretion of chromogranin A by peptide-producing endocrine neoplasms. N Engl J Med 314:1145, 1986.
14. Lam KY, Lo CY: C-erb-2 protein expression in oesophageal squamous epithelium from oesophageal squamous cell carcinomas, with special reference to histological grade of carcinoma and pre-invasive lesion. Eur J Surg Oncol 23:36, 1997.
15. Lam KY, Lo CY, Fan ST, Luk JM: Telomerase activity in pancreatic endocrine tumours: A potential marker for malignancy. Mol Pathol 53: 133, 2000.
16. Straus E, Raufman JP, Samuel S, et al: Endoscopic cure of the Zollinger-Ellison syndrome. Gastrointest Endosc 38:709, 1992.
17. Modlin IM, Lawton GP: Duodenal gastrinoma: The solution to the pancreatic paradox [editorial]. J Clin Gastroenterol 19:184, 1994.
18. Cadiot G, Vuagnat A, Doukhan I, et al: Prognostic factors in patients with Zollinger-Ellison syndrome and multiple endocrine neoplasia type 1. Groupe d'Étude des Neoplasies Endocriniennes Multiples (GENEM and Groupe de Recherche et d'Étude du Syndrome de Zollinger-Ellison (GRESZE). Gastroenterology 116:286, 1999.
19. Howard TJ, Zinner MJ, Stabile BE, Passaro E: Gastrinoma excision for cure: A prospective analysis. Ann Surg 211:9, 1990.
20. Hirasawa K, Yamada M, Kitagawa M, et al: Ovarian mucinous cystadenocarcinoma as a cause of Zollinger-Ellison syndrome: Report of a case and review of the literature. Am J Gastroenterol 95:1348, 2000.
21. Wu PC, Alexander HR, Bartlett DL, et al: A prospective analysis of the frequency, location, and curability of ectopic (nonpancreaticoduodenal, non-nodal) gastrinoma. Surgery 122:1176, 1997.
22. Smyrniotis V, Kehagias D, Kostopanagiotou G, et al: A primary hepatic gastrinoma [letter]. Am J Gastroenterol 94:3380, 1999.
23. Kehagias D, Moulopoulos L, Smirniotis V, et al: Imaging findings in primary carcinoid tumour of the liver with gastrin production. Br J Radiol 72:207, 1999.
24. Terada T, Matsunaga Y, Maeta H, et al: Mixed ductal-endocrine carcinoma of the pancreas presenting as gastrinoma with Zollinger-Ellison syndrome: An autopsy case with a 24-year survival period. Virchows Arch 435:606, 1999.
25. Noda S, Norton JA, Jensen RT, Gay WA, Jr: Surgical resection of intracardiac gastrinoma. Ann Thorac Surg 67:532, 1999.
26. Hirschowitz BI: Zollinger-Ellison syndrome: Pathogenesis, diagnosis, and management. Am J Gastroenterol 92(4 Suppl):44S, 1997.
27. Boden G: Insulinoma and glucagonoma. Semin Oncol 14:253, 1987.
28. Vinayek R: Zollinger-Ellison syndrome. Recent advances in the management of the gastrinoma. Gastroenterol Clin North Am 19:197, 1990.
29. van Heerden JA: Management of the Zollinger-Ellison syndrome in patients with multiple endocrine neoplasia type I. Surgery 100:971, 1986.
30. Fishbeyn VA, Norton JA, Benya RV, et al: Assessment and prediction of long-term cure in patients with the Zollinger-Ellison syndrome: The best approach. Ann Intern Med 119:199, 1993.
31. Mignon M, Cadiot G: Diagnostic and therapeutic criteria in patients with Zollinger-Ellison syndrome and multiple endocrine neoplasia type I. J Intern Med 243:489, 1998.
32. Gordon JN: An unusual cause of watery diarrhoea. Diagnosis: Metastatic Zollinger-Ellison syndrome. Postgrad Med J 76:512, 2000.
33. Baffy G, Boyle JM: Association of Zollinger-Ellison syndrome with pancreatitis: Report of five cases. Dig Dis Sci 45:1531, 2000.
34. Day JP, Richter JE: Medical and surgical conditions predisposing to gastroesophageal reflux disease. Gastroenterol Clin North Am 19:587, 1990.
35. Sarosiek J, Jensen RT, Maton PM, et al: Salivary and gastric epidermal growth factor in patients with Zollinger-Ellison syndrome: Its protective potential. Am J Gastroenterol 95:1158, 2000.
36. Metz DC, Starr JA: A retrospective study of the usefulness of acid secretory testing. Aliment Pharmacol Ther 14:103, 2000.
37. Pisegna JR: The effect of Zollinger-Ellison syndrome and neuropeptide-secreting tumors on the stomach. Curr Gastroenterol Rep 1:511, 1999.
38. Feldman M, Dickerman RM, McClelland RN, et al: Effect of selective proximal vagotomy on food-stimulated gastric acid secretion and gastrin release in patients with duodenal ulcer. Gastroenterology 76:926, 1979.
39. Straus E, Gerson CD, Yalow RS: Hypersecretion of gastrin associated with the short bowel syndrome. Gastroenterology 64:175, 1974.
40. Schjonsby H, Willassen Y: Renal extraction of endogenous gastrin in patients with normal renal function. Scand J Gastroenterol 12:205, 1977.
41. Corleto VD, Minisola S, Moretti A, et al: Prevalence and causes of hypergastrinemia in primary hyperparathyroidism: A prospective study. J Clin Endocrinol Metab 84:4554, 1999.
42. Romeo DP: Misdiagnosis of Zollinger-Ellison syndrome due to hyperlipidemia. Gastroenterology 99:1511, 1990.
43. Cadiot G, Jais P, Mignon M: Diagnosis of Zollinger-Ellison syndrome. From symptoms to biological evidence. Ital J Gastroenterol Hepatol Suppl 2:S147, 1999.
44. Jowell PS, Robuck-Mangum G, Mergener K, et al: A double-blind, randomized, dose-response study testing the pharmacological efficacy of synthetic porcine secretin. Aliment Pharmacol Ther 14:1679, 2000.
45. Takasu A, Shimosegawa T, Fukudo S, et al: Duodenal gastrinoma—clinical features and usefulness of selective arterial secretin injection test. J Gastroenterol 33:728, 1998.
46. Tang C, Biemond I, Lamers CB: Expression of peptide receptors in human endocrine tumours of the pancreas. Gut 40:267, 1997.
47. Ellison EC, O'Dorisio MS, O'Dorisio T: Failure of secretin to stimulate gastrin release and adenylate cyclase activity in gastrinoma in vitro. Surgery 96:1019, 1984.
48. Kato M, Imamura M, Hosotani R, et al: Curative resection of microgastrinomas based on the intraoperative secretin test. World J Surg 24: 1425, 2000.
49. Metz DC: Diagnosis of non-Zollinger-Ellison syndrome, non-carcinoid syndrome, enteropancreatic neuroendocrine tumours. Ital J Gastroenterol Hepatol 31 Suppl 2:S153, 1999.
50. McNamara D, Lewis T, O'Moran C: Zollinger-Ellison syndrome with fasting hypoglycaemia. J R Soc Med 91:92, 1998.
51. Chandrasekharappa SC, Guru SC, Manickam P, et al: Positional cloning of the gene for multiple endocrine neoplasia-type 1. Science 276: 404, 1997.
52. Guru SC, Goldsmith PK, Burns AL, et al: Menin, the product of the MEN I gene, is a nuclear protein. Proc Natl Acad Sci USA 95:1630, 1998.
53. Komminoth P, Heitz PU, Kloppel J: Pathology of MEN-I: Morphology, clinicopathologic correlations and tumor development. J Intern Med 243:455, 1998.
54. Guru SC, Manickam P, Crabtree JS, et al: Identification and characterization of the multiple endocrine neoplasia type I (MEN I) gene. J Intern Med 243:433, 1998.
55. Roijers JF, Apel T, Neumann HP, et al: Internally shortened menin protein as a consequence of alternative RNA splicing due to a germline deletion in the multiple endocrine neoplasia type I gene. Int J Mol Med 5:611, 2000.
56. Ikeo Y, Sakurai A, Suzuki R, et al: Proliferation-associated expression of the MEN I gene as revealed by in situ hybridization: Possible role of the menin as a negative regulator of cell proliferation under DNA damage. Lab Invest 80:797, 2000.
57. Maruyama K, Tsukada T, Hosono T, et al: Structure and distribution of rat menin mRNA. Mol Cell Endocrinol 156:25, 1999.
58. Maruyama K, Tsukada T, Honda M, et al: Complementary DNA

structure and genomic organization of *Drosophila* menin. Mol Cell Endocrinol 168:135, 2000.
59. Olufemi SE, Green JS, Manickam P, et al: Common ancestral mutation in the MEN I gene is likely responsible for the prolactinoma variant of MEN I (MEN Ibruin) in four kindreds from Newfoundland. Hum Mutat 11:264, 1998.
60. Burgess JR, Greenaway TM, Shepherd JJ: Expression of the MEN-I gene in a large kindred with multiple endocrine neoplasia type I. J Intern Med 243:465, 1998.
61. Wermer P: Genetic aspects of adenomatosis of endocrine glands. Am J Med 16:363, 1954.
62. Marx SJ, Agarwal SK, Kester MB, et al: Multiple endocrine neoplasia type I: Clinical and genetic features of the hereditary endocrine neoplasias. Recent Prog Horm Res 54:397. Discussion 438, 1999.
63. Dackiw AP, Cote GJ, Fleming JB, et al: Screening for MEN I mutations in patients with atypical endocrine neoplasia. Surgery 126:1097. Discussion 1103, 1999.
64. Kraimps JL: Hyperparathyroidism in multiple endocrine neoplasia syndrome. Surgery 112:1080, 1992.
65. Norton JA: Effect of parathyroidectomy in patients with hyperparathyroidism, Zollinger-Ellison syndrome, and multiple endocrine neoplasia type I: A prospective study. Surgery 102:958, 1987.
66. Gogel HK, Buckman MT, Cadieux D, McCarthy DM: Gastric secretion and hormonal interactions in multiple endocrine neoplasia type I. Arch Intern Med 145:855, 1985.
67. Ray JM, Squires PE, Curtis SB, et al: Expression of the calcium-sensing receptor on human antral gastrin cells in culture. J Clin Invest 99:2328, 1997.
68. Cheng I, Qureshi I, Chattopadhyay N, et al: Expression of an extracellular calcium-sensing receptor in rat stomach. Gastroenterology 116: 118, 1999.
69. Mitsuma T, Rhue N, Kayama M, et al: Distribution of calcium-sensing receptor in rats: An immunohistochemical study. Endocrinol Regul Jun 33:55, 1999.
70. Meichsner CL, Lee FP, Hobson SA, et al: Identification of a functional $Ca2^{+}$-sensing receptor in normal human gastric mucous epithelial cells. Am J Physiol 277(3 Pt 1):G662, 1999.
71. Yazawa K, Kuroda T, Watanabe H, et al: Multiple carcinoids of the duodenum accompanied by type I familial multiple endocrine neoplasia. Surg Today 28:636, 1998.
72. Debelenko LV, Emmert-Buck MR, Zhuang Z, et al: The multiple endocrine neoplasia type I gene locus is involved in the pathogenesis of type II gastric carcinoid. Gastroenterology 113:773, 1997.
73. Teh BT, Zedenius J, Kytola S, et al: Thymic carcinoids in multiple endocrine neoplasia type I. Ann Surg 228:99, 1998.
74. Pack SD, Kirschner LS, Pak E, et al: Genetic and histologic studies of somatomammotropic pituitary tumors in patients with the "complex of spotty skin pigmentation, myxomas, endocrine overactivity and schwannomas" (Carney complex). J Clin Endocrinol Metab 85:3860, 2000.
75. Pack S, Turner ML, Zhuang Z, et al: Cutaneous tumors in patients with multiple endocrine neoplasia type I show allelic deletion of the MEN I gene. J Invest Dermatol 110:438, 1998.
76. Schulte KM, Simon D, Dotzenrath C, et al: Sequence analysis of the MEN I gene in two patients with multiple cutaneous lipomas and endocrine tumors. Horm Metab Res 32:76, 2000.
77. Doherty GM, Olson JA, Frisella MM, et al: Lethality of multiple endocrine neoplasia type I. World J Surg 22:581, 1998.
78. Fishbeyn VA, Norton JA, Benya RV, et al: Assessment and prediction of long-term cure in patients with the Zollinger-Ellison syndrome. Ann Intern Med 119:199, 1993.
79. Goebel SU, Vortmeyer AO, Zhuang Z, et al: Identical clonality of sporadic gastrinomas at multiple sites. Cancer Res 60:60, 2000.
80. Karges W, Schaaf L, Dralle H, Boehm BO: Concepts for screening and diagnostic follow-up in multiple endocrine neoplasia type I (MEN I). Exp Clin Endocrinol Diabetes 108:334, 2000.
81. Pisegna JR: The effect of Zollinger-Ellison syndrome and neuropeptide-secreting tumors on the stomach. Curr Gastroenterol Rep 1:511, 1999.
82. Burgess JR, Nord B, David R, et al: Phenotype and phenocopy: The relationship between genotype and clinical phenotype in a single large family with multiple endocrine neoplasia type I (MEN I). Clin Endocrinol (Oxf) 53:205, 2000.
83. Jensen RT: Management of the Zollinger-Ellison syndrome in patients with multiple endocrine neoplasia type I. J Intern Med 243:477, 1998.
84. Goebel SU, Heppner C, Burns AL, et al: Genotype/phenotype correlation of multiple endocrine neoplasia type I gene mutations in sporadic gastrinomas. J Clin Endocrinol Metab 85:116, 2000.
85. Debelenko LV, Zhuang Z, Emmert-Buck MR, et al: Allelic deletions on chromosome 11q13 in multiple endocrine neoplasia type I-associated and sporadic gastrinomas and pancreatic endocrine tumors. Cancer Res 57:2238, 1997.
86. Yu F, Jensen RT, Lubensky IA, et al: Survey of genetic alterations in gastrinomas. Cancer Res 60:5536, 2000.
87. Chung DC, Brown SB, Graeme-Cook F, et al: Localization of putative tumor suppressor loci by genome-wide allelotyping in human pancreatic endocrine tumors. Cancer Res 58:3706, 1998.
88. Marx SJ, Agarwal SK, Kester MB, et al: Germline and somatic mutations of the gene for multiple endocrine neoplasia type I (MEN I). J Intern Med 243:447, 1998.
89. Agarwal SK, Debelenko LV, Kester MB, et al: Analysis of recurrent germline mutations in the MEN I gene encountered in apparently unrelated families. Hum Mutat 12:75, 1998.
90. Cetani F, Pardi E, Giovannetti A, et al: Six novel MEN I gene mutations in sporadic parathyroid tumors. Hum Mutat 16:445, 2000.
91. Uchino S, Noguchi S, Sato M, et al: Screening of the MEN I gene and discovery of germ-line and somatic mutations in apparently sporadic parathyroid tumors. Cancer Res 60:5553, 2000.
92. Kakizawa T, Sakurai A, Ikeo Y, et al: Novel deletional mutation of the MEN I gene in a kindred with multiple endocrine neoplasia type I. Clin Genet 58:61, 2000.
93. Shan L, Nakamura Y, Nakamura M, et al: Somatic mutations of multiple endocrine neoplasia type I gene in the sporadic endocrine tumors. Lab Invest 78:471, 1998.
94. Evans CO, Brown MR, Parks JS, et al: Screening for MEN I tumor suppressor gene mutations in sporadic pituitary tumors. J Endocrinol Invest 23:304, 2000.
95. Mignon M, Cadiot G: Natural history of gastrinoma: Lessons from the past. Ital J Gastroenterol Hepatol Suppl 2:S98, 1999.
96. Alexander HR, Bartlett DL, Venzon DJ, et al: Analysis of factors associated with long-term (five or more years) cure in patients undergoing operation for Zollinger-Ellison syndrome. Surgery 124:1160, 1998.
97. Jais P, Vuagnat A, Terris B, et al: Association of serum antibodies against p53 protein with poor survival in patients with Zollinger-Ellison syndrome. Gastroenterology 114:37, 1998.
98. Goebel SU, Serrano J, Yu F, et al: Prospective study of the value of serum chromogranin A or serum gastrin levels in the assessment of the presence, extent, or growth of gastrinomas [see comments]. Cancer 85:1470, 1999.
99. Bloomfeld R, Bornstein J, Jowell P: A report of a gastrinoma localized preoperatively by endoscopic ultrasound only and a review of the approach to imaging in Zollinger-Ellison syndrome. Dig Dis 17:316, 1999.
100. Sugg SL, Norton JA, Fraker DL, et al: A prospective study of intraoperative methods to diagnose and resect duodenal gastrinomas. Ann Surg 218:138, 1993.
101. Lew EA, Pisegna JR, Starr JA, et al: Intravenous pantoprazole is a novel proton pump inhibitor that rapidly and effectively controls gastric acid hypersecretion in patients with Zollinger-Ellison syndrome. Gastroenterology 118:696, 2000.
102. Pisegna JR, Norton JA, Slimak GG, et al: Effects of curative gastrinoma resection on gastric secretory function and antisecretory drug requirement in the Zollinger-Ellison syndrome. Gastroenterology 102: 767, 1992.
103. Stewart CA, Termanini B, Sutliff VE, et al: Management of the Zollinger-Ellison syndrome in pregnancy. Am J Obstet Gynecol 176: 224, 1997.
104. Metz DC, Pisegna JR, Fishbeyn VA, et al: Currently used doses of omeprazole in Zollinger-Ellison syndrome are too high. Gastroenterology 103:1498, 1992.
105. Metz DC, Pisegna JR, Ringham GL, et al: Prospective study of the efficacy and safety of lansoprazole in Zollinger-Ellison syndrome. Dig Dis Sci 38:245, 1992.
106. Welage LS, Berardi RR: Evaluation of omeprazole, lansoprazole, pantoprazole, and rabeprazole in the treatment of acid-related diseases. J Am Pharm Assoc (Wash) 40:52, 2000.
107. Maton PN: Zollinger-Ellison syndrome. Recognition and management of acid hypersecretion. Drugs 52:33, 1996.
108. Waldum HL, Brenna E, Kleveland PM, et al: Gastrin—physiological

and pathophysiological role: Clinical consequences. Dig Dis 13:25, 1995.
109. Helander HF, Rutgersson K, Helander KG, et al: Stereologic investigations of human gastric mucosa. II. Oxyntic mucosa from patients with Zollinger-Ellison syndrome. Scand J Gastroenterol 27:875, 1992.
110. Solcia E, Capella C, Fiocca R, et al: Gastric argyrophil carcinoidosis in patients with Zollinger-Ellison syndrome due to type I multiple endocrine neoplasia. A newly recognized association. Am J Surg Pathol 14:503, 1990.
111. Termanini B, Gibril F, Sutliff VE, et al: Effect of long-term gastric acid suppressive therapy on serum vitamin B_{12} levels in patients with Zollinger-Ellison syndrome. Am J Med 5:422, 1998.
112. Howden CW: Vitamin B_{12} levels during prolonged treatment with proton pump inhibitors. J Clin Gastroenterol 30:29, 2000.
113. Stewart CA, Termanini B, Sutliff VE, et al: Iron absorption in patients with Zollinger-Ellison syndrome treated with long-term gastric acid antisecretory therapy. Aliment Pharmacol Ther 12:83, 1998.
114. Keogan MT, Baker ME: Computed tomography and magnetic resonance imaging in the assessment of pancreatic disease. Gastrointest Endosc Clin North Am 5:31, 1995.
115. Pisegna JR, Doppman JL, Norton JA, et al: Prospective comparative study of ability of MR imaging and other imaging modalities to localize tumors in patients with Zollinger-Ellison syndrome. Dig Dis Sci 38:1318, 1993.
116. Marcos HB, Semelka RC, Noone TC, et al: MRI of normal and abnormal duodenum using half-Fourier single-shot RARE and gadolinium-enhanced spoiled gradient echo sequences. Magn Reson Imaging 17:869, 1999.
117. Doppman JL, Jensen RT: Localization of gastroenteropancreatic tumours by angiography. Ital J Gastroenterol Hepatol 31 Suppl 2:S163, 1999.
118. Rossi P: CT functioning tumors of the pancreas. AJR Am J Roentgenol 144:57, 1985.
119. Cherner JA, Doppman JL, Norton JA, et al: Selective venous sampling for gastrin to localize gastrinomas. A prospective assessment. Ann Intern Med 105:841, 1986.
120. Maton PN, Miller DL, Doppman JL, et al: Role of selective angiography in the management of patients with Zollinger-Ellison syndrome. Gastroenterology 92:913, 1987.
121. Roche A, Raisonnier A, Gillon-Asavouret MC, Pancreatic venous sampling and arteriography in localizing insulinomas and gastrinomas: Procedure and results in 55 cases. Radiology 145:621, 1982.
122. Gibril F, Reynolds JC, Chen CC: Specificity of somatostatin receptor scintigraphy: A prospective study and effects of false-positive localizations on management in patients with gastrinomas. J Nucl Med 40: 539, 1999.
123. Bhutani MS, Dexter D, McKellar DP, et al: Intraoperative endoscopic ultrasonography in Zollinger-Ellison syndrome. Endoscopy 29:754, 1997.
124. Benya RV, Metz DA, Hijazi YM, et al: Fine-needle aspiration cytology of submucosal nodules in patients with Zollinger-Ellison syndrome. Am J Gastroenterol 88:258, 1992.
125. Modlin IM, Cornelius E, Lawton GP: Use of an isotopic somatostatin receptor probe to image gut endocrine tumors. Arch Surg 130:367. Discussion 373, 1995.
126. Pisegna JR, Sawicki MP: Neuroendocrine pancreas. In Haskell CM (ed): Cancer Treatment. Philadelphia, WB Saunders, 2001, Chapter 69.
127. Shi W, Johnston CF, Buchanan KD: Localization of neuroendocrine tumours with [^{111}In] DTPA-octreotide scintigraphy (OctreoScan): A comparative study with CT and MR imaging. Q J Med 91:295, 1998.
128. Gibril F, Doppman JL, Reynolds JC, et al: Bone metastases in patients with gastrinomas: A prospective study of bone scanning, somatostatin receptor scanning, and magnetic resonance image in their detection, frequency, location, and effect of their detection on management. J Clin Oncol 16:1040, 1998.
129. Lebtahi R, Cadiot G, Delahaye N, et al: Detection of bone metastases in patients with endocrine gastroenteropancreatic tumors: Bone scintigraphy compared with somatostatin receptor scintigraphy. J Nucl Med 40:1602, 1999.
130. Termanini B, Gibril F, Doppman JL, et al: Distinguishing small hepatic hemangiomas from vascular liver metastases in gastrinoma: Use of a somatostatin-receptor scintigraphic agent. Radiology 202:151, 1997.
131. Gibril F, Reynolds JC, Lubensky IA, et al: Ability of somatostatin receptor scintigraphy to identify patients with gastric carcinoids: A prospective study. J Nucl Med 41:1646, 2000.
132. Jensen RT, Gibril F: Somatostatin receptor scintigraphy in gastrinomas. Ital J Gastroenterol Hepatol 31 Suppl 2:S179, 1999.
133. Wells SA, Jr: Surgery for the Zollinger-Ellison syndrome [editorial, comment]. N Engl J Med 341:689, 1999.
134. Hirschowitz BI: Surgery to cure the Zollinger-Ellison syndrome [letter, comment]. N Engl J Med 341:2096, 1999.
135. Townsend CM, Jr Thompson JC: Surgical management of tumors that produce gastrointestinal hormones. Annu Rev Med 36:111, 1985.
136. Fishbeyn VA, Norton JA, Benya RV, et al: Assesment and prediction of long-term cure in patients with the Zollinger-Ellison syndrome: The best approach. Ann Intern Med 119:199, 1993.
137. Sheppard BC, Management of islet cell tumors in patients with multiple endocrine neoplasia: A prospective study. Surgery 106:1108, 1989.
138. Thompson NW: Surgical treatment of the endocrine pancreas and Zollinger-Ellison syndrome in the MEN I syndrome. Henry Ford Hosp Med J 40:195, 1992.
139. van Heerden JA: Management of the Zollinger-Ellison syndrome in patients with multiple endocrine neoplasia type I. Surgery 100:971, 1986.
140. Park BJ, Alexander HR, Libutti SK, et al: Operative management of islet-cell tumors arising in the head of the pancreas. Surgery 124: 1056. Discussion 1061, 1998.
141. Norton JA: Aggressive resection of metastatic disease in selected patients with malignant gastrinoma. Ann Surg 203:352, 1986.
142. Frucht H: Detection of duodenal gastrinomas by operative endoscopic transillumination. A prospective study. Gastroenterology 99:1622, 1990.
143. Takasu A, Shimosegawa T, Fukudo S, et al: Duodenal gastrinoma—clinical features and usefulness of selective arterial secretin injection test. J Gastroenterol 33:728, 1998.
144. Norton JA: Curative resection in Zollinger-Ellison syndrome. Results of a 10-year prospective study. Ann Surg 215:8, 1992.
145. Norton JA, Doherty GM, Fraker DL: Surgical treatment of localized gastrinoma within the liver: A prospective study. Surgery 124:1145, 1998.
146. Owens LV, Huth JF, Cance WG: Insulinoma: Pitfalls in preoperative localization. Eur J Surg Oncol 21:326, 1995.
147. McArthur KE, Richardson CT, Barnett CC, et al: Laparotomy and proximal gastric vagotomy in Zollinger-Ellison syndrome: Results of a 16-year prospective study. Am J Gastroenterol 91:1104, 1996.
148. Scopinaro F, Schillaci O, Delle Fave G, et al: ^{111}In-pentetreotide detection of gastrinoma before and after surgery. Anticancer Res 17: 1757, 1997.
149. Jaskowiak NT, Fraker DL, Alexander HR, et al: Is reoperation for gastrinoma excision indicated in Zollinger-Ellison syndrome? Surgery 120:1055. Discussion 1062, 1996.
150. Chui AK, Jayasundera MV, Haghighi KS, et al: Octreotide scintigraphy: A prerequisite for liver transplantation for metastatic gastrinoma. Aust N Z J Surg 68:458, 1998.
151. Yu F, Venzon DJ, Serrano J, et al: Prospective study of the clinical course, prognostic factors, causes of death, and survival in patients with long-standing Zollinger-Ellison syndrome. J Clin Oncol 17:615, 1999.
152. Tennvall J, Ljungberg O, Ahren B, et al: Radiotherapy for unresectable endocrine pancreatic carcinomas. Eur J Surg Oncol 18:73, 1992.
153. Mignon M: Current approach to the management of tumoral process in patients with gastrinoma. World J Surg 10:703, 1986.
154. Moertel CG: Streptozocin alone compared with streptozocin plus fluorouracil in the treatment of advanced islet-cell carcinoma. N Engl J Med 303:1189, 1980.
155. von Schrenck T: Prospective study of chemotherapy in patients with metastatic gastrinoma. Gastroenterology 94:1326, 1988.
156. Anderson JV, Bloom SR: Treatment of malignant endocrine tumors with human leukocyte interferon. Lancet 1:97, 1987.
157. Eriksson B, Alm G, Lundqvist G, et al: Treatment of malignant endocrine pancreatic tumors with human leukocyte interferon. Lancet 2:1307, 1986.
158. Pisegna JR, Slimak GG, Metz DC, et al: An evaluation of human recombinant alpha interferon in patients with metastatic gastrinoma. Gastroenterology 105:1179, 1993.
159. Ajani J, Kavanagh J, Pratt Y, et al: Roferon and doxorubin combination against advanced islet cell or carcinoid tumors [abstract]. Proc Am Assoc Cancer Res 30:293, 1989.
160. Reubi JC, Kvols LK, Nagorney DM, et al: Detection of somato-

statin receptor in surgical and percutaneous needle biopsy of samples of carcinoid and islet cell carcinomas. Cancer Res 50:5969, 1990.

161. Redding TW, Schally AV: Inhibition of growth of pancreatic carcinomas in animal models by analogs of hypothalamic hormones. Proc Natl Acad Sci USA 84:248, 1984.
162. Saltz L, Trochanowski B, Buckley B, et al: Octreotide as an antineoplastic agent in the treatment of functional and nonfunctional neuroendocrine tumors. Cancer 72:244, 1993.
163. Arnold R, Trautmann ME, Creutzfeldt W, et al: Somatostatin analogue octreotide and inhibition of tumour growth in metastatic endocrine gastroenteropancreatic tumours. Gut 38:430, 1996.
164. Creutfeldt W, Bartsch HH, Jacubaschke U, Stockmonn F: Treatment of gastrointestinal endocrine tumors with interferon-alpha and octreotide. Acta Oncol 30:529, 1991.
165. Nold R, Frank M, Kajdan U, et al: Combined treatment of metastatic endocrine tumors of the gastrointestinal tract with octreotide and interferon-alpha. Z Gastroenterol 32:19, 1994.
166. Oh DS, Pisegna JR: A pilot study of sandostatin LAR in combination with human recombinant alpha interferon in treating patients with metastatic neuroendocrine tumors [abstract]. Gastroenterology 120: A613, 2001.
167. Chung MH, Pisegna J, Spirt M, et al: Hepatic cytoreduction followed by a novel long-acting somatostatin analog: A paradigm for intractable neuroendocrine tumors metastatic to the liver. Surgery 130:1, 2001.
168. Ruszniewski P, Malka D: Hepatic arterial chemoembolization in the management of advanced digestive endocrine tumors. Digestion 62[Suppl 1]:79, 2000.
169. Tang S-J, Jensen D, Ohning GV, Pisegna JR: The novel use of an intravenous proton pump inhibitor in a patient with short bowel syndrome: Case report and literature review. J Clin Gastroenterol 34:62, 2002.

Chapter 42

Current Role of Surgery in Peptic Ulcer Disease

Robert V. Rege and Daniel B. Jones

HISTORICAL BASIS FOR THE SURGICAL TREATMENT OF PEPTIC DISEASE

Until histamine$_2$ receptor antagonists were introduced in 1977, medical therapy for ulcer disease was limited to dietary changes and use of antacids. Primary ulcer healing rates were low, recurrence rates high, and ulcer complications common. Ulcer patients frequently required surgery for perforation, upper gastrointestinal hemorrhage, gastric outlet obstruction, or control of symptoms. Early operations removed the ulcer and large portions of stomach, frequently resulting in long-term complications. Many operated patients became nutritional cripples, developing postgastrectomy syndromes worse than their ulcer disease. Safe, effective operations for peptic ulcer disease awaited understanding of gastric physiology and pathogenesis of peptic ulcers. Careful laboratory and clinical investigation over the last century, much of it by surgeons, led to principles of gastric surgery that still hold today, and eventually provided the basis for medical control of gastric acid secretion with histamine$_2$ receptor antagonists and proton pump inhibitors.

A link between duodenal ulcer disease and higher-than-normal gastric acid output established a role for gastric acid in the formation of peptic ulcers. Not all patients with duodenal ulcer disease exhibited high gastric acid output, and many patients with gastric ulcer produced less than normal amounts of acid (although some acid production appeared to be necessary for ulcer formation). Thus, disorders of gastric acid secretion did not explain all ulcers. The concept arose that ulcers resulted from an imbalance between gastric acid production and mucosal resistance to peptic damage. A decrease in the amount of secreted acid should then improve the balance between ulcerogenic and protective forces, leading to ulcer healing.[1] Acid reduction was therefore the goal of peptic ulcer therapy until the importance of *Helicobacter pylori* was established,[2, 3] and treatments to eradicate this organism were added. Antiulcer operations were designed to balance the potential benefits for gastric acid reduction with complications of the surgical procedure. Although peptic ulcer disease is now largely treated medically, not all ulcers are associated with *H. pylori*, not all ulcers are medically controlled and, moreover, many patients develop complications of ulcers that require surgical therapy.

The goals of operative therapy today have not changed. The surgeon must effectively treat complications by controlling upper gastrointestinal hemorrhage, relieving obstruction, and closing perforations. Surgeons should consider adding an acid-reducing procedure after weighing immediate and late complications, the patient's condition, and alternative therapies. These procedures may cure the ulcer diathesis or improve subsequent medical therapy even if an ulcer recurs.

Effective medical treatment of peptic ulcer disease and improved techniques of controlling upper gastrointestinal hemorrhage nonoperatively have greatly limited the role of surgery in peptic ulcer disease. Elective peptic ulcer surgery is now rare and is most often applied to patients with gastric outlet obstruction due to long-standing ulcer disease. Emergency operations are still required, albeit less frequently. Many patients undergoing operation suffer perforation or hemorrhage as the first manifestation of their disease. Consequently, surgeons have become progressively less experienced in peptic ulcer surgery. Training of surgical residents is problematic with the present low volume of patients. Yet the patients who present for operative therapy are often more complex than in the past. They are often elderly,[4] have significant co-morbidities, are taking ulcerogenic drugs (nonsteroidal anti-inflammatory agents [NSAIDs] or glucocorticoids), are noncompliant, and have failed multiple nonoperative therapies. In choosing the proper operation, the modern surgeon must realize that the patient likely arises from a small subset of ulcer patients who do not have *H. pylori*–induced ulcers, who have not responded to medications, or who may not be able to stop NSAIDs because of the debilitating diseases for which they were prescribed. In addition, Zollinger-Ellison syndrome should currently be considered in patients with ulcers severe enough to warrant surgical treatment (see Chapter 41). Improvements in care of ulcer patients have not made decision making for the surgeons easier, and current dilemmas in surgical treatment are unlikely to be answered soon, since very few centers can assemble a large enough cohort of study patients.

This chapter describes operations available for treatment of peptic ulcer disease, complications that arise after peptic ulcer surgery, and the decision-making process used to choose an operation for the peptic ulcer patient. Correct application of operations to patients is the factor that most influences a successful outcome.

PHYSIOLOGIC BASIS FOR PEPTIC ULCER SURGERY

Several principles of gastric acid secretion were important for the development of effective operations for peptic ulcer disease. As reviewed in Chapter 38, acid secretion occurs in distinct phases.[5] In between meals and at night, low secretion of gastric acid is termed the basal phase. During the cephalic phase, the thought, sight, or smell of food triggers gastric acid secretion, preparing the digestive process for a meal. Increased secretion of acid during these first two phases may be particularly important in ulcer formation since there is no food in the stomach to buffer acid. Once food enters the stomach, gastric acid secretion increases further, causing the digestive process to begin. This phase is termed the gastric, or hormonal, phase and is mediated by local reflexes involving acetylcholine and perhaps histamine and secretion of the hormone gastrin into the circulatory system by the antrum of the stomach. Finally, hormones secreted by the duodenum and small intestine inhibit gastric acid secretion and return it to the basal state as the stomach empties its contents. Theoretically, increased secretion of acid during any of these phases may contribute to ulcer disease.

Cells secreting gastric acid are regulated through several receptor-mediated pathways.[6] The vagus nerves innervate the stomach and stimulate acid secretion through acetylcholine receptors. The vagus nerves are important in each phase of gastric acid secretion. They set the level of basal acid secretion, mediate the cephalic phase, and potentiate the effects of histamine and gastrin during other phases. Therefore, interruption of vagal fibers to the stomach lowers acid during every phase of gastric acid secretion. In addition, the vagus nerves are responsible for normal antral and pyloric motility. Division of vagal branches to the antrum results in pylorospasm and delayed gastric emptying.

Although control of gastric acid secretion is more complex and involves many other factors that refine the process, the parietal cell is in general controlled by interactions among acetylcholine, histamine, and gastrin receptors. The synergistic response of the receptors can be used to advantage by down-regulating stimulation via any of these pathways. Since vagotomy influences each phase of gastric acid secretion, it is the most important component of an operation for duodenal ulcer disease, but vagotomy is not necessary for most patients with gastric ulcer in whom antrectomy alone removes that mucosa at risk for development of ulcers, removes the gastrin-bearing portion of the stomach, and appears sufficient to treat subsequent gastric ulcer disease. Surgical interruption of vagal stimulation is straightforward, but, depending on the level of denervation, has untoward effects such as delayed gastric emptying, dumping, and postvagotomy diarrhea. Addition of antrectomy to vagotomy removes the part of the stomach responsible for gastrin secretion and interrupts the hormonal phase of gastric acid secretion. As expected, control of ulcers is enhanced, but operative and long-term complications increase.

Subtotal gastrectomy, once a popular surgical treatment for ulcer, removes the source of gastrin, mucosa at risk for ulcers, and parietal cell mass, decreasing the capacity to secrete acid, but results in an unacceptably high rate of complications. It is now reserved for the treatment of hemorrhage from diffuse gastritis not controlled medically and for gastric cancer.

OPERATIONS FOR DUODENAL ULCERS

The goal of operative therapy is long-term elimination, including avoidance of undesirable side effects and complications, of ulcer disease. Most ulcers and their complications are now treated medically or endoscopically, but operations are still required to treat hemorrhage, perforation, and obstruction not responding to medical therapy. Rarely, patients are encountered who require elective operations when they fail medical therapy. The most commonly performed operations are the Graham patch closure of perforations, vagotomy and pyloroplasty, highly selective vagotomy, and antrectomy with drainage.

GRAHAM PATCH CLOSURE OF PERFORATED DUODENAL ULCER. In general, perforating ulcers appear as small pinpoint holes on the anterior surface of the antrum, duodenum, or pylorus and now are often associated with the use of NSAIDs.[7] Graham patch closure[8] with a tongue of omentum effectively seals the perforation in most patients (Fig. 42–1). The stomach is decompressed with a nasogastric tube while

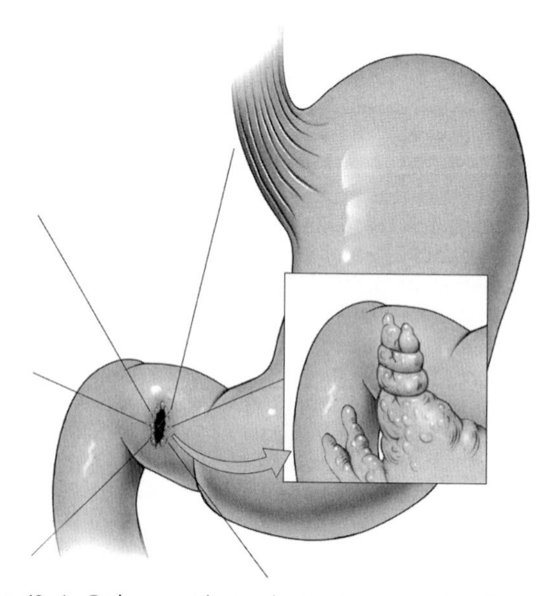

Figure 42–1. Graham patch. Lembert sutures are placed around the perforation. In some cases, the sutures may be placed to close the perforation and the closure is reinforced with an omental patch. A tongue of omentum is mobilized and placed over the perforation without tension. It is held in place by tying the previously placed sutures.

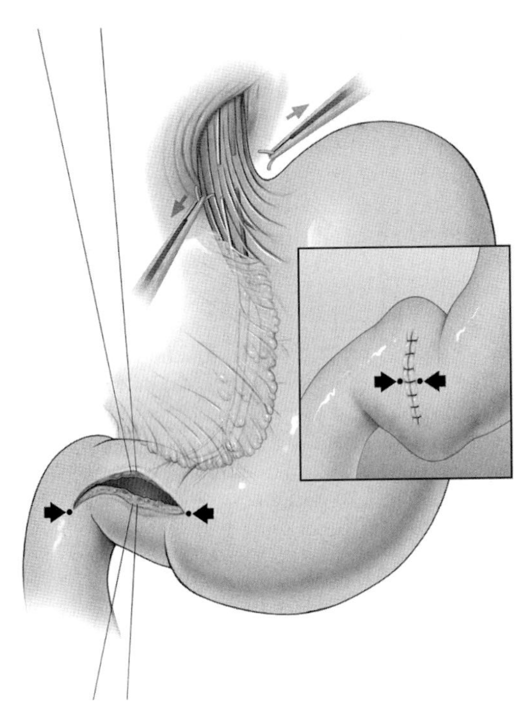

Figure 42–2. Truncal vagotomy and Heineke-Mikulicz pyloroplasty. Truncal vagotomy requires identification of both the anterior and posterior vagi at the level of the esophagus. A 2-cm segment of the left (anterior) and posterior (right) vagus nerves are excised and sent to pathology for confirmation. All tissue surrounding the esophagus must then be mobilized, and any tissue suspected to be a branch of the vagus nerves must be divided. A drainage procedure is then required, because division of vagal innervation to the antrum and pylorus results in pylorospasm. The pyloroplasty is performed after a Kocher maneuver. A full-thickness incision is begun in the stomach 2 cm proximal to the pylorus and is extended through it 1 cm into the duodenum. Stay sutures are placed, and the opening is then closed transversely using sutures or staples (*inset*), thus widening the pylorus.

the patient is aggressively resuscitated. After copious peritoneal irrigation and intravenous administration of broad-spectrum antibiotics, a vascularized tongue of omentum is mobilized to reach the site of perforation without tension. The perforation may be closed, but this often is not possible because of inflammation and edema. Instead, the omentum is secured by a ring of interrupted sutures or by imbricating sutures over the patch (see Fig. 42–1). Symptoms are relieved permanently in 75% of patients with acute perforation, but in only 25% of patients with chronic ulcer disease.[9, 10] Antiulcer operations should be considered in stable patients with minimal inflammation, especially if they suffer from chronic ulcer disease. Highly selective vagotomy is our procedure of choice (discussed later). Recurrence rate was only 3% and mortality 0% when highly selective vagotomy was added to closure of the ulcer.[10] Because of an approximate 10% risk of malignancy, gastric ulcers that perforate require resection, excision for pathologic examination, or, at a minimum, biopsy in addition to closure and/or patching.

TRUNCAL VAGOTOMY AND DRAINAGE. Truncal vagotomy requires identification of both the anterior and posterior vagi at the level of the distal esophagus. Approximately 4 to 6 cm of esophagus is mobilized below the diaphragm. The surgeon's fingers usually palpate the vagus nerves as the stomach is retracted inferiorly. The left (anterior) vagus nerve arises anterior and toward the left side of the esophagus. A 2-cm segment of nerve is bluntly elevated away from the esophagus, clipped proximally and distally, excised, and sent to the pathology laboratory for confirmation. The posterior (right) vagus lies posterior and to the right of the esophagus. It is often necessary to mobilize all the tissue between the esophagus and the aorta to locate this nerve. Again, a 2-cm segment is clipped, excised, and submitted to the laboratory. All tissue surrounding the esophagus must then be mobilized, and any tissue suspected to be a branch of the vagus nerves must also be divided. Early branching of the anterior vagus is particularly common. Pathologic confirmation that each nerve has been divided is critical since recurrent ulcer after vagotomy and pyloroplasty is frequently associated with failure to divide the posterior branch of the vagus nerve. A drainage procedure (pyloroplasty or gastrojejunostomy) is then required since division of vagal innervation to the antrum and pylorus results in pylorospasm.

The Heineke-Mikulicz pyloroplasty is performed after a Kocher maneuver mobilizes the duodenum. The pylorus is opened longitudinally with monopolar cautery (Fig. 42–2). A full-thickness incision is begun in the stomach 2 cm proximal to the pylorus and is extended through it 1 cm into the duodenum. Stay sutures are placed, and the opening is then closed transversely, by means of suture or staples, thereby widening the pylorus. The suture line is covered with omentum to prevent leakage and adhesions to the liver. Adhesions have the potential to cause angulation and obstruction of the duodenum. When the duodenum is too diseased to complete a Heineke-Mikulicz pyloroplasty, another type of pyloroplasty, such as a Finney or Jaboulay pyloroplasty, or a gastrojejunostomy, may be used instead (Fig. 42–3).

A gastrojejunostomy is performed along a dependent por-

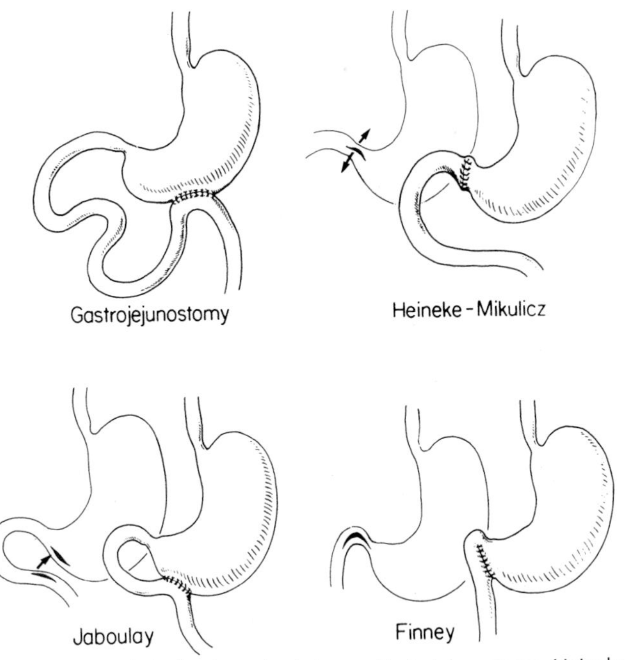

Figure 42–3. Methods of gastric drainage: Gastrojejunostomy, Heineke-Mikulicz, Jaboulay, Finney. (From Mathews JB, Silen W: Operations for peptic ulcer disease and their complications. In Sleisenger MH, Fordtran JS [eds]: Gastrointestinal Disease, 5th ed. Philadelphia, WB Saunders, 1993.)

tion of the greater curvature of the stomach. About 6 cm of stomach is freed from the gastrocolic ligament by ligating several branches of the gastroepiploic vessels. A hand-sewn or stapled anastomosis is then created at this point between the stomach and the antimesenteric surface of the jejunum, approximately 15 cm distal to the ligament of Treitz. The loop may be placed antecolic or retrocolic. It may also be placed in an iso- or antiperistaltic manner. Although there has been much controversy concerning construction of the loop, there is probably little difference between these methods of construction. More importantly, the loop of jejunum should be positioned so that the afferent and efferent loops do not twist, and the anastomosis should be big enough to accommodate two fingers easily.

HIGHLY SELECTIVE VAGOTOMY. Highly selective vagotomy, also termed parietal cell vagotomy or proximal selective vagotomy, is designed to minimize the complications and morbidity associated with other antiulcer operations. Highly selective vagotomy selectively eliminates the vagal innervation to the acid-producing parietal cells and pepsin-producing chief cells of the fundus and body of the stomach while preserving innervation to the antrum and pylorus. Thus, a drainage procedure is not needed, and the innervation of the liver and small intestine is preserved.

The anterior and posterior vagal trunks are identified at the gastroesophageal junction. Next, the junction of the body and antrum of the stomach is located by finding the point where the vagus nerves form a pattern resembling a "crow's foot" (Fig. 42–4*A*). The nerves of Latarjet are then identified in the lesser omentum, isolated, and gently retracted to the right. The stomach is retracted to the left and inferiorly, accentuating the vessels and vagal branches to the lesser curve of the stomach. Devascularization of the lesser curve of the stomach is begun by dividing the first one or two branches of the "crow's foot." [11] Devascularization is carried out proximally by dividing each vascular pedicle to the lesser curve (Fig. 42–4*B*). Since the nerves are inseparable from vessels to the lesser curve, the operation cuts all branches of the anterior and posterior vagus nerves to the stomach while preserving hepatic, celiac, and antral branches of the vagus nerve. The dissection is continued until 5 to 7 cm of esophagus is skeletonized, to ensure that all branches of the vagus, including the criminal nerve of Grassi, are divided. The devascularized lesser curve of the stomach is covered by approximating the anterior serosal surface of the stomach to the posterior surface by means of a running stitch.

Recurrence rates after highly selective vagotomy vary from 5% to 20%, depending on the surgeon's experience with the procedure.[12, 13] Complications of the operation are minimal. In experienced hands, results are similar to or better than with truncal vagotomy. Highly selective vagotomy is contraindicated for pyloric and prepyloric gastric ulcers, with 30% of patients experiencing difficult gastric emptying or recurrent ulcer after operation.[14]

TRUNCAL VAGOTOMY AND ANTRECTOMY. In 1940, in an effort to eliminate both the cephalic and gastric phases of gastric acid secretion, Farmer and Smithwick[15] and concurrently Edwards and Herrington[16] combined truncal vagotomy with antrectomy. Overall, vagotomy plus antrectomy has the lowest recurrent ulcer rate, about 2%, but has the highest complication rate. It is recommended for obstructing lesions and for selected patients at high risk for recurrence (smokers, those taking ulcerogenic medications) and may be preferable to highly selective vagotomy for pyloric and prepyloric ulcers, which have a higher likelihood of recurrence,[12, 17] and for gastric ulcers (discussed later).

Antrectomy is performed by dividing the blood supply to the distal stomach. A point is chosen along the greater curvature at the watershed between the gastroepiploic and short gastric vessels. The gastrocolic ligament is divided between this point and the duodenum, opening the lesser sac. Care is taken to avoid injury to the middle colic artery. The gastroepiploic artery is then divided proximally. A point is identi-

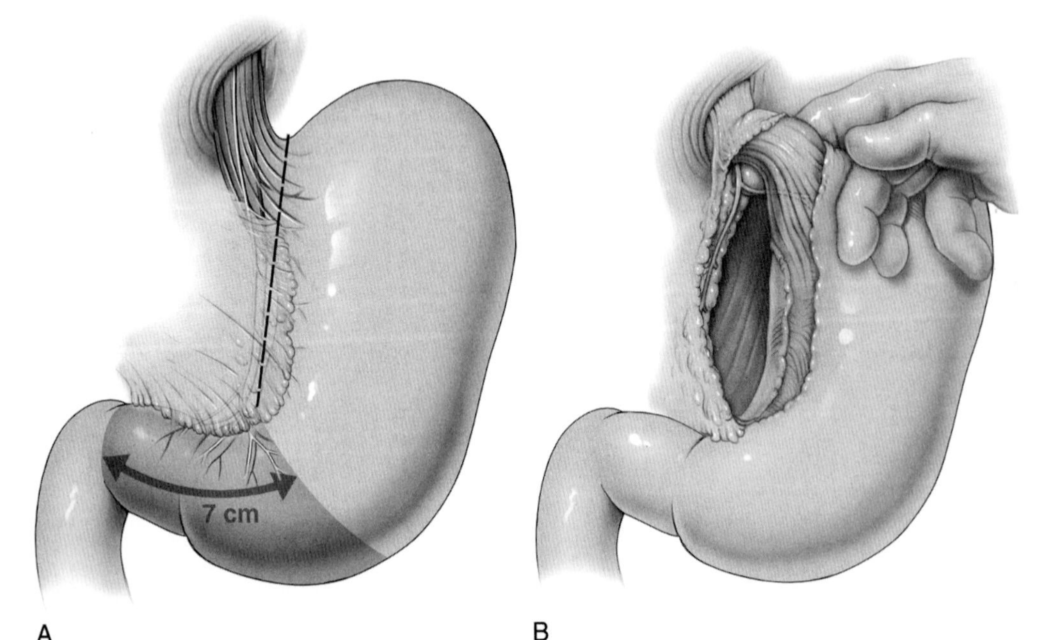

Figure 42–4. Highly selective vagotomy. *A,* The anterior and posterior vagal trunks are identified at the gastroesophageal junction, and the "crow's foot" is identified. The nerves of Latarjet are identified, isolated, and gently retracted to the right. The stomach is retracted to the left and inferiorly. Devascularization of the lesser curve of the stomach is performed by dividing the first one or two branches of the "crow's foot," and each vascular pedicle and its associated nerve to the lesser curve. *B,* Five to seven cm of esophagus are skeletonized to ensure that all branches of the vagus, including the criminal nerve of Grassi, are divided. The devascularized lesser curve of the stomach is covered by approximating the anterior serosal surface of the stomach to the posterior surface.

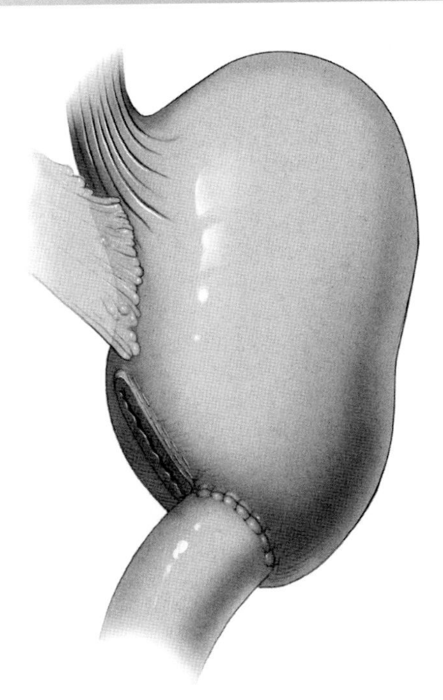

Figure 42–5. A Billroth I reconstruction. The stomach is mobilized by dividing its blood supply from the watershed between the gastroepiploic and short gastric vessels on the greater curvature and the incisura on the lesser curvature to the duodenum. Two to three cm of duodenum are mobilized, and it is divided 1 cm distal to the pylorus. Approximately 40% to 60% of the distal stomach is removed, and the proximal remnant is closed. The proximal gastric remnant is anastomosed directly to the duodenum.

fied on the lesser curvature, usually at the incisura. The blood supply from the left gastric artery to the distal antrum is then divided and carried distally so that 2 to 3 cm of duodenum are mobilized. The stomach is divided from the incisura to the greater curvature at the insertion of the gastroepiploic artery between clamps or by means of a stapling device, which simplifies gastric division. Approximately 40% to 60% of the stomach is removed with this technique. The ampulla and common bile duct must be clearly identified and protected to avoid iatrogenic injury. The duodenum is divided 1 cm distal to the pylorus to ensure that no antrum remains. Occasionally, a small gastrotomy is helpful to distinguish the pylorus from ulcer scar.

Edema and scarring of the pylorus, pancreas, and hepatoduodenal ligament may preclude safe resection of the stomach. If the surgeon is in doubt about the status of the duodenum, a vagotomy and pyloroplasty or highly selective vagotomy is favored to avoid a difficult duodenal stump closure. The difficult duodenal closure risks a fatal duodenal leak, or pancreatitis.

Reconstruction of gastrointestinal continuity may be accomplished by reconnecting the stomach directly to the duodenum (Billroth I; Fig. 42–5) or by closing the duodenal stump and creating a gastrojejunostomy. A Billroth I anastomosis requires at least 1 cm of healthy duodenal wall above the pancreas and cannot always be accomplished. However, the Billroth I reconstruction avoids the complications associated with the duodenal stump, afferent and efferent limb syndromes, and formation of marginal ulcers. In general, reconstruction with the gastroduodenostomy (Billroth I) is advocated over a gastrojejunostomy (Billroth II) because it seems to be more "physiologic," minimizing dumping and weight loss.

A Billroth II reconstruction is favored if inflammation of the duodenum makes construction of a Billroth I technically difficult. For the Billroth II, a loop of jejunum is anastomosed to the gastric remnant, as described earlier for gastrojejunostomy (Fig. 42–6). The duodenum is oversewn or stapled carefully, because leaks result in a high mortality. Nasogastric tube decompression through the gastrojejunostomy postoperatively may be protective.[18]

CLOSURE OF THE DIFFICULT DUODENAL STUMP. Occasionally, inflammation and scarring will prevent mobilization of the duodenum after the duodenum is divided. The posterior ulcer adheres to the pancreas anteriorly. As long as the anterior duodenal wall is soft and flexible, a Nissen-Cooper closure may be performed with good results. After mobilization of the distal duodenum with the Kocher maneuver, the anterior duodenum is sutured to the distal edge of the ulcer (Fig. 42–7). A second row of sutures inverts the anterior duodenum to the proximal edge of the ulcer. A duodenostomy tube with a small 14-French Foley catheter placed through the lateral duodenal wall may prevent blowout of the stump caused by increased duodenal intraluminal pressures.[19] A duodenostomy tube used alone and in lieu of stump closure is unreliable.[20]

SUBTOTAL GASTRECTOMY. Subtotal gastrectomy is rarely performed for peptic ulcers today. Gastrectomy may be fraught with duodenal stump leak, pancreatitis, retained antrum, splenic trauma, bile duct injury, and obstruction. More importantly, late complications (discussed later), such as ane-

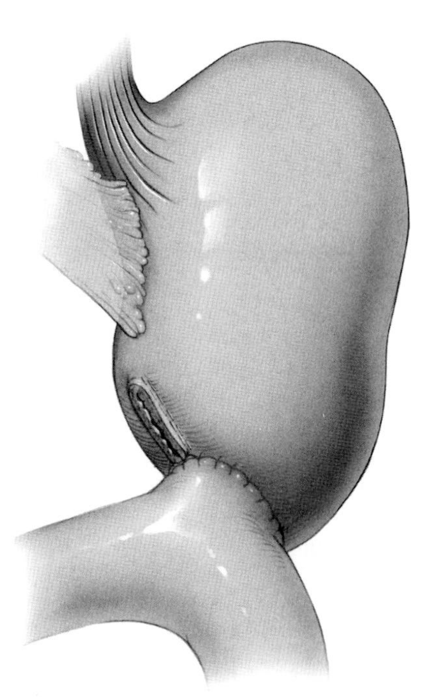

Figure 42–6. A Billroth II reconstruction after antrectomy. The duodenal stump is closed, and continuity of the gastrointestinal tract is restored by creating an anastomosis between the proximal stomach and a loop of jejunum about 15 cm distal to the ligament of Treitz. This creates afferent (duodenum to stomach) and efferent (stomach to distal bowel) loops.

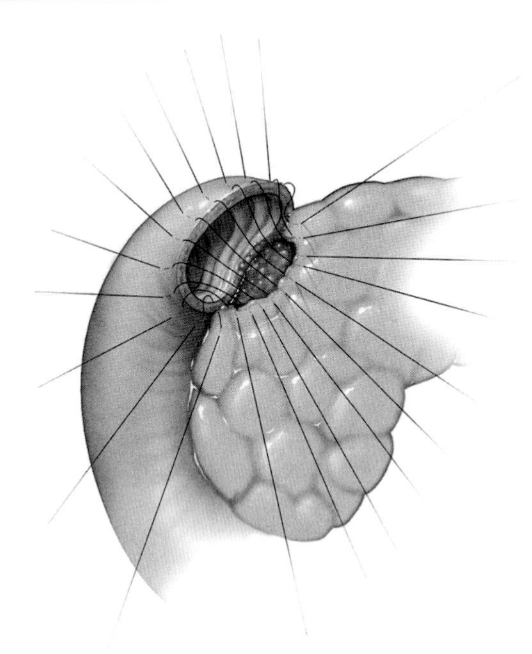

Figure 42–7. Closure of a difficult duodenal stump. Occasionally, inflammation and scarring prevent mobilization of the duodenum after the duodenum is divided. A Nissen-Cooper closure is illustrated. After mobilization of the distal duodenum with the Kocher maneuver, the anterior duodenum is sutured to the distal edge of the ulcer. A second row of sutures inverts the anterior duodenum to the proximal edge of the ulcer. A duodenostomy tube is placed through the lateral duodenal wall to prevent blowout of the stump.

mia, folic acid and cobalamin (vitamin B_{12}) deficiencies, poor calcium and vitamin D absorption, early satiety, and dumping syndromes, too often result in nutritional complications that are worse than the ulcer disease that was treated.

ROUX-EN-Y GASTROJEJUNOSTOMY

The Roux-en-Y drainage procedure is usually reserved for complications after a Billroth I or II reconstruction and is an especially effective treatment for alkaline reflux gastritis, discussed later. Essentially, the jejunum is divided about 15 cm from the ligament of Treitz. The end is closed and the loop is mobilized to reach the gastric remnant without tension. An anastomosis is performed between the stomach and the side of the loop. The proximal jejunum is then reanastomosed to the jejunal limb approximately 50 to 60 cm distal to the gastrojejunostomy (Fig. 42–8). Vagotomy, if not previously performed, is required to avoid marginal ulceration. Routine use of a Roux-en-Y operation to reconstruct patients after gastric resection is not recommended since, in some patients, it may result in delayed gastric emptying (Roux stasis syndrome).

OPERATIONS FOR BENIGN GASTRIC ULCERS

Gastric ulcers can be classified into five categories[21, 22] that are useful in determining treatment (Fig. 42–9). Type I ulcers, located in the body of the stomach usually along the lesser curve at the incisura angularis, are the most common type of gastric ulcer encountered. These patients often have low gastric acid output. Antrectomy is adequate treatment for these patients. If ulcers are found proximally along the lesser curvature, the ulcer may be excised in continuity with the antrum by extending the resection line on the lesser curve proximally without obstructing the gastroesophageal junction (Pauchet procedure) (Fig. 42–10). Similarly, type II ulcers are found in the body of the stomach but are typically preceded by an ulcer in the duodenum. Type III ulcers are found in the prepyloric region. Many patients with type II and type III ulcers are acid hypersecretors and benefit from antrectomy and vagotomy. Patients with type III ulcers appear to have very aggressive disease; results with highly selective vagotomy have been poor and it should not be performed. Since the duodenum is spared extensive fibrosis, a Billroth I can usually be reconstructed safely in patients with gastric ulcer.

Type IV gastric ulcers are ulcers lying high in the body of the stomach or near the esophagogastric junction. Their position increases the complexity of operative therapy and

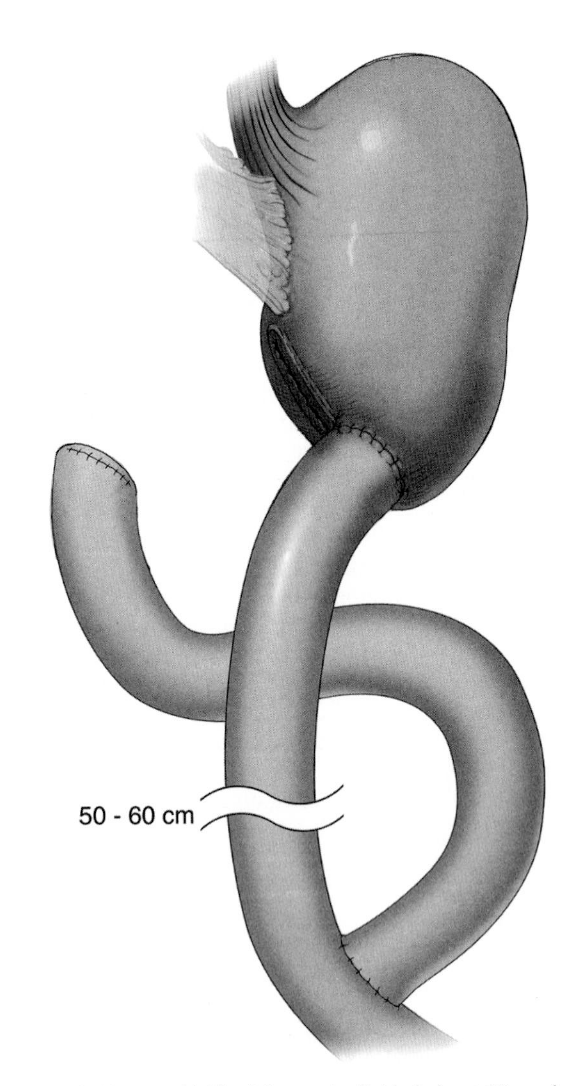

Figure 42–8. Roux-en-Y. The jejunum is divided about 15 cm from the ligament of Treitz. The end is closed, and the loop is mobilized to reach the gastric remnant without tension. An anastomosis is performed between the stomach and the side of the loop. The proximal jejunum is then reanastomosed to the jejunal limb about 50 to 60 cm distal to the gastrojejunostomy. A vagotomy, if not previously performed, is required to avoid marginal ulceration.

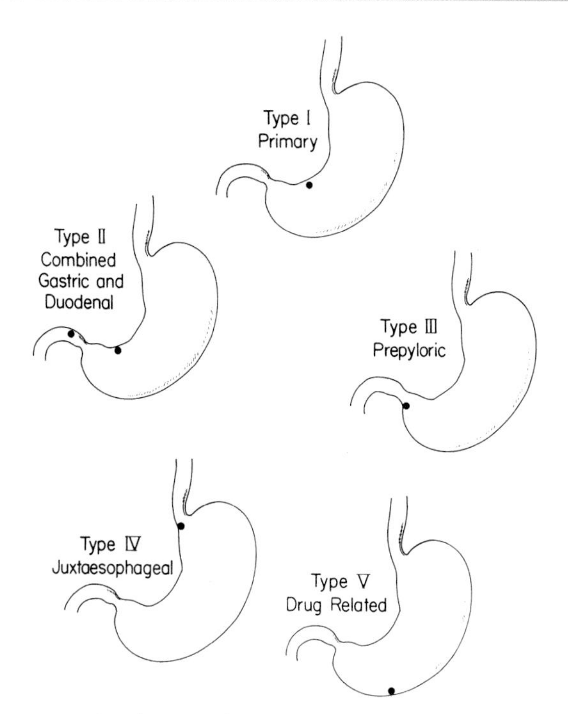

Figure 42–9. Classification of gastric ulcers. (From Mathews, JB, Silen W: Operations for peptic ulcer disease and their complications. In Sleisenger MH, Fordtran JS [eds]: Gastrointestinal Disease, 5th ed. Philadelphia, WB Saunders, 1993.)

increases surgical morbidity and mortality. After antrectomy, the proximal gastric ulcer may be left in situ (Kelling-Madlener procedure). This approach has a high recurrence rate, lacks histologic examination of the ulcer to exclude malignancy, and can be advocated only if a more definitive operation cannot be completed safely. Subtotal gastrectomy and reconstruction with a Roux-en-Y esophagogastrojejunostomy may be performed.[22, 23] The jejunum is divided 30 cm from the ligament of Treitz, the proximal end is closed, and the anastomosis is performed in one layer beginning at the level of the esophagus. Occasionally surgeons will excise only the ulcer, with a full-thickness wedge resection for juxtaesophageal ulcers. In general, "ulcerectomy" on the greater curvature is safe and achieves good results.[14] Wedge resection of a benign gastric ulcer on the lesser curve, however, risks unrecognized vagal injury. For this reason, either antrectomy or vagotomy with pyloroplasty should be performed.

Type V ulcers can be found throughout the stomach and are commonly associated with aspirin and other NSAIDs. The best treatment is to avoid the inciting irritant. Antiulcer medications and misoprostol may be useful in elderly patients and patients with a history of ulcers who require ulcerogenic medications.[7] Cyclooxygenase-2 (COX-2) selective inhibitors, such as celecoxib (Celebrex) and rofecoxib (Vioxx), cause fewer ulcers than conventional NSAIDs (Chapter 23).

EARLY POSTOPERATIVE COMPLICATIONS

In general, peptic ulcer surgery is performed with minimal morbidity and mortality. Current mortality rates range as low as 0.3% with highly selective vagotomy to about 1% for gastric resection, and patients who die often have significant co-morbidities[24] (Table 42–1). Morbidity and mortality are higher if an emergency operation is required for complicated peptic ulcer disease. Peritonitis from perforated ulcers increases the risk of intra-abdominal and subphrenic abscess. Infectious complications are more common with a long interval from perforation to surgery. Postoperative fever, elevated white blood count, and persistent ileus warrant evaluation for abscess, usually with computed tomography (CT) of the abdomen and pelvis. Abscesses must be treated promptly, either with percutaneous or operative drainage (see Chapter 24).

Massive preoperative transfusion to stabilize patients with bleeding peptic ulcers and preoperative shock increases the

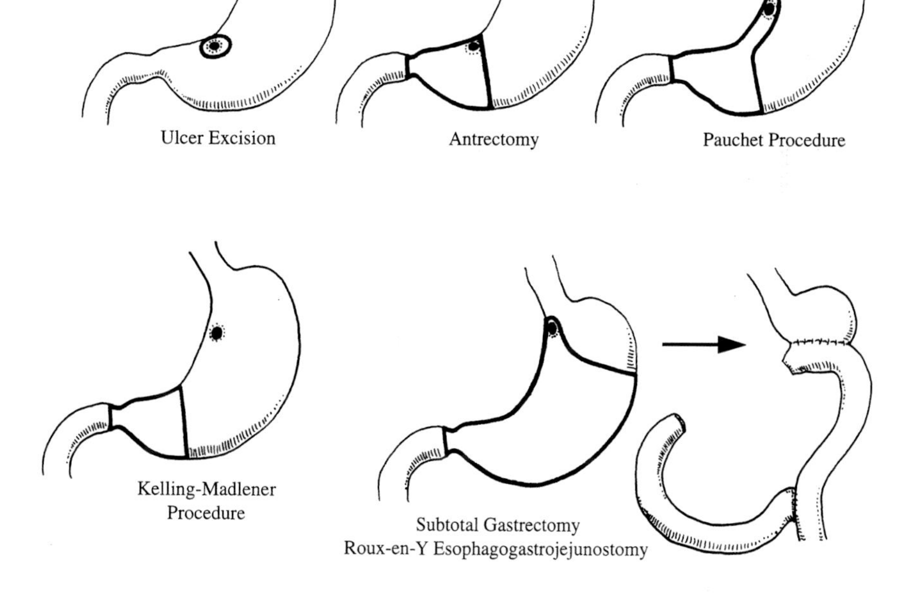

Figure 42–10. Operations for a benign gastric ulcer. Heavy lines delineate the extent of the excision. (From Seymour NE: Operations for peptic ulcer and their complications. In Feldman M, Scharschmidt BF, Sleisenger MH [eds]: Gastrointestinal Disease, 6th ed. Philadelphia, WB Saunders, 1998.)

Table 42–1 | **Operations for Peptic Ulcer Disease: Comparisons of Recurrences, Morbidity, and Mortality**

OPERATION	ULCER RECURRENCE RATES (%)	MORBIDITY (%)	MORTALITY (%)
Vagotomy and pyloroplasty	10–15	5	0.7
Vagotomy and antrectomy	0–2	5	1
Highly selective vagotomy	10–17	1	0.3

Adapted from refs. 76 and 77.

morbidity and mortality of operative therapy. Operative intervention should be instituted promptly once it is clear that hemorrhage continues despite effective attempts at nonoperative therapy. Patients with hemorrhage from peptic ulcers are also at risk for recurrent postoperative hemorrhage. Recurrent hemorrhage greatly increases morbidity and mortality and should be treated aggressively. If reoperation is required, resection of the stomach (antrectomy, including the ulcer if possible) may be necessary to control and prevent further hemorrhage.

A leak at the suture or staple line used to create a pyloroplasty, gastroenterostomy, or duodenal stump may result in abscess or, if not contained by adjacent structures, peritonitis. Well-defined, unilocular abscess cavities are amenable to percutaneous drainage, but complex abscesses and peritonitis require prompt operative therapy. In some patients, a leak at the suture line may result in a chronic draining fistula, which requires surgical closure if it persists. Patients may also experience hemorrhage at their suture lines. Most often, postoperative anastomotic hemorrhage ceases spontaneously. Transfusion and medical support usually suffice, but continued hemorrhage requires endoscopic or operative intervention.

Division of the vagal fibers to the parietal cell area of the stomach alone causes virtually no untoward physiologic effects. Therefore, complications specific to highly selective vagotomy are essentially nonexistent after a well-performed procedure. Oversewing the devascularized area on the lesser curvature of the stomach has obviated perforation of the stomach, reported in early series. Rather, complications attributable to vagotomy occur when branches of the vagus to the gastric antrum and other gastrointestinal organs are divided. Denervation of the entire stomach sometimes results in delayed gastric emptying, even with a wide-open pyloroplasty or gastroenterostomy. Most cases of delayed gastric emptying resolve spontaneously over several days to several weeks. Resolution may be facilitated by using metoclopramide (Reglan) or the motilin agonist erythromycin. Partial or complete gastric outlet obstruction must be excluded either with endoscopy or radiologically when delayed gastric emptying persists. Early gastric outlet obstruction due to edema at suture lines often resolves spontaneously, but patients with fixed obstruction require operative revision. In addition to anastomotic stenosis, patients with a gastroenterostomy are at risk for afferent loop obstruction (see later).

Early satiety and upper abdominal discomfort or pain 30 to 60 minutes after meals is the most common problem encountered by patients after gastric surgery. Episodes are usually precipitated by large meals, especially if the patient ingests large volumes of hypertonic liquids. Many patients also vomit, but vomitus is often bilious and does not contain undigested food, the expected finding with delayed gastric emptying. Rather, the problem is due to rapid gastric emptying and distention of the jejunum. In most patients, problems can be avoided by prescribing six small feedings per day and avoidance of large volumes of liquids with meals. Most patients improve over 6 to 12 weeks as they adapt to altered surgical anatomy and learn their limitations. This improvement is manifested by increasing tolerance to larger meals.

LATE POSTOPERATIVE COMPLICATIONS

Operations to treat peptic ulcer disease use division of vagal fibers to the stomach, bypass or destruction of the pylorus, and/or resection of the stomach to achieve high rates of cure and low rates of ulcer recurrence. However, these maneuvers also result in permanent anatomic and physiologic changes that allow reflux of duodenal/intestinal contents into the stomach, alter gastric adaptive relaxation, decrease gastric reservoir function, and interfere with normal gastric emptying (Fig. 42–11). Although the majority of patients have a decreased gastric capacity and rapid gastric emptying, some patients develop loss of contractile force and have delayed gastric emptying. The latter group of patients usually manifest themselves by vomiting undigested food, although vomiting is sometimes bilious, or with symptoms of alkaline bile reflux gastritis.

DISORDERS ASSOCIATED WITH DELAYED GASTRIC EMPTYING/ GASTRIC STASIS

RECURRENT/MARGINAL ULCERS. The ulcer recurrence rate after peptic ulcer surgery varies with the operation per-

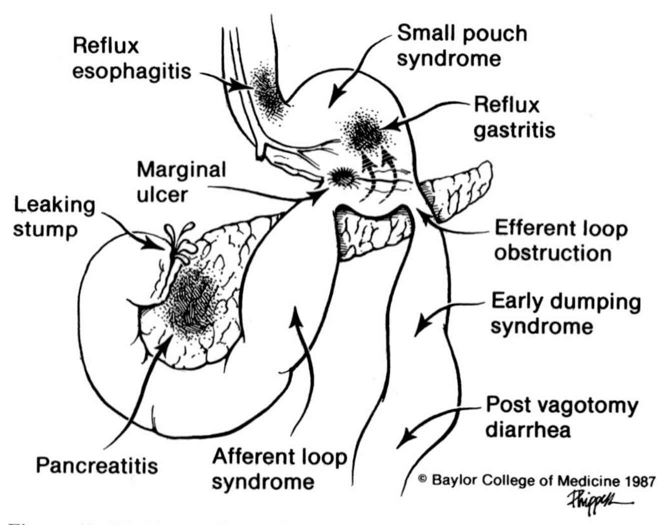

Figure 42–11. Types of complications associated with ulcer operations. (From Jordan PH Jr: Operations for peptic ulcer disease and early postoperative complications. In Sleisenger MH, Fordtran JS [eds]: Gastrointestinal Disease, 4th ed. Philadelphia, WB Saunders, 1989.)

formed. Although recurrent peptic ulcer disease is considered a failure of the operation, decreased levels of gastric acid secretion often persist, facilitating retreatment of recurrent ulcers. Revisional surgery for recurrent ulcers is rare now. Marginal ulcers that occur at a gastrojejunostomy, on the other hand, are often difficult to treat and tend to recur even if healed with medical treatment. It is felt that decreased resistance to acid digestion of the jejunum compared with the duodenum, gastric stasis, and partial obstruction of the anastomosis due to scarring or edema may contribute to marginal ulcer disease. Marginal ulcers may be due to an inadequate operation (Table 42–2) such as incomplete vagotomy, persistent hypersecretion of acid (either idiopathic or due to Zollinger-Ellison syndrome), continued use of aspirin or other NSAIDs, or ulcers related to a suture or staple at the anastomosis. A detailed medication history, gastric acid analysis, *H. pylori* test, and a fasting serum gastrin level may identify the first three causes, whereas endoscopy identifying an exposed suture can be diagnostic and therapeutic if the suture can be removed. Finally, endoscopic biopsy of the ulcer is useful in excluding a gastric carcinoma, which can sometimes mimic marginal ulcer (discussed later). Patients with marginal ulcer disease often require reresection of the stomach and revision of the anastomosis to control their problem. If possible, many surgeons advocate conversion to a Billroth I reconstruction.

GASTROPARESIS. Chronic gastroparesis, or gastric atony, is the most severe manifestation of delayed gastric emptying. Patients essentially lose all contractility in their stomach and cannot empty solids or liquids despite having a widely patent gastric outlet or anastomosis. This problem results after truncal vagotomy, but not after parietal cell vagotomy. Diabetics and patients with long-standing gastric outlet obstruction are at highest risk. It is imperative that gastric outlet or anastomotic obstruction is excluded, and this is best accomplished using upper gastrointestinal endoscopy. Unfortunately, gastroparesis after vagotomy can be refractory to treatment. Metoclopramide or erythromycin may help, but results are variable and have been less than satisfactory in the majority of patients. In unremitting cases, total gastrectomy with esophagojejunostomy or subtotal gastrectomy with a Roux-en-Y gastrojejunostomy to the small gastric remnant has been successful in returning patients to oral alimentation.

Table 42–2 | **Common Causes of Recurrent/Marginal Ulcers**

INADEQUATE OPERATION
Incomplete vagotomy
Retained antrum
Partial obstruction of the gastrojejunostomy
Gastric stasis (including afferent limb syndrome)
Exposed nonabsorbent suture/staple
MEDICATIONS
NSAIDs
Aspirin
PERSISTENT ACID HYPERSECRETION
Gastrinoma (Zollinger-Ellison syndrome)
Mastocytosis
Primary hyperparathyroidism
Idiopathic hypersecretion
GASTRIC CARCINOMA

AFFERENT LOOP SYNDROMES. This complication is peculiar to patients who undergo a gastrojejunostomy. Partial obstruction of the limb of jejunum between the ligament of Treitz and the anastomosis to the stomach causes intermittent distention of the duodenum and proximal jejunum, leading to upper abdominal/epigastric fullness and pain. Sudden emptying of the intestinal loop into the gastric remnant results in episodes of bilious vomiting followed by relief of discomfort. The obstruction of the afferent loop may be caused by stenosis at the anastomosis, by adhesions, by twisting of the intestinal loop, and rarely by tumor, cholesterol stones, or enteroliths.[3, 25–29] The diagnosis is suspected on the clinical presentation and is verified by demonstrating dilatation of the afferent loop and the site of obstruction. This has been accomplished using upper gastrointestinal barium studies, endoscopy, hepatobiliary scintigraphy,[30] CT scan,[31] or magnetic resonance cholangiography.[32] Treatment of afferent loop syndrome usually is operative, requiring revision of the gastrojejunostomy, conversion to a Billroth I or Roux-en-Y configuration, or jejunojejunostomy between the afferent and efferent loop to decompress the obstruction. Percutaneous transhepatic drainage of the duodenum to treat afferent loop obstruction has been effective in selected cases.[25, 33–35]

BILE (ALKALINE) REFLUX GASTRITIS

Reflux of duodenal contents into the stomach after pyloroplasty and gastrojejunostomy, although it occurs in almost every patient, is usually not clinically significant. However, a subset of patients exists in whom reflux of bile and pancreatic secretions damages the gastric mucosa, causing severe epigastric pain and sometimes bilious vomiting. Endoscopy supports this diagnosis when it demonstrates gastritis, either grossly or pathologically. The syndrome is difficult to distinguish from other postgastrectomy syndromes that result in epigastric pain and vomiting, but there is clearly a group of symptomatic refluxers distinguished by excessive reflux on cholecystokinin (CCK)-stimulated scintigraphy, high intragastric bile salt concentrations, and worse gastritis scores who benefit from operative therapy.[36] Conversion to a Roux-en-Y configuration using an intestinal loop that is at least 45 cm is the operation of choice (see Fig. 42–8), although some surgeons now advocate biliary diversion.[36–39] The Roux-en-Y configuration may lead to delayed gastric emptying, the so-called Roux stasis syndrome.[3, 28, 40, 41]

GASTRIC ADENOCARCINOMA

The relationships among peptic ulcer disease, surgery for peptic ulcer disease, and the risk of developing gastric adenocarcinoma have been difficult to ascertain since patients with gastric ulcer, but not patients with duodenal ulcer, are at increased risk for developing gastric cancer whether or not they undergo peptic ulcer surgery.[42–44] However, patients who have undergone gastrectomy have a twofold increase in cancer risk 15 years after resection, and cancer risk appears to increase with time.[42] The increased incidence of cancer is likely due to reflux of intestinal contents and bile into the gastric remnant, with formation of carcinogens in the gastric lumen.[44] These substances lead to increased cell proliferation rates of the gastric mucosa, especially if patients have bile reflux and *H. pylori* infection.[45] The overall risk of developing gastric carcinoma is higher in patients who had gastric ulcer, in men, and in patients who had gastrectomy rather than vagotomy and a drainage procedure.[43] The cost-effectiveness of endoscopic surveillance for gastric cancer in postgastrectomy patients has not been demonstrated. There is also a report indicating that patients who undergo peptic ulcer surgery are at higher risk for development of pancreatic cancer.[46]

SYNDROMES ASSOCIATED WITH RAPID GASTRIC EMPTYING

POSTVAGOTOMY DIARRHEA. The incidence of diarrhea after vagotomy varies from as low as 5% to as high as 50%. Most patients have intermittent episodes of diarrhea that are easily controlled by alterations in diet. Only about 10% of patients with postvagotomy diarrhea have symptoms severe enough to require medical intervention. The pathogenesis of the problem is poorly understood, but symptomatic patients clearly exhibit rapid gastric emptying. For example, symptomatic postvagotomy patients had significantly higher rates of emptying of a meal at 15 minutes (84%) measured with ^{99}mTc-diethylene compared with asymptomatic postvagotomy patients (48%) and normal controls (10%).[47] Others[48] have shown malabsorption of bile salts in symptomatic postvagotomy patients, contributing to the diarrhea. Patients with postvagotomy diarrhea should be treated conservatively with medication and dietary changes for at least 1 year since the problem may improve with time.[49] Codeine phosphate, 60 mg, and loperamide, 12 to 24 mg per day, effectively decrease transit time and malabsorption.[50] Several reports suggest that severe postvagotomy diarrhea can be treated with the somatostatin analogue octreotide (50 to 250 μg sc), but, as in treatment of dumping syndrome (discussed next) with this expensive medication, numerous side effects limit its usefulness.[51–54] Patients refractory to medical treatment may benefit from conversion to a Roux-en-Y gastrojejunostomy, because this configuration delays gastric emptying.[49]

DUMPING SYNDROME. The most severe consequence of rapid gastric emptying is dumping syndrome. Patients with early dumping syndrome experience debilitating constitutional symptoms, such as abdominal pain or cramps, diarrhea, flushing, palpitations, diaphoresis, light-headedness, tachycardia, postural hypotension, feelings of lassitude, diminished attention span, and marked weakness, symptoms that begin about 30 minutes after meals. Symptoms, although variable from patient to patient, are extremely unpleasant and markedly interfere with normal activities. Early dumping is triggered by jejunal distention as hypertonic gastric contents rapidly empty into the jejunum. Distention is caused mechanically not only by the bolus of food, but also by rapid influx of fluid into the intestinal lumen induced by its hypertonic contents. Many of the constitutional symptoms are caused by intravascular volume contraction as fluid rushes into the small intestine, while other symptoms are caused by excessive release of vasoactive hormones and autonomic reflexes triggered by the distended intestinal loop.[55, 56] In late dumping syndrome, patients experience symptoms of hypoglycemia 1 to 2 hours after meals. The pathophysiology of late dumping is not completely understood, but rapid absorption of glucose and hyperglycemia early stimulates robust insulin release that is responsible for the later, "reactive" hypoglycemia.[52]

Up to 15% of patients who undergo gastric surgery may occasionally experience symptoms of the dumping syndrome. Episodes may be avoided in most patients by dietary changes. It is advisable to place all gastric surgery patients on antidumping diets, which limit the size and increase the frequency of meals ("six small feedings" per day), restrict carbohydrate while increasing the protein content of meals, replace simple sugars with starches, avoid milk products, and encourage intake of liquids between, rather than during, meals. Restrictions may be gradually liberalized in most patients as they adapt to their operation. Only about 1% of patients develop severe, persistent, debilitating symptoms.[52]

The diagnosis of dumping syndrome is made clinically and confirmed by a simple provocative test using 50 g of glucose given orally.[56] The management of patients with persistent dumping despite dietary changes has been problematic. Operations, such as conversion to Roux-en-Y gastrojejunostomy or interposition of antiperistaltic segments of jejunum between the stomach and jejunum can be effective, but often result in new problems, such as persistent vomiting ("Roux syndrome"). More recently, both early and late dumping syndromes have been successfully treated by chronic subcutaneous administration of the somatostatin analogue octreotide (25 to 250 μg/day).[51–54, 56–59] Acute studies show that octreotide ameliorates fluid shifts causing hypovolemia, but probably mediates its primary effect by inhibiting release of intestinal peptides.[52, 56, 57, 59] In addition, in late dumping syndrome, reactive hypoglycemia is avoided because octreotide delays the onset of peak plasma glucose levels and inhibits insulin release.[52] The limitation of octreotide therapy has been side effects of the drug, including pain at the injection site, the need for long-term daily therapy, steatorrhea, diarrhea, gallstones, and decreased efficacy of treatment over time. Chronic octreotide therapy may be effective in 30% to 40% of patients. In general, patients refractory to medical therapy are probably best treated by conversion to Roux-en-Y gastrojejunostomy.

CURRENT CONTROVERSIES ON THE ROLE OF SURGERY IN PEPTIC ULCER DISEASE

PERFORATED PEPTIC ULCER. Surgeons have always had to decide whether a patient with a perforated ulcer should have simple closure of the ulcer or definitive ulcer surgery. If marked inflammation were present, simple closure with a Graham patch of omentum has always been thought safest (see Fig. 42–1). This principle still holds. In patients seeking care promptly, it was generally felt that an antiulcer operation (highly selective vagotomy or vagotomy and pyloroplasty) should be added if the patient had symptoms for greater than 2 weeks. Currently, the need for definitive therapy for perforated ulcer disease is questioned.[60–62] The availability of effective gastric acid inhibitors, and the likelihood that recurrence of ulcers can be avoided by effectively treating *H. pylori*, has decreased the chance that the patient will ever develop another surgical complication of the disease. However, in patients who have been on medical therapy or

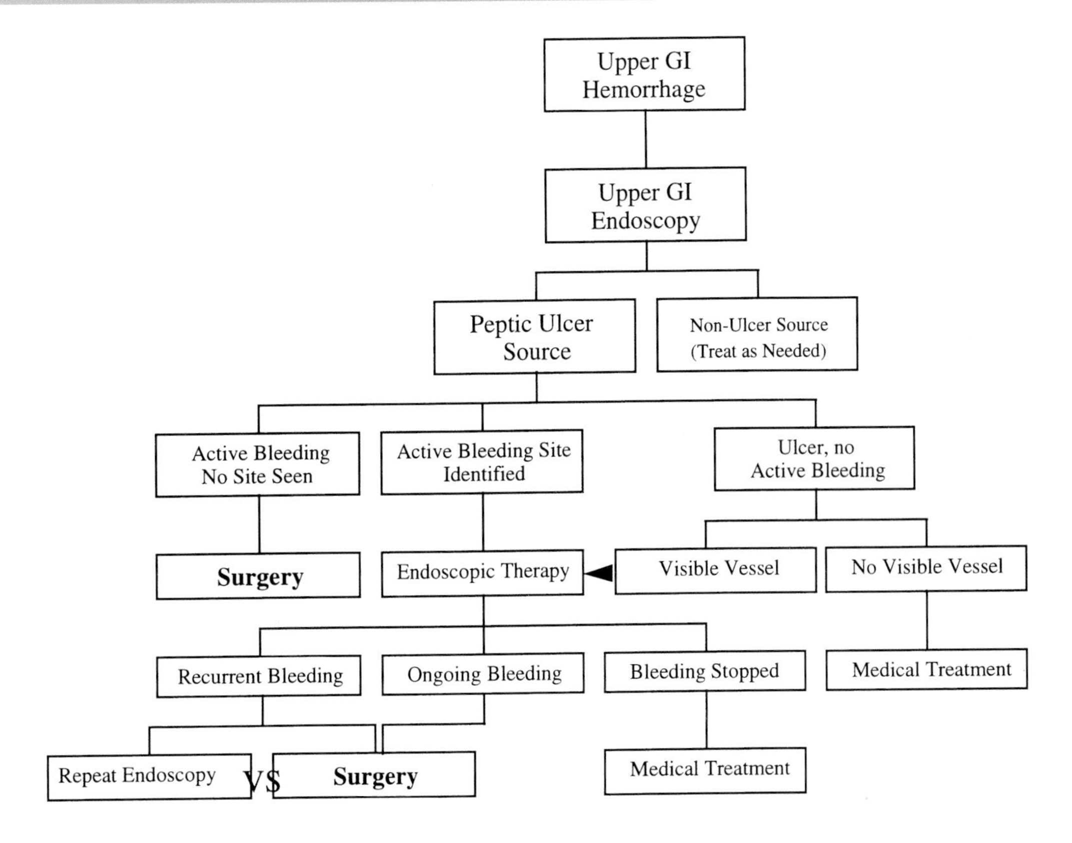

Figure 42–12. Management of bleeding peptic ulcer. (From Seymour NE: Surgery of the stomach and duodenum. In Feldman M [ed]: Gastroenterology and Hepatology: The Comprehensive Visual Reference. Philadelphia, Current Medicine, 1996.)

who require ulcerogenic drug therapy for other problems, an acid-reducing surgical procedure should be strongly considered.

Recently, laparoscopic treatment of perforated peptic ulcer has been reported in the literature.[63–65] The techniques require that the surgeon be adept with the laparoscope, including being facile with laparoscopic suturing. The operation performed includes closure of the ulcer with a Graham patch of omentum, along with careful and thorough lavage of the abdomen under direct laparoscopic observation. Laparoscopic treatment of perforated ulcers appears safe and effective, but it is not clear whether it affords benefits such as decreased length of hospital stay or decreased time to full recovery in these patients.

BLEEDING PEPTIC ULCER. Gastrointestinal hemorrhage is a life-threatening complication, with a 10% mortality, and it should be treated aggressively.[66, 67] After resuscitation, endoscopic diagnosis and therapy are usually the first line of treatment,[68, 69] since it successfully stops bleeding in 80% to 85% of patients (Fig. 42–12). Endoscopic retreatment in patients who have recurrent hemorrhage is reasonable because it may stop bleeding without the morbidity and mortality associated with operative therapy,[70] although surgery should be considered for rebleeding if the ulcer is greater than 2 cm in diameter or if the patient has associated hypotension.[70] The best results still occur if a multidisciplinary team treats the patient, if surgical therapy is undertaken as soon as the patient is transfused with 4 to 6 units of blood and shows signs of continued hemorrhage, or if the patient rebleeds on adequate medical therapy.

Typically, the source is a posterior duodenal ulcer eroding into the gastroduodenal artery, which is best approached through a longitudinal incision from the stomach, through the pylorus, and extending down the duodenum approximately 3 cm (Fig. 42–13). Proper ligation requires three sutures: a suture ligating the proximal gastroduodenal artery, a suture ligating the distal gastroduodenal artery, and most importantly, a suture deep to the bleeding vessel to ligate the transverse pancreatic artery, eliminating retrograde hemorrhage (Fig. 42–13). An antiulcer operation should be added.

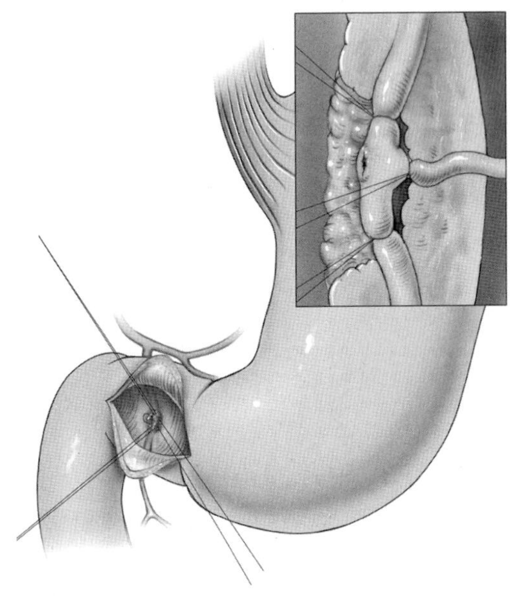

Figure 42–13. Ligation of the bleeding vessel is depicted. A gastroduodenotomy is made analogous to that used for a pyloroplasty. The bleeding site is usually located posteriorly and involves the gastroduodenal artery. The proper technique for ligation of the bleeding vessel is shown in the (*inset*).

In a multi-institutional, randomized prospective study, 137 patients underwent "conservative" therapy, consisting of underrunning the vessel or ulcer excision with ranitidine, or operative therapy, employing vagotomy and pyloroplasty or partial gastrectomy. Recurrent hemorrhage occurred in 26% versus 19% of patients after conservative therapy and antiulcer operations, respectively. More impressively, six patients died from recurrent hemorrhage after conservative therapy whereas none died from bleeding after conventional operations.[71] Some surgeons advocate gastric resection after suture ligation of the bleeding site. In another randomized study,[72] 59 patients underwent vagotomy and pyloroplasty while 61 had a gastric resection. The recurrent bleeding rate was 17% after vagotomy and pyloroplasty and only 3% after resection. Mortality was 22% and 23%, respectively. The investigators concluded that gastric resection with excision of the ulcer was better than vagotomy and pyloroplasty because of the lower rate of rebleeding and comparable mortality.[72] Certainly, patients who experience rebleeding after operative therapy require antrectomy, usually with a Billroth II reconstruction. Gastric ulcers usually require antrectomy or wedge excision of the ulcer if it is in the proximal stomach. Vagotomy is not necessary, although some surgeons add it, preferring the added protection against ulcer recurrence and marginal ulcers if a Billroth II anastomosis is performed.

GASTRIC OUTLET OBSTRUCTION. As with hemorrhage, the surgical treatment of gastric outlet obstruction has not changed.[73] If the duration of the pyloric obstruction is short, it may be treated with vagotomy and pyloroplasty. However, the cases now seen are usually quite advanced and require gastric resection. Thus, an antrectomy and truncal vagotomy is the procedure usually performed today. Truncal vagotomy and pyloroplasty or antrectomy have both been performed laparoscopically, although not in large numbers. It is not yet known whether laparoscopic approaches afford benefit to the patient.[74] Attempts at balloon dilatation of the pylorus are effective temporarily, but recurrent obstruction seems to be the rule.[75] Dilatation may be an effective bridge to surgery in patients who are malnourished.

REFERENCES

1. Mertz HR, Walsh JH: Peptic ulcer pathophysiology. Med Clin North Am 75:799–814, 1991.
2. Goldschmiedt M, Peterson WL: The role of *Helicobacter pylori* in peptic ulcer disease. Semin Gastrointest Dis 4:13–20, 1993.
3. Marshal BJ: *Helicobacter pylori*: A primer for 1994. Gastroenterologist 1:241–247, 1993.
4. Cryer B, Feldman M: Peptic ulcer disease in the elderly. Semin Gastrointest Dis 5:166–178, 1994.
5. Guyton AC, Hall JE: Secretory functions of the alimentary tract. In Guyton AC, Hall JE (eds): Textbook of Medical Physiology. Philadelphia, WB Saunders, 2000, pp 738–753.
6. Jensen RT, Gardner JD, Raufman JP, et al: Zollinger-Ellison syndrome: Current concepts and management. Ann Intern Med 98:59–75, 1983.
7. Bliss DW, Stabile BE: The impact of ulcerogenic drugs on surgery for the treatment of peptic ulcer disease. Arch Surg 126:609–612, 1991.
8. Graham RR: Technical surgical procedures for gastric and duodenal ulcer. Surg Gynecol Obstet 66:269–287, 1938.
9. Boey J, Lee NW, Wong J, et al: Perforation in acute duodenal ulcers. Surg Gynecol Obstet 155:193–196, 1982.
10. Boey J, Lee NW, Koo J, et al: Immediate definitive surgery for perforated duodenal ulcers. A prospective controlled trial. Ann Surg 196: 338–344, 1982.
11. Mistiaen W, Van Hee R, Block P, et al: Gastric emptying for solids in patients with duodenal ulcer before and after highly selective vagotomy. Dig Dis Sci 35:310–316, 1990.
12. Jordan PH, Thornby J: Should it be parietal cell vagotomy or selective vagotomy-antrectomy for treatment of duodenal ulcer? A progress report. Ann Surg 205:572–590, 1987.
13. Hoffman J, Olesen A, Jensen HE: Prospective 14 to 18 year follow-up study after parietal cell vagotomy. Br J Surg 74:1056–1059, 1987.
14. Jordan PH: Surgery for peptic ulcer disease. Curr Prob Surg 4:267–329, 1991.
15. Farmer DA, Smithwick RH: Hemigastrectomy combined with resection of the vagus nerves. N Engl J Med 247:1017–1022, 1952.
16. Edwards LW, Herrington JL Jr: Efficacy of 40 percent gastrectomy combined with vagotomy for duodenal ulcers. Surgery 41:346–348, 1957.
17. Jordan PH, Thornby J: Twenty years after parietal cell or selective vagotomy antrectomy for treatment of duodenal ulcer disease. Final Report. Ann Surg 220:283–293, 1994.
18. Passaro EJ, Bircoll M: Internal duodenal decompression. J Surg Res 13: 97–101, 1972.
19. Jones RC: Difficult closure of the duodenal stump. Arch Surg 94:690–696, 1967.
20. Burch JM, Cox CL: Management of the difficult duodenal stump. Am J Surg 162:522–526, 1991.
21. Johnson HD: Gastric ulcer: Classification, blood group characteristics, secretion patterns, and pathogenesis. Ann Surg 162:990–996, 1965.
22. Csendes A, Braghetto I, Smok G: Type IV gastric ulcer: A new hypothesis. Surgery 101:361–362, 1986.
23. Csendes A, Lazo M, Braghetto I: A surgical technique for high (cardiac and juxtacardial) benign chronic gastric ulcer. Am J Surg 135:857–858, 1978.
24. Stabile BE: Current surgical management of duodenal ulcers. Surg Clin North Am 72:335–356, 1992.
25. Caldicott DG, Ziprin P, Morgan R: Transhepatic insertion of a metallic stent for the relief of malignant afferent loop obstruction. Cardiovasc Intervent Radiol 23:138–140, 2000.
26. Wada N, Seki M, Saikawa Y, et al: Jejunal limb obstruction caused by a cholesterol stone 15 years after a total gastrectomy and 20 years after a cholecystectomy: Report of a case. Surg Today 30:181–184, 2000.
27. Tien YW, Lee PH, Chang KJ. Enterolith: An unusual cause of afferent loop obstruction. Am J Gastroenterol 94:1391–1392, 1999.
28. Carbognin G, Biasiutti C, El-Khaldi M, et al: Afferent loop syndrome presenting as enterolith after Billroth II subtotal gastrectomy: A case report. Abdom Imag 25:129–131, 2000.
29. Hui MS, Perng HL, Choi WM, et al: Afferent loop syndrome complicated by duodenal phytobezoar after a Billroth-II subtotal gastrectomy. Am J Surg 92:1550–1552, 1997.
30. Muthukrishnan A, Shanthly N, Kumar S: Afferent loop syndrome: The role of Tc-99m mebrofenin hepatobiliary scintigraphy. Clin Nucl Med 25:492–494, 2000.
31. Taylor AR, Russ PD, Lee RE, et al: Acute afferent loop obstruction diagnosed with computed tomography: Case report. Can Assoc Radiol J 50:251–254, 1999.
32. McKee JD, Raju GP, Edelman RT, et al: MR cholangiography (MRCP) in diagnosis of afferent loop syndrome presenting as cholangitis. Dig Dis Sci 24:2082–2086, 1997.
33. Kitamura H, Miwa S, Nakata T, et al: Sonographic detection of visceral adhesion in percutaneous drainage of afferent-loop small intestine obstruction. J Clin Ultrasound 28:133–136, 2000.
34. Moriura S, Takayama Y, Nagata J, et al: Percutaneous bowel drainage for jaundice due to afferent loop obstruction following pancreatoduodenectomy: Report of a case. Surg Today 29:1098–1101, 1999.
35. Yao NS, Wu CW, Tiu CM, et al: Percutaneous transhepatic duodenal drainage as an alternative approach in afferent loop obstruction with secondary obstructive jaundice in recurrent gastric cancer. Cardiovasc Intervent Radiol 21:350–353, 1998.
36. Ritchie WP: Alkaline reflux gastritis. Ann Surg 203:537–544, 1986.
37. Collard JM, Romagnoli R: Roux-en-Y jejunal loop and bile reflux. Am J Surg 179:298–303, 2000.
38. Madura JA: Primary bile reflux gastritis: Which is better, Roux-en-Y or biliary diversion? Am Surg 66:417–423, 2000.
39. Madura JA, Grosfeld JL: Biliary diversion: A new method to prevent enterogastric reflux and reverse the Roux stasis syndrome. Arch Surg 132:245–249, 1997.
40. Martinez-Ramos C, Nunez Pena J, Sanz Lopez R, et al: Roux-en-Y

syndrome after surgical treatment of alkaline reflux gastritis. Rev Espanola Enfermed Dig 91:748–758, 1999.
41. Tu BL, Kelly KA: Surgical treatment of Roux stasis syndrome. J Gastroint Surg 3:613–617, 1999.
42. Hansson LE: Risk of stomach cancer in patients with peptic ulcer disease. World J Surg 24:315–320, 2000.
43. Safatle-Ribeiro AV, Ribereiro U Jr, Reynolds JC: Gastric stump cancer: What is the risk? Dig Dis 16:159–168, 1998.
44. von Holstein CS: Long-term prognosis after partial gastrectomy. World J Surg 24:307–314, 2000.
45. Leivonen M, Nordling S, Haglund C: Does *Helicobacter pylori* in the gastric stump increase the cancer risk after certain reconstruction types? Anticancer Res 175B:38–96, 1997.
46. van Rees BP, Tascilar M, Hrubin RH, et al: Remote partial gastrectomy as a risk factor for pancreatic cancer: Potential for preventive strategies. Ann Oncol 10:204–207, 1999.
47. Parr JJ, Grime S, Brownless S, et al: Relationship between gastric emptying of liquid and postvagotomy diarrhoea. Br J Surg 75:279–282, 1988.
48. al-Hadrani A, Lavelle-Jones M, Kennedy N, et al: Bile acid malabsorption in patients with post-vagotomy diarrhoea. Ann Chir Gynaecol 81: 351–353, 1992.
49. Eagon JC, Miedema BW, Kelly KA: Postgastrectomy syndromes. Surg Clin North Am 72:445–465, 1992.
50. O'Brien JD, Thompson DG, McIntyre A, et al: Effect of codeine and loperamide on upper intestinal transit and absorption in normal subjects and patients with postvagotomy diarrhoea. Gut 29:312–318, 1988.
51. Geer R, Richards WO, O'Dorisio TM, et al: Efficacy of octreotide acetate in treatment of severe postgastrectomy dumping syndrome. Ann Surg 212:678–687, 1990.
52. Gray JL, Debas HT, Mulvhill SJ: Control of dumping symptoms by somatostatin analogue in patients after gastric surgery. Arch Surg 126: 1231–1236, 1991.
53. Tulassay Z, Tulassay T, Gupta R, et al: Long-acting somatostatin analogue in dumping syndrome. Br J Surg 76:1294–1295, 1989.
54. Vecht J, Lamers CB, Masclee AA: Long-term results of octreotide therapy in severe dumping syndrome. Clin Endocrinol 51:619–624, 1999.
55. Vecht J, Masclee AA, Lamers CB: The dumping syndrome. Current insights into pathophysiology, diagnosis, and treatment. Surg Clin North Am 223[Suppl]:21–27, 2000.
56. Vecht J, Gielkens HA, Frolich M, et al: Vasoactive substances in early dumping syndrome: Effects of dumping provocation with and without octreotide. Eur J Clin Invest 27:680–684, 1997.
57. Hasler WL, Soudah HC, Owyang C: Mechanisms by which octreotide ameliorates symptoms in the dumping syndrome. J Pharmacol Exp Ther 227:1359–1365, 1996.
58. Primrose JN: Octreotide in the treatment of dumping syndrome. Digestion 45[Suppl 1]:49–58, 1990.
59. Richards WO, Geer R, O'Dorisio TM, et al: Octreotide acetate induces fasting small bowel motility in patients with dumping syndrome. J Surg Res 49:483–487, 1990.
60. Ng EK, Lam YH, Sung JJ, et al: Eradication of *Helicobacter pylori* prevents recurrence of ulcer after simple closure of duodenal ulcer perforation. Ann Surg 231:153–158, 2000.
61. Hermansson M, Stael von Holstein C, Zilling T: Surgical approach and prognostic factors after peptic ulcer perforation. Eur J Surg 165:566–572, 1999.
62. Kulkarni SH, Kshirsagar AY: Simple closure of perforated ulcer. J Indian Med Assoc 96:309–311, 1998.
63. Azagra JS, Goergen M, DeSimone IP, et al: The current role of laparoscopic surgery in the treatment of benign gastrointestinal diseases. Hepato-Gastroenterology 46:1522–1525, 1999.
64. Gomez-Ferrer F, Ballyque JG, Azagra S, et al: Laparoscopic surgery for duodenal ulcer: First results of a multicenter study applying a personal procedure. Hepato-Gastroenterology 46:1517–1521, 1999.
65. Bergamaschi R, Marvik R, Johnsen G, et al: Open vs. laparoscopic repair of perforated peptic ulcer. Surg Endosc 13:679–682, 1999.
66. Gilbert DA, Silverstein FE, Tedesco FJ, et al: The national ASGE survey on upper gastrointestinal bleeding. Gastrointest Endosc 94:94–102, 1982.
67. Rockall TA, Logan RF, Devlin HB, et al: Incidence of and mortality from acute upper gastrointestinal haemorrhage in the United Kingdom. Br Med J 311:222–226, 1995.
68. Sacks HS, Chalmers TC, Blum AL, et al: Endoscopic hemostasis: An effective therapy for bleeding ulcers. JAMA 264:494–499, 1990.
69. Cook DJ, Guyatt GH, Salena BJ, et al: Endoscopic therapy for acute nonvariceal upper gastrointestinal hemorrhage: A meta-analysis. Gastroenterology 102:139–148, 1992.
70. Lau JYW, Sung JJY, Lam YH, et al: Endoscopic retreatment compared with surgery in patients with recurrent bleeding after initial endoscopic control of bleeding ulcers. N Engl J Med 340:571–756, 1999.
71. Poxon VA, Keighly MR, Dykes PW, et al: Comparison of minimal and conventional surgery in patients with bleeding peptic ulcer: A multicenter trial. Br J Surg 78:1344–1345, 1991.
72. Millat B, Hay J, Valleur P, et al: Emergency surgical treatment for bleeding duodenal ulcer: Oversewing plus vagotomy versus gastric resection; a controlled, randomized trial. World J Surg 17:568–574, 1993.
73. Jaffin BW, Kaye MD: The prognosis of gastric outlet obstruction. Ann Surg 201:176–179, 1985.
74. Tung W, Strasberg SM: Peptic ulcer disease. In Jones DB, Wu JS, Soper NJ (eds): Laparoscopic Surgery: Principles and Procedures. St. Louis, Quality Medical Press, 1997, pp 205–220.
75. Mentes AS: Parietal cell vagotomy and dilatation for peptic duodenal stricture. Ann Surg 212:597–601, 1990.
76. Trout HH: Ulcer recurrence, morbidity, and mortality after operations for duodenal ulcer. Am J Surg 144:570, 1982.
77. McFadden DW, Zinner MJ: Reoperations for recurrent ulcer disease. Surg Clin North Am 71:77, 1991.

Chapter

43 GASTRITIS AND OTHER GASTROPATHIES

Edward L. Lee and Mark Feldman

Patients, clinicians, endoscopists, and pathologists have different concepts of what gastritis is. Some think of it as a symptom complex, others as a description of the endoscopic appearance of the stomach, and still others use the term to describe microscopic inflammation of the stomach. This third definition of gastritis is used in this chapter. There is not a close relationship between the presence of microscopic inflammation (histologic gastritis) and gastric symptoms (epigastric pain, nausea, vomiting, bleeding). The correlation between microscopic and gastroscopic abnormalities is also poor.[1–3] In fact, most patients with histologic gastritis are asymptomatic and have normal gastroscopic findings. Certain disorders of the gastric mucosa, including erosive processes and hyperplastic disorders, may be associated with little or no inflammation (gastritis). These conditions collectively are referred to as reactive and hyperplastic gastropathies, respectively.

By the earlier definition, a gastric biopsy must be obtained to be able to diagnose gastritis. Every biopsy represents an excellent opportunity for the clinician and pathologist to communicate to correlate clinical data, endoscopic findings, and pathology. Errors may occur when the pathologist attempts to diagnose biopsies without clinical input. It is important for the pathologist to become familiar with the range of normal gastric biopsy findings, because many gastrointestinal biopsies obtained endoscopically show normal mucosa.[4]

Indications for gastroscopic biopsies include gastric erosion or ulcer, thick gastric fold(s), gastric polyp(s) or mass(es), and diagnosis of *Helicobacter pylori* infection. A set of five biopsies should be taken from patients in whom clinical or endoscopic findings are suspicious for one of the forms of chronic, nonspecific gastritis (discussed later). Preferred sites for this set of biopsies are shown in Figure 43–1. The location of the biopsy sites should be identified for the pathologist on an accessioning form.

CLASSIFICATION

Currently there is no widely accepted classification of gastritis. The Sydney System of Classifying Gastritis was an attempt to unify terminology.[5] However, the complexity of the Sydney System precluded widespread use. Failure to obtain adequate numbers of biopsies from various regions of the stomach often prevents accurate classification and often precludes a thorough assessment of the distribution of gastritis.

In this chapter, we use a combination of classifications of gastritis by three experts: Rubin,[2] Appelman,[6] and Correa.[7] The keystone of the mentioned classification is the fact that *H. pylori* and nonsteroidal anti-inflammatory drugs (NSAIDs) are the most common causes of gastritis and reactive gastropathies (acute erosive gastritis), respectively. Table 43–1 provides an etiology-based classification of gastritis and gastropathies.

CHRONIC, NONSPECIFIC GASTRITIDES

Most forms of chronic, nonspecific gastritis are clinically silent. Their importance relates to the fact that these gastritides are risk factors for other conditions such as peptic ulcer disease and gastric neoplasms. Three types of chronic, nonspecific gastritis are recognized (Fig. 43–2).

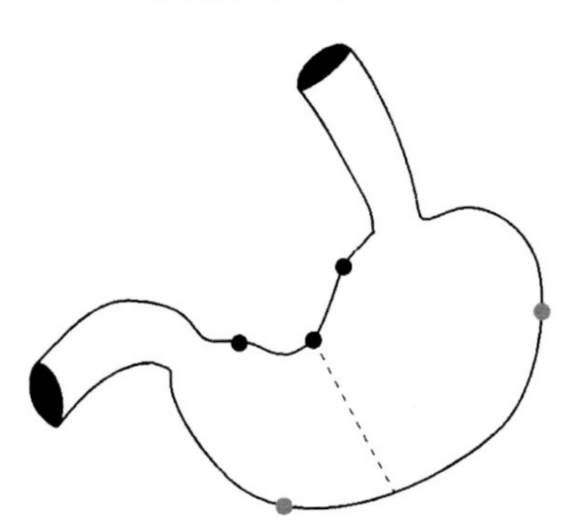

Figure 43–1. Gastric biopsy protocol. Gastric sites from which mucosal biopsies should be obtained. Biopsies from the antrum (greater and lesser curvature) and from the incisura are useful for diagnosing *Helicobacter pylori* infection. Biopsies from the gastric body (greater and lesser curvature) are useful for diagnosing diffuse corporal atrophic gastritis. Biopsies from the antrum and body in combination are useful for diagnosing multifocal atrophic gastritis. Other gastritides can also be diagnosed (see Table 43–1).

Biopsies from the antrum and the incisura are useful for diagnosing *H. pylori* infection with its diffuse antral-predominant gastritis (DAG). However, biopsies from the gastric body mucosa may be more diagnostic for *H. pylori* infection in some patients treated with proton pump inhibitors. Multifocal atrophic gastritis (MAG) is patchy and involves the antrum and body mucosa and sometimes, but not always, is associated with *H. pylori* infection. The diagnosis of diffuse corporal atrophic gastritis (DCAG; autoimmune or type A gastritis) can be confirmed with multiple biopsies from the gastric body that show atrophy and biopsies from the antrum that do not show atrophy. In most cases, biopsies are obtained at the time of endoscopy. However, gastric mucosal biopsies may be effectively obtained through a nasogastric tube under fluoroscopic guidance, a nonendoscopic method for obtaining tissue from the antral and body mucosa and for diagnosing *H. pylori* infection.[8]

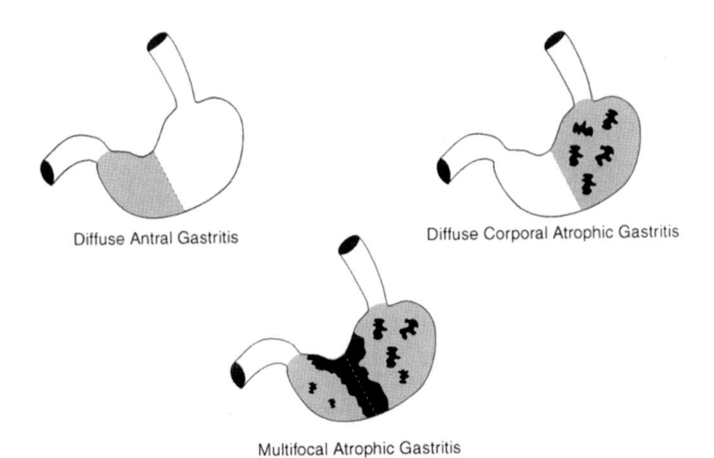

Figure 43–2. Topographic patterns of chronic, nonspecific gastritis. The black areas in the schematic of diffuse corporal atrophic gastritis and multifocal atrophic gastritis represent areas of focal atrophy and intestinal metaplasia.

Diffuse Antral-Predominant Gastritis

DAG is caused by infection of the antral mucosa with *H. pylori*.[2, 6, 7] In the United States, DAG is seen mainly in whites, and there is no increased risk of gastric cancer. Most patients with DAG are asymptomatic. In most patients the antrum appears normal to the endoscopist; some patients with active disease in the antrum may demonstrate red streaks.

A diffuse, chronic inflammatory infiltrate that may include neutrophilic infiltration expands the lamina propria and epithelium (Fig. 43–3). The presence of acute inflammatory cells is best designated an "active" gastritis and not "acute" gastritis. Additional microscopic changes include injury to the surface and foveolar epithelium with loss of apical mucin and reactive nuclear changes and erosions.[6, 9, 10] Lymphoid follicles with germinal centers are characteristic of an infection with *H. pylori*.[3, 4, 8, 11] *H. pylori* organisms lie in the superficial mucous layer along the mucosal surface and

Table 43–1 | **Gastritis and Gastropathy Classification**

Gastritides
Chronic nonspecific
Diffuse antral-predominant gastritis with *Helicobacter pylori*
Multifocal atrophic pangastritis with or without *H. pylori*
Diffuse corporal atrophic gastritis
Infectious
Viral
Bacterial
H. pylori (see Chapter 39)
Others, including mycobacterial infection
Fungal
Parasitic
Granulomatous
Crohn's disease
Sarcoidosis
Foreign bodies
Infections
Tumor associated
Distinctive forms
Collagenous
Lymphocytic
Eosinophilic
Miscellaneous
Gastritis cystica profunda
Graft-versus-host disease
Gastropathies
Reactive (erosive "gastritis")
Aspirin/NSAIDs/other medications
Alcohol
Cocaine
Stress
Radiation
Bile reflux
Ischemia
Bezoar
Prolapse/hiatal hernia
Congestive
Trauma (e.g., gastric tubes)
Hyperplastic
Ménétrier's disease and hyperplastic, hypersecretory gastropathy
Zollinger-Ellison syndrome (see Chapter 41)

Adapted from Chan Y, Hui P, Chan J, et al: Epithelial damage by *Helicobacter pylori* in gastric ulcers. Histopathology 19:47, 1991; Price A: Histologic aspects of *Campylobacter pylori* colonization and infection of gastric and duodenal mucosa. Scand J Gastroenterol 23:21, 1988; and Rosh J, Kurfist L, Benkov K, et al: *Helicobacter pylori* and gastric lymphonodular hyperplasia in children. Am J Gastroenterol 87:135, 1992.

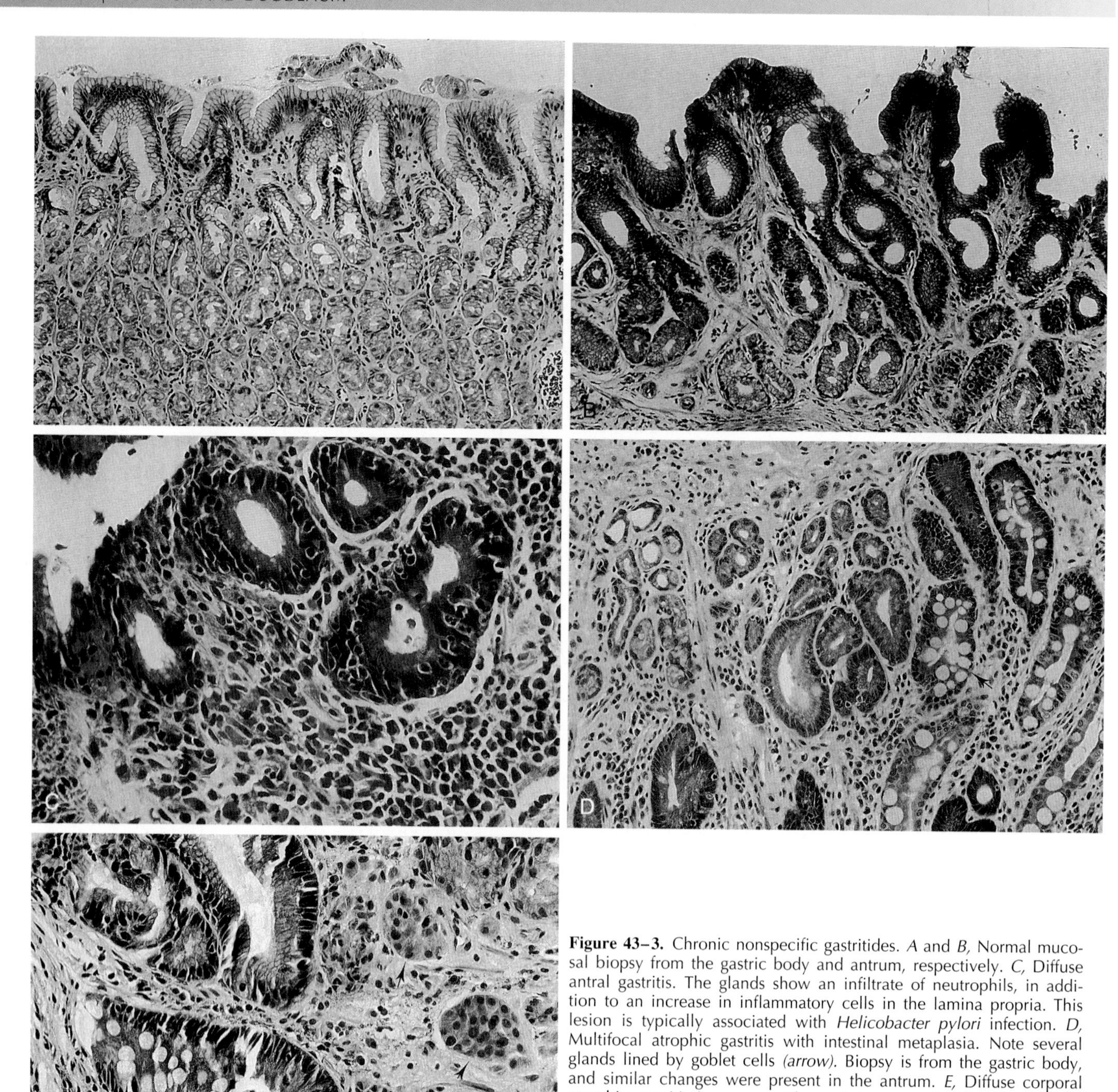

Figure 43–3. Chronic nonspecific gastritides. *A* and *B,* Normal mucosal biopsy from the gastric body and antrum, respectively. *C,* Diffuse antral gastritis. The glands show an infiltrate of neutrophils, in addition to an increase in inflammatory cells in the lamina propria. This lesion is typically associated with *Helicobacter pylori* infection. *D,* Multifocal atrophic gastritis with intestinal metaplasia. Note several glands lined by goblet cells *(arrow).* Biopsy is from the gastric body, and similar changes were present in the antrum. *E,* Diffuse corporal atrophic gastritis in a man with pernicious anemia. The gland in the lower left is lined by goblet cells. Nests of enterochromaffin-like cells are also visible *(arrows).*

within the gastric pits. Although the organisms can be seen in routine hematoxylin and eosin–stained tissue when numerous organisms are present, special stains are useful when few organisms are present. Stains that may be used to highlight the organisms are Acridine orange fluorescent stain, Giemsa stain, Warthin-Starry silver stain, Gram's stain, and immunocytochemical stains.[12–14] *Helicobacter heilmanii*–like spiral bacteria may be a less frequent cause of active gastritis.[15–17] The organisms originally known as *Gastrospirillium hominis* are longer than *H. pylori* and have multiple spirals.[15, 16] A topographic study of *H. pylori* density and distribution and the comparison of biopsy sites for the histopathologic diagnosis of *H. pylori* concludes that two antral biopsy specimens, one from the lesser and one from the greater curvature, have close to 100% sensitivity for detecting *H. pylori* infection[18] (see Fig. 43–1). Biopsy specimens from the corpus increase the diagnostic yield if extensive intestinal metaplasia is present in the antrum.[18]

Multifocal Atrophic Gastritis

MAG is characterized by the involvement of the antrum and body with mucosal atrophy and intestinal metaplasia.[7, 19–24] Endoscopy may show a pale mucosa, shiny surface, and prominent submucosal vessels.[25] The pathogenesis of MAG is multifactorial. *H. pylori* plays an important role and has been identified in about 85% of patients with MAG. Genetic and environmental factors, especially diet, are also important. Certain population groups are predisposed to MAG, including African Americans, Scandinavians, Asians, Hispanics, and immigrants from Central and South America, Japan, and China.

In patients with MAG, intestinal metaplasia is a risk factor for dysplasia and gastric cancer, usually the intestinal type[7, 21, 22, 26–30] (see Chapter 44). Inflammation in MAG destroys gastric epithelial cells and eventually the atrophic glands are replaced by metaplastic epithelium.[7, 22–24] Because criteria for gastric atrophy among pathologists are debated, intestinal metaplasia is the most reliable marker of atrophy. Intestinal metaplasia of the gastric mucosa can be classified into three types as described in Chapter 44 (Table 44–2), where their possible associations with the intestinal type of gastric cancer are discussed.

Diffuse Corporal Atrophic Gastritis

DCAG is an autoimmune destruction of fundic glands. DCAG is relatively uncommon, accounting for less than 5% of all cases of chronic gastritis. Endoscopic features of DCAG include effacement of the gastric folds and a thin fundic mucosa. DCAG is the pathologic process in patients with pernicious anemia, an autoimmune disorder usually occurring in patients of northern European or Scandinavian background.[31, 32] Patients with DCAG exhibit achlorhydria (or hypochlorhydria), hypergastrinemia secondary to achlorhydria, and antral G-cell hyperplasia, and they often have circulating parietal cell and intrinsic factor antibodies.[6, 7, 32] The incomplete (colonic) type of intestinal metaplasia may occur in DCAG and be a risk factor for gastric carcinoma in areas of the world that experience a high incidence of gastric carcinoma.[33] In the United States, the risk of gastric carcinoma in DCAG is small, and therefore screening for gastric carcinoma in patients with DCAG or pernicious anemia is not recommended.[34]

Atrophic glands with extensive intestinal metaplasia are confined to the fundus. Early in the course of this disease, atrophy may be focal and, rarely, the disease progresses to diffuse (complete) atrophy. Hypergastrinemia, a consequence of achlorhydria, is associated with an increase in enterochromaffin-like cell hyperplasia and gastric carcinoid tumors.[35–39] Gastric carcinoid tumors are discussed further in Chapter 44.

INFECTIOUS GASTRITIS

Viruses

CYTOMEGALOVIRUS[40–48]. Cytomegalovirus (CMV) may affect the esophagus, stomach, small bowel, colon, and anus. Gastrointestinal CMV infection usually occurs in the immunocompromised patient. Patients with malignant disease, immunosuppression (especially due to steroid therapy), transplants, and acquired immunodeficiency syndrome (AIDS) may experience life-threatening infections. Rarely, CMV infection may occur in an immunocompetent patient.

Patients with CMV infection of the stomach may experience epigastric pain, fever, and atypical lymphocytosis. Upper gastrointestinal tract radiographic studies may reveal a rigid and narrowed gastric antrum suggestive of an infiltrating antral neoplasm. Endoscopic studies may reveal a congested and edematous mucosa of the gastric antrum, covered with multiple ulcerations, suggestive of gastric malignancy, submucosal antral mass, or gastric ulcer (Fig. 43–4).

Examination of biopsy specimens shows inflammatory debris, chronic active gastritis, and enlarged cells with CMV inclusion bodies indicative of an active infection (see Fig. 43–4). "Owl-eye" intranuclear inclusions are the hallmark of CMV infection in routine hematoxylin and eosin histologic preparations and may be found in vascular endothelial cells, mucosal epithelial cells, and connective tissue stromal cells. Multiple, granular, basophilic, cytoplasmic inclusions may also be present. Usual treatment with intravenous ganciclovir or foscarnet is of uncertain value (see Chapter 28).

HERPESVIRUS[49–52]. Gastric involvement with herpes simplex and varicella/zoster virus is rare. Infected individuals experience the infection at an early age, and the virus remains dormant until reactivation. Activation has been related to radiation therapy, chemotherapy, lymphoma, and cancer. The typical immunocompromised patient may experience nausea, vomiting, fever, chills, fatigue, cough, and weight loss. Barium-air double-contrast radiographs show a cobblestone pattern, shallow ulcerations with a ragged contour, and an interlacing network of crevices filled with barium that correspond to areas of ulceration. Upper gastrointestinal endoscopy reveals multiple small, raised ulcerated plaques or linear, superficial ulcers in a criss-crossing pattern, giving the stomach a cobblestone appearance. Grossly, the ulcers are multiple, small, and of uniform size. Microscopically, cytologic smears and biopsy specimens show numerous single cells and clumps of cells, with ground-glass nuclei and eosinophilic intranuclear inclusion bodies surrounded by halos. Brush cytology and biopsies should be performed at the time of endoscopy. Brush cytology has the advantage of sampling a wider area of mucosa, because biopsies may not be representative. Treatment with acyclovir is reasonable but of unproven value.

Bacteria

SUPPURATIVE (PHLEGMONOUS) GASTRITIS[53–56]. Phlegmonous gastritis is a rare bacterial infection of the submucosa and muscularis propria of the stomach. Acute necrotizing gastritis (gangrene of the stomach) is a rare, often fatal disease that is now thought to be a variant of phlegmonous gastritis.[57] It has been suggested that acute necrotizing gastritis begins as phlegmonous gastritis, producing primary necrosis and gangrene. Acute necrotizing gastritis and phlegmonous gastritis have been associated with recent large intake of alcohol, upper respiratory tract infection, and AIDS, and with an infected peritoneojugular venous shunt.

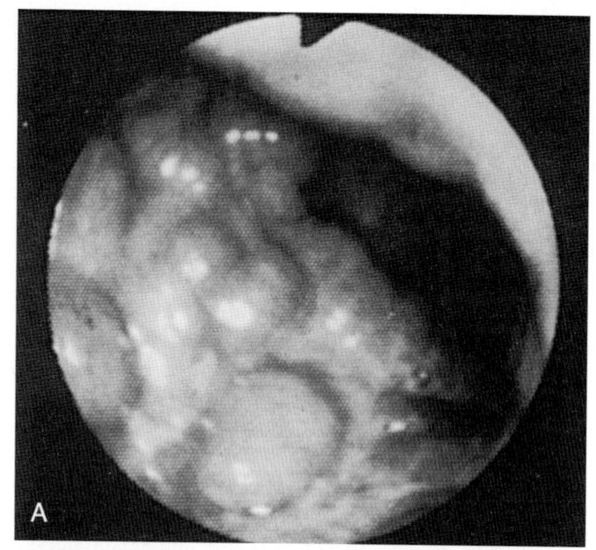

Figure 43–4. Cytomegalovirus (CMV) gastritis. *A,* Endoscopic photograph of the midbody greater curvature of a patient with AIDS and culture-proven CMV-associated gastritis. The mucosa has a thickened, bumpy appearance. *B,* Low-power histology of CMV gastritis. An acute inflammatory infiltrate is present in the lamina propria. Glandular destruction and reactive glands are present. Cystic glands are also evident. *C,* High-power view of the cystic area deep in the mucosa in *B.* There are several cytomegalic cells with the typical intranuclear and intracytoplasmic inclusions of cytomegalovirus.

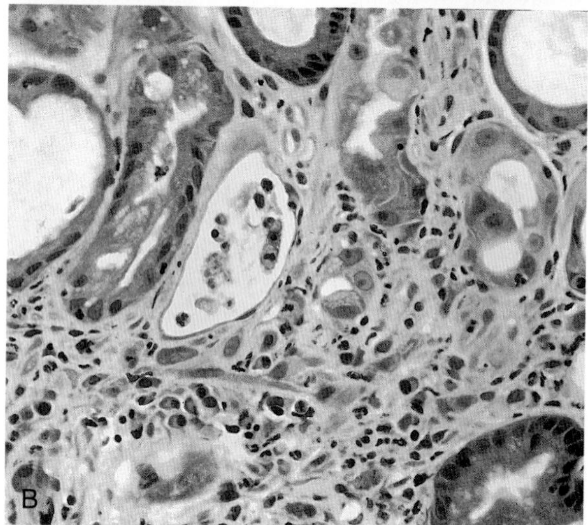

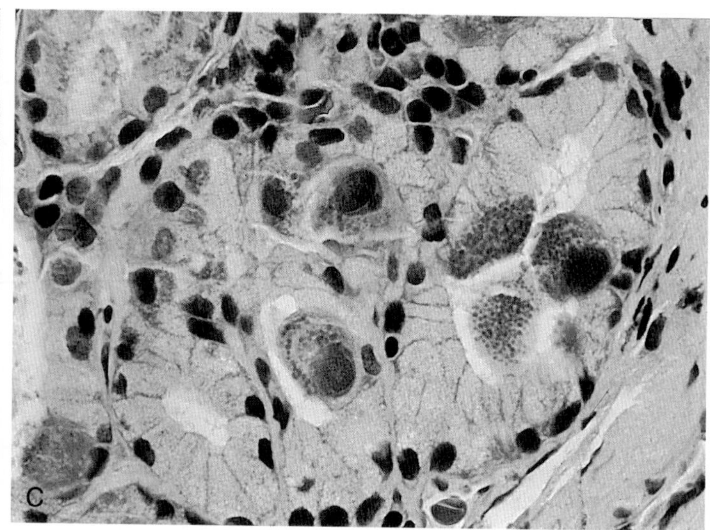

Patients typically present with acute upper abdominal pain, peritonitis, purulent ascitic fluid, fever, and hypotension. Preoperative diagnosis is rare, but gastroscopy with or without biopsy and culture of gastric contents may establish the diagnosis. Grossly, the stomach wall appears thick and edematous with multiple perforations and the mucosa may demonstrate a granular, green-black exudate. Microscopically, the edematous submucosa reveals an intense polymorphonuclear infiltrate and numerous gram-positive and gram-negative organisms as well as vascular thrombosis. The mucosa may demonstrate extensive areas of necrosis.

The mortality rate of phlegmonous gastritis is close to 60%, probably because it is so often misdiagnosed and because treatment is initiated too late. The definitive treatment is resection or drainage of the stomach, combined with large doses of systemic antibiotics, usually penicillin.

Emphysematous gastritis is a variant of phlegmonous gastritis in which the infection in the gastric wall is due to gas-forming organisms such as *Clostridium welchii*.[58, 59] Predisposing factors are gastroduodenal surgery, ingestion of corrosive materials, gastroenteritis, or gastrointestinal infarction. Radiographic studies show gas bubbles conforming to the contour of the stomach.

***MYCOBACTERIUM* TUBERCULOSIS**[60–65]. Gastric tuberculosis is a rare entity that usually occurs in association with pulmonary tuberculosis. Patients typically present with abdominal pain, nausea and vomiting, gastrointestinal bleeding, fever, and weight loss. Gastric tuberculosis may be associated with gastric outlet obstruction or with bleeding from a tuberculous gastric ulcer. Radiographic studies reveal an enlarged stomach with narrowed, deformed antrum with prepyloric ulcerations. Upper endoscopy demonstrates ulcers, masses, or gastric outlet obstruction. Grossly, the stomach may demonstrate multiple small mucosal erosions, ulcers, an infiltrating mass (hypertrophic) form, a sclerosing inflammatory form, acute miliary dissemination, and pyloric obstruction either by extension from peripyloric nodes, or by invasion from other neighboring organs. Biopsies show necrotizing granulomas with the presence of acid-fast bacilli, best demonstrated with Kinyoun acid-fast stain. Treatment is discussed in Chapter 28.

***MYCOBACTERIUM AVIUM (INTRACELLULARE)* COMPLEX**[66–71]. Although *Mycobacterium avium* complex (MAC) is the most common opportunistic bacterial infection among patients with AIDS, the stomach is rarely involved. Gastric MAC may be associated with a chronic gastric ulcer refractory to conventional antiulcer therapy. Patients may present with fever, night sweats, anorexia, weight loss, diarrhea, abdominal pain, chylous ascites, severe gastrointestinal hemorrhage, or chronic gastric ulcer. Serial computed tomographic scans of the abdomen may show mesenteric lymphadenopathy. Endoscopy may show a chronic gastric ulcer, a coarsely granular duodenal mucosa, or fine white duodenal nodules. Microscopically, the gastric mucosa demonstrates numerous foamy histiocytes containing many acid-fast bacilli. Treatment of MAC is difficult and is discussed in Chapter 28.

ACTINOMYCOSIS[72–74]. Primary gastric actinomycosis is a rare, chronic, progressive, suppurative disease characterized by formation of multiple abscesses, draining sinuses, abundant granulation, and dense fibrous tissue. Abdominal actinomycosis is more common and has a predilection for the terminal ileum, cecum, and appendix. The presenting symptoms include fever, epigastric pain, epigastric swelling, abdominal wall abscess with fistula, and upper gastrointestinal bleeding. Radiographic studies frequently suggest a malignant tumor or an ulcer. Endoscopy is suggestive of a circumscribed and ulcerated gastric carcinoma. Grossly, the resected stomach demonstrates a large, ill-defined, ulcerated mass in the wall of the stomach that measures up to 4 cm. Microscopically, multiple abscesses show the infective agent, *Actinomyces israelii*, a gram-positive filamentous anaerobic bacterium that normally resides in the mouth. A biopsy of a mass containing pus or a biopsy of a draining sinus may reveal actinomycosis. If the disease is recognized only by histologic examination, the prognosis is good. Prolonged (6- to 12-month) high-dose antibiotic treatment with penicillin or amoxicillin is indicated.

SYPHILIS[75–82]. The incidence of syphilis in the United States increased 34% from 13.7 to 18.4 cases per 100,000 persons between 1981 and 1989. Several case reports and small series emphasize the importance of the gastroenterologist and pathologist remaining alert to the protean manifestations of syphilis and familiar with the histopathologic pattern of the disease. Gastric involvement in secondary or tertiary syphilis is rarely recognized clinically, and its diagnosis by examination of endoscopic biopsy specimens has been reported infrequently. The features of syphilis in the stomach should be recognized because they can provide a window of opportunity for effective antibiotic therapy before the disease progresses and causes permanent disability. Patients typically present with symptoms of peptic ulcer disease and the most common gastric complaint is upper gastrointestinal tract bleeding. Other diseases that may mimic gastric syphilis include benign ulcer disease, gastric carcinoma, gastric lymphoma, tuberculosis, or Crohn's disease involving the stomach. The acute gastritis of early secondary syphilis produces the earliest radiologically detectable sign of the disease. Radiographs show a nonspecific gastritis, with diffusely thickened folds that may become nodular with or without detectable ulcers. Strictures in the mid-stomach ("hourglass" stomach) may be present (Fig. 43–5*A*). Endoscopy shows numerous shallow, irregular ulcers with overlying white exudate and surrounding erythema (Fig. 43–5*B*). The surrounding mucosa also demonstrates a nodular appearance. Gastroscopy may also demonstrate prominent edematous, gastric folds.

Grossly, the stomach may be thickened, contracted, and show multiple serpiginous ulcers. Partial gastrectomy specimens may show compact, thick, mucosal rugae and numerous small mucosal ulcers. Microscopically, biopsies show severe gastritis with dense plasma cell infiltrate in the lamina propria, varying numbers of neutrophils and lymphocytes, gland destruction, vasculitis, and granulomas. Warthin-Starry silver stain or modified Steiner silver impregnation stain reveals numerous spirochetes. Serum VDRL and Treponema immunofluorescence studies may be positive, and the *Treponema pallidum* gene may be detected by the polymerase chain reaction. Treatment with penicillin is highly effective (Fig. 43–5*C*).

Fungi

CANDIDIASIS[83–90]. Fungal contamination of gastric ulcers with *Candida* species is not uncommon. Data from some studies suggest that fungal colonization of gastric ulcers has little clinical significance, whereas others suggest that fungal infection aggravates and perpetuates gastric ulceration. Endoscopically, gastric ulcers associated with *Candida albicans* tend to be larger in diameter and are more often suspected to be malignant than typical gastric ulcers. Diffuse superficial erosions may be noted.

Fungal colonization of the gastrointestinal tract is frequent in patients with underlying malignancy and in immunocompromised patients who have been treated with antibiotics or corticosteroids but may occur also in immunocompetent patients. Symptoms are nonspecific. Massive growth of yeast organisms in the gastric lumen (yeast bezoar) is a potential complication of gastric surgical procedures, usually for peptic ulcer disease. *Candida* infection of the stomach may occur in alcoholic patients who ingest corrosive chemicals, such as concentrated sulfuric acid and thiocyanates. Radiologic studies show tiny aphthoid erosions, which represent the earliest detectable radiographic change in gastric candidiasis. Aphthoid ulcers progress to deep linear ulcers.

Grossly, the gastric mucosa demonstrates tiny aphthous erosions; widespread punctate, linear ulcerations; or gastric ulcers. Microscopically, the layer of necrotic fibrinoid debris demonstrates yeasts or pseudohyphae. The organisms can be seen in the hematoxylin and eosin stain; however, special stains such as periodic acid–Schiff-diastase stain or Gomori methenamine silver stain may be required. Treatment is usually not needed, but if symptomatic candidiasis is suspected, fluconazole is reasonable, but of unproven efficacy.

HISTOPLASMOSIS[91–93]. Progressive disseminated histoplasmosis is rare, occurring most frequently in the very young or elderly or in those with immunodeficiency. Although disseminated histoplasmosis can involve any portion of the gastrointestinal tract, gastric involvement is rare. Hypertrophic gastric folds or a mass that mimics a gastric carcinoma may be associated with gastric histoplasmosis. Radiographic studies may demonstrate an annular infiltrating lesion of the stomach and endoscopy may demonstrate enlarged and reddened gastric folds. Biopsy specimens show an intensive infiltration of macrophages containing *Histoplasma* capsulation. Gastric histoplasmosis has also been associated with a fatal hemorrhage from a gastric ulcer. Treatment with intravenous amphotericin B is appropriate.

PHYCOMYCOSIS[94–97]. Gastric phycomycosis (also called *zygomycosis*) is a rare and highly lethal fungal infection. Phycomycosis usually affects the sinuses, central nervous system, or lungs and is rarely confined to the gastrointestinal tract. Risk factors include malnutrition, immunosuppression, antibiotic therapy, and acidosis, usually diabetes ketoacidosis. Gastric phycomycosis can be classified as invasive or noninvasive (colonization). The former is characterized by deep invasion of the stomach wall and by blood vessel involvement with the fungus. Abdominal pain is the most frequent presenting complaint. In the noninvasive type, the fungus colonizes the superficial mucosa without causing an inflammatory response.

Grossly, surgical specimens from affected patients reveal hemorrhagic necrosis involving the mucosa and gastric wall. Microscopically, nonseptate 10- to 20-μm hyphae branched at right angles are present in the tissue, and they infiltrate into blood vessel walls. Treatment is resection of the affected necrotic portion of the stomach. Unfortunately, invasive gastric phycomycosis is almost always fatal.

Parasites (see also Chapter 99)

CRYPTOSPORIDIOSIS[98, 99]. Cryptosporidiosis may rarely involve the stomach. Gastric outlet obstruction and antral stric-

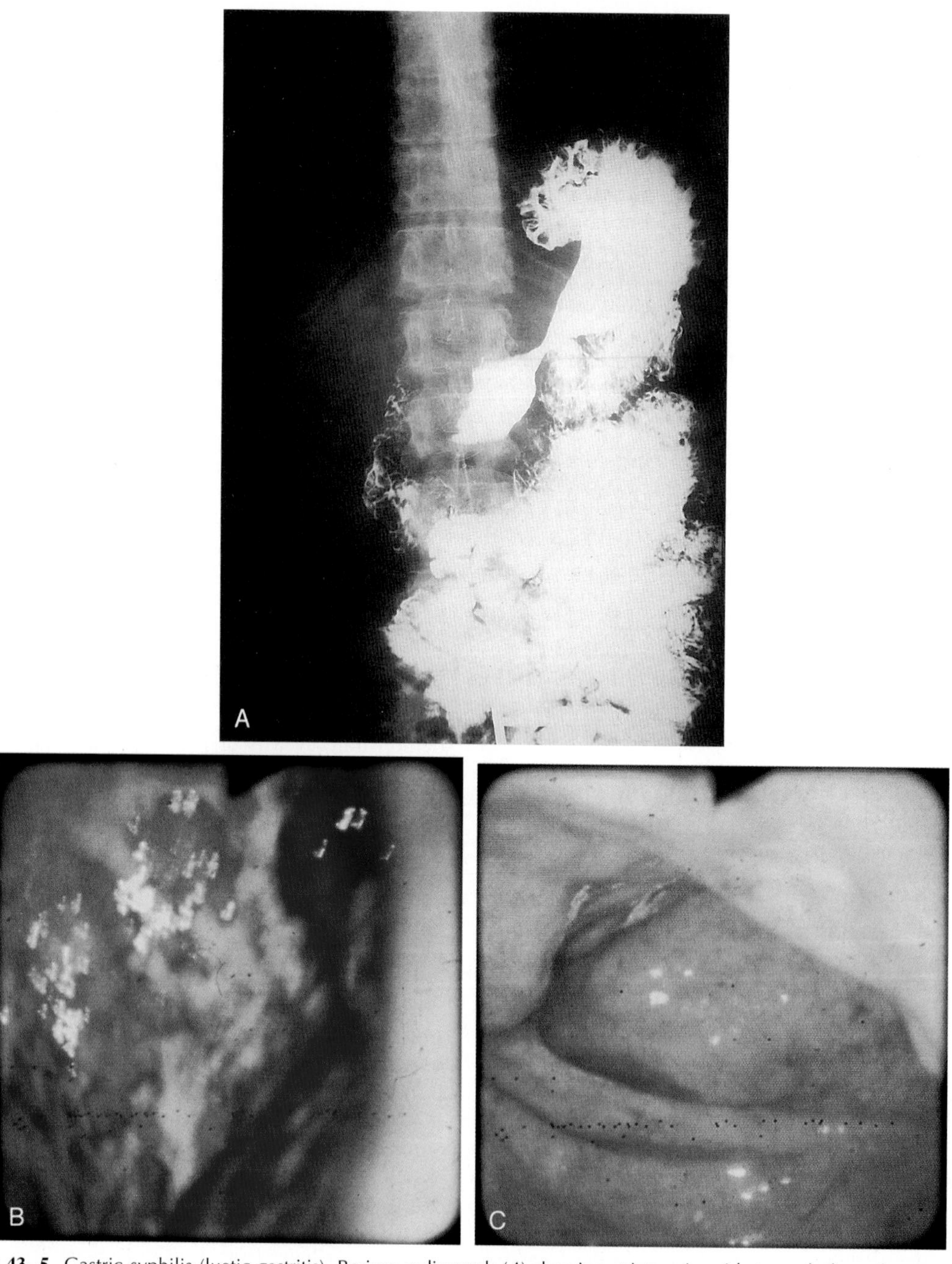

Figure 43–5. Gastric syphilis (luetic gastritis). Barium radiograph (*A*) showing stricture in mid-stomach (hourglass stomach), with antral deformity. Endoscopic appearance before (*B*) and 4 weeks after (*C*) penicillin therapy in another patient with gastric syphilis.

ture due to cryptosporidiosis have been reported in patients with AIDS and diarrhea.

STRONGYLOIDIASIS[100–103]. The stomach is rarely involved by *Strongyloides stercoralis*. However, the organisms may colonize the intact gastric mucosa and may be associated with a bleeding peptic ulcer. *S. stercoralis* hyperinfection has been associated with cimetidine therapy in an immunosuppressed patient and was diagnosed by endoscopic gastric biopsy. Diagnosis can be made by endoscopic biopsy, examination of stools, examination of duodenal aspirate, and examination of peripheral smear with elevated eosinophil count. Disseminated strongyloidiasis can be rapidly fatal. Treatment is discussed in Chapter 99.

ANISAKIASIS[104–106]. Invasive anisakiasis may occur after the ingestion of raw marine fish containing nematode larvae of the genus *Anisakis*. Hundreds of cases of anisakiasis have been diagnosed in Japan, and the number of reported cases in the United States has also increased. The parasite may migrate into the wall of the stomach, small intestine, or colon. Typically, patients present with sporadic epigastric pain or have no symptoms at all, and misdiagnosis is common. Some patients may experience a mild peripheral eosinophilia. Radiographic studies may reveal notched-shadow defects suggestive of a gastric tumor.

Grossly, the stomach demonstrates multiple erosive foci with hemorrhage and small 5- to 10-mm gastric lesions in the stomach wall. Microscopically, sections of the stomach show a marked eosinophilic granulomatous inflammatory process with intramural abscesses and granulation tissue. The eosinophilic abscess may contain a small worm measuring 0.3 mm in diameter, which can be identified as the larval form. The diagnosis may be confirmed by a serodiagnostic test for human anisakiasis on the patient's serum when the larvae may no longer be detectable by endoscopy.

ASCARIASIS[107, 108]. Although gastric ascariasis is rare, patients have experienced chronic, intermittent gastric outlet obstruction caused by roundworms *(Ascaris lumbricoides)* inhabiting the stomach. Gastric ascariasis has also been associated with upper gastrointestinal hemorrhage with endoscopic examination showing several *Ascaris* worms in the stomach and duodenum.

HOOKWORM. Endoscopic discovery and capture of *Necator americanus* in the stomach has been reported.[109]

GRANULOMATOUS GASTRITIDES

A variety of granulomatous diseases affect the stomach. The differential diagnosis of granulomatous gastritis includes Crohn's disease and sarcoidosis (discussed later), as well as foreign bodies,[110] lymphoma,[111] Whipple's disease (see Chapter 95),[112] Langerhans cell histiocytosis (gastric eosinophilic granuloma),[113] granulomatous vasculitis[114] (Churg-Strauss syndrome; see Chapter 29), and chronic granulomatous disease of childhood.[115] Isolated (idiopathic) granulomatous gastritis also occurs.[116–122]

Crohn's Disease[123–126]

In two studies, Crohn's disease was the most common disease associated with granulomatous gastritis.[116, 117] Crohn's disease of the stomach is uncommon, however, and almost always occurs together with intestinal disease (see Chapter 103). Cases isolated to the stomach have been reported. The diagnosis of isolated Crohn's disease of the stomach should be made with caution, and close follow-up is indicated for the subsequent development of Crohn's disease elsewhere in the gastrointestinal tract or of other granulomatous disease.

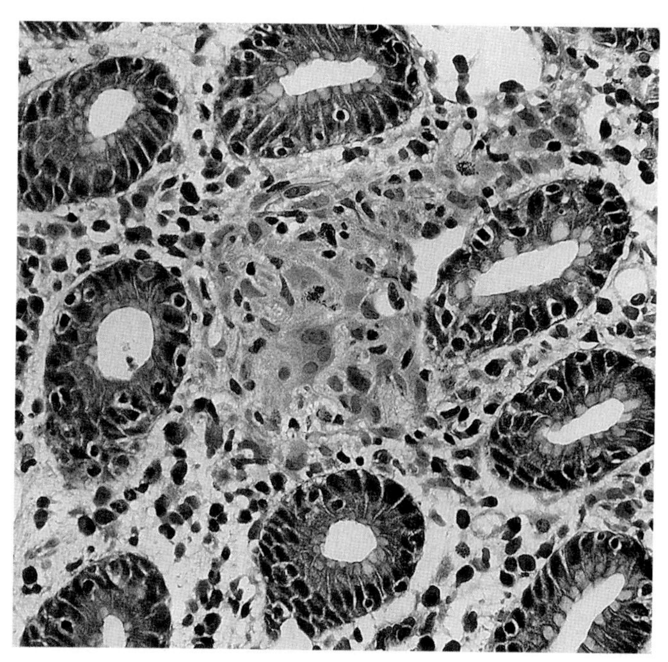

Figure 43–6. Granulomatous gastritis due to Crohn's disease. A noncaseating granuloma is present within the lamina propria.

Symptoms are nonspecific and include nausea and vomiting, epigastric pain, anorexia, and weight loss. Radiologic studies show antral fold thickening, antral narrowing, shallow ulcers (aphthae), or deeper ulcers. Involvement of the stomach from adjacent ileal or colonic disease segments is best visualized by radiologic examination. Endoscopy allows better visualization of mucosal defects and is characterized by reddened mucosa, irregularly shaped ulcers, and erosions in a disrupted mucosal pattern. Nodular lesions occur and often reveal the presence of erosions on the top of nodules. An atypical cobblestone pattern may be associated with the nodules surrounded by fissure-like ulceration. In contrast with peptic ulcers, the ulcerations and erosions of Crohn's disease are frequently serpiginous or longitudinal, rarely round or oval in shape. Ulcerations or erosions associated with Crohn's disease of the stomach typically are most commonly located in the antrum and the prepyloric region.

The microscopic features of surgical specimens of gastric Crohn's disease are similar to those in the ileum or colon (see Chapter 103). They include ulcers, granulomas, transmural chronic inflammation, and marked submucosal fibrosis (Fig. 43–6). Granulomas may be present in endoscopically normal antral mucosa. Treatment is discussed in Chapter 103.

Sarcoidosis[127–131]

Gastrointestinal manifestations of sarcoidosis are rare (see Chapter 29). Sarcoidosis is a systemic disease, and the diagnosis of sarcoidosis of the stomach should not be made in the absence of disease in other organs. More than 60 cases of gastric sarcoidosis have been reported, making the stomach the most common part of the gastrointestinal tract affected.

Affected patients, usually in the 3rd to 5th decade of life, typically present with epigastric pain, nausea, vomiting, and weight loss. Occasionally they present with massive hemorrhage. Gastric sarcoidosis may cause pyloric outlet obstruction, achlorhydria, and pernicious anemia. Radiographically, gastric sarcoidosis may mimic the diffuse form of gastric carcinoma ("linitis plastica") or Ménétrier's disease.

Endoscopy may reveal a narrow distal half of the stomach with multiple prepyloric ulcers or erosions, atrophy, thick gastric folds with a diffuse cobblestone appearance, or normal mucosa associated with microscopic granulomas.

Surgical specimens of patients with gastric sarcoidosis show a thickened stomach wall with foci of erosions and ulcers. Microscopically, mucosal biopsies show multiple noncaseating granulomas. However, the presence of noncaseating granulomas in gastrointestinal tissue is a nonspecific finding, and special stains should be performed to rule out infections, especially tuberculosis. In some cases it may be difficult to differentiate gastric sarcoidosis from gastric Crohn's disease.

Glucocorticoid therapy is the cornerstone of treatment for gastric sarcoidosis. Subtotal gastric resection is reserved for patients with obstruction and severe hemorrhage.

Xanthogranulomatous Gastritis[132]

Xanthogranulomatous gastritis is characterized by inflammation of the gastric wall by foamy histiocytes, inflammatory cells, multinucleated giant cells, and fibrosis. The destructive inflammatory process may extend into adjacent organs and simulate a neoplasm. Xanthogranulomatous gastritis has been associated with xanthogranulomatous cholecystitis.

DISTINCTIVE FORMS OF GASTRITIS

Collagenous Gastritis[133–140]

Subepithelial fibrosis has been reported in the colon (collagenous colitis), in the small bowel (collagenous sprue), and in the stomach (collagenous gastritis). Collagenous gastritis is a rare form of gastritis, and only seven cases have been reported in the literature. Collagenous gastritis may be associated with collagenous colitis and lymphocytic colitis.

Patients experience intermittent, epigastric abdominal pain, hematemesis, hematochezia, anemia, diarrhea, and hypotension. Upper gastrointestinal barium radiography may demonstrate an abnormal mucosal surface with a mosaic-like pattern in the body of the stomach, corresponding to mucosal nodularity. Endoscopy may reveal multiple, diffusely scattered, discrete submucosal hemorrhages, erosions, and nodularity of the body of the stomach along the greater curvature.

Biopsy specimens from the body and antrum of the stomach reveal a patchy, chronic, superficial gastritis, focal atrophy, and focal deposition of collagen in the subepithelial region of the lamina propria, which measures from 20 to 75 mm in thickness. Tiny areas of erosions of the surface epithelium are present, and the inflammatory infiltrate consists of mainly plasma cells and intraepithelial lymphocytes. Little is known about the etiology, natural history, and proper treatment of this rare condition.

Lymphocytic Gastritis[141–157]

Lymphocytic gastritis is a relatively new histopathologic entity characterized by a dense lymphocytic infiltration of surface and pit gastric epithelium (Fig. 43–7*A*). Studies have suggested that lymphocytic gastritis is related to an endoscopic form of gastropathy known as varioliform gastritis. Lymphocytic gastritis is also seen in *H. pylori* infection and

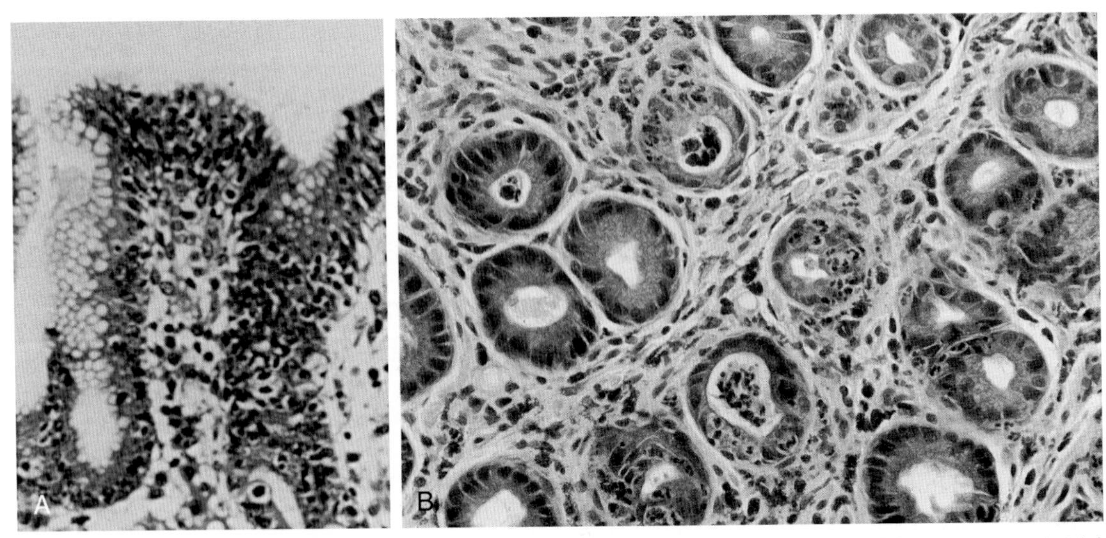

Figure 43–7. Examples of two distinctive forms of gastritis: lymphocytic gastritis *(A)* and eosinophilic gastritis *(B)*. *A*, High-power view of the oxyntic gland mucosa shows numerous dark-staining mononuclear cells within the surface and pit epithelium. *B*, Numerous leukocytes are noted within the lamina propria and within the walls and lumina of the gastric glands. Hematoxylin and eosin stains indicated that these leukocytes were eosinophils, and the patient also had peripheral blood eosinophilia.

in celiac sprue. Recent findings provide compelling evidence that lymphocytic gastritis may occur as a manifestation of celiac sprue or spruelike disease, and thus the lymphocytic infiltration of celiac sprue may affect gastric epithelial mucous cells. Lymphocytic gastritis in untreated celiac disease may be associated with functional changes such as increased permeability. Gastric biopsies from 10 of 22 patients with diarrhea or malabsorption and small bowel changes characteristic of sprue or spruelike disease showed striking lymphocytic gastritis. Following institution of a gluten-free diet, lymphocytic gastritis resolves after approximately 2 years.

Lymphocytic gastritis has also been attributed to an atypical host immune response to *H. pylori*. *H. pylori* eradication treatment in patients with lymphocytic gastritis causes significant improvement in the gastric intraepithelial lymphocytic infiltrate, corpus inflammation, and dyspeptic symptoms. *H. pylori* may be the cause of some cases of protein-losing hypertrophic lymphocytic gastritis. The disease may resolve clinically, endoscopically, and pathologically with therapeutic eradication of *H. pylori* in some patients.

Patients with gastric lymphoma have a significantly increased prevalence of lymphocytic gastritis due to *H. pylori*. As intraepithelial lymphocytes are speculated to have a role in the regulation of normal mucosal inflammatory reaction, they may also participate in the pathogenesis of mucosal lymphoma. In a 10-year follow-up study of lymphocytic gastritis, the patients with lymphocytic gastritis also appeared to have a significant increase in the grade of intestinal metaplasia in the corpus mucosa. In another study, lymphocytic gastritis was more prevalent in patients with gastric adenocarcinoma (16 of 30 cases [12.3%]) than in unselected patients undergoing endoscopy (0.83% to 2.5%).

Endoscopy in lymphocytic gastritis shows thick mucosal folds, nodularity, and aphthous erosion, historically known as "varioliform gastritis." Gastric biopsies show expansion of the lamina propria by an infiltrate of plasma cells, lymphocytes, and rare neutrophils. These findings may be seen in the antral mucosa only, body mucosa only, or in both antral and body mucosa. The surface and superficial pit epithelium shows a marked intraepithelial infiltrate with T lymphocytes, with flattening of the epithelium and loss of apical mucin secretion. Quantification of epithelial lymphocytes revealed 46.5 lymphocytes per 100 epithelial cells in lymphocytic gastritis, compared with 3.5 lymphocytes per 100 cells in normal controls and 5.1 lymphocytes per 100 cells in disease controls, including patients with *H. pylori* gastritis.

Eosinophilic Gastritis[158–161]

Eosinophilic gastroenteritis is a rare condition of unknown etiology characterized by peripheral eosinophilia, eosinophilic infiltration of the gastrointestinal tract, and gastrointestinal symptomatology. It is discussed in detail in Chapter 100. The gastric mucosa is frequently involved, and thus eosinophilic gastritis is one of the manifestations of eosinophilic gastroenteritis. Eosinophilic gastroenteritis is classified according to the layer of gastrointestinal tract involved (i.e., mucosal layer disease, muscle layer disease, and subserosal disease). Mucosal involvement may result in abdominal pain, nausea, vomiting, diarrhea, weight loss, anemia, protein-losing enteropathy, intestinal perforation, and iron deficiency anemia secondary to gastrointestinal blood loss. Patients with muscular layer disease generally have obstructive symptoms and patients with subserosal eosinophilic infiltration develop eosinophilic ascites. Patients with gastric involvement frequently present with pyloric obstruction. Radiographic studies may demonstrate thickened mucosal folds, nodularity, or ulcerations. Endoscopy may reveal normal-appearing mucosa or hyperemic edematous mucosa with surface erosions or prominent gastric folds.

Gastric mucosal biopsies are critical to the diagnosis and show marked eosinophilic infiltration, eosinophilic pit abscesses, necrosis with numerous neutrophils, and epithelial regeneration (Fig. 43–7*B*). Abnormal eosinophilic infiltration is defined as at least 20 eosinophils per high-power field either diffusely or multifocally. A full-thickness surgical biopsy is necessary for the diagnosis of muscle layer disease.

As discussed in Chapter 100, patients with disabling symptoms can be effectively treated with glucocorticoids (after other systemic disorders associated with peripheral eosinophilia have been excluded) or possibly with oral sodium chromoglycate. Surgical intervention may be required in patients with obstructive complications or refractory disease.

MISCELLANEOUS FORMS OF GASTRITIS

Gastritis Cystica Profunda[162–166]

Gastritis cystica profunda is a rare complication of partial gastrectomy with gastrojejunostomy for benign peptic ulcer disease. This entity is similar to the colonic lesion, colitis cystic profunda. Gastritis cystica profunda may also develop without an antecedent history of gastric surgery and a history of chronic gastritis may be a risk factor. Radiography and endoscopy typically demonstrate multiple exophytic gastric masses that simulate a malignancy. Grossly, the gastric mucosal surface demonstrates multiple nodules and exophytic masses. On section, the gastric wall is thick and multiple cysts are present. Microscopically, the mucosa is characterized by foveolar hyperplasia, and cystic glands extend through a disrupted muscularis mucosae into the submucosa and, rarely, the muscularis propria (Fig. 43–8). Primary gastric stump carcinoma may be associated with gastritis cystica profunda. Chronic atrophic gastritis and atypical hyperplasia may also be associated with gastritis cystica profunda and may represent precancerous conditions.

Gastric Graft-versus-Host Disease[167–169]
(see also Chapter 27)

Graft-versus-host disease (GVHD) may affect any portion of the gastrointestinal tract; therefore, both upper and lower gastrointestinal tract biopsies may provide diagnostic information not evidenced in biopsy from a single site. GVHD most often occurs after allogeneic bone marrow transplantation and rarely after solid transplantation. GVHD occurs in an acute and chronic form. Acute GVHD occurs between post-transplant days 21 and 100, whereas chronic GVHD occurs after day 100. The gastrointestinal tract is commonly affected in acute GVHD, especially the small and large intestine, and to a lesser extent the stomach and esophagus.

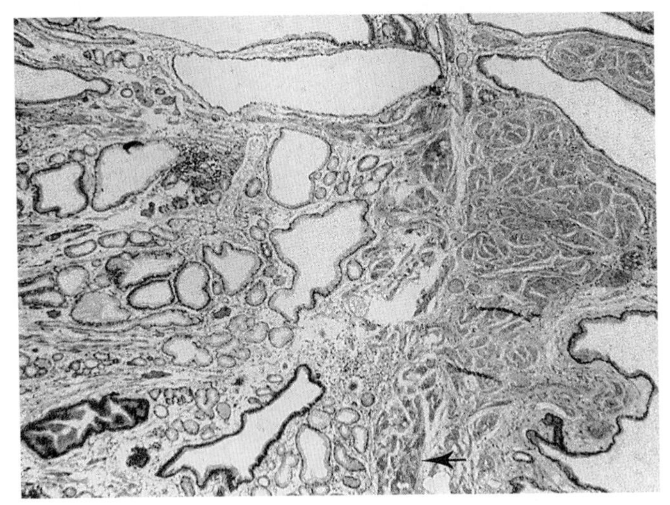

Figure 43–8. Gastritis cystica profunda. Note the cystic dilation of numerous gastric glands, which extend through the muscularis mucosae *(arrow),* simulating a gastric carcinoma.

Gastric GVHD is characterized by nausea, vomiting, and upper abdominal pain without diarrhea. Stomach biopsies may be necessary to diagnose GVHD in patients with upper gastrointestinal symptoms but no diarrhea and normal rectal biopsy specimens. The basic pathologic lesion consists of necrosis of single cells (apoptotic bodies) in the crypts of the large and small intestinal mucosa and in the neck region of the gastric mucosa. The necrosis consists of an intraepithelial vacuole filled with karyorrhectic debris and fragments of cytoplasm.

REACTIVE GASTROPATHIES (ACUTE EROSIVE GASTRITIS)

The gastric mucosa may be damaged by a variety of agents or factors that do not produce a significant inflammatory infiltrate. Because of the paucity of inflammatory cells, the mentioned lesions are best known as reactive gastropathies, as opposed to acute erosive gastritis. Risk factors for reactive gastropathy are summarized in Table 43–1.

The gastric mucosa in patients who experience a reactive gastropathy demonstrates a spectrum of hemorrhages, erosions, and ulcers. Erosions and ulcers are frequently multiple, and the base of these lesions often stains dark brown owing to exposure to acid.

Grossly, most erosions and acute ulcers appear as well-defined hemorrhagic lesions 1 to 2 mm in diameter. If the insult is severe, the mucosa between the lesions is intensely hemorrhagic. Microscopically, an erosion demonstrates necrosis to the level of the muscularis mucosa. An acute ulcer is an area of necrosis that extends beyond the muscularis mucosa. The reactive epithelial changes secondary to regeneration of the mucosa, foveolar hyperplasia (Fig. 43–9), are often associated with glands with atypical nuclei that can be misdiagnosed as dysplasia or carcinoma. The diagnosis of neoplasia in a background of necrosis, cellular debris, and granulation tissue should be made with utmost caution. The biopsy procedure may induce tissue hemorrhage; thus, subepithelial hemorrhage should involve more than one fourth of a biopsy specimen to be considered significant.[16]

Medications

Aspirin (even in low daily or less-than-daily doses) and NSAIDs that have cyclooxygenase-1 inhibitory activity are the most common cause of reactive gastropathy (see Chapter 23). Oral iron therapy may rarely cause mild endoscopic abnormalities consisting of erythema, small areas of subepithelial hemorrhage, and erosions.[170] Oral potassium chloride also may be associated with endoscopic erosions.[171] Endoscopic petechiae, erosions, and erythema have been associated with long-term fluoride ingestion.[172]

Reactive gastric epithelial atypia and gastric ulceration may be associated with hepatic arterial infusion chemotherapy for metastatic disease to the liver.[173, 174] The marked epithelial atypia that results may erroneously be interpreted as carcinoma and lead to unnecessary surgery.[26]

Alcohol

After alcohol ingestion, subepithelial hemorrhages are seen frequently at endoscopy, typically without prominent mucosal inflammation on biopsy specimens[175] (Fig. 43–10). Gastric biopsy specimens obtained from patients with chronic alcoholism have shown a higher prevalence of chronic antral gastritis due to *H. pylori,* with almost complete normalization of histologic findings after treatment.[176, 177]

The combined effects of alcohol and the NSAID ibuprofen were associated with more gastric mucosal damage by endoscopic assessment than with either agent alone.[178] The combination of alcohol and aspirin also caused more damage in the stomach than either agent alone, but not to a significant degree.[178] Alcohol appeared to be an acute triggering factor in 35% of patients admitted to an intensive care unit for massive upper gastrointestinal bleeding in Sweden.[179]

Cocaine

Gastrointestinal hemorrhage due to diffuse exudative erosion throughout the gastric fundus, body, antrum, and duodenal bulb has been reported with *crack cocaine* use. Gastrointestinal hemorrhage or pyloric perforation due to cocaine is well described.[180–182]

Stress

Erosions of the gastric mucosa may occur rapidly after major physical or thermal trauma, shock, sepsis, or head injury. These are often referred to as *stress ulcers* and are discussed in Chapter 40.

Radiation (see also Chapter 102)

Radiation effects on the stomach depend on the cell kinetics of the gastric mucosa as well as the dose of the radiation. The gastric mucosal response to radiation is unique, however, in that the most radiosensitive epithelial cells are the differentiated cells (parietal and chief cells) rather than the germinative cells in the mucous neck region.[183] Radiation injury to the stomach can be classified into acute (<6-month) and chronic (>1-year) phases. It is thought that

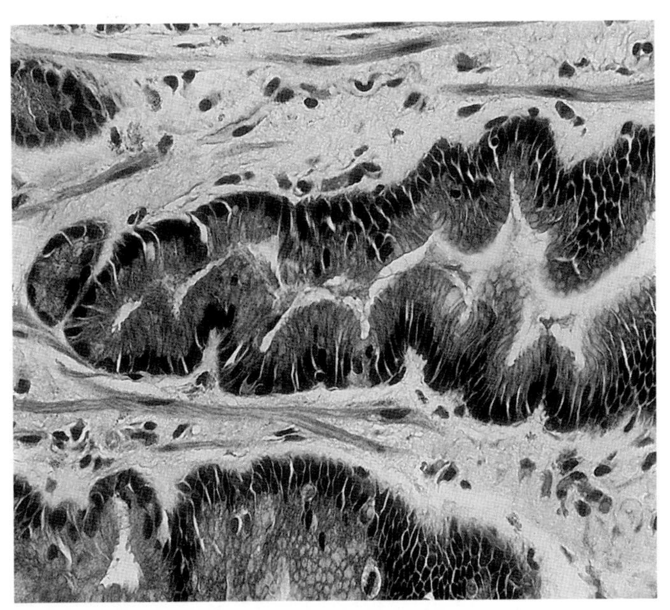

Figure 43–9. Foveolar hyperplasia. The pits show an elongated, corkscrew appearance.

the tolerance level for radiation-induced gastric ulceration is approximately 4500 cGy.[184] After a gastric dose of 5500 cGy or more, 50% of patients will develop clinical evidence of gastric ulcer formation.[185] Radiation-induced gastric ulcers are usually solitary, from 0.5 to 2 cm in diameter, and located in the antrum.

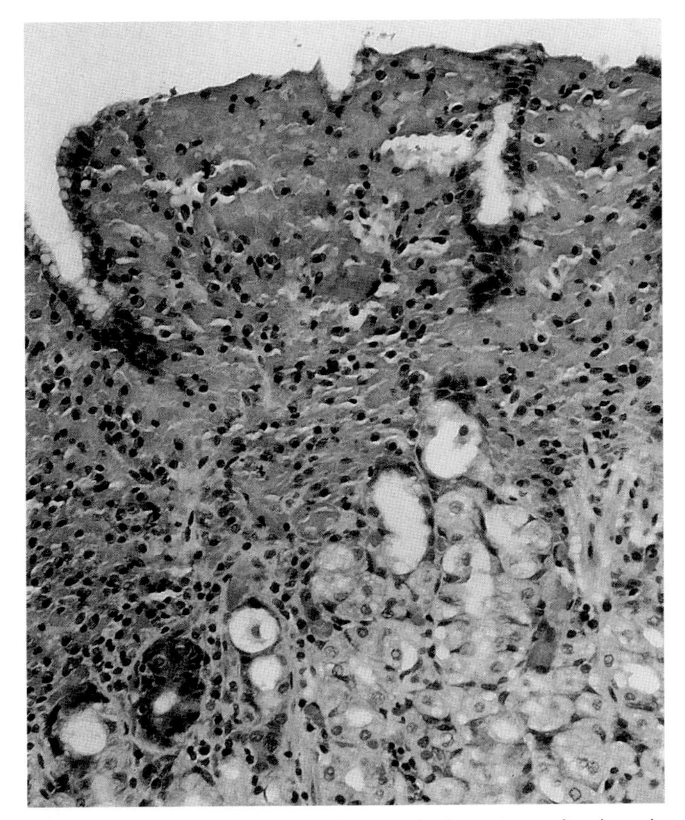

Figure 43–10. Alcoholic gastropathy. Hemorrhage is confined to the superficial portion of the mucosa, and there is a paucity of inflammatory cells.

Bile Reflux

Bile reflux into the stomach is common after partial gastrectomy with anastomosis to the duodenum (Billroth I) or jejunum (Billroth II) and after truncal vagotomy and pyloroplasty for peptic ulcer[186–191] (see Chapter 42). Bile reflux gastritis also may occur after cholecystectomy or sphincteroplasty, which allows the continuous exposure of bile to the duodenum. Occasionally, bile gastritis is observed in patients who have not had surgery[192] or who have only had highly selective vagotomy.[193] Development of bile reflux gastritis may contribute to eradication of *H. pylori,* because the prevalence of *H. pylori* infection after partial gastrectomy appears to be reduced.[193]

Endoscopy shows swelling, redness, erosions, and bile staining of the gastric mucosa. Biopsy specimens show foveolar hyperplasia, dilated cystic glands, atypical glands that may be misdiagnosed as dysplasia or carcinoma, and a paucity of acute and chronic inflammatory cells. Atrophic gastritis may result and increase the risk of carcinoma in the gastric stump (see Chapter 42).

Ischemia

Chronic ischemic gastropathy may occur secondary to chronic mesenteric insufficiency and can be reversed after a revascularization operation.[194, 195] Chronic ischemic gastropathy as well as chronic ischemic gastric ulcers may also occur in association with atheromatous embolization.[196, 197] Athletes involved in intense physical activity, especially long-distance running, may experience recurrent ischemic gastropathy and chronic gastrointestinal bleeding with anemia.[198]

Bezoar

Gastric bezoar can cause gastric injury, as discussed in Chapter 21.

Prolapse Gastropathy

The mucosa of the gastric cardia may prolapse into the esophageal lumen during retching and vomiting.[199] The mechanical injury to the cardia that results may be the cause of upper gastrointestinal hemorrhage. Esophagoscopy may demonstrate the prolapsed gastric mucosa. The congested mucosa shows erosions and superficial ulcerations.

Linear Gastric Erosions in a Hiatal Hernia (Cameron's Ulcers)[200–201]

Linear gastric erosions in a hiatal hernia are discussed in Chapters 13, 20, and 40 (see Fig. 20–4).

Congestive Gastropathy (Portal Hypertensive Gastropathy)

As discussed in more detail in Chapters 13 and 77, gastric mucosal lesions are common in portal hypertension and represent an important cause of blood loss.[202] Biopsies show vascular ectasia in the mucosal layer without a significant degree of inflammatory infiltrate. The gastric lesions in portal hypertension are associated with a congested gastric mucosa and should be renamed *congestive gastropathy* instead of *gastritis*.

HYPERPLASTIC GASTROPATHIES

Ménétrier's Disease and Hyperplastic, Hypersecretory Gastropathy[203–217]

Hyperplastic gastropathy is a rare condition characterized by giant gastric folds associated with epithelial hyperplasia. Two clinical syndromes have been identified: Ménétrier's disease and a variant of it referred to as *hyperplastic, hypersecretory gastropathy*, and Zollinger-Ellison syndrome, which is discussed in Chapter 41. Figure 43–11 (*A* and *B*) demonstrates enlarged gastric folds in these conditions.

Ménétrier's disease is typically associated with protein-losing gastropathy (see Chapter 25) and with hypochlorhydria, whereas the hyperplastic, hypersecretory variant is associated with increased or normal acid secretion and parietal and chief cell hyperplasia, with or without excessive gastric protein loss.

Other more common conditions can also cause enlarged gastric folds, including gastric neoplasm (lymphoma, carcinoma), granulomatous gastritides, gastric varices, infectious gastritis (particularly *H. pylori* and CMV), and eosinophilic

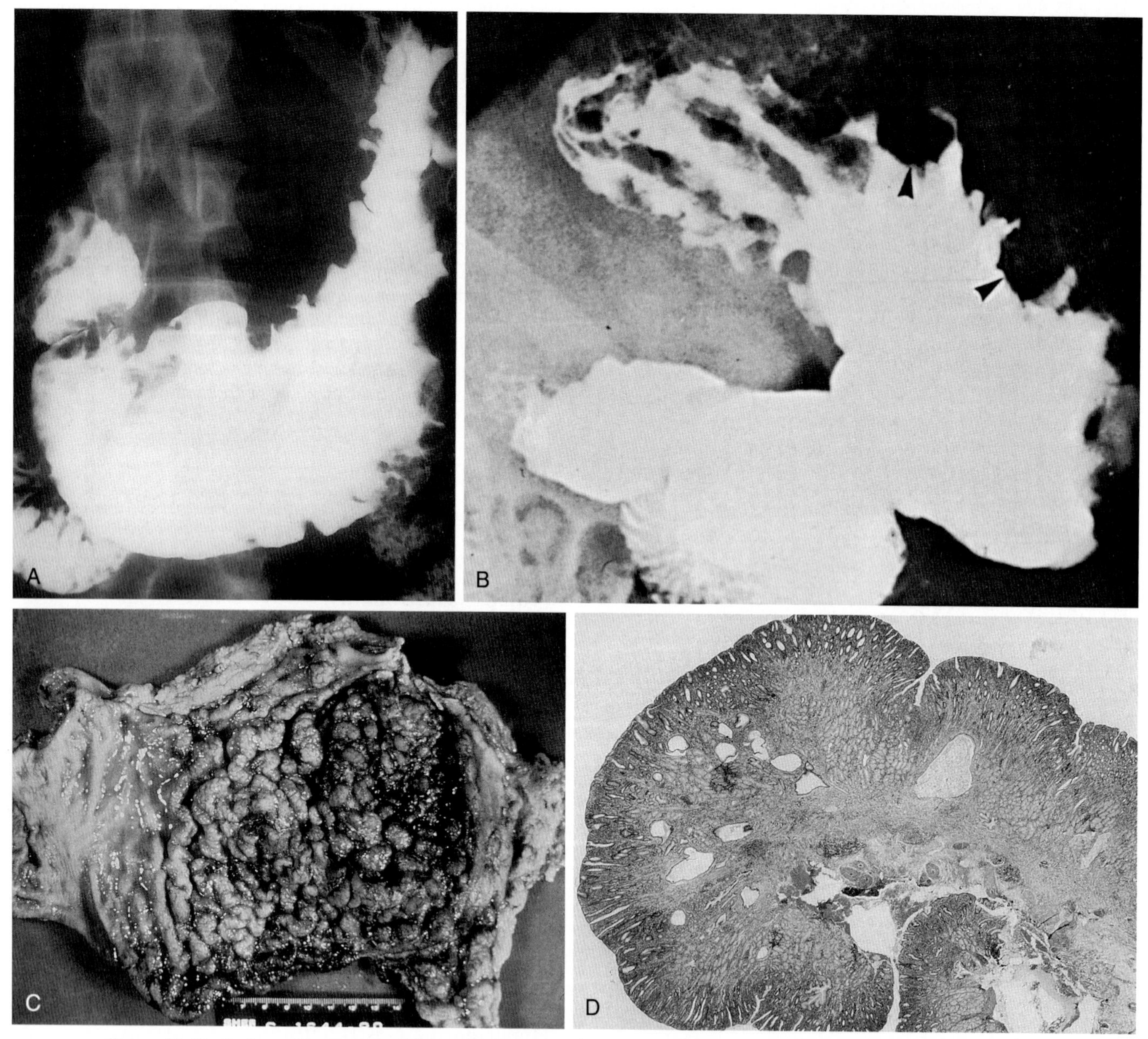

Figure 43–11. Radiographic example of hyperplastic gastropathy with giant gastric folds. *A*, Zollinger-Ellison syndrome. *B*, Ménétrier's disease. *C*, Total gastrectomy specimen in a patient with Ménétrier's disease (*right*, body, with hyperplastic mucosa and cerebriform rugal folds; *left*, antrum, with relative sparing). *D*, Histology of Ménétrier's disease showing enlarged folds with foveolar hyperplasia, cystically dilated glands, and minimal gastritis.

gastritis. Resolution of *H. pylori* hypertrophic lymphocytic gastritis with antibiotics may result in reversal of excess protein loss.

In one series, 31 patients with large gastric folds of uncertain etiology underwent full-thickness gastric mucosal biopsies. Six patients showed the features of Ménétrier's disease, 1 showed the features of hyperplastic, hypersecretory gastropathy, and 6 showed features of Zollinger-Ellison syndrome.[203] The remaining 18 (the majority) had peptic ulcer disease. The enlarged gastric folds in Ménétrier's disease are due to foveolar cell hyperplasia, edema, and variable degrees of inflammation. Patients may present with weight loss, epigastric pain, vomiting, anorexia, dyspepsia, hematemesis, and positive fecal occult blood tests. The mechanism responsible for the low gastric acid secretion is unclear, but it could be related to transforming growth factor-α (TGF-α) or its closely related peptide, epidermal growth factor (EGF).

Ménétrier's disease may be associated with hypertrophic lymphocytic gastritis and a carcinoid-like syndrome due to increased gastric mucosal production of prostaglandin E_2 concentrations. Ménétrier's disease may be self-limited and completely resolve in patients younger than 10 years of age and when it occurs in the postpartum period. The cause of Ménétrier's disease of childhood may be infection with CMV and activation of TGF-α. The risk of developing carcinoma in association with Ménétrier's disease is an open question, and some authors question whether there is a significant risk. Of the 200 cases of Ménétrier's disease reported in the literature, 30 (15%) have been associated with carcinoma.

The mucosa of patients with Ménétrier's disease demonstrates irregular hypertrophic folds that involve the entire gastric body. The mucosa also demonstrates a swollen, spongy appearance subdivided by creases creating a picture similar to cerebral convolutions. A polypoid variant of Ménétrier's disease has been described that resembles multiple hyperplastic gastric polyps (see Chapter 44).

Gastric resections from patients with Ménétrier's disease typically show large polypoid gastric folds or large cerebriform gastric folds with antral sparing (Fig. 43–11*C*). In the absence of a gastrectomy, a full-thickness gastric mucosal biopsy is required to adequately assess the gastric histology in patients with hyperplastic gastropathy. The predominant microscopic feature of Ménétrier's disease and hyperplastic, hypersecretory gastropathy is foveolar hyperplasia with cystic dilation (Fig. 43–11*D*). The parietal and chief cells may be decreased and replaced by mucous glands. Inflammation in hyperplastic gastropathies is variable and may be absent.

Ideal treatment of hyperplastic gastropathy is unclear, because the condition is rare and controlled trials are lacking. *H. pylori* infection should be treated, if present, and the entire syndrome may resolve. Symptoms may improve with antisecretory agents (histamine$_2$ [H_2] receptor antagonists, anticholinergic agents, proton pump inhibitors), especially if the patient has Zollinger-Ellison syndrome or normogastrinemic hyperplastic, hypersecretory gastropathy. It has been suggested that H_2 blockers and anticholinergics reduce gastric protein loss by strengthening intercellular tight junctions. Some patients with Ménétrier's disease have responded to corticosteroids, octreotide, antifibrinolytic agents, or monoclonal antibody against the EGF receptor. Partial or total gastric resection is reserved for severe complications, such as refractory or recurrent bleeding, obstruction, severe hypoproteinemia, or cancer development.

REFERENCES

1. Rotterdam H: Contributions of gastrointestinal biopsy to an understanding of gastrointestinal disease. Am J Gastroenterol 78:140, 1983.
2. Rubin C: Are there three types of *Helicobacter pylori* gastritis? Gastroenterology 112:2108, 1997.
3. Genta R, Wentzell H, Graham D: Gastric lymphoid follicles in *Helicobacter pylori* infection: Frequency, distribution, and response to triple therapy. Hum Pathol 24:577, 1993.
4. Genta R, Hamner H: The significance of lymphoid follicles in the interpretation of gastric biopsy specimens. Arch Pathol Lab Med 118: 740, 1994.
5. Misiewicz J: The Sydney system: A new classification of gastritis. J Gastorenterol Hepatol 6:207, 1991.
6. Appelman H: Gastritis: Terminology, etiology, and clinicopathological correlations—another biased view. Hum Pathol 25:1006, 1994.
7. Correa P: Chronic gastritis: A clinicopathological classification. Am J Gastroenterol 83:504, 1988.
8. Cryer B, Lee E, Feldman M: Gastric mucosal biopsy via a nasogastric tube: A nonendoscopic method for diagnosing fundic and antral mucosal gastritis and *Helicobacter pylori* infection in man. Gastrointest Endosc 44:317, 1996.
9. Chan Y, Hui P, Chan J, et al: Epithelial damage by *Helicobacter pylori* in gastric ulcers. Histopathology 19:47, 1991.
10. Price A: Histological aspects of *Campylobacter pylori* colonization and infection of gastric and duodenal mucosa. Scand J Gastroenterol 23:21, 1988.
11. Rosh J, Kurfist L, Benkov K, et al: *Helicobacter pylori* and gastric lymphonodular hyperplasia in children. Am J Gastroenterol 87:135, 1992.
12. Peterson W, Lee E, Feldman M: Relationship between *Campylobacter pylori* and gastritis in healthy humans after administration of placebo or indomethacin. Gastroenterology 95:1185, 1988.
13. Montgomery E, Martin D, Peura D: Rapid diagnosis of *Campylobacter pylori* by Gram's stain. Am J Clin Pathol 90:606, 1988.
14. Madan E, Kemp J, Westblom T, et al: Evaluation of staining methods for identifying *Campylobacter pylori*. Am J Clin Pathol 90:450, 1988.
15. Morris A, Ali M, Thomsen L, et al: Tightly spiral-shaped bacteria in the human stomach: Another cause of active chronic gastritis? Gut 31: 139, 1990.
16. Heilmann K, Borchard F: Gastritis due to spiral-shaped bacteria other than *Helicobacter pylori*: Clinical, histological, and ultrastructural findings. Gut 32:137, 1991.
17. Hilzenrat N, Lamoureux E, Weintrub I, et al: *Helicobacter heilmanii*–like spiral bacteria in gastric mucosal biopsies. Arch Pathol Lab Med 119:1149, 1995.
18. Genta R, Graham D: Comparison of biopsy sites for the histopathologic diagnosis of *Helicobacter pylori*: A topographic study of *H. pylori* density and distribution. Gastrointest Endosc 40:342, 1994.
19. Satoh K, Kimura K, Taniguchi Y, et al: Biopsy sites suitable for the diagnosis of *Helicobacter pylori* infection and the assessment of the extent of atrophic gastritis. Am J Gastroenterol 93:569, 1998.
20. Urakami Y, Kimura M, Seki H, et al: Gastric metaplasia and *Helicobacter pylori*. Am J Gastroenterol 92:795, 1997.
21. Rubin C: Are there three types of *Helicobacter pylori* gastritis? Gastroenterology 112:2108, 1997.
22. Genta R: Recognizing atrophy: Another step toward a classification of gastritis. Am J Surg Pathol 20:S23–S30, 1996.
23. Dixon M, Genta R, Yardley J, et al: Classification and grading of gastritis. Am J Surg Pathol 20:1161, 1996.
24. Correa P, Yardley J: Grading and classification of chronic gastritis: One American response to the Sydney system. Gastroenterology 102: 355, 1992.
25. Meshkinpour H, Orlando R, Arguello J, et al: Significance of endoscopically visible blood vessels as an index of atrophic gastritis. Am J Gastroenterol 71:376, 1979.
26. Antonioli D: Precursors of gastric carcinoma: A critical review with a brief description of early (curable) gastric cancer. Hum Pathol 25:994, 1994.
27. Stemmermann G: Intestinal metaplasia of the stomach. Cancer 74:556, 1994.

28. Ramesar K, Sander D, Hopwood D: Limited value of type III intestinal metaplasia in predicting risk of gastric carcinoma. J Clin Pathol 40:1287, 1987.
29. Fox J, Correa P, Taylor N, et al: *Campylobacter pylori*–associated gastritis and immune response in a population at increased risk of gastric carcinoma. Am J Gastroenterol 84:775, 1989.
30. Sipponen P: Intestinal metaplasia and gastric carcinoma. Ann Clin Res 13:139, 1981.
31. Wyatt J, Dixon M: Chronic gastritis—a pathogenetic approach. J Pathol 154:113, 1988.
32. Lewin K, Dowling F, Wright J, et al: Gastric morphology and serum gastrin levels in pernicious anemia. Gut 17:551, 1976.
33. Hsing A, Hansson L, McLaughlin J, et al: Pernicious anemia and subsequent cancer: A population-based cohort study. Cancer 71:745, 1993.
34. Schafer L, Larson D, Melton L, et al: Risk of development of gastric carcinoma in patients with pernicious anemia: A population-based study in Rochester, Minnesota. Mayo Clin Proc 60:444, 1985.
35. Muller J, Kirchner T, Muller-Hermelink H: Gastric endocrine cell hyperplasia and carcinoid tumors in atrophic gastritis Type A. Am J Surg Pathol 11:909, 1987.
36. Borch K, Renvall H, Kullman E, et al: Gastric carcinoid associated with the syndrome of hypergastrinemic atrophic gastritis: A prospective analysis of 11 cases. Am J Surg Pathol 11:435, 1987.
37. Mendelsohn G, de la Monte S, Dunn J, et al: Gastric carcinoid tumors, endocrine cell hyperplasia, and associated intestinal metaplasia. Cancer 60:1022, 1987.
38. Berendt R, Jewell L, Shnitka T, et al: Multicentric gastric carcinoids complicating pernicious anemia. Arch Pathol Lab Med 113:399, 1989.
39. Itsuno M, Watanabe H, Iwafuchi M, et al: Multiple carcinoids and endocrine cell micronests in type A gastritis. Cancer 63:881, 1989.
40. Chetty R, Roskell D: Cytomegalovirus infection in the gastrointestinal tract. J Clin Pathol 47:968, 1994.
41. Hinnant K, Rotterdam H, Bell E, et al: Cytomegalovirus infection of the alimentary tract: A clinicopathological correlation. Am J Gastroenterol 81:944, 1986.
42. Nowak TV, Goddard M, Batteiger B, et al: Evolution of acute cytomegalovirus gastritis to chronic gastrointestinal dysmotility in a nonimmunocompromised adult. Gastroenterology 116:953, 1999.
43. Mañez R, Kusne S, Green M, et al: Incidence and risk factors associated with the development of cytomegalovirus disease after intestinal transplantation. Transplantation 59:1010, 1995.
44. Strayer D, Phillips G, Barker K, et al: Gastric cytomegalovirus infection in bone marrow transplant patients: An indication of generalized disease. Cancer 48:1478, 1981.
45. Franzin G, Muolo A, Griminelli T: Cytomegalovirus inclusions in the gastroduodenal mucosa of patients after renal transplantation. Gut 22: 698, 1981.
46. Buckner F, Pomeroy C: Cytomegalovirus disease of the gastrointestinal tract in patients without AIDS. Clin Infect Dis 17:644, 1993.
47. Garcia F, Garau J, Sierra M, et al: Cytomegalovirus mononucleosis–associated antral gastritis simulating malignancy. Arch Intern Med 147:787, 1987.
48. Elta G, Turnage R, Eckhauser F, et al: A submucosal antral mass caused by cytomegalovirus infection in a patient with acquired immunodeficiency syndrome. Am J Gastroenterol 81:714, 1986.
49. Sperling G, Reed G: Herpetic gastritis. Dig Dis 22:1033, 1977.
50. Howiler W, Goldberg H: Gastroesophageal involvement in herpes simplex. Gastroenterology 70:775, 1976.
51. Hong J, Elgart M: Gastrointestinal complications of dermatomal herpes zoster successfully treated with famciclovir and lactulose. J Am Acad Dermatol 38:279, 1998.
52. Corey L, Spear P: Infections with herpes simplex viruses. N Engl J Med 314:749, 1986.
53. Miller A, Smith B, Rogers A: Phlegmonous gastritis. Gastroenterology 68:231, 1975.
54. Blei E, Abrahams C: Diffuse phlegmonous gastroenterocolitis in a patient with an infected peritoneojugular venous shunt. Gastroenterology 84:636, 1983.
55. Mittleman R, Suarez R: Phlegmonous gastritis associated with the acquired immunodeficiency syndrome/pre-acquired immunodeficiency syndrome. Arch Pathol Lab Med 109:765, 1985.
56. Tierney L, Gooding G, Bottles K, et al: Phlegmonous gastritis and hemophilus influenzae peritonitis in a patient with alcoholic liver disease. Dig Dis Sci 32:97, 1987.
57. Stein L, Greenberg R, Ilardi C, et al: Acute necrotizing gastritis in a patient with peptic ulcer disease. Am J Gastroenterol 84:1552, 1989.
58. de Lange E, Sluttsky V, Swanson S, et al: Computed tomography of emphysematous gastritis. J Comput Assist Tomogr 10:139, 1986.
59. Bernardino M, Lawson T: Emphysematous gastritis and gastric perforation. Gastrointest Radiol 2:107, 1977.
60. Marshall J: Tuberculosis of the gastrointestinal tract and peritoneum. Am J Gastroenterol 88:989, 1993.
61. Misra R, Agarwal S, Prakash P, et al: Gastric tuberculosis. Endoscopy 14:235, 1982.
62. Subei I, Attar B, Schmitt G, et al: Primary gastric tuberculosis: A case report and literature review. Am J Gastroenterol 82:769, 1987.
63. Tromba J, Inglese R, Rieders B, et al: Primary gastric tuberculosis presenting as pyloric outlet obstruction. Am J Gastroenterol 86:1820, 1991.
64. Weissman D, Gumaste V, Dave P, et al: Bleeding from a tuberculous gastric ulcer. Am J Gastroenterol 85:742, 1990.
65. Mathis G, Dirschmid K, Sutterlütti G: Tuberculous gastric ulcer. Endoscopy 19:133, 1987.
66. Benson C: Disease due to the *Mycobacterium avium* complex in patients with AIDS: Epidemiology and clinical syndrome. Clin Infect Dis 18:S218, 1994.
67. Gray J, Rabeneck L: Atypical mycobacterial infection of the gastrointestinal tract in AIDS patients. Am J Gastroenterol 84:1521, 1989.
68. Cappell M, Hassan T, Rosenthal S, et al: Gastrointestinal obstruction due to *Mycobacterium avium-intracellulare* associated with the acquired immunodeficiency syndrome. Am J Gastroenterol 87:1823, 1992.
69. Cappell M, Gupta A: Gastrointestinal hemorrhage due to gastrointestinal *Mycobacterium avium-intracellulare* or esophageal candidiasis in patients with the acquired immunodeficiency syndrome. Am J Gastroenterol 87:224, 1992.
70. Cappell M, Taunk J: A chronic gastric ulcer refractory to conventional antiulcer therapy associated with localized gastric *Mycobacterium avium-intracellulare* infection [letter]. Am J Gastroenterol 86:654, 1991.
71. Nguyen H, Frank D, Handt S, et al: Severe gastrointestinal hemorrhage due to *Mycobacterium avium* complex in a patient receiving immunosuppressive therapy. Am J Gastroenterol 94:232, 1999.
72. Yang S, Li A, Lin J: Colonoscopy in abdominal actinomycosis. Gastrointest Endosc 51:236, 2000.
73. Van Olmen G, Larmuseau M, Geboes K, et al: Primary gastric actinomycosis: A case report and review of the literature. Am J Gastroenterol 79:512, 1984.
74. Berardi R: Abdominal actinomycosis. Surg Gynecol Obstet 149:257, 1990.
75. Rolfs R, Nakashima A: Epidemiology of primary and secondary syphilis in the United States, 1981 through 1989. JAMA 264:1432, 1990.
76. Atten M, Altar B, Teopengco E, et al: Gastric syphilis: A disease with multiple manifestations. Am J Gastroenterol 89:2227, 1994.
77. Fyfe B, Poppiti R, Lubin J, et al: Gastric syphilis—primary diagnosis by gastric biopsy: Report of four cases. Arch Pathol Lab Med 117: 820, 1993.
78. Besses C, Sans-Sabrafen J, Badia X, et al: Ulceroinfiltrative syphilitic gastropathy: Silver stain diagnosis from biopsy specimen. Am J Gastroenterol 82:773, 1987.
79. Beckman J, Schuman B: Antral gastritis and ulceration in a patient with secondary syphilis. Gastrointest Endosc 32:355, 1986.
80. Jones B, Lichtenstein J: Gastric syphilis: Radiologic findings. Am J Radiol 160:59, 1993.
81. Morin M, Tan A: Diffuse enlargement of gastric folds as a manifestation of secondary syphilis. Am J Gastroenterol 74:170, 1980.
82. Inagaki H, Kawai T, Miyata M, et al: Gastric syphilis: Polymerase chain reaction of treponemal in DNA pseudolymphomatous lesions. Hum Pathol 27:763, 1996.
83. Loffeld R, Loffeld B, Arends J, et al: Fungal colonization of gastric ulcers. Am J Gastroenterol 83:730, 1988.
84. Katzenstein A, Maksem J: Candidal infection of gastric ulcers: Histology, incidence, and clinical significance. Am J Clin Pathol 71:137, 1979.
85. Gotlieb-Jensen K, Anderson J: Occurrence of *Candida* in gastric ulcers: Significance for the healing process. Gastroenterology 85:535, 1983.
86. Peters M, Weiner J, Whelan G: Fungal infection associated with gastroduodenal ulceration: Endoscopic and pathologic appearance. Gastroenterology 78:350, 1980.

87. Nelson R, Bruni H, Goldstein H: Primary gastric candidiasis in uncompromised subjects. Gastrointest Endosc 22:92, 1975.
88. Konok G, Haddad H, Strom B: Postoperative gastric mycosis. Surg Gynecol Obstet 150:337, 1980.
89. Cronan J, Burrel M, Trepeta R: Aphthoid ulcerations in gastric candidiasis. Diagn Radiol 134:607, 1980.
90. Khuroo M, Naik S, Sengal S, et al: *Candida* infection of the upper gastrointestinal tract superadded upon chemical injury with acids. Am J Gastroenterol 72:276, 1979.
91. Sanguino J, Rodrigues B, Baptista A, et al: Focal lesion of African histoplasmosis presenting as a malignant gastric ulcer. Hepatogastroenterology 43:771, 1996.
92. Jayalakshmi P, Soo-Hoo T, Goh K, et al: Disseminated histoplasmosis presenting as penile ulcer. Aust N Z J Med 20:175, 1990.
93. Fisher J, Sanowski R: Disseminated histoplasmosis producing hypertrophic gastric folds. Dig Dis 23:282, 1978.
94. Cherney C, Chutuape A, Fikrig M: Fatal invasive gastric mucormycosis occurring with emphysematous gastritis: Case report and literature review. Am J Gastroenterol 94:252, 1999.
95. Brullet E, Andreu X, Elias J, et al: Gastric mucormycosis in a patient with acquired immunodeficiency syndrome [letter]. Gastrointest Endosc 39:106, 1993.
96. Corley D, Lindeman N, Ostroff J: Survival with early diagnosis of invasive gastric mucormycosis in a heart transplant patient [letter]. Gastrointest Endosc 46:452, 1997.
97. Lyon D, Schubert T, Mantia A, et al: Phycomycosis of the gastrointestinal tract. Am J Gastroenterol 72:379, 1979.
98. Garone M, Winston B, Lewis J, et al: Cryptosporidiosis of the stomach. Am J Gastroenterol 81:465, 1986.
99. Forester G, Sidhom O, Nahass R, et al: AIDS-associated cryptosporidiosis with gastric stricture and a therapeutic response to paromomycin. Am J Gastroenterol 89:1096, 1994.
100. Wurtz R, Mirot M, Fronda G, et al: Gastric infection by *Strongyloides stercoralis*. Am J Trop Med Hyg 51:339, 1994.
101. Dees A, Batenburg P, Umar H, et al: *Strongyloides stercoralis* associated with a bleeding gastric ulcer. Gut 31:1414, 1990.
102. Ainley C, Clarke D, Timothy A, et al: *Strongyloides stercoralis* hyperinfection associated with cimetidine in an immunosuppressed patient: Diagnosis by endoscopic biopsy. Gut 27:337, 1986.
103. Scowden E, Schaffer W, Stone W: Overwhelming strongyloidiasis—an unappreciated opportunistic infection. Medicine 57:527, 1978.
104. Takeuchi K, Hanai H, Iida T, et al: A bleeding gastric ulcer on a vanishing tumor caused by anisakiasis. Gastrointest Endosc 52:549, 2000.
105. Pinkus G, Coolidge C, Little M: Intestinal anisakiasis: First case report from North America. Am J Med 59:114, 1975.
106. Deardorff T, Fukumura T, Raybourne R: Invasive anisakiasis: A case report from Hawaii. Gastroenterology 90:1047, 1986.
107. Choudhuri G, Saha S, Tandon R: Gastric ascariasis. Am J Gastroenterol 81:788, 1986.
108. Jacob G, Nakib A, Ruwaih A, et al: Ascariasis producing upper gastrointestinal hemorrhage. Endoscopy 15:67, 1983.
109. Dumont A, Seferian V, Barbier P, et al: Endoscopic discovery and capture of *Necator americanus* in the stomach. Endoscopy 15:65, 1983.
110. Belleza N, Lowman R: Suture granuloma of the stomach following total colectomy. Radiology 127:84, 1978.
111. Leach I, Maclennan K: Gastric lymphoma associated with mucosal and nodal granulomas: A new differential diagnosis in granulomatous gastritis. Histopathology 17:87, 1990.
112. Ectors N, Geboes K, Wynants P, et al: Granulomatous gastritis and Whipple's disease. Am J Gastroenterol 87:509, 1992.
113. Grosman GM, Rosh JR, Harpaz N: Langerhans cell histiocytosis of the stomach: A cause of granulomatous gastritis and gastric polyposis. Arch Pathol Lab Med 118:1232, 1994.
114. O'Donovan C, Murray J, Staunton H, et al: Granulomatous gastritis: Part of a vasculitic syndrome. Hum Pathol 22:1057, 1991.
115. Chin T, Stiehm R, Falloon J, et al: Corticosteroids in treatment of obstructive lesions of chronic granulomatous disease. J Pediatr 111: 349, 1987.
116. Shapiro J, Goldblum J, Petras R: A clinicopathologic study of 42 patients with granulomatous gastritis: Is there really an "idiopathic" granulomatous gastritis? Am J Surg Pathol 20:462, 1996.
117. Ectors N, Geboes K, Wynants P, et al: Granulomatous gastritis: A morphological and diagnostic approach. Histopathology 23:55, 1993.
118. Gumaste V, Janowitz H, Waye J: Granulomatous gastritis: A case report and review of the literature. Am J Gastroenterol 84:1315, 1989.
119. Hirsch B, Whitington P, Kirschner B, et al: Isolated granulomatous gastritis in an adolescent. Dig Dis Sci 34:292, 1989.
120. Khan M, Lam R, Tamoney H: Isolated granulomatous gastritis: Report of a case simulating gastric carcinoma. Am J Gastroenterol 71:90, 1979.
121. Schinella R, Ackert J: Isolated granulomatous disease of the stomach. Am J Gastroenterol 72:30, 1979.
122. Gumaste V, Janowitz H, Waye J: Granulomatous gastritis: A case report and review of the literature. Am J Gastroenterol 84:1315, 1989.
123. Rutgeerts P, Onette E, Vantrappen O, et al: Crohn's disease of the stomach and duodenum: A clinical study with emphasis on the value of endoscopy and endoscopic biopsies. Endoscopy 12:288, 1980.
124. Korelitz B, Waye J, Kreuning J, et al: Crohn's disease in endoscopic biopsies of the gastric antrum and duodenum. Am J Gastroenterol 76: 103, 1981.
125. Oren R, Harats N, Polak A, et al: Granulomatous colitis 10 years after presentation with isolated Crohn's gastritis. Am J Gastroenterol 84: 449, 1989.
126. Cary T, Tremaine W, Bands P, et al: Isolated Crohn's disease of the stomach. May Clin Proc 64:776, 1989.
127. Ona F: Gastric sarcoid: Unusual cause of upper gastrointestinal hemorrhage. Am J Gastroenterol 75:286, 1981.
128. Konda J, Ruth M, Sassaris M, et al: Sarcoidosis of the stomach and rectum. Am J Gastroenterol 73:516, 1980.
129. Tinker M, Viswanathan B, Lawfer H, et al: Acute appendicitis and pernicious anemia as complications of gastrointestinal sarcoidosis. Am J Gastroenterol 79:868, 1984.
130. Croxon S, Chen K, Davidson A: Sarcoidosis of the stomach. Digestion 38:193, 1987.
131. Stampfl D, Grimm I, Barbot D, et al: Sarcoidosis causing duodenal obstruction: Case report and review of gastrointestinal manifestations. Dig Dis Sci 35:526, 1990.
132. Guarino M, Reale D, Micoli G, et al: Xanthogranulomatous gastritis: Association with xanthogranulomatous cholecystitis. J Clin Pathol 46: 88, 1993.
133. Lee E, Schiller L, Vendrell D, et al: Subepithelial collagen table thickness in colon specimens from patients with microscopic colitis and collagenous colitis. Gastroenterology 103:1790, 1992.
134. Colletti R, Trainer T: Collagenous gastritis. Gastroenterology 97:1552, 1989.
135. Castellano V, Munoz M, Colina F, et al: Collagenous gastrobulbitis and collagenous colitis. Scand J Gastroenterol 34:632, 1999.
136. Pulimood A, Ramakrishna B, Mathan M: Collagenous gastritis and collagenous colitis: A report with sequential histological and ultrastructural findings. Gut 44:881, 1999.
137. Côté J, Handark G, Faure C, et al: Collagenous gastritis revealed by severe anemia in a child. Hum Pathol 28:883, 1998.
138. Groisman G, Meyers S, Harpaz N: Collagenous gastritis associated with lymphocytic colitis. J Clin Gastroenterol 22:134, 1996.
139. Stolte M, Ritter M, Borchard F, et al: Collagenous gastroduodenitis on collagenous colitis. Endoscopy 22:186, 1990.
140. Vesoulis Z, Lazanski G, Ravichandran P, et al: Collagenous gastritis: A case report, morphologic evaluation, and review. Mod Pathol 13: 591, 2000.
141. Haot J, Hamichi L, Wallez L, et al: Lymphocytic gastritis—a newly described entity: A retrospective endoscopic and histological study. Gut 29:1258, 1988.
142. Wu T, Hamilton S: Lymphocytic gastritis: Association with etiology and topology. Am J Surg Pathol 23:153, 1999.
143. Hayat M, Arora DS, Dixon MF, et al: Effects of *Helicobacter pylori* eradication on the natural history of lymphocytic gastritis. Gut 45:495, 1999.
144. Everett S: Lymphocytic gastritis, *Helicobacter pylori,* and gastric cancer: Is vitamin C the common link? Nutrition 15:402, 1999.
145. Niemelä S, Karttunen T, Kerola T, et al: Ten-year follow-up study of lymphocytic gastritis: Further evidence on *Helicobacter pylori* as a cause of lymphocytic gastritis and corpus gastritis. J Clin Pathol 48: 1111, 1995.
146. Miettinen A, Karttunen T, Alavaikko M: Lymphocytic gastritis and *Helicobacter pylori* infection in gastric lymphoma. Gut 37:471, 1995.
147. Groisman G, George J, Berman D, et al: Resolution of protein-losing hypertrophic lymphocytic gastritis with therapeutic eradication of *Helicobacter pylori.* Am J Gastroenterol 89:1548, 1994.

148. Dixon M, Wyatt J, Burke D, et al: Lymphocytic gastritis—relationship to *Campylobacter pylori* infection. J Pathol 154:125, 1988.
149. Haot J, Jouret A, Willette M, et al: Lymphocytic gastritis—prospective of its relationship with varioliform gastritis. Gut 31:282, 1990.
150. Crampton J, Hunter J, Neale G, et al: Chronic lymphocytic gastritis and protein-losing gastropathy. Gut 30:71, 1989.
151. Farahat K, Hainaut P, Jamar F, et al: Lymphocytic gastritis: An unusual cause of hypoproteinaemia. J Intern Med 234:95, 1993.
152. Griffiths A, Wyatt J, Jack A, et al: Lymphocytic gastritis, gastric adenocarcinoma, and primary gastric lymphoma. J Clin Pathol 47: 1123, 1994.
153. Diamanti A, Maino C, Niveloni S, et al: Characterization of gastric mucosal lesions in patients with celiac disease: A prospective controlled study. Am J Gastroenterol 94:1313, 1999.
154. Feeley K, Heneghan M, Stevens F, et al: Lymphocytic gastritis and coeliac disease: Evidence of a positive association. J Clin Pathol 51: 207, 1998.
155. Vogelsang H, Oberhuber G, Wyatt J, et al: Lymphocytic gastritis and gastric permeability in patients with celiac disease. Gastroenterology 111:73, 1996.
156. Lynch D, Sobala G, Dixon M, et al: Lymphocytic gastritis and associated small bowel disease: A diffuse lymphocytic gastroenteropathy. J Clin Pathol 48:939, 1995.
157. Wolber R, Owen D, DelBuono L, et al: Lymphocytic gastritis in patients with celiac sprue or sprue-like intestinal disease. Gastroenterology 98:310, 1990.
158. Talley N, Shorter R, Phillips S, et al: Eosinophilic gastroenteritis: A clinicopathological study of patients with disease of the mucosa, muscle layer, and subserosal tissues. Gut 31:54, 1990.
159. Lee M, Hodges W, Huggins T, et al: Eosinophilic gastroenteritis. South Med J 89:189, 1996.
160. Moots R, Prouse P, Gumpel J: Near-fatal eosinophilic gastroenteritis responding to oral sodium chromoglycate. Gut 29:1282, 1988.
161. Caldwell J, Mekhjian H, Hurtubise P, et al: Eosinophilic gastroenteritis with obstruction. Gastroenterology 74:825, 1978.
162. Koga S, Watanabe H, Enjoji M: Stomal polypoid hypertrophic gastritis: A polypoid gastric lesion at gastroenterostomy site. Cancer 43:647, 1979.
163. Franzin G, Novelli P: Gastritis cystica profunda. Histopathology 5: 535, 1981.
164. Fonde E, Rodning C: Gastritis cystica profunda. Am J Gastroenterol 81:459, 1986.
165. Matsuda I, Konno H, Maruo Y, et al: A case of triple early gastric cancer in the remnant stomach. Am J Gastroenterol 90:1016, 1995.
166. Bogomoletz W, Potet F, Barge J, et al: Pathological features and mucin histochemistry of primary gastric stump carcinoma associated with gastritis cystica polyposa: A study of six cases. Am J Surg Pathol 9:401, 1985.
167. Snover D, Weisdorf S, Vercellotti G, et al: A histopathologic study of gastric and small intestinal graft-versus-host disease following allogeneic bone marrow transplant. Hum Pathol 16:387, 1985.
168. Snover D: Graft-versus-host disease of the gastrointestinal tract. Am J Surg Pathol 14:101, 1990.
169. Snover D: Acute and chronic graft-versus-host disease: Histopathological evidence for two distinct pathogenetic mechanisms. Hum Pathol 15:202, 1984.
170. Laine L, Bentley E, Chandrasoma P, et al: Effect of oral iron therapy on the upper gastrointestinal tract: A prospective evaluation. Dig Dis Sci 33:172, 1988.
171. Moore J, Alsop W, Freston J, et al: The effect of oral potassium chloride on upper gastrointestinal mucosa in healthy subjects: Healing of lesions despite continuing treatment. Gastrointest Endosc 32:210, 1986.
172. Das T, Susheela A, Gupta I, et al: Toxic effects of chronic fluoride ingestion on the upper gastrointestinal tract. J Clin Gastroenterol 18: 194, 1994.
173. Petras R, Hart W, Bukowski R: Gastric epithelial atypia associated with hepatic arterial infusion chemotherapy: Its distinction from early gastric carcinoma. Cancer 56:745, 1985.
174. Weidner N, Smith J, LaVanway J: Peptic ulceration with marked epithelial atypia following hepatic arterial infusion chemotherapy: A lesion initially misinterpreted as carcinoma. Am J Surg Pathol 7:261, 1983.
175. Laine L, Weinstein W: Histology of alcoholic hemorrhagic "gastritis": A prospective evaluation. Gastroenterology 94:1254, 1988.
176. Parl F, Lev R, Thomas E, et al: Histologic and morphometric study of chronic gastritis in alcoholic patients. Hum Pathol 10:45, 1979.
177. Uppal R, Lateef S, Korsten M, et al: Chronic alcoholic gastritis: Roles of alcohol and *Helicobacter pylori*. Arch Intern Med 151:760, 1991.
178. Lanza F, Royer G, Nelson R, et al: Ethanol, aspirin, ibuprofen, and the gastroduodenal mucosa: An endoscopic assessment. Am J Gastroenterol 80:767, 1985.
179. Borch K, Jansson L, Sjodahl R, et al: Haemorrhagic gastritis. Incidence, etiological factors, and prognosis. Acta Chir Scand 154:211, 1987.
180. Kodali V, Gordon S: Gastrointestinal hemorrhage secondary to crack cocaine. Gastrointest Endosc 41:604, 1995.
181. Fennell D, Gandhi S, Prichard B: Gastrointestinal haemorrhage associated with free-base (crack) cocaine. Postgrad Med J 71:377, 1995.
182. Arrillaga A, Sosa JL, Najjar R: Laparoscopic patching of crack cocaine–induced perforated ulcers. Am Surg 62:1007, 1996.
183. Novak J, Collins J, Donowitz M, et al: Effects of radiation on the human gastrointestinal tract. J Clin Gastroenterol 1:9, 1979.
184. Berthrong M, Fajardo L: Radiation injury in surgical pathology: II. Alimentary tract. Am J Surg Pathol 5:153, 1981.
185. Cohen J: Surgical treatment of recalcitrant radiation-induced gastric erosions. Head Neck 22:303, 2000.
186. Valnes K, Brandtzaeg P, Stave R, et al: Local immunodefence in relation to gastritis in Billroth II–resected stomach. Scand J Gastroenterol 23:1217, 1988.
187. Bechi P, Amorosi A, Mazzanti R, et al: Gastric histology and fasting bile reflux after partial gastrectomy. Gastroenterology 93:335, 1987.
188. Rutledge P, Warshaw A: Diagnosis of symptomatic alkaline reflux gastritis and prediction of response to bile diversion operation by intragastric alkali provocation. Am J Surg 155:82, 1988.
189. Dixon M, Connor J, Axon A, et al: Reflux gastritis: Distinct histopathological entity? J Clin Pathol 39:524, 1986.
190. Weinstein W, Buch K, Elashoff J, et al: The histology of the stomach in symptomatic patients after gastric surgery: A model to assess selective pattern of gastric mucosal injury. Scand J Gastroenterol 20:77, 1985.
191. Sobala G, King R: Reflux gastritis in the intact stomach. J Clin Pathol 43:303, 1990.
192. Offerhaus G, Rieu P, Jansen J, et al: Prospective comparative study of the influence of postoperative bile reflux on gastric mucosal histology and *Campylobacter pylori* infection. Gut 30:1552, 1989.
193. Eriksson B, Szego T, Emås S: Duodenogastric bile reflux before and after selective proximal vagotomy with and without pyloroplasty. Scand J Gastroenterol 25:161, 1990.
194. Højgaard L, Krag E: Chronic ischemic gastritis reversed after revascularization operation. Gastroenterology 92:226, 1987.
195. Force T, MacDonald P, Eade O, et al: Ischemic gastritis and duodenitis. Dig Dis Sci 25:307, 1980.
196. Karalis D, Quinn V, Victor M, et al: Risk of catheter-related emboli in patients with atherosclerotic debris in the thoracic aorta. Am Heart J 131:1149, 1996.
197. Hendel R, Cuenoid H, Giansiracusa D, et al: Multiple cholesterol emboli syndrome: Bowel infarction after retrograde angiography. Arch Intern Med 149:2371, 1989.
198. Cooper B, Douglas S, Firth L, et al: Erosive gastritis and gastrointestinal bleeding in a female runner. Gastroenterology 92:2019, 1987.
199. Chen Y: Mechanical gastritis as cause of upper gastrointestinal hemorrhage. Scand J Gastroenterol 28:512, 1993.
200. Cameron AJ, Higgins JA: Linear gastric erosion: A lesion associated with large diaphragmatic hernia and chronic blood loss anemia. Gastroenterology 91:338, 1986.
201. Moskovitz M, Fadden R, Min T, et al: Large hiatal hernias, anemia, and linear gastric erosion: Studies of etiology and medical therapy. Am J Gastroenterol 87:622, 1992.
202. McCormack T, Sims J, Eyre-Brook I, et al: Gastric lesions in portal hypertension: Inflammatory gastritis or congestive gastropathy? Gut 26:1226, 1985.
203. Komorowski R, Caya J: Hyperplastic gastropathy clinicopathologic correlation. Am J Surg Pathol 15:577, 1991.
204. Sferra T, Pawel B, Qualman S, et al: Ménétrier disease of childhood: Role of cytomegalovirus and transforming growth factor data. J Pediatr 128:213, 1996.
205. Eisenstat D, Griffiths A, Cutz E, et al: Acute cytomegalovirus infection in a child with Ménétrier's. Gastroenterology 109:592, 1995.
206. Cieslak T, Mullett C, Puntel R, et al: Ménétrier's disease associated with cytomegalovirus infection in children: Report of two cases and review of the literature. Pediatr Infect Dis J 12:340, 1993.
207. Wolfsen H, Carpenter H, Talley N, et al: Ménétrier's disease: A form

of hypertrophic gastropathy or gastritis? Gastroenterology 104:1310, 1993.
208. Hoat J, Bogomoletz W, Jouret A, et al: Ménétrier's disease with lymphocytic gastritis: An unusual association with possible pathogenic implication. Hum Pathol 22:379, 1991.
209. Simson J: Hyperplastic gastropathy. BMJ 291:1298, 1985.
210. Boyd E, Julka G, Thomas J, et al: Hypertrophic gastritis associated with increased gastric mucosal prostaglandin E_2 concentrations in a patient with the carcinoid syndrome. Gut 29:1270, 1988.
211. Fieber S, Rickert R: Hyperplastic gastropathy. Am J Gastroenterol 76: 321, 1981.
212. Scharschmidt B: The natural history of hypertrophic gastropathy (Ménétrier's disease). Am J Med 63:644, 1977.
213. Meuwissen S, Ridwan B, Hasper H, et al: Hypertrophic protein-losing gastropathy: A retrospective analysis of 40 cases in The Netherlands. Paper presented at the Autumn Meeting of The Netherlands Society of Gastroenterology, Veldhoven, October 1991.
214. Davis GE, O'Rourke MC, Metz JR, et al: Hypertrophic gastropathy symptoms responsive to prednisone. J Clin Gastroenterol 13:436, 1991.
215. Yeaton P, Frierson HF: Octreotide reduces enteral protein losses in Ménétrier's disease. Am J Gastroenterol 88:95, 1993.
216. Kondo M, Ikezaki M, Kato H, et al: Antifibrinolytic therapy of giant hypertrophic gastritis (Ménétrier's disease). Scand J Gastroenterol 13: 851, 1978.
217. Burdick J, Chung E, Tanner G, et al: Treatment of Ménétrier's disease with a monoclonal antibody against the epidermal gross factor receptor. N Engl J Med 344:1697, 2000.

Chapter 44

TUMORS OF THE STOMACH

Theodore J. Koh and Timothy C. Wang

Gastric cancer remains a major cause of mortality from cancer in the world, despite declining rates of incidence in many industrialized countries. In this chapter, we discuss gastric adenocarcinoma, which makes up the majority of gastric malignancies, as well as other gastric tumors. A gastric tumor is defined as any mass lesion of the wall of the stomach. Gastric tumors can be further defined as benign or malignant depending on their metastatic potential. We review recent developments in the understanding of the pathogenesis, diagnosis, and treatment of gastric tumors.

ADENOCARCINOMA

Epidemiology

Historically, gastric adenocarcinoma has been one of the leading causes of cancer mortality in the world. Fortunately, the incidence of gastric cancer has been steadily declining since the cessation of World War II, especially in developed countries. Gastric cancer was the still the leading cause of cancer mortality in the world as recently as 1980,[1] and in 1996 gastric cancer still remained the second leading cause of cancer death in the world, resulting in 628,000 deaths per year.[2]

There is a definite geographical variation for gastric cancer, with the highest rates seen in the Far East (Fig. 44–1). Japan ranks first worldwide in gastric cancer incidence[3] and fourth in gastric cancer mortality, trailing South Korea, Costa Rica, and the former Soviet Union. Areas of low incidence include North America, Australia, Western Europe, and Africa (Fig. 44–2).

In 1930, gastric cancer was the leading cause of cancer mortality in the United States for men, and the third leading cause in women.[4] Since that time, and following worldwide trends, the incidence of gastric cancer has steadily declined. In 1997, gastric cancer was the eighth leading cause of cancer death in the United States,[2] with an estimated 22,800 newly diagnosed gastric cancers resulting in 14,000 deaths,[5] costing about $1.8 billion for health care.[6]

In the United States, the majority of patients present between the ages of 65 and 74 years,[7] with a median age at diagnosis of 70 years in men and 74 years in women. Mortality rates from gastric cancer were 6.1/100,000 for men and 2.8/100,000 in women between the years 1992 and 1996. In countries with a high incidence of gastric cancer, the age at diagnosis tends to be a decade earlier.[3] This perhaps reflects lead-time bias from better screening programs, as the percentage of early gastric cancers found in the Far East is markedly higher than that found in Western countries. When gastric cancer affects younger patients, the male:female ratio is close to one, there is a high preponderance of blood type A, there is a family history of cancer, and there is a higher proportion of the diffuse form of gastric cancer than of the intestinal form.

Since the 1960s, the American black population has had nearly double the rate of gastric cancer mortality compared with the white population.[8] Native and Hispanic Americans also have a twofold increased risk of developing gastric cancer compared with the white population.[9] This difference in mortality rates may be partly explained by the fact that several studies suggest that rates of gastric cancer mortality increase with lower socioeconomic status.[10, 11] More recently, the National Cancer Data Base has reported that the ethnic distribution of gastric cancer cases does not deviate significantly from the ethnic distribution of the national census (African Americans comprise 12.5% of gastric cancer cases and 12.5% of the national population).[12] This suggests that the increased mortality rates seen in the minority populations of the United States appear to be resolving.

In terms of gender, black and white men have nearly double the rate of gastric cancer of women,[7, 13, 14] as is true worldwide.[15, 16]

In the United States, the distribution of gastric cancer within the stomach is 39% in the proximal third, 17% in the middle third, 32% in the distal third, and 12% involving the entire stomach.[14] The decline in gastric cancer rates appears to affect primarily the distal gastric cancers; recent studies suggest that the rates of cancer of the gastric cardia have remained stable, and rates of cancer at the gastroesophageal junction have been increasing since 1970.[17–19]

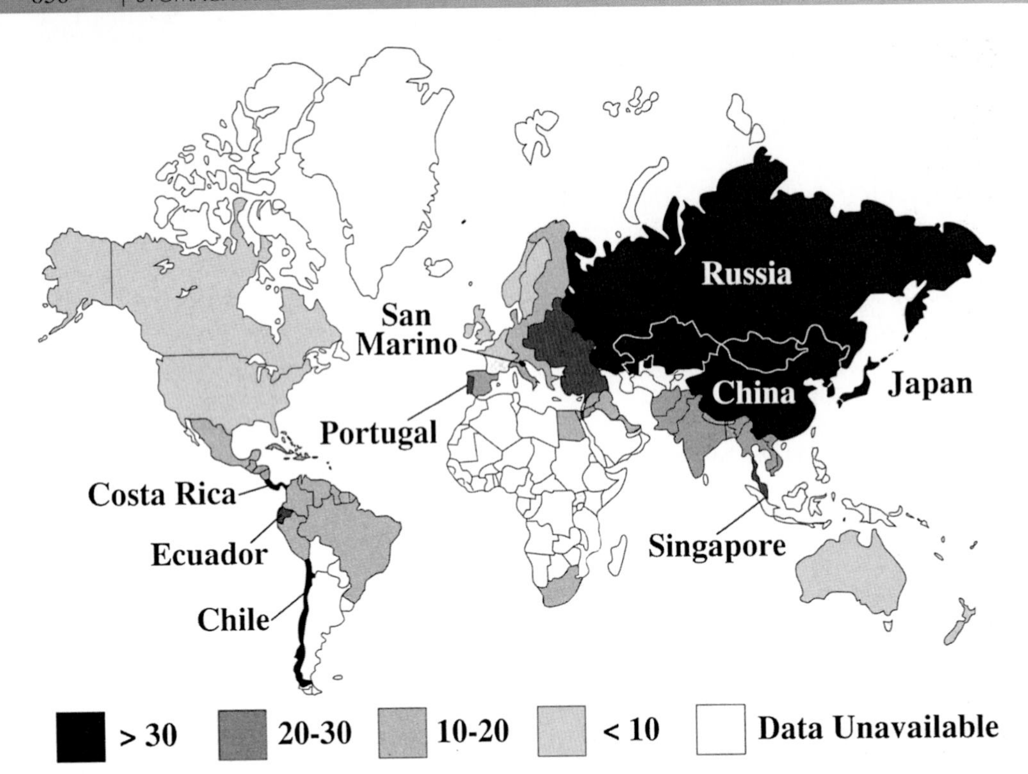

Figure 44–1. Worldwide distribution of gastric cancer age-adjusted death rates. The highest incidences are found in the Far East, Russia, and Eastern Europe, and the lowest incidences are found in North America, Africa, Australia, and New Zealand. Reliable data for comparison are not available from many countries.

Etiology

When discussing potential etiologies of gastric cancer, it is important to note that gastric cancer can be subdivided into two distinct pathologic entities that have different epidemiologic and prognostic features[20] (Fig. 44–3). The *diffuse form* of cancer is more poorly differentiated and lacks any glandular structure. It is found in the same frequency throughout the world, occurs at a younger age, and is associated with a worse prognosis than the intestinal form. The *intestinal form* of cancer is characterized by the formation of glandlike tubular structures mimicking intestinal glands.[21] This form of cancer is more closely linked to environmental and dietary risk factors, tends to occur at greater proportional rate in regions with a high incidence of gastric cancer, and is the form of cancer that is now declining worldwide.

It is now thought that the development of the intestinal type of gastric cancer is likely a multistep process, as has been well described in the pathogenesis of colon cancer, in which the normal colonic mucosa is sequentially transformed into hyperproliferative epithelium, followed by an early adenoma, late adenoma, and then carcinoma. In colon cancer, each step in the transition is associated with a specific gene mutation.[22] The contention that the pathogenesis of intestinal-type gastric cancer is a multistep process is supported by the observation that both atrophic gastritis and intestinal metaplasia are found in higher incidence in patients with intestinal-type cancer,[23] and in countries with a high incidence of gastric cancer (see Chapter 43).

This multistep model of gastric cancer, developed in large part by Correa and colleagues,[24] postulates that there is a temporal sequence of precancerous changes that eventually leads to the development of gastric cancer.[25] Initially, inflammation caused primarily by *Helicobacter pylori* infection, as well as by exposure to toxins (high salt diet, preserved food, bile salts), can result in the development of chronic active gastritis. In a subset of these patients, this inflammatory process leads to the development of atrophic gastritis (with loss of glandular tissue), followed by intestinal metaplasia, dysplasia, early gastric cancer, and eventually advanced gastric cancer (Fig. 44–4). It is thought that all stages prior to the development of high-grade dysplasia are potentially reversible, although this is still somewhat controversial. Unlike the case with colon cancer, the precise genes involved in each step of this progression are still not precisely defined. The premalignant stages of gastric cancer are not as readily identifiable endoscopically for prospective study compared with colon cancer, and many gastric carcinomas are very heterogeneous, containing a large percentage of normal stromal cells that may confound genetic analysis. This makes characterization of the timing of specific gene mutations in gastric cancer difficult at best. Currently it remains uncertain whether the diffuse type of gastric cancer follows a similar histopathologic progression.

Genetics

A number of advances have been made in our understanding of the genetic changes that occur in gastric cancer, mostly the intestinal form. The most common genetic abnormalities found in gastric cancers tend to be loss of heterozygosity (LOH) of previously described tumor suppressor genes. The gene that has garnered the most attention is the tumor sup-

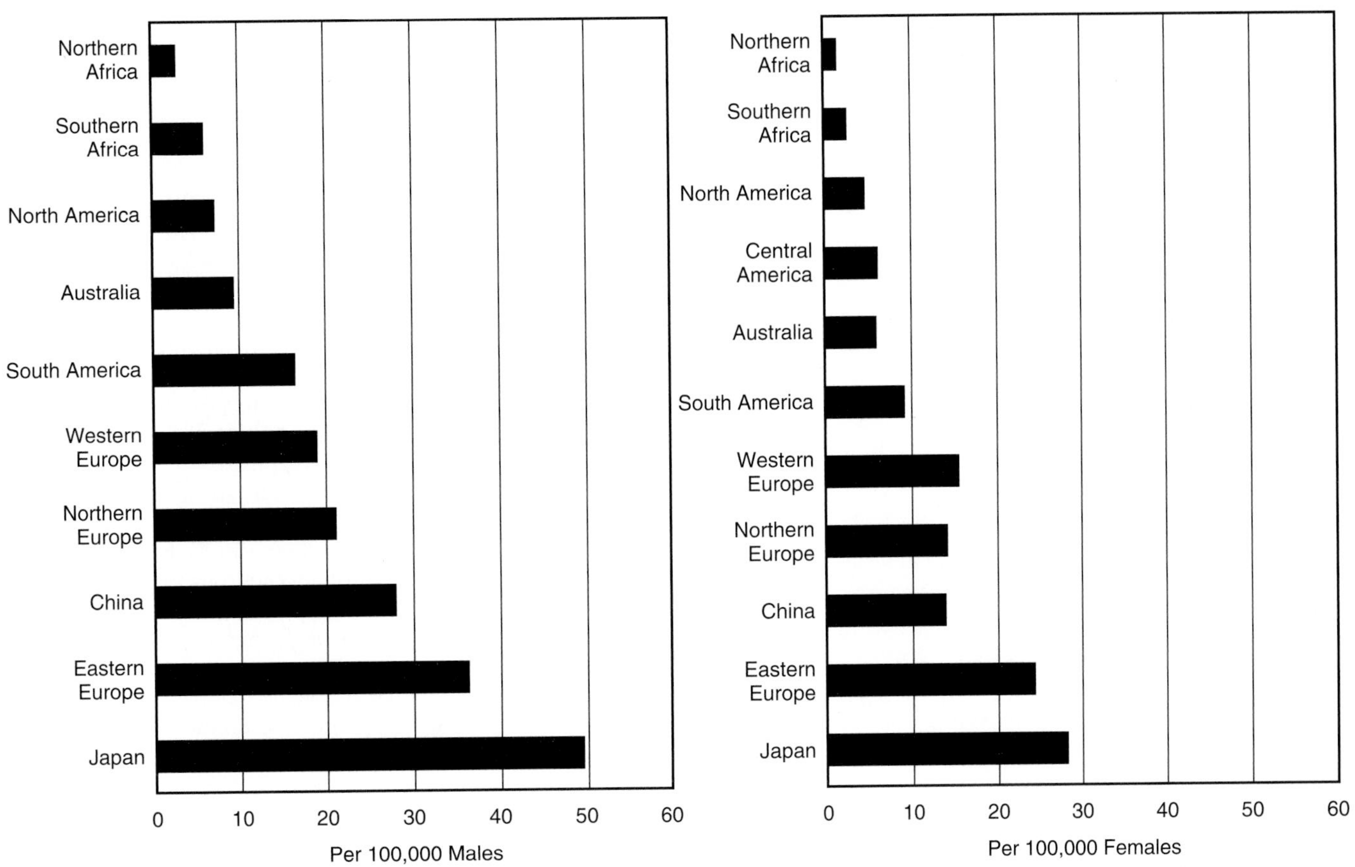

Figure 44–2. Estimates of the worldwide mortality from gastric cancer by region (1990). (Adapted from Pisani P, Parkin D, Bray F, et al: Estimates of the worldwide mortality from 25 cancers in 1990. Int J Cancer 83:18, 1999.)

pressor p53. Initial studies found that LOH (60% to 70%) and mutations (38% to 71%) of the p53 gene are quite common in gastric cancer. In addition, p53 mutations are also present in intestinal metaplasia (38%) and gastric dysplasia (58%),[26] suggesting that mutations of the p53 gene may be an early event in the pathogenesis of gastric cancer.[26–28] Further evidence for a role of p53 in the early stages of gastric cancer development comes from studies in mice that are hemizygous for p53, which exhibit an increased proliferative response to *Helicobacter* infection compared with wild-type mice.[29] Increased proliferation has generally been shown to correlate with an increased risk of developing gastric cancer.[30] Loss of p53 does not appear to confer a worse prognosis in patients with the intestinal form of cancer.[31–34] Taken together, these data suggest that inactivation of p53 is important in the early pathogenesis of gastric cancer.

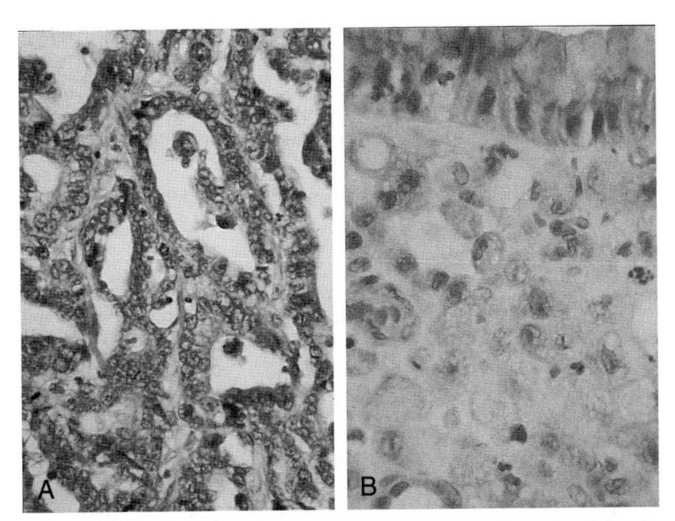

Figure 44–3. *A,* The intestinal form of cancer is characterized by the formation of gland-like tubular structures mimicking intestinal glands. *B,* In contrast, the diffuse form of gastric cancer is poorly differentiated, lacking any glandular structure. (Courtesy of Barbara Banner, MD.)

LOH at the 5q allelic locus—the site of the APC and MCC genes—occurs in over a third of gastric cancers[35] but not in gastric dysplasia,[36] with LOH being more common in the intestinal form regardless of stage.[37] Mutation of the APC gene is associated with familial adenomatous polyposis (FAP) and is an early event in the pathogenesis of colorectal cancer that is thought to be critical for the initial formation of adenomatous polyps.[38] Evidence supporting a role for APC in the pathogenesis of some forms of gastric cancer comes from the fact that FAP patients have close to a tenfold higher risk of developing gastric cancer compared with the general population.[39] Mutations of the APC gene occur in up to 20% of sporadic gastric cancers and gastric adenomas,[40] particularly in well-differentiated intestinal can-

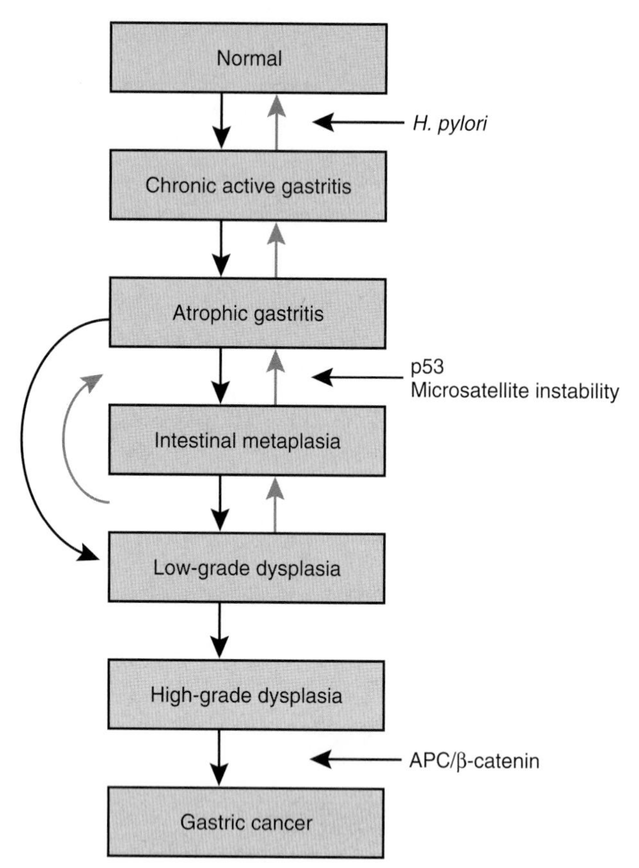

Figure 44–4. Proposed multistep pathway in the pathogenesis of gastric cancer. Infection with *Helicobacter pylori* may be a common initiating event, whereas genetic alterations (p53, APC/β-catenin pathway) or microsatellite genetic instability may play a later role. *Gray arrows* represent steps that are potentially reversible.

cers in which up to 60% may have APC mutations.[41] The mechanism of action of the APC gene product is to sequester and inactivate cytoplasmic β-catenin, preventing the formation of β-catenin/LEF, which acts as a growth-promoting transcription factor. β-Catenin mutations preventing its inactivation by APC are also found to occur in an additional 16% to 27% of sporadic intestinal-type cancers.[42, 43] The high frequency of either APC or β-catenin mutations, and/or LOH at the APC locus, suggests that APC is also important in the pathogenesis of gastric cancer. The fact that LOH of APC is seen in gastric cancer but not in gastric dysplasia suggests that suppression of APC may be involved during this late and final transition.

Genes that regulate entry into the cell cycle have been implicated in the pathogenesis of gastric cancer. The genes that inhibit entry into the cell cycle, p16 and p27, have been shown to have significantly decreased expression in nearly half of gastric cancers.[44–49] Absence of p27 expression has been associated with a poor prognosis in gastric cancer.[44, 46] Absence of p16 expression correlates with poorly differentiated carcinoma[50] but not with patient prognosis. The decreased expression of p16 and p27 occurs in the absence of detectable mutations and is thought to be secondary to hypermethylation.[48] It is difficult to ascertain the overall importance of p16 and p27 in the pathogenesis of gastric cancer in the absence of clear-cut mutations.

A number of other genes have been reported to be either mutated or suppressed in gastric cancer, although their relative importance in the pathogenesis of gastric cancer remains to be determined. These include the DCC gene, in which LOH occurs in 35%[51] and decreased expression occurs in 52%, correlating with increased rates of liver metastases.[52] FHIT (fragile histidine triad), a candidate tumor suppressor gene and a fragile locus exhibiting susceptibility to carcinogen-induced alterations, exhibits LOH in 53% and decreased expression in 62% of gastric cancers.[53, 54] There are few data on the frequency of mutations of these genes in gastric cancer, again leaving their relative importance in the pathogenesis unclear.

Conversely, amplification and/or overexpression of putative trophic factors has also been observed in gastric cancer. VEGF is a known angiogenic factor that promotes neovascularization of tumors, generally increasing the risk of invasion and metastases.[55] VEGF is overexpressed in up to 54% of gastric cancers and correlates with an increased risk of lymph node and liver metastases,[55, 56] and with disease recurrence.[33] Elevated serum levels of VEGF have also been significantly associated with adverse outcomes.[57] Thus it would appear that VEGF may play a role in the development of advanced gastric cancer, similar to that postulated for a number of other cancers.

The c-*met* gene, a proto-oncogene member of the tyrosine kinase growth factor receptors, is amplified in 10.2% and overexpressed in 46.1% of gastric cancers.[58] Its ligand, hepatocyte growth factor/scatter factor (HGF/SF), is also overexpressed in 67% of gastric cancers.[59] Amplification of the c-*met* gene is associated with increased depth of tumor invasion, lymph node metastases, and decreased survival.[58] Thus, c-*met* may be involved in the pathogenesis of gastric cancer, although the precise stage or timing of its involvement in the overall gastric cancer pathway has not been defined.

Cyclooxygenase-2 (COX-2) mRNA levels have been found to be elevated in gastric cancer.[60] There is a significant correlation between COX-2 expression and lymph node involvement.[61] Inhibition of COX-2 prevents growth of gastric cancer xenografts in nude mice,[62] and aspirin use (which inhibits both COX-1 and COX-2) decreases the risk of developing gastric cancer.[63] Thus COX-2 overexpression may also play a role in gastric carcinogenesis.[64]

A number of other genes may be overexpressed in gastric cancer, but in most cases the functional significance of such overexpression has not been directly studied. These genes are listed in Table 44–1.

Microsatellite instability (MSI) in dinucleotide repeats secondary to defects in DNA mismatch repair genes, such as MLH1 and MLH2, have been implicated in the development of colorectal cancer, and in particular the hereditary nonpolyposis colorectal cancer (HNPCC) syndrome. HNPCC patients have an 11% incidence of gastric cancer,[65] suggesting that MSI may also play a role in the development of gastric cancer. MSI is found in 15% to 50% of sporadic gastric cancers,[66–71] with a higher prevalence in the intestinal type of cancer.[68] Low-level microsatellite activity can be found in 40% in areas of intestinal metaplasia in patients with gastric cancer[71] and in 14% to 20% of adenomatous polyps.[69, 72] MSI is associated with the less frequent occurrence of p53 mutations, well-to-moderate patterns of differentiation, and distal location. Studies that have examined the effect of MSI

Table 44–1 | **Genetic Abnormalities in Gastric Adenocarcinoma**

ABNORMALITIES	GENE	APPROXIMATE FREQUENCY (%)
Deletion/suppression	p53	60–70
	FHIT	60
	APC	50
	DCC	50
	E-cadherin	<5
Amplification/overexpression	COX-2	70
	HGF/SF	60
	VEGF	50
	c-met	45
	AIB-1	40[363]
	β-catenin	25
	k-sam	20
	ras	10–15[69]
	c-erb B-2	5–7[364]
Microsatellite instability (MSI)		25–40
DNA aneuploidy		60–75

on patient survival have shown inconsistent results.[73, 74] Taken together, it would appear that MSI does play a role in the pathogenesis of gastric cancer, likely prior to the development of intestinal metaplasia (see Fig. 44–4).

The data regarding the genetics of diffuse gastric cancer are less complete. Mutations in the E-cadherin gene have been linked to the development of the diffuse type of gastric cancer. A large New Zealand kindred was recently found to carry a germ-line mutation in the E-cadherin gene.[75] Similar E-cadherin mutations have now been found in a German kindred,[76] two Korean kindreds,[77] two British kindreds,[78] and in a Japanese kindred, all with diffuse-type cancer.[79] Further evidence supporting a role for E-cadherin in the pathogenesis of gastric cancer comes from studies showing that suppression of E-cadherin occurs in 51% of cancers,[80] with a higher percentage found in the diffuse type of cancers. Furthermore, E-cadherin underexpression is associated with increased rates of lymph node metastases and decreased survival.[81, 82] The overall rates of E-cadherin mutations in gastric cancer are low, with the decreased expression of E-cadherin seen in gastric cancer likely secondary to hypermethylation of the E-cadherin promoter, which occurs in 50% of gastric cancers[83] and 83% of diffuse gastric cancers.

E-cadherin is a transmembrane protein that connects to the actin cytoskeleton through α- and β-catenin to establish cell polarity[75] and mediates homophilic cellular interactions.[76] Decreased expression of E-cadherin is thought to promote dissociation of cancer cells from their cell matrix, enhancing the migration and invasion of gastric cancer cells.[84] Expression of α-catenin is also decreased or absent in 68% of gastric cancers.[85] Taken together, E-cadherin appears to act as a tumor suppressor gene that may be important particularly in the pathogenesis of the diffuse form of gastric cancer.

In summary, the suppression/inactivation of several tumor suppressor genes, and the activation of several growth-promoting genes, appears to be important in the pathogenesis of gastric cancer. At the present time, there is no clear "gatekeeper gene" similar to APC in colon cancer, and the precise timing of the gene alterations in relation to the progression of gastric cancer remain to be defined.

Risk Factors

As is true for most malignancies, both genetic and environmental factors play important roles in the pathogenesis of gastric cancer. A recent study of twins in Scandinavia revealed that the relative risk of developing gastric cancer is 9.9 for monozygotic twins and 6.6 for dizygotic twins, suggesting that both genetic and environmental factors are involved in the pathogenesis of gastric cancer. This study further calculated that heritable factors account for 28% of gastric cancers, compared with 10% for shared environmental factors and 62% for nonshared environmental factors.[86]

Family History

Given that heritable factors account for nearly a third of gastric cancers, it is not surprising that individuals with a first-degree relative with gastric cancer have a two- to threefold increased relative risk of developing gastric cancer.[87–89] Individuals with a first-degree relative with gastric cancer are more likely to have the diffuse form of cancer and develop cancer at a younger age. Overall, 10% of cases of gastric cancer appear to exhibit familial clustering.[88] Family history remains an independent risk factor for gastric cancer, even after controlling for *H. pylori* status (which also exhibits familial clustering).[90, 91]

Individuals with a family history of gastric cancer are more likely to develop atrophic gastritis (34% vs. 5%) in the setting of *H. pylori* infection.[92] This genetic predisposition toward the development of atrophic gastritis may reflect different degrees of host immune response to infection. For example, interleukin-1 (IL-1) cluster polymorphisms have recently been identified as a risk factor for the development of atrophic gastritis and gastric cancer in *H. pylori*–infected patients but not in uninfected patients.[93]

Certain familial cancer syndromes also increase the risk of developing gastric cancer. Patients with familial adenomatous polyposis (FAP) have a prevalence of gastric adenomas ranging from 35% to 100%, and a risk of developing gastric cancer that is close to tenfold higher than that of the general population.[39] Because of the documented increased risk of gastric cancer seen with this condition, it is currently recommended to screen affected individuals every 3 to 5 years with endoscopy.[94, 95] Of note, it has also been reported that patients with FAP can also develop gastric cancer arising from fundic polyps.[39]

Patients with hereditary nonpolyposis colorectal cancer (HNPCC) have an approximately 11% chance of developing gastric cancer, predominantly of the intestinal type, with a mean age at diagnosis of 56 years and a 5-year survival rate of 15%.[65] Patients with juvenile polyposis had a 12% to 20% incidence of gastric cancer in several American kindreds.[96, 97]

Environmental Causes

HELICOBACTER PYLORI. *H. pylori* is a recently "rediscovered" pathogen of the stomach implicated in peptic ulcer disease (see Chapters 39 and 40). Virtually all patients infected with this organism develop chronic active gastritis. A subset of these patients, many of whom have high gastric acid output, will develop duodenal ulcer disease, which has been shown to be protective for gastric cancer.[98] However, another significant subset of *H. pylori*–infected patients, many of whom have low gastric acid output, will develop chronic atrophic gastritis, at a rate of 1% to 3% per year.[25, 92, 99] Atrophic gastritis is a risk factor for the development of gastric cancer (discussed later). Thus, those patients who are genetically predisposed to forming atrophic gastritis in response to *H. pylori* infection are predisposed to forming gastric cancer. *H. pylori* has been classified as a World Health Organization (WHO) class I carcinogen.[100]

Prospective case-controlled studies in the United States and England have revealed a three- to eightfold increase in gastric cancer rates in *H. pylori*–infected individuals compared with uninfected, age-matched controls.[11, 90, 101, 102] However, two recent meta-analyses of 19 and 34 trials respectively demonstrated a relative risk of gastric cancer of closer to 2 when compared with uninfected patients.[103, 104]

A number of potential mechanisms for *H. pylori*–induced gastric carcinogenesis have been proposed. A major mechanism appears to be the induction of chronic inflammation by *H. pylori* infection. Chronic inflammation has numerous consequences, and inflammation has been cited as a risk factor for a number of site-specific malignancies. Chronic inflammation leads to increased oxidative stress, with formation of oxygen-free radicals that can cause DNA damage, and to increased cytokine production, resulting in increased cell turnover and impaired DNA repair.[105] In general, it appears that the induction of a T_H1 cytokine response is most strongly linked to increased gastric cancer rates.[106]

The combination of *H. pylori* infection and the resulting inflammatory response leads to increases in gastric epithelial cell proliferation and apoptosis rates in vivo.[30, 107] While the increase in apoptosis may be related to inflammation and perhaps to direct bacterial interactions, the increase in proliferation may be secondary to *H. pylori*–induced hypergastrinemia and the induction of the mitogen-activated protein (MAP) kinase pathway.[108] In many cancer models, increased proliferation rates have been shown to be important in cancer pathogenesis. Increased gastric proliferation has been associated with an increased rate of lymph node metastases[109, 110] and worse prognosis in gastric cancer.[111]

Much attention has been given to the different virulence factors in the *H. pylori* genome, and in particular the CagA pathogenicity island. CagA is a toxin that can be injected into eukaryotic cells, resulting in host morphologic changes, increased proinflammatory cytokine production (IL-8), and gastric mucosal inflammation.[112–115] CagA-positive strains of *H. pylori* have been associated with an increased risk of developing atrophic gastritis and intestinal metaplasia.[116, 117] It remains uncertain whether *H. pylori* promotes carcinogenesis through direct host interactions, or indirectly through the induction of inflammation.

H. pylori infection, especially CagA-positive strains, has also been associated with markedly decreased levels of ascorbic acid in the gastric juice, leading to increased susceptibility to formation of *N*-nitroso compounds.[118] Acute infections result in inhibition of ascorbate secretion, whereas chronic antral-predominant gastritis also results in decreased secretion of ascorbate.[119]

Other potential effects of *H. pylori* that mediate the development of gastric cancer include the down-regulation of α-catenin and of E-cadherin.[85] *H. pylori* has also been associated with increased rates of microsatellite instability in patients with gastric cancer.[71]

A recent study of patients from Scotland and Poland suggests that specific genotypes of IL-1 (IL-1-1B-31T + and IL-1-1B-511T+) increase the risk of developing both atrophic gastritis and gastric cancer in *H. pylori*–infected individuals.[93] These genotypes are believed to enhance production of interleukin-1-beta, which is an important proinflammatory cytokine[120] and inhibitor of acid secretion.[121] The subset of *H. pylori*–infected patients that develops atrophic gastritis is more likely to be infected with a CagA-positive strain.[116, 117] In addition, those individuals who have a low acid output in response to *H. pylori* infection may be more prone to developing *H. pylori* infection beyond the antrum into the fundus, which can then lead to atrophic gastritis.[122, 123] Long-term acid suppression with proton pump inhibitors in *H. pylori*–infected individuals likewise increases the rate of gastric corpus infection and mucosal atrophy.[124] The effect of atrophic gastritis in the pathogenesis of gastric cancer is discussed in more detail later in the text.

The effect of eradicating *H. pylori* on the subsequent risk of developing gastric cancer is unclear. About 50% of patients will resolve their chronic atrophic gastritis after eradication of their *H. pylori* infection.[92] A nonrandomized trial of 132 patients with endoscopic resection of early gastric cancers (EGCs) found that none of 65 patients whose *H. pylori* infection was eradicated developed recurrent EGC in 2 years, compared with 6 of 67 patients whose *H. pylori* infection was not eradicated.[125] Eradication lowers the proliferation rate back to levels seen in noninfected controls.[126] Large, prospective, randomized controlled trials need to be performed to see whether and when eradication of *H. pylori* infection will prevent the development of gastric cancer, and whether this approach will be cost effective.

DIETARY. Numerous dietary factors have been implicated as risk factors for gastric cancer. The decline in gastric cancer rates has coincided with the widespread use of refrigeration and the concomitant increased intake of fresh fruits and vegetables and decreased intake of pickled and salted foods. Use of refrigeration for more than 10 to 20 years has been associated with a decreased risk of gastric cancer.[25, 127] Lower temperatures reduce the rate of bacterial, fungal, and other contaminants of fresh food, and the bacterial formation of nitrites. Conversely, high intake of highly preserved foods is associated with increased gastric cancer risk,[128, 129] likely because of increased content of salt, nitrates, and polycyclic aromatic amines.[130]

Much attention has been paid to the effects of high nitrate intake. When nitrates are reduced to nitrite by bacteria or macrophages,[131, 132] they can react with other nitrogenated substances to form *N*-nitroso compounds that are known mitogens and carcinogens.[133] In rats, *N*-nitroso compounds have been shown to cause gastric cancer.[134] However studies trying to link *N*-nitroso exposure to gastric cancer risk have been inconclusive, perhaps reflecting the fact that nitrate intake does not necessarily correlate with nitrosation levels.[135, 136] Recently, a large prospective cohort study of 120,852 Dutch men followed for 6.3 years failed to demonstrate an increased risk of gastric cancer with nitrate intake.[137] Although in theory nitrates can be stomach carcinogens, the overall importance of dietary nitrate intake on human gastric cancer pathogenesis remains unclear.

Another dietary factor that has been implicated in the development of gastric cancer is a diet high in salt (pickled and smoked foods, soy sauce, dried and salted fish and meat). High salt intake has been associated with increased rates of atrophic gastritis in humans and animals in the setting of *Helicobacter* infection[138] and has also been found to increase the mutagenicity of nitrosated food in animal models.[24] Populations with a relatively high salt diet have a 50% to 80% increase in gastric cancer risk in human case control studies.[129, 139] It has further been estimated that the relative risk of developing gastric cancer is about twofold[128, 140] in the upper tertile of patients. Thus, diets high in salt do appear to predispose to gastric cancer formation.

High intake of fresh fruits and raw vegetables repeatedly has been found to be protective for gastric cancer, with a 30% to 50% reduction in risk.[128, 129, 139, 141–143] A prospective cohort study of 11,907 Japanese residents of Hawaii found a risk ratio of 0.6 in those people who consumed fruit seven or more times per week.[144] It is thought that the protective effect of fresh fruits and vegetables may be secondary to increased consumption of antioxidant vitamins. These antioxidants are free radical scavengers that reduce reactive radical–induced DNA damage.[145] Ascorbate has been shown to reduce the risk of developing gastric cancer by 30% to 60%,[129, 142, 146, 147] although the protective effects seen are less than those seen of fresh fruit.[128, 142, 148] Ascorbate levels decrease with both nitrate and omeprazole ingestion.[133] The data for other vitamins, such as β-carotene,[129, 146, 149, 150] alpha-tocopherol,[137, 146] and selenium[151] have been inconclusive.

Other food problems that have been implicated as a risk factor for gastric cancer include increased intake of fried food,[129] foods high in fat,[141] high intake of red meat,[139, 152] and aflatoxins.[153] Conversely, diets with a high intake of fresh fish have been reported to be protective.[154] However, there are insufficient data to make any definitive conclusions regarding these foods.

CIGARETTE SMOKING. Cigarette smoking has consistently been found in case-control studies to be a risk factor for gastric cancer, with a risk ratio approaching 2 in heavy smokers, current smokers, and those who began smoking at a young age.[155–159]

ALCOHOL. It has previously been thought that alcohol was a risk factor for the development of gastric cancer. However, the great majority of recent trials have found that alcohol is not an independent risk factor for gastric cancer.[156, 157, 159]

ASPIRIN. Aspirin use has been associated with decreased mortality from gastric cancer, thought secondary to inhibition of cyclooxygenases involved in prostaglandin synthesis, and in particular, cyclooxygenase-2 (COX-2). As mentioned earlier, COX-2 overexpression is thought to promote the growth of tumors, and COX-2 is overexpressed in 70% of gastric cancers, although it is interesting that it is not overexpressed in those tumors with microsatellite instability.[64] A prospective mortality study of 635,031 men and women in the Cancer Prevention Study II demonstrates that regular aspirin use was protective for gastric cancer, with a risk ratio of 0.54 in men and 0.42 in women.[63] An American,[160] British,[161] and Russian[162] case-controlled study found a similar protective benefit. To date, there are no studies looking at the effect of COX-2 specific inhibitors on gastric cancer incidence.

LOW SOCIOECONOMIC STATUS. Historically, lower socioeconomic status has been linked to increased rates of gastric cancer.[163, 164] However, many potential confounding factors are associated with a low socioeconomic status, including poor sanitation, high prevalence of *H. pylori*, absence of refrigeration, and types of employment. In Western countries, the improvement of basic sanitation, widespread use of refrigeration, and decrease in *H. pylori* infection in all socioeconomic classes have resulted in a decreased correlation of socioeconomic class with gastric cancer risk in recent large studies. Although higher levels of education have been shown to have a protective effect (risk ratio of 0.6)[165] in a prospective cohort study of 58,279 Dutch men followed for 4.3 years, there was no clear association of gastric cancer with socioeconomic class. A recent retrospective study of 5645 British men likewise found that socioeconomic class was not an independent risk factor for the development of gastric cancer.[166] Thus, as basic levels of sanitation have improved regardless of socioeconomic class in Western countries, the effect of socioeconomic status on developing gastric cancer appears to have lessened.

SUMMARY OF ENVIRONMENTAL RISK/PREVENTIVE FACTORS. The major environmental risk factors for the development of gastric cancer appear to be *H. pylori* infection, diets high in salted and/or preserved foods, and cigarette smoking. Protective factors include diets high in fresh fruits and vegetables, vitamin C, and aspirin. To prevent gastric cancer, diets high in fruits and vegetables and low in salted and preserved foods should be recommended. Cigarette smoking should be discontinued. Although cost-effective analysis and large prospective studies looking at the efficacy of aspirin and/or COX-2 antagonists in preventing gastric cancer have not been performed, selective nonsteroidal anti-inflammatory drug (NSAID) use in patients at high risk for developing gastric cancer could be considered. The effect of *H. pylori* eradication on the subsequent development of gastric cancer is still unclear, and recent data have raised questions regarding the possible effect of *H. pylori* eradication on the risk of developing gastroesophageal reflux disease and/or esophageal cancer.[167] Until further studies to clarify these issues are performed, eradication of *H. pylori* for the purpose of gastric cancer prevention should be considered only in high-risk patients (i.e., positive family history, prior history of gastric cancer, atrophic gastritis, intestinal metaplasia, postantrectomy, and so on).

Premalignant Conditions

CHRONIC ATROPHIC GASTRITIS (also see Chapter 43). Chronic atrophic gastritis, which is defined as the loss of specialized glandular tissue in its appropriate region of the stomach,[168] has been associated with a nearly sixfold increased relative risk of developing the intestinal form of gastric cancer.[169–171] An increasing severity of atrophic gastritis also correlates with increased incidence of gastric cancer.[169, 170] There are two forms of atrophic gastritis. The most common form is multifocal atrophic gastritis (MAG),

Table 44–2 | **Padova International Classification System for Gastric Dysplasia**

CATEGORY	DEFINITION	HISTOLOGIC DESCRIPTION
I	*1.0.* Normal	*1.0.* Normal gastric architecture with absent or minimal inflammatory infiltrates
	1.1. Reactive foveolar hyperplasia	*1.1.* The general architecture is well preserved, with evidence of hyperproliferative epithelium, including elongated foveolae, enlarged nuclei, and mitotic figures
	1.2. Intestinal metaplasia	*1.2. Type I.* Closely resembles the morphology of the small intestine, with absorptive enterocytes, well-defined brush borders, and well-formed goblet cells
		Type II. Incomplete metaplasia with irregular mucous vacuoles, absence of brush borders, and absorptive enterocytes not easily identifiable. Predominantly secrete sialomucins
		Type III. Same as type II except predominantly secrete sulfomucins
II	Indefinite for dysplasia	Unable to discern whether cells are neoplastic or non-neoplastic. Usually in setting of inadequate biopsy specimens, and presence of architectural distortion and nuclear atypia
III	Noninvasive neoplasia	Phenotypically neoplastic epithelium confined to glandular structures inside the basement membrane. Includes adenomas. Should be divided into "low-grade" and "high-grade"
IV	Suspicious for invasive gastric cancer	Presence of neoplastic epithelium where invasion cannot be clearly identified
V	Invasive carcinoma	Invasive carcinoma

From Rugge M, Correa P, Dixon M, et al: Gastric dysplasia: The Padova International Classification, Am J Surg Pathol 24:167, 2000.

usually secondary to *H. pylori* infection. MAG is more likely to be associated with metaplasia. Gastric atrophy leads to low acid output (achlorhydria), which predisposes to increased bacterial overgrowth (with non-*Helicobacter* organisms), increased formation of *N*-nitroso compounds, and decreased ascorbate secretion into the gastric lumen.[172] Additionally, the low acid output seen in atrophic gastritis results in increased levels of gastrin, a known growth factor for the stomach and a possible risk factor for gastric cancer.[173]

Diffuse corporal atrophic gastritis is the less common form of gastritis, which is associated with antiparietal cell and intrinsic factor antibodies and is confined to the parts of the stomach where parietal cells reside (body and the fundus). It is associated with pernicious anemia and with an increased gastric cancer risk, albeit not as high as that seen with *H. pylori*–induced MAG, possibly related to lesser degrees of inflammation.[174, 175]

INTESTINAL METAPLASIA. Intestinal metaplasia can be subdivided into three categories, as classified by Filipe and Jass.[176] *Type I* is the complete form of intestinal metaplasia, containing Paneth cells, goblet cells that secrete sialomucins, and absorptive epithelium, and it does not increase risk of developing gastric cancer. *Type II* represents incomplete metaplasia, with few absorptive cells, few columnar intermediate cells, and goblet cells expressing sulfomucins (but not sialomucins). *Type III* is intermediate to type I and type II.[177] Type II or type III intestinal metaplasia occurs in almost 80% of intestinal-type cancers, whereas the incidence of intestinal metaplasia in patients with diffuse-type cancer is the same as that of the general population.[178] It has been estimated that the relative risk of developing gastric cancer in patients with type II or type III intestinal metaplasia can be as high as 20.[177] In addition, 42% of patients with type III intestinal metaplasia develop early gastric cancer within 5 years of follow-up,[177] suggesting that intestinal metaplasia may represent a precursor lesion for the intestinal form of gastric cancer. However, it remains unclear as to whether cancer arises from areas of intestinal metaplasia, or whether intestinal metaplasia simply represents a marker for increased gastric cancer risk. Screening for patients with intestinal metaplasia is problematic as it is difficult to locate areas of intestinal metaplasia or cancer endoscopically, and multiple random biopsies would be needed. The combination of low sensitivity and high cost would make screening costs prohibitive.[179]

GASTRIC DYSPLASIA. In 1971, the Japanese Research Society for Gastric Cancer proposed a classification system for gastric dysplasia.[180] Recently, an international consensus conference of gastrointestinal pathologists has agreed upon a unified classification system (Table 44–2) to facilitate comparison of research studies.[181]

Prospective studies have shown that mild dysplasia apparently can regress in up to 60% of cases, with 10% to 20% progressing to high-grade dysplasia.[182–184] Patients with moderate dysplasia can progress to severe dysplasia in 20% to 40% of cases,[183–185] Patients with high-grade dysplasia rarely regress, and 75% to 100% progress to cancer by 2 years of follow-up[182–184] (Fig. 44–5). High-grade dysplasia

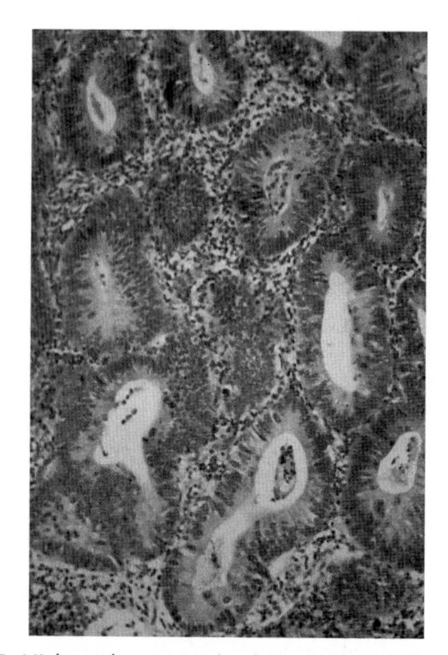

Figure 44–5. High-grade gastric dysplasia, with neoplastic epithelium confined to the glandular structures inside the basement membrane. This lesion is premalignant. (Courtesy of Barbara Banner, MD.)

is often associated with synchronous cancer and is short-lived and focal.[186] Early gastric cancer is found to have adjacent foci of high-grade dysplasia in 40% to 100% of cases, and advanced cancers are noted to have adjacent areas of high-grade dysplasia in 5% to 80%.[186] Because of these findings, it is recommended that patients with category III low to moderate-grade dysplasia undergo surveillance endoscopic screening, and patients with category III high-grade dysplasia and category IV dysplasia undergo resection by either endoscopic or surgical means.

GASTRIC POLYPS. Gastric polyps are present in less than 1% of the general population.[187] Up to 90% of them are hyperplastic polyps. They generally remain small, rarely exceeding 1.5 cm, and the rate of malignant transformation is generally quite low (<1%) and confined to polyps larger than 1 cm.[188] The rare polyps that do undergo malignant transformation often have areas of dysplasia or intestinal metaplasia and typically form well-differentiated intestinal-type cancer.[188] The majority of gastric polyps that undergo malignant transformation are adenomas. It has been documented that gastric adenomas followed by endoscopy with biopsy can progress to dysplasia and then carcinoma in situ,[189] with approximately 11% of gastric adenomas developing carcinoma in situ within 4 years of follow-up.[189] Because of this it has been suggested that patients with documented gastric adenomas have surveillance endoscopic screening examinations, with endoscopic polypectomy if adenomas are found. One recent nonrandomized study suggests that eradication of *H. pylori* may inhibit progression of gastric adenomas to gastric cancer.[190]

POSTGASTRECTOMY. It has been reported by several groups that gastric surgery for benign conditions can predispose patients to an increased risk of developing gastric cancer beginning 20 years after the surgery.[191–194] The risk is greatest for those who had their operation before the age of 50 years, perhaps reflecting the long lag period necessary between the operation and the development of cancer.[192] The cancers tend to occur at or near the surgical anastomosis, and only rarely do they reside on the intestinal side of the anastomosis.[195] Postgastrectomy cancers typically present in men over the age of 50 years, perhaps reflecting the fact that men are more likely to have peptic ulcer surgery. They represent 5% of all gastric cancers[196] and are usually advanced at the time of diagnosis, resulting in 2-year survival rates of no more than 10%.[197]

Numerous theories have been proposed to explain the increased propensity to form cancers at the surgical anastomosis site. They include hypochlorhydria resulting in bacterial overgrowth, leading to increased production of nitrites[198]; chronic reflux of bile salts and pancreatic enzymes, which are potent gastric irritants[25]; and atrophy of the remaining fundic mucosa secondary to low levels of antral hormones, including gastrin.[199] The Billroth II operation predisposes to the development of cancer at a fourfold higher rate than does a Billroth I, suggesting that bile reflux may be a significant predisposing factor.[192] It is unclear whether it would be cost effective to screen for gastric cancer in this population of patients in areas of low incidence.

MENETRIER'S DISEASE (see Chapter 43). This is a rare condition associated with hypertrophy of the surface mucus cells and atrophy of the parietal and chief cells, resulting in increased thickness of the fundic mucosa, a protein-losing enteropathy, and hypochlorhydria. It has recently been shown that this condition is associated with increased expression of the epidermal growth factor (EGF) family of ligands, most notably transforming growth factor-α. Recently it has been reported that administration of an antibody that blocks the EGF receptor can reverse gastric mucosal hypertrophy in Menetrier's disease.[200] In a review of case reports of Menetrier's, 15% mention an association with gastric cancer,[201] including several cases that document a progression from dysplasia to cancer with time.[202, 203] Because of the rarity of this condition, it has been difficult to study the relationship of Menetrier's disease and gastric cancer in any controlled fashion, and no recommendations regarding endoscopic surveillance can be made.

GASTRIC ULCER. It was previously believed that 10% of gastric ulcers would eventually progress to gastric cancer, since carcinoma would often be found at the edge of the ulcer and not at the base. With the advent of flexible endoscopy and improved radiologic techniques, it was soon recognized that many of the ulcers that were thought to transform into cancer eventually actually represent gastric cancer with ulceration.[204] More recent large cohort studies still report a risk ratio of 1.8 for patients diagnosed with a gastric ulcer eventually developing gastric cancer, after an average follow-up of close to nine years.[98] This association, if real, could be due to the association of *H. pylori* infection with both benign gastric ulcer and gastric cancer.

Screening

In Japan, there is a high prevalence of gastric cancer and, more importantly, a high proportion of early gastric cancers that have a 95% cure rate.[205] Since 1962, the Japanese have been performing mass screening, using photofluorography followed by endoscopy if any suspicious lesions were found. Photofluorography consists of images taken on 100-mm film with the patient in the prone position (anterior mucosal view and barium-filled picture), supine position (double-contrast view), right anterior oblique position, semiupright position (left anterior oblique view), and upright position (barium-filled), performed in a specially designed mobile unit.[206] Screening was also performed in more urban areas with a remote-controlled television system in special clinics where, in addition to the aforementioned views, an additional picture in the left anterior oblique position (double-contrast view) was obtained.[206] The Japanese have reported a sensitivity of 66% to 90% and a specificity of 77% to 90% using this screening approach.[207] In 1996, 6.4 million people were screened in Japan, and 6903 cases of gastric cancer were detected. There was a high prevalence (50%) of early gastric cancer (EGC) in the screened group, suggesting that treatable lesions were being found.[208, 209]

Case control studies suggest up to a 50% reduction in gastric cancer mortality in the screened population,[210] although this may reflect the overall worldwide trend toward decreased mortality from gastric cancer. A prospective case-controlled study of 24,135 Japanese patients followed for 40 months revealed a risk ratio of 0.72 of dying from gastric cancer in the patients who underwent screening.[211] Thus it would appear that routine screening in high-risk populations does have a significant survival benefit. To date, no good

Table 44–3 | **Risk Factors for Gastric Adenocarcinoma**

DEFINITE/SURVEILLANCE SUGGESTED
Familial adenomatous polyposis (FAP)
Gastric adenoma
Dysplasia
DEFINITE
Helicobacter pylori infection
Chronic atrophic gastritis
Intestinal metaplasia
Hereditary nonpolyposis colorectal cancer (HNPCC)
Postgastrectomy
First-degree relative with gastric cancer
PROBABLE
Peutz-Jeghers syndrome
Cigarette smoking
Low aspirin intake
High salt intake
Low intake of fresh fruits and vegetables
Pernicious anemia
Low ascorbate intake
POSSIBLE
Low socioeconomic status
Menetrier's disease
Gastric ulcer
QUESTIONABLE
High intake of alcohol
Hyperplastic/fundic polyps

cost-benefit analysis has been performed to estimate the cost of screening per year of life saved.

In Western countries, the prevalence of gastric cancer is much lower than in Japan, and the rate of EGC detection is lower than 20%,[212] making routine screening of asymptomatic patients questionable. In patients with a high risk of gastric cancer, such as those with low to moderate dysplasia, gastric adenomas, or a history of FAP, endoscopic screening is generally recommended, although there are no prospective randomized trials supporting this approach (Table 44–3).

Clinical Manifestations

Gastric cancers that do not penetrate into the muscularis propria (early gastric cancers or EGC) are asymptomatic in up to 80% of patients. When symptoms do occur, they tend to mimic peptic ulcer disease. Part of the reason for the poor prognosis of gastric cancer is that the disease is usually quite advanced by the time symptoms develop. At the time of diagnosis (advanced gastric cancer), the predominant symptom is weight loss, occurring in 62% of patients, followed by abdominal pain (52%). Other less frequent symptoms include nausea, vomiting, anorexia, dysphagia, melena, early satiety, and ulcer-like symptoms.[14] Pyloric outlet obstruction can occur with tumors of the antrum (Fig. 44–6*A*), presenting with early satiety and vomiting, whereas tumors affecting the cardia can cause dysphagia.[213] Feculent emesis or undigested food in the stool may represent a gastrocolic fistula secondary to the invasion of gastric cancer into the adjacent wall of the colon.[214]

Rarely, paraneoplastic syndromes occur. There have been reports of thrombophlebitis (Trousseau's sign), neuropathies,[215] nephrotic syndrome,[216] and disseminated intravascular coagulation.[217] Dermatologic paraneoplastic syndromes include hyperpigmented patches in the axilla (acanthosis nigricans) and the sudden onset of seborrheic dermatosis (senile warts) and pruritus (sign of Leser-Trélat),[220] although these findings are quite uncommon.

Physical examination is usually normal. Cachexia and signs of bowel obstruction are the most common finding. Occasionally it is possible to detect an epigastric mass, hepatomegaly, ascites, and lower extremity edema.[218] Sites of metastatic spread include infiltration of the umbilicus (Sister Joseph's nodule),[219] ovarian metastases (Krukenberg's tumor), and a mass in the pouch of Douglass (rectal shelf of Blumer).

At diagnosis, advanced cancer has usually metastasized, with the most common target organs being the liver (40%), lung, peritoneum, and bone marrow. Gastric cancer has also been reported to metastasize to the kidney, bladder, brain, bone, heart, thyroid, adrenals,[218] and skin.[219]

Diagnosis

LABORATORY STUDIES. Laboratory studies are generally unrevealing until the cancer reaches its advanced stages. Anemia and a positive test for fecal occult blood may occur owing to chronic bleeding. Hypoproteinemia can occur in patients with weight loss. Elevated liver enzyme levels can occur with hepatic metastases.

There are no reliable serum markers for gastric cancer. The gastric carcinoma–associated antigen MG7-Ag has been reported present in the serum of 82% of gastric cancer patients, compared with 8% of peptic ulcer patients.[221] Low serum pepsinogen I levels and low pepsinogen I : pepsinogen II ratios have been reported in patients with atrophic gastritis and intestinal metaplasia,[222] as has hypergastrinemia,[223] but the results for the detection of gastric cancer have been mixed, with low specificities being reported.

ENDOSCOPY. Currently, endoscopy is the procedure of choice for the diagnosis of gastric cancer (see Fig. 44–6*C* and *D*). Several studies have demonstrated the superiority of endoscopy with tissue biopsy over barium studies for the detection of gastric cancer, with a sensitivity of over 95% for advanced gastric cancer.[224, 225] When a nonhealing gastric ulcer is found, at least six to eight biopsies from the edge and base of the ulcer are recommended.[226] However, it can still be difficult to find early gastric cancers, with sensitivities of 50% to 60% reported with visual inspection alone, although the sensitivity does improve when multiple biopsies are taken.[224, 227]

The American Gastroenterological Association has recommended that an endoscopy be performed in patients who are over the age of 45 years with new-onset dyspepsia, and in patients under the age of 45 years who have alarm symptoms (weight loss, recurrent vomiting, dysphagia, evidence of bleeding, anemia). If they are under the age of 45 years and have no alarm symptoms, the Association recommends that the patient undergo *H. pylori* testing, with treatment if positive, or an empirical trial of an antisecretory or prokinetic medication if negative. If the patient is still symptomatic, an endoscopy should be considered.[228] The basis for these recommendations is the extremely low rate of gastric cancer in individuals under the age of 45 years in this population. The incidence of gastric cancer in patients under the age of 45 years with dyspepsia but without alarm symp-

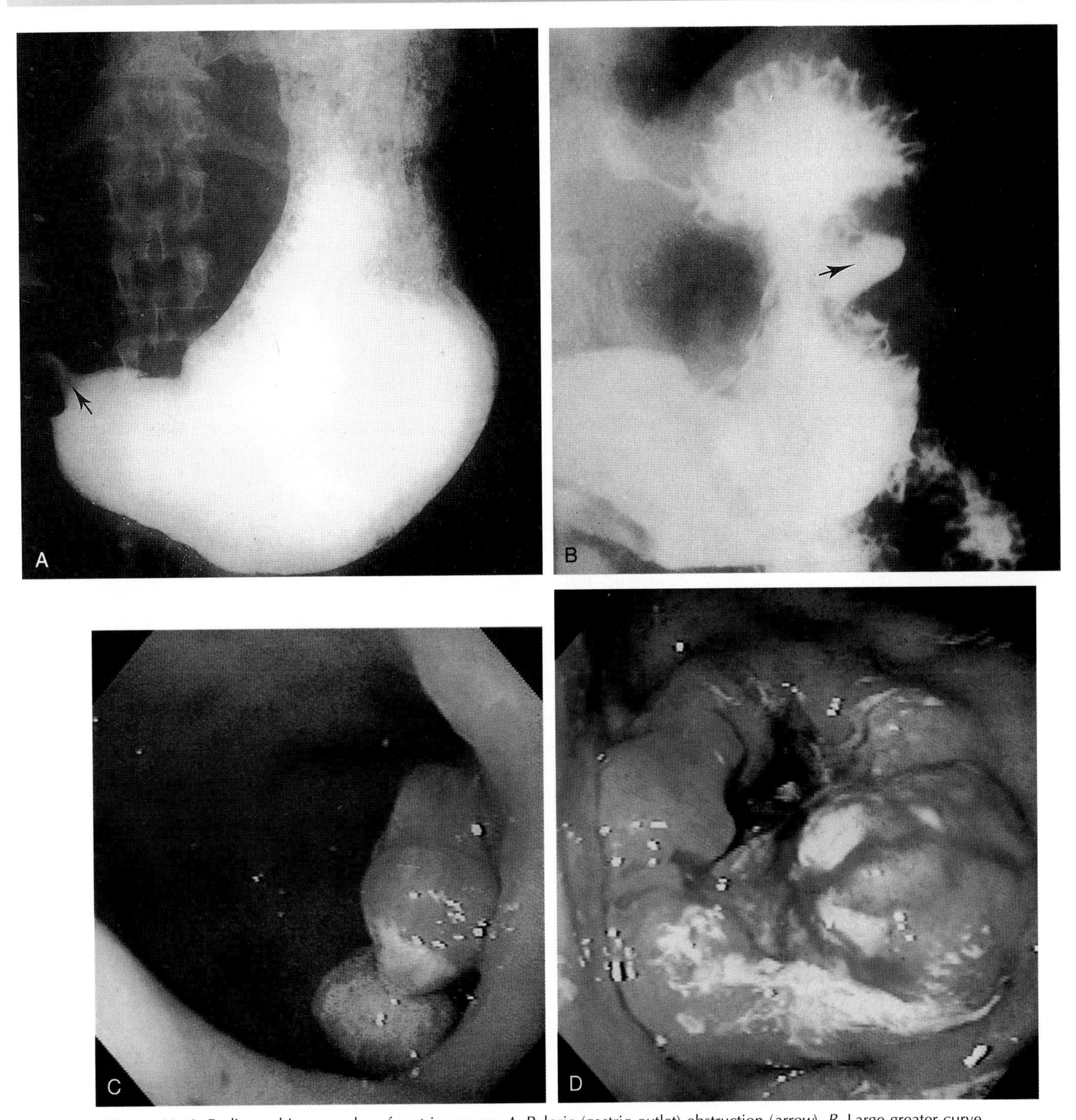

Figure 44–6. Radiographic examples of gastric cancer. *A*, Pyloric (gastric outlet) obstruction (*arrow*). *B*, Large greater curve ulcer within a mass (*arrow*). (Courtesy of Mark Feldman, MD.), *C*, Polypoid gastric cancer. Trilobed polyp at the angularis. *D*, Exophytic gastric cancer. Circumferential mass-like lesion involving the gastric body and collapsing the antrum.

toms has been estimated to be 1 in 1000.[229] The recommendations for asymptomatic patients who are fecal occult blood–positive and have a normal colonoscopy are less clear. One study of 498 asymptomatic fecal occult blood–positive patients revealed that 4 had gastric cancer, with anemia being associated with a higher probability of finding a causal source.[230]

Currently, attempts are being made to increase the sensitivity of endoscopy for the detection of early gastric cancer. The use of endoscopically administered supravital dies, and the oral administration of 5-aminolevulinic acid for the in vivo photodynamic diagnosis of premalignant and malignant lesions during endoscopy has been reported, but the sensitivity and specificity of these methods have not been well elucidated, and their use in Western countries should be confined to clinical trials.

ULTRASOUND. Transabdominal ultrasound has not been found useful for the diagnosis of gastric cancer owing to the presence of intraluminal gas throughout the abdomen that limits the transduction of ultrasound waves. Some investigators have distended the stomach with water, and although difficulties still remain with adequate visualization of the cardia, they report a 42% accuracy rate for T (tumor) staging and 66% accuracy for N (nodal) staging.[231] One problem inherent in T staging for both transabdominal and endoscopic ultrasound is that it is often difficult to distinguish the subserosal fat layer from the serosa, and thus the tendency to overstage tumors that penetrate the subserosal fat but not the serosa.[231]

ENDOSCOPIC ULTRASONOGRAPHY (EUS). Another limitation of transabdominal ultrasound is the relatively low frequency of the ultrasound transponder (higher frequencies allow better resolution but worse depth of penetration). In 1980, an ultrasound probe was affixed to the end of an endoscope, allowing placement of the probe directly against the stomach wall and the use of high-frequency transponders. High-frequency transponders provide excellent spatial resolution, allowing the visualization of the five layers of the gastric wall. The superficial gastric mucosa is represented by an echogenic first layer and the deeper mucosa by a hypoechogenic second layer. The submucosa is represented by an echogenic third layer, the muscularis propria as a hypoechogenic fourth layer, and the serosa as an echogenic fifth layer[232] (Figs. 44–7 and 44–8). The ability to distinguish among the mucosa, submucosa, and muscularis mucosa makes EUS the best imaging modality to determine depth of invasion (T stage), with an 80% accuracy rate reported.[227, 233, 234] EUS does tend to overestimate T stage because of the aforementioned difficulty distinguishing invasion through the subserosal fat (stage T2) and the serosa (stage T3).[227, 231]

EUS is 90% to 99% accurate at distinguishing between stage T1 and stage T2, which is the important criterion for the determination of early gastric cancer.[227, 235, 236] Since early gastric cancer is defined by the depth of penetration irrespective of lymph node involvement, EUS is thus an excellent modality in differentiating early from advanced gastric cancer.

The rate of detecting perigastric nodes with EUS is comparable to that of computed tomography (CT), with a diagnostic accuracy ranging around 50% to 80%.[231, 237] Much of the difficulty in N staging lies in the fact that imaging studies diagnose positive lymph nodes on the basis of size (>5 mm). However, small lymph nodes can also harbor metastases, and thus understaging can occur.[238] One study of 1253 lymph nodes in 31 gastric cancer patients found that 55% of lymph nodes containing tumor were less than 5 mm in size.[238]

The other useful application of EUS is in the identification and biopsy of submucosal lesions, such as scirrhous carcinomas and gastric lymphoma, which typically involve thickening of the submucosa and muscularis propria, and which may appear as gastric fold thickening on barium studies or endoscopy.

UPPER GI SERIES. Barium studies have reported a 60% to 70% sensitivity and a 90% specificity for the detection of advanced gastric cancer.[239] More recent technology, including digital radiography with a 4-million-pixel CCD, has improved these numbers somewhat, with overall sensitivity of 75.3% for digital radiography compared with 64.6% with conventional radiography; specificities were 90.5% and 84.5%, respectively.[240] However, their sensitivity for finding EGC is quite poor, and the ability to distinguish between a benign ulcer and a malignancy can be problematic.[241] Radiologic findings suggestive of a benign ulcer include a symmetrical ulcer with smooth margins, a radiolucent band between the ulcer and the lumen (Hampton's line), and the presence of symmetrical radiating folds around the ulcer crater (see Chapter 40). Findings suggestive of a malignancy include an asymmetrical ulcer crater, an ulcer within a mass (see Fig. 44–6*B*), the presence of an irregular mass or folds, loss of distensibility, and nodularity.[242]

COMPUTED TOMOGRAPHY. Studies looking at the role of CT in the diagnosis and staging of gastric cancer have been somewhat conflicting, partly because of the multitude of different techniques used. The shortcoming of CT lies in the need for adequate distention of the stomach to allow measurement of the thickness of the gastric wall. Currently, the modality of choice is helical CT, by which the wall of the stomach can be seen as three layers: an inner layer corre-

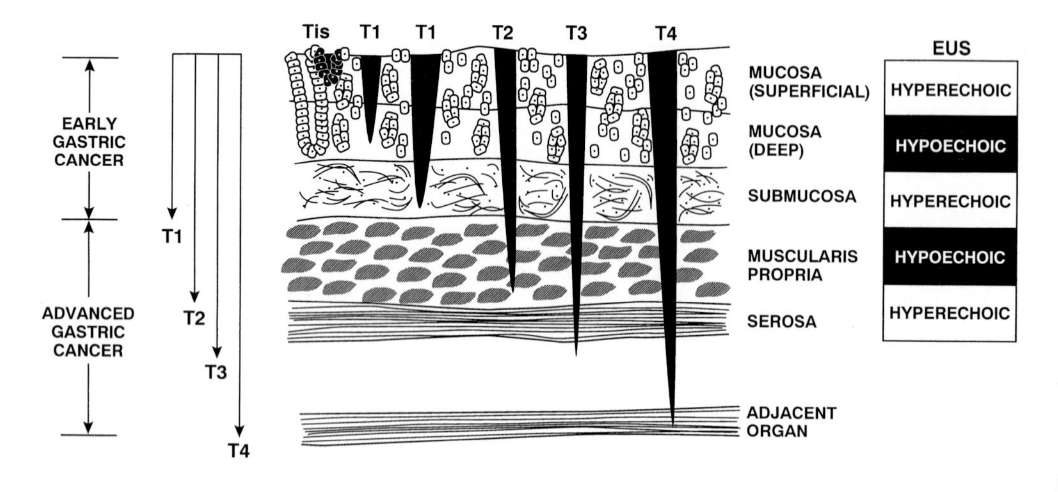

Figure 44–7. Classification of gastric adenocarcinoma by depth of invasion (T classification). In the TNM classification, T denotes depth of invasion; Tis designates carcinoma in situ; T1 tumors are confined to the mucosa and submucosa; T2 tumors penetrate the muscularis propria but not the serosa; T3 tumors penetrate the serosa without involving contiguous structures; and T4 tumors penetrate the serosa and involve adjacent organs and tissues. In early gastric cancer, the disease is confined to the mucosa and submucosa (T1), regardless of nodal involvement. Five layers shown by endoscopic ultrasonography (EUS) are also depicted.

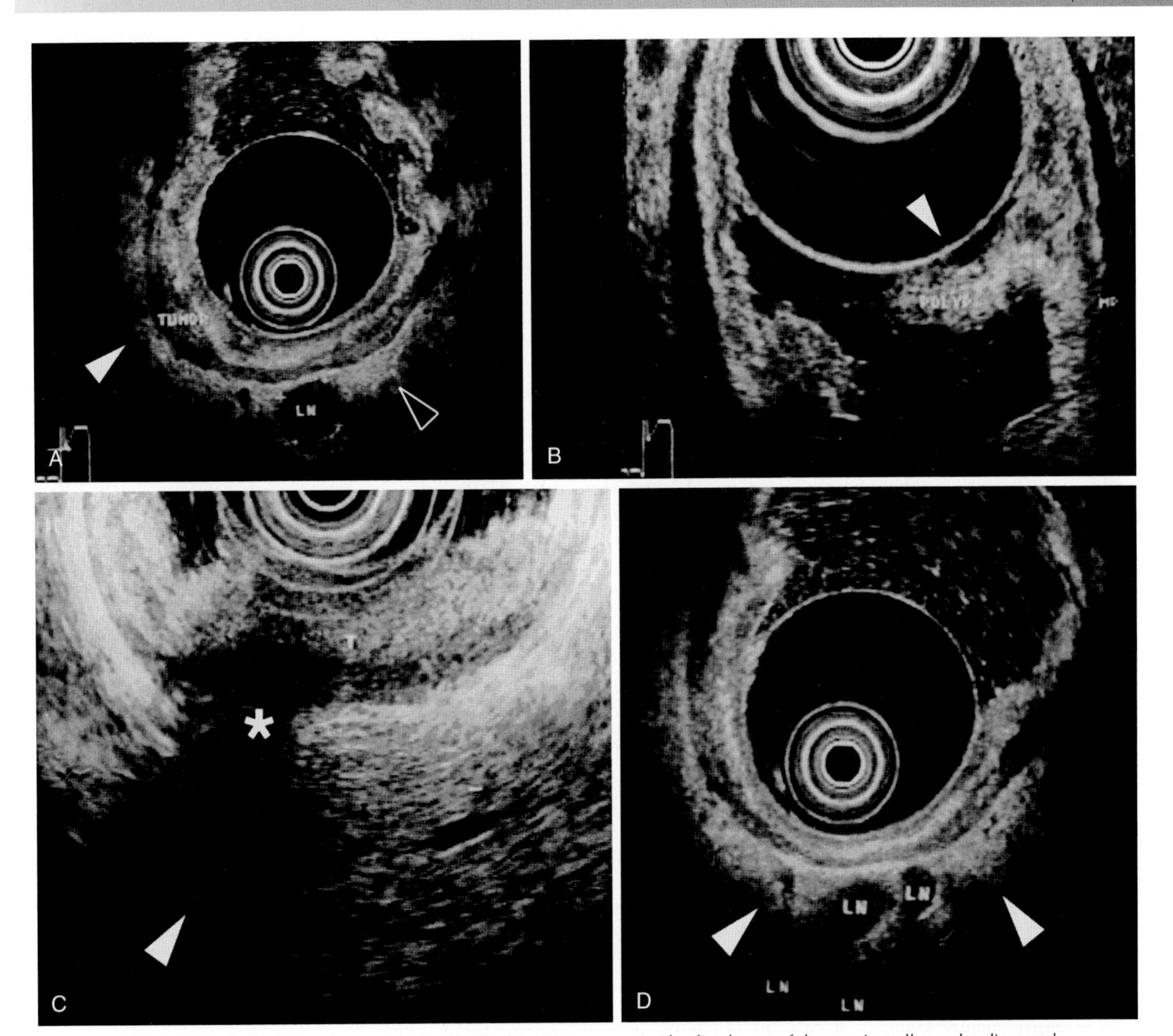

Figure 44–8. Endoscopic ultrasonography (EUS) of gastric tumors. *A,* The five layers of the gastric wall may be discerned near the bottom of the image, from the 3 o'clock position to the 6 o'clock position (*open arrowhead*). The tumor (TUMOR, *solid arrowhead*) involves the fourth hypoechoic (dark) layer, the muscularis propria, but has not encroached on the fifth hypoechoic layer, the serosa. In addition, an enlarged lymph node (LN) at the 6 o'clock position appears to be involved. The patient was found to have a T2N1 tumor. *B,* A gastric polypoid mass (POLYP, *arrowhead*) is pedunculated and involves only the first hyperechoic layer, the superficial mucosa, and has not breached deeper layers, including the muscularis propria (MP). The patient was found to have a benign, 1.5-cm pedunculated hyperplastic polyp. *C,* The tumor (*) has breached all five layers of the gastric wall, including the fifth hyperechoic (bright) layer and beyond (*arrowhead*). The patient was found to have a T4 tumor. *D,* Diffuse, hypoechoic infiltrations throughout all five layers of the gastric wall, giving a blotchy moth-eaten appearance (*arrowheads*), and four round, sharply demarcated hypoechoic lymph nodes (LN) are seen. The patient was found to have a stage IIE1 gastric lymphoma. (Courtesy of Markus Goldschmeidt, MD.)

sponding to the mucosa, an intermediate layer corresponding to the submucosa, and an outer layer of slightly higher attenuation corresponding to the muscularis and serosa.[231] The limit of detection for a discrete lesion in the stomach wall is about 5 mm. Gastric wall thickening suggests the presence of cancer, since over 90% of the normal population has a gastric wall thickness of less than a centimeter. The loss of fat planes between the gastric mass and any adjacent organ suggests invasion into that adjacent organ.[231]

CT has a 65% to 90% sensitivity for advanced gastric cancer, and 50% for early gastric cancers.[243, 244] The accuracy rate for T staging is approximately 60% to 70%,[245–247] and is between 40% and 70% for N staging.[237, 248] CT has a sensitivity of 70% for detecting peritoneal metastases and 57% for detecting hepatic metastases.[248] Again, like all other imaging modalities, CT has trouble discerning metastases less than 5 mm in size.

Thus, the role of CT is mainly for the detection of distant

metastases and as a complement to EUS for assessing regional lymph node involvement.

MAGNETIC RESONANCE IMAGING. Magnetic resonance imaging (MRI) with gadolinium has also been used for gastric cancer staging. It has similar advantages (ability to find distant metastases) and weaknesses (need for adequate gastric distention) as for CT. Several studies comparing the two techniques have found that MRI tends to be slightly better at T staging (73% to 83% vs. 67% to 73%) but slightly worse at N staging (55% to 65% vs. 59% to 73%) than spiral CT.[245–247] Given the higher cost of MRI, the superiority of EUS at T staging, and the superiority of CT at N staging, there is insufficient evidence to support the routine use of MRI in the diagnosis and staging of gastric cancer.

Classification Systems

Several classification systems further define gastric cancer and predict prognosis. As mentioned earlier, gastric cancers can be subdivided into intestinal and diffuse forms.[20] The *intestinal* (or *well-differentiated*) form consists of large, distinct cohesive cells with irregular nuclei that form glandlike tubular structures (see Fig. 44–3*A*). It is thought that intestinal cancers arise from metaplastic intestinalized gastric cells, as the intestinal form of gastric cancer is positively associated with the presence of intestinal metaplasia[23] and is associated with chronic inflammation and a prolonged precancerous phase. The intestinal form of cancer is proportionately more common in countries with a high incidence of gastric cancer,[21, 249] and in men and elderly people. It is thought that dietary and environmental factors exert a greater influence on the intestinal form of cancer. The *diffuse* (or *undifferentiated*) form consists of individual or small clusters of small cells in a nonpolarized pattern (see Fig. 44–3*B*). They are thought to rise directly from naïve gastric mucus cells and are relatively more common in low-risk populations.[196] The diffuse forms are found in roughly the same frequency throughout the world and are also associated with a younger age, with no male predominance.[250] They are more likely to occur in gastric family kindreds, have been associated with E-cadherin mutations, and are associated with a worse prognosis as they are more likely to invade transmurally.

Gastric cancer can also be divided into early and advanced cancers. *Early gastric cancer (EGC)* is defined as a cancer that does not invade beyond the submucosa regardless of lymph node involvement. This form of cancer has a much higher prevalence in the Far East, and especially Japan, and carries a very favorable prognosis, with greater than 90% 5-year survival rates being reported in Japan,[196] and 88% in Western countries.[251] Rates of EGC in Western countries have increased from less than 5% of all cases of gastric cancer ten years ago to almost 20% in more recent studies. It is unclear whether early gastric cancer is a precursor lesion for late gastric cancer, or a separate disease entity. In patients with advanced gastric cancer, early cancers are found at higher prevalence than age-matched controls. In addition, patients who have refused treatment for early gastric cancer have been documented to progress to more advanced cancer, suggesting that at least some advanced gastric cancers arise from EGCs.

Descriptive classifications of both early and advanced gastric cancer have been established based on whether the gastric cancer is a protruding, ulcerated, or superficial lesion.[251a, 252] However, the TNM staging classification system is far superior in determining prognosis. In the TNM staging system, T indicates the depth of penetration, T1 denotes a tumor confined to the mucosa or submucosa, T2 denotes involvement of the muscularis propria, T3 denotes invasion into the serosa, and T4 denotes invasion of adjacent organs or structures (see Fig. 44–7). N indicates the amount of lymph node invasion; N0 denotes no lymph node involvement, N1 denotes involvement of perigastric lymph nodes within 3 cm of the primary cancer, N2 denotes regional lymph node (left gastric, common hepatic, splenic, and celiac) involvement more than 3 cm away from the primary tumor, and N3 denotes more distant intra-abdominal lymph node involvement (duodenal, mesenteric, para-aortic, and retropancreatic) that is usually more difficult to resect surgically. M indicates the presence of metastases, with M0 denoting no metastases and M1 denoting distant metastases.[253]

The International Union Against Cancer (UICC) has come up with a new staging system for the N stage, relying on the number of positive lymph nodes rather than location. N0 denotes no lymph node metastases, N1 denotes metastases in 1 to 6 regional lymph nodes, N2 denotes metastases in 7 to 15 regional lymph nodes, and N3 denotes metastases in greater than 15 lymph nodes.[252] The new staging system correlates with clinical outcome better than the previous TNM staging system, with a more significant difference in survival between each N group and less deviation within each N classification.[254] The difference was most marked in the N1 and N2 groups. It was also found to be a more significant prognostic indicator than the Japanese classification.[255, 256] The one drawback of this classification is that patients who do not have extensive lymph node sampling may not be able to be classified in the new system. Still, the new UICC TNM classification system is now considered the classification of choice for staging patients with gastric cancer.

Prognosis

Overall, 5-year survival in the United States from gastric cancer is 18.6% in men and 25.2% in women (compared with 61.2% and 60.8% in colon cancer, respectively).[7] Untreated, median life expectancy in advanced disease with liver metastases is 4 to 6 months and 4 to 6 weeks in patients with peritoneal carcinomatosis.[257] The TNM classification can be used to stratify patients into four clinical stages (I through IV) to predict prognosis in patients treated with gastrectomy[258] (Tables 44–4 and 44–5). The survival data from the Japanese are superior to those seen in Western countries, perhaps because of their preference for extended lymphadenectomy or because of less understaging than is found in Western countries.[258]

Treatment

SURGERY. Surgical resection remains the only curative procedure for advanced gastric cancer. In addition, surgical re-

Table 44–4 | **TNM Stratification to Determine Clinical Stage of Gastric Cancer***

	N0	N1	N2	N3	M1 (any N)
Tis	0	—	—	—	—
T1	IA	IB	II	IV	IV
T2	IB	II	IIIA	IV	IV
T3	II	IIIA	IIIB	IV	IV
T4	IIIA	IIIB	IV	IV	IV
M1 (any T)	IV	IV	IV	IV	IV

*See Table 44–5 for survival by clinical stage in different countries.
Tis, tumor in situ.

section provides the most effective palliation of symptoms, particularly those of obstruction.[178] Thus, surgery should be attempted in most cases of gastric cancer. However, if linitis plastica or bulky metastatic disease is present, retroperitoneal invasion or peitoneal carcinomatosis is seen, or the patient has severe comorbid illnesses, then the prognosis is sufficiently poor to make resection questionable.[259] In some cases, surgery is required for diagnosis. Instances when surgery may be required for diagnosis include nonhealing gastric ulcers with negative biopsies, persistent pyloric outlet obstruction suggesting an antral carcinoma, and submucosal lesions such as gastric lymphoma.

The extent of margin involvement did not correlate well with local recurrence or 5-year survival in a large Italian series,[260] but in the Japanese experience, positive surgical margins were associated with a worse prognosis. After an attempt at curative surgery, recurrence tends to occur in the gastric bed, perigastric lymph nodes, liver, and peritoneal surface.

Surgery is also useful in the staging of cancer. Laparoscopy has been reported to have a diagnostic accuracy of 60% for staging with indices superior to CT,[261] and a diagnostic accuracy for the determination of resectability of over 90% with indices superior to CT, sparing 40% of unnecessary laparotomies.[262] Laparoscopic peritoneal lavage has been used to look for the presence of intraperitoneal free cancer cells. Peritoneal lavage is positive in close to 40% of patients, with a significant correlation with M status.[262, 263] In one study, all patients with positive cytology developed peritoneal metastases by 5 years, suggesting that this test is a good prognostic indicator of those patients at higher risk for peritoneal spread and thus potential candidates for intraperitoneal hyperthermic chemotherapy.[263, 264]

Several controversies regarding the extent of surgery exist. Total gastrectomy has been advocated by some groups, even in those patients whose cancer does not involve the entire stomach, since the wider margins generated by total gastrectomy may decrease the rates of metastases to regional lymph nodes.[265] In addition, patients undergoing a proximal resection will generally require a vagotomy resulting in pyloric denervation, and so it may be easier to perform a total gastrectomy rather than a pyloroplasty with a small distal pouch. Several large, randomized multicenter trials in France and Italy looking at subtotal vs. total gastrectomy for adenocarcinoma of the antrum found no difference in 5-year survival or in operative mortality.[266, 267] A retrospective study of 1704 patients in Germany found that total gastrectomy had a 35.3% 5-year survival compared with 34.5% for distal subtotal gastrectomy and 22.5% for proximal gastrectomy,[268] suggesting that total gastrectomy be reserved for patients requiring proximal gastrectomy.

Some centers have argued for performing a complete splenectomy with gastrectomy. A retrospective Mexican study of 219 patients demonstrated a 64% vs. 35.1% 5-year survival advantage with a concurrent splenectomy.[269] However, a retrospective study of 1938 Japanese patients,[270] of 328 patients in Turkey,[271] and of 243 German patients found that concurrent splenectomy has been shown to increase morbidity without affecting survival; a prospective British study showed worse prognosis with splenectomy.[272] Thus, concurrent splenectomy should not be performed unless there is direct invasion into the spleen, pancreas, or nodes along the splenic hilum or artery.[273]

Another issue regards the extent of lymphadenectomy. The Japanese advocate a more extensive lymph node dissection (D2 resection) than do their Western counterparts (D1 resection), and they do have higher published survival rates. A D2 resection entails resection of the nodes of the celiac axis and the hepatoduodenal ligament, in addition to the perigastric lymph nodes taken in a D1 procedure. This may reflect the fact that the Japanese have a much higher incidence of early gastric cancer, and the more extensive lymph node dissection performed in Japan may find more positive lymph nodes, making survival of their N0 group appear to be higher than their potentially understaged Western counterparts.

A large prospective multicenter Dutch study of 996 patients reported no significant difference in 5-year survival, with higher rates of postoperative death and complications in patients undergoing a D2 lymphadenectomy compared with those undergoing a more conservative D1 lymphadenectomy.[274] A British prospective study of 400 patients likewise showed no benefit from more extensive surgery; 5-year survival rates were 35% for D1 resection and 33% for D2 resection.[272] At present, there are insufficient data to support extended lymph node resection outside of Japan. To prevent understaging, the American Joint Committee on Cancer now recommends sampling (biopsies) of at least 15 nodes.[258]

Recently, both D1 and D2 gastrectomies have been successfully performed laparoscopically.[275] The use of laparo-

Table 44–5 | **5-Year Survival Rates in Gastric Cancer Based on Clinical Stage of Cancer***

STAGE	UNITED STATES (%)	JAPAN (%)	GERMANY (%)
IA	78	95	86
IB	58	86	72
II	34	71	47
IIIA	20	59	34
IIIB	18	35	25
IV	7	17	16

*See Table 44–4 for definition of clinical stages using TNM system.
From Hundahl S, Phillips J, Menck H: The National Cancer Data Base Report on poor survival of U.S. gastric carcinoma patients treated with gastrectomy: Fifth Edition American Joint Committee on cancer staging, proximal disease, and the "different disease" hypothesis. Cancer 88:921, 2000.

scopic surgery in the treatment of gastric cancer has not yet met with widespread acceptance; thus, it should be regarded as still in the developmental phase.

ENDOSCOPIC MUCOSAL RESECTION. Recent advances in endoscopic technique have permitted endoscopic mucosal resection (EMR) of lesions confined to the mucosa. This technique has been used widely in Japan for the intestinal-type cancers, where studies have shown that only 3.5% of patients with EGC of less than 2 to 3 cm in size have lymph node involvement, whereas those larger than 4.5 cm have a greater than 50% chance of spread into the submucosa and have positive nodes.[276] Multivariate analysis of these studies showed that lymphatic vessel invasion, histologic ulceration of the tumor, and larger size (≥3 cm) were independent risk factors for regional lymph node metastasis. The incidence of lymph node metastasis from intramucosal EGC negative for these three risk factors was only 0.36% (1 in 277 patients).[276]

From these results, four criteria have now been suggested for selecting gastric cancer patients for the limited operation: (1) the cancer is located in the mucosa and the lymph nodes are not involved, as indicated by EUS examination; (2) the maximum size of the tumor is less than 2 cm when the lesion is slightly elevated and less than 1 cm when the tumor is slightly depressed without an ulcer scar; (3) there is no evidence of multiple gastric cancers or simultaneous abdominal cancers; and (4) the cancer is the intestinal type.[277] A prospective study of 262 patients using these criteria found the same mortality rates in patients undergoing EMR compared with patients undergoing more extensive surgical resections.[277]

The strip biopsy method using a double-channel endoscope was the first method of EMR widely used. In this method, the lesion is first raised by submucosal injection of saline; the tumor is then raised by grasping forceps and then is strangulated and resected by electrocautery. This technique has been modified by using another snare in place of grasping forceps, use of concentrated epinephrine and saline instead of physiologic saline, and aspirating the lesion into a cap attached to the tip of an endoscope and then strangulating and resecting the lesion with a snare prefitted into the cap. There are insufficient data to recommend a specific method of EMR for removing the various types of EGC.[278]

Recently, it has been reported that the rate of nodal metastases in the diffuse (undifferentiated) type of early gastric cancer is also quite low.[207] The Japanese Gastric Cancer Congress has proposed guidelines stating that endoscopic mucosal resection can be attempted in undifferentiated ECG smaller than 5 mm or smaller than 10 mm in the absence of an ulcerative lesion or scarring.[207]

PHOTODYNAMIC THERAPY. Attempts at treating superficial gastric cancer with photodynamic laser therapy (PDT) with meso-tetrahydroxyphenyl-chlorin (mTHPC) as the photosensitizer in have been reported to result in complete remission in 80% of early intestinal-type cancers and 50% of diffuse cancers.[279] Studies looking at a combination of PDT with endoscopic mucosal resection have not been completed to date.

CHEMOTHERAPY. Unfortunately, in Western countries, about 75% of patients have cancer that has spread to the perigastric lymph nodes or have distant metastases at the time of diagnosis.[280] In addition, 40% of patients have recurrence of tumor at 5 years of follow-up, with 22% of tumors being local, 19% regional, and 59% distant.[14] Thus, questions have been raised about the potential value of chemotherapy in the treatment of gastric cancer. Unfortunately, gastric cancer appears to be fairly resistant to conventional chemotherapy.

Initially, single-drug therapy with 5-fluorouracil (5-FU) was used, with a response rate (defined as a 50% reduction in tumor volume) of around 20%,[281, 282] with slightly higher response rates when the drug was given as a low-dose continuous infusion.[283] Oral preparations of 5-FU have similar response rates.[284, 285] Other single-agent chemotherapeutic agents, such as mitomycin,[286] cisplatin,[287, 288] doxorubicin,[289] irinotecan (CPT-11),[290] and methotrexate,[291] also have shown less than 30% response rates. No convincing survival benefit has been seen with any single-agent chemotherapeutic regimen.

The most promising use of combination chemotherapy appears to be as an adjunct to surgical resection, with reports of significantly improved 1-year survival after surgery in node-positive patients.[292, 293, 366] (Table 44–6). None of these studies, however, are large enough to make definitive treatment recommendations. A recent meta-analysis of 13 trials of adjuvant chemotherapy after "curative resection" revealed a risk ratio of 0.94 that did not reach statistical significance.[294] At present, adjunctive chemotherapy should be limited to patients participating in randomized controlled trials.

Another interesting approach is the use of intraoperative hyperthermic peritoneal chemotherapy (IHPC) that is warmed to 43.5°C and manually distributed for advanced gastric cancer with peritoneal seeding.[295] A 41% 3-year survival has been reported with intraperitoneal mitomycin C in 42 patients with peritoneal metastases in a French nonrandomized study.[296] Two Japanese studies also reported a 26% reduction in peritoneal recurrence and significant increase in 5-year survival[297, 298] in patients undergoing IHPC. The group of patients with the greatest survival benefit from IHPC appear to be those whose tumor has invaded into the serosa (T3) at the time of initial operation.[299] Other Euro-

Table 44–6 | **Adjuvant Chemotherapy for Gastric Cancer**

DRUG(S)	RESPONSE RATE (%)	SURVIVAL BENEFIT
5-FU	20	No
Mitomycin	30	No
Irinotecan	30	No
Cisplatin	25	No
Doxorubicin	25	No
Epirubicin + LV + 5-FU	49	Yes[292]
Epirubicin + cisplatin + protracted 5-FU (ECF)	46–56	Yes[293, 365]
Epirubicin + folate + 5-FU + etoposide (ELFE)	49	Yes[366]
EEPFL	71	No[367]
5-FU + paclitaxil	66.	No[368]
5-FU, LV + cisplatin (FLP)	52	No[369]

EEPFL, etoposide + epirubicin + cisplatin + 5-FU + LV; 5-FU, 5-fluorouracil; LV, leucovorin.

pean studies have had less optimistic results, with increased morbidity and no survival benefit seen with IHPC.[300] At present, use of IHPC still should be confined to patients enrolled in clinical trials, especially in Western countries.

RADIATION THERAPY. The stomach is relatively resistant to radiation, and the administration of high doses of radiation for the treatment of gastric cancer is limited by the sensitivity of surrounding organs, such as the intestines, kidneys, spinal cord, and pancreas. It is not surprising that radiation therapy has not been shown to improve mortality when used as single therapy or as an adjunct to surgery.[301] Some recent data suggest that the response rate improves when radiation is given with a radiosensitizer such as paclitaxel, compared with chemotherapy alone.[302, 303] Until sufficiently large randomized controlled trials are performed, radiation therapy should be used only in the setting of a clinical trial.

GASTRIC LYMPHOMA (see Chapter 26)

Gastric lymphomas comprise 3% to 6% of all gastric malignancies.[304] Gastric lymphomas can be subdivided into those in which the stomach is the primary site of involvement, and those with disseminated nodal disease and secondary involvement of the stomach. Over 95% of gastric lymphomas are non-Hodgkin's lymphomas, with gastric lymphoma being the most common form of extranodal non-Hodgkin's lymphoma, accounting for over 30% of all cases of primary non-Hodgkin's lymphoma.[305, 306]

Gastric lymphoma tends to be more common in North Africa and the Middle East, where the disease tends to occur at a younger age[307] and is associated with a lower socioeconomic status.[308] In Western countries, the incidence is considerably lower, and there is not a clear geographic or socioeconomic distribution.[309, 310] In the United States, the annual occurrence of gastric lymphoma is about 1 in 150,000, with a median age at time of diagnosis of 50 to 60 years.[305, 306, 311] The male:female ratio is about 1.5:1 in the United States, although worldwide the male:female ratio varies depending on country, with rates as high as 2.8:1[309] and as low as 0.75:1.[312]

Historically, it was believed that over 90% of non-Hodgkin's gastric lymphomas were B cell lymphomas, with the majority of these being large cell, diffuse-type lymphomas. Thus, it was believed that low-grade B cell lymphomas were uncommon. However, recent years have brought the recognition that many "benign" lymphoid infiltrates were actually low-grade B cell lymphomas of mucosa-associated lymphoid tissue (MALT).[313] It is now estimated that at least 35% to 40% of all primary gastric lymphomas are MALT lymphomas.[311, 314, 315]

The normal gastric tissue does not have lymphoid tissue, but after *H. pylori* infection, a subset of patients can develop mucosa-associated lymphoid tissue,[316] with lymphoid hyperplasia and clonal expansion of B cells thought secondary to impaired T cell regulation of B cell growth.[317] It is thought that these B cell clones can then give rise to lymphoma. This has been confirmed in animal models, where it has been shown that *H. pylori* infection can induce MALT lymphomas in guinea pigs.[318] In humans, 72% to 98% of patients with MALT lymphoma have evidence of *H. pylori* infection.[304, 319] Eradication of *H. pylori* results in complete remission of early low-grade MALT lymphomas in a majority of cases.[320, 321] The relative risk of developing gastric lymphoma in those who are *H. pylori*–positive is 6,[322] with a higher risk for those individuals infected with a CagA-positive strain of *H. pylori*.[319] Gastric MALT lymphomas have also been associated with infection with *H. heilmannii*,[323] a bacterium related to *H. pylori* that is present in 0.5% of gastric biopsies,[324] also associated with the development of chronic active gastritis.[325]

Genetic analysis of gastric lymphomas reveals that the common genetic aberrations responsible for lymphomagenesis are deletions of 6q, loss of p53, loss of p16,[317] and amplification of the 3q27 and the MLL gene regions.[326] Risk factors for the development of gastric lymphoma include *H. pylori* infection (relative risk of 6.0) and HIV infection (relative risk of ≈5).[327]

Diagnosis

The clinical manifestations of gastric lymphoma are similar to that of gastric adenocarcinoma. At its early stages, and in MALT lymphomas, patients tend to be asymptomatic. With more advanced disease, patients tend to present with abdominal pain, nausea, vomiting, anorexia, weight loss, bleeding, fever, night sweats, swelling, and diarrhea.[304, 306, 311, 328]

On endoscopy, gastric lymphomas can appear to be fungating, polypoid masses, thickened gastric folds (Fig. 44–9), or ulcerating lesions, and can be difficult to distinguish from gastric adenocarcinoma. The sensitivity of endoscopy with biopsies approaches 95%.[311] Because of the involvement of the submucosa, deep biopsies may be needed for a pathologic diagnosis. EUS can be helpful in this regard, as is its

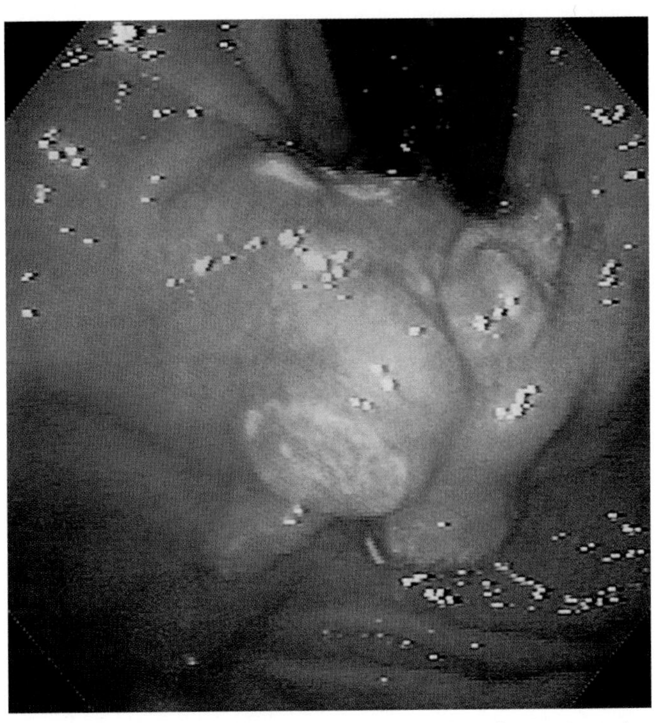

Figure 44–9. Multiple umbilicated lesions distal to the gastroesophageal junction. One large ulceration is just distal to the squamocolumnar junction.

ability to determine depth of invasion as well as regional lymph node involvement. It is estimated that a combination of endoscopy and EUS provides staging accuracy of approximately 75% to 80%.[311, 329] Other imaging modalities, such as CT or MRI, may be of value in determining involvement of the liver and spleen, as well as distant lymph nodes.

Staging

The two most widely used staging systems are the modified Ann Arbor[330] and the Musshoff modification.[331] The Musshoff staging system differs in that it subclassifies lymphomas according to the involvement of regional vs. extraregional nodes. Some evidence suggests that the involvement of extraregional nodes (stage IIE2) corresponds to a worse prognosis compared with involvement of regional nodes only (stage IIE1).[305] A summary of the staging systems and the associated prognosis is provided in Table 44–7.

In general, good prognostic indicators for gastric lymphoma include female gender,[332] younger age,[332] good performance status,[306] low-grade histology, including MALT lymphomas,[305, 306] and achievement of complete remission after therapy.[305]

Treatment

Surgery was the initial standard treatment for high-grade gastric lymphomas, since surgery was thought to be curative if the tumor was limited to the submucosa and would provide more accurate staging, better palliation, and prevention of spontaneous perforation. Debulking of tumor has also led to a modest improvement in survival in stage I-II patients.[333] However, chemotherapy plus radiation therapy has been found to have survival rates similar to those of surgery,[334] as does chemotherapy alone compared with surgery with chemotherapy.[335] The addition of radiation therapy to chemotherapy has been associated with decreased local recurrence in several studies,[336, 337] but these findings have not been reproduced by others.[338, 339] Because of its efficacy and safety, a conservative strategy (chemotherapy ± radiation therapy) should be considered as first-line treatment for high-grade primary gastric lymphomas. Gastrectomy should be indicated only for urgent cases, in which surgery followed by chemotherapy appears the best choice.[339]

The treatment of MALT lymphomas is different from that of high-grade lymphomas in that they are unlikely to involve regional or extraregional lymph nodes.[315] Several groups have shown that eradication of *H. pylori* followed by radiation therapy to the stomach results in 5-year survival rates of greater than 90%.[315] One recent study found a complete remission rate of 89% in patients with MALT lymphoma treated with *H. pylori* eradication alone.[311] Similar results have been found for MALT lymphomas thought secondary to *H. heilmannii* infection.[340] Other studies suggest that chemotherapy with chlorambucil, cyclophosphamide, or CHOP is as efficacious as radiation therapy.[304] The role of monoclonal antibodies against CD20, such as rituximab, is also being assessed. Further controlled trials need to be performed before a preferred treatment strategy for MALT lymphomas can be recommended, although *H. pylori* eradication should be a part of any treatment regimen.

Table 44–7 | **Staging Systems for Gastric Lymphoma**[305, 336]

FINDING	SYSTEM: ANN ARBOR	SYSTEM: MUSSHOFF	5-YEAR SURVIVAL (%)
Unifocal or multifocal tumors of the stomach without lymph node involvement	IE	IE	81–95
Nodal involvement below the diaphragm	IIE		38–75
Regional nodes		IIE1	80
Nonregional nodes		IIE2	53
Involvement of nodes on both sides of the diaphragm; localized invasion of associated extralymphatic organ and/or spleen	IIIE	IIIE	11–30
Nongastrointestinal extranodal involvement	IVE	IVE	5–8

GASTRIC CARCINOID TUMORS

Gastric carcinoid tumors (Fig. 44–10) account for 2% of all gastrointestinal carcinoids and 0.3% of all gastric neoplasms.[341] Carcinoid tumors arise from gastrointestinal neuroendocrine cells, and they can be subdivided into well-differentiated tumors, in which the tumor retains many of the features of neuroendocrine differentiation, and poorly differentiated tumors. In the stomach, the well-differentiated tumors are mainly of enterochromaffin-like (ECL) cell origin, with a small minority being of other endocrine cell types.[342] Although gastric carcinoids often contain neuroendocrine peptides, carcinoid syndrome does not occur unless there is hepatic involvement.

Pernicious anemia and chronic atrophic gastritis are risk factors for the development of ECL cell tumors (see Fig. 44–8). One in 25 patients with long-standing disease develops gastric carcinoids.[174, 343] This may be secondary to the hypergastrinemia caused by the absence of significant acid output in these patients, resulting in ECL cell hyperplasia.[344] Despite the initial concern that hypergastrinemia induced by long-term acid suppression by proton pump inhibitors may predispose for gastric carcinoids, there appears to be no increased risk of developing carcinoids in patients with long-term drug-induced acid suppression.[345]

ECL cell carcinoids can also be seen occasionally in the Zollinger-Ellison (ZE) syndrome, but they are much more common in those patients with multiple endocrine neoplasia, type 1 (MEN-1), than in sporadic ZE syndrome. Loss of heterozygosity (LOH) of the MEN1 gene has been found to occur in 75% of ECL cell carcinoids.[346]

The average age at diagnosis of gastric carcinoid is 62 years, with an equal male:female distribution.[341] Patients are often asymptomatic, with carcinoids found incidentally at the

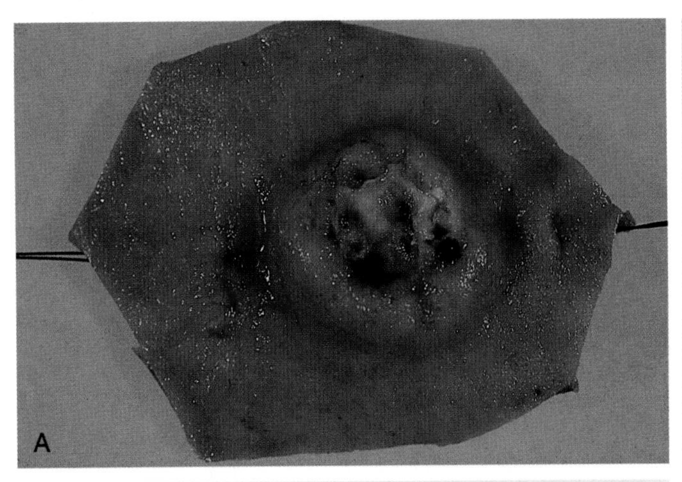

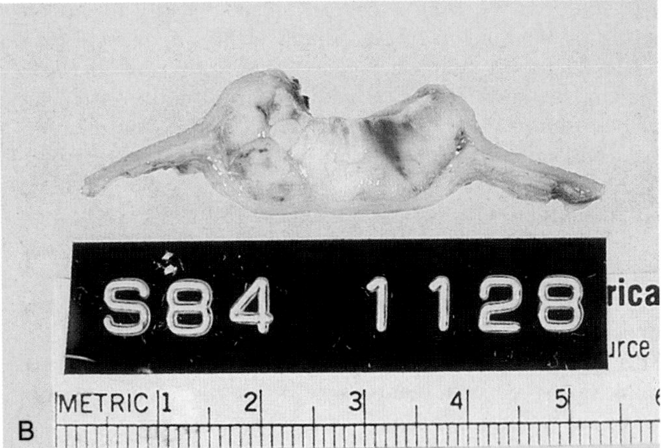

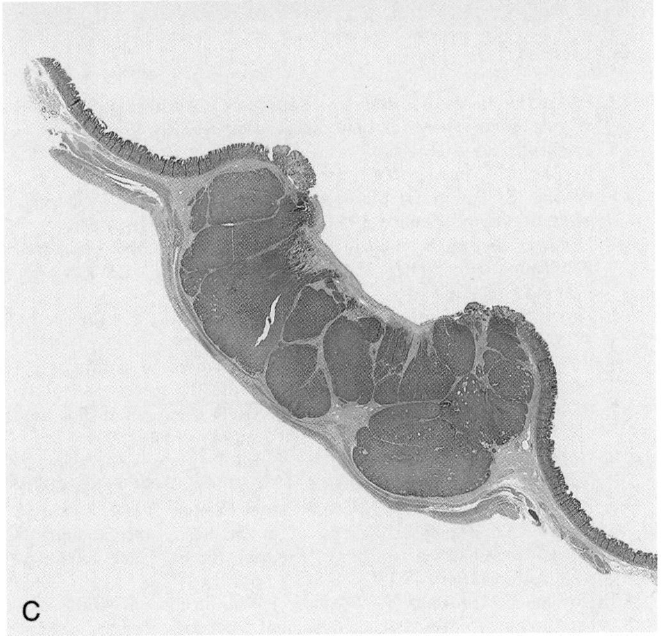

Figure 44–10. Gastric carcinoid tumor. *A*, Large, ulcerated tumor (gross). *B*, Fixed specimen (gross). *C*, Low-power histology showing a large tumor with mucosal ulceration but confined to the wall of the stomach. (Courtesy of Edward Lee, MD.)

time of upper endoscopy. When symptoms do occur, they are usually dyspeptic in nature.

The classic endoscopic finding is an irregularly shaped erythematous dimple in the center of a submucosal mass,[347] which may be confused with a pancreatic rest. As with gastric lymphoma, EUS can be helpful in defining depth of invasion and providing deep submucosal biopsies. CT and MRI may be helpful in discerning hepatic involvement. It has been reported that almost all patients with gastric carcinoids have elevated plasma chromogranin A levels, a peptide secreted by all neuroendocrine cells,[348] although prospective studies for its use as a tumor marker for carcinoids have not yet been performed.

The management of gastric carcinoids is controversial. Carcinoids secondary to pernicious anemia/atrophic gastritis and MEN-I tend to have a more benign course, with occasional spontaneous regression. In these cases, endoscopic mucosal resection for those tumors smaller than 1 to 2 cm may suffice, with surgical resection for larger tumors, especially if the tumor extends into the muscularis mucosae.[341, 349] Since gastrin may be involved in the pathogenesis of ECL cell carcinoids, some groups have reported that removal of gastrin-secreting cells by antrectomy can be effective in the treatment of small ECL cell carcinoids,[350, 351] but to date there have been no prospective trials looking at the efficacy of antrectomy. Sporadic carcinoids have higher rates of regional lymph node involvement, and thus surgical resection with lymph node sampling is generally recommended.[341, 349] Gastric carcinoids tend to have a good prognosis, with non-metastatic disease having a greater than 95% 5-year survival rate, and even those with metastases have a 5-year survival rate of over 50%.[342] However, patients with sporadic carcinoids tend to do much worse, reflecting their higher rates of metastases.[352]

GASTROINTESTINAL STROMAL TUMORS

Gastrointestinal stromal tumors (GISTs) refer to all mesenchymal tumors in the gastrointestinal tract. The majority of these tumors arise from cells that are not clearly of smooth muscle or neurogenic origin. Of all GISTs in the GI tract, 70% occur in the stomach.[353] They tend to be slow growing, indolent tumors that are usually asymptomatic until they become quite large. Virtually all GISTs have gain-of-function c-kit mutations (a proto-oncogene growth factor receptor).[354]

Patients with GISTs have a median age of 50 to 60 years at the time of diagnosis.[353] Symptoms at presentation include gastrointestinal bleeding, dyspepsia, and, with large tumors, obstructive symptoms. It is difficult to judge the malignant potential of GISTs histologically, and so only those tumors with invasion into adjacent organs, spread into regional lymph nodes, or with distant metastases (liver, lung, peritoneum) are called malignant.

Initial diagnosis is best made at the time of endoscopy. EUS is helpful in determining depth of invasion as well as regional lymph node involvement. Surgery is the treatment of choice, but because of the rarity of these tumors, there are insufficient clinical trials to make a definitive conclusion. Some advocate use of adjunctive radiation and chemotherapy. Because of the difficulty in assessing which GISTs are benign, the most useful clinical predictor of outcome is the mitotic index of the tumor. Those with a mitotic rate of greater than 2 per 10 high-power fields have a much higher risk for recurrence or metastases.[355] The size of the tumor is also a clinical predictor of outcome,[355] with those larger than 5 cm at higher risk of metastases. Asymptomatic elderly patients, or patients with serious comorbid illness, with small tumors that EUS shows have no evidence of invasion into adjacent or distant organs and have low mitotic indices may be followed by surveillance endoscopy without surgery. Recently, the tyrosine kinase inhibitor imafinib mesylate (STI571, Gleevec) has been used successfully in a metastatic GIST tumor.[356, 357]

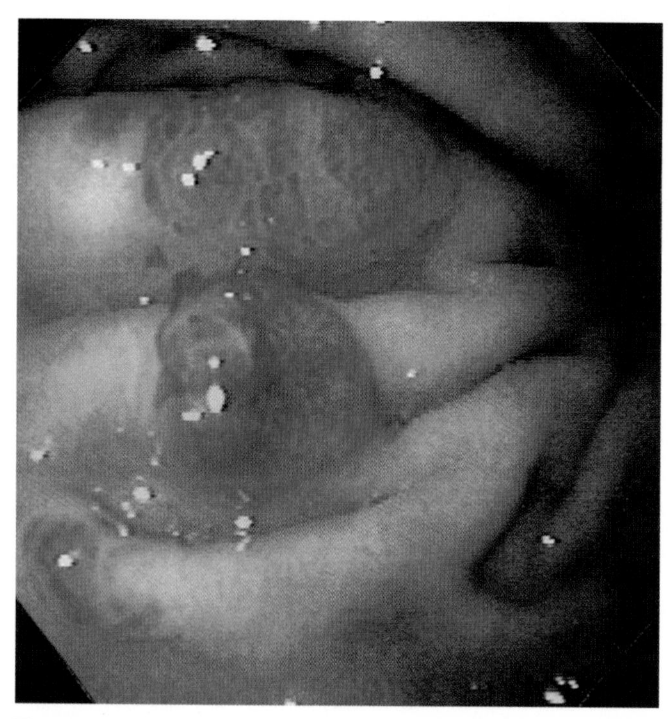

Figure 44–11. Kaposi's Sarcoma. Multiple well-demarcated violet-red lesions, some of which are flat and some elevated.

MISCELLANEOUS TUMORS

Metastatic disease to the stomach can occur with primary breast,[358] melanoma,[359] lung,[360] ovary,[361] liver,[362] colon,[363] and testicular cancer,[364] with breast cancer being the most frequent. Other rare malignant tumors that can involve the stomach include Kaposi's sarcoma[365] (Fig. 44–11), myenteric schwannoma,[366] glomus tumor,[367] small cell carcinoma,[368] and parietal cell carcinoma.[369] Benign tumors that can involve the stomach include gastric polyps, pancreatic rests,[370] xanthelasma,[371] and fundic gland cysts.[372]

REFERENCES

1. Parkin D, Laara E, Muir C: Estimates of worldwide frequency of sixteen major cancers in 1980. Int J Cancer 41:184, 1988.
2. Pisani P, Parkin D, Bray F, et al: Estimates of the worldwide mortality from 25 cancers in 1990. Int J Cancer 83:18, 1999.
3. Whelan S, Parkin D, Masuyer E: Trends in Cancer Incidence and Mortality. Lyons, France, IARC Scientific Publications, 1993.
4. Levin D, Devess S, Godwin J, et al: Cancer rates and risks. DHEW Publication No. (NIH) 75-961. Washington, DC, US Government Printing Office, 1974.
5. Parker S, Tong T, Bolden S, et al: Cancer statistics. CA Cancer J Clin 47:5, 1997.
6. Elixhauser A, Halpern M: Economic evaluations of gastric and pancreatic cancer. Hepato-Gastroenterology 46:1206, 1999.
7. Ries L, Kosary C, Hawkey B, et al: SEER Cancer Statistics Review 1973–1996. Bethesda, MD, National Cancer Institute, 1999.
8. Horm J, Asire A, Young J, et al: SEER Program: Cancer Incidence and Mortality in the United States 1973–1981. NIH Publication No. 85-1837. Bethesda, MD, National Cancer Institute, 1984.
9. Wiggins C, Becker T, Key C, et al: Stomach cancer among New Mexico's American Indians, Hispanic whites, and non-Hispanic whites. Cancer Res 49:1595, 1989.
10. Howson C, Hirayama T, Wylander E: The decline in gastric cancer: Epidemiology of an unplanned triumph. Epidemiol Rev 8:1, 1986.
11. Forman D, Eurogast Study Group: An international association between *Helicobacter pylori* infection and gastric cancer. Lancet 341: 1359, 1993.
12. Hundahl S, Menck H, Mansour E, et al: The National Cancer Data Base report on gastric carcinoma. Cancer 80:2333, 1997.
13. Haenszel W: Variation in incidence of and mortality from stomach cancer, with particular reference to the United States. J Natl Cancer Inst 21:213, 1958.
14. Wanebo H, Kennedy B, Chmiel J, et al: Cancer of the stomach: A patient care study by the American College of Surgeons. Ann Surg 218:583, 1993.
15. Haenszel W, Kurihara M: Studies of Japanese migrants. I. Mortality from cancer and other diseases among Japanese in the United States. J Natl Cancer Inst 40:43, 1968.
16. Black R, Bray F, Ferlay J, et al: Cancer incidence and mortality in the European Union: Cancer registry data and estimates of national incidence for 1990. Eur J Cancer 33:1075, 1997.
17. Blot W, Devesa S, Kneller R, et al: Rising incidence of adenocarcinoma of the esophagus and gastric cardia. JAMA 265:1287, 1991.
18. Hansson L, Sparen P, Nyren O: Increasing incidence of carcinoma of the gastric cardia in Sweden from 1970 to 1985. Br J Surg 80:374, 1993.
19. Locke G, Talley N, Carpenter H, et al: Changes in the site- and histology-specific incidence of gastric cancer during a 50 year period. Gastroenterology 109:1750, 1995.
20. Lauren R: The two histological main types of gastric carcinoma: Diffuse and so-called intestinal-type carcinoma: An attempt at a histo-clinical classification. Acta Pathol Microbiol Scand 64:31, 1965.

21. Munoz N, Correa P, Cuello C, et al: Histologic types of gastric carcinoma in high and low risk areas. Int J Cancer 3:809, 1968.
22. Fearon E: Molecular genetics of colorectal cancer. Ann NY Acad Sci 768:101, 1995.
23. Munoz N, Matko I: Histological types of gastric cancer and its relationship with intestinal metaplasia. Cancer Res 39:99, 1972.
24. Correa P: Human gastric carcinogenesis: A multistep and multifactorial process—the first American Cancer Society award lecture on cancer epidemiology and prevention. Cancer Res 52:6735, 1992.
25. Correa P, Haenszel W, Cuello C, et al: Gastric precancerous process in high risk population: Cohort follow-up. Cancer Res 50:4747, 1990.
26. Shiao Y, Rugge M, Correa P, et al: p53 alteration in gastric precancerous lesions. Am J Pathol 144:511, 1994.
27. Xiangming C, Hokita S, Natsugoe S, et al: p21 expression is a prognostic factor in patients with p53-negative gastric cancer. Cancer Lett 148:181, 2000.
28. Joypaul B, Newman E, Hopwood D, et al: Expression of p53 protein in normal, dysplastic, and malignant gastric mucosa; An immunohistochemical study. J Pathol 170:279, 1993.
29. Fox J, Li X, Cahill R, et al: Hypertrophic gastropathy in *Helicobacter felis*–infected wild-type C57BL/6 mice and p53 hemizygous transgenic mice. Gastroenterology 110:155, 1996.
30. Cahill R, Kilgallen C, Beattie S, et al: Gastric epithelial cell kinetics in the progression from normal mucosa to gastric carcinoma. Gut 38: 177, 1996.
31. Ikeguchi M, Saito H, Katano K, et al: Expression of p53 and p21 are independent prognostic factors in patients with serosal invasion by gastric carcinoma. Dig Dis Sci 43:964, 1998.
32. Kaye P, Radebold K, Isaacs S, et al: Expression of p53 and p21 waf1/cip1 in gastric carcinoma: Lack of inter-relationship or correlation with prognosis. Eur J Surg Oncol 26:39, 2000.
33. Maeda K, Kang S, Onoda N, et al: Vascular endothelial growth factor expression in preoperative biopsy specimens correlates with disease recurrence in patients with early gastric carcinoma. Cancer 86:566, 1999.
34. Maehara Y, Tomoda M, Hasuda S, et al: Prognostic value of p53 protein expression for patients with gastric cancer—a multivariate analysis. Br J Cancer 79:1255, 1999.
35. Wright P, Williams G: Molecular biology of gastric carcinoma. Gut 34:145, 1993.
36. Rhyu M, Park W, Jung Y, et al: Allelic deletions of MCC/APC and p53 are frequent late events in human gastric carcinogenesis. Gastroenterology 106:1584, 1994.
37. Wu M, Shun C, Wang H, et al: Genetic alterations in gastric cancer: Relation to histological subtypes, tumor stage, and *Helicobacter pylori* infection. Gastroenterology 112:1457, 1997.
38. Vogelstein B, Fearon E, Hamilton S, et al: Genetic alterations during colorectal tumor development. N Engl J Med 319:525, 1988.
39. Zwick A, Munir M, Ryan C, et al: Gastric adenocarcinoma and dysplasia in fundic gland polyps of a patient with attenuated adenomatous polyposis coli. Gastroenterology 113:659, 1997.
40. Tamura G, Maesawa C, Suzuki Y, et al: Mutations of the APC gene occur during early stages of gastric adenoma development. Cancer Res 54:1149, 1994.
41. Nakatsura S, Yanagisawa A, Ichii S, et al: Somatic mutations of the APC gene in gastric cancer: Frequent mutations in very well differentiated adenocarcinoma and signet-ring cell carcinoma. Hum Mol Genetics 52:3099, 1992.
42. Caca K, Kolligs Ji X, et al: Beta- and gamma-catenin mutations, but not ϵ-cadherin activation, underlie T-cell factor/lymphoid enhancer factor transcriptional deregulation in gastric and pancreatic cancer. Cell Growth Differ 10:369, 1999.
43. Park W, Oh R, Park J, et al: Frequent somatic mutations of the beta-catenin gene in intestinal-type gastric cancer. Cancer Res 59:4257, 1999.
44. Han S, Kim H, Park K, et al: Expression of p27Kip1 and cyclin D1 proteins is inversely correlated and is associated with poor clinical outcome in human gastric cancer. J Surg Oncol 71:147, 1999.
45. Kim D, Lee H, Nam E, et al: Reduced expression of the cell-cycle inhibitor p27Kip1 is associated with progression and lymph node metastasis of gastric carcinoma. Histopathology 36:245, 2000.
46. Takano Y, Kato Y, van Diest P: Cyclin D2 overexpression and lack of p27 correlate positively and cyclin E inversely with a poor prognosis in gastric cancer cases. Am J Pathol 156:585, 2000.
47. Myung N, Kim M, Chung I, et al: Loss of p16 and p27 is associated with progression of human gastric cancer. Cancer Lett 153:129, 2000.
48. Shim Y, Kang G, Ro J: Correlation of p16 hypermethylation with p16 protein loss in sporadic gastric carcinomas. Lab Invest 80:689, 2000.
49. Schneider B, Gulley M, Eagan P, et al: Loss of p16/CDKN2A tumor suppressor protein in gastric adenocarcinoma is associated with Epstein-Barr virus and anatomic location in the body of the stomach. Hum Pathol 31:45, 2000.
50. Tsujie M, Yamamoto H, Tomita N, et al: Expression of tumor suppressor gene p16(INK4) products in primary gastric cancer. Oncology 58:126, 2000.
51. Fang D, Jass J, Wang D, et al: Loss of heterozygosity and loss of expression of the DCC gene in gastric cancer. J Clin Pathol 51:593, 1998.
52. Yoshida Y, Itoh F, Endo T, et al: Decreased DCC mRNA expression in human gastric cancers is clinicopathologically significant. Int J Cancer 79:634, 1998.
53. Ohta M, Inoue H, Cotticelli M, et al: The FHIT gene, spanning the chromosome 3p14.2 fragile site and renal carcinoma-associated t(3;8) breakpoint, is abnormal in digestive tract cancers. Cell 84:587, 1996.
54. Baffa R, Veronese M, Santoro R, et al: Loss of FHIT expression in gastric carcinoma. Cancer Res 58:4708, 1998.
55. Maeda K, Chung Y, Ogawa Y, et al: Prognostic value of vascular endothelial growth factor expression in gastric carcinoma. Cancer 77: 858, 1996.
56. Yonemura Y, Endo Y, Fujita H, et al: Role of vascular endothelial growth factor C expression in the development of lymph node metastasis in gastric cancer. Clin Cancer Res 5:1823, 1999.
57. Yoshikawa T, Tsuburaya A, Kobayashi O, et al: Plasma concentrations of VEGF and bFGF in patients with gastric carcinoma. Cancer Lett 153:7, 2000.
58. Nakajima M, Sawada H, Yamada Y, et al: The prognostic significance of amplification and overexpression of c-met and c-erb B-2 in human gastric carcinomas. Cancer 85:1894, 1999.
59. Park W, Oh R, Kim Y, et al: Absence of mutations in the kinase domain of the Met gene and frequent expression of Met and HGF/SF protein in primary gastric carcinomas. APMIS 108:195, 2000.
60. Ristimaki A, Honkanen N, Jankala H, et al: Expression of cyclooxygenase-2 in human gastric carcinoma. Cancer Res 57:1276, 1997.
61. Murata H, Kawano S, Tsuji S, et al: Cyclooxygenase-2 overexpression enhances lymphatic invasion and metastasis in human gastric carcinoma. Am J Gastroenterol 94:451, 1999.
62. Sawaoka H, Kawano S, Tsuji S, et al: Cyclooxygenase-2 inhibitors suppress the growth of gastric cancer xenografts via induction of apoptosis in nude mice. Am J Physiol 274:G1061, 1998.
63. Thun M, Namboodiri M, Calle E, et al: Aspirin use and risk of fatal cancer. Cancer Res 53:1322, 1993.
64. Yamamoto H, Itoh F, Fukushima H, et al: Overexpression of cyclooxygenase-2 protein is less frequent in gastric cancers with microsatellite instability. Int J Cancer 84:400, 1999.
65. Aarnio M, Salovaara R, Aaltonen L, et al: Features of gastric cancer in hereditary non-polyposis colorectal cancer syndrome. Int J Cancer 74:551, 1997.
66. Mironov N, Aguelon A, Potapova G, et al: Alterations of (CA), DNA repeats and tumor suppression genes in human gastric cancer. Cancer Res 54:41, 1994.
67. Rhy M, Park W, Meltzer S: Microsatellite instability occurs frequently in human gastric carcinoma. Oncogene 9:29, 1994.
68. Fang D, Jass J, Wang D, et al: Infrequent loss of heterozygosity of APC/MCC and DCC genes in gastric cancer showing DNA microsatellite instability. J Clin Pathol 52:504, 1999.
69. Isogaki J, Shinmura K, Yin W, et al: Microsatellite instability and K-ras mutations in gastric adenomas, with reference to associated gastric cancers. Cancer Detect Prev 23:204, 1999.
70. Habano W, Sugai T, Nakamura S, et al: Microsatellite instability and mutation of mitochondrial and nuclear DNA in gastric carcinoma. Gastroenterology 118:835, 2000.
71. Leung W, Kim J, Kim J, et al: Microsatellite instability in gastric intestinal metaplasia in patients with and without gastric cancer. Am J Pathol 156:537, 2000.
72. Nogueira A, Carneiro F, Seruca R, et al: Microsatellite instability in hyperplastic and adenomatous polyps of the stomach. Cancer 86:1649, 1999.
73. Yamamoto H, Perez-Piteira J, Yoshida T, et al: Gastric cancers of the

microsatellite mutator phenotype display characteristic genetic and clinical features. Gastroenterology 116:1348, 1999.
74. Paulson T, Wright F, Parker B, et al: Microsatellite instability correlates with reduced survival and poor disease prognosis in breast cancer. Cancer Res 56:4021, 1996.
75. Guilford P, Hopkins J, Harraway J, et al: E-cadherin germline mutations in familial gastric cancer. Nature 392:402, 1998.
76. Keller G, Vogelsang H, Becker I, et al: Diffuse-type gastric and lobular breast carcinoma in a familial gastric cancer patient with an E-cadherin germline mutation. Am J Pathol 155:337, 1999.
77. Yoon K, Ku J, Yang H, et al: Germline mutations of E-cadherin gene in Korean familial gastric cancer patients. J Hum Genet 44:177, 1999.
78. Richards F, McKee S, Rajpar M, et al: Germline E-cadherin gene (CDH1) mutations predispose to familial gastric cancer and colorectal cancer. Hum Mol Genetics 8:607, 1999.
79. Shinmura K, Kohno T, Takahashi M, et al: Familial gastric cancer: Clinicopathological characteristics, RER phenotype and germline p53 and E-cadherin mutations. Carcinogenesis 20:1127, 1999.
80. Xiangming C, Hokita S, Natsugoe S, et al: Co-occurrence of reduced expression of alpha-catenin and overexpression of p53 is a predictor of lymph node metastasis in early gastric cancer. Oncology 57:131, 1999.
81. Kawanishi K, Doki Y, Shiozaki H, et al: Correlation between loss of E-cadherin expression and overexpression of autocrine motility factor receptor in association with progression of human gastric cancers. Am J Clin Pathol 113:266, 2000.
82. Shiozaki H, Oka H, Inoue M, et al: E-cadherin-mediated adhesion system in cancer cells. Cancer 77(8Suppl):1605, 1995.
83. Tamura G, Yin J, Wang S, et al: E-Cadherin gene promoter hypermethylation in primary human gastric carcinomas. J Natl Cancer Inst 92: 569, 2000.
84. Kanai Y, Hirohashi S: Invasion and metastasis. In Sugimura TSM (ed): Gastric Cancer. Oxford, Oxford University Press, 1997, p 109.
85. Yu J, Ebert M, Miehlke S, et al: Alpha-catenin expression is decreased in human gastric cancers and in the gastric mucosa of first-degree relatives. Gut 46:639, 2000.
86. Lichtenstein P, Holm N, Verkasalo P, et al: Environmental and heritable factors in the causation of cancer: Analyses of cohorts of twins from Sweden, Denmark, and Finland. N Engl J Med 343:78, 2000.
87. Palli D, Galli M, Caporaso N, et al: Family history and risk of stomach cancer in Italy. Cancer Epidemiol Biomarkers Prev 3:15, 1994.
88. La Vecchia C, Negri E, Franceschi S, et al: Family history and the risk of stomach and colorectal cancer. Cancer 70:50, 1992.
89. Zhanghieri G, DiGregorio C, C Sacchetti, et al: Familial occurrence of gastric cancer in the 2-year experience of a population-based registry. Cancer 66:2047, 1990.
90. Brenner H, Arndt V, Sturmer T, et al: Individual and joint contribution of family history and *Helicobacter pylori* infection to the risk of gastric carcinoma. Cancer 88:274, 2000.
91. Parsonnet J: When heredity is infectious [editorial]. Gastroenterology 118:222, 2000.
92. El-Omar E, Oien K, Murray L, et al: Increased prevalence of precancerous changes in relatives of gastric cancer patients: Critical role of *H. pylori*. Gastroenterology 118:22, 2000.
93. El-Omar E, Carrington M, Chow W, et al: Interleukin-1 polymorphisms associated with an increased risk of gastric cancer. Nature 404: 398, 2000.
94. Sarre R, Frost A, Jagelman D, et al: Gastric and duodenal polyps in familial adenomatous polyposis: A prospective study of the nature and prevalence of upper gastrointestinal polyps. Gut 28:306, 1987.
95. Sawada T, Muto T: Familial adenomatous polyposis: Should patients undergo surveillance of the upper gastrointestinal tract? Endoscopy 27: 6, 1995.
96. Howe J, Mitros F, Summers R: The risk of gastrointestinal carcinoma in familial juvenile polyposis. Ann Surg Oncol 5:751, 1998.
97. Coburn M, Pricolo V, DeLuca F, et al: Malignant potential in intestinal juvenile polyposis syndromes. Ann Surg Oncol 2:386, 1995.
98. Hansson L, Nyren O, Hsing A, et al: The risk of stomach cancer in patients with gastric or duodenal ulcer disease. N Engl J Med 335: 242, 1996.
99. Sitas F, Forman D, Yarnell J, et al: *Helicobacter pylori* infection rates in relation to age and social class in a population of Welsh men. Gut 32:25, 1991.
100. International Agency for Research on Cancers, Liver Flukes and *Helicobacter pylori*: IARC Monographs on the Evaluation of Carcinogenic Risks to Humans, Vol 61. Lyons, France, IARC, 1994.
101. Parsonnet J, Friedman G, Vanderstein D, et al: *Helicobacter pylori* infection and risk for gastric cancer. N Engl J Med 325:1127, 1991.
102. Nomura A, Stemmerman G, Chyou P, et al: *Helicobacter* infection and gastric carcinoma in a population of Japanese-Americans in Hawaii. N Engl J Med 325:1132, 1991.
103. Huang J, Srishar S, Chen Y, et al: Meta-analysis of the relationship between *Helicobacter pylori* seropositivity and gastric cancer. Gastroenterology 114:1169, 1998.
104. Eslick G, Lim L, Byles J, et al: Association of *Helicobacter pylori* infection with gastric carcinoma: A meta-analysis. Am J Gastroenterol 94:2373, 1999.
105. Ernst P: Review article: The role of inflammation in the pathogenesis of gastric cancer. Aliment Pharmacol Ther 13 Suppl 1:13, 1999.
106. Blanchard T, Czinn S: Review article: Immunological determinants that may affect the *Helicobacter pylori* cancer risk. Aliment Pharmacol Ther 12 Suppl 1:83, 1998.
107. Cahill R, Xia H, Kilgallen C, et al: Effect of eradication of *Helicobacter* infection on gastric epithelial cell proliferation. Dig Dis Sci 40: 1627, 1995.
108. Meyer-ter-Vehn T, Covacci A, Kist M, et al: *Helicobacter pylori* activates mitogen-activated protein kinase cascades and induces expression of the proto-oncogenes c-fos and c-jun. J Biol Chem 275: 16064, 2000.
109. Isozaki H, Okajima K, Ichinona T, et al: Significance of proliferating cell nuclear antigen (PCNA) expression in gastric cancer in relation to lymph node metastasis. J Surg Oncol 61:106, 1996.
110. Maeda K, Chung Y, Onoda N, et al: Association of tumor cell proliferation with lymph node metastasis in early gastric cancer. Oncology 53:1, 1996.
111. Hirose K, Iida A, Yamaguchi A, et al: Prognostic value of DNA ploidy and proliferating cell nuclear antigen in gastric cancer. Oncology 55:300, 1998.
112. Asahi M, Azuma T, Ito S, et al: *Helicobacter pylori* CagA protein can be tyrosine phosphorylated in gastric epithelial cells. J Exp Med 191: 593, 2000.
113. Odenbreit S, Puls J, Sedlmaier B, et al: Translocation of *Helicobacter pylori* CagA into gastric epithelial cells by type IV secretion. Science 287:1497, 2000.
114. Segal E, Cha J, Lo J, et al: Altered states: Involvement of phosphorylated CagA in the induction of host cellular growth changes by *Helicobacter pylori*. Proc Natl Acad Sci USA 96:14559, 1999.
115. Stein M, Rappuoli R, Covacci A: Tyrosine phosphorylation of the *Helicobacter pylori* CagA antigen after cag-driven host cell translocation. Proc Natl Acad Sci USA 97:1263, 2000.
116. Sozzi M, Valentini M, Figura N, et al: Atrophic gastritis and intestinal metaplasia in *Helicobacter pylori* infection: The role of CagA status. Am J Gastroenterol 93:375, 1998.
117. Webb P, Crabtree J, Forman D: Gastric cancer, cytotoxin-associated gene A-positive *Helicobacter pylori*, and serum pepsinogens: An international study. The Eurogast Study Group. Gastroenterology 116:269, 1999.
118. Zhang Z, Patchett S, Perrett D, et al: The relation between gastric vitamin C concentrations, mucosal histology, and CagA seropositivity in the human stomach. Gut 43:322, 1998.
119. Sipponen P, Kosunen T, Valle T, et al: *Helicobacter pylori* infection and chronic gastritis in gastric cancer. J Clin Pathol 45:319, 1992.
120. Dinarello C: Biological basis for interleukin-1 in disease. Blood 87: 2095, 1996.
121. Wallace J, Cucala M, Mugridge K, et al: Secretagogue-specific effects of interleukin-1 on gastric acid secretion. Am J Physiol 261:G559, 1991.
122. Lee A, Dixon M, Danon S, et al: Local acid production and *Helicobacter pylori*: A unifying hypothesis of gastroduodenal disease. Eur J Gastroenterol Hepatol 7:461, 1995.
123. Sipponen P, Hyvarinen H, Siurala M: *H. pylori* corpus gastritis—relation to acid output. J Physiol Pharmacol 47:151, 1996.
124. Klinkenberg-Knol E, Nelis F, Dent J, et al: Long-term omeprazole treatment in resistant gastroesophageal reflux disease: Efficacy, safety, and influence on gastric mucosa. Gastroenterology 118:661, 2000.
125. Uemura N, Mukai T, Okamoto S, et al: Effect of *Helicobacter pylori* eradication on subsequent development of cancer after endoscopic resection of early gastric cancer. Cancer Epidemiol Biomarkers Prev 6:639, 1997.

126. Rokkas T, Liatsos C, Karameris A, et al: Proliferating cell nuclear antigen (PCNA) immunostaining in *Helicobacter pylori* infection: Impact of eradication. Pathol Oncol Res 5:304, 1999.
127. Hansson L, Engstrand L, Nyren O, et al: *Helicobacter pylori* infection: Independent risk indicator of gastric adenocarcinoma. Gastroenterology 105:1098, 1993.
128. Ramon J, Serra L, Cerdo C, et al: Dietary factors and gastric cancer risk: A case-control study in Spain. Cancer 71:1731, 1993.
129. Ji B, Chow W, Yang G, et al: Dietary habits and stomach cancer in Shanghai, China. Int J Cancer 76:659, 1998.
130. Bartsch H: *N*-nitroso compounds and human cancer: Where do we stand? IARC Scientific Publications 105:1, 1991.
131. Leaf C, Wishnok J, Tannenbaum S: Mechanisms of endogenous nitrosation. Cancer Surv 8:323, 1989.
132. Marletta M: Mammalian synthesis of nitrite, nitrate, nitric oxide, and *N*-nitrosating agents. 1:249, 1988.
133. Mowat C, Carswell A, Wirz A, et al: Omeprazole and dietary nitrate independently affect levels of vitamin C and nitrite in gastric juice. Gastroenterology 116:813, 1999.
134. Sugimura T, Fujimira S, Baba T: Tumor production in the glandular stomach and alimentary tract of the rat by *N*-methyl-*N*′-nitro-*N*-nitrosoguanidine. Cancer Res 30:455, 1970.
135. Bartsch J, Ohshima H, Shuker D, et al: Human exposure to endogenous *N*-nitroso compounds: Quantitative estimates in subjects at high risk for cancer of the oral cavity, esophagus, stomach, and urinary bladder. Cancer Surv 8:335, 1989.
136. Knekt P, Jarvinen R, Dich J, et al: Risk of colorectal and other gastrointestinal cancers after exposure to nitrate, nitrite and *N*-nitroso compounds: A follow-up study. Int J Cancer 80:852, 1999.
137. van Loon A, Botterweck A, Goldbohm R, et al: Intake of nitrate and nitrite and the risk of gastric cancer: A prospective cohort study. Br J Cancer 78:129, 1998.
138. Fox J, Dangler C, Taylor N, et al: High-salt diet induces gastric epithelial hyperplasia and parietal cell loss, and enhances *Helicobacter pylori* colonization in C57BL/6 mice. Cancer Res 59:4823, 1999.
139. Ward M, Lopez-Carrillo L: Dietary factors and the risk of gastric cancer in Mexico City. Am J Epidemiol 149:925, 1999.
140. Nazario C, Szklo M, Diamond E, et al: Salt and gastric cancer: A case control study in Puerto Rico. Int J Epidemiol 22:790, 1993.
141. Cornee J, Pobel D, Riboli E, et al: A case-control study of gastric cancer and nutritional factors in Marseilles, France. Eur J Epidemiol 11:55, 1995.
142. Harrison L, Zhang Z, Karpeh M, et al: The role of dietary factors in the intestinal and diffuse histologic subtypes of gastric adenocarcinoma: A case-control study in the U.S. Cancer 80:1021, 1997.
143. Terry P, Yuen ON: Protective effect of fruits and vegetables on stomach cancer in a cohort of Swedish twins. Int J Cancer 76:35, 1998.
144. Galanis D, Kolonel L, Lee J, et al: Intakes of selected foods and beverages and the incidence of gastric cancer among the Japanese residents of Hawaii: A prospective study. Int J Epidemiol 27:173, 1998.
145. Drake I, Davies M, Mapstone N, et al: Ascorbic acid may protect against gastric cancer by scavenging mucosal oxygen radicals. Carcinogenesis 17:559, 1996.
146. Botterweck A, van den Brandt P, Goldbohm R: Vitamins, carotenoids, dietary fiber, and the risk of gastric carcinoma: Results from a prospective study after 6.3 years of follow-up. Cancer 88:737, 2000.
147. Ekstrom A, Serafini M, Nyren O, et al: Dietary antioxidant intake and the risk of cardia cancer and noncardia cancer of the intestinal and diffuse types: A population-based case-control study in Sweden. Cancer 87:133, 2000.
148. Mirvish S: Effects of vitamins C and E on *N*-nitroso compound formation, carcinogenesis, and cancer. Cancer 58:1842, 1986.
149. Santamaria C, Bianci A, Ravetto C, et al: Prevention of gastric cancer induced by MNNG in rats fed supplemental carotenoids. Hum Nutr Growth Cancer 4:175, 1987.
150. Garcia-Closas R, Gonzalez C, Agudo A, et al: Intake of specific carotenoids and flavonoids and the risk of gastric cancer in Spain. Cancer Causes Control 10:71, 1999.
151. Kobayashi M, Kogata M, Yamamura M, et al: Inhibitory effect of dietary selenium on carcinogenesis in rat glandular stomach induced by *N*-methyl-*N*′-nitro-*N*-nitrosoguanidine. Cancer Res 46:2266, 1986.
152. Tavani A, La Vecchia C, Gallus S, et al: Red meat intake and cancer risk: A study in Italy. Int J Cancer 86:425, 2000.
153. Saracci R: The diet and cancer hypothesis: Current trends. Med Oncol Tumor Pharmacol 7:99, 1990.
154. Fernandez E, Chatenoud L, La Vecchia C, et al: Fish consumption and cancer risk. Am J Clin Nutr 70:85, 1999.
155. Nomura A, Stemmermann G, Chyou P: Gastric cancer among the Japanese in Hawaii. Jpn J Cancer Res 86:916, 1995.
156. Chow W, Swanson C, Lissowska J, et al: Risk of stomach cancer in relation to consumption of cigarettes, alcohol, tea and coffee in Warsaw, Poland. Int J Cancer 81:871, 1999.
157. Lagergren J, Bergstrom R, Lindgren A, et al: The role of tobacco, snuff and alcohol use in the aetiology of cancer of the oesophagus and gastric cardia. Int J Cancer 85:340, 2000.
158. Mizoue T, Tokui N, Nishisaka K, et al: Prospective study on the relation of cigarette smoking with cancer of the liver and stomach in an endemic region. Int J Epidemiol 29:232, 2000.
159. Ye W, Ekstrom A, Hansson L, et al: Tobacco, alcohol and the risk of gastric cancer by sub-site and histologic type. Int J Cancer 83:223, 2000.
160. Coogan P, Rosenberg L, Palmer J, et al: Nonsteroidal anti-inflammatory drugs and risk of digestive cancers at sites other than the large bowel. Cancer Epidemiol Biomarkers Prev 9:119, 2000.
161. Langman M, Cheng K, Gilman E, et al: Effect of anti-inflammatory drugs on overall risk of common cancer: Case-control study in general practice research database. Br Med J 320:1642, 2000.
162. Zaridze D, Borisova E, Maximovitch D, et al: Aspirin protects against gastric cancer: Results of a case-control study from Moscow, Russia. Int J Cancer 82:473, 1999.
163. Pearce N, Howard J: Occupation, social class, and male cancer mortality in New Zealand. Int J Epidemiol 15:456, 1986.
164. Faggiano F, Partanen T, Kogevinas M, et al: Socioeconomic differences in cancer incidence and mortality. IARC Scientific Publications 138:65, 1997.
165. van Loon A, Goldbohm R, van den Brandt P: Socioeconomic status and stomach cancer incidence in men: Results from The Netherlands Cohort Study. J Epidemiol Commun Health 52:166, 1998.
166. Smith G, Hart C, Blane D, et al: Adverse socioeconomic conditions in childhood and cause-specific adult mortality: Prospective observational study. Br Med J 316:1631, 1998.
167. Labenz J, Malferheiner P: *Helicobacter pylori* in gastro-oesophageal reflux disease: Causal agent, independent or protective factor? Gut 41: 277, 1997.
168. Genta R, Rugge M: Gastric precancerous lesions: Heading for an international consensus. Gut 45 Suppl I:I5, 1999.
169. Kato I, Tominaga S, Ito Y, et al: A prospective study of atrophic gastritis and stomach cancer risk. Jpn J Cancer Res 83:1137, 1992.
170. Tatsuta M, Iishi H, Nazaizumi A, et al: Fundal atrophic gastritis as a risk factor for gastric cancer. Int J Cancer 53:70, 1993.
171. You W, Chang Y: Epidemiology of precancerous gastric lesions. J Gastroenterol Hepatol 8:375, 1993.
172. Sobala G, Schorah C, Sanderson M, et al: Ascorbic acid in the human stomach. Gastroenterology 97:357, 1989.
173. Wang T, Dangler C, Chen D, et al: Synergistic interaction between hypergastrinemia and *Helicobacter* infection in a mouse model of gastric cancer. Gastroenterology 118:36, 2000.
174. Kokkola A, Sjoblom S, Haapiainen R, et al: The risk of gastric carcinoma and carcinoid tumours in patients with pernicious anaemia. A prospective follow-up study. Scand J Gastroenterol 33:88, 1998.
175. Schafer L, Larson D, Melton L, et al: Risk of development of gastric carcinoma in patients with pernicious anemia: A population-based study in Rochester, Minnesota. Mayo Clin Proc 60:444, 1985.
176. Filipe M, Jass M: Intestinal metaplasia subtypes and cancer risk. In Filipe M, Jass J (eds): Gastric Carcinomas. Edinburgh, Churchill Livingstone, 1986, p 87.
177. Rokkas T, Felipe M, Sladen G: Detection of an increased incidence of early gastric cancer in patients with intestinal metaplasia type III who are closely followed up. Gut 32:1110, 1991.
178. Fuchs C, Mayer R: Gastric carcinoma. N Engl J Med 333:32, 1995.
179. Sipponen P: Intestinal metaplasia and gastric carcinoma. Ann Clin Res 13:139, 1981.
180. Japanese Research Society for Gastric Cancer: Japanese Classification of Gastric Carcinoma, 1st Engl ed. Tokyo, Kanehara & Co, 1995.
181. Rugge M, Correa P, Dixon M, et al: Gastric dysplasia: The Padova International Classification. Am J Surg Pathol 24:167, 2000.
182. Barranco S, Townsend C, Casartelli C, et al: Establishment and characterization of an in vitro model system for human adenocarcinoma of the stomach. Cancer Res 43:1703, 1983.

183. Rugge M, Farinati F, DiMario F, et al: Gastric epithelial dysplasia: A prospective multi-center study from the Interdisciplinary Group on Gastric Epithelial Dysplasia. Hum Pathol 22:1002, 1991.
184. Di Gregorio C, Morandi P, Fante R, et al: Gastric dysplasia. A follow-up study. Am J Gastroenterol 88:1714, 1993.
185. Kokkola A, Haapiainen R, Laxen F, et al: Risk of gastric carcinoma in patients with mucosal dysplasia associated with atrophic gastritis: A follow-up study. J Clin Pathol 49:979, 1996.
186. Sipponen P: Gastric dysplasia. Curr Top Pathol 81:61, 1990.
187. Tomasulo J: Gastric polyps. Histological types and their relationship to gastric carcinoma. Cancer 63:644, 1971.
188. Zea-Iriarte W, Sekine I, Itsuno M, et al: Carcinoma in gastric hyperplastic polyps. A phenotypic study. Dig Dis Sci 41:377, 1996.
189. Kamiya T, Morishita T, Asakura H, et al: Long-term follow-up study on gastric adenoma and its relation to gastric protruded carcinoma. Cancer 50:2496, 1982.
190. Saito K, Arai K, Mori M, et al: Effect of *Helicobacter pylori* eradication on malignant transformation of gastric adenoma. Gastrointest Endosc 52:27, 2000.
191. Caygill C, Hill M, Kirkahm J, et al: Mortality from gastric cancer following gastric surgery for peptic ulcer. Lancet 1:929, 1986.
192. Viste A, Bjornestad E, Opheim P, et al: Risk of gastric carcinoma following gastric operations for benign disease: A historical cohort study of 3470 patients. Lancet 2:502, 1986.
193. Lundegardh G, Adami H, Helmick C, et al: Stomach cancer after parietal gastrectomy for benign ulcer disease. N Engl J Med 319:195, 1988.
194. Dubrow R: Gastric cancer following peptic ulcer surgery. J Natl Cancer Inst 85:1269, 1993.
195. Domellof L, Eriksson S, Janunger K: Carcinoma and possible precancerous changes of the gastric stump after Billroth II resection. Gastroenterology 73:462, 1977.
196. Antonioli D: Gastric carcinoma and its precursors. Monogr Pathol 31: 144, 1990.
197. Schuman B, Waldaum J, Hiltz S: Carcinoma of the gastric remnant in a US population. Gastrointest Endosc 30:71, 1984.
198. Greenlee H, Vivit R Paez H, et al: Bacterial flora of the jejunum following peptic ulcer surgery. Arch Surg 102:260, 1971.
199. Dewar P, Dixon M, Johnston D: Bile reflux and degree of gastritis in patients with gastric ulcer: Before and after operation. J Surg Res 37: 277, 1984.
200. Burdick J, Chung E, Tanner G, et al: Treatment of Menetriers disease with a monoclonal antibody against the epidermal growth factor receptor. N Engl J Med 343:1697, 2000.
201. Case Records of the Massachusetts General Hospital: Case 2—1988. N Engl J Med 318:100, 1988.
202. Scharschmidt B: The natural history of hypertrophic gastropathy (Menetrier's disease): Report of a case with 16-year follow-up and review of 120 cases from the literature. Am J Med 63:644, 1977.
203. Wood G, Bates C, Brown R, et al: Intramucosal carcinoma of the gastric antrum complicating Menetrier's disease. J Clin Pathol 36: 1071, 1983.
204. Kawai K, Akasaka Y, Kohli Y: Endoscopic approach to the "malignant change of benign gastric ulcer" from follow-up studies. Endoscopy 5:53, 1973.
205. Japanese Reasearch Society for Gastric Cancer and Miwa Registry Institute for Gastric Cancer: Treatment Results of Gastric Carcinoma in Japan (1979–1982). Tokyo, Mitamura Press, 1995.
206. Murakami R, Tsukuma H, Ubukata T, et al: Estimation of validity of mass screening program for gastric cancer in Osaka, Japan. Cancer 65:1255, 1990.
207. Watanabe H, Mai M, Shimoda T, et al: Report of the meeting of the 72nd Japanese Gastric Cancer Congress. Gastric Cancer 3:1, 2000.
208. Yamakazi H, Oshima A, Murakami R, et al: A long-term follow-up study of patients with gastric cancer detected by mass screening. Cancer 63:613, 1989.
209. Committee on National Statistics: The 1996 annual report of mass screening for digestive organs. J Gastroenterol Mass Survey 37:212, 1999.
210. Hisamichi S, Sugawara N, Fukao A: Effectiveness of gastric mass screening in Japan. Cancer Detect Prev 11:323, 1988.
211. Inaba S, Hirayama H, Nagata C, et al: Evaluation of a screening program on reduction of gastric cancer mortality in Japan: Preliminary results from a cohort study. Prev Med 29:102, 1999.
212. Borchard F: Classification of gastric carcinoma. Hepato-Gastroenterology 37:223, 1990.
213. Tucker H, Snape W, Cohen S: Achalasia secondary to carcinoma: Manometric and clinical features. Ann Intern Med 89:315, 1978.
214. Malliah L, Brozinsky S, Fruchter G, et al: Malignant gastrocolic fistula: Case report and review of the literature. Am J Proctol Gastreoenterol Colon Rectal Surg 31:12, 1980.
215. Croft P, Wilkinson M: The incidence of carcinomatous neuromyopathy in patients with various types of carcinoma. Brain 88:427, 1965.
216. Wakashin M, Wakashin Y, Iesato K, et al: Association of gastric cancer and nephrotic syndrome: An immunologic study in three patients. Gastroenterology 78:749, 1980.
217. Yeh K, Cheng A: Gastric cancer associated with acute disseminated intravascular coagulation: Successful initial treatment with weekly 24-hour infusion of high-dose 5-fluorouracil and leucovorin. Br J Haematol 100:769, 1998.
218. Dupont J, Lee J, Burton G, et al: Adenocarcinoma of the stomach: Review of 1,497 cases. Cancer 41:941, 1978.
219. Ishizawa T, Mitsuhashi Y, Kondo S, et al: Sister Joseph's nodule: A case report and review of the Japanese literature. J Dermatol 24:662, 1997.
220. Yeh J, Munn S, Plunkett T, et al: Coexistence of acanthosis nigricans and the sign of Leser-Trélat in a patient with gastric adenocarcinoma: A case report and literature review. J Am Acad Dermatol 42:357, 2000.
221. Ren J, Chen Z, Juan S, et al: Detection of circulating gastric carcinoma-associated antigen MG7-Ag in human sera using an established single determinant immuno-polymerase chain reaction technique. Cancer 88:280, 2000.
222. Kitahara F, Kobayashi K, Sato T, et al: Accuracy of screening for gastric cancer using serum pepsinogen concentrations. Gut 44:693, 1999.
223. Westerveld B, Pals G, Lamers C, et al: Clinical significance of pepsinogen A isozymogens, serum pepsinogen A and C levels, and serum gastrin levels. Cancer 59:952, 1987.
224. Mori M, Sugimachi K: Clinicopathologic studies of gastric carcinoma. Semin Surg Oncol 6:19, 1990.
225. Oiwa T, Mori M, Sugimachi K, et al: Diagnostics of small gastric carcinoma. J Surg Oncol 33:170, 1986.
226. Farley D, Donohue J: Early gastric cancer. Surg Clin North Am 72: 401, 1992.
227. Yanai H, Noguchi T, Mizumachi S, et al: A blind comparison of the effectiveness of endoscopic ultrasonography and endoscopy in staging early gastric cancer. Gut 44:361, 1999.
228. American Gastroenterological Association: Medical position statement: Evaluation of dyspepsia. Gastroenterology 114:579, 1998.
229. Breslin N, Thomson A, Bailey R, et al: Gastric cancer and other endoscopic diagnoses in patients with benign dyspepsia. Gut 46:93, 2000.
230. Bini E, Rajapaksa R, Valdes M, et al: Is upper gastrointestinal endoscopy indicated in asymptomatic patients with a positive fecal occult blood test and negative colonoscopy? Am J Med 106:613, 1999.
231. Kuntz C, Herfarth C: Imaging diagnosis for staging of gastric cancer. Semin Surg Oncol 17:96, 1999.
232. Nicholson D, Shorvon P: Endoscopic ultrasound of the stomach. Br J Radiol 66:487, 1993.
233. Tio T, Schouwink M, Cikot R, et al: Preoperative TNM classification of gastric carcinoma by endosonography in comparison with the pathological TNM system: A prospective study of 172 cases. Hepatogastroenterology 36:51, 1989.
234. Sano T, Okuyama Y, Kobeori O, et al: Early gastric cancer endoscopic diagnosis of depth of invasion. Dig Dis Sci 35:1340, 1990.
235. Botel J, Lightdale C, Zauber A, et al: Preoperative staging of gastric cancer: Comparison of endoscopic US and dynamic CT. Radiology 181:426, 1991.
236. Okai T, Yamakawa O, Matsuda N, et al: Analysis of gastric carcinoma growth by endoscopic ultrasonography. Endoscopy 23:121, 1991.
237. Wang J, Hsieh J, Huang Y, et al: Endoscopic ultrasonography for preoperative locoregional staging and assessment of resectability in gastric cancer. Clin Imaging 22:355, 1998.
238. Monig S, Zirbes T, Schroder W, et al: Staging of gastric cancer: Correlation of lymph node size and metastatic infiltration. AJR Am J Roentgenol 173:365, 1999.
239. Archer A, Grant D: Recent developments in diagnostic radiology of primary and recurrent gastric cancer. Cancer Treat Rev 55:107, 1991.
240. Iinuma G, Ushio K, Ishikawa T, et al: Diagnosis of gastric cancers:

Comparison of conventional radiography and digital radiography with a 4 million-pixel charge-coupled device. Radiology 214:497, 2000.

241. Montei A, Graziani L, Pesaresi A, et al: Radiological diagnosis of early gastric cancer by routine double-contrast examination. Gastrointest Radiol 7:205, 1982.
242. Maruyama M, Baba Y: Gastric carcinoma. Radiol Clin North Am 21: 1233, 1994.
243. Minami M, Kawauchi N, Itai Y, et al: Gastric tumors: Radiologic-pathologic correlation and accuracy of T staging with dynamic CT. Radiology 185:173, 1992.
244. Paramo J, Gomez G: Dynamic CT in the preoperative evaluation of patients with gastric cancer: Correlation with surgical findings and pathology. Ann Surg Oncol 6:379, 1999.
245. Sohn K, Lee J, Lee S, et al: Comparing MR imaging and CT in the staging of gastric carcinoma. Am J Roentgenol 174:1551, 2000.
246. Kim A, Han J, Seong C, et al: MRI in staging advanced gastric cancer: Is it useful compared with spiral CT? J Comp Assist Tomog 24:389, 2000.
247. Kang B, Kim J, Kim K, et al: Value of the dynamic and delayed MR sequence with Gd-DTPA in the T-staging of stomach cancer: Correlation with the histopathology. Abdom Imaging 25:14, 2000.
248. Davies J, Chalmers A, Sue-Ling H, et al: Spiral computed tomography and operative staging of gastric carcinoma: A comparison with histopathological staging. Gut 41:314, 1997.
249. Neugut A, Hayek M, Howe G: Epidemiology of gastric cancer. Semin Oncol 23:281, 1996.
250. Correa P, Sassano N, Stemmerman G: Pathology of gastric carcinoma in Japanese populations: Comparisons between Miyagi Prefecture, Japan, and Hawaii. J Natl Cancer Inst 51:1499, 1973.
251. Hochwald S, Brennan M, Klimstra D, et al: Is lymphadenectomy necessary for early gastric cancer? Ann Surg Oncol 6:664, 1999.
251a. Japanese Research Society for Gastric Cancer: Japanese Classification of Gastric Carcinoma, 1st English ed. Toyko, Kanchora, 1995.
252. Hermanek P, Sobin L: TNM Classification of Malignant Tumors. International Union Against Cancer. Berlin, Springer-Verlag, 1992.
253. Sobin L, Wittekind C: International Union Against Cancer. TNM Classification of Malignant Tumors. New York, John Wiley, 1997.
254. Katai H, Yoshimura K, Maruyama K, et al: Evaluation of the New International Union Against Cancer TNM staging for gastric carcinoma. Cancer 88:1796, 2000.
255. Ichikura T, Tomimatsu S, Uefuji K, et al: Evaluation of the new American Joint Committee on Cancer/International Union Against Cancer classification of lymph node metastases from gastric carcinoma in comparison with the Japanese classification. Cancer 86:553, 1999.
256. Fujii K, Isozaki H, Okajima K, et al: Clinical evaluation of lymph node metastasis in gastric cancer defined by the fifth edition of the TNM classification in comparison with the Japanese system. Br J Surg 86:685, 1999.
257. Preusser P, Achterrath W, Wilke H, et al: Chemotherapy of gastric cancer. Cancer Treat Rev 15:257, 1988.
258. Hundahl S, Phillips J, Menck H: The National Cancer Data Base Report on poor survival of U.S. gastric carcinoma patients treated with gastrectomy: Fifth Edition American Joint Committee on cancer staging, proximal disease, and the "different disease" hypothesis. Cancer 88:921, 2000.
259. Buchholtz T, Welch C, Malt R: Clinical correlates of resectability and survival in gastric carcinoma. Ann Surg 188:711, 1978.
260. Bozzetti F, Bonfanti G, Bufalino R, et al: Adequacy of margins of resection in gastrectomy for cancer. Ann Surg 196:685, 1992.
261. Madden M, Price S, Learmonth G, et al: Surgical staging of gastric carcinoma: Sources and consequences of error. Br J Surg 74:119, 1987.
262. Papachristou D, Shiu M: Management by en bloc multiple organ resection of carcinoma of the stomach invading adjacent organs. Surg Gynecol Obstet 152:483, 1981.
263. Vogel P, Ruschoff J, Kummel S, et al: Prognostic value of microscopic peritoneal dissemination: Comparison between colon and gastric cancer. Dis Colon Rectum 43:92, 2000.
264. Ribeiro UJ, Gama-Rodrigues J, Safatle-Ribeiro A, et al: Prognostic significance of intraperitoneal free cancer cells obtained by laparoscopic peritoneal lavage in patients with gastric cancer. J Gastrointest Surg 2:244, 1998.
265. Shiu M, Oaochristou D, Kolsoff C, et al: Selection of operative procedure for adenocarcinoma of the mid-stomach: Twenty years' experience with implications for future treatment strategy. Int Congr Surg 542:207, 1981.
266. Gouzi J, Huguier M, Fagniez P, et al: Total versus subtotal gastrectomy for adenocarcinoma of the gastric antrum: A French prospective controlled study. Ann Surg 209:162, 1989.
267. Bozzetti F, Marubini E, Bonfanti G, et al: Subtotal versus total gastrectomy for gastric cancer: Five-year survival rates in a multicenter randomized Italian trial. Italian Gastrointestinal Tumor Study Group. Ann Surg 230:170, 1999.
268. Meyer H, Jahne J, Wilke H, et al: Surgical treatment of gastric cancer: Retrospective survey of 1,704 operated cases with special reference to total gastrectomy as the operation of choice. Semin Surg Oncol 7:356, 1991.
269. Onate-Ocana L, Aiello-Crocifoglio V, Mondragon-Sanchez R, et al: Survival benefit of D2 lymphadenectomy in patients with gastric adenocarcinoma. Ann Surg Oncol 7:210, 2000.
270. Kasakura Y, Fujii M, Mochizuki F, et al: Is there a benefit of pancreaticosplenectomy with gastrectomy for advanced gastric cancer? Am J Surg 179:237, 2000.
271. Tas F, Aykan N, Aydiner A, et al: The roles of chemotherapy and surgery in gastric carcinoma and the influence of prognostic factors on survival. Am J Clin Oncol 23:53, 2000.
272. Cuschieri A, Weeden S, Fielding J, et al: Patient survival after D1 and D2 resections for gastric cancer: Long-term results of the MRC randomized surgical trial. Br J Cancer 79:1522, 1999.
273. Schmid A, Thybusch A, Kremer B, et al: Differential effects of radical D2-lymphadenectomy and splenectomy in surgically treated gastric cancer patients. Hepatogastroenterology 47:579, 2000.
274. Bonenkamp J, Hermans J, Sasako M, et al: Extended lymph-node dissection for gastric cancer. Dutch Gastric Cancer Group. N Engl J Med 340:908, 1999.
275. Azagra J, Goergen M, Simone PD, et al: Minimally invasive surgery for gastric cancer. Surg Endosc 13:351, 1999.
276. Yamao T, Shirao K, Ono H, et al: Risk factors for lymph node metastasis from intramucosal gastric carcinoma. Cancer 77:602, 1996.
277. Fujino Y, Nagata Y, Ogino K, et al: Evaluation of endoscopic ultrasonography as an indicator for surgical treatment of gastric cancer. J Gastroenterol Hepatol 14:540, 1999.
278. Makuuchi H, Kise Y, Shimada H, et al: Endoscopic mucosal resection for early gastric cancer. Semin Surg Oncol 17:108, 1999.
279. Ell C, Gossner L, May A, et al: Photodynamic ablation of early cancers of the stomach by means of mTHPC and laser irradiation: Preliminary clinical experience. Gut 43:345, 1998.
280. Wisbeck W, Becher E, Russell A: Adenocarcinoma of the stomach: Autopsy observations with therapeutic implications for the radiation oncologist. Radiother Oncol 7:13, 1986.
281. Cocconi G, DeLisi V, Blasio BD: Randomized comparison of 5-FU alone or combined with mitomycin and cytarabine in the treatment of advanced gastric cancer. Cancer Treat Rep 66:1263, 1982.
282. Kolaric K, Potrevica V, Stanovink M: Controlled phase III clinical study of 4-EPI-doxorubicin/5-FU versus 5-FU alone in metastatic gastric and rectosigmoid cancer. Oncology 43:73, 1986.
283. Moynihan T, Hansen R, Anderson T, et al: Continuous 5-FU infusion in advanced gastric carcinoma. Am J Clin Oncol 11:461, 1988.
284. Takiguchi N, Nakajima N, Saitoh N, et al: A phase III randomized study comparing oral doxifluridine and oral 5-fluorouracil after curative resection of gastric cancer. Int J Oncol 16:1021, 2000.
285. Sugimachi K, Maehara Y, Horikoshi N, et al: An early phase II study of oral S-1, a newly developed 5-fluorouracil derivative for advanced and recurrent gastrointestinal cancers. The S-1 Gastrointestinal Cancer Study Group. Oncology 57:202, 1999.
286. Hartmann J, Kanz L, Bokemeyer C: Phase II study of continuous 120-hour-infusion of mitomycin C as salvage chemotherapy in patients with progressive or rapidly recurrent gastrointestinal adenocarcinoma. Anticancer Res 20:1177, 2000.
287. Wadler S, Green M, Muggia F: The role of anthracyclines in the treatment of gastric cancer. Cancer Treat Rev 12:105, 1985.
288. Lacave A, Izarzugaza I, Aparicio LA, et al: Phase II clinical trial of cisdichlorodiammineplatinum in gastric cancer. Am J Clin Oncol 6:35, 1983.
289. Levi J, Fox R, Tattersall M, et al: Analysis of prospective randomized comparison of doxorubicin vs. 5-FU, doxorubicin and BCNU in advanced gastric cancer: Implications for future studies. J Clin Oncol 4: 1348, 1986.
290. Bleiberg H: CPT-11 in gastrointestinal cancer. Eur J Cancer 35:371, 1999.
291. Bruckner H, Lokich J, Stablein D: Studies of Baker's antifoil, metho-

trexate, and razoxane in advanced gastric cancer: A gastrointestinal tumor study group report. Cancer Treat Rep 66:1713, 1982.
292. Neri B, de Leonardis V, Romano S, et al: Adjuvant chemotherapy after gastric resection in node-positive cancer patients: A multicentre randomised study. Br J Cancer 73:549, 1996.
293. Waters J, Norman A, Cunningham D, et al: Long-term survival after epirubicin, cisplatin and fluorouracil for gastric cancer: Results of a randomized trial. Br J Cancer 80:269, 1999.
294. Earle C, Maroun J: Adjuvant chemotherapy after curative resection for gastric cancer in non-Asian patients: Revisiting a meta-analysis of randomised trials. Eur J Cancer 35:1059, 1999.
295. Sugarbaker P, Yonemura Y: Clinical pathway for the management of resectable gastric cancer with peritoneal seeding: Best palliation with a ray of hope for cure. Oncology 58:96, 2000.
296. Sayag-Beaujard A, Francois Y, Glehen O, et al: Intraperitoneal chemo-hyperthermia with mitomycin C for gastric cancer patients with peritoneal carcinomatosis. Anticancer Res 19:1375, 1999.
297. Hirose K, Katayama K, Iida A, et al: Efficacy of continuous hyperthermic peritoneal perfusion for the prophylaxis and treatment of peritoneal metastasis of advanced gastric cancer: Evaluation by multivariate regression analysis. Oncology 57:106, 1999.
298. Fujimoto S, Takahashi M, Mutou T, et al: Successful intraperitoneal hyperthermic chemoperfusion for the prevention of postoperative peritoneal recurrence in patients with advanced gastric carcinoma. Cancer 85:529, 1999.
299. Yonemura Y, Ninomiya I, Kaji M, et al: Prophylaxis with intraoperative chemohyperthermia against peritoneal recurrence of serosal invasion–positive gastric cancer. World J Surg 19:450, 1995.
300. Samel S, Singal A, Becker H, et al: Problems with intraoperative hyperthermic peritoneal chemotherapy for advanced gastric cancer. Eur J Surg Oncol 26:222, 2000.
301. Hallissey M, Dunn J, Ward L, et al: The second British Stomach Cancer Group trial of adjuvant radiotherapy or chemotherapy in resectable gastric cancer: Five-year follow-up. Lancet 343:1309, 1994.
302. Safran H, Wanebo H, Hesketh P, et al: Paclitaxel and concurrent radiation for gastric cancer. Int J Radiat Oncol Biol Phys 46:889, 2000.
303. Weese J, Harbison S, Stiller G, et al: Neoadjuvant chemotherapy, radical resection with intraoperative radiation therapy (IORT): Improved treatment for gastric adenocarcinoma. Surgery 128:564, 2000.
304. Wotherspoon A: Gastric lymphoma of mucosa-associated lymphoid tissue and *Helicobacter pylori*. Annu Rev Med 49:289, 1998.
305. Azab M, Henry-Amar M, Rougier P, et al: Prognostic factors in primary gastrointestinal non-Hodgkin's lymphoma; A multi-variate analysis, report of 106 cases, and review of the literature. Cancer 64: 1208, 1989.
306. Amer M, El-Akkad S: Gastrointestinal lymphoma in adults: Clinical features and management of 300 cases. Gastroenterology 106:846, 1994.
307. Dajani Y, Al-Jitawi S: Primary gastrointestinal lymphoma in Jordan. Trop Geogr Med 35:375, 1983.
308. Selzer G, Sacks M, Sherman G, et al: Primary malignant lymphoma of the small intestine in Israel: Changing incidence with time. Isr J Med Sci 15:390, 1979.
309. Herrmann R, Panahon A, Barcos M, et al: Gastrointestinal involvement in non-Hodgkin's lymphoma. Cancer 46:215, 1980.
310. Back H, Gustavsson B, Ridell B, et al: Primary gastrointestinal lymphoma: Incidence, clinical presentation, and surgical approach. J Surg Oncol 33:234, 1986.
311. Fischbach W, Dragosics B, Kolve-Goebeler M, et al: Primary gastric B-cell lymphoma: Results of a prospective multicenter study. Gastroenterology 119:1191, 2000.
312. Dragosics B, Bauer P, Radaskiewicz T: Primary gastrointestinal non-Hodgkin's lymphoma: A retrospective clinicopathological study of 150 cases. Cancer 55:1060, 1985.
313. Isaacson P, Wright D: Malignant lymphoma of mucosa-associated lymphoid tissue. A distinctive type of B-cell lymphoma. Cancer 52: 1410, 1983.
314. Radaskiewicz T, Dragosics B, Bauer P: Gastrointestinal malignant lymphomas of the mucosa-associated lymphoid tissue: Factors relevant to prognosis. Gastroenterology 102:1628, 1992.
315. Fung C, Grossbard M, Linggood R, et al: Mucosa-associated lymphoid tissue lymphoma of the stomach: Long-term outcome after local treatment. Cancer 85:9, 1999.
316. Genta R, Hamner H, Graham D: Gastric lymphoid follicles in *Helicobacter pylori* infection: Frequency, distribution and response to triple therapy. Hum Pathol 24:577, 1993.
317. D'Elios MM, Amedei A, Manghetti M, et al: Impaired T-cell regulation of B-cell growth in *Helicobacter pylori*–related gastric low-grade MALT lymphoma. Gastroenterology 117:1105, 1999.
318. Shomer N, Dangler C, Whary M, et al: Experimental *Helicobacter pylori* infection induces antral gastritis and gastric mucosa-associated lymphoid tissue in guinea pigs. Infect Immun 66:2614, 1998.
319. Eck M, Schmausser B, Haas R, et al: MALT-type lymphoma of the stomach is associated with *Helicobacter pylori* strains expressing the CagA protein [see comments]. Gastroenterology 112:1482, 1997.
320. Cammarota G, Tursi A, Montalto M, et al: Prevention and treatment of low-grade B-cell primary gastric lymphoma by anti-*H. pylori* therapy. J Clin Gastroenterol 21:118, 1995.
321. Steinbach G, Ford R, Glober G, et al: Antibiotic treatment of gastric lymphoma of mucosa-associated lymphoid tissue. An uncontrolled trial. Ann Intern Med 131:88, 1999.
322. Parsonnet J, Hansen S, Rodriguez L, et al: *Helicobacter pylori* infection and gastric lymphoma. N Engl J Med 330:1267, 1994.
323. Stolte M, Kroher G, Meining A, et al: A comparison of *Helicobacter pylori* and *H. heilmannii* gastritis: A matched control study involving 404 patients. Scand J Gastroenterol 32:28, 1997.
324. Hilzenrat N, Lamoureaux E, Weintrub I, et al: *Helicobacter heilmannii*-like spiral bacteria in gastric mucosal biopsies: Prevalence and clinical significance. Arch Pathol Lab Med 119:1149, 1995.
325. Jhala D, Jhala N, Lechago J, et al: *Helicobacter heilmannii* gastritis: Association with acid peptic diseases and comparison with *Helicobacter pylori* gastritis. Mod Pathol 12:534, 1999.
326. Starostik P, Greiner A, Schultz A, et al: Genetic aberrations common in gastric high-grade large B-cell lymphoma. Blood 95:1180, 2000.
327. Dancygier H: AIDS and the gastrointestinal tract. Endoscopy 18:222, 1998.
328. Kolve M, Fischbach W, Greiner A, et al: Differences in endoscopic and clinicopathological features of primary and secondary gastric non-Hodgkin's lymphoma. German Gastrointestinal Lymphoma Study Group. Gastrointest Endosc 49:307, 1999.
329. Kolve M, Fischbach W, Wilhelm M: Primary gastric non-Hodgkin's lymphoma: Requirements for diagnosis and staging. Recent Results Cancer Res 156:63, 2000.
330. Carbone P, Kaplan H, Musshoff K, et al: Report of the Committee on Hodgkin's Disease Staging Classification. Cancer Res 31:1860, 1971.
331. Musshoff K, Schmidt-Vollmer H: Prognosis of non-Hodgkin's lymphomas with special emphasis on the staging classification. Z Krebsforsch 83:323, 1975.
332. Aozasa K, Tsujimoto M, Inoue A, et al: Primary gastrointestinal lymphoma. Oncology 42:97, 1985.
333. Romguera J, Velasquez W, Silvermintz K, et al: Surgical debulking is associated with improved survival in Stage I–II diffuse large cell lymphoma. Cancer 66:267, 1990.
334. Maor M, Velasquez W, Fuller L, et al: Stomach conservation in stages IE and IIE gastric non-Hodgkin's lymphoma. J Clin Oncol 8:266, 1990.
335. Liu H, Hsu C, Chen C, et al: Chemotherapy alone versus surgery followed by chemotherapy for stage I/IIE large-cell lymphoma of the stomach. Am J Hematol 64:175, 2000.
336. Shiu M, Nisce L, Pinna A, et al: Recent studies of multimodal therapy of gastric lymphoma. Cancer 58:1389, 1986.
337. Gospodarowicz M, Sutcliffe S, Clark R, et al: Outcome analysis of localized gastrointestinal lymphoma treated with surgery and postoperative radiation. Int J Radiat Oncol Biol Phys 19:1351, 1990.
338. Shim D, Dosoretz D, Anderson T, et al: Primary gastric lymphoma: An analysis with emphasis on prognostic factors and radiation therapy. Cancer 52:2044, 2000.
339. Ferreri A, Cordio S, Paro S, et al: Therapeutic management of stage I–II high-grade primary gastric lymphomas. Oncology 56:274, 1999.
340. Morgner A, Lehn N, Andersen LP, et al: *Helicobacter heilmannii*–associated primary gastric low-grade MALT lymphoma: Complete remission after curing the infection. Gastroenterology 118:821, 2000.
341. Gilligan C, Lawton G, Tang L, et al: Gastric carcinoid tumors: The biology and therapy of an enigmatic and controversial lesion. Am J Gastroenterol 90:338, 1995.
342. Rindi G, Bordi C, Rappel S, et al: Gastric carcinoids and neuroendocrine carcinomas: Pathogenesis, pathology, and behavior. World J Surg 20:168, 1996.
343. Muller J, Kirchner T, Muller-Hermelink H: Gastric endocrine cell hyperplasia and carcinoid tumors in atrophic gastritis type A. Am J Surg Pathol 11:909, 1987.
344. Borch K: Atrophic gastritis and gastric carcinoid tumors. Ann Med 21:219, 1989.

345. Laine L, Ahnen D, McClain C, et al: Review article: Potential gastrointestinal effects of long-term acid suppression with proton pump inhibitors. Aliment Pharmacol Ther 14:651, 2000.
346. Debelenko L, Emmert-Buck M, Zhuang Z, et al: The multiple endocrine neoplasia type I gene locus is involved in the pathogenesis of type II gastric carcinoids. Gastroenterology 113:773, 1997.
347. Nakamura S, Iida M, Yao T, et al: Endoscopic features of gastric carcinoids. Gastrointest Endosc 37:535, 1991.
348. Granberg D Wilander E, Stridsberg M, et al: Clinical symptoms, hormone profiles, treatment, and prognosis in patients with gastric carcinoids. Gut 43:223, 1998.
349. Akerstrom G: Management of carcinoid tumors of the stomach, duodenum, and pancreas. World J Surg 20:173, 1996.
350. Eckhauser F, Lloyd R, Thompson N, et al: Antrectomy for multicentric, argyrophil gastric carcinoids: A preliminary report. Surgery 104: 1046, 1988.
351. Kern S, Yardley J, Lazenby A, et al: Reversal by antrectomy of endocrine cell hyperplasia in the gastric body in pernicious anemia: A morphometric study. Mod Pathol 3:561, 1990.
352. Wilander E, El-Sathy M, Pitkanen P: Histopathology of gastric carcinoids: A survey of 42 cases. Histopathology 8:183, 1984.
353. Miettinen M, Sarlomo-Rikala M, Lasota J: Gastrointestinal stromal tumors: Recent advances in understanding of their biology. Hum Pathol 30:1213, 1999.
354. Hirota S, Isozaki K, Moriyama Y, et al: Gain of function mutations of c-kit in human gastrointestinal stromal tumors. Science 279:577, 1998.
355. Emory T, Sobin L, Lukes L, et al: Prognosis of gastrointestinal smooth muscle tumors: Dependence on anatomic site. Am J Surg Pathol 23:82, 1999.
356. Joensuu H, Roberts PJ, Sarlomo-Rikala, et al: Effect of the tyrosine kinase inhibitor STI571 in a patient with a metastatic gastrointestinal stromal tumor. N Engl J Med 344:1052, 2001.
357. Demetri GD: Targeting c-kit mutations in solid tumors: scientific rationale and novel therapeutic options. Semin Oncol 28(5 Suppl 17):19, 2001.
358. Winston C, Hadar O, Teitcher J, et al: Metastatic lobular carcinoma of the breast: Patterns of spread in the chest, abdomen, and pelvis on CT. AJR Am J. Roentgenol 175:795, 2000.
359. Blecker D, Abraham S, Furth E, et al: Melanoma in the gastrointestinal tract. Am J Gastroenterol 94:3427, 1999.
360. Kim H, Jang W, Hong H, et al: Metastatic involvement of the stomach secondary to lung carcinoma. J Korean Med Sci 8:24, 1993.
361. Spencer J, Crosse B, Mannion R, et al: Gastroduodenal obstruction from ovarian cancer: Imaging features and clinical outcome. Clin Radiol 55:264, 2000.
362. Green P, Fevre D, Barratt P: Metastatic hepatoma in the stomach masquerading as a leiomyoma. Aust N Z J Med 6:341, 1976.
363. Kondo S, Hachisuka K, Yamaguchi A, et al: Hematogenous metastasis to the stomach—a case presenting the rectosigmoid as the primary site and a review of the literature in Japan. Gan No Rinsho 28:74, 1982.
364. Fowlie S, Taylor R, Preston P, et al: Gastric and periurethral metastases from seminoma testis. Clin Radiol 38:63, 1987.
365. Chetty R, Pillay SV: Coexistent gastric MALT lymphoma and Kaposi sarcoma in an HIV-positive patient. J Clin Pathol 52:313, 1999.
366. Daimaru Y, Kido H, Hashimoto H, et al: Benign schwannoma of the gastrointestinal tract: A clinicopathologic and immunohistochemical study. Hum Pathol 19:257, 1988.
367. Imamura A, Tochihara M, Natsui K: Glomus tumor of the stomach: Endoscopic ultrasonographic findings. Am J Gastroenterol 89:271, 1994.
368. Otsuji E, Yamaguchi T, Taniguchi H, et al: Malignant endocrine carcinoma of the stomach. Hepatogastroenterology 47:601, 2000.
369. Rychterova V, Hagerstrand I: Parietal cell carcinoma of the stomach. APMIS 99:1008, 1991.
370. Mollitt DL, Golladay ES: Symptomatic gastroduodenal pancreatic rest in children. J Pediatr Surg 19:449, 1984.
371. Khachaturian T, Dinning JP, Earnest DL: Gastric xanthelasma in a patient after partial gastrectomy. Am J Gastroenterol 93:1588, 1998.
372. Cats A, Schenk BE, Bloemena E, et al: Parietal cell protrusions and fundic gland cysts during omeprazole maintenance treatment. Hum Pathol 31:684, 2000.

Section Seven

PANCREAS

Chapter 45

Anatomy, Histology, Embryology, and Developmental Anomalies of the Pancreas

David J. Magee and J. Steven Burdick

HISTORY

The pancreas was one of the last organs in the abdomen to receive the critical attention of anatomists, physiologists, physicians, and surgeons.[1, 2] It was first referred to as the "finger of the liver" in the Talmud, written between 200 **BC** and 200 **AD**. Galen named it (Ruphos, circa 100 **AD**, should probably be credited[2]) and thought the pancreas served to support and protect blood vessels. Vesalius considered it a cushion for the stomach. Little further information was available until Wirsung demonstrated the pancreatic ducts of humans in 1642 and de Graaf discovered pancreatic secretion from the pancreatic fistula of dogs in 1664.

The digestive action of pancreatic secretions was discovered almost 200 years later. Eberle in 1834, Purkinje and Pappenheim in 1836, and Valentin in 1844 observed the emulsification of fat, proteolytic activity, and digestion of starch, respectively, by pancreatic juice and extracts. Bernard subsequently demonstrated the digestive action of pancreatic juice on sugar, fats, and proteins, using secretions from pancreatic fistula preparations.

Kuhne introduced the term *enzyme* and isolated trypsin in 1876 after investigations that spanned 10 years. The concept of enzymes led shortly to the identification of pancreatic amylase and lipase. In 1889, Chepovalnikoff, a student of Pavlov, discovered enterokinase in the duodenal mucosa, an enzyme that is essential for activation of the proteolytic enzymes. Another of Pavlov's students, Dolinsky, stimulated pancreatic secretion by instilling acid into the duodenum in 1895. This led to the discovery of secretin by Bayliss and Starling, which proved to be not an enzyme but the first hormone to be identified.

The histologic structure of the pancreas was first described in 1869 by Langerhans. Shortly thereafter, Heidenhain[3] characterized the periodic postprandial changes that occurred in the histology of the dog pancreas. He found that as the granular regions of cells disappeared after feeding, the enzyme activity in pancreatic juice increased; he concluded that the granules contained the precursors of the digestive enzymes.

Pancreatic disease was rarely recorded before the 19th century. Friedreich wrote the first systematic description of pancreatic diseases in 1875. The description of acute pancreatitis by Fitz in 1889 remains a classic. Although Fitz suggested operation for pancreatitis, surgery for pancreatic neoplasms and other diseases was not popular until the 1930s, mainly as a result of the work of Whipple and Brunschwig. The pancreas was first successfully extirpated in dogs by Brunner in 1683.

NORMAL ANATOMY

The pancreas is a soft, elongated, flattened gland 12 to 20 cm in length.[4–6] The adult gland weighs between 70 and 110 g. The head lies behind the peritoneum of the posterior abdominal wall and has a lobular structure. The pancreas is covered with a fine connective tissue but does not have a true capsule. The head of the pancreas is on the right side and lies within the curvature of the duodenum. The neck, body, and tail of the pancreas lie obliquely in the posterior abdomen, with the tail extending as far as the gastric surface of the spleen (Fig. 45–1).

The second and third duodenum curvature lies around the head of the pancreas. The anterior surface of the head of the pancreas is adjacent to the pylorus, the first part of the duodenum, and the transverse colon. The posterior surface abuts the hilus and medial border of the right kidney, the inferior vena cava and the right renal vessels, the right gonadal vein, and the right crus of the diaphragm.

Some text (History, Anatomy, Normal Histology and Ultrastructure, Embryology) in this chapter was originally written by Thomas H. Ermak and James H. Grendell for the 6th edition.

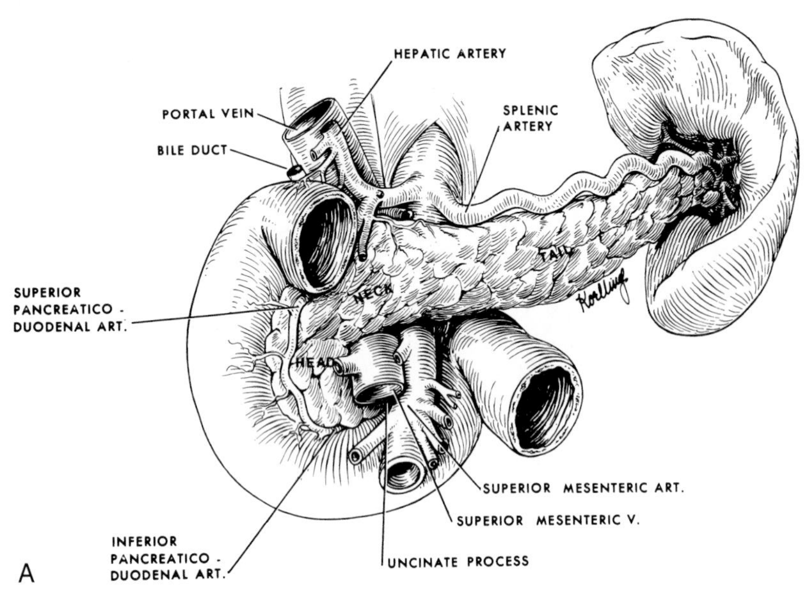

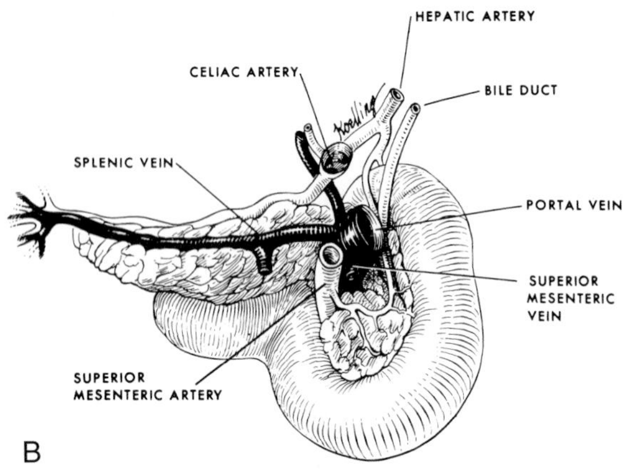

Figure 45–1. *A,* Diagrammatic representation of the anterior view of the pancreas. *B,* Diagrammatic representation of the posterior view of the pancreas.

The uncinate process is a prolongation of pancreatic tissue of variable size and shape. It projects off the lower part of the head of the pancreas. It extends upward and to the left. The uncinate process lies anterior to the aorta and inferior vena cava and is covered superiorly by the superior mesenteric vessels that emerge below the neck of the pancreas. There is much variation in the uncinate process and it may be absent altogether.

The neck of the pancreas is a constricted part of the gland extending from the head of the pancreas toward the left, joining the head with the body of the pancreas. It is 1.5 to 2.0 cm long and 3.0 to 4.0 cm wide. Posterior to the neck of the pancreas lies the confluence of the portal vein with the superior mesenteric and splenic veins. Anteriorly it is covered in part by the pylorus and peritoneum of the lesser sac. The neck extends to the right as far as the anterosuperior pancreaticoduodenal artery from the gastroduodenal artery.

The body of the pancreas runs toward the left side, anterior to the aorta. It is retroperitoneal and held against the aorta by the peritoneum of the lesser sac. The anterior surface of the body is covered by peritoneum of the omental bursa that separates the stomach from the pancreas. The antrum and body of the stomach and the transverse mesocolon contact the body anteriorly. Posterior to the body of the pancreas is the aorta, the origin of the superior mesenteric artery, the left crus of the diaphragm, the left kidney, the left adrenal gland, and the splenic vein. The midline part of the body overlies the lumbar spine, which makes this area of the pancreas most vulnerable to abdominal trauma.

The body passes laterally and merges with the tail of the pancreas without a discernible junction point. The tail is relatively mobile, with its tip usually reaching the hilus of the spleen. With the splenic artery and vein, it is contained between the two layers of the splenorenal ligament. The splenocolic ligament attaches the splenic flexure of the colon to the spleen and brings it near the tail of the pancreas. The relationship of the pancreas to important structures in the posterior abdomen is seen in Figure 45–2.

The distal end of the common bile duct, the duodenum, and the head of the pancreas form a unit. The common bile duct is located to the right of the gastroduodenal artery in the posterior wall of the duodenum. The bile duct passes through the substance of the pancreatic head, usually to join with the main pancreatic duct for some distance to reach the duodenal papilla (Fig. 45–3*A*).

The main pancreatic duct (of Wirsung) begins near the tail of the pancreas. It is formed from anastomosing ductules draining the lobules of the gland. It courses left to right and is enlarged by additional ducts. Through the tail and body the duct lies midway between the superior and inferior margins and slightly posterior. The main duct turns caudal and

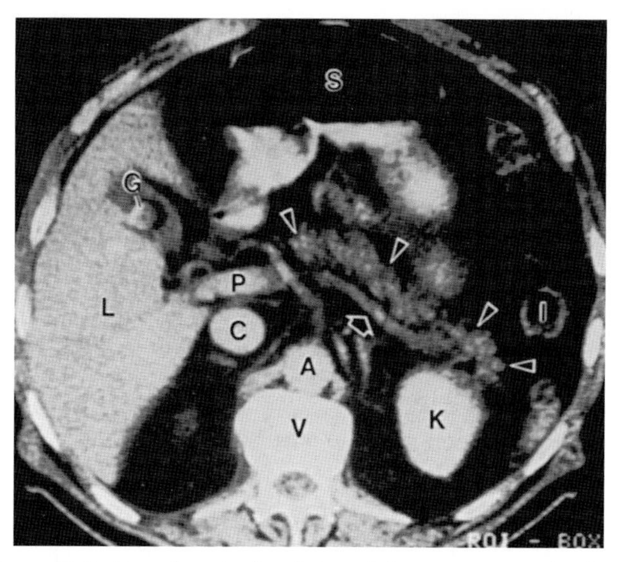

Figure 45–2. Normal anatomic relation of the pancreas to other intra-abdominal structures as shown by computed tomography. The borders of the pancreas are indicated by *arrowheads*. The splenic vein is indicated by an *arrow*. A, aorta; C, vena cava; G, incidental gallstone; I, small intestine; K, left kidney; L, liver; P, portal vein; S, stomach; V, vertebra. (Courtesy of M. P. Federle, MD.)

posterior on reaching the head of the pancreas. At the level of the major papilla, the duct turns horizontally to join usually with the common bile duct. This short common segment is the ampulla of the bile duct, which terminates in the duodenal papilla. The relationship of the common bile duct and the duct of Wirsung at the papilla is complex. The ducts may open separately at the ampulla and have an interposed septum or a common channel. A common channel for bile and pancreatic secretion ordinarily is formed by the absence of a septum between the biliary and pancreatic ducts as they approach the ampulla of Vater. In adults studied by endoscopic retrograde cholangiopancreatography (ERCP), the length of the common channel averages 4.5 mm, with a range of 1 to 12 mm.[7, 8] In various series, more than two thirds of patients had some degree of a common channel.[9–13] In a large autopsy series, 74% of patients had a common channel, 19% had separate openings, and 7% had an interposed septum.[9]

The accessory pancreatic duct of Santorini is frequently present and usually communicates with the main duct (see Fig. 45–3*A*). The accessory duct lies anterior to the bile duct and usually drains into the minor papilla, which lies proximal to the ampulla of Vater in the second duodenum. The accessory duct is patent in 70% of autopsy specimens. In about 10% of individuals there is no connection between the accessory duct and the main duct.[14] A number of variations in the two pancreatic ducts may be encountered.

The greatest diameter of the main pancreatic duct is in the head of the pancreas, and it gradually tapers, progressing to the tail of the pancreas. The main duct in the head of the pancreas ranges from 3.1 to 4.8 mm and tapers to 0.9 to 2.4 mm in the tail.[15] Specific normal limits of pancreatic duct diameter in the head (4 to 5 mm), body (3 to 4 mm) and tail (2 to 3 mm) are generally accepted. However, studies have shown an increase in pancreatic duct size with age and pancreatic disease.[16–18]

The pancreas has a rich circulation derived from branches of the celiac and superior mesenteric arteries.[18, 19] The head of the pancreas and surrounding duodenum are supplied by two pancreaticoduodenal arterial arcades. They are formed by the anterior and posterior superior arteries from the celiac artery that join a second pair of anterior and posterior inferior arteries from the superior mesenteric artery. At the neck, the dorsal pancreatic artery usually arises from the splenic artery. From this, a right branch supplies the head and usually joins the posterior arcade. It also gives off one or two left branches that pass through the body and tail of the pancreas, often making connections with branches of the splenic artery and distally with the splenic or the left gastroepiploic artery. All major arteries lie posterior to the ducts.

The gastroduodenal artery arises off the common hepatic branch of the celiac artery. It divides to form the anterior and posterior superior pancreaticoduodenal arteries. The anterior superior pancreaticoduodenal artery lies on the surface of the pancreas. It provides branches to the anterior surface of the duodenum, proximal jejunum, and pancreas. The artery enters the substance of the pancreas and, on the poster-

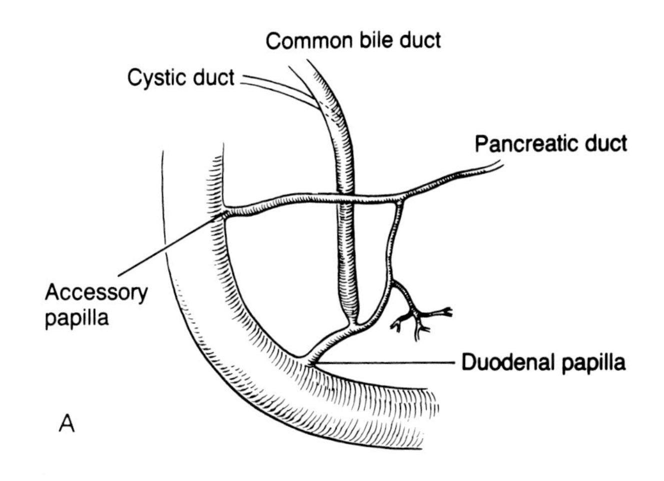

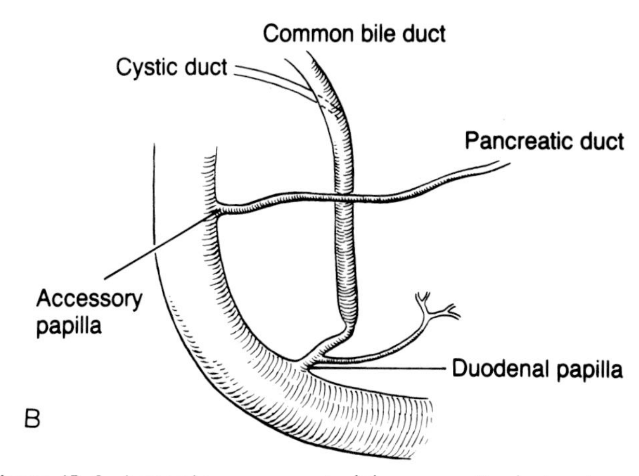

Figure 45–3. Anatomic arrangement of the pancreatic duct system. *A*, The most common arrangement. Most of the pancreatic secretion empties into the duodenum along with bile through the duodenal papilla. The proximal portion of the embryonic dorsal duct remains patent in about 70% of adults and empties through the accessory papilla. *B*, Pancreas divisum. The embryonic dorsal and ventral ducts fail to fuse. Most of the pancreatic secretion empties through the small accessory papilla. Only pancreatic secretions from the uncinate process and part of the head of the pancreas (which are derived from the embryonic ventral pancreas) drain through the duodenal papilla.

ior surface, it joins the anteroinferior pancreaticoduodenal artery from the superior mesenteric artery.

The anteroinferior pancreaticoduodenal artery arises from the superior mesenteric artery by the inferior margin of the pancreatic neck. The posteroinferior pancreaticoduodenal artery arises from the gastroduodenal artery. Its course is visible on the posterior surface of the pancreas, and branches may join with branches of the gastroduodenal artery or with a branch of the dorsal pancreatic artery. It passes posterior to the pancreatic portion of the bile duct.

The course of the splenic artery is posterior to the body and tail and loops above and below the superior margin of the pancreas. It gives off the dorsal pancreatic artery, which usually joins one of the posterior superior arcades after giving off the inferior pancreatic artery.

The caudal pancreatic artery arises from the left gastroepiploic artery or from a splenic branch at the spleen. It joins with branches of the splenic and great pancreatic arteries and other pancreatic arteries.

In general, the venous drainage of the pancreas is similar to the arterial blood supply. It flows into the portal venous system, which forms by the joining of the superior mesenteric and splenic veins at the confluence behind the neck of the pancreas. The portal vein lies behind the pancreas and in front of the inferior vena cava, with the common bile duct to the right and the hepatic artery to the left. The splenic vein originates at the hilum of the spleen and curves behind the tail of the pancreas and below the splenic artery, to the right along the posterior surface of the pancreas. The pancreatic veins drain the neck, body, and tail of the pancreas and join the splenic vein. The pancreaticoduodenal veins lie close to their corresponding arteries and empty into the splenic or portal veins. Because of the close anatomic relationship of the splenic vein with the pancreas, inflammatory or neoplastic diseases involving the body and tail can lead to splenic vein occlusion. This can result in retrograde venous drainage toward the splenic hilum and then, by way of flow through the short gastric and left gastroepiploic veins, create gastric varices.

The lymphatics, in general, drain the surface network of lymph toward regional nodes and are formed near the larger blood vessels.[20, 21] The superior lymphatic vessels run along the upper border of the pancreas closely with the splenic blood vessels. Those on the left side of the body and tail empty into nodes in the splenic hilum. Those on the right side of the body and the pancreatic neck empty into nodes near the upper border of the head. They also receive tributaries from the anterior and posterior pancreatic surfaces. The inferior lymphatic vessels run with the inferior pancreatic artery. Those that drain the lower left side of the body and tail drain toward nodes in the splenic hilum. The remaining regions of the neck and body drain toward the right.

The pancreatic head lymphatic vessel drainage is composed of an anterior and a posterior system. They generally occupy the grooves between the head of the pancreas and the duodenum, near the pancreaticoduodenal blood vessels. They each have a superior and inferior drainage system. In addition, a set of lymphatics also drains the upper portion of the head, lying on the superior border. The lymphatic drainage of the head of the pancreas and duodenum eventually flows into the celiac and superior mesenteric groups of pancreatic nodes and into the cisterna chyli. The lymphatics of the tail drain into splenic hilar nodes. The lymphatics of the body pass to the pancreaticosplenic nodes lying along the superior border, which drain into celiac nodes. Lymphatics of the upper head of the pancreas pass through subpyloric nodes. Inferiorly, lymphatics drain into retropancreatic and antepancreatic nodes, which then drain into superior mesenteric nodes.

The visceral efferent innervation of the pancreas is through the vagi and splanchnic nerves by way of the hepatic and celiac plexuses. The efferent fibers of the vagi pass through these plexuses without synapsing and terminate in parasympathetic ganglia found in the interlobular septa of the pancreas. The postganglionic fibers innervate acini, islets, and ducts. The bodies of the neurons of the sympathetic efferent nerves originate in the lateral gray matter of the thoracic and lumbar spinal cord. The bodies of the postganglionic sympathetic neurons are located in the great plexuses of the abdomen. Their postganglionic fibers innervate only blood vessels. The autonomic fibers, both efferent and afferent, are located in proximity to the blood vessels of the pancreas. Little is known about the distribution of the visceral efferent fibers in humans. They probably run through the splanchnic nerves to the sympathetic trunks and rami communicantes and through spinal nerves and ganglia. The vagi are thought to carry some visceral afferent fibers.

NORMAL HISTOLOGY AND ULTRASTRUCTURE

The pancreas is a compound, finely nodular gland that is grossly similar to but less compact than the salivary glands. It is surrounded by fine connective tissue but does not have a fibrous tissue capsule. The lobules are visible on gross examination and are connected by connective tissue septa that contain the blood vessels, nerves, lymphatics, and excretory ducts (constituting about 18% of this organ). The gland is a mixed exocrine (about 80%) and endocrine (about 2%) organ (Fig. 45–4). The endocrine portion consists of the islets of Langerhans, which are spherical clusters of light-staining cells scattered throughout the pancreas. The exocrine portion consists of numerous dark-staining acini composed of tubular and spherical masses of cells, which are the subunits of the lobule.[22, 23] Silicone casts of the duct lumen formed by retrograde injection indicate that the tubular portions of the acini are extensive and that the exocrine cells are arranged primarily as curved, branching tubules that anastomose and end blindly (Fig. 45–5).[24]

The lumen of the acinus is the origin of the secretory duct and contains centroacinar cells, which are unique to the pancreas. These cells are pale staining in histologic sections and smaller than the acinar cells. The lumen of the acinus leads into the intralobular ducts, which are covered by low columnar epithelial cells similar in appearance to the centroacinar cells. These ducts are nonstriated and anastomose to form the interlobular ducts, which are lined by a columnar epithelium (Fig. 45–6). Goblet cells and occasional argentaffin cells also are present. The interlobular ducts anastomose to become the main pancreatic duct. The larger ducts have a somewhat thick wall, consisting of connective tissue and elastic fibers (Fig. 45–6). Acinar, ductal, and islet cells can be distinguished by monoclonal antibodies specifically reactive with these cell types.[25–27]

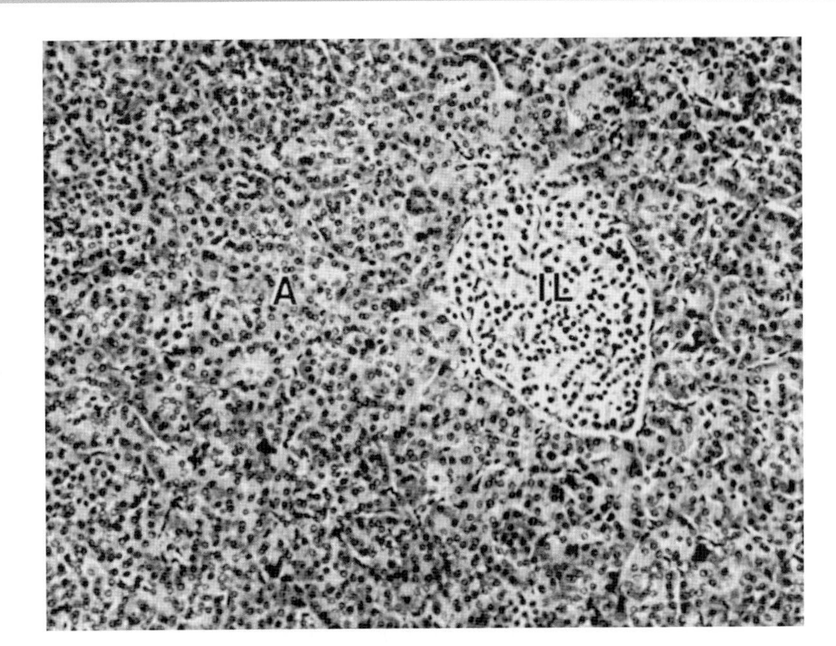

Figure 45–4. Histologic section of human pancreas obtained at autopsy shows dense-staining acinar cells (A) and a light-staining islet of Langerhans (IL). Formalin fixation, hematoxylin and eosin stain; magnification, ×140.

Acinar cells are tall, pyramidal or columnar epithelial cells, with their broad bases on a basal lamina and their apices converging on a central lumen (Fig. 45–7). In the resting state, numerous eosinophilic zymogen granules fill the apical portion of the cell. The basal portion of the cells contains one or two centrally located, spherical nuclei and extremely basophilic cytoplasm. The Golgi complex lies between the nucleus and zymogen granules and can be seen as a clear, nonstaining region (see Fig. 45–7).

The acinar cells undergo cyclic changes in morphology in response to feeding and digestion.[28, 29] After a large meal, the zymogen granule content of the cells is depleted. This apparently occurs by a decrease in both the size and the number of granules.[28] After depletion of the granules, the Golgi apparatus may be observed at the apex of the cell and appears more extensive than in the resting state. The reductions in size and in number of granules occur with a substantial increase in pancreatic enzyme secretion.

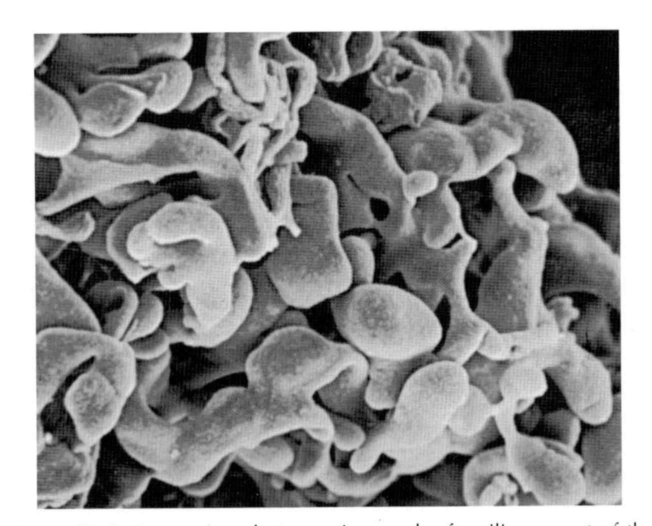

Figure 45–5. A scanning electron micrograph of a silicone cast of the acinar area of human pancreas after tissue is removed. The cast is formed by retrograde injection into the pancreatic duct and demonstrates the continuous, branching nature of the acinar pancreas. The diameter of the cast is greater than that of the original acinar lumen. Magnification, ×300. (From Bockman DE, Boydston WR, Parsa I: Architecture of human pancreas: Implications for early changes in pancreatic disease. Gastroenterology 85:55–61, 1983. Copyright 1983 by The American Gastroenterological Association.)

The subcellular structure of the acinar cells can be visualized at the electron microscopic level (Fig. 45–8). The acinar cell has several short, slender microvilli about 0.2 μm in length, which extend into the lumen of the acinus. The lumen typically contains flocculent electron-dense material, which presumably is the secreted digestive enzymes. Thin filaments form the axis of the microvilli as well as a network beneath the apical plasmalemma.[30] These microfilaments apparently play a structural role because their disruption causes expansion of the acinar lumen and loss of microvilli.[30] Adjacent cells are joined at the apical surface by electron-dense intercellular junctions. Tight junctions form a beltlike band around the apical end of the cell and are produced by the apposition of the external membrane leaflets of neighboring cells.[31] These junctions prevent the

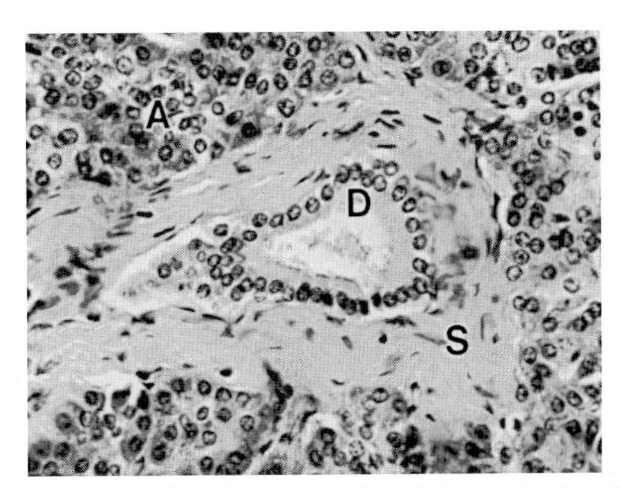

Figure 45–6. Histologic section of the interlobular duct (D) from the human pancreas showing columnar epithelium, connective tissue sheath (S), and surrounding acinar cells (A). Hematoxylin and eosin stain; magnification, ×300.

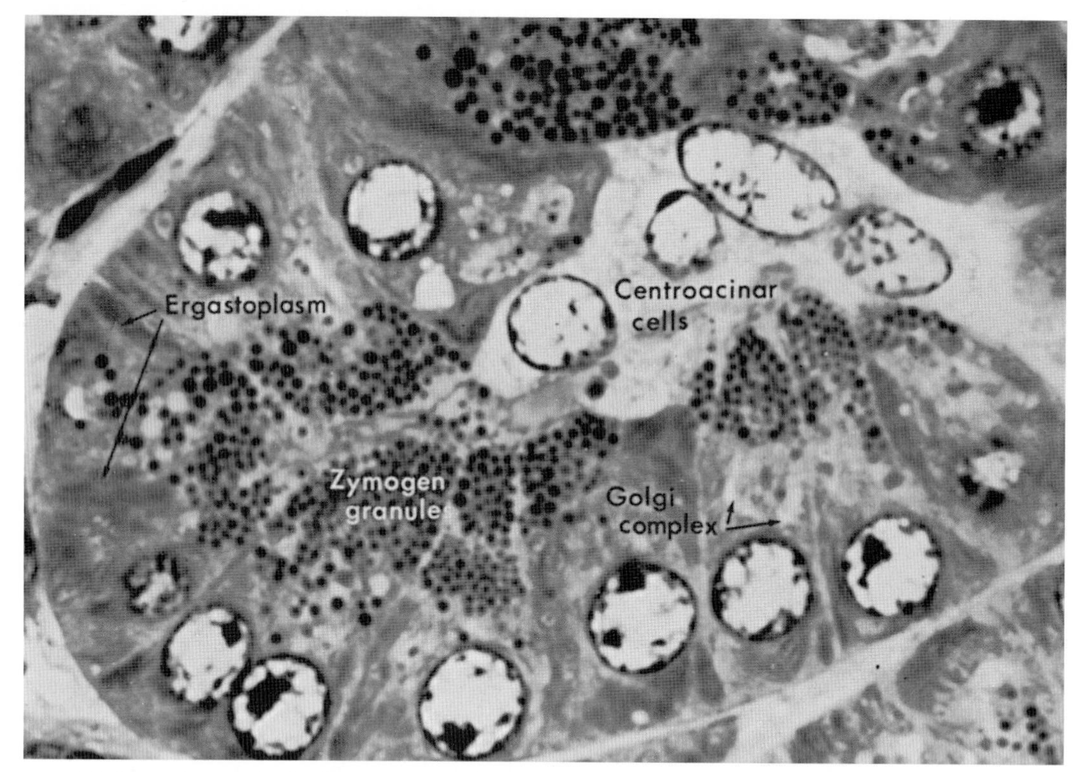

Figure 45–7. Photomicrograph of a human acinus, showing acinar and centroacinar cells. The acinar cell ergastoplasm, Golgi complex, and zymogen granules can be easily identified. Formalin stain, osmium fixation. Epon-embedded section, toluidine blue stain; magnification, ×3200. (From Bloom W, Fawcett DWA: Textbook of Histology, 11th ed. Philadelphia, WB Saunders, 1986. Courtesy of Susumu Ito, MD.)

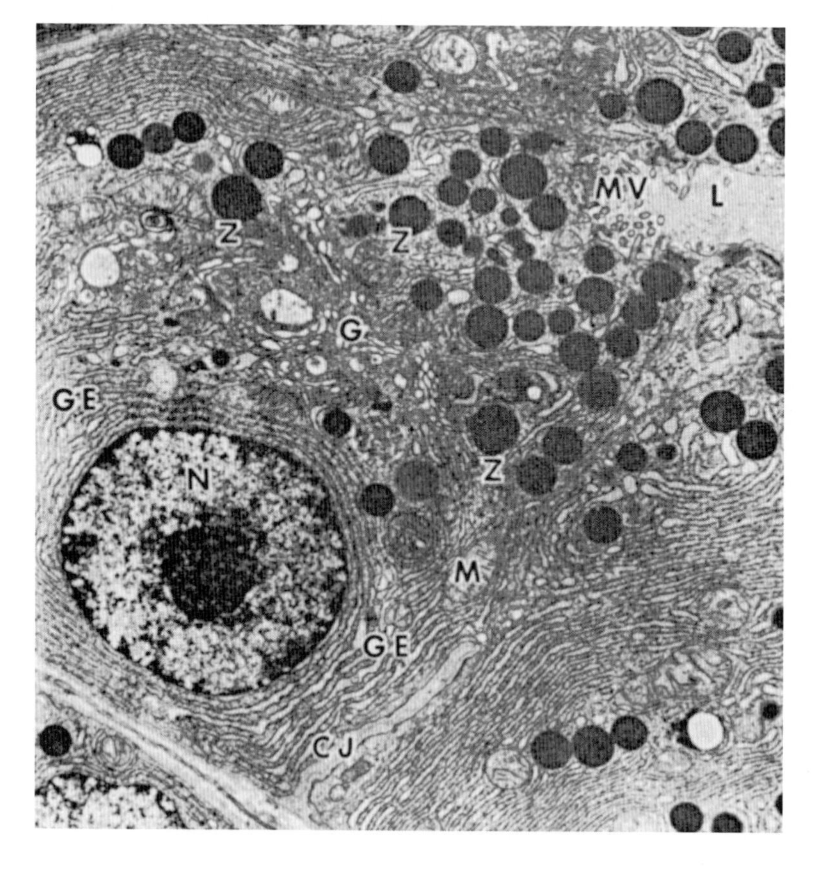

Figure 45–8. Electron micrograph of a human acinar cell. N, nucleus; GE, granular endoplasmic reticulum; G, Golgi complex; Z, zymogen granules; MV, microvilli; L, lumen of acinus; M, mitochondria; CJ, intercellular space. Magnification, ×15,000. (Courtesy of Susumu Ito, MD.)

reflux of secreted substances from the duct into the intercellular space. Gap junctions are distributed on the lateral cellular membranes and are formed by the apposition of larger, disk-shaped membrane plaques. They allow communication between cells. Below the junctions, the lateral cell borders are relatively straight and have a few, small interdigitations. Pancreatic lateral cell membranes display unique antigenic determinants that are not found on apical cell membranes.[32]

The nucleus usually is spherical, about 6 μm in diameter,[33] with one or more nucleoli in the interior and patches of dense heterochromatin along the inner nuclear membrane. Numerous conspicuous nuclear pores are located at regions where the lightly stained euchromatin makes contact with the nuclear membrane. These pores presumably are the sites where messenger and transfer RNAs are transported out of the nucleus into the cytoplasm. Binucleate cells also are seen occasionally.

Mitochondria are elongate, cylindrical structures that may appear oval in cross-section and may contain well-developed cristae and many matrix granules. They occur throughout the cytoplasm, among the granular endoplasmic reticulum or zymogen granules, and adjacent to the basolateral cell border. The cytoplasmic matrix occupies about 45% of the cell volume.[34]

Granular endoplasmic reticulum (see Fig. 45–8) occupies about 20% of the cell volume[34, 35] and fills most of the basal region of the acinar cells, although small amounts also occur in the apical region adjacent to and among the zymogen granules. It is composed of numerous parallel cisternal membranes covered with closely spaced attached ribosomes, giving the structures a granular appearance. On the basis of studies with laboratory animals, the ribosomes of the granular endoplasmic reticulum have been found to be the site of protein synthesis.[36, 37]

The Golgi complex (see Fig. 45–8) is located between the nucleus and the mass of zymogen granules present in the resting gland. It consists of flattened, membranous saccules, as well as small vesicles or vacuoles that contain flocculent electron-dense material. The Golgi saccules have been distinguished from other intracellular vesicles by enzyme cytochemistry and by immunohistochemistry using antienzyme and antireceptor antibodies.[38] The Golgi complex is believed to play an important role in the transport of secretory proteins and the formation of zymogen granules. The mechanisms by which these processes occur are still unresolved.

The secretory granules of the pancreas usually are divided into two types: electron-lucent condensing vacuoles and electron-dense zymogen granules. The condensing vacuoles typically are seen in the vicinity of the Golgi complex and, on the basis of autoradiographic data,[36, 37] are believed to be precursors of the zymogen granules. They are membrane-bound vesicles slightly larger than zymogen granules and much less numerous, occupying only about 2% of the cytoplasm.[35] Zymogen granules (see Fig. 45–8) also are spherical, membrane-bound vesicles, slightly under 1 μm in diameter,[28, 39, 40] filled with electron-dense material, which apparently represents the digestive enzymes.

Studies of the chemical composition of the zymogen granules have shown that they contain about 12 to 15 different digestive enzymes, which make up about 90% of the granule protein.[41–44] Each granule apparently contains the entire complement of secreted digestive enzymes because labeled antibodies to several different enzymes have been located over single zymogen granules from different cells.[45, 46] Individual zymogen granules can differ markedly in the concentration of specific digestive enzymes contained within the granules.[47] The digestive enzymes within the granules apparently are not in solution or suspension but in a solid state array, which exhibits specific binding between the enzymes themselves and between the enzymes and the granule membrane.[48–51] Isolated zymogen granules are stable at slightly acid pH; at alkaline pH, they release their enzymes into solution.[49, 51, 52] This behavior may account for the solubilization of digestive enzymes within the alkaline duct lumen.

Along the basal surface of the acinar cells, but not extending between adjacent cells, is a thin basal lamina, below which are collagen fibers and a rich capillary network. Efferent nerve fibers, derived from the sympathetic and parasympathetic systems, penetrate the basal lamina and terminate adjacent to the acinar cells.

The centroacinar cells (Fig. 45–9) and duct cells have electron-lucent cytoplasm containing few cytoplasmic organelles or specializations. They typically contain free ribosomes and small, round mitochondria. They contain virtually no granular endoplasmic reticulum and, therefore, are not active in protein synthesis for secretion. Farther down the ducts, the cells contain more mitochondria, but they are never associated with invaginations of the basolateral surface, as occurs in the transporting ductal epithelium of the salivary glands. Both centroacinar and duct cells apparently secrete bicarbonate and water. Carbonic anhydrase, the enzyme responsible for formation of bicarbonate, has been demonstrated in the epithelium.[23]

The islets of Langerhans number about 1 million in the human pancreas and consist of anastomosing cords of polygonal endocrine cells (see Fig. 45–4). Each islet is about 0.2 mm in diameter, much larger than an acinus, and separated from the surrounding exocrine tissue by fine connective tissue fibers, which are continuous with those of the exocrine gland.

Each islet is surrounded and penetrated by a rich network of capillaries lined by a fenestrated endothelium. The capillaries are arranged in a portal system that conveys blood from the islets to acinar cells (Fig. 45–10).[53–57] This insula-acinar portal system consists of afferent arterioles that enter the islet, form a capillary glomerulus, and leave the islet as efferent capillaries passing into the exocrine tissue. A parallel arterial system supplies blood directly to the exocrine pancreas (Fig. 45–10), and yet this portal system permits the local action of islet hormones, especially insulin, on the exocrine pancreas.[55–57] Acinar cells surrounding islets of Langerhans, termed peri-insular acini, are morphologically and biochemically different from acini situated further away (tele-insular acini).[58, 59] Peri-insular acini have larger cells, nuclei, and zymogen granule regions[58] and different ratios of specific digestive enzymes.[59]

Although the acinar cell secretes several different digestive enzymes in the exocrine pancreas, each cell type in the endocrine pancreas appears to secrete a single hormone. Four major types of cells are found: B cells, A cells, D cells, and PP cells.[60, 61] B cells, the most numerous (50% to 80%) secrete insulin.[60] A cells (5% to 20%) secrete glucagon. PP cells (10% to 35%) secrete pancreatic polypeptide.

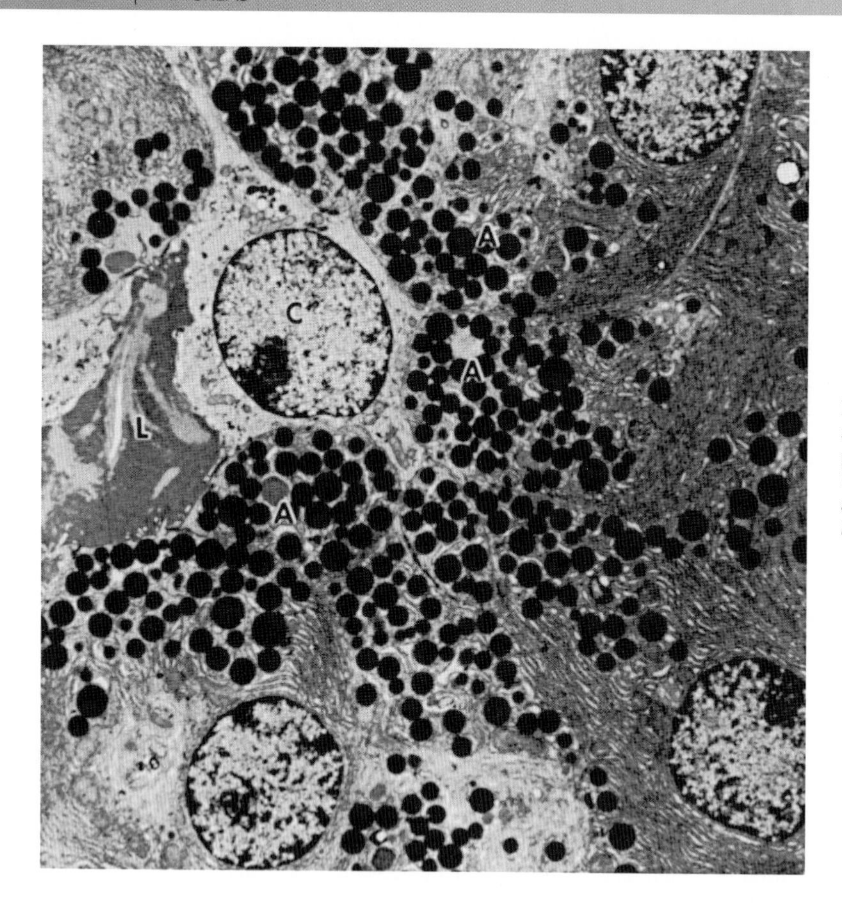

Figure 45–9. Electron micrograph of a centroacinar cell (C) and several acinar cells (A). Note the electron-lucid cytoplasm, scattered mitochondria, and lack of other membranous organelles in the centroacinar cell. L, lumen of the acinus. Magnification, ×9000. (Courtesy of Susumu Ito, MD.)

D cells (5%) secrete somatostatin. Other rare cell types occur in the islet.[62] In humans, the islets are subdivided into units, each of which exhibits a central aggregation of B cells surrounded by varying numbers of peripherally located cells that secrete the other endocrine hormones.

EMBRYOLOGY

The pancreas first appears in embryos of about 4 mm in the fourth week of gestation.[63, 64] The outpouchings from the endodermal lining of the duodenum develop at this time: the ventral pancreas and the dorsal pancreas (Fig. 45–11*A*). The dorsal anlage grows more rapidly, and by the sixth week, it is an elongated nodular structure extending into the

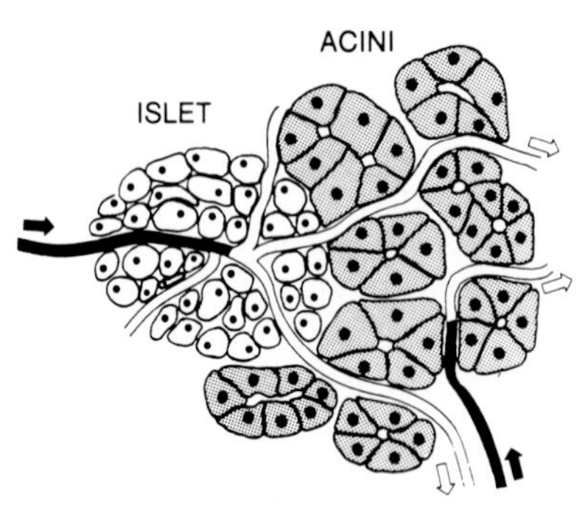

Figure 45–10. Schematic diagram of the insuloacinar portal system illustrating the dual blood supply to the exocrine pancreas. (From Goldfine ID, Williams JA: Receptors for insulin and CCK in the acinar pancreas: Relationship to hormone action. Int Rev Cytol 85:1, 1983.)

dorsal mesentery, within which its growth continues (Fig. 45–11*B*). The ventral pancreas remains smaller and is carried away from the duodenum by its connection with the common bile duct. The two primordia are brought into apposition by uneven growth of the duodenum, and they fuse by the seventh week (Fig. 45–11*C*). The tail, body, and part of the head of the pancreas are formed by the dorsal component; the remainder of the head and the uncinate process derive from the ventral pancreas. These primitive relations are still distinguishable in the adult pancreas.[64]

Both of the primitive pancreata contain an axial duct. The dorsal duct arises directly from the duodenal wall, and the ventral duct arises from the common bile duct. On fusion of the ventral and dorsal components, the ventral duct anastomoses with the dorsal one, forming the main pancreatic duct (Fig. 45–11*D*). The proximal end of the dorsal duct becomes the accessory duct of Santorini in the adult and is patent in 70% of specimens.[65] The common outlet of the bile duct and pancreatic duct observed in most adults is the result of the common origin of the bile duct and the ventral pancreas.

The pancreatic acini appear in the third month of gestation as derivatives of the side ducts and termini of the primitive ducts. The acini remain connected to the larger pancreatic ducts by small secretory ductules. The primitive pancreas is composed of relatively undifferentiated epithelial cells, similar in morphology to duct cells. Mesenchymal tissue in which the gland grows provides the thin connective tissue capsule and divides the gland into lobes and lobules.

Distinct differences in morphology, enzyme content, and secretory capacity exist between the embryonic and the adult

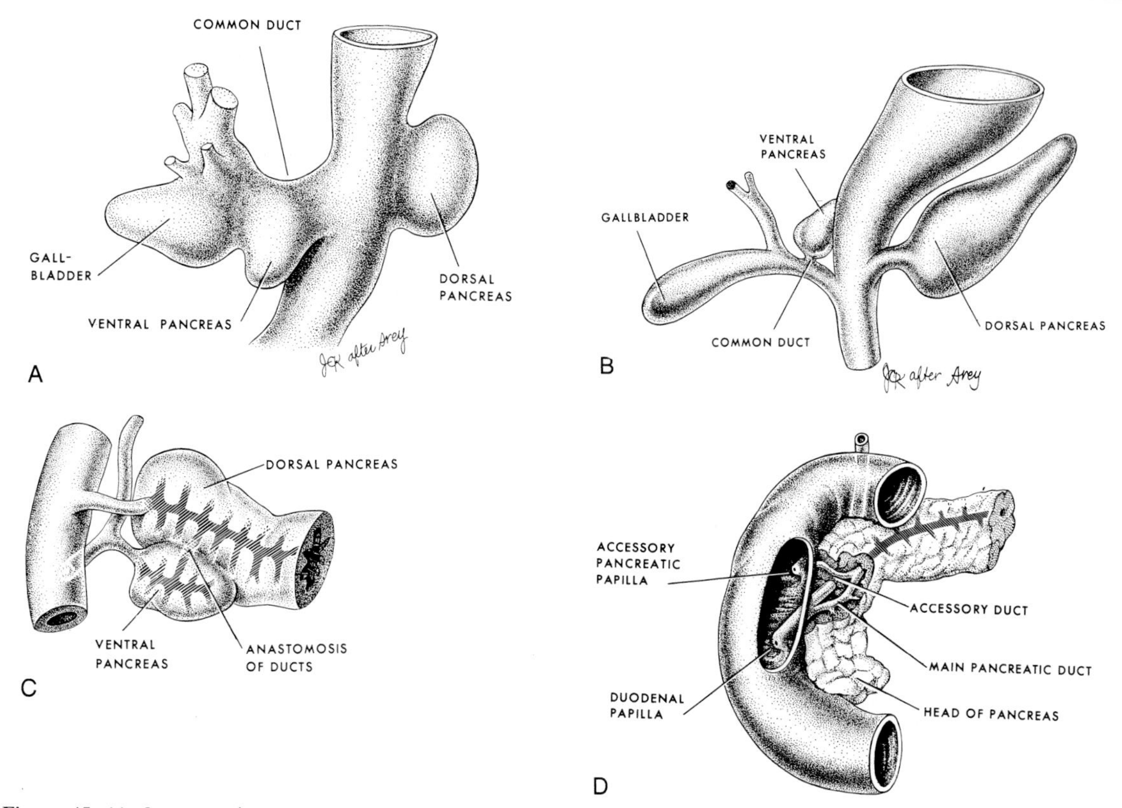

Figure 45–11. Stages in the embryonic development of the pancreas. *A*, At about 4 weeks' gestation, dorsal and ventral buds are formed from the duodenum. *B*, At 6 weeks, the ventral pancreas extends toward the larger dorsal pancreas. *C*, By about 7 weeks, fusion of dorsal and ventral pancreas has occurred and ductular anastomosis is beginning. *D*, At birth, the pancreas is a single organ, and ductular anastomosis is complete. (Modified from Arey LB: Developmental Anatomy: A Textbook and Laboratory Manual of Embryology, 7th ed. Philadelphia, WB Saunders, 1974.)

pancreas.[66–72] Early in development, the pancreas has no zymogen granules and little granular endoplasmic reticulum.[66–70] In humans, the pancreas is composed of undifferentiated epithelial cells at 9 weeks of gestation.[66] During subsequent cell differentiation, the specific activity of the digestive enzymes increases some thousandfold,[71, 72] and the granules increase in size and come to occupy most of the cytoplasm of the cells, including the basolateral regions.[67–70] At 12 weeks in humans, zymogen granules are first seen by electron microscopy. The cells also contain a Golgi complex and granular endoplasmic reticulum in relatively small amounts. By 20 weeks, larger zymogen granules typical of the adult are seen.[66] Each digestive enzyme has a characteristic rate of accumulation and increases in concentration at different times.[71, 72] At birth, the granules in laboratory animals are the largest normally found in the pancreas, being about six times the volume of the granules in adults.[73, 74] At about this time, the capacity for stimulated secretion is attained. Differentiation of the pancreas continues beyond birth with regard to the size of the zymogen granules as well as the enzyme content of the tissue.[75, 76]

The endocrine pancreas differentiates on roughly the same time course as the exocrine portion,[77, 78] and the appearance of islet hormones also precedes the appearance of secretion granules in the cells. In humans, endocrine cells are first observed singly or in small clusters along the basolateral portion of undifferentiated acinar cells (9 to 10 weeks), but by 12 to 16 weeks, distinct islets in various stages of complexity can be observed. The development of islets in the PP-rich regions lags slightly behind that of the glucagon-rich regions.[79] Insulin cells increase continuously with age, whereas glucagon cells increase during fetal life and then decrease in infants and adults. The number of somatostatin cells is elevated in fetal and infant stages, whereas pancreatic polypeptide cells are the least abundant cells during these stages.[79]

DEVELOPMENTAL ANOMALIES

Annular Pancreas

Annular pancreas is a band of pancreatic tissue encircling the second part of the duodenum and is of ventral pancreas origin.[80] Its incidence has been calculated at about 1:20,000.[81] Annular pancreas has a bimodal presentation, with peaks in neonates and in adults in the fourth and fifth decades. This entity is a common anomaly obstructing the duodenum in infancy and usually involves growth of pancreatic tissue into the wall of the duodenum. The annulus is usually proximal to the ampulla, involving the second part of the duodenum.[82] Other congenital anomalies may be associated, including trisomy 21, duodenal atresia, tracheoesophageal fistula, or cardiorenal abnormalities.[80, 81] The treatment of neonates is by surgical bypass with attention to other possible congenital anomalies. In some cases, symptoms of annular pancreas may appear for the first time in the adult. Adult presentations include duodenal stenosis, peptic ulceration, chronic pancreatitis, or as an incidental finding.[83] The most common symptom in adults is upper abdominal pain. Biliary obstruction is a rare complication. Because pancreatic tissue often extends into the duodenal wall and because the annular tissue may contain a large pancreatic duct, symptomatic cases are best treated by surgical bypass rather than by surgical resection.[82]

Pancreas Divisum

Pancreas divisum results from a failure of the ducts of the embryologic dorsal and ventral pancreata to fuse (see Fig. 45–3*B*). This leads to a situation in which most of the pancreatic exocrine secretion drains through the relatively small duct of Santorini and minor papilla, with only a small part of the pancreas emptying through the duct of Wirsung through the larger main ampulla of Vater. Normally, most pancreatic drainage is through the duct of Wirsung, and drainage through the duct of Santorini is relatively small.

Pancreas divisum has been observed in 5% to 10% of autopsy series[65, 84, 85] and in about 2% to 7% of patients undergoing ERP.[86–88] The incidence increased to 25% in one series in patients with idiopathic pancreatitis.[88] Whether pancreas divisum represents an anatomic variant of no pathologic significance or a congenital anomaly responsible for recurrent acute pancreatitis in some patients is controversial. Most patients with pancreas divisum are asymptomatic. It has been proposed that both pancreas divisum and a relatively stenotic accessory papilla must be present for clinically evident pancreatic disease to occur. Pancreas divisum is usually diagnosed by ERP (Fig. 45–12), although reports suggest that noninvasive techniques such as endoscopic ultrasound[89] and magnetic resonance cholangiopancreatography (MRCP) may be useful for diagnosis.[90]

Most series show that therapeutic interventions, either by endoscopic sphincterotomy with placement of stents through the accessory papilla[91–93] or surgical sphincteroplasty of the accessory papilla,[94, 95] show clinical benefit to patients with recurrent idiopathic pancreatitis with accessory papilla stenosis and pancreas divisum. There appears to be little beneficial effect of operative or endoscopic interventions in patients with pancreas divisum and chronic unexplained abdominal pain who do not have definable episodes of recurrent acute pancreatitis.

Ectopic Pancreatic Tissue

Ectopic pancreatic tissue and accessory pancreata are common and occur at diverse areas of the gastrointestinal tract. The frequency of ectopic pancreatic tissue has been reported from autopsy material to range from 0.55% to 13.7%.[96] The most common sites are the stomach, duodenum, proximal jejunum, and ileum. Less common sites include the umbilicus, common bile duct, gallbladder, Meckel's diverticulum, and hilus of the spleen, as well as perigastric and paraduodenal locations. Most ectopic pancreatic tissue is functional. Ectopic pancreatic tissue is usually an asymptomatic condition that is an incidental finding at endoscopy, surgery, or autopsy.

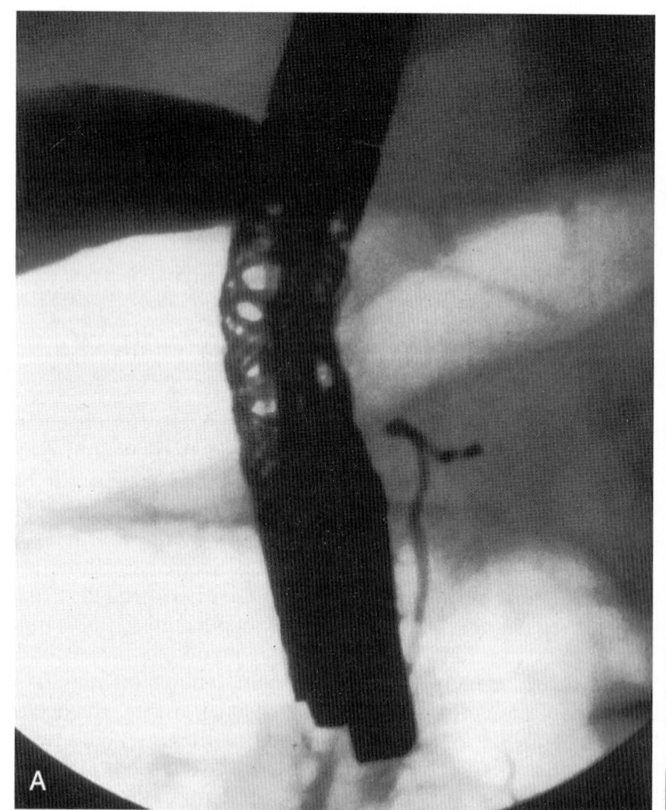

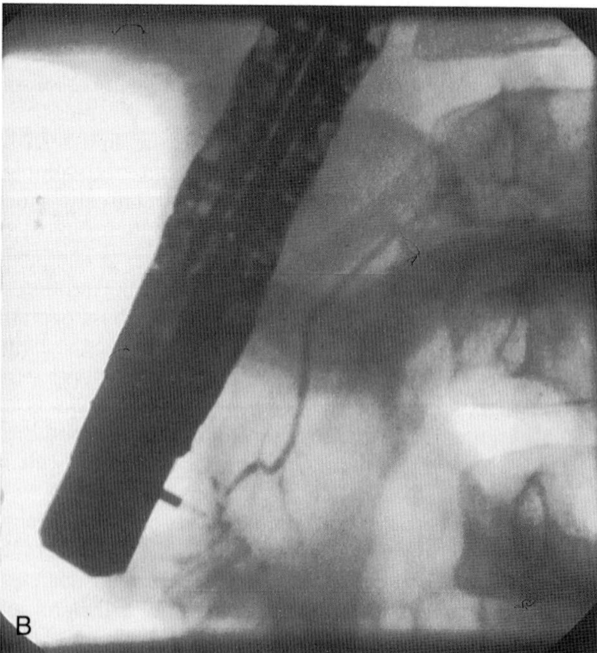

Figure 45–12. Endoscopic retrograde pancreatography in pancreas divisum. *A*, The major papilla has been cannulated. The duct terminates without communicating with the main pancreatic duct. *B*, The minor papilla has been cannulated, and the main pancreatic duct is filled. (Courtesy of Markus Goldschmiedt, MD.)

Pancreatic Agenesis

Pancreatic agenesis occurs only rarely, either in association with other anomalies or as an apparently isolated anomaly, and is associated with intrauterine growth retardation.[97, 98] Most infants affected with this condition have died soon after birth. In addition, isolated agenesis of the dorsal or, less commonly, the ventral pancreas can occur. In this situation some normal pancreatic tissue may still be formed. Pancreatic hypoplasia also has been recognized. Although the larger ducts and islands are normal, there is a reduction in the number of smaller ducts and a lack of differentiation in the terminal duct system.[99]

Congenital Cysts

Congenital cysts of the pancreas are rare and are distinguished from pseudocysts by the presence of an epithelial lining. It is believed that these cysts are caused by anomalous development of the pancreatic ductal system in which sequestered segments of a primitive ductal system give rise to microscopic or macroscopic cystic lesions.[100] Congenital cysts of the pancreas may be seen in the fetus, infant, child, or adult. Solitary congenital cysts are rare. In the pediatric cases reviewed, the majority presented before the age of 2 years, and associated anomalies were found in 30% of the cases.[101] Clinical presentations can include an asymptomatic mass, abdominal distention, vomiting, and jaundice from biliary obstruction. Symptomatic pancreatic cysts should be surgically removed whenever possible.

REFERENCES

1. Clarke ES: History of Gastroenterology. In Paulson M (ed): Gastroenterologic Medicine. Philadelphia, Lea & Febiger, 1969.
2. Major RH: A History of Medicine. Springfield, IL, Charles C Thomas, 1954.
3. Heidenhain R: Beitrage zur Kenntnis des Pankreas. Pflugers Arch 10: 557, 1875.
4. Basmajian JV: Grant's Method of Anatomy, 10th ed. Baltimore, Williams & Wilkins, 1980.
5. Clemente CD (ed): Gray's Anatomy of the Human Body, 30th ed. Philadelphia, Lea & Febiger, 1985.
6. Rottenberg N: Macroscopic and microscopic vasculature of the duodenal-biliary-pancreatic complex. Morphol Embryol 35:15, 1989.
7. Kimura K, Ohto M, Saisho H, et al: Association of gallbladder carcinoma and anomalous pancreaticobiliary ductal union. Gastroenterology 89:1258, 1985.
8. Misra SP, Gulati P, Thorat VK, et al: Pancreaticobiliary ductal union in biliary disease: An endoscopic retrograde cholangiopancreatography study. Gastroenterology 96:907, 1989.
9. Dimagno EP, Shorter RG, Taylor WF, Go VL: Relationships between pancreaticobiliary ductal anatomy and pancreatic ductal and parenchymal histology. Cancer 49:361, 1982.
10. Dowdy GS Jr, Waldron GW, Brown WG: Surgical anatomy of the pancreatobiliary ductal system. Arch Surg 84:229, 1962.
11. Newman HF, Weinberg SB, Newman EB, Northrop JD: The papilla of Vater and distal portions of the common bile duct and duct of Wirsung. Surg Gynecol Obstet 106:687, 1958.
12. Stamm BH: Incidence and diagnostic significance of minor pathologic changes in the adult pancreas at autopsy: A systematic study of 112 autopsies in patients without known pancreatic disease. Hum Pathol 15:677, 1984.
13. Sterling JA: The common channel for bile and pancreatic ducts. Surg Gynecol Obstet 98:420, 1954.
14. Kleitsch WP: Anatomy of the pancreas. A study with special reference to the duct system. Arch Surg 71:795, 1955.
15. Skandalakis LJ, Rowe JS Jr, Gray SW, Skandalakis JE: Surgical embryology and anatomy of the pancreas. Surg Clin North Am 73: 661, 1993.
16. Hastier P, Buckley MJ, Dumas R, et al: A study of the effect of age on pancreatic duct morphology. Gastrointest Endosc 48:53, 1998.
17. Kreel L, Sandin B: Changes in pancreatic morphology associated with aging. Gut 14:962, 1973.
18. Ladas SD, Tassios PS, Giorgiotis K, et al: Pancreatic duct width: Its significance as a diagnostic criterion for pancreatic disease. Hepatogastroenterology 40:52, 1993.
19. Rottenberg N: Macroscopic and microscopic vasculature of the duodenal-biliary-pancreatic complex. Morphol Embryol 35:15, 1989.
20. O'Morchoe CCC: Lymphatic system of the pancreas. Microsc Res Tech 37:456, 1997.
21. Evans BP, Ochsner A: The gross anatomy of the lymphatics of the human pancreas. Surgery 36:177, 1954.
22. Bloom W, Fawcett DW: A Textbook of Histology, 11th ed. Philadelphia, WB Saunders, 1986.
23. Tompkins RK, Traverso LW: The exocrine cells. In Keynes WM, Keith RG (eds): The Pancreas. New York, Appleton-Century-Crofts, 1981, p 23.
24. Bockman DE, Boydston WR, Parsa I: Architecture of human pancreas: Implications for early changes in pancreatic disease. Gastroenterology 85:55, 1983.
25. Shibata K, Kobayashi T, Matsuura N, et al: Production of three monoclonal antibodies specifically reactive respectively with the ductal, acinar, and islet cells of the human pancreas. Jpn J Clin Oncol 21:13, 1991.
26. Itzkowitz S, Kjeldsen T, Friera A, et al: Expression of Tn, sialosyl Tn, and T antigens in human pancreas. Gastroenterology 100:1691, 1991.
27. Soon-Shiong P, Tersaki PI, Lanza RP: Immunocytochemical identification of monoclonal antibodies with binding activity to acinar cells but not islets. Pancreas 6:318, 1991.
28. Ermak TH, Rothman SS: Zymogen granules of pancreas decrease in size in response to feeding. Cell Tissue Res 214:51, 1981.
29. Uchiyama Y, Saito K: A morphometric study of 24-hour variations in subcellular structures of the rat pancreatic acinar cell. Cell Tissue Res 226:609, 1982.
30. Bauduin H, Stock C, Vincent D, Grenier JF: Microfilamentous system and secretion of enzyme in the exocrine pancreas. Effect of cytochalasin B. J Cell Biol 66:165, 1975.
31. Metz J, Forssman WG, Ito S: Exocrine pancreas under experimental conditions. III. Membrane and cell junctions in isolated acinar cells. Cell Tissue Res 177:459, 1977.
32. De Lisle RC, Logsdon CD, Hootman SR, Williams JA: Monoclonal antibodies as probes for plasma membrane domains in the exocrine pancreas. J Histochem Cytochem 36:1043, 1988.
33. Nevalainen TJ: Effects of pilocarpine stimulation on rat pancreatic acinar cells. An electron microscopic study with morphometric analysis. Acta Pathol Microbiol Scand(Suppl)210:1, 1970.
34. Bolender RP: Stereological analysis of the guinea pig pancreas. I. Analytical model and quantitative description of nonstimulated pancreatic acinar cells. J Cell Biol 61:269, 1974.
35. Amsterdam A, Jamieson JD: Studies on dispersed pancreatic exocrine cells. I. Dissociation technique and morphologic characteristics of separated cells. J Cell Biol 63:1037, 1974.
36. Palade GE: Intracellular aspects of the process of protein synthesis. Science 189:347, 1975.
37. Jamieson JD, Palade GE: Production of secretory proteins in animal cells. In Brinkley BR, Porter KR (eds): International Cell Biology 1976–1977. New York, Rockefeller University Press, 1977.
38. Hogue-Angeletti R, Xu R-Y, Gonatas JO, et al: Identification of a novel protein (G210) specific to the Golgi apparatus. J Histochem Cytochem 37:1177, 1989.
39. Liebow C, Rothman SS: Distribution of zymogen granule size. Am J Physiol 225:258, 1973.
40. Nadelhaft I: Measurement of the size distribution of zymogen granules from rat pancreas. Biophys J 13:1014, 1973.
41. Greene LJ, Hirs CHW, Palade, GE: On the protein composition of bovine pancreatic zymogen granules. J Biol Chem 238:2054, 1963.
42. Keller PJ, Cohen E: Enzymic composition of some cell fractions of bovine pancreas. J Biol Chem 236:1407, 1961.
43. Tartakoff A, Greene LJ, Palade GE: Studies on the guinea pig pancreas. Fractionation and partial characteristics of exocrine proteins. J Biol Chem 249:7420, 1974.

44. Scheele G, Bartelt D, Bieger W: Characterization of human exocrine proteins by two-dimensional isoelectric focusing/sodium dodecyl sulfate gel electrophoresis. Gastroenterology 80:461, 1981.
45. Kraehenbuhl JP, Racine L, Jamieson JD: Immunocytochemical localization of secretory proteins in bovine pancreatic exocrine cells. J Cell Biol 72:406, 1977.
46. Geuze JJ, Slot JW, Tokuyasu KT: Immunocytochemical localization of amylase and chymotrypsinogen in the exocrine pancreatic cell, with special attention to the Golgi complex. J Cell Biol 82:697, 1979.
47. Mroz EA, Lechene, C: Pancreatic zymogen granules differ markedly in protein composition. Science 232:871, 1986.
48. Burwen SJ, Rothman SS: Zymogen granules: Osmotic properties, interaction with ions, and some structural implications. Am J Physiol 222:1177, 1972.
49. Rothman SS: The behavior of isolated zymogen granules: pH-dependent release and reassociation of protein. Biochim Biophys Acta 241: 567, 1971.
50. Rothman SS: Association of bovine alpha-chymotrypsinogen and trypsinogen with rat zymogen granules. Am J Physiol 222:1299, 1972.
51. Ermak TH, Rothman SS: Internal organization of the zymogen granule: Formation of reticular structures in vitro. J Ultrastruct Res 64:98, 1978.
52. Hokin LE: Isolation of zymogen granules of dog pancreas and a study of their properties. Biochim Biophys Acta 18:379, 1955.
53. Fujita T: Insulo-acinar portal system in the horse pancreas. Arch Histol Jpn 35:161, 1973.
54. Fujita T, Murakami T: Microcirculation of monkey pancreas with special reference to the insulo-acinar portal system. A scanning electron microscope study of vascular casts. Arch Histol Jpn 35:255, 1973.
55. Bonner-Weir S, Orci L: New perspectives on the microvasculature of the islets of Langerhans in the rat. Diabetes 31:883, 1982.
56. Williams JA, Goldfine ID: The insulin-pancreatic acinar axis. Diabetes 34:980, 1985.
57. Lifson N, Kramlinger KG, Mayrand RR, Lender EJ: Blood flow to the rabbit pancreas with special reference to the islets of Langerhans. Gastroenterology 79:466, 1980.
58. Kramer MF, Tan HT: The peri-insular acini of the pancreas of the rat. Z Zellforsch 86:163, 1968.
59. Malaisse-Lagae F, Ravazzola M, Robbercht P, et al: Exocrine pancreas: Evidence for topographic partition of secretory function. Science 190:795, 1975.
60. Stefan Y, Orci L, Malaisse-Lagae F, et al: Quantitation of endocrine cell content in the pancreas of nondiabetic and diabetic humans. Diabetes 31:694, 1982.
61. Orci L: Macro- and micro-domains in the endocrine pancreas. Diabetes 31:538, 1982.
62. Boquist L: The endocrine cells. In Keynes WM, Keith RG (eds): The Pancreas. New York, Appleton-Century-Crofts, 1981, p 31.
63. Arey LB: Developmental Anatomy. A Textbook and Laboratory Manual of Embryology, 7th ed. Philadelphia, WB. Saunders, 1974.
64. Patten BM: Human Embryology, 3rd ed. New York, McGraw-Hill, 1968.
65. Kleitsch WP: Anatomy of the pancreas. A study with special reference to the duct system. Arch Surg 71:795, 1955.
66. Laitio M, Lev R, Orlic D: The developing human fetal pancreas: An ultrastructural and histochemical study with special reference to exocrine cells. J Anat 117:619, 1974.
67. Parsa I, Marsh WH, Fitzgerald PJ: Pancreas acinar cell differentiation: I. Morphologic and enzymatic comparisons of embryonic rat pancreas and pancreatic anlage grown in organ culture. Am J Pathol 57:457, 1969.
68. Pictet RL, Clark WR, Williams RH, Rutter WJ: An ultrastructural analysis of the developing embryonic pancreas. Dev Biol 29:436, 1972.
69. Ermak TH, Rothman SS: Increase in zymogen granule volume accounts for increase in volume density during prenatal development of pancreas. Anat Rec 207:487, 1983.
70. Uchiyama Y, Watanabe M: A morphometric study of developing pancreatic acinar cells of rats during prenatal life. Cell Tissue Res 237: 117, 1984.
71. Rutter WJ, Kemp JD, Bradshaw WS et al: Regulation of specific protein synthesis in cytodifferentiation. J Cell Physiol 72(Suppl 1):1, 1968.
72. Sanders TG, Rutter WJ: The developmental regulation of amylolytic and proteolytic enzymes in the embryonic rat pancreas. J Biol Chem 249:3500, 1974.
73. Ermak TH, Rothman SS: Large decrease in zymogen granule size in the postnatal rat pancreas. J Ultrastruct Res 70:242, 1980.
74. Uchiyama Y, Watanabe M: Morphonometric and fine structural studies of rat pancreatic acinar cells during early postnatal life. Cell Tissue Res 237:123, 1984.
75. Descholdt-Lanckman M, Robberecht P, Camus J, et al: Hormonal and dietary adaptation of rat pancreatic hydrolases before and after weaning. Am J Physiol 226:39, 1974.
76. Robberecht P, Descholdt-Lanckman M, Camus J, et al: Rat pancreatic hydrolases from birth to weaning and dietary adaptation after weaning. Am J Anat 221:376, 1971.
77. Like AA, Orci L: Embryogenesis of the human pancreatic islets: A light and electron microscopic study. Diabetes 21:511, 1972.
78. Baxter-Grillo D, Blazquez E, Grillo TAI, et al: Functional development of the pancreatic islets. In Cooperstein SJ, Watkins D (eds): The Islets of Langerhans. New York, Academic Press, 1981, p 35.
79. Stefan Y, Grasso S, Perrelet A, Orci L: A quantitative immunofluorescent study of the endocrine cell populations in the developing human pancreas. Diabetes 32:293, 1983.
80. Dowsett JF, Rude J, Russell RCG: Annular pancreas: A clinical endoscopic and immunohistochemical study. Gut 30:130, 1989.
81. Salonen IS: Congenital duodenal obstruction—a review of the literature and a clinical study of 66 patients, including a histopathological study of annular pancreas and a follow-up of 36 survivors. Acta Paediatr Scand(Suppl)272:1, 1978.
82. Rantch NM: The pancreas in infants and children. Surg Clin North Am 55:377, 1975.
83. Kiernan PD, ReMine SG, Kiernan PC, ReMine WH: Annular pancreas: Mayo Clinic experience from 1957 to 1976 with review of the literature. Arch Surg 115:46, 1980.
84. Dawson W, Langman V: An anatomical-radiological study of the pancreatic duct pattern in man. Anat Rec 139:59, 1961.
85. Smanio T: Proposed nomenclature and classification of the human pancreatic ducts and duodenal papillae. Study based on 200 postmortems. Int Surg 52:125, 1969.
86. Sahel J, Cros RC, Bourry J, Sarles H: Clinico-pathological conditions associated with pancreas divisum. Digestion 23:1, 1982.
87. Delhaye M, Engelholm L, Cremer M: Pancreas divisum: Congenital anatomic variant or anomaly? Contribution of endoscopic retrograde dorsal pancreatography. Gastroenterology 89:951, 1985.
88. Cotton PB: Congenital anomaly of pancreas divisum as cause of obstructive pain and pancreatitis. Gut 21:105, 1980.
89. Bhutani MS, Hoffman BJ, Hawes RH: Diagnosis of pancreas divisum by endoscopic ultrasonography. Endoscopy 31:167, 1999.
90. Bret P, Reinhold C, Taourel P, et al: Pancreas divisum: Evaluation with MR cholangiopancreatography. Radiology 199:99, 1996.
91. Coleman SD, Eisen GM, Troughton AB: Endoscopic treatment in pancreas divisum. Am J Gastroenterol 89:1152, 1994.
92. Lans JI, Geenen JE, Johanson JF: Endoscopic therapy in patients with pancreas divisum and acute pancreatitis: A prospective, randomized, controlled clinical trial. Gastrointest Endosc 38:430, 1992.
93. Lehman GA, Sherman S, Nizi R: Pancreas divisum: Results of minor papilla sphincterotomy. Gastrointest Endosc 39:1, 1993.
94. Warshaw AL, Simeone JF, Schapiro RH: Evaluation and treatment of the dominant dorsal duct syndrome (pancreas divisum redefined). Am J Surg 159:59, 1990.
95. Richter JM, Schapiro RH, Mulley AG, Warshaw AL: Association of pancreas divisum and pancreatitis, and its treatment by sphincteroplasty of the accessory ampulla. Gastroenterology 81:1104, 1981.
96. Dolan RV, ReMine WH, Dockerty MB: The fate of heterotopic pancreatic tissue. Arch Surg 109:762, 1974.
97. Wakany J, Passarge E, Smith LB: Congenital malformations in autosomal trisomy syndromes. J Dis Child 112:502, 1966.
98. Lemons JA, Ridenour R, Orshi EN: Congenital absence of the pancreas and intrauterine growth retardation. Pediatrics 64:255, 1979.
99. Bodian M: Fibrocystic Disease of the Pancreas. New York, Grune and Stratton, 1953.
100. Cotran RS, Kumar V, Robbins SL: Robbins Pathologic Basis of Disease. Philadelphia, WB Saunders, 1989.
101. Auringer ST, Ulmer JL, Sumner TE, Turner CS: Congenital cyst of the pancreas. J Pediatr Surg 28:1570, 1993.

Chapter 46

PANCREATIC PHYSIOLOGY AND SECRETORY TESTING

Stephen J. Pandol

As has been reviewed in Chapter 45, the pancreas is both an exocrine and an endocrine organ. This chapter is devoted to the exocrine pancreas. The exocrine pancreas has been of considerable interest to physiologists and other scientists for quite some time; in fact, the first demonstration of a hormone action was in the pancreas around the turn of the 20th century.[1] The pancreas has been the major model used to demonstrate the mechanisms of synthesis and transport for exportable proteins[2] as well as the signaling pathways involved in regulated protein secretion.[3] This chapter presents a concise description of the current understanding of pancreatic physiology.

FUNCTIONAL ANATOMY

The functional unit of the exocrine pancreas is composed of an acinus and its draining ductule[4] (Fig. 46–1). The ductal epithelium extends to the lumen of the acinus with the centroacinar cell situated between the ductal epithelium and the acinus. Centroacinar cells probably act similarly to duct epithelial cells to secrete ions and water. The ductule drains into interlobular (intercalated) ducts, which, in turn, drain into the main pancreatic ductal system (see Chapter 45).

The acinus (from the Latin term meaning "berry in a cluster") can be spherical, as shown in Figure 46–1, or tubular or can have some other, irregular form.[4] The acinar cells are specialized to synthesize, store, and secrete digestive enzymes. On the basolateral membrane are receptors for hormones and neurotransmitters that stimulate secretion of the enzymes.[3] The basal aspect of the cell contains the nucleus as well as abundant rough endoplasmic reticulum for protein synthesis.[4] The apical region of the cell contains zymogen granules, the store of digestive enzymes. The apical surface of the acinar cell also possesses microvilli. In the microvilli and the cytoplasm underlying the apical plasma membrane, there is a filamentous actin meshwork that effectively excludes cell organelles such as the zymogen granules from the subapical zone. Secretion is into the lumen of the acinus. Tight junctions between acinar cells form a band around the apical aspects of the cells and act as a barrier to prevent passage of large molecules. The junctional complexes also act as permeable barriers to the passage of water and ions.

Another intercellular connection between acinar cells is the gap junction. This specialized area of the plasma membrane between adjacent cells acts as a pore to allow small (molecular weights between 500–1000 daltons) molecules to pass between cells. The gap junction allows chemical and electrical communication between cells.[3, 4, 7–9] For example, calcium signaling is coordinated between the acinar cells of an acinus with effects on digestive enzyme secretion.[8, 9]

The duct epithelium consists of cells that are cuboidal to pyramidal.[4] The duct cells as well as the centroacinar cells contain carbonic anhydrase, which is important for their ability to secrete bicarbonate.[10]

COMPOSITION OF EXOCRINE PANCREATIC SECRETIONS

Inorganic Constituents

The principal inorganic components of exocrine pancreatic secretions are water, sodium, potassium, chloride, and bicarbonate.[10] The purposes of the water and ion secretions are to deliver digestive enzymes to the intestinal lumen and to help neutralize gastric acid emptied into the duodenum.

Pancreatic juice secreted during stimulation with secretin is clear, colorless, alkaline, and isotonic with plasma.[10] The flow rate increases from 0.2 or 0.3 mL/min in the resting state to 4.0 mL/minute during stimulation.[10] The total daily volume of secretion is 2.5 L. The osmolality of pancreatic juice is independent of flow rate. However, when the pancreas is stimulated by secretin (the major mediator of the increased volume output), bicarbonate and chloride concentrations change[8] (Fig. 46–2). The changes in bicarbonate and chloride concentrations occur because secretin stimulation causes a high-volume secretion containing bicarbonate

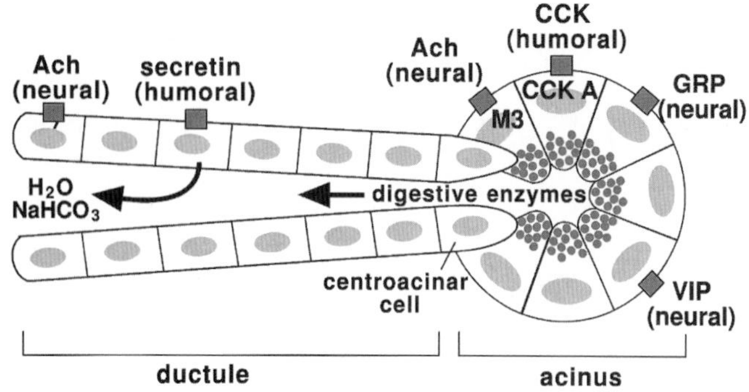

Figure 46–1. Functional unit of the exocrine pancreas. Acetylcholine (Ach), secretin, cholecystokinin (CCK), gastrin-releasing peptide (GRP), and vasoactive intestinal peptide (VIP) act as neural and humoral agonists to activate the ductule or the acinus. Acetylcholine acts through an M3 receptor and CCK through a CCK-A receptor. (Adapted from Pandol SJ, Raybould HE. The integrated response to a meal. In Alpers DH (ed): The Undergraduate Teaching Project in Gastroenterology and Liver Disease. Bethesda, MD, American Gastroenterological Association, Unit 24, 1995.) Investigations supporting this model have been derived mainly from studies using animal tissues. Of particular note, human pancreatic acinar cells do not contain CCK receptors. See text for further discussion.

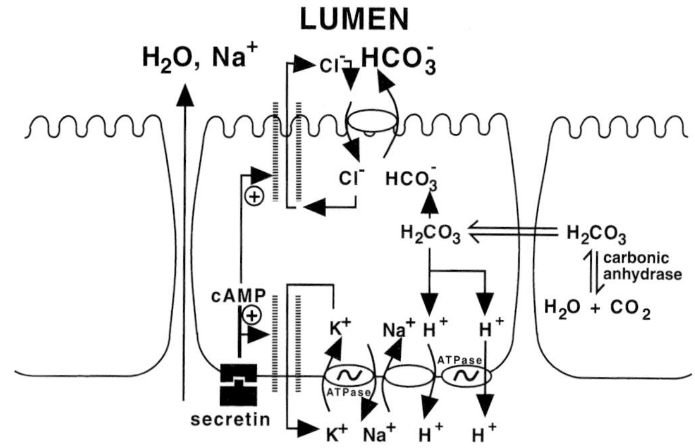

Figure 46–3. Ion transport mechanisms mediating pancreatic duct secretion. ⬭ indicates an ion channel. ⦀ indicates a transport that facilitates the movement of ions as a function of ion concentrations and electrical potential. ∿ indicates a transport that requires ATP energy input to move ions against ion concentrations and/or electrical gradients.

that originates from the pancreatic ductal system. Because the secretory flow rate from the acini is relatively small even when stimulated, the concentration of ions approaches that of ductal fluid during stimulation.

Secretin stimulates secretion by activating adenylate cyclase and increasing cyclic adenosine monophosphate (cAMP) in the ductal cell.[10–12] The mechanism by which cAMP increases bicarbonate secretion involves activation of a Cl^- channel on the luminal membrane[10,12] as well as K^+ channel activation on the basolateral membrane (Fig. 46–3). Of note, changes in intracellular calcium caused by acetylcholine, cholecystokinin (CCK), or gastrin-releasing peptide (GRP) may also stimulate these channel activities leading to augmentation of the ductal secretory response by secretin. At least one Cl^- channel is the cystic fibrosis transmembrane conductance regulator (CFTR).[11–13] The activation of both channels leads to Cl^- secretion into the lumen. The increased chloride in the lumen is coupled to a Cl^-/HCO_3^- antiport, resulting in an exchange of Cl^- for HCO_3^- in the lumen. Recent evidence also suggests a HCO_3^- channel on the apical surface mediating HCO_3^- secretion.[11] On the basolateral surface of the duct cell are a Na^+/HCO_3^- cotransport, Na^+/H^+ antiport, and Na^+/K^+-ATPase, H^+-ATPase, and K^+ channels. In combination, these transporters facilitate the HCO_3^- secretion at the apical surface as well as maintain intracellular pH.[14]

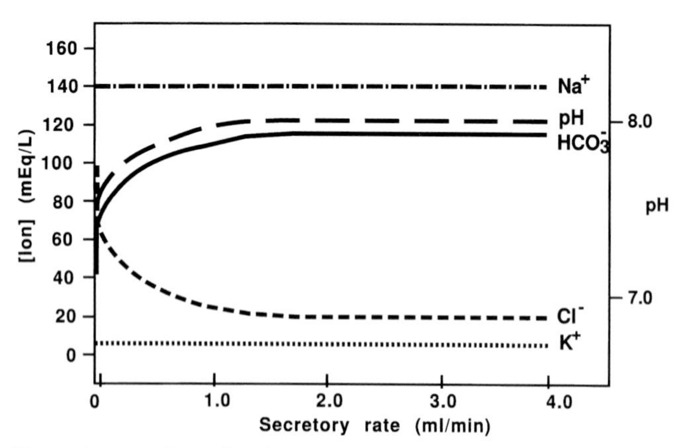

Figure 46–2. Relationship between pancreatic juice ion concentrations and secretory flow rate. (Adapted from Pandol SJ, Raybould HE: The integrated response to a meal. In Alpers DH (ed): The Undergraduate Teaching Project in Gastroenterology and Liver Disease. Bethesda, MD, American Gastroenterological Association, Unit 24, 1995.)

Organic Constituents[15, 16]

The human pancreas has a large capacity for synthesizing protein (mostly digestive enzymes). Listed in Table 46–1 are the major proteolytic, amylolytic, lipolytic, and nuclease digestive enzymes. Some of the enzymes are present in more than one form (e.g., cationic and anionic trypsinogen[15]). Enzymes that could potentially digest the pancreas are stored in the pancreas and secreted into the pancreatic duct as inactive precursor forms. As illustrated in Figure 46–4, activation of these enzymes takes place in the intestinal lumen, where a

Table 46–1 | **Digestive Enzymes in the Pancreatic Acinar Cell**

Proteolytic Enzymes
Trypsinogen
Chymotrypsinogen
Proelastase
Procarboxypeptidase A
Procarboxypeptidase B
Amylolytic Enzyme
α-Amylase
Lipolytic Enzymes
Lipase
Prophospholipase A_2
Carboxylesterase
Nucleases
Deoxyribonuclease (DNAse)
Ribonuclease (RNAse)
Others
Procolipase
Trypsin inhibitor

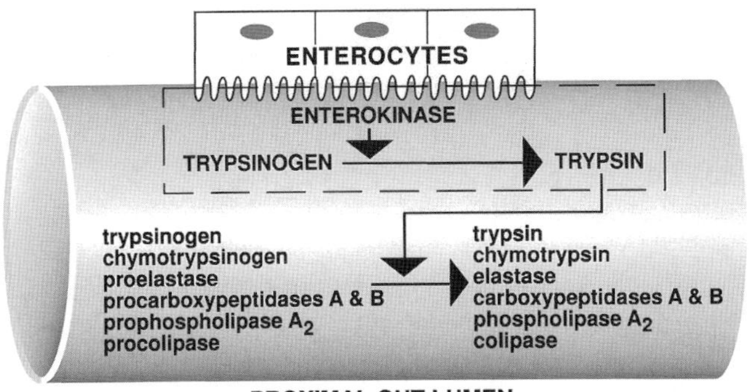

Figure 46–4. Mechanism of proenzyme activation in the intestinal lumen. (Adapted from Pandol SJ, Raybould HE: The integrated response to a meal. In Alpers DH (ed): The Undergraduate Teaching Project in Gastroenterology and Liver Disease. Bethesda, MD, American Gastroenterological Association, Unit 24, 1995.)

brush border glycoprotein peptidase, enterokinase, activates trypsinogen by removing (by hydrolysis) an N-terminal hexapeptide fragment of the molecule (Val-Asp-Asp-Asp-Asp-Lys).[15, 16] The active form, trypsin, then catalyzes the activation of the other inactive proenzymes.

In addition to the digestive enzymes, the acinar cell secretes a trypsin inhibitor, pancreatic secretory trypsin inhibitor. This 56-amino-acid peptide inactivates trypsin by forming a relatively stable complex with the enzyme near its catalytic site.[15, 17] The function of the inhibitor is to inactivate trypsins that are formed autocatalytically in the pancreas or pancreatic juice, thus preventing disorders such as pancreatitis.[18]

FUNCTIONS OF THE MAJOR DIGESTIVE ENZYMES

Amylase

Human amylase is secreted by both the pancreas and salivary glands. These enzymes digest starch and glycogen in the diet. Human salivary and pancreatic amylases have identical enzyme activities. However, they differ in molecular weight, carbohydrate content, and electrophoretic mobility.[19] Salivary amylase initiates digestion in the mouth and may account for a significant portion of starch and glycogen digestion because it is transported with the meal into the stomach and small intestine, where it continues to have activity. In the stomach, the amylase activity is protected from secreted gastric acid by buffering from the meal and by the protected alkaline environment of salivary and gastric mucus. The action of both salivary and pancreatic amylase is to hydrolyze 1,4-glycoside linkages at the junction between carbon 1 and oxygen.[12, 16] The products of amylase digestion are maltose and maltotriose (two and three α-1, 4–linked molecules, respectively) and α-dextrins containing 1,6-glycosidic linkages, because 1,6-glycosidic linkages in starch cannot be hydrolyzed by amylase. The brush border enzymes complete hydrolysis of the products of amylase digestion to glucose. The final product, glucose, is transported across the intestinal absorptive epithelial cell by a Na^+-coupled transport (see Chapter 88).[20]

Lipases

The pancreas secretes three lipases: lipase (or triglyceride lipase), phospholipase A_2, and carboxylesterase. In contrast to amylase, the most important source of these lipases is the pancreas. Salivary (lingual) and gastric lipases also contribute to fat digestion (see Chapter 38).

Pancreatic lipase hydrolyzes a triglyceride molecule to two fatty acid molecules and a monoglyceride with the fatty acid esterified to glycerol at carbon 2.[15] Lipase binds to the oil/water interface of the triglyceride oil droplet, where it acts to hydrolyze the triglyceride. Both bile acids and colipase are important for the full activity of lipase. Bile acids aid in the emulsification of triglyceride to increase surface area for lipase to act on, and they form micelles with fatty acids and monoglyceride to remove them from the oil/water interface. Colipase is thought to form a complex between itself, lipase, and bile salts. This ternary complex anchors lipase and allows it to act in a more hydrophilic environment on the hydrophobic surface of the oil droplet.

Phospholipase A_2 catalyzes the hydrolysis of the fatty acid ester linkage at carbon 2 of phosphatidylcholine.[15] This cleavage leads to the formation of free fatty acid and lysophosphatidylcholine.

Carboxylesterase has a broad specificity and will cleave cholesterol esters, lipid-soluble vitamin esters, triglycerides, diglycerides, and monoglycerides. Bile salts are also important for the full activity of this enzyme.[21]

Proteases

The pancreas secretes a variety of proteases that are activated in the duodenum. The activated forms include trypsin, chymotrypsin, and elastase. These endopeptidases cleave specific peptide bonds adjacent to certain amino acids. Also contained in pancreatic juice are the carboxypeptidases. These are exopeptidases that cleave peptide bonds at the carboxyl terminus of proteins.

The combined actions of the proteases plus pepsin from the stomach result in the release of oligopeptides and free amino acids. The oligopeptides are further digested by brush border enzymes (see Chapter 88). Both free amino acids and oligopeptides are transported by the intestinal mucosa by a group of Na^+ and H^+ coupled transporters.[22] It is interesting that only certain amino acids (mostly essential amino acids) are measured in the lumen during digestion, which indicates that the combined action of the proteases is not random and that the products result from the combined specificities of the individual proteases. These amino acids have greater effects on stimulating pancreatic secretion, inhibiting gastric emptying, regulating small bowel motility, and causing satiety. Thus, the protease actions lead to physiologic regulation of several organs in the gastrointestinal tract.

DIGESTIVE ENZYME SYNTHESIS AND TRANSPORT

Synthesis of digestive enzymes takes place in the internal space of the rough endoplasmic reticulum (RER).[2, 4] The mechanism of translation of the cell's messenger RNA (mRNA) into exportable protein is explained by the signal hypothesis.[4, 23] The main feature of the hypothesis is that a hydrophobic "signal" sequence on the NH_2-terminal of nascent proteins targets the protein being synthesized into the lumen of the RER.

Newly synthesized proteins can undergo modifications in the endoplasmic reticulum, including disulfide bridge formation, phosphorylation, sulfation, and glycosylation. Conformational changes resulting in tertiary and quaternary structure of the protein also take place in the endoplasmic reticulum.[23] Processed proteins in the RER are transported to the Golgi complex, where further post-translational modification (glycosylation) and concentration occur.[2, 23] The Golgi complex also serves an important function of sorting and targeting of newly synthesized proteins into various cell compartments. Digestive enzymes are transported to the zymogen granules.[24, 25] Lysosomal hydrolases are sorted to the lysosome.[25] For this pathway, mannose-6-phosphate groups are added to oligosaccharide chains on the protein during its presence in the *cis*-Golgi complex. The mannose-6-phosphate groups serve as a recognition site for a specific receptor. The interaction of the lysosomal enzyme mannose 6-phosphate with its receptor somehow leads to formation of vesicles that transport this complex to the lysosome, delivering the enzyme. In the lysosome the enzyme dissociates from the receptor, which, in turn, cycles back to the Golgi complex.

Secretion of the digestive enzymes occurs by exocytosis. Exocytosis includes movement of the secretory granule to the apical surface, the recognition of a plasma membrane site for fusion, and the fission of the granule membrane/plasma membrane site after fusion.[2, 4] Recent studies demonstrate roles for the actin-myosin, SNARE proteins, and guanosine triphosphate (GTP)-binding proteins in these processes.[27–32] Intracellular signals generated by agonist receptors interact with these entities to mediate digestive enzyme secretion.

Regulation of Protein Synthesis

The mechanisms involved in regulating expression of digestive enzymes in the exocrine pancreas have been partially elucidated. The investigations have addressed two questions. First, what accounts for the specific expression of digestive enzymes in the pancreas? Second, how do alterations in dietary nutrients change the synthesis of specific digestive enzymes?

Genes for digestive enzymes such as amylase, chymotrypsin, and elastase contain enhancer regions in their 5′ flanking nucleotide sequences that regulate the transcription of their mRNAs, termed the *pancreas consensus element* (PCE).[22] A transcription factor, PTF-1, is present selectively in the exocrine pancreas, binds to this region, and is essential for expression of these digestive enzymes. Thus, PTF-1 represents at least one of the differentiation-regulated factors that accounts for digestive enzyme expression in the pancreas.

Numerous studies have demonstrated that the relative synthesis rates of specific digestive enzymes change as a function of dietary intake. For example, a carbohydrate-rich diet results in an increase in synthesis of amylase and a decrease in chymotrypsinogen.[33, 34] The mechanisms responsible for this adaptation are only partially understood. Several studies have demonstrated that amylase gene expression is regulated by both insulin and diet.[33, 34]

CELLULAR REGULATION OF ENZYME SECRETION

The mechanism of neurohumoral stimulation of the acinar cell has been demonstrated with the use of in vitro preparations of dispersed acinar cells and acini from small animals. Studies involving the use of human tissue are few in number.

With the use of radiolabeled ligands and specific antagonists, receptors for cholecystokinin (CCK), acetylcholine, gastrin-releasing peptide (GRP), substance P, vasoactive intestinal peptide (VIP), and secretin have been identified in preparations from species such as guinea pigs, rats, and mice.[33] Furthermore, the molecular structure for each of these receptor types has been elucidated from cloning and sequencing.[3, 35] Each is a G-protein–coupled receptor with seven hydrophobic domains believed to be membrane-spanning segments. The receptors are on the basolateral plasma membrane of the acinar cell. Of particular note, human pancreatic acinar cells do not contain CCK receptors, suggesting that the mechanism of pancreatic secretion stimulated by CCK in humans is mediated solely by the effects of CCK on sensory neural pathways.

Receptors on acinar cells have been divided into two categories according to the mode of stimulus-secretion coupling (Fig. 46–5). In one category are VIP and secretin. The interaction of these agents with acinar cells leads to activation of adenylate cyclase and an increase in cellular cAMP, which, in turn, activates enzyme secretion through cAMP-dependent protein kinase A.[3, 36]

The pancreatic acinar cell from animal tissues contains receptors for the agonists, CCK, acetylcholine, and substance P (see Fig. 46–5).[3] As noted earlier, the human pancreatic acinar cell does not contain the CCK receptor; however, studies of the intracellular mechanism of action of these four classes of receptors have largely been investigated using

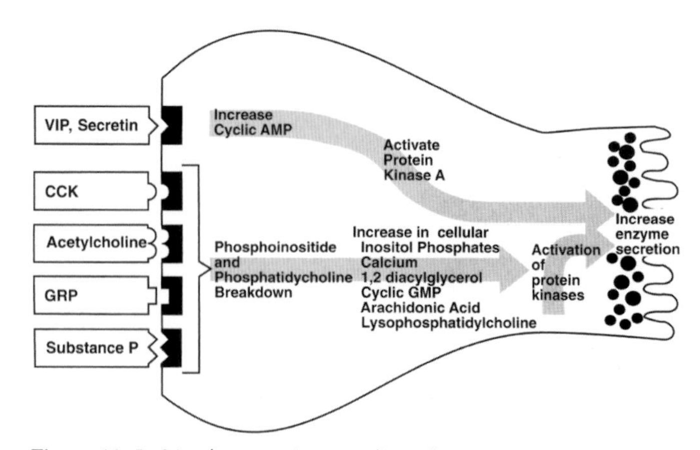

Figure 46–5. Stimulus-secretion coupling of pancreatic acinar cell protein secretion. Investigations supporting this model have been derived mainly from studies using animal tissues. Of particular note, human pancreatic acinar cells do not contain CCK receptors. See text for further discussion.

CCK in animal tissues. The actions of these agonists include stimulating cellular metabolism of membrane phosphoinositides and increasing cytoplasmic free calcium concentrations ($[Ca^{2+}]$ i).[32] The ability of these agents to cause cellular calcium mobilization results from their effect on membrane phosphoinositides.[3] Specifically, the agonist-receptor interaction leads to a phospholipase C-mediated hydrolysis of phosphatidylinositol 4, 5-bisphosphate to 1, 2-diacylglycerol and inositol 1, 4, 5-triphosphate (IP_3).[38] IP_3, in turn, releases calcium from a nonmitochondrial intracellular store that probably includes the RER. The calcium is released into the cytosol, resulting in a rapid rise in the concentration of free calcium in the cytosol. Calcium release into the cytosol is also mediated by ryanodine receptors and signals interacting with the ryanodine receptor such as calcium, fatty acid–CoA esters, and cyclic ADP-ribose.[39, 40] The mechanism by which increases in $[Ca^{2+}]$ i mediate secretion is not established but may include calmodulin-dependent protein kinases and actin-myosin interactions, SNARE proteins, and GTP-binding proteins as discussed earlier. The continued stimulation of enzyme secretion by these agents is also dependent on the influx of extracellular calcium.[3] This influx is mediated by changes in nitric oxide and cyclic guanosine monophosphate (cGMP).[41, 42] The intracellular mechanism of enzyme secretion may also be regulated by 1, 2-diacylglycerol and protein kinase C,[3, 38] as well as by arachidonic acid.[43] Specific phosphorylations and dephosphorylations of cellular proteins also occur with both cAMP agonists and calcium-phosphoinositide agonists.[3] The exact roles of these events in secretion are not established.

The enzyme secretory response of the acinar cell to a combination of an agonist that acts by cAMP and an agonist that acts by changes in calcium is greater than the additive response.[3] An example of such a combination would be VIP or secretin with CCK or acetylcholine. The mechanism of this potentiated response is not known, but it probably functions physiologically so that significant quantities of secretion occur with a combination of small increases in individual agonists.

ORGAN PHYSIOLOGY[44]

Human exocrine pancreatic secretion occurs both during the fasting (interdigestive) state and after ingestion of a meal (digestion). The interdigestive pattern of secretion begins when the upper gastrointestinal tract is cleared of food. In an individual who eats three meals per day, the digestive pattern begins after breakfast and continues until late in the day after the evening meal is cleared from the upper gastrointestinal tract.

Interdigestive Secretion

The interdigestive pancreatic secretory pattern is cyclic and follows the pattern of the migrating myoelectric complex (MMC).[44] The patterns recur every 60 to 120 minutes with bursts of enzyme secretion temporally associated with the periods of increased motor activity in the stomach and duodenum (i.e., phases II and III). In addition to pancreatic enzyme secretion, there is increased bicarbonate and bile secretion (secondary to partial gallbladder contraction) into the duodenum during phases II and III of the MMC. The underlying mechanism responsible for these responses must include cholinergic activation because cholinergic antagonists block the responses. Both motilin and pancreatic polypeptide are involved in regulation of the MMC.[44–46] The role of these secretions during the MMC is not clear but may be related to the "housekeeping" function of the MMC (see Chapter 85).

Digestive Secretion

Like gastric secretion, exocrine pancreatic secretion with ingestion of a meal is divided into three phases: cephalic, gastric, and intestinal.

The vagal nerves mediate the cephalic phase of the exocrine secretion. The extent of cephalic stimulation of exocrine pancreatic secretion in humans has been evaluated by measuring exocrine secretions stimulated by sham feeding (chewing and spitting out the food). One study indicated that sham feeding stimulated pancreatic enzyme secretion at up to 50% of the maximal secretory rate, with no increase in bicarbonate secretion when gastric secretions were prevented from entering the duodenum.[47] When gastric secretions were allowed entry into the duodenum, the rate of enzyme secretion increased to about 90% of maximal, and bicarbonate was also secreted. These results suggested that cephalic stimulation specifically stimulates acinar secretion and that a low pH in the duodenum (from gastric acid) augments this secretion as well as causes bicarbonate secretion.

Results of investigations of the mechanism of neurotransmission during cephalic stimulation are controversial. Acetylcholine is certainly a major neurotransmitter involved because atropine greatly reduces and in some cases abolishes sham feeding–stimulated pancreatic secretion in humans.[44, 48] Neural endings containing the peptides VIP, GRP, CCK, and enkephalins have been identified in the pancreas.[44] Data supporting the role of these peptides in the cephalic phase of secretion are strongest for VIP and GRP. Both are released into the venous effluent with vagal stimulation in animals.[49, 50] Furthermore, as discussed previously, acinar cells have receptors for GRP and VIP that mediate enzyme secretion. The ductal epithelium also responds to VIP with secretion of water and bicarbonate.[49]

The gastric phase of pancreatic secretion results from meal stimuli acting in the stomach. The major stimulus is gastric distention that causes predominantly secretion of enzymes with little secretion of water and bicarbonate. Balloon distention of either the gastric fundus or the antrum results in a low-volume, enzyme-rich secretion by way of a vagovagal reflex.

When gastric juice and contents of a meal enter the duodenum, a variety of intraluminal stimulants can act on the intestinal mucosa to stimulate pancreatic secretion through both neural and humoral mechanisms. Three gastric processes—gastric acid, pepsin and lipase secretion; intragastric digestion; and gastric emptying—are tightly coupled to the mechanisms of the intestinal phase of pancreatic secretion.

The intestinal phase begins when chyme first enters the small intestine from the stomach. It is mediated both by hormones and by enteropancreatic vagovagal reflexes.

The major mediator of hydrogen ion–stimulated bicarbonate and water secretion is secretin. Secretin measured by radioimmunoassay is released from the duodenal mucosa with a threshold pH of 4.5.[51] The quantity of secretin released as well as the volume of pancreatic secretion is dependent on the load of titratable acid delivered to the duodenum.[51, 52] Immunoneutralization of secretin with specific antisecretin antibody decreases pancreatic volume and bicarbonate secretion by as much as 80% in response to a mixed meal.[53] The antisecretin antibody also inhibits enzyme secretion stimulated by the mixed meal by as much as 50%, which suggests that secretin has a role in enzyme secretion, possibly by potentiating the action of agonists such as CCK and acetylcholine.

Fatty acids more than eight carbons in chain length and bile acids have also been found to increase circulating secretin and increase pancreatic exocrine secretion.[44]

If exogenous secretin is infused to reproduce the plasma concentrations of secretin during a meal, the pancreatic bicarbonate output is less than the bicarbonate output observed with a meal.[44] Secretin-induced bicarbonate secretion is augmented by CCK when both agents are infused to reproduce concentrations observed during a meal.[54] CCK alone causes no bicarbonate secretion. The bicarbonate response to secretin is also dependent on cholinergic input because atropine partially inhibits the response stimulated by exogenous secretin.[55] Thus, the complete meal-stimulated response results from a combination of mediators.

During the intestinal phase, secretion of digestive enzymes is mediated by intraluminal fatty acids more than eight carbons in length, monoglycerides of these fatty acids, peptides, amino acids, and, to a small extent, glucose.[44] The most potent amino acids for stimulating secretion in humans are phenylalanine, valine, methionine, and tryptophan.[56] The response to peptides and amino acids is related to the total load perfused into the intestine rather than the concentration.[57]

The mediators of the enzyme secretory response from intestinal stimuli are both neural and humoral (Fig. 46–6). Truncal vagotomy and atropine markedly inhibit the enzyme

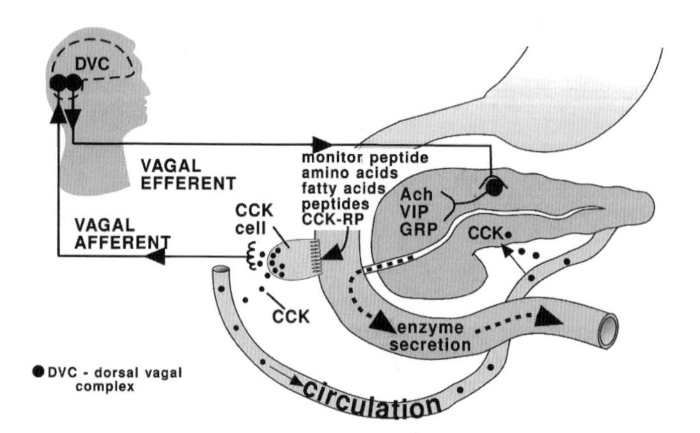

Figure 46–6. Intestinal phase of pancreatic enzyme secretion is mediated by both neural and humoral mechanisms. (Adapted from Pandol SJ, Raybould HE: The integrated response to a meal. In Alpers DH (ed): The Undergraduate Teaching Project in Gastroenterology and Liver Disease. Bethesda, MD, American Gastroenterological Association, Unit 24, 1995.)

(and bicarbonate) responses to low intestinal loads of amino acids and fatty acids.[44, 58] These results suggest a vagovagal enteropancreatic reflex that mediates enzyme secretion and augments bicarbonate secretion stimulated by secretin.

CCK is the major humoral mediator of meal-stimulated enzyme secretion. The circulating concentration of CCK is found to increase with a meal.[59] Experimenters using highly specific CCK receptor antagonists have demonstrated that a major portion of enzyme secretion with a meal is mediated by CCK.[61] CCK is released from the upper small intestinal mucosa by digestion products of fat and protein and, to a small extent, by starch digestion products.[59]

In addition to blocking meal-stimulated enzyme secretion, atropine has been reported to block the effect of physiologic concentrations of CCK on enzyme secretion.[61] Further experiments suggest that CCK activates afferent neurons in the duodenal mucosa. These afferent neurons mediate an enteropancreatic reflex that causes pancreatic enzyme secretion. Although these findings are provocative and suggest a model accounting for the relationship between neural and humoral pathways during the intestinal phase of the enzyme secretory response, the model is controversial because the CCK stimulation of the enteropancreatic reflex has been demonstrated only in the anesthetized rat and cannot be reproduced in the conscious rat.[61]

Feedback Regulation

In both animals and humans, diversion of pancreatic juice from the intestine results in augmented pancreatic secretion.[62] The augmented enzyme secretion is mediated by an increase in circulating CCK.[63] Both the increase in CCK and enzyme secretion can be inhibited by replenishing intraluminal trypsin. It is hypothesized that during a meal, when trypsin is occupied by meal proteins, there is enhanced pancreatic secretion because trypsin is not available to cause feedback inhibition. After the meal, trypsin is free and inhibits CCK release and enzyme secretion. Intraluminal CCK-releasing factors that mediate this effect of trypsin have been described. One is a protein called monitor peptide that is secreted by the pancreas.[64] Another is called luminal CCK-releasing factor (LCRF).[65] Both monitor peptide and LCRF cause CCK release from the enteroendocrine CCK cell into the blood. These releasing factors are likely mediators of the physiologic feedback mechanism for enzyme secretion. It is thought that the effects of trypsin described earlier are due to degradation of the releasing factors by trypsin when not bound to meal proteins.

A similar feedback mechanism involving a secretin-releasing factor intraluminal peptide has been described.[66] One of the secretin-releasing factors is pancreatic phospholipase A_2.

Inhibition of Pancreatic Secretion

A variety of inhibitory effects of both nutrients and gastrointestinal hormones on the stimulated pancreatic exocrine secretion have been demonstrated. However, the physiologic mechanisms underlying the effects of the nutrients have not been established.

The following nutrients have been demonstrated to cause inhibition of CCK or meal-stimulated pancreatic secretion:[44] (1) both intravenous and intrajejunal administration of amino acids; (2) hypertonic solutions of glucose infused into the duodenum or jejunum and hyperglycemia induced by intravenous glucose; and (3) intracolonic infusions of oleic acid.

Proposed mediators of the inhibition by these nutrients include glucagon, somatostatin, and peptide YY.[44] Although evidence to establish a physiologic role for each of these mediators has not been established, there is sufficient evidence of a possible role for glucagon and somatostatin in the inhibitory effect of amino acids and glucose and, for peptide YY, in the inhibitory effects of intracolonic oleic acid.

A hormone present in the islets of Langerhans, pancreatic polypeptide (PP), may also have an inhibitory role in regulating pancreatic secretion. Vagal cholinergic stimulation causes release of PP, and PP in turn inhibits pancreatic volume and bicarbonate and protein secretion via presynaptic modulation of acetylcholine release.[67] These findings suggest a feedback inhibitory loop.

PANCREATIC SECRETORY FUNCTION TESTS (Table 46–2)

Various tests have been devised to measure the secretory function of the pancreas in order to diagnose disorders such as chronic pancreatitis and pancreatic cancer. The function tests fall into two general categories: direct and indirect. Direct tests of pancreatic secretory function involve collection of pancreatic secretions after intravenous administration of a secretagogue or a combination of secretagogues. Indirect tests of pancreatic secretory function include the measurement of pancreatic enzymes in duodenal samples after nutrient ingestion; the measurement of products of digestive enzyme action on ingested substrates; the measurement of

Table 46–2 | **Pancreatic Function Tests**

TEST	DESCRIPTION	ADVANTAGES	DISADVANTAGES	CLINICAL INDICATIONS
Direct Tests				
Secretin	Measurement of volume and HCO_3^- secretion into the duodenum with IV secretin			
Cholecystokinin	Measurement of amylase, trypsin, and lipase with IV cholecystokinin	Provide the most sensitive and specific measurements of exocrine pancreatic function	Require duodenal intubation and intravenous administration of hormones; not widely available	Detection of mild, moderate, or severe exocrine pancreatic dysfunction
Secretin and cholecystokinin	Measurement of volume, HCO_3^-, and enzymes with IV secretin and cholecystokinin			
Indirect Tests Requiring Duodenal Intubation				
Lundh test meal	Measurement of duodenal trypsin concentration after oral ingestion of a test meal	Does not require IV administration of hormones	Requires duodenal intubation; requires normal anatomy, including small intestinal mucosa; not widely available	Detection of moderate or severe exocrine pancreatic dysfunction when direct tests cannot be done
Tubeless Indirect Tests				
Fecal fat	Oral ingestion of dietary fat, followed by measurement of fat in the stool	Provides a quantitative measurement of steatorrhea	Requires quantitative assessment of dietary fat and fecal fat	Detection of severe exocrine pancreatic dysfunction and steatorrhea
Fecal chymotrypsin Fecal elastase 1	Fecal measurement of chymotrypsin or elastase 1	Do not require IVs, tubes, or administration of oral substrates	Do not detect mild or moderate dysfunction; high false positive rate	Detection of severe exocrine pancreatic dysfunction especially in children
NBT-PABA	Oral ingestion of NBT-PABA with a meal, followed by measurements of PABA in serum or urinary excretion	Provide simple measurements for severe pancreatic dysfunction	Does not detect mild or moderate dysfunction; result may be abnormal with small bowel mucosal disease	Detection of severe pancreatic dysfunction
Fluorescein dilaurate	Oral ingestion of fluorescein dilaurate with a meal, followed by measurements of fluorescein in serum or urine			

NBT-PABA, *N*-benzoyl-L-tyrosyl para-aminobenzoic acid; IV, intravenous.

pancreatic enzymes in the stool; or the measurement of the plasma concentration of hormones or other markers that are altered in pancreatic insufficiency states.

The choice of which pancreatic function test to use depends on the clinical question and the characteristics and availability of the test. The exocrine pancreas has a very large functional reserve. Malabsorption does not occur until the functional capacity as measured by CCK-stimulated digestive enzyme secretion is reduced to 5% to 10% of normal.[68] Thus, many tests relying on the conversion of an ingested substrate to a product by digestive enzymes will not yield abnormal results unless moderate to severe pancreatic insufficiency is present. These tests have low sensitivity in demonstrating an abnormality in patients with mild or moderate degrees of pancreatic insufficiency. In this situation, the measurement of duodenal digestive enzymes after the intravenous administration of pancreatic secretagogues provides greater sensitivity and specificity. The major drawbacks to the more sensitive measurement techniques are the requirements for duodenal intubation and the fact that very few centers are proficient in properly performing the studies. The improved imaging techniques for diagnosing pancreatic disease have largely decreased the use of the tests. However, on certain occasions the pancreatic function tests are necessary for diagnosing pancreatic disease. The purpose of providing descriptions of the pancreatic function tests is for the reader to appreciate the relative diagnostic utility of each test.

Direct Tests

These tests provide a "gold standard" for measurement of pancreatic function. Stimulation of secretion has been described most commonly with secretin, CCK, or the combination. The combination provides the complete information about both acinar and ductular cell secretions. For these studies, both the stomach and duodenum are intubated. The gastric intubation is required to remove gastric secretions that will interfere with the ability to measure volume and bicarbonate secretions from the pancreas. Low pH may also alter pancreatic enzyme activity. The duodenal tube is used for both infusion of a nonabsorbable marker and collection of pancreatic secretions. The use of a nonabsorbable marker such as cobalamin or polyethylene glycol (PEG) allows the quantitation of secretions without the need for complete aspiration of secretions.[69]

The direct function tests are based on the principle that maximal volume, bicarbonate secretion, and enzyme secretion are related to the functional mass of the pancreas.[70] Historically, the secretin test (intravenous administration of secretin with volume and bicarbonate measurement) first provided information about the function of the pancreas in various clinical settings. CCK administration and the measurement of digestive enzyme secretion has also been used successfully to demonstrate pancreatic insufficiency. Because the combination of secretin and CCK administration provides stimulation of both functional units of the exocrine pancreas, this combination is currently the one most commonly used.[69, 71] The secretagogues are best delivered by constant intravenous infusion.[57] The dose for synthetic CCK-octapeptide (carboxy-terminal octapeptide of CCK; Squibb, Princeton, NJ) is 40 ng/kg/hour. The dose for the soon to be released synthetic secretin (Repligen, Needham, MA) will be available from the supplier.

Measurements corrected for percentage recovery are made for volume, bicarbonate, and protein concentration and for the activity of digestive enzymes. Amylase, trypsin, chymotrypsin, and lipase are the digestive enzymes most commonly measured.[69, 71]

In a discriminant analysis study of 236 subjects, continuous infusion of CCK-octapeptide (40 ng/kg/hour) and purified natural secretin (0.25 CU/kg/hour) and the measurement of mean chymotrypsin concentration and peak bicarbonate output were used to distinguish subjects with chronic pancreatitis from those without organic disease.[72] The test was 83% sensitive and 89% specific. False-positive results may occur in patients with celiac sprue and diabetes mellitus.

Indirect Tests

Lundh Test Meal[73]

As described by Lundh, the subject ingests a 300-mL liquid meal composed of dried milk, vegetable oil, and dextrose (6% fat, 5% protein, and 15% carbohydrate). After ingestion of the test meal, samples are aspirated from the intubated duodenum at intervals for measurement of digestive enzyme concentration. Usually only trypsin activity is measured; however, the additional determination of lipase or amylase may improve sensitivity.

The test is not valid in states of mucosal disease (e.g., celiac sprue) or changes in gastroduodenal anatomy (e.g., vagotomy and drainage procedure, Bilroth II gastrectomy).

Comparisons of the secretin-CCK test with the Lundh meal test demonstrate that the former is more sensitive in detecting mild forms of pancreatic disease, whereas for advanced disease they are comparable.[69]

Fecal Fat

Steatorrhea occurs when stimulated lipase output falls below 5% to 10% of normal.[68] Thus, measurement of fat in the stools collected for 72 hours in a subject ingesting a diet adequate in fat intake (70 to 100 g/day) is considered an effective means of diagnosing steatorrhea. Normally, 7% or less of ingested fat appears in the stool. A simple qualitative microscopic examination of a single stool for oil is almost as sensitive as quantitative measurements for fat.[69] Because steatorrhea occurs only with advanced pancreatic disease, measurement of fecal fat is not useful in the diagnosis of mild or moderate disease. Moreover, the test is not specific for pancreatic disease (see Chapter 89).

Fecal Chymotrypsin and Elastase 1

Chymotrypsin measurements in the stool[75] have been used as indirect tests of pancreatic function for many years, especially to establish pancreatic insufficiency in patients with cystic fibrosis.[69] They are about 85% sensitive in advanced pancreatic dysfunction and relatively insensitive in mild to moderate disease. Measurements of pancreatic elastase 1 in the stool can also detect pancreatic insufficiency. However, as with the chymotrypsin measurement, abnormal stool levels of elastase 1 are found only in severe pancreatic dysfunction. False-positive tests occur in a variety of nonpancreatic disorders.

N-Benzoyl-L-Tyrosyl-Para-Aminobenzoic Acid (NBT-PABA) Test

The NBT-PABA (bentiromide) test is the most commonly used noninvasive test of pancreatic function. The synthetic peptide NBT-PABA is specifically cleaved by the pancreatic endopeptidase, chymotrypsin, to NBT and PABA. PABA is then absorbed in the intestine, conjugated in the liver, and excreted in the urine.[69] The PABA metabolite can be measured in either the serum or the urine. Prior gastric surgery, small bowel disease, liver disease, renal insufficiency, the use of certain drugs (acetaminophen, benzocaine, chloramphenicol, lidocaine, phenacetin, procaine, sulfonamide, sulfonylurea, and thiazides), and certain foods (prunes and cranberries) may interfere with the measurements. Thus, these items should not be ingested before or during the test.

A broad range of sensitivities has been reported for the NBT-PABA test.[69] In patients with severe pancreatic insufficiency and malabsorption, the sensitivity is 80% to 90%. In those with mild to moderate impairment, sensitivity is as low as 40%. In order to improve specificity, several modifications of the NBT-PABA test have been devised. Administering free PABA on a separate day or giving ^{14}C-PABA or paraminosalicylic acid simultaneously with NBT-PABA may identify patients with abnormal NBT-PABA test result caused by mucosal disease of the small bowel.[69]

Fluorescein Dilaurate (Pancreolauryl) Test

The principle underlying this test is the same as that for the NBT-PABA test. Fluorescein dilaurate is an ester, poorly soluble in water, that is hydrolyzed by carboxylesterase into lauric acid and free water-soluble fluorescein. The fluorescein is readily absorbed into the intestine, partly conjugated in the liver, and excreted in the urine. Fluorescein dilaurate is given in the middle of a breakfast meal.[69] Urine is collected for 10 hours after breakfast, and the fluorescein excreted in the urine is measured. As with the NBT-PABA test, fluorescein can also be measured in the serum. To evaluate the subject's absorption, conjugation, and excretion, the test is repeated 2 to 3 days later with free fluorescein. The recovery rate on both days is expressed as a ratio. Like the NBT-PABA test, the pancreolauryl test is highly sensitive and specific for advanced pancreatic disease and less so for mild and moderate disease.

Other Tests

Several other indirect tubeless tests have been created in an effort to improve sensitivity for determining milder forms of exocrine pancreatic dysfunction. These include triglyceride and cholesteryl breath tests; H_2 and CO_2 breath tests; the dual label Schilling test; and plasma measurements of pancreatic polypeptide and amino acids.[69, 74–76] However, none of these tests have been shown to have increased sensitivity over the indirect tubeless tests described previously. In addition, many of these tests require radioactive isotopes or expensive equipment making their utility less desirable.

In summary, the profusion of tests of pancreatic function suggests that the ideal test has not been developed. The direct tests remain the "gold standard" and should be used to detect mild and moderate pancreatic inefficiency. To detect severe insufficiency resulting in steatorrhea, many of the tests described provide appropriate sensitivity. In this situation, the NBT-PABA test and the pancreolauryl test are preferable because of their simplicity.

REFERENCES

1. Bayliss WM, Starling EH: The mechanisms of pancreatic secretion. J Physiol 28:325, 1902.
2. Palade G: Intracellular aspects of the process of protein synthesis. Science 189:347, 1975.
3. Williams JA, Groblewski GE, Ohnishi H, Yule DI: Stimulus-secretion coupling of pancreatic digestive enzyme secretion. Digestion 58 (Suppl 1):42–45, 1997.
4. Gorelick FS, Jamieson JD: The pancreatic acinar cell. Structure-function relationships. In Johnson LR, Alpers DH, Christensen J, et al (eds): Physiology of the Gastrointestinal Tract, 3rd ed. New York, Raven, 1994, p 1353.
5. Gardner JD, Jensen RT: Receptors for secretagogues on pancreatic acinar cells. In Go VLW, Gardner JD, DiMagno EP, et al (eds): The Exocrine Pancreas: Biology, Pathobiology and Disease, 2nd ed. New York, Raven, 1993, p 151.
6. Peterson OH: Electrophysiology of acinar cells. In Go VLW, Gardner JD, DiMagno EP, et al (eds): The Exocrine Pancreas: Biology, Pathobiology and Disease, 2nd ed. New York, Raven, 1993, p 191.
7. Stauffer PL, Zhao H, Luby-Phelps K, et al: Gap junction communication modulates [Ca^{2+}]i oscillations and enzyme secretion in pancreatic acini. J Biol Chem 268:19769, 1993.
8. Chanson M, Fanjul M, Bosco D, Nelles EL, et al: Enhanced secretion of amylase from exocrine pancreas of connexin 32-deficient mice. J Cell Biol 141:1267–1275, 1998.
9. Yule DI, Stuenkel E, Williams JA: Intercellular calcium waves in rat pancreatic acini: mechanism of transmission. Am J Physiol 271:C1285–1294, 1996.
10. Argent BE, Case RM: Pancreatic ducts: Cellular mechanism and control of bicarbonate secretion. In Johnson LR, Alpers DH, Christensen J, et al (eds): Physiology of the Gastrointestinal Tract, 3rd. ed. New York, Raven, 1994, p 1473.
11. Sohma Y, Gray MA, Imai Y, Argent BE: HCO_3^- transport in a mathematical model of the pancreatic ductal epithelium. J Membrane Biol 176:77–100, 2000.
12. Gray MA, Greenwell JR, Argent BE: Secretin-regulated chloride channel on the apical plasma membrane of pancreatic duct cells. J Membrane Biol 105:131, 1988.
13. Marino CR, Matovcik LM, Gorelick FS, Cohn JA: Localization of the cystic fibrosis transmembrane conductance regulator in pancreas. J Clin Invest 88:712, 1991.
14. Stuenkel EL, Machen TE, Williams JA: pH regulatory mechanisms in rat pancreatic duct cells. Am J Physiol 254:G925, 1988.
15. Rinderknecht H: Pancreatic secretory enzymes. In Go VLW, Gardner JD, DiMagno EP, et al (eds): The Exocrine Pancreas: Biology, Pathobiology and Disease, 2nd ed. New York, Raven, 1993, p 219.
16. Kassell B, Kay J: Zymogens of proteolytic enzymes. Science 1809: 1022, 1973.
17. Pubols MH, Bartelt DC, Greene LJ: The trypsin inhibitor from human pancreas and pancreatic juice. J Biol Chem 249:2235, 1974.
18. Whitcomb DC, Gorry MC, Preston RA, et al: Hereditary pancreatitis is caused by mutation in the cationic trypsinogen gene. Nature Genet 14: 141–145, 1996.
19. Meites S, Rogols S: Amylase isoenzymes. CRRC Crit Rev Clin Lab Sci 2:103–138, 1971.
20. Chenu C, Berteloot A: Allosterism and $Na(^+)$-D-glucose cotransport kinetics in rabbit jejunal vesicles: Compatibility with mixed positive and negative cooperatives in a homodimeric or tetrameric structure and experimental evidence for only one transport protein involved. J Membrane Biol 132:95–113, 1993.
21. Tsujita T, Okuda H: Effect of bile salts on the interfacial inactivation of carboxylester lipase. J Lipid Res 31:831, 1993.

22. Kilberg MS, Stevens BR, Novak DA: Recent advances in mammalian amino acid transport. Ann Rev Nutr 13:137–165, 1993.
23. Scheele GA, Kern HF: Cellular compartmentation, protein processing, and secretion in the exocrine pancreas. In Go VOW, Gardner JD, DiMagno EP, et al (eds): The Exocrine Pancreas: Biology, Pathobiology and Disease, 2nd ed. New York, Raven, 1993, p 121.
24. Farquhar MG: Progress in unraveling pathways of Golgi traffic. Ann Rev Cell Biol 1:447, 1985.
25. Hille-Rehfeld A: Mannose 6-phosphate receptors in sorting and transport of lysosomal enzymes. Biochim Biophys Acta 1241:177–194, 1995.
26. Le Borne R, Hoflack B: Protein transport from the secretory to the endocytic pathway in mammalian cells. Biochim Biophys Acta 1404: 195–209, 1998.
27. Poucell-Hatton S, Perkins PS, Deernick TJ, et al: Myosin I is associated with zymogen granule membranes in the rat pancreatic acinar cell. Gastroenterology 113:649–658, 1997.
28. Valentijn JA, Valentijn K, Patore LM, et al: Actin coating of secretory granules during regulated exocytosis correlates with the release of rab3D. Proc Natl Acad Sci USA 97:1091–1095, 2000.
29. Hansen NJ, Antonin W, Edwardson JM: Identification of SNAREs involved in regulated exocytosis in the pancreatic acinar cell. J Biol Chem 274:22871–22876, 1999.
30. Ohnishi H, Mine T, Shibata H, et al: Involvement of Rab4 in regulated exocytosis of rat pancreatic acini. Gastroenterology 116:943–952, 1999.
31. Padfield PJ, Panesar N: The two phases of regulated exocytosis in permeablized pancreatic acini are modulated differently by heterotrimeric G-proteins. Biochem Biophys Res Commun 245:332–336, 1998.
32. Ohnishi H, Ernst SA, Yule DI, et al: Heterotrimeric G-protein Gq/11 localized on pancreatic zymogen granules is involved in calcium-regulated amylase secretion. J Biol Chem 272:16056–16061, 1997.
33. MacDonald RJ, Swift GA: Transgenic analysis of pancreatic secretion and development. In Go VLW, Gardner JD, DiMagno EP, et al (eds): The Exocrine Pancreas: Biology, Pathobiology and Disease, 2nd ed. New York, Raven, 1993, p 87.
34. Brannon PM: Adaptation of the exocrine pancreas to diet. Annu Rev Nutr 10:85–105, 1990.
35. Wank SA, Harkins R, Jensen RT, et al. Purification, molecular cloning, and functional expression of the cholecystokinin receptor from rat pancreas. Proc Natl Acad Sci USA 89:3125, 1992.
36. Pandol SJ, Sutliff VE, Jones SW, et al: Action of natural glucagon on pancreatic acini due to contamination by previously undescribed secretagogues. Am J Physiol 245:G703, 1983.
37. Pandol SJ, Schoeffield MS, Sachs G, Muallem S: Role of free cytosolic calcium in secretagogue-stimulated amylase release from dispersed acini from guinea pig pancreas. J Biol Chem 260:1008, 1985.
38. Pandol SJ, Schoeffield MS: 1,2-Diacyglycerol, protein kinase C, and pancreatic enzyme secretion. J Biol Chem 261:4438, 1986.
39. Fitzsimmons TJ, McRoberts JA, Tachiki K, Pandol SJ: The role of fatty acid-CoA esters in Ca^{2+} signaling in the pancreatic acinar cell. J Biol Chem 272:31425–31440, 1997.
40. Fitzsimmons TJ, Gukovsky I, McRoberts JA, et al: Multiple isoforms of the ryanodine receptor are expressed in rat pancreatic acinar cells. Biochem J 351:265–271, 2000.
41. Bahnson TD, Pandol SJ, Dionne VE: Cyclic GMP modulates depletion-activated Ca^{2+} entry in pancreatic acinar cells. J Biochem 268:10808–10812, 1993.
42. Gukovskaya A, Pandol SJ: Nitric oxide production regulates cGMP formation and calcium influx in pancreatic acinar cells. Am J Physiol 266:G350, 1994.
43. Pandol SJ, Hsu Y, Kondratenki NF, et al: Dual pathways for agonist-stimulated arachidonic acid release in exocrine pancreas: Possible roles in secretion. Am J Physiol 26:G423, 1991.
44. Solomon TE: Control of exocrine pancreatic secretion. In Johnson LR, Alpers DH, Christensen J, et al (eds): Physiology of the Gastrointestinal Tract, 3rd ed. New York, Raven, 1994, p 1499.
45. Itoh Z: Motilin and clinical application. Peptides 18:593–608, 1997.
46. Fox JA: Control of gastrointestinal motility by peptides: Old peptides, new tricks—new peptides, old tricks. Gastroenterol Clin North Am 18: 163–177, 1989.
47. Anagnostides A, Chadwick VS, Selden AC, Maton PN: Sham feeding and pancreatic secretion. Evidence for direct vagal stimulation of output. Gastroenterology 87:109, 1984.
48. Katschinski M, Dahmen G, Reinshagen M, et al: Cephalic stimulation of gastrointestinal secretory and motor responses in humans. Gastroenterology 103:383, 1992.
49. Holst JJ, Schaffalitzky de Muckadell OB, Fahrenkrug J: Nervous control of pancreatic exocrine secretion in pigs. Acta Physiol Scand 105: 33, 1979.
50. Holst JJ, Knuhtsen S, Skak-Nielse T: The role of gastrin-releasing peptide in pancreatic exocrine secretion. Ann NY Acad Sci 547:234, 1988.
51. Chey WY, Konturek SJ: Plasma secretin and pancreatic secretion in response to liver extract meal with varied pH and exogenous secretin in the dog. J Physiol 324:263, 1982.
52. Meyer JH, Way LW, Grossman MI: Pancreatic bicarbonate response to various acids in duodenum of dog. Am J Physiol 219:964, 1970.
53. Chey WY, Kim MS, Lee KY, Chang TM: Effect of rabbit antisecretin serum on postprandial pancreatic secretion in dogs. Gastroenterology 77:1268, 1979.
54. You CH, Rominger JM, Chey WY: Potentiation effect of cholecystokinin-octapeptide on pancreatic bicarbonate secretion stimulated by physiologic dose of secretin in humans. Gastroenterology 85:40, 1983.
55. You CH, Rominger JM, Chey WY: Effects of atropine on the action and release of secretin in humans. Am J Physiol 242:G608, 1982.
56. Go VLW, Hofmann AF, Summerskill WHJ: Pancreozymin bioassay in man based on pancreatic enzyme secretion: Potency of specific amino acids and other digestive products. J Clin Invest 49:1558, 1970.
57. Meyer JH, Kelley GA, Spingola LJ, Jones RS: Canine gut receptors mediating pancreatic responses to luminal L-amino acids. Am J Physiol 231:669, 1976.
58. Singer MV, Solomon TE, Grossman MI: Effect of atropine on secretion from intact and transplanted pancreas in the dog. Am J Physiol 238: G18, 1980.
59. Liddle RA, Goldfine ID, Rosen MS, et al: Cholecystokinin bioactivity in human plasma. Molecular forms, responses to feeding, and relationship to gallbladder contraction. J Clin Invest 75:1144, 1985.
60. Hildebrand P, Beglinger C, Gyr K, et al: Effects of a cholecystokinin receptor antagonist on intestinal phase of pancreatic and biliary responses in man. J Clin Invest 85:640, 1990.
61. Li Y, Hao Y, Owyang D: High-affinity CCK-A receptors on the vagus nerve mediate CCK-stimulated pancreatic secretion in rats. Am J Physiol 273:G679–685, 1997.
62. Green GM, Lyman RL: Feedback regulation of pancreatic enzyme secretion as mechanism for trypsin inhibitor induced hypersecretion in rats. Proc Soc Exp Biol Med 140:6, 1972.
63. Louie DS, May D, Miller P, Owyang D: Cholecystokinin mediates feedback regulation of pancreatic enzyme secretion in rats. Am J Physiol 250:G252, 1986.
64. Liddle RA: Regulation of cholecystokinin secretion by intraluminal releasing factors. Am J Physiol 269:G319, 1995.
65. Spannagel AW, Green GM, Guan D, et al: Purification and characterization of a luminal cholecystokinin-releasing factor from rat intestinal secretion. Proc Natl Acad Sci USA 93:4415–4420, 1996.
66. Li P, Chang T-M, Chey WY: Neuronal regulation of the release and action of secretin-releasing peptide and secretion. Am J Physiol 269: G305, 1995.
67. Jung G, Louie DS, Owyang D: Pancreatic polypeptide inhibits pancreatic enzyme secretion via a cholinergic pathway. Am J Physiol 253: G706, 1987.
68. DiMagno EP, Go VLW, Summerskill WHJ: Relations between pancreatic enzyme outputs and malabsorption in severe pancreatic insufficiency. N Engl J Med 288:813, 1973.
69. Niederau C, Grendell JH: Diagnosis of chronic pancreatitis. Gastroenterology 88:1973, 1985.
70. Hansky J, Tiscornia OM, Dreiling DA, Janowitz HD: Relationship between maximal secretory output and weight of the pancreas in the dog. Proc Soc Exp Biol Med 114:654, 1963.
71. Boyd EJ, Wormsley KG: Laboratory tests in the diagnosis of chronic pancreatic disease: Part 1. Secretagogues used in tests of pancreatic secretion. Int J Pancreatol 2:137, 1987.
72. Heiji HA, Obertop H, Schmitz PIM, et al: Evaluation of the secretin-cholecystokinin test for chronic pancreatitis by discriminant analysis. Scand J Gastroenterol 21:35, 1986.
73. Lundh G: Pancreatic exocrine function in neoplastic and inflammatory disease: A simple and reliable new test. Gastroenterology 42:275, 1962.
74. Newcomer AD, Hofmann AF, DiMagno EP, et al: Triolein breath test: A sensitive and specific test for fat malabsorption. Gastroenterology 76: 6, 1979.
75. Lankisch PG: Function tests in the diagnosis of chronic pancreatitis. Critical evaluation. Int J Pancreatol 14:9, 1993.

Chapter 47

Hereditary and Childhood Disorders of the Pancreas, Including Cystic Fibrosis

David C. Whitcomb

New information from the Human Genome Project, developmental biology, and molecular genetics has resulted in new discoveries and insights encompassing all aspects of pancreatic structure, function, and disease. This chapter focuses on these new findings within the context of the dynamic field of inherited and childhood disorders of the pancreas (Table 47–1). Most experts now recognize that genetic predispositions to pancreatic disorders affect both children and adults. Although genetic predispositions were historically more evident in children without the confounding factors of excessive alcohol consumption or gallstone disease commonly seen in adults, the availability of genetic testing has uncovered the importance of inherited factors in all age groups. Thus, new paradigms in the diagnosis, classification, and staging of pancreatic disorders are emerging,[1] and new strategies for prevention or early treatment of pancreatic diseases are being developed.

The primary focus of this chapter is on recent advances in our understanding of pancreatic disorders associated with mutations in key pancreatic genes and on common acquired pancreatic diseases in children. Understanding the role of developmental genes in human disease remains in its infancy, but emerging evidence suggests that altered function plays a role in developmental malformations and rare congenital disorders. The cystic fibrosis transmembrane conductance regulator gene *(CFTR)*, the cationic trypsinogen gene (*CT*, UniGene name: protease, serine, 1; *PRSS1*), and the pancreatic secretory trypsin inhibitor gene (*PSTI*, UniGene name: serine protease inhibitor, Kazal type 1; *SPINK1*) are clearly associated with human disease and are discussed in more detail. Finally, information on acute pancreatitis in children is reviewed.

GENETIC BASIS OF CONGENITAL DISORDERS OF MORPHOGENESIS

Overview of Embryology

Embryology and developmental biology play important roles in understanding many of the mechanisms that lead to human disease. This topic is covered in detail in Chapter 45. A brief review is presented here as an introduction to inherited developmental abnormalities.

In humans, the pancreas develops from two outpouchings (anlagen or buds) of the duodenal portion of the foregut during the 5th week of life.[2] As the foregut rotates, the ventral anlage and common bile duct move around to the right and behind the developing duodenum to merge with the dorsal anlage, thereby forming a single pancreas during the 7th week of gestation (see Chapter 45). The dorsal anlage therefore forms the body and tail of the pancreas,

Table 47–1 | **Hereditary and Congenital Disorders of the Exocrine Pancreas**

DISORDER	DEFECT
Exocrine Pancreatic Insufficiency	
Pancreatic agenesis	*PDXI* (recessive)
Cystic fibrosis	Two severe *CFTR* mutations (recessive)
Shwachman-Diamond syndrome	Unknown (recessive, chromosome 7 locus)
Johanson-Blizzard syndrome	Unknown (recessive)
Pearson's marrow-pancreas syndrome	Mitochondrial DNA defects
Isolated enzyme deficiency	Various
Pancreatitis	
Hereditary/familial	40% unknown
	Cationic trypsinogen (dominant)
	SPINK1 (complex)
	Mild *CFTR* mutations (recessive)
Metabolic	
Hyperlipidemias	Liproprotein lipase
	Apolipoprotein C-II
Hyperparathyroidism	
Miscellaneous	

whereas the ventral anlage forms the pancreatic head. The two duct systems usually merge to form a single pancreatic duct that joins the common bile duct at the ampulla of Vater.

The development of the pancreas from the embryonic gut depends on organized signaling between specific endodermal and mesodermal cells. Surprisingly, only a few gene products appear to direct cell differentiation toward pancreatic cells rather than duodenal, biliary, or liver cells.[3] For example, the early pancreatic bud shows uniform expression of the pancreatic and duodenal homeobox 1 gene (*PDX1*, previously known as *IPF1*[4]). This gene is clearly important because pdx1−/− (*PDX1* "knockout") mice have early developmental arrest of the pancreatic epithelium and failure of differentiation.[5, 6] In contrast, the sonic hedgehog (*Shh*) gene is expressed throughout the embryonic gut endoderm *except* in the pancreatic bud endoderm.[7, 8] When expression of the *Shh* gene is forced within the region of the future pancreas by fusing it with the *PDX1* promoter in transgenic mice, the pancreatic mesoderm develops into smooth muscle and interstitial cells of Cajal, characteristic of the intestine, rather than into pancreatic mesenchyme and spleen.[7]

Subsequent pancreatic growth and development proceed along a well-defined pathway from pancreas-committed pluripotential stem cells that can generate duct cells, acinar cells, or endocrine cells.[2, 9–14] Additional developmental genes play key roles in determining the fate of the pancreatic stem cells.[11–14] Even at birth the pancreatic exocrine function is immature[15] and may remain so through the 1st year of life.[16] Indeed, healthy infants (<6 months of age) may have physiologic steatorrhea.[16] Thus, the pathway to development of the mature pancreas extends from early gestation through infancy.

Conditions in which the pancreas or portions of the pancreas fail to develop are rare. However, they often provide insights into pancreatic development and may be an important part of defined syndromes. At other times they may be incidental findings. Examples of these syndromes include agenesis and hypoplasia of the pancreas, agenesis of the dorsal pancreas, agenesis of the ventral pancreas, and annular pancreas. A common disorder, heterotopic pancreatic tissue, is also considered here.

Pancreatic Agenesis and Hypoplasia

Agenesis of the pancreas (Online Mendelian Inheritance in Man [OMIM] No. 260370[17]) is extremely rare, with about 10 cases reported in the literature.[18, 19] In one case, genetic testing identified a homozygous nucleotide deletion in the *PDX1* gene resulting in premature termination of the *PDX1* gene production. Thus, absence of *PDX1* is a probable cause of pancreatic agenesis.[20] The clinical features of pancreatic agenesis include intrauterine growth retardation (probably from insulin deficiency), insulin-dependent diabetes, and pancreatic exocrine insufficiency. The differential diagnosis includes transient diabetes mellitus of the newborn, pancreatic hypoplasia, cystic fibrosis, Shwachman-Diamond syndrome, Johanson-Blizzard syndrome, and other rare disorders. However, with pancreatic agenesis the profound endocrine and exocrine deficiencies persist, serum C-peptide and glucagon are undetectable, and the pancreas is absent on imaging studies. These children are managed as having type 1 diabetes mellitus (treated with insulin) and severe pancreatic maldigestion (treated with pancreatic enzyme supplementation).[19, 20] Survival is possible with proper diagnosis and treatment.[19, 20]

Pancreatic hypoplasia is another genetic developmental disorder that is limited to the pancreas. The clinical features are similar to those of pancreatic agenesis, with intrauterine growth retardation, early-onset insulin-dependent diabetes mellitus, and pancreatic exocrine insufficiency, albeit in a milder form and later onset.[21] The inherited basis of this disorder was suggested by two brothers with low birth weights, early-onset insulin-dependent diabetes, and pancreatic exocrine insufficiency.[21] In contrast to the findings in pancreatic agenesis, their serum C-peptide and glucagon levels were measurable, suggesting that some endocrine cells had developed. The clinical management of these patients is that of patients with insulin-dependent diabetes mellitus and pancreatic insufficiency.

Agenesis of the Dorsal Pancreas

Agenesis of the dorsal pancreas (OMIM No. 16775517) is also extremely rare, with at least 15 cases reported.[22] A case of fatty replacement of the pancreatic body and tail was reported,[23] which may be a variant of this disorder. Unlike complete agenesis of the pancreas, patients may be asymptomatic or may present with bile duct obstruction or pancreatitis. The genetic basis of this syndrome in humans is unknown, and gene knockout experiments in mice failed to translate into answers for the human condition; that is, homeobox gene *HLXB9* knockout mice have agenesis of the dorsal pancreas,[24, 25] whereas humans with biallelic *HLXB9* gene mutations have sacral agenesis (Currarino's syndrome) and apparently normal pancreases.[26]

Agenesis of the Ventral Pancreas

Agenesis and hypoplasia of the ventral pancreas are extremely rare.[27] Agenesis of the ventral pancreas is sometimes seen in Cumming's syndrome,[28] a rare autosomal recessive disorder affecting laterality and associated with multiple developmental abnormalities.

Annular Pancreas

Annular pancreas (OMIM No. 167750[17]) is a rare congenital abnormality in which a band of pancreatic tissue encircles the second portion of the duodenum.[18] This disorder is covered in more detail in Chapters 36 and 45. Although annular pancreas is detected at a rate of only 0.03 per 1000 live births, it is commonly seen in Down syndrome with a rate of 14 per 1000 births.[29] Indeed, annular pancreas is commonly associated with other congenital abnormalities, including tracheoesophageal fistula, esophageal atresia, duodenal webs, imperforate anus, and Hirschsprung's disease,[18, 30] which are also common in Down syndrome.[29] Theories as to the origin of the annular pancreas center on fixation of the ventral pancreas before gut rotation or duplication of the ventral pancreatic bud during development, and others,[8, 18, 31] although the actual mechanism remains unproved. The observations that the risk of annular pancreas is increased 300-fold to 400-fold in the genetically confounded Down syndrome,[29, 32] that annular pancreas is usually associated with other developmental defects,[18] and that a similar phenotype is seen in mice with inactivation of genes important for pancreatic development[8] suggest that a genetic factor may contribute to development of this abnormality. Indeed, familial aggregation of annular pancreas has been reported, following both autosomal dominant[33–35] and autosomal recessive[36, 37] patterns.

The primary clinical feature of annular pancreas is abdominal pain and vomiting caused by duodenal stenosis.[18, 30] The diagnosis can be made in a vomiting infant with the "double-bubble" sign on an abdominal radiograph, caused by high-grade duodenal stenosis and air in the stomach and first portion of the (dilated) duodenum[18] (see Chapter 45). Annular pancreas is discovered during surgery for duodenal stenosis or atresia in about one third of cases.[38] However, annular pancreas can also be an incidental finding in an otherwise healthy adult or in adults with years of nausea and vomiting and a mid-duodenal stenosis. On upper gastrointestinal contrast studies, the diagnosis of annular pancreas is considered with an annular filling defect across the second portion of the duodenum, symmetrical dilation of the proximal duodenum, and reverse peristalsis of the duodenal segment proximal to the annulus[18] (Fig. 47–1). Although annular pancreas can be diagnosed by a variety of abdominal imaging techniques such as computed tomography (CT), endoscopic retrograde cholangiopancreatography (ERCP) has been considered the most useful diagnostic tool.[30] Magnetic resonance imaging (MRI) and MR cholangiopancreatography (MRCP) may play a greater diagnostic role in the future as technology continues to improve.[39]

The primary treatment for symptomatic annular pancreas is surgical. Although the pancreatic ring can be surgically divided, this approach is associated with increased complications and mortality.[18] Furthermore, strictures and webs in the distal portion of the duodenum and jejunum are also common and require specific attention. Therefore, surgical bypass of the stenosis via duodenoduodenostomy has been advocated in children with isolated duodenal stenosis,[18] with more extensive bypass procedures used when technically necessary.

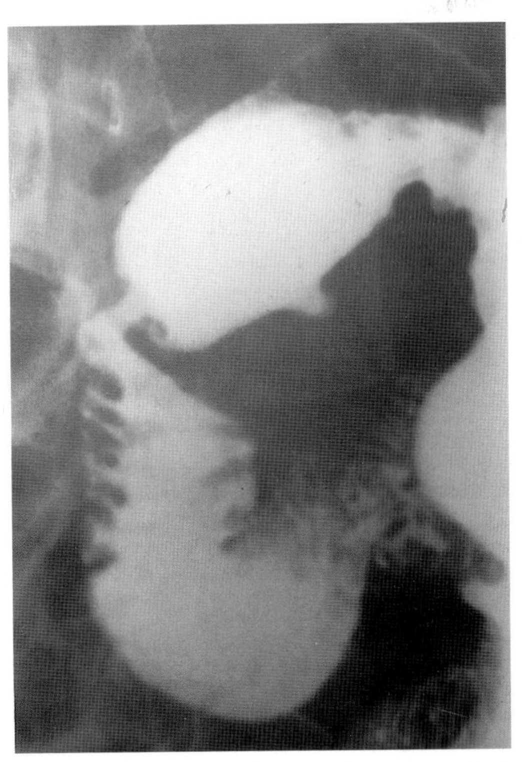

Figure 47–1. Duodenal stricture from annular pancreas. Barium contrast upper gastrointestinal tract radiographic series demonstrating a mid-duodenal stricture with proximal dilatation of the duodenum. Annular pancreas was identified on CT scan and confirmed during surgery. (Courtesy of Michael Federle, M.D.)

Heterotopic Pancreatic Tissue

Heterotopic, ectopic, or aberrant pancreatic tissue, or pancreatic rest, is defined as the presence of pancreatic tissue that lacks anatomic and vascular continuity with the main body of the pancreas.[18] Focal expression of pancreatic cells outside of the pancreatic gland appears to be relatively common in humans and is observed on careful histologic examination of 1% to 14% of autopsy cases.[18, 40, 41] It is rarely of clinical significance. Heterotopic pancreatic tissue is usually seen in the stomach (60% to 70%), duodenum, and jejunum (38% to 45%), but foci of pancreatic tissue have been reported in Meckel's diverticulum, the appendix, omentum, and other locations.[42–44] Small foci of heterotopic pancreatic tissue can also be seen in the large and medium-sized portal tracts in about 4% of human livers.[41] Pancreatic acinar tissue can also be identified with special staining of gastroesophageal junction biopsies in 16% to 24% of healthy subjects.[45]

Heterotopic pancreatic tissue usually appears as discrete, firm, yellow submucosal nodules from 2 mm to 4 cm in diameter.[18] Submucosal lesions in the stomach and duodenum usually have a central umbilication (Fig. 47–2; see also Color Fig. 47–2). However, the diagnosis must be made histologically to exclude adenomatous polyps, leiomyomas, lymphomas, carcinomas, or other entities.[18] Histologically, the heterotopic tissue contains pancreatic excretory ducts, most containing exocrine glands; islets of Langerhans are present in 33% to 84% of specimens examined.[18, 44]

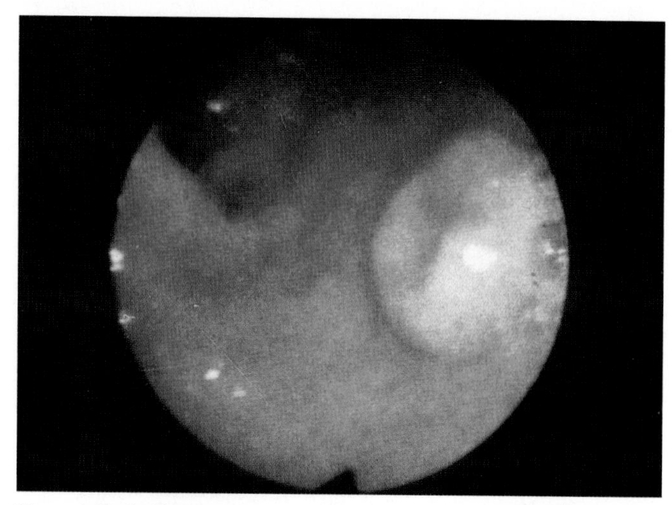

Figure 47–2. Heterotopic pancreas (pancreatic rest). Typical endoscopic image of heterotopic pancreatic tissue in the stomach. Note the submucosal location of the heterotopic pancreatic tissue mass with central umbilication.

Heterotopic pancreatic tissue is usually asymptomatic[40] and discovered during evaluation for unrelated problems. Symptoms usually arise from complications such as obstruction of the common bile duct, mucosal ulcer with hemorrhage, intussusception, or intestinal obstruction.[44] About 30 cases of pancreatic cancer arising in heterotopic pancreatic tissue have been reported.[42]

The management of heterotopic pancreatic tissue has been controversial because it is usually of no clinical significance. When complications occur, surgical excision is curative.[44] Surgical excision should be considered if there is doubt of the diagnosis or if the lesion is large.[18, 46]

DUCTAL ABNORMALITIES

During embryogenesis the main duct of the ventral pancreatic anlage (duct of Santorini) and the main duct of the dorsal pancreatic anlage (duct of Wirsung) usually fuse, after which the proximal portion of the duct of Santorini (accessory duct) involutes, resulting in a single pancreatic duct. However, this "normal" duct anatomy occurs in only about 60% to 70% of the population[18] and several variants are common.[18, 47, 48] Clinically, the most important variants are pancreas divisum, common channel syndrome, and syndromes with choledochal cysts (see Chapters 45 and 52).

INHERITED SYNDROMES WITH MAJOR PANCREATIC MANIFESTATIONS

Mutations in several known and unknown genes result in specific syndromes that affect the pancreas and other specific tissues. The most important syndrome is cystic fibrosis because of its high prevalence. Rare syndromes, including Shwachman-Diamond syndrome, Johanson-Blizzard syndrome, Pearson's marrow-pancreas syndrome, and other disorders, are also recognized and discussed here. Gene mutations that predispose patients to acquired acute and chronic pancreatitis are considered in the subsequent section.

Cystic Fibrosis

Cystic fibrosis (OMIN No. 2197000[17]) is the most common lethal genetic defect of white populations. Expected survival for typical children with cystic fibrosis born up to the early 1960s was only a matter of months. Fortunately, with digestive enzyme supplementation and improved pulmonary care and nutrition, the prognosis has dramatically improved, with median survival extending beyond 30 years of age.[49] Although cystic fibrosis affects many organs, the primary focus of this chapter is manifestations of cystic fibrosis transmembrane conductance regulator (CFTR) gene mutations in the pancreas, with brief discussions of liver and intestinal problems that are also seen by the gastroenterologist. The role of *CFTR* mutations in idiopathic chronic pancreatitis is considered in Chapter 49 as well as the following section on gene mutations predisposing to acute and chronic pancreatitis.

Clinical Features of "Typical" Cystic Fibrosis

Typical cystic fibrosis is recognized and diagnosed in about 60% of affected individuals during the first year of life and in 85% before age 5 years.[16, 50] The early clinical features are those of maldigestion or other pancreatic and intestinal manifestations of *CFTR* mutations, while the latter course is dominated by pulmonary complications. A small percentage remain undiagnosed until early adulthood.[16, 50] The presenting features during infancy include meconium ileus, malabsorption with frequent foul stools, failure to thrive, or rectal prolapse.[16] Pulmonary function is normal in patients with cystic fibrosis at birth[16] but accounts for much of the morbidity and almost all of the mortality associated with cystic fibrosis beyond the neonatal period.[16, 50] The severity of lung disease depends on known and unknown factors, including chronic infection with *Pseudomonas aeruginosa* and nutritional status, and probably the effect of unidentified modifier genes because severity of lung disease differs among patients with identical *CFTR* genotypes. The phenotype-genotype relationship between some childhood disorders and *CFTR* mutations is often striking, with severe *CFTR* mutations detected in more than 85% of all children presenting with pancreatic insufficiency and most infants presenting with meconium ileus.[51–53] In older patients, presenting symptoms of cystic fibrosis may include pulmonary disease, nasal polyps, male infertility, liver disease, recurrent acute pancreatitis, or chronic pancreatitis,[16, 50, 54] although the prevalence of *CFTR* mutations in patients these common disorders is much lower. A careful family history may also provide important clues to the diagnosis of cystic fibrosis.

Clinical confirmation of the diagnosis rests on demonstration of elevated concentrations of chloride in sweat[55] (Table 47–2) or demonstration of an abnormal nasal bioelectric response in specific testing protocols[56] reflecting abnormal *CFTR* function. When performed appropriately, these tests are reliable. However, both false-positive and false-negative results are seen in newborns, in patients with malnutrition, in the presence of some medications, or if inadequate sweat is obtained[50] (Table 47–3). Thus, most experts insist on use of standardized methods performed at cystic fibrosis centers performing the test frequently. The consensus of a Cystic

Table 47–2 | **Indications for the Sweat Test (Quantitative Pilocarpine Iontophoresis)**

Siblings with cystic fibrosis
Chronic pulmonary symptoms
  Cough
  Recurrent respiratory infection
  Bronchitis
  Bronchiectasis
  Lobar atelectasis
Failure to thrive (stunting of growth)
Rectal prolapse
Nasal polyposis
Intestinal obstruction of newborn
Meconium ileus
Jaundice in early infancy
Cirrhosis in childhood or adolescence
Portal hypertension
Adult males with aspermia or azoospermia
Heat stroke
Hypoproteinemia
Hypoprothrombinemia

Fibrosis Foundation panel suggested a diagnosis of cystic fibrosis could be made by the presence of one or more characteristic clinical features, a history of cystic fibrosis in a sibling, or a positive newborn screening test result with confirmation by laboratory evidence of *CFTR* dysfunction.[57] Furthermore, the panel suggested that either sweat chloride or nasal bioelectrical responses should be abnormal on two separate days before the diagnosis is confirmed by one of these methods.[57] Genetic testing is also commercially available to confirm the clinical diagnosis (two severe mutations must be identified), but these results cannot always be interpreted apart from the clinical context and functional testing—especially in cases with atypical symptoms.

Molecular Defects

The molecular defects underlying cystic fibrosis result in alterations in epithelial cell electrolyte transport. In a landmark series of genetic studies it was discovered that cystic fibrosis was an autosomal recessive disorder caused by severe mutations in the *CFTR* gene located on chromosome 7q32.[58] The *CFTR* gene contains more than 4300 nucleotides, divided into 24 exons that code for a single protein of 1480 amino acids.[58] The protein is a chloride channel with 12 membrane-spanning domains, two nucleotide-binding folds, and a regulatory domain (R domain) that is activated by cyclic adenosine monophosphate. *CFTR* also regulates other ion channels in the same cell, including the amiloride-sensitive epithelial sodium channel.[53, 59] Major mutations in *both CFTR* alleles result in loss of *CFTR* function. The consequences include an inability to adequately hydrate mucus and other macromolecules leading to accumulation of viscid material and inspissated glands resulting in progressive organ destruction of the respiratory system, pancreas, and dysfunction of the liver, intestine, sweat glands, and other sites where epithelial cell secretion plays an important physiologic role.

The overall clinical picture in an individual case depends on the nature of the combined *CFTR* mutations, the genetic background in which the defective genes operate (e.g., modifier genes), and environmental factors.[53] About 70% of white patients with cystic fibrosis have a three-base-pair deletion of the phenylalanine-coding codon 508 (ΔF508), although nearly 1000 other mutations have been reported.[53, 60, 61] Blacks may have their own set of common cystic fibrosis mutations that originate from the native African population, including the 3120+1G>A mutation occurring with a frequency of 12.3% in a representative population.[62] Patients with one severe *CFTR* mutation and one mild *CFTR* mutation (e.g., R117H) may have pancreatic insufficiency.[16] Cystic fibrosis patients with typical *CFTR* mutations on chromosome 7 plus a modifier gene mutation on chromosome 19 are more likely to develop meconium ileus.[63] Environmental factors such as bacterial colonization of the respiratory system, tobacco smoke,[64] and nutritional status contribute to the severity of lung disease.[65] Thus, careful consideration must be given to patients with either classic cystic fibrosis symptoms or atypical presentations resulting from less common combinations of genetic and environmental factors.

The mutations in the *CFTR* gene have been classified based on their mechanistic defect (Table 47–4). Mutations affecting synthesis (class 1), maturation and trafficking (class 2), or activation (class 3) yield little or no functional protein and are considered severe mutations.[53, 66] Mutations that alter conductance (class 4) and protein abundance (class 5) diminish, but do not eliminate, *CFTR* function are considered mild

Table 47–3 | **Conditions Reported with Elevated Sweat Electrolyte Concentrations**

Cystic fibrosis
Ectodermal dysplasia
Glycogen storage disease, type 1
Adrenal insufficiency
Familial hypoparathyroidism
Fucosidosis
Pitressin-resistant diabetes insipidus
Mucopolysaccharidosis
Familial cholestasis syndrome
Environmental deprivation syndrome
Acute respiratory disorders (croup, epiglottitis, viral pneumonia)
Chronic respiratory disorders (bronchopulmonary dysplasia, α_1-antitrypsin deficiency)

Adapted from Christoffel K, Lloyd-Still J, Brown G, Schwachman H: Environmental deprivation and transient elevation of sweat electrolytes. J Pediatr 107:231, 1985.

Table 47–4 | **Classification for *CFTR* Mutations, Defect and Degree of Pancreatic Dysfunction**

CLASS	MUTATION (EXAMPLE)	DEFECT	PANCREAS DYSFUNCTION
1	W1282X	Synthesis	Severe
2	ΔF508	Maturation	Severe
3	G551D	Activation	Severe
4	R117H	Conductance	Mild
5	5T	Abundance	Mild
6	ΔF508, G551D	Regulation of other channels	Variable

Modified from Mickle JE, Cutting GR: Genotype-phenotype relationships in cystic fibrosis. Med Clin North Am 84:597–607, 2000; and Zielinski J, Tsui LC: Cystic fibrosis: Genotypic and phenotypic variations. Annu Rev Genet 29:777–807, 1995.

Table 47–5 | **Clinical Manifestations of Cystic Fibrosis**

- Viscid secretions: small duct obstruction
- Respiratory: upper
  - Sinusitis
  - Mucous membrane hypertrophy: nasal polyposis
- Respiratory: lower
  - Atelectasis
  - Emphysema
  - Infections
    - Bronchitis
    - Bronchopneumonia, bronchiectasis, lung abscess
  - Respiratory failure, right heart failure
- Gastrointestinal
  - Gastroesophageal reflux
  - Peptic ulcer disease
  - Meconium ileus
  - Volvulus
  - Peritonitis
  - Ileal atresia
  - Distal intestinal obstruction syndrome
    - Fecal masses
    - Intussusception
    - Obstruction
  - Rectal prolapse
- Pancreas
  - Nutritional failure caused by pancreatic insufficiency
  - Diabetes
  - Calcification
  - Maldigestion
  - Vitamin deficiencies
  - Loss of bile salts
  - Steatorrhea and azotorrhea
- Hepatobiliary
  - Mucus hypersecretion
  - Gallstones, atrophic gallbladder
  - Focal biliary cirrhosis
  - Cirrhosis
  - Portal hypertension
  - Esophageal varices
    - Hypersplenism
- Reproductive system
  - Females: increased viscosity of vaginal mucus and decreased fertility
  - Males: sterility; absent ductus deferens, epididymis, and seminal vesicles
- Skeletal
  - Retardation of bone age
  - Demineralization
  - Hypertrophic pulmonary osteoarthropathy
- Eye
  - Venous engorgement
  - Retinal hemorrhage
- Other
  - Salt depletion through excessive loss of salt through skin
  - Heat stroke
  - Hypertrophy of apocrine glands

mutations and are often associated with pancreatic sufficiency or atypical cystic fibrosis.[53, 66] Some mutations affect the ability of *CFTR* to regulate other channels (class 6[53]). Finally, there are numerous silent mutations (no amino acid base change), intronic and exonic polymorphisms and mutations with unknown significance. In general, the *less* severe of the two mutations dictates the phenotype of autosomal recessive disorders such as cystic fibrosis and thus determines the phenotypic classification.

Patients with cystic fibrosis also inherit a cohort of other genes and gene mutations from their parents. Some of these genes may modify the cystic fibrosis phenotype (modifier genes). Assessing the contribution of other genes in cystic fibrosis remains difficult in human populations because of the high degree of genetic diversity.[53] However, clues from animal models have provided critical insights into some clinical features such as meconium ileus. By crossbreeding homozygous *CFTR*-mutant mice and mapping the genetic tendency toward fatal intestinal obstruction, a cystic fibrosis modifier locus for meconium ileus was localized.[67] The syntenic region to this region in humans is chromosome 19.[63] The meconium ileus modifier gene was then proved to be linked to the chromosome 19q13 region. The final identification of this modifier gene or genes will likely provide significant insight into both cystic fibrosis and intestinal pathophysiology. Likewise, mutations in other genes increase the risk of liver disease in cystic fibrosis patients. Some *CFTR* mutations may modify other *CFTR* mutations. Examples include the R553Q-ΔF508/ΔF508 phenotype, which partially reverses the ΔF508 phenotype, or the R117H-intron 8 5T allele (*in cis*), which confers tissue specific variations in expression of the mild R117H mutant *CFTR* protein.[53] Taken together, the various combinations of *CFTR* mutations, modifier genes, and environmental factors confirm significant risk for developing a variety of conditions including chronic pancreatitis, congenital bilateral absence of the vas deferens (CBAVD) with male infertility, disseminated bronchiectasis, chronic sinusitis, or other disorders without typical cystic fibrosis[53, 68, 69] (Table 47–5). The frequencies of the various gastrointestinal manifestations of cystic fibrosis are listed in Table 47–6.

Pancreatic Pathology in Cystic Fibrosis

Eighty-five percent to 90% of patients with cystic fibrosis present with evidence of exocrine pancreatic dysfunction.

Table 47–6 | **Frequency of Gastrointestinal Manifestations in Cystic Fibrosis**

ORGAN	COMPLICATION	FREQUENCY (%)
Pancreas	Total achylia	85–90*
	Partial or normal function	10–15*
	Pancreatitis	1
	Abnormal glucose tolerance	20–30
	Diabetes	4–7
Intestine	Meconium ileus	10–15
	Rectal prolapse	1–2
	Distal intestinal obstruction syndrome	3
	Intussusception	1
	Pneumatosis intestinalis	‡
	? Mucosal dysfunction	‡
Liver	Fatty liver	7†
	Focal biliary cirrhosis	2–3
	Portal hypertension	2–3
Biliary tract	Gallbladder abnormal, nonfunctional, or small	25
	Gallstones	8†
	Cholecystitis	‡
	Bile duct strictures	1–20†
Esophagus	Gastroesophageal reflux	‡
	Esophagitis	‡

*These manifestations are genotype dependent; actual prevalence is unknown.
†These percentages are primarily from unpublished series of patients (see reference 50).
‡Actual prevalence is unknown.

Although pancreatic dysfunction in an infant with cystic fibrosis may initially appear minimal, it usually progresses to pancreatic exocrine failure. When severely affected, the pancreas is shrunken, cystic, fibrotic, and fatty.[50] Histologically, hyperplasia and eventual necrosis of ductular and centroacinar cells, together with inspissated secretions, lead to blockage of pancreatic ductules and subsequently encroach on acini, causing flattening and atrophy of the epithelium (Fig. 47–3). Cystic spaces are filled with calcium-rich, eosinophilic concretions. A mild inflammatory reaction may be present around obstructed acini, and progressive fibrosis gradually separates and replaces the pancreatic lobules. The islets of Langerhans are spared in most cases until late in the process and are concentrated in the shrinking pancreas.[50] Calcification, although rare, may be apparent on radiographs. Ultrasonography, MRI, and CT scanning all can document the progression of pancreatic disease in cystic fibrosis. Radiographically the pancreas can appear normal, with incomplete or complete lipomatosis, as a cystic pancreas, macrocystic pancreas, or as atrophic pancreas.[70–72] The greatest sensitivity is provided by either MRI or CT scanning, but even with these methods the correlation of abnormalities with the degree of exocrine dysfunction is poor.[50, 70]

Exocrine Pancreas Dysfunction in Cystic Fibrosis

Fat and protein maldigestion with fecal losses are the primary manifestations of pancreatic involvement in cystic fibrosis, although there may be considerable variation in severity from one patient to another.[50] Steatorrhea and azotorrhea are generally greater with pancreatic insufficiency than with mucosal malabsorption. Exocrine pancreatic insufficiency is recognized only when the secretion of lipase and trypsin falls below 10% of normal.[73] Most patients with cystic fibrosis exhibit this pattern of pancreatic insufficiency.

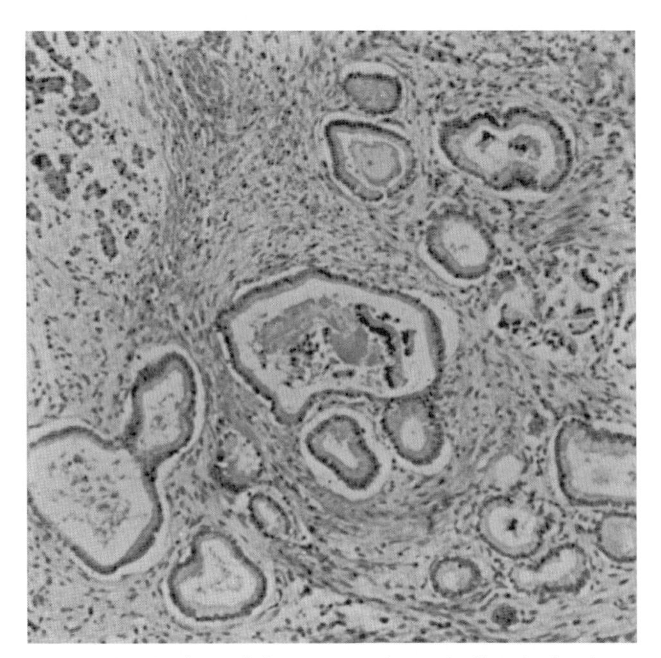

Figure 47–3. Histology of the pancreas in cystic fibrosis showing numerous ectatic ducts plugged with proteinaceous material and surrounded by fibrosis. At the top left, note acini associated with fibrosis.

Recurrent acute pancreatitis may complicate the course of cystic fibrosis in patients who do not have complete loss of pancreatic function in infancy (see also *CFTR* mutations in chronic pancreatitis in the subsequent section on gene mutations predisposing to acute and chronic pancreatitis). Pancreatitis tends to be more problematic in older patients, with the reported incidence among patients older than 30 years being about 2.4%.[74]

Endocrine Pancreas Dysfunction

Glucose intolerance has been reported in 30% to 75% of patients with cystic fibrosis, and clinically significant diabetes mellitus is reported in up to 10% of patients.[75, 76] The previously reported estimates of 1% to 2% incidence[77] may have reflected younger aged patients and poor survival among patients with cystic fibrosis before recent advances in treatment.[76] Cystic fibrosis–related diabetes mellitus develops with increasing age, being uncommon in infants, but increasing to more than 11% in patients older than 10 years[78] and 16% in adults older than 18 years of age.[76] Cystic fibrosis–related diabetes mellitus differs in etiology and presentation from typical type I or type II diabetes mellitus and may reflect destruction of the islets of Langerhans[79] as seen in other forms of chronic pancreatitis. However, the severity of the endocrine deficiency lags behind the exocrine deficiency because the islets are relatively spared until later in the course of pancreatic destruction. Cystic fibrosis–related diabetes mellitus is associated with deterioration in both respiratory and nutritional status, the development of late microvascular complications, and increased mortality.[76] No well-designed studies have addressed this significant problem. However, most experts recognize the need for multidisciplinary team approach, use of a high-energy diet (>100% of normally recommended daily intake), and appropriate adjustment of insulin doses.[76] Overnight enteral feedings may also be necessary to maintain adequate nutrition.

Treatment of Maldigestion

PANCREATIC ENZYME SUPPLEMENTS. Treatment of maldigestion from pancreatic exocrine failure in cystic fibrosis rests on the delivery of active digestive enzymes to the proximal small intestine with meals. Numerous pancreatic preparations are available commercially, but enzyme activities vary considerably from one product to another, and reduced activity of lipase remains a problem for some patients.[80] Enteric-coated microspheres are now the preferred form of replacement because they protect the digestive enzymes from destruction by gastric acid (pH <4) and are effective in treating steatorrhea.[81] The size of the microspheres must be considered. If most of the spheres are too large (>1 mm), emptying of the enzymes can be delayed until after food is well into the small intestine.[82] The use of histamine H_2-receptor blockers or proton pump inhibitors along with uncoated or enteric-coated pancreatic enzyme supplements should also be considered in patients with cystic fibrosis.[83, 84] However, even with optimized treatment, fat absorption may not return completely to normal. In contrast with other forms of pancreatic insufficiency, the bicarbonate secretion within the duodenum and biliary tree is also impaired in cystic fibrosis, resulting in a significantly lower duodenal pH.[85–87] Thus, without acid suppression, the uncoated enzymes are susceptible to inactivation by gastric acid and enteric-coated products may not release their contents.[88] The use of antacids containing calcium carbonate or magnesium hydroxide should be avoided because they may interfere with the pancreatic enzyme supplements.

Initial therapy for pancreatic exocrine insufficiency in cystic fibrosis includes pancreatic enzyme replacement at doses ranging from 500 to 2000 units of lipase activity per kilogram of body weight per meal, given just before a meal and with snacks.[89] The exact dosage depends on the age, the degree of pancreatic insufficiency, the amount of fat ingested, and the commercial preparation chosen. The response to the administered dose in terms of bowel symptoms, growth, or the coefficient of fat absorption determines adequacy. Often, additional pancreatic extract must be given in the middle of a meal.

COMPLICATIONS OF PANCREATIC ENZYME REPLACEMENT. Pancreatic enzyme replacement is not without potential complications. Perioral and perianal irritation are common in infants, although it is less common with the microsphere preparations. Because of the high purine content of pancreatic extracts, hyperuricosuria may develop in some patients taking large doses of enzyme preparations.[90] Powdered preparations of pancreatic extracts have caused immediate hypersensitivity reactions in parents of patients with cystic fibrosis.[91, 92]

Colonic strictures and fibrosing colonopathy have been reported with very-high-dose administration of pancreatic enzymes and have led to a withdrawal of all high-dose formulations of enzymes.[93, 94] Fibrosing colonopathy was first recognized in 1994[93] and nearly disappeared by 1996.[95] It usually develops as an ascending colon stricture causing intestinal obstruction and appears pathologically as postischemic ulceration with mucosal and submucosal fibrosis.[93] Nearly all patients were younger than 12 years of age, had prior gastrointestinal surgery or prior distal intestinal obstruction syndrome, or used H_2-receptor antagonists, corticosteroids, and recombinant human deoxyribonuclease.[94] However, the most striking risk was the use of high doses of lipase-containing enzyme supplements. Compared with that associated with daily doses of pancreatic enzyme supplements containing up to 2400 units of lipase per kilogram per day, the relative risk of fibrosing colonopathy was 10.9 with a daily dose of 2401 to 5000 units of lipase per kilogram per day and 199.5 for patients taking more than 5000 units per kilogram per day.[94] However, because the cases and controls were taken from the same centers where a single brand of enzyme supplement was generally used, it was never conclusively determined whether the problem was related primarily to the lipase content or to the acid-resistant coating of the many capsules that were ingested.

VITAMINS. Vitamin deficiencies may develop as a consequence of fat maldigestion and malabsorption and therefore patients with cystic fibrosis are at risk. Nearly half of all newly diagnosed cystic fibrosis patients have a deficiency of vitamin A, D, and/or E.[96, 97] Vitamin A deficiency in cystic fibrosis rarely manifests with clinical abnormalities.[50] Vitamin D levels are dependent on sunlight exposure and intake, and the bone demineralization seen in older patients with cystic fibrosis may be more a reflection of general malnutrition[50] and postcorticosteroid treatment. Chronic vitamin E deficiency is associated with hemolytic anemia (usually in infants) and neuroaxonal dystrophy with prominent neuromuscular symptoms, although these clinical symptoms appear to be rare.[50] Vitamin K deficiency and the consequent coagulopathy can be seen at any age. Its manifestation may vary from mildly increased bruisability or purpura to catastrophic intracranial hemorrhage in the neonatal period.[98] Patients with cystic fibrosis who have hepatic involvement are particularly prone to coagulation abnormalities secondary to vitamin K deficiency.[98]

Supplementation with pancreatic enzymes, a multivitamin preparation, and additional vitamin E is usually associated with rapid normalization of serum albumin, retinol, and 25-hydroxyvitamin D.[96] However, frequent and serial monitoring of the serum concentrations of fat-soluble vitamins is essential in children with cystic fibrosis because deficiencies may occur during therapy, especially with vitamin E.[97]

Intestinal Manifestations

There are a number of recognized gastrointestinal manifestations of cystic fibrosis (see Table 47–6). Although pancreatic failure and meconium ileus dominate the initial clinical picture, these other manifestations present significant problems in many patients.

PATHOLOGY. The mucosal glands of the small intestine of patients with cystic fibrosis may contain variable quantities of inspissated secretions within the lumen but rarely have increased numbers of goblet cells. Brunner's glands may show dilation, flattening of epithelial lining cells, and stringy secretions within their lumina. Severe alterations in the intestinal glands of the small bowel are found in meconium ileus.[99] However, even in patients without meconium ileus, these findings are common and appear unrelated to the severity of gastrointestinal symptoms or changes in other organs. The small intestinal mucosa in older patients with cystic fibrosis often show widely dilated crypts packed with mucus. Often, the mucus appears laminated or may extrude from a gaping crypt. Bulging goblet cells seem to crowd out the intervening columnar epithelium. Variable cellular infiltration may be present in the lamina propria. Mucus in cystic fibrosis is more abundant, stains more intensely, and contains weaker acidic groups and protein. It has now been shown to have increased fucosylation and sulfation and decreased sialylation.[100–102]

Characteristic changes of cystic fibrosis occur in the appendix. Increased numbers of goblet cells distended with mucus line dilated crypts. Eosinophilic casts of these crypts are extruded into the lumen of the appendix. The diagnosis of cystic fibrosis may be suspected on the basis of the histologic appearance of the appendix.[103] Although chronic changes in the appendix are a common finding at autopsy, the incidence of acute appendicitis is apparently not increased in cystic fibrosis, inasmuch as only about 1.5% of patients in three large series were found to have appendicitis.[104–106] The diagnosis of appendicitis in cystic fibrosis is often delayed and confused with distal intestinal obstruction syndrome, which results in higher frequency of appendiceal perforation found at the time of diagnosis. The use of chronic antibiotics may also mask typical appendiceal signs.[107, 108] A smaller subset of patients present with chronic, intermittent pain and tenderness in the right lower quadrant, which results from appendiceal distention by inspissated mucus (but there are no findings of appendicitis on histologic examination). The symptoms are relieved by appendectomy.[104] Appendicitis must be considered in all patients with cystic fibrosis who have right lower quadrant abdominal pain.

RADIOLOGY OF THE INTESTINE. Typical radiographic features of the intestine are often seen in cystic fibrosis. In approximately 80% of patients, thickened duodenal folds, nodular filling defects, mucosal smudging, dilations, and redundancy are seen.[109] The findings are not age related. Duodenal biopsies do not adequately explain the radiographic appearance. Radiographically, similar changes occur in the more distal small bowel, including thickening and distortion of jejunal folds and variable dilatation of intestinal loops from the jejunum to the rectum.[110] Pneumatosis coli, a benign condition seen with chronic pulmonary disease and fecal impaction, may be seen.

FUNCTIONAL ABNORMALITIES. Small bowel mucosal dysfunction in cystic fibrosis has been suggested by studies that demonstrate absorption defects that are apparently unexplained by exocrine pancreatic insufficiency or that persist after adequate pancreatic replacement therapy. Decreased activity of certain cytoplasmic peptide hydrolases in intestinal mucosa and reduced uptake of phenylalanine, isoleucine, and glycine have been found in patients with cystic fibrosis in comparison with control subjects.[111]

Basal and stimulated duodenal bicarbonate secretion is largely dependent on functional CFTR, and patients with cystic fibrosis suffer several consequences of diminished duodenal bicarbonate secretion. The importance of CFTR in bicarbonate secretion was first demonstrated in CFTR-deficient knockout mice.[112–115] The same abnormalities in duodenal bicarbonate secretion are also present in patients with cystic fibrosis, which partially explains the lower postprandial pH (1 to 2 units) in the proximal duodenum of cystic fibrosis patients compared with normal subjects.[85, 86] Therefore, both CFTR-dependent duodenocyte bicarbonate secretion and probably other mechanisms of alkaline secretion are defective in cystic fibrosis and contribute to the failure to maintain normal proximal duodenal pH.[87]

In contrast with the small bowel and the respiratory system, the CFTR defect in the colon cannot be compensated by any other chloride channel.[116] Therefore, the defect in colonic function closely relates to the *CFTR* genotype.

Lactase deficiency in cystic fibrosis is not related to the disease entity but merely reflects a normal ethnic- and age-related phenomenon. Young children with cystic fibrosis often have elevated lactase values in comparison with age-matched controls. This finding may be a consequence of pancreatic insufficiency with slower turnover of microvillus membrane hydrolases.[117] Xylose absorption is normal in patients with cystic fibrosis.[118]

Meconium Ileus

Meconium ileus is the presenting symptom in 10% to 20% of infants with cystic fibrosis and appears to be related, in part, to genotype.[52, 119] The meconium is characterized by a striking decrease in the content of water and the presence of undegraded serum proteins, intestinal disaccharidases, and some lysosomal enzymes. Sodium, potassium, magnesium, copper, zinc, and manganese content are reduced and calcium is greatly increased in concentration in meconium from infants with meconium ileus. Pancreatic insufficiency developing in utero could be a factor predisposing to meconium ileus. However, pancreatic involvement often appears to be mild in infants with meconium ileus, whereas the presence or absence of meconium ileus may be directly related to the severity of involvement in the intestinal glands.[99] Many infants who die of meconium ileus have a completely normal pancreas.[120] Meconium ileus rarely occurs in infants without cystic fibrosis but has been reported in infants with stenosis of the pancreatic duct or partial pancreatic aplasia and in infants with otherwise normal gastrointestinal tracts as a familial occurrence or as an isolated incident. Identification of the role of the meconium ileus modifier gene should clarify these issues.

PATHOLOGY. Uncomplicated meconium ileus characteristically demonstrates a narrow distal ileum with beaded appearance caused by waxy, gray pellets of inspissated meconium, beyond which the colon is unused.[121] Proximally, the ileal wall is hypertrophied; it then becomes greatly distended with extremely sticky, dark green to black meconium. As many as half the cases of meconium ileus are complicated by volvulus, atresia, and/or meconium peritonitis. Extravasation of meconium into the fetal peritoneal cavity causes an intense inflammatory reaction that shows variable resolution at birth (depending on when the perforation occurred); it may manifest clinically merely as intra-abdominal calcifications, a meconium pseudocyst, generalized adhesive meconium peritonitis, or meconium ascites. Fetal volvulus and vascular compromise may cause atresia.

RADIOLOGIC FEATURES. Characteristic radiologic findings may be present in meconium ileus.[122] Unevenly distended loops of bowel with absent or scarce air-fluid levels may be seen and presumably reflect the viscid nature of the intestinal secretions. Small bubbles of gas trapped in the sticky meconium may be scattered throughout the distal small bowel. Barium enema demonstrates a microcolon and may outline the obstructing meconium mass in the distal ileum. Abdominal calcification reflects meconium peritonitis, and a meconium pseudocyst may displace loops of bowel (Fig. 47–4).

CLINICAL FEATURES. Meconium ileus classically manifests with signs of intestinal obstruction within 48 hours of birth in an infant who is otherwise well; complicated meconium ileus manifests earlier, and infants appear much sicker. Hydramnios is a common prenatal finding. A family history of cystic fibrosis is helpful in establishing the diagnosis.[63] The increased frequency of meconium ileus in some families with histories of cystic fibrosis is strongly associated with a yet-to-be-identified modifier gene on chromosome 19.[63] In simple meconium ileus, no meconium passes and there is progressive abdominal distention and, eventually, bilious vomiting. Dilated, firm, rubbery loops of bowel are visible and palpable through the abdominal wall, particularly in the right lower quadrant, and rectal examination is tight, productive of only a small mucous plug or a small amount of sticky meconium.

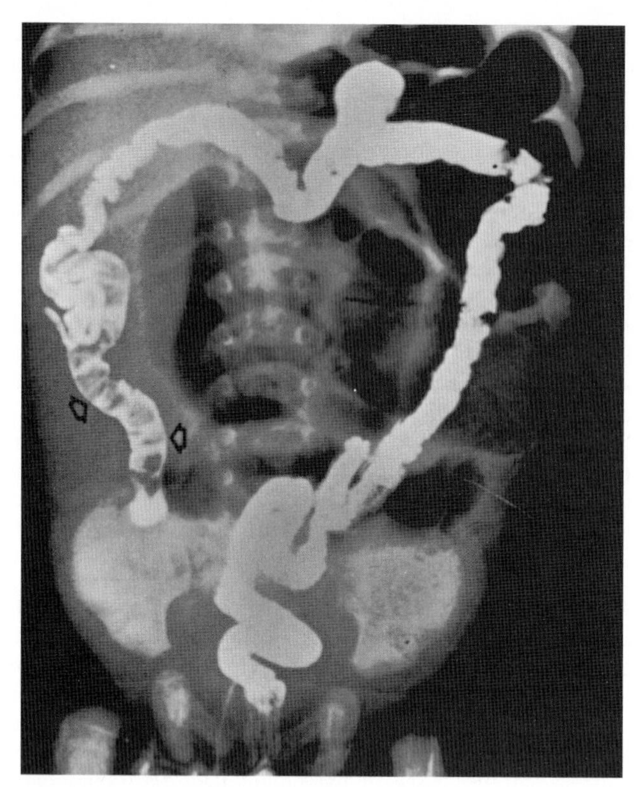

Figure 47–4. Meconium ileus. Barium enema study in an infant with meconium ileus demonstrating a microcolon as well as meconium in the distal ileum *(arrows)*. Distended small bowel loops are also noted. (From Lopez MJ, Grand RJ: Hereditary and childhood disorders of the pancreas. In Feldman M, Scharschmidt BF, Sleisenger MH (eds): Sleisenger & Fordtran's Gastrointestinal and Liver Disease: Pathophysiology/Diagnosis/Management, 6th ed. Philadelphia, WB Saunders, 1998, pp 782–808.)

Sweat tests should be performed in all infants with meconium ileus, with jejunal or ileal atresia, or with volvulus; the results are likely to be positive in 30% of patients with meconium peritonitis and in 15% to 20% of those with atresia of the small intestine.[122] Although occasional infants with meconium plug syndrome have cystic fibrosis, meconium plug syndrome and meconium ileus must be carefully differentiated.

TREATMENT. Meconium ileus was considered invariably fatal until 1948, when the first patients were successfully treated by surgery. More recent reports indicate a very low operative mortality, and long-term survival approaches 90% for uncomplicated meconium ileus.[119] Various irrigating solutions have been used during the operation and postoperatively to dissolve and dislodge the abnormal meconium. *N*-acetylcysteine (Mucomyst), which reduces the viscosity of mucoprotein solutions by cleaving disulfide bonds in the mucoprotein molecule, and polysorbate 80 (Tween 80), a mild industrial detergent and preservative, are now generally recognized as safe and effective. Nonoperative relief of obstruction with diatrizoate (Gastrografin) enemas is also possible and has virtually eliminated prolonged hospitalization and early respiratory complications for most infants with uncomplicated meconium ileus.[105, 119] Gastrografin is a radiopaque, aqueous solution that contains a small amount of polysorbate 80 and has an osmolality of 1900 mOsm. Presumably the detergent action of polysorbate 80 helps the fluid pass around and into inspissated meconium, and the hypertonicity and mild mucosal irritation draw fluid into the bowel to soften and loosen the meconium. Hypaque (also diatrizoate) enemas have also been used successfully. However, water-soluble, hypertonic enemas may cause dangerous fluid and electrolyte shifts, especially in small, sick infants. This can be avoided with the judicious use of intravenous fluids given concomitantly. Colonic perforation resulting from enemas has been reported in patients with meconium ileus. Gastrografin enemas are not appropriate therapy for infants with complicated meconium ileus, for whom surgical therapy should be performed.

A diagnostic barium enema should precede therapeutic Gastrografin enemas.[119, 120, 122] Infants with cystic fibrosis and meconium ileus who survive beyond 6 months of age have the same prognosis as for any patient with cystic fibrosis and do not tend to have more severe disease.

Distal Intestinal Obstruction Syndrome

Intestinal impaction and obstruction (distal intestinal obstruction syndrome) remain common and troublesome features in cystic fibrosis beyond the neonatal period.

PATHOGENESIS. Mechanisms other than inspissated intestinal sections and pancreatic achylia are probably operative in the pathogenesis of the distal intestinal obstruction syndrome and include undigested food residues; possible disturbances of motility; dilatation of the bowel, leading to fecal stasis; and dehydration. Intussusception and, less frequently, volvulus may complicate the distal intestinal obstruction syndrome. The incidence of distal intestinal obstruction syndrome is estimated to be as high as 10% among patients with cystic fibrosis, although more recent data show a prevalence of 3% or less.[105, 123–126] Distal intestinal obstruction syndrome may even be the presenting symptom of the disease.

CLINICAL FEATURES. A spectrum of clinical conditions results from partial or complete obstruction of the bowel by abnormal intestinal contents, including (1) abdominal pain caused by constipation or fecal impaction, (2) palpable cecal masses that may eventually pass spontaneously, and (3) complete obstruction of the bowel by firm, putty-like fecal material in the terminal ileum or right colon or both.[123, 126, 127]

Abdominal pain, usually recurrent and cramping in nature, is the most common symptom of the distal intestinal obstruction syndrome. This may be the only symptom, and it may persist for years before obstructive symptoms occur. Insufficient doses or cessation of pancreatic enzyme replacement, recent or concomitant respiratory infection, and dietary changes have been incriminated as precipitating factors.[128] Patients with inadequately controlled steatorrhea may be at higher risk for development of this problem.[126] Frequently, however, symptoms occur without warning in patients receiving presumably adequate medical management. The distal intestinal obstruction syndrome should be suspected in any patient with cystic fibrosis who has abdominal pain, a palpable mass in the right lower abdominal quadrant, or bowel obstruction. When no acute symptoms are present, the soft, indentable, nontender nature of the palpable fecal mass on examination of the abdomen may be a diagnostic aid. The plain radiograph of the abdomen characteristically shows the proximal colon and distal small bowel packed with bubbly-appearing fecal material. The fecal bolus can be identified on barium enema but may have to be differentiated from a cecal neoplasm or appendiceal abscess. It is important to consider the diagnosis of appendicitis in these patients as well.

TREATMENT. Uncomplicated distal intestinal obstruction syndrome, once a surgical problem, now usually responds to medical management. A stepwise approach with therapeutic trials of more than one modality should be used in each patient before a consideration of surgery (Table 47–7). Vigorous medical therapy includes regular oral doses of pancreatic enzymes and stool softeners, oral or rectal administration of 10% *N*-acetylcysteine, and Gastrografin enemas. Maintenance treatment with oral doses of *N*-acetylcysteine, increased doses of pancreatin, and lactulose has been successfully used to prevent recurrent episodes of the syndrome. Treatment of this disorder with balanced intestinal lavage solutions has also proved helpful.[124, 129]

Intussusception (see also Chapter 109)

Intussusception, most often ileocolic, is a complication of the distal intestinal obstruction syndrome reported in approximately 1% of patients with cystic fibrosis.[105, 130] Presumably, a tenacious fecal bolus adherent to the intestinal mucosa acts as the lead point of the intussusception. Most of the patients present acutely with intermittent, severe, cramping abdominal pain, although some experience pain for several months before the diagnosis is recognized. Only 25% of the patients note blood in their stools. Efforts should be made to reduce intussusceptions by using radiologic techniques. Intussusception has been reported as the presenting symptom of cystic fibrosis, and cystic fibrosis is a major cause of intussusception after infancy.

Rectal Prolapse (see also Chapter 118)

Rectal prolapse was once thought to be quite common in cystic fibrosis, with a frequency of about 20%. The Cystic Fibrosis Registry now reports this complication in 1% to 2% of patients.[131] Cystic fibrosis accounts for about 11% of all cases of rectal prolapse.[132] Onset of rectal prolapse is usually in the first years of life, is often the presenting symptom of cystic fibrosis, and is usually recurrent. Patients in whom cystic fibrosis is diagnosed early in life are much less likely to experience rectal prolapse than those diagnosed later in life except when stools are voluminous. Additional factors thought to be responsible for the high rate of rectal prolapse in cystic fibrosis include frequent bowel movements, varying degrees of malnutrition, and increased intra-abdominal pressure secondary to coughing. Medical management is almost always successful, and adequate replacement of pancreatic enzymes usually results in rapid improvement. However, up to 10% of affected patients may require surgical correction.

Table 47–7 | **Treatment of Distal Intestinal Obstruction Syndrome**

Acute
- Enemas (with or without Gastrografin)
- Bowel-cleansing agents (GoLytely)

Chronic
- Pancreatic enzymes
- Stool softeners
- *N*-acetylcysteine (Mucomyst)
- Mineral oil
- Lactulose

Gastroesophageal Reflux
(see also Chapter 33)

Up to 20% of patients with cystic fibrosis complain of heartburn or regurgitation.[133, 134] Esophagitis has been documented in up to 50% of patients with significant respiratory problems. Barrett's esophagus has also been seen in a number of patients.[135] It is important to recognize and treat gastroesophageal reflux in these patients, but it can be difficult because many of the complaints can be attributed to cystic fibrosis alone and are consequently ignored. Approaches to treatment should be the same as in any other patient population (see Chapter 33).

Cancer Risk in Cystic Fibrosis

Until the early 1990s, the idea of an association of cystic fibrosis with the subsequent development of cancer was controversial. Two studies reported opposite results: one including 712 patients found no increased risk,[136] whereas a second study of 412 persons suggested an increased risk of pancreatic and small intestinal tumors.[137] In a more recent study in which 38,000 persons with cystic fibrosis were observed, these discrepancies appear to be resolved. The investigators documented an increase in tumors of the digestive tract but did not observe an increase in the risk of cancer in relation to the general population for all types of cancer.[138] These cancers tended to occur in the 3rd decade and involved the esophagus, small and large intestine, stomach, liver, biliary tract, pancreas, and rectum. Their pathogenesis is uncertain, but an increased risk of pancreatic cancer has been seen in patients with chronic pancreatic inflammation from other causes including alcohol,[139] hereditary pancreatitis,[140] and tropical pancreatitis.[141] This increased risk should be kept in mind as the survival of persons with cystic fibrosis continues to increase. Adolescents and adults with unexplained complaints, especially relating to the abdominal organs, should be evaluated for occult malignancy.

Liver Disease

The frequency of hepatic abnormalities in cystic fibrosis has changed dramatically since the 1950s, with a prevalence of about 15% in newer surveys. According to older literature, hepatic involvement in cystic fibrosis varied from 20% to 50% of cases studied, although only about 5% of patients with the disease developed cirrhosis and approximately 2% progressed to clinically apparent liver disease requiring treatment.[74, 142] More recent literature suggests that most patients with mild liver abnormalities do not progress and the high frequency of abnormal liver injury test results noted in infancy spontaneously resolve.[143] Nevertheless, approximately 10% of patients develop some degree of cirrhosis, usually prior to or during puberty.[143] Although no genotypic association between liver involvement and cystic fibrosis has yet been confirmed,[144] a familial tendency to develop cirrhosis has been seen in some patients,[144] and there is now strong evidence that liver disease is associated with modifier genes.[144a] In addition, some risk factors may predispose patients to the development of biliary and liver problems. Such factors include neonatal liver disease, pancreatic insufficiency, and possibly human leukocyte antigen class.[144, 145] One study also suggested that meconium ileus may be a risk factor as well.[146] Malnutrition may also predispose patients to fatty liver and specific nutrient deficits (protein, fat-soluble vitamins, minerals, essential fatty acids, carnitine). However, a recent longitudinal 4-year study followed 124 children with cystic fibrosis; although 92% showed some evidence of liver abnormality (6% based on clinical examination; 42% had transaminitis and 35% had an abnormal ultrasound), liver abnormalities were not related to decline in nutritional status.[147] A study from Sweden, however, suggested that the presence of essential fatty acid deficiency is more common in patients with marked hepatic steatosis.[143] Altered drug metabolism in cystic fibrosis[148] is characterized mainly by increased hepatic clearance of drugs.[149]

Newer studies identify liver involvement approximately as follows: palpable liver (11%), elevated levels of liver enzymes (2.4%), abnormal serum albumin levels (7.4%), cirrhosis with portal hypertension (2.5%), fatty liver (7%), neonatal liver disease (6%), and palpable spleen (2.2%).[131] The prevalence of liver abnormalities in patients with pancreatic sufficiency is markedly lower.

PATHOLOGY. Hepatic changes may be present at any age and may be progressive.[150] Excessive biliary mucus associated with mild periportal inflammation and early fibrosis is common in infants younger than 1 year of age. Focal biliary fibrosis, characterized by inspissated granular eosinophilic material in ductules, bile duct proliferation, chronic inflammatory infiltrates, and variable fibrosis, is uncommon in infants but present in more than 20% of surviving children and adolescents (Fig. 47–5). In time, focal lesions coalesce in some patients and progress to multilobular biliary cirrhosis.[151] Bile stasis within lobules is conspicuously rare beyond the neonatal period even in advanced liver disease caused by cystic fibrosis. Cholestasis is not uncommon in neonates and young infants; it may be prolonged and associated with excessive biliary mucus and mild periportal changes. Approximately half the reported cases were associated with meconium ileus.[152]

Fatty liver, often independent of nutritional status, remains one of the most common hepatic abnormalities encountered in cystic fibrosis.[151] Unexplained hemosiderin deposits in hepatocytes, as well as Kupffer cells, may be prominent in infants and persist beyond 4 to 6 months of age.

RADIOLOGIC FEATURES. Although the abdominal flat plate may suggest splenomegaly, it should not be used for estimating the size and shape of the liver. It can help identify radiopaque gallstones, pancreatic calcification, or fecal retention. Upper gastrointestinal barium series may indicate the presence of esophageal varices.

Ultrasonography is among the best methods for identifying abnormalities of the liver in cystic fibrosis and may well reveal valuable information regarding the liver parenchyma.[153–156] Cirrhosis produces increased coarse echogenicity in many cases and, in some patients, an irregular liver margin. Fatty infiltration is associated with an increase in fine echoes within the liver, with marked attenuation of the ultrasound beam in comparison with normal. A dilated portal vein is indicative of portal hypertension.[154, 156] Enlarged hepatic veins may be seen as a consequence of congestive heart failure or poor outflow secondary to constriction of the inferior vena cava by an enlarged liver at or above the

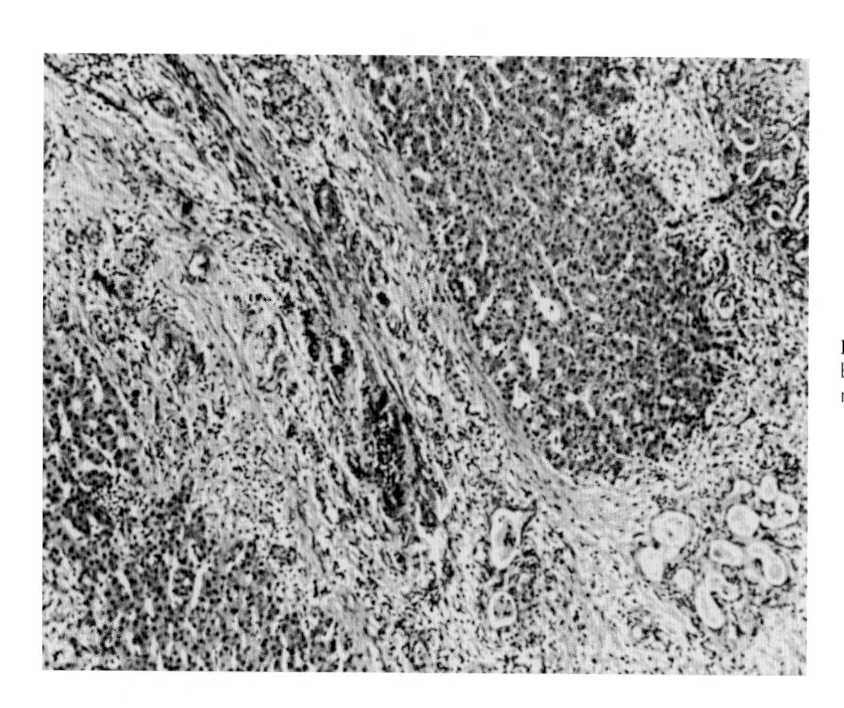

Figure 47–5. Liver histology from a patient with cystic fibrosis showing focal biliary fibrosis. Masson stain (original magnification 250 ×).

entrances of the hepatic veins. CT scanning can also be valuable in assessing the liver parenchyma and is most useful before liver transplantation.

The anatomy and morphology of the liver and spleen can be well visualized with MRI, and fatty infiltration of the liver is easily identified. Further study is needed to define its value in identifying early changes of cirrhosis in patients with cystic fibrosis. MRI with angiographic images can also be useful in assessing hepatic vasculature in the pretransplant evaluation.

Hepatobiliary scintigraphy with scanning agents derived from iminodiacetic acid is the best functional test available for imaging bile flow and can also provide valuable information about hepatocyte function, liver size, and the presence of gallbladder filling. Qualitative examination has incorporated the use of deconvolution analysis to measure the hepatic extraction fraction and the hepatic half-clearance time. The hepatic extraction fraction provides a quantitative measure of hepatocyte uptake of tracer to reflect hepatocyte function. The hepatic half-clearance time provides a quantitative measure of clearance of tracer from hepatocytes and bile flow through the ducts.[157, 158]

FUNCTIONAL ABNORMALITIES. Tests of hepatic function in cystic fibrosis may be normal even in cases of overt cirrhosis.[159] Serum enzyme levels reflecting hepatocellular injury may be moderately elevated and fluctuate over the course of the illness. As many as 20% of cystic fibrosis patients with pancreatic insufficiency have elevated serum alanine aminotransferase (ALT) values. An elevated serum alkaline phosphatase value is the next most common chemical abnormality indicative of hepatic involvement, and the high values commonly seen in normal infants and children (mainly resulting from the bone isoenzyme) may conceal increased levels of the hepatic isoenzyme.[160] Fasting bile acid levels are elevated in many patients with cystic fibrosis, and this may be among the more sensitive measures of liver function in this disease.

Prothrombin time is usually normal but may become prolonged as a consequence of reduced dietary intake of vitamin K or suppression of bowel flora by antibiotics, independent of changes in other liver function tests. Hypoalbuminemia is found in approximately 7% of patients as liver disease progresses.

Bile acid metabolism is disturbed in patients with cystic fibrosis and exocrine pancreatic insufficiency.[159, 161, 162] Fecal losses are high and may approach those of patients with ileal resection. Pancreatic enzyme replacement reduces fecal bile acid excretion and corrects steatorrhea and azotorrhea. The fractional turnover rate of the bile acid pool is increased and the total bile acid pool size diminished in the absence of pancreatic enzymes,[162] whereas the biliary lipid composition and saturation index approach those of patients with cholelithiasis.[161] Treatment with pancreatic supplements returns abnormal values toward normal.

CLINICAL FEATURES. Evidence for liver disease in patients with cystic fibrosis is often subtle; a variety of symptoms can be the presenting complaint. Although the spectrum of liver disease present in patients with cystic fibrosis is broad, there are three predominant forms: (1) neonatal cholestasis, manifesting with or without meconium ileus or intestinal atresia[163]; (2) fatty liver syndrome; and (3) cirrhosis, manifesting either as portal hypertension or as functional failure. Of importance is that asymptomatic increases in enzymes or abnormal ultrasonographic findings may be the only clinical manifestations. More commonly, hepatomegaly or splenomegaly is the initial indication of hepatic disease. Esophageal varices or ascites can also be manifestations of hepatic involvement in cystic fibrosis. These may precede evidence of functional impairment (hepatocellular failure) by many years.

Examination of the liver and spleen by percussion and palpation should be performed at each clinic visit, and the size and character of these organs should be recorded. Normal and reproducible data have been published delineating liver size in children and adolescents.[164]

In patients with suspected liver involvement, the degree of liver function and injury should be assessed at least annually by tests of synthetic capacity and reflections of liver cell damage. Synthetic capacity of the liver is most readily measured through serum protein analysis (at least total protein and albumin levels) and prothrombin time. Liver cell damage is reflected in increased levels in serum bile acids, bilirubin (direct and total), aspartate aminotransferase (AST) and ALT, and alkaline phosphatase. Elevated γ-glutamyltranspeptidase may reflect liver damage when other enzyme levels are normal.[160] Normal liver biochemistry tests at regular intervals have been proposed as a good negative predictor for liver disease.[143]

Patients with hepatomegaly, abnormal liver test results, and/or abdominal pain, even those whose complaints are not focused in the right upper quadrant, should undergo an assessment of the status of the liver and biliary system. After routine laboratory screening, the ultrasound examination is likely to be most valuable. Depending on the results, it may be appropriate to obtain scintigraphic studies or ERCP. Liver biopsy in patients with cystic fibrosis should be undertaken when indicated by the clinical course.

As with all patients with cystic fibrosis, nutritional status must be assessed regularly. Guidelines are available from the Cystic Fibrosis Foundation.[165] Carnitine levels should also be assessed.[166] Nutritional rehabilitation should be accomplished in all patients with liver and biliary disease to eliminate avoidable complications of malnutrition.[167]

TREATMENT. The treatment of symptomatic liver disease in cystic fibrosis is a challenge and usually requires a team approach. Treatment of cholestasis is probably best accomplished with ursodeoxycholic acid (20 mg/kg/day), although controlled clinical trials have not confirmed as yet that ursodeoxycholic acid can prevent the progression of liver disease. This agent also may improve liver function in patients with elevated transaminase levels but without cholestasis. The benefits of ursodeoxycholic acid have been shown to be dose dependent, and, indeed, scintigraphically evident improvement in hepatobiliary excretory function has been observed with higher doses of this bile acid.[158, 168, 169]

Nutritional rehabilitation is required in patients in whom disease activity has produced malnutrition. Preventive nutritional management in patients with early liver involvement is indicated. Attention should be paid to the provision of adequate quantities of fat-soluble vitamins. Indeed, essential fatty acid deficiency has been suggested to contribute to liver damage in cystic fibrosis.[170]

In patients with cirrhosis, infections (spontaneous bacterial peritonitis and cholangitis) necessitate treatment with appropriate antibiotics. Encephalopathy should be treated with protein restriction, lactulose, neomycin, and, when indicated, plasmapheresis, especially in preparation for liver transplantation. Gastrointestinal bleeding should be treated vigorously on diagnosis. Endoscopic banding or sclerotherapy of bleeding esophageal varices is the most effective and rapid form of therapy. Adrenergic beta blockers (e.g, propranolol [Inderal], atenolol) have not yet been widely used in patients with liver disease and cystic fibrosis.

Portosyemic shunts have been placed effectively in patients with cystic fibrosis and portal hypertension. The same indications should be applied in cystic fibrosis as in any other disorder when deciding on shunt surgery. The distal splenorenal shunt is the procedure of choice. Prophylactic shunting for varices that have never bled is not recommended. If severe lung disease is not a contraindication to surgery and the clinical status of the patient is acceptable, end-stage liver disease in cystic fibrosis is an indication for liver transplantation.[171]

Gallbladder and Biliary System

The gallbladder and biliary tract are abnormal in approximately 25% of patients with cystic fibrosis, independent of age, clinical course, or hepatic pathology.[154, 172–174] "Microgallbladders" are found in 23% and stones or sludge in 8%. Data from the Cystic Fibrosis Registry suggest that only about 2% of persons with cystic fibrosis eventually require gallbladder surgery.[131]

PATHOLOGY. Small gallbladders are commonly found, characteristically containing thick, colorless "white bile." Mucus is present within the epithelial lining cells, and numerous mucus-filled cysts may be present immediately beneath the mucosa. The cystic duct may be atrophic or occluded with mucus. Obstruction of the hepatic or common ducts by mucous plugs does not occur, but intraductal stones may cause obstructive symptoms and predispose to cholangitis.

RADIOLOGIC FEATURES. The abdominal flat plate may demonstrate gallstones. Ultrasonographic examination shows gallbladder size, content (sludge, gallstones, or bile), and wall thickness. It is excellent for estimating dilation of the biliary tract and may help in screening for cholecystitis.[154] Oral cholecystograms often identify nonfunctioning gallbladders, of which a significant fraction also fail to opacify after intravenous cholangiography. These functional and anatomic abnormalities, however, are usually not symptomatic.[172] In addition, these tests have been superseded by ultrasonography and other imaging techniques. Scintigraphy is valuable in delineating functional abnormalities in the biliary system in patients with liver disease, although test results are usually normal in cystic fibrosis patients without liver disease. ERCP reveals bile duct abnormalities in some patients with liver disease, but the prevalence of lesions such as bile duct stenosis is probably lower (approximately 1% to 10%) than originally reported.[173] It is said that these lesions are not apparent in patients with normal liver function. ERCP should be reserved for patients with one or more of the following: unexplained abdominal pain, evidence of biliary tract disease, an abnormal ultrasonogram showing intrahepatic bile duct abnormalities, and a cholangitis-like illness. ERCP may also reveal irregular filling defects throughout the biliary tree with cystic dilatations of the intrahepatic bile ducts and intrahepatic cholelithiasis. Irregularities of the smaller proximal ducts have also been noted, presumably caused by focal biliary cirrhosis. CT scanning is also valuable in the assessment of biliary abnormalities and may be useful before ERCP.

CLINICAL FEATURES. Acute or recurrent episodes of abdominal pain, whether diffuse or localized to the right upper quadrant, may be related to obstruction caused by sludge, to infection, or to common bile duct obstruction caused by pancreatic fibrosis or perhaps by sclerosing cholangitis. Jaundice and itching may indicate bile duct obstruction.

TREATMENT. In general, obstructive jaundice in infants with cystic fibrosis is not a surgical condition. Cholecystectomy is indicated in cystic fibrosis whenever clinical disease mandates it and lung disease permits. However, in patients with severe lung disease, treatment with ursodeoxycholic acid may be indicated as the first form of therapy for gallstones. Endoscopic papillotomy may be indicated as a first invasive therapeutic maneuver.

Genital Abnormalities in Male Patients

The most striking changes in the male genital tract occur in the epididymis, the vas deferens, and the seminal vesicles. The retia testis are intact. Multiple sections of spermatic cord rarely show histologic patency at more than one level. In addition to these defects, there is a striking increase in abnormalities associated with testicular descent, such as inguinal hernia, hydrocele, and undescended testes. Approximately 97% of males are sterile as a result of these changes. These abnormalities are unique; they have not been noted in any other genetic disease. These defects may be found in male infants shortly after birth and may be useful in supporting the diagnosis of cystic fibrosis in atypical cases.

Patients not clinically suspected of having cystic fibrosis but who have congenital absence of the vas deferens have a high frequency of *CFTR* mutations.[175, 176] As many as 70% of men with the sole finding of congenital absence of the vas deferens have a detectable mutation in at least one allele of *CFTR*. Other work has suggested that alterations in transcription may also be associated with this defect, inasmuch as an intronic polymorphism, 5T, that reduces functional messenger RNA transcripts of wild-type *CFTR* is found in high frequency in men with congenital absence of the vas deferens.[175, 176] This group of men, without other manifestations of cystic fibrosis, likely represents a mild form of the disease. On the other hand, the rate of *CFTR* mutations in patients with primary testicular failure is not elevated and *CFTR* gene mutations screening is not warranted.[177]

Nutrition

In the routine clinical setting, the nutritional management of patients with cystic fibrosis is based on an assessment of requirements, taking into consideration age, height, weight and anthropometrics, and severity of lung disease, as well as anorexia, pancreatic insufficiency, other intraluminal phase abnormalities, and mucosal dysfunction (Table 47–8).[167, 178] Ideally, a normal diet for age should be encouraged, with adequate pancreatic replacement therapy provided (with gastric acid suppression, if indicated) to achieve as normal a fat balance as possible.[179] However, children with end-stage lung disease may require in excess of 150% of the recommended daily allowance for age for calories and protein to promote normal growth.[180] High-calorie, high-fat, and liberal salt diets are also encouraged by many cystic fibrosis centers. Indeed, lipid levels of pancreas-insufficient adults on high-fat diets are normal or even low.[181] Medium-chain triglycerides and glucose polymers (Polycose) may be used to improve caloric intake. Several studies have suggested that improved nutritional therapy improves or at least slows progression of the pulmonary disease.[167] All centers now place an emphasis on nutritional intervention before severe malnutrition is evident. The relationship between improved nutrition (via oral, nasogastric, gastrostomic, jejunostomic, or intravenous routes) and pulmonary function will be further examined in future studies.[182]

Malnutrition in cystic fibrosis can result from a variety of factors that increase nutrient loss, reduce energy intake, and increase energy expenditure.[183] Increased losses are primarily related to underlying pancreatic insufficiency but are also influenced by conditions such as poorly controlled diabetes mellitus, vomiting and/or regurgitation, excess intestinal mucus, and inadequate bile salt secretion. Energy intake can be affected both by complications of the disease and by psychosomatic issues.[183] Severe respiratory symptoms can be accompanied by anorexia, nausea, and vomiting. Gastrointestinal symptoms or complications such as abdominal pain, gastroesophageal reflux with pain, anorexia, and vomiting can lead to reduced caloric intake. In some patients, clinical depression, physical fatigue, a disordered sense of smell (food is unappetizing), and an altered body image all can lead to reduced intake. Increased energy expenditure also frequently accompanies the severe respiratory disease of cystic fibrosis and is likely related to factors such as chronic infections, fever, increased respiratory effort, and bronchodilator medications.[183]

All patients with cystic fibrosis should receive a multivitamin preparation daily, and many require vitamin E, K, and D supplements as well.[178] Vitamin A deficiency is also seen in patients who do not take pancreatic supplements or who are not receiving a multivitamin. Serum levels of vitamin E can be low but usually respond to either water-soluble or fat-soluble forms of vitamin supplementation.

Table 47–8 | **Nutritional Therapy in Cystic Fibrosis**

- Allow a normal diet; stress high protein intake
- Pancreatic supplements with or without gastric acid suppression
- Vitamins
  - Multivitamins
  - Vitamin B complex
  - Riboflavin
  - Vitamins A, D, E, and K (aqueous preparations are preferable)
- Medium-chain triglycerides
  - Oil/spreads, cooking formula (e.g., Portagen, Pregestamil)
- Glucose polymer (Polycose)
- Defined formula diets
  - By mouth
  - By tube: nasogastric, gastrostomy, jejunostomy
- Intravenous feeding (peripheral vs. central)

Initial nutritional intervention should focus on voluntary oral intake. Initial aims should emphasize an adequate intake of food with appropriate pancreatic enzymes, multivitamins, and vitamin supplements as necessary.[184] Care should be given to monitoring of both protein and electrolytes in children. If adequate intake does not result in appropriate growth, increasing caloric intake by altering the caloric content of the meals and snacks consumed by the child or adult should be attempted. Finally, calorie-enhanced milkshakes and powders can be tried to increase caloric intake. Patients who are not growing appropriately and cannot or will not increase their intake may require nocturnal nasogastric tube or gastrostomy feedings.

A great deal has been written regarding defined-formula diets as supplements or replacement for food in patients with cystic fibrosis. Although there is no evidence that these are better than a balanced diet in providing appropriate protein, energy, and essential nutrients, liquid formulas are easy to administer by tube and may provide added nutrients when infused at night. Nutritional status should be followed carefully, and therapy should be instituted early. Some adolescents learn to pass soft Silastic feeding tubes nightly to administer nasogastric feedings. Gastrostomy feedings may be preferred by some families and patients, especially in younger children, for chronic administration of enteral supplements. Currently, gastrostomy or jejunostomy feedings are instituted at the first sign of nutritional failure.[167, 182, 184] Finally, in some cases, parenteral nutrition may be necessary, but it should be reserved for acute support, with a return to some form of enteral nutrition as soon as possible.

Prognosis of Patients with Cystic Fibrosis

More than 50% of patients with cystic fibrosis survive to 28 to 29 years of age.[49, 131] Male patients tend to live longer than females by about 4 years. Most significant morbidity and mortality are related to the chronic obstructive pulmonary disease.[131] The relative influence of nutritional support, pancreatic enzyme replacement, and aggressive treatment of pulmonary disease on improving the quality and duration of life remain under study. It has been reported that patients with intact pancreatic function have better pulmonary status than those with pancreatic insufficiency.[52] This suggests that there is a heterogeneous form of the disease (consistent with the new genetic information) and/or that survival is longer with better nutrition and treatment.

As survival improves, the problems facing these patients will become different and will begin to spill over into the domain of caretakers predominantly focused on the issues of adults. These medical problems include entities such as pancreatitis, continued difficulties with adequate nutrition, cirrhosis with portal hypertension, diabetes with its long-term complications, osteopenia, and reproductive issues, as well as all of the more common problems seen in childhood.[185, 186] In a report of the Cystic Fibrosis Registry, gallbladder disease (0.9% of patients), peptic ulcer disease (0.7%), pancreatitis (0.8%), and cirrhosis with portal hypertension (1.2%) all were more common in adults than in children.[131] Pulmonary disease is more severe in adults than in children and malnutrition continues to be a problem in about 35% of adults with cystic fibrosis.[131] Increasingly, these patients will require evaluation for potential malignancies of the digestive tract, liver disease, or other complications that will necessitate the specialized attention of a gastroenterologist. It is possible that in the near future the prognosis of these patients will be changed dramatically by new therapies aimed at recovering specific functions through either drug treatment or gene therapy.

Shwachman-Diamond Syndrome

Shwachman-Diamond syndrome (OMIM No. 260400[17]) is a rare autosomal recessive disorder characterized by exocrine pancreatic insufficiency, hematologic abnormalities, skeletal defects, short stature, and normal sweat electrolytes.[16, 187–191] However, exocrine pancreatic insufficiency and abnormalities of one or more of the bone marrow cellular elements appear to be the only universal findings.[190] Myelodysplastic syndromes and acute leukemias develop in up to a third of patients,[192, 193] and numerous other features have been reported (Table 47–9). Severe cases present in infancy with malabsorption, failure to thrive, or recurrent infections. Because of variable expression of the pancreatic, hematologic, and other features, the diagnosis in mild cases may be delayed.[190, 194] Several hundred families, most with a single affected member, have been identified.[191] Because precise diagnostic criteria or genetic markers are lacking,[190] the incidence and prevalence are unknown. Despite the imprecision in diagnosing milder cases, Shwachman-Diamond syndrome appears as the second most frequently recognized cause of pancreatic insufficiency in children.[16, 50, 195]

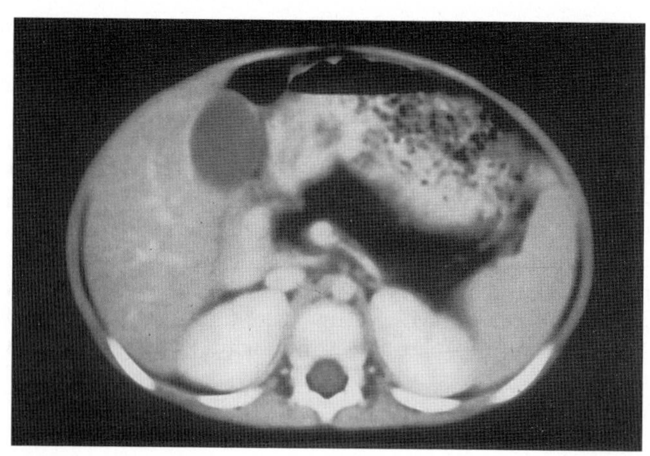

Figure 47–6. CT appearance of the pancreas in a patient with Shwachman-Diamond syndrome. Note that the pancreas retains a typical size and shape, but it is very fatty and therefore appears as a very low-density structure. (Courtesy of Professor Peter Durie.)

Table 47–9 | **Clinical Features of Shwachman-Diamond Syndrome**

CLINICAL FEATURES	PERCENTAGE AFFECTED
Pancreatic	
Exocrine pancreatic hypoplasia	91–100
Steatorrhea	55–88
Hematologic	
Neutropenia	88–100
Anemia	42–66
Thrombocytopenia	24–34
Pancytopenia	44
Leukopenia	52
Elevated fetal hemoglobin (at least once)	80
Myelodysplastic syndromes	8–33
Leukemia	12
Skeletal	
Metaphyseal dysostosis	44
Long bone tubulation defects	
Short or flared ribs	
Thoracic dystrophy	32
Others	<5
Growth	
Short stature (normal growth velocity)	Common
Other	
Psychomotor delay	Common
Mental retardation	33
Renal tubular dysfunction	
Diabetes mellitus	<5
Dental abnormalities	
Ichthyosis	Reported
Hepatomegaly	<5
Abnormal liver biochemical tests	Common
Myocardial abnormalities	50 (autopsy)

Clinical Features

PANCREATIC INSUFFICIENCY. The clinical features of Shwachman-Diamond syndrome usually present in the first year of life.[16, 190, 194, 196] Severe pancreatic insufficiency, steatorrhea, or failure to thrive is often the presenting symptom.[190, 194] A normal sweat chloride concentration or other measures of normal *CFTR* function distinguish Shwachman-Diamond syndrome from cystic fibrosis.[16] Serial assessments of exocrine pancreatic function reveal persistent deficits of enzyme secretion, but nearly half of patients showed moderate age-related improvements (at 4 years of age) leading to pancreatic sufficiency,[190, 194] some pancreatic digestive enzymes (e.g., trypsin) improving more than others (e.g., amylase). The pancreas itself may be small or even of normal size, but the acinar cells appear to have undergone fatty replacement.[16] The extensive lipomatous changes result in characteristic changes during abdominal imaging by CT scan (Fig. 47–6), MRI, or ultrasonography.[197–199]

BONE MARROW DYSFUNCTION. Neutropenia-related infections are also an early problem and are severe in at least 85%, occasionally leading to death.[50, 195] Common infections include otitis media, sinusitis, pneumonia, osteomyelitis, urinary tract infections, skin infections, and lymphadenitis.[200] Thrombocytopenia and anemia are also frequently seen.[190] The neutropenia appears cyclic in two thirds of patients, and, when tested, the neutrophils appear to have impaired chemotaxis.[192] However, one patient with severe neutropenia and recurrent infections was successfully treated with granulocyte colony-stimulating factor (GCSF) given weekly at a dose of 2 μg/kg/day.[201] However, the minimal dose needed to prevent infections is uncertain, the duration of treatment has not been defined, and concern about the use of GCSF in the context of cytogenetic alterations has been raised.[201a] Unidentified serum factors may also impair immune function.[202] Patients with hypoplasia of all three bone marrow cellular lines have the worst prognosis.[190] Indeed, the median age of survival for patients with Shwachman-Diamond syndrome is 35 years, but patients with pancytopenia have a median life expectancy of only 24 years.[200] Pancytopenia appears with a mean age of onset of 6 years and occurs in 10% to 25% of patients.[200] Up to a third of patients will develop myelodysplastic syndrome, and about 10% will develop acute myeloid leukemia or other leukemias.[190, 192, 194]

GROWTH AND DEVELOPMENT ABNORMALITIES. The birth weight of children with Shwachman-Diamond syndrome is usually low (2.9 ± 0.5 kg, 25th percentile[190]), and by 6 months of age the mean heights and weights are typically below the 5th percentile.[190] Thereafter, growth velocity appears normal.[190] The short stature is independent of nutrition.[16] Some clinically evident skeletal abnormalities may be present. For example, metaphyseal chondrodysplasia and dysostosis may be evident radiologically in 44% of patients, especially in the femoral head and proximal tibia.[16, 50] Thoracic dystrophy, short flared ribs, and other skeletal abnormalities have also been described.[16, 190, 203] Most patients remain below the 3rd percentile for height and weight, although some adults reach the 25th percentile for height.[16, 50] Although males and females are probably affected equally, males with mild disease and short stature are more likely to undergo thorough investigation than are females, leading to a mild ascertainment bias.[191, 194]

Molecular Defects

The molecular defect in Shwachman-Diamond syndrome is unknown. The pancreatic lesion appears to result in a development failure of the pancreatic acini in utero.[16] Macroscopically, the pancreas appears fatty and may be small or normal size (see Fig. 47–6). The main pancreatic ducts and islets are normal. Microscopically, there is extensive fatty replacement of the pancreatic acinar tissue.[16] Because the genetic defect also affects the bone marrow and growth plates, the defect cannot be acinar cell specific. Likewise, the hematologic disorder appears to affect cellular development and involves both the stem cells and bone marrow stroma needed to support hematopoiesis.[193] The defect appears to affect specific stem cell lineages because the hematologic deficit can be cured by bone marrow transplant[200] or improved by GCSF.[201] The long bone abnormalities appear to involve protein processing in the rough endoplasmic reticulum of cartilage chondrocytes in about 40% of patients with Shwachman-Diamond syndrome, but the exact defect remains obscure.[200, 204] Although a number of specific cytogenetic abnormalities have been reported,[192, 205–207] none are consistently observed. However, the disease gene has now been mapped to chromosome 7q near the centromere.[208] This locus matches some earlier reports,[206, 207, 209] especially those linking isochromosome 7q10 to Shwachman-Diamond syndrome.[209] The diverse speculations on the basis of this disorder include molecular defects in DNA repair, processing and/or secretion of proteins, microtubules, or microfilaments of the cytoskeleton, nuclear binding factors, or a chromosomal breakage syndrome.[192, 193, 200, 209] Discovery of the molecular defects will bring significant insight into the physiology of several important systems (including the pancreas), provide the basis for molecular testing, and possibly elucidate better treatment options.

Treatment

The treatment of the pancreatic exocrine deficiency is more straightforward with Shwachman-Diamond syndrome than in cystic fibrosis because bicarbonate secretion in the pancreas and duodenum is spared. Optimal pancreatic enzyme replacement (500 to 2000 units of lipase activity per kilogram before each meal, and half as much with snacks) should be initiated with an expectation of diminished steatorrhea and improved weight gain but not necessarily enhanced growth.[50] Fat-soluble vitamins, medium-chain triglycerides, and other high-calorie supplements may be needed, as discussed for cystic fibrosis.

During periods of granulocytopenia, febrile episodes should be evaluated and treated with particular vigor. Anecdotal information suggests that GCSF can be used in patients with severe neutropenia who have suppurative infections.[201] In the case of those with recurrent respiratory infections, humoral immunologic defects should also be considered. Episodes of bleeding or severe anemia may necessitate transfusion. Hip disease should be monitored, with intervention if progression occurs. The use of recombinant human growth hormone in this condition has not been systematically investigated, but anecdotal reports have shown efficacy in accelerating growth.

Johanson-Blizzard Syndrome

Johanson-Blizzard syndrome,[210] or nasal alar hypoplasia, hypothyroidism, pancreatic achylia, and congenital deafness syndrome (OMIM No. 243800[17]), is a rare autosomal recessive syndrome of unknown etiology. About 30 cases have been identified. It is characterized by pancreatic insufficiency and growth retardation with lipomatous transformation of the pancreas.[50] Patients with Johanson-Blizzard syndrome have preservation of ductular output of fluid and electrolytes, as in patients with Shwachman-Diamond syndrome and unlike patients with cystic fibrosis.[211] They also have decreased acinar secretion of trypsin, colipase and total lipase, and low serum immunoreactive trypsinogen levels, consistent with a primary acinar cell defect.[211] Histologically, the pancreatic ducts and islets are preserved but are surrounded by connective tissue and a total absence of acini.[212] In addition to pancreatic acinar cell defects, the syndrome is characterized by thyroid dysfunction, aplastic alae nasi, cardiac anomalies, genitourinary malformations, deafness, midline ectodermal scalp defects, dental anomalies, and imperforate or anterior anus.[210, 213] There are no skeletal or hematologic abnormalities characteristic of Shwachman-Diamond syndrome.[211] The inheritance is thought to be autosomal recessive, although no specific gene defect has been identified.

The spectrum of disease severity remains speculative while the genetic defect is being sought. The genotype-phenotype spectrum may be broad, because some patients thought to have isolated trypsinogen deficiencies may actually have a milder form of Johanson-Blizzard syndrome.[213] The treatment of the exocrine pancreas deficiencies is similar to other forms of pancreatic insufficiency.

Pearson's Marrow-Pancreas Syndrome

Pearson's marrow-pancreas syndrome (OMIM No. 55700[17]) is a rare mitochondrial DNA (mtDNA) breakage syndrome[214] characterized by refractory sideroblastic anemia with vacuolization of marrow precursors and exocrine pancreatic dysfunction.[215] The patients may have transfusion-dependent macrocytic anemia in infancy, but all of the bone marrow cell lines appear otherwise normal. The pancreatic insufficiency appears to be due to pancreatic fibrosis rather than fatty replacement of the acinar cells as in Shwachman-Diamond syndrome as well as more likely to be associated with diabetes mellitus.[216] The syndrome is generally fatal in infancy, and patients who survive develop progressive involvement of many systems, including the liver, kidney, gut, and skin, all of which have abnormal mitochondria.[50] The molecular defect in Pearson's marrow-pancreas syndrome was initially identified as a 4977-base-pair deletion of mtDNA encompassing portions of the genes coding for NADH dehydrogenase, cytochrome oxidase, and adenosine triphosphatase.[217] A variety of mitochondrial defects have now been identified,[218, 219] and these deletions appear to be flanked with nucleotide repeats.[219] The clinical features and severity of disease appear to correlate with the organ distribution and proportion of abnormal mtDNA.[218, 220] Patients who survive may develop features of other mtDNA deletion syndromes such as Kearns-Sayre syndrome.[221] No specific treatment to correct the abnormalities is known.

Other Rare Syndromes Affecting the Pancreas

A number of rare syndromes have been identified that affect the pancreas. Examples include asplenia with cystic liver, kidney, and pancreas (Iverson's syndrome, OMIM No. 208540[17]), which describes dysplasia (in the sense of disturbed development) of the kidney, liver, and pancreas without other diagnostic abnormalities.[222] Histologically, the pancreas has dilated, large, irregular-shaped ducts surrounded by concentric loose mesenchyme and prominent areas of fibrosis and atrophy of parenchyma.[222] Similar autosomal recessive renal-hepatic-pancreatic dysplasia has been described,[223] but these syndromes have little impact on clinical medicine.

GENE MUTATIONS PREDISPOSING TO ACUTE AND CHRONIC PANCREATITIS

One of the most important areas of recent progress leading to a better understanding of pancreatic diseases is molecular genetics. Through genetic linkage analysis and candidate gene studies, a number of genes have been identified that clearly predispose mutation carriers to acute and chronic pancreatitis (see Chapters 48 and 49). This has allowed for improved classification of etiologies and risk factors[1] and raises the possibility of genetic testing early in the course of the disease or even before symptoms develop.[1, 224] However, the rate of new discoveries is outpacing the development of standards and practices that balance important issues of who determines who should undergo genetic testing, when, which tests, who should provide counseling, and, from medical, ethical, and legal perspectives, what to do with the results. Genetic testing for a variety of known mutations allows for determination of *risk* (presymptomatic testing) as well as *etiology* (testing for causative factors). Finally, there is growing recognition that the severity of acute pancreatitis and the likelihood of developing chronic pancreatitis reflect the convergence of a number of important genetic and environmental factors. This section focuses primarily on the well-recognized gene mutations in the cationic trypsinogen gene, the pancreatic secretory trypsin inhibitor *(PSTI)* gene, and the *CFTR* gene. Familial hypercalcemia and hyperlipidemia are also considered.

Hereditary, Familial, and Sporadic Pancreatitis

Hereditary pancreatitis is usually recognized as an autosomal dominant disorder caused by a specific genetic defect identified in all the members of a family affected with pancreatitis.[225] *Familial pancreatitis* is a more generic term used when more family members are affected with pancreatitis than would be expected in the population. *Sporadic* and *idiopathic pancreatitis* are, in this context, terms used to differentiate individuals with unexplained pancreatitis, which may or may not have a genetic basis, from individuals with a family history of pancreatitis.

Several very large kindreds were identified during the past 50 years demonstrating that disease susceptibility was transmitted in an autosomal dominant pattern, with high penetrance (80% of gene mutation carriers affected and 20% of gene carriers unaffected) and variable expression.[226–228] These large kindreds all proved to have a pancreatitis disease gene locus on chromosome 7.[229–231] The disease gene was identified as the cationic trypsinogen gene *(PRSS1)*[232] (Fig. 47–7; see also Color Fig. 47–7). Several common mutations in the cationic trypsinogen gene are now known to be associated with hereditary pancreatitis. In addition, mutations in the *SPINK1/PSTI* gene have recently been associated with familial pancreatitis[233] and with idiopathic chronic pancreatitis.[234] Growing experience with genetic testing reveals that family history alone is not an accurate predictor of detecting or excluding specific genes or mutations that predispose to pancreatitis.[235] Thus, family history serves as an important clue to a genetic predisposition, but the final determination continues to require genetic testing.

Cationic Trypsinogen *(PRSS1)* Gene Mutations

Trypsin is the central enzyme in activation of all of the digestive proenzymes synthesized within the pancreas, with the exception of amylase and lipase, which are synthesized

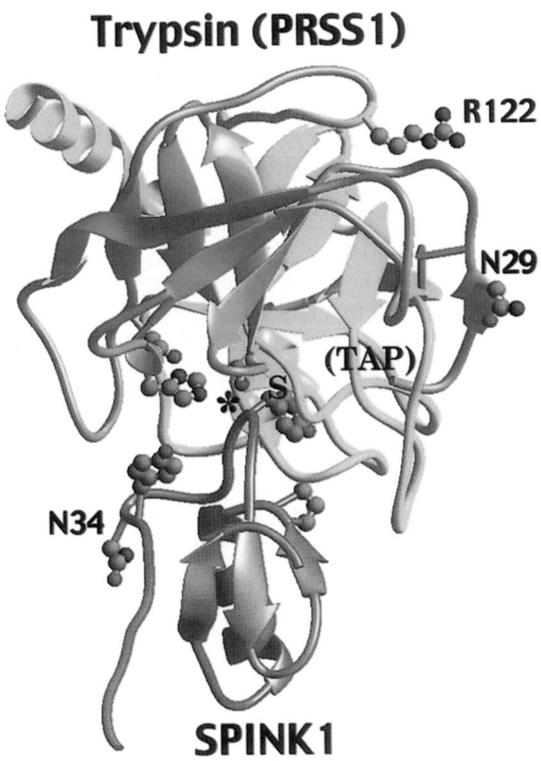

Figure 47–7. X-ray crystallography-based model of cationic trypsin (PRSS1) and pancreatic secretory trypsin inhibitor (SPINK1). The trypsin molecule contains two globular domains joined by a connecting side chain. Trypsinogen is activated to trypsin with cleavage of trypsinogen activation peptide (TAP), allowing a three-dimensional conformation change, opening of the specificity pocket (S), and high-efficiency enzyme activity at the active site (*). The location of the two major mutations associated with hereditary pancreatitis is indicated (N29, R122). Note the location of R122 in the side chain connecting the two (blue and yellow) globular domains. The SPINK1 molecule is shown bound to trypsin. The location of the major mutation associated with idiopathic and familial pancreatitis is indicated (N34). (Courtesy of Drs. Andrew Brunskill and William Furey.)

in their active form (see Chapter 46). Normally, activation of these digestive enzymes occurs within the intestinal lumen when the brush border enzyme enterokinase catalyzes the conversion of the proenzymes trypsinogen to trypsin. Trypsin then catalyzes the conversion of trypsinogen to more trypsin, and trypsin quickly activates the other proenzymes to their active form. Because of the efficiency of the rapid cascade, it is imperative that trypsinogen activation within the pancreas be greatly limited and that mechanisms exist that are capable of inactivating any trypsin within the pancreas to prevent pancreatic autodigestion and pancreatitis (Fig. 47–8).

Several mutations have been identified within one of the trypsin genes that cause acute and chronic pancreatitis. The number of mutations are limited, and the type of mutation specific, because they cause disease by altering the protein through a "gain of function" related to enhancing the activation of trypsinogen or preventing inactivation of trypsin.[236] Gain-of-function mutations often result in an autosomal dominant inheritance pattern because only one of the two alleles must be overactive to express the abnormal phenotype. Loss of function mutations are usually autosomal recessive because both copies of the gene product must be lost to cause the disease phenotype (e.g., cystic fibrosis). In the case of hereditary pancreatitis, most families have a gain-of-function mutation in the cationic trypsinogen gene.

Clinical Features

Patients with hereditary pancreatitis caused by the common trypsinogen mutations have onset of acute pancreatitis sometime between infancy and the 4th or 5th decade of life, with a median age of onset of about 10 years of age. The attacks of acute pancreatitis appear similar to other forms of pancreatitis with epigastric abdominal pain, nausea and vomiting, and elevated serum amylase and lipase levels. However, the

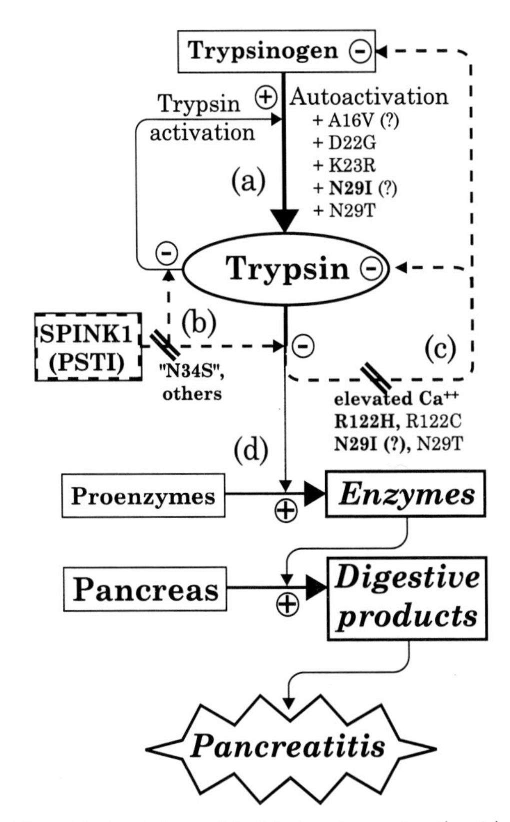

Figure 47–8. Mechanistic model of factors increasing the risk of acute pancreatitis. The current trypsin hypothesis on the initiation of acute pancreatitis is that trypsinogen becomes activated to trypsin within the pancreatic acinar cells *(bold line)*, and trypsin catalyzes *(thin lines and +)* the activation of more trypsinogen and other inactive digestive enzymes (proenzymes) to active enzymes *(bold line)*, which, in turn, cause pancreatic digestion and pancreatitis. Protective mechanisms include (a) limiting activation of trypsinogen, (b) inhibition of active trypsin by SPINK1 *(dashed lines on the left side and ⊖)*, and (c) autodigestion of trypsin and trypsinogen by trypsin beginning at R122 *(dashed lines on the right side and ⊖)*. The first mechanism of protection is reduced in the presence of active trypsin and with some trypsin mutations that enhance trypsinogen autoactivation (e.g., +D22G). The second mechanism of protection is limited by the relative amount of SPINK1 compared with that of trypsin, especially with some SPINK1 mutations (e.g., N34S haplotype, double line disrupting SPINK1 inhibitory pathway). The third fail-safe line of protection is the self-destructive, autolysis of trypsin beginning at R122. This mechanism is diminished with the trypsin R122H mutation, by elevated levels of calcium in the acinar cells, and possibly by other mutations *(double line disrupting trypsin inhibitory pathway)*.

clinical presentation can span the range of complications seen with any other type of acute pancreatitis. The treatment of an acute attack of pancreatitis is currently identical to the treatment of nonhereditary pancreatitis (see Chapter 48). Unfortunately, most patients with hereditary pancreatitis usually have recurrent episodes of acute pancreatitis. Again, there is no specific preventive treatment. Some believe that multiple small meals, avoidance of fatty meals, and use of antioxidants and vitamins are helpful; therefore, these approaches are not discouraged.[1, 237]

About half of patients with hereditary pancreatitis develop chronic pancreatitis.[224] The clinical features of chronic pancreatitis encompass all the features of other forms of chronic pancreatitis (see Chapter 49).

As discussed in Chapter 50, there are many reports of increased incidence of pancreatic cancer in patients with hereditary pancreatitis.[140, 238] Indeed, the cumulative incidence may be as high as 40% by age 70 years.[140] Even though these families are at high risk, no effective screening methods have been established.[238, 239]

Disease-Associated Mutations of Cationic Trypsinogen

Many of the specific mutations causing typical hereditary pancreatitis are known, and most involve cationic trypsinogen. Cationic trypsinogen (UniGene name: protease, serine 1; *PRSS1*) is among the most abundant molecules produced by pancreatic acinar cells.[240] Two other forms of trypsinogen are produced by the human pancreas: anionic trypsinogen and mesotrypsinogen. Anionic trypsinogen accounts for about one third of potential trypsin activity, and mesotrypsinogen accounts for about 5% of potential activity.[240] There are no current reports of mutations in these genes causing pancreatitis. Mutations in codons 29 (exon 2) and 122 (exon 3) of the cationic trypsinogen gene cause autosomal dominant forms of hereditary pancreatitis[224, 232, 236, 241] (see Figs. 47–7 and 47–8). The codon 122 mutations (amino acid 117 in an older nomenclature system) cause a substitution of the corresponding arginine (R, a target for trypsin attack) with another amino acid. The most common variant is a histidine (H) substitution: R122H.[224, 232] This substitution eliminates a "fail-safe" trypsin self-destruction site necessary to eliminate trypsin that is prematurely activated within the pancreas.[224, 232, 242] The *N29I* mutation in exon 2 (amino acid 21 in an older nomenclature system) causes a clinical syndrome identical to the R122H mutation syndrome, although the molecular mechanism causing the gain of function continues to be debated.[236, 243] Other, less common mutations at codons 29 and 122 that are associated with pancreatitis have also been identified.[244] The prevalence of cationic trypsinogen mutations in various populations varies widely, ranging from 0 to 19% among patients presumed to have idiopathic chronic pancreatitis.[245–248] This observation may reflect the settlement patterns of the descendants of early disease founders.

Mutations at codons 16, 22, and 23 within exon 2 of cationic trypsinogen appear to be associated with pancreatitis in some patients, resulting in *A16V*,[233, 234, 249] *D22G*,[250] and *K23R*[251] amino acid substitutions. The *D22G* and *K23R* mutations appear to be gain-of-function mutations by facilitating the activation of trypsinogen to trypsin.[250] They do not result in the high-penetrance hereditary pancreatitis seen with codon 29 and 122 mutations.

Genetic Testing for Cationic Trypsinogen Mutations

Before clinicians order any test, they must determine the purpose for testing, have the experience to understand and interpret the test results, and anticipate how the results will guide patient management. This is especially true for genetic testing because a genetic test result remains unchanged throughout the life of the patient; has implications for future descendants and other family members; and may impact social and reproductive choices, employment, and insurability.[252–254] Thus, the clinician must understand the implications of testing, be prepared to provide pretest and post-test counseling to the patient (or refer the patient to a genetic counselor), and ensure that informed consent is obtained before testing.[252, 252a]

Clinical and research testing is available for the major cationic trypsinogen mutations.[1] Genetic testing falls under class I U.S. Food and Drug Administration regulations, and the protocol for genetic testing must follow the guidelines of several regulatory agencies and be performed in a laboratory with a Clinical Laboratory Improvement Act license.[252, 254] Reasons for cationic trypsinogen mutation testing also vary but generally include to verify a clinical suspicion, to help a patient understand or validate his or her condition, and to assist individuals at risk of pancreatitis and eventually pancreatic cancer.[1, 140] This information may also be useful in making life decisions to minimize risk of disease (e.g., reproduction, diet, smoking[252]). Identification of an established pancreatitis-associated gene mutation can be valuable in expediting an expensive and prolonged evaluation of recurrent pancreatitis in children and precludes further evaluation of elusive causes of pancreatitis in adults. Consensus testing guidelines for the *PRSS1*, *N29I*, and *R122H* mutations have been formulated.[252a]

Interpretation of Genetic Testing for Trypsinogen Gene Mutations

The positive and negative predictive value of a genetic test in identifying specific mutations is almost perfect with properly applied modern techniques. Interpretation of test results and explanation of their meaning to the patient continue to be a central issue because the test result has implications for the patient as well as the patient's extended family. In general, 80% of individuals with either the cationic trypsinogen *R122H* or *N29I* mutation develop at least one episode of acute pancreatitis (i.e., 80% disease penetrance[255–258]). About half of clinically affected individuals with either the *R122H* or *N29I* mutation will progress to symptomatic chronic pancreatitis.[1, 259] Furthermore, patients with hereditary pancreatitis face an increased risk of eventually developing pancreatic cancer.[140] Finally, the mutation-positive individual has a 50% chance to pass on the mutation to each child. A positive test result in an unaffected person is interpreted as an increased risk of pancreatitis, with this risk *possibly* diminishing with age. A negative test result in a family with a known mutation essentially eliminates the risk of this genetic form of pancreatitis. If a mutation has *not* been previously identified in the family, then a negative test result in an *unaffected* person is considered "noninformative" because one cannot distinguish whether the tested individual is free from genetic risk or whether he or she has inherited a different pancreatitis-predisposing gene mutation.[1]

A primary concern of patients undergoing genetic testing for hereditary pancreatitis is insurance discrimination.[253] Participating in a research study, rather than going through a clinical laboratory, is attractive to patients who do not want their test results available as part of their medical record. In these cases the results are disclosed directly to the patient under IRB-approved conditions. The patient then may decide to whom to disclose the results.

Genetic Testing of Children

The genetic testing of children raises unique issues.[252a] Unlike an adult patient, a child legally cannot provide informed consent. Thus, the decision for a child is essentially left to the parents or legal guardian. For children 7 years of age and older, a parent or legal guardian may provide consent for genetic testing, although these older children should provide assent, or agreement to the testing.[260–262] The primary reason for testing of children for cationic trypsinogen gene mutations is to assist in determining the cause of unexplained pancreatitis or to confirm suspected pancreatitis in a child at risk of hereditary pancreatitis, thereby limiting further investigations. The testing of purely asymptomatic children is strongly discouraged because currently there is no clear medical benefit in identifying carriers at a young age.[252, 263] Testing for the purpose of intervention with diet, medication, or surveillance for complications of a genetic disorder (e.g., undertaking repeated colonoscopies for patients with familial adenomatous polyposis syndrome) has been advocated.[263] Because alcohol, emotional stress, and fatty foods have been reported to precipitate pancreatitis attacks,[255] and smoking increases the risk of both pancreatitis[264–266] and pancreatic cancer,[267–269] testing for the purpose of encouraging mutation-positive older children to avoid these excesses is advocated by some caregivers. However, avoidance of fatty foods, alcohol, and tobacco represents excellent general advice for all children and therefore provides no compelling reason for testing.[252] In either case, the personal desires of older children to postpone testing or to proceed with testing to relieve their own anxieties and learn more about their own personal health must also be carefully considered.[262] Ownership of test results in children must be addressed.[1]

Treatment

No specific treatment exists for the prevention or treatment of hereditary pancreatitis. However, some patients report that vitamins, antioxidants, or digestive enzyme supplements are helpful; therefore, we do not discourage their use.[237] Symptomatic treatment for pancreatic duct obstruction or other sources of pain should be handled as for other forms of pancreatitis.[270] Stronger recommendations for specific treatments await clinical evidence from well-designed trials.[237] Finally, there is an increased risk for the development of pancreatic cancer with long-standing chronic pancreatitis from any cause,[139] but especially hereditary pancreatitis.[140] Unfortunately, no good screening test exists for the early diagnosis of pancreatic cancer in high-risk groups,[238, 239] and prophylactic pancreatectomy cannot yet be advocated.

Pancreatic Secretory Trypsin Inhibitor (*SPINK1*) Gene Mutations

Pancreatic secretory trypsin inhibitor (*PSTI*, UniGene name: serine protease inhibitor, Kazal type 1; *SPINK1*) is a 56-amino-acid peptide that specifically inhibits trypsin by physically blocking its active site. *SPINK1* is synthesized by pancreatic acinar cells along with trypsinogen and it colocalizes with trypsinogen in the zymogen granules. In the mechanistic models of pancreatic acinar cell protection, *SPINK1* acts as the first line of defense against prematurely activated trypsinogen in the acinar cell.[232–234, 240, 271] However, because of a 1 : 5 stoichiometric disequilibrium between *SPINK1* and trypsinogen,[240] *SPINK1* is capable of inhibiting only about 20% of potential trypsin. Thus, within the pancreas *SPINK1* appears to act as a limited first line of defense against prematurely activated trypsinogen.

Because gain-of-function trypsin mutations cause acute pancreatitis and chronic pancreatitis, it was hypothesized that loss of trypsin inhibitor function would have similar effects. Recently, the role of *SPINK1* mutations in chronic pancreatitis emerged.[233, 234, 272] *SPINK1 N34S* and *P55S* mutations are relatively common, being present in approximately 1% of alleles tested and therefore approximately 2% of the general population.[233, 272] Families affected with pancreatitis in whom trypsinogen mutations were excluded often have *SPINK1* mutations, but the mutations do not segregate with the disease.[233, 272] Thus, *SPINK1* mutations are not sufficient to cause hereditary pancreatitis in an autosomal dominant inheritance pattern. However, the frequency of *SPINK1* mutations in populations with idiopathic chronic pancreatitis is markedly increased (approximately 25%),[233, 234] proving that these mutations are clearly associated with pancreatitis. Chronic pancreatitis occurs with heterozygous, compound heterozygous, and homozygous genotypes,[233, 234] and the severity of pancreatitis or age of disease onset among genotypes is similar.[233] Furthermore, because the *SPINK1 N34S* and *P55S* mutations are common in the general population (approximately 2%) and idiopathic chronic pancreatitis is rare (1 : 16,000[273]), the risk of an asymptomatic *SPINK1* mutation carrier developing chronic pancreatitis is approximately 1% or less. Thus, the disease mechanism is more complex than a simple autosomal recessive one. The *SPINK1* mutations appear to act as disease modifiers,[233] lowering the threshold for initiating pancreatitis or possibly worsening the severity of pancreatitis caused by other genetic and/or environmental factors. If the *SPINK1 N34S* and other mutations cause *SPINK1* loss of function,[233] then it is likely that the levels of active trypsin within the pancreas would be increased above normal basal levels. However, if the trypsin *R122* side-chain autolysis mechanism remains intact (see earlier), the pathophysiologic activation process would typically fail to progress beyond the fail-safe trypsin autolysis phase. If this were so, only patients with inherited or acquired deficiencies or impairments of other pancreatic protective mechanisms would develop pancreatitis.

With the discovery of a new disease-associated mutation, the question of presymptomatic and symptomatic testing quickly arises. Testing for *SPINK1* mutations in individuals with early-onset chronic pancreatitis may provide important information on predisposing causes of pancreatitis for the concerned patient. But because less than 1% of patients with a heterozygous *SPINK1* mutation alone are likely to develop pancreatitis, there is no reason to do presymptomatic testing. Testing is less likely to be positive in patients who develop pancreatitis after age 20.

CFTR Mutations

In 1998 two groups reported a significant association between patients with idiopathic chronic pancreatitis and various *CFTR* mutations.[274, 275] This association has been confirmed by other groups,[276–279] and key aspects of this problem have been reviewed.[280] Indeed, several mild, "pancreas-sufficient" *CFTR* mutations (e.g., *R117H* and the 5T intron 8 variant that results in a nearly 80% reduction in exon 9 expression[175, 281]) seem to be associated with isolated idiopathic chronic pancreatitis[274, 275] and CBAVD.[175, 282] Other mild *CFTR* mutations (e.g., *L997F*[279]) may also be associated with neonatal hypertrypsinemia and/or idiopathic pancreatitis, but not lung disease or an abnormal sweat chloride. These functional class 4 and 5 *CFTR* mutations probably do not cause recurrent acute or idiopathic chronic pancreatitis alone but rather are part of a compound heterozygous genotype with a functional class 1, 2, or 3 mutation (see Table 47–4). The rationale for this argument is based on at least three observations. First, parents of children with cystic fibrosis (obligate *CFTR* mutation carriers without cystic fibrosis) do not have an increased incidence of acute or chronic pancreatitis compared with the normal population.[283] Second, the prevalence of functional class 4 and 5 *CFTR* mutations (i.e., *R117H*, IV8 5T) among idiopathic chronic pancreatitis patients without a coexisting severe mutation is only about 1.5-fold above the expected number (not significant[68]). Third, the association between severe and mild *CFTR* compound heterozygous mutations in patients with idiopathic chronic pancreatitis is very strong, and most of these patients have abnormal nasal bioelectrical responses demonstrating *CFTR* dysfunction function.[68] Thus, a subset of patients with chronic pancreatitis appear to have atypical cystic fibrosis. Indeed, genetic screening infants who were thought to be heterozygous ΔF508 carriers because of a normal sweat chloride, but had elevated serum immunoreactive trypsinogen levels (associated with pancreatic injury) were frequently found to have the *R117H* mutation (9%) and IV8 5T allele (20%[284]). These data suggest that individuals with a single mutant *CFTR* allele are asymptomatic carriers, those with two severe *CFTR* alleles have classic cystic fibrosis and those who have compound heterozygous *CFTR* genotypes with a severe (classes 1 to 3) and a mild (classes 4 to 5) mutation (see Table 47–4) may be at risk of pancreatitis,[68, 274, 275] CBAVD,[175, 282, 285] sinusitis,[69] or other cystic fibrosis–associated disorders.

As noted earlier, CFTR is a large molecule with 1480 amino acids, coded for by more than 4400 nucleotides in 24 exons.[58] Furthermore, development of idiopathic chronic pancreatitis in these patients appears to be associated with some loss of CFTR function so that many combinations of *CFTR* mutations must be considered. However, mutational screening of the entire *CFTR* gene is difficult and very expensive, thereby limiting this approach to specialized research laboratories. Some commercial laboratories do offer clinical testing for a panel of mutations commonly associated with cystic fibrosis. Unfortunately, these panels may not include many of the "mild" *CFTR* mutations associated with pancreatitis.[68] Furthermore, because *CFTR* mutations are common in the population, the identification of one polymorphism does not alone prove that this is the cause of pancreatitis, nor does the identification of a *CFTR* polymorphism in an asymptomatic individual indicate a high risk of pancreatitis (e.g., if the incidence of pancreatitis is 1 : 16,000[273]) and a *CFTR* R117H genotype increases the risk 2.6-fold,[68] the overall risk becomes 2.6 : 16,000, or 0.16%). Therefore, Cohn and associates[68] suggested that, at the present time, *CFTR* testing might be considered for individuals in whom pancreatitis appears to be the earliest manifestation of classic cystic fibrosis, or in young patients with pancreatitis and borderline sweat chloride values for the purposes of referring these individuals to cystic fibrosis centers or for family planning. As continued research efforts clarify the role of *CFTR* mutations in pancreatic disease, clearer guidelines for testing and patient management will emerge.

INHERITED DISORDERS OF METABOLISM CAUSING PANCREATITIS

Familial Hyperparathyroidism with Hypercalcemia

Hypercalcemia is associated with acute pancreatitis, possibly through trypsinogen activation[286] and trypsin stabilization.[287–289] The relationship between hypercalcemia and pancreatitis became apparent in 1957 when Cope and colleagues[290] suggested that pancreatitis may be a diagnostic clue to hyperparathyroidism. Shortly thereafter, the relationship between familial hyperparathyroidism and chronic pancreatitis was noted because three of nine family members with hyperparathyroidism had chronic pancreatitis.[291] This relationship has been questioned by some[292] and verified by others[293, 294] but is now an accepted etiology.[273, 295–297]

Familial Hyperlipidemia Due to Lipoprotein Lipase Deficiency and Apolipoprotein C-II Deficiency

Familial hyperlipidemia is often associated with recurrent acute pancreatitis. Incidence proportions for associated pancreatitis are approximately 35% for familial type I, 15% for type IV, and 30% to 40% for type V.[50] The pancreatitis is usually acute and recurrent, although pancreatic insufficiency has been reported with both types I and V.[298, 299] The mechanism whereby high serum triglyceride levels lead to pancreatic injury is unknown, although the most popular and well-substantiated theory involves breakdown of excessive triglyceride within the pancreas and release of noxious free fatty acids.[300] Although hypertriglyceridemia (e.g., >500 mg/dL[301]) is associated with recurrent acute pancreatitis, the relationship between hypertryglyceridemia or other hyperlipidemias and chronic pancreatitis remains controversial. Evidence to consider includes familial lipoprotein lipase deficiency[302, 303] and apolipoprotein C-II deficiency,[304, 305] which both cause chronic hypertriglyceridemia, and bouts of pancreatitis that segregate with the disease gene. Chronic pancreatitis was seen in an extended Dutch kindred of patients with genetically deficient lipoprotein lipase catalytic activity.[306] Chronic pancreatitis was not recognized in the kindred with lipoprotein lipase deficiency reported by Wilson and coworkers.[302] Cox and associates[304] reported a kindred with apolipoprotein C-II deficiency with recurrent pancreatitis and chronic pancreatitis, although "chronic pancreatitis" was not defined (i.e., one of five pancreatitis patients had "malabsorption syndrome" and diabetes). One of three patients with apolipoprotein C-II deficiency syndrome reported by Beil and colleagues had pancreatic calcifications.[305] DiMagno and coworkers[295] noted that 5 of 462 patients evaluated for chronic pancreatitis had preexisting hyperlipidemia, but hyperlipidemia was not listed as an etiology of chronic pancreatitis in their series. Clinical series[301] and reviews[273, 307] of this topic generally recognize only acute pancreatitis with hypertriglyceridemia or do not discuss this issue,[297] whereas others note that familial chylomicronemia syndromes lead to severe pancreatic insufficiency.[303] Taken together, these data suggest that in the most severe, prolonged, and poorly controlled cases (e.g., genetic lipoprotein lipase deficiencies) with recurrent acute pancreatitis, chronic pancreatitis can develop. However, this appears to be rare.

PANCREATIC INSUFFICIENCY SYNDROMES

Isolated Enzyme Defects of the Pancreas

Isolated defects of pancreatic enzymes are rarely identified. Furthermore, some doubts about the phenotype of some of the earlier cases of isolated pancreatic enzyme deficiencies have arisen with later studies demonstrating that the "isolated" cases of trypsin deficiency reported by Morris and Fisher[308] and Townes[309] were actually patients with Johanson-Blizzard syndrome.[213] These issues will likely be resolved when the molecular causes of the various syndromes are discovered.

Lipase and Colipase Deficiencies

Congenital absence of pancreatic lipase (OMIM No. 246600[17]) is a rare disorder accompanied by variable preservation of other enzymes.[310–312] The human lipase gene has been cloned[313] and is located on the long arm of chromosome 10.[314] However, the cause of the enzyme deficiency is unknown. Both males and females are affected. The earliest and most characteristic manifestation of this disease seems to be the passage of stool with an unusual amount of readily separable oil, which is often responsible for soiling. Failure to thrive is only occasionally noted, and systemic manifestations are absent.

The concentration of pancreatic lipase activity within duodenal content is low to absent. Both trypsin and amylase activity have been somewhat diminished in some patients; however, other parameters of exocrine function, including colipase and phospholipase A_2 activities and bicarbonate and fluid secretion, are usually normal. Any residual lipase activity has been presumed to be a result of lingual or gastric lipase activity. Bile salt metabolism in this disease has not been extensively investigated.

In addition to its functional absence, no immunologically active lipase can be detected.[310] This suggests either the complete absence of pancreatic lipase or the occurrence of a major structural change affecting both immunogenicity and function. The biochemical response to exogenous pancreatic enzyme therapy is suboptimal, and limitation in dietary fat usually is necessary to avoid oily stools and incontinence. However, extensive data regarding therapy do not exist.

The colipase gene is located on the long arm of chromosome 6.[315] Colipase deficiency has been described in male offspring of consanguineous and nonconsanguineous marriages.[316, 317] These patients presented with loose stools and steatorrhea; growth and development were normal. Colipase activity was markedly reduced with otherwise normal pancreatic enzyme secretion. Fat absorption improved dramatically with the intraduodenal instillation of purified colipase. Colipase is probably secreted in the less active form, procolipase, which requires cleavage of the *N*-terminal pentapeptide by trypsin to form active colipase. Very low levels of trypsin could therefore impair colipase activity. In studies of patients with pancreatic insufficiency associated with cystic fibrosis and Shwachman-Diamond syndrome, steatorrhea occurred only when lipase and colipase secretion were diminished to less than 2% and less than 1% of mean normal values, respectively.[318]

Enterokinase Deficiency

Although few reports of congenital absence of enterokinase have appeared since the original description in 1969,[319] a familial nature was suggested by its documentation in siblings.[320] These patients presented with malabsorption, hypoproteinemia, and severe growth retardation. Evaluation findings included normal amylase and lipase activities and very low trypsin activity in the duodenum, with normal concentrations of sweat electrolytes. Luminal trypsinogen could be activated by the addition of exogenous enterokinase. Small intestinal morphology and disaccharidase levels were normal. Congenital enterokinase deficiency is recognized in 1% to 2% of infants undergoing evaluation of suspected pancreatic insufficiency.[320]

The steatorrhea associated with enterokinase deficiency may be related to a deficiency of phospholipase, the activation of which requires trypsin, which in turn is activated by enterokinase. Patients with cystic fibrosis and Shwachman-Diamond syndrome have increased intraluminal and normal mucosal enterokinase activity.[320] Enterokinase levels may also be reduced with significant mucosal injury.[320] However, even in untreated celiac sprue, normal mucosal and normal intraluminal enterokinase activities have been reported.[321]

ACQUIRED PANCREATIC DISEASE IN CHILDREN

Acquired pancreatic disease is not commonly reported in children. In addition, diagnostic criteria and the rigor with which they have been applied vary considerably.[322, 323] New etiology and risk classification systems are now being applied to chronic pancreatitis,[1] but prospective evaluations in adults and children have not been completed.

Etiology

The causes of acquired pancreatitis in children are listed in Table 47–10. Trauma, usually blunt and associated with injuries to other abdominal viscera, is responsible for pancreatitis in 13% to 33% of affected children. Onset of symptoms is usually soon after injury,[323] although injury may apparently precede the manifestation of pancreatitis by several weeks. In such an instance, a precise relationship is unclear. Perhaps of more importance is that the possibility of injury to the pancreas is often not considered in a severely injured or battered child.[254, 324]

Table 47–10 | **Reported Causes of Acquired Pancreatitis in Children**

Trauma (~14%)	Influenza A
ERCP (~3%)	Measles
Drug-induced (~11%)	Leptospirosis
Azathioprine*	Mycoplasmosis
Valproic acid*	Typhoid fever
L-Asparaginase	Ascariasis
Tetracycline*	Malaria
Mesalamine*	Rubella
Azodisalicylate†	Herpesviruses
Sulfonamides*	Rabies
Sulfasalazine*,†	AIDS-associated infections (<1%)
Cimetidine*,†	Cytomegalovirus
Cytosine arabinoside*	*Toxoplasma gondii*
Furosemide*,†	*Mycobacterium avium;* complex†
6-Mercaptopurine*	
Estrogen*	*Mycobacterium tuberculosis*†
Metronidazole*	*Cryptosporidium*†
Procainamide*,†	HIV†
Sulindac†	Biliary tract disease (~11%)
Alpha-methyldopa*,†	Pancreas divisum (~2%)
Glucocorticoids*,†	Metabolic (~8%)
Didanosine (DDI)	Protein-calorie malnutrition
Pentamidine*	Hypercalcemia
Pentavalent antimony	Reye's syndrome
Zalcitabine (DDC)†	Hypertriglyceridemia
Isoniazid (INH)*	Cystic fibrosis
Rifampin	Familial (~5%)
Erythromycin	Miscellaneous (~10%)
Lamivudine	Henoch-Schönlein purpura
Intravenous lipid emulsion	Diabetic ketoacidosis
Infections (~3%)	Systemic lupus erythematosus
Mumps virus	Perforated duodenal ulcer
Enterovirus	Kawasaki's disease
Epstein-Barr virus	Congenital partial lipodystrophy
Hepatitis A virus	Juvenile tropic pancreatitis
Coxsackievirus B	Unknown/idiopathic (34%)
Echovirus	

*Class I drug—pancreatitis occurs with rechallenge.
†Evidence of probable cause of pancreatitis.
AIDS, acquired immunodeficiency syndrome; HIV, human immunodeficiency virus; ERCP, endoscopic retrograde cholangiopancreatography.

Drugs are said to be one of the most frequent causes of pancreatitis in children, although affected children have usually been treated for significant underlying disease that is perhaps equally likely to cause pancreatitis.[325] As discussed in the literature, few drugs have been clearly incriminated, but among those used with frequency in children are azathioprine and valproic acid.[326, 327] As listed in Table 47–10, other drugs associated with pancreatitis include prednisone, L-asparaginase, thiazides, and tetracycline.[328–330] The possibility of a relationship between corticosteroid use and pancreatitis remains controversial.[329] The development of persistent abdominal pain in a child receiving any medication should suggest the possibility of drug-induced pancreatitis. This is confirmed only by documentation of pancreatic disease, improvement on drug withdrawal, and return of disease when the drug is reintroduced.

Infection

Infections, particularly with viruses, are a relatively frequent cause of childhood pancreatitis; a partial list of putative agents appears in Table 47–10. Enteroviruses, particularly coxsackievirus and echovirus, have been documented by stool isolation and concomitant serum titer rise in up to 8% of adults with "idiopathic" acute pancreatitis. As in aseptic meningitis, only about half of virus isolations are associated with an antibody rise.[331–333] Pancreatitis has been reported in children with Epstein-Barr virus infections, often appearing after an initial clinical improvement.[334, 335] Interstitial pancreatitis has been described in the congenital rubella syndrome.[336] Pancreatitis in children is often attributed to mumps virus on the basis of abdominal pain and an elevated serum amylase value, with parotitis or waxing mumps antibody titers or both.[337] Confirmation via isoamylase determinations and abdominal ultrasonography is lacking, however, and the frequency of this entity may be overestimated. Bacterial pancreatitis has been described in one patient,[338] although in that patient there may have seen other causes for development of pancreatitis, including antecedent hypotension. *Mycoplasma pneumoniae* infection, followed 1 to 2 weeks later by clinically apparent pancreatitis, has been seen in an estimated 8% of patients with this infection. Complement-fixation titers and serum immunoglobulin M values were elevated, and other causes of pancreatitis were absent.[339] Typhoid fever often manifests with abdominal pain; pancreatitis has been suggested as one possible cause.[340] Although uncommon in the United States, ascariasis is among the most frequent causes of pancreatitis in children in regions such as South Africa and India.[341–343] Worms can be found within the pancreatic duct. Malaria has also been reported to cause pancreatitis.[344]

HIV-Associated Pancreatitis

With the growing burden of human immunodeficiency virus (HIV)-related infections and the attendant drug toxicities in the pediatric population, the incidence of HIV-associated pancreatitis also grows. Pancreatitis is 35 to 800 times more common in patients with acquired immunodeficiency syndrome (AIDS).[345, 346] This extremely high risk for acute pancreatitis is attributed to several factors. A number of medications that are frequently used in HIV-infected patients are associated with pancreatitis (see Table 47–10), possibly owing to direct toxicity to pancreatic acinar cells. In addition, immunodeficiency itself predisposes patients to pancreatic infection (see Table 47–10).

The risk of acute pancreatitis in patients with asymptomatic HIV infection or CD4+ count higher than 500/mm^3 appears similar to non HIV-infected individuals.[346] However, the risk of acute pancreatitis increases with advancing stages of HIV disease, including didanosine-related pancreatitis.[347, 348] Likewise, the risk of pancreatitis in children is greatest in patients receiving pentamidine with CD4+ counts less than 100 cells/mm^3.[345]

The severity of pancreatitis and mortality in HIV-infected patients reflects the interplay of two complex and serious illnesses. Compared with non–HIV-infected patients, the hospital course is prolonged, the mortality is higher, and Ranson's criteria is a poorer predictor of outcome in HIV-infected patients.[349] However, when comorbidities are considered and Ranson's criteria are adjusted for pseudohypocalcemia and elevation in lactate dehydrogenase, the prevalence of severe pancreatitis and the sensitivity of Ranson's criteria are comparable to those in immunocompetent patients.[350]

Because drugs appear to be the most common cause of acute pancreatitis in HIV-infected patients,[349] early discontinuation of potential pancreatotoxic drugs should be considered. Treatment of acute pancreatitis in this group is mainly supportive and consists of analgesia, careful fluid management, nutritional support, and, if indicated, antibiotic or antiviral medications.

Biliary Tract Disease

Gallstone pancreatitis is less common in children than in adults and is probably a reflection of the relative infrequency of cholelithiasis in most populations before puberty. However, because almost 10% (as high as 30% in a single study) of the children with pancreatitis in some series had cystic duct stones or common bile duct disease, this diagnosis should certainly be considered, regardless of age.[323, 324] Little is known of the natural history of this disease in children.

Acquired Metabolic Derangements

Multiple metabolic derangements are associated with the development of pancreatic disease in children. Perhaps the most common of these are seen in children with protein-calorie malnutrition. In severely malnourished children, pancreatic enzyme secretion is often compromised, whereas volume and bicarbonate secretion are preserved.[351, 352] Recovery of function is said to occur more promptly after kwashiorkor than after marasmus, but in either case the pancreatic disease may contribute to malabsorption during convalescence. Vigorous early refeeding of malnourished children has been associated with the development of clinically significant pancreatitis.[353, 354] Hypercalcemia during parenteral nutrition leading to pancreatitis was first described in a child; similar reports have followed.[355] Other causes of pancreatitis were not apparent in these patients, although it has been suggested that the calcium content of the solutions infused may not have been the only factor involved in the development of hypercalcemia and pancreatic disease.[355] Histologic changes have been known to occur in the pancreas during Reye's syndrome.[356] Usually this complication has been signaled by hypotension and rapid clinical deterioration during the treatment of advanced illness. Whether the pancreatitis is a cause or a sequela of the clinical deterioration is not clear.

Several other conditions have been infrequently associated with the development of pancreatitis in children. Henoch-Schönlein purpura with pancreatitis has been reported in both children and adults,[357] which suggests another cause of abdominal pain in this syndrome. Other systemic diseases such as systemic lupus erythematosus have been reported in association with pancreatitis.[323] Pancreatitis in children has also been described with perforated duodenal ulcer and diabetic ketoacidosis. Two cases of clinically significant pancreatitis have been documented in association with Kawasaki's disease.[358] Partial lipodystrophy, accompanied by eosinophilia and renal disease, has been described with pancreatitis.[359] Tropical juvenile pancreatitis is characterized by abdominal pain, malabsorption, diabetes mellitus, and pancreatitic calcifications and seems to occur only in countries within 15 degrees of the equator. Although a nutritional cause has been proposed, this has not been confirmed.[360, 361] *SPINK1* mutations may be a common feature of tropical pancreatitis.[362]

Clinical Features

Children with pancreatitis usually present with pain of less than 2 months' duration, although longer illness can occur. Age at onset is commonly greater than 10 years, although the disease is sometimes reported in infancy. The pain is usually supraumbilical, is made worse by eating, and is often accompanied by nausea, vomiting, and occasionally jaundice. A transient fever is often present. Occasionally, affected children younger than 4 years of age present with an abdominal mass. Laboratory diagnosis centers on elevated serum amylase and lipase values. Normal amylase values increase with age, which is explained perhaps by the delayed appearance of pancreatic isoamylase, which is usually not present before the age of 3 months and often not detected until the age of 11 months; even then it is not present at adult levels until the age of 10 years. Salivary isoamylase appears and matures much sooner. The serum amylase concentration may be normal, however, despite other evidence of pancreatitis. An elevated amylase–creatinine clearance ratio may be informative in cases in which the diagnosis is unclear, although false-positive findings occur in states of diabetic ketoacidosis and burns. Other laboratory abnormalities include hypocalcemia in 27%, hyperbilirubinemia in 22%, and hyperglycemia in 15%. A "sentinel loop" is seen on abdominal radiographs in 29%.

Complications

Most often, pancreatitis is not severe in children, although hemorrhagic pancreatitis occurs in up to 13%, with a mortality rate of 86%, in comparison with 18% among those with less severe disease. Severe abdominal pain, peritoneal signs, protracted vomiting, and circulatory compromise usually suggest this complication. Such criteria as those of Ranson are poorly established in the pediatric population[286]; nonetheless, they are useful as guides for detection of complications and for monitoring severe cases of pancreatitis. In fact, the criteria advocated by Banks and colleagues may be more readily applicable in the pediatric population and serve to identify those patients with severe disease.[363]

Pancreatic pseudocysts, as diagnosed by ultrasonography, have been reported in 15% of children with pancreatitis, although the frequency is probably higher. Most of these are secondary to trauma, and the possibility of child abuse should be remembered, especially in a preschool child. Symptoms of pseudocysts include pain in two thirds, emesis in one half, and fever in one fourth: a mass is palpable in two thirds, and an elevated amylase value is found in almost 90% of the cases. An extra-abdominal location is reported in children. The location, presence or absence of infection, and, perhaps, age of the pseudocyst dictate management.

The frequency of pancreatic abscess during childhood is unknown, but the diagnosis should be considered whenever fever and clinical disease are prolonged. Disseminated fat necrosis occurs infrequently in association with pancreatitis in children. Symptoms include subcutaneous nodules, polyarthritis, fever, eosinophilia, soft tissue swelling, and bone pain. Children may display multiple osteolytic lesions occurring 3 to 6 weeks after clinical pancreatitis. These are most easily appreciated in the hands and feet and tend to heal over a period of months. The indications for performing ERCP to evaluate pancreatic disease in children are similar to those in adults. In the setting of recurrent pancreatitis, ERCP or MRCP is helpful in planning medical and surgical management. Recurrent pancreatitis should also be considered a possible manifestation of cystic fibrosis, and affected patients should be screened for this disease.

Treatment

The treatment of pancreatitis in children and adolescents is similar to that in adults (see Chapters 48 and 49).

Acknowledgments

Asif Khalid, MD, critically reviewed and made numerous suggestions and additions to various versions of this chapter. David Orenstein, MD, and Peter Durie provided critical review and suggestions for the updated cystic fibrosis sections.

The author and editors also acknowledge Drs. M. James Lopez and Richard J. Grand, who authored this chapter in the previous edition and who contributed several tables and figures in this edition.

REFERENCES

1. Etemad B, Whitcomb DC: Chronic pancreatitis: Diagnosis, classification, and new genetic developments. Gastroenterology 120:682–707, 2001.
2. Peters J, Jurgensen A, Kloppel G: Ontogeny, differentiation and growth of the endocrine pancreas. Virchows Arch 436:527–538, 2000.
3. Slack JM: Developmental biology of the pancreas. Development 121: 1569–1580, 1995.
4. Jonsson J, Carlsson L, Edlund T, et al: Insulin-promoter-factor 1 is required for pancreas development in mice. Nature 371:606–609, 1994.
5. Ahlgren U, Jonsson J, Edlund H: The morphogenesis of the pancreatic mesenchyme is uncoupled from that of the pancreatic epithelium in IPF1/PDX1-deficient mice. Development 122:1409–1416, 1996.
6. Jonsson J, Ahlgren U, Edlund T, et al: IPF1, a homeodomain protein with a dual function in pancreas development. Int J Dev Biol 39:789–798, 1995.
7. Apelqvist A, Ahlgren U, Edlund H: Sonic hedgehog directs specialised mesoderm differentiation in the intestine and pancreas [published erratum appears in Curr Biol 7:R809, 1997]. Curr Biol 7:801–804, 1997.
8. Hebrok M, Kim SK, St Jacques B, et al: Regulation of pancreas development by hedgehog signaling. Development 127:4905–4913, 2000.
9. Serup P: Panning for pancreatic stem cells. Nat Genet 25:134–135, 2000.
10. Ramiya VK, Maraist M, Arfors KE, et al: Reversal of insulin-dependent diabetes using islets generated in vitro from pancreatic stem cells. Nat Med 6:278–282, 2000.
11. Edlund H: Transcribing pancreas. Diabetes 47:1817–1823, 1998.
12. Kruse F, Rose SD, Swift GH, et al: Cooperation between elements of an organ-specific transcriptional enhancer in animals. Mol Cell Biol 15:4385–4394, 1995.
13. Madsen OD, Jensen J, Petersen HV, et al: Transcription factors contributing to the pancreatic beta-cell phenotype. Hormone Metab Res 29:265–270, 1997.
14. Cirulli V, Beattie GM, Klier G, et al: Expression and function of alpha(v)beta(3) and alpha(v)beta(5) integrins in the developing pancreas: Roles in the adhesion and migration of putative endocrine progenitor cells. J Cell Biol 150:1445–1460, 2000.
15. Lebenthal D, Lee PC: Development of the functional response in human exocrine pancreas. Pediatrics 66:556–560, 1980.
16. Durie PR: Pancreatic aspects of cystic fibrosis and other inherited causes of pancreatic dysfunction. Med Clin North Am 84:609–620, 2000.
17. McKusick-Nathans Institute for Genetic Medicine: Online Mendelian Inheritance in Man, OMIM (TM). World Wide Web URL: http://www.ncbi.nlm.nih.gov/omim/ ed: Johns Hopkins University (Baltimore, MD) and National Center for Biotechnology Information, National Library of Medicine, Bethesda, MD, 2001.
18. Hill ID, Leventhal E: Congenital abnormalities of the exocrine pancreas. In Go VLW, DiMagno EP, Gardner JD, et al (eds): The Pancreas: Biology, Pathobiology, and Disease, 2nd ed. New York, Raven, 1993, pp 1029–1049.
19. Menon PS, Khatwa UA: Diabetes mellitus in newborns and infants. Indian J Pediatr 67:443–448, 2000.
20. Stoffers DA, Zinkin NT, Stanojevic V, et al: Pancreatic agenesis attributable to a single nucleotide deletion in the human IPF1 gene coding sequence. Nature Genetics 15:106–110, 1997.
21. Winter WE, Maclaren NK, Riley WJ, et al: Congenital pancreatic hypoplasia: A syndrome of exocrine and endocrine pancreatic insufficiency. J Pediatr 109:465–468, 1986.
22. Fukuoka K, Ajiki T, Yamamoto M, et al: Complete agenesis of the dorsal pancreas. J Hepatobil Pancreat Surg 6:94-97, 1999.
23. Park CM, Han JK, Kim TK, et al: Fat replacement with absence of acinar and ductal structure in the pancreatic body and tail. J Comput Assist Tomogr 24:893–895, 2000.
24. Harrison KA, Thaler J, Pfaff SL, et al: Pancreas dorsal lobe agenesis and abnormal islets of Langerhans in Hlxb9-deficient mice. Nat Genet 23:71–75, 1999.
25. Li H, Arber S, Jessell TM, et al: Selective agenesis of the dorsal pancreas in mice lacking homeobox gene Hlxb9. Nat Genet 23:67–70, 1999.
26. Hagan DM, Ross AJ, Strachan T, et al: Mutation analysis and embryonic expression of the HLXB9 Currarino syndrome gene. Am J Hum Genet 66:1504–1515, 2000.
27. Kamisawa T, Tu Y, Egawa N, et al: Hypoplasia of ventral pancreas shows a threadlike ventral pancreatic duct [letter]. Pancreas 18:214–215, 1999.
28. Ming JE, McDonald-McGinn DM, Markowitz RI, et al: Heterotaxia in a fetus with campomelia, cervical lymphocele, polysplenia, and multicystic dysplastic kidneys: Expanding the phenotype of Cumming syndrome. Am J Med Genet 73:419–424, 1997.
29. Torfs CP, Christianson RE: Anomalies in Down syndrome individuals in a large population-based registry. Am J Med Genet 77:431–438, 1998.
30. Jadvar H, Mindelzun RE: Annular pancreas in adults: Imaging features in seven patients. Abdom Imaging 24:174–177, 1999.
31. Nobukawa B, Otaka M, Suda K, et al: An annular pancreas derived from paired ventral pancreata, supporting Baldwin's hypothesis. Pancreas 20:408–410, 2000.

32. Kallen B, Mastroiacovo P, Robert E: Major congenital malformations in Down syndrome [see comments]. Am J Med Genet 65:160–166, 1996.
33. Jackson LG, Apostolides P: Autosomal dominant inheritance of annular pancreas. Am J Med Genet 1:319–321, 1978.
34. MacFadyen UM, Young ID: Annular pancreas in mother and son [letter]. Am J Med Genet 27:987–989, 1987.
35. Rogers JC, Harris DJ, Holder T: Annular pancreas in a mother and daughter [letter]. Am J Med Genet 45:116, 1993.
36. Montgomery RC, Poindexter MH, Hall GH, et al: Report of a case of annular pancreas of the newborn in two consecutive siblings. Pediatrics 48:148–150, 1971.
37. Claviez A, Heger S, Bohring A: Annular pancreas in two sisters. Am J Med Genet 58:384, 1995.
38. Dalla Vecchia LK, Grosfeld JL, West KW, et al: Intestinal atresia and stenosis: A 25-year experience with 277 cases. Arch Surg 133:490–496; discussion 6–7, 1998.
39. Chevallier P, Souci J, Buckley MJ, et al: Annular pancreas: MR imaging including MR cholangiopancreatography (MRCP) [letter]. Pancreas 18:216–218, 1999.
40. Dolan RV, ReMine WH, Dockerty MB: The fate of heterotopic pancreatic tissue: A study of 212 cases. Arch Surg 109:762–765, 1974.
41. Terada T, Nakanuma Y, Kakita A: Pathologic observations of intrahepatic peribiliary glands in 1000 consecutive autopsy livers: Heterotopic pancreas in the liver. Gastroenterology 98:1333–1337, 1990.
42. Makhlouf HR, Almeida JL, Sobin LH: Carcinoma in jejunal pancreatic heterotopia. Arch Pathol Lab Med 123:707–711, 1999.
43. Pearson S: Aberrant pancreas: Review of the literature and report of three cases, one of which produced common and pancreatic duct obstruction. Arch Surg 63:168–184, 1951.
44. Pang LC: Pancreatic heterotopia: A reappraisal and clinicopathologic analysis of 32 cases. South Med J 81:1264–1275, 1988.
45. Popiolek D, Kahn E, Markowitz J, et al: Prevalence and pathogenesis of pancreatic acinar tissue at the gastroesophageal junction in children and young adults. Arch Pathol Lab Med 124:1165–1167, 2000.
46. Armstrong CP, King PM, Dixon JM, et al: The clinical significances of heterotopic pancreas in the gastrointestinal tract. Br J Surg 68:384–387, 1981.
47. Berman LG, Prior JT, Abramow SM, et al: A study of the pancreatic duct system in man by the use of vinyl acetate cast of postmortem preparations. Surg Gynecol Obstet 110:391–403, 1960.
48. Kozu T, Suda K, Toki F: Pancreatic development and anatomical variation. Gastrointest Endosc Clin North Am 5:1–30, 1995.
49. Anonymous: Cystic Fibrosis Patient Registry. Bethesda, MD, National Cystic Fibrosis Foundation, 1997.
50. Lopez MJ, Grand RJ: Hereditary and childhood disorders of the pancreas. In Feldman M, Scharschmidt BF, Sleisenger MH (eds): Sleisenger & Fordtran's Gastrointestinal and Liver Disease: Pathophysiology/Diagnosis/Management, 6th ed. Philadelphia, WB Saunders, 1998, pp 782–808.
51. Tsui LC: The spectrum of cystic fibrosis mutations. Trends Genet 8: 392–398, 1992.
52. Kerem E, Corey M, Kerem BS, et al: The relation between genotype and phenotype in cystic fibrosis—analysis of the most common mutation (delta F508). N Engl J Med 323:1517–1522, 1990.
53. Mickle JE, Cutting GR: Genotype-phenotype relationships in cystic fibrosis. Med Clin North Am 84:597–607, 2000.
54. McCloskey M, Redmond AO, Hill A, et al: Clinical features associated with a delayed diagnosis of cystic fibrosis. Respiration 67:402–407, 2000.
55. Shwachman G, Mahnoodian A: Pilocarpine iontophoresis sweat testing: Results of seven years' experience. Med Probl Pediatr 10:158–182, 1967.
56. Knowles MR, Paradiso AM, Brocher RC: In vivo nasal potential differences: Techniques and protocols for assessing efficacy of gene transfer in cystic fibrosis. Hum Gene Ther 6:445–455, 1995.
57. Rosenstein BJ, Cutting GR: The diagnosis of cystic fibrosis: A consensus statement. Cystic Fibrosis Foundation Consensus Panel. J Pediatr 132:589–595, 1998.
58. Riordan JR, Rommens JM, Kerem B, et al: Identification of the cystic fibrosis gene: Cloning and characterization of complementary DNA. Science 245:1066–1073, 1989.
59. Stutts MJ, Canessa CM, Olsen JC, et al: CFTR as a cAMP-dependent regulator of sodium channels. Science 269:847–850, 1995.
60. Durie PR: Pancreatitis and mutations of the cystic fibrosis gene [editorial; comment]. N Engl J Med 339:687–688, 1998.
61. Tsui LC, Durie P: Genotype and phenotype in cystic fibrosis. Hosp Pract 32:115–118, 1997.
62. Macek M, Mackova A, Hamosh A, et al: Identification of common cystic fibrosis mutations in African-Americans with cystic fibrosis increases the detection rate to 75%. Am J Hum Genet 60:1122–1127, 1997.
63. Zielenski J, Corey M, Rozmahel R, et al: Detection of a cystic fibrosis modifier locus for meconium ileus on human chromosome 19q13. Nature Genet 22:128–129, 1999.
64. Campbell PW, Parker RA, Roberts BT, et al: Association of poor clinical status and heavy exposure to tobacco smoke in patients with cystic fibrosis who are homozygous for the F508 deletion. J Pediatr 120:261–264, 1992.
65. Zemel BS, Jawad AF, FitzSimmons S, et al: Longitudinal relationship among growth, nutritional status, and pulmonary function in children with cystic fibrosis: Analysis of the Cystic Fibrosis Foundation National CF Patient Registry. J Pediatr 137:374–380, 2000.
66. Zielenski J, Tsui LC: Cystic fibrosis: Genotypic and phenotypic variations. Annu Rev Genet 29:777–807, 1995.
67. Rozmahel R, Wilschanski M, Matin A, et al: Modulation of disease severity in cystic fibrosis transmembrane conductance regulator deficient mice by a secondary genetic factor. Nat Genet 12:280–287, 1996.
68. Cohn JA, Bornstein JD, Jowell PS: Cystic fibrosis mutations and genetic predisposition to idiopathic chronic pahcreatitis. Med Clin North Am 84:621–631, 2000.
69. Wang X, Moylan B, Leopold DA, et al: Mutation in the gene responsible for cystic fibrosis and predisposition to chronic rhinosinusitis in the general population. JAMA 284:1814–1819, 2000.
70. Feigelson J, Pecau Y, Poquet M, et al: Imaging changes in the pancreas in cystic fibrosis: A retrospective evaluation of 55 cases seen over a period of 9 years. J Pediatr Gastroenterol Nutr 30:145–151, 2000.
71. Murayama S, Robinson AE, Mulvihill DM, et al: MR imaging of pancreas in cystic fibrosis. Pediatr Radiol 20:536–539, 1990.
72. Tham RT, Heyerman HG, Falke TH, et al: Cystic fibrosis: MR imaging of the pancreas. Radiology 179:183–186, 1991.
73. DiMagno EP, Go VL, Summerskill WH: Relations between pancreatic enzyme ouputs and malabsorption in severe pancreatic insufficiency. N Engl J Med 288:813–815, 1973.
74. FitzSimmons SC: The changing epidemiology of cystic fibrosis. J Pediatr 122:1–9, 1993.
75. Hardin DS, Moran A: Diabetes mellitus in cystic fibrosis. Endocrinol Metab Clin North Am 28:787–800, ix, 1999.
76. Wilson DC, Kalnins D, Stewart C, et al: Challenges in the dietary treatment of cystic fibrosis–related diabetes mellitus. Clin Nutr 19:87–93, 2000.
77. Krueger LJ, Lerner A, Katz SM, et al: Cystic fibrosis and diabetes mellitus: Interactive or idiopathic? J Pediatr Gastroenterol Nutr 13: 209–219, 1991.
78. Cotellessa M, Minicucci L, Diana MC, et al: Phenotype/genotype correlation and cystic fibrosis–related diabetes mellitus. Italian Multicenter Study. J Pediatr Endocrinol Metab 13:1087–1093, 2000.
79. Handwerger S, Roth J, Gorden P, et al: Glucose intolerance in cystic fibrosis. N Engl J Med 281:451–461, 1969.
80. Beverley DW, Kelleher J, MacDonald A, et al: Comparison of four pancreatic extracts in cystic fibrosis. Arch Dis Child 62:564–568, 1987.
81. Stern RC, Eisenberg JD, Wagener JS, et al: A comparison of the efficacy and tolerance of pancrelipase and placebo in the treatment of steatorrhea in cystic fibrosis patients with clinical exocrine pancreatic insufficiency. Am J Gastroenterol 95:1932–1938, 2000.
82. Dutta SK, Hubbard VS, Appler M: Critical examination of therapeutic efficacy of a pH-sensitive enteric-coated pancreatic enzyme preparation in treatment of exocrine pancreatic insufficiency secondary to cystic fibrosis. Dig Dis Sci 33:1237–1244, 1988.
83. Cox KL, Isenberg JN, Osher AB, et al: The effect of cimetidine on maldigestion in cystic fibrosis. J Pediatr 94:488–492, 1979.
84. Heijerman HG, Lamers CB, Bakker W: Omeprazole enhances the efficacy of pancreatin (Pancrease) in cystic fibrosis. Ann Intern Med 114:200–201, 1991.
85. Robinson PJ, Smith AL, Sly PD: Duodenal pH in cystic fibrosis and its relationship to fat malabsorption. Dig Dis Sci 35:1299–1304, 1990.
86. Allen A, Flemstrom G, Garner A, et al: Gastroduodenal mucosal protection. Physiol Rev 73:823–857, 1993.

87. Pratha VS, Hogan DL, Martensson BA, et al: Identification of transport abnormalities in duodenal mucosa and duodenal enterocytes from patients with cystic fibrosis. Gastroenterology 118:1051–1060, 2000.
88. Gan KH, Geus WP, Bakker W, et al: In vitro dissolution profiles of enteric-coated microsphere/microtablet pancreatin preparations at different pH values. Aliment Pharmacol Ther 10:771–775, 1996.
89. Borowitz DS, Grand RJ, Durie PR: Use of pancreatic enzyme supplements for patients with cystic fibrosis in the context of fibrosing colonopathy. Consensus Committee. J Pediatr 127:681–684, 1995.
90. Stapleton FB, Kennedy J, Nousia-Arvanitakis S, et al: Hyperuricosuria due to high-dose pancreatic extract therapy in cystic fibrosis. N Engl J Med 295:246–248, 1976.
91. Bergner A, Bergner RK: Pulmonary hypersensitivity associated with pancreatin powder exposure. Pediatrics 55:814–817, 1975.
92. Twarog FJ, Weinstein SF, Khaw KT, et al: Hypersensitivity to pancreatic extracts in parents of patients with cystic fibrosis. J Allergy Clin Immunol 59:35–40, 1977.
93. Smyth RL, van Velzen D, Smyth AR, et al: Strictures of ascending colon in cystic fibrosis and high-strength pancreatic enzymes. Lancet 343:85–86, 1994.
94. FitzSimmons SC, Burkhart GA, Borowitz D, et al: High-dose pancreatic-enzyme supplements and fibrosing colonopathy in children with cystic fibrosis. N Engl J Med 336:1283–1289, 1997.
95. Hasler WL, FitzSimmons SC, Lowenfels AB: Pancreatic enzymnes and colonic strictures with cystic fibrosis: A case-control study. Gastreonterology 114:609–612, 1998.
96. Sokol RJ, Reardon MC, Accurso FJ, et al: Fat-soluble vitamin status during the first year of life in infants with cystic fibrosis identified by screening of newborns. Am J Clin Nutr 50:1064–1071, 1989.
97. Feranchak AP, Sontag MK, Wagener JS, et al: Prospective, long-term study of fat-soluble vitamin status in children with cystic fibrosis identified by newborn screen. J Pediatr 135:601–610, 1999.
98. Rashid M, Durie P, Andrew M, et al: Prevalence of vitamin K deficiency in cystic fibrosis. Am J Clin Nutr 70:378–382, 1999.
99. Thomaidis T, Avey JB: The intestinal lesions in cystic fibrosis of the pancreas. J Pediatr 63:444, 1963.
100. Johansen PG, Kay R: Histochemistry of rectal mucus in cystic fibrosis of the pancreas. J Pathol 99:299–306, 1969.
101. Thiru S, Devereux G, King A: Abnormal fucosylation of ileal mucus in cystic fibrosis: I. A histochemical study using peroxidase-labeled lectins. J Clin Pathol 43:1014–1018, 1990.
102. King A, McLeish M, Thiru S: Abnormal fucosylation of ileal mucus in cystic fibrosis: II. A histochemical study using monoclonal antibodies to fucosyl oligosaccharides. J Clin Pathol 43:1019–1022, 1990.
103. Shwachman H, Holsclaw D: Examination of the appendix at laparotomy as a diagnostic clue in cystic fibrosis. N Engl J Med 286:1300–1301, 1972.
104. Coughlin JP, Gauderer MW, Stern RC, et al: The spectrum of appendiceal disease in cystic fibrosis. J Pediatr Surg 25:835–839, 1990.
105. Gross K, Desanto A, Grosfeld JL, et al: Intra-abdominal complications of cystic fibrosis. J Pediatr Surg 20:431–435, 1985.
106. Shields MD, Levison H, Reisman JJ, et al: Appendicitis in cystic fibrosis. Arch Dis Child 66:307–310, 1991.
107. Rothbaum RJ: Gastrointestinal complications. In Orenstein DM, Stern RC (eds): Treatment of the Hospitalized Cystic Fibrosis Patient. New York, Marcel Dekker, 1998, pp 166–167.
108. Orenstein DM, Rosenstein BJ, Stern RC: Cystic Fibrosis Medical Care. Philadelphia, Lippincott Williams & Wilkins, 2000.
109. Taussig LM, Saldino RM, Di Sant'Agnese PA: Radiographic abnormalities of the duodenum and small bowel in cystic fibrosis of the pancreas (mucoviscidosis). Radiology 106:369–376, 1973.
110. Grossman H, Berdon WE, Baker DH: Gastrointestinal findings in cystic fibrosis. Am J Roentgenol Radium Ther Nucl Med 97:227–238, 1966.
111. Morin CL, Roy CC, Lasalle R, et al: Small bowel mucosal dysfunction in patients with cystic fibrosis. J Pediatr 88:213–216, 1976.
112. Seidler U, Blumenstein I, Kretz A, et al: A functional CFTR protein is required for mouse intestinal cAMP-, cGMP- and Ca^{2+}-dependent HCO^{3-} secretion. J Physiol 505:411–423, 1997.
113. Hogan DL, Crombie DL, Isenberg JI, et al: Acid-stimulated duodenal bicarbonate secretion involves a *CFTR*-mediated transport pathway in mice. Gastroenterology 113:533–541, 1997.
114. Hogan DL, Crombie DL, Isenberg JI, et al: CFTR mediates cAMP- and Ca^{2+}-activated duodenal epithelial HCO^{3-} secretion. Am J Physiol 272:G872–G878, 1997.
115. Clarke LL, Grubb BR, Gabriel SE, et al: Defective epithelial chloride transport in a gene-targeted mouse model of cystic fibrosis. Science 257:1125–1128, 1992.
116. Greger R: Role of CFTR in the colon. Annu Rev Physiol 62:467–491, 2000.
117. Alpers DH, Tedesco FJ: The possible role of pancreatic proteases in the turnover of intestinal brush border proteins. Biochim Biophys Acta 401:28–40, 1975.
118. Buts JP, Morin CL, Roy CC, et al: One-hour blood xylose test: A reliable index of small bowel function. J Pediatr 92:729–733, 1978.
119. Caniano DA, Beaver BL: Meconium ileus: A fifteen-year experience with forty-two neonates. Surgery 102:699–703, 1987.
120. Oppenheimer EH, Esterly JR: Cystic fibrosis of the pancreas: Morphologic findings in infants with and without diagnostic pancreatic lesions. Arch Pathol 96:149–154, 1973.
121. Tizzano EF, Buchwald M: *CFTR* expression and organ damage in cystic fibrosis. Ann Intern Med 123:305–308, 1995.
122. Noblett H: Meconium ileus. In Ravitch M, Welch K, Benson C, et al (eds): Pediatric Surgery. Chicago, Year Book Medical, 1979, p 943.
123. Matsehe JW, Go VL, DiMagno EP: Meconium ileus equivalent complicating cystic fibrosis in postneonatal children and young adults: Report of 12 cases. Gastroenterology 72:732–736, 1977.
124. Davidson AC, Harrison K, Steinfort CL, et al: Distal intestinal obstruction syndrome in cystic fibrosis treated by oral intestinal lavage, and a case of recurrent obstruction despite normal pancreatic function. Thorax 42:538–541, 1987.
125. O'Halloran SM, Gilbert J, McKendrick OM, et al: Gastrografin in acute meconium ileus equivalent. Arch Dis Child 61:1128–1130, 1986.
126. Rubinstein S, Moss R, Lewiston N: Constipation and meconium ileus equivalent in patients with cystic fibrosis. Pediatrics 78:473–479, 1986.
127. Hubbard V: Gastrointestinal complications in cystic fibrosis. Semin Resp Med 6:299, 1985.
128. Jaffe B, Graham W, Goldman L: Postinfancy intestinal obstruction in children with cystic fibrosis. Arch Surg 92:337, 1966.
129. Cleghorn GJ, Stringer DA, Forstner GG, et al: Treatment of distal intestinal obstruction syndrome in cystic fibrosis with a balanced intestinal lavage solution. Lancet 1:8–11, 1986.
130. Holmes M, Murphy V, Taylor M, et al: Intussusception in cystic fibrosis. Arch Dis Child 66:726, 1991.
131. Board TNIE: A look at the National CF Patient Registry. N Insights Cystic Fibrosis 3:1, 1996.
132. Zempsky WT, Rosenstein BJ: The cause of rectal prolapse in children. Am J Dis Child 142:338–339, 1988.
133. Cucchiara S, Santamaria F, Andreotti MR, et al: Mechanisms of gastro-oesophageal reflux in cystic fibrosis. Arch Dis Child 66:617–622, 1991.
134. Davidson AGF, Wong LTK: Gastroesophageal reflux in cystic fibrosis. Pediatr Pulmonol 56:99, 1991.
135. Hassall E, Israel DM, Davidson AG, et al: Barrett's esophagus in children with cystic fibrosis: Not a coincidental association. Am J Gastroenterol 88:1934–1938, 1993.
136. Neglia JP, Wielinski CL, Warwick WJ: Cancer risk among patients with cystic fibrosis. J Pediatr 119:764–766, 1991.
137. Sheldon CD, Hodson ME, Carpenter LM, et al: A cohort study of cystic fibrosis and malignancy. Br J Cancer 68:1025–1028, 1993.
138. Neglia JP, FitzSimmons SC, Maisonneuve P, et al: The risk of cancer among patients with cystic fibrosis. Cystic Fibrosis and Cancer Study Group. N Engl J Med 332:494–499, 1995.
139. Lowenfels AB, Maisonneuve P, Cavallini G, et al: Pancreatitis and the risk of pancreatic cancer. International Pancreatitis Study Group. N Engl J Med 328:1433–1437, 1993.
140. Lowenfels A, Maisonneuve P, DiMagno E, et al: Hereditary pancreatitis and the risk of pancreatic cancer. J Natl Cancer Inst 89:442–446, 1997.
141. Chari ST, Mohan V, Pitchumoni CS, et al: Risk of pancreatic carcinoma in tropical calcifying pancreatitis: An epidemicologic study. Pancreas 9:62–66, 1994.
142. Park RW, Grand RJ: Gastrointestinal manifestations of cystic fibrosis. Gastroenterology 81:1143, 1981.
143. Lindblad A, Glaumann H, Strandvik B: Natural history of liver disease in cystic fibrosis. Hepatology 30:1151–1158, 1999.
144. Duthie A, Doherty DG, Williams C, et al: Genotype analysis for delta F508, G551D, and R553X mutations in children and young adults

with cystic fibrosis with and without chronic liver disease. Hepatology 15:660–664, 1992.

144a. Friedman, KJ, Ling SC, Macek M: Complex multigenic inheritance influences the development of severe CF liver disease. Pediatr Pulmonol 32(Suppl 22):340, 2001.

145. Duthie A, Doherty DG, Donaldson PT, et al: The major histocompatibility complex influences the development of chronic liver disease in male children and young adults with cystic fibrosis. J Hepatol 23:532–537, 1995.

146. Colombo C, Apostolo MG, Ferrari M, et al: Analysis of risk factors for the development of liver disease associated with cystic fibrosis. J Pediatr 124:393–399, 1994.

147. Ling SC, Wilkinson JD, Hollman AS, et al: The evolution of liver disease in cystic fibrosis. Arch Dis Child 81:129–132, 1999.

148. Knoppert D. C, Spino M, Beck R, et al. Cystic fibrosis: Enhanced theophylline metabolism may be linked to the disease. Clin Pharmacol Ther 44:254–264, 1988.

149. Kearns GL, Mallory GB, Crom WR, et al: Enhanced hepatic drug clearance in patients with cystic fibrosis. J Pediatr 117:972–979, 1990.

150. Oppenheimer EH, Esterly JR: Hepatic changes in young infants with cystic fibrosis: Possible relation to focal biliary cirrhosis. J Pediatr 86: 683–689, 1975.

151. Hultcrantz R, Mengarelli S, Strandvik B: Morphological findings in the liver of children with cystic fibrosis: A light and electron microscopical study. Hepatology 6:881–889, 1986.

152. Valman HB, France NE, Wallis PG: Prolonged neonatal jaundice in cystic fibrosis. Arch Dis Child 46:805–809, 1971.

153. McHugo JM, McKeown C, Brown MT, et al: Ultrasound findings in children with cystic fibrosis. Br J Radiol 60:137–141, 1987.

154. Wilson-Sharp RC, Irving HC, Brown RC, et al: Ultrasonography of the pancreas, liver, and biliary system in cystic fibrosis. Arch Dis Child 59:923–926, 1984.

155. Henschke CI, Teele RL: Cholelithiasis in children: Recent observations. J Ultrasound Med 2:481–484, 1983.

156. Kumari-Subaiya S, Gorvoy J, Phillips G, et al: Portal vein measurement by ultrasonography in patients with long-standing cystic fibrosis: Preliminary observations. J Pediatr Gastroenterol Nutr 6:71–78, 1987.

157. Heyman S: Hepatobiliary scintigraphy as a liver function test. J Nucl Med 35:436–437, 1994.

158. Colombo C, Castellani MR, Balistreri WF, et al: Scintigraphic documentation of an improvement in hepatobiliary excretory function after treatment with ursodeoxycholic acid in patients with cystic fibrosis and associated liver disease. Hepatology 15:677–684, 1992.

159. Strandvik B, Samuelson K: Fasting serum bile acid levels in relation to liver histopathology in cystic fibrosis. Scand J Gastroenterol 20: 381–384, 1985.

160. Kattwinkel J, Taussig LM, Statland BE, et al: The effects of age on alkaline phosphatase and other serologic liver function tests in normal subjects and patients with cystic fibrosis. J Pediatr 82:234–242, 1973.

161. Roy CC, Weber AM, Morin CL, et al: Abnormal biliary lipid composition in cystic fibrosis: Effect of pancreatic enzymes. N Engl J Med 297:1301–1305, 1977.

162. Watkins JB, Tercyak AM, Szczepanik P, et al: Bile salt kinetics in cystic fibrosis: Influence of pancreatic enzyme replacement. Gastroenterology 73:1023–1038, 1977.

163. Lykavieris P, Bernard O, Hadchouel M: Neonatal cholestasis as the presenting feature in cystic fibrosis. Arch Dis Child 75:67–70, 1996.

164. Lawson EE, Grand RJ, Neff RK, et al: Clinical estimation of liver span in infants and children. Am J Dis Child 132:474–476, 1978.

165. Borowitz D, Coburn-Miller C: Nutrition and electrolytes. In Orenstein DM, Stern RC (eds): Treatment of the Hospitalized Cystic Fibrosis Patient. New York, Marcel Dekker, 1998, pp 175–211.

166. Treem WR, Stanley CA: Massive hepatomegaly, steatosis, and secondary plasma carnitine deficiency in an infant with cystic fibrosis. Pediatrics 83:993–997, 1989.

167. Durie PR, Pencharz PB: A rational approach to the nutritional care of patients with cystic fibrosis. J R Soc Med 82(Suppl 16):11–20, 1989.

168. Colombo C, Setchell KD, Podda M, et al: Effects of ursodeoxycholic acid therapy for liver disease associated with cystic fibrosis. J Pediatr 117:482–489, 1990.

169. Colombo C, Crosignani A, Assaisso M, et al: Ursodeoxycholic acid therapy in cystic fibrosis-associated liver disease: A dose-response study. Hepatology 16:924–930, 1992.

170. Strandvik B, Hultcrantz R: Liver function and morphology during long-term fatty acid supplementation in cystic fibrosis. Liver 14:32–36, 1994.

171. Mack DR, Traystman MD, Colombo JL, et al: Clinical denouement and mutation analysis of patients with cystic fibrosis undergoing liver transplantation for biliary cirrhosis. J Pediatr 127:881–887, 1995.

172. Bass S, Connon JJ, Ho CS: Biliary tree in cystic fibrosis: Biliary tract abnormalities in cystic fibrosis demonstrated by endoscopic retrograde cholangiography. Gastroenterology 84:1592–1596, 1983.

173. Gaskin KJ, Waters DL, Howman-Giles R, et al: Liver disease and common bile duct stenosis in cystic fibrosis. N Engl J Med 318:340–346, 1988.

174. Strandvik B, Hjelte L, Gabrielsson N, et al: Sclerosing cholangitis in cystic fibrosis. Scand J Gastroenterol Suppl 143:121–124, 1988.

175. Chillon M, Casals T, Mercier B, et al: Mutations in the cystic fibrosis gene in patients with congenital absence of the vas deferens. N Engl J Med 332:1475–1480, 1995.

176. Rave-Harel N, Madgar I, Goshen R, et al: *CFTR* haplotype analysis reveals genetic heterogeneity in the etiology of congenital bilateral aplasia of the vas deferens. Am J Hum Genet 56:1359–1366, 1995.

177. Mak V, Zielenski J, Tsui LC, et al: Cystic fibrosis gene mutations and infertile men with primary testicular failure. Hum Reprod 15:436–439, 2000.

178. Ramsey BW, Farrell PM, Pencharz P: Nutritional assessment and management in cystic fibrosis: A consensus report. The Consensus Committee. Am J Clin Nutr 55:108–116, 1992.

179. Ferry G, Klish W, Borowitz D, et al: Consensus Conference: Gastrointestinal problems in CF. Concen Conf 2:35–46, 1991.

180. Bell L, Durie P, Forstner GG: What do children with cystic fibrosis eat? J Pediatr Gastroenterol Nutr 3(Suppl 1):S137–S146, 1984.

181. Slesinski MJ, Gloninger MF, Costantino JP, et al: Lipid levels in adults with cystic fibrosis. J Am Diet Assoc 94:402–408, 1994.

182. Steinkamp G, von der Hardt H: Improvement of nutritional status and lung function after long-term nocturnal gastrostomy feedings in cystic fibrosis. J Pediatr 124:244–249, 1994.

183. Stallings VA: Nutritional deficiencies in cystic fibrosis. N Insights Cystic Fibrosis 2:1, 1994.

184. Borowitz D, Coburn-Miller C: Practical guidelines to assess and monitor nutritional deficiencies in cystic fibrosis. N Insights Cystic Fibrosis 2:6, 1994.

185. Aitken ML: Managing cystic fibrosis in adults. N Insights Cystic Fibrosis 3:7, 1995.

186. Fiel SB: Unique challenges and needs of adults with cystic fibrosis. N Insights Cystic Fibrosis 3:1, 1995.

187. Shwachman H, Diamond LK, Oski AF, et al: The syndrome of pancreatic insufficiency and bone marrow dysfunction. J Pediatr 65:645–663, 1964.

188. Aggett PJ, Cavanagh NPC, Matthews DJ, et al: Schwachman's syndrome: A review of 21 cases. Arch Dis Child 55:331–347, 1980.

189. Shmerling DH, Prader A, Hitzig WH, et al: The syndrome of exocrine pancreatic insufficency, neutropenia, metaphyseal dysostosis, and dwarfism. Helv Paediatr Acta 24:547–575, 1969.

190. Mack DR, Forstner GG, Wilschanski M, et al: Shwachman syndrome: Exocrine pancreatic dysfunction and variable phenotypic expression. Gastroenterology 111:1593–1602, 1996.

191. Ginzberg H, Shin J, Ellis L, et al: Segregation analysis in Shwachman-Diamond syndrome: Evidence for recessive inheritance. Am J Hum Genet 66:1413–1416, 2000.

192. Smith OP, Hann IM, Chessells JM, et al: Haematological abnormalities in Shwachman-Diamond syndrome. Br J Haematol 94:279–284, 1996.

193. Dror Y, Freedman MH: Shwachman-Diamond syndrome: An inherited preleukemic bone marrow failure disorder with aberrant hematopoietic progenitors and faulty marrow microenvironment. Blood 94:3048–3054, 1999.

194. Ginzberg H, Shin J, Ellis L, et al: Shwachman syndrome: Phenotypic manifestations of sibling sets and isolated cases in a large patient cohort are similar. J Pediatr 135:81–88, 1999.

195. Aggett PJ, Cavanagh NP, Matthew DJ, et al: Shwachman's syndrome: A review of 21 cases. Arch Dis Child 55:331–347, 1980.

196. Hill RE, Durie PR, Gaskin KJ, et al: Steatorrhea and pancreatic insufficiency in Shwachman syndrome. Gastroenterology 83:22–27, 1982.

197. Bom EP, van der Sande FM, Tjon RT, et al: Shwachman syndrome: CT and MR diagnosis. J Comput Assist Tomogr 17:474–476, 1993.

198. MacMaster SA, Cummings TM: Computed tomography and ultrasonography findings for an adult with Shwachman syndrome and pancreatic lipomatosis. Can Assoc Radiol J 44:301–303, 1993.

199. Robberecht E, Nachtegaele P, Van Rattinghe R, et al: Pancreatic lipomatosis in the Shwachman-Diamond syndrome: Identification by sonography and CT-scan. Pediatr Radiol 15:348–349, 1985.
200. Faber J, Lauener R, Wick F, et al: Shwachman-Diamond syndrome: Early bone marrow transplantation in a high-risk patient and new clues to pathogenesis. Eur J Pediatr 158:995–1000, 1999.
201. Ventura A, Dragovich D, Luxardo P, et al: Human granulocyte colony-stimulating factor (rHuG-CSF) for treatment of neutropenia in Shwachman syndrome. Haematologica 80:227–229, 1995.
201a. Cipolli M: Shwachman-Diamond syndrome: Clinical phenotypes. Pancreatology 1:543–548, 2001.
202. Ruutu P, Savilahti E, Repo H, et al: Constant defect in neutrophil locomotion but with age decreasing susceptibility to infection in Shwachman syndrome. Clin Exp Immunol 57:249–255, 1984.
203. Dhar S, Anderton JM: Orthopaedic features of Shwachman syndrome: A report of two cases. J Bone Joint Surg Am 76:278–282, 1994.
204. Spycher MA, Giedion A, Shmerling DH, et al: Electron microscopic examination of cartilage in the syndrome of exocrine pancreatic insufficiency, neutropenia, metaphyseal dysostosis, and dwarfism. Helv Pediatr Acta 29:471–479, 1974.
205. Spirito FR, Crescenzi B, Matteucci C, et al: Cytogenetic characterization of acute myeloid leukemia in Shwachman's syndrome: A case report. Haematologica 85:1207–1210, 2000.
206. Sokolic RA, Ferguson W, Mark HF: Discordant detection of monosomy 7 by GTG-banding and FISH in a patient with Shwachman-Diamond syndrome without evidence of myelodysplastic syndrome or acute myelogenous leukemia. Cancer Genet Cytogenet 115:106–113, 1999.
207. Dror Y, Squire J, Durie P, et al: Malignant myeloid transformation with isochromosome 7q in Shwachman-Diamond syndrome. Leukemia 12:1591–1595, 1998.
208. Goobie S, Popovic M, Morrison J, et al: Shwachman-Diamond syndrome with exocrine pancreatic dysfunction and bone marrow failure maps to the centromeric region of chromosome 7. Am J Hum Genet 68:1048–1054, 2001.
209. Maserati E, Minelli A, Olivieri C, et al: Isochromosome (7q10) in Shwachman syndrome without MDS/AML and role of chromosome 7 anomalies in myeloproliferative disorders. Cancer Genet Cytogenet 121:167–171, 2000.
210. Johanson AJ, Blizzard RM: A syndrome of congenital aplasia of the alae nasi, deafness, hypothyroidism, dwarfism, absent permanent teeth, and malabsorption. J Pediatr 79:982–987, 1971.
211. Jones NL, Hofley PM, Durie PR: Pathophysiology of the pancreatic defect in Johanson-Blizzard syndrome: A disorder of acinar development. J Pediatr 125:406–408, 1994.
212. Gould NS, Paton JB, Bennett AR: Johanson-Blizzard syndrome: Clinical and pathological findings in two sibs. Am J Med Genet 33:194–199, 1989.
213. Gershoni-Baruch R, Lerner A, Braun J, et al: Johanson-Blizzard syndrome: Clinical spectrum and further delineation of the syndrome. Am J Med Genet 35:546–551, 1990.
214. Casademont J, Barrientos A, Cardellach F, et al: Multiple deletions of mtDNA in two brothers with sideroblastic anemia and mitochondrial myopathy and in their asymptomatic mother. Hum Mol Genet 3:1945–1949, 1994.
215. Pearson HA, Lobel JS, Kocoshis SA, et al: A new syndrome of refractory sideroblastic anemia with vacuolization of marrow precursors and exocrine pancreatic dysfunction. J Pediatr 95:976–984, 1979.
216. Favareto F, Caprino D, Micalizzi C, et al: New clinical aspects of Pearson's syndrome: Report of three cases. Haematologica 74:591–594, 1989.
217. Rotig A, Colonna M, Bonnefont JP, et al: Mitochondrial DNA deletion in Pearson's marrow/pancreas syndrome. Lancet 1:902–3, 1989.
218. Superti-Furga A, Schoenle E, Tuchschmid P, et al: Pearson bone marrow–pancreas syndrome with insulin-dependent diabetes, progressive renal tubulopathy, organic aciduria, and elevated fetal haemoglobin caused by deletion and duplication of mitochondrial DNA. Eur J Pediatr 152:44–50, 1993.
219. Rotig A, Cormier V, Koll F, et al: Site-specific deletions of the mitochondrial genome in the Pearson marrow-pancreas syndrome. Genomics 10:502–504, 1991.
220. Rotig A, Cormier V, Blanche S, et al: Pearson's marrow-pancreas syndrome: A multisystem mitochondrial disorder in infancy. J Clin Invest 86:1601–1608, 1990.
221. Baerlocher KE, Feldges A, Weissert M, et al: Mitochondrial DNA deletion in an 8-year-old boy with Pearson syndrome. J Inherit Metab Dis 15:327–330, 1992.
222. Bendon RW: Ivemark's renal-hepatic-pancreatic dysplasia: Analytic approach to a perinatal autopsy. Pediatr Dev Pathol 2:94–100, 1999.
223. Torra R, Alos L, Ramos J, et al: Renal-hepatic-pancreatic dysplasia: An autosomal recessive malformation. J Med Genet 33:409–412, 1996.
224. Whitcomb DC: Genetic predispositions to acute and chronic pancreatitis. Med Clin North Am 84:531–547, 2000.
225. Perrault J: Hereditary pancreatitis: Historical perspectives. Med Clin North Am 84:519–529, 2000.
226. McElroy R, Christiansen PA: Hereditary pancreatitis in a kinship associated with portal vein thrombosis. Am J Med 52:228–241, 1972.
227. Le Bodic L, Schnee M, Georgelin T, et al: An exceptional genealogy for hereditary chronic pancreatitis. Dig Dis Sci 41:1504–1510, 1996.
228. Kattwinkel J, Lapey A, Di SAP, et al: Hereditary pancreatitis: Three new kindreds and a critical review of the literature. Pediatrics 51:55–69, 1973.
229. Le Bodic L, Bignon JD, Raguenes O, et al: The hereditary pancreatitis gene maps to long arm of chromosome 7. Hum Mol Genet 5:549–554, 1996.
230. Pandya A, Blanton SH, Landa B, et al: Linkage studies in a large kindred with hereditary pancreatitis confirms mapping of the gene to a 16-cm region on 7q. Genomics 38:227–230, 1996.
231. Whitcomb DC, Preston RA, Aston CE, et al: A gene for hereditary pancreatitis maps to chromosome 7q35. Gastroenterology 110:1975–1980, 1996.
232. Whitcomb DC, Gorry MC, Preston RA, et al: Hereditary pancreatitis is caused by a mutation in the cationic trypsinogen gene. Nature Genet 14:141–145, 1996.
233. Pfützer RH, Barmada MM, Brunskil APJ, et al: *SPINK1/PSTI* polymorphisms act as disease modifiers in familial and idiopathic chronic pancreatitis. Gastroenterology 119:615–623, 2000.
234. Witt H, Luck W, Hennies HC, et al: Mutations in the gene encoding the serine protease inhibitor, Kazal type 1 are associated with chronic pancreatitis. Nature Genet 25:213–216, 2000.
235. Applebaum-Shapiro SE, Finch R, Pfützer RH, et al: Hereditary pancreatitis in North America: The Pittsburgh–Midwest Multicenter Pancreatic Study Group study. Pancreatology 1:439–443, 2001.
236. Whitcomb DC: Hereditary pancreatitis: New insights into acute and chronic pancreatitis. Gut 45:317–322, 1999.
237. Gates LK: Preventive strategies and therapeutic options for hereditary pancreatitis. Med Clin North Am 84:589–595, 2000.
238. Whitcomb DC, Applebaum S, Martin SP: Hereditary pancreatitis and pancreatic carcinoma. Ann N Y Acad Sci 880:201–209, 1999.
239. Martin SP, Ulrich CD II: Pancreatic cancer surveillance in a high-risk cohort: Is it worth the cost? Med Clin North Am 84:739–747, 2000.
240. Rinderknecht H: Pancreatic secretory enzymes. In Go VLW, DiMagno EP, Gardner JD, et al (eds): The Pancreas: Biology, Pathobiology, and Disease, 2nd ed. New York, Raven, 1993, pp 219–251.
241. Gorry MC, Gabbaizedeh D, Furey W, et al: Mutations in the cationic trypsinogen gene are associated with recurrent acute and chronic pancreatitis. Gastroenterology 113:1063–1068, 1997.
242. Varallyay E, Pal G, Patthy A, et al: Two mutations in rat trypsin confer resistance against autolysis. Biochem Biophys Res 243:56–60, 1998.
243. Sahin-Toth M: Hereditary pancreatitis–associated mutation asn-(21)→ile stabilizes rat trypsinogen in vitro. J Biol Chem 274:2699–2704, 1999.
244. Howes N, Rutherford S, O'Donnell M, et al: A new polymorphism for the *R117H* mutation in hereditary pancreatitis. Gut 48:247–250, 1999.
245. Teich N, Mossner J, Keim V: Mutations of the cationic trypsinogen in hereditary pancreatitis. Hum Mutat 12:39–43, 1998.
246. Böhm AK, Reinheckel T, Rosenstrauch D, et al: Screening for a point mutation of cationic trypsinogen in patients with pancreatic disease [abstract]. Digestion 60:369, 1999.
247. Cohn JA, Bornstein JD, Jowell PJ, et al: Molecular pathogenesis of chronic pancreatitis associated with abnormal *CFTR* genotypes. Gastroenterology 118:A159, 2000.
248. Creighton J, Lyall R, Wilson DI, et al: Mutations of the cationic trypsinogen gene in patients with chronic pancreatitis [letter]. Lancet 354:42–43, 1999.
249. Chen JM, Raguenes O, Ferec C, et al: The A16V signal peptide cleavage site mutation in the cationic trypsinogen gene and chronic pancreatitis [letter; comment]. Gastroenterology 117:1508–1509, 1999.
250. Teich N, Ockenga J, Hoffmeister A, et al: Chronic pancreatitis associated with an activation peptide mutation that facilitates trypsin activation. Gastroenterology 119:461–465, 2000.
251. Ferec C, Raguenes O, Salomon R, et al: Mutations in the cationic

trypsinogen gene and evidence for genetic heterogeneity in hereditary pancreatitis. J Med Genet 36:228–232, 1999.

252. Applebaum SE, Kant JA, Whitcomb DC, et al: Genetic testing: Counseling, laboratory, and regulatory issues and the EUROPAC protocol for ethical research in multicenter studies of inherited pancreatic diseases. Med Clin North Am 82:575–588, 2000.

252a. Ellis I, Lerch MM, Whitcomb DC, for the Concensus Committees of the European Registry of Hereditary Pancreatic Diseases, the Midwest Multi-Center Pancreatic Study Group, and the International Association of Pancreatology: Genetic testing for hereditary pancreatitis: Guidelines for indications, counselling, consent and privacy issues. Pancreatology 1:405–415, 2001.

253. Applebaum SE, O'Connell JA, Aston CE, et al: Motivations and concerns of patients with access to genetic testing for hereditary pancreatitis. Am J Gastroenterol 96:1610–1617, 2000.

254. Whitcomb D: The First International Symposium on Hereditary Pancreatitis. Pancreas 18:1–12, 1998.

255. Sibert JR: Hereditary pancreatitis in England and Wales. J Med Genet 15:189–201, 1978.

256. Perrault J: Hereditary pancreatitis. Gastroenterol Clin North Am 23: 743–752, 1994.

257. Whitcomb DC, Ulrich CD II: Hereditary pancreatitis: New insights, new directions. Baillieres Clin Gastroenterol 13:253–263, 1999.

258. Sossenheimer MJ, Aston CE, Preston RA, et al: Clinical characteristics of hereditary pancreatitis in a large family based on high-risk haplotype. Am J Gastroenterol 92:1113–1116, 1997.

259. Paolini O, Hastier P, Buckley M, et al: The natural history of hereditary chronic pancreatitis: A study of 12 cases compared to chronic alcoholic pancreatitis. Pancreas 17:266–271, 1998.

260. Anonymous: Protection of human subjects: Reports of the President's Commission for the Study of Ethical Problems in Medicine and Biomedical and Behavioral Research—Office of the Assistant Secretary for Health, HHS. Notice of availability of reports. Fed Regist 48: 34408–34412, 1983.

261. Anonymous: Protection of human subjects: Institutional Review Board: Report and recommendations of National Commission for the Protection of Human Subjects of Biomedical and Behavioral Research. Fed Regist 43:56173–56198, 1978.

262. O'Connell JA: The process of childhood genetic testing and disclosure: Parental views and intentions [master's thesis]. Pittsburgh, PA, University of Pittsburgh, 2000.

263. Clarke A: The genetic testing of children: Working Party of the Clinical Genetics Society (UK). J Med Genet 31:785–797, 1994.

264. Talamini G, Bassi C, Falconi M, et al: Cigarette smoking: An independent risk factor in alcoholic pancreatitis. Pancreas 12:131–137, 1996.

265. Talamini G, Bassi C, Falconi M, et al: Alcohol and smoking as risk factors in chronic pancreatitis and pancreatic cancer. Dig Dis Sci 44: 1301–1311, 1999.

266. Lin Y, Tamakoshi A, Hayakawa T, et al: Cigarette smoking as a risk factor for chronic pancreatitis: A case-control study in Japan. Research Committee on Intractable Pancreatic Diseases. Pancreas 21:109–114, 2000.

267. Fuchs CS, Colditz GA, Stampfer MJ, et al: A prospective study of cigarette smoking and the risk of pancreatic cancer. Arch Intern Med 156:2255–2260, 1996.

268. Stolzenberg-Solomon RZ, Albanes D, Nieto FJ, et al: Pancreatic cancer risk and nutrition-related methyl-group availability indicators in male smokers. J Natl Cancer Inst 91:535, 1999.

269. Lowenfels AB, Maisonneuve P, Whitcomb DC: Risk factors for cancer in hereditary pancreatitis. International Hereditary Pancreatitis Study Group. Med Clin North Am 84:565–573, 2000.

270. Warshaw A, Banks PA, Fernandez-del Castillo C: AGA technical review: Treatment of pain in chronic pancreatitis. Gastroenterology 115:765–776, 1998.

271. Rinderknecht H, Adham NF, Renner IG, et al: A possible zymogen self-destruct mechanism preventing pancreatic autodigestion. Int J Pancreatol 3:33–44, 1988.

272. Chen JM, Mercier B, Audrezet MP, et al: Mutational analysis of the human pancreatic secretory trypsin inhibitor (*PSTI*) gene in hereditary and sporadic chronic pancreatitis. J Med Genet 37:67–69, 2000.

273. Owyang C, Levitt M: Chronic pancreatitis. In Yamada T (ed): Textbook of Gastroenterology. Philadelphia, JB Lippincott, 1991, pp 1874–1893.

274. Sharer N, Schwarz M, Malone G, et al: Mutations of the cystic fibrosis gene in patients with chronic pancreatitis. N Engl J Med 339: 645–652, 1998.

275. Cohn JA, Friedman KJ, Noone PG, et al: Relation between mutations of the cystic fibrosis gene and idiopathic pancreatitis. N Engl J Med 339:653–658, 1998.

276. Ockenga J, Stuhrmann M, Ballmann M, et al: Mutations of the cystic fibrosis gene, but not cationic trypsinogen gene, are associated with recurrent or chronic idiopathic pancreatitis. Am J Gastroenterol 95: 2061–2067, 2000.

277. Arduino C, Gallo M, Brusco A, et al: Polyvariant mutant *CFTR* genes in patients with chronic pancreatitis. Clin Genet 56:400–404, 1999.

278. Malats N, Casals T, Porta M, et al: Cystic fibrosis transmembrane regulator (*CFTR*) deltaF508 mutation and 5T allele in patients with chronic pancreatitis and exocrine pancreatic cancer. PANKRAS II Study Group. Gut 48:70–74, 2001.

279. Gomez Lira M, Benetazzo MG, Marzari MG, et al: High frequency of cystic fibrosis transmembrane regulator mutation L997F in patients with recurrent idiopathic pancreatitis and in newborns with hypertrypsinemia. Am J Hum Genet 66:2013–2014, 2000.

280. Etemad B: Gastrointestinal complications of renal failure. Gastroenterol Clin North Am 27:875–892, 1998.

281. Strong TV, Wilkinson DJ, Mansoura MK, et al: Expression of an abundant alternatively spliced form of the cystic fibrosis transmembrane conductance regulator (*CFTR*) gene is not associated with a cAMP-activated chloride conductance. Hum Mol Genet 2:225–230, 1993.

282. Costes B, Girodon E, Ghanem N, et al: Frequent occurrence of the *CFTR* intron 8 (TG)n 5T allele in men with congenital bilateral absence of the vas deferens. Eur J Hum Genet 3:285–293, 1995.

283. Lowenfels A, Maisonneuve P, Palys BR: Re: Ockenga et al—Mutations of cystic fibrosis gene in patients with pancreatitis. Am J Gastroenterol 96:614–615, 2001.

284. Massie RJ, Wilcken B, Van Asperen P, et al: Pancreatic function and extended mutation analysis in deltaF508 heterozygous infants with an elevated immunoreactive trypsinogen but normal sweat electrolyte levels. J Pediatr 137:214–220, 2000.

285. Anguiano A, Oates RD, Amos JA, et al: Congenital bilateral absence of the vas deferens: A primarily genital form of cystic fibrosis. JAMA 267:1794–1797, 1992.

286. Mithofer K, Fernandez-Del Castillo C, Frick TW, et al: Acute hypercalcemia causes acute pancreatitis and ectopic trypsinogen activation in the rat. Gastroenterology 109:239–246, 1995.

287. Whitcomb DC: Early trypsinogen activation in acute pancreatitis. Gastroenterology 116:770–773, 1999.

288. Figarella C, Amouric M, Guy-Crotte O: Proteolysis of human trypsinogen: I. Pathogenic implications in chronic pancreatitis. Biochem Biophys Res 118:154–161, 1984.

289. Colomb E, Guy O, Deprez P, et al: The two human trypsinoens: Catalytic properties of the corresponding trypsins. Biochem Biophys Acta 525:186–193, 1978.

290. Cope O, Culver PJ, Mixer CG Jr, et al: Pancreatitis: A diagnostic clue to hyperparathyroidism. Ann Surg 145:857–863, 1957.

291. Jackson CE: Hereditary hyperparathyroidism associated with recurrent pancreatitis. Ann Intern Med 49:829–836, 1958.

292. Bess MA, Edis AJ, van Heerden JA: Hyperparathyroidism and pancreatitis: Chance or a causal association? JAMA 243:246–247, 1980.

293. Carey MC, Fitzgerald O: Hyperparathyroidism associated with chronic pancreatitis in a family. Gut 9:700–703, 1968.

294. Prinz RA, Aranha GV: The association of primary hyperparathyroidism and pancreatitis. Am Surg 51:325–329, 1985.

295. DiMagno E, Layer P, Clain J: Chronic pancreatitis. In Go V (ed): The Pancreas: Biology, Pathophysiology, and Disease. New York, Raven, 1993, pp 665–706.

296. Strum WB, Spiro HM: Chronic pancreatitis. Ann Intern Med 74:264–277, 1971.

297. Mergener K, Baillie J: Chronic pancreatitis. Lancet 340:1379–1385, 1997.

298. Krauss RM, Levy AG: Subclinical chronic pancreatitis in type I hyperlipoproteinemia. Am J Med 62:144–149, 1977.

299. Salen S, Kesseler JI, Janowitz HD: The development of pancreatic secretory insufficiency in a patient with recurrent pancreatitis and type V hyperlipoproteinemia. Mt Sinai J Med 37:103, 1970.

300. Saharia P, Margolis S, Zuidema GD, et al: Acute pancreatitis with hyperlipemia: Studies with an isolated perfused canine pancreas. Surgery 82:60–67, 1977.

301. Fortson MR, Freedman SN, Webster PD III: Clinical assessment of hyperlipidemic pancreatitis. Am J Gastroenterol 90:2134–2139, 1995.

302. Wilson DE, Hata A, Kwong LK, et al: Mutations in exon 3 of the lipoprotein lipase gene segregating in a family with hypertriglyceri-

demia, pancreatitis, and non-insulin-dependent diabetes. J Clin Invest 92:203–211, 1993.
303. Fojo SS, Brewer HB: Hypertriglyceridaemia due to genetic defects in lipoprotein lipase and apolipoprotein C-II. J Intern Med 231:669–677, 1992.
304. Cox DW, Breckenridge WC, Little JA: Inheritance of apolipoprotein C-II deficiency with hypertriglyceridemia and pancreatitis. N Engl J Med 299:1421–1424, 1978.
305. Beil FU, Fojo SS, Brewer HJ, et al: Apolipoprotein C-II deficiency syndrome due to apo C-IIHamburg: Clinical and biochemical features and HphI restriction enzyme polymorphism. Eur J Clin Invest 22:88–95, 1992.
306. Bruin T, Tuzgol S, Van DD, et al: Recurrent pancreatitis and chylomicronemia in an extended Dutch kindred. J Lipid Res 34:2109–2119, 1993.
307. Toskes PP: Hyperlipidemic pancreatitis. Gastroenterol Clin North Am 19:783–791, 1990.
308. Morris MD, Fisher DA: Trypsinogen deficiency disease. Am J Dis Child 114:203–208, 1967.
309. Townes PL: Proteolytic and lipolytic deficiency of the exocrine pancreas. J Pediatr 75:221–228, 1969.
310. Figarella C, Negri GA, Sarles H: Presence of colipase in a congenital pancreatic lipase deficiency. Biochim Biophys Acta 280:205–211, 1972.
311. Figarella C, De Caro A, Leupold D, et al: Congenital pancreatic lipase deficiency. J Pediatr 96:412–416, 1980.
312. Muller DP, McCollum JP, Trompeter RS, et al: Proceedings: Studies on the mechanism of fat absorption in congenital isolated lipase deficiency. Gut 16:838, 1975.
313. Lowe ME, Rosenblum JL, Strauss AW: Cloning and characterization of human pancreatic lipase cDNA. J Biol Chem 264:20042–20048, 1989.
314. Davis RC, Diep A, Hunziker W, et al: Assignment of human pancreatic lipase gene (PNLIP) to chromosome 10q24-q26. Genomics 11: 1164–1166, 1991.
315. Sims HF, Lowe ME: The human colipase gene: Isolation, chromosomal location, and tissue-specific expression. Biochemistry 31:7120–7125, 1992.
316. Ligumsky M, Granot E, Branski D, et al: Isolated lipase and colipase deficiency in two brothers. Gut 31:1416–1418, 1990.
317. Hildebrand H, Borgstrom B, Bekassy A, et al: Isolated co-lipase deficiency in two brothers. Gut 23:243–246, 1982.
318. Ghishan FK, Moran JR, Durie PR, et al: Isolated congenital lipase-colipase deficiency. Gastroenterology 86:1580–1582, 1984.
319. Hadorn B, Tarlow MJ, Lloyd JK, et al: Intestinal enterokinase deficiency. Lancet 1:812–813, 1969.
320. Lebenthal E, Antonowicz I, Shwachman H: Enterokinase and trypsin activities in pancreatic insufficiency and diseases of the small intestine. Gastroenterology 70:508–512, 1976.
321. Lebenthal E, Antonowicz I, Shwachman H: The interrelationship of enterokinase and trypsin activities in intractable diarrhea of infancy, celiac disease, and intravenous alimentation. Pediatrics 56:585–591, 1975.
322. Sibert JR: Pancreatitis in childhood. Postgrad Med J 55:171–175, 1979.
323. Weizman Z, Durie PR: Acute pancreatitis in childhood. J Pediatr 113: 24–29, 1988.
324. Ziegler DW, Long JA, Philippart AI, et al: Pancreatitis in childhood: Experience with 49 patients. Ann Surg 207:257–261, 1988.
325. Mallory A, Kern F: Drug-induced pancreatitis: A critical review. Gastroenterology 78:813–820, 1980.
326. Parker PH, Helinek GL, Ghishan FK, et al: Recurrent pancreatitis induced by valproic acid: A case report and review of the literature. Gastroenterology 80:826–828, 1981.
327. Sturdevant RA, Singleton JW, Deren JL, et al: Azathioprine-related pancreatitis in patients with Crohn's disease. Gastroenterology 77: 883–886, 1979.
328. Elmore MF, Rogge JD: Tetracycline-induced pancreatitis. Gastroenterology 81:1134–1136, 1981.
329. Steinberg WM, Lewis JH: Steroid-induced pancreatitis: Does it really exist? Gastroenterology 81:799–808, 1981.
330. Land VJ, Sutow WW, Fernbach DJ, et al: Toxicity of L-asparginase in children with advanced leukemia. Cancer 30:339–347, 1972.
331. Arnesjo B, Eden T, Ihse I, et al: Enterovirus infections in acute pancreatitis—a possible etiological connection. Scand J Gastroenterol 11:645–649, 1976.
332. Capner P, Lendrum R, Jeffries DJ, et al: Viral antibody studies in pancreatic disease. Gut 16:866–870, 1975.
333. Ursing B: Acute pancreatitis in coxsackie B infection. BMJ 3:524–525, 1973.
334. Lifschitz C, LaSala S: Pancreatitis, cholecystitis, and choledocholithiasis associated with infectious mononucleosis. Clin Pediatr 20:131, 1981.
335. Werbitt W, Mohsenifar Z: Mononucleosis pancreatitis. South Med J 73:1094, 1980.
336. Bunnell CE, Monif GR: Interstitial pancreatitis in the congenital rubella syndrome. J Pediatr 80:465–466, 1972.
337. Naficy K, Nategh R, Ghadimi H: Mumps pancreatitis without parotitis. BMJ 1:529, 1973.
338. Bell MJ, Ternberg JL, Feigin RD: Surgical complications of leptospirosis in children. J Pediatr Surg 13:325–330, 1978.
339. Mardh PA, Ursing B: The occurrence of acute pancreatitis in *Mycoplasma pneumoniae* infection. Scand J Infect Dis 6:167–171, 1974.
340. Russell IJ, Forgacs P, Geraci JE: Pancreatitis complicating typhoid fever: Report of a case. JAMA 235:753–754, 1976.
341. Das S: Pancreatitis in children associated with round worms. Indian Pediatr 14:81–83, 1977.
342. Marks IN, Bank S, Louw JH: Chronic pancreatitis in the Western Cape. Digestion 9:447–453, 1973.
343. Gilbert MG, Carbonnel ML: Pancreatitis in childhood associated with ascariasis. Pediatrics 33:1964, 1964.
344. Johnson RC, DeFord JW, Carlton PK: Pancreatitis complicating falciparum malaria. Postgrad Med 61:181–183, 1977.
345. Miller TL, Winter HS, Luginbuhl LM, et al: Pancreatitis in pediatric human immunodeficiency virus infection. J Pediatr 120:223–227, 1992.
346. Dutta SK, Ting CD, Lai LL: Study of prevalence, severity, and etiological factors associated with acute pancreatitis in patients infected with human immunodeficiency virus. Am J Gastroenterol 92:2044–2048, 1997.
347. Moyle GJ, Nelson MR, Hawkins D, et al: The use and toxicity of didanosine (ddI) in HIV antibody-positive individuals intolerant to zidovudine (AZT). Q J Med 86:155–163, 1993.
348. Schindzielorz A, Pike I, Daniels M, et al: Rates and risk factors for adverse events associated with didanosine in the expanded access program. Clin Infect Dis 19:1076–1083, 1994.
349. Cappell MS, Marks M: Acute pancreatitis in HIV-seropositive patients: A case control study of 44 patients. Am J Med 98:243–248, 1995.
350. Manocha AP, Sossenheimer M, Martin SP, et al: Prevalence and predictors of severe acute pancreatitis in patients with acquired immune deficiency syndrome (AIDS). Am J Gastroenterol 94:784–789, 1999.
351. Danus O, Urbina AM, Valenzuela I, et al: The effect of refeeding on pancreatic exocrine function in marasmic infants. J Pediatr 77:334–337, 1970.
352. Barbezat GO, Hansen JD: The exocrine pancreas and protein-calorie malnutrition. Pediatrics 42:77–92, 1968.
353. Gryboski J, Hillemeier C, Kocoshis S, et al: Refeeding pancreatitis in malnourished children. J Pediatr 97:441–443, 1980.
354. Keane FB, Fennell JS, Tomkin GH: Acute pancreatitis, acute gastric dilation, and duodenal ileus following refeeding in anorexia nervosa. Ir J Med Sci 147:191–192, 1978.
355. Izsak EM, Shike M, Roulet M, et al: Pancreatitis in association with hypercalcemia in patients receiving total parenteral nutrition. Gastroenterology 79:555–558, 1980.
356. Chaves-Carballo E, Menezes AH, Bell WE, et al: Acute pancreatitis in Reye's syndrome: A fatal complication during intensive supportive care. South Med J 73:152–154, 1980.
357. Puppala AR, Cheng JC, Steinheber FU: Pancreatitis—a rare complication of Schönlein-Henoch purpura. Am J Gastroenterol 69:101–104, 1978.
358. Stoler J, Biller JA, Grand RJ: Pancreatitis in Kawasaki disease. Am J Dis Child 141:306–308, 1987.
359. Smith PM, Morgans ME, Clark CG, et al: Lipodystrophy, pancreatitis, and eosinophilia. Gut 16:230–234, 1975.
360. Nwokolo C, Oli J: Pathogenesis of juvenile tropical pancreatitis syndrome. Lancet 1:456–459, 1980.
361. Pitchumoni CS: Juvenile tropical pancreatitis. Lancet 1:1028, 1980.
362. Rossi L, Pfützer RH, Parvin S, et al: *SPINK1/PSTI* mutations are associated with tropical pancreatitis in Bangladesh, a preliminary report. Pancreatology 1:242–245, 2001.
363. Bank S, Wise L, Gersten M: Risk factors in acute pancreatitis. Am J Gastroenterol 78:637–640, 1983.

Chapter 48

ACUTE PANCREATITIS

Eugene P. DiMagno and Suresh Chari

INCIDENCE AND DEFINITION

The incidence of acute pancreatitis in England, Denmark, and the United States varies from 4.8 to 24.2 per 100,000 patients.[1] However, estimates of incidence are inaccurate because the diagnosis of mild disease may be missed, and death may occur before diagnosis in 10% of patients with severe disease.[2] The two most common causes of acute pancreatitis in adults are gallstone pancreatitis, which occurs more often in women, and alcoholic pancreatitis, which occurs more often in men. The incidence increases with age and is three times higher in black men than in white men.[1] Onset in the first decade suggests a hereditary cause (e.g., hyperlipidemia or hereditary pancreatitis), infection (e.g., mumps), or trauma.

Clinical characteristics of acute pancreatitis are severe pain in the upper abdomen and at least a threefold elevation of pancreatic enzymes in the blood.[3] Abnormal exocrine and endocrine pancreatic function can occur during an acute attack.[1] Endocrine function returns to normal soon after the acute phase, whereas exocrine function may take up to a year for full recovery.[4, 5] Usually, however, the gland eventually returns to normal morphology and function if the cause of pancreatitis is eliminated and no further attacks occur. Massive pancreatic necrosis can scar the pancreas, resulting in a stricture of the main pancreatic duct with subsequent obstructive chronic pancreatitis and permanent diabetes and malabsorption.

Differentiation between acute and chronic pancreatitis is difficult because an attack of "acute pancreatitis" can occur in chronic pancreatitis with preexisting morphologic and functional abnormalities.[6] Currently, most pancreatologists use the 1992 Atlanta Symposium definition of acute pancreatitis,[3] which is *an acute inflammatory process of the pancreas with variable involvement of other regional tissues or remote organ systems*. Pancreatitis is classified as acute unless there are computed tomographic or endoscopic retrograde cholangiopancreatographic (ERCP) findings of chronic pancreatitis. Then pancreatitis is classified as chronic pancreatitis, and any episode of "acute pancreatitis" is considered an exacerbation of inflammation superimposed upon chronic pancreatitis (see Chapter 49).

At the Atlanta symposium, definitions of severe pancreatitis and associated manifestations and conditions were proposed and have been accepted generally (Tables 48–1 to 48–3). Mild acute pancreatitis consists of minimal or no organ dysfunction and an uneventful recovery. Severe pancreatitis manifests as organ failure and/or local complications such as necrosis, abscess, or pseudocyst. Other acceptable markers of severe pancreatitis include three or more of Ranson's 11 criteria (Table 48–2) and the Acute Physiology and Chronic Health Evaluation (APACHE-II) score of greater than 8.[3] In addition, there was agreement that dynamic contrast-enhanced CT scans can distinguish interstitial from necrotizing pancreatitis (Figs. 48–1 and 48–2). Pancreatic necrosis consists of focal or diffuse nonvi-

Table 48–1 | **Criteria for Severe Acute Pancreatitis**

ORGAN FAILURE
Shock: systolic blood pressure < 90 mm Hg
Pulmonary insufficiency: $PaO_2 \leq 60$ mm Hg
Renal failure: serum creatinine > 2 mg/dL
Gastrointestinal bleeding: > 500 mL/24 hr

AND/OR LOCAL COMPLICATIONS
Necrosis
Abscess
Pseudocyst

UNFAVORABLE EARLY PROGNOSTIC SIGNS
≥ 3 Ranson's signs (see Table 48–2)
≥ 8 APACHE-II points

Table 48–2 | **Ranson's 11 Criteria for Severity of Pancreatitis**

AT ADMISSION
Age > 55 yr
White blood cells > 16,000/mm^3
Glucose > 200 mg/dL
Lactate dehydrogenase > 350 IU/L
Aspartate aminotransferase > 250 U/L

DURING INITIAL 48 HR
Hematocrit decrease of > 10 mg/dL
Blood urea nitrogen increase of > 5 mg/dL
Calcium < 8 mg/dL
PaO_2 < 60 mm Hg
Base deficit > 4 mEq/L
Fluid sequestration > 6 L

able pancreatic parenchyma and usually peripancreatic fat necrosis.

An *acute fluid collection* is fluid located in or near the pancreas that lacks a definite wall and that occurs early in the course of acute pancreatitis. On CT scan it is a low attenuation mass with poor margins and no capsule. Intrapancreatic fluid collections are less than 3 cm. An acute fluid collection occurs in 30% to 50% of acute pancreatitis and most resolve spontaneously. A *pseudocyst* is a fluid collection that persists for 4 to 6 weeks and becomes encapsulated by a wall of fibrous or granulation tissue (Fig. 48–3). A *pancreatic abscess* is a circumscribed intra-abdominal collection of pus after an episode of acute pancreatitis or pancreatic trauma. It usually develops close to the pancreas and contains little pancreatic necrosis.

Finally, several terms have been replaced or deleted. *Infected pseudocyst* was replaced by *pancreatic abscess. Persistent acute pancreatitis* was replaced by *interstitial* or *necrotizing pancreatitis. Hemorrhagic pancreatitis* and *phlegmon* were deleted, the former because most cases of pancreatic necrosis occur without gross intraglandular hemorrhage, and the latter because there is confusion concerning the proper use of this term.

PATHOLOGY

Most causes of acute pancreatitis (i.e., alcohol, gallstones, and drugs) involve initial injury to peripheral acinar cells, fat necrosis, and autodigestion. The peripheral cells are distant from the arterial supply of pancreatic lobules, and some parenchymal damage likely is due to abnormalities of the microcirculation. In comparison, infectious agents are directly toxic to acinar cells and cause generalized acinar cell necrosis associated with an acute inflammatory infiltrate. By contrast, the first lesion produced by pancreatitis due to hypotension is ductal necrosis.[7]

Interstitial pancreatitis is characterized by interstitial edema associated with inflammatory cells within the parenchyma. Although parenchymal necrosis may occur, it is microscopic. Small foci of fat necrosis characteristically punctuate the surface of the gland.

The major features of necrotizing pancreatitis are macroscopic focal or diffuse necrosis of the pancreatic parenchyma, large areas of fat necrosis, and occasionally hemorrhage on the surface on the pancreas and in peripancreatic tissue. Granulocytes and macrophages demarcate areas of necrosis, which may involve acinar cells, islet cells, and the pancreatic ductal system. Pancreatic necrosis is present mostly in the periphery of the lobules, but it may progress to involve most of the gland. Severe interstitial fat necrosis involves small veins and venules, which may be infiltrated by granulocytes, leading to thrombosis, necrosis, and rupture. Arterial thrombosis is observed infrequently.

PATHOGENESIS

The initial step in the pathogenesis of acute pancreatitis is conversion of trypsinogen to trypsin within acinar cells in sufficient quantities to overwhelm normal mechanisms to remove active trypsin. Trypsin, in turn, catalyzes conversion of proenzymes, including trypsinogen and inactive precursors of elastase, phospholipase A_2, and carboxypeptidase, to active enzymes. Trypsin also may activate the complement and kinin systems. Active enzymes autodigest the pancreas and initiate a cycle of releasing more active enzymes. Normally, small amounts of trypsinogen are spontaneously activated within the pancreas, but intrapancreatic mechanisms quickly remove activated trypsin. Pancreatic secretory trypsin inhibitor (PSTI) binds and inactivates about 20% of the trypsin

Table 48–3 | **Conditions Predisposing to Acute Pancreatitis***

Gallstones
Biliary sludge and microlithiasis
Other causes of mechanical ampullary obstruction
Alcohol
Hypertriglyceridemia
Hypercalcemia
Drugs
Infections and toxins
Trauma
Pancreas divisum
Vascular disease
Pregnancy*
Post-ERCP
Postoperative pancreatitis
Hereditary pancreatitis
Structural abnormalities
- Duodenum/ampullary region
- Bile duct
- Sphincter of Oddi dysfunction
- Main pancreatic duct

*Association is not direct (see text).
ERCP, endoscopic retrograde cholangiopancreatography.

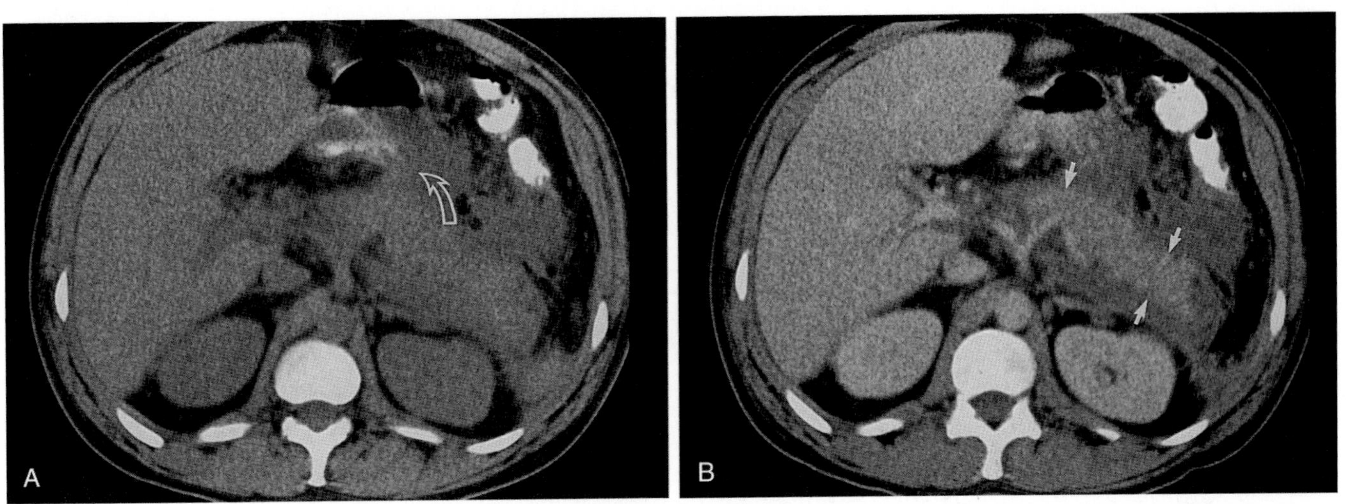

Figure 48–1. Interstitial pancreatitis. *A,* Unenhanced computed tomography (CT) scan obtained on the third day of illness. The pancreas is not clearly defined, and diffuse peripancreatic inflammation extends into the lesser sac *(curved arrow),* left anterior pararenal space, and adjacent to the left colon. *B,* Dynamic contrast-enhanced CT scan performed on the same day. There is uniform enhancement of the pancreas *(arrows)* without necrosis. The Balthazar-Ranson CT severity index is 4 (grade E pancreatitis and no necrosis; see Table 48–6).

activity. Other mechanisms for removing trypsin involve mesotrypsin, enzyme Y, and trypsin itself, which splits and inactivates trypsin. The pancreas also contains nonspecific antiproteases such as alpha-$_1$-antitrypsin and alpha-$_2$-macroglobulin. Additional protective mechanisms are the sequestration of pancreatic enzymes within intracellular compartments of the acinar cell during synthesis and transport and the separation of digestive enzymes from lysosomal hydrolases as they pass through the Golgi apparatus, which is important because cathepsin B activates trypsin from trypsinogen.

In experimental pancreatitis, activation of trypsin occurs within 10 minutes, and large amounts of trypsin[8] and increased concentrations of trypsinogen activation peptide (TAP) accumulate within the pancreas.[9, 10] TAP is cleaved when trypsinogen is activated to trypsin, and concentrations of TAP in plasma, urine, and ascites correlate with the severity of the pancreatic inflammatory response, with the highest levels associated with acinar necrosis and intrapancreatic hemorrhage.[10–12]

Co-localization of pancreatic enzymes, followed by acinar cell injury, is an attractive hypothesis for the pathogenesis of

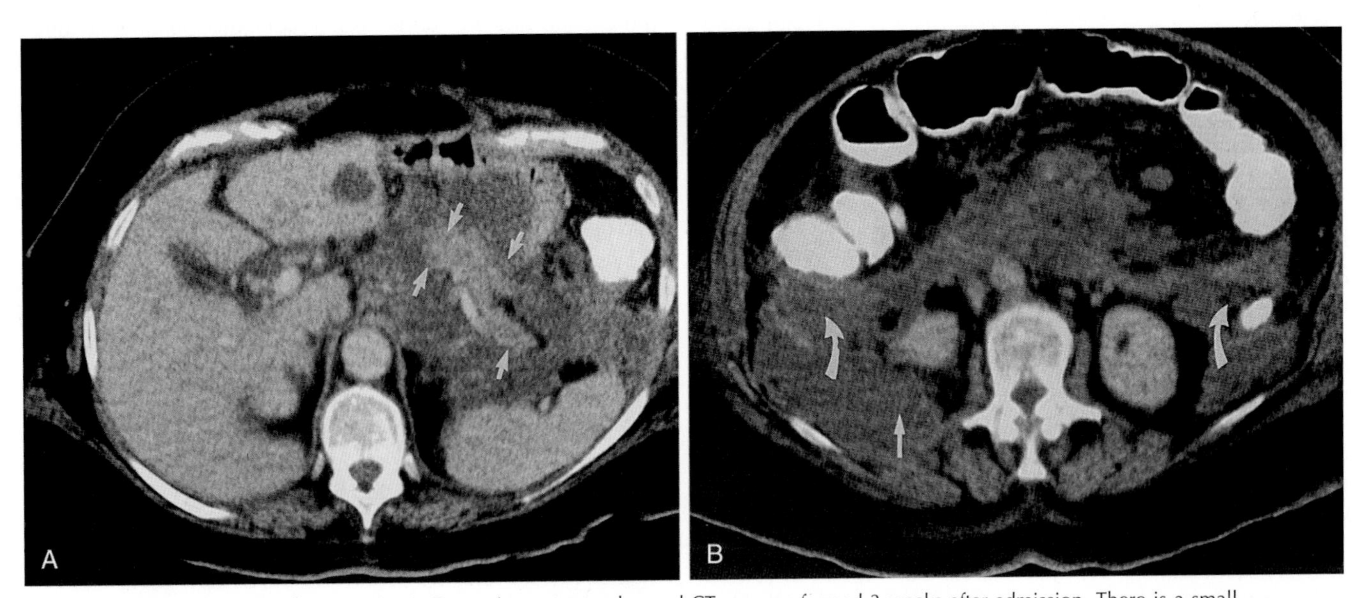

Figure 48–2. Sterile necrosis. *A,* Dynamic contrast-enhanced CT scan performed 3 weeks after admission. There is a small area of normally enhancing pancreatic parenchyma *(arrows).* Hence, pancreatic necrosis is extensive. A considerable amount of fluid and associated inflammatory changes are evident throughout the anterior pararenal space, extending to the spleen and to the region of the stomach and colon. The Balthazar-Ranson CT severity index is 10 (grade E pancreatitis plus >50% necrosis). *B,* More caudal level of CT scan depicted in *A.* There is considerable fluid in the anterior pararenal spaces bilaterally extending into the paracolic gutters *(curved arrows)* and into the right posterior pararenal space *(straight arrow).*

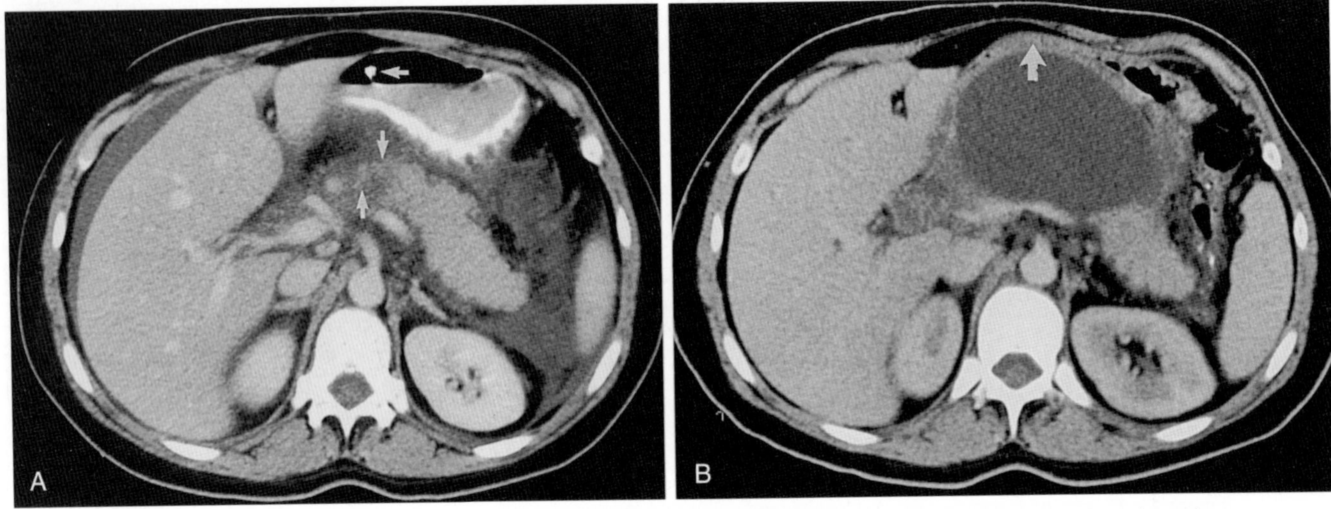

Figure 48–3. Pancreatic necrosis and pancreatic pseudocyst. *A,* Dynamic contrast-enhanced CT scan was performed on the second hospital day. There is an enlarged body and tail of the pancreas that enhances normally. Enhancement is heterogeneous in the more proximal portion of the pancreas *(vertical arrows).* Inflammatory changes are extensive in the anterior pararenal space surrounding the pancreas. A small amount of ascites surrounds the liver. A nasogastric tube is in the stomach *(horizontal arrow).* The heterogeneous enhancement of the proximal portion of the pancreas is not diagnostic of pancreatic necrosis and could represent severe interstitial edema. The CT severity index is 4 (grade E-4 points and no definite necrosis). *B,* CT scan performed 3 weeks later. There is a 12 × 8 × 15 cm low-attenuation mass that replaces the body of the pancreas and extends into the lesser sac, displacing the stomach anteriorly *(arrow).* A portion of the pancreatic tail enhances normally. The overall appearance of the mass appears homogeneous, but the absence of enhancement of the body of the pancreas indicates that this portion of the gland is necrotic and that the mass is a combination of pancreatic necrosis and fluid in the lesser sac.

acute pancreatitis, but the relevance of co-localization to the pathogenesis of acute pancreatitis is unclear. Activation of trypsinogen occurs before biochemical or morphologic injury to acinar cells, in association with co-localization of lysosomal enzymes, such as cathepsin B, and digestive enzymes, including trypsinogen within unstable vacuoles.[13, 14] Complete inhibition of pancreatic cathepsin B activity in vitro prevents trypsinogen activation induced by the cholecystokinin (CCK) analog cerulein,[15] supporting the co-localization hypothesis. Thus, complete inhibition of cathepsin B may prevent or be a treatment for acute pancreatitis. However, enzyme co-localization may occur without inducing significant acinar cell injury.[16]

Two other features of experimental acute pancreatitis are early blockade of the secretion of pancreatic enzymes while enzyme synthesis continues[8] and disruption of the paracellular barrier of acinar cells and intralobular pancreatic duct cells. The disruption facilitates the extravasation of pancreatic enzymes from acinar cells and from the duct lumen into interstitial spaces. This phenomenon may explain the rapid development of interstitial edema and the increase of pancreatic enzymes in the serum.[17]

The discovery of genetic mutations associated with hereditary pancreatitis also lends support to the hypothesis that intrapancreatic activation of pancreatic zymogens is central to the pathogenesis of acute pancreatitis[18–21] (see Chapter 47). The mutant trypsin in hereditary pancreatitis is resistant to lysis, remains active, and causes autodigestion of the pancreas and episodes of acute pancreatitis.

Another molecular pathogenic mechanism of acute pancreatitis involves mutations of the cystic fibrosis transmembrane conductance regulator (CFTR) gene. Mutations of CFTR in at least one allele occur in anywhere from 2% to 37% of patients with idiopathic chronic and acute recurrent pancreatitis,[22–26] and a similar proportion of patients with recurrent acute pancreatitis associated with pancreas divisum.[24] In contrast, the prevalence of CFTR mutations in acute biliary pancreatitis[25] and chronic pancreatitis associated with alcohol (approximately 0% to 5%)[24] is no greater than in the general population. How CFTR mutations might cause pancreatitis is unclear. Possibly, the mutations produce a more concentrated, acidic pancreatic juice leading to ductal obstruction or altered acinar cell function (e.g., reduced intracellular pH and abnormal intracellular membrane recycling or transport). The diagnostic, prognostic, and therapeutic implications of CFTR mutations are unclear. Perhaps the alleged causes of pancreatitis, such as pancreas divisum and sphincter of Oddi dysfunction, are epiphenomena and instead are due to coexisting CFTR mutations. Preliminary studies of the complete sequencing of CFTR indicate that approximately 50% of patients with unexplained pancreatitis have CFTR mutations (compound heterozygotes).[25] However, most subjects with a mutation have a normal sweat chloride and nasal mucosal potential difference, and the functional significance of the mutations is as yet unknown.

The pathogenesis of gallstone-related pancreatitis is unknown. Factors that may initiate gallstone pancreatitis include reflux of bile into the pancreatic duct[27, 28] or obstruction of the pancreatic duct at the ampulla secondary to stone(s) or to edema resulting from the passage of a stone.[29] Reflux of bile into the pancreatic duct could occur when the distal bile and pancreatic ducts form a *common channel* and a gallstone becomes impacted in the duodenal papilla (see Chapter 45). Alternatively, bile could reflux into the pancreatic duct from the duodenum through an incompetent sphincter of Oddi injured by recent passage of a gallstone.

Experimentally, reflux of bile, particularly if infected or mixed with pancreatic enzymes, causes pancreatic injury. Mixtures of bile and pancreatic enzymes increase the permeability of the main pancreatic duct, which is associated with local parenchymal inflammation.[30] The common channel theory is somewhat problematic because pancreatic duct pressure is invariably higher than common bile duct pressure, making bile reflux unlikely. Reflux of bile from the duodenum also is unlikely because pancreatitis does not occur in conditions with easily demonstrable reflux, such as after surgical sphincteroplasty or endoscopic sphincterotomy.

A popular opinion for the mechanism of gallstone pancreatitis is that an impacted gallstone in the distal common bile duct obstructs the pancreatic duct, which increases pancreatic pressure, thereby damaging ductal and acinar cells. Experiments in the opossum that support this theory are the observations that ligation of the pancreatic duct causes severe necrotizing pancreatitis[27] and that decompression of the ductal system within 3 days prevents progression to acinar cell necrosis and severe inflammation.[29]

PATHOPHYSIOLOGY

The pathophysiology of acute pancreatitis includes microcirculatory injury, leukocyte chemoattraction and release of cytokines, oxidative stress, and bacterial translocation.

The release of pancreatic enzymes damages the vascular endothelium, the interstitium, and acinar cells.[31–33] Microcirculatory changes, including vasoconstriction, capillary stasis, decreased oxygen saturation, and progressive ischemia, occur early in experimental acute pancreatitis. These abnormalities increase vascular permeability and lead to edema of the gland (edematous or interstitial pancreatitis). Vascular injury could lead to local microcirculatory failure and amplification of the pancreatic injury. It is uncertain whether ischemia-reperfusion injury occurs in the pancreas.[33] Reperfusion of damaged pancreatic tissue could lead to the release of free radicals and inflammatory cytokines into the circulation, which could cause further injury.

In early stages of animal and human pancreatitis, activation of complement and the subsequent release of C5a play significant roles in the recruitment of macrophages and polymorphonuclear leukocytes.[34–36] Active granulocytes and macrophages release proinflammatory cytokines (tumor necrosis factor, interleukins 1, 6, and 8), arachidonic acid metabolites (prostaglandins, platelet-activating factor, and leukotrienes), proteolytic and lipolytic enzymes, and reactive oxygen metabolites that overwhelm scavenging by endogenous antioxidant systems. These substances also interact with the pancreatic microcirculation to increase vascular permeability, which induces thrombosis and hemorrhage and leads to pancreatic necrosis. Because of these interactions, it is difficult to estimate the contributions of each factor. In addition, why 80% of acute pancreatitis is limited to interstitial pancreatitis is not well understood.

Translocation of bacteria from the gut into the systemic circulation does not occur normally because there is a complex barrier consisting of immunologic, bacteriologic, and morphologic components. However, during acute pancreatitis, this barrier breaks down, which can result in local and systemic infection.[37] Penetration of the gut barrier by enteric bacteria is likely due to gut ischemia secondary to hypovolemia and pancreatitis-induced arteriovenous shunting in the gut.[38] Indeed, in canine experimental pancreatitis, luminal *Escherichia coli* translocate to mesenteric lymph nodes and distant sites.[39]

Some patients with severe pancreatic damage develop systemic complications, including fever, acute respiratory distress syndrome (ARDS), pleural effusions, renal failure, shock, myocardial depression, and metabolic complications. The systemic inflammatory response syndrome (SIRS) is common and is probably mediated by activated pancreatic enzymes (phospholipase, elastase, trypsin, and so on) and cytokines (tumor necrosis factor, platelet-activating factor) released into the circulation from the inflamed pancreas.[40] ARDS, which is secondary to microvascular thrombosis, may be induced by active phospholipase A (lecithinase), which digests lecithin, a major component of lung surfactant. Acute renal failure has been explained on the basis of hypovolemia and hypotension. Myocardial depression and shock are likely secondary to vasoactive peptides and a myocardial depressant factor. Metabolic complications include hypocalcemia, hyperlipidemia, hyperglycemia with or without ketoacidosis, and hypoglycemia. The pathogenesis of hypocalcemia is multifactorial and includes calcium-soap formation, hormonal imbalances (e.g., parathyroid hormone, calcitonin, and glucagon), binding of calcium by free fatty acid–albumin complexes, and intracellular translocation of calcium. Systemic complications in acute pancreatitis are uncommon and are much less severe in interstitial pancreatitis than in necrotizing pancreatitis. However, only about 50% of patients with necrotizing pancreatitis develop organ failure, and this complication cannot be predicted from the degree of pancreatic necrosis or the presence or absence of infected necrosis.[41]

PREDISPOSING CONDITIONS

Many conditions predispose to acute pancreatitis to varying degrees (see Table 48–3). This list will undoubtedly continue to grow, and the number of cases diagnosed as "idiopathic" will decrease as our understanding of the disease improves. Gallstones and chronic alcohol abuse account for 75% of acute pancreatitis in the United States.

Gallstones

Gallstones cause 35% of acute pancreatitis in the United States.[1] Cholecystectomy and clearing the common bile duct of stones prevents recurrence, confirming the cause-and-effect relationship.[42] However, only 3% to 7% of patients with gallstones develop pancreatitis.[42]

The risk of developing acute pancreatitis due to gallstones is relatively greater in men (relative risk, 14 to 35) than in women (relative risk, 12 to 25).[42] However, more women develop gallstone pancreatitis because gallstones are more frequent in women.[42]

Acute pancreatitis occurs more frequently when stones are less than 5 mm in diameter (odds ratio, 4:5).[43] Small stones (microlithiasis) (see later) are more likely than large stones to pass through the cystic duct and cause ampullary obstruction.

Biliary Sludge and Microlithiasis

Biliary sludge is a viscous suspension in gallbladder bile that may contain small stones (<5 mm in diameter).[44] Biliary sludge is asymptomatic in most patients. It is usually composed of cholesterol monohydrate crystals or calcium bilirubinate granules.[45] On ultrasound, it is a mobile, low-amplitude echo that does not produce a shadow and that layers in the most dependent part of the gallbladder (see Chapters 55 and 58).

Typically, sludge occurs with functional or mechanical bile stasis. Common associations are a prolonged fast, total parenteral nutrition, or distal bile duct obstruction. In addition, the cephalosporin antibiotic ceftriaxone can complex with bile to form a sludge within the biliary system when its solubility in bile is exceeded, and this rarely causes stones[46, 47] that disappear after stopping the drug. Commonly, biliary sludge occurs in acute pancreatitis with no obvious cause. However, the association between biliary sludge and acute pancreatitis is unproved. There is no prospective, randomized study documenting that removing sludge or microcrystals by cholecystectomy prevents further attacks of pancreatitis. Nevertheless, results of two uncontrolled studies suggest that biliary sludge can lead to pancreatitis, and that cholecystectomy, papillotomy, or ursodeoxycholic acid therapy prevents recurrent attacks of acute pancreatitis.[45, 48] In these two studies, the incidence of biliary sludge in presumed idiopathic pancreatitis was 67% and 74%, respectively. Because of the high risk of recurrence of pancreatitis, we recommend cholecystectomy if patients have had an episode of pancreatitis and biliary sludge is present.

Other Causes of Mechanical Ampullary Obstruction

Other conditions causing obstruction of the ampulla of Vater that are associated with pancreatitis include biliary ascariasis,[49] periampullary diverticula,[50] and pancreatic and periampullary tumors.[51] These conditions are discussed in other chapters of this book.

Alcohol

Alcohol causes at least 30% of cases of acute pancreatitis in the United States. The classic teaching is that alcohol causes chronic pancreatitis, and that alcoholic patients who present with clinically acute pancreatitis have underlying chronic disease. However, a few patients with alcohol-induced acute pancreatitis by clinical criteria do not progress to chronic pancreatitis, even with continued alcohol abuse.[52, 53] By contrast, about 10% of chronic alcoholic patients develop attacks of acute pancreatitis that are indistinguishable from other forms of acute pancreatitis, but eventually develop chronic pancreatitis after 10 to 20 years of alcohol abuse. Early in the course of the disease, when attacks occur, the diagnosis of underlying chronic pancreatitis is difficult without tissue specimens because the diagnosis of chronic pancreatitis usually is made after definite signs of chronic pancreatitis appear (e.g., pancreatic calcification, exocrine and endocrine insufficiency, or typical duct changes by CT or ERCP; see Chapter 49).

The mechanism of alcohol-induced pancreatitis is unclear. Hypotheses include relaxation of the sphincter of Oddi with reflux of duodenal contents into the pancreatic duct, spasm of the sphincter of Oddi with reflux of bile into the pancreatic duct, increased permeability of the pancreatic duct, and sudden release of large amounts of enzymes that are inappropriately activated. Alcohol increases synthesis of digestive and lysosomal enzymes by pancreatic acinar cells.[54] Other hypotheses are that chronic ingestion of alcohol leads to increased protein concentration in pancreatic juice, which obstructs small ductules, and that ethanol or one of its metabolites directly injures acinar cells (the toxic-metabolic hypothesis).[55, 56]

Hypertriglyceridemia

Serum triglyceride concentrations above 1000 mg/dL (11 mmol/L) may precipitate attacks of acute pancreatitis. However, triglyceride levels of 500 to 1000 mg/dL also may induce acute pancreatitis. The average serum triglyceride concentration at presentation is approximately 4500 mg/dL (50 mmol/L). Patients have lactescent (milky) serum owing to increased concentrations of very-low-density lipoprotein (VLDL),[57] and at higher VLDL levels, owing to hyperchylomicronemia. The pathogenesis of hypertriglyceridemic pancreatitis is unclear,[58] but the release of free fatty acids may damage pancreatic acinar cells or capillary endothelium.[57]

Hypertriglyceridemia may cause 1% to 4% of acute pancreatitis.[57] The association between hypertriglyceridemia and acute pancreatitis is best defined in children with inherited disorders of lipoprotein metabolism and severe hypertriglyceridemia[59, 60] who develop acute pancreatitis in early childhood. These children are homozygous for lipoprotein lipase deficiency or APO-CII deficiency. Acute pancreatitis develops in 35%, 15%, and 30% to 40% in type I, II, and V hyperlipidemia, respectively. Lowering serum triglyceride levels to less than 200 mg/dL (2.2 mmol/L) can prevent pancreatitis.

Most adults with hyperchylomicronemia have a mild form of genetically inherited type I or type V hyperlipoproteinemia and an additional condition known to raise serum lipids (alcohol abuse, obesity, diabetes mellitus, hypothyroidism, pregnancy, estrogen or tamoxifen therapy, glucocorticoid excess, nephrotic syndrome, and beta blocker therapy).[61, 62] Typically, three types of patients develop hypertriglyceridemia-induced pancreatitis.[57] The first is a poorly controlled diabetic patient with a history of hypertriglyceridemia; administration of insulin rapidly lowers serum triglyceride. The second is an alcoholic patient with hypertriglyceridemia on hospital admission. The third (15% to 20%) is a nondiabetic, nonalcoholic, nonobese person who has drug- or diet-induced hypertriglyceridemia. Drug-induced disease is more likely to occur if there is underlying hypertriglyceridemia.[61]

Most persons who abuse alcohol have moderate, but transient, elevations of triglyceride levels. This condition is likely an epiphenomenon and not the cause of pancreatitis[63, 64] because alcohol increases serum triglyceride concentrations in a "dose-dependent" manner. For example, the prevalence of serum triglyceride concentrations above 227 mg/dL (2.5 mmol/L) at varying degrees of alcohol intake was 10%, 14%, and 20% in persons who drank 3 to 5, 6 to

8, or 9 or more drinks per day, respectively.[65] Alcoholic patients with severe hyperlipidemia often have a coexisting primary genetic disorder of lipoprotein metabolism.

The clinical manifestations of hypertriglyceridemia-associated disease are similar to other causes of acute pancreatitis; abdominal pain, nausea, and vomiting are the major symptoms.[57] However, the serum amylase may not be substantially elevated at presentation.

Hypercalcemia

Any cause of hypercalcemia can lead to acute pancreatitis.[66] Proposed mechanisms include deposition of calcium in the pancreatic duct and calcium activation of trypsinogen within the pancreatic parenchyma.[67, 68] The low incidence of pancreatitis in chronic hypercalcemia suggests that other factors (e.g., acute elevations of serum calcium) are responsible for pancreatitis, particularly since acute calcium infusion into rats leads to conversion of trypsinogen to trypsin, hyperamylasemia, and dose-dependent morphologic changes of acute pancreatitis (edema and acinar cell necrosis).[67]

Hypercalcemia due to hyperparathyroidism is a proposed cause of pancreatitis. However, primary hyperparathyroidism causes less than 0.5% of all cases of acute pancreatitis, and the incidence of acute pancreatitis in hyperparathyroidism varies among 0.4%, 0.23%, and 1.5%.[69–71] Rarely, pancreatitis occurs with other causes of hypercalcemia, including metastatic bone disease, total parenteral nutrition, sarcoidosis, vitamin D toxicity, and infusions of calcium in high doses perioperatively during cardiopulmonary bypass.[72]

Drugs

Medications are an infrequent but important and increasing cause of acute pancreatitis.[73–75] In Germany and Switzerland, 1.4% and 0.3% of cases of acute pancreatitis were related to a medication, respectively.[76, 77] Over 55 drugs have been implicated, mostly from case and anecdotal reports. Documentation of drug-induced pancreatitis is most secure if other likely causes of pancreatitis are not present, if there is recovery after drug withdrawal, and if pancreatitis recurs with reintroduction of the drug (Table 48–4).[78]

The pathogenesis of drug-induced pancreatitis is an allergic reaction (e.g., 6-mercaptopurine, aminosalicylates, sulfonamides) or direct toxicity (e.g., diuretics, sulfonamides).

Table 48–4 | **Drugs That Cause Acute Pancreatitis**

AIDS therapy—didanosine, pentamidine
Anti-inflammatory drugs—sulindac, salicylates
Antimicrobial agents—metronidazole, stibogluconate, sulfonamides, tetracycline, nitrofurantoin
Diuretics—furosemide, thiazides
Drugs used for inflammatory bowel disease—sulfasalazine, oral 5-aminosalicylic acid (5-ASA) (olsalazine [Dipentum] and mesalamine [Asacol])
Immunosuppressive agents—L-asparaginase, azathioprine, 6-mercaptopurine (6-MP)
Neuropsychiatric agents—valproic acid
Others—calcium, estrogen and tamoxifen (estrogen and tamoxifen may act by inducing hypertriglyceridemia), angiotensin-converting enzyme (ACE) inhibitors

In the past, steroids have been implicated, but evidence linking steroids to pancreatitis is weak. Many cases of pancreatitis with steroid use happened with conditions known to cause pancreatitis. None of the recent reviews classifies steroids as a definite or probable cause.[73–76] Pancreatitis associated with angiotensin-converting enzyme inhibitors likely is due to angioedema of the gland.

Drug-induced pancreatitis has no distinguishing clinical features. A high index of suspicion and careful drug history are essential for diagnosis. The time course depends upon the drug. For example, pancreatitis may develop within a few weeks after beginning a drug associated with an immunologically mediated allergic reaction and may be associated with a rash and eosinophilia. In contrast, acute pancreatitis associated with valproic acid, pentamidine, or didanosine may not develop for months of use because pancreatitis likely is due to chronic accumulation of toxic metabolites.

The prognosis of drug-induced pancreatitis is excellent. For example, of 22 cases in one study, 19 had interstitial pancreatitis, none had more than 33% necrosis of the pancreas, and none died.[76]

Infections and Toxins

Many infectious agents may cause acute pancreatitis,[79] but often reports do not meet standards for the diagnosis of pancreatitis or the infection. If modern criteria for diagnosis of pancreatitis and infection are used, pancreatitis can be associated with infectious agents with varying degrees of certainty.[79] Definite pancreatitis exists if there is surgical, autopsy, or radiologic evidence; probable pancreatitis exists if there are biochemical evidence (more than three times elevation of serum lipase or amylase) and characteristic symptoms; and possible pancreatitis exists if there is only asymptomatic biochemical evidence. The definite criterion for an infection causing pancreatitis is finding the organism in the pancreas or pancreatic duct by stain or culture. Probable criteria are culture of the organism from pancreatic juice or blood or serologic evidence combined with a characteristic clinical or epidemiologic setting. The criterion of a possible infection is culture of the organism from other body sites or serologic evidence of infection.

These criteria show that definite pancreatitis was associated with viruses (mumps, coxsackievirus, hepatitis B, cytomegalovirus, varicella-zoster, herpes simplex, Epstein-Barr, hepatitis A, and non-A, non-B hepatitis); the vaccine that contains attenuated measles, mumps, and rubella; bacteria (*Mycoplasma, Legionella, Leptospira, Salmonella*, tuberculosis,[80] and brucellosis); fungi (*Aspergillus* and *Candida albicans*[81]); and parasites (*Toxoplasma, Cryptosporidium, Ascaris, Chlonorchis sinensis*). *C. sinensis* and *Ascaris* cause pancreatitis by blocking the main pancreatic duct. In acquired immunodeficiency syndrome (AIDS), infectious agents causing acute pancreatitis include cytomegalovirus, *Candida, Cryptococcus neoformans, Toxoplasma gondii*, and possibly opportunistic organisms such as *Mycobacterium avium* complex[82] (see Chapter 28).

An infectious agent should be suspected of causing acute pancreatitis if the characteristic syndrome caused by the infectious agent is present, as this occurs 70% of the time.[79] Because an infectious agent may be in the pancreas without pancreatitis, routine search for an infection in idiopathic pancreatitis is **not** recommended. In addition, it is unknown whether treating an infectious agent reverses pancreatic pathology.

Some toxins cause acute pancreatitis. For example, the principal cause of acute pancreatitis in Trinidad is a scorpion sting. Scorpion venom releases acetylcholine from pancreatic nerves, causing prolonged hyperstimulation of pancreatic acinar cells. The same mechanism may cause acute pancreatitis after exposure to anticholinesterase insecticides. Recurrent episodes of acute pancreatitis may be due to allergy to a variety of foods, including milk, beef, potato, fish, and eggs.[83]

Trauma

Either penetrating trauma (gunshot or stab wounds) or blunt trauma can damage the pancreas, although these injuries are uncommon.[84] In most cases, there is also injury to adjacent viscera. Laparotomy is essential in all cases of penetrating trauma to assess and treat all intra-abdominal injuries, including those to the pancreas. Blunt trauma results from compression of the pancreas by the spine, such as in an automobile accident. In blunt trauma, it is important to determine preoperatively whether there is injury to the pancreas because, depending upon the severity of pancreatic injury, it will be necessary to include the pancreas in the surgical plan. Secondly, even in the absence of serious injury to adjacent organs, surgery may be necessary to treat a pancreatic ductal injury.

The diagnosis of traumatic pancreatitis is difficult and requires a high degree of suspicion. Trauma can range from a mild contusion to a severe crush injury or transection of the gland; the latter usually occurs at the point where the gland crosses over the spine. This injury can cause acute duct rupture and pancreatic ascites. Clinically, it is impossible to determine on the basis of the characteristics of the abdominal pain and tenderness whether the pancreas has been injured in addition to other intra-abdominal structures. Serum amylase activity may be increased in abdominal trauma whether or not the pancreas has been injured.

Diagnosis is highly dependent upon imaging. CT scan may show enlargement of a portion of the gland caused by a contusion or subcapsular hematoma, pancreatic inflammatory changes, or fluid within the anterior pararenal space if there is ductal disruption. The CT scan may be normal during the first 2 days despite significant pancreatic trauma. If there is a strong clinical suspicion of pancreatic injury or if the CT scan shows an abnormality, ERCP is required to determine whether there is a pancreatic duct injury. If the pancreatic duct is intact and if there is no other significant intra-abdominal injuries, surgery is not required. However, if ERCP reveals duct transection with extravasation of pancreatic fluid and there are no other intra-abdominal injuries, stenting of the pancreatic duct may be successful.[85] If there are significant intra-abdominal injuries, ERCP usually can be performed before abdominal surgery. If not, it can be performed during laparotomy once other intra-abdominal injuries have been treated. If the duct disruption cannot be treated by stenting, transection of the pancreatic duct in the body or tail of the pancreas requires distal pancreatic resection. If the duct injury is in the head of the gland, multiple drains should be used. Serious injuries to the pancreas can be treated with appropriate debridement. Injuries to the duodenum or common bile duct can be treated by biliary diversion, gastrojejunostomy, and feeding jejunostomy. External pancreatic fistulas occur in approximately one third of patients after surgery for pancreatic trauma. Thus far, octreotide has not been found to be beneficial after pancreatic injury.[86]

The prognosis of pancreatic trauma is favorable if there is no serious injury to other structures (regional blood vessels, liver, spleen, kidney, duodenum, and colon).[87, 88] However, duct injuries can scar and cause a stricture of the main pancreatic duct resulting in obstructive pancreatitis.

Pancreas Divisum

Pancreas divisum occurs in approximately 7% of autopsies and in patients undergoing ERCP for diagnosis of nonpancreatic diseases.[89] It results because the embryologic dorsal and ventral pancreases fail to fuse (see Chapter 45). Whether pancreas divisum is related to pancreatitis or abdominal pain is controversial. Some claim an association with acute pancreatitis due to relative obstruction of the flow of pancreatic juice through a narrow minor papilla, causing increased intraductal pressure. To support this hypothesis,[90–92] cessation of recurrent pancreatitis allegedly occurs with accessory papilla sphincteroplasty,[90] endoscopic minor papilla sphincterotomy,[91] or insertion of an endoscopic stent across the minor papilla.[92] For example, 60% of patients with pancreas divisum had relief of abdominal pain after surgical sphincteroplasty, and 80% of 119 patients with pancreas divisum and recurrent acute pancreatitis had no further attacks of acute pancreatitis after surgical or endoscopic papillotomy of the minor papilla.[93] In comparison, surgical sphincteroplasty and endoscopic sphincterotomy do not relieve pain among patients with chronic pain possibly of pancreatic origin or pain associated with chronic pancreatitis.

It is difficult to determine whether patients with recurrent pancreatitis will have pain relief or cessation of attacks of pancreatitis after treatment. The ultrasound secretin test may be helpful to predict success.[90] Dilation of the pancreatic duct for 15 to 30 minutes after the intravenous administration of secretin was interpreted as indicating impaired emptying of the dorsal duct and obstruction of pancreatic flow through the accessory papilla. Other investigators have not confirmed these results.

We do **not** believe there is an association between pancreas divisum, pancreatic pain, or pancreatitis because the incidence of pancreas divisum is the same in patients with and without pancreatitis.[89] Further, 95% of persons who have pancreas divisum are asymptomatic, with pancreas divisum discovered when ERCP is performed for other reasons. Also, pancreatitis in people with divisum develops in adulthood, not in childhood. In our experience, most patients with abdominal pain and pancreas divisum have irritable bowel syndrome or another unrecognized cause of abdominal pain, without any evidence of pancreatitis. Most patients with pancreatitis and pancreas divisum probably have "idiopathic" pancreatitis. This opinion is bolstered by the recent preliminary report of finding mutations of the cystic fibrosis gene in

21% of patients with pancreas divisum and pancreatitis, similar to what is observed in patients with "idiopathic pancreatitis."[24]

Unfortunately, no randomized prospective therapeutic trials have been done. In one trial, patients with recurrent pancreatitis were randomized to receive a stent across the minor papilla or no treatment.[92] However, the study was not blind, and the favorable results of stent therapy may have been influenced by the lack of blinding. Further, 50% of patients with stenting of the minor duct may incur permanent stent-induced changes in the dorsal pancreatic duct, possibly resulting in chronic pancreatitis and chronic pain.[94, 95] Thus, we urge caution and a conservative noninvasive approach for treating these patients because aggressive endoscopic therapy may be harmful.

Vascular Disease

Rarely, pancreatic ischemia causes pancreatitis. In most cases it is mild, but fatal necrotizing pancreatitis may occur. Ischemia may result from vasculitis (systemic lupus erythematosus[96] and polyarteritis nodosa[97]), atheromatous embolization of cholesterol plaques from the aorta to the pancreas after transabdominal angiography,[98, 99] intraoperative hypotension,[72] hemorrhagic shock,[100] ergotamine overdose, and transcatheter arterial embolization for hepatocellular carcinoma. Also, ischemia is one possible explanation for pancreatitis after cardiopulmonary bypass. Twenty-seven percent of patients undergoing cardiac surgery develop hyperamylasemia, and one percent develop necrotizing pancreatitis.[72] Significant risks for pancreatitis after cardiopulmonary bypass are preoperative renal insufficiency, postoperative hypotension, and giving calcium chloride perioperatively. In pigs, cardiogenic shock induced by pericardial tamponade causes vasospasm and selective pancreatic ischemia due to activation of the renin-angiotensin system.[101]

Pregnancy

Pregnancy is not a cause of acute pancreatitis. In a population-based case-control study spanning 16 years, pregnancy per se was not significantly associated with pancreatitis.[102] In this study, all ten cases of acute pancreatitis occurred postpartum, and six were associated with gallstones. In another survey of 16,000 deliveries, only 8 cases of acute pancreatitis were noted; 5 were due to gallstones and 3 were idiopathic.[103]

Pancreatitis during pregnancy may be due to hyperlipidemia.[104] Pregnancy increases serum triglyceride levels, with a peak in the third trimester. However, the total serum triglyceride level rarely exceeds 300 mg/dL (3.3 mmol/L), a concentration that does not cause pancreatitis. Hyperlipidemic gestational pancreatitis usually occurs only in women with preexisting abnormalities in lipid metabolism, although it is not clear whether preexisting hyperlipidemia significantly increases the risk of pancreatitis during pregnancy.

Management of acute pancreatitis in pregnancy is similar to that for other causes of pancreatitis. Fetal outcome is good, although there is a higher risk of prematurity. Cholecystectomy can be done without complications,[105, 106] but endoscopic sphincterotomy may be preferred to surgery during pregnancy to eliminate gallstones in the common bile duct. Because endoscopic ultrasonography is very accurate in identifying gallstones within the common bile duct, this technique may prove to be very useful in selecting patients who require ERCP.[107]

Post-ERCP

Asymptomatic hyperamylasemia occurs after 35% to 70% of ERCPs.[108] Acute pancreatitis occurs in 3% of diagnostic ERCPs, 5% of therapeutic ERCPs, and up to 25% of sphincter of Oddi manometry studies.[109] Risks for post-ERCP acute pancreatitis include the volume and pressure of contrast material that is injected, the number of injections of the pancreatic duct, ampullary trauma by multiple attempts at catheterization, overfilling of the pancreatic ducts with acinarization of the parenchyma, an underlying pathologic process of pancreatic ducts, introduction of bacteria, and properties of the contrast media that are used. Patients with a previous episode of pancreatitis after ERCP are more likely to have pancreatitis after a second ERCP, but a prior history of acute pancreatitis may ameliorate the clinical outcome of post-ERCP pancreatitis.[110]

Using an aspirating catheter during sphincter of Oddi manometry reduces the risk of pancreatitis. Endoscopic sphincterotomy after manometry does not increase the risk of pancreatitis further, unless patients have nondilated pancreatic ducts. The incidence of ERCP-induced acute pancreatitis also may be reduced by using parenteral octreotide (Sandostatin), a low osmolality and nonionic contrast agent,[111] and proteases (discussed later).

Postoperative Pancreatitis

Postoperative pancreatitis carries greater mortality than other causes of pancreatitis. The incidence of acute pancreatitis after liver transplantation is 6%, with a mortality of 33%.[112] Similar mortality occurs with pancreatitis after renal transplantation and cardiopulmonary bypass. Perhaps such a high mortality occurs postoperatively because diagnosis and treatment are delayed; postoperative pancreatitis may not be recognized because abdominal pain and tenderness is interpreted as postoperative discomfort, or analgesics mask the pain. Contributors to postoperative pancreatitis are hypotension, medications (e.g., azathioprine, cyclosporine, and perioperative calcium chloride administration), and infections.

Hereditary Pancreatitis

This is an autosomal dominant disorder with variable penetrance (see Chapter 47). It should be suspected if at least two family members have pancreatitis and episodes of abdominal pain begin in childhood.[113] Intraductal stones are usually present at the first episode of pain, but some families have intraductal radiolucent protein stones instead of calcified stones. The rate of surgery for this disease is close to 50%,[114] similar to idiopathic pancreatitis of onset in a younger than 35-year-old person.[115] Although long-term health is favorable in 75% of patients,[114] there is a markedly increased risk for pancreatic carcinoma (40% cumulative risk by age 70 years), which occurs a decade earlier than the usual ductal pancreatic cancer, particularly in families with paternal inheritance (imprinting).[116]

Structural Abnormalities

Duodenum/Ampullary Region

Annular pancreas[117] and abnormalities of the duodenum, including duodenal duplication, duodenal cysts, and intraluminal duodenal diverticula, have been implicated as causing acute pancreatitis. These abnormalities possibly cause pancreatitis by increasing pressure within the duodenum and reflux of activated pancreatic enzymes into the main pancreatic duct.

Acquired diseases of duodenum and ampulla associated with acute pancreatitis include villous adenomas and other tumors of the duodenal papilla, periampullary cysts, and duodenal Crohn's disease. Obstruction of the pancreatic duct is the common mechanism for acute pancreatitis for these entities. In Crohn's disease, other mechanisms that may cause pancreatitis include primary involvement of the pancreas,[118] fistulas into the pancreas with secondary inflammation, cholelithiasis associated with ileal disease and sclerosing cholangitis, and use of drugs that cause pancreatitis (sulfasalazine and immunosuppressives).

Bile Duct

Acute pancreatitis may occur with sclerosing cholangitis and with choledochal cysts, particularly if cysts are greater than 5 cm in diameter in patients with a long "common channel."[119] Mechanisms include regurgitation of bile and pancreatic juice into both ducts and obstruction of the pancreatic duct by large choledochal cysts.

Sphincter of Oddi Dysfunction

(see also Chapter 53)

Sphincter of Oddi dysfunction (SOD) is of two major types: (1) stenosis (fibrosis of the sphincter and increased basal pressure of the sphincter), and (2) dyskinesia (no fibrosis but increased basal pressure and at times other motility disturbances of the sphincter). Normal basal sphincter of Oddi pressure is approximately 15 mm Hg. With stenosis, the basal sphincter pressure is greater than 40 mm Hg, which is not decreased by smooth muscle relaxants such as amyl nitrate or nifedipine. The basal sphincter pressure also is greater than 40 mm Hg with dyskinesia, but it is decreased by the above-mentioned smooth muscle relaxants. Cannulation of the pancreatic duct during sphincter of Oddi manometry is associated with an incidence of pancreatitis as high as 30%. Acute pancreatitis is less frequent with common bile duct cannulation.

Most agree that stenosis of the sphincter of Oddi may cause recurrent acute pancreatitis, but this type of SOD is infrequent (less than 10% of cases) and is usually readily identifiable clinically. Whether sphincter dyskinesia causes recurrent pancreatitis is controversial. There is no association between SOD and alcoholic chronic pancreatitis.[120] However, some have claimed an association between pancreatitis and SOD because of finding structural evidence of chronic pancreatitis in 29% of patients with SOD and finding SOD in 87% of patients with chronic pancreatitis.[121] Others claim that endoscopic sphincterotomy in idiopathic pancreatitis with manometric evidence for sphincter of Oddi dyskinesia may eliminate further episodes of acute pancreatitis,[120] but this is controversial.

We maintain skepticism that sphincter of Oddi dyskinesia is related to recurrent pancreatitis. In most studies, the criteria for pancreatitis are based upon endoscopic ultrasound and nonstandard secretin pancreatic function tests. Furthermore, usually patients are not stratified as to whether they have "pancreatic pain" without evidence of pancreatitis, recurrent acute pancreatitis, or chronic pancreatitis. It is possible that most of these patients have a disorder of gut motility and pain perception. Recently two groups of investigators have emphasized that potential explanations of pain in some patients with SOD are gut dysmotility[125] and hyperalgesia.[124] In the latter study, it was pointed out that all the patients were women who had duodenal but not rectal hyperalgesia and high levels of somatization, depression, and obsessive-compulsive characteristics. Randomized prospective trials are needed to evaluate treatment in this condition.

Main Pancreatic Duct

Many benign and malignant conditions of the main pancreatic duct cause acute pancreatitis by obstructing the duct. These include parasites (*Ascaris lumbricoides* and *Clonorchis sinensis*) and tumors, including islet cell tumors,[125] adenocarcinoma of the pancreas, metastatic carcinoma, and intraductal papillary mucinous neoplasms.[126] These entities are discussed in other chapters.

Miscellaneous

Rarely, acute pancreatitis is the initial manifestation of cystic fibrosis in young adults. Other miscellaneous causes of pancreatitis include exposure to occupational chemicals, chronic renal failure, acute burn injuries,[127] and long-distance running.[128]

Idiopathic Pancreatitis

No obvious etiology is identified in approximately 30% of acute pancreatitis. After a first episode of apparent idiopathic pancreatitis, most patients have no further attacks. For example, only 1 of 31 patients with a first episode of idiopathic acute pancreatitis had another attack during a median follow-up of 36 months,[129] suggesting that extensive investigation for unusual causes of pancreatitis is not required after the first episode of idiopathic pancreatitis. We recommend laparoscopic cholecystectomy after two attacks of presumed idiopathic acute pancreatitis to exclude a biliary cause. We do not advise biliary microscopic examination for crystals because the test result will not change this recommendation.[130]

CLINICAL PRESENTATION

It is difficult to diagnose acute pancreatitis by history and physical examination because clinical features are similar to those of many acute abdominal illnesses.

History

Abdominal Pain

Abdominal pain is present at the onset of most attacks of acute pancreatitis, but the timing of abdominal pain is variable. Biliary colic may herald or progress to acute pancreatitis. Alcohol-related acute pancreatitis frequently occurs 1 to 3 days following drinking. Pain may occur the afternoon after heavy consumption of alcohol the evening before, but there may be a shorter interval between alcohol consumption and pain.

Pain in pancreatitis usually involves the entire upper abdomen. However, it may be midepigastric, in the right upper quadrant, or, infrequently, confined to the left side. Pain in the lower abdomen may arise from the rapid spread of pancreatic exudation to the left colon.

Onset of pain is rapid but not as abrupt as that of a perforated viscus. Usually it is at maximal intensity in 10 to 20 minutes. Occasionally, pain gradually increases and takes several hours to reach maximum intensity. Pain is steady and moderate to very severe in intensity. There is little pain relief with changing position. Frequently, pain is unbearable, steady, boring, and refractory to narcotics. Bandlike radiation of the pain to the back occurs in half of patients. Pain that lasts only a few hours and then disappears suggests a disease other than pancreatitis, such as biliary colic or peptic ulcer. Pain is absent in 5% to 10% of attacks, but a painless presentation may be a feature of serious fatal disease.

Nausea and Vomiting

Ninety percent of patients have nausea and vomiting. Vomiting may be severe, may last for hours, may be accompanied by retching, and may not alleviate pain. Vomiting may be related to severe pain or to inflammation involving the posterior gastric wall.

Physical Examination

Physical findings vary depending upon the severity of an attack. Patients with **mild** pancreatitis may not appear acutely ill. Abdominal tenderness may be mild, and abdominal guarding is absent. In **severe** pancreatitis, patients look severely ill and often have abdominal distention, especially epigastric, which is due to gastric ileus or dilatation of the transverse colon. Almost all patients are tender in the upper abdomen, which may be elicited by gently shaking the abdomen or by gentle percussion. Guarding is more marked in the upper abdomen. Tenderness and guarding are less than expected, considering the intensity of discomfort. Abdominal rigidity, as occurs in diffuse peritonitis, rarely is present. Bowel sounds are reduced and may be absent.

Additional abdominal findings may include ecchymosis in one or both flanks (Grey Turner's sign) or about the periumbilical area (Cullen's sign), owing to extravasation of hemorrhagic pancreatic exudate to these areas. These signs occur in 1% of cases and are associated with a poor prognosis. At times, there is a brawny erythema of the flanks caused by extravasation of pancreatic exudate to the abdominal wall. A palpable epigastric mass may appear during the disease from a pseudocyst or a large inflammatory mass.

The general physical examination, particularly in severe pancreatitis, may uncover markedly abnormal vital signs if there are third-space fluid losses and systemic toxicity. Commonly, the pulse is 100 to 150 beats/min. Blood pressure occasionally is briefly higher than normal and then lower than normal with third-space losses and hypovolemia. Initially the temperature may be normal, but within 1 to 3 days it may increase to 101 to 103°F owing to severe retroperitoneal chemical burn and the release of inflammatory mediators from the pancreas. Tachypnea and shallow respirations may be present if subdiaphragmatic inflammatory exudate causes painful breathing. Dyspnea may accompany pleural effusions, atelectasis, or congestive heart failure. Chest examination may reveal limited diaphragmatic excursion if abdominal pain causes splinting of the diaphragm, or dullness to percussion and decreased breath sounds at the lung bases if there is a pleural effusion. There may be disorientation, hallucinations, agitation, or coma, which may be due to alcohol withdrawal, hypotension, electrolyte imbalance, hypoxemia, fever, and toxic effects of pancreatic enzymes on the central nervous system. Scleral icterus may be present due to choledocholithiasis (gallstone pancreatitis), bile duct obstruction from edema of the head of the pancreas, or coexistent liver disease.

Uncommon findings include subcutaneous nodular fat necrosis, thrombophlebitis in the legs, and polyarthritis. Subcutaneous fat necroses are 0.5- to 2-cm tender red nodules that usually appear over the distal extremities but may occur over the scalp, trunk, or buttocks. They occasionally precede abdominal pain or occur without abdominal pain, but usually they appear during a clinical episode and disappear with clinical improvement. If they occur over a joint, they may be confused with arthritis.

Some physical findings point to a specific cause of acute pancreatitis. Hepatomegaly, spider angiomas, and thickening of palmar sheaths favor alcoholic pancreatitis. Eruptive xanthomas and lipemia retinalis suggest hyperlipidemic pancreatitis. Parotid pain and swelling are features of mumps. Band keratopathy (an infiltration on the lateral margin of the cornea) occurs in hypercalcemia.

LABORATORY DIAGNOSIS

Many biochemical tests have been used to diagnose acute pancreatitis. They can be classed as serum or urinary levels of pancreatic digestive enzymes, serum or urinary levels of nonenzymatic pancreatic secretions, nonspecific markers of inflammation, and miscellaneous tests.

Pancreatic Enzymes

Serum and Urine Amylase

In healthy persons, the pancreas accounts for 40% to 45% of serum amylase, and the salivary glands account for the rest (55% to 60%). Simple analytic techniques can separate pancreatic and salivary amylases. Because pancreatic diseases increase serum pancreatic (P) isoamylase, measurement of P-isoamylase improves diagnostic accuracy. In one study, P-isoamylase had the best sensitivity (90%) and specificity (92%) among all biochemical markers evaluated for the diagnosis of acute pancreatitis.[131]

However, the total serum amylase test is most frequently ordered to diagnose acute pancreatitis because it can be measured quickly and cheaply. It rises within 6 to 12 hours of onset and is cleared fairly rapidly from the blood (half-life, 10 hr). Probably less than 25% of serum amylase is removed by kidneys. It is uncertain what other processes clear amylase from the circulation. The serum amylase is increased in 75% of patients on the first day of symptoms, and it remains elevated for 3 to 5 days in uncomplicated attacks. The sensitivity of the serum amylase level for detecting acute pancreatitis is difficult to assess because an elevated amylase is often required to make the diagnosis. In mild attacks, other tests to detect pancreatic inflammation are either not sensitive enough (radiology, other biochemical markers) or not necessary (surgery).

A limitation of serum amylase is that it is not 100% sensitive or specific. The serum amylase may be normal or minimally elevated in fatal pancreatitis, during a mild attack, or an attack superimposed upon chronic pancreatitis because the pancreas has little acinar tissue and hence little enzyme, or during recovery from acute pancreatitis.[131] Serum amylase also may be normal in hypertriglyceridemia-associated pancreatitis[57] because an amylase inhibitor may be associated with triglyceride elevations. In this case, serial dilution of serum often reveals an elevated serum amylase.

Hyperamylasemia is nonspecific because it occurs in many conditions other than acute pancreatitis (Table 48–5). Half of all patients with an elevated serum amylase may not have pancreatic disease.[131] In acute pancreatitis, the serum amylase concentration is usually more than three times the upper limit of normal;[132, 133] it is usually less than this with other causes of hyperamylasemia. However, this level is not an absolute discriminator. Thus, an increased serum amylase level supports rather than confirms the diagnosis of acute pancreatitis.

Several nonpancreatic diseases cause hyperamylasemia (Table 48–5). Disease can occur in organs (e.g., salivary glands and fallopian tubes) that normally produce amylase. Some tumors, such as papillary cystadenocarcinoma of the ovary, benign cyst of the ovary, and carcinoma of the lung, cause hyperamylasemia because they secrete salivary type-isoamylase. Transmural leakage of amylase and peritoneal absorption probably explain hyperamylasemia in intestinal infarction and in perforated viscus. Renal failure increases serum amylase due to decreased renal clearance of amylase; serum levels are rarely more than three times the upper limit of normal.[132] In cholecystitis, increased serum amylase probably occurs because of subclinical or undiagnosed coexistent pancreatitis.

Chronic elevations of serum amylase (without amylasuria) occur in macroamylasemia. In this condition, normal serum amylase is bound to an immunoglobulin or abnormal serum protein to form a complex that is too large to be filtered by renal glomeruli.[134] A plasma substitute, hydroxyethyl starch, causes macroamylasemia.[135] Macroamylasemia may complicate the diagnosis of pancreatic disease, but it has no other clinical consequence.

The urinary amylase-to-creatinine clearance ratio (ACCR) increases from approximately 3% to approximately 10% in acute pancreatitis.[136] Even moderate renal insufficiency interferes with the accuracy and specificity of the ACCR. Urinary amylase excretion is not increased in macroamylasemia. Thus, other than to diagnose macroamylasemia, urinary amylase and the ACCR are not used clinically. If the urine amylase is elevated and the serum amylase is normal, deliberate contamination of urine with saliva, as in Munchausen's syndrome, should be excluded by measuring salivary amylase in the urine.

Table 48–5 | **Causes of Increased Serum Amylase Activity**

PANCREATIC DISEASES
- Acute pancreatitis
- Complications of pancreatitis
- Acute exacerbation of chronic pancreatitis
- Pancreatic tumors, cysts

OTHER SERIOUS INTRA-ABDOMINAL DISEASES
- Acute cholecystitis
- Common bile duct obstruction
- Perforation of esophagus, stomach, small bowel, or colon
- Intestinal ischemia or infarction
- Intestinal obstruction
- Acute appendicitis
- Acute gynecologic conditions such as ruptured ectopic pregnancy and acute salpingitis

DISEASES OF SALIVARY GLANDS
- Mumps
- Effects of alcohol

TUMORS
- Ovarian cysts
- Papillary cystadenocarcinoma of ovary
- Carcinoma of lung

RENAL INSUFFICIENCY

MACROAMYLASEMIA

MISCELLANEOUS
- Morphine
- Endoscopy
- Sphincter of Oddi stenosis or spasm
- Anorexia nervosa
- Head trauma with intracranial bleeding
- Diabetic ketoacidosis
- Human immunodeficiency virus

Serum Lipase

Because lipase measurements have been difficult to perform and lacked precision, they have been performed less frequently than for serum amylase.[137] Inclusion of co-lipase in the assay of commercially available kits has improved diagnostic accuracy. In addition, a radioimmunoassay has been developed to measure serum lipase. In acute pancreatitis, the magnitude of increase in serum lipase above upper normal reference limits can vary widely, depending upon the method used.[138]

The sensitivity of serum lipase for the diagnosis of acute pancreatitis is similar to that of serum amylase and is between 85% and 100%.[139] Some claim a greater specificity than with serum amylase because almost all lipase originates from the pancreas (there is a small amount of gastric lipase), and lipase is normal when serum amylase is elevated, as in salivary gland dysfunction, tumors, gynecologic conditions, and macroamylasemia. Serum lipase always is elevated on the first day of illness and remains elevated somewhat longer than does the serum amylase.[140] Consequently, some suggest combining lipase with amylase as a test for acute pancreatitis. However, others and we have found that combining enzymes does not improve diagnostic accuracy.[131, 141, 142]

Specificity of lipase suffers from some of the same problems as those of amylase. In the absence of pancreatitis, serum lipase may increase less than twofold above normal in severe renal insufficiency[132] (creatinine clearance $\leq$ 20 mL/min[128]). With intra-abdominal conditions that resemble acute pancreatitis,[133] lipase increases to levels less than threefold above normal, presumably by reabsorption through an inflamed or perforated intestine.[133]

Some believe that serum lipase measurement is preferable to that of serum amylase because it is as sensitive as amylase measurement and more specific. However, the specificity of both enzymes is very high to differentiate between painful, acute pancreatitis and a surgical condition causing abdominal pain if a cut-off of three times the upper limit of normal is used for each enzyme.[133] The cost of lipase measurement is comparable to that of amylase, and lipase is as available as amylase in most hospitals. However, we did not find a clear advantage of lipase over amylase[131] and do not routinely obtain lipase measurements in preference to those of amylase.

Other Pancreatic Enzymes

During acute pancreatic inflammation, pancreatic digestive enzymes other than amylase and lipase leak into the systemic circulation and have been used to diagnose acute pancreatitis. They include phospholipase A, trypsin, carboxylester lipase, carboxypeptidase A, co-lipase elastase, ribonuclease, and phospholipase A_2. None, alone or in combination, are better than serum amylase or lipase, and most are not available on a routine basis.[131] Urinary and serum trypsinogen-2 may be useful to detect early pancreatitis after ERCP,[143, 144] but these preliminary studies await confirmation.

Nonenzymatic Pancreatic Secretory Products

Many nonenzymatic proteins are overexpressed in acute pancreatitis. Pancreatitis-associated protein (PAP), a heat shock protein, is undetectable in the normal pancreas but markedly increases in acute pancreatitis. The sensitivity of PAP and pancreatic-specific protein (PSP) is no better than that of conventional tests[145, 146] but PAP and PSP are as accurate as serum amylase for the detection of acute pancreatitis. Serum PAP is higher in severe than mild pancreatitis in the first 24 hours of disease and thus may help in establishing prognosis.

Another potential marker of acute pancreatitis is trypsinogen-activation peptide (TAP), a five-amino acid peptide that is cleaved from trypsinogen to produce active trypsin. Since activation of trypsin is an early event in the pathogenesis of acute pancreatitis, TAP may be useful in detection of early acute pancreatitis. Elevated levels of urine TAP also may predict severe acute pancreatitis.[147]

Nonspecific Markers

C-reactive protein, neutrophil elastase, complement, tumor necrosis factor, and interleukin-6 are markers of inflammation and necrosis and may predict severity and outcome of acute pancreatitis.

Miscellaneous Tests

The methemalbumin level increases in acute pancreatitis, but it also increases in serious intra-abdominal conditions such as intestinal infarction. Serum triglyceride levels increase in acute pancreatitis but also with alcohol use, uncontrolled diabetes mellitus, or defective triglyceride metabolism.

Standard Blood Tests

The white blood cell count frequently is elevated, markedly so in severe pancreatitis. The serum glucose level also may be high and associated with high levels of serum glucagon. Aspartate transaminase, alanine transaminase, alkaline phosphatase, and serum bilirubin also may increase, particularly in gallstone pancreatitis. Presumably, calculi in the common bile duct account for these abnormalities. However, pancreatic inflammation may partially obstruct the distal common bile duct in acute pancreatitis of other causes and cause abnormalities in the liver tests. Nevertheless, transaminases may distinguish between biliary and alcoholic pancreatitis (see later).

RADIOLOGIC DIAGNOSIS

Abdominal Plain Film

Findings on a plain radiograph range from no abnormalities in mild disease to localized ileus of a segment of small intestine ("sentinel loop") or the *colon cut-off sign* in more severe disease. In addition, an abdominal plain film helps exclude other causes of abdominal pain, such as obstruction and bowel perforation.

Images of the hollow gastrointestinal tract on an abdominal plain radiograph depend upon the spread and location of pancreatic exudate. Gastric abnormalities are caused by exudate in the lesser sac producing anterior displacement of the stomach, with separation of the contour of the stomach from the transverse colon. Small intestinal abnormalities are due to exudate in proximity to small bowel mesentery and include ileus of one or more loops of jejunum (the sentinel loop), ileus of the distal ileum or cecum, or ileus of the duodenum. Generalized ileus may occur in severe disease.

Besides ileus, other abnormalities of the hollow gastrointestinal tract may be present. The descending duodenum may be displaced and stretched by an enlarged head of the pancreas. In addition, spread of exudate to specific areas of the colon may produce spasm of that part of the colon and either no air distal to the spasm, the colon cut-off sign, or dilated colon proximal to the spasm. Head-predominant pancreatitis predisposes to spread of exudate to the proximal transverse colon, producing colonic spasm and a dilated ascending colon. Uniform pancreatic inflammation predisposes spread of exudate to the inferior border of the transverse colon and an irregular haustral pattern. Exudate from the pancreatic tail to the phrenicocolic ligament adjacent to the-descending colon may cause spasm of the descending colon and a dilated transverse colon.

Other findings on plain radiography of the abdomen may give clues to etiology or severity, including calcified gallstones (gallstone pancreatitis), pancreatic stones or calcification (chronic pancreatitis with a bout of acute inflammation), and ascites (severe pancreatitis).

Chest Radiography

Abnormalities visible on the chest roentgenogram occur in 30% of patients with acute pancreatitis, including elevation of a hemidiaphragm, pleural effusion(s), basal or platelike atelectasis secondary to limited respiratory excursion, and pulmonary infiltrates. Pleural effusions may be bilateral or confined to the left side; rarely they are only on the right side.[148] During the first 7 to 10 days, there also may be signs of congestive heart failure or acute respiratory distress syndrome.[149] Pericardial effusion is rare.

Abdominal Ultrasonography

Abdominal ultrasonography is used during the first 24 hours of hospitalization to search for gallstones, dilatation of the common bile duct due to choledocholithiasis, and ascites. If the pancreas is seen (bowel gas obscures the pancreas 25% to 35% of the time) it is usually diffusely enlarged and hypoechoic. Less frequently there are focal hypoechoic areas. There also may be evidence of chronic pancreatitis, such as intraductal or parenchymal calcification and dilation of the pancreatic duct. Ultrasound is not a good imaging test to evaluate extrapancreatic spread of pancreatic inflammation or necrosis within the pancreas and consequently is not useful to ascertain severity of pancreatitis. During the course of acute pancreatitis, ultrasound can be used to evaluate progression of a pseudocyst.

Endoscopic Ultrasonography

Usually endoscopic ultrasonography (EUS) is not helpful in acute pancreatitis. However, it is more sensitive than either abdominal ultrasonography or CT to detect common duct stones.[107] One potential use of EUS is to exclude a common duct stone in patients with severe pancreatitis and jaundice (bilirubin > 5 mg%). ERCP, in this situation, may worsen pancreatitis and potentially introduce infection into necrotic areas of the pancreas. Thus, EUS might eliminate the need for urgent ERCP in severe gallstone pancreatitis.[150, 151]

Computed Tomography (CT Scan)

CT scan is the most important imaging test for the diagnosis of acute pancreatitis and its intra-abdominal complications.[152, 153] The three main indications for a CT scan in acute pancreatitis are to exclude other serious intra-abdominal conditions, such as mesenteric infarction or a perforated ulcer; to stage the severity of acute pancreatitis;[142, 153] and to determine whether complications are present, such as involvement of the gastrointestinal tract or nearby blood vessels and organs, including liver, spleen, and kidney.[153] Spiral CT is the most common technique. If possible, scanning should occur after the patient receives oral contrast, followed by intravenous contrast to identify any areas of pancreatic necrosis (unenhanced areas greater than 3 cm) (Fig. 48–4; see also Figs. 48–1 to 48–3). Note that pancreatic necrosis may not appear until 48 to 72 hours after onset of acute pancreatitis. CT or US-guided needle aspiration can confirm a suspected infection.

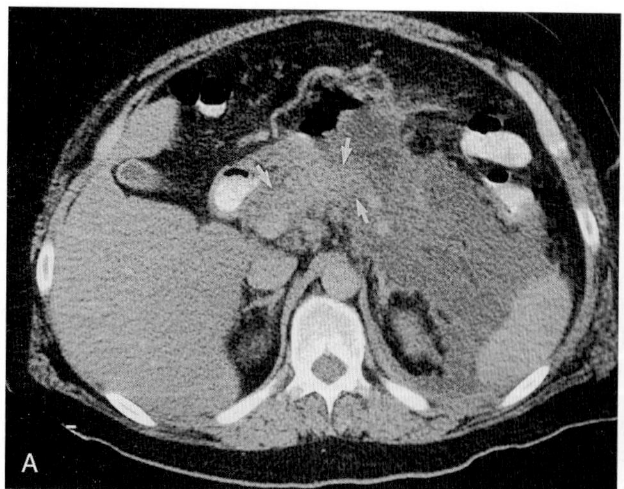

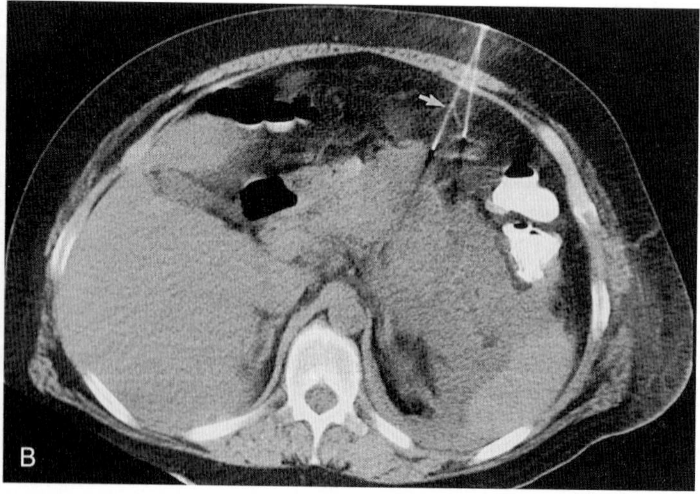

Figure 48–4. Infected necrosis. A, Dynamic contrast-enhanced CT scan performed on the 14th hospital day in a 40-year-old man with alcoholic pancreatitis. This scan reveals enhancement of the head and proximal body of the pancreas *(arrows)* but no enhancement of the distal body and tail of the pancreas. There are extensive inflammatory changes in the left anterior pararenal space. This is severe pancreatitis (Balthazar-Ranson index severity of 8 [4 points for grade E plus 4 points for 33% to 50% necrosis]). *B,* Guided percutaneous aspiration. There are two needles inserted percutaneously. The first was somewhat lateral in orientation. Accordingly, a second needle was inserted using the first as a reference guide (tandem technique) *(arrow).* Three milliliters of brownish material was aspirated from the distal body of the pancreas. A Gram stain revealed gram-positive cocci in clusters and pairs, and culture revealed *Staphylococcus aureus.*

Table 48–6 | **CT Grading System of Balthazar et al**

Grade A—Normal pancreas consistent with mild pancreatitis
Grade B—Focal or diffuse enlargement of the gland, including contour irregularities and inhomogeneous attenuation but without peripancreatic inflammation
Grade C—Abnormalities seen in grade B plus peripancreatic inflammation
Grade D—Grade C plus associated single fluid collection
Grade E—Grade C plus two or more peripancreatic fluid collections or gas in the pancreas or retroperitoneum

From Balthazar EJ, Robinson DL, Megibow AJ, et al: Acute pancreatitis: Value of CT in establishing prognosis. Radiology 174:331, 1990.

Contraindications to using intravenous contrast are a patient's history of prior severe allergy (respiratory distress or anaphylaxis) or significant renal impairment (serum creatinine greater than 2 mg/dL). If severe renal impairment requires dialysis, intravenous contrast medium may be used.[153] Hives or less severe allergic reactions with previous administration of iodinated contrast material are not contraindications, but a nonionic contrast agent should be used, and before the scan 200 mg of hydrocortisone should be administered intravenously every 6 hours for four doses and 50 mg of diphenhydramine (Benadryl) should be given intramuscularly 30 minutes prior to the scan.[153]

It has been suggested that intravenous contrast media early in the course of acute pancreatitis might increase pancreatic necrosis because iodinated contrast medium given at the onset of pancreatitis increases necrosis in experimental rat acute pancreatitis.[154] However, it did not do so in the opossum,[154] and there is little evidence in humans to support that contrast media increase necrosis.[155] Thus, contrast-enhanced CT is used clinically when needed to assess extent of disease, usually no sooner than several days after onset of the attack.

The severity of acute pancreatitis has been classified into five grades (A to E) based upon findings on unenhanced CT[156] (Table 48–6). Although the presence of gas usually ensures pancreatic infection, we have seen patients who have gas in fluid collections without signs of infection or toxicity, and they have gone on to eventual recovery. However, the great majority of pancreatic infections occur in the absence of gas on CT scan.[153, 157–159] Grade E pancreatitis represents the most severe disease. At least half of patients with grade E pancreatitis have necrotizing pancreatitis. The majority of patients with pancreatic infection have grade E pancreatitis.

A modification of this grading system quantifies the amount of pancreatic necrosis and provides a total score, the CT severity index. The higher the CT severity index, the worse the prognosis.[152, 160]

Magnetic Resonance Imaging (MRI)

MRI provides essentially the same information regarding the severity of pancreatitis as does the CT scan (just discussed). MRI is as good as CT to detect necrosis and is a better test to detect choledocholithiasis and ductal abnormalities. Experiments in rats suggest that gadolinium for MRI imaging does not increase necrosis.[161] In addition, gadolinium, unlike intravenous contrast material used for CT, is safe to use in renal failure. For these reasons, MRI, with further technical improvements and greater availability, may replace CT as the preferred imaging test in acute pancreatitis in the future.

Endoscopic Retrograde Cholangiopancreatography (ERCP)

In interstitial pancreatitis and pancreatitis associated with minimal necrosis, the main pancreatic duct usually is normal.[158, 162] Even with significant pancreatic necrosis, the main pancreatic duct is normal in half of cases.[158] The remaining patients have a blocked[158] or disrupted[162] duct. Because this information does not usually affect management of acute pancreatitis, ERCP is not used in acute pancreatitis except to remove common duct stones in severe gallstone pancreatitis.[150, 151]

DIFFERENTIAL DIAGNOSIS OF ACUTE PANCREATITIS

The differential diagnosis of acute pancreatitis includes a variety of conditions associated with severe upper abdominal pain (Table 48–7). However, the history and physical findings aid in differential diagnosis. The abdominal pain of biliary colic may simulate acute pancreatitis. It is frequently severe and epigastric, but it lasts for several hours rather than several days. Pain of perforated ulcer is sudden, becomes diffuse, and precipitates a rigid abdomen; movement aggravates pain. Nausea and vomiting occur but disappear soon after onset of pain. In mesenteric ischemia or infarction, the clinical setting often is an older person with cardiac arrhythmia or arteriosclerotic disease who develops sudden pain out of proportion to physical findings, bloody diarrhea, nausea, and vomiting. Abdominal tenderness may be mild to moderate, and muscular rigidity may not be severe despite severe pain. In intestinal obstruction, pain is cyclical, abdominal distention is prominent, vomiting persists and may become feculent, and peristalsis is hyperactive and often audible.

DISTINGUISHING ALCOHOLIC FROM GALLSTONE PANCREATITIS

Differentiation between alcoholic and gallstone pancreatitis is important because eliminating these causes may prevent further attacks. Alcoholic pancreatitis occurs more frequently in men approximately 40 years old. The first clinical episode usually occurs after 5 to 10 years of heavy alcohol consumption. By contrast, biliary pancreatitis is more frequent

Table 48–7 | **Differential Diagnosis of Acute Pancreatitis**

Biliary colic/acute cholecystitis
Perforated hollow viscus
Mesenteric ischemia or infarction
Closed-loop intestinal obstruction
Inferior wall myocardial infarction
Dissecting aortic aneurysm
Ectopic pregnancy

in women, and the first clinical episode is often after the age of 40 years. Recurrent attacks of acute pancreatitis suggest an alcoholic etiology, but unrecognized gallstones may cause recurrent pancreatitis. Among patients with acute biliary pancreatitis discharged from hospital without cholecystectomy, 30% to 50% have recurrent acute pancreatitis a mean of 108 days after discharge.[163, 164] Thus, removing the gallbladder in biliary pancreatitis is imperative.

Laboratory tests may distinguish between these two disorders. The specificity for gallstone pancreatitis of a serum alanine aminotransaminase (ALT) concentration above 150 IU/L (approximately a threefold elevation) is 96%; the positive predictive value is 95%,[140] but sensitivity is only 48%.[165] The aspartate aminotransferase (AST) concentration is nearly as useful as ALT, but the total bilirubin and alkaline phosphatase concentrations are not helpful to distinguish gallstone pancreatitis from other etiologies. A serum lipase/amylase ratio greater than 2:0 has been proposed to discriminate alcoholic pancreatitis from other causes as it is 91% sensitive and 76% specific for detecting alcoholic pancreatitis.[166] The specificity of the ratio for alcoholic pancreatitis may be greater at higher ratios.[167] However, results of other studies[168] indicate that the ratio does not reliably distinguish among causes of pancreatitis.[169] Multiple tests as a score (serum and urine amylase, AST, ALT, alkaline phosphatase, lipase-to-amylase ratio, and erythrocyte mean corpuscular volume) differentiate between biliary and alcoholic pancreatitis with a sensitivity of 92% and a specificity of 94%.[170]

Conventional transabdominal ultrasonography should be performed in every patient with a first attack of acute pancreatitis to search for gallstones in the gallbladder, common duct stones, or signs of extrahepatic biliary tract obstruction. However, common bile duct stones are frequently missed by transabdominal ultrasonography, and most stones pass during the acute attack. Our practice is to limit ERCP to patients with severe acute pancreatitis due to gallstones with persistent common bile duct obstruction and to those in whom the stone could not be removed during surgery. Thus, we image the common bile duct in most patients with biliary pancreatitis with an operative cholangiogram at the time of laparoscopic cholecystectomy performed during the same admission. EUS is the most accurate method of detecting common duct stones and has been recommended for evaluating the common duct prior to cholecystectomy.[171] However, we rarely perform EUS in this setting. If a common duct stone is found at surgery, it is either removed at operation or endoscopically after surgery. Laparoscopic exploration of the common bile duct is as safe and effective as postoperative ERCP in clearing stones from the common duct.[172]

PREDICTORS OF SEVERITY OF PANCREATITIS

Predicting severity of pancreatitis early in the course of disease is critical to maximize therapy and to prevent and minimize organ dysfunction and complications. Routine laboratory tests, clinical assessment, scoring systems, serum markers, and CT scanning have all been used.

Routine laboratory tests and observations may be abnormal in acute pancreatitis, particularly in severe disease. A hematocrit above 50%, urine output below 30 mL/hr, systolic blood pressure below 90 mm Hg, and marked tachycardia (>120 beats/min) indicate severe depletion of intravascular volume and require immediate fluid resuscitation. White blood cell count is frequently more than 16,000/mm^3. Blood urea nitrogen may increase due to prerenal azotemia and possibly acute renal injury. Metabolic acidosis indicates circulatory failure, and low oxygen saturation (< 90% by pulse oximetry) indicates respiratory insufficiency and requires a blood gas measurement and oxygen therapy.

Hypocalcemia may appear as early as the first day of disease because albumin leaks into the retroperitoneum. Increasing serum albumin proportionally increases serum calcium. Infrequently, loss of ionized calcium is due to calcium deposition within fat necrosis, hypomagnesemia, or bone refractoriness to an adequate parathyroid response. Indeed, parathyroid secretion increases in response to hypocalcemia in severe acute pancreatitis.[173] In hypertriglyceridemia, calcium binding to serum free fatty acids also may explain hypocalcemia.

Scoring Systems

Clinical Signs

Clinical evidence of severe pancreatitis includes signs of peritonitis, shock, or respiratory distress. However, use of these signs at the bedside may identify only 34% to 44% of severe acute pancreatitis cases.[174, 175] At admission, sensitivity of these signs is less than 40%, but specificity is high.[176] After 48 hours, the accuracy of clinical assessment is comparable to Ranson's and Imrie's scoring systems. Thus, with the exception of the APACHE-II system,[175] and in common with other systems (e.g., Ranson, Glasgow, Bank, and Agarwal and Pitchumoni[174, 177–179]), clinical signs are not accurate until the 48-hour mark. Other systems also can be used only once, and some include complications to be prevented (e.g., Bank) or are invasive (e.g., Leeds diagnostic peritoneal lavage[176]). For these reasons, these scoring systems usually are not used clinically.

Ranson's Signs

Ranson and colleagues identified 11 signs that had prognostic significance during the first 48 hours (see Table 48–2). Higher Ranson's scores predict more severe disease. In mild pancreatitis, the mean Ranson score is 1.6, in severe pancreatitis 2.4, and in lethal pancreatitis 5.6. Mortality is less than 5% with 0, 1, or 2 Ranson's signs, 10% with 3, 4, or 5 signs, and over 60% with 6 or more signs. More than 6 Ranson's signs also predict a high incidence of systemic complications, necrosis, and infected necrosis.

Nevertheless, Ranson's criteria have several drawbacks. First, an individual sign may be positive in 10% to 20% of all patients. Thus, it is essential to measure all 11 signs to predict severity. Second, an accurate Ranson's score takes 48 hours to compute. Although five signs are measured at admission, 5 of the 6 remaining signs are not negative unless they remain so for the full 48 hours. Third, the value of the signs is unknown beyond the first 48 hours, and they should not be used beyond this time. Fourth, the criteria are not highly sensitive and specific. For prediction of severity, sensitivity is 57% to 85%, specificity is 68% to 85%, the positive predictive value is slightly less than 50%, and the negative predictive value approximates 90%.[180] Perhaps the best use of Ranson's score is to exclude severe disease.[181]

APACHE-II Scores

APACHE-II is the most commonly used scoring system to predict severity because it can be used continuously and may be the most accurate.[175–181] In one report, it correctly identified 63% of severe attacks (versus 44% by clinical assessment).[175] However, it is complex and cumbersome.[178, 182] The APACHE-II system assigns points for 12 physiologic variables, for age, and for chronic health status, in generating a total point score. The 12 variables are temperature; heart rate; respiratory rate; mean arterial blood pressure; oxygenation; arterial pH; serum potassium, sodium, and creatinine; hematocrit; WBC; and Glasgow Coma Scale. APACHE-II scores at admission and within 48 hours help distinguish mild from severe pancreatitis and to predict death.[176, 182, 183] Most patients survive if APACHE-II scores are 9 or less during the first 48 hours. However, patients with APACHE-II scores of 13 or more have a high likelihood of dying. At admission, sensitivity is 34% to 70%, and specificity is 76% to 98%. At 48 hours, sensitivity remains less than 50%, but specificity is close to 100%.[176] Strong drawbacks are the low sensitivity at admission, and the fact that at 48 hours the score is no better than other scoring systems.[181]

Other Prognostic Systems

Other scoring systems also require 48 hours. Imrie's score incorporates nine signs[180, 183] and is as accurate as Ranson's score to distinguish mild from severe pancreatitis.[181, 183] Other investigators evaluated risk factors (cardiac, pulmonary, renal, and metabolic abnormalities) and found that the presence of one risk factor predicted serious complications and over 50% mortality.[178, 179]

Peritoneal Lavage

Percutaneous recovery of any volume of peritoneal fluid with a dark color or recovery of at least 20 mL of free intraperitoneal fluid of any color portends a high mortality (~33%). The sensitivity of peritoneal lavage is 36% to 72%, and the specificity is greater than 75%.[181] An advantage is that it can be used any time, but it has not gained wide acceptance because it is invasive.

Serum Markers

The degree of elevation of serum amylase does not distinguish mild from severe pancreatitis.[184, 185] Although not generally available clinically, levels of interleukin-6 (IL-6), polymorphonuclear leukocyte elastase, and trypsinogen activation peptide (TAP)[186–188] may prove valuable because their concentrations in blood or urine rise within 12 hours in severe acute pancreatitis, thereby providing a more rapid assessment of severity.

C-Reactive Protein

C-reactive protein (CRP) is an acute-phase reactant produced by the liver. It is elevated in severe pancreatitis and is usually higher in necrotizing pancreatitis. CRP is inexpensive to measure and readily available.[184, 189, 190] In one report of 34 patients with acute pancreatitis, in 21 of whom the disease was necrotizing,[189] the sensitivity for detecting necrotizing pancreatitis was 95%. In another series, a peak CRP level of 210 mg/L on the second, third, or fourth day was the best discriminant serum marker for severe disease.[190] However, CRP takes 48 hours to become significantly elevated, and whether it accurately predicts necrosis is uncertain. In one report, CRP was only 8% sensitive for identifying severe disease on day 1.[186]

Interleukin-6

Interleukin-6 is an acute-phase-reactant cytokine that is produced by a variety of cells and induces hepatic synthesis of C-reactive protein. In a small study of 38 patients with acute pancreatitis, 15 with severe disease,[190] the sensitivity, specificity, and diagnostic accuracy for severe pancreatitis on day one were higher with serum IL-6 (100%, 86%, and 91%, respectively) than for serum CRP (8%, 95%, and 64%). Because the peak activity of IL-6 is between 24 and 36 hours, measurement is not recommended at admission.[185]

Polymorphonuclear Leukocyte Elastase

Polymorphonuclear leukocyte elastase is higher in severe than in mild pancreatitis[187, 191, 192] and higher in necrotizing than in interstitial pancreatitis. Sensitivity and specificity of this test are very high, but the test is not generally available.

Alpha$_2$-Macroglobulin

Serum concentrations of alpha$_2$-macroglobulin decrease over time in severe acute pancreatitis, but measurement is expensive and has no advantage over CRP.[184, 189, 190] Therefore, measurement is not recommended at admission.

Urinary Trypsinogen Activation Peptide

Trypsinogen activation peptide (TAP) is the amino-terminal peptide cleaved from trypsinogen during activation of trypsin, providing a rationale for its use as a marker of acute pancreatitis. It can be measured in plasma, ascites fluid, and urine. Urinary TAP, if measured within 48 hours of onset of symptoms, distinguishes mild from severe pancreatitis.[185, 189, 193] The sensitivity, specificity, and positive and negative predictive values for severe compared with mild acute pancreatitis at 24 hours compared favorably to those for CRP (58%, 73%, 39%, and 86% versus 0%, 90%, 0%, and 75%, respectively) and when compared with the APACHE-II, Ranson, and Glasgow scores.

CT Scanning

CT scanning is used to assess severity because other methods are not as accurate.[174] CT scan is more accurate if it is combined with a Ranson score.[194] Contrast-enhanced CT distinguishes between edematous and necrotizing pancreatitis, since areas of necrosis and exudate do not contrast-enhance. CT is more accurate than ultrasonography for the diagnosis of severe pancreatic necrosis (90% versus 73% in one report).[194] In this study, 30 of 77 cases of necrotizing pancreatitis were incorrectly categorized as mild disease with the Ranson score. The finding of necrotizing pancreatitis (or even infected necrosis) does not necessarily predict the occurrence of organ failure but should alter the therapeutic approach.[41]

Summary of Scoring Systems

Most scoring systems are not routinely used in clinical practice because clinical assessment by an experienced observer is as accurate in predicting severity. If a patient has severe acute pancreatitis, as determined by clinical criteria and the APACHE-II score, contrast-enhanced CT should be performed to determine whether necrotizing pancreatitis is present.

Obesity

Obese patients with pancreatitis have a higher incidence of respiratory failure than do nonobese patients.[195] Moreover, patients with severe acute pancreatitis have a higher body mass index than those with mild disease,[196] and death in sterile necrosis is associated with a high body mass index.[182]

Chest Radiography

A pleural effusion documented within 72 hours of admission[148] by either chest radiograph or CT scan correlates with more severe disease.

Organ Failure

Organ failure profoundly influences morbidity and mortality from acute pancreatitis (see Table 48–1). Even with substantial pancreatic necrosis, mortality is low in the absence of organ failure. Conversely, mortality associated with sterile and infected necrosis is higher if organ failure is present.

Local Complications

Mortality from interstitial pancreatitis approximates 1%, whereas mortality is 10% to 15% in sterile necrosis and 30% to 35% in infected necrosis.[197] Mortality from infected necrosis is higher than that from pancreatic abscess,[198] and mortality of pancreatic pseudocyst is higher if pancreatic necrosis is present.

TREATMENT

Current medical treatment of acute pancreatitis is mostly supportive and includes fluid resuscitation, pulmonary care, and supervision in an intensive care unit. Major aims are to reduce morbidity and mortality by limiting systemic complications, preventing pancreatic necrosis and infection, treating pancreatic inflammation, and correcting any underlying predisposing factors.

Mild Pancreatitis

The prognosis of mild pancreatitis is excellent. It is treated for several days with supportive care, including intravenous fluids, pain control, and nothing by mouth. Most patients require no further therapy and recover and eat within 5 to 7 days. However, fluid resuscitation is important to replace low intravascular volume due to vomiting, diaphoresis, and third-space losses. If hypovolemia develops, the pancreatic microcirculation may become compromised, with intensification of local inflammation and evolution to necrotizing pancreatitis.

Abdominal pain is treated with 50 to 100 mg of meperidine (Demerol), given parenterally every 3 to 4 hours. More severe pain requires hydromorphone (Dilaudid), which has a longer half-life than Demerol and is given parenterally by a patient-controlled anesthesia pump. Dosing is monitored carefully and adjusted on a daily basis according to ongoing needs. Because morphine increases sphincter of Oddi tone and increases serum amylase,[199] we avoid this and other morphine-derived agents.

Nasogastric intubation is not used routinely because it is not beneficial in mild pancreatitis.[200, 201] It is used only to treat gastric or intestinal ileus or intractable nausea and vomiting. Similarly, proton pump inhibitors or H_2-receptor blocking agents[202] are not beneficial and not used. Prophylactic antibiotic therapy is not indicated in mild pancreatitis.

Severe Pancreatitis

Patients with severe pancreatitis are at risk for developing systemic complications,[3, 201] are more likely to have necrotizing than interstitial pancreatitis, and have increased mortality. Intensive care unit monitoring and support of pulmonary, renal, and hepatobiliary function may minimize systemic sequelae. Fluid resuscitation is particularly important because patients with necrotizing pancreatitis may accumulate vast amounts of fluid in the injured pancreatic bed. Cardiac filling pressures and urine output are reliable indices of adequate tissue perfusion. Inadequate hydration can lead to hypotension and acute renal tubular necrosis. In some patients, however, a low urine output may already reflect the development of oliguric renal failure from acute tubular necrosis rather than persistent volume depletion. In this setting, aggressive fluid replacement can lead to peripheral and pulmonary edema without improving the urine output.

Fluid Resuscitation

Maintaining adequate intravascular volume may require 5 to 10 liters of fluid (e.g., isotonic saline) daily for the first several days. A Swan-Ganz catheter is useful to gauge fluid resuscitation and to avoid congestive heart failure. It is also helpful when cardiovascular status is unstable or respiratory function deteriorates. Aggressive fluid replacement may not prevent pancreatic necrosis. Experimentally, hemodilution to a hematocrit of around 30% with dextran-60 improved the pancreatic microcirculation and oxygenation.[121] A controlled study is currently underway in Europe to test this treatment in humans. Until the results are known, albumin should be infused if the serum albumin falls to less than 2 g/L. When the hematocrit decreases to around 25%, packed red blood cells should be infused to maintain a hematocrit close to 30%.[203, 204]

Respiratory Care

Hypoxemia (oxygen saturation < 90%) requires oxygen, ideally by nasal prongs or by face mask if needed. If nasal oxygen fails to correct hypoxemia or if there is fatigue and borderline respiratory reserve, endotracheal intubation and assisted ventilation are required early. It is important to use a Swan-Ganz catheter to determine whether hypoxemia is due to congestive heart failure (increased pulmonary artery wedge pressure) or is a primary pulmonary problem (normal or low pulmonary artery wedge pressure).

Acute respiratory distress syndrome (ARDS) is the most serious respiratory complication of acute pancreatitis because it is associated with severe dyspnea, progressive hypoxemia, and increased mortality. It occurs between the second and seventh day of illness and consists of increased alveolar capillary permeability causing interstitial edema. Chest radiography may show multilobar pulmonary infiltrates. Treatment is endotracheal intubation with positive end-expiratory pressure ventilation. No specific treatment will prevent or affect this condition. After resolution, pulmonary structure and function usually return to normal.

Cardiovascular Care

Cardiac complications of severe acute pancreatitis include congestive heart failure, myocardial infarction, cardiac arrhythmia, and cardiogenic shock. An increase in cardiac index and a decrease in total peripheral resistance may be present and respond to infusion of crystalloids. If hypotension persists even with appropriate fluid resuscitation, intravenous dopamine may help maintain the systemic blood pressure. Dopamine does not impair the microcirculation of the pancreas as do other vasoconstrictors.

Metabolic Complications

Hyperglycemia may present during the first several days of severe pancreatitis but usually normalizes as the inflammatory process subsides. Blood sugar varies, and insulin should be administered cautiously.

Hypocalcemia due to low serum albumin causes no symptoms and requires no specific therapy. However, reduced serum ionized calcium may cause neuromuscular irritability. If hypomagnesemia co-exists, magnesium replacement should restore serum calcium to normal. Causes of magnesium depletion include vomiting, loss of magnesium in urine, or deposition of magnesium in areas of fat necrosis. When serum magnesium is normal, signs or symptoms of neuromuscular irritability require giving intravenous calcium gluconate if the serum potassium is normal and digitalis is not being given. Intravenous calcium increases calcium binding to myocardial receptors, which displaces potassium and may induce a serious arrhythmia.

Prevention of Pancreatic Infection

Bacterial infection of pancreatic and peripancreatic tissues develops in approximately 30% of severe acute pancreatitis[205] and may cause multiorgan failure and its sequelae. It usually develops late in the clinical course, particularly if there is extensive necrosis. Infection is present in 24% of patients operated on within the first 7 days and 71% of patients operated on in the third week.[206] A similar infection rate (71%) has been found by culturing a CT-guided aspirate from pancreatic necrosis.[207]

The important organisms causing infection in necrotizing pancreatitis are from the gut (*Escherichia coli*, *Pseudomonas*, *Klebsiella*, and *Enterococcus* species). Most infections (~75%) are monomicrobial. Fungi and other gram-positive organisms (besides *Enterococcus*) are uncommon but occur more frequently in the setting of antibiotic use. Gram-negative and fungal pancreatic infections have a worse prognosis than gram-positive infections.[208, 209]

Three approaches to decrease bacterial infections in acute necrotizing pancreatitis are selective decontamination of the gut with nonabsorbable antibiotics, prophylactic systemic antibiotics, and enteral feeding (see later) to avoid catheter-related infections associated with a central line, to maintain gut barrier integrity, and to decrease bacterial translocation.

Selective Decontamination of the Gut

Since the gut is the source of pancreatic bacterial infections, oral nonabsorbable antibiotics might reduce pancreatic infection. Support for this hypothesis is the result of a randomized controlled trial in severe acute pancreatitis evaluating gut decontamination with a combination of oral norfloxacin, colistin, and amphotericin.[210] Overall mortality was significantly lower with gut decontamination (22% versus 35%); reduced mortality was mostly attributed to fewer gram-negative infections (8% versus 33%). However, it is unclear whether gut decontamination alone was responsible for the results because systemic antibiotics also were used.

Systemic Antibiotics

In the 1970s it was shown that antibiotics such as ampicillin that did not penetrate the inflamed pancreas had no benefit.[211–215] Since then, investigators demonstrated adequate penetration into the pancreas for imipenem, third-generation cephalosporins, piperacillin, mezlocillin, fluoroquinolones, and metronidazole, but not for aminoglycosides, aminopenicillins, or first-generation cephalosporins.[216] Subsequently, investigators showed that use of antibiotics that penetrate the pancreas improves the outcome of severe necrotizing pancreatitis.[211–214]

In one prospective trial, 60 consecutive patients with severe acute alcoholic pancreatitis, defined as necrosis of at least one third of the pancreas by contrast-enhanced CT, were randomly assigned to the cephalosporin cefuroxime (1.5 g every 8 hours) or placebo.[211] Cefuroxime was given until occurrence of clinical recovery and normalization of the serum CRP level. Cefuroxime markedly decreased mortality (3% versus 23%) and reduced total infectious complications (30% versus 54% mostly preventing urinary tract infections and secondary infections due to *Staphylococcus epidermidis*). In another placebo-controlled study, ceftazidime, amikacin, and metronidazole, given intravenously for 10 days,[215] decreased sepsis from 58% with placebo to 0% with the antibiotics (3 in the control group died compared with 1 who received antibiotics). Imipenem reduced morbidity but had no influence on survival[212] and reduced infections when compared with pefloxacin.[214] The conclusion of a meta-analysis of eight controlled trials was that prophylactic antibiotics reduced mortality in severe acute pancreatitis when patients received broad-spectrum antibiotics that achieve therapeutic pancreatic tissue levels.[215]

Unfortunately, the use of prophylactic antibiotics has risks, such as selection of resistant organisms and development of fungal infection. Patients who develop fungal infections received antibiotics longer (~3 weeks vs. 1 week) and have increased mortality.[217] In another report, 43% mortality occurred in seven patients who developed fungal infection while receiving antibiotic prophylaxis.[208] However, the risk of fungal infections may exist only with polyantimicrobial treatment. Because of the risk of fungal infections, prophylactic antifungal therapy has been advised.

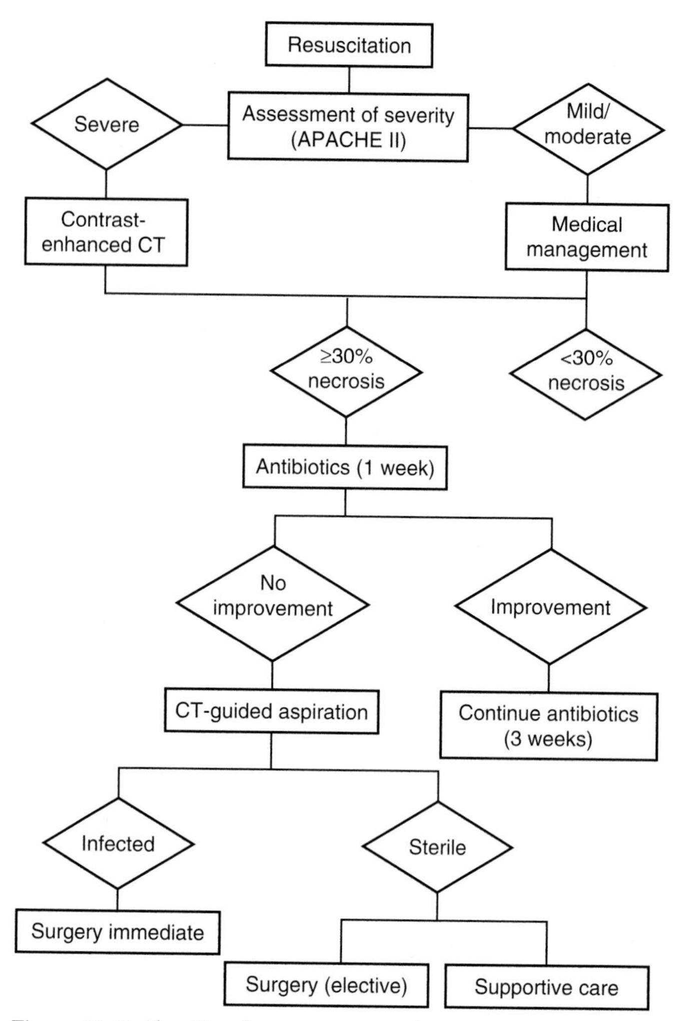

Figure 48–5. Algorithm for management of severe acute pancreatitis. CT, computed tomography.

Treatment of Pancreatic Necrosis

Pancreatic necrosis occurs in approximately 20% of acute pancreatitis cases and can be confirmed with dynamic contrast-enhanced CT scan[152, 153] (see Figs. 48–2 and 48–3). In the absence of organ failure or systemic toxicity, patients with pancreatic necrosis usually can be maintained on intravenous fluid replacement and medication for pain (Fig. 48–5). If organ dysfunction or systemic toxicity persists beyond the first 7 to 10 days, infected necrosis of the pancreas may be present.

Infected Necrosis of the Pancreas

Persisting systemic toxicity manifested by a high white blood cell count of 20,000/mm^3 or more and a temperature of 101°F to 102°F[218] or unresolved organ failure for 7 to 10 days suggests infection of necrotizing pancreatitis (infected necrosis; see Fig. 48–4). These events should trigger CT-guided percutaneous aspiration of the infected necrosis with immediate Gram stain and culture of the aspirate for aerobic and anaerobic bacteria and for fungi. With the exception of gas bubbles in the retroperitoneum on CT scan, there is no other technique for distinguishing sterile necrosis from infected necrosis.[218, 219] Guided percutaneous aspiration is safe and is an accurate method to demonstrate pancreatic infection. In almost all instances, Gram stain reveals organisms. Because guided percutaneous aspiration of necrotic tissue and fluid is so accurate, evidence of pancreatic infection on an aspirate suggests diffuse infection without pockets of sterile fluid/necrosis.[220]

Most infections are due to *Klebsiella*, *E. coli*, or *Staphylococcus aureus*. Occasionally infection is caused by a *Candida* species. In over 80% of infections, only one organism has been recovered. The prevalence of pancreatic infection likely is decreasing. Previously, the prevalence was 40% to 60% and now it is 15% to 30%. An explanation for this observation is that use of potent antibiotics may prevent or eradicate secondary pancreatic infection.

Detection of pancreatic infection requires prompt debridement,[221–224] preceded by appropriate antibiotics based on the results of Gram stain or culture. Surgical débridement is mostly by gentle blunt finger dissection of necrotic tissue rather than sharp dissection. After débridement, treatment consists of (1) closure of the abdomen by placing stuffed external Penrose and Jackson-Pratt drains; (2) closure of the abdomen with placement of large soft drains within the retroperitoneum for intermittent or continuous saline lavage; or (3) open packing of the abdomen. The last approach facilitates pancreatic débridement, which is done every 2 to 3 days. There has been no randomized prospective trial to compare techniques. Overall mortality is 10% to 48%;[198, 206, 212, 219, 221, 224] usually, mortality is 30% or less. Even though surgical débridement prolongs hospitalization, there is good quality of life after recovery.[225]

Because of the morbidity, mortality, and prolonged hospital stay associated with open surgical débridement, endoscopic drainage has been used to drain "organized" pancreatic necrosis (walled-off necrotic areas in the pancreas or peripancreatic tissue in close proximity to the gut).[226] With this endoscopic approach, the retroperitoneum is drained by several 10-French internal-diameter transgastric or transduodenal drainage catheters, and a 7-French irrigation tube is placed. Frequent irrigation of the necrotic bed through the nasocystic tube leads to a flow of solid debris around the catheters into the gut lumen. In this study, 81% of patients achieved complete resolution of necrosis without surgery. Surgery often was for complications related to endoscopy.

A similar approach has been used by interventional radiologists to place multiple large-bore irrigation catheters into necrotic areas.[227, 228] Freeny and colleagues[227] studied 34 patients with necrotizing pancreatitis and medically uncontrolled sepsis by placing catheters into the pancreatic collections. An average of three separate catheter sites per patient and four catheter exchanges per patient were necessary to remove necrotic material. Pancreatic surgery was avoided in 47%, and in another 32% elective surgery was later performed to repair external pancreatic fistulas related to catheter placement. Immediate surgery for failed percutaneous therapy was required in 32%. Death occurred in 32%. In a group of hemodynamically stable patients with infected necrosis,[228] pancreatic necrosis was débrided by placing catheters percutaneously. Complete resolution of the necrosis without surgery was achieved in all by using multiple large-bore catheters, high-volume irrigation, and stone-retrieval baskets.

The nonsurgical approaches to débridement of necrotizing pancreatitis require proper patient selection and considerable technical expertise and are associated with complications that may require emergency surgery in patients who are already quite sick. More data are needed to define the precise role and timing of these techniques in the management of necrotizing pancreatitis.

After débridement, a cutaneous or intestinal pancreatic fistula may develop.[229] Cutaneous fistulas usually close within several weeks and may be helped by octreotide. A colonic fistula usually requires a proximal colostomy; sometimes it is necessary to resect the colon containing the fistula and use 50 to 200 μg of octreotide subcutaneously every 8 hours to reduce pancreatic flow.

Sterile Necrosis of the Pancreas

Sterile necrosis of the pancreas that is clinically mild and not associated with systemic complication has a low mortality rate.[182] However, mortality is 19% to 38% in the presence of systemic complications.[182] If organ failure and systemic toxicity improve, medical treatment should be continued and may consist of systemic antibiotics to prevent secondary pancreatic infection and enteral nutrition, with oral feedings started when organ failure subsides. By contrast, absence of clinical improvement during the first 7 to 10 days indicates either severe sterile or infected necrosis. Under these circumstances, CT-guided percutaneous aspiration with Gram stain and culture should be performed to rule out infection. If aspiration does not confirm infection, most experts advise medical management for 4 to 6 weeks to allow resolution of severe systemic toxicity.[229–231] After this time, surgery may be indicated if there is persisting respiratory insufficiency with intubation and assisted ventilation, compression of the stomach causing intractable nausea and preventing oral intake, or severe recurrent pain with each effort at oral alimentation. Without randomized prospective trials comparing medical and surgical treatment or comparing early versus late surgical débridement, optimal treatment of severe sterile necrosis remains uncertain.

Nutrition (see also Chapter 16)

Mild pancreatitis often is managed with only intravenous hydration since recovery occurs rapidly. In contrast, management of severe pancreatitis requires nutritional support. In the past these patients were typically fed parenterally because they often have ileus and abdominal pain and because clinicians were fearful of stimulating the pancreas with enteral feeding. However, now there is a trend to use enteral nutrition with severe disease as soon as ileus subsides. There is increasing evidence that enteral feeding is safe and may reduce complications by maintaining the intestinal barrier and preventing or reducing bacterial translocation from the gut. Further, enteral nutrition eliminates complications of parenteral nutrition, such as catheter sepsis (2% even if the catheter is managed appropriately), and less frequent complications, such as arterial laceration, pneumothorax, vein thrombosis, thrombophlebitis, and catheter embolism.

Enteral Nutrition

Results of several controlled studies support the use of enteral nutrition. Enteral feeding (nasojejunal tube) has fewer complications than parenteral nutrition.[232] Further, nutritional requirements are fulfilled by either enteral or parenteral nutrition (7% versus 82% for the enteral and parenteral groups, respectively).[233] There are no significant differences between enteral and parenteral nutrition for mortality, pain scores, days to normalization of the serum amylase, or resumption of a normal diet. Disease severity also tends to decrease with enteral nutrition[233, 234] and to increase with parenteral nutrition during the first week of therapy, and acute-phase responses improve with enteral but not parenteral nutrition.[234] Lastly, the cost of parenteral nutrition is four times greater than that of enteral nutrition.[233] Whenever possible, radiologic or endoscopic placement of a jejunal feeding tube and enteral feeding should be attempted. We use high-protein, low-fat preparations such as Peptamen. Parenteral nutrition should be used if patients do not tolerate enteral feeding or if nutritional goals cannot be reached within 2 days. Intravenous lipids should not be withheld from parenteral feedings unless serum triglyceride levels are 500 mg/dL or more.

Initiation of Oral Feedings

Decisions about when to begin oral feedings, what to feed, and how often to feed arise for every patient with acute pancreatitis because feeding stimulates pancreatic secretion and may cause relapse of pain or recurrent acute pancreatitis. Help with answers to these questions may be derived from studies in healthy humans. The rate of pancreatic enzyme secretion directly relates to the nutrient composition of meals and to the rate of caloric delivery to the duodenum. The secretion of pancreatic enzymes decreases as more carbohydrate is ingested, particularly when carbohydrates are 50% or more of the total caloric content of the diet.[235] When nutrients are infused into the duodenum, pancreatic enzyme secretion increases as the rate of energy infused increases from 40 to 90 to 160 kcal/hr.[236]

Further, in acute pancreatitis the risk of recurrent pain is 21% if feeding is begun with diets containing 250 kcal and less than 5 g of fat on day 1, and the diet is increased gradually to 1700 kcal and 35 to 40 g of fat by day 5.[237] Half of pain relapses occurred on the first or second day of feeding, when the maximal intake was 1000 kcal and 5 to 10 g of fat. The risk of recurrent pain is greater if there is necrotizing pancreatitis, if there is a long duration of pain before feeding (11 versus 6 days), and if serum lipase is still greater than three times the upper limit of normal on the day before initiating feeding (40% versus 20%). There is no evidence that a proton pump inhibitor or H_2-receptor blocking agent is helpful in preventing an exacerbation of pain.

In mild pancreatitis, oral feeding usually can begin by the third to seventh hospital day. In mild and severe pancreatitis, we initiate oral feedings when abdominal pain and tenderness subside, if there are no complications and serum amylase is nearly normal. However, particularly in severe pancreatitis, it is not always necessary to wait for a normal serum amylase as serum amylase and lipase levels may be abnormal even at the time of hospital discharge.[159] Initiating oral feeding does not depend on CT appearance of the pancreas (see Fig. 48–3) since inflammatory changes may be present at hospital discharge and last for several months.[159]

We begin oral feedings by giving 100 to 300 mL of liquids containing no calories every 4 hours for the first 24 hours. If this diet is tolerated, we continue oral feeding by giving the same volume of liquids containing nutrients. If tolerated, feedings are then advanced gradually over 3 to 4 days to soft and finally to solid foods. All feedings contain greater than 50% carbohydrate, and the total caloric content is gradually increased from 160 to 640 Kcal per meal. However, no data in trials of acute pancreatitis support this dietary regimen.

Gallstone Pancreatitis

Gallstone pancreatitis requires separate therapeutic considerations because stones in the biliary tract or ampulla of Vater cause the pancreatitis. (See "Etiology of Acute Pancreatitis.")

Results of experimental animal studies suggest that early removal of bile duct stones by endoscopy or surgery may lessen the severity of gallstone pancreatitis. In one study, acute hemorrhagic necrotizing pancreatitis was induced in opossums by obstructing the biliopancreatic ductal system with a balloon catheter for 1, 3, or 5 days.[28] A progressive increase in the severity of pancreatitis occurred in the animals obstructed for 5 days. In contrast, decompression of the obstructed ductal system by removal of the balloon catheter after 1 or 3 days prevented progression of pancreatic injury.

These findings may apply clinically. Early endoscopic papillotomy benefits acute biliary pancreatitis.[149, 151] In one controlled trial, 195 patients with acute biliary pancreatitis were randomized to emergency ERCP with endoscopic papillotomy or to conservative therapy and selective ERCP, with or without papillotomy, if their condition deteriorated.[149] Sixty-five percent of the patients had biliary stones, and stones were present in all patients with unrelenting biliary sepsis. Early ERCP prevented biliary sepsis (0% versus 12% with conservative therapy) but had no effect on the rate of local or systemic complications.

Not all patients benefit from early ERCP and papillotomy. It does not benefit patients with acute biliary pancreatitis without obstructive jaundice or biliary sepsis. In 126 patients who had a serum bilirubin concentration below 5 mg/dL, there was no difference in survival between groups treated with or without early ERCP and papillotomy. More importantly, the early ERCP group had more severe complications.[238] Patients with a serum bilirubin concentration below 5 mg/dL already may have passed the stones and can be treated conservatively; the minority of patients who then develop progressive jaundice can undergo ERCP when needed.

Cholecystectomy should be performed after recovery but prior to hospital discharge in all patients with gallstone pancreatitis. Failure to perform cholecystectomy is associated with a 25% risk of recurrent acute pancreatitis, cholecystitis, or cholangitis within 6 weeks.[239] An additional 25% of patients may experience biliary colic without pancreatitis during the same period. Although cholecystectomy reduces the risk of acute pancreatitis to almost the same level as in the general population, the overall incidence of pancreatitis in patients with gallstones is only 3% to 7%.[42] Thus, a cholecystectomy to prevent pancreatitis is indicated only if an attack of acute pancreatitis has already occurred. A cholangiogram and clearing the common bile duct of stones either during surgery or by ERCP are mandatory to prevent recurrent pancreatitis after cholecystectomy.

Recommended Approach (see also Fig. 48–5)

After early resuscitation has been performed, and if severe pancreatitis is present by clinical assessment and by APACHE-II score, we obtain a contrast-enhanced CT scan. A CT scan is not required on the first hospital day unless there are other possible diagnoses to exclude. Pancreatic necrosis takes time to develop, and treatment will not be affected by CT findings on day 1. Although some experimental data indicate that ionic contrast material may worsen pancreatitis, the association is not strong, and the information obtained from the CT scan justifies the potential risk. If there is necrotizing pancreatitis involving more than 30% of the pancreas, we prescribe imipenem for at least a week. Fluconazole may also be used in addition to imipenem to try to reduce the incidence of fungal infection. Patients without severe necrotizing pancreatitis are managed conservatively. If there is no improvement after a week of antibiotics, we perform a percutaneous CT-guided aspiration of the pancreas.[214, 240] If there is bacterial infection or if the patient becomes unstable from pulmonary, cardiovascular, or renal complications, we recommend a necrosectomy to remove necrotic debris and pus.[207, 241] If the aspirate is sterile, we continue conservative treatment for 4 to 6 weeks since most patients do well with medical therapy. A repeat aspiration may be indicated if there is a high clinical suspicion of infection.

Experimental Agents

Pancreatic protease inhibitors have been used to treat established severe acute pancreatitis and to prevent post-ERCP pancreatitis. Gabexate mesilate is the most widely studied pancreatic protease inhibitor. A meta-analysis of five clinical trials of gabexate mesilate in acute pancreatitis found no effect on the 90-day mortality rate but a reduced incidence of complications.[242] Others used meta-analysis to evaluate the use of somatostatin, its synthetic octreotide, analog, or gabexate mesilate to prevent post-ERCP pancreatitis in 28 clinical trials and concluded that survival was better for patients treated with somatostatin or octreotide and that gabexate mesilate reduced complications.[243] However, we interpret these studies cautiously because benefits occurred in a very low proportion of patients. Furthermore, the researchers of a placebo-controlled trial (that was not included in the meta-analysis) concluded that octreotide was of no benefit.[244] Thus, the effectiveness of these treatments is uncertain, and they are unlikely to be cost-effective.

Recently, Japanese investigators suggested that pancreatic protease inhibitors and antibiotics can be better targeted to the affected regions in the pancreas with continuous regional arterial infusion (CRAI) into the celiac, splenic, inferior pancreaticoduodenal, and common hepatic arteries. Using CT, Anai and colleagues[245] showed that with CRAI the contrast was distributed to the entire pancreas in six of nine patients with inflammation of the entire pancreas; in the remaining three patients, contrast material did not penetrate the entire area of pancreatic inflammation.

In an uncontrolled study of 47 patients with necrotizing pancreatitis, Takeda and coworkers[246] used CRAI to infuse a protease inhibitor (nafamostat mesilate, 240 mg/day) and imipenem (0.5 g every 12 hr) for 5 days, starting within 7 days of hospital admission. Forty patients responded to CRAI therapy, and the mortality rate in these patients was 2.5%. Seven patients (14.9%) did not respond to CRAI. Five of seven nonresponders died of multiple organ failure, although pancreatic necrosis was persistently sterile. Even though these early results using CRAI are encouraging, double-blind randomized studies are needed to determine the benefit of this therapy.

In randomized studies, many other measures have been ineffective, including nasogastric decompression, histamine-$_2$ receptor antagonists, anticholinergics, glucagon, fresh-frozen plasma, and peritoneal lavage.[247–249]

COMPLICATIONS

Infection

Pancreatic infection is uncommon in interstitial pancreatitis,[226] but it may occur in 20% to 50% of patients with necrotizing pancreatitis.[212, 219, 221] Infection typically occurs within the first 2 weeks of illness.[218, 219] In comparison, pancreatic abscess following acute pancreatitis does not usually occur until after the first month of illness.[198] Pancreatic infection requires prompt surgical débridement. An abscess usually can be eradicated by percutaneous pigtail catheter drainage or by surgical drainage.[198]

Pancreatic Pseudocyst

A pseudocyst may occur secondary to acute pancreatitis, pancreatic trauma, or chronic pancreatitis (Chapter 49). It usually contains a high concentration of pancreatic enzymes and variable amounts of tissue debris. Most are sterile.

Regardless of size, an asymptomatic pseudocyst does not require treatment.[250, 251] It is satisfactory to monitor the pseudocyst with abdominal ultrasonography every 3 to 6 months. In two studies, there was no mortality among patients treated medically or surgically.[250, 251] New symptoms, such as abdominal pain, chills, or fever, should be reported immediately. Treatment choices include surgical, radiologic, and endoscopic methods. No randomized prospective trials compare these methods.

Surgical drainage of a pseudocyst is possible with a cystgastrostomy or cyst-duodenostomy (see Fig. 48–3) if the pseudocyst wall is broadly adherent to the stomach or duodenum. Other procedures include a Roux-en-Y cyst-jejunostomy or pancreatic resection if the pseudocyst is in the tail. Surgical mortality is 6% or less.[250–253] Pseudocyst recurrence after internal drainage occurs in 15% of cases and is more frequent if the main pancreatic duct is obstructed downstream from the surgical anastomosis. For this reason, a preoperative ERCP is usually done to determine whether there is duct obstruction. In this case, a resection of the pseudocyst is preferred.

Percutaneous catheter drainage is effective treatment to drain and close both sterile and infected pseudocysts.[152] As with surgical drainage, percutaneous catheter drainage may fail if there is obstruction of the main pancreatic duct downstream from the pseudocyst. Therefore, an ERCP is usually done before attempting catheter drainage. If contrast material enters the pseudocyst or if the main pancreatic duct fills completely without filling a pseudocyst, it is likely that catheter drainage will be successful.[253] For best results, the indwelling catheter is irrigated gently every 6 hours with sterile saline. Catheter drainage should be continued until the fluid output diminishes to 5 to 10 mL/day. If there is no reduction of flow, a CT scan should be obtained to be sure the catheter is in the pseudocyst. Fifty to 200 μg of octreotide subcutaneously every 8 hours may be beneficial.

Two endoscopic methods to decompress a pancreatic

pseudocyst are (1) an endoscopic cyst-gastrostomy or cyst-duodenostomy, or, (2) insertion of a stent through the ampulla directly into the pancreatic duct and then into the pseudocyst itself.[254–257] The former method is possible if the pseudocyst is broadly adherent to the wall of the stomach or duodenum. The endoscopist then inserts a double-pigtail stent through the hollow viscus into the cyst. Some endoscopists also insert a transpapillary pancreatic duct stent into the cyst. This is possible if ERCP shows continuity between the pseudocyst and the main pancreatic duct.[257] With either method, the catheter is removed after 3 to 4 weeks if closure of the pseudocyst is seen by CT scan. Failure of radiologic or endoscopic drainage of a pancreatic pseudocyst increases morbidity and prolongs hospitalization.[252]

There are several complications of endoscopic drainage of pseudocysts. The most important is bleeding; the risk of bleeding may be reduced if endoscopic ultrasonography is used to be certain that there are no large vessels in the drainage area. Infection may occur if the double-pigtail catheter becomes occluded. A nasocystic drain to irrigate the cyst may prevent this complication. An endoscopically placed stent in the pancreatic duct may induce ductal changes identical to those of chronic pancreatitis. For this reason, a stent should be removed after several weeks.

Pancreatic Pseudocyst Associated with Pancreatic Necrosis

If a pseudocyst accompanies considerable pancreatic necrosis, endoscopic and percutaneous catheter drainage should be used very cautiously because neither technique can evacuate the underlying particulate necrotic material, although both are successful in eliminating the fluid of the pseudocyst itself. If radiologic or endoscopic cyst drainage methods are used in this setting, it is important to provide ongoing irrigation either through the radiologically inserted catheter or through an endoscopically placed nasocystic catheter to continue the liquefaction of necrotic debris and prevent secondary infection.[258] In this situation, surgical drainage may be preferred because necrotic debris can be retrieved before completing the cyst-enteric anastomosis.

Pancreatic Abscess

A pancreatic abscess is a collection of pus near the pancreas which, on CT scan, is a poorly marginated, low-density mass that may contain diffuse air bubbles. The cause may be secondary liquefaction and secondary infection of an area of necrosis or infection of a pancreatic pseudocyst. Most pancreatic abscesses occur later than infected necrosis, at least 4 weeks after the onset of acute pancreatitis.[3, 152] Percutaneous catheter drainage and surgical drainage are effective treatments. In general, the mortality of a pancreatic abscess is less than that of infected necrosis.[198]

Systemic Complications

Central Nervous System

Pancreatic encephalopathy consists of a variety of central nervous system symptoms occurring in acute pancreatitis, including agitation, hallucinations, confusion, disorientation, and coma. A similar syndrome may be due to alcohol withdrawal, and other causes are possible, such as electrolyte disturbances (e.g., hyponatremia), hypoxia, or demyelination in the central nervous system secondary to high circulating concentrations of lipase.

Fat Necrosis

Fat necrosis occurs in subcutaneous tissue, bone, retroperitoneal tissue, peritoneum, mediastinum, pleura, and pericardium. Histologically fat cells are necrotic, associated with a diffuse inflammatory infiltration. The subcutaneous lesions are circumscribed, tender red nodules that are adherent to the skin but are moveable over deeper structures. Most commonly they are over the ankles, fingers, knees, and elbows. The lesions may drain through the skin. Rarely, there is also necrosis of adjacent tendons or involvement of joints, particularly the metatarsal, interphalangeal, wrist, knee, and ankle joints. The lesions usually resolve after days to weeks.

Gastrointestinal Bleeding

Gastrointestinal bleeding may arise secondary to stress gastropathy (acute erosive gastritis), lower esophageal or gastric varices associated with splenic vein thrombosis, or a pseudoaneurysm associated with a pancreatic pseudocyst. Splenectomy is the treatment of choice for bleeding gastric or esophageal varices. If nonbleeding varices are found, some also suggest a prophylactic splenectomy. However, a reasonable alternative is medical surveillance, reserving a splenectomy for only if the varices bleed. A pseudoaneurysm usually is well seen by dynamic contrast-enhanced CT; arteriography with embolization is the treatment of choice. Rarely, bleeding into the pancreatic duct occurs (hemosuccus pancreaticus), but this usually occurs in chronic pancreatitis caused by rupture of a splenic aneurysm. Significant coagulation abnormalities, such as disseminated intravascular coagulation, rarely occur in acute pancreatitis.

Splenic Complications

Occasionally, a pseudocyst of the tail of the pancreas or inflammation of the tail of the pancreas extends to the splenic hilum, causing a subcapsular hematoma. A small hematoma can be followed without surgery, but a large hematoma, or one causing symptoms, requires distal pancreatectomy and splenectomy.

PROGNOSIS

The mortality rate is 5% to 10% in hospitalized patients with acute pancreatitis. Some cases are not diagnosed until autopsy, so the mortality rate may be even higher. In several studies, autopsied cases represented 12% to 42% of all deaths.[2, 259] The mortality of interstitial pancreatitis, sterile necrotizing pancreatitis, and infected necrosis approximates 0%, 10%, and 30%, respectively.[224, 225] Mortality increases if there are unfavorable early prognostic signs, organ failure, and local complications, particularly pancreatic necrosis. Predictors of death include an increased serum creatinine level above 2 mg/dL and a chest radiograph showing either a pleural effusion or a pulmonary infiltrate within 24 hours of admission,[260] coma, older patients, and co-morbid disease. The great majority of deaths in acute pancreatitis occur during the first or second episode.[260] Etiology is also important; alcoholic and gallstone pancreatitis have mortality rates approximating 5%, whereas death is more frequent in idiopathic and postoperative pancreatitis.[230, 259]

REFERENCES

1. Go VLW, Everhart JE: Pancreatitis. In Everhart JE (ed): Digestive Diseases in the United States: Epidemiology and Impact. US Department of Health and Human Services, Public Health Service, National Institutes of Health, National Institute of Diabetes and Digestive and Kidney Diseases. NIH Publication no. 94–1447. Washington, DC, 1994, p 693.
2. Lankisch PG, Schirren CA, Kunze E: Undetected fatal acute pancreatitis: Why is the disease so frequently overlooked? Am J Gastroenterol 86:322, 1991.
3. Bradley EL 3rd: A clinically based classification system for acute pancreatitis. Arch Surg 128:586, 1993.
4. Büchler M, Hauke A, Malfertheiner P: Follow-up after acute pancreatitis—Morphology and function. In Beger HG, Büchler M (eds): Acute Pancreatitis; Research and Clinical Management. Berlin, Springer-Verlag, 1987, p 367.
5. Scuro AL, Angelini G, Cavallini G: Late outcome of acute pancreatitis. In Gyr K, Singer MV, Sarles H (eds): Pancreatitis: Concepts and Classifications. Proceedings of the Second International Symposium on Classification of Pancreatitis in Marseille, Paris, France, March 28–30, 1984. Excerpta Medica, 1984, p 403.
6. Sarles H: Definitions and classifications of pancreatitis. Pancreas 6: 470, 1991.
7. Klöppel G, Maillet B: Pathology of acute and chronic pancreatitis. Pancreas 8:659, 1993.
8. Steer ML: Pathogenesis of acute pancreatitis. Digestion 58(Suppl 1): 46, 1997.
9. Nakae Y, Naruse S, Kitagawa M, et al: Activation of trypsinogen in experimental models of acute pancreatitis in rats. Pancreas 10:306, 1995.
10. Bettinger JR, Grendell JH: Intracellular events in the pathogenesis of acute pancreatitis. Pancreas 6:S2, 1991.
11. Fernández-del Castillo C, Schmidt J, Warshaw AL, et al: Interstitial protease activation is the central event in progression to necrotizing pancreatitis. Surgery 116:497, 1994.
12. Steer ML: How and where does acute pancreatitis begin? Arch Surg 127:1350, 1992.
13. Lerch MM, Adler G: Experimental animal models of acute pancreatitis. Int J Pancreatol 15:159, 1994.
14. Grady T, Saluja A, Kaiser A, et al: Pancreatic edema and intrapancreatic activation of trypsinogen during secretagogue-induced pancreatitis precedes glutathione depletion. Am J Physiol 271:G20, 1996.
15. Saluja AK, Donovan EA, Yamanaka K, et al: Cerulein-induced in vitro activation of trypsinogen in rat pancreatic acini is mediated by cathepsin B. Gastroenterology 113:304, 1997.
16. Lüthen R, Niederau C, Niederau M, et al: Influence of ductal pressure and infusates on activity and subcellular distribution of lysosomal enzymes in the rat pancreas. Gastroenterology 109:573, 1995.
17. Fallon MB, Gorelick FS, Anderson JM, et al: Effect of cerulein hyperstimulation on the paracellular barrier of rat exocrine pancreas. Gastroenterology 108:1863, 1995.
18. LeBodic LL, Bignon JD, Raguenes O, et al: The hereditary pancreatitis gene maps to long arm of chromosome 7. Hum Mol Genet 5:549, 1996.
19. Whitcomb C, Preston RA, Aston CE, et al: A gene for hereditary pancreatitis maps to chromosome 7q35. Gastroenterology 110:1975, 1996.
20. Whitcomb DC, Gorry MC, Preston RA, et al: Hereditary pancreatitis is caused by a mutation in the cationic trypsinogen gene. Nat Genet 14:141, 1996.
21. Gorry MC, Gabbaizedeh D, Furey W, et al: Mutations in the cationic trypsinogen gene are associated with recurrent acute and chronic pancreatitis. Gastroenterology 113:1063, 1997.
22. Cohn JA, Friedman KJ, Noone PG, et al: Relation between mutations of the cystic fibrosis gene and idiopathic pancreatitis. N Engl J Med 339:653, 1998.
23. Sharer N, Scharz M, Malone G, et al: Mutations of the cystic fibrosis gene in patients with chronic pancreatitis. N Engl J Med 339:645, 1998.
24. Choudari CP, Yu AC, Imperiale TF, et al: Significance of heterozygous cystic fibrosis gene (cystic fibrosis transmembrane conductance regulator mutations) in idiopathic pancreatitis [abstract]. Gastroenterology 114:A447, 1998.
25. Choudari CP, Stewart T, Crabb D, et al: Yield of genetic testing in pancreatic disease as we know it in 1997 [abstract]. Gastroenterology 114:A447, 1998.
26. Castellani C, Sgarb D, Cavallini G, et al: CFTR mutations and IV658–57 prevalence in chronic and acute idiopathic pancreatitis [abstract]. Gastroenterology 114:A445, 1998.
27. Lerch MM, Saluja AK, Rünzi M, et al: Pancreatic duct obstruction triggers acute necrotizing pancreatitis in the opossum. Gastroenterology 104:853, 1993.
28. Opie EL: The etiology of acute hemorrhagic pancreatitis. Bull Johns Hopkins Hosp 12:182, 1901.
29. Rünzi M, Saluja A, Lerch MM, et al: Early ductal decompression prevents the progression of biliary pancreatitis: An experimental study in the opossum. Gastroenterology 105:157, 1993.
30. Lüthen RE, Niederau C, Grendell JH: Effects of bile and pancreatic digestive enzymes on permeability of the pancreatic duct systems in rabbits. Pancreas 8:671, 1993.
31. Prinz RA: Mechanisms of acute pancreatitis: Vascular etiology. Int J Pancreatol 9:31, 1991.
32. Klar E, Messmer K, Warshaw AL, et al: Pancreatic ischemia in experimental acute pancreatitis: Mechanism, significance, and therapy. Br J Surg 77:1205, 1990.
33. Toyama MT, Lewis MP, Kusske AM, et al: Ischaemia-reperfusion mechanisms in acute pancreatitis. Scand J Gastroenterol 31(Suppl 219):20, 1996.
34. Rinderknecht H: Fatal pancreatitis, a consequence of excessive leukocyte stimulation? Int J Pancreatol 3:105, 1988.
35. Kingsnorth A: Role of cytokines and their inhibitors in acute pancreatitis. Gut 40:1, 1997.
36. Sweiry JH, Mann GE: Role of oxidative stress in the pathogenesis of acute pancreatitis. Scand J Gastroenterol 31(Suppl 219):10, 1996.
37. Schmid SW, Uhl W, Friess H, et al: The role of infection in acute pancreatitis. Gut 45:311, 1999.
38. Andersson R, Wang XD: Gut barrier dysfunction in experimental acute pancreatitis. Ann Acad Med Singapore 28:141, 1999.
39. Kazantsev GB, Hecht DW, Rao R, et al: Plasmid labeling confirms bacterial translocation in pancreatitis. Am J Surg 167:201, 1994.
40. Agarwal N, Pitchumoni CS: Acute pancreatitis: A multisystem disease. Gastroenterology 1:115, 1993.
41. Tenner S, Sica G, Hughes M, et al: Relationship of necrosis to organ failure in severe acute pancreatitis. Gastroenterology 113:899, 1997.
42. Moreau JA, Zinsmeister AR, Melton LJ, et al: Gallstone pancreatitis and the effect of cholecystectomy. Mayo Clin Proc 63:466, 1988.
43. Diehl AK, Holleman Jr DR, Chapman JB, et al: Gallstone size and risk of pancreatitis. Arch Intern Med 157:1674, 1997.
44. Ko CW, Sekijima JH, Lee SP: Biliary sludge. Ann Intern Med 130: 301, 1999.
45. Ros E, Navarro S, Bru C, et al: Occult microlithiasis in "idiopathic" acute pancreatitis: Prevention of relapses by cholecystectomy or ursodeoxycholic acid therapy. Gastroenterology 101:1701, 1991.
46. Lopez AJ, O'Keefe P, Morrissey M, et al: Ceftriaxone-induced cholelithiasis. Ann Intern Med 115:712, 1991.
47. Ettestad PJ, Campbell GL, Welbel SF, et al: Biliary complications in the treatment of unsubstantiated Lyme disease. J Infect Dis 171:356, 1995.
48. Lee SP, Nichols JF, Park HZ: Biliary sludge as a cause of acute pancreatitis. N Engl J Med 326:589, 1992.
49. Khuroo MS, Zargar SA, Mahajan R: Hepatobiliary and pancreatic ascariasis in India. Lancet 335:1503, 1990.
50. Uomo G, Manes G, Ragozzino A, et al: Periampullary extraluminal duodenal diverticula and acute pancreatitis: An underestimated etiological association. Am J Gastroenterol 91:1186, 1996.

51. Koehler H, Lankisch PG: Acute pancreatitis and hyperamylasemia in pancreatic carcinoma. Pancreas 2:117, 1987.
52. Ammann RW, Heitz PU, Kloeppel G: Course of alcoholic chronic pancreatitis: A prospective clinicomorphological long-term study. Gastroenterology 111:224, 1996.
53. Hanck C, Singer MV: Does acute alcoholic pancreatitis exist without preexisting chronic pancreatitis? Scand J Gastroenterol 32:625, 1997.
54. Apte MV, Wilson JS, McCaughan GW, et al: Ethanol-induced alterations in messenger RNA levels correlated with glandular content of pancreatic enzymes. J Lab Clin Med 125:634, 1995.
55. Korsten MA, Haber PS, Wilson JS, et al: The effect of chronic alcohol administration on cerulein-induced pancreatitis. Int J Pancreatol 18:25, 1995.
56. Foitzik T, Fernández-del Castillo C, Rattner DW, et al: Alcohol selectively impairs oxygenation of the pancreas. Arch Surg 130:357, 1995.
57. Fortson MR, Freedman SN, Webster PD 3rd: Clinical assessment of hyperlipidemic pancreatitis. Am J Gastroenterol 90:2134, 1995.
58. Toskes PP: Hyperlipidemic pancreatitis. Gastroenterol Clin North Am 19:783, 1990.
59. Krauss RM, Levy AG: Subclinical chronic pancreatitis in type I hyperlipoproteinemia. Am J Med 62:144, 1977.
60. Salen S, Kessler JI, Janowitz HD: The development of pancreatic secretory insufficiency in a patient with recurrent pancreatitis and type V hyperlipoproteinemia. Mt Sinai J Med 37:103, 1970.
61. Glueck CJ, Lang J, Hamer T, et al: Severe hypertriglyceridemia and pancreatitis when estrogen replacement therapy is given to hypertriglyceridemic women. J Lab Clin Med 123:18, 1994.
62. Hozumi Y, Kawano M, Saito T, et al: Effect of tamoxifen on serum lipid metabolism. J Clin Endocrinol Metab 83:1633, 1998.
63. Toskes PP: Is there a relationship between hypertriglyceridemia and development of alcohol- or gallstone-induced pancreatitis? Gastroenterology 106:810, 1994.
64. Haber PS, Wilson JS, Apte MV, et al: Lipid intolerance does not account for susceptibility to alcoholic and gallstone pancreatitis. Gastroenterology 106:742, 1994.
65. Whitfield JB, Hensley WJ, Bryden D, et al: Some laboratory correlates of drinking habit. Ann Clin Biochem 15:297, 1978.
66. Brandwein SL, Sigman KM: Milk-alkali syndrome and pancreatitis. Am J Med Sci 308:173, 1994.
67. Mithofer K, Fernandez-del Castillo C, Frick TW: Acute hypercalcemia causes acute pancreatitis and ectopic trypsinogen activation in the rat. Gastroenterology 109:23, 1995.
68. Ward JB, Petersen OH, Jenkins SA, et al: Is an elevated concentration of acinar cytosolic free ionised calcium the trigger for acute pancreatitis? Lancet 346:1016, 1995.
69. Bess MA, Edis AJ, van Heerden JA: Hyperparathyroidism and pancreatitis: Chance or causal association? JAMA 243:246, 1980.
70. Prinz RA, Aranha GV: The association of primary hyperparathyroidism and pancreatitis. Am Surg 51:325, 1985.
71. Shearer MG, Imrie CW: Parathyroid hormone levels, hyperparathyroidism, and pancreatitis. Br J Surg 73:282, 1986.
72. Fernández-del Castillo C, Harringer W, Warshaw AL, et al: Risk factors for pancreatic cellular injury after cardiopulmonary bypass. N Engl J Med 325:382, 1991.
73. Ruenzi M, Layer P: Drug-associated pancreatitis: Facts and fiction. Pancreas 13:100, 1996.
74. Milminick T, Frick TW: Drug-induced pancreatitis. Drug Saf 14:406, 1996.
75. McArthur KE: Review article: Drug-induced pancreatitis. Aliment Pharmacol Ther 10:23, 1996.
76. Lankisch PG, Droege M, Gottesleben F: Drug-induced acute pancreatitis: Incidence and severity. Gut 37:565, 1995.
77. Werth B, Kuhn MK, Reinhart WH: Medikamentoes induzierte Pankreatiden: Erfahrungen der Scweizerischen Arzneimittel-Nebenswirkungenszentrale (SANZ) 1981–1993. Schweiz Med Wochenschr 125:731, 1995.
78. Mallory A, Kern F Jr: Drug-induced pancreatitis: A critical review. Gastroenterology 78:813, 1980.
79. Parenti DM, Steinberg W, King P: Infectious causes of pancreatitis. Pancreas 13:356, 1996.
80. Mourad FH, McLean A, Farthing MJG: Tuberculous pancreatitis: A diagnostic problem. J Clin Gastroenterol 20:237, 1995.
81. Chung RT, Schapiro RH, Warshaw AL: Intraluminal pancreatic candidiasis presenting as recurrent pancreatitis. Gastroenterology 104:1532, 1993.
82. Cappell MS, Hassan T: Pancreatic disease in AIDS—A review. J Clin Gastroenterol 17:254, 1993.
83. de Diego Lorenzo A, Robles Fornieles J, Herrero López T, et al: Acute pancreatitis associated with milk allergy. Int J Pancreatol 12: 319, 1992.
84. Wilson RH, Moorehead RJ: Current management of trauma to the pancreas. Br J Surg 78:1196, 1991.
85. Kozarek RA, Ball TJ, Patterson DJ, et al: Endoscopic transpapillary therapy for disrupted pancreatic duct and peripancreatic fluid collections. Gastroenterology 100:1362, 1991.
86. Nwariaku FE, Terracina A, Mileski WJ, et al: Is octreotide beneficial following pancreatic injury? Am J Surg 170:582, 1995.
87. Madiba TE, Mokoena TR: Favourable prognosis after surgical drainage of gunshot, stab, or blunt trauma of the pancreas. Br J Surg 82: 1236, 1995.
88. Degiannis E, Levy RD, Potokar T, et al: Distal pancreatectomy for gunshot injuries of the distal pancreas. Br J Surg 82:1240, 1995.
89. Delhaye M, Engelholm L, Cremer M: Pancreas divisum: Congenital anatomy or anomaly? Contribution of endoscopic retrograde cholangiopancreatography. Gastroenterology 89:951, 1985.
90. Warshaw AL, Simeone JF, Schapiro RH, et al: Evaluation and treatment of the dominant dorsal duct syndrome (pancreas divisum redefined). Am J Surg 159:59, 1990.
91. Lehman GA, Sherman S, Nisi R, et al: Pancreas divisum: Results of minor papilla sphincterotomy. Gastrointest Endosc 39:1, 1993.
92. Lans JI, Geenen JE, Johanson JF, et al: Pancreas divisum: To stent or not to stent. Gastrointest Endosc 38:430, 1992.
93. Lehman GA, Sherman S: Pancreas divisum. Diagnosis, clinical significance, and management alternatives. Gastrointest Endosc Clin North Am 5:145, 1995.
94. Sherman S, Hawes RH, Savides TJ, et al: Stent-induced pancreatic ductal and parenchymal changes: Correlation of endoscopic ultrasound and ERCP. Gastrointest Endosc 44:276, 1996.
95. Smith MT, Sherman S, Ikenberry SO, et al: Alterations in pancreatic ductal morphology following polyethylene pancreatic stent therapy. Gastrointest Endosc 44:268, 1996.
96. Takasaki M, Yorimitsu Y, Takahashi I, et al: Systemic lupus erythematosus presenting with drug-unrelated acute pancreatitis as an initial manifestation. Am J Gastroenterol 90:1172, 1995.
97. Watts RA, Isenberg DA: Pancreatic disease in the autoimmune rheumatic disorders. Semin Arthritis Rheum 19:158, 1989.
98. Molenaar W, Lamers CB: Cholesterol crystal embolization to liver, gallbladder, and pancreas. Dig Dis Sci 41:1819, 1996.
99. Orvar K, Johlin FC: Atheromatous embolization resulting in acute pancreatitis after cardiac catheterization and angiographic studies. Arch Intern Med 154:1755, 1994.
100. Warshaw AL, O Hara PJ: Susceptibility of the pancreas to ischemic injury in shock. Ann Surg 188:197, 1978.
101. Reilly PM, Toung TJ, Miyachi M, et al: Hemodynamics of pancreatic ischemia in cardiogenic shock in pigs. Gastroenterology 113:938, 1997.
102. Maringhini A, Lankisch MR, Zinsmeister AR, et al: Acute pancreatitis in the postpartum period: A population-based case-control study. Mayo Clin Proc 75:361, 2000.
103. Jouppila P, Mokka R, Larmi TK: Acute pancreatitis in pregnancy. Surg Gynecol Obstet 139:879, 1974.
104. Roberts IM: Gestational hyperlipidemic pancreatitis. Gastroenterology 104:1560, 1993.
105. Legro RS, Laifer SA: First trimester pancreatitis: Maternal and neonatal outcome. J Reprod Med 40:689, 1995.
106. Swisher SG, Hunt KK, Schmit PJ, et al: Management of pancreatitis complicating pregnancy. Am Surg 60:759, 1994.
107. Amouyal P, Amouyal G, Levy P, et al: Diagnosis of choledocholithiasis by endoscopic ultrasonography. Gastroenterology 106:1062, 1994.
108. Aliperti G: Complications related to diagnostic and therapeutic endoscopic retrograde cholangiopancreatography. Gastrointest Endosc Clin North Am 6:379, 1996.
109. Chen YK, Foliente RL, Santoro MJ, et al: Endoscopic sphincterotomy-induced pancreatitis: Increased risk associated with nondilated bile ducts and sphincter of Oddi dysfunction. Am J Gastroenterol 89: 327, 1994.
110. Chen HY, Abdulian JD, Escalante-Glorsky S, et al: Clinical outcome of post-ERCP pancreatitis: Relationship to history of previous pancreatitis. Am J Gastroenterol 90:2120, 1995.

111. Johnson GK, Geenen JE, Bedford RA, et al: A comparison of nonionic versus ionic contrast media: Results of a prospective, multicenter study. Gastrointest Endosc 42:312, 1995.
112. Camargo CA, Greig PD, Levy GA, et al: Acute pancreatitis following liver transplantation. J Am Coll Surg 181:249, 1995.
113. Comfort MW, Steinberg AG: Pedigree of a family with hereditary chronic relapsing pancreatitis. Gastroenterology 21:54, 1952.
114. Konzen KM, Perrault J, Moir C, et al: Long-term follow-up of young patients with chronic hereditary or idiopathic pancreatitis. Mayo Clin Proc 68:449, 1993.
115. Layer P, Yamamoto H, Kalthoff L, et al: The different courses of early and late onset idiopathic and alcoholic chronic pancreatitis. Gastroenterology 107:1481, 1994.
116. Lowenfels AB, Maisonneuve P, DiMagno EP, et al: Hereditary pancreatitis and the risk of pancreatic cancer. J Natl Cancer Inst 89:442, 1997.
117. Urayama S, Kozarek R, Ball T, et al: Presentation and treatment of annular pancreas in an adult population. Am J Gastroenterol 90:995, 1995.
118. Gschwantler M, Kogelbauer G, Klose W, et al: The pancreas as a site of granulomatous inflammation in Crohn's disease. Gastroenterology 108:1246, 1995.
119. Swisher SG, Cates JA, Hunt KK, et al: Pancreatitis associated with adult choledochal cysts. Pancreas 9:633, 1994.
120. Novis BH, Bornman PC, Girdwood AW, et al: Endoscopic manometry of the pancreatic duct and sphincter zone in patients with chronic pancreatitis. Dig Dis Sci 30:225, 1985.
121. Tarnasky PR, Hofman B, Aabakken L, et al: Sphincter of Oddi dysfunction is associated with chronic pancreatitis. Am J Gastroenterol 92:1125, 1997.
122. Raddawi HM, Geenen JE, Hogan WJ, et al: Pressure measurements from biliary and pancreatic segments of sphincter of Oddi. Dig Dis Sci 36:71, 1991.
123. Soffer EE, Johlin FC: Intestinal dysmotility in patients with sphincter of Oddi dysfunction. A reason for failed response to sphincterotomy. Dig Dis Sci 39:1942, 1994.
124. Desautels SG, Slivka A, Hutson WR, et al: Postcholecystectomy pain syndrome: Pathophysiology of abdominal pain in sphincter of Oddi type III. Gastroenterology 116:900, 1999.
125. Heller SJ, Ferrari AP, Carr-Locke DL, et al: Pancreatic duct stricture caused by islet cell tumors. Am J Gastroenterol 91:147, 1996.
126. Loftus EV Jr, Olivares-Pakzad BA, Batts KP, et al: Intraductal papillary-mucinous tumors of the pancreas—clinicopathologic features, outcome, and nomenclature. Gastroenterology 110:1909, 1996.
127. Ryan CM, Sheridan RL, Schoenfeld DA, et al: Postburn pancreatitis. Ann Surg 222:163, 1995.
128. Ertan A, Schneider FE: Acute pancreatitis in long-distance runners. Am J Gastroenterol 90:70, 1995.
129. Ballinger AB, Barnes E, Alstead EM, et al: Is intervention necessary after first episode of idiopathic acute pancreatitis? Gut 38:293, 1996.
130. Steinberg WM, Geenen JE, Bradley EL 3rd, et al: Controversies in clinical pancreatology. Recurrent "idiopathic" acute pancreatitis: Should a laparoscopic cholecystectomy be the first procedure of choice? Pancreas 13:329, 1996.
131. Sternby B, O'Brien JF, Zinsmeister AR, et al: What is the best biochemical test to diagnose acute pancreatitis? A prospective clinical study. Mayo Clin Proc 71:1138, 1996.
132. Seno T, Harada H, Ochi K, et al: Serum levels of six pancreatic enzymes as related to the degree of renal dysfunction. Am J Gastroenterol 90:2002, 1995.
133. Gumaste VV, Roditis N, Mehta D, et al: Serum lipase levels in nonpancreatic abdominal pain versus acute pancreatitis. Am J Gastroenterol 88:2051, 1993.
134. Sachdeva CK, Bank S, Greenberg R, et al: Fluctuations in serum amylase in patients with macroamylasemia. Am J Gastroenterol 90: 800, 1995.
135. Mishler JM, Durr GH: Macroamylasemia induced by hydroxyethyl starch—confirmation by gel filtration analysis of serum and urine. Am J Clin Pathol 74:387, 1980.
136. Johnson SG, Ellis CJ, Levitt MD: Mechanism of increased renal clearance of amylase/creatinine in acute pancreatitis. N Engl J Med 295:1214, 1976.
137. Tietz NW, Shuey DF: Lipase in serum—the elusive enzyme: An overview. Clin Chem 39:746, 1993.
138. Lessinger JM, Ferard G: Plasma pancreatic lipase activity: From analytical specificity to clinical efficiency for the diagnosis of acute pancreatitis. Eur J Clin Chem Clin Biochem 32:377, 1994.
139. Agarwal N, Pitchumoni CS, Sivaprasad AV: Evaluating tests for acute pancreatitis. Am J Gastroenterol 85:356, 1990.
140. Gwodz GP, Steinberg WM, Werner M, et al: Comparative evaluation of the diagnosis of acute pancreatitis based on serum and urine enzyme assays. Clin Chim Acta 187:243, 1990.
141. Werner M, Steinberg WM, Pauley C: Strategic use of individual and combined enzyme indicators for acute pancreatitis analyzed by receiver-operator characteristics. Clin Chem 35:967, 1989.
142. Keim V, Teich J, Fiedler F, et al: A comparison of lipase and amylase in the diagnosis of acute pancreatitis in patients with abdominal pain. Pancreas 16:45, 1998.
143. Kemppainen E, Hedstrom J, Puolakkainen P, et al: Increased serum trypsinogen-2 and trypsin 2-alpha-$_1$-antitrypsin complex values identify endoscopic retrograde cholangiopancreatography–induced pancreatitis with high accuracy. Gut 41:690, 1997.
144. Kemppainen E, Hedstrom J, Puolakkainen P, et al: Urinary trypsinogen-2 test strip in detecting ERCP-induced pancreatitis. Endoscopy 29: 247, 1997.
145. Iovanna JL, Keim V, Nordback I, et al: Serum levels of pancreatitis-associated protein as indicators of the course of acute pancreatitis. Gastroenterology 106:728, 1994.
146. Pezzilli R, Billi P, Migliori M, et al: Clinical value of pancreatitis-associated protein in acute pancreatitis. Am J Gastroenterol 92:1887, 1997.
147. Tenner S, Fernandez-del Castillo C, Warshaw A, et al: Urinary trypsinogen activation peptide (TAP) predicts severity in patients with acute pancreatitis. Int J Pancreatol 21:105, 1997.
148. Lankisch PG, Dröge M, Becher R: Pleural effusions: A new negative prognostic parameter for acute pancreatitis. Am J Gastroenterol 89: 1849, 1994.
149. Ranson JH, Turner JW, Roses DF, et al: Respiratory complications in acute pancreatitis. Ann Surg 179:557, 1974.
150. Neoptolemos JP, London NJ, James D, et al: Controlled trial of urgent endoscopic retrograde cholangiopancreatography and endoscopic sphincterotomy versus conservative treatment for acute pancreatitis due to gallstones. Lancet 2:979, 1988.
151. Fan S-T, Lai ECS, Mok FPT, et al: Early treatment of acute biliary pancreatitis by endoscopic papillotomy. N Engl J Med 328:228, 1993.
152. Balthazar EJ, Freeny PC, vanSonnenberg E: Imaging and intervention in acute pancreatitis. Radiology 193:297, 1994.
153. Freeny PC: Incremental dynamic bolus computed tomography of acute pancreatitis. Int J Pancreatol 13:147, 1993.
154. Schmidt J, Hotz HG, Foitzik T, et al: Intravenous contrast medium aggravates the impairment of pancreatic microcirculation in necrotizing pancreatitis in the rat. Ann Surg 221:257, 1995.
155. Johnson CD, Stephens DH, Sarr MG: CT of acute pancreatitis: Correlation between lack of contrast enhancement and pancreatic necrosis. Am J Radiol 156:93, 1991.
156. Balthazar EJ, Robinson DL, Megibow AJ, et al: Acute pancreatitis: Value of CT in establishing prognosis. Radiology 174:331, 1990.
157. Balthazar EJ, Freeny PC: Contrast-enhanced computed tomography in acute pancreatitis: Is it beneficial or harmful [Editorial]? Gastroenterology 106:259, 1994.
158. Angelini G, Cavallini G, Pederzoli P, et al: Long-term outcome of acute pancreatitis: A prospective study with 118 patients. Digestion 54:143, 1993.
159. Lankisch PG, Haseloff M, Becher R: No parallel between the biochemical course of acute pancreatitis and morphologic findings. Pancreas 9:240, 1994.
160. Balthazar EJ, Ranson JH, Naidich DP, et al: Acute pancreatitis: Prognostic value of CT. Radiology 156:767, 1985.
161. Werner J, Schmidt J, Warshaw AL, et al: The relative safety of MRI contrast agent in acute necrotizing pancreatitis. Ann Surg 227:105, 1998.
162. Neoptolemos JP, London NJM, Carr-Locke DL: Assessment of main pancreatic duct integrity by endoscopic retrograde pancreatography in patients with acute pancreatitis. Br J Surg 80:94, 1993.
163. Ranson JH: The timing of biliary surgery in acute pancreatitis. Ann Surg 189:654, 1979.
164. Paloyan D, Simonowitz D, Skinner DB: The timing of biliary tract operations in patients with pancreatitis associated with gallstones. Surg Gynecol Obstet 141:737, 1975.
165. Tenner S, Dubner H, Steinberg W: Predicting gallstone pancreatitis

with laboratory parameters. A meta-analysis. Am J Gastroenterol 89: 1863, 1994.
166. Gumaste VV, Dave PB, Weissman D, et al: Lipase/amylase ratio. A new index that distinguishes acute episodes of alcoholic from nonalcoholic acute pancreatitis. Gastroenterology 101:1361, 1991.
167. Tenner SM, Steinberg W: The admission serum lipase: amylase ratio differentiates alcoholic from nonalcoholic acute pancreatitis. Am J Gastroenterol 87:1755, 1992.
168. Jaakkola M, Sillanaukee P, Lof K, et al: Blood tests for detection of alcoholic cause of acute pancreatitis. Lancet 343:1328, 1994.
169. King LG, Seelig CB, Ranney JE: The lipase to amylase ratio in acute pancreatitis. Am J Gastroenterol 90:67, 1995.
170. Stimac D, Lenac T, Marusic Z: A scoring system for early differentiation of the etiology of acute pancreatitis. Scand J Gastroenterol 33: 209, 1998.
171. Aubertin JM, Levoir D, Bouillot JL, et al: Endoscopic ultrasonography immediately prior to laparoscopic cholecystectomy: A prospective evaluation. Endoscopy 28:667, 1996.
172. Rhodes M, Sussman L, Cohen L, et al: Randomised trial of laparoscopic exploration of common bile duct versus postoperative endoscopic retrograde cholangiopathy for common bile duct stones. Lancet 351:159, 1998.
173. McKay C, Beastall GH, Imrie CW, et al: Circulating intact parathyroid hormone levels in acute pancreatitis. Br J Surg 81:357, 1994.
174. Corfield AP, Cooper MJ, Williamson RC, et al: Prediction of severity in acute pancreatitis: Prospective comparison of three prognostic indices. Lancet 2:403, 1985.
175. Larvin M, McMahon MJ: Apache-II score for assessment and monitoring of acute pancreatitis. Lancet 2:201, 1989.
176. Wilson C, Health DI, Imrie CW: Prediction of outcome in acute pancreatitis: A comparative study of APACHE-II, clinical assessment and multiple factor scoring system. Br J Surg 77:1260, 1990.
177. Ranson JH, Rifkind KM, Roses DF, et al: Prognostic signs and the role of operative management in acute pancreatitis. Surg Gynecol Obstet 139:69, 1974.
178. Bank S, Wise L, Gersten M: Risk factors in acute pancreatitis. Am J Gastroenterol 78:637, 1983.
179. Agarwal N, Pitchumoni CS: Simplified prognostic criteria in acute pancreatitis. Pancreas 1:69, 1986.
180. Fan S-T, Lai ECS, Mok FPT, et al: Prediction of the severity of acute pancreatitis. Am J Surg 166:262, 1993.
181. Malfertheiner P, Dominguez-Munoz JE: Prognostic factors in acute pancreatitis. Int J Pancreatol 14:1, 1993.
182. Karimgani I, Porter KA, Langevin RE, et al: Prognostic factors in sterile pancreatic necrosis. Gastroenterology 103:1636, 1992.
183. Dominguez-Munoz JE, Carballo F, García MJ, et al: Evaluation of the clinical usefulness of APACHE-II and SAPS systems in the initial prognostic classification of acute pancreatitis: A multicenter study. Pancreas 8:682, 1993.
184. Leese T, Shaw D, Holliday M: Prognostic markers in acute pancreatitis: Can pancreatic necrosis be predicted? Ann R Coll Surg Engl 70: 227, 1988.
185. Heath DI, Cruickshank A, Gudgeon AM, et al: The relationship between pancreatic enzyme release and activation and the acute-phase protein response in patients with acute pancreatitis. Pancreas 10:347, 1995.
186. Pezzilli R, Billi P, Miniero R, et al: Serum interleukin-6, interleukin-8, and beta 2-microglobulin in early assessment of severity of acute pancreatitis. Dig Dis Sci 40:2341, 1995.
187. Gross V, Schölmerich J, Leser H-G, et al: Granulocyte elastase in assessment of severity of acute pancreatitis. Dig Dis Sci 35:97, 1990.
188. Gudgeon AM, Heath DI, Hurley P, et al: Trypsinogen activation peptides assay in the early prediction of severity of acute pancreatitis. Lancet 335:4, 1990.
189. Büchler M, Malfertheiner P, Schoetensack C, et al: Sensitivity of antiproteases, complement factors and C-reactive protein in detecting pancreatic necrosis. Results of a prospective clinical study. Int J Pancreatol 1:227, 1986.
190. Wilson C, Heads A, Shenkin A, et al: C-reactive protein, antiproteases and complement factors as objective markers of severity in acute pancreatitis. Br J Surg 76:177, 1989.
191. Dominguez-Munoz JE, Carballo F, Garcia MJ, et al: Monitoring of serum proteinase-antiproteinase balance and systemic inflammatory response in prognostic evaluation of acute pancreatitis. Dig Dis Sci 38: 507, 1993.
192. Bergenfeldt M, Berling R, Ohlsson K: Levels of leukocyte proteases in plasma and peritoneal exudate in severe, acute pancreatitis. Scand J Gastroenterol 29:371, 1994.
193. Neoptolemos JP, Kemppainen EA, Mayer JM, et al: Early prediction of severity in acute pancreatitis by urinary trypsinogen activation peptide: A multicentre study. Lancet 355:1955, 2000.
194. Block S, Mayer W, Bittner R, et al: Identification of pancreatic necrosis in severe acute pancreatitis: Imaging procedures versus clinical staging. Gut 27:1035, 1986.
195. Porter KA, Banks PA: Obesity as a predictor of severity in acute pancreatitis. Int J Pancreatol 10:247, 1991.
196. Funnell IC, Bornman PC, Weakley SP, et al: Obesity: An important prognostic factor in acute pancreatitis. Br J Surg 80:484, 1993.
197. Vesentini S, Bassi C, Talamini G, et al: Prospective comparison of C-reactive protein level, Ranson score and contrast-enhanced computed tomography in the prediction of septic complications of acute pancreatitis. Br J Surg 80:755, 1993.
198. Fedorak IJ, Ko TC, Djuricin G, et al: Secondary pancreatic infections: Are they distinct clinical entities? Surgery 112:824, 1992.
199. Mathieson DR, Gross JB, Power MH: Elevated values for serum amylase and lipase following the administration of opiates, a preliminary report. Mayo Clin Proc 26:81, 1951.
200. Sarr MG, Sanfey H, Cameron JL: Prospective, randomized trial of nasogastric suction in patients with acute pancreatitis. Surgery 100: 500, 1986.
201. Steinberg W, Tenner S: Acute pancreatitis. N Engl J Med 330:1198, 1994.
202. Regan PT, Malagelada J-R, Go VLW, et al: A prospective study of the antisecretory and therapeutic effects of cimetidine and glucagon in human acute pancreatitis. Mayo Clin Proc 56:499, 1981.
203. Hotz HG, Schmidt J, Ryschich EW, et al: Isovolemic hemodilution with dextran prevents contrast medium–induced impairment of pancreatic microcirculation in necrotizing pancreatitis of the rat. Am J Surg 169:161, 1995.
204. Klar E, Foitzik T, Buhr H, et al: Isovolemic hemodilution with dextran 60 as treatment of pancreatic ischemia in acute pancreatitis. Ann Surg 217:369, 1993.
205. Widdison AL, Karanjia ND: Pancreatic infection complicating acute pancreatitis. Br J Surg 80:148, 1993.
206. Beger HG, Bittner R, Block S, et al: Bacterial contamination of pancreatic necrosis. A prospective clinical study. Gastroenterology 91: 433, 1986.
207. Bradley EL 3rd, Allen K: A prospective longitudinal study of observation versus surgical intervention in the management of necrotizing pancreatitis. Am J Surg 161:19, 1991.
208. Grewe M, Tsiotos GG, Luque de-Leon E, et al: Fungal infection in acute necrotizing pancreatitis. J Am Coll Surg 188:408, 1999.
209. Luiten EJ, Hop WC, Lange JF, et al: Differential prognosis of gram-negative versus gram-positive infected and sterile pancreatic necrosis: Results of a randomized trial in patients with severe acute pancreatitis treated with adjuvant selective decontamination. Clin Infect Dis 25: 811, 1997.
210. Luiten EJ, Hop WC, Lange JF, et al: Controlled clinical trial of selective decontamination for the treatment of severe acute pancreatitis. Ann Surg 222:57, 1995.
211. Sanio V, Kemppainen E, Puolakkainen P, et al: Early antibiotic treatment in acute necrotizing pancreatitis. Lancet 346:663, 1995.
212. Pederzoli P, Bassi S, Vesentini S, et al: A randomized multicenter clinical trial of antibiotic prophylaxis of septic complications in acute necrotizing pancreatitis with imipenem. Surg Gynecol Obstet 176:480, 1993.
213. Delcenseire R, Yzet T, Ducroix JP: Prophylactic antibiotics in treatment of severe acute alcoholic pancreatitis. Pancreas 13:198, 1996.
214. Bassi C, Falconi M, Talamini G, et al: Controlled clinical trial of pefloxacin versus imipenem in severe acute pancreatitis. Gastroenterology 115:1513, 1998.
215. Golub R, Siddiqi F, Pohl D: Role of antibiotics in acute pancreatitis: A meta-analysis. J Gastrointest Surg 2:496, 1998.
216. Büchler M, Malfertheiner P, Friess H, et al: Human pancreatic tissue concentration of bactericidal antibiotics. Gastroenterology 103:1902, 1992.
217. Gloor B, Muller CA, Worni M, et al: Pancreatic infection in severe pancreatitis: The role of fungus and multiresistant organisms. Arch Surg 136(5):592, 2001.
218. Gerzof SG, Banks PA, Robbins AH, et al: Early diagnosis of pancre-

atic infection by computed tomography–guided aspiration. Gastroenterology 93:1315, 1987.
219. Banks PA, Gerzof SG, Langevin RE, et al: CT-guided aspiration of suspected pancreatic infection. Int J Pancreatol 18:265, 1995.
220. Banks PA, Gerzof SG, Chong FK, et al: Bacteriologic status of necrotic tissue in necrotizing pancreatitis. Pancreas 5:330, 1990.
221. Bassi C: Infected pancreatic necrosis. Int J Pancreatol 16:1, 1994.
222. Bradley EL 3rd: Necrosectomy in acute pancreatitis. J Hepat Biliary Pancreas Surg 2:152, 1994.
223. Frey CF: How I do it—Necrosectomy in acute pancreatitis. J Hepat Biliary Pancreas Surg 2:155, 1994.
224. Rattner DW, Legermate DA, Lee MJ, et al: Early surgical débridement of symptomatic pancreatic necrosis is beneficial irrespective of infection. Am J Surg 163:105, 1992.
225. Fenton-Lee D, Imrie CW: Pancreatic necrosis: Assessment of outcome related to quality of life and cost of management. Br J Surg 80:1579, 1993.
226. Baron TH, Thaggard WG, Morgan DE, et al: Endoscopic therapy for organized pancreatic necrosis. Gastroenterology 111:755, 1996.
227. Freeny PC, Hauptmann E, Althaus SJ, et al: Percutaneous CT-guided catheter drainage of infected acute necrotizing pancreatitis: Techniques and results. Am J Roentgenol 170:969, 1998.
228. Echenique AM, Sleeman D, Yrizarry J, et al: Percutaneous catheter-directed debridement of infected pancreatic necrosis: Results in 20 patients. J Vasc Interv Radiol 9:565, 1998.
229. Ho HS, Frey CF: Gastrointestinal and pancreatic complications associated with severe pancreatitis. Arch Surg 130:817, 1995.
230. de Beaux AC, Palmer KR, Carter DC: Factors influencing morbidity and mortality in acute pancreatitis: An analysis of 279 cases. Gut 37: 121, 1995.
231. Uomo G, Visconti M, Manes G, et al: Non-surgical treatment of acute necrotizing pancreatitis. Pancreas 12:142, 1996.
232. Kalfarentzos F, Kehagias J, Mead N, et al: Enteral nutrition is superior to parenteral nutrition in severe acute pancreatitis—results of a randomized prospective trial. Br J Surg 84:1665, 1997.
233. McClave SA, Greene LM, Snider HL, et al: Comparison of the safety of early enteral vs. parenteral nutrition in mild acute pancreatitis. J Parenteral Enteral Nutr 21:14, 1997.
234. Windsor AC, Kanwar S, Li AG, et al: Compared with parenteral nutrition, enteral feeding attenuates the acute phase response and improves disease severity in acute pancreatitis. Gut 42:431, 1998.
235. Boivin M, Lanspa SJ, Zinsmeister AR, et al: Are diets associated with different rates of human interdigestive and postprandial pancreatic enzyme secretion? Gastroenterology 99:1763, 1990.
236. Holtmann G, Kelly DG, DiMagno EP: Nutrients and cyclical interdigestive pancreatic enzyme secretion in humans. Gut 38:920, 1996.
237. Levy P, Heresbach D, Pariente EA, et al: Frequency and risk factors of recurrent pain during refeeding in patients with acute pancreatitis: A multivariate multicentre prospective study of 116 patients. Gut 40: 262, 1977.
238. Folsch UR, Nitsche R, Ludtke R, et al: German Study Group on Acute Biliary Pancreatitis: Early ERCP and papillotomy compared with conservative treatment for acute biliary pancreatitis. N Engl J Med 336:237, 1997.
239. Elfstrom J: The timing of cholecystectomy in patients with gallstone pancreatitis: A retrospective analysis of 89 patients. Acta Chir Scand 144:487, 1978.
240. Freeny PC, Hauptmann E, Althaus AJ, et al: Percutaneous CT-guided catheter drainage of infected acute necrotizing pancreatitis: Techniques and results. Am J Roentgenol 170:969, 1998.
241. Beger HG, Büchler M, Bittner R, et al: Necrosectomy and postoperative local lavage in patients with necrotizing pancreatitis: Results of a prospective clinical trial. World J Surg 12:255, 1988.
242. Messori A, Rampazzo R, Scroccaro G, et al: Effectiveness of gabexate mesilate in acute pancreatitis. A meta-analysis. Dig Dis Sci 40:734, 1995.
243. Andriulli A, Leandro G, Clemente R, et al: Meta-analysis of somatostatin, ocreotide and gabexate mesilate in the therapy of acute pancreatitis. Aliment Pharmacol Ther 12:237, 1998.
244. Uhl W, Büchler MW, Malfertheiner P, et al: A randomised, double blind, multicentre trial of octreotide in moderate to severe acute pancreatitis. Gut 45:97, 1999.
245. Anai H, Sakaguchi H, Uchida H, et al: Continuous arterial infusion therapy for severe acute pancreatitis: Correlation between CT arteriography and therapeutic effect. J Vasc Interv Radiol 10:1335, 1999.
246. Takeda K, Sunamura M, Shibuya K, et al: Role of early continuous regional arterial infusion of protease inhibitor and antibiotic in nonsurgical treatment of acute necrotizing pancreatitis. Digestion 1:9, 1999.
247. Steinberg WA, Schlesselman SE: Treatment of pancreatitis: Comparison of animal and human studies. Gastroenterology 93:1420, 1987.
248. Leach SD, Gorelick FS, Modlin IM: New perspectives on acute pancreatitis. Scand J Gastroenterol 27(Suppl 192):29, 1992.
249. Grendell JH: Experimental pancreatitis. Curr Opin Gastroenterol 7: 702, 1991.
250. Vitas GJ, Sarr MG: Selected management of pancreatic pseudocysts: Operative versus expectant management. Surgery 111:123, 1992.
251. Yeo CJ, Bastidas JA, Lynch-Nyhan A, et al: The natural history of pancreatic pseudocysts documented by computed tomography. Surg Gynecol Obstet 170:411, 1990.
252. Rao R, Fedorak I, Prinz RA: Effect of failed computed tomography–guided and endoscopic drainage on pancreatic pseudocyst management. Surgery 114:843, 1993.
253. Weltz C, Pappas TN: Pancreatography and the surgical management of pseudocysts. Gastrointest Endosc Clin North Am 5:269, 1995.
254. Lawson JM, Baillie J: Endoscopic therapy for pancreatic pseudocysts. Gastrointest Endosc Clin North Am 5:181, 1995.
255. Howell DA, Holbrook RF, Bosco JJ, et al: Endoscopic needle localization of pancreatic pseudocysts before transmural drainage. Gastrointest Endosc 39:693, 1993.
256. Funnell IC, Bornman PC, Krige JEJ, et al: Endoscopic drainage of traumatic pancreatic pseudocyst. Br J Surg 81:879, 1994.
257. Catalano MF, Geenen JE, Schmalz MJ, et al: Treatment of pancreatic pseudocysts with ductal communication by transpapillary pancreatic duct endoprosthesis. Gastrointest Endosc 42:214, 1995.
258. Hariri M, Slivka A, Carr-Locke DL, et al: Pseudocyst predisposes to infection when pancreatic necrosis is unrecognized. Am J Gastroenterol 89:1781, 1994.
259. Mann DV, Hershman MJ, Hittinger R, et al: Multicentre audit of death from acute pancreatitis. Br J Surg 81:890, 1994.
260. Talamini G, Bassi C, Falconi M, et al: Risk of death from acute pancreatitis. Int J Pancreatol 19:15, 1996.

Chapter 49

CHRONIC PANCREATITIS

Chris E. Forsmark

DEFINITION

Chronic pancreatitis is characterized and defined by irreversible damage to the pancreas and the development of *histologic* evidence of inflammation and fibrosis and, eventually, destruction of exocrine (acinar cell) and endocrine (islets of Langerhans) tissue. Although this definition was developed at a series of international symposia, attempts to define chronic pancreatitis based on histology have never become useful to clinicians, given the difficulty in obtaining pancreatic tissue. Another symposium[1] continued to define chronic pancreatitis on histologic grounds, but the members proposed additional definitions that relied on more readily available imaging techniques (ultrasound, computed tomography [CT], or endoscopic retrograde pancreatography [ERP]). Defining chronic pancreatitis on the basis of imaging studies is also imperfect, since the morphologic changes detected by these tests may take years to develop. Indeed, many of these imaging studies are normal in chronic pancreatitis early in its clinical course. All these systems also tend to lump together all etiologies, which obscures differences that are important to clinicians. More recent proposals for defining and classifying chronic pancreatitis have been made that recognize the importance of etiology, the difficulty of obtaining pancreatic tissue, and the lack of sensitivity of currently available diagnostic tools.[2, 3] It is not yet clear that newer systems are more useful than previous attempts.

EPIDEMIOLOGY AND NATURAL HISTORY (PROGNOSIS)

Chronic pancreatitis can be demonstrated in 0.04% to 5% of autopsies.[4, 5] Determining the prevalence of chronic pancreatitis on the basis of autopsy data is somewhat misleading, since these patients may not have had clinical symptoms of chronic pancreatitis during life. Long-standing alcohol use, for example, can lead to histologic changes of chronic pancreatitis without symptoms of chronic pancreatitis.[6–9] Similarly, aging per se can induce histologic changes within the pancreas that are difficult to distinguish from chronic pancreatitis. Making a diagnosis based solely on autopsy data may therefore overestimate the rate of clinically important (i.e., symptomatic) chronic pancreatitis. Estimates of annual incidence in several retrospective studies range from 3 to 9 cases per 100,000 population.[7, 10, 11] The only prospective study,[12] one essentially limited to alcoholic chronic pancreatitis, noted an incidence of 8.2 cases per year per 100,000 population, and an overall prevalence of 27.4 cases per 100,000 population. These limited epidemiologic data demonstrate substantial geographic variation.[7] This variation may be due partly to differences in alcohol consumption in different populations, but part of the variation in incidence rates may merely reflect different diagnostic approaches and different diagnostic criteria.

Chronic pancreatitis accounts for substantial morbidity and health care costs. Approximately 20,000 American hospital admissions with a first-listed diagnosis of chronic pancreatitis occur yearly in nonfederal hospitals,[13, 14] with more than 60,000 yearly admissions in which chronic pancreatitis is listed as one of the discharge diagnoses.

The prognosis of chronic pancreatitis is quite variable and is affected by the presence of ongoing alcoholism in those with chronic alcoholic pancreatitis. One can estimate prognosis based on such features as need for medical care, including hospitalization, or on the development of complications, changes in quality of life, or disease-related mortality. We have limited data on the quality of life of patients after surgery for chronic pancreatitis, and essentially no information on patients managed medically or endoscopically.[15] These limited data suggest that the presence of continued pain and continued alcohol abuse (in those with alcoholic chronic pancreatitis) are the dominant negative influences on quality of life. Mortality in patients with chronic pancreatitis is also substantially influenced by the presence of continued alcoholism. In one large, multicenter study,[16] the standardized mortality ratio was 3.6 (i.e., those with a diagnosis of any form of chronic pancreatitis died at 3.6 times the rate compared with age-matched controls). Older subjects and those with alcoholic chronic pancreatitis had the most significant reduction in survival. Overall, 10-year survival is about 70%, and 20-year survival is about 45%. The cause of death in patients with chronic pancreatitis is often not due to the pancreatitis itself but to other medical conditions (emphysema, coronary artery disease, stroke, cirrhosis, and extrapancreatic malignancies), continued alcohol abuse, pancreatic carcinoma, and postoperative complications.

PATHOLOGY

The different etiologies of chronic pancreatitis produce similar pathologic findings (Fig. 49–1). In early chronic pancreatitis, the damage is variable and uneven. Areas of interlobular fibrosis are seen, with the fibrosis often extending to the ductal structures. Infiltration of the fibrotic area and lobules with lymphocytes, plasma cells, and macrophages is seen.[8, 17] The ducts may contain eosinophilic protein plugs. In affected lobules, acinar cells are replaced by fibrosis. The islets are usually undamaged until very late in the course of the disease. Features of acute pancreatitis may also be seen, such as edema, acute inflammation, or acinar cell or fat necrosis (see Chapter 48). As the disease progresses, fibrosis within the lobules and between lobules becomes more widespread. The pancreatic ducts become more abnormal, with progressive fibrosis, stricture formation, and dilation. The ductal protein plugs may calcify and obstruct major pancreatic ducts.

These histologic features are found in most forms of chronic pancreatitis. Obstructive chronic pancreatitis (associated with obstruction of the main pancreatic duct by a tumor or stricture) differs slightly in that the histologic changes are limited to the gland upstream of the obstruction, and protein precipitates and intraductal stones are not seen.[18] Chronic pancreatitis associated with autoimmune diseases may demonstrate more mononuclear inflammatory cells, but the difference may not be dramatic.

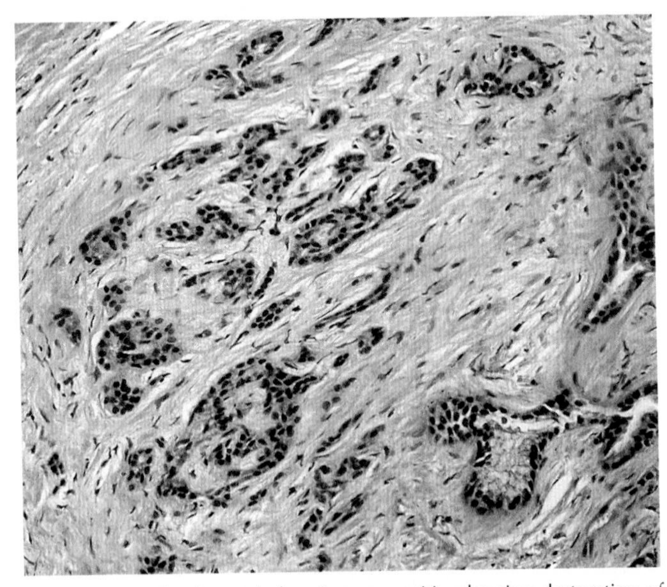

Figure 49–1. Histology of chronic pancreatitis, showing destruction of acinar tissue with replacement by extensive fibrosis.

PATHOPHYSIOLOGY

The pathophysiology of chronic pancreatitis remains incompletely understood. Studies in patients with alcoholic chronic pancreatitis have led to several different hypotheses of pathogenesis. No single theory explains adequately why only a minority of heavy alcohol users develop chronic pancreatitis and not the rest. One hypothesis, the *ductal obstruction hypothesis*, focuses on the formation of ductal protein precipitates, plugs, and stones as being the most important event. Chronic alcohol ingestion leads to the secretion of a pancreatic juice rich in protein[19] and low in volume and bicarbonate. This favors the formation of protein precipitates, and protein precipitates are present early in the evolution of alcoholic chronic pancreatitis. The hypothesis suggests that these protein plugs obstruct small ductules, leading to damage to the duct and to the parenchyma upstream of the obstruction. These precipitates may calcify, leading to the formation of pancreatic ductal stones, producing further ductal and upstream parenchymal injury.

Pancreatic ductal stones are seen in alcoholic chronic pancreatitis, tropical pancreatitis, hereditary pancreatitis, and idiopathic pancreatitis. The stones are rich in calcium carbonate. Lithostathine, a protein secreted into the pancreatic duct, is a potent inhibitor of calcium carbonate precipitation in pancreatic juice. Lithostathine levels in pancreatic juice are diminished in patients with calcifying chronic pancreatitis and also in alcoholic patients without pancreatitis.[20] This may explain the propensity for these protein precipitates to calcify. An additional protein that may be important in the formation of these stones is GP-2, a glycosyl phosphatidyl inositol (GPI)–anchored protein that is an analogue of uromodulin (Tamm-Horsfall protein, the protein responsible for the formation of urinary hyaline casts). GP-2 is a major component of pancreatic stones.[21] Thus, the effect of alcohol on the acinar cell and ductal cell appears to favor the formation of protein precipitates and the subsequent formation of calcified pancreatic stones. These changes, however, would seem to be more universal, since similar stones are seen in other forms of chronic pancreatitis. Even more importantly, it is not known whether these protein precipitates and ductal stones are causing pancreatic injury or are merely markers for the underlying pathophysiologic events.

A second hypothesis for the development of chronic pancreatitis due to alcohol is the *toxic-metabolic hypothesis*. This hypothesis holds that alcohol, or one of its metabolites, has direct injurious effects on the pancreatic ductal or acinar cells. Increased membrane lipid peroxidation, a marker of oxidative stress and free radical production, can be seen in both animal models and human alcoholic chronic pancreatitis.[22] Alcohol may also lead to abnormalities of acinar cell secretion, including an increase in the secretion of trypsinogen compared with trypsin inhibitor,[19] a situation favoring the premature activation of digestive enzymes within the acinar cell or ductal system. It appears increasingly likely that the cell most responsible for the development of pancreatic fibrosis is the pancreatic stellate cell, the analogue of the hepatic stellate cell. Alcohol and its metabolites appear to stimulate this cell to secrete proteins of the extracellular matrix.[23, 24]

A third hypothesis is the *necrosis-fibrosis hypothesis*. The theory holds that the occurrence of repeated episodes of acute pancreatitis with cellular necrosis eventually leads to the development of chronic pancreatitis as the healing process replaces necrotic tissue with fibrosis. This theory has significant supporting evidence from some natural history studies that document the more frequent development of chronic pancreatitis with more severe and more frequent acute attacks of alcoholic pancreatitis.[25, 26] There is also evidence against this theory based on studies that note that at the time of the first clinical episode of acute alcoholic pancreatitis, chronic pancreatitis is already present.[6, 9] The concept of multiple subclinical or mildly clinical attacks of acute pancreatitis leading to chronic pancreatitis is certainly being reinforced by the evolving information about hereditary pancreatitis (discussed later), and by the development of animal models of chronic pancreatitis induced by multiple attacks of mild acute pancreatitis.[27]

Careful studies of two forms of chronic pancreatitis seem to be providing new insight into this complex issue of the pathogenesis of chronic pancreatitis. First, an increase in mutations of the cystic fibrosis transmembrane conductance regulator (CFTR) has been found in patients previously believed to have idiopathic chronic pancreatitis.[28–30] Whether CFTR mutations are linked to other forms of chronic pancreatitis (e.g., alcoholic chronic pancreatitis) is not yet known. Second, a number of families with hereditary pancreatitis have been identified with mutations in the cationic trypsinogen gene (see Chapter 47).[31] These mutations appear to lead to a gain of function mutation in which trypsinogen, once activated to trypsin, is resistant to inactivation. The mutant trypsin might therefore be able to activate other proenzymes and produce clinical or subclinical episodes of acute pancreatitis, which ultimately leads to chronic pancreatitis in these patients. This presumed pathophysiology of hereditary pancreatitis provides support for the necrosis-fibrosis theory of chronic pancreatitis, in which repeated episodes of acute pancreatitis ultimately lead to chronic pancreatitis.

These theories of the pathophysiology of chronic pancreatitis are incomplete and are not mutually exclusive. They may depend on the etiology of the disease, the stage of the disease, and the genetic and environmental characteristics of the patient.

Table 49–1 | **Classification of Chronic Pancreatitis**

Alcoholic
Tropical
Tropical calcific pancreatitis
Fibrocalculous pancreatic diabetes
Genetic
Hereditary pancreatitis
Cystic fibrosis
Others?
Metabolic
Hypercalcemia
Hypertriglyceridemia, acquired or inherited (e.g.,apoprotein C-II deficiency, lipoprotein lipase deficiency)
Obstructive
Benign pancreatic duct obstruction
Traumatic stricture
Stricture after necrotizing pancreatitis
Stenosis of sphincter of Oddi
Pancreas divisum (with inadequate accessory papilla)
Sphincter of Oddi dysfunction?
Malignant pancreatic duct stricture
Pancreatic, ampullary, or duodenal carcinoma
Autoimmune
Isolated autoimmune chronic pancreatitis
Associated with autoimmune diseases (Sjögren's syndrome, primary biliary cirrhosis, primary sclerosing cholangitis)
Idiopathic
Early-onset
Late-onset
Asymptomatic pancreatic fibrosis
Chronic alcoholic patients
Aged individuals

ETIOLOGY (Table 49–1)

Alcohol

In Western countries, alcohol is the cause of 70% to 90% of all cases of chronic pancreatitis.[12, 13, 16, 32–35] The risk of alcoholic chronic pancreatitis increases logarithmically with increasing alcohol use, but there is no threshold value below which the disease does not occur.[32, 36] In countries with widespread alcohol consumption, this obviously makes it difficult to determine with certainty whether the disease is due to alcohol. In most patients, at least 5 years of alcohol intake exceeding 150 g/day is required prior to the development of chronic pancreatitis. Only 5% to 15% of heavy drinkers ultimately develop chronic pancreatitis, suggesting an important cofactor.[32] Potential cofactors that have been proposed include a diet high in fat and protein,[36, 37] a relative deficiency of antioxidants or trace elements,[38] and smoking.[32, 39] Smoking also appears to predispose to more rapid development of pancreatic calcification.[40] It remains to be studied whether mutations in the genes for trypsinogen or in CFTR are important co-factors for some patients with alcoholic chronic pancreatitis.

Many patients with alcoholic chronic pancreatitis have an early phase of recurrent attacks of acute pancreatitis, which may last 5 or 6 years, followed by the development of chronic pain or exocrine or endocrine insufficiency. In several large natural history studies, it was believed that most patients who present with their first attack of acute alcoholic pancreatitis have already developed histologic chronic pancreatitis.[6, 9, 34, 35] Up to 20% of patients presenting with acute alcoholic pancreatitis, however, will not progress to chronic pancreatitis (calcification, exocrine or endocrine insufficiency), even over prolonged follow-up.[25, 41]

Not all patients with alcoholic chronic pancreatitis will present with acute episodes of pancreatitis. Less than 10% of patients will have exocrine or endocrine insufficiency in the absence of prior abdominal pain.[33–35] Some will present with chronic pain in the absence of antecedent attacks of pain. Cessation of alcohol use after the onset of alcoholic pancreatitis appears to diminish the rate of progression to exocrine and endocrine insufficiency but does not halt it.[42] The prognosis of alcoholic chronic pancreatitis is relatively poor. Pain generally continues for years, although it may spontaneously remit. Exocrine and endocrine insufficiency develop in many patients, although this may take several years. In one large natural history study, exocrine insufficiency developed in 48% of patients at a median of 13.1 years after presentation, whereas endocrine insufficiency developed in 38% after a median of 19.8 years after presentation.[34] Diffuse pancreatic calcifications developed in 59% at a median of 8.7 years after diagnosis. Other studies have noted more rapid and more frequent development of calcifications and exocrine and endocrine insufficiency.[33]

Tropical Pancreatitis

Tropical pancreatitis is the most common form of chronic pancreatitis in certain areas of India. It has been reported from a number of other areas, including Africa, southeast Asia, and even Brazil. The disease is essentially restricted to areas within 30 degrees of latitude from the equator. Tropical pancreatitis is generally a disease of youth and early adulthood. Over 90% of patients develop the illness prior to the age of 40 years.[43] A recent field study noted an overall prevalence of 0.12% (≈1 in 830) in an endemic area, and a mean age of onset of 24 years.[44] The disease typically presents with abdominal pain, severe malnutrition, and exocrine or endocrine insufficiency. Steatorrhea is rare owing to a generally very low fat intake. Endocrine insufficiency is an inevitable consequence of tropical chronic pancreatitis and is often classified as a specific cause of diabetes called fibrocalculous pancreatic diabetes. Pancreatic calculi develop in over 90% of these patients. The pathology is characterized by large, intraductal calculi, marked dilation of the main pancreatic duct, and gland atrophy.

The pathophysiology of tropical pancreatitis is unknown. Protein-calorie malnutrition is present in the majority of these patients, but there are also many areas of the world with similar levels of malnutrition without tropical chronic pancreatitis. Some have postulated that it is the combined deficiency of trace elements and micronutrients, coupled with malnutrition, that predisposes to the disease.[43] Dietary factors have also been considered, particularly the role of cassava (tapioca). The geographic area of tropical pancreatitis is similar to the distribution of areas with high levels of consumption of cassava, and cassava is a staple of the diet in areas with the highest incidence of tropical chronic pancreatitis. Cassava contains cyanogens, which in the setting of micronutrient deficiency could produce oxidative injury. This theory is also not completely adequate, as tropical pancreatitis can occur in areas where cassava is not consumed, and some populations with high cassava consumption (west Africa) do not develop tropical chronic pancreatitis.

Hereditary Pancreatitis[45, 46]

Hereditary pancreatitis is an autosomal dominant disorder with approximately 80% penetrance. It is a rare disease, which presents typically in childhood or early adulthood with abdominal pain and recurrent acute attacks of pancreatitis. Hereditary pancreatitis accounts for only about 1% of all cases of chronic pancreatitis. It is discussed in detail in Chapter 47.

Cystic Fibrosis

Patients with classic cystic fibrosis (CF) commonly develop exocrine pancreatic insufficiency. Not all CFTR mutations are equally injurious, and the disease is highly variable.[47] This disease is discussed in detail in Chapter 47. Two recent studies of patients with idiopathic chronic pancreatitis reported CF gene mutations in 13% to 40%.[28, 29] This was far greater than the expected proportion within this population. Subsequent analysis of the genetic data suggested that the combination of a more severe mutation on one chromosome with a mild mutation on the other is particularly associated with chronic pancreatitis, but not with CF sinopulmonary disease.[48] These two studies[28, 29] examined only the most common CFTR mutations. One small study examining all known mutations noted genetic abnormalities in 10% of 16 patients, 14 of whom had "idiopathic" chronic pancreatitis.[30] There are now more than 900 known mutations, and further studies will be needed to define the contribution of these mutations to idiopathic and other forms of chronic pancreatitis and the mechanism(s) for the pancreatitis.

Obstructive Chronic Pancreatitis

Obstruction of the main pancreatic duct by tumors, scars, cysts, or stenosis of the papilla of Vater or minor papilla can produce chronic pancreatitis in the parenchyma upstream of the obstruction. Obstruction of the pancreatic ducts may also be an important contributor to other forms of chronic pancreatitis (e.g., obstruction of small ductal branches by protein precipitates in alcoholic chronic pancreatitis). Obstructive chronic pancreatitis, however, refers to a distinct entity produced by a (generally) single dominant narrowing or stricture of the main pancreatic duct. It is felt that relief of the obstruction can lead to preservation or reversal of pancreatic damage. A number of distinct entities can produce obstructive chronic pancreatitis. Acquired strictures of the main pancreatic duct can occur as a consequence of tumor obstruction (adenocarcinoma, islet cell tumor, or ampullary neoplasm). Strictures may also develop after a severe attack of acute pancreatitis, particularly with healing of a necrotic pseudocyst. Blunt and penetrating trauma to the pancreas can also lead to pancreatic duct strictures. Pancreas divisum is a common normal variant, occurring in 4% to 11% of the population (see Chapter 45). In rare patients with this congenital anomaly, the minor papilla is inadequate to allow free flow of pancreatic juice into the duodenum, possibly causing acute or chronic pancreatitis. Large studies have failed to identify a clear link between pancreas divisum and chronic pancreatitis.[49] Nonetheless, rare patients may present with pancreas divisum and substantial dilation of the dorsal pancreatic duct, associated with obstructive chronic pancreatitis.

Miscellaneous

AUTOIMMUNE PANCREATITIS. A few reports have described patients with chronic pancreatitis characterized by the presence of autoantibodies, elevated levels of immunoglobulins, enlargement of the pancreas (diffuse or focal), pancreatic duct strictures, and pathologic features of a dense lymphocytic infiltrate.[50] In 60%, the disease is associated with other autoimmune diseases such as primary sclerosing cholangitis, primary biliary cirrhosis, autoimmune hepatitis, and Sjögren's syndrome. In the small number of patients reported, the disease has responded to glucocorticoid treatment.

HYPERLIPIDEMIA. Elevations of serum triglycerides above 1000 mg/dL can produce acute pancreatitis (see Chapter 48). Rare patients will develop chronic pancreatitis after repeated episodes of acute pancreatitis.[51]

HYPERPARATHYROIDISM. Calcific chronic pancreatitis may rarely occur as a consequence of hyperparathyroidism. This has mainly been described in long-standing untreated hyperparathyroidism. This appears to be exceedingly rare today, when serum calcium is routinely checked as part of most automated chemistry panels. The pathophysiology is unknown but may be related to increases in calcium concentration in pancreatic juice and extensive precipitation of calcium carbonate in pancreatic ducts.

RADIOTHERAPY. Rare cases of chronic pancreatitis 6 or more years after abdominal radiotherapy have been reported. Marked ductal alterations, along with exocrine and endocrine insufficiency, are seen.[52]

POSTNECROTIC CHRONIC PANCREATITIS. Residual strictures of the pancreatic duct are not uncommon after severe acute pancreatitis, and this may explain the rare development of chronic pancreatitis in this group of patients.[53]

Idiopathic Chronic Pancreatitis

Idiopathic chronic pancreatitis accounts for 10% to 30% of all cases of chronic pancreatitis (see Chapter 48). Some of these patients may be mislabeled as idiopathic. Given that there is no threshold of alcohol ingestion for alcohol-induced chronic pancreatitis, some of these patients may actually suffer from alcoholic rather than idiopathic chronic pancreatitis. Similarly, it is certainly true that some of these patients may be misdiagnosed as idiopathic if appropriate genetic studies are not done, and even if done many genetic abnormalities can not be routinely screened (e.g., all of the cystic fibrosis mutations). Idiopathic chronic pancreatitis appears to occur in two forms, an early-onset type that presents in the patient's late teens or twenties and a late-onset form that presents in the patient's fifties or early sixties.[34, 54]

Early-onset idiopathic chronic pancreatitis has a mean age of onset of around 20 years. There appears to be an equal sex distribution,[34] although one series found a male predominance.[54] Pain is the predominant feature of this disease, occurring in 96% of patients, which is more frequent than in either alcoholic or late-onset chronic pancreatitis. Pancreatic calcifications, exocrine insufficiency, or endocrine insufficiency are extremely rare at presentation (<10%), and develop very slowly thereafter. The mean time to calcification in this group is 25 years, to exocrine insufficiency, 26 years, and to endocrine insufficiency, 27.5 years.[34] Complications of chronic pancreatitis (pseudocyst, abscess, biliary obstruction, and duodenal obstruction) occur in about 20%, and surgery (primarily for abdominal pain) is ultimately needed in 60%. Thus, early-onset idiopathic chronic pancreatitis is a disease characterized by severe pain but very delayed development of structural (calcifications) or functional (exocrine or endocrine insufficiency) evidence of chronic pancreatitis. This may make diagnosis quite difficult, because most available diagnostic tools rely on these structural or functional abnormalities to reach a diagnosis.

Late-onset idiopathic chronic pancreatitis presents less commonly with pain. In the best-documented series,[34] only 54% presented with pain, although three quarters of the patients ultimately experienced pain. The median age of onset was 56 years, and the disease occurred equally in men and women. Exocrine and endocrine insufficiency were present at the time of diagnosis in 22% of cases, and developed during follow-up in 46% and 41%, respectively. The median time to develop exocrine and endocrine insufficiency was 16.9 and 11.9 years, respectively. Life table analysis suggested that with very long follow-up (>30 years), exocrine insufficiency will ultimately develop in 75%, endocrine insufficiency in 50% to 60%, and diffuse pancreatic calcifications in 90%. The disease therefore tends to be one of a comparatively painless course associated with the frequent development of pancreatic calcifications and exocrine and endocrine insufficiency.

CLINICAL PRESENTATION

Abdominal Pain

Abdominal pain is the most serious clinical problem in patients with chronic pancreatitis. Severe pain decreases the appetite and limits food consumption, contributing to weight loss and malnutrition. Chronic severe pain also leads to a reduction in quality of life, loss of social functioning, and the potential for addiction to narcotic analgesics. Finally, pain is the most common reason for surgery in patients with chronic pancreatitis. There is no characteristic or diagnostic pain pattern. Pain is most commonly described as being felt in the epigastrium, often with radiation to the back. Pain is usually described as boring, deep, and penetrating and is often associated with nausea and vomiting. Pain may be relieved by sitting forward or leaning forward, by assuming the knee-chest position on one side, or by squatting and clasping the knees to the chest. Pain may increase after a meal and is often nocturnal.

The natural history of abdominal pain is variable and incompletely studied. As an example, many patients with alcoholic chronic pancreatitis initially present with episodes of pain interspersed with periods of feeling relatively well. During these more acute episodes of pain, the patient may be labeled as having acute pancreatitis. As time passes, pain may become more continuous and the diagnosis of chronic pancreatitis more obvious. Some patients may present with the more gradual onset of constant abdominal pain, and some may have no pain. Once pain develops, it commonly changes over time in its character, severity, and timing. Depending on etiology, 50% to 90% of patients will develop pain during the course of the disease.[33–35, 41, 55, 56] Many natural history studies document a decrease in pain over time in the majority of patients, although the timing and the magnitude of this decrease vary from study to study.[33–35, 55, 56] In one study, pain relief appeared to occur most commonly at the time of development of diffuse pancreatic calcifications and exocrine and endocrine insufficiency.[33] Other investigators have not found this same correlation, but many have noted a tendency for pain to "burn out" over time.[34, 35, 57, 58] Some of the pain relief is due to surgery performed during follow-up, but pain relief over prolonged follow-up is also seen in medically treated patients in similar proportions.[34, 35] The pain pattern in an individual patient, however, is not accurately predictable, and may worsen, stabilize, or improve over time. The judgment of therapeutic efficacy for any treatment for chronic pancreatitis must take into account this extremely variable natural history of pain.

Acute Pancreatic Inflammation

Superimposed episodes of acute pancreatitis may occur during the course of chronic pancreatitis. The pathophysiology of pain in this setting is unknown but may involve tissue ischemia, increases in pancreatic ductal or parenchymal pressure, neural inflammation, retroperitoneal inflammation, or other mechanisms. In general, the first clinical attack of acute pancreatitis complicating chronic pancreatitis is the most severe, with subsequent episodes becoming gradually less severe.

Increased Intrapancreatic Pressure

Several lines of clinical and experimental evidence point to increased pressure within the pancreatic duct or parenchyma as being important in the genesis of pancreatic pain. Pancreatic ductal and tissue pressures are usually elevated in patients with chronic pancreatitis undergoing surgery for chronic pain.[59–61] Elevations in pancreatic ductal pressure measured during endoscopic retrograde cholangiopancreatography (ERCP) have also been documented in a proportion of patients with chronic pancreatitis.[62] Surgical drainage of the pancreatic duct leads to an immediate reduction in pressure to normal levels and is associated with pain relief.[59, 60] In contrast, one small study of endoscopic stenting found that a reduction in pressure after stenting was not correlated with pain relief.[63]

The mechanism by which increased pressure could cause pain is speculative but may be related to pancreatic tissue ischemia. In animal models of chronic pancreatitis, increased pancreatic pressure is associated with reductions in pancreatic interstitial pH, reductions in pancreatic blood flow, and reductions in tissue oxygen tension.[64, 65] In this animal model, secretory stimulation is associated with a further decrease in pancreatic blood flow (rather than the normally expected increase), decreased capillary filling, and worsening tissue ischemia. This observation is consistent with that seen in a "compartment" type of syndrome. Small studies in humans with chronic pancreatitis undergoing surgery also demonstrate reductions in pancreatic tissue pH compared with patients without chronic pancreatitis.[65] Pancreatic blood flow, measured at ERCP using platinum electrodes, is also decreased in patients with chronic pancreatitis compared with controls.[66] The mechanism by which elevations in tissue pressure could cause pain could therefore relate to tissue ischemia that is worsened by secretory stimulation of the pancreas. Although this is an attractive hypothesis, increased pancreatic ductal and tissue pressures are not seen in all patients with painful chronic pancreatitis.[62] There is also not a predictable correlation between pancreatic duct pressure and duct appearance (dilation) or between pancreatic duct appearance and clinical symptoms.[26, 33–35, 57, 63]

Alterations in Pancreatic Nerves

Morphologic studies in patients with chronic pancreatitis demonstrate an increase in diameter and number of intrapancreatic nerves, foci of inflammatory cells associated with nerves and ganglia, and damage to the perineural sheath.[67] This disruption of the perineural sheath may allow inflammatory mediators to gain access to the neural elements. Additional studies have shown increases in substance P and calcitonin gene-related peptide (CGRP) in interlobular and intralobular nerve bundles in patients with chronic pancreatitis; both of these neurotransmitters may be involved in pain transmission. It is not known whether similar changes within pancreatic nerves occur among patients without pain.

Other Causes of Pain

A number of complications should be considered in chronic pancreatitis patients with severe pain and especially in patients who develop a worsening of a previously stable pain pattern. These complications are discussed more fully later in "Complications," but are mentioned here as contributors to the pain associated with chronic pancreatitis. The reason to evaluate for these complications is that each has specific and relatively effective therapy. These complications include pancreatic pseudocyst, mechanical obstruction of the common bile duct or duodenum, the development of pancreatic adenocarcinoma, and gastroparesis.

Steatorrhea and Weight Loss

The human pancreas has substantial exocrine reserve (see Chapter 46). Steatorrhea does not occur until pancreatic lipase secretion is reduced to less than 10% of normal.[68] Steatorrhea is therefore a feature of far-advanced chronic pancreatitis when most of the acinar cells have been injured or destroyed, but may also be seen with complete blockage of the pancreatic duct. With advanced chronic pancreatitis, maldigestion of fat, protein, and carbohydrates may occur (see Chapter 89). These patients may present with diarrhea or weight loss. Some patients may note bulky, foul-smelling stools or may even note the passage of frank oil droplets. Unlike the case in other diseases associated with malabsorption, watery diarrhea, excess gas, and abdominal cramps are uncommon. This difference may be due to better preserved carbohydrate absorption in patients with chronic pancreatitis and exocrine insufficiency compared with diseases such as celiac sprue. Even when there is significant loss of fat in stool, most patients pass only three or four stools daily.

In general, fat maldigestion occurs earlier and is more

severe than protein or carbohydrate maldigestion. There are several potential explanations for this phenomenon. Fat digestion is primarily dependent on pancreatic lipase and colipase. Gastric lipase is able to hydrolyze only 20% of dietary fat or less (see Chapter 38). Pancreatic lipase output decreases earlier and more substantially as chronic pancreatitis progresses, compared with the secretion of other pancreatic enzymes. Lipase is also more sensitive to acid destruction than are other pancreatic enzymes. As bicarbonate secretion decreases in chronic pancreatitis and duodenal pH drops, lipase is particularly inactivated. In addition to lipase inactivation, low duodenal pH also predisposes to precipitation of bile salts, thereby preventing the formation of mixed micelles and further interfering with lipid digestion and absorption. Finally, lipase is more sensitive to digestion and degradation by pancreatic proteases than other digestive enzymes. All these factors explain the predominant clinical importance of steatorrhea and the rather minor clinical problem of maldigestion of carbohydrates and protein.

The median time to development of pancreatic exocrine insufficiency has been reported to be as low as 5.6 years,[33] but most studies report a considerably longer duration of disease prior to the development of steatorrhea. In one large natural history study, the median time to development of exocrine insufficiency was 13.1 years in patients with alcoholic chronic pancreatitis, 16.9 years in patients with late-onset idiopathic chronic pancreatitis, and 26.3 years in patients with early-onset idiopathic chronic pancreatitis.[34] With prolonged follow-up, approximately 50% to 80% of patients will eventually develop exocrine insufficiency.[33–35]

Weight loss may be absent or minimal despite maldigestion. Patients generally increase their caloric intake to compensate for stool losses (hyperphagia). Weight is maintained despite the fact that the resting energy expenditure is increased in patients with chronic pancreatitis.[69] Weight loss is most commonly seen during painful flares that prevent adequate oral intake because of pain, nausea, or vomiting. Weight loss may also occur owing to the development of a concomitant disease such as small bowel bacterial overgrowth or pancreatic or extrapancreatic malignancy. Substantial weight loss should lead to an investigation of these potential causes.

Rarely, fat-soluble vitamin deficiency may develop in patients with pancreatic steatorrhea.[70] Significant vitamin D deficiency was thought to be rare, but more recent studies have documented osteopenia and osteoporosis in patients with chronic pancreatitis.[71] Water-soluble vitamin and micronutrient deficiencies are also rare and generally are seen only as a consequence of inadequate intake in chronic alcoholic patients. Despite the fact that cobalamin (vitamin B_{12}) absorption requires intact pancreatic function to degrade R-factor from dietary cobalamin (see Chapter 38), cobalamin deficiency is rare.

Diabetes Mellitus

Like exocrine insufficiency, endocrine insufficiency with secondary diabetes is a consequence of long-standing chronic pancreatitis. Islet cells appear to be relatively resistant to destruction in chronic pancreatitis. When diabetes occurs in chronic pancreatitis, both insulin-producing beta cells and glucagon-producing alpha cells are destroyed, unlike type 1 diabetes mellitus, in which beta cells are selectively destroyed. Deficiency of insulin and glucagon in chronic pancreatitis leads to a brittle type of diabetes.[72] In patients with diabetes due to chronic pancreatitis, compensatory endogenous release of glucagon in response to hypoglycemia is absent. Exogenous administration of insulin in these patients may therefore lead to prolonged and severe hypoglycemia.[73]

Diabetes mellitus appears to be nearly as common as steatorrhea in patients with far-advanced chronic pancreatitis. In one study, the median time to develop diabetes was 19.8 years, 11.9 years, and 26.3 years in patients with alcoholic, late-onset idiopathic, and early-onset idiopathic chronic pancreatitis, respectively.[34] Other studies have noted shorter median times of 6 to 10 years.[33, 56] Ultimately, 40% to 70% of patients will develop diabetes after prolonged follow-up, depending on etiology. Microangiopathic complications are as common in patients with diabetes associated with chronic pancreatitis as in patients with type 1 diabetes, if corrected for disease duration.[74]

Physical Findings

Very little on physical examination is diagnostic or specific for chronic pancreatitis. Patients generally appear well-nourished and demonstrate mild to moderate abdominal tenderness. In chronic alcoholic patients with advanced disease, weight loss and malnutrition may be more evident, or one may see signs of coexistent chronic alcoholic liver disease. Rarely, a palpable mass may be felt, indicating a pseudocyst. Jaundice may be seen in the presence of coexistent alcoholic liver disease or common bile duct compression within the head of the pancreas. A palpable spleen rarely may be felt in patients with thrombosis of the splenic vein as a consequence of chronic pancreatitis.

DIAGNOSIS

An impressive number and variety of diagnostic tests for chronic pancreatitis have been developed, which serves to point out the fact that no single test is adequate. Many tests have not been studied adequately to define their sensitivity and specificity. These diagnostic tests are usually separated into those tests that detect abnormalities of pancreatic function, discussed in Chapter 46, and those that detect abnormalities of pancreatic structure (Table 49–2). Before discussing these tests in more detail, it is useful to remember that in many patients chronic pancreatitis is a slowly progressive disease. Abnormalities of pancreatic structure or function may take years to develop or may not develop at all. All available diagnostic tests are most accurate in far-advanced disease when obvious structural or functional abnormalities have developed. Conversely, to greater or lesser degrees, all diagnostic tests are less accurate in less advanced or early chronic pancreatitis.

Structural abnormalities that can be diagnostic include changes within the main pancreatic duct (dilation, strictures, irregularity, pancreatic ductal stones), side branches of the pancreatic duct (dilation, irregularity), or pancreatic parenchyma (lobularity, hyperechoic strands, enlargement or atrophy, and others). Functional abnormalities in chronic pancre-

Table 49–2 | **Diagnostic Tests for Chronic Pancreatitis***

TESTS OF STRUCTURE	TESTS OF FUNCTION (SEE CHAPTER 46)
ERP	Direct hormonal stimulation test (secretin or secretin-CCK test)
EUS	Bentiromide test or pancreolauryl test†
MRI/MRCP	Fecal elastase or chymotrypsin
CT	Serum trypsinogen
US	Fecal fat
Plain abdominal film	Serum glucose

*Ranked in order of decreasing sensitivity (estimated).
†Not available in United States.
CCK, cholecystokinin; CT, computed tomography; ERP, endoscopic retrograde pancreatography; EUS, endoscopic ultrasonography; MRI, magnetic resonance imaging; MRCP, magnetic resonance cholangiopancreatography; US, ultrasound.

atitis include a decrease in stimulated secretory capacity, exocrine insufficiency (maldigestion and steatorrhea), and endocrine insufficiency (diabetes mellitus). Patients with alcoholic chronic pancreatitis, hereditary chronic pancreatitis, tropical pancreatitis, and late-onset idiopathic chronic pancreatitis are most prone to develop these abnormalities of structure or function, although it may still take years. Patients with early-onset idiopathic chronic pancreatitis develop these changes particularly slowly and may not develop them at all.

This has led to a general classification of chronic pancreatitis as either "big-duct" or "small-duct" disease. "Big-duct" disease implies substantial abnormalities of the pancreatic duct (generally, dilation visible on ultrasound, CT, or ERP), whereas "small-duct" disease implies the absence of these findings (e.g., a normal or near-normal US, CT, or ERP). Similarly, "big-duct" disease is usually associated with functional abnormalities, whereas "small-duct" disease is less frequently associated with exocrine or endocrine insufficiency. This distinction has both diagnostic and therapeutic implications. The diagnosis of "big-duct" disease is much simpler, the disease is usually due to alcohol abuse, and the treatment options focus on decompressing the dilated pancreatic duct. The diagnosis of "small-duct" disease is much more difficult as imaging studies and functional studies may be normal, the disease is more frequently idiopathic, and treatment options focus on medical therapy rather than surgical or endoscopic attempts to decompress the pancreatic duct.

The determination of the sensitivity, specificity, and accuracy of any of these diagnostic tests requires that the test result be compared with some gold standard, a test that gives reliable and certain evidence of the presence or absence of disease. In the case of chronic pancreatitis, this gold standard is pancreatic histology. Unfortunately, the histologic changes are not uniform throughout the gland, so that a small biopsy specimen may not give a complete picture of the presence or absence of disease. Even more important, obtaining pancreatic tissue on a routine basis is risky and seldom performed.

Given the lack of a useful gold standard, one is left with rating a new diagnostic test against some substitute for the gold standard. One such substitute is prolonged follow-up. Most series have not followed patients diagnosed with early chronic pancreatitis or possible early chronic pancreatitis (patients in whom diagnostic tests are not unequivocally positive) for long enough to establish the presence or absence of chronic pancreatitis with certainty. The second potential substitute for the gold standard is some other diagnostic test, and in fact new diagnostic tests are often compared against such tests as endoscopic retrograde pancreatography (ERP), CT, or direct pancreatic function tests.

In patients with chronic pancreatitis and far-advanced structural or functional abnormalities, little else can mimic these abnormalities and essentially all diagnostic tests are accurate. The situation is quite different in patients with early or less advanced chronic pancreatitis or in patients with possible chronic pancreatitis who lack these easily identifiable structural or functional abnormalities. In this situation, only tests of maximum sensitivity have a chance of making a diagnosis, and the lack of a gold standard can lead to diagnostic confusion and difficult decision making. In addition to choosing a diagnostic test based on sensitivity and specificity, clinicians must consider the availability, cost, and risk of each of these tests to maximize benefit and minimize risk. These issues are discussed later in relation to each of the available diagnostic tools.

Routine Laboratory Tests

Routine laboratory studies are not generally useful in making a diagnosis of chronic pancreatitis. The leukocyte count is usually normal in the absence of infection (e.g., an infected pseudocyst). Alkaline phosphatase or bilirubin may be abnormal if there is compression of the intrapancreatic bile duct by a pseudocyst or fibrosis within the head of the pancreas. Serum amylase or lipase may be elevated during acute exacerbations, but these elevations are usually only modest and are neither routinely present nor diagnostic for chronic pancreatitis. Serum amylase and lipase levels are also frequently increased in the presence of a pseudocyst, pancreatic ductal stricture, or internal pancreatic fistula. In the setting of malnutrition, serum albumin and calcium may be decreased. This is most commonly seen in chronic alcoholic patients, in whom one may also see anemia with macrocytosis, thrombocytopenia, and leukopenia. Hyperglycemia is seen when diabetes develops in advanced chronic pancreatitis.

Tests of Pancreatic Function

These tests can be divided into those that directly measure pancreatic exocrine function by measuring the output of enzymes or bicarbonate from the pancreas and those that measure the released enzymes indirectly (through the action on a substrate or the presence in stool or serum).

Direct Tests of Pancreatic Exocrine Secretion (see Chapter 46)

Although direct hormonal stimulation tests with secretin (with or without cholecystokinin [CCK]) were thought to be the most sensitive tests for chronic pancreatitis,[75] these tests are performed at only a few centers in the United States and so are not widely available. In most comparisons with pancreatography (ERP), direct hormonal stimulation tests appear to be slightly more sensitive for the diagnosis of chronic pancreatitis. The values for sensitivity in studies range from 74% to 97%, with specificity ranging from 80% to 90%.[75–80] In these studies, most patients with an abnormal pancreatogram also have an abnormal hormonal stimulation test. The two tests agree in about three quarters of patients, although some studies note higher rates of concordance.[80] Most studies also note a general correlation between increasing structural abnormalities and progressive abnormalities of hormone stimulation tests, although the relationship is not exact. Most of these studies also identify patients with discordant results: patients with abnormal pancreatograms and normal hormonal stimulation tests and patients with normal pancreatograms and abnormal hormonal stimulation tests. In four studies, the percentage of patients with an abnormal hormonal stimulation test and a normal pancreatogram ranged from 3% to 20%.[76–79]

Two small studies have followed such patients whose diagnosis was based solely on an abnormal hormonal stimulation test, and both found chronic pancreatitis developing on follow-up in 90%.[79, 81] These data point out that direct pancreatic function testing appears to be able to identify a group of patients with chronic pancreatitis who have functional abnormalities of stimulated secretion but who do not (yet) have structural abnormalities identifiable on ERCP. Conversely, most of these studies also document patients with a normal hormonal stimulation test and an abnormal pancreatogram. This group of patients is generally less common, averaging less than 10% in several studies.[76–81] Long-term follow-up in a small group of these patients noted chronic pancreatitis developing in 0% to 26%.[79, 81] These studies point out that when the two tests disagree, hormonal stimulation testing appears to be somewhat more sensitive and specific than pancreatography.

There has been little information comparing direct hormonal stimulation testing to pancreatic histology. In one study comparing histology with secretin-cholecystokinin testing in 108 patients,[82] the overall sensitivity of hormonal stimulation testing was 67% with a specificity of 90% and overall accuracy of 81%. When the analysis was restricted to the 29 patients with moderate or severe histologic changes of chronic pancreatitis, the sensitivity of hormonal stimulation testing increased to 79%. In this same group of patients, the sensitivity of pancreatography was 66%.

Like all diagnostic tests, direct pancreatic function studies are most sensitive in advanced chronic pancreatitis and less sensitive in less advanced disease. Some experts have estimated that 30% to 50% damage to the gland is necessary before these tests are reliably positive. Despite the theoretical advantages of direct pancreatic function tests, they have a number of limitations. The test has not been standardized, and the normal ranges for the test need to be established at each center performing the test. The test is available only at a very few referral centers and is not available to the majority of clinicians seeing patients with chronic pancreatitis. One of the secretagogues, natural porcine secretin, has become unavailable, although synthetic forms are now becoming available.[83] Direct hormonal stimulation tests are the most sensitive (and possibly specific) tests available, and are safe, but are moderately expensive, time consuming, and not widely available. False-positive test results have been reported in patients with diabetes, Billroth II gastrectomy, celiac sprue, cirrhosis, and those recovering from an attack of acute pancreatitis. This test is most useful in patients with presumed chronic pancreatitis who do not have easily identifiable structural and functional abnormalities on more widely available diagnostic tests such as CT.

Attempts have been made to develop variations of direct pancreatic function tests that are easier to perform. In particular, collection of secretin-stimulated pancreatic secretions at the time of ERP by placement of a catheter in the pancreatic duct (the so-called intraductal secretin test) has been proposed.[83a] This test is not standardized and does not appear to be as accurate as standard direct pancreatic function testing.

Indirect Tests of Pancreatic Exocrine Secretion (see Chapter 46)

The desire to develop indirect tests of pancreatic function is an outgrowth of the complexity, unavailability, and discomfort of direct pancreatic function testing. These tests generally can measure pancreatic enzymes (in blood or stool) or the effect of pancreatic enzymes on an orally administered substrate (with collection of metabolites in blood, breath, or urine).

Measurement of Trypsinogen in Serum

Serum trypsinogen (often called serum trypsin) is commercially available and, unlike amylase and lipase, has some diagnostic utility. Very low levels of serum trypsinogen (<20 ng/mL) are reasonably specific for chronic pancreatitis, but levels this low are seen only in advanced chronic pancreatitis with steatorrhea.[84] Serum trypsinogen levels are in the normal range in most patients with less advanced chronic pancreatitis. Serum trypsin measurement is inexpensive, widely available, and risk-free, although it is accurate only in long-standing and far-advanced chronic pancreatitis. Serum trypsin is not decreased in patients with other forms of steatorrhea, but low levels of serum trypsinogen may be seen in patients with pancreatic ductal obstruction, including malignant obstruction.

Measurement of Chymotrypsin or Elastase in Stool

Low levels of pancreatic chymotrypsin or elastase in stool reflect inadequate delivery of these enzymes to the duodenum, and hence chronic pancreatitis with exocrine insufficiency. Measurement of *fecal chymotrypsin* is abnormal in most patients with chronic pancreatitis and steatorrhea.[75] False-positive tests have been reported in other malabsorptive conditions (sprue, Crohn's disease), in diarrheal diseases when the stool is diluted, and in severe malnutrition. The test is normal in the absence of steatorrhea, so the test is positive only in advanced chronic pancreatitis. The assay is not commercially available in the United States.

Fecal elastase may have certain advantages over fecal chymotrypsin in that it is very stable in passage through stool and easy to measure. Although initial studies suggested the test could defect chronic pancreatitis in the absence of steatorrhea, more recent studies have shown the test accurate in the presence of steatorrhea but inaccurate in less advanced chronic pancreatitis.[85] In addition, the test may be falsely abnormal in other diseases causing steatorrhea, such as short bowel syndrome or small bowel bacterial overgrowth. This test is available but not widely used in the United States.

Measurement of Enzyme Actions

FECAL FAT (QUANTITATIVE/QUALITATIVE). The simplest measurement of pancreatic enzyme action is the measurement of fecal fat excretion (see Chapter 89). Maldigestion of fat occurs after 90% of pancreatic lipase secretory capacity is lost. A 72-hour collection of stool while the patient is consuming a 100 g/day fat diet provides the best evidence of fat maldigestion. Although theoretically quite simple, in practice the test is difficult to perform. The patient must be on a 100 g/day fat diet for at least 3 days prior to the test, and the complete collection of the sample is difficult to achieve. In health, less than 7 g of fat (7% of the ingested dose) should be present in stool. Measuring fecal fat requires that the dietary content of fat be known exactly, which is impossible outside a clinical research center. The qualitative analysis of fecal fat can also be performed with a Sudan III stain of a random specimen of stool. More than six globules per high-power field is considered to be positive but, again, the patient must be ingesting adequate fat to allow measurable steatorrhea. Sudan III staining of stool is positive only in patients with substantial steatorrhea.

MEASUREMENTS OF METABOLITES IN URINE. Two tests of historical importance utilized the administration of an oral substrate with measurement of urinary excretion of metabolites that are produced by the action of pancreatic digestive enzymes. The bentiromide (*N*-benzoyl-L-tyrosyl-*p*-aminobenzoic acid, or NBT-PABA) test measures the presence of pancreatic chymotrypsin within the gut lumen. The pancreolauryl test measures the presence of pancreatic arylesterases within the gut lumen. Both tests are accurate in advanced chronic pancreatitis, with sensitivities of 80% to 100%.[75] In the absence of steatorrhea, sensitivities drop to 40% to 50%. Neither test is available in the United States.

BREATH TESTS. The overall sensitivity of these tests is low,[75a] and they are not commercially available (see Chapter 89).

Tests of Pancreatic Structure

Plain Abdominal Radiography

The finding of diffuse (but not focal) pancreatic calcifications is reasonably specific for chronic pancreatitis. Calcifications occur late in the natural history of chronic pancreatitis and may take from 5[33] to 25 years[34] to develop. Calcifications are most common in alcoholic, late-onset idiopathic, hereditary, and tropical pancreatitis and far less common in early-onset idiopathic pancreatitis. Calcifications are not static and may in fact wax and wane over time.[86] The sensitivity of plain abdominal radiography, therefore, will depend on the etiology and duration of the disease. The test is inexpensive, risk-free, and widely available but can detect only long-standing and advanced disease.

Abdominal Ultrasound

Ultrasound (US) has been widely studied as a diagnostic tool for chronic pancreatitis. US is limited in that the pancreas cannot be adequately visualized in many patients because of overlying bowel gas. US findings indicative of chronic pancreatitis[1] include dilation of the pancreatic duct, shadowing pancreatic ductal stones, gland atrophy or enlargement, irregular gland margins, pseudocysts, and changes in the parenchymal echotexture (Table 49–3). Most studies suggest a sensitivity of 50% to 80%, with a specificity of 80% to 90%.[75] The true sensitivity and specificity may be different since most of these studies are older and did not use state-of-the-art equipment.

In one recent study comparing transabdominal ultrasound with CT, ERCP, and endoscopic ultrasonography (EUS), the accuracy of US was 56%.[87] In this study, 40% of patients with a normal pancreas, as defined by the other diagnostic tests, had some abnormality noted on ultrasound (such as changes in parenchymal echotexture). A large screening study of transabdominal US in Japan encompassing 130,000 examinations found increased echogenicity, mild dilation of the pancreatic duct, small cystic cavities, and even ductal calcification in the absence of chronic pancreatitis.[88] The majority of these abnormalities could not be attributed to chronic pancreatitis and were instead attributed to aging. These studies suggest that there is a large spectrum of US findings in normal individuals, and that it can be difficult to distinguish normal (or age-related) variability from chronic pancreatitis, particularly if the visualized changes are mild.

Despite this potential problem, a careful transabdominal ultrasound can be very useful in the evaluation of patients

Table 49–3 | **Grading of Chronic Pancreatitis by Ultrasound (US) or Computed Tomography (CT)**

GRADE OF CHRONIC PANCREATITIS	US OR CT FINDINGS
Normal	Good-quality study visualizing the entire gland with no abnormal findings
Equivocal	One of the following: Mild dilation of the pancreatic duct (2–4 mm) in the body of the gland Gland enlargement ≤ twofold normal
Mild to moderate	One of the above findings plus at least 1 of the following: Pancreatic duct dilation Pancreatic duct irregularity Cavities <10 mm Parenchymal heterogeneity Increased echogenicity of duct wall Irregular contour of the head or body Focal necrosis of parenchyma
Severe	Mild/moderate plus one or more of the following: Cavity >10 mm Intraductal filling defects Calculi/pancreatic calcification Ductal obstruction (stricture) Severe duct dilation or irregularity Contiguous organ invasion on US or CT

Adapted from Sarner M, Cotton PB: Classification of pancreatitis. Gut 25:756, 1984.

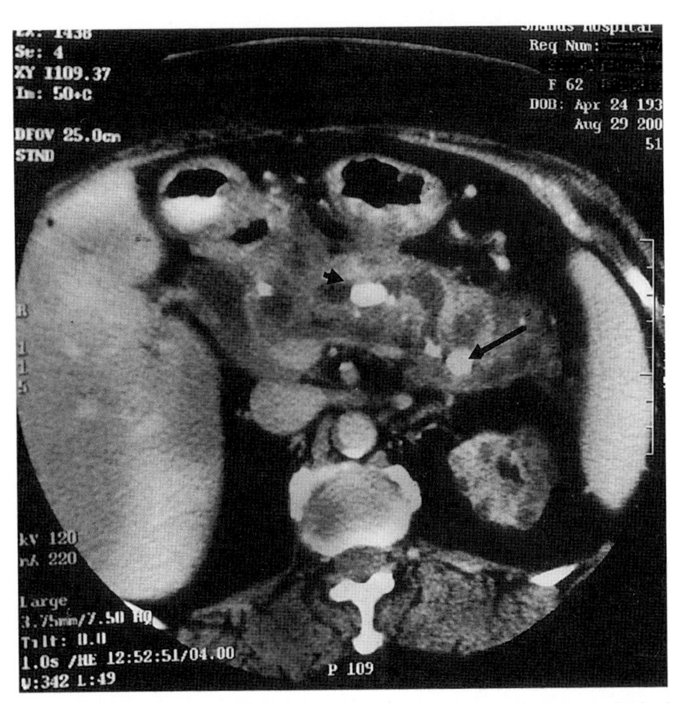

Figure 49–2. CT scan demonstrating several large, densely calcified stones *(arrows)* within a markedly dilated pancreatic duct in long-standing chronic pancreatitis.

with suspected chronic pancreatitis. The finding of a normal pancreas or moderate to marked changes of advanced chronic pancreatitis is generally definitive. Mild changes of chronic pancreatitis are less specific and need to be interpreted in light of the clinical history and the patient's age. US can also be useful in screening for complications of chronic pancreatitis (e.g., pseudocyst) and in evaluating for other conditions that might mimic the symptoms of chronic pancreatitis (i.e., biliary tract disease). Transabdominal ultrasound is widely available, rather inexpensive, and risk-free.

Computed Tomography

The overall sensitivity of CT for chronic pancreatitis is between 75% and 90%, with a specificity of 85% or more.[75] CT is able to image the pancreas in all patients and hence provides an advantage over ultrasound. CT is estimated to be 10% to 20% more sensitive than US, with a similar specificity.[75] Table 49–3 outlines the abnormalities on CT used for diagnosis. Most studies of diagnostic CT in chronic pancreatitis have not used state-of-the-art CT technology. It is likely that modern scanners produce better sensitivity.[87, 89] Like all diagnostic tests, CT is most accurate in advanced chronic pancreatitis after substantial structural changes have developed (Fig. 49–2). It is more expensive than US and exposes the patient to ionizing radiation, but it is more sensitive and probably more specific than US. Except for the rare allergic reaction to intravenous contrast, the test is very safe.

Magnetic Resonance Imaging/Magnetic Resonance Cholangiopancreatography

There is little information on MRI or MRCP in patients with chronic pancreatitis. A number of small studies suggest that MRCP provides an acceptable assessment of pancreatic ductal morphology in most patients.[89, 90] MRCP agrees with ERCP in 70% to 80% of findings, with the higher rates of agreement seen in studies using the most advanced image analysis techniques. Agreement between MRCP and ERCP is worse in areas where the pancreatic duct is small (tail of pancreas and side branches). Improvements in MR image analysis will continue to improve the image quality of MRCP and in the future it could approach ERCP in accuracy. Like ERCP, however, the test will be inaccurate in patients without significant ductal abnormalities. Whereas MRI is widely available, risk-free, and only moderately expensive, not all centers have the capacity to perform MRCP.

Endoscopic Retrograde Cholangiopancreatography

ERCP, specifically ERP, is generally considered the most specific and sensitive test of pancreatic structure, and many consider it the de facto gold standard. It is widely available so it is commonly used in the evaluation of patients with possible chronic pancreatitis. It also has the advantage over all previously discussed tests in that therapy may be administered (e.g., pancreatic duct stenting or stone extraction). It has the disadvantage that it is the riskiest diagnostic test, with complications occurring in at least 5% of patients (and as high as 20% in certain subgroups) and a mortality rate of 0.1% to 0.5%. In most studies in patients with chronic pancreatitis, the sensitivity of ERCP is between 70% and 90%, with a specificity of 80% to 100%.[75–80]

The diagnostic features for chronic pancreatitis on ERP were agreed on at an international symposium[91] (Table 49–4). The diagnosis is based on abnormalities seen in both the main pancreatic duct and in the side branches. ERP is highly sensitive and specific in patients with advanced structural abnormalities. At its most advanced, the appearance of a massively dilated pancreatic duct with alternating strictures (the chain-of-lakes appearance) is pathognomonic of chronic pancreatitis (Fig. 49–3). Less dramatic pancreatographic changes are less definitive[92] (Fig. 49–4). The interpretation in these cases may be more difficult for two main reasons: (1) similar morphologic changes of the pancreatic duct can be produced in other clinical situations, and (2) interpreta-

Table 49–4 | **Cambridge Grading of Chronic Pancreatitis by Endoscopic Retrograde Pancreatography**

GRADE	MAIN PANCREATIC DUCT	SIDE BRANCHES
Normal	Normal	Normal
Equivocal	Normal	<3 abnormal
Mild	Normal	≥3 abnormal
Moderate	Abnormal	>3 abnormal
Severe	Abnormal, with at least one of the following: Large cavity (>10 mm) Duct obstruction Intraductal filling defects Severe dilation or irregularity	>3 abnormal

Adapted from Axon ATR, Classen M, Cotton PB, et al: Pancreatography in chronic pancreatitis: International definitions. Gut 25:1107;1984.

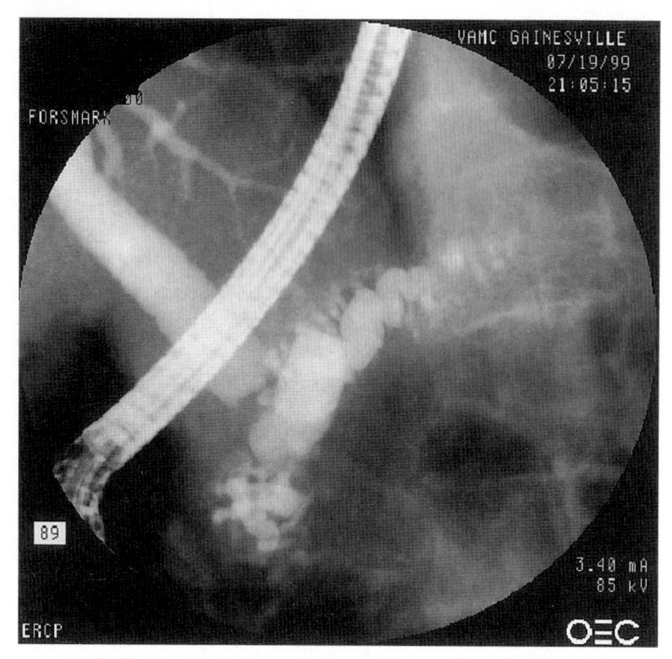

Figure 49–3. An ERCP demonstrating a markedly dilated pancreatic duct with alternating strictures and dilation. This finding of a chain-of-lakes appearance is diagnostic of chronic pancreatitis.

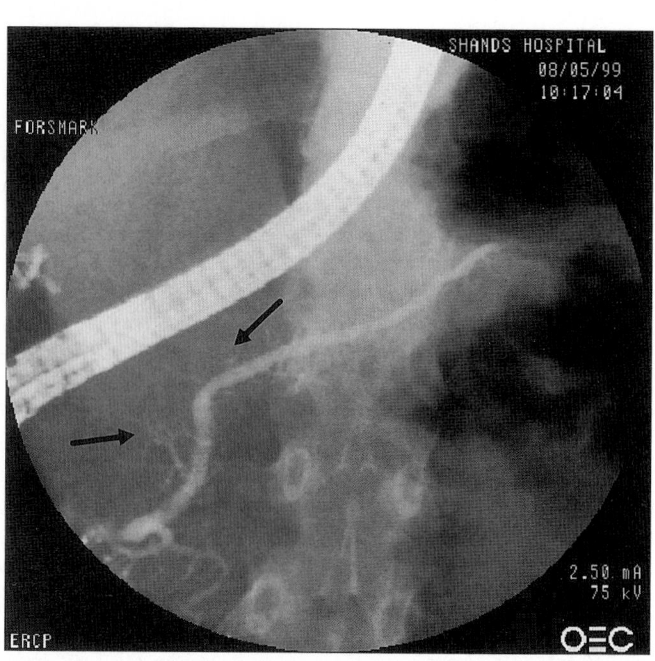

Figure 49–4. An ERCP demonstrating subtle changes limited to the side branches *(arrows)* in a patient with chronic pancreatitis demonstrated on a direct hormonal function test. Mild irregularity of the contour of the side branches can be seen. These subtle findings are generally not adequate alone to reach a diagnosis of chronic pancreatitis confidently.

tion of pancreatography is subjective, with substantial inter- and intraobserver variation. Complicating the matter still further, it is quite clear that chronic pancreatitis can exist in the absence of any changes within the pancreatic duct.[82, 92, 93]

The accurate interpretation of an ERCP requires a study of adequate quality (filled to the second generation of the side branches and without significant movement artifact). Up to 30% of pancreatograms do not meet these criteria of an adequate study.[92] An inadequate study would certainly contribute to errors in diagnosis. For example, underfilling of the pancreatic duct might produce artifactual irregularity of the main duct (leading to overdiagnosis of chronic pancreatitis) or might miss changes within the inadequately filled side branches (leading to underdiagnosis of chronic pancreatitis). The ductographic abnormalities characteristic of chronic pancreatitis are not specific. Although pancreatic function is well preserved in aging, impressive abnormalities may develop in the pancreatic duct. These changes include focal or diffuse dilation of the main pancreatic duct and its side branches, the development of cystic cavities, and even ductal calculi.[91, 92, 94, 95] In a large screening US study,[88] 50% of all calcifications and more than 80% of ductal dilation and cystic lesions seen were felt to be attributable to aging, not chronic pancreatitis. Temporary changes in the pancreatic duct may occur after an episode of acute pancreatitis[92] and may take months to resolve. Pancreatic carcinoma may produce changes within the pancreatic duct that resemble chronic pancreatitis. Finally, the placement of pancreatic duct stents can produce new abnormalities within the pancreatic duct that mimic chronic pancreatitis,[92, 96, 97] and these changes may not entirely resolve after stent removal.

There is also the potential for substantial inter- and intraobserver variability in the interpretation of pancreatography.[92] This should not be too surprising given the fact that the interpretation of an ERCP is subjective and the abnormal findings may be rather subtle. In one study of 69 pancreatograms submitted to six experienced endoscopists, there was substantial interobserver variation in interpretation.[98] Depending on the observer, between 2% and 58% of these pancreatograms were read as normal. Another study attempted to estimate intraobserver variability by submitting 51 pancreatograms to four expert endoscopists on three separate occasions.[99] The four endoscopists were unanimous in their own three reports in 47% to 95% (up to 53% intraobserver variability). Much of this interobserver and intraobserver variability is related to the interpretation of mild or subtle pancreatographic changes rather than to dramatic abnormalities. This is the most substantial clinical problem related to ERCP as a diagnostic tool; subtle or minor abnormalities of the pancreatic duct are quite nonspecific and are not reliable markers of chronic pancreatitis.

In the majority of patients, ERCP and direct pancreatic function tests reach similar conclusions. This is reassuring, because ERCP is widely available and pancreatic function tests are available at only a few centers. When using ERCP, however, astute clinicians should keep in mind the facts that other conditions may mimic the ductal changes of chronic pancreatitis, and that subtle changes of ductal contour are quite nonspecific.

Endoscopic Ultrasonography

EUS allows a highly detailed examination of the pancreatic parenchyma and pancreatic duct by overcoming the imaging problems with transabdominal ultrasonography (such as intervening gas in the bowel lumen). The diagnosis of chronic pancreatitis by EUS is based on the presence of abnormalities in the pancreatic duct and/or parenchyma. Most studies

Table 49–5 | **Criteria for Diagnosis of Chronic Pancreatitis by Endoscopic Ultrasonography**

PARENCHYMAL ABNORMALITIES	DUCTAL ABNORMALITIES
Hyperechoic foci	Main duct dilation
Hyperechoic strands	Duct irregularity
Lobularity of contour of gland	Hyperechoic ductal margins
Cysts	Dilated side branches
	Stones

have used nine features, four parenchymal and five ductular (Table 49–5). Most studies required at least three criteria, but some have required four or even five. When EUS has been compared with ERCP, the tests agree in about 80% of cases.[100–102] EUS has also been compared with standard and intraductal direct pancreatic function testing. In two studies, the tests agreed in about 75% of patients.[100–102] In two other studies, the agreement was poor.[103, 104] In one of these studies,[104] the sensitivity of EUS for advanced chronic pancreatitis (classic findings on ERCP and an abnormal pancreatic function test) was good, with a sensitivity of 73% and a specificity of 81%; three or more of the EUS criteria were used, as presented in Table 49–5. The sensitivity for less advanced chronic pancreatitis in this same study was only 10%.

In the majority of cases when EUS findings disagree with other diagnostic tests, it is the EUS that is abnormal. What remains to be determined is whether the presence of three or four EUS criteria, in the absence of corroborating information from other diagnostic tests, is adequate to reach a conclusive diagnosis of chronic pancreatitis. This will take prolonged follow-up of these patients, given the lack of a useful gold standard. This may be a substantial conundrum, as EUS changes of chronic pancreatitis are frequently encountered. In one recent study,[105] 39% of patients with dyspepsia had five or more EUS criteria for chronic pancreatitis, and 34% of controls had three or more criteria. Possibly EUS can pick up even subtle normal variation in pancreatic echotexture or can detect pancreatic fibrosis associated with aging or moderate alcohol use in the absence of clinical chronic pancreatitis. Whereas EUS abnormalities are routinely seen in those with advanced chronic pancreatitis (Fig. 49–5), and a normal EUS essentially rules out chronic pancreatitis, the sensitivity and specificity of the test in less advanced chronic pancreatitis require further study.

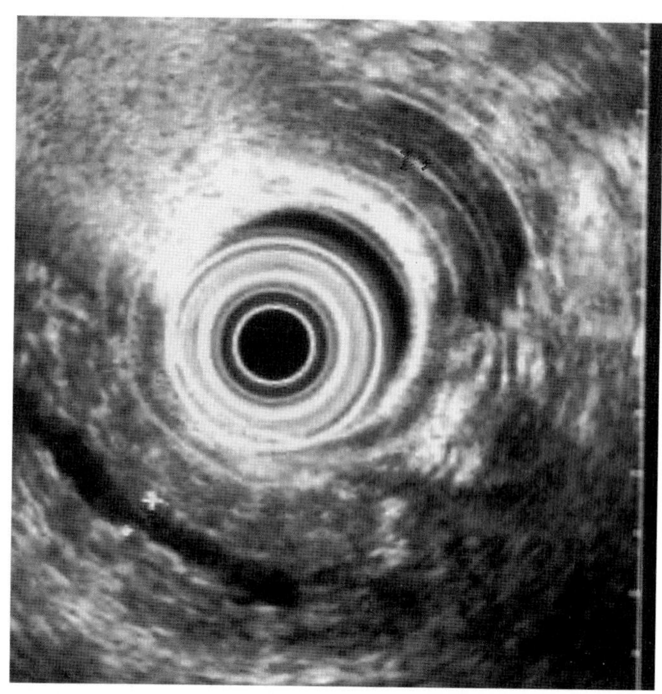

Figure 49–5. An EUS image of the pancreatic body in a patient with chronic pancreatitis. The markers on the dilated (~7 mm) pancreatic duct demonstrate hyperechoic duct margins, one of the diagnostic features of chronic pancreatitis by EUS (see Table 49–5). The parenchyma surrounding these markers demonstrates hyperechoic strands and foci, additional features of chronic pancreatitis.

Diagnostic Strategy

When choosing a diagnostic test or tests, clinicians consider not only sensitivity, specificity, and accuracy but also cost, risk, and availability. When considering chronic pancreatitis, one must also realize that the stage and etiology of the disease determine the accuracy of the diagnostic tests. One should remember that, in many cases, the clinical presentation alone is sufficiently typical to reach a tentative diagnosis, particularly in the case of chronic alcoholic pancreatitis. Each of the diagnostic tests available has strengths and weaknesses. Certain tests are inexpensive and risk free but detect only advanced disease (plain abdominal radiography, serum trypsin, fecal fat, fecal elastase, serum glucose), whereas others are more sensitive but expensive (CT, ERCP, EUS, MRCP), risky (ERCP), or not widely available (direct pancreatic function tests). The diagnostic approach should begin with tests that are safe and inexpensive and that are able to detect relatively far-advanced disease. Diagnostic tests that fit in this category include serum trypsinogen, plain abdominal radiography, and abdominal ultrasonography. If these do not lead to a diagnosis, more sensitive but more risky or expensive tests will need to be employed. The choice of test will depend in large part on availability, but CT is most commonly used as the next test. Direct pancreatic function testing, if available, could logically be used next if CT is nondiagnostic and before more expensive or invasive tests (such as ERCP) are considered. For most clinicians, however, direct pancreatic function testing is not available, and CT and then ERCP are chosen. Care must be taken to avoid overinterpretation of subtle pancreatographic changes revealed by ERCP. Additional research on EUS, MRI, and MRCP is needed to determine their sensitivity and specificity for chronic pancreatitis.

TREATMENT

Abdominal Pain

Pain is the most common symptom of chronic pancreatitis requiring medical care. The initial evaluation of pain should focus on identifying conditions for which specific therapy exists. These conditions include pancreatic pseudocyst, duodenal or bile duct compression, superimposed pancreatic car-

Table 49–6 | **Treatment of Pain**

Apply specific treatment for complications
- Pseudocyst
- Common bile duct obstruction
- Duodenal obstruction
- Gastroparesis

Give analgesics, with or without adjunctive agents (e.g., antidepressants)
Stop alcohol
Decrease intrapancreatic pressure
- Suppress pancreatic secretion (nonenteric-coated pancreatic enzymes coupled with gastric acid suppression, octreotide)
- Relieve ductal obstruction (endoscopic stent or removal of ductal stone, surgical duct decompression)

Modify neural transmission
- Celiac plexus block
- Thoracoscopic splanchnicectomy

Remove pancreatic parenchyma
- Pancreatic head resection (Beger, Frey, or Whipple resection)
- Total or subtotal pancreatectomy

cinoma, and less common conditions such as gastroparesis. This is most often done by performing a CT scan of the abdomen. CT is accurate at identifying fluid collections, pseudocysts, and mass lesions that might be consistent with pancreatic adenocarcinoma. The CT may also suggest duodenal obstruction or bile duct obstruction, although upper gastrointestinal barium radiography or ERCP, respectively, may be needed to define these processes ultimately.

In addition to identifying (or suggesting) the presence of specifically treatable complications, CT can be very useful in identifying patients with substantial abnormalities of pancreatic structure (particularly a dilated pancreatic duct). Identifying these patients with "big-duct" chronic pancreatitis and differentiating them from patients who lack these findings is very helpful in choosing therapy for pain. If one of the specific complications listed earlier is not identified, the clinician is left with choosing more nonspecific therapeutic options (Table 49–6).

Analgesics

The majority of patients with chronic pancreatitis require some form of analgesia. Some patients may be managed with acetaminophen or aspirin, but most require more potent agents, including narcotics. The risk of narcotic addiction in these patients is not defined but is estimated to be about 10% to 30%. Narcotics should not be withheld in patients with severe pain out of a concern for possible addiction, as pain relief is the first priority. Strategies to minimize the risk of overuse of narcotics and addiction include having a single physician take responsibility for prescriptions, ongoing counseling, and regular clinic visits. The use of a dedicated pain clinic is often helpful.

If non-narcotic agents fail, it is useful to begin with the least potent opioid agents, including such agents as propoxyphene napsylate; acetaminophen (Darvocet-N 100) or tramadol (Ultram). Tramadol is a dual-action analgesic, with μ-opioid agonistic and monoaminergic properties (i.e., it weakly blocks reuptake of norepinephrine and serotonin). One randomized trial compared tramadol with morphine in 25 patients with chronic calcific pancreatitis and severe pain.[106] There was no difference in pain relief, and tramadol produced fewer disturbances in orocecal and colonic transit times. The dosages used in this study were substantial, at least twice the dose used commonly in the United States. Despite this, tramadol is an excellent choice of analgesic, with fewer side effects and less potential for abuse and dependence.

More potent narcotics are required in many patients. In this situation, it is useful to increase the dosage and/or potency gradually while focusing the patient on the goal of control of pain to an acceptable level, rather than complete relief of pain. Patients requiring these agents usually benefit from referral to a pain management clinic. Adjunctive agents can also be considered in patients who require more potent narcotics. Many of these patients are depressed, and coexistent depression lowers the pain threshold. Tricyclic antidepressants can be useful adjuncts, not only by treating depression but because they have direct effects on pain and potentiate the effect of narcotics. Other antidepressants such as serotonin reuptake inhibitors (SSRIs) may also have this effect. The drug gabapentin (Neurontin) is not well studied in chronic pancreatitis but is used commonly in patients with chronic pain as an adjunct to narcotics and can be considered in patients with continued severe pain from chronic pancreatitis if other treatment options are not available.

Cessation of Alcohol

It has not been firmly established that abstinence from alcohol reduces pancreatic pain. It is clear that continued alcohol abuse hastens the development of pancreatic dysfunction,[42] although even complete abstinence does not prevent progression. It is also clear that continued alcohol abuse, along with smoking, increases mortality.[16] There are good reasons, therefore, to encourage patients to stop drinking (and smoking!) separate from any effect on abdominal pain. Any analysis of the effect of abstinence on pain is hampered by the fact that most studies are small and retrospective, did not give details on the measurement of pain, and did not confidently determine abstinence. A number of studies, but not all, have documented an apparent decrease in pain or painful relapses in patients who stop drinking. In a summary of these studies,[107] pain continued in 26% of abstinent patients compared with 53% of those who continued to drink. In another natural history study, continued alcohol abuse was associated with a higher risk of painful relapses.[108] These data suggest that abstinence might have some beneficial effect on pain, but the magnitude of the effect is not clearly defined.

Decrease of Oxidative Stress

Damage by oxygen radicals has been proposed as a cause of pain in chronic pancreatitis, and many patients with chronic pancreatitis (particularly alcoholic) may have deficiencies in micronutrients and trace elements that could be considered antioxidants. Small trials of a mixture of antioxidants (selenium, β-carotene, vitamin C, vitamin E, and methionine) have indicated that this therapy may reduce the pain of chronic pancreatitis,[108a] but these observations will require confirmation in larger numbers of patients.

Decrease of Pancreatic Pressure

Suppression of Pancreatic Secretion

The suppression of pancreatic secretion as a method to reduce pain presupposes that augmented secretion is occurring or that normal (or even subnormal) secretion is occurring in the setting of some degree of outflow obstruction. The net effect of such a situation would be to produce some degree of elevation of pancreatic ductal or parenchymal pressure. As discussed earlier, there is evidence in both animal models and humans that increases in pancreatic ductal or tissue pressure are associated with pain and at least some evidence that reduction in pressure is associated with relief or reduction in pain. A number of therapies, including suppressing pancreatic secretion, have as their goal a reduction in pancreatic pressure.

Pancreatic Enzymes

A number of studies have documented that pancreatic proteases present within the duodenum can suppress pancreatic secretion. Diversion of pancreatic juice from the duodenum stimulates the release of CCK from cells in the proximal small bowel and subsequent pancreatic enzyme secretion. Reinstallation of proteases within the duodenum suppresses CCK release and pancreatic secretion. The triggering of CCK release appears to be due to a serine protease–sensitive substance, released by the proximal small intestine, called CCK-releasing factor, or peptide. This peptide is degraded by serine proteases and has been identified in the small intestine of pigs and rats. The peptide is identical to the previously described diazepam-binding inhibitor.[109] In the fasting state, CCK-releasing peptide is thought to be largely destroyed by basal pancreatic secretion of proteases. In this situation, little CCK-releasing peptide escapes, and there is little stimulus for CCK release. After a meal, the serine proteases are competed for by dietary protein, such that CCK-releasing peptide can escape destruction and stimulate the release of CCK, which subsequently stimulates pancreatic secretion. After the meal is digested, dietary proteins no longer compete for serine proteases and the proteases destroy the CCK-releasing peptide, lowering CCK release, and returning pancreatic secretion to its basal state. In this way (along with other physiologic controls of pancreatic secretion), pancreatic enzyme secretion can be turned on for digesting a meal and turned off when this process is completed.

In patients with chronic pancreatitis, the lack of delivery of serine proteases to the duodenum could allow more CCK-releasing peptide to escape denaturing. As a result, one would expect higher levels of CCK-releasing factor within the duodenum and higher plasma levels of CCK. Higher levels of CCK would stimulate the pancreas to secrete, with this strong stimulation possibly leading to pancreatic pain. This might produce pain by raising pancreatic or tissue pressure or by forcing digestive enzymes into the interstitium if secretion is occurring against pancreatic ductal obstruction. The oral administration of pancreatic enzymes could restore normal feedback suppression of pancreatic secretion by providing active serine proteases in the duodenum, which could again denature the CCK-releasing peptide. This might relieve pain. It is clear that pancreatic secretion of volume and bicarbonate is not controlled by the presence of proteases within the duodenum. It is also clear that pancreatic secretion is under both humoral and neural control. Suppressing pancreatic enzyme release by administering oral enzyme supplements is therefore not likely to produce complete suppression of secretion, and the magnitude of the effect on secretion could vary from patient to patient.

The presence of this feedback control system, which can control pancreatic enzyme secretion, is documented in humans without chronic pancreatitis and in some patients with chronic pancreatitis. One marker of this disordered feedback system is elevations in CCK in patients with chronic pancreatitis, particularly in those with pain. Some studies demonstrate elevations in CCK in patients with chronic pancreatitis[110, 111] whereas others do not.[112] It is likely that this disordered feedback, as in all presumed causes of pain, is important only in a subgroup of patients.

Thus far, six randomized prospective double-blind trials have attempted to delineate the effectiveness of orally administered pancreatic enzymes to decrease pain in chronic pancreatitis. Two studies utilizing enzymes in nonenteric-coated (tablet) form reported a benefit.[113, 114] Four other studies using enteric-coated microsphere preparations showed no benefit.[115–118] The difference between these studies may reflect patient selection, but it may also reflect the different choice of enzyme preparations (Table 49–7). The feedback-sensitive part of the small bowel appears to be the most proximal portion, and enteric-coated preparations may not release the majority of their proteases until they reach the more distal small bowel. Nonenteric-coated enzymes might therefore be needed for adequate delivery of proteases to the duodenum.

The randomized trials assessing the effectiveness of pancreatic enzymes for pain are all rather small. High dosages of nonenteric-coated enzymes have been used in these trials (equivalent to 30,000 units of lipase with meals and at night, which has translated to 4 to 8 pills four times daily). Since these agents are inactivated by gastric acid, the concomitant use of an agent to suppress gastric acid is required. In the two studies that demonstrated effectiveness, it appears that those with less advanced disease ("small-duct" chronic pan-

Table 49–7 | **Commercially Available Enzyme Supplements**

SUPPLEMENTS	UNITS OF LIPASE/ PILL OR CAPSULE
Enteric-coated preparations	
Creon 5, 10, 20	5000, 10,000, 20,000, respectively
Pancrease MT 4, MT 10, MT 16, MT 20	4000, 10,000, 16,000, 20,000, respectively
Ultrase MT 12, MT 18, MT 20	4500, 12,000, 18,000, 20,000 respectively
Nonenteric-coated preparations*	
Viokase 8, 16	8000, 16,000, respectively
Generic pancrealipase	8000

*Require concomitant use of agents to suppress gastric acid (H_2 receptor antagonists or proton pump inhibitors).

All brand-name preparations above contain lipase, protease, and amylase.

creatitis without steatorrhea), women, and those with idiopathic chronic pancreatitis had the best response. Despite the lack of proof of clear-cut benefit, a recent consensus review recommended a trial of enzymes for pain, particularly in patients with less advanced disease who have failed other simple medical measures.[119] A trial of enzymes for pain is rarely successful in those with advanced or "big-duct" chronic pancreatitis (mainly advanced alcoholic chronic pancreatitis).

Octreotide

Octreotide, the synthetic analogue of the native hormone somatostatin, decreases pancreatic secretion and reduces plasma CCK levels. This agent, therefore, might reduce pain in chronic pancreatitis via the same mechanisms invoked for the use of enzymes for pain. In addition, octreotide has some direct antinociceptive effect on pain separate from any effect on pancreatic enzyme secretion. Four placebo-controlled studies have been performed to assess the role of octreotide. Three small studies utilizing dosages of from 100 to 250 μg thrice daily reached contradictory results.[119] A larger multicenter study compared three different dosage regimens in a dose-ranging analysis but also included a placebo group.[120] Although the goal of this study was to determine the appropriate dose for subsequent studies rather than to determine efficacy, it is possible to compare outcome in each dosage group compared with placebo. Due to the nature of the study design, statistically significant differences were not anticipated, but the group randomized to 200 μg subcutaneously three times daily had the strongest trend toward pain relief (average 60% to 65% pain relief, versus 35% to 40% for placebo). These studies do not establish the effectiveness of this drug, and additional studies will be required. Even more important, this trial demonstrated that the placebo response in these patients can average 35% to 40%, which serves to emphasize the importance of placebo-controlled trials in these patients.

Endoscopic Therapy

The general goal of endoscopic therapy is to improve drainage of the pancreatic duct by relieving obstruction. In the setting of ductal obstruction, pancreatic ductal pressures would be expected to be increased. The expected effect of endoscopic decompression of the pancreatic duct is to reduce pressures and concomitantly reduce pain. The potential application of endoscopic therapy is limited to a subgroup of patients with amenable pancreatic ductal anatomy. These are patients with "big-duct" chronic pancreatitis with advanced structural abnormalities of the pancreatic duct. For the most part, this has meant patients with a dilated pancreatic duct who also have a single dominant stricture or obstructing stone in the head of the pancreas, with dilation of the pancreatic duct upstream of the stone or stricture. It is important to remember, however, that many patients with pancreatic duct dilation have little or no clinical symptoms, and that a dilated duct appearance does not necessarily correlate with elevations in duct pressure. Strictures and calculi in the body or tail of the gland generally are not amenable to endoscopic therapy and are not discussed further here. Specific endoscopic therapies that have been studied include stent placement, stone extraction, and pancreatic sphincterotomy. The individual contribution of each of these therapies is impossible to quantify as they are often performed together. There are few placebo-controlled trials of endoscopic therapy.

Stent Therapy

Stent placement in the pancreatic duct is most often performed to bypass an obstructing calculus or stricture. A number of uncontrolled studies of stent therapy for a dominant stricture of the pancreatic duct reported pain improvement in about two thirds of patients.[121–125] Complications of therapy occurred in about 20%, with a mortality rate of 0.6%.[125] Complications most commonly reported relate to clogging of stents (producing recurrent pain, attacks of acute pancreatitis, or pancreatic sepsis), stent migration (which may require surgical extraction), and ductal perforation. Follow-up in these studies was generally less than 2 years. It would be assumed that those who respond to stent placement have high intraductal pressures and that stent therapy reduced this pressure. In one study that measured pain relief and pancreatic duct pressure after stenting, three of nine patients with normal pressure at the end of the stenting period still had pain, whereas none of four of those with continued high pressure in the pancreatic duct still had pain.[63] It is not clear that the response to stent therapy is predictable based on measurements of intraductal pressure, and the mechanism of pain relief requires further study.

The long-term management of these patients undergoing endoscopic stent therapy remains controversial. In the few studies that have examined it, about 40% of patients had resolution of the stricture after stent removal.[125] The correlation between improvement in pancreatic ductal appearance and symptom improvement is not exact, and the pancreatic duct appearance may worsen, improve, or stay the same. Symptoms may also recur after initial clinical response. About half of patients who had initially responded to stent therapy had a recurrence of symptoms over 1 to 2 years of follow-up.[122, 124] Whether long-term stent therapy with progressively larger stents will improve outcome is unknown, and the risk of such an approach remains unstudied.

In addition to the complications of pancreatic duct stenting just noted, changes reminiscent of chronic pancreatitis have been noted within the pancreatic duct that appear to be induced by stenting. These develop in about half of patients undergoing long-term pancreatic duct stenting.[92, 96, 97] The significance of these changes is not known. Changes within the pancreatic parenchyma after stenting have also been noted on EUS imaging in similar proportions of patients.[97] These studies have assessed patients with relatively normal-appearing pancreatic ducts prior to stenting. These stent-induced changes within the pancreatic duct in a patient with advanced preexisting structural abnormalities presumably are of less clinical consequence than damaging a previously normal pancreatic duct.

Pancreatic Duct Stone Removal

The endoscopic removal of pancreatic duct stones can be difficult and is possible only in a subset of patients. Those with multiple stones, stones in the body and tail of the pancreatic duct, impacted stones, or stones behind a pancreatic duct stricture generally are not manageable by endoscopic techniques. The removal of large stones often will require lithotripsy with extracorporeal or intraductal instruments. There is not a close correlation between the presence of pancreatic duct stones and pain, so many patients with pancreatic ductal stones have no pain. Most series reported success rates in carefully selected patients in whom endoscopic stone extraction seems feasible. A number of uncontrolled case series reported overall success at complete stone clearance in an average of 60% of patients.[125] Clinical improvement was seen in about 75%. The rate of symptom improvement is thus greater than the rate of complete stone clearance. Follow-up has been relatively short, between 6 and 44 months. In one recent study, 20% of patients referred for endoscopic therapy of chronic pancreatitis had ductal anatomy that allowed stone extraction.[126] Of these, half had complete clearance of ductal stones, although 95% of treated patients had complete or partial pain relief. After a mean follow-up of 2 years, less than half of the initial responders continued to have pain relief. Stones may recur after successful extraction in up to 25% of patients. Complications of stone removal occur, on average, in less than 20% of patients.[125]

Pancreatic Duct Sphincterotomy

Pancreatic duct sphincterotomy is routinely used in association with stent placement and is required for pancreatic duct stone extraction. Major papilla pancreatic sphincterotomy alone as a therapy would be applicable only in patients in whom long-standing cicatricial stenosis of the sphincter produces obstructive chronic pancreatitis. This form of chronic pancreatitis is rare, but some investigators have postulated that sphincter of Oddi hypertension might also predispose to chronic pancreatitis. Some studies have documented abnormalities of sphincter of Oddi function in patients with chronic pancreatitis whereas others have not, and this remains controversial. Surgical teaching and experience certainly discourage treatment of the sphincter alone as an effective strategy for pain control. Very rarely, patients with pancreas divisum will present with marked upstream dilation of the dorsal pancreatic duct and chronic pancreatitis. Sphincterotomy of the minor papilla for obstructive chronic pancreatitis in this setting may be useful, but minor papilla sphincterotomy for chronic pain in the absence of pancreatic ductal dilation is ineffective.[127]

Lacking controlled clinical trials, the overall efficacy and risk of endoscopic therapies for chronic pancreatitis are not defined. It is clear that only a subset of patients with chronic pancreatitis and specific ductal anatomy are even candidates for endoscopic therapy. These therapies should be considered only in patients with amenable anatomy and only in centers with substantial expertise in these techniques, hopefully as part of a randomized clinical study.

Surgical Therapy

Surgical therapy is most commonly considered for intractable abdominal pain that has failed medical therapy. Other indications for surgery in these patients include complications involving adjacent organs (duodenal, splenic vein, or biliary obstruction), pseudocysts failing endoscopic or radiologic management, internal pancreatic fistulas, and exclusion of malignancy despite an extensive work-up. The surgical approaches for these complications are discussed later, in "Complications." Surgical options for pain can include pancreatic ductal drainage, resection of all or part of the pancreas, or both. The choice of surgical procedure depends in large part on the ductal anatomy, presumed pathogenesis of pain, and associated complications, as well as local surgical preferences and expertise.

Ductal drainage procedures are the least technically demanding and preserve the most pancreatic parenchyma. The rationale for these procedures is to relieve ductal obstruction and reduce pancreatic pressures, thereby relieving pain. Pancreatic ductal drainage procedures generally require dilation of the pancreatic duct to greater than 7 mm, a size that allows relatively easy duct identification and enteric anastomosis. This operation is therefore considered in patients with "big-duct" chronic pancreatitis as documented by CT, ERCP, or other imaging procedure. The most commonly performed procedure is the lateral pancreaticojejunostomy, or modified Puestow procedure. In this procedure, the pancreatic duct is opened longitudinally and anastomosed to a defunctionalized limb of small bowel, which is connected with a Roux-en-Y anastomosis. This Roux-en-Y limb can also be used to decompress any pseudocysts that are present. At the time of the operation, any ductal strictures can be incised and any ductal stones that are present can be readily removed. The procedure can be technically performed in the absence of a dilated pancreatic duct ("normal duct" Puestow) but the efficacy for relieving pain is believed to be far less. The operative mortality of a modified Puestow procedure is extremely low.

No randomized trials exist comparing a modified Puestow procedure with other therapies. Immediate pain relief is seen in 80% of patients.[59, 119, 128–130] With long term follow-up, only 40% to 50% continue to experience pain relief.[119, 128–131] The explanation for this decline in effectiveness is unknown but may reflect closure of the anastomosis, pain originating in the undrained segments of the head of the pancreas, or the development of other sources of pain (neural inflammation, duodenal or bile duct obstruction, and so on). There is thus a trade-off between the simplicity and lack of risk of this procedure and the gradual deterioration of results over time. Exocrine and endocrine function are generally unaffected by this surgical procedure but appear to continue to deteriorate as in unoperated patients. A single study suggested that ductal drainage preserved pancreatic exocrine and endocrine function, but this has not been confirmed.[130] I have few data on overall quality of life after surgery. In one study, long-term pain relief was seen in 42% but only 24% of patients characterized their health status as "good," 42% continued to drink to excess, and 73% were unemployed.[129] The consequences of continued alcohol abuse, progression of underlying disease, and other medical conditions, rather than side effects of surgery, explain the relatively poor overall outcome.

In an attempt to overcome the modest early and substantial late failure rate of simple drainage procedures, approaches combining resection of the pancreas with drainage of the pancreatic duct have been developed. These have focused particularly on the head of the pancreas. A routine longitudinal pancreaticojejunostomy does not completely decompress the ducts in the head of the gland, the accessory duct of Santorini, and the small ducts draining the uncinate process. Similarly, many patients may have an associated inflammatory mass of the head of the pancreas, which makes drainage of the pancreatic duct within the head of the pancreas more difficult. Options to deal with this have included resection of the head of the pancreas (Whipple operation or duodenum-preserving Whipple operation) or a combination of ductal drainage with local resection of all or part of the pancreatic head. It should be noted that improved pain relief after these surgical procedures involving pancreatic resection may be partially explained by the denervation of visceral pancreatic afferents during more extensive dissection, rather than improved drainage of the pancreatic ducts in the head of the pancreas.

After a Whipple or duodenum-preserving Whipple resection, 65% to 95% of patients experience pain relief.[119, 132, 133] Whipple operations are generally considered in patients with disease limited to the head of the pancreas, particularly those with a large inflammatory mass of the pancreas in whom malignancy is also being considered. Associated biliary or duodenal obstruction, seen more commonly in these patients with inflammatory masses of the head of the pancreas, can also be dealt with at resection. These operations have higher morbidity and mortality than simple ductal drainage operations. Although the mortality in high-volume centers is less than 2%, early postoperative complications (primarily disruptions of normal motility and pancreatic duct leaks) can occur in up to 50%.[132]

Two procedures have been developed to resect all or part of the head of the pancreas, without the disruptions of gastrointestinal physiology seen with traditional Whipple operations. In the Frey procedure (named after its originator), the majority of the head of the pancreas is removed, coring out the anterior surface of the head of the pancreas but leaving a shell of pancreatic head around the duodenum, bile duct, and peripancreatic vessels.[134] This is coupled with a longitudinal incision of the pancreatic duct in the body and tail of the pancreas and the overlaying of a long jejunal anastomosis covering both the opened duct and the cored-out head. A second operation, the duodenum-preserving resection of the head of the pancreas, or Beger operation (again named after its originator), involves a more complete excision of the pancreatic head but again leaves undisturbed the duodenum, bile duct, and peripancreatic vessels.[135] These two procedures appear to have equivalent efficacy in experienced hands,[136, 137] and both have better rates of short- and long-term pain relief than a modified Puestow procedure, but at a cost of modest increases in operative morbidity and mortality.

More substantial pancreatic resection is rarely performed. In some patients with disease limited to the body and tail of the pancreas, typically after trauma to the pancreatic duct in the body of the pancreas with upstream obstructive chronic pancreatitis, resection of the body and tail may be considered. Near-total pancreatectomy is associated with unacceptable complications of severe diabetes. Improvements in islet cell transplantation might make this procedure more feasible in the future, perhaps as an alternative in refractory, painful "small-duct" chronic pancreatitis when other surgical procedures are not possible or in hereditary pancreatitis to prevent the development of malignancy.

The complications occurring after surgery for chronic pancreatitis vary with the operation chosen and include pancreatic fistula, wound infection, delayed gastric emptying, intra-abdominal abscess, pancreatitis, cholangitis, and bile leak.[133] The pre- and perioperative use of octreotide may reduce the risk of these postoperative complications, particularly pancreatic fistula.

When evaluating patients after surgery for chronic pancreatitis, it is important to remember that exocrine and endocrine insufficiency can develop both as a consequence of the surgery and of the ongoing disease process. Exocrine insufficiency in particular may escape detection, because symptoms may be mild. Steatorrhea can develop in 30% to 40% of patients undergoing simple drainage procedures and in up to 66% of those undergoing pancreatic resections.[132, 133, 137] The use of pancreatic enzyme supplements after pancreatic surgery leads to improved absorption of nutrients and should be considered for most (or all) patients after surgery for chronic pancreatitis. The development of endocrine insufficiency after pancreatic surgery is also common[133] but not invariable, and some series have even noted improvements in glucose tolerance in some patients after surgery. In general, however, diabetes mellitus still occurs after surgery, either as a consequence of pancreatic resection or from the ongoing ravages of the disease.

Interrupting Neural Transmission

The celiac plexus transmits visceral afferent impulses from the upper abdominal organs, including the pancreas. The greater, lesser, and least splanchnic nerves synapse in the celiac plexus, and these nerve fibers pass through the diaphragm to reach the spinal cord. Pancreatic nerves are sensitive to a wide variety of noxious stimuli, and it has been suggested that repeated stimulation of these nerves produces a centrally sensitized pain state, in which the threshold for stimulation is lowered and the response to stimulation is prolonged and enhanced.[138] Attempts to block the transmission of nociceptive stimuli have met with limited success.

Celiac plexus block is used rarely in patients with chronic pancreatitis, due to its very transitory effectiveness. Percutaneous injections of either alcohol or steroids have been used. In small uncontrolled studies,[119] 25% to 50% experience pain relief, which lasts on average 2 to 4 months. Repeated injections may not be effective, and the use of repeated neuroablative injections (e.g., alcohol) is discouraged owing to a risk of paraplegia. Celiac plexus block using EUS guidance may be somewhat more long-lasting than that delivered under CT guidance,[139] but the effect of even EUS-guided celiac plexus block appears to be too transitory for long-term management.

Interfering with nerve transmission through the splanchnic nerves can also block central perception of nociceptive inputs. This generally involves bilateral sectioning of the greater splanchnic nerves. Thoracotomy was used for this procedure in the past, but more recently it has been performed through a thoracoscopic approach. In a few small studies,[138, 140] an average of 50% of patients experienced pain relief after thoracoscopic splanchnicectomy. Significant complications are rare. These initial studies suggest that this therapy may be an alternative in patients who have failed medical therapy, particularly in that group with "small-duct" chronic pancreatitis in whom surgical ductal drainage procedures are not possible.

Choosing Treatment for Pain

The choice of a particular therapy for pain in chronic pancreatitis may depend on the etiology of chronic pancreatitis, the severity of the symptoms, the pancreatic ductal anatomy, and local availability of specific therapies. Few therapies have been studied in placebo-controlled trials of adequate sample size, and advocates of specific therapies often forget the substantial placebo response of 35% to 40% that can be seen in these patients.[120] The following recommendations reflect my opinion, but these are quite similar to the recommendations of a recent technical review of the topic.[119]

The first step is to make sure that the diagnosis is correct. This is straightforward in patients with advanced structural and functional derangements of the pancreas but may be difficult in patients with "small-duct" chronic pancreatitis. Administering therapy that may carry risk (i.e., celiac plexus block) without a secure diagnosis is inappropriate. If the diagnosis is secure, the second step is to search for complications and associated conditions that have specific therapy. These include pseudocysts, biliary or duodenal obstruction, coexistent pancreatic carcinoma, peptic ulcer disease, or gastroparesis. Medical therapy is appropriate in all patients and should include a low-fat diet, analgesics (non-narcotic if possible but, if not, narcotics coupled with adjunctive agents such as antidepressants), and abstinence from alcohol (if applicable). It is also worthwhile to have the patient monitor the severity and timing of pain for comparison with subsequent therapeutic response.

Failure of these simple medical therapies is not uncommon. The choice of subsequent therapy depends on differentiating "small-duct" from "large-duct" chronic pancreatitis. In those with "small-duct" chronic pancreatitis, a trial of high-dose nonenteric-coated enzyme preparations with an agent to suppress gastric acid (H_2 receptor antagonist or proton pump inhibitor) is reasonable. Enzyme therapy for pain in patients with advanced structural abnormalities (dilated pancreatic duct, diffuse calcifications) or advanced functional abnormalities (exocrine or endocrine insufficiency) is rarely effective. Treatment options for pain in patients with "big-duct" chronic pancreatitis are largely mechanical, attempting to improve ductal drainage with either endoscopic or surgical techniques. Endoscopic therapy is probably effective in a subgroup of patients with amenable ductal anatomy and in centers with appropriate expertise. In those patients with ductal anatomy not conducive to endoscopic therapy or in those who fail endoscopic therapy, surgical duct decompression with or without pancreatic resection offers the best option. In those patients with "small-duct" chronic pancreatitis, endoscopic therapy is impossible and surgical options are less attractive, often requiring extensive pancreatic resections. In these patients, octreotide is worthy of consideration, and attempts at nerve ablation can be considered in those failing medical therapy. Pancreatic resections are considered as a last resort in both groups of patients.

Maldigestion and Steatorrhea

It has been estimated that delivery of 30,000 units of lipase to the intestine with each meal should be sufficient to reduce steatorrhea to a clinically insignificant level. It would seem relatively straightforward to achieve this goal with the use of enzyme supplements but a number of factors limit the effectiveness of commercially available enzyme supplements. Much of the lipase in the nonenteric-coated supplements may not reach the small bowel in an active form, being denatured by gastric acid or destroyed by proteases. Most commercially available enteric-coated enzyme preparations use a microsphere size that is too big to empty from the stomach in synchrony with the food. These enteric-coated microspheres also may not release their enzyme contents until they reach the distal jejunum or ileum, too distal for efficient digestion and absorption. Finally, many of the enzyme preparations are of relatively low potency (see Table 49–7), so many pills or tablets must be taken. This can have a major negative influence on compliance. These factors can all interfere with the effective treatment of steatorrhea.

The first principle of managing steatorrhea is to administer 30,000 units of lipase in the prandial and postprandial portion of each meal. If nonenteric-coated preparations are chosen, concomitant suppression of gastric acid with an H_2 receptor antagonist or proton pump inhibitor is necessary (see Chapter 38 for doses). The effectiveness of enzyme supplementation is generally gauged by clinical parameters, including improvement in stool consistency, loss of visible fat in the stool, and gain in weight. Performing a 72-hour fecal fat analysis prior to and during therapy, to prove effectiveness, is rarely needed but can be considered in those who fail to respond as expected.

There are several common explanations for *failure of enzyme therapy* for steatorrhea. The most common is inadequate dose, generally due to patient noncompliance with the number of pills that must be taken. Changing to a more potent preparation to reduce the number of pills that must be taken is often helpful. It is also appropriate to make sure that an acid suppression agent has been prescribed and is being taken by patients on nonenteric-coated preparations. If the desired effect is not achieved, using more frequent, smaller meals may be helpful. It is occasionally useful to change from one formulation to another (e.g., changing from enteric-coated preparations to a combination of a nonenteric-coated plus an agent to suppress acid) or to increase the dosage above 30,000 units of lipase per meal if the response is still not satisfactory. If all these fail to achieve the desired effect, it is appropriate to search for alternative diagnoses that could also produce malabsorption, such as celiac sprue or small bowel bacterial overgrowth.[141] Finally, if all these measures fail, one can replace dietary fat with medium-chain triglycerides, which do not require lipolysis (and hence lipase) for absorption.

Diabetes Mellitus

Diabetes mellitus is an independent predictor of mortality in patients with chronic pancreatitis. Morbidity and mortality due to diabetes mellitus may occur from progressive microangiopathic complications or from more dramatic complications such as treatment-induced hypoglycemia (in those with inadequate glucagon reserve). Ketoacidosis is distinctly unusual. This may be due to the fact that insulin secretion is not entirely lost while glucagon secretion is reduced. Both effects tend to reduce the risk of ketoacidosis.

Given the risk of treatment-induced hypoglycemia and the difficulty of close follow-up in patients who continue to abuse alcohol, therapy is usually directed at controlling urinary losses of glucose rather than tight control of blood sugar. Some patients will respond to the use of oral hypoglycemics, including sulfonylureas, thiozolidenediones, and metformin. Insulin is often needed, but patients with chronic pancreatitis have lower insulin requirements than patients with type I diabetes mellitus. Overvigorous attempts at tight control are often associated with disastrous complications of treatment-induced hypoglycemia.[73] Attempts at tight control of blood sugar are indicated in one subgroup: those with hyperlipidemic pancreatitis, since the diabetes in this group is usually a primary illness, and tight control of blood sugar improves hyperlipidemia.[51] In long-standing diabetes, appropriate monitoring for nephropathy, retinopathy, and neuropathy is indicated.

Table 49–8 | **Cystic Collections Within the Pancreas**

Pseudocyst (70%–90%)
Cystic neoplasms (10%–15%)
Mucinous cystic neoplasms (cystadenoma and cystadenocarcinoma)
Serous cystadenomas
Intraductal papillary mucinous tumor (formerly, mucinous ductal ectasia)
Papillary cystic neoplasms
Rare neoplasms (acinar cell cystadenocarcinoma, choriocarcinoma, teratoma)
Neoplasms that may appear cystic rarely (islet cell tumors, adenocarcinoma)
True cysts (rare)
Polycystic disease of the pancreas (isolated, associated with polycystic disease of the kidneys, or associated with Von Hippel–Lindau disease)
Simple true cyst
Dermoid cyst
Miscellaneous cystic lesions (exceedingly rare)
Lymphoepithelial cyst
Endometrial cyst
Macrocysts associated with cystic fibrosis
Retention cyst
Parasitic cyst (echinococcus or *Taenia solium*)

COMPLICATIONS

Pancreatic Pseudocyst

Pseudocysts occur in about 25% of patients with chronic pancreatitis[33–35, 55] and are most common in alcoholic chronic pancreatitis. The most common symptom associated with a pseudocyst is abdominal pain, which occurs in 70% to 90% of patients. Less common presentations include a palpable mass, nausea and vomiting (due to compression of the stomach or duodenum), jaundice (due to compression of the bile duct), or bleeding. Elevations in serum levels of pancreatic enzymes are found in at least half these patients, and a persistent elevation in serum amylase can be a clue to the presence of a pseudocyst. The diagnosis of pseudocyst is generally easily made by imaging studies, including US, CT, MRI, or even EUS. The advantage of CT in this setting is that the capsule can be visualized, which can be used to gauge the maturity of the collection, and the relation of the pseudocyst to the stomach and duodenum can be ascertained, which can be useful in choosing therapy. ERCP is usually not required for diagnostic purposes, although around 70% of pseudocysts communicate with the pancreatic duct. ERCP is associated with an approximately 15% chance of infecting a previously uninfected pseudocyst, so ERCP should be undertaken only after giving antibiotics and only if pseudocyst therapy is imminent.

The natural history of pseudocysts complicating chronic pancreatitis is not fully defined. Overall, complications of pseudocysts occur in 5% to 41% of cases.[142–148] In one study of 75 patients with pseudocysts, around half could be managed conservatively; the size of the pseudocyst was the most important predictor of the need for intervention.[144] Only 40% of pseudocysts smaller than 6 cm required therapy, compared with 67% of those greater than 6 cm. A second retrospective analysis included 68 patients without pseudocyst complications or severe symptoms treated conservatively and followed for a mean of 46 months.[145] Complications occurred in 9%, and 19% ultimately required specific therapy. As in the previous study, those with larger pseudocysts were more likely to develop complications or require therapy. These studies suggest that patients with mature pseudocysts smaller than 6 cm and minimal symptoms may be managed conservatively if appropriate follow-up is possible (i.e., the patients are not active alcoholics). In the absence of these features, pseudocyst therapy is indicated. Unlike the acute fluid collections associated with acute pancreatitis (see Chapter 48), pseudocysts occurring in the setting of chronic pancreatitis are generally mature at diagnosis.[142] This can usually be appreciated on CT as a visible capsule around the collection.

Pseudocysts account for 90% of all cystic collections associated with the pancreas, but not all cystic collections seen on CT are pseudocysts. A number of other cystic collections can mimic the appearance of a pseudocyst, in particular cystic neoplasms (Table 49–8). Cystic neoplasms are often discovered when a CT scan or US is performed for vague abdominal symptoms or for other reasons. About one third of all cystic neoplasms have malignant potential. The appropriate therapy of these lesions is resection (not drainage as for a pseudocyst). Cystic neoplasms should be suspected when a mildly symptomatic or asymptomatic fluid collection is discovered in a patient (usually a middle-aged woman) with neither a history of pancreatitis nor risk factors for pancreatitis.[146, 147] The finding of internal septations or nodules within the wall of the collection is also highly suggestive of a cystic neoplasm[146] (Fig 49–6). The features that can assist in differentiation of a pseudocyst from a cystic neoplasm are outlined in Table 49–9. These neoplasms are generally curable and should not be mistaken for pseudocysts, even if laparotomy is required to differentiate the two.[147] Cystic neoplasms are discussed in further detail in Chapter 50.

Symptomatic, complicated, or enlarging pseudocysts require therapy that can be percutaneous, endoscopic, or surgical. Surgical therapy has been used most extensively and

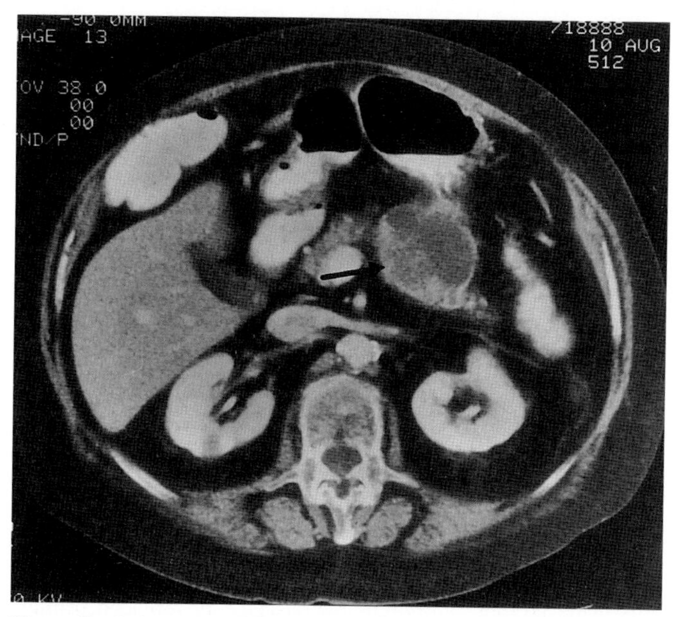

Figure 49–6. A cystic neoplasm is seen in the tail of the pancreas in an elderly female patient with no history of pancreatic disease. The loculations and mural nodules seen within the cavity *(arrow)* are most suggestive of a cystic neoplasm rather than a pseudocyst. The appropriate therapy is resection, not drainage.

Table 49–9 | **Differentiating Pancreatic Pseudocyst from Cystic Neoplasms of the Pancreas**

FEATURE	PSEUDOCYST	CYSTIC NEOPLASM
Gender	More commonly male	Usually female
Mean age	30–40 yr	60–70 yr
Alcohol abuse	Yes	No
History of acute or chronic pancreatitis	Yes	No
Ultrasound or computed tomography	Unilocular, no solid component, associated gland calcification	Uni- or multilocular, solid component, rim calcification of cyst
ERCP	Communication with duct in 70%	Rare communication with duct
Cyst fluid		
Amylase	High	Low
CEA	Low	Low or high
Cytology	Inflammatory cells	Glycogen- or mucin-containing cells, malignant cells
Biopsy of wall	Granulation tissue	Epithelial lining

CEA, carcinoembryonic antigen.

usually involves cyst decompression into a loop of small bowel or stomach; this is often coupled with a pancreatic ductal drainage procedure (e.g., modified Puestow procedure). Surgical therapy has a long-term success rate of 90% and an operative mortality of less than 3%.[144, 145, 148] Although pseudocysts recur in only about 10% of cases, pain may recur in up to half as noted by long-term follow-up.[148]

Percutaneous tube (catheter) drainage of pseudocysts is possible if a safe tract to the collection can be identified. Percutaneous drainage of pancreatic pseudocysts complicating chronic pancreatitis has been discouraged owing to the widely held view that these are associated with ductal obstruction downstream from the fluid collection and that the risk of fistula formation along the tract and pseudocyst recurrence after removal of the tube would be unacceptably high. The long-term success of percutaneous drainage is still unknown but is certainly less than with surgical techniques. Most early series reported an initial success rate of 85% or greater, with recurrence rates of less than 10%. Complications occurred in less than 10% to 15% and included bleeding, infection of the cavity, or formation of a draining fistula along the tube tract. Several more recent studies have suggested that the failure rate may be higher on long-term follow-up.[149, 150] No prospective studies exist comparing surgical with percutaneous therapy. In some reports, the addition of octreotide may hasten resolution and perhaps increase overall success rates. Failure of percutaneous tube drainage, particularly recurrence after tube removal and cutaneous fistula at the tract site, is most common in those with a stricture of the pancreatic duct downstream from the connection of the pseudocyst to the pancreatic duct.[151] ERCP can be used to identify patients with pancreatic duct strictures who may do less well with percutaneous drainage. Although not done routinely at all centers, ERCP prior to attempts at percutaneous drainage of a pseudocyst is quite reasonable.

Recurrence of a symptomatic pseudocyst after tube removal generally requires surgical therapy. The management of a chronic draining pancreaticocutaneous fistula is discussed later, in "Pancreatic Fistula."

Endoscopic therapy of pseudocysts is possible if the fluid collection can be accessed through the papilla or through the wall of the stomach or duodenum. The route chosen depends on the location of the pseudocyst. Success rates of 70% to 90% are reported in small numbers of highly selected patients, with complications reported in 10% to 20%. Most complications are related to transmural stent placement and include bleeding (which may be massive), perforation, and infection of previously uninfected collections. Antibiotic coverage and readily available surgical backup are essential if endoscopic therapy is undertaken. Perhaps half of all pseudocysts are amenable to endoscopic therapy.[152] The long-term success rate of endoscopic therapy is unknown.

Bleeding

Gastrointestinal bleeding in the setting of chronic pancreatitis may develop from a variety of causes. Some are not specific for chronic pancreatitis, such as a Mallory-Weiss tear, esophagitis, peptic ulcer disease, or varices from concomitant alcoholic cirrhosis. Others occur as a direct result of the pancreatic process, most notably bleeding from a pancreatic pseudocyst, a pseudoaneurysm, or portal or splenic vein thrombosis.

Pseudocyst Wall

Bleeding may originate from the wall of a pseudocyst. Bleeding from small vessels (vein, capillary, or arteriole) in the wall can lead to expansion of the pseudocyst and further rupture of these small vessels.[153] Blood may remain in the

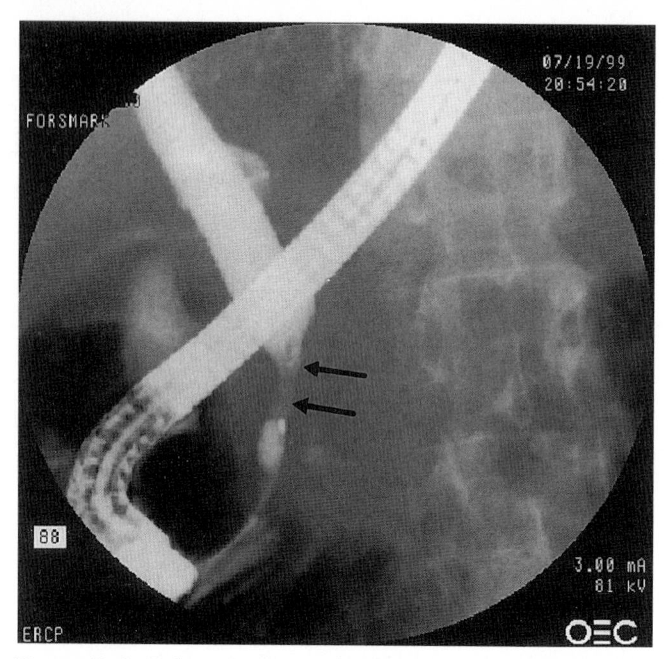

Figure 49–7. Endoscopic retrograde cholangiogram demonstrating a smooth stricture of the common bile duct *(arrows)* as it passes through the head of the pancreas.

pseudocyst; it may decompress spontaneously into the gut, or it may reach the duodenum through the pancreatic duct (hemosuccus pancreaticus). Bleeding from small vessels in the wall of the pseudocyst is generally of low volume.

Pseudoaneurysms

Pseudoaneurysms form as a consequence of enzymatic and pressure digestion of the muscular wall of an artery by a pseudocyst. The pseudoaneurysm may rupture into the pseudocyst (converting the pseudocyst into a larger pseudoaneurysm) or may rupture directly into an adjacent viscus, the peritoneal cavity, or the pancreatic duct. Pseudoaneurysmal bleeding may complicate 5% to 10% of all cases of chronic pancreatitis with pseudocysts, although pseudoaneurysms may be seen in up to 21% of patients with chronic pancreatitis undergoing angiography.[153] Many visceral arteries may be involved, but the splenic artery is most common. Once bleeding occurs, the mortality is 40% to 60%, related both to the severity of the blood loss and the presence of coexistent conditions.[153] Although death from a pseudocyst is rare, more than half the overall mortality of pseudocysts is due to hemorrhage.

Bleeding from a pseudoaneurysm may be slow and intermittent or acute and massive. Common presentations include abdominal pain (due to the enlargement of the pseudocyst), unexplained anemia, or gastrointestinal bleeding (if the blood can reach the gut lumen through the pseudocyst or via the pancreatic duct). In many cases, an initial self-limited bleed occurs, followed hours or days later with a massive exsanguinating hemorrhage. The initial self-limited bleed may be due to transient tamponade of the bleeding within the confines of the pseudocyst. The presence of unexplained blood loss or any degree of gastrointestinal bleeding in a patient with pancreatitis or a known pseudocyst should immediately raise the possibility of a pseudoaneurysm. If a pseudoaneurysm is suspected in the setting of upper gastrointestinal blood loss, an urgent upper endoscopy should be undertaken. If no obvious bleeding site is seen, consideration should be given to the possibility of pseudoaneurysm formation. Rarely, blood may be seen issuing from the ampulla (hemosuccus pancreaticus), but the absence of this finding does not rule out pseudoaneurysm.

The next step in the evaluation should be a CT scan. The finding of high-density material within a pseudocyst on noncontrast images is highly suggestive of a pseudoaneurysm, which can be confirmed by the presence of a centrally opacifying structure within the low-attenuation pseudocyst after the administration of intravenous contrast. It is prudent to avoid oral contrast so that it will not interfere with angiography if required. In most centers, such a CT finding is followed urgently by angiography to define and embolize the pseudoaneurysm. Once a pseudoaneurysm has been identified, it should be treated whether or not it has caused bleeding. Angiographic embolization has largely replaced primary surgery, with surgery reserved for failure of embolization.

Variceal Bleeding from Splenic Vein Thrombosis

Variceal bleeding may complicate patients with chronic pancreatitis owing to associated alcoholic cirrhosis or thrombosis of the splenic (and less commonly portal) vein. Thrombosis of the splenic vein is most common and produces a segmental or left-sided portal hypertension. Decompression of splenic venous outflow occurs through the short gastric veins to the coronary vein, producing prominent variceal channels in the gastric cardia and fundus. Depending on the venous anatomy, esophageal varices may also be produced, but these are generally smaller than the gastric varices.[153] The natural history of gastric varices in this setting is not known, but the overall risk of bleeding is less than with esophageal varices due to cirrhosis. Therapy is not required in the absence of bleeding, and it is not unreasonable to withhold therapy until bleeding has been documented. Should bleeding occur, splenectomy is curative.

Common Bile Duct Obstruction

The distal common bile duct is enclosed within the posterior portion of the head of the pancreas. Inflammatory and fibrotic conditions of the head of the pancreas, as well as pseudocysts in this location, can compress this intrapancreatic common bile duct, leading to abnormal liver chemistry studies, jaundice, biliary pain, or cholangitis. Symptomatic common bile duct obstruction occurs in about 10% of patients. The ductal stricture can be suspected based on a combination of cholestatic liver chemistry determinations and/or biliary ductal dilation on CT or US. ERCP characteristically demonstrates a long, tapered stenosis of the distal bile duct (Fig. 49–7).

The occurrence of cholangitis is an absolute indication for therapy. The presence of abnormal liver chemistry studies and jaundice is not so straightforward, since most of these patients are alcoholics, and alcoholic (and other intrinsic) liver disease can also produce substantial abnormalities in liver studies. The clinical, biochemical, and even radiologic features are not sufficient to distinguish biliary stenosis from intrinsic liver disease.[154] For this reason, liver biopsy is recommended prior to making a decision on therapy.

With the exception of cholangitis, guidelines for therapy remain unclear. The mere presence of a stenosis of the intrapancreatic bile duct, in the absence of symptoms or progressive abnormalities in liver chemistry studies, can usually be followed conservatively. If there is a concern for the development of secondary biliary cirrhosis, a liver biopsy should be performed. Patients with increasing jaundice or biliary pain, in the absence of alternative explanations (i.e., intrinsic liver disease) should be considered for therapy.

Therapy usually requires surgical biliary bypass, either with a cholecystojejunostomy or choledochojejunostomy. A recent small study suggested that hepatic fibrosis may actually decrease after successful surgical decompression.[155] Endoscopic therapy for biliary obstruction due to chronic pancreatitis is generally effective acutely, but the long-term success of biliary stenting is low.[156] Placement of one or more plastic stents to treat common bile obstruction is relatively simple, but the long-term management is complicated by the need for multiple stent exchanges over many months to years, and stent migration and obstruction are common. Long-term endoscopic stent therapy in alcoholic patients is particularly difficult and is associated with high complication rates due to missed appointments for scheduled stent exchanges.[157] The use of permanent metallic stents is discouraged because of the high rate of ultimate stent occlusion.

The development of a common bile duct stenosis in a patient with chronic pancreatitis may also signal the development of a pancreatic malignancy. ERCP is useful in this setting, both to define the characteristics of the stenosis for planning of therapy and also to attempt to differentiate benign from malignant stricture.

Duodenal Obstruction

Approximately 5% of patients with chronic pancreatitis experience symptomatic duodenal stenosis. The majority of these patients have chronic alcoholic pancreatitis. Fibrosis in the head of the pancreas, often associated with an inflammatory mass of the head of the pancreas, is the most common explanation. Symptoms include nausea, vomiting, weight loss, and abdominal pain. Coexistent obstruction of the common bile duct may occur. The diagnosis is best made with an upper gastrointestinal barium study, as the degree of duodenal stenosis is often underappreciated at endoscopy. Because the degree of duodenal stenosis may improve with resolution of some of the pancreatic inflammation, a trial of medical therapy may be helpful.

Surgical therapy is required for those who fail conservative management. The simplest and safest approach is a gastrojejunostomy. This may be coupled with drainage of the bile duct and/or pancreatic duct (lateral pancreaticojejunostomy). Resection of the head of the pancreas with duodenal sparing may be considered in selected patients with a large inflammatory mass of the head of the pancreas.

Pancreatic Fistula

External Pancreatic Fistula

External pancreatic fistulas occur most commonly as a consequence of surgical or percutaneous therapy for chronic pancreatitis or pseudocyst. It has been estimated that perhaps half of these will heal by keeping the patient NPO and on parenteral nutrition, but this can take a long time. There is some evidence that the addition of octreotide can hasten closure of these fistulas, using a dose of 100 μg subcutaneously every 8 hours. Successful treatment, even with octreotide, can take many weeks. The placement of an endoscopic stent across the site of ductal disruption is effective at closing these fistulas rapidly. Up to 75% of pancreaticocutaneous fistulas may be treated with endoscopic techniques.[158] In those who fail endoscopic therapy or in those in whom endoscopic therapy is not possible, surgical treatment can include pancreatic resection (if the fistula is in the tail) or a fistulojejunostomy, in which the fistula tract is "capped" with a defunctionalized limb of jejunum.[159]

Internal Pancreatic Fistulas

Internal fistulas occur mainly in the setting of chronic pancreatitis after rupture of a pseudocyst.[143] The fluid may track to the peritoneal cavity (pancreatic ascites) or into the pleural space (pancreatic pleural effusion). These patients may not complain of symptoms of chronic pancreatitis but may instead note abdominal distention or shortness of breath. Although these fistulas invariably occur in advanced chronic pancreatitis (particularly alcoholic), there may not be a clear-cut history of pancreatitis. The diagnosis can be established by documenting high levels of amylase within the respective fluid, typically greater than 4000 units/L. Conservative treatment, consisting of NPO, parenteral nutrition, paracentesis or thoracentesis, and octreotide is effective in a minority of patients. Endoscopic treatment is effective if the leak is in the body or head of the pancreas, in which case a pancreatic duct stent covering the fistula site is highly effective.[158] Endoscopic therapy is less effective if the leak is from the tail and ineffective if the leak is present upstream from a complete blockage of the pancreatic duct (excluded pancreatic tail syndrome). In this situation, resection and/or surgical drainage of the pseudocyst is required, and ERCP is used preoperatively to delineate the ductal anatomy for surgical planning.

Cancer (see also Chapter 50)

Chronic pancreatitis is a risk factor for pancreatic adenocarcinoma. The cancer risk is associated with all forms of chronic pancreatitis. The lifetime risk for pancreatic cancer in patients with chronic pancreatitis is about 4%.[160] The risk of pancreatic cancer is highest in hereditary pancreatitis, particularly in those patients who smoke. The risk of pancreatic cancer is increased 53-fold in patients with hereditary pancreatitis compared with the general population, and the cumulative lifetime risk may approach 40%.[45]

At present, there is no reliable way to differentiate chronic pancreatitis alone from chronic pancreatitis complicated by adenocarcinoma. The symptoms and signs may be similar (abdominal pain, weight loss, jaundice). In the absence of widespread metastases, imaging studies such as CT, US, and even ERCP may be unable to differentiate the two. The role of EUS is evolving, but finding a small, hypoechoic tumor within a diseased gland with preexisting altered echotexture can be difficult. EUS is probably superior to CT for detection of coexistent malignancy,[161] particularly when the lesion is small. EUS also has the advantage of allowing directed tissue biopsy of any suspicions lesions. Tumor markers may also be helpful in attempting to differentiate chronic pancreatitis from cancer. CA 19-9 is the most commonly used tumor marker for pancreatic adenocarcinoma and is elevated in 70% to 80% of patients with adenocarcinoma of the pancreas.[162] Biliary obstruction and/or cholangitis can also raise CA 19-9 levels. Mutations of K-ras are present in 90% of patients with pancreatic adenocarcinoma, but the utility of this test is diminished by the fact that similar mutations are seen in chronic pancreatitis.[163] In some patients, laparotomy is required to determine the presence or absence of coexistent pancreatic carcinoma. Proceeding to pancreatic resection in the absence of a tissue diagnosis ("blind" Whipple operation) should be done extremely rarely and only in those patients with a high likelihood of malignant disease. The use of any of these techniques for cancer surveillance is not cost-effective in the general population of patients with chronic pancreatitis.

Several reports have called attention to the development of extrapancreatic cancer in association with chronic pancreatitis.[164] These cancers, particularly those of the upper digestive tract and lungs, are probably related to the effect of concomitant tobacco and alcohol abuse. The incidence of extrapancreatic carcinomas has varied between 4% and 12%.

Dysmotility

Gastroparesis and antroduodenal dysmotility are seen in patients with chronic pancreatitis,[165, 166] possibly as a consequence of perigastric inflammation, hormonal changes associated with chronic pancreatitis (e.g., changes in CCK), or a side effect of narcotic analgesics. Gastroparesis is the most clinically important of these as it may produce symptoms occasionally indistinguishable from the disease and may interfere with the effective delivery of pancreatic enzymes.[166] Gastroparesis should be considered in patients with early satiety, nausea, vomiting, and weight loss.

REFERENCES

1. Sarner M, Cotton PB: Classification of pancreatitis. Gut 25:756, 1984.
2. Sarles H: Definitions and classification of pancreatitis. Pancreas 6:470, 1991.
3. Chari ST, Singer MV: The problem of classification and staging of chronic pancreatitis. Proposals based on current knowledge of its natural history. Scand J Gastroenterol 29:949, 1994.
4. Uys CJ, Bank S, Marks IN: The pathology of chronic pancreatitis in Cape Town. Digestion 9:454, 1973.
5. Olsen TS: The incidence and clinical relevance of chronic inflammation in the pancreas in autopsy material. Acta Pathol Microbiol Scand [A] 86(A):361, 1978.
6. Pitchumoni CS, Glasser M, Saran RM, et al: Pancreatic fibrosis in chronic alcoholics and nonalcoholics without clinical pancreatitis. Am J Gastroenterol 79:382, 1984.
7. Worning H: Incidence and prevalence of chronic pancreatitis. In Beger H, Buchler M, Ditschuneit H, Malfertheiner P (eds): Chronic Pancreatitis. Heidelberg, Germany, Springer-Verlag, 1990, p 8.
8. Kloppel G, Maillet B: Pathology of acute and chronic pancreatitis. Pancreas 8:659, 1990.
9. Suda K, Shiotsu H, Nakamura T, et al: Pancreatic fibrosis in patients with chronic alcohol abuse: Correlation with alcoholic pancreatitis. Am J Gastroenterol 89:2060, 1994.
10. O'Sullivan JN, Norbrega FT, Morlock CG, et al: Acute and chronic pancreatitis in Rochester, Minnesota, 1940–1969. Gastroenterology 62:373, 1972.
11. Andersen NN, Pedersen NT, Scheel J, et al: Incidence of alcoholic chronic pancreatitis in Copenhagen. Scand J Gastroenterol 17:247, 1982.
12. Copenhagen Pancreatitis Study: An interim report from a prospective multicentre study. Scand J Gastroenterol 16:305, 1981.
13. Everhart JE, Go VLW: Pancreatitis. In Everhart JE (ed): Digestive Diseases in the United States: Epidemiology and Impact. U.S. Department of Health and Human Services, Public Health Service, National Institutes of Health. NIH Publication No. 94-1447. Washington, DC, U.S. Government Printing Office, 1994, p 691.
14. Owings MF, Lawrence L: Detailed diagnoses and procedures. National Hospital Discharge Survey 1997, National Center for Health Statistics. Vital Health Stat 13:145, 1999.
15. Glasbrenner B, Adler G: Evaluating pain and quality of life in chronic pancreatitis. Int J Pancreatol 22:163, 1997.
16. Lowenfels AB, Maisonneuve P, Cavallini G, et al: Prognosis of chronic pancreatitis: An international multicenter study. International Pancreatitis Study Group. Am J Gastroenterol 89:1467, 1994.
17. Kloppel G, Maillet B: Pathology of chronic pancreatitis. In Beger HG, Warshaw AL, Buchler MW, et al (eds): The Pancreas. Malden, MA, Blackwell Science, 1998, p 720.
18. DeAngelis C, Valente G, Spaccapietra M, et al: Histological study of alcoholic, nonalcoholic, and obstructive chronic pancreatitis. Pancreas 7:193, 1992.
19. Sahel J, Sarles H: Modifications of pure human pancreatic juice induced by chronic alcohol consumption. Dig Dis Sci 24:897, 1979.
20. Goggin PM, Johnson CD: Pancreatic stones. In Beger HG, Warshaw AL, Buchler MW, et al (eds): The Pancreas. Malden, MA, Blackwell Science, 1998, p 711.
21. Freedman SD, Sakamoto K, Venu RP: GP2, the homologue to the renal cast protein uromodulin, is a major component of intraductal plugs in chronic pancreatitis. J Clin Invest 92:83, 1993.
22. Schoenberg MH, Buchler M, Pietrzyk C, et al: Lipid peroxidation and glutathione metabolism in chronic pancreatitis. Pancreas 10:36, 1995.
23. Bachem MG, Schneider E, Grob H, et al: Identification, culture, and characterization of pancreatic stellate cells in rats and humans. Gastroenterology 115:421, 1998.
24. Wells RG, Crawford JM: Pancreatic stellate cells: The new stars in chronic pancreatitis? Gastroenterology 115:491, 1998.
25. Ammann RW, Muellhaupt B: Progression of alcoholic acute to chronic pancreatitis. Gut 35:552, 1994.
26. Ammann RW, Heitz PU, Kloppel G: Course of alcoholic chronic pancreatitis: A prospective clinicomorphological long-term study. Gastroenterology 111:224, 1996.
27. Neuschwander-Tetri BA, Burton FR, Presti ME, et al: Repetitive self-limited acute pancreatitis induces pancreatic fibrogenesis in the mouse. Dig Dis Sci 45:665, 2000.
28. Cohn JA, Friedman KJ, Noone PG, et al: Relation between mutations of the cystic fibrosis gene and idiopathic pancreatitis. N Engl J Med 339:653, 1998.
29. Sharer N, Schwarz M, Malone G, et al: Mutations of the cystic fibrosis gene in patients with chronic pancreatitis. N Engl J Med 339: 645, 1998.
30. Bishop MD, Freedman SD: Does complete DNA analysis identify a higher percentage of cystic fibrosis gene mutations in patients with idiopathic chronic and recurrent acute pancreatitis [abstract]? Gastroenterology 116:A1113, 1999.
31. Whitcomb DC: Genetic predispositions to acute and chronic pancreatitis. Med Clin North Am 84:531, 2000.
32. Worning H: Alcoholic chronic pancreatitis. In Beger HG, Warshaw AL, Buchler MW, et al (eds): The Pancreas. Malden, MA, Blackwell Science, 1998, p 672.

33. Ammann RW, Akovbiantz A, Largiarder F, et al: Course and outcome of chronic pancreatitis. Gastroenterology 86:820, 1984.
34. Layer P, Yamamoto H, Kalthoff L, et al: The different courses of early- and late-onset idiopathic and alcoholic chronic pancreatitis. Gastroenterology 107:1481, 1994.
35. Lankisch PG, Lohr-Happe A, Otto J, et al: Natural course in chronic pancreatitis. Digestion 54:148, 1993.
36. Levy P, Mathurin P, Roqueplo A, et al: A multidimensional case-control study of dietary, alcohol, and tobacco habits in alcoholic men with chronic pancreatitis. Pancreas 10:231, 1995.
37. Durbec JP, Sarles H: Multicenter survey of the etiology of pancreatic diseases: Relationship between the relative risk of developing chronic pancreatitis and alcohol, protein, and lipid consumption. Digestion 18: 337, 1978.
38. Pitchumoni CS: Role of nutrition in chronic pancreatitis. In Beger H, Buchler M, Ditschuneit H, Malfertheiner P (eds): Chronic Pancreatitis. Heidelberg, Germany, Springer-Verlag, 1990, p 15.
39. Bourliere M, Barthet M, Berthezene P, et al: Is tobacco a risk factor for chronic pancreatitis and alcoholic cirrhosis? Gut 32:1392, 1991.
40. Cavallini G, Talamini G, Vaona B, et al: Effect of alcohol and smoking on pancreatic lithogenesis in the course of chronic pancreatitis. Pancreas 9:42, 1994.
41. Ammann RW, Muellhaupt B, Meyenberger C, et al: Alcoholic non-progressive chronic pancreatitis: Prospective long-term study of a large cohort with alcoholic acute pancreatitis (1976–1992). Pancreas 9:365, 1994.
42. Gullo L, Barbara L, Labo G: Effect of cessation of alcohol use on the course of pancreatic dysfunction in alcoholic pancreatitis. Gastroenterology 95:1063, 1988.
43. Mohan V, Pitchumoni CS: Tropical chronic pancreatitis. In Beger HG, Warshaw AL, Buchler MW, et al: (eds): The Pancreas. Malden, MA, Blackwell Science, 1998, p 688.
44. Balaji LN, Tandon RK, Tandon BN, et al: Prevalence and clinical features of chronic pancreatitis in southern India. Int J Pancreatol 15: 29, 1994.
45. Lowenfels AB, Maisonneuve P, DiMagno EP, et al: Hereditary pancreatitis and the risk of pancreatic cancer. International Hereditary Pancreatitis Study Group. J Natl Cancer Inst 89:442, 1997.
46. Whitcomb DC, Gorry MC, Preston RA, et al: Hereditary pancreatitis is caused by a mutation in the cationic trypsinogen gene. Nat Genet 14:141, 1996.
47. Mickle JE, Cutting GR: Genotype-phenotype relationships in cystic fibrosis. Med Clin North Am 84:597, 2000.
48. Cohn JA, Bornstein JD, Jowell PS: Cystic fibrosis mutations and genetic predispositions to idiopathic chronic pancreatitis. Med Clin North Am 84:621, 2000.
49. Delhaye M, Engelholm L, Cremer M: Pancreas divisum: Congenital anatomic variant or anomaly? Gastroenterology 89:951, 1985.
50. Horiuchi A, Kawa S, Akamatsu T, et al: Characteristic pancreatic duct appearance in autoimmune chronic pancreatitis: Case report and review of the Japanese literature. Am J Gastroenterol 93:260, 1998.
51. Toskes PP: Hyperlipidemic pancreatitis. Gastroenterol Clin North Am 19:783, 1990.
52. Schoo N, Broodt D, Zipf A, et al: Histological findings of chronic pancreatitis after abdominal radiotherapy. Pancreas 12:313, 1996.
53. Sarles H, Camarena-Trabous J, Gomez-Santana C, et al: Acute pancreatitis is not a cause of chronic pancreatitis in the absence of residual duct strictures. Pancreas 8:354, 1993.
54. Ammann RW, Buehler H, Muench R, et al: Differences in the natural history of idiopathic (nonalcoholic) and alcoholic chronic pancreatitis. A comparative long-term study of 287 patients. Pancreas 4:368, 1987.
55. Miyake H, Harada H, Kunichika K, et al: Clinical course and prognosis of chronic pancreatitis. Pancreas 2:378, 1987.
56. Ammann RW, Muellhaupt B, Zurich Pancreatitis Study Group: The natural history of pain in alcoholic chronic pancreatitis. Gastroenterology 116:1132, 1999.
57. Jensen AR, Matzen P, Malchow-Moller A, et al: Pattern of pain, duct morphology, and pancreatic function in chronic pancreatitis. A comparative study. Scand J Gastroenterol 19:334, 1984.
58. Lankisch PG, Seidensticker F, Lohr-Happe A, et al: The course of pain is the same in alcohol- and nonalcohol-induced chronic pancreatitis. Pancreas 10:338, 1995.
59. Ebbehoj N, Borly L, Bulow J, et al: Evaluation of pancreatic tissue fluid pressure and pain in chronic pancreatitis. Scand J Gastroenterol 25:462, 1990.
60. Ebbehoj N, Borly L, Madsen P, et al: Pancreatic tissue fluid pressure during drainage operations for chronic pancreatitis. Scand J Gastroenterol 25:1041, 1990.
61. Ebbehoj N, Borly L, Madsen P, et al: Pancreatic tissue pressure and pain in chronic pancreatitis. Pancreas 1:556, 1986.
62. Okazaki K, Yamamoto Y, Kagiyama S, et al: Pressure of papillary sphincter zone and pancreatic main duct in patients with alcoholic and idiopathic chronic pancreatitis. Int J Pancreatol 3:457, 1988.
63. Renou C, Grandval P, Ville E, et al: Endoscopic treatment of the main pancreatic duct: Correlation among morphology, manometry, and clinical follow-up. Int J Pancreatol 27:143, 2000.
64. Karanjia ND, Widdison AL, Leung FW, et al: Compartment syndrome in experimental chronic pancreatitis: Effect of decompressing the main pancreatic duct. Br J Surg 81:259, 1994.
65. Patel A, Toyama MT, Reber P, et al: Pancreatic intersititial pH in human and feline chronic pancreatitis. Gastroenterology 109:1639, 1995.
66. Lewis MP, Lo SK, Reber PU, et al: Endoscopic measurement of pancreatic tissue perfusion in patients with chronic pancreatitis and control patients. Gastrointest Endosc 51:195, 2000.
67. Bockman DE, Buchler M, Malfertheiner P, et al: Analysis of nerves in chronic pancreatitis. Gastroenterology 94:1459, 1988.
68. DiMagno EP, Go VLW, Summerskill WHJ: Relations between pancreatic enzyme outputs and malabsorption in severe pancreatic insufficiency. N Engl J Med 288:813, 1973.
69. Hebuterne X, Hastier P, Peroux J-L, et al: Resting energy expenditure in patients with chronic alcoholic pancreatitis. Dig Dis Sci 41:533, 1996.
70. Twersky Y, Bank S: Nutritional deficiencies in chronic pancreatitis. Gastroenterol Clin North Am 18:543, 1989.
71. Haaber AB, Rosenfalck AM, Hansen B, et al: Bone mineral metabolism, bone mineral density, and body composition in patients with chronic pancreatitis and pancreatic exocrine insufficiency. Int J Pancreatol 27:21, 2000.
72. Donowitz M, Hendler R, Spiro HM, et al: Glucagon secretion in acute and chronic pancreatitis. Ann Intern Med 83:778, 1975.
73. Linde J, Nilsson LH, Barany FR: Diabetes and hypoglycemia in chronic pancreatitis. Scand J Gastroenterol 12:369, 1977.
74. Levitt NS, Adams G, Salmon J, et al: The prevalence and severity of microvascular complications in pancreatic diabetes and IDDM. Diabetes Care 18:971, 1995.
75. Niederau C, Grendell JH: Diagnosis of chronic pancreatitis. Gastroenterology 88:1973, 1985.
75a. Pedersen NT: Estimation of the assimilation of simultaneously ingested ^{14}C-triolein and ^{3}H-oleic acid as a test of pancreatic digestive function. Scand J Gastroenterol 19:161, 1984.
76. Braganza JM, Hunt LP, Warwick F: Relationship between pancreatic exocrine function and ductal morphology in chronic pancreatitis. Gastroenterology 82:1341, 1982.
77. Girdwood AH, Hatfield ARW, Bornman PC, et al: Structure and function in noncalcific pancreatitis. Dig Dis Sci 29:721, 1984.
78. Malfertheiner P, Buchler M, Stanescu A, et al: Exocrine pancreatic function in correlation to ductal and parenchymal morphology in chronic pancreatitis. Hepatogastroenterology 33:110, 1986.
79. Lankisch PG, Seidensticker F, Otto J, et al: Secretin-pancreozymin test (SPT) and endoscopic retrograde cholangiopancreatography (ERCP): Both are necessary for diagnosing or excluding chronic pancreatitis. Pancreas 12:149, 1996.
80. Bozkurt T, Braun U, Lefferink S, et al: Comparison of pancreatic morphology and exocrine functional impairment in patients with chronic pancreatitis. Gut 35:1132, 1994.
81. Lambiase L, Forsmark CE, Toskes PP: Secretin test diagnoses chronic pancreatitis earlier than ERCP [abstract]. Gastroenterology 104:A315, 1993.
82. Hayakawa T, Kondo T, Shibata T, et al: Relationship between pancreatic exocrine function and histological changes in chronic pancreatitis. Am J Gastroenterol 87:1170, 1992.
83. Somogyi L, Cintron M, Toskes PP: Synthetic porcine secretin is highly accurate in pancreatic function testing in individuals with chronic pancreatitis. Pancreas 21:262, 2000.
83a. Pollack BJ, Forsmark CE: Adjunct diagnosis of pancreatic disease and pancreatic physiology. In Sivak MV (ed): Gastroenterologic Endoscopy, 2nd ed. Philadelphia, WB Saunders, 2000, p 1116.
84. Jacobsen DG, Currington C, Connery K, Toskes PP: Trypsin-like immunoreactivity as a test for pancreatic insufficiency. N Engl J Med 310:1307, 1984.

85. Amann ST, Bishop M, Currington C, Toskes PP: Fecal elastase 1 is inaccurate in the diagnosis of chronic pancreatitis. Pancreas 13:226, 1996.
86. Ammann RW, Muench R, Otto R, et al: Evolution and regression of pancreatic calcification in chronic pancreatitis: A prospective long-term study of 107 patients. Gastroenterology 95:1018, 1988.
87. Rosch T, Schusdziarra V, Born P: Modern imaging methods versus clinical assessment in the evaluation of hospital in-patients with suspected pancreatic disease. Am J Gastroenterol 95:2261, 2000.
88. Ikeda M, Sato T, Morozumi A: Morphologic changes in the pancreas detected by screening ultrasonography in a mass survey, with special reference to main duct dilation, cyst formation, and calcification. Pancreas 9:508, 1994.
89. Robinson PJ, Sheridan MB: Pancreatitis: Computed tomography and magnetic resonance imaging. Eur Radiol 10:401, 2000.
90. Sica JT, Braver J, Cooney MJ, et al: Comparison of endoscopic retrograde cholangiopancreatography with MR cholangiography in patients with pancreatitis. Radiology 210:605, 1999.
91. Axon ATR, Classen M, Cotton P, et al: Pancreatography in chronic pancreatitis. Gut 25:1107, 1984.
92. Forsmark CE, Toskes PP: What does an abnormal pancreatogram mean? Gastrointest Endosc Clin North Am 5:105, 1995.
93. Walsh TN, Rode J, Theis BA, et al: Minimal change chronic pancreatitis. Gut 33:1566, 1992.
94. Anand BS, Vic JC, Mac HS, et al: Effect of aging on the pancreatic ducts: A study based on endoscopic retrograde pancreatography. Gastrointest Endosc 35:210, 1989.
95. Nagai H, Ohtsubo K: Pancreatic lithiasis in the aged: Its clinicopathology and pathogenesis. Gastroenterology 86:331, 1984.
96. Smith MT, Sherman S, Ikenberry SO, et al: Alterations in pancreatic duct morphology following polyethylene stent therapy. Gastrointest Endosc 44:268, 1996.
97. Sherman S, Hawes RH, Savides TJ, et al: Stent-induced pancreatic ductal and parenchymal changes: Correlation of endoscopic ultrasound with ERCP. Gastrointest Endosc 44:276, 1996.
98. Schmitz-Moormann P, Himmelmann GW, Brandes JW, et al: Comparative radiological and morphological study of human pancreas. Pancreatitis-like changes in postmortem ductograms and their morphological pattern. Possible implication for ERCP. Gut 26:406, 1985.
99. Cotton PB: Progress report: ERCP. Gut 18:316, 1977.
100. Forsmark CE: The diagnosis of chronic pancreatitis. Gastrointest Endosc 52:293, 2000.
101. Catalano MF, Lahoti S, Geenan JE, et al: Prospective evaluation of endoscopic ultrasonography, endoscopic retrograde pancreatography, and secretin test in the diagnosis of chronic pancreatitis. Gastrointest Endosc 48:11, 1998.
102. Wiersma MJ, Hawes RH, Lehman GA, et al: Prospective evaluation of endoscopic ultrasonography and endoscopic retrograde pancreatography in patients with chronic abdominal pain of suspected pancreatic origin. Endoscopy 25:555, 1993.
103. Lambiase LR, Forsmark CE: Comparison of endoscopic ultrasonography and secretin testing for the diagnosis of chronic pancreatitis [abstract]. Gastrointest Endosc 45:AB175, 1997.
104. Zuccaro G, Conwell DL, Vargo JJ, et al: The role of endoscopic ultrasound in the diagnosis of early and advanced chronic pancreatitis [abstract]. Gastroenterology 118:A674, 2000.
105. Sahai AV, Mishra G, Penman ID, et al: Persistent or nonspecific dyspepsia as an atypical presentation of pancreatic disease: A prospective comparison of the endoscopic appearance of the pancreas in a consecutive series of patients with dyspepsia. Gastrointest Endosc 52: 153, 2000.
106. Wilder-Smith CJ, Hill L, Osler W, et al: Effect of tramadol and morphine on pain and gastrointestinal motor function in patients with chronic pancreatitis. Dig Dis Sci 44:1107, 1999.
107. Strum WB: Abstinence in alcoholic chronic pancreatitis. J Clin Gastroenterol 20:37, 1995.
108. Talamini G, Bassi C, Falconi M, et al: Pain relapses in the first ten years of chronic pancreatitis. Am J Surg 171:565, 1996.
108a. Uden S, Bilton D, Nathan L, et al: Antioxidant therapy for recurrent pancreatitis: Placebo-controlled trial. Aliment Pharmacol Ther 4:357, 1990.
109. Li Y, Hao Y, Owyang C: Diazepam-binding inhibitor mediates feedback regulation of pancreatic secretion and postprandial release of cholecystokinin. J Clin Invest 105:351, 2000.
110. Slaff JI, Wolfe MM, Toskes PP: Elevated fasting cholecystokinin levels in pancreatic exocrine impairment: Evidence to support feedback regulation. J Lab Clin Med 105:282, 1985.
111. Gomez Cerezo J, Codocer R, Fernandez Calle P, et al: Basal and postprandial cholecystokinin values in chronic pancreatitis with and without abdominal pain. Digestion 48:134, 1991.
112. Jansen JMBJ, Jebbink MCW, Mulders HJA, et al: Effect of pancreatic enzyme supplementation on postprandial plasma cholecystokinin secretion in patients with pancreatic insufficiency. Regul Pept 25:333, 1989.
113. Slaff J, Jacobson D, Tillman CR, et al: Protease-specific suppression of pancreatic exocrine secretion. Gastroenterology 87:44, 1984.
114. Isaksson G, Ihse I: Pain reduction by an oral pancreatic enzyme preparation in chronic pancreatitis. Dig Dis Sci 28:97, 1983.
115. Halgreen H, Pederson NT, Worning H: Symptomatic effect of pancreatic enzyme therapy in patients with chronic pancreatitis. Scand J Gastroenterol 21:104, 1986.
116. Mossner J, Secknus R, Meyer J, et al: Treatment of pain with pancreatic extracts in chronic pancreatitis: Results of a prospective placebo-controlled multicenter trial. Digestion 53:54, 1992.
117. Malesci A, Gaia E, Fioretta A, et al: No effect of long-term treatment with pancreatic extract on recurrent abdominal pain in patients with chronic pancreatitis. Scand J Gastroenterol 30:392, 1995.
118. Larvin M, McMahon MJ, Thomas WEG, et al: Creon (enteric coated pancreatin microspheres) for the treatment of pain in chronic pancreatitis: A double-blind randomised placebo-controlled crossover trial [abstract]. Gastroenterology 100:A283, 1991.
119. AGA Technical Review: Treatment of pain in chronic pancreatitis. Gastroenterology 115:763, 1998.
120. Toskes PP, Forsmark CE, Demeo MT, et al: A multicenter controlled trial of octreotide for the pain of chronic pancreatitis [abstract]. Pancreas 8:774, 1993.
121. Cremer M, Deviere J, Delhaye M, et al: Stenting in severe chronic pancreatitis: Results of medium-term follow-up in seventy-six patients. Endoscopy 23:171, 1991.
122. Smits ME, Badiga SM, Rauws EAJ, et al: Long-term results of pancreatic stents in chronic pancreatitis. Gastrointest Endosc 42:461, 1995.
123. Ashby K, Lo SK: The role of pancreatic duct stenting in obstructive ductal disorders other than pancreas divisum. Gastrointest Endosc 42: 306, 1995.
124. Ponchon T, Bory RM, Hedelius F, et al: Endoscopic stenting for pain relief in chronic pancreatitis; Results of a standardized protocol. Gastrointest Endosc 42:452, 1995.
125. Kozarek RA, Traverso LW: Endoscopic treatment of chronic pancreatitis: An alternative to surgery? Dig Surg 13:90, 1996.
126. Dumonceau J-M, Deviere J, Le Moine O, et al: Endoscopic pancreatic drainage in chronic pancreatitis associated with ductal stones: Long-term results. Gastrointest Endosc 43:547, 1996.
127. Coleman SD, Eisen GM, Troughton AB, et al: Endoscopic treatment in pancreas divisum. Am J Gastroenterol 89:1152, 1994.
128. Prinz RA, Greenlee HB: Pancreatic duct drainage in 100 patients with chronic pancreatitis. Ann Surg 194:313, 1981.
129. Adams DB, Ford MC, Anderson MC: Outcome after lateral pancreaticojejunostomy for chronic pancreatitis. Ann Surg 219:481, 1994.
130. Nealon WH, Thompson JC: Progressive loss of pancreatic function in chronic pancreatitis is delayed by main pancreatic duct decompression: A longitudinal prospective analysis of the modified Puestow procedure. Ann Surg 217:458, 1991.
131. Markowitz JS, Rattner DW, Warshaw AL: Failure of symptomatic relief after pancreaticojejunal decompression for chronic pancreatitis. Arch Surg 129:374, 1994.
132. Jimenez RE, Fernandez-del Castillo C, Rattner DW, et al: Outcome of pancreaticoduodenectomy with pylorus preservation or with antrectomy in the treatment of chronic pancreatitis. Ann Surg 231:293, 2000.
133. Saforkas GH, Farnell MB, Farley DR, et al: Long-term results after surgery for chronic pancreatitis. Int J Pancreatol 27:131, 2000.
134. Frey CF: The surgical management of chronic pancreatitis: The Frey procedure. Adv Surg 32:41, 1999.
135. Beger HG, Schlosser W, Friess HM, et al: Duodenum-preserving head resection in chronic pancreatitis changes the natural course of the disease: A single-center 26-year experience. Ann Surg 230:512, 1999.
136. Izbicki JR, Bloechle C, Knoefel WT, et al: Duodenum-preserving resection of the head of the pancreas in chronic pancreatitis. A prospective, randomized trial. Ann Surg 221:350, 1995.

137. Izbicki JR, Bloechle C, Broering DC, et al: Extended drainage versus resection in surgery for chronic pancreatitis. A prospective randomized trial comparing the longitudinal pancreaticojejunostomy combined with local pancreatic head resection with the pylorus-preserving pancreaticoduodenectomy. Ann Surg 228:771, 1998.
138. Wong GY, Saforkas GH, Tsiotsos GG, et al: Palliation of pain in chronic pancreatitis. Use of neural blocks and neurotomy. Surg Clin North Am 79:873, 1999.
139. Gress F, Schmidt C, Sherman S, et al: A prospective randomized comparison of endoscopic ultrasound- and computed tomography-guided celiac plexus block for managing chronic pancreatitis pain. Am J Gastroenterol 94:900, 1994.
140. Ihse I, Zoucas E, Gyllstedt E, et al: Bilateral thoracoscopic splanchnicectomy: Effect on pancreatic function and pain. Ann Surg 230:785, 1999.
141. Kumar A, Forsmark CE, Toskes PP: Small bowel bacterial overgrowth: The changing face of an old disease [abstract]. Gastroenterology 110:A340, 1996.
142. Crass RA, Way LW: Acute and chronic pancreatic pseudocysts are different. Am J Surg 142:660, 1981.
143. Forsmark CE, Grendell JH: Complications of pancreatitis. Semin Gastrointest Dis 2:165, 1991.
144. Yeo CJ, Bastidas JA, Lynch-Nyham A, et al: The natural history of pancreatic pseudocysts documented by computed tomography. Surg Gynecol Obstet 170:411, 1990.
145. Vitas GJ, Sarr MG: Selected management of pancreatic pseudocysts: Operative versus expectant management. Surgery 111:123, 1992.
146. Mishra G, Forsmark CE: Cystic neoplasms of the pancreas. Curr Treat Options Gastroenterol 3:355, 2000.
147. Balcolm JH, Fernandez-del Castillo C, Warshaw AL: Cystic lesions in the pancreas: When to watch, when to resect. Curr Gastroenterol Rep 2:152, 2000.
148. Lohr-Happe A, Peiper M, Lankisch PJ: Natural course of operated pseudocysts in chronic pancreatitis. Gut 35:1479, 1994.
149. Heider R, Meyer AA, Galanko JA: Percutaneous drainage of pancreatic pseudocysts is associated with a higher failure rate than surgical treatment in unselected patients. Ann Surg 229:781, 1999.
150. Criado E, De Stefano AA, Weiner TM, et al: Long-term results of percutaneous catheter drainage of pancreatic pseudocysts. Surg Gynecol Obstet 175:293, 1992.
151. Adams DB, Srinivasan A: Failure of percutaneous catheter drainage of pancreatic pseudocyst. Am Surg 66:256, 2000.
152. Beckingham IJ, Krige JE, Bornman PC, et al: Long-term outcome of endoscopic drainage of pancreatic pseudocysts. Am J Gastroenterol 94:71, 1999.
153. Forsmark CE, Wilcox CM, Grendell JH: Endoscopy-negative upper gastrointestinal bleeding in a patient with chronic pancreatitis. Gastroenterology 102:320, 1992.
154. Lesur G, Levy P, Flejou J-F, et al: Factors predictive of liver histopathological appearance in chronic alcoholic pancreatitis with common bile duct stenosis and increased serum alkaline phosphatase. Hepatology 18:1078, 1993.
155. Hammel P, Couvelard A, O'Toole D, et al: Regression of liver fibrosis after biliary drainage in patients with chronic pancreatitis and stenosis of the common bile duct. N Engl J Med 344:418, 2001.
156. Smits ME, Rauws EAJ, van Gulik TM, et al: Long-term results of endoscopic stenting and surgical drainage for biliary stricture due to chronic pancreatitis. Br J Surg 83:764, 1996.
157. Kiehne K, Folsch UR, Nitsche R: High complication rate of bile duct stents in patients with chronic alcoholic pancreatitis due to noncompliance. Endoscopy 32:377, 2000.
158. Kozarek RA: Endoscopic therapy of complete and partial pancreatic ductal disruption. Gastrointest Endosc Clin North Am 8:39, 1998.
159. Bassi C, Butturini G: A single-institution experience with fistulojejunostomy for external pancreatic fistulas. Am J Surg 179:203, 2000.
160. Lowenfels AB, Maisonneuve P, Cavallini G, et al: Pancreatitis and the risk of pancreatic cancer. N Engl J Med 328:1433, 1993.
161. Midwinter MJ, Beveridge CJ, Wilsdon JB, et al: Correlation between spiral computed tomography, endoscopic ultrasonography, and findings at operation in pancreatic and ampullary tumours. Br J Surg 86:189, 1999.
162. Steinberg W: The clinical utility of the CA 19-9 tumor-associated antigen. Am J Gastroenterol 85:350, 1990.
163. Lohr M, Maisonneuve P, Lowenfels AB: K-Ras mutations and benign pancreatic disease. Int J Pancreatol 27:93, 2000.
164. Hansen TH, Laursen M, Christensen E, et al: Chronic pancreatitis and extrapancreatic cancer. Int J Pancreatol 18:235, 1995.
165. Vu MK, Vecht J, Eddes EH, et al: Antroduodenal motility in chronic pancreatitis: Are abnormalities related to exocrine insufficiency? Am J Physiol 278:G458, 2000.
166. Newman MB, Toskes PP, Verne GN: Occurrence of idiopathic gastroparesis in patients with small duct chronic pancreatitis and refractory abdominal pain [abstract]. Gastroenterology 116:A1174, 1999.

Chapter 50

Pancreatic Cancer, Cystic Pancreatic Neoplasms, and Other Nonendocrine Pancreatic Tumors

Carlos Fernández-del Castillo and Ramon E. Jimenez

PANCREATIC CANCER

Pancreatic cancer is the second most frequent gastrointestinal malignancy, and more than 28,000 new cases are diagnosed every year in the United States.[1] It is a disease with an extremely poor prognosis: Less than 20% of affected patients survive the first year, and only 4% are alive 5 years after diagnosis.[2] Because of this, and notwithstanding its relatively low incidence compared with other malignancies, pancreatic cancer is the fourth leading cause of cancer death in both men and women. Early diagnosis, accurate preoperative staging, and better adjuvant treatment remain a challenge.

Biology and Epidemiology

Incidence

In the United States, the reported incidence of pancreatic carcinoma, which had been increasing since the 1930s, has remained unchanged since 1973 and stood at 8.8 per 100,000 in 1997, with a male-to-female ratio of 1.3:1.[2] The disease is rare before the age of 45 years, but its occurrence rises sharply thereafter. Blacks are more frequently affected, the incidence being 14.8 per 100,000 in black men.[2]

Populations at Risk

The etiology of pancreatic cancer remains unknown, but several genetic and environmental factors have been found to be associated with its development (Fig. 50–1). One of the most prominent genetic factors is *hereditary pancreatitis*, even though it accounts for only a small fraction of pancreatic cancer cases (see Chapter 47). These patients have an abnormal trypsin gene that is transmitted as an autosomal dominant trait and have a 40% estimated risk of developing pancreatic cancer by age 70 years.[3] Patients with other nonhereditary forms of *chronic pancreatitis* also have a higher likelihood of developing pancreatic cancer. A multinational study found this risk to be 2% per decade, independent of the type of pancreatitis.[4]

Aside from hereditary pancreatitis, there is also evidence that there are *genetic factors* that predispose to pancreatic cancer in some families. In several population studies, 7% to 8% of patients with pancreatic cancer have a first-degree relative with the disease.[5, 6] Germline mutations in known cancer-causing genes, such as *BRAC2* (which predisposes to hereditary breast cancer) and the tumor suppressor gene *p16* are present in some of these kindreds.[6]

Diabetes mellitus is very common in patients with pancreatic cancer. In most cases diabetes had been diagnosed within the preceding 2 years and there was no family history of diabetes.[7] Thus, recent onset of diabetes without family history may help identify patients with pancreatic cancer, particularly in individuals who are more than 50 years of age. It is unlikely there is enough destruction of the pancreas to cause endocrine insufficiency in most patients with pancreatic cancer, and it has been proposed that increased production of islet amyloid polypeptide by the tumor is responsible for the diabetogenic state. In fact, glucose tolerance frequently improves in resected patients.[8]

There are no specific recommendations for screening patients at risk for pancreatic cancer, because currently available techniques, even those that are invasive, lack sensitivity for detection of very small lesions. The timing and frequency of such screening are also uncertain. The American Gastroenterological Association suggests that screening should begin at age 35 years in hereditary pancreatitis, and 10 years before the age at which pancreatic cancer has been first diagnosed in familial pancreatic cancer. It also states that such screening is probably best done with spiral computed tomography (CT) and endoscopic ultrasonography (EUS).[9]

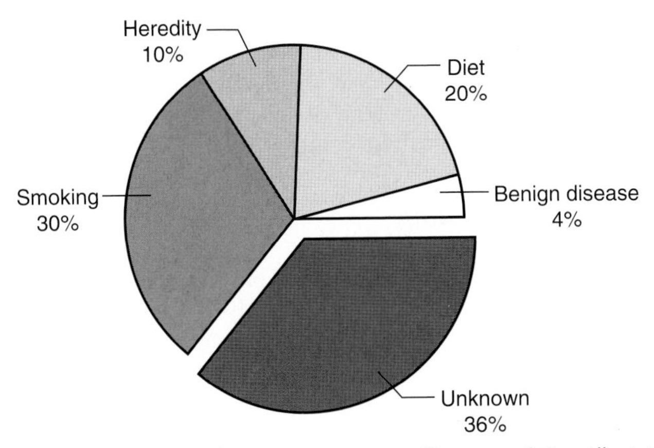

Figure 50–1. Causes of pancreatic cancer. (Courtesy of Dr. Albert P. Lowenfels.)

Environmental Factors

The most important environmental factor, and possibly the only one that has been firmly established, is cigarette smoking. Multiple cohort and case-control studies have found that the relative risk for smokers of developing pancreatic cancer is at least 1.5.[10–15] Furthermore, the risk increases with the amount of cigarette consumption,[16, 17] and the excess risk levels returns to baseline by 15 years after cessation of the habit. Experimentally, pancreatic tumors can be induced by lifetime administration of tobacco-specific nitrosamines in drinking water,[18] as well as by implantation or parenteral administration of other *N*-nitroso compounds.[19, 20] It has been suggested that these compounds reach the pancreas either through the blood or through refluxed bile in contact with the pancreatic duct.[21]

The second most important environmental risk factor associated with pancreatic cancer appears to be dietary influences. A high intake of fat and/or meat has been linked to the development of this neoplasm,[17, 22–24] and a protective effect is ascribed to fresh fruits and vegetables.[24–26] Lower serum levels of lycopene, a carotenoid present in fruits, and selenium were found in subjects who subsequently developed pancreatic cancer.[27] In the experimental setting, dietary fat and protein act as promoters of pancreatic carcinogenesis.[28]

Apart from the well-known risk of developing gastric cancer, patients with a history of peptic ulcer surgery have a higher than expected incidence of pancreatic cancer. Even after correction for smoking, there seems to be a twofold to fivefold increased risk of developing pancreatic cancer 15 to 20 years after partial gastrectomy.[29] It has been proposed that increased formation of *N*-nitroso compounds by nitrate-reductase–producing bacteria that proliferate in the hypoacidic stomach could be responsible for both the gastric and pancreatic carcinogenesis.[29] Pancreatic tumors can be induced experimentally by long-term duodenogastric reflux,[30] which is associated with increased cholecystokinin levels. Exogenous cholecystokinin promotes the growth of transplantable human pancreatic adenocarcinoma cell lines,[31] and there is some clinical evidence that cholecystectomy, after which circulating levels of this hormone are elevated, may also increase the risk of pancreatic cancer.[32]

Pathology

Three different epithelial cell types can be found in the normal pancreas: (1) acinar cells, which account for about 80% of the gland volume, (2) ductal cells comprising 10% to 15%, and (3) endocrine (islet) cells, about 1% to 2%. More than 95% of the malignant neoplasms of the pancreas arise from the exocrine elements of the gland (ductal and acinar cells) and demonstrate features consistent with adenocarcinoma. Endocrine neoplasms account for only 1% to 2% of pancreatic tumors (see Chapter 51). Nonepithelial malignancies are exceedingly rare.[33]

The World Health Organization (WHO) has proposed a classification of pancreatic tumors that is widely used today.[34] Their classification scheme for tumors of the exocrine pancreas can be found in Table 50–1.

Ductal adenocarcinoma accounts for 85% to 90% of pancreatic tumors.[35] Autopsy series have shown that 60% to 70% of tumors are localized in the head of the gland, 5% to 10% in the body, and 10% to 15% in the tail. Grossly, these tumors present as firm masses with ill-defined margins blending into the surrounding pancreatic parenchyma (Fig. 50–2). The average size of carcinomas in the head of the gland is 2.5 to 3.5 cm, compared to 5 to 7 cm for tumors in the body or tail.[33] Differences in tumor size at presentation are related to the early development of symptoms in proximal tumors as opposed to distal neoplasms.

Tumors in the head of the gland have a propensity for obstruction of the distal common bile duct and pancreatic duct. Anatomic obstruction of these structures results in jaundice and chronic obstructive pancreatitis. Pancreatic pathologic changes observed include duct dilation and fibrous atrophy of the pancreatic parenchyma. Some tumors can involve the duodenum and the ampulla of Vater. Extrapancreatic extension into the retroperitoneal tissues is almost always present at the time of diagnosis and results in invasion of the portal vein or the superior mesenteric vessels and

Table 50–1 | **World Health Organization Classification of Primary Tumors of the Exocrine Pancreas**

I. Benign
- i. Serous cystadenoma
- ii. Mucinous cystadenoma
- iii. Intraductal papillary mucinous adenoma
- iv. Mature cystic teratoma

II. Borderline (uncertain malignant potential)
- i. Mucinous cystic tumor with moderate dysplasia
- ii. Intraductal papillary mucinous tumor with moderate dysplasia
- iii. Solid-pseudopapillary tumor

III. Malignant
- i. Ductal adenocarcinoma
- ii. Osteoclast-like giant cell tumor
- iii. Serous cystadenocarcinoma
- iv. Mucinous cystadenocarcinoma (invasive/noninvasive)
- v. Intraductal papillary mucinous carcinoma (invasive/noninvasive)
- vi. Acinar cell carcinoma
- vii. Pancreatoblastoma
- viii. Solid-pseudopapillary carcinoma
- ix. Miscellaneous carcinomas

Data from Kloppel G, Solcia E, Longnecker DS, et al: Histological typing of tumors of the exocrine pancreas. In International Histological Classification of Tumors. Berlin, Springer, 1996.

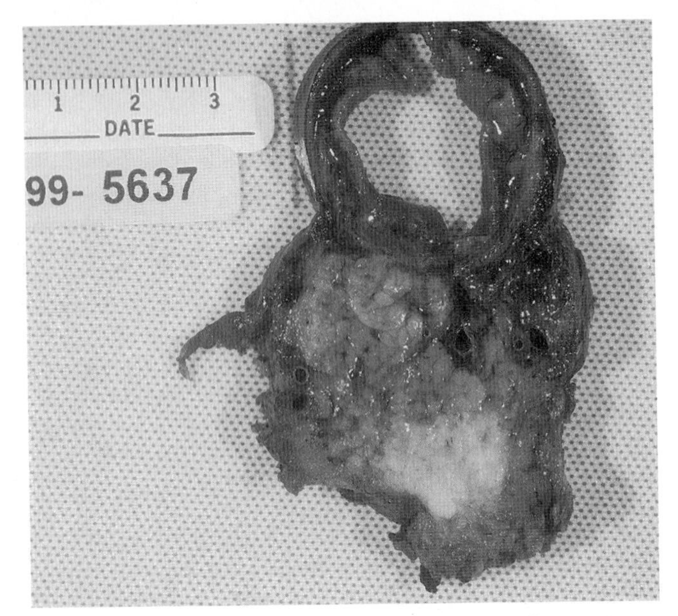

Figure 50–2. Gross pathology of pancreatic ductal adenocarcinoma. The normal pancreatic lobular archetexture is effaced by a 2-cm gray-white carcinoma. Note the overlying duodenum.

nerves. Neoplasms of the tail of the pancreas do not cause biliary or pancreatic duct obstruction. Extrapancreatic extension in distal tumors causes invasion of the spleen, stomach, and/or left adrenal gland. In patients with advanced disease, metastases to the lymph nodes, liver, and peritoneum are common; less frequently, the lung, pleura, and bone are involved.[33]

Microscopically, ductal adenocarcinomas are graded as well, moderately, or poorly differentiated. Well-differentiated tumors show irregular tubular neoplastic glands with mild cellular atypia, low mitotic activity, and significant mucin production. Loss of differentiation results from lack of cellular arrangement into glandular structures, increases in cellular atypia and mitotic figures, and cessation of mucin production. Some studies have demonstrated that histologic grading correlates with survival.[36]

Ductal adenocarcinomas elicit a strong desmoplastic reaction that is responsible for their hard consistency on gross inspection. In contrast with chronic pancreatitis, intraductal calcifications are only rarely found. Pancreatic ducts outside the area of neoplasia may demonstrate papillary hyperplasia or mucinous cell hypertrophy.[37] The significance of these findings is unknown. Microscopic tumor extension is often evident in lymphatic channels and perineural spaces.[38] Lymph node extension of tumors of the head of the gland is most common in the pancreaticoduodenal basins, with late extension into the celiac and para-aortic lymph nodes.

Several immunohistochemical markers have shown diagnostic utility in mucin-producing tumors such as pancreatic adenocarcinoma. Among the better-known markers are M1, carcinoembryonic antigen (CEA), CA 19-9, DuPan 2, CA 125, and TAG 72.[39, 40] These markers are unable to differentiate between tumors of pancreatic or extrapancreatic origin, limiting their usefulness in the evaluation of liver metastases of unknown primary. However, they are particularly useful in separating neoplastic from non-neoplastic ductal changes and in separating ductal from acinar or neuroendocrine tumors. Cytokeratins are other useful markers in differentiating between acinar, ductal, and islet cell tumors.[41] Although all ductal adenocarcinomas stain for cytokeratins 7, 8, 18, and 19, only 25% of acinar tumors and none of the neuroendocrine tumors stain for cytokeratin 7.

Molecular Pathology

As opposed to colonic neoplasms, precursor lesions in pancreatic adenocarcinomas remain largely unknown. Failure to characterize early pancreatic cancer may be the result of anatomic constraints that limit accessibility to the organ for prospective clinical examination. These shortcomings have slowed progress in the molecular characterization of pancreatic tumors when compared to colon, breast, and other carcinomas.

Three main general categories of genetic alterations have been described in pancreatic carcinogenesis[42–44]: (1) activation of oncogenes, (2) inactivation of tumor suppressor genes, (3) and defects in DNA mismatch repair genes. A long list of oncogenes and their products have been implicated in the pathogenesis of pancreatic cancer.[44] Mutations in the *K-ras* gene are a hallmark of pancreatic adenocarcinoma and appear to be present in more than 90% of tumors. Studies in intraductal papillary mucinous tumors (IPMTs) and mucinous cystic neoplasms (MCNs) of the pancreas have shown that the frequency of *K-ras* mutations correlates with the degree of microscopic dysplasia within tumors.[45, 46] Evidence suggests that *K-ras* mutation may be an early genetic event in pancreatic carcinogenesis, but mutations may even be detected in the setting of chronic pancreatitis without frank neoplasia.[47]

Loss of function in several tumor suppressor genes has also been found in pancreatic tumors, notably *p16, p53,* and *DPC4*.[44] The combination of *p16* and *K-ras* mutations in uncommon among other human tumors and may be a molecular "signature" for pancreatic adenocarcinoma.[48, 49] The most commonly mutated tumor suppressor gene in human cancer, *p53,* is present in a large percentage of pancreatic tumors.[50] Disruption of *p53* function has been linked to alterations in the cell cycle, regulation of transcription, DNA repair, and apoptosis. Another recently discovered tumor suppressor gene involved in pancreatic carcinogenesis is *DPC4*.[51] The current evidence suggests that DPC4 is a key transcription factor involved in the regulation of transforming growth factor-β expression and subsequent growth inhibition.[52] Therefore, disruption of *DPC4* could have critical effects in cell cycle regulation and cell differentiation.

Mutations in DNA mismatch repair genes, such as *MLH1* and *MSH2,* have been found in up to 4% of pancreatic tumors.[53] Disruption in the function of mismatch repair genes has been linked to some hereditary forms of pancreatic cancer and partly explain the increased risk of pancreatic cancer in some families with hereditary nonpolyposis colorectal cancer (HNPCC) syndrome.[54] In general, multiple combinations of genetic mutations are commonly found in pancreatic adenocarcinomas.[55] These data support our current understanding of carcinogenesis as an accumulation of genetic defects over time leading to a malignant phenotype.[56] A list of the most commonly mutated genes found in pancreatic cancer is given in Table 50–2 and contrasted with their mutation frequency in colorectal cancer.

Table 50–2 | **Genetic Mutations in Pancreatic Cancer***

GENE MUTATED	PANCREATIC CANCER (%)	COLORECTAL CANCER
p16	95	0
K-ras	90	50
p53	75	60
DPC4	55	15
BRAC2	7	?

*Their respective frequency in colorectal cancer is given for comparison.
Modified from Wilentz RE, Iacobuzio-Donahue CA, Argani P, et al: Loss of expression of *DPC4* in pancreatic intraepithelial neoplasia: Evidence that *DPC4* inactivation occurs late in neoplastic progression. Cancer Res 60:2002–2006, 2000.

Diagnosis

Symptoms and Signs

Most patients with pancreatic cancer develop symptoms late in the course of disease. The lack of early symptomatology leads to delays in diagnosis, and less than 20% of patients present with resectable disease.[57] Tumors of the head of the pancreas produce symptoms early in the course of disease. In contrast, tumors of the distal gland are characterized by their "silent" presentation, with physical findings appearing only after widely metastatic disease has developed. Clinical signs and symptoms can offer clues as to whether tumors will be resectable or unresectable (Table 50–3).[58]

Jaundice is often the first sign that brings patients to medical attention. Jaundice is present in more than 50% of patients and results from obstruction of the extrahepatic bile duct.[59] In less than one third of patients a palpable nontender gallbladder, referred to as *Courvoisier's sign,* can be found. Patients with concomitant obstruction of the pancreatic duct may also show pancreatic exocrine insufficiency in the form of steatorrhea and malabsorption. In the absence of jaundice, few patients present with resectable disease.

Pain in pancreatic cancer is primarily due to invasion of the celiac and superior mesenteric plexus. The pain is of low intensity, dull, and vaguely localized to the upper abdomen. In advanced disease, pain may be localized to the middle and upper back. Other common symptoms include fatigue, anorexia, and weight loss. These symptoms may or may not be associated with gastric outlet obstruction resulting from tumor involvement of the duodenum.

New-onset diabetes mellitus may also herald pancreatic cancer and can be observed in 6% to 68% of patients.[57] The mechanism of glucose intolerance remains unclear but seems to involve impaired beta cell function of the islets and decreased sensitivity of peripheral tissues to insulin related to overproduction of islet amyloid polypeptide by the tumor.[60, 61] Acute pancreatitis is occasionally the first manifestation of pancreatic cancer,[62] and this must be kept in mind especially when dealing with an elderly patient with acute pancreatitis and no obvious cause.

Computed Tomography

Although transabdominal ultrasound is frequently the first test employed in many patients with pancreatic cancer (because 50% of them present with jaundice), the method of choice for diagnosis and staging of pancreatic cancer is CT scanning.[63–66] The pancreas is ideally imaged by means of the thin-section, pancreatic protocol, helical CT.[67, 68] In large series, a correct diagnosis of pancreatic cancer can be made in up to 97% of patients.[64] Refinements in the CT resolution of peripancreatic blood vessels has rendered routine angiography obsolete in the evaluation of suspected pancreatic masses.[63, 64] The pancreas-protocol CT consists of a dual-phase scan with intravenous and oral contrast agents. The first (pancreatic) phase is obtained 40 seconds after administration of intravenous contrast agent. At this time maximum enhancement of the normal pancreas is obtained, allowing identification of nonenhancing neoplastic lesions (Fig. 50–3*A*). The second (portal vein) phase is obtained 70 seconds after injection of intravenous contrast agent and allows accurate detection of liver metastases and assessment of tumor involvement of the portal and mesenteric veins (Fig. 50–3*B*).

Current criteria for unresectablity by CT include (1) the presence of disease distant to the pancreas (e.g., liver, peritoneum); (2) contiguous invasion of adjacent organs such as the stomach or colon; and (3) arterial encasement (celiac axis or superior mesenteric artery) or venous occlusion (portal vein or superior mesenteric vein).[63–65]

Using these criteria, CT has been shown to be almost 100% accurate in predicting unresectable disease.[63] However, approximately 25% to 50% of patients predicted to have resectable disease by CT turn out to have unresectable lesions at laparotomy.[63–66, 69] These patients clearly do not benefit from surgical exploration, and their identification by preoperative imaging remains a challenge. The most common causes of unresectability are small peritoneal or liver tumor implants and vascular involvement by tumor. The advent of the helical pancreatic-protocol CT has helped improve the preoperative determination of surgical resectability, particularly in relation to vessel invasion. Recent studies have shown that assessment of the degree of circumferential vessel involvement by tumor can help predict unresectability.[70–72] Other efforts aimed at detecting small peritoneal and liver metastases beyond the resolution of CT have focused

Table 50–3 | **Presenting Symptoms and Signs in Patients with Unresectable and Resectable Pancreatic Cancer**

	PALLIATED (*N* = 256)	RESECTED (*N* = 512)
Demographics		
Age	64.0 ± 0.7 years	65.8 ± 0.5 years
Gender	57% male	55% male
Race	91% white	91% white
Symptoms and Signs		
Abdominal pain	64%	36%*
Jaundice	57%	72%*
Weight loss	48%	43%
Nausea/vomiting	30%	18%*
Back pain	26%	2%*

*$P < 0.001$ vs. palliated group.
From Sohn TA, Lillemoe KD, Cameron JL, et al: Surgical palliation of unresectable periampullary adenocarcinoma in the 1990s. J Am Coll Surg 188:658–666, 1999.

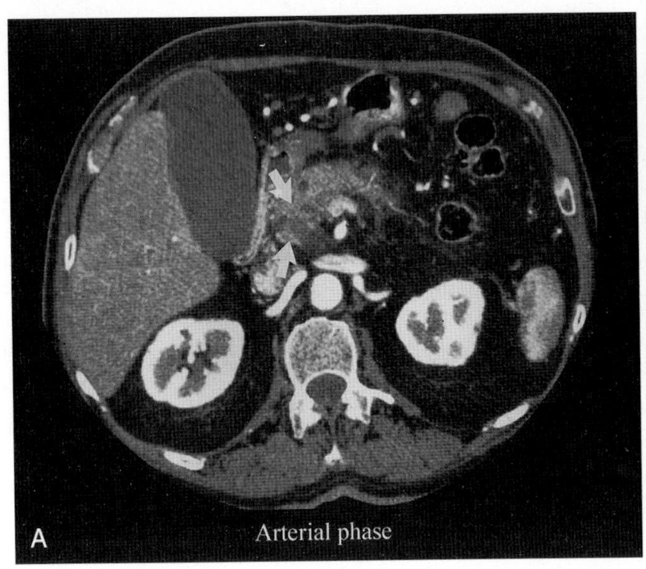

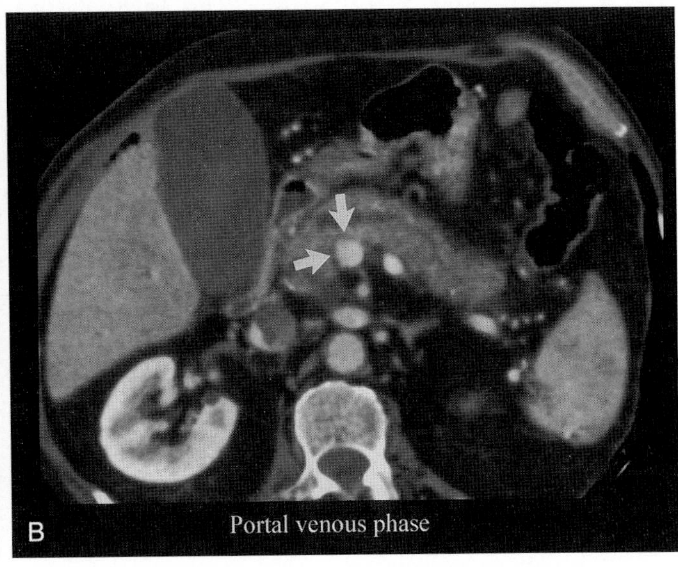

Figure 50–3. *A*, Arterial phase of a pancreatic protocol CT showing a nonenhancing lesion in the head of the pancreas (arrows). *B*, Venous phase of the same CT, showing a noninvolved fat plane around the portal vein (*arrows*).

on the development of staging laparoscopy, as discussed later.

Endoscopic Retrograde Cholangiopancreatography

Since its description by McCune and associates in 1968,[73] endoscopic retrograde cholangiopancreatography (ERCP) has become a mainstay in the differential diagnosis of the tumors of the pancreatobiliary junction. Of these 85% are pancreatic, 6% originate in the distal common bile duct, and 4% each are ampullary or duodenal carcinomas.[74] The latter two can usually be visualized and biopsied during ERCP, a welcome finding in that their 5-year survival rate of about 50% after successful resection is two to three times higher than that for pancreatic ductal carcinoma.[75] In a review of 530 ERCP examinations in pancreatic cancer, Freeny found only 15 normal pancreatograms (2.8%),[76] making it an extremely sensitive test for this diagnosis. Typically, the duct becomes encased or obstructed by the carcinoma. Other findings may include field defects (i.e., areas where no pancreatic ducts are seen), duct necrosis with extravasation, and contiguous involvement of the common bile duct.[76] A "double-duct sign," representing strictures in both the biliary and pancreatic duct, is found in many patients with pancreatic cancer (Fig. 50–4).

Current CT imaging allows for identification of pancreatic tumors in most patients with pancreatic cancer, rendering ERCP unnecessary in most cases. In practice, however, many patients with pancreatic cancer do undergo ERCP, not for the main purpose of diagnosis but rather for stenting of the biliary duct. Routine preoperative biliary stenting to relieve jaundice has not been shown to decrease postoperative morbidity and mortality, and in fact there is evidence suggesting it may increase the rate of complications.[77, 78] Therefore, its practice in resectable patients cannot be recommended, unless it is anticipated that surgery will not be done for several weeks. For patients with jaundice and unresectable or metastatic disease, endoscopic biliary stenting, preferably with expandable metal stents, offers excellent palliation.

For patients with suspected pancreatic cancer and no identifiable tumor by CT, ERCP is indicated. Increasingly, however, EUS is becoming the method of choice to identify small pancreatic tumors and assist in their differential diagnosis.

Endoscopic Ultrasonography

EUS may be the most accurate test for the diagnosis of pancreatic cancer. Several studies comparing it with CT have shown that EUS has a higher sensitivity and specificity for this diagnosis, particularly in evaluating small tumors[79, 80]) (Fig. 50–5). In addition, EUS is highly accurate for staging local invasion and nodal metastases from pancreatic cancer,[81, 82] although in direct comparison with dual-phase helical CT results are similar, and CT does give the added information regarding metastatic liver disease.[83]

EUS also allows for tissue diagnosis by fine-needle aspiration (see later). It has been found to be a highly accurate and safe approach[84] and has the added benefit of avoiding potential transperitoneal seeding of the tumor.

Magnetic Resonance Imaging

Magnetic resonance imaging (MRI) has been increasingly used in the evaluation of pancreatic tumors, and several groups have shown results that rival helical CT.[85, 86] In one study, pancreatic tumor detection was reported in 90% of patients by MRI versus 76% by helical CT.[85] Optimal MRI resolution is obtained with T1-weighted images using dynamic gadolinium enhancement. Tumors are viewed as low-signal masses against the high-signal background of normal pancreatic parenchyma. Pancreatic masses, ductal dilation,

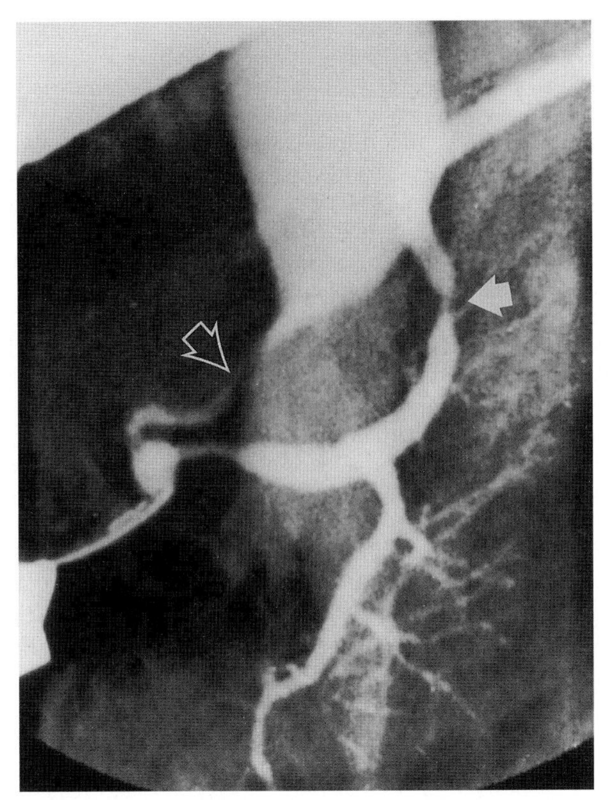

Figure 50–4. ERCP showing strictures of the biliary (*open arrow*) and pancreatic (*closed arrow*) ducts in pancreatic cancer (double-duct sign).

and liver metastasis can be demonstrated in exquisite detail. Additionally, MR angiography and MR venography techniques using gadolinium contrast can demonstrate vascular involvement with tumor and obviate the need for conventional angiography.[87] As opposed to CT, MRI does not involve radiation and employs an iodine-free contrast agent with rare renal toxicity. Limitations of MRI are related to cost, availability, and clinicians' familiarity and predilection for CT imaging.

Magnetic resonance cholangiopancreatography (MRCP) can also be obtained at the time of MRI.[88] In a recent prospective, controlled study, MRCP was found to be as sensitive as ERCP in detecting pancreatic carcinomas.[89] MRCP uses heavy T2-weighted images that emphasize fluid-containing structures such as ducts, cysts, and peripancreatic fluid collections. Images obtained are highly comparable to those after ERCP and readily demonstrate pancreatic ductal obstruction, ectasia, and calculi.

Positron Emission Tomography

Positron emission tomography (PET) is a noninvasive imaging tool that provides metabolic rather than morphologic information on tumors.[90, 91] This diagnostic method is based on greater utilization of glucose by tumor cells than normal pancreatic parenchyma. A radioactive glucose analog termed *^{18}fluorodeoxyglucose* (FDG) is administered intravenously, followed by detection of FDG uptake by the PET scanner. The normal pancreas is not usually visualized by FDG-PET. In contrast, pancreatic carcinoma appears as a focal area of increased uptake in the pancreatic bed. Hepatic metastases appear as "hot spots" within the liver. Owing to the lack of anatomic detail, PET scanning is not a principal diagnostic modality for pancreatic cancer. However, FDG-PET can be helpful in differentiating benign from malignant pancreatic masses when morphologic data is equivocal.[92] It can also be useful in assessing tumor recurrence after pancreatic resection, when scar tissue or postoperative changes may be difficult to differentiate from carcinoma. Finally, FDG-PET can be of benefit in assessing tumor response to neoadjuvant chemoradiation that may lead to alteration in clinical management.

Percutaneous and EUS-Guided Aspiration Cytology

Fine-needle aspiration cytology of the pancreas has been one of the major advances in the management of patients with pancreatic tumors. CT-guided biopsy has been used for more than 20 years and is regarded as a safe, reliable procedure, with a reported sensitivity of 57% to 96% and virtually no false-positive results.[93–96] Recent experience with EUS-guided aspiration shows similar results.[84] Whenever a patient is deemed to have unresectable or metastatic disease, CT- or EUS-guided fine-needle aspiration is indicated for histologic confirmation, unless a palliative surgical procedure is required. Even if the diagnosis of chronic pancreatitis is reasonably eliminated, proof of malignancy will exclude other rare benign conditions of the pancreas such as tuberculosis[97] and sarcoidosis.[98] Furthermore, needle-aspiration cytology can usually distinguish between adenocarcinoma and other pancreatic tumors, including those of islet cells and lymphomas. Pancreatic lymphoma has a significantly higher cure rate,[99, 100] even if unresectable, and islet cell neoplasms, many of which present as large tumors without clinically apparent endocrine dysfunction, also have a better prognosis than pancreatic adenocarcinoma (see Chapter 51).[101]

In the hands of experienced surgeons, tissue diagnosis is not a prerequisite to proceed with surgery in most patients

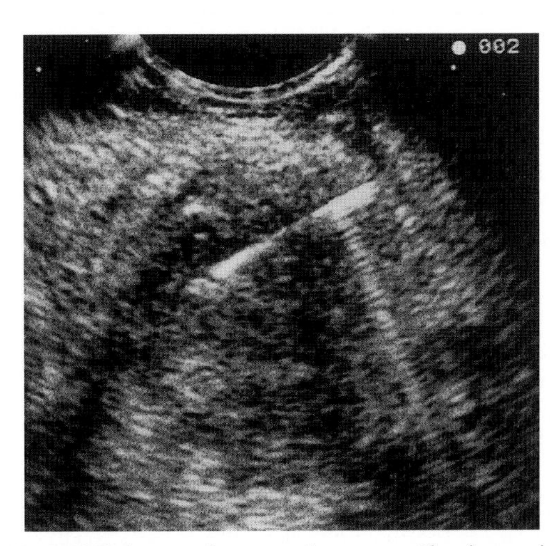

Figure 50–5. EUS image of pancreatic cancer. The figure shows the needle during biopsy.

with potentially resectable tumors. One must also keep in mind that a negative result cannot exclude malignancy even after repeated sampling; in fact, it is the smaller (i.e., more curable) tumors that are most likely to be missed by the needle.

Serum Markers

A wide variety of tumor markers have been proposed for pancreatic cancer, but currently the only one with any practical utility is CA 19-9. Although not suitable for screening, it is a valuable adjunct in the diagnosis, prognosis, and monitoring of pancreatic cancer.[102] Sensitivity and specificity vary with the cutoff values and have the caveat that in the presence of jaundice, and especially with cholangitis, very high values can be found in the absence of malignancy (false-positive results).[103] In addition, patients with a Lewis blood group phenotype (−a,−b) do not express the CA 19-9 antigen. In a recent study, using a cutoff of 37 U/mL, sensitivity and specificity were 86% and 87%, respectively.[104]

Staging

The most recent American Joint Committee on Cancer (AJCC) staging system for pancreatic cancer is shown in Table 50–4. This system has not been found to be clinically useful for several reasons. First, adequate evaluation of lymph node status cannot be performed without surgical intervention. This may lead to understaging of patients with locally advanced disease who are not candidates for laparotomy. Second, treatment options cannot be determined by a patient's TNM status. For example, patients with stage III disease may or may not be candidates for resection. Finally, patient classification by the AJCC staging system in general has not correlated to prognosis.

Appropriate treatment of patients with pancreatic cancer depends on accurate preoperative staging. Although complete resection offers the only chance for cure, surgical exploration of most of these patients is no longer necessary to establish unresectability. Patients with metastatic disease can benefit from minimally invasive percutaneous and endoscopic techniques that allow tissue sampling and treatment of malignant biliary obstruction[105, 106] without the potential morbidity and convalescence time characteristic of surgical approaches.[58] More than 95% of patients treated with only minimally invasive techniques never require a laparotomy.[107]

Staging of pancreatic cancer patients is predicated on the identification of three distinct groups. The first group includes individuals presenting with metastatic disease. Surgery is best avoided in these patients in view of their short survival, and chemotherapy is their principal treatment modality other than palliative measures.[7, 57, 108] The second group comprises those patients with advanced local disease (i.e., major vascular invasion) but without metastases. These patients can benefit from external-beam radiation therapy (EBRT) combined with chemotherapy, and according to their response, may be candidates for intraoperative radiation therapy.[109–111] A third and last subpopulation is that with resectable disease. These individuals may benefit from transfer to a tertiary referral center where pancreatic resection can be performed with low mortality rates.[112–115]

The most powerful noninvasive diagnostic test for evaluation of suspected pancreatic cancer is the high-resolution, contrast-enhanced helical CT.[64, 65] As previously discussed, CT is extremely accurate in identifying unresectable disease but fails to correctly predict resectability in 25% to 50% of patients. In most cases, lesions missed are beyond the resolution of current radiologic imaging and include small implants on the peritoneal surfaces of the liver, abdominal wall, stomach, intestine, or omentum. Additionally, micrometastases in peritoneal washings are also missed. Successful detection of such tumor dissemination depends on access to the peritoneal cavity and visual inspection, which at present can be achieved only by laparoscopy or laparotomy.

Several large studies have documented the value of staging laparoscopy in the evaluation of patients with pancreatic cancer.[66, 116–121] In our institution, the staging procedure consists of a simple diagnostic laparoscopy with collection of peritoneal washings for cytology. Patients with occult metastases detected by positive peritoneal cytology have been shown to carry a prognosis similar to those with M1 disease (stage IVB).[122–124] Other groups perform more extensive staging procedures that include extended laparoscopic dissections and laparoscopic ultrasonography.[117, 120, 125] These maneuvers allow for more thorough examination of the liver and blood vessels in the vicinity of the pancreas, but it is not clear how much of the information obtained overlaps with that from current CT imaging.

Our data show that approximately 25% of patients with localized disease by CT harbor unsuspected metastatic implants.[118, 119] A further 10% demonstrate positive peritoneal cytology despite a lack of gross metastatic disease at laparoscopy. For most of these patients, laparoscopy has prevented unnecessary surgical explorations to assess resectability.[107] The combination of CT scan and staging laparoscopy has enhanced the identification of patients with metastatic, localized-unresectable, and resectable pancreatic cancer and has helped in stratifying patients to different treatment protocols.[119] Our current algorithm for the diagnosis and staging

Table 50–4 | **TNM System and AJCC Staging of Pancreatic Cancer**

TNM System	
Tis	Carcinoma in situ
T1	Tumor limited to the pancreas 2 cm or less in greatest dimension
T2	Tumor limited to the pancreas >2 cm in greatest dimension
T3	Tumor extends directly into any of the following: duodenum, bile duct, peripancreatic tissues
T4	Tumor extends directly into any of the following: stomach, spleen, colon, adjacent large vessels
N0	No regional lymph node metastases
N1	Regional lymph node metastases
M0	No distant metastases
M1	Distant metastases

AJCC Staging			
Stage I	T1–T2	N0	M0
Stage II	T3	N0	M0
Stage III	T1–T3	N1	M0
Stage IVA	T4	Any N	M0
Stage IVB	Any T	Any N	M1

AJCC, American Joint Committee on Cancer.

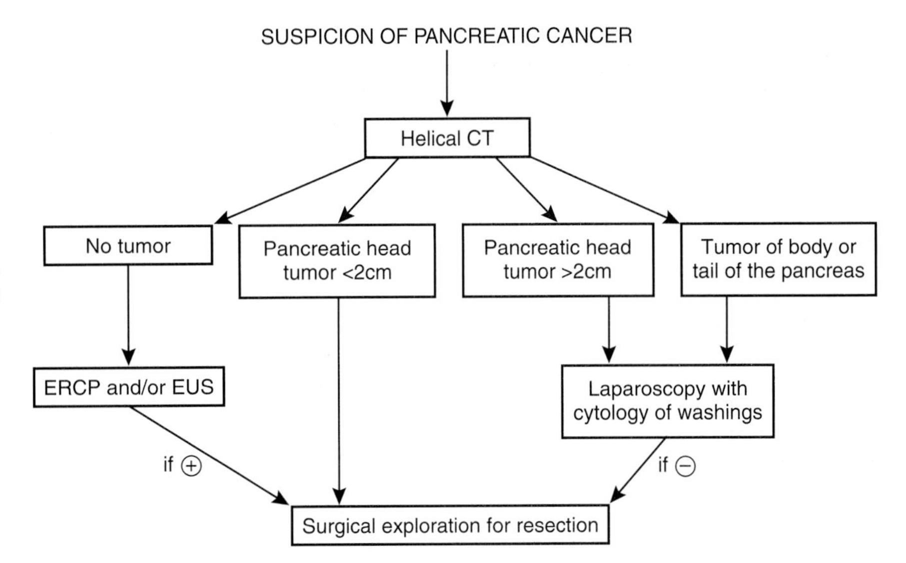

Figure 50–6. Massachusetts General Hospital algorithm for diagnosis and staging of pancreatic cancer.

of pancreatic cancer is shown in Figure 50–6. We recommend laparoscopy for all patients with tumors in the body and tail of the pancreas (in which the frequency of unsuspected metastases approaches 50%) and for patients with tumors in the head of the pancreas larger than 2 cm, because the yield of laparoscopy in smaller lesions is less than 10%.

Treatment

Surgery

Surgical resection is the only potentially curative treatment for pancreatic cancer. Because of the late presentation of the disease, only about 15% of patients are candidates for pancreatectomy. Absolute contraindications for resection include presence of metastases in the liver, peritoneum, omentum, or any extra-abdominal site. More relative contraindications are involvement of the bowel mesentery, portomesenteric vasculature, and celiac axis and its tributaries. Although under some circumstances this involvement can be dealt with from the technical standpoint, the morbidity and mortality can be substantial, and long-term outcomes may not be better than without resection.

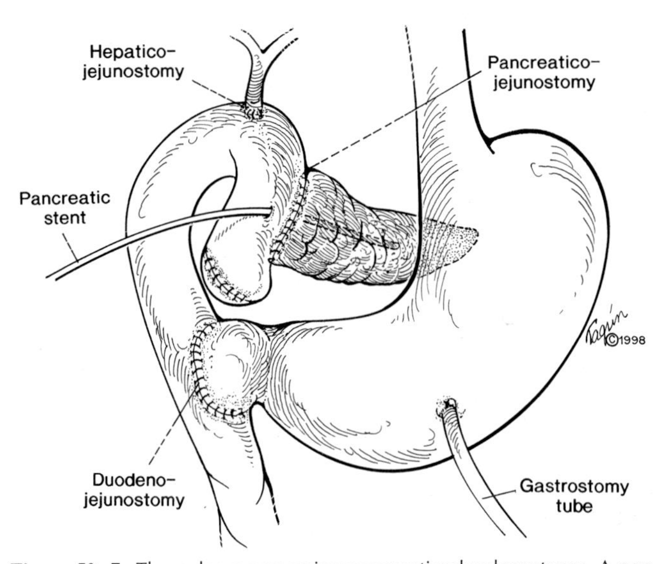

Figure 50–7. The pylorus-preserving pancreaticoduodenectomy. A pancreatic stent is shown in the pancreatic duct. (From Jimenez RE, Fernandez-del Castillo C, Rattner DW, et al: Outcome of the pancreaticoduodenectomy with pylorus preservation or with antrectomy in the treatment of chronic pancreatitis. Ann Surg 231:293–300, 2000.)

The standard operation for pancreatic cancer is pancreaticoduodenectomy, the "Whipple procedure," or a modification thereof (Fig. 50–7). This operation reflects the practical reality that with few exceptions only cancers occurring in the head of the gland prove to be resectable. Total pancreatectomy was advocated as a better operation for pancreatic cancer,[126] both to remove more potentially malignant tissue and to avoid the pancreatojejunal anastomosis, which was the source of considerable morbidity and mortality. However, results of that operation have shown no improvement over more limited resection, and it produces the additional disadvantage of obligate exocrine insufficiency and diabetes that is brittle and difficult to manage.[127–129] The so-called regional pancreatectomy also confers no survival advantage.[128, 130]

Some groups in Japan routinely complement the Whipple operation with an extensive lymph node dissection, claiming better results without an increase in postoperative morbidity.[131, 132] The single prospective trial comparing conventional versus extended lymphadenectomy showed no advantage, although post hoc analysis did demonstrate a better survival in patients with positive nodes who underwent the extensive lymphadenectomy.[133] Trials are currently underway to further address this issue. Paradoxically, the use of a lesser operation that preserves the pylorus, and thereby avoids postgastrectomy symptoms, is being increasingly used for pancreatic cancer in the United States.[134–136] No apparent compromise of long-term survival has been noted, although clearly it is not suitable for all patients.[137, 138] Adequate comparative data for these different procedures are needed before the optimal operation for resectable pancreatic cancer is established.

In the past, pancreaticoduodenectomy was associated with high morbidity and mortality rates. Many recent large series show mortality rates of less than 3%,[139–141] with concomitant decrease in complications. These changes have been attributed to the concentration of the surgery in the hands of fewer surgeons, who then develop greater expertise.[142, 143] A recent study using the Medicare database showed a fourfold increase in mortality when comparing pancreaticoduodenectomy performed in hospitals with an average of less than one case per year to those hospitals performing more than five cases per year,[115] and another study suggested that long-term outcomes are likewise improved.[144]

Even with resective surgery in appropriately selected patients, the prognosis for pancreatic cancer is not good. Large series show 5-year survival rates of 10.5% to 25% and median survival between 10.5 and 20 months.[140, 145–147] Among those variables that have been shown by multivariate analysis to be significant predictors of a better outcome are tumor size less than 3 cm, absence of lymph node metastases, negative margins, well-differentiated tumors, and intraoperative blood loss of less than 750 mL.[140, 145–148]

Palliative Procedures

Large series of patients with pancreatic cancer show that only between 5% and 22% are resectable.[149–153] The remaining majority require some form of palliation for relief of jaundice, duodenal obstruction, or pain. Operations for biliary bypass are quite effective and have the advantage of offering a preventive or therapeutic concomitant gastrojejunostomy as well as a celiac plexus block for pain control. They are, however, not exempt from risk in these debilitated patients. A recent large series shows postoperative mortality of 3.1% and a complication rate of 22%, with a median survival of 6.5 months.[58]

Relief of jaundice can also be achieved by stents placed percutaneously or endoscopically, much reducing the length of hospitalization and recovery. In experienced hands, endoscopic stent placement has a success rate of more than 85%, with a 1% to 2% procedure-related mortality,[154, 155] and has therefore become increasingly popular in the management of malignant biliary obstruction. Several randomized trials have found no difference in survival between endoscopic stent placement and surgical bypass for malignant obstructive jaundice,[156–159] but stented patients do have more frequent readmissions for stent occlusion, recurrent jaundice, and cholangitis. A recent controlled study showed that patients with malignant biliary obstruction (mostly from pancreatic cancer) did better with metal stents or with plastic stents exchanged every 3 months, when compared with patients treated with plastic stents that were only exchanged when the stent malfunctioned.[160]

Duodenal obstruction traditionally has been treated by surgery, although the real benefit for the patient has been questioned.[161, 162] Reports of the use of expandable metallic stents to relieve duodenal malignant obstruction have shown success,[163, 164] and this modality may be used increasingly in the future.

Pain in pancreatic cancer can be extremely distressing and frequently requires the use of narcotics. Randomized trials have shown that surgical and percutaneous chemical neurolysis of the celiac ganglion can offer relief to many patients,[165, 166] and radiation therapy may also significantly alleviate pain (see later).

Radiation Therapy

Radiation therapy may have a useful role in the treatment of the 40% of pancreatic cancers that are not resectable but still appear to be localized. Median survival for untreated pancreatic cancer is about 4 to 6 months.[167, 168] With the exception of one trial, conventional EBRT combined with 5-fluorouracil (5-FU) as a radiosensitizer has been shown to improve survival when compared to EBRT alone or chemotherapy alone.[111] Even though the improvement is modest (median survival of approximately 11 months and a 12% 2-year survival), this has become the standard of care, and newer radiosensitizers are under study.[7]

Intraoperative radiation therapy offers the possibility of delivering a higher dose to the cancer without increasing the injury to neighboring tissues.[169] Either before or after fractionated external radiation therapy, a 20 Gy boost is delivered by electron beam through a field-limiting cone directly to the surgically exposed tumor.[170] Its superiority over EBRT alone has not been demonstrated in controlled studies, but the reported median survival is improved by about 2 months and the 2-year survival is 20%.[111] Follow-up shows excellent local control with this modality, but patients still develop liver metastases and peritoneal seeding.

Neoadjuvant chemoradiation has also been used, and it has been suggested that preoperative chemoradiation can convert selected unresectable cases to resectable ones.[171, 172] Thus far, long-term results are no different than with postoperative chemoradiation,[173] although surgery is avoided in some patients who develop metastases during treatment.[174]

EBRT also has a role as adjuvant treatment after resective surgery. A trial by the Gastrointestinal Tumor Study Group demonstrated a significantly longer median survival time (21 months) for resected patients who received 5-FU and 40 Gy external radiation than in controls who only underwent curative resection (11 months).[175] Postoperative chemoradiation is currently routinely offered in many institutions throughout the United States. In a retrospective study from Johns Hopkins University Medical School, patients with resected pancreatic cancer treated with conventional postoperative chemoradiation had a significantly higher survival (median of 21 months) compared to no treatment (13.5 months) or an intensive chemoradiation regimen (17.5 months).[176] In a recent report of 616 resected patients by the same group, postoperative chemoradiation was found by multivariate analysis to be a strong independent predictor of survival.[140] Two trials from Europe, however, do not support its use.[177, 178]

Chemotherapy

Evaluation of the efficacy of different chemotherapy agents in pancreatic cancer has been based primarily on objective response rates.[9] In solid tumors, objective response is defined as a 50% or greater reduction in the sum of the products of all bidimensionally measurable lesions. This assessment of tumor response can be challenging in pancreatic tumors. First, pancreatic carcinomas often have an associated intense desmoplastic reaction that can greatly overestimate the malignant cell mass. Additionally, the borders of the tumor may be difficult to discern when the surrounding parenchyma is involved with acute or chronic pancreatitis. For these and other reasons, evaluation of response to chemotherapeutic agents remains a complicated problem. Better endpoints are currently needed, such as trends in serum tumor markers (i.e., CA 19-9) during chemotherapy,[179] or symptom assessment during treatment as a measure of palliation.[180]

Only two chemotherapy agents have been associated with survivals longer than 5 months in pancreatic cancer: 5-FU and gemcitabine.[7, 181, 182] Studies with 5-FU have been performed mostly using intravenous bolus administration, but current data in colorectal carcinoma suggest that antitumor activity may be enhanced by short-term continuous infusion (over 5 days) or protracted infusion (uninterrupted delivery to toxicity[183]). Multiple studies have evaluated biomodulation of 5-FU with leucovorin, interferon-α, or *N*-(phosphonacety)-L-aspartate without demonstrable improvement in survival.[9]

At this time, gemcitabine is the most efficacious single agent against pancreatic adenocarcinoma. A phase III trial by Burris and coworkers comparing 5-FU to gemcitabine in 126 patients demonstrated a statistically significant improvement in survival of 5.7 versus 4.4 months[180] (Fig. 50–8). More important, 1-year survival was 18% for patients receiving gemcitabine but only 2% for those receiving 5-FU. No patient in the studies survived 18 months, however.

Multiple combination regimens have also been used in pancreatic adenocarcinoma. Notable among these regimes are 5-FU + Adriamycin + mitomycin C (FAM),[184] 5-FU + mitomycin C + streptozocin (SMF),[185] and cisplatin + cytosine arabinoside + caffeine.[186] One study demonstrated significantly prolonged survivals for patients receiving SMF compared with those receiving cisplatin + cytosine arabinoside + caffeine.[186] However, no difference in survival can be shown between treatment with SMF compared with FAM.[187] Finally, a trial by the North Central Cancer Treatment group comparing FAM to single-agent treatment with 5-FU failed to demonstrate an advantage of combination therapy over monotherapy.[188]

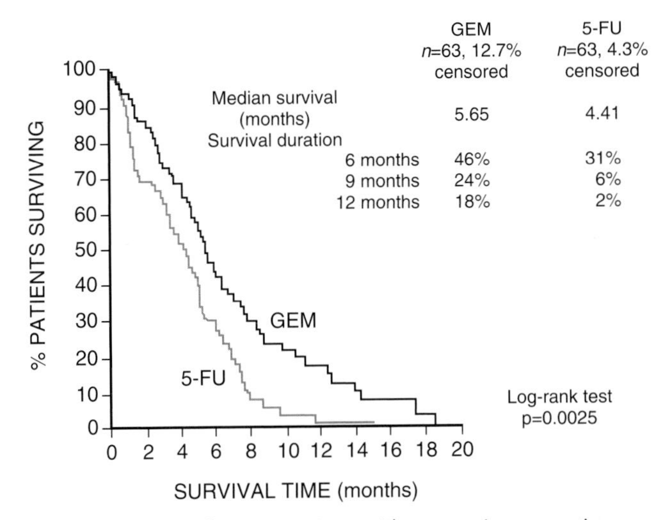

Figure 50–8. Survival in 126 patients with metastatic pancreatic cancer treated with gemcitabine or 5-FU. (From Rothenberg ML, Moore MJ, Cripps MC, et al: A phase II trial of gemcitabine in patients with 5-FU refractory pancreas cancer. Ann Oncol 7:347–353, 1996.)

Table 50–5 | **Cystic Neoplasms of the Pancreas: MGH Series**

TYPE	NUMBER (% OF TOTAL)
MCN	95 (45)
Malignant MCN	61 (29)
Serous cystadenoma	34 (16)
IPMT	38 (32)
Cystic islet cell tumor	4 (2)
Papillary cystic tumor	6 (3)
Total	**238**

MCN, mucinous cystic neoplasm; IPMT, intraductal papillary mucinous tumor; MGH, Massachusetts General Hospital.

In general, results of current chemotherapy trials in pancreatic adenocarcinoma are largely disappointing. Combination therapy does not appear to be superior to monotherapy with 5-FU, and gemcitabine is the only single agent showing an advantage over 5-FU. Studies of combination regimens involving gemcitabine are currently in progress.

CYSTIC TUMORS OF THE PANCREAS

Cystic tumors of the pancreas are relatively uncommon, accounting perhaps for only 1% of pancreatic neoplasms.[189] MCNs, serous cystadenomas, and IPMTs comprise more than 90% of the primary cystic neoplasms of the pancreas, but other tumors with cystic appearance are also known (Table 50–5). Accurate recognition of these lesions is important because of their ability to masquerade as pancreatic pseudocysts and their high cure rate following surgical treatment.

Differential Diagnosis

Patient evaluation after discovery of a cystic lesion of the pancreas should initially be directed toward exclusion of a pancreatic pseudocyst.[190, 191] As opposed to cystic neoplasms, pseudocysts lack an epithelial lining and represent collections of pancreatic secretions that have extravasated from a duct disrupted by inflammation or obstruction (see Chapters 48 and 49). Patients with pseudocysts often have a history of acute or chronic pancreatitis, or abdominal trauma, whereas most of those with cystic tumor lack such antecedent factors. Radiographic characteristics that favor a diagnosis of pseudocyst over cystic neoplasms include lack of septae, loculations, solid components, or cyst wall calcifications on CT; hypovascularity on angiography; and communication between the cyst and the pancreatic ductal system on ERCP. Aspiration of pseudocyst contents reveals high levels of amylase, which is unusual for cystic tumors. Distinction between pseudocysts and cystic neoplasms is best accomplished by EUS, which also gives better detail of the cyst's characteristics (Fig. 50–9).

If a diagnosis of pancreatic pseudocyst can be ruled out, evaluation should subsequently focus on identifying those tumors that require surgical resection due to actual or poten-

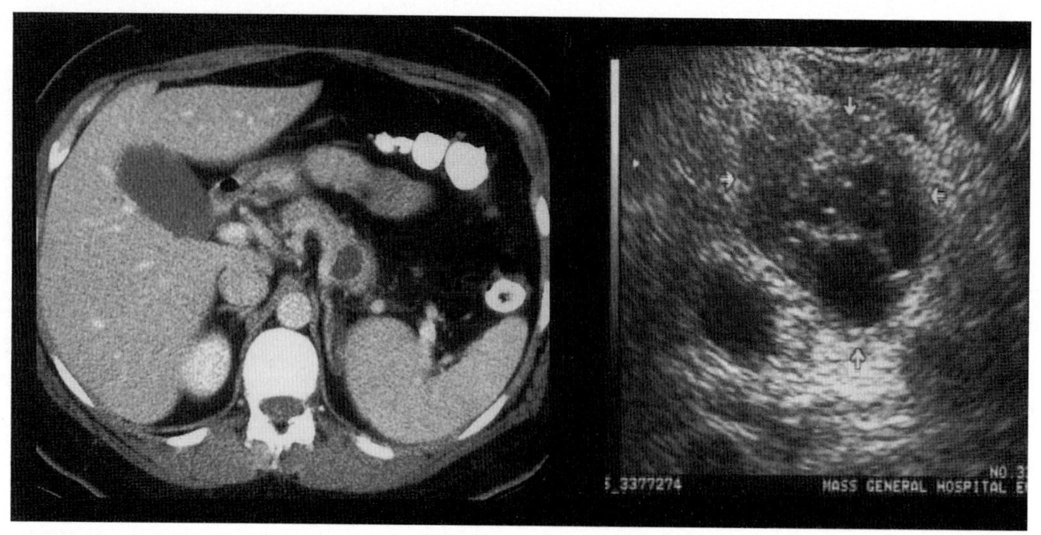

Figure 50–9. CT and EUS of a mucinous cystic neoplasm of the tail of the pancreas. EUS demonstrates septae and loculations not seen clearly by CT, and also allows for cyst fluid sampling.

tial malignancy. As opposed to ductal adenocarcinoma, cystic neoplasms with malignant potential are slow growing, and favorable prognoses have been reported even in the setting of malignant degeneration. Tumors with malignant potential include MCN, IPMT, papillary cystic neoplasms, and cystic islet cell tumors. Serous cystadenomas, in contrast, are almost universally benign. The diagnostic examination of choice is the helical CT with intravenous contrast agent enhancement, allowing tumor localization and sometimes discrimination of serous cystadenomas from other neoplasms. Our group, as well as others, has demonstrated the value of cyst fluid analysis in the evaluation of cystic neoplasms, a procedure that can be readily done with EUS.[192–194] If despite all efforts accurate diagnosis is not possible, resection rather than observation is preferred. A summary of some of the distinguishing features of the most common cystic tumors of the pancreas can be seen in Table 50–6 and are discussed later.

Mucinous Cystic Neoplasms

Mucinous cystic neoplasms (MCNs) are the most frequently encountered cystic tumors of the pancreas, accounting for 45% to 50% of tumors. MCNs display a clinical and histologic spectrum ranging from clearly benign to frankly malignant tumors.[195–197] Accurate diagnosis requires examination of extensive samples for cyst epithelium and mandates complete surgical resection and not just simple biopsy.[198] Current pathologic classification distinguishes between benign, borderline, or malignant (cystadenocarcinoma) tumors based on their maximal degree of dysplasia.[34] This classification scheme correlates with patient prognosis and suggests that all these tumors should be treated as premalignant lesions with eventual evolution to aggressive behavior if left untreated.

MCNs occur primarily in women (>80%) with a mean age of 55 years. Patients complain primarily of abdominal pain or palpable mass. Symptoms such as weight loss and jaundice are more common with malignant tumors. Today, with the more liberal application of CT scanning in medical evaluations, an increasing percentage of tumors are being diagnosed while asymptomatic.

Grossly, MCNs consist of multiloculated tumors with smooth, glistening surfaces that develop predominantly (66%) in the body or tail of the pancreas[197]) (Fig. 50–10). Cysts range in size from 2 to 26 cm in maximum diameter, large tumors being more often malignant than smaller ones. The cysts are filled with viscous mucous material, and cyst walls are dense and fibrous with occasional calcification. Abdominal ultrasound or CT successfully demonstrates many of these characteristics. CT scanning may also allow identification of solid components associated with cystic ele-

Table 50–6 | **Characteristics of Cystic Neoplasms of the Pancreas**

	MCN	SEROUS CYST-ADENOMA	IPMT
Sex	>80% female	>80% female	>50% male
Presentation	Mass, pain	Mass, pain	Pancreatitis
Location	Body and tail	Body and tail	Head
CT findings			
Septae	Yes	Yes	No
Calcifications	Yes	Yes	No
ERCP findings			
Ductal displacement	Yes	Yes	No
Ductal dilation	No	No	Yes
Filling defects	No	No	Yes
Duct-cyst communication	No	No	Yes
Patulous ampulla with mucin	No	No	Yes
Malignant potential	Yes	No	Yes
Treatment	Resection	May observe	Resection

MCN, mucinous cystic neoplasm; IPMT, intraductal papillary mucinous tumor; ERCP, endoscopic retrograde cholangiopancreatography.

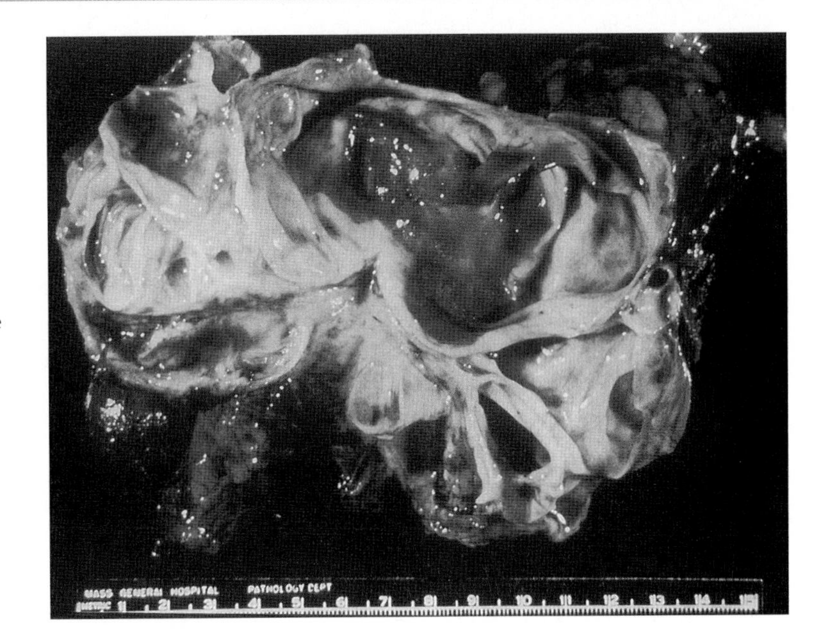

Figure 50–10. Mucinous cystic neoplasm of the tail of the pancreas. Note multiloculated cyst.

ments, features of borderline or malignant tumors but not of benign variants. ERCP rarely demonstrates cyst communication with pancreatic ducts but may show ductal obstruction or displacement by mass effect. When performed, cyst fluid analysis generally reveals high viscosity and elevated tumor markers (CEA) and may show malignant cytology (Table 50–7).

Owing to the inherent potential for malignancy in MCNs, surgical resection is advocated for all of them. In most instances this requires distal pancreatectomy with splenectomy, but pancreaticoduodenectomy is indicated for tumors of the head of the pancreas. More limited resections, such as enucleation, are not recommended owing to the risks of fistula formation and inadequate tumor margins.[199] Five-year survival rates are excellent (>95%) for benign or borderline MCN, and long-term survival rates are also expected for 50% to 75% of fully resected malignant tumors.[198, 200] In our experience, unresectable malignant tumors carry as bad a prognosis as unresected ductal adenocarcinoma.[189]

Serous Cystadenoma

Serous cystadenomas, formerly known as *microcystic adenomas,* are the second most common cystic tumor of the pancreas.[201] The clinical presentation of serous cystadenomas is similar to that of MCNs, occurring mostly in women (80%) with a mean age of 63 years. Most (50% to 70%) occur in the body or tail of the pancreas.[202] An association with von Hippel–Lindau disease has also been noted. Most patients present with vague abdominal pain or discomfort, but a significant number can present with a palpable mass when the tumor has attained a large size (1 to 25 cm). Increasingly, incidental asymptomatic tumors are being detected during evaluation for other unrelated conditions.

Macroscopically, serous cystadenomas consist of well-circumscribed pancreatic neoplasms, which on cross section show numerous tiny cysts separated by delicate fibrous septa, giving them a honeycomb appearance[203] (Fig. 50–11). The cysts are filled with clear watery fluid and are often arranged around a central stellate scar that may be calcified. The pathognomonic image by CT scan is that of a spongy mass with a central "sunburst" calcification, but this finding occurs in only 10% of patients[197] (Fig. 50–12). EUS may allow better resolution of the honeycomb structure than CT. Macrocystic variants are known that may be indistinguishable from MCN.[204]

Hypervascularity may be demonstrated by angiography, and some tumors have presented with intra-abdominal hemorrhage. Cyst fluid analysis characteristically reveals low vis cosity, low levels of CEA, and negative cytology (see Table 50–7).

As opposed to MCN, most serous cystadenomas represent benign tumors. Rare case reports of serous cystadenocarcinomas exist but constitute less than 1% of known cases.[205] Surgical resection is the treatment of choice for symptomatic lesions and may entail a Whipple procedure or distal pancreatectomy (with or without splenectomy), depending on ana-

Table 50–7 | **Cyst Fluid Analysis in Cystic Tumors of the Pancreas**

	PSEUDOCYST	SEROUS CYSTADENOMA	MCN–BENIGN	MCN–MALIGNANT
Viscosity	Low	Low	High	High
Amylase	High	Low	Low	Low
CEA	Low	Low	High	High
CA 72–4	Low	Low	Intermediate	High
Cytology	Histiocytes	Usually negative; rarely cuboidal cells	Occasionally mucinous epithelial cells	Adenocarcinomas

MCN, mucinous cystic neoplasm; CEA, carcinoembryonic antigen.

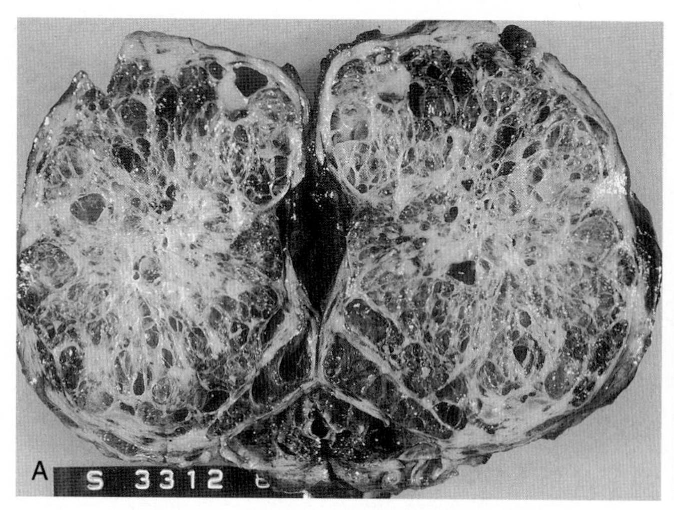

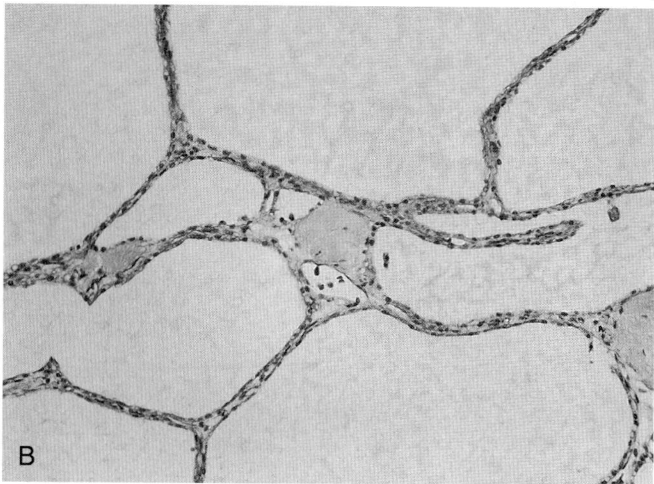

Figure 50–11. Serous cystadenoma of the tail of the pancreas. *A,* Most of the pancreatic parenchyma has been replaced by a cystic neoplasm, composed of multiple small cysts. *B,* A high power view shows cysts containing serous fluid and lined by bland cuboidal cells rich in glycogen.

tomic location. Alternatively, serous cystadenomas may be safely observed if asymptomatic. Observation carries the risk of continued growth, which may lead to complications such as hemorrhage, obstructive jaundice, pancreatic insufficiency, or gastric outlet obstruction. For these reasons, and given the safety of pancreatic resection in specialized centers, we advocate resection of all serous cystadenomas if the patient's overall medical condition allows it.

Intraductal Papillary Mucinous Tumors

Since their initial description of intraductal papillary mucinous tumors (IPMTs) in 1982, hundreds of cases of IPMT have been reported in the English literature.[206] A variety of terms have been applied in reference to these neoplasms and include mucinous ductal ectasia, intraductal mucin-producing tumor, intraductal cystadenoma, pancreatic duct villous adenoma, intraductal papillary neoplasm, and others.[207] Some

Figure 50–12. CT appearance of a serous cystadenoma of the body and tail of the pancreas. Note the spongy appearance and the calcification.

pathologists suggest that IPMTs are only a variant of MCN, but establishment of a relationship between these tumors awaits further investigation.

IPMTs represent papillary neoplasms within the main pancreatic duct that show mucin hypersecretion that often leads to duct dilation and/or chronic obstructive pancreatitis. IPMTs are considered premalignant pancreatic lesions and histologically may demonstrate areas ranging from hyperplasia to carcinoma within a single tumor.[208] Although extensive intraductal growth can be observed, they are slow to invade periductal tissues and slow to metastasize (Fig. 50–13).

Most reported case series demonstrate that IPMT occurs

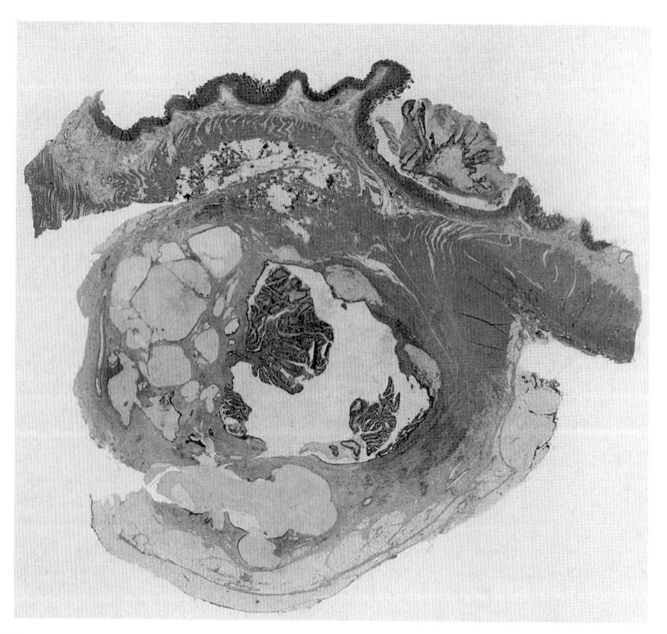

Figure 50–13. Low-power view of a malignant intraductal papillary mucinous tumor (IPMT). A papillary tumor is growing within the pancreatic duct. Note the surrounding lakes of mucin in the pancreas. At the top of the picture is the duodenum, which is focally invaded by the mucinous tumor.

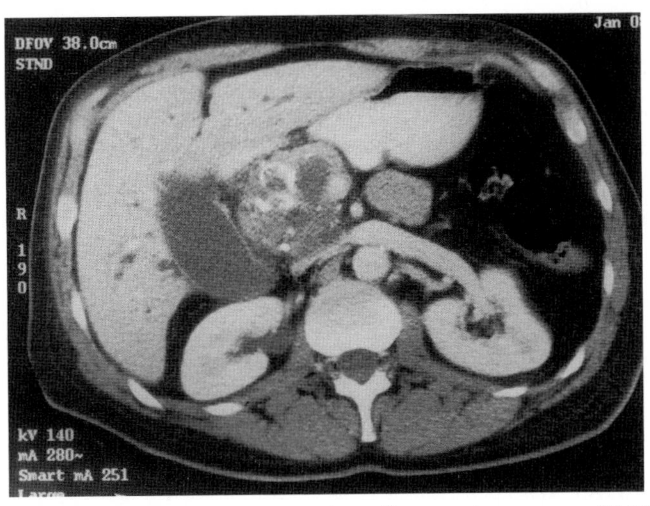

Figure 50–14. CT of an intraductal papillary mucinous tumor (IPMT) affecting the head of the pancreas.

primarily in males, with a mean age of 65 years, in contrast with the female predominance in MCN.[209–213] Patients frequently present with abdominal pain or pancreatitis and may be found to have a past history of recurrent pancreatitis. The disease is most commonly localized to the head of the pancreas but may occur at any site along the pancreatic ductal system. Duct dilation is often impressive and may mimic MCN on CT imaging[214] (Fig. 50–14). Evaluation by ERCP typically shows a patulous ampulla of Vater with extruding mucus, which is often diagnostic for IPMT. Other findings during pancreatography include main duct dilation, filling defects due to viscid mucus or tumor (Fig. 50–15), and communication between cystic areas and the main pancreatic duct in the side-branch variety of the disease.

Adequate treatment of IPMTs requires pancreatic resection, which successfully relieves symptoms and prevents tumor progression to invasive carcinoma.[210] Simpler procedures such as sphincterotomy may partially treat symptomatology but do not address the malignant potential of these tumors. Pancreaticoduodenectomy is the treatment of choice for most patients given the predominance of IPMT in the head of the pancreas, but distal pancreatectomy is indicated for lesions in the body or tail of the gland. Intraoperative frozen sections are necessary to confirm negative resection margins and may mandate extended resection if positive. When IPMT involves the entire ductal system, total pancreatectomy is the only curative surgical option. Most series report absence of recurrence and excellent 5-year survival rates after adequate pancreatic resection.[207, 209]

OTHER NONENDOCRINE PANCREATIC TUMORS

Other nonendocrine tumors of the pancreas, aside from cystic neoplasms and ductal adenocarcinoma, include acinar cell carcinomas, which are extremely rare, and often present with high serum lipase levels and peripheral fat necrosis. Nonepithelial tumors also occur and include a variety of sarcomas and lymphoma. The latter (pancreatic lymphoma) is the only one that is sufficiently common to be considered within the

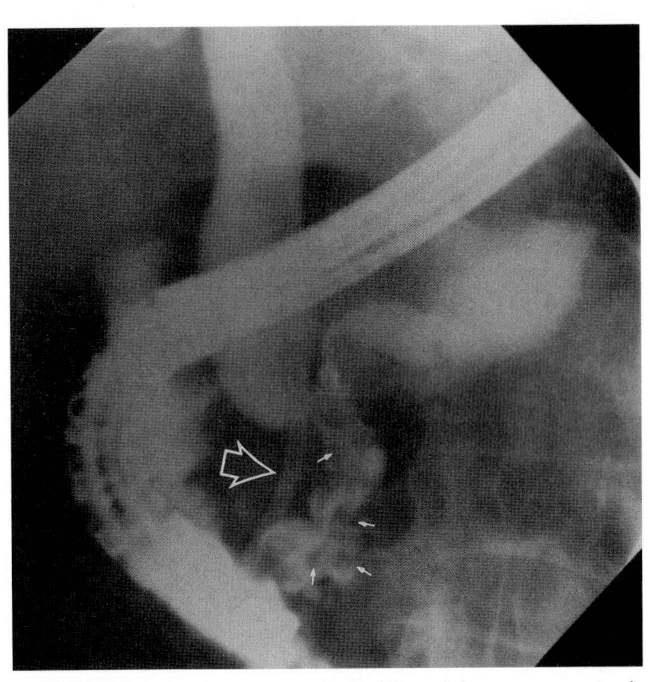

Figure 50–15. ERCP in IPMT. Multiple filling defects are seen in the proximal pancreatic duct (*small arrows*), as well as dilation of the distal duct. There is also bile duct obstruction treated with a stent (*open arrow*).

differential diagnosis. Whenever a large mass is identified in the pancreas without biliary obstruction, pain, or weight loss, the diagnosis should be contemplated, particularly in the presence of an elevated serum lactate dehydrogenase level. Pancreatic lymphoma represents less than 1% to 2% of all pancreatic malignancies and also less than 1% of all extranodal non-Hodgkin's lymphomas.[215, 216] The cure rate with combination chemotherapy and radiation therapy is very good. A few patients with small tumors, thought to represent carcinomas, have been treated with surgery alone and have had excellent survival.[216]

REFERENCES

1. Greenlee RT, Murray T, Bolden S, Wingo PA: Cancer Statistics 2000. CA Cancer J Clin 2000. 50:7–33,
2. Ries LAG, Eisner MP, Kosary CL, et al: Seer Cancer Statistics Review, 1973–1996. Bethesda, MD, National Cancer Institute, 2000.
3. Lowenfels AB, Maisonneuve P, DiMagno EP, et al: Hereditary pancreatitis and the risk of pancreatic cancer. J Natl Cancer Inst 89:442–446, 1997.
4. Lowenfels AB, Maisonneuve P, Cavallini G, et al: Pancreatitis and the risk of pancreatic cancer. N Engl J Med 328:1433–1437, 1993.
5. Lynch HT, Fusaro RM: Pancreatic cancer and the familial atypical multiple mole melanoma. Pancreas 6:127–131, 1991.
6. Hruban RH, Petersen GM, Goggins M, et al: Familial pancreatic cancer. Ann Oncol 10(Suppl 4):69–73, 1999.
7. Gullo L, Pezilli R, Morselli-Labate AM, and the Italian Pancreatic Cancer Study Group: Diabetes and the risk of pancreatic cancer. N Engl J Med 331:81–84, 1994.
8. Permert J, Larsson J, Westermark GT, et al: Islet amyloid polypeptide in patients with pancreatic cancer and diabetes. N Engl J Med 330: 313–318, 1994.
9. DiMagno EP, Reber HA, Tempero MA: AGA technical review on the epidemiology, diagnosis, and treatment of pancreatic ductal adenocarcinoma. Gastroenterology 117:1464–1484, 1999.
10. Mack TM, Yu MC, Hanisch R, Henderson BE: Pancreas cancer and

smoking, beverage consumption, and past medical history. J Natl Cancer Inst 76:49–60, 1986.
11. Falk RT, Pickle LW, Fontham ET, et al: Life-style risk factors for pancreatic cancer is Louisiana: A case-control study. Am J Epidemiol 128:324–326, 1988.
12. Doll R, Peto R: Mortality in relation to smoking: Twenty years' observations on male British doctors. BMJ 2:1525–1536, 1976.
13. Farrow DC, Davis C: Risk of pancreatic cancer in relation to medical history and the use of tobacco, alcohol, and coffee. Int J Cancer 45: 816–820, 1990.
14. Ghadirian P, Simard A, Baillargeon J: Tobacco, alcohol, and coffee and cancer of the pancreas. Cancer 67:2664–2670, 1991.
15. Cuzick J, Babiker AG: Pancreatic cancer, alcohol, diabetes mellitus, and gallbladder disease. Int J Cancer 43:415–421, 1989.
16. Howe GR, Jain M, Burch JD, Miller AB: Cigarette smoking and cancer of the pancreas: Evidence from a population-based case-control study in Toronto, Canada. Int J Cancer 47:323–328, 1991.
17. Hirayama T: Epidemiology of pancreatic cancer in Japan. Jpn J Clin Oncol 19:208–215, 1989.
18. Rivenson A, Hoffmann D, Prokopczyk B, et al: Induction of lung and exocrine pancreas tumors in F344 rats by tobacco-specific and areca-derived *N*-nitrosamines. Cancer Res 48:6912–6917, 1988.
19. Rivera JA, Graeme-Cook F, Werner J, et al: A rat model of pancreatic ductal adenocarcinoma: Targeting chemical carcinogens. Surgery 122: 82–90, 1997.
20. Rao MS: Animal models of exocrine pancreatic carcinogenesis. Cancer Metastasis Rev 6:665–676, 1987.
21. Wyner EL, Mabuchi K, Maruchi N, Fortner JG: Epidemiology of cancer of the pancreas. J Natl Cancer Inst 50:645–667, 1973.
22. Farrow DC, Davis S: Diet and the risk of pancreatic cancer in men. Am J Epidemiol 132:423–431, 1990.
23. Mills PK, Beeson L, Abbey DE, et al: Dietary habits and past medical history as related to fatal pancreas cancer risk among Adventists. Cancer 61:2578–2585, 1988.
24. Norell SE, Ahlbom A, Erwald R, et al: Diet and pancreatic cancer: A case-control study. Am J Epidemiol 124:894–902, 1986.
25. Howe GR, Jain M, Miller AB: Dietary factors and risk of pancreatic cancer: Results of a Canadian population–based case-control study. Int J Cancer 45:604–608, 1990.
26. Gold EB, Gordis L, Diener MD, et al: Diet and other risk factors for cancer of the pancreas. Cancer 55:460–467, 1985.
27. Burney J, Comstock GW, Morris JS: Serologic precursors of cancer: Serum micronutrients and the subsequent risk of pancreatic cancer. Am J Clin Nutr 49:895–900, 1989.
28. Z'Graggen K, Warshaw AL, Werner J, et al: Promoting effect of a high fat/high protein diet in DMBA-induced pancreatic cancer in rats. Ann Surg 233:688–695, 2001.
29. Offerhaus GJA, Tersmette AC, Tersmette KWF, et al: Gastric, pancreatic, and colorectal carcinogenesis following remote peptic ulcer surgery. Mod Pathol 1:352–356, 1988.
30. Taylor PR, Dowling RH, Palmer TJ, et al: Induction of pancreatic tumors by long-term duodenogastric reflux. Gut 30:1596–1600, 1989.
31. Palmer Smith J, Solomon TE, Bagheri S, Kramer S: Cholecystokinin stimulates growth of human pancreatic adenocarcinoma SW-1990. Dig Dis Sci 35:1377–1384, 1990.
32. Hyvarinen H, Partanen S: Association of cholecystectomy with abdominal cancers. Hepatogastroenterology 34:280–284, 1987.
33. Solcia E, Capella C, Kloppel G: Tumors of the exocrine pancreas. In Solcia E, Capella C, Kloppel G (eds): Tumors of the Pancreas. Washington, DC, Armed Forces Institute of Pathology, 1997, pp 145–210.
34. Kloppel G, Solcia E, Longnecker DS, et al: Histological typing of tumors of the exocrine pancreas. In International Histological Classification of Tumors. Berlin, Springer, 1996.
35. Cubilla AL, Fitzgerald PJ: Tumors of the exocrine pancreas. In Atlas of Tumor Pathology, 2nd series, fascicle 19. Washington, DC, Armed Forces Institute of Pathology, 1984, pp 109–183.
36. Kloppel G, Lingenthal G, von Bulow M, Kern HF: Histological and fine structural features of pancreatic ductal adenocarcinomas in relation to growth and prognosis: Studies in xenografted tumors and clinico-histopathological correlation in a series of 75 cases. Histopathology 9:841–856, 1985.
37. Solcia E, Capella C, Kloppel G: Tumor-like lesions of the exocrine pancreas. In Solcia E, Capella C, Kloppel G (eds): Tumors of the Pancreas. Washington, DC, Armed Forces Institute of Pathology, 1997, pp 211–236.
38. Nagai H, Kuroda A, Morioka Y: Lymphatic and local spread of T1 and T2 pancreatic cancer. Ann Surg 204:65–71, 1986.
39. Sessa F, Bonato M, Frigerio B: Ductal cancers of the pancreas frequently express markers of gastrointestinal epithelial cells. Gastroenterology 98:1655–1665, 1990.
40. Tempero M, Takasaki H, Uchida E: Co-expression of CA 19-9, DU-PAN-2, CA 125, and TAG-72 in pancreatic adenocarcinoma. Am J Surg Pathol 13:89–95, 1989.
41. Schussler MH, Skoudy A, Ramaekers F, Real FX: Intermediate filaments as differentiation markers of normal pancreas and pancreas cancer. Am J Pathol 140:559–568, 1992.
42. Hahn SA, Kern SE: Molecular genetics of exocrine pancreatic neoplasms. Surg Clin North Am 75:857–869, 1995.
43. Hruban RH, Petersen GM, Kern SE: Genetics of pancreatic cancer: From genes to families. Surg Oncol Clin North Am 7:1–23, 1998.
44. Lognecker DS: Molecular pathology of invasive carcinoma. Ann N Y Acad Sci 880:74–81, 1999.
45. Jimenez RE, Warshaw AL, Z'Graggen K, et al: Sequential accumulation of *K-ras* mutations and p53 overexpression in the progression of pancreatic mucinous cystic neoplasms to malignancy. Ann Surg 230: 501–511, 1999.
46. Z'Graggen K, Rivera JA, Compton CC, et al: Prevalence of activating *K-ras* mutations in the evolutionary stages of neoplasia in intraductal papillary mucinous tumors of the pancreas. Ann Surg 226:491–500, 1997.
47. Rivera JA, Rall CJN, Graeme-Cook F, et al: Analysis of *K-ras* oncogene mutations in chronic pancreatitis with ductal hyperplasia. Surgery 121:42–49, 1997.
48. Moskaluk CA, Hruban RH, Kern SE: *p16* and *K-ras* mutation in the intraductal precursors of human pancreatic adenocarcinoma. Cancer Res 57:2140–2143, 1997.
49. Rozenblum E, Schutte M, Goggins M, et al: Tumor-suppressive pathways in pancreatic carcinoma. Cancer Res 57:1731–1734, 1997.
50. Levine AJ, Momand J, Finlay CA: The *p53* tumor suppressor gene. Nature 351:543–546, 1991.
51. Hahn SA, Schutte M, Shamsul Hoque ATM, et al: DPC4, a candidate tumor suppressor gene at human chromosome 18q21.1. Science 271: 350–353, 1996.
52. Chiao PJ, Hunt KK, Grau AM, et al: Tumor suppressor gene Smad4/DPC4, its downstream target genes, and regulation of cell cycle. Ann N Y Acad Sci 880:31–37, 1999.
53. Goggins M, Griffin CA, Turnacioglu K, et al: Pancreatic adenocarcinomas with DNA replication errors (RER+) are associated with wild-type *K-ras* and characteristic histopathology: poor differentiation, a syncytial growth pattern, and pushing borders suggest RER+. Am J Pathol 152:1501–1507, 1998.
54. Lynch HT, Smyrk T: Hereditary nonpolyposis colorectal cancer (Lynch syndrome): An updated review. Cancer 78:1149–1167, 1996.
55. Wilentz RE, Iacobuzio-Donahue CA, Argani P, et al: Loss of expression of *DPC4* in pancreatic intraepithelial neoplasia: Evidence that *DPC4* inactivation occurs late in neoplastic progression. Cancer Res 60:2002–2006, 2000.
56. Fearon ER, Vogelstein B: A genetic model for colorectal tumorigenesis. Cell 61:759–767, 1990.
57. Warshaw AL, Fernández-del Castillo C: Medical progress: Pancreatic carcinoma. N Engl J Med 326:455–465, 1992.
58. Sohn TA, Lillemoe KD, Cameron JL, et al: Surgical palliation of unresectable periampullary adenocarcinoma in the 1990s. J Am Coll Surg 188:658–666, 1999.
59. Bakkevold KE, Kambestad B: Carcinoma of the pancreas and papilla of Vater: Presenting symptoms, signs, and diagnosis related to stage and tumour site. Scand J Gastroenterol 27:317–325, 1992.
60. Permert J, Ihse I, Jorfeldt L, et al: Pancreatic cancer is associated with impaired glucose metabolism. Eur J Surg 159:101–107, 1993.
61. Basso D, Plebani M, Fogar J, et al: B-cell function in pancreatic adenocarcinoma. Pancreas 3:332–339, 1994.
62. Mujica VR, Barkin JS, Go VLW, and Study Group Participants: Acute pancreatitis secondary to pancreatic carcinoma. Pancreas 21: 329–332, 2000.
63. Freeny PC, Marks WM, Ryan JA, Traverso LW: Pancreatic ductal adenocarcinoma: Diagnosis and staging with dynamic CT. Radiology 166:125–133, 1988.
64. Freeny PC, Traverso W, Ryan JA: Diagnosis and staging of pancreatic adenocarcinoma with dynamic computed tomography. Am J Surg 165: 600–606, 1993.

65. Megibow AJ, Zhou XH, Rotterdam H, et al: Pancreatic adenocarcinoma: CT versus MR imaging in the evaluation of resectability. Report of the Radiology Diagnostic Oncology Group. Radiology 195: 327–332, 1995.
66. Warshaw AL, Gu Z-Y, Wittenberg J, Waltman AC: Preoperative staging and assessment of resectability of pancreatic cancer. Arch Surg 125:230–233, 1990.
67. Boland GW, O'Malley ME, Saez M, et al: Pancreatic-phase versus portal vein-phase helical CT of the pancreas: Optimal temporal window for evaluation of pancreatic adenocarcinoma. AJR Am J Roentgenol 172:605–608, 1999.
68. Lu DS, Vedantham S, Krassny RM, et al: Two-phase helical CT for pancreatic tumors: Pancreatic versus hepatic phase enhancement of tumor, pancreas, and vascular structures. Radiology 199:697–701, 1996.
69. Bluemke DA, Cameron JL, Hruban RH, et al: Potentially resectable pancreatic adenocarcinoma: Spiral CT assessment with surgical and pathologic correlation. Radiology 197:381–385, 1995.
70. Lu DS, Reber HA, Krasny RM, et al: Local staging of pancreatic cancer: Criteria for unresectability of major vessels as revealed by pancreatic-phase, thin-section helical CT. AJR Am J Roentgenol 168: 1439–1443, 1997.
71. O'Malley ME, Boland GW, Wood BJ, et al: Adenocarcinoma of the head of the pancreas: Determination of surgical unresectability with thin-section pancreatic-phase helical CT. AJR Am J Roentgenol 173: 1513–1518, 1999.
72. Raptopoulos V, Steer ML, Sheiman RG, et al: The uses of helical CT and CT angiography to predict vascular involvement from pancreatic cancer: Correlation with findings at surgery. AJR Am J Roentgenol 168:971–977, 1997.
73. McCune SW, Shorb EP, Moscovitz H: Endoscopic cannulation of the ampulla of Vater: A preliminary report. Ann Surg 167:725–756, 1968.
74. Michelassi F, Erroi F, Dawson PJ, et al: Experience with 647 consecutive tumors of the duodenum, ampulla, head of the pancreas, and distal common bile duct. Ann Surg 210:544–554, 1989.
75. Tarazi RY, Hermann RE, Vogt DP, et al: Results of surgical treatment of periampullary tumors: A thirty-five-year experience. Surgery 100: 716–721, 1986.
76. Freeny PC: Radiologic diagnosis and staging of pancreatic ductal adenocarcinoma. Radiol Clin North Am 27:121–128, 1989.
77. Pitt HA, Gomes AS, Lois JF, et al: Does preoperative percutaneous biliary drainage reduce operative risk or increase hospital cost? Ann Surg 201:545–553, 1985.
78. Heslin MJ, Brooks AD, Hochwald SN, et al: A preoperative biliary stent is associated with increased complications after pancreatoduodenectomy. Arch Surg 133:149–154, 1998.
79. Rosch T, Braig C, Gain T, et al: Staging of pancreatic and ampullary carcinoma by endoscopic ultrasonography: Comparison with conventional sonography, computed tomography, and angiography. Gastroenterology 102:188–199, 1992.
80. Shoup M, Hodul P, Aranha GV, et al: Defining a role for endoscopic ultrasound in staging periampullary tumors. Am J Surg 179:453–456, 2000.
81. Brugge WR, Lee MJ, Kelsey PB, et al: The use of EUS to diagnose portal venous invasion by pancreatic cancer. Gastrointest Endosc 43: 551–567, 1996.
82. Rosch T, Lorenz R, Braig C, Classen M: Endoscopic ultrasonography in diagnosis and staging of pancreatic and biliary tumors. Endoscopy 24:304–308, 1992.
83. Legman P, Vignaus O, Dousser B, et al: Pancreatic tumors: Comparison of dual-phase helical CT and endoscopic sonography. AJR Am J Roentgenol 170:1315–1322, 1998.
84. Wiersema MJ, Vilmann P, Giovanni M, et al: Endosonography-guided fine needle aspiration biopsy: Diagnostic accuracy and complication assessment. Gastroenterology 112:1087–1095, 1997.
85. Ichikawa T, Haradome H, Hachiya J, et al: Pancreatic ductal adenocarcinoma: Preoperative assessment with helical CT versus dynamic MR Imaging. Radiology 202:655–662, 1997.
86. Semelka RC, Ascher SM: MR imaging of the pancreas. Radiology 188:593–602, 1993.
87. Shirkhoda A, Konez O, Shetty A: Mesenteric circulation: Three-dimensional MR angiography with a gadolinium-enhanced multiecho gradient-echo technique. Radiology 169:1295–1303, 1997.
88. Barish MA, Soto JA: MR cholangiopancreatography: Techniques and clinical applications. AJR Am J Roentgenol 169:1295–1303, 1997.
89. Adamek HE, Albert J, Breer H, et al: Pancreatic cancer detection with magnetic resonance cholangiopancreatography and endoscopic retrograde cholangiopancreatography: A prospective controlled study. Lancet 356:190–193, 2000.
90. Inokama T, Tamaki N, Torizuka T, et al: Evaluation of pancreatic tumors with positron emission tomography and F-18 fluorodeoxyglucose: Comparison with CT and US. Radiology 195:345–352, 1995.
91. Zimny M, Bares R, Fass J, et al: Fluorine-18 fluorodeoxyglucose positron emission tomography in the differential diagnosis of pancreatic carcinoma: A report of 106 cases. Eur J Nucl Med 24:678–682, 1997.
92. Rose DM, Delbeke D, Beauchamp D, et al: 18-Fluorodeoxyglucose–positron emission tomography in the management of patients with suspected pancreatic cancer. Ann Surg 229:729–738, 1998.
93. Athlin L, Blind PJ, Angstrom T: Fine-needle aspiration biopsy of pancreatic masses. Acta Chir Scand 156:91–94, 1990.
94. Parsons L, Palmer CH: How accurate is fine-needle biopsy in malignant neoplasia of the pancreas. Arch Surg 124:681–683, 1989.
95. DelMaschio A, Vanzulli A, Sironi S, et al: Pancreatic cancer versus chronic pancreatitis: Diagnosis with CA 19-9 assessment, US, CT, and CT-guided fine-needle biopsy. Radiology 178:95–99, 1991.
96. Al-Kaisi N, Siegler EE: Fine-needle aspiration cytology of the pancreas. Acta Cytol 33:145–152, 1989.
97. Fernández-del Castillo C, González-Ojeda A, Reyes E, et al: Tuberculosis of the pancreas. Pancreas 5:693–696, 1990.
98. Essop AR, Posen J, Path FF, et al: Isolated granulomatous pancreatitis. J Clin Gastroenterol 6:61–64, 1984.
99. Webb TH, Lillemoe KD, Pitt HA, et al: Pancreatic lymphoma: Is surgery mandatory for diagnosis or treatment? Ann Surg 209:25–30, 1989.
100. Hart MJ, White TT, Brown PC, Freeny PC: Potentially curable masses in the pancreas. Am J Surg 154:134–136, 1987.
101. Eckhauser FE, Cheung PS, Vinik AI, et al: Nonfunctioning malignant neuroendocrine tumors of the pancreas. Surgery 100:978–987, 1986.
102. Ritts RE, Pitt HA: CA 19-9 in pancreatic cancer. Surg Oncol Clin North Am 7:93–101, 1998.
103. Steinberg W: The clinical utility of the CA 19-9 tumor-associated antigen. Am J Gastroenterol 85:350–355, 1990.
104. Safi F, Schlosser W, Falkenreck S, Beger HG: CA 19-9 serum course and prognosis of pancreatic cancer. Int J Pancreatol 20:155–161, 1996.
105. Robbins DB, Katz RL, Evans DB, et al: Fine-needle aspiration of the pancreas: In quest of accuracy. Acta Cytol 39:1–10, 1995.
106. van den Bosch RP, van der Schelling GP, Klinkenbijl JH, et al: Guidelines for the application of surgery and endoprostheses in the palliation of obstructive jaundice in advanced cancer of the pancreas. Ann Surg 219:18–24, 1994.
107. Espat NJ, Brennan MF, Conlon KC: Patients with laparoscopically staged unresectable pancreatic adenocarcinoma do not require subsequent surgical biliary or gastric bypass. J Am Coll Surg 188:649–657, 1999.
108. Sener SF, Fremgen A, Menck HR, Winchester DP: Pancreatic cancer: A report of treatment and survival trends for 100,313 patients diagnosed from 1985–1995, using the National Cancer Database. J Am Coll Surg 189:1–7, 1999.
109. Gastrointestinal Tumor Study Group: Therapy of locally unresectable pancreatic carcinoma: A randomized comparison of high-dose (6000 rads) radiation alone, moderate-dose radiation (4000 rads + 5-fluorouracil), and high-dose radiation + 5 fluorouracil. Cancer 48:1705–1710, 1981.
110. Willett CG, Warshaw AL: Intraoperative electron beam irradiation in pancreatic cancer. Front Biosci 3:E207–E213, 1998.
111. Czito BG, Willett CG, Clark JW, Fernández-del Castillo C: Current perspectives on locally advanced pancreatic cancer. Oncology 14: 1535–1545, 2000.
112. Fernández-del Castillo C, Rattner DW, Warshaw AL: Standards for pancreatic resection in the 1990s. Arch Surg 130:295–300, 1995.
113. Lieberman MD, Kilburn H, Lindsey M, Brennan MF: Relation of perioperative deaths to hospital volume among patients undergoing pancreatic resection for malignancy. Ann Surg 222:638–645, 1995.
114. Sosa JA, Bowman HM, Gordon TA, et al: Importance of hospital volume in the overall management of pancreatic cancer. Ann Surg 228:429–438, 1998.
115. Birkmeyer JD, Finlayson SRG, Tosteson ANA, et al: Effect of hospital volume on in-hospital mortality with pancreaticoduodenectomy. Surgery 1255:250–256, 1999.

116. Bemelman WA, de Wit LT, van Delden OM, et al: Diagnostic laparoscopy combined with laparoscopic ultrasonography in staging of cancer of the pancreatic head region. Br J Surg 82:820–824, 1995.
117. Conlon KC, Dougherty E, Klimstra DS, et al: The value of minimal access surgery in the staging of patients with potentially resectable peripancreatic malignancy. Ann Surg 223:134–140, 1996.
118. Fernández-del Castillo C, Rattner DW, Warshaw AL: Further experience with laparoscopy and peritoneal cytology in staging for pancreatic cancer. Br J Surg 82:1127–1129, 1995.
119. Jimenez RE, Warshaw AL, Rattner DW, et al: Impact of laparoscopic staging in the treatment of pancreatic cancer. Arch Surg 135:409–415, 2000.
120. John TG, Greig JD, Carter DC, Garden OJ: Carcinoma of the pancreatic head and periampullary region: Tumor staging with laparoscopy and laparoscopic ultrasonography. Ann Surg 221:156–164, 1995.
121. Warshaw AL, Tepper JE, Shipley WU: Laparoscopy in the staging and planning of therapy for pancreatic cancer. Am J Surg 151:76–80, 1986.
122. Makary MA, Warshaw AL, Centeno BA, et al: Implications of peritoneal cytology for pancreatic cancer management. Arch Surg 133:361–365, 1998.
123. Merchant NB, Conlon KC, Saigo P, et al: Positive peritoneal cytology predicts unresectability of pancreatic adenocarcinoma. J Am Coll Surg 188:421–426, 1999.
124. Warshaw AL: Implications of peritoneal cytology for staging of early pancreatic cancer. Am J Surg 161:26–30, 1991.
125. Minnard EA, Conlon KC, Hoos A, et al: Laparoscopic ultrasound enhances standard laparoscopy in the staging of pancreatic cancer. Ann Surg 228:182–187, 1998.
126. ReMine WH, Priestley JT, Judd ES, King JN: Total pancreatectomy. Ann Surg 172:595–604, 1970.
127. Brooks JR, Brooks DC, Levine JD: Total pancreatectomy for ductal cell carcinoma of the pancreas: An update. Ann Surg 209:405–410, 1989.
128. van Heerden JA, ReMine WH, Weiland LH, et al: Total pancreatectomy for ductal adenocarcinoma of the pancreas. Am J Surg 142:308–311, 1981.
129. Andren-Sandberg A, Ihse I: Factors influencing survival after total pancreatectomy in patients with pancreatic cancer. Ann Surg 198:605–610, 1991.
130. Fortner JG: Regional pancreatectomy for cancer of the pancreas, ampulla, and other related sites. Ann Surg 199:418–425, 1984.
131. Ishikawa O, Ohhigashi H, Sasaki Y, et al: Practical usefulness of lymphatic and connective tissue clearance for the carcinoma of the pancreas head. Ann Surg 208:215–220, 1988.
132. Tsuchiya R, Tsunoda T, Yamaguchi T: Operation of choice for resectable carcinoma of the head of the pancreas. Int J Pancreatol 6:295–306, 1990.
133. Pedrazzoli S, DiCarlo V, Dionigi R, et al: Standard versus extended lymphadenectomy associated with pancreatoduodenectomy in the surgical treatment of adenocarcinoma of the head of the pancreas. Ann Surg 228:508–517, 1998.
134. Cameron JL, Crist DW, Sitzmann JV, et al: Factors influencing survival after pancreaticoduodenectomy for pancreatic cancer. Am J Surg 161:120–125, 1991.
135. Braasch JW, Rossi RL, Watkins E, et al: Pyloric and gastric preserving pancreatic resection. Ann Surg 204:411–418, 1986.
136. Grace PA, Pitt HA, Longmire WP: Pylorus preserving pancreatoduodenectomy: An overview. Br J Surg 77:968–974, 1990.
137. Sharp KW, Ross CB, Halter SA, et al: Pancreatoduodenectomy with pyloric preservation for carcinoma of the pancreas: A cautionary note. Surgery 105:645–653, 1989.
138. Boerma EJ, Coosemans JAR: Non-preservation of the pylorus in resection of pancreatic cancer. Br J Surg 77:299–300, 1990.
139. Balcom JH, Rattner DW, Warshaw AL, et al: Ten-year experience with 733 pancreatic resections: Changing indications, older patients, and decreasing length of hospitalizations. Arch Surg 136:491–498, 2001.
140. Sohn TA, Yeo CJ, Cameron JL, et al: Resected adenocarcinoma of the pancreas in 616 patients: Results, outcomes, and prognostic indicators. J Gastrointest Surg 4:567–579, 2000.
141. Trede M, Schwall G, Saeger HD: Survival after pancreatoduodenectomy. Ann Surg 211:447–458, 1990.
142. Pellegrini CA, Heck CF, Raper S, Way LW: An analysis of the reduced morbidity and mortality rates after pancreaticoduodenectomy. Arch Surg 124:778–781, 1989.
143. Crist DW, Sitzmann JV, Cameron JL: Improved hospital morbidity, mortality, and survival after the Whipple procedure. Ann Surg 206:358–365, 1987.
144. Birkmeyer JD, Warshaw AL, Finlayson SRG, et al: Relationship between hospital volume and late survival after pancreaticoduodenectomy. Surgery 126:178–183, 1999.
145. Geer RJ, Brennan MF: Prognostic indicators for survival after resection of pancreatic adenocarcinoma. Am J Surg 165:68–73, 1993.
146. Benassai G, Mastrorilli M, Quarto G, et al: Survival after pancreaticoduodenectomy for ductal adenocarcinoma of the head of the pancreas. Chir Ital 52:263–270, 2000.
147. Millikan KW, Deiel DJ, Silverstein JC, et al: Prognostic factors associated with resectable adenocarcinoma of the head of the pancreas. Am Surg 65:618–623, 1999.
148. Meyer W, Jurowich C, Reichel M, et al: Pathomorphological and histological prognostic factors in curatively resected ductal adenocarcinoma of the pancreas. Surg Today 30:582–587, 2000.
149. Rosenberg JM, Welch JP, Macaulay WP: Cancer of the head of the pancreas: An institutional review with emphasis on surgical therapy. J Surg Oncol 28:217–221, 1985.
150. Connolly MM, Dawson PJ, Michelassi F, et al: Survival in 1001 patients with carcinoma of the pancreas. Ann Surg 206:366–373, 1987.
151. Funovics JM, Karner J, Pratschner TH, Fritsch A: Current trends in the management of carcinoma of the pancreatic head. Hepatogastroenterology 36:450–455, 1989.
152. Singh SM, Longmire WP, Reber HA: Surgical palliation for pancreatic cancer: The UCLA experience. Ann Surg 212:132–139, 1990.
153. Tsuchiya R, Noda T, Harada M, et al: Collective review of small carcinomas of the pancreas. Ann Surg 203:77–81, 1986.
154. Huibregtse K, Katon RM, Coene PP, Tytgat GNJ: Endoscopic palliative treatment in pancreatic cancer. Gastrointest Endosc 32:334–338, 1986.
155. Soehendra N, Grimm H, Berger B, Nam VC: Malignant jaundice: Results of diagnostic and therapeutic endoscopy. World J Surg 13:171–177, 1989.
156. Andersen JR, Sorensen SM, Kruse A, et al: Randomised trial of endoscopic endoprosthesis versus operative bypass in malignant obstructive jaundice. Gut 30:1132–1135, 1989.
157. Smith AC, Dowsett JF, Hatfield ARW, et al: Prospective randomized trial of by pass surgery versus endoscopic stenting in patients with malignant obstructive jaundice. Gut 30:A1513, 1989.
158. Speer AG, Cotton PB, Russell RCG, et al: Randomised trial of endoscopic versus percutaneous stent insertion in malignant obstructive jaundice. Lancet 2:57–62, 1987.
159. Shepard HA, Royle G, Ross APR, et al: Endoscopic biliary endoprosthesis in the palliation of malignant obstruction of the distal common bile duct: A randomized trial. Br J Surg 75:1166–1168, 1988.
160. Prat F, Chapat O, Ducto B, et al: A randomized trial of endoscopic drainage methods for inoperable malignant strictures of the common bile duct. Gastrointest Endosc 47:1–7, 1998.
161. Doberneck RC, Berndt GA: Delayed gastric emptying after palliative gastrojejunostomy for carcinoma of the pancreas. Arch Surg 122:827–829, 1987.
162. Weaver DW, Wiencek RG, Bouwman DL, Walt AJ: Gastrojejunostomy: Is it helpful for patients with pancreatic cancer? Surgery 102:608–613, 1987.
163. Soetikno RM, Lichtenstein DR, Vandervoort J, et al: Palliation of malignant gastric outlet obstruction using an endoscopically placed Wallstent. Gastrointest Endosc 47:267–270, 1998.
164. Nevitt AW, Vida F, Kozarek RA, et al: Expandable metallic prostheses for malignant obstructions of gastric outlet and proximal small bowel. Gastrointest Endosc 47:271–276, 1998.
165. Lillemoe KD, Cameron JL, Kaufman HS, et al: Chemical splanchnicectomy in patients with unresectable pancreatic cancer. Ann Surg 217:447–457, 1993.
166. Polati E, Finco G, Gottin L, et al: Prospective randomized double-blind trial of neurolytic coeliac plexus block in patients with pancreatic cancer. Br J Surg 85:199–201, 1998.
167. Sarr MG, Cameron JL: Surgical management of unresectable carcinoma of the pancreas. Surgery 91:123–133, 1982.
168. Kalser MH, Barkin J, MacIntyre JM: Pancreatic cancer: Assessment of prognosis by clinical presentation. Cancer 56:397–402, 1985.
169. Dobelbower RR, Konski AA, Merrick HW, et al: Intraoperative electron-beam radiation therapy (IOEBRT) for carcinoma of the exocrine pancreas. Int J Radiat Oncol Biol Phys 20:113–119, 1991.

170. Heijmans HJ, Hoekstra HJ, Mehta DM: Is adjuvant intraoperative radiotherapy (IORT) for resectable and unresectable pancreatic carcinoma worthwile? Hepatogastroenterology 36:474–477, 1986.
171. Hoffman JP, Ahmad N, Coia LR, et al: Preoperative chemoradiotherapy for stage I–III adenocarcinoma of the pancreas: The Fox Chase Cancer Center experience. Cancer Bull 46:499–503, 1994.
172. Jessup JM, Steele G, Mayer RJ, et al: Neoadjuvant therapy for unresectable pancreatic adenocarcinoma. Arch Surg 127:1335–1339, 1992.
173. Spitz FR, Abbruzzese JL, Lee JE, et al: Preoperative and postoperative chemoradiation strategies in patients with pancreaticoduodenectomy for adenocarcinoma of the pancreas. J Clin Oncol 15:928–937, 1997.
174. Evans DB, Rich TA, Byrd DR, et al: Preoperative chemoradiation and pancreaticoduodenectomy for adenocarcinoma of the pancreas. Arch Surg 127:1335–1339, 1992.
175. Gastrointestinal Tumor Study Group: Further evidence of effective adjuvant combined radiation and chemotherapy following curative resection of pancreatic cancer. Cancer 59:2006–2010, 1987.
176. Yeo CJ, Abrams RA, Grochow LB, et al: Pancreaticoduodenectomy for pancreatic adenocarcinoma: Postoperative adjuvant chemoradiation improves survival. Ann Surg 225:621–636, 1997.
177. Neoptolemos JP, Baker P, Beger H, et al: Progress report: A randomized multicenter European study comparing adjuvant radiotherapy, 6-month chemotherapy, and combination therapy versus no-adjuvant treatment in resectable pancreatic cancer (ESPAC-1). Int J Pancreatol 21:97–104, 1997.
178. Klinkenbijl JHG, Jeekel J, Schmitz PIM, et al: Carcinoma of the pancreas and periampullary region: Palliation versus cure. Br J Surg 80:1575–1578, 1993.
179. Ishii H, Okada S, Sato T, et al: CA 19-9 in evaluating the response to chemotherapy in advanced pancreatic cancer. Hepatogastroenterology 44:279–283, 1997.
180. Rothenberg ML, Moore MJ, Cripps MC, et al: A phase II trial of gemcitabine in patients with 5-FU refractory pancreas cancer. Ann Oncol 7:347–353, 1996.
181. Fennely D, Kelsen DP: The role of chemotherapy in the treatment of adenocarcinoma of the pancreas. Hepatogastroenterology 43:356–362, 1996.
182. Riess H, Htun P, Loffel J, Huhn D: Chemotherapy for patients with adenocarcinoma of the pancreas: Recent results. Cancer Res 142:415–424, 1996.
183. Lokich JJ, Ahlgren JD, Gullo JJ, et al: A prospective randomized comparison of continuous infusion fluorouracil with a conventional bolus schedule in metastatic colorectal carcinoma. J Clin Oncol 7:425–432, 1989.
184. Smith FP, Hoth DF, Levin BF, et al: 5-Fluorouracil, Adriamycin, and mitomycin C (FAM) chemotherapy for advanced adenocarcinoma of the pancreas. Cancer 46:2014–2018, 1980.
185. Wiggans RG, Woolley PV, Macdonald JS, et al: Phase II trial of streptozotocin, mitomycin C, and 5-fluorouracil (SMF) in the treatment of advanced pancreatic cancer. Cancer 41:387–391, 1978.
186. Dougherty JB, Kelsen D, Kemeny N, et al: Advanced pancreatic cancer: A phase I–II trial of cisplatin, high-dose cytarabine, and caffeine. J Natl Cancer Inst 81:1735–1738, 1989.
187. Oster MW, Gray R, Panasci L, Perry MC: Chemotherapy for advanced pancreatic cancer: A comparison of 5-fluorouracil, Adriamycin, and mitomycin (FAM) with 5-fluorouracil, streptozotocin, and mitomycin (FSM). Cancer 57:29–33, 1986.
188. Cullinan SA, Moertel CG, Fleming TR, et al: A comparison of three chemotherapeutic regimens in the treatment of advanced pancreatic and gastric carcinoma. JAMA 253:2061–2067, 1985.
189. Fernández-del Castillo C, Warshaw AL: Cystic tumors of the pancreas. Surg Clin North Am 75:1001–1016, 1995.
190. Martin I, Hammond P, Scott J, et al: Cystic tumors of the pancreas. Br J Surg 85:1484–1486, 1998.
191. Warshaw AL, Rutledge PL: Cystic tumors mistaken for pancreatic pseudocysts. Ann Surg 205:393–398, 1987.
192. Alles A, Warshaw AL, Southern J, et al: Expression of CA 72-4 (TAG 72) in the fluid contents of pancreatic cysts: A new marker to distinguish malignant pancreatic cystic tumors from benign tumors and pseudocysts. Ann Surg 219:131–134, 1994.
193. Hammel P, Levy P, Voitot H, et al: Preoperative cyst fluid analysis is useful for the differential diagnosis of cystic lesions of the pancreas. Gastroenterology 108:1230–1235, 1995.
194. Sperti C, Pasquali C, Guolo P, et al: Serum tumor markers and cyst fluid analysis are useful for the diagnosis of pancreatic cystic tumors. Cancer 78:237–243, 1996.
195. Albores-Saavedra J, Angeles-Angeles A, Nadji M, et al: Mucinous cystadenocarcinoma of the pancreas: Morphologic and immunocytochemical observations. Am J Surg Pathol 11:11–20, 1987.
196. Compagno J, Oertel JE: Mucinous cystic neoplasms of the pancreas with overt and latent malignancy (cystadenocarcinoma and cystadenoma). Am J Clin Pathol 69:573–580, 1978.
197. Warshaw AL, Compton CC, Lewandrowski K, et al: Cystic tumors of the pancreas: New clinical, radiologic, and pathologic observations in 67 patients. Ann Surg 212:432–445, 1990.
198. Thompson LDR, Becker RC, Prygodzki RM, et al: Mucinous cystic neoplasm (mucinous cystadenocarcinoma of low-grade malignant potential) of the pancreas: A clinicopathological study of 130 cases. Am J Surg Pathol 23:1–16, 1999.
199. Talamini MA, Moesinger R, Yeo CJ, et al: Cystadenomas of the pancreas: Is enucleation an adequate operation? Ann Surg 227:896–903, 1997.
200. Sperti C, Pasquali C, Pedrazzoli S, et al: Expression of mucin-like carcinoma-associated antigen in the cyst fluid differentiates mucinous from nonmucinous pancreatic cysts. Am J Gastroenterol 92:672–675, 1997.
201. Compagno J, Oertel JE: Microcystic adenomas of the pancreas (glycogen-rich cystadenomas). Am J Clin Pathol 69:289–298, 1978.
202. Pyke CM, van Heerden JA, Colby TV, et al: The spectrum of serous cystadenoma of the pancreas. Ann Surg 215:132–139, 1992.
203. Albores-Saavedra J, Gould EW, Angeles-Angeles A, Henson DE: Cystic tumors of the pancreas. Pathol Annu 25:19–50, 1990.
204. Lewandrowski K, Warshaw AL, Compton CC: Macrocystic serous cystadenoma of the pancreas: A morphologic variant differing from microcystic adenoma. Hum Pathol 23:871–875, 1992.
205. Abe H, Kubota K, Mori M, et al: Serous cystadenoma of the pancreas with invasive growth: Benign or malignant? Am J Gastroenterol 93:1963–1966, 1998.
206. Ohashi K, Murakami Y, Maruyama M: [Four cases of mucin-producing cancer of the pancreas on specific findings of the papilla of Vater.] Prog Dig Endosc 20:348–351, 1982.
207. Rivera JA, Fernández-del Castillo C, Pins M, et al: Pancreatic mucinous ductal ectasia and intraductal papillary neoplasms: A single malignant clinicopathological entity. Ann Surg 225:637–646, 1997.
208. Azar C, Van de Stadt J, Rickaert F, et al: Intraductal papillary mucinous tumors of the pancreas: Clinical and therapeutic issues in 32 patients. Gut 39:457–464, 1996.
209. Fukushima N, Mukai K, Kanai Y, et al: Intraductal papillary tumors and mucinous cystic tumors of the pancreas: Clinicopathologic study of 38 cases. Hum Pathol 28:1010–1017, 1997.
210. Loftus EV, Olivares-Pakzad BA, Batts KP, et al: Intraductal papillary–mucinous tumors of the pancreas: Clinicopathologic features, outcome, and nomenclature. Gastroenterology 110:1909–1918, 1996.
211. Morohoshi T, Kanda M, Asanuma K, Kloppel G: Intraductal papillary neoplasms of the pancreas. Cancer 64:1329–1335, 1989.
212. Nagai E, Ueki T, Chijiiwa K, et al: Intraductal papillary mucinous neoplasms of the pancreas associated with so-called "mucinous ductal ectasia." Am J Surg Pathol 19:576–589, 1995.
213. Rickaert F, Cremer M, Deviere J, et al: Intraductal mucin-hypersecreting neoplasms of the pancreas. Gastroenterology 101:512–519, 1991.
214. Obara T, Maguchi H, Saitoh Y, et al: Mucin-producing tumor of the pancreas: Natural history and serial pancreatogram changes. Am J Gastroenterol 88:564–569, 1993.
215. Bouvet M, Staerkel GA, Spitz FR, et al: Primary pancreatic lymphoma. Surgery 123:382–390, 1998.
216. Koniaris LG, Lillemoe KD, Yeo CJ, et al: Is there a role for surgical resection in the treatment of early-stage pancreatic lymphoma? J Am Coll Surg 190:319–330, 2000.

Chapter 51

PANCREATIC ENDOCRINE TUMORS

Robert T. Jensen and Jeffrey A. Norton

GENERAL ASPECTS

Pancreatic endocrine tumors (PETs) are discussed in this chapter. Zollinger-Ellison syndrome due to a gastrinoma is covered in Chapter 41 and is discussed in the present chapter only in reference to the other PETs.

Historical Aspects

In 1927,[1] 5 years after the discovery of insulin, the first pancreatic hormone–producing tumor syndrome was described in a patient with a metastatic islet cell tumor and hypoglycemia; tumor extracts had hypoglycemia effects. Numerous other PETs have been described with the description of Zollinger-Ellison syndrome in 1955,[2] Verner-Morrison syndrome due to a diarrheogenic tumor in 1958,[3] glucagonoma syndrome in 1974,[4] the somatostatinoma syndrome in 1977,[5, 6] and GRFomas, pancreatic tumors secreting growth hormone–releasing factor (GRF) in 1982[7, 8] (Table 51–1). PETs secreting adrenocorticotropic hormone (ACTH), called ACTHomas, are included also (see Table 51–1) because 4% to 16% of cases of ectopic Cushing's syndrome are due to PETs.[9] PETs causing carcinoid syndrome[10, 11] and PETs causing hypercalcemia[12, 13] are also well described. Recently, PETs secreting calcitonin[14] have been proposed to cause a distinct syndrome with diarrhea; however, too few cases are well described to include this syndrome, and other causes of hypercalcitonemia such as medullary thyroid cancer are associated with diarrhea in only 25% to 42% of patients.[15]

PETs are classified as functional, if associated with a clinical syndrome due to hormone release by the tumor, or nonfunctional, if not associated with a clinical syndrome due to hormone release (see Table 51–1). In the latter category are included nonfunctional PETs that have the histologic characteristics of a PET but no associated elevation in plasma hormones or clinical syndrome, as well as PETs that release pancreatic polypeptide (PP) (called *PPomas*) or neurotensin (neurotensinomas), which do not cause a distinct clinical syndrome[16–18] (see Table 51–1).

Prevalence and Incidence

The overall prevalence of functional PETs is low, reported to be approximately 10 per 1 million population.[12, 19] In contrast, the prevalence of PETs in autopsy studies is higher, at 0.5% to 1.5%.[12, 19] The annual incidence of PETs is reported at 1 to 4 per 1 million.[12, 19] Nonfunctional PETs account for 14% to 30% of all PETs.[20] Insulinomas and

Table 51–1 | **Pancreatic Endocrine Tumors (PETs)**

TUMOR SYNDROME OR NAME(S)	ANNUAL INCIDENCE PER MILLION POPULATION	PRIMARY SYMPTOM (%)	RATE OF MALIGNANCY (%)	HORMONE CAUSING SYMPTOMS
Symptoms Due to Released Hormones (Functional PET)				
Gastrinoma, Zollinger-Ellison syndrome	0.5–1.5	Abdominal pain (76) Diarrhea (65) Dysphagia/pyrosis (10–31)	60–90	Gastrin
Insulinoma	1–2	Hypoglycemic symptoms (100)	<10	Insulin
VIPoma, Verner-Morrison syndrome, WDHA, pancreatic cholera	0.5–0.2	Diarrhea (100) Flushing (20)	>60	Vasoactive intestinal peptide
Glucagonoma	0.01–0.1	Dermatitis (70–90) Weight loss (66–96) Diarrhea (15)	50–80	Glucagon
Somatostatinoma	Rare	Diarrhea (40–90)	>70	Somatostatin
GRFoma	Unknown	Symptoms of acromegaly, abdominal pain	>30	Growth hormone–releasing factor
ACTHoma	Uncommon (4%–16% of all ectopic Cushing's syndrome)	Ectopic Cushing's syndrome	>95 (pancreatic)	ACTH
PET causing hypercalcemia	Rare	Symptoms secondary to malignant tumor, hypercalcemia	84	PTH-RP
PET causing carcinoid syndrome	<1% of all carcinoids	Carcinoid syndrome (diarrhea, flushing)	77	Serotonin, tachykinins
Symptoms not Due to Released Hormones (Nonfunctional PET)				
PPoma/nonfunctional	1–2	None	>60	None

ACTH, adrenocorticotropic hormone; GRF, growth hormone-releasing factor; PTH-RP, parathyroid hormone–related peptide; VIP, vasoactive intestinal peptide; WDHA, watery diarrhea, hypokalemia, achlorhydria.

gastrinomas in recent studies occur with an equal annual incidence of 0.5 to 3 per 1 million population.[21–23] VIPomas are 1/8 as common and glucagonomas 1/17 as common.[12] Somatostatinomas are rare,[24] and the incidence of GRFomas at present is unknown (see Table 51–1).

Origin and Histologic Features

PETs are often called *islet cell tumors*; however, it is unproven that they originate from the pancreatic islets.[25] These tumors frequently contain ductular structures,[26] produce hormones not normally present in the adult pancreas such as gastrin and vasoactive intestinal peptide (VIP), and may produce multiple hormones.[16, 25, 26] These findings suggest that PETs arise from an immature stem cell. The finding of the ductular structures in many PETs and the budding off of endocrine cells from ductules during ontogenesis of the pancreas has led to the suggestion that these tumors are ductular in origin.[27]

It was originally proposed that PETs might originate from cells that are part of the diffuse neuroendocrine cell system.[27–29] These cells share certain cytochemical properties and have been called *APUDomas* (amine precursor uptake and decarboxylation).[28, 29] Ultrastructurally, they often have electron-dense granules and produce multiple regulatory hormones and amines,[26] neuron specific enolase,[26] synaptophysin, and chromogranin A or C.[25, 30] These APUD cells are thought to give rise to carcinoid tumors, medullary carcinoma of the thyroid, melanomas, and pheochromocytomas and to explain the marked similarities in the histology of these tumors and PETs.[28, 29] Histologically, PETs consist of a relatively homogeneous sheet of small round cells with uniform nuclei and cytoplasm (see Fig. 41–1, which shows a gastrinoma; this is representative of a PET). Mitotic figures are uncommon.[25] Malignancy can be determined only by metastases or invasion and cannot be predicted by light microscopic or ultrastructural studies.[21, 26]

Most PETs produce multiple gastrointestinal hormones that can be localized by immunocytochemical methods.[25, 26] In one large series,[26] 52% of functional and 50% of nonfunctional tumors had cells immunoreactive to peptides not causing clinical symptoms. In this series,[26] 33% of insulinomas contained glucagon; 100% of glucagonomas contained insulin; and 22% of both tumors contained somatostatin, 35% PP, and 5% gastrin. At present it is unclear why usually only one or no clinical syndrome is seen despite the immunochemical occurrence of multiple hormones.[12, 21] A functional PET syndrome should be diagnosed only if the appropriate clinical symptoms are present, not based on immunocytochemistry only.

PETs frequently produce chromogranins[30] or the α- or β-subunit of human chorionic gonadotropin (HGG) which can be localized by immunocytochemistry or which circulates at elevated levels.[21, 30] Chromogranins are water-soluble acidic glycoproteins that are present in almost all endocrine or neuronal tissues.[30] Plasma chromogranin A levels are found elevated in more than 90% of patients with various PETs and carcinoid tumors.[30] Although some groups have suggested that elevations of one or the other subunit of HCG or of chromogranin A may be indicative of malignancy, this is not established.[12, 21]

In an occasional patient, a second clinical hormone tumor syndrome may be present initially or develop with time.[16, 21, 31, 32] Whereas one study reported this occurred in 7% of all patients with PETs during a 3-year follow-up,[31] another study[16] has reported that this is a rare occurrence, occurring at a rate of 2 per 100 patients followed over 10 years. However, there appears to be a high incidence of the development of Cushing's syndrome in patients with a functional PET, especially in patients with gastrinoma.[32]

Classification

PETs are classified clinically according to the functional syndrome produced (see Table 51–1). Although clinical syndromes have been attributed in some studies to patients with PETs with elevated plasma levels of either neurotensin[33] or PP,[17, 20, 33] these syndromes have not been established with certainty.[20, 21] All PETs can be associated with the multiple endocrine neoplasia type 1 (MEN I) in a variable percentage of cases. This association is important to recognize because these patients frequently have multiple tumors and may have a different natural history.[21, 34]

Pathophysiology

In patients with PETs, the symptoms due to the inappropriately released hormone are usually responsible for the initial manifestations of the disease. In general, only late in the course of the disease do symptoms due to the tumor itself, such as abdominal pain and jaundice, become dominant.

In a small percentage of the patients with a functional syndrome, no tumor is found at the time of surgery, and hyperplasia of the pancreatic islets is regarded as a possible cause of the disease.[12, 21] Beta cell hyperplasia or nesidioblastosis, which is a subtype of beta cell hyperplasia consisting of proliferation of islet cells from pancreatic ducts, is reported to be the cause of hypoglycemia and hyperinsulinemia in a number of infants and newborns.[35–37] Recently, this condition has been recognized in adolescents and adults and occurs in 5% of patients with hyperinsulinism.[35, 37, 38] It has been suggested that in up to 10% of cases gastrinoma and VIPoma syndromes are caused by hyperplasia of pancreatic ducts, but this has not been substantiated by immunocytochemical studies and thus is not generally accepted.[12, 21]

Molecular Pathogenesis

Until recently, the molecular pathogenesis of neuroendocrine tumors (NETs) (carcinoids and PETs) was largely unknown.[39] This occurred because numerous studies demonstrated that in contrast to most common nonendocrine tumors (e.g., colonic or pancreatic adenocarcinoma), neither common oncogenes (e.g., *ras, fos, myc, src, jun*) nor common tumor suppressor genes (e.g., *p53*, retinoblastoma gene) are generally important in the molecular pathogenesis of most NETs (carcinoids, PETs).[19, 39–41] Recent studies provide evidence that alterations in the *MEN1* gene, *p16/MTS1* tumor suppressor gene, *DPC4/Smad 4* gene, amplification of the *HER-2/neu* proto-oncogene, and deletions of a possible unknown tumor suppressor gene on chromosome 1 or 3p all may be important.[19, 39–44] Alterations in the *MEN1* gene occur in up to one third of sporadic (i.e., noninherited) PETs[41, 42] and alterations in the *p16/MTS1* gene occur in 50% to 92% of PETs[41, 44] and thus may be particularly important. The alterations in the *MEN1* gene are discussed in the next section.

MULTIPLE ENDOCRINE NEOPLASIA

There are three well-established MEN syndromes.[45–47] Each of these syndromes, MEN I, MEN IIa, and MEN IIb, has autosomal dominant inheritance. MEN I, or Wermer's syndrome, is considered in detail later and is characterized by hyperparathyroidism and PETs without the presence of medullary thyroid carcinoma, pheochromocytoma, or unusual phenotype.[34, 46] MEN IIa, or Sipple's syndrome, is characterized by bilateral medullary thyroid carcinoma, pheochromocytomas present in 20% to 40%, which, when they occur, are bilateral in 70%; and hyperparathyroidism in 17%, but without the occurrence of PETs or a specific phenotype.[45, 47] MEN IIb includes bilateral medullary thyroid carcinoma that often appears at an early age and appears generally more aggressive than MEN IIa. Pheochromocytomas, when they occur in MEN IIb, are bilateral in 70%. Parathyroid disease is seldom present, and the patients have a characteristic phenotype with multiple mucosal neuromas, frequently a marfanoid habitus, puffy lips, prominent jaw, pes cavus, and medullated corneal nerves, but no PETs.[45, 47]

Recent studies have localized the genetic defect in MEN I to the long arm of chromosome 11 and have shown it is due to mutations in a 10-exon gene encoding for a 610-amino acid protein, MENIN, a nuclear protein that interacts with the AP1 transcription factor, Jun D.[46] Evidence was provided from these studies that the development of MEN I endocrine tumors conformed to Knudsen's[48] two-hit model theory of neoplasm formation with a germline mutation in one chromosome inherited from one parent unmasked by a somatic deletion or mutation of the other normal chromosome, thereby removing the suppressor effect of the normal gene product. Recent studies[41, 42] showed that in PETs from patients without MEN I, up to 90% have loss of heterozygosity on chromosome 11, and 27% to 39% have mutations in the *MEN1* gene. This result suggests that sporadic PETs share a similar tumorigenesis to PETs in patients with MEN I, which principally involves deletion of a tumor suppressor gene. Recent studies indicate that the MEN II syndromes are caused by alterations in the pericentromeric region of chromosome 10 in the *RET* proto-oncogene, which is a 21-exon gene coding for a tyrosine kinase receptor.[45] Mutations in a cysteine-rich extracellular portion of the receptor primarily cause MEN IIa, whereas mutations in the gene region encoding the intracellular catalytic core of the tyrosine kinase domain cause MEN IIb.[45]

In patients with MEN I, hyperparathyroidism is the most common clinical abnormality, occurring in 88% to 97%[21, 34, 46] (Table 51–2). Functional PETs are the second most common clinical abnormality, occurring in 81% to 82% of patients. Gastrinomas occurred in 54%, whereas insulinomas, glucagonomas, and VIPomas occur in 21%, 3%, and 1% of patients, respectively[22, 34, 46] (see Table 51–2). Nonfunctional PETs and PPomas may be the most common PET in pa-

Table 51–2 | **Multiple Endocrine Neoplasia Type I**

SYMPTOM/SIGN	FREQUENCY (% OF ALL PATIENTS)
Hyperparathyroidism	88–97
Pancreatic endocrine tumors	81–82
Nonfunctional or PPomas	80–100
Gastrinomas	54
Insulinomas	21
Glucagonomas	3
VIPomas	1
Pituitary tumors	21–65
Prolactin-secreting	15–46
Growth hormone–secreting	6–20
Cushing's syndrome	16
Adrenal tumors	27–36
Cortical adenomas	
Hyperplasia, carcinoma (uncommon)	
Thyroid tumors	5–30
Adenomas	

Data from references 21, 22, 34, 46, and 47.

tients with MEN I because in histologic studies they are almost always found.[12, 34, 49] Many patients without a functional PET do not routinely undergo surgical exploration,[50, 51] and imaging studies routinely miss most small PETs (<1 cm)[52]; therefore, the true occurrence rate of asymptomatic PETs in these patients is unknown.

Pathology sudies[12, 34, 49] demonstrate that in patients with MEN I the pancreas demonstrates diffuse microadenomatosis with or without larger tumors. With immunocytochemistry[12, 34, 49] PP is most frequently seen, followed by glucagon and insulin, with gastrin rarely found. These results are consistent with clinical studies that have demonstrated that gastrinomas in 80% of patients with MEN I and Zollinger-Ellison syndrome are in the duodenum.[21, 50, 51, 53]

MEN I is present in 20% to 25% of patients with gastrinomas,[21, 54] 4% of patients with insulinomas,[34] 13% to 17% of patients with glucagonomas,[55, 56] 33% of patients with GRFomas,[12] 9% of patients with VIPomas,[57] and 7% of patients with somatostatinomas.[58] Characteristically, hyperparathyroidism is the initial manifestation of MEN I, usually presenting in the 3rd decade of life, followed by the development of a PET in the 4th or 5th decade.[34, 46, 59] It is important to recognize whether the patient has MEN I because patients with and without MEN I differ in their clinical presentation, the possibility of surgical cure, and the clinical and diagnostic approach to the tumor.[21, 34, 50, 51] In some PETs the presence of hypercalcemia due to the hyperparathyroidism may affect release of the hormones by the tumor.[21, 60] Patients with MEN I may develop more than one PET with time so that their long-term follow-up will differ from that of patients without MEN I. Screening of other family members is indicated in patients with MEN I, whereas it is not indicated in patients with sporadic disease.

OTHER INHERITED SYNDROMES ASSOCIATED WITH PANCREATIC ENDOCRINE TUMORS

Three phacomatoses have an increased occurrence of PETs: von Hippel-Lindau disease (VHL), von Recklinghausen's disease (neurofibromatosis 1 [NF1]), and tuberous sclerosis (Bourneville's disease).[61, 62] VHL is due to a defect on chromosome 3p25 encoding for a 213-amino acid protein that functions as a transcription regulator. In 10% to 17% of patients with VHL, a PET is seen that is usually nonfunctional, but occasional insulinomas and VIPomas are described.[61, 62] NF1 is due to a defect on chromosome 17q11.2 encoding for a 2845-amino acid protein, neurofibromin, which functions as a ras signaling cascade inhibitor.[61, 63] Up to 12% of NF1 patients develop a carcinoid tumor, usually (54%) in the periampullary region of the duodenum.[58, 64, 65] Most are somatostatinomas by immunocytochemistry; however, they rarely produce somatostatinoma syndrome.[58, 64, 65] NF1 has rarely been associated with Zollinger-Ellison syndrome and insulinomas.[61] Tuberous sclerosis is caused by mutations in the 1164-amino acid protein, hamartin (TSC-1), or the 1807-amino acid protein, tuberin (TSC-2).[61, 66] Both proteins affect G protein regulation.[61, 62] A few cases of nonfunctional and functional PETs (insulinomas and gastrinomas) are reported in the patients.[61, 62, 67]

INSULINOMA

Definition

Insulinomas are insulin-secreting tumors that primarily originate in the pancreas and cause symptoms due to hypoglycemia (Table 51–3).

Pathophysiology and Pathology

Almost all insulinomas (98.2%) occur in, or are attached to, the pancreas.[12, 23, 68] An occasional insulinoma presenting as a carcinoid tumor has been reported in the duodenum, ileum, and lung; however, ectopic insulinomas are rare (1% to 3%).[12, 23, 68–70] Insulinomas are evenly distributed in the pancreas, with approximately one third in the pancreatic head, body, and tail.[68, 69, 71, 72] Insulinomas are usually small. In one large series, 5% were smaller than 0.5 cm, 34% were smaller than 0.5 to 1 cm, 53% were 1 to 5 cm, and only 8% were larger than 5 cm.[71]

Insulinomas are usually solitary with multiple tumors occurring in only 2% to 13% of cases.[12, 68, 70] If multiple insulinomas are found, MEN I should be suspected. Insulinomas are generally well encapsulated, firmer than normal pancreas, and highly vascular. Only 5% to 16% of insulinomas are malignant.[23, 35, 68, 70] Malignant tumors are generally greater in size, averaging 6 cm in one series, and 5% of patients have metastases at presentation.[12, 23, 68, 72] Metastases are usually to the liver (47%), regional lymph nodes (30%), or both.[12, 23]

Among adults with hyperinsulinism and pancreatic islet cell disease, histologic studies have shown an insulinoma in 86% of cases, adenomatosis in 5% to 15%, nesidioblastosis in 4%, and hyperplasia in 1%.[35] Adenomatosis consists of multiple macroadenomas or microadenomas and occurs especially in patients with MEN I.[35] A second diffuse lesion is nesidioblastosis, a condition in which islet cells bud off from ductular structures and are mixed with globular elements. This condition previously was reported almost exclusively in infants and children[26, 35, 36] but has been recognized in 5% of

Table 51–3 | **Frequency of Clinical Symptoms and Signs in Patients with Insulinoma**

CLINICAL SYMPTOMS/SIGNS	FREQUENCY (%)
Occurrence Anytime in Clinical Course†	
Neuropsychiatric (loss of consciousness, confusion, dizziness, diplopia)	92
Confusion or abnormal behavior	80
Obesity	52
Amnesia or coma	47
Convulsions (grand mal)	12
Cardiovascular symptoms, palpitations, tachycardia	17
Gastrointestinal symptoms (hunger, vomiting, pain)	9
Occurrence During First Attack‡	
Neuroglycopenic	
Visual disturbances (diplopia, blurred vision)	59
Confusion	51
Altered consciousness	38
Weakness	32
Transient motor defects, hemiplegia	29
Dizziness	28
Fatigue	27
Inappropriate behavior	27
Speech difficulty	24
Headache	23
Seizure	23
Syncope	21
Difficulty concentrating or thinking	19
Paresthesias	17
Memory loss	15
Lethargy	12
Amnesia	8
Stupor	12
Ataxia	4
Disorientation	4
Mental change	4
Adrenergic	
Sweating	43
Tremulousness	23
Hunger, nausea	12
Palpitations	10

†Data from references 71 and 72.
‡Data modified from reference 35.

adults and adolescents with hyperinsulinism.[35, 37, 38] Diffuse islet cell hyperplasia, which consists of excessive and diffuse proliferation of beta cells in the islets, has been reported in adults.[35, 38, 71] Of 1137 cases of organic hyperinsulinism, only 6% had diffuse islet cell hyperplasia and 0.6% had both an insulinoma and diffuse islet cell disease.[71] At present it is unclear whether many of these cases are nesidioblastosis because in most cases appropriate immunofluorescent staining methods were not applied.

Insulin is synthesized and stored in beta cells of the pancreatic islets.[23] Insulin is synthesized in the rough endoplasmic reticulum as pre-proinsulin from which proinsulin is liberated and transferred to the Golgi of the cell.[73] Proinsulin consists of a 21-amino acid α chain and 30-amino acid β chain connected by a 33-amino acid connecting peptide (C-peptide).[23, 70, 73] In secretory granules, a protease excises the C-peptide and thus, when secretion occurs, the C-peptide and the double-stranded insulin molecule are released in equimolar amounts.[73] Small amounts of intact proinsulin remain in granules and are also released and can be detected in the plasma. Proinsulin contains the α and β chain of insulin, and because most insulin antibodies used in radioimmunoassays recognize moieties on these chains, they also recognize proinsulin.[70] Normal subjects have less than 25% of the serum insulin as proinsulin, whereas more than 90% of patients have an elevated proportion.[70]

Clinical Features

Insulinomas can occur at any age but are rare in adolescents, usually occurring in patients between 20 to 75 years old, with most being between 40 to 45 years old; 60% are females.[23, 35, 68, 70] Symptoms are due to hypoglycemia (see Table 51–3), characteristically associated with fasting, and thus more frequently occur when a meal is delayed or missed, or before breakfast. They may also occur during exercise. In one study,[35] 26% of patients had symptoms during or after an overnight fast delay, 27% had symptoms prior to lunch or dinner, 8% had symptoms only after a missed meal, 29% had symptoms only before lunch or dinner, and only 9% were uncertain about the timing of the symptoms. Most symptoms (82% to 92% of patients)[23, 35, 68, 71] are due to neuroglycopenia, that is, insufficient availability to the central nervous system of glucose, which is the main source of energy for the brain. Neuroglycopenia symptoms include somnolence, visual disturbances, irritability, abnormal behavior, confusion, amnesia, paresthesias, stupor, drowsiness, coma, and seizures (see Table 51–3). Symptoms can also be due to catecholamine release (adrenergic symptoms) secondary to the hypoglycemia and include anxiety, palpitations, weakness and fatigue, headache, tremor, and sweating.[68] Coma occurs in up to 53% of patients and convulsions in 12%. In one study, of the presenting symptoms of the first attack,[35] 49% of patients initially had both neuroglycopenia and adrenergic symptoms, 38% had neuroglycopenia symptoms only, 12% had adrenergic symptoms only, and 1% of patients had no symptoms (see Table 51–3). Of the neuroglycopenia symptoms, visual disturbances (57%), confusion (51%), and altered consciousness (38%) are the most common. Of the adrenergic symptoms, sweating (43%) and tremulousness (23%) are the most common (see Table 51–3). Patients frequently learn to avoid symptoms by eating frequently and obesity may result.[35] In one study,[35] 40% of patients with organic hypoglycemia were overweight. The average duration of neuroglycopenia symptoms prior to diagnosis is often prolonged, being longer than 3 years in 25% of patients and longer than 5 years in 20%.

Diagnosis and Differential Diagnosis

The key to establishing the diagnosis is suspecting by clinical history that the symptoms could be due to hypoglycemia and establishing the relationship of the symptoms to fasting.[23, 37, 70] Whipple's triad, published in 1938[74] and long used as diagnostic criteria for insulinoma, was based on this association, consisting of characteristic hypoglycemia symptoms, the presence of hypoglycemia (blood glucose < 50 mg/dL), and relief of symptoms following glucose ingestion. Unfortunately, these symptoms are not specific for insulinoma.[35]

Organic hypoglycemia is generally defined as a fasting blood glucose level of less than 40 mg/dL. In healthy individuals, after an overnight fast, plasma glucose values usually do not decrease below 70 mg/dL.[35] After an overnight fast, only 53% of patients with insulinoma are reported to have a blood glucose level of less than 60 mg/dL, and 39% have less than 50 mg/dL.[35] However, if a blood glucose determination is combined with a concomitant plasma insulin level, this level will be inappropriately elevated in 65% of patients.[35] Hypoglycemia can be classified as either a fasting hypoglycemia or as a postprandial (reactive) hypoglycemia, of which there are a number of different causes (Table 51–4). The distinction can usually be made by a careful clinical history. Because a single overnight fasting blood glucose, even when combined with a simultaneous plasma insulin level, does not establish the presence of fasting organic hypoglycemia in more than 35% of patients with organic hyperinsulinism, a fast is done with blood glucose, plasma insulin, and C-peptide levels at 3- to 6-hour intervals.[23, 35, 37, 70] Traditionally a 72-hour fast is performed, although a recent study proposes that a 48-hour fast is sufficient.[75] If at any point during the fast the patient becomes symptomatic, plasma insulin and glucose values should be obtained before intravenous glucose is given and the test stopped. Within 24 hours of starting the fast, 75% to 80% of patients with an insulinoma will have symptoms and a blood glucose level of less than 40 mg/dL; by 48 hours, 90% to 98%; and by 72 hours, virtually all patients.[12, 23, 35, 72] In nonobese normal subjects, serum insulin concentrations decrease to less than 6 μU/mL when blood glucose levels decrease to less than 40 mg/dL, and the ratio of plasma insulin (in μU/mL) to glucose (in mg/dL) remains less than 0.3.[70, 76] The test is considered positive for insulinoma if the plasma insulin glucose ratio is higher than 0.3.[70] In some normal obese subjects, because of hyperinsulinemia due to insulin resistance, the fasting plasma insulin to glucose ratio may be elevated[35] and therefore mimic the pattern in insulinoma. In these patients the fasting glucose level is normal and with fasting does not decrease to less than 55 mg/dL, as occurs with patients with insulinomas.[12, 35]

A number of conditions (see Table 51–4) in addition to insulinoma can cause fasting hypoglycemia, including organic hyperinsulinism due to pancreatic islet disease, factitious use of excessive insulin or hypoglycemic agents, or autoantibodies against the insulin receptor or insulin.[37, 70] To differentiate these conditions, measurements of plasma proinsulin, C-peptide, antibodies to insulin, and plasma sulfonylurea levels are used.[23, 35, 37, 70, 76] Plasma proinsulin level is elevated in 80% to 90% of patients with insulinoma to more than 22% of the total plasma insulin level.[35, 70, 76] In patients with surreptitious use of insulin or oral hypoglycemic agents the proinsulin level is either normal or decreased.[76] C-peptide is released in equimolar quantities to insulin into the plasma; thus, it would be expected to be proportionately elevated with insulin in insulinomas. However, it has a much longer plasma half-life than insulin and thus the plasma level shows less fluctuation than insulin.[12, 23, 37] The measurement of C-peptide has proved useful in differentiating organic hypersecretion of insulin such as in patients with insulinoma from patients surreptitiously using insulin[12, 23, 37, 76] because commercial insulin preparations contain no C-peptide. In insulinoma the characteristic findings are either an elevated or normal plasma C-peptide concentration,[76] whereas in patients surreptitiously using insulin the plasma insulin level will be high and the C-peptide level low.[76] The C-peptide level does not differentiate patients surreptitiously taking oral hypoglycemic agents from patients with insulinomas in that both have low blood glucose, elevated insulin, and C-peptide levels.[76] Measurement of plasma sulfonylurea levels helps distinguish insulinoma from surreptitious use of these drugs. Various provocative tests with tolbutamide, leucine, glucagon, and secretin and suppression tests all have been described for the diagnosis of insulinoma[12, 23, 35]; however, each has its limitations, and none is currently seldom used.

Table 51–4 | **Causes of Spontaneous Hypoglycemia**

Postprandial (Reactive) Hypoglycemia
Functional: recognizable anatomic lesion
Alimentary hyperinsulinism/usually secondary to previous gastric surgery, such as Billroth gastrectomy
Secondary to mild diabetes
Idiopathic
Due to specific hepatic enzyme deficiencies
Hereditary fructose intolerance (infants, children)
Galactosemia (infants,children)
Familial fructose and galactose intolerance (rare)
Fasting Hypoglycemia
Organic hyperinsulinism: specific anatomic lesion present
Pancreatic islet disease
Insulinoma—single or multiple
Microadenomatosis with or without macroscopic adenomas
Carcinoma
Hyperplasia
Nesidioblastosis
Nonpancreatic tumors
Severe congestive heart failure
Severe renal insufficiency in non–insulin-dependent diabetes
Due to hepatic enzyme deficiencies or decreased hepatic glucose output (primarily in infants, children)
Glycogen storage diseases
Glycogen synthetase deficiencies
Other enzyme deficiencies (fructose-1,6-diphosphate deficiencies)
Endocrine hypofunction
Anterior pituitary (in infants, children usually)
Adrenocortical (Addison's disease)
Diffuse acquired liver disease
Ethanol
Severe malnutrition, sepsis
Due to exogenous agents (factitious)
Sulfonylureas, biguanides
Insulin administration
Ingestion of ackee fruits (hypoglycine)
Other drugs (aspirin, pentamidine)
Functional hypoglycemia with no persistent anatomic defect
Autoantibodies to insulin receptor
Spontaneous autoimmune anti-insulin antibody syndrome
Transient hypoglycemia of infancy

Data from references 12, 23, 35, and 70.

Treatment

Treatment of insulinoma consists of two different approaches. Initially, treatment is directed at controlling the symptoms of hypoglycemia; then, after tumor localization studies, a surgical cure is attempted. Tumor localization of all PETs involves similar approaches and is dealt with in a later section. For the 5% to 13% patients with metastatic insulinoma, chemotherapy or other therapies directed at the tumor itself may need to be considered. This latter group is considered in a later section on treatment of metastatic PETs.

Medical Therapy

Hypoglycemia is controlled in most patients by a combination of diet and medical therapy. The use of appropriately timed feedings with a bedtime snack or midmorning, midafternoon, or 3:00 AM snack may be sufficient to control all symptoms.[35] It is generally advised not to restrict intake to simple carbohydrates because their ingestion may occasionally stimulate insulin secretion from the tumor. More slowly absorbed forms of carbohydrates such as starches, bread, potatoes, and rice are preferable.[35] During a hypoglycemic episode, rapidly absorbable forms of carbohydrate such as fruit juice with glucose or sucrose are preferable. Occasional patients with severe hypoglycemia may require the use of a continuous intravenous infusion of glucose together with increased dietary carbohydrates.

A number of drugs have been reported to control the hyperinsulinemia. Diazoxide, which is a nondiuretic benzothiazide analog, has potent hyperglycemic effects.[70, 77] It directly inhibits insulin release from beta cells through stimulation of α-adrenergic receptors and also has an extrapancreatic hyperglycemic effect that enhances glycogenolysis.[35] The major side effects of diazoxide are sodium retention (47%), gastrointestinal symptoms such as nausea, and occasional hirsutism.[35, 70, 77] Edema can result from sodium retention, and the addition of a diuretic such as trichlormethiazide, a benzothiadiazine derivative, can correct the edema as well as augment the hyperglycemic effect.[35, 70] The gastrointestinal side effects can be reduced by taking the diazoxide with a meal.[70] Diazoxide should be initiated with 150 to 200 mg per day given in two or three divided doses and if not effective, increased to a maximum of 600 to 800 mg per day.[35, 70] Side effects are dose related and may limit the ability to reach maximal doses. Approximately 60% of patients respond to the diazoxide.[70] Patients have been treated for up to 22 years with diazoxide, demonstrating it can be used long term.[77] Verapamil, propranolol, phenytoin, and glucocorticoids have been reported effective in occasional patients, but they may have only minor beneficial effects and their successes are anecdotal.[12, 35, 70, 72]

The long-acting somatostatin analog, octreotide, has controlled hypoglycemia in a number of cases of insulinoma.[70, 78–80] This compound has a half-life of 100 minutes, 33 times longer than that of native somatostatin, and thus can be self-administered two to four times a day subcutaneously. Recently, long-acting preparations of both lanreotide and octreotide that last 2 to 4 weeks have been developed.[79, 80] Octreotide controls symptoms and hypoglycemia in 40% to 60% of patients.[12, 70, 78, 80] Somatostatin analogs are thought to primarily mediate their effects on PETs such as insulinomas by interacting with high-affinity somatostatin receptors on the tumor.[12, 79–81] Five subtypes of somatostatin receptors exist, and lanreotide and octreotide have high affinity for subtypes 2 and 5, which have been shown to be present on PETs.[12, 79–82] The response rate of insulinomas to octreotide is likely lower than that of other PETs that possess high densities of receptors with high affinity for these analogs in 80% to 90% of cases.[79–82] Octreotide is generally well tolerated and is usually given in a starting dose of 50 μg two or three times per day and can be increased to doses as high as 1500 μg per day.[78, 80, 83] A recent significant advance is the availability of long-acting depot forms of octreotide (octreotide–long-acting release [LAR]).[41, 84] After a 30 mg dose, octreotide maintains a plasma level of 1 ng/mL or greater for 25 days and therefore can be given monthly. The main side effects of octreotide treatment include gastrointestinal symptoms such as bloating and abdominal cramping, and the long-term side effects include malabsorption, cholelithiasis, and, in an occasional patient, worsening of glucose tolerance.[78–80, 83] In addition to improving symptoms, octreotide decreased plasma insulin levels in 65% of patients.[83] Because somatostatin analogs also decrease glucagon and growth hormone secretion, occasionally their administration may worsen the hypoglycemia.

Surgical Therapy

Detailed tumor localization studies are important because insulinomas are frequently small and uniformly distributed throughout the pancreas and thus can be difficult to find.[23] In addition, in the fewer than 10% of patients with metastatic disease, unnecessary surgery can be avoided. Localization methods are discussed in a later section.

All authorities recommend that if metastatic disease in the liver is not present (>90% of cases), surgical exploration is indicated.[23, 70] A careful surgical exploration should be done using the results of the localization studies by a group that is experienced in treating such patients and has expertise in the use of intraoperative ultrasonography.[85] In most studies 70% to 97% of all patients are cured.[23, 69, 70] Failure to localize an insulinoma at surgery presents a difficult problem, and the role of blind distal pancreatectomy is controversial. Because insulinomas are equally distributed in the pancreas, a pancreatectomy distal to the superior mesenteric vessels gives only a 50% chance of success. To decrease the possibility of a negative laparotomy, the use of preoperative insulin venous sampling from portal venous tributaries[85, 86] and intraoperative ultrasonography should detect tumors in almost every case.

GLUCAGONOMA

Definition

Glucagonomas are PETs that secrete excessive amounts of glucagon and cause a distinct syndrome characterized by a specific dermatitis (migratory necrolytic erythema), weight loss, glucose intolerance, and anemia (Table 51–5). Although Mallinson and associates[4] specifically established the association of the rash with glucagon-producing tumors of the pancreas when they reported nine cases in 1974, the disease had been described earlier by others but the association with glucagon-release was not appreciated. In 1942 Becker and coworkers described the association of a PET with a skin rash[87]; in 1966 McGarvan and colleagues[88] reported a patient with an elevated fasting glucagon level, dermatitis, diabetes, and a PET; and in 1973 Wilkinson[89] described the rash as necrolytic migratory erythema.

Pathophysiology and Pathology

In contrast to insulinomas, most glucagonomas are large at the time of diagnosis, with the average size between 5 and

Table 51–5 | **Clinical Symptoms and Signs and Laboratory Abnormalities in Patients with Glucagonoma**

	FREQUENCY (%)
Clinical Symptoms/Signs	
Dermatitis	64–90
Weight loss	56–96
Glossitis/stomatitis/cheilitis	29–40
Diarrhea	14–15
Abdominal pain	12
Thromboembolic disease	12–35
Venous thrombosis	24
Pulmonary emboli	11
Psychiatric disturbance	Uncommon
Laboratory Abnormalities	
Diabetes/glucose intolerance	38–90
Anemia	33–85
Hypoaminoacidemia	26–100
Hypocholesterolemia	80
Renal glycosuria	Unknown

Data from references 4, 12, 55, 56, 90–94.

10 cm and a size range from 0.4 to 35 cm.[55, 90, 91] One half of glucagonomas occurred in the tail in three studies[55, 91, 92] and 80% in another study.[93] Similar to other PETs except insulinoma, 50% to 80%[55, 91–93] of glucagonomas had evidence of metastatic spread or invasion. The most common site of metastatic spread was to the liver (43% to 82%), with lymph nodes (38%), bone, and mesentery less common sites.[55, 91–93] Most glucagonomas are within the pancreas (>97%); however, a glucagonoma associated with the typical clinical syndrome was found in the proximal duodenum.[55, 93] Glucagonomas usually occur as a single tumor, although 10% to 12% of patients in one series had multiple tumors or diffuse involvement by a single mass.[91, 93]

The pathophysiology of glucagonoma syndrome is related to the known actions of glucagon. Glucagon stimulates glycogenolysis, gluconeogenesis, ketogenesis, lipolysis, and insulin secretion, as well as having effects on gut secretion, inhibiting pancreatic and gastric secretion, and inhibiting gut motility.[94] Hyperglycemia results from the increased hepatic glycogenolysis and gluconeogenesis. Because glucagon also increases secretion of insulin, which prevents lipolysis and maintains normal free fatty acid concentrations, ketonemia and ketoacidosis usually do not develop.[95] The weight loss has been attributed to the known catabolic effects of glucagon.[90, 91] However, severe anorexia and adipsia are seen in rats with transplanted glucagonomas, and studies suggest that the tumor is producing a novel anorectic substance.[96] It is not clearly established that the skin rash is due to the hyperglucagonemia because numerous patients have been given large doses of glucagon over extended periods and the skin rash did not develop.[90, 91] It is possible that the glucagon-induced hypoaminoacidemia, which develops in 80% to 90% of patients,[91–93] may cause the rash because, if amino acid deficiency is corrected, the dermatitis may improve without changing plasma glucagon levels.[12, 90] The similarity of the skin lesions to those seen in patients with zinc deficiencies has resulted in trials of zinc in some patients, with some responses.[90] However, in some patients the rash has resolved with rehydration and glucose solution; therefore, there may be differing contributing factors in different patients.[90] The severe hypoaminoacidemia is believed secondary to the hyperglucagonemia because glucagon infusions have altered amino acid metabolism by augmenting hepatic gluconeogenesis.[90, 97] This conclusion is further supported by studies that demonstrate that total pancreatectomy or somatostatin administration, which decreases plasma glucagon levels, increases plasma amino acid levels, whereas glucagon administration decreases plasma amino acid levels.[12, 91]

The role of glucagon per se in causing thromboembolic phenomena sometimes observed in this syndrome is not clear. Glucagon is known to affect coagulation parameters, but the relationship to thromboembolic events is not known.[90] The anemia often seen in patients with glucagonomas may be due to the glucagon excess because prolonged treatment with a long-acting glucagon preparation decreases erythropoiesis in animals.[98]

Immunocytochemical and histologic studies of glucagonomas show results typical of PETs. Glucagon is one of the most commonly seen peptides in immunocytochemical studies of PETs, but in most cases it is not associated with any syndrome. In one series of 1366 autopsy cases, a PET frequency of 0.8% was reported and all contained glucagon-producing cells.[12, 90] In glucagonomas, as with other PETs, multiple gastrointestinal hormones are frequently seen on immunocytochemical studies.[26, 55] The morphology of most glucagon-producing tumors demonstrates no histologic features that distinguish them from other PETs. Even though tumors are usually malignant, mitotic figures and nuclear atypia are uncommon.[12, 90, 93] With electron microscopy, readily identifiable A granules, typical of those seen in normal alpha cells, are recognizable in PETs that stain positively for glucagon and do not cause the glucagonoma syndrome, whereas in patients with a glucagonoma, atypical granules are usually seen.[12, 55, 90, 91]

Clinical Features (see Table 51–5)

Glucagonoma usually occurs in middle age or in the elderly.[55, 91–93] No cases have been reported in individuals younger than 19 years old, and only 16% of all cases occur in individuals younger than 40 years old.[91–93] Glucagonomas occur slightly more commonly (55% to 58% of all cases) in women.[55, 91, 93] Cutaneous lesions are one of the most common manifestations of the disease, occurring in 64% to 90%[56, 90–93] (see Fig. 18–26). Cutaneous lesions often precede the diagnosis of the syndrome for long periods, with a mean of 6 to 8 years and a maximum of 18 years in one study.[91] Skin lesions may wax and wane[93] and may be misdiagnosed as pemphigus foliaceous, pemphigoid, vasculitis, acrodermatitis enteropathica, psoriasis, herpes, seborrheic or contact dermatitis, eczema, pellagra, or even a chemical burn.[93] Numerous excellent descriptions of the typical rash, necrolytic migratory erythema, associated with glucagonoma have been published.[4, 89–91] Characteristically, the skin lesion starts as an erythematous area typically at periorifacial or intertriginous areas such as the groin, buttocks, thighs, or perineum and then spreads laterally. The lesions subsequently become raised with superficial central blistering. The top of the bullae frequently detaches or ruptures, leaving eroded areas that crust. The lesions tend to heal in the center while the edges continue to spread with a crusting well-defined edge. Healing is associated with the development of hyperpigmentation. This entire sequence characteristically takes 1 to 2 weeks, and while some new lesions are developing, others are healing; therefore, a mixed pattern of erythema, bulla formation with epidermal separation, crusting, and hyperpigmentation together with normal skin can occur. The histopathology can be as varied as the clinical presentation.[93] In its classic form,[4, 89, 99] early lesions demonstrate a superficial spongiosis and necrosis with subcorneal and midepidermal bullae. Fusiform keratinocytes with pyknotic nuclei are often seen, as are mononuclear inflammatory infiltrates.[4, 89] This characteristic histologic pattern is best seen in an early lesion. Glossitis or angular stomatitis is reported to occur in 34% to 68% of patients.[55, 91, 92] In addition, some patients develop a nail dystrophy with brittleness and crumbling of the nails.[93]

Glucose intolerance with or without frank diabetes mellitus occurs in 38% to 90% of cases[55, 56, 90–93] (see Table 51–5). In one series, 42% of patients required oral hypoglycemic agents and 24% required insulin.[91] The onset of the diabetes mellitus preceded the diagnosis of the glucagonoma by up to 10 years in one study, with an average time of 5 years.[91] The relationship of the diabetes mellitus to the hyperglucagonemia remains unclear. A number of patients with hyperglucagonemia do not have diabetes mellitus.[90–93] Furthermore, although correlations between plasma glucagon levels and changes in plasma glucose have been described in a few cases,[90–93] this correlation was not easily demonstrated when a number of proven cases were analyzed.[92] Tumor resection and normalization of blood glucagon may not result in normalization of the glucose intolerance.[90–93] In some patients, removal of the glucagonoma improved glucose tolerance.[4, 90] In various patients with glucagonomas plasma insulin concentrations are normal or elevated[90–93]; however, no correlation between circulating plasma insulin and glucagon levels existed.[93]

Hypoaminoacidemia occurs in 26% to 100% of patients with glucagonoma syndrome.[4, 55, 90] Plasma concentrations of amino acids are frequently less than 25% of normal, with glycogenic amino acids such as alanine or glycine most affected, whereas branched-chain amino acids are reported to be less affected.[91, 97] The intensity of the hypoaminoacidemia may vary with the intensity of the disease.[4] The hypoaminoacidemia may participate in the pathogenesis of the skin rash, as discussed in an earlier section on pathology and pathogenesis.

Weight loss is a prominent feature of the glucagonoma syndrome, occurring in 56% to 96% of patients[55, 56, 91, 93] (see Table 51–5). A number of observations suggest that the weight loss is a unique aspect of the syndrome. Weight loss is seen even in patients with small tumors without metastatic spread.[4, 90–93] The weight loss is often associated with anorexia and may be profound, with a mean weight loss of 20 kg in 44 cases and a maximal loss of 30 kg.

Thromboembolic phenomena are common in patients with glucagonoma, occurring in 12% to 35% of patients in various series.[56, 92, 93] Venous thrombosis occurred in 24% of patients and pulmonary emboli in 12%. Because this complication may be lethal, it should be carefully sought.[90] This complication is thought to be related to the glucagonoma syndrome because it is not seen in other PETs at this frequency. The mechanism is unclear. Anemia occurs in 33% to 85% of cases.[55, 56, 92, 93] The anemia is usually normochromic and normocytic (in 73% of cases in one study) and may be severe, but usually is not. When serum iron, folate, and vitamin B_{12} have been measured they are usually normal.[90] The anemia is reported to respond to successful tumor therapy.[90] Other clinical findings that have been reported to occur as part of the glucagonoma syndrome include psychiatric disturbances, abdominal pain, and diarrhea.[55, 90, 92, 93] Psychiatric symptoms, although mentioned in several reports,[4, 56, 92, 93] appear to be relatively infrequent.[93] Depression is the most commonly reported abnormality. Whether psychiatric disturbances occur with increased frequency compared to other comparable debilitating illnesses is unclear. Abdominal pain without specific identifying characteristics is reported in approximately 12% of patients. Diarrhea, weight loss, and hepatomegaly are more frequent in patients with metastatic disease.[55] Diarrhea is reported in 14% to 15% of patients,[91, 93] often with severe steatorrhea. Diarrhea is reported far more commonly than constipation (15% vs. 4% in one study),[93] and the etiology of the diarrhea remains unclear. Jejunal biopsies have been reported to be normal or to show hypertrophic folds in two different patients.[91, 93] It remains possible that other hormones may also be secreted by the tumor that could contribute to the diarrhea, but this possibility has not been extensively studied. Other abnormal laboratory findings in patients with glucagonoma include hypocholesterolemia (80%) and renal glycosuria (see Table 51–5). Renal glycosuria[4, 90, 92, 93] may occur early and may represent a direct renal effect of glucagon.

Diagnosis and Differential Diagnosis

Glucagonomas are usually suspected because of the skin rash, although occasionally the diagnosis is suspected in a patient with a pancreatic mass with weight loss or diabetes.[55, 91] The skin lesion is most frequently confused with pemphigus foliaceus, although a number of dermatologic lesions have also been misdiagnosed (see Chapter 18).[90] A number of cases of patients with a typical necrolytic migratory erythema have been described who do not have glucagonoma.[92, 93, 99] Liver disease, celiac disease or other causes of malabsorption, malignancy, and pancreatitis are the most common nonglucagonoma causes of necrolytic migratory erythema.[90, 99] In some studies, up to 20% of patients with glucagonomas also have Zollinger-Ellison syndrome (see Chapter 41), and 13% to 17% have MEN I.[55, 56]

Once the diagnosis is suspected, it can be confirmed by demonstrating an increase in plasma glucagon concentration. In most laboratories the upper limit of normal for fasting glucagon concentration (using antibody 30 K of Unger) is 150 to 200 pg/mL.[91] In one large review of 58 patients with glucagonomas, only two had a plasma glucagon level of 200 to 500 pg/mL, 4 were between 500 to 1000 pg/mL, and 52 exceeded 1000 pg/mL.[91] These results are in close agreement with another study[93] in which the mean plasma glucagon concentration in 73 cases of glucagonoma was 2110 pg/mL, with a range of 550 to 6600 pg/mL, with 30% of patients between 500 to 1000 pg/mL, and the remaining 70% greater than 1000 pg/mL. However, patients with the glucagonoma syndrome and only mildly elevated plasma glucagon levels have been described.[56, 100] Hyperglucagonemia is reported to occur in chronic renal insufficiency, diabetic ketoacidosis, prolonged starvation, acute pancreatitis, acromegaly, hypercorticism, septicemia, severe burns, severe stress (trauma, exercise), familial hyperglucagonemia, and hepatic insufficiency.[56, 88–90, 92, 101] Plasma glucagon in these conditions does not exceed 500 pg/mL.[90–92] It therefore has been recommended that a plasma glucagon concentration of greater than 1000 pg/mL is diagnostic of glucagonoma. The one reported exception to this is patients with cirrhosis.[91] Because a necrolytic migratory erythematosus-like rash has been reported in patients with hepatic disease,[90] diagnostic confusion could occasionally result. However, in one recent review of 13 cases,[90] no overlap in plasma glucagon levels was found between patients with cirrhosis or any other of the above conditions and the values seen in patients with glucagonomas.[90] Various provocative tests have been described such as the use of secretin to cause a paradoxical increase in glucagon release or a mixed or carbohydrate-rich meal.[12] However, at present none of these tests is sufficiently reliable to differentiate glucagonoma with nondiagnostic plasma glucagon elevations from these other conditions. Patients with familial hyperglucagonemia have been described.[102, 103] These patients are asymptomatic and therefore they can be distinguished from patients who have glucagonoma syndrome. In addition, fractionation of the plasma glucagon immunoreactivity gives a different pattern than seen in normal subjects or patients with glucagonoma, namely, an increased percentage of the high-molecular-weight big plasma glucagon peak.[90, 91, 102, 103]

Treatment

Because glucagonomas are generally malignant and it is not possible to predict in a given patient when metastases may develop, surgical resection should be considered in all patients if it is feasible. Similar to the considerations with other malignant functional PETs, initially treatment can be directed at controlling the symptoms, restoring nutritional status, and controlling the hyperglycemia while tumor localization studies are being performed and possible surgical curative resection is considered. Tumor localization studies are dealt with in a separate later section on this subject.

Medical Therapy

Preoperative medical control of symptoms is important in these patients, because they are generally poor operative risks. The catabolic effects of glucagon combined with glucose intolerance and diabetes mellitus (see Table 51–5) can markedly affect the nutritional status of these patients. These patients have an increased incidence of pulmonary emboli as well as venous thrombosis (see Table 51–5), increasing the postoperative surgical risk. To improve the metabolic status of these patients prior to surgery, blood transfusions in those with severe anemia and a period of extended hyperalimentation are recommended. Parenteral nutrition with restoration of plasma amino acid levels to normal is reported also to have an excellent effect in healing the dermatitis.[12]

The long-acting somatostatin analog, octreotide, has been useful in controlling symptoms in patients with glucagonoma.[56, 78, 80, 83, 91] The rash improved with octreotide treatment in 54% to 90% of patients with complete disappearance in up to 30%.[78, 83, 91] Octreotide generally improved the symptoms of weight loss, abdominal pain, and diarrhea.[78, 83] In one study diarrhea improved in four of six patients and resolved in two patients.[78] Diabetes mellitus was not improved with octreotide treatment.[78, 83] Plasma glucagon levels decreased in 80% to 90% of patients but only decreased into the normal range in 10% to 20% of patients with octreotide treatment.[78, 83, 91] In one patient the rash resolved with no change in the plasma glucagon concentration.[83] In most studies 100 to 400 μg per day of octreotide were used.[78, 83] In some patients with continued treatment, the dose had to be increased to continue to control symptoms.[83]

Surgical Therapy

Unfortunately, approximately 50% to 90% of patients with glucagonoma have metastases at the time of diagnosis.[55, 56, 90, 91, 93] Surgical resection has been successful in a number of cases, however.[89–93] The exact percentage of cases that can be cured is unknown, but with the syndrome currently recognized relatively late in most patients, cure is likely in fewer than 20% of all patients.[12] A number of patients developed recurrence with elevated plasma glucagon elevations after what was thought to be complete tumor removal.[92, 93] However, even if a patient eventually develops a recurrence, an extended disease-free interval may be attained that will be beneficial. A number of studies have reported a benefit to patients even if surgical debulking only can be done.[56, 90–93] In patients with widely metastatic disease where surgical debulking is not possible, various chemotherapeutic agents are frequently used and are dealt with in a later section on treatment of advanced disease.

VIPoma

Definition

The VIPoma syndrome is due to an NET (usually pancreatic in location in adults) that secretes excessive amounts of VIP, which causes a syndrome characterized by extreme secretory diarrhea, hypochlorhydria, and hypokalemia (Table 51–6). This association was described in 1957 by Priest and Alexander[104] and by Verner and Morrison in 1958[3] and is commonly also called *Verner-Morrison syndrome* (see Table 51–1). The absence of gastric acid secretion in these patients was later noted.[12] Because of the resemblance of the diarrhea fluid to that seen in cholera the term *pancreatic cholera* was suggested,[105] and the acronym WDHA (*w*atery *d*iarrhea, *h*ypokalemia, and *a*chlorhydria) was proposed in 1967.[106] VIP was long suspected as the mediator of this syndrome, and the ability of VIP to produce secretory diarrhea in humans at blood levels seen in VIPomas was confirmed in 1983.[107]

Pathophysiology and Pathology

In adults, more than 80% to 90% of VIPomas are pancreatic in location,[106, 108, 109] with rare cases caused by VIP-producing intestinal carcinoids, bronchial carcinomas, or pheochromocy-

Table 51–6 | **Clinical Symptoms and Signs and Laboratory Abnormalities in Patients with VIPoma Syndrome**

	FREQUENCY (%)
Clinical Symptoms/Signs	
Secretory diarrhea	89–100
Dehydration	44–100
Weight loss	36–100
Abdominal cramps, colic	10–63
Flushing	14–28
Laboratory Abnormalities	
Hypokalemia	67–100
Hypochlorhydria	34–72
Hypercalcemia	41–50
Hyperglycemia	18–50
Hyperchloremic (nongap) acidosis	Common

Data from references 57, 106, and 109–112.

tomas.[106, 108] Extrapancreatic VIPomas are reported in the retroperitoneum, liver, esophagus, and small intestine.[106, 110] VIPomas are usually large, solitary tumors.[57, 108, 109, 111] In two series[57, 109] only 2% of tumors were multiple. Within the pancreas, 42% to 75% occur in the pancreatic tail.[57, 108, 111] In various series 37% to 78% of the VIPomas[57, 106, 108, 109, 111–113] had metastases at the time of diagnosis or surgery, which is comparable to the 63% to 90% malignancy rate reported with gastrinomas, glucagonomas, and somatostatinomas. In children younger than 10 years old and rarely in adults (5% of cases), VIPoma syndrome is due to a ganglioneuroma or ganglioneuroblastoma.[106, 109] In one series 16% of all cases[109] were due to this tumor. These tumors are extrapancreatic and are less often malignant (10% of cases) than pancreatic VIPomas.[57, 109]

By immunocytochemistry, VIP was detected in 57% to 88% of VIPomas.[26, 57, 108] PP is found in 34% to 53% of VIPomas, glucagon in 19% to 27%, somatostatin in 10% to 46%, insulin in 5%, and gastrin in zero to 23%,[26, 57, 108] and 45% secrete multiple hormones.[57] VIP-producing tumors also elaborate peptide histidine methionine (PHM-27), a 27-amino acid peptide that shares with VIP a common precursor peptide (prepro VIP/PHM-27), and PHM-27–like immunoreactivity has been found in the plasma and the tumor of patients with VIPomas.[114] On conventional microscopy, VIPomas show the typical microscopic features of PETs.[108] Mitoses are uncommon (12%).[108] On electron microscopy a mixture of cells was usually seen in the same tumor, with 90% having cells with a few scattered, inconspicuous secretory granules; 89% having a few small agranular cells; and 52% having some well-differentiated endocrine cells with well-developed granules.[108] The secretory granules are small (120 to 180 nm) and resemble those of the D cells of normal gut.[57, 108] Both the histologic and electron microscopic studies do not allow VIPomas to be clearly differentiated from some other PETs; however, the presence of immunoreactive VIP is strongly suggestive for VIPoma because this is uncommonly found in other PETs (10 of 104 in one study).[26, 108]

It is now clear that VIP is the major mediator of VIPoma syndrome.[12, 106, 115] For a number of years there was considerable controversy about the mediator.[110, 115, 116] In addition to VIP, a number of other substances (including secretin, gastric inhibitory polypeptide, PP, and prostaglandins) were reported elevated in the plasma in a number of patients.[12] In early studies plasma VIP infusions in humans did not produce the syndrome.[12, 115] However, in recent studies plasma VIP is usually elevated in VIPoma syndrome.[12, 109, 110, 115] Also, a continuous infusion of VIP for 10 hours in normal human subjects to achieve plasma levels similar to that seen in patients with VIPoma syndrome produced watery diarrhea in 6 to 7 hours.[107] The ability of VIP to produce diarrhea is consistent with its known actions in the intestine (see Chapter 87).[12] Receptors for VIP have been identified on intestinal epithelial cells. VIP stimulates rat intestinal electrolyte and fluid secretion in animals, stimulates chloride secretion with increased short circuit current, and activates adenylate cyclase and cyclic adenosine monophosphate in intestinal cells that leads to intestinal secretion.[12] PHM-27–like immunoreactivity (or PHI, the porcine equivalent), which was found in 92% of VIPomas, can induce intestinal chloride secretion, and thus it could contribute to the pathogenesis of the diarrhea.[12] However, PHI was 32-fold less potent than VIP,[117] and because VIP is always present, it is likely the important peptide in most cases.

The pathogenesis of the severe hypokalemia is likely primarily due to fecal loss but also may be contributed to by the secondary hyperaldosteronism that results from VIP stimulation of renin release.[12] The mechanism of the hypercalcemia is unclear and may be partially due to the ability of VIP to stimulate bone osteolytic activity.[12] The hyperglycemia has been attributed to the glycogenolytic effect of VIP on the liver.[12] The flushing that is seen in 14% to 28% of patients with VIPoma has been attributed to the known potent vasodilatory effects of VIP.[12] The fact that only a few patients with VIPoma syndrome develop flushing despite high plasma VIP levels has been attributed to the fact that prolonged VIP infusions result in a gradual loss of flushing, suggesting tachyphylaxis.[12] The pathogenesis of the hypochlorhydria or achlorhydria that frequently occurs in patients with VIPoma syndrome is not entirely clear but has been attributed to the known inhibitory effect of VIP on gastric acid secretion.[12]

Clinical Features (see Table 51–6)

The mean age for adults at the time of diagnosis is 42 to 51 years (range, 32 to 81 years).[57, 106, 109, 111] There is a female predominance in some studies (54% to 66%)[106, 109, 110] but not others.[57, 111] In children the mean age is 2 to 4 years old[109] in two series, with a range from 10 months to 9 years.

The cardinal features of VIPoma syndrome are the presence of severe, secretory diarrhea (89% to 100%) associated with hypokalemia (67% to 100%) and dehydration (44% to 100%) (see Table 51–6). The diarrhea may be episodic[12, 105, 106, 109] and in one study[106] was intermittent in 53% of patients. The diarrhea is large in volume, with all patients having more than 1 L and most more than 3 L/day.[106, 109, 115] A stool volume of less than 700 mL per day has been proposed to rule out the diagnosis of VIPoma.[115] The diarrheal fluid is described as having the appearance of weak tea[105] and to persist during fasting.[115] Only 10% of patients have less than five bowel movements per day.[106] Gross steatorrhea is usually not present,[106, 109] and in one study none of 52 patients with VIPomas had a 24-hour fecal fat of greater than 15 g per day.[109] Weight loss is usually present (see Table 51–6), with a range from 7 to 27 kg in one study.[109] Flushing is reported in 14% to 28% of patients (see Table 51–6), is usually present in the head or trunk area, and is characteristically erythematous.[12]

The clinical laboratory studies typically demonstrate hypokalemia (67% to 100%) and, with lesser frequency, hypercalcemia (41% to 50%), hypochlorhydria (34% to 72%), and hyperglycemia (18% to 50%) (see Table 51–6). The hyperkalemia is often severe, being less than 2.5 mmol/L at some time in 93% of patients.[109] The hypercalcemia is usually not extreme, with only 8% of patients in one series[109] having a serum calcium level higher than 3 mmol/L (12 mg/dL). The hyperglycemia is usually mild.[106, 109] Tetany, attributed to hypomagnesemia from the diarrhea, has been occasionally reported.[12, 106, 113]

Diagnosis and Differential Diagnosis

The diagnosis of VIPoma syndrome requires the demonstration of an elevated plasma concentration of VIP and the establishment of the presence of a large-volume secretory diarrhea. The volume of the diarrhea[113] should suggest the diagnosis because in 70% to 85% of patients the diarrhea is more than 3 L per day and never less than 700 mL per day.[106, 109, 115] Despite the severity of the diarrhea it may be present for long periods prior to the correct diagnosis,[110] with a delay in diagnosis after symptom onset of 32 months in one study[106] and varying from 2 months to 14 years in various studies.[106, 109, 113] A large number of possible causes for the diarrhea can be excluded by fasting the patient, because in patients with VIPomas the diarrhea persists during fasting.[15, 106, 118] The diarrhea fluid should be characteristic of a secretory diarrhea[15, 106, 115, 118] (see Chapter 9), wherein the stool electrolytes can account for nearly all of the stool water osmolality [(sodium + potassium) × 2 ≐ measured osmolality].[15, 115, 118] Other diseases can give a chronic secretory diarrhea with large volumes and give rise to a syndrome called *pseudo-VIPoma syndrome,*[115, 118] with most of the clinical features of VIPoma syndrome.[115] Occasionally these patients have gastrinoma,[15, 21, 54] chronic laxative abuse,[119] and, in some cases, secretory diarrhea of unknown origin.[115, 120, 121] The diagnosis of gastrinoma can be excluded by measuring fasting serum gastrin and gastric acid secretory rate.[15, 21]

To differentiate these other conditions from VIPoma, a reliable measurement of plasma VIP concentrations is required. The fasting plasma VIP range in most laboratories is 0 to 190 pg/mL.[109, 110, 115] In one series the mean value for 29 patients with VIPomas was 956 pg/mL, with the lowest value at 225 pg/mL.[110] In another large study the mean value was 675 pg/mL, with the highest value seen in normal subjects of 53 pg/mL and the lowest value seen in a VIPoma patient being 160 pg/mL.[109] In this study the mean value[109] for patients with pancreatic VIPomas or ganglioneuromas was 702 and 539 pg/mL, respectively. Therefore, there was no overlap between patients with VIPomas and normal subjects in these large series. With current VIP radioimmunoassays, the sensitivity is reported to be 88% and its specificity 100%.[106] VIP levels are reported to fluctuate in some patients, and thus it is important to perform the measurement while the patient is having diarrhea.[115] Elevated VIP levels alone should not be the sole basis for making a diagnosis of VIPoma in a patient with diarrhea because other conditions such as prolonged fasting, inflammatory bowel disease, small bowel resection, radiation enteritis, or chronic renal failure can occasionally elevate VIP levels.[110, 122]

In a rare patient, intestinal perfusion studies may be helpful in the differential diagnosis.[106, 115] Net secretion of electrolytes and water occurs in VIPomas instead of a net absorption in perfused small intestinal segments.[106, 118] This method is reported to be particularly helpful in differentiating VIPomas from surreptitious laxative ingestion because the latter group of patients show normal perfusion results.[106, 118]

Treatment

The first objective is the replenishment of fluid and electrolyte losses to correct the profound hypokalemia, dehydration, and hyperchloremic (nongap) acidosis that is usually present (see Table 51–6). The patients may require 5 L or more per day of fluid[12, 110] and more than 350 mEq per day of potassium.[12, 123] Renal failure associated with the potassium deficiency may occur in these patients and can be a cause of death.[3, 113] Furthermore, congestive heart failure perhaps related to preexisting hypokalemia has been reported. Therefore, during rehydration, fluid and electrolyte requirements should be carefully monitored.[113] The diarrheal output should be controlled by medical therapy as discussed in the next section. Once the fluid and electrolyte abnormalities are corrected, patients should undergo imaging studies and appropriate studies to establish the diagnosis as discussed in a later section.

Medical Therapy

In the past, numerous drugs have been reported to control, to varying degrees, the diarrheal output in small numbers of patients with VIPoma, including prednisone (60 to 100 mg/day), clonidine, indomethacin, phenothiazines, lithium, propranolol, metoclopramide, loperamide, lidamidine, angiotensin II, and norepinephrine.[12, 12, 106, 109] It is proposed that these agents primarily enhanced sodium absorption in the proximal small intestine or inhibited secretion.[12]

Currently, long-acting somatostatin analogs such as octreotide or lanreotide are the agents of choice.[15, 80, 110, 124] Octreotide controls the diarrhea both short- and long-term in 78% to 87% of patients with VIPoma.[12, 57, 78, 80, 83, 106, 109] In two recent reviews, octreotide completely abolished diarrhea in 10% in one study[78] and 65% in the other[83]; it improved the diarrhea in 90% in one study[83] and 95% in the other.[78] In one study,[78] in 100% of patients it continued to be effective at 6 months, whereas in another study in 56% of patients octreotide was effective long-term and 22% required an increase in dosage.[106] In one study[106] in 17% of patients, responses have been short-lived. In nonresponsive patients or in patients whose symptoms recur, the administration of glucocorticoids concomitant with octreotide has proved effective in a small number of cases.[83] With octreotide, plasma VIP concentrations decreased in 80% to 89% of patients.[78, 83, 106] The changes in plasma VIP concentration with octreotide treatment did not always mirror the clinical responses.[83] In

Table 51–7 | **Clinical Symptoms and Signs and Laboratory Abnormalities in Patients with Somatostatinomas**

	SOMATOSTATINOMA*		FREQUENCY (%) IN SOMATOSTATINOMA SYNDROME* OVERALL
	Pancreatic	Intestinal	
Clinical Symptoms/Signs			
Gallbladder disease	94	43	68
Diarrhea	66–97	11–36	37
Weight loss	32–90	20–44	68
Laboratory Abnormalities			
Diabetes mellitus	95	21	95
Steatorrhea	83	12	47
Hypochlorhydria	86	17	26

*Somatostatinoma is the occurrence of a pancreas endocrine tumor containing somatostatin by immunocytochemistry, which can occur with (11%) or without (89%) somatostatinoma syndrome due to ectopically released somatostatin.

Data from references 12, 33, and 58.

one review,[83] of the 13 patients whose diarrhea was abolished by octreotide, plasma levels returned to normal in only 15%, decreased but not to normal ranges in 46%, decreased and then rose to pretreatment levels in 31%, and did not change in 8%. In 25% of the patients who did not respond to octreotide, plasma VIP level did not change.[83] This discrepancy in extent of clinical response and degree of change in plasma VIP levels may be partially explained by the observation that multiple forms of VIP may be elevated in the plasma and after treatment with octreotide, and only the form coinciding with the native peptide may disappear, with the remaining VIP immunoreactivity representing nonbiologic fragments.[125] In patients with unresectable or metastatic VIPomas, long-term treatment with octreotide and/or chemotherapy will need to be considered. The continuous use of octreotide decreased medical costs by 50% per year for each VIPoma patient treated.[124] There are only anecdotal studies on long-term treatment of patients with VIPomas with the new, long-acting depot form of octreotide administered monthly (octreotide-LAR)[41, 84]; therefore, it is unclear whether it will be less or more effective than the shorter-acting form currently used every 4 to 6 hours.

Surgical Therapy

After imaging studies to localize the primary VIPoma and determine the extent, possible surgical cure should be considered in all patients without metastatic disease. In one series, surgical resection of a pancreatic VIPoma relieved all symptoms in 33% of patients,[109] and 30% were cured in another series.[113] Attempted curative surgical resection was possible in only about one third of patients.[111] Surgical resection with complete control of all symptoms was possible in 78% of all patients with VIP-producing ganglioneuroblastomas.[109]

SOMATOSTATINOMA

Definition

Somatostatinomas are NETs usually originating in the pancreas or intestine that release large amounts of somatostatin and cause a distinct clinical syndrome characterized by diabetes mellitus, gallbladder disease, diarrhea, and weight loss (Table 51–7). The first two cases of somatostatinoma were described in 1977.[5, 6] Steatorrhea and hypochlorhydria were soon added as additional features.[126, 127] Somatostatinomas are the least common type of PET (see Table 51–1).

This definition of the somatostatinoma syndrome is not uniformly used in the literature. In fact, in many reports the term *somatostatinoma* is used to mean an endocrine tumor possessing somatostatin immunoreactivity and no requirement for an accompanying functional syndrome is required. For example, in a recent large review of the world literature,[58] 173 cases were found, of which only 17 had the clinical somatostatinoma syndrome. Therefore, in the remainder of the section the term *somatostatinoma* is used to refer to a somatostatin-containing tumor and the term *somatostatinoma syndrome* refers to the presence of a somatostatinoma with the accompanying clinical syndrome due to ectopically released somatostatin.

Pathophysiology and Pathology

In three reviews 46% to 75% of the somatostatinomas were in the pancreas. The distribution of the 44 tumors within the pancreas was 30:3:11 in the pancreatic head:body:tail.[33, 58, 128] Tumors not in the pancreas arise either from the duodenum in 90% of the cases in one study[58] or from the duodenum (43%), ampulla (48%), jejunum (5%), or the cystic duct (5%) in a second study.[33] This distribution in the upper gastrointestinal tract may be a consequence of the large number of somatostatin-producing D cells in this region.[33, 128] In 90% to 96% the tumors were solitary[58, 128] and varied from 1.5 to 10 cm in diameter (mean, 4.9 cm and 3.6 cm).[58, 128] The average size of pancreatic somatostatinomas was significantly larger than duodenal somatostatinomas (5.1 cm vs. 2.4 cm).[58] In two series[58, 128] 53% to 84% of all tumors had evidence of metastatic spread. In one of these studies[58] the malignancy rate of 50% was the same for pancreatic and duodenal somatostatinomas, but in another study[33] 92% of pancreatic somatostatinomas had metastases compared to 69% of intestinal somatostatinomas. Metastases occur usually in the liver (25% to 75% of patients)[58, 128] but also in lymph nodes (31%)[58, 128] and bone (4%).[33, 58] In one review,[58] both liver metastases (40% vs. 11%) and bone metastases (6% vs. 0%) occurred more frequently in pancreatic than in intestinal somatostatinomas, whereas the rate of metastases to lymph nodes was similar (25% vs. 35%). With duodenal somatostatinomas[129] the occurrence of lymph node metastases correlated with the primary tumor size. Duodenal somatostatinomas with lymph node metastases were significantly larger than those without metastases (2.9 cm vs. 1.4 cm, $P < 0.05$).[129] Using a cutoff of 2 cm in diameter, diagnostic accuracy for malignancy was 78%, with a specificity of 87% and sensitivity of 63%.[129]

With light microscopic studies, most tumors appeared as well-differentiated tumors with varying degrees of fibrous septa.[33, 128] Histologically, a specific feature of duodenal somatostatinoma is the presence of psammona bodies that are rarely found in pancreatic somatostatinomas or other types of duodenal carcinoid tumors.[24, 58, 64, 65] Electron microscopic studies reported that the secretory granules were typical of those in D cells in 52% to 89% of the tumors.[33, 58, 128] Immunocytochemical analysis[58, 128] demonstrated somatostatin-like immunoreactive (SLI) material in all tumors and, in addition, 10% to 33% contained insulin, 22% to 27% calcitonin, 8% to 13% gastrin, and 9% glucagon. Twenty-six percent of somatostatinomas were producing multiple gastrointestinal hormones.[58] Extraction of tumors and analysis for SLI material demonstrated that somatostatin-14 is usually not the predominant form.[24] Somatostatin-28 and larger forms predominated, and this heterogeneity is thought to reflect incomplete processing of precursors.[24]

The pathophysiology of the somatostatinoma syndrome can be explained by the known actions of somatostatin.[80, 130] Somatostatin exists as a tetradecapeptide (SS-14) as well as a larger form, somatostatin octapeptide (SS-28).[130] Somatostatin is found throughout the gastrointestinal tract, especially in gastric and duodenal D cells.[79, 130] It has a largely inhibitory action,[80, 130] inhibiting the release of numerous gastrointestinal hormones, inhibiting basal and stimulated acid secretion, and inhibiting stimulated pancreatic secretion as well as intestinal absorption of amino acids, sugars, and calcium.[130] Somatostatin also has both stimulatory and inhibitory effects on intestinal motility[130] and inhibitory effects on gallbladder contraction.[130] The development of diabetes mellitus in patients with somatostatinoma is likely secondary to the inhibitory action of somatostatin on insulin release and possibly by replacement of functional pancreatic endocrine tissue by the tumor.[24, 33, 80, 128, 130] Gallbladder disease may be a result of somatostatin inhibition of gallbladder emptying,[24, 80, 130, 131] as demonstrated by the occurrence of cholelithiasis or biliary sludge in patients taking octreotide.[79] Diarrhea and steatorrhea are likely due to the ability of somatostatin to inhibit pancreatic secretion of enzymes and bicarbonate,[130] gallbladder motility, and absorption of lipids[130] and occur also in patients treated with high doses of octreotide.[78, 79, 83, 130] The hypochlorhydria is likely secondary to the known ability of somatostatin to inhibit gastric acid secretion.[80, 130] The weight loss may be secondary to the malabsorption, but there may be other causative factors not identified.

Clinical Features (see Table 51–7)

The mean age of the patients with somatostatinoma is 51 to 53 years old,[33, 58, 128] with most patients aged 40 to 60. In one series[58] female patients with pancreatic tumors were older than those with duodenal tumors (55 years vs. 49 years). In one series, 66% of patients with pancreatic tumors were females, compared to 43% of those with intestinal somatostatinomas.[33] However, in another series,[58] somatostatinomas occurred equally in both genders. The youngest and oldest patients were 26 and 84 years.

In terms of symptoms with somatostatinomas, it is important to distinguish between symptoms likely due to the PET itself from those due to ectopic somatostatin release (somatostatinoma syndrome). In one large review[58] only 17 of the 173 cases of somatostatinomas from the literature were associated with the specific symptoms associated with somatostatinoma syndrome (see Table 51–7). Overall, 93% of all patients with somatostatinomas had symptoms,[58] with abdominal pain (40%), weight loss (26%), jaundice (23%), diarrhea (18%), nausea/vomiting (16%), and the detection of an abdominal tumor or hepatomegaly (22%) the most common signs and symptoms. These symptoms, in general, were due to the PET per se and not, in most cases, to the ectopic release of somatostatin.

Diabetes mellitus was present in 55% of patients with somatostatinomas in one series.[128] However, in another series the percentage with diabetes differed in patients with pancreatic tumors (95%) and those with intestinal tumors (21%) (see Table 51–7).[33] In patients with somatostatinoma syndrome, 95% had diabetes mellitus (see Table 51–7).[58] The diabetes was mild in most cases[24, 33, 128] and could be controlled with either oral hypoglycemic agents or small doses of insulin.

Gallbladder or biliary tract disease occurred in 65% of patients in one series,[128] including cholelithiasis in 35%, a massively dilated gallbladder without evidence of cholelithiasis in 10%, and obstructive jaundice due to local tumor invasion in 10%. In another series[33] gallbladder disease was present in 94% of patients with pancreatic tumors and 43% of those with intestinal tumors. Biliary calculi were present in 68% of patients with somatostatinoma syndrome[58] (see Table 51–7).

Diarrhea and steatorrhea were reported in 18% to 35% of patients.[128] Steatorrhea and diarrhea were reported in 83% and 92% of patients with pancreatic tumors, respectively,[33, 58] and in 12% and 10% to 38% of patients with intestinal tumors.[33, 58] Diarrhea characteristically consisted of 3 to 10 frequent, foul-smelling stools per day, with 20 to 76 g per day of steatorrhea.[128] In some cases the time course and severity of the diarrhea and steatorrhea paralleled that of the disease in that it worsened when metastases occurred and improved with successful tumor resection.[128] Diarrhea was present in 37% and steatorrhea in 47% of patients with somatostatinoma syndrome[58] (see Table 51–7).

Hypochlorhydria was found to be present in 70% of patients with somatostatinoma[58] and in another study in 86% of patients with pancreatic tumors and 17% with intestinal tumors.[33] Both basal and stimulated gastric acid secretion were depressed.[33] Hypochlorhydria was present in 26% of patients with somatostatinoma syndrome[58] (see Table 51–7). Weight loss ranged from 9 to 21 kg and was reported in 32% to 33% of patients with pancreatic tumors and 19% to 20% of patients with intestinal tumors.[58, 128] Mild to moderate anemia was reported in 15% to 67% of patients, with hemoglobin values of 10 to 13 g/dL.[58, 128]

Somatostatinoma syndrome was more frequently associated with pancreatic tumors than with duodenal somatostatinomas (18.5% vs. 2.5%).[58]

One half of patients with somatostatinoma have other endocrinopathies.[33] These include MEN I and MEN II.[33] Twenty percent of patients in one series[128] had hypoglycemia attacks and were diagnosed as having insulinomas.

Diagnosis and Differential Diagnosis

Most somatostatinomas (90%) do not produce the somatostatinoma syndrome, and the presenting symptoms such as abdominal pain, weight loss, jaundice, and diarrhea[58] are not specific for a somatostatinoma. The symptoms characteristic of somatostatinoma syndrome, similar to glucagonomas, are less pronounced than gastrinomas or insulinomas[128] and probably are not detected until patients develop high somatostatin blood levels, which is late in the course of the disease when the tumor is large. In most cases the somatostatinomas are found at the time of laparotomy for cholecystectomy or during gastrointestinal imaging studies for various nonspecific complaints such as abdominal pain or diarrhea.[33, 58, 128] High plasma SLI concentrations have been reported with tumors outside the pancreas or intestine, such as patients with medullary thyroid carcinoma, small cell lung cancer, pheochromocytomas, and other catecholamine producing extra-adrenal paraganglionomas.[24, 128]

The diagnosis is usually established by identifying the resected tumor as a PET containing increased numbers of D cells with somatostatin by immunocytochemistry. The diagnosis of somatostatinoma syndrome is established by the earlier findings associated with an increased plasma concentration of SLI.[128] The diagnosis of somatostatinoma syndrome requires the demonstration of elevated plasma levels of somatostatin because somatostatin can frequently be found by immunocytochemical studies, especially in duodenal tumors without elevated plasma somatostatin levels.[24, 58, 64] Modest elevations should be interpreted with caution because they can occur in nonendocrine disorders.[24] Although the plasma levels are usually elevated in pancreatic somatostatinomas, in duodenal or small intestinal tumors the plasma levels may be inconclusive or normal.[24, 64] The diagnosis of somatostatinoma at a time when plasma SLI concentrations are only marginally elevated or normal may require the development of specific provocative tests.[128] Arginine increases plasma SLI.[128] However, arginine is a well-established stimulant of somatostatin release from normal D cells and will likely not differentiate tumors from a normal response.[128] Tolbutamide stimulates somatostatin release in animals but does not change plasma SLI concentrations in normal volunteers.[128, 132] At present the key to diagnosing the somatostatinoma syndrome is to be aware of its clinical features and to consider performing plasma SLI levels on any patients with diabetes without a family history, with gallbladder disease, with a pancreatic mass, or with a history of unexplained diarrhea.[24, 126]

Duodenal somatostatin-containing NETs are being increasingly associated with von Recklinghausen's disease (NF1).[24, 58, 64, 65] Duodenal somatostatinomas in patients with von Recklinghausen's disease[58] resemble sporadic duodenal somatostatinomas in that they rarely are associated with symptoms of the somatostatinoma syndrome (2%), elevated plasma somatostatin levels are infrequent, and they frequently contain psammoma bodies (37% to 66%).[64] NF1 is found in a higher proportion of duodenal than pancreatic somatostatinomas (43% vs. 17%); furthermore, somatostatinomas in patients with NF1 are more frequently benign than are sporadic tumors (53% vs. 31%).[58]

Treatment

These patients may be severely malnourished with weight loss and require correction of the nutritional deficiencies, which may require hyperalimentation. The diabetes mellitus is usually mild, and hyperglycemia can be controlled with oral hypoglycemic agents or low doses of insulin.[128]

Medical Therapy

At present no specific drug therapy exists, and the only effective therapy is surgical resection or possibly cytotoxic drugs. Four patients with a somatostatinoma were treated with the somatostatin analog octreotide.[83, 133] Fasting plasma concentrations of SLI decreased in three patients and symptoms due to the somatostatinoma syndrome (diarrhea and diabetes) were improved in two patients.[133]

Surgical Therapy

Surgery was performed in 83% of patients in one series and in another series[128] in 60% of patients. In one series, 65% of patients underwent successful resection, but the percentage cured was not stated, as was the case in the other series. Although an occasional patient might be cured, in most series this is not possible due to the late diagnosis. Five-year survival in patients without metastases in a review[58] of 46 cases was 100%, which was significantly better than the 60% survival seen in 44 patients with metastases. Of the patients treated with a combination of surgical resection and cytotoxic therapy,[24, 33, 128] 60% were alive 6 months to 5 years after diagnosis; however, it is not clearly established whether debulking surgery extends survival. If imaging studies demonstrate possibly resectable tumor, current results suggest that these patients will benefit from surgical resection.

GRFOMA

Definition

GRFomas are tumors that frequently originate in the pancreas and secrete large amounts of growth hormone–releasing factor (GRF), which causes acromegaly. GRFomas are the most recently described type of PET, being first reported in 1982,[7, 8] and in a recent review 40 cases were reported.[134]

Pathophysiology and Pathology

GRFomas in 29% to 30% of cases originated in the pancreas, 47% to 53% in lung (with the majority in the right lung), 8% to 10% in the small intestine, and a rare case in the adrenal gland.[12, 24, 134–136] Most of the pancreatic GRFomas originated in the pancreatic tail.[134, 135] Multiple pancreatic GRFomas occurred in 30% in one series[135] and they generally occurred in patients with MEN I.[24, 135] GRFomas are generally large (>6 cm), ranging in size from 1 to 25 cm.[135] Metastases were present in 33% to 39% of all cases in two series,[12, 134, 136] in another series[135] in 30% of patients with pancreatic GRFomas, and in two of the three cases of intestinal GRFomas. Metastases were to regional lymph nodes and less frequently to the liver.[135] In one series there was no relationship among tumor size, plasma GRF levels, and the presence of metastases, with the three largest tumors not associated with metastatic disease or invasion.[135] Approximately 40% of pancreatic GRFomas occur in patients with gastrinomas, and in 40% Cushing's syndrome was also present.[12, 135]

On light microscopic studies, typical features of a PET are seen composed of trabecular or solid nests and sheets of uniform tumor cells.[135] In electron microscopic studies tumor cells containing 100- to 250-nm secretory granules are seen.[7, 12, 134] Immunochemical studies demonstrate GRF-immunoreactive (GRF-IR) material in all tumors examined with 10% to 80% of cells possessing GRF.[135] GRF-IR was seen in 31% of 45 various PETs in one study,[137] and in another study[136] in which no patients had acromegaly, GRF was present in 23% of the PETs by immunocytochemistry and in 37% using radioimmunoassay.

The known actions of GRF account for the clinical features of the syndrome. GRF is a 44-amino acid peptide[7] that is a potent stimulant of the release of growth hormone and therefore patients present with acromegaly.

Clinical Features

Patients are from 15 to 66 years old, with an average age of 38 to 39 years.[134–136] Patients with intestinal GRFomas were younger, with two of the three patients younger than 20 years old.[135] A female predominance (73%) is seen for all GRFomas as well as the patients just with pancreatic GRFomas (78%).[135, 136] The clinical features fall into three categories: acromegalic features due to the excess of GRF, clinical features due to hormones other than GRF, and local symptoms due to mass effects.[135] Acromegalic features were indistinguishable from patients with classic acromegaly and included enlargement of hands and feet, facial changes, skin changes, headache, and peripheral nerve entrapment.[24, 135, 136] The duration of time from the onset of the acromegalic changes to the diagnosis was 5.3 years in patients with pancreatic GRFomas[135] and 6 years for all GRFomas in another study.[136] Syndromes from other hormones were due to the presence of gastrinoma, Cushing's syndrome, or hyperinsulinemia hypoglycemia.[135] MEN I was present in 16% of the patients,[136] and hyperprolactinemia was observed in 70% of patients with GRFomas as compared to 50% of patients with somatotroph adenomas.[24, 136]

Diagnosis and Differential Diagnosis

The diagnosis should be suspected in any patient (1) with acromegaly without a pituitary adenoma, (2) with acromegaly associated with hyperprolactinemia, (3) with a paradoxical growth hormone response to TRH or during an oral glucose tolerance test, or (4) with acromegaly associated with an abdominal mass.[24, 134, 136] The diagnosis should also be suspected in any patient with a pancreatic or intestinal tumor who develops clinical features of acromegaly. Because as many as 33% of patients with pancreatic GRFomas have MEN I, 40% have Cushing's syndrome due to a pancreatic tumor, and 40% have Zollinger-Ellison syndrome, it should be particularly suspected in these patients. Of all patients with acromegaly, however, GRFomas are an uncommon cause, responsible for not even one case in 177 consecutive patients with acromegaly.[134] The diagnosis is established by demonstrating elevated plasma growth hormone (usually >5 μg/L in men, >10 μg/L in women) and the demonstration of elevated plasma GRF levels. In normal subjects and patients with acromegaly not due to a GRFoma, plasma GRF-IR levels are within the normal range, which in most laboratories is from 50 to 100 pg/mL.[134] The lowest level in a patient with a proven GRFoma reported was 300 pg/mL.[134] It has thus been suggested that a plasma GRF level higher than 300 pg/mL is strongly suggestive of the presence of a GRFoma.[135] Besides plasma growth hormone and GRF, plasma insulin-like growth factor 1 (IGF-1) is also elevated in patients with GRFomas.[136]

Treatment

Tumor localization studies should be performed to evaluate the extent of disease and are discussed in a later section. In patients without metastatic disease to the liver, surgical resection of the GRFoma should be carried out. Prior to surgery and in those patients with nonresectable lesions, various agents may be helpful to reduce plasma growth hormone levels. Even though dopamine agonists such as bromocriptine are widely used in patients with classic acromegaly, they are able to reduce plasma GRF levels in only 25% of patients with GRFomas.[134] Octreotide is now the agent of choice.[24, 80, 134, 136] In most cases, but not all,[12, 24, 134, 136] octreotide significantly suppressed or normalized growth hormone and IGI-1 levels and in some cases this was associated with pituitary shrinkage.[12, 136] The suppression of growth hormone secretion by octreotide was mainly due to suppression at the pituitary level because plasma GRF levels never become undetectable.[134] Surgical resection should be directed at the primary tumor, not the pituitary.[134, 136] Surgery resulted in regression of the GRFoma syndrome in a small number of cases.[7, 12, 135, 136] The actual number of patients who are cured long term is unknown.

PPOMA AND NONFUNCTIONING PANCREATIC ENDOCRINE TUMORS

Definitions

A *PPoma* is a tumor usually of the pancreas that secretes excessive amounts of PP. The clinical symptoms are due to local effects of the tumor itself, not to the actions of PP. Strictly speaking, a nonfunctioning PET is a tumor of the pancreas that has typical histologic features of a PET, is not associated with elevated plasma levels of any known peptide, and whose symptoms are entirely due to the local effects of the tumor itself. However, the term *nonfunctional PET* is most widely used to indicate a PET occurring in a patient in whom there are no clinical symptoms due to hormone overproduction. This would include PPomas, PETs secreting neurotensin, HCG subunits, or chromogranin. This is the definition that is used in the following discussion.

Pathophysiology and Pathology

Nonfunctioning PETs are usually large[17, 18, 20, 138, 139] and in one series 72% averaged more than 5 cm in diameter.[139] They are usually solitary tumors except in patients with MEN I.[49] Approximately 60% of nonfunctional PETs occur in the pancreatic head, with a ratio of 14:2:3 for pancreatic head:body:tail in one study.[139] The malignancy rate varies from 64% to 92% in different series.[17, 20, 33, 138, 139] Histologically, nonfunctioning PETs are similar and cannot be differentiated from other PETs, even by immunocytochemistry.[12, 20] In one series of 30 nonfunctioning PETs,[26] 50% had insulin-like immunoreactivity (IR), 30% glucagon IR, 43% PP IR, 13% somatostatin IR, and only 13% produced none of these peptides. With these tumors, elevated plasma levels of chromogranin A and B are found in 69% to 100%, neuron-specific enolase in 31%, PP in 50% to 75%, α-HCG in 40%, and β-HCG in 20%.[20, 33, 140] An elevated plasma PP level in a patient with a pancreatic tumor is suggestive of a PET, because none of 53 patients with adenocarcinoma of the pancreas had elevated plasma PP levels.[33]

Infusions of PP into both animals and humans have shown this peptide to have numerous biologic effects (see Chapter 1), including a net secretory effect on water and electrolytes in the small intestine; inhibitory effects on fluid, electrolyte, and enzyme secretion by the pancreas; effects on esophageal, gastric, intestinal, and gallbladder motility; and metabolic effects such as decreasing somatostatin or insulin release.[141] In various studies,[33] patients with PPomas have been reported to have symptoms that were attributed to elevated plasma levels of PP and include persistent, watery diarrhea; diabetes mellitus; weight loss; decreased gastric acid secretion; peptic disease; flushing; and acute psychosis.[12, 33] Furthermore, plasma PP is frequently elevated in other symptomatic PETs.[12, 17, 33, 142] However, the symptoms of these patients do not differ from those without elevation of plasma PP; thus, it is now generally agreed that plasma elevations of PP are not associated with specific symptoms.[16, 20, 33] At present it is unclear why patients who have elevated plasma levels of PP do not have specific symptoms.

Clinical Features and Diagnosis

Typically, the patient with a nonfunctional PET is 40 to 60 years of age.[20, 33, 138, 139] These tumors occur approximately equally in both sexes.[20, 33, 138] The median delay in the time from diagnosis to the first symptoms varies from 0.5 to 2.7 years.[20] In four different studies 36% to 56% of patients with PETs presented with abdominal pain, 28% to 40% with jaundice, 24% to 46% with weight loss, and 8% to 40% with an abdominal mass.[143] In 16% of the patients, the tumors were found incidentally at surgery, and the remaining patients presented with a variety of symptoms owing to the tumor mass.[138]

The main diagnostic challenge is differentiating the nonfunctioning PET from a nonendocrine pancreatic tumor and also in determining whether the tumor is associated with a symptomatic tumor syndrome (such as insulinoma, glucagonoma, gastrinoma). Elevated plasma levels of PP do not establish the diagnosis of a PPoma even when a pancreatic mass is present. Plasma PP levels are reported to be elevated in 22% to 71% of patients with functional PETs in various studies[12, 17, 21] as well as in nonpancreatic carcinoid tumors. In one large study,[142] plasma PP levels exceeded a value of 1000 pg/mL in 45% of patients with various PETs with such an elevation in 32% of gastrinomas, 21% of insulinomas, 57% of glucagonomas, 74% of VIPomas, 33% of somatostatinomas, and 45% of carcinoid tumors. Furthermore, elevated plasma levels of PP can occur in other situations such as old age, after bowel resection, with alcohol abuse, during certain infections, in chronic noninfective inflammatory disorders, acute diarrhea, chronic renal failure, diabetes, chronic relapsing pancreatitis, as well as hypoglycemia or after eating.[12] To increase the specificity of an elevated plasma level for a pancreatic tumor, an atropine suppression test has been proposed, because PP levels are normally under cholinergic control.[142] In one study[142] of 48 patients with elevated plasma PP levels, atropine (1 mg intramuscularly) did not suppress the levels in any of the 18 patients with PETs but did suppress the level to 50% of all patients without tumors. Somatostatin receptor scintigraphy (SRS), which is discussed in detail in the following section on tumor localization, has also been shown to be useful in distinguishing pancreatic adenocarcinoma from a nonfunctional PET.[80, 82, 144]

Treatment

With nonfunctioning PETs, treatment needs to be directed only at the tumor itself because no hormonal syndrome is present.

Surgical Therapy

In one series,[138] the diagnosis of a nonfunctioning tumor was not made in a single case preoperatively. Of 25 cases in this series, a Whipple procedure was done in 20%, partial or total pancreatectomy in 25%, and tumor excision in 10%. The remaining patients had a biopsy only. The survival rates were 60% at 3 years and 44% at 5 years.[138] In eight other studies curative resection was attempted in 26% to 79% of patients with nonfunctional PETs, with a 5-year survival of 44% to 63% and a median survival varying from 2.5 to 4.8 years.[143] The cure rate of these tumors at present is low.

OTHER PANCREATIC ENDOCRINE TUMORS

In a few studies in patients with PETs secreting the peptide neurotensin, a neurotensinoma syndrome has been proposed.[12, 16, 33, 145] Neurotensin is a 13-amino acid peptide originally isolated from bovine brain[146] that has a number of biologic effects, including tachycardia, hypotension, and cyanosis; effects on intestinal motility; and stimulation of jejunal and ileal fluid and electrolyte secretion and pancreatic protein and bicarbonate secretion.[146] Clinical features of patients with possible neurotensinomas include hypokalemia, weight loss, diabetes mellitus, cyanosis, hypotension, and flushing in a patient with a PET.[33] Recent studies[16, 145] question the existence of a specific neurotensinoma syndrome. Of 180 patients with functional PETs,[145] elevated plasma neurotensin levels were found in six patients with VIPomas, and their symptoms did not differ from those with normal neurotensin levels. In another study[16] a similar result was found in patients with gastrinomas.

Patients with PETs and Cushing's syndrome (ACTHoma) have been reported.[9, 32] In a recent review, 4% to 16% of cases of ectopic Cushing's syndrome were due to a PET.[9] Cushing's syndrome[32] was reported in 19% of patients with gastrinoma and MEN I. In these patients the disease was due to release of ACTH by a pituitary adenoma and was mild. Cushing's syndrome occurs in 4% to 5% of sporadic gastrinoma cases.[32, 147] In these patients Cushing's syndrome was severe, due to ectopic ACTH production, occurred with metastatic tumors that responded poorly to chemotherapy, and was associated with a poor prognosis.[32] In a recent large prospective study,[147] the development of Cushing's syndrome in patients with Zollinger-Ellison syndrome was shown to be an independent predictor of poor survival, with patients having a mean survival of only 1.7 years after its onset. Cushing's syndrome as the only manifestation of a PET occurs occasionally and may precede any other hormonal syndrome.[148] In every case in one series, ectopic Cushing's syndrome due to a PET occurred only in the presence of metastatic disease.[149]

Hypercalcemia, due to a PET secreting a parathyroid hormone–related peptide (PTH-RP) or to an unknown hypercalcemic substance that mimics the action of PTH and causes hyperparathyroidism, has been reported.[12, 13, 150] The tumors are usually large and metastatic to the liver by the time of diagnosis, although in one case[151] resection of a pancreatic tail tumor and subsequent treatment with chemotherapy resulted in a total remission for 5 years.

Carcinoid tumors of the pancreas are rare but have been well described in a number of studies.[10, 11] These PETs are usually large and 68% to 88% are malignant.[152] The carcinoid syndrome is present in 34% to 65% of these patients.[152] Even though foregut carcinoids, which include pancreatic PETs,[153] may lack dihydroxyphenylalanine (DOPA) decarboxylase, the enzyme that converts 5-hydroxytryptophan to serotonin (5-hydroxytryptamine [5-HT]),[153] 84% of patients with PETs causing carcinoid syndrome have increased urinary 5-HIAA levels that can be used for their detection.[152]

TUMOR LOCALIZATION

It is essential for the correct management of patients with PETs that extent of the tumor and in many cases the localization of the primary tumor be established.[12, 20, 52, 91, 106, 154] The ability of the standard imaging studies (computed tomography [CT] scan, ultrasonography, magnetic resonance imaging [MRI]) to localize the PET depends on the tumor size. CT scanning and MRI localize less than 10% of PETs

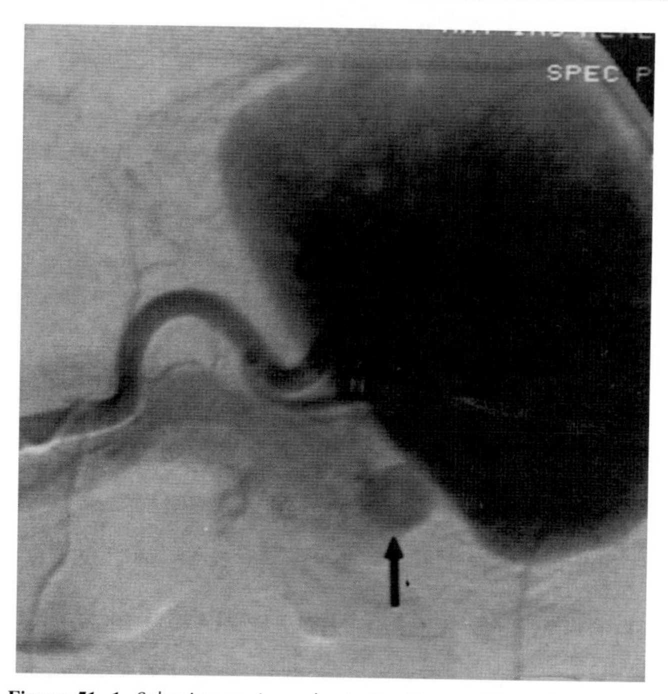

Figure 51–1. Selective angiography in insulinoma. The splenic artery injection is shown, and a 2-cm insulinoma *(arrow)* is seen that was subsequently removed at surgery.

less than 1 cm in diameter, 30% to 40% of tumors 1 to 3 cm in diameter, and greater than 50% of PETs larger than 3 cm in diameter.[12, 21, 154] All PETs are hypervascular tumors, and in terms of localization with the different conventional modalities the results with the different PETs appear to be similar and more influenced by tumor size and location than PET type.[12] Figure 51–1 shows the typical hypervascular appearance of an insulinoma characteristic of all PETs. Insulinomas are usually small (<1 cm) at the time of diagnosis, as are most duodenal gastrinomas, whereas most of the other PETs present late in their course and are large (>4 cm).[12, 22, 23, 42, 55–57, 68, 110, 155–157] Furthermore, insulinomas, nonfunctioning PETs, glucagonomas, and VIPomas in adults are almost always located in the pancreas, whereas somatostatinomas, gastrinomas, and VIPomas in children occur frequently extrapancreatically. In Table 51–8 are shown the sensitivities from different series of the ability of the different localization studies to image insulinomas and the primary and liver metastases of other PETs. The results with insulinomas are presented separately because they are almost always benign, are small (<1 cm) at presentation, and entirely within the pancreas.[23, 68–71] Because there are no systematic localization studies of the less common PETs (all but gastrinomas, insulinomas, nonfunctioning PETs) (see Table 51–1), and because gastrinomas closely resemble the other less common PETs in biologic behavior and in imaging results,[12] the results from gastrinomas were primarily used to determine the values in Table 51–8 for the other PETs. Overall, ultrasonography, CT, and MRI are not very sensitive in localizing a primary tumor, being positive in 10% to 40% of cases (see Table 51–8).[21, 154] Of the standard, invasive imaging studies, selective abdominal angiography is the most sensitive for localizing the primary tumor, identifying 60% of small PETs like insulinomas and 70% of

Table 51–8 | **Sensitivity of Imaging Studies for Localizing Pancreatic Endocrine Tumors (PETs)***

IMAGING STUDY	INSULINOMAS	OTHER PANCREATIC ENDOCRINE TUMORS	
		Primary	Liver Metastases
Ultrasonography	30 (0–64)	22 (6–70)	44 (14–76)
Computed tomography scan	31 (16–60)	42 (33–100)	70 (35–100)
Magnetic resonance imaging	10 (0–25)	27 (21–100)	80 (67–100)
Arteriography	60 (41–81)	70 (35–100)	71 (33–86)
Selective venous sampling			N/A
Portal venous sampling	80 (63–96)	71 (17–94)	N/A
Post intra-arterial calcium	88	ND	N/A
Somatostatin receptor scintigraphy (SRS)	54 (15–56)	70 (58–77)	93 (88–100)
Endoscopic ultrasonography (EUS)	81 (57–92)	70 (40–100)	N/A
Intraoperative ultrasonography	89 (80–100)	91 (80–100)	N/A

*Shown are mean values; ranges are in parentheses.
N/A, not applicable; ND, no data available.
Data from references 12, 21, 23, 52, 85, 86, 154, 158, 161, 167, and 169.

the other PETs (see Table 51–8). Among the standard imaging studies, the CT scan is generally recommended as the initial localization study because of its general availability.[12]

Metastatic disease to the liver will be detected in 44% of patients by ultrasound, 70% with CT scanning, 80% with MRI, and selective angiography will detect 71% of such patients (see Table 51–8). Recent studies[12, 52] show that improvements in MRI in the last few years have greatly improved its sensitivity in patients with PETs for the detection of metastatic disease to the liver. Metastatic liver lesions are much more easily seen on short inversion-time inversion-recovery (STIR) MR images than on CT scans. Overall, even with these improvements, a significant number (40% to 60%) of small primary tumors are missed by all of the standard imaging studies, and a proportion of patients with metastatic disease to the liver will be missed (5% to 30%).

Endoscopic ultrasound (EUS) and SRS are being increasingly used to localize PETs.[80, 158–160] PETs as well as a number of other tumors, including central nervous system tumors, lymphomas, breast cancer, and small cell lung cancer, frequently possess increased densities of somatostatin receptors and can be imaged using SRS.[80, 82, 159, 161] For SRS, both [^{111}In-DTPA-DPhe^{1}]octreotide and [^{123}I-Tyr^{3}]octreotide have been used.[159] [^{111}In-DTPA-DPhe^{1}]octreotide (OctreoScan) is approved for use in the United States and has the advantage of longer half-life (2.8 days), allowing longer imaging times and an easier labeling method using chelation instead of oxidative methods.[80, 159] In addition, it is primarily excreted in the urine instead of the bile, which allows tumors in the upper abdomen to be better visualized.[159] By in vitro autoradiography, 88% of carcinoids and 100% of gastrinomas, nonfunctional PETs, and glucagonomas, but only 67% of insulinomas and no pancreatic adenocarcinomas, have been shown to possess somatostatin receptors.[80, 82] These results are consistent with SRS results from a large combined series[82] that reported 89% of patients with carcinoid tumors positive, 77% of gastrinomas, 53% of insulinomas, 83% of nonfunctional PETs, 100% of glucagonomas, and 80% of VIPomas. Furthermore, SRS frequently identifies hepatic and extrahepatic lesions not seen on other imaging modalities. The ability of SRS compared to other imaging modalities to localize gastrinomas or insulinomas has been compared.[12, 51, 80, 82, 158, 159, 161] In patients with insulinomas, SRS detects only 54%; CT scanning, ultrasound, and MR imaging detected insulinomas in 10% to 30% of patients, whereas EUS was positive in 81% to 90%. In a number of series, in patients with Zollinger-Ellison syndrome that resembles other PETs except insulinomas in the frequency of the presence of somatostatin receptors,[82] SRS was positive in 75% of patients.[12, 51, 80, 159, 161] In one study involving 80 patients,[161] for the primary tumor SRS had the highest sensitivity (58%), which exceeded that of MRI (30%), angiography, CT, and ultrasound (10%) and was more sensitive than all the conventional imaging studies combined. SRS is now the method of choice to localize metastatic disease. Figures 51–2 and 51–3 demonstrate the enhanced sensitivity of SRS over conventional tumor localization modalities. In Figure 51–2 in a patient with a malignant PET, the CT scan was negative, but SRS detected both liver metastases and lymph node metastases. In Figure 51–3 in a patient with a malignant gastrinoma and glucagonoma, the bone scan showed a questionable left scapula/rib metastasis, whereas the SRS showed clear-cut scapula, spine, and pelvic bone metastases. SRS has the advantage of identifying distant unsuspected metastatic foci and is more sensitive than the other modalities for detecting liver or bone metastases (see Table 51–8).[51, 82, 161–163] In recent studies,[164, 165] the use of SRS after conventional imaging studies changed the clinical management in 21% to 47% of patients.

Recent studies demonstrate that EUS is a sensitive method to detect primarily PETs located in the pancreas.[12, 158, 166] In a review of more than 10 studies[166] (see Table 51–8), EUS localized an insulinoma in 81% (range 57% to 92%) and was superior to conventional imaging studies and almost as sensitive as calcium provocative testing (i.e., 88%). In patients with gastrinomas from a number of series[166] (see Table 51–8), EUS localized a gastrinoma in 67% to 70% (range 40% to 100%) and was comparable to angiography (see Table 51–8). EUS localized 90% of insulinomas compared to 54% with SRS, whereas for gastrinomas EUS and SRS each localized 70% (see Table 51–8). In a comparative study[167] involving 18 patients with foregut NETs (pancreas, duodenum, stomach), EUS had the highest sensitivity (88%), SRS had a sensitivity of 52%, and both

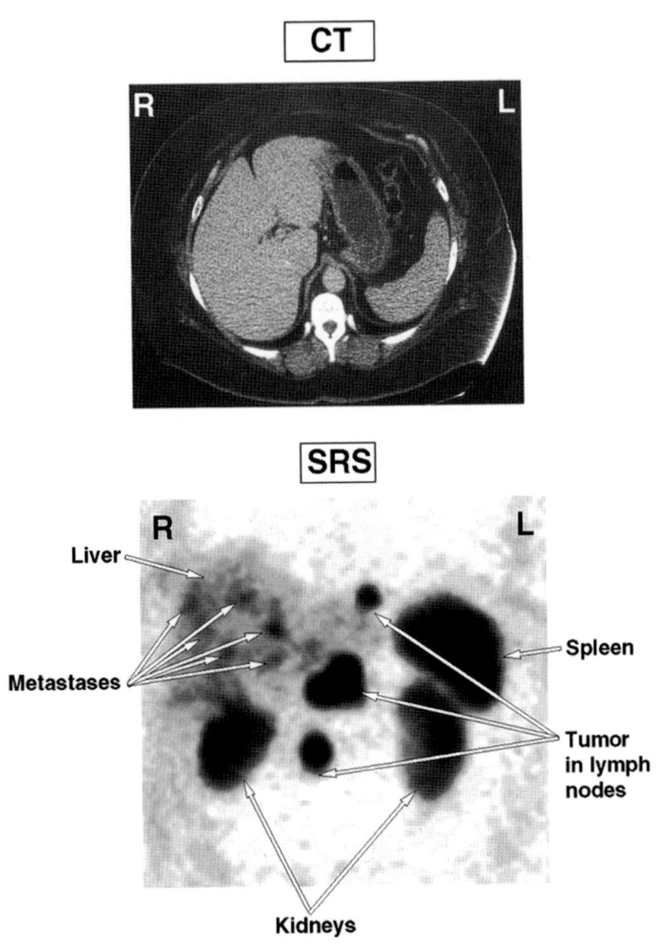

Figure 51–2. Comparison of the CT scan *(top)* and somatostatin receptor scintigraphy (SRS) *(bottom)* in a patient with a metastatic pancreatic endocrine tumor. This pancreatic endocrine tumor (PET) was secreting pancreatic polypeptide (PP), chromogranin A, and gastrin. The CT is negative, whereas the SRS shows numerous liver metastases and lymph node metastases. These results demonstrate the greater sensitivity of the SRS compared with that of conventional imaging studies (ultrasound, CT, MRI), for localizing both lymph node and liver metastases, as shown in a number of recent studies.[80, 159, 161, 165]

were more sensitive than CT scanning,[167] ultrasound, or MR imaging (24% to 36%). In this study[167] for the 17 tumors in the pancreas, EUS had a much higher sensitivity than SRS (94% vs. 47%). EUS is particularly sensitive for identifying PETs within the pancreas (>85%) and in some studies, especially for insulinomas, is more clearly sensitive than SRS. Figure 51–4 shows the ability of EUS to identify an insulinoma in the pancreatic tail. EUS, especially of the pancreas, requires considerable expertise, whereas SRS can be performed in most radiology departments. However, to obtain optimum results with SRS, single-photon emission computed tomography (SPECT) must be performed in addition to planar images.[82] Neither the SRS nor EUS appears to identify small extrapancreatic PETs, especially duodenal gastrinomas. Some studies suggest SRS in combination with EUS in patients with gastrinomas may be more sensitive than either alone.[12, 158] SRS is especially useful for identifying distant metastases, whereas EUS is not generally useful for this. With both modalities the false-positive rate has not been well defined. SRS is reported to be positive in certain thyroid disorders, granulomatous disease, accessory spleen, wound infections, and various arthritides, and in a recent study[168] had a false-positive rate of 12% for localizing a gastrinoma. However, when the clinical context was carefully considered, the percentage in whom false-positive SRS localization altered management was 3%. Similarly, there are few data on the false-positive rate of EUS, especially for PETs outside the pancreas.

Functional localization by determining the site of the maximal hormonal gradient by selective venous sampling still remains a useful technique in some situations.[86, 169] Originally this approach involved considerable expertise because transhepatic catheterization with sampling of portal venous tributaries was required. Furthermore, complications occurred in 20% of patients.[170] Recently a simplified method has been described.[169] By using various secretagogues such as secretin for gastrinomas or calcium for insulinomas, selective intra-arterial injection of these secretagogues during angiography with hepatic venous sampling has localized gastrinomas and insulinomas.[86, 169, 170] This latter procedure is easier to perform than portal venous sampling, has less complications, and has equal to greater sensitivity than portal venous sampling[169] and thus has replaced portal venous sampling. During this procedure the secretagogue is injected selectively into various arteries (superior mesenteric artery, splenic, right and left hepatic, gastroduodenal), and when the vessel supplies the area of the PET there is a sharp increase in the hepatic venous hormone concentration with the secretagogue injection.[169] Figure 51–5 shows the ability of calcium infusions to accurately localize an insulinoma to the pancreatic body, a location that was suspected from the MR imaging study. In a recent comparative study[86] in insulinomas, which are frequently less than 1 cm in diameter and difficult to localize, the intra-arterial calcium test with selective hepatic venous sampling was positive in 88% of patients, the ultrasound in 9%, the CT scan in 17%, MR imaging in 43%, selective angiography in 36%, and portal venous sampling in 67%. Calcium infusion may also increase the release of hormones from VIPomas, PPomas, glucagonomas, gastrinomas, GRFomas, or somatostatinomas, so that a similar approach may be useful with these tumors.[12]

MANAGEMENT OF METASTATIC PANCREATIC ENDOCRINE TUMORS

The treatment of all metastatic PETs is considered together because in most aspects it is similar for each of the tumors. Chemotherapeutic protocols, surgical approach, and general clinical considerations are generally the same. Metastatic PETs are relatively slow growing compared to other more common malignant nonendocrine gastrointestinal tumors.[19, 155] The long-term natural history of most functional PETs is not known because, until recently, effective treatment for the clinical syndrome was not available and therefore patients often died of complications of the hormonal excess rather than the tumor per se. However, with the recent availability of therapeutic agents such as octreotide, the natural history is changing. In contrast, with nonfunctional tumors and gastrinomas, for which effective therapy for the gastric hypersecretion has existed for more than 30 years, the natural history of the malignant tumor itself has

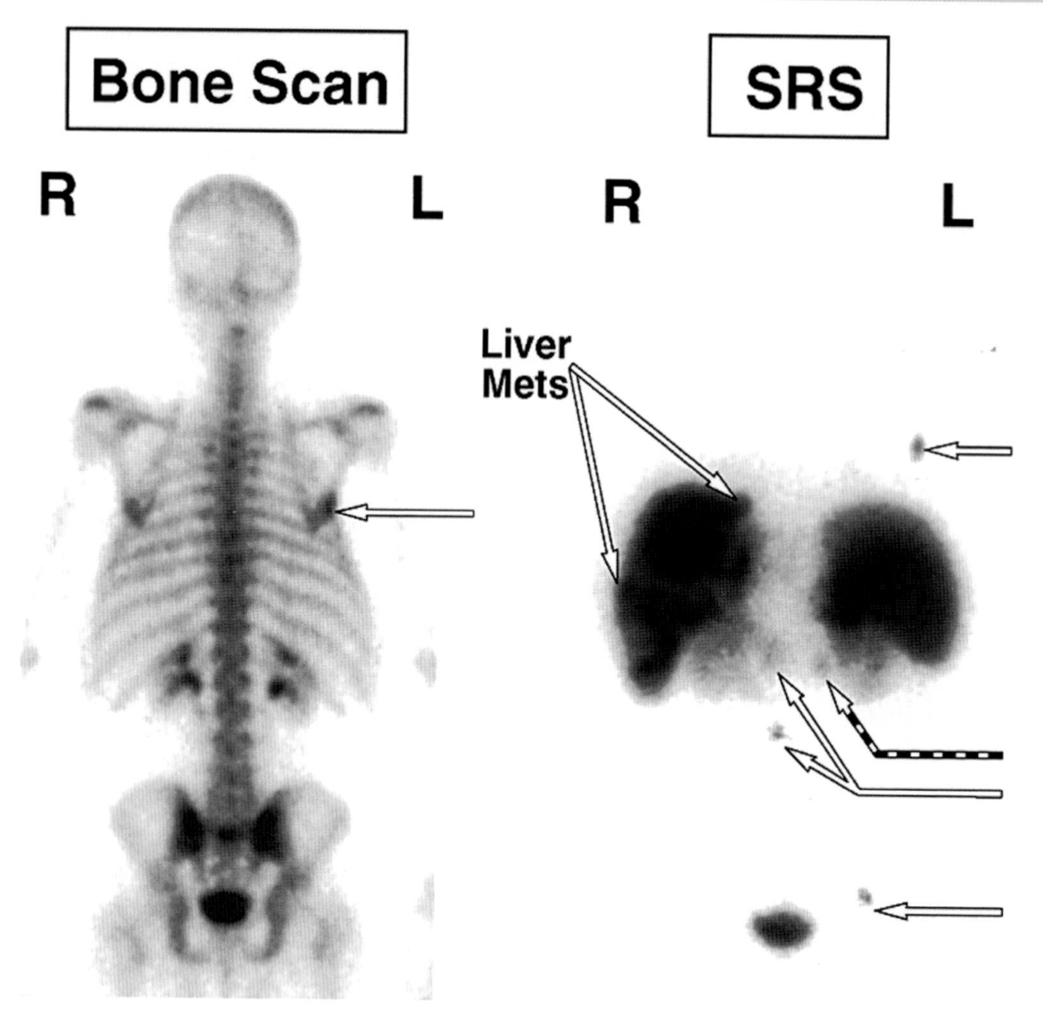

Figure 51–3. Comparison of bone scanning *(left panel)* and somatostatin receptor scintigraphy (SRS) *(right panel)* in ability to localize bone metastases in a patient with a metastatic pancreatic endocrine tumor (PET). The PET was secreting both glucagon and gastrin. This patient had bone metastases in the spine (lumbar spine), left pelvis, and left scapula. The SRS *(right panel)* demonstrates the metastases in each area *(clear arrows)*, whereas the bone scan *(left panel)* shows only a questionable metastasis in the left scapula *(clear arrow)*. The primary tumor in the pancreatic tail is shown by the *dotted arrow* on the SRS. These results demonstrate the greater sensitivity of SRS in detecting bone metastases in patients with malignant PETs.[163]

been assessed. Because of the similar biologic behavior of all PETs, the assessment of these latter tumors will likely also provide insights into the natural history of all these less common malignant PETs.[19–21, 138, 155] Recent insights into the PET biology and natural history have identified prognostic factors that determine survival.[19] An awareness of these factors is essential in planning the type and timing of treatment of advanced disease.

Tumor Biology, Prognostic Factors, and Survival

With the increased ability to control the hormone-excess state, the survival of patients with PETs is increasingly being determined by the tumor biology and natural history of the PET's growth pattern.[19, 41] Insights have been principally obtained from studies of the natural history and prognostic factors determining survival in patients with nonfunctional PETs and in patients with gastrinomas, because of the ability to medically control the gastric hypersecretion in these patients for a number of years.[19, 21, 171]

Recent studies demonstrate that PETs grow at different rates in different patients.[19, 147, 155, 172–174] In studies in patients with gastrinomas followed long term, in approximately 25% of patients the gastrinoma demonstrates aggressive growth, whereas in the remaining 75% growth was indolent or not at all.[147, 155] Similarly, even in patients with liver metastases, in only 40% did aggressive growth occur, and all deaths occurred in this subset of patients.[172] At present, the molecular basis for this difference in growth remains unclear. In different PETs a number of prognostic factors have been defined that can be clinically useful and are summarized in Table 51–9. The most important prognostic factor in all studies is the development of liver metastases. In one large study involving 221 patients with gastrinomas, the 15-year survival for all patients was 90%, for those without liver metastases was 96%, and for those with liver metastases was 26%.[147] The development of liver metastases and their extent (one lobe, both, diffuse), the presence of bone or lymph node metastases, larger primary size, primary location (pancreatic gastrinomas have a worse prognosis than duodenal), various histologic features, and laboratory and flow cytometric features all have predictive values. Two of the most important are the development of bone metastases or ectopic Cushing's syndrome, which were independent predictors of poor survival, with a mean survival from their onset of less than 2 years.[19, 147] Most authorities would therefore agree that treatment directed at metastatic disease that is increasing in size is indicated, as well as treatment to prevent the development of metastases.[12, 19] However, at present there is no agreement about what type of ther-

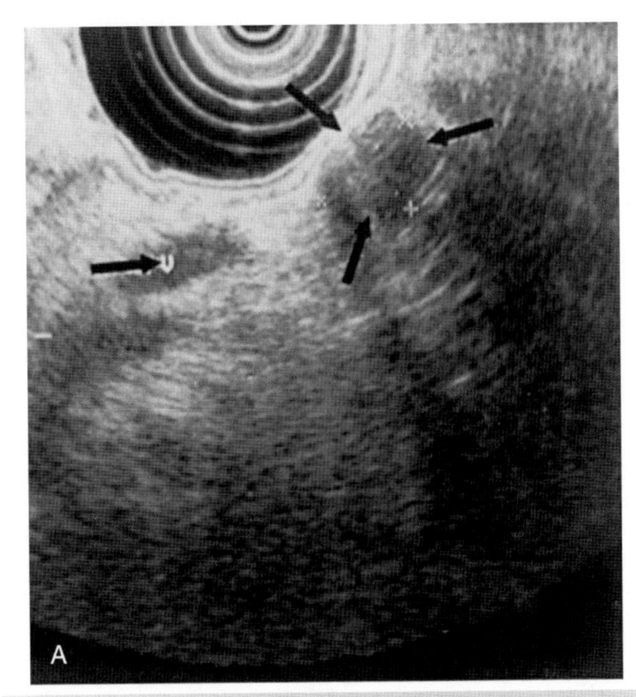

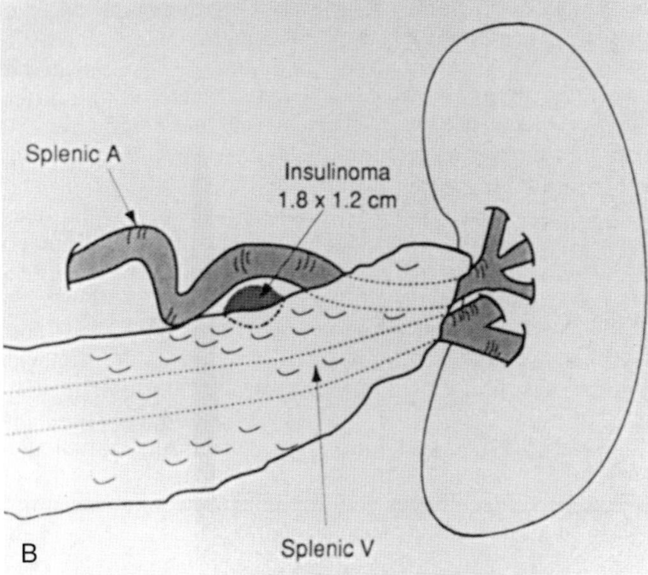

Figure 51–4. Endoscopic ultrasound localizing an insulinoma. In the *top panel (A)* the endoscopic ultrasound balloon is in the stomach. The ultrasound shows a sonolucent pancreatic endocrine tumor of 2 cm *(three arrows)* near the splenic vein (*small arrow,* labeled v). The *bottom panel (B)* is a drawing illustrating the results and location of the insulinoma. (The authors would like to thank Dr. Norman Thompson, University of Michigan, Department of Surgery, for kindly providing these pictures.)

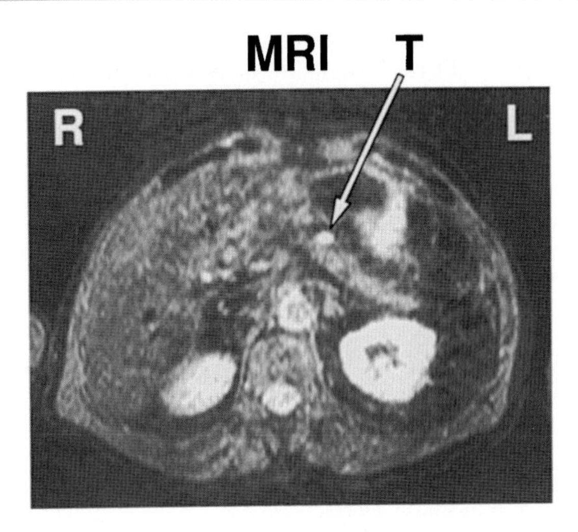

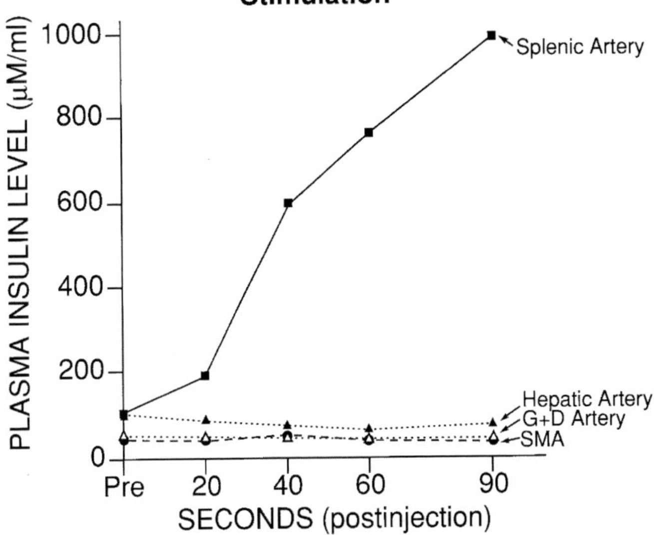

Figure 51–5. Localization of an insulinoma by magnetic resonance imaging (MRI) scanning *(top)* and by intra-arterial calcium injection and hepatic venous sampling for insulin concentrations *(bottom). (Top)* On the MRI scan a probable insulinoma *(T)* was seen in the pancreatic body, an area which the splenic artery supplies. *(Bottom)* Ca gluconate (10%) (0.025 mEq Ca/Kg) was injected into the superior mesenteric artery (SMA), gastroduodenal artery (G + D), common hepatic artery, and splenic artery, and venous samples were collected before and 20 sec, 40 sec, 60 sec, and 90 sec post injection and assayed for insulin concentration. A significant (>50%) increase in hepatic venous insulin concentration occurred at all times after injection of Ca gluconate into the splenic artery but not after calcium injection into the other vessels. At surgery, an insulinoma was found in the pancreatic body.

apy is most appropriate for patients with metastatic disease, when therapy should be started, and even the efficacy of various therapies. Chemotherapy,[12, 90, 156, 175, 176] debulking surgery with or without chemotherapy,[90, 93, 156, 175, 177] hepatic arterial embolization with or without chemoembolization,[12, 12, 12, 156, 178, 179] hormonal therapy with octreotide,[12, 41, 41, 78, 80, 83, 152, 176] interferon therapy,[41, 180] liver transplantation,[12, 41, 152, 181] and targeted radiotherapy using radiolabeled somatostatin analogs[41, 182–186] all have been reported to be useful in small numbers of cases.

Chemotherapy

Most studies of chemotherapy in metastatic PETs have included mixtures of patients with the various functional PETs as well as occasionally nonfunctional PETs and in some cases patients with carcinoid tumors.[12, 21, 156, 176] Results from these studies are limited in a number of ways. There are often small numbers of cases. Some studies suggest that responsiveness to chemotherapy is equal in the different PETs, but other observations suggest there may be important differences.[12, 21] For example, up to 93% of metastatic gluca-

Table 51–9 | **Factors in Pancreatic Endocrine Tumors (PETs) Prognostic of Decreased Survival**

Female gender
Absence of MEN I syndrome
Presence of liver metastases
Extent of liver metastases
Presence of lymph node metastases
Rate of growth of liver metastases
Bone metastases
Incomplete tumor resection
Nonfunctional tumor
Ectopic Cushing's syndrome
Increased depth of tumor invasion
Primary tumor site
Primary tumor size ≥3 cm
Various histologic features
High nuclear atypia
Poor tumor differentiation
High growth indices
Capsular invasion
Vascular or perineural invasion
Aneuploidy or flow aneuploidy
Laboratory findings
Increased serum chromogranin A (in some studies)
Increased serum gastrin level in gastrinomas
Lack of progesterone receptors
Ha-ras oncogene or *p53* overexpression

MEN, multiple endocrine neoplasia.
Data from references 80, 147, 155, 174, 230, and 231.

gonomas are reported to respond to dacarbazine (DTIC),[12, 12, 175] including some complete remissions, whereas in other PETs DTIC has a low (<10%) response rate.[187] Similarly, up to 90% of VIPomas responded to streptozotocin, whereas only 5% to 40% of metastatic gastrinomas responded to streptozotocin,[12] and no complete responses were seen.

The current recommended choice is the combination of streptozotocin and doxorubicin.[156, 156, 175, 176, 188–190] This recommendation is based on two studies from the Eastern Cooperative Oncology Group (ECOG) published in 1980[191] and 1992.[188] The study in 1980 demonstrated streptozotocin plus 5-fluorouracil was more effective than streptozotocin alone,[191] and the 1992 study[188] demonstrated that streptozotocin plus doxorubicin caused tumor regression in 69% of patients, which was significantly better than the 45% regression rate with streptozotocin plus 5-fluorouracil or 30% with chlorozotocin. Furthermore, the patients treated with streptozotocin and doxorubicin had a significantly better survival.[188] Streptozotocin, a glycosamine nitrosourea compound originally derived from a *Streptomyces* species, has been in clinical use since 1967[12] and in preclinical studies was found to have cytotoxic effects on pancreatic islets.[12] In 1968 streptozotocin was found to have clinical effectiveness against a PET[12] and since then has been used as the initial agent either alone or in combination with other agents for treating metastatic PETs. In various series streptozotocin alone gives an objective tumor response in 36% to 62%.[12, 156, 176, 189–192] In contrast, other single agents such as doxorubicin, DTIC, tubercidin, etoposide, or carboplatin have generally had a lower response rate of 6% to 33%.[12, 156, 176, 187, 190] Streptozotocin causes nausea and vomiting in almost all patients and transient dose-related renal dysfunction including proteinuria (40% to 50%)[12, 193] and a decrease in creatinine clearance, abnormalities in hepatic function, and leukopenia and thrombocytopenia in 6%.[12] In the 1992 ECOG study,[188] nine patients given streptozotocin had chronic renal failure and seven required dialysis. The nausea and vomiting can now be controlled in almost all patients using 5-HT_3 receptor antagonists such as ondansetron.[156] Chlorozotocin is structurally closely related to streptozotocin, but it causes less nausea and vomiting.[12] When given alone[12, 188] or combined with 5-fluorouracil,[12] it gives similar results to those seen with streptozotocin.[12, 156, 176, 190, 192]

Because of the limited effectiveness of single agents, various combinations have been investigated. The combination of streptozotocin and 5-fluorouracil was found to be more effective than streptozotocin alone[191]; however, in a later study it was less effective than streptozotocin and doxorubicin.[188] In the 1980 ECOG study,[191] the 42 patients treated with streptozotocin had a 36% response rate, with 12% showing a complete response, whereas with streptozotocin plus 5-fluorouracil, 63% demonstrated a response (with 33% having a complete response). Response rates in this study[191] between different functional tumors or between functional and nonfunctional tumors did not differ. In more recent prospective studies,[12, 193, 194] the response rate with streptozotocin plus 5-fluorouracil was significantly lower in two studies[193, 194] of patients with metastatic gastrinomas to the liver than in those without metastases to the liver (5% and 40%, respectively). In these recent studies,[12, 193, 194] no patient had a complete response and in one study[193] there was no difference in survival for responders and nonresponders. At present the difference in response rate between the early study[191] and the more recent ones[193, 194] remains unexplained. Streptozotocin has been used in combination with other agents such as doxorubicin or tubercidin in small numbers of cases, with response rates reported from 20% to 100%. Streptozotocin combined with 5-fluorouracil,[12, 156, 176, 188, 190–192, 194] with doxorubicin,[12, 156, 176, 187, 188, 190, 192] with both these agents,[193] with 5-fluorouracil plus tubercidin,[12] or with doxorubicin and cisplatin[12] have been used in different studies. Only the combination of streptozotocin and doxorubicin is established as superior to streptozotocin and 5-fluorouracil.[188]

Recently, the combination of etoposide and cisplatin[195] has been evaluated in patients with PETs and carcinoid tumors.[195, 196] In one study,[195] 12 of 18 of anaplastic NETs, 2 of 14 of PETs, and none of 13 of metastatic carcinoid tumors demonstrated partial to complete regression. In a second study,[196] only 1 of 12 patients with a well-differentiated NET responded, whereas 17 of the 41 patients with a poorly differentiated tumor showed an objective tumor response. Hematologic toxicity occurred in 60% and there was one treatment-related death.[196]

Surgical Therapy

Systematic removal of all resectable tumor (debulking surgery) has been recommended, if possible, for all PETs, including gastrinomas, VIPomas, glucagonomas, and somatostatinomas.[12, 33, 90, 91, 106, 156, 175, 197–202] In two studies[198, 199] involving 17 and 74 patients with metastatic NETs, the effectiveness of surgical debulking or cytoreductive surgery was assessed. In one study,[198] the tumor was completely excised at surgery in 80%, mean survival at 5 years was

74%, and patients undergoing resection had a significantly longer survival than patients with unresectable disease. In the second study,[199] 36 of 74 patients had a hemihepatectomy or extended hepatectomy and the other 38 had nonanatomic resections. Perioperative mortality was 2.7%, 4-year survival was 73%, and 90% had symptomatic improvement postresection. Both studies[198, 199] recommend that resection of metastatic disease be considered whenever possible. Unfortunately, such resection is possible in only a small proportion of patients (5% to 15%).[177, 198, 200–202] Even though this approach is recommended, at present, whether such an approach actually increases survival is not clear. This approach may be required in patients with symptomatic PETs in which octreotide or the use of chemotherapy alone is not reducing plasma hormone levels sufficiently so that symptoms are controlled.

Hepatic Artery Embolization

Hepatic artery embolization with or without postocclusion chemotherapy has been used successfully in small numbers of patients with PETs metastatic to the liver.[156, 178, 187, 203–207] Because the liver derives only 20% to 25% of its blood supply from the hepatic artery and 75% to 80% from the portal vein,[178] and because most PETs are vascular with an arterial supply, hepatic artery embolization has been used. In some studies 68% to 100% of patients have symptomatic improvement.[12, 206] Chemotherapy using doxorubicin or other chemotherapeutic agents in iodized oil combined with either gelatin or sponge particles has been reported to improve symptoms in 68% to 100% of patients and decrease tumor size and/or hormone levels in 37% to 100% of patients.[12, 41, 204, 208] In one recent study,[204] the mean duration of response was 24 months (range 6 to 63 months). This procedure is not without side effects, with almost all patients reporting abdominal pain, nausea, vomiting, and fever usually lasting 3 to 10 days,[12, 41, 204, 208] with severe complications occurring in 10% to 15% (including hepatic failure, acute renal failure, infection and sepsis, and death).[12, 178] With the availability of SRS it is now possible to easily assess the extent of metastatic disease. In a patient with diffusely metastatic disease to the liver with minimal or no bone metastases in whom hormone symptoms cannot be controlled by octreotide, chemotherapy, or other medical treatments, this therapy should be considered.

Hormonal Therapy with Somatostatin Analogs

Except for insulinomas, more than 90% of all PETs possess somatostatin receptors, and these receptors may mediate many of the effects of somatostatin analogs on these tumors.[41, 80–82, 159] The effect of octreotide on tumor growth function and size has been examined in a number of studies.[41, 80, 83, 173, 209–216] In general, octreotide causes only a decrease in PET tumor size in 17% of patients.[41] However, stabilization of progressive disease is seen in 50% to 80% of patients with metastatic PETs treated with somatostatin analogs.[41, 173, 211–216] Tumor stabilization is also reported with depot long-acting formulations of somatostatin analogs.[215] Recent studies demonstrate somatostatin analogs can induce apoptosis in NETs, and this may contribute to its tumoristatic effects.[217]

Interferon

α-Interferon has been reported to be effective at controlling symptoms in a number of patients with PETs.[180, 218–220] In a review[180] of 322 patients with various NETs treated with interferon, 43% of the patients had a biochemical response (i.e., >50% decrease in hormone levels) and 12% had a decrease in tumor size with a mean duration of 20 months (range 2 to 96 months). Disease stabilization is seen in 75% to 80% of patients with metastatic NETs.[180, 220] Recent studies[221] demonstrate that α-interferon can induce an increase in *bcl-2* expression in NETs, which may contribute to the tumoristatic effect by stabilizing cells at the G_0 phase of the cell cycle. These results suggest that interferon, similar to octreotide, may possibly extend survival by decreasing the tumor growth rate. Recently, interferon has been used in combination with somatostatin analogs.[214, 222] In one study[214] in 21 patients with progressive metastatic NETs, the combination of α-interferon and octreotide caused a decrease (6%) or tumor stabilization (61%) for a mean of 12 months.

Liver Transplantation

Liver transplantation has been carried out in a small number of patients with metastatic PETs.[41, 181, 223, 224] In a recent review of 103 cases[224] of patients with malignant NETs who underwent liver transplantation, including 43 carcinoids and 48 PETs, the 5-year survival rate was 45%. The recurrence-free survival rate was low, however (<24%).[224] It was concluded that the liver transplantation may be justified, particularly in younger patients with metastatic disease limited to the liver.[224]

Somatostatin Receptor–Directed Radiotherapy

Recently there has been an attempt to use radiolabeled somatostatin analogs for antitumor treatment.[41, 182–186] Both [^{111}In-DTPA^0]octreotide, which emits auger and conversion electrons as well as ^{90}Y-labeled somatostatin analogs coupled by a DOTA chelator (1,4,7,10-tetra-azacyclodecane-*N′*, *N″*, *N‴*) which emits β particles, are reported to inhibit tumor growth in both animal studies and in humans in preliminary tumor studies.[183, 185, 186, 225–227] In one study[182] of 20 patients primarily with advanced NETs receiving at least 20 Gbq of [^{111}-DTPA^0]octreotide, tumor stabilization occurred in 8, and in others, a decrease in tumor size was seen. In the future, with ^{90}Y-labeled somatostatin analogs, high radiation doses can be given,[228, 229] and perhaps response rates will be high.

REFERENCES

1. Wilder RM, Allan FN, Power WH, et al: Carcinoma of the islands of the pancreas: Hyperinsulinism and hypoglycemia. JAMA 89:348, 1927.

2. Zollinger RM, Ellison EH: Primary peptic ulcerations of the jejunum associated with islet cell tumors of the pancreas. Ann Surg 142:709, 1955.
3. Verner JV, Morrison AB: Islet cell tumor and a syndrome of refractory watery diarrhea and hypokalemia. Am J Med 25:374, 1958.
4. Mallinson CN, Bloom SR, Warin AP, et al: A glucagonoma syndrome. Lancet 2:1, 1974.
5. Ganda OP, Weir GC, Soeldner JS, et al: Somatostatinoma: A somatostatin-containing tumor of the endocrine pancreas. N Engl J Med 296: 963, 1977.
6. Larsson LI, Hirsch MA, Holst JJ, et al: Pancreatic somatostatinoma: Clinical features and physiological implications. Lancet 1:666, 1977.
7. Rivier J, Spiess J, Thorner M, et al: Characterization of a growth hormone–releasing factor from a human pancreatic islet tumour. Nature 300:276, 1982.
8. Thorner MD, Perryman RL, Cronin MJ, et al: Somatotroph hyperplasia: Successful treatment of acromegaly by removal of a pancreatic islet tumor secreting a growth hormone–releasing factor. J Clin Invest 70:965, 1982.
9. Becker M, Aron DC: Ectopic ACTH syndrome and CRH-mediated Cushing's syndrome. Endocrinol Metab Clin North Am 23:585, 1994.
10. Mao C, El Attaar A, Domenico DR, et al: Carcinold tumors of the pancreas. Int J Pancreatol 23:153, 1998.
11. Maurer CA, Glaser C, Reubi JC, et al: Carcinoid of the pancreas. Digestion 58:410, 1997.
12. Jensen RT, Norton JA: Endocrine tumors of the pancreas. In Feldman M, Scharschmidt BF, Sleisenger MH (eds): Gastrointestinal and Liver Disease, vol 1, 6th ed. Philadelphia, WB Saunders, 1998, p 871.
13. Mao C, Carter P, Schaefer P, et al: Malignant islet cell tumor associated with hypercalcemia. Surgery 117:37, 1995.
14. Fleury A, Flejou JF, Sauvanet A, et al: Calcitonin-secreting tumors of the pancreas: About six cases. Pancreas 16:545, 1998.
15. Jensen RT: Overview of chronic diarrhea caused by functional neuroendocrine neoplasms. Semin Gastrointest Dis 10:156, 1999.
16. Chiang HC, O'Dorisio TM, Huang SC, et al: Multiple hormone elevations in patients with Zollinger-Ellison syndrome: Prospective study of clinical significance and of the development of a second symptomatic pancreatic endocrine tumor syndrome. Gastroenterology 99:1565, 1990.
17. O'Dorisio TM, Vinik AI: Pancreatic polypeptide and mixed peptide-producing tumors of the gastrointestinal tract. In Cohen S, Soloway RD (eds): Hormone-Producing Tumors of the Gastrointestinal Tract. New York, Churchill Livingstone, 1985, p 117.
18. Soga J, Yakuwa Y: Pancreatic polypeptide (PP)-producing tumors (PPomas): A review of the literature and statistical analysis of 58 cases. J Hepatol Biliary Pancreat Surg 1:556, 1994.
19. Jensen RT: Natural history of digestive endocrine tumors. In Mignon M, Colombel JF (eds): Recent Advances in Pathophysiology and Management of Inflammatory Bowel Diseases and Digestive Endocrine Tumors. Paris, John Libbey Eurotext, 1999, p 192.
20. Eriksson B, Oberg K: PPomas and nonfunctioning endocrine pancreatic tumors: Clinical presentation, diagnosis, and advances in management. In Mignon M, Jensen RT (eds): Endocrine Tumors of the Pancreas: Recent Advances in Research and Management. Series: Frontiers in Gastrointestinal Research, vol 23. Basel, S Karger, 1995, p 208.
21. Jensen RT, Gardner JD: Gastrinoma. In Go VLW, DiMagno EP, Gardner JD, et al (eds): The Pancreas: Biology, Pathobiology, and Disease, 2nd ed. New York, Raven Press, 1993, p 931.
22. Jensen RT: Gastrinoma. Baillieres Clin Gastroenterol 10:555, 1996.
23. Grant CS: Insulinoma. Clin Gastroenterol 10:645, 1996.
24. Sassolas G, Chayvialle JA: GRFomas, somatostatinomas: Clinical presentation, diagnosis, and advances in management. In Mignon M, Jensen RT (eds): Endocrine Tumors of the Pancreas: Recent Advances in Research and Management. Series: Frontiers in Gastrointestinal Research, vol 23. Basel, S Karger, 1995, p 194.
25. Kloppel G, Schroder S, Heitz PU: Histopathology and immunopathology of pancreatic endocrine tumors. In Mignon M, Jensen RT (eds): Endocrine Tumors of the Pancreas: Recent Advances in Research and Management. Series: Frontiers in Gastrointestinal Research, vol 23. Basel, Switzerland, S Karger, 1995, p 99.
26. Heitz PU, Kasper M, Polak JM, et al: Pancreatic endocrine tumors. Hum Pathol 13:263, 1982.
27. Heitz PU, Kloppel G, Hacki WH, et al: Nesidioblastosis: The pathologic basis of persistent hyperinsulinemic hypoglycemia in infants: Morphologic and quantitative analysis of seven cases based on specific immunostaining and electron microscopy. Diabetes 26:632, 1977.
28. Pearse A: The APUD concept and hormone production. Clin Endocrinol Metab 9:211, 1980.
29. Langley K: The neuroendocrine concept today. Ann N Y Acad Sci 733:1, 1994.
30. Oberg K, Stridsberg M: Chromogranins as diagnostic and prognostic markers in neuroendocrine tumours. Adv Exp Med Biol 482:329, 2000.
31. Wynick D, Williams SJ, Bloom SR: Symptomatic secondary hormone syndromes in patients with established malignant pancreatic endocrine tumors. N Engl J Med 319:605, 1988.
32. Maton PN, Gardner JD, Jensen RT: Cushing's syndrome in patients with Zollinger-Ellison syndrome. N Engl J Med 315:1, 1986.
33. Vinik AI, Strodel WE, Eckhauser FE, et al: Somatostatinomas, PPomas, neurotensinomas. Semin Oncol 14:263, 1987.
34. Metz DC, Jensen RT, Bale AE, et al: Multiple endocrine neoplasia type 1: Clinical features and management. In Bilezekian JP, Levine MA, Marcus R (eds): The Parathyroids. New York, Raven, 1994, p 591.
35. Fajans SS, Vinik AI: Insulin-producing islet cell tumors. Endocrinol Metab Clin North Am 18:45, 1989.
36. Reinecke-Luthge A, Koschoreck F, Kloppel G: The molecular basis of persistent hyperinsulinemic hypoglycemia of infancy and its pathologic substrates. Virchows Arch 436:1, 2000.
37. Virally ML, Guillausseau PJ: Hypoglycemia in adults. Diabetes Metab 25:477, 1999.
38. Thompson GB, Service FJ, Andrews JC, et al: Noninsulinoma pancreatogenous hypoglycemia syndrome: An update in 10 surgically treated patients. Surgery 128:937, 2000.
39. Weber HC, Jensen RT: Pancreatic endocrine tumors and carcinoid tumors: Recent insights from genetic and molecular biologic studies. In Dervenis CG (ed): Advances in Pancreatic Disease: Molecular Biology, Diagnosis, and Treatment. Stuttgart, Georg Thieme Verlag, 1996, p 55.
40. Calender A: New insights in genetics of digestive neuroendocrine tumors. In Mignon M, Colombel JF (eds): Recent Advances in the Pathophysiology and Management of Inflammatory Bowel Diseases and Digestive Endocrine Tumors. Paris, John Libbey Eurotext, 1999, p 155.
41. Jensen RT: Carcinoid and pancreatic endocrine tumors: Recent advances in molecular pathogenesis, localization, and treatment. Curr Opin Oncol 12:368, 2000.
42. Goebel SU, Heppner C, Burns AD, et al: Geneotype/phenotype correlations of *MEN1* gene mutations in sporadic gastrinoma. J Clin Endocrinol Metab 85:116, 2000.
43. Muscarella P, Melvin WS, Fisher WE, et al: Genetic alterations in gastrinomas and nonfunctioning pancreatic neuroendocrine tumors: An analysis of *p16/MTS1* tumor suppressor gene inactivation. Cancer Res 58:237, 1998.
44. Serrano J, Goebel SU, Peghini PL, et al: Alterations in the p16 *INK4a/CDKN2A* tumor suppressor gene in gastrinomas. J Clin Endocrinol Metab 85:4146, 2000.
45. Hoff AO, Cote GJ, Gagel RF: Multiple endocrine neoplasias. Annu Rev Physiol 62:377, 2000.
46. Marx S, Spiegel AM, Skarulis MC, et al: Multiple endocrine neoplasia type 1: Clinical and genetic topics. Ann Intern Med 129:484, 1998.
47. Doherty GM, Jensen RT: Multiple endocrine neoplasias. In DeVita VT Jr, Hellman S, Rosenberg SA (eds): Cancer: Principles and Practice of Oncology, 6th ed. Philadelphia, Lippincott Williams & Wilkins, 2001, p 1834.
48. Knudson AG Jr: Mutation and cancer: Statistical study of retinoblastoma. Proc Natl Acad Sci U S A 68:820, 1971.
49. Thompson NW, Lloyd RV, Nishiyama RH, et al: MEN I pancreas: A histological and immunohistochemical study. World J Surg 8:561, 1984.
50. Jensen RT: Management of the Zollinger-Ellison syndrome in patients with multiple endocrine neoplasia type 1. J Intern Med 243:477, 1998.
51. Norton JA, Fraker DL, Alexander HR, et al: Surgery to cure the Zollinger-Ellison syndrome. N Engl J Med 341:635, 1999.
52. Orbuch M, Doppman JL, Strader DB, et al: Imaging for pancreatic endocrine tumor localization: Recent advances. In Mignon M, Jensen RT (eds): Endocrine Tumors of the Pancreas: Recent Advances in Research and Management. Series: Frontiers in Gastrointestinal Research, vol 23. Basel, S Karger, 1995, p 268.

53. MacFarlane MP, Fraker DL, Alexander HR, et al: A prospective study of surgical resection of duodenal and pancreatic gastrinomas in multiple endocrine neoplasia-Type 1. Surgery 118:973, 1995.
54. Roy P, Venzon DJ, Shojamanesh H, et al: Zollinger-Ellison syndrome: Clinical presentation in 261 patients. Medicine 79:379, 2000.
55. Soga J, Yakuwa Y: Glucagonomas/diabetico-dermatogenic syndrome (DDS): A statistical evaluation of 407 reported cases. J Hepatobiliary Pancreat Surg 5:312, 1998.
56. Frankton S, Bloom SR: Glucagonomas. Clin Gastroenterol 10:697, 1996.
57. Soga J, Yakuwa Y: Vipoma/diarrheogenic syndrome: A statistical evaluation of 241 reported cases. J Exp Clin Cancer Res 17:389, 1998.
58. Soga J, Yakuwa Y: Somatostatinoma/inhibitory syndrome: A statistical evaluation of 173 reported cases as compared to other pancreatic endocrinomas. J Exp Clin Cancer Res 18:13, 1999.
59. Benya RV, Metz DC, Venzon DJ, et al: Zollinger-Ellison syndrome can be the initial endocrine manifestation in patients with multiple endocrine neoplasia-type 1. Am J Med 97:436, 1994.
60. Norton JA, Cornelius MJ, Doppman JL, et al: Effect of parathyroidectomy in patients with hyperparathyroidism, Zollinger-Ellison syndrome, and multiple endocrine neoplasia Type I: A prospective study. Surgery 102:958, 1987.
61. Metz DC, Jensen RT: Carcinoids and pancreatic endocrine tumors. In Rustgi AR, Crawford J (eds): Gastrointestinal Cancers: Biology and Clinical Management, 2nd ed. Philadelphia, WB Saunders, 2002.
62. Jensen RT: Pancreatic endocrine tumors. In Braunwald E, Fauci AS, Kaspar SL, et al (eds): Harrison's Principles of Internal Medicine, 15th ed. New York, McGraw-Hill, 2001, p 593.
63. Feldkamp MM, Gutmann DH, Guha A: Neurofibromatosis type 1: Piecing the puzzle together. Can J Neurol Sci 25:181, 1998.
64. Mao C, Shah A, Hanson DJ, et al: Von Recklinghausen's disease associated with duodenal somatostatinoma: Contrast of duodenal versus pancreatic somatostatinomas. J Surg Oncol 59:67, 1995.
65. van Basten JP, van Hoek B, de Bruine A, et al: Ampullary carcinoid and neurofibromatosis: Case report and review of the literature. Neth J Med 44:202, 1994.
66. Young J, Povey S: The genetic basis of tuberous sclerosis. Mol Med Today 4:313, 1998.
67. Schwarzkopf G, Pfisterer J: Metastasizing gastrinoma and tuberous sclerosis complex. Zentralbl Pathol 139:477, 1994.
68. Soga J, Yakuwa Y, Osaka M: Insulinomas/hypoglycemic syndrome: A statistical evaluation of 1085 reported cases of a Japanese series. J Exp Clin Cancer Res 17:379, 1998.
69. Rothmund M, Angelini L, Brunt LM, et al: Surgery for benign insulinoma: An international review. World J Surg 14:393, 1990.
70. Comi RJ, Gorden P, Doppman JL: Insulinoma. In Go VLW, Lebenthal E, DiMagno EP, et al (eds): The Pancreas: Biology, Pathobiology, and Disease, 2nd ed. New York, Raven, 1993, p 979.
71. Stefanini P, Carboni M, Patrassi N, et al: Beta-islet cell tumors of the pancreas: Results of a study on 1,067 cases. Surgery 75:597, 1974.
72. Service FJ, Dale AJ, Elveback LR, et al: Insulinoma: Clinical and diagnostic features of 60 consecutive cases. Mayo Clin Proc 51:417, 1976.
73. Robbins DC, Tager HS, Rubenstein AH: Biologic and clinical importance of proinsulin. N Engl J Med 310:1165, 1984.
74. Whipple AO: The surgical therapy of hyperinsulinism. J Int Chir 3: 237, 1938.
75. Hirshberg B, Livi A, Bartlett DL, et al: Forty-eight-hour fast: The diagnostic test for insulinoma. J Clin Endocrinol Metab 85:3222, 2000.
76. Grunberger G, Weiner JL, Silverman R, et al: Factitious hypoglycemia due to surreptitious administration of insulin: Diagnosis, treatment, and long-term follow-up. Ann Intern Med 108:252, 1988.
77. Gill GV, Rauf O, MacFarlane IA: Diazoxide treatment for insulinoma: A national UK survey. Postgrad Med J 73:640, 1997.
78. Dunne MJ, Elton R, Fletcher T, et al: Therapeutic considerations in Sandostatin in the treatment of GEP endocrine tumors. In O'Dorisio TM (ed): Sandostatin and Gastroenteropancreatic Endocrine Tumors. Berlin, Springer-Verlag, 1989, p 93.
79. Lamberts SWJ, van der Lely AJ, de Herder WW, et al: Octreotide. N Engl J Med 334:246, 1996.
80. Jensen RT: Peptide therapy: Recent advances in the use of somatostatin and other peptide receptor agonists and antagonists. In Lewis JH, Dubois A (eds): Current Clinical Topics in Gastrointestinal Pharmacology. Malden, MA, Blackwell Science, 1997, p 144.
81. Reubi JC, Laissue J, Waser B, et al: Expression of somatostatin receptors in normal, inflamed, and neoplastic human gastrointestinal tissues. Ann N Y Acad Sci 733:122, 1994.
82. Krenning EP, Kwekkeboom DJ, Oei HY, et al: Somatostatin-receptor scintigraphy in gastroenteropancreatic tumors. Ann N Y Acad Sci 733: 416, 1994.
83. Maton PN, Gardner JD, Jensen RT: Use of the long-acting somatostatin analog, SMS 201-995 in patients with pancreatic islet cell tumors. Dig Dis Sci 34:28S, 1989.
84. Gillis JC, Noble S, Goa KL: Octreotide long-acting release (LAR): A review of its pharmacological properties and therapeutic use in the management of acromegaly. Drugs 53:681, 1997.
85. Norton JA: Surgical treatment of islet cell tumors with special emphasis on operative ultrasound. In Mignon M, Jensen RT (eds): Endocrine Tumors of the Pancreas: Recent Advances in Research and Management. Series: Frontiers in Gastrointestinal Research, vol 23. Basel, S Karger, 1995, p 309.
86. Doppman JL, Chang R, Fraker DL, et al: Localization of insulinomas to regions of the pancreas by intra-arterial stimulation with calcium. Ann Intern Med 123:269, 1995.
87. Becker SW, Kahn D, Rothman S: Cutaneous manifestations of internal malignant tumors. Arch Dermatol Syph 45:1069, 1942.
88. McGarvan MH, Unger RH, Recant L, et al: A glucagon-secreting alpha-cell carcinoma of the pancreas. N Engl J Med 274:1408, 1966.
89. Wilkinson DS: Necrolytic migratory erythema with carcinoma of the pancreas. Trans St Johns Hosp Dermatol Soc 59:244, 1973.
90. Holst JJ: Glucagon-producing tumors. In Cohen S, Soloway RD (eds): Hormone-Producing Tumors of the Gastrointestinal Tract. New York, Churchill Livingstone, 1985, p 57.
91. Guillausseau PJ, Guillausseau-Scholer C: Glucagonomas: Clinical presentation, diagnosis, and advances in management. In Mignon M, Jensen RT (eds): Endocrine Tumors of the Pancreas: Recent Advances in Research and Management. Series: Frontiers in Gastrointestinal Research, vol 23. Basel, S Karger, 1995, p 183.
92. Leichter SB: Clinical and metabolic aspects of glucagonoma. Medicine 59:100, 1980.
93. Stacpoole PW: The glucagonoma syndrome: Clinical features, diagnosis, and treatment. Endocr Rev 2:347, 1981.
94. Holst JJ, Orskov C: Glucagon and other proglucagon-derived peptides. In Walsh JH, Dockray GJ (eds): Gut Peptides. New York, Raven, 1994, p 305.
95. Boden G, Wilson RM, Owen OE: Effects of chronic glucagon excess on hepatic metabolism. Diabetes 27:643, 1978.
96. Madsen OD, Karlsen C, Blume N, et al: Transplantable glucagonomas derived from pluripotent rat islet tumor tissue cause severe anorexia and adipsia. Scand J Clin Lab Invest Suppl 220:27, 1995.
97. Boden G, Rezvani I, Owen OE: Effects of glucagon on plasma amino acids. J Clin Invest 73:785, 1984.
98. Naets JP, Guns M: Inhibitory effect of glucagon on erythopoiesis. Blood 55:997, 1980.
99. Mullans EA, Cohen PR: Iatrogenic necrolytic migratory erythema: A case report and review of nonglucagonoma-associated necrolytic migratory erythema. J Am Acad Dermatol 38:866, 1998.
100. Wermers RA, Fatourechi V, Wynne AG, et al: The glucagonoma syndrome: Clinical and pathologic features in 21 patients. Medicine 75:53, 1996.
101. Wermers RA, Fatourechi V, Kvols LK: Clinical spectrum of hyperglucagonemia associated with malignant neuroendocrine tumors. Mayo Clin Proc 71:1030, 1996.
102. Boden G, Owen OE: Familial hyperglucagonemia—an autosomal dominant disorder. N Engl J Med 296:534, 1977.
103. Palmer JP, Werner PL, Benson JW, et al: Dominant inheritance of large molecular weight immunoreactive glucagon. J Clin Invest 61: 763, 1978.
104. Priest WM, Alexander MK: Islet-cell tumor of the pancreas with peptic ulceration, diarrhea, and hypokalemia. Lancet 2:1145, 1957.
105. Matuchansky C, Rambaud JC: VIPomas and endocrine cholera: Clinical presentation, diagnosis, and advances in management. In Mignon M, Jensen RT (eds): Endocrine Tumors of the Pancreas: Recent Advances in Research and Management. Series: Frontiers in Gastrointestinal Research, vol 23. Basel, S Karger, 1995, p 166.
106. Matsumoto KK, Peter JB, Schultze RG: Watery diarrhea and hypokalemia associated with pancreatic islet cell adenoma. Gastroenterology 50:231, 1966.
107. Kane MG, O'Dorisio TM, Krejs GJ: Production of secretory diarrhea

by intravenous infusion of vasoactive intestinal polypeptide. N Engl J Med 309:1482, 1983.
108. Capella C, Polak JM, Buffa R, et al: Morphologic patterns and diagnostic criteria of VIP-producing endocrine tumors: A histologic, histochemical, ultrastructural, and biochemical study of 32 cases. Cancer 52:1860, 1983.
109. Long RG, Bryant MG, Mitchell SJ, et al: Clinicopathological study of pancreatic and ganglioneuroblastoma tumours secreting vasoactive intestinal polypeptide (vipomas). BMJ 282:1767, 1981.
110. Park SK, O'Dorisio MS, O'Dorisio TM: Vasoactive intestinal polypeptide-secreting tumours: Biology and therapy. Clin Gastroenterol 10: 673, 1996.
111. Smith SL, Branton SA, Avino AJ, et al: Vasoactive intestinal polypeptide secreting islet cell tumors: A 15-year experience and review of the literature. Surgery 124:1050, 1998.
112. Verner JV, Morrison AB: Non-β islet tumors and the syndrome of watery diarrhea, hypokalemia, and hypochlorhydria. Clin Gastroenterol 3:595, 1974.
113. Verner JV, Morrison AB: Endocrine pancreatic islet disease with diarrhea: Report of a case due to diffuse hyperplasia of non-β islet tissue with a review of 54 additional cases. Arch Intern Med 133:492, 1974.
114. Bloom SR, Christofides ND, Delamarter J, et al: M. diarrhoea in vipoma patients associated with cosecretion of a second active peptide (peptide histidine isoleucine) explained by single coding gene. Lancet 2:1163, 1983.
115. Krejs GJ: VIPoma syndrome. Am J Med 82:37, 1987.
116. Ginsberg AL: The VIP controversy—Stephen R. Bloom vs. Jerry D. Gardner. Dig Dis Sci 23:30, 1978.
117. Krejs GJ: Comparison of the effect of VIP and PHI on water and ion movement in the canine jejunum in vivo [abstract]. Gastroenterol Clin Biol 8:868, 1984.
118. Krejs GJ, Walsh JH, Morawski SG, et al: Intractable diarrhea: Intestinal perfusion studies and plasma VIP concentrations in patients with pancreatic cholera syndrome and surreptitious ingestion of laxatives and diuretics. Am J Dig Dis 22:280, 1977.
119. Morris AI, Turnberg LA: Surreptitious laxative abuse. Gastroenterology 77:780, 1979.
120. Read NW, Read MG, Krejs GJ, et al: A report of five patients with large-volume secretory diarrhea but no evidence of endocrine tumor or laxative abuse. Dig Dis Sci 27:193, 1982.
121. Read NW, Krejs GJ, Read MG, et al: Chronic diarrhea of unknown origin. Gastroenterology 78:264, 1980.
122. Schiller LR, Rivera LM, Santangelo WC, et al: Diagnostic value of fasting plasma peptide concentrations in patients with chronic diarrhea. Dig Dis Sci 39:2216, 1994.
123. Maton PN, O'Dorisio TM, Howe BA, et al: Effect of a long-acting somatostatin analogue (SMS 201-995) in a patient with pancreatic cholera. N Engl J Med 312:17, 1985.
124. Schonfeld WH, Elkin EP, Woltering EA, et al: The cost-effectiveness of octreotide acetate in the treatment of carcinoid syndrome and VIPoma. Int J Tech Assess Health Care 14:514, 1996.
125. Maton PN, O'Dorisio T, Malarkey WB, et al: Successful therapy of pancreatic cholera with the long-acting somatostatin analogue SMS 201-995: Relation between plasma concentrations of drug and clinical and biochemical responses. Scand J Gastroenterol 21(Suppl 119):181, 1986.
126. Krejs GJ, Orci L, Conlon JM, et al: Somatostatinoma syndrome: Biochemical, morphologic, and clinical features. N Engl J Med 301: 285, 1979.
127. Schusdziarra V, Grube D, Seifert H, et al: Somatostatinoma syndrome: Clinical, morphological, and metabolic features and therapeutic aspects. Klin Wochenschr 61:681, 1983.
128. Boden G, Shimoyama R: Somatostatinoma. In Cohen S, Soloway RD (eds): Hormone-Producing Tumors of the Gastrointestinal Tract. New York, Churchill Livingstone, 1985, p 85.
129. Tanaka S, Yamasaki S, Matsushita S, et al: Duodenal somatostatinoma: A case report and review of 31 cases with special reference to the relationship between tumor size and metastasis. Pathol Int 50:146, 2000.
130. Yamada T, Chiba T: Somatostatin. In Makhlouf GM (ed): Handbook of Physiology, Sect. 6, The Gastrointestinal Tract, vol 2: Neural and Endocrine Biology. New York, Raven, 1989, p 431.
131. Trendle MC, Moertel CG, Kvols LK: Incidence and morbidity of cholelithiasis in patients receiving chronic octreotide for metastatic carcinoid and malignant islet cell tumors. Cancer 79:830, 1997.
132. Pipeleers D, Couturier E, Gepts W, et al: Five cases of somatostatinoma: Clinical heterogeneity and diagnostic usefulness of basal and tolbutamide-induced hypersomatostatinemia. J Clin Endocrinol Metab 56:1236, 1983.
133. Angeletti S, Corleto VD, Schillaci O, et al: Use of the somatostatin analogue octreotide to localise and manage somatostatin-producing tumours. Gut 42:792, 1998.
134. Losa M, von Werder K: Pathophysiology and clinical aspects of the ectopic GH-releasing hormone syndrome. Clin Endocrinol 47:123, 1997.
135. Sano T, Asa SL, Kovacs K: Growth hormone–releasing hormone-producing tumors: Clinical, biochemical, and morphological manifestations. Endocr Rev 9:357, 1988.
136. Losa M, Schopohl J, von Werder K: Ectopic secretion of growth hormone-releasing hormone in man. J Endocrinol Invest 16:69, 1993.
137. Christofides ND, Stephanou A, Suzuki H, et al: Distribution of immunoreactive growth hormone–releasing hormone in the human brain and intestine and its production by tumors. J Clin Endocrinol Metab 59:747, 1984.
138. Kent RB, Van Heerden JA, Weiland LH: Nonfunctioning islet cell tumors. Ann Surg 193:185, 1981.
139. Eckhauser FE, Cheung PS, Vinik AI, et al: Nonfunctioning malignant neuroendocrine tumors of the pancreas. Surgery 100:978, 1986.
140. Nobels FR, Kwekkeboom DJ, Coopmans W, et al: Chromogranin A as serum marker for neuroendocrine neoplasia: Comparison with neuron-specific enolase and the alpha-subunit of glycoprotein hormones. J Clin Endocrinol Metab 82:2622, 1997.
141. Mannon P, Taylor IL: The pancreatic polypeptide family. In Walsh JH, Dockray GJ (eds): Gut Peptides. New York, Raven, 1994, p 341.
142. Adrian TE, Uttenthal LO, Williams SJ, et al: Secretion of pancreatic polypeptide in patients with pancreatic endocrine tumors. N Engl J Med 315:287, 1986.
143. Hochwald SN, Conlon KC, Brennan MF: Nonfunctional pancreatic islet cell tumors. In Doherty GM, Skogseid B (eds): Surgical Endocrinology. Philadelphia, Lippincott Williams & Wilkins, 2001, p 361.
144. van Eijck CH, Lamberts SW, Lemaire LC, et al: The use of somatostatin receptor scintigraphy in the differential diagnosis of pancreatic duct cancers and islet cell tumors. Ann Surg 224:119, 1996.
145. Blackburn AM, Bryant MG, Adrian TE, et al: Pancreatic tumours produce neurotensin. J Clin Endocrinol Metab 52:820, 1981.
146. Ferris GF: Neurotensin. In Makhlouf GM (ed): Handbook of Physiology, Sect 6, The Gastrointestinal Tract, vol 2, Neural and Endocrine Biology. Bethesda, MD, American Physiological Society, 1989, p 559.
147. Yu F, Venzon DJ, Serrano J, et al: Prospective study of the clinical course, prognostic factors, and survival in patients with long-standing Zollinger-Ellison syndrome. J Clin Oncol 17:615, 1999.
148. Clark ES, Carney JA: Pancreatic islet cell tumor associated with Cushing's syndrome. Am J Surg Pathol 8:917, 1984.
149. Doppman JL, Nieman LK, Cutler GB Jr, et al: Adrenocorticotropic hormone-secreting islet cell tumors: Are they always malignant? Radiology 190:59, 1994.
150. Wu TJ, Lin CL, Taylor RL, et al: Increased parathyroid hormone–related peptide in patients with hypercalcemia associated with islet cell carcinoma. Mayo Clin Proc 72:1111, 1997.
151. Bresler L, Boissel P, Conroy T, et al: Pancreatic islet cell carcinoma with hypercalcemia: Complete remission 5 years after surgical excision and chemotherapy. Am J Gastroenterol 86:635, 1991.
152. Jensen RT: Pancreatic endocrine tumors: Recent advances. Ann Oncol 10:170, 1999.
153. Jensen RT, Doherty GM: Carcinoid tumors and the carcinoid syndrome. In DeVita VT Jr, Hellman S, Rosenberg SA (eds): Cancer: Principles and Practice of Oncology, 6th ed. Philadelphia, Lippincott Williams & Wilkins, 2001, p 1813.
154. Orbuch M, Doppman JL, Jensen RT: Localization of pancreatic endocrine tumors. Semin Gastrointest Dis 6:90, 1995.
155. Weber HC, Venzon DJ, Lin JT, et al: Determinants of metastatic rate and survival in patients with Zollinger-Ellison syndrome: Aprospective long-term study. Gastroenterology 108:1637, 1995.
156. Fraker DL, Jensen RT: Pancreatic endocrine tumors. In DeVita VT Jr, Hellman S, Rosenberg SA (eds): Cancer: Principles and Practice of Oncology, 5th ed. Philadelphia, Lippincott-Raven, 1997, p 1678.
157. Alexander RA, Jensen RT: Pancreatic endocrine tumors. In DeVita VT Jr, Hellman S, Rosenberg SA (eds): Cancer: Principles and Practice of Oncology, 6th ed. Philadelphia, Lippincott Williams & Wilkins, 2001, p 1788.
158. Gibril F, Doppman JD, Jensen RT: Comparative analysis of tumor localization techniques for neuroendocrine tumors. Yale J Biol Med 70:481, 1997.
159. Krenning EP, Kwekkeboom DJ, Bakker WH, et al: Somatostatin re-

ceptor scintigraphy with [^{111}In-DTPA-D-Phe^{1}]- and [^{123}I-Tyr^{3}]-octreotide: The Rotterdam experience with more than 1000 patients. Eur J Nucl Med 20:716, 1993.
160. Ruszniewski P, Amouyal P, Amouyal G, et al: Endocrine tumors of the pancreatic area: Localization by endoscopic ultrasonography. In Mignon M, Jensen RT (eds): Endocrine Tumors of the Pancreas: Recent Advances in Research and Management. Series: Frontiers in Gastrointestinal Research, vol 23. Basel, S Karger, 1995, p 258.
161. Gibril F, Reynolds JC, Doppman JL, et al: Somatostatin receptor scintigraphy—its sensitivity compared with that of other imaging methods in detecting primary and metastatic gastrinomas: A prospective study. Ann Intern Med 125:26, 1996.
162. Jensen RT, Gibril F, Termanini B: Definition of the role of somatostatin receptor scintigraphy in gastrointestinal neuroendocrine tumor localization. Yale J Biol Med 70:481, 1997.
163. Gibril F, Doppman JL, Reynolds JC, et al: Bone metastases in patients with gastrinomas: A prospective study of bone scanning, somatostatin receptor scanning, and MRI in their detection, their frequency, location and effect of their detection on management. J Clin Oncol 16: 1040, 1998.
164. Termanini B, Gibril F, Reynolds JC, et al: Value of somatostatin receptor scintigraphy: A prospective study in gastrinoma of its effect on clinical management. Gastroenterology 112:335, 1997.
165. Jensen RT: Presence of somatostatin receptors on gastro-enteropancreatic endocrine tumors (GEPs): Impact on clinical management with somatostatin receptor imaging and other uses of somatostatin analogues. In Lamberts SWJ (ed): Octreotide: The Next Decade. Bristol, UK, Bioscientific, 1999, p 149.
166. Zimmer T, Scherübl H, Faiss S, et al: Endoscopic ultrasonography of neuroendocrine tumours. Digestion 62:45, 2000.
167. Zimmer T, Ziegler K, Bader M, et al: Localisation of neuroendocrine tumours of the upper gastrointestinal tract. Gut 35:471, 1994.
168. Gibril F, Reynolds JC, Chen CC, et al: Specificity of somatostatin receptor scintigraphy: A prospective study and the effects of false positive localizations on management in patients with gastrinomas. J Nucl Med 40:539, 1999.
169. Strader DB, Doppman JL, Orbuch M, et al: Functional localization of pancreatic endocrine tumors. In Mignon M, Jensen RT (eds): Endocrine Tumors of the Pancreas: Recent Advances in Research and Management. Series: Frontiers in Gastrointestinal Research, vol 23. Basel, S Karger, 1995, p 282.
170. Miller DL, Doppman JL, Metz DC, et al: Zollinger-Ellison syndrome: Technique, results and complications of portal venous sampling. Radiology 182:235, 1992.
171. Jensen RT: Use of omeprazole and other proton pump inhibitors in the Zollinger-Ellison syndrome. In Olbe L (ed): Milestones in Drug Therapy. Basel, Switzerland, Birkhauser Verlag, 1999, p 205.
172. Sutliff VE, Doppman JL, Gibril F, et al: Growth of newly diagnosed, untreated metastatic gastrinomas and predictors of growth patterns. J Clin Oncol 15:2420, 1997.
173. Arnold R, Trautmann ME, Creutzfeldt W, et al: Somatostatin analogue octreotide and inhibition of tumour growth in metastatic endocrine gastroenteropancreatic tumours. Gut 38:430, 1996.
174. Madeira I, Terris B, Voss M, et al: Prognostic factors in patients with endocrine tumours of the duodenopancreatic area. Gut 43:422, 1998.
175. Arnold R, Frank M: Systemic chemotherapy for endocrine tumors of the pancreas: recent advances. In Mignon M, Jensen RT (eds): Endocrine Tumors of the Pancreas: Recent Advances in Research and Management. Series: Frontiers in Gastrointestinal Research, vol 23. Basel, S Karger, 1995, p 431.
176. Pelley RJ, Bukowski RM: Recent advances in diagnosis and therapy of neuroendocrine tumors of the gastrointestinal tract. Curr Opin Oncol 9:68, 1997.
177. Norton JA, Sugarbaker PH, Doppman JL, et al: Aggressive resection of metastatic disease in selected patients with malignant gastrinoma. Ann Surg 203:352, 1986.
178. Arcenas AG, Ajani JA, Carrasco CH, et al: Vascular occlusive therapy of pancreatic endocrine tumors metastatic to the liver. In Mignon M, Jensen RT (eds): Endocrine Tumors of the Pancreas: Recent Advances in Research and Management. Series: Frontiers in Gastrointestinal Research, vol 23. Basel, S Karger, 1995, p 439.
179. Ruszniewski P, Malka D: Hepatic arterial chemoembolization in the management of advanced digestive endocrine tumors. Digestion 62:79, 2000.
180. Eriksson B, Oberg K: Interferon therapy of malignant endocrine pancreatic tumors. In Mignon M, Jensen RT (eds): Endocrine Tumors of the Pancreas: Recent Advances in Research and Management. Series: Frontiers in Gastrointestinal Research, vol 23. Basel, Switzerland, S Karger, 1995, p 451.
181. Azoulay D, Bismuth H: Role of liver surgery and transplantation in patients with hepatic metastases from pancreatic endocrine tumors. In Mignon M, Jensen RT (eds): Endocrine Tumors of the Pancreas: Recent Advances in Research and Management. Series: Frontiers in Gastrointestinal Research, vol 23. Basel, S Karger, 1995, p 461.
182. Krenning EP, Valkema R, Pauwels S, et al: Radiolabeled somatostatin analogue(s): Peptide receptor scintigraphy and radionuclide therapy. In Mignon M, Colombel JF (eds): Recent Advances in the Pathophysiology and Management of Inflammatory Bowel Diseases and Digestive Endocrine Tumors. Paris, John Libbey Eurotext, 1999, p 220.
183. Fjalling M, Andersson P, Forssell-Aronsson E, et al: Systemic radionuclide therapy using indium-111-DTPA-D-Phe^{1}-octreotide in midgut carcinoid syndrome. J Nucl Med 37:1519, 1996.
184. Jensen RT: Somatostatin receptor–based scintigraphy and antitumor treatment: An expanding vista? J Clin Endocrinol Metab 85:3507, 2000.
185. Janson ET, Eriksson B, Oberg K, et al: Treatment with high-dose [^{111}In-DTPA-D-PHE^{1}]-octreotide in patients with neuroendocrine tumors. Acta Oncol 38:373, 1999.
186. Krenning EP, de Jong M, Kooij PP, et al: Radiolabelled somatostatin analogue(s) for peptide receptor scintigraphy and radionuclide therapy. Ann Oncol 10:S23, 1999.
187. Moertel CG: Karnofsky Memorial Lecture: An odyssey in the land of small tumors. J Clin Oncol 5:1502, 1987.
188. Moertel CG, Lefkopoulo M, Lipsitz S, et al: Streptozotocin-doxorubicin, streptozotocin-flourouracil, or chlorozotocin in the treatment of advanced islet cell carcinoma. N Engl J Med 326:519, 1992.
189. Arnold R, Frank M: Gastrointestinal endocrine tumours: Medical management. Clin Gastroenterol 10:737, 1996.
190. Rougier P, Mitry E: Chemotherapy in the treatment of neuroendocrine malignant tumors. Digestion 62:73, 2000.
191. Moertel CG, Hanley JA, Johnson LA: Streptozotocin alone compared with streptozotocin plus fluorouracil in the treatment of advanced islet-cell carcinoma. N Engl J Med 303:1189, 1980.
192. Oberg K, Eriksson B: Medical treatment of neuroendocrine gut and pancreatic tumors. Acta Oncol 28:425, 1989.
193. von Schrenck T, Howard JM, Doppman JL, et al: Prospective study of chemotherapy in patients with metastatic gastrinoma. Gastroenterology 94:1326, 1988.
194. Ruszniewski PH, Rougier P, Andre-David F, et al: Prospective multicentric study of chemotherapy with steptozotocin (STZ) and 5-fluorouracil (5-FU) for liver metastases (LM) in Zollinger-Ellison syndrome (ZES) [abstract]. Gastroenterology 96:A431, 1989.
195. Moertel CG, Kvols LK, O'Connell MJ, et al: Treatment of neuroendocrine carcinomas with combined etoposide and cisplatin: Evidence of major therapeutic activity in the anaplastic variants of these neoplasms. Cancer 68:227, 1991.
196. Mitry E, Baudin E, Ducreux M, et al: Treatment of poorly differentiated neuroendocrine tumours with etoposide and cisplatin. Br J Cancer 81:1351, 1999.
197. Nagorney DM, Que FG: Cytoreductive hepatic surgery for metastatic gastrointestinal neuroendocrine tumors. In Mignon M, Jensen RT (eds): Endocrine Tumors of the Pancreas: Recent Advances in Research and Management. Series: Frontiers in Gastrointestinal Research, vol 23. Basel, S Karger, 1995, p 416.
198. Carty SE, Jensen RT, Norton JA: Prospective study of aggressive resection of metastatic pancreatic endocrine tumors. Surgery 112:1024, 1992.
199. Que FG, Nagorney DM, Batts KP, et al: Hepatic resection for metastatic neuroendocrine carcinomas. Am J Surg 169:36, 1995.
200. Norton JA, Doherty GD, Fraker DL, et al: Surgical treatment of localized gastrinoma within the liver: A prospective study. Surgery 124:1145, 1998.
201. Hellman P, Andersson M, Rastad J, et al: Surgical strategy for large or malignant endocrine pancreatic tumors. World J Surg 24:1353, 2000.
202. Pederzoli P, Falconi M, Bonora A, et al: Cytoreductive surgery in advanced endocrine tumours of the pancreas. Ital J Gastroenterol Hepatol 31:S207, 1999.
203. Dominguez S, Denys A, Menu Y, et al: Hepatic arterial chemoembolization in the management of advanced digestive endocrine tumours. Ital J Gastroenterol Hepatol 31:S213, 1999.
204. Kim YH, Ajani JA, Carrasco CH, et al: Selective hepatic arterial chemoembolization for liver metastases in patients with carcinoid tumor or islet cell carcinoma. Cancer Invest 17:474, 1999.

205. Eriksson BK, Larsson EG, Skogseid BM, et al: Liver embolizations of patients with malignant neuroendocrine gastrointestinal tumors. Cancer 83:2293, 1998.
206. Venook AP: Embolization and chemoembolization therapy for neuroendocrine tumors. Curr Opin Oncol 11:38, 1999.
207. Dominguez S, Denys A, Madeira I, et al: Hepatic arterial chemoembolization with streptozotocin in patients with metastatic digestive endocrine tumours. Eur J Gastroenterol Hepatol 12:151, 2000.
208. Drougas JG, Anthony LB, Blair TK, et al: Hepatic artery chemoembolization for management of patients with advanced metastatic carcinoid tumors. Am J Surg 175:408, 1998.
209. Maton PN: The use of the long-acting somatostatin analog, octreotide acetate, in patients with islet cell tumors. Gastroenterol Clin North Am 18:897, 1989.
210. Pelley RJ, Bukowski RM: Recent advances in systemic therapy for gastrointestinal neuroendocrine tumors. Curr Opin Oncol 11:32, 1999.
211. Eriksson B, Janson ET, Bax NDS, et al: The use of new somatostatin analogues, lanreotide, and octastatin, in neuroendocrine gastrointestinal tumours. Digestion 57:77, 1996.
212. Eriksson B, Renstrup J, Imam H, et al: High-dose treatment with lanreotide of patients with advanced neuroendocrine gastrointestinal tumors: Clinical and biological effects. Ann Oncol 8:1041, 1997.
213. Saltz L, Trochanowski B, Buckley M, et al: Octreotide as an antineoplastic agent in the treatment of functional and nonfunctional neuroendocrine tumors. Cancer 72:244, 1993.
214. Frank M, Klose KJ, Wied M, et al: Combination therapy with octreotide and α-interferon: Effect on tumor growth in metastatic endocrine gastroenteropancreatic tumors. Am J Gastroenterol 94:1381, 1999.
215. Tomassetti P, Migliori M, Gullo L: Slow-release lanreotide treatment in endocrine gastrointestinal tumors. Am J Gastroenterol 93:1468, 1998.
216. Ducreux M, Ruszniewski P, Chayvialle JA, et al: The antitumoral effect of the long-acting somatostatin analog lanreotide in neuroendocrine tumors. Am J Gastroenterol 95:3276, 2000.
217. Imam H, Eriksson B, Lukinius A, et al: Induction of apoptosis in neuroendocrine tumors of the digestive system during treatment with somatostatin analogs. Acta Oncol 36:607, 1997.
218. Saltz L, Kemeny N, Schwartz G, et al: A phase II trial of alpha-interferon and 5-fluorouracil in patients with advanced carcinoid and islet cell tumors. Cancer 74:958, 1994.
219. Oberg K, Eriksson B: Digestive endocrine tumor management: Medical advanced disease. In Mignon M, Colombel JF (eds): Recent Advances in the Pathophysiology and Management of Inflammatory Bowel Diseases and Digestive Endocrine Tumors. Paris, John Libbey Eurotext, 1999, p 260.
220. Öberg K: Interferon in the management of neuroendocrine GEP-tumors. Digestion 62:92, 2000.
221. Imam H, Gobl A, Eriksson B, et al: Interferon-alpha induces *bcl-2* proto-oncogene in patients with neuroendocrine gut tumor responding to its antitumor action. Anticancer Res 17:4659, 1997.
222. Oberg K, Eriksson B, Janson ET: The clinical use of interferons in the management of neuroendocrine gastroenteropancreatic tumors. Ann N Y Acad Sci 733:471, 1994.
223. Dousset B, Houssin D, Soubrane O, et al: Metastatic endocrine tumors: Is there a place for liver transplantation? Liver Transplant Surg 1:111, 1995.
224. Lehnert T: Liver transplantation for metastatic neuroendocrine carcinoma. Transplantation 66:1307, 1998.
225. deJong M, Breeman WA, Bernard HF, et al: Therapy of neuroendocrine tumors with radiolabeled somatostatin analogues. Q J Nucl Med 43:356, 1999.
226. Paganelli G, Zoboli S, Cremonesi M, et al: Receptor-mediated radionuclide therapy with ^{90}Y-DOTA-D-Phe^{1}-Tyr^{3}-octreotide: Preliminary report in cancer patients. Cancer Biother Radiopharm 14:477, 1999.
227. Krenning EP, Valkema R, Kooij PP, et al: The role of radioactive somatostatin and its analogues in the control of tumor growth. Recent Results Cancer Res 153:1, 2000.
228. deJong M, Bakker WH, Breeman WA, et al: Preclinical comparison of [DTPA^{0}] octreotide, [DTPA^{0},Tyr^{3}] octreotide and [DOTA^{0},Tyr^{3}] octreotide as carriers for somatostatin receptor–targeted scintigraphy and radionuclide therapy. Int J Cancer 75:406, 1998.
229. Leimer M, Kurtaran A, Smith-Jones P, et al: Response to treatment with yttrium-90-DOTA-lanreotide of a patient with metastatic gastrinoma. J Nucl Med 39:2090, 1998.
230. Metz DC, Kuchnio M, Fraker DL, et al: Flow cytometry and Zollinger-Ellison syndrome: Relationship to clinical course. Gastroenterology 105:799, 1993.
231. La Rosa S, Sessa F, Capella C, et al: Prognostic criteria in nonfunctioning pancreatic endocrine tumours. Virchows Arch 429:323, 1996.

Section Eight

BILIARY TRACT

Chapter 52

ANATOMY, HISTOLOGY, EMBRYOLOGY, DEVELOPMENTAL ANOMALIES, AND PEDIATRIC DISORDERS OF THE BILIARY TRACT

Frederick J. Suchy

In this chapter, the embryologic and anatomic characteristics of the bile ducts and gallbladder are reviewed with a focus on information that is useful in the diagnosis and treatment of biliary tract disease and in understanding of the anomalies and congenital malformations of these structures. Then, biliary tract disease in infants and children is considered, because many of the disorders occurring early in life are caused by abnormal morphogenesis or adversely affect the process of development.

DEVELOPMENT OF THE LIVER AND BILIARY TRACT

The human liver is formed from two primordia (Fig. 52–1): the liver diverticulum and the septum transversum.[1, 2] Close proximity of cardiac mesoderm, which expresses fibroblast growth factors (FGFs) 1, 2, and 8, causes the foregut endoderm to develop into the liver.[3] Surrounding mesoderm and ectoderm participate in the hepatic specification of the endoderm, and many transcription factors, such as cJun, retinoblastoma gene, and nuclear factor kappa B, play important roles as regulators of liver embryogenesis.[4] The liver diverticulum forms through proliferation of endodermal cells at the cranioventral junction of the yolk sac with the foregut and grows into the septum transversum in a cranioventral direction. The endodermal cells differentiate into hepatocytes and epithelial cells of the bile ducts. This early change occurs on the 18th day of gestation and corresponds to the 2.5-mm stage of the embryo. The signaling molecules that elicit embryonic induction of the liver from the mammalian gut endoderm or induction of other gut-derived organs are being defined. Members of the GATA and Hepatocyte Nuclear Factor (HNF)3/fork head transcription factor families are essential to the formation and differentiation of gut endoderm tissues.[5, 6] The septum transversum consists of mesenchymal cells and a capillary plexus formed by the branches of the two vitelline veins. At the 3- to 4-mm stage, between the third and fourth weeks of gestation, the growing diverticulum projects as an epithelial plug into the septum transversum.[2] At the 5-mm stage, a solid cranial portion (hepatic) and a hollow caudal portion of the diverticulum can be clearly distinguished. The large, hepatic portion differentiates into proliferating cords of hepatocytes and the intrahepatic bile ducts. The smaller, cystic portion, which initially is a cord of epithelial cells, forms the gallbladder, common duct, and cystic duct through a process of elongation and recanalization.

The intrahepatic bile ducts develop from primitive hepatocytes around branches of the portal vein. A ring of hepatocytes in close proximity to the portal vein branches first transforms into bile duct–type cells. A second layer of primitive hepatocytes is similarly transformed and produces a circular cleft around the portal vein that is lined on both

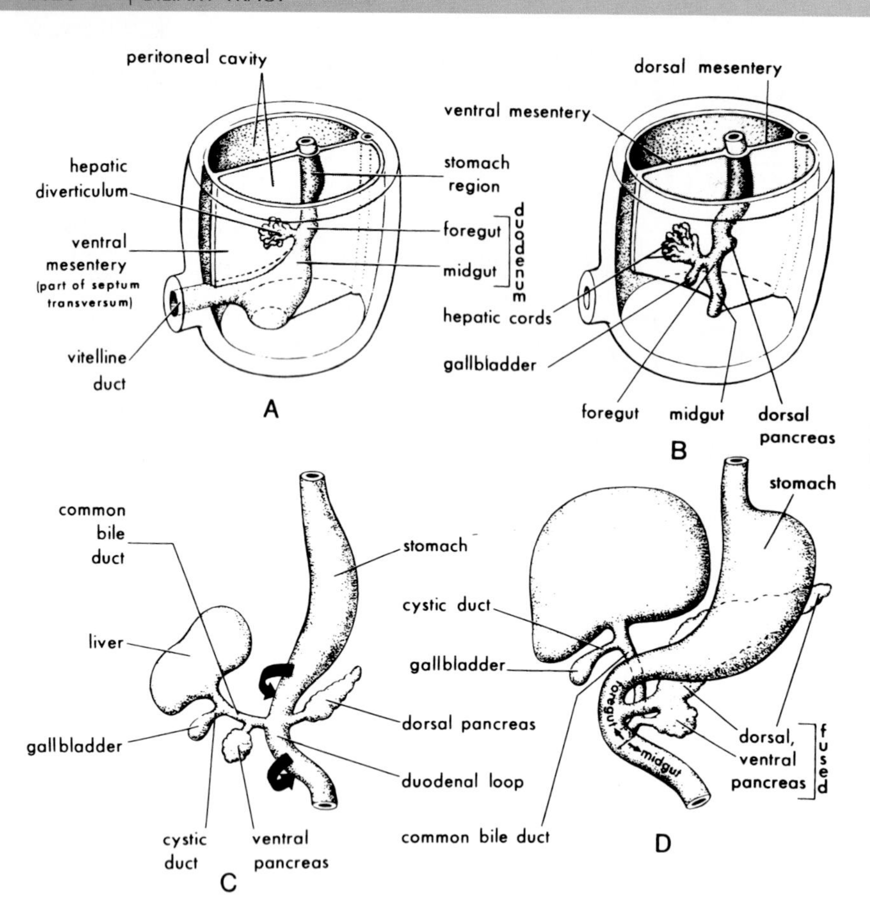

Figure 52–1. Stages in the embryologic development of the liver, gallbladder, extrahepatic ducts, pancreas, and duodenum. *A,* Four weeks. *B* and *C,* Five weeks. *D,* Six weeks. (From Moore KL: The Developing Human. Philadelphia, WB Saunders, 1973.)

sides by bile duct epithelial cells.[4] This double-walled cylinder with a slitlike lumen, the ductal plate, can be detected at 9 weeks of gestation. Thus, the entire network of interlobular and intralobular bile ductules develops from the limiting plate. Periportal connective tissue, glucocorticoid hormones, and basal laminar components may play important roles in the differentiation of bile ducts. In sections of the 10-mm embryo, many of the liver cords are traversed by double-walled canals that branch and morphologically are indistinguishable from bile capillaries of the adult. These structures differ from those of the adult in that they are bounded by six or more liver cells instead of two. The process of differentiation of bile ductular epithelial cells (cholangiocytes) from primitive hepatocytes has been documented in humans through the use of immunohistochemical staining with several anticytokeratin antibodies. During the phenotypic shift toward bile duct–type cells, hepatocytes first display increased reactivity for cytokeratins 8 and 18 and express cytokeratin 19, then at 20 to 25 weeks of gestation express cytokeratin 7.[7] The ductal plate structure requires extensive remodeling through a process of reabsorption, possibly through apoptosis, to yield the characteristic anastomosing system of biliary channels that surround the portal vein. Proteins that appear to have a role in the promotion of apoptosis, specifically fas antigen and c-myc, are consistently detected in primitive intrahepatic ductal cells.[8] Lewis antigen, which is expressed in damaged and apoptotic cells, is also present. BCL-2 protein, an inhibitor of apoptosis, is not found in early stages of intrahepatic bile duct cell development but later becomes detectable. Computed three-dimensional reconstruction of the developing ductal plate has shown that the ductal plate remodeling process starts at the porta hepatis at approximately 11 weeks of gestation and progresses toward the periphery of the liver. The process is in large part completed at term, but even at 40 weeks of gestation, some of the smallest portal vein branches may not be accompanied by an individual bile duct and may still be surrounded by a (discontinuous) ductal plate. In ductal plate malformation, which occurs in biliary disorders such as congenital hepatic fibrosis and Caroli's disease, insufficient reabsorption of ductal plates can result in the formation of large dilated segments of a primitive bile duct that surrounds the central portal vein.

Our knowledge of the early development of the extrahepatic bile ducts and gallbladder in humans remains incomplete. The gallbladder and extrahepatic bile ducts start to develop from hepatic endodermal cells and hepatoblasts immediately after formation of the liver primordium. In embryos 5 to 6 mm in length, the original hepatic diverticulum differentiates cranially into proliferating hepatic cords and bile ducts and caudally into the gallbladder. The cystic portion of the liver diverticulum is hollow initially, but the lumen is filled as cells continually migrate into it. A study in 1994 showed that the primitive extrahepatic bile duct maintains continuity with the ductal plate, from which intrahepatic bile ducts are eventually formed.[9] Contrary to long-held concepts of biliary development, no "solid stage" of endodermal occlusion of the common bile duct lumen is found at any stage of gestation. At 16 mm, the cystic duct and proximal gallbladder are hollow, but the fundus of the gallbladder is still partially obstructed by remnants of the epithelial plug. The gallbladder is patent by the third month of gestation. Further development, until birth, consists primarily of continued growth. The characteristic folds of the gallbladder are formed toward the end of gestation and are moderately developed in the neonate. Bile secretion starts at the beginning of the fourth month of gestation; thereafter, the biliary system continuously contains bile, which is secreted into the gut and imparts a dark green color to the intestinal contents (meconium).

ANATOMY OF THE BILIARY TRACT AND GALLBLADDER

Bile Ducts

The adult human liver has more than 2 km of bile ductules and ducts. These structures are far from being inert channels; they are capable of significantly modifying biliary flow and composition in response to hormones such as secretin. A general feature of bile ductules is their anatomic intimacy with portal blood and lymph vessels, which potentially allows selective exchange of materials between compartments. The functional properties of cholangiocytes are heterogeneous.[10] For example, large, but not small, intrahepatic bile ducts are involved in secretin-regulated bile ductal secretion. Correspondingly, the secretin receptor and chloride-bicarbonate exchanger messenger ribonucleic acids (mRNAs) have been detected in large, but not small, intrahepatic bile duct units.

Bile secretion begins at the level of the bile canaliculus, the smallest branch of the biliary tree.[11] Its boundaries are formed by a specialized membrane of adjacent apical poles of liver cells. The canaliculi form a meshwork of polygonal channels between hepatocytes with many anastomotic interconnections. Bile then enters the small terminal bile ductules (the canals of Hering), which have a basement membrane and are lined by three to six ductal epithelial cells. The canals of Hering provide a conduit through which bile may traverse the limiting plate of hepatocytes to enter the larger perilobular or intralobular ducts. These smallest of biliary radicles are less than 15 to 20 μm in diameter with lumens surrounded by cuboidal epithelial cells. At the most proximal level, one or more fusiform shaped ductular cells may share a canalicular lumen with a hepatocyte; gradually, the ductules become lined by two to four cuboidal epithelial cells as they approach the portal canal. Bile flows from the central lobular cells toward portal triads (from zone 3 to zone 1 of the liver acinus). The terminal bile ductules are thought to proliferate as a result of chronic extrahepatic obstruction.

The interlobular bile ducts form a richly anastomosing network that closely surrounds the branches of the portal vein[12, 13]. These bile ducts (Fig. 52–2) are initially 30 to 40 μm in diameter and are lined by a layer of cuboidal or columnar epithelium that demonstrates a microvillar architecture on its luminal surface.[11] The cells have a prominent Golgi apparatus and numerous vesicles that likely participate in the exchange of substances between cytoplasm and bile and plasma through the processes of exocytosis and endocytosis. These ducts increase in caliber and possess smooth muscle fibers within their walls as they approach the hilum of the liver. The muscular component may provide the morphologic basis for the narrowing of the ducts at this level, which can be observed on cholangiography. Furthermore, as the ducts become progressively larger, the epithelium becomes thicker, and the surrounding layer of connective tissue grows thicker and contains many elastic fibers. These ducts anastomose further to form the large hilar, intrahepatic ducts, which are 1.0 to 1.5 mm in diameter and give rise to the main hepatic ducts.

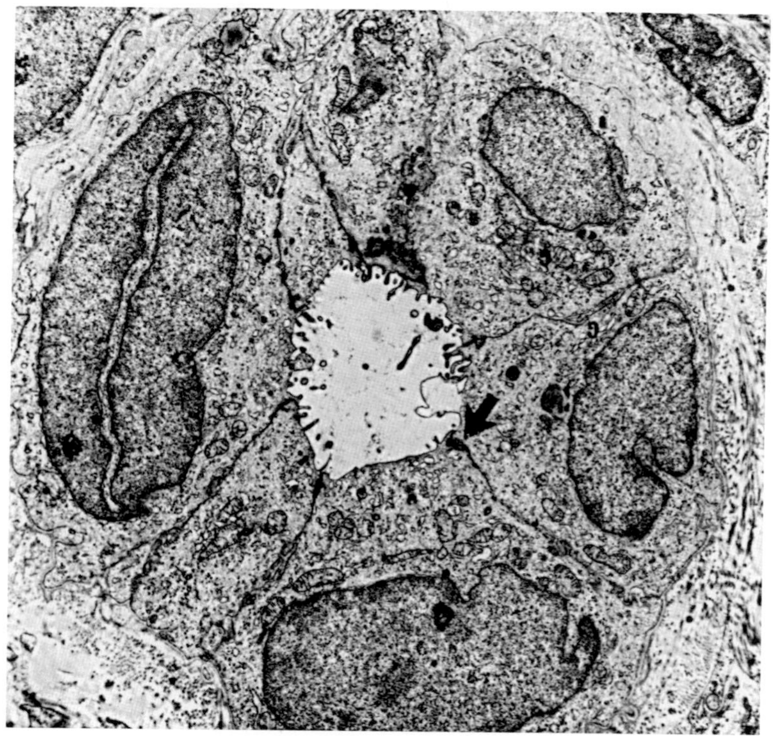

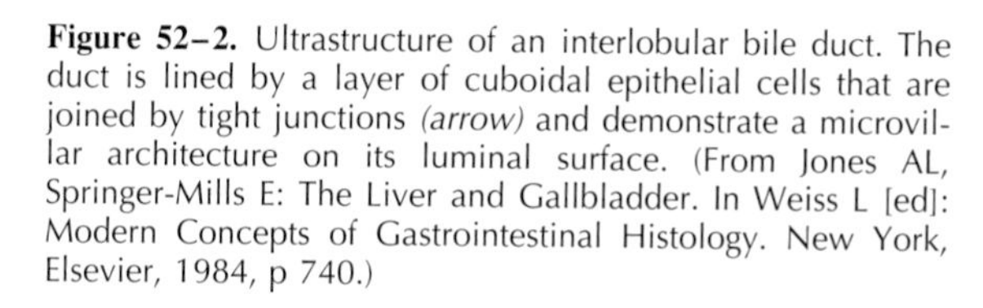

Figure 52–2. Ultrastructure of an interlobular bile duct. The duct is lined by a layer of cuboidal epithelial cells that are joined by tight junctions *(arrow)* and demonstrate a microvillar architecture on its luminal surface. (From Jones AL, Springer-Mills E: The Liver and Gallbladder. In Weiss L [ed]: Modern Concepts of Gastrointestinal Histology. New York, Elsevier, 1984, p 740.)

The common hepatic duct emerges from the porta hepatis after the union of the right and left hepatic ducts, each of which is 0.5 to 2.5 cm long (Fig. 52–3).[14] The confluence of the right and left hepatic ducts is outside the liver in approximately 95% of cases; uncommonly, the ducts merge inside the liver, or the right and left hepatic ducts do not join until the cystic duct joins the right hepatic duct.[15] As the hepatic ducts leave the porta hepatis, they lie within the two serous layers of the hepatoduodenal ligament. This sheath of fibrous tissue binds the hepatic ducts to the adjacent blood vessels. In the adult, the common hepatic duct is approximately 3 cm long and is joined by the cystic duct, usually at its right side, to form the common bile duct. However, the length and angle of junction of the cystic duct with the common hepatic duct are variable. The cystic duct enters the common hepatic duct directly in 70% of patients; alternatively, the cystic duct may run anterior or posterior to the bile duct and spiral around it before joining the bile duct on its medial side. The cystic duct may also course parallel to the common hepatic duct for 5 to 6 cm and enter it after running posterior to the first portion of the duodenum.

In humans, the large intrahepatic bile ducts at the hilum (1.0- to 1.5-mm diameter) have many irregular side branches and pouches (150- to 270-μm diameter) that are oriented in one plane, corresponding anatomically to the transverse fissure. Smaller pouches of the side branches are also found. Many side branches end as blind pouches, but others, particularly at the hilum, communicate with each other. At the bifurcation, side branches from several main bile ducts connect to form a plexus. The functional significance of these structures is not known. The blind pouches may serve to store or modify bile, whereas the biliary plexus provides anastomoses, which may allow exchange of material between the large bile ducts.

Like the intestine, the cystic, common hepatic, and common bile ducts possess mucosa, submucosa, and muscularis. The ducts are lined by a single layer of columnar epithelium. Mucus secreting tubular glands can be found at regular intervals in the submucosa, with openings to the surface of the mucosa.

The common bile duct is approximately 7 cm long, runs between layers of the lesser omentum, and lies anterior to the portal vein and to the right of the hepatic artery.[13] The common bile duct normally is approximately 0.5 to 1.5 cm in diameter.[16] The wall of the extrahepatic bile ducts is supported by a layer of connective tissue with an admixture of occasional smooth muscle fibers. The smooth muscle component is conspicuous only at the neck of the gallbladder and at the lower end of the common duct. The common bile duct passes retroperitoneally behind the first portion of the duodenum in a notch on the back of the head of the pancreas and enters the second part of the duodenum. The duct then passes obliquely through the posterior medial aspect of the duodenal wall and joins the main pancreatic duct to form the ampulla of Vater (see Fig. 52–3).[17, 18] The mucus membrane bulge produced by the ampulla forms an eminence, the duodenal papilla. In approximately 10% to 15% of patients, the bile and pancreatic ducts open separately into the duodenum. The common bile duct tapers to a diameter of 0.6 cm or less before its union with the pancreatic duct.[17]

As they course through the duodenal wall, the bile and pancreatic ducts are invested by a thickening of both the longitudinal and circular layers of smooth muscle (see Fig.

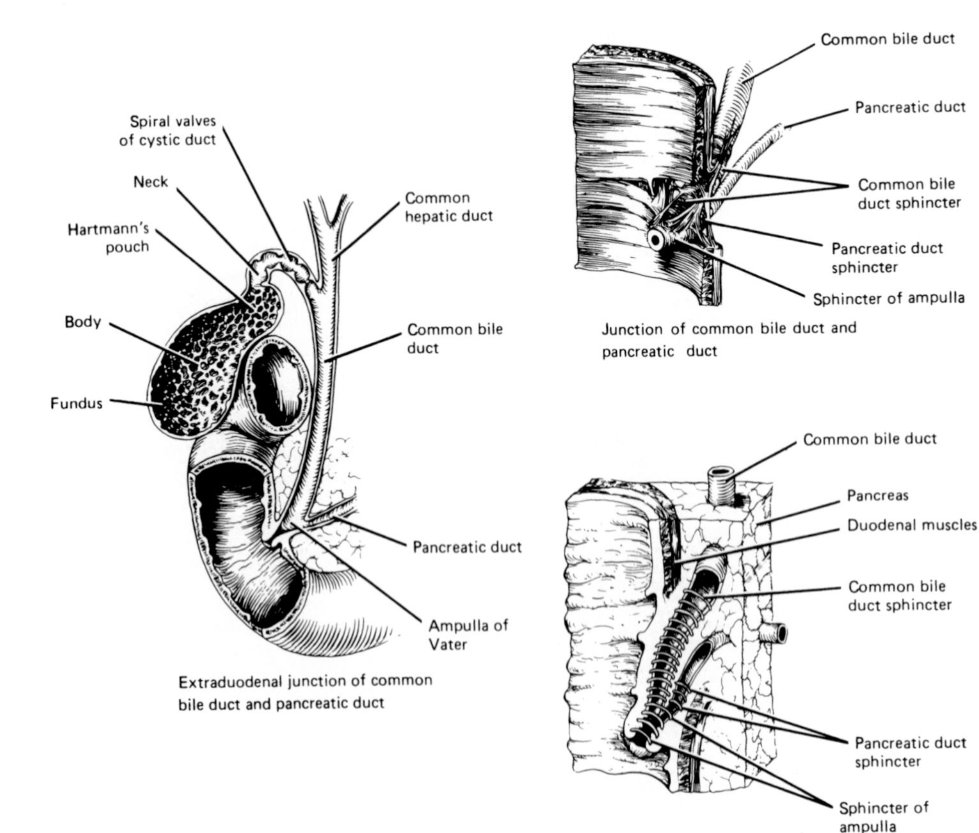

Figure 52–3. Schematic representation of the gallbladder, the extrahepatic biliary tract, and the choledochoduodenal junction. (From Lindner HH: Clinical Anatomy. East Norwalk, CT, Appleton & Lange, 1989.)

52–3) of the sphincter of Oddi.[11, 15, 17, 18] There is considerable variation in this structure, but it is usually composed of several parts: (1) the sphincter choledochus, which consists of circular muscle fibers that surround the intramural portion of the common duct immediately before its junction with the pancreatic duct; (2) a pancreatic sphincter, which is present in approximately one third of individuals and surrounds the intraduodenal portion of the pancreatic duct before its juncture with the ampulla; (3) the fasciculi longitudinales, which are composed of longitudinal muscle bundles that span intervals between the bile and pancreatic ducts; and (4) the sphincter ampullae, which consists of longitudinal muscle fibers that surround a sparse layer of circular fibers around the ampulla of Vater. The sphincter choledochus constricts the lumen of the bile duct and thus prevents the flow of bile. Contraction of the fasciculi longitudinales shortens the length of the ducts and thus promotes the flow of bile into the duodenum. The contraction of the sphincter ampullae shortens the ampulla and approximates the ampullary folds to prevent reflux of intestinal contents into the ducts. However, when both the pancreatic and common bile ducts end in the ampulla, contraction of the sphincter may cause reflux of bile into the pancreatic duct.

The arterial supply of the bile ducts arises mainly from the right hepatic artery.[16, 19] An extraordinarily rich plexus of capillaries surrounds bile ducts as they pass through the portal tracts.[13] Blood flowing through this peribiliary plexus empties into the hepatic sinusoids via the interlobular branches of the portal vein. The peribiliary plexus may modify biliary secretions through the bidirectional exchange of proteins, inorganic ions, and bile acids between blood and bile.

An abundant anastomotic network of blood vessels from branches of the hepatic and gastroduodenal arteries supplies the common bile duct.[16, 19] The supraduodenal portion of the duct is supplied by vessels running along its wall inferiorly from the retroduodenal artery and superiorly from the right hepatic artery. Injury to these blood vessels can result in bile duct stricturing.

The lymphatic vessels of the hepatic, cystic, and proximal portions of the common bile duct empty into glands at the hilum of the liver.[20] Lymphatics draining from the lower portion of the common bile duct drain into glands near the head of the pancreas.

Gallbladder

The gallbladder (see Fig. 52–3) is a storage reservoir that allows bile acids to be delivered in a high concentration and in a controlled manner to the duodenum for the solubilization of dietary lipid[13] (see Chapter 54). It lies in a fossa on the undersurface of the right lobe of the liver.[14] This distensible pear-shaped structure is 3 cm wide and 7 cm long in the adult and has a capacity of 30 to 50 mL.[21] The absorptive surface of the gallbladder is enhanced by numerous prominent folds.[13] The gallbladder is covered anteriorly by an adventitia that is fused with the capsule of the liver. On its posterior aspect and at the apex, it is covered by the visceral peritoneum. The portions of the gallbladder are the fundus, body, infundibulum, and neck. The anterior portion of the fundus is located at the level of the right lateral border of the musculus rectus abdominis and the ninth costal cartilage.[21] The posterior aspects of the fundus and body lie close to the transverse colon and duodenum, respectively. Thus, with perforation of the gallbladder, gallstones can readily penetrate into these structures. The infundibulum is an area of tapering between the gallbladder body and the neck. Hartmann's pouch is a bulging of the inferior surface of the infundibulum that lies close to the neck of the gallbladder. Gallstones can become impacted in Hartmann's pouch, thereby obstructing the cystic duct and producing cholecystitis. Extensive inflammation in Hartmann's pouch can lead to obstruction of the adjacent common bile duct (Mirizzi's syndrome).

The gallbladder is connected at its neck to the cystic duct, which empties into the common bile duct (see Fig. 52–3). The cystic duct is approximately 4 cm long and maintains continuity with the surface columnar epithelium, lamina propria, muscularis, and serosa of the gallbladder. The mucous membrane of the gallbladder neck forms the spiral valve of Heister, that is involved in regulating flow into and out of the gallbladder.

The gallbladder is supplied by the cystic artery, which usually arises from the right hepatic artery.[21] The artery divides into two branches near the neck of the gallbladder: a superficial branch that supplies the serosal surface and a deep branch that supplies the interior layers of the gallbladder wall. However, variations in the origin and course of the cystic artery are common. Because the cystic artery is an end artery, the gallbladder is particularly susceptible to ischemic injury and necrosis that result from inflammation or interruption of hepatic arterial flow.

The cystic vein provides venous drainage from the gallbladder and cystic ducts and commonly empties into the portal vein and occasionally directly into the hepatic sinusoids.[21]

The lymph vessels of the gallbladder are connected with the lymph vessels of Glisson's capsule. Subserous and submucosal lymphatics empty into a lymph gland near the neck of the gallbladder.

The sympathetic innervation of the gallbladder originates from the celiac axis and travels with branches of the hepatic artery and portal vein.[21] Visceral pain is conducted through sympathetic fibers and is frequently referred to the right subcostal, epigastric, and right scapular regions. Branches of both vagi provide parasympathetic innervation that likely contributes to the regulation of gallbladder motility.

The gallbladder is lined by a mucosa manifesting multiple ridges and folds and composed of a layer of columnar epithelial cells.[13, 22] The gallbladder wall consists of a mucosa, lamina propria, tunica muscularis, and serosa. The tunica muscularis is thick and invested with an interlocking array of longitudinal and spiral smooth muscle fibers. Tubuloalveolar glands are found in the region of the neck of the gallbladder and are involved in the production of mucus.[22] The Rokitansky-Aschoff sinuses are invaginations of the surface epithelium that may extend through the muscularis.[13] These structures can be a source of inflammation, most likely as a result of bacterial stasis and proliferation within the diverticulum. The ducts of Luschka may be observed along the hepatic surface of the gallbladder and open directly into the intrahepatic bile ducts rather than into the gallbladder cavity. These structures are thought to represent a developmental anomaly, and when they are present the gallbladder bed may have to be drained after cholecystectomy.

CONGENITAL ANOMALIES OF THE EXTRAHEPATIC DUCTS

Accessory bile ducts are aberrant ducts that drain individual segments of the liver; they may drain directly into the gallbladder, cystic duct, right and left hepatic ducts, or common bile duct.[14] In rare cases, the right hepatic duct may connect to the gallbladder or cystic duct. These anomalies must be recognized on cholangiography in order to prevent inadvertent transection or ligation of bile ducts during surgery.

Complete duplication of the common bile duct occurs rarely. In most cases, separate ducts drain the right and left lobes and open into the duodenum.

Variation in the drainage and course of the cystic duct is common.[14] Duplication of the cystic duct may also be encountered. The cystic duct is absent in most cases of agenesis of the gallbladder; rarely the duct alone may be absent, with the result that the gallbladder empties directly into the common hepatic duct.

CONGENITAL ANOMALIES OF THE GALLBLADDER

A number of structural anomalies of the gallbladder have been described.[23] Most of these defects are of no clinical importance, but occasionally the abnormal gallbladder may be a predisposing factor for bile stasis, inflammation, and formation of gallstones. Gallbladder disease in an anomalous or a malpositioned gallbladder may cause diagnostic confusion.

Congenital absence of the gallbladder may occur as an isolated anomaly or in association with other congenital malformations. The abnormality likely reflects a lack of development of the gallbladder bud or failure of the normal process of vacuolization. For example, extrahepatic biliary atresia is commonly associated with the absence of a gallbladder. Hypoplasia of the gallbladder has also been described, particularly in cystic fibrosis patients. Incomplete vacuolization of the solid endodermal cord during development can also result in congenital strictures of the gallbladder or cystic duct. Ectopic tissues of foregut endodermal origin may also be found within the gallbladder wall, including gastric, hepatic, adrenal, pancreatic, and thyroid tissues.

A double gallbladder is another rare malformation, which occurs in approximately 1 to 5 per 10,000 persons of the general population.[23, 24] The two gallbladders may share a single cystic duct, forming a Y-shaped channel, or each may have a distinct cystic duct that enters the common bile duct separately. Bilobed gallbladders and gallbladder diverticula are other rare anomalies.[23] A single gallbladder may be divided by longitudinal septa into multiple chambers, probably secondary to incomplete vacuolization of the solid gallbladder bud during morphogenesis.[25] Diverticula and septations of the gallbladder may promote bile stasis and gallstone formation.

Various malpositions of the gallbladder have also been described.[23, 26] Rarely, the gallbladder lies under the left lobe of the liver, to the left of the falciform ligament. This defect likely results from migration of the embryonic bud from the hepatic diverticula to the left rather than to the right. Some researchers have also proposed that there may be independent development of a second gallbladder from the left hepatic duct, with regression of the normal structure on the right. In other cases, a caudal bud that advances farther than the cranial bud may become buried within the cranial structure, creating an intrahepatic gallbladder. It is thought that if the caudal bud lags behind the movement of the cranial bud, a floating gallbladder results. In this setting, the gallbladder is covered completely with peritoneum and suspended from the undersurface of the liver by mesentery to the gallbladder or cystic duct. In this anomaly, the gallbladder is abnormally mobile and prone to torsion. Rarely, gallbladders have been found in the abdominal wall, falciform ligament, and retroperitoneum.

Several forms of "folded" gallbladders have been described. In one variant, the fundus appears to be bent, giving the appearance of a "Phrygian cap." The gallbladder is usually located in a retroserosal position, and the anomaly is thought to result from aberrant folding of the gallbladder within the embryonic fossa. Aberrant folding of the fossa during the early stages of development also can result in kinking between the body and the infundibulum of the gallbladder. Kinked gallbladders probably do not lead to clinical symptoms but may be a source of confusion in the interpretation of cholangiograms.

DISORDERS OF THE BILIARY TRACT IN CHILDREN

Cholestatic liver disease results from processes that interfere with either bile formation by hepatocytes or bile flow through the intrahepatic and extrahepatic biliary trees.[27] A number of these disorders result from defective ontogenesis as well as from a failure of postnatal adaptation to the extrauterine environment. This section provides a review of disorders that affect the biliary tract and occur in both infants and older children. There is a particular emphasis on neonatal cholangiopathies and the unique aspects of biliary disease in the older child (Table 52–1).[28] The general features of the many cholestatic liver diseases of the neonate are similar, and a central problem of pediatric hepatology is differentiating intrahepatic from extrahepatic cholestasis (Table 52–2). The treatment of metabolic or infective liver diseases and the surgical management of biliary anomalies require early diagnosis. Even when effective treatment is not possible, infants and children with progressive liver disease benefit from optimal nutritional support and medical management of chronic liver disease before they are referred for hepatic transplantation.

Because of the immaturity of hepatobiliary function, the number of distinct disorders that exhibit cholestatic jaundice may be greater during the neonatal period than at any other time of life (see Table 52–1). Liver dysfunction in the infant, regardless of the cause, is commonly associated with bile secretory failure and cholestatic jaundice. Although cholestasis may be traced to the level of the hepatocyte or the biliary apparatus, in practice there may be considerable over-

Table 52–1 | **Disorders of the Biliary Tract in Infants and Children**

Cholangiopathies
- Extrahepatic biliary atresia
- Choledochal cysts
- Spontaneous perforation of the common bile duct
- Mucous plug syndrome
- Sclerosing cholangitis (neonatal, inflammatory bowel disease [IBD]–associated, immunodeficiency)
- Paucity of intrahepatic bile ducts (syndromic and nonsyndromic)
- Caroli's disease
- Cystic fibrosis
- Biliary helminthiasis
- Idiopathic bile duct stricture (possibly congenital)
- Post-traumatic common duct stricture
- Bile duct tumors (intrinsic and extrinsic)
- Bile duct obstruction of pancreatic disease (inflammatory or neoplastic)
- Graft-versus-host disease
- Allograft rejection

Disorders of the Gallbladder
- Anomalies
- Cholelithiasis
- Acute cholecystitis
- Chronic cholecystitis
- Acalculous cholecystitis
- Acute hydrops of the gallbladder
- Tumors

Modified from Balistreri WF: Neonatal cholestasis: Lessons from the past, issues for the future. Semin Liver Dis 7:61, 1987.

lap among disorders with regard to the initial and subsequent sites of injury. For example, damage to the biliary epithelium often is a prominent feature of neonatal hepatitis that results from cytomegalovirus infection. Mechanical obstruction of the biliary tract invariably produces liver dysfunction and in the neonate may be associated with abnormalities of the parenchyma, such as giant cell transformation of hepatocytes. Whether giant cells, a frequent, nonspecific manifestation of neonatal liver injury, reflect the noxious effects of biliary obstruction or whether the hepatocytes and the biliary epithelium are damaged by a common agent during ontogenesis, such as a virus with tropism for both types of cells, is unknown. Furthermore, another histologic variable that often accompanies neonatal cholestasis is bile ductular paucity or a diminution in the number of interlobular bile ducts.[28] This finding may be of primary importance in patients with syndromic paucity of intrahepatic bile ducts but may also occur as an occasional feature of many other disorders, including idiopathic neonatal hepatitis, extrahepatic biliary atresia, and α_1-antitrypsin deficiency.[29] Serial liver biopsies usually show a progressive decrease in the number of bile ductules per portal tract, with a variable amount of associated inflammation.

Diagnosis of Biliary Tract Disease in Infants and Children

In most infants with cholestatic liver disease the condition appears during the first few weeks of life. Differentiating conjugated hyperbilirubinemia from the common unconjugated, physiologic hyperbilirubinemia of the neonate or the prolonged jaundice occasionally associated with breast-feeding is essential.[29] The possibility of liver or biliary tract disease must be considered in any neonate with jaundice older than 14 days. The stools of a patient with well-established biliary atresia are acholic; however, early in the course of incomplete or evolving biliary obstruction, the stools may appear normally or only intermittently pigmented. Life-threatening but treatable disorders such as bacterial infection and a number of inborn errors of metabolism must be excluded. Furthermore, the success of surgical procedures in relieving the biliary obstruction of biliary atresia or a choledochal cyst depends on early diagnosis and surgery.

The approach to the evaluation of an infant with cholestatic liver disease is outlined in Table 52–3. The initial assessment should establish promptly whether cholestatic jaundice is present and assess the severity of liver dysfunction. A more detailed investigation may be required and should be guided by the clinical features of the case. All relevant diagnostic tests need not be performed in every patient. For example, ultrasonography may promptly establish a diagnosis of a choledochal cyst in a neonate with jaundice and thus obviate the need to exclude infectious and metabolic causes of liver disease. Numerous routine and specialized biochemical tests and imaging procedures have been proposed to distinguish intrahepatic from extrahepatic cholestasis in infants and thereby preclude unnecessary surgical exploration.[30] Standard liver biochemical tests usually show variable elevations in serum direct bilirubin, aminotransferase, alkaline phosphatase, and lipid levels.[31] Unfortunately, no single test has proved to be of satisfactory discriminatory value, because at least 10% of infants with intrahepatic cholestasis have bile secretory failure sufficient to lead to an overlap in diagnostic test results with those suggestive of biliary atresia.[30] The presence of bile pigment in stools is sometimes cited as evidence against biliary atresia, but coloration of feces with secretions and epithelial cells that have been shed by the cholestatic patient may be misleading.

Ultrasonography can be used to assess the size and echogenicity of the liver. Even in neonates, high-frequency, real-time ultrasonography usually can define the presence and

Table 52–2 | **Relative Frequency of Various Forms of Neonatal Cholestasis**

DISORDER	CUMULATIVE PERCENTAGE
Idiopathic neonatal hepatitis	30–35
Extrahepatic biliary atresia	30
α_1-Antitrypsin deficiency	7–10
Intrahepatic cholestatic syndromes (Alagille's syndrome, Byler's disease, other)	5–6
Choledochal cyst	2–4
Bacterial sepsis	2
Hepatitis (cytomegalovirus, rubella, herpes, other)	3–5
Endocrinopathy (hypothyroidism, panhypopituitarism)	~1
Galactosemia	~1
Inborn errors of bile acid metabolism	~1
Other metabolic disorders	~1

Modified from Balistreri WF: Neonatal cholestasis: Lessons from the past, issues for the future. Semin Liver Dis 7:61, 1987.

Table 52–3 | **Evaluation of the Infant with Cholestasis**

History and Physical Examination
Include details of family history, pregnancy, presence of extrahepatic anomalies, and stool color
Tests to Establish the Presence and Severity of Liver Disease
Fractionated serum bilirubin analysis
Tests of liver dysfunction (AST, ALT, alkaline phosphatase, 5′ nucleotidase, gamma-glutamyl transpeptidase)
Tests of liver function (prothrombin time, partial thromboplastin time, coagulation factors, serum albumin level, serum ammonia level, serum cholesterol level, blood glucose)
Tests for Infection
Complete blood count
Bacterial cultures of blood, urine, and other sites if indicated
Paracentesis if ascites
Viral cultures
Serologic tests (HBsAg, TORCH, VDRL, EB virus, other)
Metabolic Studies
Urine for reducing substances
α_1-Antitrypsin level and phenotype
Sweat chloride analysis
Metabolic screen (urine and serum amino acids, urine organic acids)
Thyroid hormone, thyroid-stimulating hormone (evaluation of hypopituitarism as indicated)
Serum iron and ferritin
Urine and serum analysis of bile acids and bile acid precursors
Red blood cell galactose-1-phosphate uridyl transferase activity
Imaging Studies
Ultrasonography of liver and biliary tract
Hepatobiliary scintigraphy
Radiography of long bones and skull for congenital infection and chest for lung and cardiac disease
Percutaneous or endoscopic cholangiography (rarely indicated)
Procedures
Duodenal intubation to assess fluid for bile pigment
Percutaneous liver biopsy (for light and electron microscopic examination, enzymologic evaluation)
Bone marrow examination and skin fibroblast culture for suspected storage disease
Exploratory laparotomy and intraoperative cholangiography

ALT, alanine aminotransferase; AST, aspartate aminotransferase; EB, Epstein-Barr; HBsAg, hepatitis B surface antigen; TORCH, toxoplasmosis, rubella, cytomegalovirus, herpesvirus; VDRL, Venereal Disease Research Laboratory.

size of the gallbladder, detect stones and sludge in the bile ducts and gallbladder, and demonstrate cystic or obstructive dilatation of the biliary system. Extrahepatic anomalies also may be identified. A triangular cord or bandlike periportal echogenicity (3 mm or greater in thickness), which represents a cone shaped fibrotic mass cranial to the portal vein, appears to be a specific ultrasonographic finding in the early diagnosis of biliary atresia.[32]

Computed tomography provides information similar to that obtained by ultrasonography but is less suitable in patients younger than 2 years because of the paucity of intra-abdominal fat for contrast and the need for heavy sedation or general anesthesia.

Magnetic resonance cholangiography (MRC), performed with T2-weighted turbo spin echo sequences, is widely used to assess the biliary tract in all age groups. In a 1999 study, MRC reliably demonstrated the common bile duct and gallbladder in normal neonates.[33] In a small number of patients with biliary atresia, nonvisualization of the common bile duct and demonstration of a small gallbladder have been characteristic MRC findings.[33] In biliary atresia, MRC may show a triangular area of high signal intensity in the porta hepatis that may represent cystic dilatation of the fetal bile duct. Further studies are required before the reliability of MRC in evaluating the cholestatic infant can be established.

The use of hepatobiliary scintigraphic imaging agents such as ^{99m}Tc iminodiacetic acid derivatives may be helpful in differentiating extrahepatic biliary atresia from other causes of neonatal jaundice. Unfortunately, a 1997 study showed that in 50% of patients who had a paucity of interlobular bile ducts but no extrahepatic obstruction, biliary excretion of radionuclide was absent.[34] Twenty-five percent of patients who had idiopathic neonatal hepatitis also demonstrated no biliary excretion. However, the modality remains useful for assessing cystic duct patency in a patient with a hydropic gallbladder or cholelithiasis.

Percutaneous transhepatic cholangiopancreatography may be of value in visualizing the biliary tract in selected patients.[35] However, the technique is more difficult to perform in infants than in adults because the intrahepatic bile ducts are small and because most disorders that occur in infants do not result in dilatation of the biliary tree. Endoscopic retrograde cholangiography (ERCP) may be useful in evaluating children with extrahepatic biliary obstruction and has been performed successfully in a small number of cholestatic neonates.[36] Considerable technical expertise is required of the operator to complete this procedure in infants. Most neonates require general anesthesia for a satisfactory examination. The greater availability of specially designed pediatric duodenoscopes may allow the more widespread use of ERCP in infants with obstructive jaundice.

Percutaneous liver biopsy is particularly valuable in evaluating cholestatic patients and can be used for even the smallest infants with only sedation and local anesthesia.[29, 37] For example, a diagnosis of extrahepatic biliary atresia can be made on the basis of clinical and histologic criteria in 90% to 95% of patients. When doubt about the diagnosis persists, the patency of the biliary tree can be examined directly by a minilaparotomy and operative cholangiogram.

DISEASES OF THE BILE DUCTS

Extrahepatic Biliary Atresia

Extrahepatic biliary atresia is characterized by the complete obstruction of bile flow as a result of the destruction or absence of all or a portion of the extrahepatic bile ducts.[38] The disorder occurs in 1 in 10,000 to 15,000 live births and accounts for approximately one third of cases of neonatal cholestatic jaundice (see Table 52–2). It is the most frequent cause of death from liver disease and of referral for liver transplantation in children (approximately 50% of all cases).[39]

The cause of extrahepatic biliary atresia is unknown. The disease is not inherited, and there have been several reports of dizygotic and monozygotic twins discordant for biliary atresia.[38] In a study of 461 patients in France, seasonality, time clustering, and time-space clustering could not be demonstrated.[40] A significant increase in human leukocyte antigen B12 (HLA-B12) has been found among biliary atresia patients who had no associated anomalies. The HLA haplotypes -A9, -B5, -A28, and -B35 also have been found more

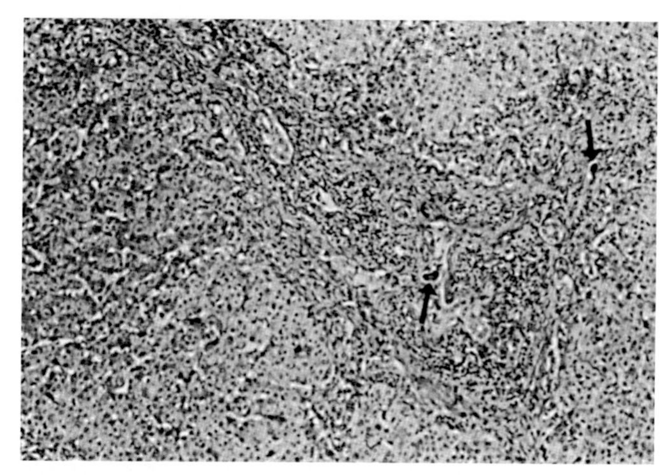

Figure 52–4. Histopathologic findings in an infant aged 4 weeks with extrahepatic biliary atresia. The portal tract is expanded by fibrous tissue, proliferating bile ductules, and a moderate inflammatory infiltrate. Bile plugs *(arrows)* are seen in several of the bile ductules. The hepatic parenchyma is well preserved.

frequently.[41] Familial cases have been reported rarely; in most a detailed histologic description of the extrahepatic biliary tree was not provided to exclude narrowing, or hypoplasia, of the common duct associated with severe intrahepatic cholestasis.[42] Rare cases of biliary atresia have been documented in stillborn or premature infants. There is no evidence that biliary atresia results from a failure in morphogenesis or recanalization of the bile duct during embryonic development. Clinical features support the concept that in most cases, injury to the biliary tract occurs after birth.[43]

Extrahepatic anomalies occur in 10% to 25% of patients and include cardiovascular defects, polysplenia, malrotation, situs inversus, and bowel atresias.[44, 45] Some patients who have heterotaxia, including an infant with biliary atresia and polysplenia, have been found to have loss of function mutations in the *CFC1* gene.[46] This gene encodes for a protein called CRYPTIC, which is involved in establishing the left-right axis during morphogenesis. A rare type of fetal biliary atresia in which congenital malformations are often found and cholestatic jaundice is present from birth has been recognized. In this disorder, a bile duct remnant cannot be found in the ligamentum hepatoduodenale at exploratory laparotomy, indicating that the extrahepatic ducts did not develop completely or were destroyed during fetal life.[38, 43]

Several mechanisms have been proposed to account for the progressive obliteration of the extrahepatic biliary tree.[47, 48] At present, there is little support for an ischemic or toxic origin of extrahepatic bile duct injury.[49] Congenital infections with cytomegalovirus, rubella virus, human herpesvirus 6, and papillomavirus occasionally have been implicated.[50] Reovirus type 3 has been implicated on the basis of the serologic evaluation of patients and immunolocalization of reovirus 3 antigens in a bile duct remnant of a patient with biliary atresia.[51, 52] The results of studies on the role of reovirus in biliary atresia have been contradictory. However, in a 1998 report, reovirus RNA was detected by reverse-transcriptase polymerase chain reaction methodology in hepatic or biliary tissues, or both, of 55% of patients who had biliary atresia and 78% of patients who had choledochal cysts.[53] Reovirus RNA also was found in extracts of hepatic or biliary tissue from 21% of patients who had other hepatobiliary diseases and 12% of autopsy cases. Initial reports of the involvement of group C rotavirus in biliary atresia have not been confirmed.[54, 55]

Pathology

Histopathologic findings on initial liver biopsy are of great importance in the management of biliary atresia patients.[43, 56] Early in the course, there generally is good preservation of the hepatic architecture with a variable degree of bile ductular proliferation, canalicular and cellular bile stasis, and portal tract edema and fibrosis (Fig. 52–4).[37, 43] The presence of bile plugs in portal triads is highly suggestive of large duct obstruction. Furthermore, bile ductules show varying injury to the biliary epithelium, including swelling, vacuolization, and even sloughing of cells into the lumen. Portal tracts may be infiltrated with inflammatory cells, and in approximately 25% of patients there may be giant cell transformation of hepatocytes to a degree more commonly observed in neonatal hepatitis. Bile ductules occasionally may assume a ductal plate configuration (Fig. 52–5), suggesting that the disease process has interfered with the process of ductular remodeling that occurs during prenatal development. Biliary cirrhosis may be present initially or may evolve rapidly over the first months of life, with or without the successful restoration of bile flow.

The morbid anatomic characteristics of the extrahepatic bile ducts in biliary atresia are highly variable. Kasai proposed a useful classification of the anatomic variants.[57] Three main types have been defined on the basis of the site of the atresia. Type I is atresia of the common bile duct with patent proximal ducts. Type II atresia involves the hepatic duct, with cystically dilated bile ducts at the porta hepatis. In type IIa atresia, the cystic and common ducts are patent, whereas in type IIb atresia, these structures also are obliterated. These forms of biliary atresia have been referred to as "surgically correctable" but unfortunately account for less than 10% of all cases. Ninety percent or more of pa-

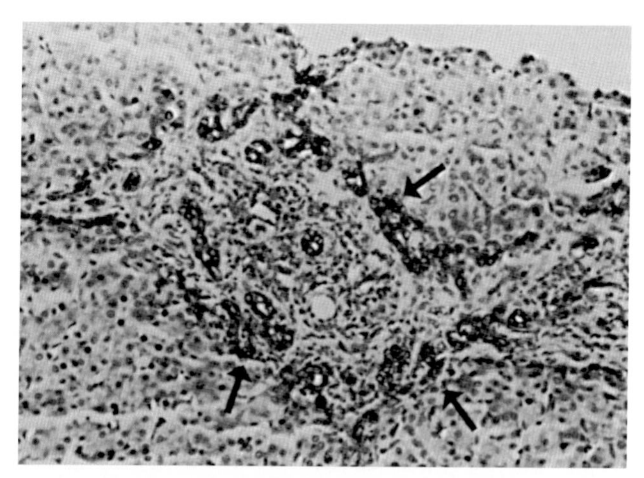

Figure 52–5. Histopathologic findings in extrahepatic biliary atresia. Immunoperoxidase stain for cytokeratin. This expanded portal tract is encircled by positively staining bile ductules *(arrows)* arranged in the pattern of the ductal plate malformation. (Photomicrograph courtesy of Dr. Brian West, University of Texas, Galveston.)

tients have type III atresia, involving obstruction of the common, hepatic, and cystic ducts, without cystically dilated hilar ducts. The entire perihilar area is in a cone of dense fibrous tissue. The gallbladder is involved to some extent in approximately 80% of patients. The type III variant has been characterized as noncorrectable, in that there are no patent hepatic or dilated hilar ducts that can be used for a biliary-enteric anastomosis.

Complete fibrous obliteration of at least a portion of the extrahepatic bile ducts is a consistent feature found on microscopic examination of the fibrous remnant.[43] Other segments of the biliary tree may demonstrate lumens with varying degeneration of bile duct epithelial cells, inflammation, and fibrosis in the periductular tissues (Fig. 52–6).[58] In most patients, bile ducts within the liver that extend to the porta hepatis are patent during the first weeks of life but are destroyed progressively, presumably by the same process that damaged the extrahepatic ducts and by the effects of biliary obstruction. In more than 20% of patients, concentric tubular ductal structures similar to those observed in ductal plate malformations are found, indicating that the disease process interfered with the normal remodeling of the biliary tract.[58, 59]

Clinical Features

Most infants with biliary atresia are born at term after a normal pregnancy and have a normal birth weight.[38] Female infants are affected more commonly than male infants. The perinatal course is typically unremarkable. Postnatal weight gain and development usually proceed normally. Jaundice is observed by the parents or the physician after the period of physiologic hyperbilirubinemia. The possibility of liver or biliary tract disease must be considered in any neonate older than 14 days with jaundice.[60] The stools of a patient with well-established biliary atresia are acholic; however, early in the course the stools may appear normally pigmented or only intermittently pigmented.[38, 61]

The liver is typically enlarged with a firm edge palpable 2 to 6 cm below the right costal margin.[38, 62] The spleen is usually not enlarged early in the course but becomes enlarged as portal hypertension develops. Ascites and edema are not present initially, but coagulopathy may result from vitamin K deficiency.

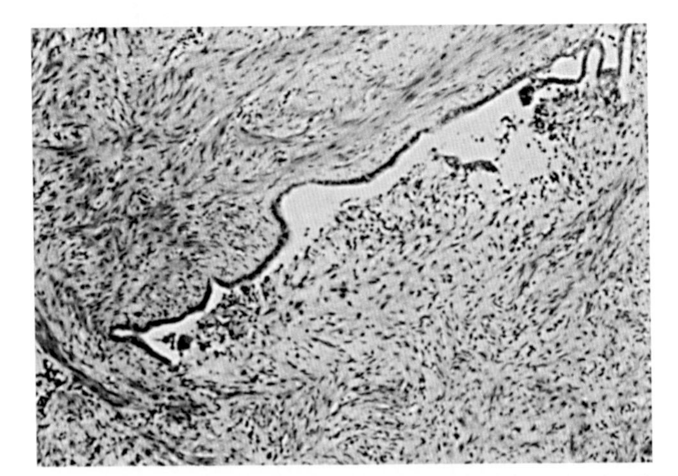

Figure 52–6. The fibrous remnant in extrahepatic biliary atresia. The common bile duct is surrounded by dense fibrous connective tissue and an inflammatory cell infiltrate. Necrosis and sloughing of a substantial portion of the epithelial lining can be observed.

Laboratory studies initially reveal evidence of cholestasis, with a serum bilirubin level of 6 to 12 mg/dL, at least 50% of which is conjugated.[61] Serum aminotransferase and alkaline phosphatase levels are moderately elevated. Serum gamma-glutamyl transpeptidase and 5′ nucleotidase levels are also elevated.[63]

Surgical Management

When the possibility of biliary atresia has been raised by clinical, pathologic, and imaging findings, exploratory laparotomy and operative cholangiography are necessary to document the site of obstruction and to direct attempts at surgical treatment.[57, 62] Sometimes, frozen sections of the transected porta hepatis are obtained to evaluate the presence and size of ductal remnants. However, the surgeon should avoid transection of the biliary tree, which may be patent but small as a result of biliary hypoplasia or markedly diminished bile flow associated with intrahepatic cholestasis. Patent proximal portions of the bile ducts or cystic structures in the porta hepatis allow conventional anastomosis with a segment of bowel in approximately 10% of patients.[38, 62] In most patients who have obliteration of the proximal extrahepatic biliary tree, the preferred surgical approach is the hepatoportoenterostomy procedure developed by Kasai.[57] The distal common bile duct is transected, and the fibrous bile duct remnant is dissected to an area above the bifurcation of the portal vein. The dissection then progresses backward and laterally at this level, and the fibrous cone of tissue is transected flush with the liver surface, thereby exposing an area that may contain residual, microscopic bile ducts. The operation is completed by the anastomosis of a Roux-en-Y loop of jejunum around the bare edge of the transected tissue to provide a conduit for biliary drainage. A number of modifications of the enteric anastomosis, most involving exteriorization of the Roux-en-Y loop with diversion of the bile to the skin, have been used in an effort to decrease the high incidence of postoperative ascending cholangitis.[38] However, there may be severe fluid and electrolyte losses from the stoma and, eventually, massive bleeding from peristomal varices.[64] There also is little evidence that the frequency of postoperative bacterial cholangitis is reduced through the use of these procedures. Many surgeons perform the original Kasai operation to prevent these complications and to permit liver transplantation, if required later.[65] Multiple attempts at reexploration and revision of nonfunctional conduits also should be avoided.[38]

Prognosis

The prognosis of untreated biliary atresia is extremely poor; death from liver failure usually occurs within 2 years. Of 88 patients in the Biliary Atresia Registry (Surgical Section, American Academy of Pediatrics) who have had either no surgery or a simple exploratory laparotomy, only 1 patient survived for more than 3 years.[66] In the same series, follow-up data from numerous pediatric surgeons and practice settings in the United States disclosed a 5-year actuarial survival rate of 48% among 670 patients who had a Kasai operation (Fig. 52–7). Several large series from Europe and Japan have demonstrated similar or slightly better results.[67, 68] With regard to long-term survival, a nationwide survey among the major pediatric centers in Japan showed that only 325 of 2013 patients survived more than 10 years, and only 157 (7.8%) remained free of jaundice with normal liver function.[68, 69] In a series of all biliary atresia patients identified in France over a period of 10 years (1986–1996), the overall survival rate of infants treated with the Kasai operation and, if necessary, liver transplantation was 68%.[70] The 10-year actuarial survival rate in patients with their native liver was 29%, a figure similar to the 31% compiled from 750 published cases by the authors.[70] Thus, children with biliary atresia derive long-term benefit from the hepatic portoenterostomy procedure, although most have some persisting liver dysfunction. Progressive biliary cirrhosis may result in death from hepatic failure or the need for liver transplantation despite an apparently successful restoration of bile flow.[70]

Several factors have been found to contribute to the varying outcome after hepatic portoenterostomy. The age of the patient at the time of surgery is most critical.[38, 40] In several series, bile flow was reestablished in 80% to 90% of infants who were referred for surgery within 60 days of birth.[38] In the series of Ohi and associates, more than 70% of patients survived for at least 10 years, albeit with varying degrees of liver disease and portal hypertension.[71] In contrast, a success rate of less than 20% was observed in infants who were at least 90 days old at the time of surgery, and few long-term survivors were observed. In the U.S. series, predictors of a poor outcome were white race, surgery at more than 60 days of age, cirrhosis indicated by the initial biopsy, totally nonpatent extrahepatic ducts, and absent ducts at the level of transection in the liver hilum.[38, 72] Independent prognostic factors for overall survival in the large French study were the performance of the Kasai operation and age at surgery less than 45 days.[40] Complete atresia of extrahepatic bile ducts and polysplenia syndrome were associated with a less favorable outcome. The experience of the surgical center was also important.[40] A normal serum bilirubin level 3 months after surgery was predictive of long-term survival.[73, 74] Prehilar bile duct structures of at least 150 to 400 μm, particularly if lined with columnar epithelium, have been associated in some studies with a favorable prognosis.[75, 76] The quantity of the bile flow has been correlated with the total area of the biliary ductules identified in the excised porta hepatis specimen.[77]

The rate of progression of the underlying bile ductular and liver disease also limits survival.[78, 79] The disorder is not limited to the extrahepatic biliary tree and can be associated with progressive inflammation, destruction of the intrahepatic bile ducts, and eventual cirrhosis.[78] Recurring episodes of ascending bacterial cholangitis, which are most frequent during the first 2 years after surgery, can contribute to the ongoing bile duct injury and even lead to reobstruction.[38, 80] Cholangitis develops primarily in infants who have some degree of bile drainage, probably because of the access to ascending infection provided by patent bile ducts in the porta hepatis. Substantial hepatocyte injury, as indicated by lobular disarray and giant cell transformation, has also been associated with a poor outcome.[79]

Liver transplantation is essential in the management of children in whom portoenterostomy does not successfully restore bile flow, referral is late (probably at 120 days of age or later), and end-stage liver disease eventually develops despite bile drainage.[81] The portoenterostomy is thought to make liver transplantation more technically difficult as a result of intra-abdominal adhesions and the various enteric conduits that are encountered.[82, 83] However, with the use of reduced-size liver allografts and living-related donors, 1-year survival rates have exceeded 90% in several series.[84]

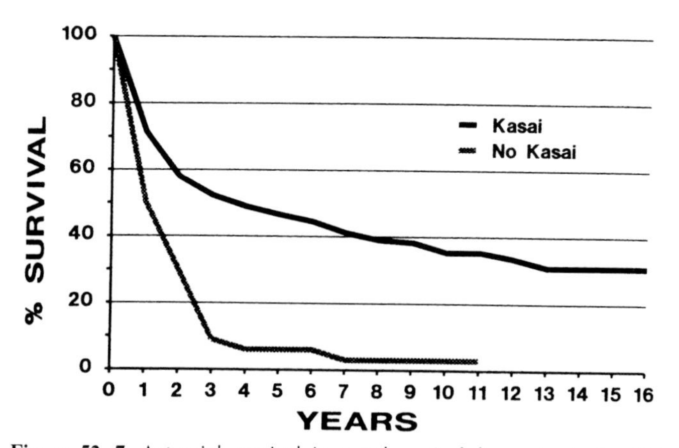

Figure 52–7. Actuarial survival in extrahepatic biliary atresia for 670 infants undergoing Kasai's portoenterostomy and 88 undergoing no operation or only an exploratory laparotomy. Average length of follow-up was 5 years. The groups are statistically different (P = .001). The mean extended length of survival in the group not undergoing the Kasai procedure is attributable to a single patient reported to be alive 11 years after exploratory laparotomy in infancy. (From Karrer FM, Lilly JR, Stewart, BA, et al: Biliary atresia registry: 1976 to 1989. J Pediatr Surg 25:1076, 1990.)

Spontaneous Perforation of the Common Bile Duct

Spontaneous perforation of the common bile duct is a rare but distinct cholestatic disorder of infancy.[85] The perforation usually occurs at the junction of the cystic and common ducts. The cause is unknown, but there may be evidence of obstruction at the distal end of the common bile duct secondary to stenosis or inspissated bile. Congenital weakness at the site of the perforation and injury produced by infection have also been suggested.

Clinical signs, including jaundice, acholic stools, dark urine, and ascites, typically occur during the first months of life.[86] The infant also may experience vomiting and lack of weight gain. Progressive abdominal distention is a usual feature; bile staining of fluid within umbilical or inguinal hernias may be observed.

Mild to moderate conjugated hyperbilirubinemia with minimal elevation of serum aminotransferase levels is typical. Abdominal paracentesis reveals clear bile-stained ascitic fluid, which usually is sterile. Ultrasonography reveals ascites or loculated fluid in the right upper quadrant; the biliary tree is not dilated. Hepatobiliary scintigraphy demonstrates the free accumulation of isotope within the peritoneal cavity.[86]

Operative cholangiography is required to demonstrate the

site of the perforation. Surgical treatment may involve simple drainage of the bilious ascites and repair of the site of the perforation. However, if the perforation is associated with obstruction of the common bile duct, drainage via a cholecystojejunostomy may be required.[86, 87]

Bile Plug Syndrome

A plug of thick, inspissated bile and mucus also may cause obstruction of the common bile duct.[86, 88] Otherwise healthy infants have been affected, but the condition occurs more commonly in sick premature infants who cannot be fed and require prolonged parenteral nutrition. The pathogenesis may involve bile stasis, fasting, infection, and an increased bilirubin load. The cholestasis associated with massive hemolysis, or the inspissated bile syndrome, may have been a variant of the bile plug syndrome but is now infrequent with measures to prevent and treat Rh and ABO blood group incompatibilities. The clinical presentation may resemble that of biliary atresia. Ultrasonography may show dilated intrahepatic bile ducts. Exploratory laparotomy and operative cholangiography usually are required for diagnosis. Simple irrigation of the common bile duct is curative.[86]

Primary Sclerosing Cholangitis

Primary sclerosing cholangitis (PSC) is an uncommon, chronic, progressive disease of the biliary tract characterized by inflammation and fibrosis of the intrahepatic and extrahepatic biliary ductal systems leading eventually to biliary cirrhosis.[89] Only aspects of PSC that are of particular importance to infants and children are discussed here (see Chapter 59 for a detailed discussion of PSC). PSC is a pathologic process that occurs in the absence of choledocholithiasis or a history of bile duct surgery. In adults, carcinoma of the bile ducts must also be excluded; however, this complication has not been reported in children. PSC is associated with inflammatory bowel disease (most often, ulcerative colitis) in 70% of adult patients.[90] However, this association is seen in fewer than one half of affected children.[89, 90] A male preponderance has been reported in some, but not all, large series of children with PSC. More than 200 cases of PSC have been reported in children, and most of these have occurred since the mid-1980s, presumably as a result of improvements in pediatric cholangiography.

The onset of PSC has been reported in the neonatal period and accounted for 15 of 56 cases in a 1994 series of children with the disorder.[89] Cholestatic jaundice and acholic stools were observed within the first 2 weeks of life. The presenting features were virtually identical to those of extrahepatic biliary atresia. However, percutaneous cholecystography disclosed a biliary system that was patent but exhibited rarefaction of segmental branches, stenosis, and focal dilatation of the intrahepatic bile ducts. The extrahepatic bile ducts were involved in six of eight patients. Jaundice subsided spontaneously within 6 months, but later in childhood all patients had clinical and biochemical features consistent with biliary cirrhosis and portal hypertension. In contrast with PSC in adults and older children, PSC in neonates has not been associated with intestinal disease.

Inflammatory bowel disease–associated PSC usually occurs in patients with ulcerative colitis, although cases have been reported in patients with Crohn's disease.[89] The bowel symptoms can precede, occur simultaneously with, or appear years after the diagnosis of PSC. As in adults, treatment of the bowel disease in infants, including colectomy, does not influence the progression of PSC.

Lesions similar to those of PSC have been defined by cholangiography in histiocytosis X (Langerhans' cell histiocytosis), but the process is caused by histiocytic infiltration and progressive scarring of portal tracts, with resulting distortion of intrahepatic bile ducts.[89] Cholestasis can occur before the diagnosis of histocytosis X has been established but most often is found later. Children with histiocytosis X may have involvement of multiple organs, including diabetes insipidus, bone lesions, skin lesions, lymphadenopathy, and exophthalmos. Chemotherapy does not affect the course of the biliary tract disease. Liver transplantation has been successful in several children who experienced progression to end-stage liver disease.[91]

In some children with a variety of immunodeficiencies, both cellular and humoral, sclerosing cholangitis appears to develop.[89] *Cryptosporidia* and *Cytomegalovirus* have been found concurrently in the biliary tract in some of these patients, as well as in adults with the acquired immunodeficiency syndrome. Treatment of the associated infection has no proven effect on the biliary tract disease.

There is no definitive diagnostic test for PSC; the diagnosis is based on a combination of biochemical, histologic, and radiologic data.[90] Typically, adult patients exhibit fatigue, weight loss, pruritus, right upper quadrant pain, and intermittent jaundice. In children, the clinical presentation is more variable; the most common symptoms are abdominal pain, jaundice, and chronic diarrhea. Physical examination sometimes reveals hepatomegaly, which may be associated with splenomegaly, scleral icterus, and, rarely, ascites.

The serum alkaline phosphatase level is often elevated in PSC, and serum aminotransferase levels may be mildly elevated. However, in a 1995 series, 15 of 32 patients had a normal alkaline phosphatase level on presentation.[90] Hyperbilirubinemia is seen in less than one half of pediatric patients. Serum autoantibodies, including antinuclear antibody and anti–smooth muscle antibodies, may be found in some patients. Antineutrophil cytoplasmic antibody may be detected.

On liver biopsy, the histologic findings may be suggestive of PSC but usually are not diagnostic. Characteristic concentric periductal fibrosis ("onion skin") may be present, but more often, only neoductular proliferation and fibrosis are found.[90] Differentiating PSC from autoimmune hepatitis, particularly in the presence of circulating non–organ-specific autoantibodies and hepatitic features on liver biopsy, may be difficult.[90, 92]

The diagnosis of PSC is established by cholangiography.[89] Endoscopic retrograde cholangiopancreatography is the method of choice for visualizing the intrahepatic and extrahepatic bile ducts. Percutaneous transhepatic cholangiography and MRC are other options. Irregularities of the intrahepatic and extrahepatic ducts can be found, including alternating strictures and areas of dilatation that produce a beaded appearance. Involvement of the intrahepatic bile ducts predominates in patients whose condition appears after the neonatal period. Occasionally, dominant strictures of the extrahepatic ducts or papillary stenosis is found.

The prognosis of PSC in children is guarded. The clinical course of the disorder is variable but usually progressive. In a 1994 series of 56 children, the median survival time from onset of symptoms was approximately 10 years, similar to that reported in adults.[89] Analysis of survival factors at presentation indicates that older age, splenomegaly, and prolonged prothrombin time predicted a poor outcome.[90] The occurrence of jaundice after the neonatal period with a persisting serum bilirubin level of more than five times the normal value was also associated with a poor outcome. Hepatocellular carcinoma also may occur, but cholangiocarcinoma, an important complication of adult PSC, has not been reported in children.

The treatment of PSC in children is unsatisfactory.[89, 90] There are no published reports of controlled trials that demonstrate convincingly that any medical therapy improves histologic characteristics and prolongs survival. Uncontrolled experience has suggested some benefit of immunosuppressive therapy with prednisone and azathioprine. Ursodeoxycholic acid therapy in adults and in a limited number of children has led to an improvement in clinical symptoms and in liver test abnormalities, but the long-term benefits of treatment are uncertain.[93] Liver transplantation is an important option for patients who experience progression to end-stage liver disease; long-term results in children appear to be excellent, with no reports of recurrent PSC in the transplanted organ.[94] In contrast, recurrent PSC has been reported in adults after liver transplantation.

Choledochal Cysts

Incidence and Classification

Choledochal cysts are congenital anomalies of the biliary tract that are manifested by cystic dilatation of the extrahepatic and intrahepatic bile ducts.[95] The incidence rate of choledochal cysts is 1 in 13,000 to 15,000 in Western countries and as high as 1 in 1000 in Japan.[96] They are not familial; female patients are more commonly affected than male patients. Cases have been described in utero and in elderly patients, but approximately two thirds of patients seek medical attention before the age of 10.

The classification proposed by Todani and others (Fig. 52–8) is cited frequently.[97, 98] Several varieties of type I cysts, accounting for 80% to 90% of cases, exhibit segmental or diffuse fusiform dilatation of the common bile duct. Type II cysts consist of a true choledochal diverticulum. Type III cysts consist of dilatation of the intraduodenal portion of the common bile duct, or choledochocele. Type IV cysts may be subdivided into type IVa, or multiple intrahe-

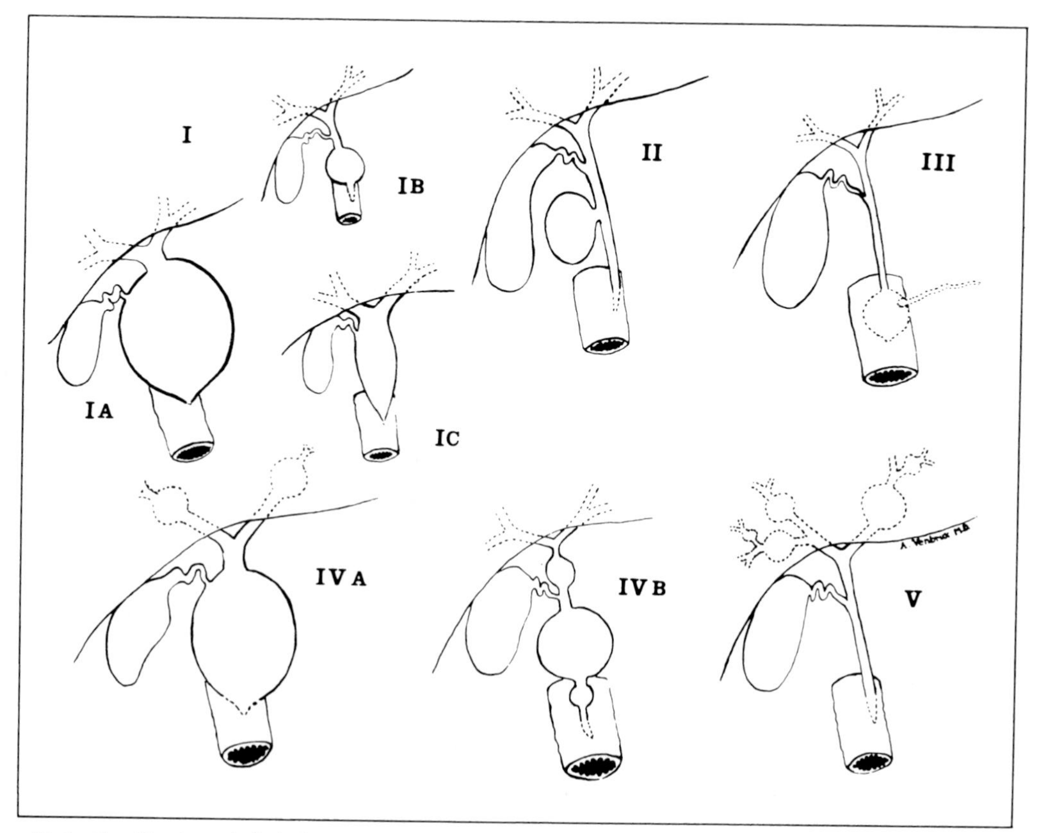

Figure 52–8. Classification of choledochal cysts according to Todani and colleagues.[97] Ia, common type; Ib, segmental dilatation; Ic, diffuse dilatation; II, diverticulum; III, choledochocoele; IVa, multiple cysts (intra- and extrahepatic); IVb, multiple cysts (extrahepatic); V, single or multiple dilatations of the intrahepatic ducts. (From Savader SJ, Benenati JF, Venbrux AC, et al: Choledochal cysts: Classification and cholangiographic appearance. AJR 156:327, 1991.)

patic and extrahepatic cysts, and type IVb, or multiple extrahepatic cysts. The type IVb variant either is uncommon or may overlap with type I. It is not settled whether type V, or Caroli's disease, which consists of a single or multiple dilatations of the intrahepatic ductal system, should be viewed as a form of choledochal cyst.

Etiology

The cause of choledochal cysts has not been established. Congenital weakness of the bile duct wall, a primary abnormality of epithelial proliferation during embryologic ductal development, and congenital obstruction of bile ducts have been suggested. A relationship to other obstructive cholangiopathies, such as biliary atresia, has been proposed but not proved.[47] Reovirus RNA has been detected by reverse-transcriptase polymerase chain reaction methodology in hepatic or biliary tissues of 78% of patients who have choledochal cysts.[53] A high incidence rate (40%) of an anomalous junction of the pancreatic and common bile ducts, which may allow reflux of pancreatic secretions into the biliary tree, has been described. This process may result in progressive injury to the developing ductal system, with subsequent weakness and dilatation.

Pathology

The cysts are composed of a fibrous wall; there may be no epithelial lining or a low columnar epithelium.[99] Mild chronic inflammation may be present. Complete, inflammatory obstruction of the terminal portion of the common bile duct is common in infants who have a choledochal cyst.

Liver biopsy in the affected neonate shows typical features of large duct obstruction.[47] Findings may mimic those observed in extrahepatic biliary atresia. Portal tract edema, bile ductular proliferation, and fibrosis may be prominent. A pattern of biliary cirrhosis may be observed in older patients with long-standing biliary obstruction. Carcinoma of the cyst wall may occur by adolescence.[95, 96]

Clinical Features

The infantile form of choledochal cyst disease must be distinguished from other forms of hepatobiliary disease of the neonate, particularly biliary atresia.[96, 100] Disease often appears during the first months of life, and as many as 80% of patients have cholestatic jaundice and acholic stools. Vomiting, irritability, and failure to thrive may occur. Examination reveals hepatomegaly and in approximately one half of patients a palpable abdominal mass. In a series of 72 patients diagnosed postnatally, 50 (69%) exhibited jaundice, which was associated with abdominal pain in 25 or with a palpable mass in 3; 13 (18%) had abdominal pain alone, and 2 (3%) had a palpable mass. Spontaneous perforation of a choledochal cyst may occur, particularly when bile flow is obstructed. Progressive hepatic injury can occur during the first months of life as a result of biliary obstruction. Portal hypertension and ascites may ensue.

In older patients, epigastric pain, which may result from pancreatitis, is the most common symptom. Intermittent jaundice and fever may result from recurrent episodes of cholangitis. The classic triad of abdominal pain, jaundice, and a palpable abdominal mass is observed in less than 20% of patients.

Diagnosis

The diagnosis of a choledochal cyst is best established by ultrasonography (Fig. 52–9).[35] In fact, several reports have demonstrated that antenatal ultrasonography can be used to detect a choledochal cyst in the fetus.[101] Sequential ultrasonographic examinations have allowed the study of the evolution of choledochal cysts during pregnancy. In the older child, percutaneous transhepatic cholangiography or ERCP may help define the anatomic features of the cyst; its site of biliary origin, including an anomalous arrangement of the pancreaticobiliary junction; and the extent of both extrahepatic and intrahepatic disease, including the presence of intraductal strictures and calculi.[35] Magnetic resonance cholangiography is being used increasingly to evaluate the extent of the cyst and defects within the biliary tree and to detect an anomalous junction of the pancreaticobiliary duct.[102] In practice, most pediatric surgeons rely on an operative cholangiogram to define the extent of intrahepatic and extrahepatic disease.

Treatment

Preferred treatment is surgical excision of the cyst with reconstruction of the extrahepatic biliary tree.[95, 96] Biliary drainage is usually accomplished by a choledochojejunostomy with a Roux-en-Y anastomosis. Excision of the cyst reduces bile stasis and the risk of cholangitis and malignancy. Simple decompression and internal drainage should be done only when the complicated anatomic characteristics do not allow complete excision. Long-term follow-up is essential, because recurrent cholangitis, lithiasis, anastomotic stricture, and pancreatitis may develop years after the initial surgery.[103]

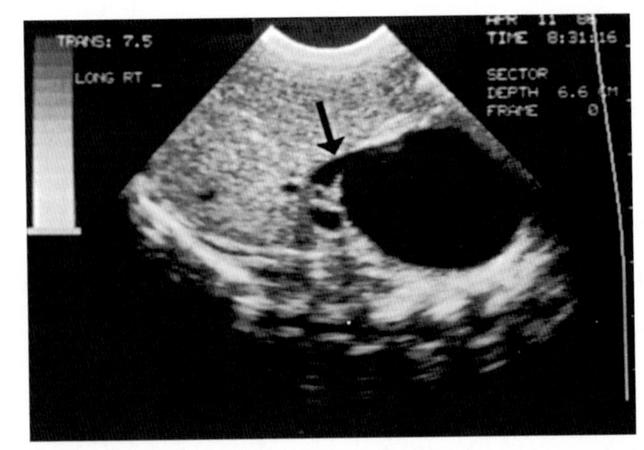

Figure 52–9. Ultrasonographic demonstration of a type I choledochal cyst in a cholestatic infant. A large cystic mass in the right upper quadrant is shown on this transverse scan. The point of juncture with the common bile duct is delineated by an arrow.

Congenital Dilatation of the Intrahepatic Bile Ducts

Nonobstructive saccular or fusiform dilatation of the intrahepatic bile ducts is a rare, congenital disorder. In the pure form, known as Caroli's disease, dilatation is classically segmental and saccular and associated with stone formation and recurrent bacterial cholangitis.[104, 105] A more common type, Caroli's syndrome, is associated with a portal tract lesion typical of congenital hepatic fibrosis (CHF). Dilatation of the extrahepatic bile ducts (choledochal cysts) also may be present. Renal disease occurs in both forms, renal tubular ectasia occurs with the simple form, and both conditions can be associated with autosomal recessive polycystic renal disease or, rarely, autosomal dominant polycystic renal disease.[106] However, the mode of inheritance of Caroli's disease is often uncertain; the form that occurs with CHF appears to be inherited as an autosomal recessive trait.

Pathology

The intrahepatic cysts are lined by epithelium that may be ulcerated and hyperplastic. The cysts may contain inspissated bile, calculi, and purulent material.

Liver biopsy may reveal normal tissue or features of acute or chronic cholangitis.[107] Portal tract edema and fibrosis may be present. In cases associated with CHF, findings associated with the ductal plate malformation can be expected; the lumen of the portal bile duct forms an epithelium lined circular cleft surrounding a central vascularized connective tissue core, or a series of bile duct lumens are arranged in a circle around a central fibrous tissue core.

Clinical Features

Patients usually seek medical attention during childhood and adolescence because of hepatomegaly and abdominal pain.[104, 106] The disorder appears in the neonate as renal disease or cholestasis.[108] Fever and intermittent jaundice may occur during episodes of bacterial cholangitis. Hepatosplenomegaly is found in cases associated with CHF; affected patients may exhibit bleeding esophageal varices. The polycystic kidneys may be palpable.

Liver biochemical tests may have normal results or show mild to moderate elevations of serum bilirubin, alkaline phosphatase, and aminotransferase levels.[106] Liver synthetic function is well preserved, but repeated episodes of infection and biliary obstruction within the cystic bile ducts eventually may lead to hepatic failure. The maximal concentrating capacity is the most frequently abnormal renal function test finding; variable elevations of blood urea nitrogen and serum creatinine levels reflect the severity of the underlying kidney disease.[106]

Diagnosis

Ultrasonography, MRC, and computed tomography are of great value in demonstrating the cystic dilatation of the intrahepatic bile ducts.[109] Renal cysts or hyperechogenicity of papillae may be detected. Percutaneous or endoscopic cholangiography (Fig. 52–10) usually demonstrates a normal common duct with segmental, saccular dilatations of the intrahepatic bile ducts.[110] Rarely, the process may be limited to one lobe of the liver.

Prognosis and Treatment

The clinical course is often complicated by recurrent episodes of cholangitis. Sepsis and liver abscess may occur. The prognosis in the setting of persistent or recurrent infection is poor. Calculi frequently develop within the cystically dilated bile ducts and can complicate the treatment of cholangitis. Patients who have extensive hepatolithiasis may experience intractable abdominal pain. Removal of stones by surgery, endoscopy, or lithotripsy usually is not feasible. Hepatic resection is indicated for disease limited to a single lobe. Surgical drainage procedures generally are not effective and may complicate later liver transplantation. Therapy with ursodeoxycholic acid has been used successfully to dissolve intrahepatic stones.[111] Cholangiocarcinoma may develop within the abnormal bile ducts. Portal hypertension and variceal bleeding may predominate in patients with CHF and Caroli's disease.[104] End-stage renal disease develops in some patients who have associated polycystic kidney disease. Liver transplantation is an option in patients who have extensive disease and frequent complications.

Paucity of the Interlobular Bile Ducts

A paucity of interlobular bile ducts may be an isolated and unexplained finding in infants and children with idiopathic cholestasis or a feature of a heterogeneous group of disorders that include congenital infections with rubella and cytomegalovirus and genetic disorders such as α_1-antitrypsin deficiency and inborn errors of bile acid metabolism.[112] The structural abnormality has also been referred to as *intrahepatic biliary atresia* or *intrahepatic biliary hypoplasia*. How-

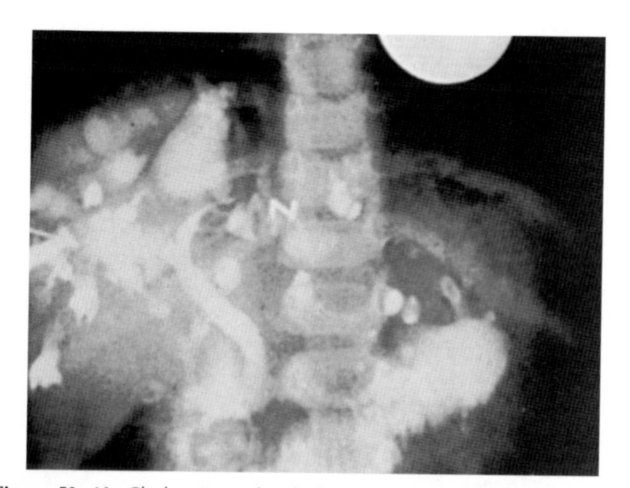

Figure 52–10. Cholangiographic findings in Caroli's disease. Percutaneous cholangiography revealed multiple cystic lesions throughout a markedly enlarged liver, which is also affected by congenital hepatic fibrosis. The cystic lesions are in continuity with the bile ducts. The extrahepatic bile ducts are normal. (From Kocoshis SA, Riely CA, Burrell M, Gryboski JD: Cholangitis in a child due to biliary tract anomalies. Dig Dis Sci 25:59, 1980.)

ever, these terms imply more insight into the pathogenesis of ductular paucity than currently prevails. Cases may arise from true biliary dysgenesis but more often result from active injury and loss of bile ducts.[113] Bile duct paucity may occur without associated developmental anomalies and without a documented intrauterine infection or genetic disorder. However, this idiopathic form of nonsyndromic bile duct paucity is likely to be heterogeneous in cause with extremely variable clinical features and prognosis. Cholestasis typically develops early in infancy and may be associated with progressive liver disease. Cholangiography of the intrahepatic bile ducts in infants with nonsyndromic paucity of bile ducts and no associated disorder demonstrates sclerosing cholangitis in at least half of patients in whom the diagnosis of "idiopathic paucity" would have been made in the past.[114]

Syndromic Paucity of Interlobular Bile Ducts (Alagille's Syndrome, or Arteriohepatic Dysplasia)

Syndromic paucity of interlobular bile ducts (Alagille's syndrome, or arteriohepatic dysplasia) is the most common form of familial intrahepatic cholestasis. This disorder is characterized by chronic cholestasis, a decreased number of interlobular bile ducts, and a variety of other congenital malformations.[115]

An autosomal dominant mode of transmission with incomplete penetrance and variable expressivity has been established from family studies.[116] A partial deletion of the short arm of chromosome 20 was detected in some patients and led to the identification of the Alagille disease gene.[116] Mutations in the jagged1 *(JAG1)* gene have been identified in approximately 70% of affected patients and include total gene deletions as well as protein truncating, splicing, and missense mutations.[117] *JAG1* encodes a ligand in the Notch signaling pathway that is involved in cell fate determination during development. There appears to be no phenotypic difference between patients with deletion of the entire *JAG1* gene and those with intragenic mutations.[116] The disorder may affect only one family member; these cases may represent spontaneous mutations of the *JAG1* gene. Alternatively, it is possible that the variability in gene expression is so great that minimally affected family members are not diagnosed. A 1994 analysis of 33 families collected through 43 probands corroborated the autosomal dominant inheritance and concluded that the rate of penetrance is 94% and that 15% of cases are sporadic. However, expressivity was variable; 26 persons (including 11 sibs) exhibited minor forms of the disease.[118]

Clinical Features

Chronic cholestasis of varying severity affects 95% of patients.[115, 116] Jaundice and clay colored stools may be observed during the neonatal period and become apparent in most patients during the first 2 years of life. Intense pruritus may be present by 6 months of age.[115] The liver and spleen are often enlarged. During the first years of life, xanthomata appear on the extensor surfaces of the fingers and in the creases of the palms and popliteal areas. Dysmorphic facies (Fig. 52–11) are usually recognized during infancy and become more characteristic with age.[114, 115] The forehead is typically broad, the eyes are deeply set and widely spaced, and the mandible is somewhat small and pointed, imparting a triangular appearance to the face. The malar eminence is flattened and the ears are prominent. Extrahepatic anomalies have been described with this syndrome, but there is considerable variability in phenotypic expression. In a 1999 series of 92 patients, cholestasis occurred in 96%, cardiac murmur in 97%, butterfly vertebrae in 51%, posterior embryotoxon in 78%, and characteristic facies in 96% of patients.[119] Short stature is a regular feature but is only partially attributed to the severity of chronic cholestasis. Growth hormone insensitivity associated with elevated circulating levels of growth hormone–binding protein has been described in these patients.[120] Mild to moderate mental retardation affects 15% to

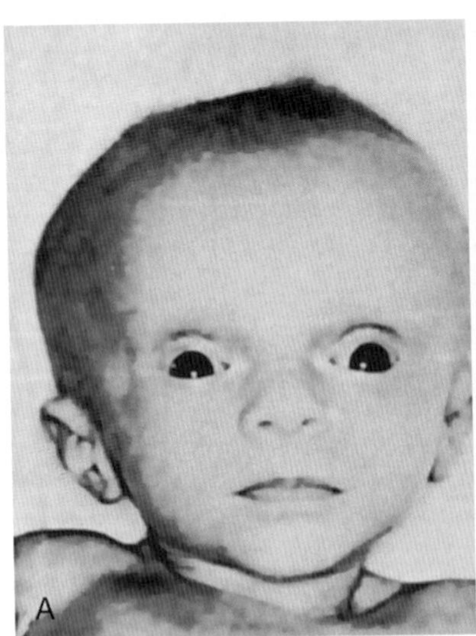

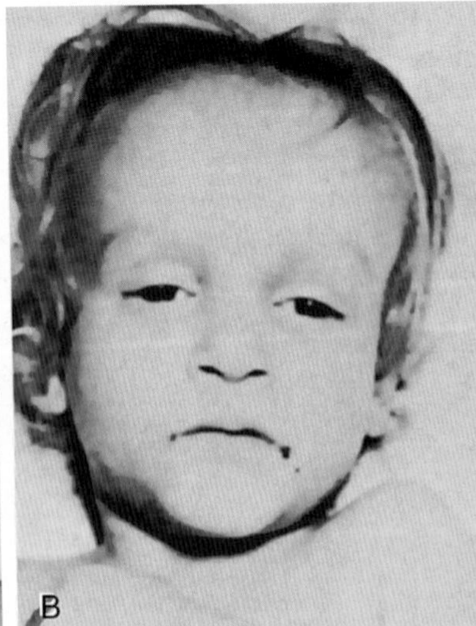

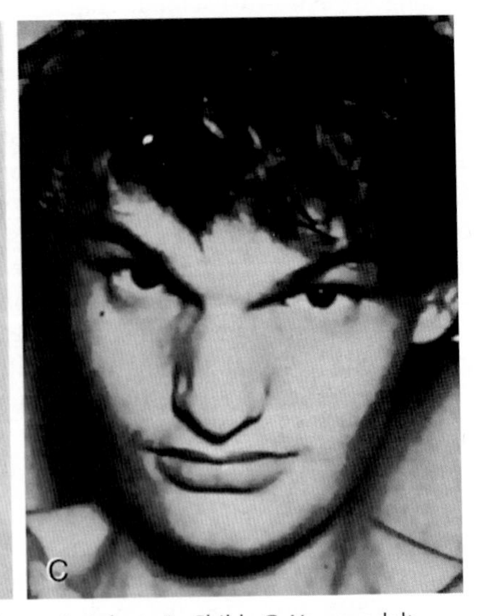

Figure 52–11. Facial appearance in syndromic paucity of the intrahepatic bile ducts. *A,* Infant. *B,* Child. *C,* Young adult. (See text for description.) (From Alagille D, Estrada A, Hadchouel M, et al: Syndromic paucity of interlobular bile ducts [Alagille's syndrome or arteriohepatic dysplasia]: Review of 80 cases. J Pediatr 110:195, 1987.)

20% of patients. Congenital heart disease occurs in most patients, and peripheral pulmonic stenosis is observed in approximately 90%.[119] Systemic vascular malformations also may be present. Osseous abnormalities include a decreased bone age, variable shortening of the distal phalanges, and vertebral arch defects (e.g., butterfly vertebrae, hemivertebrae, and a decrease in the interpedicular distance).[119] Ophthalmologic examination may reveal eye anomalies, including posterior embryotoxon (mesodermal dysgenesis of the iris and cornea), retinal pigmentation, and iris strands. Renal abnormalities and hypogonadism also have been described.[119]

Laboratory studies reveal an elevation of total serum bilirubin levels (usually 2 to 8 mg/dL) during infancy and intermittently later in life.[114, 115] Approximately 50% of the total serum bilirubin is conjugated. Serum alkaline phosphatase, gamma glutamyl transpeptidase, and 5′nucleotidase levels may be extremely high and correlate somewhat with the degree of cholestasis. Serum aminotransferase levels are mildly to moderately increased. Serum cholesterol levels may be 200 mg/dL or higher. Serum triglyceride concentrations may range from 500 to 1000 mg/dL. Total serum bile acid concentrations are markedly elevated, but the bile acid profiles in serum, urine, and bile do not differ qualitatively from those seen in other cholestatic disorders.

Pathology

The hallmark of this condition is a paucity of interlobular bile ducts.[114, 121] Paucity may be defined as a significantly decreased ratio of the numbers of interlobular portal bile ducts to portal tracts (<0.4).[121] The histologic features during the first months of life may overlap with those of neonatal hepatitis, in that there can be ballooning of hepatocytes, variable cholestasis, portal inflammation, and giant cell transformation.[121] Often, the number of interlobular bile ducts is not decreased on initial liver biopsy, but there may be evidence of bile duct injury consisting of cellular infiltration of portal triads contiguous to interlobular bile ducts, lymphocytic infiltration and pyknosis of biliary epithelium, and periductal fibrosis.[121] Serial biopsies of an individual patient may initially show bile duct proliferation, followed later in life by a paucity of bile ducts (Fig. 52–12). Paucity of interlobular bile ducts is usually apparent after 3 months. There may also be mild periportal fibrosis, but progression to cirrhosis is uncommon. The extrahepatic bile ducts are patent but usually narrowed or hypoplastic. Ultrastructural studies have demonstrated the accumulation of bile pigment in the cytoplasm near lysosomes and vesicles of the outer convex space of the Golgi apparatus. The bile canaliculi most often appear to be structurally normal, but in some cases they may appear to be dilated with blunting and shortening of microvilli.[121]

Pathogenesis

The mechanisms involved in the pathogenesis of bile duct paucity and cholestasis are not settled. Also unknown is how the hepatobiliary disease relates to the multiplicity of congenital anomalies found in other organ systems. Mice homozygous for the *JAG1* mutation die of hemorrhage early during embryogenesis and exhibit defects in remodeling of the embryonic and yolk sac vasculature.[122] The strong Jagged1 expression during human embryogenesis, both in the vascular system and in other mesenchymal and epithelial tissues, implicates abnormal angiogenesis in the pathogenesis of Alagille's syndrome and particularly the paucity of interlobular bile ducts.[123] In human embryos *JAG1* is expressed in the distal cardiac outflow tract and pulmonary artery, major arteries, portal vein, optic vesicle, otocyst, branchial arches, metanephros, pancreas, and mesocardium; around the major bronchial branches; and in the neural tube. All these structures are affected in Alagille's syndrome. Although a vascular basis for the anomalies in Alagille's syndrome seems likely, the precise mechanisms leading to bile duct paucity remain unknown. However, ischemic injury to the biliary

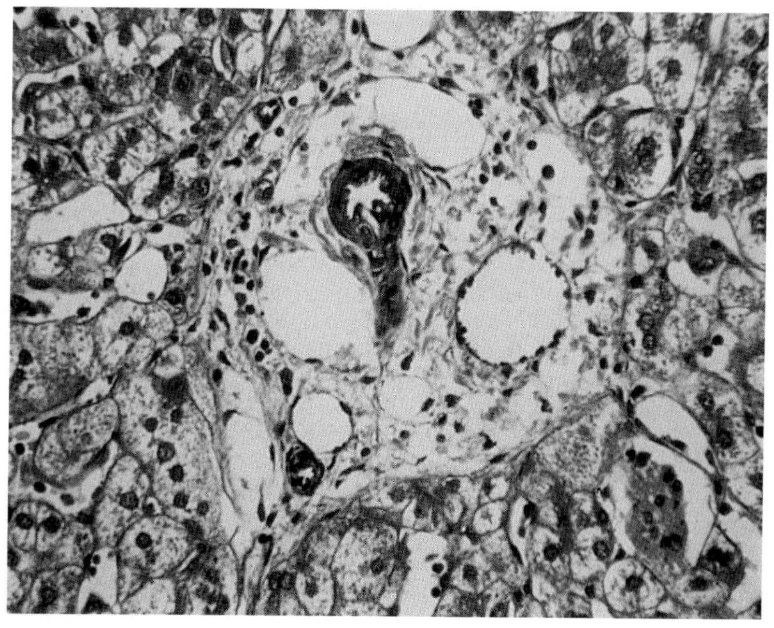

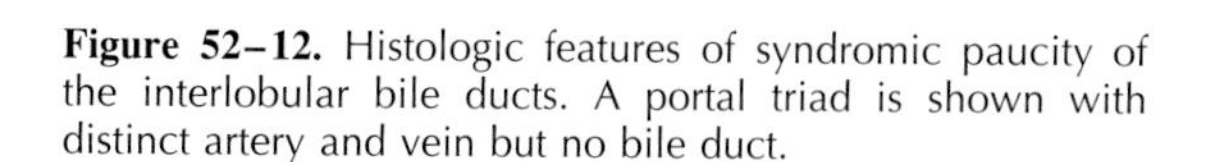

Figure 52–12. Histologic features of syndromic paucity of the interlobular bile ducts. A portal triad is shown with distinct artery and vein but no bile duct.

tree may be responsible for the progressive loss of bile ducts. It has been of great interest to note that profound cholestasis can occur in this disorder during the neonatal period even when the interlobular bile ducts are not decreased in number. In contrast, later in life, when cholestasis may be less severe as judged by clinical and biochemical criteria, interlobular bile ducts may be undetectable by liver biopsy.

Prognosis

The clinical course is marked by varying degrees of cholestasis, sometimes worsened by intercurrent viral infections. Morbidity may result from pruritus, cutaneous xanthomata, and neuromuscular symptoms related to vitamin E deficiency. Treatment involves the provision of an adequate caloric intake, prevention or correction of fat-soluble vitamin deficiencies, and symptomatic measures to relieve pruritus. The long-term prognosis depends on the severity of the liver disease and associated malformations. Of 80 patients who had this disorder and who were followed by Alagille and associates, 21 patients died, but only 4 died as a result of liver disease.[115] However, in a series of children followed for 10 years, 8 of 26 required liver transplantation for severe complications, such as bone fractures, refractory pruritus, and extensive xanthomata.[124] Progression to cirrhosis and liver failure was infrequent. Hepatocellular carcinoma was a complication. In a series of 92 patients the mortality rate was 17%.[119] The factors that contributed significantly to the mortality rate were hepatic disease or hepatic transplantation (25%), complex congenital heart disease (15%), and intracranial hemorrhage (25%). On the basis of these studies, the 20-year predicted life expectancy is approximately 75% for all patients, approximately 80% for those not requiring liver transplantation, and approximately 60% for those who require liver transplantation. Survival and candidacy for liver transplantation may be limited by the severity of associated cardiovascular anomalies. In a series of these patients who had liver transplantation, a higher than expected mortality rate of 43% was attributed to cardiac disease or a previous Kasai procedure.[125]

Medical Management of Chronic Cholestasis

In the child with chronic, and sometimes progressive, cholestatic liver disease, efforts should be directed to promoting growth and development and minimizing discomfort.

Protein-energy malnutrition leading to growth failure is an inevitable consequence of chronic liver disease in 60% of children.[126] As a result of impaired intraluminal lipolysis, solubilization, and intestinal absorption of long-chain triglycerides, steatorrhea is common in children with cholestasis.[127] Medium-chain triglycerides do not require solubilization by bile salts before intestinal absorption and thus can provide needed calories when administered orally in one of several commercial formulas or as an oil supplement.

Significant morbid conditions, resulting from fat-soluble vitamin deficiencies, can be prevented in large part in cholestatic children.[128, 129] Because metabolic bone disease, manifesting as rickets and pathologic fractures, can result from vitamin D deficiency, vitamin D should be provided as D_2 (5000 IU/day) or as 25-hydroxycholecalciferol (3 to 5 μg/kg/day).[128] Supplements of elemental calcium (50 to 100 mg/kg/day) and phosphorus (25 to 50 mg/kg/day) also may be required.

Xerophthalmia, night blindness, and thickened skin have been reported in patients who have a vitamin A deficiency. Oral supplements of vitamin A, 5000 to 25,000 IU/day, should be administered.

Vitamin K deficiency and associated coagulopathy may be treated initially with an oral water-soluble supplement administered in doses of 2.5 to 5 mg twice weekly to as much as 5 mg daily. Children who do not respond or who have significant bleeding require intramuscular injections of vitamin K.

Chronic deficiency of vitamin E may produce a disabling, degenerative neuromuscular syndrome characterized by areflexia, ophthalmoplegia, cerebellar ataxia, peripheral neuropathy, and posterior column dysfunction. The onset can be observed within the first 2 years of life. Because serum vitamin E levels may be elevated spuriously in the presence of hyperlipidemia, the ratio of serum vitamin E to total serum lipids is most useful in monitoring the vitamin E status; deficiency in a child less than 12 years old, for example, is indicated by a ratio less than 0.6. The child may not respond to massive doses of standard vitamin E preparations (150 to 200 IU/kg/day). Therapy with intramuscular *dl*-alpha-tocopherol (50 mg/day) or the water-soluble form of vitamin E, *d*-alpha-tocopherol polyethylene glycol-1000-succinate (15 to 25 IU/kg/day), is effective.

Xanthomata and pruritus may cause substantial discomfort.[130] Pruritus may be observed by 3 months of age. Regression of the symptoms may follow efforts to increase the conversion of cholesterol to bile acids, thereby reducing the regurgitation of biliary constituents into the systemic circulation and enhancing the elimination of bile acids and cholesterol. The success of most therapies depends on the presence of patent bile ducts that allow bile acids and other biliary constituents to reach the gut lumen.[131] Biliary diversion has been used as a successful alternative to relieve intractable pruritus in some intrahepatic cholestasis patients.[132] The antibiotic rifampin, through undefined mechanisms, and the choleretic bile acid ursodeoxycholic acid are under investigation for the treatment of pruritus.[131]

The nonabsorbable anion exchange resin cholestyramine may be used to bind bile acids, cholesterol, and presumably other potentially toxic agents in the intestinal lumen.[131] This medication may lower serum lipid levels and bind the substances involved in the pathogenesis of pruritus. A dose of 0.25 to 0.5 g/kg/day is administered before breakfast or in divided doses before meals to relieve severe pruritus and xanthomata. However, cholestyramine is relatively unpalatable and carries modest risks for intestinal obstruction, caused by inspissation of the drug, and hyperchloremic acidosis. Pruritus also has been treated with exposure to ultraviolet B light.

DISEASES OF THE GALLBLADDER

Cholelithiasis

Cholelithiasis is uncommon in otherwise healthy children and usually occurs in patients who have a predisposing condition.[133, 134] An ultrasonographic survey of 1570 subjects (ages 6 to 19 years) detected gallstones in only two female subjects, aged 13 and 18 years.[135] None of the subjects in the study population had undergone cholecystectomy. The overall prevalence of gallstone disease was 0.13% (0.27% in female subjects). Most cases come to light near the time of puberty, but gallstones have been reported at any age, including during fetal life. Pigmented gallstones predominate in infants and children.[134] The conditions associated with an increased risk of cholelithiasis are listed in Table 52–4. An underlying cause of the cholelithiasis can be identified in more than one half of children with calculous cholecystitis.

An in depth discussion of the pathogenesis of gallstones can be found in Chapter 55. However, certain factors may assume greater importance during infancy and childhood.[135] For example, an increased incidence of calculous cholecystitis is reported in sick premature infants, who often undergo a period of prolonged fasting without frequent stimulation of gallbladder contraction and who require periods of prolonged parenteral nutrition. Many of these patients have complicated medical courses that include frequent blood transfusions, episodes of sepsis, abdominal surgery, and use of diuretics and narcotic analgesics.[136] Limited analyses of gallstones in such cases generally have shown the presence of mixed cholesterol–calcium bilirubinate stones.[134] In the critically ill infant there may be a continuum from the common occurrence of an enlarged, distended gallbladder filled with sludge to the eventual development of cholelithiasis. As in adults, the incidence of gallstones is increased in children with disease or prior resection of the terminal ileum.[137]

Black pigment gallstones occur commonly in patients who have chronic hemolytic disorders.[134, 138] These stones are composed predominantly of calcium bilirubinate, with substantial amounts of crystalline calcium carbonate and phosphate. In sickle cell disease, the risk of gallstones increases with age and occurs in at least 14% of children younger than 10 years and 36% of those between 10 and 20 years.[138]

Obstructive jaundice in infants also may be caused by brown pigment cholelithiasis.[139] Brown pigment stones are composed of varying proportions of calcium bilirubinate, calcium phosphate, calcium palmitate, cholesterol, and organic material.[139] Unconjugated bilirubin accounts for a large percentage of the total bile biliary pigments. In several cases, bile has had high β-glucuronidase activity and on culture grew an abundant population of several bacteria.[140] It is postulated that pigment gallstones formed spontaneously in these infants, who had bacterial infections of the biliary tract.

Patients who have no identifiable cause of cholelithiasis are more likely to be female, older, and obese patients; have a family history of gallbladder disease; and have a greater likelihood of adult-like symptoms.[134] Cholesterol gallstones predominate in these patients. Insights into the pathogenesis of gallstones have been gained through careful studies of Pima Indians, who have an extraordinarily high prevalence of cholesterol gallstones. Highly saturated bile has not been detected among Pima Indians younger than 13 years, but bile saturation increases significantly in both sexes during pubertal growth and development.[141] In this population the sex-related difference in the size of the bile acid pool begins during puberty; young men show a significant rise in the size of the bile acid pool with age, whereas young women show only a slight rise. Because cholesterol gallstones are associated with smaller bile acid pools, the divergence in bile acid pool size between the two sexes also may account for the sex-related difference in the frequency of gallstones, which begins during adolescence.

Prolonged use of high-dose ceftriaxone, a third-generation cephalosporin, has been associated with the formation of calcium-ceftriaxone salt precipitates in the gallbladder.[142] The process, also called *biliary pseudolithiasis*, was observed in 16 of 37 children treated with the drug for severe infections.[143] In a prospective study of patients under treatment for borreliosis, 20 of 43 children (46.5%) aged 4 months to 16 years were found to have ultrasonographic evidence of ceftriaxone-induced cholelithiasis after treatment for at least 10 days.[144] Two of the patients had signs of intrahepatic cholestasis, three experienced severe abdominal pain, and another five (11.6%) had sludge in the gallbladder without evidence of cholelithiasis. In all patients, the "pseudocholelithiasis" resolved spontaneously within 2 months of discontinuation of the drug.

Table 52–4 | **Conditions Associated with Cholelithiasis in Children According to Age**

0–12 MO (%)	1–5 YR (%)	6–21 YR (%)
None (36.4)	Hepatobiliary disease (28.6)	Pregnancy (37.2)
Parenteral nutrition (29.1)	Abdominal surgery (21.4)	Hemolytic disease (5.5)
Abdominal surgery (29.1)	Artificial heart valve (14.3)	Obesity (8.1)
Sepsis (14.8)	None (14.3)	Abdominal surgery (5.1)
Bronchopulmonary dysplasia (12.7)	Malabsorption (7.1)	None (3.4)
Hemolytic disease (5.5)		Hepatobiliary disease (2.7)
Malabsorption (5.5)		Parenteral nutrition (2.7)
Necrotizing enterocolitis (5.5)		Malabsorption (2.8)
Hepatobiliary disease (3.6)		

Modified from Friesen CA, Roberts CC: Cholelithiasis: Clinical characteristics in children: Case analysis and literature review. Clin Pediatr (Phila) 28:294, 1989.

Clinical Features

Most stones are found in the gallbladder.[134] Children have a lower incidence of common duct stones than adults. Most patients are asymptomatic; the gallstones are discovered either incidentally during the investigation of another problem or during screening because the patient has a condition associated with a high risk for cholelithiasis.[145] Patients may complain of intermittent abdominal pain of variable severity; the pain may be localized to the right upper quadrant in older children but is generally poorly localized in infants. The physical examination findings are usually unremarkable. Tenderness in the right upper quadrant suggests cholecystitis, as occurs when a stone migrates to the neck of the gallbladder and obstructs the cystic duct. Infants may exhibit irritability, cholestatic jaundice, and acholic stools.[146]

Liver biochemical test results are usually normal.[145] Plain films of the abdomen may reveal calculi, depending on the calcium content of the stone. Ultrasonography is considered the most sensitive and specific imaging technique for the demonstration of gallstones.[147] Hepatobiliary scintigraphy is a valuable adjunct, in that failure to visualize the gallbladder provides evidence of acute cholecystitis.

Management

Cholecystectomy remains the treatment of choice in patients who have symptoms or a nonfunctioning gallbladder.[147] Laparoscopic cholecystectomy is done frequently in children and infants as young as 10 months.[148, 149] Operative cholangiography and exploration of the common duct may be indicated on the basis of clinical imaging and operative findings.

In asymptomatic patients without biochemical abnormalities ("silent gallstones"), management poses a more difficult problem. Epidemiologic studies and radiocarbon dating of gallstones in adults indicate a lag time of more than a decade between initial formation of a stone and development of symptoms.[150] In patients who have underlying disorders such as hemolysis or ileal disease, cholecystectomy may be carried out at the same time as another surgical procedure.[149] In cases associated with hepatic disease, severe obesity, or cystic fibrosis, the surgical risk of cholecystectomy may be substantial, and clinical judgment must be applied.[151] In these cases, the patient should be counseled about the nature of the disease and the potential symptoms that may develop. Spontaneous resolution of cholelithiasis and even common duct stones has been reported in infants.[152] Because recurrence of lithiasis is rare in infants, cholecystectomy may not be required. However, patients with obstructive cholestasis are at risk for sepsis and cholangitis and should undergo surgery.

There is little experience in children with alternative therapies for gallstones such as medical dissolution with oral bile acid administration or shock wave lithotripsy. Ursodeoxycholic acid therapy is of no value in the treatment of the predominantly pigment stones found in this age group. Furthermore, ursodeoxycholic acid failed to dissolve radiolucent gallstones in 10 children with cystic fibrosis.[153]

Calculous Cholecystitis

Cholelithiasis may be associated with acute or chronic inflammation of the gallbladder.[134, 146] Acute cholecystitis is often precipitated by impaction of a stone in the cystic duct.[145] A progressive increase in pressure in the gallbladder secondary to fluid accumulation, the presence of stones, and the chemical irritant effects of bile acids can lead to progressive inflammation, congestion, and vascular compromise. Infarction, gangrene, and perforation can occur. Proliferation of bacteria within the obstructed gallbladder lumen can contribute to the process and lead to biliary sepsis.

Chronic calculous cholecystitis is more common than acute cholecystitis.[145] It may develop insidiously or after several attacks of acute cholecystitis. The gallbladder epithelium commonly becomes ulcerated and scarred.

Clinical Features

The acute onset of colicky right upper quadrant pain is a constant feature of acute cholecystitis.[145] The pain may be poorly localized in infants. Nausea and vomiting are frequent. Children have a higher incidence of jaundice (50%) than adults. The patient may appear acutely ill with shallow respirations and may be febrile, particularly if there is superimposed bacterial infection. Guarding of the abdomen is common, and palpation usually elicits tenderness in the right upper quadrant. Murphy's sign may be present.

The onset of chronic cholecystitis is usually more indolent.[134] The clinical course may be marked by recurrent episodes of upper abdominal discomfort. Older patients may experience intolerance to fatty foods. In one series, episodes of right upper quadrant pain developed in 64% of children with cholelithiasis and no ductal obstruction and was most likely a consequence of chronic cholecystitis.[154] Physical examination may yield negative findings or may disclose local tenderness over the gallbladder.

In acute cholecystitis, there often is an elevation in the white blood cell count with a predominance of polymorphonuclear leukocytes.[147, 154] Serum bilirubin and alkaline phosphatase levels may be increased. Serum aminotransferase levels may be normal, but high elevations, suggestive of hepatocellular disease, can occur early with acute obstruction of the common duct.

In chronic cholecystitis, results of the complete blood count and liver biochemical tests are usually normal. In patients with an acute or chronic presentation, a plain film of the abdomen may demonstrate calcifications in the right upper quadrant.[147] Abdominal ultrasonography is extremely useful in documenting the presence of stones in the gallbladder, may show thickening of the gallbladder wall, and may demonstrate dilatation of the biliary tract secondary to obstruction of the common bile duct by a stone that has migrated from the gallbladder. Hepatobiliary scintigraphy rarely is necessary in the acutely ill patient but may be of value in demonstrating a malfunctioning gallbladder in chronic cholecystitis patients.[155]

Treatment

The acutely ill patient should be treated with intravenous fluids, analgesics, and broad-spectrum antibiotics.[145, 147] Cholecystectomy should be performed as soon as fluid deficits are corrected and infection is controlled.[148, 156] High-risk, acutely ill patients may benefit from percutaneous drainage via a transhepatic cholecystostomy. The results of surgery are excellent. Care should be taken to exclude common duct stones by surgical cholangiography and, if necessary, exploration of the duct.

Cholecystectomy is also the treatment of choice for chronic calculous cholecystitis. Laparoscopic cholecystectomy is the preferred approach for most patients.[148, 156]

Acute Acalculous Cholecystitis

Acute acalculous cholecystitis is an acute inflammation of the gallbladder without gallstones (see also Chapter 58).[157]

The disorder is uncommon in children but has been associated with infection or systemic illness. Pathogens have included streptococci (groups A and B); *Leptospira interrogans;* gram-negative organisms such as *Salmonella* and *Shigella* species and *Escherichia coli*; and parasitic infestations with *Ascaris* species or *Giardia lamblia*.[157] In immunocompromised patients, pathogens such as *Isospora belli* and *Cytomegalovirus*, *Cryptosporidium, Aspergillus,* and *Candida* species should be considered. Acalculous cholecystitis may follow abdominal trauma and has been observed in patients with systemic vasculitis, including periarteritis nodosa, and mucocutaneous lymph node (Kawasaki's) disease. However, in these conditions, gallbladder distention without inflammation also may occur. Congenital narrowing or inflammation of the cystic duct or external compression by enlarged lymph nodes has been associated with the disorder in children.

Clinical features of acute acalculous cholecystitis include right upper quadrant or epigastric pain, nausea, vomiting, fever, and occasionally jaundice.[157] Right upper quadrant guarding and tenderness are present; a tender gallbladder is sometimes palpable. The findings may be less apparent in infants or critically ill patients, because the presentation may be obscured by the underlying illness.

Laboratory evaluation may reveal elevated serum levels of alkaline phosphatase and conjugated bilirubin.[157] Leukocytosis may occur.[157] Ultrasonography discloses an enlarged, thick-walled gallbladder that may be distended with sludge but has no calculi.

The diagnosis is confirmed at laparotomy. The gallbladder is usually inflamed, and cultures of bile may yield positive findings for the offending bacteria or contain parasites. The gallbladder may become gangrenous.[158] Cholecystectomy and treatment of the systemic infection are required in most cases.[157, 159] Cholecystostomy drainage may be an alternative approach in a critically ill patient.

Acute Hydrops of the Gallbladder

Acute noncalculous, noninflammatory distention of the gallbladder may be observed in infants and children.[160] The gallbladder is not acutely inflamed, and cultures of the bile are usually sterile. The absence of gallbladder inflammation and generally benign prognosis distinguish acute hydrops from acute acalculous cholecystitis. There may be a generalized mesenteric adenitis of lymph nodes near the cystic duct without mechanical compression. A temporal relationship to other infections, including scarlet fever and leptospirosis, has been observed in some cases. Acute hydrops also has been associated with Kawasaki's disease and Henoch-Schönlein purpura.[161] Like acalculous cholecystitis, the disorder can occur in children on prolonged parenteral nutrition. In some cases, a cause is not identified.

Acute hydrops is associated with the acute onset of crampy abdominal pain and, often, nausea and vomiting.[160] Fever and jaundice may be present. The right upper quadrant is usually tender, and the distended gallbladder may be palpable.

Liver biochemical test levels may be mildly elevated. The white blood cell count may be elevated. Some of these changes can be attributed to the associated disorders such as scarlet fever or Kawasaki's disease. Ultrasonography reveals an enlarged, distended gallbladder without calculi.

The diagnosis of acute hydrops is confirmed in many patients at laparotomy.[160] Cholecystectomy obviously is required if the gallbladder appears gangrenous. Pathologic examination of the gallbladder wall usually shows edema and mild inflammation. Cultures of the bile are usually sterile. These benign findings have led some surgeons to treat acute hydrops by a simple cholecystostomy instead of a cholecystectomy.[161] However, the treatment of gallbladder hydrops frequently is nonsurgical with a focus on supportive care and management of the intercurrent illness. In most patients, particularly in children on total parenteral nutrition in whom enteral feeding has been initiated, the process subsides spontaneously. Ultrasonography has been useful in establishing the diagnosis and following the spontaneous resolution of gallbladder distention.[161] The prognosis is excellent. Gallbladder function can be expected to return to normal in most cases.

REFERENCES

1. Elias H: Origin and early development of the liver of various vertebrates. Acta Hepatol 3:1–56, 1955.
2. Moore KL: The Developing Human: Clinically Oriented Embryology, 4th ed. Philadelphia, WB Saunders, 1988.
3. Zaret KS: Liver specification and early morphogenesis. Mech Dev 92: 83–88, 2000.
4. Bezerra JA: Liver development: A paradigm for hepatobiliary disease in later life. Semin Liver Dis 18:203–216, 1998.
5. Zaret K: Early liver differentiation: Genetic potentiation and multilevel growth control. Curr Opin Genet Dev 8:526–531, 1998.
6. Zaret K: Developmental competence of the gut endoderm: Genetic potentiation by GATA and HNF3/fork head proteins. Dev Biol 209:1–10, 1999.
7. Van Eyken P, Sciot R, Callea F, et al: The development of the intrahepatic bile ducts in man: A keratin-immunohistochemical study. Hepatology 8:1586–1595, 1988.
8. Terada T, Nakanuma Y: Detection of apoptosis and expression of apoptosis-related proteins during human intrahepatic bile duct development. Am J Pathol 146:67–74, 1995.
9. Tan CE, Moscoso GJ: The developing human biliary system at the porta hepatis level between 29 days and 8 weeks of gestation: A way to understanding biliary atresia. Part 1. Pathol Int 44:587-599, 1994.
10. Kanno N, LeSage G, Glaser S, et al: Functional heterogeneity of the intrahepatic biliary epithelium. Hepatology 31:555–561, 2000.
11. Jones AL, Schmucker DL, Renston RH, Murakami T: The architecture of bile secretion: A morphological perspective of physiology. Dig Dis Sci 25:609–629, 1980.
12. Healey JJ, Paul CS: The anatomy of the biliary ducts within the human liver: Analysis of the prevailing pattern of branching and the major variations of the biliary ducts. Arch Surg 66:599–616, 1953.
13. Jones AL, Spring-Mills E: The liver and gallbladder. In Weiss L (ed): Modern Concepts of Gastrointestinal Histology. New York, Elsevier, 1983, p 738.
14. Adkins RB Jr, Chapman WC, Reddy VS: Embryology, anatomy, and surgical applications of the extrahepatic biliary system. Surg Clin North Am 80:363–379, 2000.
15. Dowdy GSJ, Waldron GW, Brown WG: Surgical anatomy of the pancreato-biliary ductal system. Arch Surg 84:229–246, 1962.
16. Strasberg SM: Terminology of liver anatomy and liver resections: Coming to grips with hepatic Babel. J Am Coll Surg 184:413–434, 1997
17. Keddie NC, Taylor AW, Sykes PA: The termination of the common bile duct. Br J Surg 61:623–625, 1974.
18. Avisse C, Flament JB, Delattre JF: Ampulla of Vater: Anatomic, embryologic, and surgical aspects. Surg Clin North Am 80:201–212, 2000.
19. Northover JM, Terblanche J: A new look at the arterial supply of the

bile duct in man and its surgical implications. Br J Surg 66:379–384, 1979.
20. Trutmann M, Sasse D: The lymphatics of the liver. Anat Embryol (Berl) 190:201–209, 1994.
21. Clemente CD: Gray's Anatomy of the Human Body, 13th ed. Philadelphia, Lea & Febiger, 1985, pp 1501–1503.
22. Frierson HF Jr: The gross anatomy and histology of the gallbladder, extrahepatic bile ducts, Vaterian system, and minor papilla. Am J Surg Pathol 13:146–162, 1989.
23. Meilstrup JW, Hopper KD, Thieme GA: Imaging of gallbladder variants. AJR Am J Roentgenol 157:1205–1208, 1991.
24. Ozgen A, Akata D, Arat A, et al: Gallbladder duplication: Imaging findings and differential considerations. Abdom Imaging 24:285–288, 1999.
25. Saimura M, Ichimiya H, Naritomi G, et al: Multiseptate gallbladder: Biliary manometry and scintigraphy. J Gastroenterol 31:133–136, 1996.
26. Naganuma S, Ishida H, Konno K, et al: Sonographic findings of anomalous position of the gallbladder. Abdom Imaging 23:67–72, 1998.
27. Arrese M, Ananthananarayanan M, Suchy FJ: Hepatobiliary transport: Molecular mechanisms of development and cholestasis. Pediatr Res 44:141–147, 1998.
28. Birnbaum A, Suchy FJ: The intrahepatic cholangiopathies. Semin Liver Dis 18:263–269, 1998.
29. Balistreri W: Neonatal cholestasis. J Pediatr 105:171–185, 1985.
30. D'Agata ID, Balistreri WF: Evaluation of liver disease in the pediatric patient. Pediatr Rev 20:376–390, 1999.
31. Rosenthal P: Assessing liver function and hyperbilirubinemia in the newborn: National Academy of Clinical Biochemistry. Clin Chem 43: 228–234, 1997.
32. Park WH, Choi SO, Lee HJ: The ultrasonographic "triangular cord" coupled with gallbladder images in the diagnostic prediction of biliary atresia from infantile intrahepatic cholestasis. J Pediatr Surg 34:1706–1710, 1999.
33. Jaw TS, Kuo YT, Liu GC, et al: MR cholangiography in the evaluation of neonatal cholestasis. Radiology 212:249–256, 1999.
34. Gilmour SM, Hershkop M, Reifen R, et al: Outcome of hepatobiliary scanning in neonatal hepatitis syndrome. J Nucl Med 38:1279–1282, 1997.
35. Paltiel HJ: Imaging of neonatal cholestasis. Semin Ultrasound CT MR 15:290–305, 1994.
36. Ohnuma N, Takahashi H, Tanabe M, et al: Endoscopic retrograde cholangiopancreatography (ERCP) in biliary tract disease of infants less than one year old. Tohoku J Exp Med 181:67–74, 1997.
37. Zerbini MC, Gallucci SD, Maezono R, et al: Liver biopsy in neonatal cholestasis: A review on statistical grounds. Mod Pathol 10:793–799, 1997.
38. Bates MD, Bucuvalas JC, Alonso MH, et al: Biliary atresia: Pathogenesis and treatment. Semin Liver Dis 18:281–293, 1998.
39. Whitington PF, Balistreri WF: Liver transplantation in pediatrics: Indications, contraindications, and pretransplant management. J Pediatr 118:169–177, 1991.
40. Chardot C, Carton M, Spire-Bendelac N, et al: Epidemiology of biliary atresia in France: A national study 1986–96. J Hepatol 31:1006–1013, 1999.
41. Silveira TR, Salzano FM, Donaldson PT, et al: Association between HLA and extrahepatic biliary atresia. J Pediatr Gastroenterol Nutr 16: 114–117, 1993.
42. Smith BM, Laberge JM, Schreiber R, et al: Familial biliary atresia in three siblings including twins. J Pediatr Surg 26:1131–1333, 1991.
43. Lefkowitch JH: Biliary atresia. Mayo Clin Proc 73:90–95, 1998.
44. Davenport M, Savage M, Mowat AP, et al: Biliary atresia splenic malformation syndrome: An etiologic and prognostic subgroup. Surgery 113:662–668, 1993.
45. Tanano H, Hasegawa T, Kawahara H, et al: Biliary atresia associated with congenital structural anomalies. J Pediatr Surg 34:1687–1690, 1999.
46. Bamford RN, Roessler E, Burdine RD, et al: Loss-of-function mutations in the EGF-CFC gene CFCI are associated with human left-right laterality defects. Nat Genet 26:365–369, 2000.
47. Landing BH: Considerations of the pathogenesis of neonatal hepatitis, biliary atresia and choledochal cyst—the concept of infantile obstructive cholangiopathy. Prog Pediatr Surg 6:113–139, 1975.
48. Tan CE, Moscoso GJ: The developing human biliary system at the porta hepatis level between 11 and 25 weeks of gestation: A way to understanding biliary atresia. Part 2. Pathol Int 44:600–610, 1994.
49. Bates MD, Bucuvalas JC, Alonso MH, Ryckman FC: Biliary atresia: Pathogenesis and treatment. Semin Liver Dis 18:281–293, 1998.
50. Jevon GP, Dimmick JE: Biliary atresia and cytomegalovirus infection: A DNA study. Pediatr Dev Pathol 2:11–14, 1999.
51. Morecki R, Glaser JH, Johnson AB, et al: Detection of reovirus type 3 in the porta hepatis of an infant with extrahepatic biliary atresia: Ultrastructural and immunocytochemical study. Hepatology 4:1137–1142, 1984.
52. Morecki R, Glaser JH, Cho S, et al: Biliary atresia and reovirus type 3 infection. N Engl J Med 310:1610, 1984.
53. Tyler KL, Sokol RJ, Oberhaus SM, et al: Detection of reovirus RNA in hepatobiliary tissues from patients with extrahepatic biliary atresia and choledochal cysts. Hepatology 27:1475–1482, 1998.
54. Riepenhoff-Talty M, Gouvea V, Evans MJ, et al: Detection of group C rotavirus in infants with extrahepatic biliary atresia. J Infect Dis 174:8–15, 1996.
55. Bobo L, Ojeh C, Chise D, et al: Lack of evidence for rotavirus by polymerase chain reaction/enzyme immunoassay of hepatobiliary samplesftom children with biliary atresia. Pediatr Res 41:229–234, 1997.
56. Hays DM, Woolley MM, Snyder WH Jr, et al: Diagnosis of biliary atresia: Relative accuracy of percutaneous liver biopsy, open liver biopsy, and operative cholangiography. J Pediatr 71:598–607, 1967.
57. Kasai M: Treatment of biliary atresia with special reference to hepatic portoenterostomy and its modifications. Prog Pediatr Surg 6:5–52, 1974.
58. Raweily EA, Gibson AA, Burt AD: Abnormalities of intrahepatic bile ducts in extrahepatic biliary atresia. Histopathology 17:521–527, 1990.
59. Ito T, Horisawa M, Ando H: Intrahepatic bile ducts in biliary atresia—a possible factor determining the prognosis. J Pediatr Surg 18: 124–130, 1983.
60. Hussein M, Howard ER, Mieli-Vergani G, et al: Jaundice at 14 days of age: Exclude biliary atresia. Arch Dis Child 66:1177–1179, 1991.
61. McEvoy C, Suchy FJ: Biliary tract disease in children. Pediatr Clin North Am 43:75–98, 1996.
62. Middlesworth W, Altman RP: Biliary atresia. Curr Opin Pediatr 9: 265–269, 1997.
63. Fung KP, Lau SP: Differentiation between extrahepatic and intrahepatic cholestasis by discriminant analysis. J Paediatr Child Health 26: 132–135, 1990.
64. Smith S, Wiener ES, Starzl TE, Rowe MI: Stoma-related variceal bleeding: An under-recognized complication of biliary atresia. J Pediatr Surg 23:243–245, 1988.
65. Meister RK, Esquivel CO, Cox KL, et al: The influence of portoenterostomy with stoma on morbidity in pediatric patients with biliary atresia undergoing orthotopic liver transplantation. J Pediatr Surg 28: 387–390, 1993.
66. Karrer FM, Lilly JR, Stewart BA, Hall RJ: Biliary atresia registry, 1976 to 1989. J Pediatr Surg 25:1076–1080, 1990.
67. Howard ER, Davenport M: The treatment of biliary atresia in Europe 1969–1995. Tohoku J Exp Med 181:75–83, 1997.
68. Miyano T, Fujimoto T, Ohya T, Shimomura H: Current concept of the treatment of biliary atresia. World J Surg 17:332–336, 1993.
69. Ibrahim M, Miyano T, Ohi R, et al: Japanese Biliary Atresia Registry, 1989 to 1994. Tohoku J Exp Med 181:85–95, 1997.
70. Chardot C, Carton M, Spire-Bendelac N, et al: Prognosis of biliary atresia in the era of liver transplantation: French national study from 1986 to 1996. Hepatology 30:606–611, 1999.
71. Ohi R, Nio M, Chiba T, et al: Long-term follow-up after surgery for patients with biliary atresia. J Pediatr Surg 25:442–445, 1990.
72. Karrer FM, Price MR, Bensard DD, et al: Long-term results with the Kasai operation for biliary atresia. Arch Surg 131:493–496, 1996.
73. Subramaniam R, Doig CM, Bowen J, Bruce J: Initial response to portoenterostomy determines long-term outcome in patients with biliary atresia. J Pediatr Surg 35:593–597, 2000.
74. Ohhama Y, Shinkai M, Fujita S, et al: Early prediction of long-term survival and the timing of liver transplantation after the Kasai operation. J Pediatr Surg 35:1031–1034, 2000.
75. Chandra RS, Altman RP: Ductal remnants in extrahepatic biliary atresia: A histopathologic study with clinical correlation. J Pediatr 93: 196–200, 1978.
76. Langenburg SE, Poulik J, Goretsky M, et al: Bile duct size does not predict success of portoenterostomy for biliary atresia. J Pediatr Surg 35:1006–1007, 2000.
77. Schweizer P, Kirschner HJ, Schittenhelm C: Anatomy of the porta hepatis (PH) as rational basis for the hepatoportoenterostomy (HPE). Eur J Pediatr Surg 9:13–18, 1999.

78. Gautier M, Valayer J, Odievre M, Alagille D: Histological liver evaluation 5 years after surgery for extrahepatic biliary atresia: A study of 20 cases. J Pediatr Surg 19:263–268, 1984.
79. Vazquez-Estevez J, Stewart B, Shikes RH, et al: Biliary atresia: Early determination of prognosis. J Pediatr Surg 24:48–50, 1989.
80. Ecoffey C, Rothman E, Bernard O, et al: Bacterial cholangitis after surgery for biliary atresia. J Pediatr 111:824–829, 1987.
81. Ryckman FC, Alonso MH, Bucuvalas JC, Balistreri WF: Long-term survival after liver transplantation. J Pediatr Surg 34:845–849, 1999.
82. Sandler AD, Azarow KS, Superina RA: The impact of a previous Kasai procedure on liver transplantation for biliary atresia. J Pediatr Surg 32:416–419, 1997.
83. Ryckman FC, Alonso MH, Bucuvalas JC, Balistreri WF: Biliary atresia—surgical management and treatment options as they relate to outcome. Liver Transpl Surg 4(suppl 1):S24–S33, 1998.
84. de Ville de Goyet J, Reding R, Lerut J, et al: Paediatric orthotopic liver transplantation: Lessons from a 532 transplant single centre experience with 532 transplants in 446 children. Acta Gastroenterol Belg 62:290–294, 1999.
85. Chardot C, Iskandarani F, De Dreuzy O, et al: Spontaneous perforation of the biliary tract in infancy: A series of 11 cases. Eur J Pediatr Surg 6:341–346, 1996.
86. Holland RM, Lilly JR: Surgical jaundice in infants: Other than biliary atresia. Semin Pediatr Surg 1:125–129, 1992.
87. Spigland N, Greco R, Rosenfeld D: Spontaneous biliary perforation: Does external drainage constitute adequate therapy? J Pediatr Surg 31: 782–784, 1996.
88. Bernstein J, Braylan R, Brough AJ: Bile-plug syndrome: A correctable cause of obstructive jaundice in infants. Pediatrics 43:273–276, 1969.
89. Debray D, Pariente D, Urvoas E, et al: Sclerosing cholangitis in children. J Pediatr 124:49–56, 1994.
90. Wilschanski M, Chait P, Wade JA, et al: Primary sclerosing cholangitis in 32 children: Clinical, laboratory, and radiographic features, with survival analysis. Hepatology 22:1415–1422, 1995.
91. Zandi P, Panis Y, Debray D: Pediatric liver transplantation for Langerhans' cell histiocytosis. Hepatology 2:129–133, 1995.
92. Mieli-Vergani G, Vergani D: Immunological liver diseases in children. Semin Liver Dis 18:271–279, 1998.
93. Gilger MA, Gann ME, Opekun AR, Gleason WA Jr: Efficacy of ursodeoxycholic acid in the treatment of primary sclerosing cholangitis in children. J Pediatr Gastroenterol Nutr 31:136–141, 2000.
94. Goss JA, Shackleton CR, Farmer DG, et al: Orthotopic liver transplantation for primary sclerosing cholangitis: A 12-year single center experience. Ann Surg 225:472–481, 1997.
95. Altman RP: Choledochal cyst. Semin Pediatr Surg 1:130–133, 1992.
96. Miyano T, Yamataka A: Choledochal cysts. Curr Opin Pediatr 9:283–288, 1997.
97. Todani T, Watanabe Y, Narusue M, et al: Congenital bile duct cysts: Classification, operative procedures, and review of thirty-seven cases including cancer arising from choledochal cyst. Am J Surg 134:263–269, 1977.
98. Savader SJ, Benenati JF, Venbrux AC, et al: Choledochal cysts: Classification and cholangiographic appearance. AJR Am J Roentgenol 156:327–331, 1991.
99. Karrer FM, Hall RJ, Stewart BA, Lilly JR: Congenital biliary tract disease. Surg Clin North Am 70:1403–1418, 1990.
100. Todani T, Urushihara N, Morotomi Y, et al: Characteristics of choledochal cysts in neonates and early infants. Eur J Pediatr Surg 5:143–145, 1995.
101. Bancroft JD, Bucuvalas JC, Ryckman FC, et al: Antenatal diagnosis of choledochal cyst. J Pediatr Gastroenterol Nutr 18:142–145, 1994.
102. Irie H, Honda H, Jimi M, et al: Value of MR cholangiopancreatography in evaluating choledochal cysts. AJR Am J Roentgenol 171:1381–1385, 1998.
103. Saing H, Han H, Chan KL, et al: Early and late results of excision of choledochal cysts. J Pediatr Surg 32:1563–1566, 1997.
104. Summerfield JA, Nagafuchi Y, Sherlock S, et al: Hepatobiliary fibropolycystic diseases: A clinical and histological review of 51 patients. J Hepatol 2:141–156, 1986.
105. Forbes A, Murray-Lyon IM: Cystic disease of the liver and biliary tract. Gut Suppl:S116–S122, 1991.
106. D'Agata ID, Jonas MM, Perez-Atayde AR, Guay-Woodford LM: Combined cystic disease of the liver and kidney. Semin Liver Dis 14: 215–228, 1994.
107. Desmet VJ: Congenital diseases of intrahepatic bile ducts: Variations on the theme of ductal plate malformation. Hepatology 16:1069–1083, 1992.
108. Keane F, Hadzic N, Wilkinson ML, et al: Neonatal presentation of Caroli's disease. Arch Dis Child Fetal Neonatal Ed 77:F145–F146, 1997.
109. Jung G, Benz-Bohm G, Kugel H, et al: MR cholangiography in children with autosomal recessive polycystic kidney disease. Pediatr Radiol 29:463–466, 1999.
110. Miller WJ, Sechtin AG, Campbell WL, Pieters PC: Imaging findings in Caroli's disease. AJR Am J Roentgenol 165:333–337, 1995.
111. Ros E, Navarro S, Bru C, et al: Ursodeoxycholic acid treatment of primary hepatolithiasis in Caroli's syndrome. Lancet 342:404–406, 1993.
112. Desmet VJ: Vanishing bile duct disorders. Prog Liver Dis 10:89–121, 1992.
113. Bosman C, Renda F, Boldrini R: Intrahepatic cholestasis by paucity of interlobular bile ducts in infancy. Recenti Prog Med 85:375–383, 1994.
114. Hadchouel M: Paucity of interlobular bile ducts. Semin Diagn Pathol 9:24–30, 1992.
115. Alagille D, Estrada A, Hadchouel M, et al: Syndromic paucity of interlobular bile ducts (Alagille syndrome or arteriohepatic dysplasia): Review of 80 cases. J Pediatr 110:195–200, 1987.
116. Krantz ID, Piccoli DA, Spinner NB: Clinical and molecular genetics of Alagille syndrome. Curr Opin Pediatr 11:558–564, 1999.
117. Oda T, Elkahloun AG, Pike BL, et al: Mutations in the human Jagged1 gene are responsible for Alagille syndrome. Nat Genet 16:235–242, 1997.
118. Dhome-Pollet S, Deleuze JF, Hadchouel M, Bonaiti-Pellie C: Segregation analysis of Alagille syndrome. J Med Genet 31:453–457, 1994.
119. Emerick KM, Rand EB, Goldmuntz E, et al: Features of Alagille syndrome in 92 patients: Frequency and relation to prognosis. Hepatology 29:822–829, 1999.
120. Bucuvalas JC, Hom JA, Carlsson L, et al: Growth hormone insensitivity associated with elevated circulating growth hormone–binding protein in children with Alagille syndrome and short stature. J Clin Endocrinol Metab 76:1477–1482, 1993.
121. Kahn E: Paucity of interlobular bile ducts. Arteriohepatic dysplasia and nonsyndromic duct paucity. Perspect Pediatr Pathol 14:168–215, 1991.
122. Xue Y, Gao X, Lindsell CE, et al: Embryonic lethality and vascular defects in mice lacking the Notch ligand Jagged1. Hum Mol Genet 8: 723–730, 1999.
123. Crosnier C, Attie-Bitach T, Encha-Razavi F, et al: JAGGEDI gene expression during human embryogenesis elucidates the wide phenotypic spectrum of Alagille syndrome. Hepatology 32:574–581, 2000.
124. Hoffenberg EJ, Narkewicz MR, Sondheimer JM, et al: Outcome of syndromic paucity of interlobular bile ducts (Alagille syndrome) with onset of cholestasis in infancy. J Pediatr 127:220–224, 1995.
125. Tzakis AG, Reyes J, Tepetes K, et al: Liver transplantation for Alagille's syndrome. Arch Surg 128:337–339, 1993.
126. Protheroe SM: Feeding the child with chronic liver disease. Nutrition 14:796–800, 1998.
127. Ramaccioni V, Soriano HE, Arumugam R, Klish WJ: Nutritional aspects of chronic liver disease and liver transplantation in children. J Pediatr Gastroenterol Nutr 30:361–367, 2000.
128. Sokol RJ: Fat-soluble vitamins and their importance in patients with cholestatic liver diseases. Gastroenterol Clin North Am 23:673–705, 1994.
129. Shetty AK, Schmidt-Sommerfeld E, Udall JN Jr: Nutritional aspects of liver disease in children. Nutrition 15:727–729, 1999.
130. Jones EA, Bergasa NV: The pruritus of cholestasis. Hepatology 29: 1003–1006, 1999.
131. Luketic VA, Sanyal AJ: Medical therapy of pruritus of cholestasis. Gastroenterologist 3:257–260, 1995.
132. Whitington PF, Whitington GL: Partial external diversion of bile for the treatment of intractable pruritus associated with intrahepatic cholestasis. Gastroenterology 95:130–136, 1988.
133. Friesen CA, Roberts CC: Cholelithiasis: Clinical characteristics in children: Case analysis and literature review. Clin Pediatr (Phila) 28: 294–298, 1989.
134. Holcomb GW Jr, Holcomb GW III: Cholelithiasis in infants, children, and adolescents. Pediatr Rev 11:268–274, 1990.
135. Palasciano G, Portincasa P, Vinciguerra V, et al: Gallstone prevalence and gallbladder volume in children and adolescents: An epidemiological ultrasonographic survey and relationship to body mass index. Am J Gastroenterol 84:1378–1382, 1989.
136. Wilcox DT, Casson D, Bowen J, et al: Cholelithiasis in early infancy. Pediatr Surg Int 12:198–199, 1997.

137. Davies BW, Abel G, Puntis JW, et al: Limited ileal resection in infancy: The long-term consequences. J Pediatr Surg 34:583–587, 1999.
138. Walker TM, Hambleton IR, Serjeant GR: Gallstones in sickle cell disease: Observations from the Jamaican Cohort Study. J Pediatr 136: 80–85, 2000.
139. Descos B, Bernard O, Brunelle F, et al: Pigment gallstones of the common bile duct in infancy. Hepatology 4:678–683, 1984.
140. Treem WR, Malet PF, Gourley GR, Hyams JS: Bile and stone analysis in two infants with brown pigment gallstones and infected bile. Gastroenterology 96(pt 1):519–523, 1989.
141. Bennion LJ, Knowler WC, Mott DM, et al: Development of lithogenic bile during puberty in Pima Indians. N Engl J Med 300:873–876, 1979.
142. Papadopoulou F, Efremidis S, Karyda S, et al: Incidence of ceftriaxone-associated gallbladder pseudolithiasis. Acta Paediatr 88:1352–1355, 1999.
143. Schaad UB, Wedgwood-Krucko J, Tschaeppeler H, et al: Reversible ceftriaxone-associated biliary pseudolithiasis in children. Lancet 2: 1411–1413, 1988.
144. Riccabona M, Kerbl R, Schwinger W, et al: Ceftriaxone-induced cholelithiasis—a harmless side-effect? Klin Padiatr 205:421–423, 1993.
145. Rescorla FJ: Cholelithiasis, cholecystitis, and common bile duct stones. Curr Opin Pediatr 9:276–282, 1997.
146. Debray D, Pariente D, Gauthier F, et al: Cholelithiasis in infancy: A study of 40 cases. J Pediatr 122:385–391, 1993.
147. Rescorla FJ, Grosfeld JL: Cholecystitis and cholelithiasis in children. Semin Pediatr Surg 1:98–106, 1992.
148. Holcomb GW III, Morgan WM III, Neblett WW III, et al: Laparoscopic cholecystectomy in children: Lessons learned from the first 100 patients. J Pediatr Surg 34:1236–1240, 1999.
149. Waldhausen JH, Benjamin DR: Cholecystectomy is becoming an increasingly common operation in children. Am J Surg 177:364–367, 1999.
150. Mok HY, Druffel ER, Rampone WM: Chronology of cholelithiasis: Dating gallstones ftom atmospheric radiocarbon produced by nuclear bomb explosions. N Engl J Med 314:1075–1077, 1986.
151. Miltenburg DM, Schaffer R III, Breslin T, Brandt ML: Changing indications for pediatric cholecystectomy. Pediatrics 105:1250–1253, 2000.
152. Stringer MD, Lim P, Cave M, et al: Fetal gallstones. J Pediatr Surg 31:1589–1591, 1996.
153. Colombo C, Bertolini E, Assaisso ML, et al: Failure of ursodeoxycholic acid to dissolve radiolucent gallstones in patients with cystic fibrosis. Acta Paediatr 82:562–565, 1993.
154. Reif S, Sloven DG, Lebenthal E: Gallstones in children: Characterization by age, etiology, and outcome. Am J Dis Child 145:105–108, 1991.
155. Roca I, Ciofetta G: Hepatobiliary scintigraphy in current pediatric practice. Q J Nucl Med 42:113–118, 1998.
156. Holcomb GW III: Laparoscopic cholecystectomy. Semin Pediatr Surg 2:159–167, 1993.
157. Tsakayannis DE, Kozakewich HP, Lillehei CW: Acalculous cholecystitis in children. J Pediatr Surg 31:127–130, 1996.
158. Fernandes ET, Hollabaugh RS, Boulden TF, Angel C: Gangrenous acalculous cholecystitis in a premature infant. J Pediatr Surg 24:608–609, 1989.
159. Schwesinger WH, Diehl AK: Changing indications for laparoscopic cholecystectomy: Stones without symptoms and symptoms without stones. Surg Clin North Am 76:493–504, 1996.
160. Crankson S, Nazer H, Jacobsson B: Acute hydrops of the gallbladder in childhood. Eur J Pediatr 151:318–320, 1992.
161. Suddleson EA, Reid B, Woolley M, Takahashi M: Hydrops of the gallbladder associated with Kawasaki syndrome. J Pediatr Surg 22: 956–959, 1987.

Chapter 53

Motility and Dysmotility of the Biliary Tract and Sphincter of Oddi

Grace H. Elta

ANATOMY AND PHYSIOLOGY

The biliary tree begins in the liver with canaliculi that converge to form hepatic ducts, which in turn converge to form the common hepatic duct (see Chapter 52). In these ducts there are few small smooth muscle cells, which are oriented circumferentially. The cystic duct also contains a thin layer of muscle that is continuous with the muscle layer of the gallbladder, with most of the cells oriented circumferentially. The common bile duct (CBD) has only sparse longitudinal muscle fibers, which become more prominent in the distal duct, but very few circularly oriented fibers. The gallbladder wall has a muscular layer with bundles oriented mainly along the longitudinal axis in the body and along the circular axis in the neck. Of gallbladder emptying, 20% to 30% actually occurs during the interdigestive period during phase II of the migrating motor complex (MMC). It is hypothesized that this interdigestive gallbladder emptying may serve a housekeeping function to decrease the risk of stones. Meal induced cholecystokinin (CCK) stimulates gallbladder contraction and sphincter of Oddi (SO) relaxation. Continuous CCK infusion leads to 55% to 75% emptying of the normal gallbladder volume of 20 to 30 mL.

The SO is composed of layers of smooth muscle that is embedded in, but functionally separate from, the muscle of the duodenal wall. There are three portions of SO: a small segment that covers the common channel (when one is present), a second small portion that surrounds the beginning of the main pancreatic duct, and the largest portion of the sphincter muscle, which covers the distal CBD (Fig. 53–1). Baseline sphincter pressures in the biliary and pancreatic portions of the sphincter are discordant in up to 20% of patients.[1] In humans, SO functions primarily as a resistor, with tonic contraction that limits bile flow during the interdigestive period. However, it also is a pump, with phasic contractions that facilitate flow into the duodenum, perhaps serving a housekeeping function for the distal bile duct. The SO also participates in the MMC, with a motilin-induced increase in the frequency and amplitude of sphincter contractions shortly before and during the burst of intense duodenal contractions.

There is complex neurohormonal control of biliary motility that involves sympathetic, parasympathetic, and enteric nerves. Almost every neurotransmitter in the enteric nervous system has been found in the biliary tree. Vasoactive intestinal polypeptide (VIP) and nitric oxide play roles in SO relaxation.

GALLBLADDER DYSKINESIA

In light of the distribution of muscle fibers in the biliary tree, it is not surprising that biliary dysmotility, or clinical problems related to motility, is focused on either the gallbladder or the SO. Although it is clear that gallbladder stasis predisposes to sludge and stone formation, it is not clear that gallbladder dysfunction, or delayed emptying of the gallbladder in the absence of stones or sludge, causes biliary symptoms. Patients who experience typical biliary pain and who have no evidence of gallstones may be studied with scintigraphic imaging of the gallbladder during CCK infusion. Although pain during infusion may be reported, CCK also stimulates intestinal motility, so it is unlikely that the production of pain is diagnostic of biliary pain. Delayed gallbladder emptying has been reported to be predictive of pain relief after cholecystectomy,[2] although this finding remains controversial.[3] It is known that delayed gallbladder emptying is more common in patients with functional bowel disease than in control subjects.[4] In many of these patients, symptoms are probably caused by the functional bowel disorder, and the gallbladder dysmotility is incidental. Some of them actually have gallstones or sludge overlooked on prior imaging studies and truly benefit from surgery. The histologic diagnosis of chronic cholecystitis in resected gallbladders has been proposed as confirmation of a gallbladder source of

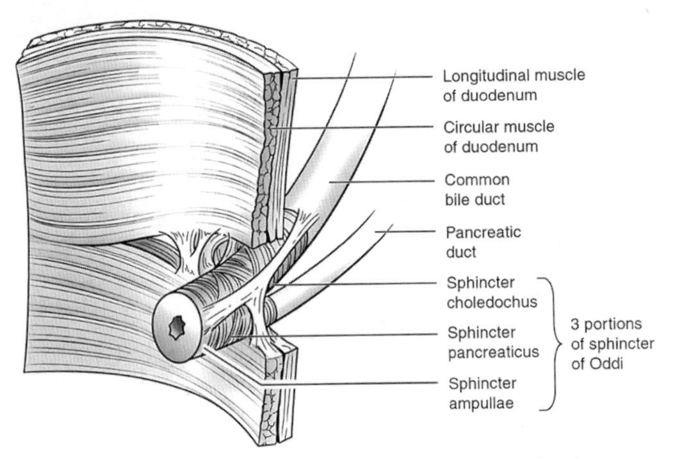

Figure 53–1. Anatomy of the sphincter of Oddi. Note the three portions of the sphincter of Oddi: the sphincter ampullae (surrounding the short common channel), the sphincter choledochus (the largest portion), and the sphincter pancreaticus.

symptoms.[2] However, in light of the high incidence of asymptomatic gallbladder stones and inflammation, the validity of this conclusion remains uncertain. Caution should be exercised when using delayed gallbladder emptying as an indication for cholecystectomy because it appears that many of these patients remain symptomatic or have recurrent symptoms postoperatively (see also Chapter 58).

SPHINCTER OF ODDI DYSFUNCTION

Definition

SO dysfunction (SOD) is a benign, noncalculous obstructive disorder that occurs at the level of the SO. The pathogenesis of SOD relates either to passive obstruction at the SO caused by fibrosis and/or inflammation or to active obstruction caused by sphincter muscle spasm. These two mechanisms of functional obstruction at the SO are not mutually exclusive. Less precise terms for SOD in the medical literature include *papillary stenosis*, *biliary dyskinesia*, and *postcholecystectomy syndrome*.

Frequency

The frequency of manometrically detected SOD in patients with an intact gallbladder has received limited study. Elevated basal sphincter pressure was reported in 4.1% of patients with biliary pain, normal serum alkaline phosphatase levels, and gallstones in the gallbladder before cholecystectomy.[5] When abnormal liver enzymes were present, 40% of 25 similar patients without ductal stones had an elevated basal sphincter pressure. In contrast, no basal sphincter pressure elevation above 30 mm Hg was found in 50 asymptomatic volunteers.[6] Ruffolo and coworkers reported that 50% of 81 patients with biliary-type pain, intact gallbladders, and no evidence of gallstones had delayed gallbladder emptying, SOD, or both.[7]

The frequency of SOD in postcholecystectomy patients with persistent or recurrent biliary-type pain depends on the criteria for patient selection. Postcholecystectomy pain resembling preoperative biliary colic occurs in 10% to 20% of patients.[8] The most common explanation is that the symptoms before surgery were not caused by gallstones. The most likely diagnosis in this group of patients is a functional gastrointestinal disorder such as irritable bowel syndrome or nonulcer dyspepsia. SOD is reported in 9% to 14% of consecutive patients who are evaluated for postcholecystectomy pain.[9, 10] When other causes of postcholecystectomy pain are excluded and SO manometry (SOM) is performed in a more carefully screened group, the frequency is 30% to 60%.[11, 12] When these patients are classified by the Milwaukee classification for possible SOD (Table 53–1), the frequencies of elevated basal sphincter pressure are 86%, 55%, and 28% for patients with types I, II, and III suspected SOD, respectively.

Table 53–1 | **Milwaukee Classification for Possible Biliary Sphincter of Oddi Dysfunction**

PATIENT GROUP	CLINICAL CRITERIA
Biliary type I	• Biliary-type pain • Serum AST or ALP level >2 times normal on ≥2 occasions • Delayed ERCP contrast drainage >45 minutes • Dilated CBD >12 mm
Biliary type II	• Biliary-type pain • One or two of the other three criteria
Biliary type III	• Biliary-type pain alone

ALP, alkaline phosphatase; AST, aspartate aminotransferase; CBD, common bile duct; ERCP, endoscopic retrograde cholangiopancreatography.

Modified from Venu RP, Geenen JE, Hogan WJ: Sphincter of Oddi stenosis and dysfunction. In Sivak MV (ed): Gastroenterologic Endoscopy, 2nd ed. Philadelphia, WB Saunders, 2000, p 1023.

Clinical Presentation

SOD is a possible cause of three clinical conditions: (1) persistent or recurrent biliary pain following cholecystectomy in the absence of structural abnormalities, (2) idiopathic recurrent pancreatitis, and (3) biliary pain in patients with intact gallbladders but without cholelithiasis (the least studied and most controversial clinical association) (Table 53–2). SOD also has been described in patients who have had liver transplantation,[13] have the acquired immunodeficiency syndrome,[14] and have hyperlipidemia.[15]

Although biliary SOD has been diagnosed in all age

Table 53–2 | **Clinical Associations for Sphincter of Oddi Dysfunction**

Best studied
Biliary-type pain postcholecystectomy
Less well studied
Idiopathic acute recurrent pancreatitis
Biliary-type pain in a patient with an intact gallbladder
Possible associations
Chronic pancreatitis
After liver transplantation
Acquired immunodeficiency syndrome-associated viral/protozoal infections*
Hyperlipidemia

*Cytomegalovirus infection, cryptosporidiosis, microsporidiosis.

groups, it is most common in middle-aged women. The female predominance among patients varies from 75% to 90%. The pain is typical of biliary colic, is epigastric or occurs in the right upper quadrant, and may radiate to the back or right shoulder blade. The pain is usually episodic and severe but may be continuous with episodic exacerbations. Less than one half of patients have abnormal liver biochemical test results, although transient elevation of serum aminotransferase levels with attacks of pain supports the diagnosis of SOD.

Diagnosis

NONINVASIVE EVALUATION. Evaluation of patients suspected of having SOD is initiated with liver biochemical testing, serum amylase and lipase measurements, and often abdominal imaging by either ultrasonography or computed tomographic scanning. Serum aminotransferase level elevations, if present, are mild, less than three to four times the upper limit of normal. Physical examination findings are usually normal, although mild right upper quadrant tenderness may be present. Standard evaluation and therapeutic trials for more common causes of abdominal pain, such as gastroesophageal reflux, fatty liver, and irritable bowel syndrome, are usually undertaken as well.

Noninvasive tests for SOD have included the morphine-neostigmine (Prostigmin) provocative test (also called the Nardi test), fatty meal or secretin-stimulated ultrasonography, and biliary scintigraphy. Reproduction of the patient's typical pain and an increase in levels of liver and pancreatic enzymes after subcutaneous injection of morphine and neostigmine methylsulfate constitute a positive test result. However, the sensitivity and specificity of this challenge test for SOD are poor, and the test is of only historical interest.[16] After a lipid-rich meal or administration of CCK, the common bile duct may dilate under pressure if SO is dysfunctional. Similarly, after secretin stimulation, the pancreatic duct may dilate, and this change can be detected by transcutaneous ultrasonography. Pain provocation also can be monitored. Compared with manometry, secretin-stimulated ultrasonography testing has a sensitivity of 88% and a specificity of 82% in patients with recurrent acute pancreatitis.[17] Biliary scintigraphy also has been used to assess bile flow into the duodenum[18] and has been proposed as a safe screening test before biliary manometry. However, although scintigraphy findings are usually positive in patients with dilated ducts and high-grade obstruction, scintigraphy lacks sufficient sensitivity in patients with lower-grade obstruction (Milwaukee classification types II and III). Therefore, none of these noninvasive tests is generally recommended for clinical use in the diagnosis of SOD.

CLASSIFICATION OF POSSIBLE SPHINCTER OF ODDI DYSFUNCTION. Patients with suspected biliary SOD are classified into three categories, depending on the clinical data that support the diagnosis (see Table 53–1). Bile duct dilation is one of these criteria, although considerable overlap in the diameter of the common bile duct of patients with SOD and asymptomatic postcholecystectomy patients exists, and the value of this criterion has been questioned.[19] The common cutoff for an abnormal bile duct diameter following cholecystectomy is 12 mm, although the standard varies from 10 to 15 mm in several studies. Elevated levels of liver enzymes, especially when associated with attacks of pain, appear to be predictive of pain relief after sphincterotomy.[19] The Milwaukee criterion is that both serum alkaline phosphatase and aminotransferase levels be elevated (2 times normal) on two occasions, whereas the criterion in the modified Milwaukee classification system is that any liver enzyme level be abnormal (1.1 times normal) on one occasion.[20] Neither classification system requires that the enzyme level elevations be timed with attacks of pain, although such an association may be a predictor of response to treatment. Delayed drainage of bile into the duodenum at cholangiography (more than 45 minutes) is the third criterion for suspected SOD, although this criterion appears to lack specificity, because delayed drainage may occur in normal persons following cholecystectomy.[21] Additionally, few endoscopists take the time to obtain this measurement. In fact, some researchers have suggested that the Milwaukee classification be modified further to consider only bile duct diameter and elevated serum aminotransferase levels as criteria for SOD[20] (Table 53–3). Despite these problems with the clinical criteria, however, these classification systems have remained useful because of their ability to predict outcome of biliary sphincter ablation.[22]

Lehman and colleagues have devised a similar classifica-

Table 53–3 | **Modified Milwaukee Classification for Possible Biliary Sphincter of Oddi Dysfunction**

PATIENT GROUP	CLINICAL CRITERIA	APPROXIMATE FREQUENCY OF ABNORMAL MANOMETRY	PROBABILITY OF PAIN RELIEF BY SPHINCTEROTOMY IF MANOMETRY FINDING IS	
			Abnormal	Normal
Biliary I	Biliary-type pain Serum ALT, AST, or ALP level 1.1 times normal on one occasion Common bile duct >10 mm	65%–85%	90%–95%	90%–95%
Biliary II	Biliary-type pain One of two additional criteria	65%	85%	35%
Biliary III	Biliary-type pain only	59%	55%–60%	<10%

ALP, alkaline phosphatase; ALT, alanine aminotransferase; AST, aspartate aminotransferase.

Modified from Eversman D, Fogel EL, Rusche M, et al: Frequency of abnormal pancreatic and biliary sphincter manometry compared with clinical suspicion of sphincter of Oddi dysfunction. Gastrointest Endosc 50:637, 1999.

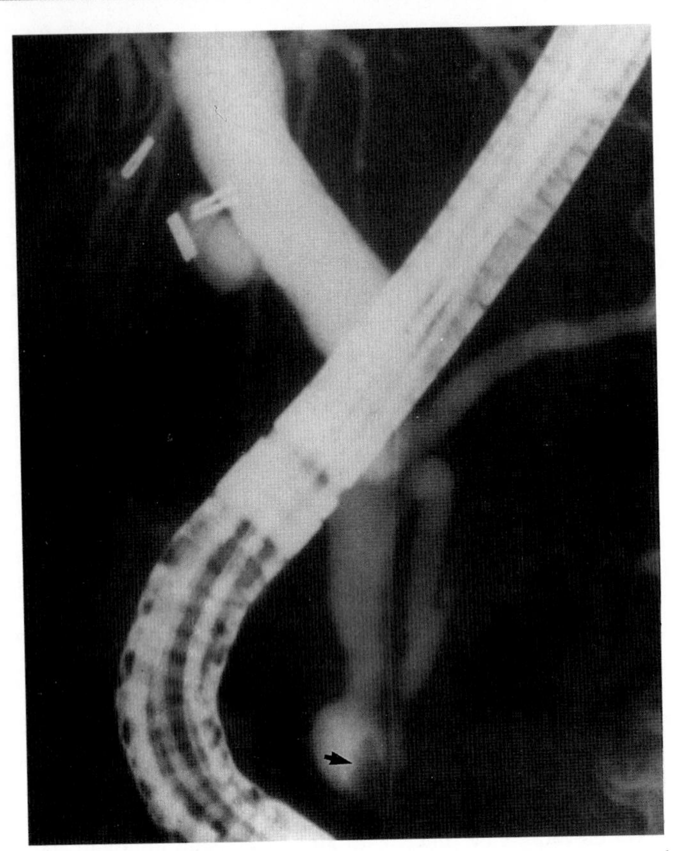

Figure 53–2. Intra-ampullary adenoma *(arrow)* presenting as suspected sphincter of Oddi dysfunction

tion system for possible pancreatic SOD.[20] Pancreatic type I patients have pancreatic-type pain, a serum amylase or lipase level of 1.1 times normal on one occasion, and pancreatic duct dilation (>6 mm in the head and >5 mm in the body); pancreatic type II patients have pain and one of the preceding criteria; type III patients have pancreatic-type pain only. Several studies have demonstrated a high frequency (60% to 72%) of sphincter hypertension in patients with idiopathic pancreatitis, and a 50% to 87% frequency in those with chronic pancreatitis.[23, 24] The utility of this pancreatic classification system will depend on outcome studies of the symptomatic response to pancreatic sphincter ablation.

INVASIVE EVALUATION. Patients with suspected SOD have the highest complication rates for endoscopic retrograde cholangiopancreatography (ERCP) and sphincterotomy. Rates of pancreatitis of 20% have been reported in this group.[25] Therefore, ERCP with manometry should be reserved for persons who have severe or debilitating symptoms. Cholangiography is essential to rule out stones or tumors as the cause of biliary obstruction and associated symptoms. Alternative biliary imaging studies, such as magnetic resonance cholangiopancreatography (MRCP) or endoscopic ultrasonography, are safer methods than ERCP for excluding stones or tumors, although they cannot diagnose SOD.

Occasionally, an intra-ampullary neoplasm may simulate SOD (Fig. 53–2). If there appears to be excess tissue in the ampulla after sphincterotomy, biopsy specimens of the area should be obtained.[26]

SPHINCTER MANOMETRY: THE TECHNIQUE. SOM is usually performed during ERCP, although it can be done in the operating room or via a percutaneous approach.[27] All drugs that relax (nitrates, calcium channel blockers, and anticholinergics) or stimulate (narcotics and cholinergics) the SO should be avoided for 12 hours prior to manometry. Benzodiazepams[28] and meperidine (the latter in a dose of 1 mg/kg) do not affect basal sphincter pressure,[29] although meperidine does increase phasic wave frequency. Anecdotal evidence indicates that droperidol may also be used as a preanesthetic. Glucagon should be avoided, although some authorities use it if necessary to achieve cannulation and wait at least 8 to 10 minutes until sphincter function is restored before measuring pressures.

SOM utilizes pressure recording equipment and infusion systems similar to those used for esophageal motility studies. Important differences are that the infusion system for SOM should be disinfected and use bubble-free sterile water. The infusion rate is 0.25 mL per channel using a low-compliance pump. Performance of manometry requires a two-person approach with one person stationed at the recorder. Triple-lumen number 5 French catheters are produced by several manufacturers in long-nose and short-nose types. The long-nose catheter has the advantage in the biliary duct of allowing several pull-throughs without losing cannulation, although in tortuous pancreatic ducts the nose occasionally is too long for free cannulation. The three orifices are spaced 2 mm apart and are oriented radially (Fig. 53–3). The middle port is used for aspiration, which has been shown in a controlled trial to lower the risk of pancreatitis.[30] This port also allows the cannulated duct to be identified easily by the color of the aspirate. The middle port can accept a 0.018 guidewire, thereby allowing wire exchange in difficult cannulations.

When manometry is clinically indicated, many experts begin ERCP with the manometry catheter, because the duodenum has less motility if contrast medium has not been given. The duodenal or zero pressure should be measured before cannulation and at the end of the manometry. The catheter is withdrawn across the sphincter at 1- to 2-mm intervals by using a standard station pull-through technique (Fig. 53–4). Abnormalities of the basal sphincter pressure should be observed on at least two pull-throughs. Depending on the clinical indication, pancreatic SOM may then be performed by the same technique. Abnormal basal sphincter pressures are usually concordant for the two ducts but may occur in only one portion of the sphincter.[31] If the clinical indication for SOM is biliary pain, rather than idiopathic

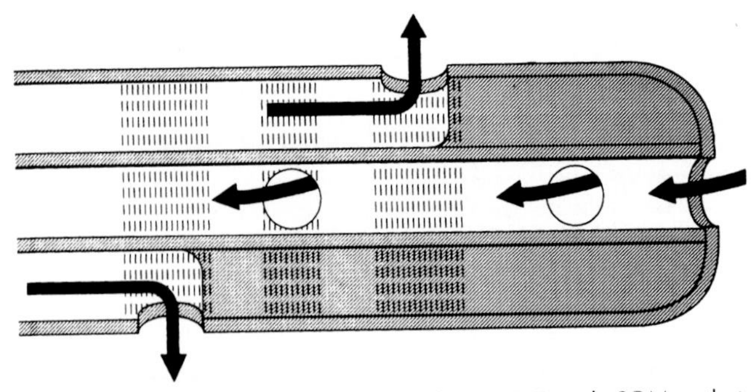

Figure 53–3. Aspiration manometry catheter: 5 French SOM catheter (Wilson Cook model no. SOM-21-S-Lehman, Wilson Cook, Winston-Salem, NC). The arrows depict direction of fluid movement; outward flow represents perfusion, and inward flow represents aspiration.

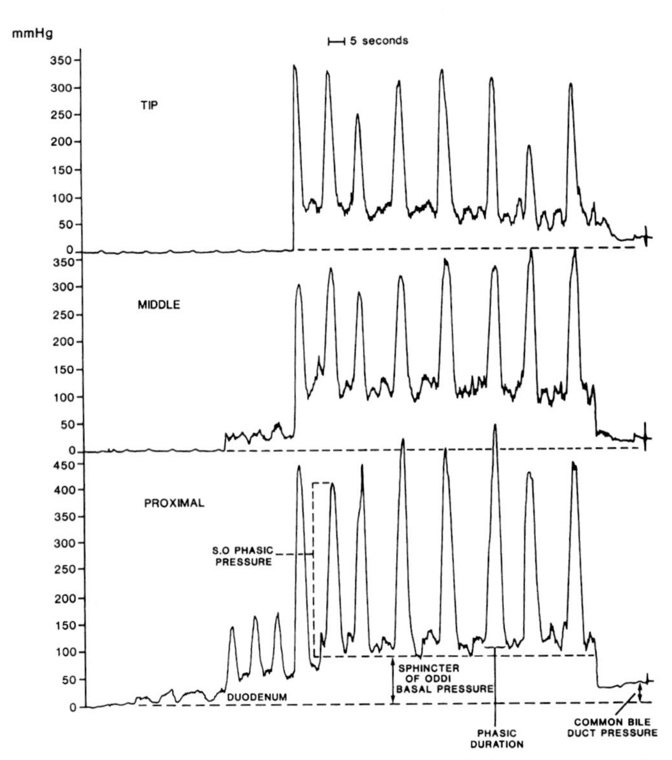

Figure 53–4. Station pull-through tracing of triple-lumen catheter for sphincter of Oddi (biliary) manometry. This tracing shows abnormal mean basal pressure of 70 mm Hg.

pancreatitis, and biliary SOM produces normal findings, some authorities avoid pancreatic cannulation entirely with the goal of decreasing the frequency of pancreatitis. Other experts advise studying both ducts in all patients. It has been shown that increased basal sphincter pressure is more likely to be confined to the pancreas in patients with pancreatitis and more likely confined to the bile duct in persons with elevated levels of serum liver enzymes.[32] When the biliary SOM result is abnormal and biliary sphincterotomy is performed, placement of a pancreatic duct stent, when there is associated pancreatic sphincter hypertension, lowers the risk of procedure-induced pancreatitis.[33] When the clinical indication for SOM is idiopathic recurrent pancreatitis, pancreatic manometry is mandatory. After the tracings are completed, glucagon or additional meperidine may be given to facilitate subsequent contrast injection or endoscopic therapy. If a simple cholangiogram is desired, the aspirating port can be used for contrast injection.

The method of averaging interpretable tracings and the number of leads used to take these measurements vary from center to center, although interobserver differences appear to be minimal.[34] The standard upper limit of normal for baseline sphincter pressure is 35 to 40 mm Hg. The reproducibility of these measurements was proved in an important study of normal volunteers by Guelrud and associates.[6] The phasic wave frequency, propagation direction of waves, and amplitude of the waves also can be determined, although the clinical significance of these measurements remains unclear. Additional pharmacologic maneuvers, such as provocation with CCK, are also of uncertain value at this time.

SPHINCTER MANOMETRY: DIAGNOSTIC USE. The landmark randomized, controlled study of patients with suspected type II biliary SOD by Geenen and colleagues established SOM as predictive of responsiveness of pain to sphincterotomy.[35] Patients with an elevated basal SO pressure of greater than 40 mm Hg had a clinical response rate of 91% compared with a 25% rate in patients with a high basal pressure in whom a sham sphincterotomy was performed. For patients with a normal SO pressure, the response to sphincterotomy was only 42% and similar to that after the sham procedure (33%). These results were confirmed in 2000 in a controlled study of patients with type II SOD and elevated sphincter pressures.[36] In this study clinical improvement was demonstrated in 11 of 13 patients treated with sphincterotomy compared with 5 of 13 control subjects treated with sham sphincterotomy.[36] There was no difference in pain response between sphincterotomy and sham sphincterotomy in patients with manometric abnormalities other than elevated basal SO pressure, namely, tachyoddia, increased retrograde contractions, or a paradoxical response to CCK.

Despite the findings of these studies, the use of SOM as a diagnostic tool remains somewhat controversial. Some uncontrolled studies suggest that more easily measurable criteria such as elevated liver enzyme levels or biliary dilatation are superior in predicting a response to sphincter ablation.[37] Alternatively, manometry may be highly specific in diagnosing SOD but may lack sensitivity; lack of sensitivity may account for the symptom response rate to sphincterotomy of 42% in biliary type II patients with normal manometry results.[35] A lack of sensitivity may also explain the relatively low rate of abnormal SOM (65% to 85%) in type I patients, who have a response rate to sphincterotomy greater than 90%.[38] It is hypothesized that the relatively low frequency of sphincter hypertension in type I patients is the result of a different pathogenesis of sphincter obstruction, namely, sphincter stenosis rather than sphincter hypertension. Another possible explanation for the insensitivity of SOM is that short-term observation of sphincter pressure may not detect the underlying pathophysiologic process. An additional problem with manometry is the high rate of procedure-related morbidity, especially pancreatitis, which occurs in 10% to 25% of patients who have SOM.[39] SOM is a difficult technique that is not widely available and has success rates of only 75% to 92% in the most experienced hands.

In biliary type III patients SOD appears to be less common than in type II patients, and the response to sphincter ablation is only 39% to 60%.[12, 22] A response to sphincter ablation in type III patients with normal SOM findings is rare. Obviously, pain is a poor indicator of any specific regional disorder. Abnormal small bowel interdigestive motor activity[40] and duodenal visceral hyperalgesia in response to duodenal (but not rectal) distention[41, 42] have been demonstrated in SOD type III patients. As in other functional gastrointestinal disorders, somatization disorder is more common in these patient populations than in the general population.[43]

OTHER DIAGNOSTIC METHODS. Placement of a pancreatic or biliary stent on a trial basis with the goal of achieving pain relief and thereby predicting a response to subsequent sphincterotomy has been suggested to be superior to manometry.[44] Although relief of pain with placement of a biliary stent is predictive of long-term relief after biliary sphincterotomy,[45] the high rate of pancreatitis in the stented patients has dampened enthusiasm for this technique. Pancreatic duct stents are strongly discouraged as a therapeutic trial because of their propensity to cause ductal injury if left in place for more than a few days.[46]

Injection of botulinum toxin into the SO decreases basal sphincter pressure by about 50%.[47] Its use also has been proposed as a therapeutic trial to assess the likelihood of success of subsequent sphincterotomy.[48] However, because this approach requires a repeat ERCP, with its attendant risks, it is not likely to become popular.

Microlithiasis, or biliary crystals, has been associated with idiopathic pancreatitis.[49] The question arises as to whether some cases of postcholecystectomy pain relate to bile duct microlithiasis, analogous to choledocholithiasis. However, detection of bile duct crystals at ERCP in postcholecystectomy patients is rare and is not associated with abnormal SOM results.[50]

Pain after biliary injection of contrast medium at ERCP may be dramatic in some patients but unfortunately has not been shown to be predictive of SOD.[51]

Therapy

MEDICAL THERAPY. Dietary or medical therapy for suspected or documented SOD has received limited study. A low-fat diet is recommended for reducing pancreaticobiliary stimulation. A trial of therapy with smooth muscle relaxants appears warranted. Nifedipine, nitrates, and antispasmodics lower basal SO pressure.[52] Two short-term placebo controlled, cross-over studies showed that 75% of suspected or documented SOD patients who used oral nifedipine experienced statistically less pain.[53, 54] In light of the safety of medical therapy and the benign nature of SOD, medical therapy should be tried in all patients with suspected type III SOD and in patients with less severe type II SOD before invasive sphincter ablation is attempted. Type II patients with more severe pain are less likely to respond to medical therapy, and in these patients a trial of medical therapy is optional.

SPHINCTEROTOMY. Historically, surgical biliary sphincterotomy and sphincteroplasty were used successfully for sphincter ablation. Endoscopic techniques have largely replaced open surgery for both biliary and pancreatic ablation. Most data on endoscopic sphincterotomy relate to biliary sphincter ablation alone.

The most common indication for SOM is biliary-type pain in a postcholecystectomy patient. If manometry findings are abnormal, relief of abdominal pain after sphincterotomy occurs in 90% to 95% of biliary type I patients, 85% of biliary type II patients, and 55% to 60% of biliary type III patients.[12, 35] When the manometry result is normal, pain relief after sphincterotomy still occurs in 90% to 95% of type I patients. Because findings of manometry may be misleading in these cases (they are normal in 14% to 35% of type I patients), manometry is not clinically indicated. Pain relief after sphincterotomy occurs in 35% to 42% of patients with biliary type II pain with normal manometry results. Although this response rate is similar to that in controls, it is likely that a true clinical response occurs in a few patients. Sphincterotomy is clearly indicated in biliary type II patients with abnormal manometry findings, although it remains controversial as to whether manometry is required to justify sphincterotomy in this group. In biliary type III patients with normal manometry findings, the clinical response rate to sphincterotomy is less than 10%, and an abnormal manometry result is mandatory before sphincterotomy.

Few studies have addressed SOD in patients with biliary-type pain, intact gallbladders, and no gallstones. One possibility is to evaluate such patients for abnormal gallbladder ejection fraction and fatty meal stimulated bile duct dilation before SOM. If there is ductal dilation, proceed to SOM and possible sphincterotomy.[55] If the stimulated meal does not cause duct dilatation and scintigraphy shows delayed gallbladder emptying, proceed to cholecystectomy. An abnormal quantitative cholescintigraphy or SOM result is present in up to 70% of these patients.[7] However, as previously discussed, the response to cholecystectomy is variable.[2, 3] Of patients with documented SOD and intact gallbladders treated with sphincterotomy first, only 43% have long-term pain relief; some additional patients eventually respond to cholecystectomy.[56] Clearly, more information is needed on how to assess and treat this challenging group of patients.

SPHINCTER OF ODDI DYSFUNCTION IN PANCREATITIS

Idiopathic Acute Recurrent Pancreatitis

SOD has been found in 25% to 60% of patients with idiopathic recurrent pancreatitis.[57] Recurrent attacks of pancreatitis appear to be prevented by pancreatic sphincterotomy in 60% to 80% of affected patients, although only preliminary uncontrolled studies are available.[58] Endoscopic pancreatic therapy carries an increased risk of complications.[59] For patients with intact gallbladders and idiopathic pancreatitis, some authors advocate either biliary sphincterotomy or treatment with ursodeoxycholic acid, with the implication that microlithiasis is the cause.[60] Other authors report that biliary sphincterotomy alone benefits only one third of these patients, whereas dual sphincterotomies benefit 80%, suggesting that pancreatic sphincter therapy must be included.[61] More studies are required to sort out the preferred approach (biliary, pancreatic, or dual sphincterotomies) and to clarify the rates of success and complication of these approaches.

Chronic Pancreatitis

SOD has been described in up to 87% of patients with chronic pancreatitis.[24] Whether SOD is the result of the chronic inflammation or plays a role in the pathogenesis of chronic pancreatitis is not known. Endoscopic pancreatic sphincterotomy improves pain scores in 60% to 65% of patients, although controlled studies are not available.[62, 63] In some cases pancreatic sphincterotomy may be performed to facilitate other therapeutic maneuvers, such as stone extraction and stricture dilation.[64] The role of sphincter manometry in chronic pancreatitis remains unclear.

FAILURE TO RESPOND TO BILIARY SPHINCTEROTOMY IN SPHINCTER OF ODDI DYSFUNCTION

There are several possible explanations for the lack of response to biliary sphincterotomy of patients with SOD (Ta-

Table 53-4 | **Possible Causes for Failure to Achieve Pain Relief after Biliary Sphincterotomy in Sphincter of Oddi Dysfunction**

- Nonpancreaticobiliary pain, especially functional gastrointestinal disease
- Inadequate initial sphincterotomy or occurrence of restenosis
- Residual pancreatic sphincter hypertension
- Subtle chronic pancreatitis with a normal pancreatographic result

ble 53-4). Perhaps the most likely explanation is that the pain was not of pancreatobiliary origin and was caused by altered gut motility or visceral hypersensitivity.[41] Alternatively, the biliary sphincterotomy may have been inadequate or restenosis may have occurred.[65] The clinical success of further biliary endoscopic treatment in such cases is unknown.

The role of residual pancreatic sphincter hypertension as a source of continuing pain is unclear. Symptomatic improvement after pancreatic sphincter ablation is reported in two thirds of these patients.[66] This finding has led some experts to advocate initial dual sphincterotomies, although the outcome of this approach is unknown.

Finally, some patients with suspected SOD who have not responded to biliary sphincterotomy may have subtle chronic pancreatitis and normal pancreatographic findings. Endoscopic ultrasonography may demonstrate parenchymal changes consistent with chronic pancreatitis in these cases.[67]

REFERENCES

1. Silverman W, Ruffolo T, Sherman S, et al: Correlation of basal sphincter pressures measured from the bile duct and the pancreatic duct in patients with suspected sphincter of Oddi dysfunction. Gastroenterology 101:786, 1991.
2. Yap L, Wycherley A, Morphett A, et al: Acalculous biliary pain: Cholecystectomy alleviates symptoms in patients with abnormal cholescintigraphy. Gastroenterology 101:786, 1991.
3. Westlake PJ, Hershfield NB, Kelly JK, et al: Chronic right upper quadrant pain without gallstones: Does HIDA scan predict outcome after cholecystectomy? Am J Gastroenterol 85:986, 1990.
4. Sood GK, Baijal SS, Lahoti D, et al: Abnormal gallbladder function in patients with irritable bowel syndrome. Am J Gastroenterol 88:1387, 1993.
5. Guelrud M, Mendoza S, Mujica V, et al: Sphincter of Oddi (SO) motor function in patients with symptomatic gallstones. Gastroenterology 104: A361, 1993.
6. Guelrud M, Mendoza S, Rossiter G, et al: Sphincter of Oddi manometry in healthy volunteers. Dig Dis Sci 35:38, 1990.
7. Ruffolo TA, Sherman S, Lehman GA, et al: Gallbladder ejection fraction and its relationship to sphincter of Oddi dysfunction. Dig Dis Sci 39:289, 1994.
8. Luman W, Adams WH, Nixon SN, et al: Incidence of persistent symptoms after laparoscopic cholecystectomy: A prospective study. Gut 39: 863, 1996.
9. Neoptolemos JA, Bailey IS, Carr-Locke D: Sphincter of Oddi dysfunction: Results of endoscopic sphincterotomy. Br J Surg 75:454, 1988.
10. Bar-Meir S, Halpern Z, Bardan E, et al: Frequency of papillary dysfunction among cholecystectomized patients. Hepatology 4:328, 1984.
11. Sherman S, Troiano FP, Hawes RH, et al: Frequency of abnormal sphincter of Oddi manometry compared with the clinical suspicion of sphincter of Oddi dysfunction. Am J Gastroenterol 86:586, 1991.
12. Botoman VA, Kozarek RA, Novell LA, et al: Long-term outcome after endoscopic sphincterotomy in patients with biliary colic and suspected sphincter of Oddi dysfunction. Gastrointest Endosc 40:165, 1994.
13. Douzdjian V, Abecassis MM, Johlin FC: Sphincter of Oddi dysfunction following liver transplantation: Screening by bedside manometric evaluation. Dig Dis Sci 39:253, 1994.
14. Cello JP, Chan MF: Long-term follow-up of endoscopic retrograde cholangiopancreatography sphincterotomy for patients with acquired immune deficiency syndrome papillary stenosis. Am J Med 99:600, 1995.
15. Szilvassy Z, Nagy I, Madacsy L, et al: Beneficial effect of lovastatin on sphincter of Oddi dyskinesia in hypercholesterolemia and hypertriglyceridemia. Am J Gastroenterol 92:900, 1997.
16. Steinberg WM, Salvato RF, Toskes PP: The morphine-Prostigmin provocative test—is it useful for making clinical decisions? Gastroenterology 78:728, 1980.
17. Di Francesco V, Brunori MP, Rigo L, et al: Comparison of ultrasound-secretin test and sphincter of Oddi manometry in patients with recurrent acute pancreatitis. Dig Dis Sci 44:336, 1999.
18. Cicala M, Scopinaro F, Corazziari E, et al: Quantitative cholescintigraphy in the assessment of choledochoduodenal bile flow. Gastroenterology 100:1106, 1991.
19. Lin OS, Soetikno RM, Young HS: The utility of liver function test abnormalities concomitant with biliary symptoms in predicting a favorable response to endoscopic sphincterotomy in patients with presumed sphincter of Oddi dysfunction. Am J Gastroenterol 93:1833, 1998.
20. Eversman D, Fogel EL, Rusche M, et al: Frequency of abnormal pancreatic and biliary sphincter manometry compared with clinical suspicion of sphincter of Oddi dysfunction. Gastrointest Endosc 50:637, 1999.
21. Elta GH, Barnett JL, Ellis JH, et al: Delayed biliary drainage is common in asymptomatic post-cholecystectomy volunteers. Gastrointest Endosc 38:435, 1992.
22. Wehrmann T, Wiemer K, Lembcke B, et al: Do patients with sphincter of Oddi dysfunction benefit from endoscopic sphincterotomy? A 5-year prospective trial. Eur J Gastroenterol Hepatol 8:251, 1996.
23. Vestergaard H, Kruse A, Rokkjaer M, et al: Endoscopic manometry of the sphincter of Oddi and the pancreatic and biliary ducts in patients with chronic pancreatitis. Scand J Gastroenterol 29:188, 1994.
24. Tarnasky PR, Hoffman B, Aabakken L, et al: Sphincter of Oddi dysfunction is associated with chronic pancreatitis. Am J Gastroenterol 92: 1125, 1997.
25. Freeman ML, Nelson DB, Sherman S, et al: Complications of endoscopic biliary sphincterotomy. N Engl J Med 335:909, 1996.
26. Ponchon T, Aucia N, Mitchell R, et al: Biopsies of the ampullary region in patients suspected to have sphincter of Oddi dysfunction. Gastrointest Endosc 42:296, 1995.
27. Sherman S, Hawes RH, Madura JA, et al: Comparison of intraoperative and endoscopic manometry of the sphincter of Oddi. Surg Gynecol Obstet 175:410, 1992.
28. Rolny P, Arleback A: Effect of midazolam on sphincter of Oddi motility. Endoscopy 25:381, 1993.
29. Elta GH, Barnett JL: Meperidine need not be proscribed during sphincter of Oddi manometry. Gastrointest Endosc 40:7, 1994.
30. Sherman S, Troiano FP, Hawes RH, et al: Sphincter of Oddi manometry: Decreased risk of clinical pancreatitis with use of a modified aspirating catheter. Gastrointest Endosc 36:462, 1990.
31. Chan Y-K, Evans PR, Dowsett JF, et al: Discordance of pressure recordings from biliary and pancreatic duct segments in patients with suspected sphincter of Oddi dysfunction. Dig Dis Sci 42:1501, 1997.
32. Raddawi HM, Geenen JE, Hogan WJ, et al: Pressure measurements from biliary and pancreatic segments of sphincter of Oddi: Comparison between patients with functional abdominal pain, biliary, or pancreatic disease. Dig Dis Sci 36:71, 1991.
33. Tarnasky PR, Palesch YY, Cunningham JT, et al: Pancreatic stenting prevents pancreatitis after biliary sphincterotomy in patients with sphincter of Oddi dysfunction. Gastroenterology 115:1518, 1998.
34. Thune A, Scicchitano J, Roberts-Thomson I, et al: Reproducibility of endoscopic sphincter of Oddi manometry. Dig Dis Sci 36:1401, 1991.
35. Geenen JE, Hogan WJ, Dodds WJ, et al: The efficacy of endoscopic sphincterotomy after cholecystectomy in patients with sphincter of Oddi dysfunction. N Engl J Med 320:82, 1989.
36. Toouli J, Roberts-Thomson IC, Kellow J, et al: Manometry based randomized trial of endoscopic sphincterotomy for sphincter of Oddi dysfunction. Gut 46:98, 2000.
37. Viceconte G, Micheletti A: Endoscopic manometry of the sphincter of Oddi: Its usefulness for the diagnosis and treatment of benign papillary stenosis. Scand J Gastroenterol 30:797, 1995.
38. Rolny P, Geenen JE, Hogan WJ, et al: Clinical features, manometric findings and endoscopic therapy results in group I patients with sphincter of Oddi dysfunction. Gastrointest Endosc 37:252, 1991.
39. Maldonado ME, Brady PG, Mamel JJ, et al: Incidence of pancreatitis in

patients undergoing sphincter of Oddi manometry (SOM). Am J Gastroenterol 94:387, 1999.
40. Evans PR, Bak Y-T, Dowsett JF, et al: Small bowel dysmotility in patients with postcholecystectomy sphincter of Oddi dysfunction. Dig Dis Sci 42:1507, 1997.
41. Desautels SG, Slivka A, Hutson WR, et al: Postcholecystectomy pain syndrome: Pathophysiology of abdominal pain in sphincter of Oddi type III. Gastroenterology 116:900, 1999.
42. Chun A, Desautels S, Slivka A, et al: Visceral algesia in irritable bowel syndrome, fibromyalgia, and sphincter of Oddi dysfunction, type III. Dig Dis Sci 44:631, 1999.
43. Abraham HD, Anderson C, Lee D: Somatization disorder in sphincter of Oddi dysfunction. Psychosom Med 59:553, 1997.
44. Rolny P: Endoscopic bile duct stent placement as a predictor of outcome following endoscopic sphincterotomy in patients with suspected sphincter of Oddi dysfunction. Eur J Gastroenterol Hepatol 9:467, 1997.
45. Goff JS: Common bile duct sphincter of Oddi stenting in patients with suspected sphincter dysfunction. Am J Gastroenterol 90:586, 1995.
46. Kozarek RA: Pancreatic stents can induce ductal changes consistent with chronic pancreatitis. Gastrointest Endosc 36:93, 1990.
47. Pasricha PJ, Miskovsky EP, Kalloo AN: Intrasphincteric injection of botulinum toxin for suspected sphincter of Oddi dysfunction. Gut 35: 1319, 1994.
48. Wehrmann T, Seifert H, Seipp M, et al: Endoscopic injection of botulinum toxin for biliary sphincter of Oddi dysfunction. Endoscopy 30:702, 1998.
49. Ros E, Navarro S, Bru C, et al: Occult microlithiasis in "idiopathic" acute pancreatitis: Prevention of relapse by cholecystectomy or ursodeoxycholic acid therapy. Gastroenterology 101:1701, 1991.
50. Stern M, Barnett J, Elta GH: Do bile duct crystals contribute to postcholecystectomy syndrome? Gastrointest Endosc 49:AB185, 1999.
51. Schmalz MJ, Geenen JE, Hogan WJ, et al: Pain on common bile duct injection during ERCP: Does it indicate sphincter of Oddi dysfunction? Gastrointest Endosc 36:458, 1990.
52. Brandstatter G, Schinzel S, Wurzer H: Influence of spasmolytic analgesics on motility of sphincter of Oddi. Dig Dis Sci 41:1814, 1996.
53. Sand J, Nordback I, Koskinen M, et al: Nifedipine for suspected type II sphincter of Oddi dyskinesia. Am J Gastroenterol 88:530, 1993.
54. Khuroo MS, Zargar SA, Yattoo GN: Efficacy of nifedipine therapy in patients with sphincter of Oddi dysfunction: A prospective, double-blind, randomized, placebo-controlled, cross over trial. Br J Clin Pharmacol 33:477, 1992.
55. American Motility Society: Position Paper: Sphincter of Oddi manometry. Gastrointest Endosc 45:342, 1997.
56. Choudhry U, Ruffolo T, Jamidar P, et al: Sphincter of Oddi dysfunction in patients with intact gallbladder: Therapeutic response to endoscopic sphincterotomy. Gastrointest Endosc 39:492, 1993.
57. Chen JWC, Saccone GTP, Toouli J: Sphincter of Oddi dysfunction and acute pancreatitis. Gut 43:305, 1998.
58. Toouli J, Francesco V, Saccone G, et al: Division of the sphincter of Oddi for treatment of dysfunction associated with recurrent pancreatitis. Br J Surg 83:1205, 1996.
59. Waye JD: Endoscopic therapy for pancreatic disease: Are we breaking the third rule of surgery? Gastrointest Endosc 52:134, 2000.
60. Testoni PA, Caporuscio S, Bagnolo F, et al: Idiopathic recurrent pancreatitis: Long-term results after ERCP, endoscopic sphincterotomy, or ursodeoxycholic acid treatment. Am J Gastroenterol 95:1702, 2000.
61. Guelrud M, Plaz J, Mendoza B, et al: Endoscopic treatment in type II pancreatic sphincter dysfunction. Gastrointest Endosc 41:398, 1999.
62. Elton E, Howell DA, Parsons WG, et al: Endoscopic pancreatic sphincterotomy: Indications, outcome, and a safe stentless technique. Gastrointest Endosc 47:240, 1998.
63. Okolo PI, Pasricha PJ, Kalloo AN: What are the long-term results of endoscopic pancreatic sphincterotomy? Gastrointest Endosc 52:15, 2000.
64. Ell C, Rabenstein T, Schneider T, et al: Safety and efficacy of pancreatic sphincterotomy in chronic pancreatitis. Gastrointest Endosc 48:244, 1998.
65. Manoukian AV, Schmalz MJ, Geenen JE, et al: The incidence of post-sphincterotomy stenosis in group II patients with sphincter of Oddi dysfunction. Gastrointest Endosc 39:496, 1993.
66. Soffer EE, Johlin FC: Intestinal dysmotility in patients with sphincter of Oddi dysfunction: A reason for failed response to sphincterotomy. Dig Dis Sci 39:1942, 1994.
67. Sahai AV, Mishra G, Penman ID, et al: EUS to detect evidence of pancreatic disease in patients with persistent or nonspecific dyspepsia. Gastrointest Endosc 52:153, 2000.

Chapter 54

Bile Secretion and the Enterohepatic Circulation of Bile Acids

Paul A. Dawson

Bile formation is essential for normal intestinal lipid digestion and absorption, cholesterol homeostasis, and the excretion of lipid-soluble xenobiotics, drugs, and heavy metals. The process of bile formation is dependent on hepatic synthesis and canalicular secretion of bile acids, the predominant organic anions in bile, and maintenance of hepatic bile formation is essential for normal liver function. Most of the bile acids secreted by the hepatocyte were previously secreted into the small intestine and have undergone an enterohepatic cycling. As a result, disturbances in bile acid synthesis, biliary secretion, and enterohepatic cycling all have profound effects on hepatic and gastrointestinal physiology. The recent cloning and functional analysis of many of the important hepatic, biliary, and intestinal transporters has helped define the molecular mechanisms involved in bile formation and advanced our understanding of genetic and acquired disorders of bile formation and secretion. Mutations have been identified in genes corresponding to many of these transport proteins in previously defined inherited clinical phenotypes such as Dubin-Johnson syndrome, several forms of progressive familial intrahepatic cholestasis (PFIC), and primary bile acid malabsorption. This chapter will review the current knowledge of the hepatic synthesis, biliary secretion, and enterohepatic circulation of bile acids.

Bile is a complex lipid-rich micellar solution that is isoosmotic with plasma and composed primarily of water, inorganic electrolytes, and organic solutes such as bile acids, phospholipids (mostly phosphatidylcholine), cholesterol, and bile pigments (Table 54–1). The relative proportions of the major organic solutes in bile are illustrated in Figure 54–1. The volume of hepatic bile secretion is estimated to be between 500 and 600 mL per day. Bile acids are the dominant components of biliary secretion and are synthesized from cholesterol in the liver. Bile acids are actively secreted across the canalicular membrane into bile and induce the secretion of other biliary constituents. In healthy humans, canalicular secretion is efficient and remarkably concentrative, as the intracellular monomeric concentration of bile acid is less than 5 μmol/L in the hepatocyte and more than 1000 μmol/L in canalicular bile. Bile acids travel down the biliary tree and are stored in the gallbladder. Following a meal, the gallbladder contracts and empties its contents into the duodenum, where they facilitate absorption of cholesterol and fat-soluble vitamins. Bile acids are poorly absorbed in the proximal small intestine but are almost quantitatively absorbed by the terminal ileum. Then the bile acids are returned to the liver in the portal circulation, actively absorbed at the hepatocyte sinusoidal membrane, and resecreted into bile.[1]

The functions of bile acids in the liver and gastrointestinal tract are multifold. First, bile acids induce bile flow and biliary lipid (phospholipid and cholesterol) secretion. The carrier-mediated active transport of bile acids into the bile canaliculus generates an osmotic water flow and is the major factor regulating bile formation and secretion. This process influences secretion of the major bile components: bilirubin, cholesterol, and phospholipid. Second, bile acids are essential for intestinal absorption of cholesterol and fat-soluble vitamins and play an important role in digestion of dietary fats. Bile acids promote intestinal absorption by solubilizing dietary lipids and their digestion products as mixed micelles to facilitate their aqueous diffusion across the intestinal mucosa. Fat-soluble vitamins (A, D, E, and K1) are not absorbed in the absence of bile acid micelles, and disturbances in the secretion or enterohepatic cycling of bile acids may lead to fat-soluble vitamin deficiency. Third, bile acids play a complex role in maintaining cholesterol homeostasis. On one hand, bile acids increase cholesterol input by facilitating

Table 54–1 | **Composition of Hepatic Bile**

COMPONENT	CONCENTRATION (MMOL/L)
Electrolytes	
Na^+	141–165
K^+	2.7–6.7
Cl^-	77–117
HCO_3^-	12–55
Ca^{2+}	2.5–6.4
Mg^{2+}	1.5–3.0
Organic anions	
Bile acids	3–45
Bilirubin	1–2
Lipids	
Lecithin	140–810 (mg/dL)
Cholesterol	97–320 (mg/dL)
Protein	2–20 (mg/mL)
Peptides and amino acids	
Glutathione	3–5
Glutamate	0.8–2.5
Aspartate	0.4–1.1
Glycine	0.6–2.6

Adapted with permission from Mosely RH: Bile secretion. In Yamada T (ed): Textbook of Gastroenterology, 3rd ed. Philadelphia, Lippincott Williams & Wilkins, 1999, p 381.

intestinal absorption of biliary and dietary cholesterol. On the other hand, bile acids function through several mechanisms to promote cholesterol elimination. Bile acids are water-soluble products of cholesterol catabolism and a major route for cholesterol elimination via fecal excretion. Bile acids also promote hepatic cholesterol secretion into bile by inducing bile flow and solubilizing biliary cholesterol, thereby enabling cholesterol ultimately to move from the hepatocyte to the intestinal lumen for elimination. Fourth, bile acids bind calcium and act to prevent calcium gallstone and oxalate kidney stone formation.[2]

BILE ACID SYNTHESIS AND SECONDARY METABOLISM

Bile acids are synthesized from cholesterol in the pericentral hepatocytes. In this process, cholesterol, a lipophilic compound, is converted into a water-soluble product. In humans the newly synthesized (primary) bile acids are cholic acid (CA), a trihydroxy–bile acid with hydroxy groups at the C-3, C-7, and C-12 positions; and chenodeoxycholic acid (CDCA), a dihydroxy–bile acid with hydroxy groups at the C-3 and C-7 positions (Fig. 54–2). The kinetics of primary bile acid synthesis in humans are summarized in Table 54–2. Hepatic bile acid synthesis was originally thought to involve one major pathway, the "classical" neutral pathway (cholesterol 7α-hydroxylase pathway) that favors CA biosynthesis. This paradigm was later modified by the discovery of a second pathway, the "alternative" acidic pathway (oxysterol 7α-hydroxylase pathway) that favors CDCA biosynthesis.[3, 4] The acidic pathway is now known to be even more complex and involves at least three distinct microsomal oxysterol hydroxylases.[5, 6]

Each pathway differs in the initial step and involves distinct sterol 7α-hydroxylase enzymes that add an essential hydroxy group to the C-7 position of the sterol ring. The overall process of bile acid biosynthesis is complex and involves as many as 20 different enzymes divided into two broad groups. The first group performs modifications to the sterol ring structure, whereas the second group modifies the sterol side chain.[3] In the classical neutral pathway that favors CA biosynthesis, sterol ring modifications precede side chain changes, whereas the side chain modifications occur before or during changes to the sterol ring structure in the acidic pathways favoring CDCA. Of the two major biosynthetic pathways, the neutral pathway is thought to be quantitatively more important.[7, 8] However, the acidic pathway is also a significant contributor and may be the major biosynthetic pathway in neonatal humans, as suggested by the finding of severe liver disease in an infant with an oxysterol 7α-hydroxylase gene defect in the acidic pathway.[4, 9]

The rate-limiting step for the classical neutral pathway is the enzyme cholesterol 7α-hydroxylase (Cyp7A1). The transcription of the Cyp7A1 gene is under a negative feedback repression by bile acids, and the molecular mechanism responsible for the regulation has recently been elucidated. Excess bile acids indirectly feed back to suppress expression

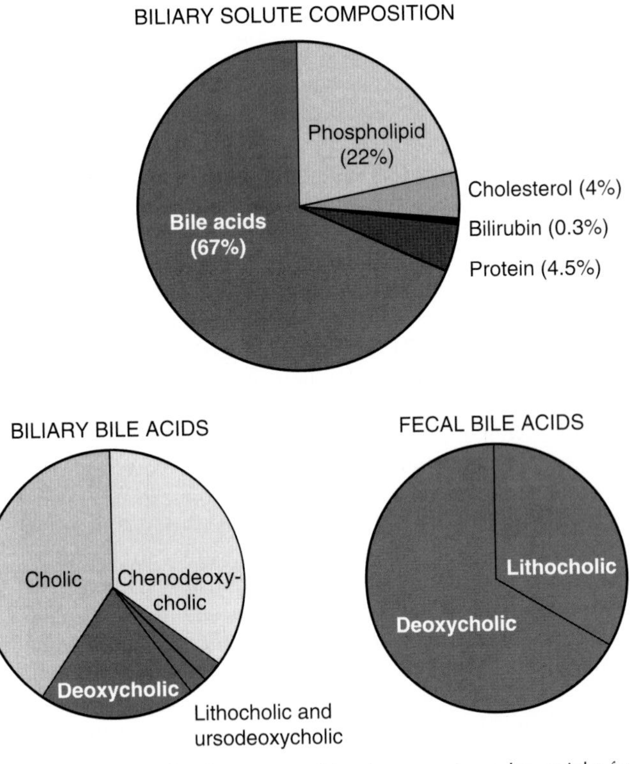

Figure 54–1. Typical solute composition in percentages by weight for hepatic and gallbladder bile in healthy humans (*top*). Bile acids are the primary solute in bile, constituting approximately 67% of bile by weight. Bile acid composition of bile is shown in the *bottom left*, and bile composition of feces is shown in the *bottom right*. Cholic acid, chenodeoxycholic acid, and deoxycholic acid constitute more than 95% of the biliary bile acids, and virtually all the biliary bile acids are in conjugated form. The proportion of biliary ursodeoxycholic acid and lithocholic acid is highly variable but rarely above 5%. The majority of lithocholic acid in bile is present in sulfated form. Fecal bile acids are almost all unconjugated as a result of bacterial deconjugating enzymes in the distal small intestine and consist of the dehydroxylated bile acids, deoxycholic acid and lithocholic acid. Ursodeoxycholic acid is usually present in trace quantities in the healthy adult. However, when administered in therapeutic doses, the proportion of ursodeoxycholic acid in bile may increase to as much as 40%.

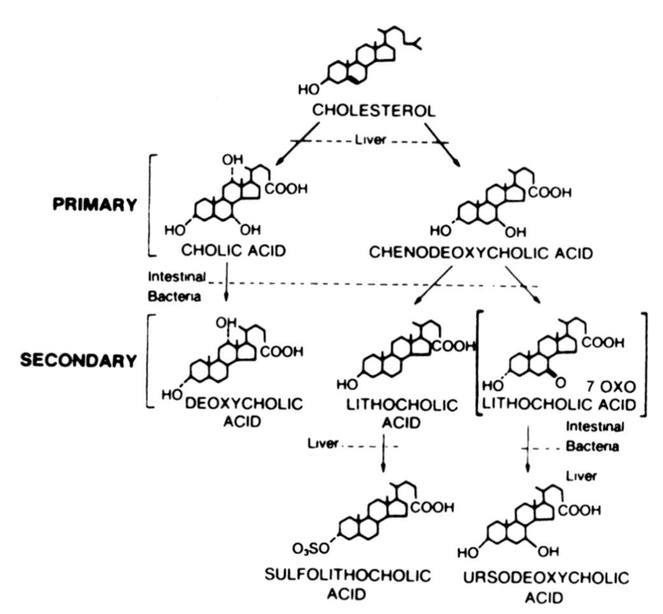

Figure 54–2. Major primary and secondary bile acids, and their sites of synthesis and metabolism. Secondary and tertiary metabolism of bile acids includes 7α-dehydroxylation by the intestinal flora, deconjugation by the intestinal flora, sulfation by the liver and kidney, and hepatic reduction of the 7-oxo derivative of chenodeoxycholic acid by the liver. (Adapted with permission from Mosely RH: Bile secretion. In Yamada T (ed): Textbook of Gastroenterology, 3rd ed. Philadelphia, Lippincott Williams & Wilkins, 1999, p 382.)

of Cyp7A1 by acting as ligands for the nuclear hormone receptor FXR.[10, 11] The bile acid receptor FXR transcriptionally activates the gene for the orphan nuclear receptor small heterodimer partner (SHP). SHP then represses the transcription of the CYP7A1 gene by antagonizing yet another orphan nuclear receptor, LRH-1 (liver receptor homolog-1), which is required for expression of the Cyp7A1 gene. This complex molecular titration allows bile acid synthesis to be linked to hepatic bile acid levels.

Before secretion into the bile canaliculus, both CA and CDCA are conjugated via their carboxyl group to the amino group of taurine or glycine. Conjugation enhances the hydrophilicity of the bile acid and the acidic strength of the side chain, in essence converting a weak acid (pKa ~ 5.0) to a strong acid (pKa ~ 3.9 for the glycine conjugate; pKa ~ 2.0 for the taurine conjugate). The major function of conjugation to glycine or taurine is to decrease the passive diffusion of bile acids across cell membranes during their transit through the biliary tree and small intestine. As a result, conjugated bile acids are absorbed only if a specific membrane carrier is present. Conjugated bile acids are also more soluble at acidic pH and more resistant to precipitation in the presence of high concentrations of calcium than their corresponding unconjugated derivatives. The net effect of conjugation is to maintain high intraluminal concentrations of bile acids down the length of the small intestine to facilitate fat digestion and absorption.[12] The importance of bile acid conjugation is clearly illustrated by a rare case of an inherited defect in bile acid conjugation in which the patient presented clinically with fat-soluble vitamin malabsorption and steatorrhea.[13]

Most of the conjugated bile acids secreted into the small intestine are efficiently absorbed intact. However, bile acids are also metabolized during their passage down the intestine by the endogenous bacterial flora. A fraction, perhaps 15%, are deconjugated by the bacterial flora in the distal small intestine. The unconjugated bile acids are absorbed passively or actively and returned to the liver, where they are reconjugated and mixed with newly synthesized bile acids to be resecreted into bile. This process of intestinal deconjugation and hepatic reconjugation is a normal part of bile acid metabolism. In the colon, the action of bacterial 7α-dehydroxylase gives rise to the secondary bile acids deoxycholic acid (DCA) and lithocholic acid (LCA) (see Fig. 54–2). An additional bacterial modification is epimerization of the C-7 hydroxy group of CDCA to form the 3α,7β-dihydroxy bile acid, ursodeoxycholic acid (UDCA). UDCA is conjugated in the liver, circulates with the pool of primary bile acids, and normally constitutes less than 5% of biliary bile acids. In addition to endogenous formation, UDCA is used as a therapeutic agent in cholestatic liver disease. When administered in therapeutic does, the proportion of UDCA in bile may increase to as much as 40% of the total. Tertiary bile acids are formed in the liver and by intestinal bacteria from secondary bile acids. These reactions include hepatic sulfation and hydroxylation of LCA and reduction of 7-oxo-lithocholate to CDCA or its 7β-epimer UDCA.

A small fraction of bile acids escapes absorption from the small intestine and passes into the colon where deconjugation is completed. The unconjugated bile acids are substrates for bacterial 7α-dehydroxylation, an anaerobic bacteria-mediated process that occurs only in the colon. The 7α-dehydroxylation converts CA to DCA, a dihydroxy bile acid with hydroxy groups at the C-3 and C-12 positions, and converts CDCA to LCA, a monohydroxy bile acid with a hydroxy group at C-3 position (see Fig. 54–2). Dehydroxylation of the primary bile acids CA and CDCA reduces their aqueous solubility so that DCA is quite insoluble at the pH of the cecum and LCA is insoluble at body temperature. The colon

Table 54–2 | **Kinetics of Individual Bile Acids in Healthy Subjects**

BILE ACID	POOL SIZE (MG)	FRACTIONAL TURNOVER RATE (DAYS^{-1})	DAILY SYNTHESIS (MG)	DAILY INPUT (MG)
Cholate	500–1500	0.20–0.50	180–360	—
Deoxycholate	200–1000	0.20–0.30	—	40–200
Chenodeoxycholate	500–1400	0.2–0.3	100–250	—
Lithocholate	50–100	1.0	100–250	40–100
Total	1250–4000	—	280–610	80–300

Adapted from Carey MC, Duane WC: Enterohepatic circulation. In Arias IM, Boyer JL, Shafritz DA (eds): The Liver: Biology and Pathobiology, 3rd ed. New York, Raven Press, 1994, pp 719–767.

absorbs approximately 50% of the DCA formed as well as a small fraction of the LCA. Following return to the liver, DCA is reconjugated with glycine or taurine and circulates with the primary bile acids. As a result, biliary bile acids always contain DCA. Hepatic conjugation of the circulating bile acids is extremely efficient, so virtually all the biliary bile acids (primarily CA, CDCA, and DCA) are in conjugated form. Bacterial deconjugation and dehydroxylation in the colon are also very efficient, so that fecal bile acids are all unconjugated and composed primarily of the secondary bile acids DCA and LCA. A comparison of the bile acid composition of bile and feces in humans is shown in Figure 54–1.

As a tertiary modification, LCA is also sulfated at the C-3 position and reconjugated to taurine or glycine. This dual conjugation blocks uptake by the ileal bile acid transporter as well as passive intestinal absorption, and the conjugated LCA is rapidly lost from the circulating pool of bile acids. Sulfation of LCA plays an important protective role because unmodified LCA is intrinsically hepatoxic and accumulation of LCA causes liver disease in experimental animal models. In addition to sulfation, LCA is detoxified and eliminated via 6-hydroxylation. The molecular mechanism for this tertiary modification has recently been elucidated and involves the orphan nuclear receptor, SXR (steroid and xenobiotic receptor; also called PXR, pregnane X receptor) and the cytochrome P-450 enzyme CYP3A4.[14, 15] LCA, as well as other xenobiotic inducers, binds to and activates SXR in the hepatocyte. SXR then induces expression of the CYP3A enzymes that confer resistance to LCA toxicity. Animal models that lack SXR/PXR are extremely sensitive to LCA-induced liver damage with the appearance of necrotic foci and elevated serum alanine aminotransferase levels, whereas pretreatment with SXR/PXR ligands, such as the anti-pruritic agent rifampicin, are protective against LCA-induced liver damage. The anticholestatic effects of rifampicin in patients may also be mediated by activation of the SXR/PXR pathway, and this is a promising new area of investigation.

THE ENTEROHEPATIC CIRCULATION

The anatomic components of the enterohepatic circulation are the liver, biliary tract, intestine, portal venous circulation, and, to a lesser extent, the colon, systemic circulation, and kidney (Fig. 54–3). At a fundamental level, the enterohepatic circulation of bile acids can be thought to consist of a series of storage chambers (gallbladder, small intestine), valves (sphincter of Oddi, ileocecal valve), mechanical pumps (canaliculi, biliary tract, small intestine), and chemical pumps (hepatocyte, cholangiocyte, and ileocyte). Remarkable progress has been made recently in identifying the transport proteins that function to maintain the enterohepatic circulation of bile acids.[16, 17] The major bile acid carriers in the human hepatocyte, cholangiocyte, ileal enterocyte, and renal proximal tubule cells are labeled in Figure 54-3, and the general properties of these carriers are listed in Table 54–3.

Efficient intestinal reabsorption and hepatic extraction of bile acids permit a very effective recycling and conservation mechanism that largely restricts bile acids to the intestinal and hepatobiliary compartments. During fasting, bile acids traverse the biliary tract and are concentrated approximately 10-fold in the gallbladder. After an overnight fast, most of the bile acids are sequestered in the gallbladder, thereby resulting in low levels of bile acids in the intestine,

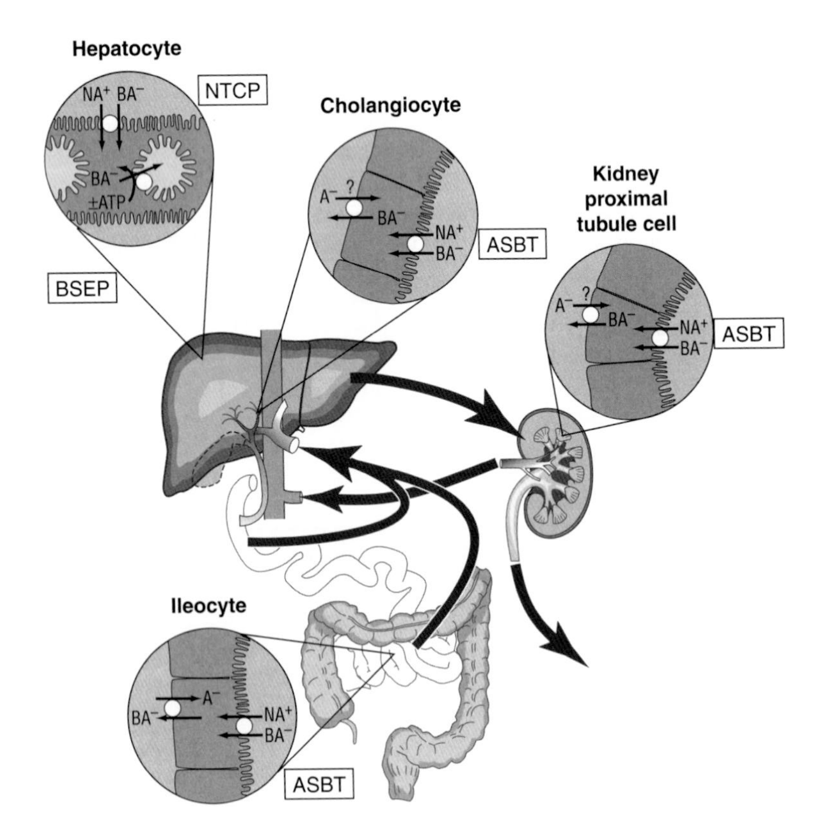

Figure 54–3. Enterohepatic circulation of bile acids showing the individual transport proteins responsible for bile acid transport across various epithelia including hepatocytes, cholangiocytes, ileal enterocytes, and renal proximal tubule cells. NTCP (SLC10A1), Na^+-taurocholate cotransporting polypeptide; BSEP (ABCB11), bile salt export pump; ASBT (SLC10A2), apical sodium bile acid transporter. (Adapted with permission from Shneider BL, Setchell KD, Crossman MW: Fetal and neonatal expressions of the apical sodium-dependent bile acid transporter in the rat ileum and kidney. Pediatr Res 42: 189, 1997.)

Table 54–3 | **Function of Transport Proteins in Bile Formation and the Enterohepatic Circulation of Bile Acids**

TRANSPORTER (GENE SYMBOL)	LOCATION	FUNCTION
Hepatocyte		
Bile Acid–dependent Bile Flow		
NTCP (*SLC10A1*)	Basolateral membrane	Na^+-dependent bile acid uptake
OATP-A (*SLC21A3*)	Basolateral membrane	Na^+-independent bile acid uptake
OATP-C (*SLC21A6*)	Basolateral membrane	Na^+-independent bile acid uptake
OATP8 (*SLC21A8*)	Basolateral membrane	Na^+-independent bile acid uptake
Na^+, K^+-ATPase	Basolateral membrane	Secretion of 2 Na^+ in exchange for 3 K^+ creating a favorable Na^+ gradient
BSEP (*ABCB11*)	Canalicular membrane	ATP-dependent bile acid export
MDR3 (*ABCB4*)	Canalicular membrane	ATP-dependent phosphatidylcholine export
FIC1 (*ATP8B1*)	Canalicular membrane	ATP-dependent aminophospholipid transport
Bile Acid–independent Bile Flow		
MRP2 (*ABCC2*)	Canalicular membrane	ATP-dependent canalicular transport of glucuronide-, GSH-, and sulfate-conjugates
OATP (A, C, 8)	Basolateral membrane	Na^+-independent organic anions, neutral steroids, organic cations
Cholangiocyte		
Ductular Secretion		
Aquaporin 1	Apical membrane	Water transport
Aquaporin 4	Basolateral membrane	Water transport
Cl^-/HCO_3^- exchanger	Apical membrane	HCO_3^- secretion in exchange for Cl^-
Cl^- channels (*CFTR*)	Apical membrane	Cl^- secretion
ASBT (*SLC10A2*)	Apical membrane	Bile acid uptake (cholehepatic shunt)
Ileal Enterocyte		
ASBT (*SLC10A2*)	Apical membrane	Bile acid uptake

ASBT, apical Na^+ bile acid transporter; CFTR, cystic fibrosis transmembrane conductance regulator; GSH, glutathione; MDR, multidrug resistance protein; MRP, MDR-related protein; NTCP, Na^+-taurocholate cotransporting polypeptide; OATP, organic anion transporting polypeptide. (For classification and nomenclature of the bile acid transporters, see http://www.med.rug.nl/mdl/mdlmm.htm.)

portal vein, serum, and liver. In response to a meal, cholecystokinin is released from the intestinal mucosa and travels to the biliary tree to relax the sphincter of Oddi and stimulate gallbladder contraction. A concentrated solution of mixed micelles (bile acids, phospholipids, and cholesterol) in gallbladder bile is emptied from the gallbladder into the small intestine, where the micelles facilitate fat absorption by stimulating the action of pancreatic lipase on triglyceride, solubilizing hydrolytic products, and delivering fat-soluble lipids to the mucosal surface. The physical-chemical events of micelle formation require that the intraluminal bile acid concentration be greater than 1.5 mmol/L. The bile acid concentration varies among different compartments and is highest in the biliary tract (20–50 mmol/L) and gallbladder (50–200 mmol/L).

During the digestion of a large meal, the gallbladder remains contracted, and bile acids secreted by the liver bypass the gallbladder and pass directly into the duodenum. During this period, the bile acid concentration in the small intestine is approximately 5 to 10 mmol/L. After a meal, the sphincter of Oddi contracts and the gallbladder relaxes, causing a larger fraction of the secreted bile acid to enter the gallbladder for storage. Thus, the enterohepatic cycling of bile acids increases during digestion and slows between meals and during overnight fasting. This rhythm of bile acid secretion is maintained even after cholecystectomy. When the gallbladder is absent, bile acids are stored in the proximal small intestine. Following ingestion of a meal, small intestinal contractions propel the stored bile acids to the distal ileum, where they are actively reabsorbed.[12]

The enterohepatic circulation of bile acids is an extremely efficient process; less than 10% of the intestinal bile acids escape reabsorption and are eliminated in the feces. Thus, most of the bile acids secreted by the hepatocyte were previously secreted into the small intestine and returned to the liver in the portal circulation. In humans, less than 5% of bile acids present in hepatic bile is newly synthesized.

In the small intestine, bile acids are absorbed predominantly by an active transport system restricted to the terminal ileum and, to a lesser extent, by passive absorption down the length of the intestine. Of all the conjugated anions secreted into bile, only bile acids are actively absorbed in conjugated form by the small intestine and undergo an enterohepatic circulation. In adult humans, the enterohepatic circulation maintains a bile acid pool size of 50 to 60 μmol per kg body weight, corresponding to approximately 2 to 4 g. The bile acid pool cycles two to three times per meal, resulting in 6 to 10 cycles per day. Thus, the intestine may reabsorb between 10 and 30 g of bile acids per day. Approximately 0.2 to 0.6 g of bile acids escape reabsorption and are eliminated in the stool each day. Hepatic conversion of cholesterol to bile acid balances fecal excretion, and this process represents an important route for the elimination of cholesterol from the body. The kinetics of bile acid turnover in humans is summarized in Table 54–2.

An enterohepatic circulation of bile acids is advantageous because it results in the accumulation of a large mass of detergent molecules that can be used repeatedly during the digestion of a single meal or multiple meals throughout the day. The presence of an ileal active transport system and enterohepatic circulation of bile acids dissociates hepatic bile acid secretion from bile acid synthesis, thereby improving the efficiency of intestinal absorption. Because secretion of bile acids induces hepatic bile flow, maintenance of the enterohepatic circulation (via the mechanical and chemical pumps) also permits continuous secretion of bile. The dissociation of bile acid biosynthesis from intestinal delivery is also promoted by the presence of a gallbladder, because the availability of a concentrative storage reservoir permits bile acids to be delivered in a high concentration and in a controlled fashion to the duodenum. The ileal bile acid transporter and gallbladder are complementary rather than redundant and together function to conserve bile acids. In the presence of a gallbladder but the absence of an active ileal bile acid transporter, the secreted bile acids would not be reabsorbed efficiently. Emptying of the gallbladder contents would necessarily be followed by a refractory period during which the bile acid supply would not be sufficient to aid in lipid digestion and absorption. The refractory period would last until hepatic synthesis could restore the bile acid pool. The existence of an ileal bile acid transporter and an enterohepatic circulation permits the bile acid pool to be used repeatedly during the digestion of a single meal.

HEPATIC BILE ACID TRANSPORT AND BILE SECRETION

Overview

Bile formation by hepatocytes involves secretion of osmotically active inorganic and organic anions into the canalicular lumen, followed by passive water movement. Canalicular bile formation has been studied with metabolically inert markers such as mannitol and erythritol and traditionally divided into two components: bile acid–dependent bile flow (bile flow relating to bile acid secretion) and bile acid–independent flow (bile flow attributed to active secretion of inorganic electrolytes and other solutes). Hepatic ATP-dependent carriers actively secrete bile acids into the canalicular lumen where they are too large to diffuse back across the paracellular junctions that line the canaliculi. Solutes such as the conjugated bile acids that are actively pumped across the canalicular membrane generate bile flow and are termed primary solutes. Other primary solutes include conjugated bilirubin, glutathione, heavy metals, and conjugates of various metabolites and xenobiotics. Water, plasma electrolytes, calcium, glucose, amino acids, bicarbonate, and other low-molecular-weight solutes that flow into the canaliculus in response to the osmotic gradient are termed secondary solutes. The choleretic activity of each primary solute is defined as the amount of bile flow induced per amount of solute secreted. The choleretic activity varies for different bile acid species and ranges from 8 to 30 μL of bile flow induced per micromole of bile acid secreted. In humans most canalicular bile flow is generated by bile acid secretion; however, secretion of other solutes by the hepatocyte and biliary epithelium is also an important determinant of bile flow. Newly secreted hepatic bile is modified further during its transit in the biliary tract via the action of ductule epithelial cells (cholangiocytes). These modifications include the movement of water through specific channels (aquaporins), the secretion of solutes such as bicarbonate and chloride, and the absorption of solutes such as glucose, amino acids, and bile acids.[18, 19]

Bile Acid–Independent Bile Flow

Canalicular bile flow is generated by active secretion of primary solutes in addition to bile acids. The ATP-dependent canalicular secretion of the tripeptide gluthathione (GSH) via the multidrug resistance protein 2 (MRP2) provides part of the driving force for canalicular bile acid–independent bile flow. GSH plays a particularly important role. In addition to being secreted at high concentrations into bile, the intraluminal catabolism of GSH by γ-glutamyl transpeptidase further increases the solute concentration and contributes to the osmotic driving force for canalicular bile formation. Besides the ATP-dependent secretion of organic anions into bile, ATP-independent secretion of bicarbonate via the HCO_3^-/Cl^- anion exchanger AE2 on the canalicular membrane also contributes to bile acid–independent bile flow.

Cholehepatic Shunt Pathway

The term cholehepatic shunt was coined to describe the cycle whereby unconjugated dihydroxy bile acids secreted into bile are passively absorbed by cholangiocytes, returned to the hepatocyte via the periductular capillary plexus, and resecreted into bile. Absorption of the protonated unconjugated bile acid molecule generates a bicarbonate anion, resulting in a bicarbonate-rich choleresis. Premature absorption and resecretion of the bile acid also induces bile acid–dependent bile flow. This cycle explains the hypercholeresis observed for unconjugated C-24 dihydroxy bile acid such as UDCA and drugs such as the nonsteroidal anti-inflammatory drug sulindac.[20] However, the physiologic significance of the cholehepatic shunt pathway for hepatic bile secretion is less clear because as originally proposed the cholehepatic shunt included only a passive absorption component. Unlike exogenously administered UDCA, which may be poorly reconjugated in the hepatocyte, most endogenous bile acids are conjugated efficiently to taurine or glycine before their biliary secretion. The majority of the biliary bile acid pool is thus ionized and unable to diffuse passively across the biliary epithelium. Recently, the biliary epithelial cells that line the large intrahepatic bile ducts were found to express the apical sodium-dependent bile acid transporter (ASBT; gene symbol *SLC10A2*). Expression of the ASBT provides a mechanism for conjugated bile acids to be absorbed by cholangiocytes and returned to the hepatocyte for resecretion into bile.[21–23] Because most bile acids are ultimately secreted from the biliary tree, the quantitative significance of this pathway is assumed to be small except under certain pathophysiologic conditions.[24] Indeed, the major function of the ASBT in biliary epithelium may be to permit cholangiocytes to sample biliary bile acid concentrations in order to activate cellular signaling pathways rather than to transport significant quantities of bile acids.[23]

Overview of Hepatic Bile Acid Transport

Approximately 95% of bile acids secreted into bile are derived from the recirculating pool. To maintain this process, liver parenchymal cells must transport bile acids efficiently from the portal blood into bile. This vectorial trans-hepatocellular movement of bile acids is a concentrative transport process that is driven by a distinct set of primary (ATP-dependent), secondary (Na^+-gradient dependent), and tertiary (OH^- or HCO_3^--dependent anion exchange) active transport systems at the sinusoidal and canalicular plasma membranes.[25] Bile acid flux through the liver and the number of

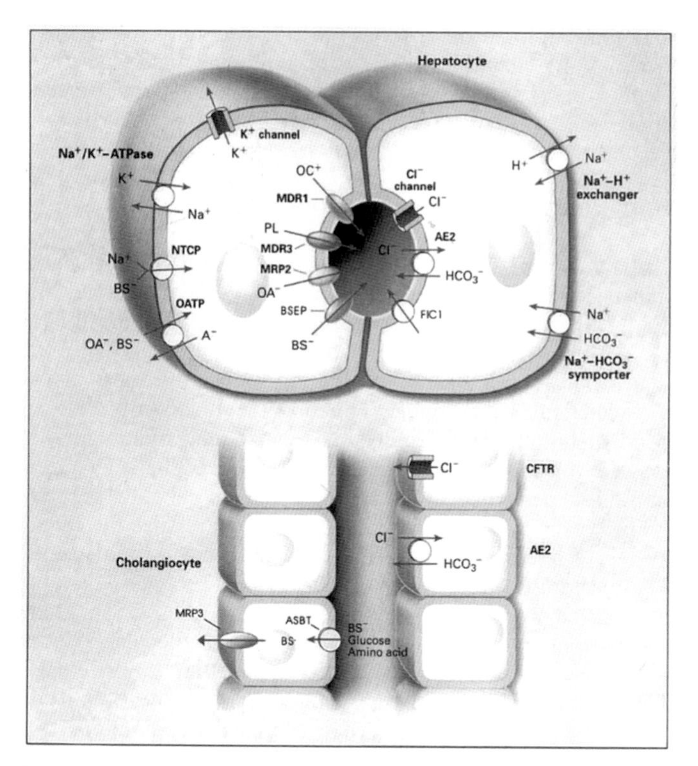

Figure 54–4. Hepatocyte and cholangiocyte transporters important for bile acid secretion. At the sinusoidal membrane, the Na^+-taurocholate cotransporting polypeptide (NTCP; *SLC10A1*) mediates the uptake of conjugated bile acids. Sodium-dependent uptake of bile acids through the NTCP is driven by an inwardly directed sodium gradient generated by the Na^+/K^+-ATPase and the membrane potential generated in part by a potassium channel. The Na^+-independent bile acid uptake is mediated by organic anion transporting polypeptide (OATP)-C (*SLC21A6*) and to a lesser extent by OATP-A (*SLC21A3*) and OATP8 (*SLC21A8*). The sinusoidal membrane also contains a sodium-hydrogen exchanger and a sodium-bicarbonate symporter. At the canalicular membrane, bile acids are pumped into bile through the bile salt export pump (BSEP; ABCB11). Excretion of sulfated or glucuronidated bile acids is mediated by the multidrug resistance protein 2 (MRP2; ABCC2). The canalicular membrane also expresses additional ATP-dependent export pumps such as the multidrug protein 1 (MDR1, ABCB1) and the multidrug resistance protein 3 (MDR3; ABCB4) that transports phospholipid into bile, ATP-independent transporters, including chloride channels, and the chloride-bicarbonate anion exchanger isoform 2 (AE2) for secretion of bicarbonate. FIC1 (gene symbol ATP8B1) is a P-type ATPase mutated in progressive familial intrahepatic cholestasis type 1. Within the bile ducts, conjugated bile acids are absorbed by the apical sodium-dependent bile acid transporter (ASBT; *SLC10A2*) expressed on the apical membrane of cholangiocytes in the large bile ducts. Bile acid may then exit at the basolateral surface into the hepatic arterial circulation through an ATP-dependent carrier, the multidrug resistance protein 3 (MRP3; ABCC3), or possibly, an anion exchange mechanism. Cholangiocytes also express a variety of other carriers important for modifying bile, including the cystic fibrosis transmembrane regulator (CFTR), the chloride-bicarbonate anion exchanger isoform 2 for secretion of bicarbonate, the sodium-glucose cotransporter (SGLT1; *SLC5A1*), and numerous aquaporin isoforms to facilitate water movement. (BS^-, bile salt; OA^-, organic anion; OC^+, organic cation). (Adapted with permission from Trauner M, Meier PJ, Boyer JL: N Engl J Med 339:1217, 1998. Copyright 1998 Massachusetts Medical Society. All rights reserved.)

participating hepatocytes are variable. In the fasting state, bile acids are taken up predominantly by the periportal hepatocytes (the first hepatocytes of the liver acinus), whereas during feeding, more hepatocytes in the liver acinus participate in bile acid uptake. In periportal hepatocytes, bile acid synthesis is repressed whereas perivenous hepatocytes actively synthesize bile acids. Thus, periportal hepatocytes primarily absorb and secrete recirculating bile acids, and perivenous cells secrete predominantly newly synthesized bile acids. Thus, the transport of recirculating bile acids through periportal hepatocytes drives the majority of bile flow.[25]

The concentration of bile acids in the portal blood of healthy humans is 20 to 50 μmol/L. Uptake by the liver is typically expressed as fractional extraction or first-pass extraction and represents the percent of bile acids removed during a single passage through the hepatic acinus. The first-pass extraction of bile acids from sinusoidal blood ranges from 50% to 90% but remains constant irrespective of systemic bile acid concentrations. The fractional extraction is related to bile acid structure and albumin binding and is greatest (80% to 90%) for conjugated hydrophilic bile acids such as conjugated CA and least (50% to 60%) for unconjugated hydrophobic protein-bound bile acids such as CDCA. The concentration of total bile acids in the systemic circulation reflects this efficient hepatic extraction and averages 3 to 4 μmol/L in the fasting state.

The major hepatic and biliary transporters important for bile formation are indicated in Figure 54–4 and listed in Table 54–3. Because of their importance for bile secretion, the bile acid transporters are highlighted. However, the hepatocyte sinusoidal and canalicular membranes also express specialized transport proteins for a wide spectrum of lipophilic endogenous and exogenous compounds besides bile acids.[26, 27]

Hepatic Sinusoidal Na^+-Dependent Bile Acid Uptake

Hepatocellular uptake of bile acids occurs against an unfavorable electrochemical ion gradient and results in a more than 10-fold concentration in hepatocytes. The uptake of conjugated bile acids at the sinusoidal (basolateral) membrane is mediated predominantly (>80%) by a secondary active Na^+-dependent transport system. The driving force for this Na^+-dependent uptake is generated by the basolateral Na^+, K^+-ATPase that maintains the prevailing out-to-in Na^+ gradient. In contrast to conjugated bile acids, Na^+-dependent uptake accounts for less than one half the uptake of unconjugated bile acids such as CA or UDCA. The hepatic sinusoidal Na^+-dependent bile acid transporter (NTCP, gene symbol *SLC10A1*) was originally identified using an expression cloning strategy and encodes a 45-kDa membrane glycoprotein.[28] The properties of NTCP satisfied all the functional criteria for hepatocytic Na^+-coupled bile acid uptake. These properties include (1) preferential high affinity transport of conjugated bile acids, (2) kinetics for taurocholate transport similar to those of isolated hepatocytes, (3) electrogenic Na^+-taurocholate uptake, (4) appropriate tissue-specific expression in the liver, and (5) similar ontogeny for Na^+-dependent bile acid uptake and NTCP during development.[16] The presence of additional sinusoidal Na^+-dependent bile acid transporters has been suggested; however, the evidence for such transport systems is thus far equivocal. The overwhelming evidence indicates that NTCP accounts for most, if not all, hepatic Na^+-dependent bile acid transport.[16, 17]

NTCP mRNA and protein expression is decreased in various animal models of cholestasis and liver disease.[29, 30] In addition, recent studies have also shown similar decreased

NTCP expression in percutaneous liver biopsy specimens of patients with various cholestatic liver diseases.[31] An inherited defect in NTCP has not yet been reported, and it is possible that an isolated NTCP gene defect may be asymptomatic because the liver also expresses Na^+-independent bile acid transporters. A rare disorder characterized by a relatively isolated hypercholanemia has been described; however, NTCP expression was found to be normal in affected patients, and the underlying defect remains to be identified.[32, 33]

Hepatic Sinusoidal Na^+-Independent Bile Acid Uptake

Unconjugated bile acids such as cholate are taken up predominantly by hepatic Na^+-independent transport systems. Whereas all the properties of hepatocellular Na^+-dependent bile acid transport is accounted for by NTCP, Na^+-independent bile acid transport was initially thought to require several different transport systems. Identification of Na^+-independent hepatic transport systems was originally confounded by their extremely broad substrate specificity, and the multiplicity of substrates could not be easily reconciled with the properties of known hepatic transport systems. The list of substrates that share apparently common transport pathways included conjugated and unconjugated bile acids, Bromsulphalein (BSP), cardiac glycosides and other neutral steroids, linear and cyclic peptides, and numerous drugs. This conundrum was resolved with discovery of the organic anion transporting polypeptide (OATP) transporter gene family.[34] Hepatocellular uptake of albumin-bound organic molecules is mediated by a limited number of multi-specific transport systems with partially overlapping specificities rather than many highly specific transport systems.[16, 17] Because members of the OATP family also transport uncharged compounds such as oubain or aldosterone and even bulky organic cations such as ADP-ajmalinium, the name organic "anion" transporter is overly restrictive.

The OATP genes encode 12 potential transmembrane domain proteins that share no sequence identity with the Na^+-dependent bile acid transporters. The driving force for OATP-mediated organic anion uptake is anion exchange, with coupling of bile acid uptake to either HCO_3^- or GSH efflux.[35, 36] The OATP-type transporters constitute a large gene family (the designation within the gene super-family of solute carriers is *SLC21A*) with over 14 members identified in human and rat tissues. Most of the previous functional data has been obtained for the rat and mouse orthologues; however, several of the major human OATP family members have recently been identified. The human carriers, OATP-B (gene symbol *SLC21A9*), OATP-C (gene symbol *SLC21A6*), and OATP8 (gene symbol *SLC21A8*) exhibit partially overlapping substrate specificities and may account for the majority of hepatic Na^+-independent bile acid, organic anion, and drug clearance. These human OATPs transport BSP, bilirubin monoglucuronide, steroid metabolites such as estradiol-17β-glucuronide and estrone-3-sulfate, arachidonic acid products such as prostaglandin E2, thromboxane B2, and leukotriene C4, and a wide variety of drugs such as pravastatin, digoxin, and fexofenadine.[37] Because the majority of hepatic bile acid uptake is sodium-dependent, the major physiologic role of these broad specificity solute carriers may be hepatic clearance of non–bile acid substrates such as endogenous amphipathic metabolites and xenobiotics.

Canalicular Bile Acid Transport

Canalicular secretion is the rate-limiting step in the hepatic transport of bile acids from blood into bile. Whereas bile acid concentrations within the hepatocyte are in the micromolar range, canalicular bile acid concentrations are more than 1000-fold higher, necessitating active transport across the canalicular membrane. Functional evidence of ATP-dependent bile acid transport by the canalicular membrane has existed for more than a decade. Moreover, characterization of ATP-dependent taurocholate transport in canalicular membrane vesicles suggested the presence of a specific carrier system that was distinct from the canalicular multispecific organic anion transporter (MOAT, MRP2; gene symbol *ABCC2*) that transports organic anions such as GSH, glutathione conjugates, and bile acid sulfates.[38] Molecular identification of the canalicular bile acid transporter proved elusive until members of the ABC (ATP binding cassette) family of transporters were investigated more closely. Functional expression and characterization studies revealed that a novel ABC transporter closely related to the MDR1/P-glycoprotein gene is the canalicular bile acid transporter.[39] This 160-kDa protein (originally named "sister of P-glycoprotein," or Spgp) has been shown to transport conjugated bile acids efficiently and was subsequently renamed the bile salt export pump (BSEP, gene symbol *ABCB1*). The human BSEP gene locus on chromosome 2q24 is linked to progressive familial intrahepatic cholestasis type 2 (PFIC2), a hepatic disorder characterized by biliary bile acid concentrations less than 1% of normal and an absence of BSEP from the canalicular membrane. Finally, the role of BSEP as the major canalicular bile acid export pump was confirmed by the identification of dysfunctional mutations in the BSEP gene in PFIC2 patients (see Chapter 65).[40, 41]

INTESTINAL AND RENAL BILE ACID TRANSPORT

Overview

Bile acids enter the small intestine along with other biliary constituents and facilitate the absorption of dietary lipids and fat-soluble vitamins. The intestinal absorption of bile acids is extremely efficient, and less than 10% of the intestinal bile acids escape reabsorption and are eliminated in the feces. Bile acids are absorbed by a combination of passive absorption in the proximal small intestine and active absorption in the distal ileum. Numerous observations indicate that the terminal ileum is the major site of bile acid reabsorption. For example, there is little decrease in intraluminal bile acid concentration proximal to the ileum, and bile acid malabsorption occurs after ileal resection. Studies using in situ perfused intestinal segments to measure bile acid absorption have also demonstrated that ileal bile acid transport is a high-capacity system sufficient to account for the biliary output of bile acids. The consensus from this work is that the ileal active transport system is the major route for conjugated bile acid uptake. A fraction of the glycine conjugated bile acids are protonated in the duodenum when the intraluminal pH becomes transiently acidic during digestion, and these nonionized bile acids may be absorbed by passive or facilitative diffusion.[42] In the distal small intestine and large intestine, bile acids are deconjugated by the intestinal flora. The unconjugated bile acids are weak acids and can be absorbed passively if they remain in solution.

A fraction (10%–50%, depending on the bile acid species) of the bile acids returning in the portal circulation escapes hepatic extraction and spills into the systemic circulation. The binding of bile acids to plasma proteins decreases their glomerular filtration and minimizes urinary excretion. In healthy humans, the kidney filters approximately 100 μmol of bile acids each day. Remarkably, only 1 to 2 μmol are excreted in the urine because of a highly efficient tubular reabsorption. Even in patients with cholestatic liver disease in whom plasma bile acid concentrations are significantly elevated, the 24-hour urinary excretion of nonsulfated bile acids is significantly less than the quantity that undergoes glomerular filtration. Subsequent studies have shown that bile acids in the glomerular filtrate are actively reabsorbed from the renal tubules, and this process contributes to the increase in bile acid concentrations found in the peripheral blood of patients with obstructive liver disease. As in the ileum, the renal proximal tubule epithelium expresses an Na^+-gradient driven transporter that functions as a salvage mechanism to conserve bile acids.

Ileal and Renal Na^+-dependent Bile Acid Uptake

Bile acids are actively transported across the ileal brush border membrane by the well-characterized ileal apical sodium bile acid transporter (ASBT, gene symbol *SLC10A2*).[43, 44] The relationship between the hepatic, cholangiocyte, ileal, and renal Na^+-bile acid cotransport systems was resolved with the cloning of the bile acid carriers from these tissues.[21, 28, 43] The liver (NTCP; *SLC10A1*) and ileal (ASBT; *SLC10A2*) Na^+-bile acid cotransporters are related gene products that share considerable amino acid identity and structural similarity. In contrast, the ileal, renal, and cholangiocyte carriers are all products of the same gene. The inwardly directed Na^+ gradient maintained by the basolateral Na^+, K^+-ATPase as well as the negative intracellular potential provide the driving force for ASBT-mediated bile acid uptake. The ASBT transports all major species of bile acids but favors trihydroxy (CA) over dihydroxy bile acids and conjugated over unconjugated species. The properties of ASBT satisfy all the functional criteria for ileal active bile acid uptake. These properties include (1) a strict sodium-dependence for bile acid transport, (2) narrow substrate specificity encompassing only conjugated and unconjugated bile acids with negligible uptake of other organic anions, (3) specific intestinal expression in the terminal ileum, and (4) similar ontogeny for ileal sodium-dependent taurocholate uptake and ASBT expression. Finally, inherited mutations in the human ASBT gene cause primary bile acid malabsorption, an idiopathic intestinal disorder associated with interruption of the enterohepatic circulation of bile acids and fat malabsorption.[44] This last finding clearly demonstrates that most intestinal bile acid absorption in humans is mediated by the ASBT.

Intracellular transport of bile acids in ileal enterocytes may be facilitated by a cytosolic carrier protein, the ileal lipid binding protein (ILBP, also called the ileal bile acid binding protein, IBABP; gene symbol *FABP6*). ILBP is a member of the fatty acid binding protein family and is a major ileal enterocyte cytosolic protein. The mechanism of bile acid secretion across the basolateral membrane of the ileal enterocyte (and of the cholangiocyte or renal proximal tubule cell) is still poorly understood and may involve an anion exchange process or an ATP-dependent transporter, MRP3 (gene symbol *ABCC3*).

DISORDERS OF THE ENTEROHEPATIC CIRCULATION

Cholestasis is defined as interruption of the normal process of bile formation and is classically subdivided into intrahepatic cholestasis, a functional defect in bile formation at the level of the hepatocyte, and extrahepatic cholestasis, an obstruction to bile flow within the biliary tract. Impaired hepatic transport of bile acids and other organic solutes is a prominent feature of both inherited and acquired forms of cholestatic liver injury. Disorders of the enterohepatic circulation are generally classified into four categories: (1) defects in bile acid formation (synthesis and conjugation), (2) defects in membrane transport of bile acids (uptake and secretion), (3) disturbances involving bacterial transformation (deconjugation and dehydroxylation), and (4) disturbances in movement through or between organs (bile acid circulation).

Defects in Bile Acid Synthesis

Continuous bile acid synthesis from cholesterol is required to maintain the bile acid pool in the enterohepatic circulation. The maximal rate of bile acid synthesis is 4 to 6 g per day. Although inherited defects in biosynthesis are extremely rare, these disorders serve to illustrate the importance of bile acid synthesis for normal hepatic function. The effects of a cessation in bile acid synthesis include depletion of the bile acid pool by fecal excretion, loss of bile acid–dependent bile flow, decreased biliary excretion of cholesterol and xenobiotics, and reduced intestinal absorption of cholesterol and fat-soluble vitamins. In most cases, a single enzyme defect is not sufficient to eliminate all bile acid biosynthesis because there are multiple biosynthetic pathways.[4–8] For example, cerebrotendinous xanthomatosis (CTX) is a rare inherited disease caused by mutations in the mitochondrial enzyme sterol 27-hydroxylase. In CTX, the alternative (acidic) pathway is blocked, and bile acid synthesis is diminished but not eliminated. There is no associated liver disease, and CTX is characterized by progressive neurologic disturbances, premature atherosclerosis, cataracts, and tendinous xanthomas. Bile acid therapy with CDCA has been reported to suppress the biochemical abnormalities in CTX and to slow disease progression.[45]

The most commonly reported defect in bile acid synthesis

is 3β-hydroxy-C27-steroid dehydrogenase deficiency, and this enzyme defect affects the classical (neutral) pathway for bile acid biosynthesis.[46] The disease is characterized by progressive intrahepatic cholestasis and accumulation of abnormal bile acids.[9] These unusual conjugates of dihydroxy- and trihydroxy-5-cholenoic acid are poorly transported by the BSEP across the canalicular membrane and also interfere with the ATP-dependent secretion of other bile acids. Clinical manifestations include unconjugated bilirubinemia, jaundice, elevated serum aminotransferase levels, steatorrhea, pruritus, and poor growth. The progression of the disease is variable but ultimately results in cirrhosis and hepatic failure in a high proportion of the reported cases. Treatment with exogenous primary bile acids such as UDCA reverses the biochemical abnormalities and may be lifesaving.[9]

Defects in Membrane Transport of Bile Acids

There is a growing list of diseases caused by inherited transporter gene defects that affect the enterohepatic circulation. These disorders include a variety of liver and intestinal diseases such as progressive familial intrahepatic cholestasis (PFIC) types 1 to 3, cystic fibrosis, Zellweger syndrome, adrenoleukodystrophy, Dubin-Johnson syndrome, and primary bile acid malabsorption (PBAM). Inherited disorders associated with mutations in the bile acid transporter or biliary organic solute transporter genes are listed in Table 54–4.

PFIC type 1 is an example of a secondary bile acid transport defect. The gene defect in many patients with PFIC and normal serum gamma glutamyltranspeptidase levels maps to chromosome 18. The same locus had previously been mapped in patients with the similar but milder phenotype of benign recurrent intrahepatic cholestasis. The gene responsible for PFIC type 1 has been cloned and encodes a P-type ATPase designated FIC1 (gene symbol, *ATP8B1*). P-type ATPases are transporters that are distinct from ABC transporters and constitute a large family that includes ion pumps such as the Na^+, K^+-ATPase, Ca^{2+}-ATPase, and the copper transporting Wilson's disease gene (gene symbol *ATP7B*). FIC1 is assumed to be an aminophospholipid (phosphatidylserine) transporter on the basis of its similarity to a previously identified aminophospholipid translocase; however, the exact function of FIC1 is unknown. In humans, FIC1 is highly expressed in pancreas, small intestine, urinary bladder, stomach, and prostate. This expression in extrahepatic tissues may help explain the increased frequency of diarrhea and pancreatitis in these patients; however, the mechanism responsible for the cholestasis remains to be elucidated.[47]

PFIC type 2 is characterized by progressive cholestasis, lobular and portal fibrosis, giant cell transformation, normal serum gamma glutamyltranspeptidase levels, and no bile duct proliferation. The disease was mapped to chromosome 2q24, and the defective gene was later shown to be the canalicular BSEP.[40] Mutations in the BSEP gene may impair synthesis, cellular trafficking, or stability of the protein, as canalicular staining with anti-BSEP antibodies is negative in patients with PFIC type 2.[41] It is interesting to note that bile acids are not completely absent in the biliary bile of these patients, suggesting an alternative efflux pathway. Evidence for another efflux pathway has also been shown in a mouse model with a defective BSEP gene.[48] However, it is not clear whether this putative alternative bile acid efflux pathway plays any role in bile acid efflux in healthy humans. Patients with PFIC type 2 do not appear to respond to UDCA therapy.[49]

PIC type 3 is quite different from the other PFIC subtypes. Serum gamma glutamyltranspeptidase levels are markedly elevated in these patients, and liver histology shows extensive bile duct proliferation and portal and periportal fibrosis. The gene defect in PFIC type 3 lies in MDR3 (gene symbol *ABCB3*), a canalicular phosphatidylcholine (PC) transporter that belongs to the ABC transporter superfamily.[50] In PFIC type 3, bile acid transport is unimpaired, but PC transport is greatly diminished. In bile, PC normally forms mixed micelles with bile acids and acts to buffer their cytotoxic detergent properties. In the absence of biliary phospholipid, the bile acid monomers are highly toxic and cause cholestatic liver damage.

Disturbances in Bile Acid Biotransformation (Deconjugation and Dehydroxylation)

Bile acid deconjugation normally begins in the distal small intestine and presumably is mediated by bacteria that spill across the ileocecal valve. In patients with intestinal stasis and bacterial overgrowth, bile acid deconjugation also occurs in the proximal intestine. The unconjugated bile acids are absorbed passively, and the extensive bacterial deconjugation can decrease intraluminal bile acid concentrations and impair micelle formation in the small intestine. Increased bile acid deconjugation can be detected indirectly by demonstrating an increased concentration of unconjugated bile acids in the systemic venous plasma or by using a breath test. However, these tests are not widely used because the presence of increased anaerobic bacteria in the small intestine can easily be detected by a hydrogen breath test following a glucose-containing meal (see Chapter 90).

In the large intestine, bile acids are first deconjugated and then 7-dehydroxylated. In healthy humans, bile acids eventually undergo nearly complete 7-dehydroxylation to yield the secondary bile acids DCA and LCA. However, in a subset of patients with cholesterol gallstones, CA undergoes rapid 7-dehydroxylation, and these patients have an increased proportion of DCA in bile. The increased DCA accumulation is related primarily to a prolonged colonic transit time and involves multiple mechanisms. In these patients can be found (1) slow colonic transit, an increased concentration of gram-positive bacteria in the colon, and greater 7α-dehydroxylase activity increase DCA formation; (2) slow transit-induced increases in distal colonic pH increase DCA solubility; and (3) slow colonic transit increases DCA absorption.[51] Because accumulation of DCA in bile can contribute indirectly to cholesterol cholelithiasis, strategies to accelerate colonic transit or acidify the colonic luminal contents may be useful in preventing cholesterol gallstones.

Table 54–4 | **Disorders of the Enterohepatic Circulation: Inherited Transporter Defects**

PHENOTYPE	TRANSPORT DEFECT	DEFECTIVE TRANSPORTER (GENE)	CHARACTERISTIC FEATURES
Defects in Hepatic Canalicular Transport			
Progressive familial intrahepatic cholestasis type 1	Canalicular aminophospholipids	FIC1 (*ATP8B1*)	Progressive cholestasis, elevated serum bile acids, pruritus, normal GGT, malabsorption
Progressive familial intrahepatic cholestasis type 2	Canalicular bile acids	BSEP (*ABCB11*)	Progressive cholestasis, no bile duct proliferation, lobular and portal fibrosis, normal GGT
Progressive familial intrahepatic cholestasis type 3	Canalicular phosphatidylcholine	MDR3 (*ABCB4*)	Cholestasis, extensive bile duct proliferation, periportal fibrosis, elevated GGT
Intrahepatic cholestasis of pregnancy	Canalicular phosphatidylcholine	MDR3 (*ABCB4*)	Cholestasis in third trimester of pregnancy, associated with fetal loss and prematurity
Dubin-Johnson syndrome	Canalicular organic anion conjugates	MRP2 (*ABCC2*)	Conjugated hyperbilirubinemia
Defects in Intestinal Transport			
Primary bile acid malabsorption	Ileal brush border bile acids	ASBT (*SLC10A2*)	Chronic diarrhea, steatorrhea, fat-soluble vitamin malabsorption

ND, not determined; GGT, gamma glutamyl transpeptidase.

Disturbances in the Bile Acid Circulation

Biliary Obstruction and Biliary Fistula

Biliary obstruction caused, for example, by a stone that obstructs the common duct leads to retention of hepatic bile acids and ultimately hepatocyte necrosis or apoptosis. A portion of the bile acids are modified by sulfation, and both sulfated and unsulfated bile acids are regurgitated from the hepatocyte into the systemic circulation. Despite increased urinary excretion, plasma concentrations of bile acids rise as much as 20-fold. When biliary obstruction is incomplete, secretion of bile acids into the intestine is decreased, and efficient ileal absorption continues to return the cytotoxic bile acids to the liver via the portal circulation. In this case, administration of bile acid sequestrants decreases the intestinal absorption of cytotoxic bile acids and may slow the progression of liver damage. With complete biliary obstruction, bile acids are not secreted into the small intestine, and malabsorption of fat-soluble vitamins and steatorrhea results. Secondary bile acids are not formed, and fecal bile acid output is decreased.

In patients with a biliary fistula, bile acids are diverted instead of entering the small intestine. Because bile acid biosynthesis is controlled by negative feedback, bile acid synthesis increases markedly, up to 20-fold. Hepatic function is not impaired, although the flux of bile acids through the liver is decreased significantly because maximal bile acid synthesis (3–6 g per day) is less than the normal flux in the presence of an intact enterohepatic circulation (12–18 g per day). As in biliary obstruction, decreased bile acid concentrations in the small intestine result in malabsorption of fat-soluble vitamins. Absorption of dietary fats, especially dietary triglycerides that contain longer chain fatty acids, is also decreased.

Cholecystectomy

Despite removal of a major storage pool of bile acids, the overall effect of cholecystectomy on biliary secretion is small, and daily bile acid secretion is not altered significantly.[52] In the absence of a gallbladder, the bile acid pool is stored in the proximal small intestine during the fasting state. Following ingestion of a meal, the bile acid pool moves to the terminal ileum, where it is actively absorbed and returned to the liver in the portal circulation. Changes in the composition of the bile acid pool have been reported with increased dehydroxylation of CA to DCA. In a small subset of patients with postcholecystectomy diarrhea, the movement of the bile acid pool to the small intestine may overwhelm the ileal transporter system, leading to bile acid malabsorption. The diarrhea may be only transitory, and affected patients generally respond to administration of a bile acid sequestrant.

Ileal Resection

Resection of the terminal ileum causes bile acid malabsorption. If the resected segment is short, the effect on bile acid metabolism is minimal because increased biosynthesis balances increased fecal loss. With longer resections, hepatic bile acid synthesis is increased more dramatically to compensate for the increased loss. The unabsorbed bile acids enter the colon in greater amounts and inhibit water absorption or induce secretion, thereby resulting in mild, watery diarrhea. Symptomatic response is obtained with administration of a bile acid sequestrant. When the length of ileum resected is greater than 100 cm, including the ileocecal valve, bile acid secretion decreases because the bile acid biosynthetic potential is well below the normal hepatic secretion rate. The bile acid pool becomes progressively depleted during the day, and fat malabsorption appears because of the lack of micelles and loss of intestinal mucosal surface. Increased dihydroxy bile acid and fatty acid flux through the colon inhibits water absorption. The loss of water and electrolyte conservation by the distal small intestine results in severe diarrhea. If the diarrhea is of sufficiently large volume and accompanied by malabsorption of other nutrients, the patient may be diagnosed as having short-bowel syndrome. Therapy is complex and has only limited success. In some patients, fecal weight and frequency are reduced by elimination of fat from the diet. Other therapies include bile acid replacement, glutamine, and growth factors (see Chapter 92).

Bile Acid Malabsorption and Diarrhea

The enterohepatic circulation conserves bile acids efficiently, thereby maintaining bile flow and adequate intraluminal bile acid concentrations to allow micellar solubilization and absorption of lipids. Impaired intestinal absorption of bile acids may play a role in the pathogenesis of a number of gastrointestinal disorders, including idiopathic chronic diarrhea, chronic ileitis, gallstone disease, postcholecystectomy diarrhea, Crohn's disease, irritable bowel syndrome, and primary bile acid malabsorption. Symptomatic bile acid malabsorption results from failure of the active intestinal transport component, and three types of bile acid malabsorption are classically recognized. Type 1 bile acid malabsorption (secondary bile acid malabsorption) is the most common form and is caused by ileal resection, ileal disease such as Crohn's disease, ileal bypass, and radiation enteritis. Type 3 bile acid malabsorption is also common and associated with conditions such as cholecystectomy, peptic ulcer surgery, chronic pancreatitis, celiac sprue, diabetes mellitus, cystic fibrosis, and the use of various drugs. In contrast, Type 2 bile acid malabsorption (primary or idiopathic bile acid malabsorption) is a rare disorder and is not associated with obvious ileal disease. The diarrhea in these patients responds immediately to treatment with bile acid sequestrants such as cholestyramine. A rare congenital form of Type 2 bile acid malabsorption associated with diarrhea, steatorrhea, and growth failure has been described and is caused by inherited mutations in the ileal ASBT gene.[44]

Bile acid malabsorption permits increased concentrations of dihydroxy bile acids to reach the colon, where they alter water and electrolyte movement, thereby leading to diarrhea. Water transport in the colon is critical for the regulation of intestinal fluid and electrolyte balance and is the ultimate determinant of diarrhea (fecal water excretion). Bile acids play a role in colonic water transport apparently by blocking sodium transport in the perfused colon and altering fluid and electrolyte movement. Whereas trihydroxy bile acids have no effect, dihydroxy bile acids induce net fluid secretion at high concentrations. At low concentrations, dihydroxy bile acids block absorption of fluid and water. To induce net secretion, bile acids must (a) have an appropriate structure (hydrophobic dihydroxy bile acids, DCA, or CDCA), (b) be present in high concentrations ($>$1.5 mM) in the aqueous phase, and (c) exist at the appropriate pH (alkaline, 7.5–8.0). An additional consequence of bile acid malabsorption and steatorrhea is an increase in renal oxalate excretion. In bile acid malabsorption, the concentration of long-chain fatty acids is increased in the colon, and they form insoluble calcium soaps. Consequently, less calcium is available for precipitation of unabsorbed dietary oxalate as calcium oxalate. Oxalate is hyperabsorbed from the colon because the luminal soluble oxalate concentration is higher and the colonic permeability is increased. This hyperoxaluria contributes to the prevalence of kidney stones in these patients. Therapeutic approaches to the fat malabsorption and diarrhea are discussed in Chapters 9 and 89.

BILE ACID THERAPY, SEQUESTRANTS, TRANSPORT INHIBITORS

Bile Acid Therapy

Bile acid therapy is divided into two types: displacement and replacement. The goal of displacement therapy is to alter the composition of the bile acid pool in order to decrease the cytotoxicity of endogenous bile acids or decrease biliary cholesterol secretion, whereas the aim of replacement therapy is to correct a bile acid deficiency. UDCA is used most widely because of its safety and lack of hepatotoxicity. Following oral administration, UDCA accumulates in the circulating bile acid pool and displaces endogenous bile acids. The bile acid pool becomes enriched (up to 40%) with UDCA conjugates, but there is little change in total bile acid secretion. UDCA was originally administered and approved by the U.S. Food and Drug Administration (FDA) for gallstone dissolution, but it is not widely used today for this purpose because of the success of laproscopic cholecystectomy. More recently, bile acid therapy has been approved by the FDA for the treatment of primary biliary cirrhosis (PBC), in which UDCA delays the progression of liver fibrosis and improves survival (see Chapter 76).[53] UDCA therapy also has favorable effects in other cholestatic conditions such as cholestasis associated with pregnancy and cholestasis associated with parenteral nutrition.[54]

Bile acid replacement therapy is used to treat inborn errors of bile acid biosynthesis. In affected patients, administration of a mixture of UDCA and CA suppresses the synthesis of cytotoxic bile acid precursors and restores the input of primary bile acids into the enterohepatic circulation.[9] Another indication for bile acid replacement therapy is in patients with severe bile acid malabsorption or short-bowel syndrome in which a deficiency of bile acids in the proximal intestine leads to impaired micellar solubilization and fat malabsorption. Desiccated bile preparations and cholylsarcosine, a deconjugation-dehydroxylation–resistant conjugated bile acid analog, have been shown to improve lipid absorption and provide clinical benefit in these patients.[55]

Bile Acid Sequestrants and Transport Inhibitors

The bile acid sequestrants are positively charged polymeric resins that bind bile acids in the intestinal lumen to decrease the aqueous concentration and reduce the efficiency of intestinal conservation. These agents were originally developed to treat hypercholesterolemia, but they have also been shown to be of value in the treatment of patients with liver and intestinal disease. In patients with mild bile acid malabsorption, bile acid sequestrants reduce diarrhea by decreasing the concentration of free bile acids in the colon. Bile acid sequestrants have also been used to decrease pruritus in patients with cholestasis, presumably by decreasing the concentration of bile acids (or other anionic biliary constituents) in the systemic circulation. Efficacy is only moderate because of the weak bile acid binding efficiency of the resins and poor patient compliance. In addition to the older preparations, cholestyramine and colestipol, more potent sequestrants with superior bile acid binding properties have been developed. Colesevelam HCl is a new bile acid sequestrant that was recently approved by the FDA for treatment of hypercholesterolemia. An alternative to luminal sequestration of bile acids by binding resins is direct inhibition of the ileal ASBT. Several such inhibitors have recently been developed and evaluated in animal models. Although these agents are being targeted primarily for the treatment of hypercholesterolemia, they may also prove useful for blocking the inappropriate ileal conservation of bile acids that contributes to hepatocellular damage and pruritus in cholestatic liver disease.

REFERENCES

1. Carey MC, Duane WC: Enterohepatic circulation. In Arias IM, Boyer JL, Shafritz DA (eds): The Liver: Biology and Pathobiology, 3rd ed. New York, Raven Press, 1994, pp 719–767.
2. Hofmann AF: Bile secretion and the enterohepatic circulation of bile acids. In Feldman M, Scharschmidt BF, Sleisenger MH (eds): Sleisenger and Fordtran's Gastrointestinal and Liver Disease, 6th ed. Philadelphia: WB Saunders, 1998, pp 937–948.
3. Russell DW, Setchell KDR: Bile acid biosynthesis. Biochemistry 31: 4737–4749, 1992.
4. Setchell KDR, Schwarz M, O'Connell NC, et al: Identification of a new inborn error in bile acid synthesis: Mutations of oxysterol 7α-hydroxylase gene cause severe neonatal liver disease. J Clin Invest 102: 1690–1703, 1998.
5. Li-Hawkins J, Lund EG, Bronson AD, et al: Expression cloning of an oxysterol 7α-hydroxylase selective for 24-hydroxycholesterol. J Biol Chem 275:16543–16549, 2000.
6. Russell DW: Oxysterol biosynthetic enzymes. Biochim Biophys Acta 1629:126–135, 2000.
7. Li-Hawkins J, Lund EG, Turley SD, et al: Disruption of the oxysterol 7α-hydroxylase gene in mice. J Biol Chem 275:16536–16542, 2000.
8. Schwarz M, Lund EG, Setchell KDR, et al: Disruption of cholesterol 7α-hydroxylase gene in mice. II. Bile acid deficiency is overcome by induction of oxysterol 7α-hydroxylase. J Biol Chem 271:18024–18031, 1996.
9. Bove KE, Daugherty CC, Tyson W, et al: Bile acid synthetic defects and liver disease. Pediatr Dev Path 3:1–16, 2000.
10. Lu TT, Makishima M, Repa JJ, et al: Molecular basis for feedback regulation of bile acid synthesis by nuclear receptors. Mol Cell 6:507–515, 2000.
11. Goodwin B, Jones SA, Price RR, et al: A regulatory cascade of the nuclear receptors FXR, SHP-1, and LRH-1 represses bile acid biosynthesis. Mol Cell 6:517–526, 2000.
12. Hofmann AF: The continuing importance of bile acids in liver and intestinal disease. Arch Intern Med 159:2647–2658, 1999.
13. Setchell KDR, Heubi JE, O'Connell NC, et al: Identification of a unique inborn error in bile acid conjugation involving a deficiency in amidation. In Paumgartner G, Stiehl A, Gerok E (eds): Bile Acids in Hepatobiliary Diseases: Basic Research and Clinical Applications. Boston, Kluwer, 1997, pp 43–47.
14. Xie W, Radominska-Pandya A, Shi Y, et al: An essential role for nuclear receptors SXR/PXR in detoxification of cholestatic bile acids. Proc Natl Acad Sci U S A 98:3375–3380, 2001.
15. Staudinger JL, Goodwin B, Jones SA, et al: The nuclear receptor PXR is a lithocholic acid sensor that protects against liver toxicity. Proc Natl Acad Sci U S A 98:3369–3374, 2001.
16. Kullack-Ublick GA, Stieger B, Hagenbuch B, et al: Hepatic transport of bile salts. Semin Liver Dis 20:273–292, 2000.
17. St. Pierre MV, Kullak-Ublick GA, Hagenbuch B, et al: Transport of bile acids in hepatic and non-hepatic tissues. J Exp Biol 204:1673–1686, 2001.
18. Marinelli RA, LaRusso NF: Solute and water transport pathways in cholangiocytes. Semin Liver Dis 16:221–229, 1996.
19. Baiocchi L, LeSage G, Glaser S, et al: Regulation of cholangiocyte bile secretion. J Hepatol 31:179–191, 1999.
20. Bolder U, Trang NV, Hagey LR, Schteingart CD, et al: Sulindac is excreted into bile by a canalicular bile salt pump and undergoes a cholehepatic circulation in rats. Gastroenterology 117:962–971, 1999.
21. Lazaridis KN, Pham L, Tietz P, et al: Rat cholangiocytes absorb bile acids at their apical domain via the ileal sodium-dependent bile acid transporter. J Clin Invest 100:2714–2721, 1997.
22. Alpini G, Glasser SS, Rodgers R, et al: Functional expression of the apical Na^+-dependent bile acid transporter in large but not small rat cholangiocytes. Gastroenterology 113:1734–1740, 1997.
23. Chingnard N, Mergey M, Veissiere D, et al: Bile acid transport and regulating functions in the human biliary epithelium. Hepatology 33: 496–503, 2001.
24. Soroka CJ, Lee JM, Azzaroli F, et al: Cellular localization and up-regulation of multidrug resistance-associated protein 3 in hepatocytes and cholangiocytes during obstructive cholestasis in rat liver. Hepatology 33:783–791, 2001.
25. Muller M, Jansen PLM: Molecular aspects of hepatobiliary transport. Am J Physiol 272:G1285–G1303, 1997.
26. Suzuki H, Sugiyama Y: Transport of drugs across the hepatic sinusoidal membrane: Sinusoidal drug influx and efflux in the liver. Semin Liver Dis 20:251–263, 2000.
27. Keppler D, Konig J: Hepatic secretion of conjugated drugs and endogenous substances. Semin Liver Dis 20:265–272, 2000.
28. Hagenbuch B, Steiger B, Foquet M, et al: Functional expression cloning and characterization of the hepatocyte Na^+/bile acid cotransport system. Proc Natl Acad Sci U S A 88:10629–10633, 1991.
29. Trauner M, Meier PJ, Boyer JL: Molecular pathogenesis of cholestasis. N Engl J Med 339:1217–1227, 1998.
30. Lee J, Boyer JL: Molecular alterations in hepatocyte transport mechanisms in acquired cholestatic liver disorders. Semin Liver Dis 20:373–384, 2000.
31. Zoller G, Fickert P, Zenz R, et al: Hepatobiliary transporter expression in percutaneous liver biopsies of patients with cholestatic liver diseases. Hepatology 33:633–646, 2001.
32. Shneider BL, Fox VL, Schwarz KB, et al: Hepatic basolateral sodium-dependent-bile acid transporter expression in two unusual cases of hypercholanemia and in extrahepatic biliary atresia. Hepatology 25:1176–1183, 1997.
33. Morton DH, Salen G, Batta AK, et al: Abnormal hepatic sinusoidal bile acid transport in an Amish kindred is not linked to FIC1 and is improved by Ursodiol. Gastroenterology 119:188–195, 2000.
34. Jacquemin E, Hagenbuch B, Steiger B, et al: Expression cloning of a rat liver Na^+-independent organic anion transporter. Proc Natl Acad Sci U S A 91:133–137, 1994.
35. Li L, Lee TK, Meier PJ, et al: Identification of glutathione as a driving force and leukotriene C4 as a substrate for Oatp1, the hepatic sinusoidal organic solute transporter. J Biol Chem 273:16184–16191, 1998.
36. Li L, Meier PJ, Ballatori N: Oatp2 mediates bidirectional organic solute transport: A role for intracellular glutathione. Mol Pharmacol 58:335–340, 2000.
37. Kullak-Ublick GA, Ismair MG, Steider B, et al: Organic anion-transporting polypeptide B (OATP-B) and its functional comparison with three other OATPs of human liver. Gastroenterology 20:525–533, 2001.
38. Paulusma CC, Kool M, Bosma PJ, et al: A mutation in the human canalicular multispecific organic anion transporter gene causes the Dubin-Johnson syndrome. Hepatology 25:1539–1542, 1997.
39. Gerloff T, Stieger B, Hagenbuch B, et al: The sister-P-glycoprotein represents the canalicular bile salt export pump of mammalian liver. J Biol Chem 273:10046–10050, 1998.
40. Strautnieks SS, Bull LN, Knisely AS, et al: A gene encoding a liver-specific ABC transporter is mutated in progressive familial intrahepatic cholestasis. Nat Genet 20:233–238, 1998.
41. Jansen PL, Stautnieks SS, Jacquemin E, et al: Hepatocanalicular bile salt export pump deficiency in patients with progressive familial intrahepatic cholestasis. Gastroenterology 117:1370–1379, 1999.
42. Walters HC, Craddock AL, Fusegawa H, et al: Expression, transport properties, and chromosomal location of organic anion transporter subtype 3 (oatp3). Am J Physiol 279:G1188–G1200, 2000.
43. Craddock AL, Love MW, Daniel RW, et al: Expression and transport properties of the human ileal and renal sodium-dependent bile acid transporter. Am J Physiol 274:G157–G169, 1998.
44. Oelkers P, Kirby LC, Heubi JE, et al: Primary bile acid malabsorption caused by mutations in the ileal sodium-dependent bile acid transporter gene (SLC10A2) J Clin Invest 99:1880–1887, 1997.

45. Björkhem I, Boberg KM: Inborn errors in bile acid biosynthesis and storage of sterols other than cholesterol. In Scriver CR, Beaudet AL, Sly WS, Valle D (eds): The Metabolic and Molecular Basis of Inherited Disease, 7th ed. New York, McGraw-Hill, 1995, pp 2073–2099.
46. Schwarz M, Wright AC, Davis DL, et al: The bile acid synthetic gene 3β-hydroxy-Δ^5-C_{27}-steroid oxidoreductase is mutated in progressive intrahepatic cholestasis. J Clin Invest 106:1175–1184, 2000.
47. Thompson R, Jansen PLM: Genetic defects in hepatocanalicular transport. Semin Liver Dis 20:365–372, 2000.
48. Wang R, Salem M, Yousef IM, et al: Targeted inactivation of sister of P-glycoprotein gene (spgp) in mice results in nonprogressive but persistent intrahepatic cholestasis. Proc Natl Acad Sci U S A 98:2011–2016, 2001.
49. Jansen PLM, Muller M: The molecular genetics of familial intrahepatic cholestasis. Gut 47:1–5, 2000.
50. Jacquemin E, De Vree JML, Cresteil D, et al: The wide spectrum of multidrug resistance 3 deficiency: From neonatal cholestasis to cirrhosis of adulthood. Gastroenterology 120:1448–1458, 2001.
51. Thomas LA, Versey MJ, Bathgate T, et al: Mechanism for the transit-induced increase in colonic deoxycholic acid formation in cholesterol cholelithiasis. Gastroenterology 119:806–815, 2000.
52. Kullak-Ublick GA, Paumgartner G, Berr F: Long-term effects of cholecystectomy on bile acid metabolism. Hepatology 21:41–45, 1995.
53. Angulo P, Batts KP, Therneau TM, et al: Long-term ursodeoxycholic acid delays histological progression in primary biliary cirrhosis. Hepatology 29:644–647, 1999.
54. Beurs U, Boyer JL, Paumgartner G: Ursodeoxycholic acid in cholestasis: Potential mechanisms of action and therapeutic applications. Hepatology 28:1449–1453, 1998.
55. Gruy-Kapral C, Little KH, Fordtran JS, et al: Conjugated bile acid replacement therapy for short bowel syndrome. Gastroenterology 116: 15–21, 1999.

Chapter 55

GALLSTONE DISEASE AND ITS COMPLICATIONS

Jay D. Horton and Lyman E. Bilhartz

EPIDEMIOLOGY, RISK FACTORS, PATHOGENESIS, AND NATURAL HISTORY OF GALLSTONES

Cholecystectomy is the most common elective abdominal operation in the United States and is overwhelmingly necessitated by the presence of gallstones. Given the enormous cost incurred in the management of gallstone disease, it is appropriate that substantial resources continue to be directed to the elucidation of the pathogenesis and natural history of this common clinical problem. This chapter reviews our current understanding of the pathogenesis, natural history, and complications of gallstone disease. Treatment of gallstones is covered in Chapter 56, Chapter 57, and Chapter 61.

Prevalence and Incidence

A summary of several large studies that estimated the prevalence of gallstone disease in different populations is shown in Table 55–1. Whereas earlier studies had principally used necropsy data, a more recent study in 1999 used ultrasonographic data.[1] Although ultrasonographic screening cannot distinguish cholesterol from pigment stones, it can be assumed that 70% to 80% of those stones detected are cholesterol gallstones in the populations presented in Table 55–1. Several interesting points can be derived from these data. There is clearly a modest difference reported in gallstone prevalence among different populations, which may reflect real genetic or environmental factors or differences in the populations chosen in different studies. In general, gallstones are approximately two times more common in women than in men, and at least 10% of the general population have gallstones. Most series indicate that the prevalence for women between the ages of 20 and 55 varies from 5% to 20% and is 25% to 30% after the age of 50. The prevalence for men is approximately half that for women in a given age group.

Ethnic Predisposition

The genetic predisposition to gallstone formation is not fully understood. Clearly, certain genetic factors play a key role in the pathogenesis of gallstone disease. These are likely to be multifactorial and to vary among populations because many physiologic factors are also determinants of gallstone formation. Within a given population, in first-degree relatives of index cases with gallstone disease, gallstones are 4.5 times more likely to develop than in age- and gender-matched controls,[2] implying a strong genetic influence. Several genes that are associated with gallstone formation or resistance have been identified in mice.[3, 4] To date, the importance of these genes in human gallstone formation has not been established.

The well-studied Pima Indians in southern Arizona are an example of an extremely high-risk population in which 70% of women older than 25 years have gallstones. Another high-risk population are the Scandinavians, in 50% of whom gallstone disease develops by age 50. Other high-risk populations include other American Indian groups in Alaska, Canada, the continental United States, and Bolivia, and all persons living in Chile.[5]

Populations at the lowest risk reside in sub-Saharan Africa[6] and Asia.[7] African Americans have a lower prevalence than whites and a rate of hospitalization for gallstone-related problems that is only 40% that of whites in the United States.[8, 9]

True Incidence

The true incidence of gallstones in a given population has been much harder to elucidate than the prevalence. The largest study to date is of the Danish population and was published in 1991.[10] The 5-year incidence of gallstones in men aged 30, 40, 50, and 60 years was 0.3%, 2.9%, 2.5%, and 3.3%, respectively. The corresponding rates for women were 1.4%, 3.6%, 3.1% and 3.7%. Women clearly had a higher incidence than men at 30 and 40 years of age, but

Table 55–1 | **Gallstone Prevalence by Age in Women and Men from Defined Populations***

POPULATION	AGE (YR)				
	20–29	30–39	40–49	50–59	>60
Brazil	3.0 (1.8)	11 (2.9)	13 (6.3)	23 (7.8)	30 (16)
Cuban Americans		11 (0)		19 (19)	(22)
Denmark		5 (2)	6 (2)	14 (7)	20 (13)
Germany	1.9 (1.4)	5.6 (4.3)	9.5 (10.5)	14 (10)	
Italy	3 (2)	9 (3)	17 (8)	22 (12)	28 (17)
Mexico	11 (1)	13 (5)	20 (7)	22 (10)	27 (14)
Mexican Americans		14 (3)		26 (10)	(16)
Norway	6 (5)	15 (13)	25 (18)	29 (25)	41 (37)
Nova Scotia	15	33	14		
Puerto Rico		9 (9)		21 (21)	(12)
Sweden			17	22	
United States	4.4 (1.3)	5.2 (1.1)	8.2 (5.9)	12 (7.3)	16 (17)

*Prevalence represents the percentage of women (or men) of various ages.

this difference disappeared with increasing age. These incidence figures are in accordance with estimated incidence rates derived from prevalence data reported for Denmark and other populations.[11]

Morphology and Composition

Gallstones are categorized as cholesterol, black pigment, or brown pigment stones, largely on the basis of their composition. Each category has unique epidemiologic features and characteristic risk factors.

Cholesterol stones, the most common type of gallstones, are composed purely of cholesterol or have cholesterol as the major chemical constituent. These stones can often be identified by inspection; stones that are composed entirely of cholesterol are generally large and yellow white in appearance. Microscopically, pure cholesterol stones are composed of many long, thin cholesterol monohydrate crystals bound together by a matrix of mucin glycoproteins with a black core composed of a calcium salt of unconjugated bilirubin. Mixed cholesterol gallstones consist of more than 50% cholesterol and are slightly more common than pure cholesterol stones. Mixed stones tend to be smaller than pure cholesterol stones and are often multiple.

Black pigment stones are composed of either pure calcium bilirubinate or polymer-like complexes with calcium, copper, and large amounts of mucin glycoproteins. A regular crystalline structure is not present. Black gallstones are more common in patients who have cirrhosis and chronic hemolytic states.

Brown pigment stones are composed of calcium salts of unconjugated bilirubin, with varying amounts of cholesterol and protein. These stones are usually associated with infection. Bacteria present in the biliary system produce ß-glucuronidases that hydrolyze glucuronic acid from conjugated bilirubin[12] to form calcium salts of unconjugated bilirubin, deconjugated bile acids, and saturated long-chain fatty acids.[13] Microscopically, brown stones contain cytoskeletons of bacteria, which is consistent with the notion that bacterial infection is a prerequisite for brown stone formation.

Epidemiology and Risk Factors

Within a population, gallstones occur sporadically but not randomly; specific risk factors that result in a predisposition for gallstone formation have been identified. Table 55–2 delineates these risk factors and lists the proposed physiologic abnormalities that may account for the increased risk.

Table 55–2 | **Risk Factors Associated with Cholesterol Gallstone Formation**

RISK FACTOR	PROPOSED METABOLIC ABNORMALITY
Age	Increased cholesterol secretion into bile and decreased bile acid synthesis
Female gender	Increased cholesterol secretion into bile and increased intestinal transit time
Obesity	Cholesterol hypersecretion into bile and increased cholesterol synthesis via increased HMG-CoA reductase activity
Weight loss	Cholesterol hypersecretion into bile, reduced bile acid synthesis, and gallbladder hypomotility
Total parenteral nutrition	Gallbladder hypomotility
Pregnancy	Increased cholesterol secretion and gallbladder hypomotility
Drugs	
Clofibrate	Decreased bile acid concentration as a result of suppression of 7-α-hydroxylase activity and decreased acyl-CoA:cholesterol acyltransferase (ACAT) activity, resulting in increased free cholesterol secretion into bile
Oral contraceptives	Increased cholesterol secretion
Estrogen treatment in women	Cholesterol hypersecretion into bile and reduced bile acid synthesis
Estrogen treatment in men	Cholesterol hypersecretion into bile
Progestogens	Diminished ACAT activity, increased cholesterol secretion, and gallbladder hypomotility
Ceftriaxone	Precipitation of an insoluble calcium-ceftriaxone salt
Octreotide	Decreased gallbladder motility
Genetic predisposition	
Native Americans	Increased cholesterol synthesis and reduced conversion of cholesterol into bile salts
Scandinavians	Increased cholesterol secretion into bile
Apolipoprotein E4/E4 alleles	Unknown
Diseases of the terminal ileum	Hyposecretion of bile salts caused by diminished bile acid pool
Decreased HDL	Increased activity of HMG-CoA reductase
Increased triglycerides	Increased activity of HMG-CoA reductase

HDL, high-density lipoprotein; HMG-CoA, 3-hydroxy-3-methylglutaryl-coenzyme A.

Age and Gender

Because gallstones rarely dissolve spontaneously, the cumulative prevalence of gallstones increases with age (see Table 55–1). In addition, cholesterol secretion into bile increases with age, whereas bile acid formation may decrease. As a result, bile becomes more lithogenic with increasing age.

Gender is a prominent risk factor for gallstone formation: most studies report a two- to threefold higher risk in women than in men. The increased incidence in women is present through the fifth decade, after which the incidence rates in men and women become essentially equal. That trend suggests that estrogen may have a role in the increased secretion of cholesterol into bile in younger women.[10]

Obesity, Weight Loss, and Total Parenteral Nutrition

Obesity is a well-known risk factor for cholelithiasis. A large prospective study of obese women found a strong linear association between body mass index (expressed in kilograms per square meter [kg/m^2]) and the reported incidence of cholelithiasis.[14] In this study, those with the highest body mass index (greater than 45 kg/m^2) had a seven-fold increased risk of development of gallstones compared to nonobese controls. This same population had a yearly incidence of gallstone formation of approximately 2%. The relationship between the body mass index and the risk for development of gallstones is also present in men, although it is somewhat weaker than for that in women.[15]

The association between obesity and gallstone formation may result from increased secretion of cholesterol into the bile as a result of higher 3-hydroxy-3-methylglutaryl-coenzyme A (HMG-CoA) reductase (the rate-limiting enzyme in cholesterol synthesis) activity, which would lead to high levels of cholesterol biosynthesis by the liver. No studies comparing nucleating with antinucleating factors from bile of obese and nonobese subjects have been performed.

In studies of gallbladder motility of obese patients no impairment in gallbladder contraction has been documented.[16] Abnormal processing of the cholecystokinin receptor gene has been reported in one obese patient who had gallstones.[17] Such an abnormality could lead to gallbladder stasis and ultimately to cholelithiasis. However, such an abnormality is not likely to be a common cause of gallstone disease in nonobese or obese patients.

Rapid weight loss is a recognized risk factor for cholesterol gallstone formation. Gallstones develop in approximately 25% of obese patients who are on strict dietary restriction, and in up to 50% of patients who have gastric bypass, gallbladder sludge or gallstones develop within 6 months of surgery.[18] As many as 40% of these patients experience symptoms caused by gallstones in the same 6-month period. A 1997 epidemiologic study showed that men and women who reported being on a slimming diet were at increased risk of gallstone disease.[15]

The physiologic alterations that lead to gallstone formation as a result of rapid weight loss are multiple. Many investigators have shown that hepatic cholesterol secretion increases during caloric restriction.[19] Additional factors may include increased production of mucin (a potent stimulator of cholesterol crystal nucleation) and decreased gallbladder motility.[20] Gallstone formation may be prevented in this high-risk population possibly through prophylactic administration of ursodeoxycholic acid. Shiffman and associates[21] reported a decrease in incidence of gallstone formation from 28% to 3% in obese patients on a very low-calorie diet who also received 600 mg/day of ursodeoxycholic acid.

Total parenteral nutrition (TPN) is associated with the development of acalculous cholecystitis as well as cholelithiasis and cholecystitis. In as many as 45% of adults[22] and 43% of children,[23] gallstones develop after 3 to 4 months of TPN. The incidence of gallbladder sludge is even higher and can occur as early as 3 weeks after initiation of TPN.[24] The primary physiologic defect is gallbladder hypomotility with bile stasis, which results from prolonged fasting. In addition, if there is failure of the sphincter of Oddi to relax, preferential flow of bile into the gallbladder may result. In general, patients who receive TPN have serious medical problems and are not good candidates for abdominal surgery; therefore, prophylactic treatment should be employed if possible. Administration of cholecystokinin-octapeptide 50 ng/kg intravenously over 10 minutes once daily has been shown to prevent gallbladder sludge and gallstone formation in patients on TPN[24] and should be done prophylactically in patients who are receiving long-term TPN in the absence of contraindications.

Pregnancy and Parity

Pregnancy is a clear risk factor for the development of biliary sludge and gallstones. Bile becomes more lithogenic during pregnancy, possibly as a result of increased estrogen levels, which result in increased cholesterol secretion and supersaturation of bile.[25] In addition, gallbladder volume doubles and stasis develops, thereby promoting sludge and gallstone formation,[26] probably as a result of higher progesterone levels, which impair gallbladder motility. The frequency of new sludge and gallstone formation during pregnancy is approximately 30% and 2%, respectively.[27] Both sludge and gallstones are usually silent, but when biliary pain does develop, it is generally associated with the presence of stones and not sludge. Women who have gallstones before they become pregnant are more likely to experience biliary pain during pregnancy than they are when not pregnant.[27] After delivery, gallbladder motility returns to its normal state and bile returns to the prepregnancy state.[26] Sludge disappears in 60% to 70% and stones in 20% to 30% of women after delivery.[27, 28]

Parity is frequently touted as a risk factor for development of gallstones. In several studies, fecundity was associated with an increased prevalence of gallstones.[29, 30] However, the absolute increase in risk seems to be small.

Drugs

Estrogen is the most extensively studied drug or hormone that is associated with gallstone formation. The observation that gallstones occur more frequently in women during their reproductive years led to the initial hypothesis that estrogen may promote gallstone formation. The relationship between exogenous estrogens and gallstone formation in men is clearly established. Men who take estrogens have an increased incidence of both symptomatic gallstones and cholecystectomy.[31] Exogenous estrogen increases biliary cholesterol secretion by 40%, causing cholesterol supersaturation of bile.[32] Estrogen therapy also decreases plasma low-density lipoprotein (LDL) cholesterol concentrations and increases plasma high-density lipoprotein (HDL) cholesterol concentrations in men.[33] The decrease in plasma LDL concentrations is a result of increased hepatic LDL receptor expression, which increases the clearance of plasma LDL.[34] Therefore, it is postulated that increased uptake of LDL by the liver results in increased secretion of cholesterol into bile.

In women, exogenous estrogen enhances lipoprotein uptake in the liver, increases cholesterol secretion into the bile, and inhibits bile acid synthesis.[35] Reported effects of estrogens on gallbladder motility have been mixed and may vary with the drug formulation studied.[35, 36] Women who take conjugated estrogens (Premarin) have at least a twofold increased risk of development of gallstones.[37] Oral contraceptive use also has been associated with an increased incidence of gallstone formation, and an estrogen dose response has been demonstrated.[38] However, a 1997 study using new oral contraceptives showed no increased risk,[15] presumably because of the lower estrogen content of newer oral contraceptives.[39]

Lipid lowering drugs as a class may be expected to alter the propensity to form gallstones because they alter key pathways in cholesterol and bile acid synthesis and metabolism. Clofibrate has the greatest association with increased gallstone formation of any lipid lowering drug. The drug induces cholesterol supersaturation in bile and diminishes bile acid concentrations by reducing the activity of cholesterol 7-α-hydroxylase, the rate limiting enzyme in the classic pathway of bile acid synthesis (see Chapter 54).[40] Cholestyramine and nicotinic acid have no significant association with gallstone formation. HMG-CoA reductase inhibitors (statins) reduce the biliary cholesterol saturation index, but their role in prevention or therapy of gallstone disease has not been clearly established.[41]

Octreotide, a somatostatin analog, increases the incidence of gallstones in patients who are treated with the drug for acromegaly. The frequency of new formation of gallstones after initiation of treatment with octreotide in an Italian population was 28%.[42] Formation of gallbladder sludge in previously normal gallbladders was documented in patients with acromegaly who received treatment with high-dose octreotide for 1 year.[43] Decreased gallbladder motility and bile stasis are associated with administration of octreotide and are likely the major defects responsible for sludge and stone formation.[44]

Ceftriaxone (Rocephin) is a third-generation cephalosporin with a long duration of action. The drug is generally excreted in the urine, but up to 40% is secreted unmetabolized into bile, reaches 100 to 200 times the concentration in serum, and exceeds its saturation level.[45] Once the saturation level is exceeded, ceftriaxone complexes with calcium and forms an insoluble salt.[46] Biliary sludge formation has been reported in 43% of children who receive high-dose ceftriaxone (60 to 100 mg/kg/day), and symptoms referable to the biliary tract were reported in 19% of these patients.[47] The sludge usually disappears spontaneously after ceftriaxone is withdrawn.

Diet and Lipid Profile

A high serum cholesterol level does not seem to be a risk factor for development of gallstones. In fact, some studies have shown an inverse relationship between serum cholesterol level and the risk of gallstones.[15] On the other hand, hypertriglyceridemia is positively associated with an increased incidence of gallstones.[15] HDL cholesterol levels are inversely correlated with the presence of gallstones and biliary cholesterol saturation in some studies,[48] whereas no association has been detected in others.[8, 15] These seemingly independent variables may be related, because serum triglyceride levels tend to increase with increasing body mass and are inversely correlated with HDL levels. Therefore, obese persons who have hypertriglyceridemia and low HDL levels are at greatest risk for development of gallstones.

Differences in diet may account for some of the discrepancies in gallstone prevalence rates reported from various countries; however, results of studies to date have been conflicting, especially in regard to fat consumption. Dietary cholesterol increases cholesterol secretion and decreases the bile salt pool, but only in people who already have gallstones.[49] Moreover, a 1999 large population-based study actually showed an inverse relationship between dietary cholesterol intake and the presence of gallstones.[50]

The ingestion of refined sugars and decreased physical activity are both positively associated with the presence of gallstones in some studies, but no clear physiologic mechanism has been shown to explain this association.[50] In addition, no association between alcohol, tobacco, or caffeine ingestion and development of gallstones has been found.[51]

Systemic Disease

It is believed that diabetics are more prone than nondiabetics to the development of complications associated with cholelithiasis. It has long been believed that patients with insulin resistant diabetes are at an increased risk of development of gallstones, because insulin resistant diabetes is also associated with hypertriglyceridemia, obesity, and gallbladder hypomotility, known risk factors for gallstone formation.[52] However, it has been difficult to prove that insulin resistant diabetes is an independent risk factor for the development of gallstones, although studies in 1997 reported an increased prevalence of gallstones in patients who had evidence of insulin resistance.[15, 53]

Diseases of the ileum are recognized risk factors for the development of gallstones. Crohn's disease is the most common systemic illness that affects the terminal ileum. Patients with Crohn's disease have a two- to threefold increased risk of formation of gallstones.[54] The classic explanation for this increased risk is that specific bile acid receptors in the terminal ileum are lost, and that excessive bile salt excretion and diminished bile acid pool size are the results. These changes ultimately lead to the formation of lithogenic bile. However, there is debate about whether the gallstones that form are principally cholesterol or pigment stones. An insightful 1999 study of patients with Crohn's disease showed that bilirubin concentrations were increased in bile and that the biliary bilirubin concentrations correlated positively with the extent of ileal disease.[55] The mechanism proposed is that the diseased ileum cannot reabsorb bile salts, and as a result bile salt concentrations increase in the colon. The colonic bile salts solubilize unconjugated bilirubin, thereby promoting the absorption of bilirubin and subsequent enterohepatic cycling.

Spinal cord injuries are associated with a high prevalence of gallstones. Moonka and associates[56] reported a prevalence of gallstones of 31% and an annual incidence of biliary complications of 2.2% in persons who had a spinal cord injury. Although the complication rate associated with gallstones in patients who have spinal cord injuries is at least twofold higher than that reported for the general population, the relative risk is still low enough that prophylactic cholecystectomy is probably not justified. The mechanism responsible for the association between spinal cord injuries and gallstone formation is not known. Gallbladder relaxation is impaired in these patients, but gallbladder contraction in response to a meal is normal. Therefore, it seems unlikely that the increased risk is due merely to biliary stasis.

Pathogenesis

Three principal defects are intimately involved in gallstone formation (Fig. 55–1): cholesterol supersaturation, accelerated nucleation, and gallbladder hypomotility. Initially, cholesterol supersaturation was thought to be sufficient for gallstone formation, but this explanation proved to be too simple after it was discovered that supersaturated bile is commonly secreted, at least intermittently, in most persons who do not have gallstones.[57] Subsequently, cholesterol crystal formation was shown to be an important factor in gallstone formation, and after an assay to measure crystal nucleation time was developed, a variety of factors were found to promote or

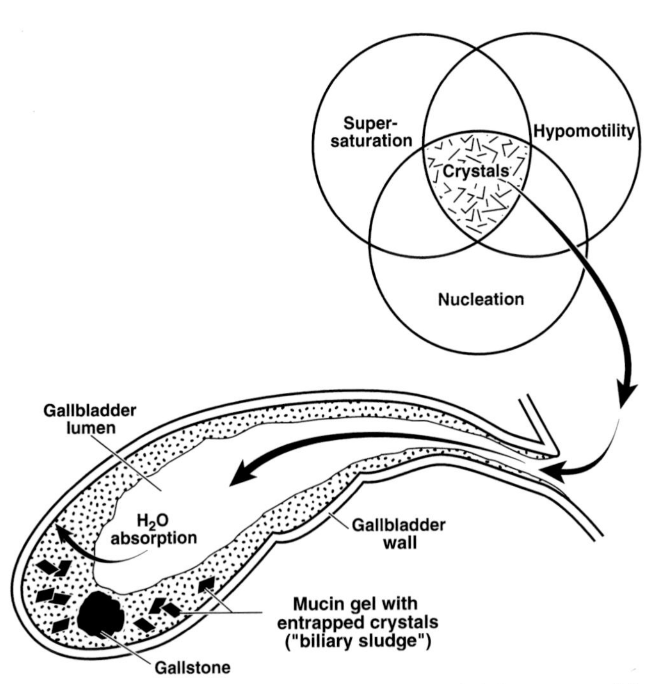

Figure 55–1. Venn diagram of the three principal defects required for cholesterol gallstone formation. Cholesterol crystals form in and are trapped by the mucin gel, which accumulates from hypersecretion in the gallbladder and defective evacuation (hypomotility). Mucin glycoprotein molecules also appear to act as annealing agents in the agglomeration of crystals to form gallstones.

inhibit crystal nucleation.[58] Gallbladder hypomotility clearly plays an important role, because small crystals should pass readily through the bile duct and into the intestine before the crystals have time to develop into a stone.

Cholesterol Supersaturation

Cholesterol is essentially insoluble in water and therefore relies on the detergent activity of bile salts and the polar phospholipids (lecithin) to stay in solution. Cholesterol, phospholipids, and bile acids are the major lipid components in bile. The degree of cholesterol saturation in gallbladder bile is the most important single determinant of crystal formation in humans.[59] Because cholesterol metabolism is intimately linked to cholesterol secretion into bile and to bile acid formation (see Chapter 54), a basic understanding of hepatic cholesterol metabolism is beneficial.

The liver is the primary organ responsible for regulating cholesterol homeostasis. It is able to vary endogenous cholesterol synthesis over the greatest range, and it is the only organ that can permanently eliminate cholesterol from the body. Unesterified cholesterol can be secreted directly into bile through an as yet unidentified process. Cholesterol is also the precursor for all bile acids, and bile acid synthesis and secretion into bile eliminate cholesterol from the body.

Newly formed cholesterol is synthesized in the endoplasmic reticulum from acetyl-coenzyme A through a sequence of highly regulated enzymatic steps. HMG-CoA reductase is the rate limiting enzyme.[60] In addition to endogenous cholesterol synthesis, the liver takes up several grams of cholesterol associated with all classes of lipoproteins via a variety of primarily endocytic pathways. The storage form of cholesterol in the liver is a fatty acid ester that is produced by the enzymatic action of hepatic acyl-CoA cholesterol acyltransferase (ACAT).[4] Although chemically inert, the cholesteryl ester pool serves as a continual supply of free cholesterol for bile acid formation and lipoprotein assembly in the endoplasmic reticulum.

It is tempting to assume that alterations in cholesterol metabolism may directly affect the rate of bile acid and cholesterol secretion into bile, thus producing potentially lithogenic bile. Some studies have shown that patients with gallstone have higher activities of HMG-CoA reductase and higher rates of cholesterol synthesis than control subjects.[61] Lovastatin, a competitive inhibitor of HMG-CoA reductase, blocks gallstone formation in the prairie dog[62] and may also inhibit crystal formation in humans.[63] However, in other animal models cholesterol synthesis can be varied over a large range with no change in the rate of biliary secretion of cholesterol.[64] Additionally, only a small percentage (~20%) of cholesterol in the bile is newly synthesized.[65]

Rates of cholesterol esterification may influence the lithogenicity of bile because drugs that reduce esterification (e.g. progesterone and clofibrate) tend to increase the secretion of cholesterol.[66] Decreased as well as normal ACAT activity levels have been reported in patients who have gallstones.[67, 68] The potential importance of ACAT activity is suggested by the observation that a pool of free cholesterol ultimately mediates the regulation of cholesterol synthesis and uptake. This pool of free cholesterol may be altered by either high or low ACAT activity. Therefore, low ACAT activity in the liver may increase the free cholesterol pool and thus stimulate cholesterol secretion into bile. A mouse with the genetic deletion of ACAT2, the principal ACAT isoform present in liver and intestine, was generated and characterized in 2000.[4] Interestingly, this mouse is actually resistant to diet-induced gallstone formation. This resistance, however, is likely the result of the markedly lower rates of intestinal absorption of cholesterol as a result of reduced ACAT activity in the intestine and not a direct result of the loss of ACAT activity from the liver. Therefore, this mouse model neither proves nor disproves the ACAT hypothesis but illustrates the potential importance of the intestine in regulating cholesterol absorption as a possible factor in gallstone formation.

The mechanism responsible for cholesterol secretion into bile is not yet fully understood. However, understanding of this process has been augmented by a study of a genetically altered mouse that lacks the multiple drug resistance 2 (mdr2) gene. The protein produced by the mdr gene is a member of the adenosine triphosphate (ATP)-binding cassette (ABC) transporter family that has recently been renamed *ABCB4*. ABCB4 normally acts as a translocase, or "flippase," that flips phosphatidylcholine molecules across the canalicular membrane. Biliary phospholipids make up 15% to 25% of the solute in bile, 95% of which is diacylphosphatidylcholines (lecithins).[69] Lecithins are needed to ensure cholesterol solubilization; they also help protect the biliary tree from the detergent effects of bile salts and are important in regulating overall bile composition. In mice lacking mdr2, severe liver disease results from inability of the liver to secrete phospholipids into bile.[70] These animals also have a marked reduction in the secretion of cholesterol into bile that suggests that cholesterol molecules normally co-flip across the canicular membrane with phospholipids.

Although virtually insoluble in water, cholesterol is made soluble in bile by associating with bile salts and phospholipids. In a classic set of experiments, Carey and Small investigated the solubility limits of cholesterol in relation to varying amounts of lecithin and bile salts as triangular phase diagrams.[71] Using the phase diagrams, it is possible to determine the phase in which cholesterol is likely to exist in a given bile (i.e., in micelles, vesicles, or both micelles and vesicles). It is also possible to determine the cholesterol saturation index (CSI) by using the phase diagrams. If the CSI is greater than 1, saturated bile is present and cholesterol can precipitate out of solution to form crystals.

In unsaturated bile, cholesterol is present predominantly in simple and mixed micelles. Micelles are lipid aggregates that have the polar phosphate or hydroxyl groups directed outward toward the aqueous phase and the nonpolar hydrocarbon chains directed inward. As cholesterol saturation increases in bile, more cholesterol is carried in the form of vesicles.[72] Vesicles are approximately 10 times larger than micelles and have phospholipid bilayers but contain no bile salts. The polar groups in vesicles also are directed outward, and the hydrophobic hydrocarbon chains are directed in toward the bilayer. This arrangement allows cholesterol to be dissolved in the core. Unilamellar vesicles can coalesce into multilamellar vesicles, which tend to be less stable, thereby allowing the growth of cholesterol crystals from the surface. Compared with control subjects, patients who have cholesterol gallstones secrete vesicles in the canalicular lumen that are 33% more enriched with cholesterol and more prone to aggregate and to nucleate.[73, 74]

Bile salts, which are the most abundant solutes in bile, are critical in determining cholesterol solubilization. The pathways responsible for the synthesis of bile acids from cholesterol are discussed in Chapter 54. Only two primary bile acids are synthesized in humans: cholate and chenodeoxycholate; each represents approximately 35% of the total bile acid pool. The secondary bile acids, deoxycholic acid and lithocholic acid represent approximately 24% and 1% to 3%, of the pool, respectively. Ursodeoxycholic acid is a tertiary bile acid that contributes up to 4% of the bile acid pool. All bile acids are conjugated with glycine or taurine in approximately a 2:1 ratio prior to secretion.

The secretion of bile acids into the canaliculus across a concentration gradient is an active process that appears to be independent of cholesterol and phospholipid molecules.[75] A bile acid transporter of the ABC transporter family was identified and characterized in 1998.[76] The bile acid transporter was initially designated "sister of P-glycoprotein" (SPGP) but has since been renamed *ABCB11*. It is expressed almost exclusively in the liver and is responsible for the canalicular secretion of bile salts.

The composition of the bile acid pool is also an important determinant of bile lithogenicity. The more hydrophobic the bile acid, the greater is its ability to induce cholesterol secretion and suppress bile acid synthesis.[77] The combination of increased cholesterol secretion and decreased bile acid synthesis leads to more lithogenic bile. The relative concentration of each bile acid also influences the CSI and the propensity of cholesterol to precipitate and form crystals. Patients with gallstones have smaller pools of cholic acid and larger pools of the bacterial bile acid metabolite deoxycholic acid.[78] Deoxycholic acid, which is very hydrophobic, increases the CSI by increasing cholesterol secretion and reducing nucleation time. Furthermore, the deoxycholic acid pool size is positively correlated with the production of arachidonic acid,[79] which is the precursor for prostaglandin synthesis. Prostaglandins stimulate secretion of mucin, a pronucleator (see the following section) and thus may contribute to the formation of lithogenic bile. At the opposite end of the spectrum is the hydrophilic bile acid ursodeoxycholic acid, which dissolves and prevents the formation of cholesterol gallstones (see Chapter 57). Ursodeoxycholic acid decreases the CSI and prolongs nucleation time, possibly as a result of a decrease in the concentration of pronucleating proteins in bile.[80]

Nucleating and Antinucleating Factors

In supersaturated bile, the first step in gallstone formation is nucleation: the condensation or aggregation process by which a propagable submicroscopic crystal or amorphous particle is formed from supersaturated bile.[57] After nucleation, crystallization occurs, producing cholesterol monohydrate crystals that can agglomerate to form macroscopic gallstones.[81] Since the development of an assay to measure rates of nucleation in native bile, specific factors that alter these rates have been sought. Initially, it was shown that bile from patients who have gallstones has a faster nucleation time than bile from control subjects.[58] Also, biliary protein is increased in bile with cholesterol crystals compared with bile without crystals.[82] A large number of potential pronucleators as well as nucleation inhibitors have been identified and studied. The physiologic relevance of these proposed factors (with the exception of mucin) continues to be debated.

Mucin glycoproteins are the most important pronucleators to be identified. The core of these proteins contains hydrophobic regions that can bind to cholesterol, phospholipids, and bilirubin.[83] The binding of cholesterol rich vesicles to the hydrophobic regions seems to mediate the observed accelerated nucleation. Also, vesicle fusion and aggregation are markedly accelerated in the presence of physiologic concentrations of mucin, and this phenomenon may also account for the pronucleating properties of mucin.[84] Because mucin and bilirubin are frequently found in the core of cholesterol gallstones, this complex may serve as a nidus for stone formation. In addition to having pronucleating effects, mucin has been shown to accelerate cholesterol monohydrate crystal growth.[85]

Mucin glycoproteins are normally secreted continuously from the gallbladder; however, mucin secretion is excessive in lithogenic bile.[73] Mucin hypersecretion precedes cholesterol crystal formation in animal models. Secretion of mucin is mediated, at least in part, by prostaglandins, which are synthesized from arachidonic acid. Therefore, nonsteroidal anti-inflammatory drugs (NSAIDs) may inhibit the secretion of mucin. Administration of aspirin prevents gallstone formation in prairie dogs and reduces mucin secretion in humans.[86, 87] However, patients who chronically ingest NSAIDs have the same prevalence of gallstone disease as those who do not.[88] Therefore, NSAIDs do not appear to offer any substantial protective effect.

A large number of other pronucleators have been isolated in model bile systems by lecithin chromatography using concanavilin A sepharose.[89] These pronucleators include immunoglobulin G (IgG) and IgM,[90] aminopeptidase N,[91] haptoglobin,[92] and α1-acid glycoprotein.[93]

Antinucleating proteins that have been identified in model bile systems include apolipoproteins A-I and A-II[94] and a biliary glycoprotein.[95] As a result of research that has defined five separate crystallization pathways, more detailed and rigorous methods can be employed to assess the physiologic role of proposed pro- and antinucleating factors.[96]

Biliary calcium concentration plays a role in bilirubin precipitation and gallstone formation because calcium salts are present in most cholesterol gallstones. Patients with gallstones may have increased concentrations of calcium in bile with supersaturation of calcium carbonate.[97] Calcium carbonate as well as calcium bilirubinate and calcium phosphate can each serve as a potential nidus for cholesterol crystallization.

Gallbladder Hypomotility

The contribution of the gallbladder to the pathogenesis of gallstones is widely recognized. The mucosa of the gallbladder has one of the highest rates of water absorption in the body. The volume of bile residing in the gallbladder decreases by 80% to 90% as a result of active sodium transport coupled with passive water absorption.[98] The gallbladder also acidifies the bile by bicarbonate absorption and secretion of hydrogen ions.[99] The concentration of bile affects vesicle formation, and bile is often saturated after an overnight fast or prolonged TPN. On the other hand, acidification of bile increases the solubility of calcium salts, thereby making precipitation less favorable.[100] The true physiologic role that is played by acidification is not clear. Patients who have uncomplicated cholelithiasis acidify bile normally,[101] but acidification is impaired in inflamed gallbladders.[102]

Neural control of gallbladder emptying is mediated by both parasympathetic and sympathetic innervation; the former increases gallbladder contractility, and the latter causes relaxation. The motility defects of gallstone patients are manifested by increased fasting and residual volumes.[73] Inhibiting the cholinergic input with atropine increases fasting volumes and reduces emptying after meals in response to cholecystokinin (CCK).[103] However, it is uncertain whether patients who have had a vagotomy are at increased risk of gallstone formation.

CCK is the most potent physiologic stimulator of gallbladder contraction. Patients with gallstones have a diminished gallbladder contractile response to intravenously administered CCK.[104] The observed abnormality is not due merely to the presence of stones, because the diminished response remains after the stones have been cleared by lithotripsy.[105] Interestingly, there is a positive correlation between the degree of impairment of gallbladder contraction and the cholesterol content in bile, even in healthy persons without stones.[106] The physiologic mechanism responsible for gallbladder hypomotility in gallstone disease remains unknown.

The stimulants of CCK release are, in order of decreasing potency, long-chain fatty acids, amino acids, and carbohydrates. The inability of patients who have cystic fibrosis and pancreatic insufficiency to produce these stimulants is the proposed cause of the higher incidence of gallstones in these patients.[107] Other hormones such as motilin, somatostatin, and pancreatic polypeptide can affect gallbladder motility, but their physiologic role remains to be determined.

A potential complication of gallbladder stasis is the formation of sludge, which can occur in patients who have high spinal cord injuries, prolonged use of TPN, or prolonged treatment with octreotide, who are pregnant, or who experience rapid weight loss.[108] Biliary sludge is the result of precipitates in bile and is composed largely of cholesterol monohydrate crystals, calcium bilirubinate granules, and mucus. The pathogenesis of biliary sludge is generally thought to be similar to that of gallstones. In patients with sludge who were followed prospectively for 38 months, asymptomatic gallstones developed in 8%, and symptomatic stones requiring cholecystectomy developed in 6%. In 18% of the patients, the sludge disappeared spontaneously; in 60%, the sludge disappeared and reappeared.[109] Complications such as acute cholecystitis have been reported to occur in as many as 20% of patients with biliary sludge.[110] It is clear from these and other studies that sludge can be a precursor to stone formation and can be a source of potential complications.

Pigment Stones

Epidemiology of Pigment Stones

Pigment stones account for 10% to 25% of all gallstones in the United States but represent a much higher percentage in

Asians.[111] As the name implies, the stones are pigmented as a result of bilirubin precipitation. As for cholesterol gallstones, the prevalence of pigment stones increases with age and is generally higher in women than in men.

Black pigment stones form in the gallbladder as a result of increased production of unconjugated bilirubin, which then precipitates as calcium bilirubinate to form stones. Therefore, black pigment stone formation is typically associated with chronic hemolysis (e.g., β-thalassemia, hereditary spherocytosis, sickle cell hemoglobinopathy), cirrhosis, and pancreatitis.[111] The risk of development of pigment stones is increased in persons who have cirrhosis, although the reported prevalence rates vary widely. Whether the risk of stone formation is higher for alcoholic cirrhosis than for other forms of cirrhosis is controversial.

Brown pigment stones are more common in areas where biliary infections are more prevalent. They can occur in the gallbladder or in the biliary tree. Brown stones are almost always associated with colonization of the bile by enteric organisms and ascending cholangitis.[112] As the incidence of biliary infections has decreased in populations prone to development of pigment stones, the ratio of cholesterol to pigment stones has increased. The percentage of pigment stones in the Japanese population fell from 60% to 24% between 1940 and 1980[113] and similar changes are being reported in other countries, such as Taiwan.[114] Brown pigment stones also are associated with duodenal diverticula and are more likely to form de novo in bile ducts than are other types of stones.[115]

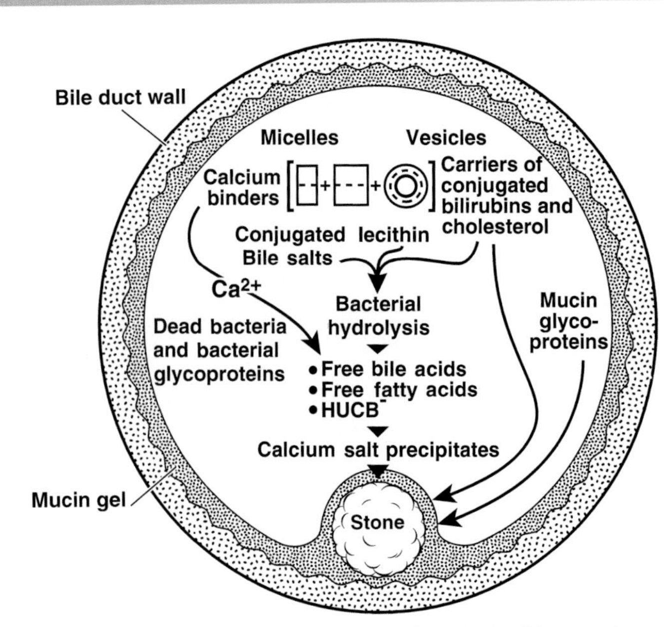

Figure 55–2. Proposed schema for the pathogenesis of brown pigment gallstones in human bile ducts. $HUCB^-$, hydrolyzed unconjugated bilirubin.[13]

Pathogenesis of Pigment Stones

Black pigment stones are composed primarily of calcium bilirubinate but also contain calcium carbonate and calcium phosphate. As much as 20% of the weight of black stones is mucin glycoprotein.[13] The unifying characteristic of the conditions that predispose to black stone formation is the hypersecretion of bilirubin conjugates (especially monoglucuronides) into the bile.[116] In the presence of hemolysis, the output of these bilirubin conjugates increases 10-fold.[117] Unconjugated monohydrogenated bilirubin is formed by the action of endogenous β-glucuronidase, which can then coprecipitate with calcium as a result of supersaturation.[118] An acidification defect has also been documented, possibly as a result of inflammation or of the buffering capacity of sialic acid and sulfate moieties of the mucus gel.[118] This buffering effect facilitates the supersaturation of calcium carbonate and phosphate, which would not occur at a more acidic pH, and allows precipitation. No gallbladder motility defects were found in patients who had black stones,[119] but mucin hypersecretion may result from increased levels of unconjugated bilirubin.[120]

Brown pigment stone formation is a result of anaerobic infection of the bile, as demonstrated by the finding of bacterial cytoskeletons in the stones.[121] A postulated schema for brown stone formation is illustrated in Figure 55–2. Stasis facilitates bacterial infection as well as accumulation of mucus and bacterial cytoskeletons in the bile ducts. The enteric bacteria produce β-glucuronidase, phospholipase A, and conjugated bile acid hydrolase. β-Glucuronidase activity results in the production of unconjugated bilirubin; phospholipase A produces palmitic and stearic acids from phospholipids; and bile acid hydrolases produce unconjugated bile acids. The anionic products of these enzymatic processes can complex with calcium to produce insoluble calcium salts, thereby resulting in stone formation.[13]

Natural History

The natural history of gallstones is typically defined in two separate groups of patients: those who have symptomatic gallstones and those who are asymptomatic. Autopsy studies clearly show that most gallstones are asymptomatic and remain asymptomatic. The true incidence of complications in persons with asymptomatic stones (as well as symptomatic stones) is critical to providing rational, cost-effective recommendations for therapy. Unfortunately, the information available has been rather sparse and somewhat varied.

Asymptomatic Stones

The study that changed our concepts about therapy for gallstone disease was that of Gracie and Ransohoff,[122] who followed 123 Michigan faculty members who had been found to have gallstones on routine screening for a period of 15 years. At 5, 10, and 15 years of follow-up, 10%, 15%, and 18% became symptomatic and none experienced complications. The authors suggested that the rate of development of biliary pain in persons with asymptomatic gallstones is approximately 2% per year for 5 years and then decreases over time. Biliary complications developed in only three patients in this study, and in all three the complications were preceded by episodes of biliary pain. Several studies have suggested that in 90% of people with asymptomatic gallstones in whom symptoms develop the initial clinical presentation is biliary pain and not a biliary complication.[122] Thus, the incidence of complications in patients who have asymptomatic stones is low, and prophylactic removal of the gallbladder for this condition is not necessary.

Subsequent studies have shown slightly higher incidence rates of biliary pain and complications,[123] but only one has been a long-term prospective study. The Group for Epidemiology and Prevention of Cholelithiasis (GREPCO) in Rome followed the natural history of 151 subjects with gallstones, 118 of whom were asymptomatic on entering the study. In those who were initially asymptomatic, the incidence of development of biliary colic, at 2, 4, and 10 years was 12%, 17%, and 26%, respectively, and the cumulative rate of biliary complications was 3% at 10 years.[124]

Symptomatic Stones

The natural history of symptomatic gallstones follows a more aggressive course. The National Cooperative Gallstone Study showed that of those patients who had an episode of uncomplicated biliary pain in the year before entering the study, 38% per year had recurrent biliary pain.[125] Others have reported an incidence of recurrent biliary pain as high as 50% per year in persons with symptomatic gallstones.[126] Patients who have symptomatic gallstones also are more likely to experience biliary complications as a result of the gallstones. The risk of development of biliary complications is estimated to be 1% to 2% per year and is thought to remain relatively constant over time.[127] Therefore, cholecystectomy should be offered to patients only after significant biliary symptoms develop. Depending on the patient, a reasonable approach may also include observing the pattern of pain before deciding on therapy, because up to 30% of patients who have one episode of pain do not have a later episode.

Diabetes Mellitus

Diabetic patients with incidental cholelithiasis were long considered to have an increased risk of serious complications even though the gallstones were asymptomatic. More recent studies have shown that the natural history of gallstones in diabetics follows the same pattern observed in nondiabetics. A prospective study of non-insulin-dependent diabetics with asymptomatic gallstones showed that after 5 years of follow-up, symptoms developed in 15%.[128] This frequency is roughly the same as that reported for nondiabetics. More importantly, the complication and mortality rates also were comparable in diabetics and nondiabetics. Therefore, prophylactic cholecystectomy is generally not recommended in diabetics.

CLINICAL MANIFESTATIONS OF GALLSTONE DISEASE

Overview

The hepatobiliary tract is a low-pressure—low-flow hydraulic excretory pathway for hydrophobic, water-insoluble waste products.[129] Because of the low-flow nature of the hydraulic system and the tenuous solubility of the constituents,[130] bile is vulnerable to precipitation and the formation of crystals. Once formed, the crystals or stones rarely dissolve spontaneously.[59]

The clinical manifestations of gallstones are shown schematically in Figure 55–3 and are summarized in more detail in Table 55–3.[127, 131–134]

In essence, a gallstone can cause symptoms by only two mechanisms: it can obstruct the cystic duct or common bile duct,[131] or, much more rarely, it can erode through the gallbladder wall. The specific syndromes produced by gallstones[135] are discussed in detail later. Acute pancreatitis caused by gallstones is detailed in Chapter 48, and the relationship between gallstones and gallbladder cancer is discussed in Chapter 60. The surgical and medical treatments of gallstone disease are discussed in Chapters 56 and 57, respectively.

It should be emphasized once again that most gallstones never cause symptoms,[136] and the purely incidental discovery of cholelithiasis rarely warrants specific intervention. Possible exceptions to this general dictum include the following:

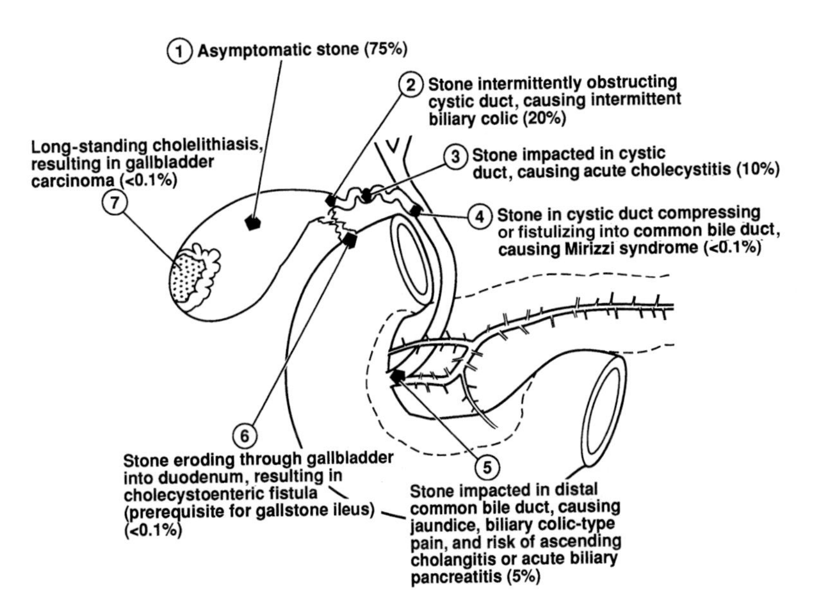

Figure 55–3. Schematic depiction of the complications of gallstones. The percentages (%) approximate the frequency of that complication occurring in untreated patients, based on natural history data. As shown, the most frequent outcome is for the stone to remain asymptomatic throughout life. Biliary colic, acute cholecystitis, and cholangitis are the most common complications, and the Mirizzi syndrome, cholecystoenteric fistula, and gallbladder cancer are relatively rare. (The total of the percentages is >100% because patients with acute cholecystitis generally have prior episodes of biliary colic.)

Table 55–3 | **Common Clinical Manifestations of Gallstone Disease**

	BILIARY COLIC	ACUTE CHOLECYSTITIS	CHOLEDOCHO-LITHIASIS	CHOLANGITIS
Pathophysiologic condition	Intermittent obstruction of cystic duct No inflammation of gallbladder mucosa	Impacted stone in cystic duct Acute inflammation of gallbladder mucosa Secondary bacterial infection in ≈50%	Intermittent obstruction of CBD	Impacted stone in CBD causing bile stasis Bacterial superinfection of stagnant bile Early bacteremia
Symptoms	Severe, poorly localized epigastric or RUQ visceral pain growing in intensity over 15 min and remaining constant for 1–6 hr, often with nausea Frequency of attacks varies from days to months Gas, bloating, flatulence, dyspepsia *not* related to stones	75% Preceded by attacks of biliary colic Visceral epigastric pain gives way to moderately severe, localized pain in RUQ, back, shoulder, or (rarely) chest Nausea with some emesis-frequent Pain lasting >6 hr suggests cholecystitis (vs. colic)	Often asymptomatic Symptoms (when present) indistinguishable from biliary colic symptoms Predisposes to cholangitis and acute pancreatitis	Charcot's triad (pain, jaundice, fever) present in 70% May be mild, transient pain often accompanied by chills Mental confusion, lethargy, and delirium suggestive of bacteremia
Physical findings	Mild to moderate gallbladder tenderness during attack with mild residual tenderness lasting days Often completely normal examination result	Febrile, usually <102°F unless complicated by gangrene or perforation Right subcostal tenderness with inspiratory arrest (Murphy's sign) Palpable gallbladder in 33%, especially in first attack Mild jaundice in 20%, higher frequency in elderly	Often completely normal examination result if obstruction intermittent Jaundice with pain suggestive of stones; painless jaundice and palpable gallbladder suggestive of malignancy	Fever in 95% RUQ tenderness in 90% Jaundice in 80% Peritoneal signs in 15% Hypotension with mental confusion in 15% suggestive of gram-negative sepsis
Laboratory findings	Usually normal In patients with findings of only uncomplicated biliary colic, elevated bilirubin, alkaline phosphatase, or amylase level suggestive of coexisting CBD stones	Leukocytosis of 12,000–15,000/mm³ with left shift common Serum bilirubin may be 2–4 mg/dL and aminotransferase and alkaline phosphatase levels may be elevated, even in absence of CBD stone or hepatic infection Mild serum amylase elevation even in absence of pancreatitis If bilirubin >4 mg/dL or amylase >1000 U/L suspect CBD stone	Elevated serum bilirubin and alkaline phosphatase levels seen with CBD obstruction Serum bilirubin level >10 mg/dL suggestive of malignant obstruction or coexisting hemolysis Transient spike in serum aminotransferase or amylase levels suggestive of stone passage	Leukocytosis in 80%; normal WBC count with left shift may be only hematologic finding in 20% Serum bilirubin level >2 mg/dL in 80%, but when <2 mg/dL diagnosis may be missed Serum alkaline phosphatase level usually elevated Blood culture results usually positive, especially during chills or fever spike; grow two organisms in one half of patients
Diagnostic tests (see Table 55–4 for details)	Ultrasonography OCG Meltzer-Lyon test	Ultrasonography Hepatobiliary scintigraphy (DISIDA, HIDA scans) Abdominal CT	ERCP THC	ERCP THC
Natural history	After initial attack, no further symptoms in 30% In remainder development of symptoms at rate of 6%/year and of severe complications at rate of 1%/year	Spontaneous resolution in 50% in 7–10 days without surgery Untreated, 10% complicated by localized perforation, 1% by free perforation and peritonitis	Natural history not well defined, but complications more frequent and severe than for asymptomatic (gallbladder) stones	High mortality rate if unrecognized with death from septicemia Dramatic improvement of survival rate with emergent decompression of CBD (usually by ERCP)
Treatment (see Chap. 56)	Elective laparoscopic cholecystectomy with IOC ERCP for stone removal if stones on IOC	Cholecystectomy with IOC If stones on IOC, then CBD exploration or ERCP for stone removal	Stone removal at time of ERCP followed by early laparoscopic cholecystectomy	Emergency ERCP with stone removal or at least biliary decompression Antibiotics to cover gram-negative organisms Interval cholecystectomy

CBD, common bile duct; CT, computed tomography; DISIDA, diisopropyl iminodiacetic acid; ERCP, endoscopic retrograde cholangiopancreatography; HIDA, hydroxy iminodiacetic acid; IOC, intraoperative cholangiography; OCG, oral cholecystography; RUQ, right upper quadrant; THC, transhepatic cholangiography; WBC, white blood cell.

1. A young patient with sickle cell anemia and incidental cholelithiasis in whom an abdominal pain crisis would be difficult to distinguish from biliary colic or acute cholecystitis[137, 138] (see Chapter 82)
2. A young woman of American Indian ancestry with incidental cholelithiasis[30] in whom prophylactic cholecystectomy may be warranted to prevent the delayed complication of gallbladder cancer[139]
3. Any patient with gallbladder wall calcification (porcelain gallbladder) who is an acceptable surgical risk for the purpose of preventing gallbladder carcinoma as a late complication[140]
4. A patient with incidental cholelithiasis who is planning prolonged space travel or other extremely remote assignments

Some investigators have proposed that patients with incidental cholelithiasis who are awaiting heart transplantation[141] have a prophylactic cholecystectomy irrespective of biliary tract symptoms, but a 1998 retrospective study that directly addressed the issue in renal transplant recipients concluded that complications of gallstones can be managed safely after symptoms emerge.[142]

Imaging Studies of the Biliary Tract

As shown in Table 55–4, a wide array of imaging technologies is available to evaluate the biliary tract.[1, 143, 144] Each test has strengths and limitations, and the tests available vary widely in relative cost and risk to the patient. With the possible exception of ultrasonography, none of the tests should be ordered routinely in the evaluation of a patient with suspected gallstone disease; rather, the diagnostic evaluation should proceed in a rational stepwise fashion based on the individual patient's symptoms, signs, and laboratory results.

Notably absent from the list of imaging studies of the biliary tract is the plain abdominal film. Although occasionally useful in evaluating patients who have abdominal pain, plain abdominal films lack both sensitivity and specificity. Only 50% of pigment stones and 20% of cholesterol stones contain enough calcium to be visible on a plain abdominal film. Because 80% of all gallstones in Western populations are of the cholesterol type, it follows that only 25% of stones are detected on plain radiographs. Plain abdominal films have their greatest utility in evaluating patients who have unusual complications of gallstones, such as emphysematous cholecystitis, cholecystoenteric fistula, and a porcelain gallbladder.

Ultrasonography

Since its introduction in the 1970s, ultrasonographic examination of the biliary tract has become the principal imaging modality for the diagnosis of cholelithiasis. Ultrasonography requires no special preparation of the patient, involves no ionizing radiation, is simple to perform, and provides accurate anatomic information. It has the additional advantage of being portable and thus available at the bedside of a critically ill patient.[145]

Ultrasonography of the gallbladder should follow a fast of at least 8 hours, because gallstones are best seen in a distended, bile filled gallbladder. The diagnosis relies on the finding of echogenic objects within the lumen of the gallbladder (see Fig. 55–4) that produce an acoustic shadow.[146] The stones are mobile and generally congregate in the dependent portion of the gallbladder. Modern ultrasonographic equipment can routinely detect stones as small as 2 mm in diameter. Stones less than 2 mm in diameter may be missed or confused with biliary sludge, which is defined as layering echogenic material that does not cast acoustic shadows. Sludge, despite its colloquial name, has been well defined from a chemical standpoint (precipitated calcium bilirubinate granules, cholesterol monohydrate crystals, and glycoproteins), and its natural history is similar to that of macroscopic cholelithiasis in that it often exhibits typical biliary pain, acute cholecystitis, or pancreatitis.[108]

The overall sensitivity of ultrasonography for the detection of gallstones in the gallbladder is greater than 95% for stones larger than 2 mm in diameter.[147] The specificity is greater than 95% when stones are seen with an accompanying acoustic shadow. Rarely, advanced scarring and contraction of the gallbladder around gallstones make it impossible to locate the gallbladder or the stones; this finding also should raise the possibility of gallbladder cancer. The contracted gallbladder filled with stones may give a "double-arc-shadow" or "wall-echo-shadow" sign, with the gallbladder wall, echogenic stones, and acoustic shadowing seen in immediate proximity. If the gallbladder cannot be identified at all by ultrasonography, then a complementary test such as oral cholecystography (OCG) or abdominal computed tomographic (CT) scan is warranted.

Although ultrasonography is the gold standard for the diagnosis of stones in the gallbladder, it is distinctly less powerful for the detection of stones in the CBD.[148] Because of the proximity of the distal CBD to the duodenum, luminal bowel gas often interferes with the ultrasonographic image, and the entire length of the CBD cannot be examined.[149] As a result, only approximately 50% of CBD stones are actually seen on ultrasonography.[143] However, the presence of an obstructing CBD stone can be inferred by the finding of a dilated CBD. As endoscopic retrograde cholangiopancreatography (ERCP) has uncovered an increasing frequency of falsely negative ultrasonographic findings, the upper limit of normal for the diameter of the CBD has declined from 10 mm to the currently accepted limit of 6 mm. Even so, inferring choledocholithiasis on the basis of a dilated CBD by ultrasonography has a sensitivity of only 75%.

Finally, ultrasonography has substantial utility in the diagnosis of acute cholecystitis.[150] Pericholecystic fluid, when seen in the absence of ascites, and thickening of the gallbladder wall to greater than 4 mm (in the absence of hypoalbuminemia) are nonspecific findings that are suggestive of acute cholecystitis. Unfortunately, in the critical care setting, these nonspecific findings are frequently seen in patients who have no evidence of gallbladder disease.[150] A more specific finding is the so-called ultrasonographic Murphy's sign, in which the ultrasonographer elicits focal gallbladder tenderness under the transducer. Although somewhat operator dependent and requiring an alert patient, an ultrasono-

Table 55–4 | **Imaging Studies of the Biliary Tract**

TECHNIQUE	CONDITION TESTED FOR	FINDINGS/COMMENTS
Ultrasonography	Cholelithiasis	Stones that appear as mobile, dependent echogenic foci in gallbladder lumen with acoustic shadowing Sludge that appears as layering echogenic material without shadows Sensitivity >95% for stones >2 mm Specificity >95% for stones with acoustic shadows Rarely stone-filled gallbladder contracted and difficult to see with "wall-echo-shadow" sign Best single test for stones in gallbladder
	Choledocholithiasis	Stones in CBD only seen sonographically in ≈50% of cases; can be inferred by finding of dilated CBD (>6 mm diameter) in ≈75%; ultrasonography able to confirm but not exclude CBD stones
	Acute cholecystitis	Sonographic Murphy's sign (focal gallbladder tenderness under the transducer) has positive predictive value >90% for detecting acute cholecystitis when stones seen Pericholecystic fluid (in absence of ascites) and gallbladder wall thickening to >4 mm (in absence of hypoalbuminemia) nonspecific findings that suggest acute cholecystitis
EUS	Choledocholithiasis	Highly accurate for excluding or confirming stones in CBD Sensitivity of 93%, specificity of 97% Concordance of EUS and ERCP diagnoses of 95% EUS (vs. ERCP) used by experienced operators in excluding CBD stones
OCG	Cholelithiasis	Stones that appear as mobile filling defects in opacified gallbladder Sensitivity and specificity >90% when gallbladder opacified; nonvisualization in 25% of tests that may be due to many causes other than stones Opacification of gallbladder that demonstrates patency of cystic duct (prerequisite for medical dissolution therapy or lithotripsy) Potential use in evaluation of acalculous gallbladder diseases (e.g., cholesterolosis, adenomyomatosis) (see Chap. 58)
Cholescintigraphy (hepatobiliary scintigraphy, HIDA, DISIDA scans)	Acute cholecystitis	Assessment of cystic duct patency On normal scan radioactivity in gallbladder, CBD, and small bowel in 30–60 min Positive scan defined as nonvisualization of gallbladder with preserved excretion into CBD or small bowel Sensitivity ≈95%, specificity ≈90%, with false-positive results in fasting, critically ill patients With CCK stimulation, gallbladder "ejection fraction" determined and may help evaluate patients with acalculous biliary pain (see Chap. 58) *Normal scan result virtually excludes acute cholecystitis*
ERCP	Cholelithiasis	With contrast medium flow retrograde into gallbladder, stones that appear as filling defects detectable with sensitivity of ≈80%; ultrasonography mainstay to confirm cholelithiasis
	Choledocholithiasis	ERCP gold standard test for stones in CBD, with sensitivity and specificity rates ≈95% Ability to extract stones (or drain infected bile) lifesaving in severe cholangitis, reducing need for CBD exploration
CT/MRI	Complications	Not well suited for detecting uncomplicated stones; standard CT excellent test for detecting complications (e.g., abscess formation, gallbladder perforation, or CBD stone) or pancreatitis Spiral CT and MR cholangiography potentially useful as noninvasive means of excluding CBD stones

CBD, common bile duct; CCK, cholecystokinin; CT, computed tomography; DISIDA, diisopropyl iminodiacetic acid; ERCP, endoscopic retrograde cholangiopancreatography; EUS, endoscopic ultrasonography; HIDA, hydroxy iminodiacetic acid; MRI, magnetic resonance imaging; OCG, oral cholecystography.

graphic Murphy's sign has a positive predictive value greater than 90% for detecting acute cholecystitis if gallstones are present.[151]

In addition to providing accurate anatomic localization of biliary tract abnormalities, ultrasonography can localize other sites of abdominal abnormalities such as abscesses or pseudocysts that may be in the differential diagnosis.

Endoscopic Ultrasonography

Inherently more invasive and expensive than standard ultrasonography, endoscopic ultrasonography (EUS) has the advantage of being able to visualize the CBD and thus confirm or exclude the presence of choledocholithiasis with a high degree of accuracy. In preliminary studies, EUS findings had a positive predictive value of 98% and a negative predictive value of 88% for the diagnosis of CBD stones, when ERCP was used as the gold standard for diagnosis.[152, 153] Of course, if CBD stones are found on EUS, the next step ordinarily is endoscopic removal of the stones, so it could be argued that ERCP should be the initial study if choledocholithiasis is strongly suspected. Nonetheless, a 1998 study[154] in which EUS and ERCP were compared directly found that both techniques are accurate means of confirming or excluding choledocholithiasis but that EUS is safer and less expensive.

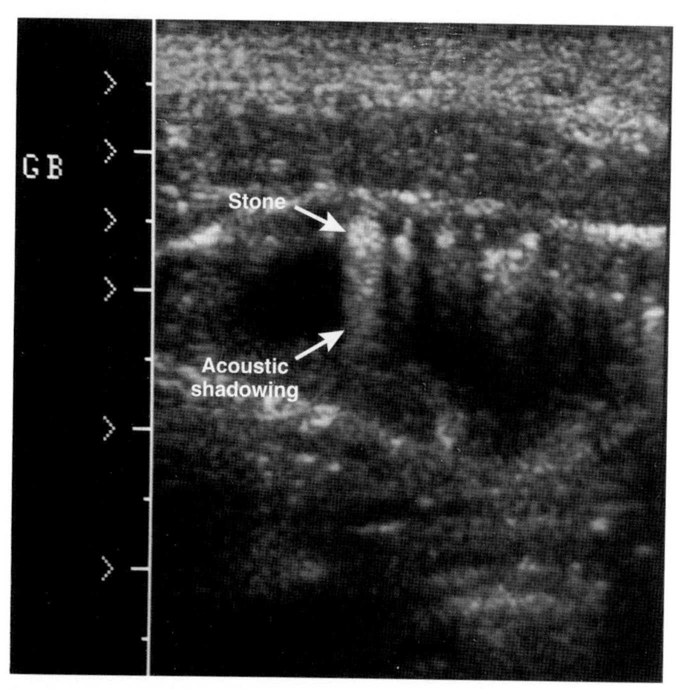

Figure 55–4. Typical ultrasonographic appearance of cholelithiasis showing multiple gallstones within the lumen of the gallbladder casting an acoustic shadow. With repositioning of the patient, the stones will move, thereby excluding the possibility of gallbladder polyps.

Therefore, EUS is an appropriate method of excluding CBD stones, especially if the pretest probability of finding stones is low.

Oral Cholecystography

Once the mainstay of imaging of the gallbladder, oral cholecystography (OCG) now has more limited application as a secondary means of identifying stones in the gallbladder.[147] The ease, reliability, and rapidity with which stones can be detected by ultrasonography as well as the lack of ionizing radiation have made ultrasonography the imaging study of choice. There are, however, unusual cases in which the gallbladder cannot be identified ultrasonographically (as in a contracted gallbladder full of stones)[155] and in which an OCG is able to demonstrate cholelithiasis. Additionally, when medical dissolution of stones or lithotripsy is under consideration,[156] it is useful to know whether the cystic duct is obstructed, and visualization of the gallbladder by OCG excludes cystic duct obstruction. Because complete OCG requires up to 48 hours, OCG has little usefulness in patients suspected of having acute cholecystitis or other complications of gallstone disease. On occasion, an OCG may diagnose unsuspected disease of the gallbladder such as adenomyomatosis or cholesterolosis of the gallbladder (see Chapter 58).

Cholescintigraphy (Hepatobiliary Scintigraphy)

Cholescintigraphy is a radionuclide based imaging test of the gallbladder and biliary tract that has its greatest utility in the evaluation of patients suspected of having acute cholecystitis.[157] By demonstrating patency of the cystic duct, cholescintigraphy can rapidly (within 90 minutes) exclude acute cholecystitis from the differential diagnosis in a patient exhibiting abdominal pain.

The test can be performed on an emergency basis in a nonfasting patient after the intravenous administration of a gamma emitting ^{99}Tc-labeled iminodiacetic acid derivative (e.g., hydroxy iminodiacetic acid [HIDA], diisopropyl iminodiacetic acid [DISIDA]) that is rapidly taken up by the liver and excreted into the bile. As shown in Figure 55–5, serial scans after injection should normally show radioactivity in the gallbladder, CBD, and small bowel within 30 to 60 minutes.[158] Historically, the ability to image jaundiced patients with this technique has been limited; however, use of DISIDA may allow imaging of the biliary tree in patients who have a serum bilirubin level as high as 20 mg/dL.

An abnormal or positive scan result is defined as nonvisualization of the gallbladder with preserved excretion into the CBD or small bowel. The sensitivity of the test is approximately 95% and the specificity approximately 90%; false-positive results are seen primarily in fasting or critically ill patients. Although nonvisualization of the gallbladder due to cystic duct obstruction is the hallmark of acute cholecystitis, pericholecystic hepatic uptake has been shown to be a useful secondary sign of acute cholecystitis.[159]

In some patients (e.g., those with chronic cholecystitis, liver disease, or choledocholithiasis) delayed imaging of the gallbladder may be seen after several hours, and scanning

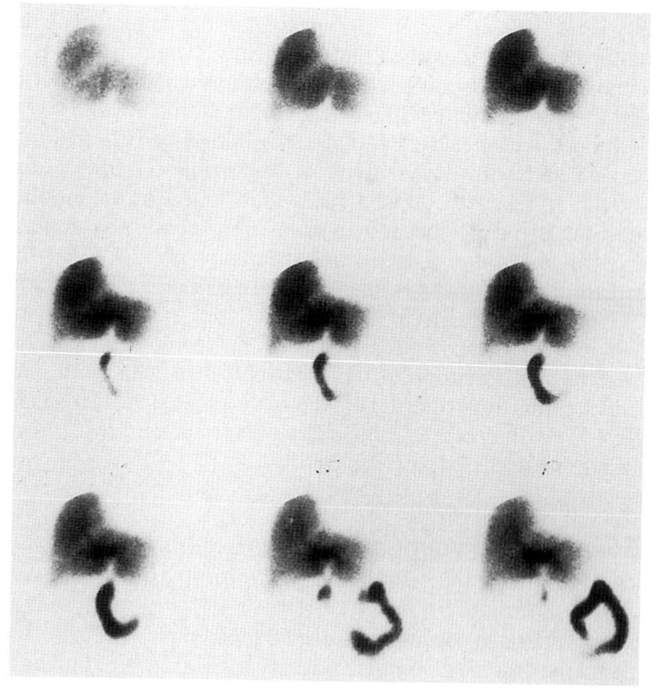
Figure 55–5. Cholescintigraphy demonstrating an obstructed cystic duct characteristic of acute cholecystitis. The gamma-emitting radioisotope DISIDA is injected intravenously and rapidly taken up by the liver and excreted into bile. Sequential images show the isotope quickly entering the duodenum and passing distally in the small intestine without ever being concentrated in the gallbladder. The failure of the gallbladder to visualize as a hot spot indicates a positive scan and implies obstruction of the cystic duct.

may have to be repeated at 4 or more hours. This delay in diagnosis creates problems in the acutely ill patient but has largely been overcome by the use of intravenous morphine sulfate in patients in whom the gallbladder does not visualize within 60 minutes. Morphine increases pressure within the sphincter of Oddi, thereby leading bile to flow preferentially into the gallbladder unless the cystic duct is obstructed. An additional scan is taken 30 minutes after injection of morphine, and if the gallbladder visualizes, cystic duct obstruction, and hence acute cholecystitis, is excluded. The gallbladder still may not visualize in critically ill patients even after morphine injection, leading to false-positive cholescintigraphy results in approximately one half of these patients.

Although primarily a tool for evaluating acutely ill patients with suspected acute cholecystitis, cholescintigraphy also may be useful in identifying patients with chronic acalculous biliary pain who are likely to benefit from empirical cholecystectomy.[160] Acalculous biliary pain and the use of CCK stimulated cholescintigraphy are discussed in Chapter 58.

Endoscopic Retrograde Cholangiopancreatography

Just as ultrasonography is the gold standard for the diagnosis of cholelithiasis, ERCP has now become the gold standard for the diagnosis of choledocholithiasis.[161] The technique of ERCP is discussed in more detail in Chapter 61. Briefly, the patient is placed in the prone position on a fluoroscopy table; while the patient is sedated, a side viewing endoscope is passed into the second portion of the duodenum, and the major papilla is identified and selectively cannulated. Water-soluble iodinated contrast material is injected into the CBD and the pancreatic duct, and radiographs are obtained.

Stones within the CBD appear as filling defects and can be detected with a sensitivity of approximately 95%. Care should be taken to prevent inadvertent injection of air into the biliary tract,[162] because bubbles may mimic the appearance of gallstones. The overall specificity of ERCP for the detecting CBD stones is approximately 95%.

Not only has ERCP become the gold standard for the diagnosis of CBD stones, but also its therapeutic applications have revolutionized the treatment of patients with choledocholithiasis[163] and those who have other bile duct disorders. The endoscopic and radiologic treatment of biliary disease is discussed in Chapter 61.

Computed Tomographic Cholangiography and Magnetic Resonance Cholangiography

Both computed tomographic cholangiography (CTC) and magnetic resonance cholangiography (MRC) are powerful imaging techniques for evaluating patients with intra-abdominal abnormalities. With respect to the biliary tract, however, their main utility to date has been not in diagnosing cholelithiasis or choledocholithiasis (which can be readily diagnosed by ultrasonography or ERCP, respectively), but rather in detecting complications of gallstones such as pericholecystic fluid in acute cholecystitis, gas in the gallbladder wall in emphysematous cholecystitis, perforation of the gallbladder, and abscess formation. As such, these studies have been useful in determining which patients need urgent surgical intervention and which patients can be treated supportively and have elective surgery at a later time.

With the advent of laparoscopic cholecystectomy, there has been an increasing need for an easy, quick, and preferably noninvasive means of excluding CBD stones. Studies in 1998 and 1999 showed that through the use of improved scanners and sophisticated computer processing of raw CT[164] or MRI[165, 166] data, a three-dimensional image of the CBD can be constructed with a high sensitivity for the detection of CBD stones. In most of these studies, patients also had ERCP (generally as the standard), and the correlation between the findings of MRC and ERCP was greater than 90%. Nonetheless, it is not yet clear that this new technology will supplant ERCP as the most sensitive means of excluding choledocholithiasis. CTC and MRC have the advantage of being noninvasive but obviously offer no therapeutic potential. Therefore, they may be most useful in excluding choledocholithiasis (either preoperatively or postoperatively) in patients thought to have a low probability of having stones in the CBD, and ERCP may be reserved for those with a higher probability of having CBD stones.

Biliary Colic and Chronic Cholecystitis

Biliary colic is the most common symptom of cholelithiasis.[135] Approximately 75% of symptomatic patients with gallstone disease seek medical attention as a result of episodic abdominal pain.[132] Even when patients have a complication of gallstones such as acute cholecystitis, a history of recurrent episodes of abdominal pain in the months preceding the complication often can be elicited.

Pathogenesis

The syndrome of biliary colic is caused by intermittent obstruction of the cystic duct by one or more gallstones. It is not necessary that inflammation of the gallbladder accompany the obstruction—only that symptoms be caused by it. The term *chronic cholecystitis* should be avoided, because it implies the presence of a chronic inflammatory infiltrate that may or may not be present in a given patient. Indeed, there is little correlation between the severity and frequency of colic and the pathologic changes in the gallbladder.[167]

The most common histologic changes observed are mild fibrosis of the gallbladder wall with a round cell infiltration and an intact mucosa. However, recurrent episodes of biliary colic may be associated with a scarred, shrunken gallbladder and Rokitansky-Aschoff sinuses (intramural diverticula). Bacteria can be cultured from gallbladder bile or gallstones themselves in approximately 10% of patients, but bacterial infection is not thought to contribute to the symptoms.

Clinical Manifestations

The pain of biliary colic is visceral in origin and therefore is poorly localized.[168] In a typical case, the patient experiences episodes of upper abdominal pain, usually in the epigastrium or right upper quadrant but sometimes in other abdominal locations.[132] The pain may be precipitated by eating a meal, but more commonly there is no inciting event; pain may even begin during sleep. The onset of biliary colic is more frequent during periods of weight reduction and marked physical inactivity such as prolonged bed rest.

The pain of biliary colic is steady rather than intermittent as would be suggested by the word *colic*. The pain gradually increases over a period of 15 minutes to 1 hour and then remains at a plateau for 1 hour or more before slowly resolving. In one third of patients, the pain has a more sudden onset and on rare occasions may cease abruptly. Pain lasting more than 6 hours suggests acute cholecystitis rather than simple biliary colic.

In order of decreasing frequency, the pain is felt maximally in the epigastrium, right upper quadrant, left upper quadrant, and various parts of the precordium or lower abdomen. It is therefore incorrect to consider pain that is located in an area other than the right upper quadrant as atypical of gallstone disease. Radiation of the pain to the scapula, right shoulder, or lower abdomen occurs in one half of patients. Diaphoresis and nausea with some vomiting are common; however, the emesis is less protracted than in intestinal obstruction or acute pancreatitis. As with other kinds of visceral pain, the patient with biliary colic is usually restless and active during an attack.[132]

Physical examination findings are usually normal with only mild to moderate gallbladder tenderness during an attack and perhaps mild residual tenderness that lasts several days after an attack.

It should be emphasized that symptoms of gas, bloating, flatulence, and dyspepsia, although frequent in patients with gallstones, are probably not related to the stones themselves, but rather are nonspecific symptoms that occur with similar frequency in people without gallstones. Accordingly, patients with gallstones whose only clinical manifestations are dyspepsia and other nonspecific upper gastrointestinal tract symptoms are not appropriate candidates for cholecystectomy.[132]

The natural history of biliary colic is cause for concern but not alarm. Approximately 30% of patients who have an initial attack of classic biliary colic experience no additional attacks over the next 24 months. Thus, a reasonable approach would be to offer cholecystectomy to those with recurring episodes of biliary colic.[169] In the 70% with recurring attacks, the frequency of recurrent attacks varies, but the pattern remains relatively similar over time for an individual patient. In patients with an initial attack of biliary colic, symptoms sufficient to warrant cholecystectomy develop at a rate of approximately 6% per year on average.[169] Fortunately, the probability that a severe complication requiring urgent surgical intervention will develop in these patients is only approximately 1% per year.

Diagnosis

In a patient with uncomplicated biliary colic, results of laboratory studies are usually completely normal. Elevations of serum bilirubin, alkaline phosphatase, or amylase levels suggest coexisting choledocholithiasis.

In general, the first (and in most cases only) imaging study to be performed on patients with biliary colic is an ultrasonographic examination of the right upper quadrant. As outlined in Table 55–4, ultrasonography is a rapid, noninvasive, highly sensitive, and highly specific means of establishing the presence or absence of stones in the gallbladder. Despite the impressive diagnostic accuracy of ultrasonography, because of the large number of patients suspected of having gallstone disease, a clinically important stone is occasionally overlooked, and the correct diagnosis is delayed.[170] In light of the relatively benign natural history of biliary colic, it is probably safe to follow patients who have negative ultrasonographic results and proceed to other diagnostic modalities if symptoms recur.[171]

OCG is generally viewed as a secondary imaging study of the gallbladder. It is reserved for patients in whom medical dissolution therapy or lithotripsy of the gallstones is planned. In such cases, it is essential to establish that the cystic duct is patent before therapy, and OCG can be used for this purpose. On rare occasions, OCG may demonstrate a layer of small floating gallstones that were missed by ultrasonography.

Long before the advent of ultrasonography and even OCG, examination of aspirated duodenal bile for the presence of cholesterol or calcium bilirubinate crystals was an established means of inferring the presence of macroscopic stones in the gallbladder. Although supplanted by modern imaging tests, the Meltzer-Lyon test now has had a modest resurgence in popularity because of the ease with which bile can be obtained at the time of upper endoscopy or ERCP. The Meltzer-Lyon test is described in more detail in Chapter 58. Briefly, gallbladder bile is aspirated from the duodenum (or CBD during ERCP) after stimulation of the gallbladder with an intravenous injection of CCK. Detection of either cholesterol crystals or calcium bilirubinate crystals on microscopic examination of the bile is highly suggestive of stones in the gallbladder.[57] The Meltzer-Lyon test is usually added to another diagnostic procedure such as an upper endoscopy or ERCP as a final effort to exclude microlithiasis as a cause of persistent symptoms in a patient who has normal ultrasonographic results.

Differential Diagnosis

The most common diseases to be considered in the differential diagnosis of a patient with recurrent, episodic upper abdominal symptoms are reflux esophagitis, peptic ulcer, pancreatitis, renal colic, colonic disorders such as diverticulitis and carcinoma, radiculopathy, and angina pectoris. Careful history taking is critical in sorting out the differential diagnosis of recurrent upper abdominal pain. For example, relief of pain with food, antacids, or antisecretory drugs suggests acid-peptic disease, whereas cramping pain suggests an intestinal disorder. Renal stones usually are associated with typical findings on urinalysis, and the pain of angina pectoris usually is precipitated by exercise and does not last for hours.

The irritable bowel syndrome, like biliary colic, is common in young women, but abdominal pain in this disorder has a distinct relationship with bowel movements (see Chapter 5). Finally, shingles or a radiculopathy from osteoarthritis may produce symptoms that resemble biliary colic.

Treatment

The treatment of recurrent, uncomplicated biliary colic in a patient with documented gallstones is generally an elective laparoscopic cholecystectomy and is discussed in Chapter 56.

Acute Cholecystitis

Acute cholecystitis is considered the most frequent complication of gallstone disease. Inflammation of the gallbladder wall that is associated with a clinical picture of abdominal pain, right upper quadrant tenderness, fever, and leukocytosis is the hallmark of acute cholecystitis. In approximately 90% of cases of acute cholecystitis, the underlying cause is a gallstone that obstructs the cystic duct.[172] In the remaining 10% of cases, cholecystitis occurs in the absence of gallstones and is termed *acute acalculous cholecystitis.* Whereas cholecystitis caused by gallstones frequently is seen in young, otherwise healthy women and has a generally favorable prognosis, acute acalculous cholecystitis is more common in critically ill elderly men and is associated with high morbidity and mortality rates. Acute acalculous cholecystitis is discussed in detail in Chapter 58.

Pathogenesis

Whereas biliary colic is caused by intermittent obstruction of the cystic duct by a gallstone, acute cholecystitis generally occurs when a stone becomes impacted in the cystic duct and causes chronic obstruction.[172] Stasis of bile within the gallbladder lumen results in damage of the gallbladder mucosa with consequent release of intracellular enzymes and activation of a cascade of inflammatory mediators.

Experimentally, if one ligates the cystic duct of an animal, the usual result is gradual absorption of the gallbladder contents without the development of inflammation.[173] In animals, installation of a luminal irritant, such as concentrated bile or lysolecithin, or trauma from an indwelling catheter is required to trigger acute cholecystitis in an obstructed gallbladder.

Lecithin, a normal constituent of bile, is converted to lysolecithin by phospholipase A, an enzyme present in gallbladder mucosa cells. There is evidence that phospholipase A may be released by gallstone-induced mucosal trauma, followed by conversion of lecithin to lysolecithin. Although normally absent from gallbladder bile, lysolecithin is present in the gallbladder contents of patients with acute cholecystitis.[174] In animal models, installation of lysolecithin into the gallbladder produces acute cholecystitis, with increased protein secretion, decreased water absorption, and white blood cell invasion associated with elevated production of prostaglandins E and $F_{1\alpha}$.[174] Administration of indomethacin, a cyclooxygenase inhibitor, has been shown to block this inflammatory response.

Studies of human tissue obtained at cholecystectomy have demonstrated enhanced prostaglandin production in the inflamed gallbladder. Additionally, intravenous indomethacin and oral ibuprofen decrease luminal pressure and the pain of acute cholecystitis in affected patients.[175]

Supporting evidence for the role of prostaglandins in the development of acute cholecystitis comes from a prospective study in which patients exhibiting biliary colic were given diclofenac, a prostaglandin synthetase inhibitor.[176] Whereas in 9 of 40 patients who received placebo acute cholecystitis developed, episodes of biliary colic resolved in all 20 patients who received the diclofenac. These data suggest a chain of events in which obstruction of the cystic duct in association with one or more intraluminal factors damages the gallbladder mucosa and stimulates prostaglandin synthetase. The resulting fluid secretion and inflammatory changes promote a cycle of further mucosal damage and inflammation.[176]

Enteric bacteria can be cultured from gallbladder bile in approximately one half of patients with acute cholecystitis, but[177] bacteria are not thought to contribute to the onset of acute cholecystitis. Generally, antibiotics are used in cases of suspected gallbladder perforation or gangrene or in a particularly toxic presentation of acute cholecystitis including fever greater than 102°F.

Pathology

If the gallbladder is examined in the initial days of an attack of acute cholecystitis, distention is usually noted, with impaction of a stone in the cystic duct.[178] On opening of the gallbladder, inflammatory exudate and, rarely, pus are present. Later in the attack, bile pigments that are normally present have been absorbed and replaced by thin mucoid fluid, pus, or blood. If the attack of acute cholecystitis is untreated for a long period and the cystic duct remains obstructed, the lumen of the gallbladder may become distended with clear mucoid fluid, so-called hydrops of the gallbladder.

Histologic changes range from mild acute inflammation with edema to necrosis and perforation of the gallbladder wall. There is surprisingly little correlation between the severity of histologic changes and the patient's symptoms.[178] When the gallbladder is resected for acute cholecystitis and no stones are found, the specimen should be carefully examined histologically for evidence of vasculitis or cholesterol emboli, because these systemic disorders may be manifested by acalculous cholecystitis.

Clinical Manifestations

As outlined in Table 55–3, three fourths of patients with acute cholecystitis report having had prior attacks of biliary colic.[179] Often the patient is alerted to the possibility that the attack is more severe than a simple recurrence of biliary colic by the duration of the pain. The pain of biliary colic usually lasts more than 1 hour but rarely more than 6 hours. If the pain has been constant for more than 6 hours, uncomplicated biliary colic is unlikely.

As inflammation in the gallbladder wall progresses, the poorly localized visceral pain gives way to moderately severe parietal pain that usually becomes localized to the right upper quadrant.[179] Less commonly, the back may be the site of maximal pain; rarely the chest is the site.

Nausea with some vomiting is characteristic of acute cholecystitis, but these symptoms almost invariably follow

Table 55–5 | **Uncommon Complications of Gallstone Disease**

COMPLICATION	PATHOGENESIS	CLINICAL MANIFESTATIONS	DIAGNOSIS/TREATMENT
Emphysematous cholecystitis	Secondary infection of gallbladder wall with gas-forming organisms (*Clostridium welchii, Escherichia coli,* anaerobic streptococci) More common in elderly and diabetic men; often occurs in absence of stones (see Chap. 58)	Similar symptoms and signs to acute cholecystitis but more toxic presentation	Plain abdominal series that may show gallbladder fossa gas Ultrasonography and CT sensitive for confirming gas Treatment with intravenous antibiotics including anaerobic coverage and early cholecystectomy Morbidity and mortality rates high
Cholecystoenteric fistula	Erosion of (usually large) stone through gallbladder wall into adjacent bowel, most often duodenum, and less often hepatic flexure, stomach, and jejunum	Similar symptoms and signs to acute cholecystitis; fistula potentially clinically silent Lingering symptoms that suggest persistence of gallbladder stones Stones >25 mm, especially in elderly women, that may produce bowel obstruction or "gallstone ileus"; terminal ileum most frequent site of obstruction	Plain abdominal series that may show biliary tree gas and SBO in gallstone ileus Contrast GI series that may demonstrate fistula Fistula from solitary stones that pass that may close spontaneously Cholecystectomy and bowel closure curative Gallstone ileus requiring emergency laparotomy; diagnosis often delayed; resulting mortality rate ≈20%
Mirizzi's syndrome	Impacted stone in gallbladder neck or cystic duct with extrinsic compression of CBD by accompanying inflammation	Jaundice and RUQ pain	ERCP that demonstrates extrinsic CBD compression Preoperative diagnosis important to guide surgical approach and minimize CBD injury risk
Porcelain gallbladder	Intramural calcification of gallbladder wall, usually associated with stones	No symptoms attributable to calcified wall, but gallbladder carcinoma late complication in ≈20% (see Chap. 60)	Plain abdominal series or CT that shows intramural gallbladder wall calcification Prophylactic cholecystectomy indicated to prevent carcinoma

CBD, common bile duct; CT, computed tomography; ERCP, endoscopic retrograde cholangiopancreatography; GI, gastrointestinal; RUQ, right upper quadrant; SBO, small bowel obstruction.

rather than precede the onset of pain. Emesis is less persistent or severe than in intestinal obstruction or acute pancreatitis.

In contrast to uncomplicated biliary colic, acute cholecystitis is in many cases suggested by the physical examination. Fever is common (because of active inflammation in the gallbladder mucosa) but is usually less than 102°F unless gangrene or perforation of the gallbladder has occurred. Mild jaundice is present in 20% of patients and 40% of elderly patients. The jaundice is often subtle, and serum bilirubin concentrations usually are less than 4 mg/dL.[180] Higher bilirubin levels suggest the possibility of CBD stones, which may be found in one half of patients who have acute cholecystitis and jaundice. Another cause of pronounced jaundice in acute cholecystitis is Mirizzi's syndrome, which is discussed later (Table 55–5).

The abdominal examination often reveals right subcostal tenderness, with a palpable gallbladder in one third of patients. A palpable gallbladder is more common in patients who are having a first attack of acute cholecystitis, because repeated attacks usually result in a scarred fibrotic gallbladder that is unable to distend. For unclear reasons, the gallbladder is usually palpable lateral to its normal anatomic location.

A relatively specific finding for acute cholecystitis is Murphy's sign.[179] During palpation in the right subcostal region, pain and inspiratory arrest may occur when the patient takes a deep breath that moves the inflamed gallbladder into contact with the examiner's hand. A positive Murphy's sign in the appropriate clinical setting is a reliable predictor of acute cholecystitis, although confirmation of gallstones by ultrasonography is still warranted.

In some cases, symptoms of acute cholecystitis are nonspecific, with only a mild ache and anorexia; some patients may have toxic manifestations, including fever, severe right upper quadrant pain, guarding, and localized rebound tenderness.

The natural history of untreated acute cholecystitis is characterized by resolution of the pain in 7 to 10 days.[181] It is not uncommon for symptoms to remit within 48 hours of hospitalization. Left untreated, approximately 10% of cases are complicated by localized perforation and 1% by free perforation and peritonitis.

Diagnosis

Perhaps because acute cholecystitis is so common, the diagnosis is often at the top of the differential diagnosis of acute abdominal pain, and the condition is actually overdiagnosed on the basis of clinical criteria alone. In a prospective series of 100 patients who had right upper quadrant pain and tenderness and suspected acute cholecystitis, this diagnosis proved to be correct in only two thirds of cases. The clinician must therefore use laboratory and imaging studies to confirm the presence of acute cholecystitis, exclude complications such as gangrene or perforation, and look for alternative causes of the clinical findings.

Table 55–3 details the most common laboratory findings in acute cholecystitis.[181] Leukocytosis with a left shift is common. Because CBD stones with cholangitis are usually in the differential diagnosis, attention often is directed to liver biochemical testing.[180] Even without detectable CBD obstruction, acute cholecystitis often causes mild elevations in the serum aminotransaminase and alkaline phosphatase levels. The serum bilirubin concentration also may be mildly elevated in the range of 2 to 4 mg/dL, and even serum amylase and lipase levels may be elevated nonspecifically. A serum bilirubin level greater than 4 mg/dL or an amylase level greater than 1000 U/dL usually indicates coexisting CBD obstruction or acute pancreatitis and warrants further evaluation.

When the degree of leukocytosis exceeds 15,000 cells/mm^3, particularly in the setting of worsening pain, high fever (greater than 102°F), and chills, suppurative cholecystitis (empyema of the gallbladder) or perforation should be suspected, and urgent surgical intervention may be required. Advanced gallbladder disease may be present even if the local and systemic clinical manifestations are unimpressive.

Ultrasonography is the single most useful imaging study in acutely ill patients who have right upper quadrant pain and tenderness. Not only can it accurately establish the presence or absence of gallstones, but as discussed previously and indicated in Table 55–4, ultrasonography is also a highly specific extension of the physical examination. An ultrasonographic Murphy's sign is defined as focal gallbladder tenderness under the transducer, and with a skillful operator and an alert patient, the positive predictive value of an ultrasonographic Murphy's sign is greater than 90% in detecting acute cholecystitis if gallstones are also present.[151]

Additionally, ultrasonography can detect nonspecific findings of acute cholecystitis, such as pericholecystic fluid and thickening of the gallbladder wall to more than 4 mm. Both findings lose specificity for acute cholecystitis if ascites or hypoalbuminemia (less than 3.2 g/dL) is present.[151]

Because gallstones are prevalent in the background population, many patients who have nonbiliary tract diseases that exhibit acute abdominal pain (such as acute pancreatitis or complications of peptic ulcer disease) may have incidental and clinically irrelevant gallstones. The greatest utility of cholescintigraphy in these patients is to exclude acute cholecystitis and allow the clinician to focus on nonbiliary causes of acute abdominal pain.[147] As outlined in Table 55–4, a normal cholescintigraphy scan result shows radioactivity in the gallbladder, CBD, and small bowel within 30 to 60 minutes of injection of the isotope. With only rare exceptions, a normal scintigraphic finding excludes acute cholecystitis caused by gallstones, because virtually all patients who have acute calculous cholecystitis have a gallstone obstructing the cystic duct at the time of the attack. If a positive scan result is defined as the absence of isotope in the gallbladder, then a falsely negative scan result indicates that the gallbladder fills with dye in the setting of acute cholecystitis, a situation that almost never occurs. In contrast, false-positive scan results, defined as the absence of isotope in the gallbladder in patients who do not have acute cholecystitis, occur regularly, especially in fasting or critically ill patients who are receiving TPN. Thus, scintigraphy should not be used as the initial imaging study for suspected cholecystitis but rather should be used as a secondary imaging study in patients known to have gallstones whose clinical features suggest the possibility of a nonbiliary cause of acute abdominal pain.[158]

To reduce the frequency of falsely positive cholescintigraphy scan results, augmentation with morphine is often performed if the gallbladder has not visualized after 60 minutes. Morphine increases pressure within the sphincter of Oddi, thereby directing bile into the gallbladder unless the cystic duct is obstructed. Additional scans obtained 30 minutes after morphine is injected occasionally cause the gallbladder to fill with isotope, thereby excluding cystic duct obstruction. Unfortunately, despite use of morphine augmentation, cholescintigraphy continues to have a 60% rate of false-positive results in critically ill patients.

In summary, cholescintigraphy is a secondary imaging test used to determine whether the cystic duct is obstructed. The test can exclude acute cholecystitis caused by gallstones but cannot confirm the diagnosis.[158]

With respect to acute cholecystitis, abdominal CT is most useful not in confirming the presence of acute cholecystitis but in detecting complications such as emphysematous cholecystitis or perforation of the gallbladder and in excluding other intra-abdominal abnormalities that may have a similar clinical picture. For example, abdominal CT is highly sensitive for detecting pneumoperitoneum, acute pancreatitis, pancreatic pseudocyst, hepatic or intra-abdominal abscesses, appendicitis, or obstruction or perforation of a hollow viscus. In a straightforward case of acute cholecystitis, an abdominal CT scan usually is not warranted; however, if the diagnosis is less certain or the optimal timing of surgery is in doubt, CT may be invaluable.

Differential Diagnosis

Because acute cholecystitis is common, even an inexperienced diagnostician often makes a correct diagnosis in cases of right upper quadrant pain, fever, and leukocytosis. However, a lengthy list of other conditions may exhibit similar clinical features. The principal conditions to consider in the differential diagnosis are appendicitis, acute pancreatitis, pyelonephritis or renal stone, peptic ulcer disease, acute hepatitis, pneumonia, hepatic abscess or tumor, and gonococcal perihepatitis. An astute clinician should consider all of these possibilities before recommending a cholecystectomy.

Acute appendicitis is the disease most often confused with acute cholecystitis because the initial diagnostic impression is based largely on right abdominal tenderness, which may be localized lower than expected in cholecystitis or higher than expected in appendicitis. In general, fever, leukocytosis, and tenderness progress more inexorably in appendicitis. Complete abdominal ultrasonography can usually distinguish these two entities.

Acute pancreatitis also may be difficult to distinguish from acute cholecystitis on the basis of the history and physical examination alone. Generally, vomiting is more prominent in acute pancreatitis, and hyperamylasemia is more profound.

Diseases of the right kidney may produce pain and tenderness similar to that of acute cholecystitis, but the urinalysis and ultrasound usually distinguish the two. Whereas the pain of uncomplicated peptic ulcer disease is usually chronic in nature and seldom confused with the pain of acute cholecystitis, a perforated ulcer may, at least initially, mimic severe acute cholecystitis. Signs of generalized peritonitis or a pneumoperitoneum strongly suggest a perforated viscus or at least the need for an emergency laparotomy.

Pneumonia with pleurisy may cause abdominal pain and tenderness, but the pleuritic nature of the pain and the chest radiographic result should be helpful in diagnoses.

In some instances, acute hepatitis, especially when caused by alcohol, may be accompanied by rather severe right upper quadrant pain and tenderness. Fever and leukocytosis add to diagnostic confusion with acute cholecystitis. In such cases, careful assessment of liver biochemical test results over time and ultrasonographic or cholescintigraphic findings may serve to exclude acute cholecystitis. Rarely, a liver biopsy may be warranted.

Gonococcal perihepatitis (Fitz-Hugh–Curtis syndrome) produces right upper quadrant pain, tenderness, and leukocytosis, which often overshadow any pelvic complaints. Nevertheless, adnexal tenderness is present on physical examination, and Gram stain of the cervical smear should show gonococci.

Hepatic abscesses and tumors usually can be differentiated from acute cholecystitis on the basis of ultrasonographic findings. Previously undiagnosed gallbladder perforation may be accompanied by fever caused by a subhepatic abscess. Finally, pseudolithiasis as a result of treatment with ceftriaxone may cause symptoms resembling those of acute cholecystitis, although the gallbladder is histologically normal.

Treatment

The patient suspected of having acute cholecystitis should be hospitalized for evaluation and treatment. Volume contraction caused by vomiting and poor oral intake is frequent, and fluids and electrolytes should be repleted intravenously. Oral feeding should be withheld and a nasogastric tube inserted if the patient's abdomen is distended or if there is persistent vomiting.

In uncomplicated cases, antibiotics may be withheld. Antibiotics are warranted if the patient's condition appears toxic or if a complication such as perforation of the gallbladder or emphysematous cholecystitis is suspected. Antibiotics that cover gram-negative enteric bacteria are effective. Coverage with a single agent such as cefoxitin is appropriate for mild cases, whereas more severely ill patients should receive broader coverage with a combination of ampicillin and an aminoglycoside or a third-generation cephalosporin and metronidazole.

Definitive therapy for acute cholecystitis is cholecystectomy, and the safety and effectiveness of a laparoscopic approach have been established.[182] Surgical management of gallstone disease and postoperative complications are discussed Chapter 56.

Choledocholithiasis

Choledocholithiasis is defined as the occurrence of stones in the CBD. As do stones in the gallbladder, choledocholithiasis by itself may remain asymptomatic for years, and the clinically silent passage of stones from the CBD into the duodenum is known to occur, perhaps frequently. Unlike stones in the gallbladder, which usually are manifested by relatively benign episodes of recurrent biliary colic, stones in the CBD, when they do cause symptoms, may lead to life-threatening complications such as cholangitis or acute pancreatitis (see Chapter 48). Thus, demonstration of choledocholithiasis generally warrants intervention to remove the stones, whereas the incidental finding of cholelithiasis can be followed expectantly.

Etiology

Gallstones may pass from the gallbladder into the CBD or form de novo in the duct. Generally, all gallstones in one patient, whether from the gallbladder or CBD, are of the same type, either cholesterol or pigment. Cholesterol stones form only in the gallbladder; cholesterol stones found in the CBD must have migrated there from the gallbladder. Likewise, black pigment stones, which are seen with old age, hemolysis, alcoholism, and cirrhosis, also form only in the gallbladder and only rarely migrate into the CBD. Most pigment stones in the CBD are the softer, so-called brown pigment stones that form de novo in the CBD as a result of bacterial action on the phospholipid and bilirubin in bile.[183] They often are found proximal to biliary strictures and frequently are associated with cholangitis. Brown pigment stones also are associated with recurrent pyogenic cholangitis[184] (oriental cholangiohepatitis) (see Chapter 59).

Fifteen percent of patients who have gallbladder stones also have stones in the CBD. Conversely, of patients who have ductal stones, 95% also have gallbladder stones.[185] In patients who have choledocholithiasis months or years after a cholecystectomy, it may be impossible to determine whether the stones were overlooked at the earlier operation or have formed since then. Obviously, if the chemical composition of the CBD stones is determined, it can be surmised that cholesterol or black pigment stones were left behind after the original operation, whereas brown pigment stones presumably could have formed de novo in the interval after cholecystectomy.[185]

Stones in the CBD usually come to rest at the lower end of the ampulla of Vater. Obstruction of the CBD increases bile pressure proximally and causes the ducts to dilate. Normal pressure in the duct is 10 to 15 cm H_2O and rises to 25 to 40 cm H_2O with complete obstruction. When pressure exceeds 15 cm H_2O, bile flow decreases, and at 30 cm H_2O it stops.

The bile duct dilates to the point that it can be detected by either ultrasonography or abdominal CT in approximately 75% of cases. In patients who have had recurrent episodes of cholangitis, the bile duct may become fibrotic and thus unable to dilate. Moreover, dilatation is sometimes absent in choledocholithiasis because obstruction is low-grade and intermittent.

An iatrogenic form of choledocholithiasis is emerging as a late complication of endoscopic sphincterotomy.[183] In a study of the long-term consequences of endoscopic sphincterotomy in more than 400 patients, the cumulative frequency of recurrent CBD stones was 12%. Interestingly, all of the recurrent stones were of the pigment type (bilirubinate), irrespective of the chemical composition of the original gallstones. The findings suggest that sphincterotomy may permit chronic bacterial colonization of the CBD with resulting deconjugation of bilirubin and precipitation of pigment stones.

Clinical Manifestations

Little information is available on the natural history of asymptomatic CBD stones. Although it is clear that in many patients such stones remain asymptomatic for months or years, the available evidence suggests that the natural history of asymptomatic CBD is less benign than that of asymptomatic gallstones.[186]

The morbidity of choledocholithiasis stems principally from biliary obstruction, which increases biliary pressure and diminishes bile flow. The rate of onset of obstruction, its degree, and the amount of bacterial contamination of the bile are the major factors that determine the resulting symptoms. Thus, acute obstruction usually causes biliary colic and jaundice, whereas obstruction that develops gradually over several months may present initially as pruritus or jaundice alone.[186] If bacteria proliferate, life-threatening cholangitis (discussed later) may result.

The physical examination is usually normal if obstruction of the CBD is intermittent. Mild to moderate jaundice may be seen when obstruction has been present for several days to a few weeks. Deep jaundice, particularly with a palpable gallbladder, suggests neoplastic obstruction of the CBD even when the patient has stones in the gallbladder. With longstanding obstruction, secondary biliary cirrhosis may result and lead to physical findings associated with chronic liver disease.

As shown in Table 55–3, laboratory studies may provide the only suggestion that choledocholithiasis is present.[187] With bile duct obstruction, serum levels of both bilirubin and alkaline phosphatase increase. Bilirubin levels rise as a result of blocked excretion, whereas alkaline phosphatase levels rise as a result of increased synthesis of the enzyme by the canalicular epithelium. The rise in alkaline phosphatase level[188] is more rapid than and precedes the rise in bilirubin level. The absolute height of the bilirubin concentration is proportional to the degree of obstruction, whereas the height of the alkaline phosphatase level bears no relationship to either the degree of obstruction or its cause. In cases of choledocholithiasis, the bilirubin level typically is in the range of 2 to 5 mg/dL[186] and rarely exceeds 12 mg/dL. Transient spikes in serum aminotransferase or amylase levels suggest passage of a CBD stone into the duodenum.

Diagnosis

Ultrasonography actually visualizes CBD stones in only approximately 50% of cases,[148] whereas dilatation of the CBD to a diameter greater than 6 mm in is seen in approximately 75% of cases. Thus, ultrasonography can confirm or at least suggest the presence of CBD stones but cannot definitively exclude them.

EUS, although clearly more invasive than standard ultrasonography, has the advantage of visualizing the CBD better. In preliminary studies, EUS has been reported to exclude or confirm choledocholithiasis with sensitivity and specificity rates of approximately 95%.[149]

ERCP is the standard for the diagnosis of CBD stones,[189] with sensitivity and specificity rates of approximately 95%.

Percutaneous transhepatic cholangiography (PTC) is also an accurate means of confirming the presence of choledocholithiasis. PTC is most readily accomplished when the intrahepatic bile ducts are dilated and is now used primarily when ERCP is unavailable or unsuccessful.

Laparoscopic ultrasonography is a new imaging modality employed in the surgical suite immediately before mobilization of the gallbladder during cholecystectomy. Preliminary studies suggest that laparoscopic ultrasonography may be as accurate as operative cholangiography in detecting CBD stones and therefore obviate the need for the latter.[190]

Endoscopic and radiologic treatment of biliary disease is discussed in Chapter 61.

Differential Diagnosis

The symptoms caused by obstruction of the CBD cannot be distinguished from those caused by obstruction of the cystic duct. Thus, biliary colic is included in the differential diagnosis of choledocholithiasis. Of course, the presence of jaundice or abnormal liver biochemical test results strongly point to the bile duct rather than the gallbladder as the source of the problem.

In patients who have jaundice, malignant obstruction of the bile duct or obstruction from a choledochal cyst may be clinically indistinguishable from choledocholithiasis.

Acute passive congestion of the liver, associated with cardiac decompensation, may cause intense right upper quadrant pain, tenderness, and even jaundice with serum bilirubin levels as high as 10 mg/dL or more. In this condition, however, the temperature is normal, and the white blood cell count is normal or only slightly elevated. The patient typically has other obvious signs of cardiac decompensation. Constrictive pericarditis and cor pulmonale also may cause acute congestion of the liver with only subtle cardiac findings.

Acute viral hepatitis rarely may cause severe right upper quadrant pain with tenderness and fever. The white blood cell count, however, is usually not elevated, whereas serum aminotransferase levels are markedly elevated.

Acquired immunodeficiency syndrome (AIDS) cholangiopathy[191] and papillary stenosis must be considered in patients infected with human immunodeficiency virus who have right upper quadrant pain and abnormal liver biochemical test findings (see Chapter 28).

Treatment

Because of the propensity for serious complications such as cholangitis and acute pancreatitis, choledocholithiasis warrants treatment in almost all cases.[192] The optimal therapy for a given patient depends on the severity of symptoms, coexisting medical problems, and local expertise, as well as on whether the gallbladder is intact.

CBD stones that are discovered at the time of a laparoscopic cholecystectomy present a dilemma to the surgeon. The operation can be converted to an open cholecystectomy with a CBD exploration, but this approach results in a greater morbidity rate and a more prolonged hospital stay. Alternatively, the laparoscopic cholecystectomy can be carried out as planned, and the patient can return for endoscopic removal of the CBD stones by ERCP. Such an approach, if successful, cures the disease but entails the risk of necessitating a third procedure, namely, a CBD exploration if the ERCP is unsuccessful in removing the stones. In general, the greater the level of expertise of the therapeutic endoscopist, the more inclined the surgeon should be simply to complete the laparoscopic cholecystectomy and have the CBD stones removed endoscopically at a later date.[192]

In especially high-risk patients, endoscopic removal of CBD stones may be performed without cholecystectomy. This approach is particularly appropriate for elderly patients who have other severe illnesses.[193] Studies indicate that subsequent cholecystectomy for symptoms of cholelithiasis is required in only 10% of patients treated in this manner.

The surgical and endoscopic management of gallstones is a complex topic that is discussed in detail in Chapters 56 and 61.

Cholangitis (Bacterial Cholangitis)

Of all the complications of gallstones, cholangitis kills most swiftly. Pus under pressure in the bile ducts leads to rapid spread of bacteria, via the liver, into the blood, and resulting septicemia. Moreover, the diagnosis of cholangitis is often problematic (especially in the critical early phase of the disease) because clinical features pointing to the biliary tract as the source of sepsis are absent.[194] Table 55–3 delineates the symptoms, signs, and laboratory findings that can aid in an early diagnosis of cholangitis.

Etiology and Pathophysiology

In approximately 85% of cases, cholangitis is caused by an impacted stone in the CBD that causes bile stasis.[194] Other causes of bile duct obstruction that may result in cholangitis include neoplasms (see Chapter 60), biliary strictures (see Chapter 61), parasitic infections (see Chapter 59), and congenital abnormalities of the bile ducts (see Chapter 52). The discussion that follows deals specifically with cholangitis caused by gallstones in the CBD.

Bile duct obstruction is necessary, but not sufficient, to cause cholangitis. Cholangitis is relatively common in patients with choledocholithiasis, nearly universal in patients who have post-traumatic bile duct stricture, but seen in only 15% of patients who have neoplastic obstruction. It is most likely to occur when a bile duct that already contains bacteria becomes obstructed, as occurs in most patients who have choledocholithiasis or a stricture but in few patients who have neoplastic obstruction. Because malignant obstruction is more often complete than obstruction caused by stricture or CBD stones, malignant obstruction is less likely to permit the reflux of bacteria from duodenal contents into the bile ducts.[194]

The bacterial species most commonly cultured are *Escherichia coli,* enterococci, and *Klebsiella, Pseudomonas,* and *Proteus* species. Anaerobic species such as *Bacteroides fragilis* or *Clostridium perfringens* are found in about 15% of appropriately cultured bile specimens. Anaerobes usually accompany aerobes, especially *E. coli.*

The shaking chills and fever of cholangitis are caused by bacteremia from bile duct organisms. The degree of regurgitation of bacteria from bile into hepatic venous blood is directly proportional to the biliary pressure and hence the degree of obstruction.[194] For this reason, decompression alone often treats the illness promptly and effectively.

Clinical Manifestations

As shown in Table 55–3, classic Charcot's triad of pain, jaundice, and fever is the hallmark of cholangitis. Unfortunately, the full triad is present in only 70% of cases.[194] The pain of cholangitis may be surprisingly mild and transient but is often accompanied by chills and rigors. Mental confusion, lethargy, and delirium may be the only features of the history obtainable, particularly in elderly patients.

On physical examination fever is nearly universal, occurring in 95% of cases. Right upper quadrant tenderness occurs in approximately 90% of patients, whereas jaundice is clinically detectable in only 80%. Peritoneal signs are found in only 15%. In severe cases, hypotension and mental confusion may coexist, indicating gram-negative septicemia. Overlooked cases of severe cholangitis may be accompanied by intrahepatic abscesses as a late complication.

Laboratory studies are often helpful in pointing to the biliary tract as the source of sepsis. In particular, the serum bilirubin level exceeds 2 mg/dL in 80% of cases. When the bilirubin level is initially normal, the diagnosis of cholangitis may be overlooked.[187] The white blood cell count is elevated in 80% of patients but normal in the remainder. However, in many patients who have a normal white blood cell count, examination of the peripheral blood smear reveals a dramatic shift to immature neutrophil forms. The serum alkaline phosphatase level is usually elevated, and the serum amylase level also may be elevated if pancreatitis is also present.

In most cases, blood culture results are positive for enteric organisms, especially if cultures are obtained during chills and fever spikes. The organism found in the blood is invariably the same as that found in the bile.

Diagnosis

The principles of radiologic diagnosis are the same as those for choledocholithiasis. As shown in Table 55–4, stones in the CBD are seen ultrasonographically in only approximately 50% of cases[148] but can be inferred by the finding of a dilated CBD in approximately 75%. Because of this lack of sensitivity, a normal ultrasonographic result does not exclude the possibility of choledocholithiasis in a patient whose clinical presentation suggests cholangitis.[194]

Similarly, abdominal CT is an excellent means of excluding complications of gallstones such as acute pancreatitis and abscess formation, but a standard abdominal CT scan is not capable of excluding CBD stones. CT or MRC, as noted earlier, may prove useful for excluding stones in the CBD.

ERCP is the standard test for the diagnosis of CBD stones. Moreover, the ability of ERCP to confirm the presence of CBD stones and establish drainage of infected bile under pressure can be life-saving. If ERCP is unsuccessful, PTC can be employed (see Chapter 61).

Treatment

In cases of suspected bacterial cholangitis, blood cultures should be obtained immediately and the patient started on antibiotics effective against the likely causative organisms discussed previously.[194] For mild cases, treatment can be initiated with a single drug, such as cefoxitin, 2.0 g intravenously every 6 to 8 hours. In severe cases, more intensive therapy (e.g., gentamicin, ampicillin, and metronidazole) is indicated.

Improvement should be expected within 6 to 12 hours, and in most cases the infection is controlled within 2 to 3 days, with defervescence, relief of discomfort, and a fall in the white blood cell count. In these cases definitive therapy can be planned on an elective basis. If, however, after 6 to 12 hours of observation, the patient's clinical status declines, with worsening fever, pain, mental confusion, or hypotension, then the CBD must be decompressed emergently.[194] If available, ERCP with stone extraction, or at least decompression of the bile duct, is the treatment of choice. Controlled studies in which ERCP with decompression of the bile duct was compared with emergency surgery and CBD exploration have shown dramatically lower morbidity and mortality rates in the patients treated endoscopically.[192]

Surgical and endoscopic management of patients with cholangitis is a complex topic,[192] which is discussed in detail in Chapters 56 and 61.

Uncommon Complications of Gallstone Disease

Table 55–5 delineates the clinical manifestations, diagnosis, and treatment of several uncommon complications of gallstone disease.

Emphysematous Cholecystitis

Patients who have emphysematous cholecystitis present with the same clinical manifestations as do patients with uncomplicated acute cholecystitis, but in emphysematous cholecystitis gas forming organisms have secondarily infected the gallbladder wall and pockets of gas are evident in the area of the gallbladder fossa on ultrasonography, plain abdominal films, or abdominal CT scan.[195] Emergency administration of antibiotics with anaerobic coverage and early cholecystectomy are warranted because the risk of perforation is high. Emphysematous cholecystitis often occurs in diabetics or older men who do not have gallstones, in whom atherosclerosis of the cystic artery with resulting ischemia may be the initiating event. Acalculous cholecystitis is discussed in Chapter 58.

Cholecystoenteric Fistula

Cholecystoenteric fistula occurs when a stone erodes through the gallbladder wall (usually the neck) and into a hollow viscus. The most common entry point into the bowel is the duodenum, followed by the hepatic flexure of the colon, stomach, and jejunum. Symptoms are initially similar to those of acute cholecystitis, although at times, the stone may pass into the bowel and be excreted without causing any symptoms.[196] Because the biliary tract is decompressed, the frequency of cholangitis is not high despite gross seeding of the gallbladder and bile ducts with bacteria. The diagnosis is suggested by radiographic evidence of pneumobilia and may be confirmed by barium contrast studies of the upper or lower GI tract, although the precise anatomic location of the fistula often is not identified until surgery.

If the gallstone exceeds 25 mm in diameter, especially in elderly women, it may cause a small bowel obstruction (gallstone ileus).[197] The ileocecal area is the most common site of obstruction. In such cases, a plain abdominal film may show the pathognomonic features of pneumobilia, dilated small bowel, and a large gallstone in the right lower quadrant. Unfortunately, the diagnosis of a gallstone ileus is often delayed, with a resulting mortality rate of approximately 20%.

Mirizzi's Syndrome

Mirizzi's syndrome is a rare complication in which a stone becomes impacted in the neck of the gallbladder or the cystic duct and extrinsically compresses the CBD with resulting jaundice and bile duct obstruction or fistulizes into the CBD.[198, 199] ERCP usually demonstrates the characteristic extrinsic compression of the CBD. Treatment is generally an open cholecystectomy, although endoscopic stent placement and laparoscopic cholecystectomy have been utilized successfully. Preoperative diagnosis of Mirizzi's syndrome is important, so that CBD injury can be prevented.[200]

Porcelain Gallbladder

Strictly speaking, a porcelain gallbladder, defined as intramural calcification of the gallbladder wall, is not necessarily a complication of gallstones but is mentioned here because of the remarkable tendency of carcinoma to develop as a late complication of calcified gallbladders. The diagnosis of a porcelain gallbladder can be made with a plain abdominal film or abdominal CT, which shows intramural calcification of the gallbladder wall. Prophylactic cholecystectomy is indicated to prevent the subsequent development of carcinoma, which may occur in up to 20% of cases.[140, 201]

REFERENCES

1. Kratzer W, Mason RA, Kachele V: Prevalence of gallstones in sonographic surveys worldwide. J Clin Ultrasound 27:1, 1999.
2. Sarin SK, Negi VS, Dewan R, et al: High familial prevalence of gallstones in the first-degree relatives of gallstone patients. Hepatology 22:138, 1995.
3. Lammert F, Wang DQ, Paigen B, et al: Phenotypic characterization of Lith genes that determine susceptibility to cholesterol cholelithiasis in inbred mice: Integrated activities of hepatic lipid regulatory enzymes. J Lipid Res 40:2080, 1999.
4. Buhman KK, Accad M, Novak S, et al: Resistance to diet-induced hypercholesterolemia and gallstone formation in ACAT2-deficient mice. Nat Med 6:1341, 2000.
5. Egbert AM: Gallstone symptoms: Myth and reality. Postgrad Med 90: 119, 1991.

6. Adedeji A, Akande B, Olumide F: The changing pattern of cholelithiasis in Lagos. Scand J Gastroenterol Suppl 124:63, 1986.
7. Su CH, Lui WY, P'eng FK: Relative prevalence of gallstone diseases in Taiwan: A nationwide cooperative study. Dig Dis Sci 37:764, 1992.
8. Everhart JE, Khare M, Hill M, et al: Prevalence and ethnic differences in gallbladder disease in the United States. Gastroenterology 117:632, 1999.
9. Sichieri R, Everhart JE, Roth H: A prospective study of hospitalization with gallstone disease among women: Role of dietary factors, fasting period, and dieting. Am J Public Health 81:880, 1991.
10. Jensen KH, Jorgensen T: Incidence of gallstones in a Danish population. Gastroenterology 100:790, 1991.
11. Lowenfels AB, Velema JP: Estimating gallstone incidence from prevalence data. Scand J Gastroenterol 27:984, 1992.
12. Skar V, Skar AG, Bratlie J, et al: Beta-glucuronidase activity in the bile of gallstone patients both with and without duodenal diverticula. Scand J Gastroenterol 24:205, 1989.
13. Carey MC: Pathogenesis of gallstones. Am J Surg 165:410, 1993.
14. Stampfer MJ, Maclure KM, Colditz GA, et al: Risk of symptomatic gallstones in women with severe obesity. Am J Clin Nutr 55:652, 1992.
15. Attili AF, Capocaccia R, Carulli N, et al: Factors associated with gallstone disease in the MICOL experience: Multicenter Italian Study on Epidemiology of Cholelithiasis. Hepatology 26:809, 1997.
16. Acalovschi M, Badea R: Ultrasonographic study of gallbladder emptying in obese patients. Int J Obes Relat Metab Disord 16:313, 1992.
17. Miller LJ, Holicky EL, Ulrich CD, et al: Abnormal processing of the human cholecystokinin receptor gene in association with gallstones and obesity. Gastroenterology 109:1375, 1995.
18. Shiffman ML, Sugerman HJ, Kellum JM, et al: Gallstone formation after rapid weight loss: A prospective study in patients undergoing gastric bypass surgery for treatment of morbid obesity. Am J Gastroenterol 86:1000, 1991.
19. Marks JW, Bonorris GG, Albers G, et al: The sequence of biliary events preceding the formation of gallstones in humans. Gastroenterology 103:566, 1992.
20. Inoue K, Fuchigami A, Higashide S, et al: Gallbladder sludge and stone formation in relation to contractile function after gastrectomy: A prospective study. Ann Surg 215:19, 1992.
21. Shiffman ML, Kaplan GD, Brinkman-Kaplan V, et al: Prophylaxis against gallstone formation with ursodeoxycholic acid in patients participating in a very-low-calorie diet program. Ann Intern Med 122: 899, 1995.
22. Pitt HA, King WD, Mann LL, et al: Increased risk of cholelithiasis with prolonged total parenteral nutrition. Am J Surg 145:106, 1983.
23. Roslyn JJ, Berquist WE, Pitt HA, et al: Increased risk of gallstones in children receiving total parenteral nutrition. Pediatrics 71:784, 1983.
24. Sitzmann JV, Pitt HA, Steinborn PA, et al: Cholecystokinin prevents parenteral nutrition induced biliary sludge in humans. Surg Gynecol Obstet 170:25, 1990.
25. Lynn J, Williams L, O'Brien J, et al: Effects of estrogen upon bile: Implications with respect to gallstone formation. Ann Surg 178:514, 1973.
26. Van Bodegraven AA, Bohmer CJ, Manoliu RA, et al: Gallbladder contents and fasting gallbladder volumes during and after pregnancy. Scand J Gastroenterol 33:993, 1998.
27. Maringhini A, Ciambra M, Baccelliere P, et al: Biliary sludge and gallstones in pregnancy: Incidence, risk factors, and natural history. Ann Intern Med 119:116, 1993.
28. Valdivieso V, Covarrubias C, Siegel F, et al: Pregnancy and cholelithiasis: Pathogenesis and natural course of gallstones diagnosed in early puerperium. Hepatology 17:1, 1993.
29. Tsimoyiannis EC, Antoniou NC, Tsaboulas C, et al: Cholelithiasis during pregnancy and lactation: Prospective study. Eur J Surg 160: 627, 1994.
30. Miquel JF, Covarrubias C, Villaroel L, et al: Genetic epidemiology of cholesterol cholelithiasis among Chilean Hispanics, Amerindians, and Maoris. Gastroenterology 115:937, 1998.
31. Everson RB, Byar DP, Bischoff AJ: Estrogen predisposes to cholecystectomy but not to stones. Gastroenterology 82:4, 1982.
32. Henriksson P, Einarsson K, Eriksson A, et al: Estrogen-induced gallstone formation in males: Relation to changes in serum and biliary lipids during hormonal treatment of prostatic carcinoma. J Clin Invest 84:811, 1989.
33. Wallentin L, Varenhorst E: Changes of plasma lipid metabolism in males during estrogen treatment for prostatic carcinoma. J Clin Endocrinol Metab 47:596, 1978.
34. Erickson SK, Jaeckle S, Lear SR, et al: Regulation of hepatic cholesterol and lipoprotein metabolism in ethinyl estradiol–treated rats. J Lipid Res 30:1763, 1989.
35. Everson GT, McKinley C, Kern F Jr: Mechanisms of gallstone formation in women: Effects of exogenous estrogen (Premarin) and dietary cholesterol on hepatic lipid metabolism. J Clin Invest 87:237, 1991.
36. Braverman DZ, Johnson ML, Kern F Jr: Effects of pregnancy and contraceptive steroids on gallbladder function. N Engl J Med 302:362, 1980.
37. The Boston Collaborative Drug Surveillance Program, Boston University Medical Center: Surgically confirmed gallbladder disease, venous thromboembolism, and breast tumors in relation to postmenopausal estrogen therapy. N Engl J Med 290:15, 1974.
38. Scragg RK, McMichael AJ, Seamark RF: Oral contraceptives, pregnancy, and endogenous oestrogen in gall stone disease—a case-control study. BMJ Clin Res Ed 288:1795, 1984.
39. Strom BL, Tamragouri RN, Morse ML, et al: Oral contraceptives and other risk factors for gallbladder disease. Clin Pharmacol Ther 39:335, 1986.
40. Stahlberg D, Reihner E, Rudling M, et al: Influence of bezafibrate on hepatic cholesterol metabolism in gallstone patients: Reduced activity of cholesterol 7 alpha-hydroxylase. Hepatology 21:1025, 1995.
41. Chapman BA, Burt MJ, Chisholm RJ, et al: Dissolution of gallstones with simvastatin, an HMG CoA reductase inhibitor. Dig Dis Sci 43: 349, 1998.
42. Montini M, Gianola D, Pagani MD, et al: Cholelithiasis and acromegaly: Therapeutic strategies. Clin Endocrinol 40:401, 1994.
43. Newman CB, Melmed S, Snyder PJ, et al: Safety and efficacy of long-term octreotide therapy of acromegaly: Results of a multicenter trial in 103 patients—a clinical research center study. J Clin Endocrinol Metab 80:2768, 1995.
44. Van Liessum PA, Hopman WP, Pieters GF, et al: Postprandial gallbladder motility during long term treatment with the long-acting somatostatin analog SMS 201-995 in acromegaly. J Clin Endocrinol Metab 69:557, 1989.
45. Arvidsson A, Alvan G, Angelin B, et al: Ceftriaxone: Renal and biliary excretion and effect on the colon microflora. J Antimicrob Chemother 10:207, 1982.
46. Shiffman ML, Keith FB, Moore EW: Pathogenesis of ceftriaxone-associated biliary sludge: In vitro studies of calcium-ceftriaxone binding and solubility. Gastroenterology 99:1772, 1990.
47. Schaad UB, Wedgwood-Krucko J, Tschaeppeler H: Reversible ceftriaxone-associated biliary pseudolithiasis in children. Lancet 2:1411, 1988.
48. Thornton J, Symes C, Heaton K: Moderate alcohol intake reduces bile cholesterol saturation and raises HDL cholesterol. Lancet 2:819, 1983.
49. Kern FJ: Effects of dietary cholesterol on cholesterol and bile acid homeostasis in patients with cholesterol gallstones. J Clin Invest 93: 1186, 1994.
50. Misciagna G, Centonze S, Leoci C, et al: Diet, physical activity, and gallstones—a population-based, case-control study in southern Italy. Am J Clin Nutr 69:120, 1999.
51. Kratzer W, Kachele V, Mason RA, et al: Gallstone prevalence in relation to smoking, alcohol, coffee consumption, and nutrition: The Ulm Gallstone Study. Scand J Gastroenterol 32:953, 1997.
52. Shaw SJ, Hajnal F, Lebovitz Y, et al: Gallbladder dysfunction in diabetes mellitus. Dig Dis Sci 38:490, 1993.
53. De Santis A, Attili AF, Ginanni Corradini S, et al: Gallstones and diabetes: A case-control study in a free-living population sample. Hepatology 25:787, 1997.
54. Lapidus A, Bangstad M, Astrom M, et al: The prevalence of gallstone disease in a defined cohort of patients with Crohn's disease. Am J Gastroenterol 94:1261, 1999.
55. Brink MA, Slors JF, Keulemans YC, et al: Enterohepatic cycling of bilirubin: A putative mechanism for pigment gallstone formation in ileal Crohn's disease. Gastroenterology 116:1420, 1999.
56. Moonka R, Stiens SA, Resnick WJ, et al: The prevalence and natural history of gallstones in spinal cord injured patients. J Am Coll Surg 189:274, 1999.
57. Sedaghat A, Grundy SM: Cholesterol crystals and the formation of cholesterol gallstones. N Engl J Med 302:1274, 1980.
58. Holan KR, Holzbach RT, Hermann RE, et al: Nucleation time: A key factor in the pathogenesis of cholesterol gallstone disease. Gastroenterology 77:611, 1979.
59. Miquel JF, Nunez L, Amigo L, et al: Cholesterol saturation, not proteins or cholecystitis, is critical for crystal formation in human gallbladder bile. Gastroenterology 114:1016, 1998.

60. Brown MS, Goldstein JL: Receptor-mediated control of cholesterol metabolism. Science 191:150, 1976.
61. Salen G, Nicolau G, Shefer S, et al: Hepatic cholesterol metabolism in patients with gallstones. Gastroenterology 69:676, 1975.
62. Saunders KD, Cates JA, Abedin MZ, et al: Lovastatin and gallstone dissolution: A preliminary study. Surgery 113:28, 1993.
63. Smit JW, van Erpecum KJ, Renooij W, et al: The effects of the 3-hydroxy, 3-methylglutaryl coenzyme A reductase inhibitor pravastatin on bile composition and nucleation of cholesterol crystals in cholesterol gallstone disease. Hepatology 21:1523, 1995.
64. Turley SD, Dietschy JM: Regulation of biliary cholesterol output in the rat: Dissociation from the rate of hepatic cholesterol synthesis, the size of the hepatic cholesteryl ester pool, and the hepatic uptake of chylomicron cholesterol. J Lipid Res 20:923, 1979.
65. Turley SD, Dietschy JM: The contribution of newly synthesized cholesterol to biliary cholesterol in the rat. J Biol Chem 256:2438, 1981.
66. Nervi FO, Del Pozo R, Covarrubias CF, et al: The effect of progesterone on the regulatory mechanisms of biliary cholesterol secretion in the rat. Hepatology 3:360, 1983.
67. Smith JL, Hardie IR, Pillay SP, et al: Hepatic acyl-coenzyme A: cholesterol acyltransferase activity is decreased in patients with cholesterol gallstones. J Lipid Res 31:1993, 1990.
68. Reihner E, Angelin B, Bjorkhem I, et al: Hepatic cholesterol metabolism in cholesterol gallstone disease. J Lipid Res 32:469, 1991.
69. Busch N, Matern S: Current concepts in cholesterol gallstone pathogenesis. Eur J Clin Invest 21:453, 1991.
70. Smit JJ, Schinkel AH, Oude Elferink RP, et al: Homozygous disruption of the murine mdr2 P-glycoprotein gene leads to a complete absence of phospholipid from bile and to liver disease. Cell 75:451, 1993.
71. Carey MC, Small DM: The physical chemistry of cholesterol solubility in bile: Relationship to gallstone formation and dissolution in man. J Clin Invest 61:998, 1978.
72. Donovan JM, Carey MC: Separation and quantitation of cholesterol "carriers" in bile. Hepatology 12:94S, 1990.
73. Lamont JT, Carey MC: Cholesterol gallstone formation. 2. Pathobiology and pathomechanics. Prog Liver Dis 10:165, 1992.
74. Harvey PR, Somjen G, Lichtenberg MS, et al: Nucleation of cholesterol from vesicles isolated from bile of patients with and without cholesterol gallstones. Biochim Biophys Acta 921:198, 1987.
75. Carey MC, LaMont JT: Cholesterol gallstone formation. 1. Physical-chemistry of bile and biliary lipid secretion. Prog Liver Dis 10:139, 1992.
76. Gerloff T, Stieger B, Hagenbuch B, et al: The sister of P-glycoprotein represents the canalicular bile salt export pump of mammalian liver. J Biol Chem 273:10046, 1998.
77. Spady DK, Cuthbert JA: Regulation of hepatic sterol metabolism in the rat. J Biol Chem 267:5584, 1992.
78. Berr F, Mayer M, Sackmann MF, et al: Pathogenic factors in early recurrence of cholesterol gallstones. Gastroenterology 106:215, 1994.
79. Marcus SN, Heaton KW: Deoxycholic acid and the pathogenesis of gall stones. Gut 29:522, 1988.
80. Van Erpecum KJ, Portincasa P, Eckhardt E, et al: Ursodeoxycholic acid reduces protein levels and nucleation-promoting activity in human gallbladder bile. Gastroenterology 110:1225, 1996.
81. Small DM: Cholesterol nucleation and growth in gallstone formation [editorial]. N Engl J Med 302:1305, 1980.
82. Jungst D, Lang T, von Ritter C, et al: Role of high total protein in gallbladder bile in the formation of cholesterol gallstones. Gastroenterology 100:1724, 1991.
83. Smith BF: Human gallbladder mucin binds biliary lipids and promotes cholesterol crystal nucleation in model bile. J Lipid Res 28:1088, 1987.
84. Afdhal NH, Niu N, Nunes DP, et al: Mucin-vesicle interactions in model bile: Evidence for vesicle aggregation and fusion before cholesterol crystal formation. Hepatology 22:856, 1995.
85. Afdhal NH, Niu N, Gantz D, et al: Bovine gallbladder mucin accelerates cholesterol monohydrate crystal growth in model bile. Gastroenterology 104:1515, 1993.
86. Lee SP, Carey MC, LaMont JT: Aspirin prevention of cholesterol gallstone formation in prairie dogs. Science 211:1429, 1981.
87. Sterling RK, Shiffman ML, Sugerman HJ, et al: Effect of NSAIDs on gallbladder bile composition. Dig Dis Sci 40:2220, 1995.
88. Pazzi P, Scagliarini R, Sighinolfi D, et al: Nonsteroidal antiinflammatory drug use and gallstone disease prevalence: A case-control study. Am J Gastroenterol 93:1420, 1998.
89. Groen AK, Ottenhoff R, Jansen PL, et al: Effect of cholesterol nucleation-promoting activity on cholesterol solubilization in model bile. J Lipid Res 30:51, 1989.
90. Upadhya GA, Harvey PR, Strasberg SM: Effect of human biliary immunoglobulins on the nucleation of cholesterol. J Biol Chem 268: 5193, 1993.
91. Offner GD, Gong D, Afdhal NH: Identification of a 130-kilodalton human biliary concanavalin A binding protein as aminopeptidase N. Gastroenterology 106:755, 1994.
92. Yamashita G, Corradini SG, Secknus R, et al: Biliary haptoglobin, a potent promoter of cholesterol crystallization at physiological concentrations. J Lipid Res 36:1325, 1995.
93. Abei M, Nuutinen H, Kawczak P, et al: Identification of human biliary alpha 1-acid glycoprotein as a cholesterol crystallization promoter. Gastroenterology 106:231, 1994.
94. Kibe A, Holzbach RT, LaRusso NF, et al: Inhibition of cholesterol crystal formation by apolipoproteins in supersaturated model bile. Science 225:514, 1984.
95. Ohya T, Schwarzendrube J, Busch N, et al: Isolation of a human biliary glycoprotein inhibitor of cholesterol crystallization. Gastroenterology 104:527, 1993.
96. Wang DQ-H, Carey MC: Complete mapping of crystallization pathways during cholesterol precipitation from model bile: Influence of physical-chemical variables of pathophysiologic relevance and identification of a stable liquid crystalline state in cold, dilute and hydrophobic bile salt—containing systems. J Lipid Res 37:606, 1996.
97. Moore EW: Biliary calcium and gallstone formation. Hepatology 12: 206S, 1990.
98. Wood JR, Svanvik J: Gall-bladder water and electrolyte transport and its regulation. Gut 24:579, 1983.
99. Plevris JN, Bouchier IA: Defective acid base regulation by the gall bladder epithelium and its significance for gall stone formation. Gut 37:127, 1995.
100. Rege RV, Nahrwold DL, Moore EW: Absorption of biliary calcium from the canine gallbladder: Protection against the formation of calcium-containing gallstones. J Lab Clin Med 110:381, 1987.
101. Magnuson TH, Lillemoe KD, Zarkin BA, et al: Patients with uncomplicated cholelithiasis acidify bile normally. Dig Dis Sci 37:1517, 1992.
102. Nilsson B, Friman S, Thune A, et al: Inflammation reduces mucosal secretion of hydrogen ions and impairs concentrating function and luminal acidification in feline gallbladder. Scand J Gastroenterol 30: 1021, 1995.
103. Gullo L, Bolondi L, Priori P, et al: Inhibitory effect of atropine on cholecystokinin-induced gallbladder contraction in man. Digestion 29: 209, 1984.
104. Pomeranz IS, Shaffer EA: Abnormal gallbladder emptying in a subgroup of patients with gallstones. Gastroenterology 88:787, 1985.
105. Spengler U, Sackmann M, Sauerbruch T, et al: Gallbladder motility before and after extracorporeal shock-wave lithotripsy. Gastroenterology 96:860, 1989.
106. Van der Werf SD, van Berge Henegouwen GP, Palsma DM, et al: Motor function of the gallbladder and cholesterol saturation of duodenal bile. Neth J Med 30:160, 1987.
107. Watkins JB, Tercyak AM, Szczepanik P, et al: Bile salt kinetics in cystic fibrosis: Influence of pancreatic enzyme replacement. Gastroenterology 73:1023, 1977.
108. Ko CW, Sekijima JH, Lee SP: Biliary sludge. Ann Intern Med 130: 301, 1999.
109. Lee SP, Maher K, Nicholls JF: Origin and fate of biliary sludge. Gastroenterology 94:170, 1988.
110. Janowitz P, Kratzer W, Zemmler T, et al: Gallbladder sludge: Spontaneous course and incidence of complications in patients without stones. Hepatology 20:291, 1994.
111. Trotman BW: Pigment gallstone disease. Gastoenterol Clin North Am 20:111, 1991.
112. Cetta F: The role of bacteria in pigment gallstone disease. Ann Surg 213:315, 1991.
113. Nagase M, Hikasa Y, Soloway RD, et al: Gallstones in Western Japan: Factors affecting the prevalence of intrahepatic gallstones. Gastroenterology 78:684, 1980.
114. Ho KJ, Lin XZ, Yu SC, et al: Cholelithiasis in Taiwan: Gallstone characteristics, surgical incidence, bile lipid composition, and role of beta-glucuronidase. Dig Dis Sci 40:1963, 1995.
115. Sandstad O, Osnes T, Skar V, et al: Common bile duct stones are

mainly brown and associated with duodenal diverticula. Gut 35:1464, 1994.
116. Fevery J, Verwilghen R, Tan TG, et al: Glucuronidation of bilirubin and the occurrence of pigment gallstones in patients with chronic haemolytic diseases. Eur J Clin Invest 10:219, 1980.
117. Trotman BW, Bernstein SE, Bove KE, et al: Studies on the pathogenesis of pigment gallstones in hemolytic anemia: Description and characteristics of a mouse model. J Clin Invest 65:1301, 1980.
118. Cahalane MJ, Neubrand MW, Carey MC: Physical-chemical pathogenesis of pigment gallstones. Semin Liver Dis 8:317, 1988.
119. Behar J, Lee KY, Thompson WR, et al: Gallbladder contraction in patients with pigment and cholesterol stones. Gastroenterology 97: 1479, 1989.
120. Trotman BW, Bernstein SE, Balistreri WF, et al: Hemolysis-induced gallstones in mice: Increased unconjugated bilirubin in hepatic bile predisposes to gallstone formation. Gastroenterology 81:232, 1981.
121. Leung JW, Sung JY, Costerton JW: Bacteriological and electron microscopy examination of brown pigment stones. J Clin Microbiol 27: 915, 1989.
122. Gracie WA, Ransohoff DF: The natural history of silent gallstones: The innocent gallstone is not a myth. N Engl J Med 307:798, 1982.
123. Friedman GD, Raviola CA, Fireman B: Prognosis of gallstones with mild or no symptoms: 25 Years of follow-up in a health maintenance organization. J Clin Epidemiol 42:127, 1989.
124. Attili AF, De Santis A, Capri R, et al: The natural history of gallstones: The GREPCO experience: The GREPCO Group. Hepatology 21:655, 1995.
125. Thistle JL, Cleary PA, Lachin JM, et al: The natural history of cholelithiasis: The National Cooperative Gallstone Study. Ann Intern Med 101:171, 1984.
126. Newman HF, Northup JD, Rosenblum M, et al: Complications of cholelithiasis. Am J Gastroenterol 50:476, 1968.
127. Ransohoff DF, Gracie WA: Treatment of gallstones. Ann Intern Med 119:606, 1993.
128. Del Favero G, Caroli A, Meggiato T, et al: Natural history of gallstones in non-insulin-dependent diabetes mellitus: A prospective 5-year follow-up. Dig Dis Sci 39:1704, 1994.
129. Donovan JM: Physical and metabolic factors in gallstone pathogenesis. Gastroenterol Clin North Am 28:75, 1999.
130. Ko CW, Lee SP: Gallstone formation: Local factors. Gastroenterol Clin North Am 28:99, 1999.
131. Traverso LW: Clinical manifestations and impact of gallstone disease. Am J Surg 165:405, 1993.
132. Fenster LF, Lonborg R, Thirlby RC, et al: What symptoms does cholecystectomy cure? Insights from an outcomes measurement project and review of the literature. Am J Surg 169:533, 1995.
133. Cox MR, Wilson TG, Luck AJ, et al: Laparoscopic cholecystectomy for acute inflammation of the gallbladder. Ann Surg 218:630, 1993.
134. Strasberg SM, Clavien PA: Overview of therapeutic modalities for the treatment of gallstone diseases. Am J Surg 165:420, 1993.
135. Berger MY, van der Velden JJ, Lijmer JG, et al: Abdominal symptoms: Do they predict gallstones? A systematic review. Scand J Gastroenterol 35:70, 2000.
136. Angelico F, Del Ben M, Barbato A, et al: Ten-year incidence and natural history of gallstone disease in a rural population of women in central Italy: The Rome Group for the Epidemiology and Prevention of Cholelithiasis (GREPCO). Ital J Gastroenterol 29:249, 1997.
137. Ware RE, Kinney TR, Casey JR, et al: Laparoscopic cholecystectomy in young patients with sickle hemoglobinopathies. J Pediatr 120:58, 1992.
138. Winter SS, Kinney TR, Ware RE: Gallbladder sludge in children with sickle cell disease. J Pediatr 1994.
139. Grimaldi CH, Nelson RG, Pettitt DJ, et al: Increased mortality with gallstone disease: Results of a 20-year population-based survey in Pima Indians. Ann Intern Med 118:185, 1993.
140. Sheth S, Bedford A, Chopra S: Primary gallbladder cancer: Recognition of risk factors and the role of prophylactic cholecystectomy. Am J Gastroenterol 95:1402, 2000.
141. Menegaux F, Dorent R, Tabbi D, et al: Biliary surgery after heart transplantation. Am J Surg 175:320, 1998.
142. Melvin WS, Meier DJ, Elkhammas EA, et al: Prophylactic cholecystectomy is not indicated following renal transplantation. Am J Surg 175:317, 1998.
143. Houdart R, Perniceni T, Darne B, et al: Predicting common bile duct lithiasis: Determination and prospective validation of a model predicting low risk. Am J Surg 170:38, 1995.
144. Barkun AN, Barkun JS, Fried GM, et al: Useful predictors of bile duct stones in patients undergoing laparoscopic cholecystectomy: McGill Gallstone Treatment Group. Ann Surg 220:32, 1994.
145. Bortoff GA, Chen MY, Ott DJ, et al: Gallbladder stones: Imaging and intervention. Radiographics 20:751, 2000.
146. Scanlan KA: Sonographic artifacts and their origins. AJR Am J Roentgenol 156:1267, 1991.
147. Shea JA, Berlin JA, Escarce JJ, et al: Revised estimates of diagnostic test sensitivity and specificity in suspected biliary tract disease. Arch Intern Med 154:2573, 1994.
148. Einstein DM, Lapin SA, Ralls PW, et al: The insensitivity of sonography in the detection of choledocholithiasis. AJR Am J Roentgenol 142:725, 1984.
149. Amouyal P, Amouyal G, Levy P, et al: Diagnosis of choledocholithiasis by endoscopic ultrasonography. Gastroenterology 106:1062, 1994.
150. Boland GW, Slater G, Lu DS, et al: Prevalence and significance of gallbladder abnormalities seen on sonography in intensive care unit patients. AJR Am J Roentgenol 174:973, 2000.
151. Ralls PW, Colletti PM, Lapin SA: Real-time sonography in suspected acute cholecystitis. Radiology 155:767, 1985.
152. Prat F, Amouyal G, Amouyal P: Prospective controlled study of endoscopic ultrasound and endoscopic retrograde cholangiography in patients with suspected common bile duct stones. Lancet 347:75, 1996.
153. Benson MD, Gandhi MR: Ultrasound of the hepatobiliary-pancreatic system. World J Surg 24:166, 2000.
154. Canto MI, Chak A, Stellato T, et al: Endoscopic ultrasonography versus cholangiography for the diagnosis of choledocholithiasis. Gastrointest Endosc 47:439, 1998.
155. Beswick JS, Hughes PM, Martin DF: Ultrasonic evaluation of gallbladder function prior to non-surgical treatment of gallstones. Br J Radiol 64:321, 1991.
156. Maglinte DD, Torres WE, Laufer I: Oral cholecystography in contemporary gallstone imaging: A review. Radiology 178:49, 1991.
157. Prevot N, Mariat G, Mahul P, et al: Contribution of cholescintigraphy to the early diagnosis of acute acalculous cholecystitis in intensive-care-unit patients. Eur J Nucl Med 26:1317, 1999.
158. Marton KI, Doubilet P: How to image the gallbladder in suspected cholecystitis. Ann Intern Med 110:722, 1988.
159. Swayne LC, Ginsberg HN: Diagnosis of acute cholecystitis by cholescintigraphy: Significance of pericholecystic hepatic uptake. AJR Am J Roentgenol 152:1211, 1989.
160. Klieger PS, O'Mara RE: The clinical utility of quantitative cholescintigraphy: The significance of gallbladder dysfunction. Clin Nucl Med 23:278, 1998.
161. Ott DJ, Gilliam J, d Zagoria RJ, et al: Interventional endoscopy of the biliary and pancreatic ducts: Current indications and methods. AJR Am J Roentgenol 158:243, 1992.
162. Braun MA, Collins MB: A simple method to reduce air-bubble artifacts during percutaneous extraction of biliary stones. AJR Am J Roentgenol 158:309, 1992.
163. Enns R, Baillie J: Review article: The treatment of acute biliary pancreatitis. Aliment Pharmacol Ther 13:1379, 1999.
164. Masui T, Takehara Y, Fujiwara T, et al: MR and CT cholangiography in evaluation of the biliary tract. Acta Radiol 39:557, 1998.
165. Fulcher AS, Turner MA, Capps GW: MR cholangiography: Technical advances and clinical applications. Radiographics 19:25, 1999.
166. Hochwalk SN, Dobryansky MB, Rofsky NM, et al: Magnetic resonance cholangiopancreatography accurately predicts the presence or absence of choledocholithiasis. J Gastrointest Surg 2:573, 1998.
167. Nahrwold DL, Rose RC, Ward SP: Abnormalities in gallbladder morphology and function in patients with cholelithiasis. Ann Surg 184: 415, 1976.
168. Middelfart HV, Jensen P, Hojgaard L, et al: Pain patterns after distension of the gallbladder in patients with acute cholecystitis. Scand J Gastroenterol 33:982, 1998.
169. Friedman GD: Natural history of asymptomatic and symptomatic gallstones. Am J Surg 165:399, 1993.
170. Walker J, Chalmers RT, Allan PL: An audit of ultrasound diagnosis of gallbladder calculi. Br J Radiol 65:581, 1992.
171. Farrell T, Mahon T, Daly L, et al: Identification of inappropriate radiological referrals with suspected gallstones: A prospective audit. Br J Radiol 67:32, 1994.
172. Glenn F: Acute cholecystitis. Surg Gynecol Obstet 143:56, 1976.
173. Roslyn JJ, DenBesten L, Thompson JE Jr, et al: Roles of lithogenic

bile and cystic duct occlusion in the pathogenesis of acute cholecystitis. Am J Surg 140:126, 1980.
174. Kaminski DL: Arachidonic acid metabolites in hepatobiliary physiology and disease. Gastroenterology 97:781, 1989.
175. Kaminski DL, Deshpande Y, Thomas C: Effect of oral ibuprofen on formation of prostaglandin E and F by human gallbladder muscle and mucosa. Dig Dis Sci 30:933, 1985.
176. Goldman G, Kahn PJ, Alon R, et al: Biliary colic treatment and acute cholecystitis prevention by prostaglandin inhibitor. Dig Dis Sci 34: 809, 1989.
177. Claesson BE, Holmlund D, Matzsch TW: Microflora of the gallbladder related to duration of acute cholecystitis. Surg Gynecol Obstet 162:531, 1986.
178. Edlund Y, Zettergen L: Histopathology of the gallbladder in gallstone disease related to clinical data. Acta Chir Scand 116:450, 1959.
179. Raine PAM, Gunn AA: Acute cholecystitis. Br J Surg 62:697, 1975.
180. Dumont AE: Significance of hyperbilirubinemia in acute cholecystitis. Surg Gynecol Obstet 142:855, 1976.
181. Edlund Y, Olsson O: Acute cholecystitis: Its aetiology and course, with special reference to the timing of cholecystectomy. Acta Chir Scand 120:479, 1961.
182. Lujan JA, Parrilla P, Robles R, et al: Laparoscopic cholecystectomy in the treatment of acute cholecystitis. J Am Coll Surg 181:75, 1995.
183. Tanaka M, Takahata S, Konomi H, et al: Long-term consequence of endoscopic sphincterotomy for bile duct stones. Gastrointest Endosc 48:465, 1998.
184. Lim JH: Oriental cholangiohepatitis: Pathologic, clinical, and radiologic features. AJR Am J Roentgenol 157:1, 1991.
185. Soloway RD, Trotman BW, Ostrow JD: Pigment gallstones. Gastroenterology 72:167, 1977.
186. Way LW: Retained common duct stones. Surg Clin North Am 53: 1139, 1973.
187. Goldman DE, Gholson CF: Choledocholithiasis in patients with normal serum liver enzymes. Dig Dis Sci 40:1065, 1995.
188. Thornton JR, Lobo AJ, Lintott DJ, et al: Value of ultrasound and liver function tests in determining the need for endoscopic retrograde cholangiopancreatography in unexplained abdominal pain. Gut 33:1559, 1992.
189. Chijiiwa K, Kozaki N, Naito T, et al: Treatment of choice for choledocholithiasis in patients with acute obstructive suppurative cholangitis and liver cirrhosis. Am J Surg 170:356, 1995.
190. Greig JD, John TG, Mahadaven M, et al: Laparoscopic ultrasonography in the evaluation of the biliary tree during laparoscopic cholecystectomy. Br J Surg 81:1202, 1994.
191. Nash JA, Cohen SA: Gallbladder and biliary tract disease in AIDS. Gastoenterol Clin North Am 26:323, 1997.
192. Cotton PB: Endoscopic retrograde cholangiopancreatography and laparoscopic cholecystectomy. Am J Surg 165:474, 1993.
193. Hill J, Martin DF, Tweedle DE: Risks of leaving the gallbladder in situ after endoscopic sphincterotomy for bile duct stones. Br J Surg 78:554, 1991.
194. Pitt HA, Cameron JL: Acute cholangitis. In Way LW, Pellegrini CA (eds): Surgery of the Gallbladder and Bile Ducts. Philadelphia, WB Saunders, 1987, p 295.
195. Lorenz RW, Steffen HM: Emphysematous cholecystitis: Diagnostic problems and differential diagnosis of gallbladder gas accumulations. Hepatogastroenterol 37(Suppl 2):103, 1990.
196. Glenn F, Reed C, Grafe WR: Biliary enteric fistula. Surg Gynecol Obstet 153:527, 1981.
197. Clavien PA, Richon J, Burgan S, et al: Gallstone ileus. Br J Surg 77: 737, 1990.
198. Meng WC, Kwok SP, Kelly SB, et al: Management of Mirizzi syndrome by laparoscopic cholecystectomy and laparoscopic ultrasonography. Br J Surg 82, 1995.
199. Toursarkissian B, Holley DT, Kearney PA, et al: Mirizzi's syndrome. South Med J 87:471, 1994.
200. Yip AW, Chow WC, Chan J, et al: Mirizzi syndrome with cholecystocholedochal fistula: Preoperative diagnosis and management. Surgery 111:335, 1992.
201. Polk C: Carcinoma and the calcified gall bladder. Gastroenterology 50:582, 1966.

Chapter 56

Surgical Management of Gallstone Disease and Postoperative Complications

Robert E. Glasgow and Sean J. Mulvihill

Many options are available for the management of patients with symptomatic gallstone disease. Improvements in endoscopic, radiologic, and chemical therapies for gallstones have enhanced the overall treatment of these patients (see Chapters 55 and 57). Nevertheless, surgery remains the most important therapeutic option. Laparoscopic cholecystectomy has become the standard method for the elective treatment of patients with biliary colic and complications of gallstone disease, such as acute cholecystitis, gallstone pancreatitis, and choledocholithiasis. In this chapter, surgical management of patients with symptomatic and asymptomatic gallstones is discussed, with particular emphasis on indications for surgery, patient selection, and outcome.

SURGERY FOR CHOLELITHIASIS

Approximately 700,000 cholecystectomies are performed for gallstone disease in the United States each year. Currently, the vast majority of these operations are performed using minimally invasive techniques. For example, 40,571 patients underwent cholecystectomy in California in 1996; in 74% of these patients, the operation was done laparoscopically, and in 26%, an open technique was used.[1] Patients with complicated gallstone disease, including acute cholecystitis, gallstone pancreatitis, and choledocholithiasis, were more likely to require an open procedure or conversion from a laparoscopic to an open approach than were patients with uncomplicated disease (biliary colic). Despite the increased reliance on minimally invasive techniques, open cholecystectomy remains an important operation in the management of complications of gallstones.

Open Cholecystectomy

Karl Langenbuch, a surgeon in Berlin, is credited with performing the first cholecystectomy in 1882. Until recently, this operation was the main therapeutic option for treating patients with gallstones, largely because of its remarkable success in relieving symptoms and its low morbidity. In prospective studies, 90% to 95% of patients who undergo cholecystectomy are substantially relieved or cured of their symptoms.[2] Cholecystectomy is more effective in relieving biliary colic than in relieving other symptoms such as dyspepsia and flatulence, which correlate less strongly with gallstone disease.

Technique

The technique of open cholecystectomy has not changed significantly since its first description. With the surgeon standing on the patient's right side, a right subcostal (Kocher) incision is made two fingerbreadths below the right costal margin. Alternatively, a midline incision may be used. After exploring the abdomen and dividing adhesions to the gallbladder, the gallbladder is dissected from its hepatic fossa from the fundus down to the infundibulum. Once the gallbladder has been mobilized from the liver, the cystic artery and cystic duct are readily identified as the only remaining attachments. A cholangiogram may be performed to evaluate for common duct stones or to confirm the anatomy. The cystic duct and artery are ligated and divided. An alternative strategy is to dissect the structures in the triangle of Calot, as is done in laparoscopic cholecystectomy, before

Table 56–1 | **Mortality Rates for Open Cholecystectomy in Large Series as a Function of Clinical Setting**

AUTHOR(S)	YEAR(S)	NO. OF PATIENTS	CLINICAL SETTING OF CHOLECYSTECTOMY		
			Biliary Colic	Acute Cholecystitis	CBDE
McSherry and Glenn[5]	1932–1978	11,808	0.5 %	2.9%	3.5%
Arnold[8]	1962–1966	28,621	1.5%	3.5%	–
Bredesen et al.[7]	1977–1981	13,854	0.4%	1.6%	2.3%
Roslyn et al.[6]	1989	42,474	0.02%	0.05%	–

CBDE, common bile duct exploration.

removing the gallbladder from the liver. The abdominal incision is then closed. Drainage of the gallbladder fossa is not indicated after routine cholecystectomy.

Results

The risk of open cholecystectomy has declined over the years. The overall mortality rate of cholecystectomy in 35,373 patients who underwent surgery before 1932 was 6.6%.[3] The rate decreased to 1.8% by 1952.[4] Since then, the overall mortality rate for cholecystectomy has averaged 1.5%. The rate is considerably lower in patients who underwent elective surgery for biliary colic, with an average less than 0.5% (Table 56–1).[5–8] The risk of death is several-fold higher when the operation is performed in the emergency setting for acute cholecystitis and when common bile duct exploration is required (see Table 56–1). Additionally, the mortality rate is directly proportional to age (Fig. 56–1). In a report of the entire Danish experience with cholecystectomy from 1977 to 1981, patients under age 50 had a risk of death of 0.028% from elective cholecystectomy.[7] This rate rose to 5.56% in patients over age 80. The experience in the

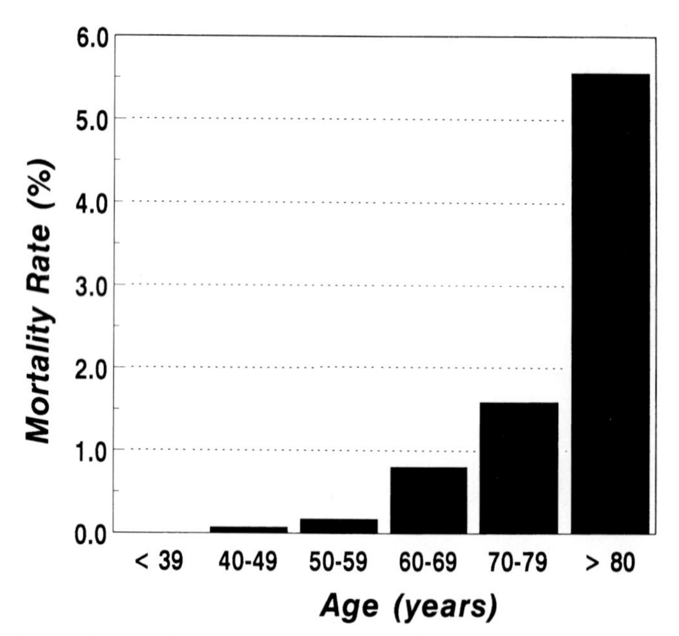

Figure 56–1. Relationship between age and risk of death from cholecystectomy. Data are from Denmark and include all patients operated on between 1977 and 1981.[7] This was in the era of open cholecystectomy.

United States has been similar. Of 11,808 patients who underwent cholecystectomy at the New York Hospital-Cornell Medical Center from 1932 to 1978, the risk of death from elective cholecystectomy for chronic cholecystitis was 0.1% and 0.8% in patients under and over age 50, respectively.[5] More recently, the overall mortality rate in 42,474 patients who underwent cholecystectomy in 1989 in California and Maryland was 0.17%.[6] In this series,[6] the mortality rate in patients under age 65 was 0.03%, compared to over 0.5% in patients over age 65. Similarly, the morbidity rate, length of hospital stay, and hospital charges were significantly higher in the older population. Most mortality following cholecystectomy is related to cardiac disease, particularly myocardial infarction.

Major complications following open cholecystectomy are rare. In a large survey of 28,621 patients who underwent cholecystectomy in the 1960s, complications occurred in 4.0% of patients.[8] Smaller, single-institution experiences before the institution of laparoscopic cholecystectomy reported similar complication rates of 4.5% in Seattle and 4.9% in Los Angeles.[2, 9] Most complications are relatively minor, such as wound infections or seromas, urinary retention or infection, and atelectasis. Complications related specifically to cholecystectomy include bile leak, bile duct injury, and acute pancreatitis. Of these, bile duct injury is the most serious because it often requires complicated and technically difficult surgical repair. If not recognized and managed optimally, bile duct injury can lead to biliary stricture, bile duct obstruction, and, rarely, secondary biliary cirrhosis and liver failure. The frequency of bile duct injury during open cholecystectomy is not known precisely but has been estimated to be one in every 200 to 600 cases.[10, 11] In recent series, two ductal injuries occurred in 1200 cholecystectomies at the Cedars-Sinai Medical Center in Los Angeles from 1982 to 1988,[9] and no bile duct injuries occurred in 1252 elective cholecystectomies at two large North American and European centers.[12] In general, bile duct injuries are preventable complications and are commonly the result of an inadequately trained surgeon, unrecognized variations in bile duct anatomy, or misidentification of normal anatomy.[10, 13] Excessive bleeding, severe inflammation, and emergency operations do not play as great a role in these injuries as might be intuitively supposed.

Laparoscopic Cholecystectomy

Since the first reports in the late 1980s, laparoscopic cholecystectomy has rapidly gained acceptance as the technique of choice in the treatment of the typical patient with biliary colic. The driving force behind the rapid development of laparoscopic cholecystectomy initially was patient demand. The benefits of this minimally invasive approach, including minimal scarring, reduced pain, and quicker return to normal activities, were quickly recognized by the lay public. Laparoscopic cholecystectomy was introduced and gained acceptance not through organized and carefully conceived clinical trials, as was the case in the United States for hip replacement surgery, but by acclamation.

Historically, laparoscopic cholecystectomy was an outgrowth of diagnostic laparoscopy and the early efforts of gynecologists at operative laparoscopy. The development of laparoscopic cholecystectomy was predicated on technical advances in miniaturized video cameras and other specialized equipment. Few other operations are as dependent on the safe and reliable function of instruments. Rapid advances are currently being made in instrument and equipment design and manufacture. Future availability of three-dimensional video systems and robotic assist devices may improve the technical dimensions of laparoscopic surgery dramatically.

Technique

The operative team for laparoscopic cholecystectomy generally consists of a surgeon, assistant surgeon, scrub nurse, circulating nurse, and anesthesiologist. The patient is asked to void immediately before entering the operating room to empty the bladder. Prophylactic antibiotics are not routinely administered to patients with uncomplicated gallstone disease, including biliary colic. Patients with potential infectious complications of gallstones, including acute cholecystitis and cholangitis, should receive antibiotics if not already prescribed before surgery. Sequential compression stockings are used in high-risk patients to reduce lower extremity venous stasis and deep venous thrombosis.

To view the abdominal contents and provide room for the instruments, a space is developed in the abdomen by inducing a pneumoperitoneum with a nonflammable gas such as carbon dioxide. After the pneumoperitoneum has been established, a trocar is placed at the umbilicus and a telescope is introduced. Three additional trocars are placed in the upper abdomen under direct vision for inserting operating instruments and retractors. The technique of laparoscopic cholecystectomy is illustrated in Figure 56–2. The assistant retracts the gallbladder fundus cephalad, anterior to the liver, and the infundibulum laterally. The surgeon, operating through the epigastric port, identifies and dissects the cystic duct and cystic artery circumferentially. Special care must be taken to identify the junction of the cystic duct and gallbladder, to ensure that the common bile duct has not been isolated inadvertently. Cholangiography is performed by cannulation of the cystic duct. If the anatomy is clear and no evidence of choledocholithiasis is seen, the cholangiocatheter is removed, and the cystic duct and cystic artery are divided between small metal clips. The gallbladder is then dissected from the liver bed and delivered through the umbilical incision. Care is taken to avoid perforation of the gallbladder during its dissection from the liver because the spillage of gallstones and bile has been shown to increase the risk of postoperative fever and intraabdominal abscess formation.[14, 15] The operation concludes with evacuation of the pneumoperitoneum and closure of the incisions.

Rationale for Cholangiography

Cholangiography during laparoscopic cholecystectomy has two main purposes. First, the cholangiogram may detect unsuspected common bile duct stones. Second, the cholangiogram confirms the surgeon's impression of the anatomy of the bile ducts. In the era before laparoscopic cholecystectomy, the value of routine cholangiography during cholecystectomy was debated, with some authorities arguing for its selective use.[16] Routine cholangiography has been criticized because of its relatively low yield, failure to identify all retained stones, occasional false-positive results, cost, and risk. Overall, 8% to 16% of all patients with cholelithiasis harbor common bile duct stones. Routine use of operative cholangiography detects unsuspected common bile duct stones in approximately 5% of patients who undergo cholecystectomy and anatomic ductal abnormalities in 12%.[17] Detection of abnormal ductal anatomy is important because during laparoscopic cholecystectomy, the two-dimensional video image and inability to palpate structures of the porta hepatitis make identification of the cystic duct-common bile duct junction a problem. Cholangiography permits identification of the bile duct anatomy before division of any important structures. A recent large population study from Australia demonstrated the importance of routine intraoperative cholangiography in decreasing the frequency of major bile duct injuries.[18]

Results

Several published series have now described the experience with laparoscopic cholecystectomy (Table 56–2).[19–29] A recent review of the literature describing the results of laparoscopic cholecystectomy in the United States showed an operative mortality rate of 0.06%.[29] In international series, the operative mortality rate has ranged from 0% to 0.15%. Conversion to an open procedure was required in 2.2% of patients in the United States and 3.6% to 8.2% of the international patients. Conversion is required most commonly when inflammation or adhesions make safe dissection of the porta hepatis difficult. Major morbidity occurs in approximately 5% of patients. In large series, bile duct injuries have occurred in 0.14% to 0.5% of patients. Operating time ranges from 1 to 2 hours. At first, most patients were observed overnight after laparoscopic cholecystectomy, but same-day discharge has become standard for elective cases. Most patients return to full activities, including work, within 1 week.

Randomized, prospective trials that compare the results of laparoscopic cholecystectomy with open cholecystectomy have not been performed in the United States, nor are any likely. Patient enthusiasm for the laparoscopic approach and the rapid acceptance of the procedure by surgeons has made direct, controlled comparison of the two procedures difficult. Nonrandomized data from the United States and small randomized trials from other countries support the contention

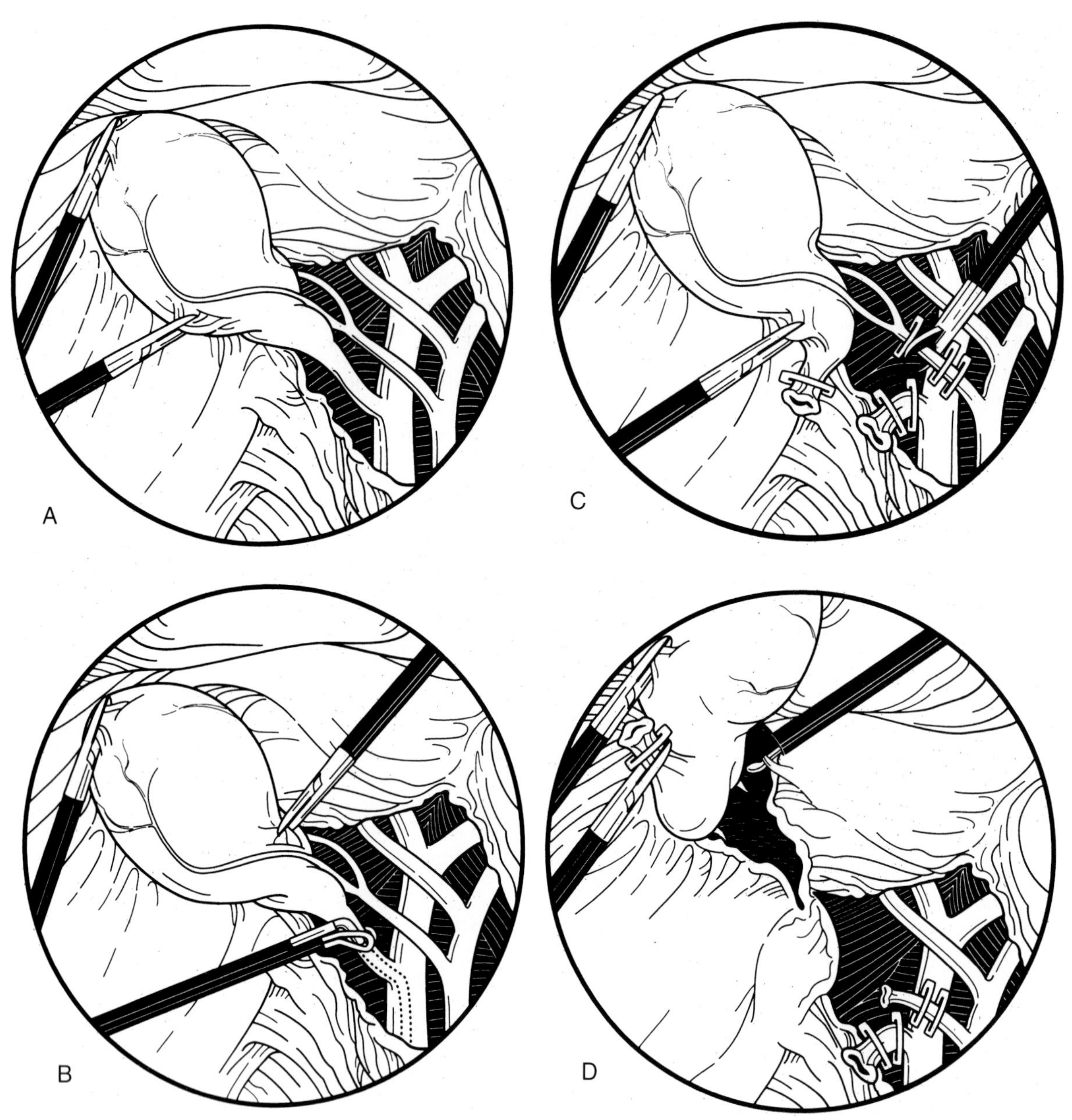

Figure 56–2. Steps in laparoscopic cholecystectomy. In all patients, the view is toward the liver through a telescope placed at the umbilicus. *A,* With appropriate retraction by the assistant surgeon, the structures of the hepatobiliary triangle are exposed. *B,* After identification and isolation of the cystic duct, a cholangiogram is obtained through direct catheterization of the cystic duct. *C,* Following cholangiography, the cystic duct and artery are ligated with small metal clips and divided. *D,* The gallbladder is dissected from the liver bed with electrocautery. The gallbladder is removed from the abdomen via the umbilical trocar incision.

that the laparoscopic approach is superior to the open approach.[30–33] In these analyses, the main benefits of the laparoscopic approach have included shortened hospital stay, decreased pain, reduced disability, and reduced costs. Population studies show a substantial decline in cholecystectomy-related mortality following the introduction of the laparoscopic technique (Table 56–3).[34]

In contrast to the perceived benefits of laparoscopic cholecystectomy over the open approach is the concern that complication rates, especially bile duct injury, are unacceptably high. Although the exact worldwide frequency of bile duct injury is not known, two lines of evidence suggest that the rate is declining. First, regional studies have demonstrated a decrease in the rate of bile duct injury as surgeon experience with laparoscopic cholecystectomy has increased (Fig. 56–3).[35] Curiously, however, the frequency of bile duct injury does not continue to decrease with increasing experience[36–38]; it plateaus. Although bile duct injuries are more common early in an individual surgeon's experience, such injuries still occur in the hands of seasoned surgeons, albeit at a lower rate. As the overall experience of surgeons has increased, the rate of bile duct injury for laparoscopic cholecystectomy has approximated the rate of bile duct injury seen with open cholecystectomy.[18] Second, the number of patients with bile duct injury treated at tertiary referral medical centers has declined since the early days of laparo-

Table 56–2 | **Experience with Laparoscopic Cholecystectomy**

GROUP	NO. OF PATIENTS	MORBIDITY RATE (%)	MORTALITY RATE (%)	BILE DUCT INJURY (%)	CONVERSION RATE (%)
Southern Surgeons[19]	1518	5.1	0.07	0.5	4.7
European[20]	1236	3.6	0	0.3	3.6
Louisville[21]	1983	4.4	0.1	0.25	4.5
SAGES[22]	1771	4.5	0.06	0.2	4.6
Canadian[23]	2201	4.3	0	0.14	4.3
Netherlands[24]	6076	4.3	0.12	0.86	6.8
Connecticut[25]	4640	8.6	0.13	0.32	6.9
British Isles[26]	3319	6.7	0.15	0.33	5.2
Brazil[160]	33,563	8.5	0.09	0.2	3.5
Hungary[27]	13,833	4.3	0.14	0.59	5.3
Switzerland[28]	10,174	10.4	0.2	0.31	8.2
United States[29]	114,005	5.4	0.06	0.5	2.2

scopic cholecystectomy.[39] The introduction of laparoscopic cholecystectomy in the United States was rapid and may have exceeded the capability of the medical educational system to train all practitioners adequately. The initial relatively high rates of bile duct injury have been ascribed to a "learning curve" and provide a cautionary example for other new technologies that are introduced into medical practice.

Of some concern are two recent reports that suggest use of laparoscopic cholecystectomy is increased when compared to historical rates of open cholecystectomy. First, in a defined health maintenance organization population in Pennsylvania, the rate of cholecystectomy increased from 1.35 per 1000 enrollees in 1988, just before the introduction of the laparoscopic approach, to 2.15 per 1000 enrollees in 1992, just after its introduction.[40] No significant changes in the rates of herniorrhaphy or appendectomy were observed during the same period. Similarly, statewide data from Maryland show that the rate of cholecystectomy increased from 1.69 per 1000 residents in 1987 to 1989 to 2.17 per 1000 residents in 1992.[34] The reasons for this increase in utilization are not yet clear. The consensus of experts in the field is that selection of patients for cholecystectomy should not be altered by the availability of the laparoscopic approach.[41]

INDICATIONS FOR CHOLECYSTECTOMY

Asymptomatic Gallstones

Decisions regarding the treatment of a patient with asymptomatic gallstones must be predicated on a knowledge of the natural history of the condition, as discussed in Chapter 55. In general, patients with asymptomatic gallstones should be reassured that life-threatening complications are rare and that symptoms related to the stones develop in only a minority of patients.[42–44] When symptoms develop in a previously asymptomatic patient, the initial presentation is most often as uncomplicated biliary colic. In fact, most patients in whom complications of gallstones develop have antecedent biliary colic.[1] Decision analysis has suggested that the risks of cholecystectomy approximate the potential benefit of preventing future serious sequelae of gallstones.[45] This determination was based on historical data regarding the outcome of open cholecystectomy. The rate of serious sequelae of gallstones was determined from long-term follow-up of a group of male faculty members at a major midwestern university. It is not known whether these data are applicable to a female patient considering laparoscopic cholecystectomy today. Nevertheless, it is doubtful that a strategy of prophylactic cholecystectomy in all asymptomatic patients with gallstones has any major advantage over the recommendation for cholecystectomy in symptomatic patients only.[46, 47]

In certain subgroups, the benefits of prophylactic cholecystectomy for asymptomatic gallstones may outweigh the

Table 56–3 | **Cholecystectomy-Related Mortality in Maryland before and after the Introduction of Laparoscopic Cholecystectomy**

VARIABLE	1989	1992	PERCENT CHANGE
Number of cholecystectomies	7416	9993	+35
Crude rate per 1000 population	1.57	2.04	+30
Operative mortality rate (%)	0.84	0.56	−33
Number of deaths	62	56	−10

Data adapted from Steiner CA, Bass EB, Talamini MA, et al: Surgical rates and operative mortality for open and laparoscopic cholecystectomy in Maryland. N Engl J Med 330:403–408, 1994.

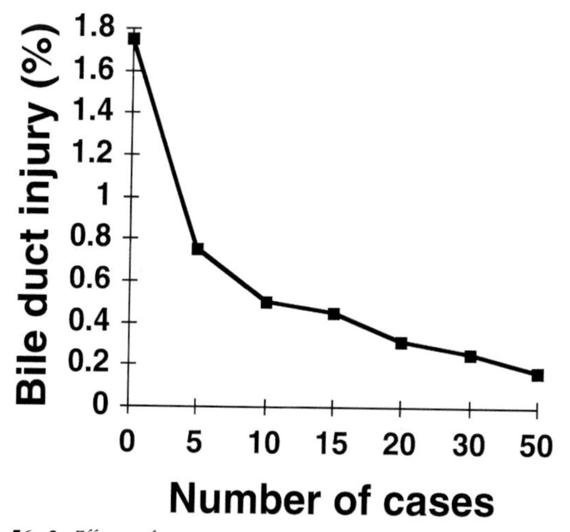

Figure 56–3. Effect of surgeon experience on risk of bile duct injury during laparoscopic cholecystectomy. The dramatic decline in risk as experience is gained has been attributed to a "learning curve." (Data from Moore MJ, Bennett CL: The learning curve for laparoscopic cholecystectomy. The Southern Surgeons Club. Am J Surg 170:55–59, 1995.)

risks. For example, American Indians appear to have a rate of gallstone-associated gallbladder cancer that is high enough to justify prophylactic cholecystectomy.[48] In patients who are morbidly obese or who have had a heart and lung transplant, complications of gallstone disease carry a high morbidity, and prophylactic cholecystectomy may be indicated.[49] Similarly, the risks of complications of gallstone disease in children may outweigh the risk of cholecystectomy. Renal transplant recipients with asymptomatic gallstones have a low risk of developing complications related to gallstone disease and therefore should not be considered for prophylactic cholecystectomy.[50, 51] (These issues are also discussed later.)

It formerly was thought that diabetic patients are particularly prone to developing both gallstones and complications resulting from the stones. The morbidity and mortality rates for diabetic patients who undergo emergency operations for complications of gallstone disease also appeared to be excessive. These perceptions have not been borne out when confounding variables, such as hyperlipidemia, obesity, cardiovascular disease, and renal insufficiency, are taken into account.[52] Thus, prophylactic cholecystectomy in an asymptomatic diabetic patient with gallstones does not appear warranted.[53]

Biliary Colic

Patient Selection

The majority of operations performed for biliary tract disorders are intended to relieve symptoms related to intermittent obstruction of the cystic duct by gallstones. The associated constellation of symptoms, which includes intermittent epigastric or right upper quadrant pain, nausea, and vomiting, has been termed *biliary colic*. Histologically, the gallbladders from patients who experience repeated attacks of biliary colic usually, but not always, show fibrosis and mononuclear cell infiltration characteristic of chronic cholecystitis. Complications of gallstones are more likely to develop in patients with biliary colic than in patients with asymptomatic stones. Therefore, cholecystectomy is indicated in these patients to relieve their symptoms and prevent complications of gallstones. As with any operation, these potential benefits must be weighed against the risk of surgery. Fortunately, the physiologic stress of cholecystectomy is minimal, and the operation may be undertaken safely even in the elderly and infirm. However, the risk of cholecystectomy rises substantially in the poorly compensated cirrhotic patient.[54] Surgery in this setting is justified only if the symptoms are severe, complications arise, or the severity of cirrhosis and portal hypertension is minimal.[55, 56]

Diagnostic Evaluation

The diagnosis of biliary colic is generally suspected from the clinical history (see Chapter 55). Few important findings specific to gallstone disease will be elicited on physical examination. Symptoms and signs of heart disease, especially congestive heart failure, should be sought during the preoperative evaluation, because heart failure increases the risk of surgery substantially.[57] Few routine preoperative laboratory tests are necessary, but liver biochemical testing should be performed to screen for unsuspected choledocholithiasis. Radiologic evaluation may be limited to ultrasonography in most patients with biliary colic. Ultrasound has high rates of sensitivity (95%) and specificity (98%) in this setting and may also be useful for detecting signs of gallbladder inflammation, including thickening of the wall, pericholecystic fluid, and dilation of the bile ducts. Ancillary tests, including oral cholecystography, magnetic resonance cholangiography (MRCP), endoscopic retrograde cholangiography, or cholecystokinin scintigraphy are used to confirm the diagnosis of gallstones in the unusual patient in whom gallstones are suspected but ultrasonography is negative. In patients with atypical symptoms, endoscopy or upper gastrointestinal contrast radiography is performed to exclude other disorders such as esophagitis or peptic ulcer disease.

Acute Cholecystitis

Treatment of the patient with acute cholecystitis begins with intravenous hydration and restoration of tissue perfusion and electrolyte balance. Vomiting is prominent in most patients, and nasogastric suction may be required. Intravenous antibiotics are indicated because culture specimens of the bile or gallbladder wall grow bacteria in over 40% of patients.[58] Cephalosporins are satisfactory for most patients. If gangrenous or emphysematous cholecystitis is suspected, an agent effective against anaerobic organisms should be added (see later).

Subsequent management depends on the severity of the attack, general condition of the patient, and confidence in the diagnosis. If cholecystitis is severe and complications such as perforation appear imminent, cholecystectomy should be undertaken early. Similarly, if the nature of the symptoms is uncertain, exploratory laparotomy may be indicated for diagnosis. Conversely, the elderly patient with concurrent illnesses such as congestive heart failure may benefit from an initial nonoperative approach.

In the past, the timing of cholecystectomy for the average patient with acute cholecystitis was controversial. Six randomized, controlled clinical trials have compared the strategies of early (within days of presentation) versus delayed (after 6 to 8 weeks) operation for acute cholecystitis (Table 56–4).[59–64] These trials indicate that, for the average patient, early operation is preferable because total hospitalization and costs are reduced, morbidity is less, and deaths related to progressive acute cholecystitis are prevented. Early operation does not appear to increase the major risks of cholecystectomy, such as bile duct injury, substantially.

Although acute cholecystitis was initially considered to be a contraindication to laparoscopic cholecystectomy, it now is clear that this approach is feasible in the majority of cases. Technical problems are occasionally encountered because of a gangrenous gallbladder, coagulopathy, or severe inflammation that obscures the structures of the hepatobiliary triangle. In these settings, an open approach is warranted. Cholangiography is particularly valuable with a laparoscopic approach to confirm the ductal anatomy. Current studies indicate that the benefits of laparoscopic cholecystectomy for biliary colic, especially decreased incisional pain, shortened hospital stay, and more rapid return to work, also apply when the operation is performed for acute cholecystitis.[65–67]

Table 56–4 | **Early versus Delayed Surgery for Acute Cholecystitis: Combined Results from Six Randomized Trials**

TIMING OF CHOLECYSTECTOMY	NO. OF PATIENTS	MORTALITY RATE (%)	BILE DUCT INJURIES	TOTAL MEAN HOSPITAL STAY (DAYS)	FAILURE OF REGIMEN*
Early	304	0	0	9.8	—
Delayed	293	2.0	0	17.1	20%

*Failure is defined as progressive acute symptoms requiring early surgery.
Data from references 59–64.

For a high-risk patient with severe concurrent illnesses, such as liver, pulmonary, or heart failure, tube cholecystostomy is preferable to cholecystectomy. Operative cholecystostomy has given way to a percutaneous approach under radiologic guidance in the majority of such cases.[68–70] Following recovery from the attack of acute cholecystitis, laparoscopic cholecystectomy should be performed if the patient's overall condition permits.[71] Alternatively, residual stones can be removed via the cholecystostomy, and subsequently the patient may be treated expectantly. However, approximately one half of all such patients will experience recurrent biliary symptoms.

Acute cholecystitis in the diabetic patient is associated with a significantly higher frequency of infectious complications, such as sepsis, than in nondiabetic controls.[72, 73] This observation supports the need for expeditious cholecystectomy in diabetic patients with acute cholecystitis. Similarly, acute cholecystitis in elderly patients may have a deceptively benign clinical presentation, but these patients have a high rate of developing empyema, gangrene, or perforation.[74–76] As in the diabetic population, early cholecystectomy is warranted in this group to ensure prompt control of infection.

Acalculous Cholecystitis

Acute cholecystitis may occur in the absence of gallstones. This clincal entity has been termed *acalculous cholecystitis* (see Chapter 58). Most commonly, acalculous cholecystitis occurs in a patient hospitalized for other serious illnesses, such as trauma, burns, or major surgery. It also may develop in outpatients, and in this setting elderly male patients with peripheral vascular disease appear to be at highest risk.[77] Acalculous cholecystitis also may complicate the treatment of patients with acquired immunodeficiency syndrome (see Chapter 28).[78]

The pathophysiology of acalculous cholecystitis is unclear, but biliary stasis caused by fasting, alterations in gallbladder blood flow, activation of factor XII, prostaglandins, and endotoxin all may play a role.[78–82] Sludge is generally present in the gallbladder and may obstruct the cystic duct. Gangrene, empyema, and perforation are more likely to complicate the course of acalculous cholecystitis than that of acute calculous cholecystitis. In some series, the frequency of these complications has approached 75%.[83, 84]

Cholecystectomy has been the mainstay of therapy for acalculous cholecystitis. Prompt removal of the gallbladder is particularly important when gangrene or empyema is suspected and when perforation is imminent. In some patients, however, the risk of surgery is high because of the gravity of their underlying illness. These patients may be treated initially with placement of a percutaneous tube cholecystostomy under ultrasound guidance. Most patients who are treated with tube cholecystostomy will recover. Those in whom evidence of intra-abdominal sepsis or persistent obstruction of the cystic duct on cholangiography develops require cholecystectomy (see also Chapter 61).

Emphysematous Cholecystitis

Emphysematous cholecystitis is an unusual condition characterized by infection of the gallbladder wall by gas-forming bacteria, particularly anaerobes. Diabetes mellitus has been cited as a risk factor.[83, 85] Gangrene and perforation commonly complicate the course of patients with emphysematous cholecystitis. The treatment of emphysematous cholecystitis is prompt cholecystectomy following restoration of fluid and electrolyte balance. Antibiotics are indicated, with coverage directed specifically against gram-negative rods and anaerobic bacteria.

Gallstone Pancreatitis

The pathophysiology and clinical presentation of gallstone pancreatitis have been discussed in Chapters 48 and 55. Initial treatment of patients with gallstone pancreatitis includes appropriate fluid resuscitation, bowel rest, and monitoring for complications. The majority of patients have a relatively mild illness that clinically resolves within 1 week with this conservative treatment strategy.

The presence of cholelithiasis should be determined by ultrasonography early in the course of acute pancreatitis. If cholelithiasis is present, laparoscopic cholecystectomy should be performed before discharge in the typical patient. In the past, cholecystectomy early in the course of gallstone pancreatitis carried significant risk. For that reason, the timing of cholecystectomy was delayed for 1 to 2 months to allow resolution of the inflammatory process. A major disadvantage of this delayed approach is that up to one half of the patients will have further attacks of pancreatitis during the observation period. It is now recognized that cholecystectomy may be performed safely during the same hospitalization after the clinical signs of pancreatitis have resolved.[86–88] This approach shortens the total duration of illness and hospitalization. Additionally, it prevents subsequent recurrent pancreatitis. Cholangiography should be performed during the cholecystectomy to exclude residual common bile duct stones. Laparoscopic cholecystectomy is safe in patients with gallstone pancreatitis.[89, 90]

A small group of patients with severe gallstone pancreatitis appear to benefit from early endoscopic sphincterotomy and clearance of the common bile duct.[91, 92] Common bile duct stones are found in a substantial fraction of patients with severe gallstone pancreatitis when sphincterotomy is performed within the first 24 to 48 hours of hospitalization. The morbidity of this approach is less than that of early surgery with common bile duct exploration. Most patients undergoing endoscopic sphincterotomy for gallstone pancreatitis should have elective cholecystectomy when the pancreatitis has subsided. In elderly patients, or those at high risk for surgery, cholecystectomy may be deferred, but further symptoms of gallstone disease may be expected in up to 25% on long-term follow-up.[93] The risk of recurrent symptoms is even higher in patients with cystic duct obstruction at cholangiography.[94]

Special Problems

Management of Biliary Colic During Pregnancy

Gallbladder disease occasionally is first noted or more troublesome during pregnancy. The most common clinical presentations during pregnancy are worsening biliary colic and acute cholecystitis. Jaundice and acute pancreatitis caused by choledocholithiasis are less common presentations. Radiologic evaluation of symptoms suggestive of biliary tract disease can almost always be limited to ultrasonography. The potential teratogenic effects of conventional radiography and radionuclide scanning make routine use of these techniques unjustified in the pregnant patient.

Therapeutic options for gallstone disease in pregnancy are limited. In the past, cholecystectomy during pregnancy had been discouraged because of fear of fetal loss. Complications such as spontaneous abortion and preterm labor were common in operated women in the first and third trimesters of gestation, respectively. Recent improvements in anesthesia and tocolytic agents appear to have made cholecystectomy during pregnancy safer. Several series of patients published in recent years have suggested that cholecystectomy may be undertaken during pregnancy with minimal fetal and maternal morbidity.[95–97] Pregnancy was formerly considered to be an absolute contraindication to a laparoscopic approach to cholecystectomy because of concern for potential trocar injury to the uterus and the unknown effects of pneumoperitoneum on the fetal circulation. Recent case series suggest that laparoscopic cholecystectomy may be performed safely.[95, 97] Until more is known about the relative safety of this approach, however, laparoscopic cholecystectomy during pregnancy should be considered only when absolutely necessary and in a carefully controlled clinical setting.

Management of Childhood Gallstone Disease

Gallstone disease in the pediatric population appears to be increasing in frequency. Chronic hemolysis leading to pigment gallstones is the cause in approximately 20% of patients.[98] A history of prolonged fasting in a patient on total parenteral nutritional support is an increasingly important risk factor.[99] Ileal disease and previous bowel resection increase the risk of gallstone development. The management of childhood cholelithiasis must take into account the type of stone (pigment or cholesterol), presence or absence of symptoms, and additional factors such as total parenteral nutrition. Cholecystectomy is indicated for all symptomatic patients. The management of asymptomatic gallstones is less clear. Gallstones in infants on total parenteral nutrition occasionally resolve following reinstitution of oral feedings. It thus seems reasonable to observe an asymptomatic infant in this setting for up to 12 months. Persistent gallstones and asymptomatic pigment stones (that do not resolve spontaneously) are best treated with cholecystectomy. Laparoscopic cholecystectomy is feasible in the pediatric population.[100]

Mirizzi Syndrome

Mirizzi syndrome refers to stricture and obstruction of the common hepatic duct as a result of compression by a gallstone impacted in the cystic duct. Two types of Mirizzi syndrome have been described.[101] In type I, the hepatic duct is compressed by a large stone impacted in the cystic duct or Hartman's pouch. Associated inflammation may contribute to the stricture. In type II, the calculus has eroded into the hepatic duct to produce a cholecystocholedochal fistula. The syndrome is rare, occurring in 1% of all patients undergoing cholecystectomy. Most patients present with repeated bouts of abdominal pain, fever, and jaundice. Ultrasonography generally reveals gallstones in a contracted gallbladder and moderate intrahepatic ductal dilation. Endoscopic retrograde cholangiography is useful in delineating the hepatic duct anatomy. The stricture may be mistaken for a bile duct tumor.[102]

Recognition of Mirizzi syndrome is important during a difficult cholecystectomy to reduce the likelihood of hepatic duct injury. Management of type I strictures includes cholecystectomy with or without common bile duct exploration. When inflammation is severe and identification of the anatomy is difficult, partial cholecystectomy with postoperative endoscopic sphincterotomy to ensure clearance of bile duct stones is preferable. Management of type II strictures complicated by a cholecystocholedochal fistula is best accomplished by partial cholecystectomy and cholecystocholedochoduodenostomy.[103, 104] Frozen section examination of the gallbladder wall may be necessary to exclude carcinoma. Rarely, a Roux-en-Y hepaticojejunostomy is required to repair large defects in the common hepatic duct.

Gallstone Ileus

Gallstone ileus is an unusual form of bowel obstruction caused by a large gallstone impacted in the intestinal lumen. It represents a true mechanical obstruction rather than a defect in motility, as the name would suggest. The median age of patients is over 70 years and most are women. Gallstone ileus is the cause of intestinal obstruction in less than 1% of patients under age 70, but in nearly 5% of those over age 70.[105] Symptoms are typical of mechanical intestinal obstruction, including crampy abdominal pain, vomiting, and abdominal distention. Only a minority of patients have symptoms suggestive of acute cholecystitis, but one half have a history of gallstones.[106] Liver biochemical test results are abnormal in 40% of cases, but overt jaundice is rare. Abdominal radiographs reveal an intestinal gas pattern compatible with intestinal obstruction in most patients. Pneumobilia is present in approximately one half of patients, and the aberrant gallstone is visible in a minority. Upper or lower gastrointestinal contrast studies occasionally may identify the site of obstruction or the fistula but are unnecessary in most cases. Ultrasonography is useful to confirm the presence of cholelithiasis and may identify the fistula.

The pathophysiology of gallstone ileus involves erosion of a gallstone, which is generally over 2.5 cm in diameter, into the intestinal lumen via a cholecystoenteric fistula. Most commonly, the fistula occurs in the duodenum and less often in the colon. As the gallstone is passed down the length of the gut, it intermittently obstructs the lumen. Characteristically, complete obstruction occurs in the ileum, where the lumen is narrowest. The obstruction has been described as "tumbling," because the symptoms wax and wane during the stone's distal passage.

Management should be directed initially at restoration of fluid and electrolyte balance, followed by exploratory laparotomy. Removing the stone via a small enterotomy relieves the obstruction. A search should be made for additional stones. Bowel resection is necessary only for intestinal perforation or ischemia. It is not necessary to deal with the cholecystoenteric fistula at the initial operation, because many such fistulas close spontaneously.[107] Cholecystectomy and closure of the fistula are indicated, on an elective basis, if symptoms of chronic cholecystitis persist on follow-up. The mortality rate in this high-risk patient population is high, with an average of 15% to 18%. Recurrent gallstone ileus occurs in approximately 5% of patients.

Incidental Cholecystectomy

Occasionally, gallstones are identified unexpectedly before or during another operation; when this happens, consideration is given to incidental cholecystectomy in addition to the original, planned procedure. The rationale for incidental cholecystectomy is to prevent the later development of symptomatic gallstone disease, including early postoperative acute cholecystitis. Conversely, addition of a cholecystectomy would be expected to increase the risk of postoperative complications somewhat. The decision to proceed with an incidental cholecystectomy is based on an assessment of the expected benefit versus risk; some data are available to assist in quantifying these factors.

In the typical patient, asymptomatic stones tend to remain asymptomatic. The rate of development of symptoms on long-term follow-up ranges from 18% to 35%.[44, 46, 47] Certain groups, however, are at higher risk. In morbidly obese patients, for example, gallstones tend to have a more aggressive natural history, making incidental cholecystectomy at the time of gastric bypass surgery appealing.[108] Patients with large (>2.5 cm) gallstones and those with calcification of the gallbladder wall (porcelain gallbladder) have a greater risk for the development of acute cholecystitis and gallbladder cancer and warrant incidental cholecystectomy.[109, 110] Patients with sickle cell disease and chronic hemolysis are at risk for the development of pigment gallstones, and it may be difficult to distinguish the clinical presentation of a sickle cell crisis from that of acute cholecystitis (see Chapter 82). Incidental cholecystectomy is indicated to avoid this dilemma.[111] Similarly, patients with other hemolytic anemias, such as beta thalassemia, are at high risk for the development of gallstones, and a high percentage of such patients become symptomatic.[112] Cholecystectomy appears warranted for asymptomatic stones if splenectomy is considered for the hemolytic anemia. Finally, laparotomy for other indications is associated with a high frequency of postoperative biliary symptoms if a gallbladder that contains stones is left in situ. In one recent study, of 68 patients with asymptomatic gallstones who underwent laparotomy, 54% experienced biliary symptoms postoperatively and 22% required cholecystectomy within 30 days.[113]

The risk of adding an incidental cholecystectomy to another abdominal procedure appears to be low.[114, 115] If the patient is otherwise in reasonable health, the primary operation has proceeded smoothly, and exposure is adequate, incidental cholecystectomy can be done safely with a number of other operations.[116, 117] The risk does not appear to be increased in the elderly. It appears, however, that in some "clean" operations, the risk of postoperative wound infection may be increased by the addition of an incidental cholecystectomy.[118]

SURGERY FOR CHOLEDOCHOLITHIASIS

Choledocholithiasis may be detected concurrently with gallbladder stones during an evaluation of biliary tract symptoms, intraoperatively in the course of cholecystectomy, or after cholecystectomy. Several management options are available, including dissolution therapy, interventional radiologic and endoscopic techniques, and surgery (see Chapters 57 and 61). The decision regarding which management strategy is most appropriate for a given patient depends on the clinical context in which the stones have been identified (i.e., jaundice, cholangitis, pancreatitis, asymptomatic), the status of the gallbladder, and the age and general condition of the patient. Additional factors to be considered are the expertise of the available surgical, endoscopic, and radiologic specialists.

Choledocholithiasis Known Before Surgery

When choledocholithiasis is known to exist before surgery, an acceptable option is to clear the common bile duct with an initial endoscopic sphincterotomy, followed by laparoscopic cholecystectomy.[119, 120] Alternative approaches include open or laparoscopic cholecystectomy with common bile duct exploration. The results of small, randomized trials suggest that there are no important differences in efficacy and safety between precholecystectomy endoscopic sphincterotomy and open common bile duct exploration.[121, 122] A more recent randomized trial has shown equivalent efficacy and safety between precholecystectomy endoscopic sphincterotomy and laparoscopic cholecystectomy with laparoscopic

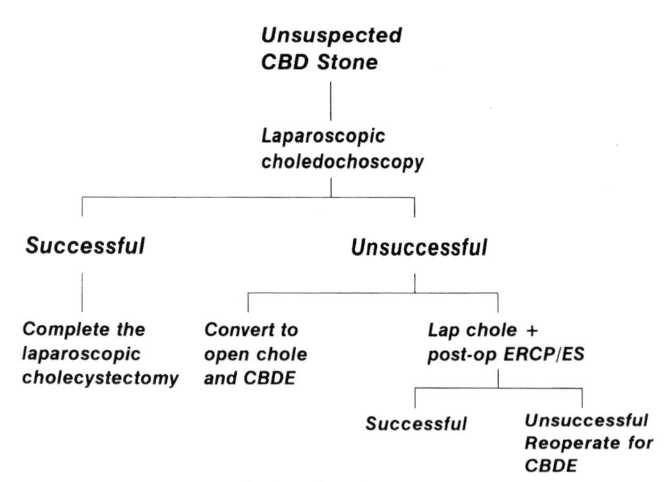

Figure 56–4. A suggested algorithm for the management of common bile duct (CBD) stones found unexpectedly during laparoscopic cholecystectomy. CBDE, common bile duct exploration; ERCP/ES, endoscopic retrograde cholangiopancreatography/endoscopic sphincterotomy.

bile duct exploration.[123] The laparoscopic approach resulted in fewer procedures and a shorter overall hospital stay.

Choledocholithiasis Identified During Cholecystectomy

If unsuspected choledocholithiasis is identified by cholangiography during laparoscopic cholecystectomy, three options are available: (1) conversion to an open operation with common bile duct exploration; (2) laparoscopic common bile duct exploration; or (3) completion of the laparoscopic cholecystectomy followed by postoperative endoscopic sphincterotomy and stone extraction. An algorithm of these options is shown in Figure 56–4. Factors influencing the decision include the number and location of common duct stones, associated ductal pathology, and skill and experience of the involved surgeon and endoscopist. Completion of the laparoscopic cholecystectomy followed by postoperative endoscopic sphincterotomy is satisfactory for most patients and has the advantage of preserving the minimally invasive approach. It must be recognized, however, that endoscopic sphincterotomy may be technically unsuccessful in 5% to 10% of patients, even in the hands of a skilled endoscopist, and complete bile duct clearance of stones is possible in only 70% to 80% of cases.[123–125] In this small group of patients, a third procedure may be required. Increasing experience has shown that laparoscopic common bile duct exploration is safe and effective. Stone clearance rates average 95%, with an operative mortality rate of 0.5%.[123, 125–129] Laparoscopic common bile duct exploration compares favorably to endoscopic sphincterotomy with regard to efficacy, cost, and safety.[123, 125, 126]

Choledocholithiasis Identified After Cholecystectomy

Choledocholithiasis identified in patients who have undergone cholecystectomy is best managed with endoscopic sphincterotomy and stone extraction. If a T-tube is still present from a recent common bile duct exploration, radiologic extraction of the stone via the T-tube tract is usually possible. These techniques are discussed in Chapter 61. Surgery is rarely required in this situation.

BILE DUCT STRICTURE

The majority of benign bile duct strictures are the result of iatrogenic injury during cholecystectomy. A minority are the sequelae of chronic pancreatitis, sclerosing cholangitis, trauma, hepatic transplantation, and choledocholithiasis. Operative injury to the bile duct during cholecystectomy may occur as a result of inaccurate placement of clips or sutures to control hemorrhage, misidentification of the common bile duct for the cystic duct, and tenting of the common bile duct during ligation of the cystic duct. During laparoscopic cholecystectomy, an additional hazard is excessive use of cautery or laser to control troublesome hemorrhage.[130] These injuries commonly occur during an otherwise uneventful cholecystectomy and may not be noticed by the surgeon.

Bile duct injury has three patterns of presentation. If the bile duct has been completely occluded, jaundice develops rapidly in the early postoperative period after cholecystectomy. In some patients, the injury is manifested by the development of bile ascites, often in association with an infected bile collection in the subhepatic space. In other patients, partial duct obstruction leads to intermittent episodes of pain, jaundice, or cholangitis, usually within 2 years of the cholecystectomy. In the early postoperative period following laparoscopic cholecystectomy, the clinician should suspect the possibility of bile duct injury in any patient with persistent abdominal pain. The differential diagnosis of cholangitis in a patient with a history of cholecystectomy is mainly bile duct stricture and choledocholithiasis. Stricture and choledocholithiasis may be difficult to differentiate on clinical grounds because the symptoms, signs, and results of liver biochemical tests may be identical.

The radiologic evaluation of a patient with a suspected bile duct stricture usually begins with ultrasonography to identify dilated ducts or a subhepatic fluid collection. In the early postoperative period, a ^{99m}Tc-labeled radionuclide scan may expeditiously and noninvasively demonstrate patency of the biliary tree and exclude a bile leak. If these studies suggest bile injury, endoscopic retrograde cholangiography (ERCP) is indicated to define the lesion. The initial goals in management include control of the subhepatic infection, usually via percutaneous drainage of any fluid collection, and biliary drainage, either via the endoscopic or transhepatic route (see Chapter 61).

Most patients with a benign postoperative stricture are best treated with surgical repair. Although numerous operations have been described, the best results are obtained with resection of the stricture and an end-to-side Roux-en-Y choledochojejunostomy or hepaticojejunostomy. The principles of a successful repair include complete dissection of the strictured segment, a tension-free anastomosis, accurate mucosa-to-mucosa approximation with fine absorbable suture material to unscarred proximal ductal tissue, and preservation of the ductal blood supply. The mortality rate of operations to correct benign biliary strictures averages less than 2% in modern series.[131–134] The risk of surgery is related directly to the presence of factors such as cirrhosis, renal failure, uncontrolled cholangitis, age, and malnutrition.[135, 136] The long-term results of biliary reconstruction for a benign bile duct stricture are good, with a cure achieved in 85% to 98% of patients. Results are worse with high strictures and in the setting of cirrhosis. In high strictures, special techniques may be necessary to obtain healthy ductal tissue uninvolved in the inflammatory process for anastomosis. Recurrent strictures pose technical difficulties, but satisfactory results are still achieved in approximately 75% of patients.[131, 132, 137]

Postoperative strictures may be treated with endoscopic or percutaneous balloon dilatation with or without stent placement. No randomized, prospective trials comparing surgical, endoscopic, and radiologic approaches have been performed. In one nonrandomized trial, long-term bile duct patency was achieved in 88% of patients treated with hepaticojejunostomy versus 55% of patients treated with balloon dilatation.[138] No procedure-related mortality was observed. In view of the excellent long-term results of hepaticojejunostomy and its low mortality rate in experienced hands, surgery should be offered as the initial treatment to all fit patients with a bile duct stricture. Nonoperative management is best reserved for patients with biliary cirrhosis, significant comorbid illness, or high recurrent strictures.

Table 56–5 | **Causes of Pain after Cholecystectomy**

Causes
Biliary
Choledocholithiasis
Biliary stricture
Cystic duct remnant
Papillary stenosis
Sphincter of Oddi dysfunction
Biliary tract malignancy
Choledochocele
Pancreatic
Pancreatitis
Pancreatic pseudocyst
Pancreatic malignancy
Pancreas divisum
Other Gastrointestinal Disorders
Gastroesophageal reflux disease
Esophageal motility disorders
Peptic ulcer disease
Mesenteric ischemia
Intestinal adhesions
Intestinal malignancy
Irritable bowel syndrome
Extraintestinal Disorders
Psychiatric disorders
Coronary artery disease
Intercostal neuritis
Wound neuroma
Neurologic disorders

POSTCHOLECYSTECTOMY SYNDROME

The *postcholecystectomy syndrome* refers to the occurrence of abdominal symptoms following cholecystectomy. Although widely cited in the medical literature, the term is inaccurate in that it encompasses a wide spectrum of biliary and nonbiliary disorders that are rarely related to the operation itself. The frequency of these symptoms after cholecystectomy ranges from 5% to 40%.[2, 139, 140] The most common postoperative symptoms noted are dyspepsia, flatulence, and bloating, which usually antedate the cholecystectomy. Other patients have persistence of right upper quadrant or epigastric abdominal pain. A small percentage of patients with postcholecystectomy symptoms present with severe abdominal pain, jaundice, or emesis. Investigation is much more likely to reveal a distinct, treatable cause in these latter patients than in those with mild or nonspecific symptoms. In patients with severe symptoms, bile peritonitis secondary to iatrogenic biliary injury must be suspected.[141]

The differential diagnosis of symptoms following cholecystectomy includes extraintestinal disorders such as cardiac ischemia, nonbiliary gastrointestinal conditions such as peptic ulcer disease, biliary disorders such as choledocholithiasis, functional illnesses such as irritable bowel syndrome, and psychiatric disorders. The breadth of possibilities is described in Table 56–5. The clinician must carefully consider the possibility of nonbiliary causes of pain and direct the evaluation appropriately. The most common biliary causes are described below.

Choledocholithiasis

Common bile duct stones are the most common cause of postcholecystectomy symptoms. They may be residual stones overlooked at the time of cholecystectomy or, less frequently, stones that have formed primarily in the duct. The natural history of choledocholithiasis is not known, but it is clear that in some patients these stones can cause pain similar to biliary colic, jaundice, pancreatitis, or cholangitis. The diagnosis of choledocholithiasis will be suggested by the clinical picture. Levels of liver biochemical tests, particularly the serum alkaline phosphatase, may be elevated. Ultrasonography may reveal indirect signs, such as a dilated common bile duct, but direct visualization of the stone is uncommon. MRCP and ERCP are important diagnostic tools to confirm the presence of ductal stones and exclude other possibilities such as bile duct stricture or tumor. ERCP has the added advantage of allowing endoscopic sphincterotomy with stone extraction, which is curative in most patients.[142]

Cystic Duct Remnant

In some patients, the cause of postcholecystectomy symptoms has been attributed to pathology in the cystic duct remnant.[143, 144] The described abnormalities include cystic duct stones, fistulas, granulomas, and neuromas. Associated common bile duct stones are common. Although the existence of such a syndrome has been controversial, in one randomized trial, complete excision of the cystic duct during cholecystectomy was associated with fewer postoperative sequelae than was a standard operative technique in which a portion of the cystic duct was left in situ.[145] ERCP is useful in delineating the biliary anatomy in patients with suspected cystic duct remnant pathology. The treatment of a cystic duct remnant is excision.

Sphincter of Oddi Dysfunction

As many as 10% of patients with postcholecystectomy pain are found to have a structural or functional abnormality of the sphincter of Oddi (see also Chapter 53).[146–148] Structural problems have been referred to as papillary stenosis, which is characterized by a fixed narrowing of the sphincter in association with an elevated basal sphincter pressure. The stenosis may result from trauma caused by passage of gallstones, instrumentation, pancreatitis, or infection. Functional, or motility, disorders have been referred to as biliary or sphincter of Oddi dyskinesia and ampullary spasm. Biliary manometry in these patients reveals an elevated sphincter pressure caused by abnormal tonic or phasic smooth muscle contractions. The etiology of this disorder is unknown. In a recent study of patients with a postcholecystectomy pain syndrome thought to be secondary to sphincter of Oddi dysfunction, many were shown to have duodenal hyperalgesia in response to duodenal stretch.[149]

Clinical manifestations of sphincter of Oddi dysfunction include biliary-type pain, jaundice, and pancreatitis. ERCP findings of a dilated common bile duct and delayed (>45 minutes) drainage of contrast medium from the common bile duct are typical. These cholangiographic findings coupled with biliary-type pain and repeatedly abnormal liver biochemical tests are highly reliable in predicting successful treatment.[150] In patients in whom the diagnosis is not as clear, biliary manometry is indicated. The treatment is endoscopic sphincterotomy. Selected patients may require transduodenal sphincteroplasty, septoplasty, or both.[151]

GALLSTONES, CHOLECYSTECTOMY, AND CANCER

A number of reports have demonstrated associations between either gallstones or cholecystectomy and the development of cancers in organs as diverse as the gallbladder, bile ducts, stomach, colon, breast, and uterus. It is not clear that any causal relationship exists between gallbladder disease or its treatment and the development of these malignancies. It is possible that shared environmental factors, perhaps dietary, influence the rates of all these diseases. On the other hand, patients with gallstones have alterations in bile that could influence the development of carcinoma, and cholecystectomy increases the enterohepatic circulation of bile acids, which increases mucosal exposure to potentially carcinogenic secondary bile acids such as deoxycholate.[152]

Gallstones and Biliary Tract Cancer

The strongest association between gallstones and cancer lies in cancers of the biliary tree itself, particularly gallbladder carcinoma. Most patients with gallbladder cancer have gallstones, and epidemiologic data show a strong relationship between the two diseases. The risk of gallbladder cancer is greatest in patients with large gallstones and in American Indians.[110, 153, 154] A weaker statistical association exists between gallstones and bile duct cancer, but a causal relationship is suggested by a reduction of risk in patients who have undergone cholecystectomy as compared with those with untreated gallstones (see also Chapter 60).[155, 156]

Gallstones and Colorectal Cancer

Studies from the early 1980s identified a statistical association between cholecystectomy and the subsequent development of colorectal cancer, particularly in the right colon.[157–159] The magnitude of the risk of colorectal cancer, although statistically significant, was low (relative risk 1.5–2.0) compared to that for patients with intact gallbladders. Subsequent studies have disputed the association or attributed it to the gallstones rather than the cholecystectomy.[160] These findings should not represent a deterrent to cholecystectomy in a patient with clear indications for the procedure.

REFERENCES

1. Glasgow RE, Cho M, Hutter MM, Mulvihill SJ: The spectrum and cost of complicated gallstone disease in California. Arch Surg 135: 1021–1027, 2000.
2. Gilliland TM, Traverso LW: Modern standards for comparison of cholecystectomy with alternative treatments for symptomatic cholelithiasis with emphasis on long term relief of symptoms. Surg Gynecol Obstet 170:39–44, 1990.
3. Heuer GJ: The factors leading to death in operations upon the gallbladder and bile ducts. Ann Surg 99:881–892, 1934.
4. Glenn F, Hayes DM: The causes of death following biliary tract surgery for nonmalignant disease. Surg Gynecol Obstet 94:282–296, 1952.
5. McSherry CK, Glenn F: The incidence and causes of death following surgery for nonmalignant biliary tract disease. Ann Surg 191:271–275, 1980.
6. Roslyn JJ, Binns GS, Hughes EF, et al: Open cholecystectomy. A contemporary analysis of 42,474 patients. Ann Surg 218:129–137, 1993.
7. Bredesen J, Jorgensen T, Andersen TF, et al: Early postoperative mortality following cholecystectomy in the entire female population of Denmark, 1977–1981. World J Surg 16:530–535, 1992.
8. Arnold DJ: 28,621 cholecystectomies in Ohio. Results of a survey in Ohio hospitals by the Gallbladder Survey Committee, Ohio Chapter, American College of Surgeons. Am J Surg 119:714–717, 1970.
9. Morgenstern L, Wong L, Berci G: Twelve hundred open cholecystectomies before the laparoscopic era. A standard for comparison. Arch Surg 127:400–403, 1992.
10. Hermann RE: A plea for a safer technique of cholecystectomy. Surgery 79:609–611, 1976.
11. Kune GA: Bile duct injury during cholecystectomy: Causes, prevention and surgical repair in 1979. Aust NZ J Surg 49:35–40, 1979.
12. Clavien PA, Sanabria JR, Mentha G, et al: Recent results of elective open cholecystectomy in a North American and a European center. Comparison of complications and risk factors. Ann Surg 216:618–626, 1992.
13. Andren-Sandberg A, Johansson S, Bengmark S: Accidental lesions of the common bile duct at cholecystectomy. II. Results of treatment. Ann Surg 201:452–455, 1985.
14. Rice DC, Memon MA, Jamison RL: Long-term consequences of intraoperative spillage of bile and gallstones during laparoscopic cholecystectomy. J Gastrointest Surg 1:85–91, 1997.
15. Schafer M, Suter C, Dlaiber C, et al: Spilled gallstones after laparoscopic cholecystectomy. A relevant problem? A retrospective analysis of 10,174 laparoscopic cholecystectomies. Surg Endosc 12:305–309, 1998.
16. Gregg RO: The case for selective cholangiography. Am J Surg 155: 540–545, 1988.
17. Kakos GS, Tompkins RK, Turnipseed W, Zollinger RM: Operative cholangiography during routine cholecystectomy: A review of 3,012 cases. Arch Surg 104:484–488, 1972.
18. Fletcher DR, Hobbs MS, Tan P, et al: Complications of cholecystectomy: Risks of the laparoscopic approach and protective effects of operative cholangiography: A population-based study. Ann Surg 229: 449–457, 1999.
19. Anonymous: A prospective analysis of 1518 laparoscopic cholecystectomies. N Engl J Med 324:1073–1078, 1991.
20. Cuschieri A, Dubois F, Mouiel J, et al: The European experience with laparoscopic cholecystectomy. Am J Surg 161:385–387, 1991.
21. Larson GM, Vitale GC, Casey J, et al: Multipractice analysis of laparoscopic cholecystectomy in 1,983 patients. Am J Surg 163:221–226, 1992.

22. Berci G, Sackier JM: SAGES laparoscopic cholecystectomy study [abstract]. Surg Endosc 6:97, 1992.
23. Litwin DE, Girotti MJ, Poulin EC, et al: Laparoscopic cholecystectomy: Trans-Canada experience with 2201 cases. Can J Surg 35:291–296, 1992.
24. Go PM, Schol F, Gouma DJ: Laparoscopic cholecystectomy in The Netherlands. Br J Surg 80:1180–1183, 1993.
25. Orlando Rd, Russell JC, Lynch J, Mattie A: Laparoscopic cholecystectomy. A statewide experience. The Connecticut Laparoscopic Cholecystectomy Registry. Arch Surg 128:494–498, 1994.
26. Dunn D, Nair R, Fowler S, McCloy R: Laparoscopic cholecystectomy in England and Wales: Results of an audit by the Royal College of Surgeons in England. Ann R Coll Surg Engl 76:269–275, 1994.
27. Ihasz M, Hung CM, Regoly-Merei J, et al: Complications of laparoscopic cholecystectomy in Hungary: A multicentre study of 13,833 patients. Eur J Surg 163:267-274, 1997.
28. Z'Graggen K, Wehrli H, Metzger A, et al: Complications of laparoscopic cholecystectomy in Switzerland. A prospective 3-year study of 10,174 patients. Swiss Association of Laparoscopic and Thoracoscopic Surgery. Surg Endosc 12:1303–1310, 1998.
29. MacFadyen Jr BV, Vecchio R, Ricardo AE, Mathis CR: Bile duct injury after laparoscopic cholecystectomy. The United States experience. Surg Endosc 12:315–321, 1998.
30. McMahon AJ, Russell IT, Baxter JN, et al: Laparoscopic versus minilaparotomy cholecystectomy: A randomised trial. Lancet 343:135–138, 1994.
31. Trondsen E, Reiertsen O, Andersen OK, Kjaersgaard P: Laparoscopic and open cholecystectomy. A prospective, randomized study. Eur J Surg 159:217–221, 1993.
32. Soper NJ, Barteau JA, Clayman RV, et al: Comparison of early postoperative results for laparoscopic versus standard open cholecystectomy. Surg Gynecol Obstet 174:114–118, 1992.
33. Barkun JS, Barkun AN, Sampalis JS, et al: Randomised controlled trial of laparoscopic versus mini cholecystectomy. The McGill Gallstone Treatment Group. Lancet 340(8828):1116–1119, 1992.
34. Steiner CA, Bass EB, Talamini MA, et al: Surgical rates and operative mortality for open and laparoscopic cholecystectomy in Maryland. N Engl J Med 330:403–408, 1994.
35. Moore MJ, Bennett CL: The learning curve for laparoscopic cholecystectomy. The Southern Surgeons Club. Am J Surg 170:55–59, 1995.
36. Windsor JA, Pong J: Laparoscopic biliary injury: More than a learning curve problem. Aust NZ J Surg 68:186–189, 1998.
37. Richardson MC, Bell G, Fullarton GM: Incidence and nature of bile duct injuries following laparoscopic cholecystectomy: An audit of 5913 cases. West of Scotland Laparoscopic Cholecystectomy Audit Group. Br J Surg 83:1356–1360, 1996.
38. Jones-Monahan K, Gruenberg JC: Bile duct injuries during laparoscopic cholecystectomy: A community's experience. Am Surg 64: 638–642, 1998.
39. Woods MS, Traverso LW, Kozarek RA, et al: Characteristics of biliary tract complications during laparoscopic cholecystectomy: A multi-institutional study. Am J Surg 167:27–33, 1994.
40. Legorreta AP, Silber JH, Costantino GN, et al: Increased cholecystectomy rate after the introduction of laparoscopic cholecystectomy. JAMA 270:1429–1432, 1993.
41. Anonymous: NIH Consensus conference. Gallstones and laparoscopic cholecystectomy. JAMA 269:1018–1024, 1993.
42. McSherry CK, Ferstenberg H, Calhoun WF, et al: The natural history of diagnosed gallstone disease in symptomatic and asymptomatic patients. Ann Surg 202:59–63, 1985.
43. Gracie WA, Ransohoff DF: The natural history of silent gallstones: The innocent gallstone is not a myth. N Engl J Med 307:798–800, 1982.
44. Attili AF, De Santis A, Capri R, et al: The natural history of gallstones: The GREPCO experience. The GREPCO Group. Hepatology 21:655–660, 1995.
45. Ransohoff DF, Gracie WA, Wolfenson LB, Neuhauser D: Prophylactic cholecystectomy or expectant management for silent gallstones. A decision analysis to assess survival. Ann Intern Med 99:199–204, 1983.
46. Ransohoff DF, Gracie WA: Treatment of gallstones. Ann Intern Med 119:606–619, 1993.
47. Gibney EJ: Asymptomatic gallstones. Br J Surg 77:368–372, 1990.
48. Weiss KM, Ferrell RE, Hanis CL, Styne PN: Genetics and epidemiology of gallbladder disease in New World native peoples. Am J Hum Genet 36:1259–1278, 1984.
49. Gupta D, Sakorafas GH, McGregor CG, et al: Management of biliary tract disease in heart and lung transplant patients. Surgery 128:641–649, 2000.
50. Melvin WS, Meier DJ, Elkhammas EA, et al: Prophylactic cholecystectomy is not indicated following renal transplantation. Am J Surg 175:317–319, 1998.
51. Greenstein SM, Katz S, Sun S, et al: Prevalence of asymptomatic cholelithiasis and risk of acute cholecystitis after kidney transplantation. Transplantation 63:1030–1032, 1997.
52. Sandler RS, Maule WF, Baltus ME: Factors associated with postoperative complications in diabetics after biliary tract surgery. Gastroenterology 91:157–162, 1986.
53. Friedman LS, Roberts MS, Brett AS, Marton KI: Management of asymptomatic gallstones in the diabetic patient. A decision analysis. Ann Intern Med 109:913–919, 1988.
54. Aranha GV, Kruss D, Greenlee HB: Therapeutic options for biliary tract disease in advanced cirrhosis. Am J Surg 155:374–377, 1988.
55. Poggio JL, Rowland CM, Gores GJ, et al: A comparison of laparoscopic and open cholecystectomy in patients with compensated cirrhosis and symptomatic gallstone disease. Surgery 127:405–411, 2000.
56. Sleeman D, Namias N, Levi D, et al: Laparoscopic cholecystectomy in cirrhotic patients. J Am Coll Surg 187:400–403, 1998.
57. Goldman L: Cardiac risk in noncardiac surgery: An update. Anesth Analg 80:810–820, 1995.
58. Thompson J, Jr., Bennion RS, Doty JE, et al: Predictive factors for bactibilia in acute cholecystitis. Arch Surg 125:261–264, 1990.
59. Linden WVD, Sunzel H: Early versus delayed operation for acute cholecystitis. A controlled clinical trial. Am J Surg 120:7–13, 1970.
60. McArthur P, Cuschieri A, Sells RA, Shields R: Controlled clinical trial comparing early with interval cholecystectomy for acute cholecystitis. Br J Surg 62:850–852, 1975.
61. Lahtinen J, Alhava EM, Aukee S: Acute cholecystitis treated by early and delayed surgery. A controlled clinical trial. Scand J Gastroenterol 13:673–678, 1978.
62. Jarvinen HJ, Hastbacka J: Early cholecystectomy for acute cholecystitis: A prospective randomized study. Ann Surg 191:501–505, 1980.
63. Lai PB, Kwong KH, Leung KL, et al: Randomized trial of early versus delayed laparoscopic cholecystectomy for acute cholecystitis. Br J Surg 85:764–767, 1998.
64. Lo CM, Liu CL, Fan ST, et al: Prospective randomized study of early versus delayed laparoscopic cholecystectomy for acute cholecystitis. Ann Surg 227:461–467, 1998.
65. Peters JH, Miller J, Nichols KE, et al: Laparoscopic cholecystectomy in patients admitted with acute biliary symptoms. Am J Surg 166: 300–303, 1993.
66. Bender JS, Zenilman ME: Immediate laparoscopic cholecystectomy as definitive therapy for acute cholecystitis. Surg Endosc 9:1081–1084, 1995.
67. Cuschieri A: Approach to the treatment of acute cholecystitis: Open surgical, laparoscopic or endoscopic? Endoscopy 25:397–398, 1993.
68. Melin MM, Sarr MG, Bender CE, van Heerden JA: Percutaneous cholecystostomy: A valuable technique in high-risk patients with presumed acute cholecystitis. Br J Surg 82:1274-1277, 1995.
69. Patel M, Miedema BW, James M, Marshall JB: Percutaneous cholecystostomy is an effective treatment for high-risk patients with acute cholecystitis. Am Surg 66:33–37, 2000.
70. Borzellino G, de Manzoni G, Ricci F, et al: Emergency cholecystostomy and subsequent cholecystectomy for acute gallstone cholecystitis in the elderly. Br J Surg 86:1521–1525, 1999.
71. Berber E, Engle K, String A, et al: Selective use of tube cholecystostomy with interval laparoscopic cholecystectomy in acute cholecystitis. Arch Surg 135:341–346, 2000.
72. Ikard RW: Gallstones, cholecystitis and diabetes. Surg Gynecol Obstet 171:528–532, 1990.
73. Aucott JN, Cooper GS, Bloom AD, Aron DC: Management of gallstones in diabetic patients. Arch Intern Med 153:1053–1058, 1993.
74. Laycock WS, Siewers AE, Birkmeyer CM, et al: Variation in the use of laparoscopic cholecystectomy for elderly patients with acute cholecystitis. Arch Surg 1354:457–462, 2000.
75. Lo CM, Lai EC, Fan ST, et al: Laparoscopic cholecystectomy for acute cholecystitis in the elderly. World J Surg 20:983–986, 1996.
76. Morrow DJ, Thompson J, Wilson SE: Acute cholecystitis in the elderly: A surgical emergency. Arch Surg 113:1149–1152, 1978.
77. Savoca PE, Longo WE, Zucker KA, et al: The increasing prevalence of acalculous cholecystitis in outpatients. Results of a 7-year study. Ann Surg 211:433–437, 1990.
78. Bonacini M: Hepatobiliary complications in patients with human immunodeficiency virus infection. Am J Med 92:404–411, 1992.

79. Babb RR: Acute acalculous cholecystitis. A review. J Clin Gastroenterol 15:238–241, 1992.
80. Kaminski DL, Andrus CH, German D, Deshpande YG: The role of prostanoids in the production of acute acalculous cholecystitis by platelet-activating factor. Ann Surg 212:455–461, 1990.
81. Kaminski DL, Feinstein WK, Deshpande YG: The production of experimental cholecystitis by endotoxin. Prostaglandins 47:233–245, 1994.
82. Warren BL: Small vessel occlusion in acute acalculous cholecystitis. Surgery 111:163–168, 1992.
83. Sharp KW: Acute cholecystitis. Surg Clin North Am 68:269–279, 1988.
84. Johnson LB: The importance of early diagnosis of acute acalculus cholecystitis. Surg Gynecol Obstet 164:197–203, 1987.
85. Hunt DR, Chu FC: Gangrenous cholecystitis in the laparoscopic era. Aust NZ J Surg 70:428–430, 2000.
86. Burch JM, Feliciano DV, Mattox KL, Jordan G Jr: Gallstone pancreatitis. The question of time. Arch Surg 125:853–859, 1990.
87. Kelly TR, Wagner DS: Gallstone pancreatitis: A prospective randomized trial of the timing of surgery. Surgery 104:600–605, 1988.
88. Kim U, Shen HY, Bodner B: Timing of surgery for acute gallstone pancreatitis. Am J Surg 156:393–396, 1988.
89. Soper NJ, Brunt LM, Callery MP, et al: Role of laparoscopic cholecystectomy in the management of acute gallstone pancreatitis. Am J Surg 167:42–50, 1994.
90. Tang E, Stain SC, Tang G, et al: Timing of laparoscopic surgery in gallstone pancreatitis. Arch Surg 130:496–499, 1995.
91. Carr-Locke DL: Role of endoscopy in gallstone pancreatitis. Am J Surg 165:519–521, 1993.
92. Fan ST, Lai EC, Mok FP, et al: Early treatment of acute biliary pancreatitis by endoscopic papillotomy. N Engl J Med 328:228–232, 1993.
93. Rosseland AR, Solhaug JH: Primary endoscopic papillotomy (EPT) in patients with stones in the common bile duct and the gallbladder in situ: A 5–8-year follow-up study. World J Surg 12:111–116, 1988.
94. Worthley CS, Toouli J: Gallbladder non-filling: An indication for cholecystectomy after endoscopic sphincterotomy. Br J Surg 75:796–798, 1988.
95. Glasgow RE, Visser BC, Harris HW, et al: Changing management of gallstone disease during pregnancy. Surg Endosc 12:241–246, 1998.
96. Dixon NP, Faddis DM, Silberman H: Aggressive management of cholecystitis during pregnancy. Am J Surg 154:292–294, 1987.
97. Lanzafame RJ: Laparoscopic cholecystectomy during pregnancy. Surgery 118:627–631, 1995.
98. Holcomb G Jr, Holcomb GD: Cholelithiasis in infants, children, and adolescents. Pediatr Rev 11:268–274, 1990.
99. Roslyn JJ, Berquist WE, Pitt HA, et al: Increased risk of gallstones in children receiving total parenteral nutrition. Pediatrics 71:784–789, 1983.
100. Holcomb Gr, Sharp KW, Neblett WR, et al: Laparoscopic cholecystectomy in infants and children: Modifications and cost analysis. J Pediatr Surg 29:900–904, 1994.
101. Csendes A, Diaz JC, Burdiles P, et al: Mirizzi syndrome and cholecystobiliary fistula: A unifying classification. Br J Surg 76:1139–1143, 1989.
102. Wetter LA, Ring EJ, Pellegrini CA, Way LW: Differential diagnosis of sclerosing cholangiocarcinomas of the common hepatic duct (Klatskin tumors). Am J Surg 161:57–62, 1991.
103. Baer HU, Matthews JB, Schweizer WP, et al: Management of the Mirizzi syndrome and the surgical implications of cholecystocholedochal fistula. Br J Surg 77:743–745, 1990.
104. Yip AW, Chow WC, Chan J, Lam KH: Mirizzi syndrome with cholecystocholedochal fistula: Preoperative diagnosis and management. Surgery 111:335–338, 1992.
105. Clavien PA, Richon J, Burgan S, Rohner A: Gallstone ileus. Br J Surg 77:737-742, 1990.
106. Deitz DM, Standage BA, Pinson CW, et al: Improving the outcome in gallstone ileus. Am J Surg 151:572–576, 1986.
107. Reisner RM, Cohen JR: Gallstone ileus: A review of 1001 reported cases. Am Surg 60:441–446, 1994.
108. Shiffman ML, Sugerman HJ, Kellum JM, et al: Gallstone formation after rapid weight loss: A prospective study in patients undergoing gastric bypass surgery for treatment of morbid obesity. Am J Gastroenterol 86:1000–1005, 1991.
109. Lo TS, Okada M: Images in clinical medicine. Porcelain gallbladder. N Engl J Med 330:10, 1994.
110. Diehl AK: Gallstone size and the risk of gallbladder cancer. JAMA 250:2323–2326, 1983.
111. Serafini AN, Spoliansky G, Sfakianakis GN, et al: Diagnostic studies in patients with sickle cell anemia and acute abdominal pain. Arch Intern Med 147:1061–1062, 1987.
112. Goldfarb A, Grisaru D, Gimmon Z, et al: High incidence of cholelithiasis in older patients with homozygous beta-thalassemia. Acta Haematol 83:120–122, 1990.
113. Bragg LE, Thompson JS: Concomitant cholecystectomy for asymptomatic cholelithiasis. Arch Surg 124:460–462, 1989.
114. McSherry CK, Glenn F: Biliary tract surgery concomitant with other intra-abdominal operations. Ann Surg 193:169–175, 1981.
115. Thompson JS, Philben VJ, Hodgson PE: Operative management of incidental cholelithiasis. Am J Surg 148:821–824, 1984.
116. Wolff BG: Current status of incidental surgery. Dis Colon Rectum 38: 435–441, 1995.
117. Juhasz ES, Wolff BG, Meagher AP, et al: Incidental cholecystectomy during colorectal surgery. Ann Surg 219:467-472, 1994.
118. Green JD, Birkhead G, Hebert J, et al: Increased morbidity in surgical patients undergoing secondary (incidental) cholecystectomy. Ann Surg 211:50–54, 1990.
119. Miller RE, Kimmelstiel FM, Winkler WP: Management of common bile duct stones in the era of laparoscopic cholecystectomy. Am J Surg 169:273–276, 1995.
120. Duensing RA, Williams RA, Collins JC, Wilson SE: Managing choledocholithiasis in the laparoscopic era. Am J Surg 170:619–623, 1995.
121. Neoptolemos JP, Carr-Locke DL, Fossard DP: Prospective randomised study of preoperative endoscopic sphincterotomy versus surgery alone for common bile duct stones. Br Med J Clin Res Ed 294:470–474, 1987.
122. Stiegmann GV, Goff JS, Mansour A, et al: Precholecystectomy endoscopic cholangiography and stone removal is not superior to cholecystectomy, cholangiography, and common duct exploration. Am J Surg 163:227–230, 1992.
123. Cuschieri A, Lezoche E, Morino M, et al: E.A.E.S. multicenter prospective randomized trial comparing two-stage vs single-stage management of patients with gallstone disease and ductal calculi. Surg Endosc 13:952–957, 1999.
124. Cotton PB, Lehman G, Vennes J, et al: Endoscopic sphincterotomy complications and their management: An attempt at consensus. Gastrointest Endosc 37:383–393, 1991.
125. Rhodes M, Sussman L, Cohen L, Lewis MP: Randomised trial of laparoscopic exploration of common bile duct versus postoperative endoscopic retrograde cholangiography for common bile duct stones. Lancet 351:159–161, 1998.
126. Memon MA, Hassaballa H, Memon MI: Laparoscopic common bile duct exploration: The past, the present, and the future. Am J Surg 179:309–315, 2000.
127. DePaula AL, Hashiba K, Bafutto M: Laparoscopic management of choledocholithiasis. Surg Endosc 8:1399–1403, 1994.
128. Berci G, Morgenstern L: Laparoscopic management of common bile duct stones. A multi-institutional SAGES study. Society of American Gastrointestinal Endoscopic Surgeons. Surg Endosc 8:1168–1174, 1994.
129. Franklin M Jr, Pharand D, Rosenthal D: Laparoscopic common bile duct exploration. Surg Laparosc Endosc 4:119–124, 1994.
130. Davidoff AM, Pappas TN, Murray EA, et al: Mechanisms of major biliary injury during laparoscopic cholecystectomy. Ann Surg 215: 196–202, 1992.
131. Lillemoe KD, Melton GB, JL C, et al: Postoperative bile duct strictures: management and outcome in the 1990s. Ann Surg 232:430–441, 2000.
132. Chapman WC, Halevy A, Blumgart LH, Benjamin IS: Postcholecystectomy bile duct strictures. Management and outcome in 130 patients. Arch Surg 130:597–602, 1995.
133. Braasch JW, Rossi RL: Reconstruction of the biliary tract. Surg Clin North Am 65:273–283, 1985.
134. Roslyn JJ, Tompkins RK: Reoperation for biliary strictures. Surg Clin North Am 71:109–116, 1991.
135. Pitt HA, Cameron JL, Postier RG, Gadacz TR: Factors affecting mortality in biliary tract surgery. Am J Surg 141:66–72, 1981.
136. Pellegrini CA, Allegra P, Bongard FS, Way LW: Risk of biliary surgery in patients with hyperbilirubinemia. Am J Surg 154:111–117, 1987.
137. Stewart L, Way LW: Bile duct injuries during laparoscopic cholecys-

tectomy. Factors that influence the results of treatment. Arch Surg 130:1123–1128, 1995.

138. Pitt HA, Kaufman SL, Coleman J, et al: Benign postoperative biliary strictures. Operate or dilate? Ann Surg 210:417–425, 1989.
139. Bates T, Ebbs SR, Harrison M, A'Hern RP: Influence of cholecystectomy on symptoms. Br J Surg 78:964–967, 1991.
140. Fenster LF, Lonborg R, Thirlby RC, Traverso LW: What symptoms does cholecystectomy cure? Insights from an outcomes measurement project and review of the literature. Am J Surg 169:533-538, 1995.
141. Lee CM, Stewart L, Way LW: Postcholecystectomy abdominal bile collections. Arch Surg 135:538–542, 2000.
142. Traverso LW, Kozarek RA, Ball TJ, et al: Endoscopic retrograde cholangiopancreatography after laparoscopic cholecystectomy. Am J Surg 165:581–586, 1993.
143. Larmi TK, Mokka R, Kemppainen P, Seppala A: A critical analysis of the cystic duct remnant. Surg Gynecol Obstet 141:48-52, 1975.
144. Woods MS, Farha GJ, Street DE: Cystic duct remnant fistulization to the gastrointestinal tract. Surgery 111:101–104, 1992.
145. Jonson G, Nilsson DM, Nilsson T: Cystic duct remnants and biliary symptoms after cholecystectomy. A randomised comparison of two operative techniques. Eur J Surg 157:583–586, 1991.
146. Chuttani R, Carr-Locke DL: Pathophysiology of the sphincter of Oddi. Surg Clin North Am 73:1311–1322, 1993.
147. Hogan WJ, Geenen JE: Biliary dyskinesia. Endoscopy 1:179–183, 1988.
148. Tzovaras G, Rowlands BJ: Diagnosis and treatment of sphincter of Oddi dysfunction. Br J Surg 85:558–595, 1998.
149. Desautels SG, Slivka A, Hutson WR, et al: Postcholecystectomy pain syndrome: Pathophysiology of abdominal pain in sphincter of Oddi type III. Gastroenterology 116:900–905, 1999.
150. Geenen JE, Hogan WJ, Dodds WJ, et al: The efficacy of endoscopic sphincterotomy after cholecystectomy in patients with sphincter-of-Oddi dysfunction. N Engl J Med 320:82–87, 1989.
151. Nussbaum MS, Warner BW, Sax HC, Fischer JE: Transduodenal sphincteroplasty and transampullary septotomy for primary sphincter of Oddi dysfunction. Am J Surg 157:38–43, 1989.
152. Schottenfeld D, Winawer SJ: Cholecystectomy and colorectal cancer. Gastroenterology 85:966–967, 1983.
153. Lowenfels AB, Lindstrom CG, Conway MJ, Hastings PR: Gallstones and risk of gallbladder cancer. J Natl Cancer Inst 75:77–80, 1985.
154. Lowenfels AB, Walker AM, Althaus DP, et al: Gallstone growth, size, and risk of gallbladder cancer: An interracial study. Int J Epidemiol 18:50–54, 1989.
155. Walden DT, Soloway RD, Crowther RS: Cholecystectomy protects against extrahepatic bile duct cancer: Is this a result of the removal of gallstones? Hepatology 19:1533–1534, 1994.
156. Ekbom A, Hsieh CC, Yuen J, et al: Risk of extrahepatic bileduct cancer after cholecystectomy. Lancet 342:1262–1265, 1993.
157. Linos D, Beard CM, O'Fallon WM, et al: Cholecystectomy and carcinoma of the colon. Lancet 2:379–381, 1981.
158. Turunen MJ, Kivilaakso EO: Increased risk of colorectal cancer after cholecystectomy. Ann Surg 194:639–641, 1981.
159. Vernick LJ, Kuller LH: Cholecystectomy and right-sided colon cancer: An epidemiological study. Lancet 2:381–383, 1981.
160. Savassi-Rocha PR, Ferreira RH, Diniz MT, Sanches SR: Laparoscopic cholecystectomy in Brazil: Analysis of 33,563 cases. Int Surg 82:208–213, 1997.

Nonsurgical Management of Gallstone Disease

Chapter 57

Gustav Paumgartner

The treatment of gallstones without surgery has long been a goal of medical therapy. Toward the end of the 19th century, Schiff,[1] who had emigrated from Germany to Florence, Italy, suggested that patients with gallstone disease be treated with bile acids. Dabney[2] of Charlottesville, Virginia, was one of the first to report that bile salts were effective in the treatment of gallstone disease. In 1937, Rewbridge,[3] a member of the Department of Surgery at the University of Minnesota, reported the disappearance of gallstone shadows after the administration of bile salts. Unfortunately, these observations were forgotten, and many years passed before it was clearly demonstrated that therapy with chenodeoxycholic acid[4] or ursodeoxycholic acid[5] dissolves cholesterol gallstones. Extracorporeal shock-wave lithotripsy[6] was added later as another treatment modality that is less invasive than cholecystectomy.

When cholecystectomy was the sole effective treatment for gallstone disease, the only relevant decision was whether to treat the patient. Since the introduction of nonsurgical therapies for cholecystolithiasis, it has been necessary to recommend the most suitable type of treatment. Cholecystectomy is the standard and definitive treatment for symptomatic gallbladder stones and can be performed regardless of the type, number, and size of the stones. However, some patients are reluctant to undergo open or laparoscopic surgery or general anesthesia, despite the low morbidity and mortality rates, and insist on the least invasive treatment. In a small number of patients, nonsurgical therapy may be suitable when there is a high surgical risk.

The nonsurgical treatments that are discussed in this chapter are oral bile acid dissolution therapy and extracorporeal shock-wave lithotripsy. With the introduction of laparoscopic cholecystectomy, direct-solvent dissolution of gallstones was abandoned. Therefore, this investigational therapy as well as other approaches that have not gained sufficient acceptance, such as percutaneous cholecystolithostomy and the crushing of stones through percutaneous introduction of an impeller, are not discussed in this chapter.

Both oral bile acid dissolution therapy and extracorporeal shock-wave lithotripsy are successful only in patients whose gallstones are composed predominantly of cholesterol.[7] Significant admixtures of pigment or calcium salts render the stones indissoluble; no effective nonsurgical therapy exists for pigment stones.

Nonsurgical approaches represent a long-term solution only for patients in whom the disturbance that led to the formation of gallstones is transient. Gallstones recur within approximately 5 years in 30% to 50% of the patients whose stones are eliminated nonsurgically,[8–10] presumably because of the persistence of an underlying disturbance in biliary lipid excretion or other factors that contribute to gallstone formation.[11]

The choice of gallstone treatment should be individualized, and the following criteria should be considered. First, objective criteria, based on the type and severity of symptoms as well as on gallstone and gallbladder characteristics, should be used to select patients for a specific therapy. These criteria allow predictions regarding the risks and outcome of the different treatments. Second, patient preference is an important subjective element in the selection process. Because there often is more than one treatment option, the pros and cons of the different treatment modalities must be discussed with the patient. Proper counseling of the patient requires that the physician be familiar with the different treatment options for gallstones and their respective selection criteria.

GENERAL ASPECTS

Before a decision can be made regarding the appropriate therapeutic approach, the stage of gallstone disease must be defined. There are three stages of cholelithiasis: (1) the asymptomatic stage, (2) the symptomatic stage without complications, and (3) the symptomatic stage with complications, such as acute cholecystitis, choledocholithiasis, biliary pancreatitis, gallbladder cancer, and gallstone ileus (see Chapter 55).

The various stages of gallstone disease differ with regard to the natural history of the disease and therefore require different therapeutic approaches. The natural history of asymptomatic gallstones is generally benign.[12] Therefore, expectant management is generally indicated for patients with asymptomatic gallbladder stones that are detected during routine ultrasonographic examinations.[12, 13] Patients with a history of biliary colic are at a substantially higher risk of recurrent biliary pain and complications than are patients with asymptomatic stones. Most of these patients experience recurring pain, and the risk of biliary complications is 1% to 2% per year; the risk of complications is higher in patients who have frequent and severe symptoms. Approximately 30% of patients who have had only one attack of biliary pain have no additional episodes of pain.[12] A therapeutic intervention should be recommended for most patients with symptomatic gallstones. However, if after appropriate counseling the patient with a first attack of biliary pain wants to try a period of watchful waiting to see whether pain recurs, this approach is acceptable.[12] The complicated forms of cholecystolithiasis usually require prompt and invasive therapy.

ORAL BILE ACID DISSOLUTION THERAPY

Modern bile acid therapy began at the Mayo Clinic with chenodeoxycholic acid[4] and was improved in Japan by the introduction of ursodeoxycholic acid.[5]

Pathophysiologic Considerations and Rationale

Therapy with bile acids is aimed at reversing the condition that is the prerequisite to the formation of cholesterol gallstones, namely, supersaturation of bile with cholesterol.[11] Stones dissolve if the surrounding medium is capable of solubilizing the cholesterol in the stones. Originally, the rationale for the use of chenodeoxycholic acid in gallstone dissolution[4] was to expand the bile acid pool, which was found to be reduced in patients with cholesterol gallstones. Subsequently, it was shown that expansion of the bile acid pool, per se, was not sufficient, because cholic acid increased the size of the bile acid pool but did not desaturate bile and did not dissolve gallstones. Of the physiologic bile acids, only chenodeoxycholic acid and ursodeoxycholic acid, the 3β-epimer of chenodeoxycholic acid, dissolve gallstones. Both desaturate bile by decreasing biliary cholesterol secretion.[14]

Removal of cholesterol from a stone can occur through micellar solubilization, formation of a liquid crystalline phase, or both (see Chapters 54 and 55). Micellar solubilization is the major mechanism responsible for gallstone dissolution by chenodeoxycholic acid, whereas the formation of a liquid crystalline phase appears to play an important additional role in gallstone dissolution by ursodeoxycholic acid.[14] The rate at which stones dissolve depends not only on the degree to which bile is unsaturated, and possibly on the content of ursodeoxycholic acid (thermodynamic factors), but also on the surface-to-volume ratio of the stones[15] and on stirring of the bile (kinetic factors). Because stone volume is proportional to the third power but stone surface is proportional only to the second power of the radius, multiple small stones have a favorable surface-to-volume ratio and therefore dissolve more rapidly than a solitary large stone. Analysis of the kinetics of stone dissolution with bile acid therapy has shown a linear decrease in the stone diameter with time in most patients.[15] A deviation from these dissolution kinetics with an initial delay of dissolution occurs if insoluble material is deposited on the surface of the stone. Although the primary goal of bile acid dissolution therapy is to change thermodynamic factors (e.g., cholesterol saturation), the use of lithotripsy as adjuvant treatment influences kinetic factors (e.g., surface-to-volume ratio). Methods of influencing the dissolution kinetics by enhancing gallbladder emptying (e.g., with dietary regimens or prokinetic drugs) or lowering the viscosity of bile (e.g., by decreasing the mucin concentration) have not been studied sufficiently.

Therapeutic Regimens

Ursodeoxycholic acid (ursodiol) in a dose of 10 to 15 mg/kg of body weight per day is the preferred drug for gallstone dissolution.[13] Bedtime administration has been advocated, the rationale being to enhance bile acid secretion during the night when it normally is lowest and cholesterol saturation is highest.[16]

Chenodeoxycholic acid (chenodiol), the first bile acid introduced for gallstone dissolution, is no longer recommended. The doses required for sufficient desaturation of bile and dissolution of cholesterol gallstones (14 to 16 mg/kg per day) frequently cause side effects such as elevations in serum aminotransferase levels, diarrhea, and elevations in serum cholesterol levels.[17] When low doses of chenodeoxycholic acid and ursodeoxycholic acid are combined, side effects are infrequent. It has been suggested, but not proven, that the combination of ursodeoxycholic acid (5 mg/kg per day) and chenodeoxycholic acid (5 mg/kg per day) causes a higher gallstone dissolution rate than monotherapy with ursodeoxycholic acid (10 mg/kg per day).[18] However, for the dissolution of stone fragments after shock-wave lithotripsy, combination therapy (7 mg/kg per day of each bile acid) and monotherapy with ursodeoxycholic acid (11 mg/kg per day) are equally effective.[19] Because the combination causes diarrhea significantly more often than ursodeoxycholic acid alone, monotherapy with ursodeoxycholic acid appears to be the preferable treatment.

Patient Selection

STAGE OF GALLSTONE DISEASE. Oral bile acid dissolution therapy is appropriate only for patients with uncomplicated gallstone disease (Table 57–1).[13] Patients with acute cholecystitis, evidence of biliary obstruction, acute cholangitis, or acute biliary pancreatitis must be excluded. Episodes of biliary colic should be mild and infrequent.

GALLBLADDER FUNCTION. The cystic duct must be patent to allow filling and emptying of unsaturated bile. Oral cholecystography has been the most widely used method to docu-

Table 57-1 | **Selection Criteria for Oral Bile Acid Dissolution Therapy**

Stage of gallstone disease
- Symptomatic stage without complications and without frequent and severe biliary pain

Gallbladder
- Opacification on oral cholecystogram or ultrasonographic evidence of patency of the cystic duct and of gallbladder emptying (gallbladder contraction following a test meal)

Stones
- Radiolucent on radiography
- Computed tomography: isodense or hypodense to bile, no calcification
- Stone diameter ≤5 mm (optimal), 6–10 mm (acceptable)

ment patency of the cystic duct. This technique also permits evaluation of gallbladder emptying after a test meal. Opacification of the gallbladder proves that the concentrating function of the gallbladder is preserved and that severe pathology of the gallbladder wall is unlikely. Increasingly, functional ultrasonography, which measures changes in gallbladder volume in response to a standard test meal, is used to document gallbladder emptying, patency of the cystic duct, and absence of pathology of the gallbladder wall (see Table 57–1).[13]

STONE CHARACTERISTICS. Because oral bile acid therapy leads to the dissolution of only cholesterol material in the stones, radiolucency of the stones on radiography is required to exclude calcifications (see Table 57–1). Success of bile acid dissolution therapy is best assured if the stones are hypodense or isodense to bile and stone calcification is absent, as determined by computed tomography (CT).[20] An excellent indicator that stones are composed of cholesterol is the buoyancy (flotation) of the stones in bile during oral cholecystography (Fig. 57–1), because the specific gravity of cholesterol stones is close to that of bile enriched by radiographic contrast material.[21]

The efficacy of bile acid therapy decreases markedly when stone diameters are larger than 5 to 10 mm. Although bile acid therapy is acceptable for patients with stones up to 10 mm in diameter (see Table 57–1), it is reasonable to restrict this therapy to patients with stones that are 5 mm or less (these patients are the optimal candidates) and to fragment larger stones before bile acid therapy if shock-wave lithotripsy is available.[22] The number of stones does not limit oral bile acid dissolution therapy, as long as less than half of the gallbladder volume is occupied by the stones.

Efficacy

The success of treatment is defined as complete stone disappearance, which should be documented during continued bile acid treatment by two consecutive ultrasonographic examinations performed at least 1 month apart. With ursodeoxycholic acid, complete dissolution is achieved in 20% to 70% of patients. The wide variation in the reported response rate

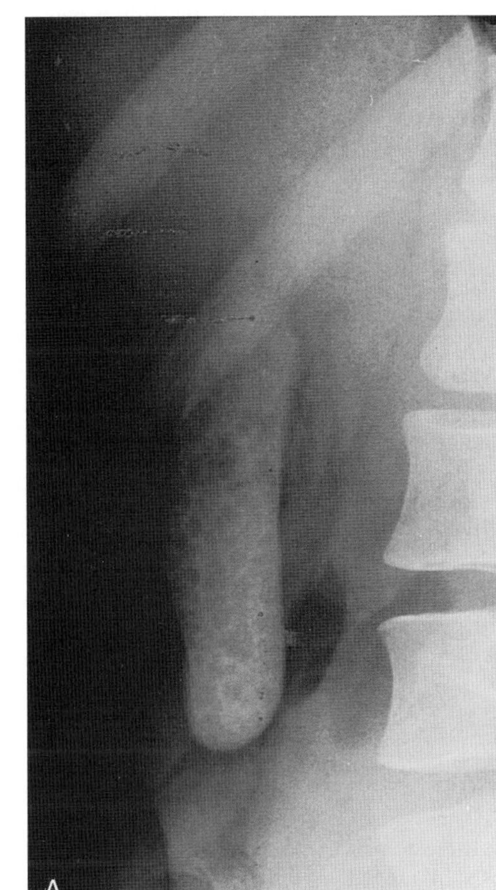

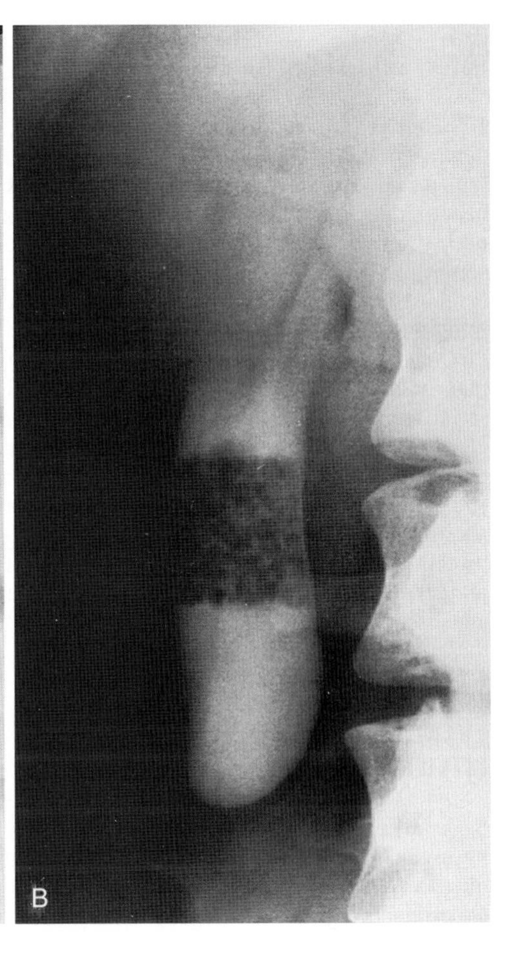

Figure 57-1. Optimal stones for oral bile acid dissolution therapy. *A,* The oral cholecystogram in a recumbent position shows multiple, small radiolucent stones. *B,* The oral cholecystogram in an upright position shows flotation of the stones. Within 1 year of oral bile acid dissolution therapy, all stones had disappeared.

can be attributed to differences in patient selection, doses of bile acid, treatment times, and the diagnostic techniques used to document complete stone dissolution.[16, 18, 23, 24] A recent meta-analysis[24] included all randomized trials of gallstone dissolution therapy in patients with radiolucent gallstones in a visualizing gallbladder with the documentation of complete stone dissolution by oral cholecystography or ultrasonography. Ursodeoxycholic acid completely dissolved the stones in 37% of all patients. In patients with gallstones no more than 10 mm in diameter, the dissolution rate was 49%. Only 29% of stones larger than 10 mm dissolved.[24] The best results—complete dissolution in more than 70% of the patients—were observed in patients with floating stones smaller than 5 mm in diameter. The time required for complete stone dissolution shows wide variation. In most patients who respond, the gallstone diameter decreases linearly with duration of treatment. The rate of decrease varies considerably among patients, with a median rate of 0.7 mm per month.[15]

Symptomatic improvement often occurs before disappearance of the gallstones. Long-term bile acid therapy has been reported to result in a reduced risk of biliary pain and acute cholecystitis, regardless of gallstone dissolution.[25] This benefit may relate to clearing of cholesterol crystals from the bile, effects on gallbladder motility, or other effects of ursodeoxycholic acid.

Treatment should be withdrawn if compliant patients show no radiologic evidence of gallstone dissolution after 6 months or if partial gallstone dissolution after 6 months does not progress to complete dissolution within 2 years.

Safety and Side Effects

Ursodeoxycholic acid is practically free of side effects. In contrast to chenodeoxycholic acid, its use is not associated with hepatotoxicity. It is a hydrophilic bile acid that exhibits hepatoprotection against hydrophobic bile acids such as chenodeoxycholic acid.[26] Ursodeoxycholic acid does not elevate serum cholesterol levels, because it does not inhibit bile acid synthesis; it lowers biliary cholesterol secretion mainly by inhibiting intestinal cholesterol absorption.

Chenodeoxycholic acid is a hydrophobic bile acid that may be toxic to cell membranes and may cause elevations in serum aminotransferase levels. Diarrhea was observed in 20% to 40% of the patients in the National Cooperative Gallstone Study.[17] Doses of chenodeoxycholic acid required for gallstone dissolution increase serum cholesterol levels by about 10%. This increase is mainly in the low-density lipoprotein fraction and is caused by the inhibition of the two major routes of cholesterol elimination: bile acid synthesis and biliary cholesterol secretion. Because of its side effects, therapy with chenodeoxycholic acid has been abandoned.

EXTRACORPOREAL SHOCK-WAVE LITHOTRIPSY

Soon after the introduction of lithotripsy for kidney stones by extracorporeally generated shock waves, the same principle was tested for the destruction of gallstones in animal experiments by Brendel and Enders.[27] The technique was first applied to patients with gallbladder or bile duct stones by Sauerbruch and associates in 1985.[6]

Background and Rationale

Extracorporeal shock-wave lithotripsy is intended to eliminate gallbladder stones by two mechanisms. As an adjunct to oral bile acid dissolution therapy, lithotripsy increases the surface-to-volume ratio of the stones and thereby enhances dissolution of cholesterol stones. By creating small stone fragments that can pass into the intestine, it also achieves clearance of stone material without prior dissolution.[28] An analysis of stone fragments in the feces of patients who underwent extracorporeal shock-wave lithotripsy has shown that 3-mm fragments can pass into the intestine without causing symptoms.[29]

Physical and Technical Aspects of Shock Waves

Shock waves are high-pressure waves that follow the laws of acoustics, but they differ from sound waves and conventional ultrasound waves by being highly distorted compared with the normal representation of sinusoidally varying acoustic pressure waves.[30] To create a limited area of high pressure at the location of the stone while keeping the pressure in the surrounding tissue relatively low, the shock waves are focused. This focusing minimizes tissue damage outside the focal area.[30]

Different lithotripters vary with respect to shock-wave generation, focusing, and targeting.[30] Shock waves can be generated by the use of an underwater spark-gap (electrohydraulic principle), piezoelectric crystals, or electromagnetic membrane. Shock waves in spark-gap lithotripters are focused by an ellipsoid metal reflector. To focus piezoelectrically generated shock waves, the piezoelectric crystals are mounted on a spherical dish. Electromagnetically generated shock waves are usually focused by acoustic lenses, but a metal reflector also can be used. In all types of lithotripters, the shock waves are generated under water. They travel through the water with little loss of energy and are transmitted into the human body by a compressible, water-filled bag that is interfaced with the skin by an ultrasonic coupling gel or by various types of water basins. The shock-wave pulse travels with little attenuation through the water and the soft tissues of the body. When it hits the anterior surface of the stone and again when it leaves the posterior surface, the changes in acoustic impedance lead to the liberation of compressive and tensile forces. In addition, cavitation phenomena occur at the anterior surface of the stone. Together, these effects result in the fragmentation of the stone. The size, microcrystalline structure, and architecture of the stone, rather than its chemical composition, determine its fragmentability.

Procedure

Patients usually are treated in the prone position.[28, 30, 31] In this position, the gallbladder is closest to the abdominal wall with no interposition of intestinal gas and most distant from the right costal margin. With lithotripters that are equipped with an overhead shock-wave generator, a supine oblique position is used. Ultrasonography is used for stone imaging and targeting and for monitoring the process of fragmentation.[28, 30, 31]

Sufficient energy per shock-wave pulse is required to obtain satisfactory results.[31] High energies generally must be used if the stones are large. With electrohydraulic lithotripters, such high energies usually cause pain, and the intravenous administration of an analgesic with or without a sedative is needed.[31] Piezoelectric lithotripters, in general, do not cause pain and do not require intravenous analgesia, but a higher number of shock-wave discharges per treatment session and multiple treatment sessions are required to achieve comparable results.[32–34] An electromagnetic lithotripter that transmits the shock-wave energy over a larger body surface area also causes less pain and requires intravenous analgesia in only a small percentage (2%) of patients.[35] A strategy, commonly called the "pulverization strategy," applies higher numbers of shock waves in repeated sessions, if necessary, to obtain very fine fragments. It has been reported that this method results in higher stone-free rates, especially within the first 3 months after lithotripsy.[33, 36, 37]

Even if the stone fragments are small enough (2 to 3 mm) to pass the cystic duct, they all cannot be expected to be eliminated from the gallbladder, because many patients with gallstone disease have disturbed motility of the gallbladder.[38, 39] In a study in which optimal fragmentation was not achieved in a high percentage of patients, adjuvant bile acid treatment with ursodeoxycholic acid improved the results of lithotripsy.[40] In a double-blind, randomized study, the rates of fragment clearance during monotherapy with ursodeoxycholic acid (11 mg/kg per day) and during combination therapy with ursodeoxycholic acid (7 mg/kg per day) plus chenodeoxycholic acid (7 mg/kg/day) did not differ.[19] Because the two-drug combination caused diarrhea more often, ursodeoxycholic acid (11 mg/kg per day) alone is recommended for the dissolution of stone fragments that remain after lithotripsy. However, complete clearance of stones can also be achieved by biliary lithotripsy without adjuvant bile acid therapy when the resulting fragments are very small (<2 mm or sludge) and the gallbladder contracts well.[33, 37, 41]

Patient Selection

SYMPTOMS AND GENERAL CRITERIA. To be a candidate for treatment, a patient should have symptoms that are typical of biliary pain. However, complications of gallstone disease, such as cholecystitis, biliary pancreatitis, and bile duct stones, must be absent (Table 57–2). Because of the risk of hematoma, patients with a coagulopathy or taking a medication with anticoagulant effects must be excluded. Female patients must not be pregnant.

STONE CHARACTERISTICS. To ensure a sufficiently high efficacy rate, shock-wave lithotripsy should be limited to patients with a solitary radiolucent stone with a maximum diameter of 20 mm (see Table 57–2). The use of CT to exclude calcified stones has been suggested, but this approach has not gained wide acceptance. Ultrasonographic echo patterns that are suggestive of a pure cholesterol stone may be valuable in selecting optimal candidates for shock-wave lithotripsy.[42]

Table 57–2 | **Selection Criteria for Extracorporeal Shock-Wave Lithotripsy**

Stage of gallstone disease
- Symptomatic stage without complications

Gallbladder
- Opacification on oral cholecystogram or ultrasonographic evidence of patency of the cystic duct (gallbladder contraction following a test meal)
- Gallbladder emptying > 60% of fasting volume

Stones
- Radiolucency on radiography
- Stone number: 1
- Stone diameter ≤ 20 mm

GALLBLADDER FUNCTION. The patency of the cystic duct must be documented by oral cholecystography or ultrasonography. Although a quantitative assessment of gallbladder motor function has not been used to select patients for shock-wave lithotripsy in most studies,[28] gallbladder emptying is a major determinant of stone clearance.[43] Therefore, it is advisable to determine gallbladder emptying following a test meal and to select patients for extracorporeal shock-wave lithotripsy in whom gallbladder emptying is more than 60% of the fasting volume.[43]

Efficacy

The efficacy of extracorporeal shock-wave lithotripsy is defined as the percentage of patients with a stone-free gallbladder at specific time points (e.g., 6 and 12 months) after extracorporeal shock-wave lithotripsy. The gallbladder may be considered stone-free if ultrasonography shows absence of echogenic foci with acoustic shadowing or gravity dependence and if this finding is confirmed on follow-up examination 1 to 3 months later (Fig. 57–2).[31] The extent of fragmentation[31] and gallbladder emptying[43] are the most important determinants of efficacy. The degree of fragmentation depends mainly on stone characteristics (e.g., quantitative factors, including size and number of the stones, and qualitative factors, including structure and calcifications)[31, 42, 44] and the shock-wave dose (energy of shock waves, number of shock waves administered per session, number of treatment sessions).[28, 31] Adjuvant bile acid therapy is a determinant of outcome when fragments are larger than 3 mm[40] but plays no significant role during the first 3 to 6 months when a fine disintegration ("pulverization") to fragments smaller than 2 mm or to sludge has been achieved with repeated lithotripsy.[33, 37, 41] Differences in the efficacy of extracorporeal shock-wave lithotripsy reported in the literature largely can be attributed to differences in patient selection and treatment modality.[28]

The largest study with the longest follow-up after extracorporeal shock-wave lithotripsy and adjuvant bile acid therapy comprises 711 patients followed for up to 5 years.[31] The highest success rate was obtained in patients with a solitary radiolucent stone less than 20 mm in diameter. Patients were not selected according to gallbladder emptying. In this study, 68% and 84% of patients were stone-free at 6 and 12

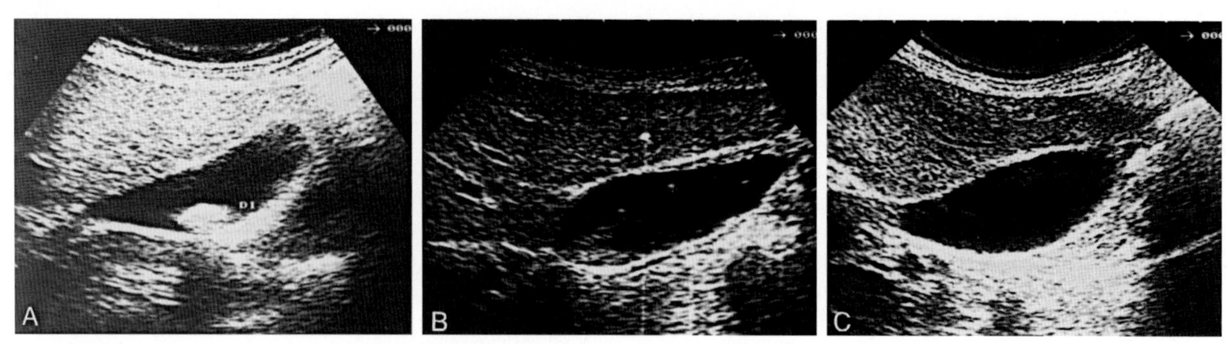

Figure 57–2. Ultrasonogram of a gallbladder with a single stone before *(A)*, 1 day after *(B)*, and 6 weeks after *(C)* extracorporeal shock-wave lithotripsy. At 1 day after treatment, multiple, small fragments are visible; these fragments had disappeared 6 weeks after lithotripsy and adjuvant bile acid therapy.

months after high-energy shock-wave lithotripsy with adjuvant bile acid therapy. When only patients in whom gallbladder emptying of more than 60% of the fasting gallbladder volume are selected, 66% are free of stones within 3 months after lithotripsy.[43] The stone-free rate decreases with increases in the number and size of stones,[31] the presence of a calcified rim,[44] and reduced gallbladder emptying.[43] Any comparison of results obtained by different groups must take into account stone characteristics and gallbladder function. Table 57–3 shows the results reported by different investigators for the treatment of solitary radiolucent gallbladder stones 20 mm or less in diameter. The percentage of patients with a stone-free gallbladder ranged from 47% to 77% at 6 months after lithotripsy and from 68% to 84% at 12 months after lithotripsy.[31–35, 41, 45, 46]

Patient characteristics and treatment modalities also determine the economic outcome. In one study,[47] extracorporeal shock-wave lithotripsy was marginally cost-effective compared with open cholecystectomy. Lithotripsy was more cost-effective for elderly than young patients and considerably less cost-effective for multiple stones than single stones. In another study,[48] lithotripsy with adjuvant bile acid therapy was at least as cost-effective as open cholecystectomy for patients with small stones but less cost-effective for those with large stones. Laparoscopic cholecystectomy appears to be more cost-effective than lithotripsy with adjuvant bile acid therapy, if long-term cost is considered.[49]

Safety and Side Effects

Complications directly related to extracorporeal shock-wave lithotripsy have been minimal. Sackmann and associates[31] have observed petechiae of the skin at the site of shock-wave entry in 8%, transient gross hematuria in 4%, and liver hematoma in 0.1% of the patients. Neither short-term (1 to 2 months after lithotripsy) nor long-term (5 to 18 months after lithotripsy) post-treatment laboratory values (alanine or aspartate aminotransferase, alkaline phosphatase, and bilirubin levels; white blood cell count) differed from pretreatment values.[19, 31] Approximately one third of the patients experienced one or more episodes of biliary colic that were related to the presence of stone fragments. The symptoms were usually mild and disappeared once the gallbladder was free of all fragments. Mild biliary pancreatitis developed in 2% of the patients, and transient cholestasis developed in 1%.[31] These events were not related directly to the application of shock waves but rather to the passage of stone fragments

Table 57–3 | **Efficacy of Extracorporeal Shock-Wave Lithotripsy in Patients with Radiolucent Solitary Gallbladder Stones 20 mm or Less in Diameter**

AUTHOR	YEAR	NO. OF PATIENTS	DEVICE*	STONE-FREE PATIENTS (%) 6 Months	STONE-FREE PATIENTS (%) 12 Months
McSherry et al[45]	1991	175	PE	47	68
Pelletier et al[46]	1991	147	PE‡	46	69
Sackmann et al[31]	1991	122†	EH‡	68	84
Benninger et al[32]	1992	98	PE‡	60	76
Elewaut et al[34]	1993	169	PE‡	61	84
Wehrmann et al[35]	1993	79	EM§	68	80
Tsuchiya et al[33]	1995	49	PE‡	63	—
		44	PE§	66	—
Sauter et al[41]	1997	34	EH‡	77	—
		27	EH§	63	—

*Device: PE, piezoelectric lithotripter; EH, electrohydraulic lithotripter; EM, electromagnetic lithotripter.
†Patients who received high-energy treatment.
‡With adjuvant bile acid therapy.
§Without adjuvant bile acid therapy.

and usually occurred during the first weeks after lithotripsy. Endoscopic sphincterotomy was only rarely (1%) necessary to remove prepapillary stone fragments from the common bile duct. Cystic duct obstruction, which usually was asymptomatic and resolved spontaneously, was observed in 5% of the patients. Elective cholecystectomy was performed because of persistence of fragments and symptoms in approximately 3% of all patients.[31] In published trials involving several thousands of patients, no fatalities attributable to lithotripsy have been reported.

EXTRACORPOREAL SHOCK-WAVE LITHOTRIPSY OF BILE DUCT STONES

Nonsurgical therapy of bile duct stones is primarily endoscopic (see Chapter 61). In about 5% of the patients, bile duct stones cannot be removed by routine endoscopic techniques (including endoscopic sphincterotomy and, if necessary, mechanical lithotripsy) because the stones are too large, impacted, or located intrahepatically or proximal to a bile duct stricture. In addition to endoscopically performed mechanical lithotripsy, several methods, such as laser lithotripsy and contact electrohydraulic lithotripsy, have been introduced to disintegrate bile duct stones. These techniques require that the lithotripter probe be brought close to or in direct contact with the bile duct stone, under either endoscopic control or fluoroscopic guidance. These procedures are technically difficult, especially in the case of bile duct stenosis or intrahepatic stones. Often, the stones are not accessible to any of these techniques, especially if they are located intrahepatically. In these situations, extracorporeal shock-wave lithotripsy has been useful for disintegrating bile duct stones. Since the first report of extracorporeal shock-wave lithotripsy of bile duct stones in 1986,[6] many trials[50–55] have shown that this treatment is highly effective in patients with bile duct stones in whom routine endoscopic measures and mechanical lithotripsy have failed. The method is safe and easier to perform than intracorporeal techniques.

Procedure

Shock-wave lithotripsy of bile duct stones differs from that of gallbladder stones with respect to stone location and shock-wave entry. In general, shock waves are applied from the back to avoid the gas-filled intestine, which is usually interposed between the anterior abdominal wall and the bile duct. Treatment of intrahepatic stones may be an exception to this rule. In general, fluoroscopy is used to locate the stones and monitor the fragmentation. To visualize the stones, a radiographic contrast medium is instilled into the common duct via a nasobiliary tube or percutaneous drain.[50, 51, 53–55] Patients receive general or epidural anesthesia or intravenous sedation and analgesia with drugs such as alfentanil or pentazocine and midazolam. Because septic complications have been reported, prophylactic antibiotics are administered intravenously. In patients with septic cholangitis, the bile duct should be drained with a nasobiliary tube before shock-wave lithotripsy is performed. If the first session of shock-wave lithotripsy fails, the treatment can be repeated within approximately 1 week.[51, 55]

Patient Selection

Extracorporeal shock-wave lithotripsy should be considered if routine endoscopic measures and mechanical lithotripsy fail to remove bile duct stones (e.g., because stones are impacted, too large, or located intrahepatically or above a bile duct stricture), if access to the bile ducts has been established with a nasobiliary tube or transhepatic catheter, and if the orifice of the common bile duct in the intestine is large enough for spontaneous passage or extraction of fragments. Patients with a coagulopathy or who are taking a medication with anticoagulant effects must be excluded.

Efficacy

In most studies involving 50 patients or more, the bile ducts have been cleared of all stones in 70% to 90% of patients undergoing lithotripsy.[50–55] Repeated sessions are required in approximately one third of the patients. Endoscopic extraction of fragments is necessary in 70% to 90% of the patients because the fragments are usually larger than after lithotripsy of gallbladder stones.

Safety and Side Effects

Mortality directly related to the procedure has not been reported. The reported 30-day mortality rate is 0 to 1%.[51, 53, 54] Thus, shock-wave lithotripsy compares favorably with open surgery in this group of elderly, high-risk patients. Mild and mostly transient hemobilia has been observed in less than 10% of cases. Additional complications that may be caused directly by the shock waves include hematoma of the liver and macrohematuria. Despite the proximity of pancreatic tissue to the shock-wave focus in patients with prepapillary stones, mild attacks of pancreatitis are rare. The most important complication after extracorporeal shock-wave lithotripsy has been sepsis related to the biliary tree in 4% of patients.[51] Therefore, prophylactic antibiotics should be started before treatment and continued until the biliary tree is cleared completely of stones.

In patients with major comorbidities in whom routine methods of endoscopic or surgical removal of bile duct stones have failed, extracorporeal shock-wave lithotripsy facilitates stone clearance in up to 90% of patients, with very low morbidity and mortality rates. Lithotripsy has proved to be a valuable nonsurgical treatment modality for difficult bile duct stones.

RECURRENCE OF GALLSTONES

Patients who have undergone a gallbladder-preserving treatment are at risk of stone recurrence. The overall recurrence rate is about 50% within 5 years after dissolution of the stones by bile acid therapy.[8] The risk of recurrence is highest in the first 2 years. The risk of gallstone recurrence appears to be lower in patients who have had a solitary stone than in those with multiple stones.[8] The rate of gallstone recurrence after successful shock-wave lithotripsy is 6%[10] to 7%[9] after 1 year and increases to 31%[9] to 44%[10] at

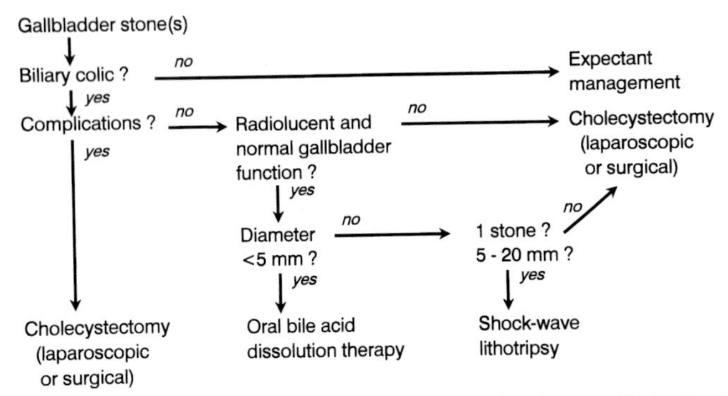

Figure 57–3. Algorithm for the management of gallstones if the least invasive approach that is possible and can be justified from a medical point of view is to be chosen.

5 years. The lower recurrence rate, as compared with oral bile acid dissolution therapy, may be explained by the fact that in 82%[10] to 89%[9] of the patients undergoing lithotripsy, the stone is initially solitary, and the risk of stone recurrence is lower in this group. There were no significant differences in age, sex, and body mass index between patients with and without stone recurrence in one study,[9] but body mass index was a risk factor for stone recurrence in another study. Incomplete emptying of the gallbladder[56, 57] and a high proportion of deoxycholic acid in the bile acid pool[57] may also be risk factors for stone recurrence. After lithotripsy, the recurrent stones were usually small (mean diameter, 6 mm) and multiple in 60% of the patients at the time of detection and caused recurrent biliary pain in about 60%.[9] Repeat treatment with ursodeoxycholic acid (combined with shock-wave lithotripsy if the stones are > 5 to 10 mm in diameter) may be considered if the recurrent gallstones cause biliary pain, but many patients with recurrent stones after lithotripsy respond poorly to repeated nonsurgical therapy,[9] and laparoscopic cholecystectomy is recommended. Low-dose therapy with ursodeoxycholic acid to prevent stone recurrence after lithotripsy has had little or no efficacy.[8, 58] Maintenance therapy with a full dose of ursodeoxycholic acid, even if proved to be effective in subgroups of patients, would not be cost-effective and, in general, cannot be recommended.

CHOICE OF TREATMENT

When patients have the options of surgical or laparoscopic cholecystectomy or a gallbladder-preserving treatment, they frequently ask for the least invasive treatment that can be justified from a medical point of view. With this in mind, our current approach is provided in a simplified algorithm (Fig. 57–3). This algorithm is based on the selection and exclusion criteria for the most commonly used treatments.

REFERENCES

1. Schiff, M: Il coleinato di soda nella cura dei calcoli biliari. L'Imparziale 13:97, 1873.
2. Dabney WC: The use of choleate of soda to prevent the formation of gallstones. Am J Med Sci 71:410, 1876.
3. Rewbridge AG: The disappearance of gallstone shadows following the prolonged administration of bile salts. Surgery 1:395, 1937.
4. Danzinger RG, Hofmann AF, Schoenfield LS, et al: Dissolution of cholesterol gallstones by chenodeoxycholic acid. N Engl J Med 286:1, 1972.
5. Makino I, Shinozaki K, Yashino K, et al: Dissolution of cholesterol gallstones by ursodeoxycholic acid. Jpn J Gastroenterol 72:690, 1975.
6. Sauerbruch T, Delius M, Paumgartner G, et al: Fragmentation of gallstones by extracorporeal shock waves. N Engl J Med 314:818, 1986.
7. Sauerbruch T, Paumgartner G: Gallbladder stones: Management. Lancet 338:1121, 1991.
8. Villanova N, Bazzoli F, Taroni F, et al: Gallstone recurrence after successful oral bile acid treatment. Gastroenterology 97:726, 1989.
9. Sackmann M, Niller H, Klueppelberg U, et al: Gallstone recurrence after shock-wave therapy. Gastroenterology 106:225, 1994.
10. Carrilho-Ribeiro L, Pinto-Correira A, Velosa J, et al: Long-term gallbladder stone recurrence and risk factors after successful lithotripsy. Eur J Gastroenterol Hepatol 12:209, 2000.
11. Paumgartner G, Sauerbruch T: Gallstones: Pathogenesis. Lancet 338: 1117, 1991.
12. Ransohoff DF, Gracie WA: Treatment of gallstones. Ann Intern Med 119:606, 1993.
13. Roda E, Festi D, Lezoche E, et al: Strategies in the treatment of biliary stones. Gastroenterol Int 13:7, 2000.
14. Hofmann AF: Medical treatment of cholesterol gallstones by bile desaturating agents. Hepatology 4:199S, 1984.
15. Senior JR, Johnson MF, DeTurck DM, et al: In vivo kinetics of radiolucent gallstone dissolution by oral dihydroxy bile acids. Gastroenterology 99:243, 1990.
16. Jazrawi RP, Pigozzi MG, Galatola G, et al: Optimum bile acid treatment for rapid gallstone dissolution. Gut 33:381, 1992.
17. Schoenfield LJ, Lachin JM, et al: Chenodiol (chenodeoxycholic acid) for dissolution of gallstones: The National Cooperative Gallstone Study: A controlled trial of efficacy and safety. Ann Intern Med 95:257, 1981.
18. Podda M, Zuin M, Battezzati PM, et al: Efficacy and safety of a combination of chenodeoxycholic acid and ursodeoxycholic acid for gallstone dissolution: A comparison with ursodeoxycholic acid alone. Gastroenterology 96:222, 1989.
19. Sackmann M, Pauletzki J, Aydemir U, et al: Efficacy and safety of ursodeoxycholic acid for dissolution of gallstone fragments: Comparison with the combination of ursodeoxycholic acid and chenodeoxycholic acid. Hepatology 14:1136, 1991.
20. Petroni ML, Jazrawi RP, Grundy A, et al: Prospective, multicenter study on value of computerized tomography (CT) in gallstone disease in predicting response to bile acid therapy. Dig Dig Sci 40:1956, 1995.
21. Dolgin SM, Schwartz S, Kressel HY, et al: Identification of patients with cholesterol or pigment gallstones by discriminant analysis of radiographic features. N Engl J Med 304:808, 1981.
22. Strasberg SM, Clavien PA: Cholecystolithiasis: Lithotherapy for the 1990s. Hepatology 16:820, 1992.
23. Erlinger S, Le Go A, Husson JM, et al: Franco-Belgian cooperative study of ursodeoxycholic acid in the medical dissolution of gallstones: A double-blind, randomized, dose-response study, and comparison with chenodeoxycholic acid. Hepatology 4:308, 1984.
24. May GR, Sutherland LR, Shaffer EA: Efficacy of bile acid therapy for gallstone dissolution: A meta-analysis of randomized trials. Aliment Pharmacol Ther 7:139, 1993.
25. Tomida S, Abei M, Yamaguchi T, et al: Long-term ursodeoxycholic acid therapy is associated with reduced risk of biliary pain and acute cholecystitis in patients with gallbladder stones: A cohort analysis. Hepatology 30:6, 1999.
26. Beuers U, Boyer JL, Paumgartner G: Ursodeoxycholic acid in cholestasis: Potential mechanisms of action and therapeutic applications. Hepatology 28:1449, 1998.
27. Brendel W, Enders G: Shock waves for gallstones: Animal studies. Lancet 1:1054, 1983.
28. Paumgartner G: Extracorporeal shock-wave lithotripsy. Eur J Gastroenterol Hepatol 6: 867, 1994.
29. Greiner L, Münks C, Heil W, Jakobeit C: Gallbladder stone fragments in feces after biliary extracorporeal shock-wave lithotripsy. Gastroenterology 98:1620, 1990.
30. Paumgartner G: Shock-wave lithotripsy of gallstones. AJR Am J Roentgenol 153:235, 1989.
31. Sackmann M, Pauletzki J, Sauerbruch T, et al: The Munich Gallbladder Lithotripsy Study: Results of the first 5 years with 711 patients. Ann Intern Med 114:290, 1991.

32. Benninger J, Schneider HT, Blaufub M, et al: Piezoelektrische Lithotripsie von Gallblasensteinen: Akut- und Langzeitergebnisse. Dtsch Med Wochenschr 117:1350, 1992.
33. Tsuchiya Y, Ishihara F, Kajiyama G, et al: Repeated piezoelectric lithotripsy for gallstones with and without ursodeoxycholic acid dissolution: A multicenter study. J Gastroenterol 30:768, 1995.
34. Elewaut A, Crape A, Afschrift M, et al: Results of extracorporeal shock-wave lithotripsy of gallbladder stones in 693 patients: A plea for restriction to solitary radiolucent stones. Gut 34:274, 1993.
35. Wehrmann T, Hurst A, Lembcke B, et al: Biliary lithotripsy with a new electromagnetic shock-wave source: A 2-year clinical experience. Dig Dis Sci 38:2113, 1993.
36. Boscaini M, Piccinni-Leopardi M, Andreotti F, et al: Gallstone pulverisation strategy in patients treated with extracorporeal lithotripsy and follow-up results of maintenance treatment with ursodeoxycholic acid. Gut 35:117, 1994.
37. Soehendra N, Nam VC, Binmoeller KF, et al: Pulverisation of calcified and non-calcified gallbladder stones: Extracorporeal shock-wave lithotripsy used alone. Gut 35:417, 1994.
38. Festi D, Frabboni R, Bazzoli F, et al: Gallbladder motility in cholesterol gallstone disease: Effect of ursodeoxycholic acid administration and gallstone dissolution. Gastroenterology 98:1779, 1990.
39. Spengler U, Sackmann M, Sauerbruch T, et al: Gallbladder motility before and after extracorporeal shock-wave lithotripsy. Gastroenterology 96:860, 1989.
40. Schoenfield LJ, Berci G, Carnovale RL, et al: The effect of ursodiol on the efficacy and safety of extracorporeal shock-wave lithotripsy of gallbladder stones. The Dornier National Biliary Lithotripsy Study. N Engl J Med 323:1239, 1990.
41. Sauter G, Kullak-Ublick GA, Schumacher R, et al: Safety and efficacy of repeated shock-wave lithotripsy of gallstones with and without adjuvant bile acid therapy. Gastroenterology 112:1603, 1997.
42. Tsuchiya Y, Saito H, Saito N, et al: Sonographic pattern of radiolucent gallbladder stones for predicting shock-wave lithotripsy. J Gastroenterol Hepatol 10:426, 1995.
43. Pauletzki J, Sailer C, Klueppelberg U, et al: Gallbladder emptying determines early gallstone clearance after shock-wave lithotripsy. Gastroenterology 107:1496, 1994.
44. Sackmann M, Pauletzki J, Delius M, et al: Noninvasive therapy of gallbladder calculi with a radiopaque rim. Gastroenterology 102:988, 1992.
45. McSherry CK: EDAP Investigators Group: The results of the EDAP multicenter trial of biliary lithotripsy in the United States. Surgery 173: 461, 1991.
46. Pelletier G, Delmont J, Capdeville R, et al: Treatment of gallstones with piezoelectric lithotripsy and oral bile acid: A multicenter study. J Hepatol 12:327, 1991.
47. Bass EB, Steinberg EP, Pitt HA, et al: Cost-effectiveness of extracorporeal shock-wave lithotripsy versus cholecystectomy for symptomatic gallstones. Gastroenterology 10:189, 1991.
48. Nicholl JP, Brazier JE, Milner PC, et al: Randomized controlled trial of cost-effectiveness of lithotripsy and open cholecystectomy as treatments for gallbladder stones. Lancet 340:801, 1992.
49. Sonnenberg A, Benninger J, Ell C: Kostenvergleich zwischen der laparoskopischen Cholecystektomie und der extrakorporalen Stoßwellenlithotripsie in der Behandlung von Gallenblasensteinen. Dtsch Med Wochenschr 119:1532, 1994.
50. Moody FG, Amerson JR, Berci G, et al: Lithotripsy for bile duct stones. Am J Surg 158:241, 1989.
51. Sauerbruch T, Holl J, Sackmann M, et al: Fragmentation of bile duct stones by extracorporeal shock-wave lithotripsy: A five-year experience. Hepatology 15:208, 1992.
52. Adamek HE, Buttmann A, Wessbecher R, et al: Clinical comparison of extracorporeal piezoelectric lithotripsy (EPL) and intracorporeal electrohydraulic lithotripsy (EHL) in difficult bile duct stones: A prospective randomized trial. Dig Dis Sci 40:1185, 1995.
53. Meyenberger C, Meierhofer U, Michel-Harder C, et al: Long-term follow-up after treatment for common bile duct stones by extracorporeal shock-wave lithotripsy. Endoscopy 28:411, 1996.
54. Neuhaus H, Zillinger C, Born P, et al: Randomized study of intracorporeal laser lithotripsy versus extracorporeal shock-wave lithotripsy for difficult bile duct stones. Gastrointest Endosc 47:327, 1998.
55. Sackmann M, Holl J, Sauter GH, et al: Extracorporeal shock-wave lithotripsy for clearance of bile duct stones resistant to endoscopic extraction. Gastrointest Endosc 53:27, 2001.
56. Pauletzki J, Althaus R, Holl J, et al: Gallbladder emptying and gallstone formation: A prospective study on gallstone recurrence. Gastroenterology 111:765, 1996.
57. Berr F, Mayer M, Sackmann MF, et al: Pathogenic factors in early recurrence of cholesterol gallstones. Gastroenterology 106:215, 1994.
58. Hood KA, Gleeson D, Ruppin DC, et al: Gallstone recurrence and its prevention: The British/Belgian Gallstone Study Group's post-dissolution trial. Gut 34:1277, 1993.

Chapter 58

ACALCULOUS CHOLECYSTITIS, CHOLESTEROLOSIS, ADENOMYOMATOSIS, AND POLYPS OF THE GALLBLADDER

Lyman E. Bilhartz

Although gallstones and their complications account for most cholecystectomies,[1] a persistent 15% of these operations are performed in patients without gallstones.[2] Misdiagnosis is not the explanation for this finding; rather, patients without gallstones may still develop important symptoms or pathology that warrants cholecystectomy. In general, one of two clinically distinct syndromes occur in these patients: acalculous biliary pain or acute acalculous cholecystitis.

As shown in Table 58–1, acalculous biliary pain is generally a disorder of young, predominantly female ambulatory patients and mimics biliary colic. Acute acalculous cholecystitis is typically a disease of immobilized and critically ill older men with coexisting vascular disease. Although the pathologic findings in the resected gallbladder specimen may be similar in the two groups, the clinical manifestations and prognosis are quite different, and the two entities are considered separately in this chapter.

ACALCULOUS BILIARY PAIN

Definition

Intense epigastric or right upper quadrant pain, starting suddenly, rising in intensity over a 15-minute period, and continuing at a steady plateau for several hours before slowly subsiding is the classic description of biliary colic. Localization of the pain to the right hypochondrium or radiation to the right shoulder is the most specific finding for a biliary tract origin.[3] The attacks of pain are frequently, but not always, precipitated by a meal and may be accompanied by restlessness and vomiting. Between attacks, the physical examination is usually normal, with the possible exception of residual upper abdominal tenderness.

When a patient presents with such a history and ultrasonography confirms the presence of gallstones, the management is straightforward, namely, elective cholecystectomy (or perhaps an attempt at medical dissolution of the stones) (see Chapters 55 to 57).

Acalculous biliary pain is a syndrome in which patients have clinical features identical to those of patients with cholelithiasis and biliary colic but a normal gallbladder by ultrasonography and normal serum levels of liver and pancreatic enzymes.[4, 5]

Epidemiology and Pathophysiology

Acalculous biliary pain is predominantly a disorder of young women.[6] In one series of more than 100 patients, 83% were female, and the mean age was approximately 30 years.[5]

The cause of the acalculous biliary pain syndrome is not

Table 58–1 | **Comparison of Acalculous Biliary Pain and Acute Acalculous Cholecystitis**

	ACALCULOUS BILIARY PAIN	ACUTE ACALCULOUS CHOLECYSTITIS
Epidemiology	Female predominance (≈80%) Young to middle age Ambulatory patient Risk factors similar to those for cholelithiasis, i.e., obesity and multiparity	Male predominance (≈80%) Elderly Critically ill patient in intensive care unit Risk factors are preexisting atherosclerosis, recent surgery, and hemodynamic instability
Clinical features	Episodic right upper quadrant or epigastric pain identical to biliary colic Physical examination is usually normal Laboratory tests are usually normal	Unexplained sepsis with few localizing signs; rapid progression to gangrene and perforation Physical examination may show fever, but right upper quadrant tenderness is only present in ≈25% Leukocytosis and hyperamylasemia may be present
Diagnostic tests	Ultrasonography shows no stones and usually a normal gallbladder Biliary drainage (Meltzer-Lyon test) typically demonstrates crystals Stimulated cholescintigraphy using cholecystokinin to measure gallbladder ejection fraction may predict which patients are likely to improve with cholecystectomy	See Table 58–2
Treatment	Elective cholecystectomy for patients with classic biliary colic symptoms and either bile crystals or a gallbladder ejection fraction <35%	Urgent cholecystostomy or emergent cholecystectomy for gangrene or perforation
Prognosis	Prognosis is good; continued attacks without cholecystectomy	Prognosis is poor with a mortality rate ranging from 10–50%

known, but indirect evidence suggests that there may be multiple different etiologies that culminate in the same clinical presentation. Stimulated duodenal bile from patients with acalculous biliary pain is more dilute with respect to both bile acids and phospholipids than bile from patients with gallstones or from control women without biliary symptoms.[7] The dilute nature of the bile is consistent with other observations showing sluggish and incomplete gallbladder contraction,[8] and the lower molar percentage of phospholipid is consistent with the hypothesis that biliary phospholipids are hydrolyzed to inflammation-producing free fatty acids.

The striking preponderance of patients with acalculous biliary pain who are young, fertile women closely parallels the epidemiology of cholelithiasis, an observation suggesting that the risk factors may be similar in the two conditions. Indeed, some studies[9] have shown that up to one half of patients with acalculous biliary pain actually have microscopic cholelithiasis in resected gallbladder specimens, a finding which indicates that the original ultrasonogram was falsely negative. Examination of a bile specimen for microlithiasis (Meltzer-Lyon test, discussed later) would be helpful in identifying these patients.

Several studies have consistently shown that a subset of patients with acalculous biliary pain have histologic evidence of cholesterolosis in their resected gallbladders.[10–12] Although usually thought to be an incidental pathologic finding, cholesterolosis of the gallbladder may, in some patients, disrupt normal gallbladder contraction and result in clinical features that are identical to biliary colic.

Finally, acalculous biliary pain is listed as a functional gastrointestinal disorder by a multinational working committee of gastrointestinal investigators (Rome classification) with the implication that a pathologic lesion is not required for the diagnosis.[4]

Clinical Manifestations, Diagnosis, and Treatment

As described earlier, the clinical manifestations of acalculous biliary pain are identical to those of biliary colic. A careful review of the patient's complaints should confirm that the symptoms are genuinely suggestive of biliary colic[3] rather than dyspepsia, heartburn, crampy abdominal pain, or flatulence. If the symptoms suggest biliary colic, then a careful review of the ultrasonogram with the radiologist is warranted. Although gallstones larger than 2 mm are unlikely to have been missed (the sensitivity of ultrasonography for detecting stones exceeds 95%), other ultrasonographic evidence of gallbladder disease may have been overlooked if the primary focus was to exclude stones. Patients with adenomyomatosis of the gallbladder or small cholesterol polyps may have symptoms identical to those of biliary colic that are relieved by cholecystectomy.

EXAMINATION OF THE BILE FOR CHOLESTEROL CRYSTALS (MELTZER-LYON TEST). If the ultrasonogram is normal, then a reasonable approach may be to examine the bile for evidence of cholesterol crystals. Long before the advent of ultrasonography, biliary drainage was used to identify patients who were likely to harbor gallstones.[13] The test has been modified so that the bile is now aspirated during an upper endoscopy after stimulation of gallbladder contraction with intravenous cholecystokinin (CCK).[14] The bile should be kept at room temperature and examined immediately under the microscope for the presence of characteristic birefringent, notched rhomboid cholesterol crystals, or calcium bilirubinate crystals.

Limited clinical studies[10, 11] in patients with acalculous biliary pain have shown that approximately one third will have crystals in their bile. If operated on, most of these patients have both microlithiasis and pathologically confirmed cholecystitis and will become symptom free after cholecystectomy. The two thirds of patients who do not have crystals in their bile generally pursue a benign course and rarely return with evidence of biliary tract disease.

STIMULATED CHOLESCINTIGRAPHY. A second approach to selecting patients with acalculous biliary pain who would likely benefit from surgery involves calculation of a gallbladder ejection fraction (GBEF) using cholescintigraphy. A radiolabeled hepatobiliary agent (e.g., ^{99m}Tc-diisopropyl iminodiacetic acid) is concentrated in the gallbladder, and a computer-assisted gamma camera measures activity before and after stimulation of gallbladder contraction with a slow intravenous infusion of CCK over 30 minutes. The GBEF is defined as the change in activity divided by the baseline activity. Studies in healthy volunteers have shown that the average GBEF is 75% and that virtually all exceed 35%.[5]

Ironically, as the test gains clinical acceptance, the predictive value of a positive test is likely to fall. When stimulated cholescintigraphy was first developed, most patients referred for testing had been followed for years with biliary pain, allowing ample time for other conditions accounting for the pain to become manifest. Therefore, the pretest probability of having a primary gallbladder motility derangement was high, and the specificity of the test appeared to be excellent. Now, the test is employed earlier in the evaluation of patients with biliary pain (sometimes immediately following an ultrasonogram that is negative for stones), and patients with nonbiliary or self-limiting diseases have not been weeded out. Hence, the earlier cholescintigraphy is employed, the lower the pretest probability of acalculous biliary pain and, unfortunately, the lower the predictive value of a positive result.[15]

In patients with acalculous biliary pain, much less than one half have a depressed GBEF, but virtually all of those who do will continue to have symptoms when followed for as long as 3 years. If a cholecystectomy is performed in these patients,[12] histologic evidence of chronic cholecystitis is found in approximately 90%, cystic duct narrowing in 80%, and cholesterolosis in 30%. The long-term outcome, with respect to relief of symptoms, has varied, but two recent studies[16, 17] have shown that between 67% and 80% of these patients are cured of their symptoms following cholecystectomy.

The patients with acalculous biliary pain and a normal GBEF pursue a variable (but generally benign) course; many ultimately are found to have nonbiliary causes of their symptoms. Thus, the combination of an examination of bile for cholesterol crystals and stimulated cholescintigraphy, when applied to patients with classic biliary colic but without ultrasonographically demonstrable gallstones, is a useful means of selecting patients who may benefit from empiric cholecystectomy. If the bile contains no crystals and the gallbladder contracts normally, then the patient is not likely to benefit from cholecystectomy.

ACUTE ACALCULOUS CHOLECYSTITIS

Definition

Acute acalculous cholecystitis is acute inflammation of the gallbladder in the absence of stones.[18] Acute cholecystitis resulting from calculi is discussed in Chapter 55. This review focuses on the clinical features that are unique to acalculous cholecystitis. In fact, the name *acalculous cholecystitis* has been questioned as incorrectly suggesting that the disease is simply cholecystitis without stones. Instead, the term *necrotizing cholecystitis* has been proposed to reflect the distinct etiology, pathology, and prognosis of the disease.[19]

Epidemiology

Acute acalculous cholecystitis accounts for 5% to 10% of cholecystectomies performed in the United States. In fact, of the cholecystectomies performed on postoperative or hospitalized patients recovering from trauma or burns, more than one half are for acalculous disease.[20]

Less commonly, acute acalculous cholecystitis may occur in the absence of antecedent trauma or stress, especially in children,[21] elderly patients with coexisting vascular disease,[22] bone marrow transplant recipients,[23] and patients with acquired immunodeficiency syndrome.[24, 25] In some cases, specific infectious etiologies can be identified, such as *Salmonella*[26] or cytomegalovirus in immunocompromised patients.[27] Systemic vasculitides such as polyarteritis nodosa or systemic lupus erythematosus may present as acute acalculous cholecystitis caused by ischemic injury to the gallbladder.[28, 29] Finally, acute acalculous cholecystitis is being recognized increasingly in otherwise healthy people without any risk factors.[30]

As a group, patients with acute acalculous cholecystitis[31] are more likely to be men and old than are patients with cholecystitis caused by calculi, which clusters in younger women.

Pathogenesis

Most cases of acute acalculous cholecystitis occur in the setting of prolonged fasting, immobility, and hemodynamic instability. The gallbladder epithelium, although normally a robust tissue, is exposed to one of the most noxious environments in the body: a concentrated solution of bile acid detergents designed to solubilize lipids. In the course of a normal day, the gallbladder empties the concentrated bile several times and is replenished with dilute (and presumably less noxious) hepatic bile. With prolonged fasting, the gallbladder never receives a CCK stimulus to empty, and, thus, the concentrated bile stagnates in the gallbladder lumen.[32] Additionally, the gallbladder epithelium has relatively high metabolic energy requirements to absorb electrolytes and water from the bile. Thus, in an immobile, fasting patient with splanchnic vasoconstriction resulting from septic shock (often, a patient in the intensive care unit), the stage is set for an ischemic and chemical injury to the gallbladder epithelium.[33] A recent study[34] that compared the microcirculation of gallbladders removed because of either gallstone disease or acalculous cholecystitis showed that, in acalculous cholecystitis, the capillaries barely filled, indicating that disturbed microcirculation may play an important role in the pathogenesis of acute acalculous cholecystitis.

Specific mediators that have been implicated in the tissue injury associated with acalculous cholecystitis include the inappropriate activation of factor XII[35] (demonstrated to initiate gallbladder inflammation in animals) and release of prostaglandins locally in the gallbladder wall.[36, 37] In animal models, tissue destruction can be attenuated by inhibiting prostaglandin synthesis with indomethacin. Infection of the gallbladder mucosa with bacteria, usually gram-negative enteric organisms and anaerobes,[38] is thought to be a secondary event in acute acalculous cholecystitis and follows rather than causes the initial injury in most cases.

Clinical Manifestations

The clinical features of acute acalculous cholecystitis differ from those of acute cholecystitis caused by stone disease. Although right upper quadrant pain, fever, localized tenderness overlying the gallbladder, and leukocytosis may be evident in classic presentations, some or all of these features are frequently lacking in elderly, postoperative patients.[39] Often, unexplained fever or hyperamylasemia is the only clue that anything is amiss. Symptoms or signs referable to the right upper quadrant are initially absent in three fourths of cases.

When compared with typical calculous cholecystitis, the clinical course of acute acalculous cholecystitis is more fulminant. By the time the diagnosis has been made, at least one half of the patients have experienced a complication of cholecystitis, such as gangrene or a confined perforation of the gallbladder.[40] Empyema and ascending cholangitis may further complicate cases in which bacterial superinfection of the gallbladder has occurred. Because the disease often occurs in debilitated patients and because the clinical course is fulminant, with rapid, early complications, the mortality rate of acute acalculous cholecystitis is high, ranging from 10% to 50%, much greater than the expected 1% mortality rate seen in patients with calculous cholecystitis. Such high mortality rates have led some investigators to propose that empiric cholecystostomy be considered in gravely ill patients in the intensive care unit for whom no source of sepsis can be found.[41]

Diagnosis

The rapid development of complications in acute acalculous cholecystitis makes early diagnosis critical for avoiding excessive mortality. Unfortunately, the lack of specific clinical findings pointing to the gallbladder, combined with a confusing clinical picture related to antecedent surgery or trauma, makes an early diagnosis difficult. For elderly patients at risk, a high index of suspicion for biliary tract sepsis is the best hope for early recognition and treatment. Table 58–2 delineates several diagnostic criteria for acute acalculous cholecystitis.

Table 58–2 | **Diagnostic Criteria for Acute Acalculous Cholecystitis**

TECHNIQUE	FINDINGS
Clinical examination	Right upper quadrant tenderness and Murphy's sign are helpful if present but are lacking in three fourths of cases Unexplained fever, leukocytosis, or hyperamylasemia are frequently the only signs
Ultrasonography	Thickened gallbladder wall, defined as >4 mm thickness in the absence of ascites or hypoalbuminemia (<3.2 g/dL) Sonographic Murphy's sign, defined as maximum tenderness over the ultrasonographically localized gallbladder Pericholecystic fluid collection • *Bedside availability is major advantage*
Computed tomography	Thickened gallbladder wall, defined as >4 mm thickness in the absence of ascites or hypoalbuminemia (<3.2 g/dL) Pericholecystic fluid, subserosal edema (in the absence of ascites), intramural gas, or sloughed mucosa • *Best test for excluding other intra-abdominal pathology but requires moving patient to scanner*
Hepatobiliary scintigraphy	Nonvisualization of the gallbladder with normal excretion of dye into the bile duct and duodenum is defined as a positive test for acute cholecystitis Critically ill immobilized patients may have false-positive scans because of viscus bile Morphine augmentation may reduce the number of false-positive results • *Better at excluding acute cholecystitis than confirming it*

ULTRASONOGRAPHY. In evaluating patients with suspected acute acalculous cholecystitis, ultrasonography offers the distinct advantages of being widely available and easily transportable to the bedside.[42] Three ultrasonographic findings that point to gallbladder disease include a thickened gallbladder wall (defined as >4 mm) in the absence of ascites or hypoalbuminemia, a sonographic Murphy's sign (defined as maximum tenderness over the sonographically localized gallbladder), and a pericholecystic fluid collection.

Although a thickened gallbladder wall (Fig. 58–1) is not specific for cholecystitis, in the proper clinical setting it is suggestive of gallbladder involvement and should prompt further evaluation. A sonographic Murphy's sign is operator dependent and requires a cooperative patient but, when positive, is a reliable indicator of gallbladder inflammation.[43] A pericholecystic fluid collection indicates advanced disease. The overall sensitivity of ultrasonography for detecting acute acalculous cholecystitis has been reported to range from 67% to 92%, with a specificity of more than 90%.[42] Investigators have proposed an ultrasonographic scoring system[44] to improve the diagnostic accuracy of ultrasonography in critically ill patients. Two points are given for distention of the gallbladder or thickening of the gallbladder wall, and one point each is given for striated thickening of the gallbladder wall, sludge, or pericholecystic fluid. Scores of six or higher accurately predict acalculous cholecystitis.

COMPUTED TOMOGRAPHY (CT). CT findings suggestive of cholecystitis include wall thickening (>4 mm), pericholecystic fluid, subserosal edema (in the absence of ascites), intramural gas, and sloughed mucosa. The sensitivity and specificity of these findings for predicting acute acalculous cholecystitis at surgery have been reported to exceed 95%. CT is superior to ultrasonography in detecting pathology

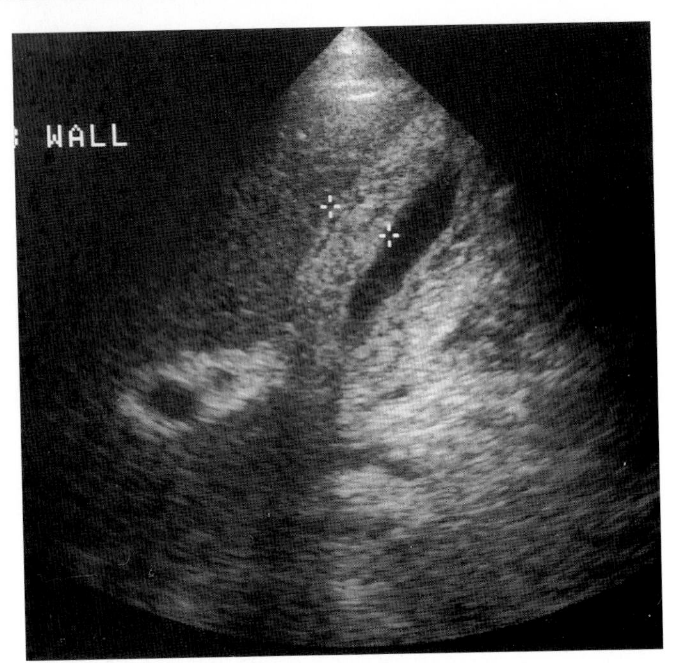

Figure 58–1. A gallbladder ultrasonogram demonstrating thickening of the gallbladder wall to 17 mm (denoted by marks) characteristic of acute acalculous cholecystitis. Point tenderness was noted when the transducer was pressed onto the gallbladder (sonographic Murphy's sign). The diagnosis was confirmed at laparotomy. (Courtesy of David Hurst, MD, Baylor Hospital, Dallas, TX.)

elsewhere in the abdomen that could be the cause of the patient's fever or pain.[45] An obvious disadvantage of CT is that it cannot be performed at the bedside, which is necessary in many critically ill patients. Several investigators have emphasized that CT is complementary to ultrasonography and often detects gallbladder disease in high-risk patients who have a negative ultrasonogram.

HEPATOBILIARY SCINTIGRAPHY. Hepatobiliary scintigraphy has proven useful in excluding cystic duct obstruction in patients with other clinical features suggestive of acute cholecystitis. Under normal conditions, the radionuclide is taken up by the liver, secreted into bile, concentrated in the gallbladder (where it produces a "hot spot"), and emptied into the duodenum. A positive scan for cystic duct obstruction is defined as failure to fill the gallbladder despite the normal passage of radionuclide into the duodenum. In suspected calculous cholecystitis, in which the pathogenesis involves obstruction of the cystic duct by a stone, filling of the gallbladder on scintigraphy virtually excludes cholecystitis as the cause of the patient's symptoms.[46]

Unfortunately, patients with acute acalculous cholecystitis have often fasted for prolonged periods. Fasting results in concentrated, viscous bile and frequently a false-positive hepatobiliary scan. Moreover, patients with acute acalculous cholecystitis (in contrast to those with calculi) often do not have an obstructed cystic duct; hence, hepatobiliary scans can be falsely negative as well,[47] although false-negative results are not as frequent as false-positive results. The sensitivity of the test may exceed 90%, but the lack of specificity in fasted, critically ill patients limits the usefulness of the test primarily to excluding acute acalculous cholecystitis rather than confirming the diagnosis. A recent study[48] in which ultrasonography and cholescintigraphy were performed in critically ill patients found cholescintigraphy to be useful for the early diagnosis of acute acalculous cholecystitis, whereas ultrasonography alone did not permit an early decision regarding the need for surgery.

In an effort to improve the accuracy of biliary scintigraphy, investigators[49] have proposed the use of *morphine-augmented cholescintigraphy* in which morphine sulfate is administered intravenously (0.05 to 0.1 mg/kg) to patients in whom the gallbladder did not visualize on standard cholescintigraphy. The rationale for this test is that morphine increases resistance to the flow of bile through the sphincter of Oddi and thus forces filling of the gallbladder if the cystic duct is patent, thereby reducing the problem of false-positive results. In approximately 60% of critically ill patients with possible biliary tract sepsis and a nonvisualizing gallbladder on standard cholescintigraphy, the gallbladder will visualize after morphine augmentation, and, therefore, acute cholecystitis will be excluded as the source of sepsis.

Treatment

In light of rapid progression of acute acalculous cholecystitis to gangrene and perforation, early recognition and intervention are required. Supportive medical care should include restoration of hemodynamic stability and antibiotic coverage for gram-negative enteric organisms and anaerobes if biliary tract infection is suspected.

SURGICAL CHOLECYSTECTOMY AND CHOLECYSTOSTOMY. For definitive therapy, the traditional approach has been urgent laparotomy and cholecystectomy.[50] In patients too unstable to tolerate anesthesia, a tube cholecystostomy has been placed surgically as a temporizing measure before definitive cholecystectomy when the patient is stable.

PERCUTANEOUS CHOLECYSTOSTOMY. Recently, several investigators[41, 51–53] have reported favorable results with the sonographically guided percutaneous transhepatic placement of a cholecystostomy drainage tube, coupled with administration of antibiotics, as definitive therapy in patients at high surgical risk. Studies suggest that most patients with acute acalculous cholecystitis can be treated with percutaneous drainage; if the postdrainage cholangiogram is normal, the catheter can be removed, and cholecystectomy is not necessary.[51, 54, 55]

TRANSPAPILLARY ENDOSCOPIC CHOLECYSTOSTOMY. Because of massive ascites or uncorrectable coagulopathy, some critically ill patients with suspected acute acalculous cholecystitis are poor candidates for even the minimally invasive, ultrasonographically guided percutaneous cholecystostomy described earlier. Such patients may benefit from a recently described endoscopic approach in which the cystic duct is selectively cannulated during endoscopic retrograde cholangiopancreatography with an obliquely angled guidewire that tracks along the lateral wall of the common bile duct and facilitates cannulation of the cystic duct.[56] If the wire can successfully negotiate the spiral valves within the cystic duct, then a nasobiliary catheter is introduced over the guidewire into the gallbladder, the contents are aspirated, and the gallbladder is lavaged with 1% *N*-acetylcysteine in saline to dissolve mucus and sludge. The nasocholecystostomy catheter is placed to gravity drainage for several days and easily removed when the crisis is over.

Preliminary studies in approximately 20 patients have shown that successful intubation of the gallbladder can be achieved in 90% of the attempts and that drainage and lavage of the viscous black bile and sludge from the gallbladder results in clinical resolution in most of these critically ill patients. The investigators acknowledge that the technique is more cumbersome and expensive than an ultrasonographically placed cholecystostomy tube and should be reserved for patients who would not tolerate a percutaneous approach.[57]

Prevention

Daily stimulation of gallbladder contraction with intravenous CCK has been shown to prevent the formation of gallbladder sludge in patients receiving total parenteral nutrition.[58] Because prolonged fasting with the resulting biliary sludge is a known risk factor for acute acalculous cholecystitis,[59] it may be possible to prevent this complication in high-risk patients through daily stimulation of gallbladder contraction with CCK. The efficacy and cost-effectiveness of such prophylaxis remain to be established.

CHOLESTEROLOSIS OF THE GALLBLADDER

Definition

Cholesterolosis is an acquired histologic abnormality of the gallbladder epithelium that results in an excessive accumulation of cholesterol esters within epithelial macrophages (Fig. 58–2).[60] Clinicians generally encounter the lesion only as an incidental pathologic finding after surgical resection of the gallbladder, although, in certain patients, the diagnosis may be suspected before surgery.

Cholesterolosis, as well as adenomyomatosis of the gallbladder, has been classified as one of the *hyperplastic cholecystoses,* a term introduced in 1960 to describe several diseases of the gallbladder thought to share the common features of mucosal hyperplasia, hyperconcentration and hyperexcretion of dye on cholecystography, and absence of inflammation.[61] The proponents of this concept believed that biliary colic, in the absence of gallstones, could often be explained by the presence of one of the hyperplastic cholecystoses, whereas other investigators, citing the lack of a common etiology and the nonspecificity of the clinical features, have recommended that the term hyperplastic cholecystoses be abandoned.

Incidence and Prevalence

Although recognized as a distinct pathologic entity for almost a century, the actual prevalence of cholesterolosis remains a matter of some dispute. Depending on whether gross or microscopic criteria were used for diagnosis, the prevalence of cholesterolosis in necropsy specimens has ranged from 5% to 40%. A large autopsy series involving more than 1300 cases in which each gallbladder was examined microscopically found the prevalence of cholesterolosis to be 12%.[62] When surgically resected gallbladders were examined, the prevalence was, not surprisingly, about 50% higher (18%) than that found in necropsy material.[63] The incidence of cholesterolosis has not been calculated, because the entity is usually only an incidental pathologic finding, and the onset is rarely known.

The epidemiology of cholesterolosis is analogous to that of cholesterol gallstone disease[64] in that similar groups of persons are predisposed; however, the two lesions occur independently and do not usually coexist in the same individual. Like gallstone disease, cholesterolosis is uncommon in children (the youngest reported patient was a 13-year-old girl) and shows a marked predilection for women as old as 60 years of age. After that, the sex differences are less pronounced. No racial, ethnic, or geographic differences in prevalence have been described, although if the analogy with

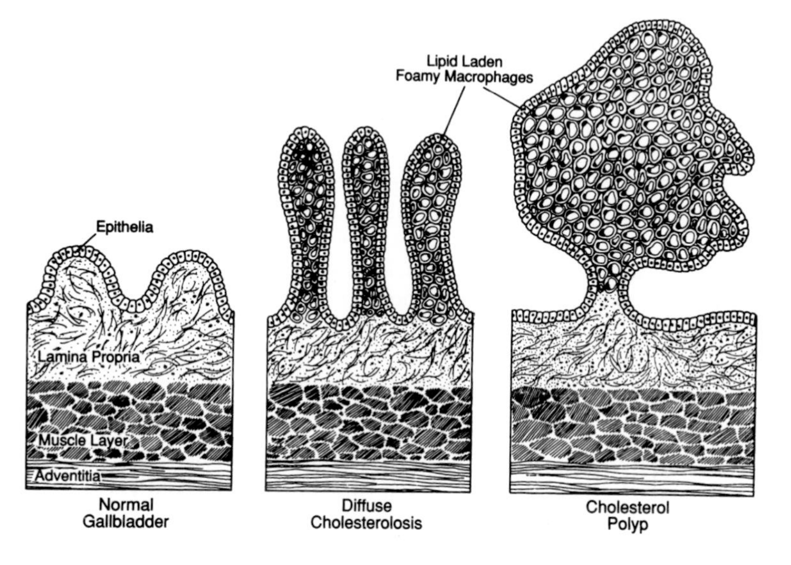

Figure 58–2. Schematic representation of the distribution of lipid-laden foamy macrophages in cholesterolosis. The diffuse form of cholesterolosis accounts for 80% of cases and generally causes no symptoms. Cholesterol polyps, present in 20% of the cases, are typically small, fragile excrescences that have a tendency to ulcerate or detach spontaneously from the mucosa. Although usually asymptomatic, the polyps have been associated with biliary colic and even acute pancreatitis.

cholesterol gallstone disease is extended, the prevalence would be expected to be higher in Western than non-Western societies.

Pathology

Cholesterolosis is defined pathologically by the accumulation of lipid (cholesterol esters and triglyceride) within the gallbladder mucosa. The following are four patterns of lipid deposition[60]:

1. Diffuse—the lipid is distributed throughout the epithelial lining of the gallbladder and ends abruptly at the cystic duct. This pattern accounts for 80% of all cases.
2. Cholesterol polyps—the excess lipid is confined to one or more areas of the epithelium that eventually form an excrescence into the lumen of the gallbladder. Isolated cholesterol polyps in the absence of diffuse cholesterolosis account for about 10% of the total cases.
3. Combined diffuse cholesterolosis and cholesterol polyps—cholesterol polyps occur on a background of diffuse cholesterolosis. This pattern accounts for about 10% of cases.
4. Focal cholesterolosis—excess lipid deposition is limited to a small area of the mucosa.

GROSS APPEARANCE. When the gallbladder is visually inspected at the time of laparotomy (or laparoscopy), a diagnosis of cholesterolosis can be made in one fifth of the cases on the basis of the gross appearance of the gallbladder mucosa as seen through the translucent serosal surface. When the gallbladder is opened, the mucosa characteristically has pale, yellow linear streaks running longitudinally, giving rise to the term *strawberry gallbladder* (although the mucosa is usually bile stained rather than red). When cholesterolosis is diagnosed at the time of surgical resection of the gallbladder, gallstones are also present in one half of cases. If the diagnosis is made at autopsy, stones are present in only 10%,[62] demonstrating that the two disease processes are independent of each other.

MICROSCOPIC APPEARANCE. Hyperplasia of the mucosa is invariably present and is described as marked in one half of cases. Usually, the hyperplasia is of the villous type. The most prominent feature is an abundance of macrophages within the elongated villi. Each macrophage is stuffed with lipid droplets and has a characteristic appearance of a "foam cell" (Fig. 58–3). In milder cases, the foam cells are limited to the tips of the villi (accounting for the linear streaks seen grossly); with more severe involvement, the foam cells may fill the entire villi and spill over into the underlying submucosa. Although extracellular deposits of lipid are rare, small yellow particles ("lipoidic corpuscles") representing detached masses of foam cells are occasionally seen floating in the bile.

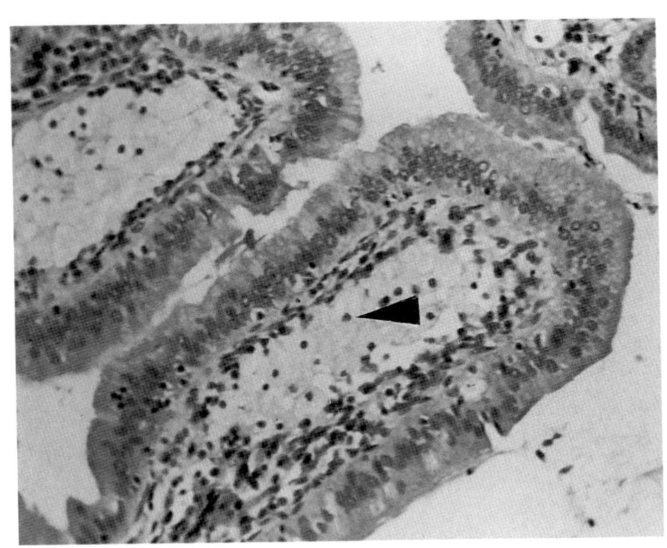

Figure 58–3. Photomicrograph (hematoxylin and eosin stain) of diffuse cholesterolosis. Note the hyperplastic, elongated villi and the foamy macrophages *(arrow)*. (Courtesy of E. L. Lee, MD, Veterans Affairs Hospital, Dallas, TX.)

Pathogenesis

The cause of the accumulation of cholesterol esters and triglyceride[65] in cholesterolosis remains obscure. Several hypotheses have been put forth suggesting that the cholesterol is derived from the blood[66] or that mechanical factors that impede emptying of the gallbladder lead to the deposition of lipid.[67] More recent data have unequivocally shown that the gallbladder epithelium is capable of absorbing cholesterol from the bile, as might be expected in epithelium that is embryologically and histologically similar to intestinal absorptive cells.[68, 69] Moreover, the cholesterol in gallbladder bile is already in the ideal physical state for absorption (i.e., a mixed micelle). The question remains as to why, in some patients, resorbed biliary cholesterol is esterified and then stored in foamy macrophages as cholesterolosis.[70] The lesion is frequently, but not always, found in gallbladders exposed to bile that is supersaturated with cholesterol,[71] just as cholesterol stones frequently, but not always, form under the same circumstances. These two disorders, both of which lead to the ectopic accumulation of cholesterol, probably share common pathogenic mechanisms (such as the secretion of an abnormal bile) but progress independently in a given patient, depending on other factors such as the presence of nucleating proteins in bile and the rate of mucosal esterification.[72]

Clinical Manifestations

Cholesterolosis usually does not cause symptoms, as demonstrated by autopsy specimens that show the lesion in patients who never had biliary symptoms. On occasion, however, individual patients may have dull, vague, right upper quadrant or epigastric pain that resembles biliary colic, and, at the time of cholecystectomy, they are found to have no stones, no gallbladder inflammation, and only incidental cholesterolosis. In those patients who undergo cholecystectomy for the syndrome of acalculous biliary pain and have incidental cholesterolosis on pathologic examination of the gallbladder, the prognosis is better in terms of resolution of pain than if cholesterolosis is not found.[73]

A retrospective surgical series looking at almost 4000 gallbladders removed by cholecystectomy identified 55 patients with acalculous cholesterolosis.[74] The investigators found that almost one half of these patients had presented with recurrent pancreatitis of unknown etiology and speculated that small cholesterol polyps had detached from the gallbladder wall and transiently obstructed the sphincter of Oddi, thereby provoking the acute pancreatitis. After 5 years of follow-up, the pancreatitis did not recur. These authors and others[75, 76] have suggested that cholesterolosis (or more specifically, cholesterol polyps) should be considered in the differential diagnosis of idiopathic pancreatitis.

Diagnosis

Diffuse cholesterolosis (which, as noted earlier, constitutes 80% of cases) is only rarely detectable by either ultrasonography or oral cholecystography. However, in the polypoid form, if the polyps are of sufficient size, there is a characteristic appearance on ultrasonography of single or multiple nonshadowing, fixed echoes projecting into the lumen of the gallbladder.[77] Most of the polyps are small (2 to 10 mm). On oral cholecystography, the polyps appear as small, round radiolucencies in the lumen of the opacified gallbladder and are best demonstrated after the gallbladder has been partially emptied and compression has been applied.

Treatment

Because cholesterolosis is only rarely diagnosed before resection of the gallbladder, the issue of treatment is usually irrelevant. In the rare case of polypoid cholesterolosis diagnosed by ultrasonography or cholecystography, the absence of biliary tract symptoms argues against any intervention. If the patient has symptoms consistent with biliary colic or pancreatitis,[74] a cholecystectomy is indicated. There is no medical therapy for cholesterolosis.

ADENOMYOMATOSIS OF THE GALLBLADDER

Definition

Adenomyomatosis (an unwieldy term that obscures its meaning) is defined as an acquired, hyperplastic lesion of the gallbladder characterized by excessive proliferation of surface epithelium with invaginations into the thickened muscularis or beyond.[78] Despite the prefix *adeno-*, the lesion is entirely benign and unrelated to adenomatous epithelia elsewhere in the gastrointestinal tract. Adenomyomatosis is not thought to have potential for malignant transformation.

The literature on this obscure topic is made all the more difficult to understand by the proliferation of different terms used to describe the same condition. One author[79] notes that adenomyomatosis has been described by at least 18 different names, the more common of which include *adenomyoma* (used when the lesion is localized to the gallbladder fundus), *diverticulosis of the gallbladder* (ignores the hyperplasia), *cholecystitis glandularis proliferans* (overemphasizes the role of inflammation), *Rokitansky-Aschoff sinuses* (familiar but anatomically incorrect), *adenomyosis*, and *adenomyomatous hyperplasia*. Some terms are used in the radiologic literature, whereas others are used exclusively by pathologists; none are familiar to most gastroenterologists.

Incidence and Prevalence

The prevalence of adenomyomatosis of the gallbladder varies greatly depending on the criteria used for diagnosis and whether resected gallbladders or necropsy specimens were examined. In a large series of more than 10,000 cholecystectomy specimens, Shepard and associates[80] found only 103 cases of adenomyomatosis, for a prevalence of about 1%. The lesion is more common in women than men, by a 3:1 ratio, and the prevalence increases with age. Neither ethnic nor geographic differences in prevalence have been described.

Pathology

To understand the pathology of adenomyomatosis, it is useful to consider briefly the normal histologic architecture of the gallbladder as well as the entity of Rokitansky-Aschoff sinuses (Fig. 58–4). Unlike the small intestine, the gallbladder has no muscularis mucosa; thus, the lamina propria abuts directly on the muscular layer. In childhood, the epithelial layer is cast up into folds and supported by the lamina propria. As the gallbladder ages, the valleys of the epithelial layer may deepen so that they penetrate into the muscular layer and form Rokitansky-Aschoff sinuses. These sinuses are acquired lesions and are present in about 90% of resected gallbladders. If the Rokitansky-Aschoff sinuses are

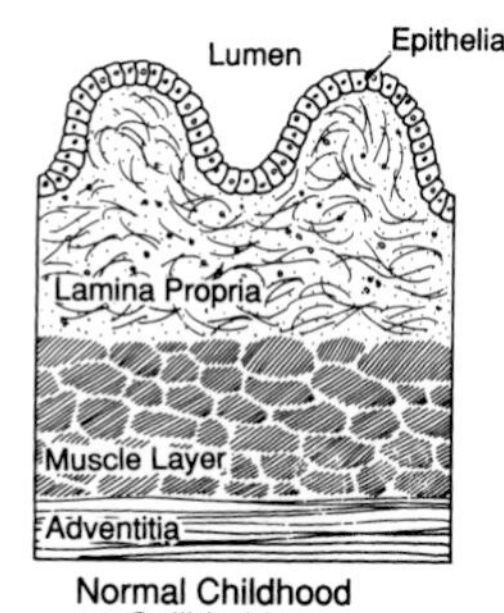

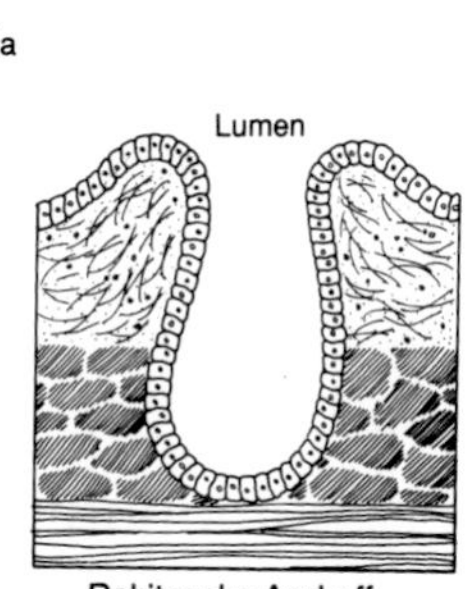

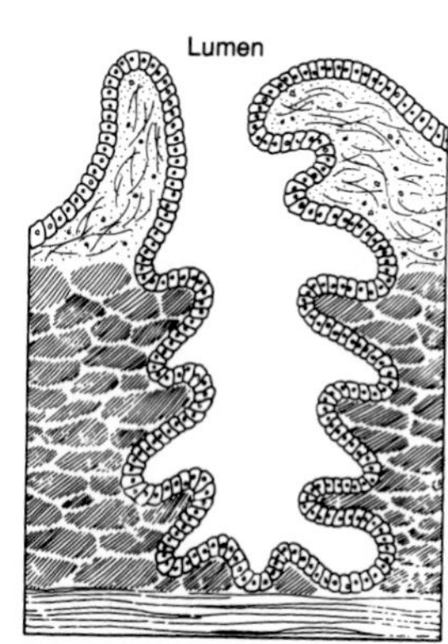

Figure 58–4. Schematic representation of a normal gallbladder, Rokitansky-Aschoff sinuses, and adenomyomatosis. Rokitansky-Aschoff sinuses, which are present in about 90% of resected gallbladders, consist of invaginations of the epithelial layer into the muscle layer, producing tiny mural diverticula. By themselves, they have no clinical significance. A histologic diagnosis of adenomyomatosis requires that the Rokitansky-Aschoff sinuses be deep and branching and accompanied by hyperplasia of the muscle layer.

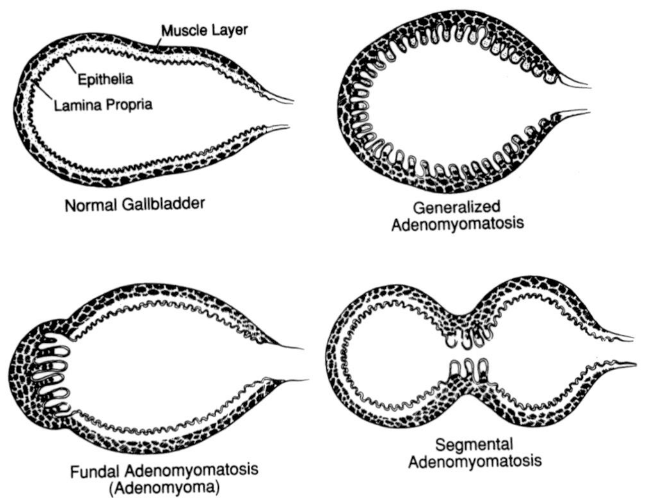

Figure 58–5. Schematic representation showing the different patterns of adenomyomatosis. Most of the cases are localized to the fundus of the gallbladder (in which case the lesion is termed an *adenomyoma*); generalized and segmental patterns are much less common. An adenomyoma is usually 10 to 20 mm in diameter and may be largely confined to the wall (as depicted here) or may project into the lumen to produce a polypoid lesion.

deep and branching and accompanied by thickening (hyperplasia) of the muscular layer, then a diagnosis of adenomyomatosis can be made.[78]

GROSS APPEARANCE. Adenomyomatosis may involve the entire gallbladder (generalized adenomyomatosis) or, more commonly, may be localized to the gallbladder fundus, in which case the lesion is often termed an *adenomyoma*. On rare occasion, the process may be limited to only an annular segment of the gallbladder wall and give rise to a luminal narrowing and a "dumbbell-shaped" gallbladder (Fig. 58–5). In any case, the involved portion of the gallbladder wall is thickened to 10 mm or more, and the muscle layer is three to five times its normal depth. On cut sections, cystic dilations of the Rokitansky-Aschoff sinuses are evident and may be filled with pigmented debris or calculi.

MICROSCOPIC APPEARANCE. Hyperplasia of the muscle layer is invariably present, and the epithelial lining occasionally undergoes intestinal metaplasia. Mild chronic inflammation is often present.

Pathogenesis

The pathogenesis of adenomyomatosis is unknown. Increased intraluminal pressure from mechanical obstruction (e.g., from an obstructing calculus, kink in the cystic duct, or congenital septum) has been postulated to result in cystic dilation of the Rokitansky-Aschoff sinuses, subsequent hyperplasia of the muscle layer, and adenomyomatosis.[78] Like pressure-related colonic diverticula, Rokitansky-Aschoff sinuses are most likely to be found where the muscle layer is weakest (at the site of a penetrating blood vessel). However, evidence for outflow obstruction is not always found; for example, calculi are present in only about 60% of the cases of adenomyomatosis.[80] Although some investigators have proposed that adenomyomatosis is a consequence of chronic inflammation, inflammation is not always present, particularly when the lesion is localized to the fundus.[81] Finally, several investigators have noted an association between adenomyomatosis and anomalous pancreaticobiliary ductal union. In one study,[82] one half of patients with adenomyomatosis had anomalous pancreaticobiliary ductal union, and, in another study,[83] one third of patients with anomalous pancreaticobiliary ductal union had adenomyomatosis. The pathogenic link between these two peculiar entities is unclear.

Clinical Manifestations

Adenomyomatosis, like cholesterolosis, usually causes no symptoms but is rather an incidental finding at autopsy or surgical resection. As noted earlier,[80] gallstones are present in more than one half of the resected gallbladders that are found to have adenomyomatosis, in which case the symptoms can be ascribed to the stones. The symptoms that have been ascribed to acalculous adenomyomatosis are indistinguishable from biliary colic caused by cholelithiasis.

On rare occasions, adenocarcinoma of the gallbladder has been found in association with adenomyomatosis[84]; however, the malignancy is often far removed from the localized area of adenomyomatosis, and the association has been thought to be coincidental rather than causal. Nonetheless, several recent reports[85, 86] of adenocarcinoma occurring in an area of gallbladder wall involved with adenomyomatosis have created diagnostic uncertainty on ultrasonography or cholecystography. In particular, a retrospective review[87] of more than 3000 resected gallbladders revealed a significantly higher frequency (6.4%) of gallbladder cancer in gallbladders with the segmental form of adenomyomatosis than would have been expected by chance alone, and the investigators proposed that segmental adenomyomatosis should be considered a potentially premalignant lesion.

When simple adenomyomatosis of the gallbladder is discovered incidentally, the lesion is likely to be benign. However, if there is any suspicion of an associated mass lesion, particularly one greater than 10 mm in size, or if segmental adenomyomatosis is found, then a thorough radiologic evaluation of the gallbladder is warranted.

Diagnosis

As noted previously, adenomyomatosis is frequently not diagnosed before resection and direct examination of the gallbladder. However, there are several specific radiologic and ultrasonographic findings that may, if present, allow a diagnosis to be made preoperatively.

On oral cholecystography, the mural diverticula constituting the Rokitansky-Aschoff sinuses may fill with contrast material and produce characteristic radiopaque dots paralleling the margin of the gallbladder lumen.[88] Any portion of the gallbladder wall may be involved (Fig. 58–6). Localized, fundal adenomyomatosis (adenomyoma) may present as a filling defect in the fundus, whereas segmental adenomyomatosis may present as a circumferential narrowing of the gallbladder lumen. As is the case with cholesterolosis, the radiologic findings of adenomyomatosis are best appreciated when the gallbladder has partially emptied of contrast material and pressure has been applied during radiography.[88]

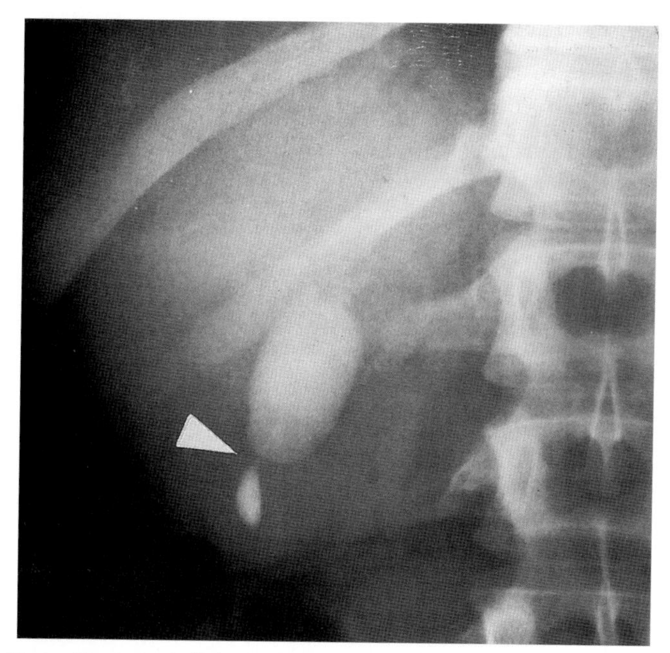

Figure 58–6. Oral cholecystogram of a 28-year-old man with postprandial epigastric pain radiating through to his back. The film demonstrates an annular segment of the gallbladder wall *(arrow)* involved with adenomyomatosis, which has produced a constriction of the lumen. Although no gallstones were present, a cholecystectomy was performed, and the patient's symptoms were relieved. (Courtesy of W. J. Kilman, MD, Parkland Hospital, Dallas, TX.)

Although ultrasonography has largely replaced oral cholecystography in the evaluation of the gallbladder, the ultrasonographic findings of adenomyomatosis are less specific than the radiographic findings.[89] A thickened gallbladder wall (>4 mm) is not specific for gallbladder disease and is seen in many other conditions, particularly liver diseases resulting in hypoalbuminemia or ascites.[90] Carefully done studies in which radiologic and ultrasonographic findings of adenomyomatosis were correlated with pathologic findings have determined that diffuse or segmental thickening of the gallbladder wall in association with intramural diverticula (seen as round anechoic foci) accurately predicts adenomyomatosis.[91] If the intramural diverticula (dilated Rokitansky-Aschoff sinuses) are filled with sludge or small calculi, then the lesions may appear echogenic with acoustic shadowing or a reverberation artifact.[92]

Finally, CT and magnetic resonance findings of adenomyomatosis have been described[93] and include differential enhancement of gallbladder wall layers, detection of Rokitansky-Aschoff sinuses within a thickened wall,[94] and subserosal fatty proliferation.[95]

Treatment

In the absence of biliary tract symptoms, adenomyomatosis requires no treatment. If the patient has biliary colic and radiographic or ultrasonographic evidence of adenomyomatosis with calculi, then a cholecystectomy is indicated. A more difficult clinical problem arises when a patient is symptomatic with suspected adenomyomatosis but no stones.[85] In such cases, the more extensive or severe the adenomyomatosis appears to be, the more confident the clinician can be that the symptoms are related to the lesion and the more likely the patient will be to benefit from cholecystectomy. Fear of malignant transformation is not a reason to operate,[96] unless an ultrasonographic or radiologic image is worrisome for a mass or perhaps the segmental form of adenomyomatosis.

POLYPS OF THE GALLBLADDER

Definition

The term *polyps of the gallbladder* is used here to describe any mucosal projection into the lumen of the gallbladder, whether neoplastic or not.[97] Ideally, histologic confirmation would allow rational treatment, but because the gallbladder is hidden from direct inspection, the clinician usually must base treatment decisions on imperfect information provided by ultrasonography and radiography. As it turns out, most gallbladder polyps are not true neoplasms but rather the result of lipid deposits or inflammation.[98] True neoplasms of the gallbladder, both benign and malignant, are discussed in more detail in Chapter 60.

Incidence and Prevalence

The prevalence of gallbladder polyps, defined either pathologically or radiologically,[99] ranges from 1% to 4%. Often, gallbladder polyps are encountered clinically as an incidental finding at the time of cholecystectomy.

Pathology

Polyps of the gallbladder may be classified as shown in Table 58–3[100] into either non-neoplastic lesions (which comprise 95% of all gallbladder polyps) or neoplastic lesions (of which adenomas comprise the vast majority).

CHOLESTEROL POLYPS. Cholesterol polyps (also known as *papillomas of the gallbladder,* although the term should be discarded) are the most common type of gallbladder polyp. They are not true neoplasms but rather variants of cholesterolosis resulting from infiltration of the lamina propria with lipid-laden foamy macrophages. The pathogenesis of cholesterol polyps is discussed in detail in the section on cholesterolosis (see earlier). Cholesterol polyps are typically small, pedunculated polyps that are less than 10 mm in diameter and attached to the mucosa by a thin, fragile stalk.[100] Frequently, detached tiny cholesterol polyps[101] are noted to be floating in the bile when the gallbladder is opened in the operating room. Although they may be solitary in one fifth of cases, the mean number of cholesterol polyps present in one series was eight.[102]

ADENOMYOMA. Adenomyomatosis of the gallbladder that is localized to the fundus may produce a hemispheric projection into the lumen that resembles a polyp. Such a lesion has come to be known as an adenomyoma, although it is not neoplastic in origin. The pathogenesis of an adenomyoma is discussed in the section on adenomyomatosis (see earlier). The lesions are usually approximately 15 mm in size, and the bulk of the adenomyoma is confined to the muscular wall of the gallbladder.[100]

Table 58–3 | **Histologic Types of Gallbladder Polyps**

HISTOLOGIC TYPE	RELATIVE FREQUENCY (%)	NEOPLASTIC	SIZE RANGE (mm)	NUMBER	COMMENTS
Cholesterol polyp (a polypoid form of cholesterolosis)	60	No	2–10	Multiple (average of 8)	May detach and behave clinically as stones and cause biliary colic or bile duct obstruction May be the unsuspected cause of some cases of idiopathic pancreatitis Surgery not required unless symptomatic
Adenomyoma (a localized form of adenomyomatosis)	25	No	10–20	Solitary	Always localized to the gallbladder fundus Forms hemispheric projection into lumen with the bulk confined to the muscular wall Surgery not required unless symptomatic or confused with a neoplasm
Inflammatory polyp	10	No	5–10	Solitary in half (2–5 in remainder)	Consists of granulation tissue and fibrous tissue with lymphocytes and plasma cells infiltrating Surgery not required
Adenoma	4	Yes	5–20	Solitary in two thirds (2–5 in remainder)	Rare lesion, found in only 0.15% of resected gallbladders Usually pedunculated (compare with adenomyoma) and coexists with stones in half of cases Only polyp in the gallbladder with a premalignant potential, and the frequency of progression from adenoma to carcinoma is much lower than that for colon polyps Virtually all adenomas with a focus of carcinoma have been >12 mm in diameter; thus lesions ≤10 mm can be followed ultrasonographically For lesions 10–18 mm, consider laparoscopic cholecystectomy in good surgical candidates For lesions >18 mm, consider open cholecystectomy, because invasive cancer is more likely and extended resection may be required
Miscellaneous polyps	1	Yes	5–20	Solitary	Extremely rare lesions with a frequency of <0.10% in resected gallbladders Histologic type cannot be predicted before surgery Histology includes leiomyoma, fibroma, lipoma, heterotropic gastric glands, neurofibroma, carcinoid, and other even rarer lesions Decision for surgery should be based on symptoms or size >10 mm

INFLAMMATORY POLYPS. Inflammatory polyps are small sessile lesions consisting of granulation and fibrous tissue infiltrated with lymphocytes and plasma cells. The average size is 5 to 10 mm. A solitary polyp is found in one half of the cases, and two to five are found in the remainder.[100] When discovered at the time of cholecystectomy, inflammatory polyps are almost always an incidental finding.

ADENOMAS. In light of the high frequency of adenomatous polyps in the tubular gastrointestinal tract, it is surprising how uncommon adenomas are in the gallbladder. Their incidence in resected gallbladder specimens is only about 0.15%.[103]

Adenomas are typically solitary, pedunculated masses from 5 to 20 mm in diameter. They may occur anywhere in the gallbladder. When multiple, as they are in approximately one third of cases, two to five polyps are usually found. Histologically, they are classified as either papillary or nonpapillary: The former consists of a branching, treelike skeleton of connective tissue covered with tall columnar cells, whereas the latter consists of a proliferation of glands encased by a fibrous stroma. On rare occasions, the entire gallbladder mucosa may undergo adenomatous transformation resulting in innumerable tiny mucosal polyps termed *multicentric papillomatosis*. Notably, gallstones are present in one half of cases of adenomatous polyps.[100]

Unlike colonic adenomas, which are much more common than adenocarcinoma of the colon, gallbladder adenomas are much less common than gallbladder carcinoma (by a 1:4 margin), and thus the frequency of progression from adenoma to adenocarcinoma is unclear.

In a series of more than 1600 consecutive cholecystectomies from Japan,[104] 18 patients were found to have gallbladder adenomas. Of these, 7 adenomas contained foci of carcinoma. In the same series, 79 cases of invasive carcinoma were found, and 15 (19%) of these were thought to have residual adenomatous tissue within the cancer, thereby suggesting that the initial lesion may have been an adenoma. Notably, all the adenomas that contained foci of carcinoma were larger than 12 mm in diameter. Thus, this study seems to contradict the prevailing opinion that adenomas rarely progress to carcinoma but rather suggests that adenomas, at least those larger than 12 mm in diameter, are premalignant lesions. Unfortunately, the clinician has no way of knowing whether a polyp (usually noted on an ultrasonogram) is a potentially premalignant adenoma or one of the other more common non-neoplastic polyps. In good surgical candidates, a prudent approach would be to resect a gallbladder containing polyps larger than 10 mm in diameter electively to minimize the chance of overlooking a premalignant lesion.

MISCELLANEOUS POLYPS. Although a wide variety of benign lesions may present as polyps in the gallbladder, all such lesions are rare. Fibromas, leiomyomas, and lipomas of the gallbladder are extraordinarily rare, especially compared to how common they are elsewhere in the gastrointestinal tract. Even less frequent are neurofibromas, carcinoids,[105] and heterotropic gastric glands.[106] Taken together, the combined incidence of nonadenomatous neoplastic polyps of the gallbladder is considerably less than 1 per 1000 resected specimens.[100]

Clinical Manifestations

Except in unusual cases, polyps of the gallbladder do not cause symptoms; their presence is noted only as an incidental finding during a cholecystectomy for coexisting gallstones. In the exceptional case in which a polyp (but not gallstones) is identified ultrasonographically or radiographically before surgery, the clinical symptomatology may resemble that of biliary colic, although several of the classic features (e.g., intense epigastric or right upper quadrant pain starting suddenly, rising in intensity over a 15-minute period, and continuing at a steady plateau for several hours before slowly subsiding) may be missing. Rare instances of acute acalculous cholecystitis and even hemobilia have been ascribed to benign gallbladder polyps.[107]

On clinical grounds alone, it is not possible to distinguish the histologic types of gallbladder polyp,[96] nor can the ultrasonogram or cholecystogram reliably predict histology[90] (Fig. 58–7). Thus, the clinician must decide, without knowing the pathology in advance, whether the symptoms, along with the ultrasonographic finding, warrant surgery. Endoscopic ultrasound may prove useful in distinguishing neoplastic from the more common non-neoplastic polyps. A recent study[108] compared conventional ultrasonography with endoscopic ultrasonography and found that the latter technique improved diagnostic accuracy when the former was equivocal.

The few studies that have attempted to define the natural history of untreated gallbladder polyps can serve to reassure the clinician who adopts a conservative "wait-and-see" approach. Based on records at the Mayo Clinic,[109] approximately 200 patients were identified who had cholecystograms that demonstrated gallbladder polyps and who did not undergo immediate cholecystectomy. After 15 years of follow-up, less than 10% of the patients subsequently developed symptoms sufficient to warrant surgery, and none of the patients available for follow-up had evidence of gallbladder cancer.

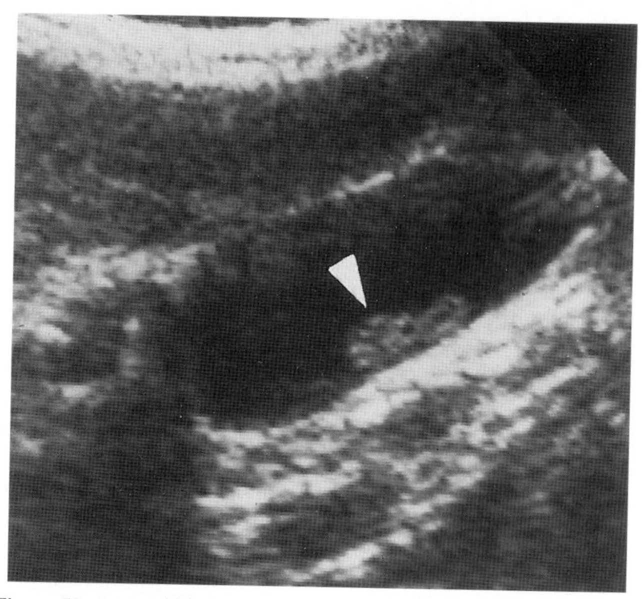

Figure 58–7. A gallbladder ultrasonogram (right longitudinal view) of a 55-year-old woman with mild biliary colic. The ultrasonogram demonstrates two luminal filling defects. The larger is 10 mm *(arrow)*; neither casts an acoustic shadow, and both are fixed to the same point on the gallbladder wall. These findings are consistent with gallbladder polyps, although the histology cannot be predicted from the ultrasonogram. A cholecystectomy was performed and revealed multiple cholesterol polyps, two of which were unusually large. (Courtesy of R. S. Harrell, MD, Parkland Hospital, Dallas, TX.)

Another study[110] (albeit with a much shorter follow-up period) identified 224 patients with gallbladder polyps, 95% of which were predicted to be cholesterol polyps on the basis of the ultrasonographic appearance and the remainder of which were classified as "polypoid lesions of uncertain benignity." After an average follow-up of 9 months, all the polyps initially thought to be benign remained the same size or were proven to be benign at resection. Two thirds of the polypoid lesions of uncertain benignity were found to be adenomas or carcinomas when resected. These studies serve to emphasize that 95% of gallbladder polyps are not neoplastic in origin.

Treatment

Patients who are symptomatic with biliary colic and have ultrasonographic demonstration of both polyps and stones should undergo an elective cholecystectomy, just as they would if there were no polyps. For patients whose ultrasonograms show polyps in the gallbladder but no stones, the decision to operate depends on the severity of the symptoms, the confidence of the clinician that the symptoms are indeed biliary in origin, and the ultrasonographic features (particularly the size) of the polyp.

Polyps smaller than 10 mm in diameter pose no immediate risk of cancer, and the decision to operate depends on the nature and severity of the symptoms.

Larger polyps between 10 and 18 mm in diameter raise the specter (albeit remote) of cancer in an adenoma and should prompt an elective laparoscopic cholecystectomy[111–113] if the patient is an acceptable surgical candidate. If the patient is a poor surgical risk, the polyp may be followed by ultrasonography or cholecystography (perhaps every 6 to 12 months) to see if it enlarges.[111, 114]

Polyps larger than 18 mm in diameter pose a significant risk of being malignant and should be resected. Moreover, one study[115] has shown that lesions of this size often contain advanced, invasive cancer that involves the serosal surface of the gallbladder and requires a more extensive dissection than can be accomplished by laparoscopy. Thus, these investigators advocated an open cholecystectomy for polypoid lesions of the gallbladder that are larger than 18 mm.

REFERENCES

1. Traverso LW, Lonborg R, Pettingell K, Fenster LF: Utilization of cholecystectomy—a prospective outcome analysis in 1325 patients. J Gastrointest Surg 4:1, 2000.
2. Fenster LF, Lonborg R, Thirlby RC, Traverso LW: What symptoms does cholecystectomy cure? Insights from an outcomes measurement project and review of the literature [review]. Am J Surg 169:533, 1995.
3. Festi D, Sottili S, Colecchia A, et al: Clinical manifestations of gallstone disease: Evidence from the multicenter Italian study on cholelithiasis (MICOL). Hepatology 30:839, 1999.
4. Drossman DA: Diagnosing and treating patients with refractory functional gastrointestinal disorders. Ann Intern Med 123:688, 1995.
5. Yap L, Wycherley AG, Morphett AD, Toouli J: Acalculous biliary pain: Cholecystectomy alleviates symptoms in patients with abnormal cholescintigraphy. Gastroenterology 101:786, 1991.
6. Jourdan JL, Stubbs RS: Acalculous gallbladder pain: A largely unrecognised entity. N Z Med J 112:152, 1999.
7. Venkataramani A, Strong RM, Anderson DS, et al: Abnormal duodenal bile composition in patients with acalculous chronic cholecystitis. Am J Gastroenterol 93:434, 1998.
8. Siegel A, Kuhn JC, Crow H, Holtzman S: Gallbladder ejection fraction: Correlation of scintigraphic and ultrasonographic techniques. Clin Nucl Med 25:1, 2000.
9. Herrera BA, Canelles GP, Medina CE, et al: [Cholecystectomy: A choice technique in biliary microlithiasis]. [Spanish]. An Med Interna 12:111, 1995.
10. Susann PW, Sheppard F, Baloga AJ: Detection of occult gallbladder disease by duodenal drainage collected endoscopically: A clinical and pathologic correlation. Am Surg 51:162, 1985.
11. Porterfield G, Cheung LY, Berenson M: Detection of occult gallbaldder disease by duodenal drainage. Am J Surg 134:702, 1977.
12. Halverson JD, Garner BA, Siegel BA, et al: The use of hepatobiliary scintigraphy in patients with acalculous biliary colic. Arch Intern Med 152:1305, 1992.
13. Lyon BBV: Diagnosis and treatment of diseases of the gallbladder and biliary ducts. JAMA 73:980, 1919.
14. Moskovitz M, Min TC, Gavaler JS: The microscopic examination of bile in patients with biliary pain and negative imaging tests. Am J Gastroenterol 81:329, 1986.
15. Ziessman HA: Cholecystokinin cholescintigraphy: Victim of its own success? J Nucl Med 40:2038, 1999.
16. Khosla R, Singh A, Miedema BW, Marshall JB: Cholecystectomy alleviates acalculous biliary pain in patients with a reduced gallbladder ejection fraction. South Med J 90:1087, 1997.
17. Goncalves RM, Harris JA, Rivera DE: Biliary dyskinesia: Natural history and surgical results. Am Surg 64:493, 1998.
18. Glenn F: Acute cholecystitis following the surgical treatment of unrelated disease. Ann Surg 126:411, 1947.
19. Barrett DS, Chadwick SJ, Fleming JA: Acalculous cholecystitis—a misnomer. J R Soc Med 81:11, 1988.
20. Barie PS, Fischer E: Acute acalculous cholecystitis [review]. J Am Coll Surg 180:232, 1995.
21. Fernandes ET, Hollabaugh RS, Boulden TF, Angel C: Gangrenous acalculous cholecystitis in a premature infant. J Pediatr Surg 24:608, 1989.
22. Savoca PE, Longo WE, Zucker KA, et al: The increasing prevalence of acalculous cholecystitis in outpatients: Results of a 7-year study. Ann Surg 211:433, 1990.
23. Wiboltt KS, Jeffrey RB Jr: Acalculous cholecystitis in patients undergoing bone marrow transplantation. Eur J Surg 163:519, 1997.
24. Nash JA, Cohen SA: Gallbladder and biliary tract disease in AIDS. Gastroenterol Clin North Am 26:323, 1997.
25. Wind P, Chevallier JM, Jones D, et al: Cholecystectomy for cholecystitis in patients with acquired immune deficiency syndrome. Am J Surg 168:244, 1994.
26. Winkler AP, Gleich S: Acute acalculous cholecystitis caused by *Salmonella typhi* in an 11-year old. Pediatr Infect Dis J 7:125, 1988.
27. Cappell MS: Hepatobiliary manifestations of the acquired immune deficiency syndrome. Am J Gastroenterol 86:1, 1991.
28. Kamimura T, Mimori A, Takeda A, et al: Acute acalculous cholecystitis in systemic lupus erythematosus: A case report and review of the literature. Lupus 7:361, 1998.
29. Parry SW, Pelias ME, Browder W: Acalculous hypersensitivity cholecystitis: Hypothesis of a new clinicopathologic entity. Surgery 104: 911, 1988.
30. Parithivel VS, Gerst PH, Banerjee S, et al: Acute acalculous cholecystitis in young patients without predisposing factors. Am Surg 65:366, 1999.
31. Kalliafas S, Ziegler DW, Flancbaum L, Choban PS: Acute acalculous cholecystitis: Incidence, risk factors, diagnosis, and outcome. Am Surg 64:471, 1998.
32. Lee SP: Pathogenesis of biliary sludge. Hepatology 12:200s, 1990.
33. Warren BL: Small vessel occlusion in acute acalculous cholecystitis. Surgery 111:163, 1992.
34. Hakala T, Nuutinen PJ, Ruokonen ET, Alhava E: Microangiopathy in acute acalculous cholecystitis. Br J Surg 84:1249, 1997.
35. Becker CG, Dubin T, Glenn F: Induction of acute cholecystitis by activation of factor XII. J Exp Med 151:81, 1980.
36. Kaminski DL, Andrus CH, German D, Deshpande YG: The role of prostanoids in the production of acute acalculous cholecystitis by platelet-activating factor. Ann Surg 212:455, 1990.
37. Kaminski DL, Feinstein WK, Deshpande YG: The production of experimental cholecystitis by endotoxin. Prostaglandins 47:233, 1994.
38. Claesson BE: Microflora of the biliary tree and liver—clinical correlates. Dig Dis 4:93, 1986.
39. Cornwell E, Rodriguez A, Mirvis SE, Shorr RM: Acute acalculous cholecystitis in critically injured patients: Preoperative diagnostic imaging. Ann Surg 210:52, 1989.
40. Johnson LB: The importance of early diagnosis of acute acalculous cholecystitis. Surg Gynecol Obstet 164:197, 1987.
41. Boland GW, Lee MJ, Leung J, Mueller PR: Percutaneous cholecystostomy in critically ill patients: Early response and final outcome in 82 patients. AJR Am J Roentgenol 163:339, 1994.
42. Mirvis SE, Vainright JR, Nelson AW, et al: The diagnosis of acute acalculous cholecystitis: A comparison of sonography, scintigraphy, and CT. AJR Am J Roentgenol 147:1171, 1986.
43. Laing FC, Federle MP, Jeffrey RB, Brown TW: Ultrasonic evaluation of patients with acute right upper quadrant pain. Radiology 140:449, 1981.
44. Helbich TH, Mallek R, Madl C, et al: Sonomorphology of the gallbladder in critically ill patients: Value of a scoring system and follow-up examinations. Acta Radiol 38:129, 1997.
45. Blankenberg F, Wirth R, Jeffrey RJ, et al: Computed tomography as an adjunct to ultrasound in the diagnosis of acute acalculous cholecystitis. Gastrointest Radiol 16:149, 1991.
46. Shuman WP, Rogers JV, Rudd TG, et al: Low sensitivity of sonography and cholescintigraphy in acalculous cholecystitis. AJR Am J Roentgenol 142:531, 1984.
47. Schneider PB: Acalculous cholecystitis: A case with variable cholescintigram. J Nucl Med 25:64, 1984.
48. Prevot N, Mariat G, Mahul P, et al: Contribution of cholescintigraphy

to the early diagnosis of acute acalculous cholecystitis in intensive-care-unit patients. Eur J Nucl Med 26:1317, 1999.
49. Flancbaum L, Choban PS, Sinha R, Jonasson O: Morphine cholescintigraphy in the evaluation of hospitalized patients with suspected acute cholecystitis. Ann Surg 220:25, 1994.
50. Pellegrini CA, Way LW: Acute cholecystitis. In Pellegrini CA, Way LW (eds): Surgery of the Gallbladder and Bile Ducts. Philadelphia, WB Saunders, 1987, p 251.
51. Shirai Y, Tsukada K, Kawaguchi H, et al: Percutaneous transhepatic cholecystostomy for acute acalculous cholecystitis. Br J Surg 80:1440, 1993.
52. Kiviniemi H, Makela JT, Autio R, et al: Percutaneous cholecystostomy in acute cholecystitis in high-risk patients: An analysis of 69 patients. Int Surg 83:299, 1998.
53. Kim KH, Sung CK, Park BK, et al: Percutaneous gallbladder drainage for delayed laparoscopic cholecystectomy in patients with acute cholecystitis. Am J Surg 179:111, 2000.
54. Tierney S, Pitt HA, Lillemoe KD: Physiology and pathophysiology of gallbladder motility [review]. Surg Clin North Am 73:1267, 1993.
55. Sugiyama M, Tokuhara M, Atomi Y: Is percutaneous cholecystostomy the optimal treatment for acute cholecystitis in the very elderly? World J Surg 22:459, 1998.
56. Johlin FC, Neil GA: Drainage of the gallbladder in patients with acute acalculous cholecystitis by transpapillary endoscopic cholecystostomy. Gastrointest Endosc 39:645, 1993.
57. Brugge WR, Friedman LS: A new endoscopic procedure provides insight into an old disease: Acute acalculous cholecystitis. Gastroenterology 106:1718, 1994.
58. Sitzmann J, Pitt H, Steinborn P: Cholecystokinin prevents parenteral nutrition induced biliary sludge in humans. Surg Gynecol Obstet 170: 25, 1990.
59. Roslyn JJ, Pitt HA, Mann LL, et al: Gallbladder disease in patients on long-term parenteral nutrition. Gastroenterology 84:148, 1983.
60. Weedon D: Cholesterolosis. In Pathology of the Gallbladder. New York, Masson, 1984, p 161.
61. Jutras JA, Longtin JM, Levesque HP: Hyperplastic cholecystoses. AJR Am J Roentgenol 83:795, 1960.
62. Feldman M, Feldman M Jr: Cholesterolosis of the gallbladder: An autopsy study of 165 cases. Gastroenterology 27:641, 1954.
63. Elfving G, Palmu A, Asp K: Regional distribution of hyperplastic cholecystoses in the gallbladder wall. Ann Chir Gynaecol Fenn 58: 204, 1969.
64. Mendez-Sanchez N, Tanimoto MA, Cobos E, et al: Cholesterolosis is not associated with high cholesterol levels in patients with and without gallstone disease. J Clin Gastroenterol 25:518, 1997.
65. Sahlin S, Stahlberg D, Einarsson K: Cholesterol metabolism in liver and gallbladder mucosa of patients with cholesterolosis. Hepatology 21:1269, 1995.
66. Juvonen T, Savolainen MJ, Kairaluoma MI, et al: Polymorphisms at the apoB, apoA-I, and cholesteryl ester transfer protein gene loci in patients with gallbladder disease. J Lipid Res 36:804, 1995.
67. Behar J, Lee KY, Thompson WR, Biancani P: Gallbladder contraction in patients with pigment and cholesterol stones. Gastroenterology 97: 1479, 1989.
68. Jacyna MR, Ross PE, Bakar MA, et al: Characteristics of cholesterol absorption by human gallbladder: Relevance to cholesterolosis. J Clin Pathol 40:524, 1987.
69. Tilvis RS, Aro J, Strandberg TE, et al: Lipid composition of bile and gallbladder mucosa in patients with acalculous cholesterolosis. Gastroenterology 82:607, 1982.
70. Satoh H, Koga A: Fine structure of cholesterolosis in the human gallbladder and the mechanism of lipid accumulation. Microsc Res Tech 39:14, 1997.
71. Braghetto I, Antezana C, Hurtado C, Csendes A: Triglyceride and cholesterol content in bile, blood, and gallbladder. Am J Surg 156:26, 1988.
72. Watanabe F, Hanai H, Kaneko E: Increased acyl CoA-cholesterol ester acyltransferase activity in gallbladder mucosa in patients with gallbladder cholesterolosis. Am J Gastroenterol 93:1518, 1998.
73. Kmiot WA, Perry EP, Donovan IA, et al: Cholesterolosis in patients with chronic acalculous biliary pain. Br J Surg 81:112, 1994.
74. Parrilla PP, Garcia OD, Pellicer FE, et al: Gallbladder cholesterolosis: An aetiological factor in acute pancreatitis of uncertain origin. Br J Surg 77:735, 1990.
75. Miquel JF, Rollan A, Guzman S, Nervi F: Microlithiasis and cholesterolosis in "idiopathic" acute pancreatitis [letter; comment]. Gastroenterology 102:2188, 1992.
76. Neoptolemos JP, Isgar B: Relationship between cholesterolosis and pancreatitis. HPB Surg 3:217, 1991.
77. Price RJ, Stewart ET, Foley WD, Dodds WJ: Sonography of polypoid cholesterolosis. AJR Am J Roentgenol 139:1197, 1982.
78. Weedon D: Adenomyomatosis. In Pathology of the Gallbladder. New York, Masson, 1984, p 185.
79. Ram MD, Midha D: Adenomyomatosis of the gallbladder. Surgery 78: 224, 1975.
80. Shepard VD, Walters W, Dockerty MB: Benign neoplasms of the gallbladder. Arch Surg 45:1, 1942.
81. Young TE: So-called adenomyoma of the gallbladder. Am J Clin Pathol 31:423, 1959.
82. Wang HP, Wu MS, Lin CC, et al: Pancreaticobiliary diseases associated with anomalous pancreaticobiliary ductal union. Gastrointest Endosc 48:184, 1998.
83. Tanno S, Obara T, Maguchi H, et al: Association between anomalous pancreaticobiliary ductal union and adenomyomatosis of the gall-bladder. J Gastroenterol Hepatol 13:175, 1998.
84. Kurihara K, Mizuseki K, Ninomiya T, et al: Carcinoma of the gallbladder arising in adenomyomatosis. Acta Pathol Jpn 43:82, 1993.
85. Aldridge MC, Gruffaz F, Castaing D, Bismuth H: Adenomyomatosis of the gallbladder: A premalignant lesion? Surgery 109:107, 1991.
86. Katoh T, Nakai T, Hayashi S, Satake T: Noninvasive carcinoma of the gallbladder arising in localized type adenomyomatosis. Am J Gastroenterol 83:670, 1988.
87. Ootani T, Shirai Y, Tsukada K, Muto T: Relationship between gallbladder carcinoma and the segmental type of adenomyomatosis of the gallbladder. Cancer 69:2647, 1992.
88. Berk RN, van der Vegt JH, Lichtenstein JE: The hyperplastic cholecystoses: Cholesterolosis and adenomyomatosis. Radiology 146:593, 1983.
89. Brambs HJ, Wrazidlo W, Schilling H: [The sonographic image of gallbladder adenomyomatosis]. [German.] Rofo Fortschr Gebiete Rontgenstrahl Nuklearmed 153:633, 1990.
90. Cooperberg P: Imaging of the gallbladder. Radiology 163:605, 1987.
91. Raghavendra BN, Subramanyam BR, Balthazar EJ, et al: Sonography of adenomyomatosis of the gallbladder: Radiologic-pathologic correlation. Radiology 146:747, 1983.
92. Hwang JI, Chou YH, Tsay SH, et al: Radiologic and pathologic correlation of adenomyomatosis of the gallbladder. Abdom Imaging 23:73, 1998.
93. Yoshimitsu K, Honda H, Jimi M, et al: MR diagnosis of adenomyomatosis of the gallbladder and differentiation from gallbladder carcinoma: Importance of showing Rokitansky-Aschoff sinuses. AJR Am J Roentgenol 172:1535, 1999.
94. Clouston JE, Thorpe RJ: Case report—CT findings in adenomyomatosis of the gallbladder. Australas Radiol 35:86, 1991.
95. Miyake H, Aikawa H, Hori Y, et al: Adenomyomatosis of the gallbladder with subserosal fatty proliferation: CT findings in two cases. Gastrointest Radiol 17:21, 1992.
96. Nahrwold DL: Benign tumors and pseudotumors of the biliary tract. In Way LW, Pellegrini CA (eds): Surgery of the Gallbladder and Bile Ducts. Philadelphia, WB Saunders, 1987, p 459.
97. Okamoto M, Okamoto H, Kitahara F, et al: Ultrasonographic evidence of association of polyps and stones with gallbladder cancer. Am J Gastroenterol 94:446, 1999.
98. Zhang XH: Polypoid lesions of the gallbladder: Clinical and pathological correlations. [Chinese]. Chung Hua Wai Ko Tsa Chih 29:211, 1991.
99. Jorgensen T, Jensen KH: Polyps in the gallbladder: A prevalence study. Scand J Gastroenterol 25:281, 1990.
100. Weedon D: Benign mucosal polyps. In Pathology of the Gallbladder. New York, Masson, 1984, p 195.
101. Takii Y, Shirai Y, Kanehara H, Hatakeyama K: Obstructive jaundice caused by a cholesterol polyp of the gallbladder: Report of a case. Surg Today 24:1104, 1994.
102. Selzer DW, Dockerty MB, Stauffer MH, Priestly JT: Papillomas (so-called) in the non-calculous gallbladder. Am J Surg 103:472, 1962.
103. Swinton NW, Becker WF: Tumors of the gallbladder. Surg Clin North Am 28:669, 1948.
104. Kozuka S, Tsubone M, Yasui A, Hachisuka K: Relation of adenoma to carcinoma in the gallbladder. Cancer 50:2226, 1982.
105. Tanaka K, Iida Y, Tsutsumi Y: Pancreatic polypeptide-immunoreactive gallbladder carcinoid tumor. Acta Pathol Jpn 42:115, 1992.

106. Vallera DU, Dawson PJ, Path FR: Gastric heterotopia in the gallbladder: Case report and review of literature [review]. Pathol Res Pract 188:49, 1992.
107. Cappell MS, Marks M, Kirschenbaum H: Massive hemobilia and acalculous cholecystitis due to benign gallbladder polyp [review]. Dig Dis Sci 38:1156, 1993.
108. Sugiyama M, Atomi Y, Yamato T: Endoscopic ultrasonography for differential diagnosis of polypoid gall bladder lesions: Analysis in surgical and follow-up series. Gut 46:250, 2000.
109. Eelkema HH, Hodgson JR, Stauffer MH: Fifteen-year follow-up of polypoid lesions of the gallbladder diagnosed by cholecystography. Gastroenterology 42:144, 1962.
110. Heyder N, Gunter E, Giedl J, et al: Polypoid lesions of the gallbladder [German]. Deutsche Med Wochenschrift 115:243, 1990.
111. Mainprize KS, Gould SW, Gilbert JM: Surgical management of polypoid lesions of the gallbladder. Br J Surg 87:414, 2000.
112. Kubota K, Bandai Y, Otomo Y, et al: Role of laparoscopic cholecystectomy in treating gallbladder polyps. Surg Endosc 8:42, 1994.
113. Edelman DS: Carcinoma of a gallbladder polyp: Treated by laparoscopic laser cholecystectomy. Surg Laparosc Endosc 3:142, 1993.
114. Sheth S, Bedford A, Chopra S: Primary gallbladder cancer: Recognition of risk factors and the role of prophylactic cholecystectomy. Am J Gastroenterol 95:1402, 2000.
115. Kubota K, Bandai Y, Noie T, et al: How should polypoid lesions of the gallbladder be treated in the era of laparoscopic cholecystectomy? Surgery 117:481, 1995.

Chapter 59

Sclerosing Cholangitis and Recurrent Pyogenic Cholangitis

Uma Mahadevan and Nathan M. Bass

SCLEROSING CHOLANGITIS

Definition and Differential Diagnosis

Sclerosing cholangitis encompasses a spectrum of chronic, cholestatic diseases of the intrahepatic and extrahepatic bile ducts characterized by patchy inflammation, fibrosis, and stricturing. The natural history of sclerosing cholangitis includes progressive obliteration of the bile ducts, biliary cirrhosis, hepatic failure, and cholangiocarcinoma. Delbet is credited with the first description of this disorder in 1924.[1] At the time, the entity was considered a rarity, usually found during surgical exploration of the abdomen for obstructive jaundice. The introduction and widespread use of endoscopic retrograde cholangiopancreatography (ERCP) in the 1970s led to the current understanding of the prevalence and associations of this group of biliary diseases.

The biliary system possesses a limited repertoire of responses to a variety of pathologic insults. The radiologic appearance of diffuse stricturing and segmental dilatation of the biliary system may be encountered in association with a broad array of local and systemic diseases. Primary sclerosing cholangitis (PSC) is the commonest, and refers to an idiopathic disorder that can occur independently or in association with other diseases or syndromes, most commonly inflammatory bowel disease. The term secondary sclerosing cholangitis specifically refers to sclerosing cholangitis that results from a known pathogenesis or injury. There are also several categories of sclerosing cholangitis that fall between the convenient bookends of primary and secondary varieties of sclerosing cholangitis (Table 59–1).

Table 59–1 outlines a classification scheme for sclerosing cholangitis. PSC, the most common type, is defined as sclerosing cholangitis that (1) lacks any apparent etiology or disease association; (2) occurs in association with inflammatory bowel disease; (3) is associated with systemic fibrosing conditions; or (4) is associated with other autoimmune disorders. Sclerosing cholangitis also can occur in the setting of alloimmunity (liver transplant rejection and graft-versus-host-disease) and infiltrative liver disease. Immunodeficiency-related sclerosing cholangitis is the second major category. Opportunistic infections are thought to be responsible for the observed biliary changes. In the acquired immunodeficiency syndrome (AIDS), infectious agents such as cytomegalovirus (CMV) have been associated with cholangiopathy, and improvement is seen with an increase in the $CD4^+$ count. Abdominal pain and fever are often accompanying symptoms.[2, 3] AIDS cholangiopathy shows a characteristic pattern of papillary stenosis, common bile duct dilatation, and possibly intrahepatic ductal stricturing. Patients often respond symptomatically to endoscopic sphincterotomy (see also Chapter 28).[4]

Secondary sclerosing cholangitis represents disease for which the etiology is well established or widely accepted. Diffuse biliary stricturing may occur as a result of obstruction, stasis, or recurrent bacterial cholangitis in the setting of postoperative biliary strictures, choledocholithiasis, parasites, congenital biliary anomalies, or cystic fibrosis.[5] Toxic insults to the biliary tree may occur from the leakage of formaldehyde during extirpation of an echinococcal cyst or via the instillation of chemotherapeutic agents such as fluorodeoxyuridine (FUDR) into the hepatic arterial system.[6, 7] FUDR causes both direct toxic damage to the biliary tree as well as ischemic damage from toxic vasculitis. Ischemic injury resulting in biliary stricturing also may occur from trauma to the biliary vascular supply during surgery or from hepatic artery thrombosis in hepatic allografts.

Systemic fungal infections may colonize or invade the biliary tree and produce cholestatic liver disease with a PSC-like cholangiogram.[8] Affected patients may be immunocompromised or have systemic manifestations of fungal disease, but sometimes a tissue diagnosis may be made only at lapa-

Table 59–1 | **Classification of Sclerosing Cholangitis**

PRIMARY (PSC)

Without Associated Diseases or Syndromes

Associated with Inflammatory Bowel Disease
Ulcerative colitis
Crohn's disease

Associated with Systemic Idiopathic Fibrosis
Retroperitoneal fibrosis and retractile mesenteritis (Weber-Christian disease)
Reidel's thyroiditis
Mediastinal fibrosis
Pseudotumor of the orbit
Inflammatory pseudotumor
Peyronie's disease

Associated with Idiopathic Autoimmune or Collagen Vascular Diseases
Systemic lupus erythematosus
Systemic sclerosis
Type I diabetes mellitus
Sjögren's syndrome
Celiac sprue
Autoimmune hemolytic anemia
Membranous nephropathy
Rapidly progressive glomerulonephritis
Rheumatoid arthritis
Chronic sclerosing sialadenitis

ALLOIMMUNE TYPE
Hepatic allograft rejection
Graft-versus-host disease in bone marrow transplantation

INFILTRATIVE TYPE
Histiocytosis X
Sarcoidosis
Systemic mastocytosis
Hypereosinophilic syndrome (eosinophilic cholangitis)

IMMUNODEFICIENCY TYPE

Congenital Immunodeficiency
Combined immunodeficiency
Dysgammaglobulinemia
X-linked agammaglobulinemia

Acquired Immunodeficiency
Selective IgA deficiency
Acquired immunodeficiency syndrome (AIDS)
Angioimmunoblastic lymphadenopathy

SECONDARY

Obstructive Cholangitis
Choledocholithiasis
Surgical stricture
Biliary parasites
Recurrent pyogenic cholangitis
Fungal infection
Cystic fibrosis
Pancreatitis
Congenital disorders
  Caroli's disease
  Choledochal cyst

Toxic
Intraductal formaldehyde or hypertonic saline (Echinococcal cyst removal)
Intra-arterial floxuridine (FUDR)

Ischemic
Vascular trauma
Toxic vasculitis (FUDR)
Hepatic allograft arterial occlusion
Paroxysmal nocturnal hemoglobinuria

Neoplastic
Cholangiocarcinoma
Hepatocellular carcinoma
Metastatic cancer
Lymphoma

rotomy or autopsy. Idiopathic, focal, isolated stricturing of the common bile duct is unlikely to be caused by PSC, and other causes such as chronic pancreatitis or periampullary tumors should be sought by abdominal imaging and cholangiography.

A number of diseases may produce distortion or stricturing of the bile ducts that, to varying degrees, mimic the cholangiographic patterns of PSC. In cirrhosis, the major cholangiographic findings are crowding of the bile ducts and marked pruning of the intrahepatic biliary tree.[9] Metastatic liver cancer may produce a biliary appearance similar to that of PSC; however, careful radiographic imaging of the biliary tree will often confirm the diagnosis.[10] As discussed in detail later, cholangiocarcinoma developing as a complication of PSC may be extremely difficult to differentiate from completely benign disease. Multiple liver abscesses from portal pyemia may communicate with the biliary tree and produce diffuse irregularity of the intrahepatic ducts.[11] A history of intra-abdominal sepsis as well as a characteristic pattern of peripheral, saccular dilatations and normal extrahepatic ducts on cholangiography should distinguish multiple liver abscesses from PSC. Abscess formation, however, may also complicate the course of bacterial cholangitis in PSC, producing a similar picture of multiple saccular communications within the biliary tree.

Primary biliary cirrhosis (PBC) rarely has been reported in association with inflammatory bowel disease.[12] The distinction from PSC is made readily on cholangiography, with which PBC may show smooth tapering and narrowing of the intrahepatic bile ducts without ductal irregularity. Also, the presence of high titers of antimitochondrial antibodies and the occurrence of the disease in middle-aged women suggest PBC. Antimitochondrial antibody-negative primary biliary cirrhosis (autoimmune cholangitis) may be more difficult to differentiate from small-duct PSC, although histologic features in the former are usually far more suggestive of PBC.[13]

Autoimmune hepatitis may also be difficult to distinguish from PSC. It rarely may occur in association with inflammatory bowel disease or as an overlap syndrome with PSC.[14, 15] In children, PSC often manifests with strong features of autoimmune hepatitis, and cholangiography is necessary before the latter diagnosis is accepted in a pediatric patient.[16] Distinguishing characteristics of autoimmune hepatitis include the occurrence primarily in women, a hepatocellular pattern of liver enzyme elevations, hyperglobulinemia, high titers of antinuclear and anti-smooth muscle antibodies, a histologic picture of periportal necroinflammation, and clinical response to glucocorticoids.[15] An overlap syndrome between PSC and autoimmune hepatitis can be diagnosed in the presence of a mixed cholestatic/hepatocellular liver chemistries, the presence of autoantibodies including antineutrophil cytoplasmic antibodies (ANCA), a cholangiogram consistent with PSC, and periductular fibrosis and necroinflammatory activity of the portal tracts consistent with autoimmune hepatitis.[14]

Viral or drug-induced hepatitis may occur incidentally in a patient with inflammatory bowel disease, especially in the setting of therapy with immunosuppressive medications such as methotrexate and 6-mercaptopurine. Hepatitis can usually be distinguished on the basis of clinical, histologic, and biochemical parameters, although cholangiography may be required on occasion.

Unusual entities in the differential diagnosis of sclerosing cholangitis include cholangitis glandularis proliferans[17] and eosinophilic cholangitis.[18] Cholangitis glandularis proliferans is a rare disorder that occurs mainly in women. Histologically, it resembles adenomyomatosis of the gallbladder. It is treated by surgical biliary bypass. Eosinophilic cholangitis is an extremely rare cause of biliary obstruction. Histiocytosis X is another infiltrative disease that can involve the biliary system, but it has cholangiographic features that are essentially indistinguishable from those of PSC.[19] Sarcoidosis[20] and chronic sclerosing sialadenitis[21] also can mimic the cholangiographic findings of PSC. Inflammatory pseudotumor is a rare benign inflammatory condition that normally occurs in the lung; when it occurs in the liver, it can mimic cholangiocarcinoma and sclerosing cholangitis.[22]

In general, in the setting of inflammatory bowel disease and a typical cholangiogram, the diagnosis will be PSC. However, in the absence of ulcerative colitis, Crohn's disease, or even nonspecific colitis, a more careful consideration of the differential diagnosis should be undertaken.

This chapter will focus on two of the commonest yet least well understood spontaneously occurring chronic biliary disorders: PSC and recurrent pyogenic cholangitis (RPC). The latter may occasionally give rise to a form of secondary sclerosing cholangitis.

PRIMARY SCLEROSING CHOLANGITIS

Epidemiology

The prevalence of PSC in Western populations has been estimated to be six to eight cases per 100,000 persons.[23, 24] Approximately 80% of patients with PSC have concomitant inflammatory bowel disease. PSC occurs more commonly in patients with ulcerative colitis (which occurs in 90% of the affected patients with inflammatory bowel disease) than in those with Crohn's disease.[25] Conversely, PSC is fairly uncommon in patients with inflammatory bowel disease, with a frequency of 3% to 5.6% of patients with ulcerative colitis and 1.2% of those with Crohn's disease.[26, 27] The association of inflammatory bowel disease with PSC may vary with race. Only 23% of Japanese patients with PSC also have inflammatory bowel disease.[28] However, a small study has suggested that PSC may be more likely to develop in African and Caribbean women with ulcerative colitis than in other groups with ulcerative colitis.[26]

Although there is a strong association between the presence of inflammatory bowel disease and PSC, the diseases appear to progress independently of each other. In patients with PSC, histologic evidence of inflammatory bowel disease, including colonic mucosal dysplasia, may precede the onset of symptoms by as many as 7 years.[29] Ulcerative colitis may run a milder course in patients with PSC than in those without PSC.[30] Inflammatory bowel disease can even develop after liver transplantation for PSC, in the setting of immunosuppression.[31]

The median age of diagnosis is 39, and there is a preponderance of men.[25] As in ulcerative colitis, there appears to be an inverse relationship between smoking and the incidence of PSC.[33] The majority of affected patients have both intrahepatic and extrahepatic disease, although in some patients, the disease is predominantly intrahepatic (27%) or extrahepatic (6%). Up to 44% of patients will be asymptomatic at the time of diagnosis. Although controversial, it is thought that survival does not differ significantly between patients who are symptomatic and those who are asymptomatic at the time of diagnosis.[25, 32]

Prognosis

The median survival from diagnosis to death or liver transplantation has been estimated to be 12 years.[25, 34–36] A population-based study in Sweden found that the overall 10-year survival rate in patients with PSC was 68.8%. Survival appears to be better in patients who have both PSC and inflammatory bowel disease than in those with PSC alone.[38] However, this apparent difference may reflect lead-time bias in the diagnosis of PSC.

Prognostic Models

A number of mathematical models have been developed to predict survival and optimal timing of liver transplantation. Selected models are outlined in Table 59–2. Unfortunately, most of these models are cumbersome and often limited to research settings. A natural history model for PSC was initially developed in 1989 by investigators at the Mayo

Table 59–2 | **Prognostic Models Used for Primary Sclerosing Cholangitis**

MODEL	VARIABLE	REFERENCE
Child-Turcotte-Pugh score	Encephalopathy grade Ascites Serum albumin Prothrombin time Bilirubin	41
Modified Mayo natural history model	R = 0.03 × age (yrs) + 0.54 × $\log_e$ (t. bili) − 0.84 × albumin + 0.54 × $\log_e$ AST + 1.24 × (1) if history of variceal bleeding	39
Cox regression model	Inflammatory bowel disease Previous abdominal surgery Ascites Serum creatinine Biliary tree malignancy	40
Swedish prognostic index	PI = 0.24 × histologic stage + 0.03 × age + 0.49 × $\log_2$ bilirubin	25

AST, serum aspartate aminotransferase level; PI, prognostic index; t. bili, serum total bilirubin level.

Clinic.[39] The five variables used were age, serum bilirubin level, blood hemoglobin concentration, histologic stage on liver biopsy, and presence or absence of inflammatory bowel disease. Recently, this model was revised to omit factors that are highly variable or difficult to obtain. The revised model uses age, serum total bilirubin level, albumin level, aspartate aminotransferase (AST) level, and a history of variceal bleeding to predict survival up to 4 years.[40]

A multivariate analysis of a Swedish population found that age, serum bilirubin concentration, and histologic stage at the time of diagnosis were independent predictors of a poor outcome. These factors were then used to develop a prognostic index for timing of transplantation.[25] Neuberger and associates[41] developed a multiple Cox regression model for optimizing the timing of transplantation. Significant variables were the type of inflammatory bowel disease (worse outcome with Crohn's disease than with ulcerative colitis), ascites, previous upper abdominal surgery, serum creatinine level, and biliary tree malignancy.

The Child-Turcotte-Pugh classification is used by the United Network for Organ Sharing (UNOS) to determine minimal listing criteria for liver transplantation (see Chapters 77 and 83). Shetty and associates[42] found that Kaplan-Meier 7-year survival rates for patients with Child-Turcotte-Pugh class A, B, and C cirrhosis caused by PSC were 89.8%, 68%, and 24.9%, respectively. This is mathematically the easiest model to use, and the most familiar to physicians. However, although the Child-Turcotte-Pugh score is excellent for advanced disease, a wide degree of variability in survival was found by other investigators for patients early in the course of their disease.[43] Unfortunately, PSC is a difficult disease to model because of its highly variable, although generally progressive, course.

Etiology and Pathogenesis

The etiology and pathogenesis of PSC are unknown. A variety of causative mechanisms have been proposed, including toxins, infectious processes, ischemia, and genetic and autoimmune factors. A reasonable hypothesis is that a self-perpetuating illness develops in a genetically susceptible host exposed to a variety of insults.

Enterohepatic Toxins

The strong association between PSC and inflammatory bowel disease, in particular ulcerative colitis, has led to speculation that the inflamed colonic mucosa allows the transmigration of bacterial products or toxic bile acids into the biliary tree via the portal circulation, thereby leading to an inflammatory response and chronic cholangitis.[44] Models for toxic damage leading to sclerosing cholangitis can be found in both humans and rats. Intraluminal instillation of formaldehyde or hypertonic saline[45] or arterial instillation of chemotherapeutic agents such as FUDR[6] produce reactions morphologically similar to PSC in humans. Administration of the biliary toxin α-naphthylisothiocyanate to rats leads to the development of a chronic cholangitis similar to sclerosing cholangitis in humans.[46] Also, the biliary epithelial cells of patients with PSC have demonstrated strong immunostaining for endotoxin.[47]

However, there is no established correlation between the course, duration, or severity of ulcerative colitis and PSC. PSC may develop many years before the development of ulcerative colitis or after colectomy has been performed.[29, 48] In addition, patients with PSC but without inflammatory bowel disease display a disease course remarkably similar to that of patients who have both inflammatory bowel disease and PSC.[49] Therefore, the strong association between inflammatory bowel disease and PSC likely represents two variable organ responses to a common insult or susceptibility, as opposed to a direct causal relationship between the two diseases.

Infectious Agents

The biliary tree is considered to be a sterile system. In the absence of surgical or endoscopic instrumentation, it is unusual for bacterial cholangitis to develop in patients with PSC. However, secondary infections can cause a sclerosing cholangitis type of picture that is difficult to distinguish from PSC. This occurrence is best demonstrated in the setting of AIDS. In patients with a low $CD4^+$ count, the radiographic image of the biliary tree can mimic PSC. *Cryptosporidium*, microsporidia, and CMV have been isolated from the bile ducts of these patients (see Chapter 28).[2, 50, 51]

However, there is no convincing evidence of a causative role for bacterial or viral infection in patients with PSC. In a study of explanted livers from patients with PSC, a wide range of positive bacterial cultures was noted from bile duct isolates. However, the number of bacterial strains was inversely related to the time interval since the most recent ERCP.[52] Systematic attempts to isolate viral and opportunistic pathogens in a cohort of patients with PSC have failed.[53]

Genetic and Immunologic Factors

A genetic predisposition to the development of PSC is supported by human leukocyte antigen (HLA) associations and the occurrence of PSC in multiple family members. Familial clustering of PSC has been documented in the past and may occur more often in families with other autoimmune diseases than in those without such disorders.[54, 55] HLA-encoded susceptibility seems to be associated to varying degrees with HLA antigens B8, DR52a and class II alleles DRB1*0301, DRB1*1301, DRB3*0101, and Cw*0701 to date. However, the strongest class II association accounts for only 53% of the patients.[56–60] Recently, a tumor necrosis factor (TNF) polymorphism in the class III HLA region was found to be associated with PSC with a similar frequency.[61] The DR4 allele may be a marker of more rapid disease progression.[62] The HLA phenotypes associated with PSC are not found in excess in patients with ulcerative colitis alone but are strongly associated with PSC, either with or without concomitant inflammatory bowel disease.

The frequency of serum autoantibodies is also increased in PSC patients. A study by Angulo and associates[63] found that 97% of patients with PSC were positive for at least one autoantibody, and 81% were positive for more than three autoantibodies. The rate of positivity was not different between those with PSC and inflammatory bowel disease and those with PSC alone. The most common autoantibodies were ANCA in 84%, antibody against cardiolipin in 66%, and antibody against nuclear antigens (ANA) in 53% of patients. Only anticardiolipin antibody levels correlated significantly with the histologic stage of disease and the Mayo risk score, thereby suggesting a role as a prognostic marker.

Multiple cellular and humoral abnormalities also have been described in patients with PSC. Elevated levels of circulating immune complexes have been found in 80% to 88% of patients with PSC, and clearance of these immune complexes is markedly impaired.[64] Levels of circulating complement fragments C3d and C4d are increased, indicating activation of the complement system via the classical pathway.[65] Evidence of exaggerated humoral immunity includes elevated serum levels of interleukins 8 and 10.[65]

Disordered cellular immune function also has been implicated in the pathogenesis of PSC. In the liver, T lymphocytes predominate within portal mononuclear cell infiltrates. The number of gamma-delta T cells, which are associated with autoimmunity, have been found to be increased in the peripheral blood as well as the portal areas of the liver of patients with PSC.[66] Recent experiments in a rat model found that when sclerosing cholangitis is chemically induced with α-naphthylisothiocyanate, the hepatic cytokine profile becomes increasingly T-helper 1 (Th1) in nature. Th1 cytokines initiate and maintain the inflammatory response; Th2 cytokines are involved in humoral and mucosal immunity.[46] It is thought that an imbalance between the two sets of helper T cells plays a pivotal role in both ulcerative colitis and Crohn's disease.[67] In a genetically susceptible host, such an imbalance toward a proinflammatory state could also lead to the progressive inflammation seen in PSC.

Ischemia

The concept that ischemic damage to the biliary tree contributes to the etiopathogenesis of PSC is gaining favor. Evidence for this theory is intertwined with data to support the role of autoimmunity. Ischemia as a result of surgical trauma to the biliary arterial supply[68] or arterial intimal damage and proliferation secondary to hepatic allograft rejection[69] can cause a picture similar to PSC.

ANCA in serum are found in patients with vasculitides such as Wegener's granulomatosis, polyarteritis nodosa, and crescentic glomerulonephritis. Among patients with PSC, 65% to 84% are ANCA-positive.[63, 70] However, there has been a lack of correlation between the presence of ANCA in serum and clinical parameters of disease activity.[63, 70] Anti-endothelial cell antibody (AECA), a marker of vascular damage, was found in 35% of patients with PSC.[71] Angulo and associates[63] found that 66% of patients with PSC were positive for anticardiolipin antibody, another marker of vascular damage. In this study, serum levels of this autoantibody correlated with histologic stage and the Mayo risk score. The strong association between PSC and the presence of ANCA, AECA, and anticardiolipin antibody supports the theory that immune-mediated vascular injury plays a pathogenic role in PSC.

Diagnosis

The diagnosis of PSC is based on typical cholangiographic findings; consistent, although nonspecific, clinical, biochemical, and hepatic histologic findings; and exclusion of secondary causes of sclerosing cholangitis (see Table 59–1).[34] Making a diagnosis of PSC may be difficult. ERCP is considered the gold standard for the diagnosis of PSC. Percutaneous transhepatic cholangiography (PTC) also can demonstrate typical ductal changes but is often difficult to perform in the setting of nondilated intrahepatic ducts. Patients with inflammatory bowel disease and a cholestatic pattern of liver enzyme abnormalities should undergo further investigation of the hepatobiliary system, because they are the group with the highest likelihood of having PSC. When the clinical suspicion of PSC is high, it is reasonable to proceed directly to ERCP, because other modalities have limited specificity in diagnosing PSC. However, in an asymptomatic patient with stable liver test abnormalities, ERCP may not be indicated unless medical or endoscopic therapy is planned. In such cases magnetic resonance cholangiography (MRCP) may prove to be diagnostic, although experience with this technique in patients with PSC is limited (see later).

Once secondary causes of sclerosing cholangitis are excluded, other diseases in the differential diagnosis may be more difficult to distinguish from PSC. Biliary stones and cholangiocarcinoma were once thought invariably to occur independently of PSC, but are now recognized as complications of the disease. Serial cholangiograms in some patients with PSC have demonstrated progressive stricturing and development of cholangiocarcinoma over time, thereby indicating that malignancy occurs as part of the natural history of the disease.[72] Biliary calculi may be found in up to 33% of patients with PSC and do not exclude a diagnosis of PSC.[73]

In the absence of associated inflammatory bowel disease, the diagnosis of PSC must be made with caution. Although abnormal liver biochemical tests and a typical cholangiogram remain the key to diagnosis, a more thorough evaluation is warranted. Careful history-taking and physical examination should be performed with routine laboratory tests, a liver biopsy, and additional investigations as dictated by the clinical circumstances. Radiologic imaging studies may be indicated to exclude other potential diagnoses.

Pathology

Large Ducts

At laparotomy, the common bile duct appears grossly as a thickened, hardened cord. Inflammatory adhesions may be present around the duct and in the porta hepatis, with enlarged lymph nodes occupying the hilum and gastrohepatic ligament.[74] Histologically, the duct wall is thickened with fibrosis extending from the subepithelial to adventitial layers. Mixed inflammatory infiltrates are present, but not prominent, near the epithelium and around biliary glands.[75] Biliary sludge and soft pigment stones may be found in the major ducts.[27] Biliary sludge may form casts of the ducts. The gallbladder may show similar fibrous thickening and chronic inflammatory changes.

Livers removed from patients with PSC who undergo liver transplantation show changes in the large intrahepatic ducts that are considered to be pathognomonic for PSC.[75, 76] These changes are (1) thin-walled, tubular, or saccular dilatations of the large ducts (cholangiectases) with semicircular or annular fibrous crests; and (2) transformation of bile ducts into fibrous cords with complete or partial obliteration of the ductal epithelium and lumen (Fig. 59–1*A*). These lesions

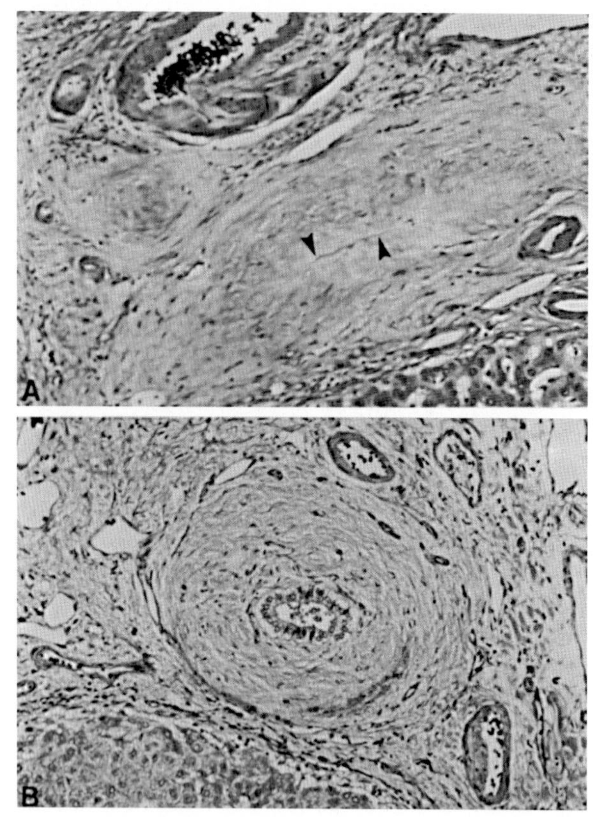

Figure 59–1. Histopathology of the bile ducts in primary sclerosing cholangitis. *A*, A segmental bile duct and an accompanying smaller septal duct are completely obliterated by fibrosis. An occluded cleft in the center of the large duct scar *(arrowheads)* marks the remains of the duct lumen. Hematoxylin and eosin stain; magnification, ×125. *B*, A large septal duct shows the typical lesion of fibrous cholangitis. Concentric fibrosis with minimal inflammation surrounds the duct in an onion skin pattern. Hematoxylin and eosin stain; magnification, ×200. (Courtesy of Linda D. Ferrell, M.D., Department of Pathology, University of California, San Francisco.)

correspond, respectively, to the appearances of "beading" and "pruning" of ducts seen on cholangiograms.

Liver Biopsy

A variety of histopathologic changes are seen in the livers of patients with primary sclerosing cholangitis. The most common characteristic feature is "onion skin" fibrosis, which describes the appearance of periductal concentric fibrosis around the interlobular and septal bile ducts (Fig. 59–1*B*).[74, 77] This appearance, however, is present in only one half of all biopsy specimens from patients with otherwise typical PSC, whereas concentric fibrosis with obliteration of the small ducts (obliterative fibrous cholangitis)—a virtually diagnostic histopathologic lesion (see Fig. 59–1*A*)—is found in fewer than 10% of specimens.[78]

Periductal fibrosis may be accompanied by infiltrates of inflammatory cells. Inflammation, usually a pleomorphic mix of lymphocytes, neutrophils, plasma cells, and eosinophils, may predominate.[78] The portal tracts may expand with edema, inflammatory cells, and fibrosis, and spillover of inflammation into the parenchyma is common and gives rise to the appearance of piecemeal necrosis typically seen in chronic hepatitis.[79] Chronic hepatitis has been a common misdiagnosis in patients with PSC when reliance has been placed on the liver biopsy without cholangiography. Complicating matters is the uncommon but real occurrence of an overlap syndrome between PSC and autoimmune hepatitis (see earlier discussion) that may respond dramatically to glucocorticoid treatment. A histologic classification scheme for PSC has been developed by Ludwig and associates.[77] In stage I, portal hepatitis with or without bile duct abnormalities and cholangitis is seen. In stage II, periportal fibrosis or hepatitis develops. Stage III is characterized by septal fibrosis or bridging necrosis, and stage IV is biliary cirrhosis.

Peribiliary glands around the extrahepatic and intrahepatic ducts can demonstrate proliferation, nonspecific inflammation, fibrosis, and destruction on liver biopsy.[80] Despite the attractive hypothesis of an ischemic process in the pathogenesis of PSC, pathologic involvement of blood vessels is either absent or seen uncommonly. The parenchyma of the liver displays nonspecific cholestatic changes that may include considerable copper staining. The impairment of biliary copper excretion in PSC can lead to parenchymal accumulation of copper comparable to that seen in Wilson disease.[81]

The histologic stage of PSC does not always correlate with symptoms. Patients may be asymptomatic and present with marked fibrosis.[82] Angulo and associates[83] found that 42% of patients with stage II disease show histologic progression of the disease at 1 year. However, only 14% of those with stage III disease show progression at 1 year; in paired biopsy specimens, 15% of the patients actually demonstrated regression. This finding illustrates the high degree of sampling variability seen in liver biopsy specimens from patients with PSC.

Small-Duct Primary Sclerosing Cholangitis

A small proportion of patients with inflammatory bowel disease and cholestatic liver test abnormalities may show histologic lesions typical of PSC on needle biopsy of the liver, without characteristic abnormalities on radiologic studies and cholangiography.[75, 84] A careful study of patients with inflammatory bowel disease and cholestatic liver tests in whom both liver histologic findings and cholangiography were performed suggested that small-duct PSC (sometimes referred to in the older literature as "pericholangitis") comprises less than 5% of the PSC disease spectrum. There is considerable overlap between the syndrome of small-duct PSC and autoimmune hepatitis, which also may be associated with inflammatory bowel disease.[84]

Radiologic Features

Noninvasive abdominal imaging can be suggestive but not diagnostic of PSC. Ultrasonography may detect extrahepatic and intrahepatic ductal dilatation, lymphadenopathy, evidence of cirrhosis, or a mass lesion. One study noted that gallbladder volume was greatly enlarged in patients with PSC compared with healthy control subjects, patients with primary biliary cirrhosis, and patients with other types of cirrhosis.[85]

Computed tomography (CT) of the abdomen can be informative, but is nonspecific. Typically, scattered, dilated intrahepatic ducts with no appreciable connection to the main bile ducts are seen. Lymphadenopathy has been found on CT scan in 66% of patients with PSC; however, there is no association with the presence of malignancy.[86] Dodd and associates[87] identified six CT findings that are found more frequently in patients with PSC than in patients with cirrhosis from other causes. These findings were (1) mild-to-moderate lobulation; (2) mild-to-moderate lateral segment atrophy; (3) mild-to-moderate or (4) severe caudate lobe hypertrophy; (5) dilated ducts; and (6) caudate pseudotumor (a low attenuation rindlike appearance of the right lobe of the liver in the presence of hypertrophy of the caudate lobe). This last finding was found only in patients with PSC.

Newer imaging modalities may have more success in diagnosing PSC. Compared with ERCP, MRCP has the advantage of imaging involved organs more extensively. When compared with ERCP, MRCP has detected the presence of PSC with a positive predictive value between 85% and 94%. Sensitivity and specificity rates for detecting extrahepatic ductal disease were 83%; for intrahepatic disease the sensitivity rate was 87%.[88] In the patient who may have contraindications to sedation and analgesia or to ERCP, MRCP is a reasonable alternative for making the diagnosis of sclerosing cholangitis.

Positron emission tomography (PET) is an imaging method that assesses metabolism in various organs by means of positron-emitting radioactive-labeled tracers. A study by Keiding and associates[89] found that PET scanning with (^{18}F) fluoro-2-deoxy-D-glucose was able to detect small cholangiocarcinomas, a notoriously difficult lesion to find by noninvasive imaging, in patients with PSC. This test shows promise in the screening of patients evaluated for orthotopic liver transplantation.

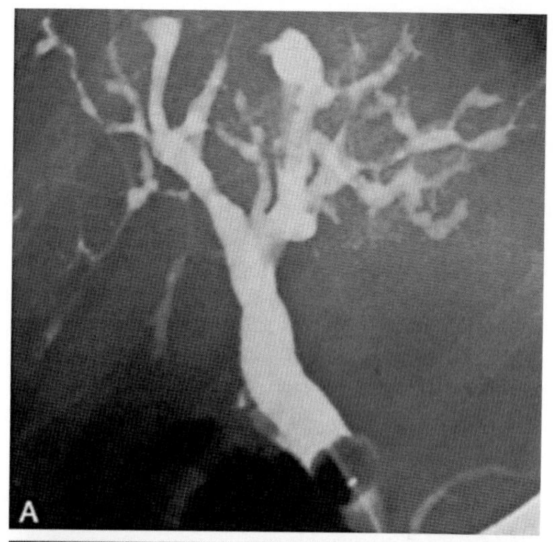

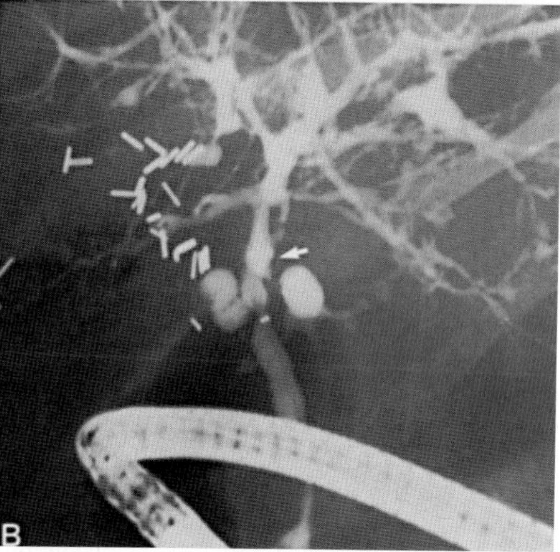

Figure 59–2. Cholangiogram in PSC. *A,* ERCP with contrast injected through a balloon catheter (seen in lower common duct). The intrahepatic ducts are mainly affected and show diminished arborization (pruning), with diffuse segmental strictures alternating with normal-caliber or mildly dilated duct segments (cholangiectases), resulting in a beaded appearance. *B,* ERCP in a patient with PSC and a history of a cholecystectomy. Radiologic features include the clips from the previous surgery, diffuse irregularity of the intrahepatic ducts comprising multiple short strictures and cholangiectases, and small diverticula in the wall of the common hepatic duct *(arrow).*

Cholangiographic Features

Cholangiographic imaging of the biliary tree, usually by ERCP, not only confirms the diagnosis of sclerosing cholangitis, but also provides information about the distribution of the disease and the presence of dominant strictures that may be amenable to interventional therapy. Adequate visualization of the intrahepatic ducts is necessary when PSC is suspected, and the use of a balloon catheter for the injection of contrast material may be required to opacify the intrahepatic ducts (Fig. 59–2*A*). However, this approach must be undertaken with care because elevation of the serum bilirubin level and cholangitis after diagnostic ERCP may be caused by the increased pressure of contrast dye in a partially obstructed ductal system.[90]

Cholangiography in PSC usually reveals a diffuse abnormality of both the intrahepatic and extrahepatic bile ducts. Abnormalities confined to the intrahepatic ducts alone are found in 15% to 30% of patients,[23, 25, 91–93] whereas involvement of the extrahepatic ducts alone is found in less than 10% of patients.[37, 92] This pattern of extrahepatic duct involvement may be more common in PSC that occurs in the absence, rather than the presence, of inflammatory bowel disease.[49] Regional patterns of duct involvement may remain stable for prolonged periods of time, but progression of disease from exclusive intrahepatic ductal involvement to disease affecting the entire biliary system has also been observed on serial cholangiography.[93]

The typical cholangiographic abnormalities of PSC consist of diffusely distributed multifocal strictures that are usually short (0.2 to 2 cm), annular, and bandlike with intervening segments of normal or dilated ducts, thereby producing a highly characteristic beaded appearance (see Fig. 59–2). Dilated segments may appear as saccular or diverticular outpouchings. Mural irregularities of the ducts are common and may impart a shaggy appearance, particularly in the common bile duct. The small branches of the intrahepatic ductal system may fill poorly, giving rise to a pruned appearance. The diffuse abnormalities of PSC, however, are usually readily distinguished from the "pruned-tree" appearance of the cholangiogram commonly produced by cirrhosis. Major, localized areas of narrowing, or dominant strictures, may be seen in the biliary system. These strictures occur with greatest frequency (75%) in the area where the hepatic duct bifurcates into the right and left main hepatic ducts.[94]

Although the gallbladder and cystic duct are affected in at least 15% to 20% of cases of PSC,[95] abnormalities of these structures are less frequently discerned on cholangiography than are abnormalities of the bile ducts. Gallstones and mucosal filling defects may be seen in the gallbladder.[95]

An association of PSC with pancreatic duct abnormalities is controversial. Studies have reported pancreatic duct involvement in 5% to 77% of cases.[96–101] Diffuse irregularity, stricturing, and beading of the main pancreatic duct may be seen in a pattern reminiscent of the biliary lesions of PSC. Subtle irregularities of the pancreatic duct side branches are a more common finding.[101]

Clinical Features

Age and Sex

Although PSC has been diagnosed in neonates and in adults in the eighth decade of life, most patients present between the ages of 25 and 45 years.[16, 23, 25, 91, 93] There is a clear male predominance, with a male-to-female ratio of 1.5:1 to 2:1.[23, 25, 35, 49, 91] In patients without associated inflammatory bowel disease, the disease is equally common among men and women.[49]

Symptoms

The most common symptoms at the time of presentation (Table 59–3) are jaundice, pruritus, and abdominal pain.[12, 25, 91, 93, 103] The pain localizes to the right upper quadrant and can be severe. The onset and progression of symptoms are usually insidious; however, in rare cases, PSC can manifest initially as an acute, hepatitis-like illness.[104] Loss of weight may occur at an alarming rate, usually secondary to intestinal malabsorption and anorexia. In a patient with previously stable disease, however, such weight loss should raise concern for cholangiocarcinoma. Patients often experience chronic fatigue. Febrile episodes may occur and can vary from recurrent bouts of low-grade fever to spiking fevers with bacterial cholangitis, jaundice, chills, and right upper quadrant pain. In patients with prior biliary reconstruction or surgical manipulation, the frequency of acute cholangitis ranges from 45% to 65%.[91, 92] Acute cholangitis, usually of lesser severity, occurs spontaneously in a smaller proportion of patients without a history of biliary surgery.

An important feature of PSC is the often extreme variability of its clinical course. Symptoms and signs such as jaundice, pruritus, abdominal pain, and fever may remit spontaneously and for prolonged periods.[27, 93, 103] Some authorities attribute this phenomenon to biliary microlithiasis and sludge, which produces sporadic, self-limiting obstruction within the diffusely strictured biliary tree.[73] Another mechanism may be low-grade, intermittent, and self-limiting bacterial cholangitis, which produces an acute inflammatory reaction in the already narrowed ductal system.[102] In unusual instances, patients with PSC present initially with complications of cirrhosis and portal hypertension. Of these complications, variceal bleeding is the most frequent.[35, 44, 91]

Patients with asymptomatic PSC constitute 20% to 44% of all patients in large series.[25, 35, 92, 93] This relatively high percentage reflects the increasingly common practice of screening patients with ulcerative colitis for liver test abnormalities and performing ERCP in those in whom the serum alkaline phosphatase level is elevated. Even with severe cholangiographic abnormalities, asymptomatic patients with PSC may remain free of symptoms for many years. However, despite increased suspicion for PSC in patients with inflammatory bowel disease, a median delay of 52 months between the onset of biochemical symptoms or signs and the diagnosis of PSC has been noted in one large series.[25]

Table 59–3 | **Clinical Presentation of Primary Sclerosing Cholangitis**

SYMPTOM	PERCENTAGE OF PATIENTS
Jaundice	30–72
Pruritus	28–69
Abdominal pain	24–72
Weight loss	29–79
Fatigue	65–66
Fever/cholangitis	13–45
Asymptomatic	7–44

Physical Findings

Jaundice and hepatomegaly are the most common abnormal physical findings, and the spleen is enlarged in about one third of patients. Stigmata of end-stage liver disease, including spider angiomata and loss of muscle mass, may be found in patients who present late in the course of the disease.

Laboratory Findings

Typically, the serum alkaline phosphatase level is increased three- to five-fold in PSC. Values up to 20 times the upper limit of normal are not uncommon.[91] Elevations in the serum alkaline phosphatase level are usually matched by increases in serum gamma glutamyl transpeptidase and 5′-nucleotidase levels. An estimated 6% of patients with PSC have normal serum alkaline phosphatase levels, which may reflect hypophosphatasia, hypothyroidism, or zinc or magnesium deficiency.[105, 106] Serum aminotransferase levels are usually increased but rarely exceed three to four times the normal values. Levels of serum bilirubin, mainly the conjugated fraction, are increased in jaundiced patients but may be normal. A low serum albumin level suggests advanced disease or nutritional failure, and prolongation of the prothrombin time reflects either vitamin K malabsorption or, more often, advanced liver disease.

The white blood cell count is usually normal but is increased with a polymorphonuclear leukocytosis during episodes of bacterial cholangitis. A small proportion of patients exhibit eosinophilia, which may be striking[57]; its significance remains unclear.

Levels of immunoglobulin (Ig) in the serum are often elevated in PSC, most frequently IgM, followed by IgG and IgA.[57, 92, 93] Patients with PSC are ANCA-positive in 65% to 84% of cases.[63, 70] Anti-endothelial cell antibody (AECA), a marker of vascular damage, has been found in 35% of patients with PSC.[71] Angulo and associates[63] found that 97%

of patients with PSC have at least one autoantibody, and 81% have three or more. The most common are ANCA (84%), anticardiolipin (66%), and ANA (53%). Antimitochondrial antibodies are typically absent. Serum levels of amino-terminal propeptide of type III collagen (S-PIIINP), a by-product of collagen synthesis and a possible marker of hepatic fibrosis, are elevated in patients with both PSC and ulcerative colitis when compared with those with ulcerative colitis alone.[107]

Nonspecific markers of cholestasis such as increased serum cholesterol and lipoprotein X levels can be found. Also, patients may have abnormal test results for trace elements and minerals, including increased serum and hepatic copper levels, increased urinary copper excretion, and low serum selenium levels.[81, 108]

Complications

Nutritional

The chronic cholestasis of PSC leads to malabsorption of fat and fat-soluble vitamins, which may result in steatorrhea, malabsorption of calcium, calorie loss, and fat-soluble vitamin deficiency.[109, 110] Significant biochemical deficiencies of vitamins A, D, K, and E may be found in patients with advanced precirrhotic and cirrhotic liver disease.

Night blindness and osteoporosis are the most common clinical consequences of fat-soluble vitamin deficiencies. Bone mineral density has been found to be below the fracture level in 8.6% of patients with PSC[111] and in 40% to 50%[110, 111] of patients with PSC who undergo liver transplantation. Risk factors for osteoporosis include older age, a longer duration of inflammatory bowel disease (itself a risk factor for bone loss), and advanced liver disease. Although patients may be vitamin K–deficient, paradoxically, hypercoagulability has been found in patients with PSC. Thromboelastography has found that 43% of patients with PSC meet the definition of hypercoagulability compared with only 5% of those with parenchymal liver disease.[112] The clinical significance of this observation is unknown.

Secondary Biliary Cirrhosis

The natural history of PSC is one of indolent progression. As in most types of chronic cholestasis, progressive damage to the liver parenchyma occurs as a result of poorly understood factors that may include retention of bile salts and copper in the parenchymal cells of the liver and extension of the fibroinflammatory process involving the bile ducts into the liver parenchyma. Eventually, portal-to-portal bridging fibrosis occurs and evolves into a biliary pattern of cirrhosis. Complications of advanced liver disease in these patients include portal hypertension with variceal hemorrhage, ascites, and liver failure, the last being the most common cause of death in PSC.[25, 27, 35, 91, 103]

Bleeding

In patients with PSC who have undergone a proctocolectomy and ileostomy for ulcerative colitis, varices may develop around the ileostomy stoma and can become a problematic source of bleeding.[113] However, perianastomotic bleeding from varices is reportedly not a problem in patients who have undergone an ileal pouch anal anastomosis.[114] Patients with PSC and cirrhosis who undergo colectomy for complications of ulcerative colitis have an increased risk of postoperative death.[115] The major perioperative complication associated with colectomy is intraoperative and postoperative bleeding, with transfusions required in 47% of cases,[114] mostly because of portal hypertension. In some cases, a transhepatic portosystemic shunt is done before colectomy to decrease the risk of surgical bleeding.

Biliary Tract Calculi

Gallstones and choledocholithiasis in the setting of sclerosing cholangitis were once thought to exclude the diagnosis of PSC; however, their development is clearly a part of the clinical spectrum of the disease. There is no difference in outcome between patients who have choledocholithiasis in the setting of PSC and those who do not.[116] In a small study of 22 patients, biliary calculi developed after the diagnosis of PSC in 77% of patients. Thirty-two percent had cholelithiasis, 41% had choledocholithiasis, and 27% had both.[73] Pigment stones may develop in the setting of cholestasis and biliary obstruction and can cause attacks of cholangitis. Affected patients may benefit from endoscopic intervention to relieve the obstruction and remove any stones (see Chapter 61).

Pancreatic Disease

The association of pancreatic duct abnormalities with PSC is controversial, with a range of reported frequencies from 5% to 77%.[96–101] However, most of the studies were retrospective and involved small numbers of patients. The abnormalities in pancreatic ductal morphology are not paralleled by impairment in pancreatic exocrine function, which, for the most part, is well preserved in PSC.[102] In addition, patients with inflammatory bowel disease without PSC have at least an 8% frequency of pancreatic duct abnormalities on pancreatography,[96] and patients with primary biliary cirrhosis have higher rates of abnormal pancreatograms when compared with patients with PSC (43% to 15%, respectively).[100]

Cholangiocarcinoma

Much support exists for the concept that PSC is a premalignant condition. Serial cholangiograms in patients with PSC have demonstrated progressive stricturing and development of cholangiocarcinoma over time, indicating that cholangiocarcinoma is part of the natural history of the disease.[72] Cholangiocarcinoma can occur in patients known to have PSC for many years. In light of the dismal natural history of cholangiocarcinoma after diagnosis, with a median survival of 5 months,[117] it is extremely unlikely that the malignancy preceded the development of sclerosing cholangitis.

The frequency of cholangiocarcinoma in series of patients with PSC studied either retrospectively or prospectively has ranged from 3% to 20%.[25, 36, 84, 92, 117, 118] The frequency on autopsy is much higher, with cholangiocarcinoma reported in 30% to 40% of patients with PSC[91, 103, 117] and in 23%

to 33% of patients with PSC undergoing liver transplantation.[36, 119] In the majority of the latter patients, the tumor was not suspected preoperatively. Tumors arise most commonly around the common hepatic duct and its bifurcation and less frequently in the common bile duct, gallbladder, cystic duct, and intrahepatic ducts.[117]

It is not possible to predict who will develop cholangiocarcinoma, and as yet, a good screening method for the tumor has not been developed. Difficulty stems in part from the lack of an association between the occurrence of cholangiocarcinoma and the duration and severity of PSC or the duration or frequency of inflammatory bowel disease.[38, 120, 121] It has been suggested that increased alcohol consumption[121] and use of tobacco[120] may increase the risk of developing cholangiocarcinoma.

Metastatic disease with spread mainly to regional lymph nodes is present in approximately two thirds of patients at the time of diagnosis of cholangiocarcinoma.[117] Although a sudden inexplicable deterioration in clinical course of PSC with the onset and rapid progression of jaundice, weight loss, and abdominal discomfort should raise suspicion of cholangiocarcinoma and warrants a diagnostic workup, studies have shown that the clinical and biochemical presentation of patients with PSC with and without hepatobiliary carcinoma do not differ during the year before the diagnosis of cancer.[120] Radiologic imaging is also of limited value in detecting small tumors, although PET scanning shows some promise.[89] Cholangiographic appearances suspicious for the development of cholangiocarcinoma include marked ductal dilatation, progressive ductal dilatation, and progressive stricture formation on serial cholangiography, as well as a polypoid mass lesion more than 1 cm in diameter (Fig. 59–3).[122]

Serum tumor markers such as CA 19-9 and carcinoembryonic antigen (CEA) may aid in the diagnosis. A serum CA 19-9 level greater than 100 U/mL had a 75% sensitivity and 80% specificity for cholangiocarcinoma in one study.[121] Using both CA 19-9 and CEA in an index {CA 19-9 + (CEA x 40)} resulted in an accuracy of 86%, including detection of 6 of 11 occult tumors.[123] However, a prospective study of patients with PSC without known cholangiocarcinoma found that serum tumor markers such as CEA, CA 19-9, CA 50, and CA 242 were of limited value because of their low specificity and the low rate of occurrence of cholangiocarcinoma over a 3-year period (3%).[118]

Cytologic brushings during ERCP have a sensitivity of approximately 50% for detectiong malignancy.[49, 124–126] Genetic defects in tumor suppression have been detected in patients with PSC. An allelic loss at the locus for the tumor suppressor gene *p*16 as well as inactivation of *p*16 has been found in patients with PSC and cholangiocarcinoma.[127] K-*ras* mutations and accumulation of p53 protein were found in 33% and 31%, respectively, of patients with cholangiocarcinoma and PSC.[128] In one study, expression of p53 protein was found in 78% of patients sampled, including one bile duct epithelial brushing.[129] However, a study of 47 brushing samples did not find an improvement in sensitivity or specificity for the detection of cholangiocarcinoma with the addition of p53 or K-*ras* analysis. This study did find that the specificity (89%) and negative predictive value (89%) of cytologic brushings were better than expected, although the sensitivity (60%) and positive predictive value (59%) were suboptimal.[126]

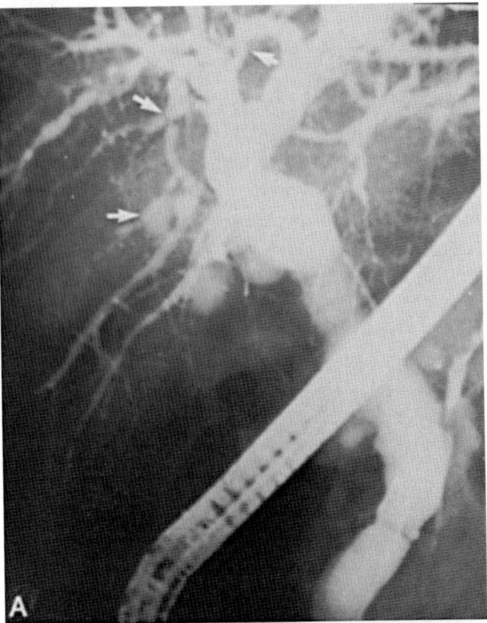

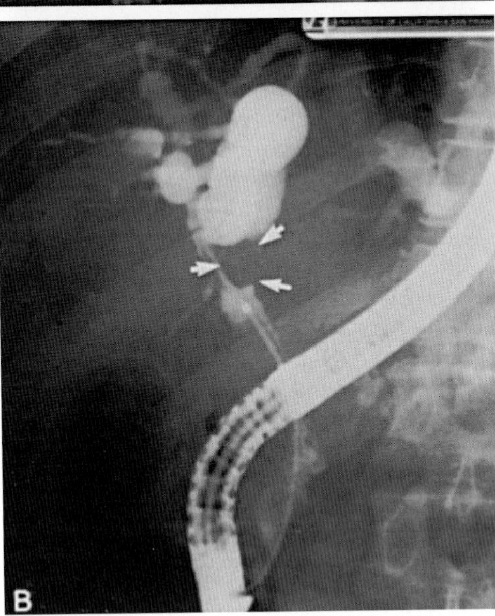

Figure 59–3. Progression of cholangiocarcinoma complicating PSC. The patient, a 43-year-old man with a history of mild ulcerative colitis for 3 years, presented with pruritus and an elevated serum alkaline phosphatase level. *A*, Initial ERCP revealed mild, diffuse changes compatible with uncomplicated PSC. Several short, annular strictures and cholangiectases are present in the intrahepatic ducts *(arrows)*, with a single, short, annular stricture of the common duct. The cystic duct is not filled, and it is possible that it was already obstructed by tumor. *B*, Repeat ERCP performed 7 months later after progressive jaundice and weight loss developed rapidly. There is now a 2-cm mass projecting into, and obstructing, the common hepatic duct *(arrows)*. A catheter has been passed beyond the obstructing mass. There is marked dilatation of the left main duct proximal to the obstruction; the right main duct is completely occluded.

Unfortunately, as noted earlier, the development of cholangiocarcinoma is not predictable, and the tumor is often detected at a late stage. Establishing the diagnosis is difficult without exploratory laparotomy, and treatment does not improve the poor survival rates. Liver transplantation in the setting of cholangiocarcinoma is often done without appreciation that a neoplasm is present and is associated with significantly decreased long-term survival.[130] A pilot study from the Mayo Clinic found that in a highly selected group of patients with early stage, unresectable cholangiocarcinoma, a combination of preoperative external beam radiation and chemotherapy with 5-fluorouracil resulted in increased post-transplant disease-free survival.[131]

Hepatocellular Carcinoma

Hepatocellular carcinoma (HCC) may be more common in PSC than originally thought. Isolated cases of the fibrolamellar variant of HCC occurring in patients with PSC have been reported.[132] However, in a study of 134 patients with PSC who underwent orthotopic liver transplantation, HCC was found in 2%.[133] This finding suggests that patients with PSC who undergo evaluation for liver transplantation should be screened for both cholangiocarcinoma and HCC.

Colonic Neoplasia

An increased risk of colorectal neoplasia in patients with both PSC and ulcerative colitis compared with ulcerative colitis alone is well recognized.[117, 134–139] Although considerable evidence has supported this association, not all studies have found an increased risk.[140, 141] Broome and associates[117] found that patients with both ulcerative colitis and PSC had an absolute cumulative risk of developing colorectal cancer or dysplasia at 10, 20, and 25 years of 9%, 31%, and 50%, respectively; in matched controls with ulcerative colitis alone, the corresponding risk was 2%, 5%, and 10%, respectively. Another study found that colorectal carcinoma or dysplasia developed in 25% of patients with PSC and ulcerative colitis as compared with only 5.6% of patients with ulcerative colitis alone. In addition, the patients with PSC and ulcerative colitis were more likely to have proximal neoplasia (76%), present at a more advanced stage (35%), and die from colorectal cancer (4.5%) than were those with ulcerative colitis alone.[134] Patients undergoing liver transplantation for PSC also may be at increased risk for the development of colorectal neoplasia,[142, 143] although there are studies that refute this finding.[31, 144, 145] The mechanism of this increased neoplastic potential is poorly understood. The high frequency of right-sided colonic neoplasia in patients with PSC supports the theory that secondary bile acids, which are increased in patients with cholestatic liver disease, may act as carcinogens in patients with an underlying predisposition to colonic malignancy, such as ulcerative colitis.[138] Further support comes from reports that ursodeoxycholic acid, which, when taken orally, displaces other bile acids from the enterohepatic circulation, has been associated with a decrease in the rate of both low- and high-grade colonic dysplasia in patients with ulcerative colitis and PSC.[146]

Pouchitis

Pouchitis is an inflammatory condition of the continent ileal reservoir in patients who have undergone a proctocolectomy.[147] It is the most common long-term complication of ileal pouch anal anastomosis (IPAA) in patients with ulcerative colitis (see Chapter 105).[148] Patients with PSC have higher rates of pouchitis than do patients without PSC.[113, 114, 149, 150] A study by Penna and associates[150] found that 63% of patients with ulcerative colitis and PSC had one or more episodes of pouchitis, as compared with only 32% of patients with ulcerative colitis alone. The cumulative risk of pouchitis at 1, 2, 5, and 10 years was 22%, 43%, 61%, and 79%, respectively, for patients with ulcerative colitis and PSC, compared with 15.5%, 22.5%, 36%, and 45.5%, respectively, for patients with ulcerative colitis alone. The disease course of pouchitis does not appear to be altered by orthotopic liver transplantation for PSC.[151, 152]

In 1991, Lofberg and associates[153] reported the case of a patient with intractable ulcerative colitis who underwent a colectomy, mucosal proctectomy, and IPAA. No dysplasia was noted in the colectomy specimen. The patient suffered from chronic pouchitis, and four years later he was noted to have low-grade dysplasia on mucosal biopsy of the pouch with DNA aneuploidy by flow cytometry. This was the first reported case of dysplasia in an IPAA. Subsequently, five additional cases have been reported by the same group.[154] The initial patient went on to develop high-grade dysplasia 5 years later, the only reported case thus far. Within 1 year, he was admitted to the hospital with abdominal pain, and a diagnosis of primary cholangiocarcinoma with likely underlying subclinical PSC was made. The patient expired 3 months later.[155] This case demonstrates the poorly understood, but repeatedly observed, connection between ulcerative colitis and PSC and the increased neoplastic potential in patients who have both diseases.

Management

There is no medical, endoscopic, or surgical therapy, except for liver transplantation, that has been shown to impact positively on the course of primary sclerosing cholangitis. Management is directed toward palliating symptoms, treating complications, and determining the optimal timing of liver transplantation.

Treatment of the Disease Process

A variety of treatments, listed in Table 59–4, have been used in patients with PSC on the basis of the various theo-

Table 59–4 | **Medical Therapy for Primary Sclerosing Cholangitis**

NO PROVEN BENEFIT	POSSIBLE BENEFIT
Antibiotics	Ursodeoxycholic acid (?High dose)
Azathioprine	
Cholestyramine	
Colchicine	
Glucocorticoids	
Budesonide	
Cyclosporine	
D-penicillamine	
Methotrexate	
Tacrolimus	
Transdermal nicotine	
Pentoxifylline	

ries of the etiopathogenesis of the disease. Immunosuppressive therapy seems to be a rational choice in light of the possible autoimmune pathogenesis; however, the results of therapeutic trials have been disappointing to date. Glucocorticoids have not shown a consistent benefit. Reports of positive results in one small study [156] were not reproduced in another,[157] and concern about side effects of glucocorticoids has stemmed enthusiasm for a large controlled trial. Budesonide, a glucocorticoid with increased first-pass hepatic metabolism, not only had no effect on the liver biochemistries, the Mayo risk score, or histologic stage of disease, but also resulted in a marked loss of bone mass from the femoral neck and lumbar spine in patients treated for one year.[158, 159] Other immunosuppressive agents such as cyclosporine[160] and azathioprine[161] have also failed to demonstrate a consistently beneficial effect. Methotrexate, when used alone, demonstrated no significant improvement in liver histology or biochemical markers except for an improvement in the serum alkaline phosphatase level.[162] When used in combination with ursodeoxycholic acid (UCDA),[163] methotrexate was associated with toxicity but with no further improvement in liver biochemistry when compared with UDCA alone. In a small study of 15 patients, the combination of azathioprine, prednisolone, and UDCA resulted in a decrease in liver enzymes and improvement in liver histologic studies in six of 10 patients.[164] A study of tacrolimus in 10 patients demonstrated a marked improvement in liver biochemical tests without related nephrotoxicity.[165] However, these results need confirmation in larger controlled trials.

Increased hepatic copper levels in patients with PSC led to the study of D-penicillamine, a cupruretic agent, in a randomized, placebo controlled trial of 70 patients.[166] Although serum copper levels improved, no benefit in biochemical or histologic parameters was noted, and 21% of patients had to discontinue the drug because of side effects. Antibiotics also have been tried for PSC. A case report of three children with PSC described an improvement in liver biochemistries and symptoms with oral vancomycin.[167] The inverse association between smoking and PSC[33] has led to trials of oral nicotine[168] and transdermal nicotine.[169] However, no beneficial effects on liver biochemistries were noted, and there was a high medication discontinuation rate because of side effects. Because tumor necrosis factor (TNF) has been postulated to have a role in the hepatic injury in PSC, a study of pentoxifylline, which prevents production of cytokines including TNF-α, was conducted. However, no beneficial effects on symptoms, liver biochemistries, or serum TNF-α levels were noted.[170]

Much of the study of medical therapy for PSC has centered on UDCA. UDCA displaces natural, toxic, and endogenous bile salts from the enterohepatic circulation. Theoretically, this displacement results in improvement in hepatic excretion of bile acids, a cytoprotective effect with prevention of bile acid–induced cytolysis and apoptosis, a membrane-protective effect, an antioxidative effect, and an immunomodulating effect.[171, 172] These effects lead to a decrease in cholestasis and improvement in liver function and histology. Randomized controlled trials have shown that UDCA can improve serum levels of alkaline phosphatase, gamma glutamyl transpeptidase, aspartate aminotransferase, bilirubin, and albumin, but no beneficial effect on symptoms of fatigue and pruritus, histologic progression, survival, or time to transplantation has been documented.[173–175] However, when UDCA was used in conjunction with endoscopic dilation of major stenoses, a survival benefit was seen.[176] Despite the lackluster results, trials of UDCA are ongoing and various strategies are being studied, including initiation of treatment early in the disease course, use of higher doses of UDCA, or use of UDCA in combination with other agents.

Medical Management of Complications

Medical measures in the treatment of the complications of PSC are aimed at providing relief from pruritus, correcting nutritional deficiencies, and treating and preventing bacterial cholangitis. Patients with pruritus initially may benefit from some simple measures, including general skin care with topical emollients, wearing comfortable cotton garments, and bathing in tepid rather than hot water. Treatment with antihistamines may provide relief, but oral cholestyramine, 4 to 8 g three times daily just before meals, is often more effective. Cholestipol hydrochloride, another anion-exchange resin, may be useful in patients who are intolerant of cholestyramine.[177] Rifampin is also an effective and usually safe therapy for patients who do not respond to the above measures.[178] Opiate antagonists such as naloxone and nalmefene have been used with some success.[35] Patients who are unresponsive to these measures and who do not obtain relief from endoscopic therapy of dominant strictures should be considered for liver transplantation.

In patients with steatorrhea, medium-chain triglycerides may be given orally to improve calorie assimilation. In rare cases, associated pancreatic insufficiency may contribute to malabsorption and can be treated with pancreatic enzyme supplementation. Fat-soluble vitamin deficiencies should be sought by measuring serum carotene and serum 25-hydroxyvitamin D levels and the prothrombin time.[109] Deficiencies are corrected by vitamin supplements given orally or, in patients with severe malabsorption, parenterally. Administration of vitamin A is effective in correcting usually subclinical vitamin A deficiency, but the value of correcting vitamin D deficiency, with or without calcium supplements, on the development and progression of bone disease in PSC is unclear. Similarly, the use of bisphosphonates and other agents to promote bone formation requires further study in patients with PSC and osteoporosis. In patients with PSC, prolongation of the prothrombin time is more likely to be secondary to end-stage liver disease than to vitamin K deficiency.

Acute episodes of bacterial cholangitis necessitate treatment with antibiotics that are effective against gram-negative bacilli, enterococci, bacteroides, and clostridia.[179] Ciprofloxacin or levofloxacin alone may be as effective as triple antibiotic therapy. Antibiotic prophylaxis is indicated in any patient with PSC who undergoes manipulation of the biliary tree endoscopically, percutaneously, or surgically. Recurrent episodes of cholangitis are a disabling problem for a few patients with PSC. Long-term antibiotic prophylaxis may be helpful in these cases, although the efficacy of this approach is unproven. Prophylaxis can be attempted with one antibiotic agent at a time, given for 3 to 4 weeks, after which the drug should be changed. Choices of antibiotics include ampicillin, trimethoprim-sulfamethoxazole, cephalexin, and ciprofloxacin. Ciprofloxacin is particularly favored because of its broad spectrum and high biliary concentrations. A serious drawback to this approach is that cholangitis resulting from resistant bacterial strains may emerge. Recurrent bacterial cholangitis may become difficult to prevent and treat in patients with PSC and constitutes an indication for liver transplantation.

Radiologic Intervention

Percutaneous intervention for the management of dominant strictures in PSC has been described. Difficulty arises from the lack of intrahepatic ductal dilatation in most patients and the frequent need to use chronic indwelling catheters. High rates of bacterial cholangitis and other complications such as bleeding and peritonitis make it a less desirable method of accessing the biliary tree than endoscopic methods.[180] However, when the biliary tree becomes obstructed by a mass lesion, such as an advanced cholangiocarcinoma or an ampullary growth that makes retrograde access impossible, the percutaneous approach may be the only way to drain the biliary system.

Endoscopic Intervention

It has been postulated that back pressure from dominant strictures and debris may lead to worsening liver function in patients with PSC.[181] Relief of that back pressure by endoscopic sphincterotomy, balloon dilation, and stent placement may, by relieving the pressure, impact favorably on the disease course. In 1983, Siegel described the first use of endoscopic hydrostatic balloon catheter dilation for the treatment of dominant strictures in PSC.[182] Since then, multiple reports have confirmed the efficacy of endoscopic balloon dilation or temporary stenting of biliary strictures in alleviating symptoms of cholestasis and improving liver biochemical abnormalities.[122, 183–189]

In a patient with increasing jaundice, severe pruritus, or recurrent cholangitis, aggressive endoscopic intervention to treat strictures or biliary calculi is warranted. The presence of dominant strictures improves the chances of benefit from endoscopic therapy. A sphincterotomy is often done to facilitate access of catheters to the biliary tree and to decrease back pressure. Then 4 to 6 mm Gruentzig-type balloons are used to dilate strictures in the common bile duct, common hepatic duct, right and left main hepatic ducts, and sometimes secondary duct branches in patients with advanced disease. Some patients require serial dilation. Debris and stones are cleared from the accessible ducts.

The use of temporary stents for dominant strictures is controversial. Some authors have noted rates of cholangitis of 48% to 80% with such stents.[183, 185, 187] In a more recent series of 32 patients who underwent short-term stenting for a mean of 11 days, clinical improvement occurred in 83%, with an 80% intervention-free rate at 1 year, but a 15% complication rate. Although cholangitis was not a complication, perforations, pancreatitis, and hydrops of the gallbladder occurred.[189] Many experts avoid stenting of dominant strictures in PSC, and if a stent is placed, recommend short-term stenting of 7 to 14 days only.

Endoscopic therapy is not believed to affect disease progression in PSC; however, there are some reports that survival is improved by endoscopic therapy. Stiehl and associates[176] reported on 23 patients with PSC who were treated with UDCA (shown in controlled trials not to affect survival) and serial endoscopic balloon dilation. The Kaplan-Meier survival probability after combined treatment was significantly improved compared with the predicted survival rates on the basis of the original Mayo model. In a study of 27 patients, we noted a trend toward decreased progression of disease based on the rate of change in the Child-Pugh and Mayo scores in patients who underwent frequent serial dilation as compared with those managed medically. No stents were used and no episodes of cholangitis were observed in 161 ERCPs. The complication rate was less than 1%, with only one episode of moderate, self-limited pancreatitis.[190] Further work in this area needs to be done. At the very best, endoscopic therapy for PSC is a safe and valuable palliative tool that can improve acute exacerbations of jaundice, pruritus, and cholangitis in patients with these complications of PSC.

Surgical Management

Colectomy

Proctocolectomy should be undertaken in patients with ulcerative colitis and PSC for indications relevant to the underlying colitis, such as colonic mucosal dysplasia or refractory colitis. A prospective study of 45 patients found that there was no beneficial effect on the course of PSC in patients who underwent colectomy as compared with those who did not undergo colectomy.[48] Moreover, PSC may develop years after colectomy.[104]

Biliary Tract Surgery

The role of biliary surgery has diminished with increasing predominance of endoscopic therapy and liver transplantation. Surgical resection of dominant bile duct strictures, sometimes accompanied by intraoperative dilation of more proximal intrahepatic ducts and followed by a choledochojejunostomy or hepaticojejunostomy, has been done in the past.[191, 192] However, surgical therapy is associated with relatively high morbidity and mortality rates, especially in patients who have progressed to cirrhosis, and has the potential to affect future liver transplantation adversely.[193]

Liver Transplantation

Liver transplantation is the treatment of choice for patients with end-stage liver disease (see Chapter 83). Transplantation is indicated for patients with PSC who experience complications of portal hypertension, hepatic protein synthetic dysfunction, severe or worsening cholestasis with cirrhosis, and recurrent cholangitis refractory to medical or interventional therapy. The prognostic models discussed earlier may help determine the optimal timing of transplantation but have not yet been fully validated. The surgical procedure differs in patients with PSC in that a choledochojejunostomy with a Roux-en-Y biliary anastomosis is usually performed instead of the usual direct donor-to-recipient duct-to-duct biliary anastomosis. This variation is undertaken to avoid using the recipient's common duct, which is often diseased.

Survival after liver transplantation for PSC is excellent. A study of 150 patients who underwent transplantation at one center reported patient survival rates at 1, 2, 5, and 10 years of 93.7%, 92.2%, 86.4%, and 69.8%, respectively. Graft survival rates for the same time periods were 83.4%, 83.4%, 79%, and 60.5%, respectively.[194] A poor survival rate after hepatic retransplantation was associated with retransplantation more than 30 days after the first transplant, suggesting that patients should be screened carefully.[195] The main indication for retransplantation was hepatic artery thrombosis, and the major cause of death was severe infection. Patients with PSC were also noted to have higher rates of acute cellular and chronic ductopenic rejection when compared with non-PSC transplant recipients. Biliary strictures occurred at the anastomosis in 16.2% of patients and at nonanastomotic sites in 27.2% of patients.[194] Patients with PSC were also noted to have higher rates of enterococcal bacteremia post-transplantation.[196]

If cholangiocarcinoma is found, even serendipitously at the time of liver transplantation, survival is dismal, with rates as low as 30% at 1 year.[197] However, some success has been reported in a highly selected group of patients with early stage, unresectable cholangiocarcinoma, with use of a combination of preoperative external beam radiation and chemotherapy with 5-fluorouracil.[131]

PSC recurs after liver transplantation in 15% to 20% of patients.[198, 199] A study from the Mayo Clinic defined recurrence of PSC as a confirmed diagnosis of PSC before transplantation and a cholangiogram consistent with PSC more than 90 days after transplantation or consistent histologic findings (fibrous cholangitis or fibro-obliterative lesions, with or without ductopenia, biliary fibrosis, or biliary cirrhosis). Criteria that exclude a diagnosis of recurrent PSC (Table 59–5) are the presence of hepatic artery thrombosis or stenosis, established ductopenic rejection, anastomotic strictures alone, nonanastomotic strictures before post-transplantation day 90, or ABO blood-type incompatibility between donor and recipient.[199] On the basis of these strict criteria, a 20% post-transplantation recurrence rate was found in 120 patients with PSC. No specific clinical risk factors were identified, and overall patient and graft survival was not affected by the presence of recurrence.

There is a strong impression, as yet unproven, that the risk of developing colon cancer in inflammatory bowel disease may be increased in the setting of immunosuppression following liver transplantation. For the present, in patients undergoing liver transplantation for PSC in whom the colon remains in situ, yearly colonoscopy is strongly advocated.

Studies of the quality of life in patients with PSC who undergo liver transplantation have demonstrated improvement in up to 80% of patients[200] as well as improvement in all aspects studied—physical, social, and emotional function and health perceptions.[201]

Table 59–5 | **Causes of Biliary Strictures after Liver Transplantation**

ABO graft incompatibility
Hepatic artery thrombosis
Ductopenic/arteriopathic rejection
Preservation-related ischemia
Roux-en-Y anastomosis-associated bacterial cholangitis
Recurrent primary sclerosing cholangitis

RECURRENT PYOGENIC CHOLANGITIS

Definition

Recurrent pyogenic cholangitis (RPC) is a syndrome of unclear etiology characterized by intrahepatic pigment stone formation with biliary strictures and dilatation and recurrent bouts of suppurative cholangitis. Digby first described this disease among the Chinese in 1930.[202] Other names for this entity include oriental cholangiohepatitis and hepatolithiasis.

RPC is found almost exclusively in Southeast Asia. The relative incidence, or frequency of intrahepatic stone disease among all patients with gallstone disease, varies by country: 54% in Taiwan, 5% in Japan, 3.1% in Hong Kong, and 1.7% in Singapore.[203, 204] The incidence in the West is increasing, largely because of immigration from endemic Asian countries; however, there are isolated case reports in occidentals.[205] The disease occurs with equal frequency in both genders[206] and has a peak prevalence in the third and fourth decades. It is more common in rural than urban populations and in lower socioeconomic groups.[204]

Pathology

The extrahepatic and larger intrahepatic bile ducts are dilated, and focal areas of stenosis are found in the intrahepatic biliary tree. The wall of the bile ducts is fibrotic, and inflammatory cell infiltration is noted.[207] Typically, the left hepatic duct, particularly the left lateral segmental duct, is affected most severely and is often involved early in the course of the disease. The papilla of the sphincter of Oddi may be hypertrophied and fibrosed from the repeated passage of stones. Macroscopically, the liver is enlarged and scarred with numerous capsular adhesions and distorted by deep and subcapsular abscesses.[208] After multiple attacks of pyogenic cholangitis, the liver may atrophy. Atrophy predominantly affects the lateral segment of the left lobe, which may consist of little more than fibrous tissue and dilated ducts. Histologically, bile duct proliferation and acute inflammatory cell infiltrates are seen in the portal tracts. Portal thrombophlebitis may be evident, and inflammatory cells may extend into the hepatic parenchyma with suppuration.

The bile ducts contain sludge and debris composed of bile pigment, desquamated epithelial cells, bacteria, and pus. Stones, often innumerable, are found in both intrahepatic and extrahepatic ducts. In one study of 16 patients, 100% had left hepatic duct stones, 73% had right hepatic duct stones, and 53% had stones in the extrahepatic duct.[209] The majority of the intrahepatic duct stones are composed of calcium bilirubinate, although changing diets have been implicated in a shift toward greater cholesterol content in the stones.[204] The stones range in size from 3 to 7 mm, although larger stones have been noted. Their color ranges from orange-brown to black, and their consistency varies from hard to mud-like. They may pack the intrahepatic ducts or be confined to a single segment, usually the left lateral segment.

Although biliary stones are a typical feature of RPC, they are absent in 20% to 25% of patients diagnosed with this disease.[207] This occurrence may reflect the earliest stages of the disease or complete passage of biliary stones. The gallbladder often shows acute or chronic inflammation and contains stones in 50% to 70% of patients.[207]

Etiology and Pathogenesis

The recurrent episodes of cholangitis reflect pyogenic infection within the biliary tree, often induced by bile stasis and stone formation proximal to biliary strictures. The most common organism cultured from the bile in RPC is *Escherichia coli*, followed by *Klebsiella*, *Pseudomonas*, and *Proteus* species and infrequently anaerobes.[210, 211] Infection with more than one organism is not unusual. Transient portal bacteremia is thought to convey enteric bacteria to the bile ducts, although, under normal circumstances, this does not lead to infection. Some underlying abnormality, such as stasis or ductal epithelial disruption, must favor the seeding of bacteria in the biliary system and the subsequent initiation of infection, suppuration, and secondary pigment stone formation. Stone formation, in turn, produces further obstruction and infection in a self-perpetuating cycle of recurrent cholangitis.

The mechanisms underlying the initiation of biliary sepsis are unknown. The distribution of the disease in Southeast Asia and among rural, lower socioeconomic groups suggests that environmental factors predominate. To this end, the leading theories are that parasitic infection and malnutrition play a role. Parasitic infestation of the biliary tree, mostly by liver flukes and roundworms, may initiate the epithelial damage and biliary obstruction that ultimately lead to RPC. Support for this theory comes from the overall similarity in the geographic distribution of RPC in Asia and that of the prevalent liver flukes—predominantly *Clonorchis sinensis*, but also *Opisthorchis viverrini* and *O. felineus* (see Chapters 69 and 99).[211–213] Infection is acquired by eating freshwater fish infested with the encysted cercariae of the parasite. Infestation with *Clonorchis* is extremely common in Southeast Asia, with an estimated 19 million cases. The worm can live for up to 30 years in the biliary system.[214] Damage to the biliary epithelium by the flukes, as well as obstruction of the ducts by parasites, ova, and debris, may be the initial insult in the pathogenesis of RPC. Evidence of active fluke infestation or a history of infestation is found in 20% to 45% of patients with RPC,[208, 210, 211] whereas cases of RPC outside Asia have shown a strong association with biliary infestation with *Ascaris lumbricoides*.[207, 213] Analysis of the pigment stones in RPC has also shown the presence of parasite debris and ova, which may act as a nidus for stone formation.[207, 213]

It is clear that heavy infestation with *Clonorchis* can produce extensive damage to the bile ducts, with a predilection for the left-sided ducts,[214] and that ductal obstruction by parasites and parasitic debris can lead to acute suppurative cholangitis and RPC in a small proportion of patients. However, infection with *Clonorchis* is extremely common in Asia, and the prevalence of the parasite in RPC is no greater than in the control population from the same geographic area. Although clonorchiasis shows a male preponderance, the sexes are equally affected by RPC.[208] Finally, RPC is well described in certain areas of China, Taiwan, and Japan that are virtually free of *Clonorchis*.[216]

The malnutrition theory was suggested initially by the observation that RPC was diagnosed mainly in patients from poor socioeconomic conditions. Repeated attacks of bacterial gastroenteritis that lead to episodes of portal bacteremia in this population were postulated to result in frequent seeding of bacteria in the biliary system.[207, 208, 216] In addition, the low-protein diet consumed by the indigent population may result in a relative deficiency in bile of glucaro-1:4-lactone, an inhibitor of the enzyme β-glucuronidase.[207, 208, 216] β-Glucuronidase is produced by bacteria that infect the bile and deconjugates water-soluble bilirubin glucuronides. The unconjugated bilirubin precipitates with calcium ions to form insoluble calcium bilirubinate, the major component of pigment stones. Stone formation leads to biliary obstruction with further stasis and obstructive cholangitis.

Other, less likely theories have been proposed as well. The young age at which hepatolithiasis develops has led some authorities to speculate that congenital anomalies of the biliary tree may predispose to stone formation, although this theory is not well supported by the literature.[204] In a small group of five patients with RPC, marked lymphopenia and a reduction in the number of $CD4^+$ cells were found, suggesting immune depression.[217] However, more work needs to be done in this area, and the leading theories of pathogenesis remain parasites and malnutrition. The decline in incidence of RPC in Asia and among the offspring of Asian immigrants to Western countries[218] lends further support to these theories by reflecting either improved standards of living and diet, lower rates of parasitic infection, or both.

Clinical Manifestations

The incidence of RPC peaks between the third and fifth decades of life, but the disease is frequently encountered in patients older than age 60 years.[207, 208, 210, 213] Attacks are characterized by Charcot's triad: right upper quadrant pain, fever with or without rigors, and jaundice. A study of 41 patients with RPC found that 44% presented with cholangitis, 32% with abdominal pain, and 17% with pancreatitis.[218] Patients may have a history of recurrent attacks, at a rate of one or two per year, although 15% to 30% of patients present with a first episode.[207, 219] Many patients have had prior biliary tract surgery.

Physical examination may reveal jaundice, tenderness in the upper abdomen, and hepatomegaly. In about one third of patients, the gallbladder is palpable, reflecting acute empyema of the gallbladder or involvement by calculous or acalculous cholecystitis.[207, 212] Laboratory findings usually show an elevated white blood cell count with a polymorphonuclear leukocytosis and an increase in liver biochemical tests, specifically alkaline phosphatase and bilirubin levels, reflecting an obstructive pattern.

Complications

Acute attacks of pyogenic cholangitis may be complicated by gram-negative septicemia manifested by shock and obtundation. Local complications include rupture of an obstructed,

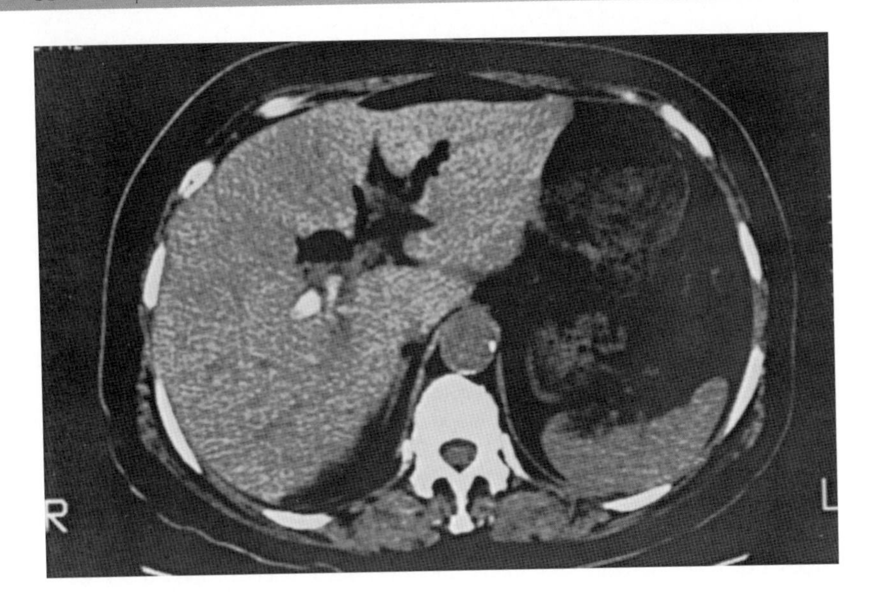

Figure 59–4. Hepatic computed tomographic (CT) scan in RPC. The patient had a history of recurrent attacks of cholangitis for 10 years and had previously undergone a cholecystectomy and common duct exploration with a Roux-en-Y choledochojejunostomy. The scan, performed without contrast, shows air in the bile ducts from the biliary-enteric anastomosis. The air cholangiogram reveals marked dilatation of the central bile ducts with rapid peripheral tapering, producing the classic arrowhead sign. The high-density foci in the right posterior ducts are calcified stones. (Courtesy of Jean M. LaBerge, M.D., Department of Radiology, University of California, San Francisco.)

pus-filled bile duct into the peritoneum or fistulization into the gastrointestinal tract, abdominal wall, pericardium, or vascular structure.[208, 210, 218] Portal vein thrombosis and hemobilia may occur, and metastatic sepsis may result in abscesses in the lungs and brain.[208, 211] Acute pancreatitis occurs in 10% to 17% of patients with RPC.[218, 220] Although clinically apparent chronic pancreatitis is rare, chronic dilatation of the pancreatic ducts has been observed in up to 8% of patients.[221]

Secondary biliary cirrhosis and cholangiocarcinoma are also complications of RPC. A study by Jan and associates of 427 patients with hepatolithiasis found that secondary biliary cirrhosis developed in 6.8% of patients and cholangiocarcinoma developed in 2.8%. The overall mortality rate from the disease was 10.3%.[222] A few patients have gone on to orthotopic liver transplantation for cirrhosis related to RPC, and as this therapy becomes increasingly available on a global basis, more transplants for this disease will likely be performed.[219] Cholangiocarcinoma has long been recognized as a complication of RPC, and the risk is felt to be independent of the risk of cholangiocarcinoma associated with chronic *Clonorchis* infestation.[214] Rates varying from 2.8% to 8.8% have been reported in cohorts of patients with RPC,[223, 224] and the tumor often arises in the atrophied left lobe of the liver.

Diagnosis

The clinical manifestations of pyogenic cholangitis, particularly in a native of Southeast Asia with a history of previous attacks, should suggest the diagnosis of RPC. Radiologic imaging studies, however, are essential for establishing the diagnosis and for directing treatment. Examination by ultrasonography is useful as a screening procedure and can reveal ductal dilatation and ductal stones in 85% to 90% of cases and localize hepatic abscesses.[207, 225] Contrast-enhanced CT scanning is the noninvasive procedure of choice and should be obtained in all patients. The CT examination is an essential supplement to cholangiography, which may fail to visualize severely affected ductal segments because of obstruction and hence may fail to delineate the full extent of the disease.[207, 210] CT scanning often reveals a characteristic pattern of dilated central intrahepatic ducts with acute tapering of the peripheral ducts (Fig. 59–4). Duct wall enhancement may be seen, and disease localized to the left lobe with lobar atrophy, hepatic abscesses, bilomas, and stones are features typical of RPC that are often best demonstrated by CT scan.[226] Calcified stones are readily detected by CT scan, but biliary mud, casts, or stones that contain little calcium may be isodense or hypodense on CT scan and missed. Recently, magnetic resonance imaging (MRI) of the liver and biliary tree has been used in patients with pancreaticobiliary disease, especially those with comorbid conditions that make ERCP a high-risk procedure. As in CT scanning, bile duct dilation, decreased branching with abrupt tapering, and stenosis or stricturing of the peripheral ducts is seen. On MRI, unlike CT, noncalcified stones can be visualized as discrete filling defects. Pneumobilia, however, is more difficult to distinguish on MRI, and CT scanning may be needed to distinguish pneumobilia from stones in the postoperative patient.[227]

Definitive imaging of the ducts and their contents is achieved by cholangiography. Preoperative cholangiography is performed most frequently via ERCP, which is preferred over the percutaneous route in RPC because it achieves better visualization of the often more severely involved lower biliary tract, is not accompanied by the risks of spilling pus into the peritoneal cavity, and has the therapeutic advantage of permitting drainage and clearance of the lower biliary tract via endoscopic sphincterotomy. Nevertheless, the procedure carries a significant risk of precipitating cholangitis in patients with quiescent RPC and should be performed with antibiotic prophylaxis.[220, 221] Cholangiography shows a spectrum of diagnostic abnormalities in RPC (Fig. 59–5), including dilatation of the intra- and extrahepatic ducts, the latter often disproportionately widened. Because of extensive periductal fibrosis, the intrahepatic ducts are typically straightened with less acute or right-angled branching patterns. There is decreased arborization and acute tapering of the more peripheral ducts, producing a classic "arrowhead" sign.[220, 228] Stones may fill the ducts or be confined to either the extrahepatic or, more commonly, intrahepatic ducts.

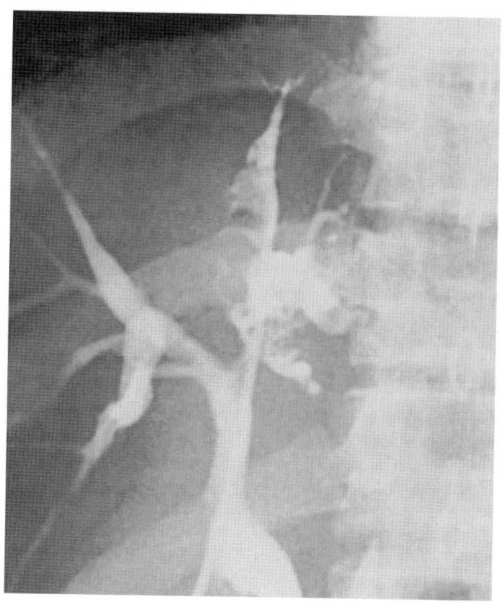

Figure 59–5. Cholangiogram in RPC. The patient had previously undergone a side-to-side choledochojejunostomy with placement of a proximal limb of a Roux loop in the subcutaneous tissues of the abdominal wall in order to facilitate repeated radiologic removal of stones. A tube has been inserted through the proximal Roux limb into the left main intrahepatic duct. Features typical of RPC include marked reduction in ductal arborization, straightening of the ducts, widening of the branching angles, and abrupt peripheral tapering. Also typical is the more severe involvement of the left ductal system, which is dilated, packed with stones, and strictured near its origin. (Courtesy of Jean M. LaBerge, M.D., Department of Radiology, University of California, San Francisco.)

They may completely obstruct segmental or subsegmental ducts ("missing duct" sign).

Differential Diagnosis

RPC differs in its clinical and radiologic aspects from the Western pattern of choledocholithiasis and acute suppurative cholangitis that complicates retained common duct stones, but in a chronic stone former, distinguishing the two entities may be difficult. Gallstones in the common duct usually produce some degree of dilatation proximal to the obstruction, whereas in RPC, ductal dilatation is usually massive and often unrelated to the level of the stones.[207] Ductal obstruction produced by periampullary tumors, including carcinoma of the pancreas and bile duct, often can be distinguished by the fact that they produce long, high-grade strictures of the bile ducts with resulting dilatation of the entire biliary tree proximal to the stricture, including the peripheral bile ducts.[207, 220]

Although there is a difference of opinion regarding the role of clonorchiasis in the pathogenesis of RPC, infestation with this parasite may certainly coexist with RPC. However, heavy infestation with *Clonorchis* produces biliary disease that is in several respects quite distinct from RPC.[214, 220] The parasites are seen on cholangiography as round, elliptical, filamentous, or wavy filling defects. Clonorchiasis produces diffuse dilatation of the intrahepatic ducts, whereas the extrahepatic ducts are often unaffected. Scalloped indentation of the duct walls is often seen, and extensive tortuosity and deformity producing a mulberry-like appearance of the extrahepatic duct system is virtually pathognomonic for clonorchiasis. As in RPC, however, early *Clonorchis* infection shows a predilection for the left hepatic ductal system. Eosinophilia may be present, and ova are invariably found in the stool.

PSC is readily differentiated from RPC by the features of global ductal narrowing and diffuse strictures that characterize PSC. Ductal stones may be present in PSC but not to the extent observed in RPC. Also, diffuse extrahepatic ductal stricturing may be an unusual occurrence in RPC,[211] and true PSC is rare in the Orient. Caroli's disease can be distinguished by its occurrence in younger patients and by the characteristic saccular or cystic dilatations present in the intrahepatic bile ducts.

Management

The goal of management of RPC is to bring the acute attack of pyogenic cholangitis under control and to prevent future attacks. Although the role of *Clonorchis* and other parasites in the pathogenesis of RPC will undoubtedly continue to generate debate, the high incidence of concurrent parasitosis in patients with RPC mandates that patients be evaluated for a parasitic infection, including examination of the stool for ova, and treated if necessary. The majority of patients with RPC and acute cholangitis respond to a conservative regimen of broad-spectrum antibiotics and intravenous fluids. Conservative treatment fails in approximately 15% of patients,[229] in whom emergency surgery is required. Persistent pain and fever, increasing jaundice, signs of peritonitis, a palpable tender gallbladder, and gram-negative septicemia indicate the need for emergent surgical treatment. Surgery often consists of common duct exploration and T-tube drainage, with cholecystectomy if the gallbladder is affected. In selected patients, emergency decompression may be accomplished by endoscopic sphincterotomy with stent placement or by percutaneous transhepatic drainage.[220, 228–230]

The prevention of future attacks of cholangitis is based on removal of all biliary stones and debris, dilation or resection of strictures, and establishment of optimal biliary drainage to allow the passage of residual stones and debris. Treatment is planned according to CT and cholangiographic findings, the latter most commonly obtained by ERCP or via a T tube inserted at the time of emergency surgery. Surgery is clearly indicated for patients with gallbladder stones or disease, stones within the intrahepatic ducts, and disease localized predominantly to the left hepatic ductal system.[231] A left hepatic lobectomy is preferred to a left lateral segmentectomy, because there is a lower rate of residual stone disease with the former approach.[234]

Surgical clearance of stones from the ducts has been aided considerably by the intraoperative use of the choledochoscope and electrohydraulic lithotripsy.[229] Drainage procedures performed by the surgeon depend on the extent and location of stones and strictures. In patients with extensive intrahepatic ductal stones, an increasingly favored approach is to construct a Roux-en-Y hepaticojejunostomy with the proximal limit of the Roux loop buried in the abdominal wall or externalized as a cutaneous stoma.[231, 232] An end-to-side anastomosis is preferred over a side-to-side anastomosis, because the latter approach may lead to "sump syndrome," in which the bile duct distal to the hepaticojejunostomy accumulates food debris and sludge, leading to cholangitis.[233]

In many cases, surgery is not adequate to remove all the stones, and patients must undergo repeated procedures by the interventional radiologist to clear the stones. The surgically created cutaneous stoma or the T-tube tract is used to access the biliary tree. In a study by Cheng and colleagues of 245 patients with hepatolithiasis, surgical choledocholithotomy failed to remove stones completely in 190 patients.[223] These patients then underwent biliary dilation and stenting via the T-tube tract as well as choledochoscopy (cholangioscopy) and electrohydraulic lithotripsy. Complete stone removal was achieved in 88.4% of patients. Failure was more common in patients with right-sided stone disease and in those with a difficult anatomy such as sharp angulations of the biliary tree.[223] If percutaneous transhepatic cholangioscopic lithotomy with stone removal is done without hepatic resection, complete stone removal can be achieved, but with higher rates of residual biliary strictures and higher 5-year recurrence rates than in patients who also undergo left lobectomy.[237] Also, patients who undergo hepatectomy rather than percutaneous transhepatic cholangioscopic lithotomy alone have a better quality of life and may have lower rates of secondary biliary cirrhosis, cholangiocarcinoma, and mortality.[222]

The use of metal stents in patients with RPC with biliary strictures and recurrent stones is controversial. One study of 18 patients (7 with metal stents) found that placement of a metal stent was associated with less recurrent stone disease, fewer procedures, and a shorter hospital stay than repeated endoscopic or percutaneous plastic stent or tube placement.[235] However, another study of 23 patients who underwent placement of a metal stent concluded that metal stents are not effective long-term therapy because of a high rate of occlusion from debris and intimal overgrowth. The patency rate at 2 years was only 67%.[236]

Endoscopic sphincterotomy and stone extraction by a balloon catheter or basket has been used in conjunction with surgery or as definitive treatment for patients with RPC. Use of these techniques is preferred in patients who are elderly or considered poor surgical candidates and in whom stones are confined to the common bile duct. However, as for all therapeutic modalities in RPC, when stones are not removed completely, patients are at risk of further attacks of cholangitis.[220, 230, 238]

REFERENCES

1. Delbet M: Retrecissement du choladogue cholecysto-duodenostomie. Bull Mem Soc Nation Chirugie 50, 1924.
2. Forbes A, Blanshard C, Gazzard B: Natural history of AIDS related sclerosing cholangitis: A study of 20 cases. Gut 34:116, 1993.
3. Blanshard C, Shanson D, Gazzard B: Pilot studies of azithromycin, letrazuril and paromomycin in the treatment of cryptosporidiosis. Int J STD AIDS 8:124, 1997.
4. Gremse D, Bucuvalas J, Bongiovanni G: Papillary stenosis and sclerosing cholangitis in an immunodeficient child. Gastroenterology 96: 1600, 1989.
5. Durieu I, Pellet O, Simonot L, et al: Sclerosing cholangitis in adults with cystic fibrosis: A magnetic resonance cholangiographic prospective study. J Hepatol 30:1052, 1999.
6. Pozniak MA, Babel SG, Trump DL: Complications of hepatic arterial infusion chemotherapy. Radiographics 11:67, 1991.
7. Ludwig J, Kim CH, Wiesner RH, et al: Floxuridine-induced sclerosing cholangitis: An ischemic cholangiopathy? Hepatology 9:215, 1989.
8. Bucuvalas JC, Bove KE, Kaufman RA, et al: Cholangitis associated with *Cryptococcus neoformans*. Gastroenterology 88:1055, 1985.
9. Terada T, Nakanuma Y: Intrahepatic cholangiographic appearance simulating primary sclerosing cholangitis in several hepatobiliary diseases: A postmortem cholangiographic and histopathological study in 154 livers at autopsy. Hepatology 22:75, 1995.
10. Vilgrain V, Erlinger S, Belghiti J, et al: Cholangiographic appearance simulating sclerosing cholangitis in metastatic adenocarcinoma of the liver. Gastroenterology 99:850, 1990.
11. Steinhart AH, Simons M, Stone R, et al: Multiple hepatic abscesses: Cholangiographic changes simulating sclerosing cholangitis and resolution after percutaneous drainage. Am J Gastroenterol 85:306, 1990.
12. Wiesner RH, LaRusso NF, Ludwig J, et al: Comparison of the clinicopathologic features of primary sclerosing cholangitis and primary biliary cirrhosis. Gastroenterology 88:108, 1985.
13. Goodman ZD, McNally PR, Davis DR, et al: Autoimmune cholangitis: A variant of primary biliary cirrhosis. Clinicopathologic and serologic correlations in 200 cases. Dig Dis Sci 40:1232, 1995.
14. Gohlke F, Lohse AW, Dienes HP, et al: Evidence for an overlap syndrome of autoimmune hepatitis and primary sclerosing cholangitis. J Hepatol 24:699, 1996.
15. McNair AN, Moloney M, Portmann BC, et al: Autoimmune hepatitis overlapping with primary sclerosing cholangitis in five cases. Am J Gastroenterol 93:777, 1998.
16. Wilschanski M, Chait P, Wade JA, et al: Primary sclerosing cholangitis in 32 children: Clinical, laboratory, and radiographic features, with survival analysis. Hepatology 22:1415, 1995.
17. Graham SM, Barwick K, Cahow CE, et al: Cholangitis glandularis proliferans. A histologic variant of primary sclerosing cholangitis with distinctive clinical and pathological features. J Clin Gastroenterol 10: 579, 1988.
18. Ichikawa N, Taniguchi A, Akama H, et al: Sclerosing cholangitis associated with hypereosinophilic syndrome. Intern Med 36:561, 1997.
19. Thompson HH, Pitt HA, Lewin KJ, et al: Sclerosing cholangitis and histiocytosis X. Gut 25:526–530, 1984.
20. Alam I, Levenson SD, Ferrell LD, et al: Diffuse intrahepatic biliary strictures in sarcoidosis resembling sclerosing cholangitis. Case report and review of the literature. Dig Dis Sci 42:1295, 1997.
21. Tsuneyama K, Saito K, Ruebner BH, et al: Immunological similarities between primary sclerosing cholangitis and chronic sclerosing sialadenitis: Report of the overlapping of these two autoimmune diseases. Dig Dis Sci 45:366, 2000.
22. Nonomura A, Minato H, Shimizu K, et al: Hepatic hilar inflammatory pseudotumor mimicking cholangiocarcinoma with cholangitis and phlebitis—a variant of primary sclerosing cholangitis? Pathol Res Pract 193:519, 1997.
23. Olsson R DA, Jarnerot G: Prevalence of primary sclerosing cholangitis in patients with ulcerative colitis. Gastroenterology 100:1319, 1991.
24. Boberg KM, Aadland E, Jahnsen J, et al: Incidence and prevalence of primary biliary cirrhosis, primary sclerosing cholangitis, and autoimmune hepatitis in a Norwegian population. Scand J Gastroenterol 33: 99, 1998.
25. Broome U, Olsson R, Loof L, et al: Natural history and prognostic factors in 305 Swedish patients with primary sclerosing cholangitis. Gut 38:610, 1996.
26. Kelly P, Patchett S, McCloskey D, et al: Sclerosing cholangitis, race and sex. Gut 41:688, 1997.
27. Tobias R, Wright J, Kottle R, et al: Primary sclerosing cholangitis associated with inflammatory bowel disease in Cape Town, 1975–1981. S Afr Med J 63:229, 1981.
28. Okada H, Mizuno M, Yamamoto K, et al: Primary sclerosing cholangitis in Japanese patients: Association with inflammatory bowel disease. Acta Med Okayama 50:227, 1996.
29. Broome U, Lofberg R, Lundqvist K, et al: Subclinical time span of inflammatory bowel disease in patients with primary sclerosing cholangitis. Dis Colon Rectum 38:1301, 1995.
30. Lundqvist K, Broome U: Differences in colonic disease activity in patients with ulcerative colitis with and without primary sclerosing cholangitis: A case control study. Dis Colon Rectum 40:451, 1997.
31. Papatheodoridis GV, Hamilton M, Mistry PK, et al: Ulcerative colitis has an aggressive course after orthotopic liver transplantation for primary sclerosing cholangitis. Gut 43:639, 1998.

32. Harewood G, Loftus E, Tremaine W, et al: "PSC-IBD": A unique form of inflammatory bowel disease associated with primary sclerosing cholangitis. Gastroenterology 116:A732, 1999.
33. Loftus EV Jr, Sandborn WJ, Tremaine WJ, et al: Primary sclerosing cholangitis is associated with nonsmoking: A case-control study. Gastroenterology 110:1496, 1996.
34. Porayko MK, LaRusso NF, Wiesner RH: Primary sclerosing cholangitis: A progressive disease? Semin Liver Dis 11:18, 1991.
35. Wiesner RH: Current concepts in primary sclerosing cholangitis. Mayo Clin Proc 69:969, 1994.
36. Farrant JM, Hayllar KM, Wilkinson ML, et al: Natural history and prognostic variables in primary sclerosing cholangitis. Gastroenterology 100:1710, 1991.
37. Porayko MK, Wiesner RH, LaRusso NF, et al: Patients with asymptomatic primary sclerosing cholangitis frequently have progressive disease. Gastroenterology 98:1594, 1990.
38. Kornfeld D, Ekbom A, Ihre T: Survival and risk of cholangiocarcinoma in patients with primary sclerosing cholangitis. A population-based study. Scand J Gastroenterol 32:1042, 1997.
39. Wiesner RH, Grambsch PM, Dickson ER, et al: Primary sclerosing cholangitis: Natural history, prognostic factors and survival analysis. Hepatology 10:430, 1989.
40. Kim R, Therneau T, Wiesner RH, et al: A revised natural history model for primary sclerosing cholangitis. Mayo Clin Proc 75:688, 2000.
41. Neuberger J, Gunson B, Komolmit P, et al: Pretransplant prediction of prognosis after liver transplantation in primary sclerosing cholangitis using a Cox regression model. Hepatology 29:1375, 1999.
42. Shetty K, Rybicki L, Carey WD: The Child-Pugh classification as a prognostic indicator for survival in primary sclerosing cholangitis. Hepatology 25:1049, 1997.
43. Kim WR, Poterucha JJ, Wiesner RH, et al: The relative role of the Child-Pugh classification and the Mayo natural history model in the assessment of survival in patients with primary sclerosing cholangitis. Hepatology 29:1643, 1999.
44. Lee YM, Kaplan MM: Primary sclerosing cholangitis. N Engl J Med 332:924, 1995.
45. Castellano G, Moreno-Sanchez D, Gutierrez J, et al: Caustic sclerosing cholangitis. Report of four cases and a cumulative review of the literature. Hepatogastroenterology 41:458, 1994.
46. Tjandra K, Sharkey KA, Swain MG: Progressive development of a Th1-type hepatic cytokine profile in rats with experimental cholangitis. Hepatology 31:280, 2000.
47. Sasatomi K, Noguchi K, Sakisaka S, et al: Abnormal accumulation of endotoxin in biliary epithelial cells in primary biliary cirrhosis and primary sclerosing cholangitis. J Hepatol 29:409, 1998.
48. Cangemi JR, Wiesner RH, Beaver SJ, et al: Effect of proctocolectomy for chronic ulcerative colitis on the natural history of primary sclerosing cholangitis. Gastroenterology 96:790, 1989.
49. Rabinovitz M, Gavaler JS, Schade RR, et al: Does primary sclerosing cholangitis occurring in association with inflammatory bowel disease differ from that occurring in the absence of inflammatory bowel disease? A study of sixty-six subjects. Hepatology 11:7, 1990.
50. Cello JP: Acquired immunodeficiency syndrome cholangiopathy: Spectrum of disease. Am J Med 86:539, 1989.
51. McWhinney PH, Nathwani D, Green ST, et al: Microsporidiosis detected in association with AIDS-related sclerosing cholangitis [letter]. AIDS 5:1394, 1991.
52. Olsson R, Bjornsson E, Backman L, et al: Bile duct bacterial isolates in primary sclerosing cholangitis: A study of explanted livers. J Hepatol 28:426, 1998.
53. Mehal WZ, Hattersley AT, Chapman RW, et al: A survey of cytomegalovirus (CMV) DNA in primary sclerosing cholangitis (PSC) liver tissues using a sensitive polymerase chain reaction (PCR) based assay. J Hepatol 15:396, 1992.
54. Jorge AD, Esley C, Ahumada J: Family incidence of primary sclerosing cholangitis associated with immunologic diseases. Endoscopy 19: 114, 1987.
55. Quigley E, Larusso NF, Ludwig, J et al: Familial occurrence of primary sclerosing cholangitis and ulcerative colitis. Gastroenterology 85: 1160, 1983.
56. Schrumpf E, Fausa O, Forre O, et al: HLA antigens and immunoregulatory T cells in ulcerative colitis associated with hepatobiliary disease. Scand J Gastroenterol 17:187, 1982.
57. Chapman R, Varghese Z, Gaul R, et al: Association of primary sclerosing cholangitis with HLA-B8. Gut 24:38, 1983.
58. Donaldson PT, Wilkinson ML, Hayllar K, et al: Dual association of HLA DR2 and DR3 with primary sclerosing cholangitis. Hepatology 13:129, 1991.
59. Olerup O, Olsson R, Hultcrantz R et al: HLA-DR and HLA-DQ are not markers for rapid disease progression in primary sclerosing cholangitis. Gastroenterology 108:870, 1995.
60. Prochazka EJ, Park MS, Goldstein LI, et al: Association of primary sclerosing cholangitis with HLA-DRw52a. N Engl J Med 322:1842, 1990.
61. Bernal W, Moloney M, Underhill J, et al: Association of tumor necrosis factor polymorphism with primary sclerosing cholangitis. J Hepatol 30:237, 1999.
62. Mehal WZ, Lo YM, Wordsworth BP, et al: HLA DR4 is a marker for rapid disease progression in primary sclerosing cholangitis. Gastroenterology 106:160, 1994.
63. Angulo P, Peter JB, Gershwin ME, et al: Serum autoantibodies in patients with primary sclerosing cholangitis. J Hepatol 32:182, 2000.
64. Boberg KM, Lundin KE, Schrumpf E: Etiology and pathogenesis in primary sclerosing cholangitis. Scand J Gastroenterol Suppl 204:47, 1994.
65. Bansal AS, Thomson A, Steadman C, et al: Serum levels of interleukins 8 and 10, interferon gamma, granulocyte-macrophage colony stimulating factor and soluble CD23 in patients with primary sclerosing cholangitis. Autoimmunity 26:223, 1997.
66. Martins EB, Graham AK, Chapman RW, et al: Elevation of gamma delta T lymphocytes in peripheral blood and livers of patients with primary sclerosing cholangitis and other autoimmune liver diseases. Hepatology 23:988, 1996.
67. Groux H, O'Garra A, Bigler M, et al: A CD4+ T-cell subset inhibits antigen-specific T-cell responses and prevents colitis. Nature 389:737, 1997.
68. Terblanche J, Allison HF, Northover JM: An ischemic basis for biliary strictures. Surgery 94:52, 1983.
69. Sebagh M, Farges O, Kalil A, et al: Sclerosing cholangitis following human orthotopic liver transplantation. Am J Surg Pathol 19:81, 1995.
70. Bansi D, Chapman R, Fleming K: Antineutrophil cytoplasmic antibodies in chronic liver diseases: Prevalence, titre, specificity and IgG subclass. J Hepatol 24:581, 1996.
71. Gur H, Shen G, Sutjita M, et al: Autoantibody profile of primary sclerosing cholangitis. Pathobiology 63:76, 1995.
72. MacCarty RL, LaRusso NF, May GR, et al: Cholangiocarcinoma complicating primary sclerosing cholangitis: Cholangiographic appearances. Radiology 156:43, 1985.
73. Kaw M, Silverman WB, Rabinovitz M, et al: Biliary tract calculi in primary sclerosing cholangitis. Am J Gastroenterol 90:72, 1995.
74. Lefkowitch J: Primary sclerosing cholangitis. Arch Intern Med 142: 1157, 1982.
75. Ludwig J: Surgical pathology of the syndrome of primary sclerosing cholangitis. Am J Surg Pathol 13:43, 1989.
76. Harrison RF, Hubscher SG: The spectrum of bile duct lesions in end-stage primary sclerosing cholangitis. Histopathology 19:321, 1991.
77. Ludwig J, Barham SS, LaRusso NF, et al: Morphologic features of chronic hepatitis associated with primary sclerosing cholangitis and chronic ulcerative colitis. Hepatology 1:632, 1981.
78. Ludwig J, Czaja AJ, Dickson ER, et al: Manifestations of nonsuppurative cholangitis in chronic hepatobiliary diseases: Morphologic spectrum, clinical correlations and terminology. Liver 4:105, 1984.
79. Barbatis C, Grases P, Shepherd HA, et al: Histological features of sclerosing cholangitis in patients with chronic ulcerative colitis. J Clin Pathol 38:778, 1985.
80. Terasaki S, Nakanuma Y, Unoura M, et al: Involvement of peribiliary glands in primary sclerosing cholangitis: A histopathologic study. Intern Med 36:766, 1997.
81. Gross JB, Jr., Ludwig J, Wiesner RH, et al: Abnormalities in tests of copper metabolism in primary sclerosing cholangitis. Gastroenterology 89:272, 1985.
82. Kawai H, Aoyagi Y, Nomoto M, et al: Asymptomatic primary sclerosing cholangitis with marked hepatic fibrosis. Dig Dis Sci 45:680, 2000.
83. Angulo P, Larson DR, Therneau TM, et al: Time course of histological progression in primary sclerosing cholangitis. Am J Gastroenterol 94:3310, 1999.
84. Boberg KM, Schrumpf E, Fausa O, et al: Hepatobiliary disease in ulcerative colitis. An analysis of 18 patients with hepatobiliary lesions classified as small-duct primary sclerosing cholangitis. Scand J Gastroenterol 29:744, 1994.

85. van de Meeberg PC, Portincasa P, Wolfhagen FH, et al: Increased gall bladder volume in primary sclerosing cholangitis. Gut 39:594, 1996.
86. Johnson KJ, Olliff JF, Olliff SP: The presence and significance of lymphadenopathy detected by CT in primary sclerosing cholangitis. Br J Radiol 71:1279, 1998.
87. Dodd GD 3rd, Baron RL, Oliver JH 3rd, et al: End-stage primary sclerosing cholangitis: CT findings of hepatic morphology in 36 patients. Radiology 211:357, 1999.
88. Fulcher AS, Turner MA, Franklin KJ, et al: Primary sclerosing cholangitis: Evaluation with MR cholangiography—a case-control study. Radiology 215:71, 2000.
89. Keiding S, Hansen SB, Rasmussen HH, et al: Detection of cholangiocarcinoma in primary sclerosing cholangitis by positron emission tomography. Hepatology 28:700, 1998.
90. Beuers U, Spengler U, Sackmann M, et al: Deterioration of cholestasis after endoscopic retrograde cholangiography in advanced primary sclerosing cholangitis. J Hepatol 15:140, 1992.
91. Chapman RW, Arborgh BA, Rhodes JM, et al: Primary sclerosing cholangitis: A review of its clinical features, cholangiography, and hepatic histology. Gut 21:870, 1980.
92. Helzberg JH, Petersen JM, Boyer JL: Improved survival with primary sclerosing cholangitis. A review of clinicopathologic features and comparison of symptomatic and asymptomatic patients. Gastroenterology 92:1869, 1987.
93. Stockbrugger RW, Olsson R, Jaup B, et al: Forty-six patients with primary sclerosing cholangitis: Radiological bile duct changes in relationship to clinical course and concomitant inflammatory bowel disease. Hepatogastroenterology 35:289, 1988.
94. Cameron JL, Gayler BW, Sanfey H, et al: Sclerosing cholangitis. Anatomical distribution of obstructive lesions. Ann Surg 200:54, 1984.
95. Brandt DJ, MacCarty RL, Charboneau JW, et al: Gallbladder disease in patients with primary sclerosing cholangitis. AJR 150:571, 1988.
96. Heikius B, Niemela S, Lehtola J, et al: Hepatobiliary and coexisting pancreatic duct abnormalities in patients with inflammatory bowel disease. Scand J Gastroenterol 32:153, 1997.
97. Schimanski U, Stiehl A, Stremmel W, et al: Low prevalence of alterations in the pancreatic duct system in patients with primary sclerosing cholangitis. Endoscopy 28:346, 1996.
98. MacCarty RL, LaRusso NF, Wiesner RH, et al: Primary sclerosing cholangitis: Findings on cholangiography and pancreatography. Radiology 149:39, 1983.
99. Borkje B, Vetvik K, Odegaard S, et al: Chronic pancreatitis in patients with sclerosing cholangitis and ulcerative colitis. Scand J Gastroenterol 20:539, 1985.
100. Epstein O, Chapman RW, Lake-Bakaar G, et al: The pancreas in primary biliary cirrhosis and primary sclerosing cholangitis. Gastroenterology 83:1177, 1982.
101. Palmer KR, Cotton PB, Chapman M: Pancreatogram in cholestasis. Gut 25:424, 1984.
102. Grijm R, Huibregtse K, Bartelsman J, et al: Therapeutic investigations in primary sclerosing cholangitis. Dig Dis Sci 31:792, 1986.
103. Aadland E, Schrumpf E, Fausa O, et al: Primary sclerosing cholangitis: A long-term follow-up study. Scand J Gastroenterol 22:655, 1987.
104. Shepherd HSW, Chapman R, Nolan D, et al: Ulcerative colitis and persistent liver dysfunction. Q J Med 52:503, 1983.
105. Cooper JF, Brand EJ: Symptomatic sclerosing cholangitis in patients with a normal alkaline phosphatase: Two case reports and a review of the literature. Am J Gastroenterol 83:308, 1988.
106. Balasubramaniam K, Wiesner RH, LaRusso NF: Primary sclerosing cholangitis with normal serum alkaline phosphatase activity. Gastroenterology 95:1395, 1988.
107. Leidenius MH, Risteli LT, Risteli JP, et al: Serum aminoterminal propeptide of type III procollagen (S-PIIINP) and hepatobiliary dysfunction in patients with ulcerative colitis. Scand J Clin Lab Invest 57:297, 1997.
108. Aaseth J, Thomassen Y, Aadland E, et al: Hepatic retention of copper and selenium in primary sclerosing cholangitis. Scand J Gastroenterol 30:1200, 1995.
109. Jorgensen RA, Lindor KD, Sartin JS, et al: Serum lipid and fat-soluble vitamin levels in primary sclerosing cholangitis. J Clin Gastroenterol 20:215, 1995.
110. Hay JE, Lindor KD, Wiesner RH, et al: The metabolic bone disease of primary sclerosing cholangitis. Hepatology 14:257, 1991.
111. Angulo P, Therneau TM, Jorgensen A, et al: Bone disease in patients with primary sclerosing cholangitis: Prevalence, severity and prediction of progression. J Hepatol 29:729, 1998.
112. Ben-Ari Z, Panagou M, Patch D, et al: Hypercoagulability in patients with primary biliary cirrhosis and primary sclerosing cholangitis evaluated by thrombelastography. J Hepatol 26:554, 1997.
113. Kartheuser AH, Dozois RR, LaRusso NF, et al: Comparison of surgical treatment of ulcerative colitis associated with primary sclerosing cholangitis: Ileal pouch–anal anastomosis versus Brooke ileostomy. Mayo Clin Proc 71:748, 1996.
114. Kartheuser AH, Dozois RR, Wiesner RH, et al: Complications and risk factors after ileal pouch–anal anastomosis for ulcerative colitis associated with primary sclerosing cholangitis. Ann Surg 217:314, 1993.
115. Post AB, Bozdech JM, Lavery I, et al: Colectomy in patients with inflammatory bowel disease and primary sclerosing cholangitis. Dis Colon Rectum 37:175, 1994.
116. Pokorny CS, McCaughan GW, Gallagher ND, et al: Sclerosing cholangitis and biliary tract calculi—primary or secondary? Gut 33:1376, 1992.
117. Broome U, Lofberg R, Veress B, et al: Primary sclerosing cholangitis and ulcerative colitis: Evidence for increased neoplastic potential. Hepatology 22:1404, 1995.
118. Hultcrantz R, Olsson R, Danielsson A, et al: A 3-year prospective study on serum tumor markers used for detecting cholangiocarcinoma in patients with primary sclerosing cholangitis. J Hepatol 30:669, 1999.
119. Abu-Elmagd KM, Selby R, Iwatsuki S, et al: Cholangiocarcinoma and sclerosing cholangitis: Clinical characteristics and effect on survival after liver transplantation. Transplant Proc 25:1124, 1993.
120. Bergquist A, Glaumann H, Persson B, et al: Risk factors and clinical presentation of hepatobiliary carcinoma in patients with primary sclerosing cholangitis: A case-control study. Hepatology 27:311, 1998.
121. Chalasani N, Baluyut A, Ismail A, et al: Cholangiocarcinoma in patients with primary sclerosing cholangitis: A multicenter case-control study. Hepatology 31:7, 2000.
122. Van Laethem JL, Deviere J, Bourgeois N, et al: Cholangiographic findings in deteriorating primary sclerosing cholangitis. Endoscopy 27:223, 1995.
123. Ramage JK, Donaghy A, Farrant JM, et al: Serum tumor markers for the diagnosis of cholangiocarcinoma in primary sclerosing cholangitis. Gastroenterology 108:865, 1995.
124. Pugliese V, Conio M, Nicolo G, et al: Endoscopic retrograde forceps biopsy and brush cytology of biliary strictures: A prospective study. Gastrointest Endosc 42:520, 1995.
125. Mansfield JC, Griffin SM, Wadehra V, et al: A prospective evaluation of cytology from biliary strictures. Gut 40:671, 1997.
126. Ponsioen CY, Vrouenraets SM, van Milligen de Wit AW, et al: Value of brush cytology for dominant strictures in primary sclerosing cholangitis. Endoscopy 31:305, 1999.
127. Ahrendt SA, Eisenberger CF, Yip L, et al: Chromosome 9p21 loss and p16 inactivation in primary sclerosing cholangitis-associated cholangiocarcinoma. J Surg Res 84:88, 1999.
128. Boberg KM, Schrumpf E, Bergquist A, et al: Cholangiocarcinoma in primary sclerosing cholangitis: K-*ras* mutations and Tp53 dysfunction are implicated in the neoplastic development. J Hepatol 32:374, 2000.
129. Rizzi PM, Ryder SD, Portmann B, et al: p53 Protein overexpression in cholangiocarcinoma arising in primary sclerosing cholangitis. Gut 38:265, 1996.
130. Abu-Elmagd KM, Malinchoc M, Dickson ER, et al: Efficacy of hepatic transplantation in patients with primary sclerosing cholangitis. Surg Gynecol Obstet 177:335, 1993.
131. De Vreede I, Steers JL, Burch PA, et al: Prolonged disease-free survival after orthotopic liver transplantation plus adjuvant chemoirradiation for cholangiocarcinoma. Liver Transpl 6:309, 2000.
132. Snook JA, Kelly P, Chapman RW, et al: Fibrolamellar hepatocellular carcinoma complicating ulcerative colitis with primary sclerosing cholangitis. Gut 30:243, 1989.
133. Harnois DM, Gores GJ, Ludwig J, et al: Are patients with cirrhotic stage primary sclerosing cholangitis at risk for the development of hepatocellular cancer? J Hepatol 27:512, 1997.
134. Shetty K, Rybicki L, Brzezinski A, et al: The risk for cancer or dysplasia in ulcerative colitis patients with primary sclerosing cholangitis. Am J Gastroenterol 94:1643, 1999.
135. Brentnall TA, Haggitt RC, Rabinovitch PS, et al: Risk and natural history of colonic neoplasia in patients with primary sclerosing cholangitis and ulcerative colitis. Gastroenterology 110:331, 1996.
136. D'Haens GR, Lashner BA, Hanauer SB: Pericholangitis and sclerosing cholangitis are risk factors for dysplasia and cancer in ulcerative colitis. Am J Gastroenterol 88:1174, 1993.
137. Kornfeld D, Ekbom A, Ihre T: Is there an excess risk for colorectal

cancer in patients with ulcerative colitis and concomitant primary sclerosing cholangitis? A population based study. Gut 41:522, 1997.
138. Marchesa P, Lashner BA, Lavery IC, et al: The risk of cancer and dysplasia among ulcerative colitis patients with primary sclerosing cholangitis. Am J Gastroenterol 92:1285, 1997.
139. Leidenius MH, Farkkila MA, Karkkainen P, et al: Colorectal dysplasia and carcinoma in patients with ulcerative colitis and primary sclerosing cholangitis. Scand J Gastroenterol 32:706, 1997.
140. Loftus EV Jr, Sandborn WJ, Tremaine WJ, et al: Risk of colorectal neoplasia in patients with primary sclerosing cholangitis. Gastroenterology 110:432, 1996.
141. Nuako KW, Ahlquist DA, Sandborn WJ, et al: Primary sclerosing cholangitis and colorectal carcinoma in patients with chronic ulcerative colitis: A case-control study. Cancer 82:822, 1998.
142. Knechtle SJ, D'Alessandro AM, Harms BA, et al: Relationships between sclerosing cholangitis, inflammatory bowel disease, and cancer in patients undergoing liver transplantation. Surgery 118:615, discussion 619; 1995.
143. Bleday R, Lee E, Jessurun J, et al: Increased risk of early colorectal neoplasms after hepatic transplant in patients with inflammatory bowel disease. Dis Colon Rectum 36:908, 1993.
144. Shaked A, Colonna JO, Goldstein L, et al: The interrelation between sclerosing cholangitis and ulcerative colitis in patients undergoing liver transplantation. Ann Surg 215:598, discussion 604; 1992.
145. Loftus EV Jr, Aguilar HI, Sandborn WJ, et al: Risk of colorectal neoplasia in patients with primary sclerosing cholangitis and ulcerative colitis following orthotopic liver transplantation. Hepatology 27:685, 1998.
146. Tung B, Emond, M., Haggitt, R., et al: Protective effect of ursodiol on neoplastic progression in ulcerative colitis patients with primary sclerosing cholangitis. Gastroenterolgy 118:A706, 2000.
147. Kock NG, Darle N, Hulten L, et al: Ileostomy. Curr Probl Surg 14:1, 1977.
148. Pemberton JH, Kelly KA, Beart RW Jr, et al: Ileal pouch–anal anastomosis for chronic ulcerative colitis. Long-term results. Ann Surg 206:504, 1987.
149. Aitola P, Matikainen M, Mattila J: Hepatobiliary changes in patients with ulcerative colitis, with special reference to the effect of proctocolectomy. Scand J Gastroenterol 33:113, 1998.
150. Penna C, Dozois R, Tremaine W, et al: Pouchitis after ileal pouch-anal anastomosis for ulcerative colitis occurs with increased frequency in patients with associated primary sclerosing cholangitis. Gut 38:234, 1996.
151. Zins BJ, Sandborn WJ, Penna CR, et al: Pouchitis disease course after orthotopic liver transplantation in patients with primary sclerosing cholangitis and an ileal pouch–anal anastomosis. Am J Gastroenterol 90:2177, 1995.
152. Rowley S, Candinas D, Mayer AD, et al: Restorative proctocolectomy and pouch anal anastomosis for ulcerative colitis following orthotopic liver transplantation. Gut 37:845, 1995.
153. Lofberg R, Liljeqvist L, Lindquist K, et al: Dysplasia and DNA aneuploidy in a pelvic pouch. Report of a case. Dis Colon Rectum 34: 280, discussion 283; 1991.
154. Gullberg K, Stahlberg D, Liljeqvist L, et al: Neoplastic transformation of the pelvic pouch mucosa in patients with ulcerative colitis. Gastroenterology 112:1487, 1997.
155. Stahlberg D, Lofberg R: Underlying cholangiocarcinoma in a patient with high-grade dysplasia in the pelvic pouch [letter]. Inflamm Bowel Dis 5:150, 1999.
156. Burgert SL, Kirkpatrick RB, LaBrecque DR: Positive corticosteroid respone in early primary sclerosing cholangitis. Gastroenterology 86: A1037, 1984.
157. Lindor KD, Wiesner RH, Colwell LJ, et al: The combination of prednisone and colchicine in patients with primary sclerosing cholangitis. Am J Gastroenterol 86:57, 1991.
158. van Hoogstraten HJ, Vleggaar FP, Boland GJ, et al: Budesonide or prednisone in combination with ursodeoxycholic acid in primary sclerosing cholangitis: A randomized double-blind pilot study. Belgian-Dutch PSC Study Group. Am J Gastroenterol 95:2015, 2000.
159. Angulo P, Batts KP, Jorgensen RA, et al: Oral budesonide in the treatment of primary sclerosing cholangitis. Am J Gastroenterol 95: 2333, 2000.
160. Wiesner RH, STeiner B, LaRusson FN, et al: A controlled clinical trial evaluating cyclosporine in the treatment of primary sclerosing cholangitis. Hepatology 14:63A, 1991.
161. Mitchell SA, Chapman RW: Review article: The management of primary sclerosing cholangitis. Aliment Pharmacol Ther 11:33, 1997.
162. Knox TA, Kaplan MM: A double-blind controlled trial of oral-pulse methotrexate therapy in the treatment of primary sclerosing cholangitis. Gastroenterology 106:494, 1994.
163. Lindor KD, Jorgensen RA, Anderson ML, et al: Ursodeoxycholic acid and methotrexate for primary sclerosing cholangitis: A pilot study. Am J Gastroenterol 91:511, 1996.
164. Schramm C, Schirmacher P, Helmreich-Becker I, et al: Combined therapy with azathioprine, prednisolone, and ursodiol in patients with primary sclerosing cholangitis. A case series. Ann Intern Med 131: 943, 1999.
165. Van Thiel DH, Carroll P, Abu-Elmagd K, et al: Tacrolimus (FK 506), a treatment for primary sclerosing cholangitis: Results of an open-label preliminary trial. Am J Gastroenterol 90:455, 1995.
166. LaRusso NF, Wiesner RH, Ludwig J, et al: Prospective trial of penicillamine in primary sclerosing cholangitis. Gastroenterology 95:1036, 1988.
167. Cox KL, Cox KM: Oral vancomycin: Treatment of primary sclerosing cholangitis in children with inflammatory bowel disease. J Pediatr Gastroenterol Nutr 27:580, 1998.
168. Angulo P, Bharucha AE, Jorgensen RA, et al: Oral nicotine in treatment of primary sclerosing cholangitis: A pilot study. Dig Dis Sci 44: 602, 1999.
169. Jorgensen G, Waldum HL: Lack of effect of transdermal nicotine on 3 cases of primary sclerosing cholangitis [letter]. Dig Dis Sci 44:2484, 1999.
170. Bharucha AE, Jorgensen R, Lichtman SN, et al: A pilot study of pentoxifylline for the treatment of primary sclerosing cholangitis. Am J Gastroenterol 95:2338, 2000.
171. Stiehl A, Benz C, Sauer P: Mechanism of hepatoprotective action of bile salts in liver disease. Gastroenterol Clin North Am 28:195, 1999.
172. Mitsuyoshi H, Nakashima T, Sumida Y, et al: Ursodeoxycholic acid protects hepatocytes against oxidative injury via induction of antioxidants. Biochem Biophys Res Commun 263:537, 1999.
173. van Hoogstraten HJ, Wolfhagen FH, van de Meeberg PC, et al: Ursodeoxycholic acid therapy for primary sclerosing cholangitis: Results of a 2-year randomized controlled trial to evaluate single versus multiple daily doses. J Hepatol 29:417, 1998.
174. Lindor KD: Ursodiol for primary sclerosing cholangitis. Mayo Primary Sclerosing Cholangitis–Ursodeoxycholic Acid Study Group. N Engl J Med 336:691, 1997.
175. De Maria N, Colantoni A, Rosenbloom E, et al: Ursodeoxycholic acid does not improve the clinical course of primary sclerosing cholangitis over a 2-year period. Hepatogastroenterology 43:1472, 1996.
176. Stiehl A, Rudolph G, Sauer P, et al: Efficacy of ursodeoxycholic acid treatment and endoscopic dilation of major duct stenoses in primary sclerosing cholangitis. An 8-year prospective study. J Hepatol 26:560, 1997.
177. Kaplan MM: Medical approaches to primary sclerosing cholangitis. Semin Liver Dis 11:56, 1991.
178. Yerushalmi B, Sokol RJ, Narkewicz MR, et al: Use of rifampin for severe pruritus in children with chronic cholestasis. J Pediatr Gastroenterol Nutr 29:442, 1991.
179. Gumaste V: Antibiotics and cholangitis. Gastroenterology 109:323, 1995.
180. May G, LaRusso NF, Wiesner RH: Nonoperative dilatation of dominant strictures in primary sclerosing cholangitis. AJR 145:1061, 1985.
181. Cotton PB, Nickl N: Endoscopic and radiologic approaches to therapy in primary sclerosing cholangitis. Semin Liver Dis 11:40, 1991.
182. Siegel JH, Guelrud M: Endoscopic cholangiopancreatoplasty: Hydrostatic balloon dilation in the bile duct and pancreas. Gastrointest Endosc 29:99, 1983.
183. Johnson GK, Geenen JE, Venu RP, et al: Endoscopic treatment of biliary duct strictures in sclerosing cholangitis: Follow-up assessment of a new therapeutic approach. Gastrointest Endosc 33:9, 1987.
184. Johnson GK, Geenen JE, Venu RP, et al: Endoscopic treatment of biliary tract strictures in sclerosing cholangitis: Larger series and recommendations for treatment. Gastrointest Endosc 37:38, 1991.
185. Lombard M, Farrant M, Karani J, et al: Improving biliary-enteric drainage in primary sclerosing cholangitis: Experience with endoscopic methods. Gut 32:1364, 1991.
186. Lee JG, Schutz SM, England RE, et al: Endoscopic therapy of sclerosing cholangitis. Hepatology 21:661, 1995.
187. van Milligen de Wit AW, van Bracht J, Rauws EA, et al: Endoscopic stent therapy for dominant extrahepatic bile duct strictures in primary sclerosing cholangitis. Gastrointest Endosc 44:293, 1996.
188. van Milligen de Wit AW, Rauws EA, van Bracht J, et al: Lack of complications following short-term stent therapy for extrahepatic bile

duct strictures in primary sclerosing cholangitis. Gastrointest Endosc 46:344, 1997.
189. Ponsioen CY, Lam K, van Milligen de Wit AW, et al: Four years experience with short term stenting in primary sclerosing cholangitis. Am J Gastroenterol 94:2403, 1999.
190. Mahadevan U, Bass N, Ostroff J: Endoscopic management of primary sclerosing cholangitis. Am J Gastroenterol 95:A237, 2000.
191. Martin FM, Rossi RL, Nugent FW, et al: Surgical aspects of sclerosing cholangitis. Results in 178 patients. Ann Surg 212:551, discussion 556; 1990.
192. Myburgh JA: Surgical biliary drainage in primary sclerosing cholangitis. The role of the Hepp-Couinaud approach. Arch Surg 129:1057, 1994.
193. Ahrendt SA, Pitt HA, Kalloo AN, et al: Primary sclerosing cholangitis: Resect, dilate, or transplant? Ann Surg 227:412, 1998.
194. Graziadei IW, Wiesner RH, Marotta PJ, et al: Long-term results of patients undergoing liver transplantation for primary sclerosing cholangitis. Hepatology 30:1121, 1999.
195. Kim WR, Wiesner RH, Poterucha JJ, et al: Hepatic retransplantation in cholestatic liver disease: Impact of the interval to retransplantation on survival and resource utilization. Hepatology 30:395, 1999.
196. Patel R, Badley AD, Larson-Keller J, et al: Relevance and risk factors of enterococcal bacteremia following liver transplantation. Transplantation 61:1192, 1996.
197. Nashan B, Schlitt HJ, Tusch G, et al: Biliary malignancies in primary sclerosing cholangitis: Timing for liver transplantation. Hepatology 23: 1105, 1996.
198. Jeyarajah DR, Netto GJ, Lee SP, et al: Recurrent primary sclerosing cholangitis after orthotopic liver transplantation: Is chronic rejection part of the disease process? Transplantation 66:1300, 1998.
199. Graziadei IW, Wiesner RH, Batts KP, et al: Recurrence of primary sclerosing cholangitis following liver transplantation. Hepatology 29: 1050, 1999.
200. Saldeen K, Friman S, Olausson M, et al: Follow-up after liver transplantation for primary sclerosing cholangitis: Effects on survival, quality of life, and colitis. Scand J Gastroenterol 34:535, 1999.
201. Gross CR, Malinchoc M, Kim WR, et al: Quality of life before and after liver transplantation for cholestatic liver disease. Hepatology 29: 356, 1999.
202. Digby K: Common duct stones of liver origin. Br J Surg 17:578, 1930.
203. Nakayama F, Soloway RD, Nakama T, et al: Hepatolithiasis in East Asia. Retrospective study. Dig Dis Sci 31:21, 1986.
204. Kim MH, Sekijima J, Lee SP: Primary intrahepatic stones. Am J Gastroenterol 90:540, 1995.
205. Wilson M, Stephen, MS, Mathur, M, et al: Recurrent pyogenic cholangitis or "oriental cholangiohepatitis" in occidentals: Case reports of four patients. Aust N Z J Surg 66:649, 1996.
206. Nagase M, Hikasa Y, Soloway RD, et al: Gallstones in Western Japan. Factors affecting the prevalence of intrahepatic gallstones. Gastroenterology 78:684, 1980.
207. Lim JH: Oriental cholangiohepatitis: Pathologic, clinical, and radiologic features. AJR 157:1, 1991.
208. Chou S: Recurrent pyogenic cholangitis: A necropsy study. Pathology 21:415, 1980.
209. Cosenza CA, Durazo F, Stain SC, et al: Current management of recurrent pyogenic cholangitis. Am Surg 65:939, 1999.
210. Carmona RH, Crass RA, Lim RC, Jr., et al: Oriental cholangitis. Am J Surg 148:117, 1984.
211. Seel DJ, Park YK: Oriental infestational cholangitis. Am J Surg 146: 366, 1983.
212. Reynolds WR, Brinkman JD, Haney BD, et al: Oriental cholangiohepatitis. Mil Med 159:158, 1994.
213. Yellin AE, Donovan AJ: Biliary lithiasis and helminthiasis. Am J Surg 142:128, 1981.
214. Lim JH: Radiologic findings of clonorchiasis. AJR 155:1001, 1990.
215. Khuroo MS, Zargar SA: Biliary ascariasis. A common cause of biliary and pancreatic disease in an endemic area. Gastroenterology 88:418, 1985.
216. Nakayama F, Koga A: Hepatolithiasis: Present status. World J Surg 8: 9, 1984.
217. Khan TF, Norazmi MN: Recurrent pyogenic cholangitis: Is immune depression a feature? [letter]. Trop Doct 28:187, 1998.
218. Sperling RM, Koch J, Sandhu JS, et al: Recurrent pyogenic cholangitis in Asian immigrants to the United States: Natural history and role of therapeutic ERCP. Dig Dis Sci 42:865, 1997.
219. Harris HW, Kumwenda ZL, Sheen-Chen SM, et al: Recurrent pyogenic cholangitis. Am J Surg 176:34, 1998.
220. Choi TK, Wong J: Endoscopic retrograde cholangiopancreatography and endoscopic papillotomy in recurrent pyogenic cholangitis. Clin Gastroenterol 15:393, 1986.
221. Lam SK, Wong KP, Chan PK, et al: Recurrent pyogenic cholangitis: A study by endoscopic retrograde cholangiography. Gastroenterology 74:1196, 1978.
222. Jan YY, Chen MF, Wang CS, et al: Surgical treatment of hepatolithiasis: Long-term results. Surgery 120:509, 1996.
223. Cheng YF, Lee TY, Sheen-Chen SM, et al: Treatment of complicated hepatolithiasis with intrahepatic biliary stricture by ductal dilatation and stenting: Long-term results. World J Surg 24:712, 2000.
224. Kubo S, Kinoshita H, Hirohashi K, et al: Hepatolithiasis associated with cholangiocarcinoma. World J Surg 19:637, 1995.
225. Lim JH, Ko YT, Lee DH, et al: Oriental cholangiohepatitis: Sonographic findings in 48 cases. AJR 155:511, 1990.
226. Chan FL, Man SW, Leong LL, et al: Evaluation of recurrent pyogenic cholangitis with CT: Analysis of 50 patients. Radiology 170:165, 1989.
227. Kim MJ, Cha SW, Mitchell DG, et al: MR imaging findings in recurrent pyogenic cholangitis. AJR 173:1545, 1999.
228. Khuroo MS, Dar MY, Yattoo GN, et al: Serial cholangiographic appearances in recurrent pyogenic cholangitis. Gastrointest Endosc 39: 674, 1993.
229. Fan ST, Choi TK, Wong J: Recurrent pyogenic cholangitis: Current management. World J Surg 15:248, 1991.
230. Tanaka M, Ikeda S, Ogawa Y, et al: Divergent effects of endoscopic sphincterotomy on the long-term outcome of hepatolithiasis. Gastrointest Endosc 43:33, 1996.
231. Stain SC, Incarbone R, Guthrie CR, et al: Surgical treatment of recurrent pyogenic cholangitis. Arch Surg 130:527, discussion 532; 1995.
232. Sun WB, Han BL, Cai JX: The surgical treatment of isolated left-sided hepatolithiasis: A 22-year experience. Surgery 127:493, 2000.
233. Gott PE, Tieva MH, Barcia PJ, et al: Biliary access procedure in the management of oriental cholangiohepatitis. Am Surg 62:930, 1996.
234. Leow CK, Lau WY: Re: Biliary access procedure in the management of oriental cholangiohepatitis [letter; comment]. Am Surg 64:99, 1998.
235. Otani K, Shimizu S, Chijiiwa K, et al: Comparison of treatments for hepatolithiasis: Hepatic resection versus cholangioscopic lithotomy. J Am Coll Surg 189:177, 1999.
236. Jeng KS, Sheen IS, Yang FS: Are expandable metallic stents better than conventional methods for treating difficult intrahepatic biliary strictures with recurrent hepatolithiasis? Arch Surg 134:267, 1999.
237. Yoon HK, Sung KB, Song HY, et al: Benign biliary strictures associated with recurrent pyogenic cholangitis: Treatment with expandable metallic stents. AJR 169:1523, 1997.
238. Lam SK: A study of endoscopic sphincterotomy in recurrent pyogenic cholangitis. Br J Surg 71:262, 1984.

Chapter 60

TUMORS OF THE GALLBLADDER, BILE DUCTS, AND AMPULLA

Taylor A. Sohn and Keith D. Lillemoe

Neoplasms that arise in the gallbladder, bile ducts, and ampulla of Vater pose significant clinical challenges. The majority of these tumors are malignant, although benign neoplasms may be encountered. There are similarities among tumors at each of these sites, including the clinical presentation, which may include biliary obstruction. Furthermore, these tumors are often asymptomatic early in their course and frequently present at an advanced stage of disease, thereby precluding potentially curative resection. Nevertheless, the prognosis for malignant ampullary neoplasms is markedly better than that for cancers of the gallbladder and bile duct.

GALLBLADDER TUMORS

Malignant Tumors

Epidemiology and Clinical Features

Gallbladder carcinoma occurs with an incidence of 2.5 cases per 100,000 population and accounts for 6500 deaths per year in the United States. Gallbladder carcinoma is the fifth most common carcinoma of the gastrointestinal tract; it accounts for 3% to 4% of all gastrointestinal tumors and is the most common carcinoma of the biliary tree (Table 60–1).[1]

Gallbladder carcinoma occurs primarily in the elderly and is three to four times more common in women than in men. Other risk factors for gallbladder carcinoma include the presence of gallstones, a porcelain gallbladder, a long common channel where the pancreatic and common bile ducts join, and the chronic typhoid carrier state. At least 80% to 90% of patients with gallbladder carcinoma have gallstones, and approximately 20% of patients with a porcelain gallbladder are found to have a cancer at cholecystectomy. Histologically, approximately 80% of gallbladder carcinomas are adenocarcinomas. Infrequently, squamous cell carcinomas, cystadenocarcinomas, small-cell carcinomas, and adenoacanthomas are identified.

The clinical presentation of gallbladder carcinoma ranges from an incidental finding at cholecystectomy for symptomatic gallstones to a rapidly progressive disease that affords little opportunity for effective treatment. The symptoms of gallbladder carcinoma are often indistinguishable from those of benign gallbladder disease and include biliary colic and acute cholecystitis. Symptoms and signs associated with gallbladder cancer are often nonspecific and include abdominal pain, nausea, fatty food intolerance, anorexia, weight loss, fever, and chills. The most common presenting symptom is right upper quadrant pain, which is present in more than 80% of patients. As the disease advances, the pain is often continuous; and as the gallbladder carcinoma grows to obstruct the common bile duct, jaundice develops. Physical findings in advanced cases may include right upper quadrant tenderness, a palpable mass, hepatomegaly, and ascites. Laboratory studies are often unremarkable until obstructive jaundice develops, and, unfortunately, there are no reliable tumor markers for early detection of this disease.

Diagnosis

The lack of reliable diagnostic criteria and the nonspecific presentation often make preoperative diagnosis of gallbladder carcinoma difficult. For those patients who present with symptoms suggestive of benign gallbladder disease, ultrasonography is usually the initial diagnostic procedure. A thickening of the gallbladder or a polypoid mass (Fig. 60–1) should increase the suspicion of a gallbladder neoplasm; however, the ultrasonographic findings often suggest benign gallbladder disease (cholelithiasis) as the cause of the symptoms, and the carcinoma is diagnosed only at exploration or on pathologic examination of the resected gallbladder. Less subtle findings include invasion of the liver by tumor, hilar lymphadenopathy, or vascular invasion associated with advanced disease.

Computed tomography (CT) is more sensitive than ultrasound in identifying gallbladder carcinoma. CT better delineates a gallbladder mass (Fig. 60–2), with sensitivity and specificity rates of nearly 90%.[2] However, it may be difficult to distinguish a gallbladder carcinoma from a carcinoma of the extrahepatic biliary tree. CT is the diagnostic procedure

Table 60–1 | **Malignant Tumors of the Gallbladder, Bile Ducts, and Ampulla**

	CLINICAL PRESENTATION						TREATMENT		
	Incidence or Prevalence	**Pathology**	**Risk Factors**	**Major Symptoms**	**Physical Findings**	**Laboratory Data**	**Surgery**	**Palliation (Stent, Chemo, RT)**	**Prognosis (Survival)**
Malignant tumors of gallbladder	1%–2% of resected gallbladders 0.5% autopsies	Adenocarcinoma: 80%: scirrhous, papillary Other: 20% squamous, cystadenocarcinoma, adenoacanthoma	Chronic cholecystitis Age > 50 yr Female sex Gallstones Porcelain gallbladder	Abdominal pain Jaundice Pruritus Weight loss	Discovered at cholecystectomy Mass (RUQ) Jaundice Hepatomegaly	*Usual:* Mildly elevated ALT, alkaline phosphatase, bilirubin *Occasional:* Markedly elevated alkaline phosphatase and bilirubin	Curative (10%) for incidental CA found at cholecystectomy Clinically evident tumors typically not resectable	Jaundice/cholangitis: ERCP or transhepatic stenting Usually poor response to chemotherapy and/or radiation therapy	5% 5-year survival Curative surgery for "incidental" gallbladder CA found at routine cholecystectomy
Malignant tumors of extrahepatic bile ducts	Incidence of 1 per 100,000 per year in US	Adenocarcinoma: 90%: scirrhous, nodular, papillary Squamous cell: 10% Rare: cystadeno CA, sarcoma, metastases (usually nodal), lymphoma	Primary sclerosing cholangitis Parasites: *Clonorchis, Ascaris* Congenital diseases: choledochal cysts, Caroli's disease	Jaundice Pruritus Abdominal pain Weight loss Cholangitis	Jaundice Hepatomegaly Palpable mass (tumor or gallbladder)	*Usual:* Markedly elevated alkaline phosphatase Variable increase in bilirubin Rarely elevated ALT	Curative (10%) for small (<2 cm) distal lesions	Jaundice/cholangitis: ERCP or transhepatic stenting Variable response to RT: wire (iridium) or external beam RT Poor response to chemotherapy	5% 5-yr survival Curative surgery for small, distal bile duct tumors
Malignant tumors of ampulla	Incidence of 2.9 per million	Adenocarcinoma (virtually all)	Adenoma of the papilla/ampulla Genetic diseases: familial polyposis, Gardner's syndrome	Jaundice/pruritus (variable) Acholic or "silver" stool Melena Cholangitis/pancreatitis, pain	Jaundice Pallor Abdominal tenderness Palpable gallbladder Occult blood	*Usual:* Elevated alkaline phosphatase, bilirubin *Occasional:* Elevated aminotransferases and iron deficiency anemia	Curative: (pancreaticoduodenectomy): 25%–40% Resectable: overall 75%	Jaundice/cholangitis: sphincterotomy/ERCP stenting, transhepatic stenting Poor response to RT and/or chemotherapy	25%–40% 5-yr survival Excellent survival for small (<2 cm) adenocarcinoma

ALT, alanine aminotransferase; CA, cancer; ERCP, endoscopic retrograde cholangiopancreatography; RT, radiation therapy; RUQ, right upper quadrant.

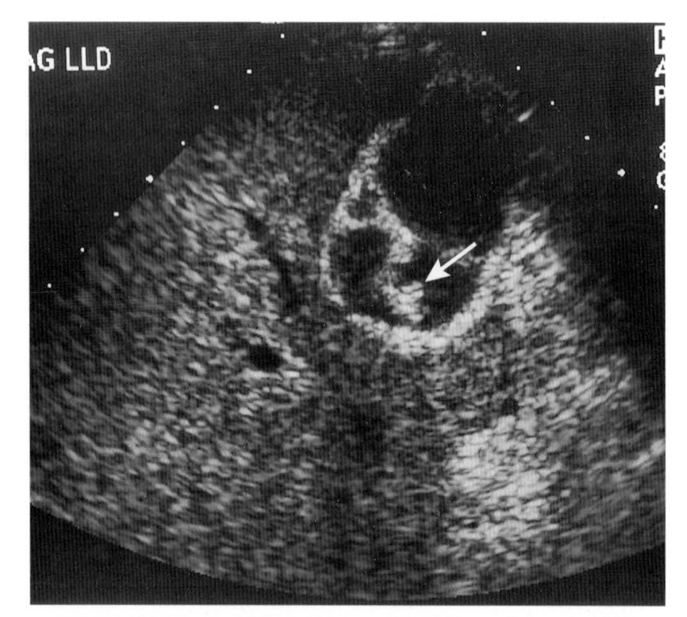

Figure 60–1. Ultrasound image of a gallbladder carcinoma showing a polypoid mass *(arrow)* and a thickened gallbladder wall.

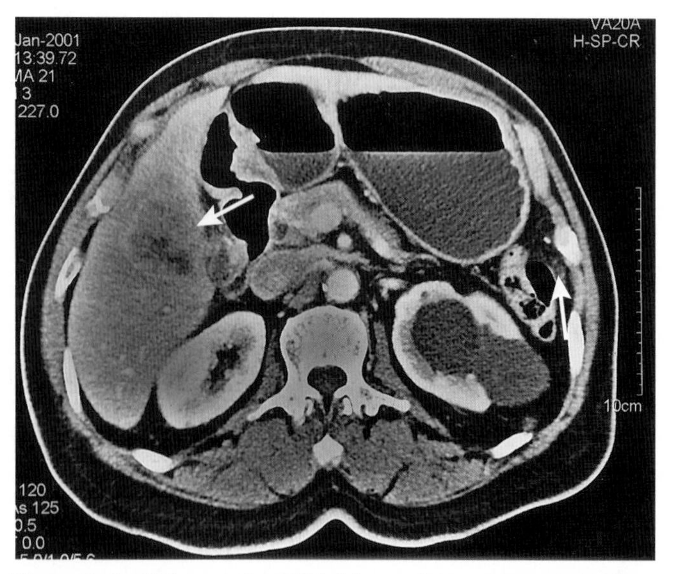

Figure 60–2. CT image of a gallbladder carcinoma demonstrating invasion of the liver *(arrow)*.

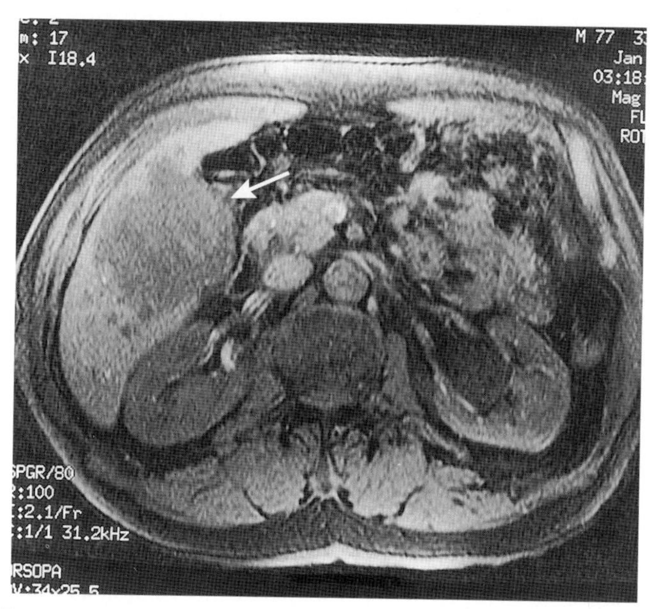

Figure 60–3. MRI of a gallbladder carcinoma with invasion of liver parenchyma *(arrow)*.

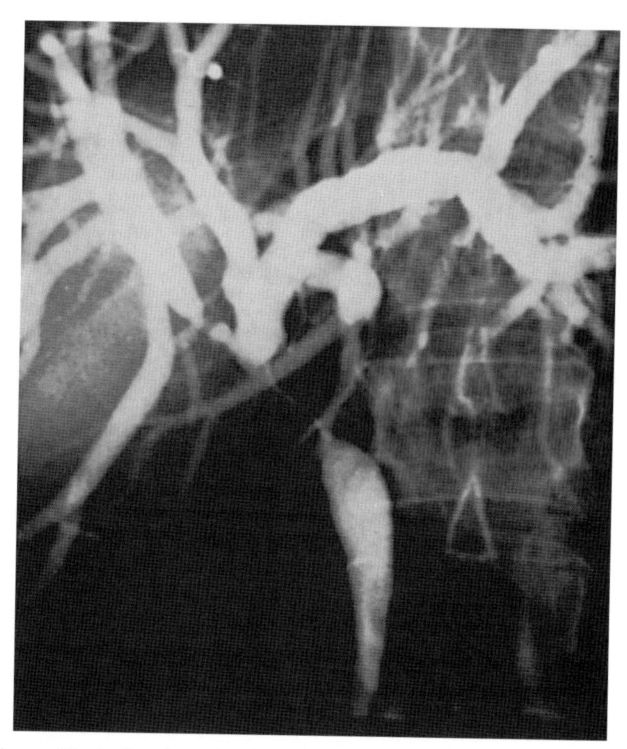

Figure 60–4. Transhepatic cholangiogram demonstrating a long stricture of the common hepatic duct caused by carcinoma of the gallbladder. (Courtesy of E. Ring, M.D., University of California, San Francisco.)

of choice in patients who present with obstructive jaundice. CT is critical for determining resectability, the extent of local disease, and the presence of lymphadenopathy, hepatic metastases, and invasion of the portal vein and hepatic artery by tumor. Recently, magnetic resonance imaging (MRI), specifically magnetic resonance cholangiopancreatography (MRCP), has permitted complete noninvasive assessment of the hepatic parenchyma, biliary tree, vasculature and lymph nodes (Fig. 60–3). Endoscopic ultrasound also has been useful, especially for demonstrating the extent of tumor invasion and lymph node metastases.

In patients who present with obstructive jaundice, either endoscopic retrograde cholangiopancreatography (ERCP) or percutaneous transhepatic cholangiography (PTC) can identify the level and extent of biliary obstruction. The typical finding in a patient with gallbladder carcinoma is a long stricture involving the common hepatic duct (Fig. 60–4). In contrast, cholangiocarcinomas tend to occur in the most distal portion of the bile duct or at the bifurcation (Klatskin tumors, Fig. 60–5). Both endoscopic and transhepatic catheters can be placed through the obstruction, but percutaneous catheters are more effective for relieving jaundice secondary to gallbladder cancer and may facilitate operative management. Noninvasive imaging of the biliary tree with MRCP may provide images similar in quality to those provided by ERCP or PTC, but does not offer the opportunity for therapeutic drainage.

Management

The management of gallbladder carcinoma depends largely on the presenting symptoms and the stage at the time of presentation (Fig. 60–6). The tumor is typically detected in one of three ways: 1) as an incidental finding during or after cholecystectomy for suspected benign disease, 2) as a suspected or confirmed lesion that appears to be resectable after preoperative evaluation, or 3) as an advanced, unresectable

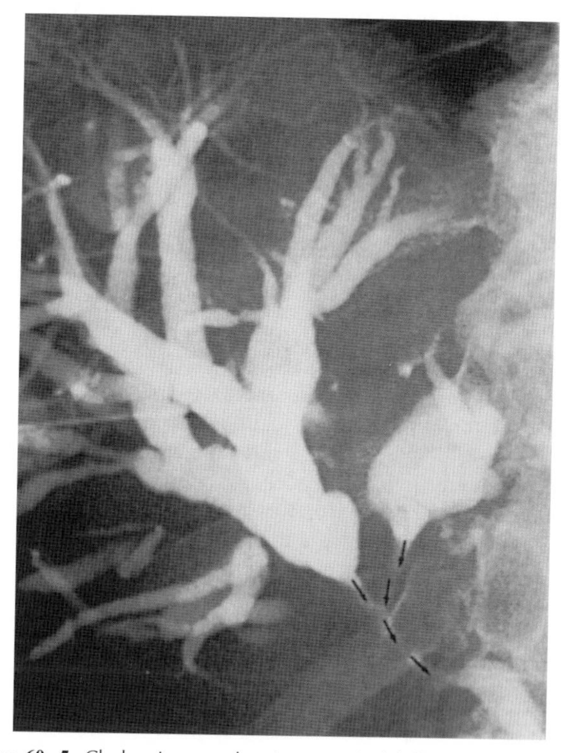

Figure 60–5. Cholangiogram showing a typical hilar carcinoma of the bile duct at the bifurcation of the common hepatic duct. The arrows indicate the bile duct lumen, which is obstructed by the tumor. (Courtesy of E. Ring, M.D., University of California, San Francisco.)

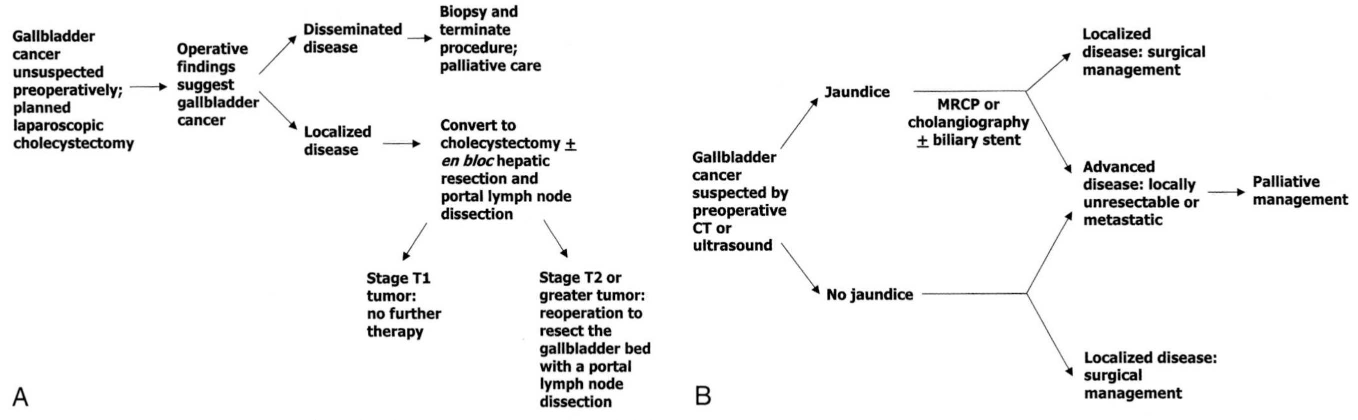

Figure 60–6. Algorithms for the management of gallbladder carcinoma unsuspected (*A*) and suspected preoperatively (*B*). (MRCP, magnetic resonance cholangiopancreatography; CT, computed tomography.)

intra-abdominal malignancy. Each of these presentations requires a different management strategy. Because resection offers the only hope of long-term survival, an aggressive approach toward surgical resection is appropriate. The extent of resection that should be carried out for each stage of the disease, however, remains controversial.

Surgical Resection

Many patients with gallbladder cancer present with symptoms and signs of benign gallbladder disease. However, if preoperative evaluation suggests gallbladder carcinoma, laparoscopic cholecystectomy should be avoided. More commonly, carcinoma is not suspected preoperatively, and the cancer is found at the time of laparoscopy (see Fig. 60–6*A*). In this case, biopsy of the gallbladder mass should be avoided, and conversion to open laparotomy should be performed unless liver metastases or carcinomatosis are identified. Recurrence of cancer at laparoscopic trochar sites has been described,[3] and diffuse peritoneal tumor dissemination has been associated with disruption of the gallbladder wall and spillage of bile. If cancer is diagnosed on histologic examination of the gallbladder after laparoscopic resection, further management is based on the stage of the tumor. If reoperation is performed, all trochar sites should be excised in their entirety.

The American Joint Committee on Cancer (AJCC) staging system for gallbladder carcinoma is shown in Table 60–2. In patients with stage I gallbladder cancer (T1N0M0), disease is confined to the gallbladder wall, and a simple cholecystectomy is usually adequate, provided that the cystic duct margin is negative for tumor. Although most surgeons believe that the morbidity and mortality of an extended resection are not justified for stage I disease,[4–6] some centers advocate a more extensive resection, especially for lesions invading the muscular layer of the gallbladder wall.[7, 8] The 5-year survival in these studies has ranged from 78% to 100% for stage I disease. In an American series, the 5-year survival rate was 88% for carcinoma in situ and 60% for T1N0M0 disease.[9]

Patients with a higher T-stage disease (T2–T4) have a higher rate of lymph node metastases and therefore pose a greater therapeutic challenge (see Fig. 60–6*B*). Fong and colleagues from Memorial Sloan-Kettering Cancer Center reported associated lymph node involvement in 33% of T2 lesions, 58% of T3 lesions, and 69% of T4 lesions.[10] The management of T2 and T3 lesions is generally accepted to include extended or radical cholecystectomy, which consists of en bloc resection of the gallbladder and nonanatomic wedge resection of the gallbladder bed (segments IV and V of the liver), with at least a 3 to 4 cm margin of normal liver parenchyma. Regional lymphadenectomy of the choledochal, periportal, hilar, and high pancreatic lymph nodes should be performed. Depending on the location of the tumor relative to the junction of the cystic duct and common bile duct, the extrahepatic biliary tree may need to be resected. Patients with T2 lesions who undergo simple cholecystectomy have reported 5-year survival rates of 36% to 40%,[11, 12] compared with 83% to 100% in those who undergo radical cholecystectomy.[8, 11, 12] Radical liver resections may be necessary for more extensive lesions and in cases requiring repeat surgery, in which it may be difficult to distinguish tumor from inflammation.

Table 60–2 | **American Joint Committee on Cancer Staging of Gallbladder Carcinoma**

Primary tumor (T stage)
- T1 Tumor invades lamina propria or muscle layer
  - T1a: Tumor invades lamina propria
  - T1b: Tumor invades muscle layer
- T2 Tumor invades perimuscular connective tissue
- T3 Tumor perforates serosa or directly invades one adjacent organ (extension 2 cm or less into liver)
- T4 Tumor extends more than 2 cm into liver and/or into two or more adjacent organs

Regional lymph nodes (N stage)
- N0 No regional lymph node metastasis
- N1 Metastasis in cystic duct, pericholedochal and/or hilar lymph nodes
- N2 Metastasis in peripancreatic, periduodenal, periportal, celiac, and/or superior mesenteric lymph nodes

Distant metastases (M stage)
- M0 No distant metastasis
- M1 Distant metastasis

TNM stage grouping

Stage	T	N	M	
Stage I	T1	N0	M0	
Stage II	T2	N0	M0	
Stage III	T3	N0	M0	or
	T1-3	N1	M0	
Stage IVA	T4	N0-2	M0	
Stage IVB	T1-4	N0-2	M1	

The management of T4 lesions remains controversial. Conservative thinking supports the idea that the morbidity and mortality of a major resection is not justified in these patients because their prognosis is poor regardless of intervention. The Memorial Sloan-Kettering Cancer Center, however, has demonstrated a 28% 5-year actuarial survival rate in 27 selected patients who underwent radical cholecystectomy for T4N0M0 disease.[10] The results suggest that an aggressive approach may be warranted in the absence of gross nodal disease, if a negative resection margin can be achieved.

Several series have demonstrated that radical resections for gallbladder cancer can be performed with mortality rates of less than 4%. In these series, at least 50% of patients had advanced T-stage disease (T3–T4), and the 5-year survival rates ranged from 31% to 65%.[6, 10, 12–14]

Palliation

If unresectable local disease is found at the time of exploration, a biliary bypass (hepaticojejunostomy) can be performed to relieve extrahepatic biliary obstruction and the associated pruritus, jaundice, and progressive liver dysfunction. If disseminated disease is found at laparotomy, laparoscopy, or preoperatively, biliary drainage can be achieved with placement of either a percutaneous or endoscopic stent. Metallic expandable Wallstents can provide permanent internal decompression of biliary obstruction in patients with a life expectancy of only a few months (Fig. 60–7).

Chemotherapy and Radiation Therapy

Gallbladder carcinoma is believed to be resistant to most standard chemoradiation regimens in the neoadjuvant, adjuvant, and palliative settings. The most commonly used chemotherapeutic agent has been 5-flourouracil (5-FU), with associated response rates ranging from 5% to 30% in most series.[15] Both cisplatin and adriamycin have been shown to have an effect, but their toxicities are greater than that of 5-FU, and most reports of efficacy are anecdotal.

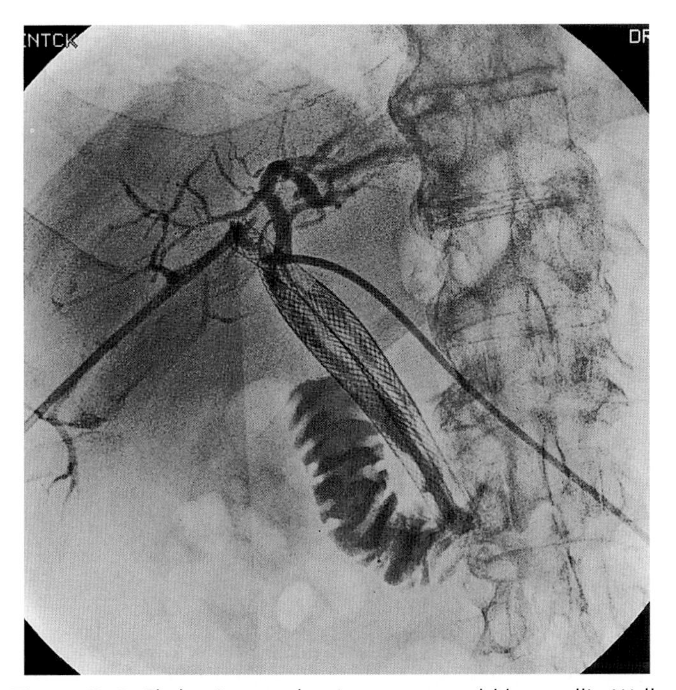

Figure 60–7. Cholangiogram showing two expandable metallic Wallstents placed through an obstruction caused by a gallbladder cancer involving the hepatic hilum.

In the adjuvant setting, radiation therapy is used to control microscopic residual foci of carcinoma in the tumor bed. Approaches have included standard external beam radiation therapy, intraoperative external beam radiation therapy (IORT), and brachytherapy. External beam radiation treats the tumor bed with a 2- to 3-cm margin around the primary tumor and the regional nodal basins. Because intolerance of the liver, kidneys, spinal cord, and duodenum occurs, doses above 54 Gy must be avoided, and usually a dose of 45 Gy is delivered. Because this dose is unlikely to kill gross tumor, brachytherapy and IORT have been attempted, but the data on these techniques are limited.

The benefit of radiation in the palliative setting is modest. Most series report a median survival of less than 2 months after biopsy only and 6 months following palliative surgery.[16] The addition of palliative radiation therapy improves the median survival to 4 months after biopsy alone[17–19] and to more than 8 months after palliative surgery.[19]

Overall Results

The overall 5-year survival rate for patients with gallbladder carcinoma is less than 5%, with a median survival of less than 6 months. In the United States, the overall survival rate in series of patients staged according to the AJCC system was 88% for carcinoma in situ, 60% for stage I, 24% for stage II, 9% for stage III, and 1% for stage IV.[9] Although aggressive surgical resection in large centers has offered some improvement in these results, most patients still present with advanced-stage disease that is unlikely to be amenable to cure.

Benign Tumors

Benign tumors of the gallbladder present most commonly as polyps or polypoid lesions. Polyps can be adenomas, pseudotumors, or hyperplastic inflammatory lesions. These lesions are usually detected on right upper quadrant ultrasound or at cholecystectomy. In general, these tumors should be resected, particularly if enlarging or greater than 1 cm, because the distinction between benign and malignant disease is difficult to determine preoperatively.

Adenomas of the gallbladder are extremely rare and can be sessile or polypoid. Both carcinoma in situ and invasive adenocarcinomas have been found in association with these lesions, suggesting that they are premalignant. The etiologic factors for the development of gallbladder adenomas are unknown. Tumors of the supporting tissues such as hemangiomas, leiomyomas, lymphomas, and lipomas can also occur.

Cholesterolosis, or pseudotumors, is manifested by yellow spots visible on the surface of the gallbladder mucosa that give the appearance of a "strawberry gallbladder" (see Chapter 58). These spots are formed by the proliferation of macrophages filled with cholesterol in the lamina propria and can result in the formation of cholesterol polyps. Inflammatory polyps are composed of a vascular connective tissue stalk with a single layer of columnar epithelial cells.

Adenomyomatosis of the gallbladder is characterized by the proliferation of the mucosa and hypertrophy of the underlying muscular layers. The cause of this condition is unknown, but it is postulated that biliary dyskinesia or functional cystic duct obstruction is responsible for the muscular hypertrophy associated with this condition (see Chapter 58).

TUMORS OF THE EXTRAHEPATIC BILIARY TREE

Benign tumors of the extrahepatic biliary tree are exceedingly rare and include adenomas and tumors of the supporting structures such as leiomyomas, lipomas, carcinoids, angioleiomyomas, and fibromas. These tumors are virtually impossible to distinguish from malignant tumors and should be resected. The remainder of this section will focus on cholangiocarcinoma of the extrahepatic biliary tree.

Cholangiocarcinoma

Epidemiology and Clinical Features

Cholangiocarcinomas are rare cancers that arise from the biliary epithelium (see Table 60–1). They occur with an incidence of 1 per 100,000 people per year in the United States.[20] Cholangiocarcinomas are classified most practically as intrahepatic, perihilar, or distal.[21] Intrahepatic cholangiocarcinomas make up only a minority of cholangiocarcinomas, are treated as primary liver tumors, and will not be discussed further in this chapter (see Chapter 81). Perihilar cholangiocarcinomas (Klatskin tumors) account for 60% to 80% of cholangiocarcinomas seen at tertiary referral centers, whereas distal bile duct cancers make up 10% to 30%.

Approximately two thirds of cholangiocarcinomas occur in patients between 50 and 70 years of age, with a slight male predominance. Important risk factors for cholangiocarcinoma include primary sclerosing cholangitis, ulcerative colitis, choledochal cysts, biliary infection with *Clonorchis sinensis* (a liver fluke), intrahepatic stones and choledocholithiasis, and exposure to the radiologic contrast agent thorium dioxide (Thorotrast). Up to 30% of patients with primary sclerosing cholangitis are found to have a cholangiocarcinoma at autopsy.[22]

The clinical presentation depends largely on the location of the tumor. More than 90% of patients present with obstructive jaundice. However, patients with early perihilar cancers that have not yet obstructed the bile duct may present with vague abdominal pain and abnormal liver biochemical tests. Other common presenting symptoms include weight loss, anorexia, acholic stool, pruritus, and fatigue. Cholangitis can occur, but usually only after percutaneous or endoscopic biliary manipulation. On physical examination, patients often have jaundice. In advanced cases, hepatomegaly or a distended palpable (Courvoisier's) gallbladder in patients with a distal cholangiocarcinoma may be present.

Diagnosis and Staging

At presentation, patients with cholangiocarcinoma typically show a pattern of liver biochemical abnormalities consistent with obstructive jaundice, including elevation of serum bilirubin, alkaline phosphatase, and gamma glutamyl transpeptidase levels. Minimal elevations of the serum aminotransferase levels may be seen, but high elevations typically do not occur until the tumor is advanced and progressive liver damage has occurred. In addition, patients with prolonged disease and resulting liver failure may have an elevated prothrombin time. Both carcinoembryonic antigen (CEA) levels and CA 19-9 levels may be elevated in serum in patients with cholangiocarcinoma, but neither test is sensitive or specific enough to be used as a screening tool.

The initial imaging study in a patient with obstructive jaundice is usually a CT or ultrasound. Findings depend on the location of the tumor. Distal bile duct carcinomas cause dilatation of the entire extrahepatic biliary tree and may be difficult to distinguish from pancreatic, ampullary, and duodenal carcinomas. A mass typically is not seen with distal bile duct carcinomas. In contrast, perihilar lesions typically cause dilatation of the intrahepatic biliary tree with a collapsed extrahepatic biliary tree and gallbladder. Contrast-enhanced, helical CT can facilitate accurate staging of most cases of cholangiocarcinoma and help identify both metastatic disease and invasion of major visceral blood vessels by tumor.

MRCP has become a commonly used noninvasive technique for imaging the biliary tree. It is useful for defining both the extent of disease and the biliary anatomy proximal to the obstruction, which is important in planning surgical reconstruction (Fig. 60–8). Previously, ERCP and PTC have been considered the gold standards for evaluating patients with obstructive jaundice (see Fig. 60–5). Both techniques can relieve biliary obstruction via placement of biliary stents. PTC is particulary useful in defining the anatomy proximal to the obstruction. For perihilar lesions, it is important to define the proximal extent of tumor in both the right and left hepatic ducts because this provides information regarding

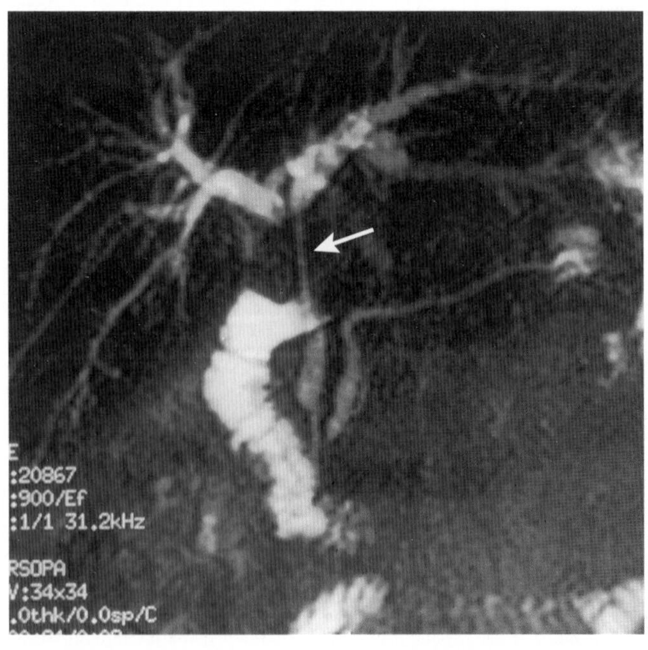

Figure 60–8. MRCP image of a perihilar cholangiocarcinoma demonstrating obstruction at the hepatic duct bifurcation *(arrow)*.

Table 60–3 | **Proposed T Stage Criteria for Hilar Cholangiocarcinoma**

STAGE	CRITERIA
T1	Tumor involving biliary confluence +/− unilateral extension to 2° biliary radicles
T2	Tumor involving biliary confluence +/− unilateral extension to 2° biliary radicles and *ipsilateral* portal vein involvement +/− *ipsilateral* hepatic lobar atrophy
T3	Tumor involving biliary confluence + bilateral extension to 2° biliary radicles;
	or unilateral extension to 2° biliary radicles with *contralateral* portal vein involvement
	or unilateral extension to 2° biliary radicles with *contralateral* hepatic lobar atrophy
	or main or bilateral portal venous involvement

From Jarnagin WE, Fong Y, DeMatteo RP, et al: Staging, resectability, and outcome in 225 patients with hilar cholangiocarcinoma. Ann Surg 234:507–519, 2001.

resectability and the potential need for associated liver resection.

Currently, the AJCC and modified Bismuth-Corlette[23] staging systems fail to account for all the local tumor-related factors that influence therapy for cholangiocarcinoma. Jarnigin and coworkers from the Memorial Sloan-Kettering Cancer Center proposed a staging system that classifies tumors according to three factors that relate to local tumor extent: (1) the location and extent of bile duct involvement (according to the Bismuth-Corlette system), (2) the presence or absence of portal venous invasion, and (3) the presence or absence of hepatic lobar atrophy (Table 60–3).[24] This proposed staging system predicts survival accurately. Increasing T stage significantly reduces the resectability rate and the likelihood of a negative resection margin. In addition, as the T stage increases, the need for partial hepatectomy increases, with 65% of T1 tumors and 100% of T2 lesions requiring hepatectomy.

Management

Resectability of cholangiocarcinomas is determined by the absence of metastatic disease, lack of local invasion of major vascular structures by tumor, and ability to achieve negative surgical margins (Fig. 60–9). Some groups advocate laparoscopy first to exclude metastatic disease, which may be undetectable on preoperative imaging studies. An alternative approach is to perform a limited laparatomy through a right subcostal incision during which the peritoneal cavity can be examined. If metastatic disease is noted, a cholecystectomy can be performed. If no metastatic disease is noted, the excision can be extended to allow the exposure necessary to complete the resection.

The use of preoperative biliary stents remains controversial. Advocates argue that preoperative drainage provides increased visualization of the biliary tree, the ability to perform biopsies, relief of jaundice, and easy access to the biliary tree after surgical reconstruction. Opponents of preoperative drainage prefer to avoid the infectious complications associated with biliary manipulation,[25, 26] as well as less common problems such as hemobilia, fistula formation, and pancreatitis.

The technical approach to resection of a cholangiocarcinoma depends entirely on the location of the primary tumor and its relationship to surrounding structures. Distal cholangiocarcinomas confined to the distal bile duct and head of the pancreas are resected by pancreaticoduodenectomy. The treatment of perihilar carcinomas is individualized on the basis of preoperative imaging studies and intraoperative findings.

Perihilar Cholangiocarcinoma

The perihilar region or common hepatic duct bifurcation is the most common site for cholangiocarcinomas (see Fig. 60–9*A*). Tumors in this location are surgically challenging because of their proximity to major vascular structures and the potential for extension into the right and left hepatic ducts.

Once metastatic disease is ruled out, the distal common bile duct is isolated and divided just cephalad to the duodenum. It is then retracted upward and dissected from the portal vein posteriorly and from the hepatic artery medially. The gallbladder is removed en bloc or as a separate specimen. The portacaval lymphatics are also removed en bloc with the specimen. Exposure of the bile duct bifurcation is accomplished, and the individual right and left hepatic ducts

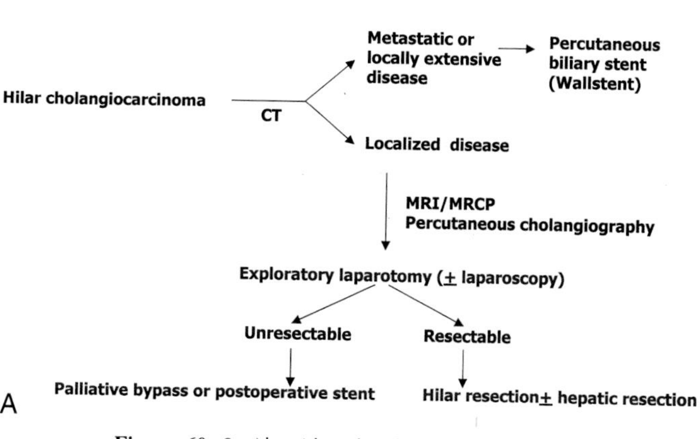

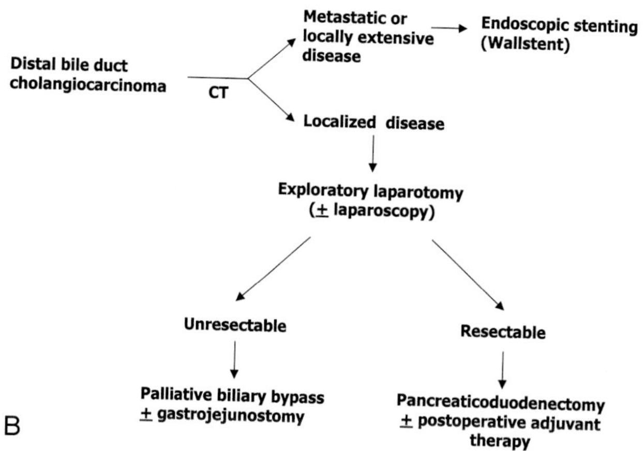

Figure 60–9. Algorithm for the management of hilar (*A*) and distal (*B*) cholangiocarcinoma. (CT, computed tomography, MRI, magnetic resonance imaging; MRCP, magnetic resonance cholangiopancreatography.)

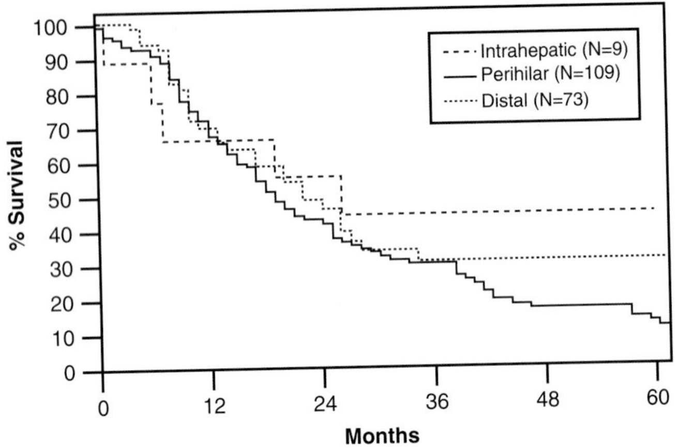

Figure 60–10. Survival of patients with resected intrahepatic, perihilar, and distal cholangiocarcinomas. (From Nakeeb A, Pitt HA, Sohn TA, et al: Cholangiocarcinoma. A spectrum of intrahepatic, perihilar, and distal tumors. Ann Surg 224:469, 1996.)

are dissected to determine the visible extent of disease. In most patients, the left hepatic duct is dissected proximal to the tumor, identified with stay sutures, and divided. If a frozen section is negative for tumor, the right hepatic duct is dissected and divided in a similar fashion. The status of the resection margin should be determined, and if both proximal margins are histologically negative on frozen section, the resection is complete. Reconstruction is accomplished by individual anastomoses (hepaticojejunostomies) usually to a Roux-en-Y loop of jejunum. Some groups favor the use of silastic biliary stents in the reconstruction.

Because survival results correlate closely with the ability to achieve negative proximal resection margins, most groups advocate performing either central lobectomies (segments IV and V) or lobectomies of the right or left side as determined by the margin status.[27] With the addition of liver resection, these groups achieve negative surgical margins in 49% to 83% of patients and have demonstrated trends toward improved survival rates, with margin-negative 5-year survival rates ranging from 21% to 56%. Another approach based on demonstrable caudate lobe involvement in 96% of perihilar cholangiocarcinomas[31] has led several groups to advocate caudate lobectomy in conjunction with resection of the extrahepatic biliary tree.[31, 32] The addition of hepatic resection increases the rates of perioperative morbidity (30%–50%) and mortality (5%–10%) for the surgical treatment of hilar cholangiocarcinoma, although significant improvement in perioperative results has been reported at major centers.[24, 27, 28]

Although orthotopic liver transplantation has been used to treat both resectable and unresectable perihilar cholangiocarcinomas, the high incidence of associated lymph node metastases has limited its use. In a series by Pichlmayr and colleagues,[33] 125 patients who underwent resection for cholangiocarcinoma were compared with 25 patients who underwent liver transplantation. Resection yielded superior or equivalent results for all stages. A later report from the same institution noted that only four of 32 patients with cholangiocarcinoma survived 5 years after transplantation.[34] Liver transplantation may be appropriate in selected cases of cholangiocarcinoma but should not be considered the standard therapy.

Distal Bile Duct Cholangiocarcinoma

The distal bile duct is the second most common site for cholangiocarcinoma (see Fig. 60–9*B*) and the third most common resected periampullary adenocarcinoma.[35] Distal bile duct carcinomas are resected via pancreaticoduodenectomy, as are other periampullary malignancies. A series of 80 distal bile duct cancers from the Johns Hopkins Hospital was reported in 1996.[21] Negative pathologic margins of resection were attained in 90% of resectable patients, and the 5-year survival rate of 28% compared favorably with that for resection of perihilar lesions (Fig. 60–10). Pancreaticoduodenectomy is generally performed in major tertiary referral centers with a perioperative mortality of less than 5%.[36–40] Postoperative complications are frequent (approximately 30%) but are seldom life-threatening.

Palliation

If advanced local or metastatic disease is identified preoperatively or at the time of surgical exploration, therapy is directed toward palliation of biliary obstruction and its associated symptoms. In patients with unresectable hilar cholangiocarcinoma on the basis of preoperative imaging, therapeutic biliary drainage should be accomplished via a percutaneous transhepatic route. This external system can be converted later to an expandable metallic Wallstent to provide internal drainage (see Fig. 60–7). For perihilar cholangiocarcinomas associated with cholangitis, multiple stents may be necessary to relieve all obstructed biliary radicles. In the absence of cholangitis, the entire liver does not require drainage because only 30% of the functioning hepatic mass needs decompression to relieve jaundice. For distal bile duct cancers, endoscopic drainage techniques are usually preferred. Following adequate decompression, jaundice usually resolves quickly.

Chemotherapy and Radiation Therapy

The use of chemotherapy as the sole modality for the treatment of cholangiocarcinoma has not been well established. 5-FU, streptozotocin, lomustine (CCNU), mitomycin C, epirubicin, methotrexate, leucovorin, and carboplatin have been used in single agent and combination regimens. Only four small phase II trials of chemotherapy as primary treatment for bile duct cancer have been undertaken, with response rates of 10% to 21% or less.[41–44]

Even when negative resection margins are obtained after surgery for cholangiocarcinoma, the margins are minimal, and local failure is an important problem. Therefore, it is reasonable to consider adjuvant radiation to destroy residual tumor at resection margins. Studies to date have been nonuniform, with a mixture of resected and unresected patients[17, 45–53] and no prospective randomized data that compare surgery alone with surgery plus adjuvant radiation therapy. In several series from the Johns Hopkins Hospital,[46, 48, 49] no significant survival advantage was noted with the addition of adjuvant radiation therapy, but the three 5-year survivors in the series had received radiation therapy. However, this group of patients was heterogeneous, with some receiving brachytherapy in addition to standard external beam radiation. Kamada and colleagues in 1996 reported on the outcomes of 59 patients who received postoperative brachytherapy in combination with external beam radiation[45] and demonstrated improved survival with the addition of brachytherapy, with a median survival of 21.5 months. At least one report, however, has shown that the combination of brachytherapy and external beam radiation can be detrimental to survival.[53]

Adjuvant chemoradiation protocols have also been used. In a series of 24 patients treated with external beam radiation, brachytherapy, and either 5-FU or 5-FU, adriamycin, and mitomycin C (FAM), survival was improved (25 months vs 6 months) in those receiving adjuvant therapy.[54] Foo and colleagues from the Mayo Clinic also showed promising results with a similar regimen, with two of nine patients in the adjuvant therapy group surviving 5 years.[55]

Several trials of preoperative, or neoadjuvant, chemoradiation have been reported. In the largest series, by Urego and colleagues, chemoradiation was followed by either complete resection or liver transplantation.[56] They reported an initial response rate of 38% and a 20-month median survival for those with negative resection margins. In addition, a number of patients who were considered unresectable at initial evaluation were down-staged by chemoradiation. McMaster and coworkers reported the results of nine patients receiving neoadjuvant chemoradiation for the purpose of down-staging and observed a 33% complete response rate and a median survival of 22 months.[57]

Overall Results

The outcome for patients with cholangiocarcinoma depends on both the stage and location of the tumor. Hilar cholangiocarcinomas often present late in the course with either metastatic disease or local extension into major portal vascular structures. Proximal extension into both the right and left hepatic ducts may also preclude resection. In a series of 197 perihilar cholangiocarcinomas treated at the Johns Hopkins Hospital, only 56% were resectable, with an overall 5-year survival rate of 11%.[21] Aggressive hepatic resection to obtain negative surgical margins has been shown to increase survival rates to 21% to 56%.[27–30]

The resectability rate is higher for distal bile duct cancers than for hilar tumors. The survival rate after resection also exceeds that for perihilar cholangiocarcinoma (see Fig. 60–10). Of the periampullary adenocarcinomas, the 5-year survival rate for bile duct cancer (28%) generally exceeds that for pancreatic cancer but does not compare favorably with that for resected ampullary or duodenal cancer.[35]

TUMORS OF THE AMPULLA OF VATER

The ampulla of Vater is a complex anatomic site that represents the junction of the duodenum, pancreatic ductal system, and biliary ductal system. Although less than 1 cm in diameter, this area of the small bowel has the highest incidence of neoplastic transformation and malignancy. The high incidence of malignancy is likely the result of production of local carcinogens through the combined interactions of the components of bile, pancreatic juice, and duodenal contents. Both benign and malignant tumors of the ampulla of Vater occur. Benign tumors include adenomas, gastrointestinal stromal tumors (GISTs), lipomas, and neuroendocrine tumors. Tumors metastatic from other primary sites have also been reported.

Ampullary Adenoma and Adenocarcinoma

Epidemiology and Clinical Features

Adenocarcinoma is the most common malignant tumor of the ampulla of Vater (see Table 60–1). Adenocarcinoma of the ampulla of Vater accounts for less than 10% of all periampullary adenocarcinomas, but for up to 25% of those that are resectable. The incidence of ampullary adenocarcinoma is 2.9 cases per million population.[58] Ampullary adenocarcinomas arise from the mucosal cells of the ampulla of Vater and undergo an adenoma-carcinoma progression sequence similar to that described for colon cancer. Benign adenomas become dysplastic, with subsequent progression to adenocarcinoma. Evidence for this sequence has been demonstrated in studies in which adenomas were observed over time; 80% to 90% of adenocarcinomas were surrounded by benign adenomas, and in many cases a transition from benign to malignant histology was noted.[59, 60]

Risk factors for ampullary adenocarcinoma include familial adenomatous polyposis (FAP) and Peutz-Jehgers syndrome. Patients with FAP have a markedly increased frequency of ampullary adenomas that ranges from 50% to 86%[61, 62] (see Chapter 114).

The average age of patients with ampullary adenoma is the mid-50s, whereas that for ampullary adenocarcinoma is the mid-60s. Patients present most commonly with obstructive jaundice, seen in approximately 80%, because the tumors tend to obstruct the bile duct early in the course. Weight loss occurs in 75% of patients, and abdominal pain in 50%. Occult gastrointestinal bleeding is common and is seen in up to one third of patients. Nonspecific symptoms such as anorexia, dyspepsia, and malaise can also occur. Rarely, patients with ampullary adenocarcinoma present with pancreatitis secondary to pancreatic duct obstruction or with features of sphincter of Oddi dysfunction. Typical findings on physical examination include scleral or cutaneous icterus, and less commonly, hepatomegaly, a distended gallbladder, or positive results on a fecal occult blood test. Very rarely, the combination of obstructive jaundice and bleeding from the tumor gives rise to distinctive silver stools, which result from a combination of the absence of bilirubin and the presence of blood.

Diagnosis and Staging

The earliest and most common laboratory abnormality is an increase in the serum alkaline phosphatase level, followed by hyperbilirubinemia as the tumor obstructs the bile duct. No tumor markers have been identified that are either sensitive or specific for ampullary adenocarcinoma.

Early diagnosis of ampullary adenocarcinoma requires a high level of clinical suspicion and prompt evaluation of the patient with obstructive jaundice. As for any patient with obstructive jaundice, the first imaging modality should be ultrasound or CT to determine the level of biliary obstruction. Dual-contrast helical CT is the most informative and cost-effective imaging technique. CT can detect a periampullary mass greater than 1 cm in size (Fig. 60–11) and pro-

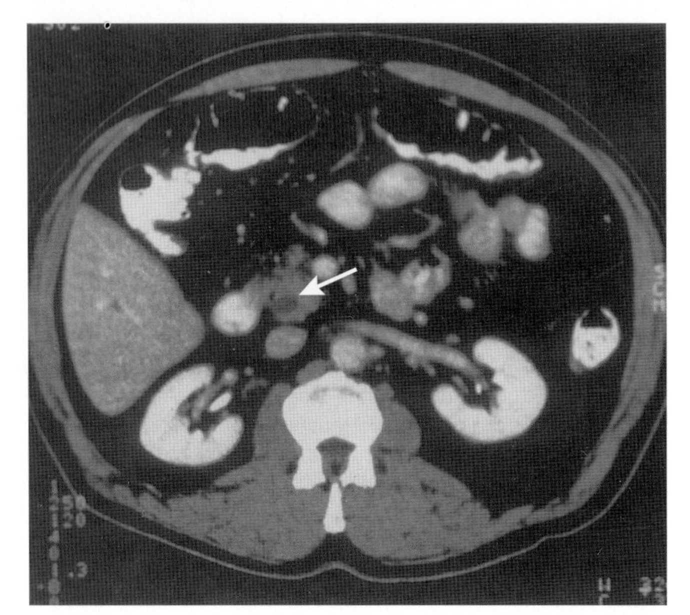

Figure 60–11. CT scan of an ampullary adenocarcinoma demonstrating a dilated common bile duct *(arrow)* extending into the pancreatic head.

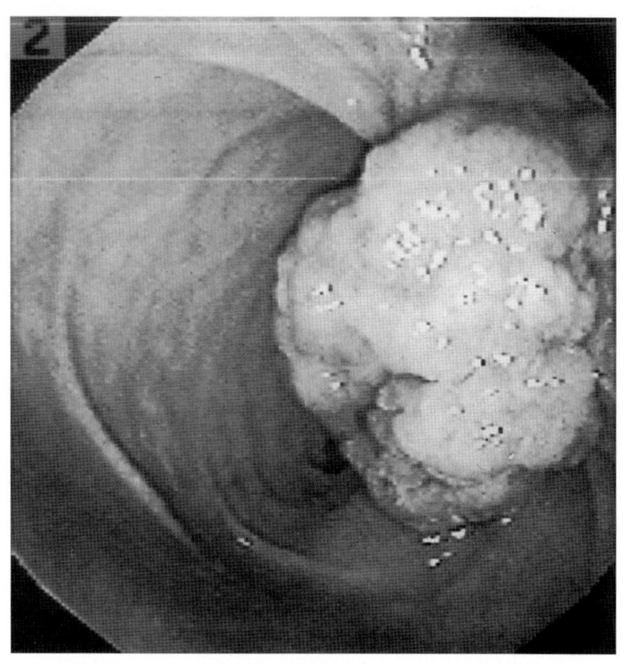

Figure 60–12. Endoscopic view of an ampullary adenocarcinoma.

vides information regarding the level of biliary obstruction, relationship of the mass to surrounding vascular structures, and presence or absence of liver metastases. For patients with ampullary cancer, the entire extrahepatic biliary tree extending into the pancreatic parenchyma and gallbladder will be dilated.

Upper gastrointestinal barium studies can be used to visualize duodenal mucosal abnormalities but have been replaced by upper endoscopy and ERCP. After confirming biliary obstruction, ERCP is often the next procedure for patients with a suspected ampullary malignancy. The endoscopic component of the examination will define the extent, size, and gross morphology of the lesion and allow endoscopic biopsy or cytology brushings (Fig. 60–12). Endoscopic biopsies may yield false-negative results, especially with a large adenoma that contains a focus of adenocarcinoma, in which sampling error is likely.[63] Therefore, complete resection of the lesion is warranted to relieve biliary obstruction and detect (or prevent) a potentially malignant lesion.

The choice of ERCP or PTC to image the biliary tree in patients with obstructive jaundice is largely a function of local expertise, the level of obstruction, the presence of coagulopathy, and the patient's gastrointestinal anatomy. For patients with an ampullary lesion, however, visualization of the tumor and the ability to perform a biopsy make the endoscopic route preferable. A biliary tract stent can be placed by ERCP or PTC to relieve obstructive jaundice, but stenting is not routinely indicated. In the future, MRCP may replace invasive cholangiography in the diagnosis of ampullary cancer. MRCP permits visualization of the biliary tree and provides information on the size and extent of the tumor and on the relationship of the tumor to the surrounding vasculature.

Endoscopic ultrasound (EUS) has been reported to be both reliable and accurate in the diagnosis and staging of ampullary cancer. Real-time EUS enables the viewer to evaluate mucosal, vascular, ductal, nodal, and parenchymal abnormalities with a single examination (Fig. 60–13). In one prospective study, 93% of ampullary tumors were correctly diagnosed by EUS, compared with only 7% and 29% by ultrasound and CT, respectively.[64] EUS can also provide a method of selecting cases for local resection or pancreaticoduodenectomy. Although EUS can identify T3 and T4 lesions, it cannot distinguish T1 lesions (limited to the mucosa) from adenomas.[65, 66]

The staging of ampullary carcinoma is based on tumor size, extent of tumor invasion, presence or absence of lymph

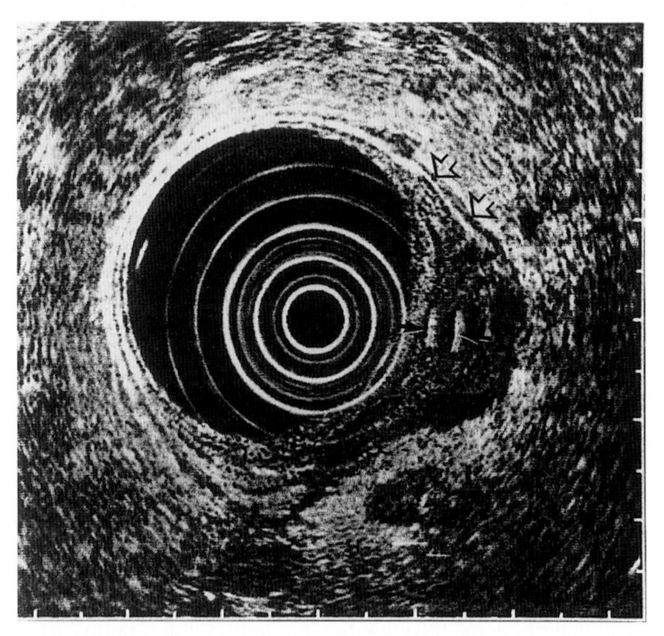

Figure 60–13. Endoscopic ultrasound of an ampullary neoplasm, represented by a hypoechoic area on the right. An endoprosthesis *(small black arrows)* can be seen passing through the tumor. The tumor infiltrates beyond the muscularis propria *(open arrows)* into the pancreas.

Table 60–4 | **TNM Staging of Ampullary Adenocarcinoma**

Primary tumor (T stage)
- T1 Tumor limited to ampulla of Vater
- T2 Tumor invades duodenal wall
- T3 Tumor invades ≤ 2 cm into pancreas
- T4 Tumor invades > 2 cm into pancreas and/or adjacent organs

Regional lymph nodes (N stage)
- N0 No regional lymph node metastasis
- N1 Regional lymph node metastasis

Distant metastasis (M stage)
- M0 No distant metastasis
- M1 Distant metastasis

TNM stage grouping

Stage	T	N	M
Stage I	T1	N0	M0
Stage II	T2-3	N0	M0
Stage III	T1-3	N1	M0
Stage IVA	T4	N0-1	M0
Stage IVB	T1-4	N0-1	M1

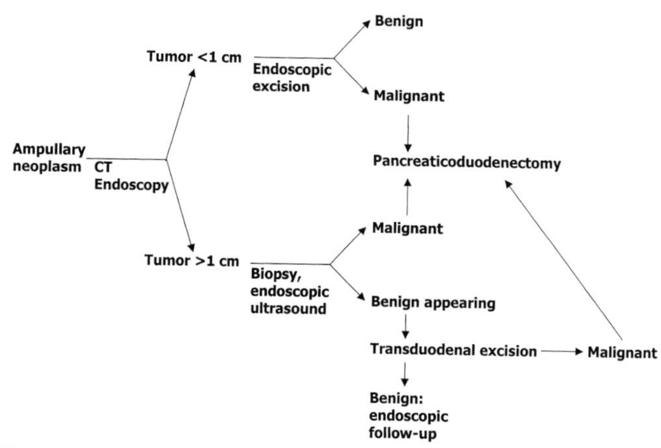

Figure 60–14. Algorithm for the management of an ampullary neoplasm.

node metastases, and presence or absence of distant metastases. The TNM system currently used is shown in Table 60–4. Because the majority of ampullary adenocarcinomas are resectable and associated with a good prognosis when resected, many surgeons feel that extensive preoperative staging is unnecessary. Dual-contrast helical CT will detect liver metastases greater than 1 cm, major vascular invasion, and ascites. Patients who are good operative risks and have no evidence of distant metastases should undergo surgical exploration and resection when possible. Nonoperative palliation should be considered in patients who are not operative candidates and those with metastatic disease at the time of presentation.

Management

Local Excision

The first local resection of an ampullary tumor was performed by William S. Halsted in 1899.[67] Currently, local resection of ampullary tumors is reserved for patients with benign adenomas, ampullary neuroendocrine tumors, and highly selected patients with ampullary adenocarcinoma (Fig. 60–14). The options for local treatment include endoscopic snare removal, endoscopic ablation, and surgical ampullectomy. Pedunculated, tubular adenomas less than 1 cm without severe dysplasia can be managed endoscopically, usually by snare excision and sphincterotomy. However, the risk of incomplete resection and recurrence is as high as 20% with this method.[68]

For adenomas greater than 1 cm, operative resection is indicated once metastatic disease is excluded. A longitudinal duodenotomy centered over the ampulla of Vater is made, and the tumor is excised completely with the full thickness of the duodenal wall and segments of both the bile and pancreatic ducts. The duodenal mucosa is approximated, and the pancreatic and common duct orifices are reimplanted. Postoperative morbidity following local ampullectomy is low, and mortality rates of less than 2% have been reported.[69–73]

In a review of the recent literature, Beger and colleagues identified 62 patients who had undergone ampullectomy for benign neoplasms. Of these 62 patients, all were free of disease with follow-up ranging from 1 to 156 months.[74] In contrast, Branum and colleagues reported that 5 of 19 patients with a benign neoplasm resected by ampullectomy had recurrence at a mean of 35 months (range, 8–72 months)[71]; two of these patients also had FAP. More concerning, however, is a recent report from the Mayo Clinic,[73] which suggests that these patients may be at risk for the development of adenocarcinoma at the site of recurrence. Fifty patients with a benign villous tumor were treated by local excision. Seventeen tumors recurred, with actuarial recurrence rates of 32% at 5 years and 43% at 10 years. Four of the recurrences (24%) were adenocarcinomas, and in one of the affected patients, the recurrent tumor was unresectable. In this series, a known polyposis syndrome, but not tumor size, increased the likelihood of recurrence. These results led these authors to recommend annual endoscopic surveillance with biopsy following local excision of benign ampullary neoplasms and to consider removing all mucosa at risk (i.e., the duodenum) by pancreaticoduodenectomy in patients with FAP.

Some groups have advocated local excision for patients with stage T1 cancers. However, this technique is limited by the potential for inadequate resection and uncertainty regarding the extent of invasion of the duodenal wall and pancreas. In addition, up to 10% of patients with stage T1 cancers have lymph node metastases, and local ampullectomy provides no nodal clearance.[75] In recent series, reported 5-year survival rates following ampullectomy for adenocarcinoma have been approximately 40%.[71, 75, 76]

The detection of carcinoma in an adenoma at the time of local ampullectomy usually alters management. Most surgeons advocate pancreaticoduodenectomy if malignancy is found at the time of exploration, because adequate staging may not be achieved by frozen section analysis. If postoperative histologic findings show invasive malignancy, most patients should return for pancreaticoduodenectomy.

Pancreaticoduodenectomy

Pancreaticoduodenectomy (Whipple's procedure) is the treatment of choice for patients with ampullary adenocarcinoma. Classic pancreaticoduodenectomy, which includes a distal gastrectomy, and the pylorus-preserving modification are appropriate alternatives. Local lymph node resection is adequate because there are no data to support N2 lymph node dissection for ampullary adenocarcinoma.

Pancreaticoduodenectomy can be performed safely, with many centers reporting operative mortality rates of less than 5%.[36-39] Morbidity rates associated with this procedure remain high, from 25% to 50%.[36-39] The frequency of a pancreatic fistula appears higher with surgery for ampullary adenocarcinoma than for pancreatic carcinoma, probably because of the increased risk of a pancreatic anastomotic leak associated with the "soft" gland frequently found in neoplasms of the duodenum and ampulla in the absence of obstructive pancreatitis.[40]

In 1997, the group at the Johns Hopkins Hospital reported the largest single institution experience in the management of adenocarcinoma of the ampulla of Vater.[77] One hundred twenty patients with adenocarcinoma were treated over a 28-year period. Resection was performed in 106 patients (88%), and 105 of them (99%) underwent either a pancreaticoduodenectomy (n = 103) or total pancreatectomy (n = 2). The overall operative mortality rate was 3.8%. One or more complications occurred in 49 patients for an overall morbidity rate of 47%. The most common complication was pancreatic fistula, which occurred in 23 patients (25%).

Chemotherapy and Radiation Therapy

Although combined modality adjuvant chemoradiation improves survival in patients with pancreatic adenocarcinoma,[78-80] there are no data to support its use for ampullary adenocarcinoma. It is tempting to extrapolate the data for pancreatic cancer to ampullary cancer because the number of patients with ampullary cancers is too small to perform a good randomized, controlled trial. Limited data demonstrate that adjuvant chemotherapy with 5-FU, doxorubicin, and mitomycin C delays tumor recurrence in patients with ampullary adenocarcinoma, but more data are needed.[81]

Palliation

Resection is possible in more than 85% of patients with ampullary adenocarcinoma.[77] In some patients, however, metastatic disease or unresectable local disease is found at the time of surgical exploration. In such cases, operative palliation of obstructive jaundice with a Roux-en-Y hepaticojejunostomy is appropriate. A gastrojejunostomy should also be performed in patients with a compromised duodenal lumen to prevent gastric outlet obstruction before death. If identified preoperatively, biliary decompression can be accomplished using endoscopic or percutaneous techniques.

Overall Results

Survival in patients with unresectable ampullary adenocarcinoma is similar to that for other types of unresectable periampullary cancers, with median survival from 5 to 9 months.[77, 82, 83] The overall 5-year survival rate for patients with resected ampullary cancer ranges from 25% to 55%.[35, 36, 77, 83-85] The 5-year survival rate is significantly better than that for pancreatic adenocarcinoma (Fig. 60–15).[35] In the

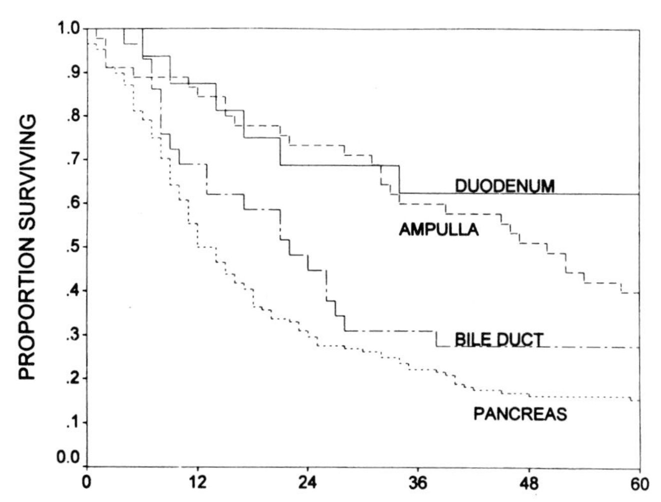

Figure 60–15. Tumor-specific actual 5-year survival curves for a cohort of 242 patients treated by pancreaticoduodenectomy for periampullary adenocarcinoma. (From Yeo CJ, Sohn TA, Cameron JL, et al: Periampullary adenocarcinoma: Analysis of 5-year survivors. Ann Surg 227:824, 1998. By permission.)

1997 Johns Hopkins series, lymph node status, degree of differentiation, and operative blood loss were signficant predictors of survival.[77] Tumor diameter had no effect on survival, nor did adjuvant therapy, although the number of patients receiving adjuvant therapy was small. In a series of 101 patients who underwent resection for ampullary adenocarcinoma at Memorial Sloan-Kettering Cancer Center,[83] the 5-year survival rate was 46%, and resection margin status, nodal status, and tumor differentiation were predictive of survival. As in the experience at Johns Hopkins,[56] the survival rate for patients with ampullary adenocarcinoma was second only to duodenal cancer among the periampullary adenocarcinomas.

Acknowledgment

The authors thank Richard D. Schulick, MD, for his contribution to this chapter.

REFERENCES

1. Landis SA, Murra T, Bolden S, Wingo PA: Cancer statistics. CA Cancer J Clin 49:8–31, 1999.
2. Shinka H, Kimura W, Muto T: Surgical indications for small polypoid lesions of the gallbladder. Am J Surg 175:114–117, 1998.
3. Lundberg O, Kristoffersson A: Port site metastases from gallbladder cancer after laparoscopic cholecystectomy. Results of a Swedish survey and review of published reports. Eur J Surg 165:215–222, 1999.
4. Shirai Y, Yoshida K, Tsukuda K, et al: Early carcinoma of the gallbladder. Eur J Surg 158:545–548, 1992.
5. Yamaguchi K, Tsuneyoshi M: Subclinical gallbladder carcioma. Am J Surg 163:382–386, 1992.
6. Donohue JH, Nagorney DM, Grant CS, et al: Carcinoma of the gallbladder. Arch Surg 125:237–241, 1990.
7. Ogura Y, Mizumoto R, Isaji S, et al: Radical operations for carcinoma of the gallbladder: Present status in Japan. World J Surg 15:337–343, 1991.
8. Matsumoto Y, Fujii H, Aoyama H, et al: Surgical treatment of primary carcinoma of the gallbladder based on the histologic analysis of 48 surgical specimens. Am J Surg 163:239–245, 1992.
9. American Joint Committee on Cancer: Manual of Staging of Cancer, 4th ed. Philadelphia, Lippincott-Raven, 1992.
10. Fong Y, Jarnagin W, Blumgart L: Gallbladder cancer: Comparison of

patients presenting initially for definitive operation with those presenting after prior noncurative intervention. Ann Surg 232:557–569, 2000.
11. Shirai Y, Yoshida K, Tsukada K, et al: Inapparent carcinoma of the gallbladder: An appraisal of a radical second operation after simple cholecystectomy. Ann Surg 215:326–331, 1992.
12. Bartlett DL, Fong Y, Fortner JV, et al: Long-term results after resection for gallbladder cancer. Ann Surg 224:639–646, 1996.
13. Shirai Y, Yoshida K, Tsukada K, et al: Radical surgery for gallbladder carcinoma. Long-term results. Ann Surg 216:565–568, 1992.
14. Chijiiwa K, Tanaka M: Carcinoma of the gallbladder: An appraisal of surgical resection. Surgery 115:751–756, 1994.
15. Falkson G, MacIntyre JM, Moertel CG: Eastern Cooperative Oncology Group experience with chemotherapy for inoperable gallbladder and bile duct cancer. Cancer 54:965–969, 1984.
16. Douglass HO, Tepper J, Leichman L: Neoplasms of the gallbladder. In Holland JF, Frei E, Bast RC, et al (eds): Cancer Medicine. Philadelphia, Lea and Febiger, 1993, pp 1448–1454.
17. Kraybill WG, Lee H, Pincus J, et al: Multidisciplinary treatment of biliary tract cancers. J Surg Oncol 55:239–245, 1994.
18. Flickenger JC, Epstein AH, Iwatsuki S, et al: Radiation therapy for primary carcinoma of the extrahepatic biliary system. Cancer 68:289–294, 1991.
19. Mahe M, Romestaing P, Talon B, et al: Radiation therapy in extrahepatic bile duct carcinoma. Radiother Oncol 21:121–127, 1991.
20. Callery MR, Meyers WC: Bile duct cancer. In Cameron JL (ed): Current Surgical Therapy, 6th ed. Baltimore, Mosby, 1998, pp 455–461.
21. Nakeeb A, Pitt HA, Sohn TA, et al: Cholangiocarcinoma. A spectrum of intrahepatic, perihilar, and distal tumors. Ann Surg 224:463–475, 1996.
22. Rosen CB, Nagorney DM, Weisner RH, et al: Cholangiocarcinoma complicating primary sclerosing cholangitis: Report of six cases and review of the literature. Ann Surg 213:21–25, 1991.
23. Bismuth H, Corlette MB: Intrahepatic cholangioenteric anastomosis in carcinoma at the hilus of the liver. Surg Gynecol Obstet 140:170–176, 1975.
24. Jarnagin WR, Fong Y, DeMatteo RP, et al: Staging, analysis of resectability and outcome in 225 patients with hilar cholangiocarcinoma. Ann Surg 234:507–519, 2001.
25. Sohn TA, Yeo CJ, Cameron JL, et al: Do preoperative biliary stents increase postpancreaticoduodenectomy complications? J Gastrointest Surg 4:258–268, 2000.
26. Hochwald SN, Burke EC, Jarnagin WR, et al: Association of preoperative biliary stenting with increased postoperative infectious complications in proximal cholangiocarcinoma. Arch Surg 134:261–266, 1999.
27. Kosuge T, Yamamoto J, Shimada K, et al: Improved surgical results for hilar cholangiocarcinoma with procedures including major hepatic resection. Ann Surg 230:663–671, 1991.
28. Burke ED, Jarnagin WR, Hochwald SN, et al: Hilar cholangiocarcinoma: Patterns of spread, the importance of hepatic resection for curative operation, and a presurgical clinical staging system. Ann Surg 228: 385–394, 1998.
29. Miyazaki M, Ito H, Nakagawa K, et al: Aggressive surgical approaches to hilar cholangiocarcinoma: Hepatic or local resection? Surgery 123: 131–136, 1998.
30. Su C, Tsay S, Wu C, et al: Factors influencing postoperative morbidity, mortality, and survival after resection for hilar cholangiocarcinoma. Ann Surg 223:384–394, 1996.
31. Nimura Y, Hayakawa N, Kamiya J, et al: Hepatic segmentectomy with caudate lobe resection for bile duct carcinoma of the hepatic hilus. World J Surg 14:535–544, 1990.
32. Mizumoto R, Suzuki H: Surgical anatomy of the hepatic hilum with special reference to the caudate lobe. World J Surg 12:2–10, 1998.
33. Pichlmayr R, Weimann A, Klempnauer J, et al: Surgical treatment in proximal bile duct cancer. A single-center experience. Ann Surg 224: 628–638, 1996.
34. Klempnauer J, Ridder GJ, Werner M, et al: What constitutes long term survival after surgery for hilar cholangiocarcinoma? Cancer 79:26–34, 1997.
35. Yeo CJ, Sohn TA, Cameron JL, et al: Periampullary adenocarcinoma: Analysis of 5-year survivors. Ann Surg 227:821–831, 1998.
36. Yeo CJ, Cameron JL, Sohn TA, et al: Six hundred fifty consecutive pancreaticoduodenectomies in the 1990s: Pathology, complications, and outcomes. Ann Surg 226:248–260, 1997.
37. Trede M, Schwall G, Saeger H-D: Survival after pancreatidoduodenectomy: 118 consecutive resections without an operative mortality. Ann Surg 211:447–458, 1990.
38. Cameron JL, Pitt HA, Yeo CJ, et al: One hundred and forty-five consecutive pancreaticoduodenectomies without mortality. Ann Surg 217:430–438, 1993.
39. Fernandez-del Castillo C, Rattner DW, Warshaw AL: Standards for pancreatic resection in the 1990s. Arch Surg 130:295–300, 1995.
40. Yeo CJ, Cameron JL, Lillemoe KD, et al: Does prophylactic octreotide decrease the rates of pancreatic fistula and other complications after pancreaticoduodenectomy? Results of a prospective randomized placebo-controlled trial. Ann Surg 232:419–429, 2000.
41. Sanz-Altamira PM, Ferante K, Jenkins RL, et al: A phase II trial of 5-fluorouracil, leucovorin, and carboplatin in patients with unresectable biliary tree carcinoma. Cancer 82:2321–2325, 1998.
42. Patt YZ, Jones DV, Hoque A, et al: Phase II trial of intravenous flourouracil and subcutaneous interferon alpha-2b for biliary tract cancer. J Clin Oncol 14:2311–2315, 1996.
43. Ravry MJ, Omura GA, Bartolucci AA, et al: Phase II evaluation of cisplatin in advanced hepatocellular carcinoma and cholangiocarcinoma: A Southeastern Cancer Study Group trial. Cancer Treat Resp 70:311–312, 1986.
44. Bukowski RM, Leichman LP, Rivkin SE: Phase II trial of m-AMSA in gallbladder and cholangiocarcinoma: A Southwest Oncology Group study. Eur J Cancer Clin Oncol 19:721–723, 1983.
45. Kamada T, Saitou H, Takamura A, et al: The role of radiotherapy in the management of extrahepatic bile duct cancer: An analysis if 145 consecutive patients treated with intraluminal and/or external beam radiotherapy. Int J Radiation Oncol Biol Phys 34:767–774, 1996.
46. Abrams RA, Grochow LB, Chakravarthy A, et al: Intensified adjuvant therapy for pancreatic and periampullary adenocarcinoma: Survival results and observations regarding patterns of failure, radiotherapy dose and CA 19-9 levels. Int J Radiation Oncology Biol Phys 44:1039–1046, 1999.
47. Gunderson LL, Haddock MG, Burch P, et al: Future role of radiotherapy as a component of treatment in biliopancreatic cancers. Ann Oncol 10:S291–S295, 1999.
48. Pitt HA, Nakeeb A, Abrams RA, et al: Perihilar cholangiocarcinoma. Ann Surg 221:788–798, 1995.
49. Cameron JL, Pitt HA, Zinner MJ, et al: Management of proximal cholangiocarcinomas by surgical resection and radiotherapy. Am J Surg 159:91–98, 1990.
50. Verbeek PCM, van Leeuwen DJ, van Der Heyde MN, et al: Does additive radiotherapy after hilar resection improve survival of cholangiocarcinoma? Ann Chir 45:350–354, 1991.
51. Veeze-Kujpers B, Meerwaldt JH, Lameris JS, et al: The role of radiotherapy in the treatment of bile duct carcinoma. Int J Radiation Oncology Biol Phys 18:63–67, 1989.
52. Fogel TD, Weissberg JB: The role of radiation therapy in carcinoma of the extrahepatic bile ducts. Int J Radiation Oncology Biol Phys 10: 2251–2258, 1984.
53. Gonzalez DG, Gouma DJ, Rauws EAJ, et al: Role of radiotherapy, in particular intraluminal brachytherapy, in the treatment of proximal bile duct carcinoma. Ann Oncol 18:S215–S220, 1999.
54. Alden ME, Mohiuddin M: The impact of radiation dose in combined external beam and intraluminal IR-192 brachytherapy for bile duct cancer. Int J Radiation Oncology Biol Phys 28:945–951, 1994.
55. Foo ML, Gunderson LL, Bender CE, et al: External radiation therapy and transcatheter iridium in the treatment of extrahepatic bile duct carcinoma. Int J Radiation Oncology Biol Phys 39:929–935, 1997.
56. Urego M, Flickinger JC, Carr BI: Radiotherapy and multimodality management of cholangiocarcinoma. Int J Radiation Oncology Biol Phys 44:121–126, 1999.
57. McMaster KM, Tuttle TM, Leach SD, et al: Neoadjuvant chemoradiation for extrahepatic cholangiocarcinoma. Am J Surg 174:605–609, 1997.
58. Anderson JB, Cooper MJ, Williamson RCN: Adenocarcinoma of the extrahepatic biliary tree. Ann R Coll Surg Engl 67:139–143, 1985.
59. Cattell RB, Braasch J, Kahn F: Polypoid epithelial tumors of the bile ducts. N Engl J Med 266:57–61, 1962.
60. Baczakok, Büchler M, Beger HG, et al: Morphogenesis and possible precursor lesions of invasive carcinoma of the papilla of Vater: Epithelial dysplasia and adenoma. Hum Pathol 16:305–310, 1985.
61. Yao T, Iida M, Ohsato K, et al: Duodenal lesions in familial polyposis of the colon. Gastroenterology 73:1086–1092, 1977.
62. Offerhaus GJA, Giardiello FM, Krush AJ, et al: The risk of upper gastrointestinal cancer in familial adenomatous polyposis. Gastroenterology 102:1080–1982, 1992.
63. Ryan DP, Schapiro RH, Warshaw AL: Villous tumors of the duodenum. Ann Surg 203:301–306, 1986.
64. Rosch T, Braig C, Gain T, et al: Staging of pancreatic and ampullary

carcinoma by endoscopic ultrasongraphy. Comparison with conventional sonography, computed tomography, and angiography. Gastroenterology 102:188–199, 1992.
65. Mukai H, Nakajima M, Yasuela K, et al: Evaluation of endoscopic ultrasonography in the preoperative staging of carcinoma of the ampulla of Vater and common bile duct. Gastrointest Endosc 38:676–683, 1992.
66. Quirk DM, Rattner DW, Castillo, FC, et al: The use of endoscopic ultrasonography to reduce the cost of treating ampullary tumors. Gastrointest Endosc 46:334-337, 1997.
67. Halsted WS: Contributions to the surgery of the bile passages, especially of the common bile duct. Boston Med J 141:645–654, 1899.
68. Binmoeller KF, Boaventura S, Ramsperger K, et al: Endoscopic snare excision of benign adenomas of the papilla of Vater. Gastrointestin Endosc 39:127–131, 1993.
69. Rattner DW, Fernandez-del Castillo C, Brugge WR, et al: Defining the criteria for local resection of ampullary neoplasms. Arch Surg 131:366–371, 1996.
70. Asburn HJ, Rossi RL, Munson JL: Local resection for ampullary tumors: Is there a place for it. Arch Surg 128:515–520, 1993.
71. Branum GD, Pappas TN, Meyers WC: The management of tumors of the ampulla of Vater by local resection. Ann Surg 224:621–627, 1996.
72. Bjork KJ, Davis CJ, Nagorney DM, et al: Duodenal villous tumors. Arch Surg 125:961–965, 1990.
73. Farnell MB, Sakorafas GH, Sarr MG, et al: Villous tumors of the duodenum: Reappraisal of local versus extended resection. J Gastrointest Surg 4:13–21, 2000.
74. Beger HG, Treitschke F, Poch P, et al: Adenoma of the ampulla of Vater: Operative treatment and results. In Beger HG, Warshaw AL, Buchler MW, Carr-Locke DL, Russell C, Sarr MG (eds): The Pancreas. Oxford, Blackwell Sciences, 1998, pp 1324–1327.
75. Tarazi RY, Hermann RF, Voyt DP: Results of surgical management of periampullary tumors: A 35-year experience. Surgery 100:716–723, 1986.
76. Klein P, Reingruber B, Kart LS, et al: Is local excision of $_pT_1$ ampullary carcinomas justified? Eur J Surg Oncol 22:366–371, 1996.
77. Talamini MA, Moesinger RC, Pitt HA, et al: Adenocarcinoma of the ampulla of Vater: A 28 year experience. Ann Surg 225:590–600, 1997.
78. Kalser MH, Ellenberg SS: Pancreatic cancer. Adjuvant combined radiation and chemotherapy following curative resection. Arch Surg 120: 899–903, 1985.
79. Gastrointestinal Tumor Study Group: Further evidence of effective adjuvant combined radiation and chemotherapy following curative resection of pancreatic cancer. Cancer 59:2006–2020, 1987.
80. Yeo CJ, Abrams RA, Grochow LB, et al: Pancreaticoduodenectomy for pancreatic adenocarcinoma: Postoperative adjuvant chemoradiation improves survival. A prospective, single-institution experience. Ann Surg 225:621–636, 1997.
81. Bakkevold KE, Arnesjo B, Dahl O, Kambestad B: Adjuvant combined chemotherapy (AMF) following radical resection of carcinoma of the pancreas and papilla of Vater—results of a controlled prospective, randomized multicentre trial. Eur J Cancer 29A:698–703, 1993.
82. Sohn TA, Lillemoe KD, Cameron JL, et al: Surgical palliation of unresectable periampullary adenocarcinoma in the 1990's. J Am Coll Surg 188:658–669, 1999.
83. Howe JR, Klimstra DS, Moccia RD, et al: Factors predictive of survival in ampullary carcinoma. Ann Surg 228:87–94, 1998.
84. Allema JH, Reinders ME, van Gulik TM, et al: Results of pancreaticoduodenectomy for ampullary carcinoma and analysis of prognostic factors for survival. Surgery 117:247–253, 1995.
85. Willett CG, Warshaw AL, Convery K, Compton CC: Patterns of failure after pancreaticoduodenectomy for ampullary carcinoma. Surg Gynecol Obstet 176:33-38, 1993.

Chapter 61

ENDOSCOPIC AND RADIOLOGIC TREATMENT OF BILIARY DISEASE

James W. Ostroff and Jeanne M. LaBerge

Since the early 1980s, there have been dramatic advances in the treatment of biliary disease. While traditional surgical approaches have been refined, new nonoperative techniques have been developed that have supplanted surgery in many situations. The subspecialties of interventional radiology and interventional gastroenterology have emerged in response to these technical developments, and biliary centers have been formed to foster an interdisciplinary approach to complicated problems.[1]

GENERAL PRINCIPLES

Endoscopic Versus Radiologic Approaches

The appropriate therapy for an individual patient depends on a number of factors, including the severity of the symptoms, location and extent of disease, age and health of the patient, and the patient's personal preference. The aims of nonoperative intervention typically include relief of symptomatic biliary obstruction, diversion of bile flow, and extraction of tissue for biopsy. Frequently, these aims can be accomplished with either percutaneous or endoscopic techniques. For example, biliary drainage, stricture dilation, and stone removal can be performed with either approach. Strict guidelines for selecting an endoscopic or radiologic approach are difficult to establish because technology is evolving rapidly and the success of each approach is greatly influenced by operator expertise.[2, 3] Table 61–1 summarizes selected advantages and disadvantages of each approach.

An Algorithm for Choosing Endoscopic Retrograde Cholangiopancreatography or Percutaneous Transhepatic Cholangiography

Local availability and expertise have a great impact on the method of diagnosis and therapy. Ideally, diagnostic methods should have minimal morbidity and great accuracy and should not restrict palliative or curative therapy. Therapy should be based solely on appropriateness and safety, taking into consideration the patient's expectations and preferences.

The traditional initial imaging methods of evaluating the patient with elevated liver biochemical tests and jaundice (extracorporal ultrasound [US], computed tomography with "thin-cut" sections [CT], endoscopic ultrasound [EUS], endoscopic retrograde cholangiopancreatography [ERCP], and percutaneous transhepatic cholangiography [PTC]) should be replaced by magnetic resonance cholangiopancreatography (MRCP) (see also Chapters 14 and 64). MRCP is becoming the preferred imaging technique for diagnosing possible biliary obstruction and for staging tumor size, assessing vascular invasion, and determining the level and degree of ductal obstruction. The current availability of MRCP is limited to larger medical centers, but the sensitivity with absence of morbidity associated with MRCP is apparent, and MRCP should replace diagnostic ERCP and PTC. MRCP provides three-dimentional images similar to those of ERCP and also visualizes intrasegmental bile duct dilation in liver segments.

ERCP remains the preferred invasive imaging modality because of its relatively low rate of serious morbidity (3% to 5%) and its ability to image and treat diseases of the bile duct, ampulla, pancreas, and duodenum. PTC is indicated only after a failed ERCP and in situations in which the anatomy precludes an ERCP, such as a long Roux-en-Y choledochojejunostomy. PTC may also be the preferred procedure or may serve as a complementary examination to ERCP when there is the need to evaluate the intrahepatic biliary tree above a high-grade biliary obstruction.

MRCP is the best and most sensitive noninvasive test for biliary obstruction. On some occasions, the patient can be taken directly for surgical therapy after MRCP. The use of MRCP as the sole preoperative examination will increase with the availability of MRCP. On some occasions, a patient will subsequently have a postoperative ERCP or PTC for

Table 61–1 | **Endoscopic versus Radiologic Diagnosis and Treatment**

CLINICAL VARIABLE	ENDOSCOPIC	PERCUTANEOUS
Visualization of ampulla	Preferred	—
Pancreatography	Preferred	—
Stenting neoplasms	Equal	Equal
Recovery time	Less	Greater
Morbidity	Less	Greater
Roux-en-Y choledocho-jejunostomy	—	Preferred
Complex intrahepatic stricture	—	Preferred

palliation of advanced disease found at surgery, treatment of choledocholithiasis, or management of a postoperative complication (Fig. 61–1).

Radiation Safety

In most cases, radiation exposure during ERCP or PTC is small; however, in some difficult cases with a prolonged procedure time, the radiation dose to the patient may be substantial and can produce symptoms. Immediate or delayed effects such as hair loss, skin burns, and blistering have been reported following procedures that require prolonged or continuous fluoroscopy exceeding several hours.[4] The effects of the radiation exposure during fluoroscopy depend on the total duration of fluoroscopy or the volume of tissue exposed and the sensitivity of the exposed organs to radiation. Exposure is quantified as the absorbed dose at the skin and is measured in grays (Gy).[5] Temporary hair loss is observed approximately 3 weeks following a single dose of 3 Gy, and transient erythema can be seen within several hours following a dose of 2 Gy. Radiation-induced cataracts can occur with a single direct dose of 2 Gy to the lens of the eye. The lifetime risk of radiation-induced neoplasia from low-level radiation exposure is more difficult to quantify. The mortality rate from radiation-induced leukemia may be as high as 0.050% for a 0.1-Gy exposure.

Radiation exposure to medical personnel comes chiefly from radiation scattered from the patient and is affected by the fluoroscopy time, volume of patient tissue exposed, distance from the patient, and amount and type of external shielding. Cumulative occupational dose is usually measured in rem or milliSieverts (mSv). (There is a mean natural background dose of 3 mSv in the United States from radon and other natural sources of radiation.) The National Council on Radiation Protection recommends an occupational dose limit of 50 mSv per year. Reported occupational radiation exposure among interventional radiologists varies from 0.37 to 10.1 mSv per year (Table 61–2).[6, 7]

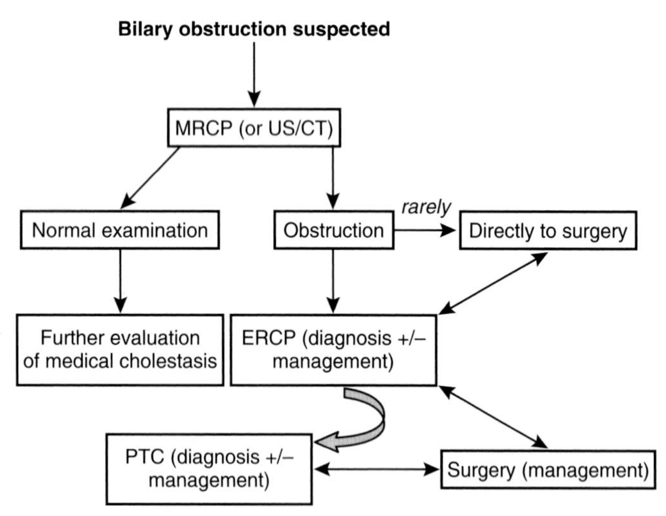

Figure 61–1. MRCP is the best initial diagnostic test for suspected biliary obstruction. If the biliary system is shown to be obstructed and further nonoperative diagnostic testing or therapy is warranted, then ERCP should be performed. If this is not possible, then a PTC is performed. On some occasions, an ERCP or PTC is required in the postoperative period for palliative therapy or for treatment of a surgical complication. As MRCP is further validated, patients may go directly to surgery after MRCP. (CT, computed tomography; ERCP, endoscopic retrograde cholangiopancreatography; MRCP, magnetic resonance cholangiopancreatography; PTC, percutaneous transhepatic cholangiopancreatography; US, ultrasound.)

Table 61–2 | **Measures to Reduce Radiation Exposure**

- Tightly collimate radiation beam to minimize exposed patient tissue.
- Limit fluoroscopy time: avoid continuous fluoroscopy.
- Stand as far as possible from patient.
- Implement quality improvement programs for equipment and radiation exposure.[141]

PROCEDURAL TECHNIQUES

Radiologic Intervention

A C-arm fluoroscopy unit with a tilting table is desirable for performing complex biliary intervention. Iodinated contrast material is used to opacify the biliary tree, and intravenous sedation and analgesia are routinely employed.[8] Intravenous antibiotics are generally administered prophylactically for most percutaneous biliary interventions.[9]

Percutaneous Transhepatic Cholangiography (PTC)

PTC was first attempted in the 1930s. Complications of bile leak, peritonitis, and sepsis frequently necessitated emergency biliary surgery. The risks of the procedure were markedly reduced with the substitution of a 22-gauge needle for the larger sheathed needle.[10] "Skinny needle" (22-gauge) PTC is now a widely accepted procedure.

When cholangiography is necessary, it is usually performed endoscopically. Diagnostic PTC is still required in special circumstances, such as complex hilar obstructions, failed ERCP, or the presence of a biliary-enteric anastomosis that precludes ERCP.

TECHNIQUE. With the patient lying supine, a 22-gauge needle is introduced into the liver parenchyma from a percutaneous puncture through the 10th or 11th intercostal space in the right midclavicular line. The needle is aimed toward the

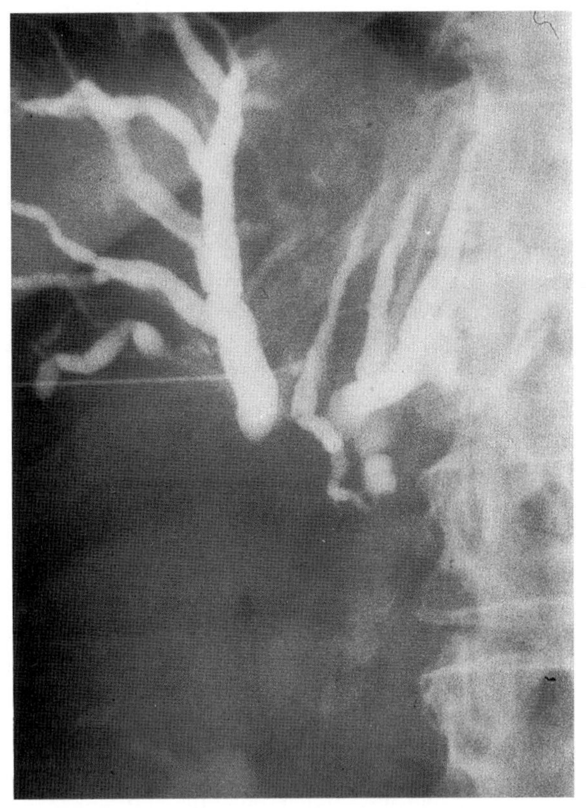

Figure 61–2. Percutaneous transhepatic cholangiography from a right transhepatic approach shows right-sided ductal obstruction in a 65-year-old woman with jaundice and a hilar mass on completed tomography that proved to be a cholangiocarcinoma on biopsy.

xiphoid and advanced through the liver parenchyma. As the needle is slowly withdrawn, contrast medium is injected under fluoroscopic observation (Fig. 61–2). Percutaneous cholangiography can also be accomplished by thin-needle opacification of the left hepatic duct using an epigastric approach (Fig. 61–3). A transcholecystic approach to opacify the biliary tree may be appropriate when transhepatic opacification is not possible. For example, in patients with anomalous biliary anatomy or nondilated ducts, injection of contrast material into the gallbladder may be used to opacify the intra- or extrahepatic biliary tree.[11]

RESULTS. The biliary tree can be visualized successfully in 99% of patients with dilated bile ducts and in 40% to 90% of those in whom the bile ducts are not dilated.[12] The overall rate of serious complications, including sepsis, bile leakage, and intraperitoneal hemorrhage, is approximately 2% to 4%.[13] The risk of bile leak and peritonitis may be greater with a transcholecystic approach. The frequency of sepsis is markedly reduced if the obstruction is relieved by subsequent percutaneous transhepatic drainage. High intercostal punctures may lead to pleural complications such as pneumothorax or bilious pleural effusions.

Percutaneous Transhepatic Biliary Drainage (PTBD)

PTBD was first undertaken in the early 1970s in an attempt to prevent the complications of bile leakage following needle sheath cholangiography in patients with biliary obstruction.[14, 15] A more secure catheter position is achieved by advancing an angiographic wire through the needle sheath into the biliary tree and then advancing the catheter over the wire into the bile duct.[16]

PTBD may be performed as a primary drainage procedure, or it may be performed as a prelude to another interventional procedure such as stricture dilation or stone removal. Temporary drainage is indicated in patients with sepsis or cholangitis. Permanent drainage is indicated for malignant biliary obstruction. Contraindications to PTBD include massive ascites and coagulopathy.

TECHNIQUE. Preprocedural CT, US, or ERCP may be helpful in determining the optimal transhepatic access route. Thin-needle PTC is usually performed at the beginning of

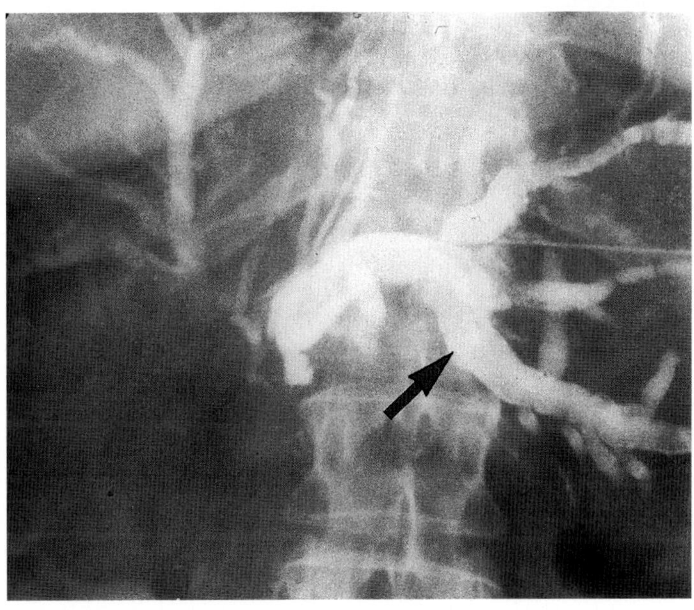

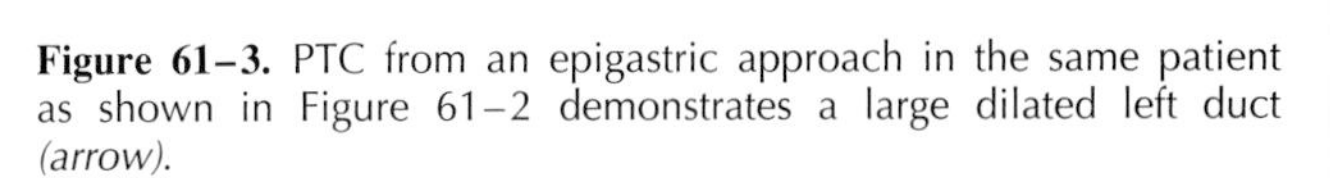

Figure 61–3. PTC from an epigastric approach in the same patient as shown in Figure 61–2 demonstrates a large dilated left duct *(arrow)*.

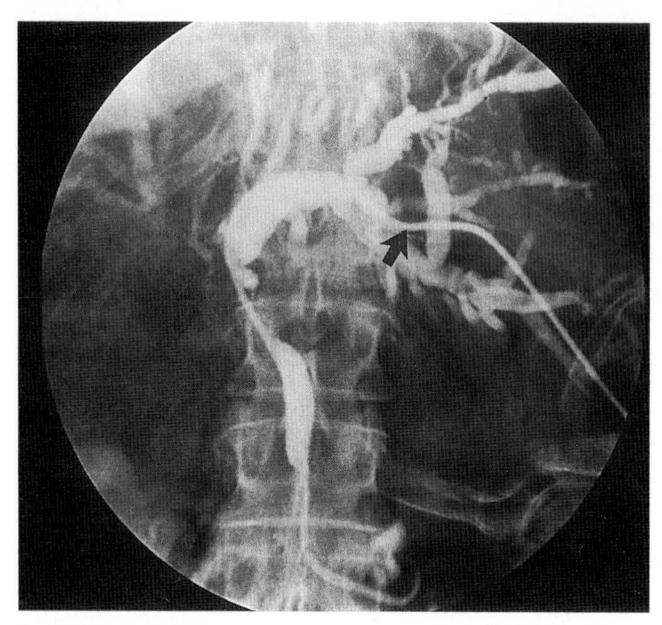

Figure 61–4. Transhepatic biliary drainage was performed in the patient depicted in Figures 61–2 and 61–3 using an epigastric approach to the left duct. A temporary internal external drain was placed *(arrow)*. Subsequently, a Wallstent was deployed to provide internal drainage.

the drainage procedure. Overdistention of an infected biliary system must be avoided. Real-time US guidance is used to facilitate duct selection.[17] A No. 5 French needle sheath is advanced into the duct, and a torquable wire is advanced within the biliary tree, through any obstructing lesions, into the duodenum. A drainage catheter is then advanced over the wire and positioned so that sideholes extend above and below the obstructing lesion. External drainage is achieved by connecting the catheter to an external drainage bag. Internal drainage into the duodenum can be achieved by capping the external portion of the catheter (Fig. 61–4).

The advantage of an external drainage catheter is that the catheter can easily be flushed and exchanged for a new one when necessary; however, the external portion is annoying to the patient, the skin entry is a site for potential infection, and the catheter inadvertently may be pulled out.

Access to the biliary tree is usually obtained by puncturing the right or left intrahepatic duct,[18] or both systems. Alternatively, both independently obstructed right and left systems can be drained from a single percutaneous access.[19]

Complications of PTBD include cholangitis, sepsis, bleeding, and bile leakage.[20–22] The most serious complication of PTBD is sepsis, which may occur in up to 10% of patients, although septic shock is unusual. Transient hemobilia is common, but severe bleeding is uncommon. Severe bleeding usually reflects injury to the hepatic artery, a complication that can be treated by angiographic embolization. Other complications observed in fewer than 1% of cases include bile leakage, hepatic abscesses, pancreatitis, and pleural effusion. Late complications of PTBD include skin infection and granuloma formation at the skin entry site. Carcinomatous extension along the catheter tract is exceedingly rare.[23]

Endoprosthesis

In 1978, Pereiras and colleagues reported on the successful insertion of a plastic endoprosthesis positioned above the ampulla.[24] Subsequently, a wide variety of plastic stents were developed in varying lengths, sizes, and shapes designed for placement either above or across the ampulla into the duodenum.[25] The major disadvantages of plastic endoprosthesis are discomfort because of the large size of the transhepatic tract necessary for stent placement (Nos. 12 to 14 French) and subsequent stent occlusion. The search for an improved endoprosthesis led to the development of the expandable metallic endoprosthesis in the 1990s.[26] These devices have the advantage that they can be placed through a small transhepatic tract (Nos. 8 to 10 French) but when deployed in the liver open to a large diameter (Nos. 24 to 30 French). Preliminary results suggest that the duration of patency of metallic stents is greater than that of plastic stents.[27]

Indwelling metallic endoprostheses are used for palliative treatment of malignant biliary obstruction. More recently, metallic endoprostheses have gained acceptance for the treatment of inoperable benign biliary strictures.[28–30] A variety of metallic stent designs are now in widespread use.[31] We have favored the Gianturco stent (Figs. 61–5, 61–6*A* and *B*) for patients with a benign biliary stricture and the Wallstent (Figs. 61–7, 61–8*A* and *B*) in patients with malignant biliary obstruction. Metallic stents are considered permanent and cannot be removed easily.

TECHNIQUE. The obstructed biliary segment is first delineated cholangiographically to determine the appropriate length and position for the endoprosthesis, which is then advanced over a transhepatic guidewire, positioned across the obstructing lesion, and deployed. A temporary drainage catheter is usually left in place for 24 hours to evacuate debris or thrombus. If repeat cholangiography performed 1 or 2 days after stent placement confirms adequate internal drainage, the external drain may be removed. The transhepatic tract heals within several days. Endoprostheses can be placed in patients with independently obstructed right and left ducts.[32]

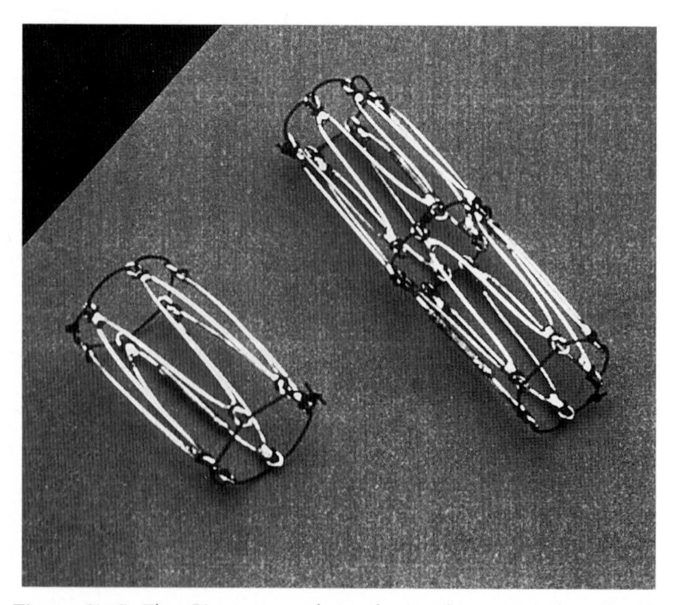

Figure 61–5. The Gianturco endoprosthesis. This stent is less flexible but has less wire mesh and improved radial force when compared with the Wallstent. It is very radiopaque and easy to position fluoroscopically.

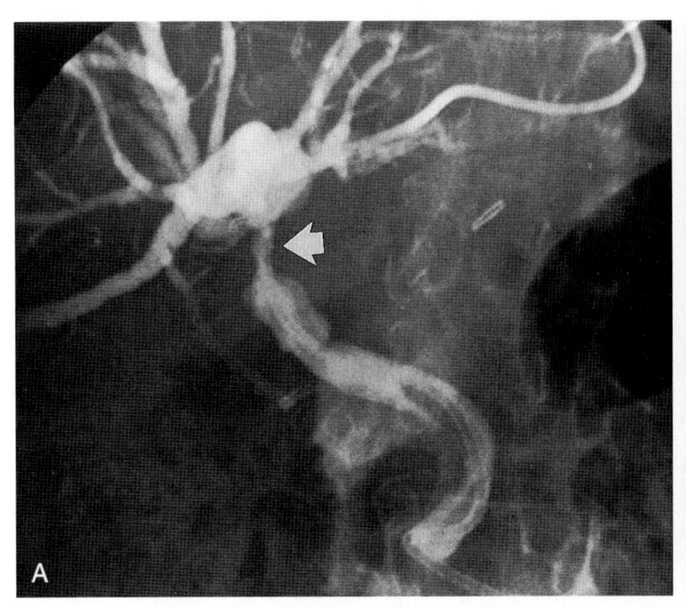

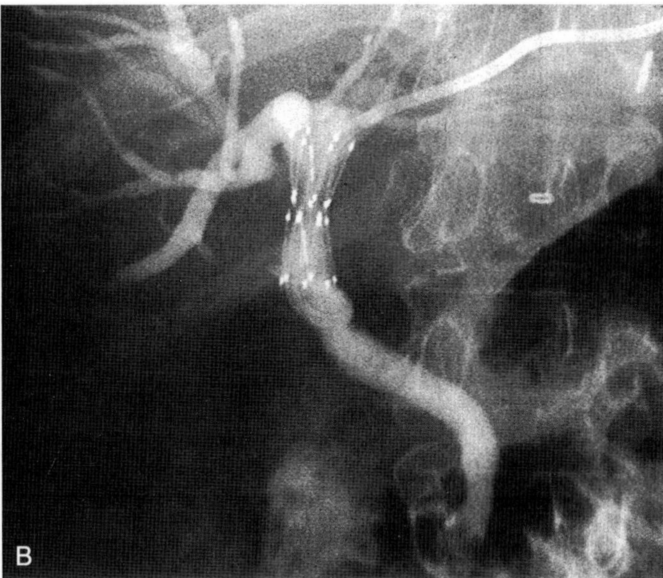

Figure 61–6. *A,* Cholangiogram showing an ischemic stricture of the common hepatic duct *(arrow)* in a liver transplantation patient. *B,* This patient was treated by placement of a single Gianturco stent. Postdeployment cholangiography shows a widely patent duct with restoration of normal luminal diameter.

RESULTS. Endoprostheses can be placed successfully in almost all patients with biliary obstruction. The average patency of both plastic and metallic stents appears to exceed 6 months.[33–35] Major complications, including sepsis, bleeding, and abscess formation, occur in 5% to 10% of patients.[36] The 30-day mortality rate has been reported to be 8%. Specific stent complications include occlusion, migration, and duodenal perforation. Occlusion may be caused by the accumulation of inspissated bile, sludge, and debris within the stent or growth of tumor through or around the stent.[37] Stent occlusion, leading to recurrent symptoms of jaundice, fever, and pruritus, develops in approximately one fourth of patients[27, 37] and is usually treated by repeat intervention and restenting. Stent migration is more common with plastic endoprostheses (up to 6%) than with metallic ones. Duodenal perforation is rare following placement of either plastic or metallic stents.

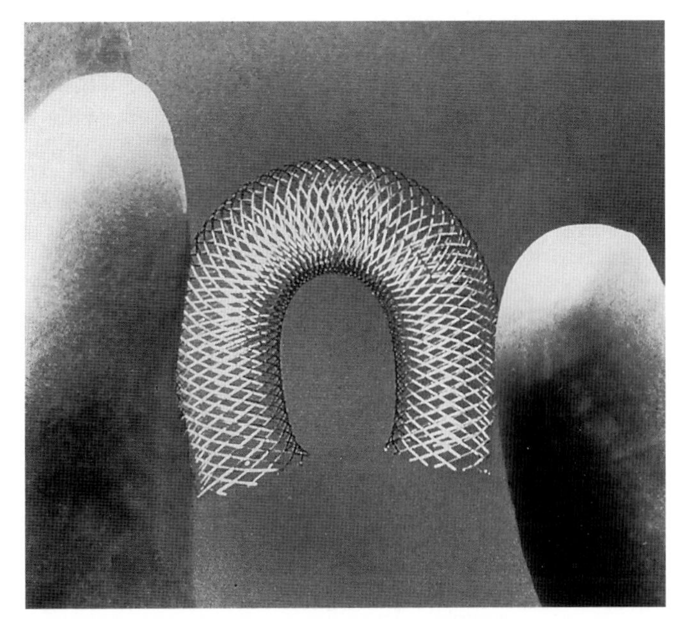

Figure 61–7. The Wallstent endoprosthesis. This is a flexible wire mesh stent that expands to a preset diameter.

Covering metallic stents with a synthetic material may lower the rate of tumor ingrowth and extend patency in patients treated for malignant biliary obstruction. Clinical trials with these "covered" metal stents are under way, but results to date are limited.[38]

Stricture Dilation

A nonoperative alternative to surgical resection was first introduced in 1978, when a Teflon-caged balloon was used successfully to dilate choledochoenterostomy strictures in 13 patients.[39] Subsequently, Gruntzig-type balloons were adapted for this purpose. Although success was achieved in some patients with a single dilation technique, a high frequency of restenosis led some investigators to incorporate repetitive dilations and long-term stenting with large-bore external catheters into the treatment regimen.[40] A new alternative strategy for the treatment of recurrent benign strictures is internal stenting with expandable metallic endoprostheses.[29]

Nonoperative management of benign biliary strictures should be considered in the following situations: intrahepatic strictures that are not amenable to operative repair, strictures that recur after operative repair, and strictures in patients at high operative risk. Stricture dilation should be avoided in the setting of cholangitis.

TECHNIQUE. Once the biliary tree has been catheterized, a wire is manipulated across the stricture. An angioplasty balloon catheter is then passed over the wire and centered across the stenotic area. Balloon size is chosen to match the size of the duct: 4- to 8-mm balloons are used in the intrahepatic system, and 6- to 10-mm balloons are used for extrahepatic stenosis. If a stricture is too tight to allow passage of an angioplasty balloon, the lesion can be predilated

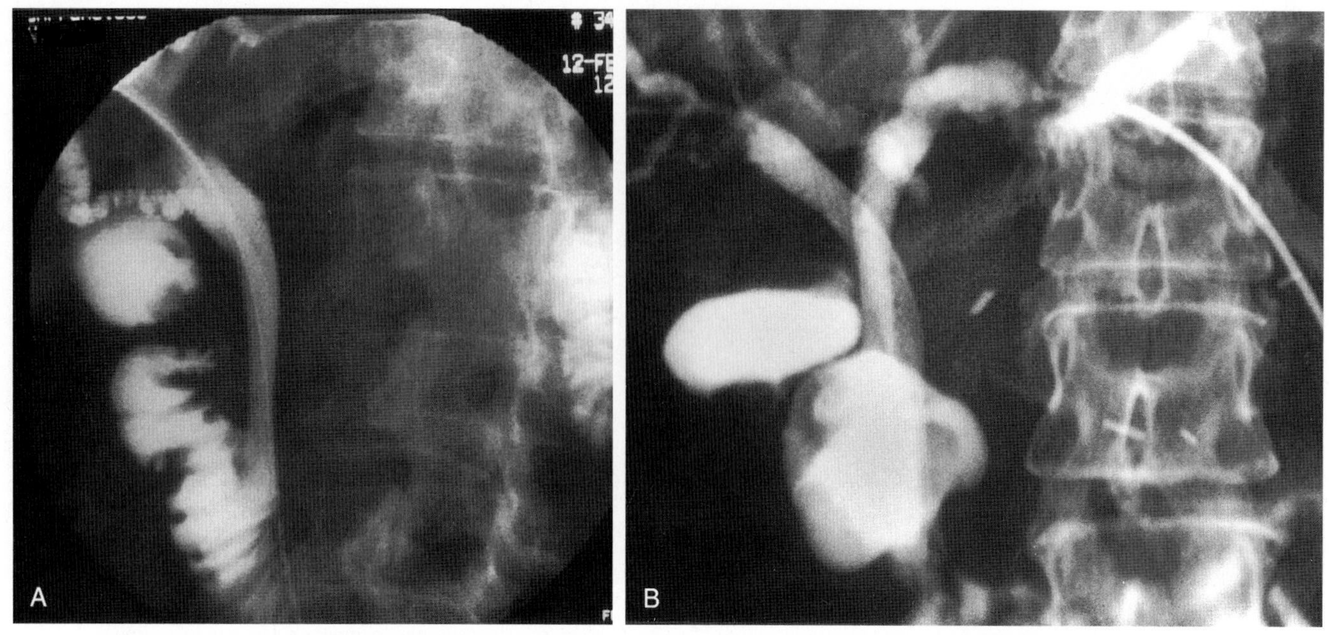

Figure 61–8. *A,* A single Wallstent is deployed in this patient with malignant obstruction of the distal duct. *B,* Bilateral Wallstents were deployed in this patient with malignant hilar obstruction.

with semirigid Teflon dilators. If long-term stenting is desired, a No. 12 to 18 French external biliary catheter is placed across the lesion. Alternatively, a permanent metallic stent can be deployed across the stenosis following balloon dilation.

RESULTS. Three-year patency rates of 67%, 76%, and 42% have been reported for anastomotic strictures, iatrogenic strictures, and sclerosing cholangitis, respectively.[41] Bleeding is an acute complication of stricture dilation but is usually self-limited. Pain occurs during balloon inflation but resolves following deflation.

When possible, surgical repair of a benign biliary stricture is preferrable to nonoperative dilation. In a comparative study, Pitt and colleagues[42] demonstrated that long-term patency was superior after surgery than after dilation (88% versus 55%).

Stone Removal

Percutaneous stone extraction through a T-tube tract was first described in the 1960s.[43] A modified angiographic technique for percutaneous stone removal with a retrieval basket and a steerable catheter is still used today. Additional adjunctive measures that have been employed include T-tube tract dilation, ultrasonic or electrohydraulic lithotripsy, and chemical stone dissolution.

Radiologic stone extraction is preferred for patients with an existing T-tube tract, whereas endoscopic sphincterotomy with stone extraction is preferred in patients without T-tube access. Transhepatic stone removal[44–46] or extracorporeal shock-wave lithotripsy (ESWL)[47, 48] may be employed if endoscopic therapy is unsuccessful in patients without T-tube access.

TECHNIQUE. Standard postcholecystectomy T-tube stone extraction is performed 4 to 6 weeks after surgery to allow time for the T-tube tract to mature. The T tube is withdrawn, and the tract is catheterized with a blunt-tipped steerable catheter (Meditech, Watertown, MA). Dilute contrast material is injected through the catheter to identify the stone(s). A Dormia-type retrieval basket is manipulated to entrap the stone, which is then withdrawn through the T-tube tract. Stone(s) larger than the diameter of the T-tube tract can be extracted by a variety of techniques: the tract can be dilated with an angioplasty balloon; a stone can be fragmented mechanically with a stone basket; or lithotripsy probes can be introduced through the T-tube tract to fragment the stone. Chemical dissolution with methyl-tert-butyl ether (MTBE)[51] is an investigational alternative therapy for large retained stones but is rarely used.

Techniques for stone extraction performed through a surgical jejunal loop are similar to those described earlier.[49] The large diameter of the jejunal access facilitates use of large-bore instruments such as a choledochoscope or ultrasonic/electrohydraulic lithotripsy probes.[50] Transhepatic stone removal is accomplished through an existing transhepatic biliary drainage tract. Using standard basket or balloon catheters, the stone is pushed into the duodenum. If the stone is large and cannot be pushed easily into the duodenum, the ampulla may be predilated with an angioplasty balloon.

RESULTS. The overall success rate of stone removal performed through a T-tube tract approaches 95%.[43] Failures of conventional technique may occur when a stone is impacted or larger than 1 cm. Success with transhepatic stone removal has been reported in over 90% of cases in recent studies when adjunctive ampullary dilation or chemical dissolution is used.[44, 45]

A complication rate of less than 5% has been reported for conventional T-tube stone extraction. Cholangitis and pancreatitis occur infrequently. Bleeding and subscapular hematoma can result from transhepatic stone removal. Systemic absorption of MTBE can result in sedation and pain, but if properly administered, side effects from MTBE are minor.[51] Complications of ESWL, which occur in 8% to 25% of patients treated for common bile duct (CBD) stones, include hemobilia, biliary sepsis, abdominal pain, liver hematoma, skin ecchymosis, and hematuria[47, 48]; however, complications requiring further therapy are uncommon.

Percutaneous Cholecystostomy

Percutaneous cholecystostomy (PC) was first performed under fluoroscopic guidance in the 1960s for emergency decompression of gallbladders that had been punctured inadvertently during PTC. However, fear of bile leak and peritonitis delayed broad acceptance of this procedure. In the 1980s, several large series of successful PCs established the safety of this technique.[52–54] Modifications in catheter design and increased familiarity with the procedure have improved the ease and safety of the procedure. Although most patients with acute gallbladder disease undergo surgical cholecystectomy, PC is indicated in specific circumstances, such as acute cholecystitis in a patient who is at high risk for operative cholecystectomy. PC also may be performed as a means of biliary decompression in patients in whom standard PTBD is difficult (i.e., patients with nondilated intrahepatic bile ducts).[55]

TECHNIQUE. The procedure can be performed at the bedside under US guidance alone or, preferably, a combination of US and fluoroscopic guidance. Two approaches may be used to puncture the gallbladder: an anterior transperitoneal approach is used if there is no bowel between the skin and gallbladder, and a transhepatic route is used if there is intervening bowel. The gallbladder is initially localized with real-time US guidance, and a puncture site is selected. The gallbladder is then punctured with either a 22- or 18-gauge needle. Bile is aspirated through the needle, and then a wire is coiled into the gallbladder. Fluoroscopy is used to confirm the position of the wire within the gallbladder and to monitor the subsequent placement of a drainage catheter. A No. 10 or 12 French pigtail catheter with multiple sideholes is inserted over the wire and secured to the skin. A removable metallic anchor can be used to affix the gallbladder to the anterior abdominal wall.

RESULTS. The procedure can be performed in almost all patients. Technical success can be expected in 95% to 100%.[52] PC is an effective means of gallbladder decompression and appears to be a beneficial therapy for acute calculous and acalculous cholecystitis.[56] Progression of gallbladder disease has been reported but is rare.[53] Because of the difficulty of making a definitive diagnosis of acute cholecystitis without surgery, the effectiveness of this therapy in treating patients with acute cholecystitis is not well defined; however, the technique is gaining popularity in the treatment of debilitated or severely ill patients with acalculous cholecystitis.[57–59] Patients with pericholecystic fluid and symptoms referable to the gallbladder appear to have the highest response rate.[60]

The overall complication rate is low (8%)[56]; complications include bile leak, pain, hemorrhage, and catheter dislodgement. Bile peritonitis from a bile leak—the most common complication of this procedure—has occurred only after a cholecystostomy catheter had been dislodged inadvertently; the use of a locking pigtail catheter can prevent this complication. Additionally, an anchoring device designed to afix the gallbladder to the abdominal wall may diminish the risk of bile leak.[61] Sepsis can be prevented by not overdistending the gallbladder during catheter placement.

Endoscopic Intervention

ERCP was first described by McCune and coworkers in 1968.[62] Technologic advances in video endoscopy have improved image resolution, facilitated the teaching of advanced procedures, and permitted the digitization of radiographic and endoscopic images. Endoscopic intervention is performed with sedation and analgesia and only rarely under general anesthesia. The side-viewing duodenoscope has a viewing field that is perpendicular to the long axis of the instrument to permit better visualization of the medial wall of the descending duodenum, the usual location of the duodenal papilla. The ability to cannulate the biliary tree selectively and perform diagnostic ERCP is the first step in all therapeutic procedures.[63, 64] Various diagnostic and therapeutic duodenoscopes are available with channels of different sizes. "Mother-daughter" scopes and cholangioscopes that can be inserted through a 4.2-mm channel are available. Although forward-viewing instruments may permit localization of the papilla more easily in a patient with a Billroth II gastrojejunostomy,[65–67] a side-viewing duodenoscope is still preferred because of its elevator. The most versatile approach is to use a small-diameter duodenoscope with a 4.2-mm channel for all interventions. Reliable reusable accessories will keep costs down.[68, 69]

Complications associated with diagnostic and therapeutic endoscopic cholangiography include infection, bleeding, pancreatitis,[70–74] retroduodenal perforation,[75] and an impacted stone or basket. Complications of varying severity occur in 5% to 10% of endoscopic biliary interventions, and experience results in fewer complications.[76] It is likely that perforation and pancreatitis occur more frequently in patients with papillary stenosis, and bleeding is more frequent in patients with papillary tumors. The use of somatostatin or gabexate mesilate to prevent pancreatitis may have some benefit, but many concerns limit their use, including efficacy, choice of patient, ease of administration, and cost.[77] In general, there does not appear to be an increased risk of complications in patients with a duodenal diverticulum.[75] It is possible that patients with an obstructed cystic duct are at increased risk of developing acute cholecystitis after endoscopic sphincterotomy (ES) for CBD stones.[76] Late complications of ERCP and ES include acute cholecystitis, stenosis of the papilla, cholangitis, and retained or new stones.[77] Previous surgery, such as a Billroth II gastrojejunostomy or Roux-en-Y choledochojejunostomy, makes ERCP difficult or impossible.[65, 67] There can be a greater major complication rate in patients with a Billroth II anastomosis, in particular bowel perforation in the afferent limb, which may require surgical intervention.[78] Uncorrectable coagulopathy also is associated with an increased risk and may represent a contraindication to ERCP and ES. It is likely that inexperience of the biliary endoscopist who performs the procedure (<200 cases per year) and the use of a "pre-cut" technique to gain access to the bile duct are independent risk factors for major complications.[79] The routine use of antibiotics prior to ERCP is controversial,[79] but it appears that oral antibiotic prophylaxis in patients undergoing therapeutic ERCP is both safe and less costly than intravenous antibiotics.[80, 81] Adequate sedation is of the utmost importance, and if standard sedation and analgesia are not possible or too dangerous, general anesthesia must be considered. Midazolam (a benzodiazepine) and meperidine (a narcotic) are generally employed. The addition of droperidol is often useful in the patient who is difficult to sedate[83] (see also Chapter 30).

The duodenal papilla is usually identified without difficulty. In patients with a normal anatomy, cannulation is usually successful, but to approach a 95% success rate, a pre-cut papillotomy may be needed to unroof the bile duct.[83–87] Neither cholangitis nor pancreatitis is a contraindication to ERCP if a therapeutic modality is being considered. Competence in therapeutic ERCP requires additional specialized training with continued mentoring[88] and proctoring. When an attempt at ERCP fails, the patient should be referred to a more experienced biliary endoscopist; success rates of over 96% with a complication rate of approximately 10% should be expected.[89, 90] The storing of data and images is particularly important with these therapeutic procedures in order to delineate the precise anatomy for surgical and radiologic colleagues. Usually, a patient can be discharged home after a therapeutic ERCP. Persons who have pain after the procedure, a history of pancreatitis, suspected sphincter of Oddi dysfunction, or cirrhosis or who had a difficult cannulation of the bile duct or underwent a "pre-cut" sphincterotomy appear to be at higher risk for a complication and can be hospitalized overnight for observation.[91, 92]

Endoscopic Sphincterotomy

ES is the preferred therapy for retained CBD stones and is successful in more than 90% of cases.[93–96]

TECHNIQUE. The sphincter muscle is cut at the ampulla with a unipolar blended current applied through a sphincterotome (a Teflon catheter with a threaded piece of conducting wire at its end). Sphincterotomes have different configurations: pull, push, and needle-knife, depending on their use.[84]

The landmark that helps determine the safe extent of the cut is the intraduodenal portion of the CBD. As a general rule, the incision of the sphincterotomy is stopped when it reaches the transverse fold located superior to the papilla. There can be variability of the blood supply to this area, especially in the presence of a diverticulum.[97, 98] The cut is performed with short bursts of current, so that the disruption is accomplished with minimal transmural burn and good coagulation. Most sphincterotomes accept a guidewire, which provides greater security. The size of the sphincterotomy is determined by the therapeutic objectives (i.e., when a large stone is to be removed, the cut required is larger than that required when the papillary opening must be enlarged slightly to permit ease of placement of an endoprosthesis). Occasionally a pre-cut sphincterotomy is performed to assist passage of the diagnostic catheter, and on some occasions a needle-knife is employed in place of a sphincterotome to gain access to a totally obstructed duct system or one that cannot be cannulated otherwise. Rarely, a choledochoduodenal fistula may be created in the supra-ampullary area when the ampulla is totally occluded by a tumor or stone (Figs. 61–9 to 61–13).

COMPLICATIONS. In most cases, complications of sphincterotomy resolve spontaneously. Cholangitis and acute cholecystitis may require drainage, decompression, or surgery. Bleeding that requires blood transfusions is unusual and typically stops spontaneously, although endoscopic, angiographic, or surgical hemostasis may be required. Endoscopic approaches, including electrocautery, tamponade, and epinephrine injection, are usually successful.[70, 98] A small contained retroduodenal perforation is best managed nonoperatively with nasogastric suction and antibiotics.[99] If a free perforation is present, surgical repair should be considered.

Nasobiliary Drainage

Nasobiliary drainage involves placement of a specialized catheter, which is "anchored" in the biliary tree via a pigtail-like end; the other end is brought out through the duodenal papilla via the stomach to the mouth and then the nose. This procedure is employed when the therapeutic objectives are to divert the bile flow away from a leak, drain an obstructed or infected system until definitive therapy can be performed, or visualize the biliary tree to access a leak or before ESWL. A nasobiliary catheter can be used for the instillation of various agents to dissolve stones[100] or for the insertion of radioactive wires for radiotherapy.[101–106] It is particularly useful for relieving biliary obstruction. The advantages of a nasobiliary catheter over a stent are that it permits later injection of contrast material so that the biliary tree can be studied, it can be removed without the need for repeat endoscopy, and it can be gently irrigated if it occludes. Unfortunately, some persons do not tolerate a tube coming out through the nose, and a confused or agitated patient may remove it inadvertently (Fig. 61–14).

TECHNIQUE. Nasobiliary catheters are 5 to 7 French in diameter and do not require ES or even a special therapeutic duodenoscope for placement. A guidewire is placed into the biliary tree above the leak or proximal obstruction, and the nasobiliary catheter is advanced over this guidewire and initially brought out through the mouth; a naso-oral catheter is then used to redirect the nasobiliary catheter through the nose. The catheter is generally placed to dependent drainage until definitive therapy is carried out.

Endoprosthesis Placement

Biliary endoprostheses are usually placed for malignant obstruction, to palliate pruritus, and occasionally to permit chemotherapy or chemoembolization, which may be precluded by jaundice. Other indications may include prevention of stone impaction, dilation of benign strictures, and bridging disruptions in the bile duct. The prostheses are usually plastic and can be straight or curved in a hockey-stick, pigtail, or double pigtail configuration to prevent displacement.[107–111] Recently, expandable metal stents have become popular. Their major advantage is that they can be

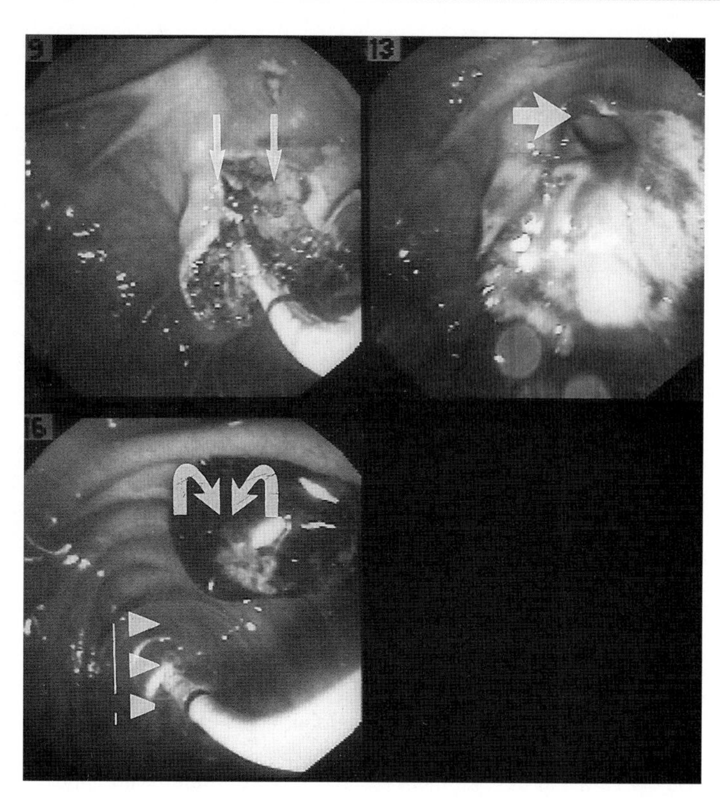

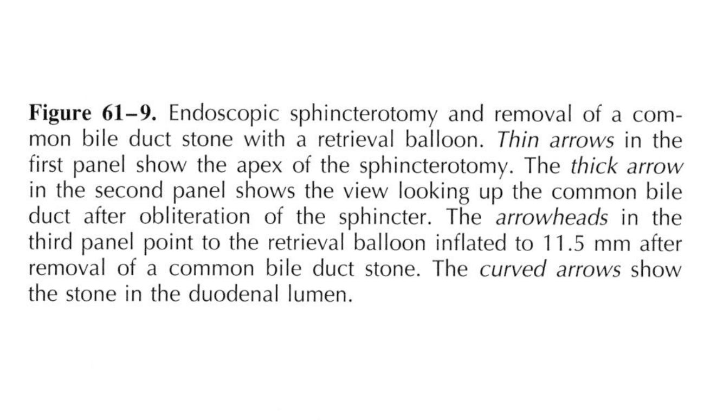

Figure 61–9. Endoscopic sphincterotomy and removal of a common bile duct stone with a retrieval balloon. *Thin arrows* in the first panel show the apex of the sphincterotomy. The *thick arrow* in the second panel shows the view looking up the common bile duct after obliteration of the sphincter. The *arrowheads* in the third panel point to the retrieval balloon inflated to 11.5 mm after removal of a common bile duct stone. The *curved arrows* show the stone in the duodenal lumen.

inserted with a relatively small delivery system yet produce a large-diameter stent.[112, 113] Disadvantages of metal stents include the potential for ingrowth of neoplastic tissue, accumulation of debris, and the inability to be removed. They remain patent longer than plastic stents but are more costly. Recently developed coiled stents may be removable. The development of a coated metal stent that might prevent tumor ingrowth has been hampered by the tendency of these stents to migrate out of the ducts. Patients with a distal bile duct neoplasm and limited life expectancy are probably served equally well with a plastic stent.[114, 115] Occlusions of metal stents are managed by removal of debris with baskets and snares as well as placement of new stents within the existing stents[116] (Figs. 61–15 and 61–16).

TECHNIQUE. Dilation or a small papillotomy may be necessary to facilitate insertion of the prosthesis. Stents of varying

Figure 61–10. Cholangiogram in a patient with choledocholithiasis. The *arrows* point to multiple stones in the common bile duct. The common bile duct is dilated to nearly 11.3 mm, the same size as the shaft of the duodenoscope.

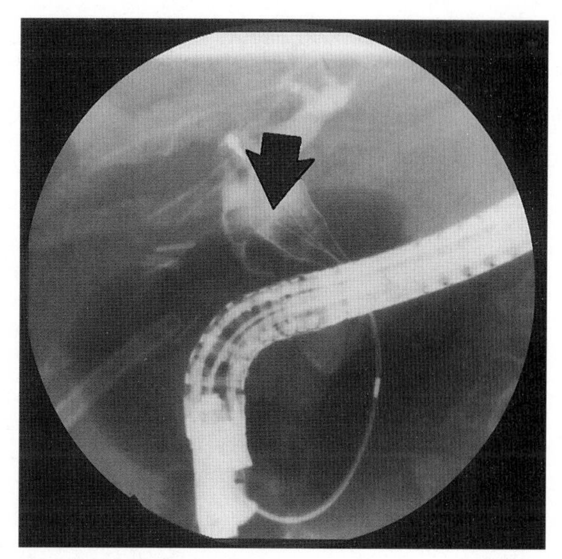

Figure 61–11. Another patient with choledocholithiasis in whom cholangiography shows multiple stones as dark irregular objects in the common bile duct. There is a basket in the common bile duct *(arrow)*.

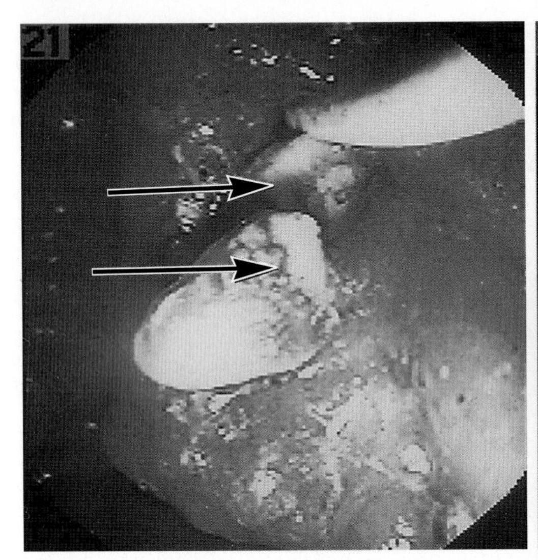

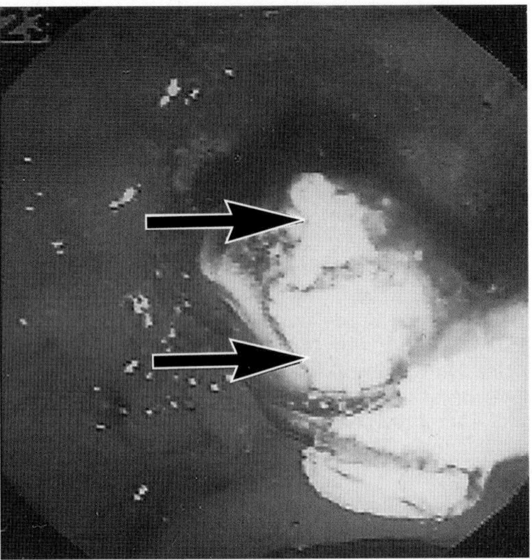

Figure 61–12. Extraction of stones from the bile duct after endoscopic sphincterotomy. *Thin arrows* in the left panel point to several stones being brought into the duodenum. The *thick arrows* in the right panel point to the stone trapped in the basket in Figure 61–11.

sizes (No. 10 to 12 French) are available. There is no proven advantage to a No. 11.5 or 12 French stent over a No. 10 stent with respect to drainage or the frequency of occlusion or subsequent complications, and a No. 10 French stent is easier to insert.[117] It is possible that new materials may permit the development of stents with thinner walls and a larger internal diameter.

Impregnation of the stent with antibiotics has been advocated, but the efficacy of this technique in preventing plugging has not been proved. Occlusion of the stent is assumed to be secondary to a bacterial biofilm. Some evidence suggests that elimination of sideholes may decrease colonization of the stent and prolong patency. Placement of the stent entirely within the bile duct, with no papillotomy, may also improve stent survival.[118, 119]

Figure 61–13. Large stone measuring 2 cm within a basket *(arrows)* in the bile duct before mechanical lithotripsy.

Larger plastic stents require a large-channel endoscope, and a 4.2-mm channel is generally required to place stents with an outer diameter of No. 11.5 French. Improvements in the handling characteristics of large therapeutic video duodenoscopes have permitted the diagnostic ERCP, papillotomy, and stent placement to be done easily with the same scope (Figs. 61–17 and 61–18).

RESULTS. Early complications of stent placement are usually related to the papillotomy. The most common complication

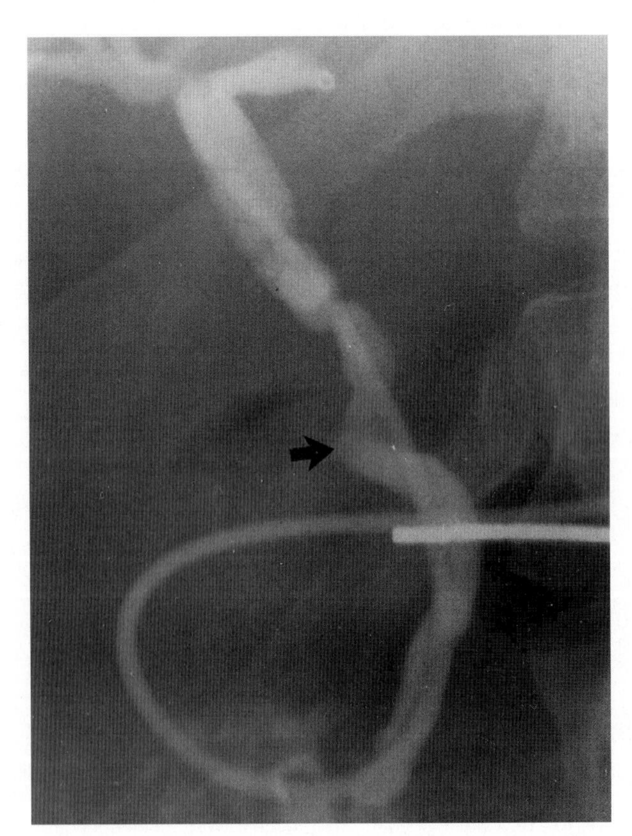

Figure 61–14. A nasobiliary catheter in the common bile duct. The *arrow* points to an earlier leak at a T-tube insertion site that closed after 3 days of biliary diversion.

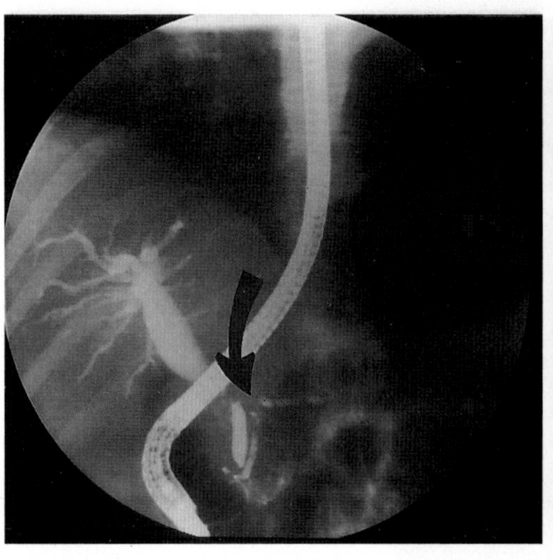
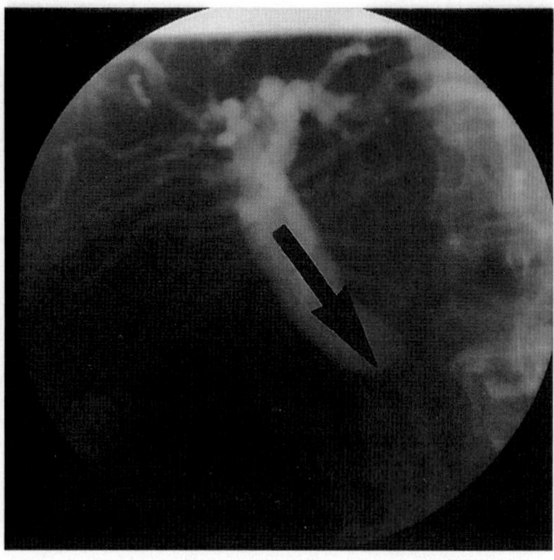

Figure 61–15. Placement of a plastic stent in a patient with carcinoma of the pancreas obstructing the common bile duct. Note the pancreatic duct stricture at the *curved arrow* at the same level as a biliary obstruction, the double-duct sign. The *straight arrow* reveals the shelf of the extrinsically obstructing cancer with a plastic stent placed through the obstructing lesion.

is sepsis secondary to occlusion and displacement of the endoprosthesis. When the patient has benign disease or a slowly growing neoplasm, stent occlusion may occur, and the stent must be changed periodically. Some endoscopists change stents routinely after several months to prevent obstruction and sepsis; others wait for symptoms to develop. We advocate the latter approach in malignant disease, because the average patency of 6 months (ranging from less than 1 month to more than 12 months) often exceeds the mean survival time for patients with advanced malignant disease. Our experience is that occlusion usually presents with mild "sentinel" manifestations, including a rising serum alkaline phosphatase level, low-grade fever, and chills, which signal the need for antibiotics and removal of the obstructed prosthesis.

The success rate of endoprosthesis placement approaches 90%. The success in establishing effective drainage with a single stent is higher for distal than proximal lesions; that is, a lesion at the biliary bifurcation is more difficult to drain effectively than a periampullary lesion. Cholangitis that is associated with endoprosthesis placement is more likely to occur with hilar than distal tumors.

Stricture Dilation

TECHNIQUE. The stent is passed over a guidewire through the obstructed lesion. A tight stricture may prevent passage of a No. 5 French diagnostic ERCP catheter or even the standard guidewire. Often a soft "high-torque" wire has to be advanced through the stricture followed by a hollow catheter and then an exchange for a standard guidewire before dilation can actually be started. A dilating catheter (up to 11.5 French) is used initially, followed by a Gruntzig-type balloon for further dilation up to about No. 30 French

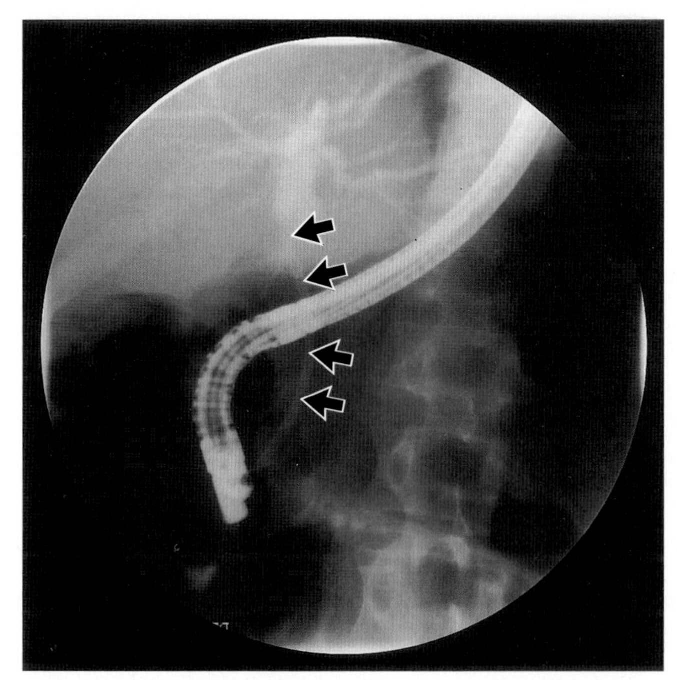

Figure 61–16. *Arrows* along the length of a No. 10 French 9-cm straight stent that is draining the biliary tree.

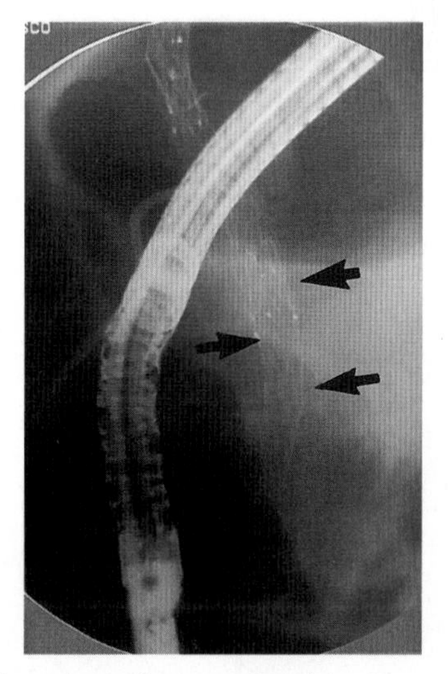

Figure 61–17. Several metal stents placed in an overlapping manner (*arrows*) in a patient with retroperitoneal adenopathy from an advanced breast cancer and with deep jaundice and severe pruritus. The bile duct was obstructed along most of its extrahepatic course and was braced open with these stents.

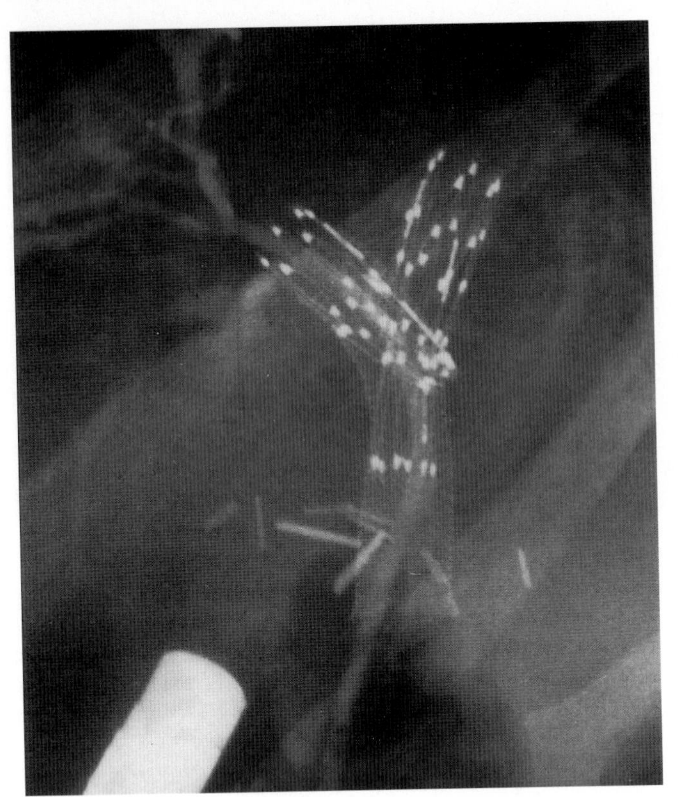

Figure 61–18. Multiple metal and plastic stents in the bile duct of a patient with cholangiocarcinoma who survived for 2 years. Each stent was placed after bouts of obstruction from tumor overgrowth and stasis.

(10 mm), which is performed at 4 to 6 atm pressure.[120–122] With inflation, the "waist" of the balloon disappears. Following dilation, the stricture may be stented temporarily with a stent having a diameter smaller than the maximum diameter of the balloon (Fig. 61–19).

Stone Removal

Except under exceptional circumstances (aberrant anatomy or uncorrectable coagulopathy), an ES is performed as the initial procedure in removing stones in the biliary tree. Stones in the CBD may pass spontaneously with the initial gush of bile, or they may be easily retrieved with an occlusion balloon.[93, 123, 124] When the bile duct cannot be entered, a needle-knife is used to cut into the duct. The safety of this technique is operator-dependent; bleeding, perforation, and incomplete cuts occur more commonly in inexperienced hands. With dilation of the bile duct and increasing size of the intraduodenal ductal segment, the risk of using the needle-knife is lower (Fig. 61–20*A* and *B*).

Balloon dilation of the papilla prior to removal of small stones has achieved some popularity because of uncertainty about the long-term effects of ES and the desire to eliminate its associated risks. The papilla is dilated, the stone is extracted, and the competence of the papilla is preserved.[125]

The practicality of long-term use of an endoprosthesis for stone disease is questionable, particularly when the projected survival of the patient exceeds 1 year. There is a risk of sepsis despite the use of oral ursodeoxycholic acid to prolong patency of plastic stents. The use of metal stents for stone disease is untested; they typically occlude within 1 year and cannot be removed.[126, 127]

Treatment of very large stones (larger than 1.5 cm) may require more sophisticated techniques, such as (1) mechanical lithotripsy,[128] (2) laser lithotripsy[129] with a cholangioscope to visualize the stone prior to laser lithotripsy, or (3) ESWL after placement of a nasobiliary catheter to target the stone correctly. If a stone is left behind, it is often advisable to leave a short stent or nasobiliary catheter in place to prevent impaction in the ampulla until definitive therapy is undertaken.[108] Very large stones that cannot be removed from a low-risk patient represent an indication for surgery. Generally, in patients in whom choledocholithiasis and cholecystolithiasis coexist, the common bile duct stones are removed via ERCP, and a laparoscopic cholecystectomy is then performed. In persons who have not subsequently undergone a cholecystectomy after an ERCP and ES, the risk of acute cholecystitis is approximately 5.9% after a mean follow-up of 7.7 years (see Chapter 56).[130]

Combined Endoscopic-Radiologic Approach

Endoscopic intervention requires successful cannulation of the CBD, which sometimes is not possible. Large duodenal

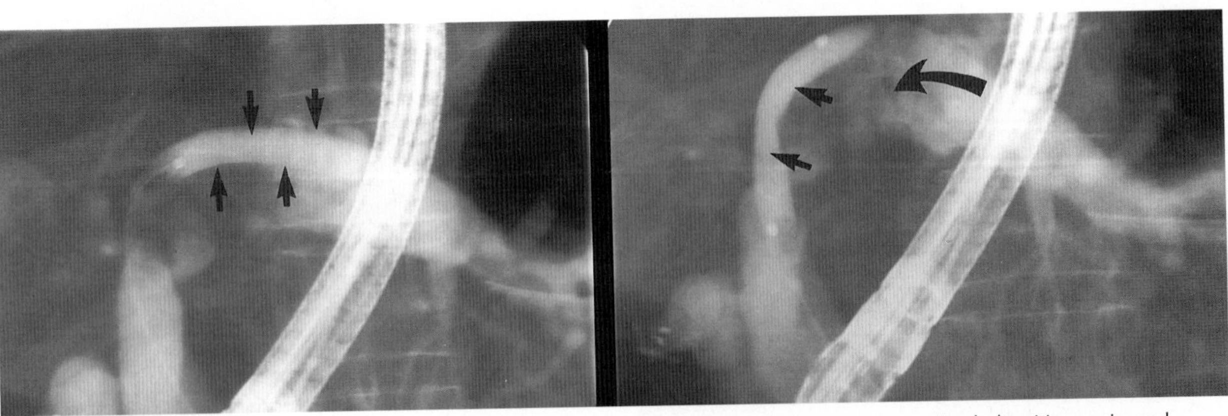

Figure 61–19. In the left panel, balloon dilation of a stricture in a patient with recurrent pyogenic cholangitis, sepsis, and jaundice. A high-grade stricture was present at the take-off of the left hepatic duct. A 4-mm dilating balloon *(short arrows)* is inflated across the stricture. In the right panel, the balloon exhibits a waist at the level of the stricture *(short arrows)*. The *curved arrow* points to multiple stones proximal to the stricture in the left main hepatic duct.

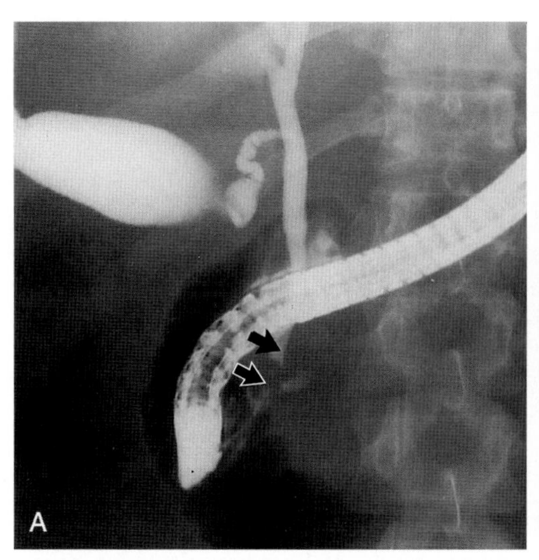

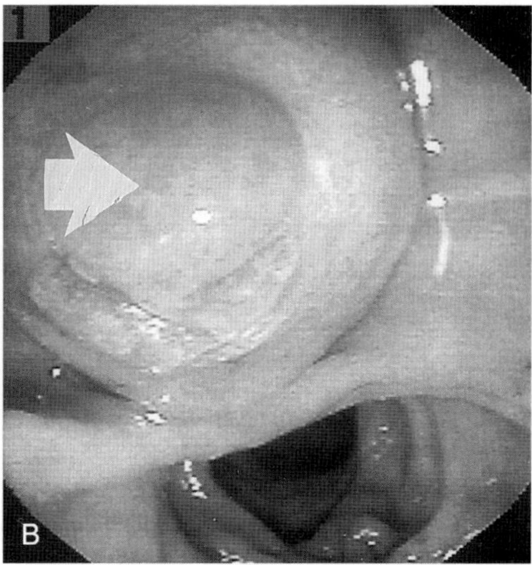

Figure 61–20. *A*, Impacted common bile stone in a common channel *(straight arrows)* in a patient who presented with severe acute pancreatitis. The stone is obstructing both the biliary tree and the pancreatic duct. The serum amylase level remained elevated. *B*, On duodenoscopy, the papilla is markedly enlarged and edematous *(short white arrow)* because of an impacted stone. A needle-knife was used to enter the bile duct.

diverticula, postoperative alteration of anatomy (Billroth II or Roux-en-Y anastomosis), exophytic ampullary tumors, and tight strictures of the distal CBD may preclude cannulation. When endoscopic catheterization is not possible, a combined transhepatic and endoscopic approach may be successful. This approach has been used to facilitate sphincterotomy, stone removal, and stent placement.[1, 132] Occasionally a combined procedure may be needed to reposition, remove, or clean out a previously placed percutaneous stent.[132–136]

TECHNIQUE. With the patient in a supine position, transhepatic biliary drainage is performed in the standard fashion. Once a guidewire has been advanced into the duodenum, a No. 5 French sheath is advanced over the wire so that the tip is within the biliary tree. A long exchange wire is then placed into the duodenum. The catheter entry site is covered with a sterile dressing, and the patient is placed in the prone, oblique position. A duodenoscope is passed in the usual manner and advanced until the ampulla and the angiographic exchange wire are visible. The endoscopist then engages the tip of the wire with a snare and pulls it out as the wire is fed in through the transhepatic catheter with sterile technique. Once the free end of the wire has been pulled out through the biopsy channel of the endoscope, the wire can be used for sphincterotomy, stone removal, or stent placement in the standard fashion. Following completion of the endoscopic procedure, the patient is returned to the supine position. A No. 5 or 6 French drainage catheter is positioned within the biliary tree to provide temporary drainage for 24 to 28 hours. The transhepatic catheter may be removed the following day if cholangiography demonstrates free flow of contrast material into the duodenum.

RESULTS. Combined procedures can be accomplished successfully in most cases. Robertson and colleagues have reported a success rate for stent insertion with this technique of 90%.[131] The chief disadvantages of the combined approach are the combined morbidity of transhepatic catheterization and endoscopic intervention and the requirement for temporary external biliary drainage. Fortunately, the small size of the transhepatic catheter required for a combined procedure minimizes the pain and risk associated with transhepatic catheterization, and complications are infrequent.

TREATMENT OF SPECIFIC DISEASES

Benign Diseases

Postoperative Complications

Complications of biliary surgery include strictures, bile leaks, and sump syndrome (see Chapter 56). The initial management of a suspected bile duct injury must begin with diagnostic cholangiography. The type and extent of nonoperative intervention will be determined by the anatomic site of the bile duct injury.

STRICTURES. The most common cause of benign biliary strictures is previous biliary tract surgery (Fig. 61–21). Symptoms of cholangitis or jaundice caused by strictures usually occur within 2 years of surgery. Surgical repair is successful in 90% of cases but is difficult in patients with multiple previous operations or intrahepatic strictures.[137] Nonoperative therapy is indicated in patients who are at high risk for surgery (e.g., patients with cirrhosis and portal hypertension) or who have a stricture in a nonoperable site (e.g., high in the porta hepatis or in the intrahepatic ducts).

Radiologic intervention for postoperative strictures consists of a combination of balloon dilation, external stenting with large-bore catheters (No. 12 to 20), and more recently, stenting with internal metallic endoprostheses (No. 24 to 30). Long-term clinical improvement has been reported in several series in over 50% of cases.[41] Biliary-enteric anastomotic strictures may respond better than nonanastomotic strictures of the duct to dilation. If restenosis occurs following dilation and external stenting, stenting with a metallic endoprosthesis may be indicated.[30] Complications associated with metallic endoprostheses include stent migration and occlusion caused by mucosal hyperplasia within the stent.

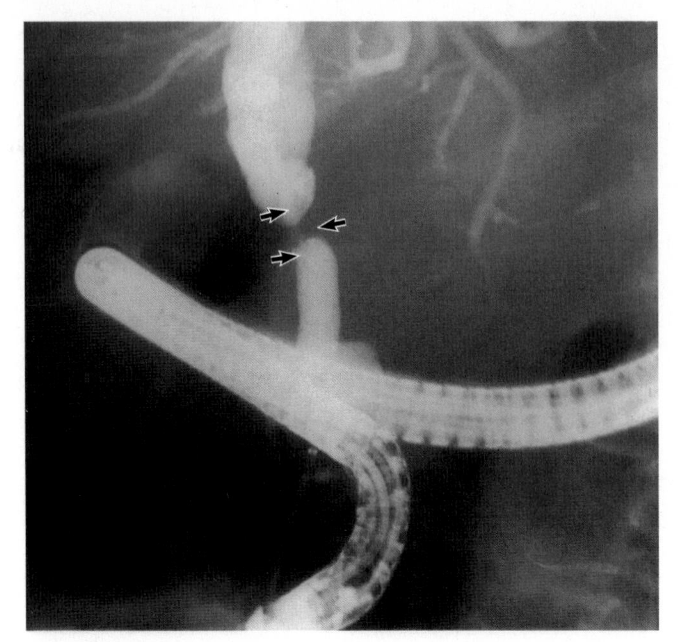

Figure 61–21. A high-grade stricture at the level of the common hepatic duct *(arrows)* in a patient who had undergone a laparoscopic cholecystectomy 2 months earlier.

Patients with an inoperable recurrent benign biliary stricture often require recurrent biliary interventions. In these patients repeated and convenient access to the biliary tree can be achieved via a jejunal loop affixed surgically to the abdominal wall.[49]

Endoscopic intervention requires negotiating a wire through the stricture, followed by dilation with a Sonde- or a Gruntzig-type balloon. The stricture is stented for a variable period of time. Repeat dilation may be necessary following stent removal.[138–140] Some groups advocate endoscopic balloon dilation and stent placement for benign strictures and report excellent results (approaching 88%) after several years. There is controversy, however, about the value of repeated stricture dilation and long-term stenting of benign operable lesions. The authors advocate long-term endoscopic stenting of benign lesions only when it is unlikely that an operative approach would provide definitive therapy[14] or when it would be hazardous, as with significant portal hypertension.

FISTULAS. Operative bile duct injury may lead to the development of a biliary fistula or biloma. Diagnostic cholangiography will frequently reveal the location of the bile leak.[142] If an extrahepatic biliary leak is detected, a nasobiliary catheter or stent may be placed across the disruption in the bile duct to divert bile temporarily from the site of injury and allow time for the injury to heal.[100–103] If the bile leak is small, ES alone may permit spontaneous fistula closure. Alternatively, bile leaks may be treated by diversion of bile via a percutaneous transhepatic drainage catheter. If the fistula does not resolve following simple biliary diversion, transcatheter occlusion techniques may be used to close the leak[143, 144] (Fig. 61–22).

SUMP SYNDROME. This entity is an infrequent complication of a side-to-side choledochoduodenostomy. Stenosis of the surgical anastomosis is a prerequisite. As food, stones, and other debris accumulate in the CBD distal to the stenotic anastomosis and proximal to the papilla, overgrowth of bacteria results in suppurative cholangitis. Sump syndrome can be treated by the combination of ES and passage of a balloon through the distal CBD to sweep out debris from the duct.[145] Alternatively, it may be possible to extract debris and stones via the choledochoduodenostomy, obviating the need for a papillotomy; however, without a papillotomy and with a strictured choledochoduodenostomy, the sump syndrome may recur.

Sclerosing Cholangitis (see also Chapter 59)

The treatment of sclerosing cholangitis depends on the location and extent of biliary involvement. In the past, surgical therapy consisted of hepaticoenteric anastomosis for patients with predominantly extrahepatic disease. The recently improved results of liver transplantation have led some investigators to advocate transplantation as the treatment of choice in patients with primary sclerosing cholangitis and cirrhosis. The emergence of liver transplantation and the disappointing results of surgery have led to increased use of nonoperative therapy in symptomatic patients before liver transplantation[146] (Fig. 61–23).

Radiologic therapy for sclerosing cholangitis includes balloon dilation, stenting, and placement of internal metallic endoprostheses. Transhepatic stenting for prolonged periods is undesirable, because the drainage catheter frequently obstructs the biliary tree in these patients with diffusely small ducts. An alternative approach is to perform radiologic inter-

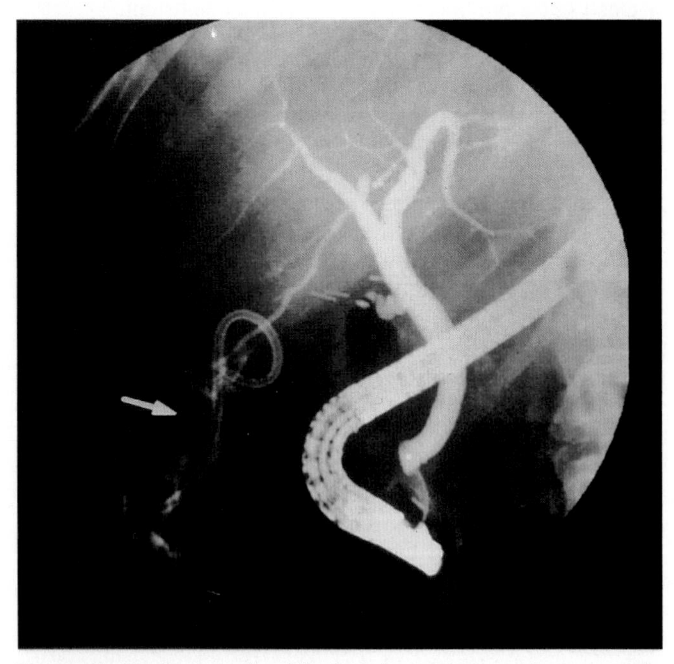

Figure 61–22. Postoperative bile leak in a 76-year-old woman who presented with pain and fever 2 weeks after a laparoscopic cholecystectomy. Ultrasonography revealed a subhepatic fluid collection. The collection was evacuated by percutaneous placement of a No. 10 French pigtail catheter *(arrow)*. An ERCP was performed, which demonstrated a leak from a small peripheral duct (duct of Luschka) in the bed of the gallbladder. Sphincterotomy was performed. The external biloma drainage catheter was pulled out 2 weeks after the leak had sealed completely.

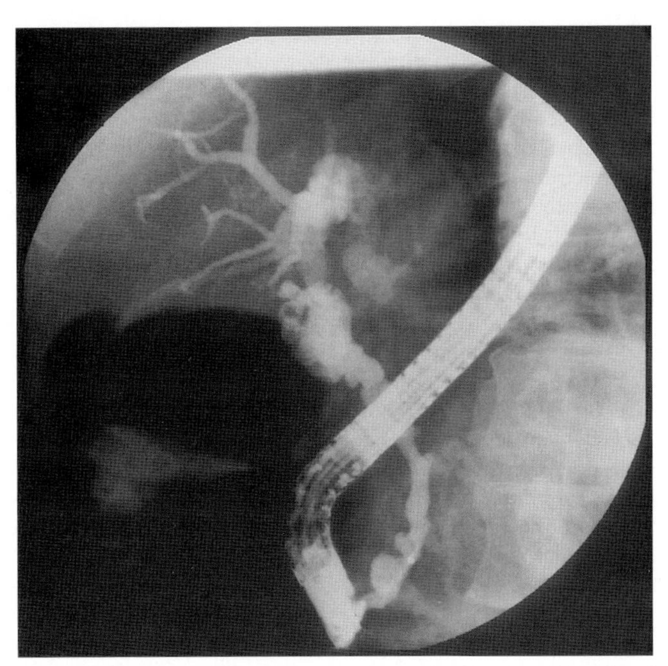

Figure 61–23. Moderately severe sclerosing cholangitis associated with idiopathic ulcerative colitis. Note involvement with ulcerations and strictures of the entire extrahepatic biliary tree.

vention through a jejunal access loop affixed to the anterior abdominal wall.[149] With this technique, the biliary tree can be accessed repeatedly, and the need to place a long-term transhepatic catheter is obviated. However, because of the complexity of transjejunal interventions and the problems associated with transhepatic intervention, nonoperative management in sclerosing cholangitis is now performed almost exclusively by endoscopic means.

Endoscopic balloon dilation may be beneficial for patients with jaundice secondary to dominant extrahepatic strictures.[141] Additionally, ES can be used to relieve back-pressure and facilitate bile flow through a fixed stricture. Dilation of a dominant stricture should be preceded by cytologic brushing and biopsy to exclude a neoplasm. Care must be exercised in interpreting brush cytology because false-positive and false-negative results are routinely observed. Preservation and sphincterotomy artifacts may make interpretation particularly tricky. There also is the possibility of seeing cytologically dysplastic cells even in the absence of malignancy.[146] The long-term benefits of biliary dilation are uncertain in patients with this progressive disease. Stricture dilation can be labor intensive and technically difficult if branches must be treated to reverse cholestasis.[147] Some evidence suggests that endoscopic management of sclerosing cholangitis with periodic balloon dilation without the use of stents results in slowing of disease progression, with a low complication rate.[148] Complications of biliary drainage and stricture dilation include acute and chronic cholangitis (Fig. 61–24).

Papillary Stenosis

Scarring of the duodenal papilla may produce mechanical biliary obstruction. Papillary stenosis can be treated by ES, stenting, or balloon dilation. The risk of retroduodenal perforation from a sphincterotomy is increased after a previous sphincterotomy when the bile duct is not dilated, because the intraduodenal segment of the bile duct is small.[76]

Biliary Sepsis

Biliary sepsis is the result of biliary obstruction and infection (see Chapter 55). The severity of this condition varies from mild fever and slight chills, which can be treated temporarily with antibiotics, to the full-blown picture of right upper quadrant pain, jaundice, sepsis, obtundation, and consumptive coagulopathy (Charcot's triad[149] and Reynold's pentad[150]), which requires immediate biliary decompression. Because emergency surgical decompression is associated with a high mortality rate (up to 50%), nonsurgical approaches are appropriate. The treatment of biliary sepsis requires experience, judgment, and skill in establishing drainage.[151, 152]

Percutaneous decompression can be achieved using standard PTBD techniques. A catheter is left either above the obstruction or across it (with the tip in the duodenum). The

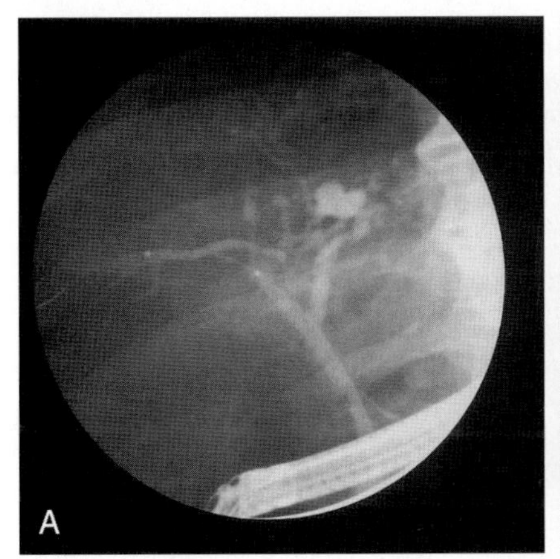

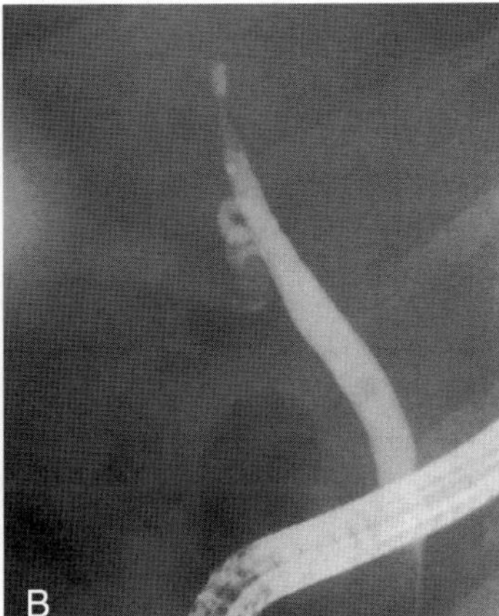

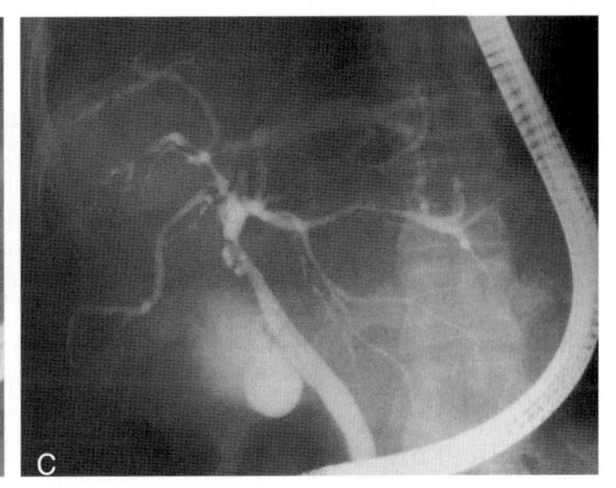

Figure 61–24. Sclerosing cholangitis with both intrahepatic and extrahepatic stricturing. The patient was deeply jaundiced and responded to dilation of the extra-hepatic right and left main ductal systems. Dilation of this type is used as a bridge to hepatic transplantation until a donor liver becomes available.

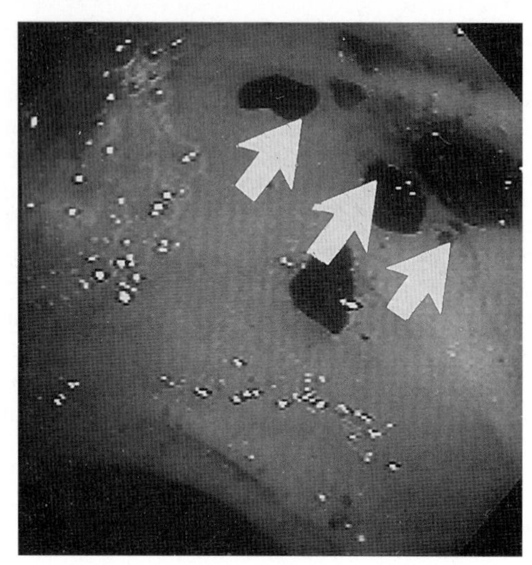

Figure 61–25. Multiple bilirubin (black pigment) stones *(arrows)* removed from a patient who had sickle cell disease and was deeply jaundiced.

procedure is performed expeditiously with minimal catheter manipulation to avoid exacerbation of sepsis. Using this approach, Kadir and colleagues reported a mortality rate of only 17% in patients with acute obstructive cholangitis treated by percutaneous drainage.[153] Some authors have advocated cholecystostomy as a less morbid percutaneous technique for biliary decompression in patients with low CBD obstruction.[55] However, transhepatic biliary drainage is a more reliable drainage technique and thus generally preferred at our institution.

Because of its lower morbidity rate, endoscopic drainage may be preferred over transhepatic drainage in patients with cholangitis. In a nonrandomized trial, Sugiyama and Atomi reported morbidity and mortality rates of 16.7% and 5.6%, respectively, in elderly patients treated for acute cholangitis by endoscopic drainage, but morbidity and mortality rates of 36.4% and 9.1%, respectively, in those treated by PTBD.[154]

Endoscopic biliary decompression is accomplished through a combination of ES[150, 151] and stent placement. Sphincterotomy provides immediate drainage, and stent placement prevents obstruction of the papillary orifice by debris or stones. A wide sphincterotomy (10- to 15-mm diameter) provides more effective drainage than can be achieved with a thin (2 to 3 mm) stent; however, stents prevent impaction of any residual stones and allow purulent material to drain through as well as around the stent. It is advisable not to perform complete cholangiography at the time of ERCP but to visualize just enough of the biliary system to perform sphincterotomy safely, remove any stones, and place an endoprosthesis. The endoprosthesis can be a single or multiple stents or a nasobiliary catheter. At a later time, after the duct has been decompressed and the patient's general medical condition has improved, the biliary tree can be evaluated thoroughly for stones, strictures, or neoplasms.

Biliary Tract Stones

In the United States, biliary tract stones are seen most commonly in association with gallbladder stones (see Chapter 55). The advent of laparoscopic cholecystectomy has resulted in increased utilization of endoscopic stone removal. Percutaneous stone removal techniques are utilized only in the rare case in which T-tube access is available. Specific techniques employed to treat retained stones following cholecystectomy in patients with and without T-tube access have been discussed in detail earlier.[108, 124] Less common causes of biliary stones are recurrent pyogenic cholangitis and sclerosing cholangitis (see Chapter 59). Diffuse intrahepatic stone disease in patients with recurrent pyogenic cholangitis or sclerosing cholangitis is frequently complicated by biliary strictures or intrahepatic abscesses. These two associated conditions make removal of intrahepatic stones difficult and increase the likelihood of stone recurrence. Proper management depends on the extent and location of disease.[155] When stone disease is localized to a single hepatic lobe, curative surgical resection may be possible,[156] but when the disease is diffuse, nonoperative techniques must be employed. Nonoperative stone extraction and stricture dilation can be facilitated by the creation of a subcutaneous jejunal access loop.[50] New techniques such as choledochoscopy and percutaneous lithotripsy have also proved valuable in treating diffuse intrahepatic stone disease.[157] Endoscopic stone removal and sphincterotomy may also be employed in this disease (Figs. 61–25 and 61–26).

Acute Cholecystitis

Although acute cholecystitis is usually caused by obstruction of the cystic duct by a stone, an increasing frequency of acalculous cholecystitis has been reported in patients with severe debilitating disease (see Chapter 55). Initial management of patients with acute cholecystitis includes intravenous

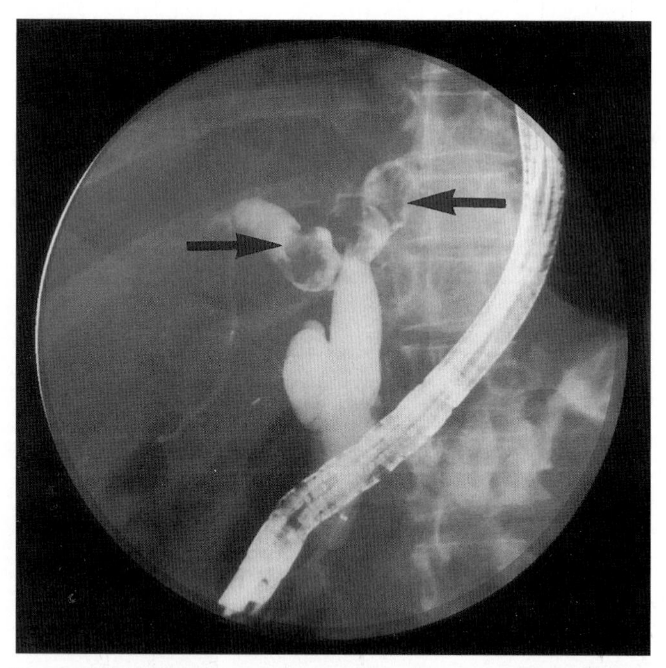

Figure 61–26. Cholangiogram in a patient with recurrent pyogenic cholangitis. Large stone collections appear in the right and left main hepatic ducts *(arrows)*. Balloon dilation and mechanical lithotripsy were employed to remove the stones after an ample endoscopic sphincterotomy.

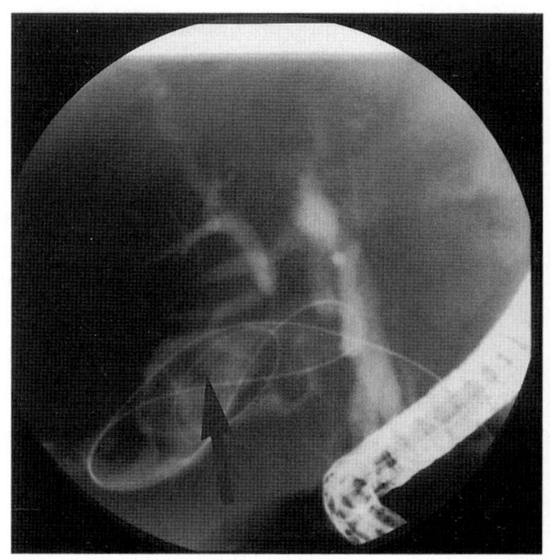
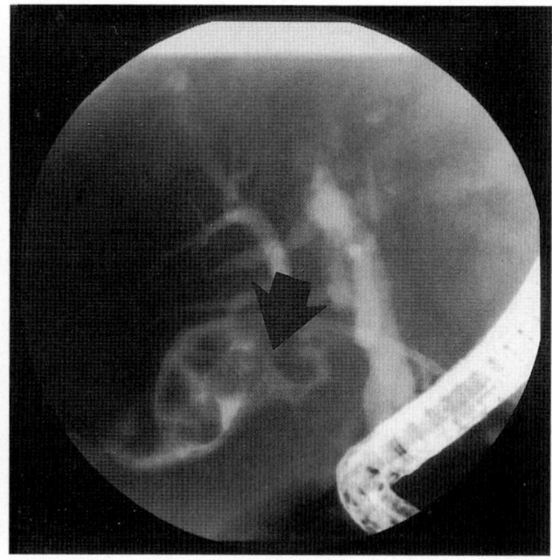

Figure 61–27. Because of disseminated intravascular coagulation caused by cholecystitis and ascites secondary to pre-existing alcoholic cirrhosis, an operation or percutaneous drainage was not possible. Therefore, a guidewire was placed into the necrotic stone-filled gallbladder *(arrow)* via a transpapillary route (left panel). The right panel shows a transpapillary cholecystostomy tube draining the gall bladder *(short arrow)*.

hydration and antibiotics. The objectives of further treatment are relief of pain and prevention of potentially lethal complications such as empyema and gallbladder perforation. Although cholecystectomy is the definitive treatment, nonoperative therapy is gaining acceptance in patients who are at high operative risk.[158–160]

RADIOLOGIC TECHNIQUE. The effectiveness of cholecystostomy in treating acute cholecystitis is difficult to determine because a definitive diagnosis of acute cholecystitis requires surgical confirmation. However, Lee et al. reported clinical improvement in 58% of septic patients in an intensive care unit who were treated by PC.[161] England et al.[60] reported that in 59 patients the factors predictive of a positive response to PC included clinical symptoms referable to the gallbladder and the presence of pericholecystic fluid. Gallstones in patients with acute calculous cholecystitis can be removed percutaneously, or elective cholecystectomy can be performed. This therapeutic decision is determined by the perioperative risk of the patient and by personal preference.

ENDOSCOPIC APPROACH. There is little role for endoscopic therapy of acute cholecystitis. For patients with concomitant biliary obstruction from an impacted CBD stone, sphincterotomy may be indicated. A transpapillary stent or nasocholecystic catheter is useful in rare cases of acalculous cholecystitis in severely ill patients with a coagulopathy. The cystic duct is entered with a soft high-torque guidewire, which is then exchanged for a more rigid guidewire. A nasocholecystic catheter has a slight advantage, because the small size (No. 7) and length (10 cm) of the standard stent do not permit effective drainage of the gallbladder into the duodenum. The use of stents for drainage of the gallbladder is most efficacious when the cystic duct is patent and there is acalculous cholecystitis[162] (Fig. 61–27).

Malignant Diseases

Nonoperative intervention in patients with malignant biliary disease is usually performed to palliate pruritus that accompanies jaundice. Nonoperative drainage, whether performed endoscopically or radiologically, results in a decrease in serum bilirubin levels, and pruritus usually resolves within 24 to 48 hours of drainage. In the past, nonoperative drainage was performed to lower the serum bilirubin level before definitive surgical resection, but preoperative drainage has not been shown to improve outcome and is not utilized today under ordinary circumstances,[163, 164] although it still is occasionally employed to decrease the bilirubin level so that chemotherapy or chemoembolization can be employed.

Therapy for malignant biliary obstruction should be initiated for pruritus when prolonged survival is anticipated. There have been no validated quality of life measurements for persons in whom biliary obstruction has been relieved. If both biliary and duodenal obstruction are present and endoscopic stent therapy for the duodenal obstruction is being considered, then the biliary obstruction should be relieved first.

Endoscopic stenting is now widely accepted as the preferred method of palliation for malignant obstruction when the lesion is inoperable. Percutaneous stenting is reserved for situations in which endoscopic stenting is not possible or has failed to relieve jaundice or sepsis. Percutaneous stenting often requires temporary external drainage and is associated with an increased risk of sepsis and hemorrhage. The need for a combined ERCP and percutaneous procedure is rare and subjects the patient to the combined morbidity of both approaches (see earlier).

Endoscopic plastic stenting has a success rate comparable to that of surgical bypass (95% versus 94%), with lower rates of procedure-related death (3% versus 14%, $P = 0.01$) and major complications (11% versus 29%, $P = 0.02$) and a shorter mean hospital stay and fewer days spent in the hospital from the time of randomization until death. As expected, late complications are more common in stented patients. There is a clear short-term advantage to stenting, although for the patient with a longer survival, much of this advantage may be lost because of stent obstruction[165] (Fig. 61–28).

Metal expandable biliary stents occlude less frequently than plastic No. 10 or 11.5 French stents, with consequently lower rates of repeat ERCPs and hospitalizations. Mean stent patency usually exceeds 9 months. The stents are expensive, with a cost to the institution of more than $1000. Long-term follow-up has shown that some of these stents will remain patent for as long as 1.5 years. If the patient is still alive

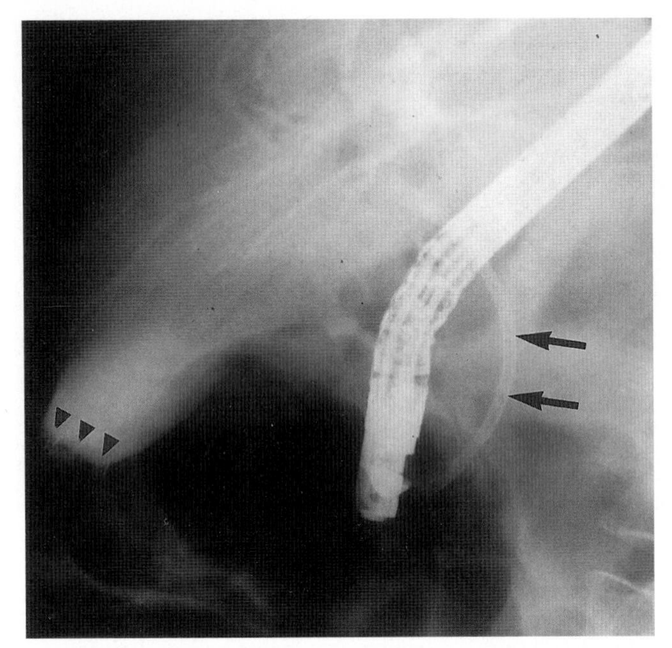

Figure 61–28. This 65-year-old man underwent an exploratory laporatomy for carcinoma of the pancreas, which was found to be inoperable for cure. He underwent a cholecystojejunostomy, which became occluded after 3 months *(arrowheads)*. A plastic No. 10 French 7-cm straight stent *(arrows)* was placed through the obstructing neoplasm to re-establish biliary drainage.

after this period, he or she will experience recurrent bouts of sepsis, because the metal struts and bile duct remain infected. The ideal strategy for treating occluded metal stents is unknown; options include placement of another metal stent, mechanical cleaning, and placement of a plastic stent. The most cost-effective strategy in the initial choice of stent (metal versus plastic) has not been established. It has been suggested that a plastic stent should be placed first, and when it occludes, a metal stent should be placed in long-term survivors[166–169] (Fig. 61–29).

Metal stents can be removed at surgery, but they do damage the involved duct. Endoscopic removal is usually not possible after 1 to 2 weeks. Covered stents employed to prevent tumor ingrowth have had mixed results and can occlude both the pancreatic and the cystic ducts if not placed carefully with an ample sphincterotomy.[170, 171] Covered stents may be retrievable and may also be useful in treating benign strictures.[172, 173]

The duration of palliation afforded by nonoperative stenting depends on the nature and location of the underlying disease as well as the type of stent used to relieve the obstruction. An average patency of 6 months is expected for a No. 10 French plastic stent, and a patency of a few months longer is expected for a metallic endoprosthesis.

Distal Common Bile Duct Lesions

Pancreatic carcinoma, ampullary carcinoma, and metastatic disease to the peripancreatic nodes can result in distal CBD obstruction. The primary approach to palliation of distal CBD lesions is endoscopic stenting.[96, 174] It also is important to make every effort to obtain biopsy specimens.

Successful endoscopic intervention can be performed when the duodenum and the duodenal papilla are not distorted. The CBD is entered with standard cannulation techniques, and an endoprosthesis is placed through the obstructing lesion. When there is marked distortion of the duodenum or papilla, the intraduodenal segment of the CBD may be entered above the papilla. This technique, which is more hazardous than a standard endoscopic sphincterotomy, involves use of a needle-knife to bore a passageway into the CBD.[175] When an endoscopic approach is not possible, a stent may be inserted transhepatically. Our metallic stent of choice for malignant disease is the Wallstent.

Proximal Common Bile Duct and Common Hepatic Duct Lesions

The lesions encountered most commonly in the proximal common bile duct and common hepatic duct are cholangiocarcinomas, extrinsic metastatic nodal diseases, and gallbladder carcinomas. An endoscopically placed endoprosthesis can be positioned across an obstruction, and a large plastic

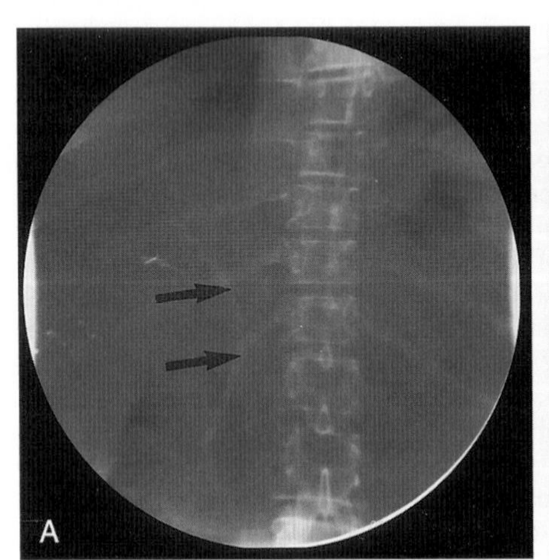

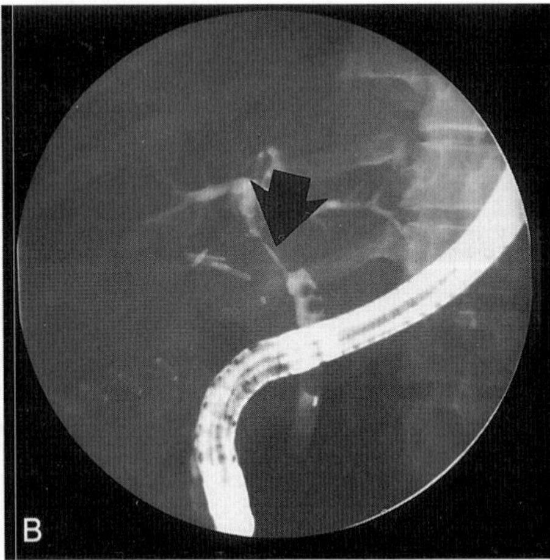

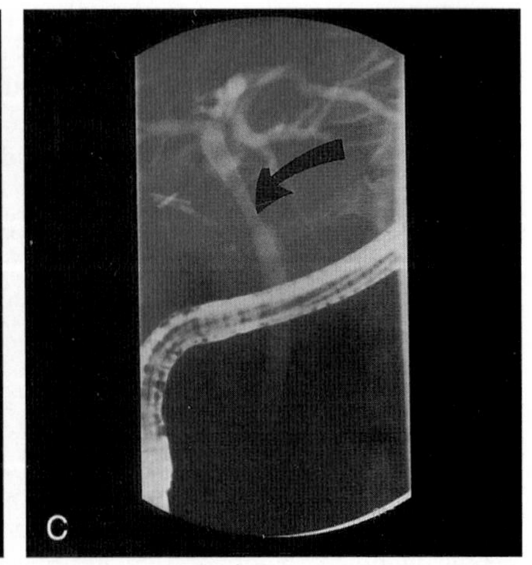

Figure 61–29. *A,* A plastic stent placed for advanced cholangiocarcinoma in a patient who became febrile and jaundiced after 8 months. No. 10 French 12-cm straight stent is indicated by *arrows*. *B,* After removal of the plastic stent a 2-cm stricture was noted at the level of the common hepatic duct *(short arrow)*. *C,* The biliary system was then drained with serial expandable metal stents *(curved arrow)*.

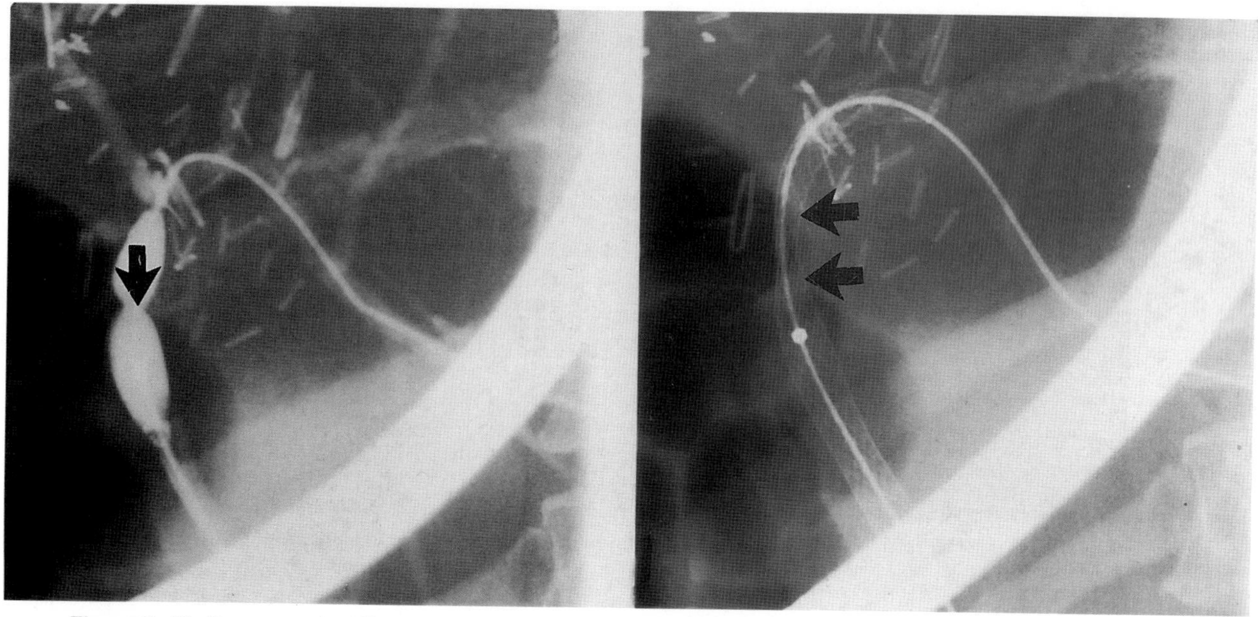

Figure 61–30. Treatment of a hilar tumor (recurrent hepatocellular carcinoma after right lobectomy). The left panel shows a dilating balloon passed over a guidewire with the waist of the balloon at the tumor *(arrow)*. The right panel shows a Wallstent in place with a narrowed area *(arrows)* at the tumor.

or metallic expandable endoprosthesis can be inserted across a tumor. When endoscopic stenting is not possible, transhepatic stenting is performed in the standard fashion. Transhepatic endoprostheses are usually positioned above the ampulla, to minimize reflux of duodenal contents through the stent.

Hilar and Intrahepatic Lesions

Tumors at the hepatic hilum pose a challenge for nonoperative intervention, because they frequently grow into the liver, thereby isolating both the right and left ducts. Stenting of hilar obstructions is accomplished most easily by percutaneous techniques.[176, 177] Endoscopic stent insertion is more difficult because of the long distances and acute angles involved.

Draining a single system usually provides adequate palliation of jaundice. In patients with cholangitis, both obstructed systems must be drained. When only one system is to be drained, we favor draining the left duct. Compared to the right duct, the left duct has fewer branches near the hilum and thus permits a greater potential for long-term palliation as malignant tumor spreads into the hilum. If the left lobe is atrophic because of long-term obstruction, the right duct is drained. Percutaneous stenting of hilar malignancy can be accomplished with either a plastic or metallic endoprosthesis. Alternatively, long-term external drainage can be employed.

Expandable metal stents can be delivered effectively by a transhepatic approach and can be overlapped so that the intrahepatic biliary radicles are drained into the duodenum. Very proximal lesions may be drained into the common bile duct rather than into the duodenum, or an ES can be performed. The stent should not be placed close to the ampulla, in order to avoid mechanical obstruction. It is possible to place parallel expandable stents in each main duct. There is a risk of entrapment when the metal stent is placed into a small proximal duct and the delivery system does not release.[178]

Endoscopic stenting of a hilar malignancy can be accomplished with both plastic and metallic endoprostheses.[180, 181] Results with endoscopic stenting are best when the disease is confined to the biliary confluence and does not extend into the liver parenchyma. The longest standard plastic stents are 15 cm. These stents are usually long enough to reach from the papilla to several centimeters above the bifurcation. It is necessary for the distal end of the plastic stent to extend through the papilla so that it can be removed if it becomes occluded. If a plastic stent is not sufficiently long to meet this requirement, an expandable metallic stent can be used. Expandable metallic stents can be "overlapped" with each other to reach through the papilla. They also may drain other ducts via their sideholes. Occlusion of metal stents can be treated by placing another expandable or plastic stent inside the occluded stent (Figs. 61–30 and 61–31).

Other Conditions

Complications Relating to Liver Transplantation

Despite high overall survival following liver transplantation, the postoperative morbidity rate is significant (see Chapter 83). Biliary complications, including bile leaks, obstruction, and T-tube–related problems, are seen in 10% to 30% of patients.[181] T-tube cholangiography is a simple method for evaluating patients with suspected biliary complications. However, because of their high complication rate, T tubes are no longer used routinely in most patients with duct-to-duct anastomoses. Postoperative surgical re-exploration or retransplantation may be necessary in some patients with biliary complications, but nonoperative intervention is useful as a temporizing measure or as a definitive procedure.[15, 102]

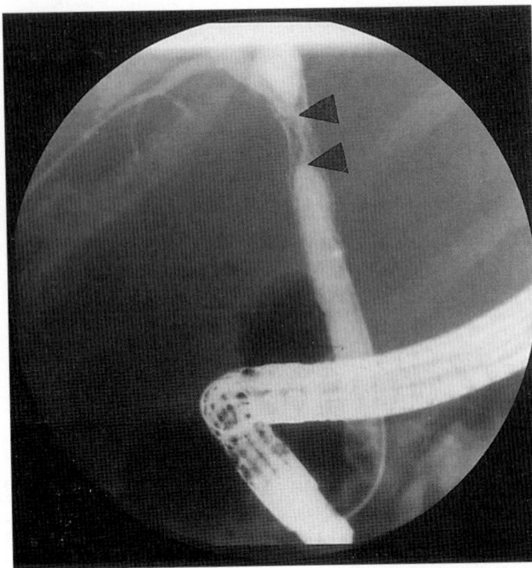

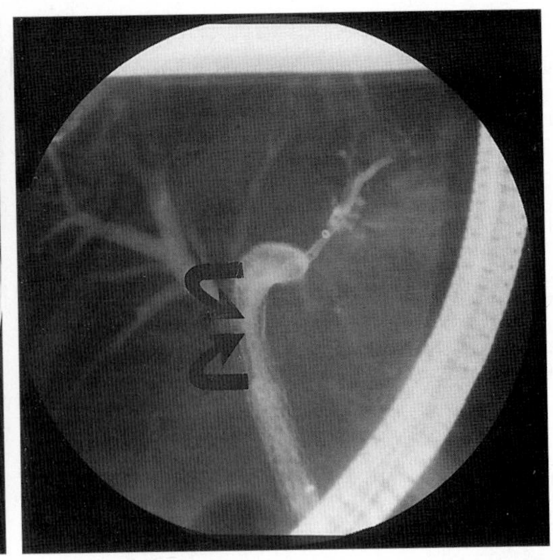

Figure 61–31. *Left,* Internal narrowing of a metal stent caused by tumor ingrowth and debris *(arrowheads). Right,* A wire and another metal stent were placed across the stricture so as to extend proximal to the previous stent *(curved arrows).*

TREATMENT OF BILIARY OBSTRUCTION. Obstruction usually results from formation of a biliary stricture, either at the biliary anastomotic site or in the more proximal biliary tree. Anastomotic strictures result from technical complications or postoperative scarring. Nonanastomotic strictures result from chronic rejection, ischemia, or cytomegalovirus (CMV) infection. Another less well defined cause of obstruction is dysfunction of the sphincter of Oddi, which can lead to intermittent obstruction or a bile leak. Rarely, a choledochocele can cause biliary obstruction. High intrahepatic strictures and choledochojejunostomy strictures are treated with percutaneous techniques. More distal strictures are treated endoscopically. In patients without T tubes, the authors are treating many anastomotic strictures endoscopically with balloon dilation (Fig. 61–32).

Figure 61–32. An anastomotic biliary stricture *(between arrows)* in a patient who underwent orthotopic liver transplantation with a duct-to-duct anastomosis and became jaundiced 3 months later.

The long-term benefit of dilation of transplant strictures appears to be less than that of nontransplant-related strictures. Nonanastomotic strictures, which occur within 3 months of transplantation and are not associated with rejection or CMV infection, are the lesions that respond best to balloon dilation.[182] Anastomotic strictures are usually treated surgically. In nonoperative patients who fail balloon dilation, stenting with a metallic endoprosthesis may be considered. Culp et al.[28] reported excellent immediate results using metal stents for post-transplant biliary strictures, but strictures recurred in almost all patients. Therefore, use of stents in transplant patients is not broadly advised.

TREATMENT OF BILE LEAKS. Bile leaks can occur at either a biliary duct anastomosis or a nonanastomotic site. Anastomotic leaks are more common in patients with choledochojejunostomy than in those with duct-to-duct anastomoses. Nonanastomotic leaks may occur at the T-tube insertion site or in the donor bile duct. Leaks in the donor duct should suggest the possibility of hepatic artery thrombosis or operative trauma.

The treatment for bile leaks is twofold: (1) drainage of any associated bilomas and (2) diversion of bile flow.[184, 185] Biloma drainage is accomplished by percutaneous insertion of a drainage catheter under US guidance. Bile diversion can be accomplished in a variety of ways: T-tube drainage may be adequate if the leak is small and a T tube is in place; a nasobiliary catheter or stent may be placed across the leak; or a percutaneous biliary drain may be positioned within the ducts to divert bile from the location of the leak. In some patients, bile leakage is aggravated by sphincter of Oddi dysfunction, and in such patients sphincterotomy may be beneficial as the sole therapy.

TREATMENT OF MALPOSITIONED T-TUBES. The T tube itself can be the cause of significant morbidity. Bile leaks can occur at the T-tube insertion site; the limbs of the tube can be malpositioned into the cystic duct; or the tube can be pulled out inadvertently. When a T tube is pulled partially

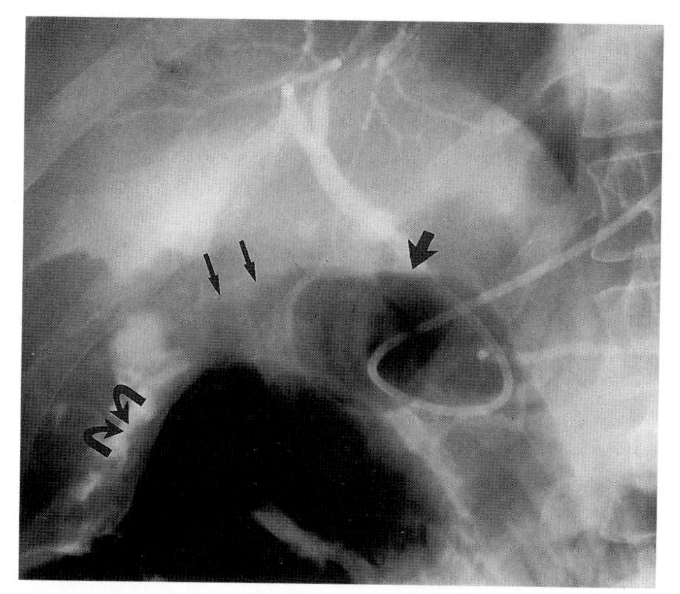

Figure 61–33. A bile leak in a liver transplant recipient developed several hours after removal of a T tube in a patient who had undergone an orthotopic liver transplant 2 months earlier with a duct-to-duct anastomosis. The *thin arrows* show the former T-tube tract, and the *curved arrows* reveal a free leak into the peritoneum. There is a nasobiliary catheter in the bile duct *(thick arrow)*.

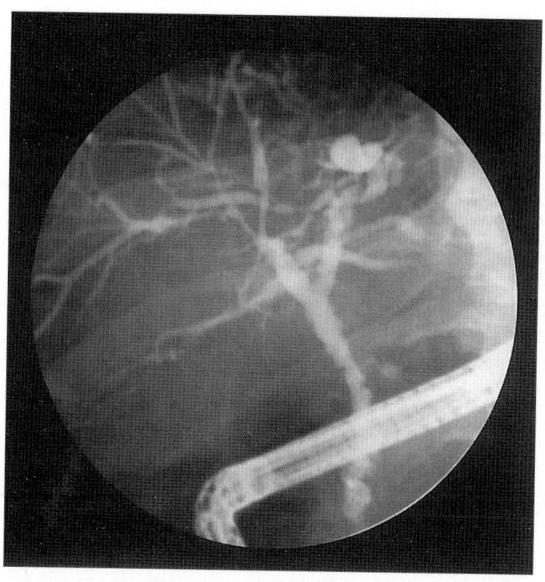

Figure 61–35. A cholangiogram in a patient with AIDS cholangiopathy. The findings are similar to those of primary sclerosing cholangitis. The entity has virtually disappeared since the aggressive use of multiple antiviral agents to treat AIDS.

out of the biliary tree, it can be replaced with another percutaneous catheter in the following manner: a wire is manipulated into the biliary tree through the existing T tube; the T tube is withdrawn; and a new drainage catheter is inserted over the wire so that the tip lies in the intrahepatic duct system. The replacement catheter drains the biliary tree and prevents leakage at the choledochotomy site. If a T tube is inadvertently pulled entirely out of the biliary tree, fluoroscopically guided replacement often is not possible, because T-tube tract formation is delayed by immunosuppression. Therefore, a nasobiliary catheter or stent is inserted or sphincterotomy is performed[103] (Fig. 61–33).

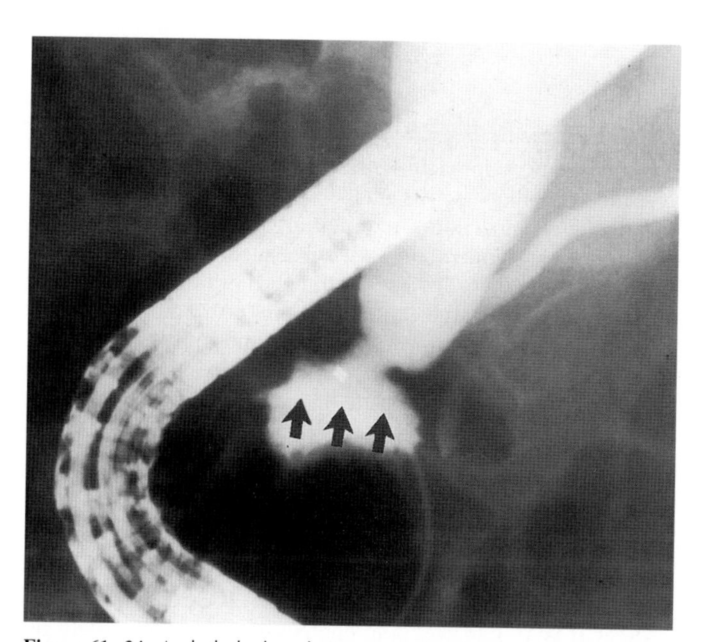

Figure 61–34. A choledochocele *(arrows)* near the ampulla in a patient with postoperative jaundice after an orthotopic liver transplant. The obstruction responded to a long endoscopic sphincterotomy with unroofing of the choledochocele.

OBSTRUCTION AT THE PAPILLA. Selective dilation of the liver transplant recipient's CBD and obstruction at the papilla are occasionally noted and can result in jaundice. The cause is unknown, although opportunistic infections and an achalasia-like denervation have been suggested. Satisfactory therapy can be achieved by ES, which also can treat an obstructing choledochocele (Fig. 61–34).

Sphincter of Oddi Dysfunction

The evaluation of sphincter of Oddi dysfunction is usually undertaken in young patients with persistent pain following cholecystectomy (see Chapter 53). When the sphincter of Oddi pressure is elevated, ES may be performed. The results of such therapy vary, and to some degree probably reflect the accuracy of sphincter of Oddi measurements.[186] The CBD typically is not dilated with this condition, the frequency of retroduodenal perforation after sphincterotomy is probably greater for this group of patients than for those with choledocholithiasis.[186]

Acquired Immunodeficiency Syndrome (AIDS)

AIDS CHOLANGIOPATHY (INFECTIOUS SCLEROSING CHOLANGITIS). Patients with AIDS cholangiopathy typically present with pain and elevated serum alkaline phosphatase levels but rarely with jaundice.[187, 188] Cholangiographic findings resemble those of sclerosing cholangitis and include beading and ulceration along the intra- and extrahepatic biliary system (Fig. 61–35). Endoscopic sphincterotomy is fre-

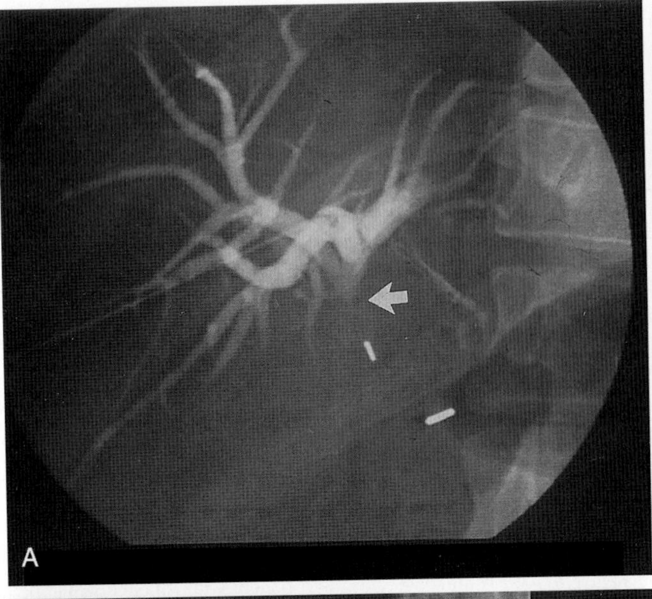

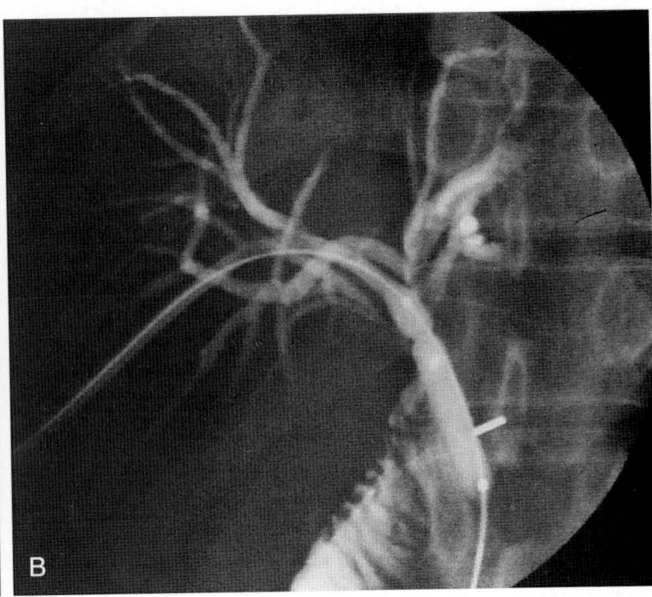

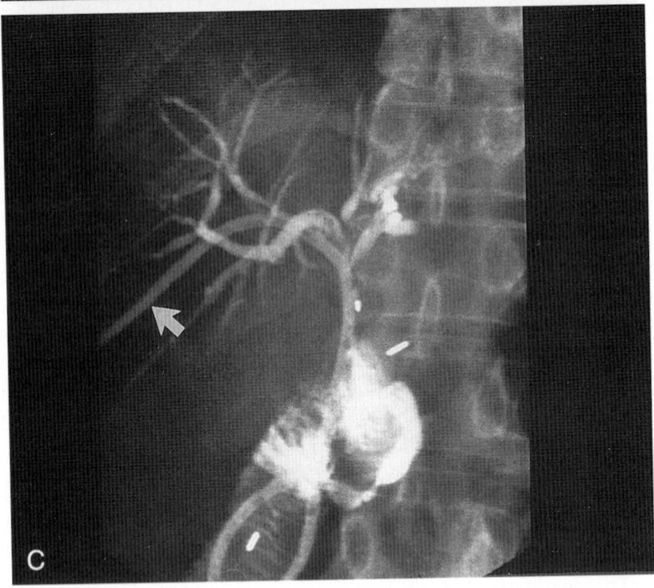

Figure 61–36. Percutaneous cholangiogram in a 30-year-old woman who complained of jaundice following laparoscopic cholecystectomy and Roux-en-Y hepaticojejunostomy. *A,* The cholangiogram shows dilated intrahepatic ducts and obstruction at the Roux anastomosis *(arrow)*. *B,* Percutaneous transhepatic biliary drainage was performed, the stricture was negotiated, and a balloon was inflated across the stricture. *C,* A No. 12-French catheter *(arrow)* was positioned across the stricture, and the result was evaluated cholangiographically 6 weeks later.

quently beneficial for relieving the pain, and at the time of the sphincterotomy biopsies and cultures the area around the duodenal papilla or the distal CBD can be obtained to exclude a medically treatable infection. This entity is rarely seen now since the advent of highly active antiretroviral therapy (see Chapter 28).

Laparoscopic Cholecystectomy

Before the advent of laparoscopic cholecystectomy there was no substantive evidence that preoperative ES was superior to operative removal of CBD stones in patients undergoing cholecystectomy. With the advent of laparoscopic cholecystectomy, the treatment of concomitant CBD stones has changed dramatically.[190]

ROLE OF ERCP. Advances in laparoscopic technique have permitted the management of small common duct stones via a transcystic approach, although solitary stones larger than 1 cm or multiple large stones at present are best handled via an endoscopic approach with ES and stone retrieval. The presence of biliary sepsis and obstructive jaundice or worsening biliary pancreatitis requires urgent endoscopic decompression after stabilization and, subsequently, semielective or urgent laparoscopic cholecystectomy. If intraoperative stone removal is not feasible and there are no complicating circumstances (e.g., Roux-en-Y gastrojejunostomy), we do not recommend that the surgeon convert to an open procedure. Rather, it is best to complete the case and perform endoscopic stone removal later during that hospitalization. A certain percentage of the smaller stones pass spontaneously, and the remainder are removed endoscopically. In the future, intraoperative endoscopically assisted sphincterotomy may be used.[190, 191]

COMPLICATIONS FOLLOWING LAPAROSCOPIC CHOLECYSTECTOMY. Laparoscopic cholecystectomy has largely replaced "open" surgical cholecystectomy because laparoscopic cholecystectomy results in a shorter hospital stay, faster recovery, and lower overall morbidity rate. Unfortunately, the frequency of complications resulting from bile duct injury has increased with the advent of laparoscopic cholecystectomy. Bile duct injury, which was observed in 0.1% of open cases, may occur in as many as 0.2% to 0.5% of laparoscopic cases.[192, 193] In addition, laparoscopic bile duct injuries tend to be more severe and more difficult to treat than biliary injuries produced by open surgery.[194]

Bile duct injury that occurs during laparoscopic cholecystectomy results in two basic problems: (1) bile leak with biloma formation and (2) biliary obstruction caused by stricture formation. Patients may present with pain and fever from a biloma or jaundice because of biliary obstruction. Bile leaks result from incomplete clipping of the cystic duct or laceration or transection of central or peripheral bile ducts. Failure to recognize variant bile duct anatomy, particularly an aberrant low insertion of a segmental right duct, is a common cause of bile duct transection.[195] Strictures tend to occur in the common hepatic duct owing to thermal injury to the hilum from cautery and dissection probes. Strictures or obstruction can also result from inadvertent ligation of aberrant ducts.

The initial work-up of patients with presumed bile duct injury includes cholangiography to assess the biliary anatomy and a cross-sectional imaging study such as CT or US to investigate the presence and location of biloma. Cholangiography is performed via an endoscopic approach when possible. Biliary tract disruption results in decompression of the bile ducts, and the ducts may actually be decreased in caliber, making percutaneous cannulation difficult or even hazardous. When endoscopic cannulation of the duct is not possible or when contrast material cannot be directed into the intrahepatic ducts, PTC may be necessary. In patients with possible laparoscopic cholecystectomy injury, it is particularly important to opacify all the intrahepatic ducts by cholangiography. Inadvertent ligation of peripheral ducts may result in incomplete opacification of the biliary tree, which is difficult to notice immediately.

The treatment of bile duct injury following laparoscopic cholecystectomy depends on the nature and extent of injury.[178, 196] Small to moderate bile duct leaks at the cystic duct stump or peripheral ducts may be cured with nonoperative therapy alone, but large leaks or transection of the main ducts often requires surgery. The treatment of small bile duct leaks includes percutaneous drainage of large or symptomatic bilomas coupled with a biliary drainage procedure to divert bile from the site of injury. The drainage catheter is initially placed into the biloma under US or CT guidance, and then the collection is evacuated. External biloma drainage is continued until biliary output through the drain ceases. Biliary diversion is usually achieved endoscopically by sphincterotomy and placement of a temporary plastic endoprosthesis. Although the leak may require several stent changes to achieve complete closure, most leaks will close within 6 weeks.[197]

Strictures after laparoscopic cholecystectomy may occur after an uneventful operation and may not be recognized until many months to several years after surgery. The treatment of these strictures is usually surgical—creation of a Roux-en-Y hepaticojejunostomy.[198] In selected patients who cannot undergo this surgery because of severe medical problems or cirrhosis with portal hypertension, nonoperative management by means of balloon dilation or placement of a metallic endoprosthesis may be appropriate. Lillemoe and colleagues reported a success rate of 100% in the treatment of bile duct strictures using a combination of surgery and percutaneous dilation. However, the cost of treating these patients was quite high, with mean cost of $51,000[198] (Fig. 61–36).

REFERENCES

1. Chespak LW, Ring EJ, Shapiro HA, et al: Multidisciplinary approach to complex endoscopic biliary intervention. Radiology 70:995, 1989.
2. Shorvon P, Dowsett J: Internal biliary stenting-up or down the bile duct? J Intervent Radiol 4:3, 1989.
3. Stanley J, Gobien RP, Cunningham J, et al: Biliary decompression: An institutional comparison of percutaneous and endoscopic methods. Radiology 158:195, 1986.
4. Shope TB: Radiation induced skin injuries from fluoroscopy. Radiographics 16:1195, 1998.
5. Wagner LK, Eifel PJ, Geise RA: Potential biological effects following high x-ray dose interventional procedures. J Vasc Interv Radiol 5:71–84, 1994.
6. Niklason LT, Marx MV, Chan H-P: Interventional radiologists: Occupational radiation doses and risks. Radiology 187:729–733, 1993.
7. Brateman L: Radiation safety considerations for diagnostic radiology personnel. Radiographics 19:1037, 1999.
8. Vogelzang RL, Nemcek AA: Toward painless percutaneous biliary procedures: New strategies and alternatives. J Intervent Radiol 3:131, 1988.
9. McDermott VG, Schuster MG, Smith TP: Antibiotic prophylaxis in vascular and interventional radiology. AJR 169:31, 1997.
10. Okuda K, Tanikawa K, Imura T, et al: Non-surgical percutaneous transhepatic cholangiography. Am J Dig Dis 19:21, 1974.
11. Teplick SK, Haskin PH, Sammon JK, et al: Common bile duct obstruction: Assessment by transcholecystic cholangiography. Radiology 161:135, 1986.
12. Jacques PF, Mauro MA, Schtliff JH: The failed transhepatic cholangiogram. Radiology 134:33, 1980.
13. Burke DR, Lewis CA, Cardella JF, et al: Quality improvement guidelines for percutaneous transhepatic cholangiography and biliary drainage. J Vasc Interv Radiol 8:677–681, 1997.
14. Kaude JV, Weidenmier CT, Agee OF: Decompression of bile ducts with the percutaneous transhepatic technique. Radiology 93:69, 1969.
15. Molnar W, Stockum AE: Relief of obstructive jaundice through percutaneous transhepatic catheter—a new therapeutic method. AJR 122: 356, 1974.
16. Ring EJ, Oleaga JA, Freiman DB, et al: Therapeutic applications of catheter cholangiography. Radiology 128:333, 1978.
17. Hayashi N, Sakai T, Kitagawa M, et al: US-guided left-sided biliary drainage: Nine-year experience. Radiology 204:119–122, 1997.
18. Mueller PR, Ferrucci JT, van Sonnenberg E, et al: Obstruction of the left duct: Diagnosis and treatment by selective fine-needle cholangiography and percutaneous biliary drainage. Radiology 145:297, 1987.
19. Burke DR, McLean GK: Obstructions of the hepatic duct confluence: Internal drainage of bilateral lesions with a single catheter. Radiology 172:1035, 1989.
20. Mueller PR, van Sonnenberg E, Ferrucci JT: Percutaneous biliary drainage: Technical and catheter related problems in 200 procedures. AJR 138:17, 1983.
21. Hamlin JA, Friedman M, Stein MG, et al: Percutaneous biliary drainage: Complications of 118 consecutive catheterizations. Radiology 158:199, 1986.
22. Dawson SL, Neff CC, Mueller PR, et al: Fatal hemothorax after inadvertent transpleural biliary drainage. AJR 141:33, 1983.
23. Miller GA, Heaston DK, Moore AV, et al: Peritoneal seeding of cholangiocarcinoma in patients with percutaneous biliary drainage. AJR 141:561, 1983.
24. Pereiras R, Rheingold OJ, Huston D, et al: Relief of malignant obstructive jaundice by percutaneous insertion of a permanent prosthesis in the biliary tree. Ann Intern Med 89:589, 1978.
25. McLean GK, Burke DR: Role of endoprosthesis in the management of malignant biliary obstruction. Radiology 170:961, 1989.

26. Gillams A, Dick R, Dooley JS, et al: Self-expandable stainless steel braided endoprosthesis for biliary strictures. Radiology 174:137, 1990.
27. Lammer J, Hausegger KA, Fluckiger F, et al: Common bile duct obstruction due to malignancy: Treatment with plastic versus metal stents. Radiology 201:167–172, 1996.
28. Culp WC, McCowan TC, Lieberman RP, et al: Biliary strictures in liver transplant recipients: Treatment with metal stents. Radiology 199: 339–346, 1996.
29. Rossi P, Salvatori FM, Bezzi M, et al: Percutaneous management of benign biliary strictures with balloon dilation and self-expanding metallic stents. Cardiovasc Intervent Radiol 13:231, 1990.
30. Bonnel DH, Liguory CL, Lefebvre JF, Cornud FE: Placement of metallic stents for treatment of postoperative biliary strictures: Long-term outcome of 25 patients. AJR 169:1517–1522, 1997.
31. Tesdal IK, Adamus R, Poeckler C, et al: Therapy for biliary stenoses and occlusions with use of three different metallic stents: Single-center experience J Vasc Intervent Radiol 8:869, 1997.
32. LaBerge JM, Doherty M, Gordon RL, et al: Hilar malignancy treatment with an expandable metallic transhepatic biliary stent. Radiology 177:793, 1990.
33. Lammer J, Neumayer K: Biliary drainage endoprosthesis: Experience with 201 placements. Radiology 159:625, 1986.
34. Gordon RL, Ring EJ, LaBerge JM, et al: Treatment of malignant biliary obstruction with expandable metallic Wallstent: Follow-up of 50 consecutive patients. Radiology 182:697, 1992.
35. Lee BH, Choe DH, Lee JH, et al: Metallic stents in malignant biliary obstruction: Prospective long-term clinical results. AJR 168:741, 1997.
36. Mueller PR, Ferrucci JT, Teplick SK, et al: Biliary stent endoprosthesis: Analysis of complications in 113 patients. Radiology 156:637, 1985.
37. Lee JM, Mueller PR, Saini S, et al: Occlusion of biliary endoprosthesis: Presentation and management. Radiology 176:531, 1990.
38. Hausegger KA, Thurnher S, Bodendorfer G, et al: Treatment of malignant biliary obstruction with polyurethane-covered Wallstents. AJR 170:403–408, 1998.
39. Molnar W, Stockum AB: Transhepatic dilation of choledochoenterostomy strictures. Radiology 129:59, 1978.
40. Gallacher DJ, Kadir S, Kaufman SL, et al: Nonoperative management of benign postoperative biliary strictures. Radiology 156:625, 1985.
41. Mueller PR, van Sonnenberg E, Ferrucci JT, et al: Biliary stricture dilatation: Multicenter review of clinical management in 73 patients. Radiology 160:17, 1986.
42. Pitt HA, Kauffman SL, Coleman J, et al: Benign postoperative biliary strictures. Ann Surg 210:417, 1989.
43. Burhenne HJ: Percutaneous extraction of retained biliary tract stones: 661 patients. AJR 134:888, 1980.
44. Graziani L, Fabrizzi G, Manfrini E, et al: Percutaneous transhepatic Oddi-sphincter dilation for bile duct stone removal. AJR 152:73, 1989.
45. Berkman WA, Bishop AF, Palagallo GL, et al: Transhepatic balloon dilation of the distal common bile duct and ampulla of Vater for removal of calculi. Radiology 167:453, 1988.
46. Stokes KR, Falchuk KR, Clause ME: Biliary duct stones: Update on 54 cases after percutaneous transhepatic removal. Radiology 170:999, 1989.
47. Saverbruch T, Stern M: Fragmentation of bile duct stones by extracorporeal shock waves. Gastroenterology 96:146, 1989.
48. Moody FG, Amerson JR, Berci G, et al: Lithotripsy for bile duct stones. Am J Surg 158:241, 1989.
49. McPherson SJ, Gibson RN, Collier NA, et al: Percutaneous transjejunal biliary intervention: 10-year experience with access via Roux-en-Y loops. Radiology 206:665, 1998.
50. Gott PE, Tieva MH, Barcia PJ, LaBerge JM: Biliary access procedure in the management of oriental cholangiohepatitis. Am Surg 62:930, 1996.
51. Brandon JC, Teplick SK, Haskin PH, et al: Common bile duct calculi: Updated experience with dissolution with methyl tertiary butyl ether. Radiology 166:665, 1988.
52. McGahan JP, Lindfors KK: Percutaneous cholecystostomy: An alternative to surgical cholecystostomy for acute cholecystitis? Radiology 173:481, 1989.
53. Vogelzang RL, Nemcek AA: Percutaneous cholecystostomy: Diagnostic and therapeutic efficacy. Radiology 168:29, 1988.
54. Teplick SK: Diagnostic and therapeutic interventional gallbladder procedures. AJR 152:913, 1989.
55. van Sonnenberg E, D'Agostino HB, Casola G, et al: The benefits of percutaneous cholecystostomy for decompression in selected cases of obstructive jaundice. Radiology 176:15, 1990.
56. Lo LD, Vogelzang RL, Braun MA, Memcek AA Jr: Percutaneous cholecystostomy for the diagnosis and treatment of acute calculous and acalculous cholecystitis. J Vasc Intervent Radiol 6:629–634, 1995.
57. Lee MJ, Saini S, Brink JA, et al: Treatment of critically ill patients with sepsis of unknown cause: Value of percutaneous cholecystostomy. AJR 156:1163, 1991.
58. Boland GW, Lee MJ, Leung J, Mueller PR: Percutaneous cholecystostomy in critically ill patients: Early response and final outcome in 82 patients. AJR 163:339–342, 1994.
59. Hamy A, Visset J, Likholatnikov D, et al: Percutaneous cholecystostomy for acute cholecystitis in critically ill patients. Surgery 121:398–401, 1997.
60. England RE, McDermott VG, Smith T, et al: Percutaneous cholecystostomy: Who responds. AJR 168:1247–1251, 1997.
61. Cope C: Percutaneous subhepatic cholecystostomy with removable anchor. AJR 151:1129, 1988.
62. McCune WS, Shorb PE, Moscowitz H: Endoscopic cannulation of the ampulla of Vater: A preliminary report. Ann Surg 167:752, 1968.
63. Kozarek RA, Sanowski RA: Nonsurgical management of extrahepatic obstructive jaundice. Ann Intern Med 96:743, 1982.
64. Schuman BM: The evolution of diagnostic ERCP. Gastrointest Endosc 36:155, 1990.
65. Katon RM, Bilbao MK, Parent JA, Smith FW: Endoscopic retrograde cholangiopancreatography in patients with gastrectomy and gastrojejunostomy (Billroth II): A case for the forward look. Gastrointest Endosc 21:164, 1975.
66. Osnes M, Rosseland AR, Aabakken L: Endoscopic retrograde cholangiography and endoscopic papillotomy in patients with a previous Billroth-II resection. Gut 27:1193, 1986.
67. Goldschmidt M, Marcon N, Kandel P, et al: A review of 160 endoscopic retrograde cholangiopancreatographies (ERCP) in patients with Billroth II anastomosis (abstract). Gastrointest Endosc 37:247, 1991.
68. Kim-Deobald J, Kozarek RA, Ball TJ, et al: Prospective evaluation of costs of disposable accessories in diagnostic and therapeutic ERCP. Gastrointest Endosc 39:763, 1993.
69. O'Connor KW: Disposable versus reusable ERCP equipment: The tip of the regulatory iceberg (editorial). Gastrointest Endosc 39:846, 1993.
70. Krasinski E, Zuccaro G, Ferguson JS, et al: The necessary level of aftercare for endoscopic sphincterotomy (abstract). Gastrointest Endosc 37:282, 1991.
71. Ostroff JW, Shapiro HA: Complications of endoscopic sphincterotomy. In Jacobson IM (ed): ERCP Diagnostic and Therapeutic Applications. New York, Elsevier, 1989.
72. Okuno M, Himeno S, Kurakawa M, et al: Changes in serum levels of pancreatic isoamylase, lipase, trypsin and elastase 1 hour after endoscopic retrograde pancreatography. Hepatogastroenterology 32:87, 1985.
73. Tulassay Z, Papp J: The effect of long-acting somatostatin analogue on enzyme changes after endoscopic pancreatography. Gastrointest Endosc 37:49, 1991.
74. Guelrud M, Mendoza S, Viera L, et al: Somatostatin prevents acute pancreatitis after pancreatic duct sphincter hydrostatic balloon dilation in patients with idiopathic recurrent pancreatitis. Gastrointest Endosc 37:45, 1991.
75. Shemesh E, Klein E, Czerniak A, et al: Endoscopic sphincterotomy in patients with gallbladder in situ: The influence of periampullary duodenal diverticula. Surg 107:268, 1990.
76. Worthley CS, Toouli J: Gallbladder non-filling: An indication for cholecystectomy after endoscopic sphincterotomy. Br J Surg 75:796, 1988.
77. Escourrou J, Cordova JA, Lazorthes F, et al: Early and late complications after endoscopic sphincterotomy and hilar lithiasis with and without the gallbladder "in situ." Gut 25:598, 1984.
78. Soehendra N: Billroth II sphincterotomy. Can J Gastroenterol 4:588, 1990.
79. Loperfido SL, Angelini G, Benedetti G, et al: Major early complications from diagnostic and therapeutic ERCP: A prospective multicenter study. Gastrointest Endosc 48:1–10, 1998.
80. Harris A, Chan CH, Torres-Viera C, et al: Meta-analysis of antibiotic prophylaxis in endoscopic retrograde cholangiopancreatography (ERCP) endoscopy. Endoscopy 31:718–724, 1999.
81. Tanchel M, Adkisson KW, Prince DR, et al: Oral Antiobiotic Prophy-

laxis for Therapeutic ERCP Is Cost Effective and Safe: Results of Randomized Clinical Trial. ASGE Poster Session, May 22, 2001.
82. Ostroff JW: The use of ERCP in pancreatic and biliary tract disease. In Jacobson IM (ed): ERCP and Its Application. Lippincott-Raven, Philadelphia, 1998.
83. Cotton PB: Precut papillotomy: A risky technique for experts only. Gastroenterology 35:578, 1989.
84. Huibregtse K, Katon HJ, Tytgat GNJ: Precut papillotomy via fine-needle knife papillotomy: A safe and effective technique. Gastrointest Endosc 32:403, 1986.
85. Liguory CM, Lefevre JF, Bonnel D, et al: Cutting the difficult papilla: Ancillary techniques in the performance of endoscopic sphincterotomy. Can J Gastroenterol 4:564, 1990.
86. Weisberg MF, Miller GL, McCarthy JH: Needle knife papillotomy: A valuable yet dangerous technique (abstract). Gastrointest Endosc 37: 267, 1991.
87. Dowsett JF, Polydorou AA, Vaira D, et al: Needle knife papillotomy: How safe and how effective? Gut 31:905, 1990.
88. Jowell PS: Endoscopic retrograde cholangiopancreatography: Toward a better understanding of competence (editorial). Endoscopy 31:755, 1999.
89. Kumar S, Sherman S, Hawes RH, Lehman GA: Success and yield of second attempt ERCP. Gastrointest Endosc 41:445, 1995.
90. Choudari CP, Sherman S, Fogel EL, et al: Success of ERCP at a referral center after a previously unsuccessful attempt. Gastrointest Endosc 52:478, 2000.
91. Ho KY, Montes H, Sossenheimer MJ, et al: Features that may predict hospital admission following outpatient therapeutic ERCP. Gastroint Endosc 49:587–592, 1999.
92. Freeman ML, Nelson DB, Sherman S, et al: Same-day discharge after endoscopic biliary sphincterotomy: Observations from a prospective multicenter complication study. Gastroint Endsoc 49:580–586, 1999.
93. Cotton PB: Endoscopic management of bile duct stones: Apples and oranges. Gut 25:587, 1984.
94. Classen M, Safrany L: Endoscopic papillotomy and removal of gallstones. Br Med J 4:371, 1975.
95. Zimmon DS: Endoscopic sphincterotomy—the basics. Can J Gastroenterol 4:559, 1990.
96. Concensus Opinion: Endoscopic therapy of biliary tract and pancreatic disease. Gastrointest Endosc 37:117, 1991.
97. Waye JD, Geenen JE, Fleischer D, Venu PR: Techniques in therapeutic endoscopy. Philadelphia, WB Saunders, 1987, pp 66–92.
98. Guelrud M, Plaz J, Mendoza S, et al. Can endoscopic sphincterotomy be done at the endoscopy unit (abstract)? Gastrointest Endosc 37:251, 1991.
99. Dunham F, Bourgeois N, Gelin M, et al: Retroperitoneal perforation following endoscopic sphincterotomy: Clinical course and management. Endoscopy 14:92, 1982.
100. Kortan P: Nasobiliary drainage. Can J Gastroenterol 4:588, 1990.
101. Cotton PB, Burney PG, Mason RR: Transnasal bile duct catheterization after endoscopic sphincterotomy. Gut 20:285, 1979.
102. Ostroff JW, Roberts JP, Gordon RL, et al: The management of T-tube leaks in orthotopic liver transplant recipients with endoscopically placed nasobiliary catheters. Transplantation 5:922, 1990.
103. Ponchon T, Gallez JF, Valeete PJ: Endoscopic treatment of biliary tract fistulas. Gastrointest Endosc 35:490, 1989.
104. Venu RP, Geenen JE, Hogan JH, et al: Intraluminal radiation therapy for biliary tract malignancy—an endoscopic approach. Gastrointest Endosc 36:610, 1991.
105. Levitt MD, Laurence BM, Cameron F, et al: Transpapillary iridium-192 wire in the treatment of malignant bile duct obstruction. Gut 29: 149, 1988.
106. Lebovics E, Mittelman A, Del Guercio L, et al: Pancreaticobiliary fistula and obstructive jaundice complicating ^{125}I interstitial implants for pancreatic cancer: Endoscopic diagnosis and management. Gastrointest Endosc 36:610, 1991.
107. Burcharth F, Jensen LI, Oleson K: Endoprosthesis for internal drainage of the biliary tract. Gastroenterology 77:133, 1979.
108. Siegel JH, Yatto RP: Biliary endoprosthesis for management of retained common bile duct stones. Am J Gastroenterol 79:50, 1984.
109. Huibregtse K, Haverkamp HJ, Tytgat GNJ: Transpapillary positioning of a large 3.2 mm biliary endoprosthesis. Endoscopy 13:217, 1981.
110. Huibregtse K, Katon RM, Coene PP, Tytgat GNJ: Endoscopic palliative treatment in pancreatic cancer. Gastrointest Endosc 32:334, 1986.
111. Hoffman BJ, Cunningham JT, Marsh WH: Multiple stent placement with a new steerable guidewire. Gastrointest Endosc 36:696, 1991.
112. Vanabguas A, Ehrenpreis E: Endoscopic evacuation of hematobilia induced by large bore self-expanding biliary mesh stent (letter). Gastrointest Endosc 37:117, 1991.
113. Neuhaus H, Hagenmuller F, Griebel M, et al: Percutaneous cholangioscopic or transpapillary insertion of self-expanding biliary metal stents. Gastrointest Endosc 37:31, 1991.
114. Smits M, Huibregtse K, Tytgat G: Results of the new Nitinol self-expandable stents for distal biliary strictures. Endoscopy 27:505, 1995.
115. Kawase Y, Takemura T, Hashimoto T: Endoscopic implantation of expandable metal Z stents for malignant biliary strictures. Gastrointest Endosc 39:65, 1993.
116. Mixon T, Goldschmid S, Brady PG, Boulay J: Endoscopic management of expandable metallic biliary stent occlusion. Gastrointest Endosc 39:82, 1993.
117. Kadakia S: Comparison of 10-F gauge stent with 11.5-F gauge stent in biliary tract disease (abstract). Gastrointest Endosc 37:25, 1991.
118. Leung JWC, Ling TKW, Kung JLS, et al: The role of bacteria in the blockage of biliary stents. Gastrointest Endosc 34:19, 1988.
119. Coene P, Groen AK, Cheng J, et al: Clogging of biliary endoprosthesis. Gut 31:913, 1990.
120. Geenen DJ, Geenen JE, Hogan WJ, et al: Endoscopic therapy for benign bile duct strictures. Gastrointest Endosc 5:367, 1989.
121. Berkelhammer C, Kortran P, Haber GB: Endoscopic biliary prosthesis as treatment for benign post-operative bile duct strictures. Gastrointest Endosc 35:95, 1989.
122. Pitt HA, Kaufman SL, Coleman J, et al: Benign post-operative biliary strictures: Operate or dilate? Ann Surg 210:417, 1989.
123. Sivak MV: Endoscopic management of bile duct stones. Am J Surg 158:228, 1989.
124. Baillie J, Cairns SR, Cotton PB: Endoscopic management of choledocholithiasis during pregnancy. Surg 171:1, 1990.
125. May GR, Cotton PB, Edmunds EJ, Chong W: Removal of stones from the bile duct at ERCP without sphincterotomy. Gastrointest Endosc 39:749, 1993.
126. Bergman J, Rauws AJ, Tijssen J, et al: Biliary endoprostheses in elderly patients with endoscopically irretrievable common bile duct stones, report on 117 patients. Gastrointest Endosc 42:195, 1995.
127. Cotton P: Stents for stones: Short-term good, long term uncertain (editorial). Gastrointest Endosc 42:272, 1995.
128. Chung SCS, Leung JWC, Leong HT, et al: Endoscopic extraction of large common duct stones using a mechanical lithotripsy basket (abstract). Gastrointest Endosc 37:252, 1991.
129. Cotton PB, Kozarek RA, Schapiro RH, et al: Endoscopic laser lithotripsy of large bile duct stones. Gastroenterology 99:1128, 1990.
130. Saito M, Tsuyuguchi T, Yamaguchi T, et al: Long-term outcome of endoscopic papillotomy for choledocholithiasis with cholecystolithiasis. Gastrointest Endosc 51:540, 2000.
131. Robertson AF, Hacking CN, Birch S, et al: Experience with a combined percutaneous and endoscopic approach to stent insertion in malignant obstructive jaundice. Lancet 2:1449, 1987.
132. Ponchon T, Valette P-J, Borg R, et al: Evaluation of a combined percutaneous-endoscopic procedure for the treatment of choledocholithiasis and benign papillary stenosis. Endoscopy 19:164, 1987.
133. Mason R, Hall MA: A complication of combined percutaneous and endoscopic biliary stenting. J Intervent Radiol 4:13, 1989.
134. Dowsett JF, Vaira D, Hatfield ARW, et al: Endoscopic biliary therapy using the combined percutaneous and endoscopic technique. Gastroenterology 96:1180, 1989.
135. Robertson DAF, Hacking LN, Birch S, et al: Experience with a combined percutaneous and endoscopic approach to stent insertion in malignant obstructive jaundice. Lancet 2:1149, 1987.
136. Marshall L, Aliperti G, Picus D, et al: Combined endoscopic retrograde sphincterotomy and percutaneous cholecystolithotomy in the management of complicated biliary stone disease in the elderly (abstract). Gastrointest Endosc 37:249, 1991.
137. Lillemoe KD, Melton GB, Cameron JL, et al: Postoperative bile duct strictures: Management and outcome in the 1990s. Ann Surg 232:430, 2000.
138. Huibregtse K, Katon RM, Tytgat GNJ: Endoscopic treatment of post-operative biliary strictures. Endoscopy 18:133, 1986.
139. Berkelhammer C, Kortran P, Haber GB: Endoscopic biliary prosthesis as treatment for benign post-operative bile duct strictures. Gastrointest Endosc 35:95, 1989.
140. Way LW, Biliary stricture. In Way LW, Pelligrini CA (eds): Surgery of the Gallbladder and Bile Ducts. Philadelphia, WB Saunders, 1987, pp 419–419.

141. Geenen DJ, Geenen JE, Hogan WJ, et al: Endoscopic therapy for benign bile duct strictures. Gastrointest Endosc 5:367, 1989.
142. Johnson GK, Geenen JE, Venue RP, et al: Endoscopic treatment of biliary duct strictures in sclerosing cholangitis: Follow-up assessment of a new therapeutic approach. Gastrointest Endosc 33:9, 1987.
143. Rappoport AS, Diamond AB: Cholangiographic demonstration of post-operative bile leakage from aberrant biliary ducts. Gastrointest Radiol 6:273, 1981.
144. Berge H, Weinzierl M, Neville ES, Pratschke E: Percutaneous transcatheter occlusion of the cystic duct stump in post-cholecystectomy bile leakage. Gastrointest Radiol 14:334, 1989.
145. Shaw DW, Bertino RE, Mulholland MW, et al: Use of tetracycline for sclerosis of a biliary-cutaneous fistula. AJR 153:65, 1989.
146. Eckhauser FE, Colleti LM, Knol JA: The changing role of surgery for sclerosing cholangitis. Dig Dis 14:180, 1996.
147. Gibbons JC, Williams SJ: Progress in the endoscopic management of benign biliary strictures. J Gastro Hepatol 13:116–124, 1998.
148. Mahadevan U, Bass NM, Ostroff JW: Endoscopic management of primary sclerosing cholangitis: Results in slowing of disease progression (abstract). Am J Gastroenterol 95:252, 2000.
149. Charcot JM: Lecons sur les Maladies du foie, des Voies Billares et des Reins. Paris, Faculte de Medicine de Paris, 1887, p 194.
150. Reynolds BM, Dargan EL: Acute obstructive cholangitis: A distinct clinical syndrome. Ann Surg 150:299, 1959.
151. Carr-Locke DL, Cotton PB: Biliary tract and pancreas. Br Med Bull 42:257, 1986.
152. Lai ESC, Patterson IA, Tam PC, et al: Severe acute cholangitis: The role of emergency nasobiliary drainage. Surgery 268:107, 1990.
153. Kadir S, Baassiri A, Barth K; et al: Percutaneous biliary drainage in the management of biliary sepsis. AJR 138:25, 1982.
154. Sugiyama M, Atomi Y: Treatment of acute cholangitis due to choledocholithiasis in elderly and younger patients. Arch Surg 132:1129, 1997.
155. Harris HW, Kumwenda ZL, Sheen-Chen SM, et al: Recurrent pyogenic cholangitis. Am J Surg 176:34, 1998.
156. Choi TK, Wong J: Partial hepatectomy for intrahepatic stones. World J Surg 10:281, 1986.
157. Picus D, Weyman PJ, Marx MV: Role of percutaneous intracorporeal electrohydraulic lithotripsy in the treatment of biliary tract calculi. Radiology 170:989, 1989.
158. Berber E, Engle KL, String A, et al: Selective use of tube cholecystostomy with interval laparoscopic cholecystectomy in acute cholecystitis. Arch Surg 135:341, 2000.
159. Davis CA, Landercasper J, Gundersen LH, Lambert PJ: Effective use of percutaneous cholecystostomy in high-risk surgical patients: Techniques, tube management, and results. Arch Surg 134:727, 1999.
160. Borzellino G, de Manzoni G, Ricci F, et al: Emergency cholecystostomy and subsequent cholecystectomy for acute gallstone cholecystitis in the elderly. Br J Surg 86:1521, 1999.
161. Lee MJ, Saini S, Brink JA, et al: Treatment of critically ill patients with sepsis of unknown cause: Value of percutaneous cholecystostomy. AJR 156:1163, 1991.
162. Kalloo AN, Thuluvath PJ, Pasricha PJ: Treatment of high-risk patients with symptomatic cholelithiasis by endoscopic gallbladder stenting. Gastrointest Endosc 40:608, 1994.
163. Gobien RP, Stanley JH, Sovcek CD, et al: Routine pre-operative biliary drainage: Effect on management of obstructive jaundice. Radiology 152:353, 1984.
164. McPherson GAD, Benjamin IS, Hodgson HJ, et al: Preoperative percutaneous biliary drainage: The results of a controlled trial. Br J Surg 71:371, 1984.
165. Smith AC, Dowsett JF, Russell RC, et al: Randomized trial of endoscopic stenting versus surgical bypass in malignant low bile duct obstruction. Lancet 344:1655–1660, 1994.
166. Carr-Locke DL, Ball TJ, Connors PJ et al: Multicenter randomized trial of Wallstent biliary endoprosthesis versus plastic stents (abstract). Gastrointest Endosc 39:310A, 1993.
167. Hoepffner N, Foerster EC, Hogemann B, et al: Long-term experience in Wallstent therapy for malignant choledochal stenosis. Endoscopy 26:597–602, 1994.
168. Yeoh KG, Zimmerman MJ, Cunningham JT, et al: Comparative costs of metal versus plastic stent strategies for malignant obstructive jaundice by decision analysis. Gastrointest Endosc 49:466–471, 1999.
169. Cvetkovski B, Gerdes H, Kurtz RC: Outpatient therapeutic ERCP with endobiliary stent placement for malignant common bile duct obstruction. Gastrointest Endosc 50:63–66, 1999.
170. Costamagna G: Therapeutic biliary endoscopy. Endoscopy 32:209–216, 2000.
171. Fogel EL, Sherman S, Devereaux BM, et al: Therapeutic biliary endoscopy. Ther Biliary Endosc 33:31–38, 2001.
172. Seo DW, Cheon YK, Moon JH, et al: Treatment of benign intrahepatic duct stricture using polyurethane-covered retrievable nitinol stent. Gastrointest Endosc 51:AB97, 2000.
173. Meier PN: ERCP topics. Endoscopy 32:863–873, 2000.
174. McPherson GAD, Benjamin IS, Hodgson HJ, et al: Pre-operative percutaneous biliary drainage: The results of a controlled trial. Br J Surg 71:371, 1984.
175. Aabakken L, Osnes M: Endoscopic choledochoduodenostomy as palliative treatment of malignant periampullary obstruction of the common duct. Gastrointest Endosc 32:41, 1986.
176. Little JM: Hilar biliary cancer: Are we getting it right? HPB Surg 1: 93, 1989.
177. Ahrendt SA, Cameron JL, Pitt HA: Current management of patients with perihilar cholangiocarcinoma. Adv Surg 30:427, 1996.
178. Jowell PS, Cotton P, Huibregtse K, et al: Delivery catheter entrapment driving deployment of expandable metal stents. Gastrointest Endosc 39:199, 1993.
179. Cremer M, Devier J: Bifurcation tumors: Is endoscopic drainage sufficient? Can J Gastroenterol 4:576, 1990.
180. Deviere J, Baize M, de Toeuf J, et al: Long-term follow-up of patients with hilar malignant stricture treated by endoscopic internal biliary drainage. Gastrointest Endosc 34:95, 1988.
181. Ward EM, Kiely JM, Maus TP, et al: Hilar biliary stricture after liver transplantation: Cholangiography and percutaneous treatment. Radiology 177:259, 1991.
182. Zajko AB, Sheng R, Zetti GM, et al: Transhepatic balloon dilation of biliary strictures in liver transplant patients: A 10-year experience. J Vasc Intervent Radiol 6:79, 1995.
183. Zajko AB, Campbell WL, Bron KM, et al: Diagnostic and interventional radiology in liver transplantation. Gastroenterol Clin North Am 43:47, 1987.
184. Stratta RJ, Wood RP, Langnas AN, et al: Diagnosis and treatment of biliary tract complications after orthotopic liver transplantation. Surgery 106:675, 1989.
185. Ostroff JW: Post-transplant biliary complications. Gastrointest Endosc Clin North Am 11:163, 2001.
186. Venu RP, Geenen JE: Diagnosis and treatment of diseases of the papilla. Clin Gastroenterol 15:439, 1986.
187. Roulot D, Valla D, Brun-Vezinet F, et al: Cholangitis in the acquired immunodeficiency syndrome: Report of two cases and review of the literature. Gut 27:1193, 1986.
188. Schneiderman DJ, Cello JP, Laing FC: Papillary stenosis and sclerosing cholangitis in the acquired immunodeficiency syndrome. Ann Intern Med 106:546, 1987.
189. Edmundowiz S: Diagnosis and management of choledocholithiasis in the era of laparoscopic cholecystectomy: An endoscopist's perspective. Endoscopy 27:443, 1995.
190. Feretis C, Kalliakmanis B, Benakis P, Apostolidis N: Laparoscopic transcystic papillotomy under endoscopic control for bile duct stones. Endoscopy 26:697–700, 1994.
191. Cox MR, Wilson TG, Toouli J: Preoperative endoscopic sphincterotomy during laparoscopic cholecystectomy for choledocholithiasis. Br J Surg 82:257, 1995.
192. Trerotola SO, Savader SJ, Lund GB, et al: Biliary tract complications following laparoscopic cholecystectomy: Imaging and intervention. Radiology 184:195–200, 1992.
193. Slanetz PJ, Boland GW, Mueller PR: Imaging and interventional radiology in laparoscopic injuries to the gallbladder and biliary system. Radiology 201:595, 1996.
194. Savader SJ, Lillemoe KD, Prescott CA, et al: Laparoscopic cholecystectomy-related bile duct injuries: A health and financial disaster. Ann Surg 228:268, 1997.
195. Suhocki PV, Meyers WC: Injury to aberrant bile ducts during cholecystectomy: A common cause of diagnostic error and treatment delay. AJR 172:955, 1999.
196. Wright TB, Bertino RB, Bishop SF, et al: Complications of laparoscopic cholecystectomy and their radiologic management. Radiographic 13:119, 1993.
197. Ryan ME, Geenen JE, Lehman GA, et al: Endoscopic intervention for biliary leaks after laparoscopic cholecystectomy: A multicenter review. Gastrointest Endosc 47:261–266, 1998.
198. Lillemoe KD, Martin SA, Cameron JL, et al: Major bile duct injuries during laparoscopic cholecystectomy. Follow-up after combined surgical and radiologic management. Ann Surg 225:459, 1997.

INDEX

Note: Page numbers followed by f and t refer to figures and tables, respectively.